AF877669

Foye's

PRINCIPLES OF MEDICINAL CHEMISTRY

9TH EDITION

Foye's

PRINCIPLES OF MEDICINAL CHEMISTRY

9TH EDITION

MARC W. HARROLD, PHD
Professor of Medicinal Chemistry
School of Pharmacy
Duquesne University
Pittsburgh, Pennsylvania

KIMBERLY BECK, PHD
Pharmacy Program Director/Associate Professor
College of Health Professions
Butler University
Indianapolis, Indiana

VICTORIA F. ROCHE, PHD
Professor Emerita
School of Pharmacy and Health Professions
Creighton University
Omaha, Nebraska

S. WILLIAM ZITO, PHD
Professor Emeritus
College of Pharmacy and Health Sciences
St. John's University
Jamaica, New York

THOMAS L. LEMKE, PHD
Professor Emeritus
College of Pharmacy
University of Houston
Houston, Texas

DAVID A. WILLIAMS, PHD
Professor Emeritus
School of Pharmacy
MCPHS University
Boston, Massachusetts

Wolters Kluwer

Philadelphia • Baltimore • New York • London
Buenos Aires • Hong Kong • Sydney • Tokyo

Acquisitions Editor: Matt Hauber
Development Editor: Deborah Bordeaux
Editorial Coordinator: Janet Jayne
Senior Production Specialist: Bridgett Dougherty
Marketing Manager: Kirsten Watrud
Manager, Graphic Arts & Design: Steve Druding
Art Director: Jennifer Clements
Prepress Vendor: S4Carlisle Publishing Services

Ninth Edition

Copyright © 2026 Wolters Kluwer.

Copyright © 2020 Wolters Kluwer. Copyright © 2013 Lippincott Williams & Wilkins, a WOLTERS KLUWER BUSINESS. Copyright © 2008, 2002 Lippincott Williams & Wilkins. Copyright © 1995 Williams & Wilkins. Copyright © 1989, 1981, 1974 Lea & Febiger. All rights reserved. This book is protected by copyright. No part of this book may be reproduced or transmitted in any form or by any means, including as photocopies or scanned-in or other electronic copies, or utilized by any information storage and retrieval system without written permission from the copyright owner, except for brief quotations embodied in critical articles and reviews. Materials appearing in this book prepared by individuals as part of their official duties as U.S. government employees are not covered by the above-mentioned copyright. To request permission, please contact Wolters Kluwer at Two Commerce Square, 2001 Market Street, Philadelphia, PA 19103, via email at permissions@lww.com, or via our website at shop.lww.com (products and services).

9 8 7 6 5 4 3 2 1

Printed in Mexico

Library of Congress Cataloging-in-Publication Data

Names: Harrold, Marc W., editor.
Title: Foye's principles of medicinal chemistry / [edited by] Marc W. Harrold, Kimberly Beck, Victoria F. Roche, S. William Zito, Thomas L. Lemke, David A. Williams.
Other titles: Principles of medicinal chemistry
Description: 9th edition. | Philadelphia : Wolters Kluwer Health, [2026] | Includes bibliographical references and indexes. | Summary: "Foye's Principles of Medicinal Chemistry, 9th Edition, remains the most complete and respected medicinal chemistry text available. Whether used in traditional course structures or integrated into systems-based modules, this streamlined edition makes content more approachable than ever, providing expert perspectives to clarify the chemical basis of drug action, emphasizing the structure-activity relationships, physicochemical-pharmacokinetic properties, and metabolic profiles of the most commonly used drugs"—Provided by publisher.
Identifiers: LCCN 2024057455 (print) | LCCN 2024057456 (ebook) | ISBN 9781975218720 (paperback) | ISBN 9781975218737 (ebook)
Subjects: MESH: Chemistry, Pharmaceutical | Pharmaceutical Preparations—chemistry
Classification: LCC RS403 . F695 2026 (print) | LCC RS403 (ebook) | NLM QV 744 | DDC 616.0756–dc23/eng/20250714
LC record available at https://lccn.loc.gov/2024057455
LC ebook record available at https://lccn.loc.gov/2024057456

This work is provided "as is," and the publisher disclaims any and all warranties, express or implied, including any warranties as to accuracy, comprehensiveness, or currency of the content of this work.

This work is no substitute for individual patient assessment based upon healthcare professionals' examination of each patient and consideration of, among other things, age, weight, gender, current or prior medical conditions, medication history, laboratory data and other factors unique to the patient. The publisher does not provide medical advice or guidance and this work is merely a reference tool. Healthcare professionals, and not the publisher, are solely responsible for the use of this work including all medical judgments and for any resulting diagnosis and treatments.

Given continuous, rapid advances in medical science and health information, independent professional verification of medical diagnoses, indications, appropriate pharmaceutical selections and dosages, and treatment options should be made and healthcare professionals should consult a variety of sources. When prescribing medication, healthcare professionals are advised to consult the product information sheet (the manufacturer's package insert) accompanying each drug to verify, among other things, conditions of use, warnings and side effects and identify any changes in dosage schedule or contraindications, particularly if the medication to be administered is new, infrequently used or has a narrow therapeutic range. To the maximum extent permitted under applicable law, no responsibility is assumed by the publisher for any injury and/or damage to persons or property, as a matter of products liability, negligence law or otherwise, or from any reference to or use by any person of this work.

QUADM0925

This textbook is dedicated to students of all ages who seek to master the complexity and elegance of medicinal chemistry and its role in therapeutic decision-making within the profession of pharmacy. It is also dedicated to colleagues who have inspired us in our academic careers, who have contributed to this text, and who have served as our educational and scientific role models.

Marc W. Harrold

Kimberly Beck

Victoria F. Roche

S. William Zito

Thomas L. Lemke

David A. Williams

Dedication to William O. Foye

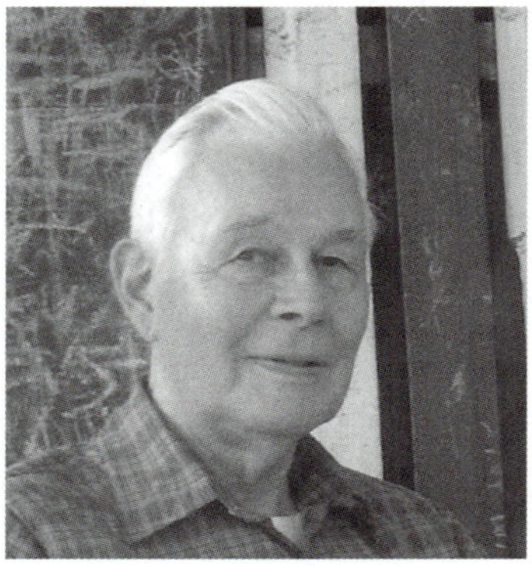

William O. Foye, Sawyer Professor of Medicinal Chemistry at the MCPHS University (formerly Massachusetts College of Pharmacy), Boston, MA, was born in 1923 in western Massachusetts. He received his BA (1944) in chemistry from Dartmouth College and PhD in organic chemistry (M. Carmack) from Indiana University (1948). He served in the U.S. Navy during World War II as a chemical warfare instructor. He joined DuPont (Delaware) as a research scientist, then in 1950 joined the School of Pharmacy at the University of Wisconsin as assistant professor of pharmaceutical chemistry. In 1955, he moved to MCPHS University, Boston, as professor of chemistry, where he brought a new vision of pharmaceutical chemistry (medicinal chemistry) to the pharmacy curriculum. As department chair, he advocated for organic medicinal chemistry in the pharmacy curriculum.

The impetus for a new text in medicinal chemistry, grounded on Alfred Burger's two-volume *Medicinal Chemistry*, came from Dr. Norman Doorenbos, College of Pharmacy, University of Maryland (Baltimore), who had made arrangements with Lea & Febiger (forerunner of Wolters Kluwer) for publishing a companion text to Wilson & Gisvold's *Textbook of Organic Medicinal and Pharmaceutical Chemistry*. Because Dr. Doorenbos was moving to chair the new Pharmacognosy Department at the School of Pharmacy, University of Mississippi, he relinquished the job of editing this text to Dr. Foye. During this time, a number of teachers and researchers in medicinal chemistry felt that a text on drugs that included biochemical mechanisms of action, aimed primarily at professional students, should be written. Although other pharmaceutical and medicinal chemistry books had been written during this time (*The Chemistry of Organic Medicinal Products*, Jenkins and Hartung, and *Textbook of Organic Medicinal and Pharmaceutical Chemistry*, Wilson and Gisvold), these authors organized their books according to the accepted scheme of chemical classification of the more important organic medicinal compounds, their methods of synthesis, their properties and descriptions, and their uses and modes of administration. Therefore, this "Principles" text provided a contemporary basis for the biochemical understanding of drug action that included the principles of structure-activity relationships (SAR) and drug metabolism. Dr. Foye assembled authors who were experts in their respective fields and published the first edition of *Principles of Medicinal Chemistry* in 1972.

The authors of the ninth edition of *Foye's Principles of Medicinal Chemistry* have embraced Dr. Foye's original concept of a textbook of significant value to pharmacy students. Today, even more than when the original text appeared in 1972, the complex nature of disease states and their biochemical/physiologic origins need to be explored and understood at the molecular level for health care professionals to ensure maximal benefits for patients. All editions of this text have had a primary goal to both meet students' short-term need for a contemporary medicinal chemistry education and stimulate a lifelong desire to know more about how the chemicals we call drugs work.

Dr. Foye had a long and creative career in medicinal chemistry with more than 150 refereed scientific publications, book chapters, and serving as the editor of *Cancer Chemotherapeutic Agents* (ACS Monograph Series). His research focused on numerous areas, especially the SAR of antiradiation organosulfur compounds, anticancer agents, and chelation as a mechanism of drug action. He was elected Fellow of the AAPS and Fellow of APhA, received the APhA Foundation Research Achievement Award in Medicinal Chemistry, and was an emeritus member of AAAS, ACS, APhA, and AAPS. He was one of the founding members of the Medicinal Chemistry Group of the Northeast Section of the American Chemical Society (1968). He retired in 1995.

In addition to being Chair of the Department of Chemistry, he was also the Dean of Faculties and Dean of Graduate Studies at the MCPHS University. Dr. Foye traveled widely and was an invited participant at numerous meetings.

Not only was Dr. Foye a distinguished scientist, he was also an avid fly fisherman, outdoorsman, and environmentalist. He published several books about the western Massachusetts wilderness, *Trout Waters: Reminiscence with Description of the Upper Quabbin Valley* (1992) and *North Quabbin Wilds: A Populous Solitude* (2005). He was a dedicated supporter of the arts in Boston. He married Lila Siddons in 1974 and has a son Owen and stepson Kenneth. Dr. Foye died in 2014.

David A. Williams, PhD

Preface

FOYE'S PRINCIPLES OF MEDICINAL CHEMISTRY: AN EDUCATIONAL TREASURE FOR OVER 50 YEARS

William O. Foye, for whom this textbook is named, was a groundbreaking pioneer in medicinal chemistry education. Committed to the concept that drug structure and the biochemical environments in which they act are intricately interwoven, in 1972, he launched the first edition of a principles-focused teaching and learning resource that has both stood the test of time and evolved with it. Many readers will be familiar with the academic life and reputation of Bill Foye, but we encourage those who aren't to read the excellent tribute that precedes this preface, authored by his devoted friend and MCPHS colleague, editor David A. Williams.

Dr. Foye's goal for the first edition of the *Principles of Medicinal Chemistry* text that would ultimately bear his name was "to present a coherent and scientifically correct account of the principles that determine the course of a drug molecule when it enters the complex world of the cell." The ninth edition continues to build on his vision, and all editions in between have successfully honored this worthy goal thanks to the scholarly and learner-centered writings of the many contributors who have participated over the past 52 years. More than 170 authors from 70 U.S. colleges and schools of pharmacy, 16 industrial and private organizations, and 7 international institutions of higher learning have brought their expertise to bear in educating the next generations of professional and graduate students through the authoring of one or more chapters. The English version of the text is available to everyone, regardless of country of residence, and the last five editions have been fully translated into Italian. A partial Japanese translation was initially published as a three-volume set, with the eighth edition fully translated. Clearly, *Foye's Principles of Medicinal Chemistry* has something valuable to say to learners worldwide.

In this golden jubilee era of *Foye's Principles of Medicinal Chemistry*, the editors would like to acknowledge everyone who has helped make this textbook the outstanding success it has been for the duration of its existence. The publisher has described it as a "gold standard" in medicinal chemistry education. The editors clearly believe it is a "gold mine" of cutting-edge scholarship presented in a way that permits research scientists and pharmacy practitioners alike to understand how a drug's structure dictates its activity in all environments and to apply that understanding to advance their own work in the laboratory or clinic.

THE EVOLUTION OF MEDICINAL CHEMISTRY EDUCATION

The senior editors can recall a time when medicinal chemistry coursework and the textbooks that supported it organized drugs according to their functional groups (eg, alcoholic, amine-containing, acidic, basic) and emphasized topics such as drug synthesis, chemical stability, analytical methods, pharmacognosy, and the rote memorization of drug structures. Medicinal chemistry was then commonly taught as a stand-alone foundational course early in the curriculum, usually concurrent with pharmacology and pharmaceutics. In fact, it wasn't until the 1960s that departments of medicinal chemistry began to appear. Prior to this time, faculty involved in design and synthesis of potential drug candidates were usually found in pharmaceutical chemistry departments.

Regardless of their department, medicinal chemistry faculty were often eager to stimulate interest in graduate studies rather than emphasize how a drug's chemistry could provide insight on its potential value in treating patients; clinical utility analyses were left exclusively to pharmacy practice colleagues. In our collective memory, once these densely scientific medicinal chemistry courses were successfully passed, they were rarely (if ever) thought about again by students, nor were the concepts revisited or reinforced by other faculty as the curriculum progressed.

The 1980s saw the beginning of a shift to incorporate clinical applications in medicinal chemistry teaching. Medicinal chemistry faculty realized that a critical evaluation of drug structure and the interpretation of structure-activity relationship (SAR) data could be correlated to topics that pharmacy students could apply to clinical decision-making. Key chemical parameters such as receptor affinity, pKa, logP, and metabolism directly affect potency, routes of administration, systemic distribution, duration of action, and the potential for metabolism-based drug-drug interactions and other adverse effects. Every drug carries its scientific and therapeutic profile within its structure. Of all the health care team members, only pharmacists understand and speak the language that decodes those profiles and translates them into a wealth of foundational and clinical information relevant to drug action in vitro and in vivo.

The first published discussion of incorporating clinical relevance in medicinal chemistry coursework appeared in 1985, with medicinal chemistry case studies formally introduced in 1993. Originally, case studies were "pen and paper" exercises that required students to mine a select number of unnamed drug structures for clinically relevant information and use it to make a straightforward therapeutic decision or solve a fairly simple clinical problem. A similar approach, the structurally based therapeutic evaluation (SBTE), was published in 1997, which was also the year when more complex computerized medicinal chemistry case studies were first shared with the academy. This latter learning tool involved multifaceted and interconnecting decision trees that took learners step-by-step through the analysis of the structure-dependent impact of potential therapies on physiologic parameters and therapeutic outcomes that could be desired or detrimental in a specific patient care scenario. As before, students had only the drug structures to evaluate in order to emphasize critical thinking and analytical skills versus memorized facts.

The 21st century saw the continued evolution of medicinal chemistry professional education, as many schools and colleges experimented with blocked curricula (where one or two subjects were intensely taught in their entirety over a fairly short period of time) or, conversely, by fully integrating the subject with pharmacology, physiology, and therapeutics in disease state–specific modules that often spanned two or more academic years. Each approach depended significantly on faculty solidarity, exemplified by reinforcing intensely learned "blocked" content in future coursework or allowing each discipline appropriate lesson time and examination emphasis in the integrated disease state approach. True team-teaching in integrated course models also demanded sustained, time-intensive faculty collaboration. Some programs never deviated from the single-subject approach to course organization, and some reverted back to that model after a few years on the blocked or combined content curricular model.

Through the years, the *Foye* text has adapted to these changing curricular models so that faculty and students would find the resource to be on the cutting-edge of contemporary pedagogy. The fifth edition, published in 2002, was the first to include case study exercises at the end of each Pharmacodynamic Agents chapter. This tradition continued through the seventh edition, expanding to include a clinical scenario exercise option in the eighth edition and additional capstone learning assessment choices in the current edition. The eighth edition also included three chapters written in a Disease State Management format, where interprofessional authorship was encouraged. An editorial decision was made to eliminate those chapters from the ninth edition since, despite efforts to emphasize an integrated approach to coverage, their content was viewed as redundant with related Pharmacodynamic Agents chapters.

Celebrating and Honoring Our Colleagues

The years between editions of this text invariably bring the loss of valued medicinal chemistry educators, scientists, and friends, and the 6 years since the eighth edition was published is no different. Every loss is keenly felt, and every life is celebrated for the good brought to our discipline and to so many academic and personal communities.

The senior editors would like to pay special tribute to the recent passing of colleagues whose death was personally poignant or impactful. We honor them always in our hearts.

- **Dave Williams:** Donald Robb (2021) and John Midgley (2022), British mentors during my sabbatical leave at Strathclyde University in Glasgow, Scotland.
- **Tom Lemke:** John Neumeyer (2023), a mentor directing me during my undergraduate days. Bob Wiley (2009) and Don Witiak (1998), mentors in my graduate and early academic days.
- **S. William (Sandy) Zito:** James E. Wynn (2012), outstanding and inspiring medicinal chemistry teacher/researcher, national leader, and best friend. A loss to our profession.
- **Victoria Roche:** Edward B. (Ted) Roche (2022), beloved husband and inspirational chemistry education role model. Patrick M. Woster (2023), world-renowned scientist-educator, dear friend, and Ted's PhD student.

Transitions

The ninth edition of *Foye* will be the last for long-standing editors Tom Lemke and Dave Williams, who began their editorial leadership with the fourth edition, and for Sandy Zito and Victoria Roche, who joined the editorial team with the sixth edition. When discussing to whom we could pass the cherished baton with confidence in the future quality of this seminal resource, the first person who came to our collective mind was Duquesne University colleague Marc W. Harrold. Marc's outstanding chapters on dyslipidemia and other cardiovascular-related therapies have graced the pages of previous editions of *Foye*, and his dedication, professionalism, and student-focused educational writing skills made him a natural choice to become the next lead editor. The senior editors also valued the conscientious input and literature-based inquiries of Kimberly Beck (Butler) Universityon various elements of previous editions and were extremely pleased to invite her to work with Marc as a *Foye* editor. Our labor of love is in exceptionally qualified hands, and we are excited to see where they will take future editions of *Foye* to showcase the critical importance of our discipline to the pharmacy profession and to meet the needs of those who teach and study it.

David A. Williams, PhD
Thomas L. Lemke, PhD
S. William Zito, PhD
Victoria F. Roche, PhD

Acknowledgments

The editorial team gratefully acknowledges the dedicated collaboration of our publication partners at Wolters Kluwer, in particular Janet Jayne (editorial coordinator), Deborah Bordeaux (development editor), and Matt Hauber (acquisitions editor). Their unfailing support and assistance throughout this major undertaking have been truly noteworthy and did much to ensure the quality of the final product. In addition, the support of colleagues and administrators at the Schools of Pharmacy at Duquesne and Butler Universities is recognized with sincere appreciation. Of course, this book would not exist without the commitment of our chapter authors to craft contemporary narratives that are scholarly yet readable, comprehensive yet focused, as well as effectively organized and engagingly illustrated. Our clinical contributors who wrote the "Clinical Significance" sections are also acknowledged for their important contribution to the goal of making this text explicitly relevant to patient care.

The editors acknowledge with love and gratitude the support and patience of our spouses through a sometimes exhausting and intense 2.5 years: Barbara Harrold, Steve Beck, Julie Zito, Patricia Lemke, and Gail Williams. Finally, the editors acknowledge the support and dedication of Edward (Ted) Roche. Ted was a valued contributor to this text and an excellent teacher. He died in March of 2022 and left behind a lifelong legacy of commitment to the discipline and the profession.

Marc W. Harrold, PhD
Kimberly Beck, PhD
Victoria F. Roche, PhD
S. William Zito, PhD
Thomas L. Lemke, PhD
David A. Williams, PhD

Contributors

Rami A. Al-Horani, PhD
Xavier University of Louisiana
New Orleans, Louisiana

Kimberly Beck, PhD
College of Health Professions
Butler University
Indianapolis, Indiana

Swati Betharia, PhD
School of Pharmacy
MCPHS University
Boston, Massachusetts

Stacy D. Brown, PhD
East Tennessee State University
Johnson City, Tennessee

Clinton E. Canal, PhD
College of Pharmacy
Mercer University
Atlanta, Georgia

Christopher W. Cunningham, PhD
School of Pharmacy
Concordia University
Mequon, Wisconsin

Gregory D. Cuny, PhD
College of Pharmacy
University of Houston
Houston, Texas

Stephen J. Cutler, PhD
College of Pharmacy
University of South Carolina
Columbia, South Carolina

James T. Dalton, PhD
University of Alabama
Tuscaloosa, Alabama

Patrick T. Flaherty, PhD
Associate Professor
School of Pharmacy
Duquesne University
Pittsburgh, Pennsylvania

Carolyn Friel, PhD
MCPHS University
Worcester, Massachusetts

Helmut B. Gottlieb, PhD
Feik School of Pharmacy
University of the Incarnate Word
San Antonio, Texas

Marc W. Harrold, PhD
School of Pharmacy
Duquesne University
Pittsburgh, Pennsylvania

Peter J. Harvison, PhD
St. Joseph's University
Philadelphia, Pennsylvania

Kirk E. Hevener, PharmD, PhD
University of Tennessee Health Science Center
Memphis, Tennessee

David A. Johnson, PhD
School of Pharmacy
Duquesne University
Pittsburgh, Pennsylvania

Stephen G. Kerr, PhD
School of Pharmacy
MCPHS University
Boston, Massachusetts

Dan Kiel, PhD
School of Pharmacy
MCPHS University
Boston, Massachusetts

Srikanth Kolluru, PhD
Thomas J. Long School of Pharmacy
University of the Pacific
Stockton, California

Vijaya L. Korlipara, PhD
College of Pharmacy and Health Sciences
St. John's University
Queens, New York

Sonali Kurup, PhD
Ferris State University
Big Rapids, Michigan

Thomas L. Lemke, PhD
College of Pharmacy
University of Houston
Houston, Texas

Francisco León, PhD
University of South Carolina
Columbia, South Carolina

Michael L. Mohler, PharmD, PhD
Veru Inc.
Miami, Florida

Nader H. Moniri, PhD
College of Pharmacy
Mercer University
Atlanta, Georgia

Bob M. Moore II, PhD
University of Tennessee Health Science Center
Memphis, Tennessee

Marilyn E. Morris, PhD
School of Pharmacy and Pharmaceutical Sciences
The State University of New York at Buffalo
Buffalo, New York

Bridget L. Morse, PharmD, PhD
Eli Lilly and Company
Indianapolis, Indiana

Ramesh Narayanan, PhD
College of Pharmacy
University of Tennessee Health Science Center
Memphis, Tennessee

Lauren A. O'Donnell, PhD
Graduate School of Pharmaceutical Sciences
Duquesne University
Pittsburgh, Pennsylvania

Sushma Ramsinghani, PhD
University of the Incarnate Word
San Antonio, Texas

Victoria F. Roche, PhD
School of Pharmacy and Health Professions
Creighton University
Omaha, Nebraska

David P. Rotella, PhD
Sokoi Professor of Chemistry and Biochemistry
Montclair State University
Montclair, New Jersey

Jozef Stec, PhD
Marshall B. Ketchum University
Fullerton, California

Tanaji T. Talele, PhD
College of Pharmacy and Health Sciences
St. John's University
Queens, New York

Abby Weldon, PhD
School of Pharmacy
William Carey University
Biloxi, Mississippi

Dave Weldon, PhD
School of Pharmacy
William Carey University
Biloxi, Mississippi

David A. Williams, PhD
School of Pharmacy
MCPHS University
Boston, Massachusetts

Raghunandan Yendapally, PhD
Feik School of Pharmacy
University of the Incarnate Word
San Antonio, Texas

Sabesan Yoganathan, PhD
College of Pharmacy and Health Sciences
St. John's University
Queens, New York

Robin M. Zavod, PhD
Chicago College of Pharmacy
Midwestern University
Downers Grove, Illinois

S. William Zito, PhD
College of Pharmacy and Health Sciences
St. John's University
Jamaica, New York

Clinical Contributors

Emily M. Ambizas, PharmD, MPH
College of Pharmacy and Health Sciences
St. John's University
Queens, New York

Jarrett R. Amsden, PharmD
College of Health Professions
Butler University
Indianapolis, Indiana

Ahlam Ayyad, PharmD
College of Pharmacy
Xavier University of Louisiana
New Orleans, Louisiana

Jill S. Borchert, PharmD
College of Pharmacy
Midwestern University
Downers Grove, Illinois

Lauren Czosnowski, PharmD
College of Health Professions
Butler University
Indianapolis, Indiana

Danielle Ezzo, PharmD
St. John's University
College of Pharmacy and Health Sciences
Queens, New York

Bradi L. Frei, PharmD, MSc, BCPS, BCOP
Feik School of Pharmacy
University of the Incarnate Word
San Antonio, Texas

Anthony J. Guarascio, PharmD, BCPS, BCIDP
School of Pharmacy
Duquesne University
Pittsburgh, Pennsylvania

Brandon Hawkins, PharmD
College of Pharmacy
University of Tennessee Health Science Center
Memphis, Tennessee

Rick Hess, PharmD, CDE, BC-ADM, BCACP
Bill Gatton College of Pharmacy
East Tennessee State University
Johnson City, Tennessee

Emily L. Knezevich, PharmD, BCPS, CDCES, FCCP
School of Pharmacy and Health Professions
Creighton University
Omaha, Nebraska

Lindey Lane, PharmD
College of Pharmacy
University of Tennessee Health Science Center
Memphis, Tennessee

Holly Lassila, DrPH, MSEd, RPh, LPC
School of Pharmacy
Duquesne University
Pittsburgh, Pennsylvania

Elizabeth A. Laubach, PharmD, BCPS, DABAT
School of Pharmacy
Concordia University
Mequon, Wisconsin

Kathleen A. Lusk, PharmD, BCPS, BCCP
Feik School of Pharmacy
University of the Incarnate Word
San Antonio, Texas

Katelynn Mayberry, PharmD
College of Pharmacy
Mercer University
Macon, Georgia

Marsha McFalls, PharmD, MSEd
School of Pharmacy
Duquesne University
Pittsburgh, Pennsylvania

Susan W. Miller, PharmD, BCGP, FASCP
College of Pharmacy
Mercer University
Macon, Georgia

Courtney A. Montepara, PharmD, BCCP
School of Pharmacy
Duquesne University
Pittsburgh, Pennsylvania

Joseph Nosser, PharmD, BCACP, BCMTMS
School of Pharmacy
William Carey University
Biloxi, Mississippi

Christine K. O'Neil, PharmD, BCPS, BCGP
School of Pharmacy
Duquesne University
Pittsburgh, Pennsylvania

Claire Saadeh, PharmD
College of Pharmacy
Ferris State University
Big Rapids, Michigan

Jeffrey T. Sherer, PharmD, MPH, BCPS, BCGP
College of Pharmacy
University of Houston
Houston, Texas

Jordan Wulz, PharmD, MPH, BC-ADM
School of Pharmacy
Concordia University
Mequon, Wisconsin

Dinesh Yogaratnam, PharmD
School of Pharmacy
MCPHS University
Boston, Massachusetts

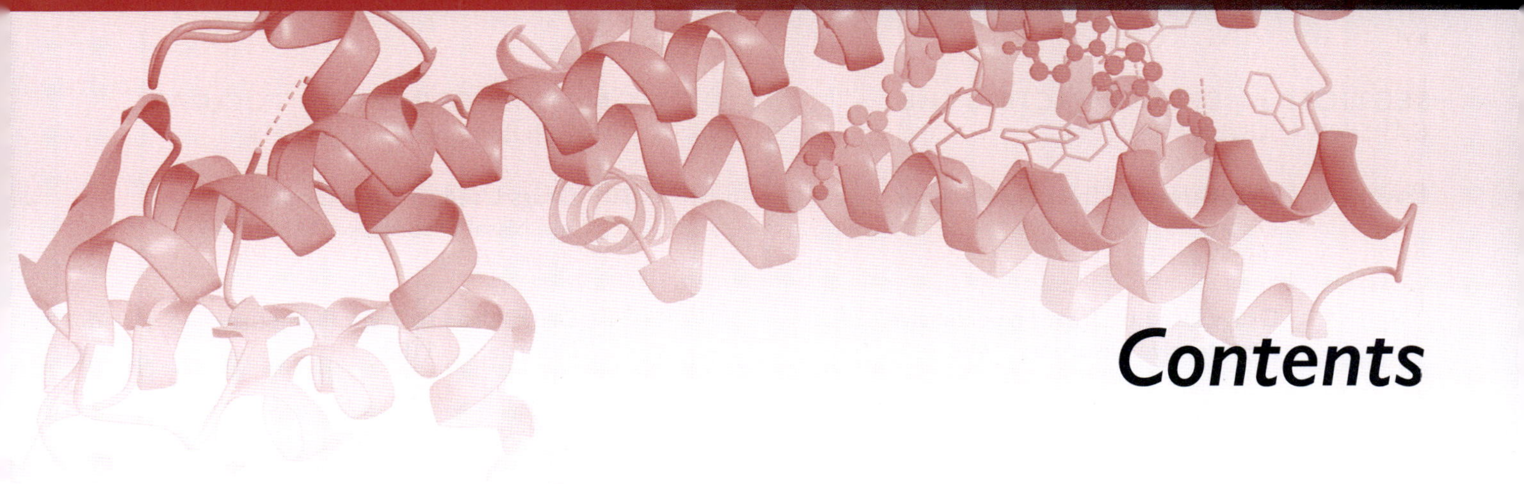

Contents

SECTION 3 DRUGS IMPACTING THE CARDIOVASCULAR SYSTEM

SECTION 4 DRUGS IMPACTING HORMONAL SYSTEMS

SECTION 5 DRUGS IMPACTING IMMUNE, GASTROINTESTINAL AND GENITOURINARY SYSTEMS

SECTION6 DRUGS IMPACTING OCULAR, NASAL, AND PULMONARY SYSTEMS

SECTION 7 DRUGS IMPACTING INFECTIOUS AND NEOPLASTIC DISEASE PROCESSES

SECTION 8 THERAPEUTIC BIOLOGICS

PART I

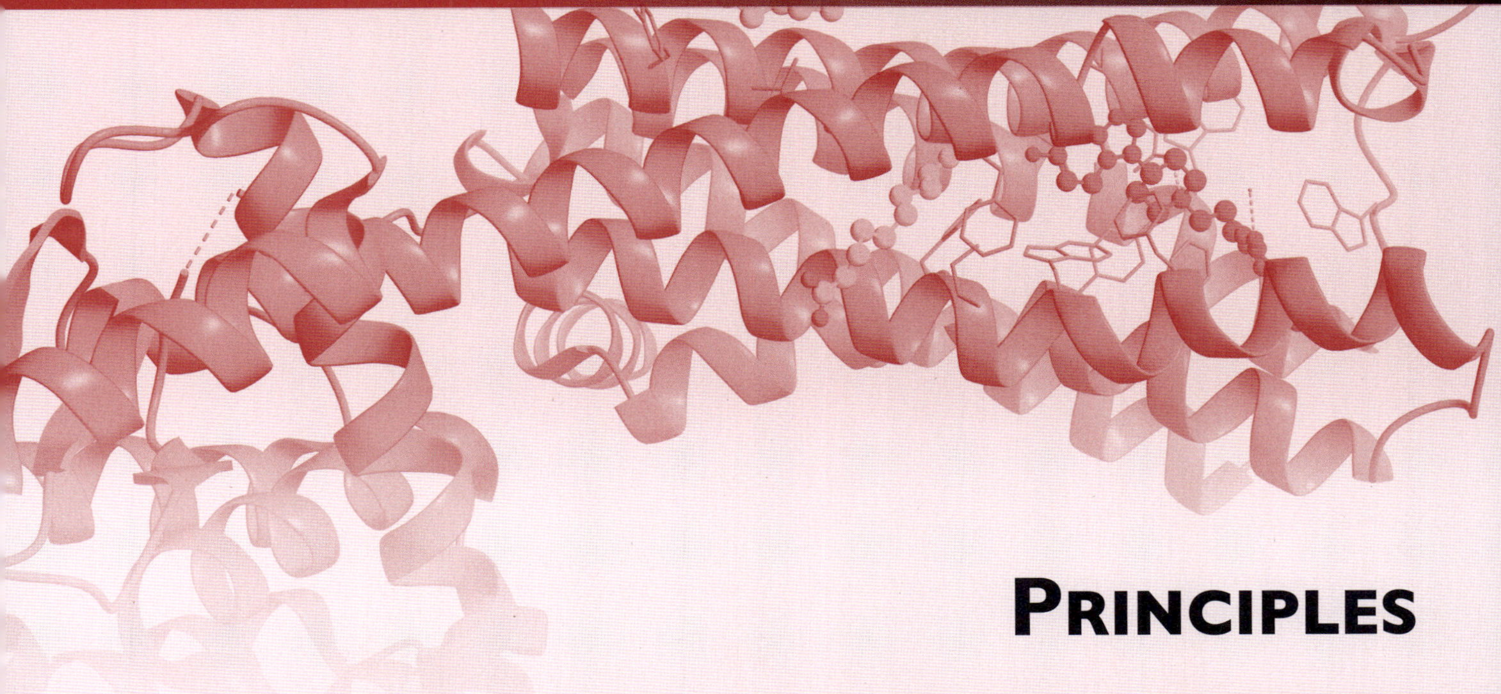

PRINCIPLES

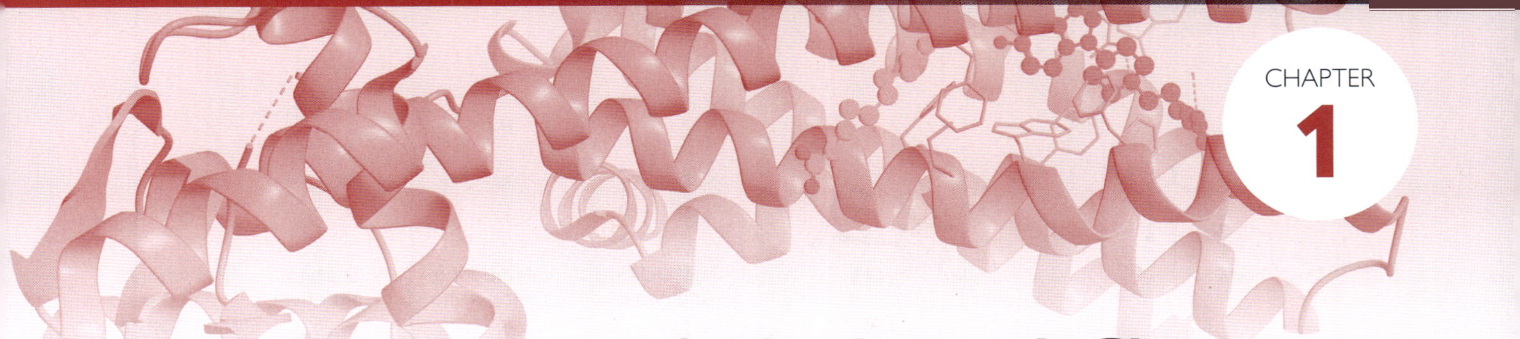

CHAPTER 1

The Evolution of Medicinal Chemistry

David P. Rotella

Abbreviations

ATP adenosine triphosphate
CNS central nervous system
DMSO dimethyl sulfoxide
DNA deoxyribonucleic acid
FDA U.S. Food and Drug Administration
GPCR G protein–coupled receptor
HIV human immunodeficiency virus
HTS high-throughput screening
NMR nuclear magnetic resonance
PCR polymerase chain reaction
PROTAC proteolysis-targeting chimera
RNA ribonucleic acid
SAR structure-activity relationship

Discovery and Chemistry of Biologically Active Substances

As the term implies, medicinal chemistry involves the study of the chemistry of biologically active substances. This includes synthesis, characterization, and measurement of physical properties and biologic investigation of these molecules. A recent definition was offered by Khan et al[1] that says, "Medicinal chemistry is defined as an independent mature science that is a combination of applied (medicine) and basic (chemistry) sciences." The interdisciplinary nature of the field requires a medicinal chemist to understand chemistry and biology, along with the limitations inherent in the methods in each, and how and when to apply appropriate techniques for the activity/function of interest. These technologies, like the discipline, evolved significantly over time to enable a better understanding of how and why a particular molecule can exert biologic activity. In spite of improved capabilities of molecular-level interaction between a ligand and a target, gaps remain in our understanding of many biologic processes from both a chemical and biologic perspective. This creates the need for continued growth and development in medicinal chemistry; thus, the Khan definition of medicinal chemistry as a mature science might be better defined as an evolving science. This chapter will survey examples to illustrate where this growth contributed to advances in the field.

Interest in and the use of biologically active substances has been a central feature as civilization developed.[2] Much of this was based on random exploration of natural product sources, primarily plant-based because of their ready availability and comparative ease of preparation as a drink or topical formulation. Efficacy was assessed based on individual responses to a preparation and could be recorded either verbally or in some more permanent form.[3] From this inauspicious beginning, medicinal chemistry as a distinct discipline developed and was recognized for the ability to demonstrate a connection between chemical structure and biologic activity as the science associated with these features advanced.

Most frequently, the evaluation of biologic activity in animals or humans was based on responses to historical models lacking a mechanism or target. Quantitation and dose-response effects were limited at best and controls were often not employed, making comparison of results and compounds challenging, if not impossible. In the mid- to late 19th century, the remarkable and distinct biologic activity of digitalis, morphine, and quinine furnished a strong stimulus to understand how these chemically distinct molecules could produce their useful biologic activity (Fig. 1.1). This began to change when Paul Ehrlich in 1885 proposed a "side chain theory" that hypothesized the need for receptors to express biologic activity of compounds.[4] This concept took root by recognizing a connection between biology in the body and a substance that was administered to produce an effect. A short time later, in 1891, Ehrlich coined the term "chemotherapy" to formalize this concept.[5] Contemporaneously, Emil Fischer developed a lock and key theory to explain enzyme action and the interaction of enzymes with substrates.[6] This concept was a pivotal advance in explaining how biologic macromolecules such as enzymes could selectively act on small molecules. At this same time, the concept of receptors as a means of expression of biologic activity

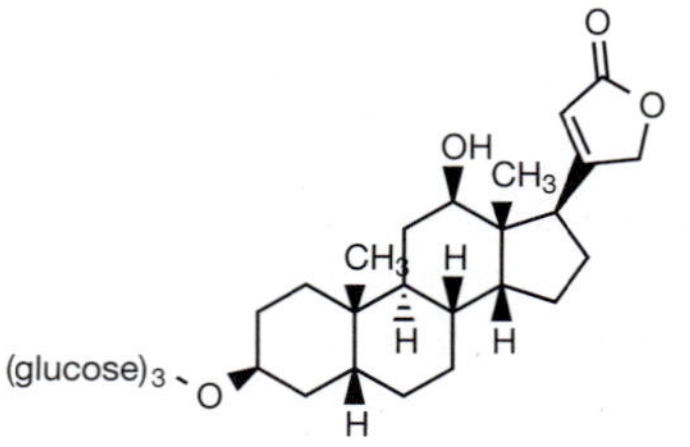

1
Digoxin
influences cardiac
contractility

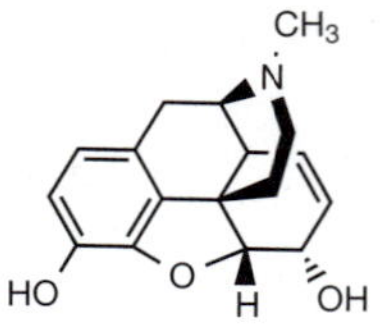

2
Morphine
analgesic

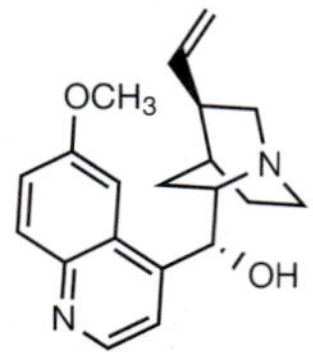

3
Quinine
antimalarial

Figure 1.1 Natural products with diverse structure and biologic activity.

gained experimental evidence by virtue of work carried out by John Langley[7] who showed that the actions of pilocarpine could be antagonized by atropine.

Synthetic medicinal chemistry began to play a more important role in the discipline during this same period of time. For example, acetanilide, antipyrine, barbital, and aspirin were prepared and demonstrated antipyretic, analgesic, and sedative activity (Fig. 1.2). A detailed summary of medicinal chemistry's early history was published.[8] In the early 20th century, the concept of structure-activity began to take shape as the effects of chemical structure and biologic activity of ephedrine derivatives were reported.[9]

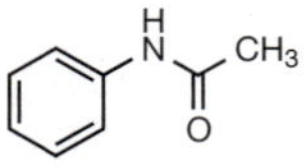

4
Acetanilide
analgesic

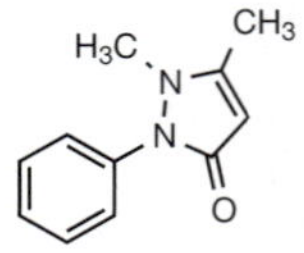

5
Antipyrine
antipyretic

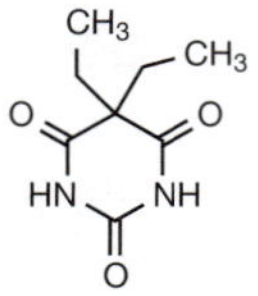

6
Barbital
sedative

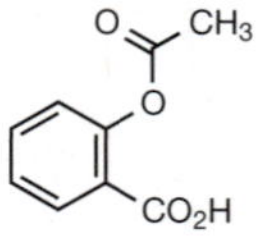

7
Aspirin
analgesic
anti inflammatory
antipyretic

Figure 1.2 Early synthetic molecules with biologic activity.

Chemically enabled investigation of anti-infective agents was another very active area of research, leading to the identification of organometallics with antiparasitic activity. Topical anti-infectives such as benzethonium and the antimalarial quinacrine were prepared and showed good activity (Fig. 1.3). The discovery of an antibacterial sulfonamide Prontosil (2,4-diaminoazobenzene-4′-sulfonamide, Fig. 1.3) used to treat gram-positive bacterial infections demonstrated that it was possible to selectively kill bacteria compared to human cells.[10] A few years later, it was discovered that the actual biologically active material was sulfanilamide, and perhaps this is the first documented example of a prodrug. During the 1940s, antibiotics such as penicillin, tetracycline, and chloramphenicol were characterized and widely employed to treat bacterial infections. The ability to safely treat infectious disease played a significant part in raising life expectancy and remains an objective of great significance (but unfortunately little progress) even today. Alfred Burger provided an illustrative summary of many of these important discoveries in medicinal chemistry (shown in Table 2.1 of the published work of Langley[7] cited earlier).

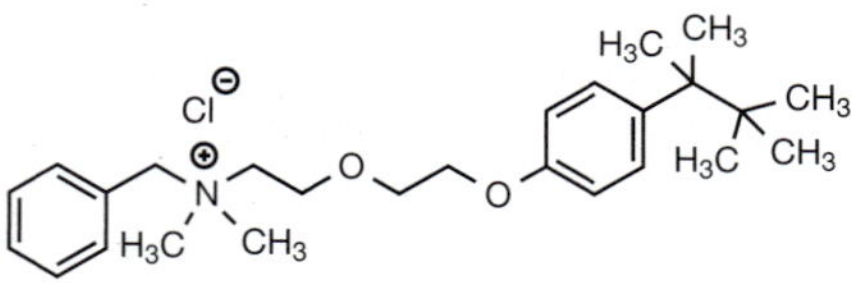

7
Benzethonium

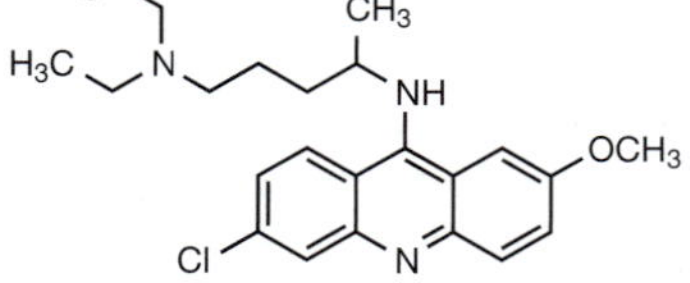

8
Quinacrine

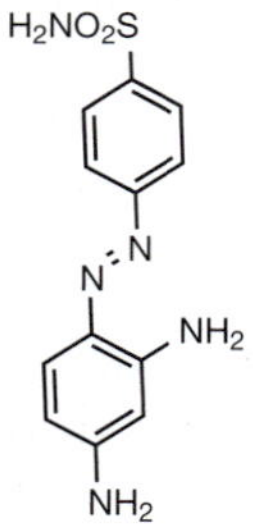

9
Prontosil

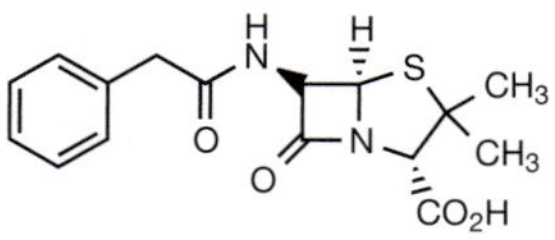

10
Penicillin G

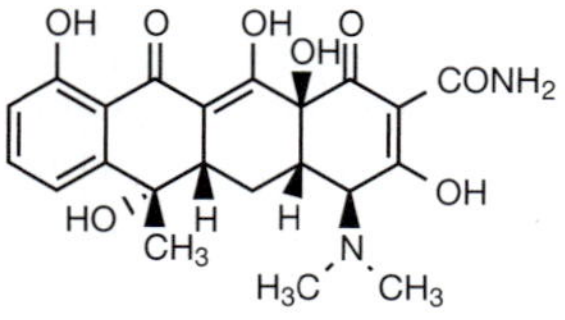

11
Tetracycline

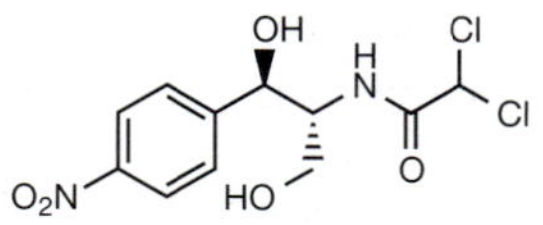

12
Chloramphenicol

Figure 1.3 Early synthetic antiparasitic and antibiotic compounds.

Evolution From Art to Science

As mentioned earlier, the ability to synthesize and evaluate different structures for biologic activity was an important advance in medicinal chemistry. The discovery of new compounds during the period extending from the mid-20th century until the 1980s was a slow, labor-intensive process. Chemists were limited by a comparatively (by today's standards) small variety of chemical reactions and starting materials. However, with perhaps the exception of antibiotics, in vivo evaluation was the primary means by which biologic activity was measured. This was (and remains) a time-consuming, labor-intensive, and low-throughput process that can produce unclear results. These limitations were technologic in nature and the solution was assisted by developments in areas outside of chemistry and biology, such as improved computational capabilities and automated compound handling to dispense compounds and to analyze and store experimental data. Coupled with the rapid progress in genetics and deoxyribonucleic acid (DNA) modification and the ability to express and characterize both enzymes and receptors, there was a pressing need to improve the rate of biologic assessment by developing reliable, scalable, and reproducible in vitro methods.

These advances enabled the development high-throughput screening (HTS) assays using simpler in vitro systems where the effect of compounds on receptors or enzymes could be studied.[11,12] In the earliest formats, compounds dissolved in dimethyl sulfoxide (DMSO) distributed in 96-well plates were exposed to aqueous reaction media (enzymes and/or cells) at comparatively high concentrations (eg, 1 and 10 μM) to provide an initial survey of thousands of compounds in a comparatively short period of time. Some of the earliest screens were carried out on natural products or natural product extracts. As this technology advanced, more compounds could be screened by increasing the number of wells on a plate to 384, and subsequently to 1,536. Today, HTS of a million compounds can be routinely accomplished. The time frame for such an effort varies, depending on the complexity of the system. Some screens can be completed in a few months, others require a year or more.[13,14]

This gave rise to the need to provide more compounds and a desire to expand the diversity of structures to offer distinct chemotypes for exploration. The need to feed a substantially higher capacity biology engine provided a powerful impetus for chemists to develop and implement more rapid methods for synthesis, purification, and analysis of new compounds in solution and on a solid support. Within a short period of time, parallel and combinatorial synthesis technologies developed. This resulted in an explosion of the number of compounds that could be evaluated. To accomplish this, chemists took advantage of a subset of transformations that reliably proceeded in moderate to high yield, such as amide formation and reductive amination that offered a wide range of aromatic and aliphatic reaction components (eg, carboxylic acids, ketones, aldehydes, amines). Soon, a single chemist could set up a library that could provide tens to hundreds of compounds that could be characterized by automated analytical methods, then screened immediately and/or plated for future use.

Medicinal chemists soon realized some of the limitations of both HTS and parallel/combinatorial chemistry. These observations resulted in a more considered perspective on the utility of HTS methodology and the accompanying high-throughput chemistry. It is accurate to say that parallel and combinatorial synthesis have their place in contemporary medicinal chemistry under the right circumstances. For example, rather than make one analog at a time to develop structure-activity relationship (SAR), a series can be developed more rapidly if related analogs are prepared and studied together. A downside to this approach is the bias imparted on chemical starting points that are more suitable for parallel synthesis. It is also accurate to state that this technology has not greatly accelerated the discovery of new drug candidates. A full discussion of the chemical advances, benefits, and limitations of parallel and combinatorial synthesis is beyond the scope of this chapter.

The benefits of HTS are also somewhat mixed as a result of difficulties that were encountered, accompanied by unrealistic expectations associated with the theory that by screening huge numbers of compounds, a useful hit and/or a drug candidate will emerge from the effort. Nonetheless, HTS campaigns were instrumental in the discovery of several approved drugs.[15] Difficulties with HTS include the quality and identity of samples in the screening deck, and the resultant confidence in the results. There can be technical issues associated with converting an assay from a laboratory format to one that can be effectively miniaturized and automated. Furthermore, there are cost and time factors to consider when accumulating reagents and protein or cells for the campaign.

Another technologic advance that developed during this same period of time is structure-based drug design and computational chemistry.[16,17] The ability to identify how a small molecule interacted with a target was viewed as a major advance because it could be directly applied to the design of new molecules with improved affinity. Coupled with this was the development of computational models to predict a variety of properties such as biologic activity, physical properties such as solubility, and pharmacokinetic features such as oral bioavailability and metabolic stability.[18] These models were applied in an effort to speed up an inherently complicated process such as drug discovery and were widely employed in the pharmaceutical industry, where time and cost are precious commodities. A major limiting feature of any computational model is the quality and quantity of data available to build and train it for predictive use. Often these models are limited to a specific chemical series, making their applicability across divergent structures much less valuable.

One example illustrates the complexity based in part on the now well-known Lipinski guidelines for oral bioavailability.[19] The "rules" state that, to maximize the possibility of oral bioavailability, no more than one violation of the following characteristics is permitted: (1) molecular weight less than 500, (2) no more than five hydrogen bond donors, (3) cLogP less than 5, (4) no more than 10 hydrogen bond acceptors. These guidelines were based on analysis of compounds studied at Pfizer. Many exceptions were known at the time, and many examples of molecules that followed all four were not orally bioavailable. Subsequent development of other models, such as the Veber[20] variation, evaluated other features and ranges. In 2018, a review article[21] assessed the predictive value of these and other approaches to predict oral bioavailability and concluded that an "accurate prediction is challenging." It is important to point out that, while the generality of such models may be limited, a high-quality dataset based on a specific group of molecules can provide useful predictions for not only oral bioavailability, but also subsets of other pharmaceutical properties.

This brief survey of some important advances in medicinal chemistry and drug discovery in the 1980s and 1990s demonstrates that capabilities and tools expanded significantly. The accumulated experience with these new tools revealed their strengths and limitations. Medicinal chemists in both academia and industry have a better understanding of these features and this stimulated continued development in all of these areas with the aim to improve the utility, validity, and reliability of these tools.

Biology-Enabled Chemistry and Vice Versa

The technologies highlighted in the previous section proved to be assets in a new medicinal chemistry phase in the late 1990s and early 2000s, when a need arose to identify novel targets along with an expansion of the chemical probes to evaluate those targets. This arose from advances in genetics to enable in vivo functional analysis of manipulation of the human genome. The ability to delete a gene and study the animals using behavior and/or physiologic measurement gives science a tool to evaluate in cells and in animals many previously unstudied proteins and other biologic macromolecules. This gave rise to the exciting possibility that known cell surface G protein–coupled receptors (GPCRs), selected ion channels, enzymes, and known antibacterial and antiviral proteins represented only a small proportion of potential drug targets. This excitement continues today with the development of additional technologies discussed later.

One example of biology-enabled chemistry was the explosion of interest in discovery of kinase inhibitors. Kinases were found to be important regulators of many aspects of cell growth and function.[22,23] Analysis of the human genome indicated there were hundreds of these enzymes in the genome, many of them with unknown or poorly understood function. This created a circumstance in which medicinal chemistry and biology had to work closely to develop tools and methods of analysis for this important class of proteins. Using HTS and other methods, kinase inhibitors were identified and investigated for properties such as selectivity, cell permeability, and efficacy in both cellular and animal disease models. Distinct classes of kinases were characterized to include substrate classification such as tyrosine or serine/threonine and cellular localization such as receptor-associated or soluble. In 1995, the first kinase inhibitor, fasudil, was approved in China and Japan for use in cerebral vasospasm. A few years later, imatinib was approved by the U.S. Food and Drug Administration (FDA), and, by the end of 2023, a total of 80 kinase inhibitors were approved for cardiovascular, oncology, immunology, infectious disease, and other applications (Fig. 1.4).[24] This remains a highly active area of research in both industry and academia. From a medicinal chemistry perspective, kinase inhibitors expanded from molecules that are adenosine triphosphate (ATP)-competitive to include those that bind at allosteric sites. Within these larger groups, there are different conformationally based classifications accompanied by distinct structural classes in each set.[25] Each class of kinase inhibitors has its own distinct structural characteristics because of the nature of the binding site changes. This gives rise to structural diversity and new avenues for both chemical and therapeutic investigation.

A second area driven by chemistry was the discovery and use of DNA-encoded chemical libraries to provide an enormous diversity of candidates for biologic examination.[26,27] Originally derived in the 2000s using DNA to encode a large library of peptides, this technique permits encoding of molecules using DNA bases and polymerase chain reaction (PCR)-based signal amplification to identify molecules with affinity for a target. Synthesis is often carried out by a combinatorial split/pool method using generally reliable chemistry (eg, amide formation, reductive amination, selected organometallic couplings, and condensation reactions). This approach can provide a large number of compounds (often in the millions), depending on the variety of building blocks and number of steps. Complex structures can be prepared using this methodology and often include stereochemical features as well. A primary advantage of this technique is structural diversity. Like all screening methods, hits must be confirmed and in all cases require resynthesis to confirm not only structure, but also to establish that the potential hit can be efficiently prepared in the laboratory. Because hits are identified by a PCR-based method, it requires tiny amounts of compound whose signal is amplified enzymatically based on binding to the target. This large array of compound enables screening of many targets using small amounts of compound and protein.

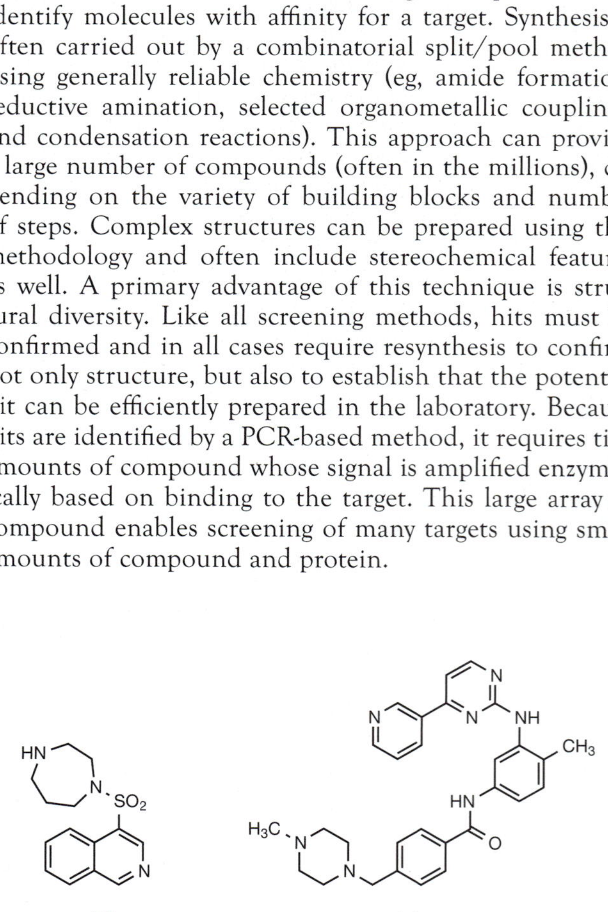

Figure 1.4 Early kinase inhibitors approved as drugs.

Selected Technology-Based Examples of Medicinal Chemistry Development

Among the many advances in science and medicinal chemistry, one that employs technology that continues to develop is computational and structure-based drug discovery. The human immunodeficiency virus (HIV) crisis that began in the mid-1980s created substantial needs in both chemistry and biology to identify and characterize the causative agent, accompanied by tools to evaluate their effect on what was found to be a ribonucleic acid (RNA) virus. A key advance came when an enzyme essential for viral replication was identified as an aspartic protease.[28] HIV-1 protease inhibitors could be designed and evaluated based on long-standing knowledge of other aspartic protease inhibitors. This class of enzymes uses two aspartic acid residues to activate a water molecule as a nucleophile to create a gem-diol intermediate that subsequently breaks down to the hydrolyzed peptide. A natural product, pepstatin, is used as a diagnostic inhibitor for this class of enzymes because it includes a hydroxyethylamine isostere of the amide bond (Fig. 1.5).

This information allowed medicinal chemists to design inhibitors based on this and other templates with the assistance of x-ray crystal structures of compounds bound within the active site of HIV-1 protease.[29] Structural information was used to guide new compound design, and this was extended to assist in the discovery of HIV-1 protease inhibitors that were active against mutant enzymes that developed during the course of therapy with first-generation agents.[30] Examples of these compounds are shown in Figure 1.6.

Technology is advancing in several ways, and one of the most impactful is the ability to carry out structure determination in much more of a higher throughput manner.[31] In a manner similar to the benefits of HTS, being able to evaluate more ligand-protein structures more rapidly assists with optimization. This is particularly relevant to the evaluation and development of fragment-based screening hits. Fragment screening is a technology that employs ligands with low molecular weight (generally <300). Hits have comparatively low affinity, with micromolar concentrations often in the tens or hundreds; however, because of their simplicity, they offer multiple opportunities for optimization.[32] With a detailed picture of how these low-affinity ligands interact with a protein, design hypotheses can be rapidly identified, tested, and validated. While this paradigm can enable identification of high-affinity ligands, there are limitations, including the need for comparatively large amounts of protein for initial screening and comparatively complex and low-throughput screening methods such as nuclear magnetic resonance (NMR) and surface plasmon resonance. Different methods can be applied to carry out this process, including linking two fragments that bind to different pockets on a protein as well as simply building additional features into a structure to interact with a protein.

A conceptually very different approach to affecting protein function is to promote their degradation. The two major routes are lysosomal and ubiquitin-mediated proteosomal degradation. The latter was first investigated approximately 20 years ago and has progressed rapidly.[33] A noteworthy benefit is the ability to expand the range of proteins with biologically relevant functions beyond receptors, enzymes, and ion channels. Targeted protein degradation involves binding a small molecule ligand to both the protein of interest and a ubiquitin ligase. This enables the ligase to more efficiently traffic the protein to the degradation machinery, and by its nature is catalytic rather than stoichiometric. Once a protein is directed toward the degradative pathway, the small molecule ligand dissociates and can repeat the process. This approach is more commonly known as proteolysis-targeting chimera (PROTAC) and is being widely investigated in several therapeutic areas including oncology and immunology. At least 20 different clinical trials are underway,[34] and one

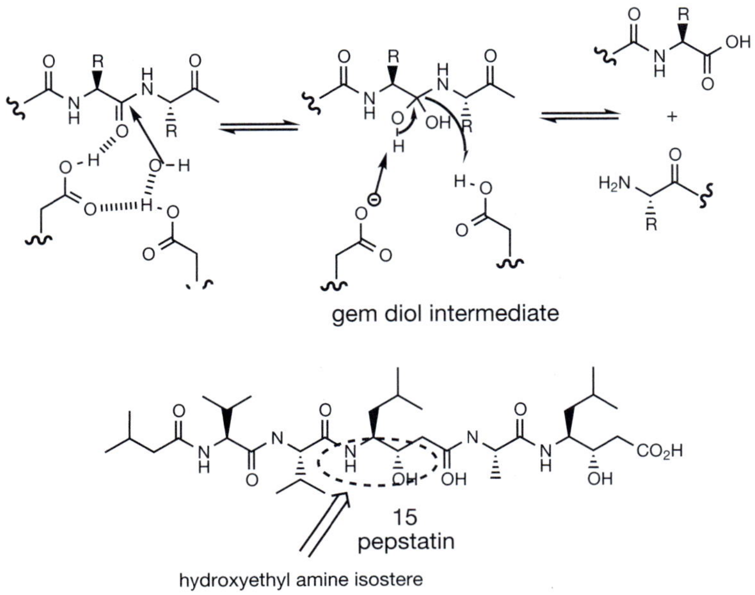

Figure 1.5 Mechanism of aspartyl protease hydrolysis and pepstatin.

Examples of First Generation HIV-1 Protease Inhibitors

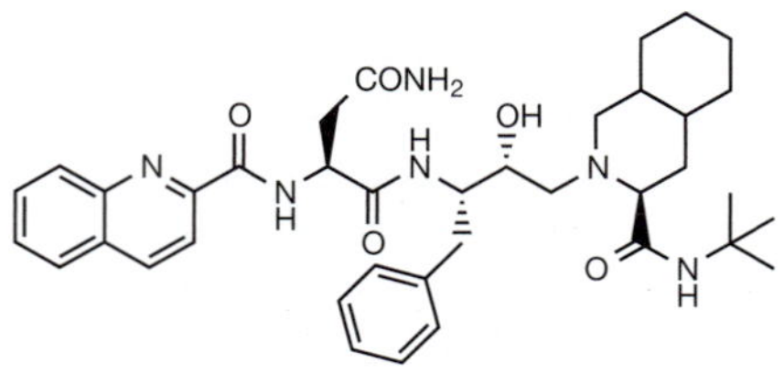

16
Saquinavir

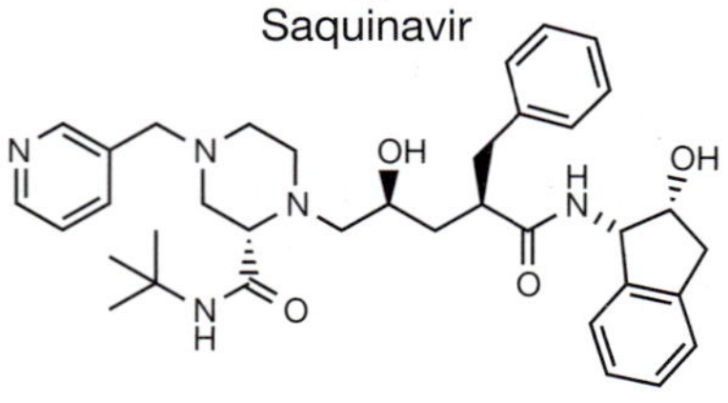

17
Indinavir

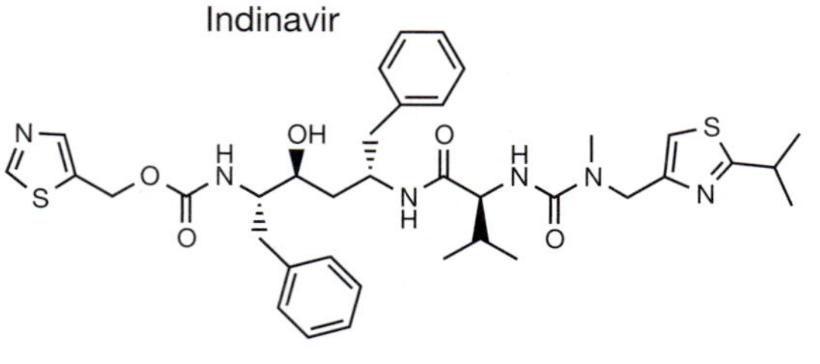

18
Ritonavir

HIV-1 Protease Inhibitor Active against mutant enzyme

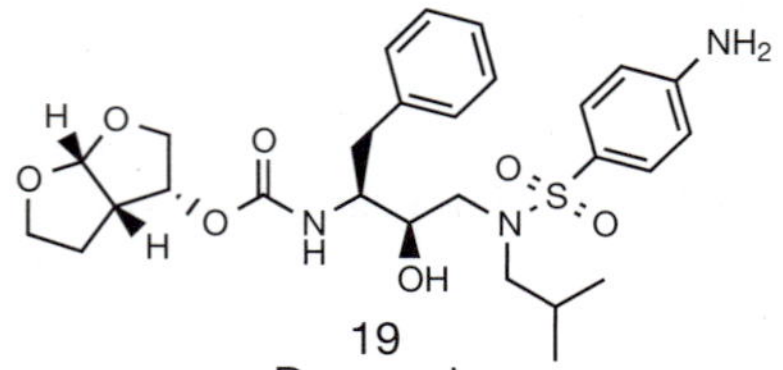

19
Darunavir

Figure 1.6 Human immunodeficiency virus-1 protease inhibitors.

compound, vepdegestrant (ARV-471, Fig. 1.7) is currently in phase 3 trials for the treatment of breast cancer.

Compounds with targeted protein degradation activity are designed to be multitarget ligands, one portion of the structure has affinity for a specific ligase such as cereblon, and another region of the molecule binds with the target protein. These two fragments are joined by a linker (Fig. 1.7). Multiprotein targeting in this manner helps to create a degree of specificity for the protein of interest. This can be tuned by traditional structure-activity studies to achieve the desired profile. In spite of their structural complexity, this class of drug candidates exhibits sufficient cell penetration and oral bioavailability to demonstrate efficacy in their respective disease models. In the phase 3 trial mentioned earlier, 200 mg of vepdegestrant is administered once daily, in combination with palbociclib, a serine/threonine cyclin-dependent kinase inhibitor.

The remarkable activities demonstrated by PROTACs stimulated additional research in protein degradation with one aim being to simplify the complexity of the molecule,

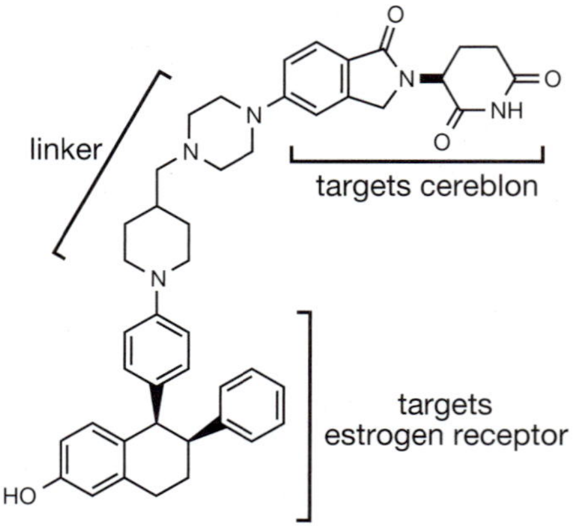

20
Vepdegestrant
(ARV-471)

Figure 1.7 Proteolysis-targeting chimera in phase 3 clinical trials.

leading to the advent of molecular glues, compounds that modulate protein function by virtue of protein-protein interactions.[34,35] Modulation can involve either inhibition or stimulation of function as well as degradation similar to PROTACs. Examples of compounds that act in this manner are shown in Figure 1.8. These approved drugs led to the inhibition of protein function and are used in the treatment of cardiovascular, immunologic, and oncology-related diseases.

In the subset of glues whose mechanism of action is based on protein degradation, there are similarities to PROTACs as well as notable differences.[36] Both groups induce protein degradation, can be targeted to specific proteins, and involve a catalytic (non-stoichiometric) mode of action. Glues tend to be of lower molecular weight, do not contain a linker, and originally were discovered serendipitously. More recently, with the development of improved screening assays, it is possible to carry out more focused discovery and screening for

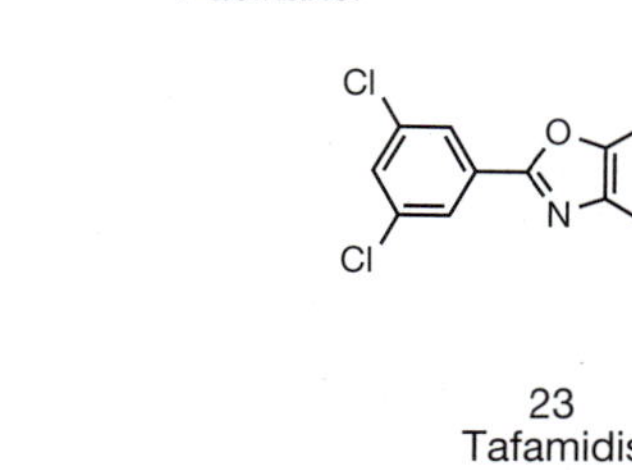

21
Paclitaxel

22
Pomalidomide

23
Tafamidis

Figure 1.8 U.S. Food and Drug Administration–approved molecular glues.

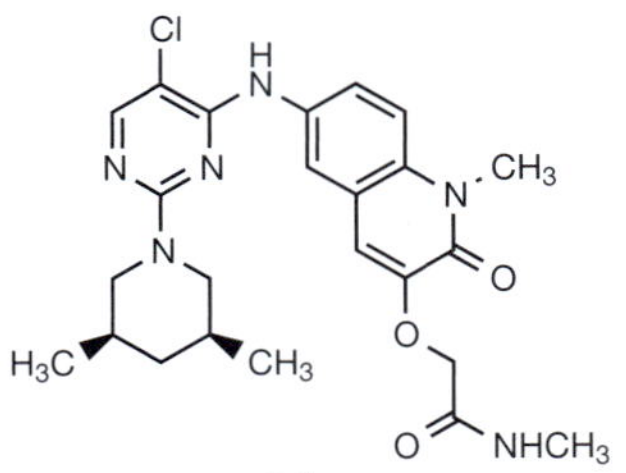

24
BI-3812

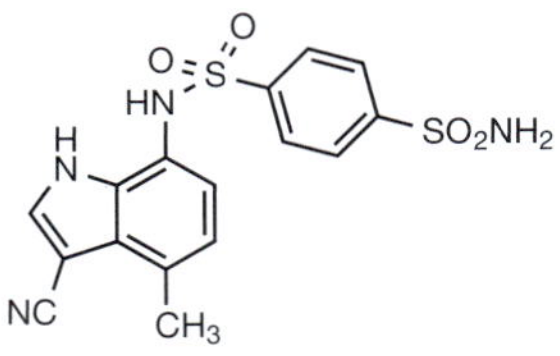

25
Indisulam

Figure 1.9 New molecular glues.

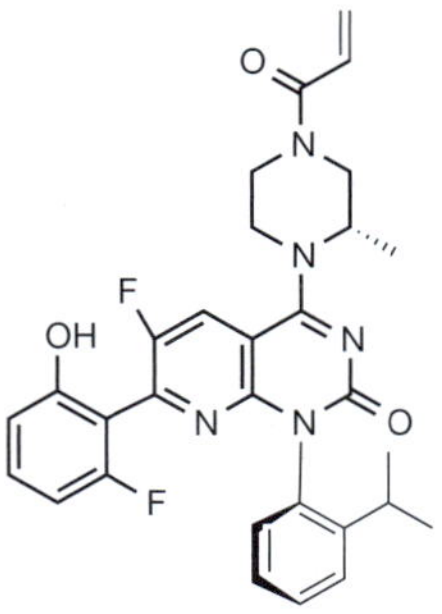

26
AMG-510
Sotorasib

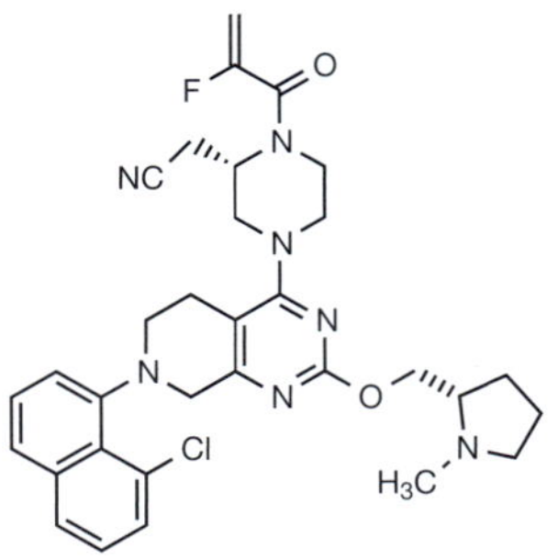

27
MRTX849
Adagrasib

Figure 1.10 U.S. Food and Drug Administration–approved mutant KRAS inhibitors.

potential glues. This work is aided greatly by structure-based optimization once a hit is identified. This field is expanding rapidly from a focus on cancer and immunology to other therapeutic areas, in particular central nervous system (CNS)-based drug discovery. Examples of more recently discovered molecular glues are shown in Figure 1.9, and these compounds were reported to have anticancer activity.

Where Will Medicinal Chemistry Be in 2050?

Medicinal chemistry, like other branches of science, is continuing to evolve in response to needs and discoveries. Looking back over the last 40 years, technologies that were originally touted as groundbreaking and revolutionary are now recognized more appropriately to be useful in selected circumstances. For example, screening methods such as high-throughput, fragment-based, and DNA-encoded libraries created a wealth of diverse structures that are now available for use to influence macromolecular function. These benefits are offset by limitations that were identified by experience. The same can be said of structure-based drug design, PROTACs, and molecular glues. With the benefit of experience, improvements have been made in all of these areas to more productively enable their use.

Medicinal chemists, and by extension the discipline, must work to better understand the advantages and weaknesses of these techniques in order to apply them most appropriately to solve the important questions being asked. It is appropriate at this stage to recall the definition cited previously: "Medicinal chemistry is defined as an independent mature science that is a combination of applied (medicine) and basic (chemistry) sciences." Said another way, the discipline investigates the chemistry of biologically active molecules. This requires molecules to interrogate a biologic system of interest. The ability to understand a biologic system, to measure a response in a reliable, appropriate manner, and to create molecules that interact with that system illustrate the multidisciplinarity of the field.

A key area of ongoing development is the application of machine learning and artificial intelligence.[37-39] These computational techniques employ data to guide a field, and medicinal chemistry is an area where applications abound, such as which molecule(s) to make, how to make them, and what target(s) are relevant to a disease of interest. Advances in processing speed and computer power enable rapid evaluation of enormous amounts of data to provide answers to questions of interest. Like any other data analysis tool, the value of the answer is critically dependent on the quality of inputs used to create the model. Extension of results from one question to another can be risky, particularly if those questions involve biology. Nevertheless, this approach has been shown to speed up the identification of biologically active molecules, with recent examples in antibiotic,[40] kinase inhibitor,[41] and oncology targets.[42]

The concept of "undruggable" targets (proteins with no known conventional drug ligand) is another area of rapid development and significant growth.[43] This is a large chemical space that includes proteins that function in nonenzymatic roles and, more recently, has been modified to refer to targets that have not been successfully drugged. An early report described a method to carry out proteome-wide covalent modification of proteins using a library of fragment-size molecules.[44] Perhaps the most recent example is found in the approval of two molecules for the treatment of cancer that target mutant KRAS (Fig. 1.10). This protein was known for many years as a key regulator of uncontrolled cell growth; however, molecules that could beneficially alter its function were few and far between. These two molecules covalently react with a cysteine residue present in mutant KRAS found in some lung, pancreatic, and colorectal cancers, providing a significant degree of selectivity over wild-type KRAS needed for normal cell growth and division.

Summary

In summary, medicinal chemistry is a multidisciplinary field that requires understanding of synthetic, analytical, biologic, and physical chemistry as well as biology. Practitioners in the field must remain current in the rapidly developing aspects of interest to them. The number of unanswered questions in these areas provides the stimulus for continued expansion and growth in the discipline.

REFERENCES

1. Khan FMO, Deimling MJ, Philip A. Medicinal chemistry and the pharmacy curriculum. *Am J Pharm Educ.* 2011;75(8):161.
2. Delgado JN, Remers WA. Introduction. In: Beale JM Jr, Wilson CO, Gisvold O, eds. *Wilson and Gisvold's Textbook of Organic Medicinal and Pharmaceutical Chemistry*. 9th ed. J. B. Lippincott Co; 1991:1-2.
3. Sneader W. *Drug Discovery: A History*. John Wiley and Sons; 2005.
4. Witbesky E. Ehrlich's side chain theory in the light of present immunology. *Ann N Y Acad Sci.* 1954;59(2):168-191.
5. Ceresia GB, Brusch CA. An introduction to the history of medicinal chemistry. *Am J Pharm Sci.* 1955;127(11):384-395.
6. Koshland DE Jr. The key-lock theory and induced fit. *Angew Chem Int Ed Engl.* 1995;33:2375-2378.
7. Langley JN. On the physiology of salivary secretion. Part II. On the mutual antagonism of atropine and pilocarpine, having especial reference to their relations in the sub-maxillary gland of the cat. *J Physiol.* 1878;1:339-369.
8. Burger A. The history and economics of medicinal chemistry. In: Burger A, ed. *Medicinal Chemistry*. 3rd ed. John Wiley and Sons; 1970:4-19.
9. Barger G, Dale HH. Chemical structure and sympathomimetic action of amines. *J Physiol.* 1910;41(1-2):19-59.
10. Rubin RP. A brief history of great discoveries in pharmacology: in celebration of the centennial anniversary of the founding of the American Society of Pharmacology and Experimental Therapeutics. *Pharmacol Rev.* 2007;59(4):289-359.
11. Mayr LM, Fuerst P. The future of high-throughput screening. *J Biomol Screen.* 2008;13(6):443-448.
12. Pereira DA, Williams JA. Origin and evolution of high throughput screening. *Br J Pharmacol.* 2007;152:53-61.
13. Cox B, Denyer JC, Binnie A, et al. Application of high-throughput screening techniques to drug discovery. *Prog Med Chem.* 2000;37:84-132.
14. Blay V, Tolani B, Ho SP, et al. High-throughput screening: today's biochemical and cell-based approaches. *Drug Discov Today.* 2020;25(10):1807-1821.
15. Macarron R, Banks MN, Bojanic D, et al. Impact of high-throughput screening in biomedical research. *Nat Rev Drug Discov.* 2011;10:188-195.
16. Klebe G. Recent developments in structure-based drug design. *J Mol Med.* 2000;78:269-281.
17. Blaney J. A very short history of structure-based design: how did we get here and where do we need to go? *J Comput Aided Mol Des.* 2012;26:13-14.
18. Bassani D, Moro S. Past, present and future perspectives on computer-aided drug design methodologies. *Molecules.* 2023;28(9):3906.
19. Lipinski CA, Lombardo F, Dominy BW, et al. Experimental and computational approaches to estimate solubility and permeability in drug discovery and development settings. *Adv Drug Deliv Rev.* 2001;46(1-3):3-26.
20. Veber DF, Johnson SR, Cheng HY, et al. Molecular properties that influence oral bioavailability of drug candidates. *J Med Chem.* 2002;45(12):2615-2623.
21. Cabrera-Perez MA, Pham-The H. Computational modeling of human oral bioavailability: what will be next? *Expert Opin Drug Discov.* 2018;13(6):509-521.
22. Roskowski R Jr. A historical overview of protein kinases and their targeted small molecule inhibitors. *Pharmacol Res.* 2015;100:1-23.
23. Lightfoot HL, Goldberg FW, Sedelmeier J. Evolution of small molecule kinase drugs. *ACS Med Chem Lett.* 2019;10(2):153-160.
24. Roskowski R Jr. Properties of FDA-approved small molecule protein kinase inhibitors: a 2024 update. *Pharmacol Res.* 2023;200:107059. doi:10.1016/j.phrs.2024.107059
25. Roskowski R Jr. Classification of small molecule protein kinase inhibitors based on the structures of their drug-enzyme complexes. *Pharmacol Res.* 2016;103:26-48.
26. Gartner ZJ, Liu DR. The generality of DNA-templated synthesis as a basis for evolving non-natural small molecules. *J Am Chem Soc.* 2001;123(28):6931-6933.
27. Kleiner RE, Dumelin CE, Liu DR. Small-molecule discovery from DNA-encoded chemical libraries. *Chem Soc Rev.* 2011;40(12):5707-5717.
28. Brik A, Wong CH. HIV-1 protease: mechanism and drug discovery. *Org Biomol Chem.* 2003;1(1):5-14.
29. Kempf DJ, Sham HJ. HIV protease inhibitors. *Curr Pharm Des.* 1996;2:225-246.
30. Ghosh AK, Chapsal BD, Weber IT, et al. Design of HIV protease inhibitors targeting protein backbone: an effective strategy for combating drug resistance. *Acc Chem Res.* 2008;41(1):78-86.
31. Blundell TL, Patel S. High-throughput X-ray crystallography for drug discovery. *Curr Opin Pharmacol.* 2004;4(5):490-496.
32. Rees DC, Congreve M, Murray CW, et al. Fragment-based lead discovery. *Nat Rev Drug Discov.* 2004;4:660-672.
33. Békés M, Langley DR, Crews CM. PROTAC targeted protein degraders: the past is the prologue. *Nat Rev Drug Discov.* 2022;21:181-200.
34. Liu Z, Hu M, Yang Y, et al. An overview of PROTACs: a promising drug discovery paradigm. *Mol Biomed.* 2022;3:46.
35. Dewey JA, Delalande C, Azizi S-A, et al. Molecular glue discovery: current and future approaches. *J Med Chem.* 2023;66:9278-9296.
36. Dong G, Ding Y, He S, et al. Molecular glues for targeted protein degradation. *J Med Chem.* 2021;64(15)10606-10620.
37. Ivanenkov Y, Zagribelnyy B, Malyshev A, et al. The hitchhiker's guide to deep learning driven generative chemistry. *ACS Med Chem Lett.* 2023;14(7):901-915.
38. Blanco-González A, Cabezón A, Seco-González A, et al. The role of AI in drug discovery: challenges, opportunities and strategies. *Pharmaceuticals (Basel).* 2023;16(6):891.
39. Tyrchan C, Nittinger E, Gogishvili D, et al. Approaches using AI in medicinal chemistry. In: Akitsu T, ed. *Computational and Data-Driven Chemistry Using Artificial Intelligence*. Elsevier; 2022:111-159.
40. Ali T, Ahmed S, Aslam M. Artificial intelligence for antimicrobial resistance prediction: challenges and opportunities towards practical implementation. *Antibiotics (Basel).* 2023;12(3):523.
41. Gupta R, Srivastava D, Sahu M, et al. Artificial intelligence to deep learning: machine intelligence approach for drug discovery. *Mol Divers.* 2021;25:1315-1360.
42. Zhu J, Wang J, Wang X, et al. Prediction of drug efficacy from transcriptional profiles with deep learning. *Nat Biotechnol.* 2021;39:1444-1452.
43. Xie X, Yu T, Li X, et al. Recent advances in targeting the "undruggable" proteins: from drug discovery to clinical trials. *Signal Transduct Target Ther.* 2023;8:335.
44. Backus KM, Correia BE, Lum KM, et al. Proteome-wide covalent ligand discovery in native biological systems. *Nature.* 2016;534(7608):570-574.

CHAPTER 2

Foundational Principles and Functional Group Impact on Activity

Robin M. Zavod

Abbreviations

ACE angiotensin-converting enzyme
ACh acetylcholine
BBB blood-brain barrier
BCRP breast cancer–resistance protein
CIP Cahn, Ingold, Prelog
GI gastrointestinal
HCl hydrochloric acid
HIV human immunodeficiency virus
HPT-1 human peptide transporter 1
IM intramuscular
IV intravenous
MRP2, MRP3 multidrug resistance–associated proteins 2 and 3
MW molecular weight
NaOH sodium hydroxide
OATP organic anion transporting polypeptide
OCTP organic cation transporting polypeptide
PABA *p*-aminobenzoic acid
PEPT1 peptide transporter 1
P-gp P-glycoprotein
QSAR quantitative structure-activity relationship
SAR structure-activity relationship
SC subcutaneous
USP U.S. Pharmacopeia

Medicinal chemistry is an interdisciplinary science at the intersection of organic chemistry, biochemistry (bio-organic chemistry), computational chemistry, pharmacology, pharmacognosy, molecular biology, and physical chemistry. This branch of chemistry is involved with the identification, design, synthesis, and development of new drugs that are safe and suitable for therapeutic use in humans and animals. It includes the study of marketed drugs, their biologic properties, and their quantitative structure-activity relationships (QSARs).

Medicinal chemists study how chemical structure influences biologic activity. As such, it is necessary to understand not only the mechanism by which a drug exerts its effect but also how the molecular and physicochemical properties of the molecule influence the drug's pharmacokinetics (absorption, distribution, metabolism, toxicity, and elimination) and pharmacodynamics (what the drug does to the body). The term "physicochemical properties" refers to how the functional groups present within a molecule influence its acid-base properties, water solubility, partition coefficient, crystal structure, stereochemistry, and ability to interact with biologic systems, such as enzyme active sites and receptor binding sites. To design better medicinal agents, the relative contribution that each functional group makes to the overall physicochemical properties of the molecule must be evaluated. Studies of this type involve modification of the molecule in a systematic fashion followed by a determination of how these changes affect biologic activity. Such studies are referred to as structure-activity relationships (SARs)—that is, the relationship of how structural features of the molecule contribute to, or take away from, the desired biologic activity. Because of the foundational nature of the content of this chapter, there are numerous case studies presented throughout the chapter (as boxes).

Introduction

Chemical entities, usually derived from plants and other natural sources, have been used by humans for thousands of years to alleviate pain, diarrhea, infection, and various other maladies. Until the 19th century, these "remedies" were primarily crude preparations of plant material of unknown constitution. The revolution in synthetic organic chemistry during the 19th century produced a concerted effort toward identification of the structures of the active constituents of these naturally derived medicinals and synthesis of what were hoped to be more efficacious agents. By determining the molecular structures of the active components of these complex mixtures, it was thought that a better understanding of how these components worked could be elucidated.

Relationship Between Molecular Structure and Biologic Activity

Early studies of the relationship between chemical structure and biologic activity were conducted by Crum-Brown and Fraser[1] in 1869. They demonstrated that many molecules containing tertiary amine groups exhibited activity as muscle relaxants when converted to quaternary ammonium molecules. Molecules with widely differing pharmacologic properties, such as strychnine (a convulsant), morphine (an analgesic), nicotine (a deterrent, insecticide), and atropine (an anticholinergic), could be converted to muscle relaxants with properties similar to those of tubocurarine when methylated (Fig. 2.1). Crum-Brown and Fraser therefore concluded that muscle relaxant activity required the presence of a quaternary ammonium group within the structure. This initial hypothesis was later disproven by the discovery of the natural neurotransmitter and activator of muscle contraction, acetylcholine (ACh), as shown in Figure 2.2. Even though Crum-Brown and Fraser's initial hypothesis that related chemical structure with action as a muscle relaxant was incorrect, it demonstrated the concept that molecular structure influences the biologic activity of chemical entities and that alterations in structure produce changes in biologic action.

With the discovery by Crum-Brown and Fraser that quaternary ammonium groups could produce molecules with muscle relaxant properties, scientists began to look for other functional groups that produce specific biologic responses. At the time, it was thought that specific chemical groups, or nuclei (rings), were responsible for specific biologic effects. This led to the postulate, which took some time to disprove, that "one chemical group gives one biological action."[2] Even after the discovery of ACh by Loewi and Navrati,[3] which effectively dispensed with Crum-Brown and Fraser's concept of all quaternary ammonium molecules being muscle relaxants, this was still considered to be dogma and took a long time to refute.

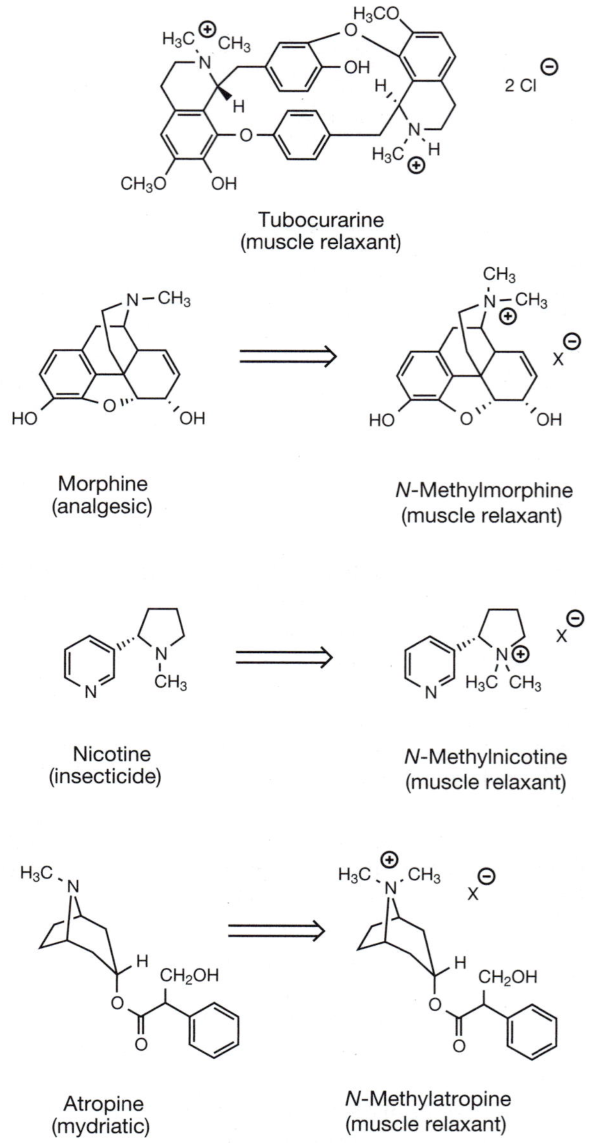

Figure 2.1 Effects of methylation on biologic activity.

Selectivity of Drug Action and Drug Receptors

Although the structures of many drugs or xenobiotics, or at least their functional group composition, were known at the start of the 20th century, how these molecules exerted their effects was still a mystery. Using his observations with regard to the staining behavior of microorganisms, Ehrlich[4] developed the concept of drug receptors. He postulated that certain "side chains" on the surfaces of cells were "complementary" to the dyes (or drug) and suggested that the two could therefore interact with one another. In the case of antimicrobial molecules, interaction of the chemical with the cell surface "side chains" produced a toxic effect. This concept was the first description of what later became known as the receptor hypothesis for explaining the biologic action of chemical entities. Ehrlich also discussed selectivity of drug action via the concept of a "magic bullet." He suggested that this selectivity permitted eradication of disease states without significant harm coming to the organism being treated (ie, the patient). This was later modified by Albert[5] and today is referred to as "selective toxicity." An example of poor selectivity was demonstrated when Ehrlich developed arsenic (As)-containing compounds that were toxic to trypanosomes due to their irreversible reaction with thiol groups (-SH) on vital proteins. The formation of As-S bonds resulted in death of the target organism. Unfortunately, these molecules were toxic not only to the target organism but also to the host once certain blood levels of arsenic were achieved.

The "paradox" that resulted after the discovery of ACh—that is, how one chemical group can produce two different biologic effects (ie, muscle relaxation and muscle contraction)—was explained by Ing,[6] using the actions of ACh and tubocurarine as his examples. Ing hypothesized that both ACh and tubocurarine act at the same receptor, but that

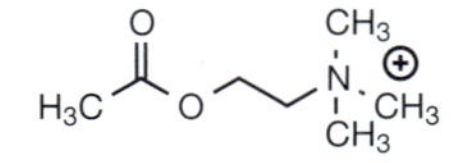

Figure 2.2 Acetylcholine, a neurotransmitter and muscle relaxant.

one molecule fits the receptor in a more complementary manner and "activates" it, causing muscle contraction. (Ing did not elaborate just how this activation occurred.) The blocking effect of the larger molecule, tubocurarine, could be explained by its occupation of part of the receptor, thereby preventing ACh, the smaller molecule, from interacting with the receptor. With both molecules, the quaternary ammonium functional group is a common structural feature and interacts with the same region of the receptor. In examining the structures of other molecules with opposing effects on the same pharmacologic system, this appears to be a common theme: Molecules that block the effects of natural neurotransmitters, such as norepinephrine, histamine, dopamine, or serotonin, for example, are called antagonists and are usually larger in size than the native molecule. This is not the case for antagonists of peptide neurotransmitters and hormones such as cholecystokinin, melanocortin, or substance P. Antagonists to these peptide molecules are usually smaller in size. However, regardless of the type of neurotransmitter (biogenic amine or peptide), both agonists and antagonists share common structural features with the neurotransmitter that they influence. This provides support to the concept that the structure of a molecule, its composition and arrangement of functional groups, determines the type of pharmacologic effect that it possesses (ie, SAR). For example, molecules that are muscle relaxants acting via the cholinergic nervous system possess a quaternary ammonium or protonated tertiary ammonium group and are larger than ACh (compare ACh in Fig. 2.1 with tubocurarine in Fig. 2.2).

SARs are the underlying principle of medicinal chemistry. Similar molecules exert similar biologic actions in a qualitative sense. A corollary to this is that structural elements (functional groups) within a molecule most often contribute in an additive manner to the physicochemical properties of a molecule and, therefore, to its biologic action. One need to only peruse the structures of drug molecules in a particular pharmacologic class to become convinced (eg, histamine H_1 antagonists, histamine H_2 antagonists, β-adrenergic antagonists). In the quest for better medicinal agents (drugs), it must be determined which functional groups within a specific structure are important for its pharmacologic activity and how these groups can be modified to produce more potent, more selective, and safer molecules.

An example of how different functional groups can yield chemical entities with similar physicochemical properties is demonstrated by the sulfanilamide antibiotics. In Figure 2.3, the structures of sulfanilamide and *p*-aminobenzoic acid (PABA) are shown. In 1940, Woods[7] demonstrated that PABA reverses the antibacterial action of sulfanilamide (and other sulfonamide-based antibacterials) and both PABA and sulfanilamide have similar steric and electronic properties. Both molecules contain acidic functional groups, with PABA containing an aromatic carboxylic acid (Ar-COOH) and sulfanilamide an aromatic sulfonamide (Ar-SO_2NH_2). When ionized at physiologic pH, both molecules have a similar electronic configuration, and the distance between the ionized acid and the weakly basic amino group is also very similar. It should be no surprise that sulfanilamide acts as an antagonist to PABA metabolism in bacteria.

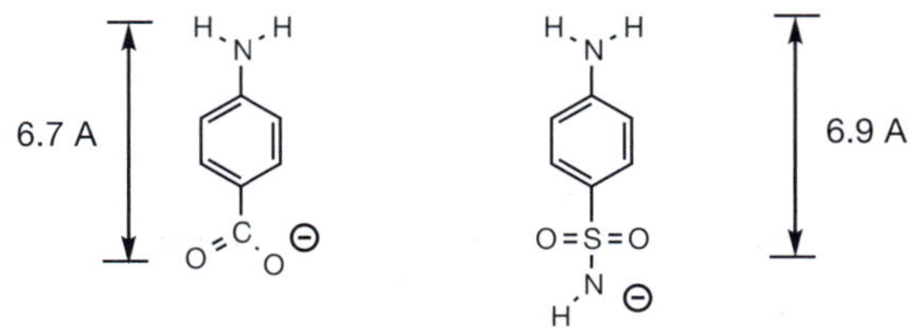

p-Aminobenzoic acid

Sulfanilamide

Figure 2.3 Ionized forms of *p*-aminobenzoic acid (PABA) and sulfanilamide, with comparison of the distance between amine and ionized acids of each molecule. Note how closely sulfanilamide resembles PABA.

Biologic Targets for Drug Action

In order for drug molecules to exhibit their pharmacologic activity, they must interact with a biologic target, typically a receptor, enzyme, nucleic acid, excitable membrane, or other biopolymers. These interactions occur between the functional groups found in the drug molecule and those functional groups found within each biologic target. The relative fit of each drug molecule with its target is a function of a number of physicochemical properties including acid-base chemistry and related ionization, functional group shape and size, and three-dimensional spatial orientation. The quality of this "fit" has a direct impact on the biologic response produced. In this chapter, functional group characteristics are discussed to better understand overall drug molecule absorption, distribution, metabolism, and excretion as well as potential interaction with a biologic target.

Physicochemical Properties of Drugs

Acid-Base Properties

The human body is 70% to 75% water, which amounts to approximately 51 to 55 L of water for a 160-lb (73-kg) individual. For an average drug molecule with a molecular weight (MW) of 200 g/mol and a dose of 20 mg, this leads to a solution concentration of approximately 2×10^{-6} M (2 μM). The solution behavior of a drug within the body is that of a dilute solution, for which the Brönsted-Lowry[8] acid-base theory is most appropriate to explain and predict acid-base behavior. This is a very important concept in medicinal chemistry, because the acid-base properties of drug molecules determine the ionization state of the molecule at a given pH, therefore directly affecting absorption, excretion, and compatibility with other drugs in solution.

According to the Brönsted-Lowry theory, an "acid" is any substance capable of yielding a proton (H^+), and a "base" is any substance capable of accepting a proton. When an acid gives up a proton to a base, it is converted to its "conjugate base." Similarly, when a base accepts a proton, it is converted to its "conjugate acid" (Equations 2.1 and 2.2):

Eq. 2.1 $CH_3COOH + H_2O \rightleftharpoons CH_3COO^{\ominus} + H_3O^{\oplus}$

CH_3COOH	H_2O	$CH_3COO^{\ominus}$	$H_3O^{\oplus}$
Acid (acetic acid)	Base (water)	Conjugate Base (acetate)	Conjugate Acid (hydronium ion)

Eq. 2.2 $CH_3NH_2 + H_2O \rightleftharpoons CH_3NH_3^{\oplus} + {}^{\ominus}OH$

CH_3NH_2	H_2O	$CH_3NH_3^{\oplus}$	${}^{\ominus}OH$
Base (methylamine)	Acid (water)	Conjugate Acid (methyl ammonium ion)	Conjugate Base (hydroxide ion)

Note that when an acidic functional group loses its proton (often referred to as having undergone "dissociation"), it is left with an extra electron and becomes negatively charged. This is the "ionized" form of the acid. The ability of the ionized functional group to participate in an ion-dipole interaction with water (see the "Water Solubility of Drugs" section) enhances its water solubility. Many functional groups behave as acids (Table 2.1). The ability to recognize these functional groups and their relative acid strengths helps predict absorption, distribution, excretion, and potential incompatibilities between drugs.

When a basic functional group is converted to the corresponding conjugate acid, it too becomes ionized. In this instance, however, the functional group becomes positively charged due to the extra proton. Most drugs that contain basic functional groups contain primary, secondary, or tertiary amines or imino amines, such as guanidines and amidines.

Table 2.1 Common Acidic Organic Functional Groups and Their Ionized (Conjugate Base) Forms

Acids (pK_a)			Conjugate Base
Phenol (9-11)	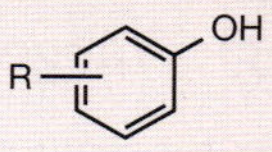	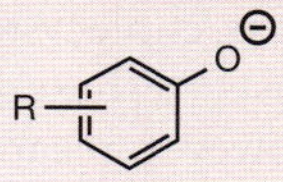	Phenolate
Sulfonamide (9-10)	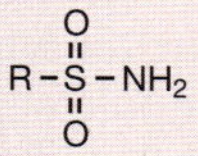	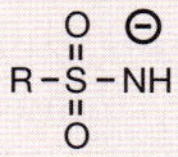	Sulfonamidate
Imide (9-10)	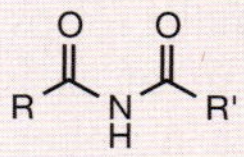	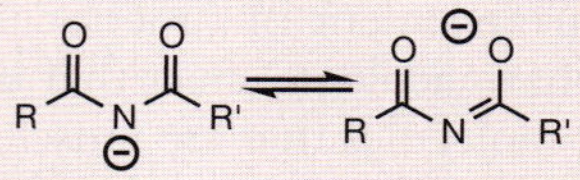	Imidate
Alkyl thiol (10-11)	R-SH	$R{-}S^{\ominus}$	Thiolate
Thiophenol (6-7)	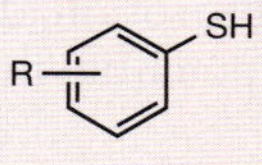	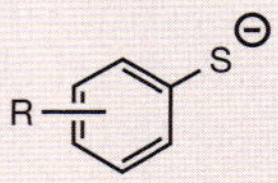	Thiophenolate
N-Arylsulfonamide (6-7)	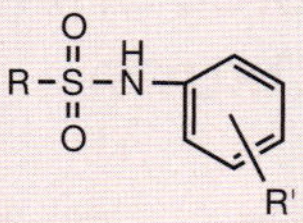	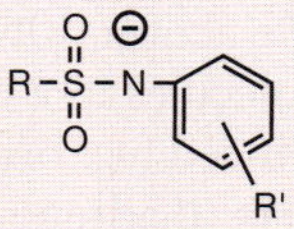	*N*-Arylsulfonamidate
N-Acylsulfonamide (5-6)	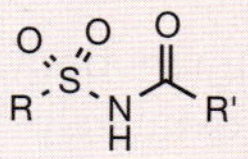	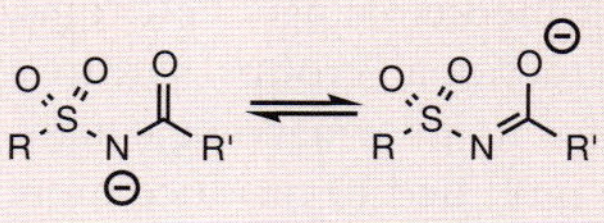	*N*-Acylsulfonamidate
Alkylcarboxylic acid (5-6)	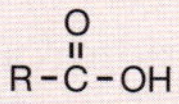	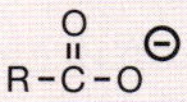	Alkylcarboxylate
Arylcarboxylic acid (4-5)	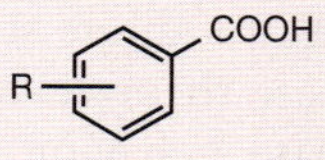	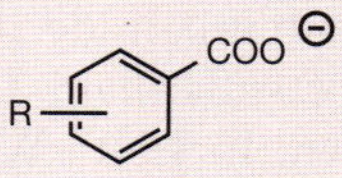	Arylcarboxylate
Sulfonic acid (0-1)	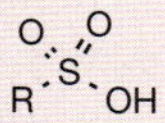	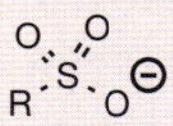	Sulfonate

Acid strength increases down the table.

Table 2.2 Common Basic Organic Functional Groups and Their Ionized (Conjugate Acid) Forms

Base			Conjugate Acid (p*K*a HB⁺)
Imine	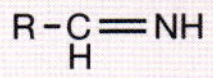	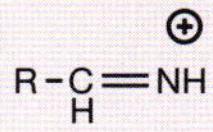	Iminium (3-4)
Arylamine	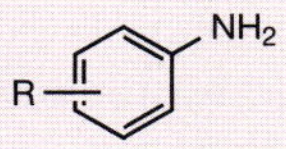	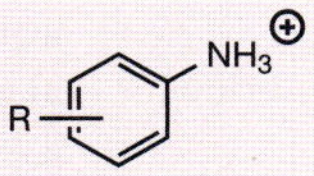	Arylammonium (4-5)
Aromatic amine	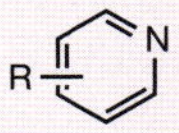	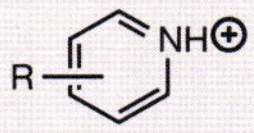	Aromatic ammonium (5-6)
Alkylamines	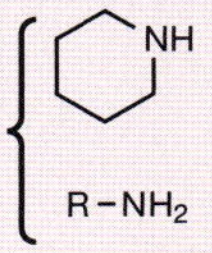	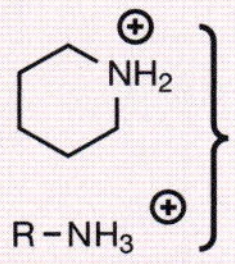	Alkylammonium (1°—9-10) (2°—10-11)
Amidine	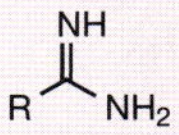	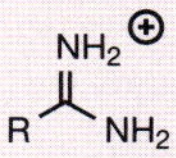	Amidinium (10-11)
Guanidine	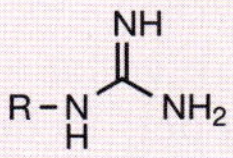	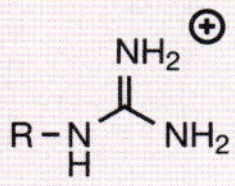	Guanidinium (12-13)

Other functional groups that are basic are shown in Table 2.2. As with the acidic groups, it is important to become familiar with these functional groups and their relative strengths.

Functional groups that cannot lose/donate or accept a proton are considered to be "neutral" (or "nonelectrolytes") with respect to their acid-base properties. Common neutral functional groups are shown in Table 2.3. Quaternary ammonium molecules are neither acidic nor basic and are not electrically neutral. Additional information about the acid-base properties of the functional groups listed in Tables 2.1 through 2.3 can be found in Lemke.[9]

A molecule can contain multiple functional groups with acid-base properties and, therefore, can possess both acidic and basic character. For example, ciprofloxacin (Fig. 2.4), a fluoroquinolone antibacterial agent, contains a secondary alkylamine, one tertiary arylamine (aniline-like amine), and a carboxylic acid. The arylamine is weakly basic and, therefore, does not contribute significantly to the acid-base properties of ciprofloxacin under physiologic conditions. Depending on the pH of the physiologic environment, this molecule will either accept a proton (secondary alkylamine) or donate a proton (carboxylic acid), or do both. Thus, it is described as amphoteric (both acidic and basic) in nature. Figure 2.5 shows the acid-base behavior of ciprofloxacin in two different environments. Note that at a given pH (eg, pH 1.0-3.5), only one of the functional groups (the alkylamine) is significantly ionized. To be able to make this prediction,

Table 2.3 Common Organic Functional Groups That Are Considered Neutral Under Physiologic Conditions

$R-CH_2-OH$ Alkyl alcohol	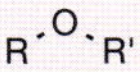 Ether	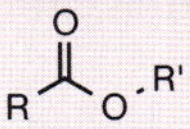 Ester	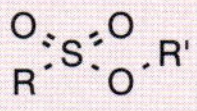 Sulfonic acid ester
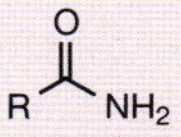 Amide	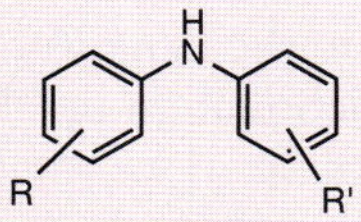 Diarylamine	R−C≡N Nitrile	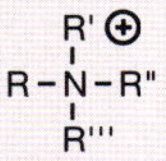 Quaternary ammonium
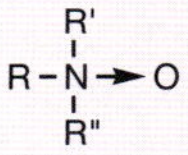 Amine oxide	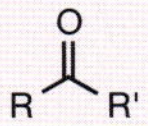 Ketone and aldehyde	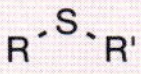 Thioether	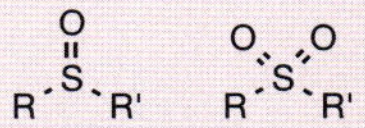 Sulfoxide sulfone

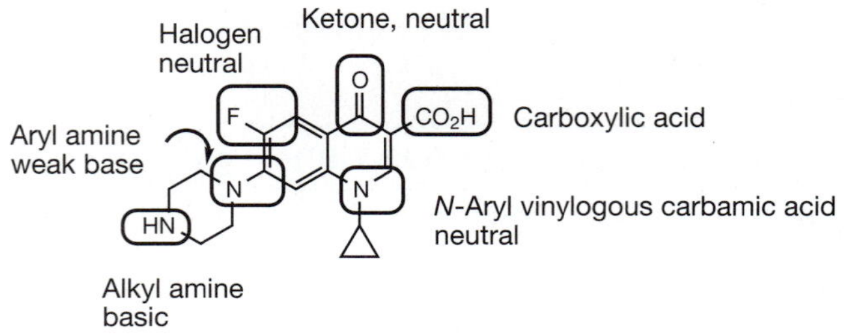

Figure 2.4 Chemical structure of ciprofloxacin showing the various organic functional groups.

an appreciation for the relative acid-base strength of both the acidic and basic functional groups is required. Thus, knowing which acidic or basic functional group within a molecule containing multiple functional groups is the strongest and which acidic or basic functional group is the weakest are necessary. The concept of pK_a not only describes relative acid-base strength of functional groups but also allows one to calculate, for a given pH, the relative percentages of the ionized and unionized forms of the drug. As stated, this helps predict relative water solubility, absorption, and excretion for a given chemical entity.

RELATIVE ACID STRENGTH (pK_A)

Strong acids and bases completely donate (dissociate) or accept a proton (associate) in aqueous solution to produce their respective conjugate bases and acids. For example, mineral acids, such as hydrochloric acid (HCl), or bases, such as sodium hydroxide (NaOH), undergo 100% dissociation in water, with the equilibrium between the ionized and unionized forms shifted completely to the right (ionized), as shown in Equations 2.3 and 2.4:

Eq. 2.3 $$HCl + H_2O \rightleftharpoons Cl^{\ominus} + H_3O^{\oplus}$$

Eq. 2.4 $$NaOH + H_2O \rightleftharpoons Na^{\oplus} + OH^{\ominus} + H_2O$$

Acids and bases of intermediate or weak strength, however, incompletely donate (dissociate) or accept a proton (associate), and the equilibrium between the ionized and unionized forms lies somewhere in the middle, such that all possible species can exist at any given time. Note that in Equations 2.3 and 2.4, water acts as a base in one instance and as an acid in the other. Water is therefore *amphoteric*—that is, it can act as an acid or a base, depending on the prevailing pH of the solution. From a physiologic perspective, drug molecules are always present as a dilute aqueous solution. The strongest base that is present is OH^-, and the strongest acid is H_3O^+. This is known as the "leveling effect" of water. Thus, some functional groups that have acidic or basic character do not behave as such under physiologic conditions in aqueous solution. For example, alkyl alcohols, such as ethyl alcohol, are not sufficiently acidic to become significantly ionized in an aqueous solution at a physiologic pH. Water is not sufficiently basic to remove the proton from ethyl alcohol to form the ethoxide ion (Equation 2.5). Therefore, under physiologic conditions, alcohols are neutral with respect to acid-base properties:

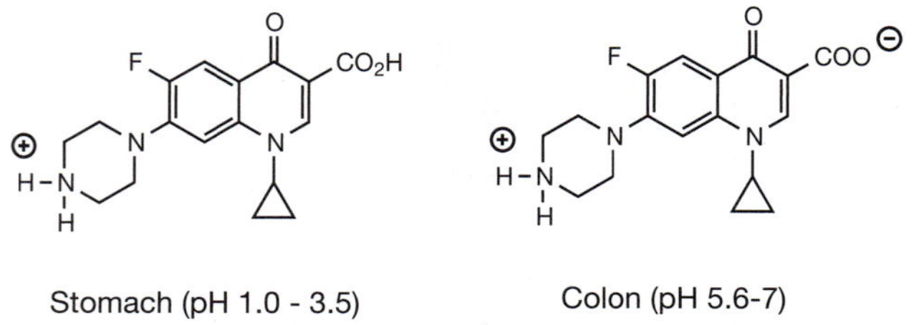

Figure 2.5 Predominate forms of ciprofloxacin at two different locations within the gastrointestinal tract.

Eq. 2.5 $$CH_3CH_2OH + H_2O \not\rightleftharpoons CH_3CH_2O^- + H_3O^{\oplus}$$

Predicting the Degree of Ionization of a Molecule

By knowing if there are acidic and/or basic functional groups present in a molecule, one can predict whether a molecule is going to be predominantly ionized or unionized at a given pH. To be able to quantitatively predict the degree of ionization of a molecule, the pK_a values of each of the acidic and basic functional groups present and the pH of the environment in which the molecule will be located must be known. It is also necessary to know if a given functional group is acidic or basic in character. The magnitude of the pK_a value is a measure of relative acid or base strength, and the Henderson-Hasselbalch equation (Equation 2.6) can be used to calculate the percent ionization of a molecule at a given pH (this equation was used to calculate the major forms of ciprofloxacin in Fig. 2.5):

Eq. 2.6 $$pK_a = pH + \log \frac{[\text{acid form}]}{[\text{base form}]}$$

The key to understanding the use of the Henderson-Hasselbalch equation for calculating percent ionization is to realize that this equation relates a constant, pK_a, to the ratio of the acidic form of a functional group to its conjugate base form (and conversely, the conjugate acid form to its base). Because pK_a is a constant for any given functional group, the ratio of acid to conjugate base (or conjugate acid to base) will determine the pH of the solution. A sample calculation is shown in Figure 2.6 for the sedative hypnotic amobarbital.

When dealing with a basic functional group, one must recognize the conjugate acid represents the ionized form of the functional group. Figure 2.7 shows the calculated percent ionization for the decongestant phenylpropanolamine. It is very important to understand that for a base, the pK_a refers to the conjugate acid or ionized form of the molecule. To thoroughly comprehend this relationship, calculate the percent ionization of an acidic functional group and a basic functional group at different pH values and carefully observe the trend.

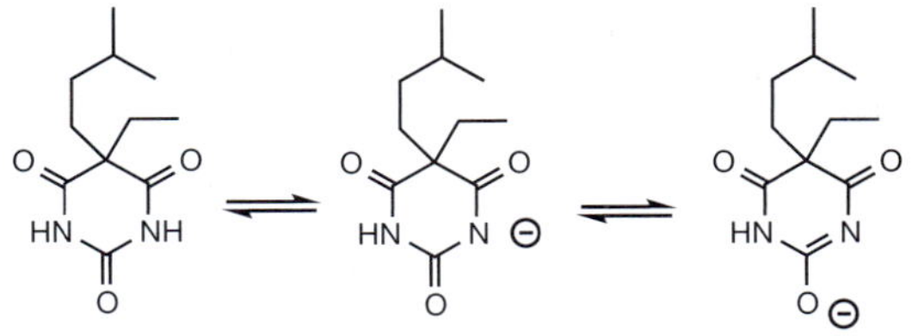

Acid form
pK_a 8.0

Conjugate base

Question: What percent of amobarbital is ionized at pH=7.4?

Answer:

$$8.0 = 7.4 + \log \frac{[\text{acid}]}{[\text{base}]}$$

$$0.6 = \log \frac{[\text{acid}]}{[\text{base}]}$$

$$10^{0.6} = \frac{[\text{acid}]}{[\text{base}]} = \frac{3.98}{1}$$

$$\%\text{ acid form} = \frac{3.98 \times 100}{4.98} = 79.9\%$$

$$\%\text{ ionization} = 100\% - 79.9\% = 20.1\%$$

Figure 2.6 Calculation of percent ionization of amobarbital. Calculation indicates that 80% of the molecules are in the acid (or protonated) form, leaving 20% in the conjugate base (ionized) form.

Water Solubility of Drugs

The solubility of a drug molecule in water greatly affects the routes of administration that are available, as well as its absorption, distribution, and elimination. Two key concepts to keep in mind when considering the water (or fat) solubility of a molecule are the potential for hydrogen bond formation and ionization of one or more functional groups within the molecule.

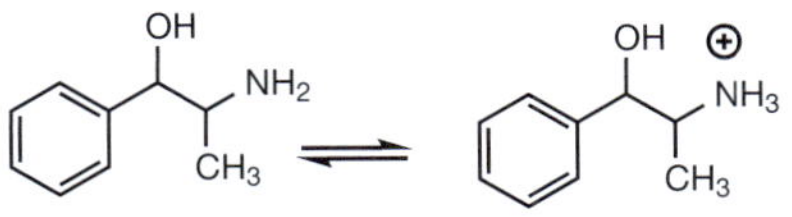

Base form

Conjugate acid form
pK_a 9.4

Question: What is the % ionization (acid form) of phenylpropanolamine at pH 7.4?

Answer:

$$7.4 = 9.4 + \log \frac{[\text{acid}]}{[\text{base}]}$$

$$2.0 = \log \frac{[\text{acid}]}{[\text{base}]}$$

$$10^2 = \frac{[\text{acid}]}{[\text{base}]} = \frac{100}{1}$$

$$\%\text{ ionization} = \frac{100 \times 100}{101} = 99\%$$

Figure 2.7 Calculation of percent ionization of phenylpropanolamine. Calculation indicates that 99% of the molecules are in the conjugate acid form, which is the same as the percent ionization.

Hydrogen Bonds

Each functional group capable of donating or accepting a hydrogen bond contributes to the overall water solubility of the molecule and increases the hydrophilic (water-loving) nature of the molecule. Conversely, functional groups that cannot form hydrogen bonds do not enhance hydrophilicity and will contribute to the hydrophobic (water-fearing) nature of the molecule. Hydrogen bonds are a special case of what are usually referred to as dipole-dipole interactions. A permanent dipole occurs as a result of an unequal sharing of electrons between two atoms within a covalent bond. This unequal sharing of electrons only occurs when these two atoms have significantly different electronegativities. When a permanent dipole is present, a partial charge is associated with each of these atoms along a single bond (one atom has a partial negative charge, and one atom has a partial positive charge). The atom with a partial negative charge has higher electron density than the other atom. When two functional groups containing one or more permanent dipoles approach one another, they align such that the negative end of one dipole is electrostatically attracted to the positive end of the other. When the positive end of the dipole is a hydrogen atom, this interaction is referred to as a "hydrogen bond" (or H-bond). Thus, for a hydrogen bonding interaction to occur, at least one functional group must contain a dipole with an electropositive hydrogen. The hydrogen atom must be covalently bound to an electronegative atom, such as oxygen (O), nitrogen (N), sulfur (S), or selenium (Se). Of these four elements, only oxygen and nitrogen atoms contribute significantly to the dipole, and we will therefore concern ourselves only with the hydrogen bonding capability (specifically as hydrogen bond donors) of functional groups that contain a bond between oxygen and hydrogen atoms (eg, alcohols) and functional groups that contain a bond between nitrogen and hydrogen atoms (eg, primary and secondary amines and amides) (eg, NH and CONH groups).

Even though the energy associated with each hydrogen bond is small (1-10 kcal/mol/bond), it is the additive nature of multiple hydrogen bonds that contributes to the overall water solubility of a given drug molecule. This type of interaction is also important in the interaction between a drug and its biologic target (eg, receptor). Figure 2.8 shows several types of hydrogen bonding interactions that can occur with a couple of functional groups and water. As a general rule, the more hydrogen bonds that are possible between a drug molecule and water, the greater the water solubility of the molecule. Table 2.4 lists several common functional groups and the number of hydrogen bonds in which they can potentially participate. Note that this table does not account for the possibility of intramolecular hydrogen bond formation. Each intramolecular hydrogen bond decreases water solubility (and increases lipid solubility) because there is one less interaction possible with water.

Ionization

In addition to the hydrogen bonding capacity of a molecule, another type of interaction plays an important role in determining water solubility: the ion-dipole interaction. This type of interaction can occur with organic salts. Ion-dipole

Case Study 2.1

ABSORPTION/ACID-BASE CASE

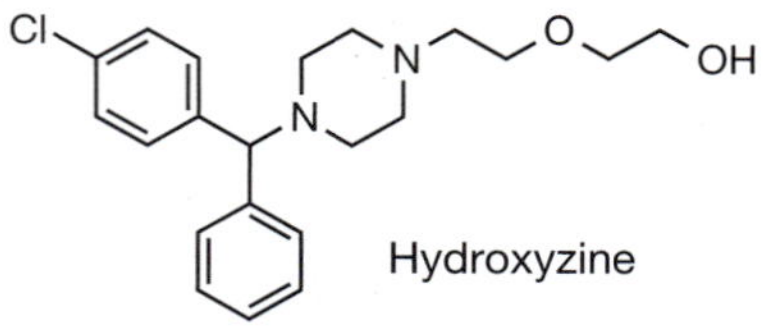

Hydroxyzine

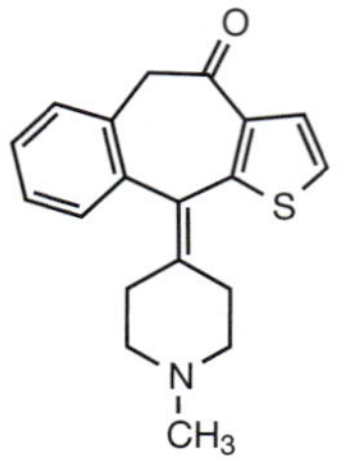

Ketotifene

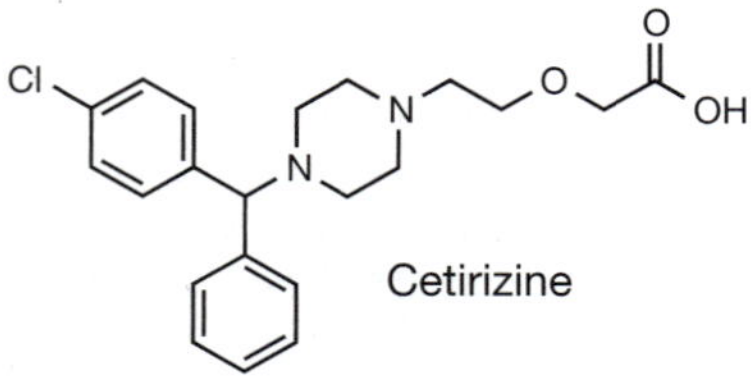

Cetirizine

Marcus, a horse used for equine therapy for special needs individuals, has seasonal allergies and is miserable in the summer. The barn director Ms L limits the hives that Marcus experiences by administering powdered hydroxyzine in his morning feed grain. During the afternoon riding therapy, Marcus is slow to move, appears lethargic, and is constantly trying to chew/scratch his legs. The veterinarian recommends that Ms L switch to powdered Zyrtec to see if it would offer better antihistaminergic action. Within a week, she notices that Marcus seems more alert during lessons but is still constantly chewing/scratching his legs.

1. Identify the functional groups present in hydroxyzine and cetirizine and evaluate the effect of each functional group on the ability of the drug to cross lipophilic membranes (eg, blood-brain barrier [BBB]). Based on your assessment of each agent's ability to cross the BBB (and, therefore, potentially cause drowsiness), provide a rationale for why Marcus is lethargic during afternoon therapy sessions.
2. For her own allergies, Ms L uses Systane Zaditor (ketotifen), an ophthalmic eye drop that is sold as an aqueous solution of the fumarate salt. Modify the structure present in the box to show the appropriate salt form of this agent. This agent is applied to the eye to relieve itching associated with allergies. Describe why this agent is soluble in water and what properties make it able to be absorbed into membranes that surround the eye.

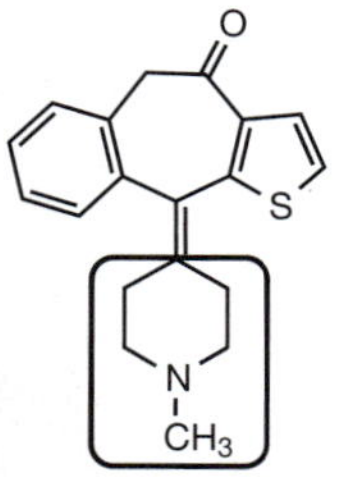

Ketotifene

3. Consider the structural features of hydroxyzine and cetirizine. In which compartment of the horse digestive system (stomach [pH 2] or hindgut [pH 6.5-7]) will each of these two drugs be best absorbed?
4. Horses that do not continuously forage, such as those that are stabled, can develop an acidic hindgut (pH 5). Based on your answer to question 3, determine whether Marcus will get the full antihistaminergic effect if he is given the antihistamine while experiencing an acidic hindgut. Provide a rationale for your answer.

Case Solution found immediately after References.

Case Study 2.2

ACID-BASE CHEMISTRY/COMPATIBILITY CASE

The intravenous (IV) technician in the hospital pharmacy gets an order for a patient that includes the two drugs shown. She is unsure if she can mix the two drugs together in a Y-site and is not certain how water soluble the agents are.

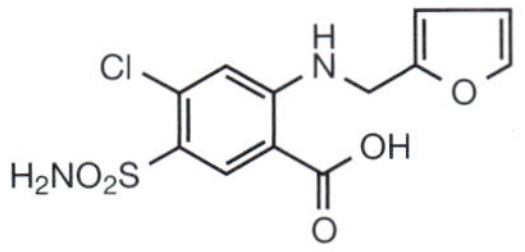

Furosemide

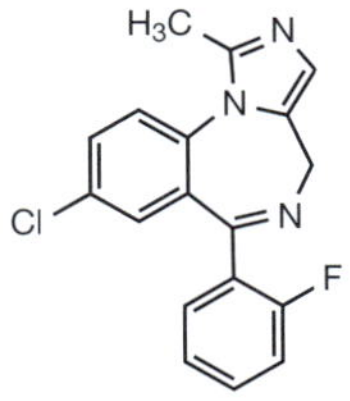

Midazolam

1. Determine the acid-base character of each of the functional groups in the two molecules shown. Modify the structures to show the form of the drug at pH 7.4 and reevaluate the acid-base character of these functional groups.
2. As originally drawn, which of these two agents is more water soluble? Provide a rationale for your selection that includes appropriate structural properties. Is the salt form of midazolam more or less water soluble than the free base form of the drug? Provide a rationale for your answer based on the structural properties of the salt form of midazolam.
3. What is the chemical consequence of mixing aqueous solutions of each drug in a Y-site? Provide a rationale that includes an acid-base assessment.

Case Solution found immediately after References.

interactions occur between either a cation and the partially negatively charged atom found in a permanent dipole (eg, the oxygen atom in water) or an anion and the partially positively charged atom found in a permanent dipole (eg, the hydrogen atoms in water), as shown in Figure 2.9.

Organic salts are composed of a drug molecule in its ionized form and an oppositely charged counterion. For example, the salt of a carboxylic acid is composed of the carboxylate anion (ionized form of the functional group) and a positively charged ion (eg, Na^+), and the salt of a secondary amine is composed of the ammonium cation (ionized form of the functional group and a negatively charged ion, eg, Cl^-). Not all organic salts are very water soluble. To associate with enough water molecules to become soluble, the salt must be highly dissociable; in other words, the cation and anion must be able to separate and interact independently with water molecules. Highly dissociable salts are those formed from strong acids with strong bases (eg, sodium chloride), weak acids with strong bases (eg, sodium phenobarbital), or strong acids with weak bases (eg, atropine sulfate). Examples of strong acids (strong acids are 100% ionized in water [ie, no ionization constants or pK_a values >1]) include the hydrohalic (hydrochloric, hydrobromic, and hydrofluoric), sulfuric, nitric, and perchloric acids. All other acids (eg, phosphoric, tartaric, acetic, and other organic acids and phenols) are partially ionized with pK_a values from 1 to 14 and are, therefore, considered to be moderate or weak acids. Hydroxides of sodium, potassium, and calcium are strong bases because they are 100% ionized, whereas other bases, such as amines, are of moderate or weak strength. The salt formed by a carboxylic acid with an alkylamine is the salt of a weak acid and weak base, respectively. This salt does not dissociate appreciably and cannot significantly contribute to the overall water solubility of a given drug molecule.

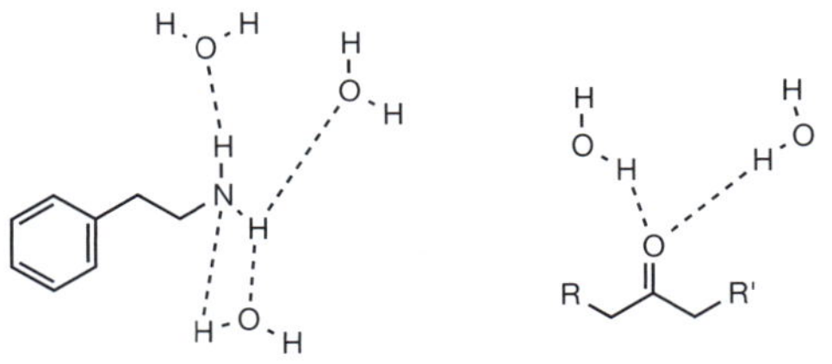

Figure 2.8 Examples of hydrogen bonding between water and hypothetical drug molecules.

Table 2.4 Common Organic Functional Groups and Their Hydrogen Bonding Potential

Functional Groups	Number of Potential H-Bonds
R-OH	3
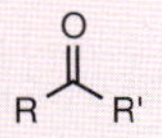	2
$R-NH_2$	3
R-NH with R'	2
R-N-R" with R'	1
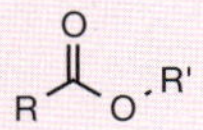	2

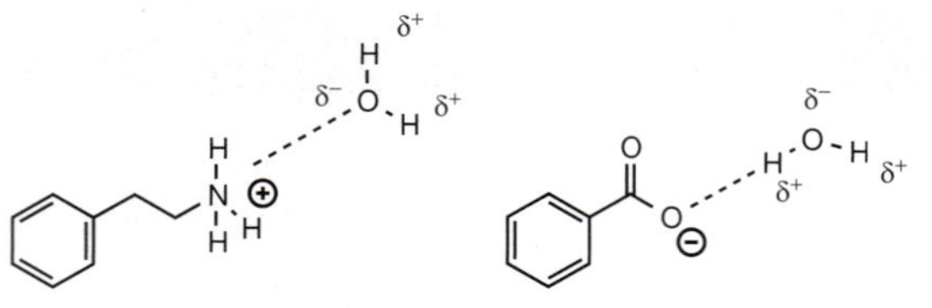

Figure 2.9 Examples of ion-dipole interactions.

In general, low-molecular-weight salts are water soluble, and high-molecular-weight salts are water insoluble. Examples of common organic salts used in pharmaceutical preparations are provided in Figure 2.10.

The extent to which ionized molecules are soluble in water is also dependent on the presence of intramolecular ionic interactions. Molecules with ionizable functional groups of opposite charge have the potential to interact with each other rather than with water molecules. When this occurs, these molecules often become water insoluble. A classic example is the amino acid tyrosine (Fig. 2.11). Tyrosine contains three very polar functional groups, two of which are ionizable (the alkylamine and carboxylic acid) depending on the pH of the environment.

The phenolic hydroxyl group is also ionizable (pK_a 9-10); however, it does not contribute significantly to the ionization of tyrosine under pharmaceutically or physiologically

Case Study 2.3

ABSORPTION/BINDING INTERACTIONS CASE

A 32-year-old woman comes into the pharmacy and asks you to recommend a treatment for the itching and burning she has recently noticed on both feet. She indicates that she would prefer a cream rather than a spray or a powder. You recommend Tinactin (tolnaftate), a very effective topical antifungal agent sold over the counter.

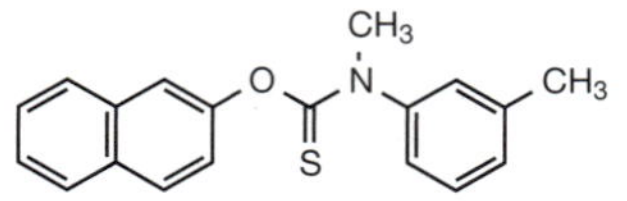

Tolnaftate (Tinactin)

1. Identify the structural characteristics and the corresponding properties that make tolnaftate an agent that can be used topically.
2. A biologic target for drug action for tolnaftate is squalene epoxidase. Consider each of the structural features of this antifungal agent and describe the type of interactions that the drug will have with the target for drug action. Which amino acids are likely to be present in the active site of this enzyme?

Case Solution found immediately after References.

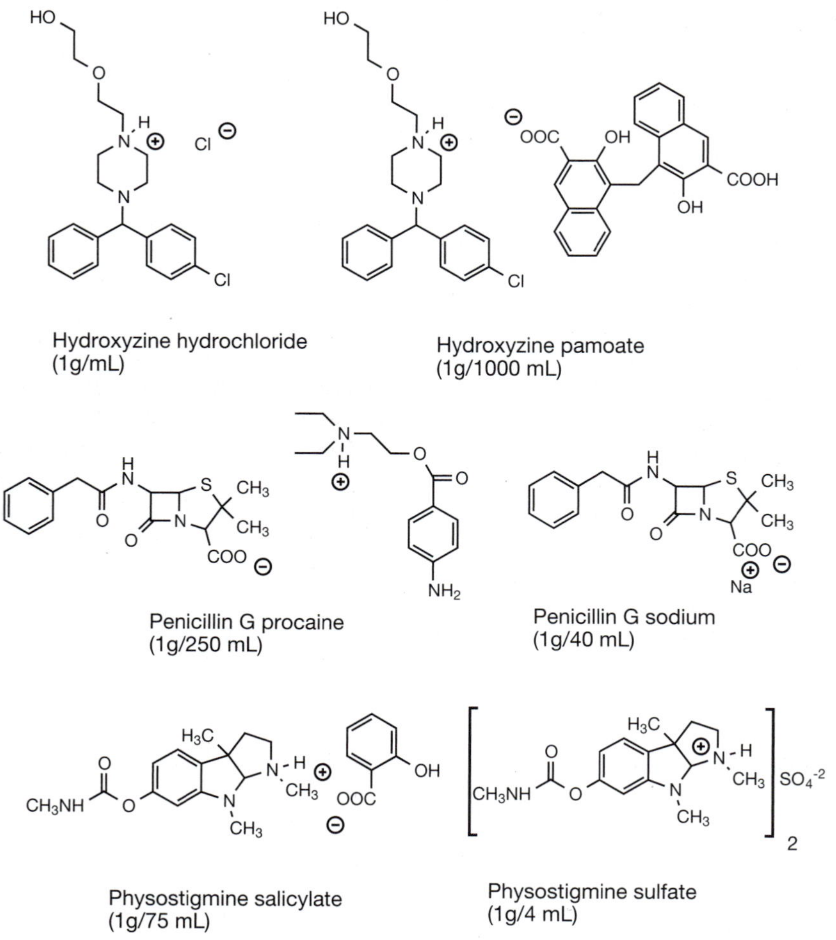

Figure 2.10 Water solubilities of different salt forms of selective drugs.

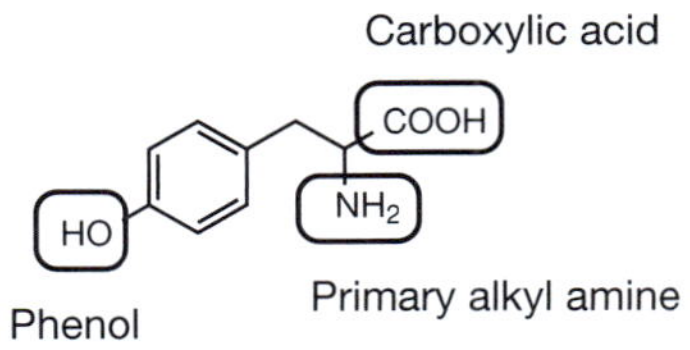

Figure 2.11 Functional groups present in tyrosine (see text for pK_a values).

relevant conditions (<1% ionized at pH 7). Because of the presence of three very polar functional groups (two of them being ionizable), one would expect tyrosine to be very soluble in water, yet its solubility is only 0.45 g/1,000 mL. The basic alkylamine (pK_a (HB^+) 9.1 for the conjugate acid) and the carboxylic acid (pK_a 2.2) are both ionized at physiologic pH, and a zwitterionic molecule results. These two charged groups are sufficiently close that a strong ion-ion interaction occurs, thereby keeping each group from participating in ion-dipole interactions with surrounding water molecules. This lack of interaction between the ions and the dipoles found in water results in a more water-insoluble molecule (Fig. 2.12). Not all zwitterions or multiply charged molecules demonstrate this behavior; only those that contain ionized functional groups close enough for an ionic interaction to occur will be poorly soluble. Generally, the greater the separation between charges, the more highly water soluble one anticipates the molecule will be. This is only true, however, up to a certain number of carbon atoms. This will be discussed in more detail later.

Predicting Water Solubility: Empirical Approach

Lemke[9] developed an empirical approach to predicting the water solubility of molecules based on the carbon-solubilizing potential of several functional groups. In his approach, if the solubilizing potential of the functional groups exceeds the total number of carbon atoms present, then the molecule is considered to be water soluble. Otherwise, it is considered to be water insoluble. Participation in intramolecular hydrogen bonding or ionic interactions decreases the solubilizing potential of a given functional group. It is difficult to quantitate how much such interactions will decrease a molecule's overall water solubility.

Table 2.5 shows the water-solubilizing potential for several functional groups common to many drugs. Because most drug molecules contain more than one functional group (ie, are polyfunctional), the second column in the table will be of more utility. To demonstrate Lemke method, consider the structure of anileridine. Anileridine (Fig. 2.13) is an opioid analgesic containing three functional groups that contribute to water solubility: an aromatic amine (very weak base), a tertiary alkylamine (weak base), and an ester

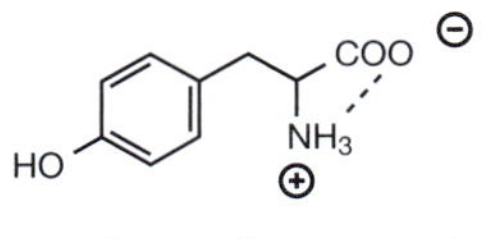

Figure 2.12 Zwitterionic form of tyrosine showing ion-ion bond.

Table 2.5 Water-Solubilizing Potential of Organic Functional Groups in a Mono- or Polyfunctional Molecule

Functional Group	Monofunctional Molecule	Polyfunctional Molecule
Alcohol	5-6 carbons	3-4 carbons
Phenol	6-7 carbons	3-4 carbons
Ether	4-5 carbons	2 carbons
Aldehyde	4-5 carbons	2 carbons
Ketone	5-6 carbons	2 carbons
Amine	6-7 carbons	3 carbons
Carboxylic acid	5-6 carbons	3 carbons
Ester	6 carbons	3 carbons
Amide	6 carbons	2-3 carbons
Urea, carbonate, carbamate		2 carbons

Water solubility is defined as >1% solubility.[9]

(neutral). There are a total of 22 carbon atoms in the molecule and a solubilizing potential from the three functional groups of nine carbon atoms. Since the solubilizing potential of the functional groups is less than the total number of carbons present, it is predicted that anileridine is insoluble in water. This is, indeed, the case: The solubility of anileridine is reported in the U.S. Pharmacopeia (USP) as 1 g/10,000 mL, or 0.01%. Now consider the hydrochloride salt of anileridine. Not only do the three functional groups contribute a solubilizing potential of nine carbon atoms, the positive charge of the alkylammonium also contributes to its water solubility. Lemke[9] estimates that each ionized functional group (cationic or anionic) found within a drug molecule contributes a solubilizing potential of 20 to 30 carbon atoms. Thus, the solubilizing potential for all of the functional groups in anileridine hydrochloride is 29 to 39 carbon atoms, which is more than the total number of carbon atoms in the molecule. This salt should therefore be soluble in water, and it is to the extent of 0.2 g/mL, or

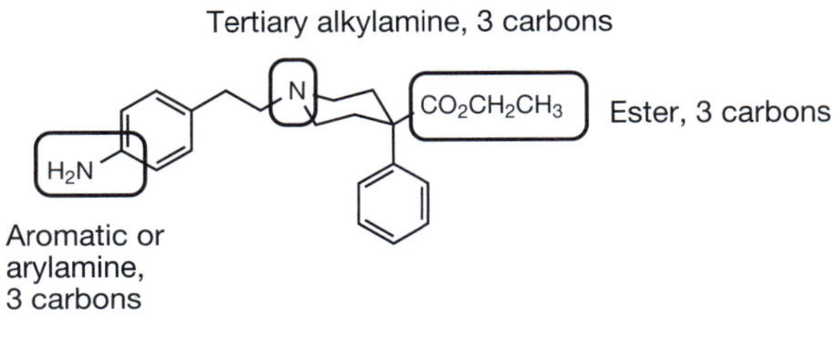

Figure 2.13 Identification of functional groups in anileridine.

Case Study 2.4

BINDING INTERACTIONS CASE

Each of these drug molecules interacts with a different biologic target and elicits a unique pharmacologic response. For each of the three molecules, list the types of interactions that are possible with a biologic target. For each type of interaction, provide one example of an amino acid that could participate in that interaction.

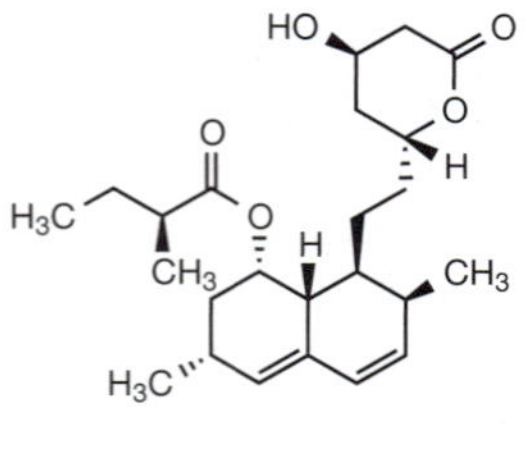

Lovastatin (Mevacor)

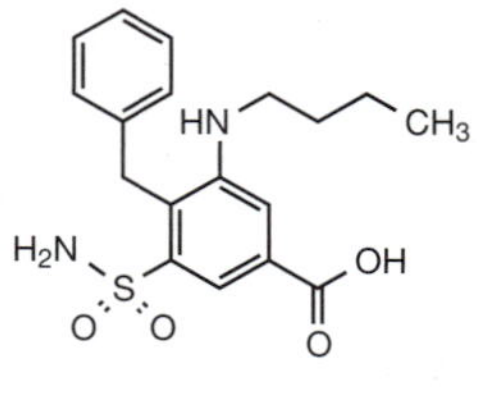

Bumetamide (Bumex)

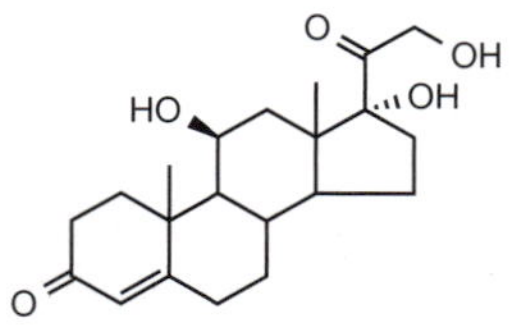

Hydrocortisone (Hydrocort)

Case Solution found immediately after References.

Case Study 2.5

WATER/LIPID SOLUBILITY CASE

When you look at any drug molecule, a number of functional groups are present that contribute to the properties of that drug molecule. Identify the types of functional groups in each molecule and to which physical properties (water/lipid solubility) each contributes.

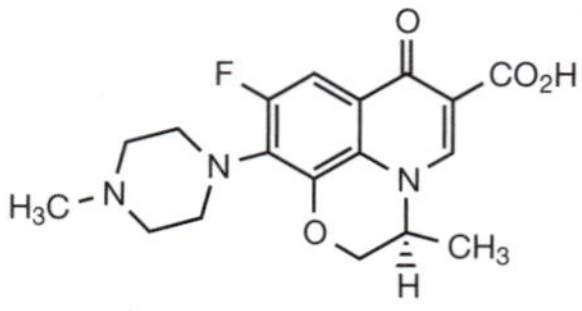

Levofloxacin (Levaquin)

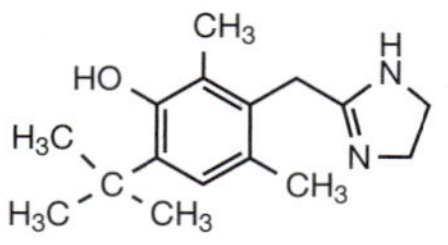

Oxyometazoline (Afrin)

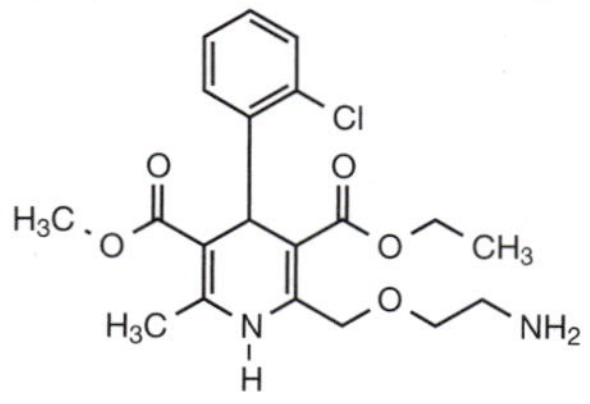

Amlodipine (Norvasc)

Case Solution found immediately after References.

Case Study 2.6

INTERACTIONS/SOLUBILITY CASE STUDY

L.A. presents a prescription for her 16-year-old daughter for Bromfed DM. She wants to know if this medication will have an effect on her daughter's alertness.

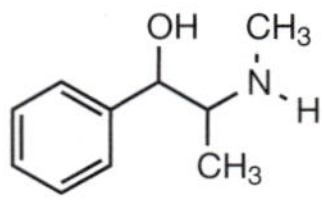

Pseudoephedrine

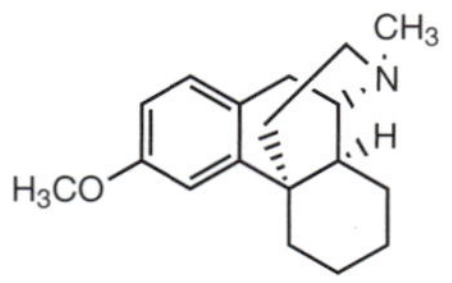

Dextromethorphan

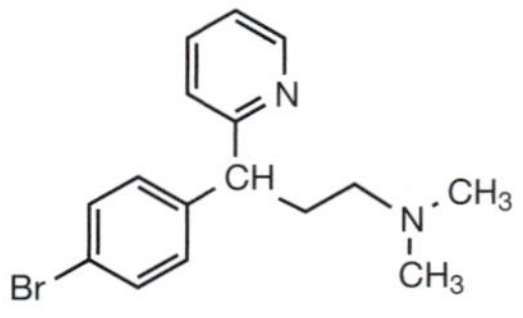

Brompheniramine

COMPONENTS OF BROMFED DM:

1. Identify the structural features/functional groups of pseudoephedrine and brompheniramine that contribute to improved water solubility (medication administered as a liquid). List the type(s) of interactions that these groups have with water and draw an example of these interactions (with appropriate labels).
2. Evaluate each of the three molecules and determine if each molecule contains any functional groups that will allow the drug to cross the BBB and have an effect on this child's alertness (create a list of relevant functional groups for each molecule). Based on your evaluation, which agent is likely to have the most significant effect? Identify what property is necessary for these agents to cross this biologic membrane.
3. Identify the binding interactions that brompheniramine and dextromethorphan could have with their respective targets for drug action. Be sure to identify which functional groups will participate in each of these binding interactions.

Case Solution found immediately after References.

20%. Solubility data for drug molecules can be found in the USP. In most instances, discrepancies between approximate and actual water solubilities can be rationalized by careful inspection of the chemical structure.

Predicting Water Solubility: Analytical/Quantitative Approach

Another method for predicting water solubility involves calculation of an approximate logP, or log of the partition coefficient for a molecule. This approach is based on an approximation method developed by Cates[10] and discussed in Lemke.[9] In this approach, one sums the hydrophobic or hydrophilic properties of each functional group present in the molecule. Before we can calculate logP values, a brief explanation of the concept of partition coefficient is necessary.

In its simplest form, the partition coefficient, *P*, refers to the ratio of drug concentration in octanol (C_{oct}) to that in water (C_{water}) (Equation 2.7). Octanol is used to mimic the amphiphilic nature of lipids, because it has a polar head group (primary alcohol) and a long hydrocarbon chain, or tail, similar to the fatty acid tail that makes up part of a lipid membrane. Because *P* is logarithmically related to free energy,[11] *P* is generally expressed as logP and is, therefore, the sum of the hydrophobic and hydrophilic characteristics of the functional groups that make up the structure of a molecule. Thus, logP is a measure of the lipid/water solubility characteristics of the entire molecule. Because each functional group contained within the molecule contributes to its overall hydrophilic/hydrophobic character, a hydrophilic/hydrophobic value (the hydrophobic substituent constant, π) can be assigned to each functional group. Equation 2.8 defines this relationship:

$$P = C_{oct}/C_{water}$$

$$\text{LogP} = \sum \pi(\text{fragments})$$

When calculating logP from hydrophobic substituent constants, the sum is usually referred to as logP_{calc} or ClogP (for software sources to calculate ClogP, see Ref[15]) to distinguish it from an experimentally determined value (MlogP or logP_{meas}). Over the years, extensive tables of π values have been compiled for organic functional groups and molecular fragments.[11-14] Table 2.6 is a highly abbreviated summary of π values from Lemke,[9] based largely on the manuscript by Cates.[10] Using the values in this table, a fairly reasonable estimate for the water solubility of many organic molecules (shown as logP) can be determined.

Again, we will consider the structure of the opioid analgesic anileridine to demonstrate the calculation of logP

Table 2.6 Hydrophilic-Lipophilic Values (πV) for Organic Fragments

Functional Group	π Value (Aliphatic)	π Value (Aromatic)
H		0.00
Alkane	0.50	0.56 (CH_3); 1.02 (CH_2CH_3)
Alkene		0.82
C_6H_5 (phenyl)	2.15	1.96
Br, Cl, F, I	0.60; 0.39; −0.17; 1.00	0.86; 0.71; 0.14; 1.12
NO_2	−0.85	−0.28
NH_2 (primary amine)	−1.19	−1.23
NHR (secondary amine)	−0.67	0.47
NR_2 (tertiary amine)	−0.30	0.18
-NHC=OR (amide)	−0.97	
SC_6H_5	2.32	
OH	−1.12	−0.67
OCH_3		−0.02
-OC=OR (ester)	−0.27	−0.64
CHO (aldehyde)		−0.65
C=OCH_3 (ketone)		−0.55
CO_2H		−0.32
SO_2 NH_2 (sulfonamide)		−1.82

Based on Cates LA. Calculation of drug solubilities by pharmacy students. *Am J Pharm Educ.* 1981;45:11-13.

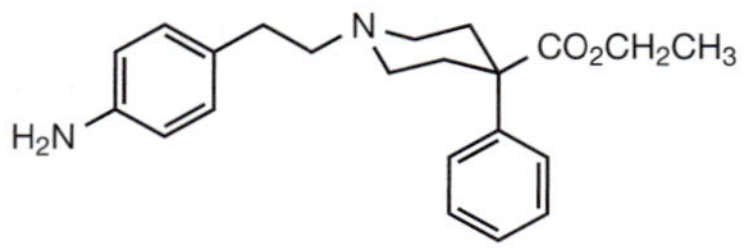

Fragments	≠
1 primary arylamine	-1.23
1 tertiary alkylamine	-0.30
9 aliphatic carbons	+4.5
2 phenyl rings	+4.30
1 ester	-0.27
logP	+7.0

Figure 2.14 Calculation of logP for anileridine.

(Fig. 2.14). This molecule has a total of 22 carbon atoms, some aliphatic and some aromatic. We need to distinguish between the aliphatic and aromatic carbon atoms because the delocalized π orbitals for the sp^2-hybridized aromatic carbon atoms make them more polar than aliphatic carbons. The molecule also contains one tertiary alkylamine, one aromatic or arylamine, and one ester. Evaluation of esters and amides requires that the oxygen, nitrogen, and ester/amide carbon atoms are counted in this π value. The remaining aliphatic carbons are then counted. Figure 2.14 summarizes the logP calculation for anileridine. The calculation gives a ClogP value for anileridine of +7.0. Water solubility as defined by the USP is solubility greater than 3.3%, which equates to an approximate logP of +0.5. LogP values less than +0.5 are therefore considered to be water soluble, and those greater than +0.5 are considered to be water insoluble. According to our calculation, anileridine would be predicted to be insoluble in water. This calculation agrees with the empirical procedure discussed earlier.

Other sample calculations are shown in Figure 2.15. In Figure 2.15, MlogP values (when available) and ClogP values[15] are included for comparison purposes (see Appendix A for additional ClogP values). Even though the π values from Table 2.6 are not as extensive as those in the computer program, there is good general agreement with most of these molecules with respect to their solubility (or insolubility) in water. In addition, other programs besides ClogP are available to predict logP values; some of these programs are available on the internet. One must keep in mind that due to the assumptions made in these programs, they cannot produce results that are in total agreement with measured values or other prediction programs. ClogP values calculated from ACDLogP[15] are generally considered to be more accurate. Other programs for calculating logP values, such as Molinspiration,[16] use different methods and assumptions and, therefore, do not always agree with ClogP predictions or experimentally determined values. This is not to say that other programs do not give accurate results. Often, one or all of the available programs will have reasonable agreement with measured values, but greater disagreement tends to occur as the number of functional groups in the molecule that participate as hydrogen bond acceptor and/or hydrogen bond donor groups increases. This increases the likelihood that intramolecular interactions will occur—something that is not always taken into account with these programs.

The ability to predict the percent ionization or water solubility of a molecule should not be viewed as an exercise in arithmetic, but rather to understand the solution behavior of molecules, especially as it relates to admixtures and the pharmacokinetic differences among molecules. The ionization state of a molecule not only influences its water solubility but also its ability to traverse membranes, and therefore, its ability to be absorbed. The distribution of the drug and its ability to bind to proteins other than its target are also greatly influenced by the ionization state and the hydrophilic/hydrophobic nature of the molecule.

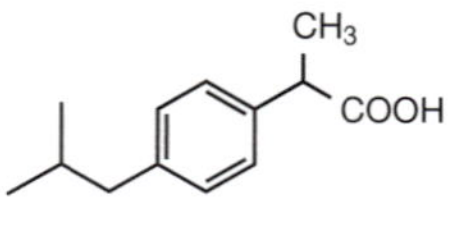

Ibuprofen

Fragments	≠
6 carbons	+3.0
1 phenyl	+2.0
1 carboxyl	-0.7
logP	+4.3

MlogP +3.5;
ClogP +3.68

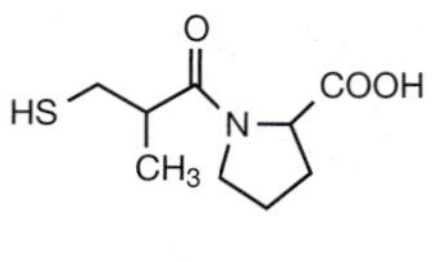

Captopril

Fragments	≠
7 carbons	+3.5
1 sulfur	0.0
1 carboxyl	-0.7
1 amide	-0.7
logP	+2.1

ClogP +1.16

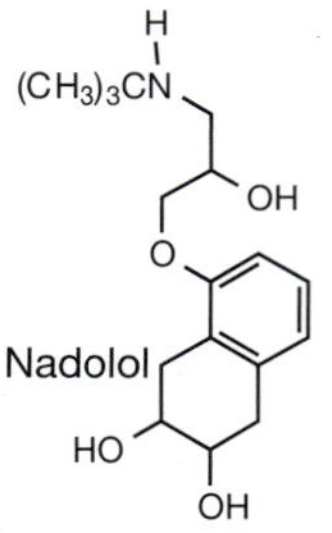

Nadolol

Fragments	≠
11 carbons	+5.5
1 phenyl	+2.0
2 IMHB	+1.3
1 amine	-1.0
1 ether	-1.0
3 alcohols	-3.0
logP	+3.8

MlogP +0.71;
ClogP +0.23

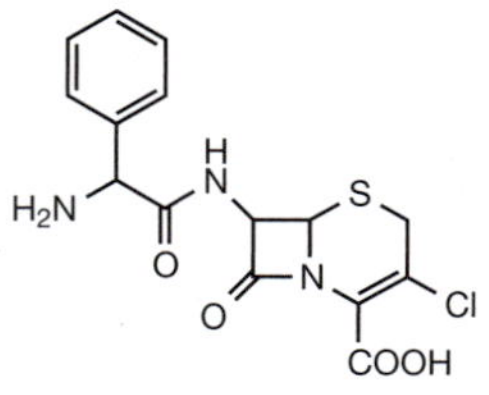

Cefaclor

Fragments	≠
6 carbons	+3.0
1 phenyl	+2.0
1 chloride	+0.5
1 amine	-1.0
1 sulfur	0.0
2 amides	-1.4
1 carboxyl	-0.7
logP	+2.4

MlogP -1.69;
ClogP -1.79

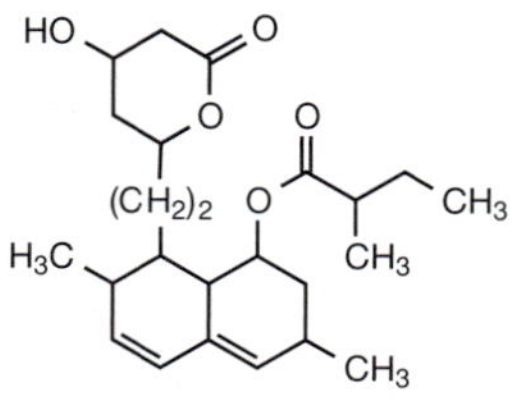

Lovastatin

Fragments	≠
22 carbons	+11.0
1 alcohols	-1.0
2 carboxyls	-1.4
logP	+ 8.6

MlogP +4.26;
ClogP +4.08

Figure 2.15 ClogP calculations for selected molecules.

Drug Absorption

A variety of routes for administration of drugs exist varying from IV, subcutaneous (SC), and intramuscular (IM) injection. Nasal, buccal, inhalation, and rectal administration have also been used. By far the most common, and desirable from a compliance point of view, is that of oral administration: swallowing a tablet, capsule, liquid, or syrup. Each of these approaches to delivery of medications has its advantages and disadvantages, but from a patient perspective the oral route is preferred. As a result, the physicochemical properties of the medication greatly influence the absorption properties of the molecule as well as its stability as it traverses the gastrointestinal (GI) tract. The type of formulation is also influenced by the physicochemical properties of the molecule and will enhance absorption, protect from degradation, or affect the rate of absorption. Because the oral route of drug administration is so important and desirable for drug delivery, a discussion of GI physiology is necessary in order to understand the complexities of the conditions encountered by the medication as it passes through this region.

Gastrointestinal Physiology

When administered orally, a drug molecule encounters many physical and chemical barriers to its absorption into the systemic circulation. Figure 2.16 is a diagram of these barriers to absorption and the complexities involved.[17] The stomach is divided into two major anatomic regions: the body of the stomach and the pylorus. The former region secrets pepsin and HCl and is also muscular, and contractions of these muscles allow for mechanical breakdown of ingested food. By breaking food particles into smaller pieces, a larger surface area is obtained allowing for additional digestion to occur with pepsin and HCl. The pyloric region is the mucus-secreting area. This mucus serves as a protective layer preventing damage to the stomach lining by pepsin and HCl. That is, it helps prevent the stomach from digesting itself. It also lubricates the GI tract allowing freer movement of solid material. Within the stomach the dosage form begins to disaggregate, and some dissolution of the drug may begin to occur, except in the case of enteric-coated formulations that do not break down under acidic conditions and pass through the stomach. These types of formulations will be discussed in later chapters with specific molecules. Depending upon the physicochemical properties of the molecule, some dissolution may occur within the stomach. Significant absorption generally does not occur within the stomach due to the low surface area, acidity, and possible association with other contents of the stomach such as fiber and metal ions.

Passage into the small intestine is accompanied by a significant change in pH and in the anatomic structure of the region. The small intestine comprises three distinct regions: duodenum, jejunum, and ileum. Within this region the pH changes from approximately 5 (duodenum) to 7 to 8 (ileum)

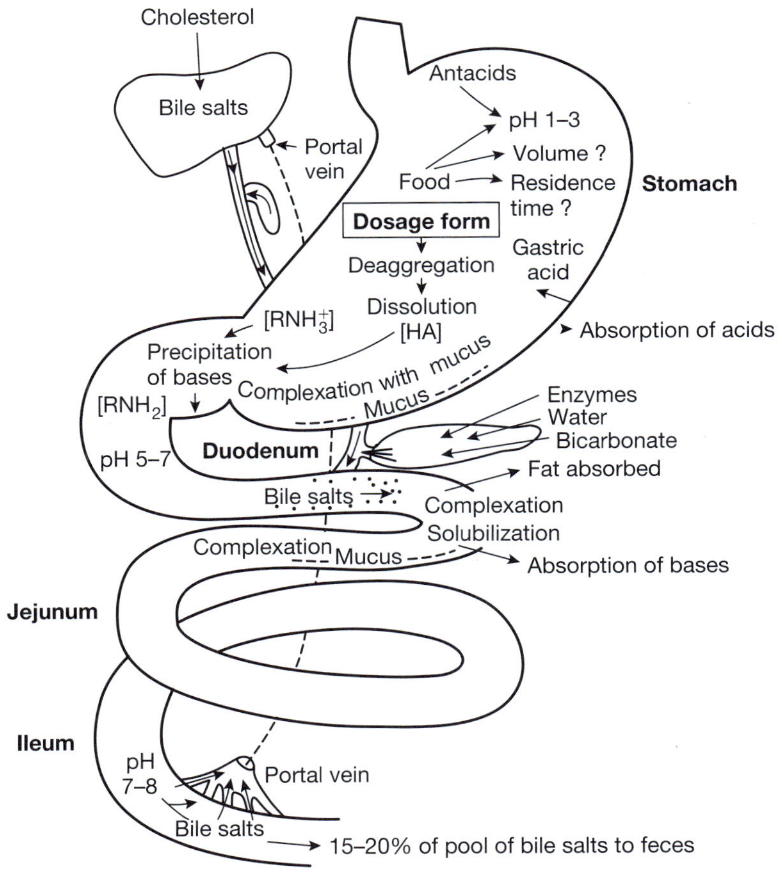

Figure 2.16 Processes occurring along with drug absorption when drug molecules travel down the gastrointestinal tract and the factors that affect drug absorption. (Reprinted with permission from Florence AT, Attwood D. *Physiochemical Principles of Pharmacy*. 5th ed. Chapman & Hall; 2011.)

and significantly affects the solubility of drugs. Acidic molecules now become ionized and more water soluble, while basic molecules become less ionized and may even begin to precipitate. Because the epithelium of the small intestine is highly convoluted, the nutrients (and drugs) here are efficiently absorbed due to the large surface area that results. Because bases are less ionized within this region, they are more lipophilic and therefore able to cross the cell membranes more efficiently. Basic molecules therefore undergo more rapid absorption in the small intestine. All is not perfect, however. The presence of bile acids, mucus, and food particles can prevent absorption by forming complexes or adsorbing the drug. Such an action results in some drugs passing through the GI tract and being excreted in the feces.

In order to get to the systemic circulation, the drug must traverse the biomembranes of the epithelial cells lining the lumen of the intestine, pass through the cells and through another membrane to reach the blood. This requires the drug to be hydrophilic enough to be soluble in water (the major constituent within the GI tract) to be able to come into contact with the membrane and hydrophobic enough to be able to cross the membrane. Thus, there is a delicate balance between being too hydrophilic or too hydrophobic to be able to be absorbed into the systemic circulation. To complicate matters even more, the presence on the drug of functional groups that are acidic, basic, or both will influence solubility and therefore absorption. Obviously, these barriers can be overcome; otherwise, we would not have orally administered medications in our formularies.

The processes of disaggregation and dissolution of drug formulations are beyond the scope of this chapter, and the reader will become acquainted with this area of physical pharmacy in other parts of the curriculum. For now, we will concentrate on what occurs once the drug is in solution within the GI tract and how even ionized molecules are able to cross biologic membranes. We will mainly concentrate on the process of passive diffusion of drugs across membranes. Other processes will also be mentioned but will be discussed in more detail in other chapters within this text.

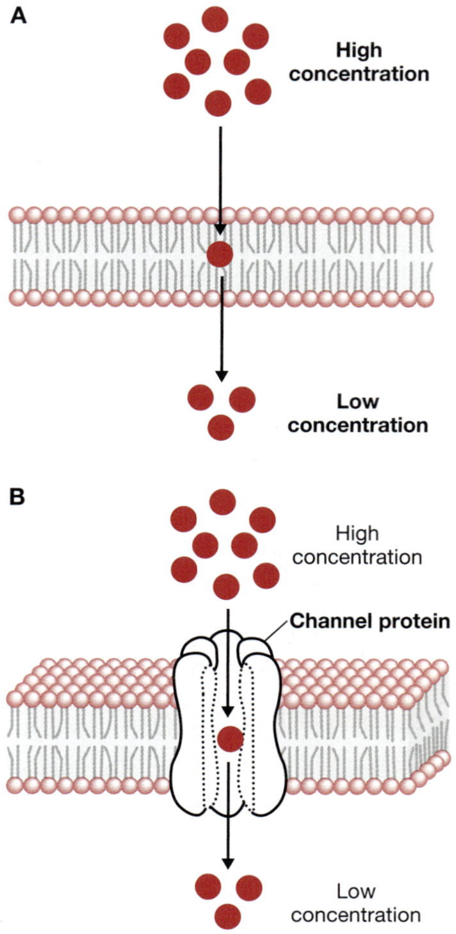

Figure 2.17 A. Simple diffusion. B. Membrane channels. (Adapted with permission from Smith C, Marks A, Lieberman M, eds. *Basic Medical Biochemistry*. 2nd ed. Lippincott Williams & Wilkins; 2004.)

Passive Diffusion

Nonionized Drugs

The simplest case to consider is that of a drug that is neither basic nor acidic with sufficient water solubility to have contact with the membranes of epithelial cells lining the intestine. With this process the molecule is simply undergoing diffusion across the membrane from a region of high drug concentration to that of low concentration. Such diffusion may occur through the membrane lipid layer (Fig. 2.17A) or via a channel protein (Fig. 2.17B). In either case, no energy expenditure is involved, and this is referred to as passive diffusion (Fig. 2.17).[18]

Acidic Drugs

Acidic drugs encounter an increasingly basic environment as they pass through the GI tract, resulting in an increase in the percentage of ionized drug. Absorption of the acidic drug occurs within the stomach primarily due to the protonated unionized species predominating there. However, the greatest absorption occurs just below the stomach, in the duodenum, due to the greater surface area of the microvilli of the brush border. Efficient absorption can occur even though a significant amount of drug may be ionized due to the equilibria shown in Figure 2.18, with HA representing the protonated, unionized drug and A^- the deprotonated ionized species.

In the duodenum, the molecule is ionized with the equilibrium shifted toward A^-. However, there is always some HA present that can partition through the membrane into the epithelial cell of the brush border. Once through the membrane, another equilibrium is established within the cytoplasm of the cell due to the pH (~7.4). As HA partitions through the membrane and into the cell, the equilibrium in the intestinal lumen must shift to form more HA. This is an example of Le Chatelier principle from a typical first-year chemistry course. The equilibrium within the lumen of the duodenum must be maintained. More HA forms can now cross the membrane into the cytoplasm of the epithelial cell. But something else must be occurring to keep HA partitioning across the membrane. For this, we now need to consider what is happening within the epithelial cell of the brush border.

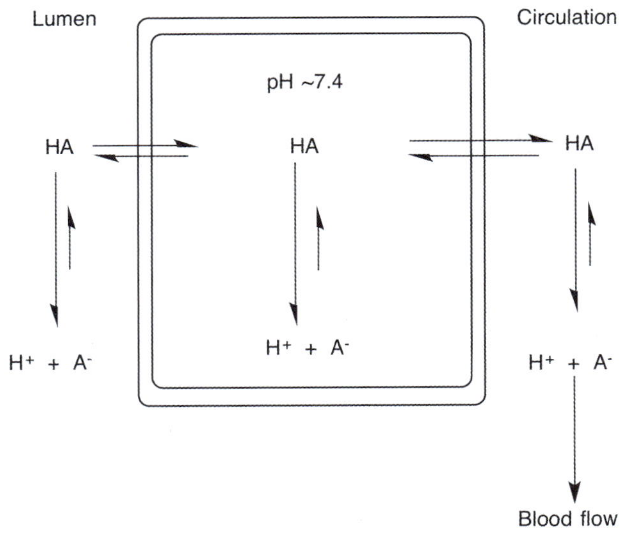

Figure 2.18 Equilibria involved in absorption of an acidic drug from the gastrointestinal tract.

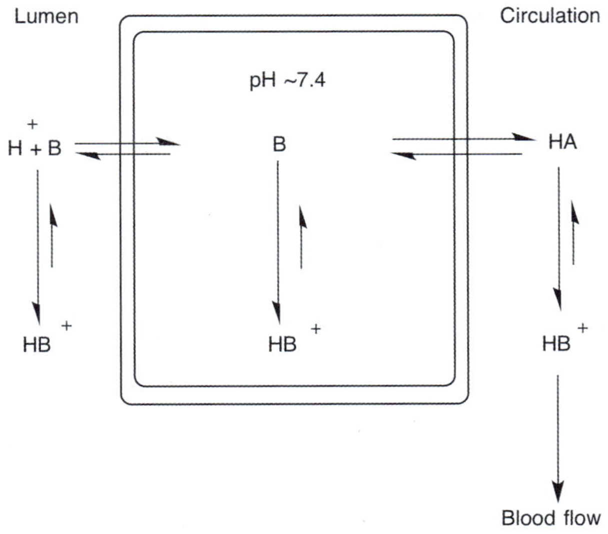

Figure 2.19 Equilibria involved in absorption of a basic drug from the gastrointestinal tract.

Within the cell the pH causes deprotonation of the drug, resulting in a second equilibrium that is shifted toward A^-. This decreases the amount of HA within the cell, causing a shift in the equilibrium across the cell membrane. The HA within the cytoplasm can pass through the membrane of the epithelial cell into the circulation where two things occur. First, due to the pH of the blood, a fourth equilibrium occurs between HA and A^- and is shifted toward A^-. Second, the circulation carries both HA and A^- away, which causes the equilibrium across the membrane to shift, allowing more HA to cross into the circulation. In summary, Le Chatelier principle is at play here. As the equilibria shift in response to changes in pH and relative concentrations of unionized and ionized drug, absorption of the drug into the systemic circulation occurs.

Basic Drugs

With the increasing basicity in the jejunum and ileum, the absorption of basic drugs becomes more efficient. As shown in Figure 2.19, as the pH increases, the equilibrium between the conjugate acid (BH^+) and free base (B) form shifts to favor the latter. Following the same line of reasoning as with acidic drugs, the free base form crosses the membranes and reestablishes equilibria with the conjugate acid form within the cytoplasm and subsequently within the circulation. As the equilibria shift to form more B, and as HB^+ and B are removed by the circulation, diffusion of the drug from high to low concentration occurs.

Active Transport (Influx and Efflux Transporters)

As discussed, passive diffusion is the passage of a drug from a region of high concentration to that of low concentration and is an energy neutral process. Active transport requires energy and is generally a process of transporting the drug against a concentration gradient. Because active transport requires the drug to be "recognized" by a transport protein that normally mediates movement of a molecule of similar structure across the membrane, it is also a saturable process. That is, at high drug concentrations, the ability to transport the drug plateaus due to the limited number of transport proteins available. Another difference is that the structural specificity required to be recognized and transported can result in competition with other molecules of similar structure. These could be natural substances that normally are transported by these proteins, or other drugs.[19] These will be discussed in more detail later (Fig. 2.20).

Some membrane transporters enhance the passage of drugs across membranes (influx), while others reverse absorption (efflux transporters). All transporters (influx and efflux) are membrane-associated proteins that have multiple transmembrane regions and require energy for the process. Some transporters recognized a broad range of structures, while others are very specific.

Influx Transporters

Several types of influx transporters with differing substrate selectivity exist within the luminal surface of the intestinal mucosa and can influence the rate of oral absorption (see Chapter 4 for more discussion). Peptide transporters such as the peptide transporter 1 (PEPT-1) and human peptide transporter 1 (HPT-1) are responsible for the transport of many diverse peptide and peptide mimetic substrates such as β-lactam antibiotics, angiotensin-converting enzyme (ACE) inhibitors, and amino acid conjugated drugs (eg, valacyclovir). Other transporters within the intestinal tract include the bile acid, nucleoside, organic cation/anion (OCTP and OATP, respectively), and fatty acid transporters. Just as with PEPT-1 and HPT-1, drugs that structurally resemble the natural substrates for these may have enhanced absorption in addition to passive diffusion. Throughout this text, the influence of influx transporters on intestinal absorption of specific drugs will be discussed when relevant.

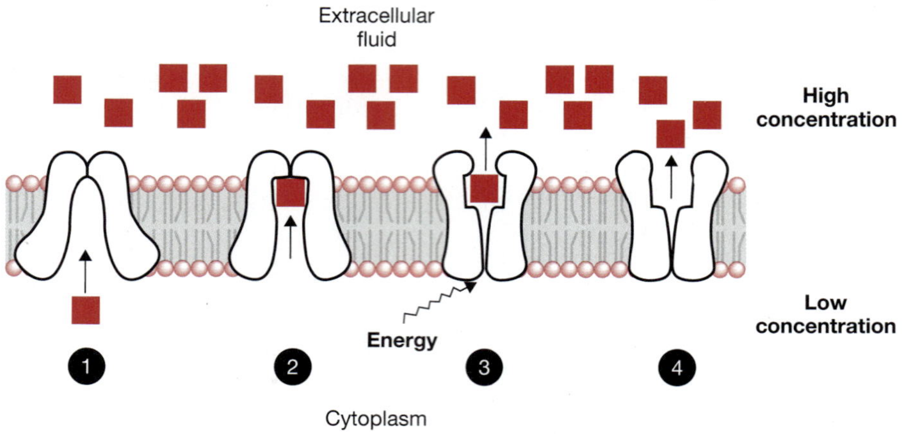

Figure 2.20 Active transport. (Adapted with permission from Smith C, Marks A, Lieberman M, eds. *Basic Medical Biochemistry*. 2nd ed. Lippincott Williams & Wilkins; 2004.)

Efflux Transporters

Drug efflux into the intestinal lumen is influenced by P-glycoprotein (P-gp), multidrug resistance–associated proteins 1 and 2 (MRP1 and MRP2), and breast cancer–resistance protein (BCRP) (see Chapter 4). These transporters prevent the influx and accumulation of many drugs into the general circulation as well as specific organs: for example, transport into bile, preventing BBB penetration, and tumor tissue. P-gp appears to be the most ubiquitous of these efflux proteins, returning a portion of drug entering the intestinal mucosa back to the lumen in a concentration-dependent manner. Two types of P-gp have been shown to exist in mammals: drug-transporting and phospholipid-transporting P-gp. Localization of P-gp in the intestine, kidney, and liver suggests that it is a leading player in excreting xenobiotics into the intestinal lumen, urine, and bile. The number of drugs shown to be substrates increases each year and includes human immunodeficiency virus (HIV) protease inhibitors and verapamil. The latter also acts as an inhibitor of P-gp, increasing intestinal permeabilities.

PRODRUGS

Prodrugs are molecules that undergo metabolic or chemical conversion to produce a biologically active substance. That is, the ingested molecule is not pharmacologically active and must first be converted via action of an enzyme or chemical degradation to produce the active species. Some prodrugs have been developed because the pharmacologically active form has poor oral bioavailability, usually due to poor absorption in the GI tract. Other prodrugs are highly water-soluble derivatives of molecules that are too hydrophobic to be dissolved in an aqueous solution to be given intravenously. Examples of well-known prodrugs include omeprazole, simvastatin, lovastatin, enalapril, clopidogrel, valacyclovir, acyclovir, and oseltamivir (Fig. 2.21).

Other reasons for developing prodrugs may be chemical instability, unacceptable odor or taste, gastric irritation, inadequate BBB permeability, presystemic metabolism, or toxicity. The most common approach to prodrug design is to use an ester linkage to the drug (eg, lovastatin, simvastatin, oseltamivir, clopidogrel, valacyclovir, and enalapril in Fig. 2.21). As detailed in Chapter 3, esters are readily hydrolyzed by ubiquitous esterases within the systemic circulation. The rates at which these esters are hydrolyzed can be influenced via steric or electronic effects of substituents on either side of the ester bond following basic organic chemical principles. The ester may be hydrophobic (ie, alkyl esters) to improve diffusion across membranes; ionizable (eg, succinates or amino acids) to improve aqueous solubility; or sterically hindered to slow hydrolysis, providing an acceptable rate for "release" of the active drug.

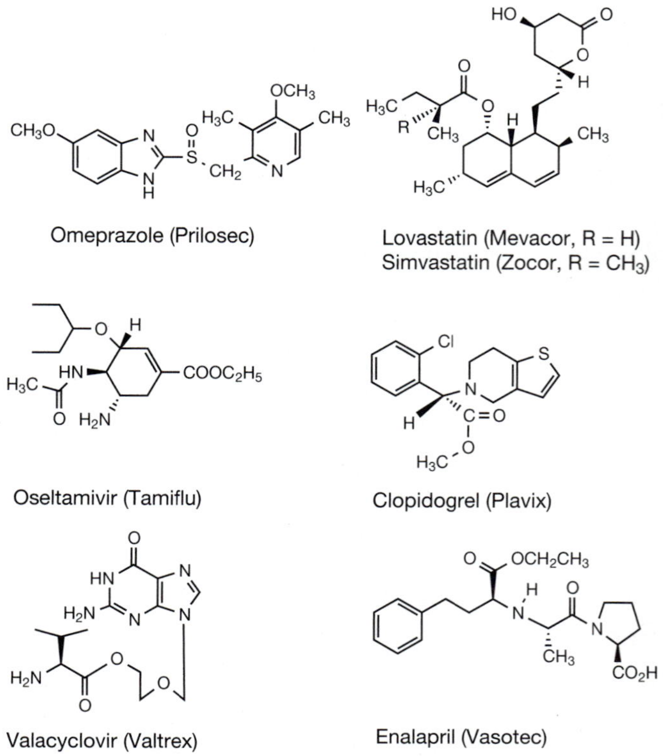

Figure 2.21 Commercially available blockbuster prodrugs and their structures.

Stereochemistry and Drug Action

Stereoisomers are molecules that contain the same number and kinds of atoms, the same arrangement of bonds, but different three-dimensional structures; in other words, they only differ in the three-dimensional arrangement of atoms in space. There are two types of stereoisomers: enantiomers and diastereoisomers. Enantiomers are pairs of molecules for which the three-dimensional arrangement of atoms represents nonsuperimposable mirror images. Diastereoisomers represent all of the other stereoisomeric molecules that are not enantiomers. Thus, the term "diastereoisomer" includes molecules that contain double bonds (geometric isomers) and ring systems. Unlike enantiomers, diastereoisomers exhibit different physicochemical properties, including, but not limited to, melting point, boiling point, solubility, and chromatographic behavior. These differences in physicochemical properties allow the separation of individual diastereoisomers from mixtures with the use of standard chemical separation techniques, such as column chromatography or crystallization. Enantiomers cannot be separated using such techniques unless a chiral environment is provided or if they are first converted to diastereoisomers (eg, salt formation with another enantiomer). Examples of enantiomers and diastereoisomers are provided in Figure 2.22.

The physicochemical properties of a drug molecule are dependent not only on what functional groups are present in the molecule but also on the spatial arrangement of these groups. This becomes an especially important factor when the environment that a molecule is in is asymmetric, such as the human body. Proteins and other biologic targets are asymmetric in nature. How a particular drug molecule interacts with these macromolecules is determined by the three-dimensional orientation of the functional groups present. If critical functional groups in the drug molecule do not occupy the proper spatial region, then productive interactions with the biologic target will not be possible. As a result, it is possible that the desired pharmacologic activity will not be achieved. If, however, the functional groups within a drug molecule are located in the proper three-dimensional orientation, then the drug can participate in multiple key interactions with its biologic target. It is important to understand not only which functional groups contribute to the pharmacologic activity of a drug, but also the importance of the three-dimensional nature of these functional groups in predicting drug potency and potential side effects.

Approximately one in every four drugs currently on the market is some type of isomeric mixture. For many of these drugs, the biologic activity may reside in one isomer (or at least predominate in one isomer). The majority of these isomeric mixtures are termed "racemic mixtures" (or "racemates"). A racemic mixture is comprised of equal amounts of both possible drug enantiomers. As mentioned earlier in this chapter, when enantiomers are introduced into an asymmetric, or chiral, environment, such as the human body, they display different physicochemical properties. This

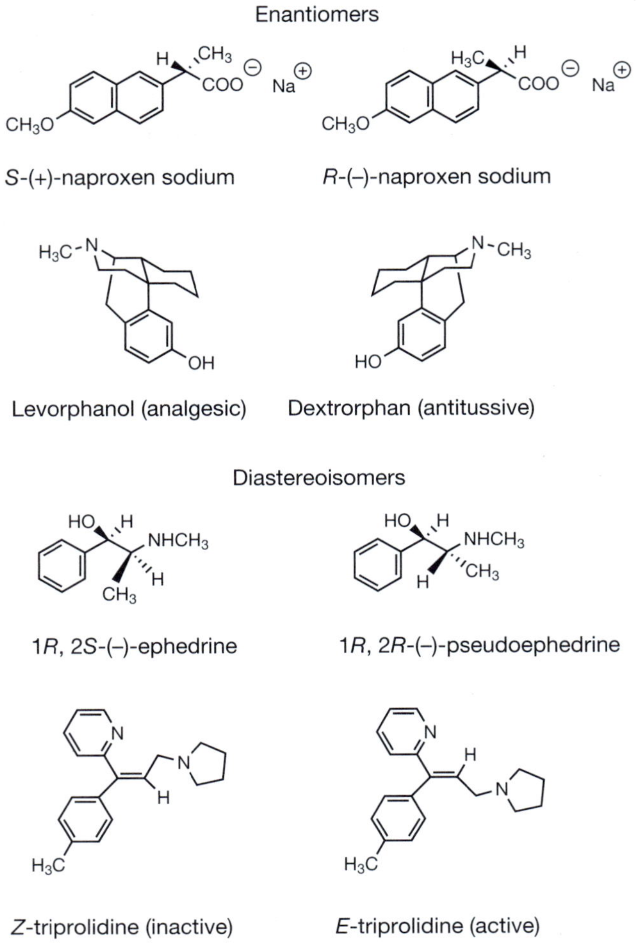

Figure 2.22 Examples of stereoisomers.

can lead to significant differences in their pharmacokinetic and pharmacodynamic behavior, resulting in adverse side effects or toxicity. For example, individual isomers in a racemic mixture can exhibit significant differences in absorption (especially active transport), serum protein binding, and metabolism. As it relates to drug metabolism, it is certainly possible that only one of the isomers can be converted into a toxic substance or can influence the metabolism of another drug (see Chapter 3). Since stereochemistry can have a profound effect on both the pharmacokinetic and pharmacodynamic properties of a drug, it is important to review the foundational concepts.

Stereochemical Definitions

Designation of Absolute Configuration

At first, enantiomers were distinguished by their ability to rotate the plane of polarized light. Isomers that rotate the plane of polarized light to the right, or in a clockwise direction, were designated as dextrorotatory, indicated by a (+) sign before the chemical name (eg, (+)-amphetamine or dextroamphetamine). The opposite designation, levorotatory or (−), was assigned to molecules that rotate the plane of polarized light to the left, or in a counterclockwise direction. The letters *d*- and *l*- are also used to indicate (+) and (−), respectively. A racemate (racemic mixture)—that is, a 1:1 mixture of enantiomers—is indicated by placement of a (±) before the molecule's name. This nomenclature is based on a physical property of the molecule and does not describe the absolute configuration or three-dimensional arrangement of atoms around the chiral center.

In the late 19th century, Fisher and Rosanoff developed a system of nomenclature based on the structure of glyceraldehyde (Fig. 2.23). Since there were no methods at that time to determine the absolute three-dimensional arrangement of atoms in space, the two isomers of glyceraldehyde were arbitrarily assigned the designation of D-(+) and L-(−). It was not until the 1950s that the absolute configurations of these molecules were determined (Fisher had fortuitously guessed correctly). The configurations of other molecules were then assigned based on their relationship to D- or L-glyceraldehyde via synthetic methods or chemical degradation. Thus, via chemical degradation, it was possible to determine that (+)-glucose, (−)-2-deoxyribose, and (−)-fructose had the same terminal configuration as D-(+)-glyceraldehyde and, therefore, were assigned the D-absolute configuration. Amino acid configurations were assigned based on their relationship to D-(+)- and L-(−)-serine (Fig. 2.23). Unfortunately, this system becomes very cumbersome with molecules that contain more than one chiral center.

In 1956, a new system of stereochemical nomenclature was introduced by Cahn et al[20] (CIP) and is known as the CIP sequence rules. With this system, atoms attached to a chiral center are ranked based on their atomic number. Highest priority is given to the atom with the highest atomic number, and subsequent atoms are ranked accordingly, from highest to lowest. When a decision cannot be made in the assignment of priority—for example, two atoms with the same atomic number attached to the chiral center—this evaluation extends to the next atom until a priority can be established. When the molecule is then viewed from the side opposite to the lowest priority atom, the priority sequence from highest to lowest can then be determined. If the priority sequence proceeds to the right, or in a clockwise direction, the chiral center is designated with an *R*-absolute configuration. The designation is *S* when the priority sequence proceeds to the left, or in a counterclockwise direction. An example of this is seen in the neurotransmitter norepinephrine.

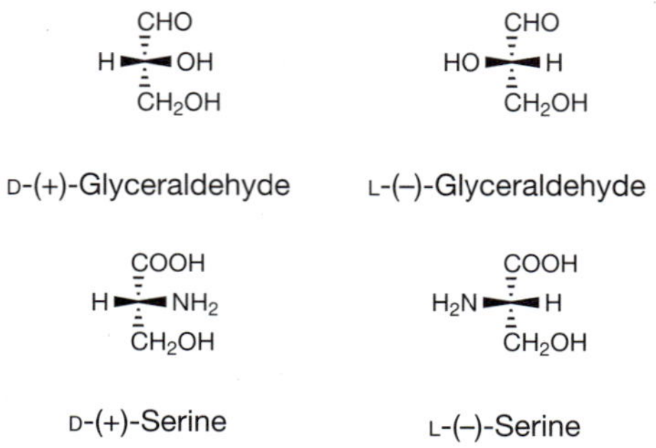

Figure 2.23 Relationship of optical isomers of serine to D- and L-glyceraldehyde.

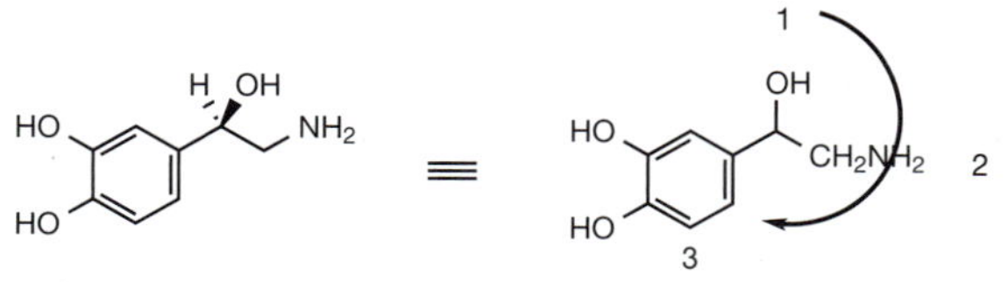

Norepinephrine

R

Degradation studies demonstrate that (−)-norepinephrine is related to D-(−)-mandelic acid; therefore, it was given the D-designation using the Fisher system. With the CIP system, norepinephrine is assigned the *R*-absolute configuration.

It should be noted that the CIP nomenclature system uses a set of arbitrary rules and, therefore, should be viewed as a system that tracks absolute configuration only. In many instances, two molecules can have different absolute configurations as designated by the CIP system, but the same relative orientation of the functional groups relevant for biologic activity. An example of this is demonstrated when the absolute configuration of the nonselective β-adrenergic antagonist propranolol is compared to norepinephrine. Because of the presence of the ether oxygen atom, the priority

QUESTIONS WE CAN NOW ANSWER ABOUT ANY DRUG MOLECULE

- Based on your knowledge of acid-base chemistry, from where will this drug primarily be absorbed?
- What is the solubility of the drug in the stomach, plasma, or an aqueous IV?
- What are the possible interactions that the drug could have with its respective target for drug action?
- What is the compatibility of the drug if mixed with other drugs?
- How should this drug be delivered? Is it stable in stomach acid?

LEARNING THE LINGO: DRUG MOLECULE EVALUATION

Analysis of individual functional groups:
Name of functional group
Shape of functional group
Hydrophobic vs hydrophilic character
Polar vs nonpolar character
Acidic vs basic (pK_a) character
Binding interactions
Chemical/enzymatic stability
Analysis of the whole drug molecule:
Looking for functional group balance: water solubility and absorption
Ionization issues: effect on solubility and absorption
Drug combinations: acid-base interactions
Drug interactions with biologic target: good fit or not?
Stability and bioavailability: route of administration

sequence of the functional groups about the chiral center results in the assignment of the *S*-absolute configuration for the more active enantiomer of propranolol. Close inspection of both *R*-norepinephrine and *S*-propranolol, however, shows that the hydroxy group, basic amine, and aromatic rings of both molecules occupy the same regions in three-dimensional space.

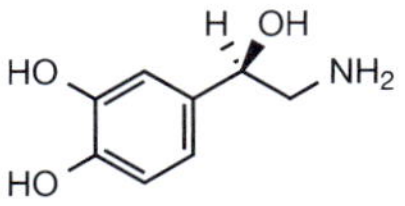

(*R*)-Norepinephrine

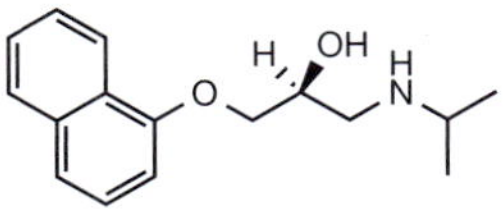

(*S*)-Propranolol

Stereochemistry and Biologic Activity

Easson-Stedman Hypothesis

In 1886, Piutti[21] reported different physiologic actions for the enantiomers of asparagine, with (+)-asparagine having a sweet taste and (−)-asparagine a bland one. This was one of the earliest observations that enantiomers can exhibit differences in biologic action. In 1933, Easson and Stedman[22] reasoned that differences in biologic activity between enantiomers resulted from selective interactivity of one enantiomer with its receptor. They postulated that such interactions require a minimum of a three-point fit to the receptor. This is demonstrated in Figure 2.24 for two hypothetical enantiomers. In Figure 2.24, the letters A, B, and C represent hypothetical functional groups that can interact with complementary sites on the hypothetical receptor surface, represented by A′, B′, and C′. Only one enantiomer is capable of attaining the correct special orientation to enable all three functional groups to interact with their respective sites on the receptor surface. The inability of the other enantiomer to achieve the same number of interactions with the hypothetical receptor surface explains its reduced biologic activity. The Easson-Stedman hypothesis states that the more potent enantiomer must be involved in a minimum of three intermolecular interactions with the surface of the biologic target and that the less potent enantiomer only interacts with two sites. This can be illustrated by looking at the differences in vasopressor activity of *R*-(−)-epinephrine, *S*-(+)-epinephrine, and the achiral *N*-methyldopamine (Fig. 2.25). With *R*-(−)-epinephrine, the three points of interaction with the receptor site are the substituted aromatic ring, β-hydroxyl group, and the protonated secondary ammonium group. All three functional groups interact with their complementary sites on the receptor surface, resulting in receptor stimulation (in this case). With *S*-(+)-epinephrine, only two interactions are possible (the protonated secondary ammonium and the substituted aromatic ring). The β-hydroxyl group is located in the wrong place in space and, therefore, cannot interact properly with the receptor. *N*-methyldopamine can achieve the same interactions with the receptor as *S*-(+)-epinephrine; therefore, it is not surprising that its vasopressor response is the same as that of *S*-(+)-epinephrine and less than that of *R*-(−)-epinephrine.

Not all stereoselectivity seen with enantiomers can be attributed to differences in the ability of the drug molecule to interact with its biologic target. Differences in biologic activity can also result from differences in the ability of each enantiomer to reach the biologic target. Because the biologic system encountered by the drug is asymmetric, each enantiomer can experience selective penetration into membranes, metabolism, absorption at sites of loss (eg, adipose tissue), and/or excretion. Figure 2.26 shows various phases that enantiomers can encounter before reaching the biologic target. An enantiomer may not encounter stereoselective environments at each of these points; however, enantioselectivity at any point can provide enough of an influence to cause one enantiomer to produce a significantly better pharmacologic effect than the other. Conversely, such processes can also contribute to untoward effects of a particular enantiomer. Differences in pharmacologic action among stereoisomers provide an excellent example of how not all pharmacologic effects of a drug are necessarily beneficial to the patient. Although there is no regulatory prohibition on the development of racemic agents, it is reasonable that single enantiomer drugs will become the overwhelming therapeutic choice in the future.

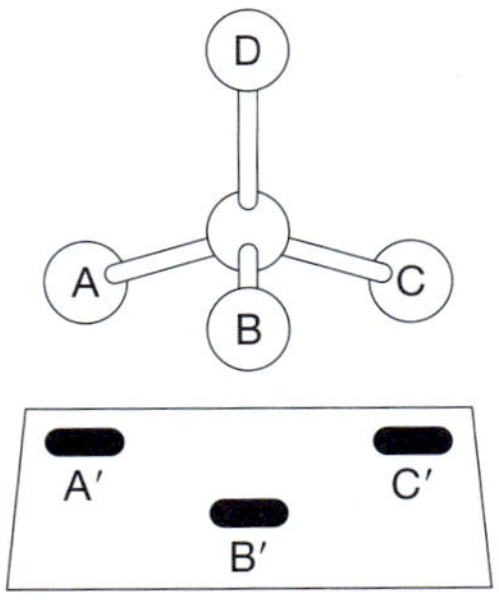

Compound 6

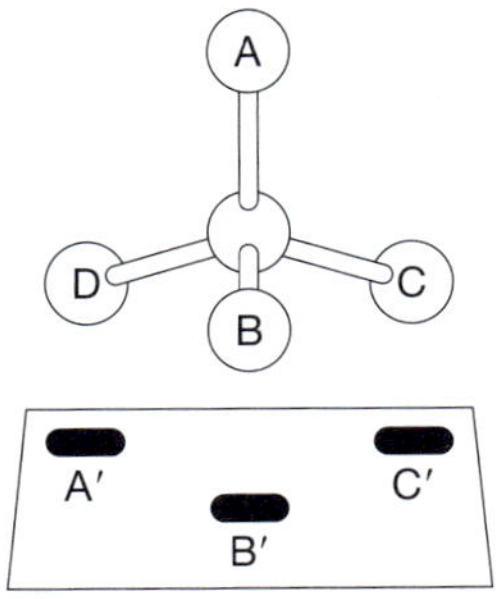

Compound 7

Figure 2.24 Optical isomers. Only in molecule 6 do the functional groups A, B, and C align with the corresponding sites of binding on the asymmetric surface.

Diastereomers

As mentioned earlier, diastereoisomers are molecules that are nonsuperimposable, nonmirror images. This type of isomer can result from the presence of more than one chiral center in the molecule, double bonds, or ring systems. These isomers have different physicochemical properties, and as a result, it is possible that they can have differences in biologic activity.

Molecules that contain more than one chiral center probably are the most common type of drug-based

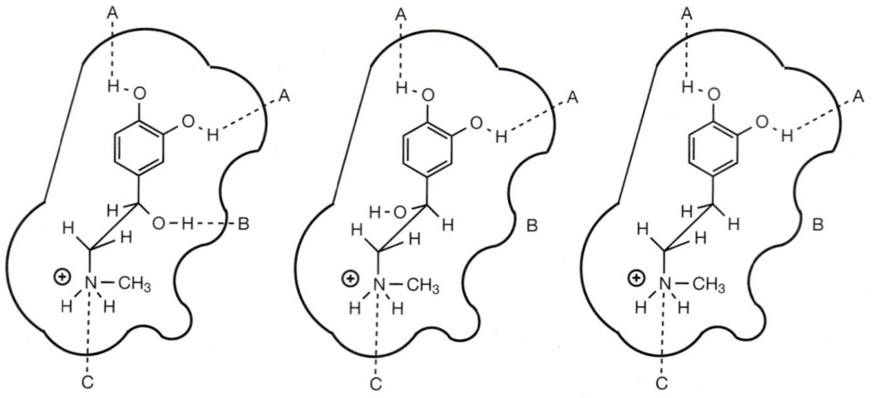

(R)-(–)-Epinephrine (S)-(+)-Epinephrine N-Methyldopamine

Figure 2.25 Drug receptor interaction of R-(−)-epinephrine, S-(+)-epinephrine, and N-methyldopamine.

diastereoisomers. Classic examples are the diastereoisomers ephedrine and pseudoephedrine (Fig. 2.27). When a molecule contains two chiral centers, there can be as many as four possible stereoisomers consisting of two sets of enantiomeric pairs. When considering an enantiomeric pair of molecules, there is inversion of all chiral centers. In diastereomers, there is inversion of one or more, but not all chiral centers. Figure 2.28 shows several examples that contain two or more chiral centers and, therefore, are diastereoisomeric.

Restricted bond rotation caused by carbon-carbon double bonds (alkenes or olefins) and similar systems, such as imines (C=N), can produce stereoisomers. These are also referred to as geometric isomers, although they more properly are classified as diastereoisomers. In this situation, substituents can be oriented on the same side or on opposite sides of the double bond. The alkene 2-butene is a simple example.

cis or *Z* isomer *trans* or *E* isomer

With 2-butene, it is readily apparent that the methyl groups can be on the same or on opposite sides of the double bond. When they are on the same side, the molecule is defined as the *cis*- or *Z*-isomer (from the German *zusammen*, meaning "together"); when they are on opposite sides, the designation is *trans*- or *E*-isomer (from the German *entgegen*, meaning "opposite"). With simple molecules, such as 2-butene, it is easy to determine which groups in the molecule are *cis* or *trans* to one another. This becomes more difficult to determine, however, with more complex structures, where it is less obvious which substituents should be referred to when naming the molecule. In 1968, Blackwood et al[23] proposed a system for the assignment of "absolute" configuration with respect to double bonds. Using the CIP sequence rules, each of the two substituents attached to the carbon atoms comprising the double bond is assigned a priority of 1 or 2, depending on the atomic number of the atom attached to the double bond. When two substituents of higher priority are on the same side of the double bond, this isomer is given the designation of *cis* or *Z*. When the substituents are on opposite sides, the designation is *trans* or *E*. The histamine H_1-receptor antagonist triprolidine (Fig. 2.29) is a good example for demonstrating how this nomenclature system works. The *E*-isomer of triprolidine is more active both in vitro and in vivo, indicating that the distance between the pyridine and pyrrolidine rings is critical for binding to the receptor.

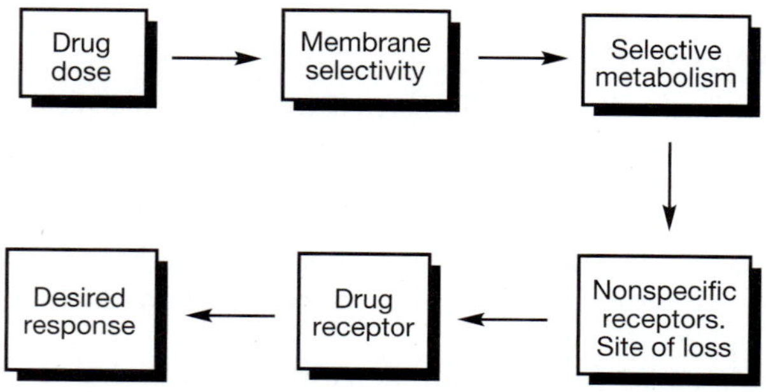

Figure 2.26 Selective phases to which optical isomers can be subjected before biologic response.

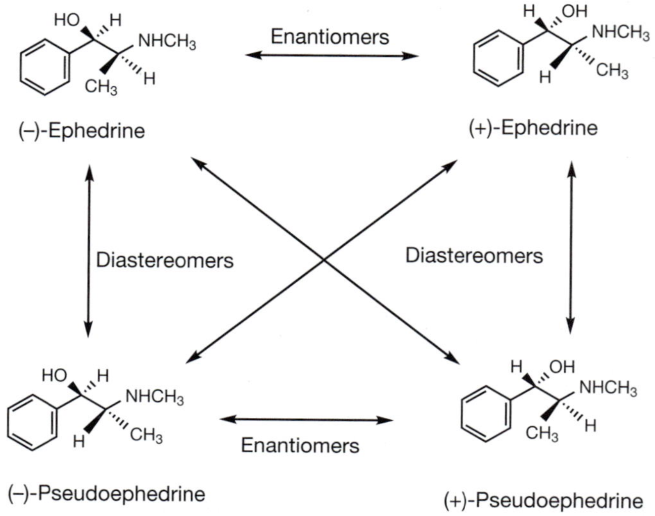

Figure 2.27 Relationship between the diastereomers of ephedrine and pseudoephedrine.

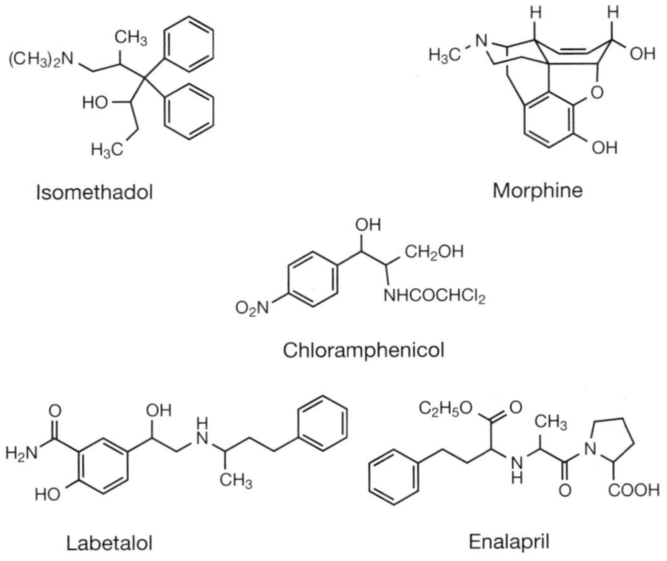

Figure 2.28 Examples of chiral drugs with two or more asymmetric centers.

Diastereoisomers (as well as enantiomers) can also be found in cyclic molecules. For example, the cyclic alkane 1,2-dimethylcyclohexane can exist as *cis/trans*-diastereoisomers, and the *trans*-isomer can also exist as an enantiomeric pair. In Figure 2.30, each of the *trans*-enantiomers is depicted in the two possible chair conformations for the cyclohexane ring. Since cyclohexane rings can exhibit significant conformational freedom, this allows for the possibility of conformational isomers. Isomers of this type will be discussed in the next section. When two or more rings share a common bond (eg, decalin), rotation around the bonds is even more restricted. This prevents ring "flipping" from occurring, and as a result, diastereoisomers and enantiomers are generated.

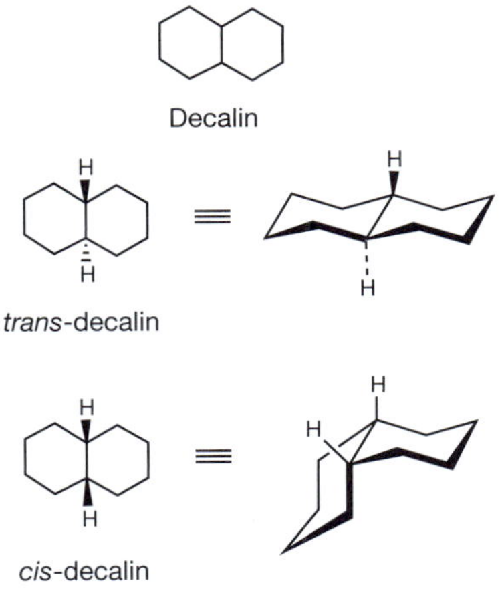

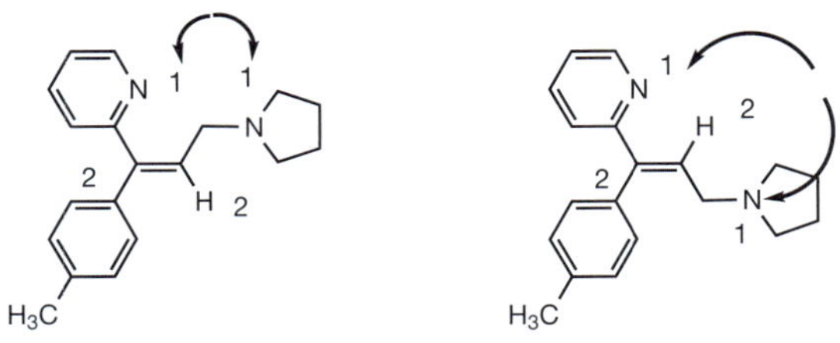

Figure 2.29 Geometric isomers of triprolidine.

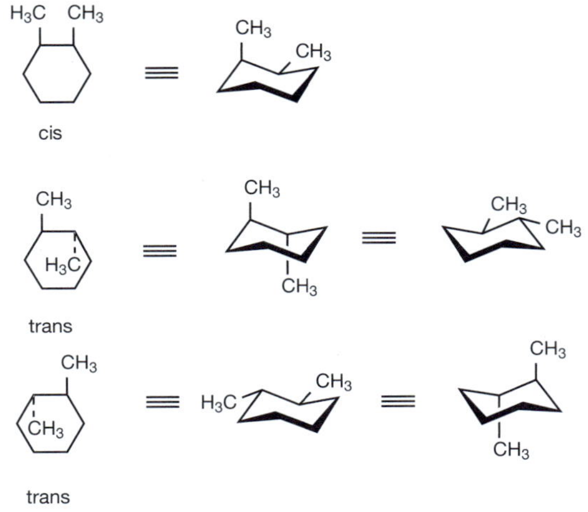

Figure 2.30 Diastereomers of 1,2-dimethylcyclohexane.

In the case of decalin, a two-ring system, the rings are fused together via a common bond in either the *trans* or *cis* configuration as shown. Steroids, a class of medicinally important molecules that consist of four fused rings (three cyclohexanes and one cyclopentane), exhibit significantly different biologic activity when the first two cyclohexane rings are fused into different configurations, referred to as the 5α- or 5β-isomers (Fig. 2.31). The α-designation indicates that the hydrogen atom in the 5-position is below the "plane" of the ring system; the β-designation refers to the hydrogen atom being above this plane. What appears to be a very minor change in orientation for the substituent results in a very drastic change in the three-dimensional shape of the molecule and in its biologic activity. Figure 2.31 shows the diastereoisomers 5α-cholestane and 5β-cholestane as examples. The chemistry and pharmacology of steroids will be discussed in more detail in later chapters.

Conformational Isomerism

Conformational isomerism takes place via rotation about one or more single bonds. Such bond rotation results in nonidentical spatial arrangement of atoms in a molecule. This type of isomerism does not require much energy because no

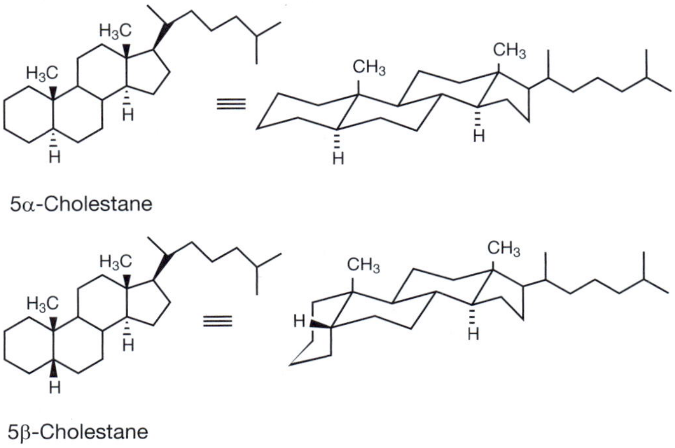

Figure 2.31 The 5α and 5β conformations of the steroid nucleus cholestane.

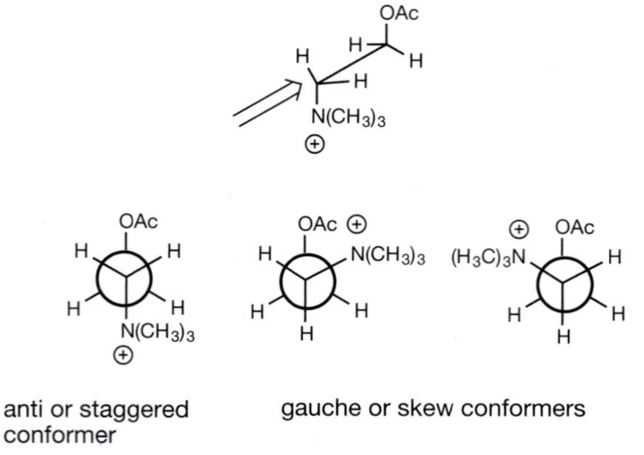

Figure 2.32 Anti- and gauche conformations of acetylcholine.

bonds are broken. In the conversion of one enantiomer into another (or diastereoisomer), bonds are broken, which requires significantly more energy. The neurotransmitter ACh can be used to demonstrate the concept of conformational isomers.

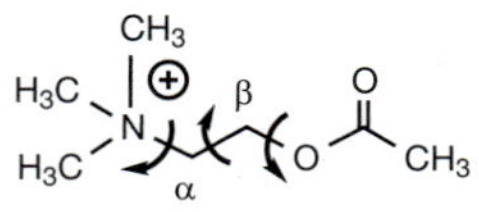

Acetylcholine

Each single bond within the ACh molecule is capable of undergoing rotation, and at room temperature, such rotations readily occur. Rotation around single Cα-Cβ bond of ACh was shown by Kemp and Pitzer[24] in 1936 not to be free but, rather, to have an energy barrier, which is sufficiently low that at room temperature ACh exists in many interconvertible conformations. Rotation around the central Cα-Cβ bond produces the greatest spatial rearrangement of atoms compared to rotation around any other bond. Since the atoms at the end of some of the bonds within ACh are identical, rotation about several of these bonds produces redundant structures when viewed along the Cα-Cβ bond and can be depicted in the sawhorse or Newman projections, as shown in Figure 2.32. When the ester and trimethylammonium groups are 180° apart, the molecule is said to be in the anti-, or staggered, conformation (or conformer or rotamer). This conformation allows maximum separation of the functional groups and is the most stable conformation energetically. It is possible that other conformations are more stable if factors other than steric interactions are considered (eg, intramolecular hydrogen bonds). Rotation of one end of the Cα-Cβ bond by 120° or 240° results in the two gauche, or skew, conformations shown in Figure 2.32. These are less stable than the anticonformer, although some studies suggest that an electrostatic attraction between the electron-poor trimethylammonium and electron-rich ester oxygen atom stabilizes this conformation. Rotation by 60°, 180°, and 240° produces the least stable conformations in which all of the atoms overlap, what are referred to as eclipsed conformations.

Drug Design: Discovery and Structural Modification of Lead Molecules

Process of Drug Discovery

The process of drug discovery begins with the identification of new, previously undiscovered, biologically active molecules, often called "hits," which are typically found by screening many molecules for the desired biologic properties. We will next explore the various approaches used to identify "hits" and how these are converted into "lead" molecules and, subsequently, into drug candidates suitable for clinical trials. Sources of "hits" can originate from natural sources, such as plants, animals, or fungi; from synthetic chemical libraries, such as those created through combinatorial chemistry or historic chemical molecules' collections; from chemical and biologic intuition from years of chemical-biologic training; from targeted/rational drug design; or from computational modeling of a target site such as an enzyme. Chemical or functional group modifications are then performed in order to improve the pharmacologic, toxicologic, physiochemical, and pharmacokinetic properties of a "hit" molecule to ultimately obtain a "lead" molecule. The lead molecule to be optimized should be of a known chemical structure and possess a known mechanism of action, including knowledge of its functional groups (pharmacophoric groups) that are recognized by the receptor/active site and are responsible for that molecule's affinity at the targeted receptor site. "Lead optimization" is the process whereby modifications of the functional groups of the lead molecule are carried out in order to improve its recognition, affinity, and binding geometries of the pharmacophoric groups for the targeted site (a receptor or enzyme); its pharmacokinetics; or its reactivity and stability toward metabolic degradation. The final step of the drug discovery process involves rendering the lead molecule into a drug candidate that is safe and suitable for use in human clinical trials, including the preparation of a suitable drug formulation.

Natural Product Screening

Perhaps the most difficult aspect of drug discovery is that of lead discovery. Until the late 19th century, the development of new chemical entities for medicinal purposes was achieved primarily through the use of natural products, generally derived from plant sources. As the colonial powers of Europe discovered new lands in the Western Hemisphere and colonized Asia, the Europeans learned from the indigenous peoples of the newly discovered lands of remedies for many ailments derived from plants and animals. Salicylic acid was isolated from the bark of willow trees after learning that Native Americans brewed the bark to treat inflammatory ailments. Structural optimization of this lead molecule (salicylic acid) by the Bayer Corporation of Germany resulted in acetylsalicylic acid, or aspirin, the first nonsteroidal anti-inflammatory agent. South American natives used a tea obtained by brewing Cinchona bark to treat chills and fever. Further study in Europe led to the isolation of quinine and quinidine, which subsequently were used to treat malaria and cardiac arrhythmias, respectively. Following "leads" from folklore medicine, chemists of the late 19th and early 20th centuries began to seek new medicinals from plant sources and to assay them for many types of pharmacologic actions. This approach to drug discovery is often referred to as "natural product screening." Before the mid-1970s, this was one of the major approaches to obtaining new chemical entities as "leads" for new drugs. Unfortunately, this approach fell out of favor and was replaced with the rational approaches to drug design developed during that period (see the next section). Heightened awareness of the fragility of ecosystems, especially the rainforests, has fueled a resurgence of screening products from plants before they become extinct. A new field of pharmacology, called "ethnopharmacology," which is the discipline of identifying potential natural product sources with medicinal properties based on native lore, has emerged as a result.

Molecules isolated from natural sources are usually tested in one or more bioassays for the ailment(s) that the plant material has been purported to treat. Interestingly, the treatment of different ailments can require different methods of preparation (eg, brewing, chewing, or direct application to wounds) or different parts of the same plant (eg, roots, stem, leaves, flowers, or sap). As it turns out, each method of administration or part of the plant used can produce one or more different molecules that are necessary to generate the desired outcome.

Drug Discovery via Random Screening of Synthetic Organic Molecules

The random screening of synthetic organic molecules approach to the discovery of new chemical entities for a particular biologic action began in the 1930s, after the discovery of the sulfonamide class of antibacterials. All molecules available to the investigator (natural products, synthetic molecules), regardless of structure, were tested in the pharmacologic assays available at the time. This random screening approach was also applied in the 1960s and 1970s in an effort to find agents that were effective against cancer. Some groups did not limit their assays to identify a particular type of biologic activity but, rather, tested compounds in a wide variety of assays. This large-scale screening approach of drug "leads" is referred to as high-throughput screening, which involves the simultaneous bioassay of thousands of molecules in hundreds to thousands of bioassays. These types of bioassays became possible with the advent of computer-controlled robotic systems for the assays and combinatorial chemistry techniques for the synthesis of large numbers of molecules in small (milligram) quantities.

Drug Discovery From Targeted Dedicated Screening and Rational Drug Design

Rational drug design is a more focused approach that uses greater knowledge (structural information) about the drug receptor (targets) or one of its natural ligands as a basis to design, identify, or create drug "leads." Testing is usually done with one or two models (eg, specific receptor systems or enzymes) based on the therapeutic target. The drug design component often involves molecular modeling and the use of QSARs to better define the physicochemical properties and the pharmacophoric groups that are essential for biologic activity. The development of QSARs relies on the ability to examine multiple relationships between physical properties and biologic activities. In classic QSAR (eg, Hansch-type analysis), an equation defines biologic activity as a linear free-energy relationship between physicochemical and/or structural properties. It permits evaluation of the nature of interaction forces between a drug and its biologic target, as well as the ability to predict activity in molecules. These approaches are better for the development of a lead molecule into a drug candidate than for the discovery of a lead molecule.

Drug Discovery via Drug Metabolism Studies

New drug entities have been "discovered" as drug leads through investigation of the metabolism of drug molecules that already are clinical candidates or, in some instances, are already on the market. In this method, metabolites of known drug entities are isolated and assayed for biologic activity using either the same target system or broader screen target systems. The broader screening systems are more useful if the metabolite under evaluation is a chemical structure that was radically altered from the parent molecule through some unusual metabolic rearrangement reaction. In most cases, the metabolite is not radically different from the parent molecule and, therefore, would be expected to exhibit similar pharmacologic effects. One advantage of evaluating this type of drug candidate is that a metabolite can possess better pharmacokinetic properties, such as a longer duration of action, better oral absorption, or less toxicity with fewer side effects (eg, terfenadine and its antihistaminic hydroxylated metabolite, fexofenadine). As it turns out, the sulfonamide antibacterial agents were discovered in this way. The azo dye prontosil was found to have only antibacterial action in vivo. It was soon discovered that this molecule required metabolic activation via reduction of the diazo group to produce the active metabolite 4-aminobenzenesulfonamide (Fig. 2.33). The sulfonamide mimics the physicochemical properties of PABA, a crucial component in microbial metabolism. It is no surprise that the sulfonamide acts as a competitive inhibitor of the enzyme for which PABA is a substrate.

Drug Discovery From the Observation of Side Effects

An astute clinician or pharmacologist can detect a side effect in a patient or animal model that could lead, on further development, to a new therapeutic use for a particular chemical entity. Discovery of new lead molecules via exploitation of side-effect profiles of existing agents is discussed further.

One of the more interesting drug development scenarios is that of the phenothiazine antipsychotics (see Chapter 11).

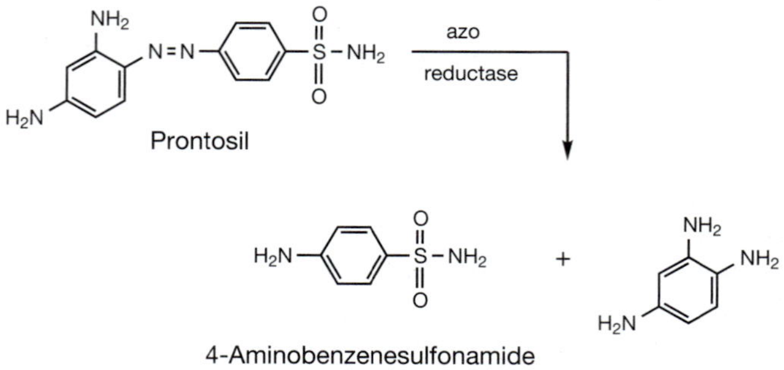

Figure 2.33 Metabolic conversion of prontosil to 4-aminobenzenesulfonamide.

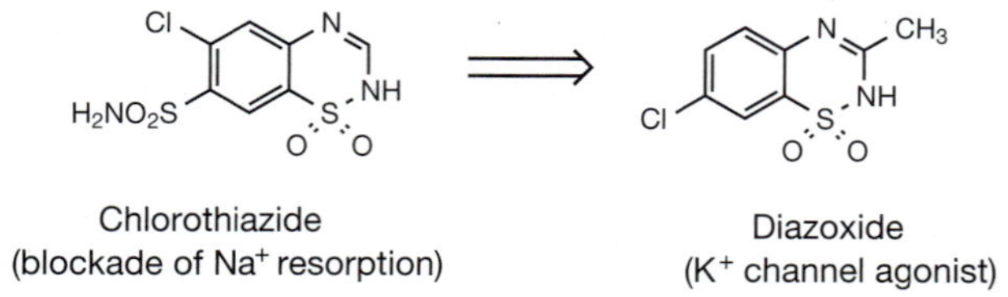

Figure 2.35 Structural similarity of chlorothiazide (a diuretic) and diazoxide (an antihypertensive that acts via opening of K+ channels).

Molecules with this type of biologic activity can be traced back to the first histamine H_1-receptor antagonists developed in the 1930s. In 1937, Bovet and Staub[25] were the first to recognize that it should be possible to antagonize the effects of histamine and, thereby, treat allergic reactions. They tested molecules that were known to act on the autonomic nervous system and, eventually, discovered that benzodioxanes (Fig. 2.34) significantly antagonized the effects of histamine. During an attempt to improve the antihistaminergic action of the benzodioxanes, it was discovered that phenyl-substituted ethanolamines also demonstrated significant antihistaminergic activity. Further development of this class generated two different classes of antihistamines: the diphenhydramine class of antihistamines represented by diphenhydramine and the ethylenediamine class, represented by tripelennamine (Fig. 2.34; see also Chapter 29).

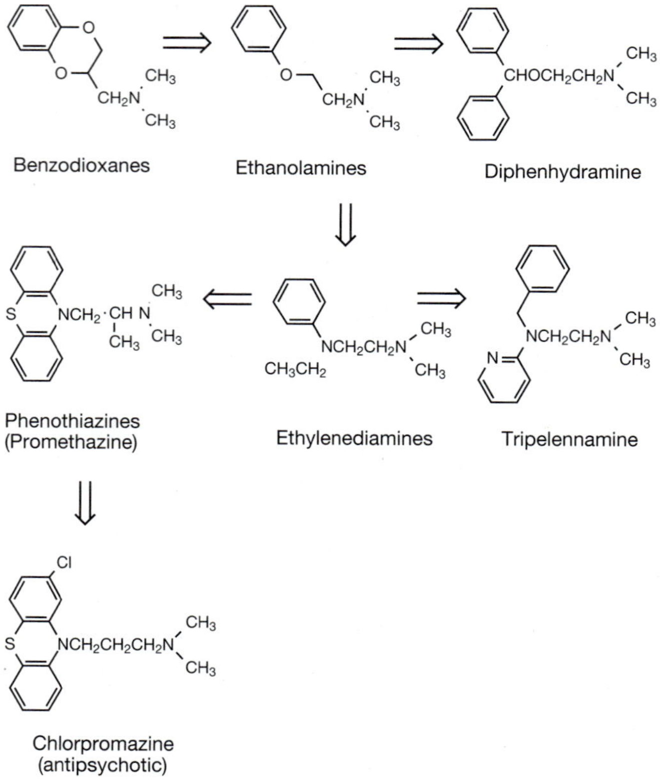

Figure 2.34 Development of phenothiazine-type antipsychotic drugs.

Incorporation of the aromatic rings of the ethylenediamines into the rigid and planar tricyclic phenothiazine structure produced molecules (eg, promethazine) with good antihistaminergic action and relatively strong sedative properties (see also Chapter 11). At first, these molecules were found to be useful as antihistamines, but their very strong sedative properties led to their use as potentiating agents for anesthesia.[26] Further development to increase the sedative properties of the phenothiazines resulted in the development of chlorpromazine in 1950.[27]

Chlorpromazine was found to produce a tendency for sleep, but unlike the antihistamine phenothiazines, it also produced a disinterest in patients with regard to their surroundings (ie, tranquilizing effects). In patients with psychiatric disorders, an ameliorative effect on the psychosis and a relief of anxiety and agitation were noted. These observations suggested that chlorpromazine had potential for the treatment of psychiatric disorders. Thus, what started out as an attempt to improve antihistaminergic activity ultimately resulted in an entirely new class of chemical entities useful in the treatment of an unrelated disorder.[28]

Another example of how new chemical entities can be derived from biologically unrelated molecules is illustrated by the development of the potassium channel agonist diazoxide (Fig. 2.35). This molecule was developed as a result of the observation that the thiazide diuretics, such as chlorothiazide, not only exhibited diuretic activity, due to inhibition of sodium absorption in the distal convoluted tubule, but also demonstrated a direct effect on the renal vasculature. Structural modification to enhance this direct effect led to the development of diazoxide and related potassium channel agonists for the treatment of hypertension (see Chapter 19).

Refinement of the Lead Structure

Determination of the Pharmacophore

Once a "hit" molecule has been discovered for a particular therapeutic use, the next step is to identify the pharmacophoric groups. The pharmacophore of a drug molecule is that portion of the molecule that contains the essential functional group(s) that directly interact with the active site of the biologic target to produce the desired biologic activity. Because drug-target interactions can be very specific (think of a lock [receptor] and key [drug] relationship), the pharmacophore can constitute a small portion of the molecule. In many cases, a very structurally complex molecule can be "stripped down" to a simpler structure with retention of the pharmacophoric groups while maintaining the desired biologic action. An example of this is the opioid analgesic morphine, a tetracyclic molecule with five chiral centers. Not only would structure simplification possibly provide molecules with fewer side effects, but a reduction in the number of chiral centers would greatly simplify the synthesis of morphine derivatives. Figure 2.36 shows how the morphine structure has been simplified in the search for molecules with fewer deleterious side effects, such as respiratory depression and addiction potential. Within each class are analogues that are less potent, equipotent, and many times more potent than morphine. As shown in the figure, the pharmacophore of morphine consists of a tertiary alkylamine that is at least four atoms away from an aromatic ring. A more detailed discussion of the chemistry and pharmacology of morphine can be found in Chapter 16.

Alterations in Alkyl Chains: Chain Length, Branching, and Rings

An increase or decrease in the length of an alkyl chain (homologation), branching, and alteration of ring size can have a profound effect on the potency and pharmacologic activity of the molecule. A change in the length of an alkyl chain by one CH_2 unit or branch alters the lipophilic character of the molecule and, therefore, its properties of absorption, distribution, and excretion. If the alkyl chain is directly involved in an interaction with the biologic target, then this type of alteration can influence the quality of those interactions. Molecules that are conformationally flexible can become less flexible if branching is introduced at a key position of an alkyl chain or the alkyl chain is incorporated into a ring equivalent. Changes in conformation can alter the spatial relationship between the pharmacophoric (functional) groups in the molecule and thereby influence interactions with the biologic target. Small structural changes are important to consider in the design of structural analogues.

An example that demonstrates how an increase in hydrocarbon chain length has significant effects not only on potency but also on drug action (agonist vs antagonist) is provided by a series of *N*-alkyl morphine analogues (Fig. 2.37). In this series, homologation of $R=CH_3$ (morphine) to $R=CH_2CH_2CH_3$ (*N*-propylnormorphine) produces a pronounced decrease in agonist activity and an increase in antagonist activity. When further homologated by one methylene unit $R=CH_2CH_2CH_2CH_3$ (*N*-butylnormorphine), the resulting analogue is totally devoid of agonist or antagonist activity (ie, the molecule is inactive). Additional increases in chain length ($R=CH_2CH_2CH_2CH_2CH_3$ and $R=CH_2CH_2CH_2CH_2CH_2CH_3$) produce molecules with increasing potency as agonists. When R is β-phenylethyl, the molecule is a full agonist, with a potency approximately 14-fold that of morphine.[29,30]

Branching of alkyl chains can also produce drastic changes in potency and pharmacologic activity. If the mechanism of action is closely related to the lipophilicity of the molecule, then hydrocarbon chain branching will result in a less lipophilic molecule and a significant alteration in biologic effect. This decrease in lipophilicity is a result of the alkyl chain becoming more compact and causes less disruption of the hydrogen bonding network of water. If the hydrocarbon chain is directly involved in interactions with its biologic target, then branching can produce major changes in pharmacologic activity. For example, consider the phenothiazines promethazine and promazine.

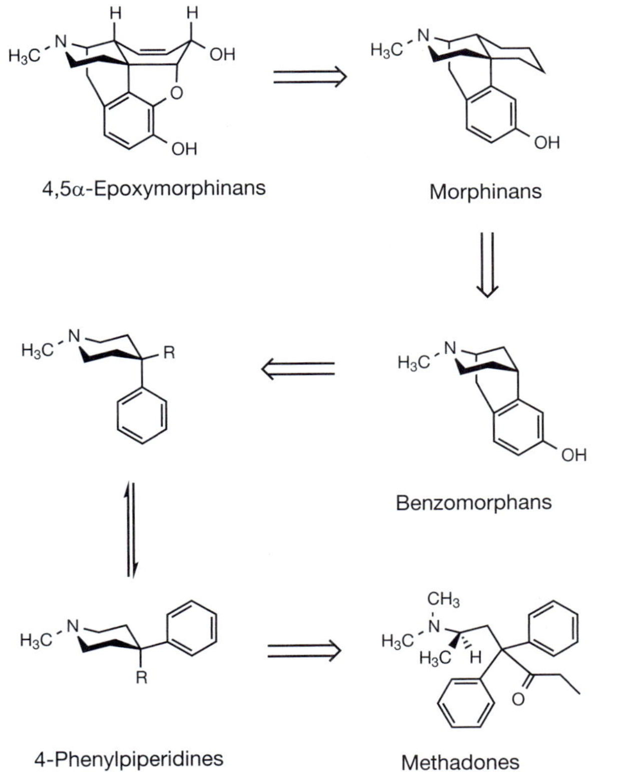

Figure 2.36 Morphine pharmacophore and its relationship to analgesic derivatives.

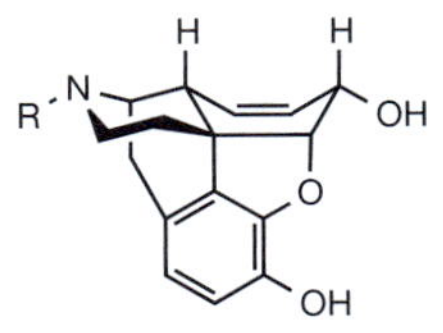

R	Pharmacological activity
$-CH_3$	Analgesic (morphine)
$-CH_2CH_3$	Opioid agonist activity decreased
$-CH_2CH_2CH_3$	Opioid antagonist activity increased
$-CH_2CH_2CH_2CH_3$	Inactive as opioid agonist or antagonist
$-CH_2CH_2CH_2CH_2CH_3$	Opioid antagonist activity increased
$-CH_2CH_2CH_2CH_2CH_2CH_3$	Opioid antagonist activity increased
$-CH_2CH_2-$ 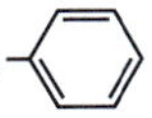	14X potency of morphine

Figure 2.37 Effect of alkyl chain length on bioactivity of morphine.

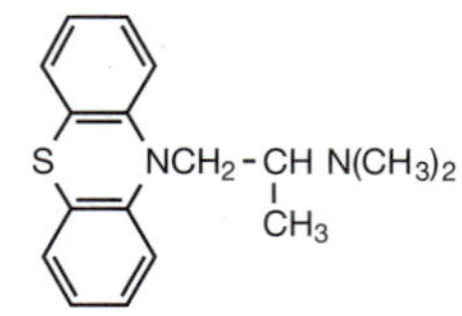

Promethazine

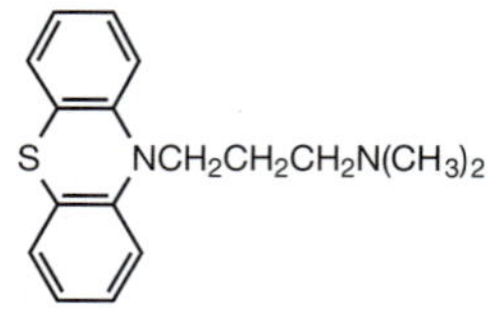

Promazine

The primary pharmacologic activity of promethazine is that of an antihistamine, whereas promazine is an antipsychotic. The only difference between the two molecules is the alkylamine side chain. In the case of promethazine, there is an isopropylamine side chain, whereas promazine contains an *n*-propylamine. In this case, simple modification of one carbon atom from a branched to a linear hydrocarbon radically alters the pharmacologic activity.

Positional isomers of aromatic ring substituents can also possess different pharmacologic properties. Substituents on aromatic rings can alter the electron distribution throughout the ring, which, in turn, can influence how the ring interacts with the biologic target. Aromatic ring substituents can also influence the conformation of the flexible portion of a molecule, especially if the substituents are located ortho to the same carbon attached to the flexible side chain. Ring substituents influence the conformations of adjacent substituents via steric interactions and can significantly alter interactions with the biologic target.

Functional Group Modification: Bioisosterism

Bioisosterism

When a lead molecule is first discovered, it often lacks the required potency and pharmacokinetic properties suitable for making it a viable clinical candidate. These can include undesirable side effects, physicochemical properties, other factors that affect oral bioavailability, and adverse metabolic or excretion properties. These undesirable properties are often the result of the presence of specific pharmacophoric (functional) groups in the molecule. Successful modification of the molecule to reduce or eliminate these undesirable features without losing the desired biologic activity is the goal. Replacement or modification of specific pharmacophoric (functional) groups with other groups having similar properties is known as "isosteric replacement" or "bioisosteric replacement."

In 1919, Langmuir[31,32] first developed the concept of chemical isosterism to describe the similarities in physical properties among atoms, functional groups, radicals, and molecules. The similarities among atoms described by Langmuir resulted primarily from the fact that these atoms contained the same number of valence electrons and came from the same columns within the periodic table. This concept of isosterism was limited to elements in adjacent rows and columns, inorganic molecules, ions, and small organic molecules, such as diazomethane and ketene. Table 2.7 shows a comparison of the physical properties of N_2O and CO_2 to illustrate the Langmuir concept.

Table 2.7 Comparison of Physical Properties of N_2O and CO_2

Property	N_2O	CO_2
Viscosity at 20 °C	148×10^6	148×10^6
Density of liquid at 10 °C	0.856	0.858
Refractive index of liquid, D line 16 °C	1.193	1.190
Dielectric constant of liquid at 0 °C	1.593	1.582
Solubility in alcohol at 15 °C	3.250	3.130

To account for similarities between functional groups with the same number of valence electrons but different numbers of atoms, Grimm[33] developed his hydride displacement law. This is not a "law" in the strict sense but, rather, more an illustration of similar physical properties among closely related functional groups. Table 2.8 presents an example of Grimm hydride displacement. Descending diagonally from left to right in the table, hydrogen atoms are progressively added to maintain the same number of valence electrons for each group of atoms within a column (thus the term "hydride"). Within each column, the groups are considered to be "pseudoatoms" with respect to each another. Thus, NH_2 is considered to be isosteric to OH, and so on. This early view of isosterism did not consider the actual location, motion, and resonance of electrons within the orbitals of these functional group replacements. Careful observation of this table reveals that some groups do share similar physicochemical properties, but others have very different properties, despite having the same number of valence electrons. For example, OH and NH_2 share similar hydrogen bonding properties and, therefore, should be interchangeable if that is the only important criterion. The NH_2 group is basic, whereas the OH is neutral. Hence, at physiologic pH, the NH_2 group exists in its protonated or conjugate acid form and the molecule becomes positively charged. If OH is being replaced by NH_2, the

Table 2.8 Grimm's Hydride Displacement "Law"

C	N	O	F	Ne
	CH	NH	OH	FH
		CH_2	NH_2	OH_2
			CH_3	NH_3

additional positive charge could have a significant effect on the overall physicochemical properties of the molecule in which it is being introduced. The difference in physicochemical properties of the CH_3 group relative to the OH and NH_2 groups is even greater. In addition to acid-base character, this "law" fails to take into account other important physicochemical parameters, such as electronegativity, polarizability, bond angles, size, shape of molecular orbitals, electron density, and partition coefficients, all of which contribute significantly to the overall physicochemical properties of a molecule.

Instead of considering only partial structures, Hinsberg[34] applied the concept of isosterism to entire molecules. He developed the concept of "ring equivalents"—that is, functional groups that can be exchanged for one another in aromatic ring systems without drastic changes in physicochemical properties relative to the parent structure. Benzene, thiophene, and pyridine illustrate this concept (Fig. 2.38). A-CH=CH- group in benzene is replaced by the divalent sulfur, -S-, in thiophene, and a -CH= is replaced by the trivalent -N= to give pyridine. The physical properties of benzene and thiophene are very similar. For example, the boiling point of benzene is 81.1 °C, and that of thiophene is 84.4 °C (at 760 mm Hg). Pyridine, however, deviates, with a boiling point of 115 °C to 116 °C. Hinsberg, therefore, concluded that divalent sulfur (-S- or thioether) must resemble -C=C- in shape, and these groups were considered to be isosteric. Note that hydrogen atoms are ignored in this comparison. Today, this isosteric relationship is seen in many drugs (eg, H_1-receptor antagonists) (Fig. 2.38).

It is difficult to relate biologic properties to physicochemical properties of individual atoms, functional groups, or entire molecules, because many physicochemical parameters are involved simultaneously and, therefore, are difficult to quantitate. Simple relationships as described earlier often do not hold up across the many types of biologic systems seen with medicinal agents. That is, what can work as an isosteric replacement in one biologic system cannot work in another. Because of this, it was necessary to introduce the term "bioisosterism" to describe functional groups related in structure that have similar biologic effects. Friedman[35] introduced the term bioisosterism and defined it as follows: "Bioisosteres are (functional) groups or molecules that have chemical and physical similarities producing broadly similar biological properties." Burger[36] expanded this definition to take into account biochemical views of biologic activity: "Bioisosteres are molecules or groups that possess near equal molecular shapes and volumes, approximately the same distribution of electrons, and which exhibit similar physical properties such as hydrophobicity. Bioisosteric molecules affect the same biochemically associated systems as agonist or antagonists and thereby produce biological properties that are related to each other."

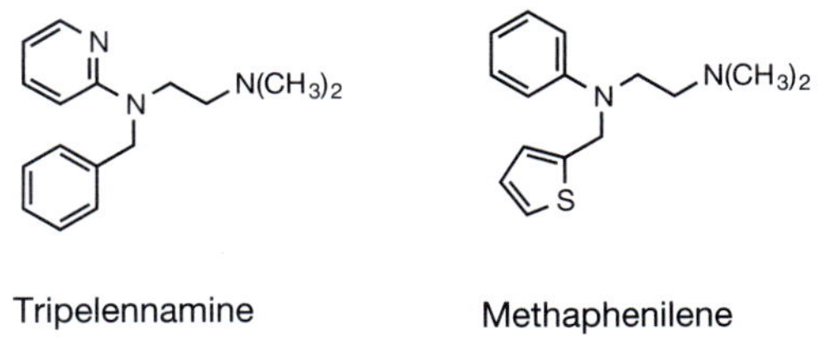

Figure 2.38 Isosteric substitution of thiophene for benzene and benzene for pyridine.

Classical and Nonclassical Bioisosteres

Bioisosteric groups can be subdivided into two categories: classical and nonclassical bioisosteres. Functional groups that satisfy the original conditions of Langmuir and Grimm are referred to as classical bioisosteres. Nonclassical bioisosteres do not obey steric and electronic definitions of classical bioisosteres and do not necessarily have the same number of atoms as the functional group that they replace. A wider set of molecules and functional groups are encompassed by nonclassical bioisosteres that produce, at the molecular level, qualitatively similar agonist or antagonist action. In animals, many hormones and neurotransmitters with very similar structures and biologic actions can be classified as bioisosteres.

What can be a successful bioisosteric replacement for a given molecule that interacts with a particular biologic target quite often has no effect or abolishes biologic activity in another. Thus, the use of bioisosteric replacement (classical or nonclassical) in the design of new chemical entities (drug discovery) is highly dependent on the biologic system under investigation. No hard-and-fast rules exist to determine which bioisosteric replacement is going to work with a given molecule, although as the following tables and examples demonstrate, some generalizations are possible. Each category of bioisostere can be further subdivided as shown in the following list, and examples are provided in Tables 2.9 and 2.10:

1. Classical bioisosteres
   a. Monovalent atoms and groups
   b. Divalent atoms and groups
   c. Trivalent atoms and groups
   d. Tetrasubstituted atoms
   e. Ring equivalents
2. Nonclassical bioisosteres
   a. Exchangeable groups
   b. Rings versus noncyclic structure

Classical Bioisosteres

Substitution of hydrogen with fluorine is a common monovalent isosteric replacement. Sterically, hydrogen and fluorine are quite similar, with their van der Waals radii measuring 1.2 and 1.35 Å, respectively. Because fluorine is the most electronegative element in the periodic table, any differences in biologic activity resulting from replacement of hydrogen with fluorine can be attributed to this property.

A classic example of hydrogen replacement by fluorine is development of the antineoplastic agent 5-fluorouracil from uracil. Another example is shown in Figure 2.39, in which the chlorine of chlorothiazide has been replaced with bromine or a trifluoromethyl group. For each of the

Table 2.9 Classical Bioisosteres (Groups Within the Row Can Replace Each Other)

Monovalent bioisosteres
F, H
OH, NH
F, OH, NH, or CH_3 for H
SH, OH
Cl, Br, CF_3

Divalent bioisosteres
—C=S, —C=O, —C=NH, —C=C—

Trivalent atoms or groups:
—CH=, —N=
—P=, —As=

Tetrasubstituted atoms:

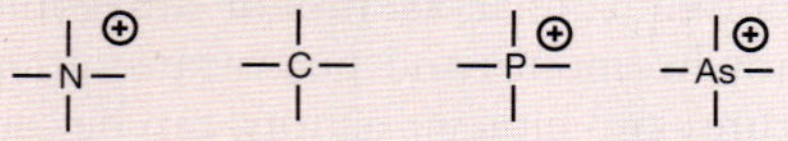

Ring equivalents:

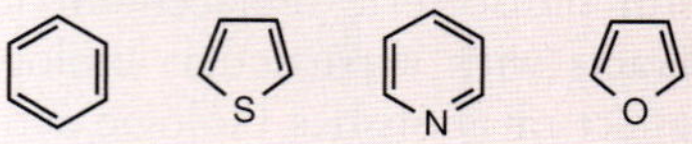

substitutions, the electronic (σ, where σ+ is electron withdrawing and σ− is electron donating) and hydrophobic (π) properties of each group are maintained relatively constant, but the size of each group varies significantly, as indicated by the Taft steric parameter (E_s).

Figure 2.40 shows an example of classical isosteric substitution of an amino group for a hydroxyl group in folic acid. The amino group is capable of mimicking the tautomeric forms of folic acid and providing the appropriate hydrogen bonds to the enzyme active site.

A tetravalent bioisosteric replacement study was conducted by Grisar et al[37] with a series of α-tocopherol analogues (Fig. 2.41). α-Tocopherol has been shown to scavenge lipoperoxyl and superoxide radicals that accumulate in heart tissue. This is thought to be part of its mechanism of action

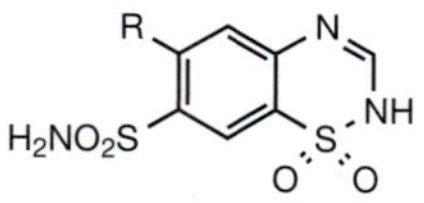

R =	Cl	Br	CF_3
σ	+0.23	+0.23	+0.54
π	+0.71	+0.86	+0.88
E_s	-0.97	-1.16	-2.40

Figure 2.39 Isosteric replacement of chlorine in thiazide diuretics. Comparison of physicochemical properties of the substituents.

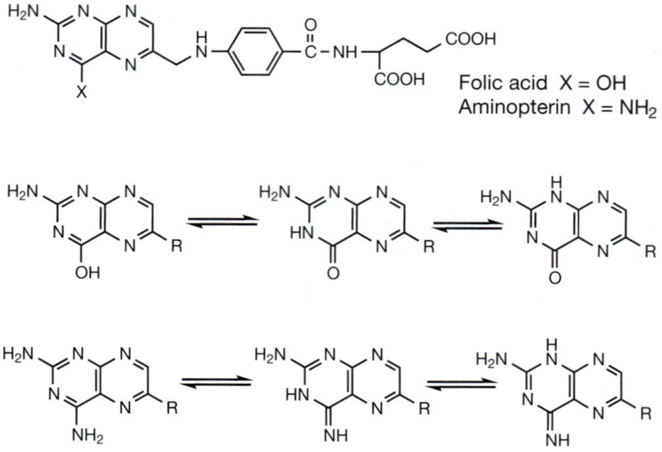

Figure 2.40 Isosteric replacement of OH by NH_2 in folic acid and possible tautomers of folic acid and aminopterin.

to reduce cardiac damage resulting from myocardial infarction. All of the bioisosteric analogues were found to produce similar biologic activity.

Nonclassical Bioisosteres

As mentioned earlier, nonclassical bioisosteres are replacements of functional groups not defined by classical definitions. Some of these groups, however, mimic spatial arrangements, electronic properties, or some other physicochemical property of the molecule or functional group critical for biologic activity. One example is the use of a double bond to position essential functional groups into a particular spatial configuration critical for activity. This is shown in Figure 2.42 with the naturally occurring hormone estradiol and the synthetic analogue diethylstilbestrol. The *trans*-isomer of diethylstilbestrol has approximately the same potency as estradiol, whereas the *cis*-isomer is only one-fourteenth as active. In the *trans* configuration, the phenolic hydroxy groups mimic the correct orientation of the phenol and alcohol in estradiol.[38,39] This is not possible with the *cis*-isomer, and more flexible analogues (Fig. 2.42) have little or no activity.[40,41]

Another example of a nonclassical replacement is that of a sulfonamide group for a phenol in catecholamines (Fig. 2.43). With this example, steric factors appear to have less influence on receptor binding than acidity and

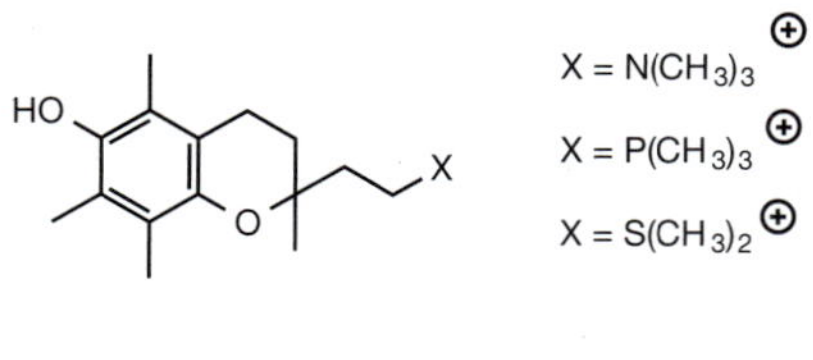

α-Tocopherol X = $C_{14}H_{29}$

Figure 2.41 Tetravalent bioisosteres of α-tocopherol.

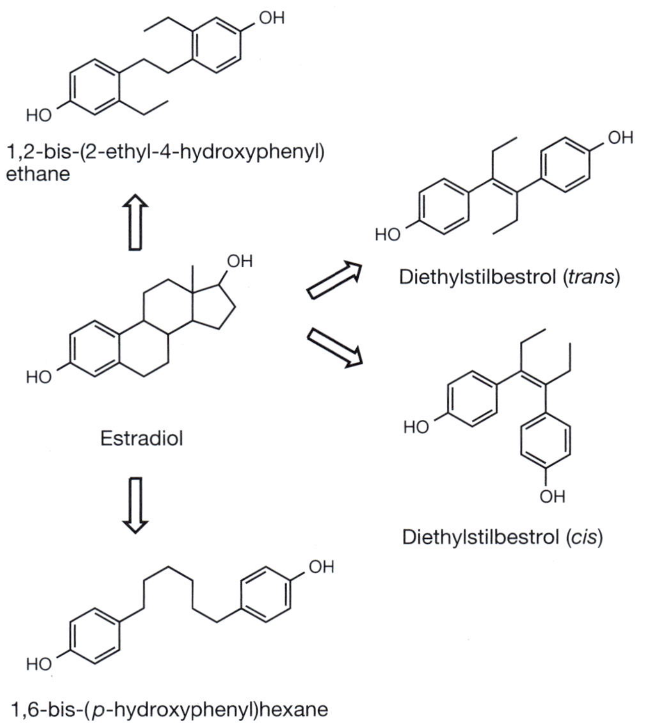

Figure 2.42 Noncyclic analogues of estradiol.

hydrogen bonding potential of the functional group on the aromatic ring. Both the phenolic hydroxyl of isoproterenol and the acidic proton of the arylsulfonamide have nearly the same pK_a (~10).[42] Both groups are weakly acidic and capable of losing a proton and interacting with the biologic target as anions (Fig. 2.43). Because the replacement is not susceptible to metabolism by catechol O-methyltransferase, it has also the added advantage of increasing the duration of action and making the molecule orally active. Other examples of successful bioisosteric replacements are shown in Table 2.10, and a more detailed description of the role of bioisosterism can be found in the review by Jayashree et al.[43]

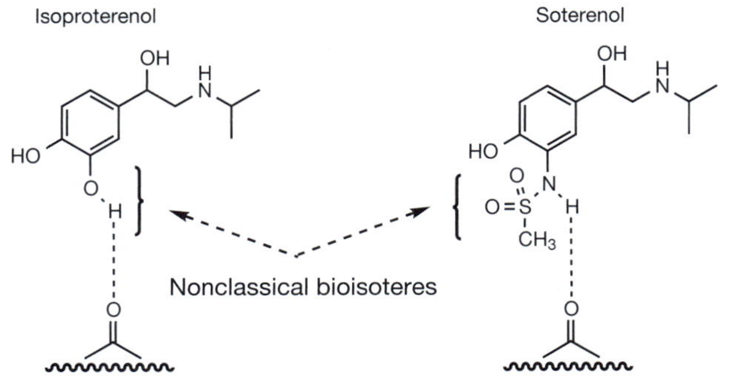

Figure 2.43 Bioisosteric replacement of *m*-OH of isoproterenol with a sulfonamide group and similar hydrogen bonding capacity to a possible drug receptor.

Table 2.10 Nonclassical Bioisosteric Replacements

Molecules	Bioisosteric Replacement	References
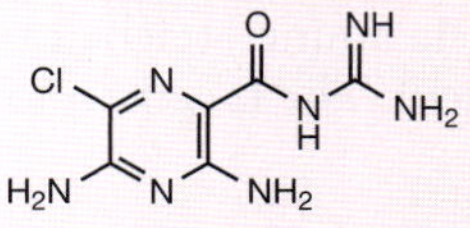	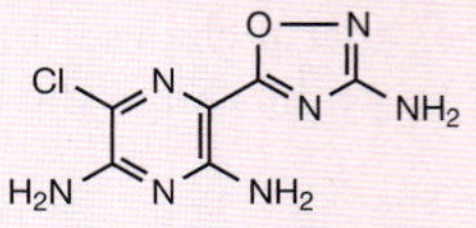	40
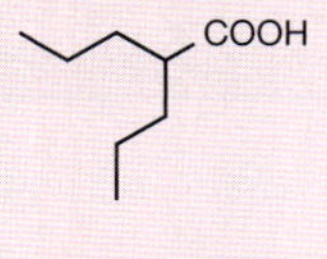	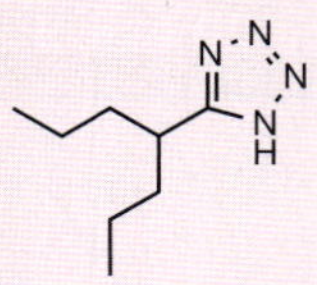	41
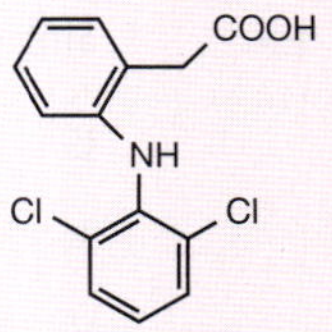	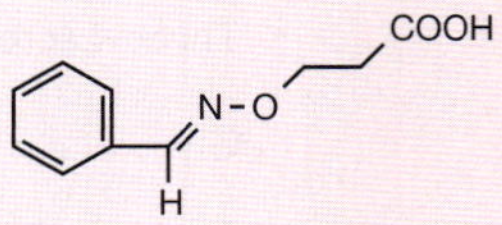	42
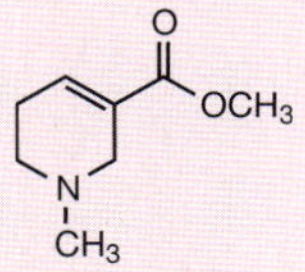	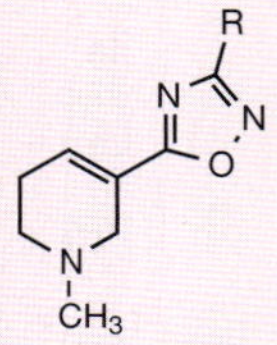	43
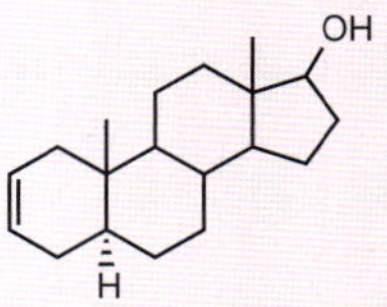	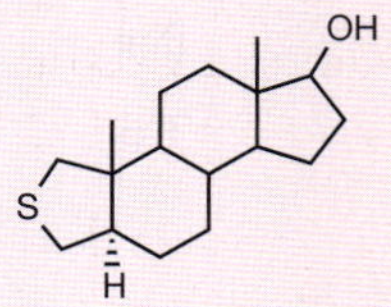	44
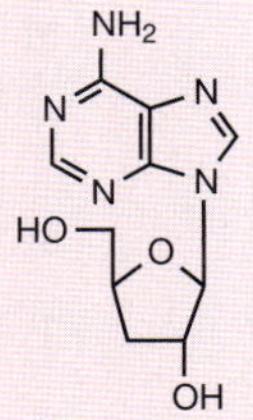	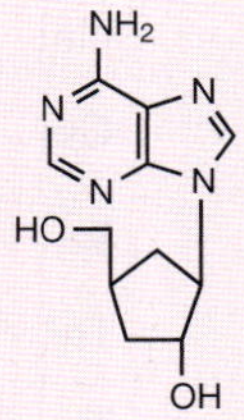	45
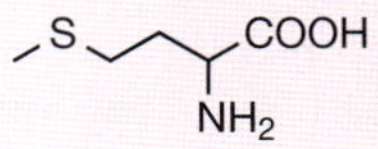	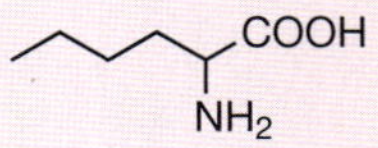	46

Peptide and Protein Drugs

Not all drugs are small molecules as described thus far. Some very important therapeutic agents are peptidic in nature (eg, insulin, calcitonin) and, due to their physicochemical properties, generally cannot be delivered orally and must be administered parenterally. Peptides and proteins are very similar in that they are made up of units, or residues, of amino acids that are linked by amide bonds, also referred to as peptide bonds. There is no definitive number of amino acid residues that delineate a peptide from a protein.

However, the term "peptide" refers generally to molecules that contain 15 to 50 amino acids. Molecules composed of more than 50 residues are generally referred to as proteins.

There are 20 naturally occurring amino acids that serve as the building blocks for both peptide and protein drugs (Table 2.11). Each amino acid contains a common functional group "backbone" that includes a basic amine attached to the α-carbon of an acidic carboxylic acid. The α-carbon for each amino acid is substituted with a unique side chain. The amino acid side chains contribute significantly to the physicochemical properties of the peptide that is formed from a unique sequence of amino acids.

As mentioned, the amino acid residues are linked by amide bonds, as shown in Figure 2.44. Each carboxylic acid forms an amide bond with the amine group of the next amino acid in the sequence. As with other amide bonds,

Table 2.11 The 20 Natural Occurring Amino Acids

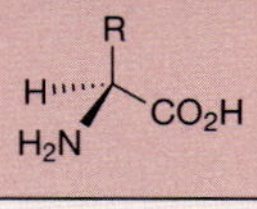			**General Structure**	
Name	Three-Letter Code	Single-Letter Code	Structure R=	pK_a of Side Chain
Glycine	Gly	G	-H	None
Alanine	Ala	A	-CH_3	None
Valine	Val	V	-$CH(CH_3)_2$	None
Isoleucine	Ile	I	-$CH(CH_3)CH_2CH_3$	None
Leucine	Leu	L	-$CH_2CH(CH_3)_2$	None
Proline	Pro	P	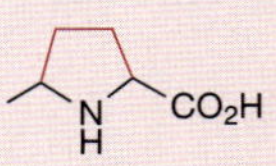	None
Phenylalanine	Phe	F	-CH_2-C_6H_5	None
Tryptophan	Trp	W	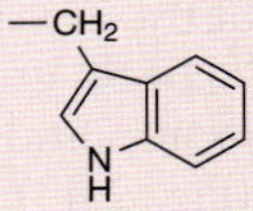	None
Methionine	Met	M	-$CH_2CH_2SCH_3$	None
Cysteine	Cys	C	-CH_2SH	(Acidic) ~8
Serine	Ser	S	-CH_2OH	None
Threonine	Thr	T	-$CH(CH_3)OH$	None
Tyrosine	Tyr	Y	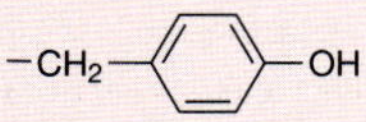	(Acidic) ~10
Arginine	Arg	R	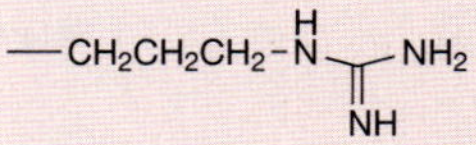	(Basic) ~12.5
Lysine	Lys	K	-$CH_2CH_2CH_2NH_2$	(Basic) ~10.5
Histidine	His	H	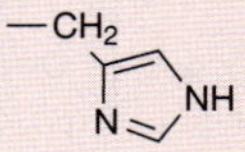	(Basic) ~6
Asparagine	Asn	N	-CH_2CONH_2	None
Glutamine	Gln	Q	-$CH_2CH_2CONH_2$	None
Aspartic acid	Asp	D	-CH_2COOH	(Acidic) ~3.8
Glutamic acid	Glu	E	-CH_2CH_2COOH	(Acidic) ~4

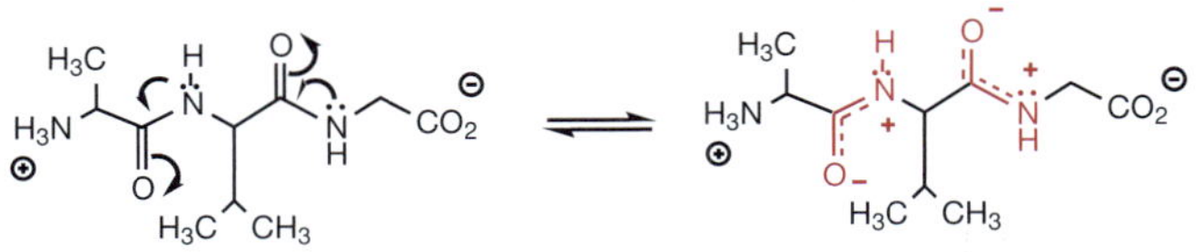

Figure 2.44 Tripeptide, Ala-Val-Gly, indicating the planarity of the peptide bonds caused by the restricted rotation around the amide bond.

conjugation between the lone pair of electrons on the nitrogen atom and the adjacent carbonyl group results in the amide bond having partial double bond character due to a resonance structure as shown in Figure 2.44. This property has two major consequences: (1) the amide bond is therefore co-planar; and (2) there is restricted rotation around the C-N bond (Fig. 2.44). Because of this restricted rotation, there are two conformations possible, *cis* and *trans* (Fig. 2.45). The *trans*-conformation is lower in energy due to fewer steric interactions (similar to that found with a carbon-carbon double bond) and is favored. When proline is one of the amino acid residues, the *cis*-conformation can be favored as a result of the amine group being part of a pyrrolidine ring. For this reason, the presence of proline in peptides and proteins is associated with a "kink" or bend in the overall conformation of the peptide chain.

Physicochemical Properties of Peptides

Since the α-amine and α-carboxylic acid of each amino acid are involved in the peptide backbone (except at each terminus of the chain), the basic and acidic nature of these functional groups does not contribute to the overall physicochemical properties of the molecule. The functional groups found within the amino acid side chains are what are integral to the physicochemical properties of the peptide or protein and represent important points of interaction with the corresponding biologic target. Examination of Table 2.11 shows that the functional groups found within the amino acid side chains can be basic (eg, amine, guanidine, imidazole), acidic (eg, carboxylic acid, phenol, thiol), neutral (eg, thioether, amide), or hydrocarbon (eg, alkyl, aromatic rings) in nature. All of the functional groups found in amino acid side chains were discussed previously as components of small-molecule drugs. The primary differences in physicochemical properties between peptides and small molecules are due to their large size (MW) and, as a result, the sheer number of different side chains (ie, functional groups) present in a given structure. As might be expected, the types and number of functional groups present in the side chains dictate how much more or less polar the peptide is compared to a small-molecule drug. It is certainly plausible that peptide-based drugs will not have optimal logP values for passive absorption across membranes and, given their large MW, will not readily cross membranes.

Metabolism/Degradation of Peptide and Protein Drugs

Peptides and proteins are metabolized extensively by enzymes in the GI tract, blood, interstitial fluid, vascular bed, and cell membranes, which results in very poor oral absorption and a short half-life for these molecules. The primary route of metabolism of peptides and proteins involves hydrolysis of the peptide bonds that link the amino acids by enzymes called peptidases. Some of these peptidases exhibit specificity for certain amino acid sequences or have specificity for either the amino or carboxyl terminus of the peptide (exopeptidase). For example, carboxypeptidases cleave off one C-terminal residue, dipeptidyl carboxypeptidases cleave dipeptides from the C-terminus, aminopeptidases cleave off one N-terminal residue, and amidases (endopeptidases) cleave internal peptide bonds. There are also peptidase subclasses that exhibit specificity for certain amino acid sequences within the peptide or at either of the termini. Some peptidases (eg, dipeptidyl peptidase IV) have been found to catalyze the degradation of naturally occurring peptides (eg, Glucagon-like peptide 1) (Fig. 2.46) (see also Chapters 5 and 22).

Summary

Medicinal chemistry involves the discovery of new chemical entities and the systematic study of the SARs of these molecules for disease state management. Such studies provide the basis for development of better and therapeutically safer medicinal agents from lead molecules found from natural sources, random screening, systematic screening, and focused rational design. Drug design goals include increasing the potency and duration of action of newly discovered molecules and decreasing adverse side effects.

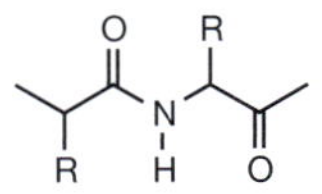

Trans peptide bond

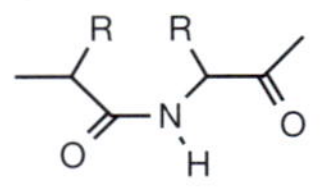

Cis peptide bond

Figure 2.45 *Cis/trans* peptide bond configuration.

Subject to proteolytic degradation
catalyzed by dipeptidyl peptidase

↓

His-Ala-Glu-Gly-Thr-Phe-Thr-Ser-Asp-Val-Ser-Ser-Tyr-Leu-Glu—

Gly-Gln-Ala-Ala-Lys-Glu-Phe-Ile-Ala-Trp-Leu-Val-Lys-Gly-Arg

GLP-1

Figure 2.46 Glucagon-like peptide 1 degradation by dipeptidyl peptidase IV.

For the pharmacist, it is also important to understand how the physicochemical properties influence the pharmacokinetic properties of the medicinal agents being dispensed. Such knowledge will help the pharmacist not only to better understand the clinical properties of these molecules but also to anticipate the properties of newly marketed agents. An understanding of the chemical properties of the molecule will allow the pharmacist to anticipate formulation problems (especially IV admixtures), as well as potential adverse interactions with other drugs as the result of serum protein binding and metabolism.

Acknowledgments

The author wishes to acknowledge the work of Jim Knittel, PhD, who authored content used within this chapter in a previous edition of this text.

REFERENCES

1. Crum-Brown A, Fraser TR. On the connection between chemical constitution and physiological action. Part 1: on the physiological action of the ammonium bases derived from Strychia, Brucia, Thebia, Codeia, Morphia, and Nicotia. *Trans R Soc Edinb.* 1869;25:257-274.
2. Ariëns EJ. A general introduction to the field of drug discovery. In: Ariëns EJ, ed. *Drug Design.* Academic Press; 1971:689-696.
3. Loewi O, Navrati E. Über humorale übertragbarkeit der herznervenwirkung XI mitteilung. über den mechanismus der vaguswirkung von physostigmin und ergotamine. *Plugers Arch Ges Physiol Menshen Tiere.* 1926;214:689-696.
4. Ehrlich P. On immunity with special reference to cell life. In: Himmelweit F, ed. *Collected Papers of Paul Ehrlich.* Pergamon; 1957:178-195.
5. Albert A. The long search for valid structure–action relationships in drugs. *J Med Chem.* 1982;25:1-5.
6. Ing HR. The curariform action of onium salts. *Physiol Rev.* 1936;16:527-544.
7. Woods DD. The relation of p-aminobenzoic acid to the mechanism of the action of sulfanilamide. *Br J Exp Pathol.* 1940;21:74-90.
8. Kauffman GB. The Brönsted-Lowry acid-base concept. *J Chem Ed.* 1988;85:28-31.
9. Lemke TL. *Review of Organic Functional Groups: Introduction to Medicinal Organic Chemistry.* 5th ed. Lippincott Williams & Wilkins; 2012.
10. Cates LA. Calculation of drug solubilities by pharmacy students. *Am J Pharm Ed.* 1981;45:11-13.
11. Fujita T. The extrathermodynamic approach to drug design. In: Hansch C, ed. *Comprehensive Medicinal Chemistry.* Vol 4. Pergamon Press; 1990:497-560.
12. Tute MS. Principles and practice of Hansch analysis: a guide to structure-activity correlation for the medicinal chemist. In: Harper NJ, Simons AB, eds. *Advances in Drug Research.* Academic Press; 1971:1-77.
13. Hansch C, Leo A. *Substituent Constants for Correlation Analysis in Chemistry and Biology.* John Wiley; 1979.
14. Hansch C, Leo A. *Exploring QSAR: Hydrophobic, Electronic, and Steric Constants.* American Chemical Society; 1995.
15. ClogP. BioByte Corp, Claremont, CA; ACDLogP®, Advanced Chemistry Development, Toronto, Canada; KOWWIN®, Chemaxon, Budapest, Hungary; CSLogP, ChemSilico, Tewksbury, MA.
16. Molinspiration Chemoinformatics. Accessed November 20, 2023. http://www.molinspiration.com
17. Florence AT, Attwood D. *Physiochemical Principles of Pharmacy.* 5th ed. Chapman & Hall; 2011.
18. Smith C, Marks A, Lieberman M, eds. *Basic Medical Biochemistry.* 2nd ed. Lippincott Williams & Wilkins; 2004.
19. Kunta JR, Sinko PJ. Intestinal drug transporters: in vivo function and clinical importance. *Curr Drug Metab.* 2004;5:109-124.
20. Cahn RS, Ingold CK, Prelog V. The specification of asymmetric configuration in organic chemistry. *Experientia.* 1956;12:81-94.
21. Piutti A. Su rune nouvelle espec d'asparagine. *C R.* 1886;103:134-138.
22. Easson LH, Stedman E. Studies on the relationship between chemical constitution and physiological action. V. Molecular dissymmetry and physiological activity. *Biochem J.* 1933;27:1257-1266.
23. Blackwood JE, Gladys CL, Loening KL, et al. Unambiguous specification of stereoisomerism about a double bond. *J Am Chem Soc.* 1968;90:509-510.
24. Kemp JD, Pitzer KS. Hindered rotation of the methyl groups in ethane. *J Chem Phys.* 1936;4:749.
25. Bovet D, Staub A. Action protectice des ethers phenoliques au cours de l'intoxication histaminique. *C R Soc Biol (Paris).* 1937;124:547-549.
26. Laborit H, Huguenard P, Alluaume R. Un nouveau stabilisateur vegetatif, le 4560 RP. *Presse Med.* 1952;60:206-208.
27. Charpentier P, Gaillot P, Jacob R, et al. Recherches sur les dimethylaminopropyl N-phenothiazines. *C R Acad Sci (Paris).* 1952;325:59-60.
28. Delay J, Deniker P, Hurl JM. Utilisation en thirapeutique psychiatrique d'une phenothiazine d'action centrale elective. *Ann Med Psychol (Paris).* 1952;110:112-117.
29. McCawley EL, Hart ER, Marsh DF. The preparation of N-allylnormorphine. *J Am Chem Soc.* 1941;63:314.
30. Clark RL, Pessolano AA, Weijlard J, et al. N-substituted epoxymorphinans. *J Am Chem Soc.* 1953;75:4964-4967.
31. Langmuir I. The arrangement of electrons in atoms and molecules. *J Am Chem Soc.* 1919;41:868-934.
32. Langmuir I. Isomorphism, isosterism, and covalence. *J Am Chem Soc.* 1919;41:1543-1559.
33. Grimm HG. Über ban und grösse der nichtmetallhydride. *Z Elektrochem.* 1925;31:474-480.
34. Hinsberg O. The sulfur atom. *J Prakt Chem.* 1916;93:302-311.
35. Friedman HL. Influence of isosteric replacements upon biological activity. In: *Symposium on Chemical-Biological Correlation.* Publication 206. Vol 206. National Academy of Science; 1951:295-358.
36. Burger A. Isosterism and bioisosterism in drug design. *Prog Drug Res.* 1991;37:288-371.
37. Grisar JM, Marciniak G, Bolkenius FN, et al. Cardioselective ammonium, phosphonium, and sulfonium analogues of α-tocopherol and ascorbic acid that inhibit in vitro and ex vivo lipid peroxidation and scavenge superoxide radicals. *J Med Chem.* 1995;38:2880-2886.
38. Dodds EC, Goldberg L, Lawson W, et al. Estrogenic activity of certain synthetic compounds. *Nature.* 1938;141:247-248.
39. Walton E, Brownlee G. Isomers of stilbestrol and its esters. *Nature.* 1943;151:305-306.
40. Blanchard EW, Stuart AH, Tallman RC. Studies on a new series of synthetic estrogenic substances. *Endocrinology.* 1943;32:307-309.
41. Baker BR. Some analogues of hexestrol. *J Am Chem Soc.* 1943;65:1572-1579.
42. Larsen AA, Gould WA, Roth HR, et al. Sulfonanilides. II. Analogues of catecholamines. *J Med Chem.* 1967;10:462-472.
43. Jayashree BS, Nikhil PS, Paul S. Bioisosterism in drug discovery and development—an overview. *Med Chem.* 2022;18:915-925.
44. Foinard A, Décaudin B, Barthélémy C, et al. Impact of physical incompatibility on drug mass flow rates: example of furosemide-midazolam incompatibility. *Ann Intensive Care.* 2012;2:28.

Case Study 2.1

ABSORPTION/ACID-BASE CASE SOLUTION

1.

Name of Functional Group	Drug(s) in Which Functional Group Is Present	Character: Hydrophilic or Hydrophobic	Function: ↑ Aqueous Solubility or Drug Absorption	Character: Acidic, Basic, or Neutral	Function: Contributes to Ability of Drug to Cross BBB?
Aromatic hydrocarbon	Cetirizine; Hydroxyzine	Hydrophobic	↑ Absorption	Neutral	Yes
Halogenated aromatic hydrocarbon	Cetirizine; Hydroxyzine	Hydrophobic	↑ Absorption	Neutral	Yes
Tertiary amine	Cetirizine; Hydroxyzine	Hydrophobic (R) Hydrophilic (N)	↑ Absorption ↑ Solubility	Basic (pK_a 9-11)	Yes (in unionized form to a limited extent via R groups); No (in ionized form)
Ether	Cetirizine; Hydroxyzine	Hydrophobic (R) Hydrophilic (O)	↑ Absorption ↑ Solubility (limited)	Neutral	Yes (via R groups)
Primary alcohol	Hydroxyzine	Hydrophobic (R) Hydrophilic (OH)	↑ Absorption ↑ Solubility (limited)	Neutral	Yes (via R group)
Carboxylic acid	Cetirizine	Hydrophilic	↑ Solubility	Acidic (pK_a 2-5)	No (in ionized form); Yes (in unionized form to a limited extent via R groups)

R, alkyl group.

Cetirizine is a second-generation H_1 antagonist and is purported to be nonsedating. Hydroxyzine is a first-generation H_1 antagonist and is considered to be a sedating antihistamine. Based on the structure evaluation process, both cetirizine and hydroxyzine contain several hydrophobic functional groups that would facilitate their passive diffusion across the blood-brain barrier (BBB). Both molecules contain an ionizable amine that will be predominantly ionized in the plasma (pH 7.4). A key structural difference between these drug molecules is the presence of a carboxylic acid in cetirizine. This functional group is very hydrophilic and will also be predominantly ionized in the plasma (pH 7.4) and therefore may limit the extent of absorption across the BBB. Though both of these drugs will be predominantly ionized at pH 7.4, it is important to remember that ionizable functional groups exist in equilibrium with their unionized forms. In the case of hydroxyzine, it is possible that for a small fraction of time there will be some unionized drug available to cross the BBB. In the case of cetirizine, with multiple ionizable functional groups, it is highly unlikely that the drug will exist in its unionized form. In order to limit his lethargy, it would be appropriate to recommend cetirizine (Zyrtec) for Marcus.

2.

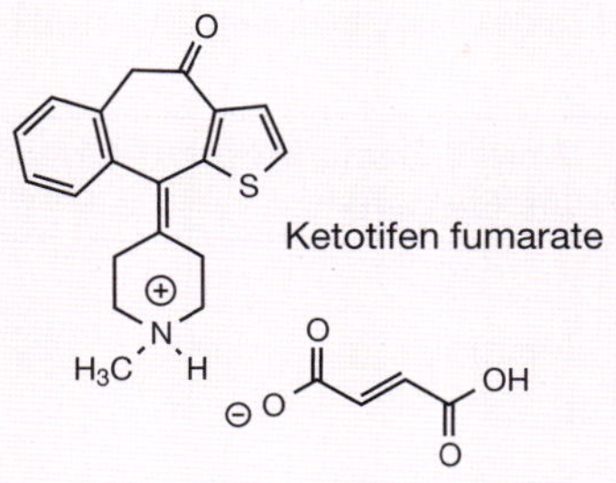

(continued)

Case Study 2.1 (continued)

Ketotifen contains functional groups (eg, aromatic hydrocarbons, alkene, R groups of ketone, and thiophene) with hydrophobic character. Since hydrophobic character contributes to the ability of a drug to cross lipophilic membranes (eg, the membranes that surround the eye) passively, then it is no surprise based on our evaluation thus far that there is the potential for this agent to be absorbed.

The next set of functional groups to evaluate are those that exist predominantly in their ionized form at physiologic pH. Ketotifen contains an ionizable amine (pK_a = 9-11) that will be predominantly ionized in the ocular fluid. This ionizable functional group contributes to the drug's ability to be soluble in an aqueous environment, including in the aqueous eye drop formulation. This same functional group limits the ability of the drug to be absorbed passively into the membranes of the eye.

3.

Assumptions:	pK_a (tertiary amine) = 9.5	
	pK_a (carboxylic acid) = 3.0	
	pH = 2 (stomach)	*pH = 6.5-7 (hindgut)*
Tertiary amine (basic)	Predominantly ionized	Predominantly ionized
Carboxylic acid (acidic)	Unionized	Predominantly ionized

Cetirizine: In the hindgut the tertiary amine and carboxylic acid functional groups will both be predominantly ionized. This will significantly limit the extent of cetirizine absorption from this compartment. In the stomach only one of these two functional groups (the tertiary amine) will be predominantly found in its ionized form. Only a small percentage of cetirizine will be in its unionized form in the stomach. Since it is the unionized form of the drug that is absorbed, cetirizine is probably absorbed best from the stomach.

Hydroxyzine: In both compartments the amine functional groups will be predominantly ionized. It will be slightly better absorbed in the hindgut where the % of unionized drug is slightly greater at any given time.

4. If the horse is experiencing an acidic hindgut from a lack of prolonged foraging, then the hindgut pH will decrease from 6.5-7 to pH = 5. For hydroxyzine, there will be an even lower % of unionized drug in an acidic hindgut. This means that there will be less hydroxyzine absorbed from an acidic hindgut and the horse may not receive the maximal antihistaminergic effect. For cetirizine, there is really little appreciable change in the % of drug that is in its unionized form when the horse is experiencing an acid hindgut and therefore there is little to no change in the amount of drug that is absorbed from that compartment. One could anticipate no change in the antihistaminergic effect experienced by the horse.

Assumptions:	pK_a (tertiary amine) = 9.5	
	pK_a (carboxylic acid) = 3.0	
	pH = 6.5-7 (hindgut)	*pH = 5 (hindgut)*
Tertiary amine (basic)	Predominantly ionized	Predominantly ionized
Carboxylic acid (acidic)	Predominantly ionized	Predominantly ionized

Case Study 2.2

ACID-BASE CHEMISTRY/COMPATIBILITY CASE SOLUTION

1. Acid-base evaluation of furosemide and midazolam as drawn and at pH 7.4.

Name of Functional Group	Acidic/Basic/Neutral Character (as Drawn)	Acidic/Basic/Neutral Character (at pH 7.4)
Furosemide		
Halogenated aromatic hydrocarbon	Neutral	Neutral
Aniline	Basic	Basic
Furan	Neutral	Neutral
Sulfonamide	Acidic	Acidic
Carboxylic acid	Acidic	Basic

Case Study 2.2 (continued)

Midazolam		
Halogenated aromatic hydrocarbon	Neutral	Neutral
Imine	Basic	Basic
Imidazole	Basic	Acidic

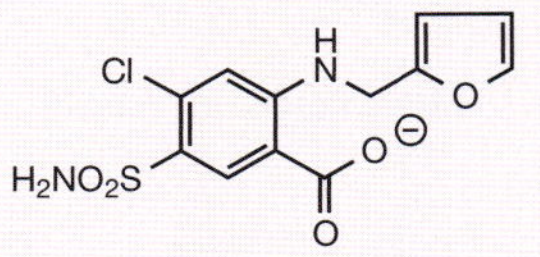

Furosemide

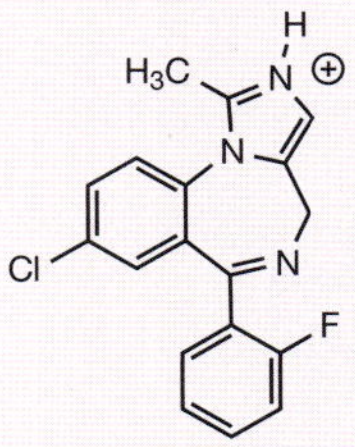

Midazolam

2. Furosemide contains several hydrophilic (polar) functional groups (aniline, sulfonamide, carboxylic acid, furan [O]) and only a moderate amount of hydrophobic character (halogenated aromatic hydrocarbon, furan [C]). Midazolam contains an imine and an imidazole that are hydrophilic in character. It has a functional group that has mixed hydrophobic/hydrophilic character (halogenated [F] aromatic hydrocarbon) and a functional group with hydrophobic character (halogenated [Cl] aromatic hydrocarbon). In order for a drug to be water soluble it must be able to interact with water via hydrogen bonding or an ion/dipole interaction. Hydrophilic functional groups can typically participate in these types of interactions. Considering the structural features of both agents, furosemide will be more water soluble due to the presence of several hydrophilic functional groups, including the ionizable carboxylic acid. The ionized form of midazolam is much more water soluble than the free base/parent form since the ionized imidazole can participate in ion/dipole interactions with water (a strong interaction).

3. Furosemide solution for injection has a pH of ~8.7. Therefore, in the solution for injection, furosemide exists predominantly in the ionized state and is water soluble. Midazolam solution for injection has a pH of ~3.2. Therefore, in the solution for injection, midazolam exists predominantly in the ionized state and is water soluble. When both solutions are mixed together in a Y-site, the pH of the solution is ~5.6 such that less of both furosemide and midazolam is ionized, which decreases their water solubility and one or both may precipitate out of solution.[44] Additionally, it is certainly possible that these drugs (acid + base) could form a complex (ionic). This complex is not likely to be particularly water soluble and may very well form a precipitate.

Case Study 2.3

ABSORPTION/BINDING INTERACTIONS CASE SOLUTION

Name of Functional Group	Character: Hydrophilic and/or Hydrophobic	Function: ↑ Aqueous Solubility or Drug Absorption	Function: Contributes to Ability of Drug to Penetrate Skin	Binding Interactions Possible With Enzyme	Examples of Amino Acids That Could Interact With Group
Aromatic hydrocarbon	Hydrophobic	↑ Absorption	Yes	Hydrophobic Stacking interactions	Phenylalanine Tyrosine
Mono thiocarbamic ester	Hydrophobic (R) Hydrophilic (N-C=S-O)	↑ Absorption (R) ↑ Solubility (N-C=S-O)	Yes (via the R groups)	H-bonding Dipole-dipole Ion-dipole	Serine Threonine Cysteine Tyrosine Glutamic acid

R, alkyl group.

1. Those functional groups that are hydrophobic in character will facilitate the absorption of this medication into the skin.

2. Selection of the amino acids is based on the types of interactions that are possible with the particular functional group. The mono thiocarbamic ester can participate as a hydrogen bond acceptor only. For the ion-dipole interaction the mono thiocarbamic ester is participating as the dipole when coupled with ionized amino acids.

Case Study 2.4

BINDING INTERACTIONS CASE SOLUTION

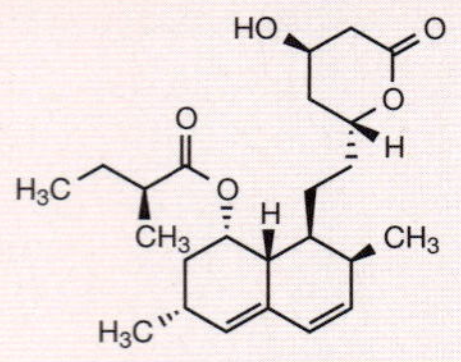

Lovastatin (Mevacor)

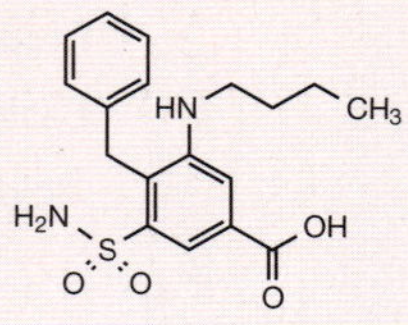

Bumetamide (Bumex)

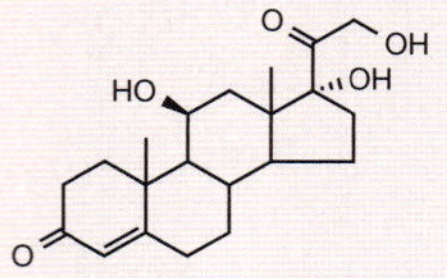

Hydrocortisone (Hydrocort)

Name of Functional Group	Drugs in which Functional Group is Present	Binding Interactions Possible with Enzyme	Examples of Amino Acids that could Interact with Group
Aromatic hydrocarbon	Bumetanide	Hydrophobic stacking interaction	Phenylalanine, Tyrosine
Cycloalkene	Lovastatin	Hydrophobic	Isoleucine, Leucine
Cycloalkane	Hydrocortisone	Hydrophobic	Isoleucine, Leucine
Alkane	Lovastatin, Bumetanide	Hydrophobic	Isoleucine, Leucine
Ether	Bumetanide	H-bonding, Dipole/dipole, Hydrophobic	Serine, Threonine, Valine
Ketone	Hydrocortisone	H-bonding, Dipole/dipole, Ion/dipole	Cysteine, Lysine, Glutamate
Aniline	Bumetanide	H-bonding, Dipole/dipole, Ion/dipole, Ionic	Histidine, Glutamine, Cysteine, Aspartic acid
Carboxylic acid	Lovastatin	H-bonding, Dipole/dipole, Ion/dipole, Ionic	Serine, Cysteine, Glutamine, Lysine
Ester/lactone	Lovastatin	H-bonding, Dipole/dipole, Ion/dipole, Ionic	Serine, Threonine, Arginine
Sulfonamide	Bumetanide	H-bonding, Dipole/dipole, Ion/dipole, Ionic	Tyrosine, Threonine, Cysteine, Lysine
Primary alcohol	Hydrocortisone	H-bonding, Dipole/dipole, Ion/dipole, Ionic	Glutamic acid, Glutamine, Arginine
Secondary alcohol	Lovastatin, Hydrocortisone	H-bonding, Dipole/dipole, Ion/dipole, Ionic	Aspartic acid, Glutamine, Lysine
Tertiary alcohol	Hydrocortisone	H-bonding, Dipole/dipole, Ion/dipole, Ionic	Glutamic acid, Asparagine, Arginine

Name of Functional Group	Drug(s) in Which Functional Group Is Present	Binding Interactions Possible With Enzyme	Examples of Amino Acids That Could Interact With Group
Aromatic hydrocarbon	Bumetanide	Hydrophobic Stacking interactions	Phenylalanine Tyrosine
Cycloalkene	Lovastatin Hydrocortisone	Hydrophobic	Isoleucine Leucine
Cycloalkane	Hydrocortisone	Hydrophobic	Isoleucine Leucine
Alkane	Lovastatin Bumetanide	Hydrophobic	Leucine Isoleucine
Ether	Bumetanide	H-bonding Dipole-dipole Hydrophobic	Serine Threonine Valine
Ketone	Hydrocortisone	H-bonding Dipole-dipole Ion-dipole	Cysteine Lysine Glutamic acid (in ionized form)
Aniline	Bumetanide	H-bonding Dipole-dipole Ion-dipole	Histidine Glutamine Cysteine Aspartic acid (in ionized form)
Carboxylic acid	Lovastatin	H-bonding Dipole-dipole Ion-dipole Ionic	Serine Cysteine Glutamine Lysine (in ionized form)

Case Study 2.4 (continued)

Name of Functional Group	Drug(s) in Which Functional Group Is Present	Binding Interactions Possible With Enzyme	Examples of Amino Acids That Could Interact With Group
Ester lactone	Lovastatin	H-bonding Dipole-dipole Ion-dipole	Serine Threonine Arginine (in ionized form)
Sulfonamide	Bumetanide	H-bonding Dipole-dipole Ion-dipole	Tyrosine Threonine Cysteine Lysine (in ionized form)
Primary alcohol	Hydrocortisone	H-bonding Dipole-dipole Ion-dipole	Glutamic acid (in ionized form) Glutamine Arginine (in ionized form)
Secondary alcohol	Lovastatin Hydrocortisone	H-bonding Dipole-dipole Ion-dipole	Aspartic acid (in ionized form) Glutamine Lysine (in ionized form)
Tertiary alcohol	Hydrocortisone	H-bonding Dipole-dipole Ion-dipole	Glutamic acid (in ionized form) Asparagine Arginine (in ionized form)

Case Study 2.5

WATER/LIPID SOLUBILITY CASE SOLUTION

Name of Functional Group	Drug(s) in Which Functional Group Is Present	Character: Hydrophilic and/or Hydrophobic	Function: ↑ Aqueous Solubility or Drug Absorption
Halogenated aromatic hydrocarbon	Levofloxacin (F) Amlodipine (Cl)	Hydrophobic Hydrophilic (F)	↑ Absorption ↑ Solubility (F)
Phenol	Oxymetazoline	Hydrophobic Hydrophilic (O)	↑ Absorption ↑ Solubility (O)
Ether	Levofloxacin Amlodipine	Hydrophobic (R) Hydrophilic (O)	↑ Absorption (R) ↑ Solubility (O)
Ester	Amlodipine	Hydrophobic (R) Hydrophilic (COO)	↑ Absorption (R) ↑ Solubility (COO)
Carboxylic acid	Levofloxacin	Hydrophobic (R) Hydrophilic (COOH)	↑ Absorption (R) ↑ Solubility (COOH)
Ketone	Levofloxacin	Hydrophobic (R) Hydrophilic (CO)	↑ Absorption (R) ↑ Solubility (CO)
Alkene	Levofloxacin	Hydrophobic	↑ Absorption (R)
Alkane	Oxymetazoline	Hydrophobic	↑ Absorption (R)
Aniline	Levofloxacin	Hydrophobic (R) Hydrophilic (N)	↑ Absorption (R) ↑ Solubility (N)
Amidine	Oxymetazoline	Hydrophobic (R) Hydrophilic (N-C=N)	↑ Absorption (R) ↑ Solubility (N-C=N)
Primary amine	Amlodipine	Hydrophobic (R) Hydrophilic (NH_2)	↑ Absorption (R) ↑ Solubility (NH_2)
Tertiary amine	Levofloxacin	Hydrophobic (R) Hydrophilic (N)	↑ Absorption (R) ↑ Solubility (N)
Dihydropyridine	Amlodipine	Hydrophobic (R) Hydrophilic (NH)	↑ Absorption (R) ↑ Solubility (NH)

R, alkyl group.

Case Study 2.6

INTERACTIONS/SOLUBILITY CASE SOLUTION

Evaluation of pseudoephedrine and brompheniramine for aqueous solubility.

Name of Functional Group	Drugs in Which Functional Group Is Present	Character: Hydrophilic and/or Hydrophobic	Function: ↑ Aqueous Solubility and/or ↑ Absorption Across BBB	Binding Interactions Possible With Target of Drug Action
Aromatic hydrocarbon	Pseudoephedrine Dextromethorphan	Hydrophobic	↑ Absorption	Hydrophobic π-π stacking interactions
Halogenated aromatic hydrocarbon (Br)	Brompheniramine	Hydrophobic	↑ Absorption	Hydrophobic π-π stacking interactions Dipole-dipole
Cycloalkane	Dextromethorphan	Hydrophobic	↑ Absorption	Hydrophobic
Pyridine	Brompheniramine	Hydrophobic (R) Hydrophilic (N)	↑ Absorption (R) ↑ Solubility (N)	H-bonding Dipole-dipole Ion-dipole Ionic
Piperidine	Dextromethorphan	Hydrophobic (R) Hydrophilic (N)	↑ Absorption (R) ↑ Solubility (N)	H-bonding Dipole-dipole Ion-dipole Ionic
Ether	Dextromethorphan	Hydrophobic (R) Hydrophilic (O)	↑ Absorption (R) ↑ Solubility (O)	H-bonding Dipole-dipole Ion-dipole
Secondary or tertiary amine	Pseudoephedrine (2°) Brompheniramine (3°) Dextromethorphan (3°)	Hydrophobic (R) Hydrophilic (N)	↑ Absorption (R) ↑ Solubility (N)	H-bonding Dipole-dipole Ion-dipole Ionic
Secondary alcohol	Pseudoephedrine	Hydrophobic (R) Hydrophilic (OH)	↑ Absorption (R) ↑ Solubility (OH)	H-bonding Dipole-dipole Ion-dipole

R, alkyl group.

Functional groups that contribute to aqueous solubility are hydrophilic in character and interact with water via hydrogen bonding or dipole-dipole interactions. If the functional group is ionizable (eg, secondary and tertiary amines, pyridine, piperidine), then the group can participate in an ion-dipole interaction with water.

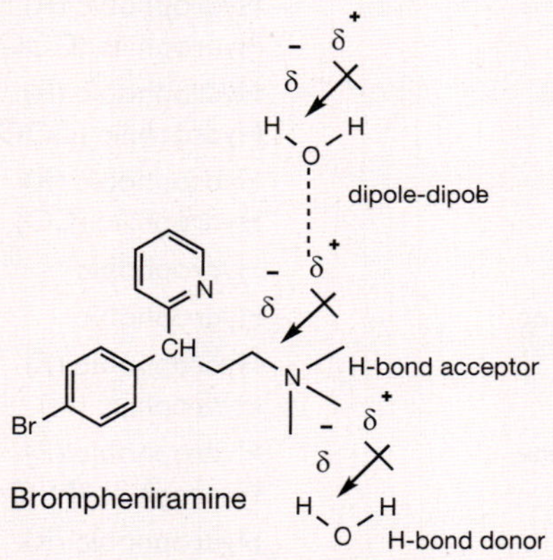

The agent that has the most hydrophobic character is the one that is most likely to cross the lipophilic blood-brain barrier (BBB) and has an effect on the child's alertness. Of these agents, dextromethorphan has the most hydrophobic character (see list of structural features mentioned earlier).

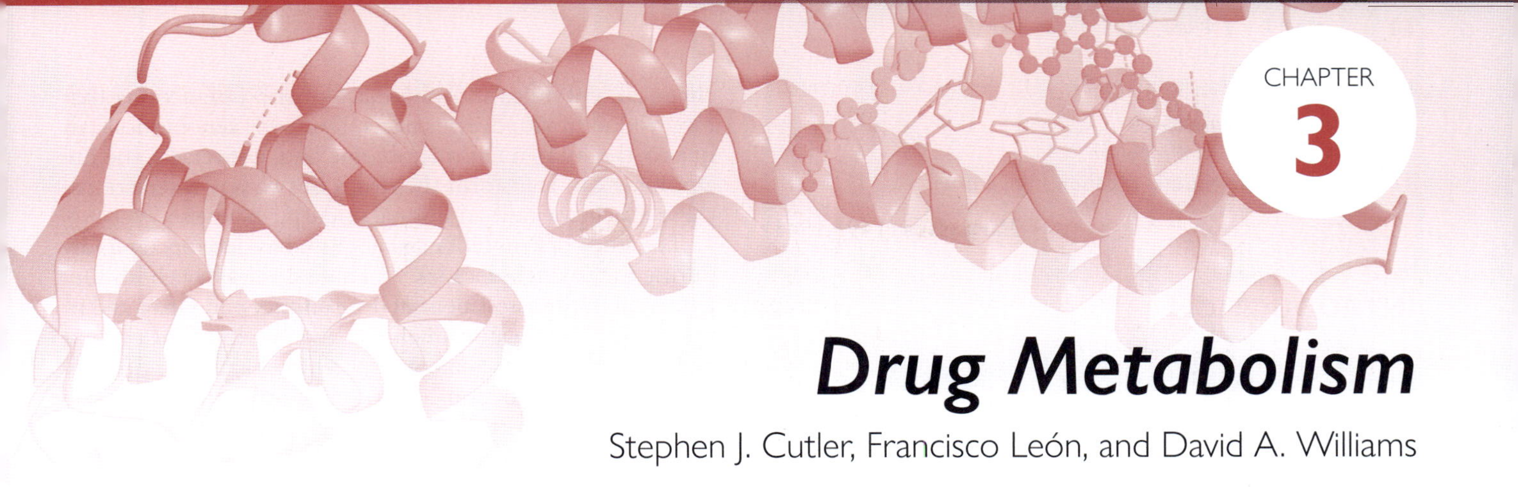

CHAPTER 3

Drug Metabolism

Stephen J. Cutler, Francisco León, and David A. Williams

Abbreviations

ABC ATP-binding cassette
ADH alcohol dehydrogenase
AhR aromatic hydrocarbon receptor
ALDH aldehyde dehydrogenase
ALT alanine aminotransferase
AOX aldehyde oxidase
AST aspartate aminotransferase
ATP adenosine triphosphate
AUC area under the curve
BBB blood-brain barrier
CAR constitutive androstane receptor
CES carboxylesterase
CNS central nervous system
CoA coenzyme A
COMT catechol-*O*-methyltransferase
COX cyclooxygenase
DDI drug-drug interaction
DHEA dehydroepiandrosterone
DILI drug-induced liver injury
EPO eosinophil peroxidase
EHC enterohepatic recirculation
EM extensive metabolizer
ER endoplasmic reticulum
FAD flavin dinucleotide
FDA U.S. Food and Drug Administration
FMN flavin mononucleotide
FMO flavin-containing monooxygenase
GI gastrointestinal
GST glutathione *S*-transferase
HAT hydrogen atom abstraction
HMG-CoA hydroxymethylglutaryl coenzyme A
HOCl hypochlorous acid
IDR idiosyncratic drug reaction
IM intermediate metabolizer
LPO lactoperoxidase
MAO monoamine oxidase
MDMA 3,4-methylenedioxy-methamphetamine
MDR medium-chain dehydrogenase/reductase
MIC metabolite-intermediate complex
MPO myeloperoxidase
MPP$^+$ 1-methyl-4-phenylpyridinium ion
MPTP 1-methyl-4-phenyl-1,2,3,6-tetrahydropyridine
mRNA messenger RNA
NAD$^+$ nicotinamide adenine dinucleotide
NADH reduced form of nicotinamide adenine dinucleotide
NADP$^+$ nicotinamide adenine dinucleotide phosphate
NADPH reduced form of nicotinamide adenine dinucleotide phosphate
NAT *N*-acetyltransferase
NSAID nonsteroidal anti-inflammatory drug
OTC over-the-counter
P450 cytochrome P450 monooxygenase (P450 genes are in italics)
PAH polycyclic aromatic hydrocarbon
PAPS 3′-phosphoadenosine-5′-phosphosulfate
P-gp P-glycoprotein
PGG2 prostaglandin G_2
PM poor metabolizer
PPAR peroxisome proliferator–activated receptor
PXDN peroxidasin
PXDNL peroxidasin-like protein
PXR pregnane X receptor
RM rapid or ultra-rapid metabolizer
ROS reactive oxygen species
SET single-electron transfer
SNP single-nucleotide polymorphism
SSRI selective serotonin reuptake inhibitor
SULT sulfotransferase
TMT thiol methyltransferase
TPMT thiopurine *S*-methyltransferase
TPO thyroid peroxidase
UDP uridine diphosphate
UDPGA UDP-glucuronic acid
UGT UDP-glucuronosyltransferase
XDH xanthine dehydrogenase
XO xanthine oxidase
XOR xanthine oxidoreductase

What is a poison?
All substances are poisons;
There is none that is not a poison.
The right dose differentiates a poison from a drug.

Paracelsus (1493-1541)

Introduction

Humans are exposed throughout their lives to a large variety of drugs and nonessential exogenous (foreign) compounds (collectively termed "xenobiotics") that can pose health hazards. Drugs taken for therapeutic purposes, as well as exposures to vapors and/or smokes of volatile chemicals or solvents, pose possible health risks; smoking, vaping, and drinking lead to the absorption of large amounts of xenobiotics with potentially adverse health effects. Furthermore, ingestion of natural toxins in vegetables and fruits, pesticide residues in food, and carcinogenic pyrolysis products from fats and protein formed during the charbroiling of meat pose additional health risks. Most of these exogenous substances undergo enzymatic biotransformations by xenobiotic-metabolizing enzymes in the liver and extrahepatic tissues and are eliminated by excretion as hydrophilic metabolites. In some cases, especially during oxidative metabolism, numerous chemical procarcinogens form reactive metabolites capable of covalently binding to critical biomolecules, such as proteins or nucleic acids, which can lead to mutagenicity, cytotoxicity, and carcinogenicity. Therefore, insight regarding the biotransformation and bioactivation of xenobiotics becomes an irrefutable requirement to assess drug safety and estimate risks linked with chemicals and drugs.

Detoxication and toxic effects of drugs and other xenobiotics have been studied extensively in various vertebrate species. Frequently, differences in sensitivity to these toxic effects were observed and can now be attributed to genetic differences between species in the isoenzyme/isoforms of cytochrome P450 monooxygenases (P450). The level of expression of the P450 enzymes is regulated by genetics and by a variety of endogenous factors such as hormones, gender, age, and disease, as well as the presence of environmental factors, such as inducing agents. Prior to the 21st century, drugs were developed and prescribed under the old paradigm that "one dose fits all," which largely ignored the fact that humans (both adults and children) are genetically and metabolically different, resulting in variable responses to drugs and risks of drug-drug interactions (DDIs). Some of today's health disparities can be attributed to this outdated paradigm.

Drugs can no longer be regarded as chemically stable entities that elicit the desired pharmacologic responses and then are excreted from the body. Drugs undergo a variety of chemical changes in humans brought about by enzymes of the liver, intestine, kidney, lung, and other tissues, with subsequent alterations of their pharmacologic activities, durations of activity, and toxicities. Thus, the pharmacologic and toxicologic activities of a drug (or xenobiotic) are, in many ways, consequences of its metabolism.

The practice of simultaneous prescriptions of several drugs has become common. Thus, an awareness of possible DDIs is essential to avoid catastrophic synergistic effects and chemical, enzymic, and pharmacokinetic interactions that can produce toxic adverse effects. Drugs (or xenobiotics) can impact the human gut microbiome and, conversely, the microbiome can transform the drugs in two-way interactions; these effects warrant additional scientific studies.

The study of xenobiotic metabolism has developed rapidly during the past few decades.[1-10] These studies have been fundamental in the assessment of drug efficacy and safety and in the design of dosage regimens; in the development of food additives and the assessment of potential hazards of contaminants; in the evaluation of toxic chemicals; and in the safe development of pesticides and herbicides and the assessment of their metabolic fates in insects, other animals, and plants. The metabolism of drugs and other xenobiotics is fundamental to many toxic processes, such as carcinogenesis, teratogenesis, and tissue necrosis. Often the same enzymes involved in drug metabolism also carry out the regulation and metabolism of endogenous substances such as steroids, vitamin D, prostaglandins, and lipids. Consequently, the inhibition and induction of these enzymes by drugs and xenobiotics can have a profound effect on the normal processes of intermediary metabolism, such as tissue growth and development, hematopoiesis, calcification, and lipid metabolism.

Familiarity with the mechanisms of drug metabolism can often aid the prediction of the consequences of DDIs, drug-food interactions, drug-herbal interactions, drug-dietary supplement interactions, and microbiota-drug interactions and help explain patients' adverse responses to drug regimens. Incorporating pharmacogenomics into the selection of drug regimens will change the way in which drugs are prescribed. Selection based on a patient's individual genetic makeup could eliminate previously unpredictable responses to drug treatment caused by genetic polymorphisms that affect metabolism, clearance, and tolerance. Pharmacogenomic testing to determine a patient's phenotype (ie, poor metabolizer [PM]) and thus, their ability to metabolize drugs, will become common in the future. Such knowledge will ensure improved selection of proper drug regimens and doses before therapy begins.

The increased knowledge of drug metabolism, fed by the need for better safety evaluations of drugs and chemicals, has resulted in a proliferation of publications (eg, *Drug Metabolism Reviews*, *Drug Metabolism and Disposition*, *Journal of Xenobiotics*, and *Xenobiotica*) and a series of monographs that present the current state of knowledge of foreign compound metabolism from biochemical and pharmacologic viewpoints.[5-9]

Pathways of Metabolism

The goals of drug metabolism are to change/terminate the physical and pharmacologic properties of a drug/xenobiotic through metabolic biotransformations (and therefore its action and effectiveness) and to effectively remove these apparently chemically stable drugs from the body. The metabolite thus becomes less lipophilic, more water soluble (hydrophilic), and possibly more easily eliminated (increased body clearance) by multiple routes (eg, urine, feces).

To achieve these goals, drug metabolism changes the molecular structure and shape of the drug/xenobiotic by the addition or exposure of a "handle" so that the substance no longer binds to its receptors/enzymes. The "handle" often increases molecular hydrophilicity to ensure increased water solubility by oxidation and conjugation and ensures elimination from the body by one or more routes. Common handles include alcoholic or phenolic hydroxyl groups, ionic carboxyl groups, ionic glucuronides, ionic sulfate esters, and ionic mercapturates.

The term "detoxication" describes the result of these metabolic biotransformations. Although, as a rule, drug metabolism leads to detoxication, the processes of oxidation, reduction, glucuronidation, sulfonation (sulfoconjugation), and other enzyme-catalyzed reactions can lead to the formation of metabolites having therapeutic or toxic effects from inactive parent drugs. This process is often referred to as "bioactivation." One of the earliest discoveries of bioactivation to an active metabolite was the reduction of prontosil to the antibacterial agent sulfanilamide. The N-demethylation of the antidepressant imipramine to form desipramine, the P450-mediated conversion of the anticancer drug tegafur-uracil to 5-fluorouracil, and conversion of the anxiolytic diazepam to desmethyldiazepam are other examples. The insecticide parathion is desulfurized by both insects and mammals to form the toxic metabolite paraoxon.

Most drugs and other xenobiotics are metabolized by enzymes normally associated with the metabolism of endogenous constituents (eg, steroids and biogenic amines). The liver is the primary site of drug metabolism, although other xenobiotic-metabolizing enzymes are found in nervous tissue, kidney, lung, plasma, and in the digestive secretions, bacterial flora, and wall of the gastrointestinal (GI) tract.

Although hepatic metabolism continues to be the most important route of metabolism for xenobiotics and drugs, other biotransformation pathways play a significant role in the metabolism of these substances. Among the more active extrahepatic tissues capable of metabolizing drugs are the intestinal mucosa, kidney, and lung (see "Extrahepatic Metabolism" section). The ability of the liver and extrahepatic tissues to metabolize substances to either pharmacologically inactive or bioactive metabolites before they achieve systemic blood levels is termed "first-pass metabolism" or the "presystemic first-pass effect." Other metabolic reactions occurring in the GI tract are associated with the microbiota in the tract. The gut microbiome can affect metabolism through: (1) production of toxic metabolites, (2) formation of carcinogens from inactive precursors, (3) detoxication, (4) species differences in drug metabolism, (5) exhibition of individual differences in drug metabolism, (6) production of pharmacologically active metabolites from inactive precursors, and (7) production of metabolites not formed by animal tissues.

Phase 1 Reactions

The pathways of xenobiotic metabolism are divided into three major categories. Phase 1 reactions (biotransformations) include oxidation, hydroxylation, reduction, and hydrolysis. In each of these enzymatic reactions, a new functional group is introduced into the substrate molecule, an existing functional group is modified, or a functional group or acceptor site for phase 2 transfer reactions is exposed, thus making the xenobiotic more polar and, therefore, more readily excreted.

Phase 2 Reactions

Phase 2 reactions (conjugation) are enzymatic syntheses whereby a functional group, such as an alcohol, a phenol, an amine, or a carboxylic acid, is masked by the addition of a new group, such as acetyl, sulfate, glucuronic acid, or certain amino acids, which usually increases the polarity of the drug or xenobiotic. Most substances undergo both phase 1 and phase 2 reactions sequentially.

Those xenobiotics that are resistant to metabolizing enzymes or are already hydrophilic are excreted largely unchanged. This basic pattern of xenobiotic metabolism is common to all animal species, including humans, but species can differ in details of the reaction and enzyme control.

Phase 3 Transporters

Once xenobiotics have been converted into low-toxicity and water-soluble metabolites by the combination of phase 1 and phase 2 reactions, these metabolites must be transported against a concentration gradient out of the cell into the interstitial space between cells, and then into the bloodstream for filtration by the kidneys. The biggest hurdle is the transport of these hydrophilic metabolites out of the cell. Charged phase 2 metabolites will be effectively "ion-trapped" in the cell, as the cell membrane is highly lipophilic and is an effective barrier to the exit, as well as entry, of most hydrophilic molecules. In addition, failure to remove the hydrophilic products of conjugation reactions can lead to toxicity.

Consequently, an array of multipurpose membrane-bound transport carrier systems has evolved, which can actively remove hydrophilic metabolites and many other low-molecular-weight drugs and toxins from cells (see Chapter 4). Thus, the term "phase 3 metabolism" has been applied to the study of this essential arm of the detoxification process. Efflux transporters move hydrophilic substrates out of cells into interstitial fluid, blood, kidneys, and the GI tract. Influx transporters transport hydrophilic substrates into cells from the bloodstream.

Factors Affecting Metabolism

Drug therapy is becoming more oriented toward controlling metabolic, genetic, and environmental illnesses rather than short-term therapy associated with infectious diseases. In most cases, drug therapy lasts for months or even years, and the problems of DDIs and chronic toxicity from long-term drug therapy have become more serious. Therefore, a greater knowledge of drug metabolism is essential. Several factors influencing xenobiotic metabolism include:

- *Genetic factors.* Genetic polymorphisms of drug-metabolizing enzymes give rise to distinct subgroups in the population that differ in their ability to perform certain drug biotransformation reactions. Polymorphisms are generated by mutations in the genes for these enzymes, which cause decreased, increased, or absent enzyme expression or activity by multiple molecular mechanisms. Individual differences in drug effectiveness (drug sensitivity or drug resistance), DDIs, and drug toxicity can depend on racial and ethnic characteristics impacting the population frequencies of the many polymorphic genes and the expression of the metabolizing enzymes. Pharmacogenetics focuses primarily on genetic polymorphisms (mutations) responsible for interindividual differences in drug metabolism and disposition. Genotype-phenotype correlation studies have validated that inherited mutations result in two or more distinct phenotypes causing very different responses following drug administration. The genes encoding for CYP2A6, CYP2C9, CYP2C19, and CYP2D6 are functionally polymorphic; therefore, at least 30% of P450-dependent metabolism is performed by polymorphic enzymes. For example, mutations in the CYP2D6 gene result in PM, intermediate (IM), or rapid/ultra-rapid (RM) metabolizers of more than 30 cardiovascular and central nervous system (CNS) drugs. Thus, each of these phenotypic subgroups experience different responses to drugs extensively metabolized by the CYP2D6 pathway ranging from severe toxicity to complete lack of efficacy (see "Genetic Polymorphism" section).

- *Physiologic factors.* Age is a factor, as both very young and old have impaired metabolism. Hormones (including those induced by stress), sex differences, pregnancy, changes in intestinal microflora, diseases (especially those involving the liver), and nutritional status can also influence drug and xenobiotic metabolism.

Because the liver is the principal site for xenobiotic and drug metabolism, liver disease can modify the pharmacokinetics of drugs hepatically metabolized. Liver disease affects the elimination half-life of some drugs but not of others, even if they all undergo hepatic biotransformation. Some studies have shown that the capacity for drug metabolism is impaired in chronic liver disease, which could lead to unintentional drug overdose by increasing drug bioavailability. Because of the unpredictability of drug effects in the presence of liver disorders, drug therapy in these circumstances is complex and extra caution is needed.

Protein deficiency leads to reduced hepatic microsomal protein and lipid metabolism, and oxidative metabolism is decreased due to an alteration in endoplasmic reticulum (ER) membrane permeability affecting electron transfer. Protein deficiency would increase the toxicity of drugs and xenobiotics by reducing their oxidative P450 metabolism and clearance from the body.

- *Pharmacodynamic factors.* Dose, frequency, and route of administration, plus tissue distribution and protein binding of a drug, affect its metabolism.
- *Environmental factors.* Competition of ingested environmental substances for metabolizing enzymes and poisoning of enzymes by toxic chemicals such as carbon monoxide can alter drug and other xenobiotic metabolism. Induction of enzyme expression (in which the number of enzyme molecules is increased, while the activity is constant) by other drugs and xenobiotics is another consideration. Environmental factors can change not only the kinetics of an enzyme reaction but also the whole pattern of metabolism, thereby altering bioavailability, pharmacokinetics, pharmacologic activity, and/or toxicity of a xenobiotic. Interspecies differences in response to xenobiotics must be considered in the extrapolation of pharmacologic and toxicologic data from animal experiments to predict effects in humans.

DRUG BIOTRANSFORMATION PATHWAY (PHASE 1)

Human Hepatic Cytochrome P450 Enzyme System

Introduction

Oxidation, the most common reaction in xenobiotic metabolism, is catalyzed by a group of membrane-bound monooxygenases found in the smooth ER of the liver and other extrahepatic tissues, termed the cytochrome P450 monooxygenase enzyme system, CYP450 or simply P450 (P450). P450 has also been called a mixed-function oxidase or microsomal hydroxylase. The tissue homogenate fraction containing the smooth ER is called the microsomal fraction. P450 functions as a multicomponent electron transport system, responsible for the oxidative metabolism of a variety of endogenous substrates (eg, steroids, fatty acids, prostaglandins, and bile acids) and xenobiotics including drugs, carcinogens, insecticides, plant toxins, environmental pollutants, and other foreign chemicals. Central to the functioning of this unique superfamily of heme proteins is an iron protoporphyrin. Iron protoporphyrin is coordinated to the sulfur of cysteine and can form a complex with carbon monoxide, resulting in a complex that has its primary absorption maximum at 450 nm (thus the title of these metabolizing P450 enzymes). P450 has an absolute requirement for NADPH (the reduced form of nicotinamide adenine dinucleotide phosphate) and molecular oxygen (dioxygen). The rate at which various compounds are metabolized by this system depends on the animal species, strain, nutritional status, type of tissue, age, and pretreatment of animals. P450 can catalyze the C-H oxidation of a wide range of structurally dissimilar functional groups. All these reactions have a common characteristic: H atom abstraction (HAT) from C-H, with the resultant formation of a hydroxyl group via oxygen rebound.[11] The same active enzyme site binds to structurally dissimilar substrates, resulting in indiscriminate substrate binding. The variety of reactions catalyzed by P450 (Table 3.1) include the oxidation of alkanes and aromatic compounds; the epoxidation of alkenes, polycyclic hydrocarbons, and halogenated benzenes; the dealkylation of secondary and tertiary amines, ethers, and thioethers; the deamination of amines; the conversion of amines to *N*-oxides, hydroxylamine, and nitroso derivatives; and the dehalogenation of halogenated hydrocarbons. It also catalyzes the oxidative cleavage of organic thiophosphate esters, the sulfoxidation of some thioethers, and the reduction of azo and nitro compounds to primary aromatic amines. A nonheme, microsomal flavoprotein monooxygenase is

Table 3.1 Hydroxylation Mechanisms Catalyzed by Cytochrome P450

Aromatic hydroxylation	
	$CH_3CO-\overset{H}{N}-C_6H_5 \xrightarrow{[OH]} CH_3CO-\overset{H}{N}-C_6H_4\text{-}OH$
Aliphatic hydroxylation	
	$R-CH_3 \xrightarrow{[OH]} R-CH_2\text{-}OH$
Deamination	
	$R-CH(NH_2)\text{-}CH_3 \xrightarrow{[OH]} (R-C(OH)(NH_2)\text{-}CH_3) \longrightarrow R-CO\text{-}CH_3 + NH_3$
O-Dealkylation	
	$R\text{-}O\text{-}CH_3 \xrightarrow{[OH]} (R\text{-}O\text{-}CH_2\text{-}OH) \longrightarrow R-OH + CH_2O$
N-Dealkylation	
	$R-N(CH_3)_2 \xrightarrow{[OH]} (R-N(CH_2OH)(CH_3)) \longrightarrow R-\overset{H}{N}-CH_3 + CH_2O$
	$R-NH\text{-}CH_3 \xrightarrow{[OH]} (R-NH\text{-}CH_2OH) \longrightarrow R-NH_2 + CH_2O$
N-Oxidation	
	$(CH_3)_3-N \xrightarrow{[OH]} ((CH_3)_3-NOH) \longrightarrow (CH_3)_3-NO + H^{\oplus}$
Sulfoxidation	
	$R-S-R' \xrightarrow{[OH]} (R-\overset{+}{\underset{\mid\atop O}{S}}-R') \longrightarrow R-\underset{\|\atop O}{S}-R' + H^{\oplus}$

responsible for the oxidation of certain nitrogen- and sulfur-containing organic compounds. Substrate and inhibitor promiscuity have an impact on DDIs.

While all P450 enzymes share a common tertiary protein structure, the flexibility and functional amino acids around the active site account for the ability of P450 enzymes to accommodate a vast number of structurally dissimilar substrates and support a wide range of selective oxidations. The P450 superfamily has a remarkable adaptability (plasticity) for substrate recognition and regio- and stereoselectivity in catalytic chemistry. This is possibly due to secondary protein structural features surrounding the P450 active site. Not only do these features differ between enzymes, but they change even between different states of individual enzymes.

The most important function of P450 is to activate molecular oxygen (dioxygen) to a ferric iron-oxene intermediate, permitting the incorporation of one atom of oxygen into an organic substrate molecule concomitant with the reduction of the other atom of oxygen to water. The introduction of a hydroxyl group into the hydrophobic substrate provides a site for subsequent conjugation with hydrophilic compounds (phase 2), thereby increasing the aqueous solubility of the product for transport and excretion from the body. The P450 enzyme system not only catalyzes xenobiotic transformations in ways that lead typically to detoxication but, in some cases, in ways that lead to products having greater cytotoxic, mutagenic, or carcinogenic properties.

Components of P450

P450 consists of at least two protein components: a heme protein called P450 and a flavoprotein called NADPH-P450 reductase, containing both flavin mononucleotide (FMN) and flavin dinucleotide (FAD). P450 is the substrate- and oxygen-binding site of the enzyme system, whereas the reductase serves as an electron carrier, shuttling electrons from NADPH to P450. A third component essential for electron transport from NADPH to P450 is a phospholipid, phosphatidylcholine, which facilitates the transfer of electrons from NADPH-P450 reductase to P450.[5] Although the phospholipid does not function in the system as an electron carrier, it has a great influence on the P450 monooxygenase system. The phospholipid constitutes approximately a third of the hepatic ER and contributes to a negatively charged environment at physiologic pH.

Of the three components involved in microsomal oxidative xenobiotic metabolism, P450 is important due to its vital role in oxygen activation and substrate binding. P450 is an integral protein embedded in the membrane matrix. The electron components of P450 are located on the cytoplasmic side of the ER membrane, and the hydrophobic active site is oriented toward the lumen of the ER.[5] The active site of P450 consists of a hydrophobic substrate–binding domain in which is embedded an iron protoporphyrin (heme) prosthetic group. This group is exactly like that of hemoglobin, peroxidase, and the *b*-type cytochromes. The iron in the iron protoporphyrin is coordinated with four nitrogens via a tetradentate link to the porphyrin ring. X-ray studies reveal that in the ferric state, the two nonporphyrin ligands are water and cysteine (Fig. 3.1). The cysteine thiolate ligand (proximal) is absolutely essential for the formation of the reactive ferric-oxenoid intermediate. The sixth (distal) coordination position is occupied by an easily exchangeable ligand, most likely water, which is labile and readily displaced by stronger drug or xenobiotic ligands. The ferrous form loses the water ligand completely, leaving the sixth position open for binding ligands such as oxygen and carbon monoxide. The process is highly dynamic and amino acid residues have been found to be involved in the catalytic process.[12]

The vast array of xenobiotics presents a unique challenge to the human body to metabolize these many lipophilic foreign compounds. This makes it impractical to have one enzyme to metabolize each compound or each class of compounds. Therefore, whereas most cellular functions are normally very specific, oxidation of xenobiotics necessitates P450s with diverse substrate specificities and regioselectivities (ie, multiple sites of oxidation). Several types of P450 enzymes can be found in a single animal species. Humans have 57 functional genes and more than 59 pseudogenes divided among 18 families and 43 subfamilies of P450 genes, each coding for a different version of the enzyme (isoform) so that, together, the P450s can metabolize almost any lipophilic compound to which the individual is exposed.

Classification of the P450 Multigene Family

Nebert and colleagues[13,14] classified the P450 supergene family based on amino acid sequence similarity and structural (evolutionary) relationships. P450 monooxygenases resulting from this supergene family have been subdivided into families, which possess at least 40% identity (amino acid homology), and subfamilies possessing greater than 55% homology.[14-16] The P450s are named with the root symbol CYP followed by an Arabic numeral designating the family (eg, CYP1, CYP2, or CYP3), a letter denoting the subfamily (eg, CYP1A, CYP2C, CYP2D, or CYP2E), and another Arabic numeral representing the individual gene (eg, CYP3A4). Names of genes are written in italics. The nomenclature system is based solely on sequence similarity among the P450s and does not indicate the properties or functions of individual P450s (eg, drug metabolism vs homeostasis). Recently, through a global proteomics study, 17 P450 isoforms have been identified in the liver (Fig. 3.2), with the CYP2E isoenzyme family being the most abundant with 21% of the total P450s expressed in the liver.[17]

P450s initially evolved for the regulation of endogenous substances, such as the metabolism of cholesterol necessary to maintain membrane integrity, and for steroid biosynthesis and metabolism, rather than for metabolizing toxic xenobiotics. P450s are either located in the inner mitochondrial membrane and involved in highly specific steroid hydroxylations or bound to the ER of the cell and have broad substrate specificity. In evolutionary terms, P450s evolved from a common ancestor, and only more recently (during the last 100 million years) have P450 genes taken on the role of producing enzymes to metabolize a vast array of lipophilic foreign compounds. The xenobiotic P450 genes probably emerged from the steroidogenic P450s to enhance animal survival by synthesizing new P450s to metabolize plant, fungal, and bacterial toxins concentrated in the food chain. It is not surprising that animals and humans possess a vast array of P450 enzymes capable of handling a multitude of xenobiotics. Thus, there is a continuous evolution of gene expression (up- or downregulation) based on environmental changes.[14] Interindividual variation in the expression of xenobiotic P450 genes (genetic polymorphism) or in their inducibility can be associated with differences such as individual susceptibilities to cigarette smoke–induced carcinogenesis. Certain P450 isoforms that clearly exhibit genetic polymorphisms are known to metabolize therapeutic agents. The extent of P450 polymorphism in humans is being investigated to determine the potential for protection against cancers. Specific forms of P450 in hepatic microsomes are regulated by hormones (eg, the CYP3A subfamily) and are induced or inhibited by drugs, food toxins, or other environmental xenobiotics (see "Induction and Inhibition of Cytochrome P450 Isoforms" section). Identification of a specific P450 isoform as the primary form responsible for the metabolism of a specific drug in humans permits reconciliation of the drug's toxicity and/or other pharmacologic effects.

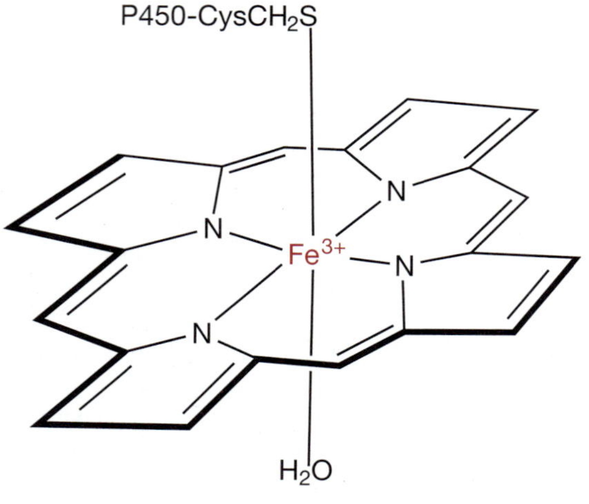

Figure 3.1 Ferric heme thiolate catalytic center of P450. The porphyrin side chains are deleted for clarity.

Substrate Specificity

The substrate specificities, affinities, regioselectivities, and rates of hydrogen abstraction are most likely consequences of the conformational changes resulting from ligand binding at the site of hydroxylation. Protein-protein interactions and amino acid side chains play a key role in substrate cooperativity as well as flexible and dynamic arrangements that change depending upon the presence of substrate, cofactor, and oxidation state.[18,19] Because a primary function of these enzymes is the metabolism of hydrophobic substrates, it is likely that hydrophobic forces are important in the binding of many substrates to these apoproteins. Nonspecific binding is consistent with the observation of multiple substrate

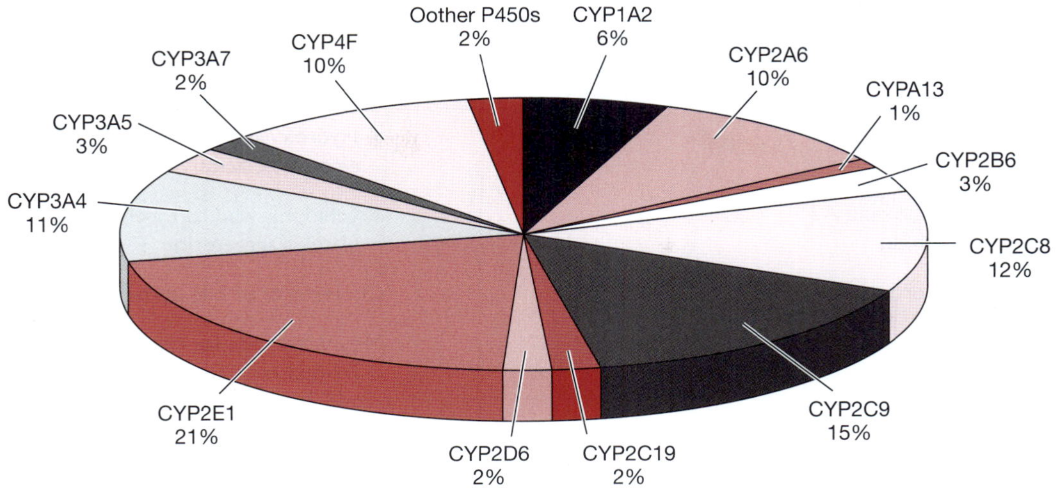

Figure 3.2 Total human P450 isoforms expressed in the liver.

orientations at the active site of these enzymes, emphasizing broad regioselectivity. In other words, a specific binding requirement would decrease the diversity of potential substrates. Some P450 isoforms have constrained binding sites, thus they metabolize only small organic molecules (eg, CYP2E1). CYP1A1/2 isoforms have planar binding sites and metabolize only aromatic planar compounds, for example, polycyclic aromatic hydrocarbons (PAHs). CYP2D6 exhibits high affinity for specific apoprotein interactions (hydrogen bonds, ion-pair formation) with specific substrates such as lipophilic amines. CYP3A4 has a broader affinity for a variety of lipophilic substrates with molecular weights of 200 to 1,200 Da. If P450 isoforms are tightly membrane bound, substrate access to the active sites is limited to compounds that can diffuse through the membranes. P450 isoforms that are less tightly bound will metabolize hydrophilic compounds.

The site of hydroxylation is determined by accessibility to, and topography of, the active site of the protein, the degree of steric hindrance encountered by substrate to the heme ferric-oxenoid species at the site of reaction, the ease of HAT or electron transfer from the compound (metabolic soft spot), and the stability of the carbon center radical, which follows the carbocation (C^+) stability: tertiary > secondary > primary > CH_3.[18,20] Alkyl groups are electron donating so they neutralize the positive charge on the C^+. The more alkyl substituents attached to the C^+, the greater the surface area over which to spread the positive charge. The lower charge density translates to greater stability. Since the tertiary carbons are electron donating, this will stabilize a partial negative charge on an electronegative atom.[21]

The P450s were often referred to as having broad and overlapping specificities, but it became apparent that the broad substrate specificity could be attributed to multiple isoenzymic forms of P450. The phenotype of an individual with respect to the forms and amounts of individual P450s expressed in the liver can determine the rate and pathway of the metabolic clearance of a compound (see "Genetic Polymorphism" section). Significant differences exist between humans and other animal species with respect to the catalytic activities and regulation of expression of hepatic drug-metabolizing P450s. These differences often make it difficult to extrapolate results of P450-mediated metabolism studies performed experimentally in animal species to humans. Caution is warranted in the extrapolation of rodent data to humans, as some isoforms are similar between species (eg, CYP1A and CYP3A subfamilies) whereas others are different (eg, CYP2A, CYP2B, CYP2C, and CYP2D subfamilies).

Other P450 Isoforms

Other P450 isoforms catalyzing the oxidation of steroids, bile acids, fat-soluble vitamins, and other endogenous substances are shown in Table 3.2.

Cytochrome P450 Isoforms Metabolizing Drugs/Xenobiotics

Figure 3.3 shows the percent participation of the hepatic P450 isoforms in drug metabolism.[15] P450s are the most important enzymes responsible for phase 1 drug metabolism.[5] The polymorphic nature of the P450s influences individual drug responses and DDIs and induces adverse drug reactions. There has been a continuous increase in the number of reported crystal structures of human P450s and redox partners, which have provided understanding of their active sites and functional roles. Currently, more than a hundred crystal structures of human CYPs interacting with various substrates have been resolved and published. Representative examples are: CYP1A1, CYP1A2, CYP2A6, CYP2C8, CYP2C9, CYP2D6, CYP3A4, CYP3A5.[16,19,22] Approximately one-third of all drugs are metabolized by one isoform, CYP3A4, increasing the potential for DDIs.[5] When two drugs are metabolized by the same isoform, only one drug can serve as a substrate at a time at an individual enzyme active site, increasing the likelihood of a DDI, especially if one drug has a narrow therapeutic window.

Table 3.2 Other Cytochromes With Indicated Specificities and Actions

P450s	Activity	Location	Actions
CYP4	ω-Hydroxylases		ω-Hydroxylation of fatty acids, leukotrienes, eicosanoic acids
CYP5	Thromboxane A2 synthase		Arachidonic acid to thromboxane A_2 effecting platelet aggregation
CYP7A	7α-Hydroxylase		Cholesterol to bile acids formation
CYP7B	7α-Hydroxylase	Brain	Neurosteroids formation: 7α-hydroxydehydroepiandrosterone and 7α-hydroxypregnenolone
CYP8A	Prostacyclin synthase		Synthesis of prostaglandin I2 regulating hemostasis
CYP8B	12α-Hydroxylase		Catalyzes bile acid biosynthesis
CYP11A1	Steroid 20α-/22-hydroxylase	Adrenal mitochondria	Catalyzes mitochondrial steroid biosynthesis via 17-side chain cleavage of cholesterol to pregnenolone—lack of leads to feminization and hypertension
CYP11B1	11β-Hydroxylase	Adrenal cortex	Catalyzes 11-deoxycortisol to hydrocortisone or 11-deoxycorticosterone to corticosterone
CYP11B2	18-Hydroxylase	Adrenal zona glomerulosa	Hydroxylates corticosterone at the 18-position leading to aldosterone
CYP17A1	17α-Hydroxylase and 17,20-lyase	ER of adrenal cortex	Production of testosterone and estrogen—lack of it affects sexual development
CYP19A	Aromatase	ER of gonads, brain, adipose tissue	Aromatization of ring A of testosterone leading to estrogen—lack of it causes estrogen deficiency
CYP21A1	C_{21} steroid hydroxylase	Adrenal cortex	17-Hydroxyprogesterone to cortisol
CYP24	24-Hydroxylase	Mitochondria	Catalyzes the degradation/inactivation of vitamin D metabolites
CYP26A1	*Trans*-retinoic acid hydroxylase		Terminates retinoic acid signal
CYP26B1	Retinoic acid hydroxylase		Catalyzes the hydroxylation of *cis*-retinoic acids
CYP26C	Retinoic acid hydroxylase		Unknown
CYP27A1	27-Hydroxylase		Catalyzes the oxidation of the cholesterol in bile acid biosynthesis
CYP27B1	Vitamin D_3 1-α-hydroxylase	Mitochondria	Activates vitamin D3
CYP27C1			Unknown
CYP39			Catalyzes the 7-hydroxylation of 24-hydroxy cholesterol
CYP46	Cholesterol 24-hydroxylase		Unknown
CYP51	Lanosterol 14α-demethylase		Converts lanosterol into cholesterol

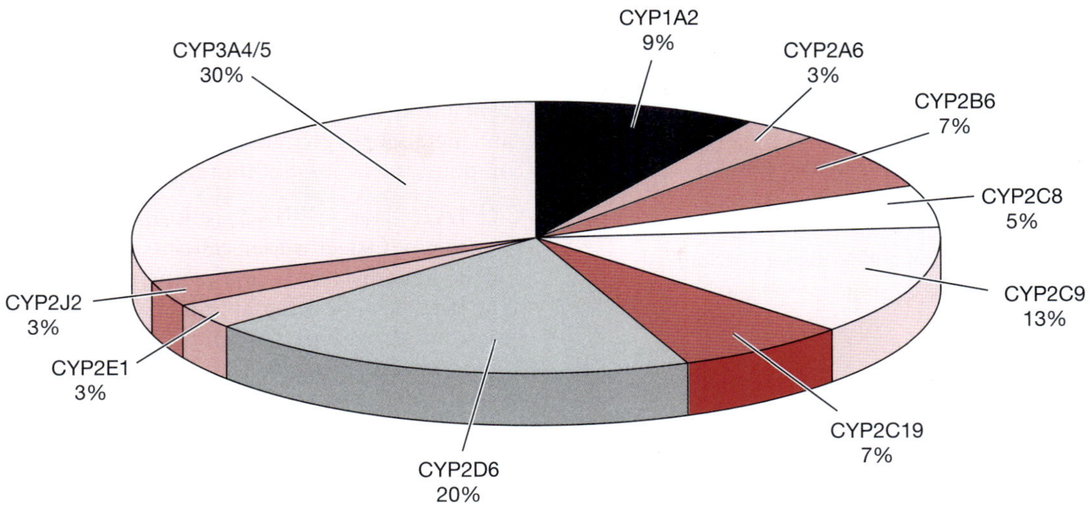

Figure 3.3 Percentage of clinically important drugs metabolized by human P450 isoforms.

Family 1

CYP1 consists of three isoforms, CYP1A1, CYP1A2, and CYP1B1, encoded by three genes, and one isoform encoded as a pseudogene, CYP1D1. The human CYP1A subfamily has an integral role in the metabolism of estrogens and important classes of environmental carcinogens, including halogenated aromatic hydrocarbons, PAHs, and arylamines (Tables 3.3 and 3.4). PAHs are commonly present in the environment through industrial combustion processes and tobacco products. Several potent carcinogenic arylamines result from the pyrolysis of amino acids in cooked meats and cause colon cancer in rats. Environmental and genetic factors can alter the expression of this subfamily of enzymes.

CYP1A1. The CYP1A1 isoform (previously called aromatic hydrocarbon hydroxylase or aryl hydrocarbon hydroxylase) is expressed primarily in extrahepatic tissues, the small intestine, placenta, skin, heart, brain, lung, and, to a lesser extent, liver. Levels increase in the presence of CYP1A1 inducers such as PAHs (in cigarette smoke and the carcinogen 3-methylcholanthrene), α-naphthoflavone (a noncarcinogenic inducer related to dietary flavones), and indole-3-carbinol (found in Brussels sprouts and related vegetables). CYP1A1 metabolizes a range of PAHs, including many procarcinogens and promutagens (Table 3.4). Interindividual variations in the inducible expression of CYP1A1 might be related to genetic differences in aromatic hydrocarbon receptor (AhR) expression, which could explain differences in individual susceptibilities to cigarette smoke–induced lung cancer. Therefore, genetic factors appear to be important in the expression of the *CYP1A1* gene in humans. There are more than a thousand single-nucleotide polymorphic (SNP) variants generating the 12 known allelic isoforms for CYP1A1 that are linked to human carcinogenesis. Women who smoke are at greater risk than men to develop lung cancer (adenocarcinoma) and chronic obstructive pulmonary disease.[23,24] Several *CYP1A1* polymorphic variants are

Table 3.3 Some Substrates for Human Subfamily CYP1A2
Acetaminophen (oxidation to iminoquinone)
Aminopyrine (*N*-demethylation)
Amitriptyline (*N*-demethylation)
Caffeine (N_1- and N_3-demethylation)
Chlordiazepoxide
Clomipramine (*N*-demethylation)
Clopidogrel
Clozapine (*N*-demethylation, *N*-oxidation)
Cyclobenzaprine
Dacarbazine (*N*-demethylation)
Desipramine (*N*-demethylation)
Diazepam
Duloxetine (4,5,6-hydroxylation)
Erlotinib
Estradiol (2- and 4-hydroxylation)
Flutamide (2-hydroxylation)
Fluoroquinolones (3′-hydroxylation of piperazine ring)
Fluvoxamine
Haloperidol
Imipramine (*N*-demethylation)
Leflunomide (*N-O* bond cleavage)
Levobupivacaine

(*continued*)

Table 3.3 Some Substrates for Human Subfamily CYP1A2 (*continued*)

Lidocaine
Melatonin (6-hydroxylation and *O*-demethylation)
Mexiletine
Mirtazapine (8-hydroxylation and *N*-demethylation)
Nabumetone
Naproxen
Nortriptyline
Olanzapine (*N*-demethylation and 7-hydroxylation)
Ondansetron
Phenacetin (*O*-deethylation and *C*-hydroxylation)
Promazine (*N*-demethylation and 5-sulfoxidation)
Propafenone
Propranolol (*N*-deisopropylation and 4,5-hydroxylation)
Ramelteon (Aliphatic hydroxylation)
Rasagiline (*N*-dealkylation and hydroxylation)
Riluzole (*N*-hydroxylation)
Ropinirole (*N*-depropylation)
Ropivacaine (hydroxylation)
Tacrine (hydroxylation)
Theophylline
Tizanidine
Triamterene
Verapamil
R-Warfarin
Zileuton
Zolmitriptan

CYP1A2 metabolized a minimum of 25% by this isoform.
Drugs in bold italic have been reported to cause drug-drug interactions.

associated with an increased risk of prostate cancer.[25] The *CYP1A1* and *CYP1A2* genes are located on chromosome 15. These encode functional proteins that possess 71% homology and molecular masses of 58 kDa with 512 and 516 amino acids, respectively.[24]

The mechanism for induction of the *CYP1A1* gene begins with binding of the inducing agent to a cytosolic receptor protein, the AhR, which is then translocated to the nucleus where it binds to the DNA of the *CYP1A1* gene, thus enhancing the rate of transcription. The presence of the AhR in hepatic and intestinal tissues can have implications beyond xenobiotic metabolism and can have a role in the induction of other genes for the control of cellular growth and differentiation. On the other hand, CYP1A1 can metabolize procarcinogens to hydroxylated inactive compounds that are not mutagenic.

CYP1A2. The CYP1A2 isoform (previously known as phenacetin *O*-deethylase, caffeine demethylase, or antipyrine *N*-demethylase) is one of the major P450s in the human liver, metabolizing approximately 9% of the clinically important drugs (see Fig. 3.3). This isoform catalyzes the oxidation (and in some cases the bioactivation) of arylamines, nitrosamines, and aromatic hydrocarbons, and the bioactivation of promutagens and procarcinogens, estrogens, and other substances (see Table 3.4). CYP1A2 is expressed in the liver (6%) (see Fig. 3.2), intestine, and stomach, and is induced by smoking, coffee consumption, and PAHs. CYP1A2 is primarily responsible for caffeine metabolism and largely responsible for the activation of the food carcinogen aflatoxin B1 found in contaminated peanuts. CYP1A2 is subject to reversible and/or irreversible inhibition by several drugs, natural substances, and other compounds. Examples include ciprofloxacin and several azole antifungal agents, among others, increasing the risk of DDIs.[23,26]

The CYP1A2 structure exhibits a relatively compact and planar active site cavity that is highly adapted for the size and shape of its substrates. A large interindividual variability in the expression and activity of CYP1A2 has been observed, which is largely caused by genetic, epigenetic, and environmental factors (eg, smoking). CYP1A2 is primarily regulated by the AhR. Induction or inhibition of CYP1A2 may provide a partial explanation for some clinical drug interactions. More than 33 variant alleles of the *CYP1A2* gene have been identified and some of them have been associated with altered drug clearance and response and disease susceptibility. Evidence for polymorphism of this isoform has been reported, and it is likely that low CYP1A2 activity will be associated with altered susceptibility to the bioactivation of procarcinogens, promutagens, and other xenobiotic substrates. The polymorphism of CYP1A2 has been linked with different types of cancers;[23] however, recent reports have not confirmed this association.[27,28]

Family 2

The human CYP2 family comprises 13 subfamilies and 16 isoforms, CYP2A6, CYP2A7, CYP2A13, CYP2B6, CYP2C8, CYP2C9, CYP2C18, CYP2C19, CYP2D6, CYP2E1, CYP2F1, CYP2J2, CYP2R1, CYP2S1, CYP2U1, CYP2W1, 16 genes and 16 pseudogenes. CYP2A7 is nonfunctional.

CYP2A6. CYP2A6 has a high level of hepatic expression and represents approximately 10% of the total of hepatic P450 isoforms (see Fig. 3.2). It is also expressed at low levels in lung and nasal epithelium and exhibits high interindividual variability (polymorphism). Lung CYP2A6 bioactivates many tobacco smoke–specific carcinogens, procarcinogens, and nitrosoamines. Mutant alleles of this isoenzyme have been associated with an elevated risk for small cell lung

Table 3.4 Some Procarcinogens and Other Toxins Activated by Human Cytochrome P450s

CYP1A1	CYP1A2	CYP2E1	CYP3A4
Benzo[a]pyrene and other polycyclic aromatic hydrocarbons	4-Aminobiphenyl	Benzene	Aflatoxin B1
	2-Naphthylamine	Styrene	Aflatoxin G1
	2-Aminofluorene	Acrylonitrile	Estradiol
	2-Acetylaminofluorene	Vinyl bromide	6-Aminochrysene
	2-Aminoanthracene	Trichloroethylene	Polycyclic hydrocarbons
	Heteropolycyclic amines (2-aminoquinolines)	Carbon tetrachloride	Dihydrodiols
		Chloroform	
	Aflatoxin B1	Methylene chloride	
	Ipomeanol	1,2-Dichloropropane	
	Thiolated arsenicals	Ethyl carbamate	

cancer. Hepatic CYP2A6 catalyzes the 4-hydroxylation of ifosfamide and the C5 oxidation of nicotine to cotinine (nicotine C-oxidase) (Table 3.5). Other substrates include the prodrug tegafur, aflatoxin B1, naproxen, tacrine, clozapine, mexiletine, letrozole, and cyclobenzaprine. In vitro studies with human microsomes expressing human CYP2A6 have shown that selegiline and its desmethyl metabolite are mechanism-based CYP2A6 inhibitors of nicotine metabolism, and inhibition of nicotine metabolism by selegiline could increase plasma nicotine in vivo. CYP2A6 exhibits high polymorphism, including around 40 alleles in multiple populations. A CYP2A6 allele variant is associated with the drug response of the sedative dexmedetomidine.[29] Smokers with a defective *CYP2A6* gene smoke fewer cigarettes, implicating a genetic factor in nicotine dependence.[30]

CYP2A13. CYP2A13 exhibits the highest levels of expression in nasal epithelium, followed by lung and trachea with high interindividual variability. CYP2A13 activates tobacco smoke–specific carcinogens, procarcinogens, and nitrosoamines into DNA-altering compounds that cause lung cancer. Individuals with a high level of CYP2A13 expression could likely have an increased risk of developing tobacco smoke–related lung cancers. Although CYP2A13 and CYP2A6 are 93.5% identical in amino acid sequence, CYP2A13 exhibits higher affinity for metabolizing tobacco smoke carcinogens than does CYP2A6. A comparison of the crystal structures of CYP2A13 and CYP2A6 has shown them to be very similar and, like CYP2A6, the CYP2A13 active site cavity is small and highly hydrophobic with a cluster of phenylalanine residues. Amino acid differences between CYP2A6 and CYP2A13 at key positions could be the cause of the significant variations observed in ligand binding and catalysis.[31]

CYP2B6. CYP2B6 is the only member of the 2B subfamily expressed in humans. It represents approximately 3% of the total of hepatic P450 isoforms (see Fig. 3.2), and it is expressed mainly in the liver with small amounts in the brain, kidneys, lungs, and nasal mucosa. CYP2B6 metabolizes approximately 7% of important clinically used drugs (Table 3.6; also see Fig. 3.3). CYP2B6 also metabolizes arachidonic acid, lauric acid, 17β-estradiol, estrone, ethinyl estradiol, and testosterone, and can also bioactivate several procarcinogens and toxicants. CYP2B6 is closely regulated by the androstane receptor, which can activate CYP2B6 expression upon ligand binding. Pregnane X receptor (PXR) and glucocorticoid receptor also have a role in the regulation of CYP2B6. This enzyme exhibits polymorphic and ethnic differences in expression and therefore could be important in DDIs. There is great interest to know the structure-function relationship within the active site of CYP2B6 and its allelic variants.[32]

Induction of CYP2B6 may partially explain some clinically relevant DDIs observed. For example, coadministered carbamazepine decreases the blood levels of bupropion. There is a wide interindividual variability in the expression and activity of CYP2B6. Such a large variability is the result of genetic polymorphisms and exposure to drugs that are inducers or inhibitors of CYP2B6. CYP2B6 substrates are by and large small nonplanar molecules, unionized or weakly basic, highly lipophilic with one or two hydrogen bond acceptors, and frequently active in the CNS. The barbituric phenobarbital (Sezaby) induced its formation through androstane receptors and hepatocyte nuclear factors.

CYP2C. The CYP2C subfamily is one of the most complex, consisting of four isoforms, CYP2C8, CYP2C9, CYP2C18, and CYP2C19, metabolizing approximately 25% of the

Table 3.5 Some Substrates for CYP2A6

Acetaminophen	Methoxsalen
Artemisinin	Nicotine
Caffeine	Omeprazole
Carbamazepine	Phenytoin
Cisapride	Pilocarpine
Clomethiazole	Promazine
Cyclophosphamide	Propofol
Disulfiram	Tamoxifen
Efavirenz	Tretinoin
Etodolac	Valproic acid
Fluoropyridine	Vortioxetine
Halothane	Zidovudine
Ifosfamide	

Table 3.6 Some Substrates for Human Subfamily CYP2B6

Amitriptyline	Diazepam	Methadone	Sevoflurane
Artemisinin	Diclofenac	Methoxyflurane	Siponimod
Atomoxetine	Diphenhydramine	Metoprolol	S-mephenytoin
Bupropion	Disulfiram	Mianserin	S-mephobarbital
Carbamazepine	Efavirenz	Nevirapine	Tamoxifen
Carbaryl	Fluoxetine	Nicotine	Temazepam
Clobazam	Haloperidol	Ospemifene	Thiotepa
Clomethiazole	Ifosfamide	Prasugrel	Tramadol
Clopidogrel	Imipramine	Promazine	Tretinoin
Cyclophosphamide	Ketamine	Propofol	Valproic acid
Desmethylselegiline	Meperidine	Selegiline	Verapamil
Dextromethorphan		Sertraline	

clinically important drugs (Table 3.7; also see Fig. 3.3). Not a single drug is completely metabolized by members of this subfamily, instead several CYP2C or other P450 enzymes can contribute to the catabolism of drugs. The CYP2C subfamily represents approximately 30% of the total of P450 isoforms in the liver (Fig. 3.2). CYP2C8 is expressed primarily in extrahepatic tissues (kidney, adrenal, brain, uterus, breast, ovary, and intestine) and metabolizes the tricyclic antidepressants diazepam and verapamil. CYP2C18 has a minor contribution to the metabolism of warfarin, diclofenac, acenocoumarol, and clobazam. CYP2C9 and CYP2C19 isoforms are highly expressed in hepatic tissue and metabolize several therapeutic agents (Table 3.7).[33]

CYP2C9 metabolizes approximately 13% of clinically relevant drugs (see Table 3.7) being the second most expressed P450 in the liver (see Fig. 3.2). CYP2C9, a highly polymorphic isoform, also metabolizes endogenous compounds such as steroids, melatonin, retinoids, and arachidonic acid. Many CYP2C9 substrates are weak acids, but CYP2C9 also has the capacity to metabolize unionized, highly lipophilic compounds. Ligand-based, structure-based, and homology models of CYP2C9 have been reported, which have provided insights into how its substrates are bound to the active site and, therefore, in drug design. So far, more than 10 resolved crystal structures of CYP2C9 have confirmed the importance of substrate specificity and ligand orientation.[33] CYP2C9 is subject to induction by rifampin, phenobarbital, and dexamethasone, indicating the involvement of PXR, the androstane receptor, and the glucocorticoid receptor in the regulation of CYP2C9.

Several compounds inhibit CYP2C9, which could provide an explanation for some clinically important DDIs. Tienilic acid, suprofen, and silibinin are mechanism-based inhibitors of CYP2C9. Phytocannabinoids, including tetrahydrocannabinol and cannabidiol, can inhibit the enzymatic activity of CYP2C9 at low micromolar range. Given the importance of CYP2C9 in drug metabolism and the presence of polymorphisms, it is important to identify drugs as potential substrates, inducers, or inhibitors of CYP2C9.

CYP2C19 is found primarily in the liver and intestine. The expression of CYP2C19 in the liver is less than that of CYP2C9 and exhibits polymorphism. Differences in the DNA sequence for the *CYP2C* gene change the enzyme's ability to metabolize substrates (ie, PM phenotype). Because of this genetic difference in expressing CYP2C isoforms, it is important to be aware of a person's race when prescribing and/or dispensing drugs that are commonly metabolized differently by different racial populations (see "Genetic Polymorphism" section). This allows pharmacists to be proactive in evaluating the potential risk to patients who may be of the PM phenotype by assessing a patient's pharmacogenomics and their reaction to previously prescribed CYP2C substrates and encouraging communication if the patient experiences adverse reactions. CYP2C19 conserves a high sequence identity with CYP2C9 (~91.2%), and studies on their crystal structures revealed the difference of two residues within the active site.[33]

CYP2D6. CYP2D6 is responsible for at least 30 different drug oxidations, representing approximately 20% of clinically important drugs (see Fig. 3.3). Currently, special recommendations for at least 72 CYP2D6 drugs/substrates are included on the pharmacogenomic clinical guidelines.[34] Only 2% of CYP2D6 is expressed in the liver and minimally expressed in the intestine, brain, and lymphoid cells, and it does not appear to be inducible. This isoform metabolizes a wide variety of lipophilic amines (Table 3.8) and is probably the only P450 for which a charged or ion-pair interaction is important for substrate binding. Genetic polymorphisms in the CYP2D6 gene (~140 allelic variations) include SNPs and minor insertions and/or deletions, as well as major structural variations including duplications, deletions, tandem arrangements, and hybridizations with nearby nonfunctional pseudogenes. This wide range of genetic

Table 3.7 Some Substrates and Reaction Type for Human Subfamily CYP2C

CYP2C8	CYP2C9	CYP2C9 (cont.)	CYP2C19
Amiodarone	Δ^1-THC (7-hydroxylation)	*R*-Mephenytoin	Acenocoumarol
Amodiaquine	Acenocoumarol	Mestranol	Amitriptyline
Atorvastatin	Amitriptyline	Methoxyflurane	Atomoxetine
Benzphetamine	Bosentan	Montelukast	Bupropion
Carbamazepine	Buprenorphine	Naproxen	Cannabidiol
Docetaxel	Candesartan	Nateglinide	Carisoprodol
Fluvastatin	Cannabidiol	Nevirapine	Cilostazol
Isotretinoin	Carvedilol	Nilotinib	Citalopram
Mycophenolic acid	Celecoxib	Omeprazole	Clomipramine
Paclitaxel	Chloramphenicol	Ospemifene	***Clopidogrel***
Phenytoin	Chlorpheniramine	Pazopanib	Cyclophosphamide
Pioglitazone	Chlorpropamide	Phenobarbital	Desipramine
Ponatinib	Clobazam	Phenylbutazone (4-hydroxylation)	***Diazepam*** (*N*-demethylation)
Repaglinide	Clopidogrel	***Phenytoin*** (4′-hydroxylation)	Doxepin
Retinol	Clozapine	Piroxicam	Escitalopram
Rosiglitazone	Cyclophosphamide	Prasugrel	Esomeprazole
Simvastatin	Dapsone	Propofol	Formoterol
Sorafenib	Dasatinib	***Ramelteon***	Hexobarbital
Tolbutamide	Desogestrel	Rosiglitazone	Imipramine (*N*-demethylation)
Torsemide	***Diazepam***	Rosuvastatin	Indomethacin
Verapamil	Diclofenac (4′-hydroxylation)	Sertraline	Lansoprazole
Zopiclone	Diphenhydramine	Sildenafil	Loratadine (*N*-decarboxylation)
	Donepezil	Siponimod	*R*-Mephenytoin (*N*-demethylation)
	Dorzolamide	Sulfamethoxazole	*S*-Mephenytoin (4′-hydroxylation)
	Dronabinol	Sulfinpyrazone (aromatic hydroxylation)	*R*-Mephobarbital
	Eletriptan	Suprofen	Methadone
	Etodolac	Tamoxifen	Mitotane
	Fluoxetine	Tenoxicam	Moclobemide
	Flurbiprofen (4′-hydroxylation)	Terbinafine	Nelfinavir
	Fluvastatin	Testosterone (16α-hydroxylation)	Nilutamide
	Formoterol	Tienilic acid (thiophene ring hydroxylation)	Omeprazole (hydroxylation)
	Glibenclamide	Tolbutamide (*p*-methyl-hydroxylation)	Ospemifene
	Gliclazide	Tolterodine	Pantoprazole
	Glimepiride	Torsemide	Pentamidine
	Glipizide	Trimethadione	Phenobarbital
	Glyburide	Valdecoxib	***Phenytoin*** (ring hydroxylation)
	Haloperidol	Valproic acid	Prasugrel
	Halothane	Valsartan	Progesterone
	Hexobarbital (3′-hydroxylation)	Vardenafil	Proguanil (cyclization)
	Hydrocodone	Voriconazole	Propranolol (side chain hydroxylation)
	Ibuprofen (i-butylmethyl-hydroxylation)	*S*-Warfarin (7′-hydroxylation)	Rabeprazole
	Ifosfamide	Zafirlukast	Teniposide
	Imipramine	Zidovudine	***Thioridazine***
	Indomethacin	Zileuton	Tolbutamide
	Irbesartan	Zopiclone	Venlafaxine
	Irinotecan		***Voriconazole***
	Ketamine		Vortioxetine
	Lornoxicam		*R*-Warfarin
	Losartan (hydroxymethyl to carboxylic acid)		
	Mefenamic acid		
	Meloxicam		

Drugs in bold italic have been reported to cause drug-drug interactions.

Table 3.8 Some Substrates and Reaction Type for Human CYP2D6 Isoform

Alprenolol (4-Hydroxylation)	Dexfenfluramine	Lidocaine (3-Hydroxylation)	Pindolol
Amitriptyline (10-hydroxylation)	***Dextromethorphan*** (*O*-demethylation)	Maprotiline	Promethazine (ring hydroxylation, *S*-oxidation, *N*-demethylation)
Amphetamine	Diphenhydramine (*N*-demethylation, ring hydroxylation, cleavage ether bond)	***Meperidine***	***Propafenone*** (4-hydroxylation)
Aripiprazole	Dolasetron (hydroxylation of indole ring)	***Methadone***	***Propoxyphene***
Atenolol	***Donepezil***	Methamphetamine	Propranolol (4′-hydroxylation)
Atomoxetine			
Brexpiprazole	***Doxepin***	Methoxyamphetamine (4-hydroxylation, *N*-demethylation)	Quetiapine
Bisoprolol	***Duloxetine***	Metoclopramide	Quinidine (hydroxylation)
Bufuralol (1′-hydroxylation)		***Eliglustat***	
Captopril	Encainide (*N*-demethylation, *O*-demethylation)	Metoprolol (*O*-demethylation)	Ranolazine
Carvedilol	Fenfluramine	***Mexiletine*** (4-hydroxylation and methyl hydroxylation)	Risperidone
Cevimeline	Fluphenazine	Minaprine	Ritonavir
Citalopram			
Chlorpheniramine (*N*-demethylation, ring hydroxylation, deamination)	***Fentanyl***	Mirtazapine	Sertraline
Chlorpromazine	***Flecainide*** (*O*-dealkylation)	Morphine	*S*-Metoprolol
Chlorpropamide	Fluoxetine (*N*-dealkylation)	Nebivolol	Sparteine (*N*-oxidation)
	Fluphenazine		
Clemastine	***Fluvoxamine***	***Nortriptyline*** (10-hydroxylation)	Tamoxifen
Clomipramine (hydroxylation)	Formoterol	Olanzapine	**Thioridazine** (aromatic hydroxylation)
Clozapine (aromatic hydroxylation)	Galantamine	Ondansetron (hydroxylation of indole ring)	Timolol (*O*-dealkylation)
	Gefitinib		
Codeine (*O*-demethylation)	Guanoxan (6- and 7-hydroxylation)	***Oxycodone*** (*O*-demethylation)	Tolterodine (2-hydroxylation)
Cyclobenzaprine	***Haloperidol***	Paroxetine	***Tramadol*** (*O*-demethylation)
Darifenacin	***Hydrocodone***	Perhexiline (4′-hydroxylation)	***Trazodone***
Debrisoquine (4-hydroxylation)	Hydroxyzine (ring hydroxylation)	Perphenazine (aromatic hydroxylation)	Tripelennamine
Desipramine	***Imipramine*** (2-hydroxylation)	Pimozide	Tropisetron (hydroxylation of indole ring)
Disopyramide	Indoramin (6-hydroxylation)		Venlafaxine
	Zuclopenthixol		

Drugs in bold italic have been reported to cause drug-drug interactions.

polymorphisms has made the CYP2D6 isoform the most extensively studied of the CYP family.[35] Because there might not be any other way to clear drugs metabolized by CYP2D6 from the system, polymorphism of CYP2D6 substrates can put patients at severe risk for adverse drug reactions, drug overdoses, and DDIs. For example, consider atomoxetine, a drug prescribed for attention-deficit/hyperactivity disorder metabolized largely by CYP2D6. In a population with deficient DYP2D6 activity (different polymorphic variants), as is the case with 7% of the Caucasian population, the blood concentration levels of the drug will be augmented, dramatically increasing the risk of adverse effects.[36]

Quinidine is an inhibitor of CYP2D6 and its concurrent administration with CYP2D6 substrates results in increased blood levels and toxicities for these substrates. If the pharmacologic action of the CYP2D6 substrate depends on the formation of active metabolites, 2D6 inhibition results in a lack of a therapeutic response. The competition of two substrates for CYP2D6 can prompt a number of varying clinical responses. For example, when substrates have unequal affinities for CYP2D6, the first-pass hepatic metabolism of a substrate (drug) with high affinity for CYP2D6 will inhibit binding of a second substrate that has a lower affinity for this enzyme. The result will be a rapid absorption of the second nonmetabolized substrate leading to a higher plasma concentration and to the increased potential for an adverse reaction or toxicity.[37]

CYP2E1. Despite the fact that CYP2E1 is most abundantly expressed in the liver at approximately 21% (see Fig. 3.2), few drugs are metabolized by this isoform. Even so, this isoform plays a major role in the metabolism of numerous halogenated hydrocarbons, including volatile general anesthetics such as halothane, isoflurane, sevoflurane, enflurane, and desflurane, and a range of low-molecular-weight organic compounds including dimethylformamide, acrylamide, acetonitrile, glycerol, acetone, ethanol, *N*,*N*-dimethylnitrosamine, and benzene. CYP2E1 is also the key enzyme in the activation of acetaminophen to its reactive metabolite *N*-acetyl-*p*-benzoquinoneimine, and in the metabolism of salicylic acid and valproic acid (Table 3.9). CYP2E1 is of high interest because of the oxidation of ethanol into its reactive products, acetaldehyde and 1-hydroxyethyl radicals, and its ability to activate low-molecular-weight products into electrophilic reactive metabolites, which result in toxicity and carcinogenicity. It also is involved in the activation of procarcinogenic nitrosamines into carcinogenic agents. This isoform is expressed also in the kidney, intestine, and lung.

The CYP2E1 isoform is inducible under diverse pathophysiologic conditions including diabetes, obesity, fasting, cancer, and fatty liver disease, and by xenobiotics including ethanol, isoniazid, and 4-methylpyrazole, among others (Table 3.9). CYP2E1 exhibits oxidase activity without substrate because it can reduce dioxygen to superoxide and hydrogen peroxide. Thus, lipid peroxidation generates reactive aldehydes, which activate immune cells for cytokine production, as well as collagen formation from adipocytes/lipocytes. CYP2E1 reacts with the hydrogen in the hydroxyl moiety on ethanol, generating hydroxyl radicals, which can be oxidized to spontaneously produce acetaldehyde, and the same process can happen with short chain alcohols. Consequently, the production of reactive oxygen species (ROS) by CYP2E1 will also increase the number of antioxidants, including heme oxygenase and glutathione (GSH) transferase, so there will be a mechanistic equilibrium to remove the oxidants generated by CYP2E1. So far, the contribution of CYP2E1 to alcoholic liver disease is still not well understood.[38]

The *CYP2E1* gene has at least 10 SNPs, some of which are associated with an elevated risk of cancer. Most of the compounds that induce CYP2E1 are also substrates for this enzyme. The induction of this enzyme in humans can cause enhanced susceptibility to the toxicity and carcinogenicity of CYP2E1 substrates. Some evidence shows interindividual variation in the in vitro liver expression of this isoform. The mechanism of induction appears to be a combination of an increase in CYP2E1 transcription, messenger RNA (mRNA) translation

Table 3.9 Some Substrates and Reaction Type for Human CYP2E1 Isoform

Acetaminophen (*p*-benzoquinoneimine)
Caffeine
Chlorzoxazone (hydroxylation)
Disulfiram
Halogenated hydrocarbons
Dehalogenation of chloroform, methylene chloride
Isoniazid
Lidocaine
Styrene (epoxidation)
Theophylline (8-oxidation)
Volatile anesthetics (fluorinated hydrocarbons)
Enflurane, halothane, methoxyflurane, sevoflurane, desflurane
Miscellaneous organic solvents
Acetone
Acetonitrile (hydroxylation to cyanohydrin)
Aniline (hydroxylation)
Benzene (hydroxylation)
Diethylether
Dimethylformamide (*N*-demethylation)
Ethanol (to acetaldehyde)
Glycerin
Pyridine (hydroxylation)

Drugs in bold italics have been reported to cause drug-drug interactions.

efficiency, and stabilization of CYP2E1 against proteolytic degradation. The induction of CYP2E1 resulting from ketosis (ie, due to starvation, a high-fat diet, uncontrolled diabetes, or obesity) or from exposure to alcoholic beverages or other xenobiotics can be detrimental to individuals simultaneously exposed to halogenated hydrocarbons (increased hepatotoxicity because of exposure to halothane or chloroform). Chronic alcohol intake is known to enhance the hepatotoxicity of halogenated hydrocarbons, which was found to be influenced by proapoptotic enzymes caspase 8 and 9.[39] Testosterone appears to regulate CYP2E1 levels in the kidney, and pituitary growth hormone regulates hepatic levels of CYP2E1.

Family 3

The human CYP3 family comprises one subfamily, four isoforms, CYP3A4, CYP3A5, CYP3A7, CYP3A43, four genes, and two pseudogenes. CYP3A members play an important role in bile acid and steroid (testosterone) metabolism.

CYP3A4/5. CYP3A4 is an abundant CYP enzyme in the liver, representing about 11% of the CYP hepatic content (see Fig. 3.2). It is expressed in the intestine, esophagus, duodenum, and colon. CYP3A4 is almost non-expressed in fetal liver, but after the second trimester the level of CYP3A4 begins to increase. Contrary to this, CYP3A7 is expressed in fetal liver and then the levels decrease over time. Meanwhile, CYP3A5 shows a wider distribution in extrahepatic tissue and represents 85% sequence identity to CYP3A4. CYP3A4 and CYP3A5 are generally functionally redundant; nonetheless, they do display modifications in their regulation and mRNA expression. CYP3A4 and CYP3A5 account for the metabolism of approximately 30% of the current drugs (Table 3.10; also see Fig. 3.3) and are inhibited by a number of xenobiotics (Table 3.11). CYP3A4 and CYP3A5 show extensive interindividual and ethnic variation in expression and activity.

Binding to CYP3A4 is predominantly a lipophilic interaction. Drugs known to be substrates for CYP3A4 have low and variable oral bioavailabilities, which might be explained by prehepatic metabolism by a combination of intestinal CYP3A4 and P-glycoprotein (P-gp) in the enterocytes of the intestinal wall (see "First-Pass Metabolism" section). Therefore, it is the expression and function of CYP3A4 that govern the rate and extent of metabolism of the substrates for the CYP3A subfamily. The induction of the CYP3A subfamily by phenobarbital in humans could ultimately be responsible for many of the well-documented interactions between barbiturates and other drugs. CYP3A4 appears also to activate aflatoxin B1 and, possibly, to metabolize benzo[a]pyrene. The interindividual differences reported for metabolism of nifedipine, cyclosporine, triazolam, and midazolam are related to changes in induction and not to polymorphism. Results from a comparison of CYP3A4 and CYP3A5 enzyme kinetics indicate that they have different characteristics in some CYP3A-catalyzed reactions. The enzyme kinetics of CYP3A5 suggests faster substrate turnover than that observed with CYP3A4.

Strong inhibitors of CYP3A enzymes include antifungals, anticancer agents, macrolide antibiotics, antivirals (used for HIV infection), and atypical antidepressants. This has a high impact in DDIs, for example, in the case of the antifungal ketoconazole. A well-known strong CYP3A inhibitor, coadministered ketoconazole will impact the metabolism of the antipsychotic risperidone, the sedative midazolam, the kinase inhibitors fostamatinib and midostaurin, and the contraceptive drospirenone, among others. Many SNPs at the CYP3A locus show large differences in allele frequency across populations. There have been shown to be ethnic differences in the expression of CYP3A5 and its primary functional variants. The *CYP3A5*3* (PM) allele frequency ranges from 50% to 55% in African Americans to 91% in Caucasians. This nonfunctional form is present in 85% of Japanese, 65% of Chinese, 67% of Mexican, and 40% of Native American populations. CYP3A enzymes function intricately since the effects of activation of their genes are determined by an extensive variety of endogenous and exogenous ligands and by a unique regulatory system that involves CYP3A enzymes in many physiologic and pathologic processes. Most recently, several studies have linked higher intratumoral expression of CYP3A4 and CYP3A5 with tumor resistance to therapy in pancreatic ductal adenocarcinoma, breast cancer, and colorectal cancer.[40]

CYP3A7 is predominantly expressed in fetal liver (~50% of total fetal P450 enzymes) but is also found in some adult livers and extrahepatically. CYP3A7 has a specific role in the hydroxylation of retinoic acid, 16α-hydroxylation of steroids, and hydroxylation of allylic and benzylic carbons, and therefore, it is relevant in both normal development and carcinogenesis.

Family 4

The human CYP4 family consists of six subfamilies of *CYP4* genes, including CYP4A, B, F, V, X, and Z, comprising a total of 13 CYP4 proteins. CYP4 family is implicated in several physiologic functions and their enzymes are involved in endogenous metabolism, acting on fatty acids and signaling molecules including eicosanoids, or in the modification of xenobiotics and therapeutic drugs. CYP4 family members are linked in pathologic processes and in the development of diseases including, among others, inflammation processes, cardiovascular disease, and several cancers. The CYP4A subfamily, and specifically CYP4A11, catalyzes the hydroxylation of the terminal ω-carbon and, to a lesser extent, the ω-1 position of saturated and unsaturated fatty acids (C10-C16), as well as the ω-hydroxylation of various prostaglandins. The other member of this subfamily, CYP4A22, is expressed at low levels and seems to be an orphan CYP. In rodents, induction of CYP4A expression by fibrate antihyperlipidemic agents is due to transcriptional activation, mediated possibly via peroxisome proliferator–activated receptors (PPARs). CYP4A gene expression is hormonally regulated. There is a close association between microsomal CYP4A1 induction, peroxisome proliferation, and induction of the peroxisomal fatty acid–metabolizing system. The immune suppressant tacrolimus is metabolized to an inactive form by CYP4A11.

The single member of the human CYP4B subfamily that is well expressed at the RNA level in the lung microsomes is CYP4B1; however, it is catalytically inactive and exhibits no

Table 3.10 Substrates and Reaction Type for Human CYP3A4 Isoform

Alfentanil	Clomipramine	Dronabinol	Isradipine	***Ondansetron***	***Solifenacin***	Δ1-THC
Alfuzosin	Clonazepam	Dutasteride	(aromatization)	***Omeprazole***	Sorafenib	(6β-hydroxylation)
Almotriptan	***Clopidogrel***	Efavirenz	***Itraconazole***	***Oral contraceptives/***	Steroids	Theophylline
Alprazolam	Clozapine	***Eplerenone***	***Ketoconazole***	***progestins***	Testosterone	(8-oxidation)
Amitriptyline	Cocaine	***Ergotamine***	Lansoprazole	Oxybutynin	(6β-hydroxylation)	***Tiagabine***
Amiodarone	Codeine	***Erlotinib***	Letrozole	***Paclitaxel***	Progesterone	Tinidazole
(*N*-deethylation)	(*N*-demethylation)	***Erythromycin***	***Lidocaine***	Pantoprazole	(6β-hydroxylation)	***Tipranavir***
Amlodipine	***Colchicine***	(*N*-demethylation)	(*N*-deethylation)	Pioglitazone	***Estradiol*** (2- and	***Tolterodine***
Amprenavir	Cyclophosphamide	Esomeprazole	Lopinavir	Prasugrel	4-hydroxylation)	(*N*-demethylation)
Aprepitant	***Cyclosporine*** (*N*-de-	***Eszopiclone***	Loratadine	Propranolol	***17α-ethinyl es-***	Toremifene
Aripiprazole	methylation and	***Ethinyl estradiol***	***Lovastatin***	***Quetiapine***	***tradiol*** (2- and	Tramadol
Astemizole	methyl oxidation)	***Ethosuximide***	(6-hydroxylation)	***Quinidine***	4-hydroxylation)	***Trazodone***
Atazanavir	Dapsone (*N*-oxide)	Etonogestrel	***Methadone***	(3-hydroxylation)	***Norethisterone***	***Triazolam***
Atorvastatin	***Darifenacin***	***Etoposide***	***Midazolam*** (methyl	Quinine	(2-hydroxylation)	Trimetrexate
"Azole" antifungals	Delavirdine	Exemestane	hydroxylation)	Rabeprazole	Hydrocortisone	Valdecoxib
Bepridil	Desogestrel	***Felodipine***	***Mifepristone***	***Ramelteon***	(6-hydroxylation)	Valproic acid (hy-
Bromocriptine	Dextromethorphan	***Fentanyl***	***Mirtazapine***	***Ranolazine***	Methylprednisolone	droxylation and
Budesonide	(*N*-demethylation)	Fexofenadine	***Modafinil***	Repaglinide	***Prednisone***	dehydrogenation)
Buprenorphine	Diazepam (C_7	Finasteride	***Mometasone***	Rifampin, ***rifabutin***, and	(6β-hydroxylation)	***Vardenafil***
Buspirone	hydroxylation)	Flutamide	***Montelukast***	related compounds	***Prednisolone***	***Verapamil***
Cafergot	***Dihydroergotamine***	***Fluticasone***	Nateglinide	***Ritonavir***	(6β-hydroxylation)	(*N*-demethylation)
Caffeine	***Disopyramide***	Galantamine	***Nelfinavir***	Salmeterol	Dexamethasone	***Vinblastine***
Cannabinoids	***Diltiazem***	Gleevec	Nevirapine	***Saquinavir Sertraline***	***Sunitinib***	***Vincristine***
Carbamazepine	(*N*-deethylation)	Haloperidol	***Nicardipine***	Sibutramine	***Tacrolimus***	***Voriconazole***
(epoxidation)	Docetaxel	Hydrocodone	(aromatization)	***Sildenafil***	***Tadalafil***	***R-Warfarin***
Cevimeline	Dofetilide	Imatinib	***Nifedipine***	***Simvastatin***	***Tamoxifen***	Zaleplon
Chlorpheniramine	Dolasetron	Imipramine	***Nisoldipine***	***Sirolimus***	(*N*-demethylation)	***Zileuton***
Cilostazol	(*N*-oxide)	(*N*-demethylation)	Nitrendipine		***Telithromycin***	***Ziprasidone***
Citalopram	Domperidone	***Indinavir***	Norethindrone		Temazepam	Zolpidem
Clarithromycin	Donepezil	Irinotecan				***Zonisamide***
Clindamycin	Doxorubicin					

Drugs in bold italic have been reported to cause drug-drug interactions.

Table 3.11 Cytochrome P450 Inhibitors

CYP1A2	CYP2B6	CYP2C8	CYP2C19	CYP2C9	CYP2D6	CYP2E1	CYP3A4/5/7
Amiodarone	Amiodarone	***Alectinib***	***Cabozantinib***	***Amiodarone***	***Amiodarone***	Diethyl dithiocarbamate	***Alectinib***
Atazanavir	Amlodipine	Anastrozole	Cimetidine	Atazanavir	***Binimetinib***	Disulfiram	***Amiodarone***
Axitinib	Azelastine	***Axitinib***	Citalopram	***Binimetinib***	Bupropion	***Midostaurin***	***Amprenavir***
Binimetinib	Citalopram	***Cabozantinib***	Delavirdine	***Cabozantinib***	Celecoxib	Pazopanib	***Aprepitant***
Cimetidine	Clotrimazole	***Gemfibrozil***	Efavirenz	***Cimetidine***	Chloroquine	Ribociclib	***Atazanavir***
Ciprofloxacin	***Crizotinib***	Glitazones	Felbamate	Clopidogrel	Chlorpheniramine		***Cabozantinib***
Citalopram	Desipramine	***Midostaurin***	Fluconazole	Cotrimoxazole	Chlorpromazine		***Cimetidine***
Clarithromycin	Disulfiram	Montelukast	***Fluoxetine***	Delavirdine	***Cimetidine***		Ciprofloxacin
Diltiazem	Doxorubicin	Nicardipine	Fluvastatin	Disulfiram	***Cinacalcet***		***Clarithromycin***
Enoxacin	Ethinyl estradiol	Pazopanib	***Fluvoxamine***	Efavirenz	Citalopram		***Cobicistat***
Erythromycin	Fluoxetine	Sulfinpyrazone	Gefitinib	Escitalopram	Clemastine		***Cobimetinib***
Ethinyl estradiol	Fluvoxamine	Topiramate	Indomethacin	***Etravirine***	Clomipramine		***Crizotinib***
Fluoroquinolones	Isoflurane	Trimethoprim	Isoniazid	Fenofibrate	***Cobicistat***		***Cyclosporine***
Fluvoxamine	Ketoconazole		Ketoconazole	***Fluconazole***	***Cobimetinib***		Danazol
Interferon	Mestranol		Lansoprazole	Fluorouracil	Cocaine		***Delavirdine***
Isoniazid	Methimazole		Leflunomide	***Fluoxetine***	***Darifenacin***		Diethyl dithiocarbamate
Ketoconazole	Miconazole		Lovastatin		Desipramine		***Diltiazem***
Methoxsalen	***Midostaurin***		Methoxsalen	Fluphenazine	Diphenhydramine		***Efavirenz***
Mibefradil	Nelfinavir		***Metronidazole***	Fluvastatin	Doxepin		Erlotinib
Midostaurin	Orphenadrine		Mexiletine	***Fluvoxamine***	Doxorubicin		***Erythromycin***
Pazopanib	Paroxetine		***Midostaurin***	Gemfibrozil	***Duloxetine***		Ethinyl estradiol
Ribociclib	Sertraline		Modafinil	Halofantrine	***Etravirine***		***Fluconazole***
Rucaparib	Sorafenib			Haloperidol	***Gefitinib***		Fluoxetine
Thiotepa	Tamoxifen		Nalidixic acid	Hydroxychloroquine	***Midostaurin***		***Fluvoxamine***
Ticlopidine	Ticlopidine		Norethindrone	Hydroxyzine	***Pazopanib***		Gestodene
Venlafaxine			Norfloxacin	Imatinib	***Sorafenib***		***Idelalisib***
			Omeprazole				Imatinib
				Itraconazole			***Indinavir***
			Oral contraceptives	Ketoconazole			***Isoniazid***
			Oxcarbazepine	Levomepromazine			***Itraconazole***
			Paroxetine	Methadone			***Ketoconazole***
			Pazopanib	Metoclopramide			***Lorlatinib***

	Mibefradil	Methylprednisolone
Phenylbutazone	Midodrine	***Metronidazole***
Probenecid	***Midostaurin***	Mibefradil
	Moclobemide	***Miconazole***
Sertraline	Norfluoxetine	***Midostaurin***
Sorafenib	***Paroxetine***	Mifepristone
Sulfamethoxazole	Perphenazine	***Nelfinavir***
Sulfaphenazole	Propafenone	Nicardipine
Sulfonamides	Propoxyphene	***Nifedipine***
Tacrine	***Propranolol***	***Nilotinib***
Teniposide	Quinacrine	Norethindrone
Ticlopidine	***Quinidine***	***Norfloxacin***
	Ranitidine	Norfluoxetine
Tipranavir	Ranolazine	Osimertinib
Troleandomycin	***Ritonavir***	Oxiconazole
Voriconazole	***Sertraline***	***Palbociclib***
Zafirlukast	Sorafenib	***Pazopanib***
Zileuton	Terbinafine	Prednisone
	Thioridazine	***Quinine***
	Ticlopidine	***Ranolazine***
	Tipranavir	***Ribociclib***
	Tripelennamine	***Rilpivirine***
		Ritonavir
		Roxithromycin
		Saquinavir
		Sertraline
		Sorafenib
		Telithromycin
		Troleandomycin
		Verapamil
		Voriconazole
		Zafirlukast
		Zileuton
		Zolpidem

P450 isoform inhibitors presented in bold italics have been associated with drug-drug interactions of clinical relevance or with drug-drug interaction warnings that can require dosage adjustment.
Data from *Stockley's Drug Interactions: A Source Book of Interactions, Their Mechanisms, Clinical Importance and Management.* 11th ed. Pharmaceutical Press; 2016.[81,86]

expression in hepatic tissues. There are interspecies differences because, in several mammals, this enzyme is highly active and metabolizes some procarcinogens and xenobiotics.

The human CYP4F subfamily consists of seven members CYP4F2, CYP4F3A, CYP4F3B, CYP4F8, CYP4F11, CYP4F12, and CYP4F22, which function as eicosanoid regulators and ω-hydroxylases. This family is responsible for inactivating the vascular effects of leukotrienes, omega-3 fatty acids, and tocopherols (vitamin E analogs). CYP4F2 and CYP4F11 are implicated in the metabolism of vitamin K, accelerating its inactivation and elimination. Similarly, CYP4F11 has shown catalytic activity against erythromycin, benzphetamine, and chlorpromazine. CYP4F12 slowly metabolized ebastine and terfenadine.[41,42]

Clearly, no single animal model or combination of animal models represents the metabolic capabilities of humans. By having a complete understanding of the factors (eg, inducers, inhibitors, and effects of disease states) that alter the expression and activity of an enzyme responsible for the metabolism of a particular compound, and by a determination of responsible isoforms and patient phenotyping, it might be possible to predict DDIs and metabolic clearance.

An alphabetic listing of the clinically important drugs and the P450 isoforms catalyzing their oxidative metabolism is presented in Table 3.12.

Oxygen Activation

Elemental oxygen (dioxygen) is a relatively unreactive form of oxygen that exists as an unpaired diradical in the triplet form. Dioxygen activation by P450s requires the sequential addition of two single electrons to the P450 from NAD(P)H through the flavin or iron-sulfur protein redox partners, as in the following equation:

$$\text{R-H} + O_2 + 2\ \text{NAD(P)H} + 2\text{H}^{\oplus} \rightarrow \text{R-OH} + H_2O + 2\text{NADP}^{\oplus}$$

Although the function of P450 monooxygenases is mostly oxidation of a substrate, several examples of substrates are recognized in the literature. A reactive radical like iron-oxenoid intermediate is generated that is reactive enough to split aliphatic C-H bonds, add to C-H bonds α to heteroatoms, or remove single electrons from heteroatoms to produce radical cations.[43,44]

Catalytic Cycle of Cytochrome P450: Steps of the Catalytic Cycle

Many variant P450 isoforms that have been isolated show a remarkable uniformity for the catalytic mechanism. The net C-H hydroxylation reaction is an insertion of oxygen with a ferric-oxenoid complex into a C-H bond to

Table 3.12 Some Substrates for the Main P450 Isoforms Catalyzing Their Metabolism

Acetaminophen	1A2, 2E1, 3A4, 2C9	Caffeine	1A2
Albendazole	3A4, 1A2	Cannabinoids	3A4
Alfentanil	3A4	Carbamazepine	2C8, 3A4, 2B6
Alprazolam	3A4	Carisoprodol	2C19
Amiodarone	3A4, 2C9	Carvedilol	2C9, 2D6
Amitriptyline	1A2, 2C9, 2D6, 3A4, 2C19	Celecoxib	2C9
Amlodipine	3A4	Cevimeline	2D6
Amphetamine	2D6	Chlordiazepoxide	1A2
Aripiprazole	2D6, 3A4	Chloroquine	3A4
Anastrozole	3A4	Chlorpromazine	2D6, 3A4
Astemizole	3A4	Chlorzoxazone	2E1
Atomoxetine	2D6	Cimetidine	3A4
Atorvastatin	3A4	Cisapride	3A4
Bepridil	3A4	Citalopram	2C19, 3A4
Bisoprolol	2D6	Clarithromycin	3A4
Bosentan	2C9	Clindamycin	3A4
Bupropion	2C9, 2B6, 2A6, 1A2	Clomipramine	1A2, 2C9, 2C19, 2D6, 3A4
Busulfan	3A4	Clopidogrel	2C19, 2C9, 1A2, 3A4/5
Clonazepam	3A4	Estrogens, oral	3A4

Table 3.12 Some Substrates for the Main P450 Isoforms Catalyzing Their Metabolism (*continued*)

Clozapine	1A2, 2D6, 2C19, 3A4	Ethanol	2E1
Cocaine	3A4	Ethinyl estradiol	3A4
Codeine	2D6, 3A4	Etodolac	2C9
Cyclobenzaprine	1A2, 2A6, 2D6, 3A4	Etoposide	3A4
Cyclophosphamide	2B6, 2C19, 3A4	Felodipine	3A4
Cyclosporine	3A4	Fenfluramine	2D6
Dapsone	2C9, 3A4	Fentanyl	2D6, 3A4
Delavirdine	3A4	Fexofenadine	3A4
Desipramine	1A2, 2C19, 2D6	Finasteride	3A4
Desogestrel	2C9	Flecainide	2D6
Dexamethasone	3A4	Fluconazole	3A4
Dexfenfluramine	2D6	Flurbiprofen	2C9
Dextromethorphan	2D6, 3A4	Fluoxetine	2C9, 2D6, 2B6
Diazepam	1A2, 2C19, 2C9, 3A4	Fluvastatin	2C8, 2C9
Diclofenac	2C8, 2C9	Fluphenazine	2D6
Diltiazem	3A4	Flutamide	1A2, 3A4
Diphenhydramine	2C9	Fluvoxamine	1A2, 2D6
Disopyramide	3A4	Formoterol	2C9, 2C19, 2D6
Divalproex sodium	2C19	Galantamine	2D6
Docetaxel	2C8, 3A4	Glimepiride	2C9
Dolasetron	2D6, 3A4	Glipizide	2C9
Donepezil	2D6, 3A4, 2C9	Glyburide	2C9, 3A4
Dorzolamide	2C9	Granisetron	3A4
Doxepin	2D6	Halofantrine	3A4
Doxorubicin	3A4	Haloperidol	1A2, 2D6
Dronabinol	2C9	Halothane	2E1, 2C9
Efavirenz	2B6	Hydrocodone	2D6, 3A4
Eletriptan	2C9	Hydrocortisone	2D6, 3A4
Enalapril	3A4	Ibuprofen	2C9
Encainide	2D6	Ifosfamide	2B6, 3A4
Enflurane	2E1	Imipramine	1A2, 2C19, 2C9, 2D6, 3A4
Ergot alkaloids	3A4	Indinavir	2D6, 3A4
Erythromycin	3A4	Indomethacin	2C9, 2C19
Esomeprazole	2C19	Irbesartan	2C9
Estradiol	1A2	Isoflurane	2E1, 2B6
Isotretinoin (retinoids)	1A2, 2C8, 3A4	Nelfinavir	2B6, 3A4
Isradipine	3A4	Nevirapine	3A4

(continued)

Table 3.12 Some Substrates for the Main P450 Isoforms Catalyzing Their Metabolism (*continued*)

Itraconazole	3A4	Nicardipine	3A4
Ketamine	2B6, 2C9	Nicotine	2A6, 2B6, 2A13
Ketoconazole	3A4	Nifedipine	3A4/5
Labetalol	2D6	Nilutamide	2C19
Lansoprazole	2C19, 3A4	Nimodipine	3A4
Lidocaine	2D6, 3A4	Nisoldipine	3A4
Leflunomide	1A2, 2C9, 2C19	Nitrendipine	3A4
Losartan	2C9, 3A4	Nortriptyline	1A2, 2D6
Lovastatin	3A4	Olanzapine	1A2, 2D6, 3A4
Maprotiline	2D6	Omeprazole	2C19, 2C9, 3A4
Moclobemide	2C19	Ondansetron	1A2, 2D6, 2E1, 3A4
Mefenamic acid	2C9	Oral contraceptives	3A4
Mefloquine	3A4	Oxycodone	2D6
Meloxicam	2C9	Paclitaxel	2C8, 3A4
Meperidine	2D6, 2B6	Pantoprazole	2C19
Mephenytoin	2C19	Paroxetine	2D6
Mephobarbital	2C9, 2B6	Perphenazine	2D6
Mestranol	2C9	Phenol	2E1
Methadone	1A2, 2D6, 2B6	Phenobarbital	2B6, 2C9
Methamphetamine	2D6	Phenytoin	2C19, 2C8, 2C9
Metoprolol	2D6	Pimozide	3A4
Mexiletine	1A6, 2D6, 2A6	Pindolol	2D6, 3A4
Mibefradil	3A4	Pioglitazone	2C8, 3A4
Miconazole	3A4	Piroxicam	2C18, 2C9
Midazolam	3A4	Prasugrel	3A4, 2B6, 2C9
Mirtazapine	1A2, 2D6, 3A4	Pravastatin	3A4
Modafinil	3A4	Praziquantel	2B6, 3A4
Montelukast	2C9	Prednisone	3A4
Morphine	2D6	Progesterone	3A4, 2C19
Naproxen	1A2, 2C18, 2C9, 2A6	Proguanil	2C18, 2C19
Nateglinide	2C9	Propafenone	1A2, 2D6, 3A4
Navelbine	3A4	Propofol	2B6, 2C9
Nefazodone	3A4	Propoxyphene	2D6
Propranolol	1A2, 2C18, 2C19, 2D6	Terfenadine	3A4
Quetiapine	3A4	Testosterone	3A4
Quinidine	3A4	Δ9-THC	2C9
Quinine	3A4	Thiabendazole	1A2

Table 3.12 Some Substrates for the Main P450 Isoforms Catalyzing Their Metabolism (*continued*)

Rabeprazole	2C19	Timolol	2D6
Repaglinide	2C8	Tolbutamide	2C8, 2C9, 2C19
Retinoic acid	2C8	Tolterodine	2D6, 2C9
Rifabutin	3A4	Torsemide	2C9
Rifampin	3A4	Tramadol	2D6
Riluzole	1A2	Trazodone	2D6
Risperidone	2D6, 3A4	Tretinoin	2C8, 3A4
Ritonavir	2A6, 2C19, 2C9, 2D6, 2E1, 3A4	Triazolam	3A4
Ropinirole	1A2	Troleandomycin	3A4
Ropivacaine	1A2, 2D6	Tropisetron	2D6
Rosiglitazone	2C8, 2C9	Valsartan	2C9
Rosuvastatin	2C9	Valproic acid	2C9, 2A6, 2B6
Salmeterol	3A4	Valdecoxib	2C9
Saquinavir	3A4	Vardenafil	3A4
Selegiline	2D6, 2B6, 2A6	Venlafaxine	2D6
Sertindole	2D6	Verapamil	1A2, 3A4, 2C8
Sertraline	2D6, 2C19, 3A4, 2B6	Vinblastine	3A4
Sevoflurane	2E1	Vincristine	3A4
Sildenafil	2C9, 3A4	Voriconazole	2C9
Simvastatin	3A4	Warfarin	2C18, 2C9
Sufentanil	3A4	*R*-Warfarin	1A2
Suprofen	2C9	*S*-Warfarin	2C9, 2C18
Sulfamethoxazole	2C9	Yohimbine	2D6
Tacrine	1A2, 2A6	Zafirlukast	2C9
Tacrolimus	3A4	Zaleplon	3A4
Tamoxifen	1A2, 2A6, 2B6, 2D6, 2E1, 3A4	Zileuton	1A2, 2C9, 3A4
Temazepam	3A4	Zolpidem	3A4
Teniposide	3A4, 2C19	Zopiclone	2C8, 2C9, 3A4
Terbinafine	2C9		

produce an alcohol or phenol. The ease with which P450 enzymes perform hydroxylation in unreactive substrates such as hydrocarbons indicates a highly reactive enzyme intermediate capable of mediating such chemistry. A major determinant in the regioselectivity of hydroxylation is the HAT and the stability of the radical intermediate being formed.[45]

The current view illustrating the cyclic ("wheel") mechanism for reduction and oxygenation of P450 with stepwise interactions with substrate molecules, electron donors, and oxygen is shown in Figure 3.4 and can be summarized as follows.[45-49]

The Catalytic P450 Cycle

Step 1. The resting [Fe^{III}-P450-OH] complex binds reversibly with a molecule of the substrate (R-H) displacing the distal water, resulting in a complex resembling enzyme-substrate complex [Fe^{III}-P450*RH]. RH is bound near the heme iron (but not directly to it). The binding of the substrate triggers/facilitates the first one-electron reduction step from NADPH.

Step 2. The substrate complex of [Fe^{III}-P450*RH] undergoes reduction to a [Fe^{II}-P450*RH] substrate complex by an electron originating from its redox partner by the flavoprotein [NADPH-P450 reductase $FNMH_2$-FADH complex].

Step 3. The reduced [Fe^{II}-P450*RH] substrate complex readily binds dioxygen as the sixth ligand of Fe^{2+} to form a [O_2-Fe^{II}-P450*RH] substrate complex.

Step 4. The complex [O_2-Fe^{II}-P450*RH] is subjected to a second electron from its redox partner to form the [Fe^{III}-P450*RH-superoxide anion O_2^(-1)] complex.

Step 5. The [Fe^{III}-P450*RH-superoxide anion O_2^(-1)] is protonated to form the ferric hydroperoxo state [HOO-Fe^{III}-P450*RH]. This complex is termed compound 0 and is believed to be implicated in oxidation reactions.

Step 6. The [HOO-Fe^{III}-P450*RH] complex is protonated, and a water molecule is released by heterolytic cleavage of peroxide anion upon protonation to form water and a highly electrophilic porphyrin-radical cation intermediate (ferryl-oxenoid species, [P450-Fe^{IV}=O*RH]) (compound 1, the more favorable oxygen-cysteine-porphyrin radical cation resonance-stabilized complex). The Fe^{IV}=O species is the catalytically active oxygenation species. One role of the cysteine sulfur ligand is thought to be electron donation (push) that weakens the peroxide O-O bond, causing peroxide bond scission to produce a highly reactive and strong oxidizing intermediate (compound 1). It has also been suggested that there are various oxidizing species (ie, FeO complexes) and that different ones can be referred to various oxidation reactions.[50-52]

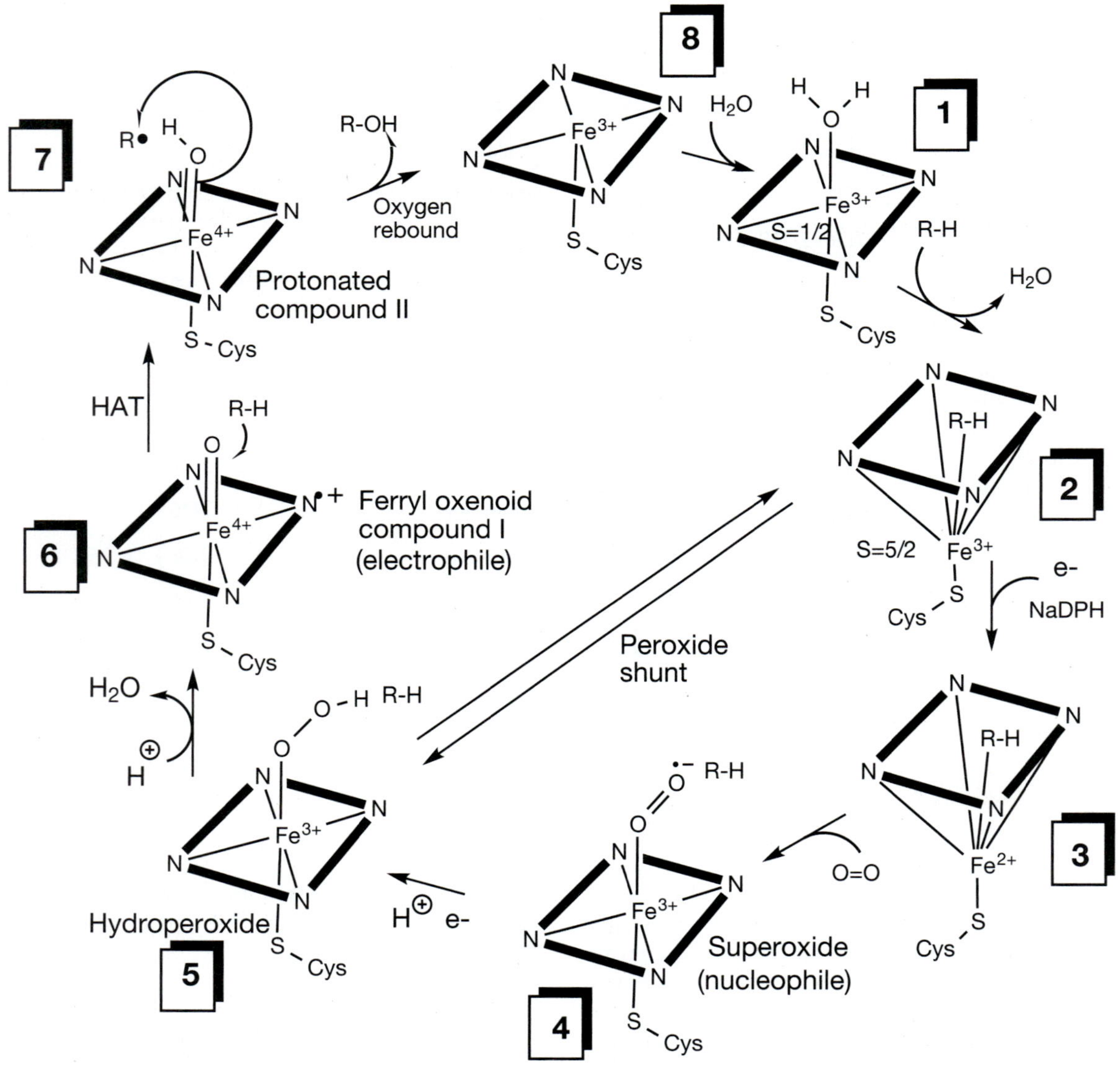

Figure 3.4 Generalized cyclic mechanism for P450.

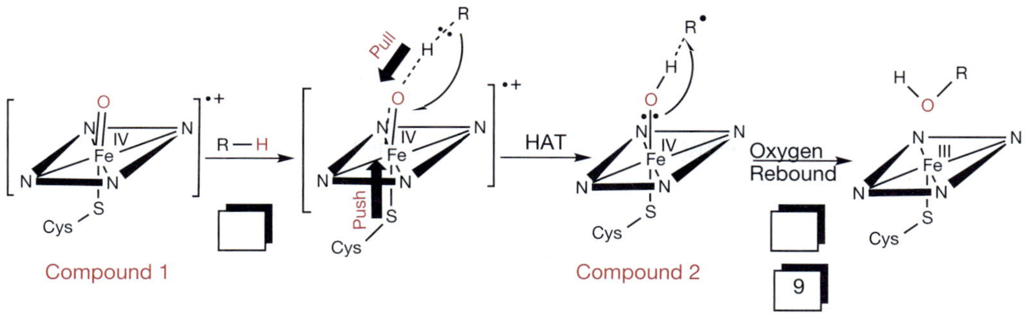

Figure 3.5 Oxygen rebound: a two-step mechanism: the electrophilic ferryl-oxenoid species [$Fe^{4+}=O$] abstracts a hydrogen (step 7) from the substrate (R-H) to give a carbon radical intermediate (R•) that recombines with the ferric-bound hydroxyl radical [Fe^{4+}*OH] (step 8/9) to give the final hydroxyl product.

Step 7. The unstable compound 1 [P450-Fe^{IV}=O*RH] can abstract a hydrogen atom from a substrate when it is in spatial proximity to form [P450-Fe^{IV}=OH*R•], the carbon-oxidized hydroxylated product compound 2.

Step 8. The [P450-Fe^{IV}=OH*R•] complex can undergo a radical recombination, in a "caged" reaction in an oxygen rebound, yielding the oxygenated product [P450-Fe^{III*}OHR].[50]

Step 9. The [P450-Fe^{III*}OHR] complex releases R-OH through one of the exit channels on the distal side and is replaced by a water molecule to regenerate the initial [Fe^{III}-P450-OH] enzyme complex (Fig. 3.5).[53,54]

Until the final step, the oxidizable substrate has been an inactive spectator in the chemical events of oxygen activation. None of the peroxide or superoxide intermediates in the cycle are sufficiently reactive to abstract hydrogen from the substrate. The ferryl-oxenoid complex (step 6) is a good hydrogen abstractor, even for relatively inert terminal methyl groups on hydrocarbon chains. The ferric-oxenoid complex exhibits regioselectivity in its choice of hydrogen atoms, balancing stability of the resulting carbon radical with stereochemical constraints. The reactivity of C-H abstraction depends on carbon radical stability. Some of the factors that stabilize carbon radicals include neighboring carbon atoms, neighboring carbon-carbon multiple bonds, and neighboring heteroatoms with lone pairs of electrons, for example, oxygen and nitrogen. Carbon radicals are electron deficient and are seeking electrons and therefore are stabilized by nearby electron-donating groups. Because the inert aliphatic region of the substrate has been converted to a highly reactive radical, the process is described as substrate activation.[5]

Oxidations Catalyzed by Cytochrome P450 Isoforms

Aliphatic and Alicyclic Hydroxylations

The accepted mechanism of hydroxylation of alkane C-H bonds is shown in Figure 3.6 and has been reviewed in detail elsewhere.[48,55-57] The principal metabolic pathway of the methyl group is oxidation to the hydroxymethyl derivative followed by microsomal oxidation to the carboxylic acid (eg, tolbutamide) (Fig. 3.7). On the other hand, some methyl groups are oxidized only to the hydroxymethyl derivative, without further oxidation to the acid. Where there are several equivalent methyl groups, as a rule only one methyl group is oxidized. In the case of aromatic methyl groups, *p*-methyl is the most vulnerable because it is less sterically hindered.

Alkyl side chains exhibit regioselectivity and are often hydroxylated on the terminal or penultimate (secondary) carbon atoms (eg, pentobarbital) (see Fig. 3.7). The isopropyl group is an interesting side chain that is hydroxylated at the tertiary carbon and at either of the equivalent methyl groups (eg, ibuprofen) (see Fig. 3.7). Hydroxylation of alkyl side chains attached to an aromatic ring does not follow the general rules for alkyl side chains, because the aromatic ring activates the α-position of hydroxylation (see Fig. 3.7). Oxidation occurs preferentially on the benzylic methylene group and, to a lesser extent, at other positions on the side chain.

The methylene groups of an alicycle are readily hydroxylated, usually at the least hindered position or at an activated position, for example, α to a carbonyl (cyclohexanone), α to a double bond (cyclohexene), or α to a phenyl ring (tetralin).

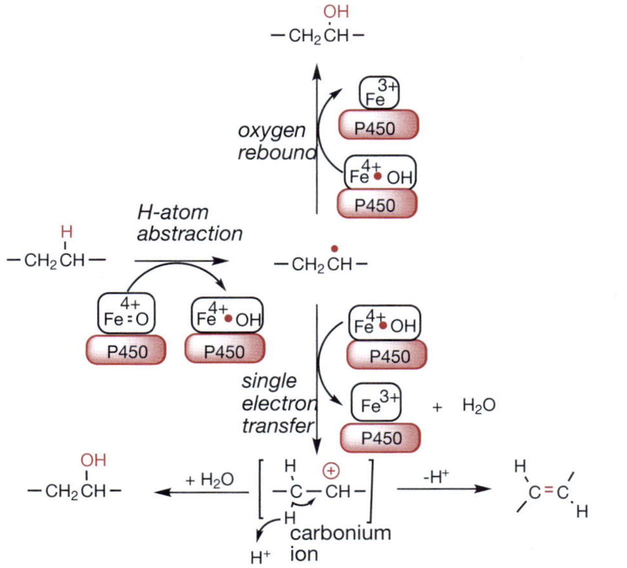

Figure 3.6 Proposed mechanisms for the hydroxylation and dehydrogenation of alkanes.

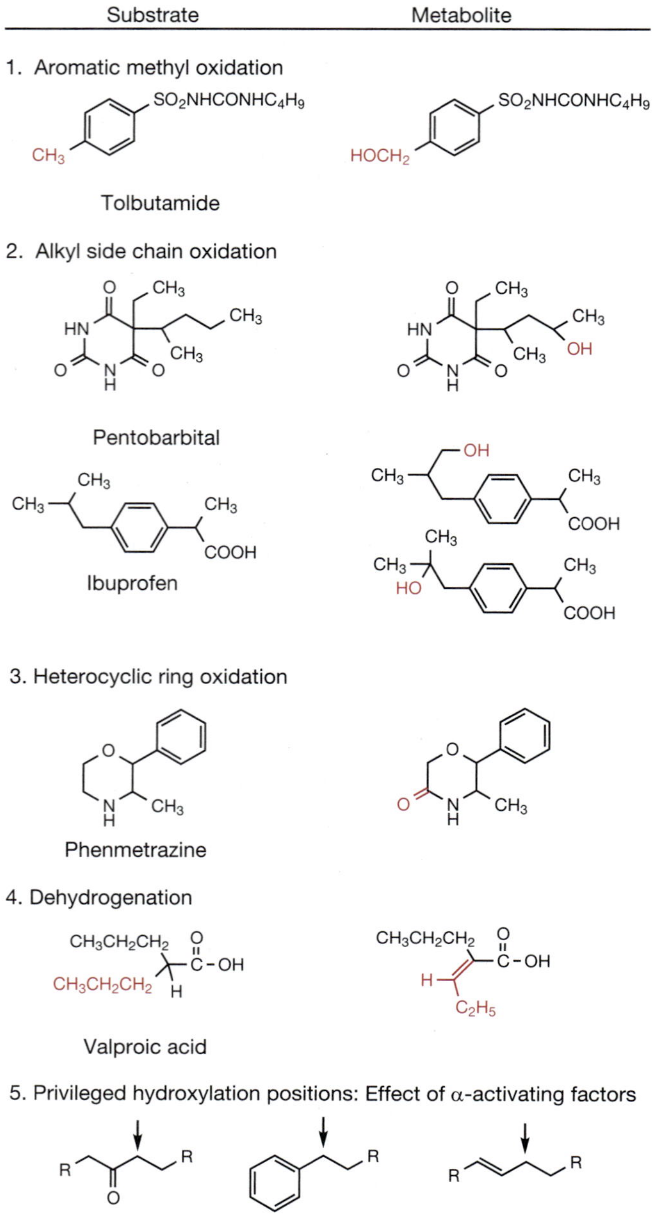

Figure 3.7 Examples of oxidative metabolism of aliphatic and alicyclic hydrocarbons catalyzed by P450.

The products of hydroxylation often show regioselectivity and stereoisomerism. Nonaromatic heterocycles normally undergo oxidation at the α-carbon adjacent to the heteroatom (see Fig. 3.7).[55]

In addition to hydroxylation reactions, P450s can catalyze the dehydrogenation of an alkane to an alkene (olefin). The reaction is thought to involve formation of a carbon radical and electron transfer to the ferryl complex of P450, which produces a carbocation that is deprotonated to a dehydrogenated product alkene (see Fig. 3.7).[5,51] An example of the ability of P450 to function as both a dehydrogenase and a monooxygenase has been demonstrated with the antiseizure drug valproic acid. Whereas the major metabolic products in humans are formed by β-oxidation and phase 2 acyl glucuronidation, several alkenes are also formed, including the (*E*)2-ene isomer (Fig. 3.7). CYP2C9, CYP2A6, and CYP2B6 are the enzymes that catalyze these reactions.[58] The factors that determine whether P450 catalyzes hydroxylation (oxygen rebound/recombination) or dehydrogenation (electron transfer) remain unknown, but hydroxylation is usually favored. In some instances, the product of dehydrogenation can be the primary product (eg, 6,7-dehydrogenation of testosterone).

Alkene and Alkyne Hydroxylation

The proposed mechanism for the oxidation of π-bonds in alkenes is a stepwise sequence of one-electron transfers between the radical complex and the ferryl-oxenoid intermediate [Fe^{+4}=O], leading to alkene oxidation (Fig. 3.8).[55] Following the initial formation of an unsaturated P450 π-complex, the one-electron transfer (1) yields a radical σ-complex that can collapse either to an alkene or an arene epoxide (step a or d, Fig. 3.8), (2) undergoes a 1,2-group migration to form a carbonyl product (steps a and b, Fig. 3.8), or (3) produces a vinyl hydroxylated product (step c, Fig. 3.8) or a σ-complex, which can break down to a phenol (step e, Fig. 3.8). The presence of a hydroxyl radical in the porphyrin ring allows some substrate radicals to covalently bond by *N*-alkylation of a pyrrole nitrogen rather than recombination with $(Fe\text{-}OH)^{+3}$ radical. An alternative mechanism was proposed as "chameleon theory" where different electronic distributions of compound I (see Fig. 3.4) participate in the formation of different products.[51] This deviation from the normal course of reaction explains the suicide inhibition exhibited by some xenobiotics, such as the oral contraceptives erythromycin and paroxetine.

The oxidation of alkenes yields primarily epoxides and a series of products derived from 1,2-migration (see Fig. 3.8). The stereochemical configuration of the alkene is retained during epoxidation. The epoxides can differ in reactivity. Those that are highly reactive undergo either pH-catalyzed hydrolysis to excretable vicinal dihydrodiols or covalent reactions (alkylation) with macromolecules such as proteins or nucleic acids, which lead to tissue necrosis or carcinogenicity. Moreover, the ubiquitous epoxide hydrolase can catalyze the rapid hydrolysis of epoxides to nontoxic vicinal dihydrodiols. Several drugs (carbamazepine, cyproheptadine, and protriptyline), however, were found to form stable epoxides at the 10,11-position during biotransformation (Fig. 3.9). The fact that these epoxides could be detected in the urine indicates that these oxides are not particularly reactive and should not readily react covalently with macromolecules.

The epoxidation of terminal alkenes is accompanied by the mechanism-based ("suicide") *N*-alkylation of the heme-porphyrin ring. If the π-complex attaches to the alkene at the internal carbon, the terminal carbon of the double bond can irreversibly *N*-alkylate the pyrrole nitrogen of the porphyrin ring.[59] The heme adduct formation is observed mostly with monosubstituted, unconjugated alkenes (ie, 17α-ethylenic steroids [steroid D-ring homoannulation] and 4-ene metabolite of valproic acid)[60,61] (see Fig. 3.9).

In addition to the formation of epoxides, heme adducts, and hydroxylated products, carbonyl products are also created. These latter products result from the migration of atoms to adjacent carbons (ie, 1,2-group migration). For

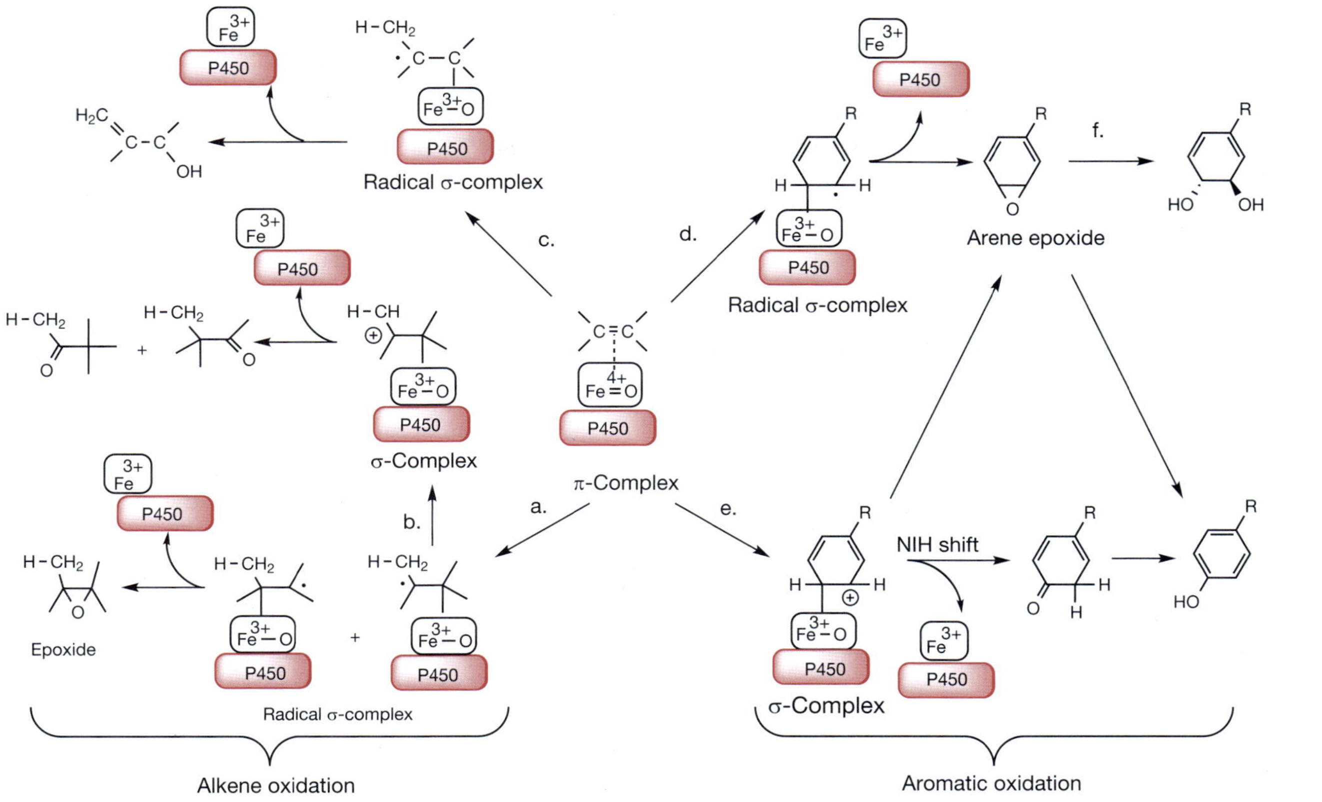

Figure 3.8 Proposed mechanisms for the oxidation of alkene and aromatic compounds.

example, during the P450-catalyzed oxidation of trichloroethylene, a 1,2-shift of chloride occurs to yield chloral (see Fig. 3.9).

Like the alkenes, alkynes (acetylenes) are readily oxidized, but usually faster.[59,61] Depending on which of the two alkyne carbons are attacked, different products are obtained. If attachment of P450 occurs on the terminal alkyne carbon, a R2 group migrates, forming a ketene intermediate that readily hydrolyzes with water to form an acid or that alkylates nucleophilic protein side chains (ie, lysinyl or cysteinyl) to form a protein adduct (Fig. 3.10). The effect of attaching the ferryl oxygen at the internal alkenyl carbon is *N*-alkylation of a pyrrole nitrogen in the porphyrin ring by the terminal acetylene carbon, with the formation of a keto heme adduct. This mechanism has been proposed for the irreversible inactivation of CYP3A4 with the anticancer drug erlotinib and similarly the irreversible effect with the monoamine oxidase inhibitor selegiline.[61]

Aromatic Hydroxylation

In the case of aromatic oxidations (see Fig. 3.8),[5,62,63] following the initial formation of an arene P450 π-complex, one-electron transfer yields either a π-complex or a radical σ-complex. The radical σ-complex can collapse to the arene epoxide (see Fig. 3.8, step d) or the π-complex can proceed to a σ-complex followed by an NIH shift (1,2-group migration) to a phenolic product (see Fig. 3.8, step e). Arene oxides are highly unstable entities and rearrange (NIH shift) nonenzymatically to phenols or hydrolyze enzymatically with epoxide hydrolase to 1,2-dihydrodiols (*trans* configuration) (see Fig. 3.8, step f), which subsequently are dehydrogenated to

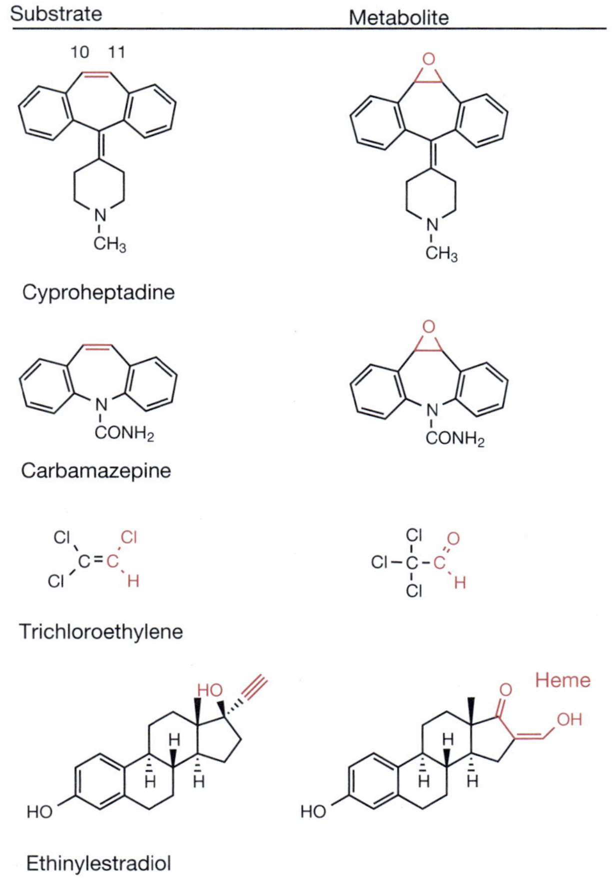

Figure 3.9 Examples of oxidative metabolism of alkenes and alkynes catalyzed by P450.

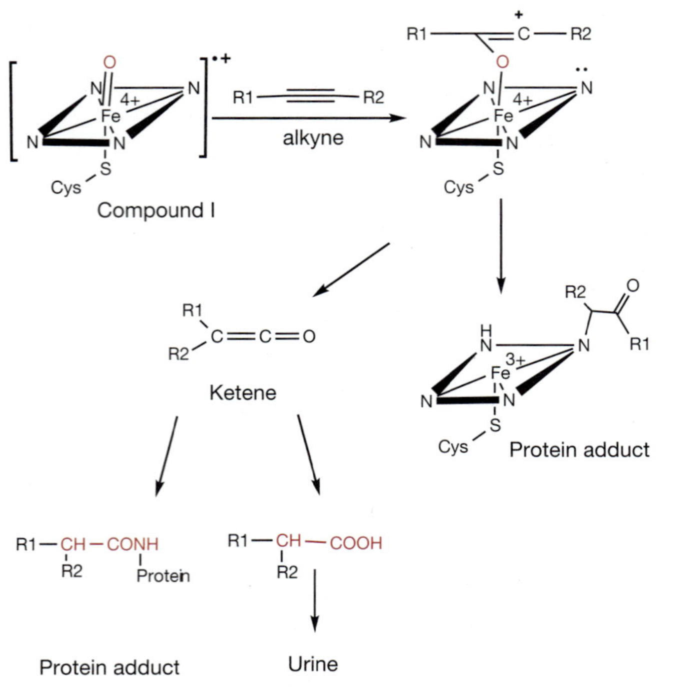

Figure 3.10 Alkyne oxidation catalyzed by P450.

1,2-diphenols (catechols). The oxidation of aromatic compounds can be highly specific to individual P450 isoforms, suggesting that substrate binding and orientation at the active site can dominate the mechanism of oxidative catalysis.

The metabolic oxidation of aromatic carbon atoms by P450 depends on both the isoform catalyzing the oxidation and the oxidation potential of the aromatic compound. The products are typically phenolic, and the position of hydroxylation can be activated/deactivated by the type of substituents on the ring, according to the theories of aromatic electrophilic substitution (see Fig. 3.8). For example, electron-donating substituents enhance *o*- and *p*-hydroxylation, whereas electron-withdrawing substituents reduce or prevent *o*- or *p*-hydroxylation. Moreover, steric factors must also be considered since oxidation occurs mostly at the least hindered position. For monosubstituted benzene compounds, *p*-hydroxylation frequently predominates, with some ortho product also formed (Fig. 3.11). When more than one phenyl ring is present, only one ring is typically hydroxylated (eg, phenytoin).

Traditionally, hydroxylation of aromatic compounds by P450 has been thought to be mediated by an arene oxide (epoxide) intermediate, followed by the NIH shift as discussed previously[5] (see Fig. 3.8). The formation of phenols and the isolation of urinary dihydrodiols, catechols, and phase 2 GSH conjugates (mercapturic acid derivatives) implicate arene oxides as intermediates in the metabolism of both benzene and substituted benzenes. Arene oxides are also prone to conjugate with GSH to form pre-mercapturic acids (see "Glutathione Conjugation and Mercapturic Acid Synthesis" section).

The CYP1A and CYP3A subfamilies are important contributors to 2- and 4-hydroxylation of estradiol, and CYP3A4 is an important contributor to 2-hydroxylation of the synthetic estrogens (eg, 17α-ethinyl estradiol). The principal metabolite (as much as 50%) of estradiol is 2-hydroxyestradiol, with 4-hydroxy and 16α-hydroxyestradiol (estriol) as minor

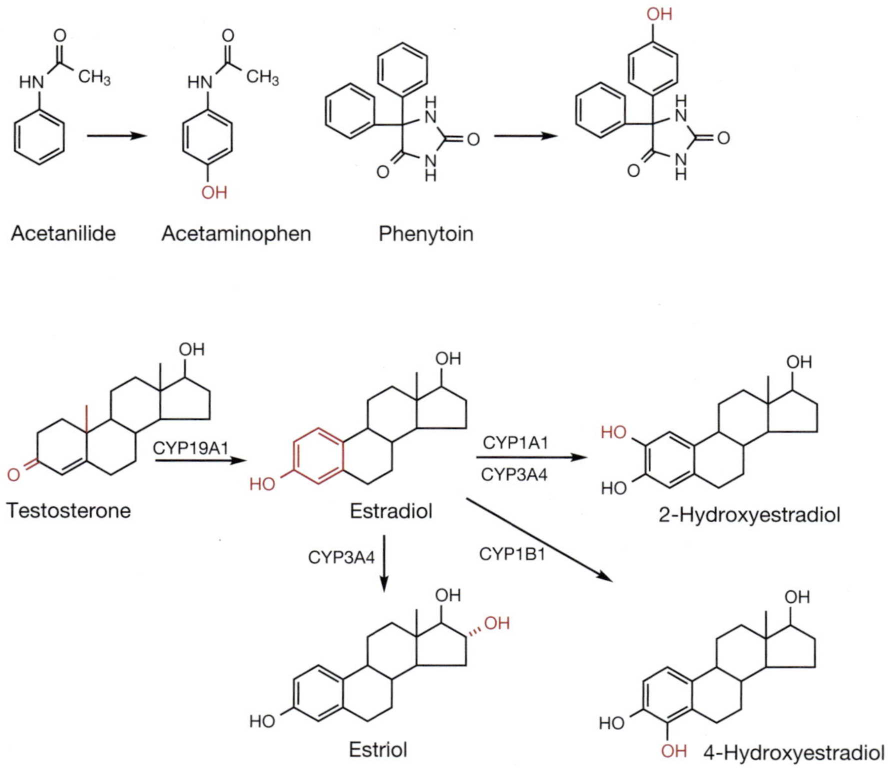

Figure 3.11 Examples of oxidative metabolism of aryl compounds catalyzed by P450.

metabolites (see Fig. 3.11). The 2-hydroxy metabolite of both estradiol and ethinyl estradiol have limited or no estrogenic activity, whereas the C_4 and C_{16} α-hydroxy metabolites have a potency like that of estradiol. In humans, estriol is the primary estrogen metabolite both in pregnancy and in breast cancer. The metabolites 16α-hydroxyestrone and 4-hydroxyestrone can be carcinogenic in specific cells since they are capable of damaging cellular proteins and DNA after activation to quinone intermediates.

Xenobiotic-metabolizing enzymes not only detoxify xenobiotics but also cause the formation of active intermediates (bioactivation), which in certain circumstances can elicit a multitude of toxicities, including mutagenesis, carcinogenesis, and hepatic necrosis. Approximately 66% of all bioactivators of carcinogenics are the P450 enzymes, primarily CYP1A1, CYP1A2, CYP1B1, CYP2A6, CYP2E1, and CYP3A4.[64] In addition to GSH, some nucleophiles such as other sulfhydryl compounds (most effective), alcohols, and phosphates can react with arene oxides. Many of these nucleophiles are found in proteins and nucleic acids. The covalent binding of these bioactive epoxides to intracellular macromolecules provides a molecular basis of these toxic effects.

N-Dealkylation, Oxidative Deamination, and *N*-Oxidation

The accepted mechanism of oxidative *N*-, *O*-, and *S*-dealkylations involves two competing mechanisms: single-electron transfer (SET) or HAT (Fig. 3.12).[5,59] Heteroatom-containing substrates most commonly undergo hydroxylation adjacent (α) to the heteroatom, as compared to other positions. Reactions of this type include *N*-, *O*-, and *S*-dealkylations, as well as dehydrohalogenations and oxidative deamination reactions. The SET pathway involves abstraction of an electron from the heteroatom to produce a radical cation, while the HAT pathway involves hydrogen abstraction. Both pathways are followed by the loss of the α-proton from the more labile α-carbon to generate a carbon radical that can recombine with the ferric hydroxyl radical intermediate (oxygen rebound) to generate an unstable geminal hydroxy heteroatom-substituted intermediate (eg, carbinolamine, halohydrin, hemiacetal, hemiketal, or hemithioketal) that breaks down, releasing the dealkylated heteroatom and forming a carbonyl compound. The resultant carbon radical is stabilized by the heteroatom. However, if the recombination reaction with the ferric hydroxyl radical intermediate (oxygen rebound) is faster than the deprotonation of the α-proton from the adjacent α-carbon, the oxidation will simply result in oxidation of the heteroatom, as in the formation of *N*-oxides or oxidation of sulfides to sulfoxides and/or sulfones. Therefore, whether *N*-dealkylation metabolism occurs by HAT or SET depends on the substrate. A comprehensive compilation of the *N*-dealkylation and *N*-oxidation in drugs has been published.[65]

Xenobiotics containing heteroatoms (*N* and *S*) can also be metabolized by P450-catalyzed oxidation to their corresponding heteroatom oxides (tertiary amines to *N*-oxides, sulfides to sulfoxides and/or sulfones). Heteroatom oxidation can also be attributed to a microsomal flavin-containing monooxygenase (FMO). As is the case with heteroatom α-hydroxylation, one-electron oxidation of the heteroatom occurs as the first step to form the heteroatom ferric hydroxide radical intermediate. This reaction is favored by the absence of α-hydrogens and by the stability of the heteroatom radical cation, which cannot lose a proton, and collapses to generate the heteroatom oxide.[65]

N-DEALKYLATION. Dealkylation of secondary and tertiary amines to yield primary and secondary amines, respectively, is one of the most important and frequently encountered

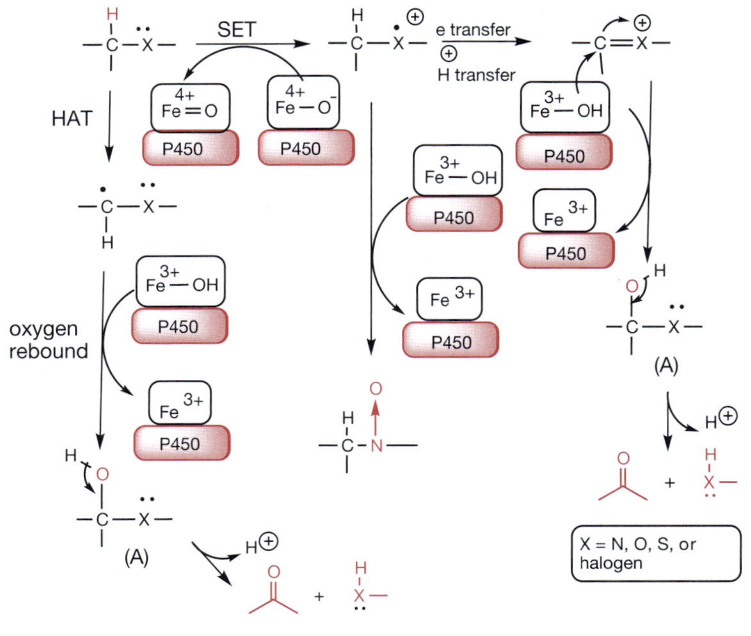

Figure 3.12 Proposed mechanism for heteroatom-compound oxidation, dealkylation, and dehalogenation.

reactions in drug metabolism.[5,65] The proposed mechanism of oxidative *N*-dealkylation involves α-hydrogen abstraction or an electron abstraction from the nitrogen by the ferryl-oxenoid and has been previously discussed (Fig. 3.12).

Typical *N*-substituents removed by oxidative dealkylation are methyl, ethyl, *n*-propyl, isopropyl, *n*-butyl, allyl, and benzyl. Dealkylation occurs most readily with a smaller alkyl group. Substituents that are more resistant to dealkylation include *t*-butyl (no α-hydrogen) and cyclopropylmethyl. In general, tertiary amines are dealkylated to secondary amines faster than secondary amines are dealkylated to primary amines. This rate difference has been correlated with lipid solubility. Appreciable amounts of secondary and primary amines accumulate as metabolites, which are more polar than the parent amine, thus slowing the rate at which the amines diffuse across membranes and reducing their accessibility to receptors. Frequently, these amine metabolites contribute to the pharmacologic activity of the parent substance, as in the case of imipramine in which the major metabolite produced by CYP3A/12A is desipramine (Fig. 3.13), or they produce unwanted side effects, such as hypertension that results from the *N*-dealkylation of *N*-isopropylmethoxamine to methoxamine. The design of an analogous drug without these unwanted metabolites can be achieved by proper choice of replacement substituents, such as substitution of the *N*-isopropyl group in *N*-isopropylmethoxamine with a metabolically stable tert-butyl (*N*-tert-butylmethoxamine or butoxamine).

N-dealkylation of substituted amides and aromatic amines occurs in a similar manner to aliphatic amines. *N*-substituted nonaromatic nitrogen heterocycles undergo oxidation on the α-carbon to a cyclic amide or lactam (eg, nicotine to cotinine), in which the main P450 involved is 2A6. Cotinine is the major nicotine metabolite (~75%) but *N*-dealkylation via CYP2A6 occurs as well (eg, nicotine to nornicotine and cotinine to norcotinine) (see Fig. 3.13).[66] The "nor" in the nomenclature of nornicotine and norcotinine translates to "minus methyl" and is a common prefix in many dealkylated drug metabolites.

OXIDATIVE DEAMINATION. The mechanism of oxidative deamination follows a pathway like that of N-dealkylation. Initially, oxidation to the iminium ion occurs, followed by decomposition to the carbonyl metabolite and ammonia. Oxidative deamination can occur with α-substituted amines, as in the case of amphetamine in which CYP2C catalyzes the formation of the oxidized metabolite (see Fig. 3.13). Some secondary and tertiary amines, as well as amines substituted with bulky groups, can undergo deamination directly without *N*-dealkylation (eg, fenfluramine, diphenhydramine, promethazine). Apparently, this behavior is associated with increased lipid solubility.[65]

***N*-OXIDATION.** In general, *N*-oxygenation of amines forms stable *N*-oxides with tertiary amines, and amides and hydroxylamines with primary and secondary amines. This reaction predominates when no α-hydrogens are available (eg, mephentermine and arylamines) (see Fig. 3.13). Tertiary amines having one or more hydrogens on the adjacent carbon dealkylate via the *N*-oxide. Rearrangement of the

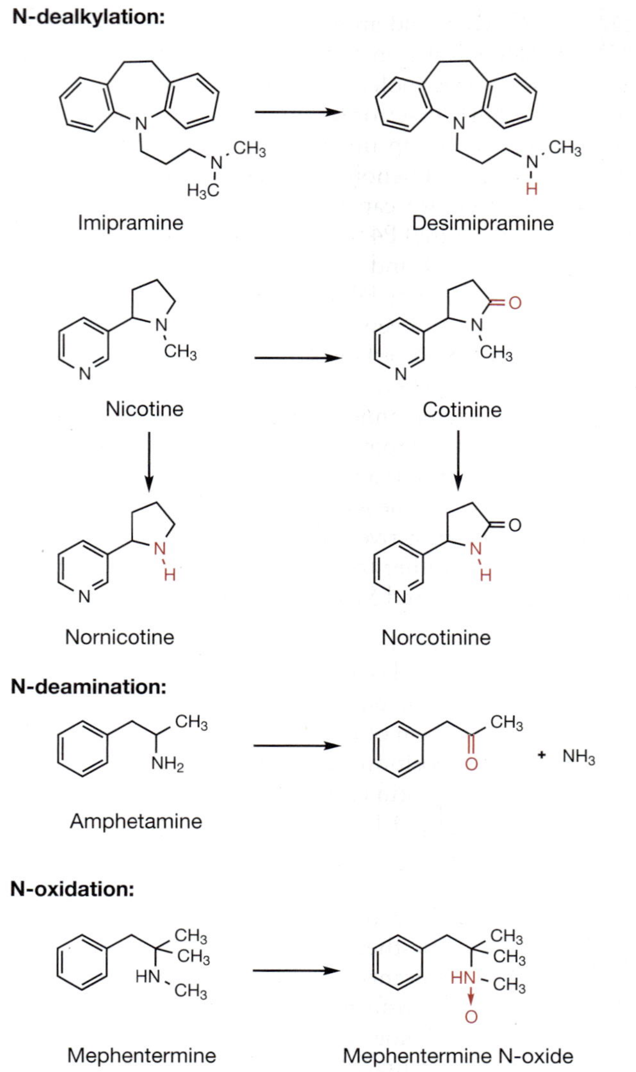

Figure 3.13 Examples of *N*-dealkylation, oxidative deamination, and *N*-oxidation reactions catalyzed by P450.

N-oxide forms a carbinolamine, which subsequently collapses to produce the secondary amine. Amine metabolites can be *N*-conjugated with polar endogenous molecules such as glucuronic acid, increasing their rate of excretion.[65]

***O*- AND *S*-DEALKYLATION.** Oxidative *O*-dealkylation of ethers is a common metabolic reaction with a mechanism analogous to *N*-dealkylation: oxidation of the α-carbon and subsequent decomposition of the unstable hemiacetal to an alcohol (or phenol) and a carbonyl product. *S*-dealkylation of thioethers to hemithioacetals is a minor pathway in comparison to the major direct P450 oxidation of sulfur to sulfoxides and/or sulfones. Sulfone formation can be explained as a result of density functional energies.[67]

Most ether groups in drug molecules are aromatic ethers (eg, codeine, prazosin, and verapamil). For example, codeine is *O*-demethylated to morphine by CYP2D6 (Fig. 3.14). The rate of *O*-dealkylation is a function of chain length, as increasing chain length or branching reduces dealkylation rate. Steric factors and aromatic ring substituents influence the rate of dealkylation but are complicated by electronic effects. Some drug molecules contain more than one ether group, in which case, only one ether is dealkylated. The methylenedioxy group undergoes variable rates of dealkylation to the 1,2-diphenolic metabolite. The metabolism of such a group is also capable of forming a stable complex with (and inhibiting) P450.

By analogy to *O*- and *N*-dealkylations, esters and amides can also be oxidized by P450. In these reactions, the carbon next to the ether-oxygen of an ester or the nitrogen of an amide (termed the α-carbon) is attacked by the enzyme. This reaction is minor due to the significantly more common hydrolysis of esters and amides.

Aliphatic and aromatic methyl thioethers undergo *S*-dealkylation to thiols and carbonyl compounds. For example, 6-methylthiopurine is demethylated by a cocktail of P450 enzymes to give the active anticancer drug 6-mercaptopurine (see Fig. 3.14).[68] Other thioethers are oxidized to sulfoxides or sulfones (see *N*- and *S*-oxidations).

C-DEALKYLATION. While uncommon in drug metabolism, *C*-dealkylation (C-C bond cleavages, methyl oxidations) is also catalyzed by P450 enzymes via *C*-oxidation and elimination. The metabolism of testosterone involves the demethylation of the C_{19} position, and the methyl group is removed and aromatized to form estradiol by the action of CYP19A1 (aromatase) (see Fig. 3.11).[69]

Oxidative Dehalogenation

Many halogenated hydrocarbons, such as insecticides, pesticides, general anesthetics, plasticizers, flame retardants, and commercial solvents, undergo a variety of different dehalogenation biotransformations.[70,71] Because of potential exposure to these halogenated compounds as drugs and environmental pollutants in air, soil, water, or food, it is important to understand the interactions between metabolism and toxicity.

When the carbon bearing the halogen also contains one hydrogen, carbon-centered hydroxylation (C-OH) occurs. The hydroxylated products are unstable and react with loss

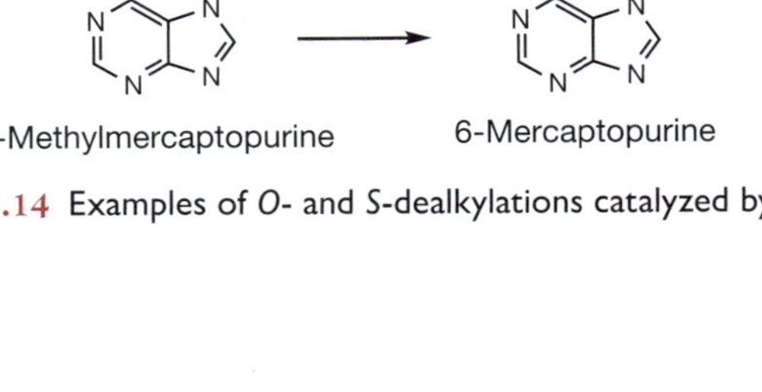

Figure 3.14 Examples of *O*- and *S*-dealkylations catalyzed by P450.

of the halogen to give an aldehyde or a ketone, as in the case of solvent carbon tetrachloride. Halogenated hydrocarbons differ in their chemical reactivity because of the electron-withdrawing properties of the halogens on adjacent carbon atoms, resulting in the α-carbon developing electrophilic character that promotes carbon-centered oxidation (C-OH). The halogen atoms also could stabilize α-carbon cations, free radicals, carbanions, and carbenes. If other halogens are also present in the molecule, then acyl halides result (see Fig. 3.12). Acyl halides can react with macromolecules (protein) and cause hepatotoxicity or immunogenicity. These acyl halides have been implicated in the toxicity of chloroform and halothane. Some halogenated hydrocarbons form GSH or mercapturic acid conjugates, whereas others undergo oxidative dehydrohalogenation (elimination of hydrogen halide such as HCl) and reductive dehalogenation catalyzed by CYP2E1. In many cases, reactive intermediates, including radicals, anions, and cations, are produced that, like acyl halides, can react with a variety of molecules in tissues, resulting in hepatotoxicity or immunogenicity.[72]

Oxidative dehydrohalogenation is a common metabolic pathway of many halogenated hydrocarbons. P450-catalyzed oxidative dehydrohalogenation generates the transient *gem*-halohydrin (analogous to alkane hydroxylation) that can eliminate the hydrohalic acid to form carbonyl derivatives (aldehydes, ketones, acyl halides, and carbonyl halides) (Fig. 3.15). This reaction requires the presence of at least one halogen and one α-hydrogen. *gem*-Trihalogenated hydrocarbons are more readily oxidized than *gem*-dihalogenated and monohalogenated compounds. The acyl and carbonyl halides formed are reactive metabolites that can react either with water to form carboxylic acids that can be conjugated and excreted, or nonenzymatically with tissue molecules, which presents a toxicity risk.[72,73]

The fluranes (see Fig. 3.15) are metabolized by CYP2E1 to reactive intermediates that produce trifluoroacetylated immunogenic protein adducts. The severity of hepatotoxicity is associated with the degree of hepatic metabolism. The hepatotoxicity of halothane and the other fluranes is related to their metabolism to either an acid chloride (or fluoride) or a trifluoroacetate intermediate.[70] The hydroxylated intermediate decomposes spontaneously to reactive intermediates, an acid halide (chloride or fluoride) or trifluoroacetate, that can either react with water to form halide anions and a fluorinated carboxylic acid, or bind covalently to tissue proteins to produce an acylated protein. The acylated protein becomes a hapten, stimulating an immune response and a hypersensitivity reaction. Halothane has received the most attention because of its ability to cause "halothane-associated" hepatitis. This immunologic reaction occurs after repeated exposure in surgical patients to a trifluoroacetylated protein. After subsequent exposure to a fluorinated anesthetic, the antigenic trifluoroacetylated protein stimulates an immunogenic response, producing halothane-like hepatitis. For this reason, halothane is no longer used in general anesthesia in humans.

Because of the common metabolic pathway involving CYP2E1 for enflurane, isoflurane, desflurane, and

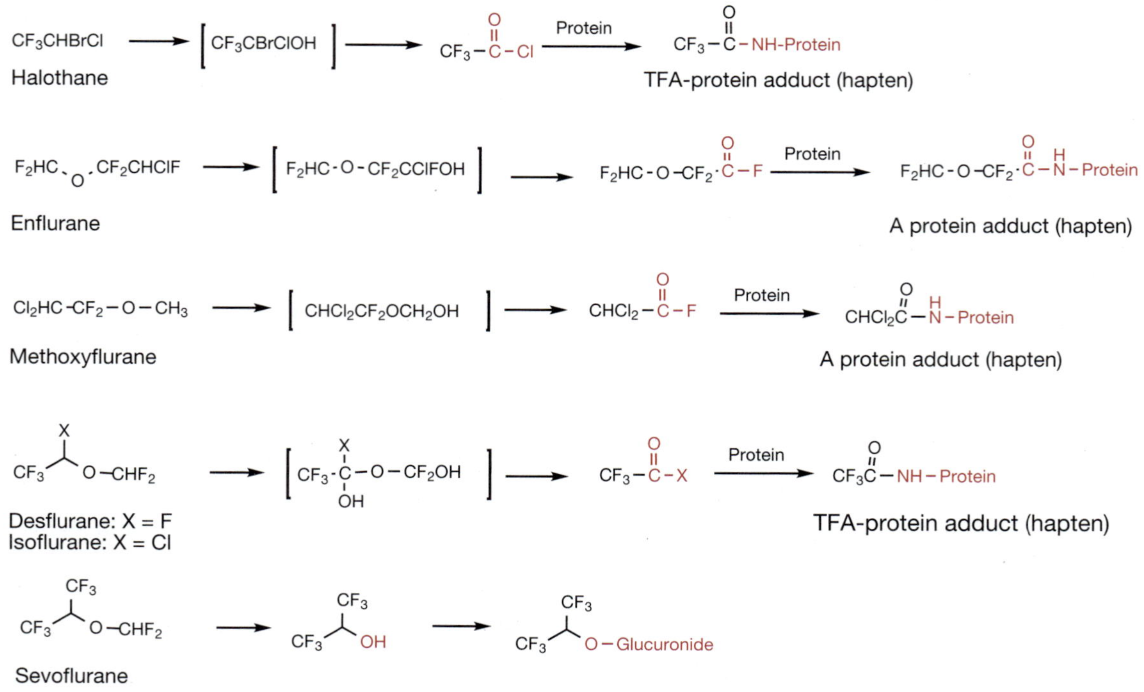

Figure 3.15 CYP2E1-catalyzed metabolism of fluorinated volatile anesthetics to antigenic proteins.

methoxyflurane, patients exposed to halothane who have halothane hepatitis can show cross-sensitivity to one of the other fluranes, triggering an idiosyncratic hepatotoxicity. The formation of antigenic protein is related to the amount of CYP2E1-catalyzed metabolism of each agent: halothane (20%-40%) > enflurane (2%-8%) > isoflurane (0.2%-1.0%) > desflurane (<0.1%). Enough fluoride ion is generated from oxidative dehalogenation during flurane anesthesia to produce subclinical nephrotoxicity. For patients with preexisting liver dysfunction, isoflurane, desflurane, or sevoflurane may be better choices of general anesthetic.[70,74]

Unlike halothane and the other halogenated anesthetics, sevoflurane is not significantly metabolized to hepatotoxic trifluoroacetylated proteins but, rather, is metabolized by O-dealkylation to hexafluoroisopropanol and readily eliminated as the glucuronide (see Fig. 3.15). Approximately 90% of administered sevoflurane is eliminated intact in the patient's expired air. The glucuronide is mostly excreted in urine within 12 hours after anesthesia, whereas trifluoroacetic acid is detectable in urine for up to 12 days after anesthesia.[75]

In today's environment, most humans have been exposed to many CYP2E1-inducing agents (including recreational, industrial, and agricultural chemicals and alcohol). This exposure has an unknown effect on hepatic toxicity from administered volatile anesthetics. Enhanced activity of CYP2E1 has been observed in the case of obesity, isoniazid therapy, ketogenic diets, and alcohol use disorder.

Azo and Nitro Reduction

In addition to the oxidative systems, liver microsomes also contain enzyme systems that catalyze the reduction of azo and nitro compounds to primary amines. A number of azo compounds, such as sulfasalazine (Fig. 3.16), are converted to aromatic primary amines by azoreductase, an NADPH-dependent enzyme system in the liver microsomes.[76] Evidence exists for the participation of P450 in some reductions.[77] Nitro compounds (eg, chloramphenicol and nitrobenzene) are reduced to aromatic primary amines by a nitroreductases, presumably through nitrosamine and hydroxylamine intermediates.[78] Some evidence has been shown for the participation of the P450 enzymes in the reduction to amines.[72,79] These reductases are not solely responsible for reduction of azo and nitro compounds; reduction by the bacterial flora in the anaerobic environment of the intestine can also occur.

In addition to the examples of metabolism of common therapeutic agents listed earlier, other non-canonical or uncommon reactions in which P450 is involved include ring expansion, for example, the metabolism of the antiviral drug efavirenz in which the cyclopropyl ring is converted to a cyclobutenyl ring (Fig. 3.17).[61] Dimerizations are unusual but, in the case of raloxifene (a drug used to treat osteoporosis), a C-C dimerization was generated by the action of CYP3A4. Also, by the action of CYP2C19, an atypical Diels-Alder-type dimer was found as a metabolite of the antiplatelet drug ticlopidine (Fig 3.17).[51,61]

In summary, all known oxidative reactions catalyzed by P450 monooxygenases can be described in the context of a mechanistic scheme that involves the ability of a high-valent ferric iron–oxenoid species to bring about the stepwise one-electron oxidation through the abstraction of hydrogen atoms, abstraction of electrons from heteroatoms, or addition to π-bonds. A series of radical recombination reactions completes the oxidation process.

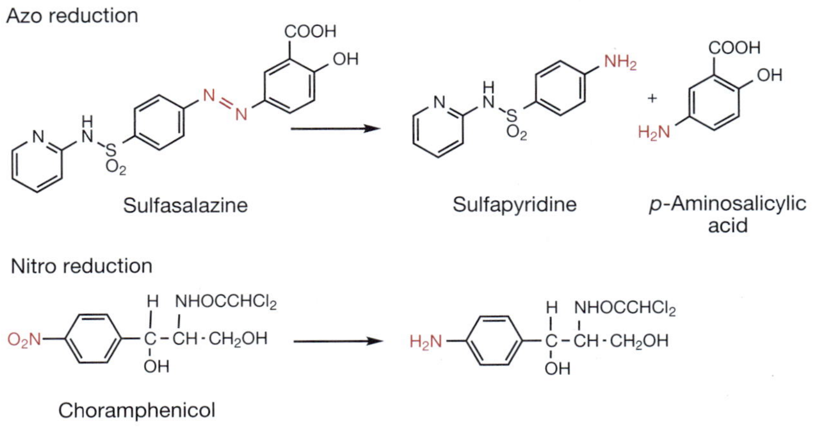

Figure 3.16 P450-catalyzed reduction of azo and nitro compounds.

Induction and Inhibition of Cytochrome P450 Isoforms

Induction

Many of the enzymes involved in drug metabolism can be upregulated by exposure to drugs and environmental chemicals or by other coingested/inhaled compounds. This leads to increased rates of drug metabolism, thereby altering pharmacologic and toxicologic effects.[80-82] Prolonged administration of some drugs or xenobiotics can enhance their own metabolism, along with a wide variety of other compounds. This phenomenon is known as enzyme induction, a dose-dependent phenomenon. Drugs and xenobiotics exert this effect by inducing transcription of P450 mRNA and synthesizing xenobiotic-metabolizing enzymes in the smooth ER of the liver and other extrahepatic tissues. Besides the transcriptional factors, other nontranscriptional mechanisms, including stabilization of mRNA and inhibition of protein degradation routes, have been described.[82] Enzyme induction is an adaptive response associated with increases in liver weight, induction of gene expression, and morphologic changes in hepatocytes. Induction is the process whereby the rate of enzyme synthesis is increased relative to the rate of enzyme synthesis in the uninduced organism. In many older studies of mammalian systems, the term "induction" was inferred from an increase in enzyme activity, but the amount of enzyme protein had not been determined.

Enzyme induction is important to the interpretation of chronic toxicity, mutagenicity, or carcinogenesis events, and to explain certain unexpected DDIs. Enzyme inducers trigger pathways involving the constitutive androstane receptor (CAR), PPAR, AhR, and PXR.[81,82] PXR and CAR are members of the nuclear receptor superfamily and upregulate the expression of P450 proteins responsible for the metabolism and excretion of these xenobiotics. Thus, it is a key regulator of xenobiotic P450 metabolism.

Predictions and in vitro evaluation on the inducers and inhibitors of the P450 enzymes are a functional part of the drug discovery paradigm. Currently, FDA guidelines require the evaluation of CYP1A2, CYP2B6, CYP2C8, CYP2C9, CYP2C19, and CYP3A4 for a potential drug induction.[83]

Many drugs and xenobiotics induce/stimulate the upregulation of P450 isoforms, as shown in Table 3.13. These inducers have nothing in common so far as their pharmacologic activities or chemical structures are concerned, but they are all metabolized by one or more of the P450 isoforms. Most of them are lipid soluble at physiologic pH. PAHs in cigarette smoke, xanthines and flavones in foods, several herbal products, halogenated hydrocarbons in insecticides, polychlorinated biphenyls, and food additives are but a few of the environmental chemicals that alter the activities of P450 enzymes.[80,81]

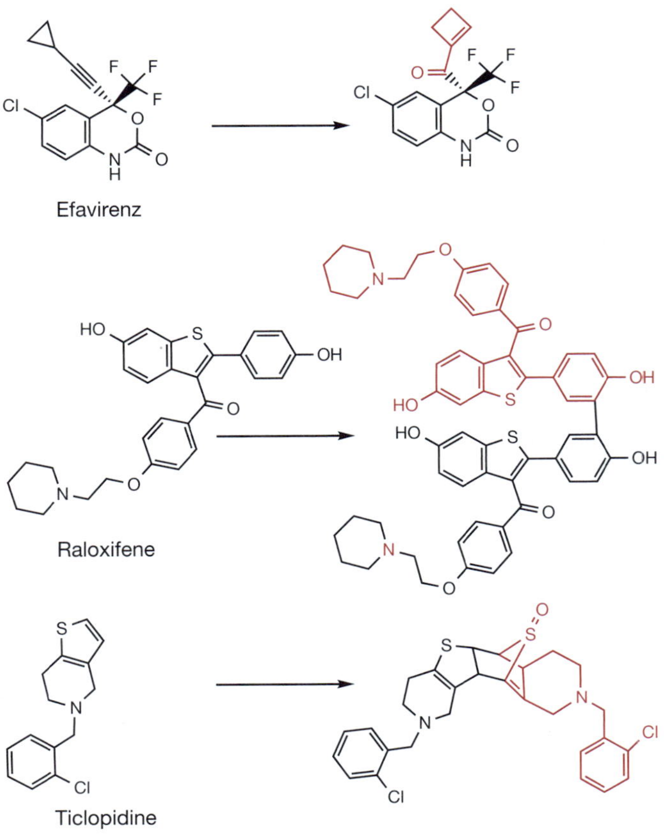

Figure 3.17 P450 miscellaneous reactions.

Table 3.13 Drugs That Induce the Expression of P450 Isoforms

Drug	Enzymes
Abemaciclib	1A2, 2B6, 3A4
Amprenavir	3A4
Aprepitant	2C9
Barbiturates	3A4, 2C9, 2C19, 2B6
Cabozantinib	1A1
Carbamazepine	1A2, 3A4, 2C8, 2C9, 2D6, 2B6
Charbroiled meats	1A1/2
Cigarette smoke	1A1/2
Clotrimazole	1A1/2, 3A4
Dabrafenib	2B6, 2C9, 3A4
Efavirenz	3A4
Encorafenib	2B6, 2C9, 3A4
Erlotinib	3A4
Erythromycin	3A4
Ethanol	2D6, 2E1
Ethosuximide	3A4
Glucocorticoids (Dexamethasone, prednisone)	3A4, 2A6, 2C19
Griseofulvin	3A4
Lansoprazole	1A1/2, 3A4
Lorlatinib	2A6, 2B6
Mephenytoin	2B6
4-Methylpyrazole	2E1
Midostaurin	1A2, 2B6, 3A4
Modafinil	1A2, 2B6, 3A4
Nevirapine	3A4, 2B6
Norethindrone	2C19
Olaparib	2B6
Omeprazole	1A1/2, 3A4
Oxcarbazepine	3A4
Palbociclib	1A2, 2B6
Phenobarbital	3A4, 2C, 2B6, 2D6, 1A2
Phenytoin	3A4, 1A2, 2B6, 2C8, 2C19, 2D6
Polycyclic aromatic hydrocarbons	1A1/2
Primidone	3A4, 2C9, 1A2, 2B6, 2D6
Psoralen	1A1/2
Rifabutin	2C8, 3A4
Rifampin	2C8, 2C9, 2C19, 2D6, 3A4, 2B6
Rifapentine	3A4
Ritonavir	1A2, 2B6, 2C8, 2C9, 2C19
St. John's wort	1A2, 2C9, 3A4
Topiramate	3A4

Drugs in bold italic have been reported to cause drug-drug interaction.

Enzyme induction, which can last as long as 1 to 3 weeks before drug blood levels decrease, can alter the pharmacokinetics and pharmacodynamics of a drug, with clinical implications for the therapeutic actions of the drug as well as increased potential for DDIs. Because of induction, a drug can be metabolized more rapidly to metabolites that are more potent, more toxic, or less active than the parent drug. Induction can also enhance the activation of procarcinogens or promutagens.

Not all inducing agents enhance their own metabolism; for example, phenytoin induces CYP3A4 but is hydroxylated by CYP2C9. Some of the more common enzyme inducers of P450 subfamilies, which can also be substrates for the same P450 isoforms, include phenobarbital (CYP2B6, CYP2C, and CYP3A4), rifampicin (CYP3A4), and cigarette smoke (CYP1A1/2) (see Table 3.13). The broad range of drugs metabolized by these P450 subfamilies (see Table 3.12) that are also affected by these enzyme inducers raise the issue of clinically significant DDIs and their clinical implications. Examples of a clinically significant P450 DDI and an herbal-drug interaction are rifampin and oral contraceptives, and St. John's wort and oral contraceptives, respectively. Both rifampin and St. John's wort induce the expression of CYP3A4. This reduces the serum levels of the oral contraceptive due to increased oxidative metabolism of the oral contraceptives by CYP3A4 to form less active metabolites, thereby increasing the risk for pregnancy. Drugs poorly metabolized by P450 enzymes are less affected by enzyme induction.

Rifampin, a strong human PXR agonist, provides an example of a drug whose actions and metabolism are closely connected. PXR protein level is regulated by mRNA, which in turn affects the expression levels of *CYP3* and *CYP2* genes. Rifampin is metabolized by many members of the CYP2 and CYP3 families and, therefore, the rifampin target protein and metabolizing enzyme levels are simultaneously impacted by the same RNA stimulus.[84]

Inducers of P450 isoforms can stimulate oxidative metabolism of endogenous substances: for example, the hydroxylation of androgens, estrogens, progestational steroids (synthetic oral contraceptives), and glucocorticoids, which decreases their biologic activity. These enzyme inducers might also be implicated in deficiencies associated with these steroids. For example, the induction of C_2 hydroxylation of estradiol and synthetic estrogens by phenobarbital, dexamethasone, or cigarette smoking in women results in the increased formation of the principal (and less active) metabolite of these estrogenic substances, reducing their effectiveness. Thus, along with other serious health risks, cigarette smoking in premenopausal women could result in an estrogen deficiency, increasing the risks of osteoporosis and early menopause. Postmenopausal women who smoke and take estrogen replacement therapy risk decreasing the effectiveness of the estrogen.

In addition to enhancing the metabolism of other drugs, many compounds, when chronically administered, stimulate their own metabolism, thereby decreasing their therapeutic activity and producing a state of apparent tolerance. This self-induction can explain some of the changes in drug toxicity observed during prolonged treatments. The duration of the sedative action of phenobarbital, for example, becomes shorter with repeated doses, and this can be explained, in part, on increased inactivating metabolism via enzyme induction.

The time course of induction varies with different inducing agents and with different P450 isoforms. AhR is activated by several environmental contaminants and some drugs, including omeprazole. It also regulates the expression of the CYP1 family, of which only CYP1A2 plays an important role in hepatic metabolism. Increased transcription of P450 mRNA has been detected as early as 1 hour after administration of phenobarbital, with maximum induction occurring after 48 to 72 hours. After administration of PAH such as 3-methylcholanthrene and benzo[a]pyrene, maximum induction of the CYP1A subfamily is reached within 24 hours. Less potent inducers of hepatic drug metabolism can take as long as 6 to 10 days to produce maximum induction.[84]

Exposure to a variety of different xenobiotics can increase the hepatic content of specific isoforms of P450. Therefore, the process of enzyme induction involves the adaptive increase in the content of specific enzymes in response to the enzyme-inducing agent. Inducible phase 2 metabolizing enzymes include uridine diphosphate (UDP)-glucuronosyltransferase (UGT) and GSH transferase (see "Drug Conjugation Pathways [Phase2]" section).

Specific Inducers

PHENOBARBITAL AND RIFAMPIN. Phenobarbital and rifampin are the most extensively studied enzyme inducers. Phenobarbital is an indirect CAR activator, involving repression of epidermal growth factor receptor and reduction of activated C kinase 1 phosphorylation. These drugs alter the pharmacokinetics and pharmacodynamics of many concurrently administered drugs listed in Tables 3.7 (CYP2C) and 3.10 (CYP3A4), which raises the issue of clinically significant DDIs.

CIGARETTE SMOKE. Cigarette smoke has been shown to induce the activity of CYP1A1, CYP1A2, and UGT enzymes, mostly due to the high content of PAHs. A stimulation of the CYP1A1/2 metabolism of several drugs, and a decrease in their pharmacologic action, is the result. Cigarette smoking has been reported to lower blood levels of drugs metabolized by CYP1A1/2, including the antipsychotics clozapine and olanzapine; the antidepressants fluvoxamine, duloxetine, and imipramine; and several steroidal contraceptives, among others. Smoking also decreases urinary excretion of nicotine and the drowsiness caused by chlorpromazine, diazepam, and chlordiazepoxide.[85]

ALCOHOL. Alcoholics show an increase in CYP2E1 enzyme activity, leading to more rapid clearance of drugs and xenobiotics that are substrates for this isoform. As discussed previously, hepatic CYP2E1 oxidizes ethanol, and chronic ethanol intake increases the activity of CYP2E1 by enzyme induction through PPAR downregulation. Ethanol also can cause intestinal CYP3A induction. The changes in drug metabolism in alcoholics can also be attributed to other factors, such as malnutrition, coadministered drugs, and the trace chemicals that are sources of flavors and odors of alcoholic beverages. Heavy drinkers metabolize phenobarbital, tolbutamide, and phenytoin more rapidly, which can be clinically important when adjusting drug therapies for those with alcohol use disorder.

Inhibition

Another pathway to altered in vivo effects of xenobiotics metabolized by P450s is the concomitant use of inhibitors (see Table 3.11). The P450 inhibitors can be divided broadly into two large categories according to their mechanisms of action: reversible inhibition and irreversible inhibition.[86] The polysubstrate nature of P450 is responsible for the large number of documented interactions associated with the inhibition of drug oxidation and biotransformation. Clinically significant inhibitors for notable P450s have been published.[81] As with induction, inhibition plays an important part in the drug discovery paradigm, and FDA drug approval requires evaluation in silico and in vitro for CYP1A2, CYP2B6, CYP2C8, CYP2C9, CYP2C19, CYP2D6, CYP3A4, and CYP3A5 inhibition.[83,87]

Reversible Inhibition

Reversible inhibition of P450 is the result of reversible interactions at the heme iron active center of P450, the lipophilic sites on the apoprotein, or both. The interaction occurs before the oxidation steps of the catalytic cycle and the effects dissipate quickly when the inhibitor is discontinued. These inhibitors act quickly without destroying the enzyme. The most effective reversible inhibitors are those that interact strongly with both the apoprotein and the heme iron. Reversible inhibition can be competitive, noncompetitive, uncompetitive, and mixed. If two drugs compete for the same active site on the enzyme as independent substrates, it is known as competitive inhibition. In a noncompetitive relationship, one drug must be bound in a separate enzyme site, for example, an allosteric site, while the other binds to the orthosteric (active) site. In uncompetitive inhibition, one drug will bind only in a complex between the enzyme and the drug substrate.

It is widely accepted that inhibition has an important impact on the oxidative metabolism and pharmacokinetics of drugs that have a metabolism that overlaps with that of an inhibitor (see Tables 3.3 and 3.7-3.10).[84,86] Some drugs that interact reversibly with P450 are shown in Table 3.11. The imidazole-based azole antifungals are potent inhibitors of CYP3A4 and of the P450-mediated biosynthesis of endogenous steroid hormones. The azole antifungals noted in this table exert their fungistatic effects through inhibition of fungal P450, inhibiting the oxidative biosynthesis of lanosterol to ergosterol, thereby affecting the integrity and permeability of the fungal membranes.

Irreversible Inhibition

Irreversible inhibition of P450 is the result of an interaction of a drug with the enzyme, resulting in a tight or irreversible (covalent) binding within the active site or other site (eg, allosteric), leading to its inactivation or formation of a more potent inhibitory species. Irreversible inhibition is time dependent and includes different mechanisms such as metabolite complexation, formation of inhibitory product, and true mechanism-based inhibition. Another mechanism, termed "tight binding inhibition," was differentiated due to its slow reversibility.[49,86]

P450 COMPLEXATION INHIBITION. Some alkylamine drugs can undergo P450-mediated oxidation to nitrosoalkane metabolites, which have high affinities for the P450 heme iron active center and form stable complexes with the reduced (ferrous form) heme-P450 intermediates of the CYP2B, CYP2C, and CYP3A subfamilies. Thus, the P450 isoform is unavailable for further oxidation, and synthesis of the new enzyme is required to restore P450 activity. The process relies on at least one iteration of the P450 catalytic cycle to generate the required heme intermediate.[49] The macrolide antibiotics troleandomycin, erythromycin, and clarithromycin, as well as their analogs, are selective inhibitors of CYP3A4 and are capable of inducing expression of hepatic and extrahepatic CYP3A4 mRNA and of inducing their own biotransformation into nitrosoalkane metabolites that covalently bind to the CYP3A4 active site. The clinical significance of this inhibition with CYP3A4 is the perpetual impairment of metabolism of many coadministered substrates of this isoform, and the potential for DDIs and time-dependent nonlinearities in their pharmacokinetics upon long-term administration (Tables 3.11 and 3.12). A second example is methylenedioxyphenyl compounds (ie, the antidepressant paroxetine, the insecticide synergist piperonyl butoxide, and the flavoring agent isosafrole), which generate metabolic intermediates that form stable complexes with both the ferric and ferrous state of P450.

TRUE MECHANISM-BASED INHIBITION. Certain drugs that are not direct inhibitors of P450 contain functional groups that, when oxidized by P450, generate metabolites that irreversibly bind to the enzyme.[49] This process is termed "mechanism-based inhibition" ("suicide inhibition") and requires at least one catalytic P450 cycle, either during or subsequent to the oxygen transfer step, when the drug is activated to the inhibitory species. This is distinguished from the generation of reactive products in that a reactive entity is generated in the course of the reaction but does not leave the enzyme. Alkenes and alkynes were the first functionalities found to inactivate P450 by generation of a radical intermediate that alkylates the heme structure (see "Alkene and Alkyne Hydroxylation" section). Iron is lost from the heme and abnormal *N*-alkylated porphyrins are produced. Drugs that are mechanism-based inhibitors of P450 include: (1) the 17α-acetylenic estrogen 17α-ethinyl estradiol, the 17α-acetylenic progestin norethindrone (norethisterone), and their radical intermediates that *N*-alkylate the heme of CYP3A4; (2) cyclophosphamide and its acrolein and phosphoramide mustard decomposition products that alkylate CYP2B6 apoprotein; (3) spironolactone and its 7-thio metabolite that alkylates heme; (4) 8-methoxypsoralen (a furocoumarin) and its epoxide metabolite that alkylates the P450 apoprotein of CYP2A6; (5) nicotine that inactivates CYP1A6 and CYP1A13 isoforms; (6) isoniazid that alkylates CYP1A2, CYP2A6, CYP2C19, and CYP3A4 isoforms; (7) 21-halosteroids; (8) halocarbons; and (9) secobarbital. The selectivity of P450 isoform destruction by several of these inhibitors indicates involvement of specific isoforms in the bioactivation of such drugs.

P450 GENERATION OF REACTIVE METABOLITES. A reactive product or metabolite generated by P450 can covalently modify other endogenous biomolecules to produce an antigenic determinant called a neoantigen. Activated quinones, quinone imines, epoxides, and other electrophilic species are examples of these. Hydroxylation of a -$CHCl_2$ moiety in chloramphenicol yields a *gem*-halohydrin (-CH(OH)Cl) and then an acyl chloride (-C(O)Cl), which reacts with lysine residues in various biomolecules.

Oxidations Catalyzed by Flavin Monooxygenase

FMO oxidizes drugs, xenobiotics, and environmental chemicals containing a soft nucleophile, usually nitrogen or sulfur. A soft nucleophile is a group that has a weak tendency to donate or share its electrons and, thus, a low charge density and large polarizable orbitals. FMO is a monooxygenase but, unlike P450, utilizes the two electron-reducing equivalents of NADPH (as hydride anion) in one step to reduce one atom of molecular oxygen to water while the other oxygen atom is used to oxidize the substrate. Because oxygen activation occurs in two steps before substrate addition, any compound binding to 4α-hydroperoxyflavin, the enzyme-bound monooxygenating FMO intermediate, is a potential substrate. The products formed from FMO-catalyzed oxidation are consistent with a two-electron oxidation of the heteroatom. Unlike P450, FMO does not catalyze epoxidation reactions or hydroxylation reactions at unactivated carbon atoms of xenobiotics. FMO and P450 also exhibit similar tissue and cellular locations, molecular weights, and substrate specificities, and exist as multiple enzymes.

Humans express five different flavin monooxygenases (FMO1, FMO2, FMO3, FMO4, and FMO5) in a tissue-specific manner, each with different substrate specificities. Unlike P450, the human FMO functional gene family consists of five families each expressing a single protein. Three of the five expressed human FMO genes, *FMO1*, *FMO2*, and *FMO3*, exhibit genetic polymorphisms. FMO1 is the major form expressed in the liver and kidney during neonatal development and in the small intestine in adults. FMO2 is expressed mainly in human lungs. Importantly, FMO3 is the prominent form in adult human liver and likely associated with the bulk of FMO-mediated metabolism (>50%). It also contributes to the disease known as trimethylaminuria. Because of their low expression, little is known about the substrate specificity for FMO4 and FMO5. Thus, these enzymes do not contribute significantly (<5%) to human drug metabolism.[88]

The catalytic cycles of FMO and P450 are very different. For example, FMO does not require a reductase to transfer electrons from NADPH. Another distinction is the lack of induction of FMOs by xenobiotics. In general, P450 is the major contributor to oxidative xenobiotic metabolism.

However, FMO activity may be of significance in several reactions involving *N*- or *S*-oxygenation and should not be overlooked. FMO and P450 have overlapping substrate specificities but often yield different metabolites with potentially diverse toxicologic/pharmacologic consequences.

The physiologic functions of FMO are poorly understood, although recently FMO1 has been identified as a regulator of energy balance, promoting metabolic efficiency through *FMO* knockout mouse lines.[89] Unlike P450, which exhibits interindividual variation in expression to both genetic and environmental factors, FMO is not regulated by environmental factors, and interindividual variability in FMO enzyme expression would be predominately genetic in origin.

N- and *S*-Oxygenations

FMO constitutes an alternative biotransformation pathway for converting *N*- and *S*-containing lipophilic drugs and xenobiotics to more polar metabolites that are more efficiently excreted in the urine. Typically, FMO catalyzes oxygenation of the *N*- and *S*-heteroatoms (soft nucleophiles) (Fig. 3.18), excluding heteroatom dealkylation reactions. FMO is not normally inducible by phenobarbital, nor is it affected by P450 inhibitors. With few exceptions, however, xenobiotic substrates of FMO are also substrates of the P450 isoforms, producing similar oxidation products. Which monooxygenase is responsible for the oxidation can be readily determined because FMO is thermally labile in the absence of NADPH, whereas P450 is stable.

Of the many nitrogens-containing functional groups in xenobiotics, only secondary and tertiary acyclic, cyclic, and arylamines, as well as hydroxylamines and hydrazines, are oxidized by FMO and excreted in urine (see Fig. 3.18). The tertiary amines form stable amine oxides (*N*-oxides) that are highly polar, hydrophilic, and less basic compounds, and that can be reduced back to the parent tertiary amine in the GI tract. On the other hand, secondary amines are sequentially oxidized to the potentially toxic hydroxylamines, nitrones, and a complex mixture of products, oximes, and nitroso compounds. Secondary *N*-alkylarylamines can be *N*-oxygenated to reactive *N*-hydroxylated metabolites, which are responsible for the toxic, mutagenic, and carcinogenic activity of these compounds. For example, the chemically unstable hydroxylamine intermediates of aromatic amines degrade into bladder carcinogens (see "Glucuronic Acid Conjugation" section), and the hydroxamic acid intermediates of *N*-arylacetamides are bioactivated into liver carcinogens. Hepatic FMO, however, will not catalyze the oxidation of primary alkyl- or arylamines, except for the carcinogenic *N*-hydroxylated derivatives of 2-aminofluorene, 2-aminoanthracene, and other amino PAHs.

S-oxidation occurs almost exclusively by FMO (see Fig. 3.18). Sulfides are oxidized to sulfoxides and sulfones; thiols to disulfides and thiocarbamates; mercaptopyrimidines and mercaptoimidazoles (ie, the antithyroid drug methimazole) via sulfenate anions (RSO^-) to sulfinate anions (R-SO-O), all of which are eliminated in the urine. FMO *S*-oxygenates a number of sulfur-containing substrates. The hepatotoxicity of thioureas (eg, the antimycobacterial drug ethionamide) is the result of metabolic bioactivation through FMO3-dependent *S*-oxidation to produce toxic sulfinic acid metabolites. Other heteroatoms including boron, phosphorous, selenium, and iodine can be oxidized by the action of FMO enzymes.[90] In contrast, primary aromatic amines and amides, aromatic heterocyclic amines and imines, and the aliphatic primary amine phentermine are *N*-oxidized by P450 to hydroxylamines.

Catalytic Cycle for Flavin Monooxygenase

The major steps in the catalytic cycle for FMO are shown in Figure 3.19.[88,89,91] Like most of the other monooxygenases, FMO requires NADPH and oxygen as cofactors to catalyze the oxidation of the xenobiotic substrate. Unlike P450, however, the xenobiotic being oxidized does not need to be bound to the 4α-hydroperoxyflavin intermediate (FAD-OOH) for oxygen activation to occur. FMO is present within the cell in its enzyme-bound activated hydroperoxide (Enz-FAD-OOH) state, ready to oxidize any suitable lipophilic substrate that binds to it. The FMO uses a nonradical, nucleophilic displacement type of mechanism binding dioxygen with a reduced flavin. The reactive oxygen intermediate is a reactive derivative of hydrogen peroxide, flavin-4α-hydroperoxide (see Fig. 3.19), which is reactive enough to successfully attack a lone electron pair on a heteroatom, such as nitrogen or sulfur, but not reactive enough to abstract a hydrogen atom from a typical C-H bond. Studies suggest the xenobiotic substrate interacts with the 4α-hydroperoxyflavin form of FMO and is oxidized by oxygen transfer from Enz-FAD-OOH to form the oxidized product. Steps 2 through 5 in Figure 3.19 simply regenerate the oxygenating agent Enz-FAD-OOH from Enz-FAD-OH, NADPH, oxygen, and a proton. If there is no substrate that can be oxygenated nearby in step 5, it will release peroxide and $NADPH^+$. Any compound readily crossing cell membranes and penetrating to the FMO-bound hydroperoxyflavin intermediate is a potential substrate, thus explaining the broad substrate specificity exhibited by FMO. The fact that the xenobiotic substrate is not required for activation of the FMO-hydroperoxyflavin state distinguishes FMO from P450 monooxygenases, in which substrate binding initiates the P450 catalytic cycle and activation of oxygen to the ferryl-oxenoid intermediate. It is not unusual for FMO oxidation products to undergo reduction to the parent xenobiotic, which can enter into repeated redox reactions (termed "metabolic cycling").

Results of substrate specificity studies suggest that the number of ionic groups on an endogenous substrate is an important factor in enabling FMO to distinguish between xenobiotic and endogenous substrates, thus preventing the indiscriminate oxidation of physiologically important amine and sulfur compounds. Without exception, FMO readily catalyzes the oxidation of uncharged amines or sulfur compounds (in equilibrium with its respective monocation or monoanion; for sulfur compounds, the charge is on sulfur atom). The FMO will not catalyze the oxidation of dianions (eg, thiamine pyrophosphate), dications (eg, polyamines), dipolar ions (eg, amino acids and peptides), or other polyionic compounds with one or more anionic

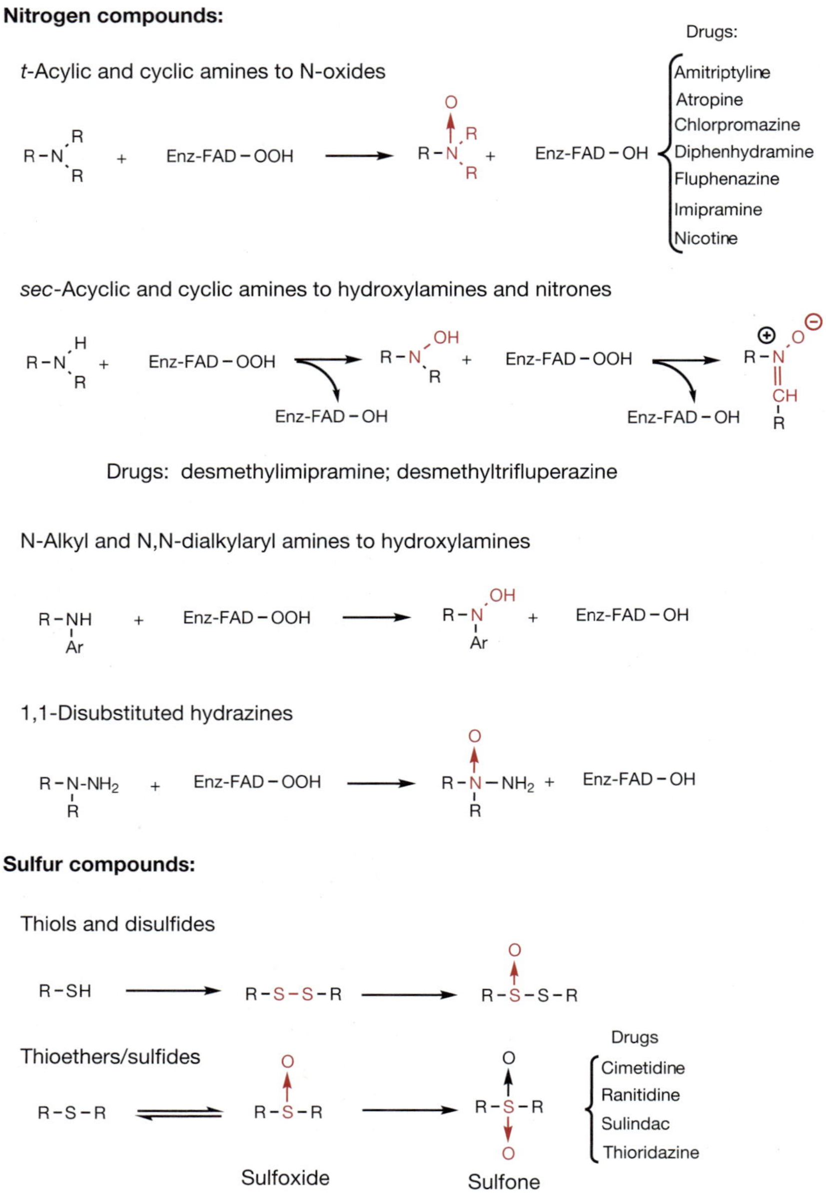

Figure 3.18 Examples of flavin monooxygenase oxidations.

groups (eg, COO^-) distal to the heteroatom (eg, coenzyme A [CoA]). For *N*- or *S*-oxygenations, FMO5 is capable of adding an oxygen atom in the carbon-carbon bond adjacent to a carbonyl to form an ester or lactone in a Baeyer-Villiger oxidation.[48,88]

All five isoforms of hepatic FMO have been characterized in the adult human liver.[92] As noted, FMO1 is the major form in fetal liver. The availability of different forms of FMO can be of clinical importance in the pharmacologic and toxicologic properties of FMO-dependent drug oxidations.

FMO3 specifically *N*-oxygenates primary, secondary, and tertiary amines, whereas FMO1 is only efficient at *N*-oxygenating tertiary amines. FMO3, the most important isoform in adult metabolism, is sensitive to steric features of the substrate, and aliphatic amines with linkages of at least five carbons between the nitrogen atom and a large aromatic group (eg, phenothiazines) are *N*-oxygenated significantly more efficiently than substrates with a two- or three-carbon spacer. Amines with smaller aromatic substituents (eg, phenethylamines) are often efficiently *N*-oxygenated by FMO3. Interindividual variation in FMO3-dependent metabolism of drugs, xenobiotics, and environmental chemicals is more likely because of genetic differences, rather than environmental effects.

Certain mutations of the *FMO3* gene have been associated with deficient *N*-oxygenation of trimethylamine, which results in a rare inherited genetic condition called trimethylaminuria (fish odor syndrome). Allelic variations of FMO3 might cause abnormal metabolism of drugs, which has clinical implications for human drug metabolism. For example,

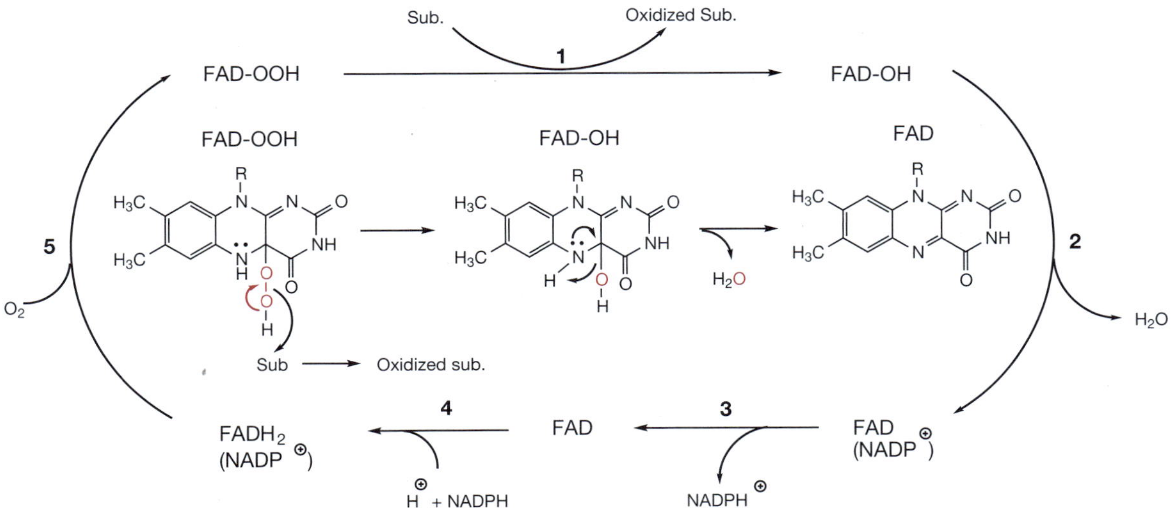

Figure 3.19 Flavin monooxygenase (FMO) catalytic cycle. Oxygenated substrate is formed by nucleophilic attack of a substrate (Sub.) by the terminal oxygen of the enzyme-bound hydroperoxyflavin (FAD-OOH), followed by heterolytic cleavage of the peroxide (1). The release of H_2O (2) or of $NADP^+$ (3) is rate limiting for reactions catalyzed by liver FMO. Reduction of flavin by NADPH (4) and addition of oxygen (5) complete the cycle by regeneration of the oxygenated FAD-OOH. $NADP^+$, nicotinamide adenine dinucleotide phosphate; NADPH, reduced form of nicotinamide adenine dinucleotide phosphate.

(S)-Nicotine N_1'-oxide formation is a highly stereoselective product of FMO3 in adult humans who smoke cigarettes, inducing a reduction in nicotine dependence without reducing cigarette consumption.[93] Thus, *FMO3* gene polymorphism and PM phenotype in certain human populations could contribute to adverse drug reactions or exaggerated clinical response to certain medications.[94] *FMO3* may be another example of an environmental gene that participates in a protective mechanism to help shield humans from potentially toxic exposure to chemicals.[95]

Peroxidases and Other Monooxygenases

Peroxidases are hemoproteins that are closely related enzymes to P450 monooxygenase. Peroxidases belong to the phylogenetic peroxidase-cyclooxygenase (COX) superfamily of heme peroxidases: myeloperoxidase (MPO), COX, eosinophil peroxidase (EPO), lactoperoxidase (LPO), thyroid peroxidase (TPO), peroxidasin (PXDN), and peroxidasin-like protein (PXDNL) are the six members of this superfamily.[96,97] There are also pseudo-peroxidases that interact with peroxide indirectly, as their active sites are not designed to catalyze the reduction of peroxide to water.[97] The differences between peroxidase and P450 include replacement of the cysteine axial ligand of P450 with a histidine residue and the inclusion of polar amino acids within proximity of the heme-active site. These polar amino acid differences allow the peroxidase to rapidly catalyze the reduction of hydroperoxides to alcohol (water in the case of hydrogen peroxide) and the simultaneous reoxidation of peroxidase. The normal course of peroxide (ROOH)-catalyzed oxidation involves the formation of the ferryl-oxo intermediate, analogous to the ferryl-oxenoid complex in P450.

Figure 3.20 shows a basic mechanism for peroxidases, which is simpler than that of P450. Unlike P450, which can abstract a hydrogen atom from almost any type of substrate, peroxidase-catalyzed oxidation of drugs and xenobiotics is limited to electron-rich substrates that are easily oxidized (eg, heteroatom oxygenation, aromatization [oxidation] of 1,4-dihydropyridines [calcium channel blockers] and arylamines). Another important role of heme peroxidases is the oxidation of halogenated compounds under physiologic conditions.[98]

COX (also known as prostaglandin synthase or prostaglandin endoperoxide synthetase) is a widely distributed heme-peroxidase enzyme responsible for the formation of important biologic mediators, called prostanoids, from arachidonic acid. These essential prostanoids include prostaglandins, prostacyclin, and thromboxane. COX catalyzes the

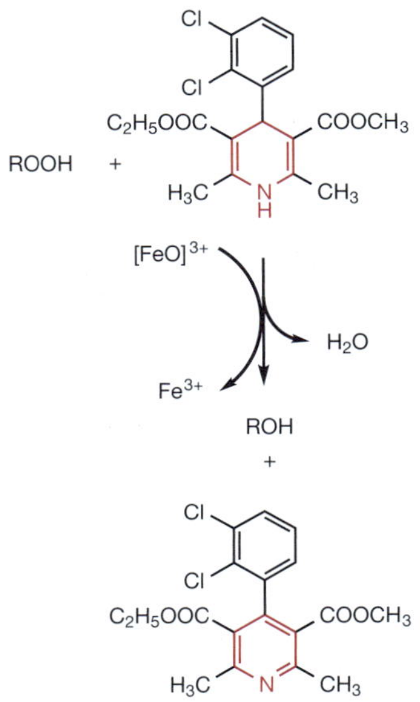

Figure 3.20 Simplified mechanism for peroxidases.

heme-peroxidation of arachidonic acid by means of HAT by a tyrosine radical generated by a ferryl-oxo-heme intermediate to hydroperoxy endoperoxide prostaglandin G_2 (PGG_2), which is then reduced to prostaglandin H_2, regenerating the COX. Two oxygen molecules react with the arachidonic acid radical to produce PGG_2. During the reduction of PGG_2 to prostaglandin H_2, drug substrates can be oxidized. Three COX isoenzymes are known: COX-1, COX-2, and COX-3; however, COX-3 seems nonfunctional in humans. Inhibitors of COX-1 and COX-2 are used therapeutically as nonsteroidal anti-inflammatory drugs (NSAIDs; see Chapter 17).[99]

MPO is a heme-peroxidase enzyme most abundantly present in neutrophil granulocytes (a subtype of white blood cells). MPO differs from P450 and other peroxidases in that the substrates are hydrogen peroxide and chloride anion. The chloride anion is oxidized to hypochlorous acid (HOCl) in the granulocyte, which is cytotoxic and very effective in killing bacteria, viruses, and other pathogens, which is the natural function of neutrophils. HOCl can oxidize drugs to reactive intermediates (eg, nitrenium ions), which can cause agranulocytosis. Examples of HOCl-generated reactive intermediates associated with agranulocytosis are the atypical antipsychotic clozapine, the antimalarial amodiaquine, and the phosphodiesterase cardiotonic vesnarinone. Chronic activation of MPO can induce several disease-like states, including chronic inflammation and cardiovascular issues, among others. The high level of DNA damage observed at high concentration of topoisomerase 2 inhibitors, as in the case of the anticancer drug etoposide, is due to the formation of etoposide radical by the action of MPO.[100]

In addition to those already described, other peroxidases include horseradish peroxidase (found in plants), LPO found in breast milk, and TPO found in the thyroid gland to produce thyroid hormones from iodide. Other monooxygenases catalyzing oxidation reactions similar to P450 include dopamine β-monooxygenase, a mammalian copper-containing enzyme catalyzing carbon hydroxylation, epoxidation, *S*-oxygenation, and *N*-dealkylation reactions, and nonheme iron–containing enzymes from bacteria and plants.

Nonmicrosomal Oxidations

In addition to the microsomal monooxygenases, other oxidases and dehydrogenases that catalyze oxidation reactions are present in the mitochondrial and soluble fractions of tissue homogenates.

Oxidation of Alcohols

Belonging to the superfamily of medium-chain dehydrogenases/reductases (MDRs), alcohol dehydrogenases (ADHs) are nicotinamide adenine dincucleotide (NAD)-specific zinc-containing dehydrogenases that occur in many organisms and are responsible for catalyzing the oxidation of primary and secondary alcohols to aldehydes and ketones, respectively, with concurrent reduction of NAD^+ to reduced form of nicotinamide adenine dinucleotide (NADH). ADHs can also catalyze the reverse reaction, oxidizing NADH to NAD^+. In humans and many other animals, genetic evidence suggests that, early on in evolution, ADHs were effective for metabolizing endogenous and exogenous formaldehyde and metabolizing naturally occurring toxic alcohols contained in foods or produced by bacteria in the digestive tract.

In humans, ADHs exist as dimeric proteins with a mass around 80 kDa, which are encoded by at least seven different genes. There are five classes of ADH enzymes (I-V). Class I consists of three *ADH* genes, *ADH1A*, *ADH1B*, and *ADH1C*. The human genes that encode class II, III, IV, and V ADHs are *ADH4*, *ADH5*, *ADH7*, and *ADH6*, respectively. The hepatic forms of ADH primarily present in humans are ADH1 and ADH4. ADH5 is expressed extensively in several organs, including liver, kidney, intestine, and heart, and ADH7 is found in the GI tract. The large number of ADH classes and enzymes gives the body the capability to metabolize/detoxify a variety of primary and secondary alcohols.[101,102]

Human ADH is present at high levels in the liver and the lining of the stomach and exhibits a broad specificity for alcohols. Most primary alcohols are readily oxidized to their corresponding aldehydes. Some secondary alcohols are oxidized to ketones, whereas other secondary and tertiary alcohols are excreted either unchanged or as their phase 2 glucuronide conjugate metabolite. Some secondary alcohols show mixed activity due to steric factors and a lack of substrate affinity for the enzyme. The mechanism of dehydrogenation involves abstraction and transfer of a hydride anion from the alcohol to NAD^+, reducing NAD^+ to NADH, with the subsequent formation of an aldehyde. ADH contains two Zn^{+2} ions in each subunit (Fig. 3.21). One of the Zn ions is located at the catalytic site and binds the hydroxyl group of the alcohol in place for dehydrogenation to occur. ADH is in the soluble fraction of tissue homogenates.

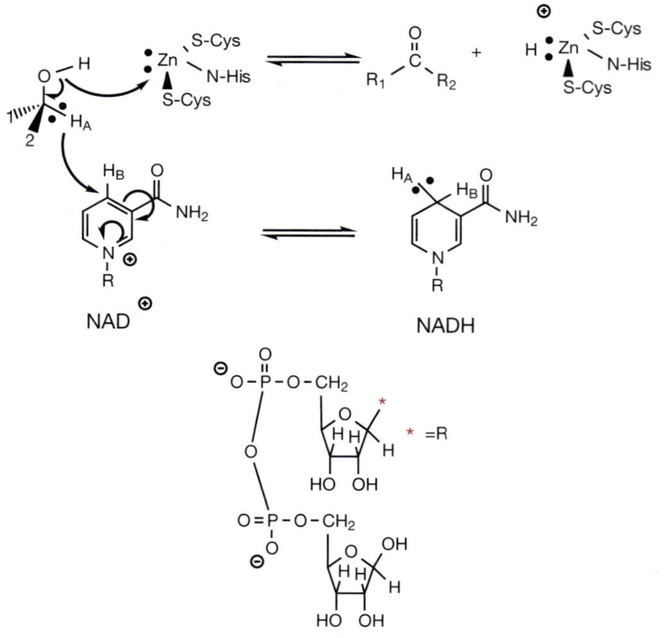

Figure 3.21 Alcohol dehydrogenase oxidation mechanism.

Oxidation by ADH is the principal pathway for ethanol metabolism, but the microsomal isoform CYP2E1 also has a significant role in ethanol metabolism and tolerance, along with minor catalase contributions. Two-thirds of ingested ethanol is oxidized by ADH and the remainder by CYP2E1 and catalase (Fig. 3.22). During intoxication, however, ethanol induces the expression of CYP2E1. The induction of CYP2E1 contributes to the activation of other drugs and xenobiotics, increasing the vulnerability of heavy drinkers to anesthetic drugs, over-the-counter (OTC) analgesics (including those used to treat hangover symptoms), prescription drugs, and chemical carcinogens. In turn, the excessive amounts of acetaldehyde generated cause hepatotoxicity, lipid peroxidation of membranes, formation of protein adducts, and other hepatocellular changes. Polymorphisms with physiologic consequence happen for *ADH1B* and *ADH1C* genes, as these polymorphisms generate differences in the efficacy of the enzymes to oxidize ethanol. For example, most African American individuals possess the *ADH1B*3* gene, which allows for faster ethanol metabolism than in people without this gene. Another variant of *ADH1B* is associated with a protective effect and this is often seen in European and Asian heritage populations.[103,104]

The toxicity of methanol and ethylene glycol in humans has long been recognized, but frequent reports of such toxicity are not surprising given the number of consumer products containing these alcohols (eg, automotive antifreeze). Methanol (wood alcohol or methyl alcohol) is commonly used as a solvent in organic synthetic procedures and is available to consumers in a variety of products, ranging from solid fuels (Sterno), paint removers, motor fuels, antifreeze, to alcoholic beverages (an adulterant in wines or an unintentional ingredient). Oral methanol toxicity in humans is characterized by its rapid absorption from the gut, followed by a latent period of many hours before metabolic acidosis (lowered blood pH and bicarbonate levels) and ocular toxicity are evident. Metabolic acidosis and blindness result from the excessive accumulation of formic acid and the inability of the hepatic tetrahydrofolate pathway to oxidize formate to carbon dioxide. The rate of elimination of methanol from the blood is relatively slow compared to the rapid rate for ethanol, accounting for its long latency period. Its half-life ranges from 2 to 3 hours at low blood concentration to 27 hours at high blood concentration. Research supports the singular role of liver ADH in the metabolism of methanol to formaldehyde, although it is oxidized slowly by ADH (approximately one-sixth the rate of ethanol).[105]

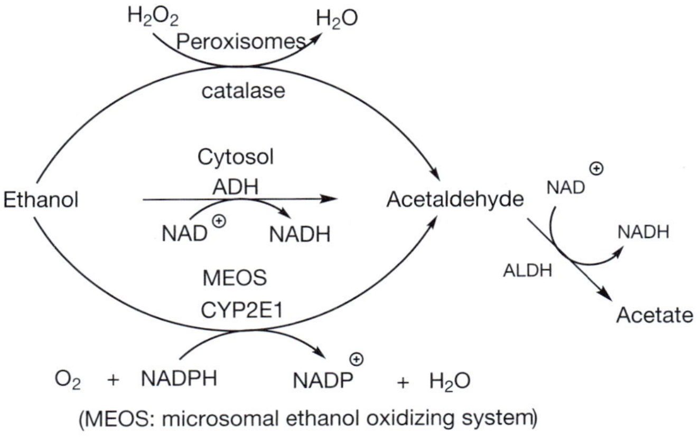

Figure 3.22 Ethanol metabolism in humans.

The fact that methanol is a substrate for ADH provides a rational basis for the use of ethanol in the treatment of methanol toxicity. Ethanol depresses the rate of methanol oxidation by acting as a competitive substrate for ADH, reducing the formation of formaldehyde. On the other hand, formaldehyde is not customarily detected in the blood because of its rapid metabolism by ADH to formate. Although human exposure to methanol vapor is less prevalent, methanol is rapidly absorbed through the skin or by inhalation, and depending on the severity of exposure, this can result in methanol poisoning.

Ethylene glycol is oxidized to hydroxyacetaldehyde and glyoxal and, subsequently, to oxalate by ADH. When eliminated into the urine, oxalate forms calcium oxalate crystals that can block the renal tubules. 4-Methylpyrazole (fomepizole) is an ADH inhibitor that is used as an antidote for the treatment of methanol or ethylene glycol poisoning. 1,4-Butanediol is a solvent that has become known to the public as a date rape drug and drug of abuse due to its metabolism to γ-hydroxybutyrate. The oxidized metabolite binds to the γ-hydroxybutyrate receptor, which in turn produces CNS sedation with amnesia.[105] ADHs also play an important role in the oxidative metabolism of different drugs, including abacavir, acyclovir, celecoxib, cyclophosphamide, felbamate, and fluvoxamine, posing a risk for DDIs.[101]

As noted earlier, ADH functions as a reductase when it catalyzes the reduction of an aldehyde or ketone to an alcohol. In addition, other nicotinamide adenine dinucleotide phosphate (NADP)- or NAD-dependent dehydrogenases in the cytosol are capable of reducing a variety of ketones. Ketones are stable to further oxidation and, consequently, yield reduction products as major metabolites. Examples of ADH-catalyzed reduction include the sedative-hypnotic chloral hydrate to trichloroethanol, the opioid antagonist naltrexone to 6β-naltrexol, the opioid analgesic methadone to α-methadol, the antipsychotic haloperidol to hydroxyhaloperidol, and the antiemetic dolasetron to dihydrodolasetron. These alcohol metabolites are all pharmacologically active.

Aldehyde Dehydrogenase

Aldehyde dehydrogenases (ALDHs), not to be confused with aldehyde oxidase (AOX), are a family of polymorphic NAD^+-specific enzymes that catalyze the NAD^+-dependent oxidation (dehydrogenation) of aldehydes to carboxylic acids, which are subsequently metabolized by the body's muscle and heart. ALDHs are implicated in several functions including structural and regulatory mechanisms, and detoxification. Its role in biosynthesis is also recognized. In total, the human ALDH superfamily is comprised of 19 isoforms categorized into three mammalian classes: class 1 (low K_m, cytosolic ALDH1), class 2 (low K_m, mitochondrial ALDH2), and class 3 (high K_m, cytosolic, such as those expressed in tumors, stomach, and cornea). In all the three classes, constitutive (an enzyme whose activity is constant and active) and inducible forms exist. Cytosolic ALDH1A1 and mitochondrial ALDH2 are the most important enzymes for aldehyde oxidation, and both are homotetrameric enzymes composed of 50 to 60 kDa subunits. These enzymes are found in many tissues of the body but are at the highest concentration in the liver.[106]

ALDH1A1, along with ADH, is responsible for the metabolism of retinol to retinoic acid. ALDH2 possesses nitrate reductase activity, catalyzing the bioactivation of nitroglycerin (glyceryl trinitrate) in blood vessels, resulting in vasodilation by nitric oxide. Some ALDHs can carry out esterease activity. ALDH2 has a major role in the hepatic detoxication of acetaldehyde and other aldehydes produced from oxidation of ethanol and other primary alcohols, and the oxidation of endogenous aldehydes, such as those produced by the oxidation of the biogenic amines norepinephrine, serotonin, and dopamine. These aldehydes can be toxic, and health problems arise when the aldehyde cannot be cleared. For example, the accumulation of unmetabolized acetaldehyde in the blood has been shown to be carcinogenic.

When high levels of acetaldehyde occur in the blood, symptoms of facial flushing, light-headedness, palpitations, nausea, and general "hangover" occur. These symptoms can be indicative of a disorder known as alcohol flush reaction, which is due to a mutant form of ALDH2 termed *ALDH2*2*. In the protein expressed by this mutant, a lysine residue replaces a glutamate in the active site, yielding an enzyme with about 8% of the activity of the wild-type (normal) *ALDH2* allele. The mutant allele shows a higher K_m for NAD^+ than the wild-type allele. This mutation is common in Japan, where 41% of a control group were *ALDH2* (wild-type) deficient, and where only 2% to 5% of a group with alcohol use disorder were wild-type deficient. In Taiwan, the numbers are similar, with 30% of the control group showing the wild-type deficiency and 6% of those with alcohol use disorder displaying the deficiency. The ALDH2 wild-type deficiency is manifested by slow acetaldehyde removal and low alcohol tolerance, which may explain the lower frequency of alcoholism in *ALDH2*2* carriers. These acetaldehyde toxicity symptoms are like those observed in people who drink ethanol while being treated with the drug disulfiram (Antabuse), which is why it is used to treat alcohol use disorder in patients seeking recovery but at risk for relapse. These patients show higher blood levels of acetaldehyde and become violently ill upon consumption of even small amounts of alcohol. Several other drugs (eg, metronidazole) cause a similar reaction known as "disulfiram-like reaction." It has also been shown that the concomitant use of alcohol and cigarettes is related to a high risk of cancer, mainly for carriers of the *ALDH2*2* (PM) allele.[107]

Molybdenum Hydroxylases

Molybdenum hydroxylases are non-P450 enzymes capable of catalyzing the oxidation of drugs. The molybdenum hydroxylases, which include AOX, xanthine oxidoreductase (XOR), sulfite oxidase, and mitochondrial amidoxime reducing component, are more commonly found in the cytosol of mammalian liver and carry out the oxidation and detoxification of several xenobiotics, mainly heteroaromatic compounds (Fig. 3.23).[88] The efficient oxidation of endogenous purine nucleosides suggests that their metabolism and detoxification might be an important physiologic role of the molybdenum hydroxylases. Among the azaheterocycles metabolized are derivatives of pyridine, quinoline, pyrimidine, purine, quinazoline, and pteridines. These hydroxylases, as a rule, oxidize the carbon α to the nitrogen of the azaheterocycle to oxo metabolites (also known as lactams).

The molybdenum hydroxylases are cytosolic with a common electron transfer system in each enzyme subunit: a molybdopterin (a pyranopteridine ligand) cofactor that binds the single molybdenum ion, two iron-sulfur centers, and an FAD molecule. Molybdenum is an essential component of the enzyme and, along with FAD, is required for enzyme catalysis. The enzyme is biologically inactive until it becomes complexed by the pterin to form the pteridine complex (termed Moco). Moco is coordinated with a sulfido ligand that is essential for the catalytic activity. The pterin moiety positions the catalytic molybdenum correctly within the active site of the enzyme to participate in electron transfer to and from the molybdenum atom. The molybdenum hydroxylases catalyze their reactions differently than P450 and other hydroxylase enzymes, requiring water rather than molecular oxygen as the source of the oxygen atom incorporated into the metabolite, and with the concomitant reduction of molecular oxygen to superoxide.[88,108] The active sites possess a catalytically labile Mo^{VI} group that is transferred to the substrate during the hydroxylation reaction to produce a Mo^{IV}.

ALDEHYDE OXIDASE. AOX is an enzyme located in the cytosol of cells and is similar to the XOR family of molybdoenzymes that require a molybdenum cofactor (Moco) for catalytic activity. AOX plays an important role in the clearance of xenobiotics, including drug compounds containing aldehydes and *N*-containing heterocyclic aromatic compounds. It generates carboxylic acids from aldehydes in the presence of oxygen. Although aldehydes are not often present in drug compounds, they can be a product of biotransformation reactions by P450s and monoamine oxidase (MAO), which can be subsequently oxidized to a carboxylic acid by AOX. At least 13% of drugs on the market are potential substrates for AOX. In addition to metabolizing some aldehydes,

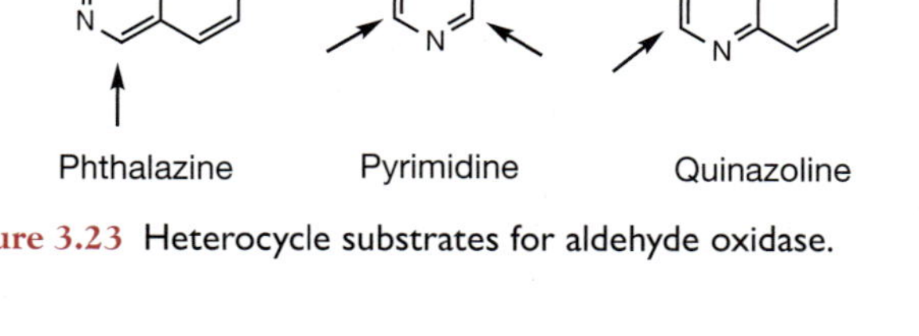

Figure 3.23 Heterocycle substrates for aldehyde oxidase.

AOX also oxidizes a variety of azaheterocycles, but excludes thia- or oxaheterocycles. Of the various purine nucleoside AOX substrates, the 2-hydroxy and 2-amino derivatives are more efficiently metabolized. The typical order of N_9 substituent preference of the acyclic nucleosides is as follows: 9-[(hydroxy-alkyloxy)methyl]-purines > 2′-arabinofuranosyl > H. The kinetic rate constants for purine analogs reveal that the pyrimidine portion of the purine ring system is more important for substrate affinity than the imidazole portion. AOX is inhibited by potassium cyanide and menadione (synthetic vitamin K).[102,109]

AOX metabolizes an assortment of azaheterocycles, including the short-acting sedative-hypnotic drug zaleplon (a pyrazolo[1,5α] pyrimidine derivative) to its 5-oxo metabolite; the anticancer drug thioguanine to 8-oxothioguanine; the α_2-adrenergic agonist brimonidine (a pyrimidine derivative) to its 2-oxo-, 3-oxo-, and 2,3-dioxo metabolites; quinine and quinidine to their 2-quinolone metabolites; the pro-antiviral drug famciclovir (a purine derivative) to its active 6-oxo metabolite (penciclovir); O6-benzylguanine to its 8-oxo metabolite (also formed primarily from CYP3A4); and the antiseizure drug zonisamide (a 1,2-benzisoxazole derivative), primarily by reductive cleavage of the 1,2-benzisoxazole ring to 2-sulfamoylacetylphenol. Although the azaheterocycles thiazole and oxazole are not metabolized by AOX, their carbocyclic analogs benzothiazole, benzoxazole, and 1,2-benzisoxazole are. On the other hand, the heterocycles, benzothiophene and benzofuran, which do not contain a nitrogen atom, are not metabolized by, nor do they inhibit, AOX. At high doses, the renal toxicity of methotrexate (a 2,4-diaminopteridine) is associated with the AOX metabolite, 7-hydroxymethotrexate, which is poorly water soluble.[88]

Potent inhibitors of AOX include the selective estrogen receptor modulators raloxifene, tamoxifen, estradiol, and ethinyl estradiol. Other classes of drugs that demonstrate inhibition of AOX include phenothiazines, tricyclic antidepressants, tricyclic atypical antipsychotic agents, dihydropyridine calcium channel blockers, loratadine, ondansetron, propafenone, domperidone, quinacrine, verapamil, and salmeterol. Thus, the possibility of clinically relevant drug interactions mediated by the inhibition of AOX could be observed between these drugs and drugs for which AOX is the primary route of metabolism.[88]

Xanthine oxidoreductase. The properties of AOX and XOR are closely related. Both enzymes are present in the cytosol. The primary difference between the two enzymes is that XOR can exist in two interconvertible forms, xanthine oxidase (XO) and xanthine dehydrogenase (XDH), while AOX exists only in the oxidase form. AOX utilizes only molecular oxygen as an electron acceptor in contrast to XOR, which can transfer electrons to both oxygen for XO and NAD^+ for XDH. The key physiologic function of XOR has been recognized as the oxidative metabolism of purines into the terminal metabolite uric acid (Fig. 3.24).[88,102]

XO and XDH represent different forms of the same gene product. XDH can be interconverted to XO by reversible sulfhydryl oxidation. XOR is the rate-limiting enzyme in human purine catabolism of hypoxanthine to uric acid and can also generate ROS. XOR is a cytosolic, homodimeric molybdoflavoenzyme approximately 300 kDa in size, although it can also be found on the outer surface of cell membranes that require a Moco center, two iron-sulfur centers, and FAD site.[110]

Both XO and XDH have important roles in the metabolism of purine anticancer drugs to their active and inactive metabolites. Although XOR is strongly inhibited by the antigout drug allopurinol, AOX also oxidizes allopurinol to oxypurinol. Only XDH requires NAD^+ as an electron acceptor for the oxidation of azaheterocycles. 6-Mercaptopurine is metabolized by XO and XDH to 6-thiouric acid (see Fig. 3.24). In humans, XOR is normally found in the liver but not in the blood unless hepatotoxicity is present. Xanthinuria I and II is a rare genetic disorder where the lack of XOR activity leads to high concentrations of xanthine in blood and can cause health problems such as renal failure.[88,110] There is no specific treatment for this disorder except to avoid foods high in purine and to maintain a high fluid intake.

Oxidative Deamination of Amines

MAO catalyzes the oxidative deamination of amines to aldehydes in the presence of oxygen. The aldehyde products can be metabolized further to the corresponding acid or alcohol by AOX or ADH.

Monoamine Oxidase

MAO is a mitochondrial membrane flavin-containing enzyme that catalyzes the oxidative deamination of monoamines, where oxygen is used to remove an amine group from a monoamine substrate resulting in the formation of the corresponding aldehyde and ammonia (Fig. 3.25). MAO participates in approximately 4% of the metabolism of xenobiotics, including drugs, and endogenous molecules.[88]

Substrates for this enzyme include primary, secondary, and tertiary amines in which the amine substituents are methyl groups. The amine must be attached to an unsubstituted methylene group. Compounds having a single

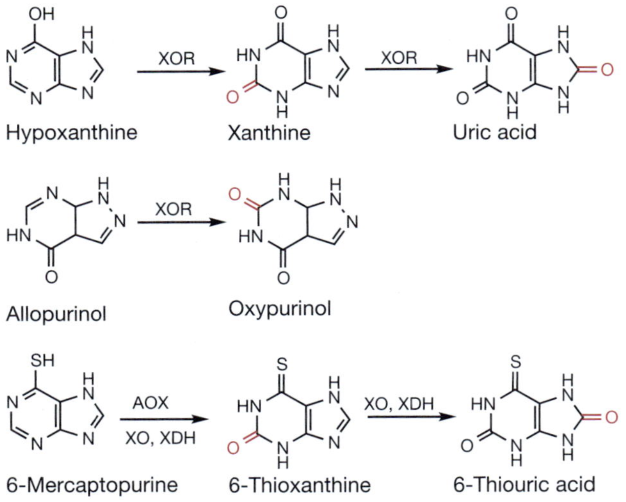

Figure 3.24 Xanthine oxidase reactions.

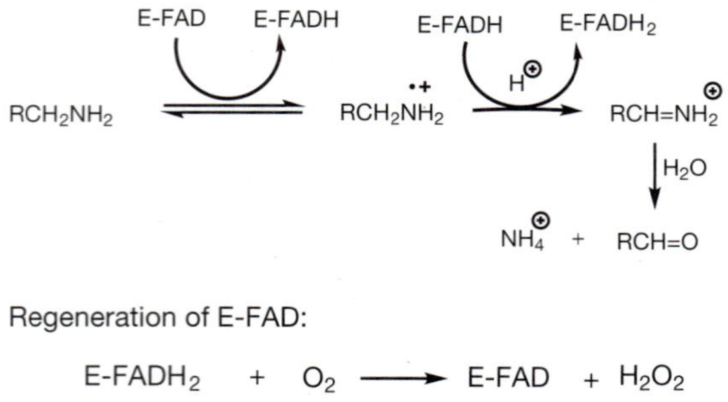

Figure 3.25 Monoamine oxidase oxidation of monoamines.

MPTP MPP+

Figure 3.26 Chemical structures for MPTP (1-methyl-4-phenyl-1,2,3,6-tetrahydropyridine) and MPP^+ (1-methyl-4-phenylpyridinium ion).

substitution at the α-carbon atom are poor substrates for MAO (eg, aniline, amphetamine, and ephedrine) but can be oxidized by the microsomal P450 enzymes. For secondary and tertiary amines, alkyl groups larger than a methyl and branched alkyl groups (ie, isopropyl, *t*-butyl, or β-phenylisopropyl) inhibit MAO oxidation, but such substrates can function as reversible inhibitors of this enzyme. Nonselective irreversible inhibitors of MAO that include phenelzine and tranylcypromine; the MAO-A irreversible clorgyline; the irreversible MAO-B selective inhibitors pargyline, selegiline, and rasagiline; and the selective MAO-B reversible inhibitor safinamide are some drugs available on the market. MAO is important in regulating the metabolic degradation of catecholamines and serotonin in neural tissues. Hepatic MAO has a crucial defensive role in inactivating circulating monoamines, or those originating in the GI tract and absorbed into the systemic circulation (eg, tyramine).[111]

As alluded to earlier, there are two types of MAO: MAO-A and MAO-B. They show dissimilar substrate preferences and different sensitivities to inhibitors due to different structural patterns in the active site. MAO-A, found mainly in peripheral adrenergic nerve terminals but also in the liver, GI tract, and placenta, shows substrate preference for 5-hydroxytryptamine, norepinephrine, and epinephrine. MAO-B is found principally in platelets and shows selectivity for nonphenolic, lipophilic β-phenethylamines. Common substrates to both MAO-A and MAO-B are dopamine, tyramine, and other monophenolic phenylethylamines.[111]

A contaminant in the synthesis of reversed esters of meperidine, 1-methyl-4-phenyl-1,2,3,6-tetrahydropyridine (MPTP), was discovered to be a highly selective neurotoxin for dopaminergic cells, producing parkinsonism.[112] The neurotoxicity of MPTP is associated with cellular destruction in the substantia nigra along with severe reductions in the concentration of dopamine, norepinephrine, and serotonin. The remarkable neurotoxic action for MPTP involves a sequence of events beginning with the metabolic activation of MPTP to the toxic metabolite MPP^+ (1-methyl-4-phenylpyridinium ion) by MAO-B, followed by specific uptake and accumulation of MPP^+ in the nigrostriatal dopaminergic neurons and ending with the inhibition of oxidative phosphorylation (Fig. 3.26). This inhibition results in mitochondrial injury, depriving the sensitive nigrostriatal cells of oxidative phosphorylation with their eventual death (neurotoxic actions of MPP^+). The MAO-B inhibitors (eg, deprenyl) blocked this biotransformation. More than 50 years of studies investigating MPTP and its role on dopaminergic neurons have led to the identification of numerous molecular and cellular pathways critical in the origins of Parkinson disease.[113]

Because of the vital role that MAOs have in the inactivation of neurotransmitters, MAO dysfunction (too much or too little MAO activity) is thought to be responsible for a number of neurologic disorders. For example, unusually high or low levels of MAOs in the body have been associated with depression, schizophrenia, substance abuse, attention-deficit disorder, and migraines. MAO inhibitors are one of the major classes of drugs prescribed for the treatment of depression, although they are last-line treatment due to risk of the drug's interaction with dietary constituents (eg, tyramine) or other drugs. Excessive levels of catecholamines (epinephrine, norepinephrine, and dopamine) may lead to a hypertensive crisis, and excessive levels of serotonin may lead to serotonin syndrome, both of which are potentially fatal.[111]

Carbonyl Reduction

Various studies on the biotransformation of xenobiotic ketones have established that ketone reduction is an important metabolic pathway in mammalian tissue.[114] Because carbonyl compounds are lipophilic and can be retained in tissues, their reduction to hydrophilic alcohols and subsequent conjugation is critical to their elimination. Although carbonyl reductases can be closely related to ADHs, they have distinctly different properties, use NADPH as the cofactor, and are NADP-dependent enzymes. Carbonyl reductase participates in the transformation of carbonyl-containing parent compounds or metabolites, for example, in arachidonic acid metabolism. They are also able to transform adducts (aldehydes) produced by GSH and lipid peroxidation. The metabolism of xenobiotic ketones to free alcohols or conjugated alcohols has been demonstrated for aromatic, aliphatic, alicyclic, and unsaturated ketones (eg, naltrexone, naloxone, hydromorphone, and daunorubicin). Carbonyl reductases are distinguished by the stereospecificity of their alcohol metabolites.[114,115]

Hydrolysis

In general, esters and amides are hydrolyzed by enzymes in the blood, liver microsomes, intestine, kidneys, and other tissues. Esters and certain amides are rapidly hydrolyzed by a group of enzymes termed carboxylesterase (CES). The more lipophilic the amide, the more favorable it is as a substrate for this enzyme. In most cases, the hydrolysis of an ester or amide results in bioinactivation to two hydrophilic metabolites that are readily excreted. Some of these metabolites can yield conjugated phase 2 metabolites (ie, glucuronides). Proteins and peptides in meat contain multiple amide bonds, and so, not surprisingly, there are a large number of proteolytic enzymes in the GI tract called amino endopeptidases and amino exopeptidases that hydrolyze ingested proteins into smaller peptides or individual amino acids.

CES include cholinesterase (pseudocholinesterase), arylcarboxyesterases, liver microsomal CESs, and other unclassified liver CESs. These enzymes play an important role in drug metabolism; they are responsible for hydrolyzing around 20% of marketed drugs and activating about 50% of prodrugs (drugs designed to depend on metabolism for bioactivation). Cholinesterase hydrolyzes choline-like esters (eg, actylcholine, succinylcholine) and procaine, as well as acetylsalicylic acid. Genetic variant forms of cholinesterase have been identified in human serum; toxicity results when succinylcholine is administered as a ganglionic blocker for muscle relaxation to patients with the variant form of cholinesterase. Meperidine is hydrolyzed only by liver microsomal CESs, and diphenoxylate is hydrolyzed to its active metabolite diphenoxylic acid within 1 hour. Presumably, the lack of a central pharmacologic action of diphenoxylate is attributed to the formation of a zwitterionic diphenoxylic acid, which is readily eliminated in the urine (Fig. 3.27). It has been also reported that CES inhibitors can lead to DDIs and drug-herbal interactions.[116]

Sterically hindered esters are hydrolyzed slowly and can appear unchanged in the urine. For example, approximately 50% of a dose of atropine, whose ester linkage is shielded by a bulky azabicyclic ring system, appears unchanged in the urine of humans, and the remainder consists of unhydrolyzed biotransformed products.

As a rule, amides are more stable to hydrolysis than esters, and it is not surprising to find amide drugs excreted largely unchanged. This fact has been exploited in developing the antiarrhythmic drug procainamide. Procaine is not useful as an antiarrhythmic because of its rapid esterase-catalyzed hydrolysis, but 60% of a dose of procainamide was recovered unchanged from the urine of humans, with the remainder being mostly *N*-acetylprocainamide (a phase 2 metabolite). On the other hand, the deacylated metabolite of indomethacin (a tertiary amide) is one of the major metabolites detected in human urine. Amide hydrolysis of phthalylsulfathiazole and succinylsulfathiazole by bacterial enzymes in the colon releases the antibacterial agent sulfathiazole.

Summary

In summary, phase 1 metabolic transformations introduce new polar functional groups into the molecule, which can produce one or more of the following changes:

1. Decreased pharmacologic activity (deactivation)
2. Increased pharmacologic activity (activation)
3. Increased toxicity (carcinogenesis, mutagenesis, cytotoxicity)
4. Altered pharmacologic activity

Phase 1 metabolites usually undergo further phase 1 metabolism and/or phase 2 conjugation, most commonly resulting in deactivation and excretion of the inactive conjugates in urine or bile.

Drug Conjugation Pathways (Phase 2)

Conjugation reactions (Fig. 3.28) represent probably the most important xenobiotic biotransformation. Xenobiotics are, as a rule, lipophilic, well absorbed into tissues from the blood, but excreted slowly in the urine.[117] Only after conjugation (phase 2) reactions have added an ionic hydrophilic moiety, such as glucuronic acid, sulfate ester, or glycine, to the xenobiotic is water solubility significantly increased and lipid solubility decreased enough to make urinary elimination possible. Enhancing hydrophilicity enables metabolite transport into the aqueous compartments of the cell and

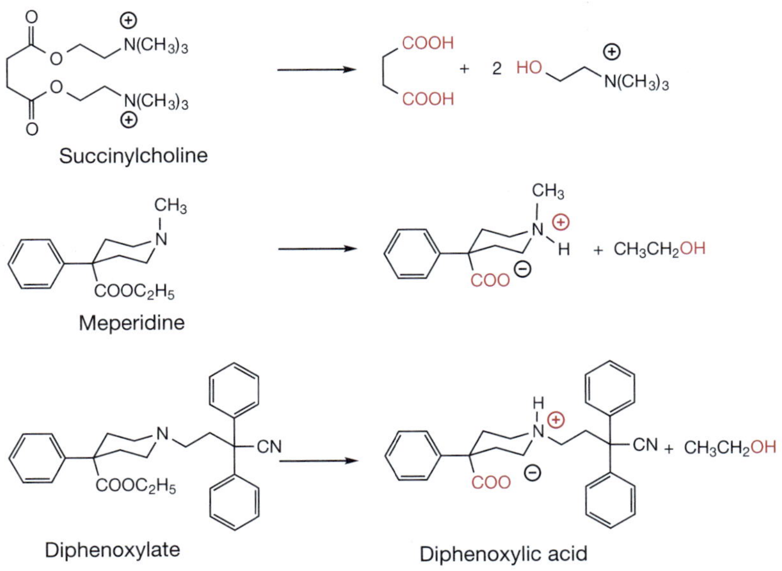

Figure 3.27 Examples of hydrolysis reactions.

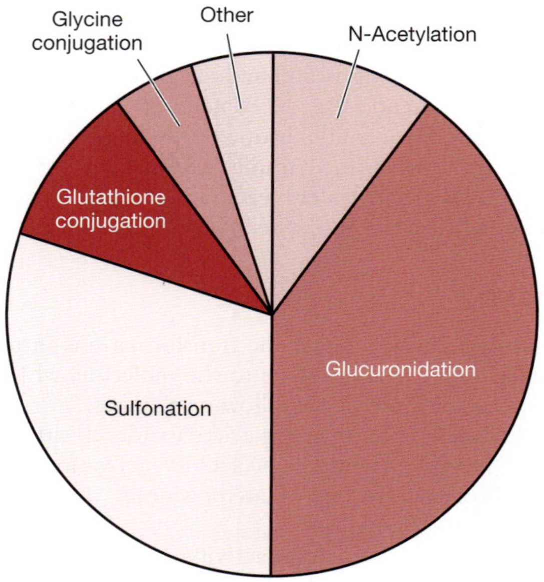

Figure 3.28 Phase 2 pathways contributing to drug metabolism.

the body. The major proportion of the administered drug dose is excreted as conjugates into the urine and bile. Conjugation reactions can be preceded by phase 1 reactions. For xenobiotics with a functional group available for phase 2 metabolism, direct conjugation can be its fate.

Common Features of Phase 2 Pathways

Phase 2 conjugation commonly creates anionic metabolites (eg, glucuronides, sulfate esters, glycine conjugates, GSH conjugates) that are then actively excreted into the bile via biliary transporters or into the renal proximal tubules by renal transporters.[7,117] Conjugated metabolites often have higher elimination clearance than the parent drug, due in part to active excretion/transport into urine and/or bile, and are expected to have a half-life shorter than that of the parent drug. Cofactors that provide the endogenous polar structure to be transferred to (ie, conjugated with) the drug substrate are required for phase 2 reactions, and cofactor depletion can occur at high drug doses. Biliary excretion of glucuronide and sulfate ester conjugates with higher molecular weight (eg, >325) is increased compared to lower molecular weight metabolites.

The major conjugation reactions (glucuronidation and sulfonation) were traditionally thought to terminate pharmacologic activity by transforming the parent drug or phase 1 metabolite into readily excreted ionic products with presumably poor cellular diffusion and low affinity for the active drug's receptor. This long-established view has changed with the discoveries that morphine-6-glucuronide has more analgesic activity than morphine in humans, and that minoxidil sulfate is the active metabolite for the antihypertensive minoxidil. Some glucuronides are cleaved in vivo to regenerate the active drug species (eg, propranolol, estradiol, statin antihyperlipidemics). For most xenobiotics, however, conjugation is an inactivating and detoxification mechanism. It bears noting that some compounds can form reactive intermediates that have been implicated in carcinogenesis, allergic reactions, and tissue damage.

Competing conjugation pathways for the same drug substance produces multiple conjugated products (eg, *p*-aminosalicylic acid in Fig. 3.29). Thus, the drug or xenobiotic can be a substrate for more than one metabolizing enzyme. Different conjugation pathways could compete for the same functional group with the outcome being an array of metabolites excreted in the urine or feces. Factors determining the outcome of this interplay include availability of cofactors, enzyme kinetics (V_{max}), affinity of the drug/xenobiotic (K_m) for the metabolizing enzyme, and type of tissues (eg, hepatic, kidney, lung). When a cofactor level is low or depleted, the competing conjugation reactions can take control. The reactivity of the functional group is determined also by all subsequent conjugation reactions. For example, major competing conjugation reactions are sulfonation, ether glucuronidation, and methylation for the phenolic hydroxyl groups; acetylation, sulfonation, and glucuronidation for amine groups; and amino acid conjugation, CoA conjugation, and ester glucuronidation for carboxyl groups.

Conjugation enzymes can show enantiomeric stereospecificity when a racemic drug is administered. The metabolic pattern of a drug administered orally can be different compared to the same drug administered intravenously because of the avoidance of presystemic intestinal conjugation via the latter route.

Glucuronic Acid Conjugation

Glucuronide formation is the most common route for phase 2 metabolism to water-soluble metabolites, accounting for approximately 40% of drug conjugation and the major share of the conjugated metabolites found in the urine and bile. The predominance of glucuronidation lies in the available supply of glucuronic acid (oxidized glucose) in the liver and in the many heteroatomic functional groups capable of forming glucuronide conjugates, such as nitrogen (eg, amines) and oxygen (eg, phenols, alcohols, carboxylic acids) to form *N*-glucuronides and *O*-glucuronides, respectively. *S*-glucuronidation is rare.[90]

Mechanism of Glucuronide Conjugation

Glucuronide conjugation involves the direct condensation of the xenobiotic (or its phase 1 metabolite) with the activated form of glucuronic acid, UDP-glucuronic acid (UDPGA). The overall scheme of the glucuronide conjugation reaction is shown in Figure 3.30. The S_N2 reaction between UDPGA and drug substrate requires a nucleophilic target on the drug or xenobiotic acceptor

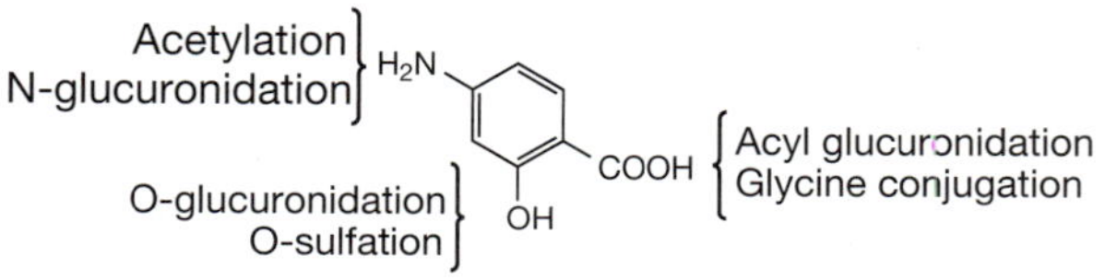

Figure 3.29 Competing conjugation pathways for *p*-aminosalicylic acid.

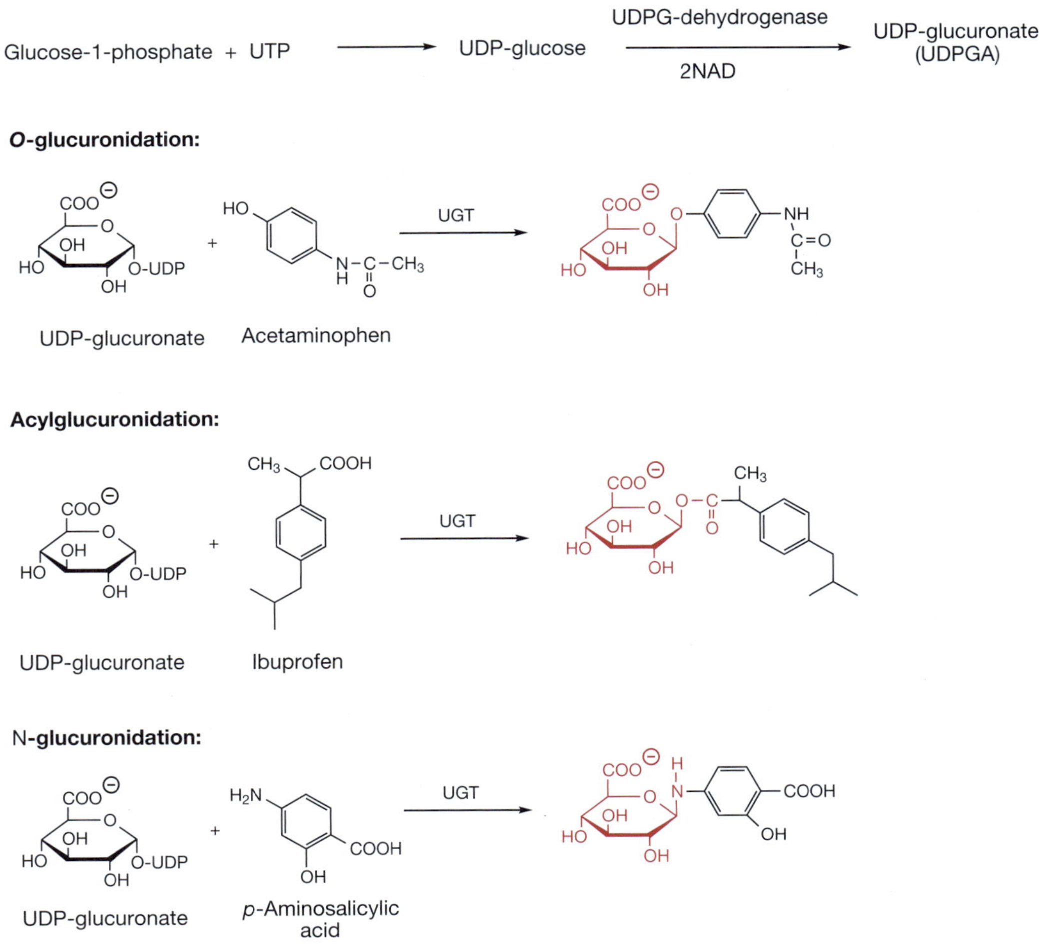

Figure 3.30 Glucuronidation pathways catalyzed by UDP-glucuronosyltransferases (UGTs).

compound, and is catalyzed by a family of UGTs, a multigene family of isozymes located along the ER of the liver, epithelial cells of the intestine, and other extrahepatic tissues.[118,119] Its unique location in the ER, along with the P450 isoforms, has important physiologic effects in the conjugation of reactive metabolites generated by the P450 isoforms and in controlling the levels of reactive metabolites present in these tissues. Transporters carry the UDPGA and xenobiotics from the cytosol into the ER lumen and then transport the glucuronide metabolite from the ER lumen into the cytosol. The presence of the active site for UGT toward the ER lumen catalyzes the reaction between the substrate and UDPGA.[119]

Glucuronidation is a low-affinity (a higher concentration of the xenobiotic is required for full enzyme activity) and high-capacity (high rate of xenobiotic turnover) phase 2 reaction. The resultant glucuronide has the β-configuration about carbon 1 of glucuronic acid since the drug substrate attacks from the β-face of the hexose when displacing UDP-OH. With the attachment of the hydrophilic carbohydrate moiety containing a readily ionizable carboxyl group (pK_a = 3-4), a lipid-soluble substance is converted into an anionic conjugate that is reabsorbed poorly by the renal or biliary system and is simply excreted in urine or feces.

Endogenous substances that readily conjugate with glucuronic acid include catecholamines, steroids, bilirubin, and thyroxine. As noted, not all glucuronides are excreted by the kidneys. Some are excreted into the intestinal tract with bile (enterohepatic cycling), where β-glucuronidase in the intestinal flora hydrolyzes the C_1-O-glucuronide to the aglycone (xenobiotic or their metabolites) for reabsorption into the portal circulation (see "Enterohepatic Circulation of Drugs" section). A summary of drug functional groups commonly glucuronidated is provided in Figure 3.31.

Uridine Diphosphate Glucuronosyltransferase Families

UGTs have been classified into families according to similarities in amino acid sequences, analogous to the P450 family.[118] The human UGT family is divided into subfamilies UGT1A (UGT1A1, UGT1A3, UGT1A4, UGT1A5, UGT1A6, UGT1A7, UGT1A8, UGT1A9, and UGT1A10), UGT2A (UGT2A1, UGT2A2, and UGT2A3), UGT2B (UGT2B4, UGT2B7, UGT2B10, UGT2B11, UGT2B15, UGT2B17, and UGT2B28), UGT3A (UGT3A1, UGT3A2), and UGT8A1.[117,118] Not all UGTs are involved in substrate metabolism. UGT1A1, UGT1A3, UGT1A4, UGT1A6, UGT1A9, UGT2B4, UGT2B7, UGT2B10, UGT2B15, and UGT2B17 are expressed in human liver.[17] Considerable overlap in substrate specificities exists between subfamilies UGT1A and UGT2B. The UGT1A1 isoform is primarily

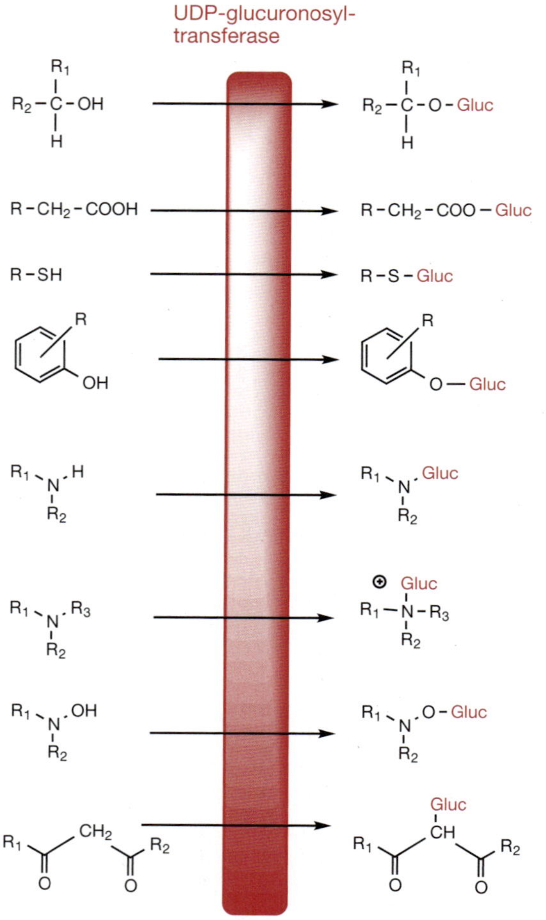

Figure 3.31 Phase 2 glucuronidation pathways contributing to drug metabolism.

responsible for the glucuronidation of bilirubin, estradiol, carvedilol, etoposide, ezetimibe, and other estrogenic steroids; UGT1A3 and UGT1A4 catalyze the glucuronidation of drugs with tertiary amines to form quaternary glucuronides and hydroxylated xenobiotics, and UGT1A3 also forms the acyl glucuronide of telmisartan; UGT1A6 exhibits limited substrate specificity for planar phenolic substances while UGT1A9 has a wide range of substrate specificity and can glucuronidate nonplanar phenols, plant substances (eg, anthraquinones and flavones), steroids, and other phenolic drugs. UGT1A10 glucuronidates mycophenolic acid, an inhibitor of inosine monophosphate dehydrogenase. Human family 2 isoform UGT2B4 is homologous to UGT2B7 and catalyzes the glucuronidation of the 6α-hydroxyl group of bile acids; UGT2B7 glucuronidates the largest number of substrates including the 3- and 6-glucuronidation of morphine and 6-glucuronidation of codeine; UGT2B11 glucuronidates a wide range of planar phenols, bulky alcohols, and polyhydroxylated estradiol metabolites; and UGT2B15 catalyzes the glucuronidation of the 17α-hydroxyl group of dihydrotestosterone and other steroidal compounds. UGT1A isoforms are inducible with 3-methylcholanthrene and cigarette smoking and the UGT2B family is induced by barbiturates.[118]

Uridine Diphosphate Glucuronosyltransferase Distribution

The human liver is the most important tissue for all routes of phase 1 and phase 2 metabolism. The UGT family is primarily expressed in the liver, with the exception of UGT1A8 and UGT1A10, which are principally found in the small intestine, colon, and bladder. Moreover, UGT1A7 is particularly expressed in the stomach. Substrate specificities of intestinal UGT isoforms are comparable to those in the liver. The UGT isoforms in the intestine can glucuronidate orally administered drugs, such as morphine, acetaminophen, α- and β-adrenergic agonists, and other phenolic phenethanolamines, as well as other dietary xenobiotics, reducing their oral bioavailability (first-pass metabolism).[119] Deficiencies in the expression of functional UGT1A1, which conjugates hepatic bilirubin, results in the inherited genetic disorder known as Gilbert syndrome, which is characterized by high serum concentrations of free (unconjugated) bilirubin.[118]

O-, *N*-, and *S*-Glucuronides

The xenobiotics that contain electron-rich nucleophilic oxygen, nitrogen, and sulfur (heteroatoms) or extremely electrophilic carbon atoms form glucuronides. In humans, almost 40% to 70% of clinically used drugs are subjected to *O*-glucuronidation, with alcohols and phenols producing ether *O*-glucuronides. *O*-phenolic glucuronides predominate over nonaromatic alcohol *O*-glucuronidation because of the greater nucleophilicity of ionizable phenols (pK_a = 7-10), reaction efficiencies, and turnover rates. Aromatic and some aliphatic carboxylic acids form ester (acyl) glucuronides. Aromatic amines form *N*-glucuronides and sulfhydryl compounds form *S*-glucuronides, both of which are more labile to acid as compared with the *O*-glucuronides. Some tertiary amines (eg, tripelennamine) have been reported to form quaternary ammonium *N*-glucuronides. Substances containing a 1,3-dicarbonyl structure (eg, phenylbutazone) can undergo formation of *C*-glucuronides by direct conjugation without previous metabolism because the central carbon is capable of becoming anionic. The acidity of the methylene C-H of the 1,3-dicarbonyl group, which generates the carbanion when the hydrogen is donated as proton, determines the degree of *C*-glucuronide formation.[117,120]

Acyl Glucuronides

Drug-acyl glucuronides are reactive conjugates of carboxylic acids at physiologic pH. The acyl group of the C_1-acyl glucuronide can migrate via transesterification from the original C_1 position of the glucuronic acid to the OH-substituted C_2, C_3, or C_4 positions (see Fig. 3.30). The resulting positional isomers are not hydrolyzed by β-glucuronidase, giving the appearance of a new unknown conjugate. However, under physiologic or weakly alkaline conditions, the C_1-acyl glucuronide can hydrolyze in the urine to produce the parent substance (aglycone) or undergo acyl migration to an acceptor macromolecule, forming an immunoreactive hapten. The pH-catalyzed migration of the acyl group from the drug C_1-*O*-acyl glucuronide to a protein or other cellular constituent occurs with the formation of a covalent bond to the protein. The acylated protein becomes a hapten and could stimulate an immune response against the drug, resulting in the expression of a hypersensitivity reaction or other forms of immunotoxicity. A high incidence of idiosyncratic/immunotoxic reactions have been reported for several NSAIDs, for example, benoxaprofen, zomepirac, indoprofen, alclofenac, ticrynafen, and ibufenac. All of these NSAIDs were metabolized to acyl glucuronides, and all have been removed from the market. Similar reactions have been reported for currently marketed NSAIDs, including tolmetin, sulindac, ibuprofen, ketoprofen, and acetylsalicylic acid. The frequency of the immunotoxic response can be related to the stability of the acyl glucuronide, the chemical rate kinetics for the migration of the acyl group, and the concentration and stability/half-life of the antigenic protein.[120]

When the acyl glucuronide is the primary metabolite in patients with decreased renal function (ie, older adults) or when probenecid is coadministered, renal cycling of the unconjugated (aglycone) parent drug or metabolite is likely to occur, resulting in the plasma accumulation of the active aglycone. The reduced elimination of the acyl glucuronide increases its hydrolysis to either the aglycone or the migration of the C_1-O-acyl group to an acceptor macromolecule, as previously described.

Bioactivation and Toxic Glucuronides

Generally, glucuronides are biologically and chemically less reactive than their parent molecules and are readily eliminated without interaction with intracellular substances. However, some glucuronide conjugates are more pharmacologically active than the parent drug. Morphine, for example, forms the 3-O- and 6-O-glucuronides in the intestine and in the liver. The 3-O-glucuronide is the primary glucuronide metabolite of morphine with a blood concentration 20-fold that of morphine. Pharmacologically, it is an opioid antagonist. On the other hand, 6-O-glucuronide is a more potent μ-receptor agonist than morphine and, whether administered orally or parentally, is 650-fold more analgesic than morphine in humans. Thus, the analgesic effects of morphine are the result of a complex interaction of the drug and its two glucuronide metabolites with the opioid receptor. The 6-O-glucuronide is transported into the brain via an anion-transport system.[121]

Glucuronidation is also capable of causing hepatotoxicity and carcinogenesis by facilitating the formation of reactive electrophilic (electron-deficient) intermediates and their transport into target tissues. As previously described, the major metabolic biotransformations for carboxylic acids include conjugation with glucuronic acid, which are bioactivated via UGT-catalyzed conjugation with glucuronic acid to acyl glucuronides. The reactive acyl glucuronides are electrophilic and, therefore, can contribute to the acylation of target proteins (see "Reactive Metabolites Resulting From Bioactivation" section), resulting in idiosyncratic reactions.

The induction of bladder cancer by aromatic amines can result from the O-glucuronidation of the N-hydroxylarylamine (Fig. 3.32). These O-glucuronides become concentrated in the urine, where they either hydrolyze in the acidic pH of the urine to produce N-hydroxylarylamines or eliminate water from the N-hydroxylarylamine under these acidic conditions to form an electrophilic arylnitrenium species (Fig. 3.32, metabolite 4). This reactive species binds covalently with endogenous cellular constituents (eg, nucleic acids and proteins), initiating carcinogenesis.[122] The negative role of the UGTs, either directly or indirectly, in cancer is expanded for patients with deficiencies in wild-type UGT1A1 or who carry the PM UGT1A1*28 allele, as these patients may be at high risk for severe toxicity since irinotecan is metabolized by this enzyme.[123] Irinotecan doses are commonly reduced in patients with cancer who are homozygous for UGT1A1*28.

Sulfonation and glucuronidation occur side by side, often competing for the same substrate (most commonly phenols, ie, acetaminophen). The balance between sulfonation and glucuronidation is influenced by factors such as animal species, dose, availability of cofactors, and inhibition and induction of the respective transferases.

Sulfonation (Sulfoconjugation)

Sulfonation (sulfoconjugation) is an important conjugation reaction in the biotransformation of steroid hormones, catecholamine neurotransmitters, thyroxine, bile acids, phenolic drugs, and other xenobiotics.[117,120,124] The major physiologic consequence of sulfonation of a drug or xenobiotic is its increased aqueous solubility and excretion. Because the pK_a of the sulfate group is approximately 1, sulfate esters are completely ionized in physiologic solution and possess a smaller volume of distribution than unconjugated steroids and drugs. Thus, a lipid-soluble substance is converted into a conjugate that is reabsorbed poorly by the renal system. For some drugs, sulfonation can result in their bioactivation to reactive electrophiles (molecules that accept an electron pair to make a covalent bond) or therapeutically active conjugates (eg, minoxidil sulfate). Cytosolic sulfotransferases (SULTs) are, in general, associated with the sulfonation of phenolic steroids, neurotransmitters, and xenobiotics. Membrane-bound SULTs are localized in the Golgi apparatus of most cells and are responsible for the sulfonation of glycosaminoglycans, glycoproteins, and the tyrosinyl group of peptides and proteins, but are usually not associated with xenobiotic metabolism.[120]

Mechanism of Sulfonation

Xenobiotics are sulfonated by the transfer of a sulfonic group ($-SO_3^-$) from 3′-phosphoadenosine-5′-phosphosulfate

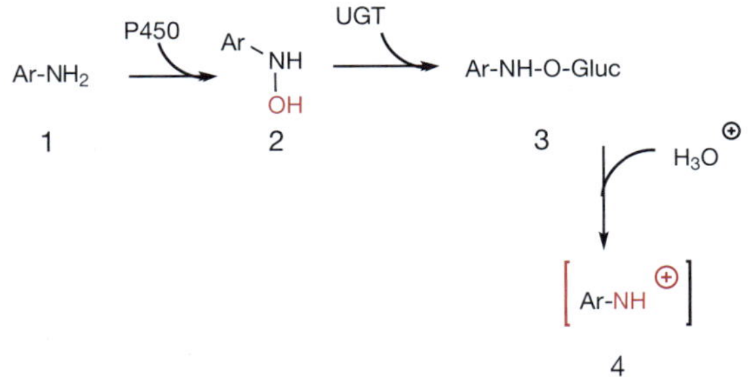

Figure 3.32 Bioactivation of arylamines.

(PAPS) to the acceptor molecule, a cytosolic reaction catalyzed by a family of multigene SULTs (Fig. 3.33). PAPS is formed enzymatically from adenosine triphosphate (ATP) and inorganic sulfate. Sulfonation is a reaction principally of phenols, and to a lesser extent of alcohols, to form highly ionic and hydrophilic sulfate esters (R-O-SO_2H). The availability of PAPS and its precursor inorganic sulfate determines the sulfonation reaction rate.

The total pool of sulfate is frequently limited and can be readily exhausted due to the large number of substrates.

Sulfonation is a high-affinity and low-capacity phase 2 reaction, which works in conjunction with glucuronidation on overlapping substrates. Thus, sulfonation predominates at low substrate concentrations and glucuronidation at high substrate concentrations. When sulfonation becomes saturated from increasing doses of a drug, sulfonation becomes a less predominant pathway and the rate of glucuronidation increases until it reaches saturation. At that point, either the drug is excreted unchanged or other metabolism pathways become activated. For example, at high doses of acetaminophen, glucuronidation predominates over sulfonation, which prevails at low doses. When PAPS, inorganic sulfate, or the sulfur amino acids are low or depleted, or when a substrate for sulfonation is given in high doses, competing reactions with glucuronidation can take control. Additionally, O-methylation is a competing reaction for a catechol.[120]

Sulfotransferase Family

In humans, the superfamily cytosolic SULTs are divided into four families, SULT1, SULT2, SULT4, and SULT6. SULT enzymes are broadly expressed, and metabolically important subfamilies of SULT1 and SULT2 are known.[125] SULTs catalyze the sulfonation of many phenolic drugs, catecholamines, hormones, aromatic amines, and other xenobiotics. SULT1A1 plays an important role in metabolizing phenolic compounds. SULT1A3 displays stereoselectivity in the sulfonation of chiral phenolic phenethanolamines. This isoform can be responsible, in part, for the enantiomer-specific metabolism observed for the β-adrenergic agonists. For example, the (+)-enantiomers of terbutaline and isoproterenol and the (−)-enantiomer of albuterol are selectively sulfonated.

SULTs were named based on their presumed function prior to the mid-1990s, for example, SULT1A1 and SULT1A2 were formerly known as phenol SULT. The crystal structures for SULT1A1 and SULT1A2 have provided insights into this enzyme's substrate specificity and catalytic function, including its role in the sulfonation of endogenous substrates such as estrogens. SULT1A3 selectively sulfonates the catecholamines dopamine, norepinephrine, and epinephrine, as well as the *N*-oxide of minoxidil, thyroid hormones, but not estrogenic steroids and other hydroxy steroids. SULT1B1 catalyzes the sulfonation of the thyroid hormones, while SULT1C subfamily is involved with the bioactivation of procarcinogens via sulfonation, as in the case of *N*-hydroxy-2-acetylaminofluorene. SULT1C4 catabolizes xenobiotic phenolic compounds. SULT1E1 (formerly known as estrogen SULT) preferentially sulfonates estradiol in the nanomolar range, playing a critical role in steroid homeostasis. SULT2A1 (formerly known as dehydroepiandrosterone [DHEA] SULT) conjugates DHEA, estradiol (micromolar range), synthetic estrogens, and androgens and bile acids. Finally, SULT2B1 (formerly known as hydroxysteroid SULT) sulfonates DHEA and pregnenolone.[124] A summary of drug functional groups commonly sulfonated is provided in Figure 3.34.

Sulfonation is an important reaction in the transport and metabolism of steroids. Sulfonation decreases the biologic activity of steroids because steroid sulfate esters are not capable of binding to their receptors. It provides for the transport of an inactive form of the steroid to its target tissue, where the active steroid is regenerated by sulfatases at the target tissue.

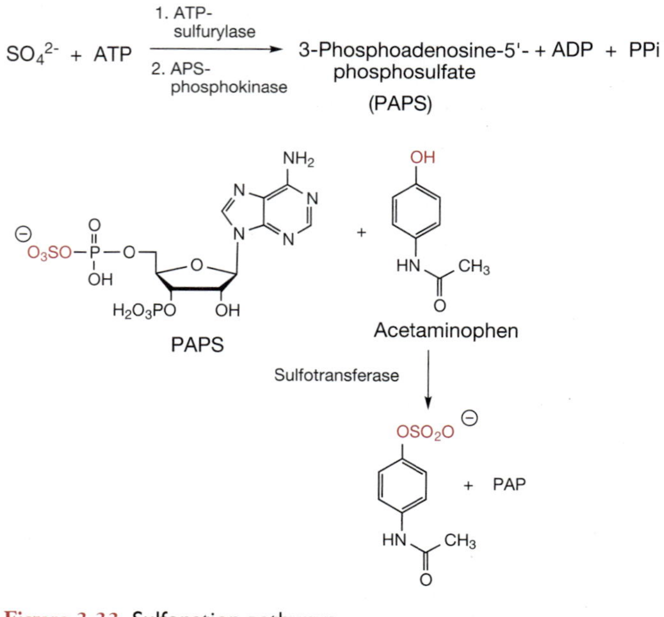

Figure 3.33 Sulfonation pathways.

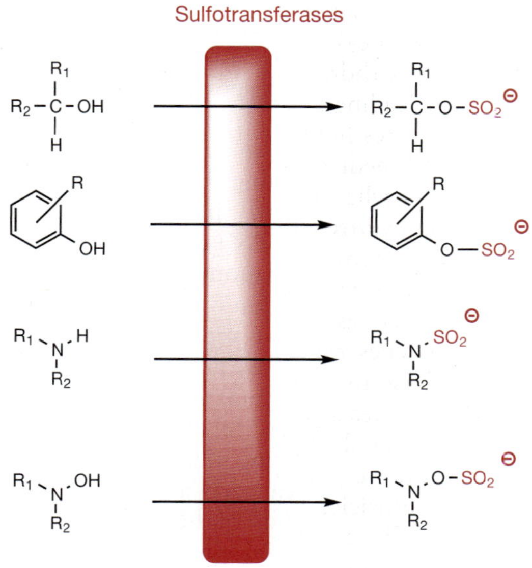

Figure 3.34 Phase 2 sulfonation pathways contributing to drug metabolism.

Sulfotransferase Distribution

The SULT1A subfamilies are abundantly expressed in the liver, small intestine, brain, kidneys, and platelets. SULT1A1 is mainly expressed in the liver as opposed to SULT1A3, which is practically undetected in the liver. For example, phenol is sulfonated by a SULT in the liver, kidneys, and intestines, whereas steroids are sulfonated only in the liver. The broad diversity of compounds sulfonated in human tissues results, in part, from the multi-isoforms of the cytosolic SULTs and their overlapping substrate specificities. Sulfate esters are almost totally ionized and, therefore, are excreted mostly in the urine via transporters, but biliary elimination is common for steroids. When biliary sulfate esters are hydrolyzed in the intestine by sulfatases, the parent drug (or xenobiotic) or its metabolites can be reabsorbed into the portal circulation to be resulfonated for eventual elimination in the urine as a sulfate ester (enterohepatic cycling). The rate of sulfonation appears to be age dependent, decreasing with age.[126]

An important site of sulfonation, especially after oral administration, is the intestine. The result is a presystemic first-pass effect, decreasing drug bioavailability of several drugs for which the primary route of conjugation is sulfonation. Drugs such as isoproterenol, albuterol, steroid hormones, α-methyldopa, acetaminophen, and fenoldopam are sulfonated in the gut. Competition for intestinal sulfonation between coadministered substrates can influence their bioavailability with either an increase or decrease in therapeutic effects. An example would be the coadministration of a 500-mg dose of acetaminophen and 0.03-mg dose of the oral contraceptive ethinyl estradiol. This interaction could result in increased toxicity of ethinyl estradiol because of less sulfonation in the gut.[126]

Bioactivation and Toxicity

Sulfonation is a common final step in the biotransformation of xenobiotics and is traditionally associated with inactivation, although sulfate esters have been reported to be pharmacologically active (eg, minoxidil sulfate, DHEA sulfate, and morphine-6-sulfate). However, the sulfate ester group is electron-withdrawing and may be cleaved off in some molecules, leading to an electrophilic cation forming reactive intermediates implicated in carcinogenesis and tissue damage. SULT-mediated toxicity has been demonstrated for numerous benzylic alcohols derived from PAHs and various aromatic hydroxylamines. For example, 1′-hydroxysafrole (an allylic/benzylic alcohol) is bioactivated to reactive metabolites by SULTs. SULT1A1 can also sulfonate procarcinogens such as hydroxymethyl PAHs, producing reactive intermediates capable of forming DNA adducts, potentially resulting in mutagenesis. Sulfonation of an alcohol moiety generates a good leaving group and can be an activation process for alcohols to produce a reactive electrophilic species. However, like the *N*-glucuronides, *N*-sulfates can promote cytotoxicity by facilitating the formation of reactive electrophilic intermediates. Sulfonation of *N*-oxygenated aromatic amines is an activation process for some arylamines, which can eliminate sulfate to produce an electrophilic species capable of reacting with proteins or DNA (eg, 2-acetylaminofluorene). *N*-sulfonation of arylamines to arylsulfamic acids ($R\text{-}NHSO_3H$) is a minor pathway.[127]

Conjugation With Amino Acids

Conjugation with amino acids is an important route in the metabolism of drugs or xenobiotic carboxylic acids before elimination. The reaction involves the formation of CoA thioesters, with CoA serving as the carboxylic acid–activating cofactor. Glycine and taurine are the most common amino acids that form water-soluble ionic conjugates with aromatic, arylaliphatic, and heterocyclic carboxylic acids. These conjugates are usually less toxic than their precursor acids and are readily excreted into the urine and bile. The reactions involve the formation of an amide or peptide bond between the xenobiotic carboxylic acid and the amino group of the amino acid. The xenobiotic is first activated to its CoA thioester before reacting with the amino group (Fig. 3.35). The formation of the xenobiotic acyl CoA thioester is of critical importance in intermediary metabolism of lipids, as well as medium and long-chain fatty acids.[128]

The major metabolic biotransformations for xenobiotic carboxylic acids include conjugation with either glucuronic acid or glycine. Carboxylic acids can be bioactivated via two distinct pathways: UGT-catalyzed conjugation with glucuronic acid to acyl glucuronides, or acyl CoA synthetase–catalyzed formation of acyl CoA thioesters.[128] The reactive acyl glucuronides and CoA thioester intermediates of carboxylic acids are electrophilic and, therefore, can contribute to the acylation of target proteins (see "Reactive Metabolites Resulting From Bioactivation" section). The acyl CoA

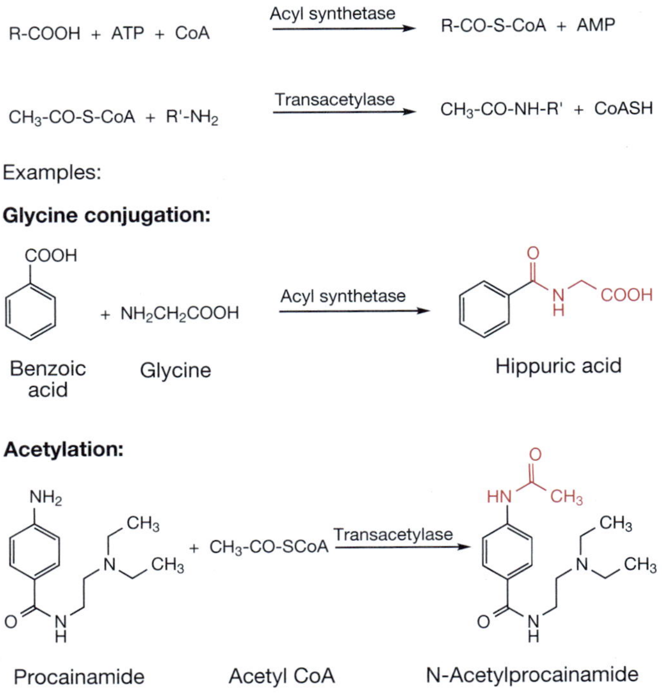

Figure 3.35 Amino acid conjugation pathway of carboxylic acids with glycine and acetylation pathway catalyzed by acetyltransferases.

thioester serves as an obligatory intermediate in the formation of glycine conjugates and carnitine esters, which are involved in mitochondrial acyl transfer or elimination of acyl groups into urine. Therefore, their appearance in metabolism studies and urine is of significance because they serve as biomarkers for the formation of acyl CoA thioesters, which can provide the link between protein-reactive acyl CoA thioesters and rare and unpredictable idiosyncratic drug reactions (IDRs) in humans. Unlike CYP and UGT, which are localized in the smooth ER, the enzymes of amino acid conjugation reside in mitochondria of the liver and kidney.[128]

Glycine conjugation has generally been assumed to be a detoxification mechanism, increasing the water solubility of organic acids in order to facilitate their urinary excretion. However, glycine conjugation does not significantly increase the water solubility of aromatic acids. In this case, the role of glycine conjugation is to dispose of the end products of benzoic acid metabolism into hippuric acid products.[129]

The metabolic fate of carboxylic acids depends on the size and type of substituents adjacent to the carboxyl group. Most unbranched aliphatic acids are completely oxidized by β-oxidation to acetic acids and do not typically form conjugates. Branched aliphatic and arylaliphatic acids are resistant to β-oxidation and form glycine or acyl glucuronide conjugates, and substitution of the α-carbon favors glucuronidation over glycine conjugation. Benzoic and heterocyclic aromatic acids are mostly conjugated with glycine. Glycine conjugation is preferred for xenobiotic carboxylic acids at low doses, and glucuronidation is preferred at high doses with broad substrate selectivity. In humans, glutamine can also form a conjugate with phenylacetic acids and related arylacetic acids. Bile acids form conjugates with glycine and taurine by the action of enzymes in the microsomal fraction rather than in the mitochondria.

In contrast to the enhanced reactivity and toxicity of some glucuronides, sulfate ester, acetyl and GSH conjugates, amino acid conjugates have not been proven to be toxic. However, organic acids can be toxic if they are not a substrate for glycine conjugation with CoA.[130] Carboxylic acids have been associated with adverse reactions linked to the metabolic activation of the carboxylic acid moiety of the compounds. It has been proposed that amino acid conjugation is a detoxication pathway for reactive acyl CoA thioesters. Several carboxylic acid–containing drugs (eg, zomepirac and benoxaprofen) have been implicated in rare but serious adverse reactions. These carboxylic acids were withdrawn in the late 1980s from the market as a result of unpredictable idiosyncratic reactions that could have been caused by carboxylic acid–protein adducts formed by reaction of their reactive acyl glucuronide or acyl CoA thioesters with endogenous proteins.

Acetylation

Acetylation is principally a reaction of amino groups involving the transfer of acetyl CoA to primary aliphatic and aromatic amines, amino acids, hydrazines, or sulfonamide groups, but at first glance seems contradictory because the metabolites produced by the acetylation are less water soluble. The liver is the primary site of acetylation, although extrahepatic sites have been identified. Antimicrobial sulfonamides (eg, sulfisoxazole), being bifunctional, can form either N_1 or N_4 acetyl derivatives. Secondary amines are not acetylated. Acetylation can produce conjugates that retain the pharmacologic activity of the parent drug (eg, *N*-acetylprocainamide) (see Fig. 3.35).

Acetylation, a nonmicrosomal form of metabolism, also exhibits polymorphisms that were first demonstrated in the acetylation of isoniazid.[131] Two *N*-acetyltransferases (NAT1 and NAT2) occur in humans, they have distinct substrate specificity and differ in organ and tissue distribution. NAT1 (arylamine NAT) is widely distributed and catalyzes the *N*-acetylation of acidic arylamines, such as *p*-aminobenzoic acid, *p*-aminosalicylic acid, and *p*-aminobenzoyl glutamic acid; therefore, its expression levels in the body have toxicologic importance regarding drug toxicity and cancer risk (eg, bladder cancer and colorectal cancer). The large distribution of NAT1 throughout several body tissues indicates an endogenous function beyond the metabolism of xenobiotics. Since it uses acetyl CoA as a cofactor, this implies it being a critical player in the regulation of the cell cycle and it is proposed to be an epigenetic regulator in folate metabolism.

NAT2 is found predominantly in the liver, intestine, and prostate. Clinically used drugs that undergo NAT2-catalyzed *N*-acetylation include isoniazid, sulfamethazine, procainamide, hydralazine, phenelzine, dapsone, caffeine, and the carcinogenic secondary *N*-alkylarylamines (2-aminofluorene, benzidine, and 4-aminobiphenyl). Substituents ortho to the amino group sterically block acetylation.[117,132] Polymorphisms in the NAT2 gene in human populations can be segregated into fast, intermediate, and slow acetylator phenotypes. Acetylation polymorphism has been associated with differences in human drug toxicity between slow and fast acetylator phenotypes. Slow acetylators are more prone to drug-induced toxicities and accumulate higher blood concentrations of the unacetylated drug than do fast acetylators. Examples of toxicities that can result include hydralazine- and procainamide-induced lupus erythematosus,[130] isoniazid-induced peripheral nerve damage, and sulfasalazine-induced hematologic disorders. Fast acetylators eliminate a drug more rapidly by conversion to its relatively nontoxic *N*-acetyl metabolite. However, for some drug substances, fast acetylators can pose a greater risk of liver toxicity than slow acetylators because fast acetylators produce toxic metabolites more rapidly. Interestingly, intestinal NAT appears not to be polymorphic (ie, 5-aminosalicylic acid).

Polymorphisms in NAT2 are associated with higher incidences of cancer. The possibility arises that genetic differences in acetylation capacity can confer differences in susceptibility to chemical carcinogenicity from arylamines.[133] The tumorigenic activity of arylamines can be the result of a complex series of sequential metabolic reactions commencing with *N*-hydroxylation by CYP1A2 or CYP2E1, followed by *N*-acetylation by NATs to form the *N*-acetoxy derivative (Fig. 3.36). The acetoxyarylamine can eventually eliminate the acetoxy group to form the reactive arylnitrenium ion which is capable of covalently binding to nucleic acids and proteins, thus increasing the risk for development of bladder and liver tumors. The rapid acetylator phenotype

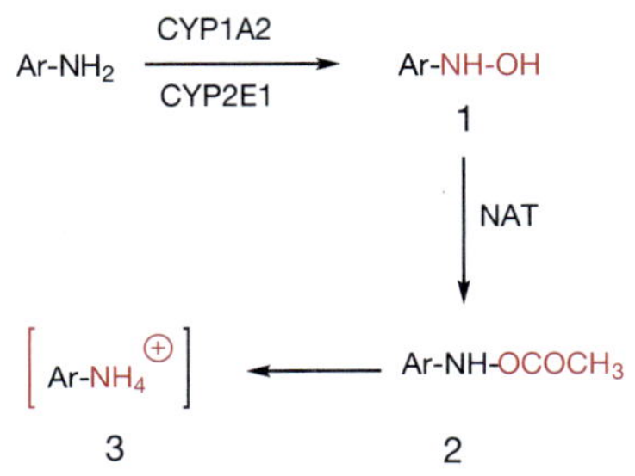

Figure 3.36 Bioactivation of acetylated arylamines.

is expected to form the acetoxyarylamine metabolite at a faster rate than the slow acetylator phenotype and, thereby, to present a greater risk for the development of tumors.[134]

Glutathione Conjugation and Mercapturic Acid Synthesis

Mercapturic acids are *S*-derivatives of *N*-acetyl-L-cysteine synthesized from GSH.[135,136] The mercapturic acid pathway appears to have evolved as a protective (scavenger) mechanism against xenobiotic-induced hepatotoxicity or carcinogenicity, serving to detoxify a large number of noxious substances (particularly electrophiles) that we inhale or ingest, or that are produced daily in the human body. Several enzymes of the mercapturic acid pathway are named "moonlighting" proteins (involved in various biochemical and biophysical functions).[135] Most xenobiotics that are metabolized to mercapturic acids first undergo conjugation with GSH catalyzed by the enzyme glutathione *S*-transferase (GST), a multigene isoenzyme superfamily that is abundant in the soluble supernatant liver fractions. In humans, there are three different GST superfamilies, cytosolic GST (17 members), mitochondrial kappa-class GST (1 member), and microsomal MAPEG (6 members). The GST cytosolic superfamily is the most involved in xenobiotics and consists of seven classes: alpha (five members, A1-A5), mu (five members, M1-M5), omega (two members, O1-O2), pi (one member, P1), theta (two members, T1-T2), zeta (one member, Z1), and sigma (one member, S1). The principal drug substrates for the mu family are the nitrosourea and mustard-type anticancer drugs. The theta isoform metabolizes small organic molecules, such as solvents, halocarbons, and electrophilic compounds (eg, α,β-unsaturated carbonyl compounds). The GSH conjugation reaction to mercapturic acid metabolites is depicted in Figure 3.37.

GST increases the ionization of the thiol group of GSH, increasing its nucleophilicity toward electrophiles (a group or ion that accepts an electron pair to make a covalent bond such as a carbocation or acyl ion) and thereby increasing the rate of conjugation with these potentially harmful electrophiles. In this way, GSH conjugation protects other vital nucleophilic centers in the cell, such as nucleic acids and proteins, from these electrophiles. GSH is also capable of reacting nonenzymatically with nucleophilic sites on some drugs and chemicals (see Fig. 3.37). Once conjugated with GSH, electrophiles are excreted in the bile and urine.

A range of functional groups yield thioether conjugates of GSH as well as products other than thioethers (see Fig. 3.37). The nucleophilic attack by GSH occurs on electrophilic carbons with leaving groups (eg, halogen [alkyl, alkenyl,

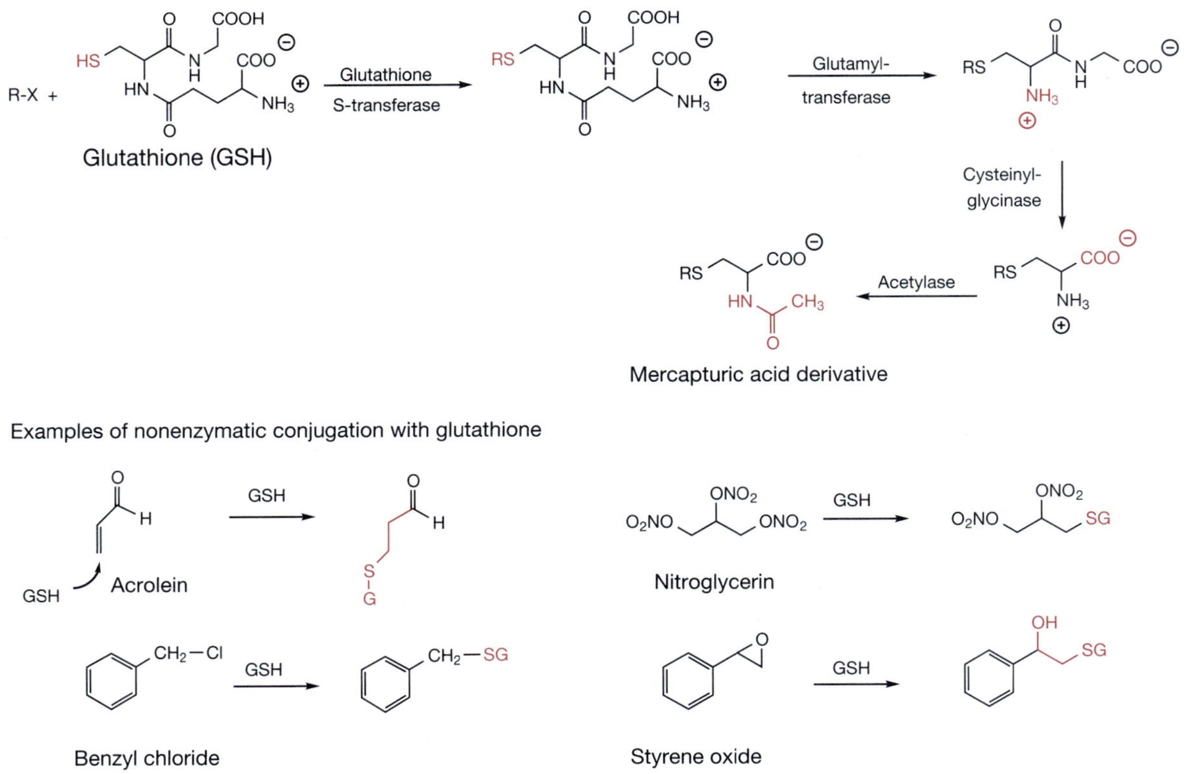

Figure 3.37 Glutathione and mercapturic acid conjugation pathways.

aryl, or aralkyl halides], sulfonates [alkylmethanesulfonates], and nitro [alkyl nitrates] groups), ring opening of small cyclic ethers (epoxides and β-lactones, eg, β-propiolactone), and the Michael-type addition to the activated β-carbon of an α,β-unsaturated carbonyl compound (eg, acrolein) (see "Reactive Metabolites Resulting From Bioactivation" section). The lack of substrate specificity provides a basis to further support the presumption that GSH transferase has undergone adaptive changes to accommodate the variety of xenobiotics to which it is exposed. The conjugation of an electrophilic compound with GSH is usually a reaction of detoxication, but in some cases carcinogens have been activated through conjugation with GSH.[136]

The enzymatic conjugation of GSH with epoxides provides a mechanism for protecting the liver from injury caused by certain bioactivated intermediates (see "Reactive Metabolites Resulting From Bioactivation" section). Not all epoxides are substrates for this enzyme, but the more chemically reactive epoxides appear vulnerable. Important among the epoxides that are substrates for this enzyme are those produced from halobenzenes and PAHs through the action of a P450 monooxygenase. Epoxide formation represents bioactivation because the epoxides are reactive and potentially toxic, whereas their GSH conjugates are inactive. Conjugation of GSH with the epoxides of aryl hydrocarbons eventually results in the formation of hydroxymercapturic acids (pre-mercapturic acids), which undergo acid-catalyzed dehydration to the mercapturic acids. The halobenzenes are typically conjugated in the *p*-position.[136]

Monohalogenated, *gem*-dihalogenated, and vicinal dihalogenated alkanes undergo GSH transferase–catalyzed conjugation reactions to produce *S*-substituted GSH derivatives that are metabolically transformed into the more stable and less toxic mercapturic acids. This common route of metabolism occurs through nucleophilic displacement of a halide ion by the thiolate anion of GSH. The mutagenicity of the 1,2-dihaloethanes (eg, the pesticide and fumigant ethylene dibromide) has been attributed to GSH displacing bromide with the formation of the *S*-(2-haloethyl) GSH, which subsequently rearranges to a reactive episulfonium ion electrophile that, in turn, alkylates DNA. Many of the halogenated hydrocarbons exhibiting nephrotoxicity undergo the formation of similar *S*-substituted cysteine derivatives.[137]

A correlation exists between the hepatotoxicity of acetaminophen and levels of GSH in the liver. The probable mechanism of toxicity that has emerged from animal studies is that acetaminophen is oxidized by CYP1A2 and CYP2E1 to the *N*-acetyl-*p*-benzoquinoneimine intermediate, which conjugates with and depletes hepatic GSH levels (Fig. 3.38). This action allows the benzoquinoneimine to bind covalently to tissue macromolecules. The mercapturic acid derivative of acetaminophen represents approximately 2% of the administered dose. Thus, the possibility exists that the toxic metabolites that are mostly detoxified by conjugating with GSH exhibit their hepatotoxicity (or, perhaps, carcinogenicity) because the liver has been depleted of GSH and is incapable of inactivating them. Pretreatment of animals with phenobarbital often hastens the depletion of GSH by increasing the formation of epoxides or other reactive intermediates.[138]

Methylation

Methylation is a common biochemical reaction but appears to be of greater significance in the metabolism of endogenous compounds and epigenetics than for drugs and other xenobiotics. Methylation differs from other conjugation processes in that the *O*-methyl metabolites formed can sometimes have as great or greater pharmacologic activity and lipophilicity than the parent molecule (eg, the conversion of norepinephrine to epinephrine). Methionine is involved in the methylation of endogenous and exogenous substrates, transferring a methyl group via the activated intermediate *S*-adenosylmethionine to the substrate under the influence of methyltransferases (Fig. 3.39). Methylation results principally in the formation of *O*-methylated, *N*-methylated, and *S*-methylated products.

O-Methylation

O-methylation is commonly, but not exclusively, catalyzed by the magnesium-dependent enzyme catechol-*O*-methyltransferase (COMT), which transfers a methyl group primarily to the *meta* (*m*)- or 3-hydroxy group of the catechol moiety (3,4-dihydroxylphenyl moiety) of norepinephrine, epinephrine, or dopamine, resulting in inactivation. Less frequently, the *p*- or 4-hydroxy group of these catecholamines and their deaminated metabolites is methylated (ie, the reaction is regioselective). COMT does not methylate monophenols or other dihydroxy non-catechol phenols. The *m*/*p* product ratio depends greatly on the type of

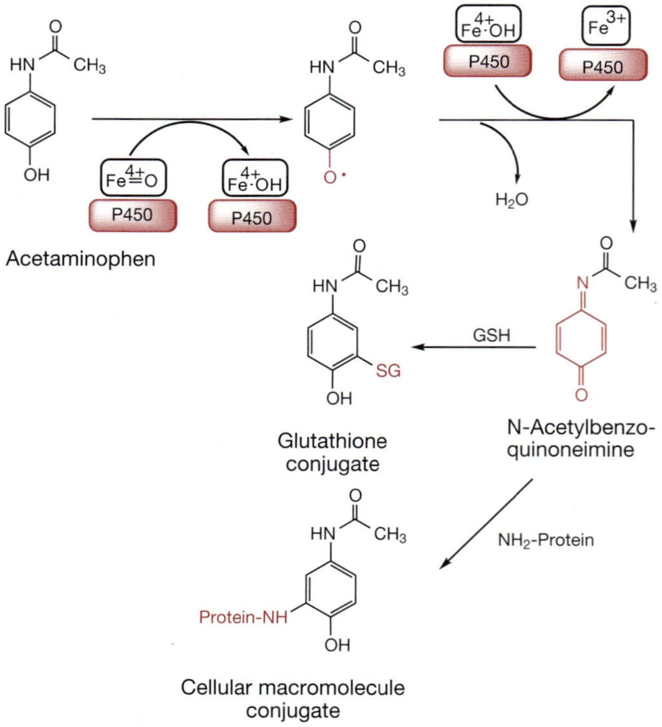

Figure 3.38 Proposed mechanism for the P450-catalyzed oxidation of acetaminophen to its *N*-acetyl-*p*-benzoquinoneimine intermediate, which can further react with either glutathione (GSH) or cellular macromolecules (NH_2-protein).

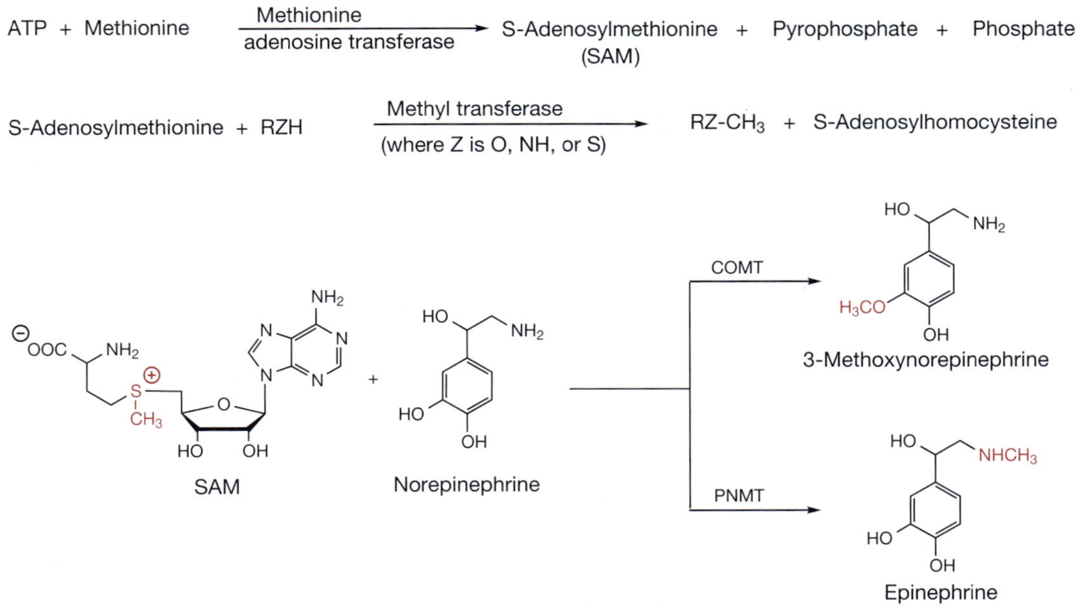

Figure 3.39 Methylation pathways.

substituent attached to the catechol ring. Substrates specific for COMT include the catecholamines norepinephrine, epinephrine, and dopamine, the catechol amino acids L-DOPA and α-methyl-DOPA, and 2- and 4-hydroxyestradiol (catechol-like) metabolites of estradiol. COMT is found in the liver, kidneys, nervous tissue, and other tissues.

Hydroxyindole-O-methyltransferase (also known as N-acetylserotonin O-methyltransferase), which O-methylates N-acetylserotonin, serotonin, and other hydroxyindoles, is found in the pineal gland and is involved in the formation of melatonin, a hormone associated with the dark-light diurnal cycle in humans. This enzyme differs from COMT in that it does not methylate catecholamines and has no requirement for magnesium ion.

N-Methylation

N-Methylation is among several conjugation options for metabolizing amines. Specific *N*-methyltransferases catalyze the transfer of activated methyl groups from *S*-adenosylmethionine to the acceptor substance. Phenylethanolamine-*N*-methyltransferase methylates several endogenous and exogenous phenylethanolamines (eg, normetanephrine, norepinephrine, and norephedrine) but does not methylate phenylethylamines. Histamine-*N*-methyl transferase methylates specifically histamine, producing the inactive metabolite N_1-methylhistamine. Indolethylamine *N*-methyltransferase (also known as amine-*N*-methyltransferase, nicotine *N*-methyltransferase, tryptamine *N*-methyltransferase, and arylamine *N*-methyltransferase) will *N*-methylate a variety of primary and secondary amines from a number of sources, including endogenous biogenic amines (serotonin, tryptamine, tyramine, and dopamine) and drugs (desmethylimipramine, amphetamine, and normorphine). Indolethylamine *N*-methyltransferase seems to have a role in recycling *N*-demethylated drugs.

S-Methylation

As a rule, thiols are toxic, and the role of thiol methyltransferases (TMTs) is a nonoxidative detoxification pathway of these compounds. *S*-methylation of sulfhydryl compounds also involves a microsomal enzyme requiring *S*-adenosylmethionine. Although a wide range of exogenous sulfhydryl compounds are *S*-methylated by this microsomal enzyme, none of the endogenous sulfhydryl compounds (eg, cysteine and GSH) can function as substrates. Dialkyldithiocarbamates (eg, disulfiram) and the antithyroid drugs (eg, 6-propyl-2-thiouracil), mercaptans, and hydrogen sulfide (from thioglycosides as natural constituents of foods, mineral sulfides in water, fermented beverages, and bacterial digestion) are *S*-methylated. Other drugs undergoing *S*-methylation include captopril, thiopurine, azathioprine, penicillamine, and 6-mercaptopurine.

Thiopurine methyltransferase or thiopurine *S*-methyltransferase (TPMT) catalyzes the *S*-methylation of thiopurine drugs, such as 6-mercaptopurine. Interindividual variations in sensitivity and toxicity to thiopurine are correlated with TPMT genetic polymorphisms. Mercaptopurine is a prodrug, and its activation cannot occur if the SH group is methylated; dosing regimens are designed for patients who carry the wild-type TPMT allele (normal methylation rate). Patients who are TPMT PMs cannot effectively methylate the drug and will essentially activate the entire dose of mercaptopurine, leading to potentially fatal bone marrow suppression. Interestingly, if *S*-methylation takes place after drug activation, the metabolite has an estimated 10-fold increase in potency. This can result in the anomaly of TPMT extensive metabolizers (EMs) also being at risk for toxicity, since they will rapidly convert any activated mercaptopurine molecules to the super-potent *S*-methyl metabolite. Approximately 5% of all thiopurine therapies will fail due to toxicity related to TPMT polymorphism.

Elimination Pathways

Most xenobiotics are lipid soluble and are altered chemically by the metabolizing enzymes, usually into less toxic and more water-soluble substances, before being excreted into the urine or bile. The formation of conjugates with sulfonate, amino acids, and glucuronic acid is particularly effective in increasing the hydrophilicity of drug molecules. The principal route of excretion of drugs and their metabolites is via the urine. If drugs and other compounds foreign to the body are not metabolized in this manner, substances with a high lipid-water partition coefficient could be reabsorbed readily from the urine through the renal tubular membranes and returned to the plasma. Therefore, such substances would continue to be recirculated and their pharmacologic or toxic effects would be prolonged. Very polar or highly ionized drug molecules often are excreted in the urine unchanged. The bile and biliary efflux transporters have been recognized as major routes of excretion for many endogenous and exogenous compounds. Other elimination routes include saliva, lungs, sweat, and milk.

Enterohepatic Circulation of Drugs

The liver is the principal organ for the metabolism and eventual elimination of xenobiotics from the human body in either the urine or the bile. When eliminated in the bile, steroid hormones, bile acids, drugs, and their respective conjugated metabolites are available for reabsorption from the duodenal-intestinal tract into the portal circulation, undergoing the process of enterohepatic recirculation (EHC) (Fig. 3.40).[139] Nearly all drugs are excreted in the bile, but only a few are concentrated in the bile. For example, the bile salts are efficiently concentrated in the bile and reabsorbed from the GI tract, such that the entire body pool of bile acids/salts is recycled multiple times per day. Therefore, EHC is responsible for the conservation of bile acids, steroid hormones, thyroid hormones, and other endogenous substances.

In humans, compounds excreted into the bile typically have a molecular weight greater than 500 Da, and metabolites with a molecular weight between 300 and 500 Da are excreted in both urine and bile. Compounds excreted into bile are, as a rule, hydrophilic substances that can be either charged (anionic) or uncharged (eg, cardiac glycosides and steroid hormones). Biotransformation of these compounds by means of phase 1 and phase 2 reactions would produce a conjugated metabolite, which is anionic and hydrophilic with a molecular weight greater than that of the parent compound. The conjugated metabolites in bile are most often glucuronides, because glucuronidation adds 176 Da to the molecular weight of the parent compound. Unchanged drug in the bile is excreted with the feces, metabolized by the bacterial flora in the intestinal tract, or reabsorbed into the portal circulation via EHC.[139,140]

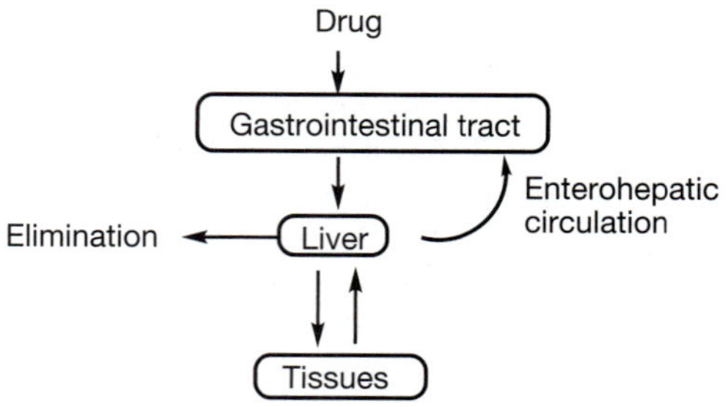

Figure 3.40 Enterohepatic cycling.

The intestinal microbiota is directly involved in EHC and the recycling of drugs through the portal circulation. A conjugated drug and metabolites excreted via the bile can be hydrolyzed by enzymes of the bacterial flora, releasing the parent drug or its phase 1 or 2 metabolite for reabsorption into the portal circulation. Among the numerous compounds metabolized in the EHC process are estrogen- and progestin-based steroids, digitoxin, indomethacin, diazepam, pentaerythritol tetranitrate, mercurials, arsenicals, and morphine. The oral ingestion of xenobiotics inhibiting the gut flora can affect the pharmacokinetics of drugs.[141]

The impact of EHC on the pharmacokinetics and pharmacodynamics of a drug depends on the importance of biliary excretion relative to renal clearance and on the efficiency of GI reabsorption. The EHC becomes dominant when biliary excretion is the major clearance mechanism for the drug. Because most of the bile is stored in the gallbladder and released upon the ingestion of food, intermittent spikes in the plasma drug concentration are observed following reentry of the drug from the bile via EHC, resulting in a multiple peak phenomenon. From a pharmacodynamic point of view, the net effect of EHC is to increase the duration of a drug in the body and to prolong its pharmacologic action.[139,140]

Drug Metabolism and Age

Metabolism in Older Adults

The widespread use of medications in older adults, as well as the complex process of aging, increase the potential for drug-related interactions, which can be related to changes in drug metabolism and clearance from the body (Table 3.14). The interpretation of the age-related alteration in drug response must consider the contributions of absorption, distribution, metabolism, and excretion. Drug therapy in older adults is one of the more significant problems for clinical medicine. It has been well documented that the metabolism of many drugs and their elimination is impaired in older adults.[142-144]

The decline in drug metabolism due to advancing age is associated with physiologic changes that have pharmacokinetic implications affecting the steady-state plasma concentrations and renal clearance for the parent drug and its metabolites. Changes relevant to the bioavailability of drugs in older adults are decreases in hepatic blood flow, glomerular filtration rate, hepatic P450 activity, plasma protein binding, and body mass. Because the rate of a drug's elimination from the blood through hepatic metabolism is determined by hepatic blood flow, protein binding, and intrinsic clearance, a reduction in hepatic blood flow can

Table 3.14 Effect of Age on the Clearance of Some Drugs

No Change	Decrease
Acetaminophen[a]	Alprazolam
Aspirin	Amitriptyline
Diclofenac	Chlordiazepoxide
Diphenhydramine	Chlormethiazole
Ethanol	Diazepam
Flunitrazepam	Labetalol
Midazolam	Lidocaine
Nitrazepam	Lorazepam
Oxazepam	Morphine
Phenytoin[a]	Meperidine
Prazosin	Nifedipine and other dihydropyridines
Propylthiouracil	Norepinephrine
Temazepam	Nortriptyline
Thiopental[a]	Phenytoin
Tolbutamide[a]	Piroxicam
Warfarin	Propranolol
	Quinidine
	Quinine
	Theophylline
	Verapamil

[a]Drugs for which clearance is disputable but can be increased.

lead to an increase in drug bioavailability and decreased clearance, with the symptoms of drug overdose and toxicity as the outcome (eg, warfarin in patients with congestive heart failure[145]). Those orally administered drugs exhibiting a reduction in first-pass metabolism in older adults include antihypertensives, diuretics, and antidepressants.

Age-related changes in drug metabolism are a complicated interplay between the age-related physiologic changes, genetics, environmental influences (diet and nutritional status, smoking, and enzyme induction), concomitant disease states, and drug intake. In most studies, older adults appear to be just as responsive to drug-metabolizing enzyme activity (phase 1 and phase 2) as younger individuals. Given the number of factors that determine the rate of drug metabolism, it is not surprising that the effects of aging on drug elimination by metabolism have yielded variable results, even for the same drug. The fact that drug elimination can be altered in old age suggests that doses of metabolized drugs should be initially reduced in elderly patients and then adjusted according to the clinical response. A decrease in hepatic drug metabolism coupled with age-related alterations in clearance, volume of distribution, and receptor sensitivity can lead to prolonged plasma half-life and increased drug toxicity. Thus, pharmacodynamic changes and their mechanism of action for the elderly are much more difficult to study and to predict.[144]

Drug Metabolism in the Fetus and During Pregnancy

Over two-thirds of patients receive prescription drugs while pregnant, with treatment and dosing strategies based on data from healthy male volunteers and nonpregnant females, and with little adjustment for the complex physiology of pregnancy and its unique potential disease states. Hormone levels, volume of distribution, cardiac output, renal clearance, and protein binding are some of the physiologic changes that occur during pregnancy. Hormone levels in the plasma, which rise during pregnancy, are capable of regulating expression of hepatic drug-metabolizing enzymes. These hormones include estrogens, progesterone, cortisol, and prolactin. Studies are needed to examine the role of pregnancy hormones in altered drug metabolism during pregnancy. Pharmacogenomic aspects must also be taken into consideration.[146-149]

The activities of CYP3A4, CYP2B6, CYP2D6, CYP2C8, CYP2E1, and CYP2C9 are all increased during pregnancy. Enhancement of CYP3A4 activity leads to increased metabolism of many drugs (Table 3.10). By contrast, CYP1A2 and CYP2C19 decrease in activity with advancing gestation, though with uncertain effects on drug therapy.[147,148] The activity of phase 2 enzymes, including UGTs (particularly UGT1A1 and UGT1A4), is also altered during pregnancy, with a 200% increase in UGT1A4 activity during the first and second trimesters. This change leads to lower concentrations of UGT1A4 substrates such as lamotrigine, leading directly to poorer seizure control with advancing gestation in the absence of appropriate dose titration. Moreover, other factors such as UGT1A4 polymorphism and/or estradiol upregulation can be important in pregnancy.[147]

Knowledge of drug transporter function during pregnancy is necessary for a complete understanding of drug absorption, distribution, elimination, and effect. In addition, fetal development is dependent upon the transport of nutrients by the placenta toward the fetal side and the transport of fetal metabolic products away from the fetus for subsequent elimination by the mother. The placenta produces and secretes hormones that affect the maternal physiology and endocrine state. Compounds transported between the mother and the fetus are carried by maternal circulation within the uterine vasculature.

The ability of the human fetus and placenta to metabolize xenobiotics is well established. Drug-metabolizing enzymes expressed in the placenta include CYP1A1, CYP2E1, CYP3A4/5, CYP3A7, CYP4B1, epoxide hydrolase, ADH, GST, UGT, SULTs, and NAT. Many of the drugs used in pregnancy readily cross the placenta, thus exposing the fetus to a large number of xenobiotic agents. The human fetus is at special risk from these substances due to the presence of the P450 system, which is capable of metabolizing xenobiotics during the first part of gestation. Placentas of those who smoke tobacco have shown a significant increase in the rate of placental CYP1A activity. There is cause for concern because this enzyme system is known to catalyze the formation of reactive metabolites capable of covalently binding to macromolecules, producing permanent effects (eg, teratogenicity, hepatotoxicity, or carcinogenicity) in the fetus and newborn. Adding to the concern is the fact that conjugation enzymes (ie, UGT, GST, and SULT), which are important for the formation of phase 2 conjugates of these reactive metabolites, are found in low to negligible levels in the fetus and newborn, increasing the exposure of these infants to these potentially toxic metabolites.[147]

The placenta is not a barrier protecting the fetus from xenobiotics; almost every drug present in the maternal circulation will cross the placenta and reach the fetus. For some drugs, however, the placental efflux transport (ATP-binding cassette [ABC] transporters) protein P-gp functions as a materno-fetal barrier, pumping drugs and P-gp substrates out of the fetal circulation back into the maternal circulation and protecting the fetus from exposure to potentially harmful teratogenic xenobiotics/drugs and endogenous substances that have been absorbed through the placenta.[150] Before administration to patients who are pregnant, drugs that are P-gp inhibitors should be carefully evaluated for their potential to increase fetal susceptibility to drug/chemical-induced teratogenesis. On the other hand, selective inhibition of P-gp could be used clinically to improve pharmacotherapy of the unborn infant.

Because metabolites are usually more water soluble than the parent substance, drug metabolites formed in the fetus can be trapped and accumulate on the fetal side of the placenta. Such accumulation can result in drug-induced toxicities or developmental defects. The activity of CYP3A isoenzymes in the human fetal liver is like that seen in adult liver microsomes. The fetal activity for CYP3A7 is unusual, as most other fetal isoenzymes of P450 exhibit activity 5% to 40% of the adult isoenzymes. Fetal and neonatal drug-metabolizing enzyme activities can differ from those in adults.[146,147]

Most xenobiotics cross the placental barrier by simple diffusion. Protein binding, degree of ionization, lipid solubility, and molecular weight can affect placental transport. In fact, small, lipid-soluble, ionized, and poorly protein-bound molecules cross the placenta easily. For other substrates, the placenta facilitates maternal to fetal transport through the expression of various transporters. Transporters enable influx or efflux of specific endogenous substrates (such as cytokines, nucleoside analogs, and steroid hormones); however, exogenous compounds with similar structures may also interact.[146]

From the day of birth, the neonate is exposed to drugs and other foreign compounds persisting from pregnancy as well as those transferred via breast milk. Fortunately, many of the drug-metabolizing enzymes are operative in the neonate, developed during the fetal period. The routine use of therapeutic agents during labor and delivery, as well as during pregnancy, is widespread, and consideration must be given to the fact that potentially harmful metabolites can be generated by the fetus and newborn. Consequently, the use of drugs capable of forming reactive metabolic intermediates should be avoided during pregnancy, delivery, and the neonatal period. The activity of phase 1 and phase 2 drug-metabolizing enzymes is high at birth but decreases to normal levels with increasing age. Evidence suggests increased activity of drug-metabolizing enzymes in liver microsomes of neonates resulting from treatment of the mother during the pregnancy with enzyme inducers (eg, phenobarbital).

Genetic Polymorphism

The reality of drug therapy is that many drugs do not work in all patients.[151,152] By current estimates, the percentage of patients who will react favorably to a drug ranges from 20% to 80%. Drugs have been developed and dosage regimens prescribed under the old paradigm that "one dose fits all," which largely ignores the fact that humans are genetically different, resulting in interindividual differences in drug metabolism and disposition. It is widely accepted that genetic factors have an important impact on the oxidative metabolism and pharmacokinetics of drugs.[153] Genotype-phenotype correlation studies (pharmacogenetics) have shown that inherited mutations in P450 genes (alleles) result in distinct phenotypic subgroups. For example, mutations in the *CYP2D6* gene result in poor (PM), intermediate (IM), normal (NM), and rapid (RM) metabolizers of CYP2D6 substrates (see Table 3.8).[154,155] Each of these phenotypic subgroups experiences different responses to drugs extensively metabolized by the CYP2D6 pathway, ranging from severe toxicity to complete lack of efficacy. Genetic studies confirm that "one dose does not fit all," leaving the question of why we would continue to develop and prescribe drugs under the old paradigm. Regulatory agencies have recognized that identifying genetic polymorphisms might allow the safe dosing, marketing, and approval of drugs that would otherwise not be approved and advised pharmaceutical companies to incorporate the knowledge of genetic polymorphisms into drug development. In fact, the FDA has genomic biomarker data on approximately 500 drugs used in the United States.[34] Importantly, pharmacogenomic testing (the study of heritable traits affecting patient response to drug treatment) can significantly increase the likelihood of developing drug regimens that benefit most patients without severe adverse events. Pharmacists play a vital role in the development of patient-specific dosing regimens based on metabolizing phenotype.[153] In the era of the "omics," pharmacogenomics is a corner stone in precision medicine.[156]

Polymorphisms are expressed for several metabolizing enzymes, but the polymorphic P450 isoforms that are most important include CYP2A6, CYP2B6, CYP2C8, CYP2C9, CYP2C19, CYP2D6, CYP3A4, and CYP3A5.[155,157] Most gene variants are expressed into inactive, truncated proteins or they fail to express any protein. These polymorphic isoforms give rise to phenotypic subgroups in the population differing in their ability to perform clinically significant biotransformation reactions with obvious clinical ramifications. Metabolic polymorphism can have several consequences; for example, when enzymes that metabolize drugs to inactive metabolites are deficient, therapeutic or recreational usage of these drugs can pose the risk of adverse or toxic drug reactions in these individuals.[152]

The discovery of genetic polymorphism resulted from the observation of increased frequency of adverse effects or no drug effects after normal doses of drugs to some patients (eg, hyper-CNS response from the administration of the antihistamine doxylamine or no analgesic response with codeine). Polymorphism is a difference in DNA sequence found at 1% or greater in a population and expressed as an amino acid substitution in the protein sequence of an enzyme resulting in changes in its rate of activity (V_{max}) or affinity (K_m). Thus, mutant DNA sequences can lead to interindividual differences in drug metabolism. Furthermore, polymorphisms do not occur with equivalent frequency in all racial or ethnic groups. Because of these differences, it is important to be aware of a person's race and ethnicity when giving drugs that are metabolized differently by different populations, although practitioners must guard against stereotyping, For example, CYP2A6 PMs (33%) and IMs (49%) are predominate in the East Asian population, while, for the Middle Eastern population, only 2% are PMs.[91] Because no other way may exist to adequately clear these drugs from the body, PMs can be at greater risk for adverse drug reactions or toxic overdoses. The signs and symptoms of these overdoses are primarily extensions of the drug's common adverse effects or pharmacologic effects (Table 3.15).[152] The level of adverse reactions or overdosage depends very much on the overall contribution of the mutant isoform to the drug's metabolism. Perhaps the most interesting explanation for the various mutant isoforms is that they evolved as protective mechanisms against alkaloids and other common substances in the food chain for the different ethnicities.

Occasionally, one derives benefit from an unusual P450 phenotype. For example, cure rates for peptic ulcer treated with omeprazole are substantially greater in individuals with defective CYP2C19 due to the sustained high plasma levels achieved.

CYP3A4

CYP3A4 is of particular importance due to it being one of the major drug-metabolizing enzymes and because it is considered the CYP most responsible for drug/herbal/dietary supplement interactions. The differences in metabolic phenotypes for this enzyme are low. For example, in the European population 10% are IMs and the rest appear to be normal metabolizers (EM).[155] These data concur with the low number of missense mutations found for the *CYP3A4* gene (1.5%).[158] Drug interactions for the Parkinson disease drug istradefylline can be related to the use of the vasodilator nimodipine and various CYP3A4 polymorphisms.[159]

CYP2A6

CYP2A6 is of particular importance because it activates several procarcinogens to carcinogens and is the major isoform metabolizing nicotine and various commercial drugs.[160] It also has a high difference in metabolic phenotypes across ethnic groups.[155] CYP2A6 is exceptionally polymorphic, since approximately 33% of Asian populations are PMs as compared to 5% of Europeans. PM phenotype is correlated with the presence of the alleles *CYP2A6*4* (prevalent in the Asian population[161]) and *CYP2A6*7*, both of which heavily diminish the nicotinic metabolic ratio. Alleles *CYP2A6*1A*, **2*, **9*, and **12* also result in low-functioning enzymes and lower the nicotinic metabolic ratio. A benefit from being a PM of CYP2A6 substrates might be the protection against some carcinogens, including cigarette smoke, due to the high plasma levels of nicotine achieved with fewer cigarettes.

CYP2B6

CYP2B6 is of special interest due to its wide interindividual variability in expression and activity.[155,162] Such a large variability for an enzyme that is 3% expressed in liver (see Fig. 3.2) is probably because of genetic polymorphisms and exposure to drugs that are inducers or inhibitors of CYP2B6, which induce several DDIs.[163] Variant alleles resulting from splicing defects or gene deletions have been identified in individuals with PM with altered metabolic activity or impaired enzyme function. Of the approximately 48 different alleles currently described in PharmVar consortium, at least 28 allelic variants and some subvariants of *CYP2B6* have been shown to influence drug clearance and drug response. For example, HIV-infected individuals with a defective variant of *CYP2B6*6* are PMs of efavirenz and have plasma levels approximately 3-fold higher than individuals with the normal *CYP2B6* gene, increasing the risk of adverse reactions for those patients. On the other hand, patients with *CYP2B6*6* allele showed the lowest response to treatment with cyclophosphamide due to the inability to metabolize cyclophosphamide to the carbinolamine that nonenzymatically generates the active DNA-alkylating structure. Those with the *CYP2B6*6* allele also showed less mechanism-related toxicity in the cyclophosphamide treatment group, although other pathways to nonspecific toxicity are still functional. A different variant, *CYP2B6*18*, is associated with approximately 2-fold greater plasma levels of nevirapine in patients infected with HIV. A benefit of being a PM of CYP2B6 antiviral drugs might be enhanced HIV protection because of the higher plasma levels of the antiviral drugs achieved with lower dosages. Smokers with PM variants of *CYP2B6* may be more vulnerable to abstinence symptoms and relapse following treatment with bupropion (a CYP2B6 substrate) as a smoking cessation agent.[162,164]

CYP2C9

CYP2C9 is highly polymorphic with at least 80 variants identified. It is also the third highest P450 enzyme involved in drug metabolism, biotransforming 13% of clinically used drugs (see Fig. 3.3), including phenytoin, warfarin, sulfonylureas, and NSAIDs. Due to low-function protein, the *CYP2C9*2* allele is clinically significant, resulting in IM (when heterozygous with wild-type *1) or PM (when homozygous) phenotypes. It is frequently found among Caucasian-European (~13%), Asian (11%), Middle Eastern (13%), and Latino (8%) populations. Another clinically important allele is the nonfunctional *CYP2C9*3* variant found most frequently in Central/South Asian populations (11%).[165,166]

Table 3.15 **Impact of Human P450 Polymorphisms on Drug Treatment in Poor Metabolizers**

Polymorphic Enzyme	Decreased Clearance	Adverse Effects (Overdosage)	Reduced Activation of Coadministered Prodrug
CYP2C9	S-warfarin	Bleeding	Losartan
	Phenytoin	Ataxia	
	Losartan		
	Tolbutamide	Hypoglycemia	
	NSAIDs	GI bleeding	
CYP2C19	Omeprazole		Proguanil
	Diazepam	Sedation	
CYP2D6	Tricyclic antidepressants	Cardiotoxicity	Tramadol
	SSRIs	Serotonin syndrome	Codeine
	Antiarrhythmic drugs	Arrhythmias	Ethylmorphine
	Perhexiline	Neuropathy	
	Haloperidol	Parkinsonism	
	Perphenazine		
	Zuclopenthixol		
	S-Mianserin		
	Tolterodine		
CYP2A6	Nicotine		

GI, gastrointestinal; NSAID, nonsteroidal anti-inflammatory drug; SSRI, selective serotonin reuptake inhibitor.

Clinical studies have addressed the importance of the *CYP2C9*2* and *3 alleles as a determining factor for drug clearance and drug response. Individuals with any of the above IM/PM alleles have an increased area under the curve (AUC) for the NSAIDs ibuprofen, flurbiprofen, and celecoxib. It is currently recommended to initiate NSAID therapy with lower doses to avoid gastric bleeding and/or cardiovascular adverse effects or to choose alternative NSAIDs less dependent on CYP2C9 inactivation (eg, meloxicam and piroxicam).[167] Individuals with the PM phenotype who possess this deficient isoform variant are ineffective in clearing *S*-warfarin (so much so that they can be fully anticoagulated on just 0.5 mg of warfarin per day) and in the clearance of phenytoin, which can be potentially very toxic due to its narrow therapeutic range. On the other hand, the prodrug losartan will be poorly activated and ineffective. Along with *CYP2C9*2* and *3, the African allele *CYP2C9*11* was recently found to be a PM phenotype, with a 50% decrease in enzymatic activity compared to the wild type.[168]

CYP2C19

CYP2C19 metabolizes approximately 7% of clinically used drugs. Although CYP2C19 metabolizes fewer drugs than CYP2D6, the drugs that CYP2C19 does metabolize are clinically important (Table 3.7). The deficit of CYP2C19 found in the PM phenotype secondary to nonfunctional *CYP2C19*2*, 19*3, and 19*4 alleles is present in 15% and 12% of East Asian and South Asian populations, respectively. The allele *CYP2C19*7* is predominant in RMs, and this variant is found to a high extent in European/Caucasian (34%) and Middle Eastern (36%) populations.[155] The large interindividual variability observed in the therapeutic response to the antiseizure drug mephenytoin is attributed to CYP2C19 polymorphism, which catalyzes the *p*-hydroxylation of the *S*-stereoisomer. The *R*-enantiomer is *N*-demethylated by CYP2C8 with no difference in its metabolism between 2C19 PMs and NMs.[169] *CYP2C19*2* and *19*17* alleles are also implicated in the bioactivation of clopidogrel, voriconazole, tamoxifen, several antidepressants, and proton pump inhibitors.[153,170] A combined effect of CYP2C9 and CYP2C19 polymorphism is especially clinically significant with the sulfonylurea hypoglycemic agent gliclazide, which is biotransformed by both enzymes.[171]

CYP2D6

Even though CYP2D6 accounts for merely ~2% of the P450 content in liver (see Fig. 3.2), it is of specific importance because it metabolizes a wide range of commonly prescribed drugs, which translates to approximately 20% of drugs used clinically (see Fig. 3.3). The substrates of CYP2D6 include antidepressants, antipsychotics, β-adrenergic blockers, and antiarrhythmics (see Table 3.8).[157] Approximately 170 allelic variants have been characterized for CYP2D6 (PharmVar), making *CYP2D6* the most polymorphic P450 gene. This fact, along with the phenomenon called phenoconversion (in which an individual's drug response phenotype is conflicting with its genotype metabolizer due to nongenetic factors), gives insight into the complexity of CYP2D6 pharmacogenetics.[172]

CYP2D6 deficiency is a clinically relevant genetic determinant of drug metabolism. About 5% to 7% of Caucasians/Europeans have gene variants that result in a functionally deficient CYP2D6 enzyme, and these PMs often respond inadequately to drugs, such as codeine, that are activated by CYP2D6. The PM phenotype is inherited as an autosomal recessive trait, with 5 of 30 of the known *CYP2D6* gene mutations leading to either zero expression or the expression of a nonfunctional enzyme. At the other end, RMs are notably found in Oceania (21%), Jewish (11%), and Middle Eastern (9%-11%) populations.[151,172,173]

*CYP2D6*4, D6*10, D6*17,* and *D6*29* are all decreased function (PM) alleles, with *4 being nonfunctional.[151,172] Approximately 18% of Caucasians/Europeans and 22% of Ashkenazi Jews express the *CYP2D6*4* allele. *CYP2D6*17* and 6*29 alleles are highly expressed in Central/East African groups (14% of Hausa, 14% of Igbo, and 22% of Yoruba ethnic groups) and are also common in African Americans, with approximately 34% expressing these alleles. Between 35% and 79% of Asian populations express *CYP2D6*10* allele, but relatively low expression is observed in European (3%) and sub-Saharan African (6%) populations.[151,172] In contrast, 7% of Middle Eastern, 4.7% of European/Caucasian, and 5.6% of Ashkenazi Jew populations who carry the *CYP2D6*1xN* and/or *2D6*2xN* alleles are known as RMs of CYP2D6 substrates because they express excess enzyme due to functional gene duplications.[155] Inasmuch as CYP2D6 is not inducible, many individuals of Middle Eastern and sub-Saharan descent have developed a genetically different strategy to cope with the traditionally high load of alkaloids and other 2D6 substrates in their diet, thus the high expression of CYP2D6 using multiple copies of the gene.[174]

Individuals who are deficient in CYP2D6 will be predisposed to adverse effects or drug toxicity from antidepressants or neuroleptics caused by inadequate metabolism, leading to long half-lives, but the metabolism of CYP2D6-dependent prodrugs in these patients will be ineffective due to lack of activation (eg, codeine, which must be metabolized by O-demethylation to morphine). It can be anticipated that large differences in steady-state concentration for CYP2D6 substrates will occur between individuals of different phenotypes when they receive the same dose. It has been estimated that, depending on the drug and reaction type, a 10- to 30-fold difference in blood concentrations can be observed due to PM phenotype polymorphism.[172] Individuals with the PM phenotype also lose CYP2D6 stereoselectivity in hydroxylation reactions.

In contrast, individuals with the Ultrarapid metabolism (UM) phenotype will require a dose of drugs inactivated by CYP2D6 that is higher than normal to attain therapeutic drug plasma concentrations, and a lower dose for prodrugs that require 2D6-catalyzed activation. It is now recommended that analgesics other than the prodrug codeine be used in children to reduce the risk of severe toxicity in the event of an undisclosed UM phenotype. Individuals with the PM phenotype are also characterized by loss of CYP2D6 stereoselectivity in hydroxylation reactions.

Other Polymorphic-Metabolizing Enzymes

CYP2E1 polymorphism is expressed more frequently in individuals of Chinese ancestry than in Caucasians. Those with the CYP2E1 PM phenotype exhibit tolerance to alcohol and less toxicity from halohydrocarbon solvents. It is not clear whether a particular polymorph of CYP2E1 shows a significant effect with increasing or decreasing enzyme activity, thus the differentiation based on genotype is not well supported. Environmental factors (diet, lifestyle) might exert a significant effect on CYP2E1 phenotype.[175]

CYP1A enzymes play a fundamental role in influencing a multitude of endogenous processes. Polymorphic variability in these enzymes may be triggered by xenobiotics and carcinogens. For example, cigarette or coffee consumption may cause modification in the expression of these enzymes and/or the processes they regulate, possibly contributing to adverse effects, including ROS imbalance, carcinogen activation, endocrine disruption, and different drug pharmacokinetics. Several variants of these enzymes have been linked with cancer.[24,176]

Polymorphism has been associated with serum cholinesterases, ADH, ALDH, epoxide hydrolase, and XO. Approximately 50% of the East Asian population lacks ALDH, resulting in high levels of acetaldehyde following ethanol ingestion and causing nausea and flushing. People with genetic variants of cholinesterase respond abnormally to succinylcholine, procaine, and other related choline esters. The clinical consequence of reduced enzymatic activity of cholinesterase is that succinylcholine and procaine are not hydrolyzed in the blood, resulting in prolongation of their pharmacologic activities (eg, skeletal muscle paralysis in the case of succinylcholine).

First-Pass Metabolism

Although hepatic metabolism continues to be the most important route for xenobiotics, the ability of the liver and intestine to metabolize substances to either pharmacologically inactive or bioactive metabolites before reaching the systemic circulation is called presystemic first-pass metabolism. This metabolic process results in low systemic availability for orally susceptible drugs. Some drugs experience substantial first-pass metabolism and, in those cases, a different route of administration should be explored.[177] Sulfonation and glucuronidation are major pathways of presystemic intestinal first-pass metabolism in humans. For example, oral acetaminophen, phenylephrine, terbutaline, albuterol, fenoterol, or isoproterenol exhibit approximately 5% bioavailability because of sulfonation and glucuronidation in the GI tract.

The discovery that CYP3A4 is found in the mucosal enterocytes of the intestinal villi signifies its role as a key determinant in the oral bioavailability of its numerous drug substrates (see Table 3.10). Drugs known to be substrates for CYP3A often have a low and/or variable oral bioavailability that can be explained by presystemic first-pass metabolism by the small intestine P450 isoforms.[178] The concentration of functional intestinal CYP3A is influenced by genetic disposition, induction, and inhibition, which to a great extent determines drug blood levels and therapeutic response. Xenobiotics, when ingested orally, can change the activity of intestinal CYP3A enzymes by induction and inhibition. Through modulation of the isoform pattern in the intestine, a xenobiotic could alter its own metabolism and that of others in a time- and dose-dependent manner.

The concentration of CYP3A in the intestine is comparable to that of the liver. The oral administration of dexamethasone induces the formation of CYP3A, and erythromycin inhibits it. Glucocorticoid inducibility of CYP3A4 can also be a factor in differences of metabolism between males and females. Studies have suggested that intestinal CYP3A4 promotes C_2 hydroxylation of estradiol, contributing to the oxidative metabolism of endogenous estrogens circulating with the enterohepatic recycling pool.[179] Norethisterone has a low oral bioavailability of 42% due to oxidative CYP3A first-pass metabolism, but levonorgestrel is completely available in women, having no conjugated metabolites.[180]

Several clinically relevant DDIs between orally coadministered drugs and CYP3A4 can be explained by a modification of drug metabolism at the P450 level. If a drug has high presystemic elimination (low bioavailability) and is metabolized primarily by CYP3A4, then coadministration with a CYP3A4 inhibitor can be expected to alter the drug's pharmacokinetics by reducing its metabolism, thus increasing its plasma concentration. Drugs and some foods (eg, grapefruit juice) that are known inhibitors, inducers, or substrates for intestinal CYP3A4 can potentially impact the metabolism of a coadministered drug, affecting its AUC and rate of clearance (see Tables 3.10-3.12). Inducers can reduce absorption and oral bioavailability, whereas these same factors are increased by inhibitors. For example, erythromycin can enhance the oral absorption of another drug by inhibiting its metabolism in the small intestine by CYP3A4. Because they are competitive substrates for CYP3A4, prednisone, prednisolone, and methylprednisolone (but not dexamethasone) are competitive inhibitors of synthetic glucocorticoid metabolism. This is because a major metabolic pathway for synthetic glucocorticoids involves CYP3A4. The use of corticosteroids, with significant metabolism by the CYP3A enzymes, is not recommended with the concurrent use of the antiviral ritonavir, a CYP3A4 inhibitor. In addition to coadministered drugs, metabolic interactions with exogenous CYP3A4 substrates secreted in the bile are possible. The poor oral bioavailability of cyclosporine is attributed to a combination of intestinal metabolism by CYP3A4 and efflux by P-gp.[181]

Because the intestinal mucosa is enriched with UGT, SULT, and GST enzymes, presystemic first-pass metabolism for orally administered drugs susceptible to these conjugation reactions results in their low oral bioavailability. Presystemic metabolism often exceeds hepatic metabolism for some drugs. For example, more than 80% of intravenously administered albuterol is excreted unchanged in urine, with the remainder presenting as glucuronide conjugates, while when albuterol is administered orally, less than 5% is systemically absorbed because of intestinal sulfonation and glucuronidation. Presystemic metabolism is a major pathway in humans for most β-adrenergic agonists, such as glucuronide or sulfate esters of terbutaline, fenoterol, albuterol and isoproterenol, morphine (3-O-glucuronide), acetaminophen (O-sulfate and O-glucuronide), and estradiol (3-O-sulfate). The bioavailability of orally administered estradiol or ethinyl estradiol in females is approximately 50% because of conjugation. Mestranol (3-methoxyethinyl estradiol) has greater oral bioavailability because, as a nonphenol, it is not significantly conjugated. Levodopa has a low oral bioavailability because of its metabolism by intestinal L-aromatic amino acid decarboxylase. Drugs subject to first-pass metabolism are included in Table 3.16.

The extensive presystemic first-pass sulfonation of phenolic drugs can lead to increased bioavailability of other drugs by competing for the available sulfate pool, resulting in the possibility of drug toxicity. Concurrent oral administration of acetaminophen with phenolic drugs could result

Table 3.16 Examples of Drugs Exhibiting Presystemic Metabolism

Acetaminophen	Isoproterenol	Oxprenolol
Albuterol	Lidocaine	Pentazocine
Alprenolol	Meperidine	Propoxyphene
Aspirin	Methyltestosterone	Propranolol
Cyclosporin	Metoprolol	Salicylamide
Desmethylimipramine	Dihydropyridines (nifedipine)	Terbutaline
Fluorouracil	Nortriptyline	Verapamil
Hydrocortisone	Organic nitrates	
Imipramine		

in an increase in drug blood levels. Ascorbic acid, which is sulfonated, also increases the bioavailability of concurrently administered phenolic drugs. Sulfonation and glucuronidation occur side by side, often competing for the same substrate, and the balance between sulfonation and glucuronidation is influenced by several additional factors, such as species, doses, availability of alternative substrates, inhibition, and induction of the respective transferases.

Extrahepatic Metabolism

Because the liver is the primary tissue for xenobiotic metabolism, it is not surprising that current understanding of mammalian P450 monooxygenase is based chiefly on hepatic studies. Although the tissue content of P450s is highest in the liver, P450 enzymes are found in the lung, nasal epithelium, GI tract, kidney, adrenal tissues, and brain. It is possible that the expression of the polymorphic genes and induction of the isoforms in the extrahepatic tissues can affect the activity of the P450 isoforms in the metabolism of endogenous steroids, drugs, and other xenobiotics. Therefore, characterization of P450, UGT, SULT, and other polymorphic drug-metabolizing enzymes in extrahepatic tissues is important to the overall understanding about the biologic importance of these isoform families to improved drug therapy, design of new drugs and dosage forms, toxicity, and carcinogenicity.

The mucosal surfaces of the GI tract, the nasal passages, and the lungs are major portals of entry for xenobiotics into the body and, as such, are continuously exposed to a variety of orally ingested or inhaled airborne xenobiotics, including drugs, plant toxins, environmental pollutants, and other chemical substances. Because of this exposure, these tissues represent a major target for tumorigenesis and other chemically induced toxicities. Many of these toxins and chemical carcinogens are relatively inert substances that must be bioactivated to exert cytotoxicity and tumorigenicity. The epithelial cells of these tissues can metabolize a wide variety of exogenous and endogenous substances, and these cells supply the principal and initial source of biotransformation for these xenobiotics during the absorptive phase. The consequences of such presystemic biotransformation are either (1) a decrease in the amount of xenobiotics available for systemic absorption by facilitating the elimination of polar metabolites or (2) toxification by activation to carcinogens, which can be one determinant of tissue susceptibility for the development of intestinal cancer. The risk of colon cancer can depend on dietary constituents that contain either procarcinogens or compounds modulating the response to carcinogens.

Intestinal Metabolism

As noted earlier, many of the clinically relevant aspects of P450 can, in fact, occur at the level of the intestinal mucosa and can account for differences among patients in dosing requirements. The intestinal mucosa is enriched especially with the CYP3A4 isoform, UGT, SULT, and GST enzymes, making it particularly important for orally administered drugs susceptible to oxidation and/or phase 2 glucuronidation, sulfonation, or GSH conjugation. In the human intestine CYP3A4 (77%-78%) is most highly expressed, followed by CYP4F2 (7%-12%). CYP2C9 and CYP2C19 were also found in 5% to 10% and 1% to 2.6% abundance, respectively. CYP2J2, CYP3A5, and CYP2D6 were also found in lower amounts (0.7%-2.6%). The contribution of the other P450 members is minor. The highest concentrations of P450s occur in the duodenum, with gradual tapering into the ileum. CYP3A4 is the predominant in all intestinal sections, with a lower expression of CYP2C9 and CYP2C19 in the ileum.[182] In the jejunum, CYP1A1, CYP1A2, CYP1B1, CYP4A11, and CYP51A1 were detected in lower concentrations.[183] Therefore, intestinal P450 isoforms provide potential presystemic first-pass metabolism of ingested xenobiotics affecting their oral bioavailability or the bioactivation of carcinogens or mutagens.

It is not surprising that dietary factors can affect the intestinal P450 isoforms. For example, a 2-day dietary exposure to cooked Brussels sprouts decreased the 2α-hydroxylation of testosterone, yet induced CYP1A2 activity for PAH metabolism. An 8-oz glass of grapefruit juice inhibited the sulfoxidation metabolism of omeprazole (CYP3A4) but not its hydroxylation (CYP2C19), thus increasing its systemic blood concentrations. These types of interactions between a drug and a dietary inhibitor could result in a clinically significant drug interaction.

Intestinal UGT isoforms can glucuronidate orally administered drugs, such as morphine, acetaminophen, α- and β-adrenergic agonists, and other phenolic phenethanolamines and dietary xenobiotics, resulting in a reduction of their oral bioavailability (increasing first-pass metabolism), thus altering their pharmacokinetics and pharmacodynamics. The UGTs expressed in the intestine include UGT1A1, UGT1A3, UGT1A4, UGT1A6, UGT1A8, UGTA10, UGT1B4, UGT2B17, and UGT2B7. Substrate specificities of intestinal UGT isoforms are comparable to those in the liver. Glucuronidase hydrolysis of biliary glucuronide conjugates in the intestine can contribute to EHC of the parent drug.[183,184]

Likewise, the SULTs in the small intestine can metabolize orally administered drugs and xenobiotics for which the primary route of conjugation is sulfonation (eg, isoproterenol, albuterol, steroid hormones, α-methyldopa, acetaminophen, and fenoldopam), decreasing their oral bioavailability and, thus, altering their pharmacokinetics and pharmacodynamics. The SULTs expressed in the intestine include SULT1A1, SULT1A3, and SULT2A1. Competition for intestinal sulfonation between coadministered substrates can influence their bioavailability with either an enhancement or a decrease of therapeutic effects. Sulfatase hydrolysis of biliary sulfate esters in the intestine can contribute to EHC of the parent drug.[184] In addition to P450s, UGTs, and SULTs, other enzymes have been identified in the intestine, including CES1 and CES2, and the NADPH-P450 reductase.[183,184]

Plants contain a variety of protoxins, promutagens, and procarcinogens, and the occurrence of intestinal P450 enzymes and bacterial enzymes in the microflora allows the metabolic conversion of relatively stable environmental pollutants and food-derived xenobiotics into mutagens and carcinogens. For example, cruciferous vegetables (Brussels sprouts, cabbage, broccoli, cauliflower, and spinach) are all rich in indole compounds (eg, indole 3-carbinol), which, with regular and chronic ingestion, can induce some intestinal P450s (CYP1A subfamily) and inhibit others (CYP3A subfamily). It is likely that these vegetables would also alter the metabolism of food-derived mutagens and carcinogens. For example, heterocyclic amines produced during the charbroiling of meat are *N*-hydroxylated by P450 and become carcinogenic in the manner of arylamines (see Fig. 3.36).

Intestinal Microflora

When drugs are orally ingested, or there is considerable biliary excretion of a drug or its metabolites into the GI tract, such as with a parentally administered drug (EHC or recirculation), the intestinal bacterial microflora can have a significant metabolic role. It is believed that between 300 and 500 different bacterial strains populate the human gut microbiota ecosystem, exposing individuals to more than 2 million bacterial genes, also called the microbiome.[185] Current estimates have shown that all gut bacterial strains can use drugs or xenobiotics as substrates. A recent study found that 60% of drugs can be metabolized by at least one bacterial strain, which has the capability to metabolize between 11 and 95 different drugs.[186] The microflora has an important role in drug pharmacokinetics and in the EHC of xenobiotics via their conjugated metabolites (eg, digoxin, the oral contraceptives norethisterone and ethinyl estradiol and chloramphenicol) and endogenous substances (steroid hormones, bile acids, folic acid, and cholesterol), which reenter the gut via the bile. Compounds eliminated in the bile are conjugated with glucuronic acid, glycine, sulfate, and GSH and, once secreted into the small intestine, the bacterial β-glucuronidases, sulfatases, nitroreductases, and various glycosidases catalyze the hydrolysis of the conjugates.[187,188] The activity of orally administered conjugated estrogens involves the hydrolysis of sulfate esters by sulfatases, releasing estrogens to be reabsorbed from the intestine into the portal circulation. The clinical use of oral antibiotics (eg, erythromycin, penicillin, clindamycin, and aminoglycosides) has a profound effect on the gut microflora and the enzymes responsible for the hydrolysis of drug conjugates undergoing EHC. Bacterial reductions include nitro reduction of nitroimidazole, azo reduction of azides (sulfasalazine to 5-aminosalicylic acid and sulfapyridine), and reduction of the sulfoxide to its sulfide. Brivudine is metabolized by bacterial strain to the bromo vinyl uracil, which can induce hepatotoxicity. Levodopa is transformed to dopamine in the intestine causing diminished bioavailability. Subsequently, it is converted into *m*-tyramine, which causes toxicity. The sulfoxide of sulindac is reduced by both gut microflora and hepatic P450s.[189]

Other ways in which bacterial flora can affect metabolism include the following: (1) production of toxic metabolites, (2) formation of carcinogens from inactive precursors, (3) detoxication, (4) exhibition of species differences in drug metabolism, (5) exhibition of individual differences in drug metabolism, (6) production of pharmacologically active metabolites from inactive precursors, and (7) production of metabolites not formed by animal tissues.

In contrast to the predominantly hepatic oxidative and conjugative metabolism of the liver, gut microflora is largely degradative, hydrolytic, and reductive, with a potential for both metabolic activation and detoxication of xenobiotics.[190] The impact of the microbiome diverges across the human population. Host genetics, host immune response, diet, infections, diurnal rhythm, environmental microbial exposures, diseases, allergies, and association with other bacterial strains are some of the factors that can influence the intestinal microbiome.[191]

Lung Metabolism

Some of the hepatic xenobiotic biotransformation pathways are also operative in the lung. Because of the differences in organ size, the total content of the pulmonary xenobiotic-metabolizing enzyme systems is lower than in the liver, creating the impression of a minor role for the lung in xenobiotic elimination. The most important P450 drug metabolizers in the liver can also be found in the lungs, including CYP1A1, CYP1A2, CYP1B1, CYP2A6, CYP2B6, CYP2E1, CYP2F1, CYP2R1, and CYP3A5. CES1, the flavin-dependent monooxygenase FMO2, and ADH1B and ADH1C can also be found in the lungs. Fewer phase 2 enzymes can be found in the lungs, for example, SULT1A1 and UGT2A1. Thus, the lungs can have a significant role in the metabolic elimination or activation of low-molecular-weight inhaled xenobiotics.

Numerous PAHs are altered to mutagens and/or carcinogens by members of the CYP1 family, which are highly inducible by PAHs in the lung. Several inhaled glucocorticoids are metabolized in different tissue in the lungs, for example, beclomethasone dipropionate is converted by esterase to beclomethasone monopropionate, which can be further metabolized by CYP3A into 6-hydroxy beclomethasone monopropionate.[192] When drugs are injected intravenously, intramuscularly, or subcutaneously, or after skin absorption or inhalation, the drug initially enters the pulmonary circulation, after which the lung becomes the organ of first-pass metabolism for the drug. The blood levels and therapeutic response of the drug are influenced by genetic disposition, induction, and inhibition of the pulmonary metabolizing enzymes. By modulation of the P450 isoform pattern in the lung, a xenobiotic could alter its own metabolism and that of others in a time- and dose-dependent manner. Because of its position in the circulatory system, the lung provides a second-pass metabolism option for xenobiotics and their metabolites exiting from the liver, but it is also susceptible to the cytotoxicity or carcinogenicity of hepatic activated metabolites. Antihistamines, β-blockers, opioids, and tricyclic antidepressants are among the basic amines known to accumulate in the lungs because of their binding (in cationic conjugate acid form) to anionic surfactant phospholipids in lung tissue.[193]

Nasal Metabolism

The nasal olfactory mucosa is recognized as a first line of defense for the lung against airborne environmental xenobiotics because the mucosa is constantly exposed to the airborne external environment. Drug metabolism in the olfactory nasal epithelium represents a major metabolic pathway for protecting the CNS against the entry of drugs, inhaled environmental pollutants, or other volatile chemicals. Thus, the olfactory pathway is known to be a gateway to the brain for foreign compounds.[194] In some instances, these enzymes can biotransform a given drug or environmental or airborne xenobiotic into more reactive and potentially toxic metabolites, increasing the risk of carcinogenesis in the nasopharynx and lung (eg, procarcinogens and nitrosamines in cigarette smoke). P450 activity is high in olfactory tissue and olfactory-specific isoforms have been found, including 21 different P450s. Highly expressed enzymes include CYP1A2, CYP2A6, CYP2A13, CYP2E1, CYP3A4, and the olfactory-specific CYP2G1 isoform as well as four ALDHs, seven ADHs, two FMOs, and other reductases and oxidases. The potential for phase 1 metabolic toxicity is exemplified by the metabolism of pulegone, a monoterpene odorant, which, after monooxygenation, can lead to the formation of menthofuran, a hepatotoxic and pneumotoxic agent at high concentrations. Phase 2 enzymes found in the olfactory mucosa include 11 UGTs and 15 GSTs, among others.[195]

The most striking feature of the nasal epithelium is that the P450 catalytic activity per gram of tissue is higher than in any other extrahepatic tissue or in the liver. Nasal decongestants, essences, anesthetics, alcohols, nicotine, and cocaine have been shown to be metabolized in vitro by P450 enzymes from the nasal epithelium/mucosa.[196] Because the P450s in the nasal mucosa are active, first-pass metabolism should be considered when delivering susceptible drugs intranasally.

The nasal mucosa is also exposed to a wide range of odorants. Odorants, which are mostly small lipophilic molecules, enter the mucosa and reach the odorant receptors on sensory neurons by a transient process requiring signal termination, which could be provided by biotransformation of the odorant in the epithelial supporting cells. Thus, metabolism of odorants could be involved in both the termination and initiation of olfactory stimuli.[194]

Brain Metabolism

The metabolism of endogenous neurochemicals and neurotransmitters by brain P450s may help explain variations in mood, aggression, personality disorders, and other psychiatric conditions.[197-199] Brain P450 metabolism in neurotoxicity may also contribute to the underlying mechanisms of Parkinson disease. Knowledge of P450 isoforms and transporter function in the blood-brain barrier (BBB) may inform the design of strategies for the selective delivery of active forms of drugs to the brain.[200]

The isoforms of P450s and their regulation in the brain are of interest in defining their possible involvement in CNS toxicity and carcinogenicity. The expression level of P450 in the brain is approximately 0.5% to 2% of that in liver, too low to significantly influence the overall pharmacokinetics of drugs and hormones in the periphery.[197,201] Brain P450s can impact acute and chronic drug response (eg, nicotine dependence), CNS drug activation, susceptibility to damage by neurotoxins, and are associated with altered personality, behavior, and risk of neurologic disease.

While hepatic P450s are expressed primarily in the ER, brain expression is found in the mitochondrial and plasma membrane fraction and other cell membrane compartments. CYP1A1, CYP2B6, CYP2D6, CYP2E1, and CYP3A are predominantly found in neurons and glial cells. CYP3A4 and CYP2C19 are expressed in human prefrontal cortex, hippocampus, and amygdala, areas that may mediate the behavioral effects of testosterone. Human CYP1B1 is found at the blood-brain interface, where it may act in conjunction with transporters, such as ABC efflux transporters, to regulate passage of xenobiotics in and/or out of the brain. The interaction of a variety of transporters, in addition to local P450-mediated metabolism, may play an important role in regulating the levels of centrally acting drugs in the brain and, thereby, their therapeutic effects.[201]

The expression of brain P450 levels varies among different brain regions. For example, in the human brain, CYP2B6 protein expression varies significantly among brain regions with a 2.5-fold range. Brain CYP2D6 can metabolize endogenous neurochemicals, such as tyramine to dopamine and 5-methoxytryptamine to serotonin, while the metabolism of the endogenous cannabinoid anandamide, the neurosteroid progesterone, and testosterone (to 16α-hydroxytestosterone) is catalyzed by CYP2B6.[199] CYP2C19 can metabolize the sex hormones testosterone, progesterone, and estradiol that are known to affect brain function and personality traits, such as aggression and anxiety, and is notably found in several brain regions including the amygdala.[201] CYP19 aromatase found in brain converts testosterone to estradiol. CYP2E1 can metabolize the fatty acid neural signaling molecule arachidonic acid, which is abundant in the brain and is required for neurologic health. The differences in expression of specific brain P450s can cause shifts in the neurochemical homeostasis in the brain.[200]

Individuals with a CYP2D6 PM genotype are at greater risk for parkinsonism, and this risk is even greater with exposure to neurotoxic pesticides.[199] CYP2D6 metabolizes and inactivates a number of compounds that can cause parkinsonian symptoms, including MPTP, a Parkinson-causing compound, and its neurotoxic metabolite MPP+ (discussed previously). CYP2D6 is expressed in human brain regions affected by Parkinson disease, such as the substantia nigra. The impaired ability of CYP2D6 PMs to inactivate these neurotoxic metabolites may contribute to their increased risk for Parkinson disease. In contrast to CYP2D6 PMs, those who smoke are at lower risk for Parkinson disease since nicotine is neuroprotective. In humans, CYP2D6 expression levels are higher in the brains of those who smoke. Therefore, induction of brain CYP2D6 by nicotine or smoking may reduce an individual's relative risk for the disease. These data support a contributing role for lower brain expression levels of CYP2D6 for an increased risk for Parkinson disease, likely through modulation of local neurotoxin metabolism.[199,201]

Nicotine is the main component of cigarette smoke that causes tobacco dependence, and genetic variation in brain CYP2B6, CYP2D6, and CYP2E1 can affect smoking behaviors.[198,199] CYP2B6 PMs and IMs progress to tobacco dependence more quickly and have more difficulty quitting than normal (EM) metabolizers. Brain CYP2B6 metabolizes nicotine and other endogenous substrates, such as serotonin and neurosteroids. Nicotine and smoking induce the brain's expression of CYP2B6, CYP2D6, and CYP2E1, all of which affect smoking behaviors. Smokers have higher levels of brain CYP2D6, but unchanged levels of hepatic CYP2D6. Individuals exposed to nicotine through smoking or through nicotine replacement therapy are likely to have increased CYP2D6-mediated brain metabolism of centrally acting drugs, neurotoxins, and endogenous neurochemicals, increasing the risk of drug interactions and neurotoxicity. Brain levels of CYP2D6 enzymes and activity may be contributing factors to the clinical observations of personality differences with chronic nicotine administration between CYP2D6 EM and PM phenotypes. Preliminary data suggest that reducing brain CYP2B and CYP2D6 activity increases the rewarding properties of nicotine by altering brain levels of nicotine and its metabolites.[201]

Metabolism in Other Tissues

P450s in the kidney and adrenal tissues include isoforms primarily involved in the hydroxylation of steroids, arachidonic acid, and 25-hydroxycholecalciferol. In tumors, the P450 expression is abnormal compared with normal tissue, which plays a role in tumorigenesis, progression, and also in the mechanism of drug resistance.[202]

Stereochemical Aspects of Drug Metabolism

In addition to the physicochemical factors that affect xenobiotic metabolism, stereochemical factors have an important role in the biotransformation of drugs. This involvement is not unexpected, because the xenobiotic-metabolizing enzymes are also the same enzymes that metabolize certain endogenous substrates, which, for the most part, are chiral molecules. Most of these CYP isoforms show stereoselectivity but not stereospecificity; in other words, one stereoisomer enters into biotransformation pathways preferentially, but not exclusively. Metabolic stereochemical reactions can be categorized as follows: substrate stereoselectivity, in which two enantiomers of a chiral substrate are metabolized by the same or different CYP isoforms at different rates; product stereoselectivity, in which a new chiral center is created in a symmetric molecule and one enantiomer is generated preferentially; and substrate-product stereoselectivity, in which a new chiral center of a chiral molecule is metabolized preferentially to one of two possible diastereomers.

An example of substrate stereoselectivity is the preferred decarboxylation of (*S*)-α-methyldopa to (*S*)-α-methyldopamine, with almost no reaction for (*R*)-α-methyldopa. Another example is the (*S*)-ketamine enantiomer, which is preferentially *N*-demethylated by CYP2B6 to (*S*)-norketamine, whereas the (*R*) enantiomer is *N*-demethylated by CYP3A4. The reduction of ketones to stereoisomeric alcohols and the hydroxylation of enantiotropic carbons by P450 are examples of product stereoselectivity. For example, phenytoin undergoes aromatic *p*-hydroxylation of only one of its two phenyl rings to create a chiral center at C_5 of the hydantoin ring, methadone's ketone group is reduced preferentially to its α-diastereomeric alcohol, and naltrexone is reduced to its 6-β-alcohol. Two examples of substrate-product stereoselectivity are the reduction of the enantiomers of warfarin and the β-hydroxylation of (*S*)-α-methyldopamine to (1*R*,2*S*)-α-methylnorepinephrine ((*R*)-α-methyldopamine is hydroxylated only to a negligible extent). In vivo studies often can be confounded by the further biotransformation of one stereoisomer, giving the false impression that only one stereoisomer from the original metabolic reaction was formed preferentially. Moreover, some compounds show stereoselective absorption, distribution, and excretion, which proves the importance of performing in vitro studies.

Although studies regarding the stereoselective biotransformation of drug molecules are not yet extensive, those that have been done indicate that stereochemical factors have an important role in drug metabolism. In many cases, stereoselective biotransformation could account for the differences in pharmacologic activity and duration of action between enantiomers.

Metabolic Bioactivation: Role in Hepatotoxicity, Idiosyncratic Reactions, and Chemical Carcinogenesis

Drug-Induced Hepatotoxicity

Drug-induced hepatotoxicity is the leading cause of hepatic injury, accounting for approximately half of all cases of acute liver failure in the United States. Recent studies have shown that drug-induced hepatotoxicity represents a larger percentage of adverse drug reactions than reported previously, and that the incidence and severity of drug-induced liver injury (DILI) are underestimated among the general population.

Acetaminophen overdose is the leading cause for calls to poison control centers (>100,000 calls/year) and accounts for more than 56,000 emergency room visits, 2,600 hospitalizations, and an estimated 500 deaths from acute liver failure each year.[203] Among the listed drugs in Table 3.17, acetaminophen is the most often implicated hepatotoxic agent and can cause extensive hepatic necrosis with as little as 10 to 12 g (30-40 tablets). Watkins reported that a third of 106 patients taking a maximum daily acetaminophen dose of 4 g for 8 days, either alone or in combination with hydrocodone, exhibited a 3-fold increase in liver enzymes associated with acetaminophen-induced liver injury.[204] This 3-fold increase in transaminase levels is a signal for potential liver safety concerns in those individuals who are at risk of acetaminophen-induced liver toxicity. Chronic alcohol intake enhances acetaminophen hepatotoxicity more than 5 times as compared to acute alcohol intake, yet acetaminophen is heavily marketed for its safety as compared to analgetic NSAIDs.

U.S. drug manufacturers continue to market and promote extra-strength acetaminophen products (500-750 mg/tablet) and a variety of extra-strength acetaminophen-drug combination products. Self-poisoning with acetaminophen

Table 3.17 Some Drugs Causing Hepatic Injury

Acarbose	*Felbamate*	Methotrexate	Ritonavir
Acetaminophen	Fenofibrate	Methsuximide	Rosiglitazone
Allopurinol	*Fluconazole*	Methyldopa	Rosuvastatin
Amiodarone	*Flutamide*	Nabumetone	*Saquinavir*
Amprenavir	Fluvastatin	Naproxen	Simvastatin
Anagrelide	Gemfibrozil	**Nefazodone (2005)**	Sulindac
Atomoxetine	Gemtuzumab	*Nevirapine*	*Tacrine*
Atorvastatin	Griseofulvin	Niacin (SR)	Tamoxifen
Azathioprine	*Halothane*	Nitrofurantoin	**Tasosartan (1998)**
Bicalutamide	Imatinib	Olanzapine	*Terbinafine*
Bosentan	Indinavir	Oxaprozin	Testosterone
Bromfenac (1998)	*Infliximab*	**Pemoline (2005)**	Thioguanine
Carbamazepine	Isoflurane	Pentamidine	Tizanidine
Celecoxib	Isotretinoin	Pioglitazone	*Tolcapone*
Dapsone	Itraconazole	Piroxicam	**Troglitazone (2000)**
Diclofenac	*Ketoconazole*	Pravastatin	*Trovafloxacin*
Disulfiram	*Ketorolac*	*Pyrazinamide*	*Valproic acid*
Duloxetine	Lamivudine	Ribavirin	Voriconazole
Efavirenz	*Leflunomide*	Rifabutin	**Ximelagatran (2004)**
Ethotoin	Lovastatin	*Rifampin*	*Zileuton*
Ethosuximide	Meloxicam	Riluzole	*Zafirlukast*

Drugs in **bold** have exhibited severe drug-induced hepatotoxicity and were withdrawn either voluntarily or by a regulatory agency (year given). Drugs in *italics* have exhibited moderate-severe drug-induced hepatotoxicity requiring a black box warning restricting their use. The other drugs have exhibited mild to moderate drug-induced hepatotoxicity that can need frequent liver transaminase testing for those at risk (see Table 3.18).

(paracetamol) is also a common cause of hepatotoxicity in other parts of the Western world. To reduce the number of acetaminophen poisonings in the UK, OTC sales of acetaminophen are limited to 16 tablets per packet.

Drug-induced hepatotoxicity is also the most frequent reason that new therapeutic agents are not approved by the FDA (eg, ximelagatran in 2004) and the most common adverse drug reaction leading to withdrawal of a drug from the market (see Table 3.17). Hepatotoxicity almost always involves metabolism with phase 1 P450 enzymes rather than phase 2 enzymes. More than 600 drugs, chemicals, and herbal remedies can cause hepatotoxicity, of which more than 30 drugs have either been withdrawn from the U.S. market because of hepatotoxicity or have carried a black box warning for hepatotoxicity since 1990. Table 3.17 includes some of the more common drugs that have exhibited drug-induced hepatotoxicity ranging from severe, requiring the drug's regulatory withdrawal from the market; moderate to severe, requiring black box warning restrictions; or mild to moderate, requiring frequent liver function monitoring.

The most frequently used indicators of hepatotoxicity (ie, liver injury) are increased levels of the liver transaminases, aspartate aminotransferase (AST) and alanine aminotransferase (ALT). Although drug-induced liver damage commonly occurs after a prolonged period of drug administration, it can sometimes develop rapidly, often before abnormal laboratory tests are noticed; tests are characterized by rapid elevations in ALT and AST of 8 to 500 times the upper normal limit, with variable elevations in bilirubin. Drugs causing acute liver injury (hepatocellular necrosis) exhibit elevations in hepatic transaminases ranging from 50 to 100 times higher than the normal level. On the other hand, the elevations of ALT and AST in alcoholic liver disease are 2 to 3 times higher than normal. Some hepatotoxins, however, do not elevate transaminases, whereas nonhepatic toxins can elevate ALT.[205]

DILI (also known as drug-induced hepatotoxicity) is an injury of the liver that occurs when taking certain drugs, and it is classified intrinsic (dose related) and idiosyncratic (unpredictable). Intrinsic hepatotoxicity results from the intact drug or toxin while idiosyncratic toxicity is induced by metabolites. Most drug-induced hepatotoxicity is of an idiosyncratic nature, occurring in a small percentage of patients (1 in 10,000) who ingest the drug.[206,207] These reactions tend to be of two distinct types: (1) hypersensitivity reactions that are immune mediated, occurring within the first 4 to 6 weeks, and associated with fever, rash, eosinophilia, and a hepatitis-like picture (eg, phenytoin, sulindac, and allopurinol); and (2) metabolic idiosyncratic reactions that tend to occur at almost any time during the first year of treatment (eg, troglitazone). The incidence of overt idiosyncratic liver diseases varies with the drug, ranging from approximately 1 in 1,000 with phenytoin, to 1 in 10,000 or more with sulindac and troglitazone, to 1 in 100,000 with diclofenac. To detect a single case of drug-induced hepatotoxicity with 95% confidence requires the number of patients studied to be triple the incidence of the reaction (ie, for one adverse drug reaction in 10,000 patients, at least 30,000 patients need to be evaluated). Thus, many drugs are approved before liver toxicity is observed. It is the responsibility of postmarketing surveillance and monitoring of liver transaminases to identify potential cases of liver adverse drug reactions.

Risk factors for DILI, such as age, gender, genetic predisposition, multiple drugs, or dietary supplements and degree of alcohol consumption, appear to increase the susceptibility to drug-induced hepatotoxicity (Table 3.18).[207,208] The drugs in Table 3.17 should be used with caution in these high-risk patients, because such patients can have altered metabolism of these drugs and, therefore, can be at increased risk for liver injury. The coadministration of drugs in Table 3.17 with enzyme inducers, such as phenobarbital, phenytoin, ethanol, and/or cigarette smoke, can induce hepatic enzymes, resulting in the enhancement of hepatotoxicity.

Most hepatic adverse effects associated with drugs occur in adults rather than children. DILI occurs at a higher rate in patients older than 50 years, and drug-associated jaundice occurs also more frequently in the geriatric population.[206] This age-related risk can be the result of increased frequency of drug exposure, multidrug therapy, and age-related changes in drug metabolism.

For reasons that are unclear, DILI affects females more than males. Females accounted for approximately 79% of all reactions to acetaminophen and 73% of all idiosyncratic drug-induced reactions. Females exhibit increased risk of hepatic injury from drugs such as atorvastatin, nitrofurantoin, methyldopa, and diclofenac.[209]

Genetic factors resulting in enzyme polymorphism in affected individuals can decrease the ability to metabolize or eliminate drugs, thus increasing their duration of action and drug exposure and/or decreasing the ability to modulate the immune response to drugs or metabolites. Chronic ingestion of alcohol can also predispose many patients to

Table 3.18 Risk Factors for Drug-Induced Liver Injury

Ethnicity	Some drugs exhibit different toxicities based on ethnicity because of individual P450 polymorphism. For example, Black and Hispanic individuals can be more susceptible to isoniazid toxicity.
Age	Older adults are at increased risk of hepatic injury due to decreased clearance, drug-drug interactions, reduced hepatic blood flow, variation in drug binding, and lower hepatic volume. In addition, poor diet, infections, and multiple hospitalizations are important reasons for drug-induced hepatotoxicity. Hepatic drug reactions are rare in children (eg, acetaminophen, halogenated general anesthetics).
Gender	Although the reasons are unknown, hepatic drug reactions are more common in females. Females are more susceptible to hepatotoxicity from acetaminophen, halothane, nitrofurantoin, diclofenac, and sulindac.
Alcohol	Alcoholics are susceptible to drug toxicity because alcohol induces liver injury and cirrhotic changes that alter drug metabolism. Alcohol causes depletion of glutathione (hepatoprotective) stores, making the person more susceptible to toxicity by drugs (eg, acetaminophen, statins).
Liver disease	Patients with chronic liver disease are not uniformly at increased risk of hepatic injury. Although the total P450 level is reduced, some patients can be affected more than others. The modification of doses in persons with liver disease should be based on knowledge of the specific P450 isoform involved in the metabolism. Patients with HIV infection who are coinfected with hepatitis B or C virus are at increased risk for hepatotoxic effects. Similarly, patients with cirrhosis are at increased risk to hepatotoxic drugs (eg, methotrexate, methyldopa, valproic acid).
Genetic factors	Genetic (polymorphic) differences in the formation of P450 isoforms (2C family and 2D6) can result in abnormal reactions to drugs, including idiosyncratic reactions.
Other comorbidities	Patients with AIDS, renal disease, and diabetes mellitus; persons who are malnourished; and persons who are fasting can be susceptible to drug reactions because of low glutathione stores.
Pharmacokinetics	Long-acting and sustained release formulation drugs can cause more injury than short-acting drugs.
Drug adulterants	Contaminants are often found in noncertified herbal supplements (eg, hepatitis C).

increased hepatotoxicity from drugs by lowering the stores of GSH (a detoxifying mechanism), which prevents trapping of the toxic metabolites as mercapturate conjugates that are excreted in the urine.

The common trigger for both mild and severe forms of hepatotoxicity is bioactivation of relatively inert functional groups to reactive electrophilic intermediates, which is an obligatory event in the etiology of many drug-induced idiosyncratic hepatotoxicities.[207,210] Research now shows that reactive metabolites are formed from drugs known to cause idiosyncratic hepatotoxicity, but how these toxic species initiate and propagate tissue damage remains poorly understood. Clearly, the relationship between bioactivation and the occurrence of hepatic injury is not simple. For example, many drugs at therapeutic doses undergo bioactivation in the liver but are not hepatotoxic. The tight coupling of bioactivation with bioinactivation pathways can be one reason for the lack of hepatotoxicity with these drugs. Examples of bioinactivation (detoxification) pathways include GSH conjugation of quinones by GSTs and hydration of arene oxides to dihydrodiols by epoxide hydrolases. When reactive metabolites are poor substrates for such detoxifying enzymes, they can escape bioinactivation and, thereby, damage proteins and nucleic acids, prompting hepatotoxicity.

Most drugs, however, are not directly chemically reactive but, through the normal process of drug metabolism, can form electrophilic, chemically reactive metabolites. Formation of chemically reactive metabolites is mainly catalyzed by P450 enzymes (phase 1), but products of phase 2 metabolism (eg, acylglucuronides, acyl CoA thioesters, or *N*-sulfates) can also lead to toxicity. However, if phase 1 drug bioactivation is closely coupled with phase 2 bioinactivation (eg, GSH conjugation to mercapturates), then the net chemical process is one of detoxification if the final product is rapidly cleared.

Toxicity can accrue when accumulation of a chemically reactive metabolite leads to covalent modification of biologic macromolecules. The identity of the target macromolecule and the functional consequence of its modification or destruction will dictate the resulting toxicologic response. P450 enzymes are present in many organs, mainly the liver, but also the kidney and lung, and thus can bioactivate chemicals to cause organ-specific toxicity. Evidence for the formation of reactive metabolites was found for five of the six drugs that have been withdrawn from the market since 1995, and for 8 of the 15 drugs that have black box warnings (see Table 3.17). Evidence for reactive metabolite formation has been found for acetaminophen, bromfenac, diclofenac, clozapine, tamoxifen, and troglitazone. As noted previously, acetaminophen is the most studied hepatotoxin.[207,211]

The current hypothesis of how reactive metabolites lead to liver injury suggests that hepatic (target) proteins can be modified by reactive metabolites. Much more clinically important is the identification of the target proteins modified by these toxic metabolites and how these reactions alter the function of those proteins. Additionally, it is important to note that the toxicity of reactive metabolites can also be mediated by noncovalent (in addition to covalent) binding mechanisms, which can have profound effects on normal liver physiology. Such information should dramatically improve understanding of drug-induced hepatotoxic reactions.

While it is important to identify targets for reactive metabolites that covalently modify biomolecules, no simple rules predict the target macromolecules for a particular chemically reactive metabolite or the biologic consequences of a particular modification. As noted earlier, noncovalent interactions also have a role, because covalent binding of hepatotoxins is not indiscriminate with respect to proteins. Even within a single protein, there can be selective modification of an amino acid side chain found repeatedly in the primary structure. Thus, the microenvironment (eg, pK_a and hydrophobicity) of the amino acid in the tertiary structure appears to be the crucial determinant of selective binding and, therefore, the impact of covalent binding on protein function. In turn, the extent of binding and the biochemical role of the protein will determine the toxicologic insult of drug bioactivation. The resulting pathologic consequences will be a balance between the rates of protein damage and the rates of protein replacement and cellular repair.

Drug-Induced Idiosyncratic Reactions

IDRs (type B adverse drug reactions) occur with a frequency between 1 in 1,000 and 1 in 50,000 patients. IDRs are not predictable from the known pharmacology or toxicology of the drug, are not produced experimentally in vitro and in vivo, and are dose independent. The occurrence of IDRs during late clinical trials or after a drug has been released can lead to severe restriction of its use or even its withdrawal. IDRs do not, as a rule, result from the drug itself because most people can tolerate the drug, but rather from a unique set of patient characteristics, including gender, age, genetic predisposition, and a lack of drug-metabolizing enzymes that can increase the risk of these adverse drug reactions. Most IDRs are caused by hypersensitivity reactions and can result in hepatocellular injury. Hepatic injury occurs within 1 week to 12 months after initiation of drug therapy and is often accompanied by systemic characteristics of allergic drug reactions, such as rash and fever. Signs of hepatic injury reappear with subsequent administration of only one or two doses of the same drug.

Hypersensitivity reactions can be severe and associated with fatal reactions, such as a multiorgan clinical syndrome characterized by the following: (1) fever, (2) rash, (3) GI symptoms (eg, nausea, vomiting, diarrhea, or abdominal pain), (4) generalized malaise, fatigue, or achiness, and (5) respiratory symptoms (eg, dyspnea, cough, or pharyngitis). Examples of drugs causing IDRs through a hypersensitivity mechanism include penicillin, methyldopa, chlorpromazine, erythromycin, azathioprine toxicity in TPMT-deficient individuals, sulfonamide and acetaminophen hepatotoxicity in alcoholics, perhexiline hepatotoxicity in CYP2D6-deficient individuals, phenytoin toxicity in CYP2C9-deficient individuals, and valproic acid hepatotoxicity.[212]

The metabolism of drugs largely occurs in hepatic tissue, so it makes sense that the most frequent type of IDRs takes place in the liver. This type of IDR is called idiosyncratic DILI, which is a subset of the DILI pathology. The clinical features of some cases of idiosyncratic DILI strongly suggest an involvement of the immune system. These clinical characteristics include the following: (1) concurrence of rash, fever, high ALT values, and eosinophilia, (2) delay of the initial reaction (5-90 days) or requirement of repeated exposure to the culprit drug (exceptional cases can delay onset as long as 1 year after therapy), (3) rapid recurrence of toxicity on reexposure to the drug (challenge), and (4) presence of antibodies specific for native or drug-modified hepatic proteins.[213,214] Current understanding of drug-induced adaptive immune response is largely based on the hapten hypothesis and the complementary theory, the "danger hypothesis."[213]

IDRs that are connected with hepatotoxicity involve the formation of reactive metabolites. Current bioanalytical technology has enabled the in vivo identification of reactive metabolite formation, as evidenced by the detection of biomarkers (ie, mercapturate or cysteine adducts) in urine, drug-specific antibodies, GSH conjugate formation, or antibodies to P450 isoforms. Most of the idiosyncratic toxins listed in Table 3.19 that have been studied to date produce reactive metabolites.[212] Some drugs known to cause hepatic injury are still in use to this day because the drug's benefit outweighs the risks, and no alternative efficacious drug exists.

Current hypotheses regarding IDRs suggest that metabolic activation of a drug to a reactive metabolite is a necessary step in the generation of an idiosyncratic reaction, but not the only precursor to idiosyncratic DILIs. Evidence for this hypothesis comes from drugs that are associated with idiosyncratic hepatotoxicity (Table 3.19) and the detection of drug-metabolite-specific antibodies in affected patients. For the other drugs that have been associated with idiosyncratic hepatotoxicity but that do not have black box warnings, either evidence for hepatotoxicity was not available or suitable studies had not been carried out. High doses increase the risk for an IDR (eg, clozapine at 300 mg/d vs olanzapine 20 mg/d). There are some examples of drugs and biologics that do not undergo bioactivation, yet produce idiosyncratic DILIs. In general, the reactive metabolite, where it is produced, and what it binds to are likely to have a key function in whether IDRs result, and what kind of IDR is produced.

The hapten hypothesis proposes that the reactive metabolites of hepatotoxic drugs do just that (act as haptens) and bind covalently to endogenous proteins to form immunogenic drug-protein adducts, triggering either antibody or cytotoxic T-cell responses. The hapten hypothesis is supported by the detection of antibodies that recognize drug-modified hepatic proteins in the serum of patients with DILI. For example, antibodies that recognize trifluoroacetate-altered hepatic proteins have been detected in the sera of patients with halothane-induced hepatitis. Such drug-specific antibodies that recognize native liver proteins have also been found in patients with liver injury caused by other drugs, such as diclofenac. Most drugs are small molecules and are unlikely to form haptens. Nonetheless, not only hapten binding to a macromolecule can trigger an immune response, but it also requires something to activate antigen-presenting cells, which upregulate costimulatory molecules on the antigen-presenting cells. This generates an additional signal from the antigen-presenting cells; without this there will be either nonimmune response or immune tolerance. A reactive metabolite can both act as a hapten and cause some type of cell damage to produce a danger signal (danger hypothesis) that activates neoantigens. The association of reactive metabolites with human lymphocyte antigens plays an important role in IDRs and how they interact can generate different physiologic outcomes.[213,215]

Table 3.19 Some Examples of Idiosyncratic Toxins

Abacavir	Hypersensitivity
Acetaminophen	Hepatotoxicity
Amiodarone	Hepatotoxicity
Aromatic anticonvulsants	Hypersensitivity
Cefaclor	Hepatotoxicity
Clozapine	Agranulocytosis
Diclofenac	Hepatotoxicity
Felbamate	Aplastic anemia
Fibrates	Hepatotoxicity
Halothane	Hepatotoxicity
Indomethacin	Hepatotoxicity
Isoniazid	Hepatotoxicity
Levamisole	Hepatotoxicity
Nefazodone	Hepatotoxicity
Nevirapine	Agranulocytosis
Oral contraceptives	Hepatotoxicity
Paroxetine	Hepatotoxicity
Penicillamine[a]	Hypersensitivity
Phenytoin	Hepatotoxicity
Statins	Hepatotoxicity
Sulfonamides	Stevens-Johnson syndrome
Tamoxifen	Hepatotoxicity
Tacrine	Hepatotoxicity
Tienilic acid	Hypersensitivity
Ticlopidine	Agranulocytosis
Troglitazone	Hepatotoxicity
Valproic acid	Hepatotoxicity
Vesnarinone	Agranulocytosis

[a]Does not produce reactive metabolites.

Electrophilic acylators can react with the lysine ω-amino residues of the target protein or guanosine residues of DNA. Halothane is the most studied molecule for supporting the hapten hypothesis regarding IDRs. Therefore, it is not surprising that irreversible chemical modification of a protein, which has a profound effect on function, is a mechanism of idiosyncratic hepatotoxicity. However, it is important to note that several drugs (eg, penicillins, aspirin, and omeprazole) rely on covalent binding to proteins for their efficacy; thus, prevention of their covalent binding through chemical modification of the compound can also, inadvertently, lead to loss of efficacy.

Reactive Metabolites Resulting From Bioactivation

Electrophiles

The concept that small organic molecules can undergo bioactivation to electrophiles (an electron-deficient group or ion, such as carbocations and acyl ions, that accepts an electron pair to make a covalent bond) and free radicals, and can elicit toxicity by chemical modification of cellular macromolecules has its basis in chemical carcinogenicity and the pioneering work of the Millers[216], Park et al and Rendiac et al.[217,218] and Gillette et al.[216-218] Electrophiles are reactive because they possess electron-deficient centers (polarization-activated double bonds or positive charge acylators) (Fig. 3.41) and can form covalent bonds with electron-rich biologic nucleophiles such as the thiol groups in either GSH or cysteine residues within proteins. A number of different types of reactive metabolites exist; however, they can be broadly classified as either electrophiles (Fig. 3.41) or free radicals (Fig. 3.42).[219,220] These reactive metabolites are short-lived, with half-lives of usually less than 1 minute, and they are not normally detectable in plasma or urine except as phase 2 conjugates or other biomarkers.

Activated double bonds are electrophilic intermediates. Examples of activated double bond electrophiles include α,β-unsaturated carbonyl compounds, quinones, quinoneimines, quinonemethides, and diiminoquinones as shown in Figure 3.43. These electrophilic intermediates are highly polarized and can react with nucleophiles in a 1,4-Michael-type addition at the more electrophilic β-carbon of the activated double bond intermediate to generate the addition product (Fig. 3.43A). Specific examples of activated double bond electrophiles that have been proposed for the anticancer drug leflunomide, acetaminophen, the antiandrogen flutamide, the anticonvulsant felbamate, and the cytotoxic cyclophosphamide are shown in Figure 3.43C. The bioinactivation pathways for these electrophilic intermediates can involve direct addition, with or without catalysis by GSH or epoxide transferases, depending upon the degree of polarization and reactivity of the electrophilic intermediate.[220]

Other commonly found electrophilic metabolic intermediates for drug molecules in Figure 3.41 include ketenes from the bioactivation of acetylenic groups (eg, ethinyl estradiol) (2 in Fig. 3.41); isocyanates from thiazolidinediones (eg, the "glitazones") (4 in Fig. 3.41); acylium ions from halogenated hydrocarbons (eg, halothane) (3 in Fig. 3.41) and carboxylic acids; β-dicarbonyl from furans (eg, furosemide) (5 in Fig. 3.41); activated thiophene-*S*-oxide from thiophenes, such as ticlopidine and tenoxicam, which cause an IDR, agranulocytosis (6 in Fig. 3.41); and epoxides and arene oxides from olefins and aromatic compounds (7 in Fig. 3.41).

Drugs containing structural features prone to metabolic epoxidations are abundant. Therefore, the incidence of epoxide metabolites in mediating adverse biologic effects has aroused concern about clinically used drugs known to be metabolized to epoxides. Metabolically produced epoxides have been reported for allobarbital, secobarbital, protriptyline, carbamazepine, and cyproheptadine, and are implicated with 8-methoxypsoralen and other furanocoumarins (6,7-dihydroxybergamottin in grapefruit juice), phenytoin, phensuximide, phenobarbital, mephobarbital, lorazepam, and imipramine.[64,218,221] The alarming biologic effects of some epoxides, however, do not imply that all epoxides have similar effects. Epoxides vary greatly in molecular geometry, stability, electrophilic reactivity, and relative activity as substrates for epoxide-transforming enzymes (eg, epoxide hydrolase, GST, and others).

Some carboxylic acid–containing drugs have been implicated in rare IDRs, which was the basis for the market withdrawal of the NSAIDs zomepirac and benoxaprofen. These drugs can be bioactivated to acyl glucuronides or acyl CoA thioesters (1 and 5 in Fig. 3.44). These products are electrophilic acylators that can acylate target proteins if they escape inactivation by *S*-GSH-thioester formation.[222] A crucial factor is the concentration of acyl glucuronides in hepatocytes due to their transport by conjugate export pumps, since acylglucuronides can selectively acylate hepatic membrane proteins. Acyl CoA esters can be either rapidly hydrolyzed or further metabolized in hepatocytes. Evidence is accumulating that acyl glucuronides can alter cellular function by haptenation of peptides, target protein acylation or glycation, or direct stimulation of neutrophils and macrophages. The role of acyl CoA reactive metabolites is less clear. It should be noted that some noncarboxylic acid drugs can be biotransformed by oxidative metabolism in the liver to the respective carboxylic acids.[222]

Free Radicals

P450 activates molecular dioxygen to generate ROS, such as singlet oxygen ($^1O_2$) or superoxide. Reactive metabolites that possess an odd unpaired electron are free radicals that can react with molecular oxygen (ground state triplet) to generate intracellular oxidative stress damage.[218,220] Free radicals abstract a hydrogen atom from other molecules rather than becoming covalently bound. Free radical reactions can be self-propagated by abstracting a hydrogen atom from the double bond of a lipid that initiates a chain reaction leading to lipid peroxidation, oxidative stress, or other types of modification of biologic molecules.

Selected examples of free radicals generated by the bioactivation of drug molecules are shown in Figure 3.42. Isoniazid is acetylated to its major metabolite acetylisoniazid, which is hydrolyzed to acetylhydrazine and isonicotinic acid (1 in Fig. 3.42). Acetylhydrazine is further metabolized by CYP2E1 to an *N*-hydroxy intermediate that hydrates into an acetyl radical, which can then initiate the process that leads to hepatic necrosis. Other carbon-centered radicals are formed from hydrazines, such as the antihypertensive hydralazine and thio-radicals from the angiotensin-converting enzyme inhibitor captopril (3 in Fig. 3.42).

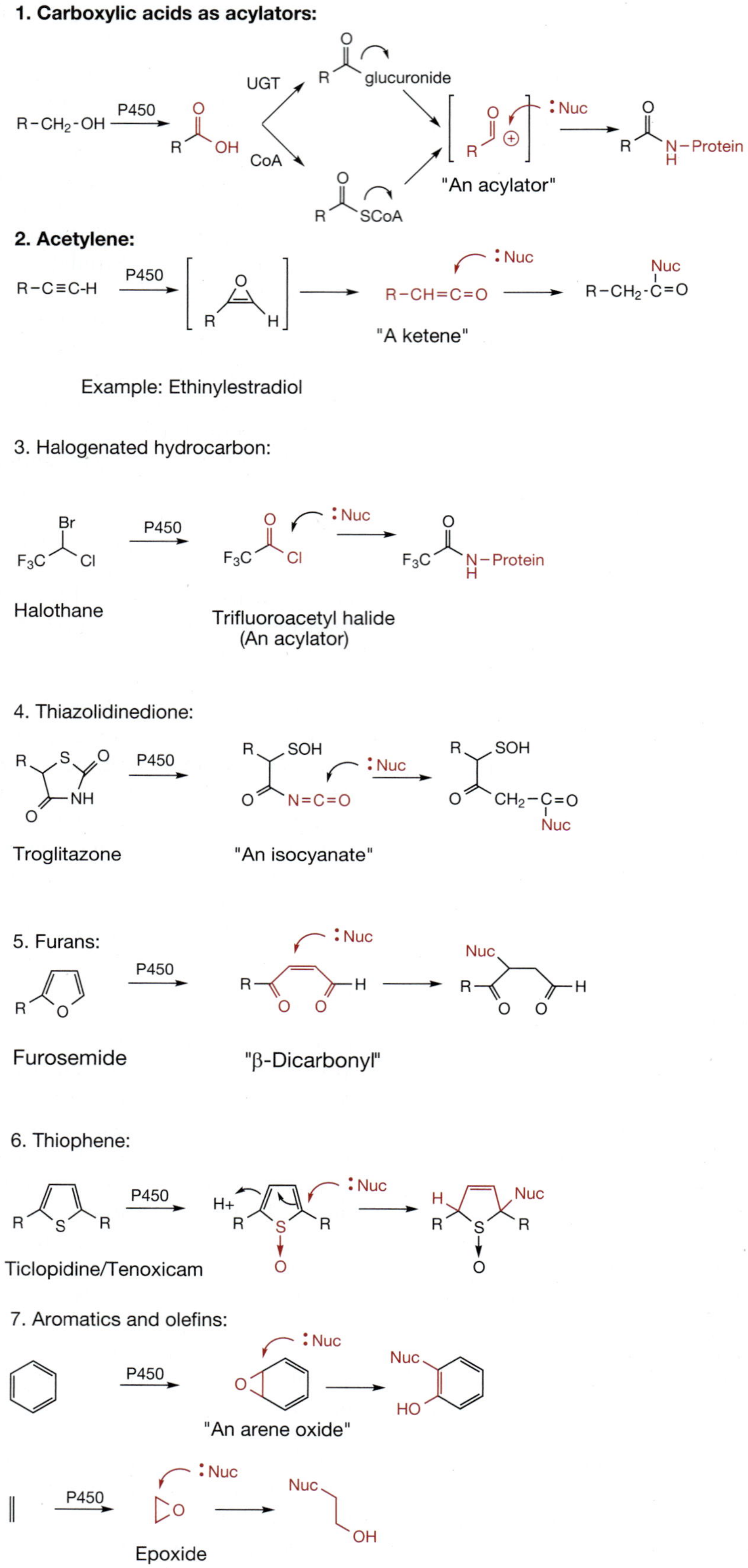

Figure 3.41 Some examples of electrophilic intermediates resulting from bioactivation. *Nuc*, nucleophiles.

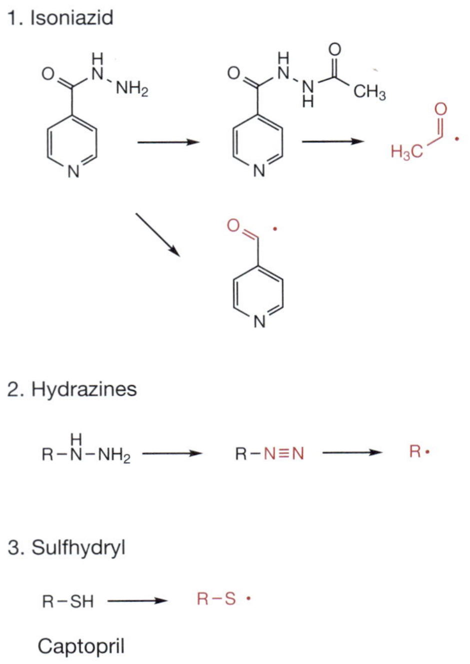

Figure 3.42 Drug bioactivation to free radicals.

Bioinactivation Mechanisms

Several enzyme systems exist as cellular defense (detoxification) pathways against the chemically reactive metabolites generated by P450 metabolism. These include GST, epoxide hydrolase, and quinone reductase, as well as catalase, GSH peroxidase, and superoxide dismutase, which detoxify the peroxide and superoxide by-products of metabolism. The efficiency of the bioinactivation process is dependent on the inherent chemical reactivity of the electrophilic intermediate, its affinity and selectivity for the bioinactivation enzymes, the tissue expression of these enzymes, and the rapid upregulation of these enzymes and cofactors mediated by the cellular sensors of chemical stress. The reactive metabolites that can evade these defense systems can damage target proteins and nucleic acids by either oxidation or covalent modification.

The most abundant agents of cellular defense are thiols. GSH will only react noncatalytically with electrophiles, such as activated double bonds (see Fig. 3.43). GSH conjugation to mercapturates is one of the most important defenses against hepatocellular injury.[223] GSH protects cellular enzymes and membranes from toxic metabolites, and its inadequate storage can compromise efficient detoxification of the reactive metabolites. The subsequent inability to detoxify the reactive metabolites can result in hepatocellular injury. The rate-limiting factor for GSH synthesis is the intracellular concentration of cysteine. *N*-acetylcysteine is often used as an alternative to GSH to trap the iminoquinone intermediate in the treatment of acute acetaminophen toxicity and in preventing nephrotoxicity from ifosfamide-generated chloroacetaldehyde. The molecule excreted after these toxic metabolites react with clinically administered *N*-acetylcysteine is the same as the endogenous GSH-inactivated toxin. GSH has a protective role in the hepatic tissue injury produced by acetaminophen, but not by furosemide.

The relationship between bioactivation, bioinactivation, and DNA adduct formation has been well established for a number of hepatocarcinogens. GSH conjugation of carcinogens becomes more efficient when catalyzed by GSTs, an important example being the detoxification of the hepatocarcinogen aflatoxin. Aflatoxin, a hepatocarcinogen and a hepatotoxin found in mold growing on peanuts, is converted into aflatoxin B1 epoxide in rodents, which is more readily detoxified by GST enzymes than by epoxide hydrolase. The balance between these transferase reactions explains the greater DNA damage in humans compared with rodents, because human forms of GST are less able to catalyze the conjugation of aflatoxin epoxide compared with the rodent forms. Transgenic knockout mice have been used to establish the role of bioactivation by P450 and bioinactivation by GSTs for a number of carcinogenic polyaromatic hydrocarbons.[224,225]

Substances that detoxify free radicals include the antioxidants vitamin C, vitamin E, and carotene, which scavenge free radicals, including reactive metabolites and ROS generated as a consequence of chemical stress.

Specific Examples

Some examples of bioactivation to hepatotoxic or IDR-inducing electrophilic intermediates are shown in Figure 3.44. Bioactivation can occur by both oxidation and conjugation reactions, for example, diclofenac, which undergoes the formation of an acyl glucuronide to produce iminoquinones via formation of a phenol intermediate (1 in Fig. 3.44). The anticonvulsant carbamazepine is 2-hydroxylated, and the elimination of the amide group yields the reactive quinoneimine intermediate (2 in Fig. 3.44). The antidepressant paroxetine and other xenobiotics with the common methylenedioxyphenyl nucleus undergo methylene oxidation to a *p*-quinoid intermediate (3 in Fig. 3.44). The nitro group of the COMT inhibitor tolcapone, used in the treatment of parkinsonism, is first reduced to an amine, then oxidized to an *o*-quinoneimine (4 in Fig. 3.44). The mitochondrial/hepatotoxicity of the anticonvulsant valproic acid results from the formation of an activated α, β-unsaturated CoA thioester via mitochondrial β-oxidation, most commonly associated with the oxidation of fatty acids (5 in Fig. 3.44). The agranulocytosis resulting from the ingestion of the antipsychotic clozapine is bioinitiated by oxidation by HOCl in neutrophils to a nitrenium intermediate (6 in Fig. 3.44).[88,218]

The effect of structure modification for troglitazone that reduced its hepatotoxicity is shown in Figure 3.45. The *p*-dihydroxy groups of the chroman ring nucleus (outlined in red in Fig. 3.45) of troglitazone are bioactivated to an activated double bond (*p*-quinone) and replaced with a pyridine ring that is not bioactivated, although the thiazolidinone ring can be bioactivated to an isocyanate (Fig. 3.45).

The oxidation of acetaminophen to the chemically reactive *N*-acetyl-*p*-benzoquinoneimine (Fig. 3.38) is catalyzed by the isoforms CYP1A2 and CYP2E1. The reactive quinoneimine can react covalently either with GSH to form an inactive product

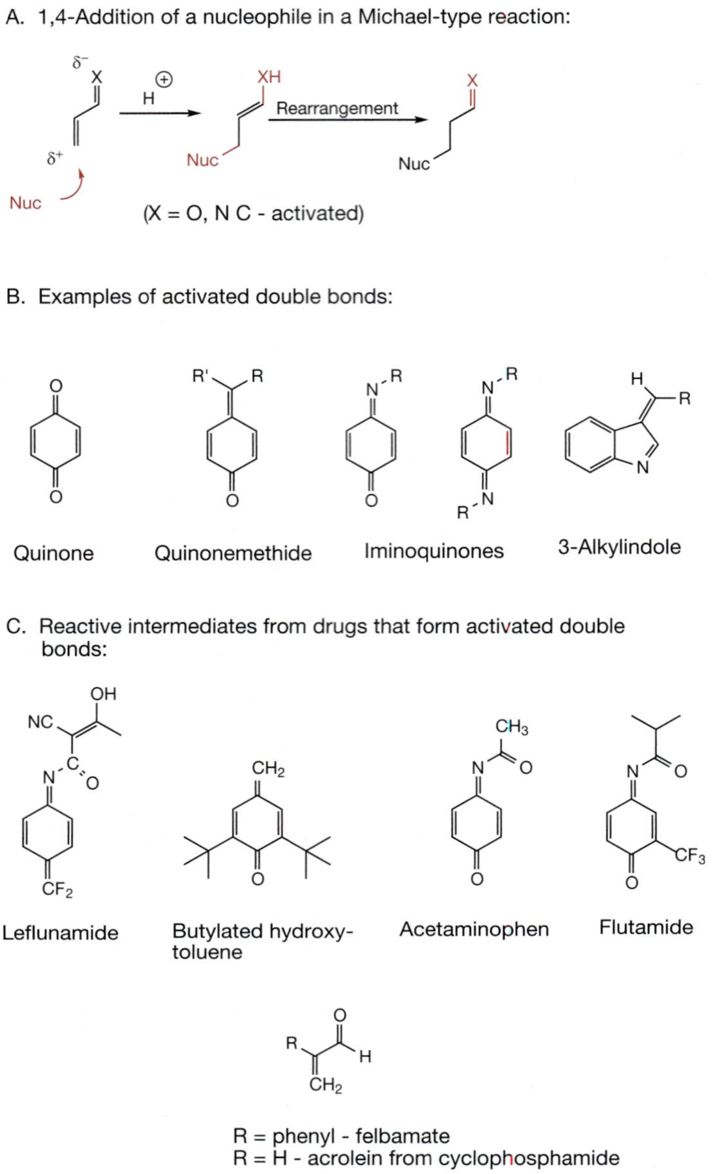

Figure 3.43 Examples of activated double bonds to electrophilic reactive intermediates.

or with cellular macromolecules, initiating the processes leading to hepatic necrosis (see Fig. 3.38).[218] The usual route for acetaminophen metabolism is glucuronidation. If insufficient UDPGA is present, then bioactivation will dominate.

Furosemide, an often used diuretic drug, is reportedly a human hepatocarcinogen. The hepatic toxicity apparently results from metabolic activation of the furan ring to a β-dicarbonyl intermediate (5 in Fig. 3.41). Ticlopidine and tenoxicam, reported to cause agranulocytosis, do so via metabolic activation of the thiophene ring to an S-oxide (6 in Fig. 3.41). The agranulocytosis resulting from the ingestion of clozapine is via its bioactivation to a nitrenium ion intermediate (6 in Fig. 3.44).[226]

Drug-Induced Chemical Carcinogenesis

The mechanism whereby xenobiotics are transformed into chemical carcinogens is usually accepted as bioactivation to reactive metabolites responsible for initiating carcinogenicity.[227] Many carcinogens elicit their cytotoxicity through a covalent linkage to DNA. This process can lead to mutations and, potentially, to cancer. The carcinogens of greatest concern are chemically inert but require activation by the xenobiotic-metabolizing enzymes before they can undergo reaction with DNA or proteins (cytotoxicity). There are many ways to bioactivate procarcinogens, promutagens, plant toxins, drugs, and other xenobiotics (Fig. 3.46).[227-229]

Oxidative bioactivation reactions are by far the most studied and common. Conjugation reactions (phase 2), however, are also capable of activating these xenobiotics to produce electrophiles, in which the conjugating derivative acts as a leaving group. These reactive metabolites are mostly electrophiles, such as epoxides, quinones, or free radicals formed by the P450 enzymes or FMO.[230,231] The reactive metabolites tend to be oxygenated in sterically hindered positions, making them poor substrates for subsequent bioinactivation enzymes, such as epoxide hydrolase and GST. Therefore, their principal fate is formation of covalent linkage to

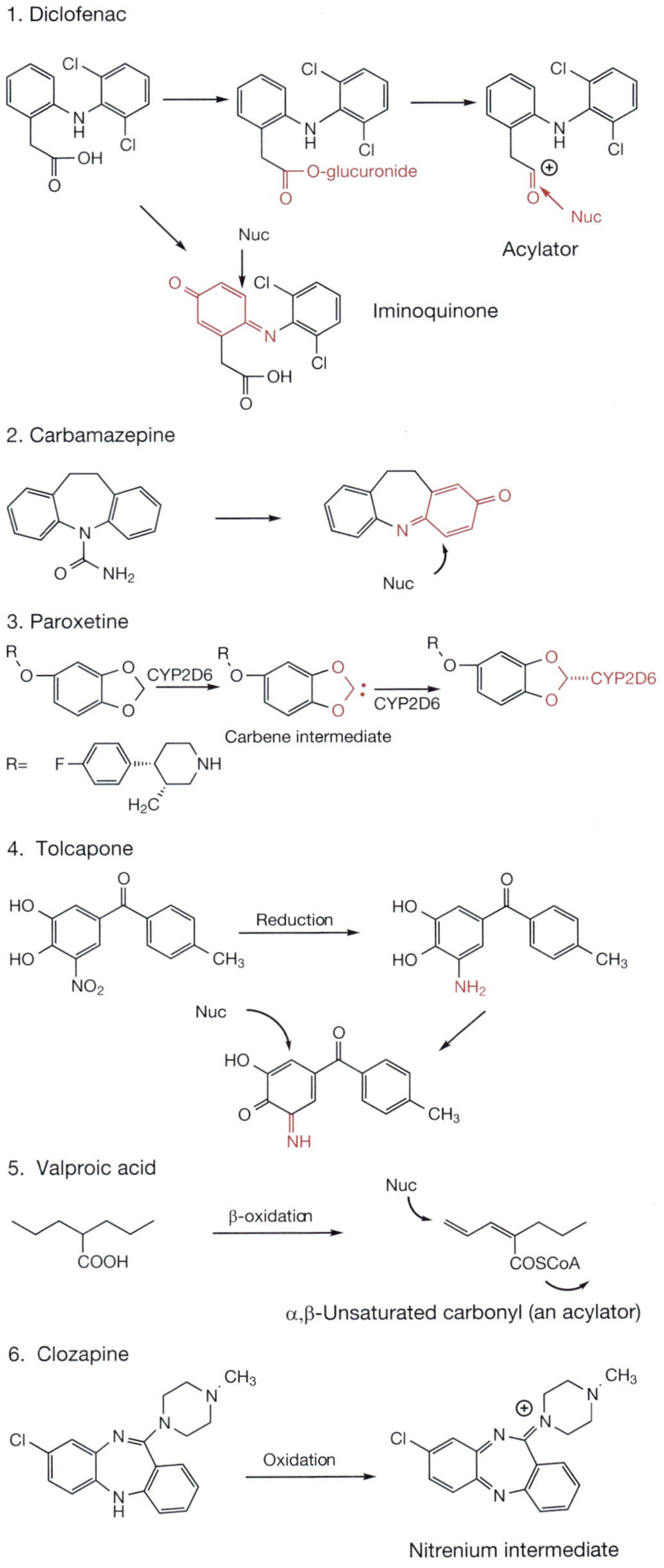

Figure 3.44 Examples of drug bioactivation to hepatotoxic intermediates.

intracellular macromolecules, including enzyme proteins and DNA. Experimental studies indicate that the CYP1A subfamily can oxygenate aromatic hydrocarbons (eg, PAHs) in sterically hindered positions to arene oxides. Activation by *N*-hydroxylation of polycyclic aromatic amines (eg, aryl *N*-acetamides) appears to depend on either FMO or P450 isoforms.[230] The formation of chemically reactive metabolites is important because they frequently cause a number of different toxicities, including tumorigenesis, mutagenesis, tissue necrosis, and hypersensitivity reactions.

A scheme illustrating the complexities of drug-induced chemical carcinogenesis is shown in Figure 3.46. Reactions that proceed via the open arrows eventually lead to neoplasia. Some carcinogens can form the ultimate carcinogen entity directly through P450 isoform bioactivation. Others, like the PAHs (eg, benzo[a]pyrene), appear to involve a multistep reaction sequence forming an epoxide, reduction to a diol by epoxide hydrolase, and perhaps the formation of a second epoxide group on another part of the molecule. Other procarcinogens form the *N*-hydroxy intermediate that requires transferase-catalyzed conjugation (eg, *O*-glucuronide and *O*-sulfate) to form the ultimate carcinogen entity. The quantity of the ultimate carcinogen entity formed should relate directly to the proportion of the dose that binds or alkylates DNA.[229,231]

The solid-arrow reaction sequences in Figure 3.46 are intended to show detoxification mechanisms, which involve several steps: (1) the original chemical can form fewer active products (phenols, diols, mercapturic acids, and other conjugates), (2) the ultimate carcinogen entity can rearrange to be prevented from its reaction with DNA and/or other target macromolecules, (3) the covalently bound DNA can be repaired, and (4) immunologic removal of the tumor cells can occur. Several mechanisms within this scheme could regulate the quantity of covalently bound carcinogen: (1) activity of the rate-limiting enzyme, such as epoxide hydrolase, P450 isoform, or one of the transferases could be involved; (2) availability of cofactors, such as GSH, UDPGA, or PAPS may be rate limiting; (3) relative P450 activities for detoxification and activation could be considered; (4) availability of alternate reaction sites for the ultimate carcinogen (eg, RNA and protein) could be involved; (5) specific transport mechanisms that deliver either the procarcinogen or its ultimate carcinogen to selected molecular or subcellular sites may be possible.[229]

It is well established that numerous organic compounds that are essentially nontoxic as long as their structure is preserved can be converted into cytotoxic, teratogenic, mutagenic, or carcinogenic compounds by normal biotransformation pathways in both animals and humans. The reactive electrophilic intermediate involves reaction with cellular DNA constituents forming either detoxified products or covalent bonding with essential macromolecules, initiating processes that eventually lead to the toxic effect. A better understanding of the mechanisms underlying these reactions can lead to more rational approaches to the development of nontoxic therapeutic drugs. Special attention to risk factors is required for drugs that will be used for long periods in the same patient.

Drug-Drug Interactions

DDIs represent a common clinical problem that has been compounded by the introduction of many new drugs and the expanded use of herbal medicines. Such interactions do significant harm and prompted 6.1 per 1,000 patient visits

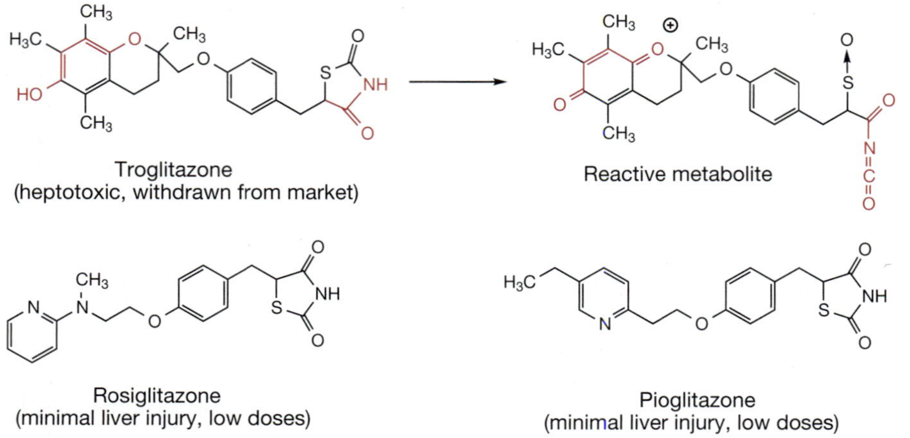

Figure 3.45 Effect of structure modification on drug-induced hepatotoxicity of troglitazone.

to hospital emergency departments per year between 2017 and 2019.[232] Approximately 50% of these serious DDIs involved P450 inhibition. The problem is likely to grow in the future as the population ages and more people take multiple medications.[233]

DDIs occur when the efficacy or toxicity of a medication is changed by coadministration of another substance, drug, food (ie, grapefruit), or herbal product. Pharmacokinetic interactions often occur because of a change in drug metabolism. For example, CYP3A4 oxidizes more than 30% of the clinically used drugs with a broad spectrum of structural features, and its location in the small intestine and liver allows an effect on both presystemic and systemic drug disposition. Some DDIs with CYP3A4 substrates/inhibitors can also involve inhibition of P-gp. Other clinically important consequences due to DDIs resulting from coadministration of CYP3A4 substrates or inhibitors include rhabdomyolysis with the coadministration of some 3-hydroxy-3-methylglutaryl-CoA reductase inhibitors (statin antihyperlipidemics),

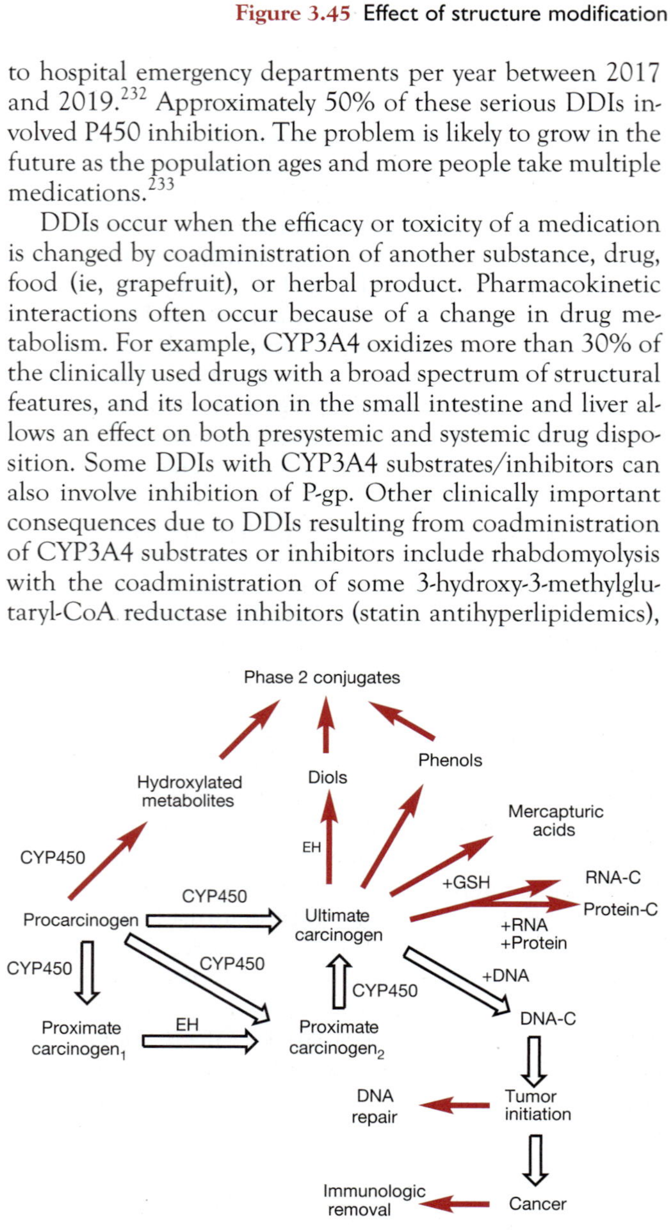

Figure 3.46 Bioactivation of procarcinogens and a proposed mechanism of chemical carcinogenesis. Red arrows indicate detoxification mechanisms

symptomatic hypotension with some dihydropyridine calcium antagonists, excessive sedation from benzodiazepine or nonbenzodiazepine sedative-hypnotics, ataxia with carbamazepine, and ergotism with ergot alkaloids.[230]

The clinical importance of any DDI depends on factors that are drug-, patient-, and administration related. Drugs with low oral bioavailability or high first-pass metabolism are particularly susceptible to DDIs when inhibitors that alter absorption, distribution, and elimination are coadministered. In general, a doubling or more of the plasma drug concentration has the potential for an enhanced adverse and/or beneficial drug response. Less pronounced pharmacokinetic drug interactions can still be clinically important for drugs with a steep concentration-response relationship or narrow therapeutic index. In most cases, the extent of drug interaction varies markedly among individuals, likely dependent on interindividual differences in P450 content (polymorphism), preexisting medical conditions, and possibly age. DDIs can occur under single-dose conditions or at steady state. The pharmacodynamic consequences may or may not closely follow pharmacokinetic changes. DDIs can be most apparent when patients are stabilized on the affected drug and the P450 substrates or inhibitors are then added to the regimen. One reason for the increased incidence of DDIs is the practice of simultaneously prescribing several potent drugs as well as concurrently ingesting nonprescription products and herbal products that compete for, inhibit, or induce metabolizing enzymes.[234]

Although DDIs constitute only a small proportion of adverse drug reactions, they have become an important issue in health care. Many DDIs can be explained by alterations in the metabolic enzymes in the liver and extrahepatic tissues, and many of the major pharmacokinetic interactions between drugs are caused by hepatic P450 isoenzymes being affected by coadministration of other drugs. Some drugs act as potent enzyme inducers, whereas others are inhibitors. DDIs involving enzyme inhibition, however, are much more common. Understanding these mechanisms of enzyme inhibition or induction is extremely important to appropriately administer multidrug therapies. Individuals at greatest risk for DDIs and adverse events need to be identified and treated based upon their specific pharmacogenomic-related needs.[234]

P450s have a dominant role in the metabolism and elimination of drugs from the body, and their substrates are shown in Tables 3.3 and 3.7 to 3.10. Drugs in bold italics have been associated with clinically relevant DDIs. Inhibitors of P450 are shown in Table 3.11. Pharmacokinetic interactions can arise when the biotransformation and elimination of a drug are impaired by coadministered drugs. Thus, drugs can compete for biotransformation by a common P450. Adverse drug reactions, including toxicity, can occur if elimination is dependent on a P450 that exhibits defective gene variants. Thus, the genetic makeup of the individual (see "Genetic Polymorphism" section) has a major influence on the duration of drug action, as well as on drug efficacy and safety. Thus, the future safe use of drug combinations in patients can require genotyping and phenotyping of individuals before the commencement of therapy, particularly when there is risk for morbidity/mortality-related toxicity. Identification of subjects who metabolize drugs differently from patients with wild-type enzyme function (eg, PMs, IMs, RMs) should minimize the impact of pharmacogenetic variation on drug pharmacokinetics.

DDIs and drug-food interactions have been expanding and the methods of predictions have been increasing with the use of deep learning, machine learning, and artificial intelligence being implemented earlier in the drug discovery process.[235-237]

Metabolism-Based Enzyme Inhibition

Many DDIs are the result of inhibition or induction of P450 enzymes. Metabolism-based enzyme inhibition involves mostly reversible competition between two drugs for the enzyme's active site. Metabolic DDIs occur when drug A (or its metabolite) alters the pharmacokinetics of a coadministered drug B by inhibiting, activating, or inducing the activity of the enzymes that metabolize drug B. Inhibitory DDIs could result in serious adverse effects, including fatalities in patients receiving multiple medications. This process is competitive and begins with the first dose of the inhibitor, with the extent of inhibition correlating with their relative affinities for the shared enzyme(s) and the metabolic half-lives of the drugs involved. Metabolism-based inhibition is distinct from mechanism-based (irreversible) inhibition, which results from a metabolite that binds irreversibly to the enzyme through a covalent bond, rendering the enzyme inactive (detailed further).

Enzyme-specific P450 inhibitors, including metabolism- and mechanism-based inhibitors, can present a significant challenge when considered for new drug development. Not only is CYP3A4 one of the most abundant isoforms in human liver (Fig. 3.2), but it also metabolizes around 30% of the drugs in clinical use (see Fig 3.3), which renders CYP3A4 highly susceptible to both metabolism- (reversible) and mechanism-based inhibition. The CYP3A subfamily is involved in many clinically significant DDIs and therefore metabolism-based inhibition of CYP3A can cause clinically significant DDIs, such as those involving nonsedating antihistamines and the GI motility stimulant cisapride (no longer available in the United States) that posed a significant risk for cardiac dysrhythmias. Likewise, life-threatening ventricular arrhythmia associated with QT prolongation (torsades de pointes) occurred when CYP3A4 substrates or inhibitors were coadministered with terfenadine, astemizole, cisapride, or pimozide. This potentially lethal drug interaction led to the withdrawal of CYP3A4 substrates terfenadine and cisapride from clinical use and to the approved marketing of fexofenadine, the active metabolite of terfenadine that is not metabolized by CYP and does not have this interaction.

Inhibitors of CYP3A4 can increase the risk of toxicity from many drugs, including carbamazepine, cyclosporine, ergot alkaloids, lovastatin, protease inhibitors, rifabutin, simvastatin, tacrolimus, and vinca alkaloids. Furthermore, inhibitors of CYP1A2 can increase the risk of toxicity from clozapine or theophylline. Inhibitors of CYP2C9 can increase the risk of toxicity from phenytoin, tolbutamide, and oral anticoagulants (eg, warfarin). Inhibitors of CYP2D6 can increase the risk of toxicity of many antidepressants, opioid analgesics, and psychotherapeutic agents.

While this discussion is focused on enzyme inhibition, it bears repeating that P450 enzymes can also be induced by some drugs and environmental chemicals. Examples of drug-based enzyme inducers include barbiturates, carbamazepine, glutethimide, griseofulvin, phenytoin, primidone, rifabutin, and rifampin. Cigarette smoke is the classic example of an environmental enzyme inducer. Some drugs, such as ritonavir, can act as either an enzyme inhibitor or an enzyme inducer, depending on the situation. Drugs metabolized by CYP3A4 or CYP2C9 are particularly susceptible to enzyme induction,[238] while CYP2D6 is generally considered to be induction resistant.

Mechanism-Based Enzyme Inhibition

Mechanism-based inhibition differs from metabolism-based (reversible) inhibition in that the inhibitors require enzymatic activation by the target enzyme prior to exerting their inhibitory effect. This initial activation step leads to the formation of an active inhibitor, often referred to as the metabolite-intermediate complex (MIC).[239] MIC can then exert its inhibitory effect by either forming a direct covalent link with the enzyme or forming a noncovalent tight binding complex. Mechanism-based inhibition is characterized by NADPH-, time-, and concentration-dependent enzyme inactivation, occurring when some drugs are converted by P450s to reactive metabolites. Mechanism-based inactivation of CYP3A4 by drugs can be the result of chemical modification of the heme, the apoprotein, or both when covalent binding of the modified heme to the protein occurs. The clinical pharmacokinetic effect of a mechanism-based CYP3A4 inhibitor is a function of its enzyme kinetics (ie, K_m and V_{max}) and the rate of synthesis of new or replacement enzyme. Predicting DDIs involving CYP3A4 inactivation is possible when pharmacokinetic principles are followed. Such prediction can become difficult, however, because the clinical outcomes of CYP3A4 inactivation depend on many factors associated with the enzyme, the drugs, and the patients.

Some of the clinically important drugs that have been identified to be mechanism-based CYP3A4 inhibitors include antibacterials (eg, clarithromycin, erythromycin, isoniazid), anticancer drugs (eg, irinotecan, tamoxifen, raloxifene), antidepressants (eg, fluoxetine and paroxetine), anti-HIV agents (eg, ritonavir and delavirdine), antihypertensives (eg, dihydralazine and verapamil), steroids and their receptor modulators (eg, ethinyl estradiol, gestodene, and raloxifene), dihydrotestosterone reductase inhibitors (eg, finasteride), and some herbal constituents (eg, bergamottin and glabridin). Drugs inactivating CYP3A4 often possess several common moieties such as a tertiary amine, furan ring, or an acetylene group. The chemical properties of a drug critical to CYP3A4 inactivation include formation of reactive metabolites by P450 isoenzymes, P450 inducers, P-gp substrates, or inhibitors and the occurrence of clinically significant pharmacokinetic interactions with coadministered drugs.

Compared to the more common metabolism-based (reversible) inhibition, mechanism-based inhibitors of CYP3A4 more frequently cause pharmacokinetic-pharmacodynamic DDIs that can be serious and/or prolonged because the inactivated CYP3A4 must be replaced by newly synthesized CYP3A4 protein.[240] The resultant drug interactions may lead to adverse (sometimes fatal) events. For example, raloxifene, a drug approved for the treatment of osteoporosis and chemoprevention of breast cancer in postmenopausal women at high risk for invasive disease, acts as a mechanism-based inhibitor of CYP3A4 by forming adducts with the apoprotein. It has been established that 3′-hydroxyraloxifene is produced exclusively via CYP3A4-mediated oxygenation to produce a reactive diquinone methide, in lieu of the alternative arene oxide pathway (eg, 7 in Fig. 3.41).[241]

Predicting DDIs involving CYP3A4 inactivation is difficult, since the clinical outcomes depend on a number of factors that are associated with drugs and patients. The apparent pharmacokinetic effect of a mechanism-based inhibitor of CYP3A4 would be a function of its enzyme kinetics and the synthesis rate of new or replacement enzyme. Most CYP3A4 inhibitors are also P-gp substrates/inhibitors, confounding the in vitro to in vivo extrapolation. The clinical significance of CYP3A inhibition for drug safety and efficacy warrants an in-depth understanding of the mechanisms for each inhibitor. Furthermore, such inactivation may be exploited for therapeutic gain in certain circumstances. Clinicians should have an in-depth knowledge about CYP3A4 inhibitors and avoid their combination with potentially toxic substrates.

Although CYP2D6 constitutes a relatively minor fraction of the total hepatic P450 content (see Fig. 3.2), the contribution of this isoform is significant because of its role in the metabolism and clearance of many therapeutic agents that target the cardiovascular system and the CNS (see Fig. 3.3 and Table 3.8). In addition, clinically significant polymorphisms in the CYP2D6 gene have been identified in a variety of populations with altered metabolic activity, such as PMs or individuals with impaired enzyme function resulting from splicing defects or gene deletions. On the other hand, EMs (individuals with normal enzyme function) are heterozygous for the wild-type allele or homozygous but without a PM second allele. In vivo clearance of CYP2D6 substrates in PMs (especially those homozygous for a nonfunctional allele) is usually much lower than in EMs, leading to higher plasma concentrations and the potential for clinical toxicities with therapeutic doses. For example, paroxetine is a selective serotonin reuptake inhibitor (SSRI) that is both a substrate for and an inhibitor of CYP2D6. Paroxetine is metabolized by CYP2D6 via the formation of a carbene intermediate of the methylenedioxy group yielding an irreversible complex with CYP2D6 (3 in Fig. 3.44). Also, an in vitro study with 3,4-methylenedioxy-methamphetamine (MDMA, "ecstasy") suggested that a typical recreational MDMA dose could inactivate most hepatic CYP2D6 within an hour, and the return to a basal level of CYP2D6 could take at least 10 days, impacting its pharmacokinetics.

Because of the pivotal role of P450 isoenzymes in drug metabolism, significant inactivation of these isoforms, and particularly the major human hepatic and intestinal CYP3A4 and hepatic CYP2D6, could result in DDIs and adverse drug reactions. As noted earlier, mechanism-based inhibitors of CYP3A4 and CYP2D6 cause pharmacokinetic/pharmacodynamic DDIs more frequently than reversible inhibitors, as the inactivated isoenzyme must be replaced by newly synthesized P450 protein. Pharmacokinetic interactions often occur because of a change in drug metabolism. For example, macrolide antibiotics increase the plasma concentrations of therapeutic agents that are substrates of CYP3A4. Diltiazem has been shown to inhibit the metabolism of a variety of coadministered drugs including carbamazepine, quinidine, midazolam, and lovastatin (see Table 3.10). Inhibition of CYP3A by ritonavir explains, in part, the remarkable elevation of blood concentrations and area under the plasma concentration-time curve of other concomitantly administered drugs that are extensively metabolized by CYP3A4 and have significant first-pass metabolism. These drugs include rifabutin (400%), clarithromycin (77%), ketoconazole, saquinavir (5,000%), amprenavir (210%), nelfinavir (152%), lopinavir (7,700%), and indinavir (380%).[96] Furthermore, such inactivation can be exploited for therapeutic gain in certain circumstances, for example, extended duration of action of the protease inhibitors ritonavir/indinavir used in the treatment of AIDS.

Beneficial Drug-Drug Interactions

By understanding the unique functions and characteristics of P450 isoenzymes, health care practitioners can better anticipate and manage DDIs. They can also predict or explain an individual's response to a particular therapeutic regimen. A beneficial drug interaction, for example, is the coadministration of a CYP3A4 inhibitor with cyclosporine. By inhibiting CYP3A4, the plasma concentrations of cyclosporine (a CYP3A4 substrate) are increased which allows a reduction of the cyclosporine dosage, thereby improving clinical efficacy and reducing cost. Similarly, certain HIV protease inhibitors, such as saquinavir, have a low oral bioavailability due to intestinal CYP3A4 metabolism. The oral bioavailability of saquinavir can be profoundly increased by the addition of a low dose of the mechanism-based CYP3A4 inhibitor, ritonavir. This concept of altering drug pharmacokinetics by adding a low, subtherapeutic dose of a mechanism-based CYP3A4 inhibitor (ritonavir) to increase the oral bioavailability of another protease inhibitor, lopinavir (CYP3A4 substrate), led to the marketing of Kaletra, a drug combination of lopinavir and ritonavir.

Another beneficial mechanism-based inhibition is of the P2Y12 receptor (a protein found on the surface of blood platelet cells and an important regulator in blood clotting) by the platelet anti-aggregating prodrugs clopidogrel and prasugrel. Clopidogrel is bioactivated to its reactive metabolite by CYP2C19, CYP1A2, and CYP3A4, whereas prasugrel is bioactivated by CYP3A4 and CYP2B6. The bioactivated metabolites can then react with the P2Y12 receptor protein to attenuate clotting and lower the risk of myocardial infarction or stroke.

Grapefruit Juice–Drug Interactions

Historical Significance of Grapefruit Juice

The discovery that grapefruit juice can markedly increase the oral bioavailability of CYP3A4-vulnerable drugs was based on an unexpected observation from an interaction study between the dihydropyridine calcium channel antagonist felodipine (a CYP3A4 substrate) and ethanol, in which grapefruit juice was used to mask the taste of the ethanol. Subsequent investigations confirmed that grapefruit juice significantly increased the oral bioavailability of felodipine by reducing presystemic felodipine metabolism through selective inhibition of CYP3A4 expression in the intestinal wall.[242]

Grapefruit juice is a beverage often consumed at breakfast for its health benefits and to mask the taste of drugs or foods. Unlike other citrus fruit juices, however, grapefruit juice can significantly increase the oral bioavailability of drugs that are metabolized primarily by intestinal CYP3A4, causing an elevation in their serum concentrations (Table 3.20). Those drugs with high oral bioavailabilities (>60%), however, are all likely safe to be taken with grapefruit juice because their high oral bioavailability leaves little room for elevation by grapefruit juice. The importance of the interaction appears to be influenced by individual patient susceptibility, type and amount of grapefruit juice, and administration-related factors.

Grapefruit juice can alter oral drug pharmacokinetics by different mechanisms. Irreversible inactivation of intestinal CYP3A4, which can persist up to 24 hours while new enzyme is synthesized, is produced by grapefruit juice given as a single, normal, 200- to 300-mL drink or by whole fresh fruit segments (see Table 3.20). As a result, presystemic metabolism is reduced and oral drug bioavailability increased

Table 3.20 Some CYP3A4 Substrates and Interactions With Grapefruit Juice

Drug	Interaction[a]	Drug	Interaction[a]	Drug	Interaction[a]
Calcium channel blockers		**HIV protease inhibitors**		**CNS drugs**	
Amlodipine	Y	Indinavir	N?	Buspirone	Y
Felodipine	Y	Nelfinavir	N?	Carbamazepine	Y
Nifedipine	Y	Ritonavir	N?	Diazepam	Y
Nimodipine	Y	Saquinavir	Y	Midazolam	Y
Nisoldipine	Y	**Macrolides**		Triazolam	Y
Nitrendipine	Y	Clarithromycin	N	**Immunosuppressants**	
Pranidipine	Y	**HMG-CoA reductase inhibitors**		Cyclosporine	Y
Antiarrhythmics		Atorvastatin	Y	Tacrolimus	Y?
Diltiazem	N	Fluvastatin	N?	**Other**	
Verapamil	N	Lovastatin	Y	Methadone	Y
Quinidine	N	Pravastatin	N?	Sildenafil	Y
Antihistamines		Simvastatin	Y		
Ebastine	Y?				
Loratadine	Y?				

CNS, central nervous system; HMG-CoA, hydroxymethylglutaryl coenzyme A.

[a]Y (yes) and N (no) indicate published evidence of the presence or absence of an interaction with grapefruit juice. Y? and N? indicate expected findings based on available data. Those drugs with Y or Y? should not be consumed with grapefruit juice in an unsupervised manner.

for drugs with low-moderate bioavailability. Enhanced oral drug bioavailability can occur up to 24 hours after juice consumption, so taking CYP3A4-vulnerable drugs with water or other liquids within 24 hours of consuming grapefruit juice can still result in an interaction. Inhibition of P-gp is a possible mechanism by which grapefruit juice, and perhaps the nutraceutical grapefruit oil, increases oral drug bioavailability by reducing intestinal and/or hepatic efflux transport. Inhibition of organic anion–transporting polypeptides by grapefruit juice and apple juice has been observed; intestinal uptake transport appeared to decrease as oral drug bioavailability was reduced.

Numerous medications used in the prevention or treatment of coronary artery disease and its complications have been observed or predicted to interact with grapefruit juice. Such DDIs can increase the risk of rhabdomyolysis when dyslipidemia is treated with the hydroxymethylglutaryl coenzyme A (HMG-CoA) reductase inhibitors (statins). Excessive vasodilation when hypertension is managed with the dihydropyridines amlodipine, felodipine, nicardipine, nifedipine, nisoldipine, or nitrendipine has been documented, although incidence and severity with some agents can be unpredictable. The therapeutic effect of the angiotensin II type I receptor antagonist losartan can be reduced by grapefruit juice with a subsequent loss of its blood pressure–lowering effect. Grapefruit juice interacting with the antidiabetic agent repaglinide can cause hypoglycemia, and interaction with the appetite suppressant sibutramine can cause elevated blood pressure and heart rate. In angina pectoris, administration of grapefruit juice could result in atrioventricular conduction disorders with verapamil or attenuated antiplatelet activity with clopidogrel. Grapefruit juice can enhance the drug toxicity for antiarrhythmic agents, such as amiodarone, quinidine, disopyramide, or propafenone, and for the congestive heart failure drug carvedilol. Some drugs used for the treatment of peripheral or central vascular disease also have the potential to interact with grapefruit juice. Interaction with sildenafil, tadalafil, or vardenafil for erectile dysfunction can cause serious systemic vasodilation, especially when combined with nitrate. In stroke, interaction with nimodipine can cause systemic hypotension.

If a drug has low inherent oral bioavailability from presystemic metabolism by CYP3A4 or efflux transport by P-gp and the potential to produce serious overdose toxicity, avoidance of grapefruit juice entirely during pharmacotherapy appears mandatory. Although altered drug response is variable among individuals, the outcome is difficult to predict and avoiding the combination will guarantee that this potential toxicity pathway is prevented.

The mechanism by which grapefruit juice produces its effect is through inhibition of the enzymatic activity and a decrease in the intestinal expression of CYP3A4. The P-gp efflux pump also transports many CYP3A4 substrates; thus, the presence of inhibitors of P-gp in grapefruit juice (eg, 6′,7′-dihydroxybergamottin and other furanocoumarins) could be a related factor for drug-grapefruit juice interactions.[243] Numerous studies have shown that grapefruit juice consumed in normal (single glass) quantities acts on intestinal CYP3A4, not at the hepatic level.

Does the quantity of juice matter? The majority of the presystemic CYP3A4 inhibition is obtained following ingestion of one glass of grapefruit juice; however, 24 hours after ingestion of a glass of grapefruit juice, 30% of its effect is still present. The reduction in intestinal CYP3A4 concentration is rapid: a 47% decrease occurred in a healthy volunteer within 4 hours after consuming grapefruit juice. Daily ingestion of grapefruit juice results in a loss of CYP3A4 from the small intestinal epithelium. Consumption of very large quantities of grapefruit juice (six to eight glasses/day) can lead to inhibition of hepatic CYP3A4.[243]

The active constituents found in grapefruit juice originally thought responsible for its effects on CYP3A4 include the flavonoids naringenin and naringin and the furanocoumarins bergamottin and 6′,7′-dihydroxybergamottin (Fig. 3.47). The flavonoids were initially believed to be the causative agents for the effect of grapefruit juice on CYP3A4. However, it was later determined through in vivo studies that furanocoumarins were the actual mediators of drug-grapefruit juice interactions.[242]

Many studies to date have used freshly squeezed grapefruit juice, reconstituted frozen juice, commercial grapefruit juice, grapefruit segments, or grapefruit extract; all are capable of causing DDIs with CYP3A4 substrates (blended grapefruit juices have not yet been investigated). The active constituents in grapefruit juice are present not just in the juice but also in the pulp, peel, and core of the fruit and are responsible for its flavor. Bergamottin and 6′,7′-dihydroxybergamottin are potent mechanism-based inhibitors of CYP3A4 and naringenin isomers are competitive inhibitors of CYP3A4. Higher concentrations of 6′,7′-dihydroxybergamottin are present in grapefruit segments. Thus, any therapeutic concern for a drug interaction with grapefruit juice should now be extended to include whole fruit and other products derived from the grapefruit peel. The interaction of grapefruit juice with P450 pushed the study of other natural juices.[244] The difference in the in vitro CYP3A4 inhibition between grapefruit juice and orange juice is that orange juice contained no measurable amounts of 6′,7′-dihydroxybergamottin. The nutraceutical grapefruit oil contains minor amounts of bergamottin; therefore, grapefruit oil has the potential to cause drug interactions with CYP3A4 substrates.

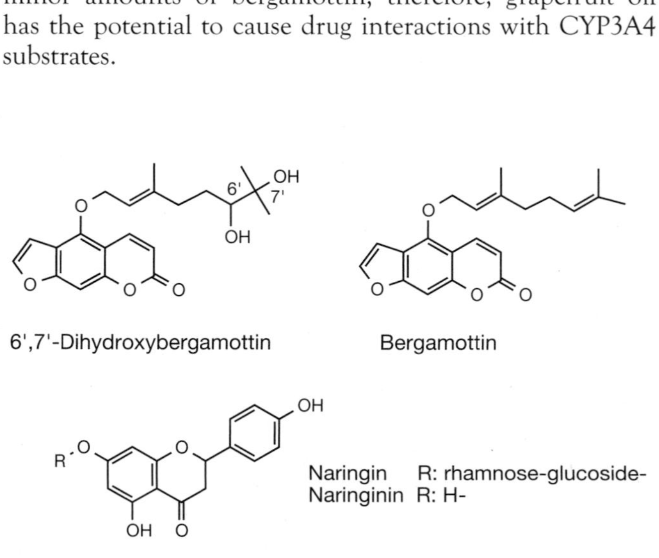

Figure 3.47 Active constituents of grapefruit juice.

If a patient has been taking medication with grapefruit juice for some time without ill effects, is it safe to continue to do so? Much of this unpredictability results from the inconsistency of the juice concentrations and the sporadic way grapefruit juice is consumed, suggesting that this approach cannot be entirely safe. Given the unpredictability of the effect of grapefruit juice on the oral bioavailability of the drugs in Table 3.20, patients should be advised to avoid this combination, thus preventing the onset of potential adverse effects. Each patient's situation should be considered, and advice should be based on consumption history and the specific medications involved. The benefits of increased and controlled drug bioavailability by grapefruit juice may, in the future, be achieved through either standardizing the constituents or coadministration of the isolated active ingredients. This would then lead to a safe, effective, and cost saving means to enhance the absorption of many therapeutic agents.

P-Glycoprotein-Drug Interactions

P-gp-mediated transport has an important role in pharmacokinetic-mediated DDIs. The effect of P-gp inhibition is to increase the oral bioavailability of CYP3A4 substrates so that the later actions of CYP3A4 inhibition will be increased. One of the best examples is the interaction between digoxin and quinidine. Quinidine blocks P-gp in the intestinal mucosa and in the proximal renal tubule; thus, digoxin elimination into the intestine and urine is inhibited, increasing the plasma digoxin concentration to toxic levels. Another example is loperamide, which is an opioid antidiarrheal normally kept out of the brain by the P-gp efflux pump. Inhibition of P-gp allows accumulation of loperamide in the brain, leading to respiratory depression as a result of central μ opioid receptor agonism.

The components of grapefruit juice reportedly inhibit P-gp, and this can be one of the mechanisms for the increase in bioavailability of drugs that are substrates for P-gp.[238]

Drug-Dietary Supplement Interactions

The increasing use of dietary supplements presents a special challenge in health care, and there is an increasing need to predict and avoid these potential adverse drug-dietary supplement interactions.[245-247] The present interest and widespread use of herbal remedies has created the possibility of interaction with OTC or prescription drugs if they are used simultaneously. As herbal medicines become more popular, herbal hepatotoxicity is being increasingly recognized. Females appear to be predisposed to hepatotoxicity, and coadministered agents that induce P450 enzymes (eg, St. John's wort) can also increase individual susceptibility to some dietary supplements. Nearly one in five adults taking prescription medicines is also taking at least one dietary supplement. The mechanisms for drug-dietary supplement interactions are similar to those for DDIs affecting the pharmacokinetics of the respective drug. Little is known regarding the pharmacokinetic properties of many of the substances in dietary supplements. Therefore, the potential for drug-dietary supplement interactions has greatly increased.[245]

A reported drug-dietary supplement interaction is between St. John's wort and HIV protease inhibitors (indinavir, ritonavir), leading to drug resistance and treatment failure. St. John's wort is a popular dietary supplement often used for depression. Of the two substances found in St. John's wort, hypericin and hyperforin, hyperforin appears to be the main constituent, with in vitro SSRI activity. Hyperforin appears also to be the more potent inducer of CYP3A enzymes based on in vitro and in vivo studies.[248] St. John's wort also decreases the therapeutic activity of other CYP3A4 substrates, including warfarin, simvastatin, digoxin, and oral contraceptives.

Other Dietary Supplements

DHEA and androstenedione are dietary testosterone precursors that have been associated with hepatic toxicity and should not be taken by those with hepatic disease. Coingestion with other potentially hepatotoxic products or enzyme inducers that might increase the risk of liver damage should also be avoided.

Black cohosh (*Actaea racemosa*), commonly used by women for menopausal symptoms, including hot flashes and sleep disorders, forms potentially hepatotoxic quinone metabolites in vitro, but no mercapturate conjugates were detected in urine samples from women who consumed multiple oral doses of up to 256 mg of a standardized black cohosh extract. At moderate doses of black cohosh, the risk of liver injury is minimal.

Silybum marianum (milk thistle) is used in the treatment of chronic or acute liver disease, as well as in protecting the liver against toxicity. *Silybum* is cited as one of the oldest known herbal medicines. The active constituents of milk thistle are flavonolignans, which are known collectively as silymarin.

Besides the aforementioned plants, the bioactive components of several others can interact with drugs including *Aloe vera*, *Curcuma longa*, *Hydrastis canadensis*, *Gingko biloba*, *Panax quinquefolius*, *Valeriana officinalis*, *Cannabis sativa*, etc. Clinicians should have a good understanding on herb-drug interactions and avoid their combinations when warranted.[245,246]

Miscellaneous Drug-Drug Interactions

The ability of drugs and other foreign substances to induce metabolism of other drugs has been discussed. Phenobarbital, for example, stimulates metabolism of a variety of drugs (eg, phenytoin and coumarin anticoagulants). Stimulation of bishydroxycoumarin metabolism can create a problem in patients undergoing anticoagulant therapy. If phenobarbital administration is stopped, the rate of metabolism of the anticoagulant decreases, resulting in greater plasma concentrations of bishydroxycoumarin and enhanced anticoagulant activity, increasing the possibility of hemorrhage. Serious side effects have resulted from this type of interaction. These observations indicate that combined therapy of a potent drug (eg, bishydroxycoumarin) and an inducer of drug metabolism (eg, phenobarbital) can create a hazardous situation if the enzyme inducer is withdrawn and therapy with the potent drug is continued without an appropriate decrease in dose.

Serious reactions have been reported in patients treated with an MAO inhibitor such as tranylcypromine because they are, as a rule, sensitive to a subsequent dose of a sympathomimetic amine (eg, amphetamine) or a tricyclic antidepressant (eg, amitriptyline), which is metabolized by MAO. An increase in the duration and therapeutic impact of the sympathomimetic would result.

Allopurinol, an XO inhibitor used for the treatment of gout, inhibits metabolism of 6-mercaptopurine and other drugs metabolized by this enzyme. A serious drug interaction results from the concurrent use of allopurinol for gout and 6-mercaptopurine to block the immune response from a tissue transplant or as antimetabolite in neoplastic diseases.

GENDER DIFFERENCES IN DRUG METABOLISM

Although numerous gender differences have been described in humans, so far most clinical research has been conducted with the limited view that the male can fulfill the function of being representative for the whole human species. However, in spite of the increasing evidence pointing out physiologic and pathologic differences between the sexes beyond those related to reproduction, women differ from men in gene expression and regulation, in the susceptibility to and risk for many medical conditions, and in the response to numerous drugs.[249,250] Gender difference in drug response may explain, at least in part, the interindividual variations occurring in therapeutic response and toxicity, especially considering that female sex has been shown to be a risk factor for the development of adverse drug reactions. Nonetheless, current studies indicate that gender differences in pharmacologic response are more widespread than originally believed and involve pharmacogenomics, pharmacodynamics, and pharmacokinetics, with pharmacokinetic determinants being the most investigated.[250]

The role of pharmacokinetics versus pharmacodynamics is not yet completely appreciated, and only a few contributions have evaluated the impact of genetics, hormonal variations, and their relative interactions.[249] The role of gender as a contributor to variability in xenobiotic metabolism and IDRs, which are more common in females, is not clear, but increasing numbers of reports show differences in metabolism between males and females, raising the possibility that endogenous sex hormones, hydrocortisone, or their synthetic equivalents can influence the activity of inducible CYP3A. *N*-demethylation of erythromycin was significantly higher in females than males, which was persistent throughout adulthood. In contrast, males had unchanged *N*-demethylation values.

Gender-dependent differences of metabolic rates have been detected for some drugs. Side chain oxidation of propranolol was 50% faster in males than in females. Propranolol metabolism is stimulated by testosterone but not by estrogens, resulting in an up to 80% difference in plasma drug levels between males and females. No differences between genders were noted in propranolol aromatic ring hydroxylation. CYP1A2 shows a higher activity in males, and therefore, clearance of antidepressants, antipsychotics, and theophylline is faster in males. CYP1A2 activity is decreased during pregnancy. Although CYP1A2 does not catalyze meperidine *N*-demethylation, meperidine's metabolism by other CYP isoforms, including 3A4, 2B6, and 2C19, was depressed during pregnancy and in females taking oral contraceptives.

CYP3A4 activity is generally higher in females. Drugs such as cyclosporine, erythromycin, nimodipine, and cortisol are substrates of CYP3A4, showing faster clearance among females. Although CYP3A4 is also responsible for about 60% of CYP-mediated metabolism of zolpidem, its overall clearance is actually slower in females, requiring an FDA-recommended 50% dose reduction. Other examples of drugs cleared by CYP3A4 more rapidly in males include chlordiazepoxide and lidocaine. Diazepam, prednisolone, caffeine, and acetaminophen are metabolized slightly faster by females. No gender differences have been observed in the clearance of phenytoin, nitrazepam, and trazodone, which interestingly are not substrates for the CYP3A subfamily.

Gender differences in the rate of glucuronidation have been noted. Males show a faster clearance of drugs that are primarily eliminated by glucuronidation. Thus, oxazepam, metabolized mainly by UGT2B15, has a longer half-life in females, although the kinetic difference is also connected to the *D85Y* polymorphic variant. Gender differences are also found in other pharmacokinetic parameters such as drug absorption, drug distribution, and excretion.

Historically, females were less frequently enrolled in clinical trials because both the pharmacokinetics and pharmacodynamics of a drug can be influenced by menstrual cycle phases, hormonal fluctuations, use of oral contraceptives, and hormonal therapy. There was also concern about life events such as pregnancy and lactation, including the potential negative impact of investigational drugs on the fetus or nursing neonate. The number of trials enrolling females has increased after an FDA request to include a fair representation of both genders as participants, but overall, women are still underrepresented. Females are generally treated with doses that essentially reflect the results obtained by trials carried out mainly in males.

Despite the differences in drug pharmacokinetics, sex-specific recommendations in dosage do not exist for most drugs. Pharmacists need to recognize the underrepresentation of females in clinical trials and take the responsibility to inform consumers and emphasize to clinicians that females can differ significantly from males with respect to metabolism, absorption, distribution, and excretion of drugs. Pharmacists also need to be aware that pregnancy, oral contraceptive use, and hormone replacement therapy can significantly change drug metabolism and drug clearance. If a female patient consistently experiences more adverse drug events or less therapeutic effect from a particular drug, it may be necessary to discuss with their physician the possibility of changing the dosing regimen or switching to a different medication. Even postmenopausally, CYP3A function can be altered and influenced by the lack of estrogen or the presence of androgens. In the past decades, there has been a significant and focused effort from the Office of Women's Health/National Institutes of Health to include gender equality in clinical trials.[251,252]

Compared to males, there are more females in the U.S. population, more females with chronic diseases, and more females visiting physicians. It is, therefore, obvious that there needs to be a greater interest in understanding how they react to drugs. Ultimately, a better understanding of sex-related influences on drug responses will help to improve drug safety and efficacy and will also permit practitioners to tailor pharmacologic treatments in both males and females.

Major Pathways of Metabolism

Table 3.21 contains an extensive list of commonly used drugs and the P450 isoforms that catalyze their metabolism. In addition, phase 1 and phase 2 metabolic pathways for some common drugs are listed in Table 3.21.

Table 3.21 Metabolic Pathways of Common Drugs

Drug	Pathway	Drug	Pathway
Amphetamines 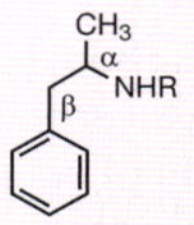	Deamination (followed by oxidation and reduction of the ketone formed) *N*-oxidation *N*-dealkylation Hydroxylation of the aromatic ring Hydroxylation of the β-carbon atom Conjugation with glucuronic acid of the acid and alcohol products from the ketone formed by deamination	Barbiturates 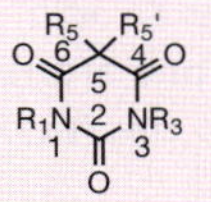	Oxidation and complete removal of substituents at carbon 5 *N*-dealkylation at *N*1 and *N*3 Desulfuration at carbon 2 (thiobarbiturates) Scission of the barbiturate ring at the 1:6 bond to give substituted malonylureas
Phenothiazines 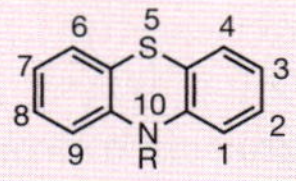	*N*-dealkylation in the N_{10} side chain *N*-oxidation in the N_{10} side chain Oxidation of the heterocyclic S atom to sulfoxide or sulfone Hydroxylation of one or both aromatic rings Conjugation of phenolic metabolites with glucuronic acid or sulfate Scission of the N_{10} side chain	Sulfonamides 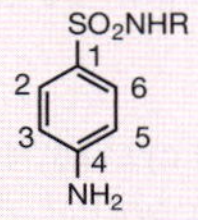	Acetylation at the N_4 amino group Conjugation with glucuronic acid or sulfate at the N_4 amino group Acetylation or conjugation with glucuronic acid at the N_1 amino group Hydroxylation and conjugation in the heterocyclic ring, R
Phenytoin 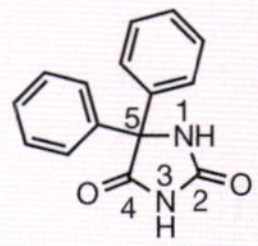	Hydroxylation of one aromatic ring Conjugation of phenolic products with glucuronic acid or sulfate Hydrolytic scission of the hydantoin ring at the bond between carbons 3 and 4 to give 5,5-diphenylhydantoic acid	Meperidine 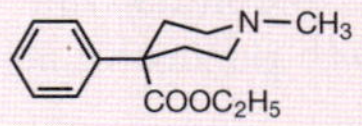	Hydrolysis of ester to acid *N*-dealkylation Hydroxylation of aromatic ring *N*-oxidation Both *N*-dealkylation and hydrolysis Conjugation of phenolic products
Pentazocine 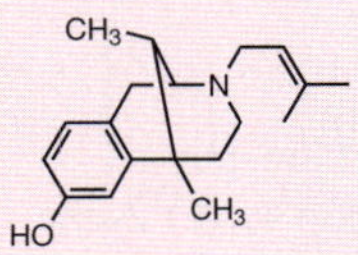	Hydroxylation of terminal methyl groups of the alkenyl side chain to give *cis* and *trans* (major) alcohols Oxidation of hydroxymethyl product of the alkenyl side chain to carboxylic acids Reduction of alkenyl side chain and oxidation of terminal methyl group	Cocaine 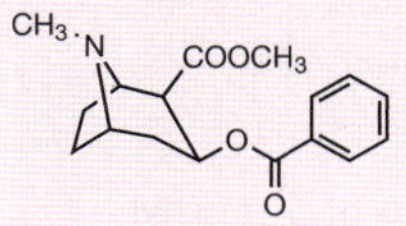	Hydrolysis of methyl ester Hydrolysis of benzoate ester *N*-dealkylation Both hydrolysis and *N*-dealkylation

(continued)

Table 3.21 Metabolic Pathways of Common Drugs (*continued*)

Drug	Pathway	Drug	Pathway
Phenmetrazine 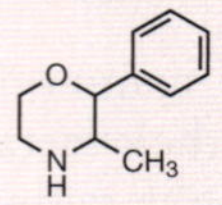	Oxidation to lactam Aromatic hydroxylation *N*-oxidation Conjugation of phenolic products	Ephedrine 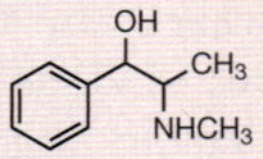	*N*-dealkylation Oxidative deamination Oxidation of deaminated product to benzoic acid Reduction of deaminated product to 1,2-diol
Propranolol 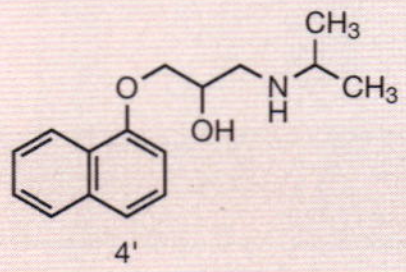	Aromatic hydroxylation at C4′ *N*-dealkylation Oxidative deamination Oxidation of deaminated product to naphthoxyacetic acid Conjugation with glucuronic acid *O*-dealkylation	Indomethacin 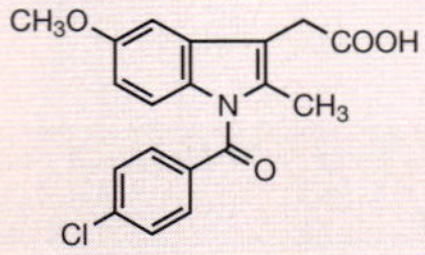	*O*-demethylation *N*-deacylation (hydrolysis) of p-chlorobenzoyl group Both *O*-dealkylation and *N*-deacylation (hydrolysis) Conjugation of phenolic products with glucuronic acid Other conjugation products
Diphenoxylate 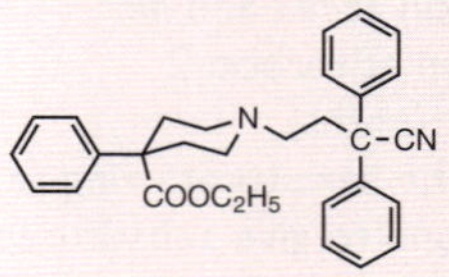	Hydrolysis of ester to acid Hydroxylation of one aromatic ring attached to the *N*-alkyl side chain	Diazepam 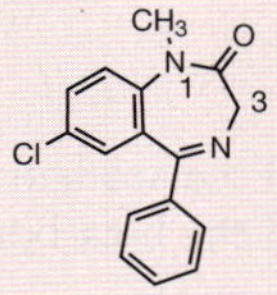	*N*-dealkylation at N_1 Hydroxylation at carbon 3 Conjugation with glucuronic acid Both *N*-dealkylation of N_1 and hydroxylation at carbon 3
Prostaglandins 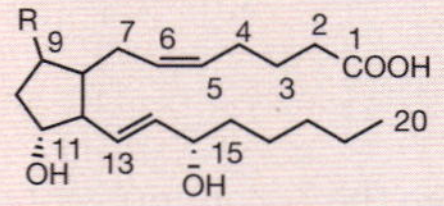	Reduction of double bonds at carbons 5 and 6 and 13 and 14 Oxidation of 15-hydroxyl to ketone β-Oxidation of carbons 3, 5, and 7 ω-Oxidation of carbon 20 to acid	Cyproheptadine 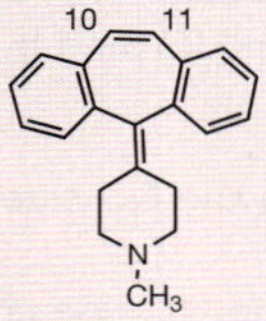	*N*-dealkylation 10,11-epoxide formation Both *N*-dealkylation and 10,11-epoxidation
Hydralazine 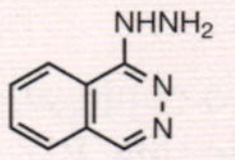	*N*-acetylation with cyclization to a methyl-*S*-triazolophthalazine *N*-formylation with cyclization to an *S*-triazolophthalazine Aromatic hydroxylation of benzene ring Oxidative loss of hydrazinyl group to 1-hydroxy Hydroxylation of methyl of methyl-*S*-triazolophthalazine Conjugation with glucuronic acid	Methadone 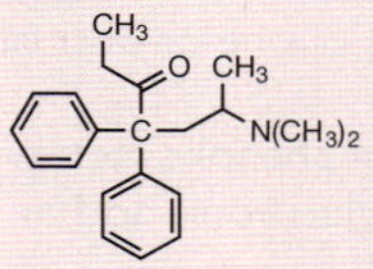	Reduction of ketone to hydroxyl Aromatic hydroxylation of one aromatic ring *N*-dealkylation of alcohol product *N*-dealkylation with cyclization to pyrrolidine
Lidocaine 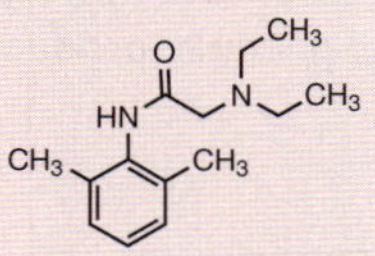	*N*-dealkylation Oxidation of amine N Aromatic hydroxylation ortho to methyl Benzylic (aromatic methyl) hydroxylation followed by oxidation to carboxylic acid Hydrolysis of amide	Imipramine 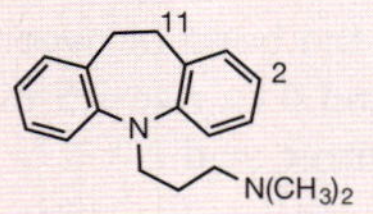	*N*-dealkylation Hydroxylation at C_{11} Aromatic hydroxylation (C_2) *N*-oxidation Both *N*-dealkylation and hydroxylation
Cimetidine 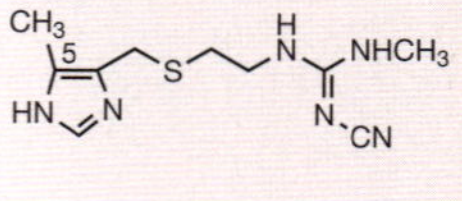	*S*-oxidation Hydroxylation of 5-methyl	Valproic acid 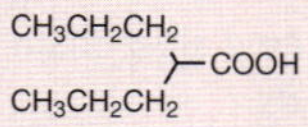	Coenzyme A thioester Dehydrogenation to (*E*) 2-ene Dehydrogenation to (*E*) 2,4-diene Dehydrogenation to 4-ene 3-Hydroxylation

Table 3.21 Metabolic Pathways of Common Drugs (*continued*)

Drug	Pathway	Drug	Pathway
Piroxicam 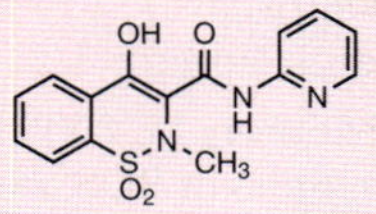	Pyridine 3′-hydroxylation Hydrolysis of amide Decarboxylation of hydrolysis product	Caffeine 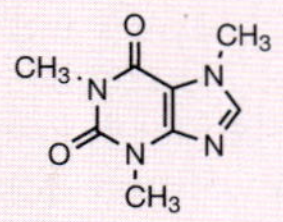	N_3-demethylation N_1-demethylation N_7-demethylation to theophylline C_8 oxidation to uric acids Imidazole ring opening
Theophylline 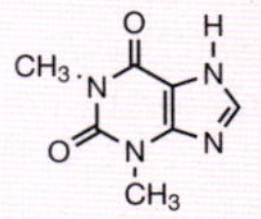	N_3-demethylation N_1-demethylation C_8 oxidation to uric acids Imidazole ring opening	Nicotine 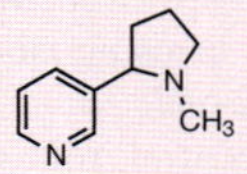	Pyrrolidine 5′-hydroxylation to cotinine Pyrrolidine *N*-oxidation *N*-demethylation (nornicotine and norcotinine) Pyridine *N*-methylation 3′-Hydroxylation of cotinine
Ibuprofen 8 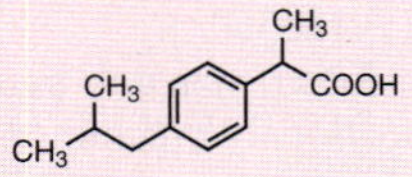	Coenzyme A thioester and epimerization of R− to S+ enantiomer Methyl hydroxylation followed by oxidation to carboxylic acid Acylglucuronide	Tamoxifen 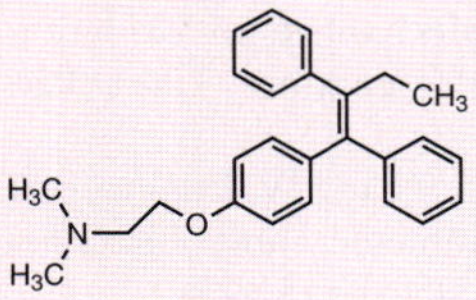	*N*-demethylation 4′-Hydroxylation *N*-oxidation 4′-*O*-sulfate 4′-*O*-glucuronide
Lovastatin 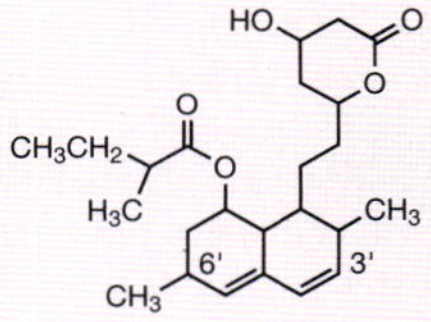	6′-Hydroxylation 3′-Side chain hydroxylation 3′-Hydroxylation β-oxidation of lactone *O*-glucuronide	Ciprofloxacin 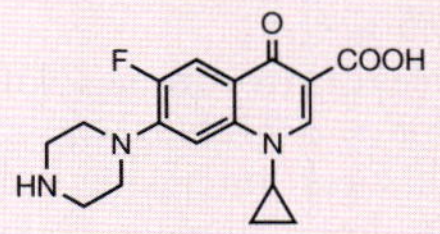	Piperazine 3′-hydroxylation *N*-sulfonation
Labetalol 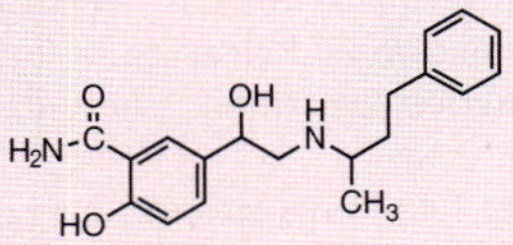	*O*-sulfate (major) *O*-glucuronide	Acetaminophen 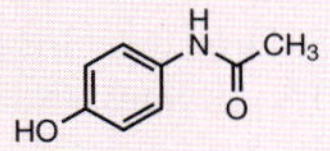	*O*-glucuronide *O*-sulfate Oxidation to *N*-acetyl-*p*-benzoquinoneimine Conjugation of *N*-acetyl-*p*-benzoquinoneimine with glutathione
Tripelennamine 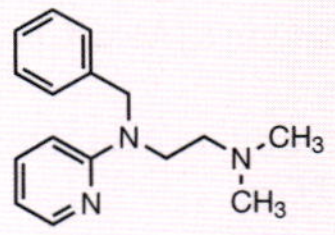	*p*-Hydroxylation Benzylic C-hydroxylation *N*-depyrimidination *N*-debenzylation	Felodipine 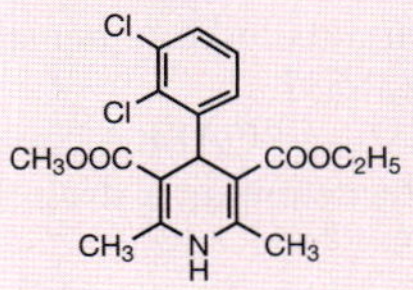	Aromatization Ester hydrolysis Methyl hydroxylation

REFERENCES

1. Williams RT. Detoxication mechanisms in man. *Clin Pharmacol Ther*. 1963;4(2):234-254.
2. Anders MW. *Bioactivation of Foreign Compounds*. Academic Press; 1985.
3. Bend JR, Caldwell J, Jakoby WB. *Metabolic Basis of Detoxication: Metabolism of Functional Groups*. Academic Press; 1982.
4. Hodgson E. *Enzymatic Basis of Detoxication*. Vols 1 and 2. William B. Jakoby-ed. Academic Press; 1981.
5. De Montellano PRO. *Cytochrome P450: Structure, Mechanism, and Biochemistry*. Vol 3. Springer; 2005.
6. Testa B, Krämer S-D. *The Biochemistry of Drug Metabolism: Volume 1: Principles, Redox Reactions, Hydrolyses*. Helvetica Chimica Acta Wiley-VCH; 2008.
7. Testa B, Krämer S-D. *The Biochemistry of Drug Metabolism: Volume 2: Conjugations, Consequences of Metabolism, Influencing Factors*. Helvetica Chimica Acta Wiley-VCH; 2010.
8. Rodrigues AD. *Drug-Drug Interactions*. CRC Press; 2019.
9. Pearson PG, Wienkers LC. *Handbook of Drug Metabolism*. CRC Press; 2019.
10. Groves JT. Models and mechanisms of cytochrome P450 action. In: Ortiz de Montellano PR, ed. *Cytochrome P450: Structure, Mechanism, and Biochemistry*. Springer; 2005:1-43.
11. Huang X, Groves JT. Beyond ferryl-mediated hydroxylation: 40 years of the rebound mechanism and C-H activation. *J Biol Inorg Chem*. 2017;22(2-3):185-207.
12. Poulos TL, Follmer AH. Updating the Paradigm: redox partner binding and conformational dynamics in cytochromes P450. *Acc Chem Res*. 2022;55(3):373-380.

13. Nelson DR, Koymans L, Kamataki T, et al. P450 superfamily: update on new sequences, gene mapping, accession numbers and nomenclature. *Pharmacogenetics*. 1996;6(1):1-42.
14. Dornburg A, Mallik R, Wang Z, et al. Placing human gene families into their evolutionary context. *Hum Genomics*. 2022;16(1):56.
15. Zhao M, Ma J, Li M, et al. Cytochrome P450 enzymes and drug metabolism in humans. *Int J Mol Sci*. 2021;22(23):12808.
16. Wu J, Guan X, Dai Z, et al. Molecular probes for human cytochrome P450 enzymes: recent progress and future perspectives. *Coord Chem Rev*. 2021;427:213600.
17. Couto N, Al-Majdoub ZM, Achour B, Wright PC, Rostami-Hodjegan A, Barber J. Quantification of proteins involved in drug metabolism and disposition in the human liver using label-free global proteomics. *Mol Pharm*. 2019;16(2):632-647.
18. Esteves F, Rueff J, Kranendonk M. The central role of cytochrome P450 in xenobiotic metabolism—a brief review on a fascinating enzyme family. *J Xenobiot*. 2021;11(3):94-114.
19. Guengerich FP, Waterman MR, Egli M. Recent structural insights into cytochrome P450 function. *Trends Pharmacol Sci*. 2016;37(8):625-640.
20. Meunier B, de Visser SP, Shaik S. Mechanism of oxidation reactions catalyzed by cytochrome p450 enzymes. *Chem Rev*. 2004;104(9):3947-3980.
21. Li Z, Jiang Y, Guengerich FP, Ma L, Li S, Zhang W. Engineering cytochrome P450 enzyme systems for biomedical and biotechnological applications. *J Biol Chem*. 2020;295(3):833-849.
22. Machalz D, Pach S, Bermudez M, Bureik M, Wolber G. Structural insights into understudied human cytochrome P450 enzymes. *Drug Discov Today*. 2021;26(10):2456-2464.
23. Kwon Y-J, Shin S, Chun Y-J. Biological roles of cytochrome P450 1A1, 1A2, and 1B1 enzymes. *Arch Pharm Res*. 2021;44:63-83.
24. Kukal S, Thakran S, Kanojia N, et al. Genic-intergenic polymorphisms of CYP1A genes and their clinical impact. *Gene*. 2023;857:147171.
25. Zhu W, Liu H, Wang X, et al. Associations of CYP1 polymorphisms with risk of prostate cancer: an updated meta-analysis. *Biosci Rep*. 2019;39(3):BSR20181876.
26. Klomp F, Wenzel C, Drozdzik M, Oswald S. Drug-drug interactions involving intestinal and hepatic CYP1A enzymes. *Pharmaceutics*. 2020;12(12):1201.
27. Vukovic V, Ianuale C, Leoncini E, et al. Lack of association between polymorphisms in the CYP1A2 gene and risk of cancer: evidence from meta-analyses. *BMC Cancer*. 2016;16:83.
28. Fekete F, Mangó K, Minus A, Tóth K, Monostory K. CYP1A2 mRNA expression rather than genetic variants indicate hepatic CYP1A2 activity. *Pharmaceutics*. 2022;14(3):532.
29. Fang C, Ouyang W, Zeng Y, et al. CYP2A6 and GABRA2 gene polymorphisms are associated with dexmedetomidine drug response. *Front Pharmacol*. 2022;13:943200.
30. El-Boraie A, Chenoweth MJ, Pouget JG, et al. Transferability of ancestry-specific and cross-ancestry CYP2A6 activity genetic risk scores in African and European populations. *Clin Pharmacol Ther*. 2021;110(4):975-985.
31. Vrzal R. Genetic and enzymatic characteristics of CYP2A13 in relation to lung damage. *Int J Mol Sci*. 2021;22(22):12306.
32. Angle ED, Cox PM. Multidisciplinary insights into the structure-function relationship of the CYP2B6 active site. *Drug Metab Dispos*. 2023;51(3):369-384.
33. Mustafa G, Nandekar PP, Bruce NJ, Wade RC. Differing membrane interactions of two highly similar drug-metabolizing cytochrome P450 isoforms: CYP 2C9 and CYP 2C19. *Int J Mol Sci*. 2019;20(18):4328.
34. U.S. Food and Drug Administration. Table of pharmacogenomic biomarkers in drug labeling. Accessed August 2023. https://www.fda.gov/drugs/science-and-research-drugs/table-pharmacogenomic-biomarkers-drug-labeling
35. Taylor C, Crosby I, Yip V, Maguire P, Pirmohamed M, Turner RM. A review of the important role of CYP2D6 in pharmacogenomics. *Genes (Basel)*. 2020;11(11):1295.
36. Schoretsanitis G, de Leon J, Eap CB, Kane JM, Paulzen M. Clinically significant drug-drug interactions with agents for attention-deficit/hyperactivity disorder. *CNS Drugs*. 2019;33(12):1201-1222.
37. McLaughlin LA, Paine MJ, Kemp CA, et al. Why is quinidine an inhibitor of cytochrome P450 2D6? The role of key active-site residues in quinidine binding. *J Biol Chem*. 2005;280(46):38617-38624.
38. Harjumäki R, Pridgeon CS, Ingelman-Sundberg M. CYP2E1 in alcoholic and non-alcoholic liver injury. Roles of ROS, reactive intermediates and lipid overload. *Int J Mol Sci*. 2021;22(15):8221.
39. Ijiri Y, Kato R, Sadamatsu M, et al. Contributions of caspase-8 and-9 to liver injury from CYP2E1-produced metabolites of halogenated hydrocarbons. *Xenobiotica*. 2018;48(1):60-72.
40. Klyushova LS, Perepechaeva ML, Grishanova AY. The role of CYP3A in health and disease. *Biomedicines*. 2022;10(11):2686.
41. Jarrar YB, Lee SJ. Molecular functionality of cytochrome P450 4 (CYP4) genetic polymorphisms and their clinical implications. *Int J Mol Sci*. 2019;20(17):4274.
42. Zhou M, Li J, Xu J, Zheng L, Xu S. Exploring human CYP4 enzymes: physiological roles, function in diseases and focus on inhibitors. *Drug Discov Today*. 2023;28(5):103560.
43. Batabyal D, Richards LS, Poulos TL. Effect of redox partner binding on cytochrome P450 conformational dynamics. *J Am Chem Soc*. 2017;139(37):13193-13199.
44. Rendic S, Guengerich FP. Survey of human oxidoreductases and cytochrome P450 enzymes involved in the metabolism of xenobiotic and natural chemicals. *Chem Res Toxicol*. 2015;28(1):38-42.
45. Makris TM, Denisov I, Schlichting I, Sligar SG. Activation of molecular oxygen by cytochrome P450. In: *Cytochrome P450: Structure, Mechanism, and Biochemistry*. 3rd ed. Springer; 2005:149-182.
46. Hargrove TY, Lamb DC, Smith JA, Wawrzak Z, Kelly SL, Lepesheva GI. Unravelling the role of transient redox partner complexes in P450 electron transfer mechanics. *Sci Rep*. 2022;12(1):16232.
47. Behrendorff J. Reductive cytochrome P450 reactions and their potential role in bioremediation. *Front Microbiol*. 2021;12:649273.
48. Guengerich FP, Yoshimoto FK. Formation and cleavage of C-C bonds by enzymatic oxidation-reduction reactions. *Chem Rev*. 2018;118(14):6573-6655.
49. Guengerich FP. Roles of cytochrome P450 enzymes in pharmacology and toxicology: past, present, and future. *Adv Pharmacol*. 2022;95:1-47.
50. Guengerich FP, Tateishi Y, McCarty KD. C-C bond cleavage reactions catalyzed by cytochrome P450 enzymes. *Med Chem Res*. 2023;32:1263-1277.
51. Guengerich FP. Mechanisms of cytochrome P450-catalyzed oxidations. *ACS Catal*. 2018;8(12):10964-10976.
52. Munro AW, McLean KJ, Grant JL, Makris TM. Structure and function of the cytochrome P450 peroxygenase enzymes. *Biochem Soc Trans*. 2018;46(1):183-196.
53. Groves JT. Enzymatic C-H bond activation: using push to get pull. *Nat Chem*. 2014;6(2):89-91.
54. Shaik S, Dubey KD. The catalytic cycle of cytochrome P450: a fascinating choreography. *Trends Chem*. 2021;3(12):1027-1044.
55. Ortiz de Montellano PR. Cytochrome P-450 catalysis: radical intermediates and dehydrogenation reactions. *Trends Pharmacol Sci*. 1989;10(9):354-359.
56. Guengerich FP. Mechanisms of cytochrome P450 substrate oxidation: MiniReview. *J Biochem Mol Toxicol*. 2007;21(4):163-168.
57. Furge LL, Guengerich FP. Cytochrome P450 enzymes in drug metabolism and chemical toxicology: an introduction. *Biochem Mol Biol Educ*. 2006;34(2):66-74.
58. Kiang TKL, Ho PC, Anari MR, Tong V, Abbott FS, Chang TKH. Contribution of CYP2C9, CYP2A6, and CYP2B6 to valproic acid metabolism in hepatic microsomes from individuals with the CYP2C9*1/*1 Genotype. *Toxicol Sci*. 2006;94(2):261-271.
59. Guengerich FP, Macdonald TL. Mechanisms of cytochrome P-450 catalysis. *FASEB J*. 1990;4(8):2453-2459.

60. Fabre G, Briot C, Marti E, et al. Delta 2-valproate biotransformation using human liver microsomal fractions. *Pharm Weekbl Sci.* 1992;14(3a):146-151.
61. Ortiz de Montellano PR. Acetylenes: cytochrome P450 oxidation and mechanism-based enzyme inactivation. *Drug Metab Rev.* 2019;51(2):162-177.
62. Ullrich R, Hofrichter M. Enzymatic hydroxylation of aromatic compounds. *Cell Mol Life Sci.* 2007;64(3):271-293.
63. Bathelt CM, Ridder L, Mulholland AJ, Harvey JN. Mechanism and structure–reactivity relationships for aromatic hydroxylation by cytochrome P450. *Org Biomol Chem.* 2004;2(20):2998-3005.
64. Rendic S, Guengerich FP. Contributions of human enzymes in carcinogen metabolism. *Chem Res Toxicol.* 2012;25(7):1316-1383.
65. Eh-Haj BM. Metabolic *N*-dealkylation and *N*-oxidation as elucidators of the role of alkylamino moieties in drugs acting at various receptors. *Molecules.* 2021;26(7):1917.
66. Murphy SE. Biochemistry of nicotine metabolism and its relevance to lung cancer. *J Biol Chem.* 2021;296:100722.
67. Rydberg P, Ryde U, Olsen L. Sulfoxide, sulfur, and nitrogen oxidation and dealkylation by cytochrome P450. *J Chem Theory Comput.* 2008;4(8):1369-1377.
68. Watanabe Y, Numata T, Iyanagi T, Oae S. Enzymatic oxidation of alkyl sulfides by cytochrome P-450 and hydroxyl radical. *Bull Chem Soc Jpn.* 1981;54(4):1163-1170.
69. Guengerich FP. Drug metabolism: a half-century plus of progress, continued needs, and new opportunities. *Drug Metab Dispos.* 2023;51(1):99-104.
70. Thummel KE, Kharasch ED, Podoll T, Kunze K. Human liver microsomal enflurane defluorination catalyzed by cytochrome P-450 2E1. *Drug Metab Dispos.* 1993;21(2):350-357.
71. Mohn WW. Biodegradation and bioremediation of halogenated organic compounds. In: Singh A, Ward OP, eds. *Biodegradation and Bioremediation.* Springer Berlin Heidelberg; 2004:125-148.
72. Guengerich FP. Common and uncommon cytochrome P450 reactions related to metabolism and chemical toxicity. *Chem Res Toxicol.* 2001;14(6):611-650.
73. Guengerich FP. Cytochrome P450 2E1 and its roles in disease. *Chem Biol Interact.* 2020;322:109056.
74. Kharasch ED, Hankins DC, Thummel KE. Human kidney methoxyflurane and sevoflurane metabolism. Intrarenal fluoride production as a possible mechanism of methoxyflurane nephrotoxicity. *Anesthesiology.* 1995;82(3):689-699.
75. De Hert S, Moerman A. Sevoflurane. *F1000Res.* 2015;4:626.
76. Misal SA, Gawai KR. Azoreductase: a key player of xenobiotic metabolism. *Bioresour Bioprocess.* 2018;5(1):1-9.
77. Zbaida S, Levine WG. Characteristics of two classes of azo dye reductase activity associated with rat liver microsomal cytochrome P450. *Biochem Pharmacol.* 1990;40(11):2415-2423.
78. Ramirez M, Joseph Srinivasan S, Cleary S, Todd P, Reeve H, Vincent K. H2-driven reduction of flavin by hydrogenase enables cleaner operation of nitroreductases for nitro-group to amine reductions. *Front Catal.* 2022;2:906694.
79. Harada N, Omura T. Participation of cytochrome P-450 in the reduction of nitro compounds by rat liver microsomes. *J Biochem.* 1980;87(5):1539-1554.
80. Williams SN, Dunham E, Bradfield CA. Induction of cytochrome P450 enzymes. In: *Cytochrome P450: Structure, Mechanism, And Biochemistry.* 3rd ed. Springer; 2007:323-346.
81. Hakkola J, Hukkanen J, Turpeinen M, Pelkonen O. Inhibition and induction of CYP enzymes in humans: an update. *Arch Toxicol.* 2020;94(11):3671-3722.
82. Manikandan P, Nagini S. Cytochrome P450 structure, function and clinical significance: a review. *Curr Drug Targets.* 2018;19(1):38-54.
83. U.S. Food and Drug Administration. In vitro drug interaction studies—cytochrome P450 enzyme- and transporter-mediated drug interactions guidance for industry. January 2020. Accessed August 2023. https://www.fda.gov/regulatory-information/search-fda-guidance-documents/in-vitro-drug-interaction-studies-cytochrome-p450-enzyme-and-transporter-mediated-drug-interactions
84. Pelkonen O, Turpeinen M, Hakkola J, Honkakoski P, Hukkanen J, Raunio H. Inhibition and induction of human cytochrome P450 enzymes: current status. *Arch Toxicol.* 2008;82(10):667-715.
85. Kroon LA. Drug interactions with smoking. *Am J Health Syst Pharm.* 2007;64(18):1917-1921.
86. Guengerich FP. Inhibition of cytochrome P450 enzymes by drugs-molecular basis and practical applications. *Biomol Ther (Seoul).* 2022;30(1):1-18.
87. Kato H. Computational prediction of cytochrome P450 inhibition and induction. *Drug Metab Pharmacokinet.* 2020;35(1):30-44.
88. Rendić SP, Crouch RD, Guengerich FP. Roles of selected non-P450 human oxidoreductase enzymes in protective and toxic effects of chemicals: review and compilation of reactions. *Arch Toxicol.* 2022;96(8):2145-2246.
89. Phillips IR, Shephard EA. Endogenous roles of mammalian flavin-containing monooxygenases. *Catalysts.* 2019;9(12):1001.
90. Öeren M, Walton PJ, Suri J, Ponting DJ, Hunt PA, Segall MD. Predicting regioselectivity of AO, CYP, FMO, and UGT metabolism using quantum mechanical simulations and machine learning. *J Med Chem.* 2022;65(20):14066-14081.
91. Deng Y, Zhou Q, Wu Y, Chen X, Zhong F. Properties and mechanisms of flavin-dependent monooxygenases and their applications in natural product synthesis. *Int J Mol Sci.* 2022;23(5):2622.
92. Scott F, Gonzalez Malagon SG, O'Brien BA, et al. Identification of flavin-containing monooxygenase 5 (FMO5) as a regulator of glucose homeostasis and a potential sensor of gut bacteria. *Drug Metab Dispos.* 2017;45(9):982-989.
93. Teitelbaum AM, Murphy SE, Akk G, et al. Nicotine dependence is associated with functional variation in FMO3, an enzyme that metabolizes nicotine in the brain. *Pharmacogenomics J.* 2018;18(1):136-143. doi:10.1038/tpj.2016.92
94. Zhou J, Shephard EA. Mutation, polymorphism and perspectives for the future of human flavin-containing monooxygenase 3. *Mutat Res.* 2006;612(3):165-171.
95. Cashman JR, Zhang J. Interindividual differences of human flavin-containing monooxygenase 3: genetic polymorphisms and functional variation. *Drug Metab Dispos.* 2002;30(10):1043-1052.
96. Sirokmány G, Geiszt M. The relationship of NADPH oxidases and heme peroxidases: Fallin' in and out. *Front Immunol.* 2019;10:394.
97. Vlasova, II. Peroxidase activity of human hemoproteins: keeping the fire under control. *Molecules.* 2018;23(10):2561.
98. Arnhold J, Malle E. Halogenation activity of mammalian heme peroxidases. *Antioxidants (Basel).* 2022;11(5):890.
99. Rouzer CA, Marnett LJ. Cyclooxygenases: structural and functional insights. *J Lipid Res.* 2009;50(suppl):S29-S34.
100. Atwal M, Lishman EL, Austin CA, Cowell IG. Myeloperoxidase enhances etoposide and mitoxantrone-mediated DNA damage: a target for myeloprotection in cancer chemotherapy. *Mol Pharmacol.* 2017;91(1):49-57.
101. Di L, Balesano A, Jordan S, Shi SM. The role of alcohol dehydrogenase in drug metabolism: beyond ethanol oxidation. *AAPS J.* 2021;23(1):20.
102. Pang X, Tang C, Guo R, Chen X. Non-cytochrome P450 enzymes involved in the oxidative metabolism of xenobiotics: focus on the regulation of gene expression and enzyme activity. *Pharmacol Ther.* 2022;233:108020.
103. Edenberg HJ, McClintick JN. Alcohol dehydrogenases, aldehyde dehydrogenases, and alcohol use disorders: a critical review. *Alcohol Clin Exp Res.* 2018;42(12):2281-2297.
104. Jiang Y, Zhang T, Kusumanchi P, Han S, Yang Z, Liangpunsakul S. Alcohol metabolizing enzymes, microsomal ethanol oxidizing system, cytochrome P450 2E1, catalase, and aldehyde dehydrogenase in alcohol-associated liver disease. *Biomedicines.* 2020;8(3):50.
105. Lee SL, Shih HT, Chi YC, Li YP, Yin SJ. Oxidation of methanol, ethylene glycol, and isopropanol with human alcohol dehydrogenases and the inhibition by ethanol and 4-methylpyrazole. *Chem Biol Interact.* 2011;191(1-3):26-31.

106. Shortall K, Djeghader A, Magner E, Soulimane T. Insights into aldehyde dehydrogenase enzymes: a structural perspective. *Front Mol Biosci*. 2021;8:659550.
107. Matsumura Y, Stiles KM, Reid J, et al. Gene therapy correction of aldehyde dehydrogenase 2 deficiency. *Mol Ther Methods Clin Dev*. 2019;15:72-82.
108. Kitamura S, Sugihara K, Ohta S. Drug-metabolizing ability of molybdenum hydroxylases. *Drug Metab Pharmacokinet*. 2006;21(2):83-98.
109. Hall WW, Krenitsky TA. Aldehyde oxidase from rabbit liver: specificity toward purines and their analogs. *Arch Biochem Biophys*. 1986;251(1):36-46.
110. Bortolotti M, Polito L, Battelli MG, Bolognesi A. Xanthine oxidoreductase: one enzyme for multiple physiological tasks. *Redox Biol*. 2021;41:101882.
111. Chaurasiya ND, Leon F, Muhammad I, Tekwani BL. Natural products inhibitors of monoamine oxidases—potential new drug leads for neuroprotection, neurological disorders, and neuroblastoma. *Molecules*. 2022;27(13):4297.
112. Singer TP, Ramsay RR. Mechanism of the neurotoxicity of MPTP. An update. *FEBS Lett*. 1990;274(1-2):1-8.
113. Ferrucci M, Fornai F. MPTP neurotoxicity: actions, mechanisms, and animal modeling of Parkinson 's disease. In: Kostrzewa RM, ed. *Handbook of Neurotoxicity*. Springer; 2023:443.
114. Malátková P, Wsól V. Carbonyl reduction pathways in drug metabolism. *Drug Metab Rev*. 2014;46(1):96-123.
115. Barracco V, Moschini R, Renzone G, et al. Dehydrogenase/reductase activity of human carbonyl reductase 1 with NADP(H) acting as a prosthetic group. *Biochem Biophys Res Commun*. 2020;522(1):259-263.
116. Song YQ, Jin Q, Wang DD, Hou J, Zou LW, Ge GB. Carboxylesterase inhibitors from clinically available medicines and their impact on drug metabolism. *Chem Biol Interact*. 2021;345:109566.
117. Jančová P, Šiller M. Phase II drug metabolism. In: Paxton J, ed. *Topics on Drug Metabolism*. InTech; 2012:35-60.
118. Rowland A, Miners JO, Mackenzie PI. The UDP-glucuronosyltransferases: their role in drug metabolism and detoxification. *Int J Biochem Cell Biol*. 2013;45(6):1121-1132.
119. Fujiwara R, Yokoi T, Nakajima M. Structure and protein-protein interactions of human UDP-glucuronosyltransferases. *Front Pharmacol*. 2016;7:388.
120. Coleman MD. *Human Drug Metabolism*. John Wiley & Sons; 2020.
121. Ouzzine M, Gulberti S, Ramalanjaona N, Magdalou J, Fournel-Gigleux S. The UDP-glucuronosyltransferases of the blood-brain barrier: their role in drug metabolism and detoxication. *Front Cell Neurosci*. 2014;8:349.
122. Shahab U, Moinuddin, Ahmad S, et al. Genotoxic effect of N-hydroxy-4-acetylaminobiphenyl on human DNA: implications in bladder cancer. *PLoS One*. 2013;8(1):e53205.
123. Allain EP, Rouleau M, Lévesque E, Guillemette C. Emerging roles for UDP-glucuronosyltransferases in drug resistance and cancer progression. *Br J Cancer*. 2020;122(9):1277-1287.
124. Kurogi K, Rasool MI, Alherz FA, et al. SULT genetic polymorphisms: physiological, pharmacological and clinical implications. *Expert Opin Drug Metab Toxicol*. 2021;17(7):767-784.
125. Isvoran A, Peng Y, Ceauranu S, Schmidt L, Nicot AB, Miteva MA. Pharmacogenetics of human sulfotransferases and impact of amino acid exchange on Phase II drug metabolism. *Drug Discov Today*. 2022;27(11):103349.
126. Gamage N, Barnett A, Hempel N, et al. Human sulfotransferases and their role in chemical metabolism. *Toxicol Sci*. 2006;90(1):5-22.
127. Coughtrie MWH. Function and organization of the human cytosolic sulfotransferase (SULT) family. *Chem Biol Interact*. 2016;259(Pt A):2-7.
128. Darnell M, Weidolf L. Metabolism of xenobiotic carboxylic acids: focus on coenzyme A conjugation, reactivity, and interference with lipid metabolism. *Chem Res Toxicol*. 2013;26(8):1139-1155.
129. Beyoğlu D, Idle JR. The glycine deportation system and its pharmacological consequences. *Pharmacol Ther*. 2012;135(2):151-167.
130. Skonberg C, Olsen J, Madsen KG, Hansen SH, Grillo MP. Metabolic activation of carboxylic acids. *Expert Opin Drug Metab Toxicol*. 2008;4(4):425-438.
131. Sim E, Abuhammad A, Ryan A. Arylamine N-acetyltransferases: from drug metabolism and pharmacogenetics to drug discovery. *Br J Pharmacol*. 2014;171(11):2705-2725.
132. Hernández-González O, Herrera-Vargas DJ, Martínez-Leija ME, Zavala-Reyes D, Portales-Pérez DP. The role of arylamine N-acetyltransferases in chronic degenerative diseases: their possible function in the immune system. *Biochim Biophys Acta Mol Cell Res*. 2022;1869(9):119297.
133. Mitchell SC. N-acetyltransferase: the practical consequences of polymorphic activity in man. *Xenobiotica*. 2020;50(1):77-91.
134. Wang S, Hanna D, Sugamori KS, Grant DM. Primary aromatic amines and cancer: novel mechanistic insights using 4-aminobiphenyl as a model carcinogen. *Pharmacol Ther*. 2019;200:179-189.
135. Vašková J, Kočan L, Vaško L, Perjési P. Glutathione-related enzymes and proteins: a review. *Molecules*. 2023;28(3):1447.
136. Hanna PE, Anders MW. The mercapturic acid pathway. *Crit Rev Toxicol*. 2019;49(10):819-929.
137. Cho SH, Guengerich FP. In vivo roles of conjugation with glutathione and O6-alkylguanine DNA-alkyltransferase in the mutagenicity of the bis-electrophiles 1,2-dibromoethane and 1,2,3,4-diepoxybutane in mice. *Chem Res Toxicol*. 2013;26(11):1765-1774.
138. Dahlin DC, Miwa GT, Lu AY, Nelson SD. N-acetyl-p-benzoquinone imine: a cytochrome P-450-mediated oxidation product of acetaminophen. *Proc Natl Acad Sci U S A*. 1984;81(5):1327-1331.
139. Malik MY, Jaiswal S, Sharma A, Shukla M, Lal J. Role of enterohepatic recirculation in drug disposition: cooperation and complications. *Drug Metab Rev*. 2016;48(2):281-327.
140. Gao Y, Shao J, Jiang Z, et al. Drug enterohepatic circulation and disposition: constituents of systems pharmacokinetics. *Drug Discov Today*. 2014;19(3):326-340.
141. Klaassen CD, Cui JY. Review: mechanisms of how the intestinal microbiota alters the effects of drugs and bile acids. *Drug Metab Dispos*. 2015;43(10):1505-1521.
142. Andres TM, McGrane T, McEvoy MD, Allen BFS. Geriatric pharmacology: an update. *Anesthesiol Clin*. 2019;37(3):475-492.
143. Klotz U. Pharmacokinetics and drug metabolism in the elderly. *Drug Metab Rev*. 2009;41(2):67-76.
144. Drenth-van Maanen AC, Wilting I, Jansen PAF. Prescribing medicines to older people—how to consider the impact of ageing on human organ and body functions. *Br J Clin Pharmacol*. 2020;86(10):1921-1930.
145. Koyanagi T, Nakanishi Y, Murayama N, et al. Age-related changes of hepatic clearances of cytochrome P450 probes, midazolam and R-/S-warfarin in combination with caffeine, omeprazole and metoprolol in cynomolgus monkeys using in vitro-in vivo correlation. *Xenobiotica*. 2015;45(4):312-321.
146. Kazma JM, van den Anker J, Allegaert K, Dallmann A, Ahmadzia HK. Anatomical and physiological alterations of pregnancy. *J Pharmacokinet Pharmacodyn*. 2020;47(4):271-285.
147. Pinheiro EA, Stika CS. Drugs in pregnancy: pharmacologic and physiologic changes that affect clinical care. *Semin Perinatol*. 2020;44(3):151221.
148. Pariente G, Leibson T, Carls A, Adams-Webber T, Ito S, Koren G. Pregnancy-associated changes in pharmacokinetics: a systematic review. *PLoS Med*. 2016;13(11):e1002160.
149. Betcher HK, George AL Jr. Pharmacogenomics in pregnancy. *Semin Perinatol*. 2020;44(3):151222.
150. Kozlosky D, Barrett E, Aleksunes LM. Regulation of placental efflux transporters during pregnancy complications. *Drug Metab Dispos*. 2022;50(10):1364-1375.
151. Johansson I, Ingelman-Sundberg M. Genetic polymorphism and toxicology—with emphasis on cytochrome p450. *Toxicol Sci*. 2011;120(1):1-13.

152. Tomalik-Scharte D, Lazar A, Fuhr U, Kirchheiner J. The clinical role of genetic polymorphisms in drug-metabolizing enzymes. *Pharmacogenomics J*. 2008;8(1):4-15.
153. Pirmohamed M. Pharmacogenomics: current status and future perspectives. *Nat Rev Genet*. 2023;24(6):350-362.
154. Gaedigk A, Sangkuhl K, Whirl-Carrillo M, Klein T, Leeder JS. Prediction of CYP2D6 phenotype from genotype across world populations. *Genet Med*. 2017;19(1):69-76.
155. Zhou Y, Lauschke VM. The genetic landscape of major drug metabolizing cytochrome P450 genes-an updated analysis of population-scale sequencing data. *Pharmacogenomics J*. 2022;22(5-6):284-293.
156. Primorac D, Bach-Rojecky L, Vađunec D, et al. Pharmacogenomics at the center of precision medicine: challenges and perspective in an era of Big Data. *Pharmacogenomics*. 2020;21(2):141-156.
157. Waring RH. Cytochrome P450: genotype to phenotype. *Xenobiotica*. 2020;50(1):9-18.
158. Cao X, Durairaj P, Yang F, Bureik M. A comprehensive overview of common polymorphic variants that cause missense mutations in human CYPs and UGTs. *Biomed Pharmacother*. 2019;111: 983-992.
159. Hu X, Ni J, Gao N, et al. The effect of CYP3A4 genetic polymorphism and drug interaction on the metabolism of istradefylline. *Chem Biol Interact*. 2022;366:110123.
160. Kato K, Nakayoshi T, Nokura R, et al. Deciphering structural alterations associated with activity reductions of genetic polymorphisms in cytochrome P450 2A6 using molecular dynamics simulations. *Int J Mol Sci*. 2021;22(18):10119.
161. Perez-Paramo YX, Lazarus P. Pharmacogenetics factors influencing smoking cessation success; the importance of nicotine metabolism. *Expert Opin Drug Metab Toxicol*. 2021;17(3):333-349.
162. Langmia IM, Just KS, Yamoune S, Brockmöller J, Masimirembwa C, Stingl JC. CYP2B6 functional variability in drug metabolism and exposure across populations-implication for drug safety, dosing, and individualized therapy. *Front Genet*. 2021;12:692234.
163. Di Paolo V, Ferrari FM, Poggesi I, Quintieri L. Quantitative prediction of drug interactions caused by cytochrome P450 2B6 inhibition or induction. *Clin Pharmacokinet*. 2022;61(9):1297-1306.
164. Desta Z, El-Boraie A, Gong L, et al. PharmVar GeneFocus: CYP2B6. *Clin Pharmacol Ther*. 2021;110(1):82-97.
165. Sangkuhl K, Claudio-Campos K, Cavallari LH, et al. PharmVar GeneFocus: CYP2C9. *Clin Pharmacol Ther*. 2021;110(3):662-676.
166. Sukprasong R, Chuwongwattana S, Koomdee N, et al. Allele frequencies of single nucleotide polymorphisms of clinically important drug-metabolizing enzymes CYP2C9, CYP2C19, and CYP3A4 in a Thai population. *Sci Rep*. 2021;11(1):12343.
167. Kathuria A, Roosan MR, Sharma A. CYP2C9 polymorphism and use of oral nonsteroidal anti-inflammatory drugs. *US Pharm*. 2021;54(3):23-30.
168. Wanounou M, Shaul C, Abu Ghosh Z, Alamia S, Caraco Y. The impact of CYP2C9*11 allelic variant on the pharmacokinetics of phenytoin and (S)-warfarin. *Clin Pharmacol Ther*. 2022;112(1):156-163.
169. Tamminga WJ, Wemer J, Oosterhuis B, et al. Mephenytoin as a probe for CYP2C19 phenotyping: effect of sample storage, intra-individual reproducibility and occurrence of adverse events. *Br J Clin Pharmacol*. 2001;51(5):471-474.
170. Sienkiewicz-Oleszkiewicz B, Wiela-Hojeńska A. CYP2C19 polymorphism in relation to the pharmacotherapy optimization of commonly used drugs. *Pharmazie*. 2018;73(11):619-624.
171. Kang P, Cho CK, Jang CG, et al. Effects of CYP2C9 and CYP2C19 genetic polymorphisms on the pharmacokinetics and pharmacodynamics of gliclazide in healthy subjects. *Arch Pharm Res*. 2023;46(5):438-447.
172. Kehinde O, Ramsey LB, Gaedigk A, Oni-Orisan A. Advancing CYP2D6 pharmacogenetics through a pharmacoequity lens. *Clin Pharmacol Ther*. 2023;114(1):69-76.
173. Ingelman-Sundberg M. Genetic polymorphisms of cytochrome P450 2D6 (CYP2D6): clinical consequences, evolutionary aspects and functional diversity. *Pharmacogenomics J*. 2005;5(1):6-13.
174. Alali M, Ismail Al-Khalil W, Rijjal S, Al-Salhi L, Saifo M, Youssef LA. Frequencies of CYP2D6 genetic polymorphisms in Arab populations. *Hum Genomics*. 2022;16(1):6.
175. Neafsey P, Ginsberg G, Hattis D, Johns DO, Guyton KZ, Sonawane B. Genetic polymorphism in CYP2E1: population distribution of CYP2E1 activity. *J Toxicol Environ Health B Crit Rev*. 2009;12(5-6):362-388.
176. Lu J, Shang X, Zhong W, Xu Y, Shi R, Wang X. New insights of CYP1A in endogenous metabolism: a focus on single nucleotide polymorphisms and diseases. *Acta Pharm Sin B*. 2020;10(1):91-104.
177. Herman TF, Santos C. First pass effect. In: *StatPearls*. StatPearls Publishing; 2023.
178. Kato M. Intestinal first-pass metabolism of CYP3A4 substrates. *Drug Metab Pharmacokinet*. 2008;23(2):87-94.
179. Kaminsky LS, Fasco MJ. Small intestinal cytochromes P450. *Crit Rev Toxicol*. 1991;21(6):407-422.
180. Thummel KE. Gut instincts: CYP3A4 and intestinal drug metabolism. *J Clin Invest*. 2007;117(11):3173-3176.
181. Van Matre ET, Satyanarayana G, Page 2nd RL, Levi ME, Lindenfeld J, Mueller SW. Pharmacokinetic drug-drug interactions between immunosuppressant and anti-infective agents: antimetabolites and corticosteroids. *Ann Transplant*. 2018;23:66-74.
182. Grangeon A, Clermont V, Barama A, Gaudette F, Turgeon J, Michaud V. Determination of CYP450 expression levels in the human small intestine by mass spectrometry-based targeted proteomics. *Int J Mol Sci*. 2021;22(23):12791.
183. Miyauchi E, Tachikawa M, Declèves X, et al. Quantitative atlas of cytochrome P450, UDP-glucuronosyltransferase, and transporter proteins in jejunum of morbidly obese subjects. *Mol Pharm*. 2016;13(8):2631-2640.
184. Zhang H, Wolford C, Basit A, et al. Regional proteomic quantification of clinically relevant non-cytochrome P450 enzymes along the human small intestine. *Drug Metab Dispos*. 2020;48(7):528-536.
185. Quigley EMM. Gut bacteria in health and disease. *Gastroenterol Hepatol (N Y)*. 2013;9(9):560-569.
186. Zimmermann M, Zimmermann-Kogadeeva M, Wegmann R, Goodman AL. Mapping human microbiome drug metabolism by gut bacteria and their genes. *Nature*. 2019;570(7762): 462-467.
187. Clarke G, Sandhu KV, Griffin BT, Dinan TG, Cryan JF, Hyland NP. Gut reactions: breaking down xenobiotic–microbiome interactions. *Pharmacol Rev*. 2019;71(2):198-224.
188. Enright EF, Gahan CGM, Joyce SA, Griffin BT. The impact of the gut microbiota on drug metabolism and clinical outcome. *Yale J Biol Med*. 2016;89(3):375-382.
189. Weersma RK, Zhernakova A, Fu J. Interaction between drugs and the gut microbiome. *Gut*. 2020;69(8):1510-1519. doi:10.1136/gutjnl-2019-320204
190. Sun C, Chen L, Shen Z. Mechanisms of gastrointestinal microflora on drug metabolism in clinical practice. *Saudi Pharm J*. 2019;27(8):1146-1156.
191. Lynch SV, Pedersen O. The human intestinal microbiome in health and disease. *N Engl J Med*. 2016;375(24):2369-2379.
192. Enlo-Scott Z, Bäckström E, Mudway I, Forbes B. Drug metabolism in the lungs: opportunities for optimising inhaled medicines. *Expert Opin Drug Metab Toxicol*. 2021;17(5):611-625.
193. Oesch F, Fabian E, Landsiedel R. Xenobiotica-metabolizing enzymes in the lung of experimental animals, man and in human lung models. *Arch Toxicol*. 2019;93:3419-3489.
194. Heydel JM, Faure P, Neiers F. Nasal odorant metabolism: enzymes, activity and function in olfaction. *Drug Metab Rev*. 2019;51(2):224-245.
195. Kornbausch N, Debong MW, Buettner A, Heydel JM, Loos HM. Odorant metabolism in humans. *Angew Chem Int Ed Engl*. 2022;61(35):e202202866.
196. Zhang H, Prisinzano TE, Donovan MD. Permeation and metabolism of cocaine in the nasal mucosa. *Eur J Drug Metab Pharmacokinet*. 2012;37(4):255-262.

197. Toselli F, Dodd PR, Gillam EMJ. Emerging roles for brain drug-metabolizing cytochrome P450 enzymes in neuropsychiatric conditions and responses to drugs. *Drug Metab Rev.* 2016;48(3):379-404.
198. McMillan DM, Tyndale RF. CYP-mediated drug metabolism in the brain impacts drug response. *Pharmacol Ther.* 2018;184:189-200.
199. Miksys S, Tyndale RF. Cytochrome P450-mediated drug metabolism in the brain. *J Psychiatry Neurosci.* 2013;38(3):152-163.
200. Silva-Adaya D, Garza-Lombó C, Gonsebatt ME. Xenobiotic transport and metabolism in the human brain. *Neurotoxicology.* 2021;86:125-138.
201. Kuban W, Daniel WA. Cytochrome P450 expression and regulation in the brain. *Drug Metab Rev.* 2021;53(1):1-29.
202. Song Y, Li C, Liu G, et al. Drug-metabolizing cytochrome P450 enzymes have multifarious influences on treatment outcomes. *Clin Pharmacokinet.* 2021;60(5):585-601.
203. Agrawal S, Khazaeni B. Acetaminophen toxicity. In: *StatPearls.* StatPearls Publishing; 2023.
204. Watkins PB. Role of cytochromes P450 in drug metabolism and hepatotoxicity. *Semin Liver Dis.* 1990;10(4):235-250. doi: 10.1055/s-2008-1040480
205. Andrade RJ, Robles M, Fernández-Castañer A, López-Ortega S, López-Vega MC, Lucena MI. Assessment of drug-induced hepatotoxicity in clinical practice: a challenge for gastroenterologists. *World J Gastroenterol.* 2007;13(3):329-340.
206. Park BK, Kitteringham NR, Maggs JL, Pirmohamed M, Williams DP. The role of metabolic activation in drug-induced hepatotoxicity. *Annu Rev Pharmacol Toxicol.* 2005;45:177-202.
207. Andrade RJ, Chalasani N, Björnsson ES, et al. Drug-induced liver injury. *Nat Rev Dis Primers.* 2019;5(1):58.
208. Navarro VJ, Senior JR. Drug-related hepatotoxicity. *N Engl J Med.* 2006;354(7):731-739.
209. Williams DP, Kitteringham NR, Naisbitt DJ, Pirmohamed M, Smith DA, Park BK. Are chemically reactive metabolites responsible for adverse reactions to drugs? *Curr Drug Metab.* 2002;3(4):351-366.
210. Hussaini SH, Farrington EA. Idiosyncratic drug-induced liver injury: an update on the 2007 overview. *Expert Opin Drug Saf.* 2014;13(1):67-81.
211. Srivastava A, Maggs JL, Antoine DJ, Williams DP, Smith DA, Park BK. Role of reactive metabolites in drug-induced hepatotoxicity. *Handb Exp Pharmacol.* 2010;196:165-194.
212. Uetrecht J. Idiosyncratic drug reactions: past, present, and future. *Chem Res Toxicol.* 2008;21(1):84-92.
213. Uetrecht J. Idiosyncratic drug reactions: a 35-year *Chemical Research in Toxicology* perspective. *Chem Res Toxicol.* 2022;35(10):1649-1654.
214. Hoofnagle JH, Björnsson ES. Drug-induced liver injury—types and phenotypes. *N Engl J Med.* 2019;381(3):264-273.
215. Mosedale M, Watkins PB. Understanding idiosyncratic toxicity: lessons learned from drug-induced liver injury. *J Med Chem.* 2020;63(12):6436-6461.
216. Miller EC, Miller JA. Mechanisms of chemical carcinogenesis. *Cancer.* 1981;47(5 suppl):1055-1064.
217. Park BK, Boobis A, Clarke S, et al. Managing the challenge of chemically reactive metabolites in drug development. *Nat Rev Drug Discov.* 2011;10(4):292-306.
218. Rendic SP, Guengerich FP. Human family 1-4 cytochrome P450 enzymes involved in the metabolic activation of xenobiotic and physiological chemicals: an update. *Arch Toxicol.* 2021;95(2):395-472.
219. Kalgutkar AS, Gardner I, Obach RS, et al. A comprehensive listing of bioactivation pathways of organic functional groups. *Curr Drug Metab.* 2005;6(3):161-225.
220. Walsh JS, Miwa GT. Bioactivation of drugs: risk and drug design. *Annu Rev Pharmacol Toxicol.* 2011;51:145-167.
221. Testa B, Pedretti A, Vistoli G. Reactions and enzymes in the metabolism of drugs and other xenobiotics. *Drug Discov Today.* 2012;17(11-12):549-560.
222. Mitra K. Acyl glucuronide and coenzyme A thioester metabolites of carboxylic acid-containing drug molecules: layering chemistry with reactive metabolism and toxicology. *Chem Res Toxicol.* 2022;35(10):1777-1788.
223. Cooper A, Hanigan M. Metabolism of glutathione S-conjugates: multiple pathways. *Comprehensive Toxicology.* 2018:363-406.
224. Ziglari T, Allameh A. The significance of glutathione conjugation in aflatoxin metabolism. In: Razzaghi-Abyaneh M, ed. *Aflatoxins–Recent Advances and Future Prospects.* InTech; 2013:267-286.
225. Cummins I, Dixon DP, Freitag-Pohl S, Skipsey M, Edwards R. Multiple roles for plant glutathione transferases in xenobiotic detoxification. *Drug Metab Rev.* 2011;43(2):266-80.
226. Jee A, Sernoskie SC, Uetrecht J. Idiosyncratic drug-induced liver injury: mechanistic and clinical challenges. *Int J Mol Sci.* 2021;22(6):2954.
227. Loeb LA, Harris CC. Advances in chemical carcinogenesis: a historical review and prospective. *Cancer Res.* 2008;68(17):6863-6872.
228. Cohen SM, Arnold LL. Chemical carcinogenesis. *Toxicol Sci.* 2011;120(suppl_1):S76-S92.
229. Reed L, Arlt VM, Phillips DH. The role of cytochrome P450 enzymes in carcinogen activation and detoxication: an in vivo–in vitro paradox. *Carcinogenesis.* 2018;39(7):851-859.
230. Guengerich FP. A history of the roles of cytochrome P450 enzymes in the toxicity of drugs. *Toxicol Res.* 2021;37(1):1-23.
231. Penning TM. *Chemical Carcinogenesis.* Springer Science & Business Media; 2011.
232. Budnitz DS, Shehab N, Lovegrove MC, Geller AI, Lind JN, Pollock DA. US Emergency Department visits attributed to medication harms, 2017-2019. *JAMA.* 2021;326(13):1299-1309.
233. Merel SE, Paauw DS. Common drug side effects and drug-drug interactions in elderly adults in primary care. *J Am Geriatr Soc.* 2017;65(7):1578-1585.
234. Clarke SE, Jones BC. Human cytochromes P450 and their role in metabolism-based drug-drug interactions. In: David Rodrigues A, ed. *Drug-Drug Interactions.* CRC Press; 2019:53-85.
235. Jang HY, Song J, Kim JH, et al. Machine learning-based quantitative prediction of drug exposure in drug-drug interactions using drug label information. *NPJ Digit Med.* 2022;5(1):88.
236. Ryu JY, Kim HU, Lee SY. Deep learning improves prediction of drug-drug and drug-food interactions. *Proc Natl Acad Sci U S A.* 2018;115(18):E4304-E4311.
237. Chen S, Li T, Yang L, et al. Artificial intelligence-driven prediction of multiple drug interactions. *Brief Bioinform.* 2022;23(6):bbac427.
238. Pal D, Mitra AK. MDR-and CYP3A4-mediated drug–drug interactions. *J Neuroimmune Pharmacol.* 2006;1:323-339.
239. Deodhar M, Al Rihani SB, Arwood MJ, et al. Mechanisms of CYP450 inhibition: understanding drug-drug interactions due to mechanism-based inhibition in clinical practice. *Pharmaceutics.* 2020;12(9):846.
240. Zhou S, Chan E, Li X, Huang M. Clinical outcomes and management of mechanism-based inhibition of cytochrome P450 3A4. *Ther Clin Risk Manag.* 2005;1(1):3-13.
241. Davis JA, Greene RJ, Han S, Rock DA, Wienkers LC. Formation of raloxifene homo-dimer in CYP3A4, evidence for multi-substrate binding in a single catalytically competent P450 active site. *Arch Biochem Biophys.* 2011;513(2):110-118.
242. Won CS, Oberlies NH, Paine MF. Influence of dietary substances on intestinal drug metabolism and transport. *Curr Drug Metab.* 2010;11(9):778-792.
243. Bailey DG, Dresser GK, Kreeft JH, Munoz C, Freeman DJ, Bend JR. Grapefruit-felodipine interaction: effect of unprocessed fruit and probable active ingredients. *Clin Pharmacol Ther.* 2000;68(5):468-477.
244. Petric Z, Žuntar I, Putnik P, Bursać Kovačević D. Food-drug interactions with fruit juices. *Foods.* 2020;10(1):33.
245. Asher GN, Corbett AH, Hawke RL. Common herbal dietary supplement-drug interactions. *Am Fam Physician.* 2017;96(2):101-107.

246. Loretz C, Ho MD, Alam N, Mitchell W, Li AP. Application of cryopreserved human intestinal mucosa and cryopreserved human enterocytes in the evaluation of herb-drug interactions: evaluation of CYP3A inhibitory potential of grapefruit juice and commercial formulations of twenty-nine herbal supplements. *Drug Metab Dispos*. 2020;48(10):1084-1091.
247. Ronis MJJ, Pedersen KB, Watt J. Adverse effects of nutraceuticals and dietary supplements. *Annu Rev Pharmacol Toxicol*. 2018;58:583-601.
248. Nicolussi S, Drewe J, Butterweck V, Meyer Zu Schwabedissen HE. Clinical relevance of St. John's wort drug interactions revisited. *Br J Pharmacol*. 2020;177(6):1212-1226.
249. Mauvais-Jarvis F, Berthold HK, Campesi I, et al. Sex- and gender-based pharmacological response to drugs. *Pharmacol Rev*. 2021;73(2):730-762.
250. Franconi F, Campesi I. Pharmacogenomics, pharmacokinetics and pharmacodynamics: interaction with biological differences between men and women. *Br J Pharmacol*. 2014;171(3):580-594.
251. Zucker I, Prendergast BJ. Sex differences in pharmacokinetics predict adverse drug reactions in women. *Biol Sex Differ*. 2020;11(1):32.
252. Elahi M, Eshera N, Bambata N, et al. The Food and Drug Administration Office of Women's Health: impact of science on regulatory policy: an update. *J Womens Health (Larchmt)*. 2016;25(3):222-234.

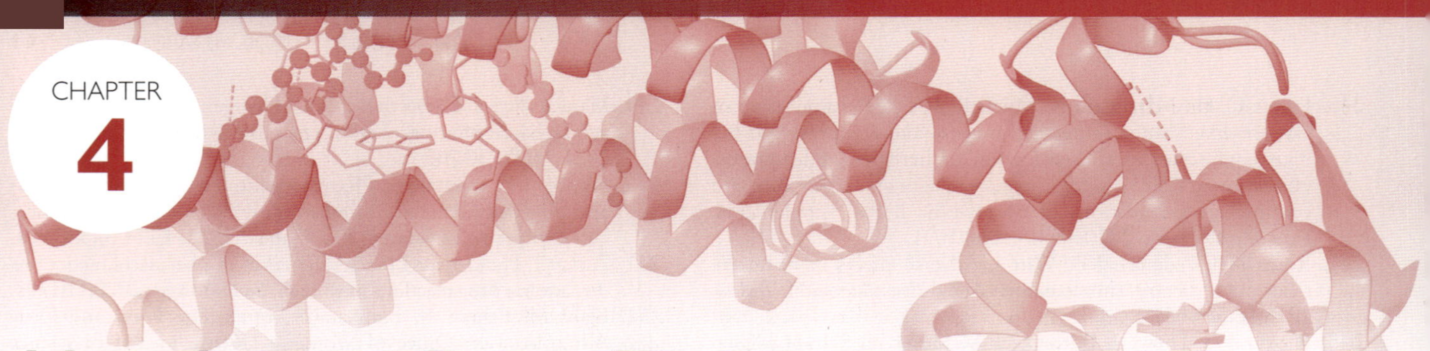

CHAPTER 4

Membrane Drug Transporters

Marilyn E. Morris and Bridget L. Morse

Abbreviations

ABC ATP-binding cassette
ACE angiotensin-converting enzyme
ASBT sodium-dependent bile acid transporter
ATP adenosine triphosphate
AUC area under the curve
BBB blood-brain barrier
BCRP breast cancer–resistance protein
BSEP bile salt export pump
CNT concentrative-nucleoside transporter
CPI coproporphyrin 1
CSF cerebrospinal fluid
ENT equilibrative-nucleoside transporter
FR fraction of unchanged drug
FXR farnesoid X receptor
GHB γ-hydroxybutyrate
HMG-CoA 3-hydroxy-3-methyl-glutaryl-coenzyme A
LAT L-type amino acid transporter
MATE multidrug and toxin extrusion protein
MCT monocarboxylate transporter
MDR multidrug resistance
MRP multidrug resistance–associated protein
NMN N1-methylnicotinamide
NTCP sodium-taurocholate cotransporting polypeptide
OAT organic-anion transporter
OATP organic anion–transporting polypeptide
OCT organic cation transporter
OCTN organic cation/carnitine transporter
OSTα/β organic solute transporter alpha/beta
P-gp P-glycoprotein
RNA ribonucleic acid
PEPT peptide transporter
PHT peptide/histidine transporter
PXR pregnane X receptor
SLC solute carrier
SMCT sodium-coupled monocarboxylate transporter
SNP single-nucleotide polymorphism

Introduction

Transporters have fundamental roles in cell homeostasis and physiologic function by facilitating the movement of molecules across biologic membranes. Transporters are responsible for maintaining ionic and osmotic gradients necessary for normal cell activity. Transporters facilitate the oxygen binding and release in red blood cells, and they are necessary for the transport of nutrients to vital organs. The primary function of transporters is to transport endogenous substances, such as hormones, glucose, and amino acids; however, many of these transporters also transport xenobiotics. It is these drug transporters that are of importance when considering drug disposition and drug response.

Drug transporters are localized to barrier membranes of the body responsible for xenobiotic entry and exit. They are expressed in organs of absorption, such as the intestine, and in clearance organs, including the liver and kidney. Transporters are also expressed on membranes that separate particularly susceptible organs from the rest of the body, including the blood-brain and blood-placenta barriers, where they facilitate the influx of nutrients and efflux of potentially harmful xenobiotics. Because of their location on barrier membranes, transporters have an important role in drug pharmacokinetics and pharmacodynamics. Transporters can have a role in drug absorption and can facilitate or prevent drug entry into the body. Transporters also have a role in drug distribution, as they facilitate the movement of drugs between the blood and peripheral tissues. The role of transporters in drug distribution can also affect drug response by allowing or preventing drug access to the site of action. One of the most interesting roles of drug transporters is their indirect effects on drug metabolism. Transporters can restrict or allow a drug's distribution into organs that contain drug-metabolizing enzymes, particularly the liver and the intestine. In this regard, there can be extensive transport-metabolism interplay, and transport or metabolism can be the rate-limiting process controlling drug elimination. Transporters are also responsible for transport and removal of drug metabolites. Finally, transporters have a significant role in drug excretion, as they are present in the kidney and on the canalicular membrane of the liver, where they can facilitate drug elimination into the urine or bile, respectively.

Because transporters can have a significant effect on drug absorption, distribution, and clearance, changes in the function of these transporters can significantly alter drug pharmacokinetics and pharmacodynamics. Factors leading to changes in transporter function include interactions with other drugs, disease states, and genetic variability in expression. Understanding transporter effects and the effects of changes in transporter function is important for effective therapeutic use of drugs that interact with transporters.

Note that throughout this chapter, the Human Genome Organisation–approved designations for transporter genes and proteins are used, with human genes and proteins designated by all capitals, and nonhuman genes and proteins with the first letter being a capital letter, followed by lower-case letters. Gene names are designated in italics.

Mechanisms of Membrane Transport

Membrane transport is essential for almost every drug to be therapeutically effective. This can be achieved by different mechanisms of transport (Fig. 4.1). Passive diffusion is the simplest way for a drug to pass through a membrane and depends only on the existence of a concentration gradient for a molecule across the membrane. Because of the lipophilicity of biologic membranes, diffusion is energetically unfavorable for drugs that are relatively hydrophilic, particularly for drugs that are predominantly ionized at physiologic pH, and these molecules require facilitated transport. Facilitated transport refers to any transport aided by a facilitating protein. Similar to diffusion, passive facilitated transport depends only on the existence of a concentration gradient and involves movement of molecules down this gradient. Active transport uses a separate energy source to move molecules against their concentration gradient. Drug transporters can use either passive or active transport mechanisms. Paracellular transport (transfer of substances between cells of an epithelial cell layer) and transcytosis (vesicular transfer of substances across the interior of a cell) are less commonly used mechanisms of membrane transport. Mannitol can pass through membranes via paracellular transport and can be used as a probe for this type of transport. Transcytosis is often receptor mediated and is a mechanism of transport for endogenous substances such as insulin and transferrin.

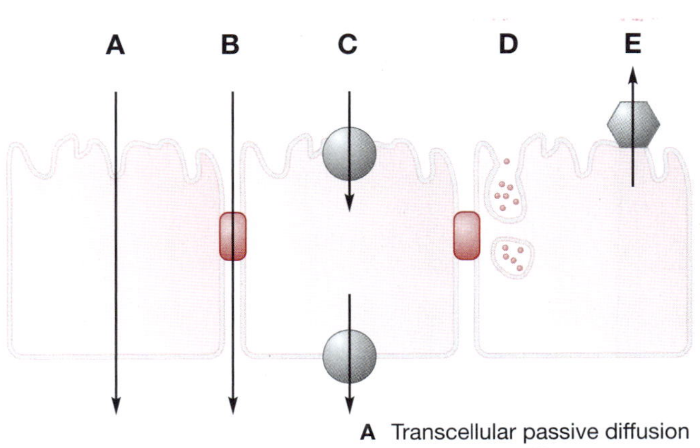

Figure 4.1 Mechanisms of membrane transport. Transport mechanisms most commonly affecting therapeutic agents include passive diffusion, facilitated transport, and active efflux.

Molecules can use one or more of these mechanisms to cross biologic membranes. Transporter processes are saturable, and substrates are often lipophilic and capable of passive diffusion; therefore, drug transport can often be described with the following equation:

$$J = \frac{V_{max} \times C}{K_m + C} + P \times C$$

where J is the rate of total drug transport, V_{max} is the maximum rate of the saturable transporter system, K_m reflects the affinity of a drug substrate for the transporter system, P is the rate of nonsaturable transport or passive diffusion, and C is the drug concentration. The importance of a transporter depends on to what extent transporter-mediated transport (V_{max}/K_m) is responsible for membrane passage of a drug compared to other mechanisms like passive diffusion (P). Transporter-mediated transport becomes particularly important when the need is present to move a molecule against its concentration gradient, as this type of transport can only be achieved by active transporters.

When considering drug transport, it is important to consider the polarization of biologic membranes, in that different membranes can have different properties relating to their function as a barrier, including the expression of different transporters. The membrane facing the systemic circulation is referred to as the basolateral membrane, or the sinusoidal membrane in the liver. The membrane facing the exterior, such as the gut lumen, is referred to as the apical membrane. The apical membrane is also called the brush border membrane in the kidney or intestine and the canalicular membrane in the liver. Transport across membranes is a two-step process in which molecules must be transported across the apical then basolateral membrane or vice versa. Drug transport is a concerted action between transporters expressed on both membranes.

Classification of Transporters

Facilitative Versus Active Transporters

Although all transporters are facilitating proteins, the terms facilitative and active transporters refer to transporters that transport substrates down their concentration gradients and against their concentration gradients, respectively. Transporters that are classified as facilitative transporters only move molecules down their concentration gradient, without the use of a separate energy source. The transporters of this type should not be confused with channels. Channels also facilitate the movement of ions and hydrophilic molecules across membranes and down their concentration gradient; however, channels control transport or flow of substrates by gating mechanisms, whereas transporters bind to their substrates and undergo a conformational change to transport the substrate across a membrane.

Primary Versus Secondary Active Transporters

Most drug transporters are active transporters that use an energy source other than the drug's concentration gradient to transport substrates across membranes from a region of lower concentration to a region of higher concentration (ie, against its concentration gradient). Active transporters are further classified as primary or secondary active transporters. Primary active transporters most commonly use adenosine triphosphate (ATP) as an energy source for substrate transport. Secondary active transporters use the concentration gradient of another substance, such as protons or sodium ions, but also other ionic endogenous substances, as energy sources to drive transport. The concentration gradients that drive secondary active transport are generally created by primary active transporters; an example of interplay between the two types of transporters is depicted in Figure 4.2. As shown, primary active transport by the Na^+/K^+-ATPase results in a concentration gradient of Na^+ ions. This concentration gradient drives secondary active transport by the Na^+/H^+ exchanger, and the resulting proton gradient drives transport of the drug substrate against its concentration gradient. The Na^+/K^+-ATPase and Na^+/H^+ exchanger do not transport drug substrate but are involved in drug transport by producing the sodium and proton gradients used as driving forces. Molecules used to drive secondary active transport are also substrates for the secondary active transporter and are simultaneously transported across the membrane. This simultaneous transport may be in the same direction, referred to as *symport*, or in opposite directions, referred to as *antiport*.

Influx Versus Efflux Transporters

Influx transporters transport substrates from extracellular spaces into cells and are also referred to as uptake transporters. Efflux transporters transport substrates out of cells. Transporters are usually responsible for either drug influx or drug efflux, but, in some cases, facilitate both types of transport, depending on the direction of the driving force.

ATP-Binding Cassette Versus Solute-Carrier Transporters

Drug transporters have been classified into two families, namely the ABC (ATP-binding cassette) and SLC (solute carrier) families. Members of the ABC family are primary active transporters that use ATP as an energy source. Most

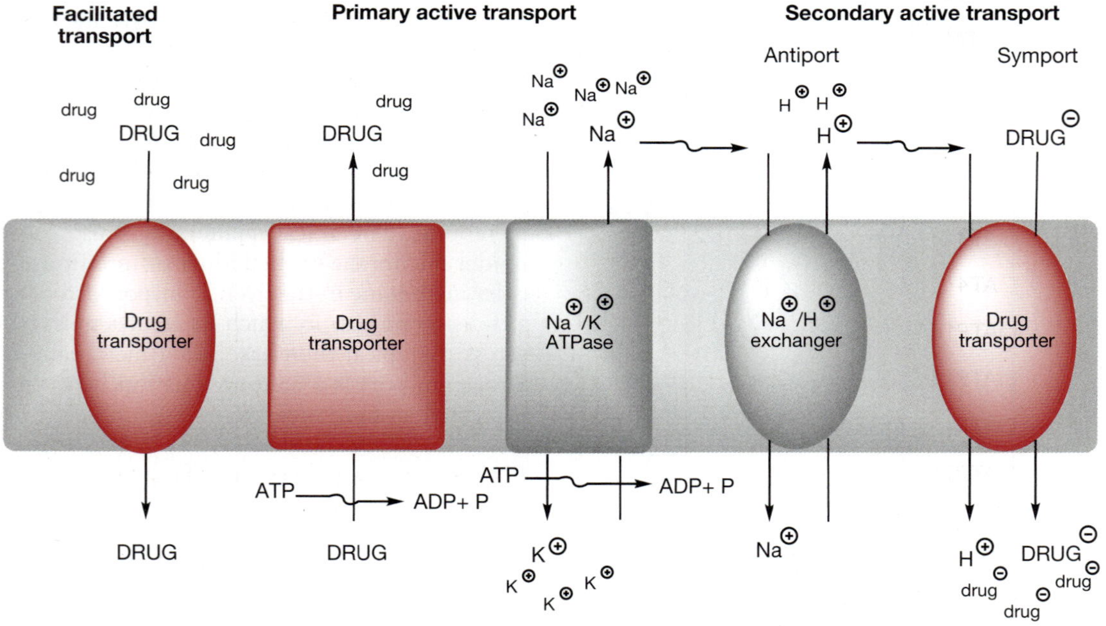

Figure 4.2 Types of drug transporters. Primary active transporters use adenosine triphosphate (ATP) and have the ability to transport substrates against their concentration gradient. Secondary active transporters use gradients created by primary active transport to transport drug substrates. Facilitated transporters only transport substrates down their concentration gradient. Transporters that transport drug substrates are shown in *red*, whereas those shown in *gray* provide driving forces for drug transport.

SLC transporters are secondary active transporters, using the concentration gradients of several different molecules as a driving force for transport. The SLC family also includes a handful of facilitative transporters. Many members of each family have a role in drug disposition, and these transporters are summarized in Table 4.1.

ATP-Binding Cassette Transporters

ABC transporters are efflux transporters, many of which are located on the apical side of biologic membranes, facilitating drug secretion. ABC transporters are primary active transporters and use ATP as an energy source. The widespread physiologic expression of ABC transporters

Table 4.1 Drug Transporters

Transporter Family	Family Member	Gene Name	Location	Role in Drug Disposition
MDR	MDR1	*ABCB1*	Intestine, liver, kidneys, brain, heart, placenta	Role in oral absorption, biliary clearance, renal secretion, and drug penetration of blood-brain barrier Role in multidrug resistance
MRP	MRP1	*ABCC1*	Intestine, brain	Role in multidrug resistance Facilitates basolateral membrane drug efflux
	MRP2	*ABCC2*	Intestine, liver, kidney	Role in oral absorption, biliary clearance, and renal secretion of drugs and drug conjugates
	MRP3	*ABCC3*	Liver, intestine, brain	Facilitates sinusoidal membrane efflux of bile acids, drugs and drug conjugates
	MRP4	*ABCC4*	Kidney, liver, brain	Facilitates renal secretion and sinusoidal membrane efflux of bile acids, drugs, and drug conjugates
BCRP	BCRP1	*ABCG2*	Intestine, liver, brain, heart, placenta	Role in oral absorption, biliary secretion, and drug penetration of blood-brain barrier Role in multidrug resistance
OCT	OCT1	*SLC22A1*	Liver	Facilitates sinusoidal membrane uptake
	OCT2	*SLC22A2*	Kidney	Facilitates renal secretion
OCTN	OCTN1	*SLC22A4*	Kidney, intestine	Role in oral absorption and renal reabsorption
	OCTN2	*SLC22A5*	Kidney, intestine, liver, brain, muscle, lung	Role in oral absorption and renal reabsorption
OAT	OAT1	*SLC22A6*	Kidney	Facilitates renal secretion
	OAT2	*SLC22A7*	Liver	Facilitates sinusoidal membrane uptake and renal secretion
	OAT3	*SLC22A8*	Kidney	Facilitates renal secretion
	OAT4	*SLC22A11*	Kidney	Facilitates renal reabsorption
OATP	OATP1A2	*SLCO1A2*	Brain	Role in brain uptake
	OATP1B1	*SLCO1B1*	Liver	Facilitates sinusoidal membrane uptake
	OATP1B3	*SLCO1B3*	Liver	Facilitates sinusoidal membrane uptake
	OATP2A1	*SLCO2A1*	Intestine, liver	Role in oral absorption and sinusoidal membrane uptake
	OATP2B1	*SLCO2B1*	Kidney	Facilitates renal secretion
	OATP4C1	*SLCO4C1*	Kidney, liver	Role in renal and biliary secretion
MATE	MATE1	*SLC47A1*	Kidney	Facilitates renal secretion
	MATE2-K	*SLC47A2*	Kidney	Facilitates renal secretion

(*continued*)

Table 4.1 Drug Transporters (*continued*)

Transporter Family	Family Member	Gene Name	Location	Role in Drug Disposition
MCT	MCT1	*SLC16A7*	Ubiquitous	Facilitates oral absorption
PEPT	PEPT1	*SLC15A1*	Kidney	Facilitates renal reabsorption
	PEPT2	*SLC15A2*	Intestine, kidney, liver	Role in absorption and disposition of nucleoside analogues
CNT	CNT1	*SLC28A1*	Intestine, kidney, liver	Role in absorption and disposition of nucleoside analogues
	CNT2	*SLC28A2*	Kidney, brain, placenta	Role in distribution and renal reabsorption of nucleoside analogues
	CNT3	*SLC28A3*	Ubiquitous	Role in absorption and disposition of nucleoside analogues
ENT	ENT1	*SLC29A1*	Ubiquitous	Role in absorption and disposition of nucleoside analogues
	ENT2	*SLC29A2*	Liver	Role in biliary secretion of bile acids
Bile acid	BSEP	*ABCB11*	Liver	Sinusoidal membrane uptake of bile acids
	NTCP	*SLC10A1*	Liver, Intestine	Basolateral/sinusoidal membrane efflux of bile acids
	OSTα/β	*OSTA/B*	Intestine	Role in absorption of bile acids
	ASBT	*SLC10A2*	Intestine, liver, kidneys, brain, heart, placenta	Role in oral absorption, biliary clearance, renal secretion, and drug penetration of blood-brain barrier Role in multidrug resistance

and their extensive range of substrates make it inevitable for these transporters to have effects on drug pharmacokinetics and elicit clinically significant drug interactions. Substrates and inhibitors for ABC transporters are given in Table 4.2.

Multidrug-Resistance Proteins (*ABCB*)

MDR1 (ABCB1). Multidrug-resistance protein-1 (MDR1), more commonly known as P-glycoprotein (P-gp), is the most extensively characterized of all drug transporters. The structure of P-gp consists of two homologous halves, each with

Table 4.2 Relevant Drug Substrates and Inhibitors of Adenosine Triphosphate–Binding Cassette Transporters

Transporter	Substrates	Inhibitors
MDR1	Atorvastatin, cyclosporine, dabigatran etexilate, daunorubicin, digoxin, diltiazem, docetaxel, doxorubicin, erythromycin, etoposide, fexofenadine, loperamide, methadone, morphine, paclitaxel, quinidine, simvastatin, tacrolimus, talinolol, verapamil, vinblastine, vincristine	Clarithromycin, cyclosporine, elacridar, quinidine, verapamil
MRP2	Ampicillin, ceftriaxone, daunomycin, doxorubicin, etoposide, fluorouracil, glucuronide conjugates, glutathione conjugates, irinotecan, methotrexate, mitoxantrone, olmesartan, pravastatin, rosuvastatin, SN-38-glucuronide	Cyclosporine, probenecid, efavirenz, emtricitabine
MRP3	Bile acids, fexofenadine, glucuronide conjugates, methotrexate, rosuvastatin	Efavirenz, emtricitabine
MRP4	Adefovir, furosemide, methotrexate, rosuvastatin, tenofovir, topotecan	Diclofenac
BCRP	Atorvastatin, ciprofloxacin, imatinib, irinotecan, methotrexate, mitoxantrone, nitrofurantoin, rosuvastatin, sulfasalazine, sorafenib, topotecan	Elacridar

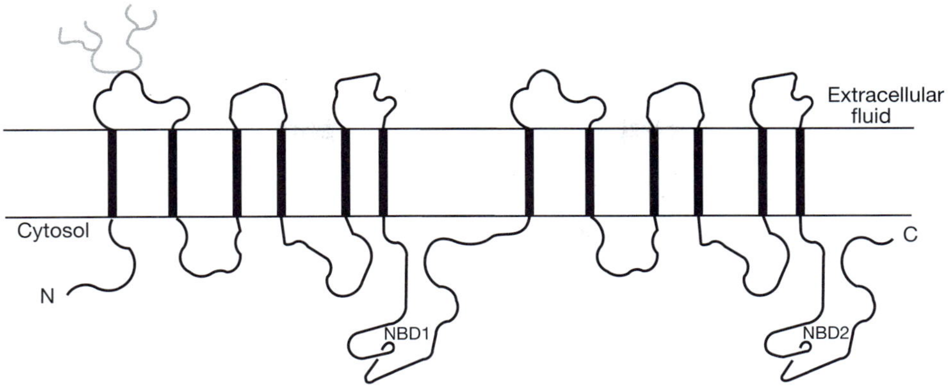

Figure 4.3 Structure of P-glycoprotein including 12 transmembrane-spanning domains and two nucleotide-binding domains (NBDs).

six transmembrane-spanning domains and one ATP-binding site (Fig. 4.3). Transport by P-gp is notably complicated, with at least two binding sites and three different proposed mechanisms by which it transports substrates.[1,2]

P-gp is expressed in most tissues and has involvement in drug transport in the intestine, liver, kidney, brain, and placenta as well as in tumor cells. This ubiquitous expression is one reason P-gp remains a transporter of clinical interest. The ability of P-gp to transport a wide range of substrates is another remarkable feature, and its substrates span many therapeutic areas and drug classes. Much progress on the structure-activity relationship for P-gp–mediated transport has been made in recent years.[3] Digoxin serves as a probe for P-gp in both in vitro and in vivo studies.[4] Other substrates include many chemotherapeutic drugs, other cardiovascular agents, and HIV protease inhibitors. One common feature of P-gp substrates is that they are generally lipophilic (Fig. 4.4). The relative lipophilicity of these substrates implies that most P-gp substrates may also have high rates of passive diffusion. This means that P-gp transport must be efficient to have an effect on the passage of its substrates across membranes, and P-gp-mediated transport does not always result in clinically relevant effects on drug disposition or drug interactions. P-gp substrates are rarely specific and are also often substrates of other transporters and drug-metabolizing enzymes, particularly CYP3A4 and BCRP, making it difficult to attribute in vivo pharmacokinetic effects or interactions entirely to P-gp alone. Mouse models of P-gp knockout indicate that intestinal efflux by P-gp contributes to the low bioavailability of many compounds.[5] Accordingly, significant drug-drug interactions have also been demonstrated involving P-gp in humans at the intestine, as well as in the kidneys.[6,7] P-gp is also likely important in pregnancy in that it protects the fetus from xenobiotics by effluxing them back into the maternal blood circulation.[8] In addition, as the original name "multidrug-resistance protein" implies, P-gp is also recognized as a potential factor for chemotherapeutic drug resistance due to its overexpression in tumor cells; while clinical studies evaluating P-gp inhibition to overcome resistance have had varying results, this continues to be considered as potential concurrent treatment with chemotherapy.[9] Similarly, while single-nucleotide polymorphisms (SNPs) in the *MDR1* gene have been identified, the impact of these on drug disposition remains controversial.[10]

TRANSPORTER-DRUG INTERACTIONS: P-GP AND DIGOXIN

Digoxin undergoes little metabolism in humans, and transport by P-gp is the primary determinant of digoxin pharmacokinetics. One of the first drug interactions noted with digoxin was that with cyclosporine, leading to decreased digoxin clearance and digoxin-associated arrhythmias.[11] It was later discovered that cyclosporine and other therapeutic agents decrease digoxin clearance due to inhibition of P-gp–mediated renal secretion.[12] Nonrenal clearance of digoxin is minimal; however, P-gp inhibitors have similarly been demonstrated to decrease digoxin biliary excretion.[13] P-gp function also affects digoxin absorption, and concomitant oral administration of clarithromycin was demonstrated to increase digoxin bioavailability along with decreasing digoxin renal clearance.[6] Because in vivo P-gp inhibition can affect both absorption and clearance, there exists substantial risk of elevated digoxin plasma concentrations and digoxin-associated toxicity with concomitant inhibitor administration.

P-gp induction can also affect digoxin pharmacokinetics. In a study of human volunteers, chronic rifampin administration resulted in a 3.5-fold increase in duodenal P-gp expression, leading to a decrease in digoxin bioavailability.[14] P-gp expression correlated well with digoxin area under the curve (AUC) in this study, emphasizing the significance of intestinal P-gp on digoxin.

Multidrug Resistance–Associated Proteins (*ABCC*)

MRP2 (*ABCC2*). Multidrug resistance–associated protein 2 (MRP2) is primarily localized to three apical membrane barriers, the liver canalicular membrane, the brush border membrane in the kidney, and the apical membrane of the gut, where it serves to excrete substrates into the bile, urine, and back into the gut lumen, respectively. The major substrates of MRP2 are conjugates, including glucuronide, glutathione, and sulfate conjugates, and the primary endogenous function of MRP2 is the secretion of bilirubin and bile acid conjugates across the canalicular membrane into the bile. MRP2 substrates also include phase 2 drug metabolites and many unconjugated therapeutic drugs, including vinca alkaloids. Glutathione symport is often required for

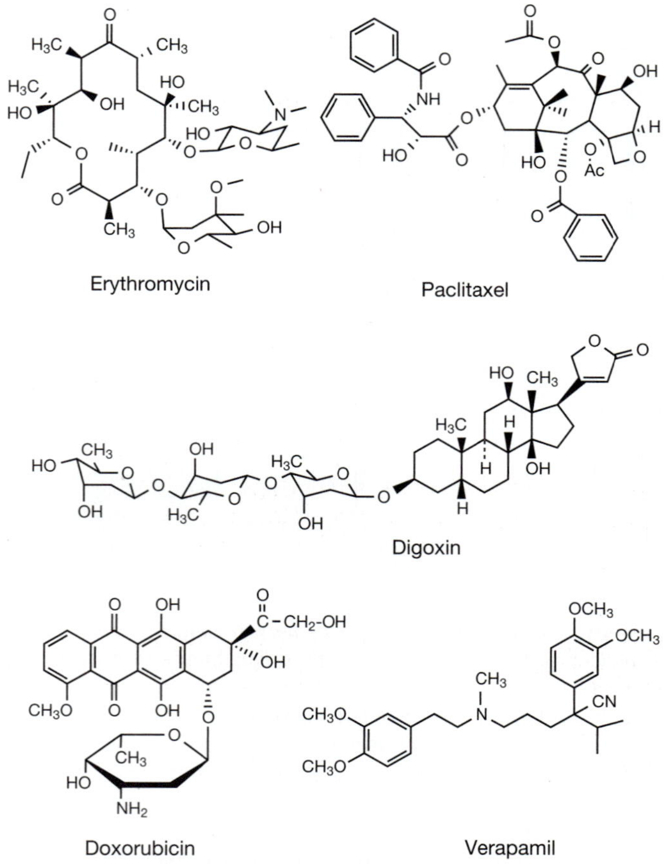

Figure 4.4 Examples of P-gp substrates/inhibitors.

transport of unconjugated substances.[15] MRP2 can contribute to the renal secretion of some drug substrates; however, the main role of MRP2 in drug disposition appears to be hepatobiliary transport.[1,16] Due to transport of drug conjugates, MRP2 has an important role in enterohepatic cycling. MRP2 transports conjugates into the bile, which empties into the gut lumen. Bacteria in the gut metabolize the conjugate back to the parent drug, which can then be reabsorbed back into the systemic blood circulation. In this way, MRP2 can be responsible for maintaining plasma concentrations of drugs that are not substrates, due to transport of their conjugated metabolites. P-gp is also expressed on the canalicular membrane, although it does not appear to play a primary role in biliary secretion of drug conjugates. Because of overlapping specificity of MRP2 substrates and inhibitors with P-gp, as well as overlapping tissue expression of these transporters, it can sometimes be difficult to attribute in vivo pharmacokinetic effects to MRP2 alone. SNPs in MRP2 have been identified, leading to a condition called Dubin-Johnson Syndrome. While not leading to severe pathology, subjects with this condition display increased plasma levels of endogenous MRP2 substrates such as conjugated bilirubin.[17]

Other Multidrug Resistance–Associated Proteins. In contrast to the apical expression of MRP2, MRPs 1, 3, 4, 5, and 6 are basolateral membrane efflux transporters. MRP1 is another ABC transporter that can be overexpressed in cancer cells, resulting in resistance to chemotherapy.[15] MRP3 has an important role in the transport of conjugated drug metabolites in the liver, particularly glucuronide conjugates. Located on the sinusoidal membrane, MRP3 serves to efflux metabolites out of hepatocytes into the plasma, resulting in conjugate excretion into the urine. Although the bile acid transporters discussed later play a primary adaptive role to cholestasis, MRP3 also transports conjugated bile acids and can be induced in cholestatic conditions.[18] MRP3 protein has also been detected in the intestine.[19] MRP4 is expressed on the brush border membrane of the kidney and has a role in anionic drug secretion into the urine.[16] Similar to MRP3, it has a postulated compensatory role in effluxing substrates from the liver during cholestasis or other forms of liver injury.[20] MRP4 and MRP5 also transport cGMP and cAMP and therefore play a role in maintaining the intracellular concentrations of these molecules.[21]

Breast Cancer–Resistance Protein

BCRP (*ABCG2*). Breast cancer–resistance protein (BCRP) is actually a "half" transporter, in that it consists of only six transmembrane-spanning domains and one ATP-binding site (Fig. 4.5). Like P-gp, BCRP expression is widespread. Its highest expression is in the placenta, and it is present in the intestine, liver, kidney, brain, heart, testes, and ovaries.[22] Also, similar to P-gp, multiple binding sites have also been proposed for BCRP. As its name implies, BCRP has also been attributed with causing chemotherapeutic drug resistance due to overexpression in tumor cells, and among its substrates are several chemotherapeutic agents. BCRP shares many substrates with P-gp and is commonly localized with P-gp, making it difficult to attribute drug transport or inhibition to BCRP. However, the use of BCRP inhibitors, Bcrp knockout animals, and identification of SNPs in the *ABCG2* gene have demonstrated the importance of BCRP in drug disposition (see "Transporter Polymorphisms: Role in Statin Disposition" section). Significant effects of BCRP transport have been demonstrated on drug absorption, biliary clearance, and interestingly on drug transport in the mammary gland, mediating the transport of some drugs into breast milk.[23-25] BCRP has a role similar to that of P-gp in pregnancy, as it is highly expressed at the blood-placenta barrier, where it also serves a protective function to efflux potentially harmful xenobiotics.[8] Likewise, given their co-localization and shared substrate specificity,

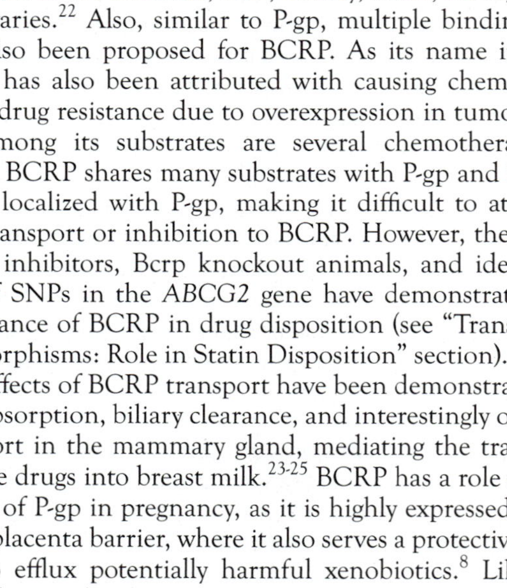

Figure 4.5 Structure of breast cancer–resistance protein (BCRP). BCRP is regarded as a half transporter due to its structure, including only six transmembrane-spanning domains and one nucleotide-binding domain (NBD).

synergism between P-gp and BCRP has been demonstrated at other particularly vulnerable physiologic barriers, such as that in the brain and testes in P-gp/Bcrp knockout animal models.[26]

Solute-Carrier Transporters

Members of the SLC transporter family are secondary active transporters and, as such, use the concentration gradients of many other substances to transport drug substrates. The concentration gradients of these other substances generally facilitate drug uptake, although in some physiologic locations, they can facilitate efflux, and some transporters can be capable of transport in both directions. Like the ABC transporters, SLC transporters are physiologically expressed throughout the body. They transport many different xenobiotics along with many endogenous substances, leading to effects on drug disposition and drug interactions. Substrates and inhibitors of SLC transporters are given in Table 4.3.

Organic Anion–Transporting Polypeptides (*SLCO*)

OATP1B1 (*SLCO1B1*). This transporter is one of the most clinically relevant transporters in that its substrates include drugs such as the 3-hydroxy-3-methyl-glutaryl-coenzyme A (HMG-CoA) reductase inhibitors, or statins, which are widely prescribed. This transporter is localized specifically on the sinusoidal membrane of the liver, where it serves to uptake substrates into hepatocytes, following which they can be metabolized or transported into bile. The driving force of organic anion transporter polypeptide (OATP) 1B1 and other OATPs is unclear, but it is proposed that they are antiporters, potentially using the high intracellular concentration of bicarbonate or reduced glutathione as a driving force. Although the name implies anion transport, OATPs are also capable of transporting cationic and neutral compounds, with OATP1B1 displaying the broadest substrate specificity overall. OATP1B1 transports many endogenous substrates, including conjugates of bilirubin and

Table 4-3. Relevant Drug Substrates and Inhibitors of Solute-Carrier Transporters

Transporter	Substrates	Inhibitors
OATP1B1	Atorvastatin, bosentan, cerivastatin, fexofenadine, fluvastatin, methotrexate, olmesartan, pitavastatin, pravastatin, repaglinide, rosuvastatin, simvastatin, SN-38, valsartan	Cyclosporine, rifampin, ritonavir, saquinavir
OATP1B3	Digoxin, docetaxel, fexofenadine, olmesartan, paclitaxel, statins, telmisartan	Cyclosporine, rifampin, ritonavir
OATP1A2	Fexofenadine, imatinib, levofloxacin, methotrexate, pitavastatin, rocuronium, rosuvastatin, sumatriptan	Fruit juices, rifampin, ritonavir, saquinavir, verapamil
OATP2B1	Fexofenadine, pravastatin, rosuvastatin, sulfasalazine	Fruit juices, cyclosporine, gemfibrozil
OAT1	Acyclovir, adefovir, cidofovir, ciprofloxacin, lamivudine, methotrexate, penicillins, tenofovir, zidovudine	Probenecid, NSAIDs
OAT2	Ketoprofen, theophylline	NSAIDs
OAT3	Bumetanide, cefaclor, ceftizoxime, furosemide, methotrexate, NSAIDs, penicillins	Probenecid, NSAIDs
OCT1	Metformin, morphine, ondansetron, oxaliplatin, sumatriptan	Erlotinib, propranolol, quinidine, verapamil
OCT2	Cisplatin, lamivudine, metformin, oxaliplatin, procainamide	Cimetidine, pyrimethamine, vandetanib, dolutegravir
MATE1	Cisplatin, metformin, oxaliplatin	Cimetidine, cobicistat, famotidine, quinidine, pyrimethamine, trimethoprim, vandetanib
MCT1	Salicylic acid, valproic acid, γ-hydroxybutyric acid	Dietary flavonoids, AZD3965, α-cyano-4 hydroxycinnamate
PEPT1	Captopril, cefadroxil, cephalexin, enalapril, valacyclovir	Glycyl-proline, zinc
PEPT2	Captopril, cefadroxil, cephalexin, enalapril, valacyclovir	Fosinopril
CNT/ENT	Clofarabine, ribavirin, other nucleoside analogues	Dipyridamole
NTCP	Atorvastatin, pravastatin, rosuvastatin	Bosentan, cyclosporine, gemfibrozil

NSAIDs, nonsteroidal anti-inflammatory drugs.

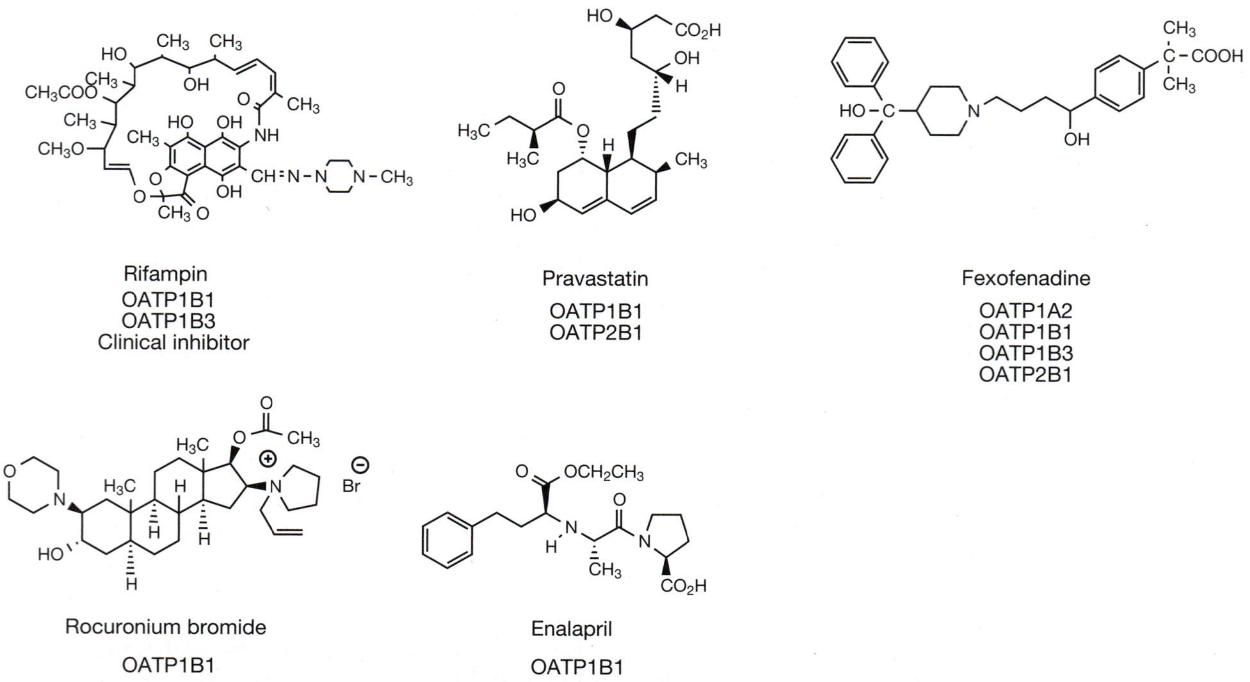

Figure 4.6 Common OATP substrates/inhibitors.

estrogen. Common drug substrates of OATP1B1 and other OATPs are given in Figure 4.6. Rifampin and cyclosporine potently inhibit OATP1B1 in vivo and are used in the clinic for assessment of interactions with potential OATP substrates. Interactions with these inhibitors can result in very large increases in substrate exposure, the largest of any transporter-mediated interactions. Recent findings may help explain the large magnitude of these interactions in that long-lasting inhibition has been demonstrated in vitro and in vivo, at least in rats, particularly for cyclosporine.[27,28] This long-lasting inhibition is dependent on incubation time and suggested to be due to trans-inhibition driven by intracellular concentrations of cyclosporine.[29] This transporter has also gained attention due to the recognition that it is highly polymorphic, with a large number of SNPs having been identified in the *SLCO1B1* gene. Many of these SNPs translate into decreased hepatic uptake in vivo, resulting in decreased clearance of OATP1B1 substrates (see "Transporter Polymorphisms: Role in Statin Disposition" section).[30]

TRANSPORTER POLYMORPHISMS: ROLE IN STATIN DISPOSITION

The effect of OATP1B1 polymorphisms on statin pharmacokinetics further emphasizes the significance of OATP-mediated uptake for the hepatic clearance of these compounds. Studies of subjects with the common *SLCO1B1* c.521CC genotype have reported increases in plasma AUC from 65% with rosuvastatin to 221% with simvastatin, compared to subjects carrying the wild-type allele.[30] Likely the most prominent finding with regard to statin myopathy was the genome-wide association study, which found this polymorphism to be the strongest predictor of the toxicity of simvastatin.[31] A more recent genome-wide association study also reported that this polymorphism was associated with atorvastatin intolerance and increased muscular symptoms.[32] Given that many statins are also substrates for BCRP and there are known polymorphisms in *ABCG2*, studies have also evaluated the effect of the *ABCG2* c.421CA polymorphism on statin exposure. The greatest effect of 144% increased exposure has been demonstrated for rosuvastatin, which may involve increased bioavailability and/or decreased biliary secretion by BCRP.[33] Increased effect of rosuvastatin has also been demonstrated in subjects with this polymorphism.[34] Alterations in the function of both OATPs and BCRP can significantly affect the safe and effective use of statins. Algorithms for statin dosing incorporating *SLCO1B1* and *ABCG2* genotyping are currently proposed for individualizing statin therapy.[35]

Other OATPs. OATP1B3 is expressed like OATP1B1 exclusively on the sinusoidal membrane of the liver. The substrates and inhibitors for OATP1B3 are generally shared by OATP1B1; therefore, the two transporters are collectively referred to as OATP1B regarding drug interactions. There are compounds, such as telmisartan, to which OATP1B3 transport is attributed to be predominant,[36] and OATP1B3 acts as a compensatory transport mechanism when transport by OATP1B1 is deficient due to genetic polymorphisms. The other OATPs with identified drug substrates and effects on drug disposition include OATP1A2, 2B1, and 4C1. OATP1A2 is expressed in the brain and may be responsible for blood-brain barrier (BBB) transport of drugs and endogenous substances. OATP2A1 is thought to be a primary transport mechanism for endogenous prostaglandins and has particularly high expression in the lungs.[37] OATP2B1 is also expressed on the sinusoidal membrane of the liver with OATP1B1 and 1B3; however, unlike these transporters, it is also expressed in other tissues, including the intestine.[19] Due to its intestinal localization, it is important for drug absorption and for drug-drug and diet-drug interactions of orally administered drugs. Ingestion of grapefruit or apple juice produces inhibition of OATP2B1 substrates, due to the flavonoid content of these juices.[38] OATP4C1 is expressed on the basolateral membrane of the kidney and is thought to be responsible for uptake of these drugs into the proximal tubule cell. Among its substrates are digoxin and the antidiabetic drug sitagliptin; however, the role of this transporter in in vivo drug interactions of these substrates is as of yet unclear.[39]

Organic-Anion Transporters (*SLC22A*)

The organic-anion transporters (OATs) are highly expressed in the kidney, where they have a significant role in the renal clearance of many anionic drugs. The driving forces and polarized renal expression of OATs support renal secretion of drug substrates from the blood circulation into the urine. OAT1 is expressed primarily in the kidney, on the basolateral membrane of renal tubule cells, along with OAT2 and OAT3. These transporters facilitate anion transport into renal tubule cells, through antiport with intracellular dicarboxylates such as α-ketoglutarate. Located on the apical membrane, OAT4 can transport drugs from the tubule cells into the urine, but it is likely primarily responsible for renal reabsorption.[40] OATs transport an expansive range of drugs, and the importance of OAT expression in the kidney has been demonstrated with numerous clinically relevant drug interactions. OAT2 has been identified as the predominant mechanism of renal proximal tubule uptake of three antiviral drugs: acyclovir, ganciclovir and penciclovir.[41] Coadministration of OAT inhibitors can lead to decreased renal secretion of OAT substrates, including penicillin antibiotics and diuretic agents (Tables 4.3 and 4.4).[16] However, clinical drug-drug interaction (DDI) studies of acyclovir and ganciclovir with the prototypical OAT1/3 inhibitor, probenecid, showed no to little decrease ($\leq$30% decrease) in the renal clearance of these OAT2-substrate drugs, indicating that probenecid is not an inhibitor or is a weak inhibitor of OAT2.[42,43] Along with renal transport, OAT2 is also located on the liver sinusoidal membrane, where it facilitates anion uptake into hepatocytes. OATs are also present on the choroid plexus (a structure in the brain where cerebrospinal fluid [CSF] is produced), where they can have a role in transfer of drugs between the blood and CSF.[44] Pharmacologic inhibition with probenecid results in the increased CSF concentration of the OAT substrate bumetanide, supporting their function in removal of anionic substrates from CSF into choroid plexus.[44]

Organic-Cation/-Carnitine Transporters (*SLC22A*)

Organic cation transporters (OCTs) are electrogenic uniporters, which use only the negative membrane potential as a driving force and require no co-substrate. OCT1 is expressed primarily in the liver, and OCT2 in the kidney, both on the basolateral membrane. Although they are named cation transporters, these transporters are also capable of transporting some anionic and neutral compounds. SNPs in OCT1 have demonstrated effects on the plasma exposure of multiple OCT1 substrates.[45] In Oct1/2 knockout mice, the hepatic clearance and liver partitioning of sumatriptan and fenoterol is significantly decreased, indicating importance of Oct1 in the hepatic uptake of these OCT1 substrates.[46] Drug interactions and drug toxicity have been attributed to OCT2-mediated transport, due to a substrate range that includes commonly prescribed therapeutic agents, such as metformin (see Table 4.3). Coadministration of OCT2 inhibitors and genetic variation in OCT2 have been demonstrated to increase plasma concentrations of metformin due to its decreased renal secretion (see Table 4.4).[47-49] Renal transport of cisplatin by OCT2 has also been identified as a significant factor in cisplatin-induced nephrotoxicity (see "Renal Clearance by OCT2/MATE: Cisplatin Toxicity" section).[50] OCT3 transports monoamines and is located in the brain and placenta, where its primary role can be to eliminate catecholamines from the fetal blood circulation.[51] Decreased OCT3 transport has also been suggested to be related to cases of preeclampsia.[52] Recently, OCT3 has been shown to play a role in the uptake of doxorubicin into cardiomyocytes; inhibition of OCT3 resulted in prevention of doxorubicin-mediated cardiac damage, without altering its antitumor efficacy.[53] These studies suggest the importance of OCT3-mediated uptake of doxorubicin in its cardiac toxicity.

Organic-cation/-carnitine transporter (OCTN) 1 and OCTN2 are involved in the bidirectional transport of cations and zwitterions. Multiple transport mechanisms have been reported, depending on the substrate. OCTN transporters can function as uniporters or sodium-dependent cotransporters. Both OCTN1 and OCTN2 are highly expressed in the kidney, where they are localized on the apical membrane.[54] OCTN2 is responsible for carnitine transport into tissues and is widely expressed, including in the kidney, skeletal muscle, liver, brain, small intestine, and lung.[55] It predominantly functions as a high-affinity sodium-dependent L-carnitine transporter. These transporters share substrates with OCTs, and their apical expression may allow for the concerted movement of these substrates across membranes in which they are co-expressed. OCTNs are of particular importance in the placenta, as they are responsible for transporting carnitine to the fetus.[51] Some antiepileptics, like valproate, inhibit OCTNs, and it has been suggested that inhibition of carnitine transport can be partly responsible for teratogenicity and other adverse effects associated with valproate use.[56] Mutations in OCTN2 lead to systemic carnitine deficiency syndrome, causing early-onset cardiomyopathy, including congestive heart failure.[57] The anticholinergic drugs ipratropium and tiotropium are transported primarily by OCTN2 and, to a lesser extent, by OCTN1, into bronchial epithelial cells.[58] These findings are consistent with the pharmacologic activity of the drugs after administration via inhalation. OCTN2 has been a target for drug delivery to increase intestinal, lung, kidney, and BBB permeability. Multiple carnitine-conjugated prodrugs have been developed. One example is for the chemotherapeutic

Table 4.4 Select Clinically Relevant Drug Interactions Involving Transporters

Transporter	Substrate	Inhibitor(s)	Effect on Substrate Pharmacokinetics
MDR1	Digoxin	Clarithromycin, cyclosporine, dronedarone, ritonavir, verapamil	↑ plasma AUC 70-150% (↓ Cl_r, ↓ Cl_{bile}, and/or ↑ F)
		Rifampin (multiple dose), St. John's wort	↓ plasma AUC 20-30%, (↓ F due to induction)
	Dabigatran etexilate	Dronedarone, ketoconazole	↑ plasma AUC 110-150% (of dabigatran), ↑ F
		Rifampin (multiple dose)	↓ plasma AUC 60-70%, (↓ F due to induction)
BCRP	Topotecan	Elacridar	↑ plasma AUC 140%, ↑ F
	Rosuvastatin	Fenebrutinib	↑ plasma AUC 150% (↑ F and/or ↓ Cl_{bile})
MRP2	Mycophenolic acid (glucuronide conjugates)	Cyclosporine	↓ plasma AUC 20-40% (↓ Cl_{bile} of conjugates leading to ↓ enterohepatic circulation)
OATP1B1/1B3	Atorvastatin	Rifampin (single dose)	↑ plasma AUC 680%, ↓ Cl
	Pitavastatin	Cyclosporine	↑ plasma AUC 360%, ↓ Cl
	Rosuvastatin	Rifampin (single dose)	↑ plasma AUC 230%, ↓ Cl
OATP2B1	Rosuvastatin	Ronacaleret	↓ plasma AUC 50%, ↓ F
OAT1/3	furosemide	Probenecid	↑ plasma AUC 200%, ↓ Cl_r 75%
OCT2/MATE1	Metformin	Cimetidine, dolutegravir, pyrimethamine, vandetanib	↑ plasma AUC 30-150%, ↓ Cl_r
	Dofetilide	Cimetidine	↑ plasma AUC 50%, ↓ Cl_r 30%

AUC, area under the curve; Cl, clearance; Cl_{bile}, biliary clearance; Cl_r, renal clearance; F, bioavailability.

agent gemcitabine, where carnitine-conjugated gemcitabine exhibited 5-fold increased oral bioavailability over gemcitabine.[59]

Multidrug and Toxin Extrusion Transporters (*SLC47A*)

Multidrug and toxin extrusion transporter (MATE) 1 and MATE2-K are cation transporters that use proton antiport as a driving force. MATE1 is located primarily on the apical membrane of the kidney and canalicular membrane of the liver. MATE2-K is kidney specific, and recently, it was found that expression even in human proximal tubule cells of kidney is low, leading to ambiguity of its in vivo relevance given that substrates are often shared with MATE1.[60] The significance of MATE1 transport in metformin pharmacokinetics was characterized in Mate1 knockout mice, in which the renal clearance of metformin was decreased to less than 20% that of controls, indicating the importance of this transporter for metformin renal secretion.[61] Drug interactions with metformin and other substrates in humans involve MATE inhibition in the kidney (see Table 4.4).[62] Inhibition of Mate1 in mice increased the liver accumulation of metformin, and SNPs with decreased function in the *SLC47A* gene have been associated with increased metformin response.[63,64] MATE1 has a role in the renal secretion and nephrotoxicity of platinum agents, where MATE1 secretion appears protective due to the prevention of renal cell accumulation (see "Renal Clearance by OCT2/MATE: Cisplatin Toxicity" section).[65,66] Many drug substrates and inhibitors of these transporters have been identified and can be cationic, neutral, or anionic at physiologic pH.[62] MATE substrates and inhibitors are often shared with those of OCT2, and sometimes with those of OAT1 or OAT3, which can lead to DDIs involving both uptake and efflux into proximal tubule cells, discussed in further detail later.[67]

Monocarboxylate Transporters (*SLC16A* and *SLC5A*)

The first discovered monocarboxylate transporters (MCTs 1-4) were proton-coupled, transporting monocarboxylates via symport. Because the transport of substrates by MCTs is driven by the proton gradient, these transporters can influx or efflux substrates depending on this gradient. MCT1 is ubiquitously expressed, and its role in the transport of endogenous substances, including lactate, pyruvate, butyrate and ketone bodies, has been extensively characterized.[68] Many therapeutic agents have also been identified as substrates; however, the clinical relevance of transport by

MCT1-4 of these agents is unclear (see Table 4.3). A relevant therapeutic aspect of MCT1 is its high expression in the intestine, making this transporter a target as a means for oral drug absorption (see box MCT1 and oral drug delivery).[69] MCT1 has also been identified to be overexpressed in tumor cells, and inhibition of this transporter represents a possible therapeutic strategy for some cancers.[70] The drug of abuse γ-hydroxybutyrate (GHB) has been identified as a MCT substrate, and the relevance of MCT transport of this drug has been established. Inhibition of the MCT-mediated renal reabsorption of GHB has been demonstrated to increase its renal and total clearance, making MCT inhibition a possible strategy for the treatment of GHB overdose.[71,72] Other MCTs have been less well studied, but MCT8 has demonstrated affinity for thyroid hormones,[73] MCT10 for thyroid hormones and amino acids, MCT6 for bumetanide, nateglinide, and prostaglandin F2α (carboprost), and MCT7 for ketone bodies, MCT9 for carnitine, and MCT12 for creatine.[74]

MCT1 AND ORAL DRUG DELIVERY

The antiepileptic agent, gabapentin, has unfavorable oral pharmacokinetics, with low, dose-dependent bioavailability and poor rates of clinical response. In an effort to improve the oral delivery of gabapentin, a prodrug, gabapentin enacarbil, was designed to target absorption by MCT1. In a pilot study comparing the pharmacokinetics of gabapentin to the prodrug, gabapentin displayed dose-dependent bioavailability ranging from 27% to 65%, whereas gabapentin enacarbil displayed bioavailability above 68% for all doses and dose-proportional oral exposure.[75] Gabapentin enacarbil resulted in higher plasma concentrations of gabapentin at similar doses compared with gabapentin itself. This case emphasizes the utility of high-capacity transporters like MCT1 for facilitating oral drug delivery and achieving clinically desirable drug pharmacokinetics.

Another subset of MCTs has been identified that use sodium for monocarboxylate symport and are referred to as sodium-coupled MCTs (SMCTs). Expression of SMCTs is also widely distributed, including the apical membranes of the intestine and kidney, where they likely act in conjunction with proton-coupled MCTs to transport monocarboxylates across membranes.

Peptide Transporters (*SLC15A*)

Peptide transporters (PEPTs) mediate the transport of di- and tripeptides via proton symport. PEPT1 has been identified as a transporter of emerging importance for drug pharmacokinetics and DDIs for peptide drugs, including β-lactam antibiotics and angiotensin-converting enzyme (ACE) inhibitors (see Table 4.3). PEPT1 has very high expression on the apical membrane of the intestine and, as such, is used for drug delivery.[19] Transport mediated by PEPT1 facilitates sufficient oral absorption to allow oral administration for many therapeutic drugs and prodrugs structurally designed to target this transporter (Fig. 4.7; also see Table 4.3).[69] PEPT1

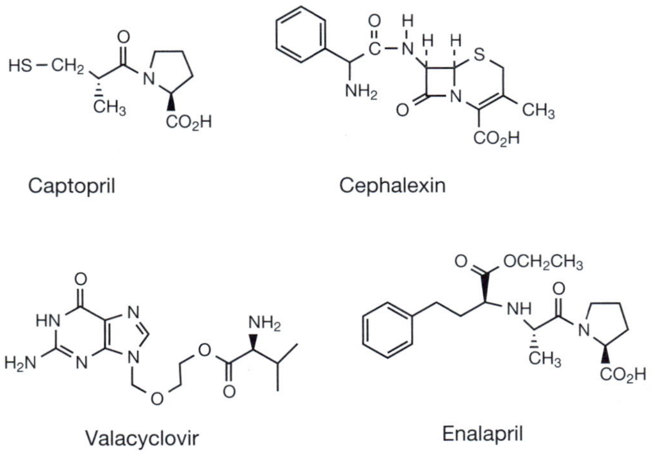

Figure 4.7 Drug substrates of peptide transporters.

is also present at lower levels on the brush border membrane of the kidney; however, PEPT2 is the major peptide transporter at this site. PEPT2 is also localized to the apical membrane, where it serves mainly to reabsorb peptides from the urine in renal tubule cells, facilitating transport of drug substrates similar to PEPT1.[76] Two peptide/histidine transporters (PHTs) were recently identified, PHT1 and PHT2. Expression of these transporters has been demonstrated in the intestine, and they likely have a role in peptide absorption, along with PEPT1. Expression of mRNA for these transporters has also been identified in several other human tissues.[77] The role of the PHTs in drug disposition has yet to be elucidated.

Nucleoside Transporters (*SLC28* and *SLC29*)

Two nucleoside transporter groups exist: the concentrative-nucleoside transporters (CNTs) and the equilibrative-nucleoside transporters (ENTs). CNTs are present on the apical membrane of cells and are sodium dependent, whereas ENTs are facilitative and located primarily on basolateral membranes.[78] These two groups of transporters work together to achieve vectorial transport of purines and pyrimidines. The expression of both groups of transporters is widespread, and although their primary function is to facilitate cellular uptake of nucleosides, they also transport many nucleoside analogues (Fig. 4.8), and these transporters are associated with toxicity and therapeutic response to these drugs (see Table 4.3).[78,79] For example, ENT1 is important for the distribution of the antiretroviral drug abacavir across the placenta, and therefore, a determinant of the efficacy of this drug that is used to prevent transfer of HIV from mother to fetus.[80]

Bile Acid Transporters (*ABCB11, SLC10A,* and *OSTA/B*)

The human in vivo bile acid pool is highly conserved due to their enterohepatic recirculation; therefore, the bile acid transporters involved in this process have been well-characterized.[81]

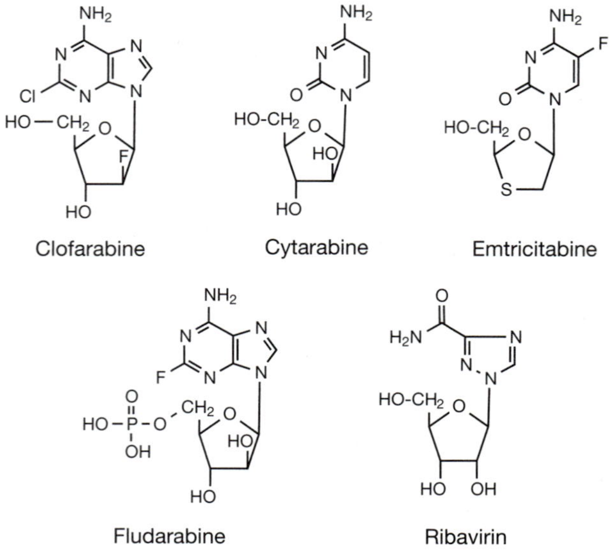

Figure 4.8 Drug substrates of nucleoside transporters.

It has been recently demonstrated, however, that these transporters can also transport xenobiotics. Sodium-taurocholate cotransporting polypeptide (NTCP) is primarily responsible for the hepatic uptake of bile acids, and this transporter has been demonstrated to transport some of the statins, and many drugs are also known to inhibit NTCP.[82] The bile salt export pump (BSEP) is likely the most notable bile acid transporter that interacts with drugs, as it has been shown that inhibitors of this transporter often lead to hepatotoxicity.[83] Recently, other transporters in the liver have also been recognized to be involved in bile acid–induced hepatotoxicity such as MRP3/4 and OSTα/OSTβ. These transporters are expressed on the basolateral membrane of the liver, and their role is compensatory to BSEP inhibition in that bile acid accumulation leads to their upregulation.[18,84] Many inhibitors of BSEP also inhibit these compensatory transporters, which may explain the resulting hepatotoxicity observed with these compounds.[85] There are also bile acid transporters in the intestine, including apical sodium-dependent bile acid transporter (ASBT) and MRP2 on the apical membrane and OSTα/β and MRP3 on the basolateral membrane, which are responsible for reabsorption of bile acids in the gut following their export by BSEP into the bile; additionally, drugs can also interact with these transporters, both as substrates and inhibitors. Inhibition of ASBT in the gut, in particular, has been postulated as potential therapy for hypercholesterolemia and diabetes by preventing the conservation of bile acids.[86]

EVALUATING TRANSPORTER EFFECTS IN VIVO

Many transporters share substrates with other transporters and with drug-metabolizing enzymes, making it difficult to attribute in vivo effects to a specific transporter. The use of probe substrates and specific inhibitors makes this identification easier, but these are not available for most transporters or may not be suitable for in vivo use. Knockout animals can be used to assess the effects of a specific transporter in vivo, whereas transfected cell lines or oocytes and specific silencing of a transporter using small interfering double-stranded RNA or clustered regularly interspaced short palindromic repeats (CRISPR)-associated protein 9 technology can be useful to assess effects in vitro. Assessment of the effects of transporter polymorphisms can be useful to allow some determination of a transporter's role in the disposition of a drug in humans. When evaluating the effects of drug transport on bioavailability, it can be difficult to attribute effects to transport in the intestine alone, as changes in both bioavailability and clearance can affect plasma concentrations after oral administration. It is necessary to assess plasma concentrations of substrates administered both orally and intravenously, with and without an inhibitor, to determine if transport primarily affects substrate bioavailability or systemic clearance. Often both parameters are affected by changes in transport because the same transporters are responsible for both processes. Significant effects on absorption cannot always be demonstrated with efflux transporter substrates in vivo. This can be due to the very high luminal concentrations of substrate causing transporter saturation and to the passive membrane permeability of these compounds. A lack of effect can also be due to shared transporter substrates, allowing compensatory transport by one transporter when another is inhibited.

Effect of Transport on Drug Pharmacokinetics and Drug-Drug Interactions

Intestinal Transport

The importance of transporter-mediated uptake or efflux in the intestine depends primarily on two factors. The first is the contribution of transporter-mediated transport compared to the other mechanisms of drug passage across the gut wall. The second is drug concentration. Drug concentrations are generally much higher in the gut lumen compared to the systemic blood circulation due to a lower volume of distribution in the gut. This causes the concentration gradient driving diffusion to be very large, but more importantly, can lead to transporter saturation. This can result in low bioavailability due to saturation of uptake transporters and nonlinearity in drug absorption. Transporter saturation can also aid in drug absorption in that high drug concentrations in the enterocyte can saturate efflux transporters. High drug concentrations in the gut also increase the risk of drug interactions affecting oral absorption of other drugs. The Biopharmaceutics Classification System recommended by the U.S. Food and Drug Administration names solubility and permeability as determining factors of oral absorption,[87] factors that can be translated into effects on drug concentration (C) and passive diffusion (P) in the intestine. Considering these factors, the predicted effects of drug transporters on oral absorption are given in Figure 4.9.[88]

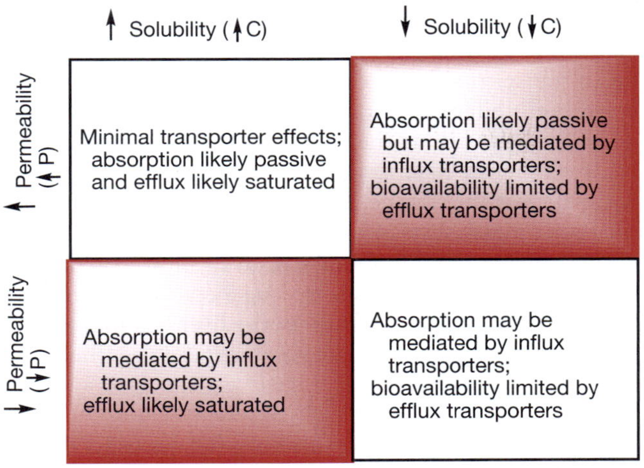

Figure 4.9 Role of transporters in drug absorption. High aqueous drug solubility will result in high luminal drug concentrations, allowing for possible transporter saturation. High permeability results in high passive diffusion, allowing these drugs to be orally absorbed without dependence on transporters. (Adapted from Shugarts S, Benet LZ. The role of transporters in the pharmacokinetics of orally administered drugs. *Pharm Res.* 2009;26:2039-2054.)

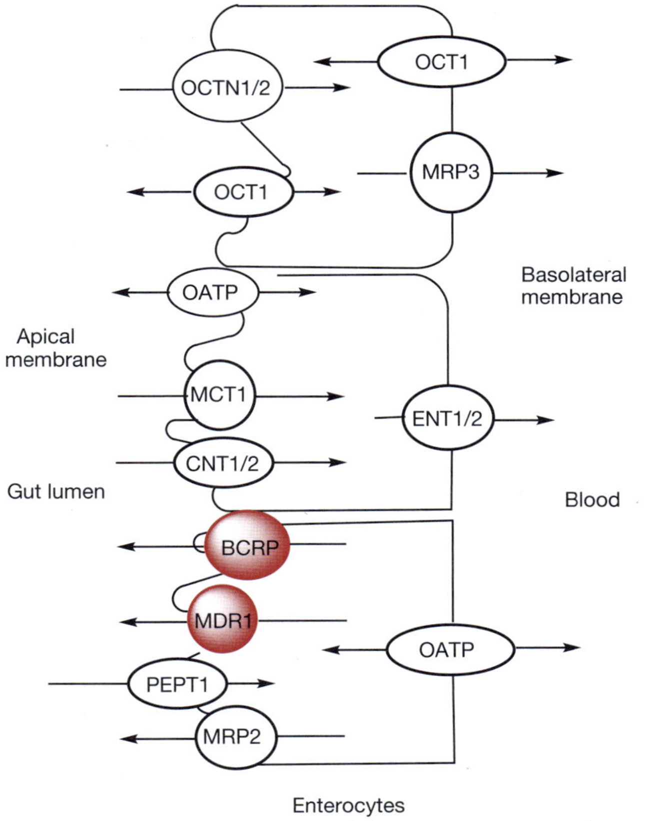

Figure 4.10 Polarized expression of drug transporters in the intestine. Transporters most relevant to drug disposition are shown in *red*.

The polarized expression of relevant drug transporters in the intestine is illustrated in Figure 4.10. Clinical relevance of drug transport is determined not only by the presence of transporters on a biologic membrane, but also by their relative expression. Drug transporters with high expression throughout the intestine include PEPT1, MCT1, P-gp, BCRP, and MRP2/3/4.[89] High expression of influx transporters, such as PEPT1 and MCT1, allows the use of these high-capacity transporters as a drug delivery mechanism. High expression of efflux transporters makes these transporters important in limiting drug bioavailability.

Along with drug transporters, drug-metabolizing enzymes are also present in the enterocytes forming the gut wall, including phase 1 and phase 2 enzymes. First-pass metabolism in the gut can be a reason for low oral bioavailability. Transporters often share substrates with drug-metabolizing enzymes, and the intestine is one site in which substantial transport-metabolism interplay has been purported. In particular, P-gp shares many substrates with the enzyme CYP3A4, and it is proposed that P-gp can prevent oral absorption through drug efflux and by facilitating drug metabolism by CYP3A4.[90] Interplay between transporters and intestinal metabolism likely occurs by multiple mechanisms, including decreasing intracellular substrate concentrations preventing saturation of metabolism, and by the cycling of substrates through the gut lumen and enterocytes, allowing enzymes such as CYP3A4 multiple opportunities to metabolize their substrates.[91] This interplay is depicted in Figure 4.11.

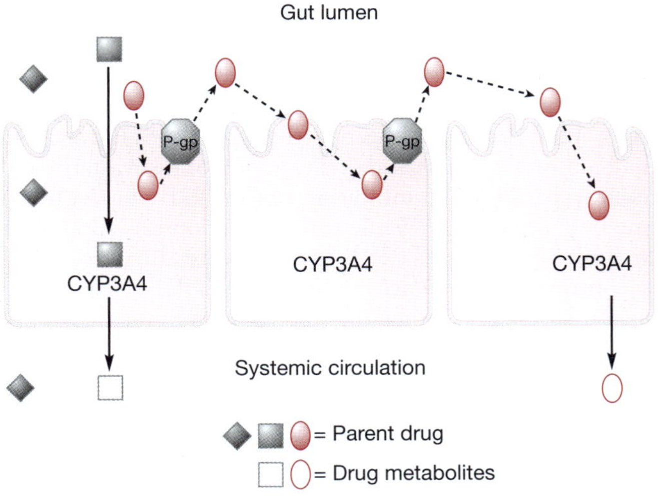

Figure 4.11 Transport-metabolism interplay in the intestine. Drugs may be orally absorbed without undergoing metabolic conversion. Drugs may undergo metabolism in the gut, and this may occur upon initial entry into the enterocyte or after cycling between the gut lumen and the enterocyte. P-gp facilitates CYP3A4 metabolism by decreasing intracellular substrate concentrations preventing enzyme saturation and by allowing the enzyme multiple opportunities for drug metabolism, as demonstrated by the molecule shown in red. (Adapted from Benet LZ. The drug transporter-metabolism alliance: uncovering and defining the interplay. *Mol Pharm.* 2009;6:1631-1643.)

Efflux Transporters and Drug Bioavailability

Studies using specific P-gp inhibitors and Mdr1 knockout animals have demonstrated the importance of P-gp in the oral bioavailability of drugs, including HIV protease inhibitors, β-receptor antagonists, morphine, and many other therapeutic agents.[92] Most drug interactions in the intestine with P-gp or other efflux transporters involve inhibition of transport, resulting in increased bioavailability of the transporter substrate. Efflux transporters, specifically P-gp, may also be induced, resulting in decreased bioavailability (see "Transporter-Drug Interactions: Pgp and Digoxin" section and Table 4.4). Administration of P-gp inhibitors and inducers has demonstrated clinically significant effects on the bioavailability of P-gp substrates, including digoxin, paclitaxel, and dabigatran.[12,14] Drug bioavailability can also be limited by BCRP. Administration of the P-gp/BCRP inhibitor elacridar increased the bioavailability of topotecan 6-fold in Mdr1 knockout mice, and oral coadministration with elacridar has been shown to increase the bioavailability of topotecan in humans to almost 100%.[23,24] Similarly, oral coadministration of the statin rosuvastatin, a clinical BCRP substrate, and known inhibitors of BCRP can significantly increase rosuvastatin exposure in humans, due to inhibition of BCRP-mediated intestinal efflux and/or biliary secretion.[93] Polymorphisms in the *ABCG2* gene can also affect the plasma exposure of rosuvastatin and other BCRP substrates (see "Transporter Polymorphisms: Role in Statin Disposition" section).

Uptake Transporters and Drug Bioavailability

Select uptake transporters in the intestine have been used to facilitate oral absorption. The high expression of PEPT1 has made it a target for oral drug delivery, and among its substrates are ACE inhibitors, β-lactam antibiotics, and the antiviral drug valacyclovir.[76] Nonlinearity in the oral pharmacokinetics of valacyclovir can be attributed to saturable PEPT1-mediated absorption.[94] Other uptake transporters reported to be involved in oral drug delivery include MCT1, OATP2B1, OCTN2, and nucleoside transporters.[69]

Influx transporters can also be responsible for drug interactions in the intestine, although fewer drug interactions have been noted compared with efflux transporters. Specifically, interactions have been attributed to OATP transport in the intestine. Decreased oral exposure of rosuvastatin was recently attributed to inhibition of OATP2B1 in the intestine by ronacaleret.[95] While this interaction was supported by inhibition of OATP2B1 by ronacaleret in vitro, there is controversial evidence regarding OATP2B1 expression on the basolateral rather than apical membrane, leaving a potential for interaction with another transporter prior to rosuvastatin reaching the basolateral membrane.[96] Plasma concentrations of fexofenadine, rosuvastatin, and other OATP substrates are decreased with concomitant ingestion of grapefruit juice.[97] This is most likely due to OATP2B1 inhibition by the naringin and other flavonoids in fruit juices, to which drug interactions with intestinal P-gp have also been attributed.[98] Flavonoids are also present in other fruit juices, which can affect the disposition of OATP2B1 substrates.

Hepatic Transport

As a clearance organ, the liver can eliminate drug through two pathways: metabolism and biliary excretion. Uptake into the liver is necessary for both of these processes, and for hydrophilic drugs; primarily ionized at blood pH, this is often a transporter-mediated process. Active transport is also necessary for biliary excretion, as diffusion of drugs into the bile is unlikely due to the low volume of the bile canaliculus, resulting in high drug concentrations on this side of the canalicular membrane. As with the intestine, there exists transporter-metabolism interplay in the liver because transporters regulate the distribution of drug substrates into the liver and therefore their access to drug-metabolizing enzymes. The intrinsic clearance of drugs in the liver has traditionally been thought of as simply the rate of metabolism, therefore:

$$Cl_{int} = Cl_{met}$$

That is, the hepatic intrinsic clearance (Cl_{int}) can be defined as solely the intrinsic ability of the liver to metabolize a drug (metabolic clearance, Cl_{met}). It is now recognized that for drugs that undergo active uptake by drug transporters, multiple processes need to be incorporated to define its intrinsic clearance, namely those in the "extended clearance" equation:

$$Cl_{int} = Cl_{met/bile} \bullet \frac{Cl_{active} + Cl_{passive}}{Cl_{passive} + Cl_{met/bile}}$$

where $Cl_{met/bile}$ is the combined metabolic and biliary clearances, and Cl_{active} and $Cl_{passive}$ represent the active transporter-mediated and passive diffusion clearances in the liver, respectively.[99] This Cl_{int} can then be incorporated into a hepatic clearance model incorporating other physiologic parameters to derive the in vivo hepatic clearance from Cl_{int}.[100] The transporters facilitating both drug uptake and biliary excretion in the liver are depicted in Figure 4.12. As shown in the figure, while it is known that efflux transporters are present not only on the canalicular membrane but also on the sinusoidal membrane of hepatocytes, there is as

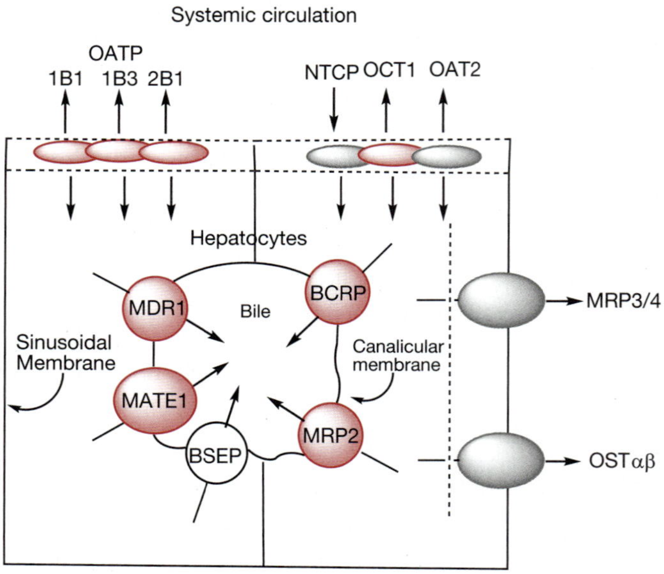

Figure 4.12 Drug transporter expression in hepatocytes. Transporters most relevant to drug disposition are shown in *red*.

of yet limited clinical relevance known of the role of these transporters in drug disposition or DDIs.

Role of Transporters in Hepatic Clearance and Drug Interactions at the Sinusoidal Membrane

Of the transporters present on the sinusoidal membrane, the greatest number and greatest magnitude of drug-drug interactions have been demonstrated with the OATPs. One of the first interactions noted was the several-fold increase in cerivastatin plasma concentrations following gemfibrozil administration, resulting in severe cases of rhabdomyolysis.[101,102] This drug interaction was determined to be due to inhibition of OATP1B1 and CYP2C8 by gemfibrozil and its glucuronide metabolite and eventually contributed to cerivastatin being withdrawn from market.[102] Gemfibrozil increases the plasma AUC of other statins, which undergo little metabolism, indicating the significance of OATP-mediated transport.[30,103] Similar effects on statin pharmacokinetics have also been demonstrated with other OATP1B inhibitors, including cyclosporine and single-dose rifampin.[104-106] The relevance of OATP-mediated hepatic uptake may not only relate to the pharmacokinetics of drugs, but is also an instance in which transporters are involved in pharmacodynamics as well, given they allow the statins access to their site of action, the liver. Drug interactions through OATP1B inhibition and polymorphisms in the *SLCO1B1* gene also lead to decreased clearance of other OATP substrates, including repaglinide, methotrexate, and the active metabolite of irinotecan, SN-38 (see "Transporter Polymorphisms: Role in Statin Disposition" section).[30,107] While OATP-mediated transport put the concept of uptake rate-limited hepatic clearance on the map, more recently clinical relevance of other hepatic transporters has surfaced, specifically that of OCT1. Polymorphisms have been identified in the *SLC22A1* gene that have reduced or no functional uptake of OCT1 substrates.[45] Clinical studies have shown that homozygous carriers of OCT1 variants have increased plasma exposure of sumatriptan, morphine, and 5HT-3 antagonists.[108-110] While metformin is not eliminated by metabolism or biliary clearance and, therefore, is cleared completely by the kidneys, OCT1-mediated uptake of metformin is another example of hepatic transporters having a role in pharmacodynamics. Some studies have shown that carriers of reduced function *SLC22A1* variants have reduced response to metformin, although there exist conflicting reports.[111] Few drug interactions affecting OCT1 substrate plasma exposure have been assessed; therefore, no clinically relevant drug interactions via OCT1 are known. However, one study did show a change in metformin pharmacodynamics reportedly through OCT1 inhibition by verapamil.[112]

Role of Transporters in Biliary Drug Excretion and the Effect of Drugs on Canalicular Membrane Transport

It can be difficult to attribute clearance to biliary excretion in vivo, given that sampling bile is very technically challenging, and in the absence of this, drug excreted into bile ends up in the feces and is therefore undistinguishable from unabsorbed drug following oral absorption. Drug excreted into the bile may also be completely reabsorbed into the intestine, negating biliary elimination as an actual clearance pathway. Fecal drug amounts following IV administration can be evaluated and other methods for sampling drug in the duodenum and/or via noninvasive imaging methods are becoming useful. Accordingly, bile duct-cannulated mice, including transporter knockout mice, are often relied upon to identify this route of elimination for drugs and the mechanism. Some of the first drug interactions discovered to affect biliary clearance of drugs in humans involved the ABC transporter P-gp. It was demonstrated that quinidine and verapamil, known P-gp inhibitors, significantly decreased the biliary clearance of digoxin, resulting in increased digoxin plasma concentrations.[13,113] P-gp efflux also has a role in the biliary excretion of doxorubicin, as demonstrated by an 80% to 90% decrease in doxorubicin biliary clearance in Mdr1 knockout mice[114]; fecal excretion is also a significant elimination pathway for doxorubicin in humans, suggesting biliary clearance. MRP2 also mediates biliary excretion of doxorubicin, along with that of other therapeutic agents including pravastatin and valsartan (see Table 4.3).[115-117] MRP2 has a significant role in the biliary excretion of drug conjugates, resulting in their enterohepatic cycling. There is a clear in vivo DDI between cyclosporine and mycophenolic acid, which has been attributed to inhibition of MRP2-mediated biliary secretion of the glucuronide conjugate leading to decreased hydrolysis of the conjugate in the intestinal tract and reabsorption of mycophenolic acid itself.[118] BCRP has a more significant role in the excretion of sulfate conjugates, along with its role in secreting unconjugated drugs. Decreased biliary excretion of acetaminophen sulfate and other sulfate conjugates has been reported in mice lacking Bcrp but not in those lacking Mdr2.[119,120] Bcrp knockout or inhibition results in decreased biliary clearance of therapeutic agents in mice, including topotecan, nitrofurantoin, and ciprofloxacin.[24,25,121] In addition, polymorphisms in the ABCG2 gene have been shown to correlate with increased response to rosuvastatin, which may be explained by increased concentrations in the liver, the site of action, due to decreased biliary excretion by BCRP, along with increased absorption[34] (see "Transporter Polymorphisms: Role in Statin Disposition" section). As mentioned above, efflux transporters MRP2 and BSEP are also primarily responsible for the biliary secretion of endogenous substances, and drug interactions may also interfere with these processes through inhibition of these transporters (see Table 4.3).

Renal Transport

Renal clearance is mediated by three primary pathways: glomerular filtration, tubular secretion, and renal reabsorption. Small molecules that are not protein bound will be filtered at the glomerulus. Drugs that undergo glomerular filtration can have negligible renal clearance if they are sufficiently lipophilic to be passively reabsorbed from the tubular lumen back into systemic circulation. Drugs that undergo filtration and are hydrophilic or ionized will be excreted into the urine unless they are actively reabsorbed by transporters.

Drugs can have extensive renal clearance, sometimes much greater than the glomerular filtration rate, if they undergo renal secretion. The following equation can be used to determine renal clearance, considering the possibility of all three processes:

$$Cl_r = (GFR \times f_{up} + Cl_{rs})(1 - FR)$$

where GFR is the glomerular filtration rate; f_{up} is the fraction unbound in the plasma; Cl_{rs} is the clearance by renal secretion; and FR is the fraction of unchanged drug that is filtered and secreted in the urine, which is reabsorbed. Given that urine is a biological sample easily collected, renal clearance and the net contribution of active secretion or reabsorption are readily calculable; transporters are involved whenever active secretion or active reabsorption occur. Secretion and reabsorption require transport of drug across both apical and basolateral membranes, and the polarized expression of organic anion and OCTs on both membranes allows directional transport of ionized substrates. The transporters responsible for active secretion and active reabsorption and their polarized expression in the kidney are illustrated in Figure 4.13.

Renal Clearance of Anions

Tubular secretion of anions across the basolateral membrane is mediated primarily by OAT1, OAT2, and OAT3. Substrates of these transporters include β-lactam antibiotics, nonsteroidal anti-inflammatory drugs, and many other anionic therapeutic agents (see Table 4.3). Probenecid is a known inhibitor of OAT1/3, and coadministration with OAT substrates leads to decreased renal clearance of these substrates. One of the most highly recognized transporter interactions is that between probenecid and penicillin derivatives, and coadministration of probenecid has been demonstrated to decrease the renal clearance of numerous drugs of this class, including piperacillin, nafcillin, ticarcillin, and others.[16] Inhibition of OAT transport by probenecid also causes decreased renal clearance of diuretics like furosemide and results in diminished diuretic effect due to decreased tubular drug concentrations.[122,123] OAT-mediated drug interactions affect renal secretion of many other OAT substrates, including methotrexate, acyclovir, and zidovudine.[16] Secretion of anions across the renal brush border membrane is primarily mediated by MRP2 and MRP4. Probenecid is also an MRP2 inhibitor, and some of its effects on renal clearance can be due to combined inhibition of OATs and MRP2. MRP4 is present at levels similar to those of MRP2 in human kidney and Mrp4 knockout mice display significant renal cell accumulation of the nucleotide phosphonates adefovir and tenofovir.[60,124] Additionally, case reports exist in which administration of MRP4 inhibitors have been associated with nephrotoxicity of tenofovir.[125] Interestingly, cidofovir does not appear to be transported by MRP4, and this may be a reason for the significant nephrotoxicity associated with this drug. These drugs are also OAT substrates, and OAT inhibition may have therapeutic potential for preventing renal accumulation and toxicity with these agents.[124] OATP4C1, which is localized in the basolateral membrane of the proximal tubule, is the first member of the OATP family found to be predominantly expressed in the kidney. OATP4C1 has a wide substrate specificity and is involved in the renal clearance of endogenous compounds, including cAMP, thyroid hormones, estrone 3-sulfate and glycocholic acid, as well as drugs such as the cardiac glycosides digoxin and ouabain, methotrexate, sitagliptin, and remdesivir.[126,127] Protein expression of OATP4C1 in the human kidney cortex is high and similar to that of P-glycoprotein and MATE1.[128] Based

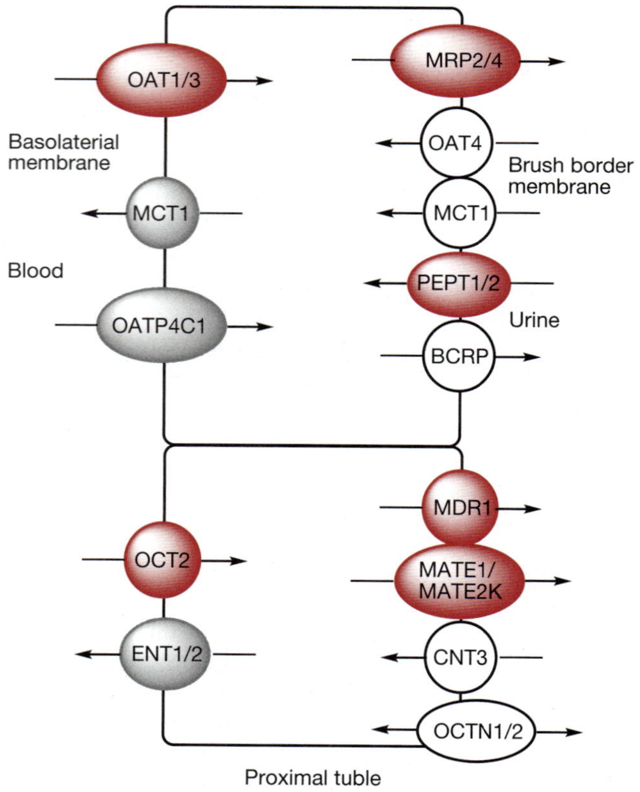

Figure 4.13 Drug transporter expression in the renal proximal tubule. Transporters most relevant to drug disposition are shown in *red*.

RENAL CLEARANCE BY OCT2/ MATE: CISPLATIN TOXICITY

The platinum agents are used clinically for treatment of a variety of cancers. Treatment with cisplatin has been limited by its adverse effects, including nephrotoxicity, ototoxicity, and neurotoxicity.[129] Transport by OCT2 has been attributed with facilitating cisplatin toxicity in the kidney, demonstrated by decreased nephrotoxicity with coadministration of OCT2 inhibitors and in Oct2 knockout animals.[130] Genetic polymorphism in OCT2 has also been correlated with decreased serum creatinine concentrations in patients undergoing cisplatin treatment, suggesting decreased nephrotoxicity.[50] Oxaliplatin, another OCT2 substrate, is not associated with severe nephrotoxicity. Oxaliplatin is efficiently transported by MATE1 and MATE2-K, allowing for secretion of this drug from tubule cells into the urine.[66] Cisplatin is a poor MATE substrate, and cisplatin has been demonstrated to accumulate in renal tubule cells.[131] Carboplatin, another platinum-based agent, is a substrate for neither OCT2 or MATE transporters and, similarly to oxaliplatin, does not display nephrotoxicity.[66] It is apparent that the effects of cisplatin in the kidney can be attributed to OCT2-mediated influx followed by inefficient apical efflux, resulting in renal cell accumulation and toxicity. Recently, OCT2 was also found to be present in the cochlea, and Oct2 knockout prevented cisplatin-induced ototoxicity, along with reducing nephrotoxicity in mice.[132] OCT2 inhibition represents a potentially clinically relevant therapy for the prevention of both toxicities during cisplatin therapy; however selective inhibition of OCT2 over MATE1 is essential.

on limited data, the potential for clinically relevant DDIs appears to be low.

Renal Clearance of Cations

Renal secretion of cations generally involves transport across the basolateral membrane by OCT2 followed by transport across the brush border membrane by MATE1 or possibly P-gp. Cations can be substrates of OATs as well, and MATE1 can also be involved in the secretion of anions.[62] Metformin is a substrate of both OCT2 and MATE1, and drug interactions involving either or both of these transporters results in significant decreases in metformin renal clearance (see Table 4.4).[47,133] As mentioned, inhibitor specificity is often, but not always, shared between OCT2 and MATEs. Genetic variants of both OCT2 and MATE1 have also been correlated with decreased metformin clearance and/or increased glucose-lowering effects with metformin treatment, although conflicting reports exist.[49,64,134] Platinum-based chemotherapeutic agents also use the OCT2/MATE transport system, and this transport is a factor in toxicity of these agents (see "Renal Clearance by OCT2/MATE: Cisplatin Toxicity" section). A highly relevant topic related to drug development is the inhibition of OCT2 or MATEs by compounds leading to increased serum creatinine, due to its decreased active secretion. Creatinine serum concentrations or renal clearance have traditionally been used as a surrogate for measurement of glomerular filtration rate (GFR) and kidney injury. However, it has been recognized that changes in serum creatinine and creatinine clearance can occur without changes in other biomarkers of renal injury or without change in other markers of GFR, such as iohexol or cystatin C, and that renal clearance of creatinine is greater than fup*GFR when measured using these other methods. Creatinine has been shown to be taken up by cationic renal transporters OCT2, MATE1, and MATE-2K, and there are multiple clinical examples in which the administration of drugs that inhibit these transporters result in an elevation of serum creatinine or decrease in creatinine clearance.[135] Therefore, for in vivo inhibitors of OCT2/MATEs, a "pseudotoxicity" of elevated serum creatinine levels without change in kidney function may occur.

ENDOGENOUS SUBSTRATES AS BIOMARKERS OF IN VIVO TRANSPORTER ACTIVITY

Due to lack of specific substrates and inhibitors for use in clinical drug interaction studies, understanding the role of transporters in drug interactions can be challenging. Owing to this, recently, there has been much interest in exploring potential endogenous substrates as selective and sensitive biomarkers of in vivo transporter activity, for understanding drug interactions as well as other factors that may contribute to intersubject variability in in vivo transporter activity. By far, the most clinical data generated to date is that evaluating coproporphyrin 1 (CPI) as a biomarker for OATP1B activity. CPI is metabolically stable and excreted unchanged in bile and, to a lesser extent, in urine. Basal CPI concentrations are higher in subjects with *SLCO1B1* polymorphisms, and several clinical studies have also demonstrated a correlation between change in CPI exposure and that of our clinical OATP1B substrates of interest, primarily the statins.[136-138] Although less clinical data exists, other endogenous substances (including certain bile acid conjugates) also show promise as additional biomarkers for OATP1B activity.[136,139] Biomarkers for both the anionic and cationic renal transporters have also been explored. N1-methylnicotinamide (NMN) is an endogenous substrate for OCT2/MATEs and change in NMN renal clearance has been demonstrated, similar with that of our clinically relevant OCT2/MATE substrate metformin.[140] Although creatinine is also an endogenous OCT2/MATE substrate, and inhibitors may increase serum creatinine, there is still controversy over the role of other transporters, such as OAT2, in creatinine renal secretion.[141] Additionally renal secretion only accounts for 10% to 40% of creatinine renal clearance. Therefore, while inhibition of OCT2/MATE may mildly increase serum creatinine levels, it is not considered a selective or sensitive biomarker for OCT2/MATE function. Potential biomarkers of renal OATs include cortisol metabolites and bile acid conjugates (which are also OATP1B substrates).[142] Therefore, an important stipulation in the measurement of certain renal transporter biomarkers should be noted, specifically the need to collect urine and assess renal clearance since inhibitors may affect nonrenal elimination of the biomarkers.

Blood-Brain Barrier and Blood-Cerebrospinal Fluid Barrier Transport

The BBB serves an important protective function for the central nervous system (CNS) and presents both structural and metabolic barriers for xenobiotic penetration into the brain. The endothelial cells of the BBB form tight junctions with minimal fenestrations, limiting BBB penetration to drug molecules that are capable of transcellular diffusion. For entry of polar or charged essential nutrients such as amino acids and glucose, transport processes are necessary. Transporters present on the BBB for this function have been exploited to facilitate brain penetration of agents like levodopa, one of the most commonly used agents in Parkinson disease, which is transported into the brain by the L-type amino acid transporter (LAT) 1.[143] MCT1 is also expressed at the BBB and along with its role in the renal reabsorption of GHB; it is responsible for distribution of GHB into the brain, where it elicits its euphoric effects.[144] Other influx transporters expressed at the BBB include ENTs and OCTs, which have known drug substrates and may therefore be involved in brain distribution of these drugs.[44] It should be noted that drug concentrations in the brain are not easily measured and changes in brain concentrations do not generally result in any changes in plasma concentrations of the drug, making it difficult to assess the in vivo importance of transporters at the BBB using plasma concentration-time relationships. However, preclinical knockout models are particularly useful in this case, although extrapolation to humans is uncertain because knockout models represent an extreme scenario, and there is the potential for interspecies differences in transporters. These models have aided in assigning a clear limitation of brain penetration to transport by efflux transporters expressed at the BBB, including P-gp, BCRP, and MRPs. Mdr1 knockout mice display substantially higher brain/plasma concentration ratios for many P-gp substrates, with over 10-fold increases exhibited for digoxin, paclitaxel, and protease inhibitors compared to wild-type animals.[145,146] Inhibition of P-gp has been used as a strategy to increase BBB penetration and has been demonstrated to be effective in animal models.[146,147] The use of P-gp inhibitors in studies with human subjects shows similar but much more modest effects on brain penetration. This decreased effect is, in part, due to the lower inhibitor concentrations reached at doses used in human subjects.[148] Bcrp knockout animals have demonstrated the ability of this efflux transporter to limit brain penetration of drugs such as sorafenib.[149] Many anticancer drugs are co-substrates for P-gp and BCRP, and knockout of both transporters has demonstrated synergistic effects on brain accumulation of these drugs.[26,149,150] The use of co-inhibitors represents a potential strategy for improving treatment of brain tumors with these agents.[147] The blood-cerebrospinal fluid (BCSFB) is formed from the choroid plexus, with epithelial cells joined by tight junctions. There are various influx and efflux transporters present on the BCSFB as well, including P-gp and MCT1, as well as others not present at the BBB, such as PEPT2.[44] Given that the CSF occasionally sampled in clinical studies as a surrogate for the rest of the CNS, it is important to recognize there are differences in transporter expression at the BBB and the BCSFB, and even those transporters expressed on both barriers may be present to different extents and may serve different functions. For example, for P-gp substrates it has been shown that P-gp serves to keep drug out of the brain at the BBB, however pumps drug into the CSF, resulting in a disparity in the CSF-to-plasma and brain-to-plasma ratios for P-gp substrates.[44,151,152]

Regulation of Transporters and Interindividual Variability

Extrinsic and intrinsic factors can result in interindividual variability in transporter activity and drug exposure. Drug interactions discussed above are examples of extrinsic factors. Pharmacokinetic variability can also be a result of intrinsic factors such as genetics, gender, age, and disease status. While inherent polymorphisms in transporter genes can be one factor in the interindividual variability of certain transporter substrate pharmacokinetics (see "Transporter Polymorphisms: Role in Statin Disposition" section), other factors such as transcriptional regulation of transporters can also contribute. While there is little evidence of in vivo induction with most transporters, there are nuclear receptors implicated to affect transporter expression in vitro or in human tissue samples.[153,154] One exception among these is P-gp, for which there are multiple examples of in vivo DDIs as a result of induction. Rifampin, a strong agonist of the nuclear receptor pregnane X (PXR), induces the expression of several enzymes and transporters, including CYP3A4 and MDR1. During rifampin treatment, decreased drug exposure is observed with CYP3A4/MDR1 co-substrates such as cyclosporine, calcium-channel blockers, and chemotherapeutic agents, leading to a complete loss of response for some of these substrates.[155,156] Rifampin and other PXR agonists also result in interactions with P-gp substrates that are not metabolized by CYP3A4, such as digoxin (see "Transporter-Drug Interactions: Pgp and Digoxin" section), dabigatran, talinolol, and fexofenadine, demonstrating the in vivo relevance of intestinal P-gp induction.[14,157-159] In vitro and in vivo evidence suggest insignificant induction of OATPs by rifampin.[160] (Note that inhibitor vs inductive effects of rifampin can be determined with single- and multiple-dose rifampin administration, respectively.) Limited evidence suggests constitutive androstane receptor (CAR) activation may induce BCRP and MRP2, as evidenced by expression in the presence of CAR agonists carbamazepine and phenobarbital.[160] While effects at nuclear receptors may be mediated by concomitant drugs, interesting effects on transporter and enzyme regulation also occur in the presence of disease states. As mentioned earlier, during cholestasis, hepatic transporter expression changes to facilitate bile acid secretion into the plasma by MRPs and OSTα/β and decrease secretion into the bile by MRP2 and BSEP. This change in transporter function has been attributed to the effect of bile acids on the farnesoid X receptor (FXR), as well as PXR, causing upregulation of sinusoidal efflux transporters and downregulation of those at the canalicular membrane.[161] Changes in transporter expression and/or activity have also been demonstrated in chronic disease states, including cancer, chronic kidney disease, hepatic insufficiency, inflammation, and epilepsy, which display considerable interindividual variability.[162-164] Current literature supports the involvement of select nuclear receptors in the regulation of affected proteins in some of these conditions.[162] For many disease states, comparative tissue transporter expression data in humans are limited; therefore, changes in activity are interpreted by altered pharmacokinetics of clinical transporter substrates. The identification of endogenous biomarkers has provided additional conclusive evidence regarding certain changes in transporter activity in vivo. Chronic liver disease leads to changes in the expression/activity of many hepatic transporters, and these changes appear to be heterogenous in concordance with the heterogeneity of liver diseases.[165] In particular, it was recently demonstrated the activity of OATP1B is decreased in accordance with liver disease severity, as evidenced by basal levels of OATP1B endogenous biomarkers CPI, which were increased up to 8-fold in severe hepatic impairment.[166] Increased exposure of numerous OATP1B clinical substrates has also been observed in subjects with hepatic impairment.[166] CPI also appears to be mildly elevated in chronic kidney disease, elucidating an effect of renal disease on hepatic transporter function; basal CPI concentrations increase up to about 2-fold in end-stage renal disease, as does exposure to statins.[167] Liver disease can also affect kidney transporter function, as it was recently demonstrated that expression of various renal transporters was affected in kidneys from subjects with varying liver diseases.[168] Chronic renal disease can also affect renal transporter activity, potentially through changes in transporter expression or inhibition of activity by uremic toxins. This has been evidenced by change in the renal secretory clearance for several therapeutic renal OAT substrates in subjects with renal impairment.[169] Interestingly, in subjects with severe renal insufficiency, the decline in secretory clearance was shown to exceed the decline in GFR, demonstrating deviance from the intact nephron hypothesis and suggesting GFR alone may not accurately support dosing adjustments in this population.[169] Along with changes in gene expression or structure, transporter function can also be affected by post-translational modifications, such as glycosylation or phosphorylation, which can lead to rapid changes in transporter activity.[81] Understanding the mechanisms by which transporter functions are altered, including the role of posttranscriptional modifications and regulatory effects with the aforementioned diseases, is continuing to evolve and will aid in the accurate dosing of drugs in patient populations.

Conclusions

Transporters have important roles in the pharmacokinetics of many therapeutic agents. Effects on drug transport can result in drug-drug interactions, nonlinear pharmacokinetics, and interindividual variability. Changes in transporter function can translate into drug toxicity, although transporter interactions also have the potential to be beneficial for drug therapy by increasing bioavailability or decreasing clearance. Application of transport principles and understanding the effects of transport on drug substrate concentrations promote the safe and effective use of therapeutic agents. Further investigation of transporter effects in vivo and mechanisms in vitro is expected to reveal additional significant effects of drug transporters on drug disposition.

References

1. Hoffmann U, Kroemer HK. The ABC transporters MDR1 and MRP2: multiple functions in disposition of xenobiotics and drug resistance. *Drug Metab Rev*. 2004;36(3-4):669-701.
2. Zhou SF. Structure, function and regulation of P-glycoprotein and its clinical relevance in drug disposition. *Xenobiotica*. 2008;38(7-8):802-832.
3. Liu H, Ma Z, Wu B. Structure-activity relationships and in silico models of P-glycoprotein (ABCB1) inhibitors. *Xenobiotica*. 2013;43(11):1018-1026.
4. Giacomini KM, Huang SM, Tweedie DJ, et al. Membrane transporters in drug development. *Nat Rev Drug Discov*. 2010;9(3):215-236.
5. Chan LM, Lowes S, Hirst BH. The ABCs of drug transport in intestine and liver: efflux proteins limiting drug absorption and bioavailability. *Eur J Pharm Sci*. 2004;21(1):25-51.
6. Rengelshausen J, Göggelmann C, Burhenne J, et al. Contribution of increased oral bioavailability and reduced nonglomerular renal clearance of digoxin to the digoxin-clarithromycin interaction. *Br J Clin Pharmacol*. 2003;56(1):32-38.
7. Ding R, Tayrouz Y, Riedel KD, et al. Substantial pharmacokinetic interaction between digoxin and ritonavir in healthy volunteers. *Clin Pharmacol Ther*. 2004;76(1):73-84.
8. Hutson JR, Koren G, Matthews SG. Placental P-glycoprotein and breast cancer resistance protein: influence of polymorphisms on fetal drug exposure and physiology. *Placenta*. 2010;31(5):351-357.
9. Joshi P, Vishwakarma RA, Bharate SB. Natural alkaloids as P-gp inhibitors for multidrug resistance reversal in cancer. *Eur J Med Chem*. 2017;138:273-292.
10. Wolking S, Schaeffeler E, Lerche H, Schwab M, Nies AT. Impact of genetic polymorphisms of ABCB1 (MDR1, P-glycoprotein) on drug disposition and potential clinical implications: update of the literature. *Clin Pharmacokinet*. 2015;54(7):709-735.
11. Dorian P, Strauss M, Cardella C, David T, East S, Ogilvie R. Digoxin-cyclosporine interaction: severe digitalis toxicity after cyclosporine treatment. *Clin Invest Med*. 1988;11(2):108-112.
12. Koren G, Woodland C, Ito S. Toxic digoxin-drug interactions: the major role of renal P-glycoprotein. *Vet Hum Toxicol*. 1998;40(1): 45-46.
13. Hedman A, Angelin B, Arvidsson A, et al. Digoxin-verapamil interaction: reduction of biliary but not renal digoxin clearance in humans. *Clin Pharmacol Ther*. 1991;49(3):256-262.
14. Greiner B, Eichelbaum M, Fritz P, et al. The role of intestinal P-glycoprotein in the interaction of digoxin and rifampin. *J Clin Invest*. 1999;104(2):147-153.
15. Schinkel AH, Jonker JW. Mammalian drug efflux transporters of the ATP binding cassette (ABC) family: an overview. *Adv Drug Deliv Rev*. 2003;55(1):3-29.
16. Masereeuw R, Russel FG. Therapeutic implications of renal anionic drug transporters. *Pharmacol Ther*. 2010;126(2):200-216.
17. Keppler D. The roles of MRP2, MRP3, OATP1B1, and OATP1B3 in conjugated hyperbilirubinemia. *Drug Metab Dispos*. 2014;42(4):561-565.
18. Scheffer GL, Kool M, de Haas M, et al. Tissue distribution and induction of human multidrug resistant protein 3. *Lab Invest*. 2002;82(2):193-201.
19. Drozdzik M, Gröer C, Penski J, et al. Protein abundance of clinically relevant multidrug transporters along the entire length of the human intestine. *Mol Pharm*. 2014;11(10):3547-3555.
20. Köck K, Ferslew BC, Netterberg I, et al. Risk factors for development of cholestatic drug-induced liver injury: inhibition of hepatic basolateral bile acid transporters multidrug resistance-associated proteins 3 and 4. *Drug Metab Dispos*. 2014;42(4):665-674.
21. Keppler D. Multidrug resistance proteins (MRPs, ABCCs): importance for pathophysiology and drug therapy. *Handb Exp Pharmacol*. 2011;(201):299-323.

22. Mao Q, Unadkat JD. Role of the breast cancer resistance protein (BCRP/ABCG2) in drug transport—an update. *AAPS J.* 2015;17(1):65-82.
23. Kruijtzer CM, Beijnen JH, Rosing H, et al. Increased oral bioavailability of topotecan in combination with the breast cancer resistance protein and P-glycoprotein inhibitor GF120918. *J Clin Oncol.* 2002;20(13):2943-2950.
24. Jonker JW, Smit JW, Brinkhuis RF, et al. Role of breast cancer resistance protein in the bioavailability and fetal penetration of topotecan. *J Natl Cancer Inst.* 2000;92(20):1651-1656.
25. Merino G, Jonker JW, Wagenaar E, van Herwaarden AE, Schinkel AH. The breast cancer resistance protein (BCRP/ABCG2) affects pharmacokinetics, hepatobiliary excretion, and milk secretion of the antibiotic nitrofurantoin. *Mol Pharmacol.* 2005;67(5):1758-1764.
26. Kodaira H, Kusuhara H, Ushiki J, Fuse E, Sugiyama Y. Kinetic analysis of the cooperation of P-glycoprotein (P-gp/Abcb1) and breast cancer resistance protein (Bcrp/Abcg2) in limiting the brain and testis penetration of erlotinib, flavopiridol, and mitoxantrone. *J Pharmacol Exp Ther.* 2010;333(3):788-796.
27. Taguchi T, Masuo Y, Kogi T, Nakamichi N, Kato Y. Characterization of long-lasting OATP inhibition by typical inhibitor cyclosporine A and in vitro-in vivo discrepancy in its drug interaction potential in rats. *J Pharm Sci.* 2016;105(7):2231-2239.
28. Shitara Y, Sugiyama Y. Preincubation-dependent and long-lasting inhibition of organic anion transporting polypeptide (OATP) and its impact on drug-drug interactions. *Pharmacol Ther.* 2017; 177:67-80.
29. Nozaki Y, Izumi S. Preincubation time-dependent, long-lasting inhibition of drug transporters and impact on the prediction of drug-drug interactions. *Drug Metab Dispos.* 2023;51(9):1077-1088.
30. Kalliokoski A, Niemi M. Impact of OATP transporters on pharmacokinetics. *Br J Pharmacol.* 2009;158(3):693-705.
31. SEARCH Collaborative Group, Link E, Parish S, et al., SLCO1B1 variants and statin-induced myopathy—a genomewide study. *N Engl J Med.* 2008;359(8):789-799.
32. Turner RM, Fontana V, Zhang JE, et al. A genome-wide association study of circulating levels of atorvastatin and its major metabolites. *Clin Pharmacol Ther.* 2020;108(2):287-297.
33. Keskitalo JE, Zolk O, Fromm MF, Kurkinen KJ, Neuvonen PJ, Niemi M. ABCG2 polymorphism markedly affects the pharmacokinetics of atorvastatin and rosuvastatin. *Clin Pharmacol Ther.* 2009;86(2):197-203.
34. Lee HK, Hu M, Lui SS, Ho CS, Wong CK, Tomlinson B. Effects of polymorphisms in ABCG2, SLCO1B1, SLC10A1 and CYP2C9/19 on plasma concentrations of rosuvastatin and lipid response in Chinese patients. *Pharmacogenomics.* 2013;14(11):1283-1294.
35. DeGorter MK, Tirona RG, Schwarz UI, et al. Clinical and pharmacogenetic predictors of circulating atorvastatin and rosuvastatin concentrations in routine clinical care. *Circ Cardiovasc Genet.* 2013;6(4):400-408.
36. Ishiguro N, Maeda K, Kishimoto W, et al. Predominant contribution of OATP1B3 to the hepatic uptake of telmisartan, an angiotensin II receptor antagonist, in humans. *Drug Metab Dispos.* 2006;34(7):1109-1115.
37. Nakanishi T, Tamai I. Roles of organic anion transporting polypeptide 2A1 (OATP2A1/SLCO2A1) in regulating the pathophysiological actions of prostaglandins. *AAPS J.* 2017;20(1):13.
38. Kashihara Y, Ieiri I, Yoshikado T, et al. Small-dosing clinical study: pharmacokinetic, pharmacogenomic (SLCO2B1 and ABCG2), and interaction (atorvastatin and grapefruit juice) profiles of 5 probes for OATP2B1 and BCRP. *J Pharm Sci.* 2017;106(9):2688-2694.
39. Chu XY, Bleasby K, Yabut J, et al. Transport of the dipeptidyl peptidase-4 inhibitor sitagliptin by human organic anion transporter 3, organic anion transporting polypeptide 4C1, and multidrug resistance P-glycoprotein. *J Pharmacol Exp Ther.* 2007;321(2):673-683.
40. Ekaratanawong S, Anzai N, Jutabha P, et al. Human organic anion transporter 4 is a renal apical organic anion/dicarboxylate exchanger in the proximal tubules. *J Pharmacol Sci.* 2004;94(3):297-304.
41. Cheng Y, Vapurcuyan A, Shahidullah M, Aleksunes LM, Pelis RM. Expression of organic anion transporter 2 in the human kidney and its potential role in the tubular secretion of guanine-containing antiviral drugs. *Drug Metab Dispos.* 2012;40(3):617-624.
42. Cimoch PJ, Lavelle J, Pollard R, et al. Pharmacokinetics of oral ganciclovir alone and in combination with zidovudine, didanosine, and probenecid in HIV-infected subjects. *J Acquir Immune Defic Syndr Hum Retrovirol.* 1998;17(3):227-234.
43. Laskin OL, de Miranda P, King DH, et al. Effects of probenecid on the pharmacokinetics and elimination of acyclovir in humans. *Antimicrob Agents Chemother.* 1982;21(5):804-807.
44. Morris ME, Rodriguez-Cruz V, Felmlee MA. SLC and ABC transporters: expression, localization, and species differences at the blood-brain and the blood-cerebrospinal fluid barriers. *AAPS J.* 2017;19(5):1317-1331.
45. Lozano E, Herraez E, Briz O, et al. Role of the plasma membrane transporter of organic cations OCT1 and its genetic variants in modern liver pharmacology. *Biomed Res Int.* 2013;2013:692071.
46. Morse BL, Kolur A, Hudson LR, et al. Pharmacokinetics of organic cation transporter 1 (OCT1) substrates in Oct1/2 knockout mice and species difference in hepatic OCT1-mediated uptake. *Drug Metab Dispos.* 2020;48(2):93-105.
47. Somogyi A, Stockley C, Keal J, Rolan P, Bochner F. Reduction of metformin renal tubular secretion by cimetidine in man. *Br J Clin Pharmacol.* 1987;23(5):545-551.
48. Song IS, Shin HJ, Shim EJ, et al. Genetic variants of the organic cation transporter 2 influence the disposition of metformin. *Clin Pharmacol Ther.* 2008;84(5):559-562.
49. Hou W, Zhang D, Lu W, et al. Polymorphism of organic cation transporter 2 improves glucose-lowering effect of metformin via influencing its pharmacokinetics in Chinese type 2 diabetic patients. *Mol Diagn Ther.* 2015;19(1):25-33.
50. Filipski KK, Mathijssen RH, Mikkelsen TS, Schinkel AH, Sparreboom A. Contribution of organic cation transporter 2 (OCT2) to cisplatin-induced nephrotoxicity. *Clin Pharmacol Ther.* 2009;86(4):396-402.
51. Ganapathy V, Prasad PD. Role of transporters in placental transfer of drugs. *Toxicol Appl Pharmacol.* 2005;207(2 suppl):381-387.
52. Ciarimboli G. Organic cation transporters. *Xenobiotica.* 2008;38(7-8):936-971.
53. Huang KM, Zavorka Thomas M, Magdy T, et al. Targeting OCT3 attenuates doxorubicin-induced cardiac injury. *Proc Natl Acad Sci U S A.* 2021;118(5):e2020168118.
54. Koepsell H, Lips K, Volk C. Polyspecific organic cation transporters: structure, function, physiological roles, and biopharmaceutical implications. *Pharm Res.* 2007;24(7):1227-1251.
55. Tamai I. Pharmacological and pathophysiological roles of carnitine/organic cation transporters (OCTNs: SLC22A4, SLC22A5 and Slc22a21). *Biopharm Drug Dispos.* 2013;34(1):29-44.
56. Wu SP, Shyu MK, Liou HH, Gau CS, Lin CJ. Interaction between anticonvulsants and human placental carnitine transporter. *Epilepsia.* 2004;45(3):204-210.
57. Tein I. Carnitine transport: pathophysiology and metabolism of known molecular defects. *J Inherit Metab Dis.* 2003;26(2-3):147-169.
58. Nakanishi T, Hasegawa Y, Haruta T, Wakayama T, Tamai I. In vivo evidence of organic cation transporter-mediated tracheal accumulation of the anticholinergic agent ipratropium in mice. *J Pharm Sci.* 2013;102(9):3373-3381.
59. Wang G, Chen H, Zhao D, et al. Combination of l-carnitine with lipophilic linkage-donating gemcitabine derivatives as intestinal

novel organic cation transporter 2-targeting oral prodrugs. *J Med Chem.* 2017;60(6):2552-2561.
60. Prasad B, Johnson K, Billington S, et al. Abundance of drug transporters in the human kidney cortex as quantified by quantitative targeted proteomics. *Drug Metab Dispos.* 2016;44(12):1920-1924.
61. Tsuda M, Terada T, Mizuno T, Katsura T, Shimakura J, Inui K. Targeted disruption of the multidrug and toxin extrusion 1 (mate1) gene in mice reduces renal secretion of metformin. *Mol Pharmacol.* 2009;75(6):1280-1286.
62. Nies AT, Damme K, Kruck S, Schaeffeler E, Schwab M. Structure and function of multidrug and toxin extrusion proteins (MATEs) and their relevance to drug therapy and personalized medicine. *Arch Toxicol.* 2016;90(7):1555-1584.
63. Hume WE, Shingaki T, Takashima T, et al. The synthesis and biodistribution of [(11)C]metformin as a PET probe to study hepatobiliary transport mediated by the multi-drug and toxin extrusion transporter 1 (MATE1) in vivo. *Bioorg Med Chem.* 2013;21(24):7584-7590.
64. Stocker SL, Morrissey KM, Yee SW, et al. The effect of novel promoter variants in MATE1 and MATE2 on the pharmacokinetics and pharmacodynamics of metformin. *Clin Pharmacol Ther.* 2013;93(2):186-194.
65. Nies AT, Koepsell H, Damme K, Schwab M. Organic cation transporters (OCTs, MATEs), in vitro and in vivo evidence for the importance in drug therapy. *Handb Exp Pharmacol.* 2011;(201):105-167.
66. Yonezawa A, Inui K. Organic cation transporter OCT/SLC22A and H(+)/organic cation antiporter MATE/SLC47A are key molecules for nephrotoxicity of platinum agents. *Biochem Pharmacol.* 2011;81(5):563-568.
67. Tanihara Y, Masuda S, Sato T, Katsura T, Ogawa O, Inui K. Substrate specificity of MATE1 and MATE2-K, human multidrug and toxin extrusions/H(+)-organic cation antiporters. *Biochem Pharmacol.* 2007;74(2):359-371.
68. Merezhinskaya N, Fishbein WN. Monocarboxylate transporters: past, present, and future. *Histol Histopathol.* 2009;24(2):243-264.
69. Varma MV, Ambler CM, Ullah M, et al. Targeting intestinal transporters for optimizing oral drug absorption. *Curr Drug Metab.* 2010;11(9):730-742.
70. Kennedy KM, Dewhirst MW. Tumor metabolism of lactate: the influence and therapeutic potential for MCT and CD147 regulation. *Future Oncol.* 2010;6(1):127-148.
71. Morris ME, Hu K, Wang Q. Renal clearance of gamma-hydroxybutyric acid in rats: increasing renal elimination as a detoxification strategy. *J Pharmacol Exp Ther.* 2005;313(3):1194-1202.
72. Morris ME, Morse BL, Baciewicz GJ, et al. Monocarboxylate transporter inhibition with osmotic diuresis increases gamma-hydroxybutyrate renal elimination in humans: a proof-of-concept study. *J Clin Toxicol.* 2011;1(2):1000105.
73. Jones RS, Morris ME. Monocarboxylate transporters: therapeutic targets and prognostic factors in disease. *Clin Pharmacol Ther.* 2016;100(5):454-463.
74. Felmlee MA, Jones RS, Rodriguez-Cruz V, Follman KE, Morris ME. Monocarboxylate transporters (SLC16): function, regulation, and role in health and disease. *Pharmacol Rev.* 2020;72(2):466-485.
75. Cundy KC, Sastry S, Luo W, Zou J, Moors TL, Canafax DM. Clinical pharmacokinetics of XP13512, a novel transported prodrug of gabapentin. *J Clin Pharmacol.* 2008;48(12):1378-1388.
76. Rubio-Aliaga I, Daniel H. Peptide transporters and their roles in physiological processes and drug disposition. *Xenobiotica.* 2008;38(7-8):1022-1042.
77. Herrera-Ruiz D, Wang Q, Gudmundsson OS, et al. Spatial expression patterns of peptide transporters in the human and rat gastrointestinal tracts, Caco-2 in vitro cell culture model, and multiple human tissues. *AAPS PharmSci.* 2001;3(1):E9.
78. Huber-Ruano I, Pastor-Anglada M. Transport of nucleoside analogs across the plasma membrane: a clue to understanding drug-induced cytotoxicity. *Curr Drug Metab.* 2009;10(4):347-358.
79. Endres CJ, Moss AM, Govindarajan R, Choi DS, Unadkat JD. The role of nucleoside transporters in the erythrocyte disposition and oral absorption of ribavirin in the wild-type and equilibrative nucleoside transporter 1-/- mice. *J Pharmacol Exp Ther.* 2009;331(1):287-296.
80. Cerveny L, Ptackova Z, Ceckova M, et al. Equilibrative nucleoside transporter 1 (ENT1, SLC29A1) facilitates transfer of the antiretroviral drug abacavir across the placenta. *Drug Metab Disp. 2018*;46(11):1817-1826.
81. Stieger B. The role of the sodium-taurocholate cotransporting polypeptide (NTCP) and of the bile salt export pump (BSEP) in physiology and pathophysiology of bile formation. *Handb Exp Pharmacol.* 2011;(201):205-259.
82. Dong Z, Ekins S, Polli JE. Structure-activity relationship for FDA approved drugs as inhibitors of the human sodium taurocholate cotransporting polypeptide (NTCP). *Mol Pharm.* 2013;10(3):1008-1019.
83. Dawson S, Stahl S, Paul N, Barber J, Kenna JG. In vitro inhibition of the bile salt export pump correlates with risk of cholestatic drug-induced liver injury in humans. *Drug Metab Dispos.* 2012;40(1):130-138.
84. Schaffner CA, Mwinyi J, Gai Z, Thasler WE, Eloranta JJ, Kullak-Ublick GA. The organic solute transporters alpha and beta are induced by hypoxia in human hepatocytes. *Liver Int.* 2015;35(4):1152-1161.
85. Morgan RE, van Staden CJ, Chen Y, et al. A multifactorial approach to hepatobiliary transporter assessment enables improved therapeutic compound development. *Toxicol Sci.* 2013;136(1):216-241.
86. Chen L, Yao X, Young A, et al. Inhibition of apical sodium-dependent bile acid transporter as a novel treatment for diabetes. *Am J Physiol Endocrinol Metab.* 2012;302(1):E68-E76.
87. Amidon GL, Lennernäs H, Shah VP, Crison JR. A theoretical basis for a biopharmaceutic drug classification: the correlation of in vitro drug product dissolution and in vivo bioavailability. *Pharm Res.* 1995;12(3):413-420.
88. Shugarts S, Benet LZ. The role of transporters in the pharmacokinetics of orally administered drugs. *Pharm Res.* 2009;26(9):2039-2054.
89. Drozdzik M, Busch D, Lapczuk J, et al. Protein abundance of clinically relevant drug transporters in the human liver and intestine: a comparative analysis in paired tissue specimens. *Clin Pharmacol Ther.* 2019;105(5):1204-1212.
90. Benet LZ. The drug transporter-metabolism alliance: uncovering and defining the interplay. *Mol Pharm.* 2009;6(6):1631-1643.
91. Shi S, Li Y. Interplay of drug-metabolizing enzymes and transporters in drug absorption and disposition. *Curr Drug Metab.* 2014;15(10):915-941.
92. Mealey KL. Therapeutic implications of the MDR-1 gene. *J Vet Pharmacol Ther.* 2004;27(5):257-264.
93. Costales C, Lin J, Kimoto E, et al. Quantitative prediction of breast cancer resistant protein mediated drug-drug interactions using physiologically-based pharmacokinetic modeling. *CPT Pharmacometrics Syst Pharmacol.* 2021;10(9):1018-1031.
94. Bolger MB, Lukacova V, Woltosz WS. Simulations of the nonlinear dose dependence for substrates of influx and efflux transporters in the human intestine. *AAPS J.* 2009;11(2):353-363.
95. Johnson M, Patel D, Matheny C, Ho M, Chen L, Ellens H. Inhibition of intestinal OATP2B1 by the calcium receptor antagonist ronacaleret results in a significant drug-drug interaction by causing a 2-fold decrease in exposure of rosuvastatin. *Drug Metab Dispos.* 2017;45(1):27-34.
96. Keiser M, Kaltheuner L, Wildberg C, et al. The organic anion-transporting peptide 2B1 is localized in the basolateral membrane

of the human jejunum and Caco-2 monolayers. *J Pharm Sci*. 2017;106(9):2657-2663.
97. Dresser GK, Kim RB, Bailey DG. Effect of grapefruit juice volume on the reduction of fexofenadine bioavailability: possible role of organic anion transporting polypeptides. *Clin Pharmacol Ther*. 2005;77(3):170-177.
98. Shirasaka Y, Suzuki K, Nakanishi T, Tamai I. Differential effect of grapefruit juice on intestinal absorption of statins due to inhibition of organic anion transporting polypeptide and/or P-glycoprotein. *J Pharm Sci*. 2011;100(9):3843-3853.
99. Varma MV, Steyn SJ, Allerton C, El-Kattan AF. Predicting clearance mechanism in drug discovery: Extended Clearance Classification System (ECCS). *Pharm Res*. 2015;32(12):3785-3802.
100. Zuegge J, Schneider G, Coassolo P, Lavé T. Prediction of hepatic metabolic clearance: comparison and assessment of prediction models. *Clin Pharmacokinet*. 2001;40(7):553-563.
101. Backman JT, Kyrklund C, Neuvonen M, Neuvonen PJ. Gemfibrozil greatly increases plasma concentrations of cerivastatin. *Clin Pharmacol Ther*. 2002;72(6):685-691.
102. Shitara Y, Hirano M, Sato H, Sugiyama Y. Gemfibrozil and its glucuronide inhibit the organic anion transporting polypeptide 2 (OATP2/OATP1B1:SLC21A6)-mediated hepatic uptake and CYP2C8-mediated metabolism of cerivastatin: analysis of the mechanism of the clinically relevant drug-drug interaction between cerivastatin and gemfibrozil. *J Pharmacol Exp Ther*. 2004;311(1):228-236.
103. Schneck DW, Birmingham BK, Zalikowski JA, et al. The effect of gemfibrozil on the pharmacokinetics of rosuvastatin. *Clin Pharmacol Ther*. 2004;75(5):455-463.
104. Kostapanos MS, Milionis HJ, Elisaf MS. Rosuvastatin-associated adverse effects and drug-drug interactions in the clinical setting of dyslipidemia. *Am J Cardiovasc Drugs*. 2010;10(1):11-28.
105. Neuvonen PJ, Niemi M, Backman JT. Drug interactions with lipid-lowering drugs: mechanisms and clinical relevance. *Clin Pharmacol Ther*. 2006;80(6):565-581.
106. Lau YY, Huang Y, Frassetto L, Benet LZ. Effect of OATP1B transporter inhibition on the pharmacokinetics of atorvastatin in healthy volunteers. *Clin Pharmacol Ther*. 2007;81(2):194-204.
107. Fahrmayr C, Fromm MF, Konig J. Hepatic OATP and OCT uptake transporters: their role for drug-drug interactions and pharmacogenetic aspects. *Drug Metab Rev*. 2010;42(3):380-401.
108. Matthaei J, Kuron D, Faltraco F, et al. OCT1 mediates hepatic uptake of sumatriptan and loss-of-function OCT1 polymorphisms affect sumatriptan pharmacokinetics. *Clin Pharmacol Ther*. 2016;99(6):633-641.
109. Tzvetkov MV, Saadatmand AR, Bokelmann K, Meineke I, Kaiser R, Brockmöller J. Effects of OCT1 polymorphisms on the cellular uptake, plasma concentrations and efficacy of the 5-HT(3) antagonists tropisetron and ondansetron. *Pharmacogenomics J*. 2012;12(1):22-29.
110. Tzvetkov MV, dos Santos Pereira JN, Meineke I, Saadatmand AR, Stingl JC, Brockmöller J. Morphine is a substrate of the organic cation transporter OCT1 and polymorphisms in OCT1 gene affect morphine pharmacokinetics after codeine administration. *Biochem Pharmacol*. 2013;86(5):666-678.
111. Shu Y, Sheardown SA, Brown C, et al. Effect of genetic variation in the organic cation transporter 1 (OCT1) on metformin action. *J Clin Invest*. 2007;117(5):1422-1431.
112. Cho SK, Kim CO, Park ES, Chung JY. Verapamil decreases the glucose-lowering effect of metformin in healthy volunteers. *Br J Clin Pharmacol*. 2014;78(6):1426-1432.
113. Angelin B, Arvidsson A, Dahlqvist R, Hedman A, Schenck-Gustafsson K. Quinidine reduces biliary clearance of digoxin in man. *Eur J Clin Invest*. 1987;17(3):262-265.
114. van Asperen J, van Tellingen O, Beijnen JH. The role of mdr1a P-glycoprotein in the biliary and intestinal secretion of doxorubicin and vinblastine in mice. *Drug Metab Dispos*. 2000;28(3):264-267.
115. Vlaming ML, Mohrmann K, Wagenaar E, et al. Carcinogen and anticancer drug transport by Mrp2 in vivo: studies using Mrp2 (Abcc2) knockout mice. *J Pharmacol Exp Ther*. 2006;318(1):319-327.
116. Yamazaki M, Akiyama S, Ni'inuma K, Nishigaki R, Sugiyama Y. Biliary excretion of pravastatin in rats: contribution of the excretion pathway mediated by canalicular multispecific organic anion transporter. *Drug Metab Dispos*. 1997;25(10):1123-1129.
117. Yamashiro W, Maeda K, Hirouchi M, Adachi Y, Hu Z, Sugiyama Y. Involvement of transporters in the hepatic uptake and biliary excretion of valsartan, a selective antagonist of the angiotensin II AT1-receptor, in humans. *Drug Metab Dispos*. 2006;34(7):1247-1254.
118. Kuypers DR, Ekberg H, Grinyó J, et al. Mycophenolic acid exposure after administration of mycophenolate mofetil in the presence and absence of cyclosporin in renal transplant recipients. *Clin Pharmacokinet*. 2009;48(5):329-341.
119. Zamek-Gliszczynski MJ, Nezasa K, Tian X, et al. The important role of Bcrp (Abcg2) in the biliary excretion of sulfate and glucuronide metabolites of acetaminophen, 4-methylumbelliferone, and harmol in mice. *Mol Pharmacol*. 2006;70(6):2127-2133.
120. Chen C, Hennig GE, Manautou JE. Hepatobiliary excretion of acetaminophen glutathione conjugate and its derivatives in transport-deficient (TR-) hyperbilirubinemic rats. *Drug Metab Dispos*. 2003;31(6):798-804.
121. Ando T, Kusuhara H, Merino G, Alvarez AI, Schinkel AH, Sugiyama Y. Involvement of breast cancer resistance protein (ABCG2) in the biliary excretion mechanism of fluoroquinolones. *Drug Metab Dispos*. 2007;35(10):1873-1879.
122. Walshaw PE, McCauley FA, Wilson TW. Diuretic and non-diuretic actions of furosemide: effects of probenecid. *Clin Invest Med*. 1992;15(1):82-87.
123. Honari J, Blair AD, Cutler RE. Effects of probenecid on furosemide kinetics and natriuresis in man. *Clin Pharmacol Ther*. 1977;22(4):395-401.
124. Imaoka T, Kusuhara H, Adachi M, Schuetz JD, Takeuchi K, Sugiyama Y. Functional involvement of multidrug resistance-associated protein 4 (MRP4/ABCC4) in the renal elimination of the antiviral drugs adefovir and tenofovir. *Mol Pharmacol*. 2007;71(2):619-627.
125. Morelle J, Labriola L, Lambert M, Cosyns JP, Jouret F, Jadoul M. Tenofovir-related acute kidney injury and proximal tubule dysfunction precipitated by diclofenac: a case of drug-drug interaction. *Clin Nephrol*. 2009;71(5):567-570.
126. Sato T, Maekawa M, Mano N, Abe T, Yamaguchi H. Role of OATP4C1 in renal handling of remdesivir and its nucleoside analog GS-441524: the first approved drug for patients with COVID-19. *J Pharm Pharm Sci*. 2021;24:227-236.
127. Sato T, Mishima E, Mano N, Abe T, Yamaguchi H. Potential drug interactions mediated by renal organic anion transporter OATP4C1. *J Pharmacol Exp Ther*. 2017;362(2):271-277.
128. Al-Majdoub ZM, Scotcher D, Achour B, Barber J, Galetin A, Rostami-Hodjegan A. Quantitative proteomic map of enzymes and transporters in the human kidney: stepping closer to mechanistic kidney models to define local kinetics. *Clin Pharmacol Ther*. 2021;110(5):1389-1400.
129. de Jongh FE, van Veen RN, Veltman SJ, et al. Weekly high-dose cisplatin is a feasible treatment option: analysis on prognostic factors for toxicity in 400 patients. *Br J Cancer*. 2003;88(8):1199-1206.
130. Katsuda H, Yamashita M, Katsura H, et al. Protecting cisplatin-induced nephrotoxicity with cimetidine does not affect antitumor activity. *Biol Pharm Bull*. 2010;33(11):1867-1871.
131. Yokoo S, Yonezawa A, Masuda S, Fukatsu A, Katsura T, Inui K. Differential contribution of organic cation transporters, OCT2 and MATE1, in platinum agent-induced nephrotoxicity. *Biochem Pharmacol*. 2007;74(3):477-487.
132. Ciarimboli G, Deuster D, Knief A, et al. Organic cation transporter 2 mediates cisplatin-induced oto- and

nephrotoxicity and is a target for protective interventions. *Am J Pathol*. 2010;176(3):1169-1180.
133. Elsby R, Chidlaw S, Outteridge S, et al. Mechanistic in vitro studies confirm that inhibition of the renal apical efflux transporter multidrug and toxin extrusion (MATE) 1, and not altered absorption, underlies the increased metformin exposure observed in clinical interactions with cimetidine, trimethoprim or pyrimethamine. *Pharmacol Res Perspect*. 2017;5(5):e00357.
134. Chen Y, Li S, Brown C, et al. Effect of genetic variation in the organic cation transporter 2 on the renal elimination of metformin. *Pharmacogenet Genomics*. 2009;19(7):497-504.
135. Chu X, Bleasby K, Chan GH, Nunes I, Evers R. The complexities of interpreting reversible elevated serum creatinine levels in drug development: does a correlation with inhibition of renal transporters exist? *Drug Metab Dispos*. 2016;44(9):1498-1509.
136. Mori D, Kimoto E, Rago B, et al. Dose-dependent inhibition of OATP1B by rifampicin in healthy volunteers: comprehensive evaluation of candidate biomarkers and OATP1B probe drugs. *Clin Pharmacol Ther*. 2020;107(4):1004-1013.
137. Mochizuki T, Zamek-Gliszczynski MJ, Yoshida K, et al. Effect of cyclosporin A and impact of dose staggering on OATP1B1/1B3 endogenous substrates and drug probes for assessing clinical drug interactions. *Clin Pharmacol Ther*. 2022;111(6):1315-1323.
138. Neuvonen M, Tornio A, Hirvensalo P, Backman JT, Niemi M. Performance of plasma coproporphyrin I and III as OATP1B1 biomarkers in humans. *Clin Pharmacol Ther*. 2021;110(6):1622-1632.
139. Neuvonen M, Hirvensalo P, Tornio A, et al. Identification of glycochenodeoxycholate 3-O-glucuronide and glycodeoxycholate 3-O-glucuronide as highly sensitive and specific OATP1B1 biomarkers. *Clin Pharmacol Ther*. 2021;109(3):646-657.
140. Muller F, Pontones CA, Renner B, et al. N(1)-methylnicotinamide as an endogenous probe for drug interactions by renal cation transporters: studies on the metformin-trimethoprim interaction. *Eur J Clin Pharmacol*. 2015;71(1):85-94.
141. Shen H, Liu T, Morse BL, et al. Characterization of organic anion transporter 2 (SLC22A7): a highly efficient transporter for creatinine and species-dependent renal tubular expression. *Drug Metab Dispos*. 2015;43(7):984-993.
142. Chu X, Liao M, Shen H, et al. Clinical probes and endogenous biomarkers as substrates for transporter drug-drug interaction evaluation: perspectives from the international transporter consortium. *Clin Pharmacol Ther*. 2018;104(5):836-864.
143. Pinho MJ, Serrão MP, Gomes P, Hopfer U, Jose PA, Soares-da-Silva P. Over-expression of renal LAT1 and LAT2 and enhanced L-DOPA uptake in SHR immortalized renal proximal tubular cells. *Kidney Int*. 2004;66(1):216-226.
144. Roiko SA, Felmlee MA, Morris ME. Brain uptake of the drug of abuse gamma-hydroxybutyric acid in rats. *Drug Metab Dispos*. 2012;40(1):212-218.
145. Schinkel AH, Wagenaar E, van Deemter L, Mol CA, Borst P. Absence of the mdr1a P-glycoprotein in mice affects tissue distribution and pharmacokinetics of dexamethasone, digoxin, and cyclosporin A. *J Clin Invest*. 1995;96(4):1698-1705.
146. Kemper EM, van Zandbergen AE, Cleypool C, et al. Increased penetration of paclitaxel into the brain by inhibition of P-glycoprotein. *Clin Cancer Res*. 2003;9(7):2849-2855.
147. Breedveld P, Beijnen JH, Schellens JH. Use of P-glycoprotein and BCRP inhibitors to improve oral bioavailability and CNS penetration of anticancer drugs. *Trends Pharmacol Sci*. 2006;27(1):17-24.
148. Eyal S, Ke B, Muzi M, et al. Regional P-glycoprotein activity and inhibition at the human blood-brain barrier as imaged by positron emission tomography. *Clin Pharmacol Ther*. 2010;87(5):579-585.
149. Agarwal S, Sane R, Ohlfest JR, Elmquist WF. The role of the breast cancer resistance protein (ABCG2) in the distribution of sorafenib to the brain. *J Pharmacol Exp Ther*. 2011;336(1):223-233.
150. Zhou L, Schmidt K, Nelson FR, Zelesky V, Troutman MD, Feng B. The effect of breast cancer resistance protein and P-glycoprotein on the brain penetration of flavopiridol, imatinib mesylate (Gleevec), prazosin, and 2-methoxy-3-(4-(2-(5-methyl-2-phenyloxazol-4-yl)ethoxy) phenyl)propanoic acid (PF-407288) in mice. *Drug Metab Dispos*. 2009;37(5):946-955.
151. Shen J, Carcaboso AM, Hubbard KE, et al. Compartment-specific roles of ATP-binding cassette transporters define differential topotecan distribution in brain parenchyma and cerebrospinal fluid. *Cancer Res*. 2009;69(14):5885-5892.
152. Venkatakrishnan K, Tseng E, Nelson FR, et al. Central nervous system pharmacokinetics of the Mdr1 P-glycoprotein substrate CP-615,003: intersite differences and implications for human receptor occupancy projections from cerebrospinal fluid exposures. *Drug Metab Dispos*. 2007;35(8):1341-1349.
153. Tirona RG. Molecular mechanisms of drug transporter regulation. *Handb Exp Pharmacol*. 2011;(201):373-402.
154. Klaassen CD, Aleksunes LM. Xenobiotic, bile acid, and cholesterol transporters: function and regulation. *Pharmacol Rev*. 2010;62(1):1-96.
155. Harmsen S, Meijerman I, Beijnen JH, Schellens JH. The role of nuclear receptors in pharmacokinetic drug-drug interactions in oncology. *Cancer Treat Rev*. 2007;33(4):369-380.
156. Niemi M, Backman JT, Fromm MF, Neuvonen PJ, Kivistö KT. Pharmacokinetic interactions with rifampicin: clinical relevance. *Clin Pharmacokinet*. 2003;42(9):819-850.
157. Härtter S, Koenen-Bergmann M, Sharma A, et al. Decrease in the oral bioavailability of dabigatran etexilate after co-medication with rifampicin. *Br J Clin Pharmacol*. 2012;74(3):490-500.
158. Westphal K, Weinbrenner A, Zschiesche M, et al. Induction of P-glycoprotein by rifampin increases intestinal secretion of talinolol in human beings: a new type of drug/drug interaction. *Clin Pharmacol Ther*. 2000;68(4):345-355.
159. Bosilkovska M, Samer CF, Déglon J, et al. Geneva cocktail for cytochrome p450 and P-glycoprotein activity assessment using dried blood spots. *Clin Pharmacol Ther*. 2014;96(3):349-359.
160. Rodrigues AD, Lai Y, Shen H, Varma MVS, Rowland A, Oswald S. Induction of human intestinal and hepatic organic anion transporting polypeptides: where is the evidence for its relevance in drug-drug interactions? *Drug Metab Dispos*. 2020;48(3):205-216.
161. Jonker JW, Liddle C, Downes M. FXR and PXR: potential therapeutic targets in cholestasis. *J Steroid Biochem Mol Biol*. 2012;130(3-5):147-158.
162. Morgan ET, Goralski KB, Piquette-Miller M, et al. Regulation of drug-metabolizing enzymes and transporters in infection, inflammation, and cancer. *Drug Metab Dispos*. 2008;36(2):205-216.
163. Dreisbach AW. The influence of chronic renal failure on drug metabolism and transport. *Clin Pharmacol Ther*. 2009;86(5):553-556.
164. Potschka H. Modulating P-glycoprotein regulation: future perspectives for pharmacoresistant epilepsies? *Epilepsia*. 2010;51(8):1333-1347.
165. Chu X, Prasad B, Neuhoff S, et al. Clinical implications of altered drug transporter abundance/function and PBPK modeling in specific populations: an ITC perspective. *Clin Pharmacol Ther*. 2022;112(3):501-526.
166. Lin J, Kimoto E, Yamazaki S, et al. Effect of hepatic impairment on OATP1B activity: quantitative pharmacokinetic analysis of endogenous biomarker and substrate drugs. *Clin Pharmacol Ther*. 2023;113(5):1058-1069.
167. Tatosian DA, Yee KL, Zhang Z, et al. A microdose cocktail to evaluate drug interactions in patients with renal impairment. *Clin Pharmacol Ther*. 2021;109(2):403-415.
168. Frost KL, Jilek JL, Sinari S, et al. Renal transporter alterations in patients with chronic liver diseases: nonalcoholic steatohepatitis, alcohol-associated, viral hepatitis, and alcohol-viral combination. *Drug Metab Dispos*. 2023;51(2):155-164.
169. Tan SPF, Scotcher D, Rostami-Hodjegan A, Galetin A. Effect of chronic kidney disease on the renal secretion via organic anion transporters 1/3: implications for physiologically-based pharmacokinetic modeling and dose adjustment. *Clin Pharmacol Ther*. 2022;112(3):643-652.

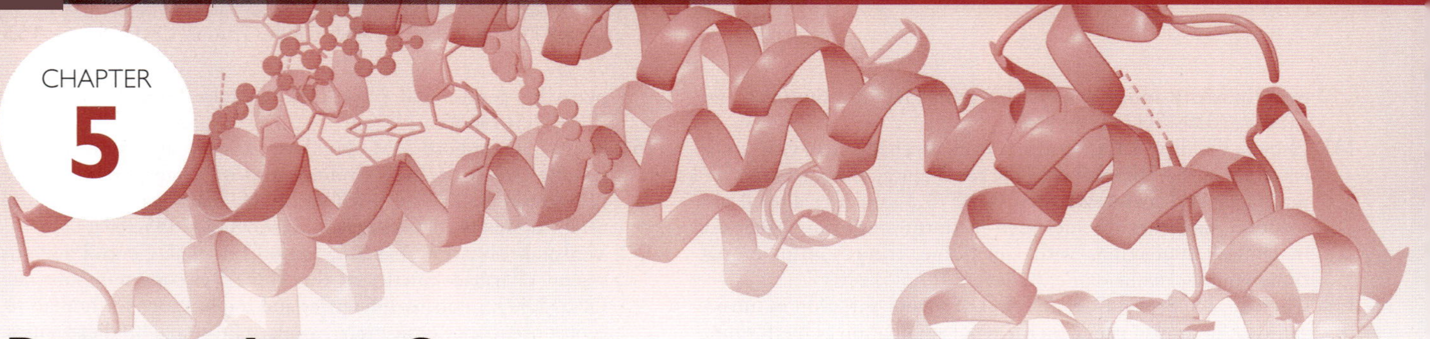

CHAPTER 5

Principles of Biotechnology-Derived Drugs

Tanaji T. Talele and Vijaya L. Korlipara

Drugs covered in this chapter:

- Abciximab
- Ado-trastuzumab emtansine
- Alemtuzumab
- Ave9633
- Axicabtagene
- Belantamab mafodotin-blmf
- Beremagene geperpavec-svdt
- Betibeglogene autotemcel
- Bevacizumab
- Brentuximab vedotin
- Brexucabtagene autoleucel
- Capromab pendetide
- Catumaxomab
- Cetuximab
- Ciltacabtagene autoleucel
- Clopidogrel
- Codeine
- Eculizumab
- Enfortumab vedotin
- Etranacogene dezaparvovec
- 5-Fluorouracil
- Gemtuzumab ozogamicin
- Idecabtagene vicleucel
- Imgn901
- Imciromab pentetate
- Infliximab
- Inotuzumab ozogamicin
- Irinotecan
- Isoniazid
- Lisocabtagene maraleucel
- Loncastuximab tesirine-lpyl
- 6-Mercaptopurine
- Mirvetuximab soravtansine
- Moxetumomab pasudotox
- Nadofaragene firadenovec-vncg
- Niraparib
- Nofetumomab
- Olaparib
- Onasemnogene abeparvovec-xioi
- Pegloticase
- Polatuzumab vedotin-piiq
- Rucaparib
- Sacituzumab govitecan
- SAR3419
- Satumomab
- Talazoparib
- Talimogene laherparepvec
- Tamoxifen
- Technetium-99m-arcitumomab
- Tisagenlecleucel
- Tisotumab vedotin-tftv
- Tolterodine
- Trastuzumab
- Trastuzumab deruxtecan
- Valoctocogene roxaparvovec-rvox
- Vemurafenib
- Voretigene neparvovec-rzyl
- Warfarin

Abbreviations

AAV adeno-associated virus
ABC ATP-binding cassette
ADC antibody-drug conjugate
BCMA B-cell maturation antigen
BRCA breast cancer–associated gene
CAR chimeric antigen receptor
CAR-T chimeric antigen receptor T cell
Cas9 CRISPR-associated protein 9
cDNA complementary DNA
CDR complementarity-determining region
CRISPR clustered regularly interspaced short palindromic repeats
DAR drug-to-antibody ratio
DPD dihydropyrimidine dehydrogenase
DSB double strand break
fAb functional human antibody
G6PD glucose-6-phosphate dehydrogenase
gDNA genomic DNA
HAMA human anti-mouse antibody
HDR homology-directed repair
HGP human genome project
IgG immunoglobulin G
MAb monoclonal antibody
MMAE monomethyl auristatin E
mRNA messenger RNA
NADH Nicotinamide adenine dinucleotide
NAT *N*-acetyl transferase
PARP poly (ADP-ribose) polymerase
PCR polymerase chain reaction
PEG polyethylene glycol
RBC red blood cell
rDNA recombinant DNA
rRNA ribosomal RNA

Abbreviations—continued

SNP single-nucleotide polymorphism
TALEN transcription activator–like effector nuclease
TPMT thiopurine methyl transferase
tRNA transfer RNA
UDP uridine diphosphate
UGT UDP glucuronyl transferase
URE upstream regulatory elements
ZFN zinc finger nuclease

Introduction

Pharmaceutical biotechnology generates basic scientific knowledge, useful therapeutic and diagnostic products, and promising methodologies for future research and clinical applications. The techniques of biotechnology lead to the development of novel therapeutics, improved methods of manufacturing pharmaceuticals, and significant contributions to our understanding of disease etiology, pathophysiology, and biochemistry. Genomics, transcriptomics, proteomics, pharmacogenomics, and metabolomics, the core approaches to pharmaceutical biotechnology, are making major contributions in the following three areas:

1. Identification of new genes
2. Identification of drug targets
3. Development of "personalized medicine"

Although many of the first biotechnology-derived therapeutics were initially used in acutely ill, hospitalized patients, the products of today's pharmaceutical biotechnology have an impact on patient populations with chronic diseases such as rheumatoid arthritis, gout, and cancer.

Pharmacogenetics

The human genome project (HGP), funded by the Department of Energy (DOE) and the National Institutes of Health (NIH), began in the early 1990s and was completed in the early 2000s.[1] The application of genetic information gained from the HGP to disease diagnosis and drug therapy is a major development that is bringing about a wealth of change, including the potential to develop drugs for hundreds of rare, inherited Mendelian disorders. A major benefit of pharmacogenetic screening is a reduction in the health care costs resulting from more effective treatments with fewer side effects and higher cure rates achieved from the patient treatments targeted to the molecular etiology of their disease. Mutations are the result of heritable, permanent changes in DNA base sequence. These usually come about by one of the following three mechanisms: substitution, addition, or deletion. The number of base pair changes involved in a single gene mutation can vary from a single base pair change or single-nucleotide polymorphism (SNP) to many gross changes in the gene structure involving insertion, deletion, or rearrangements of a very large number of base pairs.

Mutations result in a variety of changes to the gene product. If the base change occurs within the reading frame of the gene product, it may alter the amino acid sequence of the gene product (protein). SNPs have been defined as single base mutations that occur in 1% or more of the population.[2,3] Many of these SNPs may be responsible for producing a malfunctioning gene product that, in turn, is responsible for a serious disease. The well-used example is the A → T mutation in the β-globin gene, in which the GAG glutamic acid codon is changed to the GTG valine codon, resulting in abnormal aggregation of the hemoglobin molecules, and causing sickle cell anemia. Another example is one form of β-thalassemia that results from a mutation of a CAG glutamine codon to the TAG stop codon early in the DNA sequence, resulting in premature termination of the translation process and total loss of the β-subunit of the adult hemoglobin molecule.

In principle, we can manipulate the therapeutic outcome of a patient population by separating patients who will not respond normally to a particular drug therapy from those who will, based on an analysis of established genetic biomarkers related to the drug's metabolic profile (Fig. 5.1). Patients who are homozygous for the genetic biomarkers indicating poor metabolism of the recommended therapeutic agent may, depending on the therapeutic window of the drug, exhibit a response resembling an overdose to the normal drug dose and require a reduced dose to achieve therapeutic levels, whereas patients carrying the biomarkers indicating extensive metabolism may exhibit a lack of efficacy at normal doses and require an increased dose of the

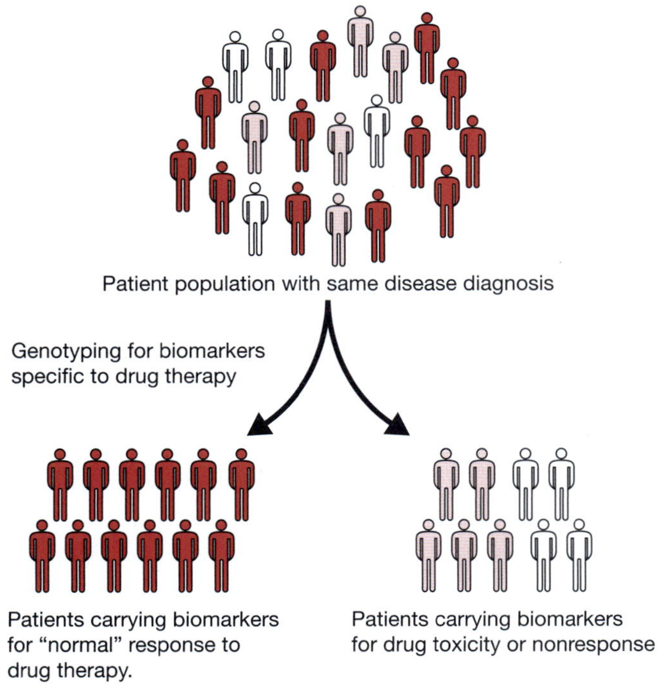

Figure 5.1 Manipulating therapeutic outcomes. Manipulating therapeutic outcomes through pharmacogenetic analysis of a population with the same disease diagnosis to eliminate patients with genetic biomarkers indicating an adverse response to a particular drug therapy.

drug to achieve therapeutic activity. The patients who are homozygous or heterozygous for the normal (wild-type) genetic biomarker may require no alteration of the "normal" dose of the drug for adequate therapeutic outcome.

The action of a drug on the body is a complex interaction involving the metabolism of drugs, the transport of drugs throughout the body, and the interaction of the drug with its target. The application of genetic variation to drug therapy centered on the variations seen in several metabolic enzymes, and much of the pharmacogenetic research has developed with the phase I and phase II metabolic enzymes. Currently, considerable data relate SNPs in the coding and regulatory regions of these genes to poor metabolism of drugs. This has the potential to result in drug overdoses in patients carrying the genetic variations and given the "normal" dose of drug. Transport proteins, such as the ATP-binding cassette (ABC) transporters, that move drugs through membrane barriers are critical in the absorption, distribution, and excretion of drugs and drug metabolites. Drug targets as well as the biochemical pathways following the drug-receptor interaction influence the drug response. Thus, the candidate genes for the therapeutic drug pathway include the genes for drug metabolism, drug transport, and drug response (Table 5.1).

Table 5.1 Specific Examples of the Application of Allelic Variation in Drug Therapy

Protein	Action	Drug	Therapy	Efficacy/Toxicity
CYP450 2D6	Drug metabolism	Codeine	Pain	Efficacy
CYP450 2C9	Drug metabolism	Warfarin	Coagulation	Toxicity (hemorrhage)
Thiopurine S-methyltransferase	Drug metabolism	Mercaptopurine	Acute lymphoblastic leukemia	Toxicity (myelotoxic)
HER2/neu	Drug target	Herceptin	Breast cancer	Efficacy
BCR/ABL	Drug target	Gleevec	Chronic myelogenous leukemia	Efficacy
EGFR	Drug target	Erbitux	Colon cancer	Efficacy
Apolipoprotein E4	Marker	Tacrine	Alzheimer disease	Efficacy
Cholesteryl ester transferase	Marker	Statins	Atherosclerosis	Efficacy
ATP-binding cassette B1	Drug transport	Saquinavir Indinavir Ritonavir Daunorubicin Etoposide	HIV Leukemia	Efficacy
UDP-glucuronosyl-transferase 1A1	Drug metabolism	Irinotecan	Cancer	Toxicity (myelotoxic)
N-Acetyltransferase 2	Drug metabolism	Isoniazid	Tuberculosis	Toxicity (hepatotoxic)
Pseudocholinesterase	Drug metabolism	Suxamethonium	Muscle relaxation during surgery	Toxicity (prolonged apnea)
CYP3A4/CYP2D6	Drug metabolism	Tamoxifen	Cancer	Efficacy
CYP2C19	Drug metabolism	Clopidogrel	Antithrombotic	Cardiovascular toxicity
CYP3A4/CYP2D6	Drug metabolism	Tolterodine	Antimuscarinic	Efficacy
Dihydropyrimidine dehydrogenase	Drug metabolism	5-Fluorouracil	Cancer	Toxicity
BRAF V600E	Drug target	Vemurafenib	Metastatic melanoma	Efficacy
BRCA-deficiency	Synthetic lethality	Olaparib, niraparib, rucaparib	BRCA-mutated cancers	Efficacy

ATP, adenosine triphosphate; BRCA, breast cancer–associated gene; EGFR, epidermal growth factor receptor; HER2, human epidermal growth factor receptor 2; HIV, human immunodeficiency virus.

Genomics

Genomics is the study of the full complement of genetic information, both coding and noncoding, in an organism's genome. The main genomics technique is the use of SNPs as biomarkers to inform clinicians about subtypes of disease that require differential treatments and provide pharmacists with information for selection of the best therapeutic methodology to effectively manage the disease as well as provide an indication of the patients at risk of experiencing adverse reactions or those who will not respond to a given drug dose. The general genotyping procedure for detecting known SNPs consists of polymerase chain reaction (PCR) amplification of the region of interest in the genome, discrimination of the alleles in that region, and detection of the discrimination products.

Transcriptomics

Transcriptomics is the technology behind the study of the full complement of messenger RNA (mRNA) transcripts in the cell's transcriptome and is also known as expression profiling. Methods of expression profiling are either "open" or "closed." Open systems do not require any advance knowledge of the sequence of the genome being examined; closed systems require some advance knowledge and usually involve the use of oligonucleotide or complementary DNA (cDNA) array hybridization technologies (the gene chip) and quantitative PCR (Fig. 5.2).

The cDNA arrays are prepared by spotting gene-specific PCR products, including full-length cDNAs, collections of partially sequenced cDNAs, or randomly chosen cDNAs from any library of interest onto a glass, silicon, gel, or bead matrix or a nylon or nitrocellulose membrane. The matrix (most often glass) is coated with polylysine, amino silanes, or amino-reactive silanes to assist in the attachment of the cDNA probes. The PCR products of the clones are purified and spotted onto the matrix by robots through contact printing or noncontact piezo or ink-jet devices. After cross-linking the probe to the matrix by ultraviolet irradiation, the probe is made single stranded by heat or alkali treatment. The mRNA target is prepared from both a test and reference sample by reverse transcription to produce cDNA, which is then labeled with fluorescent probes (one for the test and another for the reference). The fluorescent targets are pooled and hybridized to the probe array under very stringent conditions. Laser excitation of the hybridized samples on the matrix and comparison of the fluorescence intensity of the reference sample with the fluorescence intensity of the test sample using computer algorithms yield an emission characteristic of the increase or decrease of mRNA expression under test conditions.

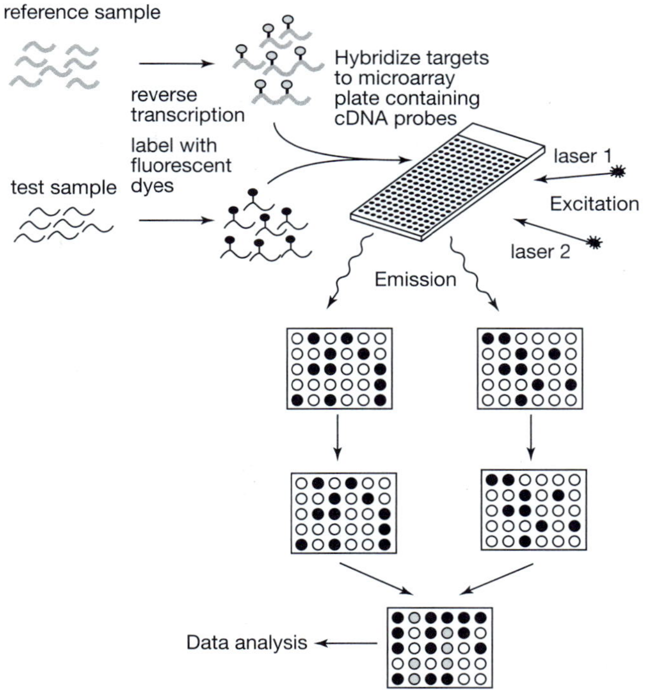

Figure 5.2 cDNA chip. Schematic representation of a cDNA microarray chip. Probes of interest are obtained from DNA clones and printed on coated glass microscope slides. Analysis of mRNA expression is carried out by taking total messenger RNA (mRNA) from both a test and control sample, fluorescently labeling the samples with either Cy3- or Cy5-dUTP during a single round of reverse transcription, pooling the fluorescent targets, and hybridizing to the immobilized probes on the array under very stringent conditions. Laser excitation of the incorporated targets yields an emission with a characteristic spectrum, which is measured using a scanning confocal laser microscope and analyzed using a computer program. (From Duggan DJ, Bittner M, Chen Y, Meltzer P, Trent JM. Expression profiling using cDNA microarrays. *Nat Genet.* 1999;21(suppl 1):10-14.)

CRISPR Technologies and Therapeutic Applications

Clustered regularly interspaced short palindromic repeats (CRISPR)–CRISPR-associated protein (Cas9) complex, a genome editing tool that holds promise for human gene therapy, was named as the "Breakthrough of the Year" by *Science* magazine in 2015.[4] CRISPR technology is composed of three components: (1) a guide RNA that targets a specific locus in the gene; (2) a Cas9 nuclease, which creates a DNA break at the locus; and (3) a DNA repair template to enable gene replacements and insertions.[5] The use of this technology offers the ability to genetically manipulate the patient-derived stem cells to generate various disease models, including cystic fibrosis, Parkinson disease, cardiomyopathy, and ischemic heart disease. CRISPRs, together with Cas9 RNA–guided endonuclease proteins, can be easily targeted to virtually any genomic location of choice by a short RNA guide. The guide sequence within these CRISPR RNAs typically corresponds to phage sequences, which constitute the natural mechanism by which CRISPR produces antiviral defense; however, it can be easily replaced by a sequence of interest to retarget the Cas9 nuclease. The principle behind CRISPR is illustrated in Figure 5.3.[6]

Some applications of CRISPR technologies include homology-directed repair (HDR), gene silencing, pooled genome-scale knockout screening, transient activation of endogenous genes (CRISPRa or CRISPRon), transient gene silencing or transcriptional repression (CRISPRi), DNA-free

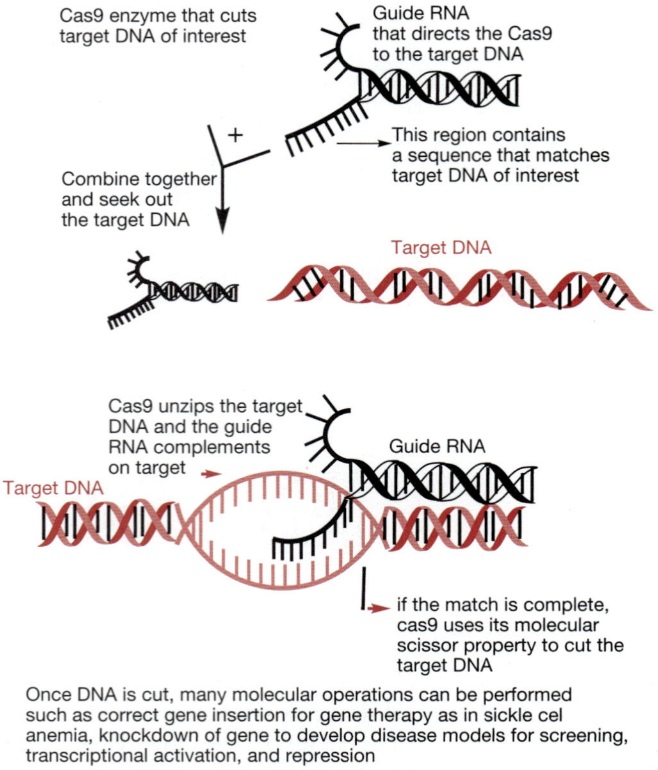

Figure 5.3 CRISPR (clustered regularly interspaced short palindromic repeats) technology.

CRISPR-cas9 gene editing, and embryonic stem cells and transgenic animals.[6]

CRISPR technology–based modified bacteriophages can be developed as a delivery vehicle for a CRISPR-cas9 gene editing system that targets and inactivates either virulence genes or the resistance genes themselves, leaving the rest of the microbiome intact. In another application, CRISPR can be used to target known bacterial resistance genes to deactivate them in situ and resensitize virulent bacteria, thus making existing antibiotics effective again.[7]

Although promising, CRISPR-based therapeutic development has several challenges that remain to be addressed. These include (1) a potential for the induction of off-target mutations at sites other than the intended target, (2) considerable safety concerns for CRISPR use in humans, (3) ethical concerns, (4) the fact that most diseases are not caused by single mutations, and (5) availability of safe carrier systems for CRISPR-cas9 delivery to human cells in vivo.

Chimeric Antigen Receptor T-Cell Therapy

Chimeric antigen receptor (CAR) T-cell therapy is a rapidly growing and evolving field leading to the approval of six products. Despite promising strategy, it has limitations such as life-threatening toxicities, limited efficacy against solid tumors, antigen escape, poor tumor infiltration, and the immunosuppressive microenvironment.[8] CARs represent modular synthetic receptors comprising four main components: (1) an extracellular target antigen-binding domain, (2) a hinge region, (3) a transmembrane domain, and (4) one or more intracellular signaling domains.[8] CARs are engineered synthetic receptors that function to redirect T cells to recognize and eliminate cells expressing a specific target antigen. CAR binding to target antigens expressed on the cell surface is independent from the major histocompatibility complex (MHC) receptor resulting in vigorous T-cell activation and powerful antitumor response.[9] These therapies involve genetically modified patient-derived (autologous) peripheral blood T cells to express a CAR directed to certain antigens present on the surface of targeted tumor cells, such as CD19 or B-cell maturation antigen (BCMA). In principle, T cells of patients are collected and genetically modified to include a new gene that targets and kills intended cancer cells. Once the cells are modified, they are infused back into the patient. The U.S. Food and Drug Administration (FDA)-approved CAR-T cell therapies include (1) axicabtagene ciloleucel (Yescarta), a cell-based gene therapy indicated for the treatment of adult patients with certain types of large B-cell lymphoma[10]; (2) brexucabtagene autoleucel (Tecartus), a CD19-directed genetically modified autologous T-cell immunotherapy indicated for the treatment of adult patients with relapsed or refractory mantle cell lymphoma (MCL); (3) ciltacabtagene autoleucel (Carvykti), a BCMA-directed genetically modified autologous T-cell immunotherapy indicated for the treatment of adult patients with relapsed or refractory multiple myeloma; (4) idecabtagene vicleucel (Abecma), a BCMA-targeted immunotherapy approved for the treatment of adult patients with relapsed or refractory multiple myeloma; and (5) lisocabtagene maraleucel (Breyanzi), a CD19-directed genetically modified autologous T-cell immunotherapy indicated for the treatment of large B-cell lymphoma (LBCL)[11]; and (6) tisagenlecleucel (Kymriah), a CD19-directed genetically modified autologous T-cell immunotherapy indicated for the treatment of pediatric and young adult lymphoblastic leukemia, large B-cell lymphoma, and follicular lymphoma.[12] To meet the increased demand for CAR T-cell cancer therapy, it is necessary to develop closed, automated, and scalable production platforms.[13]

Proteomics

The array of proteins found within the cell, their interactions, and modifications hold the key to understanding biologic systems. The proteome is defined as a protein population of a cell characterized in terms of localization, posttranslational modification, interactions, and turnover, at any given time. The complexity of the proteome surpasses that of the genome. Proteomics is the technology behind the study of the total protein complement of a genome or the complete set of proteins expressed by a cell, tissue, or organism. The presence of an open reading frame in a DNA sequence indicates the presence of a gene, but it does not indicate gene transcription, RNA editing, translation, or posttranslational modification and the presence of isoforms. Analysis of the transcriptome does not indicate alteration of protein levels by proteolysis, recycling, and sequestration. Therefore, it is important to determine protein levels, protein expression, and protein-protein interactions directly.

Proteomics is divided into three main areas[14]:

1. Microcharacterization for large-scale identification of proteins and posttranslational modifications[14]
2. Differential gel electrophoresis for comparison of protein levels[15]
3. Protein-protein interaction studies using protein chips,[16] mass spectrometry isotope-coded affinity tag technology,[17] and the yeast two-hybrid system[18]

Metabolomics

Metabolomics is the technology behind the measurement of metabolite concentrations, fluxes, and secretions in cells and tissues (metabolome). Metabolomics is at the cross-roads of genotype/phenotype interactions, where the interrelationship of metabolic pathways is considered to be the fundamental component of an organism's phenotype. Metabolomics is distinguished by the fact that metabolites are not directly linked to the genetic code but actually are products of a concerted action of many enzyme networks and other regulatory proteins.[19,20] Metabolites also are more complex than nucleic acids, which are composed of four nucleotides, or proteins, which in turn are composed of 20 different amino acids. As a result, metabolites cannot be sequenced like genes and proteins, and so their characterization requires that the structure of each metabolite be determined individually through description of elemental composition and stereochemical orientation of functional groups.

Metabolites are more than just products of enzyme-catalyzed reactions. They also are sensors and regulators of complex molecular interactions in the organism. As a result, the composition of the metabolome can be altered by changes in the individual's environment. Therefore, a study of the metabolome is complicated not only by the uniqueness of the individual's genome but also by the uniqueness of the individual's environment. Alternatively, one could consider the metabolome to be a very sensitive indicator of the individual's phenotype.[21,22]

Metabolomics can be approached by using several different but related strategies:

1. Target analysis investigates the primary metabolic effect of a genetic variation. This analysis usually is limited to the substrate and/or product of the protein expressed by the altered gene.
2. Metabolic profiling limits the investigation to several predefined metabolites, usually in a specific metabolic pathway.
3. Metabolomics is a comprehensive analysis (both identification and quantification) of metabolites in a biologic system that investigates the effect of multiple genetic variations on many different biochemical pathways.
4. Metabolic fingerprinting is a strategy to screen many metabolites for biologic relevance in diagnostic or other analytical procedures in which it is important to rapidly distinguish between individuals in a population. Metabolic fingerprinting is the ultimate characterization of an individual's phenotype for disease diagnosis and drug therapy. Once the technologic problems of high-throughput metabolic analysis are developed, it will be a major competitor of SNP analysis in pharmacogenomics.

The analytical technologies used in metabolomic investigations are nuclear magnetic resonance and mass spectrometry alone or in combination with liquid or gas chromatographic separation of metabolites. Other techniques include thin-layer chromatography, Fourier transform infrared spectrometry, metabolite arrays, and Raman spectroscopy.

Pharmaceutical Biotechnology Methods

Pharmaceutical biotechnology is defined, at its most basic level, as the manipulation of nucleic acids in the production of therapeutic and diagnostic agents. To understand both DNA and RNA, the fundamental genetic material, it is important to understand the basic process that moves information from DNA to RNA. This process starts with transcription.

Transcription

The genetic information in DNA is transcribed to the intermediate RNA molecule that moves to the cytoplasm, where it directs the synthesis of the gene product it encodes using ribosomes. RNA differs chemically from DNA in that the deoxyribose sugar molecule in DNA is replaced by ribose, and the thymine in DNA is replaced by uracil in RNA. Structurally, RNA contains both single-stranded runs and short, double helical regions.

There are several types of RNA molecules in the cell, three of which are highlighted here. Messenger RNA (mRNA) is transcribed from a particular DNA sequence. Transfer RNA (tRNA) is covalently linked to a specific amino acid and carries an anticodon triplet. The anticodon triplet recognizes a complementary trinucleotide sequence of the mRNA that is specific for the amino acid that it carries. The ribosome contains both ribosomal RNA (rRNA) and proteins.

Several differences exist in the mechanism of transcription between prokaryotes and eukaryotes. These differences are important when evaluating if recombinant expression of a protein should be carried out in a eukaryotic or prokaryotic system. For our purposes, we describe transcription in a eukaryotic system.

Transcription is carried out by RNA polymerases, which there are of three types in eukaryotes. RNA pol I catalyzes the synthesis of rRNA, RNA pol II is responsible for the synthesis of mRNA, and RNA pol III synthesizes tRNA. All three polymerases are large enzymes containing 12 or more subunits.

Each eukaryotic RNA polymerase copies DNA from the 3′ end, thus catalyzing mRNA formation in the $5' \rightarrow 3'$ direction and synthesizing RNA complementary to the antisense DNA template strand. The reaction requires the precursor nucleotides adenosine triphosphate (ATP), guanosine triphosphate (GTP), cytidine triphosphate (CTP), and uridine triphosphate (UTP) and does not require a primer for the initiation of transcription. The five stages of eukaryotic transcription include initiation, elongation and termination, capping, polyadenylation, and splicing.

Initiation

Eukaryotes have different RNA polymerase–binding promoter sequences than prokaryotes. The TATA consensus sequence of the eukaryotic promoter region is located 25 to 35 base pairs upstream from the transcription start site (Fig. 5.4). The low activity of basal promoters is greatly increased by the presence of upstream regulatory elements (UREs) located 40 to 200 base pairs upstream of the promoter sequence and includes the SP1 box, the CCAAT box, and the hormone response elements. Transcription from many eukaryotic promoters can be stimulated by control elements, called enhancers, located many thousands of base pairs away from the transcription start site.

Elongation and Termination

RNA polymerase moves along the DNA template until a terminator sequence is reached. The RNA molecule made from a protein-coding gene by RNA pol II in eukaryotes is called pre-mRNA. The pre-mRNA from a eukaryotic protein-coding gene is extensively processed within the nucleus before export to the cytoplasm.

Capping

At the end of polymerization, the 5′ end of the pre-mRNA molecule is modified by addition of an N^7-methyl guanine molecule (Fig. 5.5).

Polyadenylation

The 3′ end of the pre-mRNA is generated by nuclease-catalyzed cleavage followed by the addition of a run, or tail, of 100 to 200 adenosine nucleotides, resulting in what is called the poly (A) tail. Cleavage and polyadenylation require specific sequences in the DNA and its pre-mRNA transcript that are part of the transcription termination signal. The poly (A) tail helps stabilize the mRNA molecule, reducing its sensitivity to 3′-nuclease activity.

RNA Splicing

Splicing is the precise excision of the intron sequences and joining of exons to produce a functional mRNA molecule.

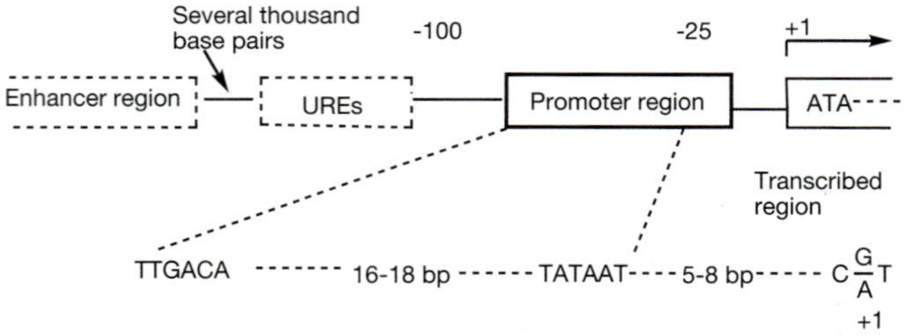

Figure 5.4 Schematic representation of the eukaryotic transcription unit showing the relationship between the promoter, upstream regulatory elements (UREs), and enhancer region. Note that transcription usually starts with a purine base in the 1 position. (Adapted from Turner PC, McLennan AG, Bates AD, White MRH. *Instant Notes in Molecular Biology*. BIOS Scientific Publishers Ltd, Springer-Verlag; 1997; with permission.)

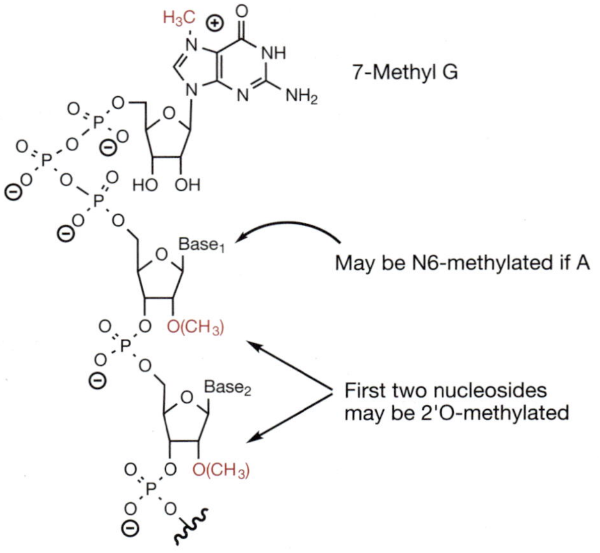

Figure 5.5 Chemical structure of the 5′-cap of mRNA (messenger RNA). Cap 0 consists of the 7-methylguanosine triphosphate attached to the 5′ end of the mRNA. Cap 1 consists of the 7-methylguanosine and 2′-*O*-methylation of the 5′ base. Cap 2 consists of the 7-methylguanosine and the 2′-*O*-methylation of the first two bases in the sequence.

Translation

Once the fully processed mRNA has been transported from the nucleus to the cytoplasm, protein synthesis occurs. The triplet genetic code carried on the mRNA is translated into a protein sequence by the ribosome. Amino acids are delivered to the ribosome by tRNAs that carry specific amino acids attached to their 3′-terminus, based on the tRNA anticodon sequence. The anticodon complements the triplet codon sequence in mRNA, and 61 triplet sequences code for the 20 amino acids (Table 5.2). Three codons are nonsense or stop codons that terminate translation. The code is degenerate with 18 of the 20 common amino acids coded for by more than one codon. Two amino acids, Met (AUG) and Trp (UGG), have one unique codon each. From a fixed start point on the mRNA (start codon, AUG), which establishes the open reading frame, each group of three bases in the coding region of the mRNA represents a codon that is recognized by a complementary triplet on the tRNA molecule.

While protein synthesis is more complex (or different) in eukaryotes, there are four common stages in both prokaryotes and eukaryotes:

1. *Initiation*—assembly of rRNA and mRNA
2. *Elongation*—repeated cycles of amino acid addition by tRNA
3. *Termination*—recognition of the stop codon, release of the new protein chain, and breakdown of the synthetic complex
4. *Posttranslational modification*—usually includes protein cleavage by carboxy or aminopeptidases and chemical modification such as acetylation, sulfonylation, phosphorylation, hydroxylation, lipidation, and/or addition of polysaccharides

Table 5.2 Genetic Code

First Position	Second Position				Third Position
	U	**C**	**A**	**G**	
U	**Phe** UUU	**Ser** UCU	**Tyr** UAU	**Cys** UGU	U
	Phe UUC	**Ser** UCC	**Tyr** UAC	**Cys** UGC	C
	Leu UUA	**Ser** UCA	**Stop** UAA	**Stop** UGA	A
	Leu UUG	**Ser** UCG	**Stop** UAG	**Trp** UGG	G
C	**Leu** CUU	**Pro** CCU	**His** CAU	**Arg** CGU	U
	Leu CUC	**Pro** CCC	**His** CAC	**Arg** CGC	C
	Leu CUA	**Pro** CCA	**Gln** CAA	**Arg** CGA	A
	Leu CUG	**Pro** CCG	**Gln** CAG	**Arg** CGG	G
A	**Ile** AUU	**Thr** ACU	**Asn** AAU	**Ser** AGU	U
	Ile AUC	**Thr** ACC	**Asn** AAC	**Ser** AGC	C
	Ile AUA	**Thr** ACA	**Lys** AAA	**Arg** AGA	A
	Met AUG	**Thr** ACG	**Lys** AAG	**Arg** AGG	G
G	**Val** GUU	**Ala** GCU	**Asp** GAU	**Gly** GGU	U
	Val GUC	**Ala** GCC	**Asp** GAC	**Gly** GGC	C
	Val GUA	**Ala** GCA	**Glu** GAA	**Gly** GGA	A
	Val GUG	**Ala** GCG	**Glu** GAG	**Gly** GGG	G

Genes

A gene is the segment of genomic DNA (gDNA) involved in producing a polypeptide chain. The mRNA assembled from the gene includes regions preceding (the leader or 5′-untranslated region) and following (the trailer or 3′-untranslated region) the coding region as well as intervening sequences such as introns that are removed in the processing of the pre-mRNA. With the discovery of other processes that contribute to the penultimate sequence of the mature mRNA, the definition of a gene is evolving.[23]

Cloning and the Preparation of DNA Libraries

Two discoveries in the early 1970s provided breakthroughs in nucleic acid chemistry: the discovery of bacterial enzymes capable of cleaving nucleic acids at specific, palindromic (symmetrical) base sequences (Figs. 5.6 and 5.7) and the discovery of bacterial plasmids as vehicles (vectors) to amplify and carry the gene fragments produced by those restriction enzymes. Plasmids are small, circular, extrachromosomal nucleic acid molecules in bacteria that replicate independently within the bacterial cell. Restriction enzymes (and now PCR) are used

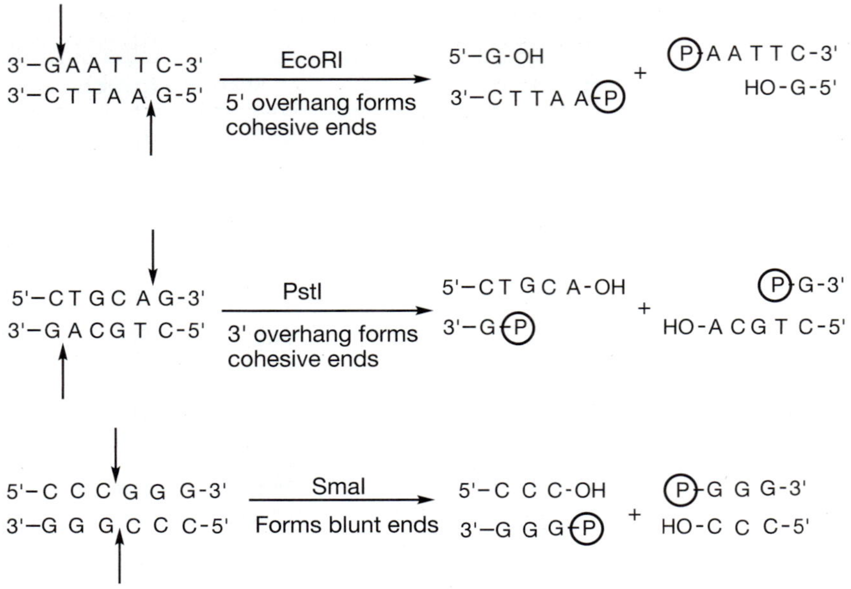

Figure 5.6 Actions of restriction endonucleases EcoRI, PstI, and SmaI at their recognition sequences. Note that EcoRI and PstI enzymes produce "sticky ends" with overlapping sequences, whereas SmaI produces "blunt ends" or nonoverlapping sequences.

to produce relatively small DNA fragments that are inserted into bacterial plasmid vectors, forming recombinant DNA (rDNA) molecules. The rDNA vectors are inserted into bacterial hosts, where the plasmid replicates with the bacteria, producing many identical rDNA molecules known as clones, thus completing the process known as DNA cloning.

SEQUENCING DNA FRAGMENTS. The two previous methods of nucleic acid sequencing, the Maxam and Gilbert method (chemical method)[24] and the Sanger dideoxy method,[25] have been superseded by the far faster massive parallel sequencing methods. In short, high-throughput sequencing involves breaking up gDNA into fragments and placing the individual fragments onto specially designed microbeads where the many copies of each fragment have been amplified. The amplified fragments are then loaded into the small wells of a substrate. As the wells are loaded with samples, reagents are pumped across the plate. The addition of the reagents results in an enzymatic reaction between complimentary bases in the DNA fragments, and a fluorescent signal is released and read by a computational sequence analyzer.[26]

SYNTHESIZING OLIGONUCLEOTIDES. The need for short oligonucleotides of known sequence has grown tremendously with the need for radiolabeled and fluorescently labeled probes to isolate and characterize nucleic acids. The phosphite triester and the phosphotriester methods are convenient solid-phase automated techniques for the synthesis of oligonucleotides (Fig. 5.8).[27]

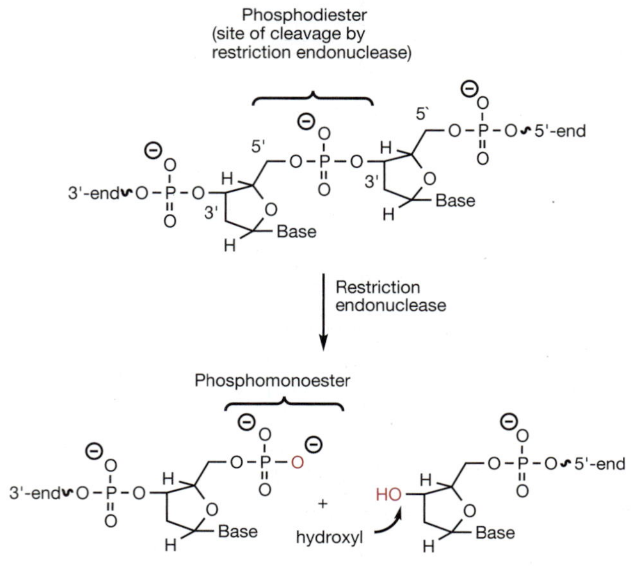

Figure 5.7 Cleavage by restriction endonuclease.

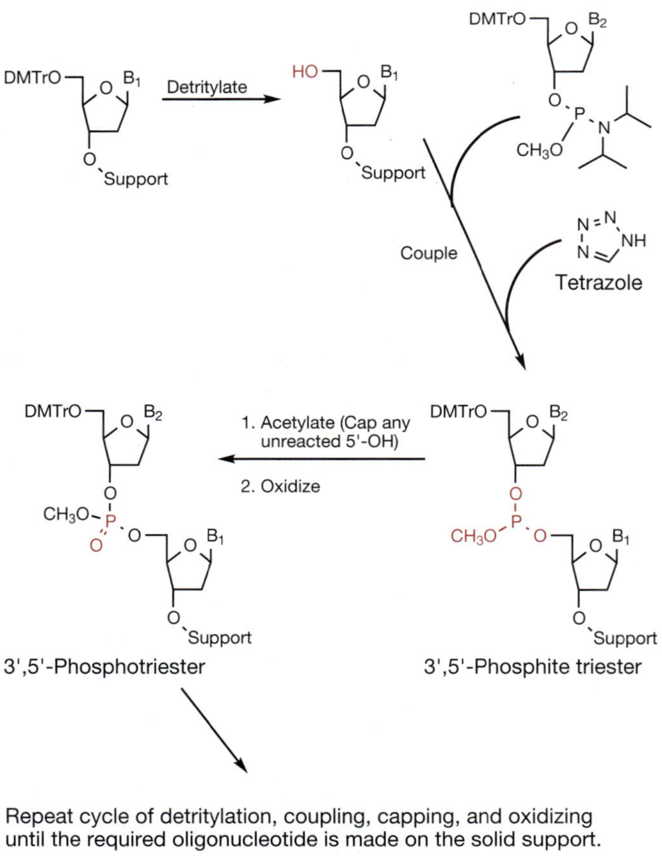

Figure 5.8 Solid-phase phosphate and phosphite triester method of oligodeoxyribonucleotide synthesis. DMTr, 4,4-dimethoxytrityl.

Polymerase Chain Reaction. Working with small quantities of nucleic acids isolated from cell and tissue sources can prove to be difficult, and there is often a need to amplify these sequences. PCR is used to amplify fragments of DNA without the need for cloning. The process can amplify samples that contain as little as a single-nucleotide fragment used as template. There is a requirement for the sequences flanking the boundaries of the fragment to be amplified so that oligonucleotide primers can be prepared.[28]

Protein Synthesis Through Recombinant DNA. Once the gene coding for the desired protein has been identified and isolated (Fig. 5.9), the genetic material is introduced into cells on a vector capable of DNA replication and initiation of transcription. A cloning vector is a carrier molecule, the vehicle that is used to insert foreign DNA into a host cell. Typically, vectors are genetic elements that can be replicated in a host cell separately from that cell's chromosomes. Bacterial plasmids are circular DNA molecules containing a few thousand base pairs. These plasmids replicate freely within the cells and are ideal for carrying the gene into the host organism. DNA fragments coding for the desired protein can be cloned from gDNA or cDNA and inserted into the vector that carries the code to synthesize the protein in the host.

The vector containing the code for the target protein is then inserted into the host. Host cells are typically bacteria (eg, *Escherichia coli*), eukaryotic yeast (eg, *Saccharomyces cerevisiae* [baker's yeast]), or mammalian cell lines. The choice of host system is influenced primarily by the type of protein to be expressed and by the key differences among the various host cells. Overall protein yields generally are much lower in mammalian cells, but in some cases, this may be the only system that produces the specific protein of interest. It should be noted that recombinant proteins produced in gram-negative bacteria may contain endotoxins.

The host cells containing the vector are grown under selection to identify a clone that contains the desired gene and

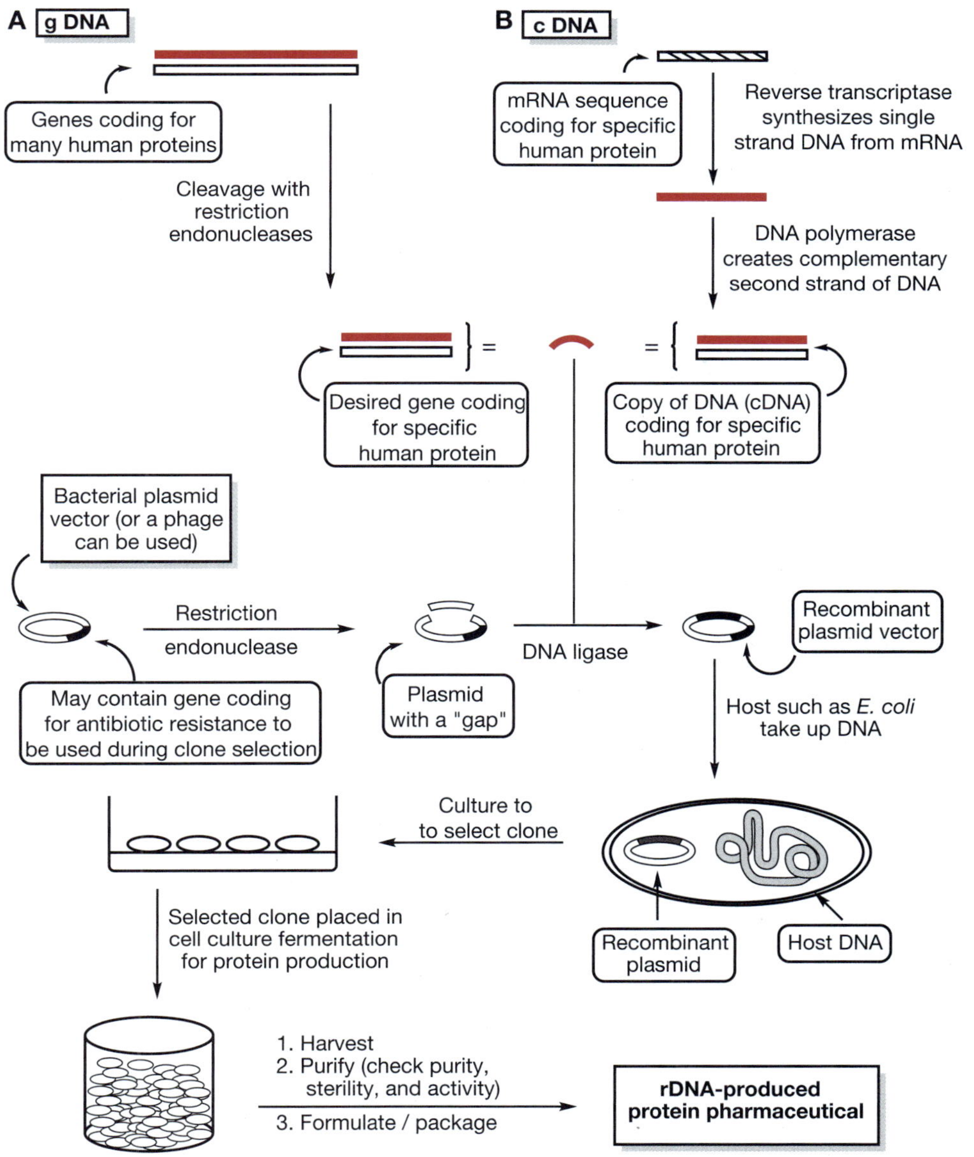

Figure 5.9 Summary of typical rDNA production of a protein from either (A) genomic DNA or (B) cDNA.

can produce the best protein. The selected cloned cells are first used as an inoculum for a small-scale cell culture/fermentation. This is then followed by larger fermentations in bioreactors. The medium is carefully controlled to enhance cell reproduction and protein synthesis. The host produces its natural proteins along with the desired protein, which may be secreted into the growth medium. The protein of interest can then be isolated from fermentation, purified, and formulated to give a potential rDNA-produced pharmaceutical.

Protein Isolation and Purification. The isolation and purification of the final protein product from the complex mixture of cells, cellular debris, medium nutrients, and other host metabolites is a challenging task. The structure, purity, potency, and stability of the recombinant protein must be considered. Often, sophisticated filtrations, phase separations, precipitation, and complex multiple-column chromatographic procedures are required to obtain the desired protein. Although isolation of the recombinant protein, produced in culture in relatively large amounts, is generally easier than isolating the native protein, ensuring the stability and retention of the bioactive three-dimensional structure (correct protein folding) of any biopharmaceutical is a more arduous task. In addition, recombinant proteins from bacterial hosts require removal of endotoxins, whereas viral particles may need to be removed from mammalian cell culture products. A discussion of these techniques is beyond the scope of this chapter; however, useful reviews on the analysis and chromatography[29] of biotechnology products are available as a resource for further information.

General Properties of Biotechnology-Produced Medicinal Agents

rDNA and hybridoma technologies have made it possible to produce large quantities of highly pure, therapeutically useful proteins. The rDNA-derived proteins and monoclonal antibodies (MAbs) are not dissimilar to the other protein pharmaceuticals or biopharmaceuticals that pharmacists have dispensed in the past. As polymers of amino acids joined by peptide bonds, the properties of these proteins differ generally from those of small organic molecule pharmaceuticals.

Stability of Biotech Pharmaceuticals

The instability of proteins, including protein pharmaceuticals, can be separated into three distinct classes. Chemical instability results from bond formation or cleavage yielding a modification of the protein and a new chemical entity. Photoinstability of protein drugs upon exposure to light results in chemical and physical instability. Physical instability involves a change to the secondary or higher order structure of the protein rather than a covalent bond–breaking modification.[30-32]

Chemical Instability

A variety of reactions give rise to the chemical instability of proteins, including hydrolysis, oxidation, racemization, β-elimination, and disulfide exchange (Fig. 5.10). Each of these changes may cause a loss of biologic activity. Proteolytic hydrolysis of peptide bonds results in fragmentation of the protein chain. It is well established that in dilute acids, aspartic acid residues in proteins are hydrolyzed at a rate at least 100-fold faster than that of other peptide bonds because of the mechanism of the reaction. An additional hydrolysis reaction is the deamidation of the neutral residue of asparagine and glutamine side chain linkages, forming the ionizable carboxylic acid residues aspartic acid and glutamic acid (Fig. 5.10A). This conversion may be considered primary sequence isomerization.[32]

Oxidative degradative reactions can occur on the side chains of sulfur-containing methionine and cysteine residues and the aromatic amino acid residues histidine, tryptophan, and tyrosine in proteins during their isolation and storage. The weakly nucleophilic thioether group of methionine ($R\text{-}S\text{-}CH_3$) can be oxidized at low pH by hydrogen peroxide as well as by oxygen in the air, to the sulfoxide ($R\text{-}SO\text{-}CH_3$) and the sulfone ($R\text{-}SO_2\text{-}CH_3$). The thiol (sulfhydryl, R-SH) group of cysteine can be successively oxidized to the corresponding sulfenic acid (R-SOH), disulfide (R-SS-R), sulfinic acid ($R\text{-}SO_2H$), and, finally, sulfonic acid ($R\text{-}SO_3H$). Several factors, including pH, influence the rate of this oxidation. Oxidation of histidine, tryptophan, and tyrosine residues is believed to occur with a variety of oxidizing agents, resulting in the cleavage of the aromatic rings.

Base-catalyzed racemization reactions may occur in any of the amino acids except achiral glycine to yield residues in proteins with mixtures of L- and D-configurations. The α-methine hydrogen is removed to form a carbanion intermediate (see Fig. 5.10B). The degree of stabilization of this intermediate controls the rate of this reaction. Racemization generally alters the physicochemical properties and biologic activity of proteins. Also, racemization generates nonmetabolizable D-configuration forms of the amino acids. Aspartate residues in proteins racemize at a 10^5-fold faster rate than when free, in contrast to the 2 to 4-fold increase for the other residues. The facilitated rate of racemization for aspartic acid residues is believed to result from the formation of a stabilized cyclic imide.

Proteins containing cysteine, serine, threonine, phenylalanine, and lysine are prone to β-elimination reactions under alkaline conditions (see Fig. 5.10C). The reaction proceeds through the same carbanion intermediate as racemization. The reaction is influenced by several additional factors, including temperature and the presence of metal ions.

The interrelationships of disulfide bonds and free sulfhydryl groups in proteins are important factors influencing the chemical and biologic properties of protein pharmaceuticals. Disulfide exchange can result in incorrect pairings and major changes in the higher order structure (secondary and above) of proteins. The exchange may occur in neutral, acidic, and alkaline media.

Photoinstability

The exposure of proteins to light and the ensuing chemical and physical degradation have been studied extensively for many years.[32] The peptide backbone, tryptophan, tyrosine, phenylalanine, and cysteine are the primary targets of photodegradation in proteins. Primary or type I photodegradation

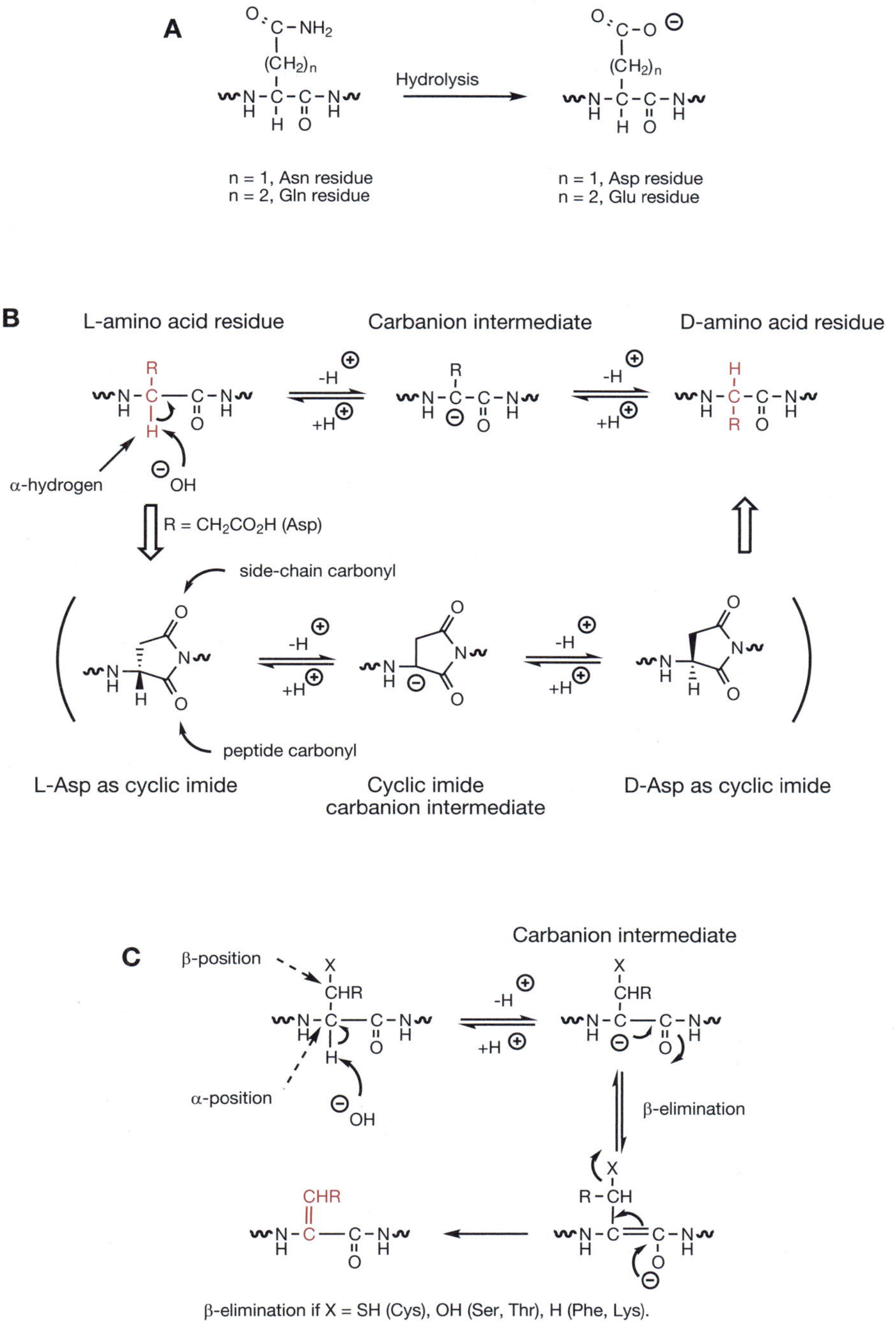

Figure 5.10 Chemical instability of protein biopharmaceuticals. (A) Hydrolysis, (B) base-catalyzed racemization, and (C) β-elimination.

begins with absorption of light, resulting in excitation of an electron to higher energy singlet states. Absorption occurs through either the peptide backbone or by the amino acid side chains of tryptophan, tyrosine, phenylalanine, and cysteine. In aqueous solution, the absorption wavelengths are 180 to 230 nm for the peptide backbone, 280 to 305 nm for tryptophan, 260 to 290 nm for tyrosine, 240 to 270 nm for phenylalanine, and 250 to 300 nm for cysteine. Although tryptophan is present in relatively low abundance in proteins, it has the highest molar absorption coefficients and is therefore a major player in the photodegradation of protein drugs.

The major photolytic pathways of tryptophan in proteins are shown in Figure 5.11. Following absorption of light, the excited state tryptophan will relax to the lowest energy singlet state followed by fluorescence, undergo intersystem crossing to the triplet state (^{3}tryptophan), or eject an electron with formation of a tryptophan radical cation that will rapidly deprotonate to form the neutral tryptophan radical. The tryptophan radical may extract hydrogen from a nearby tyrosine, repairing the tryptophan and forming a tyrosine phenoxy radical; react with oxygen, if present, forming a peroxy radical on the Trp; or react with nearby amino acids.

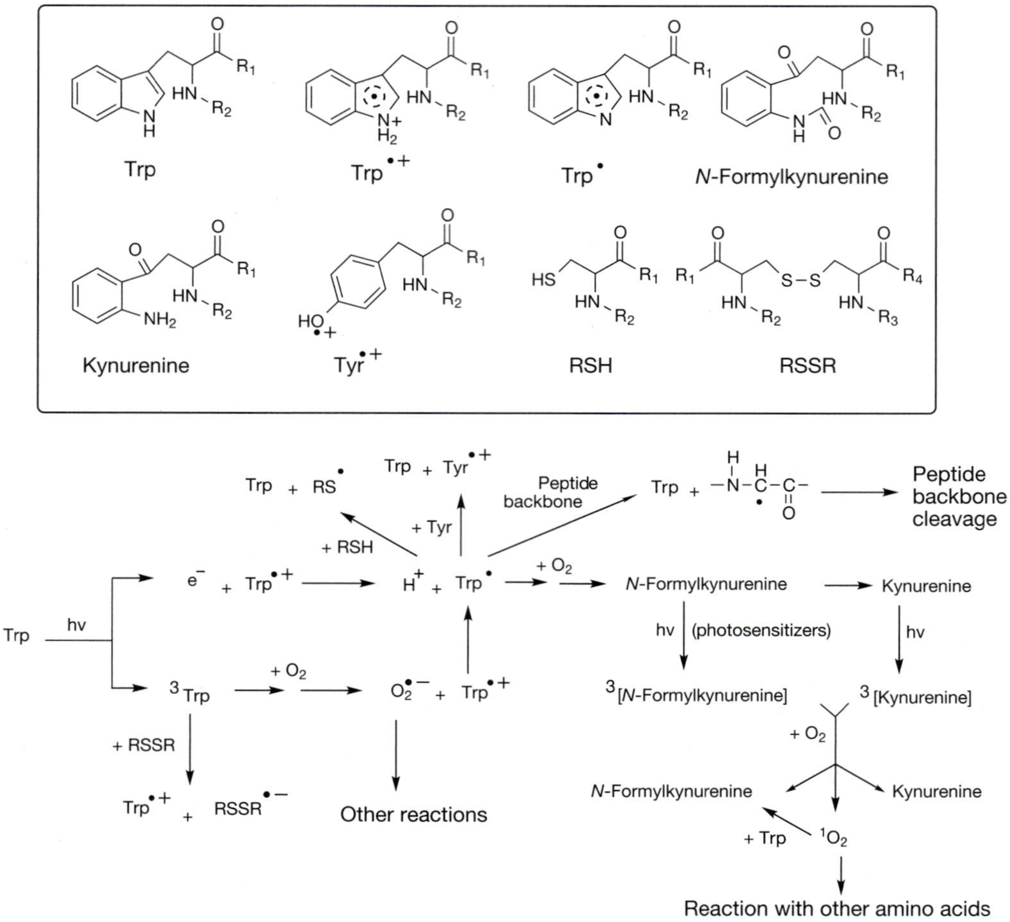

Figure 5.11 Structure of tryptophan (Trp), tyrosine (Tyr), and common photolytic pathways.

The ejected electron can become solvated forming an e^-_{aq} or migrate along the peptide backbone and react with cystine residues, forming a disulfide radical anion as discussed below. Under anaerobic conditions, the tryptophan triplet state generally either relaxes back to the ground state with formation of light at 420 to 500 nm or electron transfers to a nearby cystine with subsequent reactions as discussed earlier. In the presence of oxygen, formation of the tryptophan-based peroxy radical can undergo further reaction to produce *N*-formylkynurenine and kynurenine. Interestingly, the *N*-formylkynurenine and kynurenine absorb light at longer wavelengths than Trp, thereby acting as photosensitizers to visible light, causing additional damage to the protein. Likewise, photodegradation of tyrosine, phenylalanine, cysteine, and histidine residues in proteins can occur.

Changes in the primary structure of the protein can result in changes in the secondary and tertiary structures, impacting long-term stability, bioactivity, and immunogenicity of the peptide and protein drugs. Complete protection of the proteins from light is the only method to prevent photodegradation. This is achieved with primary and secondary packaging containers such as cardboard boxes that block incoming light to the protein. Excipients such as methionine is also added to further reduce the protein aggregation as in the case of darbepoetin alfa formulation. Methionine is known to react with peroxide to form methionine sulfoxide and likely reduces protein aggregation through its effect as a peroxide scavenger. Photodegradation reactions can occur through the generation of singlet oxygen species that are formed during the photolytic process by the reaction of molecular dioxygen. As a result, some liquid and lyophilized biopharmaceutical products are packaged in inert atmospheres.

Physical Instability

Generally not encountered in most small organic molecules, physical instability is a consequence of the polymeric nature of proteins. Proteins adopt secondary, tertiary, and quaternary structures, which influence their three-dimensional shape and, therefore, their biologic activity. Any change to the higher order structure of a protein may alter both. Physical instability includes denaturation, adsorption to surfaces, and noncovalent self-aggregation (soluble and precipitation). The most widely studied aspect of protein instability is denaturation. Noncovalent aggregation, however, is one of the primary mechanisms of protein degradation.[33]

A protein, in principle, can be folded into a virtually infinite number of conformations. Denaturation occurs by disrupting the weaker noncovalent interactions that hold a protein together in its secondary and tertiary structures. Temperature, pH, and the addition of organic solvents and solutes may cause denaturation. The process can be reversible or irreversible. In general, denaturation affects the protein by decreasing aqueous solubility, altering the three-dimensional molecular shape, increasing susceptibility to enzymatic hydrolysis, and causing the loss of the native protein's biologic activity.

Handling and Storage of Biotechnology-Produced Products

The preparation and administration of protein drugs of synthetic, recombinant, or hybridoma origin are dissimilar to the nonprotein pharmaceuticals. Proteins generally have a more limited shelf stability. The average shelf life for a biotechnology product is 12 to 18 months, compared to that for a low-molecular-weight drug, which is more than 36 months. Although each individual biotechnology drug may be different, several generalizations can be made.

Proper storage of the lyophilized and the reconstituted drug is essential. Most of these drugs are expensive; therefore, special care must be taken not to inactivate the therapeutic protein during storage and handling. Human proteins have limited chemical and physical stability, which is shortened on reconstitution. Expiration dates range from 2 hours to 30 days. The self-association of either native state or misfolded protein subunits may readily occur under certain conditions. This can lead to aggregation and precipitation and results in a loss of biologic activity. Self-association mechanisms depend on the conditions of formulation and may occur because of hydrophobic interactions.

Many of the biotechnology-produced drugs are stored refrigerated, but not frozen (2-8 °C). In general, temperature extremes must be avoided. One example is the rDNA-produced, blood clot–dissolving drug alteplase. A recombinant version of a naturally occurring human tissue-type plasminogen activator, lyophilized alteplase is stable at room temperature for several years if protected from light. Freezing or exposure to excessive heat decreases the physical stability of the protein. Anything that causes denaturation or self-aggregation, even though labile peptide bonds are not broken, may inactivate the protein. Pharmacy facilities may need to increase cold storage capacity to accommodate biotech storage needs. If the patient must travel any distance from home after receiving the medication, the pharmacist should help package the biotechnology product, according to the manufacturer instructions. This may mean supplying a reusable cooler for the patient's use. Because the protein drug should not be frozen, the cooler should contain an ice pack rather than dry ice.

Some rDNA-derived pharmaceuticals, particularly the cytokines (eg, the interferons, interleukin-2, colony-stimulating factors), require human serum albumin in their formulation to prevent adhesion of the protein drug to the glass surface of the vial, which results in loss of protein. The amount of human serum albumin added varies with the biotech product. The vials should not be shaken to prevent foaming of the albumin, which causes protein loss or inactivation of the biotechnology-derived proteins. Care must be exercised in reconstituting protein pharmaceuticals. The diluent used for reconstitution of biotechnology drugs varies with the product and is specified by the manufacturer. Diluents can include normal saline, bacteriostatic water, and 5% dextrose. For additional information about handling and storage of biotechnology drugs, interested readers are directed to.[34,35]

Pharmacokinetic Considerations of Biotechnology-Produced Proteins

The processes of absorption into, distribution within, metabolism by, and excretion from the body (ie, ADME) of biotechnology-produced pharmaceuticals are important factors affecting the time course of their pharmacologic effect. To deliver quality pharmaceutical care with biotech products, a pharmacist must be able to apply pharmacokinetic principles to establish and maintain a nontoxic, therapeutic effect. The pharmacokinetics of protein and peptide drugs differs in some pharmacokinetic aspects from those of the small-molecule organic agents with which we are most familiar. Although a lengthy discussion of this topic is beyond the scope of this chapter, a brief overview of metabolism follows. Useful reviews are also available for further information.[36,37]

The plasma half-life of most administered proteins and peptides is relatively short because they are susceptible to a wide variety of metabolic reactions. The enzymes involved in peptide bond hydrolysis and, thus, the degradation of peptides and proteins are known as peptidases and can be found in the blood, in the vascular bed, in the interstitial fluid, on cell membranes, and within cells. These enzymes include carboxypeptidases (cleaves C-terminal residues), dipeptidyl carboxypeptidases (cleaves dipeptides from the C-terminus), aminopeptidases (cleaves N-terminal residues), and amidases (cleaves internal peptide bonds). For the most part, these enzymes are all specific to the natural amino acids of the L-configuration. Overall, the metabolic products of most proteins and peptides are not considered to be a safety issue. They generally are broken down into amino acids and reincorporated into new, endogenously biosynthesized proteins.

Metabolic oxidation reactions may occur to the side chains of sulfur-containing residues, similar to that observed for in vitro chemical instability. Methionine can be oxidized to sulfoxide, whereas metabolic oxidation of cysteine residues forms a disulfide. Metabolic reductive cleavage of disulfide bridges in proteins may occur, yielding free sulfhydryl groups.

Biotechnology Drug Delivery

Protein-based pharmaceuticals, whether produced by biotechnology or isolated from traditional sources, present challenges to drug delivery because of the unique demands imposed by their physicochemical and biologic properties. Although a detailed discussion of this topic is beyond the scope of this chapter, a brief overview follows. Useful reviews also are available for further information.[38-40]

Delivery of high-molecular-weight, biotechnology-produced drugs into the body is difficult because of the poor absorption of these drugs, the acid lability of peptide bonds, and the rapid enzymatic degradation of these drugs in the body. In addition, protein pharmaceuticals are susceptible to physical instability, complex feedback control mechanisms, and peculiar dose-response relationships.

Given the limitations of today's technology, the strongly acidic environment of the stomach, the peptidases in the gastrointestinal tract, and the barrier to absorption presented by gastrointestinal mucosal cells preclude successful oral administration of most protein and peptide drugs. Therefore, administration of all the biotechnology-produced protein drugs and some natural or synthetic peptides currently is parenteral (by intravenous, subcutaneous, or intramuscular injections) to provide a better therapeutic profile. Manufacturers supply most of these drugs as sterile solutions without a preservative. In such cases, it is recommended that only one dose be prepared from each vial to prevent bacterial contamination.

Novel solutions to overcome delivery problems associated with biotechnology protein products and natural or synthetic peptide drugs are being explored. Oral drug delivery approaches in development for proteins and peptide drugs include conjugated systems (eg, PEGylation with polyethylene glycol), amino acid substitution, liposomes, microspheres, erythrocytes as carriers, and viruses as drug carriers.

PEGylation is frequently used to improve the pharmacokinetic properties of biotechnology-produced drugs.[41] This method involves the attachment of a flexible strand or strands of polyethylene glycol (PEG) to a protein. PEG is a simple, water-soluble, nontoxic polymer that is nonimmunogenic, is readily cleared from the body, and has been approved for human administration by mouth, injection, and topical application. The most common process used for PEGylation of protein is to activate the PEG with functional groups suitable for reaction with lysine and N-terminal amino groups. PEGylated proteins are broken down less rapidly by the body's enzymes than unmodified proteins. PEG can extend the duration of action of proteins and peptides in the body from minutes to hours, to days, depending on the PEG molecule used. By increasing the biologic half-life and improving the efficacy of proteins in the body, these modifications can reduce the frequency of injections a patient requires. They also reduce the rapidity and intensity of the body's immune reaction against molecules such as uricase. Several PEGylated protein products (eg, pegvisomant, certolizumab pegol, peginterferon α2a, pegloticase) are currently marketed, and many are under development.

When metabolism studies indicate a predominant cleavage site, attempts can be made to replace that residue with another that retains the receptor-binding activity of the protein/peptide drug while yielding enhanced resistance to peptidase activity. This can often be accomplished by replacing the offending L-residue with its enantiomer, the D-amino acid, or another D-residue. Many peptidases are unable to cleave peptide bonds consisting of a "fraudulent" D-amino acid, and peptides containing such changes are designed to increase their half-life. Also, the replacement of an L-amino acid with L-proline or N-methylation of the amide nitrogen offers the possibility of generating a peptide that is more resistant to enzymatic hydrolysis. The introduction of pseudopeptide bonds[42] and the design of retro-inverso peptides[43] are two examples of strategies that can afford peptidase resistance to peptide drugs.

Adverse Effects

An important consideration in the pharmaceutical care of a patient being administered a biotechnology-produced medicinal agent is the potential for adverse reactions. Many of the protein drugs are biotechnology-derived versions of endogenous human proteins normally present, on stimulus, in minute quantities near their specific site of action. Therefore, the same protein administered in much larger quantities may cause adverse effects not commonly observed at normal physiologic concentrations. Careful monitoring of patients administered biotechnology-produced drugs is critical for the health care team.

Immunogenicity

The immune system may respond to an antigen, such as a protein pharmaceutical, by triggering the production of antibodies. Biotechnology-derived proteins may possess a different set of antigenic determinants (ie, regions of a protein recognized by an antibody) because of structural differences between the recombinant protein and the natural human protein.[44] Factors that can contribute to this immunogenicity include lack of or incorrect glycosylation, amino acid modifications, and amino acid additions and deletions. Several recombinant proteins produced with bacterial vectors contain an N-terminal methionine attached to the natural human amino acid sequence. Bacterial vector-derived recombinant protein preparations may also contain small amounts of immunoreactive bacterial polypeptides as possible contaminants. Additionally, immunogenicity may result from proteins that are misfolded, denatured, or aggregated.

Production of Peptide and Protein Drugs

The production of many important peptides and proteins, via synthetic procedures as well as through biotechnology, involves the pharmaceutical industry. Of necessity, peptides of low to moderate molecular weight, chemically modified peptides, and those containing pseudopeptide bonds or fraudulent amino acids will continue to be made via synthetic procedures rather than through biotechnology. Many of these peptides and proteins are available as chemical analogs, and these also are discussed, particularly the chemical changes made and the implications of these changes to the resulting biologic action (see Chapter 38).

MONOCLONAL ANTIBODIES

Introduction to Antibodies

The cell-mediated branch of the immune system includes the antibody-secreting B cells or plasma cells.[45] Antibodies or immunoglobulins are soluble proteins produced in response to an antigenic stimulus. As part of the normal

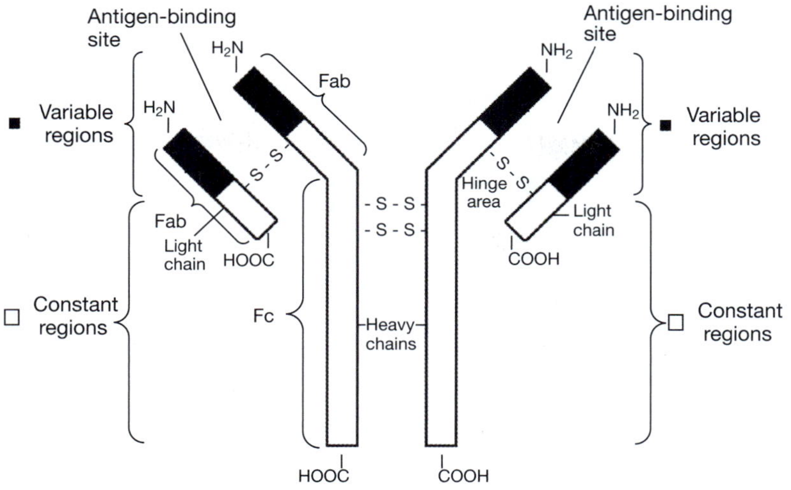

Figure 5.12 Schematic model of an antibody molecule.

immune system, each B cell produces as many as 100 million antibody proteins (polyclonal antibodies) directed against bacteria, viruses, and other foreign invaders. Antibodies act by binding to a particular antigen, thereby "tagging" it for removal or destruction by other immune system components.

The production of antigen-"neutralizing" antibodies or immunoglobulins and the detection of a sufficient antibody titer are important concepts for an understanding of vaccinations and exposure to antigens. The humoral response to an antigen involves the creation of memory B cells and the transformation of B lymphocyte into plasma cells that serve as factories to produce secreted antibodies. Approximately 4 days after initial contact with an antigen (immunization), immunoglobulin M (IgM) antibodies (one of the five types of immunoglobulin structures) appear and then peak approximately 4 hours later. Approximately 7 days after exposure to immunoglobulin G (IgG), the major class of circulating immunoglobulin, appears. The antibodies bind to the antigen and affect additional immune system–mediated events, "neutralizing" the antigen and leading to its elimination. The concentration of an immunoglobulin specific for a given antigen at a given time is referred to as the antibody titer and may be a measure of the effectiveness of the initial antigen exposure/vaccination to elicit immunologic memory.

MAbs are monovalent, meaning that they bind to the same epitope and are produced from a single B-lymphocyte clone. Some of the improvements that can be done on MAbs include minimizing immunogenicity and enhancing antigen-binding affinity, effector function, and pharmacokinetic profile.[46] One can reduce immunogenicity by minimizing nonhuman sequences by creating chimeric, humanized, or human versions of MAbs. Antigen-binding affinity can be enhanced by using phage display libraries to isolate MAbs with strong affinities to the antigen.

Antibody Structure

Antibodies are glycoproteins. The simplest structure of an immunoglobulin molecule consists of two identical long-peptide chains (the heavy chains) and two identical short-polypeptide chains (the light chains) interconnected by several disulfide bonds. The selectivity of any immunoglobulin for a particular antigen is determined by its structure and, specifically, by the variable or antigen-binding regions (Fig. 5.12). Enzymatic digestion of the antibody with papain yields the functional human antibody (Fab) fragment, which contains the antigen-binding sites, and the Fc fragment, which specifies the other biologic activities of the molecule.

Hybridoma Technology

MAbs are ultrasensitive, hybrid immune system–derived proteins designed to recognize specific antigens. Nobel Laureates Kohler and Milstein first reported MAbs in 1975.[47] MAbs have been used in laboratory diagnostics, site-directed drugs, and home test kits. The B lymphocyte produces a wide range of structurally diverse antibody proteins with varying degrees of specificity in response to a single antigen stimulus. Because of their structural diversity, these antibodies would be called polyclonal antibodies. MAbs are homogeneous hybrid proteins produced by a selected, single clone of an engineered B lymphocyte. They are designed to recognize specific sites or epitopes on antigens.

Hybridoma technology (the technology used to produce MAbs) consists of combining or fusing two different cell lines: a myeloma cell (generally from a mouse) and a plasma spleen cell (B lymphocyte) capable of producing an antibody that recognizes a specific antigen (Fig. 5.13). The resulting fused cell, or hybridoma, possesses some of the characteristics of both original cells: the ability of myeloma cells to survive and reproduce in culture (immortality) and the ability of plasma spleen cells to produce antibodies to a specific antigen.

Monoclonal antibodies are more attractive than polyclonal antibodies for diagnostic and therapeutic applications because of their increased specificity of antigen recognition. Thus, they can serve as target-directed "homing devices" to find and attach to the targeted antigen. Developments in hybridoma technology have led to highly specific diagnostic agents for home use in pregnancy testing and ovulation prediction kits; laboratory use in detection of colorectal cancer, ovarian cancer, and others; and design of site-directed therapeutic agents, such as trastuzumab to combat metastatic

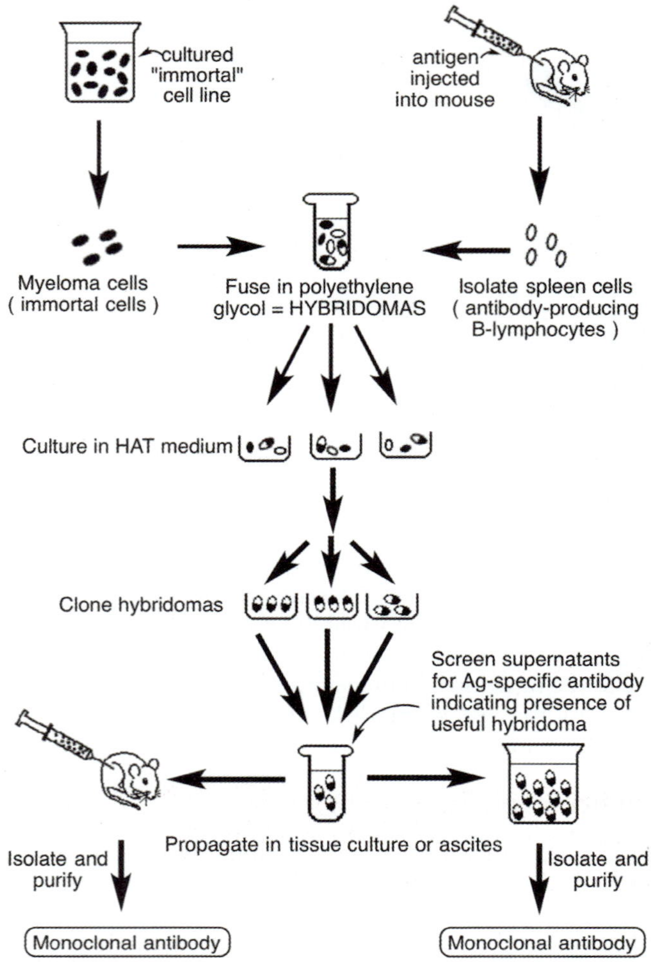

Figure 5.13 Outline of hybridoma creation and monoclonal antibody (MAb) production.

breast cancer and abciximab as an adjunct for the prevention of cardiac ischemic complications.

Monoclonal Antibody Immunogenicity

Nearly 25 years after the pioneering work of Kohler and Milstein, MAbs began to realize their therapeutic potential.[48] Until recently, most MAbs were murine proteins, based on their production. Initial clinical trials of murine MAbs showed that these mouse proteins were highly immunogenic in patients after just a single dose. Human patients formed antibodies to combat the foreign MAb that was administered. The human anti-mouse antibody response is known as HAMA. So, far from being the "magic bullets" that were proposed, immunogenic murine MAbs were useless in chronic therapy. Thus, a different approach was needed to eliminate the unwanted immune response (HAMA) in patients.

The variable regions of an immunoglobulin must be of a specific chemical structure with the ability to bind to the antigen they "recognize." The part within the variable region that forms the intermolecular interactions with the antigen is the complementarity-determining region (CDR). The variable domains of antibody light and heavy chains contain three CDRs each.

It was determined that immune responses against the mouse produced MAbs were directed against both the variable and the constant regions of the antibody. Human and murine antibodies are very homologous in chemical structure. Thus, a MAb with decreased immunogenicity can be engineered by replacing the mouse constant regions of an IgG with human constant regions, making the antibody less "mouse like." In practice, what generally occurs is that the variable heavy chain and variable light chain domains (CDRs) of human immunoglobulins are replaced with those of a murine antibody, which possesses the requisite antigen specificity. This "chimeric" MAb will retain its ability to recognize the antigen (a property of the murine MAb) and retain the many effector functions of an immunoglobulin (both murine and human) but will be much less immunogenic (a property of a human immunoglobulin). A chimeric MAb, containing approximately 70% human sequence, will have a longer half-life than its murine counterpart in a human patient. Therapeutic MAbs that are chimeric include catumaxomab (for malignant ascites), cetuximab (for colorectal cancer), and infliximab (for Crohn disease).

The discovery of the conserved structure of antibodies, particularly IgG, across many species suggested the possibility of chimeric antibodies, and the realization that the homology extended to the antigen-binding site facilitated the engineering of humanized immunoglobulins. Advances in phage display technology and the production of transgenic animals have led to the production of humanized or fully human MAbs.[43] Functional human antibody fragments (eg, Fab fragments) can be displayed on the surface of bacteriophages. A bacteriophage, also called a phage, is a virus that infects bacteria. The expression of these human antibody fragments on the phage surface has facilitated efficient screening of large numbers of phage clones (phage display) for antigen-binding specificity.[45] Once a fragment with the requisite antigen specificity is selected, it can be isolated and engineered into a humanized MAb (replacing up to 95% of the murine protein sequence) or a fully human MAb (100% human sequence). Transgenic strains of mice have been genetically engineered to possess most or all the essential human antibody genes. Thus, on immunization with a foreign antigen, the transgenic mice will develop humanized or fully human antibodies in response. Both techniques, although very complex and expensive, have yielded FDA-approved, humanized antibody pharmaceuticals, such as alemtuzumab (for lymphocytic leukemia), bevacizumab (for metastatic colorectal cancer), eculizumab (for paroxysmal nocturnal hemoglobinemia), and trastuzumab (for refractory breast cancer). The half-life of humanized antibodies is dramatically enhanced (from hours to weeks), and immunogenicity is drastically reduced.

Monoclonal Antibody Diagnostic Agents

Several ultrasensitive diagnostic MAb-based products have enjoyed great success; these include a variety of imaging agents for the detection of blood clots and cancer cells. A monoclonal Fab fragment, technetium-99m-arcitumomab (CEA-scan), can detect the presence and indicate the location of recurrent and metastatic colorectal cancer. Colorectal cancer and ovarian cancer can be detected with satumomab pendetide (OncoScint CR/OV). Capromab pendetide (ProstaScint) is used for detection, staging, and follow-up of patients with prostate adenocarcinoma. Small-cell lung cancer can be detected with nofetumomab (Verluma). The first imaging MAb for myocardial infarction is imciromab pentetate (MyoScint).

Monoclonal Antibody–Based, In-Home Diagnostic Kits

The strong trend toward self-care, coupled with a heightened awareness by the public of available technology and an emphasis on preventive medicine, has increased the use of in-home diagnostics. MAbs specifically minimize the possibilities of interference from other substances that might yield false-positive test results. The antigen being selectively detected by MAb-based pregnancy test kits is human chorionic gonadotropin, the hormone produced if fertilization occurs and that continues to increase in concentration during the pregnancy. Table 5.3 lists some examples of MAb-containing in-home pregnancy test kits as well as some examples of MAb-based, in-home ovulation prediction kits.

Antibody-Drug Conjugates

Paul Ehrlich, in the late 1800s and early 1900s, pioneered the studies in immunology as well as chemotherapy and introduced the concept of "magic bullets." It is now known that cancer cells differ from normal cells because of genomic mutations in oncogenes and/or tumor suppressor genes.[46] Consequently, certain antigens are specifically expressed on the surface of human tumor cells, which can be targeted by MAbs. Binding of MAbs to surface antigens in such tumor cells is highly specific and triggers cell death by many mechanisms, including abrogation of tumor cell signaling and apoptosis, complement-dependent cytotoxicity, and inhibition of tumor vasculature. Despite many cell-killing mechanisms, MAbs often have limited antitumor activity as single agents, particularly against solid tumors.[47] Conventional chemotherapeutic agents, on the other hand, suffer from systemic toxicity and a lack of tumor specificity. This has paved the way for the development of antibody-drug conjugates (ADCs).[48] ADCs are tripartite drugs containing a tumor-specific MAb conjugated to a potent cytotoxic agent via a stable linker. The advantage of an ADC is that it

Table 5.3 Some MAb-Based In-Home Test Kits

Manufacturer	Product Distributor	Positive End Point
Pregnancy		
Answer Plus	Carter Products	Plus in test window = +
Answer Quick and Simple	Carter Products	Plus in test window = +
Clear Blue Easy	Unipath	Blue line in large window = +
Clear Blue Easy One Min.	Unipath	Blue line in large window = +
Conceive	Quidel	Pink to purple test line = +
1 Step E.P.T.	Warner Lambert	Pink color in test and control = +
Ovulation		
Answer Quick and Simple	Carter Products	Purple stick line darker than reference = +
Conceive 1 Step	Quidel	Pink to purple test line darker than reference = +
First Response 1 Step	Carter Products	Purple test line darker than reference = +
Clear Plan Easy	Unipath	Blue test line in large window similar or darker than line in small window = +
Ovukit Self Test	Quidel	White to shades of blue compared to LH surge guide = +
OvuQuick	Quidel	Test spot appears darker than reference = +
Q Test	Quidel	Purple test line darker than reference = +

LH, luteinizing hormone; MAb, monoclonal antibody.
Data from Pray W. *Nonprescription Product Therapeutics*. 2nd ed. Lippincott Williams & Wilkins; 2006:778-780; Quattrocchi E, Hove I. Ovulation & pregnancy home testing products. *U.S. Pharmacist*. 1998;23:54-63; and Rosenthal WM, Briggs GC. Home testing and monitoring devices. In: Allen LV Jr, Berardi RR, DeSimone EM II, et al, eds. *Handbook of Nonprescription Drugs*. American Pharmaceutical Association; 2000:917-942.

selectively delivers a cytotoxic agent to the cancer cells while sparing the normal cells offering a better balance between safety and efficacy.

There has been an explosion in ADC research over the last 10 years.[49] Early attempts to develop ADCs were plagued with limited success due to low drug potency, high antigen expression on normal cells, and unstable nature of the linker used for attaching the drug to the MAb.[50] Currently 13 ADCs are approved by the FDA for the treatment of cancer: (1) ado-trastuzumab emtansine (Kadcyla) is composed of HER2-targeted antibody conjugated to a potent microtubule inhibitor maytansinoid via noncleavable linker, (2) brentuximab vedotin (Adcetris) contains CD30 targeted antibody linked to antimitotic agent MMAE via cleavable valine-citrulline dipeptide linker, (3) mirvetuximab soravtansine (Elahere) is comprised of a folate receptor α (FRα) directed antibody conjugated to a microtubule inhibitor via a glutathione-sensitive disulfide cleavable linker, (4) tisotumab vedotin-tftv (Tivdak) involves conjugation of fully humanized MAb specific for tissue factor (TF-011) to monomethyl auristatin E (MMAE), (5) Loncastuximab tesirine-lpyl (Zynlonta) is composed of CD19-directed MAb conjugated to alkylating agent (SG3199) through a protease-sensitive valine-alanine dipeptide linker, (6) belantamab mafodotin-blmf (Blenrep, withdrawn from the U.S. market in 2022), (7) Sacituzumab govitecan (Trodelvy) is a Trop-2-directed MAb conjugated to a topoisomerase I inhibitor (SN-38) through a hydrolyzable linker, (8) trastuzumab deruxtecan (Enhertu) contains humanized MAb trastuzumab covalently linked to the topoisomerase I inhibitor deruxtecan through a tetrapeptide-based cleavable linker, (9) enfortumab vedotin (Padcev) is a nectin-4-directed MAb conjugated to MMAE through cleavable valine-citrulline dipeptide linker, (10) polatuzumab vedotin-piiq (Polivy) is a CD79b-directed MAb conjugated to MMAE through a cleavable valine-citrulline dipeptide linker, (11) moxetumomab pasudotox (Lumoxiti) is composed of an anti-CD22 MAb fused to a 38 kDa *Pseudomonas* exotoxin A, PE38, (12) Inotuzumab ozogamicin (Besponsa) is a CD22-targeted MAb conjugated to calicheamicin through acid-sensitive hydrazone linker, and (13) gemtuzumab ozogamicin (Mylotarg) is composed of CD33-trageted MAb linked to a cytotoxic *N*-acetyl calicheamicin through acid-sensitive hydrazone linker. Many others are in clinical development.

Various Aspects of Designing Antibody-Drug Conjugates

The selected MAb should target a well-defined antigen that is highly expressed at the tumor site but minimally expressed in the normal tissue to ensure efficient killing of tumor cells by ADCs while limiting general toxicity. Bifunctional linkers carrying attachment sites for both the MAb and cytotoxic drug are used to join the two components. Existing linker attachment strategies typically depend on the modification of solvent-accessible cysteine or lysine residues on the MAb, which leads to heterogeneous ADC populations with variable drug/MAb ratios. While low drug-loading reduces potency, high drug-loading can negatively impact pharmacokinetics (PK). The drug: MAb can also significantly influence the efficacy of ADCs. Moreover, the linker must remain stable in systemic circulation to minimize adverse effects yet rapidly cleave once the ADC binds to its intended target antigen. Once the antigen is recognized and the ADC binds to it, the ensuing ADC-antigen complex is internalized via a receptor-mediated endocytosis.[51] Once inside the cell, the drug is released by one of several mechanisms, including nonenzymatic hydrolysis or enzymatic cleavage of the linker or via degradation of the antibody.

Linker Technology and Stability

The two major classes of linkers being widely used in ADC drug development include cleavable and noncleavable linkers that utilize different mechanisms for release of the drug payload from the MAb (Fig. 5.14). The cleavable linkers are of three types: (1) lysosomal protease–sensitive linkers, (2) acid-sensitive linkers, and (3) glutathione-sensitive linkers.

1. Lysosomal protease–sensitive linkers. Lysosomal proteases such as cathepsin B particularly recognize and cleave a dipeptide bond as in a valine-citrulline linker (Fig. 5.15) to release the free drug from the ADC.[52] Several ADCs evaluated in the clinic, including FDA-approved brentuximab vedotin (for Hodgkin lymphoma), contain such a linker because it provided optimal balance between plasma stability and subsequent cleavage by intracellular protease.[53]
2. Acid-sensitive linkers (Fig. 5.15). These types of linkers exploit the low pH (~5) in the lysosomal compartment to initiate hydrolysis of an acid-labile hydrazone group of the linker and subsequent release of the drug payload from the ADC. Hydrazone linkers have been used in the discovery and development of gemtuzumab ozogamicin (anti-CD33 calicheamicin conjugate) and in inotuzumab ozogamicin (anti-CD22 calicheamicin conjugate).[54,55] Gemtuzumab ozogamicin was approved under accelerated approval program of the FDA in 2000, withdrawn from the market voluntarily by Pfizer in 2010, and reintroduced in 2020 for newly diagnosed CD33-positive acute myeloid leukemia.
3. Glutathione-sensitive linkers (Fig. 5.15). These linkers take advantage of the higher concentration of

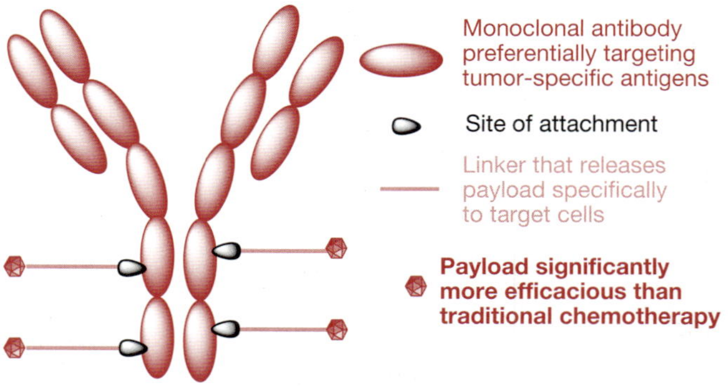

Figure 5.14 Schematic representation of key components of an antibody-drug conjugate (ADC).

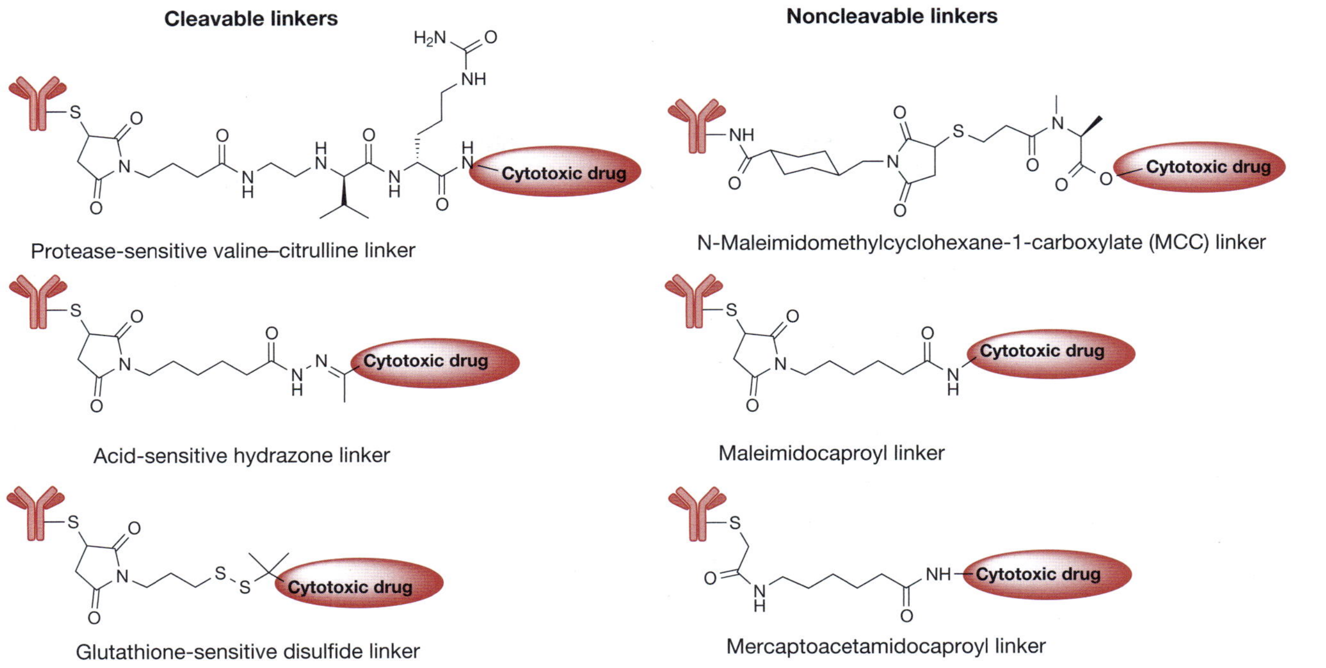

Figure 5.15 Snapshot of cleavable and noncleavable linkers used in antibody-drug conjugate (ADC) development.

glutathione inside the cell relative to that in the plasma. Therefore, a disulfide bond in these linkers is relatively stable in the bloodstream; however, it is capable of undergoing reduction by intracellular glutathione, which ultimately leads to release of the free drug from ADCs. The increased plasma stability of a disulfide bond in the circulation is a result of the insertion of a sterically crowded *gem*-dimethyl group adjacent to the disulfide bond to prevent premature cleavage in the plasma.[56,57] Similar to other linkers described above, glutathione-sensitive linkers are also used in several clinical ADC candidates, including SAR3419 (anti-CD19 maytansine conjugate), IMGN901 (anti-CD56 maytansine conjugate), and AVE9633 (anti-CD33 maytansine conjugate).[58]

The noncleavable linker strategy depends on complete degradation of the MAb upon internalization of the ADC, which results in release of free drug molecules that still carry a linker moiety and amino acid residue from the MAb (see Fig. 5.15). Noncleavable linker strategies are useful for those payloads that exert their antitumor effect despite being chemically modified. Noncleavable linker strategy has been effectively used in the development of ado-trastuzumab emtansine for metastatic breast cancer, wherein the released modified payload (lysine-MCC-DM1) demonstrated comparable potency to DM1 alone.[58] Noncleavable linkers have greater stability in the plasma as compared to cleavable linkers.

Conjugation Strategies: Chemical Conjugation

This strategy involves covalent bonding of a reactive moiety pendant to the drug-linker to the target antibody via an amino acid residue side chain, usually the ε-amine of lysine. This strategy has been successfully used for the development of gemtuzumab ozogamicin (Mylotarg; for acute myeloid leukemia).[59] Another approach involves a two-step process wherein surface lysine residues on the target antibody are first modified to insert a reactive functional group such as a maleimide, and subsequent conjugation to the drug-linker moiety containing a suitable reactive handle such as thiol group.[60] This strategy was used for the development of ado-trastuzumab emtansine (Kadcyla; for metastatic breast cancer). Yet another approach involves controlled reduction of existing disulfide bonds in the target antibody to liberate free cysteine residues, which are further reacted with a maleimide attached to the drug-linker. This approach was successfully used in development of brentuximab vedotin (Adcetris; for Hodgkin lymphoma).[61] The above-mentioned approaches are random and as a result, produce heterogeneous mixtures of conjugated antibodies with a highly variable drug-to-antibody ratio (DAR). Therefore, techniques that allow production of site-specific conjugation with robust DARs are highly desirable.

Site-Specific Conjugation

This strategy allows production of homogeneous ADCs. Three major strategies for site-specific conjugation are (1) insertion of cysteine residues in the target antibody sequence by site-directed mutagenesis, (2) insertion of an unnatural amino acid residue with a bio-orthogonal reactive handle, and (3) enzymatic conjugation. As compared to conventional conjugation-derived ADCs, ADCs generated through drug-linker conjugation with the surface cysteine residues showed minimal heterogeneity, defined DAR, and improved pharmacokinetic and pharmacodynamic parameters.

Bystander Killing by Antibody-Drug Conjugates

A bystander killing mechanism operates when cytotoxic species comes out of the tumor cell and diffuse and kill nearby cancer cells.[62]

Vaccines

There are two types of immunization: active immunization and passive immunization. Active immunization is the induction of an immune response either through exposure to an infectious agent or by deliberate immunization with a vaccine (vaccination) made from the microorganism or its products to develop protective immunity. Passive immunization involves the transfer of products produced by an immune animal or human (preformed antibody or sensitized lymphoid cells) to a previously nonimmune recipient host, usually by injection. Sufficient active immunity may take days, several weeks, or even months to induce (possibly including booster vaccinations), but it generally is long-lasting (even lifelong) through the clonal selection of genetically specific immunologic memory B and T lymphocytes. Passive immunity, although often providing effective protection against some infection, is relatively brief, lasting only until the injected immunoglobulin or lymphoid cells have disappeared (a few weeks or months). Thus, vaccines enable the body to resist diseases caused by infectious agents. In response to an injection of a vaccine, the immune system makes antibodies, which recognize surface antigens found in the vaccine. If the subject is later exposed to a virulent form of the virus, the immune system is primed and ready to eliminate it. Many viral vaccines are produced from the antigens isolated from pooled human plasma of virus carriers. Vaccinations are among the most cost-effective and widely used public health interventions. Although generally safe, the minimal risk of vaccine-produced infections can be eliminated by administration of highly purified vaccine antigens of recombinant origin. The different types of vaccines are described below, and the vaccines currently available in the Unites States are listed in Table 5.4.

Table 5.4 Some Food and Drug Administration–Approved Vaccines

Generic Name	Trade Name	Vaccine Type	Protection Against
Anthrax	BioThrax	Inactivated	Anthrax
Chicken pox	Varivax	Live attenuated	Chicken pox
Diphtheria	Pediarix	Toxoid	Diphtheria
Haemophilus influenza type b (Hib)	ActHIB, PedvaxHIB	Conjugate	*H. influenza*
Hepatitis A	Havrix, Vaqta	Inactivated	Hepatitis A
Hepatitis B	Engerix-B, Recombivax	Recombinant subunit	Hepatitis B
HepA-HepB	Twinrix	Inactivated recombinant	Hepatitis A and B
Herpes zoster	Zostavax	Live attenuated	Herpes zoster
Human papilloma virus	Gardasil, Cervarix	Recombinant	Cervical cancer
Influenza	Fluarix, Fluvirin, Fluzone, Flulaval, Afluria, Agriflu, FluMist	Inactivated live attenuated	Influenza
Japanese encephalitis	Ixiaro, JE-Vax	Inactivated	Japanese encephalitis
Measles	Attenuvax	Live attenuated	Measles
Meningococcal conjugate	Menactra, Menomune, Menveo	Inactivated	Meningococcal
Moderna	Moderna	mRNA	COVID-19
Mumps	Mumpsvax	Live attenuated	Mumps
Novavax	Novavax	Protein subunit	COVID-19
Pertussis	Boostrix	Subunit	Pertussis
Pfizer-BioNTech	Pfizer-BioNTech	mRNA	COVID-19

Table 5.4 Some Food and Drug Administration–Approved Vaccines (*continued*)

Generic Name	Trade Name	Vaccine Type	Protection Against
Pneumococcal	Prevnar, PCV13, Pneumovax23	Conjugate	Pneumococcal
Polio	Ipol	Inactivated	Polio
Sipuleucel-T	Provenge	Autologous	Prostate cancer
Rabies	Imovax, Rabavert	Inactivated	Rabies
Rotavirus	Rotarix, RotaTeq	Live attenuated	Rotavirus
Rubella	Meruvax	Live attenuated	Measles
Tetanus toxoid (TT)		Toxoid	Tetanus
Typhoid	Typherix, Vivotif Berna, Ty-phim Vi	Inactivated	Typhoid
Varicella	Varivax	Live attenuated	Varicella
Vaccinia (smallpox)	ACAM2000	Live attenuated	Smallpox
Yellow fever	YF-Vax	Live attenuated	Yellow fever

Live, Attenuated Vaccines

To make a live, attenuated vaccine, the disease-causing organism is grown under special laboratory conditions that cause it to lose its virulence or disease-causing properties.

Inactivated Vaccines

Inactivated vaccines are produced by killing the disease-causing microorganism with chemicals or heat.

Subunit Vaccines

Sometimes vaccines developed from antigenic fragments can evoke an immune response, often with fewer side effects than might be caused by a vaccine made from the whole organism.

Toxoid or Inactivated Toxins

A toxoid is an inactivated toxin, the harmful substance produced by a microbe. Many of the microbes that infect people are not themselves harmful. It is the powerful toxins they produce that can cause illness. To inactivate such powerful toxins, vaccine manufacturers treat them by chemical means (formalin solution) and irradiation to completely cripple any disease-causing ability.

Conjugate Vaccines

The bacteria that cause some diseases, such as pneumococcal pneumonia and certain types of meningitis, have special outer coats. These coats disguise antigens so that the immature immune systems of infants and younger children are unable to recognize these harmful bacteria. In a conjugate vaccine, proteins or toxins from a second type of organism, one that an immature immune system can recognize, are linked to the outer coats of the disease-causing bacteria. This enables a young immune system to respond and defend against the disease agent.

DNA Vaccines or Naked Vaccine

Genes encoding antigens of an infectious organism are expressed by own cells of the host. Genes are inserted into a bacterial plasmid under the control of a mammalian promoter. The chimeric plasmid is either directly injected into muscle or the DNA is conjugated to a solid matrix such as gold particles.

Recombinant Vector Vaccines

A vaccine vector, or carrier, is a weakened virus or bacterium into which harmless genetic material from another disease-causing organism can be inserted.

mRNA Technology Vaccines

A mRNA vaccine works by introducing a small piece of mRNA that corresponds to a viral protein found on the outer membrane of the virus. Administration of an mRNA vaccine in a series of shots trigger the immune system to generate antibodies to fight against infections such as COVID-19.

COVID-19 Vaccines

Two COVID-19 vaccines (Pfizer-BioNTech and the Moderna COVID-19) based on mRNA technology are approved by the FDA. Upon administration of these vaccines, the muscle cells make the pieces of S protein and subsequently display them on cell surfaces, leading to the production of antibodies. These antibodies protect the host during COVID-19 infection. Two COVID-19 vaccines (Janssen/Johnson & Johnson [no longer available for use in the United States] and AstraZeneca and the University of Oxford), based on vector vaccine technology, are authorized by the FDA for emergency use for people aged 18 years and older. The Novavax COVID-19 vaccine is an example of a protein subunit type of vaccine that is authorized by the FDA for emergency use for people aged 12 years and older.

Pharmacogenomics and Personalized Medicine

Personalized medicine, also known as precision medicine, is a health care approach that integrates information about an individual's genetic profile to help patients make informed decisions regarding the prevention, diagnosis, and treatment of disease. The genetic profile consists of molecular biomarkers from an individual's genome, transcriptome, proteome, and metabolome under the influence of the individual's envirome. This information is then used in the assessment of predisposition to disease, screening and early diagnosis of disease, assessment of prognosis, pharmacogenomic prediction of therapeutic drug efficacy and the risk of toxicity, and monitoring of therapeutic outcomes. Biomarkers serve as critical tools for disease detection and subsequent monitoring. For example, gene mutations, alterations in gene transcription and translation, and alterations in their protein products can all serve as specific biomarkers for disease.[63] Furthermore, mass spectrometry–driven proteomic analysis plays an important role in rapid detection of disease-specific biomarkers and proteomic patterns of various tissues and body fluids.[64]

The concept of personalized medicine was anticipated by Sir William Osler (1849-1919), a well-known Canadian physician during his time. He recognized that "variability is the law of life, and as no two faces are the same, so no two bodies are alike, and no two individuals react alike and behave alike under the abnormal conditions we know as disease." Personalized medicine has rapidly advanced the prediction of disease incidence as well as the prevention of prescribing the incorrect drug based on clinical, genetic, and environmental information of a person. The goal of personalized medicine is optimizing the medical care and outcomes for each patient.[65]

Pharmacogenomics uses genomic tools to understand the genotype effects of relevant genes on the behavior of a drug, as well as the effects of a drug on gene expression. The best examples of successful pharmacogenomic applications are presented below.

Drug efficacy is not solely influenced by variations in drug-metabolizing genes but also by polymorphisms in genes that encode drug receptors and transporters. Polymorphisms and alleles in major phase I drug-metabolizing enzymes (CYP450s) and phase II drug-metabolizing enzymes (UDP glucuronyl transferases, thiopurine *S*-methyltransferases [TPMT]) can be genotyped to aid physicians in individualizing treatment doses for patients on therapeutics metabolized through the products of these genes.

The oral anticoagulant warfarin is prescribed for the long-term treatment and prevention of thromboembolic events. An investigation of the pharmacokinetic and pharmacodynamic drug properties of warfarin indicated the additive involvement of two genes when determining the dosage. One of these genes encodes for CYP2C9, which is responsible for the metabolic clearance (~80%) of the pharmacologically potent *S*-enantiomer of warfarin (Fig. 5.16). There are three allele types, wild-type CYP2C9*1 and nonsynonymous polymorphisms CYP2C9*2 and CYP2C9*3. Both CYP2C9*2 and *3 code for CYP2C9 enzymes with reduced enzymatic activity, leading to increased warfarin half-life and subsequent significant clinical influence on warfarin sensitivity and severe bleeding events.[66] A 10-fold difference in warfarin clearance was observed between groups of individuals having the genotype of the highest metabolizer (CYP2C9*1 homozygote) and lowest metabolizer (CYP2C9*3 homozygote).[67]

Tamoxifen is a prodrug that is metabolized by members of the CYP450 family into two active metabolites: 4-hydroxy tamoxifen (4OH-TAM) and 4-hydroxyl-*N*-desmethyltamoxifen (endoxifen) (Fig. 5.17). CYP3A4/5 is responsible for the conversion of tamoxifen into *N*-desmethyltamoxifen, which is then converted into its active metabolite, endoxifen, by CYP2D6. CYP2D6 is also responsible for the conversion of tamoxifen into 4OH-TAM. In a recent study of steady-state levels of tamoxifen and active tamoxifen metabolites, there was interpatient variability for all three metabolites. A recent study investigating the *CYP2D6*4* allele (inactive enzyme), a poor metabolizer that is common in Whites, in patients being treated with tamoxifen found that individuals who were homozygous for *CYP2D6*4* had significantly lower endoxifen levels than patients who had the wild-type gene. This study clearly indicates that genotyping of patients with impaired CYP2D6 function may be beneficial in a clinical setting to determine which patients will derive the most benefit from tamoxifen therapy.[68]

Tolterodine [(*R*)-*N*,*N*-diisopropyl-3-(2-hydroxy-5-methylphenyl)-phenylpropanamine] is an antimuscarinic drug for the treatment of urinary urge incontinence and other symptoms associated with an overactive bladder. Two different oxidative metabolic pathways, hydroxylation and *N*-dealkylation, have been identified in humans (Fig. 5.18). Hydroxylation to the pharmacologically active 5-hydroxymethyl metabolite (5-HM) is catalyzed by CYP2D6, whereas the

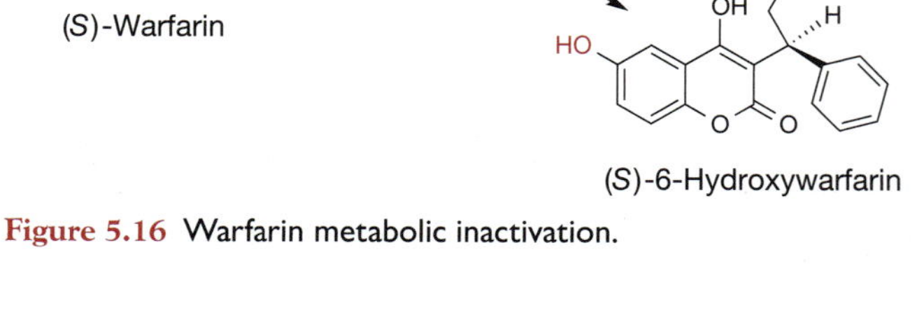

Figure 5.16 Warfarin metabolic inactivation.

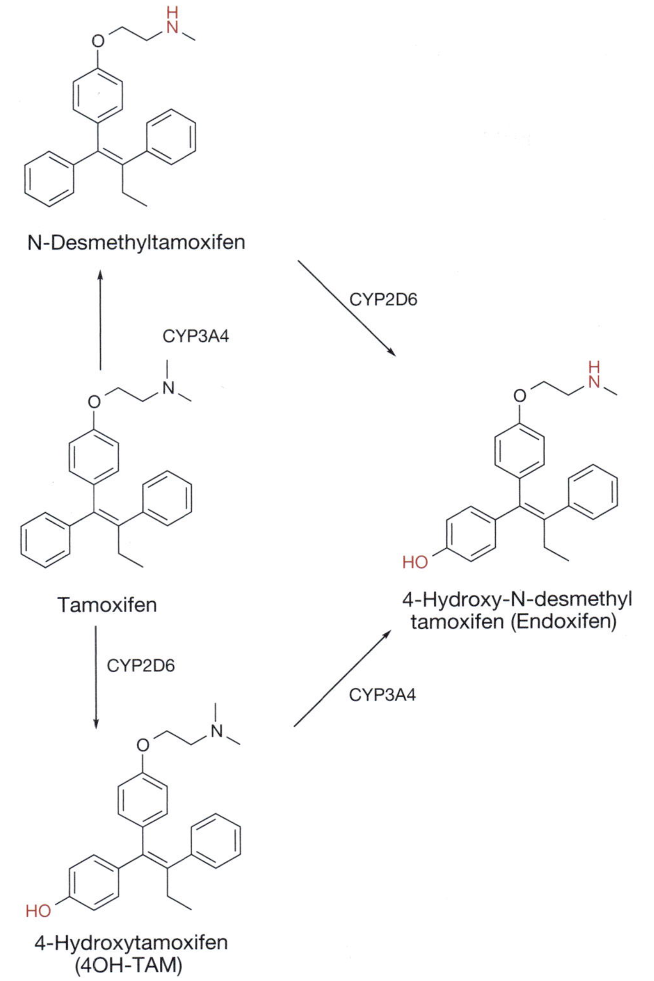

Figure 5.17 Tamoxifen metabolic pathway.

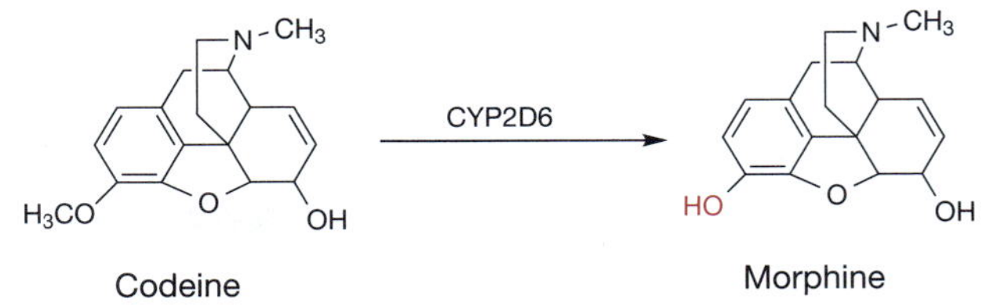

Figure 5.19 Codeine metabolism to morphine.

N-dealkylation pathway to a weakly active metabolite is catalyzed by CYP3A4. Further oxidation of 5-HM catalyzed by alcohol and aldehyde dehydrogenases yields the carboxylic acid of tolterodine and its *N*-dealkylated form, along with *N*-dealkylated 5-HM. The carboxylic acid metabolites are inactive. As described, CYP2D6 is subject to genetic polymorphism, with important implications for drugs that are metabolized by this enzyme such as tolterodine. Clinical studies have demonstrated that individuals with reduced CYP2D6-mediated metabolism represent a high-risk group in the population, with a propensity to develop adverse drug effects. In fast metabolizers, the mean systemic clearance of tolterodine was found to be 44 L/h, yielding a half-life of 2 to 3 hours. In contrast, poor metabolizers have a 5-fold lower clearance and a mean half-life of 9 hours, which results in a 7-fold higher maximum serum concentration of tolterodine at steady state.[69]

Codeine is a prodrug whose analgesic property is primarily due to its metabolic conversion to the central analgesic morphine (Fig. 5.19). This metabolic conversion is catalyzed by CYP2D6 enzyme. Loss-of-function variations in CYP2D6 can lead to a poor analgesic response, and patients carrying such a variation are considered poor metabolizers and receive little therapeutic benefit from codeine. About 5% to 10% of Whites are CYP2D6 poor metabolizers; the percentage is approximately 2% to 3% in other ethnic groups.[70] On the other hand, variations that result in increased metabolic activity of CYP2D6 will lead to enhanced conversion of codeine to morphine with concomitant increased analgesic response. Patients who carry such variations are at risk for opioid toxicity, which includes moderate to severe central nervous system depression. Because some patients are CYP2D6 ultrarapid metabolizers, drugs containing codeine carry a product label that include warnings such as "may experience overdose symptoms such as extreme sleepiness, confusion or shallow breathing, even at labeled dosage

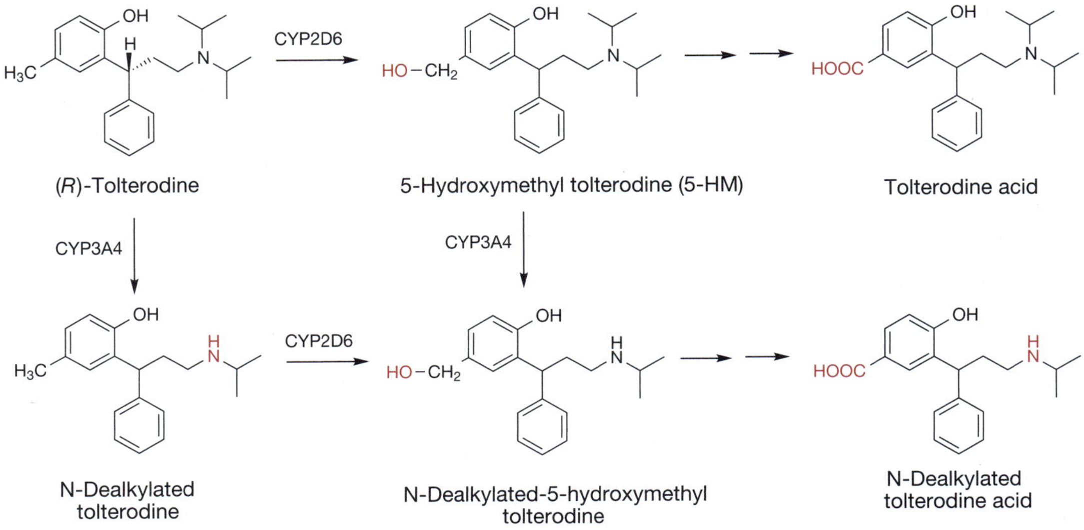

Figure 5.18 Tolterodine metabolic pathway.

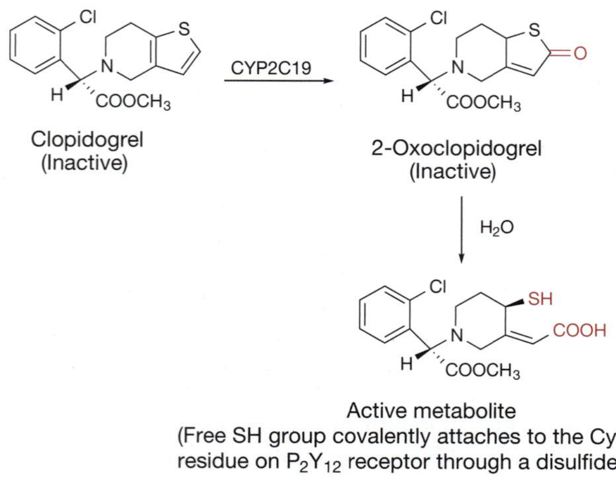

Figure 5.20 Clopidogrel metabolism to active metabolite.

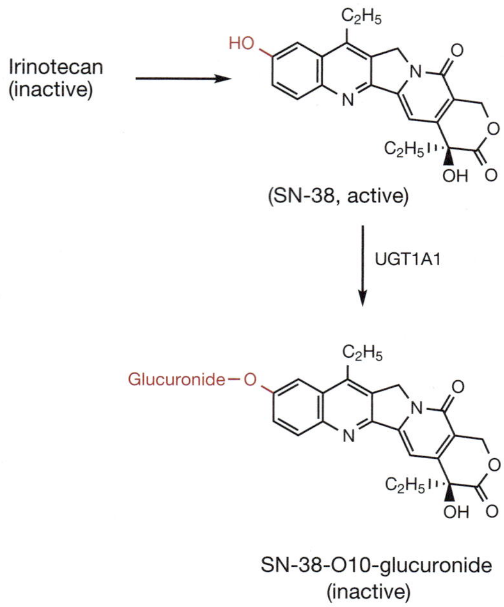

Figure 5.21 Metabolic activation of irinotecan.

regimens," and encourages physicians to "choose the lowest effective dose for the shortest period of time and inform their patients about the risks and the signs of morphine overdose."

Clopidogrel, a thienopyridine derivative, is used for the prevention of recurrent thrombosis in patients with myocardial infarction and percutaneous coronary intervention with stent implantation. Clopidogrel response has been shown to vary widely, both interindividually and interethnically. CYP2C19 metabolizes clopidogrel to its pharmacologically active metabolite (Fig. 5.20). Therefore, patients who carry the loss-of-function *CYP2C19*2* alleles are particularly at higher risk for producing major cardiovascular events such as bleeding as compared to noncarriers.[71]

Irinotecan (also known as CPT-11 or Camptosar) is an approved topoisomerase I inhibitor used to treat patients with metastatic colon cancer. Acute and delayed diarrhea and neutropenia often occur after treatment with irinotecan. Diarrhea following treatment with irinotecan occurs due to the excretion of an active metabolite (SN-38:10-hydroxy-7-ethyl-camptothecin) initially into the bile and subsequently the colon (Fig. 5.21; for more details, see Chapters 36 and 37). Irinotecan treatment is associated with an increased frequency of severe and potentially life-threatening toxicity among patients with genetic polymorphisms that markedly reduce glucuronidation of SN-38 to its inactive metabolite. Patients with decreased capacity to glucuronidate SN-38 (eg, patients homozygous for specific UDP-glucuronosyl transferase 1A1 [UGT1A1] genotypes such as UGT*1A1*28* [TA7]) are at increased risk for severe neutropenia after treatment with irinotecan or SN-38 than patients with the wild-type sequence.[72]

TPMT is a key enzyme involved in the metabolism of azathioprine (AZA) and 6-mercaptopurine (6-MP), two widely used drugs to treat leukemia, rheumatic diseases, inflammatory bowel disease, and solid organ transplantation.[73] AZA is metabolized to 6-MP, the active metabolite of AZA. 6-MP can be inactivated by either xanthine oxidase (XO) or TPMT to nontoxic metabolites (Fig. 5.22). TPMT-deficient patients carrying the nonfunctional TPMT*2, TPMT*3A, and TPMT*3C alleles are at higher risk for producing severe hematologic toxicity, and consequently TPMT-deficient patients require substantial reduction in dose.[74]

Dihydropyrimidine dehydrogenase (DPD) is the rate-limiting enzyme that metabolizes 5-fluorouracil (5-FU), a widely used anticancer drug (Fig. 5.23). A genetic deficiency of the DPD enzyme can lead to toxicity to 5-FU due to reduced clearance, and thus, this drug should not be used in patients with DPD deficiency.[75,76]

The human *N*-acetyl transferases (NATs) are responsible for the catalytic transfer of an acetyl group from acetyl coenzyme A to arylhydrazines as in isoniazid (Fig. 5.24).[77] Functional polymorphisms have been observed in two human NAT genes, NAT*1* and NAT*2*, leading to altered enzyme activity. Based on NAT activity, patients can be classified into two phenotypes: fast acetylators (wild-type NAT acetylation activity) and slow acetylators (reduced NAT enzyme

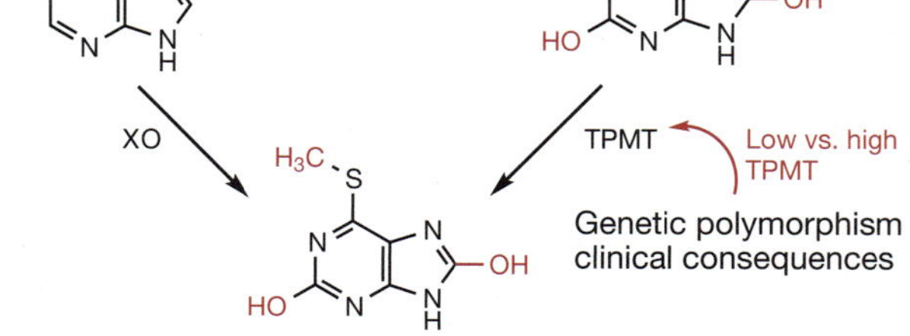

Figure 5.22 Metabolism of 6-mercaptopurine (6-MP) by thiopurine methyl transferase (TPMT) and xanthine oxidase (XO).

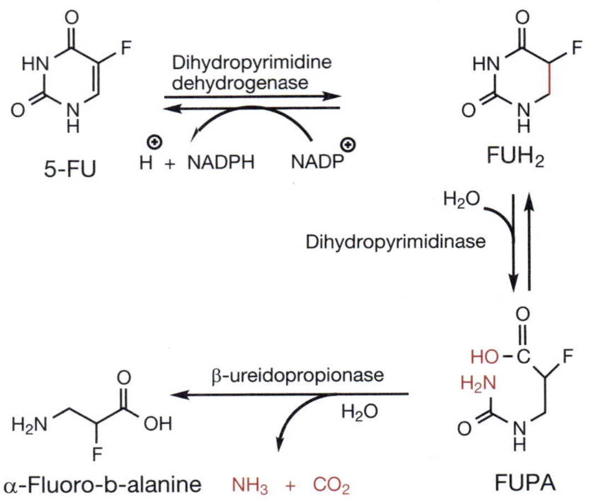

Figure 5.23 5-Fluorouracil (5-FU) inactivation by dihydropyrimidine dehydrogenase (DPD).

activity). Polymorphisms in the NAT*1* (ie, NAT*1*14*, NAT*1*15*, NAT*1*17*, NAT*1*19*, and NAT*1*22*) and NAT2 (eg, NAT2**5*, NAT2**6*, NAT2**7*, NAT2**10*, NAT2**14*, and NAT2**17*) result in slow acetylation phenotype.[78] Since NAT2 plays an important role in deactivation of isoniazid, its response is dependent on the presence/absence of a particular NAT2 genotype. Slow acetylators are presented with increased risk of isoniazid-induced hepatitis.[79]

Trastuzumab is a MAb that specifically targets breast cancers overexpressing the HER2/*neu* gene and thus is marketed solely for the subset of breast cancer patients overexpressing the HER2/*neu* gene (~10%). Because trastuzumab was developed for marker-positive individuals, who comprise a rather low proportion of breast cancer patients, trastuzumab therapy may be one of the best examples of a genomic technology paving the way for personalized medical treatment.[80]

Vemurafenib is specifically indicated for the treatment of metastatic melanoma with BRAF V600E mutation.[81] It is not indicated for patients with wild-type BRAF melanoma. A newly developed diagnostic kit, Cobas 4800 BRAF V600 mutation test, was approved by the FDA to identify patients who will respond to vemurafenib treatment.

Readers are encouraged to refer to a complete list of pharmacogenetic association of gene-drug combinations.[82]

Compounds that pharmacologically inhibit the nuclear poly (ADP-ribose) polymerase (PARP) family of enzymes are a novel class of anticancer drugs targeting the DNA repair activity of PARP-1, the principal member of the PARP family. PARP inhibitors (PARPis) as single agents are efficacious in treating tumors deficient in homologous recombination (HR) components, including breast cancer–associated genes

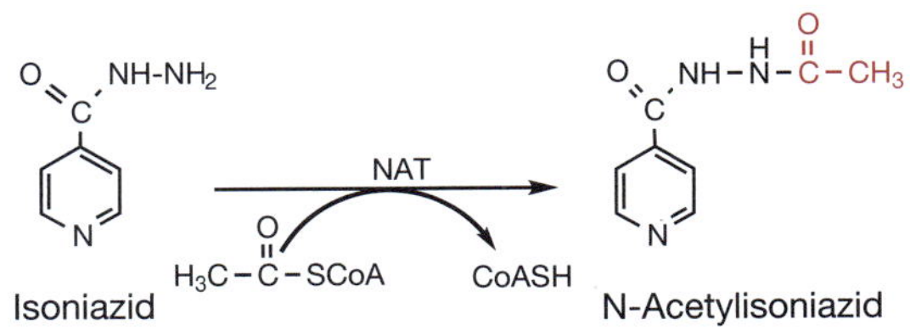

Figure 5.24 Metabolism of isoniazid by *N*-acetyltransferase (NAT).

(*BRCA*)1/2. *BRCA1/2* and other tumor suppressor genes are crucial for accurate HR-mediated DNA double strand break (DSB) repair mechanism (Fig. 5.25). Restoration of BRCA function leads to resistance to PARPi. The FDA-approved PARPis such as olaparib (Lynparza), niraparib (Zejula), rucaparib (Rubraca), and talazoparib (Talzenna) are primarily used as a single drug to treat BRCA-deficient tumors based on the synthetic lethality concept, that is, cancer cells that have lost key BRCA gene functions depend on backup DNA repair pathways such as PARP, and, by inhibiting PARP, such dependence is exploited to preferentially kill the cancer cells while sparing normal cells (Fig. 5.26).[83]

Pegloticase (Krystexxa), a pegylated uricase enzyme approved for the treatment of chronic gout, metabolizes uric acid to allantoin, a highly water-soluble product that is easily excreted by the kidney (Fig. 5.27). With each molecule of uric acid degradation, there is a simultaneous production of one molecule of hydrogen peroxide, which leads to overwhelming oxidative stress and subsequent hemolytic anemia and methemoglobinemia. Normally, oxidative stress is counteracted by the presence of glucose-6-phosphate dehydrogenase (G6PD) through production of cellular reducing equivalents such as nicotinamide adenine dinucleotide (NADH) and glutathione. Pegloticase treatment of patients with G6PD deficiency is thus precluded.[84]

Gene Therapy

Translation of gene therapy concepts to patient care began nearly three decades ago.[85] In principle, gene therapy can produce a lasting and potentially curative clinical benefit. After numerous setbacks due to therapy-related toxicities, the studies are bearing fruit with approvals of gene therapy products by the FDA beginning in 2017.[86] A major problem encountered in gene therapy was similar to the problem encountered in all forms of drug therapy—the assurance of drug efficacy through efficient delivery of the therapeutic agent to its biologic target in a fully functional form. Gene therapy is unique in the sense that it is the product of gene expression, protein, and not the gene itself that is the therapeutic agent. Hence, we must not only deliver the gene to its proper target but also assure that when the gene reaches its target, it will arrive in a form that will produce the therapeutic agent in such a form that it, too, will be assured of reaching its specified target.[87-89]

Gene therapy studies have traditionally focused on direct in vivo administration of viral vectors such as replication-defective retroviruses and adeno-associated virus (AAV). The steps (administration, delivery, and expression) involved in the delivery of the therapeutic gene are shown in Figure 5.28.[90] The field is further fueled by the availability of robust gene-editing technologies such as CRISPR, zinc finger nuclease (ZFN), and transcription activator–like effector nuclease (TALEN) and *ex vivo* approaches using genetically engineered T cells[91] and hematopoietic stem cells. Several gene therapy products have been approved by the FDA, ushering in a new approach to the treatment of serious and life-threatening diseases. For example, voretigene neparvovec-rzyl (Luxturna) is an AAV vector-based gene

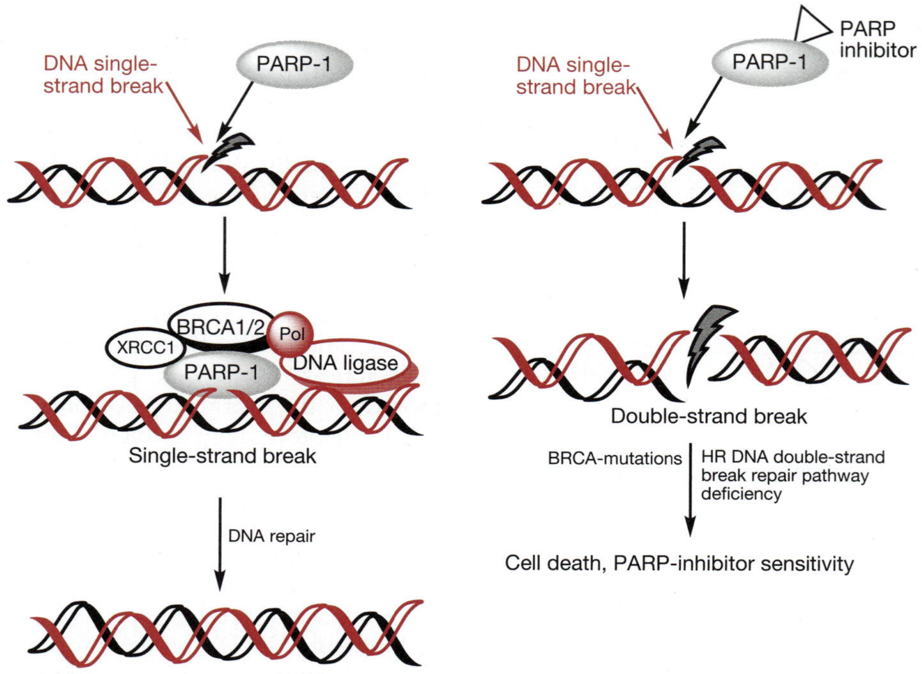

Figure 5.25 Role of poly (ADP-ribose) polymerase-1 (PARP-1) in DNA single-strand break repair and PARP-inhibitor sensitivity in patients with breast cancer–associated gene (BRCA) mutations (homologous recombination [HR] deficiency).

therapy for *the* treatment of patients with confirmed biallelic *RPE65* mutation-associated retinal dystrophy. Etranacogene dezaparvovec (Hemgenix) is an AAV vector-based gene therapy approved for the treatment of adults with hemophilia B. Onasemnogene abeparvovec-xioi (Zolgensma) is an AAV vector-based gene therapy approved for the treatment of pediatric patients age younger than 2 years with spinal muscular atrophy with biallelic mutations in the *survival motor*

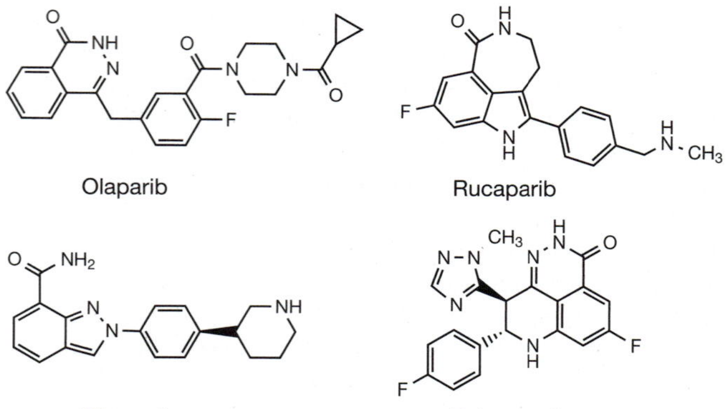

Figure 5.26 Structures of FDA-approved PARP-1 (poly [ADP-ribose] polymerase-1) inhibitors.

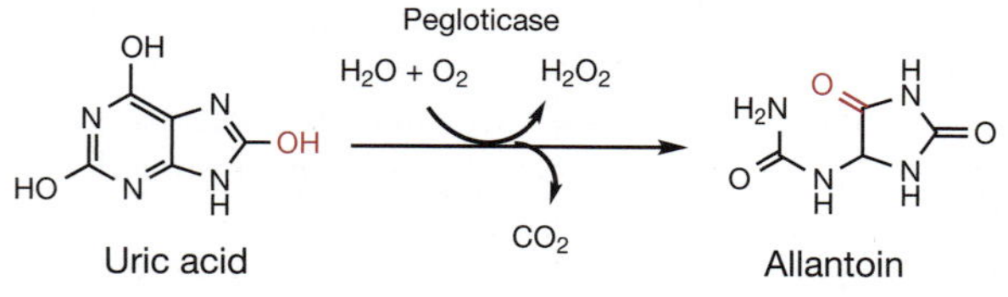

Figure 5.27 Degradation of uric acid by pegloticase.

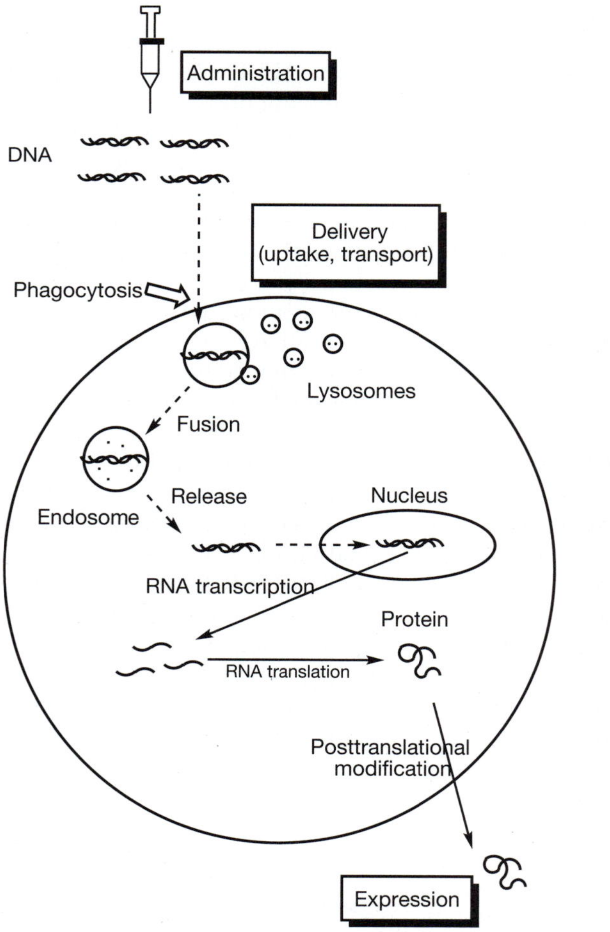

Figure 5.28 Steps in gene therapy. Gene therapy involves the steps of administration, delivery, and expression. (Note: dashed arrows represent uptake and transport.)

neuron 1 (*SMN1*) gene. Betibeglogene autotemcel (Zynteglo) is an autologous hematopoietic stem cell-based gene therapy approved for the treatment of adult and pediatric patients with β-thalassemia who require regular red blood cell (RBC) transfusions. Beremagene geperpavec-svdt (Vyjuvek) is a herpes-simplex virus type 1 vector-based gene therapy indicated for the treatment of wounds in patients 6 months of age and older with dystrophic epidermolysis bullosa with mutations in the *collagen type VII α1 chain* (*COL7A1*) gene. Valoctocogene roxaparvovec-rvox (Roctavian) is an AAV vector-based gene therapy approved for the treatment of adults with severe hemophilia A. Talimogene laherparepvec (Imlygic) is a genetically modified oncolytic viral therapy approved for the treatment of unresectable cutaneous, subcutaneous, and nodal lesions in patients with melanoma. Nadofaragene firadenovec-vncg (Adstiladrin) is a nonreplicating AAV-based gene therapy approved for the treatment of adult patients with high-risk bacillus Calmette-Guerin (BCG)-unresponsive nonmuscle-invasive bladder cancer.

Summary

Completion of the HGP in 2003 resulted in the elucidation of the entire sequence of the 3 billion base pairs in the human genome, estimated to contain some 25,000 genes. The full impact that this scientific advance will have on our lives has yet to be determined, but the social, legal, ethical, and economic issues are certain to be extensive and complex. The manipulation and analysis of the genomic information obtained from the HGP is paving the path for transformative biomedical developments. DNA-based tests are among the first commercial medical applications. Gene tests can be used to diagnose and confirm disease, provide prognostic information about the course of disease, and predict the risk of future disease in healthy individuals.

Knowledge of genes involved in diseases, disease pathways, and drug response sites will result in the discovery of novel therapeutic targets beyond the 500 or so that were known prior to the completion of the HGP, providing a tremendous opportunity for the discovery of drugs that work through previously unexplored mechanisms.

Discovery of genomic biomarkers can help determine the type of drug therapy. For example, one of the most used predictive biomarkers in cancer is immunohistochemical staining for the presence of the estrogen receptor in breast cancer. Only estrogen receptor–positive breast tumors are likely to respond to antihormonal therapy. Identification of biomarkers for various diseases can help in the selection of patients most likely to benefit from a potential drug, which in turn will speed the design of clinical trials that are more efficient and have the potential to reduce drug approval time and associated costs. Predicting toxicity is another important outcome of the availability of genomic information. For example, patients who have mutations in the TPMT gene will metabolize the chemotherapeutic mercaptopurine drugs at a reduced rate and can be overdosed on their treatment. Similarly, an SNP in the coding region of genes expressing drug-metabolizing CYP450 enzymes results in either poor (overdose) or fast (subtherapeutic dose) metabolism of drugs.

The future will see an altered form of health care using a genetic information infrastructure to contain costs and predict outcomes, create advanced personalized therapies, and develop a predict-and-manage paradigm of health care. Recent years have witnessed the introduction of a steady stream of biotechnology-derived drugs. The trend is expected to continue for the foreseeable future. The expiration of patents on biotechnology-derived drugs will introduce an era of more affordable biosimilars or follow-on biologics.[92] A biosimilar is defined by the World Health Organization as a biotherapeutic agent that is similar in terms of quality, safety, and efficacy to an already licensed biotherapeutic (innovator) product. Unlike small molecules, biologics are much more complex and produced in living cells through rDNA technologies, rendering their exact replication impossible. Consequently, the approval process of a biosimilar is highly regulated and requires a comparability exercise between biosimilar and innovator product in terms of physicochemical and biological comparability (quality studies), preclinical comparability (in vitro and in vivo studies), and clinical comparability.[93,94] The first biosimilar product, filgrastim (Zarxio), was FDA approved in 2015. Dozens of additional biosimilars were approved by July 2023, as shown in Table 5.5.

Table 5.5 Food and Drug Administration–Approved Biosimilars

Drug Name	Approval Date	Indication
Zarxio (filgrastim)	March 2015	Increases white blood cells to reduce the risk of infection
Inflectra (infliximab)	April 2016	Tumor necrosis factor (TNF) blocker to treat inflammatory diseases
Erelzi (etanercept)	August 2016	TNF blocker to treat inflammatory diseases
Amjevita (adalimumab)	September 2016	TNF blocker to treat inflammatory diseases
Renflexis (infliximab)	May 2017	TNF blocker to treat inflammatory diseases
Cyltezo (adalimumab)	August 2017	TNF blocker to treat inflammatory diseases
Mvasi (bevacizumab)	September 2017	Vascular endothelial growth factor–specific angiogenesis inhibitor to treat wide range cancers

(continued)

Table 5.5 Food and Drug Administration–Approved Biosimilars (*continued*)

Drug Name	Approval Date	Indication
Ogivri (trastuzumab)	December 2017	HER2/neu receptor antagonist for treating breast and gastric cancers
Ixifi (infliximab)	December 2017	TNF blocker to treat inflammatory diseases
Retacrit (epoetin alfa-epbx)	May 2018	Treatment of anemia
Fulphila (pegfilgrastim-jmdb)	June 2018	Reduces the risk of infection during cancer treatment
Nivestym (filgrastim-aafi)	July 2018	Leukocyte growth factor to reduce incidence of infection
Hyrimoz (adalimumab-adaz)	October 2018	TNF blocker for the treatment of rheumatoid arthritis, psoriatic arthritis, ankylosing spondylitis, adult Crohn disease, ulcerative colitis, and plaque psoriasis
Udenyca (peg-filgrastim-cbqv)	November 2018	Leukocyte growth factor to reduce incidence of infection
Truxima (rituximab-abbs)	November 2018	For the treatment of adult patients with non-Hodgkin lymphoma
Herzuma (trastuzumab-pkrb)	December 2018	For the treatment of *HER2*-overexpressing breast cancer
Ontruzant (trastuzumab-dttb)	January 2019	For the treatment of *HER2*-overexpressing breast and metastatic gastric cancer
Trazimera (trastuzumab-qyyp)	March 2019	For the treatment of *HER2*-overexpressing breast and metastatic gastric cancer
Eticovo (etanercept-ykro)	April 2019	TNF blocker for the treatment of rheumatoid arthritis, psoriatic arthritis, ankylosing spondylitis, and plaque psoriasis
Kanjinti (trastuzumab-anns)	June 2019	For the treatment of *HER2*-overexpressing breast and metastatic gastric cancer
Zirabev (bevacizumab-bvzr)	June 2019	For the treatment of metastatic colorectal cancer
Ruxience (rituximab-pvvr)	July 2019	For the treatment of non-Hodgkin lymphoma, chronic lymphocytic leukemia and granulomatosis with polyangiitis
Hadlima (adalimumab-bwwd)	July 2019	TNF blocker for the treatment of rheumatoid arthritis, psoriatic arthritis, ankylosing spondylitis, adult Crohn disease, ulcerative colitis, and plaque psoriasis
Ziextenzo (peg-filgrastim-bmez)	November 2019	Leukocyte growth factor to reduce incidence of infection
Abrilada (adalimumab-afzb)	November 2019	TNF blocker for the treatment of rheumatoid arthritis, psoriatic arthritis, ankylosing spondylitis, adult Crohn disease, ulcerative colitis, and plaque psoriasis
Avsola (infliximab-axxq)	December 2019	TNF blocker for the treatment of rheumatoid arthritis, psoriatic arthritis, ankylosing spondylitis, adult Crohn disease, ulcerative colitis, and plaque psoriasis
Nyvepria (peg-filgrastim-apgf)	June 2020	Leukocyte growth factor to reduce incidence of infection
Hulio (adalimumab-fkjp)	July 2020	TNF blocker for the treatment of rheumatoid arthritis, psoriatic arthritis, ankylosing spondylitis, adult Crohn disease, ulcerative colitis, and plaque psoriasis

Table 5.5 Food and Drug Administration–Approved Biosimilars (*continued*)

Drug Name	Approval Date	Indication
Riabni (rituximab-arrx)	December 2020	For the treatment of non-Hodgkin lymphoma, chronic lymphocytic leukemia and granulomatosis with polyangiitis
Semglee (insulin glargine-yfgn)	July 2021	For the treatment of diabetes
Byooviz (ranibizumab-nuna)	September 2021	For the treatment of macular degeneration disease and other eye conditions
Rezvoglar (insulin glargine-aglr)	December 2021	For the treatment of diabetes
Yusimry (adalimumab-aqvh)	December 2021	TNF blocker for the treatment of rheumatoid arthritis, psoriatic arthritis, ankylosing spondylitis, adult Crohn disease, ulcerative colitis, and plaque psoriasis
Releuko (filgrastim-ayow)	February 2022	Leukocyte growth factor to reduce incidence of infection
Alymsys (bevacizumab-maly)	April 2022	For the treatment of metastatic colorectal cancer
Fylnetra (pegfilgrastim-pbbk)	May 2022	Leukocyte growth factor to reduce incidence of infection
Cimerli (ranibizumab-eqrn)	August 2022	For the treatment of macular degeneration disease and other eye conditions
Stimufend (pegfilgrastim-fpgk)	September 2022	Leukocyte growth factor to reduce incidence of infection
Vegzelma (bevacizumab-adcd)	September 2022	For the treatment of metastatic colorectal cancer
Idacio (adalimumab-aacf)	December 2022	TNF blocker for the treatment of rheumatoid arthritis, psoriatic arthritis, ankylosing spondylitis, adult Crohn disease, ulcerative colitis, and plaque psoriasis
Yuflyma (adalimumab-aaty)	May 2023	TNF blocker for the treatment of rheumatoid arthritis, psoriatic arthritis, ankylosing spondylitis, adult Crohn disease, ulcerative colitis, and plaque psoriasis

Data from U.S. Food and Drug Administration. Biosimilar product information. https://www.fda.gov/drugs/biosimilars/biosimilar-product-information

REFERENCES

1. Hefti MM, Beck AH. The human genome project and personalized medicine. In: McManus LM, Mitchell RN, eds. *Pathobiology of Human Disease: A Dynamic Encyclopedia of Disease Mechanisms.* Elsevier; 2014:3418-3422.
2. Wang DG, Fan JB, Siao CJ, et al. Large-scale identification, mapping, and genotyping of single-nucleotide polymorphisms in the human genome. *Science.* 1998;280:1077-1082.
3. American Cancer Society. Cancer facts & figures 2023. 2023. https://www.cancer.org/content/dam/cancer-org/research/cancer-facts-and-statistics/annual-cancer-facts-and-figures/2023/2023-cancer-facts-and-figures.pdf
4. Travis J. Genetic engineering. Germline editing dominates DNA summit. *Science.* 2015;350:1299-1300.
5. Wang JY, Doudna JA. CRISPR technology: a decade of genome editing is only the beginning. *Science.* 2023;379: eadd8643. doi:10.1126/science.add8643
6. Hsu PD, Lander ES, Zhang F. Development and applications of CRISPR-Cas9 for genome engineering. *Cell.* 2014;157:1262-1278.
7. Greene AC. CRISPR-based antibacterials: transforming bacterial defense into offense. *Trends Biotechnol.* 2018;36:127-130.
8. Sterner RC, Sterner RM. CAR-T cell therapy: current limitations and potential strategies. *Blood Cancer J.* 2021;11(4):69.
9. Sadelain M, Brentjens R, Rivière I. The basic principles of chimeric antigen receptor design. *Cancer Discov.* 2013;3(4):388-398.
10. Neelapu SS, Locke FL, Bartlett NL, et al. Axicabtagene ciloleucel CAR T-cell therapy in refractory large B-Cell lymphoma. *N Engl J Med.* 2017;377(26):2531-2544.
11. Abramson JS, Palomba ML, Gordon LI, et al. Lisocabtagene maraleucel for patients with relapsed or refractory large B-cell lymphomas (TRANSCEND NHL 001): a multicentre seamless design study. *Lancet.* 2020;396(10254):839-852.
12. Awasthi R, Maier HJ, Zhang J, et al. Kymriah® (tisagenlecleucel)—an overview of the clinical development journey of the first approved CAR-T therapy. *Hum Vaccine Immunother.* 2023;19(1):2210046.
13. Abou-el-Enein M, Elsallab M, Feldman SA, et al. Scalable manufacturing of CAR T cells for cancer immunotherapy. *Blood Cancer Discov.* 2021;2(5):408-422.
14. Pandey A, Mann M. Proteomics to study genes and genomes. *Nature.* 2000;405:837-846.

15. Tonge R, Shaw J, Middleton B, et al. Validation and development of fluorescence two-dimensional differential gel electrophoresis proteomics technology. *Proteomics.* 2001;1:377-396.
16. Zhu H, Snyder M. Protein arrays and microarrays. *Curr Opin Chem Biol.* 2001;5:40-45.
17. Smolka MB, Zhou H, Purkayastha S, et al. Optimization of the isotope-coded affinity tag-labeling procedure for quantitative proteome analysis. *Anal Biochem.* 2001;297:25-31.
18. Uetz P, Giot L, Cagney G, et al. A comprehensive analysis of protein-protein interactions in Saccharomyces cerevisiae. *Nature.* 2000;403:623-627.
19. Saghatelian A, Cravatt BF. Global strategies to integrate the proteome and metabolome. *Curr Opin Chem Biol.* 2005;9:62-68.
20. Clish CB. Metabolomics: an emerging but powerful tool for precision medicine. *Cold Spring Harb Mol Case Stud.* 2015;1:a000588.
21. Bino RJ, Hall RD, Fiehn O, et al. Potential of metabolomics as a functional genomics tool. *Trends Plant Sci.* 2004;9:418-425.
22. Fiehn O. Metabolomics—the link between genotypes and phenotypes. *Plant Mol Biol.* 2002;48:155-171.
23. Gerstein MB, Bruce C, Rozowsky JS, et al. What is a gene, post-ENCODE? History and updated definition. *Genome Res.* 2007;17:669-681.
24. Maxam AM, Gilbert W. A new method for sequencing DNA. *Proc Natl Acad Sci U S A.* 1977;74:560-564.
25. Sanger F, Nicklen S, Coulson AR. DNA sequencing with chain-terminating inhibitors. *Proc Natl Acad Sci U S A.* 1977;74 5463-5467.
26. Tucker T, Marra M, Friedman JM. Massively parallel sequencing: the next big thing in genetic medicine. *Am J Hum Genet.* 2009;85:142-154.
27. Lonnberg H. Solid-phase synthesis of oligonucleotide conjugates useful for delivery and targeting of potential nucleic acid therapeutics. *Bioconjug Chem.* 2009;20:1065-1094.
28. Arnheim N, Erlich H. Polymerase chain reaction strategy. *Annu Rev Biochem.* 1992;61:131-156.
29. Briggs J, Panfili PR. Quantitation of DNA and protein impurities in biopharmaceuticals. *Anal Chem.* 1991;63:850-859.
30. Li S, Schoneich C, Borchardt RT. Chemical instability of protein pharmaceuticals: mechanisms of oxidation and strategies for stabilization. *Biotechnol Bioeng.* 1995;48:490-500.
31. Frokjaer S, Otzen DE. Protein drug stability: a formulation challenge. *Nat Rev Drug Discovery.* 2005;4:298-306.
32. Kerwin BA, Remmele RL Jr. Protect from light: photodegradation and protein biologics. *J Pharm Sci.* 2007;96:1468-1479.
33. Rathore N, Rajan RS. Current perspectives on stability of protein drug products during formulation, fill and finish operations. *Biotechnol Prog.* 2008;24:504-514.
34. Allen LV Jr. Compounding with biotechnology products, part 1: general considerations. *Int J Pharm Compd.* 2022;26(5):385-395.
35. Sindelar RD. Dispensing biotechnology products: handling, professional education, and product information. In: Crommelin DJA, Sindelar RD, Meibohm B, eds. *Pharmaceutical Biotechnology: Fundamentals and Applications.* Springer International Publishing; 2019: 239-251.
36. Buckley ST, Hubalek F, Rahbek UL. Chemically modified peptides and proteins—critical considerations for oral delivery. *Tissue Barriers.* 2016;4:e1156805.
37. Pisal DS, Kosloski MP, Balu-Iyer SV. Delivery of therapeutic proteins. *J Pharm Sci.* 2010;99:2557-2575.
38. Goldberg M, Gomez-Orellana I. Challenges for the oral delivery of macromolecules. *Nat Rev Drug Discovery.* 2003;2:289-295.
39. Bayley H. Protein therapy-delivery guaranteed. *Nat Biotechnol.* 1999;17:1066-1067.
40. Orive G, Hernandez RM, Rodriguez Gascon A, Dominguez-Gil A, Pedraz JL. Drug delivery in biotechnology: present and future. *Curr Opin Biotechnol.* 2003;14:659-664.
41. Dozier JK, Distefano MD. Site-specific PEGylation of therapeutic proteins. *Int J Mol Sci.* 2015;16:25831-25864.
42. Dostalek M, Gardner I, Gurbaxani BM, et al. Pharmacokinetics, pharmacodynamics and physiologically-based pharmacokinetic modelling of monoclonal antibodies. *Clin Pharmacokinet.* 2013;52:83-124.
43. Hoogenboom HR. Selecting and screening recombinant antibody libraries. *Nat Biotechnol.* 2005;23:1105-1116.
44. Bakhtiar R. Therapeutic recombinant monoclonal antibodies. *J Chem Edu.* 2012;89:1537-1542.
45. Gai SA, Wittrup KD. Yeast surface display for protein engineering and characterization. *Curr Opin Struct Biol.* 2007;17:467-473.
46. Chow AY. Cell cycle control by oncogenes and tumor suppressors: driving the transformation of normal cells into cancerous cells. *Nature Educ.* 2010;3:7.
47. Reichert JM. Monoclonal antibodies in the clinic. *Nat Biotechnol.* 2001;19:819-822.
48. Lambert JM. Drug-conjugated antibodies for the treatment of cancer. *Br J Clin Pharmacol.* 2013;76:248-262.
49. Nathan LT. Thinking small and dreaming big: medicinal chemistry strategies for designing optimal antibody-drug conjugates (ADCs). *Med Chem Rev.* 2016;52:363-381.
50. Petersen BH, DeHerdt SV, Schneck DW, et al. The human immune response to KS1/4-desacetylvinblastine (LY256787) and KS1/4-desacetylvinblastine hydrazide (LY203728) in single and multiple dose clinical studies. *Cancer Res.* 1991;51:2286-2290.
51. Ritchie M, Tchistiakova L, Scott N. Implications of receptor-mediated endocytosis and intracellular trafficking dynamics in the development of antibody drug conjugates. *mAbs.* 2013;5:13-21.
52. Dubowchik GM, Firestone RA. Cathepsin B-sensitive dipeptide prodrugs. 1. A model study of structural requirements for efficient release of doxorubicin. *Bioorg Med Chem Lett.* 1998;8:3341-3346.
53. Dubowchik GM, Firestone RA, Padilla L, et al. Cathepsin B-labile dipeptide linkers for lysosomal release of doxorubicin from internalizing immunoconjugates: model studies of enzymatic drug release and antigen-specific in vitro anticancer activity. *Bioconjug Chem.* 2002;13:855-869.
54. Hamann PR, Hinman LM, Hollander I, et al. Gemtuzumab ozogamicin, a potent and selective anti-CD33 antibody-calicheamicin conjugate for treatment of acute myeloid leukemia. *Bioconjug Chem.* 2002;13:47-58.
55. Sapra P, Hooper AT, O'Donnell CJ, et al. Investigational antibody drug conjugates for solid tumors. *Expert Opin Investig Drugs.* 2011;20:1131-1149.
56. Saito G, Swanson JA, Lee KD. Drug delivery strategy utilizing conjugation via reversible disulfide linkages: role and site of cellular reducing activities. *Adv Drug Deliv Rev.* 2003;55:199-215.
57. Talele TT. Natural-products-inspired use of the *gem*-dimethyl group in medicinal chemistry. *J Med Chem.* 2018;61:2166-2210.
58. Erickson HK, Widdison WC, Mayo MF, et al. Tumor delivery and in vivo processing of disulfide-linked and thioether-linked antibody-maytansinoid conjugates. *Bioconjug Chem.* 2010;21:84-92.
59. Bross PF, Beitz J, Chen G, et al. Approval summary: gemtuzumab ozogamicin in relapsed acute myeloid leukemia. *Clin Cancer Res.* 2001;7:1490-1496.
60. Junutula JR, Raab H, Clark S, et al. Site-specific conjugation of a cytotoxic drug to an antibody improves the therapeutic index. *Nat Biotechnol.* 2008;26:925-932.
61. Senter PD. Potent antibody drug conjugates for cancer therapy. *Curr Opin Chem Biol.* 2009;13:235-244.
62. Staudacher AH, Brown MP. Antibody drug conjugates and bystander killing: is antigen-dependent internalisation required? *Brit J Cancer.* 2017;117:1736.
63. Srinivas PR, Kramer BS, Srivastava S. Trends in biomarker research for cancer detection. *Lancet Oncol.* 2001;2:698-704.
64. Wulfkuhle JD, Liotta LA, Petricoin EF. Proteomic applications for the early detection of cancer. *Nat Rev Cancer.* 2003;3:267-275.
65. Hong KW, Oh B. Overview of personalized medicine in the disease genomic era. *BMB Rep.* 2010;43:643-648.

66. Klein TE, Altman RB, Eriksson N, et al. Estimation of the warfarin dose with clinical and pharmacogenetic data. *N Engl J Med.* 2009;360:753-764.
67. Voora D, McLeod HL, Eby C, et al. The pharmacogenetics of coumarin therapy. *Pharmacogenomics.* 2005;6:503-513.
68. Rofaiel S, Muo EN, Mousa SA. Pharmacogenetics in breast cancer: steps toward personalized medicine in breast cancer management. *Pharmgenomics Pers Med.* 2010;3:129-143.
69. Postlind H, Danielson A, Lindgren A, et al. Tolterodine, a new muscarinic receptor antagonist, is metabolized by cytochromes P450 2D6 and 3A in human liver microsomes. *Drug Metab Dispos.* 1998;26:289-293.
70. Rollason V, Samer C, Piguet V, et al. Pharmacogenetics of analgesics: toward the individualization of prescription. *Pharmacogenomics.* 2008;9:905-933.
71. Mega JL, Simon T, Collet JP, et al. Reduced-function CYP2C19 genotype and risk of adverse clinical outcomes among patients treated with clopidogrel predominantly for PCI: a meta-analysis. *JAMA.* 2010;304:1821-1830.
72. Gagne JF, Montminy V, Belanger P, et al. Common human UGT1A polymorphisms and the altered metabolism of irinotecan active metabolite 7-ethyl-10-hydroxycamptothecin (SN-38). *Mol Pharmacol.* 2002;62:608-617.
73. Eichelbaum M, Ingelman-Sundberg M, Evans WE. Pharmacogenomics and individualized drug therapy. *Annu Rev Med.* 2006;57: 119-137.
74. Whirl-Carrillo M, McDonagh EM, Hebert JM, et al. Pharmacogenomics knowledge for personalized medicine. *Clin Pharmacol Ther.* 2012;92:414-417.
75. Gonzalez FJ, Fernandez-Salguero P. Diagnostic analysis, clinical importance and molecular basis of dihydropyrimidine dehydrogenase deficiency. *Trends Pharmacol Sci.* 1995;16:325-327.
76. van Kuilenburg AB. Screening for dihydropyrimidine dehydrogenase deficiency: to do or not to do, that's the question. *Cancer Invest.* 2006;24:215-217.
77. Blum M, Grant DM, McBride W, et al. Human arylamine *N*-acetyltransferase genes: isolation, chromosomal localization, and functional expression. *DNA Cell Biol.* 1990;9:193-203.
78. Sim E, Lack N, Wang CJ, et al. Arylamine *N*-acetyltransferases: structural and functional implications of polymorphisms. *Toxicology.* 2008;254:170-183.
79. Huang YS, Chern HD, Su WJ, et al. Polymorphism of the *N*-acetyltransferase 2 gene as a susceptibility risk factor for antituberculosis drug-induced hepatitis. *Hepatology.* 2002;35:883-889.
80. Ross JS, Schenkein DP, Pietrusko R, et al. Targeted therapies for cancer 2004. *Am J Clin Pathol.* 2004;122:598-609.
81. Chapman PB, Robert C, Larkin J, et al. Vemurafenib in patients with BRAFV600 mutation-positive metastatic melanoma: final overall survival results of the randomized BRIM-3 study. *Ann Oncol.* 2017;28:2581-2587.
82. Rubinstein WS, Pacanowski M. Pharmacogenetic gene-drug associations: FDA perspective on what physicians need to know. *Am Fam Physician.* 2021;104(1):16-19.
83. Lord CJ, Ashworth A. PARP inhibitors: synthetic lethality in the clinic. *Science.* 2017;355:1152-1158.
84. Owens RE, Swanson H, Twilla JD. Hemolytic anemia induced by pegloticase infusion in a patient with G6PD deficiency. *J Clin Rheumatol.* 2016;22:97-98.
85. Keeler AM, ElMallah MK, Flotte TR. Gene therapy 2017: progress and future directions. *Clin Transl Sci.* 2017;10:242-248.
86. Dunbar CE, High KA, Joung JK, et al. Gene therapy comes of age. *Science.* 2018;359:eaan4672.
87. Terazaki Y, Yano S, Yuge K, et al. An optimal therapeutic expression level is crucial for suicide gene therapy for hepatic metastatic cancer in mice. *Hepatology.* 2003;37:155-163.
88. Goverdhana S, Puntel M, Xiong W, et al. Regulatable gene expression systems for gene therapy applications: progress and future challenges. *Mol Ther.* 2005;12:189-211.
89. Chen P, Tian J, Kovesdi I, et al. Promoters influence the kinetics of transgene expression following adenovector gene delivery. *J Gene Med.* 2008;10:123-131.
90. Ledley FD. Nonviral gene therapy: the promise of genes as pharmaceutical products. *Hum Gene Ther.* 1995;6:1129-1144.
91. Sadelain M, Riviere I, Riddell S. Therapeutic T cell engineering. *Nature.* 2017;545:423-431.
92. Dahodwala H, Sharfstein ST. Biosimilars: imitation games. *ACS Med Chem Lett.* 2017;8:690-693.
93. Agarwal AB, McBride A. Understanding the biosimilar approval and extrapolation process—a case study of an epoetin biosimilar. *Crit Rev Oncol Hematol.* 2016;104:98-107.
94. Blandizzi C, Meroni PL, Lapadula G. Comparing originator biologics and biosimilars: a review of the relevant issues. *Clin Ther.* 2017;39:1026-1039.

PART II

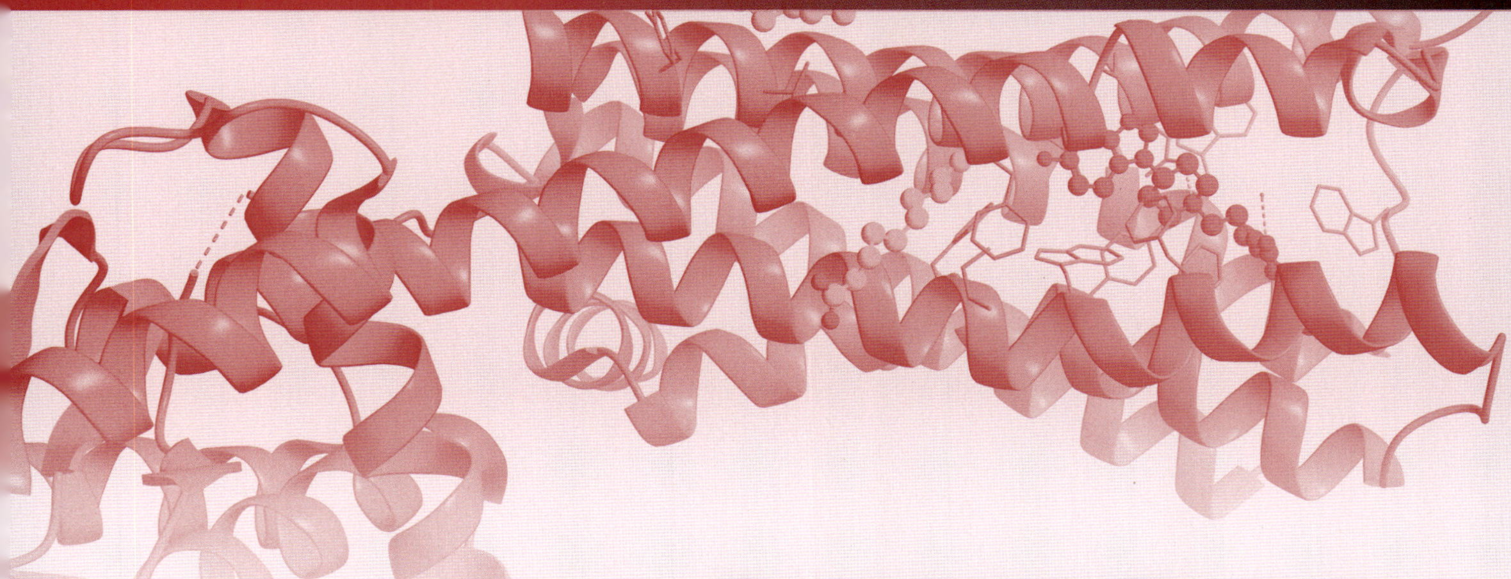

RECEPTOR TARGETS

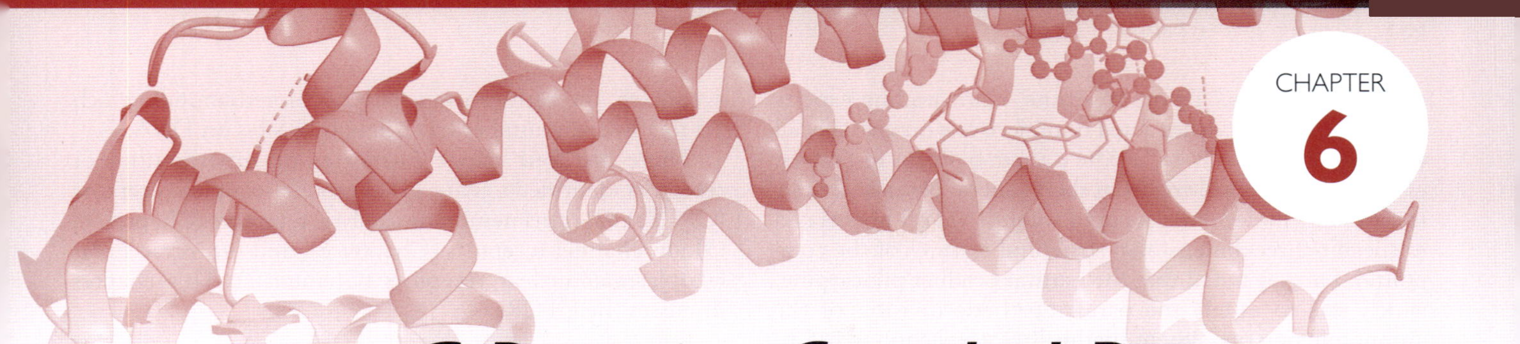

CHAPTER

6

G Protein–Coupled Receptors

Dan Kiel

Drugs covered in this chapter:

- Acetylcholine
- Atropine
- Butorphanol
- Cimetidine
- Dihydromorphinone
- Diphenhydramine
- Dopamine
- Doxepin
- Epinephrine
- Fexofenadine
- Isoproterenol
- Istradefylline
- Mechlorethamine
- Morphine
- Muscarine
- Nalbuphine
- Naloxone
- Naltrexone
- Norepinephrine
- Oliceridine
- Pentazocine
- Pilocarpine
- Pirenzepine
- Pitolisant
- Propranolol
- Ranitidine
- Risperidone
- Sufentanil

Abbreviations

βARK β-adrenoceptor kinase
5-HT 5-hydroxytryptamine
ACh acetylcholine
ADHD attention-deficit/hyperactivity disorder
ATP adenosine triphosphate
BBB blood-brain barrier
CaM calmodulin
cAMP cyclic adenosine monophosphate
cDNA complementary DNA
cGMP cyclic guanosine monophosphate
CNS central nervous system
DAG diacylglycerol
FDA U.S. Food and Drug Administration
GABA γ-aminobutyric acid
GDP guanosine diphosphate
GI gastrointestinal
GPCRs G protein–coupled receptors
GSK-3 glycogen synthase kinase 3
GTP guanosine triphosphate
IP_3 inositol 1,4,5-trisphosphate
IUPHAR International Union of Basic and Clinical Pharmacology
NOP N/OFQ peptide
PKC protein kinase C
PLC phospholipase C
SAR structure-activity relationship
TMD transmembrane domain

Introduction

Historical Perspectives

For years it had been known that some drugs were capable of producing their effects by acting at specific sites within the body. Claude Bernard was the first to demonstrate this in the mid-1800s, with his classical experiments involving curare.[1] He demonstrated that this neuromuscular blocking agent, which was used as an arrow poison by the South American natives, was capable of preventing skeletal muscle contraction following nerve stimulation but was without effect when the muscle was stimulated directly. This work demonstrated for the first time a localized site of action for a drug and, most importantly, suggested that a gap, now termed a synapse, existed between the nerve and the muscle. From these findings, he postulated that some chemical substance normally communicated the information between the nerve and the target tissue—in this case, the muscle. These findings established the foundations for what is known today as "chemical neurotransmission," a process frequently disrupted by diseases and, likewise, the target of many therapeutic agents.

Investigations by J. N. Langley[2] in the early 1900s established the initial foundations for the interaction of drugs with specific cellular components, later to be identified and termed "receptors." Before this time, many leading experts believed that most drugs acted nonselectively on virtually all the cells in the body to produce their biologic responses, with a response resulting from their general physical characteristics (eg, molecular size, lipid solubility) and not related to specific three-dimensional structural features of the compound. Langley noted that the natural product pilocarpine, which acts to mimic the parasympathetic division of the autonomic nervous system that utilizes acetylcholine (ACh) as the endogenous neurotransmitter, was very selective and also extremely potent. Additionally, the natural product atropine was capable of blocking, in a rather selective fashion, the effects of pilocarpine and parasympathetic nervous system stimulation. Importantly, he concluded that these two compounds interacted with the same component of the cell.

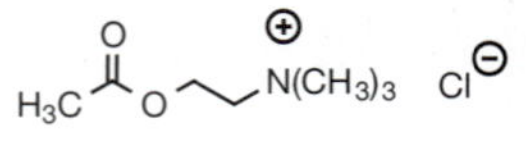

Acetylcholine chloride

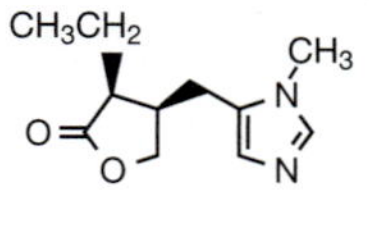

Pilocarpine

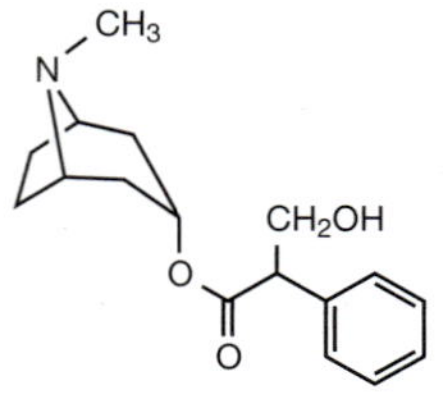

Atropine

Paul Ehrlich,[3] a noted microbiologist during the late 19th and early 20th centuries, is credited with coining the term "receptive substance," or "receptor." His observations that various organic compounds appeared to produce their antimicrobial effects with a high degree of selectivity led him to speculate that drugs produced their effects by binding to such a receptive substance. The interaction or binding of the drug with the receptor was analogous to a "lock" (the receptor) and a "key" (the drug), which gave rise to the "lock and key" fit theory for drug receptors. Thus, certain organic compounds would properly fit into the receptor and activate it, leading to a high degree of specificity. Although such a situation might be considered ideal for drug therapy, few drugs actually interact only with their intended receptors. The frequency of side effects is not always associated with a simple extension of their desired pharmacologic actions; instead, drug molecules can also bind with other receptors or nonreceptor entities on or within cells to produce a host of other—and often undesirable—effects.

A small number of drugs produce their desired therapeutic effects without interacting with a specific receptor. For example, osmotic diuretics produce their pharmacologic effects simply by creating an osmotic gradient in the renal tubules promoting the elimination of water in the urine, and antacids produce their beneficial effects by chemically neutralizing the hydrochloric acid found in the stomach. More sophisticated mechanisms can also be involved in the non–receptor-mediated actions of older antineoplastic agents (eg, the nitrogen mustard mechlorethamine), which act to alkylate a number of nucleophilic sites on DNA.

There are four major categories or superfamilies of receptors identified to date: (1) G protein–coupled receptors (GPCRs), (2) transmembrane catalytic receptors (Chapter 9), (3) ion channel receptors (Chapter 8), and (4) intracellular cytoplasmic/nuclear receptors (Chapter 7). This chapter discusses the GPCRs.

TRANSMEMBRANE G PROTEIN–COUPLED RECEPTORS

The GPCRs are a family of large membrane-bound proteins that share a well-conserved structure and transduce their signal via the activation of an intracellular guanine nucleotide-binding protein (G protein). This family of proteins has seven hydrophobic (heptahelical) transmembrane domains (TMDs) that span the plasma membrane, and its shape has a serpentine structure (Fig. 6.1). The extracellular region of the protein is composed of the amino-terminus and several loops (EC1-EC3), which comprise the ligand-binding site. The seven TMDs are composed primarily of lipophilic amino acids arranged in α-helices connected by regions of hydrophilic amino acids. The hydrophilic regions form loops on the intracellular and extracellular faces of the membrane. Smaller sized ligands tend to bind deep within the transmembrane regions, close to the plasma membrane, whereas larger sized molecules have binding sites that are more superficial.

The carboxy end of the receptor is located in the area of the protein that protrudes into the cytoplasm. The intracellular side of the receptor also includes the binding site for the G protein, which usually binds to the protein on the third loop between TMD 6 and 7. Close to the carboxy terminus are Ser and Thr residues, which are targets for adenosine triphosphate (ATP)-dependent phosphorylation.

More than 100 different GPCRs bind to a variety of ligands encompassing biogenic amines, such as norepinephrine, dopamine, serotonin, histamine, and ACh; amino acid neurotransmitters, such as glutamate and γ-aminobutyric acid (GABA); peptide neurotransmitters, neuromodulators, and hormones, such as endogenous opioids, angiotensin II, and somatostatin; and other neurotransmitters such as the endocannabinoids. There are oftentimes multiple GPCR types for a single ligand—in some cases as many as 12. The result is the possibility that a single ligand can activate a variety of transduction pathways and produce a multiplicity of cellular responses. Thus, a receptor is defined not only by which ligand binds to it but also by how the signal is transduced and the nature of the resultant physiologic response.

As an example, at least nine different adrenergic receptor (adrenoceptor) subtypes exist. Norepinephrine can bind to the β_1-adrenoceptor, which is coupled to a G protein (designated G_s). Following receptor stimulation of G_s, there is activation of the enzyme adenylyl cyclase, leading ultimately to an increase in heart rate and force of contraction. Norepinephrine binding to α_1-adrenoceptors, on the other hand,

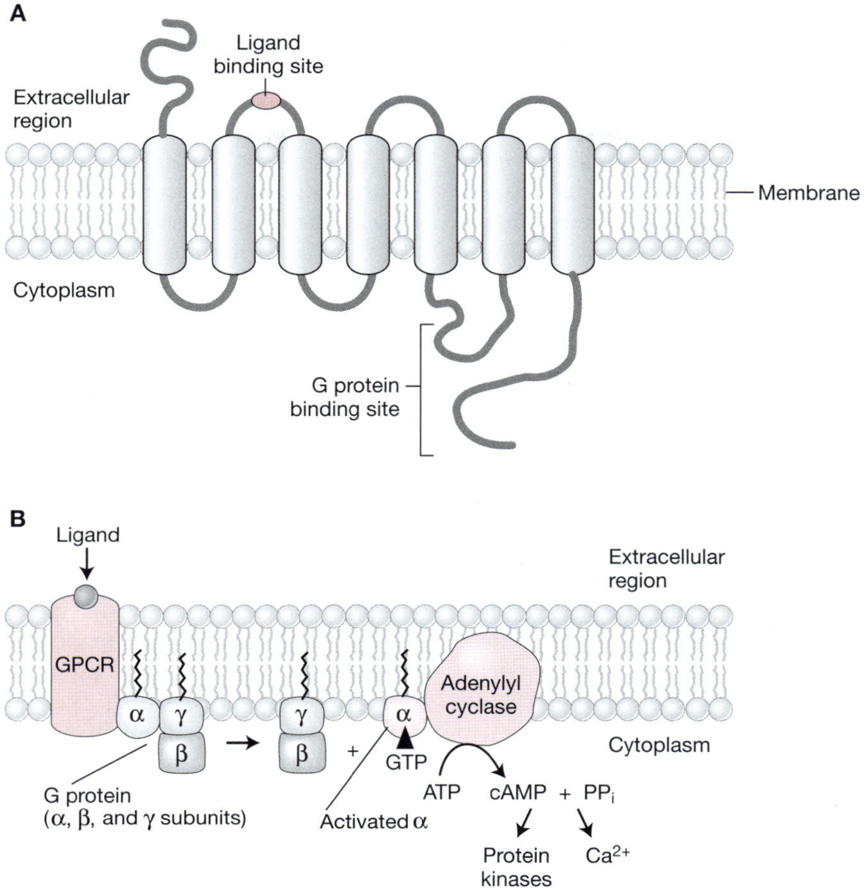

Figure 6.1 General G protein–coupled receptor (GPCR) structure and activation by agonist. A. Diagram of a GPCR showing the extracellular N-terminus, three extracellular loops (one of which binds ligands), and the seven transmembrane regions. Three intracellular loops and the C-terminus are also depicted with the interface between intracellular loop 3 and the C-terminus representing the site of G protein recognition. B. Activation of a G_s-linked GPCR leads to dissociation of the three G protein subunits and the subsequent stimulation of adenylyl cyclase by the guanosine triphosphate (GTP)-bound α-subunit. Adenylyl cyclase converts adenosine triphosphate (ATP) into cyclic adenosine monophosphate (cAMP), which activates protein kinase A. (From Pandit N, Soltis R. *Introduction to the Pharmaceutical Sciences*. 2nd ed. Lippincott Williams & Wilkins; 2011, with permission.)

results in the binding to a different G protein (G_q), which activates the enzyme phospholipase C (PLC), producing the second messengers inositol 1,4,5-trisphosphate (IP_3) and diacylglycerol (DAG), which then can initiate a cascade of intracellular events leading to smooth muscle contraction. Therefore, a single ligand can induce a wide range of responses as a consequence of activating different receptors linked to different G proteins. Which G protein is activated depends on factors such as the presence and availability of individual G proteins within a particular cell type, kinetic issues (eg, the binding affinity of the G protein for the receptor protein), and, finally, the affinity of the activated G-protein subunits for signal transduction enzymes.

A number of experimental findings over the last 30 years have demonstrated that the "lock and key" model for GPCR activation is inadequate. The demonstration that systems overexpressing GPCRs have low but measurable basal activity, and that certain ligands termed "inverse agonists" reduce this activity, cannot be explained by the "lock and key" model. Thus the "two-state" receptor model has replaced it. This postulates that a population of any GPCR exists in at least two conformations, an active and an inactive form.[4] The active form spontaneously couples to G proteins while the inactive form does not. With no ligand present, the vast majority of the receptors are in the inactive form but a small percentage is in the active form, thus generating basal activity. Agonists are defined as ligands that selectively bind to the active receptor; the more agonist added to cells, the greater the population of receptors that shifts to the active conformation and thus the greater activation of the G protein. Inverse agonists are those ligands that have affinity for the inactive conformation and not the active conformation, and as concentrations of inverse agonists are increased, the basal activity decreases as those few active receptors shift to the inactive conformation. Partial agonists are defined as having preferential affinity for the active receptor but still having some affinity for inactive receptors. Thus, as the concentration of partial agonist is increased, the cell becomes activated because the net effect is that more receptors shift into the active conformation than the inactive one. But as the ligand also binds the inactive conformation, all the receptors cannot convert to the active conformation no matter how much partial agonist is added. This results in a partial agonist activating a system but with a lower maximal effect compared to a full agonist. Some ligands bind with equal affinity for the active and inactive conformations of the receptor and are termed neutral antagonists. These ligands will not change the basal activity of the biologic system but will block the binding and actions of both agonists and inverse agonists.

G Proteins

The G proteins are heterotrimeric in structure with the subunits (in decreasing size) designated as α, β, and γ. Many types of these G proteins have been identified, with as many as 20 varieties of the α-subunits, 5 of the β-subunits, and 12 of the γ-subunits. The characteristics of the α-subunit are what largely determine the designation of the G protein and are thus the most widely studied.[5] Some of the more common α-subunits characterized are termed G_s, G_i, G_o, and $G_{q/11}$. Individual G proteins transduce the receptor activation signal via one of a number of second-messenger systems discussed later. The best understood second-messenger systems associated with each G protein family are summarized in Table 6.1.

Binding to an active receptor molecule leads to a conformational change in the associated G protein, triggering the release of bound guanosine diphosphate (GDP) from the α-subunit, which is then replaced by a molecule of guanosine triphosphate (GTP). With the binding of GTP, the α-subunit-GTP complex dissociates from the βγ-subunits and binds to a particular target enzyme, resulting in its activation or inhibition. Within a short period of time, the intrinsic phosphatase activity of the α-subunit catalyzes the dephosphorylation of the associated GTP molecule to GDP, resulting in the reassociation of the α-subunit with the βγ-subunits and, thus, the return of the G protein to the inactivated state. Variations on this scheme include the activation of proteins such as G protein–gated ion channels by dissociated βγ-subunits and the ability of receptor proteins to activate more than a single G protein. The simultaneous activation of more than one type of GPCR results in the initiation of multiple signals, which can then interact with one another (a phenomenon commonly referred to as "cross-talk"). This interaction can be of several types: If both receptors use a common signal transduction pathway, the activation can result in an additive response by the cell. Conversely, if simultaneous receptor activation triggers opposing signal transduction pathways, the outcome will be an attenuated cellular response. Other types of interactions include the desensitization or activation of other receptor proteins or second-messenger pathways. The final outcome of the activation of multiple signals is an overall integrated response by the cell (Fig. 6.2).

Table 6.1 G Protein Transducers and Second Messengers

G Protein Transducer Family	Second-Messenger System
G_s	Stimulates adenylyl cyclase activity and Ca^{2+} channels
$G_{i/o}$	Inhibits adenylyl cyclase activity and opens K^+ channels
G_q	Stimulates phospholipase C activity
G_{12}	Modulates sodium/hydrogen ion exchanger

Second-Messenger Pathways

As discussed, in response to receptor activation, G proteins activate plasma membrane–bound enzymes, which then trigger a metabolic cascade that results in a cellular response.[5] The products of these enzymatic actions are termed "second messengers" because they mobilize other enzymatic and structural proteins, which then ultimately produce the cellular response. (Although not referred to as such, the neurotransmitter or hormone that activates the GPCR is the "first messenger" to a cell.) The enzymes catalyzing the synthesis of second messengers fall generally into two categories: those that convert the purine triphosphates ATP and GTP into their respective cyclic monophosphates (eg, cyclic adenosine monophosphate [cAMP], cyclic guanosine monophosphate [cGMP]) and enzymes that synthesize second messengers from plasma membrane phospholipids (eg, DAG and IP_3). The most thoroughly studied second-messenger system is controlled by a family of 10 plasma membrane–bound isozymes of adenylyl cyclase that catalyze the conversion of ATP to cAMP (Fig. 6.1B). Adenylyl cyclase is activated by the G_s family of G proteins and inhibited by the G_i family. Following synthesis, cAMP activates cAMP-dependent protein kinases by triggering the dissociation of regulatory subunits from catalytic subunits. The catalytic subunits then activate other target proteins via phosphorylation, which then trigger the cellular response (Fig. 6.3). The magnitude of the cellular response is proportional to the concentration of cAMP. Degradation of cAMP occurs via phosphodiesterases or by reducing cAMP concentration via active transport out of the cell. The result is termination of the signal.

A similar, although less ubiquitous, second-messenger pathway is associated with guanylyl cyclase. Guanylyl cyclase is activated in response to some other non-GPCR catalytic receptors selective for ligands including atrial natriuretic factor and nitric oxide. When stimulated, guanylyl cyclase catalyzes the synthesis of cGMP from GTP. The formed cGMP subsequently activates cGMP-dependent protein kinases, which then phosphorylate other proteins. The actions of cGMP are terminated by enzymatic degradation of the second messenger by the same phosphodiesterases mentioned earlier or the dephosphorylation of substrates.

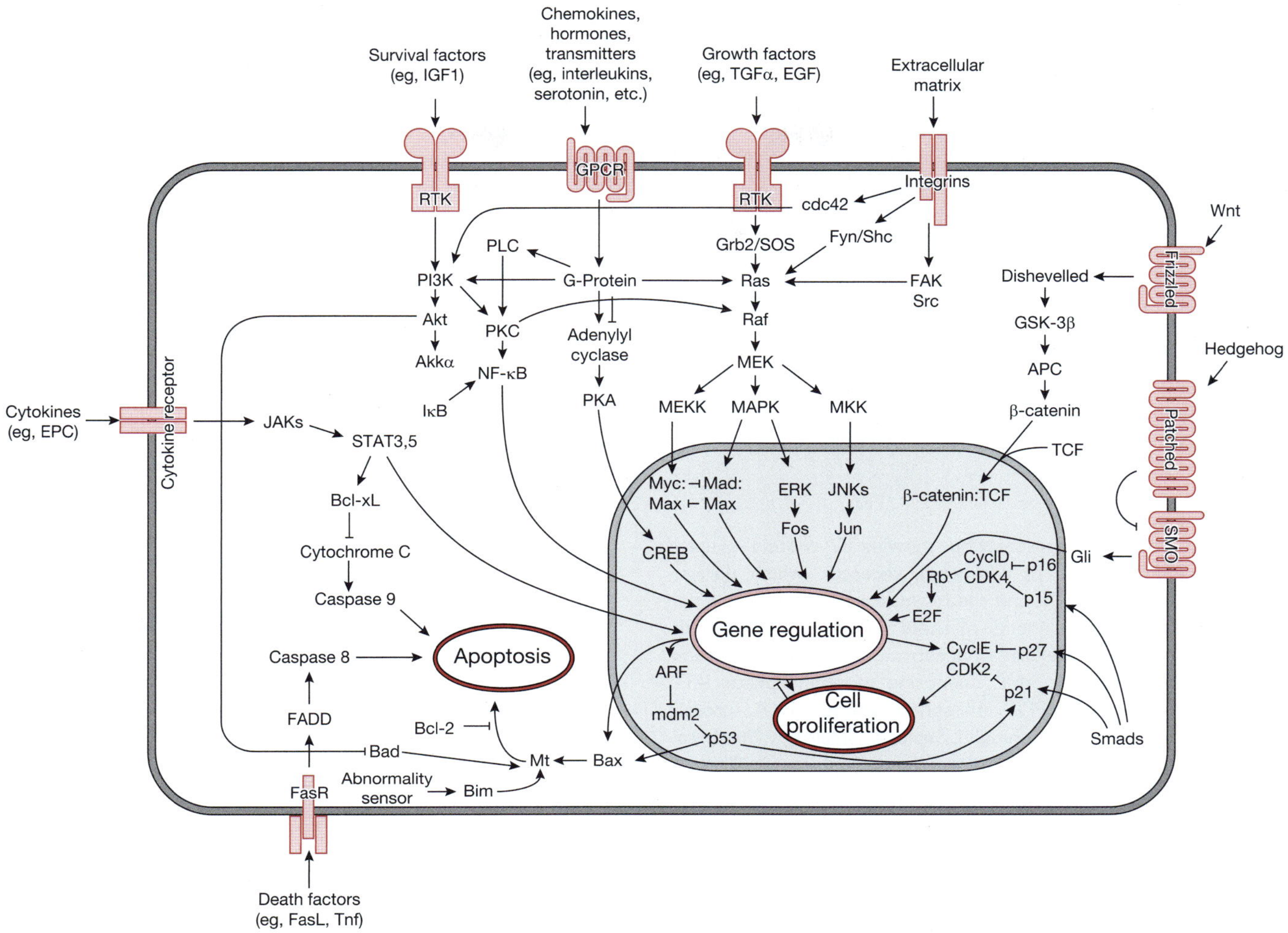

Figure 6.2 Signal transduction cascades that regulate gene expression and apoptosis. (From Wikipedia. Mitogen-activated protein kinase. https://en.wikipedia.org/wiki/Mitogen-activated_protein_kinase)

One effect of this second-messenger pathway is relaxation of smooth muscle via the dephosphorylation of myosin light chain kinases.

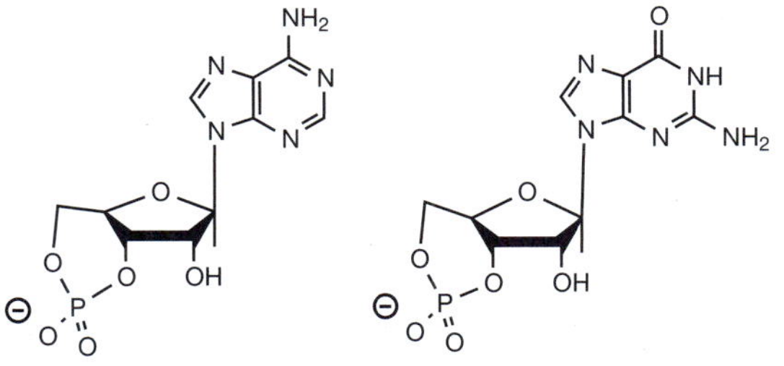

cAMP cGMP

The generation of second messengers from plasma membrane phospholipids is mediated primarily by G protein activation of PLC.[6] There are three families of PLC, designated PLC-β, PLC-γ, and PLC-δ. PLC-β can be activated by the α-subunit of the G_q family of G proteins or the βγ-subunits of other G proteins. PLC-γ is activated via tyrosine kinase receptors, but the mechanism for PLC-δ is not yet well understood.

On activation, PLC hydrolyzes phosphatidylinositol 4,5-bisphosphate to DAG and IP_3. The water-soluble IP_3 diffuses into the cytoplasm, where it triggers the release of calcium (Ca^{2+}) from intracellular stores. Intracellular calcium then binds to the protein calmodulin (CaM) and also to protein kinase C (PKC), both of which then stimulate, via protein phosphorylation, a broad range of enzymes and other proteins, including specific kinases. The other product of PLC, DAG, is lipid soluble and remains in the plasma membrane, where it facilitates the activation of PKC by calcium (Fig. 6.4). The signal is terminated via inactivation of IP_3 by dephosphorylation, whereas DAG is inactivated by phosphorylation to phosphatidic acid or deacetylation to fatty acids. The concentration of intracellular calcium is reduced by sequestration within cytoplasmic organelles or transport out of the cell. Because there are at least eight isozymes of PKC as well as numerous possible DAG species generated based on the fatty acids at the two positions, it is not surprising that some species have been shown to activate certain isozymes better than others, thus adding another layer of complexity to this signaling pathway.[7]

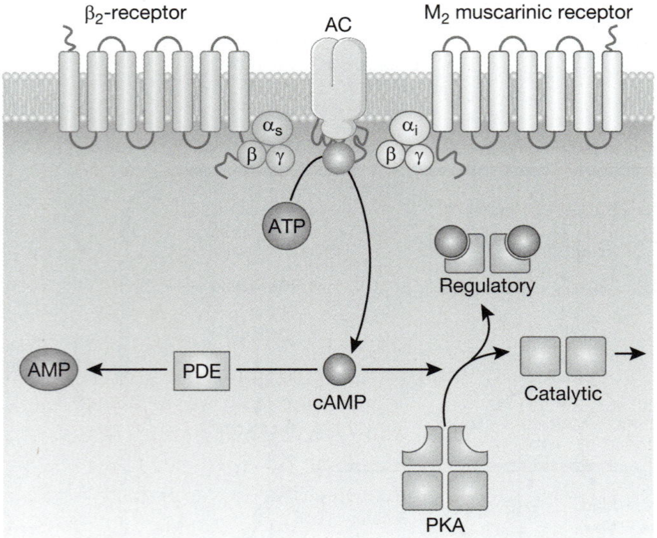

Figure 6.3 Schematic presentation showing G protein–coupled receptors (GPCRs); the β_2 adrenergic receptor, which upregulates adenylyl cyclase (AC); and the M_2 muscarinic receptor, which downregulates AC. The effects of these GPCRs are then mediated through the intercellular concentration of cyclic adenosine monophosphate (cAMP). AMP, adenosine monophosphate; ATP, adenosine triphosphate; PDE, phosphodiesterase; PKA, protein kinase A. (From Flood P, Rathmell J, Shafer S. *Stoelting's Pharmacology & Physiology in Anesthetic Practice*. 5th ed. Lippincott Williams & Wilkins; 2014, with permission.)

Activation of phospholipase D hydrolyzes phosphatidylcholine to phosphatidic acid, which can then be metabolized to DAG via phosphatidate phosphohydrolase. This pathway prolongs the duration of elevated levels of DAG. Phospholipase A_2 is activated by increased concentrations of intracellular calcium and hydrolyzes the fatty acid found at the sn-2 position of phospholipids, often arachidonic acid. Arachidonic acid then functions as a substrate for the synthesis of autacoids, including prostaglandins, thromboxane A_2, and leukotrienes.

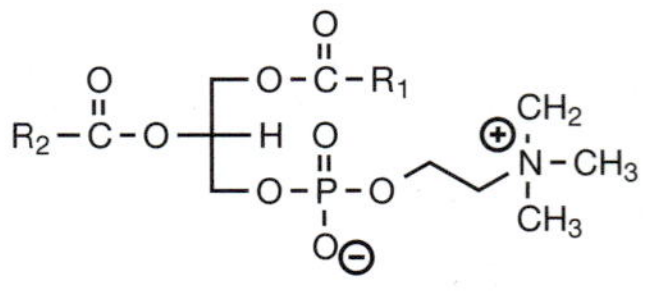

Phosphatidylcholine

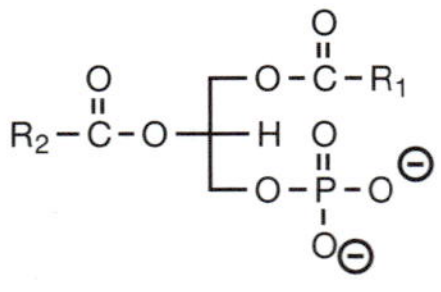

Phosphatidic acid

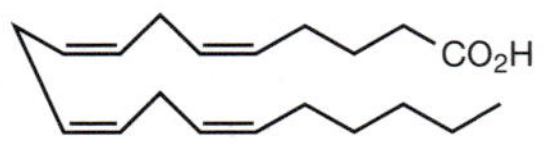

Arachidonic acid

Abundantly expressed in the brain, G_o is related to G_i and regulates various ion channels. Receptors that couple to G_i often couple to G_o as well and include somatostatin receptors and the therapeutically important opioid receptors.

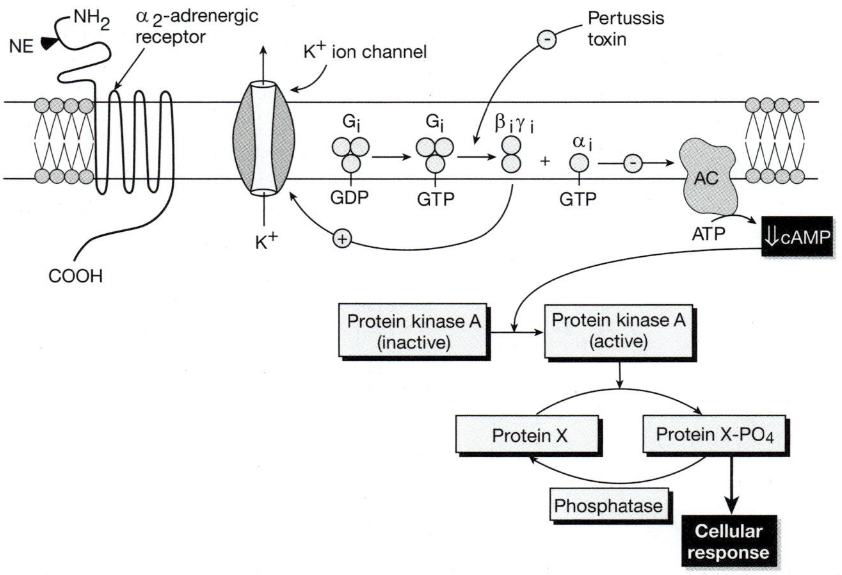

Figure 6.4 Activation of the α_2-adrenergic receptor. Stimulation of a G_i-linked receptor results in the dissociation of the G protein into the α- and $\beta\gamma$-subunits. The $\beta\gamma$-subunits bind to potassium channels increasing their open state, leading to potassium efflux and hyperpolarization of the cell. The α-subunit bound to GTP inhibits adenylyl cyclase, thus decreasing intracellular cAMP and reducing activation of protein kinase A. Pertussis toxin is used as a tool to modify subunits of G_i preventing them from inhibiting adenylyl cyclase. AC, adenylate cyclase; ATP, adenosine triphosphate; cAMP, cyclic adenosine monophosphate; GDP, guanosine diphosphate; GTP, guanosine triphosphate; NE, norepinephrine. (From Dudek R. *High-Yield Histopathology*. 2nd ed. Lippincott Williams & Wilkins; 2010, with permission.)

Activation of G_o leads to inhibition of voltage-dependent calcium channels and the opening of potassium channels. These effects result in reduced release of neurotransmitter and hyperpolarization of neurons, leading to reduced cellular activity. The effect of G_o on adenylyl cyclase may not be as clear-cut as that of G_i, but in vitro studies suggest that some species of G_o may inhibit adenylyl cyclase.

Frizzled is another family of GPCR proteins that regulate functions such as embryonic development, the formation of neural synapses, and cell polarity via a signal transduction cascade composed of protein kinases such as glycogen synthase kinase 3 (GSK-3), phosphatases, and proteolytic enzymes. A target molecule for this cascade is β-catenin, which promotes specific gene expression.

With the development of screening assays of complementary DNA (cDNA) libraries, a number of GPCRs have been identified for which there is no known endogenous ligand. These receptors are termed "orphan receptors." When the endogenous ligand is identified, the receptor is said to be "adopted." Strategies for identifying the ligand of orphan receptors include: (1) expression of the GPCR in a recombinant assay system, (2) screening candidate ligands against the receptor, (3) detecting active ligands by activation of signal transduction cascades, and (4) further testing of the ligand against other GPCRs to determine selectivity (Fig. 6.5). An example of an adopted orphan GPCR is Axor 35, which was ultimately characterized as the histamine H_4 receptor.[8]

Dynamic Nature of G Protein–Coupled Receptors

The GPCRs, as is characteristic of most individual components of living systems, are not static but, rather, are constantly in a state of dynamic adaptation (envision these protein molecules floating within the fluid mosaic of the biologic membrane, awaiting interaction with normal physiologic signals). The function of such receptors, once stimulated, involves attempts to respond to perturbations of the normal physiology of the cell or organism. The role in maintaining homeostasis within the organism requires constant adaptation of receptor number and/or sensitivity in response to the changing environment in the vicinity of the receptor.

One approach to controlling receptor activation is by regulating the concentration of neurotransmitter at the receptor-binding site. This is oftentimes accomplished by

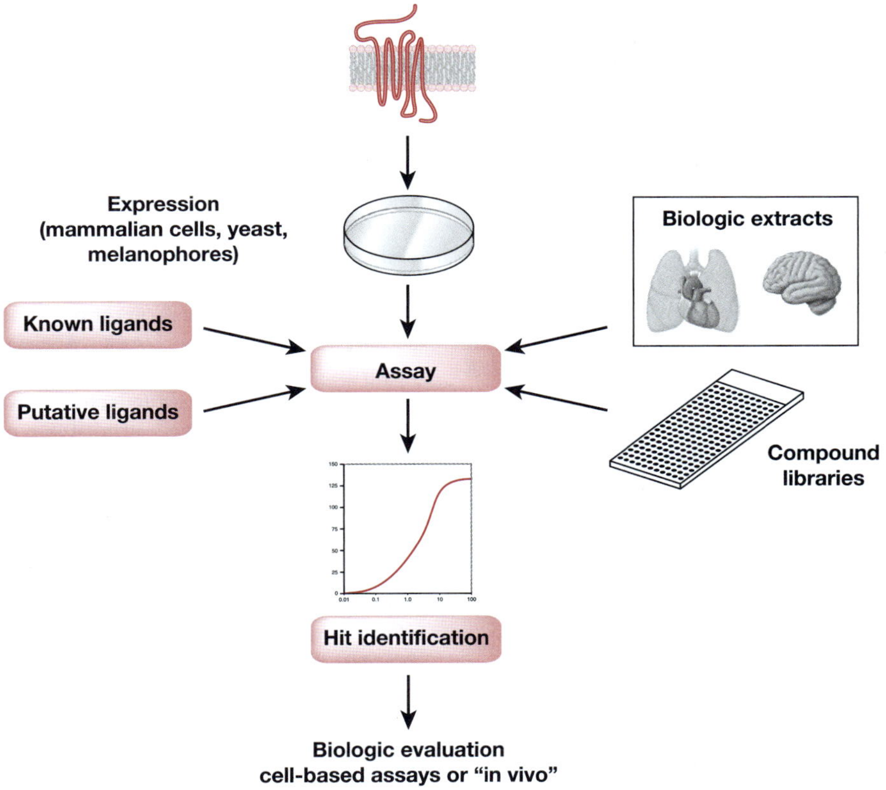

Figure 6.5 Strategy for the identification of ligands for orphan G protein–coupled receptors (GPCRs). Orphan GPCRs are expressed in a recombinant expression system, such as mammalian cells, yeast, or *Xenopus* melanophores. Following expression, it is usual to generate an assay amenable to the screening of candidate ligands in microtiter plate formats. The identification of an activating ligand is detected according to the activation of an intracellular signaling cascade. An activating ligand is identified according to its ability to cause a concentration-dependent increase in the activity of a signaling cascade. Once identified, the ligand can be further characterized against other GPCRs to determine its activity and selectivity profile prior to being used in cell-based, tissue, and, in some cases, whole-animal experiments in order to study the physiologic role of the newly liganded receptor.

the modulation of neurotransmitter release via activation of presynaptic receptors; this modulation can be either an increase or a decrease. Altering the rate of synthesis, degradation, or efficiency of the enzymes that create or degrade neurotransmitter molecules is also used to regulate neurotransmitter concentrations at the receptor. An example of this is seen when, in response to product feedback inhibition, the activity of the enzyme tyrosine hydroxylase (which catalyzes the rate-limiting step of catecholamine synthesis) is modulated via phosphorylation by protein kinases or dephosphorylation by phosphatases. This and other control mechanisms allow for a strict minute-to-minute regulation of catecholamine synthesis and, thus, neurotransmission.[9]

A second mechanism for modulating the cellular response to receptor activation is to alter postsynaptic receptor number and/or sensitivity. The process is best understood for GPCRs but has also been characterized for other receptor types, such as the ion channel nicotinic receptor. The alteration in the availability or functional capacity of a given receptor constitutes an adaptive mechanism, whereby the cell or organism is protected from agonist overload. For example, the chronic administration of a β-adrenoceptor agonist, such as isoproterenol, is known to produce a desensitization of the β-adrenoceptors in the heart.[10] During the period of overstimulation, the receptor becomes desensitized to further activation via phosphorylation by protein kinase A or G protein–coupled kinases, such as β-adrenoceptor kinase (βARK), at Ser and Thr residues on the C-terminal domain. The receptors remain in the membrane but the phosphorylation impairs their ability to couple with G_s (Fig. 6.6). Desensitization can also occur at other receptors with analogous phosphorylation sites (heterologous desensitization).

A more prolonged or powerful overstimulation typically results in a decrease in receptor number and is termed "downregulation." In these GPCRs, downregulation initiated by phosphorylation of amino acids near the intracellular C-terminal domain results in binding to β-arrestins that facilitate their internalization via a clathrin-dependent pathway. Following internalization, the receptor can either be recycled back into the plasma membrane via endosomes or degraded by lysosomes (Fig. 6.6). Reduced receptor numbers can also be accomplished via changes in the transcription and/or translation of genes that code for the receptor. The mechanisms of GPCR desensitization were largely deciphered by the laboratory of Robert Lefkowitz, for which he was awarded the 2012 Nobel Prize in Chemistry with Brian Kobilka.[11] Changes in receptor number or efficiency of receptors that lead to diminished responses and, thus, diminished efficacy of a drug with repeated or long-term use are examples of pharmacodynamic tolerance. As a general principle, the body will always attempt to maintain homeostasis, whether perturbed by environmental challenges, disease processes, or even the administration of drugs. Actually, the body interprets the administration of drugs as a perturbation of homeostasis and may attempt to counter the effects of the drug by invoking receptor adaptations. Often, however, with appropriate dosing schedules, drugs can be used with little observed receptor adaptation such that the desired pharmacologic effect continues to be observed.

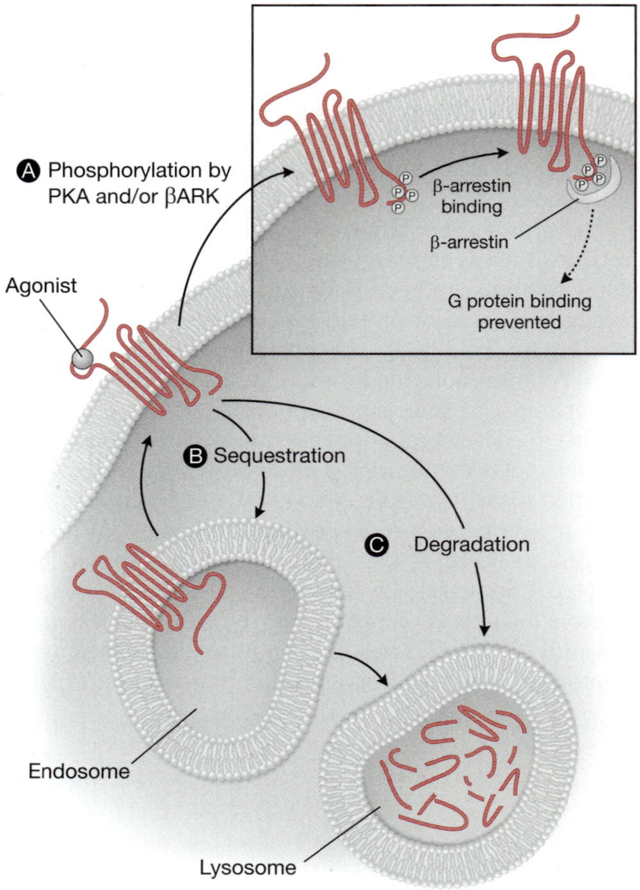

Figure 6.6 Adrenergic receptor regulation. Agonist-bound adrenergic receptors activate G proteins, which then stimulate adenylyl cyclase activity (not shown). A. Repeated or persistent stimulation of the receptor by agonist results in phosphorylation of amino acids at the C-terminus of the receptor by protein kinase A (PKA) and/or adrenergic receptor kinase (ARK). Arrestin then binds to the phosphorylated domain of the receptor and blocks G_s binding, thereby decreasing adenylyl cyclase (effector) activity. B. Binding of arrestin also leads to receptor sequestration into endosomal compartments via clathrin-mediated endocytosis (not shown), effectively neutralizing adrenergic receptor signaling activity. The receptor can then be recycled and reinserted into the plasma membrane. C. Prolonged receptor occupation by an agonist can lead to receptor downregulation and eventual receptor degradation. Cells can also reduce the number of receptors by inhibiting the transcription or translation of the gene coding for the receptor (not shown). (From Golan D. *Principles of Pharmacology*. 4th ed. Lippincott Williams & Wilkins; 2012, with permission.)

In a similar fashion to the example described, chronic administration of the β-adrenoceptor antagonist propranolol leads to a state of receptor supersensitivity or upregulation. The cells within the tissue, such as the heart, sense an alteration in the normal rate of basal β-adrenoceptor stimulation and, thus, respond by either increasing the number or the affinity of the receptors for their endogenous agonists, norepinephrine and epinephrine. Enhanced efficiency of the interaction between the receptor and its transducing systems can also account for a portion of the observed supersensitivity. The knowledge that such a receptor adaptation occurs has paramount practical therapeutic implications, as abrupt withdrawal of this class of agents can precipitate acute myocardial infarction due to activation of a very high number of β-receptors, and thus, this practice should be scrupulously avoided.

Besides their key role in GPCR downregulation, β-arrestins have also been shown to be involved in post-receptor signaling. An agonist-activated GPCR will generally bind to a G protein as well as β-arrestin, which has been demonstrated to activate various kinases leading to effects different than those stimulated by the G protein. While most agonists have been shown to stimulate both G protein and β-arrestin pathways, some compounds have been identified as "biased agonists," those that stabilize a receptor conformation that activates one pathway more than the other. The recently approved drug oliceridine is classified as a biased agonist at the μ-opioid receptors. This compound has been shown to produce analgesia like morphine does, but may be associated with fewer adverse effects.

The movement of GPCRs within the membrane allows for activated receptors to associate with one another: homodimerization in the case of two activated β-adrenergic receptors or heterodimerization where two different GPCRs associate with one another.[12] Adenosine A_{2A} receptor dimers heterodimerize with dopamine D_2 receptor dimers, and activated A_{2A} receptors negatively modulate D_2 receptor function. This approach has been exploited therapeutically with the development of istradefylline, an A_{2A} receptor antagonist recently approved for the treatment of Parkinson disease. Inhibition of the A_{2A} receptor leads to increased D_2 receptor activity in the brain.

Some pathophysiologic states are characterized by perturbations in receptor dynamics. Prinzmetal angina is thought to be characterized by an imbalance between vasodilatory β_2-adrenoceptor function and vasoconstrictor α_1-adrenoceptor function. In this disease state, the excessive α-vasoconstriction of coronary arteries leads to myocardial ischemia and pain. The inadvertent use of a β-adrenoceptor antagonist, which can be safely employed in typical angina pectoris to prevent β-adrenoceptor vasodilation, can leave unopposed α-adrenoceptor-mediated vasoconstrictor inputs and actually precipitate anginal pain. Thus, an understanding of the role that receptors have in physiology, pathophysiology, and pharmacology is essential for optimal therapeutic interventions.

Major classes of therapeutic agents interact with GPCRs to produce their desired effects. Some of these are now discussed in greater detail.

ADRENOCEPTORS

Adrenoceptors were initially subclassified by Ahlquist[13] in 1948 into α- and β-adrenoreceptors according to their responses to different adrenergic receptor agonists, principally norepinephrine, epinephrine, and isoproterenol. These catecholamines are able to stimulate α-adrenoceptors in the following descending order of potency: epinephrine > norepinephrine > isoproterenol. In contrast, β-adrenoceptors are stimulated in the following descending order of potency: isoproterenol > epinephrine > norepinephrine.

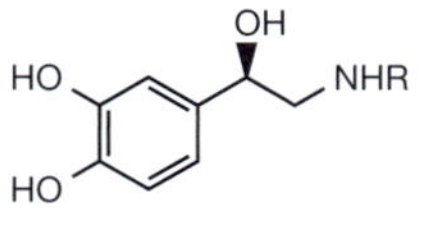

Norepinephrine, R = H
Epinephrine, R = CH_3
Isoproterenol, R = $CH(CH_3)_2$

Since this original classification, additional small-molecule agonists and antagonists have been used to allow further subclassification of α- and β-receptors into the α_1- and α_2-subtypes of α-adrenoceptors and the β_1-, β_2-, and β_3-subtypes of β-adrenoceptors. The human β_2-adrenoceptor was one of the first to be cloned and extensively studied (Fig. 6.7).[14]

The powerful tools of molecular biology have been used to clone, sequence, and identify even more subtypes of α-adrenoceptors for a total of six. Currently, three types of α_1-adrenoceptors, termed α_{1A}, α_{1B}, and α_{1D}, are known. (There is no α_{1C} because identification of a supposed α_{1C} was found to be incorrect.) Currently, three subtypes of α_2, known as α_{2A}, α_{2B}, and α_{2C}, are also known. An example of the α_2-adrenoceptor from human kidney is depicted in Figure 6.8. Currently, the α_1-, α_2-, β_1-, β_2-, and β_3-adrenoceptor subtypes are sufficiently well differentiated by their small-molecule binding characteristics to be clinically significant in pharmacotherapeutics.

Salient features of the extensively studied β_2-adrenoreceptor are indicated in Figure 6.7. Binding studies with selectively mutated β_2-adrenoceptors have provided strong evidence for binding interactions between agonist functional groups and specific residues in the TMDs of adrenoceptors. Such studies indicate that Asp113 in TMD3 of the β_2-adrenoceptor is the acidic residue that forms a bond, presumably ionic or a salt bridge, with the positively charged amino group of catecholamine agonists. An Asp residue is also found in a comparable position in all the other adrenoceptors as well as other known GPCRs that bind substrates having positively charged nitrogen atoms in their structures. Elegant studies with mutated receptors and analogues of isoproterenol demonstrated that Ser204 and Ser207 of TMD5 are the residues that form hydrogen bonds with the catechol hydroxyls of β_2-agonists.[15] Furthermore, the evidence indicates that Ser204 interacts with the *m*-hydroxyl group of the ligand, whereas Ser207 interacts specifically with the *p*-hydroxyl group. Serine residues are found in corresponding positions in TMD5 of the other known adrenoceptors. Evidence indicates that Phe on TMD6 is also involved in ligand-receptor bonding with the catechol ring. Studies such as these and others that indicated the presence of specific disulfide bridges between Cys residues of the β_2-adrenoceptor lead to receptor binding.

Structural differences exist among the various adrenoceptors with regard to their primary structure, including the actual peptide sequence and length. Each of the adrenoceptors

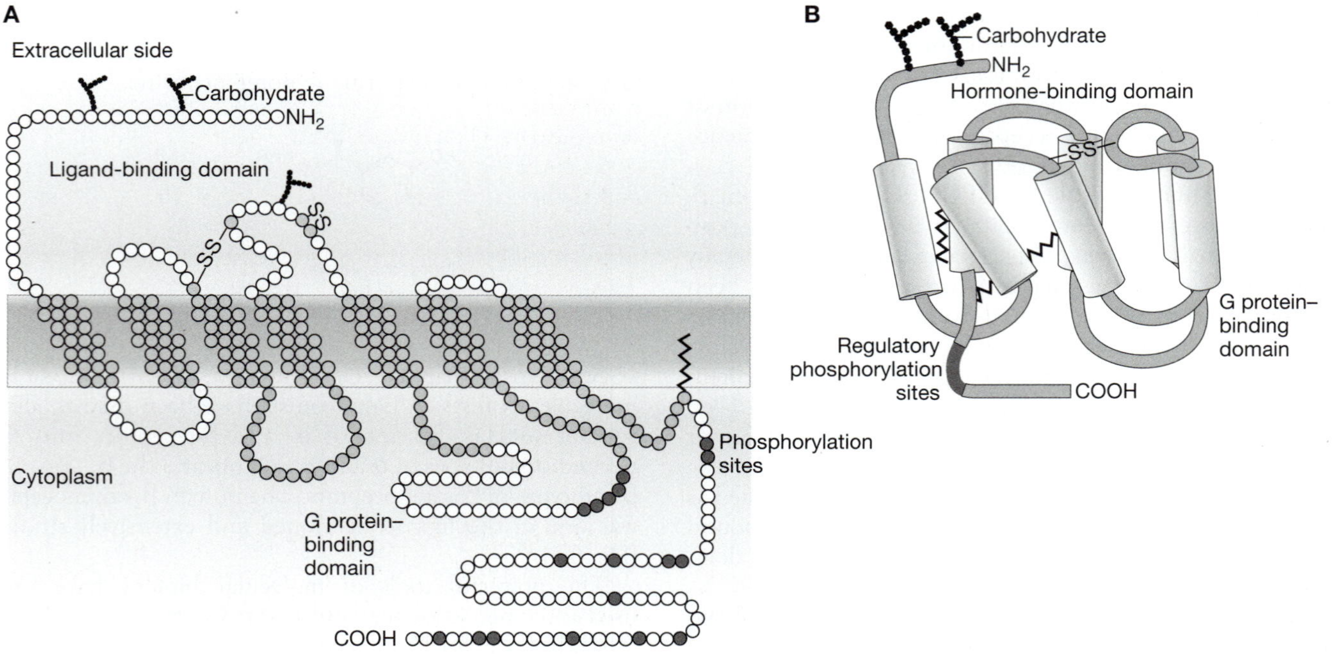

Figure 6.7 β_2-Adrenergic receptor. The receptor has seven α-helical domains that span the membrane and is therefore a member of the heptahelical class of receptors. A. The transmembrane domains are drawn in an extended form. The amino-terminus (residues 1 through 34) extends out of the membrane and has branched high-mannose oligosaccharides linked through *N*-glycosidic bonds to the amide of asparagine. Part of the receptor is anchored in the lipid plasma membrane by a palmitoyl group that forms a thioester with the -SH residue of a cysteine. The -COOH terminus, which extends into the cytoplasm, has several serine and threonine phosphorylation sites. B. The seven transmembrane helices (shown as tubes) form a cylindrical structure. Loops connecting helices form the hormone binding site on the external side of the plasma membrane, and a binding site for a G protein is on the intracellular side. (From Lieberman M. *Marks' Essentials of Medical Biochemistry*. 5th ed. Wolters Kluwer; 2017, with permission.)

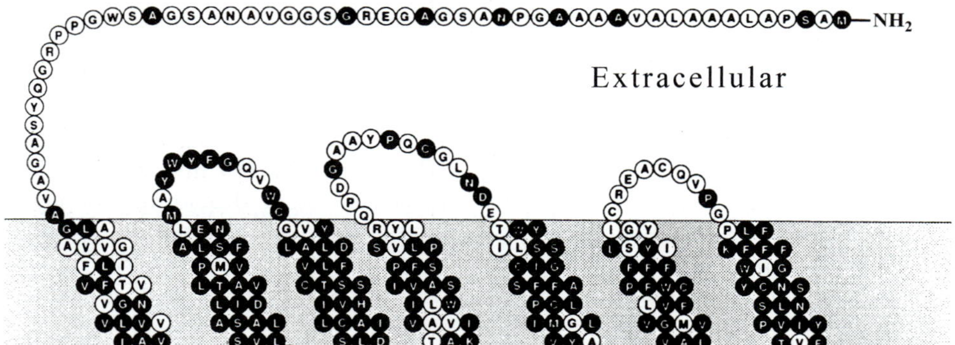

Figure 6.8 Human kidney α_2-adrenergic receptor: amino acid sequence of the human kidney α_2-receptor showing the seven transmembrane domains and the connecting intracellular and extracellular loops. Note particularly the large third intracellular loop, which is the G protein–binding site. The arrows point to the sites of glycosylation. Amino acids in black circles are those identical to the amino acids in the human platelet α_2-receptor. (From Regan JW, Kobilka TS, Yang-Feng TL, et al. Cloning and expression of a human kidney cDNA for an α_2-adrenergic receptor subtype. *Proc Natl Acad Sci U S A*. 1988;85:6301-6305, with permission.)

is encoded on a distinct gene, and this information was crucial to the proof that each adrenoceptor is, indeed, distinct (although related). The amino acids that make up the seven transmembrane regions are highly conserved among the various adrenoceptors, but the hydrophilic portions are quite variable. The largest differences occur in the third intracellular loop connecting TMD5 and TMD6, which is the site of linkage between the receptor and its associated G protein. (Compare the diagram of the β_2-receptor in Fig. 6.7 with that of the α_2-receptor in Fig. 6.8.)

Each adrenoceptor is coupled through a G protein to an effector mechanism; all the α_1-adrenoceptors are linked to $G_{q/11}$, all the α_2-adrenoceptors to $G_{i/o}$, and all the β_1- and β_2-adrenoceptors to G_s, while the β_3-adrenoreceptor is linked to either G_s (adipocytes and bladder smooth muscle) or G_i (myocardial atrial cells).

Receptor Localization

The generalization made in the past about synaptic locations of adrenoceptor subtypes was that all α_1-, β_1-, β_2-, and β_3-adrenoceptors are postsynaptic receptors linked to stimulation of biochemical processes in the postsynaptic cell. Presynaptic β-adrenoceptors, however, are known to occur, although their function is unclear. Traditionally, the α_2-adrenoceptor has been viewed as a presynaptic receptor that resides on the outer membrane of the adrenergic nerve terminus or presynaptic cell and interacts with released neurotransmitter. The α_2-adrenoceptor serves as a sensor or "autoreceptor" and modulator of the quantity of neurotransmitter present in the synapse at any given moment, and thus, during periods of rapid nerve firing and neurotransmitter release, the α_2-adrenoceptor is stimulated and causes an inhibition of further release of neurotransmitter. This is a well-characterized mechanism for modulation of neurotransmission. The α_2-adrenoceptor is also located on non-adrenergic neurons, including serotonergic neurons, where it is classified as a "heteroreceptor" whose activation reduces the release of serotonin. However, not all α_2-adrenoceptors are presynaptic, but the physiologic significance of postsynaptic α_2-receptors is less well understood.[16]

Serotonin Receptors

Initially, serotonin (5-hydroxytryptamine [5-HT]) was thought to interact with what were termed 5-HT receptors. Today, seven distinct families or populations of serotonergic receptors have been identified, 5-HT_1 through 5-HT_7, and several are divided into subpopulations (Table 6.2). With

Table 6.2 Classification and Nomenclature for the Various Populations of 5-HT Receptors

Populations and Subpopulations	Second-Messenger System[a]	Currently Accepted Name[b]	Comments
5-HT_1			
5-HT_{1A}	AC(−)	5-HT_{1A}	Cloned and pharmacologic 5-HT_{1A} receptors
5-HT_{1B}	AC(−)	5-HT_{1B}	Rodent homolog of 5-HT_{1B} receptors
$5\text{-HT}_{1B}\beta$			A mouse homolog of $h5\text{-HT}_{1B}$ receptors
5-HT_{1D}			Sites identified in binding studies using human and calf brain homogenates
$5\text{-HT}_{1D}\alpha$	AC(−)	$h5\text{-HT}_{1D}$	Cloned human 5-HT_{1D} subpopulation
$5\text{-HT}_{1D}\beta$	AC(−)	$h5\text{-HT}_{1B}$	Second cloned human 5-HT_{1D} subpopulation; human counterpart of rat 5-HT_{1B}
5-HT_{1E}	AC(−)	5-HT_{1E}	Sites identified in binding studies using brain homogenates and cloned receptors
$5\text{-HT}_{1E}\alpha$			Alternate name that has been used for cloned human 5-HT_{1E} receptors
$5\text{-HT}_{1E}\beta$	AC(−)	5-HT_{1F}	Cloned mouse homolog of 5-HT_{1F} receptors
5-HT_{1F}			Cloned human 5-HT_1 receptor population
5-HT_2			
5-HT_2	PI	5-HT_{2A}	Original "5-HT_2" (sometimes called $5\text{-HT}_2\alpha$) receptors
5-HT_{2F}	PI	5-HT_{2B}	5-HT_2-like receptors originally found in rat fundus
5-HT_{1C}	PI	5-HT_{2C}	Originally described as 5-HT_{1C} ($5\text{-HT}_2\beta$) receptors

(continued)

Table 6.2 Classification and Nomenclature for the Various Populations of 5-HT Receptors (*continued*)

Populations and Subpopulations	Second-Messenger System[a]	Currently Accepted Name[b]	Comments
5-HT_3			
5-HT_3	Ion channel	5-HT_3	Ion channel receptor
5-HT_4	AC(+)	5-HT_4	5-HT_4 population originally described in functional studies
5-HT_{4S}			Short form of cloned 5-HT_4 receptors
5-HT_{4L}			Long form of cloned 5-HT_4 receptors
$5\text{-HT}_{4(b)\text{-}4(d)}$			Recently identified human 5-HT_4 receptor isoforms
5-HT_5			
5-HT_{5A}	?	5-HT_{5A}	Cloned mouse, rat, and human 5-HT_5 receptors
5-HT_{5B}	?	5-HT_{5A}	Cloned mouse and rat 5-HT_{5A}-like receptor
5-HT_6			
5-HT_6	AC(+)	5-HT_6	Cloned rat and human 5-HT receptor
5-HT_7			
5-HT_7	AC(+)	5-HT_7	Cloned rat, mouse, guinea pig, and human 5-HT receptors

[a]AC, adenylyl cyclase; (−), negatively coupled; (+), positively coupled; PI, phospholipase coupled.

From Currently accepted names are taken from Hoyer D, Clarke DE, Fozard JR, et al. International union of pharmacology nomenclature and classification of receptors for 5-hydroxytryptamine (serotonin). *Pharmacol Rev.* 1994;46:157-203; Tekin I, Roskoski R Jr, Carkaci-Salli N, et al. Complex molecular regulation of tyrosine hydroxylase. *J Neural Transm.* 2014;121:1451-1481.

the exception of the 5-HT_3 receptor (see Chapter 8), which is an ion channel–type receptor, all of the 5-HT receptors are members of the GPCR superfamily. The discovery of the individual populations and subpopulations of 5-HT receptors follows the approximate order of their numbering and, as a consequence, more is known about 5-HT_1 and 5-HT_2 receptors than about 5-HT_6 and 5-HT_7 receptors. A factor contributing to our current lack of understanding about the function of certain 5-HT receptor populations (eg, 5-HT_{1E} or 5-HT_5 receptors) is the absence of agonists and/or antagonists with selectivity for these receptors.

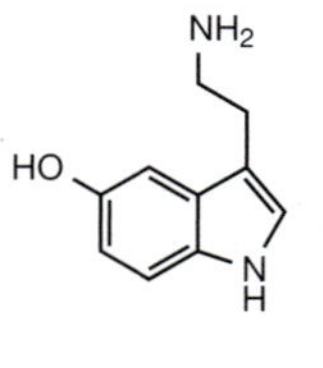

Serotonin
(5-HT)

Table 6.2 lists the receptor classification and nomenclatures that have been employed for serotonergic receptors. Care should be taken when reading the older primary literature because 5-HT receptor nomenclature has changed so dramatically and, often, can be confusing and very frustrating to comprehend.

All of the six 5-HT GPCR populations (and subpopulations) have been cloned and, together with the cloning of other neurotransmitter receptors, this has led to generalizations regarding amino acid sequence homology.[17] Any two receptors with amino acid sequences that are approximately 70% to 80% identical in their transmembrane-spanning segments are called the *intermediate-homology group*. This group of receptors could be members of the same subfamily and have highly similar to nearly indistinguishable pharmacologic profiles or second-messenger systems. A *low-homology group* (~35%-55% transmembrane homology) consists of distantly related receptor subtypes from the same neurotransmitter family, and a *high-homology group* (~95%-99% transmembrane homology) consists of species homologs from the same gene in different species.[17] Species homologs of the same gene reveal high sequence conservation in regions outside the TMDs, whereas intraspecies receptor subtypes usually are quite different.[17] Current 5-HT receptor classification and nomenclature require that several criteria be met before a receptor population can be adequately characterized. Receptor populations must be identified on the basis of drug binding characteristics (*operational* or *recognitory criteria*), receptor-effector coupling (*transductional criteria*), and gene and receptor structure sequences for the nucleotide and amino acid components, respectively (*structural criteria*).[17-19]

The 5-HT receptors are linked to G proteins as follows: $5\text{-}HT_{1A}$, $5\text{-}HT_{1B}$, $5\text{-}HT_{1D}$, $5\text{-}HT_{1E}$, $5\text{-}HT_{1F}$, and $5\text{-}HT_5$ are linked to $G_{i/o}$; $5\text{-}HT_{2A}$, $5\text{-}HT_{2B}$, and $5\text{-}HT_{2C}$ are linked to $G_{q/11}$; and $5\text{-}HT_4$, $5\text{-}HT_6$, and $5\text{-}HT_7$ are linked to G_s.

Cholinergic Muscarinic Receptors

The endogenous neurotransmitter ACh can interact with two major cholinergic receptor classes: nicotinic (see Chapter 8) and muscarinic. The cholinergic receptors at the parasympathetic neuroeffector site are termed muscarinic receptors (mAChRs) because muscarine, a natural alkaloid, demonstrated activity at these sites while having none at the nicotinic sites (neuromuscular junction and autonomic ganglia) where nicotine had activity.

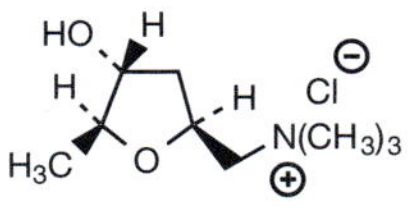

L(+)-Muscarine chloride

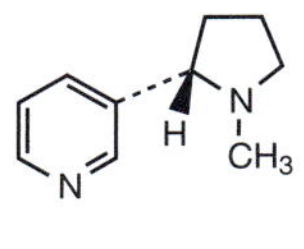

S(−)-Nicotine

Prior to the discovery that mAChRs were members of the GPCR family, early structure-activity relationship (SAR) studies regarding affinity and efficacy of cholinergic agonists provided the basis for models (as depicted in Fig. 6.9) indicating the importance of the binding of an ester functional group and a quaternary ammonium group separated by two carbons. This model depicts ionic bonding between the positively charged quaternary nitrogen of ACh and a negative charge at the anionic site of the mAChR. The negative charge was suggested to result from a carboxylate ion from the free carboxyl group of a dicarboxylic amino acid (eg, aspartate or glutamate) at the binding site on the receptor protein. This model also involved a hydrogen bond between the ester oxygen of ACh and a hydroxyl group contributed by the esteratic site of the receptor.

Although this early mAChR model accounted for two important SAR requirements for muscarinic agonists, it failed to explain the following: (1) at least two of the alkyl groups bonded to the quaternary nitrogen must be methyl groups; (2) the known stereochemical requirements for agonist binding to the receptor; and (3) the fact that all potent cholinergic agonists have only five atoms between the quaternary nitrogen and the terminal hydrogen atom. This last point is known as Ing's "Rule of Five."[20]

Heterogeneity in the mAChR population was first suggested in the late 1970s during pharmacologic studies using the muscarinic antagonist pirenzepine. At the time, pirenzepine was the only muscarinic antagonist to block gastric acid secretion at concentrations that did not block the effects of muscarinic agonists. This observation initiated research that ultimately led to the discovery of mAChR subtypes, designated as M_1, M_2, and M_3 based on their pharmacologic responses to various ligands. Rapid advances in molecular biology led to cloning of cDNAs that encoded for five mAChRs, designated as m_1 through m_5; m_1, m_2, and m_3 correspond to the respective M_1 through M_3 receptors identified

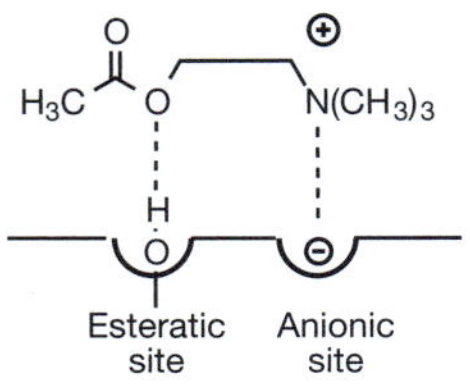

Figure 6.9 Original representation of the muscarinic acetylcholine receptor (mAChR).

by their pharmacologic specificity. The International Union of Basic and Clinical Pharmacology (IUPHAR) Committee on Receptor Nomenclature and Drug Classification has recommended that the uppercase nomenclature M_1 through M_5 be used to designate both pharmacologic and molecular subtypes.[21]

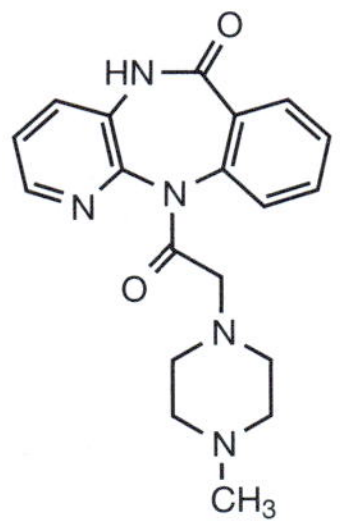

Pirenzepine

All mAChR subtypes (M_1-M_5) are found in the central nervous system (CNS), and other tissues can contain more than one. These receptors are summarized in Table 6.3. As more mAChR subtypes have been discovered, it has become apparent that there is a lack of known antagonists and agonists exhibiting very high subtype selectivity. Thus, proof for involvement of any one receptor subtype in a given system currently requires use of more than one antagonist. Additionally, if the selectivity of a novel muscarinic antagonist or putative agonist is to be assessed, it should be through use of recombinant mAChRs expressed in cell lines, rather than with native receptors.

Computer-assisted molecular modeling has made it possible to obtain three-dimensional representations of the mAChR[22]; a proposed top-view model of the M_1 mAChR is shown in Figure 6.10.[23] This model suggests that the quaternary nitrogen of ACh participates in an ionic bond with the free carboxylate group of an aspartate residue (Asp105 in TMD 3)—one of the receptor functional groups that was originally hypothesized to be involved in receptor binding of ACh.

Signal transduction at the stimulatory "odd-numbered" mAChRs (ie, M_1, M_3, and M_5) is via coupling with a $G_{q/11}$ protein that is involved with mobilization of intracellular calcium. The M_1, M_3, and M_5 receptors also stimulate phospholipase A_2 and phospholipase D. Activation of phospholipase A_2 results in release of arachidonic acid, with subsequent synthesis of eicosanoids (C_{20} fatty acids).

The "even-numbered" mAChR subtypes (ie, M_2 and M_4) are coupled to G_i/G_o proteins, whose activation inhibits

Table 6.3 Muscarinic Acetylcholine Receptor Subtypes

Receptor	G Protein	Tissue Location	Cellular Response	Function
M_1	$G_{q/11}$	CNS, gastric and salivary glands, autonomic ganglia, enteric nerves	PLC activation ($\uparrow IP_3$ and $\uparrow$DAG $\rightarrow$ $\uparrow Ca^{2+}$ and PKC); depolarization and excitation ($\uparrow$sEPSP); PLA_2 and PLD_2 activation; $\uparrow$AA	$\uparrow$ Cognitive function $\uparrow$ Seizure activity $\uparrow$ Secretions $\uparrow$ Autonomic ganglia depolarization $\downarrow$ DA release and locomotion
M_2	G_i/G_o	Autonomic nerve terminals; CNS; heart; smooth muscle	Inhibition of adenylyl cyclase ($\downarrow$cAMP) and voltage-gated Ca^{2+} channels; activation of inwardly rectifying K^+ channels	$\downarrow$ Heart rate $\uparrow$ Smooth muscle contraction Neural inhibition in periphery via autoreceptors and heteroreceptor $\downarrow$ Ganglionic transmission Neural inhibition in CNS $\uparrow$ Tremors, hypothermia, and analgesia
M_3	$G_{q/11}$	CNS (less than other mAChRs), smooth muscle, glands, heart	Same as M_1	$\uparrow$ Smooth muscle contraction (eg, bladder) $\uparrow$ Salivary gland secretion $\uparrow$ Food intake, body fat deposits Inhibits dopamine release Synthesis of nitric oxide
M_4	G_i/G_o	CNS	Same as M_2	Inhibition of autoreceptor- and heteroreceptor-mediated transmitter release in CNS Analgesia Cataleptic activity Facilitates dopamine release
M_5	$G_{q/11}$	Low levels in CNS and periphery; predominate mAChRs in dopaminergic neurons of substantia nigra and ventral tegmentum area	Same as M_1	Mediates dilation of cerebral arteries Facilitates dopamine release Augments drug-seeking behavior and reward

AA, arachidonic acid; cAMP, cyclic adenosine monophosphate; CNS, central nervous system; DA, dopamine; DAG, diacylglycerol; IP_3, inositol 1,4,5-trisphosphate; mAChRs, muscarinic acetylcholine receptor subtypes; PKC, protein kinase C; PLA, phospholipase A; PLC, phospholipase C; PLD2, phospholipase D; sEPSP, slow excitatory postsynaptic potential.

Used with permission of McGraw-Hill, from Westfall TC, Westfall DP. Neurotransmission: the autonomic and somatic motor nervous systems. In: Brunton LL, Lazo JS, Parker KL, eds. *Goodman and Gilman's the Pharmacological Basis of Therapeutics*. 11th ed. McGraw-Hill; 2006:137-181; permission conveyed through Copyright Clearance Center, Inc.

adenylyl cyclase. This results in a decrease in cAMP, inhibition of voltage-gated calcium channels, and activation of inwardly rectifying potassium channels. The result is hyperpolarization and inhibition of these excitable membranes.

The M_1 receptors are sometimes described as "neural" due to their abundance in the cerebral cortex, hippocampus, and striatum. M_1 receptors have been implicated in Alzheimer disease and are thought to be involved with memory and learning. Early studies suggested that the agonist McN-A-343 was selective for the M_1 receptor, but more recent evidence indicates otherwise. It can show moderate selectivity for M_4 receptors. Additionally, M_1 receptors are found at autonomic ganglia, enteric nerves, and salivary and gastric glands. Agonists at M_1 receptors show the greatest promise for treatment of the cholinergic deficit associated with Alzheimer disease.

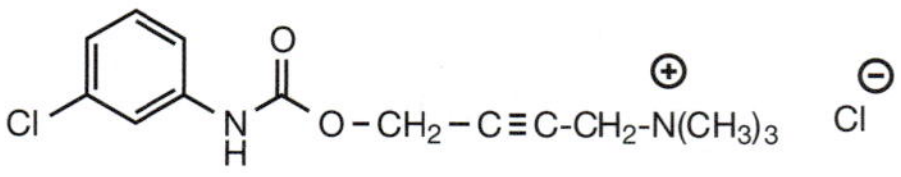

McN-A-343

M_2 receptors are found in abundance in the heart, where activation exerts both negative chronotropic and inotropic actions, and stimulates contraction of smooth muscle. Activation of M_2 autoreceptors located on nerve terminals affords neural inhibition by decreasing ACh release.

M_3 receptors are found in abundance in smooth muscle and glands, where their stimulation leads to contraction and secretion, respectively. Knowledge of this effect on smooth muscle of the bladder has led to the development and subsequent approval of several M_3 receptor antagonists for the

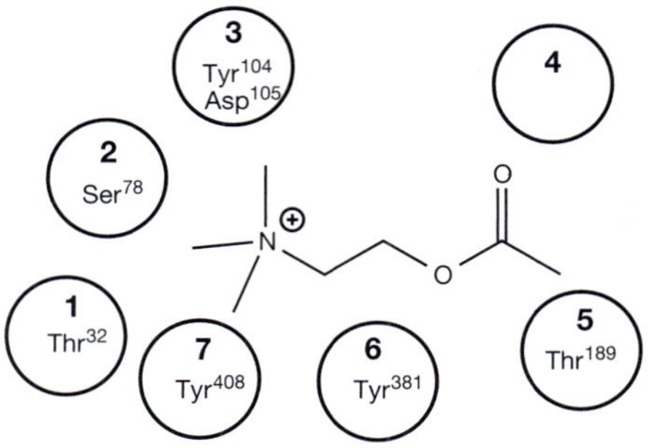

Figure 6.10 Model of acetylcholine interaction with muscarinic M_1 receptor. Circles represent seven transmembrane domains.

Met-enkephalin = Tyr-Gly-Gly-Phe-Met

Leu-Enkephalin = Tyr-Gly-Gly-Phe-Leu

β-Endorphin = Tyr-Gly-Gly-Phe-Met-Thr-Ser-Glu-Lys-Ser^{10}-Gln-Thr-Pro-Leu-Val-Thr-Leu-Phe-Lys- Asn^{20}-Ala-Ile-Ile-Lys-Asn-Ala-Tyr-Lys-Lys-Gly-GluOH^{31}

Dynorphin(dyn$^{1-17}$) = Tyr-Gly-Gly-Phe-Leu-Arg-Arg-Ile-Arg-Pro-Lys-Leu-Lys-Trp-Asp-Asn-Gln

Dynorphin(dyn$^{1-8}$) = Tyr-Gly-Gly-Phe-Leu-Arg-Arg-Ile

Dynorphin(dyn$^{1-13}$) = Tyr-Gly-Gly-Phe-Leu-Arg-Arg-Ile-Arg-Pro-Lys-Leu-Lys

α-Neoendorphin = Tyr-Gly-Gly-Phe-Leu-Arg-Lys-Tyr-Pro-Lys

β-Neoendorphin = Tyr-Gly-Gly-Phe-Leu-Arg-Lys-Tyr-Pro

Nociceptin = Phe-Gly-Gly-Phe-Thr-Gly-Ala-Arg-Lys-Ser-Ala-Arg-Lys-Leu-Ala-Asn-Gln

Figure 6.11 Precursor proteins to the endogenous opioid peptides.

treatment of overactive bladder. Although widely distributed in the CNS, their concentration in the CNS is lower than those of other mAChRs. M_3 mAChRs function to decrease neurotransmitter release.

M_4 receptors are found in the striatum and basal forebrain, where they decrease transmitter release in both the CNS and periphery. Their activation in smooth muscle and secretary glands leads to inhibition of potassium and calcium channels.

M_5 receptors are the least characterized of the mAChRs, and there is evidence for their existence in the CNS and periphery, where they can regulate dopamine release in the CNS.

Opioid Receptors

While scientists had postulated for some time, based on the rigid structural and stereochemical requirements essential for the analgesic actions of morphine and related opioids, that binding to specific receptors was required, the endogenous ligands for such receptors were unknown until the discovery by Hughes et al[24] of the two pentapeptides, Tyr-Gly-Gly-Phe-Met (Met-enkephalin) and Tyr-Gly-Gly-Phe-Leu (Leu-enkephalin), that caused the opioid activity (Fig. 6.11). Because these endogenous compounds were isolated from brain tissue they were named enkephalins after the Greek word *Kaphale*, which translates as "from the head." Shortly after this discovery additional endogenous opioids were identified including other endogenous opioid peptides β-endorphin,[25] the dynorphins,[26] and the endomorphins.[27] All of the endogenous opioid peptides are synthesized as part of the structures of large precursor proteins.[28]

Identification of multiple opioid receptors has depended on the discovery of selective agonists and antagonists, the identification of sensitive assay techniques,[29] and, ultimately, the cloning of the receptor proteins.[30] The techniques that have been especially useful are the radioligand binding assays on brain tissues and the electrically stimulated peripheral muscle preparations. Rodent brain tissue contains all three opioid receptor types, and special evaluation procedures (computer-assisted line fitting) or selective blocking (with reversible or irreversible binding agents) of some of the receptor types must be used to sort out the receptor selectivity of test compounds. The myenteric plexus-containing longitudinal strips of guinea pig ileum contain μ- and κ-opioid receptors. The contraction of these muscle strips is initiated by electrical stimulation and is inhibited by opioids. The vas deferens from mouse contains μ-, δ-, and κ-receptors and reacts similarly to the guinea pig ileum to electrical stimulation and to opioids. Homogenous populations of opioid receptors are found in rat (μ), hamster (δ), and rabbit (κ) vas deferentia, and all interact with receptors that belong to the GPCR superfamily.

All three of the receptor types have been well characterized and cloned.[30] The signal transduction mechanism for these three opioid receptor subtypes is through $G_{i/o}$ proteins resulting in inhibition of adenylyl cyclase activity, leading to decreased cAMP production, efflux of potassium ions, and closure of voltage-gated Ca^{2+} channels. The net result is cellular hyperpolarization and cell firing inhibition.[31]

As with many other receptors during the initial stages of discovery and characterization, the nomenclature usually evolves as more research is conducted. A system for consistent nomenclature, adopted by the IUPHAR in 2000, named the receptors as MOP-μ, DOP-δ, and KOP-κ. In current literature, however, the opioid receptors often are referred to as DOR (δ), KOR (κ), and MOR (μ). There is evidence for subtypes of each of these receptors; however, the failure of researchers to find genomic evidence for additional receptors indicates that the receptor subtypes are posttranslational modifications (splice variants) of known receptor types.[32] Receptor subtypes may also be known receptor types that are coupled to different signal transduction systems.

Table 6.4 lists the opioid receptor types, their known physiologic functions, and selective agonists and antagonists for each of the receptors. All three of the major opioid receptor types are located in human brain or spinal cord tissues, and each has a role in the mediation of pain. See Chapter 16 for a summary of key binding interactions of μ- and κ-receptor agonists and antagonists.

As with other GPCRs, opioid receptors can undergo dimerization to form homo- and heterodimers (eg, DOR-MOR, DOR-KOR), with a resultant lower affinity for very selective agonists. Additionally, these heterodimers tend to display an altered cellular signaling in response to agonists. Interestingly, antagonism of DOR receptors or DOR knockout animals, where no DOR dimers can exist, results in

Table 6.4 Opioid Receptors

Receptor Subtype	δ (delta, DOP)	κ (kappa, KOP)	μ (mu, MOP)	NOP (N/OFQ Peptide)
Transduction Mechanism	**Inhibition of adenylyl cyclase, activation of inwardly rectifying K^+ channels, inhibition of Ca^{2+} channels, phospholipase C stimulation**			
G protein	$G_{i/o}$	$G_{i/o}$	$G_{i/o}$	$G_{i/o}$
Localization	Olfactory bulb Nucleus accumbens Caudate putamen neocortex	Cerebral cortex Nucleus accumbens Hypothalamus	CNS (neocortex, thalamus, nucleus accumbens, hippocampus, amygdala) Vas deferens Myenteric gut neurons	Cortex, olfactory nucleus, hypothalamus, hippocampus, substantia nigra, locus coeruleus, spinal cord, amygdala
Endogenous ligand	Enkephalins β-Endorphin	Dynorphins β-Endorphin	Endomorphin 1 Endomorphin 2 β-Endorphin	N/OFQ peptide
Likely physiologic roles	Analgesia GI motility Olfaction Immune stimulation Respiratory depression (rate) Cognitive function Motor integration	Regulation of nociception Analgesia Sedation Miosis Diuresis Dysphoria Neuroendocrine secretions	Analgesia (morphine-like) Euphoria Increased gastrointestinal transit time Thermoregulation Immune suppression Respiratory depression (volume) Emetic effects Tolerance Physical dependence	Motor and balance control Reinforcement and reward Nociception Stress response Sexual behavior Aggression Autonomic control of physiologic processes
Key selective agonists	DADLE (D-Ala2-D-Leu5-enkephalin) DSLET (Tyr-D-Ser-Gly-Phe-Leu-Thr) DPDPE (D-Pen2-D-Pen5-enkephalin) DADLE (δ_2) D-Ala2-deltorphin II (δ_2)	Ethylketocyclazocine (EKC) Bremazocine Mr2034 Dyn (1-17) Trifluadom U-50,488 (κ_1) Spiradoline (U-62,066) (κ_1) U-69,593 (κ_1) PD 117302 (κ_1) Dyn (1-17) (κ_1) NalBzOH (κ_1)	Morphine Sufentanil DAMGO (Tyr-D-Ala-MePhe-NH-$(CH_2)_2$OH) PLO17 (Tyr-Pro-Me-Phe-D-Pro-NH_2) BIT (affinity label) Meptazinol (μ_1 high affinity) Etonitazene	N/OFQ peptide Nociceptin (1-13)
Key selective antagonists	ICI 174864 FIT (affinity label) SUPERFIT (affinity label) Naltrindole (NTI) BNTX Naltriben (NTB) Naltrindole isothiocyanate (NTII)	TENA nor-BNI UPHIT	Naloxone Naltrexone CTOP Cyprodime β-FNA (affinity label) Naloxonazine	(*N*-phe1)-Nociceptin (1-13) J-113397UFP-101

CNS, central nervous system; GI, gastrointestinal; nor-BNI, norbinaltorphimine.

reduced tolerance that develops on chronic administration of the MOR agonist morphine, suggesting a possible link between tolerance and opioid receptor dimerization.[33]

Mu (μ)-Opioid Receptors

Endomorphin-1 (Tyr1-Pro-Trp-Phe4-NH_2) and endomorphin-2 (Tyr1-Pro-Phe-Phe4-NH_2) are endogenous opioid peptides with a high degree of selectivity for μ (MOP) receptors. A number of therapeutically useful compounds have been found that are selective for μ-opioid receptors (Fig. 6.12). All of the opioid alkaloids and most of their synthetic derivatives are μ-selective agonists (see Chapter 16). Morphine, normorphine, and dihydromorphinone have 10- to 20-fold μ-receptor selectivity and were particularly important in early studies to differentiate the opioid receptors. Sufentanil and the peptides DAMGO and dermorphin,[34] all with 100-fold selectivity for μ over other opioid receptors,

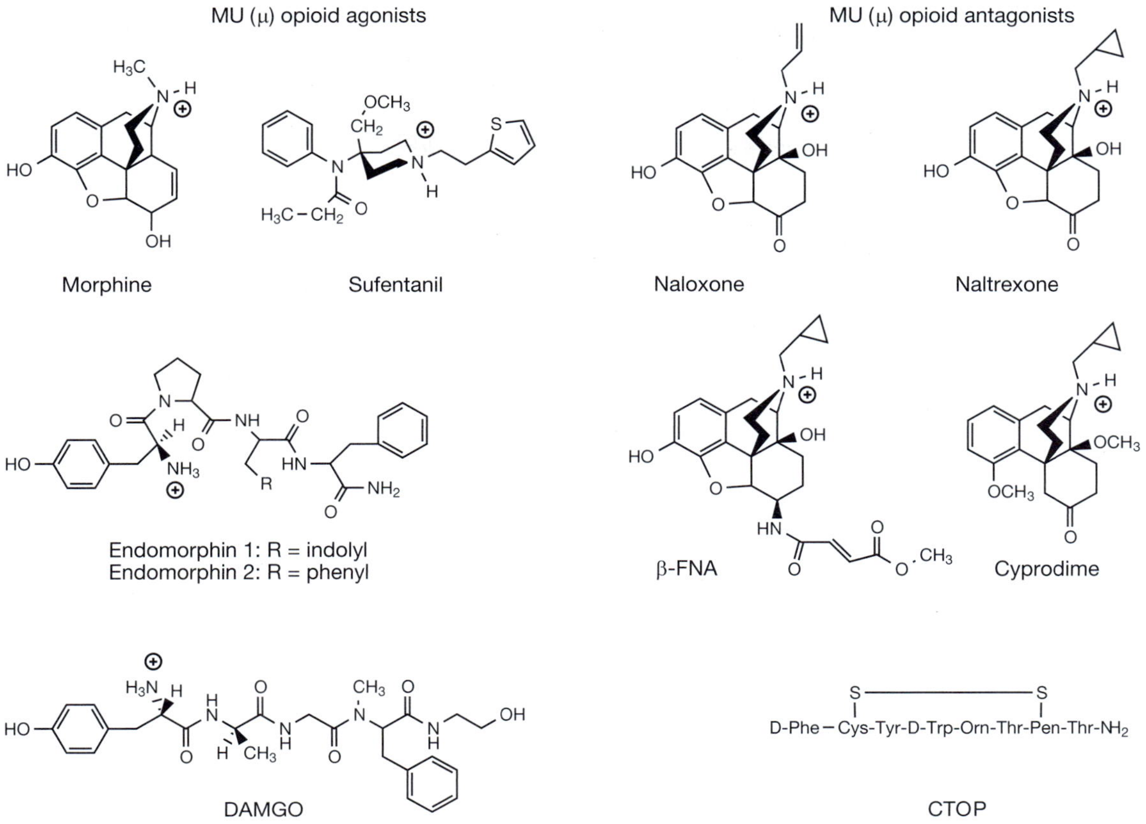

Figure 6.12 Structures of compounds selective for μ (OP3) opioid receptors.

are frequently used in laboratory studies to demonstrate μ-receptor selectivity in cross-tolerance, receptor binding, and isolated smooth muscle assays. Studies with μ-receptor knockout mice have confirmed that all the major pharmacologic actions observed on injection of morphine (eg, analgesia, respiratory depression, tolerance, withdrawal symptoms, decreased gastric motility, and emesis) occur by interactions with μ-receptors.[35]

There is evidence that μ_1-receptors are high-affinity binding sites that mediate pain neurotransmission, whereas μ_2-receptors control respiratory depression. Naloxonazine is a selective inhibitor of μ_1-opioid receptors.[36] Naloxone and naltrexone are antagonists that have weak (5- to 10-fold) selectivity for μ-receptors.

Using μ-opioid receptor ligands, investigators have demonstrated that opioid binding is generally rather superficially located and exposed to that portion of the receptor that is on the extracellular surface. This superficial binding location may help to partially account for the rather rapid dissociation half-lives of many of the potent opioids as compared with other ligands that bind to other nonopioid receptors (eg, some muscarinic and β-adrenoceptors).[37] Both agonists and antagonists bind to the μ-opioid receptor such that the OH and N^+ groups of the tyramine moiety found in alkaloid ligands interact within the binding pocket with Asp7 in TMIII and His20 in TMVI. With cyclic peptide opioids, a similar interaction with the receptor occurs, but this involves H-bonding via the Tyr found in the opioid peptides.[38]

Kappa (κ)-Opioid Receptors

Ethylketazocine and bremazocine are 6,7-benzoxazocine derivatives with κ-opioid receptor selectivity (Fig. 6.13). These two compounds were used in early studies to investigate κ (KOP) receptors, and the "k" in ethylketocyclazocine gave the κ-receptor its name. They are not highly selective, however, and their use in research has diminished. A number of arylacetamide derivatives having a high selectivity for κ- over μ- or δ-receptors have been discovered. The first of these compounds, (±)-U50488, has a 50-fold selectivity for κ- over μ-receptors and has been extremely important in the characterization of κ-opioid activity.[39] Other important agents in this class are (±) PD-117302[40] and (−) CI-977.[41] Each of these agents has 1,000-fold selectivity for κ- over μ- or δ-receptors. Evidence suggests that the arylacetamides bind to a subtype of κ-receptors.

In animals, including humans, κ-agonists produce analgesia. Other prominent effects are diuresis, sedation, and dysphoria. Compared to μ-agonists, κ-agonists were initially thought to have less respiratory depressant, constipating, and addictive (euphoria and physical dependence) properties. It was hoped that κ-agonists would become useful strong analgesics that lacked addictive properties; however, clinical trials with several highly selective and potent κ-agonists were aborted because of the occurrence of unacceptable sedative and dysphoric side effects. Pentazocine, butorphanol, and nalbuphine are κ-agonists that provide only mild analgesia (see Chapter 16). κ-Selective opioids with only a peripheral action have been shown to be effective in relieving inflammation and the pain associated with it.[42] Scientific evidence suggests there are κ_1-, κ_2-, and κ_3-subtypes of κ-receptors; however, the physiologic effects initiated by the κ-receptor subtypes are not well defined.[43]

The peptides related to dynorphin are the natural agonists for κ-receptors, but their selectivity for κ- over μ-receptors is not very high. Synthetic peptide analogues have been reported that are more potent and more selective than dynorphin for κ-receptors. The major antagonist with good selectivity for κ-receptors is norbinaltorphimine (Fig. 6.13).[44] This compound has approximately 100-fold selectivity for κ- over δ-receptors and an even greater selectivity for κ- over μ-receptors when tested during competitive binding studies in monkey brain homogenate. No medical use for a κ-antagonist has been found.

Delta (δ)-Opioid Receptors

Enkephalins, the natural ligands at δ (DOP) receptors, are only slightly selective for δ- over μ-receptors. Changes in the amino acid composition of the enkephalins can give compounds with high potency and selectivity for δ-receptors. The peptides most often used as selective δ-receptor ligands are (D-Ala2, D-Leu5) enkephalin (DADLE),[45] (D-Ser2, Leu5) enkephalin-Thr (DSLET),[46] and the cyclic peptide (D-Pen2, D-Pen5) enkephalin (DPDPE)[47] (Fig. 6.14). These and other δ-receptor selective peptides have been useful for in vitro studies, but their metabolic instability and poor distribution properties (penetration of the blood-brain barrier [BBB] is limited by their hydrophilicity) have limited their usefulness for in vivo studies.

Nonpeptide agonists that are selective for δ-receptors have been reported. Derivatives of morphindoles (eg, nor-OMI; see Fig. 6.14) were the first nonpeptide molecules to show δ-selectivity in in vitro assays.[48] SNC-80 (see Fig. 6.14) is a newer and more selective δ-opioid receptor agonist.[49] This compound produces analgesia after oral dose in several rodent models, and side effects appear minimal. Clinical trials with SNC-80 and other nonpeptide δ-receptor agonists were attempted and aborted, primarily because of the convulsant action of δ-receptor agonists.

Naltrindole[50] and naltriben[51] (see Fig. 6.14) are highly selective nonpeptide antagonists for δ-receptors. Naltrindole penetrates the CNS and displays antagonist activity that is selective for δ-receptors in in vitro and in vivo systems. The δ-opioid receptor antagonists have shown clinical potential as immunosuppressants and in the treatment of cocaine abuse.

Kappa (κ) opioid agonists

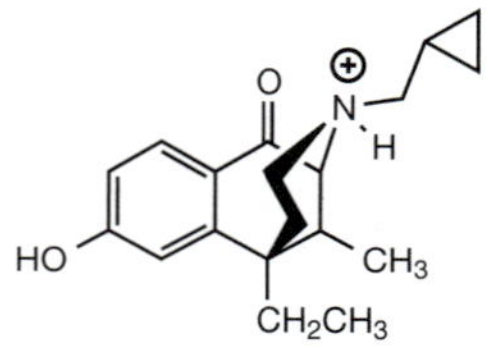

(±) Ethylketazocine

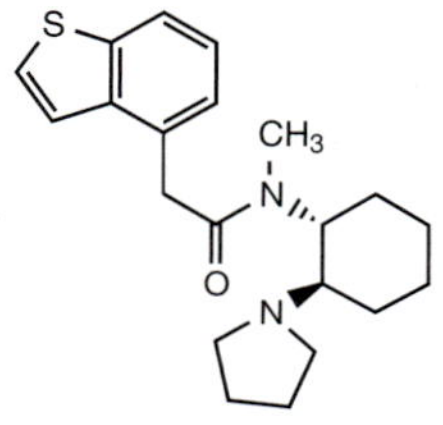

(±) PD 117302

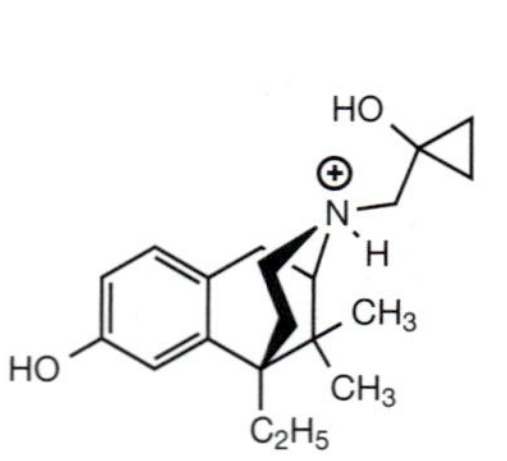

(±) Bremazocine

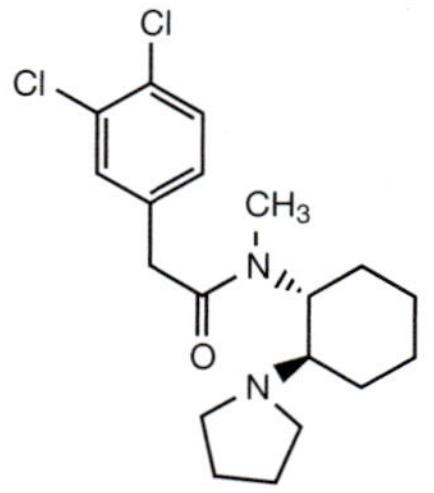

(±) U 50488

Kappa (κ) opioid antagonists

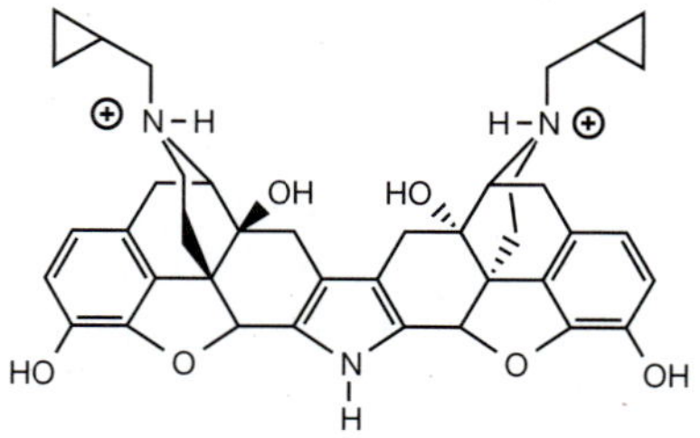

(±) Norbinaltorphimine

Figure 6.13 Structures of compounds selective for κ (OP2) opioid receptors. (−)-Stereoisomers are the most active compounds.

N/OFQ Peptide Receptor

A fourth opioid receptor named after its endogenous ligand N/OFQ peptide (NOP; OP_4) has been identified and cloned based on homology with the cDNA sequence of the known (μ, δ, and κ) opioid receptors.[52,53] Despite the homology in cDNA sequence with known opioid receptors, NOP did not bind the classical opioid peptide or nonpeptide agonists or antagonists with high affinity. Thus, the receptor was initially called the orphan opioid receptor or opioid-like receptor (OPLR-1). In subsequent studies, two research groups found a heptadecapeptide (Phe-Gly-Gly-Phe-Thr-Gly-Ala-Arg-Lys-Ser-Ala-Arg-Lys-Leu-Ala-Asn-Gln) to be the endogenous peptide for this receptor and named it nociceptin because it caused hyperalgesia (nociception) after intracerebral ventricular injection in mice.[54] Another research group[55] named the heptapeptide orphanin FQ, after its affinity for the "orphan opioid receptor" and after the first and last amino acids in the peptide's sequence (ie, F = Phe and Q = Gln). Thus, the OPRL-1 receptor was renamed the NOP or N/OFQ peptide receptor, and the current name for the endogenous ligand is N/OFQ peptide. Human NOP is derived from a precursor protein, preproN/OFQ (ppN/OFQ), which consists of 176 amino acids and resembles dynorphin A in structure, with the most notable difference being the replacement of the N-terminus Tyr1 for dynorphin A with Phe1.[55]

Conflicting results have been published regarding the ability of NOP to produce hyperalgesia versus analgesia in rodent pain assay models. One study has established this compound to be a potent initiator of pain signals in the periphery, where it acts by releasing substance P from nerve terminals.[56] NOP is thought to be an endogenous antagonist of dopamine transport that may act either directly on dopamine or by inhibiting GABA to affect dopamine levels.[57]

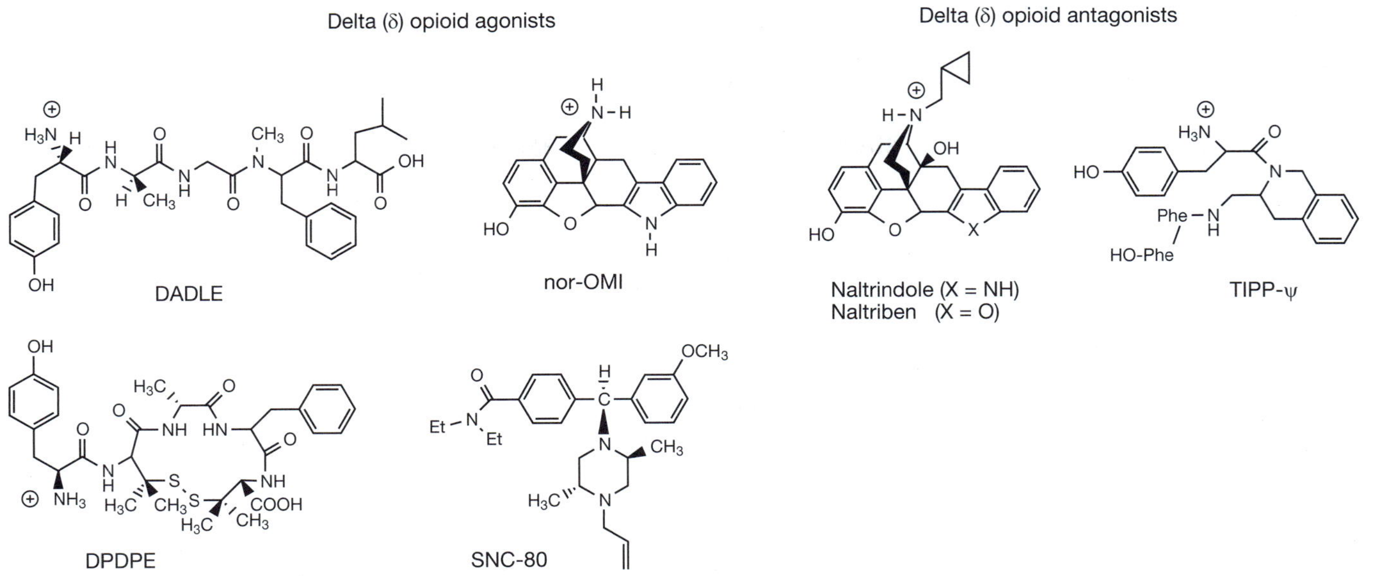

Figure 6.14 Structures of compounds selective for δ (OP1) opioid receptors.

Within the CNS, the actions of N/OFQ can be either similar or opposite to those of opioids depending on the location. It controls a wide variety of biologic functions ranging from nociception to food intake, from memory processes to cardiovascular and renal functions, from spontaneous locomotor activity to gastrointestinal (GI) motility, and from anxiety to the control of neurotransmitter release at peripheral and central sites.[54] Several commonly used opioid drugs, including etorphine and buprenorphine, have been demonstrated to bind to nociceptin receptors, but this binding is relatively insignificant compared to their binding at other opioid receptors. More recently, a range of selective ligands for NOP have been developed that show little or no affinity to other opioid receptors, which allows NOP-mediated responses to be studied in isolation.[58] Injection of an N/OFQ peptide antagonist into the brains of laboratory animals results in an analgesic effect, raising hope for the use of these agents in the management of pain.[54]

The NOP receptors are widely distributed in the brain, and it is not surprising that many central actions of N/OFQ peptide have been suggested from animal studies, including supraspinal hyperalgesia, spinal analgesia, hyperphagia, depression, and inhibitions of anxiety, epilepsy, cough, motor activity, and learning and memory as well as the regulation of cardiovascular, urogenital, GI, and immune systems. Many efforts have been expended in the development of agonists or antagonists of this novel member of the opioid receptor family. Table 6.4 identifies the major NOP receptor agonists and antagonists developed thus far.

Histamine Receptors

Histamine is an endogenous amine involved in a variety of functions in the human body. It functions peripherally as an autacoid and centrally as a neurotransmitter. Histamine produces these effects through activation of at least four different GPCRs named H_1, H_2, H_3, and H_4 receptors. The potency of histamine for activating its receptors is highest for the H_3 and H_4 receptors, followed by the H_2 receptor and lastly the H_1 receptor. The development of receptor ligands displaying selectivity for each of these receptor subtypes has helped elucidate the functions of these various receptors.

H_1 Receptors

H_1 receptors mediate the classical effects of histamine associated with allergic symptoms and are the targets of "antihistamines" that have been commercially available for more than 60 years, even though the H_1 receptor was not cloned until the early 1990s. Activation by histamine results in constriction of smooth muscle, including the airway smooth muscle during anaphylaxis. Vasodilation leading to shock is the result of H_1-mediated nitric oxide production from vascular endothelial cells. H_1 receptors are widespread throughout the brain, and receptor knockout studies in mice link these receptors to the cortical activation during waking. Thus, H_1 receptor antagonists that cross the BBB produce pronounced sedation by blocking histamine signaling in the brain.

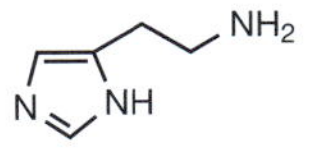

Histamine

As befitting a monoamine receptor, the H_1 receptor shares certain structural and binding features with other biogenic amine receptors, most notably the β-adrenergic receptors, including ligand binding within a pore formed by TM3, TM5, and TM6 as determined by site-directed mutagenesis studies and x-ray crystallography.[59] Coupled primarily to $G_{q/11}$ and $G_{i/o}$ in a few systems, increased intracellular calcium is the main response to H_1 receptor stimulation.

Antihistamines, or H_1 receptor inverse agonists, are classified into the older "first-generation" antihistamines and the newer "second-generation" drugs. First-generation antihistamines, characterized by diphenhydramine (Benadryl), are more lipophilic and less selective (considerable antagonism of muscarinic receptors) compared to the newer peripherally selective ("nonsedative") drugs such as fexofenadine (Allegra).

The molecular determinants of antihistamine binding to the H_1 receptor have been identified through the crystal structure of the H_1 receptor bound to the first-generation antihistamine doxepin.[60] As predicted, doxepin binds within the pore created by TM3, TM5, and TM6, which is a well-conserved binding pocket among adrenergic receptors and also the site of histamine binding. Doxepin directly interacts with Trp428, a highly conserved residue. Affinity for these binding determinants, common in many monoamine receptors, is thought to be the basis for the poor selectivity of the first-generation antihistamines. Modeling of second-generation antihistamines with the H_1 receptor shows that fexofenadine can form a salt bridge with Lys191, which is found in TM5 near the extracellular surface and is not conserved among monoaminergic receptors. This may be the basis for the greater selectivity of the second-generation antihistamines.

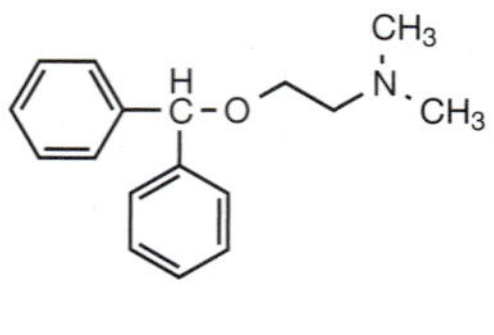

Diphenhydramine

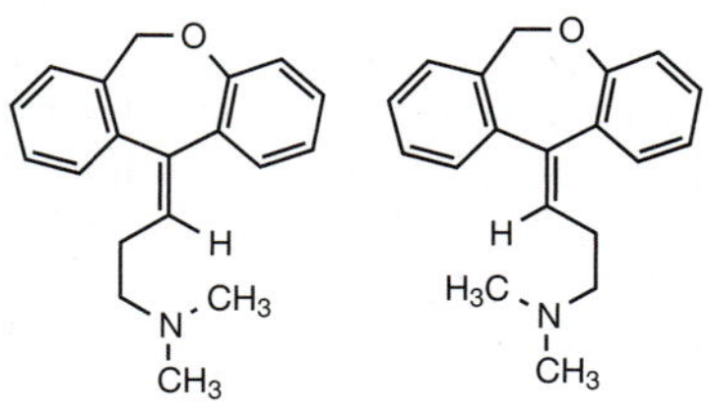

E-isomer *Z*-isomer

Doxepin (*E*/*Z* = 85/15%)

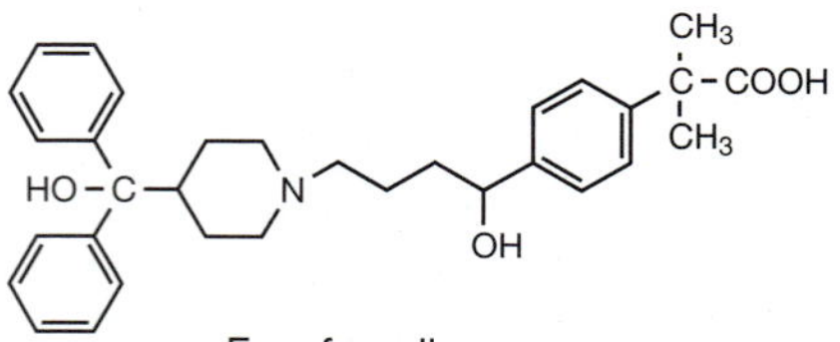

Fexofenadine

H_2 Receptors

The inability of classical antihistamines to reduce histamine-induced gastric acid secretion led to the identification of H_2 histamine receptors in the 1970s. Linked mainly to G_s, activation of H_2 receptors leads to increased cAMP. Expression is highest in the stomach and brain. H_2 antagonists such as cimetidine and ranitidine have been demonstrated to be inverse agonists as they reduce constitutive activity. Although they have been largely replaced by proton pump inhibitors recently, the development and commercialization of H_2 antagonists reduced the need for surgical intervention in the management of gastric ulcers.

The search for H_2 receptor antagonists began by modifying the structure of histamine and testing compounds in bioassays. This approach ultimately yielded cimetidine, which shares the imidazole ring of histamine but with a longer side chain. Mutagenesis data with the H_2 receptor supports a model where Asp186 in TM5 of the H_2 receptor is essential for cimetidine binding, probably through an interaction between the negatively charged amino acid and the imidazole ring.[61] This residue is not necessary for binding of histamine, but a nearby Thr190 is required for the agonist binding and activity.

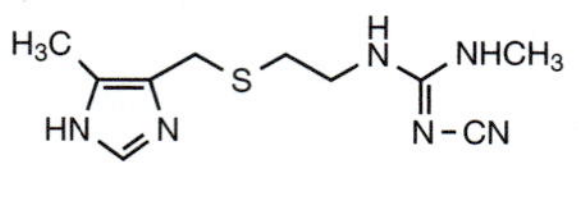

Cimetidine

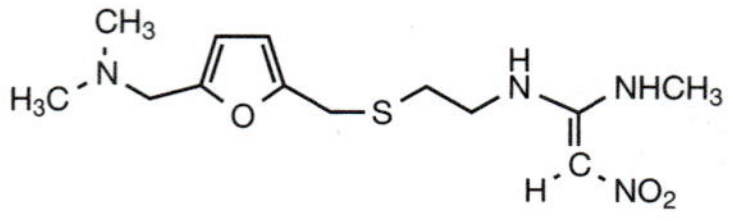

Ranitidine

H_3 Receptors

The H_3 receptors differ from the H_1 and H_2 receptors in a number of ways. There is low overall homology between the H_3 and either the H_1 or H_2 receptors; no blockbuster drugs target this receptor; and it is one of the few GPCRs that displays considerable in vivo constitutive signaling. High constitutive signaling is indicative of a receptor population where a greater than usual proportion of receptors are in the active conformation in the absence of ligands. The ability of pertussis toxin to inhibit H_3-mediated effects suggested linkage to $G_{i/o}$, and activation of H_3 receptors is coupled to a reduction in intracellular cAMP.

The H_3 receptor primarily functions as a presynaptic autoreceptor regulating histamine synthesis and release in various areas of the brain. Evidence also suggests that H_3 receptors may function as heteroreceptors regulating release of neurotransmitter from adrenergic, serotonergic, cholinergic, and dopaminergic neurons. Consequently, a number of inverse agonists at the H_3 receptor have been developed and clinically tested in a variety of neurologic disorders including sleep disorders, attention-deficit/hyperactivity disorder (ADHD), and Alzheimer disease. The inverse agonist pitolisant (aka tiprolisant) is the first H_3 ligand and has been approved by the U.S. Food and Drug Administration (FDA) to treat excessive daytime sleepiness in patients with narcolepsy, presumably by increasing the release of histamine in the brain.[62]

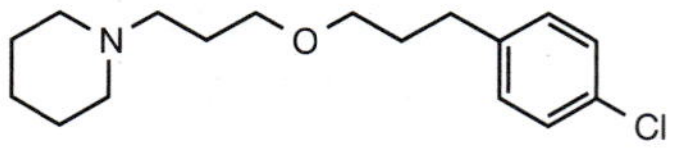

Tiprolisant

H_4 Receptors

The most recently discovered histamine receptor is the H_4 receptor. It is most similar to the H_3 receptor in terms of secondary structure, histamine binding, and G protein selectivity ($G_{i/o}$). Receptor expression seems highest in the bone marrow and hematopoietic cells. H_4 receptor antagonists have demonstrated clinical efficacy in pruritic conditions including psoriasis and atopic dermatitis.

Dopamine Receptors

Dopamine mediates a variety of central and peripheral effects including vessel tone, voluntary movement, sensory gating, and reward behavior via activation of D_1, D_2, D_3, D_4, or D_5 receptors, which are found in a wide range of central and peripheral locations. There is considerable homology between the D_1 and the D_5 receptors, and also between the D_2, D_3, and D_4 receptors. The D_1 class (D_1 and D_5 receptors) activates G_s and is primarily postsynaptic while the D_2 class (D_2 through D_4 receptors) activates G_i and includes both presynaptic and postsynaptic locations. Ligands of varying selectivity have been developed for most of the receptors with the exception of the D_5 receptor.

Agonists at the D_2 receptors have been developed to treat Parkinson disease while antagonists at this receptor are the traditional antipsychotics (eg, haloperidol) or the atypical antipsychotics (eg, risperidone). which also bind the 5-HT_{2A} receptor. The crystal structure of the D_2 receptor complexed with risperidone revealed that risperidone binds in a deep binding pocket between TM3, TM5, and TM6 and interacts with a number of amino acids in these regions.[63] Ligands that bind to the D_3 or D_4 receptors do not bind as deeply into those receptors. Importantly, many of the residues required for risperidone binding to the D_2 receptor are also present in the 5-HT_{2A} receptor.

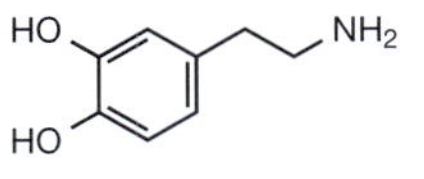

Dopamine

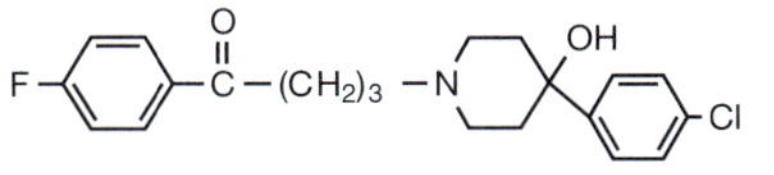

Haloperidol

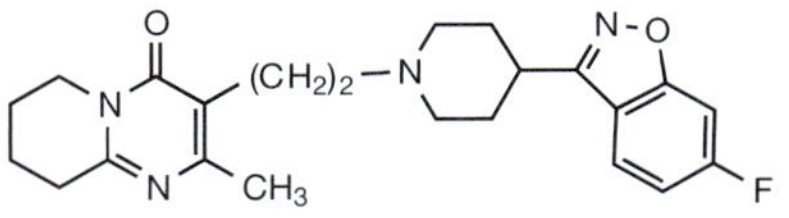

Risperidone (Risperdal)

Dopamine receptors represent another GPCR for which "biased ligands" have been developed. A number of studies have demonstrated that D_2 receptor–induced β-arrestin activation leads to stimulation of Akt/GSK3 signaling. Compounds such as UNC9975 and UNC9994, analogues of the antipsychotic aripiprazole, have been demonstrated to act as β-arrestin-biased D_2 receptor ligands.[64] These compounds promote signaling via the β-arrestin pathways while inhibiting signaling via the canonical G_i pathway. UNC9975 reportedly demonstrated antipsychotic properties in mice without the extrapyramidal adverse effects characteristic of most D_2 receptor antagonists. Thus, the development of biased ligands may improve the benefit-to-risk ratio of antipsychotics.

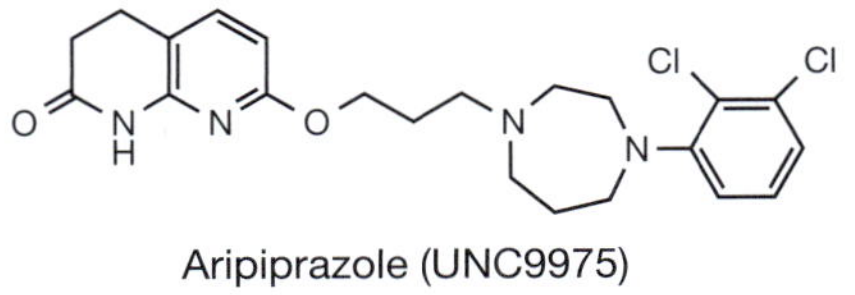

Aripiprazole (UNC9975)

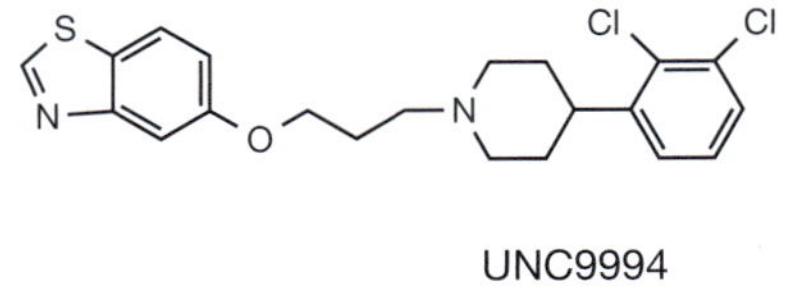

UNC9994

ACKNOWLEDGMENTS

The authors wish to acknowledge the works of Malgorzata Dukat, PhD, Richard A. Glennon, PhD, Robert K. Griffith, PhD, Wendel L. Nelson, PhD, Edward B. Roche, PhD, Victoria F. Roche, PhD, and David A. Williams, PhD who authored content used within this chapter in a previous edition of this text.

REFERENCES

1. Leake CD. *A Historical Account of Pharmacology in the 20th Century.* Charles C. Thomas; 1975.
2. Langley JN. On the reaction of cells and nerve endings to certain poisons. *J Physiol.* 1905;33:374-413.
3. Himmelweit F, ed. *Collected Papers of Paul Ehrlich.* Vol 3. Pergamon; 1957.
4. Gether U, Kobilka BK. G protein-coupled receptors: II. Mechanism of agonist activation. *J Biol Chem.* 1998;273:17979-17982.
5. Gilman AG. G proteins: transducers of receptor-generated signals. *Annu Rev Biochem.* 1987;56:615-649.
6. Berridge MJ. Inositol triphosphate and diacylglycerol: two interacting second messengers. *Ann Rev Biochem.* 1987;56:159-193.
7. Madani S, Hichami A, Legrand A, Belleville J, Khan NA. Implication of acyl chain of diacylglycerols in activation of different isoforms of protein kinase C. *FASEB J.* 2001;15(14):2595-2601.
8. Wise A, Jupe SC, Rees S. The identification of ligands at orphan G-protein coupled receptors. *Annu Rev Pharmacol Toxicol.* 2004;44:43-66.
9. Tekin I, Roskoski R Jr, Carkaci-Salli N, et al. Complex molecular regulation of tyrosine hydroxylase. *J Neural Transm.* 2014;121:1451-1481.
10. Tattersfield AD. Tolerance to β-agonists. *Bull Eur Physiopathol Respir.* 1985;21:1S-5S.
11. Lefkowitz RJ. A brief history of G-protein coupled receptors (Nobel Lecture). *Angew Chem Int Ed Engl.* 2013;52(25):6366-6378.
12. Salahpour A, Angers S, Mercier JF, Lagacé M, Marullo S, Bouvier M. Homodimerization of the β2-adrenergic receptor as a prerequisite for cell surface targeting. *J Biol Chem.* 2004;279(32):33390-33397.
13. Ahlquist RP. A study of the adrenotropic receptors. *Am J Physiol.* 1948;153:586-600.
14. Kobilka BK, Dixon RA, Frielle T, et al. cDNA for the human beta 2-adrenergic receptor: a protein with multiple membrane-spanning domains and encoded by a gene whose chromosomal location is shared with that of the receptor for platelet-derived growth factor. *Proc Natl Acad Sci U S A.* 1987;84:46-50.
15. Strader CD, Candelore MR, Hill WE, et al. Identification of two serine residues involved in agonist activation and the β-adrenergic receptor. *J Biol Chem.* 1989;264:13572-13578.
16. Starke K. Presynaptic α-autoreceptors. *Rev Physiol Biochem Pharmacol.* 1987;107:73-146.
17. Hartig PR, Branchek TA, Weinshank RI. A subfamily of 5-HT1D receptor genes. *Trends Pharmacol Sci.* 1992;3:152-159.
18. Hoyer D, Hannon JP, Martin GR. Molecular, pharmacological, and functional diversity of 5-HT receptors. *Pharmacol Biochem Behav.* 2002;71:533-534.
19. Hoyer D, Clarke DE, Fozard JR, et al. International Union of Pharmacology classification of receptors for 5-hydroxytryptamine (serotonin). *Pharmacol Rev.* 1994;46:157-203.
20. Ing HR. The structure-action relationships of the choline group. *Science.* 1949;109:264-266.
21. Caulfield JP, Birdsall NJM. International Union of Pharmacology. XVII. Classification of muscarinic acetylcholine receptors. *Pharmacol Rev.* 1998;50:279-290.
22. Nordvall G, Hacksell U. Binding-site modeling of the muscarinic m1 receptor: a combination of homology-based and indirect approaches. *J Med Chem.* 1993;36:967-976.

23. Humblet C, Mirzadegan T. Three-dimensional models of G-protein coupled receptors. *Annu Rep Med Chem*. 1992;27:291-300.
24. Hughes J, Smith TW, Kosterlitz HW, et al. Identification of two related pentapeptides from the brain with potent opiate agonist activity. *Nature*. 1975;258:577-579.
25. Li CH, Lemaire S, Yamashiro D, et al. The synthesis and opiate activity of β-endorphin. *Biochem Biophys Res Commun*. 1976;71:19-25.
26. Goldstein A, Tachibana S, Lowney LI, et al. Porcine pituitary dynorphin: complete amino acid sequence of the biologically active heptadecapeptide. *Proc Natl Acad Sci U S A*. 1979;76:6666-6670.
27. Zadina JE, Hackler L, Ge LJ, et al. A potent and selective endogenous agonist for the μ-opiate receptor. *Nature*. 1997;386:499-502.
28. Akil H, Watson SJ, Young E, et al. Endogenous opioids: biology and function. *Annu Rev Neurosci*. 1984;7:233-255.
29. Leslie FM. Methods used for the study of opioid receptors. *Pharmacol Rev*. 1987;39:197-249.
30. Satoh M, Minami M. Molecular pharmacology of the opioid receptors. *Pharmacol Ther*. 1995;68:343-364.
31. Connor M, Christie MD. Opioid receptor signaling mechanisms. *Clin Exp Pharmacol Physiol*. 1999;26:493-499.
32. Pan L, Xu J, Yu R, et al. Identification and characterization of six new alternatively spliced variants of the human mu opioid receptor gene, *Oprm*. *Neuroscience*. 2005;133:209-220.
33. Zhu Y, King MA, Schuller AG, et al. Retention of supraspinal delta-like analgesia and loss of morphine tolerance in delta opioid receptor knockout mice. *Neuron*. 1999;24:243-252.
34. Negri L, Erspamer GF, Severini C, et al. Dermorphin-related peptides from the skin of Phyllomedusa bicolor and their amidated analogs activate two mu opioid receptor subtypes that modulate antinociception and catalepsy in the rat. *Proc Natl Acad Sci U S A*. 1992;89:7203-7207.
35. Keiffer BL. Opioids: first lessons from knockout mice. *Trends Pharmacol Sci*. 1999;20:19-25.
36. Paul D, Pasternak GW. Differential blockade by naloxonazine of two mu opiate actions: analgesia and inhibition of gastrointestinal transit. *Eur J Pharmacol*. 1988;149:403-404.
37. Manglik A, Kruse AC, Kobilka TS, et al. Crystal structure of the μ-opioid receptor bound to a morphinan antagonist. *Nature*. 2012;485:321-326.
38. Pogozheva ID, Lomize AL, Mosberg HI. Opioid receptor three-dimensional structures from distance geometry calculations with hydrogen bonding constraints. *Biophys J*. 1998;75:612-634.
39. Szmuszkovicz J, Von Voigtlander PF. Benzeneacetamide amines: structurally novel non-m mu opioids. *J Med Chem*. 1982;25:1125-1126.
40. Clark CR, Halfpenny PR, Hill RG, et al. Highly selective κ opioid analgesics. Synthesis and structure-activity relationships of novel *N*-[(2-aminocyclohexyl)aryl]acetamide and *N*-[(2-aminocyclohexyl) aryloxy]acetamide derivatives. *J Med Chem*. 1988;31:831-836.
41. Hunter JC, Leighton GE, Meecham KG, et al. CI-977, a novel and selective agonist for the κ-opioid receptor. *Br J Pharmacol*. 1990;101:183-189.
42. Barber A, Bartoszyk GD, Bender HM, et al. A pharmacological profile of the novel, peripherally-selective κ-opioid receptor agonist, EMD 61753. *Br J Pharmacol*. 1994;113:843-851.
43. Rothman RB, Bykov V, de Costa BR, et al. Evidence for four opioid κ binding sites in Guinea pig brain. *Prog Clin Biol Res*. 1990;328:9-12.
44. Portoghese PS, Lipkowski AW, Takemori AE. Bimorphinans as highly selective, potent κ opioid receptor antagonists. *J Med Chem*. 1987;30:238-239.
45. James IF, Goldstein A. Site-directed alkylation of multiple opioid receptors. I. Binding selectivity. *Mol Pharmacol*. 1984;25:337-342.
46. Gacel C, Fournie-Zaluski M-C, Roques BP. D-Tyr-Ser-Gly-Phe-Leu-Thr, a highly preferential ligand for δ-opiate receptors. *FEBS Lett*. 1980;118:245-247.
47. Mosberg HI, Hurst R, Hruby VJ, et al. Bis-penicillamine enkephalins possess highly improved specificity toward δ opioid receptors. *Proc Natl Acad Sci U S A*. 1983;80:5871-5874.
48. Portoghese PS, Larson DL, Sultana M, et al. Opioid agonist and antagonist activities of morphindoles related to naltrindole. *J Med Chem*. 1992;35:4325-4329.
49. Bilsky EJ, Calderon SN, Wang T, et al. SNC 80, a selective, nonpeptidic and systemically active opioid δ agonist. *J Pharmacol Exp Ther*. 1995;273:359-366.
50. Portoghese PS, Sultana M, Takemori AE. Naltrindole, a highly selective and potent nonpeptide δ opioid receptor antagonist. *Eur J Pharmacol*. 1988;146:185-186.
51. Takemori AE, Sultana M, Nagase H, et al. Agonist and antagonist activities of ligands derived from naltrexone and oxymorphone. *Life Sci*. 1992;50:1491-1495.
52. Henderson G, McKnight AT. The orphan opioid receptor and its endogenous ligand—nociceptin/orphanin FQ. *Trends Pharmacol Sci*. 1997;18:293-300.
53. Meunier JC, Mollereau C, Toll L, et al. Isolation and structure of the endogenous agonist of opioid receptor-like OR1 receptor. *Nature*. 1995;377:532-535.
54. Zeilhofer HU, Calo G. Nociceptin/orphanin FQ and its receptor—potential targets for pain therapy. *J Pharmacol Exp Ther*. 2003;306:423-429.
55. Chiou LC, Liao YY, Fan PC, et al. Nociceptin/orphanin FQ peptide receptors: pharmacology and clinical implications. *Curr Drug Targets*. 2007;8:117-135.
56. Portoghese PS, Larson DL, Sayre LM, et al. A novel opioid receptor site directed alkylating agent with irreversible narcotic antagonistic and reversible agonistic activities. *J Med Chem*. 1980;23:233-234.
57. Calo G, Guerrini R, Rizzi A, et al. Pharmacology of nociception and its receptor: a novel therapeutic target. *Br J Pharmacol*. 2000;129:1261-1283.
58. Lambert DG. The nociceptin/orphanin FQ receptor: a target with broad therapeutic potential. *Nat Rev Drug Discov*. 2008;7:694-710.
59. Cordova-Sintjago TC, Fang L, Bruysters M, et al. Molecular determinants of ligand binding at the human histamine H1 receptor: site-directed mutagenesis results analyzed with ligand docking and molecular dynamics studies at H1 homology and crystal structure models. *J Chem Pharm Res*. 2012;4(6):2937-2951.
60. Shimamura T, Shiroishi M, Weyand S, et al. Structure of the human histamine H1 receptor complex with doxepin. *Nature*. 2011;475:65-70.
61. Gantz I, DelValle J, Wang LD, et al. Molecular basis for the interaction of histamine with the histamine H2 receptor. *J Biol Chem*. 1992;267:20840-20843.
62. Schwartz J-C. The histamine H3 receptor: from discovery to clinical trials with pitolisant. *Br J Pharmacol*. 2011;163(4):713-721.
63. Wang S, Che T, Levit A, et al. Structure of the D2 dopamine receptor bound to the atypical antipsychotic drug risperidone. *Nature*. 2018;555:269-273.
64. Allen JA, Yost JM, Setola V, et al. Discovery of β-arrestin-biased dopamine D2 ligands for probing signal transduction pathways essential for antipsychotic efficacy. *Proc Natl Acad Sci U S A*. 2011;108(45):18488-18493.

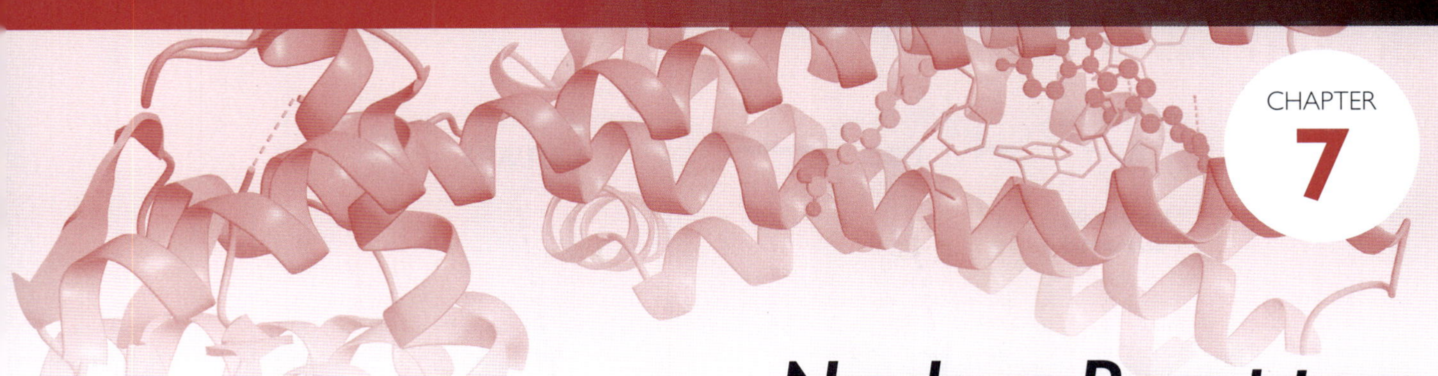

CHAPTER 7

Nuclear Receptors

David A. Johnson

Abbreviations

AF1 hormone-independent transactivation function 1
AF2 ligand-dependent activation function 2
APL acute promyelocytic leukemia
AR androgen receptor
ARE androgen response element
ATRA *all-trans* retinoic acid
BP base pair
9CRA 9-*cis* retinoic acid
DBD DNA-binding domain
DHT dihydrotestosterone
DNA deoxyribonucleic acid
DR direct repeat
ER estrogen receptor
ERE estrogen response element
ERRs estrogen-related receptors
GCNF germ cell nuclear factor
GR glucocorticoid receptor
GRE glucocorticoid response element
HSP heat shock proteins
LBD ligand-binding domain
MR mineralocorticoid receptors
NRs nuclear receptors
NTD N-terminal domain
PPAR peroxisome proliferator–activated receptors
PPARE PPAR response element
PR progesterone receptor
PRA progesterone receptor subtype A
PRB progesterone receptor subtype B
RARE retinoic receptor response element
RARs retinoic acid receptors
RNA ribonucleic acid
RXR retinoid X receptor
SF-1 steroidogenic factor 1
SHP small heterodimer partner
T testosterone
T_3 triiodothyronine
T_4 thyroxine
TR thyroid receptors
TRE thyroid response element
TRH thyrotropin-releasing hormone
TSH thyroid-stimulating hormone
VDR vitamin D receptor
VDRE vitamin D response element
WHI Women's Health Initiative

Introduction

Definitions

Nuclear receptors (NRs) are a class of intracellular proteins that function as ligand-activated transcription factors. They are involved in regulating gene expression in response to a variety of physiologic and environmental signals, including hormones, vitamins, and fatty acids. NRs typically consist of a ligand-binding domain (LBD), a deoxyribonucleic acid (DNA)-binding domain, and a transcriptional activation domain. When a ligand binds to the receptor, it undergoes a conformational change that allows it to bind to specific DNA sequences and activate or repress gene expression. NRs play important roles in many physiologic processes, including development, metabolism, and immune function, and are important targets for the development of therapeutic drugs.

Classification

There are over 300 protein molecules included in the superfamily of NRs; however, only 48 are found in humans. NRs are divided into seven subfamilies that include receptors for steroidal hormones, thyroid hormone, bile acids, and vitamins A and D. In addition, NRs include receptors discovered by screening DNA libraries called "orphan receptors" that have no known endogenous ligand.[1]

Structure and Functions

NRs are single peptide chains comprising five domains: (1) domain A/B, the N-terminal domain (NTD), that functions in the allosteric binding of coactivator and corepressor proteins that participate in receptor activation, (2) domain C, the DBD, that selectively docks the NR to specific DNA-response elements to initiate the process of gene transcription, (3) domain D, the hinge domain that links the DBD to the LBD, (4) domain E, LBD that contains the primary hormone binding site and allosteric sites for binding coactivators and repressors, and (5) domain F, whose function is not well understood (Fig. 7.1).

N-Terminal Domain and Hormone-Independent Transactivation Function 1

The NTD, domain A/B, is a highly variable amino-terminal region that contains a hormone-independent transactivation

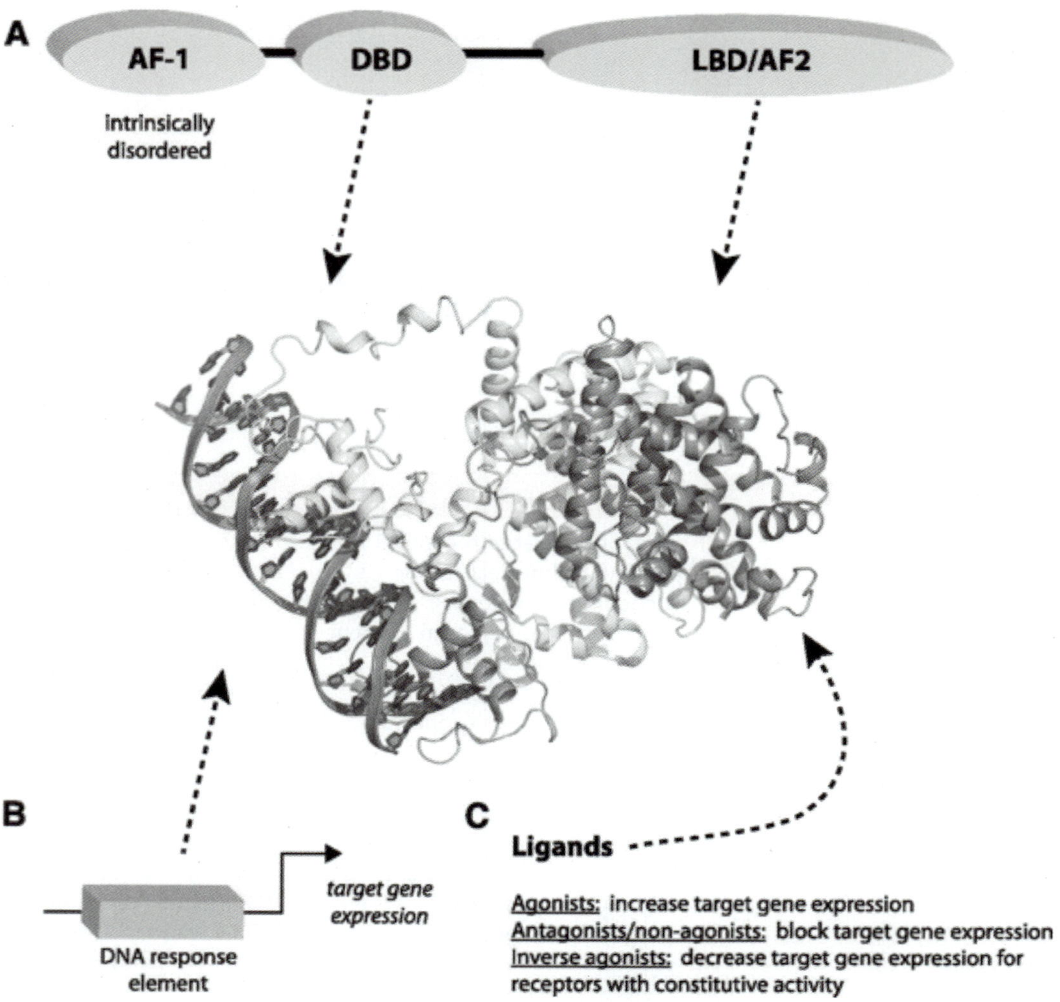

Figure 7.1 Nuclear receptor (NR) structure. A. Order and relative size of domains within the NR protein. B. NRs bind to particular response elements of DNA to trigger gene translation and expression. C. Ligands bind to the LBD domain to regulate receptor activation and gene expression.

function (AF-1). AF-1 can bind coactivator or corepressor proteins that modulate receptor activation without a ligand. In addition, the NTD contains phosphorylation sites that can facilitate or inhibit gene transcription by modulating NR dimerization and the recruitment of coactivators or corepressors and other regulators of gene expression.

DNA-Binding Domain

Domain C, the DBD, is composed of a 66-amino-acid core, including two loops coordinated by "zinc fingers" that play a key role in DNA binding[2]: a "D-box" involved in receptor dimerization, and a "P-box" that binds the NR to specific half-element DNA sequences.[3] NRs usually bind to DNA as homodimers for steroid NRs or heterodimers for nonsteroid NRs. The DBD binds to DNA-response elements. Selectivity for DNA response–element binding is achieved through variations in the arrangement of nucleotides in the response element and the degree of separation between "half-sites."

Domain D: Hinge Domain, Domain E: Ligand-Binding Domain, and Domain F

Domain D is a variable "hinge domain" that links the DBD to domain E, the LBD. The LBD includes the ligand-dependent activation function 2 (AF-2), containing the ligand-binding site of the NR. AF-2 comprises a sandwich of 12 α-helices (H1-H12), arranged in an antiparallel three-layer sandwich fold that forms a hydrophobic binding pocket comprising helices H3, H4/5, H7, and H11.[4] The binding of an agonist shifts the orientation of H12 and stabilizes the LBD in a conformation favorable for binding coactivators to AF-2. Antagonists do not stabilize AF-2 or stabilize the domain in a conformation that recruits corepressors to suppress activation. Partial agonists can recruit either coactivators or corepressors. The variability of NR response to activation in different tissues is a consequence of the differential expression of coactivators and corepressors in different cell types. Domain F is not found in every NR, and the function of this domain is not well understood.

Nuclear Receptor Activation

Unbound steroid receptors are located in the cytoplasm. Following ligand binding, they dimerize and are transported to the nucleus via molecular chaperones. Once in the nucleus, steroid NR homodimers selectively bind to DNA-response elements and recruit coactivators and other proteins involved in regulating gene transcription (Fig. 7.2). Inactive nonsteroid NRs are located in the nucleus as hetero- or homodimers bound to a response element and corepressors that inhibit gene transcription. When an agonist binds to the dimer, the corepressors are exchanged for coactivators, and gene transcription is initiated.

Transactivation and Transrepression

The binding of an NR to a DNA-response element can also facilitate the transcription of adjacent genes by enhancing the binding of coactivators or the binding of NRs to DNA-response elements. NRs can also inhibit adjacent gene expression by decreasing the availability of coactivators and transcription factors. In addition, NRs can inhibit gene expression by functioning as corepressor proteins or by slowing the degradation of corepressors.[5]

Estrogen Receptors

Estrogens are principal hormones in women involved in the regulation of the estrous cycle, pregnancy, breast development, and secondary sex characteristics. Estrogens also affect cognition and mood, bone density, fat distribution, and other functions. There are two isoforms of the estrogen receptor (ER): ERα and ERβ. The two receptors have a relatively close amino acid sequence homology in the LBD and DBD. The relative distribution of ERα and ERβ can vary both within and between tissues. Moreover, the variability of tissue responsiveness to estrogens may in part be due to the presence of differing numbers and abundance of ER subtypes and splice variants.

Ligand Binding

Activation of ERs following the binding of an agonist involves a shift in the orientation of the H12 loop in AF-2 to facilitate the binding of coactivators, while the binding of antagonists repositions H12 to sterically hinder coactivator binding and/or facilitate the binding of corepressors. For binding to the ER, estrogens are unique in having a 3-hydroxyl group on the A-ring of the steroid core. This structural distinction provides

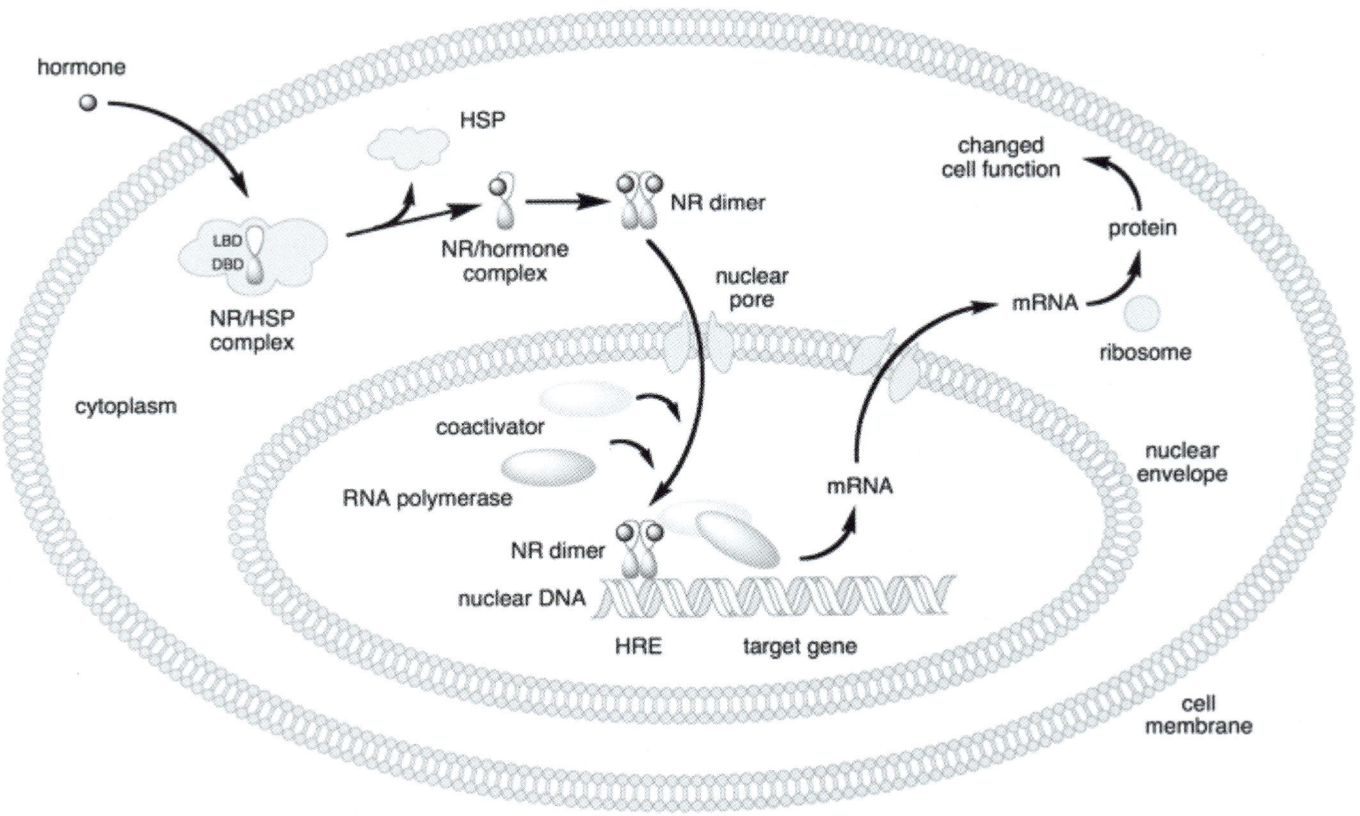

Figure 7.2 Nuclear receptor (NR)-ligand binding: translocation and DNA docking. Steps in NR activation, translocation to the nucleus, and DNA docking: (1) the steroid hormone diffuses or is transported into the cytoplasm, where it binds to the NR bound to chaperone heat shock proteins (HSP), (2) the HSP chaperones dissociate from the NR-hormone complex, (3) the NR-hormone complex is translocated to the cell nucleus, where it binds to coactivator and/or corepressor proteins, (4) the complex docks with the DNA-response element and recruits additional proteins, including RNA polymerase to initiate gene transcription.

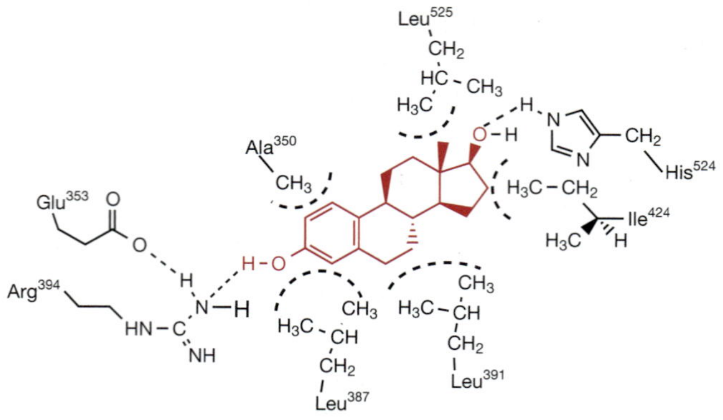

Figure 7.3 Crystal structure of the ligand-binding domain of the estrogen receptor bound to estradiol.

selectivity for ligand binding to the ER. Estrogens bind to the receptor using hydrogen bonds with the 3-hydroxyl group to glutamate-353 and arginine-394. In addition, amino acids with neutral side chains provide van der Waals interactions with rings A, B, and C of the steroid core. An additional hydrogen bond occurs between the 17-hydroxyl group of the D-ring and the δ nitrogen of histidine-524 (Fig. 7.3).[6] ERs, especially ERα, can also be activated by coactivators' binding to AF-1 independent of estrogen binding. Moreover, phosphorylation of sites in the amino-terminal region enables "cross-talk" interactions between ERs and other signal transduction pathways.

Estrogen-Receptor Binding to the DNA Estrogen Response Element

Once the ER dimer has translocated to the nucleus, it binds to the estrogen response element (ERE). Binding of the receptor to the ERE triggers the binding of nuclear coactivators, which then recruit enzymes that modify the chromatin to allow greater accessibility to DNA for transcription by ribonucleic acid (RNA) polymerase. ER dimers can also modulate the transcription of other genes via cooperativity with other NRs such as progesterone receptors (PRs) and the recruitment of enzymes to facilitate gene transcription. ERs can repress gene activation by binding to particular transcription factors and repress activation of other genes by inhibiting DNA interactions or the activity of other factors.[7]

Progesterone Receptors

Progesterone is a hormone released by the ovaries, testes, adrenal cortex, and, to a lesser extent, in brain and adipose tissue. It is a metabolic precursor for other steroids, including aldosterone, testosterone (T), and estrogens. Physiologically, progesterone is important for female reproductive organs, such as the uterus and breast, and PR antagonists are effective for treating endometriosis and benign uterine tumors. Aside from female reproductive organs, progesterone modulates neurotransmission in the brain and plays a role in smooth muscle and skin.[8] There are two PR subtypes, PRA and PRB, that share high amino acid sequence homology in the DBD and LBD domains.[9] PRA and PRB target distinct genomic sites and bind different coregulators. In normal tissues, PRA and PRB are expressed in equimolar amounts; however, knockout models demonstrate that PRA plays a significant role in mammary gland development, while PRB is predominantly involved in ovarian and uterine functions.[10] In cancer cells, there can be a variable level of expression of the PR isotypes.

Progesterone-Receptor Binding

Unlike ERs, the PR forms a hydrogen bond via glutamine-725 with the 3-keto group of the A-ring of progesterone. Analogous to the ER-binding pocket, arginine-766 serves to properly orient glutamine-725 via water-mediated hydrogen bonds, and phenylalanine-778 interacts with the A-ring of progesterone via van der Waals contacts. There is no well-defined binding of the C_{20} ketone moiety on the D-ring of progesterone (Fig. 7.4).[11]

Progesterone Receptor–ER Interactions

There is significant cross-talk between PRs and ERs. It is well established that PRs bound to either progestin agonists or antagonists can suppress ER-mediated gene expression, and PRA activation or inhibition of PR can shift ER signaling.[12] The use of progestin agonists and antagonists in breast cancer treatment is controversial. The Women's Health Initiative (WHI) found that postmenopausal women receiving hormone replacement therapy containing estrogens and progestin had a higher incidence of breast cancer.[13] Other studies found that progesterone antagonists, by suppressing ER signaling, could slow the growth of ER-positive tumors.[14]

Androgen Receptors

The androgens, T and dihydrotestosterone (DHT) are steroid hormones that promote the development of primary and secondary sex characteristics of male anatomy and physiology. Androgen effects are mediated by the androgen receptor (AR), a member of subfamily 3 of the NR superfamily (Table 7.1). The gene for AR is widely expressed across organ systems. Aside from male reproductive organs and sexual

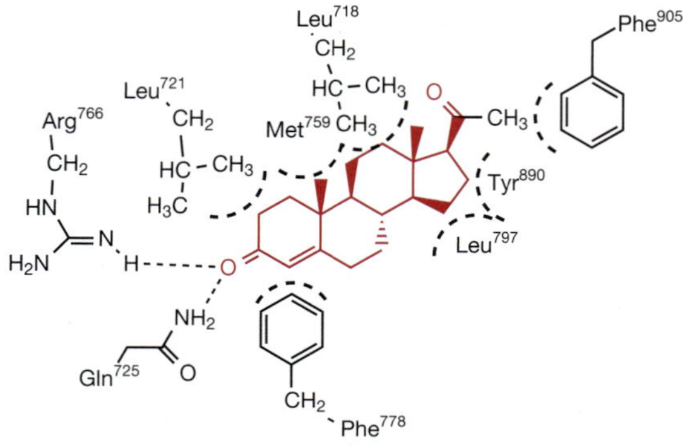

Figure 7.4 Crystal structure of the ligand-binding domain of the progesterone receptor bound to progesterone.

Table 7.1 Nuclear-Receptor Superfamily: Receptors and Ligands

Subfamily	Receptor (Including Subtypes)	Endogenous Ligands
0	NROB1 (DAX 1)	Orphan
	NROB2 Small heterodimer partner (SHP)	Orphan
1	Thyroid receptor α, β	Thyroid hormone
	Retinoic acid receptor α, β, γ	Retinoic acid
	Peroxisome proliferator–activated receptor α, β/δ, γ	Fatty acids, eicosanoids
	Vitamin D receptor	1α,25-dihydroxyvitamin D_3
	Farnesoid X receptor	Bile acids
	Liver X receptor α, β	Oxysterols
2	Retinoid X receptor α, β, γ	9-*cis*-Retinoic acid unsaturated fatty acids
3	Estrogen receptor α, β	Estrogens
	Estrogen-related receptor α, β, γ	Orphan
	Progesterone receptor A, B	Progesterone
	Androgen receptor	Testosterone, DHT
	Glucocorticoid receptor α, β	Cortisol, aldosterone
	Mineralocorticoid receptor	Aldosterone, cortisol
4	Neuron-derived orphan	Orphan
5	Steroidogenic factor 1	Orphan
6	Germ cell nuclear factor	Orphan

functions, androgens affect the skin, bone development and density, muscle, and fat distribution, and cardiovascular, neuro, and immune function.[15]

Androgen Receptor Structure

The AR, like other NRs, has a modular structure made up of NTD, DBD, hinge, and LBD domains. The NTD is relatively long and has a variable amino acid sequence that contains AF1. In addition, the NTD has polymeric glutamine repeats that can affect cellular sensitivity to androgens. The nucleotide half-site sequence for AR comprises two 6-base-pair (BP) asymmetrical elements separated by a 3-BP spacer. A C-terminal extension functions to selectively bind the androgen-response element (ARE). The LBD of the AR is similar to those of other NRs being composed of 12 α-helices. The binding of ligand changes the conformation of helix 12 to allow for binding of coactivators.

Androgen-Receptor Binding

Androgens bind to the AR with affinity in the nanomolar range, with DHT having an approximately 2-fold higher affinity than T and a dissociation rate that is 5-fold slower. The binding of T to the AR is similar to progesterone binding to the PR receptor except that the 3-keto group on the A-ring has hydrogen-binding interactions with arginine-752. In addition, the hydroxyl group on the D-ring binds to asparagine-705 and threonine-877. Aside from hydrogen binding, there are a number of van der Waals interactions between the steroid ring core structure and neutral amino acids, including methionine, tryptophan, leucine, and phenylalanine (Fig. 7.5).[16]

Androgen-Receptor Signal Transduction

The AR without ligand is located in the cytosol bound to chaperone proteins. When androgens bind to the receptor, there is a conformational change, and the receptor dissociates from chaperone proteins and translocates into the nucleus, where it binds to the ARE on the promoter region of target genes. Once bound, coregulator proteins promote transcription by remodeling histones and attracting general transcription factors to initiate gene transcription.

Clinical Applications

AR receptor antagonists are utilized clinically to treat prostate cancer. However, in later stages of the disease, tumor cells can become resistant to antiandrogen therapy.[17]

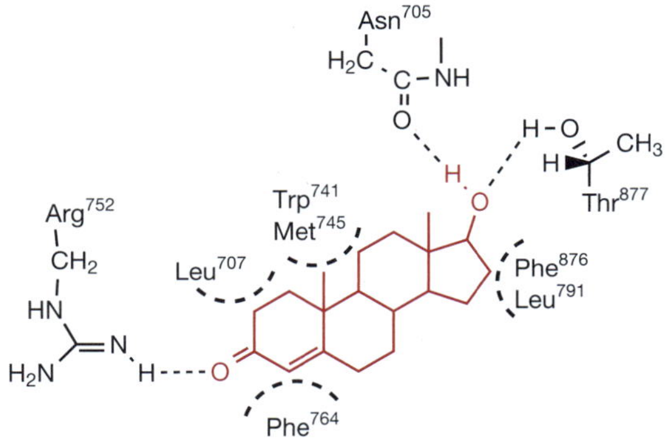

Figure 7.5 Crystal structure of the ligand-binding domain of the androgen receptor bound to testosterone.

Glucocorticoid Receptors

Cortisol is a primary human stress hormone released from the adrenal cortex. Glucocorticoids are involved in maintaining organ system and cellular homeostasis during normal function and in response to stressful physiologic challenges. Cortisol produces its effects through regulation of metabolism, and immune, reproductive, and neuronal systems. Glucocorticoid receptors (GRs) are found in almost all cell types, consistent with the wide-ranging role that glucocorticoids play in regulating physiologic functions.[18] Drugs that interact with the GR are among the most prescribed drugs in the world. Glucocorticoids are effective in treating inflammatory and autoimmune diseases, preventing organ transplant rejection, and the treatment of certain cancers. A variety of GR isoforms provide a range of responses to glucocorticoids within particular tissues and different organs.

Glucocorticoid-Receptor Structure

The GR structure is consistent with that of other steroid hormone receptors. In addition, GRs have two nuclear localization signals, NL1 and NL2, to selectively bind the receptor to the glucocorticoid response element (GRE) and an LBD that facilitates the shuttling of the GR from the cytosol to the nucleus.[19] Alternative splicing results in two isoforms: GRα and GRβ. The GRα isoform mediates the actions of glucocorticoids, while the GRβ does not bind agonists but resides constitutively in the cell nucleus. By competing for transcriptional coregulators, a GRα-GRβ heterodimer is inhibitory when bound to the GRE[20] and as a consequence, the heterodimer may play a role in glucocorticoid resistance and hypersensitivity to proinflammatory factors.[21] GRβ can also decrease the response to glucocorticoids via recruitment of histone deacetylases that repress gene expression.[22] There are eight translational isoforms of GRα that provide selectivity for gene expression. Moreover, posttranslational phosphorylation of AF-1 can increase or decrease gene transcription, depending on the particular phosphorylation site.

Glucocorticoid-Receptor Binding

The cellular response and tissue sensitivity to corticosteroids are dependent on the intracellular concentration of the hormone. Following diffusion into the cytosol, cortisol concentration is regulated by enzymes that maintain an equilibrium between cortisol and the inactive metabolite cortisone. For cortisol binding to the GR, in addition to hydrophobic interactions, cortisol has four hydrogen bonds formed between the hydrophilic groups of the steroid and the polar amino acids of the binding pocket (Fig. 7.6).[23]

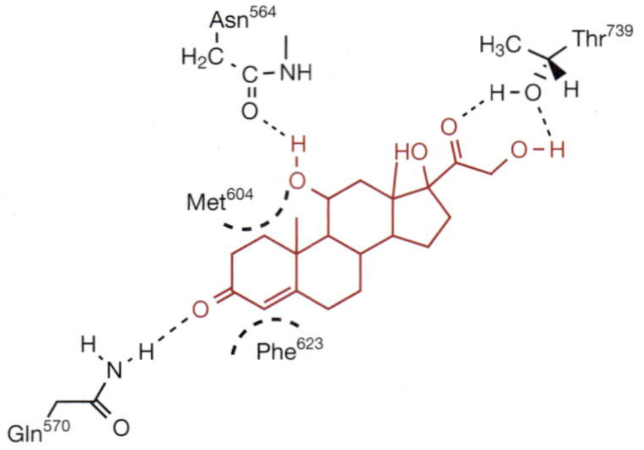

Figure 7.6 Crystal structure of the ligand-binding domain of the glucocorticoid receptor bound to cortisol.

Signal Transduction

The binding of cortisol to GR results in dissociation of chaperone proteins and translocation to the nucleus, where it binds to the GRE. As with other NRs, once GR is bound to GRE, coregulators are recruited to facilitate gene transcription. The result is the transcription of genes regulated by GRE and the potential suppression of other genes. The range of gene expression under the control of GREs varies from tissue to tissue, and hence responses to glucocorticoids are also variable. The GR can also influence the transcription of genes regulated by other NRs. As an example, GR binds to proinflammatory transcription factors AP1 and NF-κB to inhibit transfection of inflammatory cytokines and ultimately suppress inflammation.[24]

Mineralocorticoid Receptors

Mineralocorticoid receptors (MRs) were first identified in 1974. Activation of MRs by aldosterone promotes renal sodium reabsorption and potassium excretion. However, activation of MRs is also associated with a number of pathologic conditions, including promotion of inflammation and fibrosis in the aortic endothelium, proliferation of smooth muscle cells, cardiac remodeling,[25] and thermogenesis. The single gene for the MR produces several transcription isoforms and variants that provide for diverse responses to receptor activation in different tissues. Glucocorticoids can also activate MRs; however, activation is limited by enzymes that metabolize glucocorticoid hormones to structures that lack significant binding affinity for the MR. The MR antagonist spironolactone has been employed as an adjunct for patients with hypertension treated with potassium-depleting diuretic agents. More recently, spironolactone has also been prescribed for patients with heart failure to inhibit the myocardial remodeling associated with that disorder.

Mineralocorticoid-Receptor Structure

The MR has a longer NTD than other steroid receptors and contains two AF1 domains and a domain that can inhibit transactivation by AF-1.[26] There is a high degree of homology between the MR DBD domain and those of GR, PR, and AR. The DBD "D-box" facilitates homodimerization or heterodimerization with other steroid receptors especially GR and AR.[27] The LBD of the MR is structurally similar to other steroid receptors and contains a ligand-dependent AF-2 domain, which can interact with coactivator proteins. Posttranslational modifications to the MR include phosphorylation that facilitates cytoplasmic to nuclear transport and MR degradation.

Mineralocorticoid Receptor Binding

Aldosterone binding to MR is stronger than cortisol binding to GR. Hydrogen-bond interactions between aldosterone and MR include the 3-keto group and glutamine-776, the 11- and 21-hydroxyl groups with asparagine-770, the 18-aldehyde group and cysteine-942, and the 20-ketone and 21-hydroxyl group with threonine-945 (Fig. 7.7).[28]

Thyroid Receptors

Thyroid hormones are regulated by the hypothalamus through the release of thyrotropin-releasing hormone (TRH) that stimulates the release of thyroid-stimulating hormone (TSH) from the anterior pituitary gland. TSH stimulates the synthesis and release thyroid hormones triiodothyronine (T_3) and thyroxine (T_4). Following release from the thyroid gland, T_4 is peripherally converted to T_3. The T_3 released by the thyroid gland as well as that formed from T_4 circulates in the blood, enters the nucleus of cells, and binds to the thyroid nuclear receptor. Binding of T_3 to TR alters the conformation of the receptor and triggers the thyroid DNA–response element (TRE) to initiate target gene transcription. Physiologic responses to receptor activation include regulation of brain development, thermogenesis, increased cardiac function, and increased cellular metabolism.

Thyroid Receptor Structure

The structure of TR is consistent with the modular domains of other NRs. TR subtypes designated TRα and TRβ are the product of two distinct genes. Each TR transcript is subject to alternative splicing that results in three isoforms of TRα and two of TRβ.[29] As with other NRs, the binding of corepressors and activators to the AF1 region plays an important role in ligand-dependent and ligand-independent activation. Variations in the amino-terminal domain of TR isoforms provide selectivity in receptor dimerization and hence in gene transcription in different tissues.

Thyroid Receptor-Ligand Binding

The ligand-binding pockets of TRα and TRβ are largely composed of amino acids with neutral side chains. However, two polar regions of the binding pocket provide hydrogen bonding and ion-dipole bonding opportunities at the opposite ends of ligands. Histidine-435 forms a hydrogen bond with the phenolic hydroxyl of T_3, while arginine-282 provides an ion-dipole bond to the carboxylate group at the other end of the molecule (Fig. 7.8).[30]

Thyroid Receptor Signal Transduction

Thyroid receptors generally form homodimers or heterodimers with different TR isoforms or the retinoid X receptor (RXR), employing dimerization surfaces in the LBD and DBD. Dimers bind selectively to TREs of target genes. Characteristics of TRE include 4-BP spacer between half-sites arranged as direct repeats (DRs).[31] The two zinc finger modules of the DBD mediate selective DNA sequence recognition and spacing between half-sites of the TRE. The hinge regions of the two receptors provide flexibility for the dimer to bind to TREs with different half-site orientations. When not bound to ligand, TR dimers repress gene transcription by binding to the TRE while complexed with corepressors. The conformational change that results from ligand-binding facilitates the release of corepressors and the binding of coactivators, resulting in reorientation of the chromatin by coactivators and upregulation of transcription of the target gene.

Peroxisome Proliferator–Activated Receptors

Peroxisome proliferator-activated receptors (PPARs) belong to NR subfamily 1. There are three receptor isotypes designated, PPARα, PPARβ/δ, and PPARγ, each derived from a separate gene. The α isotype is abundant in brown adipose tissue, liver, heart, kidney, and intestine—organs involved in lipid catabolism.[32] The γ isotype has two isoforms γ1 and γ2; γ2 is found in high concentrations in adipose tissues, while γ1 and PPARβ/δ are broadly distributed.[33]

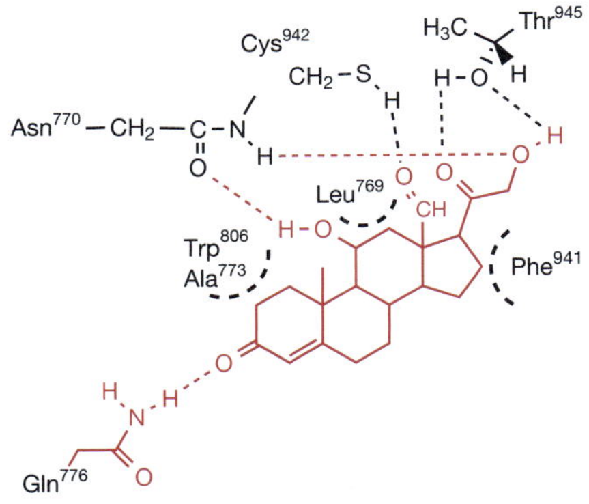

Figure 7.7 Crystal structure of the ligand-binding domain of the mineralocorticoid receptor bound to aldosterone.

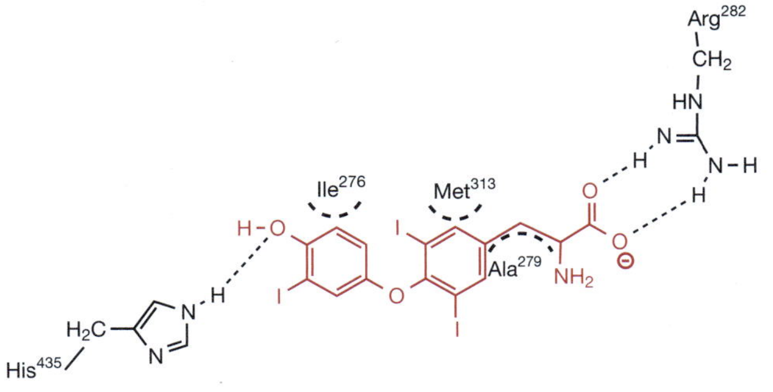

Figure 7.8 Crystal structure of the ligand-binding domain of the thyroid hormone receptor bound to T_3.

Peroxisome Proliferator–Activated Receptor Function

PPARs are involved in a wide array of functions, including carbohydrate metabolism and storage, insulin sensitivity, cell proliferation and differentiation, tissue repair, and inflammation. The primary function of PPARα is regulation of lipid metabolism, including hepatic fatty acid catabolism and gluconeogenesis.[34] In the liver, PPARα increases fatty acid oxidation, lipolysis, and high-density lipoprotein synthesis, leading to enhanced reverse cholesterol transport. It also attenuates inflammation by inhibiting leukocyte recruitment and adhesion to endothelial cells. Increased fatty acid oxidation mediated by PPARα lowers plasma triglycerides, liver, and muscle steatosis, reduces adiposity, and enhances insulin sensitivity. Fibrate drugs such as fenofibrate and gemfibrozil activate PPARα to lower plasma triglycerides and decrease the progression of atherosclerosis. PPARα also decreases the synthesis of very-low-density lipoproteins, resulting in decreased plasma triglycerides and low-density lipids. In addition, activation of PPARα enhances the release of the vasodilator nitric oxide.[35] In coronary heart disease, fibrates are effective in lowering cardiovascular disease risk in patients with type 2 diabetes. Overall, the activation of PPARα promotes vasoprotection from atherosclerosis.[36]

PPARβ/δ receptors are involved in cell proliferation, differentiation, and tissue repair.[37] Inflammation increases the expression of PPARβ/δ and the ligands that activate the receptor. Increased receptor activity decreases apoptosis following injury and facilitates the rate of wound healing. PPARγ is expressed primarily in adipose tissue and is associated with adipocyte differentiation, leading to increased numbers of adipocytes and increased cell size. Receptor activation is also associated with fluid retention and edema.

Drugs that activate PPARγ have clinical utility in treating type 2 diabetes.[38] The thiazolidinediones, pioglitazone, and rosiglitazone are PPARγ agonists and are effective for enhancing insulin sensitivity and increasing plasma glucose uptake into skeletal muscle and adipose tissues. Also, via actions at adipocytes, there is increased fatty acid clearance and reduced lipolysis. Adverse effects associated with PPARγ activation include weight gain and edema; therefore, thiazolidinediones are contraindicated in patients with heart failure.

Peroxisome Proliferator–Activated Receptor Structure

PPARs have the same general structural features common to NRs, including a highly conserved DBD and an LBD containing the binding pocket and surfaces for coactivator and corepressor binding. Interestingly, the binding cavity for PPARα and PPARγ are larger than for PPAR β/δ, which allows for binding of a wider array of ligands. PPARs also form heterodimers with the RXR receptor, independent of ligand binding.

Peroxisome Proliferator–Activated Receptor Signal Transduction

When activated, the receptor binds to a PPAR response element (PPARE) located in the promoter region of the target gene. The response element is composed of DR-binding half-sites separated by a single nucleotide spacer. Selectivity for the particular PPAR isotype is mediated by the 5′-flanking region of the PPARE. Activation of the dimer requires the binding of coactivators. Seventeen coactivators have currently been identified for PPARγ.

RETINOIC ACID RECEPTORS

Vitamin A, retinol, is metabolized via alcohol dehydrogenase to retinaldehyde, which is then oxidized to *all-trans* retinoic acid (ATRA) by retinaldehyde dehydrogenase. The ATRA metabolite is the most potent natural ligand acting at retinoic acid receptors (RARs). ATRA and metabolites regulate a number of functions during embryonic development, including organogenesis, cellular differentiation, and apoptosis.[39] The effects are mediated through one of the three RAR subtypes designated as RARα, RARβ, and RARγ. The LBD of each subtype has a single amino acid substitution that provides selectivity for subtype-specific binding (see Fig. 7.9 for receptor binding to ATRA).[40]

RARs form heterodimers with one of the three subtypes of the RXR. The dimer binds to retinoic receptor–response elements (RAREs), located in the promoter region of target genes. A RARE is composed of DR-binding half-sites and separated by one, two, or five nucleotide spacers (DR1, 2, 5). In the absence of agonist, the RXR-RAR heterodimer binds corepressors that inhibit gene transcription. When an agonist binds to the dimer, a conformational change occurs, and the corepressors are released and replaced by coactivators that facilitate gene transcription. Interestingly, while the dimer will initiate gene transcription following the binding of an RAR agonist, the binding of an RXR agonist will not result in transcription without the binding of an RAR agonist that will initiate dissociation of corepressors from the RXR receptor.[41] The RAR–RXR dimer is also subject to "cross-talk" from other signal transduction pathways via phosphorylation at AF-1 and AF-2 domains.

Abnormal signaling involving genes for RARα and genes for promyelocyte leukemia proteins results in a fusion

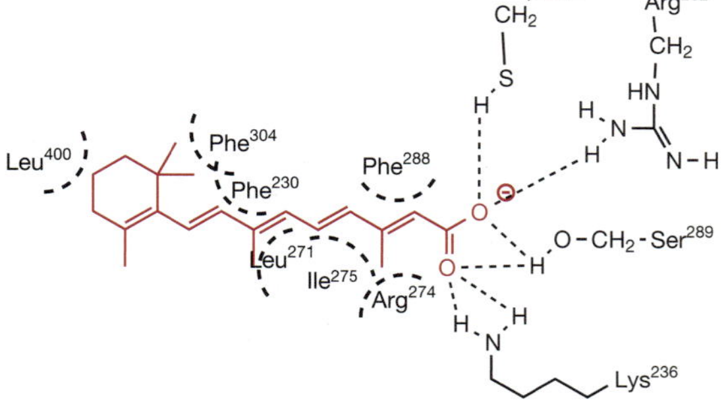

Figure 7.9 Crystal structure of the ligand-binding domain of the retinoic acid receptor bound to *all-trans*-retinoic acid.

protein with high binding affinity for corepressors. The result leads to acute promyelocytic leukemia (APL). Fortunately, APL is responsive to treatment with ATRA, which dissociates the corepressors from RAR and facilitates gene transcription and differentiation of immature leukemic promyelocytes, ultimately triggering spontaneous apoptosis. ATRA has also shown effectiveness for patients diagnosed with cutaneous T-cell malignancies and juvenile chronic myelogenous leukemia.[42] Aside from cancer, retinoids including ATRA, 9-*cis* retinoic acid (9CRA), and the synthetic compounds isotretinoin and etretinate are effective in treating dermatologic diseases such as acne and psoriasis.[43]

Retinoid X Receptors

RXRs selectively bind 9CRA with high affinity (Fig. 7.10).[44]

There are three subtypes (RXRα, RXRβ, and RXRγ) derived from different genes. The expression of RXR subtypes is dependent on cell type and the degree of cell differentiation.[45] Natural ligands for RXRα include unsaturated fatty acids, including arachidonic and oleic acids.[46] 9CRA binds with high affinity to both RAR and RXR; however, the conformations of the ligand-binding pockets between the two receptors are substantially different, which provide selectivity for ligand binding. Drugs that target RXR heterodimers are utilized in the treatment of a number of diseases, including cancer, endocrine disorders, dermatologic diseases, and metabolic syndrome.[47] RXRα is expressed in the epidermis, intestine, liver, and kidney, while RXRγ is found primarily in the brain and muscle cells. RXRβ is broadly expressed across cell types. RXR receptors can form heterodimers with a number of NRs and can also form homodimers, but the role of RXR-RXR homodimers in gene expression is not well understood. RXR facilitates the binding of heterodimer partners to response elements found in the promoter regions of target genes and is necessary for the dimer to initiate gene expression following ligand binding.[48] The specificity of the RXR heterodimer for a particular response element is dependent on the number of spacer BPs between response element half-sites. As examples, the RXRRAR heterodimer requires 5-BP spacing (DR5), while the RXRPPAR heterodimer requires a DR1 spacing. Flanking nucleotides adjacent to the response element can also enhance the selectivity of dimer binding. The activation of RXR heterodimers can be "permissive" or "nonpermissive," meaning that for certain heterodimer partners such as PPARs, activation of the dimer will occur with ligand binding to either the PPAR receptor or the RXR receptor or both. However, for nonpermissive heterodimers such as RAR and TR, ligand binding to the RXR receptor will not result in activation unless the partner is bound to an agonist as well. This phenomenon is referred to as subordination.

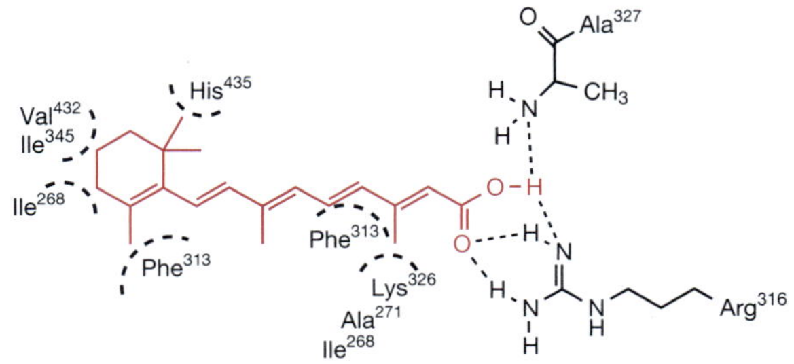

Figure 7.10 Crystal structure of the ligand-binding domain of the RXR receptor bound to 9-*cis*-retinoic acid.

Vitamin D Receptors

D vitamins include D_2, ergocalciferol, and D_3, cholecalciferol. Vitamin D is a fat-soluble vitamin with a steroid-like structure that, in addition to magnesium and phosphate, regulates blood calcium levels via facilitation of calcium absorption from the gastrointestinal tract and resorption of calcium from the bone. In addition to calcium transport, calcitriol (1,25-dihydroxycholecalciferol) is associated with a number of physiologic functions, including inhibition of the synthesis of parathyroid hormone,[49] regulation of keratinocyte differentiation, hair follicle cycling,[50] immune function,[51] cardiac function,[52] skeletal muscle,[53] breast development,[54] and lung development.[55]

Although D vitamins are constituents of the diet, a major source of the vitamin is via synthesis from 7-dehydrocholesterol in the skin following exposure to ultraviolet radiation. Vitamin D_3 is transported to the liver and metabolized to calcifediol and subsequently transported to the kidneys, where it is metabolized to the most metabolically active form, calcitriol. Calcitriol binds to the vitamin D receptor (VDR), triggering the transcription of target genes (Fig. 7.11).[56]

There are two isoforms of the receptor resulting from different transcription start sites. Individuals with the shorter isoform tend to have lower bone density than those with the longer isoform. As with other NRs, the DBD of the VDR is highly conserved with two zinc fingers: the N-terminal finger providing selectivity for binding to the vitamin D–receptor response element, and the C-terminal finger facilitating heterodimerization with RXR and other NR receptors. Although there are variations in conformation, the VDRE generally comprises two DR half-sites separated by three nucleotides. RXR binds to the upstream half-site and VDR

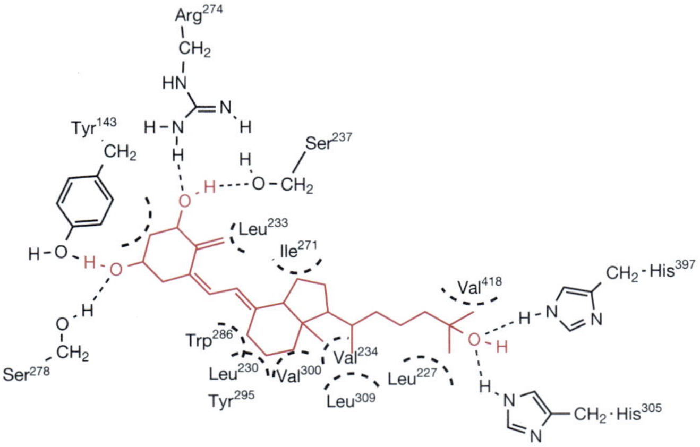

Figure 7.11 Crystal structure of the ligand-binding domain of the vitamin D receptor bound to vitamin D.

binds to the downstream site. The LBD, aside from providing surfaces for dimerization, contains AF-2, the ligand binding site for calcitriol and coactivators and corepressors.[57]

Orphan Receptors

Orphan receptors are proteins that bind to and activate DNA-response elements for which the endogenous ligand has yet to be discovered or are constitutively active. The following NRs are currently classified as orphan receptors:

Subfamily 0

DAX 1

DAX 1 receptors lack the DBD found on other NRs. It is involved in the development of hormone-releasing tissues, including the adrenal, pituitary, hypothalamic, and reproductive glands.[58]

The small heterodimer partner (SHP) plays a role in the regulation of glucose and cholesterol metabolism as well as innate immunity.[59]

Subfamily 3

Estrogen-Related Receptors

Estrogen-related receptors (ERRs) share sequence homology with ERs, but do not respond to ligands that bind to ERs. There are three subtypes of ERRs: α, β, and γ. ERRα is active without endogenous ligand binding, but activity is increased by cholesterol. ERRα plays a role in cellular metabolism,[60] and in animal models, it has been found to be a key mediator of statin and bisphosphonate actions in the bone, muscle, and macrophages.[61]

Subfamily 4

Neuron-Derived Orphan Receptor

The neuron-derived orphan receptor is involved in vascular smooth vessel function and has been shown in mouse models to enhance the effects of the hormone angiotensin II, resulting in increased inflammation.[62]

Subfamily 5

Steroidogenic Factor 1

Steroidogenic factor 1 (SF-1) is a transcription factor that plays a critical role in the regulation of steroid hormone biosynthesis. It is expressed in the adrenal gland, gonads, and hypothalamus, where it regulates the expression of key enzymes involved in steroidogenesis. SF-1 is essential for the development and function of these organs, and is required for the synthesis of all steroid hormones, including glucocorticoids, mineralocorticoids, and sex steroids. It interacts with other transcription factors and coregulators to activate or repress gene expression. Mutations in the SF-1 gene can lead to disorders of sex development and adrenal insufficiency.[63]

Subfamily 6

Germ Cell Nuclear Factor

Germ cell nuclear factor (GCNF) is a transcription factor that plays a crucial role in the development and maintenance of germ cells. It is expressed predominantly in germ cells, although it has also been found in other tissues. GCNF is involved in the regulation of gene expression during neurogenesis, spermatogenesis, and oogenesis, and is necessary for the survival and differentiation of germ cells. It is also involved in the maintenance of pluripotency in embryonic stem cells. GCNF interacts with a variety of other transcription factors and coregulators to control gene expression, and its activity is regulated by ligand binding and posttranslational modifications. Dysfunction or loss of GCNF can lead to infertility, abnormal embryonic development, and other reproductive disorders.[64]

REFERENCES

1. Aranda A, Pascual A. Nuclear hormone receptors and gene expression. *Physiol Rev.* 2001;81:1269-1304.
2. Rastinejad F. Structure and function of the steroid and nuclear receptor DNA binding domain. In: Freedman L, ed. *Molecular Biology of Steroid and Nuclear Hormone Receptors.* Birkhauser; 1998:105-131.
3. Freedman LP. Anatomy of the steroid receptor zinc finger region. *Endocr Rev.* 1992;13(2):129-145.
4. Wurtz JM, Bourguet W, Renaud JP, et al. A canonical structure for the ligand-binding domain of nuclear receptors. *Nat Struct Biol.* 1996;3:87-94.
5. Nagy L, Schwabe JW. Mechanism of the nuclear receptor molecular switch. *Trends Biochem Sci.* 2004;29:317-324.
6. Brozowski AM, Pike AC, Dauter Z, et al. Molecular basis of agonism and antagonism in the oestrogen receptor. *Nature.* 1997;389:753-758.
7. Harrington R, Sheng S, Barnett DH. Activities of estrogen receptor alpha- and beta-selective ligands at diverse estrogen responsive gene sites mediating transactivation or transrepression. *Mol Cell Endocrinol.* 2013;206(1-2):13-22.
8. Graham JD, Clarke CL. Physiological action of progesterone in target tissues. *Endocr Rev.* 1997;18:502-519.
9. Sartorius CA, Melville MY, Hovland AR, et al. A third transactivation function (AF3) of human progesterone receptors located in the unique N-terminal segment of the B-isoform. *Mol Endocrinol.* 1994;8:1347-1360.
10. Mote PA, Gompel A, Howe C, et al. Progesterone receptor A predominance is a discriminator of benefit from endocrine therapy in the ATAC trial. *Breast Cancer Res Treat.* 2015;151(2):309-318.
11. Williams SP, Sigler PB. Atomic structure of progesterone complexed with its receptor. *Nature.* 1998;393:392-396.
12. Singhal H, Greene ME, Zarnke AL, et al. Progesterone receptor isoforms, agonists, and antagonists differentially reprogram estrogen signaling. *Oncotarget.* 2018;9(4):4282-4300.
13. Chlebowski RT, Anderson GL, Gass M, et al. Estrogen plus progestin and breast cancer incidence and mortality in postmenopausal women. *JAMA.* 2010;304:1684-1692.
14. Mohammed H, Russell IA, Stark R, et al. Progesterone receptor modulates ERα action in breast cancer. *Nature.* 2015;523:313-317.
15. MacLean HE, Chu S, Warne GL, et al. Related individuals with different androgen receptor gene deletions. *J Clin Invest.* 1993;91:1123-1128.
16. Askew EB, Gampe RT, Stanley TB, et al. Modulation of androgen receptor activation function 2 by testosterone and dihydrotestosterone. *J Biol Chem.* 2007;282:25801-25816.

17. Joseph JD, Lu N, Qian J, et al. A clinically relevant androgen receptor mutation confers resistance to second-generation antiandrogens enzalutamide and ARN-509. *Cancer Discov*. 2013;3(9):1020-1029.
18. Rhen T, Cidlowski JA. Antiinflammatory action of glucocorticoids—New mechanisms for old drugs. *N Engl J Med*. 2005;353(16):1711-1723.
19. Grad I, Picard D. The glucocorticoid responses are shaped by molecular chaperones. *Mol Cell Endocrinol*. 2007;275(1-2):2-12.
20. Uhlenhaut NH, Barish GD, Yu RT, et al. Insights into negative regulation by the glucocorticoid receptor from genome-wide profiling of inflammatory cistromes. *Mol Cell*. 2013;49(1):158-171.
21. Reddy TE, Gertz J, Crawford GE, et al. The hypersensitive glucocorticoid response specifically regulates period 1 and expression of circadian genes. *Mol Cell Biol*. 2012;32(18):3756-3767.
22. Kelly A, Bowen H, Jee YK, et al. The glucocorticoid receptor beta isoform can mediate transcriptional repression by recruiting histone deacetylases. *J Allergy Clin Immunol*. 2008;121(1):203-208.
23. He Y, Yi W, Suino-Powell KM, et al. Crystal structure of cortisol-bound glucocorticoid receptor ligand binding domain. *Cell Res*. 2014;24:713-726.
24. Surjit M, Ganti KP, Mukherji A, et al. Widespread negative response elements mediate direct repression by agonist-liganded glucocorticoid receptor. *Cell*. 2011;145(2):224-241.
25. Nakamura Y, Suzuki S, Suzuki T, et al. MDM2: a novel mineralocorticoid-responsive gene involved in aldosterone-induced human vascular structural remodeling. *Am J Pathol*. 2006;169:362-371.
26. Pascual-Le Tallec L, Kirsh LMC, Lecomte MC, et al. Protein inhibitor of activated signal transducer and activator of transcription 1 interacts with the N-terminal domain of mineralocorticoid receptor and represses its transcriptional activity: implication of small ubiquitin-related modifier 1 modification. *Mol Endocrinol*. 2003;17:2529-2542.
27. Rupprecht R, Arriza JL, Spengler D, et al. Transactivation and synergistic properties of the mineralocorticoid receptor relationship to the glucocorticoid receptor. *Mol Endocrinol*. 1993;7:597-603.
28. Bledsoe RK, Madauss KP, Holt JA, et al. Mineralocorticoid receptor with bound aldosterone. *J Biol Chem*. 2005;280:31283-31293.
29. Lazar MA. Thyroid hormone receptors: multiple forms, multiple possibilities. *Endocr Rev*. 1993;14:184-193.
30. Nascimento AS, Dias SMG, Nunes FM, et al. Structural rearrangements in the thyroid hormone receptor hinge domain and their putative role in receptor function. *J Mol Biol*. 2006;360:586-598.
31. Brent GA, Williams GR, Harney JW, et al. Capacity for cooperative binding of thyroid hormone (T_3) receptor dimers defines wild type T_3 response elements. *Mol Endocrinol*. 1992;6(4):502-514.
32. Mandard S, Muller M, Kersten S. Peroxisome proliferator-activated receptor alpha target genes. *Cell Mol Life Sci*. 2004;61:393-416.
33. Chawla A, Schwarz EJ, Dimaculangan DD, et al. Peroxisome proliferator-activated receptor (PPAR) gamma: adipose-predominant expression and induction early in adipocyte differentiation. *Endocrinology*. 1994;135:798-800.
34. Reddy JK, Hashimoto T. Peroxisomal beta-oxidation and peroxisome proliferator-activated receptor alpha: an adaptive metabolic system. *Annu Rev Nutr*. 2001;21:193-230.
35. Goya K, Sumitani S, Xu X, et al. Peroxisome proliferator-activated receptor agonists increase nitric oxide synthase expression in vascular endothelial cells. *Arterioscler Thromb Vasc Biol*. 2004;24:658-663.
36. Marx N, Duez H, Fruchart JC, et al. Peroxisome proliferator-activated receptors and atherogenesis: regulators of gene expression in vascular cells. *Circ Res*. 2004;94:1168-1178.
37. Tan NS, Michalik L, Desvergne B, et al. Peroxisome proliferator activated receptor-beta as a target for wound healing drugs. *Expert Opin Ther Targets*. 2004;8:39.
38. Staels B, Fruchart JC. Therapeutic roles of peroxisome proliferator activated receptor agonists. *Diabetes*. 2005;54:2460-2470.
39. Petkovich M, Brand NJ, Krust A, et al. A human retinoic acid receptor which belongs to the family of nuclear receptors. *Nature*. 1987;330:444-450.
40. Renaud JP, Rochel N, Ruff M. Crystal structure of the RAR-gamma ligand-binding domain bound to all-trans retinoic acid. *Nature*. 1995;378:681-689.
41. Bastien J, Rochette-Egly C. Nuclear retinoid receptors and the transcription of retinoid-target genes. *Gene*. 2004;328:1-16.
42. Smith MA, Parkinson DR, Cheson BD, et al. Retinoids in cancer therapy. *J Clin Oncol*. 1992;10(5):839-864.
43. Heller EH, Siffman NJ. Synthetic retinods in dermatology. *Can Med Assoc J*. 1985;132(10):1129-1136.
44. Egea PF, Mitschler A, Rochel N. Crystal structure of the human RXR alpha ligand binding domain bound to 9-cis-retinoic acid. *EMBO J*. 2000;19:2592-2601.
45. Mangelsdorf DJ, Borgmeyer U, Heyman RA, et al. Characterization of three RXR genes that mediate the action of 9-cis retinoic acid. *Genes Dev*. 1992;6:329-344.
46. Fan Y-Y, Spencer TE, Wang N, et al. Chemopreventive n-3 fatty acids activate RXRα in colonocytes. *Carcinogenesis*. 2003;24:1541-1548.
47. Dawson MI. Synthetic retinoids and their nuclear receptors. *Curr Med Chem Anticancer Agents*. 2004;4:199-230.
48. Westin S, Kurokawa R, Nolte RT, et al. Interactions controlling the assembly of nuclear-receptor heterodimers and co-activators. *Nature*. 1998;395:199-202.
49. Cantley LK, Russell J, Lettieri D, et al. 1,25-Dihydroxyvitamin D3 suppresses parathyroid hormone secretion from bovine parathyroid cells in tissue culture. *Endocrinology*. 1985;117:2114-2119.
50. Hsieh JC, Sisk JM, Jurutka PW, et al. Physical and functional interaction between the vitamin D receptor and hairless corepressor, two proteins required for hair cycling. *J Biol Chem*. 2003;278:38665-38674.
51. van Etten E, Mathieu C. Immunoregulation by 1,25-dihydroxyvitamin D3: basic concepts. *J Steroid Biochem Mol Biol*. 2005;97:93-101.
52. Weishaar RE, Kim SN, Saunders DE, et al. Involvement of vitamin D3 with cardiovascular function. III. Effects on physical and morphological properties. *Am J Physiol*. 1990;258:E134-E142.
53. Girgis CM, Clifton-Bligh RJ, Hamrick MW, et al. The roles of vitamin D in skeletal muscle: form, function, and metabolism. *Endocr Rev*. 2013;34:33-83.
54. Lopes N, Paredes J, Costa JL, et al. Vitamin D and the mammary gland: a review on its role in normal development and breast cancer. *Breast Cancer Res*. 2012;14:211.
55. Nguyen TM, Guillozo H, Marin L, et al. 1,25-dihydroxyvitamin D3 receptors in rat lung during the perinatal period: regulation and immunohistochemical localization. *Endocrinology*. 1990;127(4):1755-1762.
56. Rochel N, Wurtz JM, Mitschler A, et al. The crystal structure of the nuclear receptor for vitamin D bound to its natural ligand. *Mol Cell*. 2000;5(1):173-179.
57. Prufer K, Racz A, Lin GC, et al. Dimerization with retinoid X receptors promotes nuclear localization and subnuclear targeting of vitamin D receptors. *J Biol Chem*. 2000;275:41114-41123.
58. Niakan KK, McCabe ER. DAX1 origin, function, and novel role. *Mol Genet Metab*. 2006;86(1-2):70-83.
59. Yuk J-M, Jin HS, Jo E-K. Small heterodimer partner and innate immune regulation. *Endocrinol Metab (Seoul)*. 2016;31(1):17-24.
60. Tripathi M, Yen PM, Singh BK. Estrogen-related receptor alpha: an under-appreciated potential target for the treatment of metabolic diseases. *Int J Mol Sci*. 2020;21(5):1645.
61. Zuo H, Wan Y. Nuclear receptors in skeletal homeostasis. *Curr Top Dev Biol*. 2017;125:71-107.
62. Cañes L, Martí-Pàmies I, Ballester-Servera C, et al. High NOR-1 (neuron-derived orphan receptor 1) expression strengthens the vascular wall response to angiotensin II leading to aneurysm formation in mice. *Hypertension*. 2021;77(2):557-570.
63. Parker KL, Schimmer BP. Steroidogenic factor 1: a key determinant of endocrine development and function. *Endocr Rev*. 1997;18(3):361-377.
64. Greschik H, Schüle R. Germ cell nuclear factor: an orphan receptor with unexpected properties. *J Mol Med*. 1998;76(12):800-810.

CHAPTER

8

Ion Channel Receptors

Swati Betharia

Drugs covered in this chapter:

- Acetylcholine
- Allopregnanolone
- Allotetrahydrodeoxycorticosterone
- Amantadine
- Anandamide
- 2-Arachidonylglycerol
- Aspartate
- Atracurium
- Bicuculline
- Brexanolone
- Bupropion
- Carbachol
- Chloroquine
- Clozapine
- Curare
- Cyclothiazide
- Cytisine
- D-(-)-2-Amino-5-phosphonopentanoic acid (D-AP5)
- Dextromethorphan
- Dextrorphan
- Diazepam
- Diltiazem
- 1,1-Dimethyl-4-phenylpiperazinium iodide (DMPP)
- Dizocilpine
- Domoic Acid
- D-Serine
- Δ9-Tetrahydrocannabinol (THC)
- Enflurane
- Etomidate
- Felbamate
- Flumazenil
- Gaboxadol
- γ-Aminobutyric acid (GABA)
- Glutamate
- Glycine
- Granisetron
- Hexamethonium
- Homoquinolinic acid
- Indiplon
- Irinotecan
- Isoguvacine
- Ivermectin
- Ketamine
- Lidocaine
- Mecamylamine
- Memantine
- Methacholine
- Methyl 4-ethyl-6,7-dimethoxy-9*H*-pyrido[5,4-b]indole-3-carboxylate (DMCM)
- MK-801
- Muscimol
- Nicotine
- *N*-Methyl-D-aspartate (NMDA)
- Ondansetron
- Palonosetron
- Pancuronium
- Perampanel
- Phaclofen
- Phencyclidine
- Picrotoxin
- Piracetam
- Pregnanolone
- Pregnenolone sulfate
- Propofol
- Quinine
- Ramosetron
- (*R*)-HA-966 (*R*-(+)-3-Amino-1-hydroxypyrrolidin-2-one)
- Ro19-4603
- Serotonin
- Spermidine
- Spermine
- Strychnine
- Succinylcholine
- (1,2,5,6-Tetrahydropyridin-4-yl)-methylphosphinic acid (TPMPA)
- Tetramethylammonium (TMA)
- Trimethaphan
- Tubocurarine
- Varenicline
- Vecuronium
- Zaleplon
- Zopiclone
- Zolpidem
- Zuranolone

Abbreviations

AMPA α-amino-3-hydroxy-5-methyl-4-isoxazole propionic acid
ATP adenosine triphosphate
cAMP cyclic adenosine monophosphate
CNS central nervous system
D-AP5 D-(-)-2-amino-5-phosphonopentanoic acid
DMPP 1,1-dimethyl-4-phenylpiperazinium iodide
EAA excitatory amino acid
FDA Food and Drug Administration`
GABA γ-aminobutyric acid
GABAA γ-aminobutyric acid receptor family A
GABAB γ-aminobutyric acid receptor family B

Abbreviations—continued

GABAC γ-aminobutyric acid receptor family C
GLU glutamate
GluR glutamate receptor
GLY glycine
GPCR G protein–coupled receptors
5-HT 5-hydroxytryptamine
5-HTRs 5-HT receptors
5-HT$_3$R 5-HT receptor subtype 3
HVA high-voltage activated
IAA inhibitory amino acid
IP$_3$ inositol-1,4,5-triphosphate
LGIC ligand-gated ion channel
LTD long-term depression
LTP long-term potentiation
LVA low-voltage activated
mAChR muscarinic acetylcholine receptor
mRNA messenger ribonucleic acid
nAChR nicotinic acetylcholine receptor
NMDA *N*-methyl-D-aspartate
NM neuromuscular
NN neuronal
NSF *N*-ethylmaleimide-sensitive fusion protein
PCP phencyclidine
PICK protein interacting with C kinase
PLC phospholipase C
TMA tetramethylammonium
TM transmembrane
ZAC zinc-activated channel

Introduction

Signal transduction can occur through various receptor types present on the cellular transmembrane surface. These include ligand-gated ion channels (LGICs), G protein–coupled receptors (GPCRs), and catalytic receptors or enzyme-coupled receptors. Voltage-gated ion channels, while also found on the transmembrane surface, are not categorized as receptors in the classical sense, as they do not require ligand binding for activation. A fourth receptor type, known as nuclear receptors, is located intracellularly and is not found on the transmembrane surface.

Ligand-Gated Ion Channels

The most rapid cellular responses to receptor activation are mediated via LGICs. The majority of LGICs are categorized into the Cys-loop family of pentameric receptors. These plasma membrane-spanning proteins are composed of five peptide subunits with a central ion-conducting pore. Each subunit is comprised of an extracellular ligand-binding N-terminus, four transmembrane loops (TM1-TM4), a large cytoplasmic domain, and an extracellular C-terminus. A characteristic Cys-loop is formed in the N-terminus when the two Cys terminal ends of an approximately 13 amino acid chain form an internal disulfide bond.[1] The nicotinic acetylcholine receptor (nAChR), serotonin (5-hydroxytryptamine, 5-HT) receptor 5-HT$_3$R, γ-aminobutyric acid (GABA) receptor, glycine (GLY) receptor, and the zinc-activated channel (ZAC) all belong to the Cys-loop family of receptors. They share a similar structural conformation and function, except for the specificity of the ligand-binding site and selectivity of the channel for particular ions. Exceptions in the LGICs are the glutamate receptor (GluR) family and the adenosine triphosphate (ATP)-gated purinergic receptors (P2X), which do not belong to the Cys-loop pentameric receptor family and are tetrameric and trimeric proteins, respectively.

The binding of a ligand (neurotransmitter, exogenous molecule, or allosteric modulator) results in a conformational change in the receptor protein structure, allowing for the central pore to conduct specific ions down their electrochemical gradient. The primary reason for the rapidity (milliseconds) of the cellular response with LGICs is that the transduction of the signal requires the activation of a single molecule. Therefore, this transduction mechanism is especially suited for physiologic processes needing an immediate response, such as the stimulation of nerves and muscle fibers. A survey of LGIC is provided in Table 8.1, and the structures of their endogenous ligands are shown in Figure 8.1.

Nicotinic Acetylcholine Receptors

Structure and Function

The nAChRs are perhaps the best characterized LGICs. These receptors are found at the skeletal neuromuscular junction, adrenal medulla, and autonomic ganglia. They are composed of five distinct subunits: two α and, depending on the receptor subtype, various combinations of additional α, β, γ, and δ subunits. A total of 17 subunit types have been identified to date (α1-α10, β1-β4, γ, δ, and ε). The five subunits of each nAChR protein are arranged around a central pore that serves as the ion channel.[2] Based on molecular modeling of the deduced primary structure of the individual subunits, it has been proposed that each subunit (α, β, γ [or ε], and δ) possesses a hydrophilic extracellular N-terminus, a hydrophilic extracellular C-terminus, and four α-helical hydrophobic transmembrane domains (TM1-TM4) (Fig. 8.2). A pentameric arrangement of these five amphipathic subunits makes up the walls of the ion channel.[3] Two binding sites for the endogenous ligand acetylcholine exist on the extracellular domain of the nAChR molecule. In Figure 8.2, one binding site is located on each α subunit at the αγ and αδ interfaces. The binding sites show a positive cooperativity, meaning that ligand binding to one site facilitates binding to the other. The ability of the sites to communicate exists even though the binding sites are not adjacent to each other in the pentameric receptor.[4] Ligand binding induces a conformational change in the receptor, opening the ion channel and allowing the passage of sodium (Na^+) and potassium (K^+) ions through the center of the protein. The result is depolarization of the surrounding plasma membrane.

Table 8.1 Survey of Ligand-Gated Receptor Subtypes

Receptor Class	Subtype	Selective Agonist	Antagonist	Effector
Nicotinic receptors	N_{muscle}	?	Decamethonium	↑Na^+/Ca^{2+}
	$N_{neuronal}$	?	Hexamethonium	↑Na^+/Ca^{2+}
Serotonin receptors (5-HT)	$5\text{-}HT_3$	m-Chlorophenylbiguanide hydrochloride	Ondansetron	↑$Na^+/K^+/Ca^{2+}$
GABA receptors	$GABA_A$	Muscimol	Bicuculline	↑Cl^-
	$GABA_c$	*cis*-4-Aminocrotonic acid	TPMPA	↑Cl^-
Glycine (GLY) receptors		Glycine	Strychnine	↑Cl^-
Zinc-activated channel (ZAC)		Copper ions	Tubocurarine	↑$Na^+/K^+/Cs^+$
Excitatory amino acid receptors	NMDA	NMDA	D-AP5	↓Na^+/Ca^{2+}
	AMPA	AMPA	CNQX	↑Na^+
	Kainate	Kainate	CNQX	↑Na^+/K^+
P2X receptors	$P2X_1$-$P2X_7$	ATP	TNP-ATP triethylammonium salt	↑$Na^+/K^+/Ca^{2+}$

?, no known selective compounds available; cloned, receptor subtype has been cloned and the amino acid structure is known.
5-HT, 5-hydroxytryptamine, serotonin; AMPA, D, L-α-amino-3-hydroxy-5-methyl-4-isoxalone propionic acid; ATP, adenosine triphosphate; CNQX, 6-cyano-7-nitroquinoxaline-2, 3-dione; D-AP5, D-amino-5-phosphonopentanoate; GABA, γ-aminobutyric acid; NMDA, *N*-methyl-D-aspartate; TPMPA, [1,2,5, 6-tetrahydropyridin-4-yl]-methylphosphinic acid.

The multiplicity of nAChRs is based on different structural requirements for agonists and antagonists acting at the autonomic ganglia and the skeletal neuromuscular junction and is supported by research in molecular biology.[5] The two types of nAChRs, namely ganglionic neuronal (NN) and neuromuscular (somatic muscle) (NM), are both classified as LGICs. The former increases neuronal firing in autonomic ganglia and causes the release of stored catecholamines from the adrenal medulla. The latter, located in skeletal neuromuscular junctions, facilitates skeletal muscle contraction. Apart from these peripheral locations, nAChRs are also found centrally in the pre- and postsynaptic junctions, where they control neurotransmitter release. Both peripheral and central nAChRs are excitatory in nature and increase permeability for Na^+ and K^+ ions.[6] The diversity of the subunits and the pentameric structure within these receptors suggest that a large number of nAChR subtypes can exist.[3]

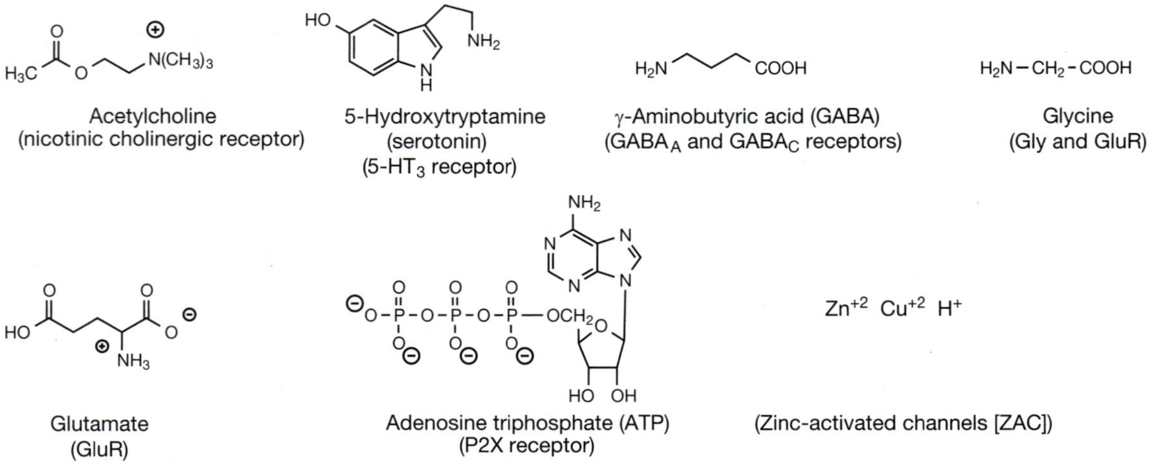

Figure 8.1 Natural ligands of ion channel receptors. Acetylcholine for nicotinic cholinergic receptors, 5-hydroxytryptamine (serotonin) for $5\text{-}HT_3$ receptors, γ-amino butyric acid (GABA) for $GABA_A$ and $GABA_C$ receptors, GLY for glycine and GluR, GLU for GluR, and ATP for P2X receptors. Zn^{2+}, Cu^{2+}, and H^+ serve as natural ligands for the zinc-activated channels.

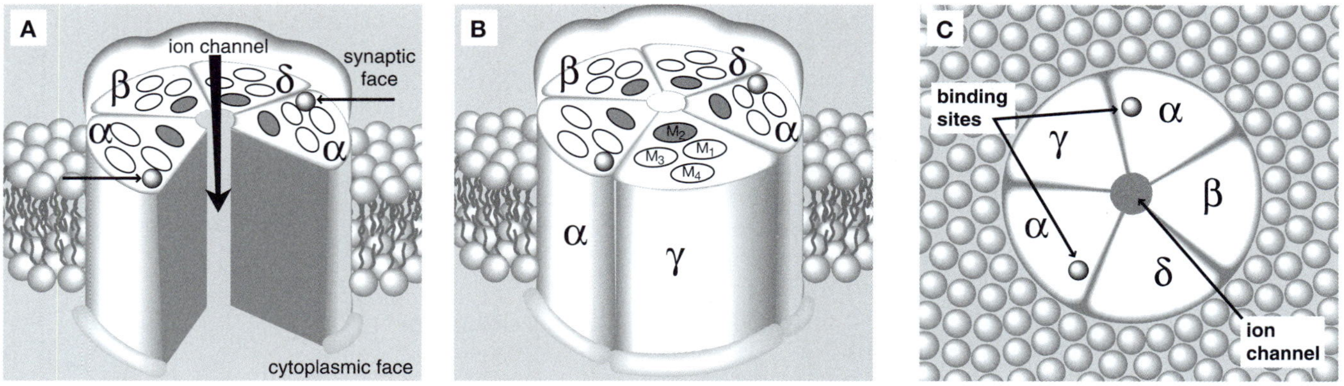

Figure 8.2 Nicotinic acetylcholine receptor (nAChR): A. Longitudinal view (γ subunit removed) showing the internal ion channel. Acetylcholine binding sites on the α subunits are indicated by the arrows. These are located at the αγ and αδ interfaces. B. Each of the five transmembrane subunits (α, α, β, δ, and γ) is composed of four hydrophobic membrane-spanning segments (M_1-M_4). C. Top view of the nAChR showing the subunits surrounding the ion channel.

Nicotinic Receptor Agonists

The nAChRs have been the focus of intensive research, even though the majority of clinically effective cholinergic medicinal agents are either muscarinic agonists or antagonists. The best-known nicotinic agonist is nicotine, which is an alkaloid obtained from the *Nicotiana tabacum* plant, with minimal effects on the cholinergic muscarinic receptors (mAChRs). Other nAChR agonists such as acetylcholine, carbachol, and methacholine are nonselective and also activate the muscarinic receptors. Full (nicotine) and partial (varenicline and cytisine) agonists for the nAChRs decrease nicotine craving and have been used in the treatment of tobacco addiction.[7]

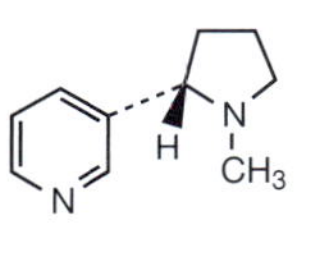

S(-)-Nicotine

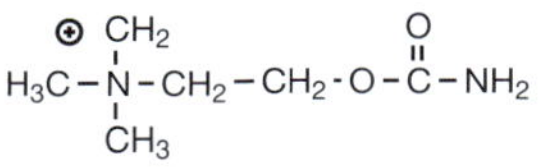

Carbachol

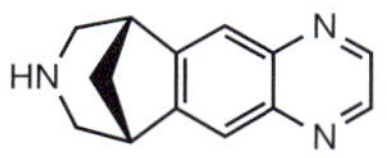

Varenicline

Nicotinic Receptor Antagonists

Nicotinic antagonists are chemical compounds that bind to nAChRs but have no intrinsic activity. All therapeutically useful nicotinic antagonists are competitive antagonists; in other words, their effects are reversible with acetylcholine. There are two subclasses of nicotinic antagonists—skeletal neuromuscular-blocking agents and ganglionic blocking agents—classified according to the two populations of nAChRs, N_M and N_N, respectively.

Neuromuscular Nicotinic Receptor–Blocking Agents. In terms of the historical perspective, tubocurarine, the first known neuromuscular-blocking drug, was as important to the understanding of nicotinic antagonists as atropine was to that of muscarinic antagonists. The neuromuscular-blocking effects of extracts of curare were first reported as early as 1510, when explorers of the Amazon River region of South America found natives using these plant extracts as arrow poisons. Early research with these crude plant extracts indicated that the active components caused muscle paralysis by effects on either the nerve or the muscle (remember that the concept of neurochemical transmission was not introduced until the late 19th century). In 1856, however, Bernard described the results of his experiments, which demonstrated unequivocally that curare extracts prevented skeletal muscle contractions by an effect at the neuromuscular junction, rather than the nerve innervating the muscle or the muscle itself.[8]

Much of the early literature concerning the effects of curare is confusing and difficult to interpret. This is not at all surprising considering that this research was performed using crude extracts, many of which came from different plants. It was not until the late 1800s that scientists recognized that curare extracts contained quaternary ammonium salts. This knowledge prompted the use of other quaternary ammonium compounds to explore the neuromuscular junction. In the meantime, curare extracts continued to be used to block the effects of nicotine and acetylcholine at skeletal neuromuscular junctions and to explore the nAChRs.

In 1935, King isolated a pure alkaloid, which he named D-tubocurarine, from a tube curare of unknown botanical origin.[9] The word "tube" refers to the container in which the South American natives transported their plant extract. It was almost 10 years later that the botanical source for D-tubocurarine was clearly identified as *Chondrodendron tomentosum*. The structure that King assigned to tubocurarine possessed two nitrogen atoms, both of which were quaternary ammonium salts (ie, a bis-quaternary ammonium compound). It was not until 1970 that the correct structure was reported by Everett et al.[10] The correct structure has only one quaternary ammonium nitrogen; the other nitrogen is a tertiary amine salt. Nevertheless, the incorrect structure of tubocurarine served as the model for the synthesis of all the neuromuscular-blocking agents in use today. These compounds have been of immense therapeutic value for surgical and orthopedic procedures and have been essential to research that led to the isolation and purification of nAChRs.

By the 1980s, important developments in the characterization of the nAChR resulted from research on two unlikely animal sources. The finding that the electric eel, *Torpedo californica*, contained a rich source of nAChR that could be isolated allowed for the purification of large quantities of the receptor for study.[11] Additionally, it was found that the venom from a snake, the Southeast Asian banded krait, *Bungarus multicinctus*, contained the 74-amino acid peptide, α-bungarotoxin, which binds competitively and almost irreversibly with very high affinity to the two α7 subunits of the nAChR to prevent channel opening. When exposed to α-bungarotoxin, the nAChRs in the skeletal muscles responsible for normal respiration are antagonized, leading to respiratory paralysis and, if not treated, death.[12] These two findings were essential to our understanding of the structure and binding requirements of the nAChR.

The potential therapeutic benefits of the neuromuscular-blocking effects of tubocurarine, as well as the difficulty in obtaining pure samples of the alkaloid, encouraged medicinal chemists to design structurally related compounds possessing nicotinic antagonist activity. Using the incorrectly assigned bis-quaternary ammonium structure of tubocurarine as reported by King[9] as a guide, a large number of compounds were synthesized and evaluated. It became apparent that a bis-quaternary ammonium compound having two quaternary ammonium salts separated by 10 to 12 carbon atoms (similar to the distance between the nitrogen atoms in tubocurarine) was a requirement for neuromuscular-blocking activity. The rationale for this structural requirement was that, in contrast to muscarinic acetylcholine receptor, nAChRs possessed two anionic-binding sites, both of which had to be occupied for a neuromuscular-blocking effect. It is important to observe that the current transmembrane model for the nAChR protein has two anionic sites in the extracellular domain.

Some of the new bis-quaternary ammonium agents such as the dicholine ester succinylcholine, produced depolarization of the postjunctional membrane at the neuromuscular junction before causing blockade; other compounds, such as tubocurarine, did not produce this initial depolarization. Thus, the structural features of the remainder of the molecule determined whether the nicotinic antagonist was a depolarizing or a nondepolarizing neuromuscular blocker.

Neuromuscular-blocking agents are used primarily as adjuncts to general anesthesia. They produce skeletal muscle relaxation that facilitates operative procedures such as abdominal surgery. Furthermore, they reduce the depth requirement for general anesthetics; this decreases the overall risk of a surgical procedure and shortens the postanesthetic recovery time. Muscles producing rapid movements are the first to be affected by neuromuscular-blocking agents. These include muscles of the face, eyes, and neck. Muscles of the limbs, chest, and abdomen are affected next, with the diaphragm (respiration) being affected last. Recovery generally is in the reverse order. Neuromuscular-blocking agents have also been used in the correction of dislocations and the realignment of fractures. Short-acting neuromuscular-blocking agents, such as the depolarizing blocker succinylcholine, are routinely used to assist in tracheal intubation. Other neuromuscular agents that act by a nondepolarizing mechanism (similar to tubocurarine) include pancuronium and vecuronium, which structurally are aminosteroids, and atracurium, a benzylisoquinoline.[13]

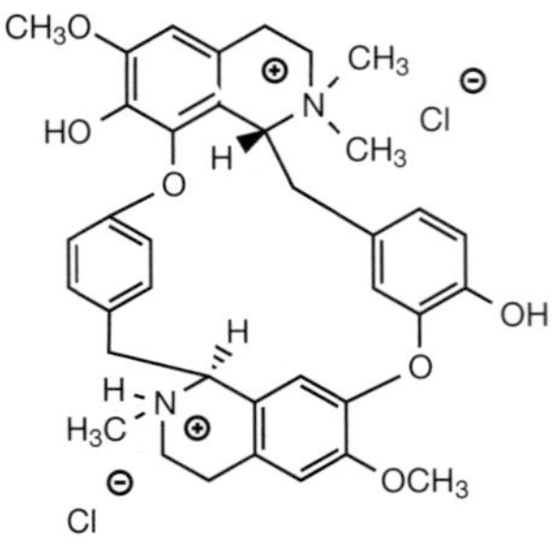

d-Tubocurarine chloride

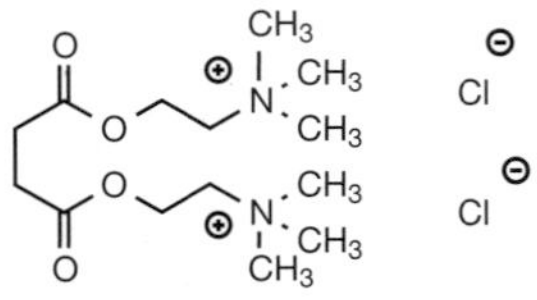

Succinylcholine chloride

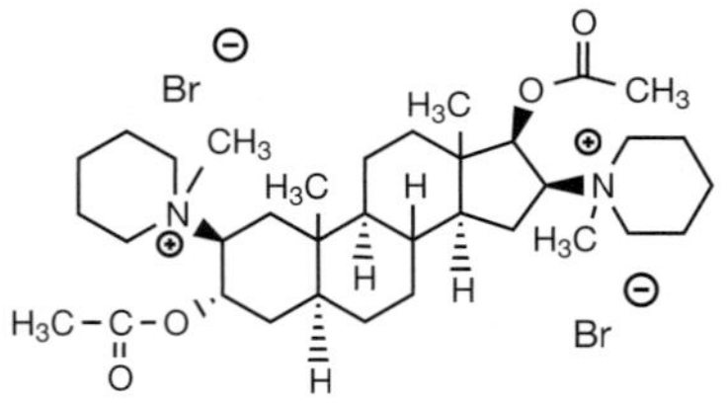

Pancuronium bromide

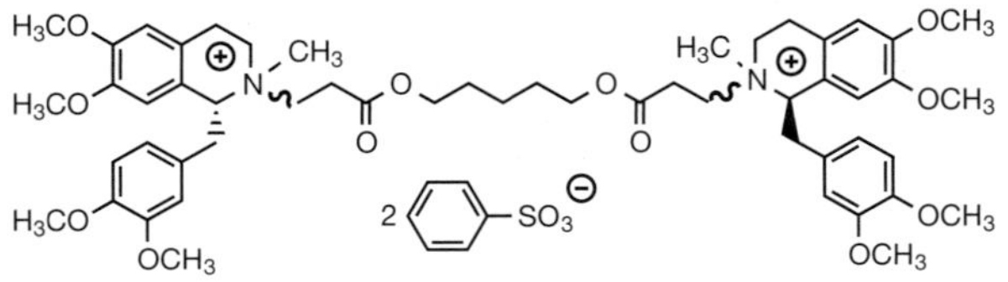

Atracurium besylate

Adverse reactions to most, but not all, of the neuromuscular-blocking agents can include hypotension, bronchospasm, and cardiac disturbances. The depolarizing agents also cause an initial muscle fasciculation before relaxation. Many of these agents cause release of histamine and subsequent cutaneous (flushing, erythema, urticaria, and pruritus), pulmonary (bronchospasm and wheezing), and cardiovascular (hypotension) effects. For more information on neuromuscular blockers, refer to Chapters 10 and 14.

Neuronal (Ganglionic) Nicotinic–Receptor Agonists and Antagonists. While the blockade of the neuromuscular nAChRs was observed to require a separation of nitrogen atoms by 10 to 12 carbons, the blockade of the neuronal nAChRs in the ganglia can be observed with a separation of six carbon atoms, indicating the differences in antagonist binding requirements. Thus, hexamethonium is rather selective for the neuronal nAChR with little activity at the neuromuscular nAChRs or the mAChRs. Other so-called ganglionic antagonists include trimethaphan and mecamylamine.

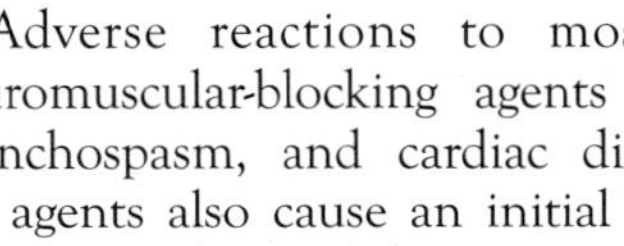

Hexamethonium bromide

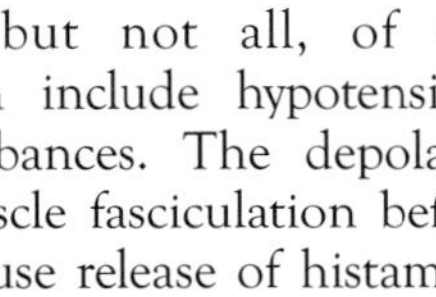

Mecamylamine

While nicotine initially acts as an agonist and stimulates the ganglionic nAChRs, which is followed by blockade, there are agonists at this site that do not also block the receptor.

These include tetramethylammonium (TMA) and 1,1-dimethyl-4-phenylpiperazinium iodide (DMPP).

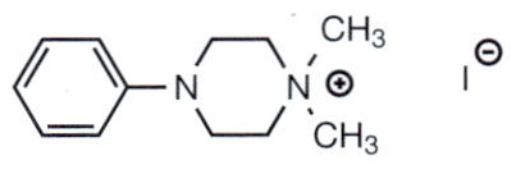

1,1-Dimethyl-4-phenylpiperazinium iodide (DMPP)

Serotonergic Receptors

Seven classes of 5-HT receptors (5-HTRs) have been identified, of which only the $5\text{-}HT_3R$ is an excitatory, cationic LGIC belonging to the Cys-loop receptor family. Five subunit types, namely $5\text{-}HT_3A$ through $5\text{-}HT_3E$, have been cloned in humans. However, the functional 5-HTRs are only found as homopentamers of subunit A, depicted as $(5\text{-}HT_3A)_5$, or as heteropentamers of subunits A and B, depicted as $5\text{-}HT_3AB$, implying that subunit A is required to constitute functional receptors.[14] Each subunit is composed of extracellular, transcellular, and intracellular domains. Binding of the natural ligand 5-HT at the orthosteric binding site (extracellular domain) results in the opening of the ion pore permeable to Na^+, K^+, and calcium (Ca^{2+}) ions. This cationic movement results in net membrane depolarization, and in the case of presynaptic $5\text{-}HT_3R$ present on GABAergic or glutamatergic neurons, the synaptic release of corresponding neurotransmitters.[15]

$5\text{-}HT_3Rs$ are located centrally in regions of the brain stem, forebrain, olfactory tract, and prefrontal cortex.[16] Activation of these receptors located in the vomiting center leads to emesis. Varenicline, a partial agonist at nAChRs noted earlier, is also a partial agonist at the $5\text{-}HT_3R$, which could explain the nausea associated with its use as a smoking cessation therapy.[14] Competitive antagonists, which also bind to the extracellular receptor domain, have therefore been used as antiemetic agents in vomiting associated with chemotherapy and pregnancy.[17] Examples include ondansetron, granisetron, ramosetron, and palonosetron ("setron" family). Some additional compounds that have also been found to have a competitive antagonistic effect at the $5\text{-}HT_3R$ include chloroquine (antimalarial), clozapine (antipsychotic), irinotecan (anticancer), and tubocurarine (neuromuscular blocker).

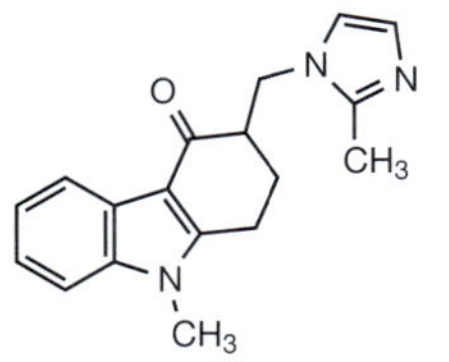

Ondansetron

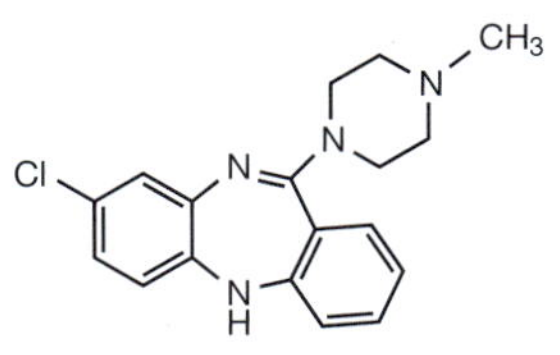

Clozapine

Noncompetitive antagonists that bind to the TM domain as opposed to the 5-HT binding extracellular domain of the receptor have also been identified. These vary in their selectivity for the homopentamer and heteropentamer $5\text{-}HT_3Rs$, based on the differences in the transmembrane amino acid residues in these two receptor subtypes. Examples of noncompetitive antagonists include picrotoxin ($GABA_A$ receptor antagonist), diltiazem (calcium-channel blocker), quinine (antimalarial), and Δ^9-tetrahydrocannabinol (cannabinoid). $5\text{-}HT_3$ receptor antagonists have been explored for their use in the treatment of irritable bowel syndrome, schizophrenia, anxiety, substance abuse, pain, and inflammation. Additionally, general anesthetics (eg, ethanol, chloroform) can bind to distinct binding sites on the extracellular or TM domains and serve as positive allosteric modulators.[14]

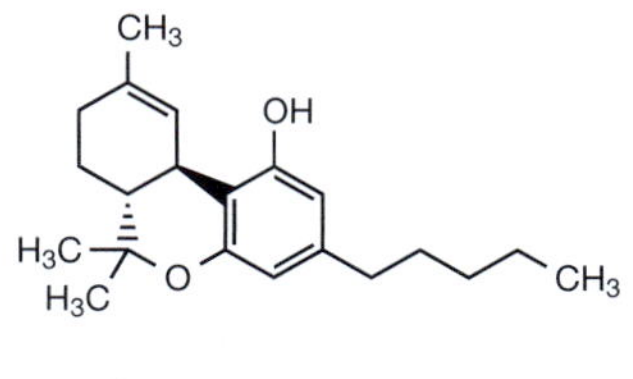

Δ^9-tetrahydrocannabinol (Δ^9-THC)

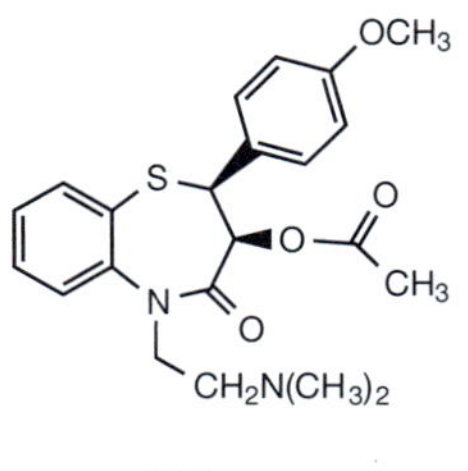

Diltiazem

GABA Receptors

The initial observations that application of GABA was capable of hyperpolarizing neurons, coupled with the lack of activity of structurally related amino acids and other compounds, suggested that a specific receptor likely mediated this response. There have been at least three different families of GABA receptors identified to date. These are referred to as $GABA_A$, $GABA_B$, and $GABA_C$. While $GABA_A$ and $GABA_C$ are LGICs, $GABA_B$ belongs to the GPCR family of receptors.

$GABA_A$ Receptors

The $GABA_A$ receptor was the first identified and found to be an LGIC that, when activated, allows for the entry of chloride ion (Cl^-) into the cell, thereby hyperpolarizing the neuron and making cell firing more difficult. The $GABA_A$ receptor is also a member of the Cys-loop family of receptors and is a heteropentamer containing various combinations of subunits termed α, β, γ, δ, ε, π, ρ, and θ. Various subunit isoforms have been identified with six αs, three βs, three γs, and three ρs (some have suggested that the ρ subunits are found only in the $GABA_C$ receptor). Each subunit is a four transmembrane-spanning protein that, when arranged pseudosymmetrically, forms the ion channel with a diameter of about 8 nm. One of the most common $GABA_A$ receptor conformations in the mammalian central nervous system (CNS) consists of a pair of $\alpha 1$ subunits, a pair of β subunits, and a single $\gamma 2$ subunit. Other identified conformations contain $\alpha 1$, $\alpha 2$, $\alpha 3$, $\alpha 5$, forms of the β subunit, and typically the $\gamma 2$ subunit, and are always in a 2:2:1 stoichiometry.[18] The binding of two molecules of GABA, probably to the individual β subunits near the α-β interface, is believed to be required for normal receptor activation.

A major class of compounds that modulate $GABA_A$ receptor function is the benzodiazepines. The binding site for benzodiazepines (eg, diazepam) is likely the α subunits in proximity to the β subunit. The form of the γ subunit appears to help determine the affinity of the individual benzodiazepine for the receptor. The benzodiazepines bind better to receptors containing γ2 than to the γ1 subunit. Similarly, very low affinity binding is observed if a receptor contains the α6 subunit. In fact, the α6 subunit seems to confer binding preference to inverse agonists such as Ro19-4603. The benzodiazepines do not bind to the GABA recognition site on the receptor and can only produce effects if presynaptic GABA has been released and is present at the receptors. Via an allosteric modulation of the $GABA_A$ receptor, the benzodiazepines appear to increase the frequency of the Cl^- channel opening when GABA is bound, which potentiates the response of exogenously released GABA.

Clinically, the benzodiazepines are very safe when used alone in the absence of CNS depressants, as they are not active on GABA receptors alone. This is in contrast to the barbiturates, which can directly activate the $GABA_A$ receptor when present in a much higher concentration than therapeutic concentrations and thus have a much lower therapeutic index. However, a benzodiazepine receptor antagonist flumazenil is available, which is used for the treatment of severe benzodiazepine overdose. Flumazenil competitively antagonizes the binding and allosteric effects of benzodiazepine agonists as well as benzodiazepine inverse agonists, such as the β-carboline DMCM (methyl 4-ethyl-6,7-dimethoxy-9*H*-pyrido[5,4-b]indole-3-carboxylate).

Using molecular biologic techniques, point mutations of the α subunits have revealed that the sedative effects of the benzodiazepines are due to an interaction with the α1 subunit, while the anxiolytic effects are due to an interaction at the α2 subunit.[19,20] Nonbenzodiazepine receptor agonists such as indiplon, zaleplon, zopiclone, and zolpidem are α1 subunit–preferring ligands that are used as sedative hypnotics.[21]

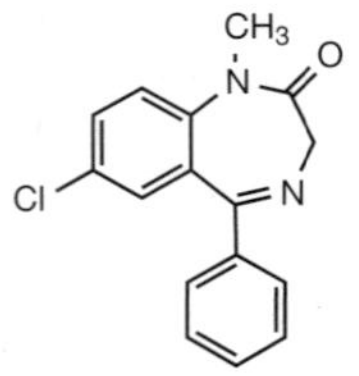

Diazepam

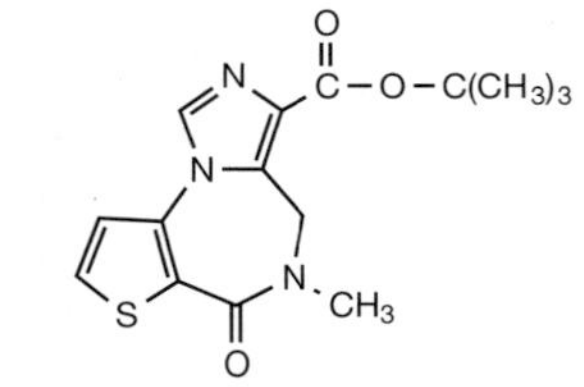

Ro19-4603

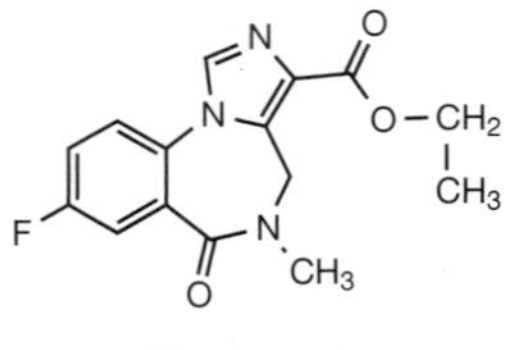

Flumazenil

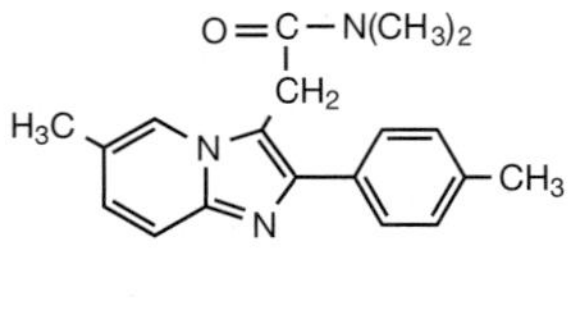

Zolpidem

An agent that acts on the $GABA_A$ receptor that does not interact with the benzodiazepine binding site is gaboxadol (previously called THIP; 4,5,6,7-tetrahydroisoxazolo[4,5-c]pyridine-3-ol). This sedative hypnotic binds with high affinity to the extrasynaptic α4β8$GABA_A$ receptor and does not alter sleep onset or rapid eye movement (REM) sleep as the benzodiazepines do. On the other hand, gaboxadol increases slow-wave sleep.[22]

The barbiturates bind to a different portion of the $GABA_A$ receptor and, similar to the benzodiazepines, enhance the activity of GABA. However, this leads to an increase in the duration of Cl^- channel opening, rather than frequency as seen with the benzodiazepines. Higher concentrations of the barbiturates can directly activate the $GABA_A$ receptor and open the Cl^- channel, explaining why overdoses of barbiturates can lead to life-threatening CNS-mediated respiratory and cardiovascular depression.

A number of compounds are known to directly activate the $GABA_A$ receptor. Of these compounds, muscimol and isoguvacine are the most well known. Unlike GABA, which does not cross the blood-brain barrier, these agents do enter the CNS and display GABA-mimetic activity following peripheral administration. Additionally, a number of compounds can bind to the $GABA_A$ receptor and antagonize the actions of GABA. Bicuculline, by binding to the GABA recognition site and preventing GABA from binding, produces convulsions in experimental animals. Picrotoxin, via its active metabolite picrotoxinin, binds in the Cl^- channel to prevent ion flow when the receptor is activated by GABA. Picrotoxin does not alter GABA binding, but instead prevents ions from flowing and is a potent convulsant.

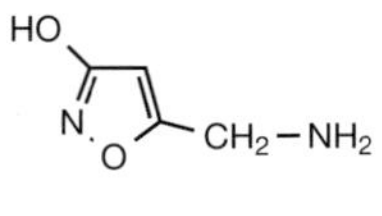

Muscimol

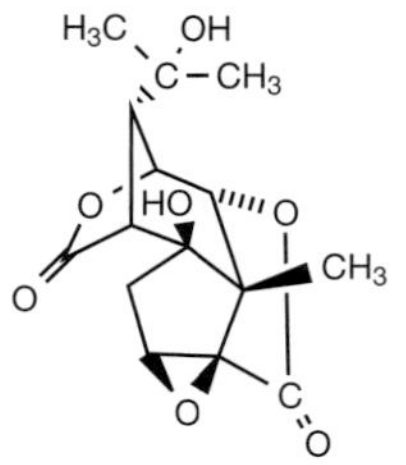

Picrotoxin

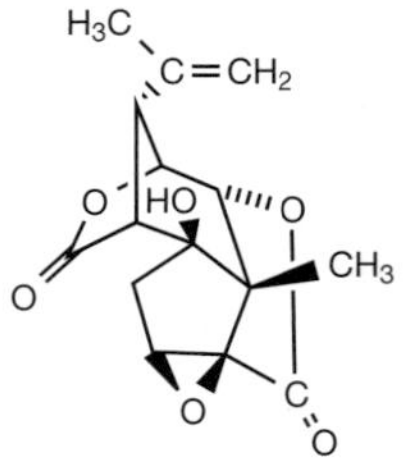

Picrotoxinin

With the many possible assembly sequences of $GABA_A$ receptors, advances in medicinal chemistry may someday be able to design compounds that target specific pentameric subunit assemblies to preferentially produce specific effects.[23] For instance, located on the base of the dendritic spines of hippocampal pyramidal cells are $GABA_A$ receptors with an α5 subunit composition. These receptors are thought to counteract the excitatory input due to glutamatergic *N*-methyl-D-aspartate (NMDA) receptor activation involved in learning and memory. Activation of $GABA_A$ receptors in this area disrupts learning and memory, while NMDA receptor activation improves these critical skills. Administration of an inverse agonist of the $GABA_A$ receptor with selectivity for the α5 subunit improves memory performance in experimental animals.[24] Additionally, α3 selective agonists may be useful in treating schizophrenia, as this subtype of $GABA_A$ receptor appears to play a role in decreasing the release of dopamine from overactive neurons in the mesolimbic system.[25]

General anesthetics also appear to have interactions with the $GABA_A$ receptor in producing their various anesthetic effects, including immobilization, respiratory depression, and hypnosis via binding to hydrophobic pockets within the receptor. Using point-mutated knockin mice, agents such as enflurane, etomidate, and propofol have been found to interact with the β3 subunit of the $GABA_A$ receptor to produce immobilization and hypnosis.[26] However, the heart rate and body temperature–depressant effects of etomidate and propofol do not appear to be mediated by the β3 subunit. Studies are underway to improve our understanding of the molecular mechanisms of this chemically varied group of agents used as general anesthetics.

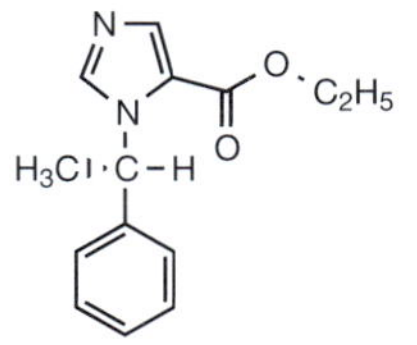

Etomidate

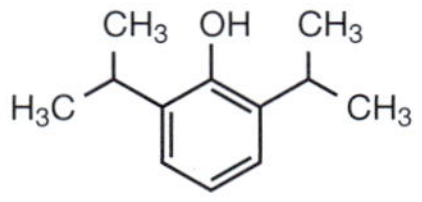

Propofol

Neurosteroids are also capable of modulating the activity of GABA at the $GABA_A$ receptor by binding to a site distinct from that utilized by GABA, benzodiazepines, and barbiturates. These steroids, including the progesterone metabolites pregnanolone (3α-hydroxy-5β-pregnan-20-one), allopregnanolone (3α-hydroxy-5α-pregnan-20-one), and allotetrahydrodeoxycorticosterone (3α,21-dihydroxy-5α-pregnan-20-one), enhance GABA-mediated inhibitory activity. The sudden drop in the levels of allopregnanolone, a natural positive allosteric modulator for $GABA_A$ receptors, is believed to be involved in the symptoms of postpartum depression. Brexanolone and the more recently approved zuranolone stabilize this fluctuation by using a similar mechanism of action and are approved for the treatment of post-partum depression (see Chapter 12 for more details).[27] The presence of the δ subunit in the pentameric $GABA_A$ receptor greatly increases the affinity of steroid binding and efficacy. High concentrations of these steroids can also result in direct activation of the receptor. Thus, it may be possible in the future to selectively target the various modulatory sites on the $GABA_A$ receptor to produce preferential pharmacological effects: for instance, benzodiazepines that are anxiolytic without sedative effects, antischizophrenic agents that lack sedation and extrapyramidal side effects, and general anesthetics that do not alter respiratory and/or heart rates.

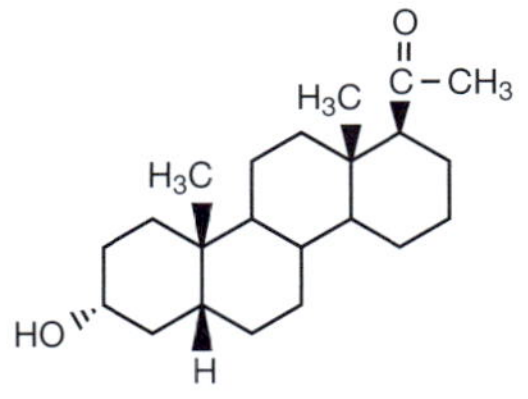

Pregnanolone

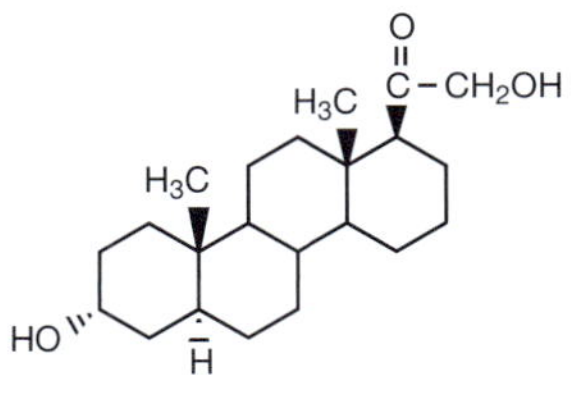

Allotetrahydrodeoxycorticosterone

$GABA_C$ Receptors

Another receptor that binds GABA, but is not antagonized by bicuculline (a $GABA_A$ antagonist) or phaclofen (a $GABA_B$ antagonist) and is not influenced by either the benzodiazepines or barbiturates, is termed the $GABA_C$ receptor. The endogenous neurotransmitter GABA is an order of magnitude more potent on the $GABA_C$ receptor as compared with the $GABA_A$ receptor, and the responses to activation of the $GABA_C$ receptor are much slower and sustained as compared with the rapid and brief responses following $GABA_A$ receptor activation. The $GABA_C$ receptor is most abundant in the retina, with significant levels in the spinal cord and pituitary gland. A pentamer of subunits form the Cl^- ion channel. As noted earlier, the ρ subunit may be unique to the $GABA_C$ receptor.[28] On the extracellular domain, there appears to be binding sites for zinc, which is a potent modulator of receptor activity.

The most well-described $GABA_C$ receptor antagonist is TPMPA ([1,2,5,6-tetrahydropyridin-4-yl]-methylphosphinic acid). Interestingly, isoguvacine, an agonist at the $GABA_A$ receptors, acts as an antagonist at the $GABA_C$ receptor. Much information regarding the location, function, and pharmacology of the $GABA_C$ receptor is needed to begin to take advantage of this receptor for therapeutic purposes.

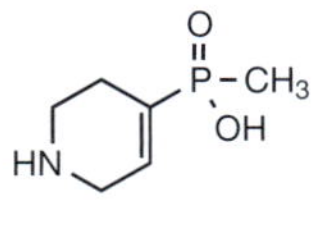

TPMPA

Glycine Receptors

The receptor mediating the actions of the inhibitory amino acid (IAA) GLY is similar to the $GABA_A$ receptor and other members of the Cys-loop family in being a pentameric ion channel that allows for the conduction of Cl^-.[29] However, unlike the GABA receptors, the inhibitory GLY receptor can be a homopentamer of α subunits or a heteropentamer composed of three α subunits and two β subunits. There have been four isoforms of the α subunit identified, while only one β subunit is known. The inhibitory neurotransmitter GLY, in addition to taurine, D-alanine, L-alanine, β-alanine, hypotaurine, L-serine, and β-aminobutyric acid, can activate the receptor by binding to any of the three α subunits. Positive modulators of the inhibitory GLY receptor include zinc, neurosteroids, propofol, ethanol, and volatile anesthetics such as isoflurane.[30]

The best described antagonist of the inhibitory GLY receptor is the convulsant strychnine. Strychnine binds to a site different from that which recognizes GLY. Sometimes the inhibitory GLY receptor is referred to as the "strychnine-sensitive" GLY receptor to distinguish it from the GLY modulatory site on the glutaminergic NMDA receptor. The $GABA_A$ receptor antagonist picrotoxin can also inhibit the GLY receptor. More recently, endocannabinoids such as anandamide and 2-arachidonylglycerol have been shown to antagonize the activity of GLY at this receptor. Agents that act as agonists at the IAA GLY receptor may find utility as anticonvulsants, muscle relaxants, sedatives, and general anesthetics.

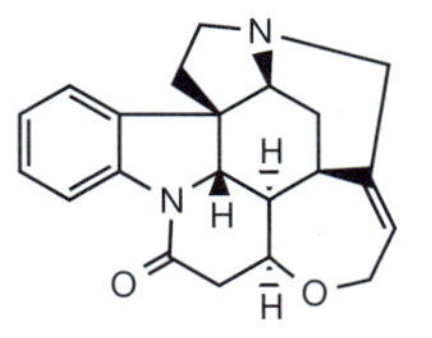

Strychnine

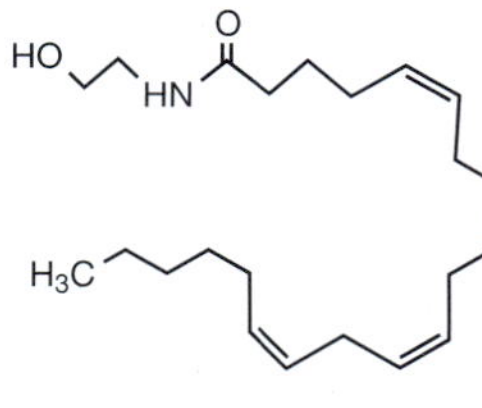

Anandamide

Zinc-Activated Channel

As another member of the Cys-loop family of receptors, the zinc-activated channel (ZAC) is yet to be fully characterized. It exists as a homopentamer with four transmembrane loops and is activated by divalent zinc (Zn^{2+}) and copper (Cu^{2+}) ions and by proton (H^+). Contrary to its name, Cu^{2+} and H^+ have been found to be more potent at activating this channel compared to Zn^{2+}. When open, the central pore of the ZAC is permeable to monovalent cations such as Na^+, K^+, and cesium (Cs^+) but is impermeable and inactivated by high concentrations of extracellular Ca^{2+} and magnesium (Mg^{2+}).[31] In the adult human brain, ZAC messenger RNA (mRNA) has been located in hippocampus, striatum, thalamus, and amygdala. In the periphery, ZAC mRNA is expressed in the lungs, trachea, thyroid, and prostate.[32] These channels show constitutive activity that can be blocked by tubocurarine, but their physiologic roles are still under investigation.[33]

Excitatory Amino Acid Receptors

The receptors for glutamate (GLU) and the other excitatory amino acids (EAAs) are categorized into two major groups: ionotropic and metabotropic. The three ionotropic receptor types are classified based on their originally preferred synthetic agonist: NMDA, α-amino-3-hydroxy-5-methyl-4-isoxazole propionic acid (AMPA), and kainate. Distinct from the pentameric Cys-loop receptor family, these LGIC receptors are composed of homo—or heterotetramers of individual subunits that confer cation selectivity. Each subunit has an extracellular N-terminus with three TM domains, an intramembrane reentrant "p-loop" between the first and third TM domains, and an intracellular C-terminus.[34] The metabotropic GluRs belong to the larger family of GPCRs (see Chapter 6). When activated, these receptors can alter the activity of effector proteins such as adenylyl cyclase and phospholipase C (PLC). To date, there appears to be at least eight distinct EAA metabotropic receptor subtypes. The EAA receptors, in balance with the receptors for the IAAs, are likely crucial for the regulation of neuronal plasticity, including long-term potentiation (LTP) and long-term depression (LTD).

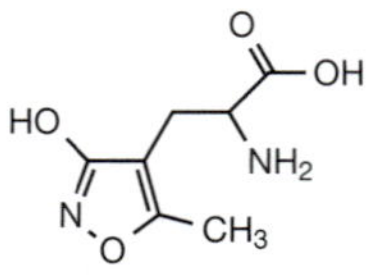

AMPA

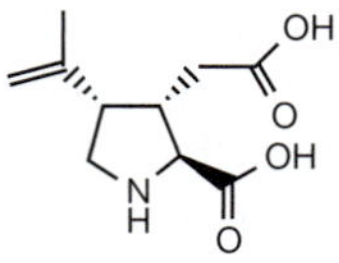

Kainic acid

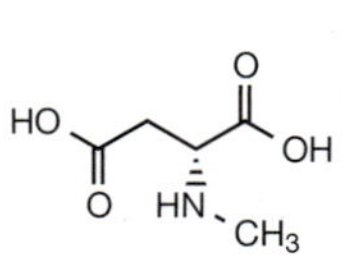

N-Methyl-D-aspartic acid (NMDA)

N-methyl-D-aspartate Receptor

The NMDA receptor is a heterotetramer composed of a number of subunit forms termed GLUN1, GLUN2A, GLUN2B, GLUN2C, GLUN2D, GLUN3A, and GLUN3B that can confer unique pharmacology to individual receptors. Additionally, splice variants can lead to a number of isoforms of the above subunits with the potential of changing the binding characteristics and functions of the receptor. Activation of the NMDA receptor requires the binding of two agonists: GLU to the GLUN2 subunit and GLY to a binding site on the GLUN1 subunit.[35] GLY appears to act as an important co-agonist-positive modulator at a unique recognition site, and unlike the actions of GLY as an IAA neurotransmitter, this recognition site is not sensitive to blockade by strychnine. Thus, this GLY binding site is often referred to as the strychnine-insensitive receptor site.

Agonists at the GLU binding site include NMDA, L-glutamate, L-aspartate, and homoquinolinic acid. The best characterized antagonist at this site is D-(-)-2-amino-5-phosphonopentanoic acid (D-AP5). In addition to GLY, D-serine is a well-known agonist at the GLY site. D-Serine, which is normally only found in glia and astrocytes, is synthesized from L-serine via serine racemase, and is thought to be one of the important modulators of NMDA receptor activity.

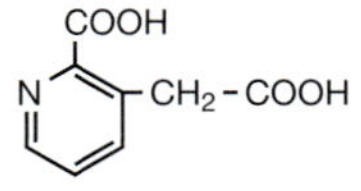

Homoquinolinic acid

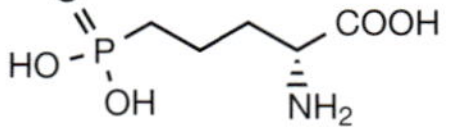

D-AP5

The NMDA receptor also has many sites for channel modulation by pharmacological agents. Endogenous inhibitory channel modulators include Mg^{2+}, Zn^{2+}, and H^+. Neurosteroids can either inhibit or potentiate NMDA receptor channel function depending upon the subunit forms comprising the tetrameric structure. For instance, pregnenolone sulfate inhibits NMDA receptors assembled as GLUN1/GLUN2C but potentiates those assembled as GLUN1/GLUN2A and GLUN1/GLUN2B.[36] Polyamines such as spermine and spermidine are known to be positive channel modulators.

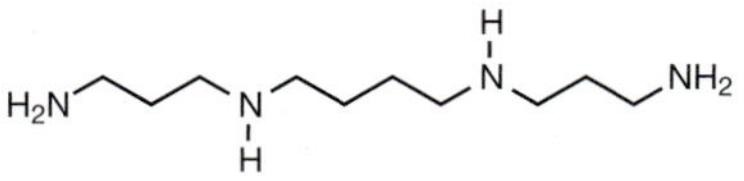

Spermine

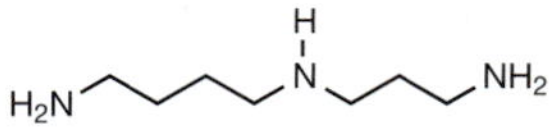

Spermidine

A number of important NMDA-channel antagonists also exist and include amantadine (an antiviral agent that also releases dopamine and is used in Parkinson disease), ketamine (a dissociative anesthetic agent that acts via the NMDA receptor), phencyclidine (a psychoactive drug of abuse also known as "PCP"), and memantine (approved for the treatment of Alzheimer disease). While the antitussive agent dextromethorphan, via its metabolite dextrorphan, is known to block the NMDA channel, its cough-suppressant activity is likely not due to its action at this site. However, the psychotomimetic effects observed with the abuse of this compound could likely be NMDA receptor mediated. The new U.S. Food and Drug Administration (FDA)-approved drug Auvelity is a combination of dextromethorphan and bupropion (a cytochrome P450 2D6 inhibitor to increase the half-life of dextromethorphan) and is used in the treatment of major depressive disorder.[37] An endogenous antagonist of the NMDA receptor is the Mg^{2+} ion, which normally prevents the flow of Ca^{2+} through the channel. However, when both glutamate (or another suitable agonist) and glycine bind, the inhibition normally maintained by Mg^{2+} is relieved, Ca^{2+} can flow, and the cell can depolarize. Some studies in experimental animals have demonstrated the NMDA receptor–mediated neuroprotective effects of Mg^{2+} in models of stroke and other CNS insults.

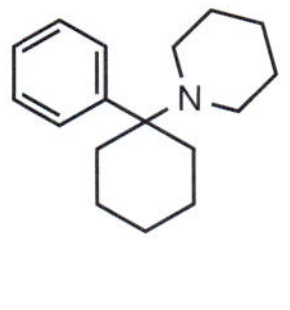

Phencyclidine (PCP)

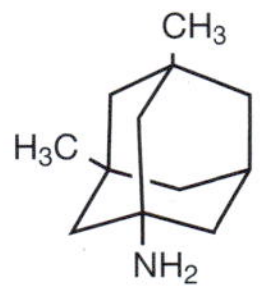

Memantine

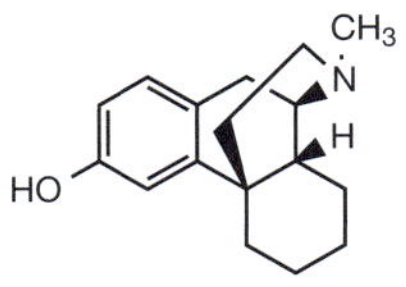

Dextrorphan

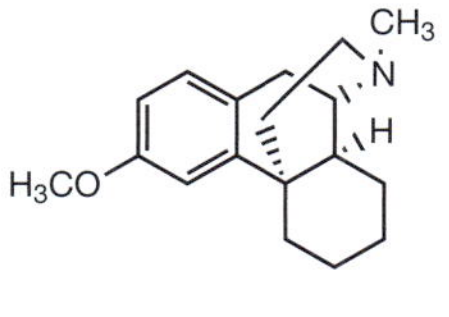

Dextromethorphan

One of the first NMDA receptor antagonists to be identified was dizocilpine, commonly known as MK-801. Much excitement was initially generated with the discovery of MK-801, as the ability to block the excessive intracellular cation flow (Ca^{2+}, Na^{+}) that follows neuronal hypoxic insults following cerebral vascular accidents (stroke) or head trauma might lead to effective treatments for such pathologic conditions. While MK-801 was very effective in decreasing infarct size in various rodent models of stroke, poor efficacy was noted in humans. Additionally, the generation of severe psychotic behaviors was deemed unacceptable.[38]

The strychnine-insensitive binding site on the NMDA receptor has also been a target for researchers, since an agent that would antagonize this binding site might be useful in preventing the neuronal damage that occurs following hypoxic insults leading to excessive GLU release or in controlling electrical neuronal dysfunction associated with epilepsy. One agent, (R)-HA-966 (*R*-(+)-3-amino-1-hydroxypyrrolidin-2-one), is a GLY receptor antagonist that, unfortunately, has not been used therapeutically due to its NMDA receptor–unrelated hepatotoxic properties. While the anticonvulsant felbamate (2-phenyl-1,3-propanedioldicarbamate) produces part of its activity by allosterically altering the binding of GLY at the NMDA GLY binding site, it also has interactions at the AMPA and kainate receptors which contribute to its anticonvulsant activity.[39]

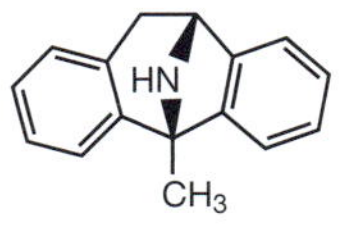

Dizocilpine

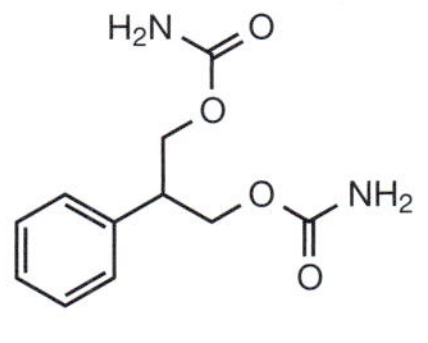

Felbamate

AMPA Receptors

Another ionotropic EAA receptor is preferentially activated by AMPA. While at one time this receptor was referred to as the quisqualate receptor, the AMPA receptor (as it is now known) mediates fast synaptic activity via the influx of Na^{+} and, in some neurons, K^{+} efflux. The AMPA receptor, in high abundance in the cerebral cortex and hippocampus, is composed of subunits GluR1, GluR2, GluR3, and GluR4. One of these subunits, GluR2, when present, prevents the formation of an ionophore that can efficiently conduct Ca^{2+}. However, when the AMPA receptor does not contain a GluR2 subunit, Ca^{2+} can be conducted through the ion channel. On the extracellular loop between TM3 and TM4, there exists a region termed the "flip-flop" that is sensitive to splice variants of the gene coding for each subunit. Such splice variants can lead to significant differences in the desensitization kinetics of the receptor.[40] Additionally, intracellular sites on the C-terminus, where modulatory proteins such as *N*-ethylmaleimide-sensitive fusion protein (NSF) and PICK (protein interacting with C kinase) can bind, allow for another important site where regulation of receptor trafficking can be influenced.

The discovery that some 2,3-benzodiazepines (eg, GYK1 53655) can selectively bind the AMPA receptor has aided in studies to understand its location and functions, especially where mixed populations of EAA receptors are present.[41] Agents known to potentiate AMPA receptor activity include piracetam (2-oxo-1-pyrrolidine acetamide), a cyclic derivative of GABA, the benzothiazide, and cyclothiazide (6-chloro-3,4-dihydro-3[2-norbornen-5-yl]-2H-1,2,4-benzothiadiazine-7-sulfonamide). Additionally, some evidence suggests that certain barbiturates and volatile anesthetics have binding sites on the AMPA receptor. Agents that positively modulate the AMPA receptor have been termed "ampakines" and have been suggested in various studies to improve memory, enhance the activity of certain antipsychotic agents, improve attention-deficit hyperactivity disorder, improve Parkinson disease symptoms, and provide neuroprotection following CNS ischemic insults.[42] Perampanel, (2-[2-oxo-1-phenyl-5-pyridin-2-yl-1,2 dyhydropyridin-3-yl] benzonitrile hydrate, is the one and only FDA-approved noncompetitive AMPA receptor antagonist used in the treatment of epilepsy.[43] Its exact mechanism of action is still unclear (see Chapter 15 for more information).

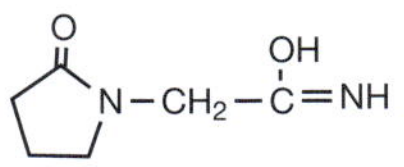

Piracetam

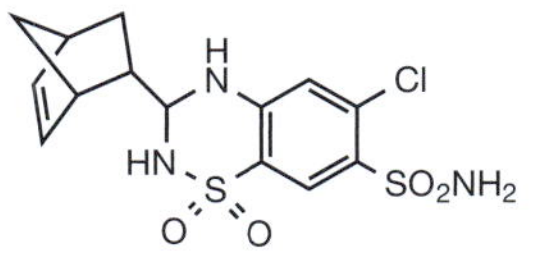

Cyclothiazide

Kainate Receptors

The ionotropic kainate receptor is a heterotetramer composed of subunits GluR5, GluR6, GluR7, KA1, and KA2.

While GluR5-7 can form functional homo and heteromeric receptors, the KA1 and KA2 subunits require the presence of the Glu5-7 subunits to assemble into functional receptors. Similarities exist between the binding characteristics of AMPA receptors and kainite receptors, such that few pharmacological agents are available that effectively differentiate between the two.[44] Kainate receptors tend to be more sensitive to the kainic acid analog domoic acid than AMPA receptors.

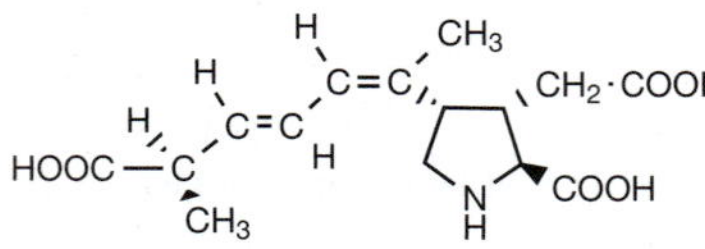

Domoic acid

While kainate receptors are located postsynaptically and mediate neuronal excitation (as do NMDA and AMPA receptors), kainate receptors have also been found presynaptically. Such presynaptic receptors appear to act to regulate the release of GABA in the hippocampus and GLU in other brain regions. Additionally, some kainate receptors have been shown to be linked to a pertussis toxin–sensitive G protein, which, via interaction with PLC, in turn, may act to influence nearby voltage-dependent Ca^{2+} channels.[45] This dual signaling capability of kainate receptors appears unique for an EAA ionotropic receptor and may facilitate the role of this receptor subtype in influencing both short- and long-term synaptic plasticity in the CNS.

P2X Receptors

Purinergic P2X receptors occur as trimeric proteins with agonist-binding extracellular domains, the pore-forming transmembrane (TM1-TM2) domains, and intracellular domains. Seven functional isoforms (P2X1-P2X7) have been identified to date in mammals, varying from homotrimers to heterotrimers.[46] These receptors are gated by ATP, at least three molecules of which are needed to open this channel, and nucleotide analogs of ATP have been found to have agonistic effects. Pore opening allows for the flow of Na^+, K^+, and Ca^{2+} ions. Prolonged ATP binding leads to receptor desensitization to varying degrees between the seven receptor subtypes. A number of allosteric modulators (eg, zinc, copper) have been found to have varying effects on receptor activation based on the modulator concentration and receptor subtype.[47] Ivermectin (an antihelminthic agent used to treat river blindness in humans and commonly used in veterinary medicine for heart worms; also known to bind to GABA and GLY receptors) interacts with P2X4 as a positive modulator potentiating ATP-gated currents.[48] Because these receptors are involved in the release of inflammatory molecules, selective antagonists for the P2X7 and P2X3 have been explored for their use in inflammatory pain with mixed results.

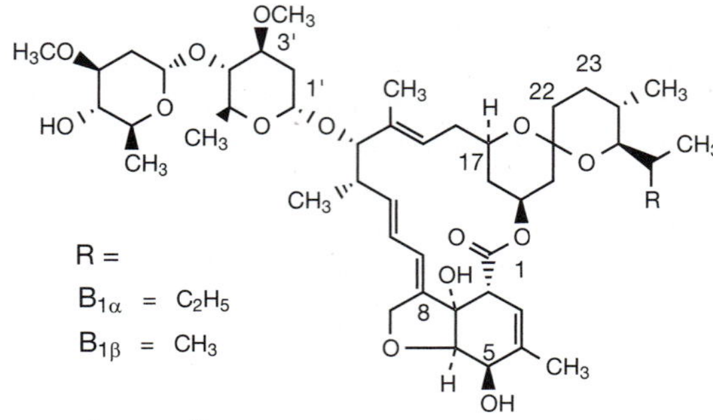

Ivermectin

Voltage-Gated and Second Messenger–Gated Channels

Although not considered receptors since they are not ligand dependent, there are other ion channels that are controlled by either voltage changes or second messenger molecules. An example of a voltage-gated channel includes the Na^+ channels responsible for impulse conduction in sensory nerve fibers that transmit information about pain and temperature. Following administration, the local anesthetic lidocaine enters the nerve cell via diffusion in its free base form. Once inside the nerve cell, lidocaine is protonated and, in this charged form, is capable of blocking the Na^+ channel from the intracellular side. Some second messenger molecules (eg, cyclic adenosine monophosphate (cAMP) and IP_3) generated following the activation of GPCRs can influence the degree of channel opening or closing. The most common channels influenced by these second messengers include those for Ca^{2+} and K^+.

Mechanisms of Calcium Movement and Storage

The regulation of cytosolic Ca^{2+} levels occurs via specific influx, efflux, and sequestering mechanisms (Fig. 8.3). The influx of Ca^{2+} can occur through receptor-operated channels (site 1), the Na^+/Ca^{2+} exchange process (site 2), "leak" pathways (site 3), and potential-dependent channels (site 4). Influx via either receptor-operated or voltage-dependent channels has been proposed to be the major entry pathway for Ca^{2+}. Receptor-operated channels have been defined as those associated with cellular membrane receptors and activated by specific agonist-receptor interactions. In contrast, potential-dependent channels, also known as voltage-dependent or voltage-gated calcium channels, have been defined as those activated by membrane depolarization. The Na^+/Ca^{2+} exchange process can promote either influx or efflux because the direction of Ca^{2+} movement depends on the relative intracellular and extracellular ratios of Na^+ and Ca^{2+}. The "leak" pathways, which include unstimulated Ca^{2+} entry as well as entry during the fast-inward Na^+ phase of an action potential, play only a minor role in Ca^{2+} influx.

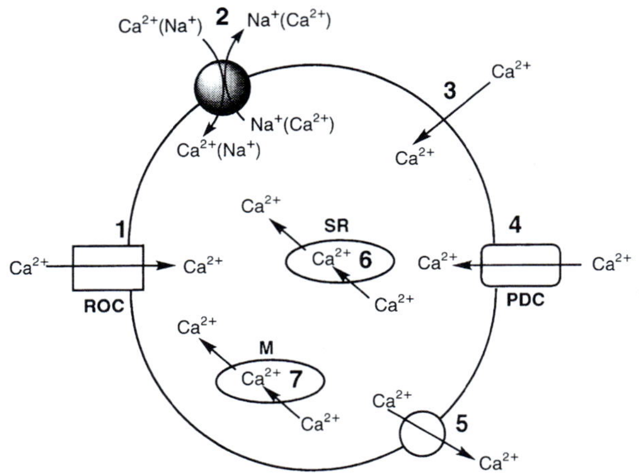

Figure 8.3 Cellular mechanisms for the influx, efflux, and sequestering of Ca^{2+}. M, mitochondria; PDC, potential-dependent Ca2+ channels; ROC, receptor-operated Ca^{2+} channels; and SR, sarcoplasmic reticulum.

Efflux can occur through either an ATP-driven membrane pump (site 5) or via the Na^+/Ca^{2+} exchange process previously mentioned (site 2). In addition to these influx and efflux mechanisms, the sarcoplasmic reticulum (site 6) and the mitochondria (site 7) function as internal storage/release sites. These storage sites work in concert with the influx and efflux processes to assure that cytosolic Ca^{2+} levels are appropriate for cellular needs. Although influx and release processes are essential for excitation-contraction coupling, efflux and sequestering processes are equally important for terminating the contractile process and for protecting the cell from the deleterious effects of Ca^{2+} overload.[49,50]

Potential-Dependent Calcium Channels

The pharmacologic class of agents known as calcium-channel blockers produces their effects through interaction with potential-dependent channels. To date, six functional subclasses, or types, of potential-dependent Ca^{2+} channels have been identified: T, L, N, P, Q, and R. These types differ in location and function and can be divided into two major groups: low-voltage-activated (LVA) channels and high-voltage-activated (HVA) channels. Of the six types, only the T (transient, tiny) channel can be rapidly activated and inactivated with small changes in the cell membrane potential. It is thus designated as an LVA channel. All of the other types of channels require a larger depolarization and are thus designated as HVA channels.

The L (long-lasting, large) channel is the site of action for currently available calcium-channel blockers and, therefore, has been extensively studied. It is located in skeletal, cardiac, and smooth muscle and, thus, is highly involved in organ and vessel contraction within the cardiovascular system. The N channel is found in neuronal tissue and exhibits kinetics and inhibitory sensitivity distinct from both L and T channels. The functions, sensitivities, and properties of the other three types of channels are not as well known. The P channel has been named for its presence in the Purkinje cells, whereas the Q and R channels have been characterized by their abilities to bind to certain polypeptide toxins.[51]

The L channel is a pentameric complex consisting of α_1, α_2, β, γ, and δ polypeptides (Fig. 8.4). The α_1 subunit is a transmembrane-spanning protein that consists of four domains and functions as the pore-forming subunit. The α_1 subunit also contains binding sites for all the currently

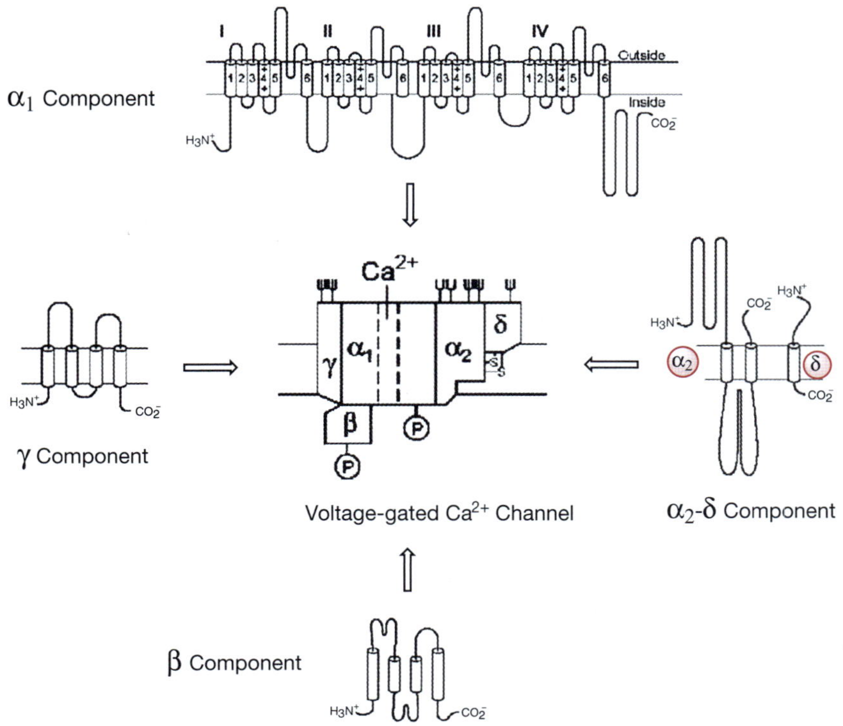

Figure 8.4 Representation of the structure of the voltage-gated Ca^{2+} channel (L channel) composed of several subunits—α_1, $\alpha_2\delta$, β, γ—organized as depicted in the central area.

available calcium-channel blockers. The other four subunits surround the α_1 portion of the channel and contribute to the overall hydrophobicity of the pentamer. This hydrophobicity is important in that it allows the channel to be embedded in the cell membrane. Additionally, the α_2, δ, and β subunits modulate the α_1 subunit.

Other types of potential-dependent channels are similar to the L channel. They all have a central α_1 subunit; however, molecular cloning studies have revealed that there are at least six α_1 genes: α_{1S}, α_{1A}, α_{1B}, α_{1C}, α_{1D}, and α_{1E}. Three of these genes, α_{1S}, α_{1C}, and α_{1D}, have been associated with L channels. The L channels found in skeletal muscle result from the α_{1S} gene; those in the heart, aorta, lung, and fibroblast result from the α_{1C} gene; and those in endocrine tissue result from the α_{1D} gene. Both α_{1C} and α_{1D} are used for L channels in the brain. Thus, there are some differences among the L channels located in different organs and tissues. Additionally, differences in α_1 genes and differences among the other subunits are responsible for the variations seen among the other five types of potential-dependent channels. As an example, the N channel lacks the γ subunit and contains an α_1 subunit derived from the α_{1B} gene.[51] A number of calcium-channel blockers are currently available for use in cardiovascular disorders.

ACKNOWLEDGMENTS

The author wishes to acknowledge the work of E. Kim Fifer, PhD, Marc Harrold, PhD, and Timothy J. Maher, PhD who authored the content used within this chapter in a previous edition of this text.

REFERENCES

1. Sparling BA, DiMauro EF. Progress in the discovery of small molecule modulators of the Cys-loop superfamily receptors. *Bioorg Med Chem Lett.* 2017;27(15):3207-3218.
2. Albuquerque EX, Pereira EF, Alkondon M, Rogers SW. Mammalian nicotinic acetylcholine receptors: from structure to function. *Physiol Rev.* 2009;89:73-120.
3. Papke RL. Merging old and new perspectives on nicotinic acetylcholine receptors. *Biochem Pharmacol.* 2014;89:1-11.
4. Taylor P, Brown JH. Nicotinic receptors. In: Siegel GJ, Agranoff BW, Albers RW, et al, eds. *Basic Neurochemistry: Molecular, Cellular and Medical Aspects.* 6th ed. Lippincott-Raven; 1999.
5. Lindstrom J, Anand R, Peng X, Gerzanich V, Wang F, Li Y. Neuronal nicotinic receptor subtypes. *Ann NY Acad Sci.* 1995;757:100-116.
6. Hogg RC, Raggenbass M, Bertrand D. Nicotinic acetylcholine receptors: from structure to brain function. *Rev Physiol Biochem Pharmacol.* 2003;147:1-46.
7. Crooks PA, Bardo MT, Dwoskin LP. Nicotinic receptor antagonists as treatments for nicotine abuse. *Adv Pharmacol.* 2014;69:513-551.
8. McIntyre AR. History of curare. In: Cheymol J, ed. *International Encyclopedia of Pharmacology and Therapeutics.* Section 14. Vol. 1. Pergamon Press; 1972:187-203.
9. King H. Curarie alkaloids. I. Tubocurarine. *J Chem Soc.* 1935;2:1381-1389.
10. Everett AJ, Lowe LA, Wilkinson S. Revision of the structures of (+)-tubocurarine chloride and (+)-chondrocurine. *J Chem Soc.* 1970;16:1020-1021.
11. Kistler J, Stroud RM. Crystalline arrays of membrane-bound acetylcholine receptor. *Proc Natl Acad Sci USA.* 1981;78:3678-3682.
12. Barnard EA, Coates V, Dolly JO, Mallick B. Binding of α-bungarotoxin and cholinergic ligands to acetylcholine receptors in the membrane of skeletal muscle. *Cell Biol Int Rep.* 1977;1:99-106.
13. Raghavendra T. Neuromuscular blocking drugs: discovery and development. *J R Soc Med.* 2002;95(7):363-367.
14. Thompson AJ. Recent developments in 5-HT3 receptor pharmacology. *Trends Pharmacol Sci.* 2013;34:100-109.
15. Gupta D, Prabhakar V, Radhakrishnan M. 5HT3 receptors: target for new antidepressant drugs. *Neurosci Biobehav Rev.* 2016;64:311-325.
16. Parker RM, Barnes JM, Ge J, et al. Autoradiographic distribution of [3H]-(S)zacopride-labelled 5 HT-3 receptors in human brain. *J Neurol Sci.* 1996;144:119-127.
17. Walstab J, Rappold G, Niesler B. 5-HT3 receptors: role in disease and target of drugs. *Pharmacol Ther.* 2010;128:146-169.
18. Rudolph U, Mohler H. GABA-based therapeutic approaches: GABAA receptor subtype functions. *Curr Opin Pharmacol.* 2006;6:18-23.
19. Rudolph U, Crestani F, Benke D, et al. Benzodiazepine actions mediated by specific gamma-aminobutyric acid(A) receptor subtypes. *Nature.* 1999;401:796-800.
20. Löw K, Crestani F, Keist R, et al. Molecular and neuronal substrates for the selective attenuation of anxiety. *Science.* 2000;290:131-134.
21. Foster AC, Pelleymounter MA, Cullen MJ, et al. In vivo pharmacological characterization of indipion, a novel pyrazolopyrimidine sedative-hypnotic. *J Pharmacol Exp Ther.* 2004;311:547-559.
22. Lancel M, Langebartels A. Gamma-aminobutyric acid(A) agonist 4,5,6,7-tetrahydroisoxazolo[4,5-c] pyridine-3-ol persistently increases sleep maintenance and intensity during chronic administration to rats. *J Pharmacol Exp Ther.* 2000;293:1084-1090.
23. Whiting PJ. GABA-A receptors: a viable target for novel anxiolytics? *Curr Opin Pharmacol.* 2006;6:24-29.
24. Sternfeld F, Carling RW, Jelley RA, et al. Selective, orally active gamma-aminobutyric acidA alpha5 receptor inverse agonists as cognition enhancers. *J Med Chem.* 2004;47:2176-2179.
25. Yee BK, Keist R, von Boehmer L, et al. A schizophrenia-related sensorimotor deficit links α3-containing GABAA receptors to a dopamine hyperfunction. *Proc Natl Acad Sci USA.* 2005;102:17154-17159.
26. Jurd R, Arras M, Lambert S, et al. General anesthetic actions in vivo strongly attenuated by point mutation in the GABA(A) receptor beta3 subunit. *FASEB J.* 2003;17:250-252.
27. Carlini SV, Osborne LM, Deligiannidis KM. Current pharmacotherapy approaches and novel GABAergic antidepressant development in postpartum depression. *Dialogues Clin Neurosci.* 2023;25(1):92-100.
28. Seighart W, Sperk G. Subunit composition, distribution and function of GABA(A) receptor subtypes. *Curr Top Med Chem.* 2002;2:795-816.
29. Breitinger H-G, Becker C-M. The inhibitory glycine receptor-simple views of a complicated channel. *Chembiochem.* 2003;3:1042-1052.
30. Lobo IA, Harris RA. Sites of alcohol and volatile anesthetic action on glycine receptors. *Int Rev Neurobiol.* 2005;65:53-87.
31. Trattnig SM, Gasiorek A, Deeb TZ, et al. Copper and protons directly activate the zinc-activated channel. *Biochem Pharmacol.* 2016;103:109-117.
32. Houtani T, Munemoto Y, Kase M, et al. Cloning and expression of ligand-gated ion-channel receptor L2 in central nervous system. *Biochem Biophys Res Commun.* 2005;335:277-285.
33. Davies PA, Wang W, Hales TG, Kirkness EF. A novel class of ligand-gated ion channel is activated by Zn^{2+}. *J Biol Chem.* 2003;278:712-717.

34. Dingdledine R, Borges K, Bowie D, et al. The glutamate receptor ion channels. *Pharmacol Rev*. 1999;51:7-61.
35. Erreger K, Chen PE, Wyllie DJ, Traynelis SF. Glutamate receptor gating. *Crit Rev Neurobiol*. 2004;16:187-224.
36. Maleyev A, Gibbs TT, Farb DH. Inhibition of the NMDA response by pregnenolone sulphate revels subtype selective modulation of NMDA receptors by sulphated steroids. *Br J Pharmacol*. 2002;135:901-909.
37. Huettner JE, Bean BP. Block of *N*-methyl-D-aspartate-activated current by the anticonvulsant MK-801: selective binding to open channels. *Proc Natl Acad Sci USA*. 1988;85:1307-1311.
38. McCarthy B, Bunn H, Santalucia M, Wilmouth C, Muzyk A, Smith CM. Dextromethorphan-bupropion (Auvelity) for the treatment of major depressive disorder. *Clin Psychopharmacol Neurosci*. 2023;21(4):609-616.
39. Subramaniam S, Rho JM, Penix L, et al. Felbamate block of the *N*-methyl-D-aspartate receptor. *J Pharmacol Exp Ther*. 1995;273:878-886.
40. Brorson JR, Li D, Suzuki T. Selective expression of heteromeric AMPA receptors driven by flip-flop differences. *J Neurosci*. 2004;24: 3461-3470.
41. Paternain AV, Morales M, Lerma J. Selective antagonism of AMPA receptors unmasks kainate receptor-mediated responses in hippocampal neurons. *Neuron*. 1995;14:185-189.
42. Lynch G. Glutamate-based therapeutic approaches: ampakines. *Curr Opin Pharmacol*. 2006;6:82-88.
43. Lerma J, Paternain AV, Rodriguez-Moreno A, López-García JC. Molecular physiology of kainate receptors. *Physiol Rev*. 2001;81: 971-998.
44. Chu H, Zhang X, Shi J, Zhou Z, Yang X. Antiseizure medications for idiopathic generalized epilepsies: a systematic review and network meta-analysis. *J Neurol*. 2023;270(10):4713-4728.
45. Lerna J. Kainate receptor physiology. *Curr Opin Pharmacol*. 2006;6:89-97.
46. North RA. Molecular physiology of P2X receptors. *Physiol Rev*. 2002;82:1013-1067.
47. Stojilkovic SS, Leiva-Salcedo E, Rokic MB, Coddou C. Regulation of ATP-gated P2X channels: from redox signaling to interactions with other proteins. *Antioxid Redox Signal*. 2014;21: 953-970.
48. Pasqualetto G, Brancale A, Young MT. The molecular determinants of small-molecule ligand binding at P2X receptors. *Front Pharmacol*. 2018;9:58.
49. Janis RA, Triggle DJ. New developments in Ca^{2+} channel antagonists. *J Med Chem*. 1983;26:775-785.
50. Swamy VC, Triggle DJ. Calcium channel blockers. In: Craig CR, Stitzel RE, eds. *Modern Pharmacology with Clinical Applications*. 6th ed. Lippincott Williams & Wilkins; 2004:218-224.
51. Varadi G, Mori Y, Mikala G, Schwartz A. Molecular determinants of Ca^{2+} channel function and drug action. *Trends Pharmacol Sci*. 1995;16:43-49.

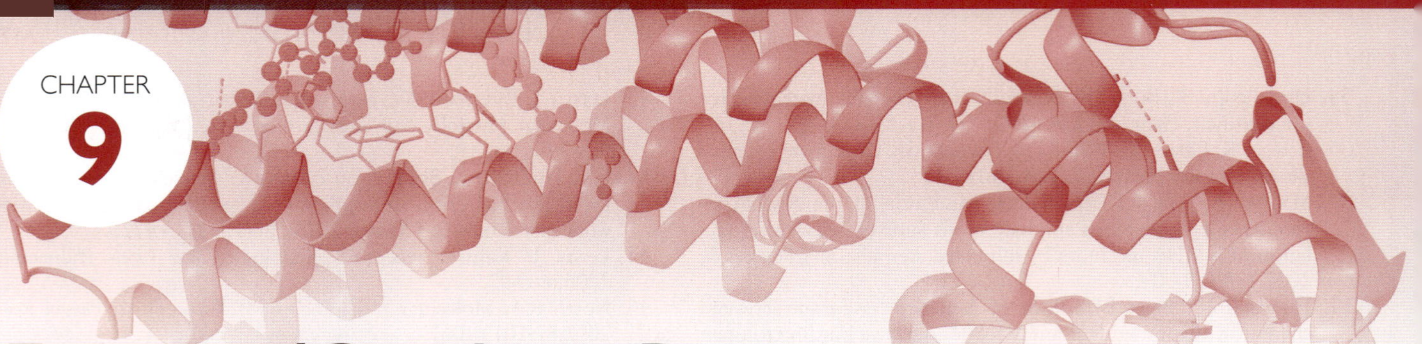

CHAPTER 9

Enzyme/Catalytic Receptors

Stephen G. Kerr

Drugs covered in this chapter:

- Abemaciclib
- Acetylcholine
- Alisertib
- Amoxicillin
- Ara-C
- Asciminib
- Avanafil
- Azidothymidine
- Barasertib
- Baricitinib
- Bosutinib
- Captopril
- Cilomilast
- Cilostazol
- Clavulanic acid
- Coformycin
- Copanlisib
- Dabrafenib
- Danusertib
- Dasatinib
- Deucravacitinib
- Deoxycoformycin
- Dideoxycytidine
- Dipyridamole
- Enalapril
- Enalaprilat
- Everolimus
- Finasteride
- Fluorodeoxyuridine monophosphate
- Fluorouracil
- Gabaculin
- Gefitinib
- Ibrutinib
- Imatinib
- Inamrinone
- Methotrexate
- Milrinone
- Nevirapine
- Palbociclib
- Penicillin
- Physostigmine
- Prontosil
- Rapamycin
- Ribociclib
- Ritlecitinib
- Roflumilast
- Ruxolitinib
- Sildenafil
- Sirolimus
- Sulfanilamide
- Sunitinib
- Taladafil
- Temsirolimus
- Thiacytidine
- Thymidine
- Tofacitinib
- Trametinib
- Vardenafil
- Vemurafenib
- Zaprinast

Abbreviations

ACE angiotensin-converting enzyme
AChE acetylcholinesterase
Akt protein kinase B
AMP adenosine monophosphate
ANP atrial natriuretic peptide
Ara-C cytosine arabinoside
ATP adenosine triphosphate
AZT azidothymidine
cAMP cyclic adenosine monophosphate
CDK cyclin-dependent kinase
cGMP cyclic guanosine monophosphate
CML chronic myelogenous leukemia
cNMP cyclic nucleoside monophosphate
COPD chronic obstructive pulmonary disease
DAG diacylglycerol
dC deoxycytidine
ddC 2′,3′-dideoxycytidine
deoxy CTP deoxycytidine triphosphate
DFG aspartate-phenyl-glycine
DHFR dihydrofolate reductase
dNTP deoxynucleotide triphosphate
E enzyme
EC Enzyme Commission
EGFR epidermal growth factor receptor
E.I. enzyme-inhibitor complex
E.S. enzyme–substrate complex
FDA U.S. Food and Drug Administration
FdUMP 5-fluorodeoxyuridine monophosphate
5-FU 5-fluorouracil
GABA-T γ-aminobutyric acid transaminase
GIST gastrointestinal stromal tumors
GMP guanosine monophosphate
GTP guanosine triphosphate
HGNC Human Genome Nominating Committee
IL interleukin
IUPHAR/BPS The International Union of Basic and Clinical Pharmacology

Abbreviations—continued

JAK Janus kinase
k_{cat} catalytic or first-order rate constant
K_d enzyme–substrate dissociation constant
k_{diff} diffusion rate constant
K_i inhibition constant
k_{inact} inactivation rate constant
KLIFS kinase–ligand interaction fingerprints and structures
K_m Michaelis-Menten constant or apparent substrate–enzyme dissociation constant
K_p partition ratio
M moles/L
MAPK mitogen-activated protein kinase
mTOR mammalian target of rapamycin
NC-IUPHAR International Union of Basic and Clinical Pharmacology
NDA new drug application
NTP nucleoside triphosphate
P product
PAP 2-phenylaminopyrimidine
PDE phosphodiesterase
PDGFR platelet-derived growth factor receptor
Pi inorganic phosphate
PI3K phosphoinositide-3-kinase
PIP_3 phosphatidylinositol-3,4,5-triphosphate
PLP pyridoxal phosphate
PTP protein tyrosine phosphatases
RT reverse transcriptase
RTK receptor tyrosine kinases
S substrate
SAR structure-activity relationship
Ser195 residue 195 of the serine protease
STAMP specifically targeting the ABL myristoyl pocket
STAT signal transducer and activators of transcription
TKI tyrosine-kinase inhibitor
TLCK tosyl-lysyl-chloromethyl-ketone
TPCK tosyl-phenylalanyl-chloromethyl- ketone
3-TC 3-thiacytidine
TYK2 tyrosine kinase 2
v velocity or rate of enzyme reaction
VEGFR vascular endothelial growth factor receptor
V_{max} maximum velocity or rate of enzyme reaction

Introduction

Overview of Catalytic Receptors and Enzymes: A Perspective

The sequencing of the human genome has resulted in an explosive growth into the research and understanding of receptors. Furthermore, it has also spawned the adoption of select nomenclature to categorize receptors.[1] The International Union of Basic and Clinical Pharmacology (IUPHAR/BPS) Guide to Pharmacology works closely with the Human Genome Nominating Committee (HGNC) to standardize the receptor nomenclature. In elementary terms, a receptor may be defined as a biomacromolecule (protein, nucleic acid, polysaccharide, or lipid aggregate) that, on binding a ligand, results in some biological effect. Receptors may be present on the cell surface, be cytoplasmic or in extracellular fluid. Those present on the cell surface, on binding a ligand, transmit a signal, resulting in some cellular action. Catalytic receptors are specifically those cell-surface receptors whose binding to a ligand causes conformational changes, such as dimeric action or oligomerization, which results in a chemical reaction (usually phosphorylation) leading to activation of downstream signaling events. The IUPHAR/BPS has described four major catalytic receptors, which include many subtypes. The major catalytic receptors are the cytokine receptors, pattern recognition receptors, receptor guanyl cyclases, receptor kinases inclusive of the tyrosine kinase and serine/threonine kinases or tyrosine-like kinases.[1] Catalytic receptors have been subdivided based on their specific catalytic reaction, and there are five major transmembrane receptors with catalytic activity. These are the receptor tyrosine kinases (RTKs)—the largest group, which, on being activated by a ligand, dimerize and phosphorylate tyrosine residues on the cytosolic side of the receptor; the tyrosine phosphatases, which can dephosphorylate (or hydrolyze) phosphorylated tyrosine residues; tyrosine-associated receptor kinases (non-receptor tyrosine kinases) that phosphorylate cytosolic proteins; the receptor serine/threonine kinases, which can phosphorylate serine/threonine residues on cytosolic proteins; and the receptor guanylyl cyclases that catalyze the formation of cyclic guanosine monophosphate (cGMP) from guanosine triphosphate (GTP) on the cytosolic side to induce signaling. Various catalytic receptors[2] are briefly depicted in Figure 9.1. More general types of receptors, however, are the biological catalysts, which are more commonly known as enzymes, since they bind substrates (ligands) and in essence transmit a "biologic signal" through product formation of the chemical reaction being catalyzed, which results in some specific action. It is often the dysregulation of these receptors either through genetic mutation or through over-/underexpression that results in various disease states (eg, cancer, autoimmune disease, diabetes) as homeostasis gets disrupted and signaling mechanisms are compromised. During infections of the host, it is the expression or presence of foreign substances—proteins, lipids, nucleic acids, and other factors, that result in the pathogenesis. For either of these scenarios, in order to ameliorate the disease state, the design of molecules (drugs) to counterbalance the dysregulation or neutralize the pathogen has long been a continuous developmental strategy.

The concept of using small molecules that specifically target one or more enzymatic systems in the body is not new. Historically, compounds that were extracted from natural products have been used as medicinal agents. Subsequently, they have been shown to have their therapeutic effect by targeting certain systemic enzymes.[3] A classic example is the bark of the willow tree, known since ancient days to have antipyretic and analgesic effects. Its active ingredient, salicin, a glycoside, is metabolized in vivo to salicylic acid, which

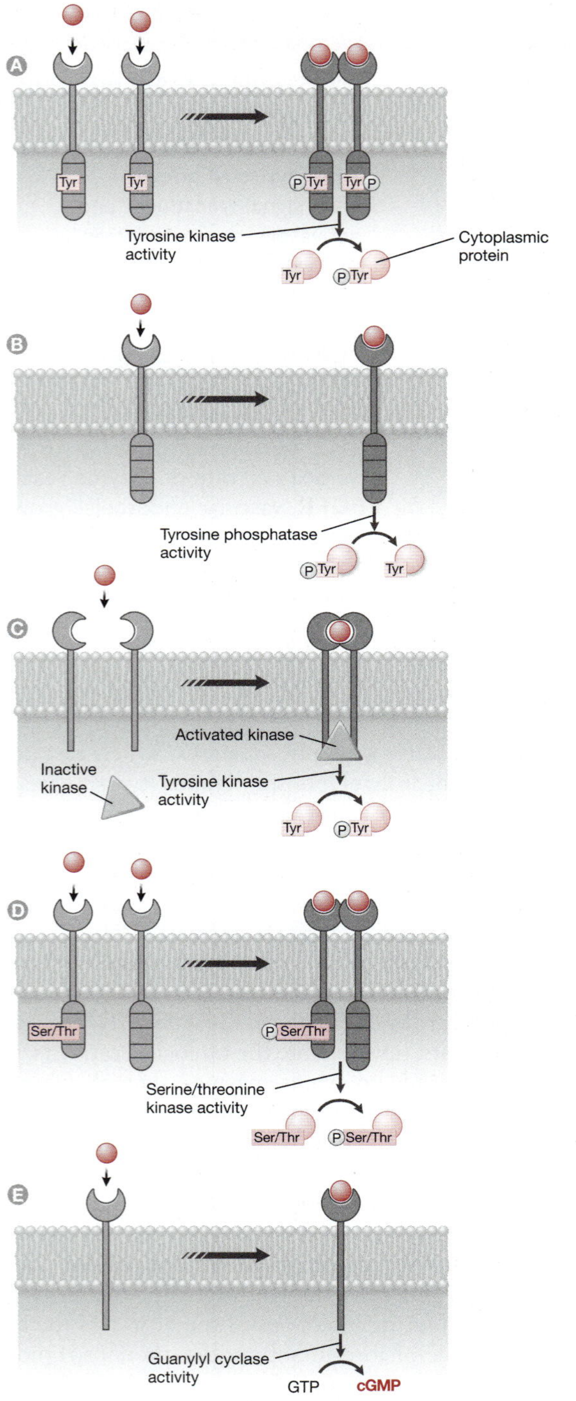

Figure 9.1 Major types of transmembrane receptors with linked enzymatic domains. A. The receptor tyrosine kinases. B. Tyrosine phosphatases. C. Tyrosine kinase-associated receptors. D. Receptor serine/threonine kinases. E. Receptor guanylyl cyclases. (Reprinted with permission from Golan DE, Armstrong EJ, Armstrong AW, eds. *Principles of Pharmacology: The Pathophysiologic Basis of Drug Therapy*. 4th ed. Wolters Kluwer; 2017:12.)

is a known inhibitor of cyclooxygenase, a key enzyme in the formation of prostaglandins, which are mediators of pain and fever. Similarly, physostigmine, isolated from the West African Calabar bean, was used as a treatment for glaucoma in the mid-1800s.

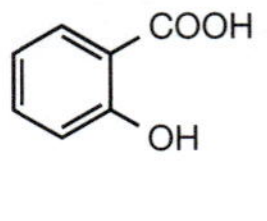

Salicylic acid

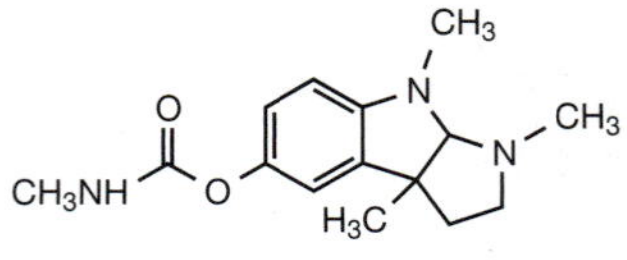

Physostigmine

Physostigmine's mechanism of action was only later determined to be inhibition of acetylcholinesterase.[3] Inhibition of acetylcholinesterase in the eye leads to improved drainage and, thus, a decrease in the intraocular pressure giving relief to glaucoma patients. It was only in the 20th century, with the concept of the "magic bullet" having selective toxicity, introduced by Ehrlich as a rational approach to chemotherapy,[4] that the concept of rational design and discovery of enzyme inhibitors followed. The discovery of the antibacterial activity of the azo dye prontosil in 1935 by Domagk,[4] and the subsequent explanation[5] of its metabolic reduction to sulfanilamide, an antimetabolite of *p*-aminobenzoic acid, in 1940 by Woods, finally paved the way for the rational design of enzyme inhibitors (Fig. 9.2). *p*-Aminobenzoic acid is an essential metabolite used in the bacterial synthesis of folic acid. Sulfanilamide, by its structural resemblance to *p*-aminobenzoic acid, competes for and selectively inhibits the bacterial enzyme dihydropteroate synthase (Fig. 9.3). In the absence of dihydropteroic acid, the bacteria are unable to synthesize tetrahydrofolic acid, an essential cofactor in one-carbon transfers that is involved in the de novo synthesis of purines and in the synthesis of thymidylate.

This concept of designing drugs as antimetabolites, or structural analogues of essential metabolites, became the hallmark for the development of enzyme inhibitors. This was especially important in cancer therapy during the early days of rational drug design.[6] As mechanisms of enzymes became better understood, the inhibitor design strategy grew more sophisticated, resulting in more potent and selective inhibitors being developed. The present-day focus on drug design through enzyme inhibition makes use of the antimetabolite theory as well as detailed kinetic and mechanistic information about the enzymatic pathways. These strategies use sophisticated assays, enzyme crystal structures and active site environments, site-directed mutagenesis experiments of catalytic residues of enzymes, and molecular docking experiments employing computers. It must be mentioned, however, that in the drug design process, designing a potent inhibitor of an enzyme is only the first step in the long and difficult process of drug development. Other factors, including pharmacokinetic profile of the inhibitor, toxicities

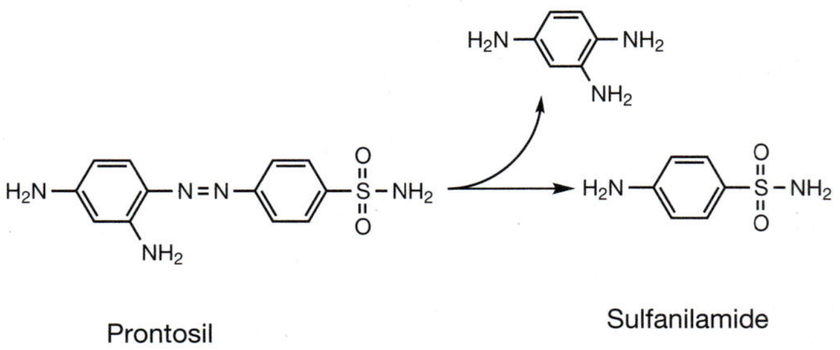

Figure 9.2 Metabolic reduction of prontosil to sulfanilamide.

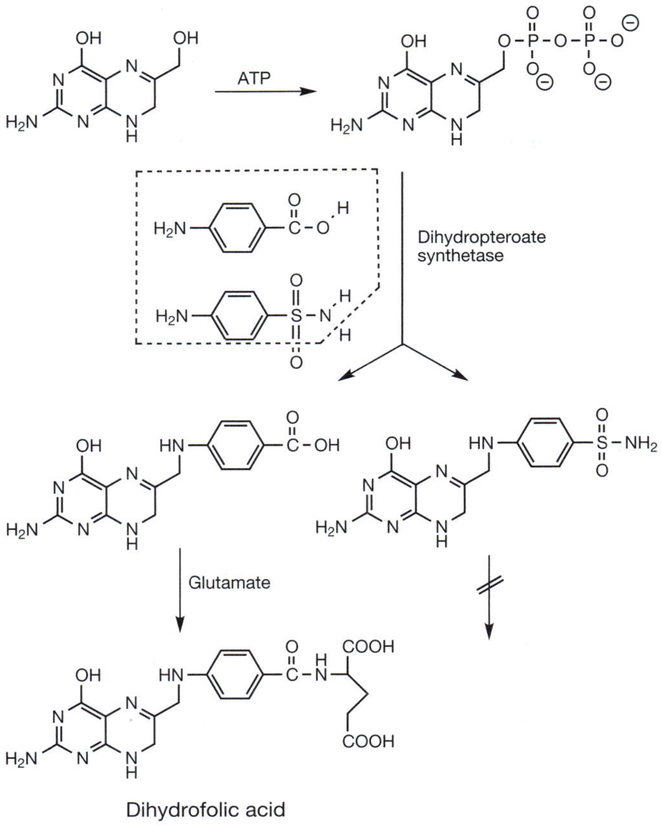

Figure 9.3 Metabolic pathway leading to dihydrofolic acid and its inhibition by sulfanilamide. This figure shows the structural resemblance to *p*-aminobenzoic acid.

and side effects, and animal and preclinical studies, must all be satisfactorily completed or addressed before the inhibitor can even enter clinical studies as a new drug candidate. Thus, even though an enormous amount of data exist regarding enzyme inhibitors, only a selected few turn out to be marketable drugs (Table 9.1).

The succeeding paragraphs provide an overview of enzymes as catalytic receptors and general concepts of enzyme inhibitors and their rational design into drugs, with selected examples. Enzymes catalyze chemical reactions involved in the biosynthesis and degradation of many cellular products. Moreover, all catalytic receptors have enzymatic activity and are involved in group transfer reactions with amino acid side chains on polypeptides, resulting in products that propagate a cellular signal. Historically, enzymes derive their name from Greek, where "enzyme" means "in yeast" and the term was used to distinguish the "whole" microorganism, such as yeast ("organized ferments"), from the "extracts" of the whole microorganisms ("unorganized ferments"). Although the vast majority of enzymes are proteins, certain nucleic acids (RNAs) also possess enzymatic activity (ie, ribozymes). Enzymes are the most efficient catalysts known in nature because they have the ability to enhance reaction rates by enormous factors.[7] Like all catalysts, enzymes have the ability to lower the activation energy of reactions, and the tremendous catalytic power they possess results from their inherent ability to provide stabilization to the reacting molecules at their activated complex states. From a preliminary enquiry, enzymatic rates for reactions in physiological solutions are limited by the diffusion rate constant of water.

Table 9.1 A Partial Listing of Enzyme Inhibitors Presently Used as Drugs

Inhibitor (Drug)	Enzyme Inhibited	Use	Organism
Caspofungin	1,3-β-Glucan synthase	Antifungal	Fungal
Trilostane	3-(or 17)β-Hydroxysteroid dehydrogenase	Breast cancer	Human
Sildenafil	3′,5′-Cyclic GMP phosphodiesterase	Erectile dysfunction	Human
Theophylline	3′,5′-Cyclic nucleotide phosphodiesterase	Asthma	Human
Nitisinone	4-Hydroxyphenylpyruvate dioxygenase	Tyrosinemia	Human
Finasteride	Steroid 5α-reductase	Benign prostatic hyperplasia	Human
Pyridostigmine	Acetylcholinesterase	Myasthenia gravis	Human
Pentostatin	Adenosine deaminase	Cancer	Human
Cycloserine	Alanine racemase	Tuberculosis	Bacterial
Fomepizole	Alcohol dehydrogenase	Alcoholism	Human
Disulfiram	Aldehyde dehydrogenase	Alcoholism	Human
Acarbose	α-Amylase	Diabetes	Human
Miglitol	α-Glucosidase	Diabetes	Human
Ethambutol	Arabinosyltransferase	Tuberculosis	Bacterial

(*continued*)

Table 9.1 A Partial Listing of Enzyme Inhibitor Presently Used as Drugs (*continued*)

Inhibitor (Drug)	Enzyme Inhibited	Use	Organism
Zileuton	Arachidonate 5-lipoxygenase	Inflammation	Human
Carbidopa	Aromatic l-amino acid decarboxylase	Parkinson disease	Human
Clavulanic acid	β-Lactamase	In combination with penicillins	Bacterial
Acetazolamide	Carbonate dehydratase (carbonic anhydrase)	Glaucoma	Human
Entacapone	Catechol O-methyltransferase	Parkinson disease	Human
Miglustat	Ceramide glucosyltransferase	Gaucher disease	Human
Methotrexate	Dihydrofolate reductase	Cancer	Human
Trimethoprim	Dihydrofolate reductase	Antibacterial	Bacterial
Sulfamethoxazole	Dihydropteroate synthase	Antibacterial	Bacterial
Topotecan	DNA topoisomerase	Cancer	Human
Ciprofloxacin	DNA gyrase	Antibacterial	Bacterial
Acyclovir	DNA-directed DNA polymerase	Antiviral (anti-HSV)	Viral
Rifampin	DNA-directed RNA polymerase	Antibacterial	Bacterial
Bacitracin	Dolichyl phosphatase	Antibacterial	Bacterial
Isoniazid	Fatty acid enoyl reductase	Tuberculosis	Bacterial
Oseltamivir	Viral neuraminidase	Anti-influenza	Viral
Fondaparinux	Factor Xa	Thrombosis	Human
Alendronate	Farnesyl-diphosphate farnesyltransferase	Osteoporosis	Human
Pyrazinamide	Mycobacterial fatty acid synthase	Tuberculosis	Bacterial
Valproic acid	Histone acetyltransferase	Seizures	Human
Nelfinavir	HIV protease	AIDS (anti-HIV)	Viral
Esomeprazole	H^+/K^+-ATPase	Gastroesophageal reflux disease	Human
Atorvastatin	HMG-CoA reductase	Hyperlipidemia	Human
Mycophenolate	IMP dehydrogenase	Immune suppression	Human
Propylthiouracil	Iodide peroxidase	Hyperthyroid	Human
Cilastatin	Renal dehydropeptidase	In combination with imipenem	Human
Eflornithine	Ornithine decarboxylase	Trypanosomes	Parasitic
Allopurinol	Xanthine oxidase	Gout	Human
Captopril	Peptidyl-dipeptidase A (angiotensin-converting enzyme)	Hypertension	Human
Pemetrexed	Phosphoribosylglycinamide formyltransferase	Cancer	Human
Aprotinin	Plasma kallikrein	Thrombosis	Human
Aminocaproic acid	Plasmin	Thrombosis	Human
Etodolac	Prostaglandin-endoperoxide synthase (cyclooxygenase)	Inflammation	Human
Bortezomib	Proteasome endopeptidase complex	Myeloma	Human

Table 9.1 A Partial Listing of Enzyme Inhibitor Presently Used as Drugs (*continued*)

Inhibitor (Drug)	Enzyme Inhibited	Use	Organism
Imatinib	Protein-tyrosine kinase	Cancer	Human
Gemcitabine	Ribonucleoside-diphosphate reductase	Cancer	Human
Ribavirin	IMP dehydrogenase	Antiviral (broad spectrum)	Viral
Azidothymidine	HIV reverse transcriptase	AIDS (anti-HIV)	Viral
Lamivudine	Reverse transcriptase	AIDS, hepatitis B	Viral
Penicillin	Serine-type d-Ala—Ala carboxypeptidase	Antibiotic	Bacterial
Digitoxin	Na^+/K^+-ATPase	Congestive heart failure	Human
Terbinafine	Squalene monooxygenase	Antifungal	Fungal
Itraconazole	Sterol 14 α-demethylase	Antifungal	Fungal
Lepirudin	Thrombin	Thrombosis	Human
Floxuridine	Thymidylate synthase	Cancer	Human
Orlistat	Triacylglycerol lipase	Obesity	Human
Metyrosine	Tyrosine 3-monooxygenase	Pheochromocytoma	Human
Fosfomycin	UDP-*N*-acetylglucosamine 1-carboxyvinyltransferase	Antibacterial	Bacterial
Aminoglutethimide	Monooxygenase	Breast cancer	Human
Acetohydroxamic acid	Urease	Gastritis	Bacterial
Dicumarol	Vitamin K epoxide reductase	Thrombosis	Human

Adapted from Robertson J. Mechanistic basis of enzyme-targeted drugs. *Biochemistry*. 2005;44:5561-5771, with permission. Copyright 2005. American Chemical Society.

This implies that the second-order rate constant of an enzyme (k_{cat}/K_m) is approximately 10^9 M^{-1} s^{-1} (diffusion rate constant of water),[8] a value that infers that every collision of a reactant molecule (substrate) with the enzyme leads to product formation. Because for many enzymes K_m (the Michaelis or apparent substrate–enzyme dissociation constant) values are in the micro- or sub-micromolar range (10^{-4} M), we can compute the k_{cat} (the catalytic or first-order rate constant) value to be approximately 10^5/s. Estimates9 for uncatalyzed reactions in water have ranged from 10^{-1} to 10^{-20}/s; thus, the rate enhancements for enzyme-catalyzed reactions over the noncatalyzed reaction (also referred to as the proficiency of an enzyme) can range from 10^6 to over 10^{25}—truly remarkable proficiencies. Moreover, enzymes display great specificity toward particular chemical bonds (bond specificity; eg, peptidases for peptide bonds) or functional groups (group specificity; eg, esterases for esters), or they display absolute specificity toward a single molecule (eg, carbonic anhydrase, which catalyzes the hydration of carbon dioxide or decomposition of carbonic acid). Furthermore, this specificity and catalytic proficiency is carried out, in most cases, at ambient temperatures and normal pressures in aqueous solutions.

Enzymes have been classified based on the type of reaction catalyzed, and six major classes (families) of enzymes, numbered from 1 to 6, have been assigned by the Enzyme Commission (EC) of the International Union of Biochemistry and Molecular Biology.[9] These classes are (1) oxidoreductases (eg, dehydrogenases), (2) transferases (group transfer enzymes; eg, kinases), (3) hydrolases (hydrolytic reactions; eg, esterases), (4) lyases (formation or removal of double bonds; eg, hydratase—addition of water across a double bond), (5) isomerases (eg, mutarotation of glucose by mutases), and (6) ligases (joining of two substrates at the expense of energy, also referred to as synthetases). All presently discovered enzymes are identified by the prefix EC followed by an Arabic numeral based on the major class of reaction catalyzed, as indicated earlier. Furthermore, this is followed by a series of three more Arabic numerals, which indicate the subclass (functionality), sub-subclass (specific bond type), and serial number of the enzyme in that class, respectively. For example, the enzyme, acetylcholinesterase has been assigned the following classification code: EC 3.1.1.7. In this example, the numeral 3 indicates that this enzyme belongs to the family of hydrolases, the first 1 indicates that the nature of the bond being hydrolyzed is an ester, the second 1 indicates that specific ester bond is a carboxylic acid ester, and the last number is the serial number of this enzyme in this sub-subclass.

Many enzymes make use of cofactors, which enable them to carry out the catalysis. These small molecules (including ions) are intimately bound to the enzyme and are essential to the functioning of the enzyme. As macromolecular receptors, enzymes have the inherent ability to bind ligands (substrates). In effecting the transformation of these substrates to products (catalyzing the chemical reaction), enzymes use all the necessary tools in the chemical bonding arsenal to hold these substrates extremely tightly as the transformation occurs. Because all chemical reactions require bond breakage and formation, the substrate must go through a transition state, or an "activated complex," which is a destabilizing event because bonds are being polarized and there is partial charge development. It is the inherent ability of the enzyme to greatly stabilize such activated complexes that give them their role in nature and allows their phenomenal catalytic power.

Pauling first proposed the stabilization theory of the activated complex by enzymes.[10] He concluded that the active site of the enzyme is complementary to the structure of the activated complex so that the binding of the enzyme to the activated complex is extremely tight. The ability to stabilize such complexes and correspondingly reduce the activation energy of the reaction and, thus, enhance the reaction rate is caused by many factors, both noncovalent and covalent.[11] Noncovalent influences include entropic effects, such as proximity and orientation; restricted motion, where enzymes, by their evolvement, have the inherent ability to bring reacting molecules closer together and in the correct orientation for bonds to form; desolvation effects, to strip solvent (water) molecules from the reactants; transition-state electrostatic stabilization, to stabilize the partial charges being developed in the activated complex; induced-fit effects, in which the flexibility of the enzyme can accommodate the substrate, intermediate, and/or product; strain and distortion effects, to increase the reactivity of compounds; and many other such ancillary effects. Moreover, covalent influences (effects) also play a vital role in the enzyme's catalytic role. "Covalent effects" imply a covalent bond being made by the enzyme (or its cofactor) to the substrate being transformed. These covalent effects would include general acid-base catalysis, in which amino acid residues partake in the overall reaction through proton donation (general acid) or proton abstraction (general base), as well as nucleophilic and electrophilic catalysis, in which there is bond formation with an amino acid side-chain residue (or cofactor) to the substrate.

It should be mentioned here that "covalent catalysis" has traditionally implied a group transfer reaction between one substrate and another being facilitated through an enzyme-residue intermediate (eg, the enzyme sucrose phosphorylase transfers a glucose residue from sucrose to phosphate giving the products glucose-1-phosphate and fructose through an enzyme-glucosyl intermediate). Many amino acid side-chain residues (ie, acidic and basic amino acids, eg, Asp, Glu, His, Lys, Arg, Tyr, and Cys) and nucleophilic amino acid residues allow such covalent effects. Recent analysis of enzyme rate enhancements has postulated that noncovalent effects allow an increase of as many as 11 orders of magnitude over the noncatalyzed reaction, whereas for those enzymes with rate enhancements exceeding 11 orders of magnitude (over noncatalyzed reactions), it is covalent catalysis in the transition state that accounts for this exceptional increase in rate enhancement.[12]

Noncovalent effects like proximity and orientation may be explained on the basis that enzymes have the inherent ability to affect the order of reactions by the "effective concentration" principle—for example, to change a second-order reaction to a first-order one by bringing the reacting molecules closer to each other so that there is a lower amount of entropic loss for the reacting substrates. In the example shown in Figure 9.4, which is taken from physical-organic chemical studies,[13,14] one can consider the hydrolysis of a nitrophenyl ester by an amine in two scenarios: reaction (A), with two individual molecules reacting (ie, amine and ester), versus reaction (B), with a single molecule having an "in-built" amine on the ester molecule. If the reaction rate constants are compared (one needs to keep in mind that we are comparing a first-order rate constant for [B], with a second-order rate constant for [A], which may not be a true comparison because mechanisms are likely to be different), however, one finds that the first-order rate reaction (reaction [B]) has a rate enhancement over the reaction [A] by a factor of ~5,000 M attributed to the fact that reaction [A] needs to give up more degrees of freedom (as compared to reaction [B]) to react (ie, form productive collision complexes, leading to product formation). This proximity effect indicates that by using such a system (bringing the reacting centers closer to each other), one can effectively increase the concentration of the reactants by this factor, resulting in a faster reaction. This enhancement factor of 5,000 M (ie, effectively changing a second-order reaction to that of a first-order one)

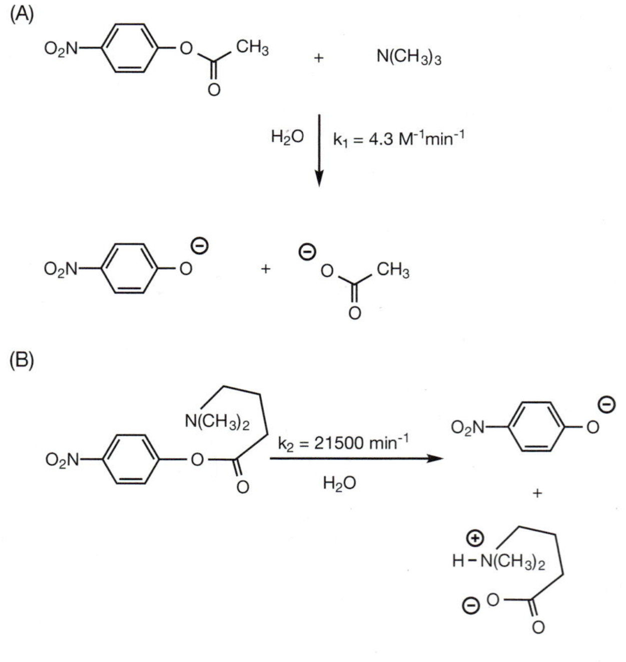

Figure 9.4 Concept of proximity and effective concentration. A. A second order reaction. B. A first order reaction.

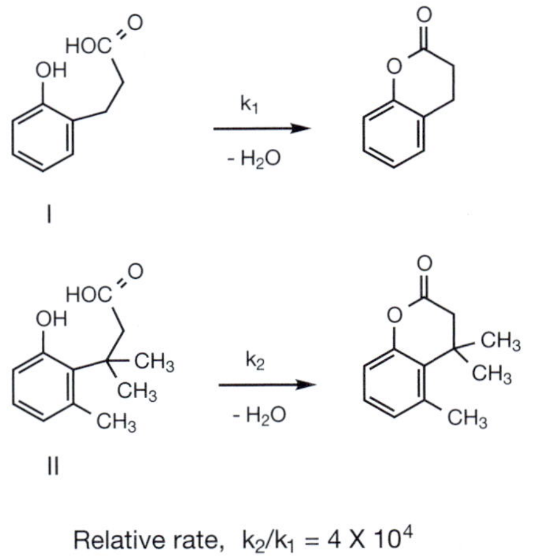

Figure 9.5 Concept of orientation.

has been termed the "effective concentration" because this is an unrealistic increase in the concentration of the reactants, which gives rise to the higher rate constant (ie, it is impossible to make a solution of 5,000 M of the reactants—consider the concentration of water is only 55 M).

The next example, which is shown in Figure 9.5, illustrates that besides the proximity factor, one can also use "orientation" effects to bring about an increase in the reaction rate constant.[14] For example, as shown in Figure 9.5, one may use alkyl groups to sterically hinder rotation about single bonds, effectively freezing the molecule in a particular conformation to provide maximum orbital overlap for bonding. Thus, using a "dimethyl lock" system in molecule II, which restricts rotation, ensures that lactonization for molecule II is faster by a factor of 4×10^4 than molecule I. Both of these effects, proximity and orientation, are thought to be part of an enzyme's arsenal of tools in allowing enzymes to lower the activation energy for reactions.

Other noncovalent effects, such as desolvation of the reactant molecules, can also be effectively achieved by enzymes. Enzymes have the capacity, by lining their exterior and/or interior surfaces with appropriately situated hydrophobic amino acids, to effectively strip away water molecules from substrates as they enter into the active site of the enzyme through such channels. Thus, no further expense of energy is required to desolvate the substrate before the reaction.

As mentioned previously, enzymes also use covalent chemistry as a means to effect catalysis. Indeed, it has been recently postulated that covalent chemistry plays a far greater role in enzyme catalysis than previously thought.[12] Nucleophilic catalysis by hydrolytic enzymes, such as the serine proteases or esterases, is a classic example of covalent effects in enzyme catalysis. In such systems, for example, as in the case of the serine protease chymotrypsin, which hydrolyzes peptide bonds containing aromatic amino acids (eg, phenylalanine and tyrosine), the covalent effects occur at the level of general acid, general base, and nucleophilic covalent catalysis. Figure 9.6 illustrates an accepted mechanism for such enzymes. It should be noted that all serine proteases contain a "catalytic triad" of the amino acids, designated as Ser195, His57, and Asp102 (numerals represent the amino acid position in the protein primary structure), which are present in the active sites of these proteases. The catalysis is effected by making the hydroxyl functionality of the serine residue more nucleophilic for attack at the carbonyl center of the peptide bond. One should recall that in general, hydroxyl groups have pK_a values in the range of greater than 14 and, as such, are not acidic and unable to ionize at physiologic pH. Because of catalytic triad, however, the proton from the serine-hydroxyl group is transferred to the aspartate residue

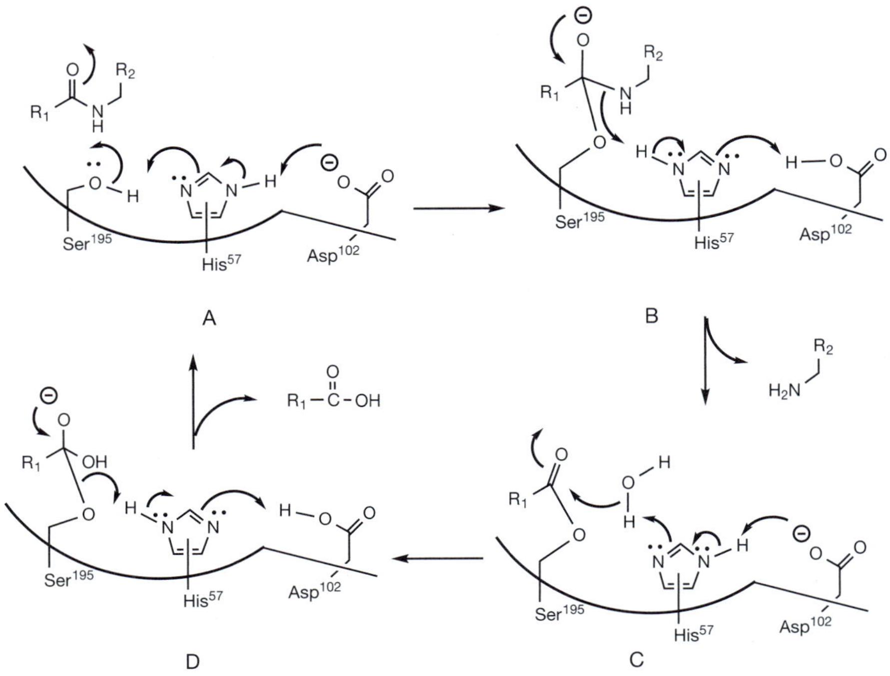

Figure 9.6 Acid, base, and nucleophilic covalent catalysis by chymotrypsin.

through the histidine residue in a "charge relay system" such that the serine-hydroxyl group can be made into the highly nucleophilic alkoxide ion. This is achieved by the aspartate residue acting as a general base to pick up the proton from histidine, which also can abstract a proton from the serine-hydroxyl group (see A in Fig. 9.6). Thus, histidine behaves as a tautomeric catalyst in this enzyme (ie, acts as both a general acid and a general base) and, in essence, relays the proton from serine to aspartate. The serine (as its alkoxide) is now a much more powerful nucleophile and can attack the peptidyl carbonyl group to generate a "tetrahedral oxy-anion intermediate" (see B in Fig. 9.6), which collapses to liberate a new amino terminus of the peptide and the acylated serine enzyme (see C in Fig. 9.6). The next part of the reaction involves a water molecule (which also is made more nucleophilic by a similar mechanism; see C in Fig. 9.6) that goes on to hydrolyze, through a tetrahedral intermediate (see D in Fig. 9.6), the serine-acyl bond to liberate the new carboxyl terminus of the peptide (R_1COOH) and the free enzyme, which can be recycled for another round of catalysis.

Knowledge of the mechanisms and interactions, both noncovalent and covalent, that allow enzymes to function as such efficient catalysts provides the medicinal chemist with insights to design molecules that achieve selective inhibition of the enzyme. Such knowledge also paves the way to the design and discovery of drugs.

General Concepts of Enzyme Inhibition

The body is composed of thousands of different enzymes, many of them acting in concert to maintain homeostasis. Although disease states may arise from the malfunctioning of a particular enzyme, or the introduction of a foreign enzyme through infection by microorganisms, inhibiting a specific enzyme to alleviate a disease state is a challenging process. Most bodily functions occur through a cascade of enzymatic systems, and it becomes extremely difficult to design a drug molecule that can selectively inhibit an enzyme and result in a therapeutic benefit. To address the problem, however, the basic mechanism of enzyme action needs to be understood. Once knowledge of a particular enzymatic pathway is determined and the mechanism and kinetics are worked out, the challenge is then to design a suitable inhibitor that is selectively used by the enzyme causing its inhibition.

As outlined, enzymes (E) represent the best-known chemical catalysts because they are uniquely designed to carry out specific chemical reactions in a highly efficient manner.[8,11] They initially act by binding a substrate (S) to form an enzyme-substrate complex [E·S], which undergoes specific chemistry (catalysis) to give the enzyme-product complex [E·P], followed by dissociation of product (P) and free enzyme (E). Equation 9.1 represents a simplified version of this scenario:

Eq. 9.1 $$E + S \underset{}{\overset{K_d\ (or\ K_m)}{\rightleftharpoons}} [E \cdot S] \overset{k_{cat}}{\rightleftharpoons} [E \cdot P] \rightleftharpoons E + P$$

where K_d is the enzyme-substrate dissociation constant and k_{cat} represents the rate constant for the catalytic step (chemical modification step or slowest step in the overall pathway). If the binding step of E + S to form [E·S] is relatively fast as compared to the catalytic step and one assumes steady-state conditions, then K_m, the Michaelis constant (the substrate concentration at half-maximum velocity $[V_{max}/2]$) may be equated to the K_d, as shown in Equation 9.2:

Eq. 9.2 $$\text{Michaelis – Menten equation}: v = \frac{V_{max}[S]}{K_m + [S]}$$

$$\text{Lineweaver – Burk equation}: \frac{1}{v} = \frac{K_m}{V_{max}} \times \frac{1}{[S]} + \frac{1}{V_{max}}$$

where v is the velocity of the reaction.

The rate of the reaction can then be derived in terms of K_m and V_{max} (or $k_{cat} = V_{max}/[E]$). From the knowledge of the dissociation constant ($K_{m[d]}$) and the rate constant for catalysis (k_{cat}), it is then possible to compare inhibitors and the dissociation constant for the inhibitors, K_i, in relation to the natural substrates and the effect on the catalytic rates. These kinetic parameters, k_{cat} and $K_{m(d)}$ (or K_i), can then give an indication as to the affinity (K_i vs $K_{m[d]}$) and specificity (k_{cat}/K_i or $k_{cat}/K_{m[d]}$) of the inhibitor for a particular enzyme. Equations 9.3a and b represent the general scheme of reversible inhibition, competitive and noncompetitive, respectively, and Figure 9.7 illustrates graphically and mathematically the relationship of the velocity of the enzyme

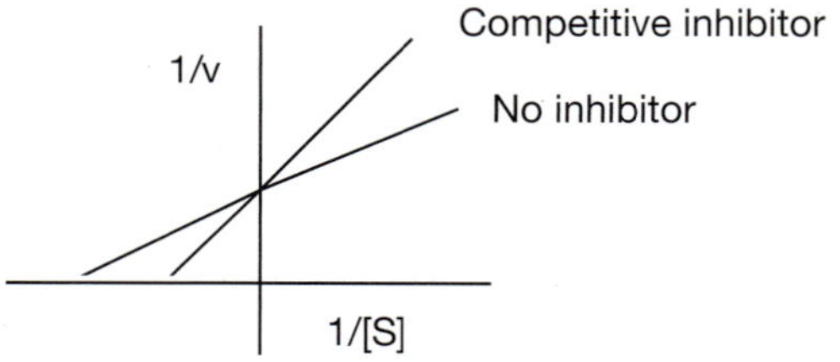

$$v = \frac{V_{max}}{1 + (K_m/[S])\,(1 + [I]/K_i)}$$

(K_m increases, V_{max} unchanged)

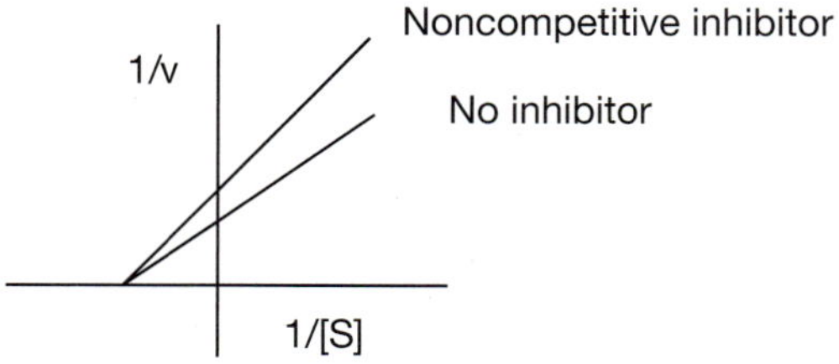

$$v = \frac{V_{max}/(1 + [I]/k_i)}{1 + (K_m/[S])}$$

(K_m unchanged, V_{max} decreases)

Figure 9.7 Graphic representation of competitive and noncompetitive enzyme inhibition.

reaction to the substrate [S] and inhibitor [I] concentration as well as the kinetic parameters K_m, K_i, and V_{max} (or $k_{cat} = V_{max}/[E]$):

Eq. 9.3a

$$E + S \underset{}{\overset{K_m}{\rightleftharpoons}} [E \cdot S] \overset{k_{cat}}{\rightleftharpoons} E + P$$

$$E + I \overset{K_i}{\rightleftharpoons} [E \cdot I] \rightarrow P$$

Inhibition of enzymes may be broadly classified under two categories—reversible and irreversible inhibitors—as shown in Equation 9.4:

Eq. 9.3b

$$\begin{array}{ccccc} E + S & \overset{K_m}{\rightleftharpoons} & [E \cdot S] & \overset{I}{\rightleftharpoons} & \\ & & & & [ESI] \\ E + I & \overset{K_i}{\rightleftharpoons} & [E \cdot I] & \overset{S}{\rightleftharpoons} & \end{array}$$

Eq. 9.4

$$E + I \overset{K_i}{\rightleftharpoons} [E \cdot I] \quad \text{(Reversible inhibition)}$$

$$E + I \overset{K_i}{\rightleftharpoons} E - I \quad \text{(Irreversible inhibition)}$$

In the presence of inhibitor, the enzyme-substrate complex, [E·S], is replaced by the enzyme-inhibitor complex, [E·I], which may block or retard the formation of product. In the presence of a reversible inhibitor, the enzyme is tied up and the reaction, retarded or stopped; however, the enzyme can be subsequently regenerated from the enzyme-inhibitor complex, [E·I], to react again with substrate and produce product (see Equation 9.3). On the other hand, irreversible inhibition implies that the enzyme cannot be regenerated, and the only way for catalysis to proceed would be if new molecules of the enzyme are generated from gene transcription and translation. Irreversible inhibition is commonly associated with covalent bond formation between inhibitor and enzyme [E—I], which *cannot* be easily broken and often is defined as a time-dependent loss of enzyme activity. Reversible inhibition, on the other hand, does not necessarily imply noncovalent bond formation. In many instances, reversible inhibition can occur through covalent bond formation, but these bonds can be hydrolyzed to regenerate free enzyme and inhibitor. Thus, for a reversible enzyme inhibitor, there is no time-dependent loss of activity, and enzyme activity can always be recovered. There are instances when reversible inhibition tends to look kinetically like irreversible inhibition. This scenario results whenever there is a tight binding of a reversible inhibitor to the enzyme; consequently, the dissociation of the enzyme from this enzyme-inhibitor complex is extremely slow. Kinetically, it is extremely difficult to distinguish this type of inhibition from an irreversible inhibitor because over time, the enzyme does tend to look like it loses its activity and, for all practical purposes, the enzyme behaves as if it were irreversibly tied up. To differentiate between tight-binding reversible and irreversible inhibitors, one can dialyze the enzyme-inhibitor complex. In case of the reversible inhibitor, on dialysis, the inhibitor will be removed from the enzyme, resulting in recovery of the enzyme activity; however, this is not so with the irreversible one.

Reversible Enzyme Inhibition

Reversible enzyme inhibition may be classified under two main headings, competitive and noncompetitive, with both following Michaelis-Menten kinetics. Competitive inhibition, by definition, requires that the inhibitor competes with the substrate for binding to the enzyme at the active site, and this binding is mutually exclusive. That is, if the inhibitor binds to the enzyme, the substrate will not be able to bind, and vice versa. Competitive inhibition also, however, suggests that the inhibition can be reversed in the presence of saturating amounts of substrate, because in this case, all enzyme active sites will be occupied by substrate-displacing inhibitor. In contrast, noncompetitive inhibition implies independent binding (ie, both inhibitor and substrate may bind to the enzyme at different sites). Because binding of the inhibitor to the enzyme is at a site other than the active site, noncompetitive inhibition cannot be reversed by increasing the concentration of substrate. Graphing the kinetics of inhibition (Fig. 9.7), the Lineweaver-Burk plot of $1/V$ versus $1/[S]$ shows distinguishing characteristics between the two types of inhibition. In competitive inhibition, there is no change in the maximum velocity of the reaction (V_{max}; the intercept on the *y*-axis remains constant in the presence of inhibitor). However, the slope of the curve (K_m/V_{max}) is different with the inhibitor present, and K_m changes because of the presence of the competitive inhibitor (see Fig. 9.7, competitive inhibition). In the case of noncompetitive inhibition, only the V_{max} of the reaction decreases, while the K_m remains unchanged (intercept on the *x*-axis unchanged with inhibitor; see Fig. 9.7, noncompetitive inhibition).

Most of the rationally designed and clinically useful reversible inhibitors are competitive inhibitors. Table 9.1 gives a listing of several currently approved drugs that act as enzyme inhibitors. The majority of enzyme inhibitors generally bear some structural resemblance to the natural substrate of the enzyme. The design of such inhibitors would thus seem to be a logical and rational task, which is uniquely suited to the medicinal chemist who can use the principles of bioisosteric modification of natural enzyme substrates and metabolites, or modification of "lead" structures and structure-activity relationships, to create selective and potent inhibitors. There are pitfalls in this endeavor, however, because even the most rationally designed drug must still overcome transport and other cellular barriers before exerting its effects. In the case of the noncompetitive inhibitors, the design is not as straightforward. These inhibitors can have widely differing structures, which in many instances bear no resemblance to the natural substrate. In general, inhibitors of the noncompetitive type have been obtained primarily through random screening of chemically novel molecules followed by further synthetic manipulation of the pharmacophore to optimize their inhibitory effects.

Examples of Reversible Inhibitors

The design of enzyme inhibitors has included random screening of synthetic chemical agents, natural products, and combinatorial libraries followed by molecular optimization or structure-activity relationships of so-called lead structures as well as bio-isosteric analogues of the enzyme substrates themselves. Drugs (eg, finasteride) also have been developed for one indication but, based on observed side effects, have led to other uses.

The rational approach in the design of enzyme inhibitors is greatly aided if the enzymatic reaction is characterized in terms of its kinetic mechanism. Such a characterization would include the knowledge of the kinetic parameters (rate constants and dissociation constants) of individual steps in the overall reaction pathway as well as the characterization of (any) intermediates involved in these individual steps. Examples of such "rational" inhibitors include both reversible and irreversible inhibitors of enzymes.

USES OF FINASTERIDE

Finasteride (Proscar), an inhibitor of steroid 5α-reductase, an enzyme involved in the catalytic reduction of testosterone to dihydrotestosterone, was originally developed as an agent to treat prostate hyperplasia. In addition to this original use, finasteride is also indicated as an agent (Propecia) to stimulate hair growth for treatment of male pattern baldness. This benefit was recognized as a useful side effect during clinical trials of finasteride as an antiprostate agent.

Antimetabolites

Antimetabolites are agents that interfere with the functioning of an essential metabolite and that most often are designed as structural analogues of the natural metabolite. As described earlier, the mechanism of action of sulfanilamide is that of a competitive inhibitor of *p*-aminobenzoic acid. In the case of sulfanilamide, however, the mechanism was only determined after the bacterial inhibitory action was noted. This often is the case when a drug is discovered to have a certain therapeutic effect and, later, this effect is "rationalized" as being caused by an enzyme-inhibitory action. Other classic examples of a competitive inhibitor acting as an antimetabolite include a number of nucleoside analogues used as antiviral and anticancer agents. These agents again bear structural resemblance to natural nucleosides, which in their triphosphate form are substrates for nucleic acid polymerases involved in the synthesis of nucleic acids. Nucleic acid polymerases catalyze the condensation of the free 3′-hydroxy end of a nucleic acid with an incoming 5′-triphosphate derivative of a nucleoside (dNTP), resulting in a 3′,5′-phosphodiester linkage. Hence, nucleoside analogues, to compete with the natural substrate in the synthesis of nucleic acid, must be converted intracellularly to their mono-, di-, and finally, triphosphate derivative before exerting their inhibitory effects on nucleic acid synthesis. Certain drug design strategies incorporate a "masked" phosphate group on the nucleoside such that once absorbed, they enter into the systemic circulation as the monophosphate.[15] The majority of these analogues are designed such that they lack the 3′-hydroxy group and are dideoxy derivatives of the natural substrate. These analogues thus ensure that once they are incorporated into nucleic acid, further extension of the nucleic acid is prevented because of the lack of a 3′-hydroxy group.

INHIBITION OF HIV-REVERSE TRANSCRIPTASE

***Azidothymidine* (AZT).** The advent of AIDS stimulated a great interest in designing inhibitors against the essential viral polymerase—HIV-reverse transcriptase (HIV-RT). AZT is a potent inhibitor of HIV-RT,[16] the retroviral polymerase that catalyzes the formation of proviral DNA from viral RNA. Structurally, AZT is similar to the natural nucleoside thymidine but has an azide group ($-N_3$) rather than a hydroxy group (–OH) at the 3′-position of the sugar deoxyribose (Fig. 9.8).

AZT is activated intracellularly to its triphosphate and competes with thymidine triphosphate for uptake by HIV-RT into DNA.[17] Once incorporated, further chain extension of the DNA is prevented because there is no 3′-hydroxyl group to continue the DNA synthesis. In this fashion, AZT is an effective chain terminator of viral DNA synthesis.

Dideoxycytidine (ddC [Zalcitabine]) and 3-thiacytidine (3-TC [Lamivudine]). 2′,3′-Dideoxycytidine is another antiretroviral agent used against HIV-RT. In this case, ddC resembles the natural metabolite, deoxycytidine (dC), and as in the case of AZT, it is a 3′-deoxy analogue of dC, where the 3′-OH group of dC is replaced by a hydrogen atom. Similarly, 3-TC is another anti-HIV agent that resembles dC. In this example, however, rather than replacing the 3′-hydroxyl functionality as in ddC, the 3′-carbon position of the sugar has been substituted by a sulfur atom. Since the early development of these reverse transcriptase inhibitors, many more have since been designed and marketed.

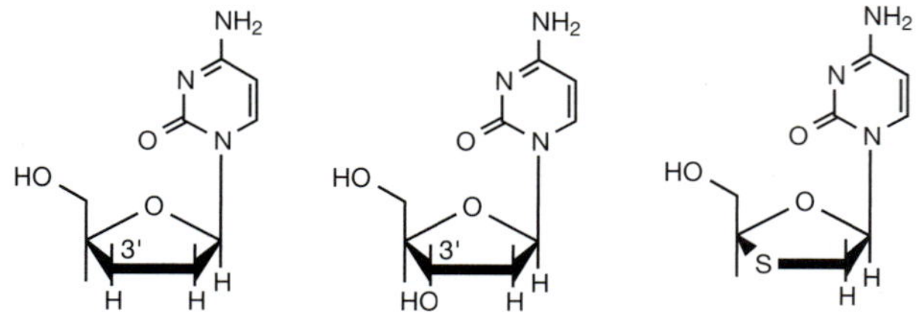

ddC dC 3-TC

HISTORICAL DEVELOPMENT OF AZIDOTHYMIDINE

Interestingly, AZT was originally synthesized as an anticancer agent to inhibit cellular DNA synthesis, but it was found to be too toxic. Subsequently, in the mid-1980s, during a random screening of nucleoside agents for potential inhibitory effects against HIV-RT, AZT was found to have selectivity for HIV-RT.[16] As such, its effects on host cell polymerases result in its dose-limiting bone marrow toxicity.

Nevirapine. An example of a potent noncompetitive inhibitor of HIV-RT is the drug nevirapine, a benzodiazepine analogue,[18] which is extremely tight-binding to the enzyme, having a K_i in the nanomolar range. As can be seen in the structure of nevirapine, the drug bears no resemblance to any of the natural nucleotide substrates and was discovered through a random screening program.

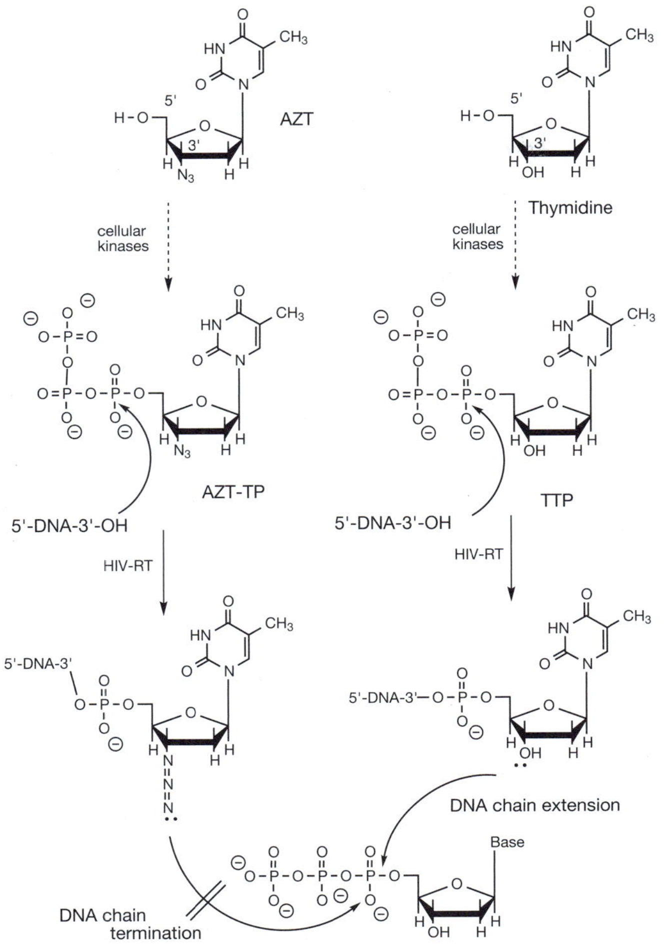

Figure 9.8 Activation, incorporation, and chain-terminating action of azidothymidine (AZT), a thymidine analogue, as a reversible inhibitor of human immunodeficiency virus-reverse transcriptase (HIV-RT).

X-ray crystallographic studies of HIV-RT complexed with nevirapine have shown it binding in a hydrophobic pocket at a site adjacent to and slightly overlapping the nucleotide-binding site of HIV-RT.[19] Kinetic studies with the enzyme have revealed an extremely slow binding rate for the drug; however, once bound, the polymerization rate for the reaction is effectively reduced.[20]

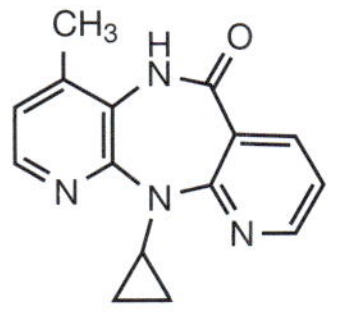

Nevirapine

A drawback for nevirapine, however, is that the virus can develop resistance very rapidly, through mutation of the amino acid residues in the binding pocket.[20,21] Thus, its usefulness is limited to combination therapy with other antiretroviral agents rather than single-drug therapy.

Reversible Inhibitors Used in Cancer Therapy

The design of several anticancer agents has been based on the antimetabolite theory. Because cancer results in overproliferation and uncontrolled cell growth, drugs designed against cancer have been based on inhibiting DNA synthesis in the cell. Thus, these drugs have been targeted against those enzymes, including nucleic acid polymerases, thymidylate synthase, and dihydrofolate reductase (DHFR), that play a role in DNA synthesis. Examples of drugs that have been designed against nucleic acid polymerases include cytosine arabinoside (Ara-C) and 5-fluorouracil (5-FU) (Fig. 9.9). Cytosine arabinoside is first converted to its triphosphate, and as such, it functions as an antimetabolite of deoxycytidine triphosphate (deoxy CTP) to inhibit DNA polymerase. As can be seen from its structure, Ara-C is the arabino isomer of cytidine. That is, the 2′-hydroxyl functionality in Ara-C is in the arabino configuration rather than the ribo configuration of cytidine. Because of this stereochemical change in the placement of the 2′-hydroxyl function, Ara-C tends to resemble deoxycytidine rather than cytidine. In this way, Ara-C inhibits DNA polymerases by competing with deoxycytidine. 5-FU is an analogue of the pyrimidine base uracil, where the hydrogen at the 5-position in uracil has been substituted by an isosteric fluorine (F) atom. This makes 5-FU look very similar to uracil. 5-FU, after conversion to 5-fluorodeoxyuridine monophosphate (FdUMP), is an inhibitor of thymidylate synthase, the enzyme involved in the de novo synthesis of thymidylate. In this case, FdUMP is an antimetabolite of deoxyuridine monophosphate.

Methotrexate is a potent inhibitor of DHFR, the enzyme responsible for the reduction of folic acid to dihydro- and

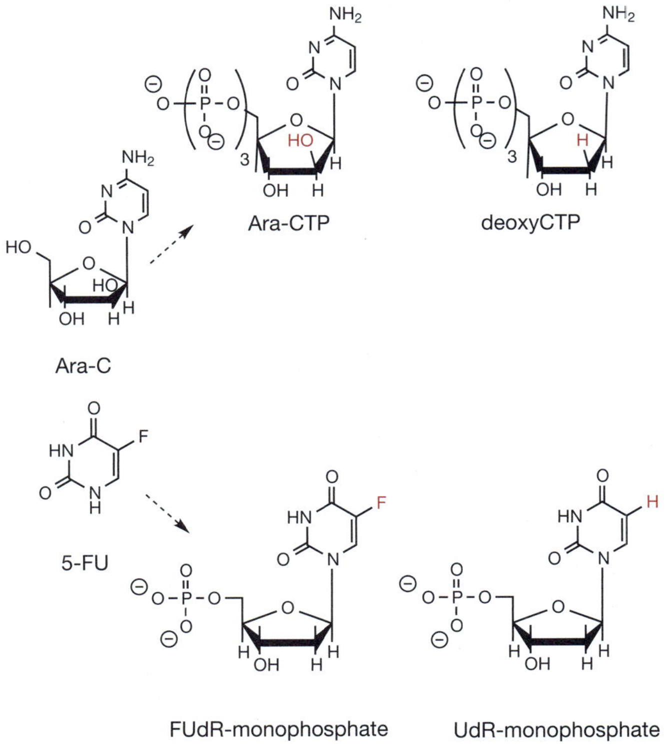

Figure 9.9 Structures of pyrimidine antimetabolites used in cancer chemotherapy.

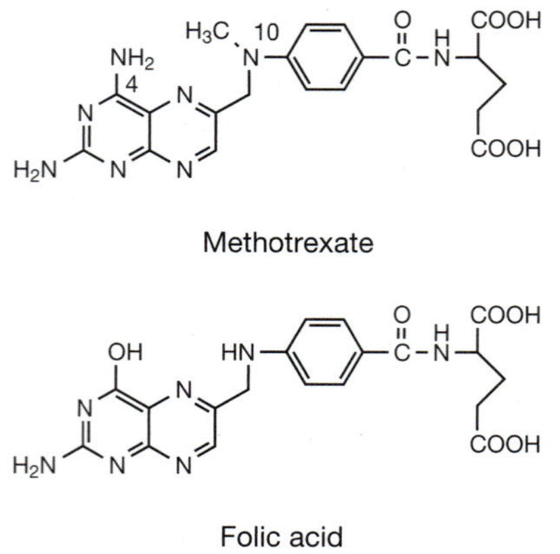

Figure 9.10 Methotrexate, the antimetabolite of folic acid.

tetrahydrofolic acid, precursors to one-carbon donation in purine and pyrimidine de novo synthesis. Methotrexate is an analogue of folic acid where the 4-hydroxyl group (–OH) on the pteridine ring of folic acid has been replaced by an amino ($-NH_2$) functionality and the nitrogen atom at the 10-position is methylated (Fig. 9.10). These substitutions led to methotrexate having an affinity for DHFR orders of magnitude greater than that for the natural metabolite, folic acid, and allow it to be an extremely potent inhibitor.

Inhibition of Acetylcholinesterase

Acetylcholinesterase (AChE) is the enzyme that catalyzes the catabolism of the neurotransmitter acetylcholine to acetate and choline. Thus, inhibition of AChE would lead to increased concentrations of acetylcholine and a prolonged action of the neurotransmitter. Inhibitors of AChE have found use in cases of myasthenia gravis, glaucoma, and Alzheimer disease. To appreciate the design of these inhibitors, it is useful to first understand the mechanism of action of AChE. AChE has an anionic site that can bind the positively charged quaternary ammonium group of the choline functionality and an active esteratic site that contains a nucleophilic serine residue involved in the hydrolysis of the ester bond (Fig. 9.11). The mechanism involves the attack of the nucleophilic serine hydroxy group on the carbonyl

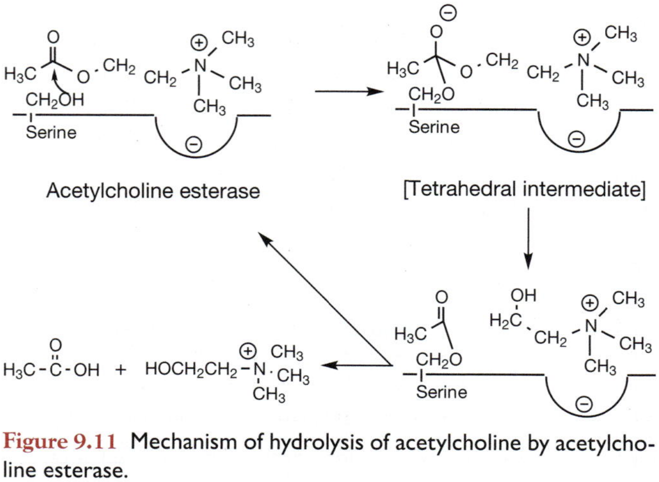

Figure 9.11 Mechanism of hydrolysis of acetylcholine by acetylcholine esterase.

group of acetylcholine to form a tetrahedral intermediate that breaks down, resulting in the release of choline and an intermediate, acetylated serine that subsequently hydrolyzes to release AChE.

Physostigmine has been used in the treatment of glaucoma. It is an alkaloid with a carbamate moiety that resembles the ester linkage of acetylcholine. Being an alkaloid, it is protonated at physiological pH and, thus, can bind to the anionic site of AChE. Following the mechanism of AChE, the serine residue of the enzyme can attack the carbonyl group of physostigmine, and in the process, the serine is carbamylated (Fig. 9.12). This carbamyl serine intermediate is more stable to enzymatic hydrolysis than is acetylated serine, and subsequent hydrolysis by water occurs extremely slowly. The carbamylated enzyme is only slowly regenerated, with a half-life of 38 minutes—more than seven orders of magnitude slower than that for the natural substrate, acetylcholine. This is an example of a reversible inhibitor involved in covalent bond formation with the enzyme that ultimately gets hydrolyzed.

Inhibitors of Angiotensin-Converting Enzyme

Angiotensin-converting enzyme (ACE) is a carboxypeptidase having a zinc ion as a cofactor and is involved in the renin-angiotensin cascade of blood pressure control.[22] The design of the antihypertensive drug captopril, a clinically important and potent reversible inhibitor of ACE, is an example of one of the early endeavors and successes of a rationally designed enzyme inhibitor (see Chapter 17). The design of captopril was based on several factors. These included the knowledge that ACE was similar in its enzymatic mechanism to carboxypeptidase A, except that ACE cleaved off a dipeptide, whereas carboxypeptidase A cleaved single amino acid residues from the carboxyl end of the protein; the discovery of l-benzylsuccinic acid as a potent inhibitor of carboxypeptidase A; and, studies of a potent pentapeptide inhibitor of ACE, $BPP_5\alpha$ (Glu-Lys-Trp-Ala-Pro), from the venom of the Brazilian viper (*Bothrops jararaca*), which showed that the N-terminal peptide fragments, including tetra-, tri-, and dipeptide fragments (Ala-Pro) of $BPP_5\alpha$, retained some inhibitory activity. Benzylsuccinic acid has been described as a by-product inhibitor of carboxypeptidase A, wherein its design was based on the combination of the products of the peptidase reaction (ie, the two peptide fragments, one with a free carboxyl end that coordinates the zinc ion of the protease and the other with a free amino terminus; Fig. 9.13).[23,24] In the case of benzylsuccinic acid, the amino ($-NH_2$) functionality is replaced by the isosteric methylene ($-CH_2-$) group. Using the above concepts, it was rationalized that succinyl amino acids could similarly behave as by-product inhibitors of ACE. Starting with a succinyl-proline moiety, the structural activity developmental effort finally resulted in captopril with the substitution of the stronger zinc coordinating mercapto functionality in place of the carboxylic residue (of succinic acid) and a stereospecific R methyl group on the succinyl function to represent the methyl group on the natural l-Ala residue in Ala-Pro (the dipeptide fragment that had previously shown inhibitory activity). Captopril soon became highly successful in

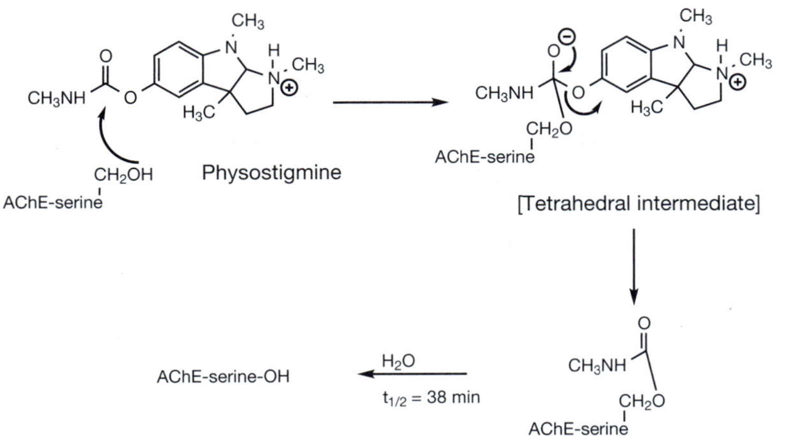

Figure 9.12 Mechanism of inhibition of acetylcholine esterase by physostigmine.

the clinic as an antihypertensive agent and, in combination with diuretics, has proved to be the treatment of choice in controlling hypertension.

Following on the heels of captopril was another by-product ACE inhibitor, enalaprilat. Enalaprilat incorporated a phenylethyl moiety with the *S*-configuration and made use of a hydrophobic binding pocket in ACE that was overlooked during the design of captopril.[25] Recalling that the tripeptide fragment of $BPP_5\alpha$ (Trp-Ala-Pro) contained

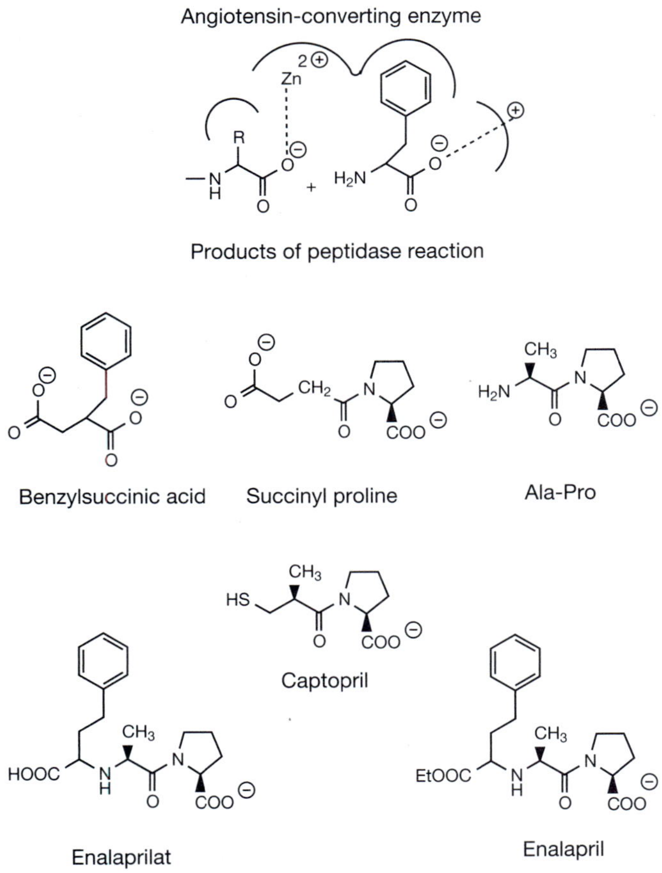

Figure 9.13 Angiotensin-converting enzyme (ACE) inhibitors and efforts that led to their development.

the aromatic tryptophan residue and showed weak inhibitory properties suggested the benefit of an aromatic binding site. Substituting the tryptophan residue with a phenyl group allowed the design of enalaprilat, which retained the carboxylic group as the coordinating ligand for zinc and resulted in a 20-fold increase in potency over captopril. However, enalaprilat, a diacid, was poorly absorbed from the gastrointestinal tract; thus, a pro-drug ethyl ester of enalaprilat, called enalapril, was developed. Enalapril had superior pharmacokinetics to enalaprilat and was rapidly metabolized to the active drug.

Transition-State Analogues

Transition-state analogues are compounds that resemble the substrate portion of the hypothetical transition state of an enzymatic reaction. All chemical reactions progressing from substrate to product must cross an energy barrier and proceed through a transition state or activated high-energy complex. This energy barrier is described as the activation energy. In the case of enzyme-catalyzed reactions, it is accepted that the enzyme reduces this energy barrier as compared to the nonenzyme-catalyzed reaction. Factors contributing to this reduced energy barrier are several and include stabilization of the transition state and intermediate forms of the reaction during the course of transition from substrate to product as well as conformational effects of distortion of the substrate while traversing toward the product. In 1948, Pauling[10] initially suggested that compounds resembling the transition state of an enzyme-catalyzed reaction would be effective inhibitors of the enzyme because the substrate transition state should have the greatest affinity for the enzyme.[10] Later, Wolfenden[26] proposed that thermodynamically, it is possible to relate the hypothetical equilibrium dissociation constants between substrate and its transition state of an enzyme-catalyzed reaction with that of the nonenzyme-catalyzed one. Using such an analysis, he showed that the ratio of the hypothetical transition-state dissociation constants of nonenzyme-catalyzed reaction to that of the enzyme-catalyzed one is equal to the ratio of the first-order rate constants of formation of transition state for enzyme-catalyzed reaction to noncatalyzed reaction. Because the ratio of the enzyme-catalyzed rate constant to that of the noncatalyzed one ranges from 10^7 to 10^{10}, it follows that the substrate transition state would bind the enzyme 10^7- to 10^{10}-fold more tightly than the substrate itself.[27] Hence, transition-state analogues that resemble the substrate would be extremely tight-binding compounds. To design a transition-state inhibitor, knowledge of the enzyme chemistry and its mechanism is a basic requirement. It must be understood, however, that these substrate transition states are, by nature, unstable transient species existing for no longer than a few picoseconds. Nevertheless, experimental evidence has shown that even crudely designed transition-state inhibitors resembling the substrate are extremely potent inhibitors.[27]

Transition-State Inhibitor of Adenosine Deaminase. Adenosine deaminase is the enzyme that hydrolyzes adenosine (or deoxyadenosine) to inosine (or deoxyinosine) and is important for purine metabolism. High levels of adenosine are toxic to B cells of the immune system and can result in an immunocompromised state. Also, people who lack the gene for adenosine deaminase have the genetic condition of severe combined immunodeficiency and are extremely susceptible to opportunistic infections. Many cancer and antiviral agents are also degraded by this enzyme; hence, there is a role for the development of inhibitors of this enzyme.[28] The mechanism proposed for adenosine deaminase is a nucleophilic attack of water at the 6-position of the purine base to form a tetrahedral intermediate (Fig. 9.14). The transition state presumably resembles this intermediate.

During the course of the deaminase reaction, the hybridization of the G-carbon changes from an sp^2-hybridized state to an sp^3 state. Subsequently, there is a loss of ammonia to give the product inosine. To develop a transition-state inhibitor for this enzyme, one would have to factor in this change in the hybridization of the substrate molecule; thus, molecules having an sp^3-hybridized carbon at this position and resembling the substrate would potentially be candidates for transition-state inhibitors. The compound 1,6-dihydro-6-hydroxymethylpurine has such geometry, and its potent inhibitory properties of adenosine deaminase ($K_i < 1\ \mu M$, as compared to a K_m for adenosine of 31 M) has been rationalized as being a transition-state inhibitor.[29] Two compounds that nature has provided, coformycin and its deoxyribose analogue, deoxycoformycin (Fig. 9.14), are extremely potent inhibitors of adenosine deaminase ($K_i = 0.002$ nM). Both of these compounds contain a seven-member ring structure, which through its flexibility is presumed to resemble the hypothesized distorted sp^2–sp^3 transition state that forms during the addition of water to adenosine.[30]

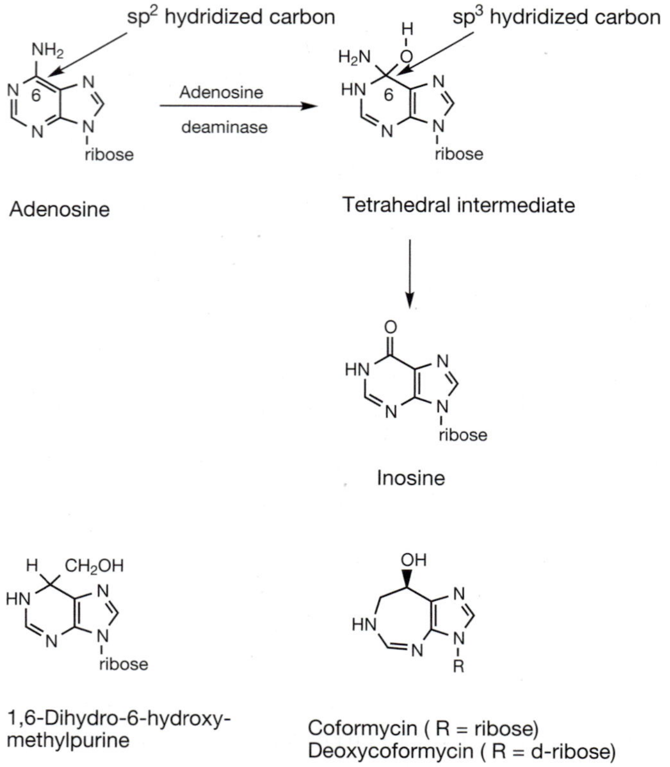

Figure 9.14 Mechanism and transition-state inhibitors of adenosine deaminase.

Irreversible Enzyme Inhibition

As previously described, irreversible enzyme inhibition is defined as "time-dependent inactivation of the enzyme," which implies that the enzyme has, in some way or form, been permanently modified, because it can no longer carry out its function. This modification is the result of a covalent bond being formed with the inhibitor and some amino acid residue in the protein. Furthermore, this bond is extremely stable and, for all practical purposes, is not hydrolyzed to give back the enzyme in its original state or structure. In most examples of irreversible inhibition, a new enzyme must be generated through gene transcription and translation for the enzyme to continue its normal catalytic action. Basically, there are two types of irreversible enzyme inhibitors, the affinity labels or active site–directed irreversible inhibitors, and the mechanism-based irreversible enzyme inactivators.

Affinity Labels and Active Site–Directed Irreversible Inhibitors. The affinity labels are those chemical entities that are inherently reactive and can target any nucleophilic residue in the enzyme, especially those residing in and around the catalytic center of the protein. These agents generally resemble the substrate so that they may bind in the active site of the enzyme. In most examples, these agents also contain an electrophilic functional group, which includes groups such as halo-methyl ketones ($X\text{-}CH_2C{=}O$, where X = halide), sulfonyl fluorides (SO_2F), nitrogen mustards ($[ClCH_2CH_2]_2NH$), diazoketones ($COCHN_2$), α, β-unsaturated carbonyls (eg, Michael acceptors), and other such reactive groups, that can "label," or alkylate, a nucleophilic amino acid residue in the enzyme. They generally tend to be indiscriminate in their action and have little therapeutic value because they are nonselective and, thus, inherently toxic. They have been used mainly as biochemical tools to probe active sites of enzyme to discern the types of amino acid residues both in and around the catalytic center of an enzyme. The classic example of an affinity label is TPCK (tosyl-phenylalanyl-chloromethyl-ketone), an irreversible inhibitor of the serine protease chymotrypsin.[31] Because TPCK resembles the amino acid phenylalanine, it can bind to the active site of the chymotrypsin, the selectivity of which is

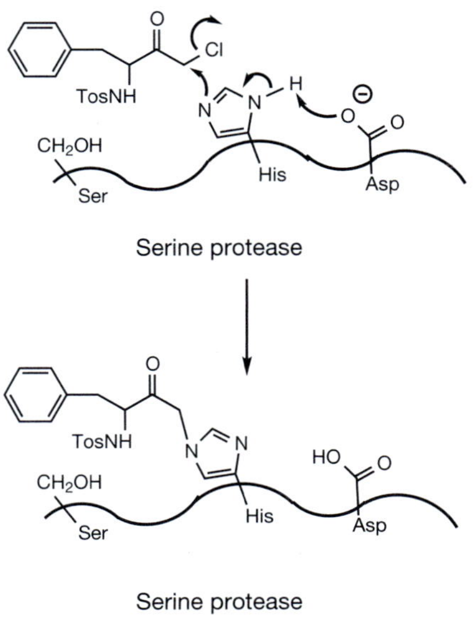

Figure 9.15 Mechanism of affinity label of serine protease with TPCK (tosyl-phenylalanyl-chloromethyl-ketone).

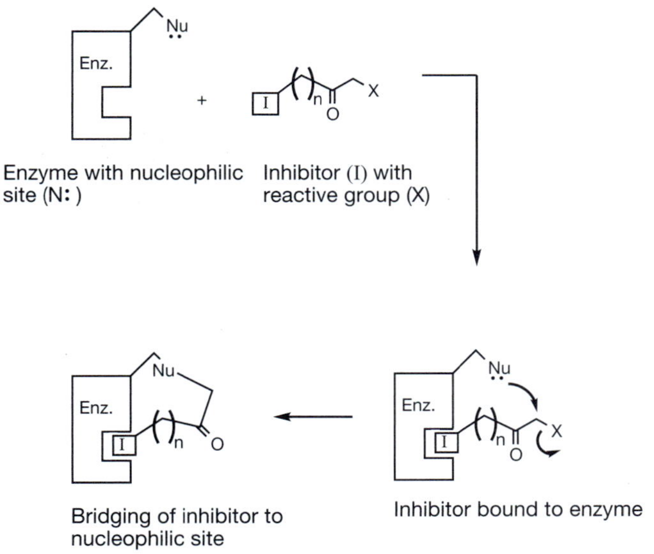

Figure 9.16 Model showing Baker[32] active site–directed irreversible inhibitors. Baker BR. *Design of Active Site Directed Irreversible Enzyme Inhibitors*. Wiley; 1967.

for such hydrophobic amino acid residues (Phe and Tyr). During the course of normal peptide hydrolysis, the reactive chloromethyl-ketone labels the nucleophilic histidine residue present as part of the catalytic triad (Ser-His-Asp) in the active site of the protease (Fig. 9.15). Another similarly designed affinity label is TLCK (tosyl-lysyl-chloromethyl-ketone), the specificity of which is for the protease trypsin. Trypsin cleaves peptide bonds adjacent to the basic amino acids, lysine, and arginine. It was found that TLCK was a specific inhibitor of trypsin but had no activity for chymotrypsin. On the other hand, TPCK, although extremely specific for chymotrypsin, showed no activity for trypsin. However, there are some examples of such molecules (eg, Michael acceptors) being developed as useful drugs—see discussion on Tyrosine Kinase Inhibitors (TKIs) (see Chapter 37).

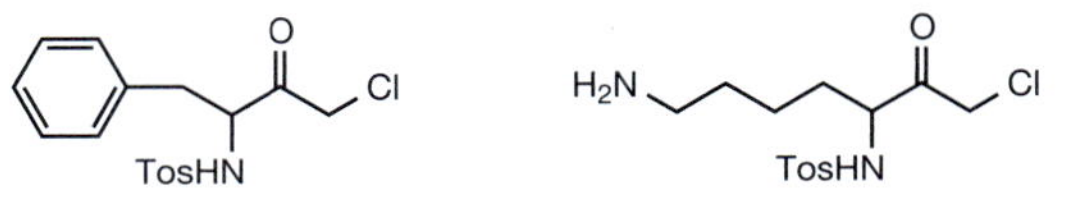

TPCK TLCK

Because of the inherent reactivity and nonselectivity of many affinity labels and their limited utility in drug therapy, B.R. Baker extended this concept to design inhibitors that would have greater selectivity and specificity and, thus, be potential drug candidates.[32] He designed several analogues, termed active site–directed irreversible inhibitors, targeted toward thymidylate synthase, a key enzyme involved in the de novo metabolism of thymidylate. These analogues contained a substrate-binding region linked to a reactive group, such as a halomethyl ketone, by a tether whose chain length could be manipulated. The substrate portion of the analogue ensures both affinity and rapid binding to the enzyme active site. Once bound, areas in and around the binding site and on the surface of the enzyme could be probed for nucleophilic amino acid residues. By manipulating the length of the tether, ideal inhibitors could then be designed such that any suitably located, sufficiently nucleophilic amino acid residue on the surface of the enzyme could potentially be alkylated by the halomethyl ketone (Fig. 9.16). Once alkylated, the tether "bridges" the active site with the labeled amino acid residue, thus "tying up" and preventing further catalysis by the enzyme.

Mechanism-Based Irreversible Enzyme Inactivators

OVERVIEW. The mechanism-based irreversible inhibitors also have been termed as "suicide substrates," "k_{cat} inhibitors," "Trojan horse inhibitors," or "latent alkylating agents." These inhibitors are inherently unreactive but, on normal catalytic processing by the enzyme, are activated into highly reactive moieties.[33-35] These reactive functionalities can then irreversibly alkylate a nucleophilic amino acid residue or cofactor in the enzyme and, in essence, cause the enzyme's death ("suicide"). Basically, these inhibitors have a latent reactive functionality that only becomes apparent after binding and acted on by the normal catalytic machinery of the enzyme. This type of inhibitor design differs from the preceding one in that these inhibitors have one more level of built-in selectivity. The kinetic scheme for such inhibition is shown in Equation 9.5, in which enzyme, E, binds with inhibitor, S, to give an [E − S] complex with dissociation constant of K_m (or K_i):

Eq. 9.5
$$E + S \overset{K_m}{\rightleftharpoons} [E \cdot S] \overset{K_{cat}}{\rightleftharpoons} [E \cdot S^*] \overset{K_{inact}}{\rightarrow} E - S^*$$
$$\downarrow k_{diff} \quad \text{(Enzyme inactivated)}$$
$$E + S^* \xrightarrow{+\ddot{N}u} Nu - S^* \text{ (Nonselective inactivation)}$$
$$K_p \text{ (partition ratio)} = k_{diff}/k_{inact}$$

Next, the [E·S] complex is converted into a highly activated complex [E·S*] by the catalytic machinery (k_{cat}) of

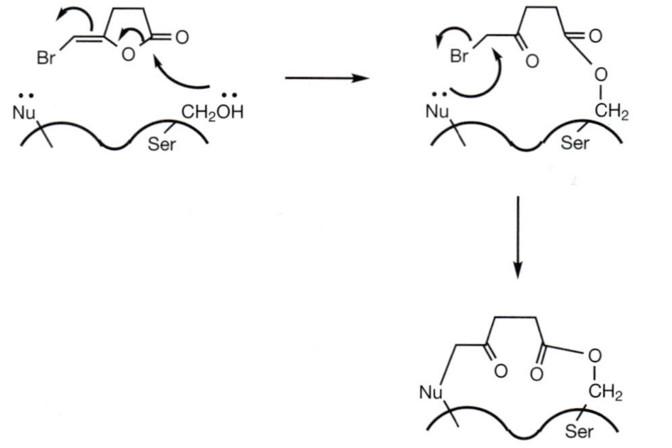

Figure 9.17 Mechanism-based inhibition of serine proteases by Katzenellenbogen halo enol lactone.

the enzyme, which can then go on to alkylate the enzyme, [E-S*]. Note that it is possible for the reactive species [S*] to diffuse (dissociate) from the enzyme and react with some other (off) target nucleophilic species (Nu), that is, the system is "leaky." If this happens, however, the inhibitor cannot be classified as a true suicide substrate, because specificity is lost.

Several requirements need to be met by these inhibitors for them to be classified as suicide substrates. These include the following: (1) inactivation should be time dependent (reaction should be irreversible), (2) kinetics should be first order, (3) the enzyme should show saturation phenomenon, (4) the substrate should be able to protect the enzyme, and (5) stoichiometry of the reaction should be 1:1 (one active site to one inhibitor), and if stoichiometry is not 1:1, then the partition ratio, ratio of the diffusion step to the inactivation step ($K_p = k_{diff}/k_{inact}$), should not change with increasing inhibitor concentrations.

Examples of Suicide Substrates. During the past three decades, besides the rational design of hundreds of molecules that have been synthesized and tested as suicide substrates, it also has come to light that nature itself has known about this mechanistic mode of enzyme inhibition and provided us with several extremely potent mechanism-based suicide inactivators. Below are a few selected examples to demonstrate the mode of action of these inhibitors.

Halo Enol Lactones. Halo enol lactones are an example of suicide inhibitors for serine proteases. These analogues were developed by Katzenellenbogen and coworkers[35] at the University of Illinois. On normal catalytic processing by the serine hydroxyl functionality, they give rise to a reactive halo-methyl ketone, which subsequently alkylates a nearby nucleophilic residue on the enzyme (Fig. 9.17). Other suicide inactivators for the serine proteases have been designed by various researchers.[34]

Clavulanic Acid. Clavulanic acid, a natural product synthesized by certain *Streptomyces* bacteria, is a potent inhibitor of bacterial β-lactamase.[36] This enzyme is a serine protease and can hydrolyze β-lactams, such as the penicillin antibiotics. It is the principal enzyme responsible for penicillin-resistant bacteria. Clavulanic acid itself is a β-lactam and, if given in combination with penicillin, is preferentially taken up by β-lactamase and hydrolyzed. During the process of hydrolysis, however, the molecule undergoes a cleavage, leading to the formation of a Michael acceptor, which subsequently alkylates a nucleophilic residue on β-lactamase, causing irreversible inhibition (Fig. 9.18). Such combinations of a β-lactamase inhibitor and a penicillin have resulted in clinically useful agents (clavulanic acid plus amoxicillin [Augmentin]).

Gabaculin. Gabaculin, a naturally occurring neurotoxin, is a potent mechanism-based inhibitor of the enzyme γ-aminobutyric acid transaminase (GABA-T) with an interesting mechanism of action.[37] GABA-T is a pyridoxal phosphate (PLP)–dependent enzyme involved in the catabolism (transamination) of the excitatory neurotransmitter, GABA, to succinate semialdehyde and pyridoxamine. As part of the normal catalytic mechanism of PLP-dependent enzymes, the amino group of gabaculin first forms a Schiff base with the aldehyde of PLP (Fig. 9.19). Next, this adduct undergoes an aromatization reaction, resulting in an extremely stable covalent bond with the cofactor, PLP. Hence, in this case, rather than an enzymatic nucleophilic residue being alkylated, the cofactor is "tied up," resulting in the inhibition.

Finasteride. Finasteride is a clinically useful agent in the treatment of prostate hyperplasia and male pattern baldness. It is a potent inhibitor of human steroid-5α-reductase, the enzyme responsible for the reduction of testosterone to dihydrotestosterone (Fig. 9.20). The inhibitory action of finasteride has been attributed both to its similarity in structure

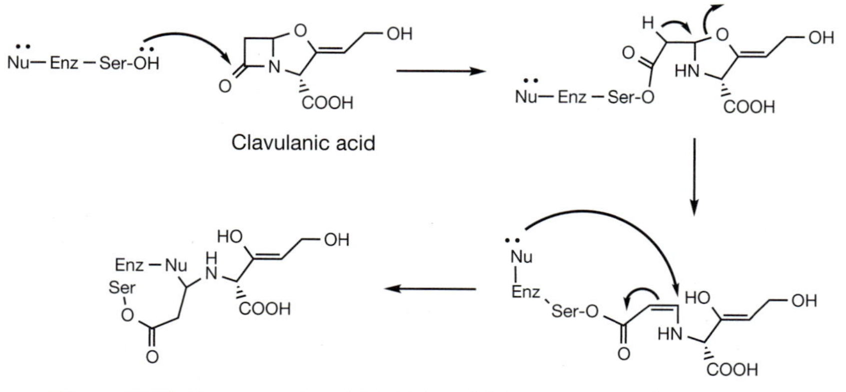

Figure 9.18 Mechanism-based inhibition of β-lactamases by clavulanic acid.

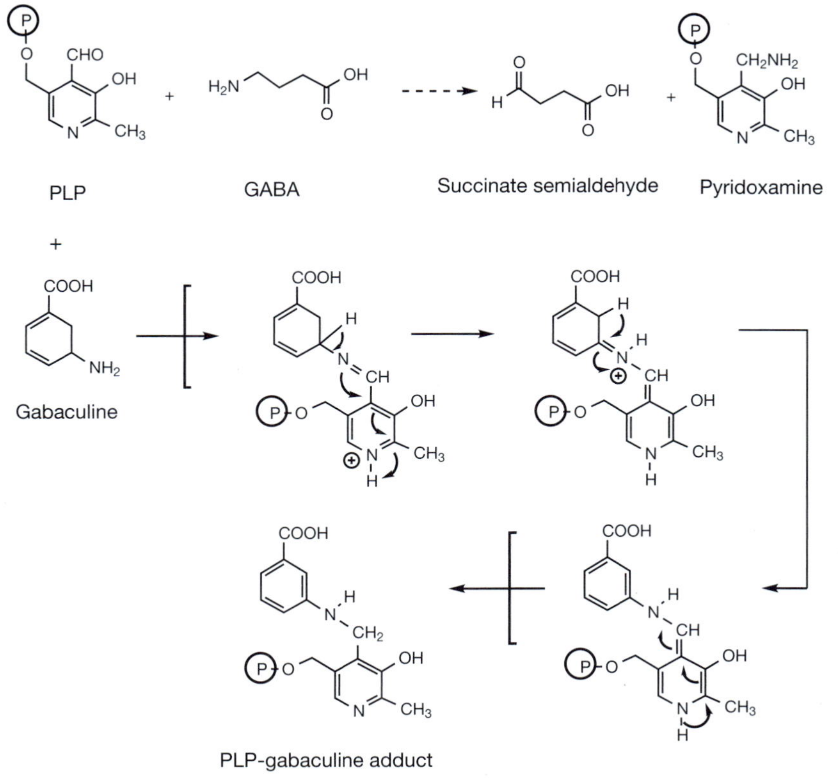

Figure 9.19 Pyridoxal phosphate–dependent γ-aminobutyric acid transaminase (GABA-T) reaction and the mechanism of suicide inhibition by gabaculin.

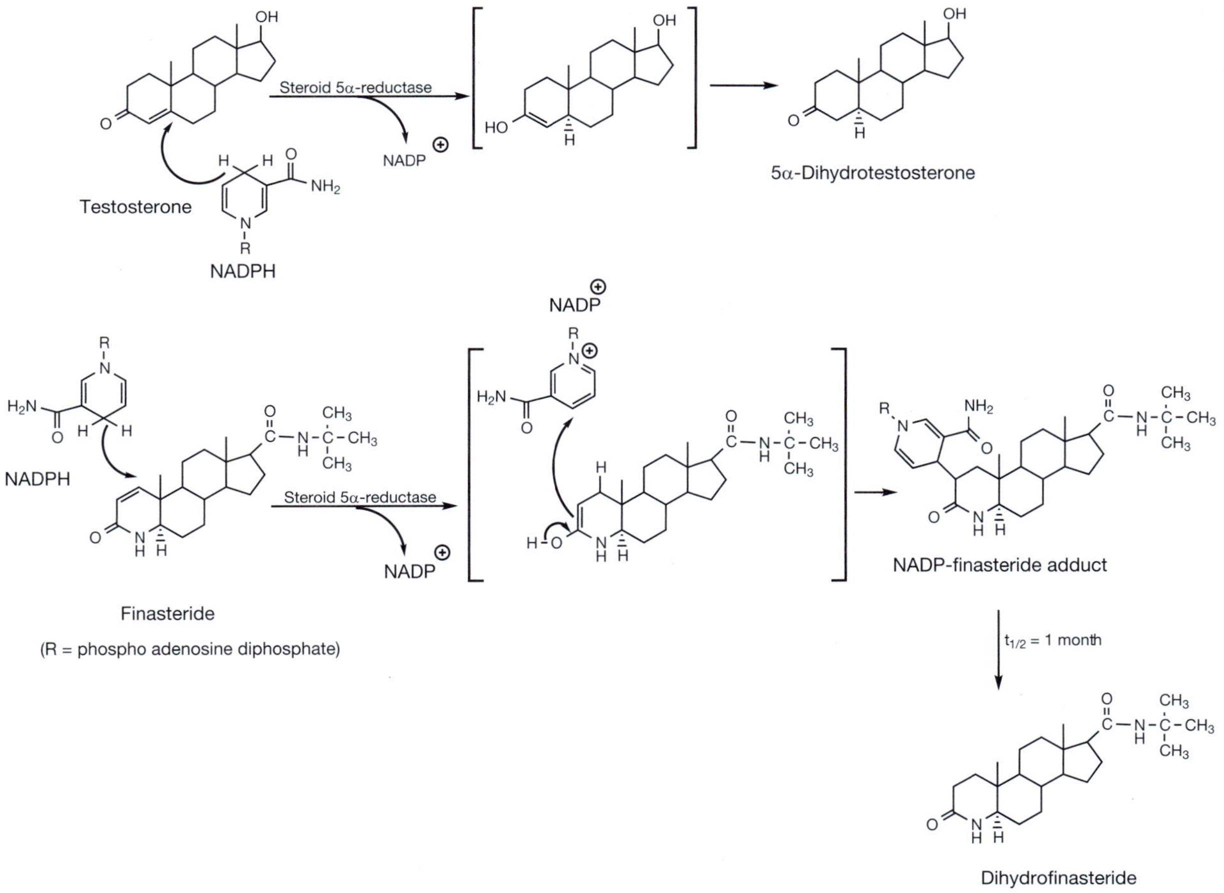

Figure 9.20 Mechanism of steroid reductase reduction on finasteride and testosterone and the structure of hypothesized NADPH-dihydrofinasteride adduct.[38] Reprinted with permission from Bull HG, Garcia-Calvo M, Andersson S, et al. Mechanism-based inhibition of human steroid 5α-reductase by finasteride: enzyme-catalyzed formation of NADP-dihydrofinasteride, a potent bisubstrate analogue inhibitor. *J Am Chem Soc.* 1996;118:2359-2365. Copyright 1996. American Chemical Society.

to testosterone, which allows it to bind to the enzyme and be reduced to dihydrofinasteride in place of testosterone, as well as to its ability to act as a mechanism-based inhibitor, during which it can tie up the cofactor, NADPH, by forming a covalent NADP-dihydrofinasteride adduct (Fig. 9.20) (see Chapter 25). This adduct very slowly releases dihydrofinasteride with a half-life of 1 month.[38]

Inhibitors of Clinically Important Enzymes

Cyclic Nucleotide Phosphodiesterase Inhibitors

Phosphodiesterases (PDEs) belong to a large family of enzymes that hydrolyze phosphate-ester bonds (viz. ester bonds between two hydroxyl functionalities with phosphoric acid). In nature, there are numerous biomolecules containing such phosphodiester bonds, including glycerol-phosphates (phosphor-lipids), sugar phosphates, inositol phosphates, nucleic acids, and nucleotides including the cyclic nucleotides. While all of these molecules are essentially hydrolyzed by a phosphodiesterase, however, the specific name of phosphodiesterase (PDE) has been reserved for enzymes that hydrolyze the cyclic nucleotide monophosphate (cNMP), viz. cyclic adenosine monophosphate (cAMP) and cyclic guanosine monophosphate (cGMP), both molecules involved in signal transduction and second messenger cell signaling (Fig. 9.21). Enzymes that hydrolyze the phosphodiester bonds other than the cyclic nucleotides are known by other names, for example, nucleases (DNAses or RNAses, for nucleic acids) and phospholipases for glycerol phosphates.

The cyclic nucleotide PDEs hydrolyze the 3′-5′ phosphodiester bond of cAMP and cGMP leading to the formation of AMP (5′-adenosine monophosphate) and guanosine monophosphate (GMP) (5′-guanosine monophosphate). The PDEs can bind either cyclic nucleotide with selectivity depending on the particular isozyme. These cyclic nucleotide (cAMP and cGMP), substrates for PDEs, are formed from their precursor nucleotide triphosphates, NTP (ATP and GTP, respectively) by nucleotide cyclases (Fig. 9.21). There are many different isoforms of the PDEs present in cells, which allow for great diversity in substrate specificity and cell regulation.

This diversity further governs specific roles for each of these PDEs in various cellular locales, physiological and pathological conditions. Currently, the PDEs have been classified into 11 different families, based upon gene products (amino acid homology) and are estimated to comprise over 100 different mRNAs from 21 different genes due to alternative splicing and transcription start sites.[39-41] The nomenclature of these PDE families is based on the species of origin, the gene, and the variant discovered. For example, HsPDE2A3 signifies that the origin is from *Homo sapiens* (Hs), PDE denotes that it is a cyclic nucleotide phosphodiesterase, the 2A indicates that it is from the PDE gene 2 family A, and 3 indicates that it is the third variant that was reported in the gene database.

The different PDEs have been shown to regulate various cellular activities, and hence because of this diverse functional ability, one could develop drugs to control these PDEs in a selective manner (Table 9.2).[42,43] Structural studies of several of these PDEs have shown that they all contain a "catalytic domain" with a consensus sequence denoting a metal ion binding site (a phosphorylase sequence, containing a signature recognition sequence for all PDEs) of two histidines and two aspartates that bind Zn^2+/Mg^2+; a "glutamine switch" that accounts for the substrate specificity (cAMP or cGMP) where an invariant glutamine amino acid residue can rotate to either H-bond with cAMP or cGMP (utilizing either cNMP as substrate) or is constrained from binding to one of the cNMPs thus favoring binding to the other nucleotide; and a "regulatory domain" based on the specific PDE family (eg, Ca^2+—calmodulin binding site for PDE1) as well as an allosteric binding sites for cGMP.[40,41]

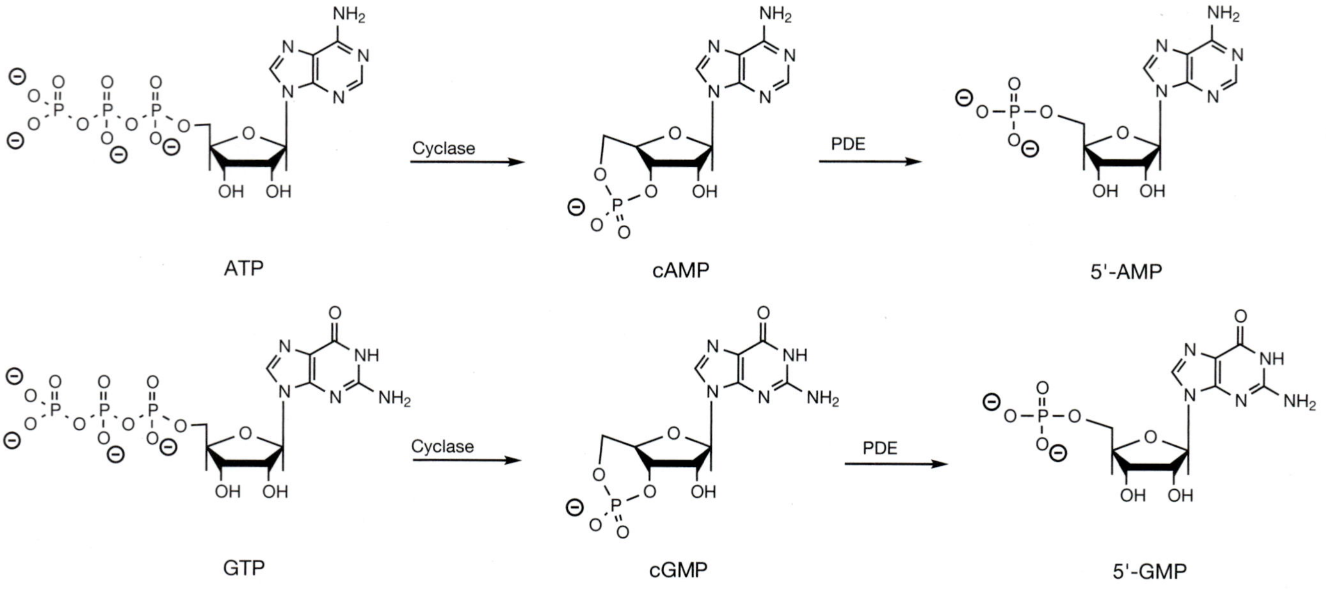

Figure 9.21 Enzymatic interconversions of cyclic and linear nucleotides.

Table 9.2 Specificity and Potency of Phosphodiesterase Inhibitors

PDE	Specificity	Inhibitor	IC_{50}[a] (nM)	PDE	Specificity	Inhibitor	IC_{50}[a] (nM)
PDE1B	Duel	Rolipram	>200,000	PDE6	cGMP	Sildenafil	50[b]
		Cilomilast	87,000			Vardenafil	11[c]
		Roflumilast	>200,000			Tadalafil	2,000[b]
		Sildenafil	1,500	PDE7B	cAMP	Rolipram	>2,000,000
		Vardenafil	300			Cilomilast	44,000
		Tadalafil	50,000			Roflumilast	>200,000
PDE2A	Duel	Rolipram	>200,000			Sildenafil	78,000
		Cilomilast	160,000			Vardenafil	1,900
		Roflumilast	>200,000			Tadalafil	74,000
		Sildenafil	35,000	PDE8A	cAMP	Rolipram	>200,000
		Vardenafil	3,100			Cilomilast	7,000
		Tadalafil	130,000			Roflumilast	>200,000
PDE3B	cAMP > cGMP	Rolipram	>200,000			Sildenafil	>200,000
		Cilomilast	87,000			Vardenafil	57,000
		Roflumilast	>200,000			Tadalafil	>200,000
		Sildenafil	15,000	PDE9A	cGMP	Rolipram	>200,000
		Vardenafil	580			Cilomilast	>200,000
		Tadalafil	280,000			Roflumilast	>200,000
PDE4B	cAMP	Rolipram	570			Sildenafil	5,600
		Cilomilast	25			Vardenafil	680
		Roflumilast	0.84			Tadalafil	150,000
		Sildenafil	20,000	PDE10A	cAMP<cGMP	Rolipram	140,000
		Vardenafil	3,800			Cilomilast	73,000
		Tadalafil	9,200			Roflumilast	>200,000
PDE4D	cAMP	Rolipram	1,100			Sildenafil	6,800
		Cilomilast	11			Vardenafil	880
		Roflumilast	0.68			Tadalafil	19,000
		Sildenafil	14,000	PDE11A	Duel	Rolipram	>200,000
		Vardenafil	3,900			Cilomilast	21,000
		Tadalafil	19,000			Roflumilast	25,000

(continued)

Table 9.2 Specificity and Potency of Phosphodiesterase Inhibitors (*continued*)

PDE	Specificity	Inhibitor	IC_{50}[a] (nM)	PDE	Specificity	Inhibitor	IC_{50}[a] (nM)
PDE5A	cGMP	Rolipram	>200,000			Sildenafil	6,100
		Cilomilast	53,000			Vardenafil	240
		Roflumilast	17,000			Tadalafil	10
		Sildenafil	2.2				
		Vardenafil	1.0				
		Tadalafil	1.2				

[a]Data are from Sutherland and Rall[41] unless stated otherwise. The numbers shown in the table are the 50% inhibition concentration (IC50). Concentrations used were far below the K_m of all the PDEs assayed except for PDE9A, in which case it was close to the K_m. The IC50s obtained are good approximations of the inhibition constant K_i. Selectivities of an inhibitor may be determined by taking ratios of the numbers given in the table.
Abbreviations: cAMP, cyclic adenosine monophosphate; cGMP, cyclic guanosine monophosphate.
[b]K_i values are from Card et al.[42]
[c]Value from Hatzelmann and Schudt.[43]

X-ray crystallographic studies with inhibitors bound with the protein have indicated that there are several binding modes for inhibition, and the active site architecture is often unique for different PDEs. Inhibitors can bind to the protein through H-bonds with amino acid residues that make up the active site for cNMP binding, with residues that line the channel leading to the active site as well as by H-bonding with water to residues that bind to the active site metal ions. Moreover, because of the order of magnitude differences in cellular concentrations of the cyclic nucleotides (as compared to its precursor, NTP molecule, <1 to 10 μM for cAMP/cGMP vs mM concentrations for ATP/GTP), these PDEs become attractive targets to design drugs[40] (since competitive inhibition for a natural substrate whose cellular concentration is 1 μM is achieved much more easily than if the substrate concentration was 1 mM). Structural knowledge of the different binding modes for inhibitors with the PDEs has given rise to the rapid development of selective PDE inhibitors to allow for specific interactions along regulatory pathways involving such PDEs. While inhibitors of PDEs have been known for quite some time, such as, caffeine and theophylline have been in use as therapeutic agents for many decades (as nonselective inhibitors of PDE), the development of drugs to selectively inhibit a particular PDE is a more recent phenomenon. Moreover, selective inhibitors would also have a better safety profile as one would expect a decreased amount of side/toxic effects. For example, theophylline, a nonselective PDE inhibitor, is known to have a narrow therapeutic index because of its interaction with multiple PDEs.

Phosphodiesterase-5 Selective Inhibitors. The impetus for the development of PDE inhibitors arose from the knowledge that vasodilation (for treatment of high blood pressure) could be achieved through the stimulation of atrial natriuretic peptide (ANP), an endogenous peptide that allows for renal excretion of sodium/water. Furthermore, it was also known that ANP stimulated the synthesis of cGMP through its activation of guanylyl cyclase. Hence, inhibition of cGMP hydrolysis (ie, PDE activity) was a rational target for the development of these vasodilators. Since ANP worked in the kidney, the idea was to target the specific PDE in the kidney. The lead compound for the development of these PDE inhibitors was a xanthine derivative, zaprinast (Fig. 9.22), previously shown to demonstrate weak PDE inhibition.[44] Analysis of the heterocyclic ring of zaprinast and comparison with the purine heterocycle of cGMP led to the development of a number of derivatives displaying PDE5 inhibitory activity, including the design of one containing a pyrazolopyrimidinone, which ultimately resulted in the development of the potent PDE5 inhibitor, sildenafil.[45] During clinical trials of sildenafil as an antihypertensive and vasodilatory agent, it was found

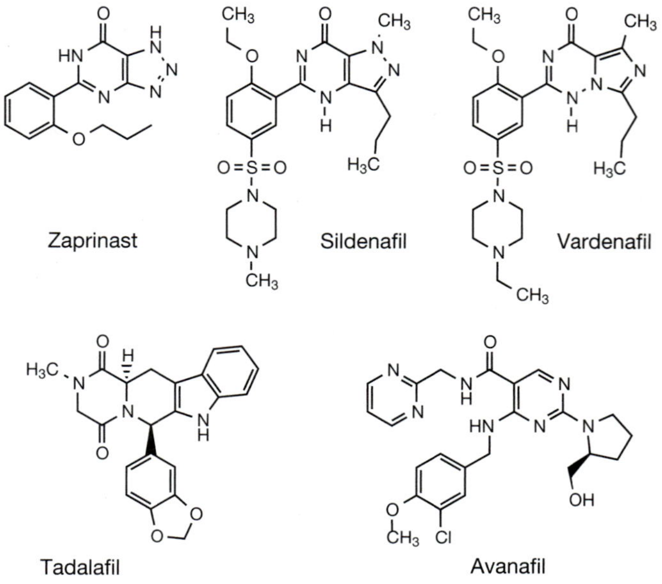

Figure 9.22 Inhibitors of phosphodiesterase (PDE)5.

to have a (beneficial) side effect in erectile dysfunction. This pharmacologic effect was recognized, appreciated, and commercialized into a new line of therapeutic agents to treat the condition, erectile dysfunction. Inhibition of cGMP hydrolysis (PDE5) in the corpus cavernosum results in elevated levels of cGMP, leading to increased smooth muscle relaxation and improved blood flow and maintenance of an erection. Presently, PDE5 selective inhibitors include the drugs sildenafil (Viagra), vardenafil (Levitra), tadalafil (Cialis), and Avanafil (Stendra). They have been one of the most widely marketed and commercially successful drugs in recent years to treat erectile dysfunction in males and, more recently, have also been approved to treat pulmonary hypertension. These drugs have high selectivity to inhibit PDE5 over the other PDE classes. PDE5 is a phosphodiesterase that specifically hydrolyzes cGMP to GMP at low substrate levels and also has a high affinity binding site for cGMP on its regulatory domain.

The enzyme, originally isolated from platelets, was later found to be a regulator in vascular smooth muscle contraction present in the lungs and brains. The drugs mentioned above act as reversible inhibitors of the enzyme PDE5, binding in the active site of the enzyme where the heterocyclic nucleus of the inhibitors bind in a pocket reserved for the purine ring of the natural substrate, cGMP. Side effects include hypotension, and also, since the active site structures of PDE5 and PDE6 are similar in architecture, some cross inhibition to PDE6 enzymes has been observed. PDE6 enzymes regulate the phototransduction cascade, where PDE6 rapidly reduces the steady-state concentration of cGMP in response to light stimuli. Thus, side effects of these PDE5 inhibitors include decreased vision in some patient populations. The drug, tadalafil, however, is about 1,000-fold more selective for PDE5 versus PDE6. Several other selective competitive PDE inhibitors are approved for use, and these include the PDE4 inhibitors, cilomilast and roflumilast for treatment of chronic obstructive pulmonary disease ([COPD] Fig. 9.23) as well as the PDE3 inhibitors, dipyridamole and cilostazol, as antiplatelet drugs (Fig. 9.24), and inamrinone and milrinone as positive inotropic agents (Fig. 9.25).

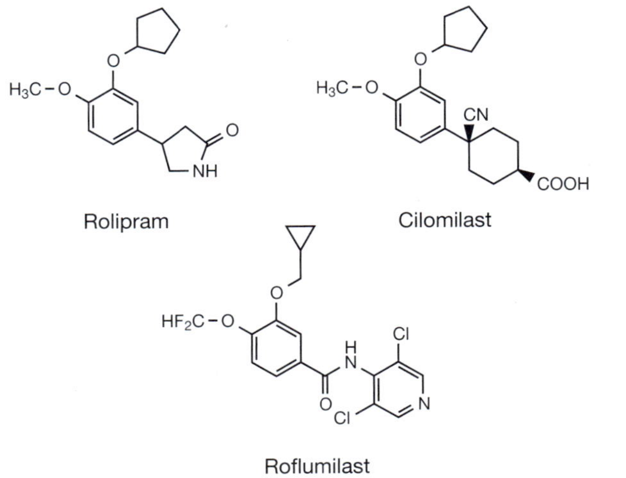

Figure 9.23 Competitive inhibitors of phosphodiesterase (PDE)4.

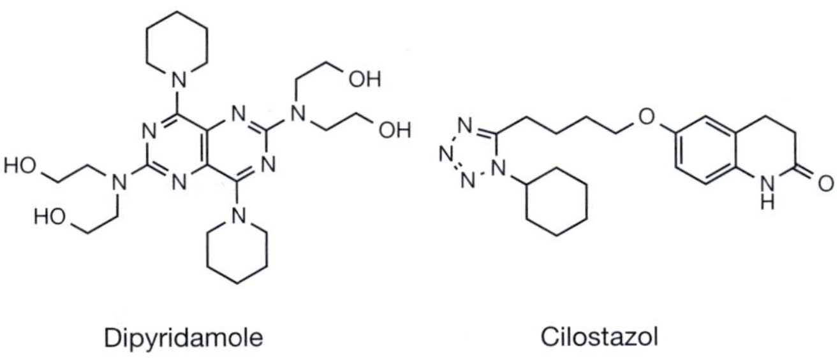

Figure 9.24 Antiplatelet inhibitors of phosphodiesterase (PDE)3.

Protein-Kinase Inhibitors

Protein kinases belong to the family of group transfer phosphorylating enzymes that transfer a phosphate group from ATP onto amino acid residues of proteins. It is estimated that there are over 500 of these kinases encoded by the human genome (the kinome), and this kinase reaction, when coupled with a phosphatase (dephosphorylation) reaction (ie, reversible phosphorylation of proteins), offers cells a precise regulatory mechanism to control its differentiation, maturation, proliferation, apoptosis, and other cellular functions.[46] The substrate amino acid residues on proteins that are phosphorylated belong largely to the hydroxyl bearing amino acids such as serine, threonine, and tyrosine. Hence, these kinases are referred to as either serine/threonine kinases or tyrosine kinases. Similarly, the phosphatases are referred to as serine/threonine or tyrosine phosphatases, of which the tyrosine phosphatases predominate. Since these proteins are involved in regulatory functions of the cell, it becomes intuitive that mutations or aberrations of expression of these proteins can lead to dysregulation of cellular functions, giving rise to tumors and cancers and other diseases. Indeed, research has shown that of the 518 kinase genes present in the human genome, 244 map to disease loci and cancer.[46] Moreover, targeting these enzymes with inhibitors would be a way to selectively target cancers without the noxious side effects seen with conventional anticancer drugs such as alkylating agents or antitumor antibiotics. Research over the last decade has provided this as a rationale to develop selective (targeted) anticancer therapy, where such kinases (which manifest themselves in certain cancers) have been specifically targeted for inhibition, resulting in dramatic declines of cancer cells and greater survival times for tpatients.[47] Examples of such targeted anticancer drugs have involved primarily the development of the tyrosine kinase inhibitors (TKIs), of which several are U.S. Food and Drug Administration (FDA) approved (see Chapter 33); however, more recently, inhibitors of serine/threonine kinases have entered the clinical market, while inhibitors of the tyrosine phosphatases are in development.

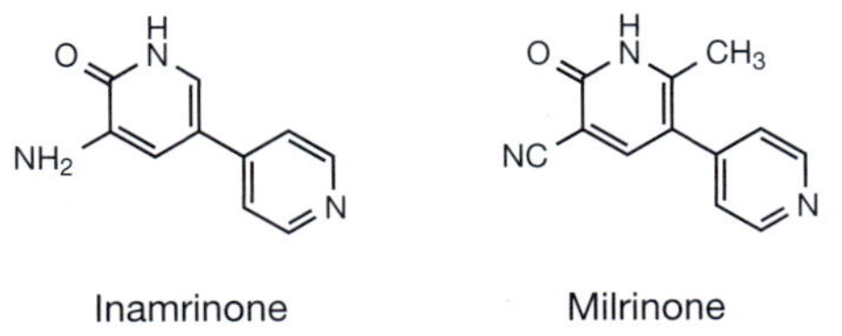

Figure 9.25 PDE3 inhibitors with cardiac and pulmonary effects.

Tyrosine-Kinase Inhibitors. The tyrosine kinases are a group of enzymes responsible for signal transduction and intracellular signaling functions, of which many are involved in cell differentiation and proliferation (see Chapter 37). They can be divided into two major types, depending upon where they act in the cell, viz. receptor tyrosine kinases (RTK), a membrane-spanning protein having an extracellular ligand binding domain and an intracellular catalytic (kinase) domain involved in the transduction of extracellular signals from the membrane to the cytoplasm, and the non-receptor tyrosine kinases involved in cytosolic signaling events.[47,48] Inhibitors for these have been developed for both types and have shown excellent and selective activity in cancers manifested by aberrant expression of these proteins. The design for selective inhibitors has been based on determining important binding regions to the protein. The kinase domain has a C-terminal domain linked via a "hinge region" to the N-terminal domain, and structural studies have indicated that ATP is known to bind to the backbone of this hinge region (ATP-binding pocket). These kinases all have an "activation loop," which contains a tyrosine residue (Tyr393), the major phosphorylated residue that allows switching the kinase from inactive to active forms and allowing for ATP binding. The large majority of the TKIs bind to this region via H-bonding. Areas of the protein that have been identified as important for the function of kinases include a glycine-rich loop (G-loop), ATP-binding pocket, a gatekeeper residue (an amino acid preceding the hinge region), and the DFG activation motif. Most of the inhibitors that have been developed tend to bind to the ATP-binding pocket and have been classified based on their binding motif. The type I inhibitors bind the "DFG-in" motif of the activation loop (the active form of the kinase, where the kinase is poised for the phosphoryl transfer) and is a more conserved region, while the type II inhibitors bind the inactive (DFG-out) motif, which is a region of less-conserved residues but would allow for greater specificity. Type III and type IV inhibitors bind to regions outside the ATP-binding pocket (distal sites) and are classified as allosteric inhibitors. The kinase-ligand interaction fingerprints and structures (KLIFS) is a useful database that identifies the binding pocket for types I to IV inhibitors, which includes the gatekeeper residues for various kinases and is often used to aid medicinal chemists in designing new kinase inhibitors.

The development of a TKI to selectively treat a cancer, chronic myelogenous leukemia (CML), was the impetus leading to the large number of presently available TKIs. CML in the majority of patients is due to a reciprocal translocation of chromosomes 9 and 22, resulting in a fusion of the *abl* (Abelson leukemia virus) gene of chromosome 9 to the *bcr* (breakpoint cluster) gene of chromosome 22 leading to the *bcr-abl* fusion gene (the Philadelphia chromosome). While the *abl* gene normally produces a non-receptor tyrosine kinase whose activity is highly regulated, the *bcr-abl* fusion gene produces a tyrosine kinase that is constitutively active and whose activity is required for the transformation of cells to become malignant.[49] The knowledge of this direct correlation between expression of the abnormal fusion protein and CML allowed for the development of specific inhibitors for this protein and other such dysregulated kinases that are overexpressed in many cancers. Using a high-throughput screening program to develop inhibitors for receptor tyrosine kinases as a possible treatment for such cancers, 2-phenylaminopyrimidine (PAP) became a lead compound. Further structure-activity optimization and refinement of this lead led to imatinib (Fig. 9.26), the first targeted drug for treatment of CML.[49-51] Note, the structure optimization to imatinib included addition of a pyridine, a methyl as well as a benzamide to enhance the potency of the basic PAP nucleus. The piperazinyl functionality helped increase water solubility, allowing for better "drug-like" properties. Imatinib also proved to be inhibitory in many other cancers with overexpressed kinases, such as gastrointestinal stromal tumors (GIST) (which overexpress *c-kit*), myelodysplastic diseases associated with platelet-derived growth factor receptor (PDGFR) as well as in Philadelphia chromosome-positive adult lymphoblastic leukemia.[50] X-ray crystallographic studies with imatinib co-crystallized with the TK expressed from *abl* showed that imatinib binds to the ATP binding site of the protein in its inactive conformation (DFG-out form—type II), and this binding prevented the kinase from achieving its productive binding conformation with ATP.[49] Studies showed that with the protein-bound imatinib, Tyr393 was not phosphorylated; however, the conformation of this activation loop in the nonphosphorylated protein resulted in one that resembled substrate (ATP) being bound to the kinase. In this way, the altered geometry brought about by imatinib binding to the protein prevented the protein from binding its true substrate, ATP.

Resistance develops to imatinib due to mutations (in the hydrophobic pocket, gate keeper residue being mutated to a larger residue) that prevent access of imatinib to the protein in the off state, thus allowing for the kinase to bind ATP and cancer to progress. TKIs dasatinib and bosutinib have been developed to bind the kinase in its "on" (active conformation, type I), where the drugs can access hydrophobic regions in the ATP-binding pocket. Moreover, drugs that can bind both "on" and "off" forms—dual mode inhibitors which are more potent than imatinib—have also been developed.[52-54] It has been more than 20 years since the introduction of imatinib, and today many other TKI drugs have been developed for related tyrosine kinases such as epidermal growth factor receptor (EGFR), platelet-derived growth factor receptor (PDGFR), vascular endothelial growth factor receptor (VEGFR) as well as related TKs such as the JAK-STAT (Janus kinase/signal-transducer activator of transcription) pathway involved in many immune related diseases including cancer. The inhibitors

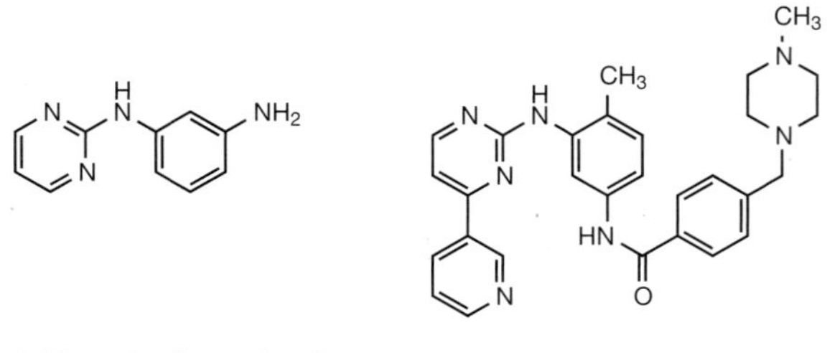

Figure 9.26 Structures of 2-phenylaminopyrimidine and imatinib.

make use of differences in the variable region of the protein surrounding the ATP-binding pocket, which allows for specific binding interactions with the various functionalities present on the individual inhibitors. Resistance to these inhibitors manifest themselves due to mutations to these variable regions on the protein as well as to cellular efflux pumps being activated. While the vast majority of these clinically used drugs are reversible inhibitors of types I and II, more recently, types III and IV inhibitors have been introduced in the clinic. Furthermore, irreversible inhibitors of type I, which employ the Michael acceptor functionality to irreversibly alkylate an active site cysteine residue have also been introduced. Examples of these inhibitors such as dasatinib (type I for imatinib resistance), sunitinib (type I, inhibitor of VEGFR), gefitinib (type I, inhibitor of EGFR), trematinib (type III, inhibitor of MEK), and the irreversible type I inhibitor, ibrutinib with the α, β unsaturated system (Michael acceptor) are shown in Figure 9.27.

Recently, asciminib, a novel TKI was developed and approved by the FDA to treat chronic phase CML with resistance or intolerance to the previously developed ATP-binding pocket inhibitors, such as imatinib. This new inhibitor is a first in-class allosteric myristoyl inhibitor and referred to as a "STAMP" (specifically targeting the ABL myristoyl pocket) inhibitor, to distinguish it from the conventional ATP-binding pocket inhibitors. The wild-type ABL protein is usually regulated through an auto-inhibitory process due to the presence of an N-terminal myristoyl group binding in the N-terminal pocket of the protein. However, in CML, the mutated BCR-ABL protein lacks this myristoyl group and thus is rendered constitutionally active. Asciminib (Fig. 9.28) works by binding the N-terminal myristoyl pocket in the mutated BCR-ABL protein and thus continues to auto-inhibit its function.[55]

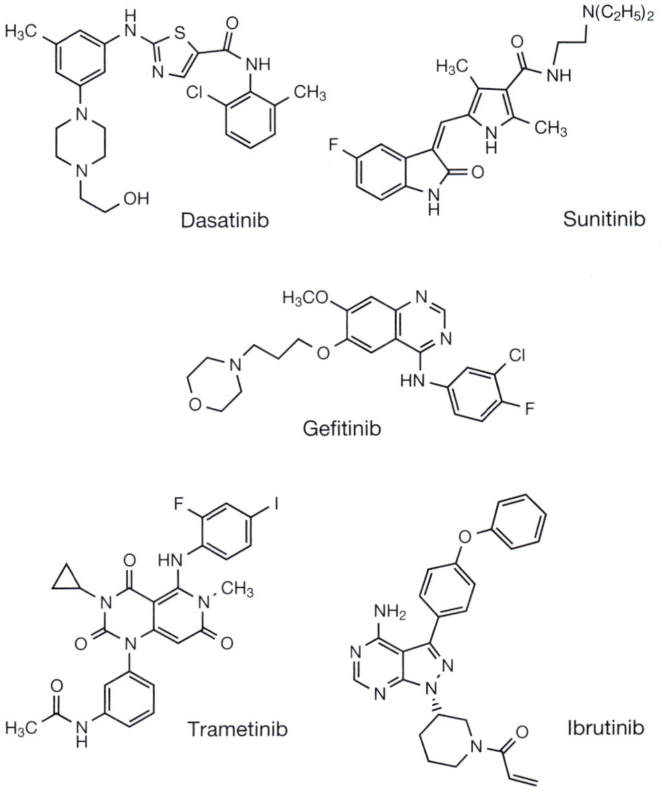

Figure 9.27 Structures of the tyrosine kinase inhibitors, dasatinib, sunitinib, gefitinib, and ibrutunib.

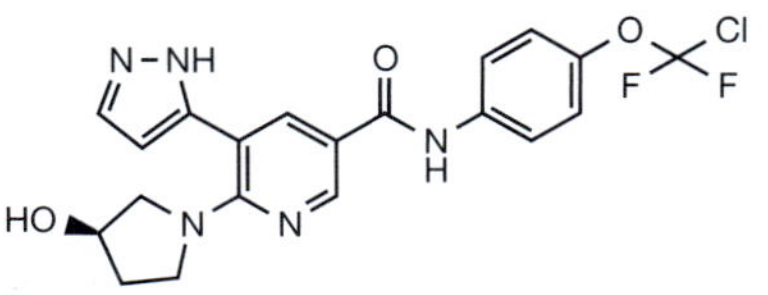

Figure 9.28 Structure of the STAMP inhibitor asciminib.

JAK/STAT and Tyrosine Kinase 2 Inhibitors. The Janus tyrosine kinases (JAK) and signal transducers and activators of transcription (STATs) family of proteins are important regulatory proteins that have profound implications in signal transduction especially pertaining to cell development, proliferation, differentiation, and apoptosis. These proteins play a vital role in many immune-related disease states, including cancer and inflammatory conditions.[56] The JAK family of proteins have been categorized as intracellular non-receptor tyrosine kinases and have four members, JAK1, JAK2, JAK3, and TYK2 (tyrosine kinase 2), while the STAT family have seven members that mainly act as transcription factors. Research has demonstrated that a number of cytokines act as transmembrane signals to stimulate activity of various members of the JAK/STAT pathway. Moreover, mutations in these proteins impact multiple cellular events and have been linked to various disease states including cancer. Research into the JAK/STAT family has demonstrated that particular cytokine receptors, interleukins, and interferons are associated with activation of specific JAK member proteins. For example, the interleukin (IL)-23 receptor specifically upregulates JAK1,2 and TYK2. Such upregulation often manifests in various immune disease states, including cancer, and thus, the JAK/STAT pathway is an attractive target to ameliorate such disease states. Specific members may be targeted to develop targeted drugs for diseases states associated with these cytokine receptors.[57]

Drug development of inhibitors for individual JAK member proteins (JAK 1-3) has resulted in the development of inhibitors that bind to the putative ATP catalytic binding site of the kinase domain as well as the allosteric regulatory domain of the kinase. These ATP-binding site inhibitors include the reversible type-I (drugs that bind the active conformation of the ATP-binding domain), and type-II inhibitors (drugs binding in the inactive conformation) as well as the irreversible inhibitors that covalently bind to the kinase. While these drugs have been designed to target a specific JAK member protein, often there has been cross-binding to the other JAK proteins because of the conserved nature of the ATP-binding pocket. This often leads to adverse effects and must be closely monitored. Over the past decade, several drugs have been FDA approved to treat a variety of immune related conditions, including alopecia, dermatitis, rheumatoid arthritis, psoriasis, and other related conditions. These inhibitors target various members of the JAK family that are believed to be activated via the cytokine involved in the signaling pathway implicated in disease pathogenesis. Examples of JAK 1 through 3 inhibitors include baricitinib approved for rheumatoid arthritis and alopecia areata, tofacitinib for

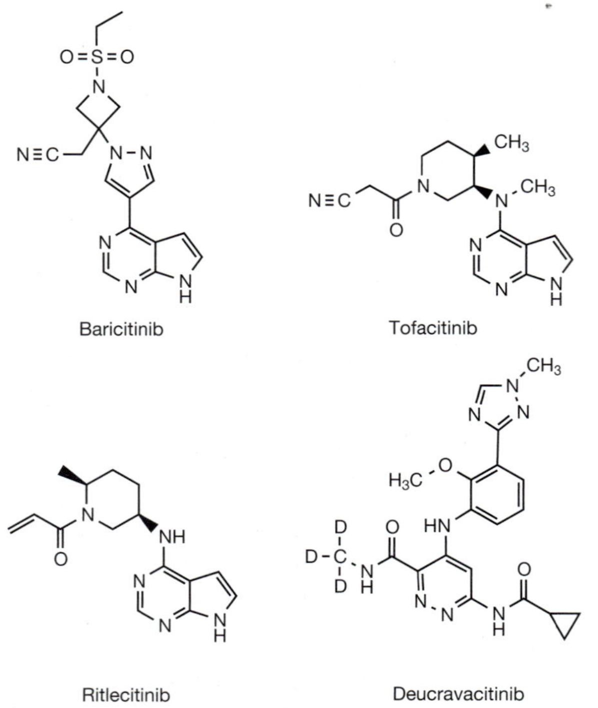

Figure 9.29 Structures of the JAK 1-3 inhibitors.

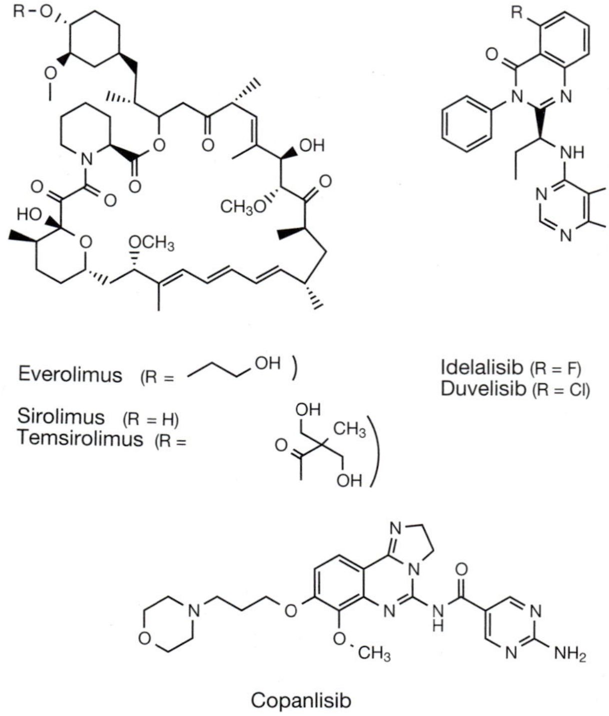

Figure 9.30 Structures of mTOR and PI3K-Akt serine/threonine kinase inhibitors.

psoriatic arthritis, ritlecitinib, a covalent inhibitor having a Michael acceptor functionality and approved for alopecia areata, ruxolitinib for myelofibrosis, and polycythemia vera and deucravacitinib, a specific TYK2 inhibitor that binds to the regulatory domain of TYK2, rather than the catalytic site, demonstrating greater selectivity and few adverse effects, for treatment of plaque psoriasis.[58] Figure 9.29 depicts the structures of these inhibitors.

Serine/Threonine-Kinase Inhibitors. The serine/threonine kinases are a family of enzymes that phosphorylate the hydroxyl groups of serine and threonine present on proteins. There are a number of such serine/threonine kinases that are important regulators of cell proliferation and survival and whose dysregulation often leads to cancer and tumorigenesis. Protein kinase C is perhaps the most well-studied system, whose activation results in the formation of diacylglycerol (DAG), phosphatidylinositol-3,4,5-triphosphate (PIP_3), and concomitant increase in intracellular calcium, leading to various signal transduction events in the cell through activation of the mitogen-activated protein kinase (MAPK) family.[59] Furthermore, other serine/threonine-kinase proteins such as PI3K (phosphoinositide-3-kinase), Akt (protein kinase B), and mTOR (mammalian target of rapamycin) are part of an intracellular signaling pathway that is important for regulation of cell proliferation, migration, and survival. Initial events leading to cell proliferation via the PI3K-Akt-mTOR have been shown to begin with growth factor or hormonal activation of a receptor tyrosine kinase, which leads to activation of PI3K. This activation results in the release of PIP_3 which in turn leads to phosphorylation and further activation of Akt and mTOR. Inhibitors of mTOR include rapamycin (sirolimus) and its derivatives everolimus and temsirolimus.[59] Rapamycin is a macrolide originally isolated from a microbe on Easter Island and primarily used as an immunosuppressant drug, while its derivatives everolimus and temsirolimus have been used to treat renal cell carcinoma.

Additional development of molecules to specifically inhibit the PI3K-Akt pathway include copanlisib, which was recently introduced to treat follicular lymphoma, and duvelisib, a first-in-class inhibitor of PI3K that was approved by the FDA in 2018 to treat chronic lymphocytic leukemia (Fig. 9.30). Additional serine/threonine kinase function is also observed during mitosis, which is a highly regulated process with multiple checkpoints encountered during the chromosomal segregation stage of cell division. The phosphorylation of specific serine/threonine residues by these mitotic kinases (also known as Aurora A and Aurora B kinases) serves as important checkpoints during mitosis. These Aurora kinases interact with many proteins, including tumor suppressors and activators from the mitotic entry stage all the way to cytokinesis. It is not surprising then that they are overexpressed in many tumors (breast, colon, gastric, ovarian, and pancreatic) and thus have become an attractive target for anticancer drug development.[60,61] Examples of some of these inhibitors include alisertib whose development was abandoned because of poor clinical trials, while danusertib, and a phosphate-based pro-drug currently under development, and barasertib is still under development (Fig. 9.31).

Other serine/threonine kinases include the RAF proteins, which are involved in the MAPK activation cascade during cell growth. B-RAF is one member of the RAF family where mutations (specifically the V600E) have resulted in dysregulation of the cascade leading to many cancers. Specific clinically used inhibitors of the V600E B-RAF mutated protein include vemurafenib and dabrafenib used to treat metastatic melanoma (Fig. 9.32).[62]

Cyclin-Dependent Kinases. The cyclin-dependent kinases (CDKs) are a subgroup of serine/threonine kinases

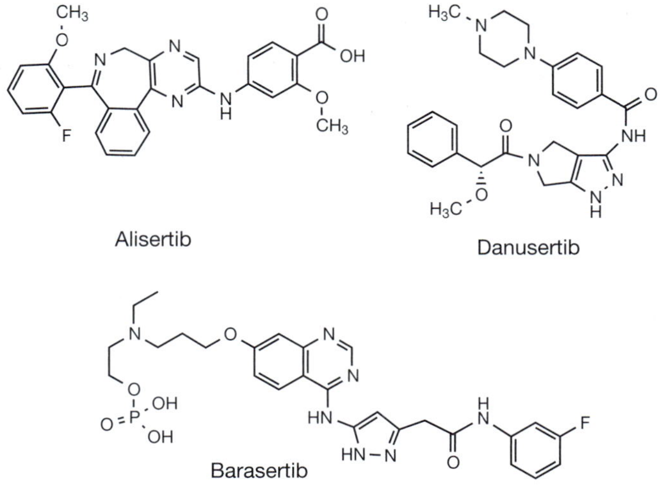

Figure 9.31 Structures of Aurora kinase inhibitors.

that exhibit both mitogenic and transcriptional control in cells and regulate cell cycle progression into the different phases of G1, S, G2, and M. These kinases are activated only when they pair with other small regulatory counterpart proteins, the cyclins. Cyclins are proteins whose levels rise and fall during progression through the cell cycle. The cyclins, in association with their kinases (CDKs), control key checkpoint processes during the cell cycle progression. Often, these protein pairs (CDKs/cyclins) work independently from other external growth signals, such as hormones in stimulating cell proliferation. The D-type cyclins and their associated cyclin-dependent kinases (CDK4 and CDK6) function as a complex to regulate cells at the G1/S check point. Research over the past several years in the treatment of hormone-positive (HR+) breast cancer, especially estrogen receptor resistance to aromatase inhibitors, has shown that the cyclin D-CDK4/6 complexes play an important component of aromatase inhibitor resistance, where their independent upregulated activity drives proliferation in breast cancers resistant to aromatase inhibitors.[63] Thus, a combination strategy involving the dual use of an aromatase inhibitor in conjunction with a CDK4/6 inhibitor has been an area of increased research activity for the past several years and has shown to have positive clinical benefit for these breast cancers.

Structural determinants of previous kinase inhibitors have aided in the development of the CDK4/6 inhibitors and have focused on inhibiting the ATP-binding site of the CDK4/6 proteins. Based upon classical TKIs developed for CML, these CDK4/6 inhibitors have been designed and developed using a similar approach with protein crystallographic data. Present clinically approved inhibitors all utilize the ATP-binding pocket for the kinase and are known as ATP-competitive inhibitors. These inhibitors generally possess a fused bicyclic heterocyclic ring system analogous to the purine ring of ATP along with functionalities to provide maximum binding. These ATP-competitive inhibitors bind to the hinge region of the kinase along with hydrophobic residues that bind to the purine ring of ATP. These drugs also contain other structural features that provide for enhanced "drug-like" properties. To date, three such inhibitors have been approved by the FDA: palbociclib, ribociclib, and abemaciclib (Fig 9.33).[63] Ongoing development in identifying ATP noncompetitive inhibitors is to achieve greater selectivity and reduced side effects.

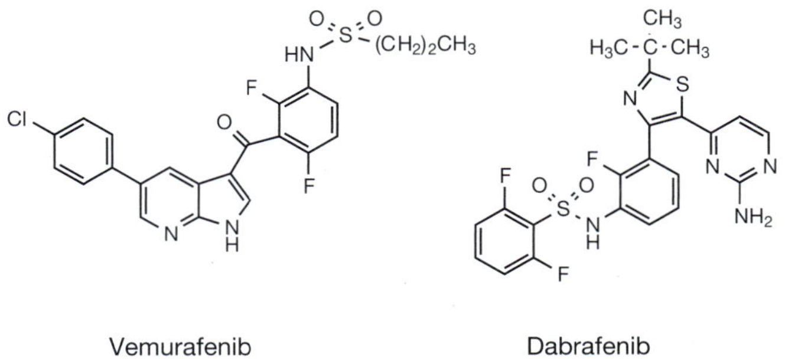

Figure 9.32 Structures of B-RAF inhibitors.

Protein Tyrosine Phosphatases. The protein tyrosine phosphatase (PTP) is another family of proteins that is important for maintaining homeostasis where levels and extent of protein phosphorylation/dephosphorylation bring about changes in cellular activity. Recent estimates from proteonomic data suggest that the bulk of cellular proteins get phosphorylated at serine/threonine and/or tyrosine residues at some time or another during their tenure. This implies that dephosphorylation (phosphatase activity) must also occur in order to control the overall level of protein phosphorylation.[64] The extent and variation of phosphorylation would result in changes at the cellular level to protein–protein interactions, protein localization, migration, protein stability, gene transcription, apoptosis, protein signaling, and other types of cellular interactions. Thus, phosphatases, in conjunction with the kinases, provide a mechanism for precise control of cellular activities. It is evident then that any dysregulation in kinase and/or phosphatase activity would likely lead to various disease states, including cancer, diabetes, and autoimmune diseases. The mechanism of action of PTPs involves nucleophilic covalent catalysis by an active site cysteine residue on the phosphorous atom of the

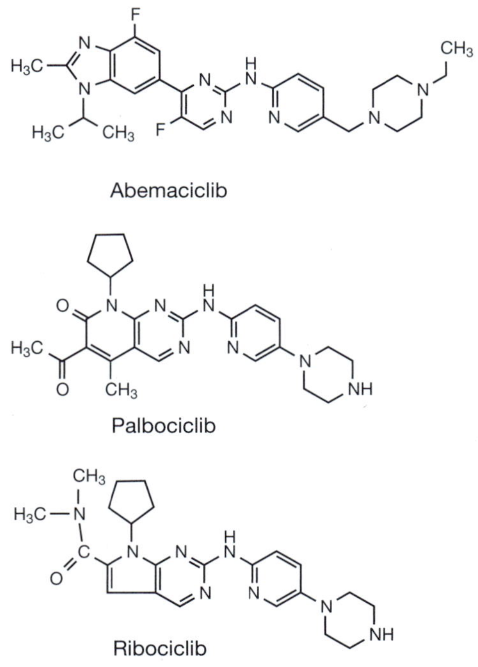

Figure 9.33 Structures of the CDK4/6 inhibitors

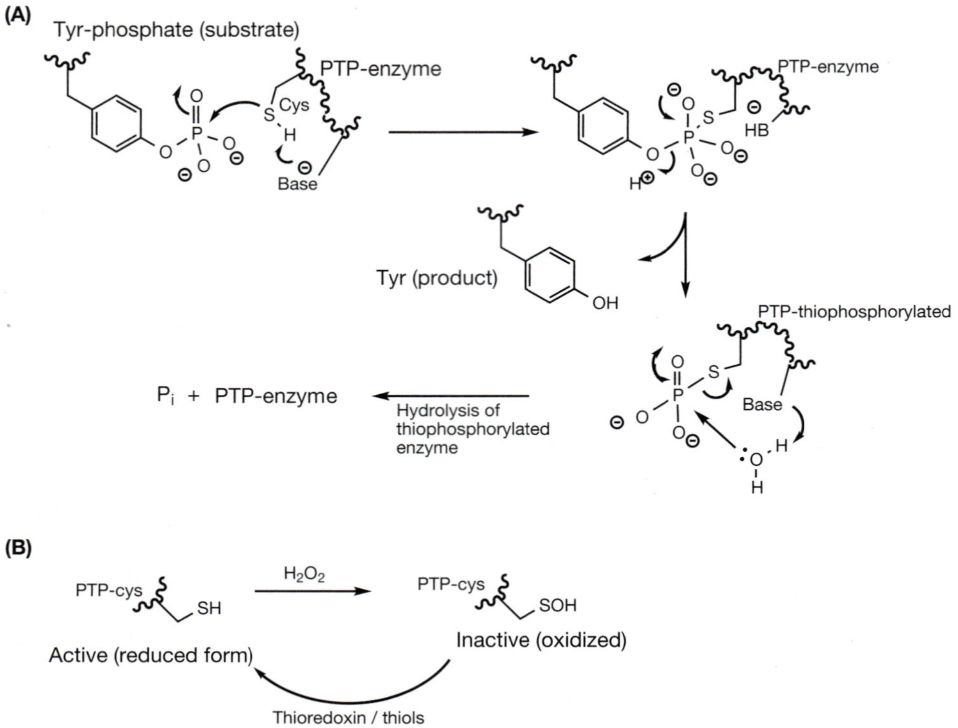

Figure 9.34 A. Mechanism of protein tyrosine phosphatase (PTP) action. B. Oxidation of free thiol of cysteine by hydrogen peroxide.

phosphorylated tyrosine to form a thiophosporyl intermediate, which is subsequently hydrolyzed by general base catalysis to release the free cysteine.[64] Moreover, the active sites of the PTPs are remarkably conserved, and so it becomes a challenge to design inhibitors directed to the active site to achieve specificity. However, studies have also shown that the activity of PTPs may be regulated by several mechanisms, including gene transcription, protein localization, and oligomerization (dimerization), as well as the oxidation state of the thiol group of the active site cysteine. Dimerization of the PTPs results in preventing the substrate from binding to the PTP active site.[64] Additionally, the catalytic activity of the active site cysteine thiol group is regulated by intracellular hydrogen peroxide. The –SH (thiol) group of the active site cysteine is easily oxidized by H_2O_2 to the nonnucleophilic, sulfenate (–SOH), thus inhibiting the phosphorylase activity. Figure 9.34A and B depicts the mechanism of the phosphatase activity as well as the redox regulation of the free cysteine. It should be remembered that the sulfenate can be easily reduced back to the active thiol by cytosolic thioredoxin or other small-molecule thiols.

This redox mechanism controlling the activity of the PTPs may then be exploited in order to design specific inhibitors. Efforts aimed to design inhibitors of the PTPs include molecules that interfere with the dimerization of the PTPs (compound 211 and SHP099) as well as those that can capture the sulfenate forms of active site cysteines (1,3-diketones and dimedone; see Fig. 9.35).[65]

Proteolysis-Targeting Chimeras. In the search for more potent inhibitors of dysfunctional proteins that contribute to disease states, developing enzyme inhibitors has been one of the more predominant strategies yielding phenomenal results in discovering selective and potent drugs with an increased safety and reduced toxicity profile. While this strategy has led to the development of highly potent inhibitors with activities in nM and pM concentrations, there is still a nagging tendency for even these excellently designed molecules to display toxicity and induce resistance. Devising strategies to control the dysfunctional effects of proteins to achieve enhanced clinical efficacy is an ongoing process. One recent strategy gaining momentum is to use small-molecule inhibitors with high binding to the aberrant protein and to simultaneously induce the natural proteosomal degradation of the protein. Such molecules being developed in this arena have been termed proteolysis-targeting chimeras (PROTACs).[63] These molecules, which have high binding domains to the offending protein, are conjugated via a flexible linker to another high affinity ligand that binds to the E3 ubiquitin ligase protein. Through this dual binding approach, the targeted protein is selected by ubiquitin for proteosomal degradation.

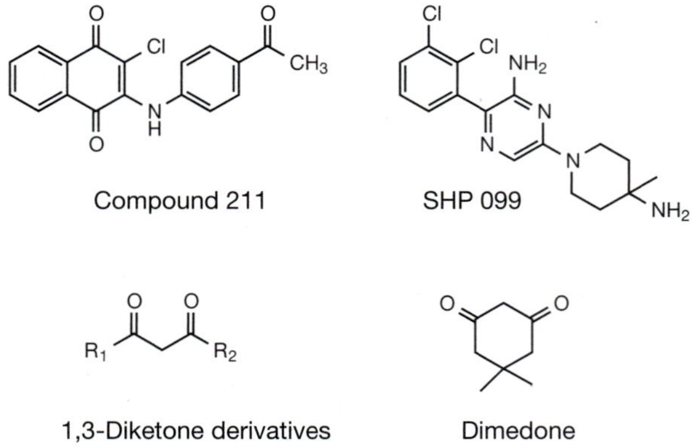

Figure 9.35 Structures of protein tyrosine phosphatase (PTP) inhibitors.

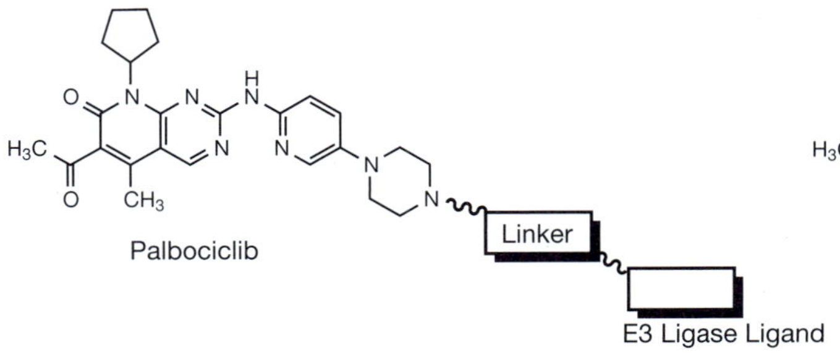

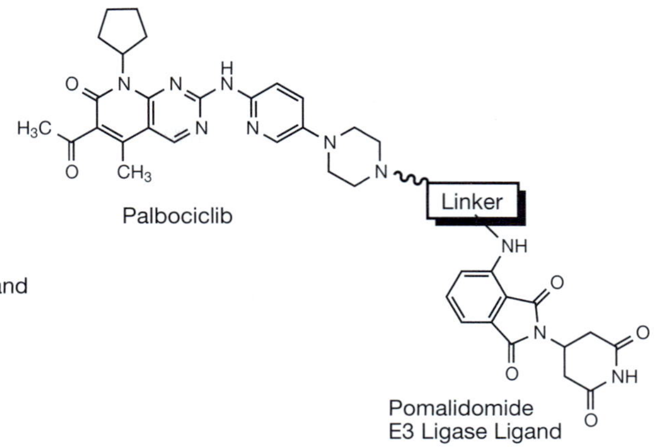

Figure 9.36 Structure of a proteolysis-targeting chimera (PROTAC).

Interestingly, these PROTACs act catalytically and may be generally applicable to target any protein for proteasomal degradation.

Examples of PROTACs used in the development for CDK4/6 inhibitors include a palbociclib conjugated to pomalidomide, a high affinity ligand for the E3 ubiquitin ligase as shown in Figure 9.36.[63]

CONCLUSION

This chapter has attempted to give the reader an overview of catalytic receptors and enzyme catalysis. Based on the properties and mechanisms of enzyme action, the essentials of the drug design process and discovery through enzyme inhibition with a few examples have been presented. The reader is referred to suggested reading material for some of the historical efforts as well as more detailed explanations and insights regarding the rationale and design strategies of enzyme inhibitors. In conclusion, catalytic receptors and enzymes continue to be an area that is exploited to develop therapies for human diseases. There will always be the need to elucidate receptor and enzyme mechanisms and based on those discoveries, to design more selective and potent inhibitors in an effort to increase therapeutic benefits to patients. The recent strategy and evolving use of PROTAC technology is likely to provide an additional tool in the overall arsenal to develop useful inhibitors that meet the health needs of the world. It is hoped that this chapter has given the reader an insightful perspective into this fascinating area of medicinal chemistry.

REFERENCES

1. Catalytic Receptors. IUPHAR/BPS guide to pharmacology. Accessed 2, August 2023. https://www.guidetopharmacology.org/GRAC/ReceptorFamiliesForward?type=CATALYTICRECEPTOR
2. Golan DE, Armstrong EJ, Armstrong AW, eds. Drug-receptor interactions. In: *Principles of Pharmacology: The Pathophysiologic Basis of Drug Therapy*. 4th ed. Wolters Kluwer; 2017:12.
3. Albert A. *Selective Toxicity–The Physicochemical Basis of Therapy*. 7th ed. Chapman & Hall; 1985.
4. Domagk G. Ein beitrag zur chemotherapie der bakteriellen infektionen. *Dtsch Med Wochenschr*. 1935;61:250-253.
5. Woods DD. Relation of p-aminobenzoic acid to mechanism of action of sulfanilamide. *Br J Exp Pathol*. 1940;21:74-90.
6. Albert A. Anti-metabolites: antagonistic analogues of coenzymes and enzymic substrates. In: *Selective Toxicity–The Physicochemical Basis of Therapy*. 7th ed. Chapman & Hall; 1985.
7. Fersht A. *Structure and Mechanism in Protein Science: A Guide to Enzyme Catalysis and Protein Folding*. 17th ed. World Scientific Press; 2017.
8. Lad C, Williams H, Wolfenden R. The rate of hydrolysis of phosphomonoester dianions and the exceptional catalytic proficiencies of protein and inositol phosphatases. *Proc Natl Acad Sci U S A*. 2003;100:5607-5610.
9. Nomenclature Committee of the International Union of Biochemistry and Molecular Biology. Enzyme nomenclature. Accessed August 6, 2023. http://www.sbcs.qmul.ac.uk/iubmb/enzyme/
10. Pauling L. The nature of forces between large molecules of biological interest. *Nature*. 1948;161:707-709.
11. Garcia-Viloca M, Gao J, Karplus M, Truhlar DG. How enzymes work: analysis by modern rate theory and computer simulations. *Science*. 2004;303:186-195.
12. Zhang X, Houk KN. Why enzymes are proficient catalysts: beyond the Pauling paradigm. *Acc Chem Res*. 2005;38:379-385.
13. Bruice TC, Benkovic SJ. A comparison of the bimolecular and intramolecular nucleophilic catalysis of the hydrolysis of substituted phenyl acylates by the dimethylamino group. *J Am Chem Soc*. 1963;85:1-8.
14. Michael C, Gaston S. Formation and hydrolysis of lactones of phenolic acids. *J Am Chem Soc*. 1980;102:4815-4821.
15. Pradere U, Garnier-Amblard EC, Coats SJ, et al. Synthesis of nucleoside phosphate and phosphonate prodrugs. *Chem Rev*. 2014;114:9154-9218.
16. Mitsuya H, Weinhold KJ, Furman PA, et al. 3′-Azido-3′-deoxythymidine (BW A509U): an antiviral agent that inhibits the infectivity and cytopathic effect of human T-lymphotropic virus type III/lymphadenopathy-associated virus in vitro. *Proc Natl Acad Sci U S A*. 1985;82:7096-7100.
17. Furman PA, Fyfe JA, St Clair MH, et al. Phosphorylation of 3″-azido-3′-deoxythymidine and selective interaction of the 5′-triphosphate with human immunodeficiency virus reverse transcriptase. *Proc Natl Acad Sci U S A*. 1986;83:8333-8337.
18. Grob PM, Wu JC, Cohen KA, et al. Nonnucleoside inhibitors of HIV-1 reverse transcriptase: nevirapine as a prototype drug. *AIDS Res Hum Retroviruses*. 1992;8:145-152.
19. Kohlstaedt LA, Wang J, Friedman JM, Rice PA, Steitz TA. Crystal structure at 3.5 A resolution of HIV-1 reverse transcriptase complexed with an inhibitor. *Science*. 1992;256:1783-1790.
20. Spence RA, Kati WM, Anderson KS, Johnson KA. Mechanism of inhibition of HIV-1 reverse transcriptase by nonnucleoside inhibitors. *Science*. 1995;267:988-993.
21. Mellors JW, Dutschman GE, Im GJ, Tramontano E, Winkler SR, Cheng YC. In vitro selection and molecular characterization of human immunodeficiency virus-1 resistant to nonnucleoside inhibitors of reverse transcriptase. *Mol Pharmacol*. 1992;41:446-451.

22. Harvison P, Harrold M. Drugs used to treat hypertensive/hypotensive disorders. In: Roche V, Zito S, Lemke T, Williams DA, eds. *Foye's Principles of Medicinal Chemistry*. 8th ed. Kluwers Wolters; 2019.
23. Cushman DW, Cheung HS, Sabo EF, Ondetti MA. Design of potent competitive inhibitors of angiotensin-converting enzyme. Carboxyalkanoyl and mercaptoalkanoyl amino acids. *Biochemistry*. 1977;16:5484-5491.
24. Byers LD, Wolfenden R. Binding of the by-product analogue benzylsuccinic acid by carboxypeptidase A. *Biochemistry*. 1973;12:2070-2078.
25. Patchett AA, Harris E, Tristram EW, et al. A new class of angiotensin-converting enzyme inhibitors. *Nature*. 1980;288:280-283.
26. Wolfenden R. Transition-state analogues for enzyme catalysis. *Nature*. 1969;223:704-705.
27. Wolfenden R. Transition-state analogues as potential affinity labeling agents. *Methods Enzymol*. 1977;46:15-28.
28. Shannon WM, Schabel FM. Antiviral agents as adjuncts in cancer chemotherapy. *Pharmacol Ther*. 1980;11:263-390.
29. Evans BE, Wolfenden RJ. A potential transition-state analogue for adenosine deaminase. *J Am Chem Soc*. 1970;92:4751-4752.
30. Nakamura H, Koyama G, Iitaka Y, Ono M, Yagiawa N. Structure of coformycin, an unusual nucleoside of microbial origin. *J Am Chem Soc*. 1974;96:4327-4328.
31. Walpole CSJ, Wrigglesworth R. Enzyme inhibitors in medicine. *Nat Prod Rep*. 1989;63:311-346.
32. Baker BR. *Design of Active Site Directed Irreversible Enzyme Inhibitors*. Wiley; 1967.
33. Walsh C. Recent developments in suicide substrates and other active site–directed inactivating agents of specific target enzymes. *Horiz Biochem Biophys*. 1977;3:36-81.
34. Abeless RH. Suicide enzyme inactivators. *Chem Eng News*. 1983;61(38):48-55.
35. Kraft GA, Katzenellenbogen JA. Synthesis of halo enol lactones. Mechanism-based inactivators of serine proteases. *J Am Chem Soc*. 1981;103:5459-5466.
36. Charnas RL, Knowles JR. Inactivation of RTEM β-lactamase from Escherichia coli by clavulanic acid and 9-deoxyclavulanic acid. *Biochemistry*. 1981;20:3214-3219.
37. Rando RR. Mechanisms of naturally occurring irreversible enzyme inhibitors. *Acc Chem Res*. 1975;8:281-288.
38. Bull HG, Garcia-Calvo M, Andersson S, et al. Mechanism-based inhibition of human steroid 5α-reductase by finasteride: enzyme-catalyzed formation of NADP-dihydrofinasteride, a potent bisubstrate analogue inhibitor. *J Am Chem Soc*. 1996;118:2359-2365.
39. Bender AT, Beavo JA. Cyclic nucleotide phosphodiesterases: molecular regulation to clinical use. *Pharmacol Rev*. 2006;58:488-520.
40. Lugnier C. Cyclic nucleotide phosphodiesterase (PDE) superfamily: a new target for the development of specific therapeutic agents. *Pharmacol Ther*. 2006;109:366-398.
41. Sutherland EW, Rall TW. Fractionation and characterization of a cyclic adenine ribonucleotide formed by tissue particles. *J Biol Chem*. 1958;232:1077-1091.
42. Card GI, England BP, Suzuki Y, et al. Structural basis for the activity of drugs that inhibit phosphodiesterases. *Structure*. 2004;12:2233-2247.
43. Hatzelmann A, Schudt C. Anti-inflammatory and immunomodulatory potential of the novel PDE4 inhibitor roflumilast in vitro. *J Pharmacol Exp Ther*. 2001;297:267-279.
44. Emmons PR, Harrison MJG, Honour AJ, Mitchell JR. Effect of dipyridamole on human platelet behavior. *Lancet*. 1965;2:603-606.
45. Terrett NK, Bell AS, Brown P, et al. Sildenafil (Viagara®), a potent and selective inhibitor of type 5 cGMP phosphodiesterase with utility for the treatment of male erectile dysfunction. *Bioorg Med Chem Lett*. 1996;6:1819-1824.
46. Manning G, Whyte DB, Martinez R, Hunter T, Sudarsanam S. The protein kinase complement of the human genome. *Science*. 2002;298:1912-1934.
47. Ferguson FM, Gray NS. Kinase inhibitors: the road ahead. *Nat. Rev*. 2018;17:353-376.
48. Sawyers C. Chronic myeloid leukemia. *N Eng J Med*. 1999;340:1330-1340.
49. Schindler T, Bornmann W, Pellicena P, Miller WT, Clarkson B, Kuriyan J. Structural mechanism for STI-571 inhibition of Abelson tyrosine kinase. *Science*. 2000;289:1938-1942.
50. Druker BJ, Tamura J, Buchdunger E, et al. Effects of a selective inhibitor of the Abl tyrosine kinase on the growth of Bcr-Abl positive cells. *Nat Med*. 1996;2:561-566.
51. Aurora A, Scholar EM. Role of tyrosine kinase inhibitors in cancer therapy. *J Pharmacol Exp Ther*. 2005;315:971-979.
52. Nagar B, Bornmann WG, Pellicena P, et al. Crystal structures of the kinase domain of c-Abl in complex with the small molecule inhibitors PD173955 and imatinib (STI-571). *Cancer Res*. 2002;62:4236-4243.
53. Wu P, Neilson TE, Cluasen MH. FDA-approved small molecule kinase inhibitors. *Trends Pharmacol Sci*. 2015;36(7):422-439.
54. Kooistra AJ, Kanev GK, van Linden OPJ, et al. KLIFS: a structural kinase-ligand interaction database. *Nucleic Acids Res*. 2016;44(Database issue):D365-D371.
55. Yeung DT, Shanmuganathan N, Hughes TP. Asciminib: a new therapeutic option in chronic-phase CML with treatment failure. *Blood*. 2022;139(24):3474-3478.
56. Bousoik E, Aliabadi HM. Do we know Jack about JAK—A closer look at JAK/STAT signaling pathway. *Front Oncol*. 2019;8:1-20.
57. Hu X, Li J, Fu M, Zhao X, Wang W. The JAK/STAT signaling pathway—from bench to clinic. *Signal Transduct Target Ther*. 2021;6:402-435.
58. Hoy SM. Deucravacitinib: first approval. *Drugs*. 2022;18:1671-1679.
59. Maoz A, Ciccone MA, Matsuzaki S, et al. Emerging serine-threonine kinase inhibitors for treating ovarian cancer. *Expert Opin Emerg Drugs*. 2019; 24(6):239-253.
60. Vader G, Lens SMA. The Aurora kinase family in cell division and cancer. *Biochim Biophys Acta*. 2008;1786:60-72.
61. Katayama H, Sen S. Aurora kinase inhibitors as anticancer molecules. *Biochim Biophys Acta*. 2010;1799:829-839.
62. Hertzman Johansson C, Egyhazi Brage S. BRAF inhibitors in cancer therapy. *Pharmacol Ther*. 2014;142:176-182.
63. Amamazzalorso A, Agamennone M, De Filippis BD, Fantacuzzi M. Development of CDK4/6 inhibitors. A five years update. *Molecules*. 2021;26:1488-1509.
64. Sharma K, D'Souza RCJ, Tyanova S, et al. Ultradeep human phosphoproteome reveals a distinct regulatory nature of Tyr and Ser/Thr-based signaling. *Cell Rep*. 2014;8:1583-1594.
65. Yu ZH, Zhang ZY. Regulatory mechanisms and novel therapeutic targeting strategies for protein tyrosine phosphatases. *Chem Rev*. 2018;118:1069-1091.

SUGGESTED READINGS

Abeless RH. Suicide enzyme inactivators. *Chem Eng News*. 1983;61(38):48-55.

Albert A. *Selective Toxicity—The Physicochemical Basis of Therapy*. 7th ed. Chapman & Hall; 1985.

Baker BR. *Design of Active Site Directed Irreversible Enzyme Inhibitors*. Wiley; 1967.

Kalman TI, ed. *Drug Action & Design—Mechanism-Based Enzyme Inhibitors*. Elsevier; 1979.

Seiler N, Jung MJ, Kock-Weser J, eds. *Enzyme-Activated Irreversible Inhibitors*. Elsevier North-Holland; 1978.

Silverman RB. *The Organic Chemistry of Enzyme Catalyzed Reactions, Revised edition*. 2nd ed. Academic Press; 2002.

Silverman RB, Holladay MW. *The Organic Chemistry of Drug Design and Drug Action*. 3rd ed. Elsevier; 2014.

Smith JS, *ed. Smith and Williams' Introduction to the Principles of Drug Design and Action*. 3rd ed. Harwood Academic Press; 1998.

Sneader W. *Drug Discovery—A History*. John Wiley & Sons; 2005.

Walpole CSJ, Wrigglesworth R. Enzyme inhibitors in medicine. *Nat Prod Rep*. 1989;63:311-346.

Wolfenden R. Transition-state analogues as potential affinity labeling agents. *Methods Enzymol*. 1977;46:15-28.

PART III

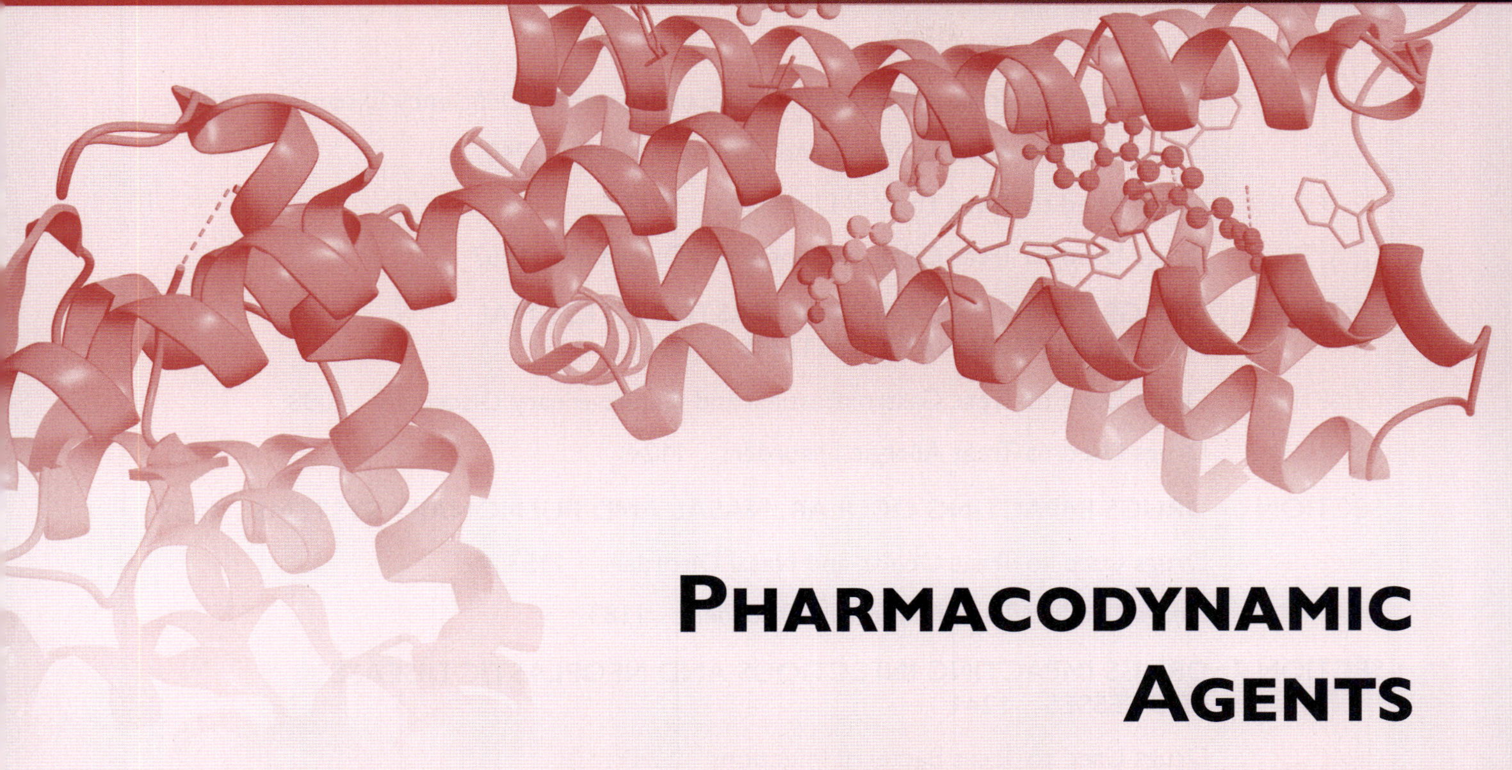

PHARMACODYNAMIC AGENTS

SECTION 1

Drugs Impacting the Central Nervous System

CHAPTER 10

Drugs Used to Treat Neuromuscular Disorders

Gregory D. Cuny

Drugs covered in this chapter:

- Alemtuzumab
- Amantadine
- Amifampridine
- Apomorphine
- Baclofen
- Botulinum toxin type A
- Bromocriptine
- Cabergoline
- Carbidopa
- Carisoprodol
- Cladribine
- Cyclobenzaprine
- Dalfampridine
- Dantrolene
- Deflazacort
- Diazepam
- Dimethyl fumarate
- Diroximel
- Edaravone
- Entacapone
- Eteplirsen
- Fingolimod
- Glatiramer
- Interferon beta-1a
- Interferon beta-1b
- Istradefylline
- L-Dopa
- Metaxalone
- Methocarbamol
- Monomethyl fumarate
- Natalizumab
- Neostigmine
- Nusinersen
- Ocrelizumab
- Omaveloxolone
- Opicapone
- Ozanimod
- Peginterferon beta-1a
- Pramipexole
- Pyridostigmine
- Rasagiline
- Riluzole
- Ropinirole
- Rotigotine
- Safinamide
- Selegiline
- Siponimod
- Sugammadex
- Teriflunomide
- Tetrabenazine
- Tizanidine
- Tofersen
- Tolcapone
- Valbenazine

Abbreviations

21-desDFZ 21-desacetyldeflazacort
AAAD aromatic L-amino acid decarboxylase
AD aldehyde dehydrogenase
ALS amyotrophic lateral sclerosis
AUC area under the (plasma concentration) curve
BBB blood-brain barrier
BCRP breast cancer resistance protein
CBR carbonyl reductase
C_{max} maximum plasma concentration
CNS central nervous system
COMT catechol-*O*-methyltransferase
CP cerebral palsy
CSF cerebral spinal fluid
CYP450 cytochrome P450
DβH dopamine β-hydroxylate
DMD Duchenne muscular dystrophy
DOPAC 3,4-dihydroxyphenylacetic acid
DOPAL 3,4-dihydroxyphenylacetaldehyde
FAD flavin adenine dinucleotide
GABA gamma-aminobutyric acid
HVA homovanillic acid
IgG immunoglobulin G

Abbreviations—continued

JAK/STAT Janus kinase/signal transducers and activators of transcription
KEAP-1 Kelch-like erythroid cell–derived associated protein 1
LEMS Lambert-Eaton myasthenic syndrome
LRRK2 leucine-rich repeat kinase 2
MAO monoamine oxidase
MBP myelin basic protein
MG myasthenia gravis
MHC major histocompatibility complex
MND motor neuron disease
MPDP⁺ 1-methyl-4-phenyl-2, 3-dihydropyridinium
MPP⁺ 1-methyl-4-phenylpyridinium
MPTP 1-methyl-4-phenyl-1,2,3, 6-tetrahydropyridine
mRNA messenger RNA
MS multiple sclerosis
MTA 3-methoxytyramine
NADP⁺ nicotinamide adenine dinucleotide phosphate
NMDA *N*-methyl-D-aspartate
Nrf2 nuclear factor (erythroid-derived 2)-like 2
OCT organic cation transporter
PD Parkinson disease
PDB Protein Data Bank
PENT phenylethanolamine-*N*-methyltransferase
PINK1 PTEN-induced putative kinase 1
PLP pyridoxal-5′-phosphate
RLS restless leg syndrome
RYR ryanodine receptor
S1P1 sphingosine-1-phosphate receptor 1
SAM S-adenosyl methionine
SMA spinal muscular atrophy
SMN survival motor neuron
SOD superoxide dismutase
SULT sulfotransferase
TDP-43 TAR DNA-binding protein 43
TH tyrosine hydroxylase
T_{max} time to maximum plasma concentration
UGT UDP-glucuronosyltransferase
VCAM-1 vascular cell adhesion molecule 1
VMA vanillylmandelic acid
VMAT2 vesicular monoamine transporter 2
VPS35 vacuolar protein sorting–associated protein 35

CLINICAL SIGNIFICANCE

The past few decades have seen progress in the development and application of drugs to treat many neuromuscular disorders including Parkinson disease (PD), multiple sclerosis (MS), amyotrophic lateral sclerosis (ALS), and more. These conditions can be debilitating and/or life-threatening. Understanding the chemistry behind these drugs' mechanisms of action is necessary for clinical practitioners for several reasons such as predicting and monitoring for potential adverse reactions. For example, hallucinations and other symptoms of psychosis are much more common with levodopa and dopamine receptor agonists than monoamine oxidase (MAO) inhibitors. Understanding how these complex agents interact with their receptors enables individuals in clinical settings to make rational drug selections as well as anticipating specific adverse effects.

Jeffrey T. Sherer, PharmD, MPH, BCPS, BCGP

Overview of Neuromuscular Disorders

Neuromuscular disorders are a broad classification of conditions for which chemotherapeutic agents are available for only a subset of maladies. This chapter will cover the neurodegenerative movement disorder PD and the autoimmune disease MS. In addition, several neuromuscular disorders for which drug treatments have only more recently become available will also be described, including ALS and Duchenne muscular dystrophy (DMD). However, pharmacotherapy for these ailments remains far from ideal. Although advances are being made in understanding the cause and pathogenesis of these diseases, prophylactic or curative therapies are not currently available.

The second group of conditions examined includes muscle spasticity disorders, which broadly cover maladies characterized by tonic stretch reflexes, flexor muscle spasms, and muscle weakness. Spasticity may accompany several disorders but is often associated with cerebral palsy (CP), MS, spinal cord injury, and stroke. A few chemotherapeutics are available to treat these ailments. But their mechanism of action, and in some cases their efficacy, is less clear. Recently approved chemotherapeutic agents for reversing anesthetic drug–induced nondepolarizing neuromuscular blockage that have also been used for treating myasthenia gravis (MG), as well as a recently approved agent to treat Lambert-Eaton myasthenic syndrome (LEMS), will be described. Finally, drugs to treat chorea associated with Huntington disease and tardive dyskinesia, which can occur in patients on long-term neuroleptic medication treatment, as well as a new drug to treat Friedreich ataxia will be presented.

Parkinson Disease

Therapeutic Context Overview

PD is a chronic and progressive movement disorder that presents with symptoms of (1) resting tremor of the hands, arms, legs, jaw, and/or face; (2) bradykinesia or slow initiation and paucity of voluntary movements; (3) rigidity of the limbs and trunk; and (4) postural instability, including impaired balance and coordination. Many patients with PD also suffer from dementia and psychiatric conditions, including hallucinations and depression.[1]

PD is a neurodegenerative disease most prominently afflicting the extrapyramidal dopaminergic neurons that have cell bodies in the substantia nigra pars compacta located in the midbrain with nerve terminals extending into the corpus striatum (Fig. 10.1). These regions of the brain play significant roles in motor control. PD results from progressive dysfunction and cell death of these neurons, causing a deficiency of dopamine in the nerve terminals in the corpus striatum.[1]

Like many other neurodegenerative diseases, PD is characterized by diagnostic histopathologic features. One of the most prominent facets is Lewy bodies, which are intracellular protein aggregates that form spherical deposits within neurons. However, Lewy bodies are not confined to the substantia nigra pars compacta or corpus striatum but can also be found in other areas of the brain. Furthermore, these aggregates are present in other neurologic conditions,[2] such as dementia with Lewy bodies and multiple system atrophy. The primary component of the aggregates is α-synuclein, an abundant protein found mainly in the brain and in lesser amounts in other tissues. The functions of α-synuclein are not well understood. However, it may play a role in regulating dopamine homeostasis, including modulation of dopamine synthesis (eg, interacting with tyrosine hydroxylase [TH]), release, and reuptake at nerve terminals.[3,4] However, its neurotoxicity may stem from synaptic dysfunction, mitochondrial impairment, defective endoplasmic reticulum function and autophagy lysosomal pathways, and nuclear dysfunction.[5] In addition, oligomeric forms of the protein are also thought to be involved in neurotoxicity mechanisms.[6]

The etiology of PD is unknown. However, in some cases, genetics appears to play a critical role. Epidemiologic studies have found age is the most prominent risk factor for developing PD followed by a family history of the disease.[7,8] Genetic forms of PD have been found in a small portion of cases (<10%), most involving early disease onset. For example, autosomal dominant mutations in the α-synuclein gene (eg, *SNCA*) have been described in several families.[9,10] Mutations in other genes have also been found to be associated with PD, including those that encode leucine-rich repeat kinase 2 (LRRK2), VPS35, parkin, PINK1, and DJ-1.[11]

Mutations in the *PARK8* gene, which encodes for LRRK2, have been linked to early-onset PD. Individuals who inherit the G2019S mutation in LRRK2 from either parent have a significant increased risk for developing PD with increasing age. In addition, up to 40% of people of North African Arab ancestry and 25% of Ashkenazi Jewish people with PD have this mutation.[12] LRRK2 is a complex protein containing domains with GTPase, kinase, and scaffolding functions. LRRK2 (wild type and mutants) has been implicated in a host of neurotoxic mechanisms, such as apoptosis induction, autophagy, and mitochondrial dysfunction, which could contribute to PD.

A mutation (D620N) in the vacuolar protein sorting–associated protein 35 (VPS35) subunit of the retromer complex, which is involved in retrograde transport of proteins from endosomes to the Golgi, was identified as a rare cause of autosomal dominant familial PD.[13,14] The VPS35 D620N mutation exhibits both gain and loss of functions that could contribute to PD.[15]

Loss-of-function mutations in the *PARK2* gene, which encodes the protein parkin, cause autosomal recessive juvenile PD. Loss of the protein may lead to synaptic damage and dysfunction resulting in dopaminergic neuron loss.[16] Parkin appears to also be recruited to impaired mitochondria where it can promote autophagy, which is an intracellular degradation system that delivers cytoplasmic constituents to the lysosome for catabolism.[17,18]

Autosomal recessive mutations have been found in the *PARK6* gene, which encodes the PTEN-induced putative kinase 1 (eg, PINK1), a mitochondrial serine/threonine protein kinase. This protein appears to function in mitochondrial quality control since mutations in this gene have been shown to compromise mitochondrial integrity.[19,20]

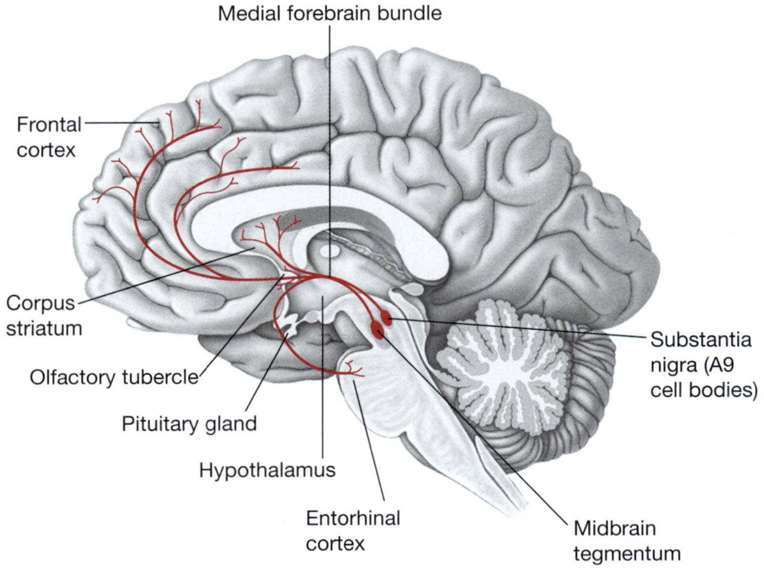

Figure 10.1 Depiction of brain regions and dopaminergic pathways involved in Parkinson disease.

Finally, autosomal recessive mutations have been reported in the *PARK7* gene (also known as the *DJ-1* gene), which encodes the protein DJ-1. In the context of PD, this protein is thought to function as a redox-dependent molecular chaperone of α-synuclein.[21,22] While its functions in cells are not fully understood, it appears to provide neurons protection against oxidative stress.[23] Although an array of protein mutations have been associated with PD, most cases are sporadic.[24]

Environmental factors also appear to play an important role in the etiology of PD. It has been well recognized that exposure to certain chemicals can cause symptoms of PD to significantly increase the risk of developing the disease. One of the most direct connections of chemical exposure and PD involves the compound MPTP (1-methyl-4-phenyl-1,2,3,6-tetrahydropyridine). This material induces a PD-like condition in humans and primates that is similar in neuropathology and motor abnormalities seen in the idiopathic form of the disease,[25] which came to light through tragic cases of illicit designer drug use involving a derivative of meperidine where the ester was reversed.[26,27] In this case, it is not the parent compound that is the culprit for the neurotoxicity, but a reactive metabolite (Fig. 10.2). Since MPTP has low molecular weight and contains a lipophilic tertiary amine, it readily crosses the blood-brain barrier (BBB), where it undergoes oxidative metabolism to the unstable intermediate 1-methyl-4-phenyl-2,3-dihydropyridinium ($MPDP^+$), which is further oxidized to 1-methyl-4-phenylpyridinium (MPP^+),[28,29] a pyridinium cation that is a reactive electrophile. The metabolism is MAO-B mediated, as inhibitors of this enzyme have been shown to block the reaction pathway.[30] Furthermore, MPP^+ is taken up by dopamine transporters present in catecholamine neurons, including those in the *substantia nigra*, and elicits neurotoxicity by inhibition of mitochondrial complex I.[31] Other chemicals have similarly been linked to PD, including the herbicide paraquat (which is structurally similar to MPP^+),[32] the natural product rotenone,[33,34] and manganese.[35]

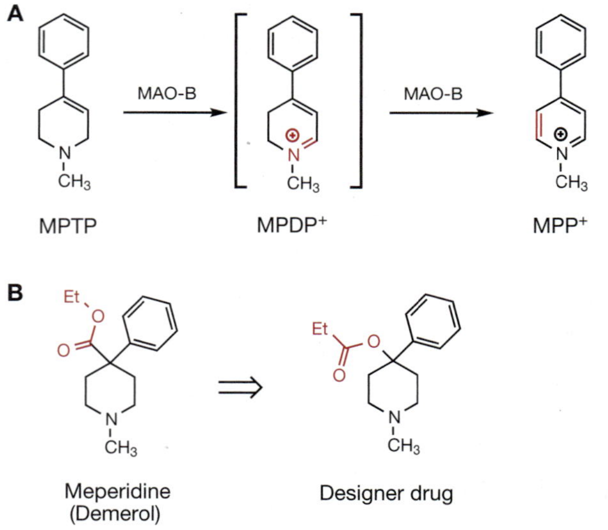

Figure 10.2 A. Metabolism of MPTP to MPP+, a neurotoxin that causes a Parkinson-like condition. B. Structures of meperidine and a designer drug where the ester of meperidine is reversed. MAO, monoamine oxidase; MPDP+, 1-methyl-4-phenyl-2, 3-dihydropyridinium; MPP+, 1-methyl-4-phenylpyridinium; MPTP, 1-methyl-4-phenyl-1,2,3,6-tetrahydropyridine.

Interestingly, some environmental factors appear to reduce the risk of developing PD. For example, cigarette smokers have a lower incidence of PD than nonsmokers.[36,37] It has been proposed that tobacco smoke may contain MAO inhibitors[38,39] or that nicotine might play a role.[40] Coffee consumption is also correlated with a lower risk of developing PD[41] possibly due to caffeine's antagonism of adenosine receptors.[42]

PD typically presents after age 55 and affects approximately 1% to 2% of the population over age 65. However, after age 84, the incidence of PD increases to 3% to 5% per year.[43] Very little prevalence differences are seen in the incidence of PD between men and women as well as geographical location.[44]

As the second most common neurodegenerative disease, PD accounts for significant national economic burdens. In the United States, the cost associated with PD exceeded US$14.4 billion in 2010 (~US$22,800 per patient). This burden is projected to grow substantially over the next few decades as the size of the older adult population increases.[45] Similar trends are likely throughout the world where the size of the older adult population is increasing. According to the Parkinson's Foundation, the estimated per patient medication cost for treating PD is US$2,500 per year.[46]

Pharmacology Overview

Since the most consequential tissue affected by PD is extrapyramidal dopaminergic neurons in the substantia nigra pars compacta and corpus striatum, it is perhaps not surprising that most current pharmacologic therapies for the treatment of PD have a connection to the neurotransmitter dopamine. However, direct administration of dopamine to patients with PD is not an effective treatment mainly due to the inability of peripheral dopamine to penetrate the BBB. Although dopamine has a low molecular weight, it is a relatively polar molecule and is not subjected to active transport into the brain.

To understand the rationale for the development of dopamine-based PD drugs, it is first important to review the biosynthesis and catabolism of this neurotransmitter (Fig. 10.3). The essential amino acid L-tyrosine is converted to L-dopa by TH, which is found peripherally and in the central nervous system (CNS).[47] The primary route of metabolism of L-dopa is decarboxylation to dopamine by an aromatic L-amino acid decarboxylase (AAAD, eg, L-dopa decarboxylase), again in both the periphery and CNS, although a minor pathway generating 3-methoxy-4-hydroxyphenyllactic acid also occurs. Dopamine is further metabolized via two primary pathways. The first route involves MAO-mediated oxidation to DOPAL (3,4-dihydroxyphenylacetaldehyde) that is further oxidized by aldehyde dehydrogenase (AD) to DOPAC (3,4-dihydroxyphenylacetic acid), which is methylated on the 3-hydroxy by catechol-O-methyltransferase (COMT) to generate homovanillic acid (HVA). Alternatively, dopamine is converted

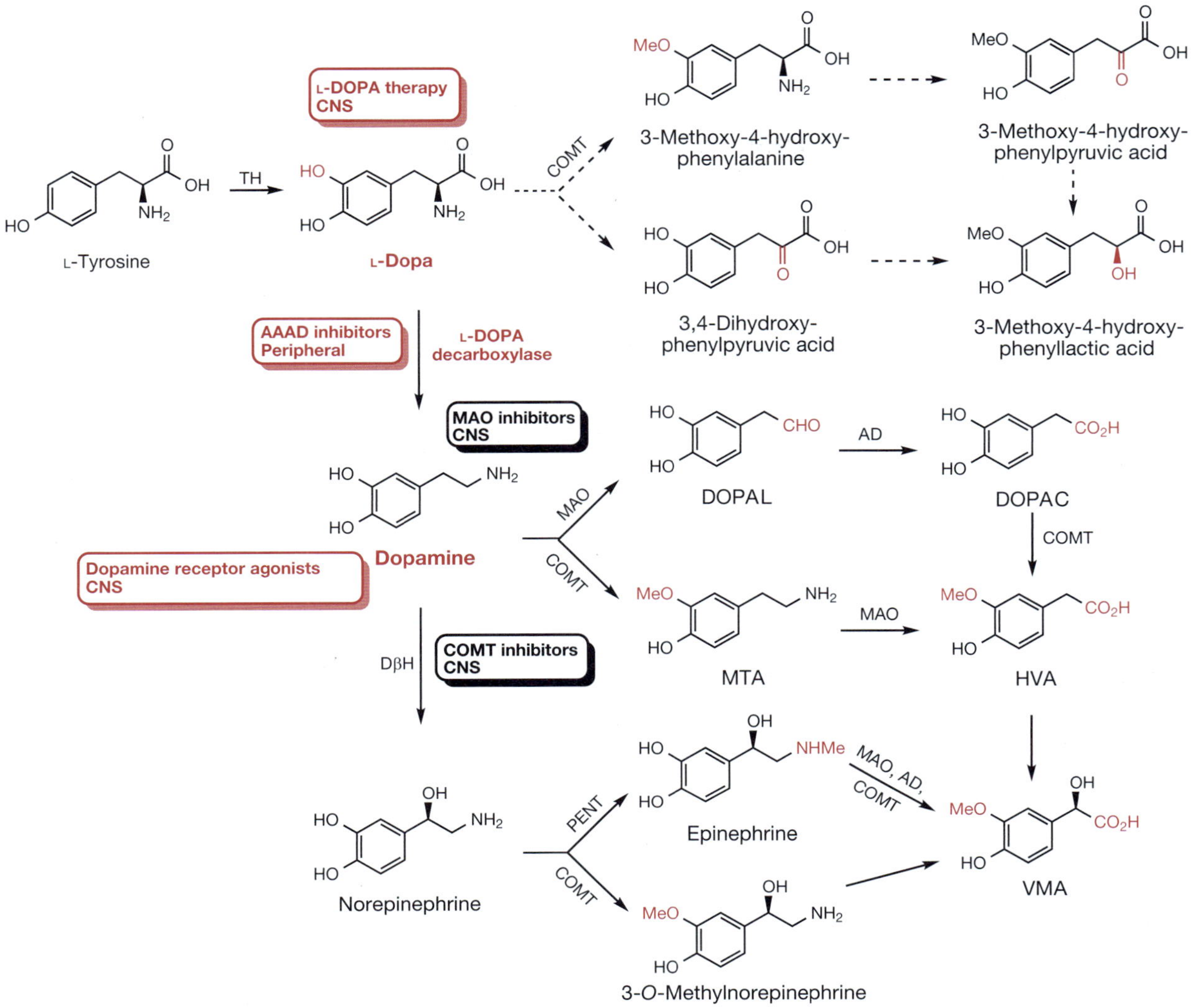

Figure 10.3 Biosynthesis and catabolism of dopamine. Intervention points to increase brain dopamine concentration and/or neurotransmitter function are highlighted. Dash arrows indicate minor routes. AAAD, aromatic L-amino acid decarboxylase; AD, aldehyde dehydrogenase; CNS, central nervous system; COMT, catechol-*O*-methyltransferase; DH, dopamine β-hydroxylase; DOPAC, 3,4-dihydroxyphenylacetic acid; DOPAL, 3,4-dihydroxyphenylacetaldehyde; HVA, homovanillic acid; MAO, monoamine oxidase; MTA, 3-methoxytyramine; PENT, phenylethanolamine-*N*-methyltransferase; VMA, vanillylmandelic acid.

to 3-methoxytyramine (MTA) via COMT and then oxidized by MAO to generate HVA. The second pathway involves dopamine β-hydroxylate (DβH) oxidation of dopamine to norepinephrine, which is converted to vanillylmandelic acid (VMA) via a series of enzyme-mediated reactions.

The nature of the oxidative metabolism of dopamine is also believed to play a contributing role in the neurotoxicity observed in PD via several different mechanisms. For example, in the synthesis of dopamine, L-tyrosine is converted to L-dopa via hydroxylation of the 3-position of the phenol. This reaction may proceed directly via C-H bond insertion, circumventing highly electrophilic and reactive intermediates (Fig. 10.4A). Alternatively, the process can generate an epoxide intermediate, as is seen in the metabolic conversion of benzene to phenol.[48] This intermediate can rearrange to a hydroxyl ketone intermediate that can tautomerize to L-dopa. However, this same intermediate can potentially be oxidized to an *ortho*-quinone intermediate. Both the epoxide and *ortho*-quinone intermediates are electrophilic and highly reactive toward nucleophilic functional groups, such as those present in proteins, RNA, DNA, or other biomolecules, which can lead to neurotoxicity.[49] In addition, dopamine can auto-oxidize to the hydroxyl ketone and *ortho*-quinone intermediates.[50,51] Finally, during MAO catalysis of dopamine (and other monoamine neurotransmitters, like norepinephrine and serotonin), hydrogen peroxide is generated (Fig. 10.4B) that can undergo a redox reaction (eg, Haber-Weiss reaction) with superoxide to form the cytotoxic hydroxyl radical (eg, OH•).

It was recognized several decades ago that dopamine concentrations in the corpus striatum of patients with PD were only 20% of normal levels.[52] Thus, the biosynthesis and catabolism of dopamine presented several intervention points to increase dopamine concentration and/or the function of the neurotransmitter in affected brain areas. One of the most direct strategies to do this was to administer L-dopa.

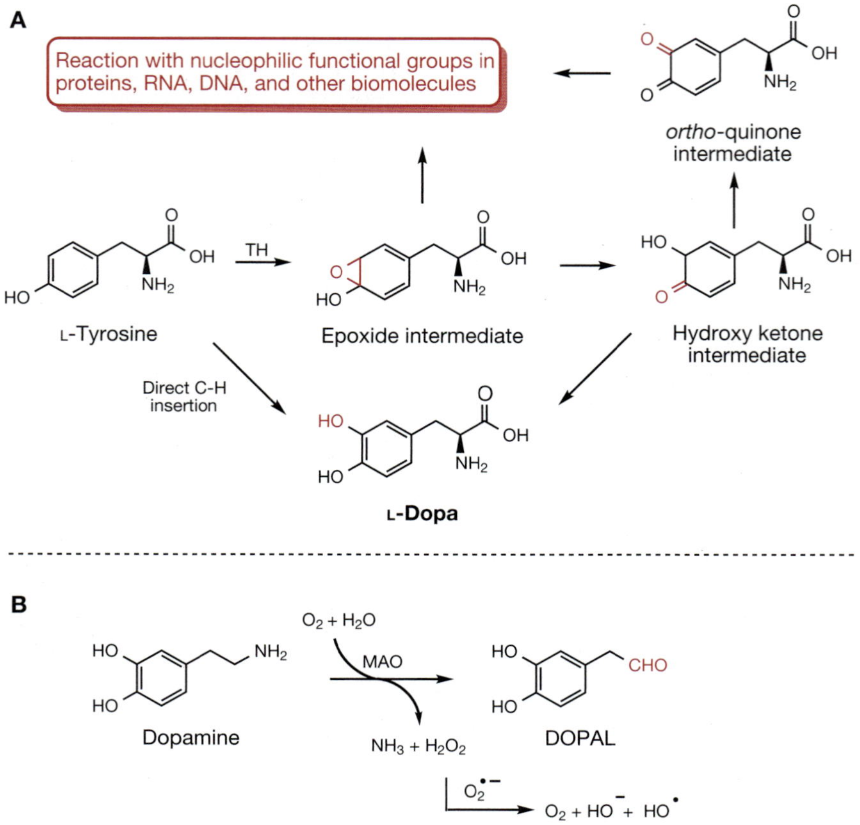

Figure 10.4 A. Potential mechanism for the conversion of L-tyrosine to L-dopa and reactive intermediates that could contribute to neurotoxicity in PD. B. Potential mechanisms for the generation of cytotoxic hydroxy radical (eg, HO•) during MAO-mediated oxidation of dopamine to DOPAL. DOPAL, 3,4-dihydroxyphenylacetaldehyde; MAO, monoamine oxidase; PD, Parkinson disease.

Birkmayer and Hornykiewicz found that high oral doses of racemic dopa to patients with PD were effective.[53] Subsequent clinical trials with racemic and enantiomeric pure L-dopa demonstrated the benefits of this therapeutic strategy.[54-56] Although L-dopa is more polar than dopamine and, based on its physicochemical properties, would not be expected to cross the BBB, it is actively transported into the brain primarily by L-type amino acid transporters and then decarboxylated to dopamine in situ.[57]

Although L-dopa can be efficacious as a single agent, only about 1% of an orally administered dose reaches the brain.[58] The remainder undergoes rapid decarboxylation in peripheral tissues to generate dopamine, which does not cross the BBB. However, the peripheral decarboxylation of L-dopa can be competitively inhibited by coadministration of a dopa decarboxylase inhibitor.[59] Furthermore, the dopa decarboxylase inhibitors were designed to restrict permeability across the BBB. Thus, these compounds prevent decarboxylation of L-dopa selectively in the periphery, but not in the CNS. Overall, this combination therapy markedly increases (by 2.5- to 30-fold) the amount of L-dopa that reaches the brain where it is converted to dopamine.[60]

Two other therapeutic strategies for the treatment of PD involve inhibition of dopamine-metabolizing enzymes. As previously mentioned, once dopamine is generated in the brain it is subjected to three routes of metabolism. One of these pathways is the conversion of dopamine to norepinephrine via benzylic oxidation by DβH. However, this is not a process for which inhibitors have been developed for the treatment of PD. But blocking the conversion of dopamine to DOPAL via MAO and to MTA via COMT has become an effective means of increasing brain levels of dopamine that provides symptomatic relief for patients with PD.

The final dopamine-related therapeutic approach is the use of dopamine agonists to mimic the actions of the depleted endogenous neurotransmitter. Although these drugs do not increase brain levels of dopamine, they bind to various dopamine receptors and act as functional agonists, stimulating signaling pathways normally activated by dopamine. Although these drugs can provide symptomatic relief for patients with PD, they do not impact the underlying disease progression.

The last common pharmacotherapy approach currently available for the treatment of PD is the use of nondopamine-related drugs. These agents have a variety of functions that may offer neuroprotective effects that can provide benefit for PD and/or the associated dyskinesias induced by L-dopa therapy. Although several genetic links have been made to PD as discussed earlier, to date, these targets and associated pathways have yet to be translated into effective pharmacotherapy. Research activities into these various molecular targets continue with the hope that new and potentially disease-modifying agents will emerge for clinical testing.

Many PD pharmacotherapies are associated with common adverse effects. For example, patients receiving drugs that increase dopamine levels or function report falling asleep while engaged in activities of daily living, including driving or operating machinery. Although many of these patients reported somnolence, some perceived that they had no warning signs. Other common adverse effects of anti-PD drugs include hyperpyrexia and confusion, impulse control and compulsive behaviors, hallucinations/psychotic-like behavior, dyskinesia, and depression. Interestingly, studies have shown that patients with PD have a higher risk (2- to 6-fold) of developing melanoma, a malignant skin cancer. It is unclear if this increased risk is due to the neurodegenerative disease or drug treatment. Also, since many drugs used to treat PD increase dopamine levels or agonize dopamine receptors, they can modulate the function of dopamine antagonists, such as antipsychotics.

In addition, some PD pharmacotherapies are associated with drug-drug interactions. For example, concomitant use of nonselective or selective MAO inhibitors with antidepressants, including selective serotonin reuptake inhibitors, serotonin/norepinephrine reuptake inhibitors, and tricyclics as well as opioid analgesics such as meperidine, tramadol, methadone, and propoxyphene, can cause serotonin syndrome. This condition can range in severity from mild to life-threatening, typically consisting of signs broadly characterized as altered mental status, abnormal neuromuscular tone, and autonomic hyperactivity.[61] These symptoms can include high body temperature (>40 °C), agitation, increased reflexes, tremor, sweating, dilated pupils, and diarrhea, potentially resulting in seizure. Another example of drug-drug interactions is the modulation of MAO and COMT that are involved in the biosynthesis and catabolism of catecholamines, as well as the metabolism of xenobiotics (see Chapter 3). Inhibitors of these enzymes can have an impact on catecholamine levels and the metabolism of concomitant drug treatment. Therefore, drugs known to be metabolized by MAO or COMT should be administered with caution in patients receiving MAO or COMT inhibitors.

Dopamine and Dopamine Receptor–Related Therapy

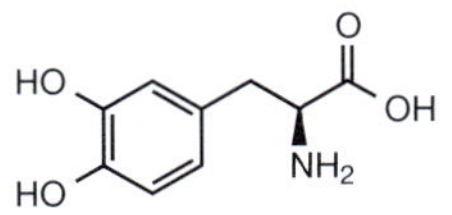

L-Dopa
(Levodopa)

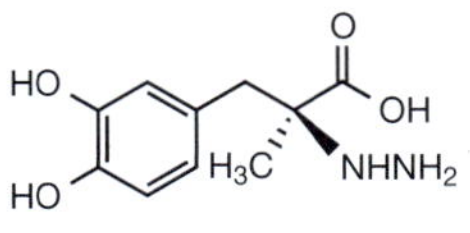

Carbidopa
(Lodosyn)

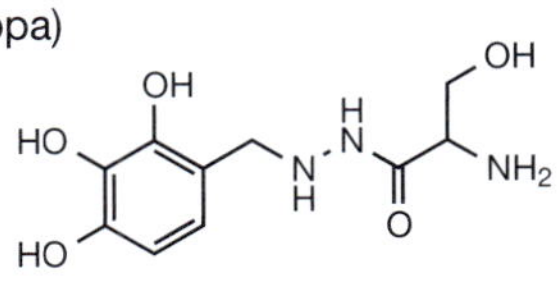

Benserazide

L-Dopa decarboxylase inhibitors

L-Dopa

L-Dopa is an amino acid ([S]-3,4-dihydroxyphenylalanine) that has been used as dopamine replacement therapy since it can cross the BBB and undergo decarboxylation to generate dopamine in the brain. However, L-dopa is currently coadministered/coformulated with a dopa decarboxylase inhibitor (eg, carbidopa or benserazide). In patients with an average age of 71, L-dopa has an oral bioavailability of 63%, a plasma clearance of 14.2 mL/min/kg, and a volume of distribution of 1.01 L/kg (Table 10.1). In the presence of carbidopa, the area under the (plasma concentration) curve (AUC) after oral administration of L-dopa significantly increases (2,926 ng h/mL to 4,530 ng h/mL) due to lower systemic clearance.[62] In addition, the plasma elimination half-life of L-dopa increases from 50 minutes to 1.5 hours. L-Dopa undergoes extensive peripheral metabolism with <1% of an oral dose being eliminated as the parent drug in the urine.[63]

Carbidopa

Carbidopa is used in combination with L-dopa for the treatment of PD. Although carbidopa is structurally similar to L-dopa, it has two notable differences. First, the amine in L-dopa has been replaced with a hydrazine moiety, while the absolute stereochemistry (eg, *S*) has been retained. Second, the carbon that the hydrazine is attached to is further substituted with a methyl group. These changes provide a hydrazine that can readily react with a cofactor in the active site of L-dopa decarboxylase. Carbidopa is formulated as a monohydrate that is a white crystalline solid and slightly soluble in water. Benserazide, although not approved for use in the United States, is another L-dopa decarboxylase inhibitor used in other countries for the same purpose. Structurally it is quite different from carbidopa. It is comprised of the racemic form of the amino acid serine linked through an acyl hydrazine, which is further substituted with pyrogallol attached through a methylene. Benserazide is readily hydrolyzed in plasma to trihydroxybenzylhydrazine that readily reacts with a cofactor in the active site of L-dopa decarboxylase.[64]

Carbidopa itself has not been demonstrated to have any additional pharmacodynamic activity in the treatment of PD. Since it does not cross the BBB, it does not affect the metabolism of L-dopa within the CNS. However, carbidopa reduces the amount of L-dopa required for therapeutic response by about 75% by increasing both the plasma level and half-life of L-dopa and decreasing plasma and urinary dopamine and HVA levels.

A cocrystal structure of a carbidopa derivative containing a hydrazone linkage to its cofactor pyridoxal-5′-phosphate (PLP) bound to L-dopa decarboxylase has been reported (Fig. 10.5).[65] The structure reveals key engagements including a hydrogen bond and an ionic-dipole interaction between the catechol and the alcohol side chain of Thr82 (eg, threonine residue 82) and the phosphate of PLP, respectively, and interactions between the carboxylate of carbidopa and the imidazole side chain of His192. A cocrystal structure of benserazide with dopa decarboxylase has not been reported.

Both carbidopa and L-dopa have relatively low plasma protein binding of 36% and 10% to 30%, respectively (Table 10.1). Carbidopa has an oral bioavailability of 60% and a terminal phase plasma elimination half-life of 2 hours. A similar terminal phase plasma elimination

Table 10.1 Pharmacokinetic Parameters of Drugs Used to Treat Parkinson Disease

Drug Class	Drug	Plasma Elimination Half-Life	Clearance	Volume of Distribution	Oral Bioavailability	Plasma Protein Binding
Dopamine and dopamine receptor–related therapy	L-Dopa	50 min-1.5 h	14.2 mL/min/kg	1.01 L/kg	63%	10%-30%
	Carbidopa	2 h			60%	36%
Monoamine oxidase inhibitors	Rasagiline	3 h		87 L	36%	88%-94%
	Selegiline	1.5 h	59 L/min	1,854 L	10%	
	Safinamide	20-26 h	4.6 L/h	165 L	95%	88%-90%
Catechol-*O*-methyl transferase inhibitors	Entacapone	2.4 h			35%	98%
	Tolcapone		7 L/h		65%	>99.9%
Dopamine receptor agonists	Apomorphine	40 min	223 L/h	218 L	–	
	Bromocriptine	4.9 h				>90%
	Cabergoline	63-109 h				40%
	Pramipexole	8-12 h	400 mL/min	500 L	>90%	15%
	Ropinirole	6 h	47 L/h	7.5 L/kg	45%-55%	40%
	Rotigotine	5-7 h		84 L/kg		90%
Nondopamine-related therapy	Amantadine	12-17 h	0.28 L/h/kg	3-8 L/kg		

half-life of L-dopa, in the presence of carbidopa, is also observed. About 30% of a carbidopa dose is eliminated unchanged in urine. Carbidopa is metabolized to generate α-methyl-3,4-dihydroxyphenylpropionic acid (Fig. 10.6) via reduction of the hydrazine.[66,67] This metabolite is then converted to α-methyl-3-methoxy-4-hydroxyphenylpropionic acid, presumably by COMT. The catechol metabolite also undergoes a rather unusual transformation of being reduced to α-methyl-3-hydroxyphenylpropionic acid. All three of these metabolites participate in conjugation with glucuronic acid with subsequent elimination in urine, although the structures of the glucuronides have not been reported. Finally, 3,4-dihydroxyphenylacetone has also been isolated from urine after administration of carbidopa. This compound may arise via oxidative decarboxylation of α-methyl-3-methoxy-4-hydroxyphenylpropionic acid. However, it may also form directly by auto-oxidation of the parent drug.[68]

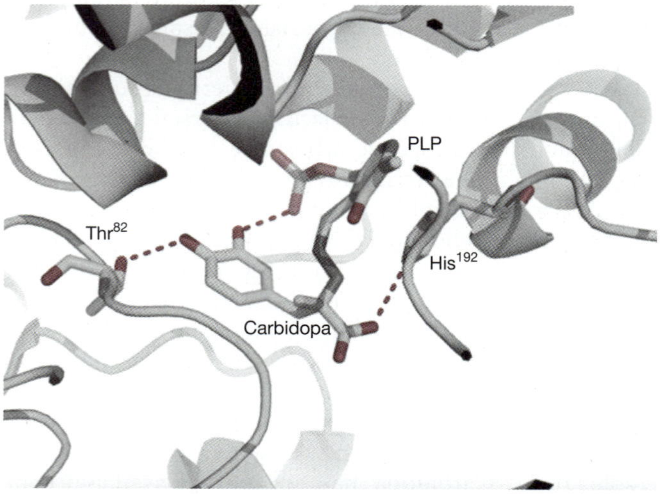

Figure 10.5 Cocrystal structure of carbidopa-pyridoxal-5′-phosphate (PLP) hydrazone with L-dopa decarboxylase (PDB: 1JS3). Hydrogen bonding interactions shown with red dashes. PDB, Protein Data Bank.

Several drug-drug interactions can occur with carbidopa. For example, iron salts (including in multivitamins) can chelate carbidopa, reducing its bioavailability.[69] Also carbidopa can have a drug-drug interaction with isoniazid since both inhibit tryptophan oxygenase and kynureninase.[70] Carbidopa concomitantly administered with L-dopa is contraindicated with nonselective MAO inhibitors. When carbidopa is administered concomitantly with L-dopa, the most common adverse reactions in early PD are nausea, dizziness, headache, insomnia, abnormal dreams, dry mouth, dyskinesia, anxiety, constipation, vomiting, and orthostatic hypotension. In advanced PD, the most common adverse events include nausea and headache.

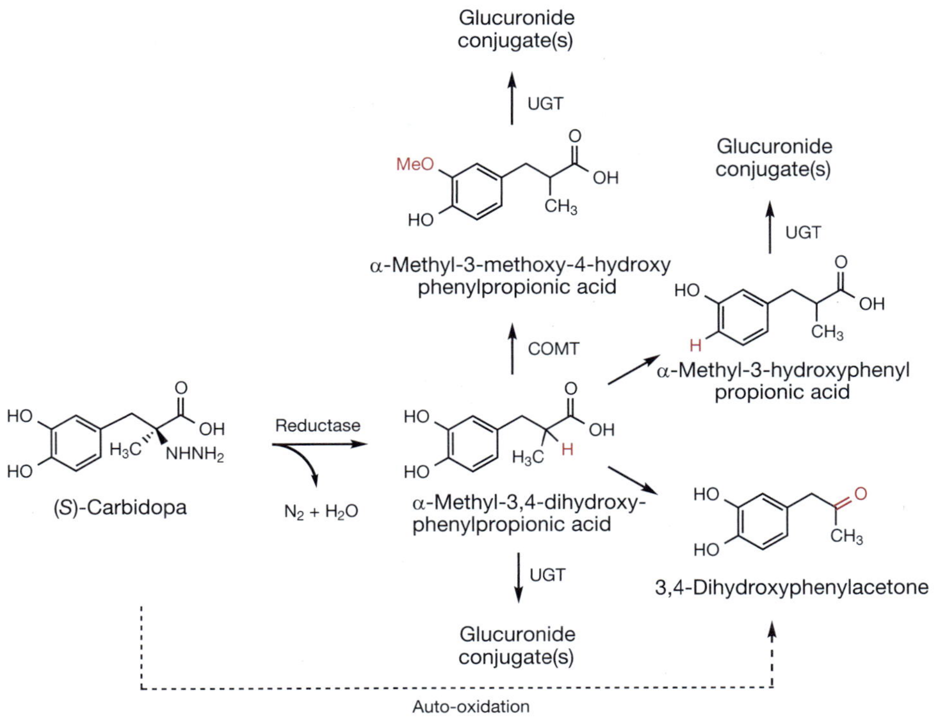

Figure 10.6 Metabolism of carbidopa.

Monoamine Oxidase Inhibitors

In addition to dopamine replacement therapy, another widely used strategy for the treatment of PD is to block the conversion of dopamine to DOPAL via inhibition of the enzyme MAO. Three drugs, rasagiline, selegiline, and safinamide, operate through this mechanism of action.

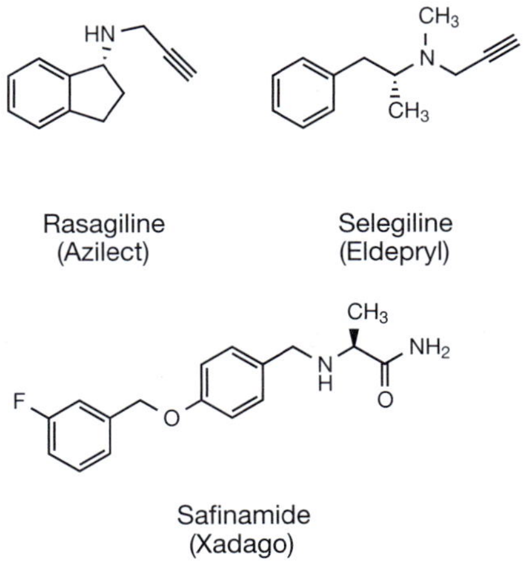

Monoamine oxidase inhibitors

Rasagiline

Rasagiline is indicated as a monotherapy or as adjunct therapy in patients with PD taking L-dopa. Rasagiline is a secondary amine that is substituted with two hydrophobic groups, a propargyl (eg, type of alkyne) and an indane. It also contains one chiral center with an (*R*)-configuration. Rasagiline is formulated as a mesylate salt and is a white powder that is freely soluble in water or ethanol, but sparingly soluble in isopropanol.

Rasagiline acts as a selective inhibitor of MAO-B. However, it does not block the enzyme activity by reversibly binding to the active site. Instead, rasagiline is initially a substrate for MAO-B and is converted to a reactive intermediate that then forms a covalent irreversible adduct with the enzyme cofactor flavin adenine dinucleotide (FAD). The chemistry is shown in Figure 10.7A.[71] MAO-B oxidation activates the propargyl amine to undergo nucleophilic attack by one of the nitrogen atoms of FAD. The resulting adduct of this reaction can be seen in a reported rasagiline·MAO-B·FAD cocrystal structure (Fig. 10.7B).[72]

Rasagiline is readily soluble and permeable, resulting in rapid absorption (T_{max} of 1 hour) following oral administration.[73] The drug is subjected to first-pass metabolism. As a result, it has an oral bioavailability of only 36% (Table 10.1). The drug's steady-state plasma elimination half-life is 3 hours. However, there is no correlation of its pharmacokinetics with its pharmacologic outcome due to its irreversible inhibition of MAO-B. Food does not affect the time to maximum plasma concentration (eg, T_{max}), but the maximum plasma concentration (C_{max}) and exposure (AUC) are decreased by approximately 60% and 20%, respectively, when the drug is taken with a high-fat meal. Rasagiline demonstrates plasma protein binding of 88% to 94% and a moderate volume of distribution of 87 L.

Rasagiline is highly metabolized and undergoes almost complete biotransformation in the liver prior to excretion. The parent drug is *N*-dealkylated to yield 1-aminoindane (Fig. 10.8). It also undergoes benzylic oxidation to form 3-hydroxy-*N*-propargyl-1-aminoindane. Both metabolites can be further oxidized to 3-hydroxy-1-aminoindane. All these metabolic reactions are cytochrome P450 (CYP450) mediated, with CYP1A2 being the major isoenzyme involved.

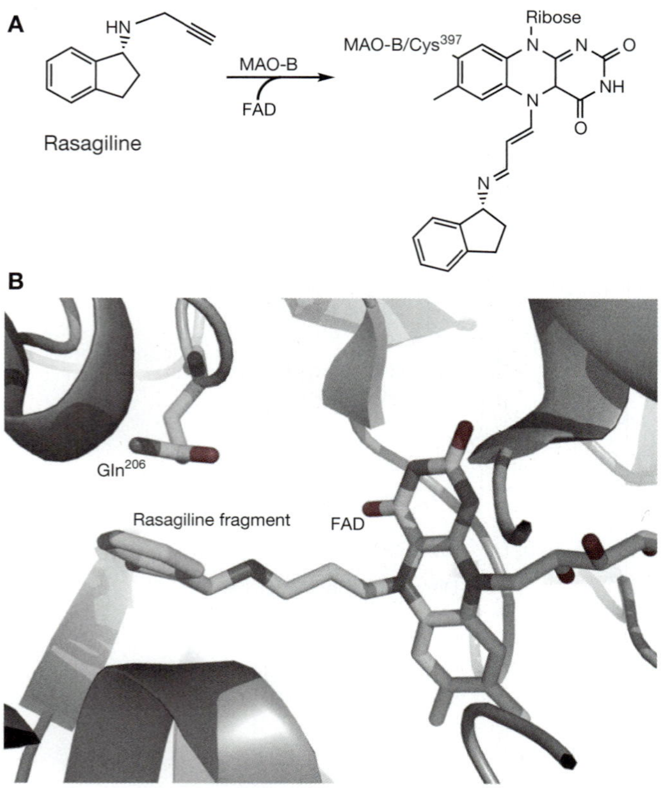

Figure 10.7 A. Covalent interaction between rasagiline, MAO-B, and FAD. B. Cocrystal structure of rasagiline covalently bonded to FAD and complexed with MAO-B (PDB: 1S2Q). FAD, flavin adenine dinucleotide; MAO, monoamine oxidase; PDB, Protein Data Bank.

These phase 1 metabolites also undergo glucuronidation before subsequent urinary excretion.

Given the extensive CYP450-mediated metabolism of rasagiline, especially via the CYP1A2 isozyme, patients taking concomitant ciprofloxacin or other CYP1A2 inhibitors are advised not to exceed a dose of 0.5 mg once daily. In addition, patients with mild hepatic impairment should also not exceed this dose. Rasagiline can also exacerbate hypertension. The most common adverse effects of rasagiline are somnolence, hypotension, dyskinesia, psychotic-like behavior, compulsive behaviors, withdrawal-emergent hyperpyrexia, and confusion.

Selegiline

Selegiline (also known as L-deprenyl) is approved as an adjunct therapy in the management of patients with PD

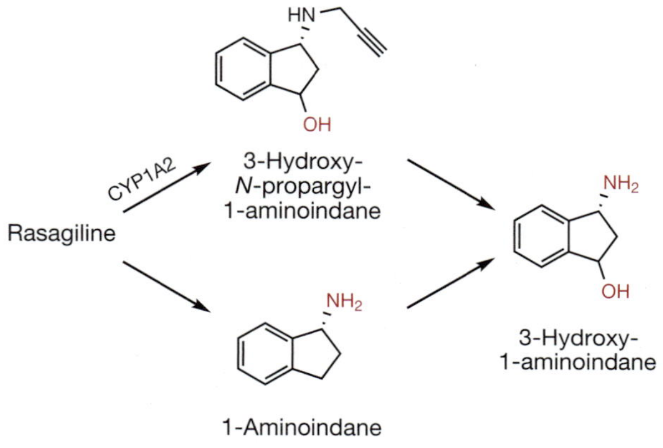

Figure 10.8 Phase 1 metabolism of rasagiline.

being treated with L-dopa/carbidopa who exhibit deterioration in the quality of their response to dopamine replacement therapy. Selegiline has not demonstrated beneficial effect in the absence of concurrent L-dopa/carbidopa therapy. It is also formulated for transdermal delivery and is used for the treatment of depression. Selegiline is structurally related to rasagiline, except that it contains a tertiary amine and a 2-phenylpropyl in place of the indane. The drug is formulated as a hydrochloride salt, which is a white crystalline solid that is readily soluble in water. Like rasagiline, selegiline is a substrate for MAO-B oxidation and subsequent reactivity with FAD to form a covalent adduct. Hence, it is a selective irreversible inhibitor of MAO-B.

Selegiline is readily soluble and permeable, resulting in rapid absorption (T_{max} <1 hour) following oral administration.[74] It is subjected to extensive first-pass metabolism. As a result, it has an oral bioavailability of only 10% (see Table 10.1). The pharmacokinetics of selegiline is highly variable. An oral 10-mg dose results in a maximum plasma concentration of 2 μg/L and plasma elimination half-life of 1.5 hours. The drug has a large volume of distribution of 1,854 L and a clearance of 59 L/min, which is higher than liver blood flow and indicative of extrahepatic elimination.[75] Following multiple administration, accumulation of both the parent drug and its metabolites has been reported.[76]

Selegiline undergoes extensive metabolism to (*R*)-methamphetamine, via oxidative dealkylation of the propargyl, as the major plasma metabolite (Fig. 10.9). A minor metabolite is *N*-desmethylselegiline, which is also an irreversible MAO-B inhibitor that is not surprising given its structural similarity to both selegiline and rasagiline.[77] *N*-Desmethylselegiline is further metabolized to (*R*)-amphetamine again via oxidative dealkylation of the propargyl. Both (*R*)-methamphetamine and (*R*)-amphetamine undergo aromatic hydroxylation to (*R*)-4-hydroxymethamphetamine and (*R*)-4-hydroxyamphetamine, respectively, which are found as their corresponding glucuronide phase II metabolites in urine.[78]

Selegiline is contraindicated for use with meperidine and other opioids due to increased risk of serotonin syndrome. CNS toxicity can occur with the combination of tricyclic antidepressants and selegiline. CNS toxicity can also be observed with the combination of selegiline and selective serotonin reuptake inhibitors. The most common adverse effects of selegiline include nausea, hallucinations, confusion, depression, loss of balance, insomnia, orthostatic hypotension, increased akinetic involuntary movements, agitation, arrhythmia, bradykinesia, chorea, delusions, hypertension, new or increased angina pectoris, and syncope.

Safinamide

Safinamide is the latest MAO-B inhibitor to be introduced for the treatment of PD.[79] It is approved as an adjunct therapy to L-dopa/carbidopa and has resulted in improved motor function without involuntary movements. The drug has not been shown to be effective as a monotherapy for PD. It is structurally different from both selegiline and rasagiline. Its composition is based on the amino acid alanine. It has a primary amide, a benzyl amine and ether, and one chiral center with an (*S*)-configuration. Safinamide is formulated as the mesylate salt, which is a white crystalline solid that is

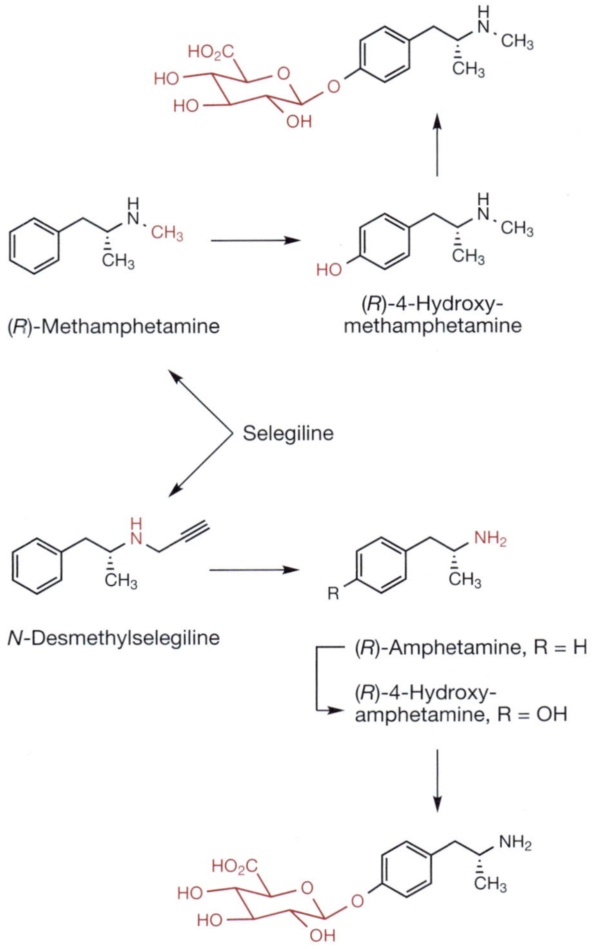

Figure 10.9 Metabolism of selegiline.

highly soluble in water. Safinamide's aqueous solubility is pH dependent, showing greatest solubility at pH 1.2 to 4.5, but with low solubility (<0.4 mg/mL) at pH ≥6.8.

The mechanism of action of safinamide for inhibition of MAO-B is also different than that of selegiline and rasagiline. It is a reversible MAO-B inhibitor and consequently does not form a covalent bond with the enzyme or the FAD cofactor. But this mode of inhibition still results in increased levels of dopamine. It has a 5,000-fold selectivity over inhibition of MAO-A. Several molecular interactions contribute to the binding of safinamide to MAO-B, which occur close to the bound FAD. These engagements include van der Waals interaction of the 3-fluorobenzyloxy moiety and hydrogen bonding of the amide and secondary amine of safinamide with Gln206 and an ordered water molecule (Fig. 10.10).[80] Safinamide inhibits glutamate release and dopamine reuptake, as well as blocks sodium and calcium channels. However, these latter two properties probably do not contribute to the drug's pharmacodynamic effects in the treatment of PD.

Safinamide is readily absorbed following oral administration and is not subjected to extensive first-pass metabolism, resulting in a bioavailability of 95% (see Table 10.1).[81] It reaches maximum plasma concentration about 2 to 3 hours after administration. The drug has plasma protein binding of 88% to 90%, a long terminal plasma elimination half-life of 20 to 26 hours, a moderate volume of distribution

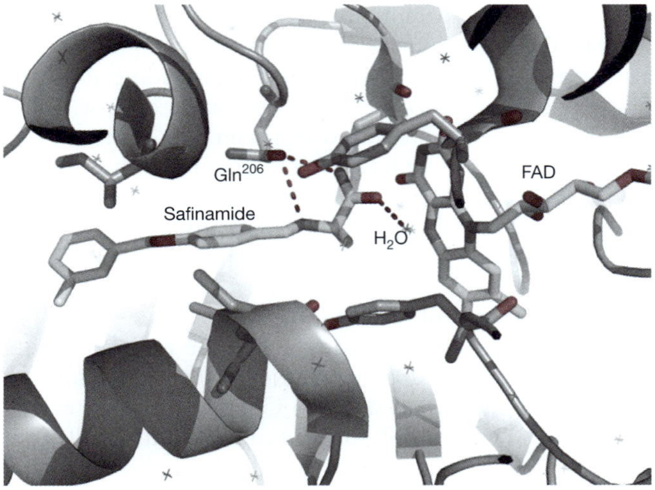

Figure 10.10 Cocrystal structure of safinamide with MAO-B and FAD (PDB: 2V5Z). Hydrogen bonding interactions are depicted with red dashes. FAD, flavin adenine dinucleotide; MAO, monoamine oxidase; PDB, Protein Data Bank.

of 165 L, and total clearance of 4.6 L/h. A slight delay in maximum plasma concentration is observed in the fed versus fasted state, but this has no effect on exposure ($AUC_{0-\infty}$) or maximum plasma concentration (C_{max}). Although safinamide avoids first-pass metabolism, it does eventually undergo extensive metabolism, with only about 8.5% of the parent drug being excreted unchanged in urine and feces. Safinamide undergoes amidase-mediated hydrolysis of the primary amide to the corresponding carboxylic acid, which is *N*-dealkylated to a primary amine (Fig. 10.11).

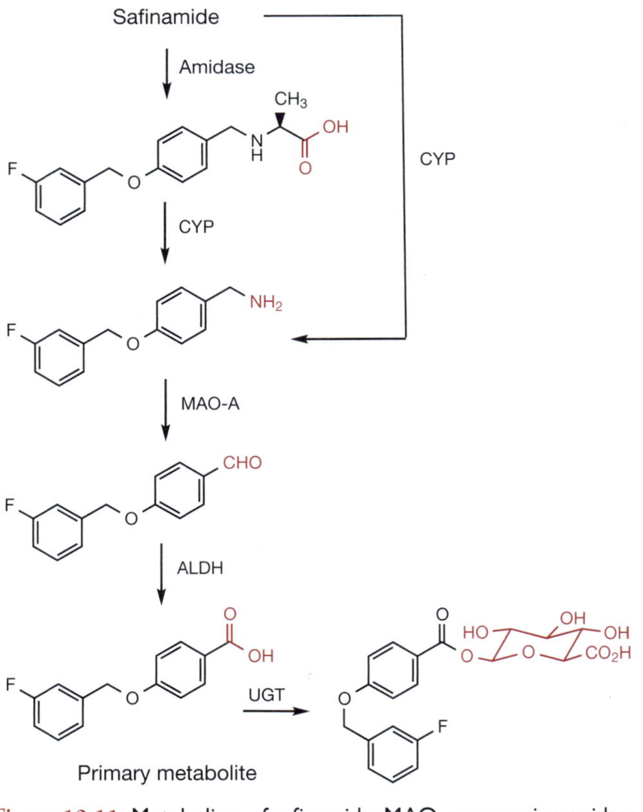

Figure 10.11 Metabolism of safinamide. MAO, monoamine oxidase; UGT, UDP-glucuronosyltransferase.

Alternatively, the parent drug is directly *N*-dealkylated to generate the same primary amine. This metabolite is deaminated via MAO-A oxidation to the corresponding aldehyde, which is oxidized via AD to the carboxylic acid, which is the primary metabolite found in plasma. In addition, this metabolite undergoes phase 2 UDP-glucuronosyltransferase (UGT)-mediated glucuronidation. The metabolites of safinamide are primarily excreted via the kidney. Furthermore, none of these metabolites appear to exhibit biologic activity responsible for the pharmacodynamic effects of the parent drug in the treatment of PD.

Animal and human studies have not revealed an increased risk of drug-drug interaction with safinamide. Although safinamide does undergo CYP450 metabolism, the prototypic CYP3A4 inhibitor ketoconazole did not alter the formation and clearance of safinamide metabolites to a clinically relevant extent.[82] However, individuals with severe liver problems as well as those using dextromethorphan, other MAO inhibitors, opioids, St. John's wort, antidepressants, or cyclobenzaprine should not use safinamide. The most common adverse effects of safinamide include uncontrolled involuntary movements, nausea, insomnia, and falls.

Catechol-*O*-Methyltransferase Inhibitors

An alternative strategy used for the treatment of PD is to block the conversion of dopamine to MTA by inhibition of the enzyme COMT. Three drugs, entacapone, tolcapone, and opicapone, operate through this mechanism of action.

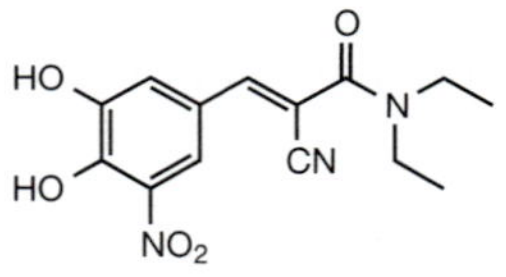

Entacapone (Comtan)

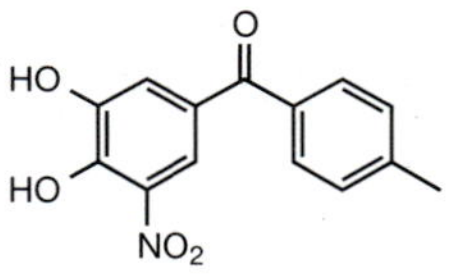

Tolcapone (Tasmar)

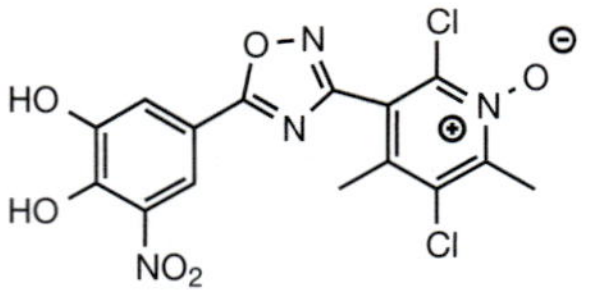

Opicapone (Ongentys)

Entacapone

Entacapone is approved for the treatment of PD as an adjunct therapy to L-dopa/carbidopa. The structure of entacapone has an (*E*)-alkene substituted with a tertiary amide, nitrile, and nitro-containing catechol. The drug is a crystalline solid that is only sparingly soluble in water. Its mechanism of action is selective and reversible inhibition of COMT.

Entacapone's pharmacokinetic properties are independent of coadministered L-dopa/carbidopa. The drug is readily absorbed following oral administration reaching maximum plasma concentrations within 1 hour.[83] However, first-pass metabolism limits oral bioavailability to 35% (see Table 10.1). Food does not affect the pharmacokinetics of entacapone. The elimination of entacapone is biphasic, with a plasma elimination half-life of 0.4 to 0.7 hours based on the β-phase and 2.4 hours based on the γ-phase. After a single 200-mg oral dose of entacapone, the maximum plasma concentration is 1.2 μg/mL. The drug's volume of distribution is low, limiting tissue concentrations due to high plasma protein binding (eg, 98%).

Entacapone is significantly metabolized prior to excretion, with only 0.2% of the parent drug found unchanged in urine and 10% in feces. Entacapone undergoes alkene isomerization to the inactive *Z*-isomer. Interestingly, (*Z*)-entacapone is the only phase 1 metabolite found in human plasma. The parent drug is also metabolized via glucuronidation predominately by UGT1A9 to generate two regioisomeric metabolites.[84] The isomerized phase 1 metabolite also undergoes glucuronidation. The resulting glucuronides from the parent and the alkene isomer represent about 70% and 25%, respectively, of the urinary metabolites (Fig. 10.12).[85] Curiously, the nitro group appears to block COMT-mediated methylation of the catechol.

One precautionary note about entacapone is that the exposure (AUC) and maximum plasma concentration (C_{max}) can significantly increase in patients with hepatic impairment. The most common adverse effects of entacapone are urine discoloration, nausea, hyperkinesia, abdominal pain, vomiting, and dry mouth.

Tolcapone

Like entacapone, tolcapone is indicated for the treatment of PD as an adjunct therapy to L-dopa/carbidopa. The two compounds also have a structural resemblance since they both contain a nitro-substituted catechol. However, tolcapone has another benzene ring linked through a ketone as

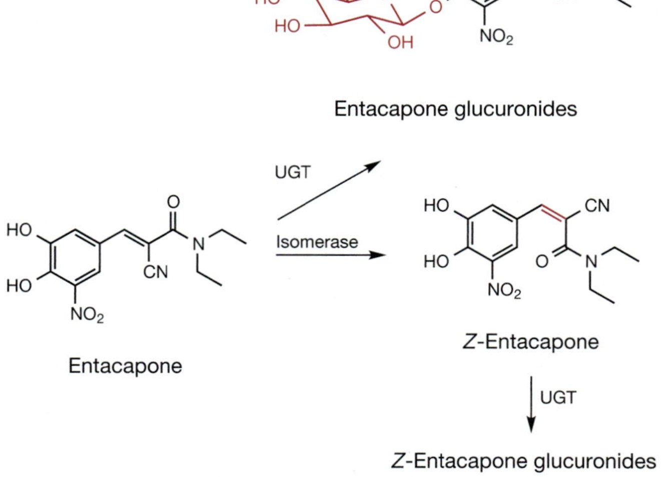

Figure 10.12 Metabolism of entacapone. UGT, UDP-glucuronosyltransferase.

opposed to an alkene. Tolcapone is a yellow crystalline solid that is poorly soluble in water.

Tolcapone is a selective and reversible inhibitor of COMT. As can be seen in the tolcapone· S-adenosyl methionine (SAM)·COMT·Mg^{+2} cocrystal structure,[86] the catechol of tolcapone forms an interaction with the Mg^{+2} ion as well as a hydrogen bond to Asn170 and an ionic-dipole interaction with Glu199 (Fig. 10.13). Furthermore, the SAM methyl group that normally is transferable to the substrate is positioned close to the para-hydroxyl group of tolcapone. However, transfer does not occur likely due to the strong electron-withdrawing effect of the nitro group, although some methylation of the other hydroxyl group is observed as a minor metabolite (see later).

Tolcapone's pharmacokinetic properties are linear and independent of L-dopa/(S)-carbidopa coadministration. The drug is readily absorbed after oral administration and demonstrates moderate bioavailability of 65%, reaching maximum plasma concentration in 2 hours (see Table 10.1).[87] Food delays and decreases the absorption of tolcapone by about 10% to 20%. After oral doses of 100 or 200 mg, maximum plasma concentrations of 3 and 6 μg/mL, respectively, are obtained. Tolcapone has high plasma protein binding (>99.9%). Consequently, it has moderate systemic clearance (7 L/h) and does not distribute widely into tissues.

Tolcapone is extensively metabolized prior to excretion, with only 0.5% of the dose found unchanged in urine and 60% and 40% of the metabolites excreted in urine and feces, respectively. The primary metabolite of tolcapone is the glucuronide of the more sterically accessible phenol (Fig. 10.14). Several minor metabolites are also formed, including oxidation of the benzylic position (via CYP3A4 and 2A6) to an alcohol that is subsequently oxidized to the corresponding carboxylic acid, reduction of the nitro to an aniline that is subsequently acetylated, and COMT-mediated methylation to 3-O-methyl-tolcapone, as mentioned.

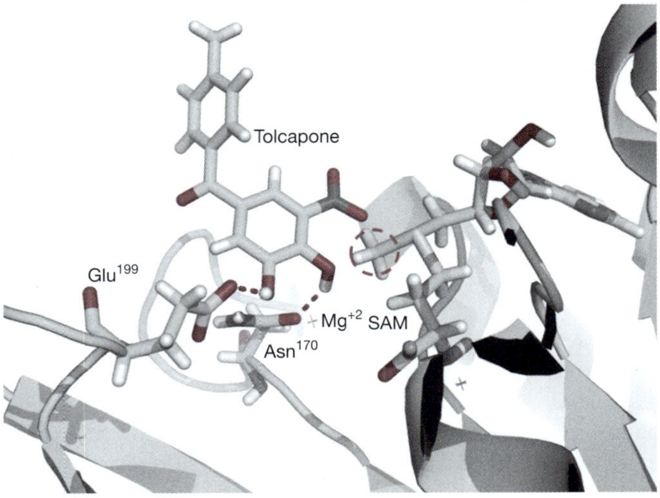

Figure 10.13 Tolcapone·SAM·COMT·Mg^{+2} cocrystal structure (PDB: 3S68). Hydrogen bonding interactions are shown with red dashes. The transferable methyl on SAM is highlighted with a red dashed circle. Residues 3 to 12 and 21 to 56 have been deleted for clarity. COMT, catechol-*O*-methyltransferase; PDB, Protein Data Bank; SAM, S-adenosyl methionine.

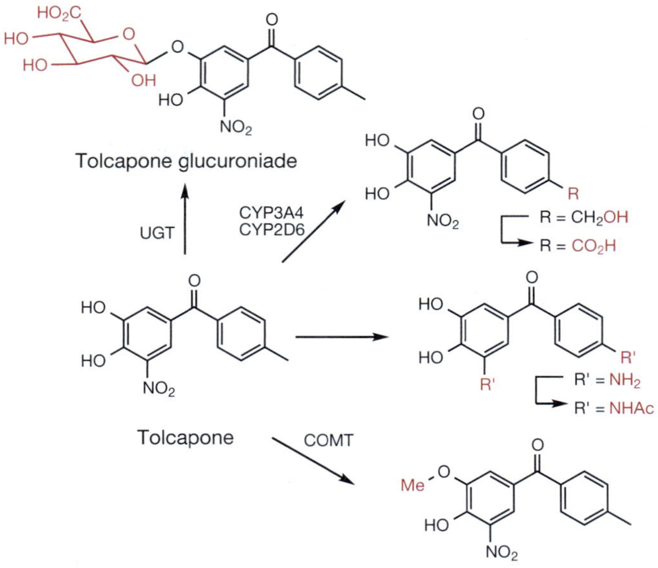

Figure 10.14 Metabolism of tolcapone. COMT, catechol-*O*-methyltransferase; UGT, UDP-glucuronosyltransferase.

Tolcapone is contraindicated in patients with liver disease or in patients who were withdrawn from tolcapone treatment because of drug-induced hepatocellular injury. Hepatic failures have been observed leading to its market withdrawal in some countries, as well as restriction in the United States to only those patients not responsive to other therapies and who can be appropriately monitored for hepatic toxicity. It is also contraindicated in patients with a history of nontraumatic rhabdomyolysis or hyperpyrexia and/or confusion possibly related to medication. The most common adverse effects of tolcapone are nausea, anorexia, sleep disorder, vomiting, urine discoloration, dystonia, and sweating.

Opicapone

Opicapone is also a reversible COMT inhibitor indicated as adjunctive treatment to levodopa/carbidopa in patients with PD experiencing "off" episodes. These are motor or non-motor symptoms that occur between doses of levodopa/carbidopa. Opicapone has structural similarities to entacapone and tolcapone, but contains a central 1,2,4-oxadiazole linked to a pyridine *N*-oxide and is a yellow solid with limited aqueous solubility.

Opicapone demonstrates dose-proportional pharmacokinetics, reaching maximum plasma levels within 2 hours of oral administration, and has a mean elimination half-life of 1 to 2 hours.[88-90] It is less metabolized than the other COMT inhibitors, with 22% recovered unchanged in feces. The primary metabolic pathway of opicapone is sulfation of the sterically more accessible phenol. Like other COMT inhibitors, opicapone is highly plasma protein bound (>99%).

Dopamine Receptor Agonists

Another strategy for the treatment of PD is through agonism of dopamine receptors, particularly postsynaptic D_2-types. Six drugs, apomorphine, bromocriptine, cabergoline, pramipexole, ropinirole, and rotigotine, work via this mode, providing symptomatic relief to patients.

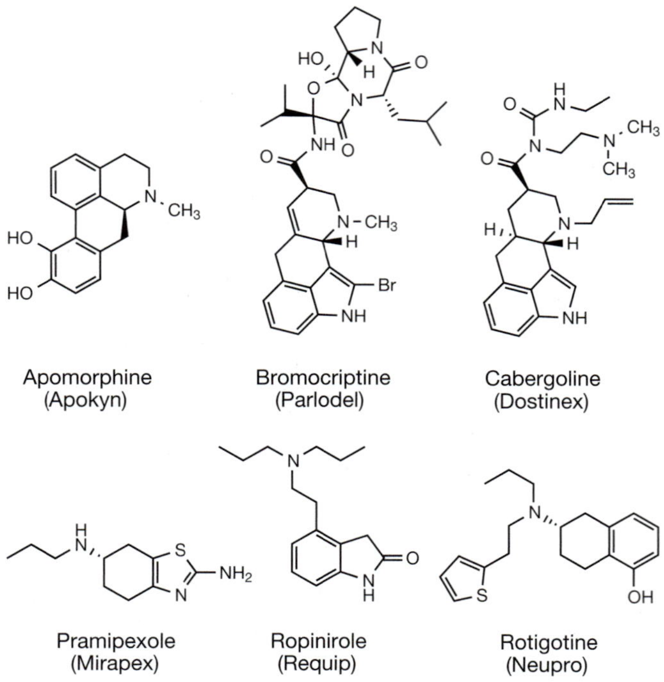

Dopamine receptor agonists

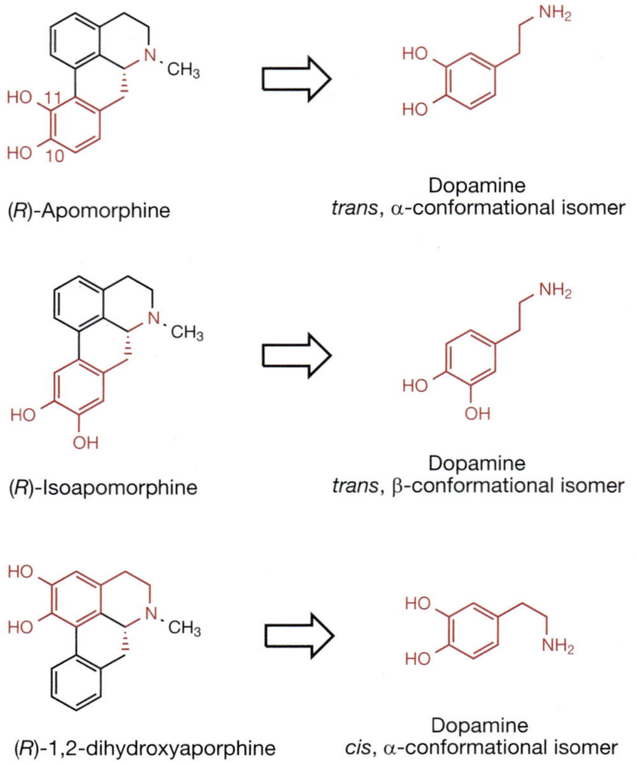

Figure 10.15 Comparison of conformational restricted dopamine analogues (*R*)-apomorphine, (*R*)-isoapomorphine, and (*R*)-1,2-dihydroxyaporphine with the *trans*-α-, *trans*-β-, and *cis*-α-conformational isomers of dopamine.

Apomorphine

Apomorphine is indicated for the acute, intermittent treatment of hypomobility, or "off" episodes (eg, times when other PD medications, such as L-dopa/carbidopa, are not working well) in patients with advanced PD. It is a synthetic compound related to a class of alkaloids called aporphines that are found in a wide variety of plants. Apomorphine contains a tertiary amine and has a catechol that makes up part of the aporphine tetracyclic scaffold and one chiral center with an (*R*)-configuration. The drug is formulated as a hydrochloride salt that forms white crystals or is a white powder. It is administered by subcutaneous injection.

Apomorphine's mechanism of action in the treatment of PD is postulated to occur via stimulation of postsynaptic dopamine D_2-type receptors within the caudate-putamen region of the brain. Apomorphine has high in vitro binding affinity for the D_4 receptor and moderate affinity for D_2, D_3, and D_5, and adrenergic α_{1D}, α_{2B}, α_{2C} receptors.[91] The rigid tetracyclic structure and hydroxyl groups at C_{10} and C_{11} of (*R*)-apomorphine mimic the *trans*-α-conformational isomer of dopamine likely representing the binding conformation (Fig. 10.15).[92] In contrast, (*R*)-isoapomorphine that displays the structure of dopamine in the *trans*-β-conformational isomer has less activity. Finally, (*R*)-1,2-dihydroxyaporphine that displays the structure of dopamine in the *cis*-α-conformational isomer is inactive as a dopamine receptor agonist.[93]

Apomorphine hydrochloride is rapidly absorbed following subcutaneous administration into the abdominal wall and reaches a maximum plasma concentration in 10 to 60 minutes.[94] The drug exhibits linear pharmacokinetics over a dose range of 2 to 8 mg following a single subcutaneous injection. It also demonstrates an apparent volume of distribution of 218 L, apparent clearance of 223 L/h, and a relatively short mean terminal plasma elimination half-life of 40 minutes (see Table 10.1). The major excreted metabolites are apomorphine sulfate and apomorphine glucuronide.[95]

Apomorphine is contraindicated in patients using concomitant 5-HT_3 antagonists, including antiemetics (eg, ondansetron, granisetron, dolasetron, palonosetron) and alosetron used to treat severe diarrhea-predominant irritable bowel syndrome, due to increased risk of hypotension that can result in loss of consciousness. The drug dose should also be reduced in patients with mild or moderate renal impairment, as well as mild or moderate hepatic impairment. In both cases apomorphine exposure can increase in these patients. The most common adverse effects of apomorphine are nausea and vomiting, coronary events, QT prolongation, proarrhythmia, and priapism.

Bromocriptine

Bromocriptine is indicated for the treatment of idiopathic or postencephalitic PD, as well as hyperprolactinemia-associated dysfunctions and acromegaly. It is a structurally complex synthetic compound related to naturally occurring ergot alkaloids. Bromocriptine contains a tertiary amine that allows the free base to be formulated as a mesylate salt. Although salt formation increases aqueous solubility, it remains low (<1 mg/mL).

Bromocriptine is a partial agonist at D_2 and D_3 receptors[96] with selectivity over D_1, D_4, and D_5 receptors.[91] It also has potent to moderate binding affinity for α_{1A}, α_{1B}, α_{1D},

α_{2A}, α_{2B}, α_{2C}, 5-HT_{1A}, and 5-HT_{1D} receptors.[91] The drug was the first direct dopamine agonist indicated for the treatment of PD, after its development for use at lower doses as a prolactin inhibitor.[97]

The enteral absorption of bromocriptine is incomplete (~30%-40% in rats and monkeys) possibly due to its high molecular weight, poor aqueous solubility, and/or permeability. Following an oral dose (2 × 2.5 mg) of bromocriptine mesylate, a maximum plasma concentration of 465 pg/mL is achieved in 2.5 hours. Bromocriptine is highly protein bound (>90%) and has a plasma elimination half-life of 4.9 hours (see Table 10.1).[98]

The drug undergoes extensive first-pass metabolism with the main route of elimination in bile (80%-93% of the absorbed dose), with little parent drug excreted in urine and feces. It appears that two primary pathways are responsible for the metabolism of bromocriptine[99,100]: hydrolysis and epimerization generating 2-bromolysergic acid and the epimer 2-bromoisolysergic acid via the intermediate amides (Fig. 10.16). The second metabolism route involves oxidation of C_8 in the proline fragment. Further oxidation of the C_9 position, as well as formation of the 8-O- and 9-O-glucuronides, occurs. These metabolites are likely also susceptible to hydrolysis and epimerization. Interestingly, the lysergic acid portion of bromocriptine and its metabolites seems quite stable to metabolism.

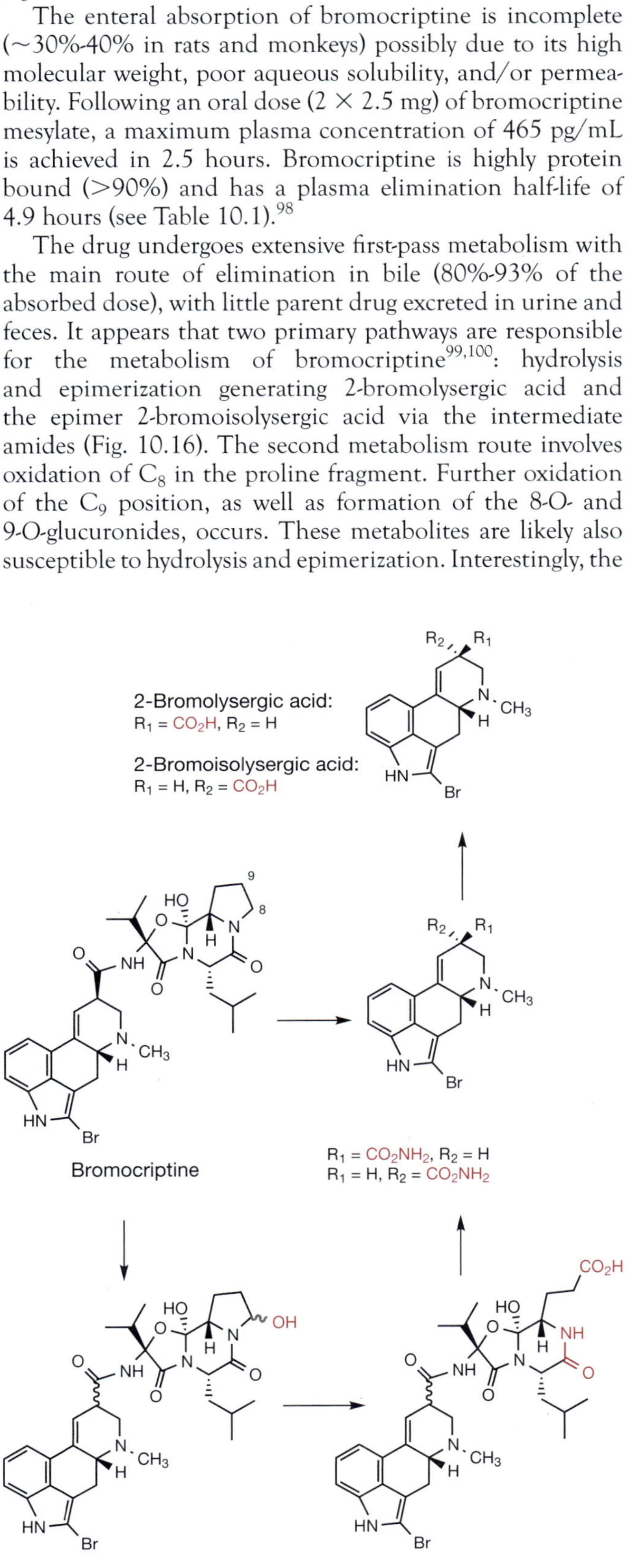

Figure 10.16 Metabolism of bromocriptine.

Caution should be used when coadministering bromocriptine with drugs that inhibit CYP3A4. The concomitant use of macrolide antibiotics, such as erythromycin, can increase the plasma levels of bromocriptine.[101] In addition, bromocriptine should not be used during the postpartum period in women with a history of coronary artery disease and other severe cardiovascular conditions due to an increased risk of vasospastic reactions. The most common adverse effects of bromocriptine with concomitant reduction in the dose of L-dopa/carbidopa are nausea, abnormal involuntary movements, hallucinations, confusion, "on-off" phenomenon, dizziness, drowsiness, faintness/fainting, vomiting, asthenia, abdominal discomfort, visual disturbance, ataxia, insomnia, depression, hypotension, shortness of breath, constipation, and vertigo.

Cabergoline

Cabergoline is indicated for the treatment of early phase PD, as well as several other conditions including hyperprolactinemic disorders (eg, idiopathic or due to pituitary adenomas). It is structurally related to bromocriptine. However, the secondary amide in cabergoline has been significantly simplified, the *N*-alkyl group has been changed, the alkene has been saturated, and the bromine on the indole has been removed. Cabergoline is a white powder slightly soluble in 0.1 N hydrochloric acid but insoluble in water. Its mechanism of action is also similar to bromocriptine, demonstrating full agonism at D_2 receptors and partial agonism at D_3 and D_4 receptors, without appreciable activity at D_1 receptors.[91,96] It also has potent binding affinity for α_{2D}, and 5-HT_{1D}, 5-HT_{2A}, and 5-HT_{2B} receptors.[91]

Following oral administration, cabergoline reaches maximum plasma levels in 2 to 3 hours and has a long elimination plasma half-life of 63 to 109 hours (Table 10.1).[102] Cabergoline is moderately bound to human plasma proteins (~40%). The drug is extensively metabolized by the liver, with fecal excretion of metabolites as the main route of elimination over a prolonged period. Two hydrolysis routes of the acylurea account for the predominate metabolism of cabergoline (Fig. 10.17). In the first, the urea moiety is hydrolyzed to generate a secondary amide. Alternatively, the acylurea bond is broken to produce the carboxylic acid. Like bromocriptine, the tetracyclic scaffold is quite resistant to metabolism.

Cabergoline is contraindicated in patients with a history of cardiac valvular disorders, as well as pulmonary, pericardial, or retroperitoneal fibrotic disorders. The drug's most common adverse effects are headache, nausea, and vomiting.

Pramipexole

Pramipexole is indicated for the treatment of PD. It is structurally distinct from bromocriptine and cabergoline in that it is unrelated to ergot alkaloids. Its structure consists of a 2-aminothiazole fused to cyclohexyl hydrocarbon that is further substituted with a secondary amine as the (S)-enantiomer. It is formulated as the dihydrochloride monohydrate salt that is a white powder with more than

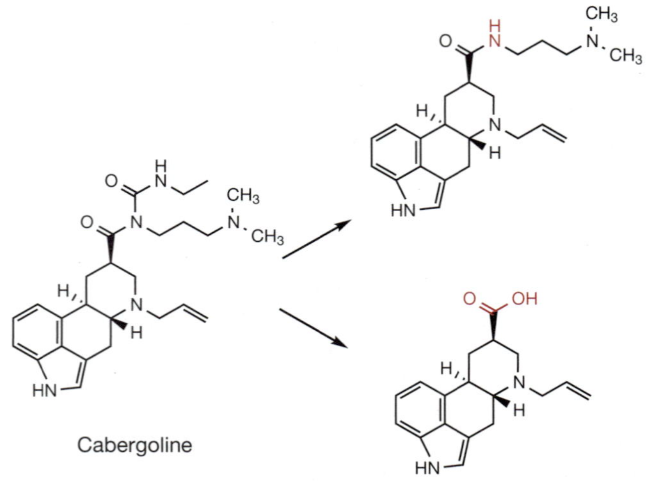

Figure 10.17 Metabolism of cabergoline.

20% by weight solubility in water. Mechanistically, it is a D_2 receptor agonist with affinity for the D_3 and D_4 receptor subtypes, but low affinity for the D_1 receptor. However, it demonstrates lower in vitro binding affinity versus adrenergic and serotonin receptors compared to apomorphine, bromocriptine, and cabergoline.[91]

Pramipexole's low molecular weight and good aqueous solubility, coupled with permeability and resistance to first-pass metabolism, result in excellent oral bioavailability of more than 90% (see Table 10.1).[103] It reaches maximum plasma concentration in 2 hours after oral administration, although this can increase to 3 hours if taken with food. Pramipexole is only about 15% bound to plasma proteins contributing to its extensive tissue distribution (eg, volume of distribution of 500 L). Pramipexole is not extensively metabolized, contributing to a long terminal plasma elimination half-life of 8 to 12 hours, with 90% excreted in urine unchanged with clearance of 400 mL/min.

Pramipexole does not significantly inhibit CYP450 enzymes and does not appear to participate in drug-drug interactions. However, given its dependence on renal clearance, elimination can be significantly lower in patients with moderate to severe kidney impairment. Finally, the most common adverse effects of pramipexole are nausea, dizziness, somnolence, insomnia, constipation, asthenia, and hallucinations.

Ropinirole

Ropinirole, which is structurally like pramipexole, is also indicated for the treatment of PD. It contains an oxindole tethered via an ethylene linker at the 4-position to a tertiary amine. This later functional group is used to formulate ropinirole as a hydrochloride salt, which is a white to yellow solid with excellent water solubility of 133 mg/mL. Ropinirole is a D_2 agonist with weaker binding affinities to D_3, D_4, 5-HT_2, and α_2 receptors.[104]

Ropinirole, with a low molecular weight and good aqueous solubility, is rapidly absorbed after oral administration reaching maximum plasma concentrations in 1 to 2 hours, which can increase to 4 hours (along with concomitant decrease in maximum plasma concentration of 25%) when taken with food.[105] However, ropinirole is more susceptible to first-pass metabolism compared to pramipexole, likely contributing to a lower absolute bioavailability of 45% to 55% (see Table 10.1). Ropinirole is modestly bound to plasma proteins (eg, 40%) with a high apparent volume of distribution of 7.5 L/kg, clearance of 47 L/h, and plasma elimination half-life of 6 hours. The primary route of elimination is in urine, with <10% of the administered dose of ropinirole excreted unchanged.

Ropinirole is extensively metabolized by the liver. The predominant route of metabolism is via *N*-depropylation.[106] This metabolite is further transformed by hydroxylation at C-7 followed by glucuronidation (Fig. 10.18). In addition, *N*-despropylropinirole is converted to a carboxylic acid metabolite and an *N*-carbamoylglucuronide, a rather uncommon type of metabolite.

The primary CYP450 isozyme responsible for the phase 1 metabolism of ropinirole is CYP1A2.[107] Consequently, coadministration with CYP1A2 inhibitors, such as ciprofloxacin, can increase exposure (eg, AUC) and maximum plasma concentration (eg, C_{max}) of ropinirole. On the other hand, cigarette smoking is expected to decrease exposure to ropinirole since CYP1A2 is known to be induced by smoking, which may require drug dose adjustment. The most common adverse effects of ropinirole are nausea, somnolence, dizziness, syncope, asthenic condition (ie, asthenia, fatigue, and/or malaise), viral infection, leg edema, vomiting, and dyspepsia.

Rotigotine

Rotigotine is indicated for the treatment of both early and advanced PD. It is administered by transdermal patch.[108] Like ropinirole and pramipexole, rotigotine does not resemble

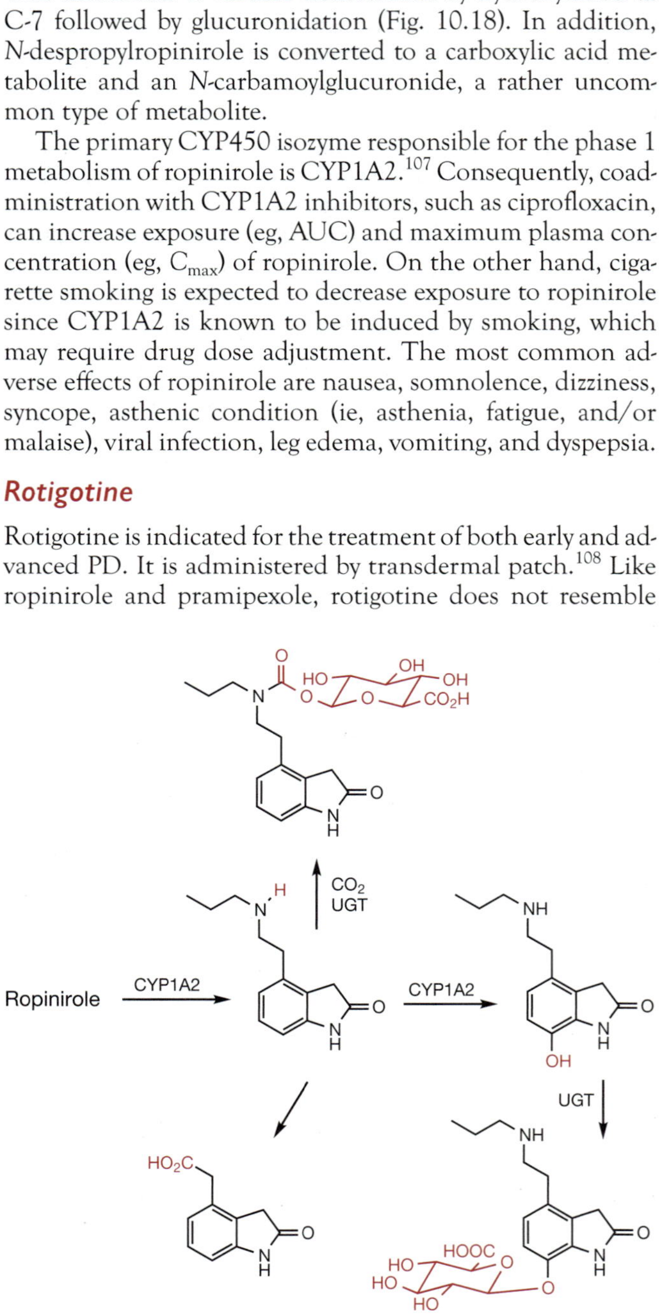

Figure 10.18 Metabolism of ropinirole. UGT, UDP-glucuronosyltransferase.

ergot alkaloids and contains a phenol fused to a cyclohexyl, which is tethered via an ethylene linker to a tertiary amine, again as the (*S*)-enantiomer. The amine is also connected to a thiophene. Rotigotine's mechanism of action is similar to ropinirole and pramipexole, specifically, D_1, D_2, and D_3 receptor agonism.[109]

Rotigotine is relatively highly bound to human plasma proteins (eg, ~90%). The drug has a high apparent volume of distribution of 84 L/kg (see Table 10.1). After removal of the patch, drug levels decrease with a terminal plasma elimination half-life of 5 to 7 hours. Rotigotine is primarily excreted in urine (~71%) and feces (~23%).[110] It is metabolized by multiple CYP450 isozymes to *N*-despropyl and *N*-desthienylethyl phase 1 metabolites, which undergo sulfonation of the phenol. The parent drug is also a substrate for sulfotransferase (SULT) and UGT, generating metabolites resulting from sulfonation and glucuronidation of the phenol (Fig. 10.19).[111]

Since rotigotine is metabolized by multiple CYP450, SULT, and UGT isoforms, it has low risk of interacting with other drugs. The most common adverse effects of rotigotine are nausea, vomiting, somnolence, application site reactions, dizziness, anorexia, hyperhidrosis, insomnia, peripheral edema, and dyskinesia.

The three dopamine agonists pramipexole, ropinirole, and rotigotine are also indicated for the treatment of restless leg syndrome (RLS), also known as Willis-Ekbom disease, which is a neuromuscular condition associated with abnormal sensations in the legs particularly during sleep. Although the cause is not known, RLS appears to involve brain iron deficiency. Surprisingly, overall brain dopamine is increased in patients with RLS. However, dopamine has a circadian activity pattern, decreasing in the evening/night and increasing in the morning. Therefore, overcompensation of postsynaptic adjustment to increased dopamine stimulation during the daytime may cause deficient dopamine response

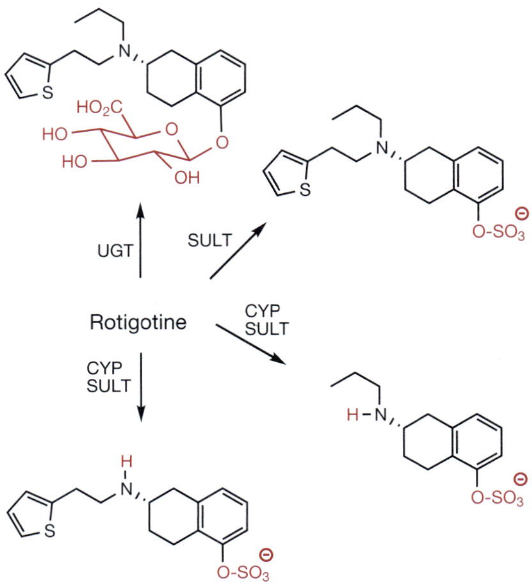

Figure 10.19 Metabolism of rotigotine. CYP, cytochrome P; SULT, sulfotransferase; UGT, UDP-glucuronosyltransferase.

at night.[112] Thus, dopamine agonists may help dampen the effects of lower nocturnal dopamine responsiveness. In addition to dopamine agonists, calcium channel α-2-δ antagonists (eg, gabapentin, gabapentin enacarbil, and pregabalin) are also used as first-line treatments and in some cases are preferred.[113]

Nondopamine-Related Therapy

The mainstay of current PD chemotherapy is focused on dopamine, through replacement, inhibition of its catabolism, or functional agonism of postsynaptic dopamine receptors. However, nondopamine-based therapies have also been assessed as alternative strategies. One drug that has been approved for the treatment of PD that does not elicit its effects via dopamine-related mechanisms is amantadine.

Amantadine

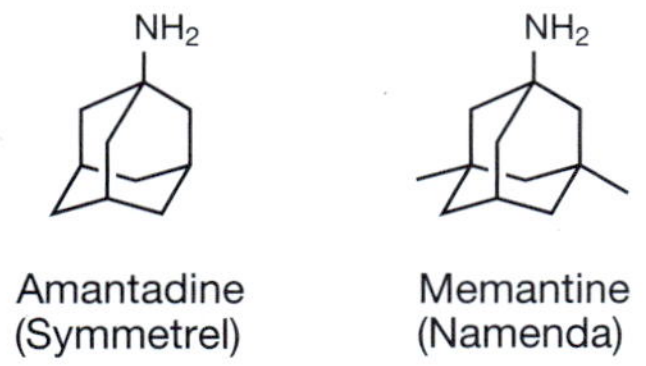

Amantadine is indicated in the treatment of PD and drug-induced extrapyramidal reactions, including to help reduce symptoms during off-episodes. Interestingly, it was originally developed and indicated for the prophylaxis and treatment of influenza A virus infections. The drug contains a primary amine attached to the bulky and hydrophobic cyclic hydrocarbon adamantane. It is formulated as the hydrochloride salt, which is a white crystalline solid that is readily soluble in water.

Amantadine is an N-methyl-D-aspartate (NMDA) glutamate receptor antagonist that might provide neuroprotective effects in PD. The drug has been shown to cause dopamine and norepinephrine release from intraneuronal storage sites and to block dopamine reuptake.[114] It may provide moderate benefit early in PD by enhancing the effects of L-dopa and limiting the severity of dyskinesias induced by L-dopa therapy.[115] Although the drug was originally developed as an antiviral agent, patients with PD appeared to have improvements of symptoms.[116] However, others have cast doubt on the efficacy of amantadine in the treatment of PD, concluding that randomized controlled clinical trials did not provide sufficient evidence of efficacy and safety in the treatment of idiopathic PD.[117] Memantine is a close structural derivative that demonstrates similar pharmacology but is indicated for the treatment of moderate to severe dementia of the Alzheimer type.

Amantadine is well absorbed following oral administration, reaching maximum plasma concentrations in about 3 hours.[118] The drug has a clearance of 0.28 L/h/kg with a large volume of distribution of 3 to 8 L/kg and a long plasma elimination half-life of 12 to 17 hours (see Table 10.1). It is primarily excreted unchanged (65%-85% of the dose) in urine. However, a number of metabolites are observed

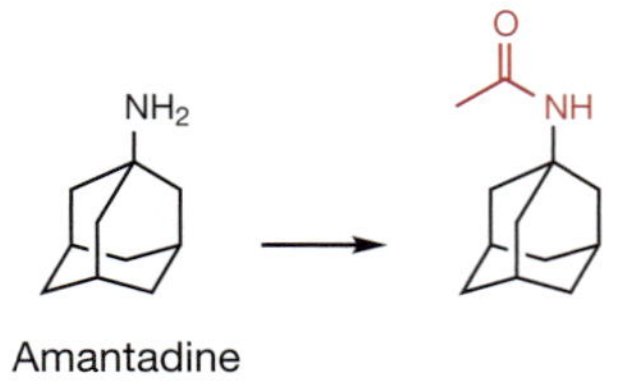

Figure 10.20 Metabolism of amantadine.

following therapeutic dosing (Fig. 10.20). The major metabolite of amantadine is the *N*-acetylated derivative (5%-15% of the dose). However, several other minor metabolites have been identified.[119]

Amantadine can accumulate in patients with renal dysfunction. However, it does not appear to interact with other drugs.[120] The most common adverse effects of amantadine are nausea, dizziness, and insomnia.

Istradefylline

A more recently approved drug indicated for adjunctive treatment to levodopa/carbidopa in adult patients with PD experiencing off-episodes is the adenosine A_{2A} receptor antagonist istradefylline. Structurally, istradefylline is a xanthine derivative containing a dimethoxystyrenyl group and a light yellow-green solid with aqueous solubility of 0.6 mg/L.[121]

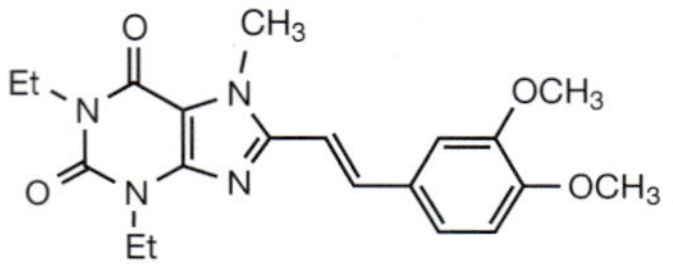

Istradefylline
(Nourianz)

Istradefylline exhibits dose-proportional pharmacokinetics, reaching maximum plasma levels within 4 hours of oral administration.[121] However, steady-state levels may not be reached until 2 weeks of once-daily dosing. In addition, the mean terminal half-life for istradefylline at steady state is approximately 83 hours. The drug also has plasma protein binding of approximately 98%. Istradefylline is extensively metabolized by CYP450s, including principally CYP1A1 and CYP3A4. Lower dose is recommended with concomitant use of CYP3A4 inhibitors and avoidance with CYP3A4 inducers. The most common adverse effects of istradefylline are dyskinesia, dizziness, constipation, nausea, hallucination, and insomnia.

Multiple Sclerosis

Therapeutic Context Overview

MS is a chronic disease that involves demyelination of nerve cells (eg, oligodendrocytes) in the brain and spinal cord. The condition leads to a variety of symptoms including vision difficulties, fatigue, coordination problems, spasticity, as well as cognitive and behavioral changes. The disease takes two forms: progressive and relapsing-remitting. This latter form of MS is most common (80%-90% of cases), with about half of the patients eventually entering a degenerative progressive phase.

Although the cause of MS is not known, there are two general hypotheses that have influenced current MS chemotherapeutic development.[122] The most widely accepted premise is the autoimmune hypothesis. According to this hypothesis, myelin basic protein (MBP) antigen-specific CD4-positive T cells are first primed by dendritic cells in peripheral CNS-draining lymph nodes. This leads to differentiation into Th17 cells by interleukin-23. Th17 cells enter the cerebral spinal fluid (CSF), where they are reactivated by major histocompatibility complex (MHC) class II–expressing macrophages or dendritic cells, followed by entry into the CNS. Here these autoreactive leukocytes initiate disease leading to neuroinflammation that results in oligodendrocyte demyelination. The other premise is the oligodendrogliopathy hypothesis, where the disease starts with oligodendroglial apoptosis initiated from undetermined causes resulting in demyelination. The associated neuroinflammation is a secondary event in response to the oligodendroglial apoptosis.[123]

MS typically presents in adults ages 20 to 50 years and is the most common cause of nontraumatic disability in young adults. The disease afflicts approximately 2 to 2.5 million people worldwide, with the highest prevalence (100-200 cases per 100,000) in populations of Northern European origin.[124] Furthermore, the prevalence ratio of MS in women to men has increased markedly during the last decades (2.3-3.5:1).[125] In the United States, the annual costs per patient of disease-modifying therapies have dramatically increased and are currently more than US$70,000 a year.[126]

Pharmacology Overview

Given the complex pathologic processes involving different cell types in both the periphery and CNS that result in MS, it is not surprising that diverse therapeutic strategies have emerged. However, the assortment of available chemotherapeutics also extends to the chemical matter that comprises MS drugs, from low-molecular-weight organic molecules to a polymeric composition to monoclonal antibodies.

The pharmacology of MS drugs falls into several categories. The first group comprises agents that either (1) replace or mimic the action of endogenous interferon beta resulting in upregulation of immunomodulatory genes or (2) enhance the production of the anti-inflammatory cytokines interleukin 4 and 5, as well as induce an antioxidative stress response. The second set of agents can broadly be defined as those altering the modulation (eg, reduced activation or proliferation, or induced lysis) of T and/or B cells through several different mechanisms. The third category of drugs either results in sequestration of lymphocytes in lymph nodes or prevents their migration from the periphery into the CNS. The fourth class of drugs does not directly target the underlying neuropathology of MS per se. Instead, it blocks potassium channels restoring axonal conduction that improved mobility of patients with MS.

Interferon beta-1a, Interferon beta-1b, and Peginterferon beta-1a

Interferon beta-1a (Avonex), interferon beta-1b (Betaseron), and peginterferon beta-1a (Plegridy) are indicated for the treatment of patients with relapsing forms of MS. Interferon beta-1a is administered via intramuscular injection, while interferon beta-1b and peginterferon beta-1a are given by subcutaneous injection. The structure of interferon beta-1a consists of a 166-amino-acid glycosylated protein (molecular weight ~22.5 kDa) that is identical to human interferon beta. Interferon beta-1b is similar, but with several modifications, including serine in place of the cysteine residue at position 17, one less amino acid, and no carbohydrate side chains, resulting in a lower molecular weight (~18 kDa). Peginterferon beta-1a is a derivative of interferon beta-1a in which a single linear 20-kDa methoxy poly(ethyleneglycol)-O-2-methylpropionaldehyde is covalently attached near the N-terminus of the protein, which reduces clearance. These drugs are manufactured using recombinant DNA technology genetically engineered into either Chinese hamster ovary cells or *Escherichia coli*. For peginterferon beta-1a, a subsequent step is needed to attach the polymer chain.

Interferon beta is an endogenous cytokine that is produced in response to biologic and chemical stimuli. It binds to type I interferon receptors that signal through the Janus kinase/signal transducers and activators of transcription (JAK/STAT) pathway, resulting in the modulation of gene expression for a host of biologic molecules culminating in immunomodulatory, antiviral, and antitumor effects.[127] With regard to the mechanism of action for interferon beta-1a, interferon beta-1b, and peginterferon beta-1a in the treatment of MS, it is the immunomodulatory role that is likely critical. These molecules reduce peripheral myeloid dendritic cells, T-cell responses, and antigen presentation by microglia and monocytes.

Interferon beta-1a reaches maximum plasma concentrations 3 to 15 hours after administration with a plasma elimination half-life of 10 hours. For interferon beta-1b, plasma concentrations are not detectable following subcutaneous administration of low dose (eg, ≤0.25 mg). At higher dose (eg, 0.5 mg) maximum plasma concentrations were reached within 1 to 8 hours. Peginterferon beta-1a reaches maximum plasma concentration within 1 to 1.5 days and has a volume of distribution of 481 L, a plasma elimination half-life of 78 hours, and a clearance of 4.1 L/h. The drugs are catabolized and excreted by the kidneys.

These drugs are contraindicated in patients sensitive to stabilizers used in the formulations, such as albumin and mannitol. Some of the most common adverse effects of these agents are flu-like symptoms including injection site reaction, myalgia, asthenia, lymphopenia, leukopenia, neutropenia, increased liver enzymes, insomnia, abdominal pain, asthenia, pyrexia, and arthralgia.

Glatiramer

Glatiramer (Copaxone) is indicated for reduction of the frequency of relapses in patients with relapsing-remitting MS. Structurally, this drug is quite unique. It consists of a synthetic polymer of L-glutamic acid, L-alanine, L-lysine, and L-tyrosine in an average molar fraction of 0.141, 0.427, 0.095, and 0.338, respectively. The material is formulated as an acetate salt (eg, $[Glu, Ala, Lys, Tyr]_x \cdot xCH_3COOH$). The polymeric drug has an average molecular weight of 5 to 9 kDa.

The polymeric drug is believed to elicit its effects in MS by mimicking MBP. In this way the drug competes with MBP, reducing the number of antigen-specific CD4-positive T cells, which interrupts the autoimmune cascade.[128] Glatiramer may also modulate the activity of MHC antigen-presenting cells.[129] These mechanisms are distinct from those elicited by interferon beta-1a, interferon beta-1b, and peginterferon beta-1a.[130]

A significant portion of the subcutaneously administered dose is partially hydrolyzed near the injection site. A portion of the injected material, either intact or partially hydrolyzed, likely enters the lymphatic circulation with some entering the systemic circulation. The most common adverse effects of glatiramer are injection site reactions, vasodilation, rash, dyspnea, and chest pain.

Ocrelizumab, Alemtuzumab, and Natalizumab

Three human monoclonal antibodies have also been developed for the treatment of MS. Ocrelizumab (Ocrevus) is indicated for the treatment of patients with relapsing form of MS. It is also the first drug approved for the treatment of the primary progressive form of MS. Ocrelizumab is a humanized anti-CD20 immunoglobulin G1 (IgG1) glycosylated monoclonal antibody with a molecular weight of 145 kDa that is administered via intravenous infusion. The antibody binds to CD20 on the cell surface of B lymphocytes, causing antibody-dependent cellular cytolysis and complement-mediated cell lysis. The efficacy of ocrelizumab in the treatment of MS highlights the important role of B lymphocytes as precursors of antibody-secreting plasma cells and as antigen-presenting cells for the activation of T cells.[131] The residence time of ocrelizumab is long, requiring maintenance doses of 600 mg every 6 months for patients with relapsing-remitting MS or two 300-mg infusions separated by 14 days every 6 months for patients with primary progressive MS.[132] The drug has a volume of distribution of 2.78 L, a clearance of 0.17 L/d, and terminal plasma elimination half-life of 26 days with metabolism via catabolism. Ocrelizumab is contraindicated for use in patients with active hepatitis B virus infection. The most common adverse effects of ocrelizumab are respiratory tract and skin infections, as well as infusion reactions.

Alemtuzumab (Lemtrada) is indicated for the treatment of patients with relapsing forms of MS. It is a recombinant humanized anti-CD52 IgG1κ monoclonal antibody with a molecular weight of 150 kDa that is administered via intravenous infusion. The drug binds to CD52, a cell surface antigen present on T and B lymphocytes, natural killer cells, monocytes, and macrophages. Binding results in antibody-dependent cellular cytolysis and complement-mediated lysis. The drug is primarily distributed to the blood and interstitial space with a volume of distribution of 14.1 L.[133] It has a plasma elimination half-life of 2 weeks and is undetectable after 30 days. Alemtuzumab is contraindicated in patients with HIV. It has several associated warnings including causing serious autoimmune conditions, life-threatening infusion reactions, and increased risk of malignancies, such as thyroid cancer and melanoma. In addition, the drug has an array of common adverse effects, such as rash, headache, pyrexia, nasopharyngitis, nausea, urinary tract infection, fatigue, insomnia, upper respiratory tract infection, herpes viral infection, urticaria, pruritus, thyroid gland disorders, fungal infection, arthralgia, pain in the extremity, back pain, diarrhea, sinusitis, oropharyngeal pain, paresthesia, dizziness, abdominal pain, flushing, and vomiting.

Natalizumab (Tysabri) is indicated for the treatment of patients with relapsing forms of MS, as well as those with moderate to severe active Crohn disease. It is a recombinant humanized anti-α4 integrin IgG1κ monoclonal antibody with a molecular weight of 149 kDa that is administered via intravenous infusion. The drug binds the α4-subunit of α4β1 and α4β7 integrins expressed on all leukocytes except neutrophils. This binding prevents the leukocytes from associating with vascular cell adhesion molecule 1 (VCAM-1) on the surface of vascular brain and spinal cord endothelial cells, blocking entry of leukocytes into the CNS.[134,135] Natalizumab has a mean plasma elimination half-life of 11 days, volume of distribution of 5.7 L, and clearance of 16 mL/h.[136] The drug should not be used concomitantly with chronic immunosuppressant or immunomodulatory therapies. It is also contraindicated in patients who have or have had progressive multifocal leukoencephalopathy. Several warnings are associated with natalizumab, including hypersensitivity reactions, increased risk for certain infections, and hepatotoxicity. The most common adverse effects of natalizumab in patients with MS are headache, fatigue, arthralgia, urinary tract infections, lower respiratory tract infections, gastroenteritis, vaginitis, depression, pain in extremities, abdominal discomfort, diarrhea, and rash.

Cladribine

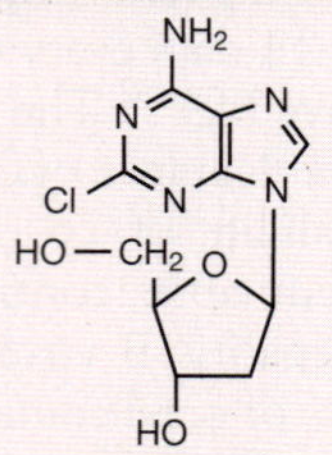

Cladribine
(Mavenclad)

Cladribine (Leustatin) is a nucleoside antimetabolite indicated for the treatment of active hairy cell leukemia and relapsed/refractory acute lymphocytic leukemia. However, cladribine (Mavenclad) is also indicated for the treatment of relapsing forms of MS.[137] This drug is not recommended for use in patients with clinically isolated forms of MS because of its safety profile. Its beneficial effects for the treatment of MS likely arise from ability to deplete B cells.[138,139]

Monomethyl Fumarate, Dimethyl Fumarate, and Diroximel Fumarate

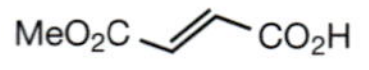

Monomethyl fumarate
(Bafiertam)

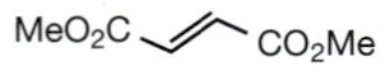

Dimethyl fumarate
(Tecfidera)

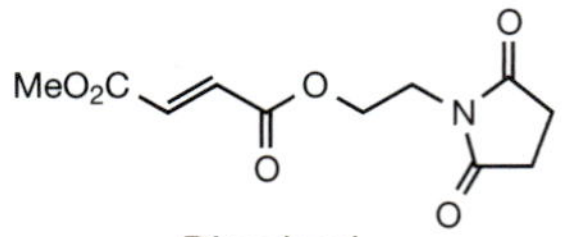

Diroximel
(Vumerity)

Monomethyl fumarate is indicated for the treatment of relapsing forms of MS, including isolated syndrome, relapsing-remitting disease, and active secondary progressive disease, in adults. The drug is structurally simple with a low molecular weight and consists of one methyl ester attached to an alkene in an E-orientation. Monomethyl fumarate is a white solid and highly soluble in water.

Monomethyl fumarate modulates several immune-related properties that could contribute to its efficacy in the treatment of relapsing forms of MS.[140] For example, it is able to enhance anti-inflammatory interleukin 4 and 5 production in stimulated peripheral mononuclear blood cells.[141] The drug also appears able to induce an antioxidative stress response that may contribute to its efficacy. It binds Kelch-like erythroid cell–derived associated protein 1 (KEAP-1), dissociating it from nuclear factor (erythroid-derived 2)-like 2 (Nrf2). This transcription factor translocates to the nucleus, resulting in transcription of antioxidative genes, including those for hemoxygenase-1 nicotinamide adenine dinucleotide phosphate ($NADP^+$), and quinoline oxidoreductase-1.[142]

Monomethyl fumarate is administered orally as delayed-release capsules with maximum plasma concentration reached in 4 hours.[143] A high-fat meal does not significantly affect drug exposure. However, it does decrease maximum plasma concentration by 20% and delays maximum plasma concentration to 11 hours. Monomethyl fumarate has relatively low plasma protein binding of 27% to 45% and a volume of distribution of 53 to 73 L. The drug does not undergo CYP450 metabolism. Instead, it enters the tricarboxylic acid cycle and is metabolized to fumaric acid, citric acid, and glucose with exhalation of CO_2 as the primary route of elimination. The plasma elimination half-life of monomethyl fumarate is 1 hour.

Dimethyl fumarate is indicated for the treatment of patients with relapsing forms of MS. It is also a white powder that is highly soluble in water. Dimethyl fumarate appears to act as a prodrug, with its hydrolysis metabolite monomethyl fumarate being the active component.

After oral administration, dimethyl fumarate undergoes rapid presystemic hydrolysis to its active metabolite monomethyl fumarate, which reaches maximum plasma concentration in 2 to 2.5 hours.[144] Taking the drug with a high-fat meal decreases maximum plasma concentrations by 40% and delays the time to reach maximum plasma concentration to 5.5 hours.

Diroximel fumarate is structurally similar to dimethyl fumarate except one of the methyl esters of the latter is replaced with a 1-(2-hydroxyethyl)pyrrolidine-2,5-dione and is indicated for the treatment of patients with relapsing forms of MS.[145] Like dimethyl fumarate, diroximel fumarate acts as a prodrug being hydrolyzed to active monomethyl fumarate. The other hydrolysis product, 2-hydroxyethyl succinimide, is inactive. Following oral administration of diroximel fumarate, maximum plasma concentration of monomethyl fumarate is reached in 2.5 to 3 hours. Taking the drug with a high-fat meal delays the time to reach maximum plasma concentration to 7 hours.

Neither dimethyl fumarate, diroximel fumarate nor their active metabolite monomethyl fumarate appear to participate in drug-drug interactions. Most common adverse effects of the three drugs are flushing, abdominal pain, diarrhea, and nausea.

Fingolimod, Siponimod, Ozanimod

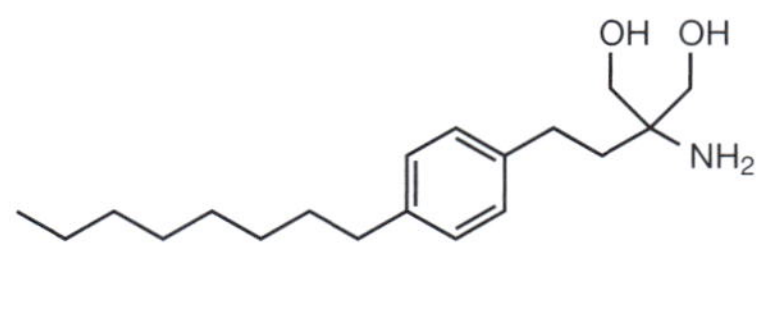

Fingolimod
(Gilenya)

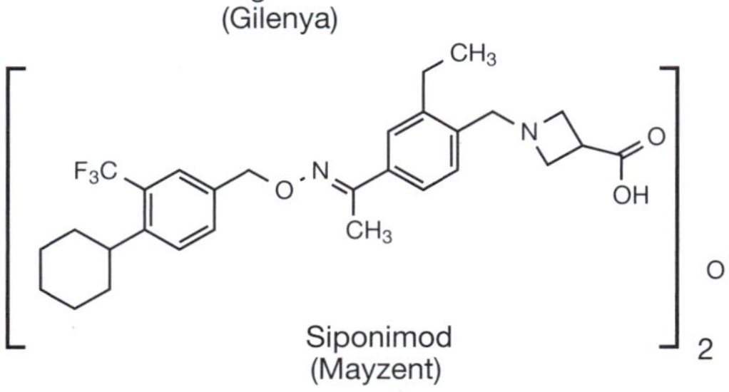

Siponimod
(Mayzent)

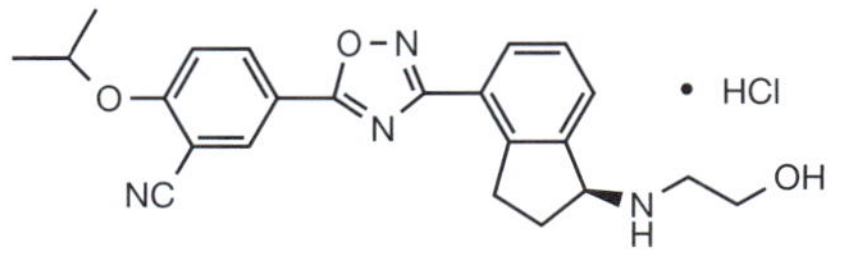

Ozanimod
(Zeposia)

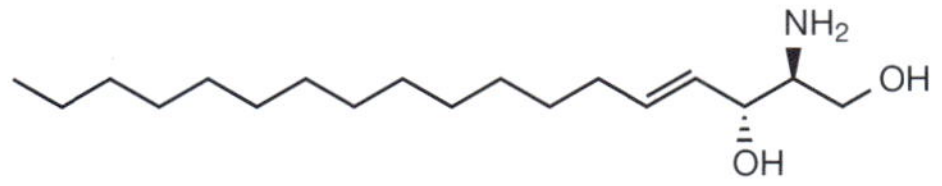

Sphingosine

Fingolimod, siponimod, and ozanimod are indicated for treating the relapsing forms of MS. The active forms of fingolimod (eg, phosphate), siponimod, and ozanimod bind to the sphingosine-1-phosphate receptor 1 ($S1P_1$) as a receptor modulator. This results in the internalization of the receptor causing sequestration of lymphocytes in lymph nodes, which prevents them from infiltrating the CNS. However, additional effects of $S1P_1$ modulation may also contribute to efficacy.[146]

Structurally fingolimod is related to sphingosine and consists of a hydrophobic *n*-octyl substituted phenyl that is connected to a hydrophilic fragment made up of a primary amine and two alcohols. Fingolimod is formulated as a hydrochloride salt that is a white powder and readily soluble in water. It acts as a prodrug that is rapidly converted to fingolimod phosphate, which modulates $S1P_1$ and lymphocytes to egress from lymph nodes.

Fingolimod is readily absorbed after oral administration with a bioavailability of >90% and is unaffected by dietary intake.[147] The drug reaches maximum plasma concentrations in 12 to 16 hours. Fingolimod and its active metabolite fingolimod phosphate are highly protein bound (>99%). In addition, the parent drug is highly distributed in red blood cells, resulting in a large volume of distribution of about 1,200 L.[148] Fingolimod and its active metabolite are cleared very slowly with a terminal plasma half-life of 5 to 6 days.[149] Fingolimod is converted to fingolimod phosphate via sphingosine kinase type 2 (Fig. 10.21). One of the metabolic pathways of fingolimod phosphate is dephosphorylation by lipid phosphate phosphohydrolases and sphingosine-1-phosphate phosphatase.[150] A second metabolic pathway is alkyl oxidation (CYP4F mediated) to produce a primary alcohol metabolite, as well as six other alkyl hydroxyl metabolites, and oxidation to a butanoic acid metabolite, which is the major metabolite found in urine.[151] Finally, fingolimod undergoes biotransformation by (dihydro)ceramide synthase to produce ceramides.

Fingolimod is contraindicated in patients with a variety of cardiovascular and related conditions, including recent myocardial infarction, unstable angina, stroke, transient ischemic attack, heart failure, history of atrioventricular block, sick sinus syndrome, or QT prolongation, since it is known to induce a transient decrease in heart rate during initial dosing possibly by enhancing cardiac parasympathetic activity.[152] The most common adverse effects of fingolimod are headache, liver transaminase elevation, diarrhea, cough, influenza, sinusitis, back pain, abdominal pain, and pain in extremities.

Siponimod contains an alkyl oxime flanked by hydrophobic disubstituted phenyl and an azetidine substituted with a carboxylic acid. The drug is formulated as a fumaric acid salt. Following oral administration, siponimod reaches maximum plasma concentration in 4 hours with an absolute oral bioavailability of 84%.[153] However, steady-state plasma concentrations are not achieved until 6 days of once-daily administrations. Siponimod has high plasma protein binding (>99%), but moderate volume of distribution of 124 L and an elimination half-life of 30 hours. Siponimod is metabolized by oxidation and conjugation (sulfation and glucuronidation) of the cyclohexyl group. In addition, a cholesterol ester conjugate with the carboxylic acid group of siponimod is also formed.[154]

Siponimod is also contraindicated in patients with a variety of cardiovascular and related conditions and those with CYP2C9 genotype. The most common adverse effects are headache, hypertension, and transaminase elevation.

Ozanimod contains a 1,2,4-oxadiazole flanked by a substituted phenyl and an amino alcohol containing indane. It is formulated as a hydrochloride salt. Ozanimod reaches maximum plasma concentration in 6 to 8 hours after oral administration and plasma elimination half-life of 21 hours.[155] Ozanimod has plasma protein binding (98.2%) and an apparent volume of distribution of 5,590 L. It is also extensively metabolized. However, two major active metabolites are formed (Fig. 10.22).[156,157]

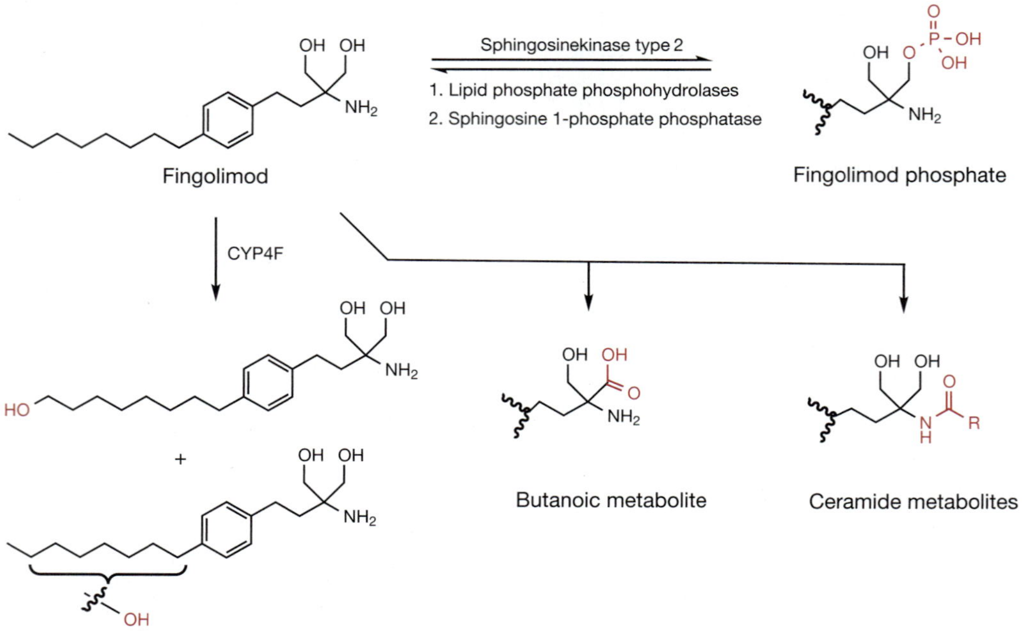

Figure 10.21 Metabolism of fingolimod.

Like fingolimod and siponimod, ozanimod is contraindicated in patients with a variety of cardiovascular and related conditions. It is also contraindicated in patients with severe untreated sleep and concomitant use of a MAO inhibitor. The most common adverse effects are upper respiratory infection, transaminase elevation, orthostatic hypotension, urinary tract infection, back pain, and hypertension.

Teriflunomide

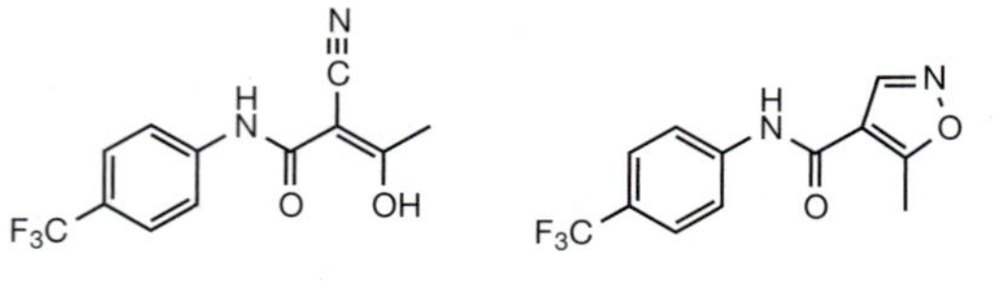

Teriflunomide (Aubagio) Leflunomide

Teriflunomide is indicated for the treatment of patients with relapsing forms of MS. The structure of the drug consists of a para-trifluoromethyl-substituted anilide that also contains a nitrile Z-substituted enol. It is the active metabolite of leflunomide, which is used in the treatment of rheumatoid and psoriatic arthritis. Teriflunomide is a white powder that is practically insoluble in water. Teriflunomide is a selective and reversible inhibitor of dihydroorotate dehydrogenase, a key mitochondrial enzyme in the de novo pyrimidine synthesis pathway. Inhibition of this enzyme leads to reduced proliferation of activated T and B lymphocytes.[158]

Teriflunomide reaches maximum plasma concentration in about 5 hours after oral administration.[159] The drug is extensively bound to plasma protein (>99%), which limits its distribution primarily to plasma with a very long plasma elimination half-life.[160] The parent drug is primary eliminated unchanged in feces. Although the drug is not extensively metabolized, 2-oxo-2-([4-(trifluoromethyl)phenyl] amino)acetic acid is a minor metabolite found in plasma with renal excretion.[161] This metabolite may be formed by hydrolysis to the corresponding aniline, which is known to be acylated and oxidized to 2-oxo-2-([4-(trifluoromethyl)phenyl]amino)acetic acid in rodents (Fig. 10.23).[162]

Teriflunomide participates in several potential drug-drug interactions. For example, it is a substrate of the efflux transporter breast cancer resistance protein (BCRP) and thus

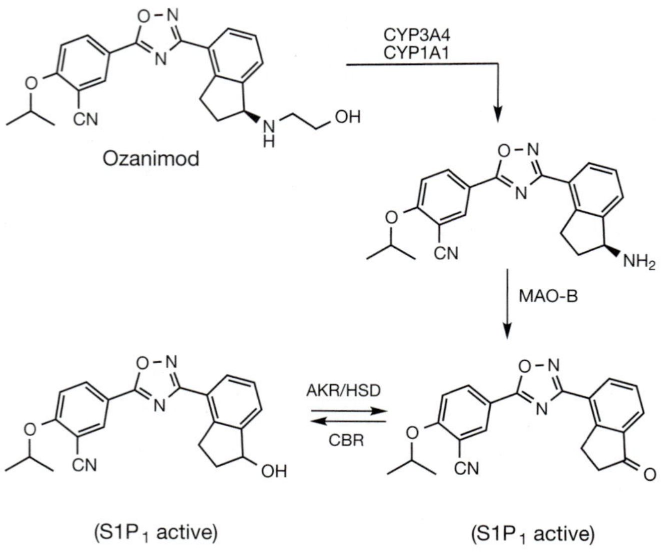

Figure 10.22 Metabolism of ozanimod. MAO, monoamine oxidase.

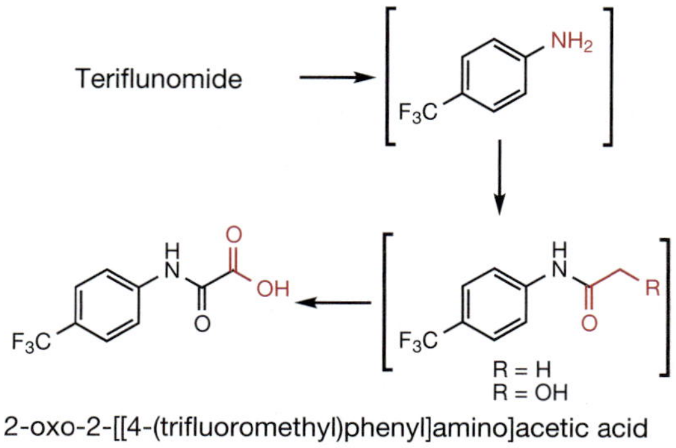

Figure 10.23 Metabolism of teriflunomide.

BCRP inhibitors may increase exposure of teriflunomide. It also can interact with drugs metabolized by CYP2C8 and 1A2. The drug is contraindicated for use in patients with severe hepatic impairment and has a significant risk to cause hepatotoxicity. Teriflunomide presents a risk of teratogenicity and should not be used during pregnancy.

Dalfampridine

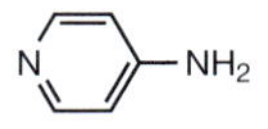

Dalfampridine
(Ampyra)

Dalfampridine is indicated to improve walking in adult patients with MS. Structurally, it is a 4-aminopyridine, which is a white powder. Dalfampridine's mechanism of action is proposed to be its ability to block potassium channels that become exposed during axonal demyelination. This blockage restores axonal conduction, resulting in improved walking speed and perceptions of walking reported by patients with MS.[163]

Dalfampridine is rapidly absorbed after oral administration with a bioavailability of 96% and reaches maximum plasma concentration in 3 to 4 hours.[164] The drug has very low plasma protein binding (≤3%), a volume of distribution of 2.6 L/kg, a plasma elimination half-life of 5 to 6 hours, and a majority of the dose is excreted in urine as parent drug. Dalfampridine does undergo CYP2E1-mediated oxidation to 3-hydroxy-4-aminopyridine, which is conjugated by SULT to 3-hydroxy-4-aminopyridine sulfate (Fig. 10.24).

Dalfampridine is contraindicated in patients taking organic cation transporter 2 (OCT2) inhibitors, such as cimetidine. The most common adverse effects of dalfampridine are urinary tract infection, insomnia, dizziness, headache, nausea, asthenia, back pain, balance disorder, MS relapse, paresthesia, nasopharyngitis, constipation, dyspepsia, and pharyngolaryngeal pain.

Amyotrophic Lateral Sclerosis

Therapeutic Context Overview

ALS, also called Lou Gehrig disease in the United States and motor neuron disease (MND) in the United Kingdom, is a neurodegenerative condition that results in the death of corticospinal neurons with cell bodies in the motor cortex region of the brain and descending axons in the brainstem and lateral spinal cord, as well as cell death of spinal motor neurons that innervate voluntary skeletal muscles. The disease initially presents with subtle cramping or weakness in limbs, which then progresses to paralysis of most skeletal muscles, ultimately resulting in death usually within 3 to 5 years after onset, most commonly from respiratory failure.

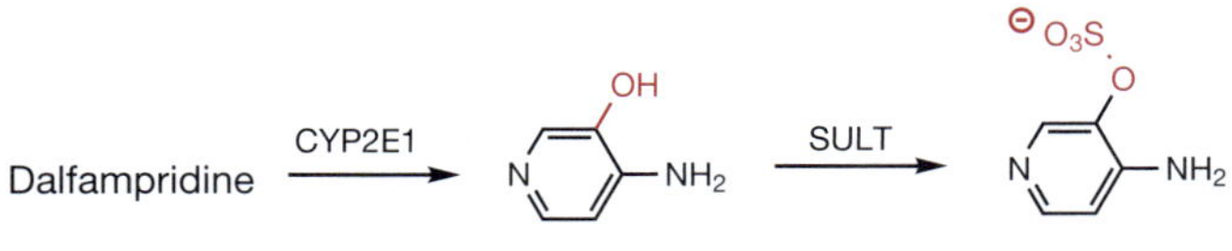

Figure 10.24 Metabolism of dalfampridine. SULT, sulfotransferase.

The prevalence of ALS in the United States is around 4 to 5 cases per 100,000. Overall, ALS is more common among Caucasians, males, and persons ages 60 to 69 years.[165] Although the disease can strike most age groups, the mean age of onset is 55 years. Like other neurodegenerative diseases, most cases of ALS appear to be idiopathic. However, about 10% of patients with ALS have a clear genetic link. In 1993, the first gene connected to ALS, superoxide dismutase-1 (*SOD1*), was reported.[166] SOD1 is a homodimeric Cu/Zn-containing enzyme that catalyzes the disproportionation of highly reactive superoxide to hydrogen peroxide and dioxygen (eg, $2O_2^{-} + 2H^{+} \rightarrow H_2O_2 + O_2$). SOD1 appears to play a prominent role in cellular response to oxidative stress. Consequently, loss of function for this enzyme (eg, by mutations) could hinder a cell's ability to cope with oxidative stress, resulting in dysfunction or death. Over 170 ALS-causing SOD1 mutations have now been identified. However, no correlation between reduced SOD enzyme activity and age of disease onset or disease progression has been found, suggesting that the toxic properties of SOD1 are due to other factors.[167]

Since the discovery of SOD1 mutations, other potential ALS genes have been proposed, including those involved in protein quality control, RNA stability, function and metabolism, as well as cytoskeletal dynamics.[168] Even in sporadic cases of ALS, 1% to 3% of patients have missense SOD1 mutations.[169] Furthermore, genetic alterations may also contribute to disease susceptibility and progression. Like other neurodegenerative diseases, aggregated protein deposits appear as inclusions in affected cells in patients with ALS. In this case, the spinal motor neurons accumulate deposits of ubiquitinated TAR DNA-binding protein 43 (TDP-43).[170] However, the clinical significance of TDP-43 neuropathology on duration of disease or rate of progression is not obvious.[171]

The economic encumbrance of ALS is significant. A study in 2015 found that the annual total cost per patient with ALS in the United States was US$69,475, with the national economic burden estimated at US$279 to US$472 million. These per patient costs were greater than for most other neurologic diseases.[172] Medication costs per year vary from US$14,400 (estimated nonsubsidized 2011 cost) for the older drug riluzole approved in the United States in 1995 compared to US$145,000 (estimated nonsubsidized 2017 cost) for the newly introduced drug edaravone.[173,174]

Pharmacology Overview

The pharmacology of most current therapies for the treatment of ALS is not particularly clear. It is possible that the drugs elicit their effects through a complex set of interactions and functions that are difficult to reduce to a few molecular targets. This is similarly reflected in the emerging array of genes and mutations associated with a subset of patients with familial ALS. The net result has been great difficulty assigning mechanism of actions for currently available drugs and for crafting therapeutic strategies necessary for the development of new chemotherapeutic approaches for treating this devastating neuromuscular degenerative disease. Two small molecules, riluzole and edaravone, and one antisense oligonucleotide, tofersen, are currently available to treat ALS.

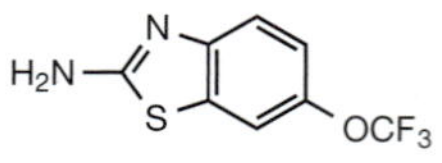

Riluzole
(Rilutek)

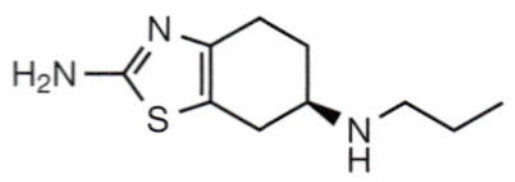

Dexpramipexole

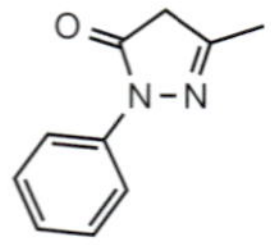

Edaravone
(Radicava)

Riluzole

Riluzole is indicated for the treatment of patients with ALS. Although riluzole extends survival and/or time to tracheostomy, measures of muscle strength and neurologic function do not show a benefit. Riluzole contains a 2-aminobenzothiazole substituted with a trifluoromethyl ether. It is a white to faintly yellow powder that is slightly soluble in water.

The mechanism of action of riluzole is unclear and may be multifactorial. It may be related to inhibitory effects on neurotransmitter (eg, glutamate) release, including interference with intracellular events that follow transmitter binding at excitatory amino acid receptors, inactivation of voltage-dependent sodium channels (eg, Na^+ current and repetitive firing), and/or potentiation of calcium-dependent K^+ current.[175] Interestingly, in 2013, a structurally related compound called dexpramipexole (the enantiomer of the PD drug (S)-pramipexole) failed in a phase 3 clinical trial for ALS due to insufficient efficacy, highlighting the continued lack of understanding for this class of therapeutic agents.

Riluzole is quite hydrophobic, which contributes to it being well absorbed (~90%) with an oral bioavailability of 60%.[176] However, intersubject variation in plasma concentrations of the drug can be large (eg, 30%-100%), likely resulting from variable first-pass metabolism. After oral administration, riluzole reaches maximum plasma concentrations within 1 to 1.5 hours and has a mean plasma elimination half-life of 12 hours. A high-fat meal decreases absorption with reduced exposure (eg, AUC and C_{max} decrease 20% and 45%, respectively).

Riluzole undergoes only limited first-pass metabolism and is excreted predominantly unchanged in urine.[177] The phase 1 reactions that do occur appear to be mediated by CYP1A2 and extrahepatic CYP1A1 isozymes. These reactions include *N*-hydroxylation, oxidation of the benzene portion of the heterocyclic system in the 4-, 5-, and 7-positions generating phenols, as well as dealkylation of the trifluoromethyl ether (Fig. 10.25). These phase 1 metabolites are subjected to phase 2 glucuronidation, with the resulting glucuronides accounting for >85% of the metabolites in urine.

Riluzole should be used with caution in patients with concomitant liver insufficiency. The most common adverse effects associated with this drug are asthenia, nausea, dizziness, decreased lung function, diarrhea, abdominal pain, pneumonia, vomiting, vertigo, circumoral paresthesia, anorexia, and somnolence.

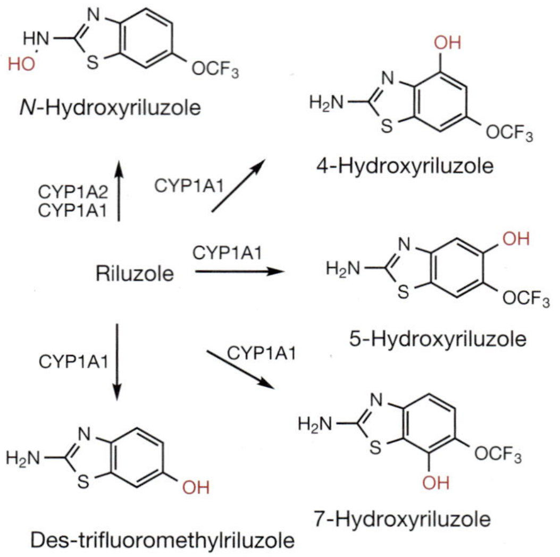

Figure 10.25 Phase 1 metabolism of riluzole.

Edaravone

Edaravone is indicated for the treatment of ALS as an intravenous infusion, receiving approval in the United States in May 2017. The drug consists of a 5-pyrazolone connected to a phenyl. It is a white crystalline powder that is only slightly soluble in water.

Although the precise mechanism of action for edaravone is not known, one potential pathway might be the ability of the compound to reduce oxidative stress. In vitro and in vivo data suggest that edaravone may possess broad free radical scavenging activity, which protects neurons, glia, and vascular endothelial cells.[178]

Edaravone has high human protein binding of 92% and a terminal plasma elimination half-life of 4.5 to 6 hours. The drug mainly undergoes phase 2 metabolism with glucuronidation and sulfonation on the oxygen atom to form the corresponding pyrazole metabolites (Fig. 10.26). The sulfonate conjugate is the primary metabolite detected in plasma. However, in the urine the drug is excreted as its glucuronide conjugate (70%-90% of the dose) and sulfonate conjugate (5%-10% of the dose) with only 1% of the parent drug remaining unchanged.[179]

Edaravone is not expected to participate in drug-drug interactions since it has not demonstrated significant effects on CYP450 isozymes, UGT enzymes, or major transporters. The most common adverse effects reported for this drug are contusion, gait disturbance, and headache.

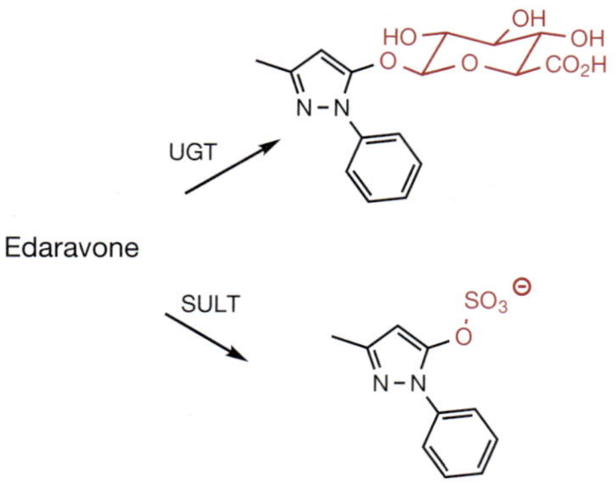

Figure 10.26 Metabolism of edaravone. SULT, sulfotransferase; UGT, UDP-glucuronosyltransferase.

Tofersen

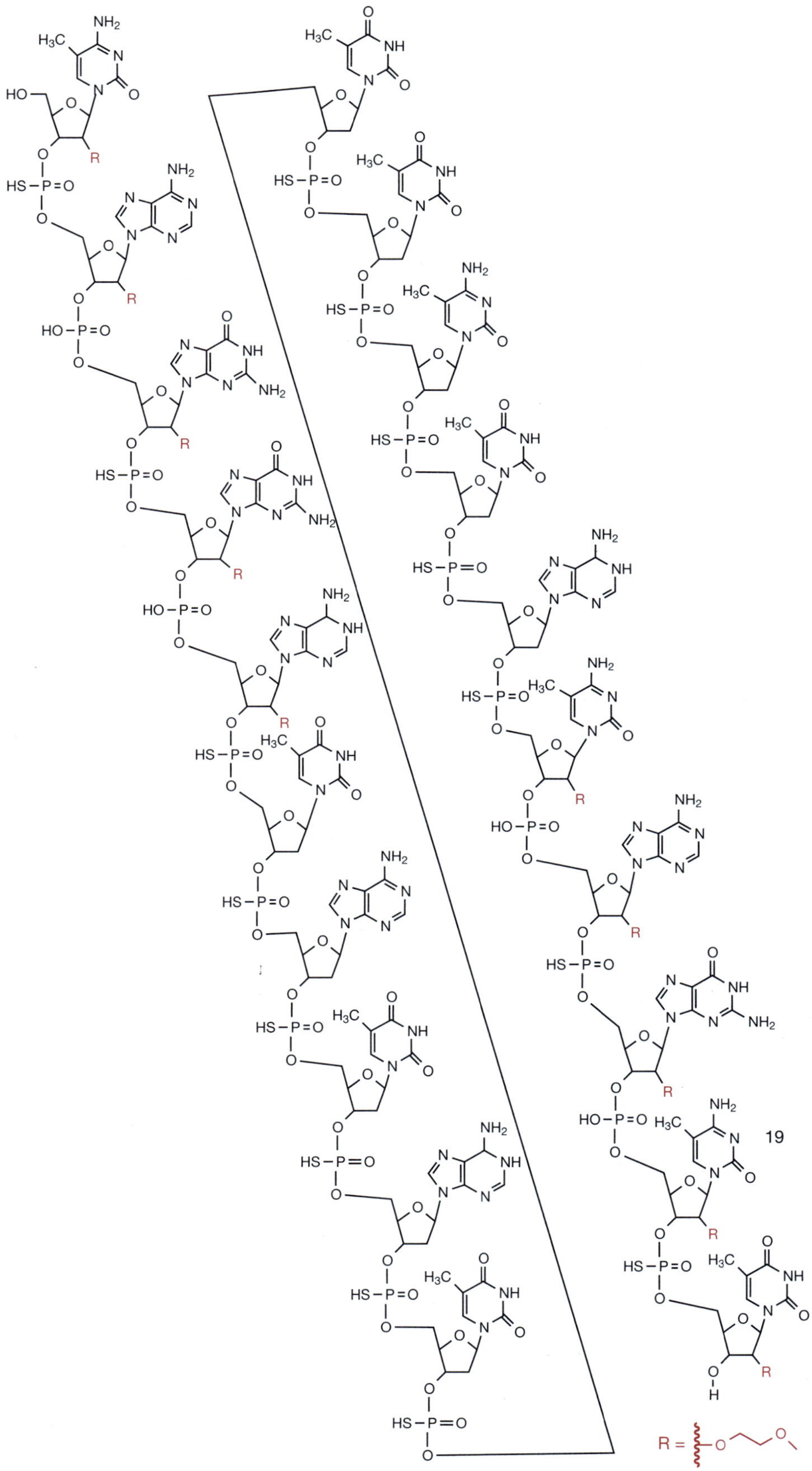

19

Tofersen
(Qalsody)

In 2023, tofersen was granted accelerated approved for the treatment of ALS in adults who have a mutation in the *SOD1* gene. Tofersen is an antisense oligonucleotide that consists of 20 subunits.[180] The first and last five residues are 2′-O-(2-methoxyethyl)-D-ribose units flanking ten 2-deoxy-D-ribose units. The 3′-O to 5′-O internucleotide linkages are either phosphorothioate diesters or phosphate diesters. In addition, the cytosine and uridine bases are methylated at the 5-position. Tofersen binds to SOD1 messenger RNA (mRNA) leading to its degradation, resulting in reduction of SOD1 protein synthesis.[181] The drug is administered intrathecally, with the first three doses given at 14-day intervals followed by maintenance doses given every 28 days. Tofersen distributes within the CNS and moves from the CSF into systemic circulation, reaching a maximum plasma concentration in 2 to 6 hours. The drug has an effective half-life in CSF estimated to be 4 weeks. Most common adverse effects are pain, fatigue, arthralgia, cerebrospinal fluid white blood cell increase, and myalgia.

Duchenne Muscular Dystrophy

Therapeutic Context Overview

DMD is a progressive neuromuscular disorder involving the gene that encodes for the protein dystrophin.[182,183] This condition severely affects males (but is mild or asymptomatic in females) and is characterized by progressive muscle degeneration and weakness. About two-thirds of cases are inherited from the mother as an X-linked mutation (eg, an exon deletion/frameshift mutation—most commonly, a point mutation or a duplication), while the remainder arises from noninherited mutations of the dystrophin gene. Symptoms usually begin to appear around age 3 to 4 years as muscle weakness of the hips, pelvis, thighs, and shoulders. As the disease progresses, voluntary skeletal muscles in the arms, legs, and trunk begin to be impacted followed by heart and respiratory muscles. Death usually occurs in the second to fourth decade of life, with the most common cause being heart failure from cardiomyopathy.

Dystrophin is a large (eg, 427 kDa) cytoplasmic protein that is part of a complex that connects the cytoskeleton of muscle fibers to the surrounding extracellular matrix. Dystrophin links actin filaments to another support protein that resides on the inside surface of the muscle fiber's plasma membrane. Functionally, dystrophin supports muscle fiber strength. Therefore, mutations in this protein can compromise functional properties of the muscle, leading to progressive muscle weakness and other pathologic conditions, including severe myocardial fibrosis and cardiac hypertrophy.

DMD is the most common muscular dystrophy, with an incidence in boys of about 200 per million births.[184] DMD presents a significant public health burden, with average annual patient health care costs of US$23,005. These costs significantly increase for patients ages 14 to 29 years to US$40,132.[185] Although drugs for the treatment of DMD have only very recently been approved in the United States, per patient costs are significant, ranging from US$35,000 to US$300,000 per year, which will certainly increase the future average annual patient health care costs.

Pharmacology Overview

Few chemotherapeutic options are available for the treatment of DMD. One approach is the use of glucocorticoids. These compounds bind to the glucocorticoid nuclear receptor and have been shown to increase muscle strength in patients with DMD.[186] However, this action is in contrast to their direct effect on myofibers, resulting in decreased protein synthesis and increased protein catabolism, causing muscle weakness and atrophy.[187] The purported explanation for these opposing mechanisms for glucocorticoids is that the clinical outcome of increased muscle strength, although mitigated to some extent by adverse effects on myofibers, provides an overall benefit to patients with DMD.[188]

A second pharmacologic approach for the treatment of DMD has been recently developed and is applicable to only a subset of patients with a specific exon deletion/frameshift mutation. The drug causes excision of an exon during pre-mRNA splicing that partially corrects the reading frame of the dystrophin mRNA, resulting in production of partially functional dystrophin protein.

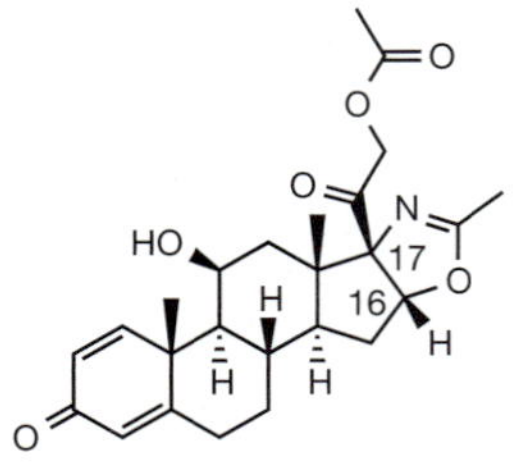

Deflazacort
(Emflaza)

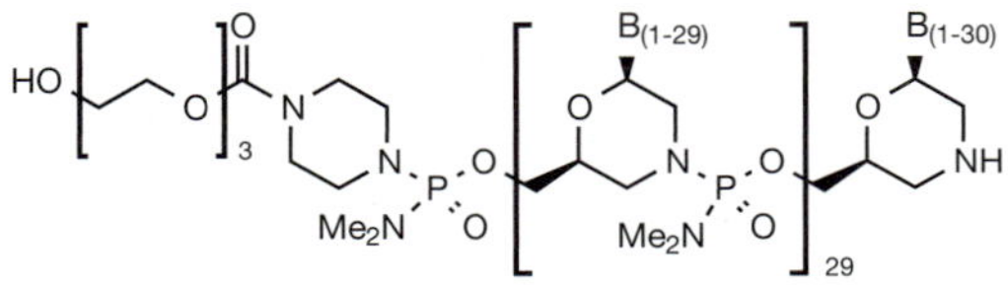

B(1-30): C-T-C-C-A-A-C-A-T-C-A-A-G-G-A
-A-G-A-T-G-G-C-A-T-T-T-C-T-A-G

(where A: adenine, C: cytosine, G: guanine, T: thymine)

Eteplirsen
(Exondys 51)

Deflazacort

Deflazacort is indicated for the treatment of DMD in patients aged ≥5 years. It consists of a glucocorticoid structure with a dihydrooxazole fused to carbons 16 and 17 and an ester-protected α-hydroxy ketone on carbon 17. Deflazacort is a white powder with poor water solubility (<1 mg/mL). However, the pharmacologically active metabolite 21-desacetyldeflazacort (21-desDFZ) is more soluble in water (1.4 mg/mL) due to the exposed primary alcohol.

Deflazacort is a prodrug that is rapidly converted by esterases to 21-desDFZ (Fig. 10.27). This metabolite likely elicits its pharmacology through the glucocorticoid receptor to exert anti-inflammatory and immunosuppressive effects, although the precise mechanism by which it exerts therapeutic properties in DMD is not entirely clear.

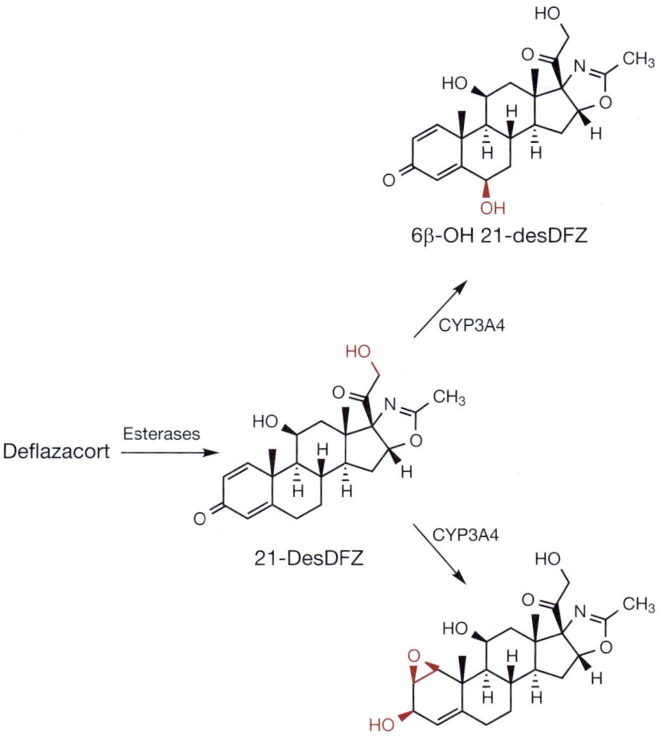

Figure 10.27 Metabolism of deflazacort. 21-desDFZ, 21-desacetyldeflazacort.

After oral administration, deflazacort is readily absorbed, reaching maximum plasma concentration within 1 hour.[189] Following a 0.65 mg/kg dose of deflazacort, the maximum plasma concentration of 21-desDFZ is 0.28 μg/mL and is reached in 2 hours. The plasma elimination half-life of this metabolite is 1.94 hours, its volume of distribution is 1.5 L, and its clearance is 0.53 L/h. The active metabolite 21-desDFZ is about 40% plasma protein bound and urinary excretion is the predominant route of elimination. 21-desDFZ is metabolized by CYP3A4 to several inactive metabolites, including oxidation to 6β-hydroxy 21-desDFZ.[190] Another interesting metabolite found in plasma and urine forms from ketone reduction and stereoselective alkene epoxidation.[191]

Deflazacort should be used with caution in patients coadministered moderate to potent CYP3A4 inhibitors and avoided in patients coadministered moderate or potent CYP3A4 inducers. The most common adverse effects of deflazacort are typical for glucocorticoids, including Cushingoid appearance, weight gain, increased appetite, upper respiratory tract infection, cough, pollakiuria, hirsutism, central obesity, and nasopharyngitis.

Eteplirsen

Eteplirsen is indicated for the treatment of DMD in patients with a confirmed mutation of the *DMD* gene that is amenable to exon 51 skipping (~13% of patients with DMD). The drug is administered by intravenous infusion. Eteplirsen is a synthetic molecule that has a complex chemical structure consisting of 30 subunits of morpholino phosphorodiamidate, each linked to an oligonucleotide, terminating in a carbamate capped piperazine. The morpholino phosphorodiamidates replace the five-membered ribofuranosyls found in DNA and RNA. Eteplirsen binds to the splice-donor region of exon 51 of dystrophin pre-mRNA, inducing skipping of exon 51 that yields an in-frame, truncated, and partially functional dystrophin protein, which causes a less severe form of the disease.[192]

The maximum plasma concentrations of eteplirsen occurred near the end of infusion. The drug has low plasma protein binding (eg, 6%-17%), with a volume of distribution of 600 mL/kg.[193] Eteplirsen is nearly eliminated within 24 hours of administration with no accumulation observed. The clearance of eteplirsen is 339 mL/h/kg following 12 weeks of therapy with 30 mg/kg/wk and a plasma elimination half-life of 3 to 4 hours. The primary route of elimination is renal clearance. Due to eteplirsen's low plasma protein binding, lack of CYP450 metabolism, and lack of interaction with drug transporters, it is expected to have a low potential for drug-drug interactions. The most common adverse effects of the drug were balance disorder and vomiting.

Spinal Muscular Atrophy

Therapeutic Context Overview

Spinal muscular atrophy (SMA) is a rare genetic neuromuscular disorder with an incidence of 1 in 6,000-10,000 live births.[194] The disease involves loss of motor neurons in the spinal cord with progressive muscle wasting. The age of symptom onset correlates with disease severity.[195] For example, children who display symptoms at birth or during infancy (referred to as type 1) usually have the most severe outcome oftentimes not surviving beyond age 5, with death most likely caused by respiratory failure, making SMA the most common genetic cause of infant death. Conversely, SMA onset in teens or adults (referred to as type 4) commonly correlates with higher levels of motor function and normal life expectancy.

The survival motor neuron 1 (*SMN1*) gene encodes for the SMN protein, which plays a key role in the subsistence of motor neurons.[196] A related gene, *SMN2*, undergoes alternative splicing with only 10% to 20% of SMN2 transcripts coding fully functional SMN protein, whereas the remaining transcripts result in a truncated protein (SMNΔ7) that is rapidly degraded. SMA is caused by homozygous mutations of the *SMN1* gene, generally showing the absence of exon 7. This results in SMN protein deficiency causing death of motor neurons in the anterior horn of the spinal cord and brain. Consequently, decreased impulse transmissions to muscles via the motor neurons lead to decreased muscle contractility and progressive muscle atrophy.

Pharmacology Overview

The principal strategy pursued for chemotherapeutic treatment of SMA has been to identify mechanisms for circumventing the alternative splicing of the SMN2 transcript to enhance the production of fully functional SMN protein.[197] This approach has been clinically successful using an antisense oligonucleotide, while additional mechanisms for achieving a similar outcome are actively being investigated. Several other approaches are also currently being pursued at the preclinical stage and in clinical trials, including activation of the *SMN2* gene, *SMN1* gene replacement, and SMN protein stabilization. Finally, the identification of potential disease-modifying factors underlying motor neuron vulnerability and subsequent muscle weakness may offer additional therapeutic modalities.[198]

Nusinersen

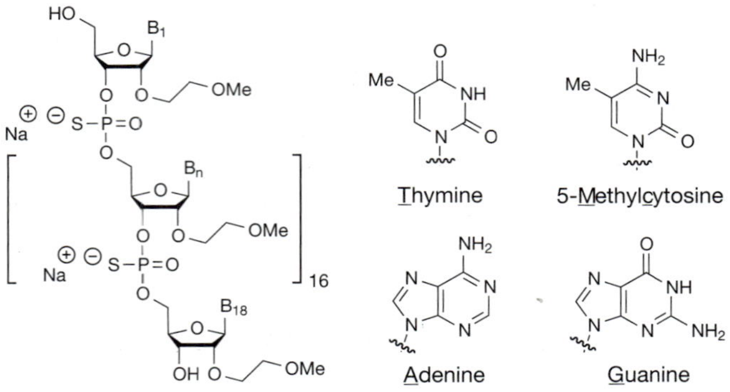

$B_{1\text{-}18}$: T-MC-A-MC-T-T-T-MC-A-T-A-A-T-G-MC-T-G-G

Nusinersen
(Spinraza)

Nusinersen is indicated for the treatment of SMA in pediatric and adult patients. The structure of nusinersen is an antisense oligonucleotide derivative consisting of 18 subunits in which the ribofuranosyl 2′-hydroxys and phosphates found in oligonucleotides are replaced with 2′-O-2-methoxyethyls and phosphorothioates, respectively. The drug is supplied as a solution for intrathecal administration. Nusinersen increases exon 7 inclusions in SMN2 mRNA transcripts, resulting in enhanced production of full-length SMN protein.

Upon intrathecal administration, nusinersen distributes to both CNS and peripheral tissues with maximum plasma concentrations reached within 1.7 to 6.0 hours.[199] The plasma terminal elimination half-life is 63 to 87 days, while the terminal elimination half-life in cerebrospinal fluid is 135 to 177 days. Nusinersen is metabolized via exonuclease (3′- and 5′)-mediated hydrolysis with elimination of the parent drug and chain-shortened metabolites via urinary excretion. Nusinersen is not an inhibitor or inducer of CYP450 enzymes.

Nusinersen increases the risk of coagulation abnormalities and thrombocytopenia, as well as renal toxicity, including fatal glomerulonephritis. The most common adverse effects of the drug are lower and upper respiratory infections, as well as constipation.

Spasticity Disorders

Therapeutic Context Overview

Spasticity is characterized by skeletal muscle spasms and an increase in tonic stretch reflexes that cause muscle stiffness. This can interfere with normal movement and gait, as well as speech. Other common symptoms can include muscle stiffness, muscle and joint deformities, muscle fatigue, and longitudinal muscle growth deficits. The origin of the spasticity is usually injury to the portion of the brain or spinal cord that controls voluntary movement.[200] This impairment can lead to changes in signaling between the nervous system and muscles, often involving damage to descending pathways in the spinal cord that results in hyperexcitability of motor neurons.[201] However, the detailed pathophysiology of spasticity is not well understood. In addition, assessing the effectiveness of antispasmodic drugs is difficult.[202,203] Since spasticity is frequently associated with pain, antispasmodic drugs may elicit efficacy via skeletal muscle relaxation as well as through analgesia.[204,205]

Spasticity disorders afflict more than 12 million people worldwide, thus representing a significant public health burden. It also commonly occurs in patients with CP and MS. For example, about 80% of patients with CP and MS have spasticity. In addition, many other maladies have associated spasticity disorders, including traumatic brain and spinal cord injuries and stroke, which contributes to its overall prevalence.

Several other conditions related to spasticity will also be covered in this chapter. This includes chemotherapeutics that reverse anesthetic drug–induced nondepolarizing neuromuscular blockage that have also been used to treat MG and an agent to treat LEMS. New agents used to treat the neuromuscular conditions of chorea associated with Huntington disease and tardive dyskinesia, which can result in some patients after long-term use of neuroleptic medications, will be presented. Finally, a new drug for the treatment of Friedreich ataxia will be discussed.

Pharmacology Overview

Several classes of drugs are used to treat spasticity disorders and can generally be categorized as those indicated for the relief of discomfort associated with musculoskeletal conditions and those indicated for the treatment of spasticity. The oldest class of skeletal muscle relaxants indicated for the relief of discomfort associated with musculoskeletal conditions are those based on 3-phenoxy-1,2-propanediol. These molecules appear to elicit muscle relaxant properties similar to that of sedative-hypnotics. However, the 3-phenoxy-1,2-propanediol class of drugs have greater selectivity for modulating effects mediated by the spinal cord, thus producing less sedation than general sedative-hypnotics. Nonetheless, this class of drugs has common side effects related to CNS depression, including sedation and dizziness, as well as muscle weakness.

Another class of skeletal muscle relaxants used in the relief of discomfort associated with musculoskeletal conditions is alkanediols and their derivatives. These molecules may modulate $GABA_A$ receptors in addition to producing benzodiazepine-like sedative and anxiolytic effects. Consequently, drugs of this class can have abuse and dependency liabilities.[206]

Several other drugs have been marketed for relief of discomfort associated with musculoskeletal conditions. For example, chlorzoxazone appears to provide skeletal muscle relaxation via CNS depression. However, it is associated with idiosyncratic hepatotoxicity and several sensitivity reactions (eg, urticaria, erythema, and pruritus) that limits it use.[203] Orphenadrine is a drug that has been used as a muscle relaxant that likely elicits its therapeutic effects through blocking acetylcholine in the central and peripheral nervous systems.

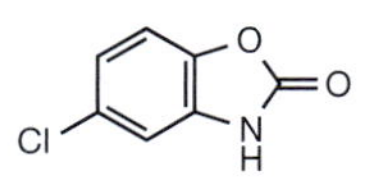

Chlorzoxazone
(Paraflex)

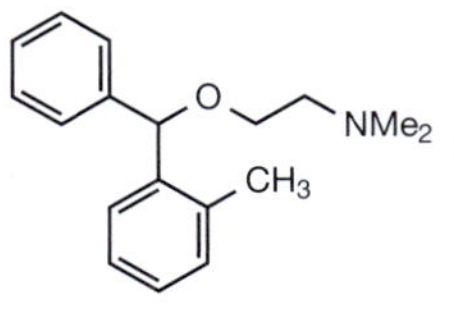

Orphenadrine citrate
(Norflex)

Several small molecule drugs, as well as a protein therapeutic, are indicated (or used off-label) for the treatment of spasticity. These drugs elicit their pharmacology through an array of mechanisms, including adrenergic receptor agonism, serotonin receptor antagonism, modulation of $GABA_B$ receptor, interfering with the release of Ca^{+2} from the sarcoplasmic reticulum (possibly due to antagonizing ryanodine receptor [RYR] channels), or blocking acetylcholine release at neuromuscular junctions. In many cases, the precise mechanism of drug action is unknown or debatable.

Finally, a drug has recently been approved to reverse the effects of neuromuscular blockade induced by the aminosteroid anesthetics rocuronium bromide and vecuronium bromide. The drug sequesters these two agents through noncovalent interactions, preventing them from binding their intended target. Peripherally acting acetylcholinesterase inhibitors have been used for the same indication, as well as for the treatment of the neuromuscular condition MG. A drug that blocks potassium channels has been approved for the treatment of LEMS. Other drugs recently introduced for the treatment of chorea associated with Huntington disease and tardive dyskinesia elicit therapeutic effects via inhibition of the vesicular monoamine transporter 2 (VMAT2). Finally, a drug for the treatment of Friedreich ataxia, which is thought to work via enhancement of the Nrf2 pathway, was recently approved.

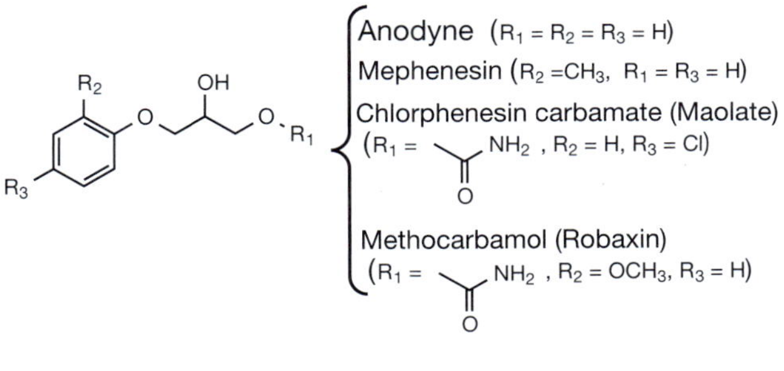

Methocarbamol

Methocarbamol is indicated for the relief of discomfort associated with acute, painful musculoskeletal conditions. Structurally it consists of a glycerol unit substituted on one terminus with a 2-methoxyphenyl ether and with a carbamate on the other. It belongs to the broader class of drugs based on 3-phenoxy-1,2-propanediol pharmacophore. The first drug recognized to exhibit spasmolytic activity from this class was anodyne. However, it had too short of plasma half-life for clinical use. The close structurally related derivative mephenesin was a widely prescribed skeletal muscle relaxant, but it is no longer used.[206] The primary alcohol is not required for antispasmolytic activity. It was replaced with a carbamate resulting in chlorphenesin carbamate and methocarbamol, although the former is no longer prescribed. Methocarbamol is chiral with the *R*-enantiomer demonstrating greater muscle relaxant activity in mice.[207] However, the drug is currently only available in racemic form. Methocarbamol is a white powder with low aqueous solubility.

The mechanism of action of methocarbamol as a skeletal muscle relaxant is not known but appears to be indirect. It seems to be a CNS depressant with sedative properties that result in musculoskeletal relaxation. Interestingly, it has no direct action on the contractile mechanism of striated muscle, the motor end plate, or nerve fibers.

Methocarbamol is readily absorbed following oral administration and reaches maximum plasma concentrations in 1.4 hours. The drug has plasma protein binding of 50%, a moderate volume of distribution of 0.48 L/kg, plasma clearance of 0.20 to 0.80 L/h/kg, and a rapid plasma elimination half-life of 1.2 hours (Table 10.2).[208] A small amount of the parent drug is excreted in the urine, while its metabolites are also eliminated by renal clearance. Methocarbamol is metabolized via demethylation of the ether and hydroxylation of the *para*-position on the benzene ring (Fig. 10.28). Extensive conjugation (eg, glucuronidation and sulfonation) of methocarbamol and its phase 1 metabolites also occurs.[209] Several of the glucuronides have been identified and characterized in rodents.[210]

The clearance of methocarbamol can be reduced in patients with renal or hepatic impairment. Since methocarbamol possesses CNS depressant effects, it may cause drowsiness and therefore should be used with caution in combination with alcohol and other CNS depressants and in situations where patients are performing activities requiring mental alertness. Other adverse effects include dizziness, ataxia, nausea, flushing, blurred vision, and fever.

Metaxalone

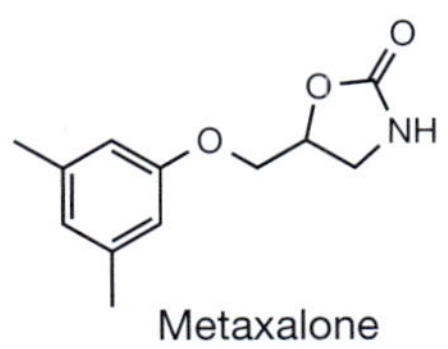

Metaxalone
(Skelaxin)

Metaxalone is indicated as an adjunct to rest, physical therapy, and other measures for relief of discomfort associated with acute, painful musculoskeletal conditions. Structurally it is closely related to methocarbamol, except that the phenyl is substituted differently, and it contains a cyclic carbamate (2-oxazolidinone), demonstrating that the secondary alcohol

Table 10.2 Pharmacokinetic Parameters of Several Drugs Used to Treat Spasticity Disorders

Drug	Plasma Elimination Half-Life	Clearance	Volume of Distribution	Oral Bioavailability
Methocarbamol	1.2 h	0.20-0.80 L/h/kg	0.48 L/kg	
Metaxalone	5 h		800 L	
Carisoprodol	1.7-2.0 h		0.93-1.3 L/kg	92%
Cyclobenzaprine	18 h	0.7 L/min		33%-55%
Baclofen	3-4 h		0.7 L/kg	70%-80%
Dantrolene	12 h			70%
Tizanidine	2.5 h		2.4 L/kg	40%
Diazepam	1-3 h; $t_{1/2}\beta$ 1-2 d		0.8-1.0 L/kg	

present in the 3-phenoxy-1,2-propanediol structure is not required. Although it does contain a chiral center, the drug is only available in racemic form. Metaxalone is a white crystalline solid with low aqueous solubility. The mechanism of action of methocarbamol again appears to be indirectly acting as CNS depressant with sedative properties that result in musculoskeletal relaxation.

After oral administration, metaxalone reaches peak plasma concentration in 3 hours.[211] The drug's very large volume of distribution of approximately 800 L is indicative of extensive tissue distribution, and its plasma elimination half-life is 5 hours (see Table 10.2). If taken with a high-fat meal, the maximum plasma concentration can increase 23% and the time to maximum plasma concentration can be 8 hours. The major route of metaxalone metabolism is benzylic oxidation to give the corresponding carboxylic acid (Fig. 10.29). In this phase 1 metabolism CYP1A2, CYP2D6, CYP2E1, and CYP3A4 are the primary isozymes involved. The carboxylic acid undergoes phase 2 conjugation to the glucuronide. A minor route of metaxalone metabolism is cleavage of the ether, which again is CYP450 mediated.[212]

Metaxalone does not significantly inhibit or induce major CYP450 enzymes. Consequently, it may not be prone to drug-drug interactions. However, the drug should be administered with caution to patients with mild to moderate hepatic and renal impairment. Metaxalone is contraindicated in patients with known tendency to drug-induced, hemolytic, or other anemias. Again, since metaxalone possesses CNS depressant effect, it should be used with caution in combination with other CNS depressants. Other adverse effects include drowsiness, dizziness, headache, nervousness, nausea, vomiting, and gastrointestinal upset.

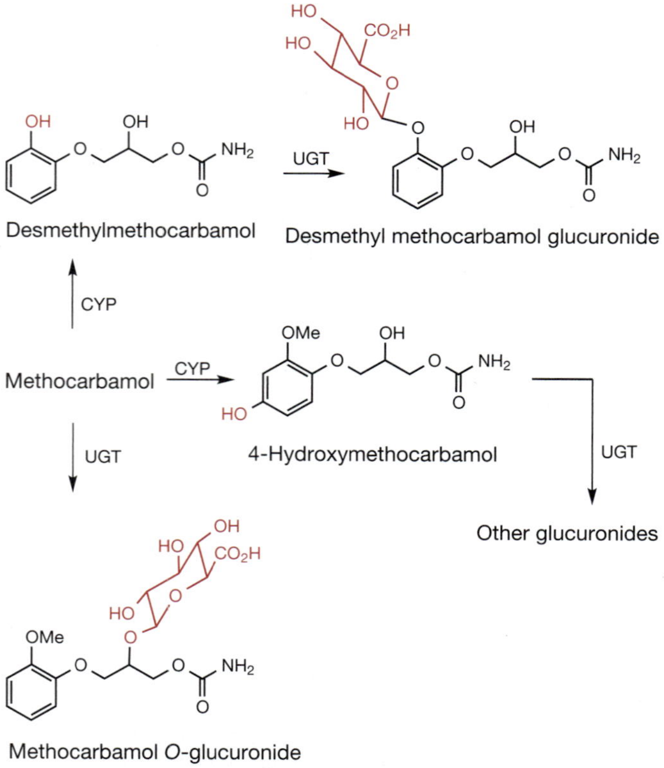

Figure 10.28 Metabolism of methocarbamol. CYP, cytochrome P; UGT, UDP-glucuronosyltransferase.

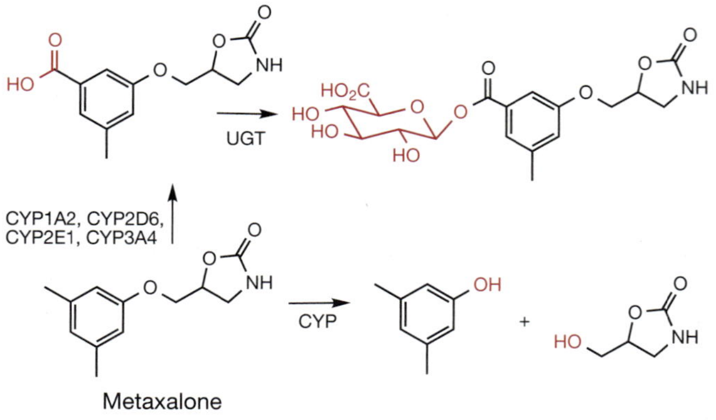

Figure 10.29 Metabolism of metaxalone. CYP, cytochrome P; UGT, UDP-glucuronosyltransferase.

Carisoprodol

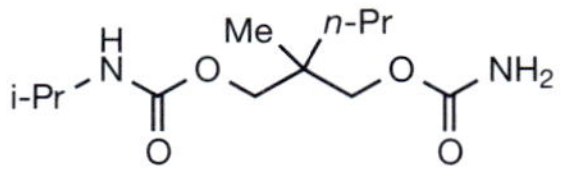

Carisoprodol
(Rela, Soma)

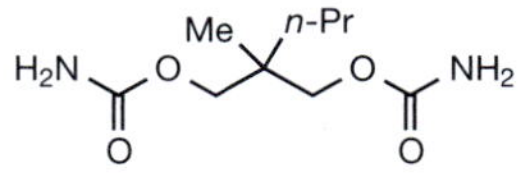

Meprobamate
(Equanil, Miltown)

Carisoprodol is indicated for the relief of discomfort associated with acute, painful musculoskeletal conditions. It is a bis-carbamate of a substituted 1,3-propanediol that is a prodrug of meprobamate. Carisoprodol is a white crystalline solid that is slightly soluble in water.

Although the mechanism of action of carisoprodol is not fully understood, its ability to modulate $GABA_A$ receptors likely plays a role in muscle relaxation.[213] In addition, the primary metabolite, meprobamate, has comparable properties producing sedative and anxiolytic effects similar to benzodiazepines.[214,215]

Carisoprodol is well absorbed and quickly reaches maximum plasma levels within 1.5 to 1.7 hours after oral administration. It is not subjected to extensive first-pass metabolism, thus providing excellent oral bioavailability of 92% (see Table 10.2). Although its terminal plasma elimination half-life is only 1.7 to 2.0 hours, terminal plasma elimination half-life for its metabolite meprobamate is 3.6 to 4.5 hours, which reaches maximum plasma levels in 9.7 hours.[216] Pharmacokinetic modeling of carisoprodol and meprobamate disposition estimates a moderate volume of distribution for the parent prodrug to be 0.93 to 1.3 L/kg and meprobamate to be 1.4 to 1.6 L/kg.[217]

Carisoprodol is metabolized via dealkylation of the isopropyl attached to the carbamate (Fig. 10.30) in the liver by CYP2C19 to meprobamate.[218] In addition, meprobamate has been shown to undergo additional metabolism in rats and rabbits, including oxidation of the *n*-propyl group to a carboxylic acid and secondary alcohol. This secondary alcohol can undergo further oxidation to the corresponding ketone and conjugation to the corresponding glucuronide. Finally, meprobamate also undergoes glucuronidation on the nitrogen atom of the carbamate.[219]

Carisoprodol can participate in drug-drug interactions. Coadministration of CYP2C19 inhibitors (eg, omeprazole or fluvoxamine) with carisoprodol can result in increased exposure of carisoprodol and decreased exposure of meprobamate. Coadministration of CYP2C19 inducers (eg, rifampin, St. John's wort, or aspirin) with carisoprodol can result in decreased exposure of carisoprodol and increased exposure of meprobamate. The drug is also contraindicated in patients with a history of acute intermittent porphyria. Given the modulation of carisoprodol and its principal metabolite on $GABA_A$ receptor and their benzodiazepine-like effects, carisoprodol has liabilities for dependence, withdrawal, and abuse with prolonged use.[203] The most common adverse effects of carisoprodol are drowsiness, dizziness, and headache.

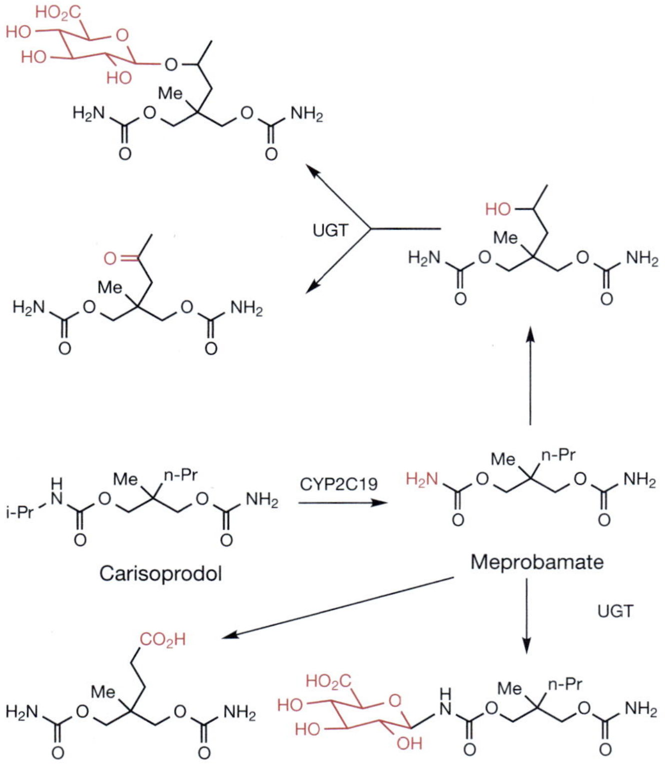

Figure 10.30 Metabolism of carisoprodol and meprobamate. CYP, cytochrome P; UGT, UDP-glucuronosyltransferase.

Cyclobenzaprine

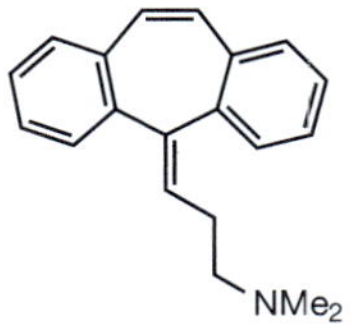

Cyclobenzaprine
(Flexeril)

Cyclobenzaprine is indicated for relief of muscle spasm associated with acute, painful musculoskeletal conditions. Structurally, it contains a dibenzo[*a*,*d*][7]annulene core, which is attached to a tertiary amine through an alkene-linked propyl group. Due to the basic amine, it is formulated as the hydrochloride salt that is a white crystalline solid with very good water solubility (eg, >200 mg/mL).

Cyclobenzaprine can provide relief from skeletal muscle spasm of local origin without interfering with muscle function. It is not effective in treating muscle spasm due to CNS disease, although the efficacy for skeletal muscle spasm is likely centrally mediated. Although the mechanism of action of cyclobenzaprine is unclear, it has been postulated to act via α_2 agonism. However, other mechanisms have been proposed, including via $5\text{-}HT_2$ antagonism.[220] Pharmacologic studies in animals show a similarity between the effects of cyclobenzaprine and structurally related tricyclic antidepressants.

Cyclobenzaprine is well absorbed after oral administration but is subject to first-pass metabolism that reduces its oral bioavailability to 33% to 55% (see Table 10.2).[221] The drug also participates in enterohepatic circulation, is highly bound to plasma proteins, and accumulates reaching steady state within 3 to 4 days upon multiple dosing. Cyclobenzaprine is eliminated slowly, with a plasma half-life of 18 hours and a plasma clearance of 0.7 L/min. The drug is metabolized by CYP450-mediated oxidation (eg, 3A4, 1A2, and, to a lesser extent, 2D6) of the alkene present in the dibenzo[*a*,*d*][7]annulene, likely to an intermediate epoxide that undergoes hydrolysis to the *cis*-10,11-dihydroxyl metabolite (Fig. 10.31).[222] Although the *trans*-diol metabolite has not been reported for cyclobenzaprine, it has been observed in the metabolism of amitriptyline, a structurally related compound.[223] Cyclobenzaprine also undergoes glucuronidation of the tertiary amine. These metabolites are excreted primarily via the kidneys.

Cyclobenzaprine should be used with caution in older adults, in whom increased exposure has been observed likely due to diminished metabolic activity, and in patients with hepatic impairment. The drug is contraindicated with concomitant use of MAO inhibitors or within 14 days after MAO inhibitor discontinuation due to increased risk of hyperpyretic crisis seizures. Cyclobenzaprine has also been associated with the development of serotonin syndrome. Given its structural similarity to tricyclic antidepressants, it also may enhance the effects of alcohol, barbiturates, and other CNS depressants. The most common adverse effects of cyclobenzaprine are drowsiness, dry mouth, and dizziness.

Baclofen

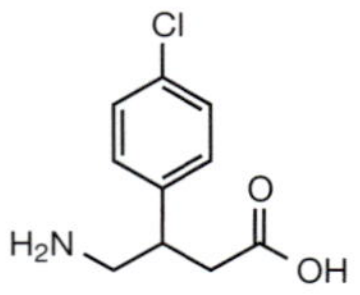

Baclofen
(Lioresal)

Baclofen is indicated for the suppression of voluntary muscle spasm in MS and spinal lesions caused by trauma, infections, degeneration, neoplasm, and unknown origins that cause skeletal hypertonus, as well as spastic and dyssynergia of the bladder. However, it is not recommended in PD or spasticity arising from stroke, CP, or rheumatoid disorders. Structurally, baclofen is related to the inhibitory neurotransmitter GABA (gamma-aminobutyric acid), except it contains a 4-chlorophenyl substituent on the β-carbon. It also contains one chiral center. Although the (*R*)-enantiomer is the more active isomer, only the racemate is approved for clinical use. Baclofen is a white crystalline solid that is slightly soluble in water.

Baclofen's antispastic activity is believed to result from receptor binding in the spinal cord, effectively reducing muscle hypertonia. In contract, its adverse effects (eg, depressant properties) are likely centrally mediated. Hence, intrathecal administration using an indwelling pump can provide direct delivery to the site of action within the spinal cord, while limiting systemic exposure potentially reducing adverse effects.[224] Baclofen depresses monosynaptic and polysynaptic reflex transmission via agonism of $GABA_B$ receptors.[225] This stimulation in turn inhibits the release of excitatory amino acids, such as glutamate and aspartate. Baclofen also displays antinociceptive activity,[226] although the clinical significance of this is not clear. In neurologic diseases associated with skeletal muscle spasm, baclofen can cause muscle relaxation and pain relief.

Despite having two ionizable functional groups, baclofen is rapidly and completely absorbed following oral administration, reaching maximum plasma concentration in 2 to 4 hours.[227] It is subjected to some first-pass metabolism resulting in an oral bioavailability of 70% to 80% (see Table 10.2). Baclofen has plasma protein binding of 30%, a moderate volume of distribution of 0.7 L/kg, and a plasma elimination half-life of 3 to 4 hours.[228] The charged state of baclofen at physiologic pH does limit its ability to cross into the CNS and spinal cord. As a result, cerebrospinal fluid concentrations are 8.5 times lower than in plasma. Approximately 70% of baclofen is eliminated in the urine unchanged, whereas 15% of the dose is metabolized in the liver and excreted in the urine and feces. The primary metabolism pathway for baclofen is deamination to β-4-chlorophenyl-γ-hydroxybutyric acid (Fig. 10.32).[229] More recently, it has been shown that this metabolic process is more extensive for the (*S*)-enantiomer.[230]

Baclofen should be used cautiously in patients with psychiatric and nervous system disorders. In addition, caution is advised in patients with epilepsy or other convulsive conditions, cortical or subcortical brain damage, or significant electroencephalography abnormalities, since the drug can lower the convulsion threshold. In addition, baclofen should be used with caution in patients with impaired renal function. The most common adverse effects for baclofen are sedation, somnolence, and nausea.

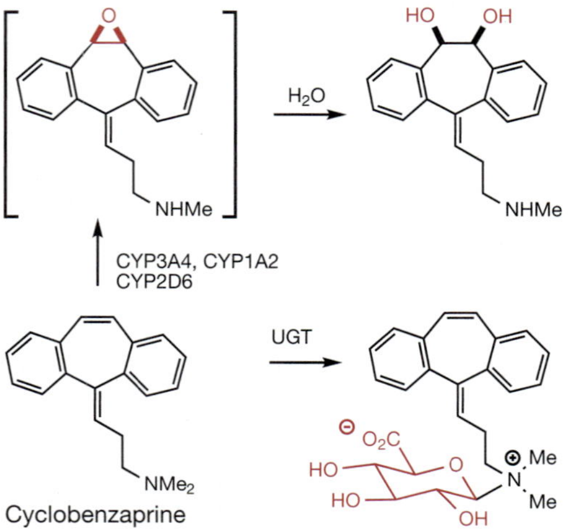

Figure 10.31 Metabolism of cyclobenzaprine. CYP, cytochrome P; UGT, UDP-glucuronosyltransferase.

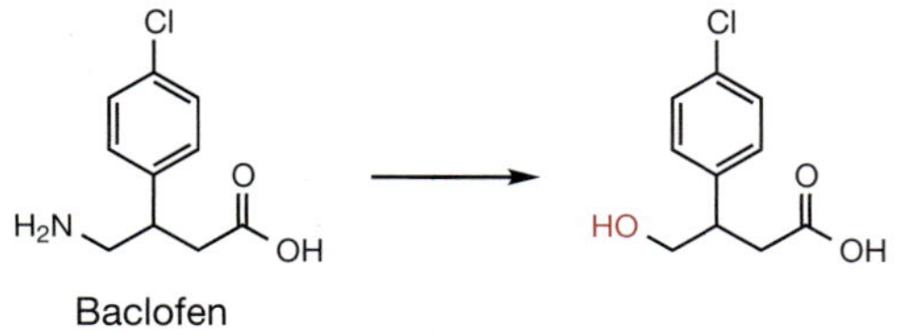

Figure 10.32 Metabolism of baclofen.

Dantrolene

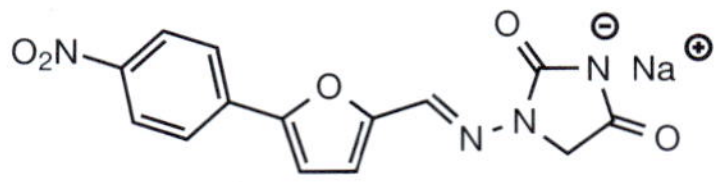

Dantrolene sodium
(Dantrium)

Dantrolene is indicated for the treatment of spasticity resulting from upper motor neuron disorders, such as spinal cord injury, stroke, CP, or MS. It is also indicated for preoperative prevention or attenuation of malignant hyperthermia. Structurally, the drug contains a *p*-nitrophenyl-substituted furan that is linked via an imine to 1-aminohydantoin. This latter component contains an imide with a pK_a of 7.5. This functional group can be deprotonated under basic conditions. Thus, dantrolene is formulated as a sodium salt, which is a hydrate (~15% water) and is an orange powder. Although it is a salt, the drug is poorly soluble in water, presenting difficulties for rapid preparation of intravenous solutions in emergency situations. In addition, intravenous formulations require a pH of 9.5 to ensure solubility, which can be highly irritating to peripheral veins, thus requiring injection into a large vein or use of a fast-running infusion.[231] Although dantrolene contains a hydantoin, it does not have local anesthetic or anticonvulsant activities.[232]

Dantrolene appears to produce skeletal muscle relaxation by affecting the contractile response beyond the myoneural junction. It dissociates the excitation-contraction coupling, probably by interfering with the release of Ca^{+2} from the sarcoplasmic reticulum and is more pronounced in fast muscle fibers. More recently, dantrolene has been shown to block RYR channels inhibiting Ca^{+2} release from sarcoplasmic reticulum. The drug displays selectivity for RYR1 (skeletal muscle) and RYR3 (brain) isoforms over RYR2 (myocardium).[233]

Dantrolene is well absorbed following oral administration, with a bioavailability of 70% and maximum plasma concentration reached in 6 hours. The plasma elimination half-life of the drug is 12 hours (see Table 10.2). Dantrolene undergoes oxidation to 5-hydroxydantrolene (Fig. 10.33), a potent skeletal muscle relaxant, which undergoes conjugation to the corresponding glucuronide and sulfate.[234] In addition, dantrolene is metabolized by nitroreductases to aminodantrolene, which is acetylated. The reduction process appears to form electrophilic intermediates that generate mercapturic acid metabolites.[235] Such intermediates could increase risk for hepatotoxicity that has resulted in a black box warning. Dantrolene and its metabolites are excreted mainly in the urine and bile.

Dantrolene is contraindicated in patients with hepatic disease, such as hepatitis and cirrhosis. It can cause idiosyncratic or hypersensitive liver disorders. The drug is also contraindicated in patients where spasticity is utilized to sustain upright posture and balance in locomotion. The most common adverse effects of dantrolene are drowsiness, dizziness, weakness, general malaise, fatigue, and diarrhea.

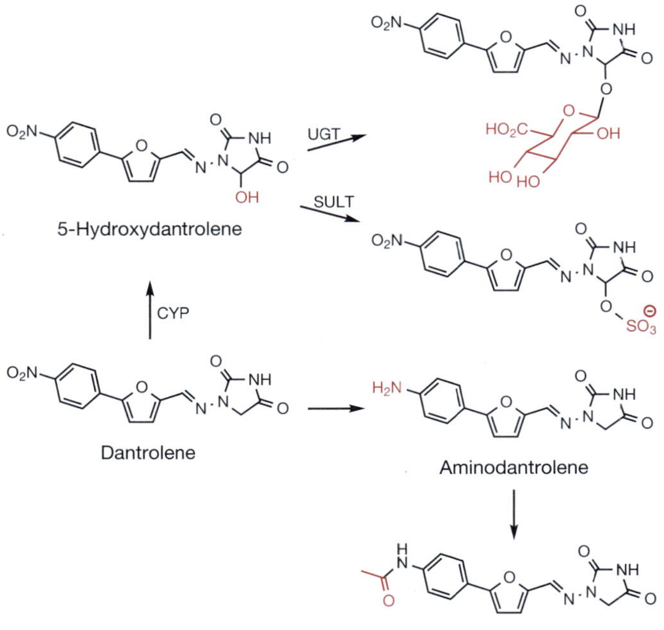

Figure 10.33 Metabolism of dantrolene. CYP, cytochrome P; SULT, sulfotransferase; UGT, UDP-glucuronosyltransferase.

Tizanidine

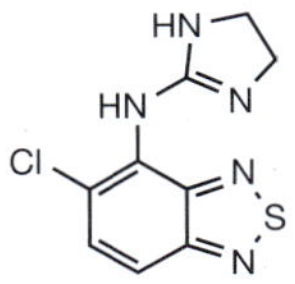

Tizanidine
(Zanaflex)

Tizanidine is indicated for the management of spasticity. This short-acting drug is comparable to baclofen or diazepam, with global tolerability data favoring tizanidine.[236] Structurally it contains a benzo[c][1,2,5]thiadiazole that is substituted with a chlorine atom and a guanidine (eg, the aminoimidazoline), a basic functional group. The drug is formulated as the hydrochloride salt that is a slight water-soluble white crystalline solid. Tizanidine readily crosses the BBB where it functions as a α_2-adrenergic agonist reducing spasticity by increasing presynaptic inhibition of motor neurons.

Tizanidine is well absorbed following oral administration. However, its absolute oral bioavailability is only 40% due to first-pass hepatic metabolism (see Table 10.2).[237] It reaches maximum plasma concentration in 1 hour, but the parent drug has a relatively short plasma elimination half-life of 2.5 hours. Tizanidine also has relatively low plasma protein binding (30%) and a large volume of distribution (2.4 L/kg) indicative of extensive tissue exposure.

Approximately 95% of an orally administered dose of tizanidine is metabolized primarily by CYP1A2. Very little parent drug is excreted unchanged (0.4% in urine). Tizanidine is oxidized to the sulfuric diamide TZD-1 (Fig. 10.34).[238] The parent compound also undergoes oxidation of the imidazoline to generate TZD-2, which is hydrolyzed to intermediate TZD-3 that is dealkylated to TZD-4.

Furthermore, the parent drug is oxidized to intermediate TZD-5, which leads to intermediate TZD-6 that is conjugated to glucuronide TZD-7 and sulfate TZD-8. Finally, the epoxide intermediate also undergoes reaction with glutathione and further enzyme-mediated processing to metabolite TZD-9. The metabolites are slowly eliminated, with plasma elimination half-lives of 20 to 40 hours, via the urine (70%) and feces (30%).

Tizanidine is contraindicated with concomitant use of CYP1A2 inhibitors, such as fluvoxamine or ciprofloxacin. Cigarette smoking is expected to decrease exposure to tizanidine, which may require drug dose adjustment. The drug should also be used with caution in patients with renal insufficiency or hepatic impairment. Since tizanidine is an α_2-adrenergic agonist, it can result in hypotension and syncope. The most frequent adverse events with tizanidine are dry mouth, somnolence/sedation, asthenia (eg, weakness, fatigue, and/or tiredness), and dizziness.

Diazepam

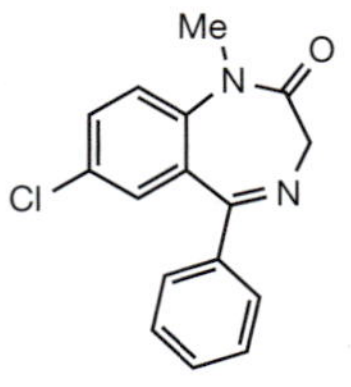

Diazepam
(Valium)

Diazepam is indicated for the management of anxiety disorders. However, it is a useful adjunct therapy for the relief of skeletal muscle spasm due to reflex spasm to local pathology (eg, inflammation of muscles) and spasticity caused by upper motor neuron disorders. In addition, it is useful for treating acute alcohol withdrawal and adjunctively in convulsive disorders. Structurally diazepam is a benzodiazepine derivative that contains a tertiary amide and substituted with a chlorine atom and phenyl, which contribute to its hydrophobicity. It is a colorless to light yellow crystalline compound that is insoluble in water. Diazepam, being a benzodiazepine, is a positive allosteric modulator of the $GABA_A$ receptor, with high affinity likely for the α2 and α3 subunits.[239,240] Consequently, binding of diazepam and GABA increases chloride ion influx that hyperpolarizes the neuron's membrane potential, increasing the difference between resting and threshold potentials. For the treatment of spasticity disorders, this likely results in decreased neuronal firing in the spinal cord.[241] However, diazepam does not appear to be more efficacious than carisoprodol, cyclobenzaprine, or tizanidine.[202,203]

Diazepam is well absorbed (>90%) after oral administration and reaches a maximum plasma concentration in 1 to 1.5 hours.[242] Taking the drug with food delays absorption and the time to reach maximum plasma concentration, while decreasing maximum plasma concentration (eg, 20% reduction in C_{max}) and exposure (eg, AUC decreased 27%). Diazepam is highly plasma protein bound (98%) and has a moderate volume of distribution of 0.8 to 1.0 L/kg and biphasic elimination with the first phase being 1 to 3 hours (Table 10.2). However, the terminal plasma elimination half-life (eg, $t_{1/2}\beta$) can be 1 to 2 days.[243]

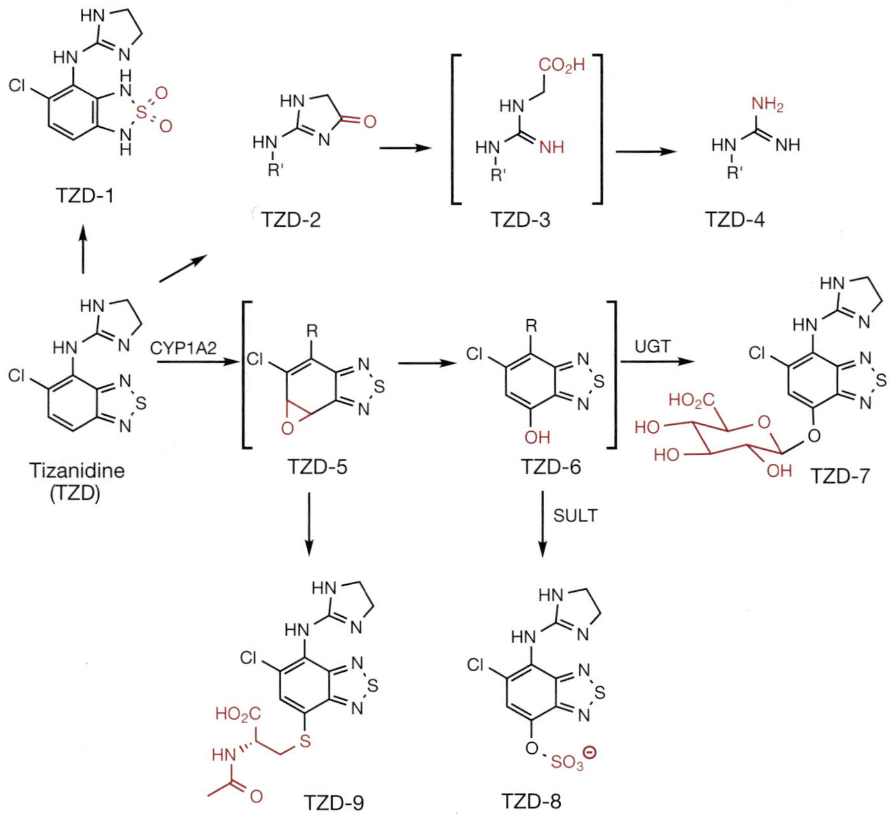

Figure 10.34 Metabolism of tizanidine. CYP, cytochrome P; SULT, sulfotransferase; UGT, UDP-glucuronosyltransferase.

The major diazepam metabolite found in plasma is *N*-desmethyldiazepam via CYP450-mediated *N*-demethylation (Fig. 10.35).[244] In addition, the parent drug also undergoes CYP450 alkyl oxidation on the carbon between the amide and imine functional groups to yield temazepam. Both metabolites can be further oxidized to oxazepam. The *N*-demethylation reactions appear to be catalyzed by 2C19 and 3A4 isozymes, whereas the hydroxylation is mediated by 3A4.[245] All three phase 1 metabolites are active as positive allosteric modulators of the $GABA_A$ receptor. In addition, temazepam and oxazepam are conjugated with glucuronic acid before renal excretion.

Diazepam has the potential to participate in drug-drug interactions with drug-modulating CYP3A and 2C19. The drug is contraindicated in patients with MG, severe respiratory insufficiency, severe hepatic insufficiency, and sleep apnea. It is also not recommended in the treatment of patients with psychosis and should not be used concomitantly with alcohol or CNS depressants.

Botulinum Toxin Type A

Botulinum toxin type A is indicated for the treatment of upper limb spasticity in adult patients, as well as prophylaxis of headaches in adult patients with chronic migraine, cervical dystonia in adult patients, severe axillary hyperhidrosis, blepharospasm associated with dystonia, and strabismus. Botulinum toxin type A is one of seven immunologically distinct forms of botulinum neurotoxin. All forms consist of a 100-kDa heavy chain and a 50-kDa light chain.[246] The C-terminal region binds to synaptic vesicle protein 2 receptors expressed on presynaptic acetylcholine motor nerve endings before being endocytosed.[247] Once in the cytoplasm, the light chain, a zinc-containing protease, targets synaptobrevin proteins that mediate fusion of acetylcholine-containing synaptic vesicles.[248,249] This process results in inhibition of acetylcholine release at the neuromuscular junction, blocking motor endplate potential[250] and causing temporary muscle denervation and relaxation, which can be used to treat involuntary muscle spasticity. Botulinum toxin type A is injected into target muscles, but generally does not diffuse beyond 2 cm,[249] although distant spreading of the toxin is a risk. Patients with compromised respiratory status being treated for upper limb spasticity should be closely monitored. The clinical effect is observed about 4 days after injection and lasts 3 to 4 months.[251] Coadministration of botulinum toxin type A and drugs that interfere with neuromuscular transmission (eg, aminoglycosides) should be done with caution, as the effect of the toxin may be potentiated. Anticholinergic drugs may also potentiate systemic anticholinergic effects of botulinum toxin type A.

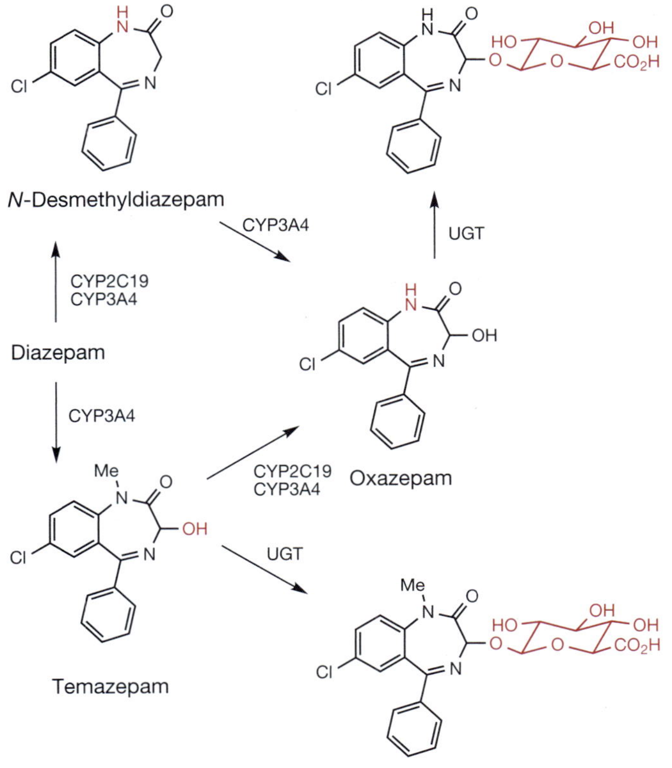

Figure 10.35 Metabolism of diazepam. CYP, cytochrome P; UGT, UDP-glucuronosyltransferase.

Sugammadex

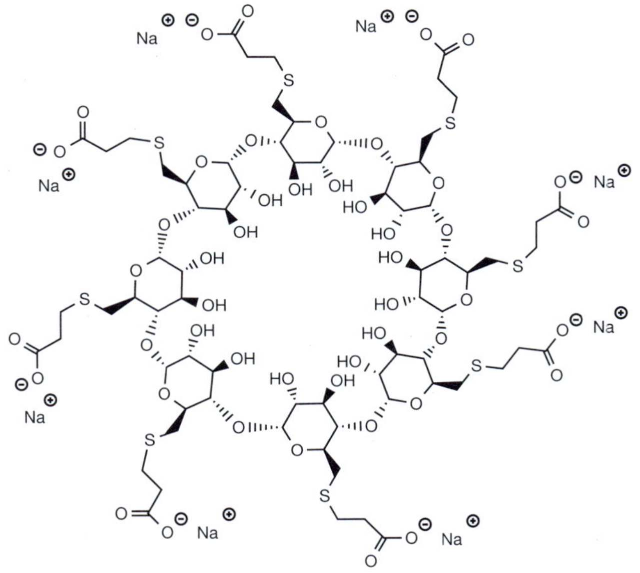

Sugammadex
(Bridion)

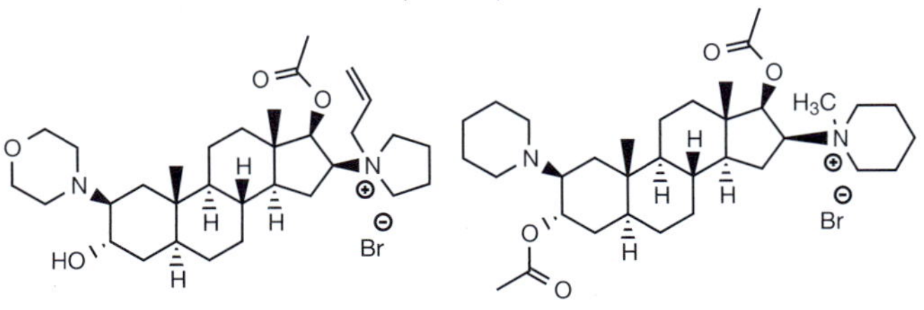

Rocuronium bromide | Vecuronium bromide

Sugammadex is indicated for intravenous use for the reversal of neuromuscular blockade by the nicotinic acetylcholine receptor antagonists rocuronium bromide and vecuronium bromide in adults undergoing surgery. The structure of this drug consists of a γ-cyclodextrin, which is made up of eight dextrose residues connected into a macrocycle that provides a lipophilic core and a hydrophilic periphery, with each sugar subunit attached to a propionate linked through thioethers. The hydroxyl and propionate groups on the outer surface of the cyclodextrin core impart excellent water solubility. Sugammadex is associated with the aminosteroids through van der Waals and ionic interactions to form stable complexes.[252] Overall, this results in a reduction of free aminosteroid concentration, which in turn allows acetylcholine binding to nicotinic acetylcholine receptors at neuromuscular junctions.[253]

Sugammadex does not have appreciable binding to plasma proteins and has a volume of distribution of 18 L.[254] In adult anesthetized patients with normal renal function, the plasma elimination half-life is 2 hours. In vivo, the drug is quite stable, does not undergo metabolism, and is primarily excreted in urine unchanged.[255] Drug-drug interactions are possible with the selective estrogen receptor modulator toremifene and hormonal contraceptives, which have relatively high binding affinities for sugammadex. Most common adverse effects of the drug are vomiting, pain, nausea, hypotension, and headache.

Neostigmine and Pyridostigmine

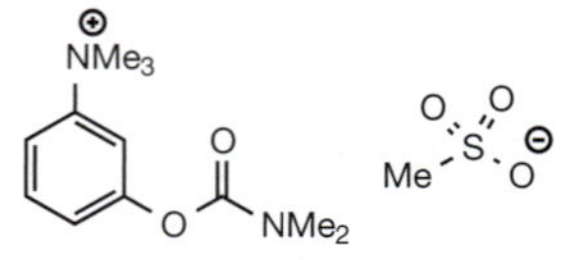

Neostigmine methylsulfate (Bloxiverz)

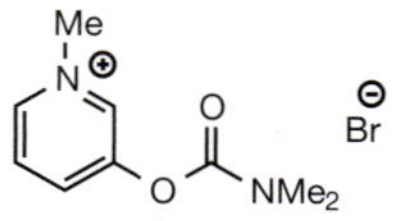

Pyridostigmine bromide (Mestinon)

Neostigmine is indicated for the reversal of the effects of nondepolarizing neuromuscular blocking agents after surgery and for the treatment of MG, both via parenteral administration. This latter condition is an autoimmune disease in which IgG1-dominant antibodies disrupt nicotinic acetylcholine receptors at neuromuscular junctions (as well as muscle-specific kinase or lipoprotein-related protein 4), resulting in muscle weakness that affects the eyes, face, head, and neck, causing difficulties swallowing, speaking, and eating. In addition, limb and respiratory muscles can also be affected. MG is associated with thymomas (eg, benign or malignant tumors arising in epithelial cells of the thymus) in 20% of patients, as well as other autoimmune diseases such as hyperthyroidism and Hashimoto disease.[256] The estimated prevalence of MG is 25 to 142 per million.[257] Neostigmine is a competitive cholinesterase inhibitor that increases acetylcholine in the neuromuscular junctions, which enhances nerve impulse transmission. As a quaternary amine, the drug does not have CNS effects due to its inability to cross the BBB.

Structurally, neostigmine consists of benzene substituted with a quaternary amine and a carbamate. It is formulated as a methyl sulfate salt that is a highly water-soluble white crystalline solid.

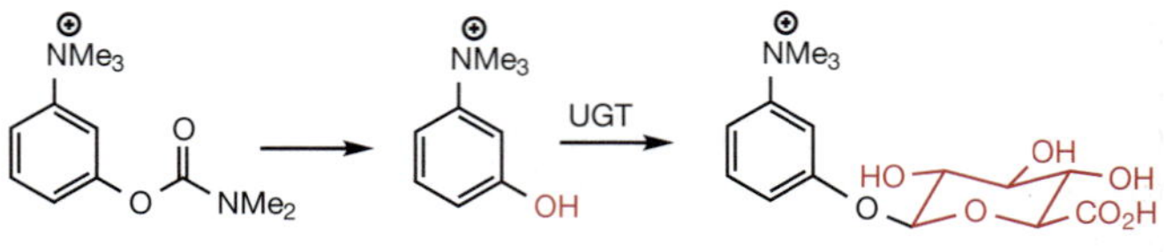

Neostigmine

Figure 10.36 Metabolism of neostigmine. UGT, UDP-glucuronosyltransferase.

Neostigmine has relatively low plasma protein binding (15%-25%). Following intravenous injection, the drug has a rapid distribution half-life of less than 1 minute,[258] plasma elimination half-life of 24 to 113 minutes, clearance of 1.14 to 16.7 mL/min/kg, and volume of distribution of 0.12 to 1.4 L/kg. The drug is metabolized to the corresponding phenol, which is subjected to glucuronidation (Fig. 10.36).[259] Neostigmine is contraindicated in patients with peritonitis or mechanical obstruction of the intestinal or urinary tract. The most common adverse effects of the drug are bradycardia, nausea, and vomiting.

Pyridostigmine is a structurally related drug with a similar mechanism of action that is also indicated for the treatment of MG. It contains an *N*-methylpyridinium substituted with a carbamate and formulated as the bromide salt that is orally or intravenously administered. The drug's oral bioavailability is 12% to 20%. Its plasma elimination half-life is 200 minutes, which is twice as long as the terminal plasma elimination half-life (97 minutes) after intravenous infusion. This suggests that absorption may proceed at a slower rate than elimination.[260] Pyridostigmine, like neostigmine, is primarily metabolized by hydrolysis of the carbamate to the corresponding phenol followed by glucuronidation.[261] This drug has the same contraindication as neostigmine, and the most common adverse effects are nausea, vomiting, upset stomach, diarrhea, abdominal cramps, increased saliva/mucus, decreased pupil size, and increased urination.

Azathioprine, Cyclosporine, Mycophenolate Mofetil, and Amifampridine

In addition to neostigmine and pyridostigmine, another chemotherapeutic treatment of MG is the use of immunomodulators. For example, both azathioprine[262] and

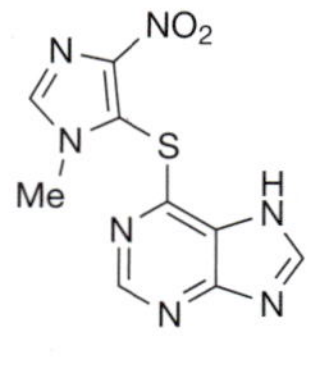

Azathioprine (Imuran)

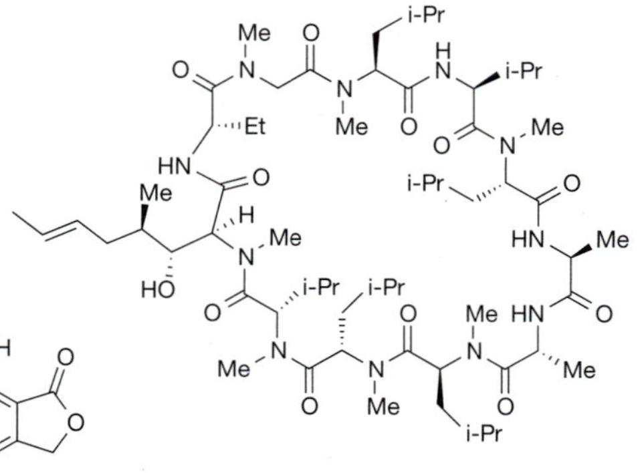

Cyclosporine (Neoral)

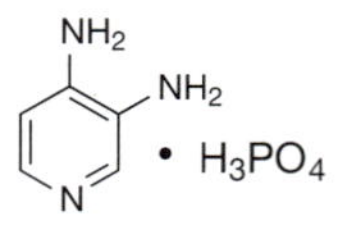

Amifampridine (Firdapse)

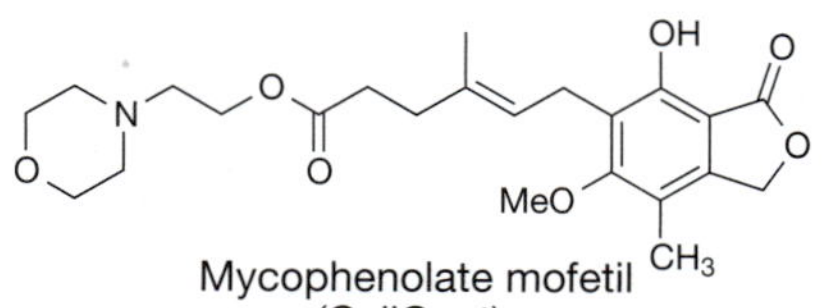

Mycophenolate mofetil (CellCept)

cyclosporine[263] have been shown to be efficacious and safe in the treatment of MG. Azathioprine is an orally bioavailable prodrug converted by reductive cleavage of the thioether to 6-mercaptopurine, which has immunosuppressive properties. Azathioprine is indicated as an adjunct for the prevention of rejection in renal homotransplantations and for the management of active rheumatoid arthritis.[264] Cyclosporine is an orally bioavailable macrocylic peptide that has potent immunosuppressive properties. It is indicated for kidney, liver, and heart transplantation; rheumatoid arthritis; and psoriasis.[265] Finally, the immunomodulator mycophenolate mofetil is used in the treatment of MG. However, its efficacy for this indication is not clear.[266] Mycophenolate mofetil is a prodrug that is readily hydrolyzed to mycophenolic acid, which is a potent inhibitor of inosine monophosphate dehydrogenase, an enzyme involved in guanine nucleotide synthesis. It is indicated for kidney, liver, and heart transplantation.[267]

LEMS is a condition like MG but involves presynaptic voltage-gated ion channels. Amifampridine is a voltage-gated potassium channel blocker indicated for the treatment of LEMS. It is a 3,4-diaminopyridine formulated as the phosphate salt. Amifampridine is rapidly absorbed after oral administration and eliminated via *N*-acetyltransferase 2 metabolism to 3-*N*-acetyl-amifampridine with a terminal half-life of 1.8 to 2.5 hours.[268]

Tetrabenazine

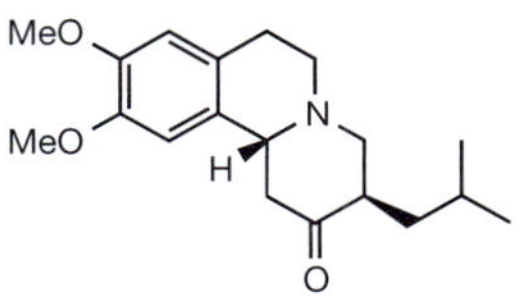

Tetrabenazine
(Xenazine)

Tetrabenazine is indicated for the treatment of chorea, an abnormal involuntary movement disorder, associated with Huntington disease. Structurally, the drug consists of a benzoquinolizine with two dimethoxyethers on the benzo-portion and a ketone on the piperidine fragment, as well as two chiral centers. The drug is currently marketed as a racemate. Although it contains a basic tertiary amine, it is formulated as the freebase that is a white to slightly yellow crystalline solid with low water solubility.

The mechanism of action of tetrabenazine and its active metabolites (eg, α- and β-dihydrotetrabenazine resulting from ketone reduction) is via reversible and selective inhibition of VMAT2. This transporter participates in the regulation of monoamine (particularly dopamine) uptake from the cytoplasm to the synaptic vesicle for storage and release.[269] Thus, the drug's efficacy for the treatment of chorea associated with Huntington disease presumably stems from blocking dopamine release via inhibition of VMAT2. The tetrabenazine eutomer has high binding affinity for VMAT2 (K_i = 4.5 nM), while the distomer demonstrates significantly less affinity (K_i = 36,400 nM). The active metabolites α- and β-dihydrotetrabenazines also bind with high affinity to VMAT2 (K_i = 4.0 and 13.4 nM, respectively).[270]

Tetrabenazine has moderate absorption (75%) after oral administration but undergoes rapid and extensive hepatic metabolism by carbonyl reductase (CBR) to α- and β-dihydrotetrabenazines (Fig. 10.37), which reach maximum plasma concentrations in 1 hour. Very little of the parent drug makes it into systemic circulation and it is not detectable in urine.[271] Tetrabenazine and α- and β-dihydrotetrabenazines have moderate plasma protein binding (59%-85%). The plasma elimination half-lives of the parent drug and the two metabolites are 2.1, 7.6, and 5.9 hours, respectively.[272] Both α- and β-dihydrotetrabenazines are further metabolized by CYP2D6 via dealkylation to the corresponding 9-O-desmethyl metabolites, with 9-O-desmethyl-β-dihydrotetrabenazine having a plasma elimination half-life of 12 hours. All four metabolites are conjugated to give an array of glucuronide and sulfonate phase 2 metabolites. The primary route of elimination of all metabolites appears to be renal.

Tetrabenazine is contraindicated in patients with hepatic impairment and those taking MAO inhibitors or reserpine. It is also not recommended in combination with other drugs that prolong the QT interval and should be used with caution with other drugs that induce CYP2D6. The drug can increase the risk for depression and suicidal thoughts, as well as lead to parkinsonism, dysphagia, and neuroleptic malignant syndrome. The most common adverse effects of tetrabenazine are sedation, somnolence, fatigue, insomnia, depression, akathisia, anxiety, and nausea.

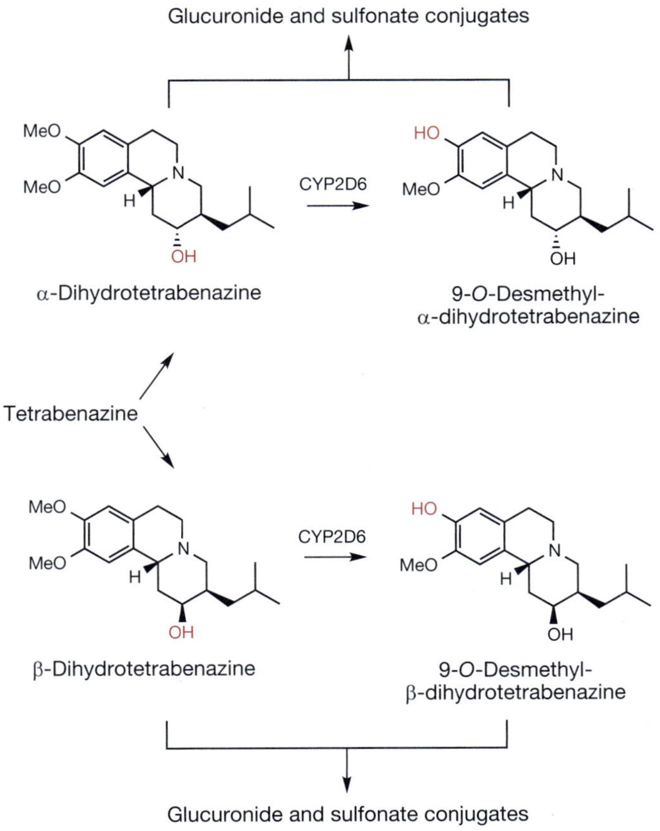

Figure 10.37 Metabolism of tetrabenazine. CYP, cytochrome P.

Valbenazine

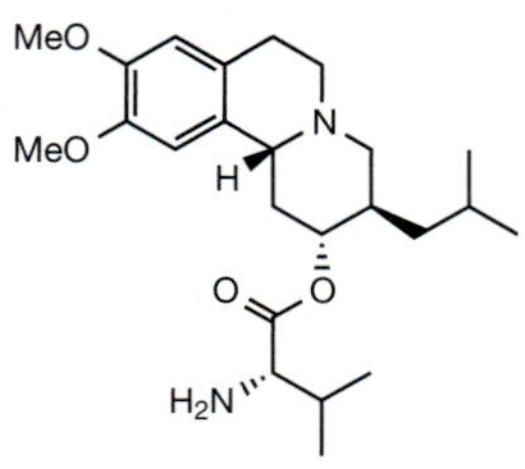

Valbenazine
(Ingrezza)

Valbenazine is indicated for the treatment of adults with tardive dyskinesia, which is believed to arise from neuroleptic-induced dopamine hypersensitivity. The drug is also being evaluated as a treatment for Tourette syndrome. Structurally, valbenazine is similar to tetrabenazine, except that the ketone is replaced with a secondary alcohol (resulting in one additional chiral center) that is formed into a valine ester prodrug. Given that the drug has two basic amines, it is formulated as a ditosylate salt that is slightly soluble in water. Like tetrabenazine, both valbenazine and its active metabolite (eg, α-dihydrotetrabenazine) are reversible and selective inhibitors of VMAT2. However, the parent drug demonstrates lower binding affinity (K_i = 150 nM).[273]

Valbenazine reaches maximum plasma concentration in 0.5 to 1 hour after oral administration with a bioavailability of 49%. The active metabolite α-dihydrotetrabenazine, formed by ester hydrolysis (Fig. 10.38), reaches maximum plasma concentration 4 to 8 hours after administration. Taking the drug with a high-fat meal decreases maximum plasma concentration (C_{max}) and exposure (AUC) of the parent drug by 47% and 13%, respectively. The parent drug is highly plasma protein bound (99%), while the active metabolite is less strongly bound (64%). Both the parent drug and active metabolite are slowly eliminated, resulting in long plasma elimination half-lives (15-22 hours). In addition to being hydrolyzed to the active metabolite, valbenazine is also subjected to CYP3A4/5-mediated oxidation on the valine ester portion of the molecule.[274]

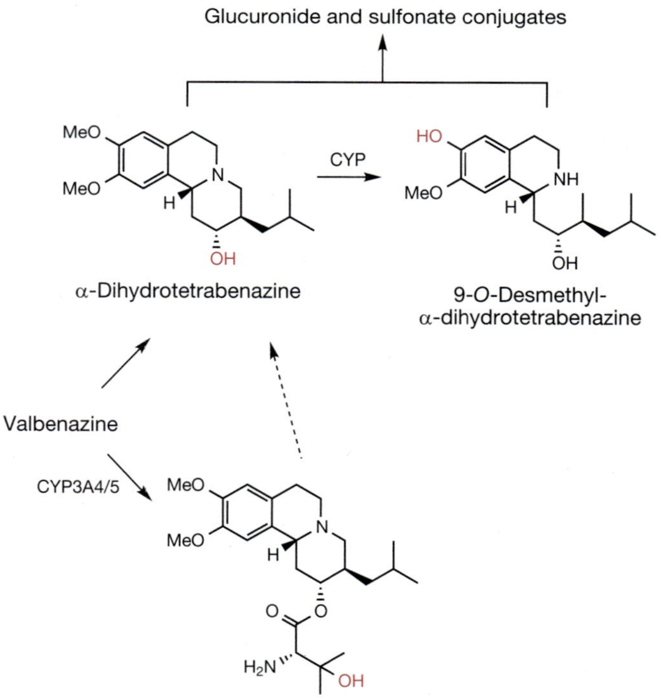

Figure 10.38 Metabolism of valbenazine. Dashed arrow indicates a presumed reaction. CYP, cytochrome P.

Valbenazine may cause an increase in the QT interval and should not be used in patients with congenital long QT syndrome or with arrhythmias associated with a prolonged QT interval. The most common adverse effect of valbenazine is somnolence.

Omaveloxolone

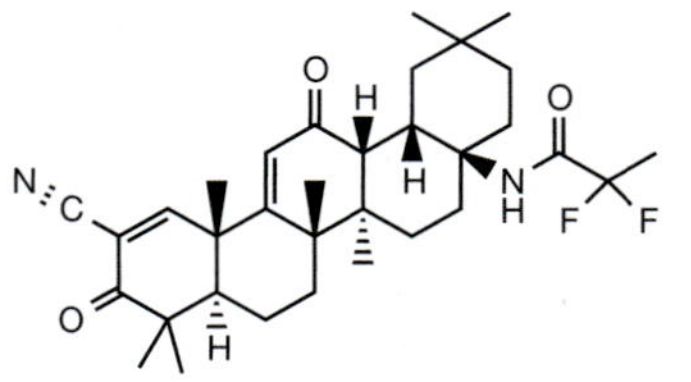

Omaveloxolone (Skyclarys)

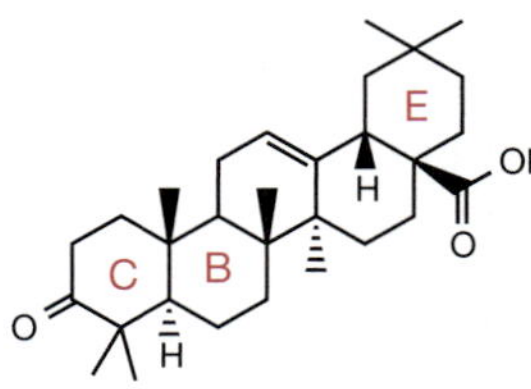

Oleanolic acid

Omaveloxolone is indicated for the treatment of Friedreich ataxia in adults and adolescents ages 16 years and older. Friedreich ataxia is an autosomal recessive genetic disease that manifests in mobility difficulties in addition to non-CNS complications. The disease is caused by loss-of-function mutations in the *FXN* gene that encodes frataxin, a mitochondrial protein that may function as an iron chaperone in iron metabolism.[275]

Structurally, omaveloxolone is related to oleanane triterpenoid natural products, such as oleanolic acid. However, rings A and C, as well as the carboxylic acid on ring E are modified. Omaveloxolone is a white amorphous solid with poor water solubility. Although the mechanism of action of this drug is not known, it may involve increasing the Nrf2 pathway that could be important for antioxidant and mitochondrial functions.[276,277]

Omaveloxolone is slowly absorbed, reaching peak plasma concentration in 7 to 14 hours.[278] Omaveloxolone has a plasma protein binding of 97%, an apparent volume of distribution of 7,361 L, a terminal half-life of 57 hours, and an apparent plasma clearance of 109 L/h. Omaveloxolone undergoes oxidative metabolism (CYP3A, and to a minor extent by CYP2C8 and CYP2J2) and is eliminated primarily in feces. The drug should not be used concomitantly with CYP3A4 inhibitors or inducers. The most common adverse reactions are elevated liver enzymes, headache, nausea, abdominal pain, fatigue, diarrhea, and musculoskeletal pain.

ACKNOWLEDGMENT

The author wishes to acknowledge the work of Raymond G. Booth, PhD, who authored content used within this chapter in a previous edition of this text.

Structure Challenge

The following are structures of eight drugs described in this chapter. For each patient described indicate (a) two drugs that would be appropriate to use based on the indication, (b) from among these two drugs, the drug of choice, and (c) your rationale for selecting the drug of choice.

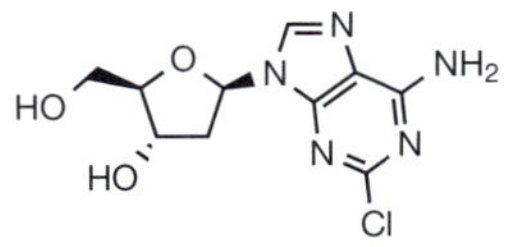

A

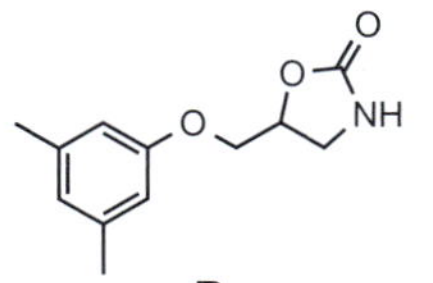

B

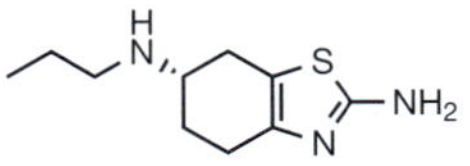

C

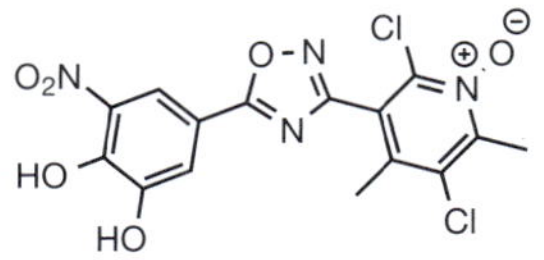

D

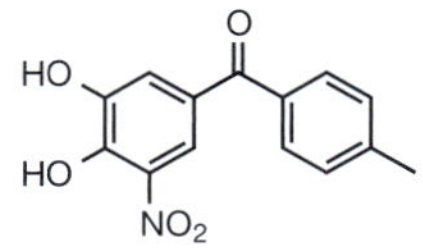

E

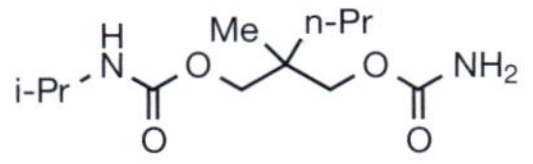

F

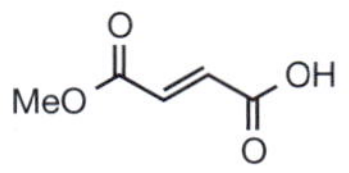

G

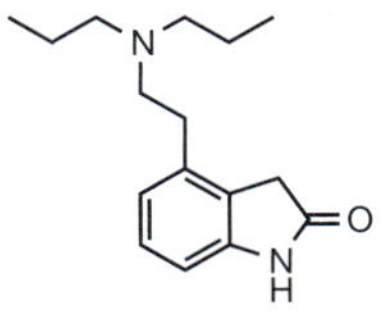

H

1. A patient with PD who would benefit from treatment for off-episodes, but has liver disease.
2. A patient who would benefit from treatment for relapsing MS who has previously been diagnosed with cancer.
3. A patient with acute musculoskeletal pain, who is also taking esomeprazole.
4. A patient with PD, who has demonstrated hypersensitivity to COMT inhibitors and has renal disease.

Structure Challenge answers found immediately after References.

REFERENCES

1. Olanow CW, Stern MB, Sethi K. The scientific and clinical basis for the treatment of Parkinson disease. *Neurology*. 2009;72(21 suppl 4):S1-S136.
2. Galasko D. Lewy body disorders. *Neurol Clin*. 2017;35(2):325-338.
3. Norris EH, Giasson BI, Lee VM. α-Synuclein: normal function and role in neurodegenerative diseases. *Curr Top Dev Biol*. 2004;60:17-54.
4. Ozansoy M, Başak AN. The central theme of Parkinson's disease: α-synuclein. *Mol Neurobiol*. 2013;47(2):460-465.
5. Wong YC, Krainc D. α-Synuclein toxicity in neurodegeneration: mechanism and therapeutic strategies. *Nat Med*. 2017;23:1-13.
6. Bengoa-Vergniory N, Roberts RF, Wade-Martins R, et al. Alpha-synuclein oligomers: a new hope. *Acta Neuropathol*. 2017;134(6):819-838.
7. Semchuk KM, Love EJ, Lee RG. Parkinson's disease: a test of the multifactorial etiologic hypothesis. *Neurology*. 1993;43:1173-1180.
8. Gwinn-Hardy K. Genetics of parkinsonism. *Mov Disord*. 2002;17:645-656.
9. Polymeropoulos MH, Lavedan C, Leroy E, et al. Mutation in the α-synuclein gene identified in families with Parkinson's disease. *Science*. 1997;276:2045-2047.
10. Kruger R, Kuhn W, Muller T, et al. Ala30Pro mutation in the gene encoding α-synuclein in Parkinson's disease. *Nat Genet*. 1998;18:106-108.
11. Lill CM. Genetics of Parkinson's disease. *Mol Cell Probes*. 2016;30(6):386-396.
12. Ozelius LJ, Senthil G, Saunders-Pullman R, et al. LRRK2 G2019S as a cause of Parkinson's disease in Ashkenazi Jews. *N Engl J Med*. 2006;354:424-425.
13. Vilariño-Güell C, Wider C, Ross OA, et al. VPS35 mutations in Parkinson disease. *Am J Hum Genet*. 2011;89(1):162-167.
14. Zimprich A, Benet-Pagès A, Struhal W, et al. A mutation in VPS35, encoding a subunit of the retromer complex, causes late-onset Parkinson disease. *Am J Hum Genet*. 2011;89(1):168-175.
15. Mohan M, Mellick GD. Role of the VPS35 D620N mutation in Parkinson's disease. *Parkinsonism Relat Disord*. 2017;36:10-18.
16. Sassone J, Serratto G, Valtorta F, et al. The synaptic function of Parkin. *Brain*. 2017;140(9):2265-2272.
17. Narendra D, Tanaka A, Suen DF, et al. Parkin is recruited selectively to impaired mitochondria and promotes their autophagy. *J Cell Biol*. 2008;183:795-803.
18. Mizushima N. Autophagy: process and function. *Genes Dev*. 2007;21:2861-2873.
19. Clark IE, Dodson MW, Jiang C, et al. Drosophila pink1 is required for mitochondrial function and interacts genetically with Parkin. *Nature*. 2006;441:1162-1166.
20. Park J, Lee SB, Lee S, et al. Mitochondrial dysfunction in Drosophila PINK1 mutants is complemented by Parkin. *Nature*. 2006;441:1157-1161.
21. Shendelman S, Jonason A, Martinat C, et al. DJ-1 is a redox-dependent molecular chaperone that inhibits alpha-synuclein aggregate formation. *PLoS Biol*. 2004;2(11):e362.
22. Zhou W, Zhu M, Wilson MA, et al. The oxidation state of DJ-1 regulates its chaperone activity toward alpha-synuclein. *J Mol Biol*. 2006;356:1036-1048.

23. Biosa A, Sandrelli F, Beltramini M, et al. Recent findings on the physiological function of DJ-1: beyond Parkinson's disease. *Neurobiol Dis*. 2017;108:65-72.
24. Gasser T. Genetics of Parkinson's disease. *Curr Opin Neurol*. 2005;18:363-369.
25. Burns RS, Chiueh CC, Markey SP, et al. A primate model of parkinsonism: selective destruction of dopaminergic neurons in the pars compacta of the substantia nigra by N-methyl-4-phenyl-1,2,3,6-tetrahydropyridine. *Proc Natl Acad Sci U S A*. 1983;80:4546-4550.
26. Davis GC, Williams AC, Markey SP, et al. Chronic parkinsonism secondary to intravenous injection of meperidine analogues. *Psychiatr Res*. 1979;1:249-254.
27. Langston JW, Ballard P, Tetrud JW, et al. Chronic parkinsonism in humans due to a product of meperidine-analog synthesis. *Science*. 1983;219:979-980.
28. Chiba K, Trevor A, Castagnoli N. Metabolism of the neurotoxic tertiary amine, MPTP, by brain monoamine oxidase. *Biochem Biophys Res Commun*. 1984;120:574-578.
29. Salach JI, Singer TP, Castagnoli N, et al. Oxidation of the neurotoxic amine 1-methyl-4-phenyl-1,2,3,6-tetrahydropyridine (MPTP) by monoamine oxidases A and B and suicide inactivation of the enzymes by MPTP. *Biochem Biophys Res Commun*. 1984;125:831-835.
30. Langston JW, Irwin I, Langston EB, et al. Pargyline prevents MPTP-induced parkinsonism in primates. *Science*. 1984;225:1480-1482.
31. Storch A, Ludolph AC, Schwarz J. Dopamine transporter: involvement in selective dopaminergic neurotoxicity and degeneration. *J Neural Transm (Vienna)*. 2004;111(10-11):1267-1286.
32. Brooks AI, Chadwick CA, Gelbard HA, et al. Paraquat elicited neurobehavioral syndrome caused by dopaminergic neuron loss. *Brain Res*. 1999;823:1-10.
33. Miller GW. Paraquat: the red herring of Parkinson's disease research. *Toxicol Sci*. 2007;100:1-2.
34. Hatcher JM, Pennell KD, Miller GW. Parkinson's disease and pesticides: a toxicological perspective. *Trends Pharmacol Sci*. 2008;29:322-329.
35. Graham DG. Catecholamine toxicity: a proposal for the molecular pathogenesis of manganese neurotoxicity and Parkinson's disease. *Neurotoxicology*. 1984;5:83-95.
36. Kessler II, Diamond EL. Epidemiologic studies of Parkinson's disease. I. Smoking and Parkinson's disease: a survey and explanatory hypothesis. *Am J Epidemiol*. 1971;94:16-25.
37. Tanner CM, Goldman SM, Aston DA, et al. Smoking and Parkinson's disease in twins. *Neurology*. 2002;58:581-588.
38. Yu PH, Boulton AA. Irreversible inhibition of monoamine oxidase by some components of cigarette smoke. *Life Sci*. 1987;41:675-682.
39. Khalil AA, Davies B, Castagnoli N. Isolation and characterization of a monoamine oxidase B selective inhibitor from tobacco smoke. *Bioorg Med Chem*. 2006;14:3392-3398.
40. Chapman MA. Does smoking reduce the risk of Parkinson's disease through stimulation of the ubiquitin-proteasome system? *Med Hypotheses*. 2009;73:887-891.
41. Hernan MA, Takkouche B, Caamano-Isorna F, et al. A meta-analysis of coffee drinking, cigarette smoking, and the risk of Parkinson's disease. *Ann Neurol*. 2002;52:276-284.
42. Trevitt J, Kawa K, Jalali A, et al. Differential effects of adenosine antagonists in two models of parkinsonian tremor. *Pharmacol Biochem Behav*. 2009;94:24-29.
43. Alves G, Forsaa EB, Pedersen KF, et al. Epidemiology of Parkinson's disease. *J Neurol*. 2008;255(suppl 5):18-32.
44. Pringsheim T, Jette N, Frolkis A, et al. The prevalence of Parkinson's disease: a systematic review and meta-analysis. *Mov Disord*. 2014;29(13):1583-1590.
45. Kowal SL, Dall TM, Chakrabarti R, et al. The current and projected economic burden of Parkinson's disease in the United States. *Mov Disord*. 2013;28(3):311-318.
46. Parkinson's Foundation. Understanding Parkinson's: statistics. Accessed June 13, 2023. https://www.parkinson.org/understanding-parkinsons/statistics
47. Nagatsu T. Tyrosine hydroxylase: human isoforms, structure and regulation in physiology and pathology. *Essays Biochem*. 1995;30:15-35.
48. Soloway AH. Potential endogenous epoxides of tyrosine: causative agents in initiating idiopathic Parkinson's disease? *Med Hypotheses Res*. 2009;5:19-26.
49. Soloway AH. Potential endogenous epoxides of steroid hormones: initiators of breast and other malignancies? *Med Hypotheses*. 2007;69:1225-1229.
50. Graham DG, Tiffany SM, Bell WR, et al. Autoxidation versus covalent binding of quinones as the mechanism of toxicity of dopamine, 6-hydroxydopamine, and related compounds toward C1300 neuroblastoma cells in vitro. *Mol Pharmacol*. 1978;14:644-653.
51. Jenner P. Oxidative stress in Parkinson's disease. *Ann Neurol*. 2003;53(suppl 3):S26-S36.
52. Ehringer H, Hornykiewicz O. Distribution of noradrenaline and dopamine(3-hydroxytyramine) in the human brain and their behavior in diseases of the extrapyramidal system. *Wien Klin Wochenschr*. 1960;38:1236-1239.
53. Birkmayer W, Hornykiewicz O. The L-3,4-dioxyphenylalanine (DOPA)-effect in Parkinson-akinesia. *Wien Klin Wochenschr*. 1961;73:787-788.
54. Barbeau A. Biochemistry of Parkinson's disease. *Proc Seventh Int Congr Neurol*. 1961;2:925.
55. Barbeau A. L-DOPA therapy in Parkinson's disease: a critical review of nine years' experience. *Can Med Assoc J*. 1969;101:59-68.
56. Cotzias GC, Papavasiliou PS, Gellene R. Modification of Parkinsonism—chronic treatment with L-DOPA. *N Engl J Med*. 1969;280:337-345.
57. Sampaio-Maia B, Serrão MP, Soares-da-Silva P. Regulatory pathways and uptake of L-DOPA by capillary cerebral endothelial cells, astrocytes, and neuronal cells. *Am J Physiol Cell Physiol*. 2001;280(2):C333-C342.
58. Vogel WH. Determination and physiological disposition of *p*-methoxyphenylethylamine in the rat. *Biochem Pharmacol*. 1970;19:2663-2665.
59. Burkard WP, Gey KF, Pletscher A. Inhibition of decarboxylase of aromatic amino acids by 2,3,4-trihydroxybenzylhydrazine and its seryl derivative. *Arch Biochem Biophys*. 1964;107:187-196.
60. Standaert DG, Young AB. Treatment of central nervous system degenerative disorders. In: Brunton LL, Lazo JS, Parker KL, eds. *Goodman and Gilman's the Pharmacological Basis of Therapeutics*. McGraw-Hill; 2006:527-546.
61. Iqbal MM, Basil MJ, Kaplan J, et al. Overview of serotonin syndrome. *Ann Clin Psychiatry*. 2012;24(4):310-318.
62. Robertson DR, Wood ND, Everest H, et al. The effect of age on the pharmacokinetics of levodopa administered alone and in the presence of carbidopa. *Br J Clin Pharmacol*. 1989;28(1):61-69.
63. Abrams WR, Coutino CB, Leon AS, et al. Absorption and metabolism of levodopa. *J Am Med Assoc*. 1971;218:1912-1914.
64. Schwartz DE, Brandt R. Pharmacokinetic and metabolic studies of the decarboxylase inhibitor benserazide in animals and man. *Arzneimittelforschung*. 1978;28:302-307.
65. Burkhard P, Dominici P, Borri-Voltattorni C, et al. Structural insight into Parkinson's disease treatment from drug-inhibited DOPA decarboxylase. *Nat Struct Biol*. 2001;8:963-967.
66. Vickers S, Stuart EK, Bianchine JR, et al. Metabolism of carbidopa (1-(-)-alpha-hydrazino-3,4-dihydroxy-alpha-methylhydrocinnamic acid monohydrate), an aromatic amino acid decarboxylase inhibitor, in the rat, rhesus monkey, and man. *Drug Metab Dispos*. 1974;2(1):9-22.
67. Vickers S, Stuart EK, Hucker HB. Further studies on the metabolism of carbidopa, (minus)-L-alpha-hydrazino-3,4-dihydroxy-alpha-methylbenzenepropanoic acid monohydrate, in the human, Rhesus monkey, dog, and rat. *J Med Chem*. 1975;18(2):134-138.

68. Chase TN, Watanabe AM. Methyldopahydrazine as an adjunct to L-dopa therapy in parkinsonism. *Neurology*. 1972;22(4):384-392.
69. Campbell NR, Hasinoff BB. Iron supplements: a common cause of drug interactions. *Br J Clin Pharmacol*. 1991;31(3):251-255.
70. Bender DA. Inhibition in vitro of the enzymes of the oxidative pathway of tryptophan metabolism and of nicotinamide nucleotide synthesis by benserazide, carbidopa and isoniazid. *Biochem Pharmacol*. 1980;29(5):707-712.
71. Hubálek F, Binda C, Li M, et al. Inactivation of purified human recombinant monoamine oxidases A and B by rasagiline and its analogues. *J Med Chem*. 2004;47(7):1760-1766.
72. Binda C, Hubálek F, Li M, et al. Crystal structures of monoamine oxidase B in complex with four inhibitors of the *N*-propargylaminoindan class. *J Med Chem*. 2004;47(7):1767-1774.
73. U.S. Food and Drug Administration. Prescribing information for Azilect. Accessed June 13, 2023. https://www.accessdata.fda.gov/drugsatfda_docs/label/2014/021641s016s017lbl.pdf
74. U.S. Food and Drug Administration. Prescribing information for Eldepryl. Accessed June 13, 2023. https://www.accessdata.fda.gov/drugsatfda_docs/label/2008/020647s006s007lbl.pdf
75. Mahmood I. Clinical pharmacokinetics and pharmacodynamics of selegiline. An update. *Clin Pharmacokinet*. 1997;33:91-102.
76. Barrett JS, Rohatagi S, DeWitt KE, et al. The effect of dosing regimen and food on the bioavailability of the extensively metabolized, highly variable drug Eldepryl(®) (selegiline hydrochloride). *Am J Ther*. 1996;3(4):298-313.
77. Heinonen EH, Anttila MI, Karnani HL, et al. Desmethylselegiline, a metabolite of selegiline, is an irreversible inhibitor of monoamine oxidase type B in humans. *J Clin Pharmacol*. 1997;37:602-609.
78. Shin HS. Metabolism of selegiline in humans: identification, excretion, and stereochemistry of urine metabolites. *Drug Metab Dispos*. 1997;25:657-662.
79. Caccia C, Maj R, Calabresi M, et al. Safinamide: from molecular targets to a new anti-Parkinson drug. *Neurology*. 2006;67(7 suppl 2):S18-S23.
80. Binda C, Wang J, Pisani L, et al. Structures of human monoamine oxidase B complexes with selective noncovalent inhibitors: safinamide and coumarin analogs. *J Med Chem*. 2007;50:5848-5852.
81. U.S. Food and Drug Administration. Prescribing information for Xadago. Accessed June 13, 2023. https://www.accessdata.fda.gov/drugsatfda_docs/label/2017/207145lbl.pdf
82. Krösser S, Marquet A, Gallemann D, et al. Effects of ketoconazole treatment on the pharmacokinetics of safinamide and its plasma metabolites in healthy adult subjects. *Biopharm Drug Disp*. 2012;33(9):550-559.
83. U.S. Food and Drug Administration. Prescribing information for Comtan. Accessed October 15, 2024. https://www.accessdata.fda.gov/drugsatfda_docs/label/2010/020796s15lbl.pdf.
84. Lautala P, Ethell BT, Taskinen J, et al. The specificity of glucuronidation of entacapone and tolcapone by recombinant human UDP-glucuronosyltransferases. *Drug Metab Dispos*. 2000;28(11):1385-1389.
85. Wikberg T, Vuorela A, Ottoila P, et al. Identification of major metabolites of the catechol-O-methyltransferase inhibitor entacapone in rats and humans. *Drug Metab Dispos*. 1993;21:81-92.
86. Ellermann M, Lerner C, Burgy G, et al. Catechol-O-methyltransferase in complex with substituted 3′-deoxyribose bisubstrate inhibitors. *Acta Crystallogr D Biol Crystallogr*. 2012;68(Pt 3):253-260.
87. U.S. Food and Drug Administration. Prescribing information for Tasmar. Accessed June 13, 2023. https://www.accessdata.fda.gov/drugsatfda_docs/label/2013/020697s004lbl.pdf
88. European Medicines Agency. Annex I: summary of product characteristics. Accessed June 26, 2023. https://www.ema.europa.eu/en/documents/product-information/ongentys-epar-product-information_en.pdf
89. U.S. Food and Drug Administration. Prescribing information for Ongentys. Accessed June 26, 2023. https://www.accessdata.fda.gov/drugsatfda_docs/label/2020/212489s000lbl.pdf
90. Rocha JF, Almeida L, Falcão A, et al. Opicapone: a short lived and very long acting novel catechol-O-methyltransferase inhibitor following multiple dose administration in healthy subjects. *Br J Clin Pharmacol*. 2013;76(5):763-775.
91. Millan MJ, Maiofiss L, Cussac D, et al. Differential actions of antiparkinson agents at multiple classes of monoaminergic receptor. I. A multivariate analysis of the binding profiles of 14 drugs at 21 native and cloned human receptor subtypes. *J Pharmacol Exp Ther*. 2002;303(2):791-804.
92. Giesecke J. The absolute configuration of apomorphine. *Acta Cryst*. 1977;B33:302-303.
93. Neumeyer JL, McCarthy M, Battista S, et al. Aporphines. 9. Synthesis and pharmacological evaluation of (±)-9,10-dihydroxyaporphine [(±)-isoapomorphine], (±)-,(−)-, and (±)-1,2-dihydroxyaporphine, and (+)-1,2,9,10-tetrahydroxyaporphine. *J Med Chem*. 1973;16:1228-1233.
94. U.S. Food and Drug Administration. Prescribing information for Apokyn. Accessed June 13, 2023. https://www.accessdata.fda.gov/drugsatfda_docs/label/2022/021264s022lbl.pdf
95. van der Geest R, van Laar T, Kruger PP, et al. Pharmacokinetics, enantiomer interconversion, and metabolism of *R*-apomorphine in patients with idiopathic Parkinson's disease. *Clin Neuropharmacol*. 1998;21(3):159-168.
96. Newman-Tancredi A, Cussac D, Audinot V, et al. Differential actions of antiparkinson agents at multiple classes of monoaminergic receptor. II. Agonist and antagonist properties at subtypes of dopamine D_2-like receptor and alpha$_1$/alpha$_2$-adrenoceptor. *J Pharmacol Exp Ther*. 2002;303:805-814.
97. Blanchet PJ. Rationale for use of dopamine agonists in Parkinson's disease: review of ergot derivatives. *Can J Neurol Sci*. 1999;26(suppl 2):S21-S26.
98. Schran HF, Bhuta SI, Schwartz HJ, et al. The pharmacokinetics of bromocriptine in man. *Adv Biochem Psychopharmacol*. 1980;23:125-139.
99. Maurer G, Schreier E, Delaborde S, et al. Fate and disposition of bromocriptine in animals and man. I: Structure elucidation of the metabolites. *Eur J Drug Metab Pharmacokinet*. 1982;7(4):281-292.
100. Maurer G, Schreier E, Delaborde S, et al. Fate and disposition of bromocriptine in animals and man. II: Absorption, elimination and metabolism. *Eur J Drug Metab Pharmacokinet*. 1983;8(1):51-62.
101. Nelson MV, Berchou RC, Kareti D, et al. Pharmacokinetic evaluation of erythromycin and caffeine administered with bromocriptine. *Clin Pharmacol Ther*. 1990;47(6):694-697.
102. Del Dotto P, Bonuccelli U. Clinical pharmacokinetics of cabergoline. *Clin Pharmacokinet*. 2003;42(7):633-645.
103. Boehringer Ingelheim. Accessed June 13, 2023. https://content.boehringer-ingelheim.com/DAM/12fba98b-0752-4fe6-99e4-af1e0125cce0/mirapex-us-pi.pdf
104. Eden RJ, Costall B, Domeney AM, et al. Preclinical pharmacology of ropinirole (SK&F 101468-A) a novel dopamine D2 agonist. *Pharmacol Biochem Behav*. 1991;38(1):147-154.
105. U.S. Food and Drug Administration. Prescribing information for Requip. Accessed June 13, 2023. https://www.accessdata.fda.gov/drugsatfda_docs/label/2014/020658s024s026s027s030s032lbl.pdf
106. Ramji JV, Keogh JP, Blake TJ, et al. Disposition of ropinirole in animals and man. *Xenobiotica*. 1999;29(3):311-325.
107. Bloomer JC, Clarke SE, Chenery RJ. In vitro identification of the P450 enzymes responsible for the metabolism of ropinirole. *Drug Metab Dispos*. 1997;25(7):840-844.
108. Hutton JT, Metman LV, Chase TN, et al. Transdermal dopaminergic D_2 receptor agonist therapy in Parkinson's disease with N-0923 TDS: a double-blind, placebo-controlled study. *Mov Disord*. 2001;16:459-463.
109. Morgan JC, Sethi KD. Rotigotine for the treatment of Parkinson's disease. *Expert Rev Neurother*. 2006;6:1275-1282.
110. U.S. Food and Drug Administration. Prescribing information for Neupro. Accessed June 13, 2023. https://www.accessdata.fda.gov/drugsatfda_docs/label/2012/021829s001lbl.pdf

111. Cawello W, Braun M, Boekens H. Absorption, disposition, metabolic fate, and elimination of the dopamine agonist rotigotine in man: administration by intravenous infusion or transdermal delivery. *Drug Metab Dispos*. 2009;37(10):2055-2060.
112. Allen RP. Restless leg syndrome/Willis-Ekbom disease pathophysiology. *Sleep Med Clin*. 2015;10(3):207-214.
113. Wijemanne S, Ondo W. Restless legs syndrome: clinical features, diagnosis and a practical approach to management. *Pract Neurol*. 2017;17(6):444-452.
114. Le DA, Lipton SA. Potential and current use of N-methyl-D-aspartate (NMDA) receptor antagonists in diseases of aging. *Drugs Aging*. 2001;18:717-724.
115. Paci C, Thomas A, Onofrj M. Amantadine for dyskinesia in patients affected by severe Parkinson's disease. *Neurol Sci*. 2001;22:75-76.
116. Schwab RS, Poskanzer DC, England AC, et al. Amantadine in the treatment of Parkinson's disease: review of more than two years' experience. *JAMA*. 1972;222:792-795.
117. Crosby N, Deane KH, Clarke CE. Amantadine in Parkinson's disease. *Cochrane Database Syst Rev*. 2003;(1):CD003468.
118. U.S. Food and Drug Administration. Prescribing information for Symmetrel. Accessed June 13, 2023. https://www.accessdata.fda.gov/drugsatfda_docs/label/2009/016023s041,018101s016lbl.pdf
119. Köppel C, Tenczer J. A revision of the metabolic disposition of amantadine. *Biomed Mass Spectrom*. 1985;12(9):499-501.
120. Aoki FY, Sitar DS. Clinical pharmacokinetics of amantadine hydrochloride. *Clin Pharmacokinet*. 1988;14(1):35-51.
121. U.S. Food and Drug Administration. Prescribing information for Nourianz. Accessed June 26, 2023. https://www.accessdata.fda.gov/drugsatfda_docs/label/2019/022075s000lbl.pdf
122. Nakahara J, Maeda M, Aiso S, et al. Current concepts in multiple sclerosis: autoimmunity versus oligodendrogliopathy. *Clin Rev Allergy Immunol*. 2012;42(1):26-34.
123. Nakahara J, Aiso S, Suzuki N. Autoimmune versus oligodendrogliopathy: the pathogenesis of multiple sclerosis. *Arch Immunol Ther Exp (Warsz)*. 2010;58(5):325-333.
124. Milo R, Kahana E. Multiple sclerosis: geoepidemiology, genetics and the environment. *Autoimmun Rev*. 2010;9(5):A387-A394.
125. Harbo HF, Gold R, Tintoré M. Sex and gender issues in multiple sclerosis. *Ther Adv Neurol Disord*. 2013;6(4):237-248.
126. Hartung DM. Economics and cost-effectiveness of multiple sclerosis therapies in the USA. *Neurotherapeutics*. 2017;14(4):1018-1026.
127. Haji Abdolvahab M, Mofrad MR, Schellekens H. Interferon beta: from molecular level to therapeutic effects. *Int Rev Cell Mol Biol*. 2016;326:343-372.
128. Fridkis-Hareli M, Teitelbaum D, Gurevich E, et al. Direct binding of myelin basic protein and synthetic copolymer 1 to class II major histocompatibility complex molecules on living antigen-presenting cells—specificity and promiscuity. *Proc Natl Acad Sci U S A*. 1994;91(11):4872-4876.
129. Weber MS, Hohlfeld R, Zamvil SS. Mechanism of action of glatiramer acetate in treatment of multiple sclerosis. *Neurotherapeutics*. 2007;4(4):647-653.
130. Yong VW. Differential mechanisms of action of interferon-beta and glatiramer aetate in MS. *Neurology*. 2002;59(6):802-808.
131. Lehmann-Horn K, Kronsbein HC, Weber MS. Targeting B cells in the treatment of multiple sclerosis: recent advances and remaining challenges. *Ther Adv Neurol Disord*. 2013;6(3):161-173.
132. U.S. Food and Drug Administration. Prescribing information for Ocrevus. Accessed June 13, 2023. https://www.accessdata.fda.gov/drugsatfda_docs/label/2022/761053s029s030lbl.pdf
133. U.S. Food and Drug Administration. Prescribing information for Lemtrada. Accessed June 13, 2023. https://www.accessdata.fda.gov/drugsatfda_docs/label/2017/103948s5158lbl.pdf
134. Yednock TA, Cannon C, Fritz LC, et al. Prevention of experimental autoimmune encephalomyelitis by antibodies against alpha 4 beta 1 integrin. *Nature*. 1992;356(6364):63-66.
135. Léger OJ, Yednock TA, Tanner L, et al. Humanization of a mouse antibody against human alpha-4 integrin: a potential therapeutic for the treatment of multiple sclerosis. *Hum Antibodies*. 1997;8(1):3-16.
136. U.S. Food and Drug Administration. Prescribing information for Tysabri. Accessed June 13, 2023. https://www.accessdata.fda.gov/drugsatfda_docs/label/2012/125104s0576lbl.pdf
137. U.S. Food and Drug Administration. Prescribing information for Mavenclad. Accessed June 26, 2023. https://www.accessdata.fda.gov/drugsatfda_docs/label/2019/022561s000lbl.pdf
138. Baker D, Marta M, Pryce G, et al. Memory B cells are major targets for effective immunotherapy in relapsing multiple sclerosis. *EBioMedicine*. 2017;16:41-50.
139. Jacobs BM, Ammoscato F, Giovannoni G, et al. Cladribine: mechanisms and mysteries in multiple sclerosis. *J Neurol Neurosurg Psychiatry*. 2018;89(12):1266-1271.
140. Bomprezzi R. Dimethyl fumarate in the treatment of relapsing-remitting multiple sclerosis: an overview. *Ther Adv Neurol Disord*. 2015;8(1):20-30.
141. de Jong R, Bezemer AC, Zomerdijk TP, et al. Selective stimulation of T helper 2 cytokine responses by the anti-psoriasis agent monomethylfumarate. *Eur J Immunol*. 1996;26(9):2067-2074.
142. Chen H, Assmann JC, Krenz A, et al. Hydroxycarboxylic acid receptor 2 mediates dimethyl fumarate's protective effect in EAE. *J Clin Invest*. 2014;124(5):2188-2192.
143. U.S. Food and Drug Administration. Prescribing information for Bafiertam. Accessed June 26, 2023. https://www.accessdata.fda.gov/drugsatfda_docs/label/2020/210296s000lbl.pdf
144. U.S. Food and Drug Administration. Prescribing information for Tecfidera. Accessed June 13, 2023. https://www.accessdata.fda.gov/drugsatfda_docs/label/2013/204063lbl.pdf
145. U.S. Food and Drug Administration. Prescribing information for Vumerity. Accessed June 26, 2023. https://www.accessdata.fda.gov/drugsatfda_docs/label/2019/211855s000lbl.pdf
146. Groves A, Kihara Y, Chun J. Fingolimod: direct CNS effects of sphingosine 1-phosphate (S1P) receptor modulation and implications in multiple sclerosis therapy. *J Neurol Sci*. 2013;328(1-2):9-18.
147. U.S. Food and Drug Administration. Prescribing information for Gilenya. Accessed June 13, 2023. https://www.accessdata.fda.gov/drugsatfda_docs/label/2019/022527s031lbl.pdf
148. David OJ, Kovarik JM, Schmouder RL. Clinical pharmacokinetics of fingolimod. *Clin Pharmacokinet*. 2012;51(1):15-28.
149. Kovarik JM, Hartmann S, Bartlett M, et al. Oral-intravenous crossover study of fingolimod pharmacokinetics, lymphocyte responses and cardiac effects. *Biopharm Drug Dispos*. 2007;28(2):97-104.
150. Zollinger M, Gschwind HP, Jin Y, et al. Absorption and disposition of the sphingosine 1-phosphate receptor modulator fingolimod (FTY720) in healthy volunteers: a case of xenobiotic biotransformation following endogenous metabolic pathways. *Drug Metab Dispos*. 2011;39(2):199-207.
151. Jin Y, Zollinger M, Borell H, et al. CYP4F enzymes are responsible for the elimination of fingolimod (FTY720), a novel treatment of relapsing multiple sclerosis. *Drug Metab Dispos*. 2011;39(2):191-198.
152. Li K, Konofalska U, Akgün K, et al. Modulation of cardiac autonomic function by fingolimod initiation and predictors for fingolimod induced bradycardia in patients with multiple sclerosis. *Front Neurosci*. 2017;11:540.
153. U.S. Food and Drug Administration. Prescribing information for Mayzent. Accessed June 26, 2023. https://www.accessdata.fda.gov/drugsatfda_docs/label/2019/209884s000lbl.pdf
154. Glaenzel U, Jin Y, Nufer R, et al. Metabolism and disposition of siponimod, a novel selective S1P1/S1P5 agonist, in healthy volunteers and in vitro identification of human cytochrome P450 enzymes involved in its oxidative metabolism. *Drug Metab Dispos*. 2018;46(7):1001-1013.
155. U.S. Food and Drug Administration. Prescribing information for Zeposia. Accessed June 26, 2023. https://www.accessdata.fda.gov/drugsatfda_docs/label/2020/209899s000lbl.pdf

156. Surapaneni S, Yerramilli U, Bai A, et al. Absorption, metabolism, and excretion, in vitro pharmacology, and clinical pharmacokinetics of ozanimod, a novel sphingosine 1-phosphate receptor modulator. *Drug Metab Dispos.* 2021;49(5):405-419.
157. Tran JQ, Zhang P, Ghosh A, et al. Single-dose pharmacokinetics of ozanimod and its major active metabolites alone and in combination with gemfibrozil, itraconazole, or rifampin in healthy subjects: a randomized, parallel-group, open-label study. *Adv Ther.* 2020;37(10):4381-4395.
158. Bar-Or A, Pachner A, Menguy-Vacheron F, et al. Teriflunomide and its mechanism of action in multiple sclerosis. *Drugs.* 2014;74(6):659-674.
159. U.S. Food and Drug Administration. Prescribing information for Aubagio. Accessed June 13, 2023. https://www.accessdata.fda.gov/drugsatfda_docs/label/2012/202992s000lbl.pdf
160. Parekh JM, Vaghela RN, Sutariya DK, et al. Chromatographic separation and sensitive determination of teriflunomide, an active metabolite of leflunomide in human plasma by liquid chromatography-tandem mass spectrometry. *J Chromatogr B Analyt Technol Biomed Life Sci.* 2010;878(24):2217-2225.
161. Wiese MD, Rowland A, Polasek TM, et al. Pharmacokinetic evaluation of teriflunomide for the treatment of multiple sclerosis. *Expert Opin Drug Metab Toxicol.* 2013;9(8):1025-1035.
162. Wilson ID, Macdonald CM, Fromson JM, et al. Species differences in the metabolism of 14C-p-trifluoromethylaniline: production of an oxanilic acid as the major metabolite by the rat. *Biochem Pharmacol.* 1985;34(11):2025-2028.
163. Blight AR, Henney HR, Cohen R. Development of dalfampridine, a novel pharmacologic approach for treating walking impairment in multiple sclerosis. *Ann N Y Acad Sci.* 2014;1329:33-44.
164. U.S. Food and Drug Administration. Prescribing information for Ampyra. Accessed June 13, 2023. https://www.accessdata.fda.gov/drugsatfda_docs/label/2021/022250s018lbl.pdf
165. Mehta P, Kaye W, Bryan L, et al. Prevalence of amyotrophic lateral sclerosis—United States, 2012-2013. *MMWR Surveill Summ.* 2016;65(8):1-12.
166. Rosen DR, Siddique T, Patterson D, et al. Mutations in Cu/Zn superoxide dismutase gene are associated with familial amyotrophic lateral sclerosis. *Nature.* 1993;362:59-62.
167. Cleveland DW, Laing N, Hurse PV, et al. Toxic mutants in Charcot's sclerosis. *Nature.* 1995;378:342-343.
168. Taylor JP, Brown RH, Cleveland DW. Decoding ALS: from genes to mechanism. *Nature.* 2016;539(7628):197-206.
169. Gamez J, Corbera-Bellalta M, Nogales G, et al. Mutational analysis of the Cu/Zn superoxide dismutase gene in a Catalan ALS population: should all sporadic ALS cases also be screened for SOD1? *J Neurol Sci.* 2006;247:21-28.
170. Neumann M, Sampathu DM, Kwong LK, et al. Ubiquitinated TDP-43 in frontotemporal lobar degeneration and amyotrophic lateral sclerosis. *Science.* 2006;314:130-133.
171. Cykowski MD, Powell SZ, Peterson LE, et al. Clinical significance of TDP-43 neuropathology in amyotrophic lateral sclerosis. *J Neuropathol Exp Neurol.* 2017;76(5):402-413.
172. Gladman M, Zinman L. The economic impact of amyotrophic lateral sclerosis: a systematic review. *Expert Rev Pharmacoecon Outcomes Res.* 2015;15(3):439-450.
173. The ALS Association. Accessed June 13, 2023. http://web.alsa.org/site/PageServer?pagename=ALSA_Ask_Dec2011
174. Forbs. The first ALS drug in 22 years is approved—and it costs 4 times what it does in Japan. Accessed June 13, 2023. https://www.forbes.com/sites/matthewherper/2017/05/05/fda-approves-first-new-drug-to-treat-als-in-22-years/#305578337fb3
175. Bellingham MC. A review of the neural mechanisms of action and clinical efficiency of riluzole in treating amyotrophic lateral sclerosis: what have we learned in the last decade? *CNS Neurosci Ther.* 2011;17(1):4-31.
176. Le Liboux A, Lefebvre P, Le Roux Y, et al. Single- and multiple-dose pharmacokinetics of riluzole in white subjects. *J Clin Pharmacol.* 1997;37(9):820-827.
177. Sanderink GJ, Bournique B, Stevens J, et al. Involvement of human CYP1A isoenzymes in the metabolism and drug interactions of riluzole in vitro. *J Pharmacol Exp Ther.* 1997;282(3):1465-1472.
178. Takei K, Watanabe K, Yuki S, et al. Edaravone and its clinical development for amyotrophic lateral sclerosis. *Amyotroph Lateral Scler Frontotemporal Degener.* 2017;18(suppl 1):5-10.
179. Komatsu T, Nakai H, Takamatsu Y, et al. Pharmacokinetic studies of 3-methyl-1-phenyl-2-pyrazolin-5-one (MCI-186): metabolism in rats, dogs and human. *Drug Metab Pharmacokinet.* 1996;11:451-462.
180. U.S. Food and Drug Administration. Prescribing information for Qalsody. Accessed June 26, 2023. https://www.accessdata.fda.gov/drugsatfda_docs/label/2023/215887s000lbl.pdf
181. Miller TM, Cudkowicz ME, Genge A, et al. Trial of antisense oligonucleotide tofersen for SOD1 ALS. *N Engl J Med.* 2022;387(12):1099-1110.
182. Monaco AP, Neve RL, Colletti-Feener C, et al. Isolation of candidate cDNAs for portions of the Duchenne muscular dystrophy gene. *Nature.* 1986;323(6089):646-650.
183. Hoffman EP, Brown RH, Kunkel LM. Dystrophin: the protein product of the Duchenne muscular dystrophy locus. *Cell.* 1987;51(6):919-928.
184. Stark AE. Determinants of the incidence of Duchenne muscular dystrophy. *Ann Transl Med.* 2015;3(19):287.
185. Thayer S, Bell C, McDonald CM. The direct cost of managing a rare disease: assessing medical and pharmacy costs associated with Duchenne muscular dystrophy in the United States. *J Manag Care Spec Pharm.* 2017;23(6):633-641.
186. Biggar WD, Politano L, Harris VA, et al. Deflazacort in Duchenne muscular dystrophy: a comparison of two different protocols. *Neuromuscul Disord.* 2004;14(8-9):476-482.
187. Hoffman EP, Nader GA. Balancing muscle hypertrophy and atrophy. *Nat Med.* 2004;10(6):584-585.
188. Hoffman EP, Reeves E, Damsker J, et al. Novel approaches to corticosteroid treatment in Duchenne muscular dystrophy. *Phys Med Rehabil Clin N Am.* 2012;23(4):821-828.
189. U.S. Food and Drug Administration. Prescribing information for Emflaza. Accessed June 13, 2023. https://www.accessdata.fda.gov/drugsatfda_docs/label/2017/208684s000,208685s000lbl.pdf
190. Assandri A, Buniva G, Martinelli E, et al. Pharmacokinetics and metabolism of deflazacort in the rat, dog, monkey and man. *Adv Exp Med Biol.* 1984;171:9-23.
191. Huber EW, Barbuch RJ. Spectral analysis and structural identification of a major deflazacort metabolite in man. *Xenobiotica.* 1995;25(2):175-183.
192. Mendell JR, Rodino-Klapac LR, Sahenk Z, et al. Eteplirsen for the treatment of Duchenne muscular dystrophy. *Ann Neurol.* 2013;74(5):637-647.
193. U.S. Food and Drug Administration. Prescribing information for Exondys 51. Accessed June 13, 2023. https://www.accessdata.fda.gov/drugsatfda_docs/label/2016/206488lbl.pdf
194. D'Amico A, Mercuri E, Tiziano FD, et al. Spinal muscular atrophy. *Orphanet J Rare Dis.* 2011;6:71.
195. Kolb SJ, Kissel JT. Spinal muscular atrophy. *Neurol Clin.* 2015;33(4):831-846.
196. Ahmad S, Bhatia K, Kannan A, et al. Molecular mechanisms of neurodegeneration in spinal muscular atrophy. *J Exp Neurosci.* 2016;23(10):39-49.
197. Parente V, Corti S. Advances in spinal muscular atrophy therapeutics. *Ther Adv Neurol Disord.* 2018;11:1756285618754501. doi:10.1177/1756285618754501
198. Tu WY, Simpson JE, Highley JR, et al. Spinal muscular atrophy: factors that modulate motor neurone vulnerability. *Neurobiol Dis.* 2017;102:11-20.
199. U.S. Food and Drug Administration. Prescribing information for Spinraza. Accessed June 13, 2023. https://www.accessdata.fda.gov/drugsatfda_docs/label/2016/209531lbl.pdf
200. American Association of Neurological Surgeons. Patients: conditions and treatment: spasticity. Accessed June 13, 2023.

http://www.aans.org/Patients/Neurosurgical-Conditions-and-Treatments/Spasticity
201. Elbasiouny SM, Moroz D, Bakr MM, et al. Management of spasticity after spinal cord injury: current techniques and future directions. *Neurorehabil Neural Repair*. 2010;24:23-33.
202. Montane E, Vallano A, Laporte JR. Oral antispastic drugs in nonprogressive neurologic diseases: a systematic review. *Neurology*. 2004;63:1357-1363.
203. Beebe FA, Barkin RL, Barkin S. A clinical and pharmacologic review of skeletal muscle relaxants for musculoskeletal conditions. *Am J Ther*. 2005;12:151-171.
204. Delgado MR, Hirtz D, Aisen M, et al. Practice parameter: pharmacologic treatment of spasticity in children and adolescents with cerebral palsy (an evidence-based review): report of the Quality Standards Subcommittee of the American Academy of Neurology and the Practice Committee of the Child Neurology Society. *Neurology*. 2010;74:336-343.
205. Chou R. Pharmacological management of low back pain. *Drugs*. 2010;70:387-402.
206. Berger FM, Bradley W. The pharmacological properties of an alpha, betadihydroxy-gamma-(2-methylphenoxy)-propane (Myanesisn). *Br J Pharmacol Chemother*. 1946;1:265-272.
207. Souri E, Sharifzadeh M, Farsam H, et al. Muscle relaxant activity of methocarbamol enantiomers in mice. *J Pharm Pharmacol*. 1999;51:853-855.
208. Forist AA, Judy RW. Comparative pharmacokinetics of chlorphenesin carbamate and methocarbamol in man. *J Pharm Sci*. 1971;60(11):1686-1688.
209. Bruce RB, Turnbull LB, Newman JH. Metabolism of methocarbamol in the rat, dog, and human. *J Pharm Sci*. 1971;60(1):104-106.
210. Thompson RM, Gerber N, Seibert RA. Metabolism of methocarbamol (robaxin) in the isolated perfused rat liver and identification of glucuronides. *Xenobiotica*. 1975;5(3):145-153.
211. U.S. Food and Drug Administration. Prescribing information for Metaxolone. Accessed June 13, 2023. https://www.accessdata.fda.gov/drugsatfda_docs/label/2022/022503s001lbl.pdf
212. Bruce RB, Turnbull L, Newman J, et al. Metabolism of metaxalone. *J Med Chem*. 1966;9(3):286-288.
213. Gonzalez LA, Gatch MB, Taylor CM, et al. Carisoprodol-mediated modulation of GABAA receptors: in vitro and in vivo studies. *J Pharmacol Exp Ther*. 2009;329(2):827-837.
214. Rho JM, Donevan SD, Rogawski MA. Barbiturate-like actions of the propanediol dicarbamates felbamate and meprobamate. *J Pharmacol Exp Ther*. 1997;280(3):1383-1391.
215. Kumar M, Dillon GH. Assessment of direct gating and allosteric modulatory effects of meprobamate in recombinant GABAA receptors. *Eur J Pharmacol*. 2016;775:149-158.
216. Simon S, D'Andrea C, Wheeler WJ, et al. Bioavailability of oral carisoprodol 250 and 350 mg and metabolism to meprobamate: a single-dose crossover study. *Curr Ther Res Clin Exp*. 2010;71(1):50-59.
217. Lewandowski TA. Pharmacokinetic modeling of carisoprodol and meprobamate disposition in adults. *Hum Exp Toxicol*. 2017; 36(8):846-853.
218. Dalén P, Alvan G, Wakelkamp M, et al. Formation of meprobamate from carisoprodol is catalysed by CYP2C19. *Pharmacogenetics*. 1996;6(5):387-394.
219. Yamamoto A, Yoshimura H, Tsukamoto H. Metabolism of drugs. 28. Metabolic fate of meprobamate. (1). Isolation and characterization of metabolites. *Chem Pharm Bull*. 1962;10:522-528.
220. Kobayashi H, Hasegawa Y, Ono H. Cyclobenzaprine, a centrally acting muscle relaxant, acts on descending serotonergic systems. *Eur J Pharmacol*. 1996;311(1):29-35.
221. U.S. Food and Drug Administration. Prescribing information for Flexeril. Accessed June 13, 2023. https://www.accessdata.fda.gov/drugsatfda_docs/label/2003/017821s045lbl.pdf
222. Hucker HB, Stauffer SC, Balletto AJ, et al. Physiological disposition and metabolism of cyclobenzaprine in the rat, dog, rhesus monkey, and man. *Drug Metab Dispos*. 1978;6(6):659-672.
223. Prox A, Breyer-Pfaff U. Amitriptyline metabolites in human urine. Identification of phenols, dihydrodiols, glycols, and ketones. *Drug Metab Dispos*. 1987;15(6):890-896.
224. Penn RD, Savoy SM, Corcos D, et al. Intrathecal baclofen for severe spinal spasticity. *N Engl J Med*. 1989;320:1517-1521.
225. Bowery NG. GABAB receptor: a site of therapeutic benefit. *Curr Opin Pharmacol*. 2006;6(1):37-43.
226. Wilson PR, Yaksh A. Baclofen is antinociceptive in the spinal intrathecal space of animals. *Eur J Pharmacol*. 1978;51:323-330.
227. National Center for Biotechnology Information. Baclofen. *StatPearls* [Internet]. Accessed June 13, 2023. https://www.ncbi.nlm.nih.gov/books/NBK526037/
228. Wuis EW, Dirks MJ, Termond EF, et al. Plasma and urinary excretion kinetics of oral baclofen in healthy subjects. *Eur J Clin Pharmacol*. 1989;37:181-184.
229. Faigle JW, Keberle H. The chemistry and kinetics of lioresal. *Postgrad Med J*. 1972;48(suppl 5):9-13.
230. Sanchez-Ponce R, Wang LQ, Lu W, et al. Metabolic and pharmacokinetic differentiation of STX209 and racemic baclofen in humans. *Metabolites*. 2012;2(3):596-613.
231. Krause T, Gerbershagen MU, Fiege M, et al. Dantrolene—a review of its pharmacology, therapeutic use and new developments. *Anaesthesia*. 2004;59(4):364-373.
232. Ward A, Chaffman MO, Sorkin EM. Dantrolene. A review of its pharmacodynamic and pharmacokinetic properties and therapeutic use in malignant hyperthermia, the neuroleptic malignant syndrome and an update of its use in muscle spasticity. *Drugs*. 1986;32:130-168.
233. Zhao F, Li P, Chen SR, et al. Dantrolene inhibition of ryanodine receptor Ca^{2+} release channels. *J Biol Chem*. 2001;276:13810-13816.
234. Ellis KO, Wessels FL. Muscle relaxant properties of the identified metabolites of dantrolene. *Naunyn Schmiedebergs Arch Pharmacol*. 1978;301(3):237-240.
235. Arnold TH, Epps JM, Cook HR, et al. Dantrolene sodium: urinary metabolites and hepatotoxicity. *Res Commun Chem Pathol Pharmacol*. 1983;39(3):381-398.
236. Kamen L, Henney HR, Runyan JD. A practical overview of tizanidine use for spasticity secondary to multiple sclerosis, stroke, and spinal cord injury. *Curr Med Res Opin*. 2008;24(2):425-439.
237. U.S. Food and Drug Administration. Prescribing information for Zanaflex. Accessed June 13, 2023. https://www.accessdata.fda.gov/drugsatfda_docs/label/2013/021447s011_020397s026lbl.pdf
238. Koch P, Hirst DR, von Wartburg BR. Biological fate of sirdalud in animals and man. *Xenobiotica*. 1989;19(11):1255-1265.
239. Crestani F, Low K, Keist R, et al. Molecular targets for the myorelaxant action of diazepam. *Mol Pharmacol*. 2001;59:442-445.
240. Basile AS, Lippa AS, Skolnick P. Anxioselective anxiolytics: can less be more? *Eur J Pharmacol*. 2004;500:441-451.
241. Date SK, Hemavathi KG, Gulati OD. Investigation of the muscle relaxant activity of nitrazepam. *Arch Int Pharmacodyn Ther*. 1984;272(1):129-139.
242. U.S. Food and Drug Administration. Prescribing information for Valium. Accessed June 13, 2023. https://www.accessdata.fda.gov/drugsatfda_docs/label/2016/013263s094lbl.pdf
243. Klotz U. Klinische Pharmakokinetik von Diazepam und seinen biologisch aktiven Metaboliten. *Klin Wochenschr*. 1978;56(18):895-904.
244. Jack ML, Colburn WA. Pharmacokinetic model for diazepam and its major metabolite desmethyldiazepam following diazepam administration. *J Pharm Sci*. 1983;72:1318-1323.
245. Jung F, Richardson TH, Raucy JL, et al. Diazepam metabolism by cDNA-expressed human 2C P450s: identification of P4502C18 and P4502C19 as low K_M diazepam *N*-demethylases. *Drug Metab Dispos*. 1997;25(2):133-139.
246. Dolly JO, Aoki KR. The structure and mode of action of different botulinum toxins. *Eur J Neurol*. 2006;13(suppl 4):1-9.
247. Dolly JO, Black J, Williams RS, et al. Acceptors for botulinum neurotoxin reside on motor nerve terminals and mediate its internalization. *Nature*. 1984;307:457-460.

248. Schiavo G, Benfenati F, Poulain B, et al. Tetanus and botulinum-B neurotoxins block neurotransmitter release by proteolytic cleavage of synaptobrevin. *Nature*. 1992;359:832-835.
249. Koussoulakos S. Botulinum neurotoxin: the ugly duckling. *Eur Neurol*. 2009;61:331-342.
250. Dolly JO, Lande S, Wray DW. The effects of in vitro application of purified botulinum neurotoxin at mouse motor nerve terminals. *J Physiol*. 1987;386:475-484.
251. Ward AB. Spasticity treatment with botulinum toxins. *J Neural Transm*. 2008;115:607-616.
252. Bom A, Bradley M, Cameron K, et al. A novel concept of reversing neuromuscular block: chemical encapsulation of rocuronium bromide by a cyclodextrin-based synthetic host. *Angew Chem Int Ed Engl*. 2002;41:266-270.
253. Tarver GJ, Grove SJ, Buchanan K, et al. 2-O-substituted cyclodextrins as reversal agents for the neuromuscular blocker rocuronium bromide. *Bioorg Med Chem*. 2002;10:1819-1827.
254. Nag K, Singh DR, Shetti AN, et al. Sugammadex: a revolutionary drug in neuromuscular pharmacology. *Anesth Essays Res*. 2013;7(3):302-306.
255. Hemmerling TM, Zaouter C, Geldner G, et al. Sugammadex: a short review and clinical recommendations for the cardiac anesthesiologist. *Ann Card Anaesth*. 2010;13:206-216.
256. Berrih-Aknin S, Frenkian-Cuvelier M, Eymard B. Diagnostic and clinical classification of autoimmune myasthenia gravis. *J Autoimmun*. 2014;48-49:143-148.
257. Silvestri NJ, Wolfe GI. Myasthenia gravis. *Semin Neurol*. 2012;32(3):215-226.
258. Calvey TN, Wareing M, Williams NE, et al. Pharmacokinetics and pharmacological effects of neostigmine in man. *Br J Clin Pharmacol*. 1979;7(2):149-155.
259. Somani SM, Chan K, Dehghan A, et al. Kinetics and metabolism of intramuscular neostigmine in myasthenia gravis. *Clin Pharmacol Ther*. 1980;28(1):64-68.
260. Breyer-Pfaff U, Maier U, Brinkmann AM, et al. Pyridostigmine kinetics in healthy subjects and patients with myasthenia gravis. *Clin Pharmacol Ther*. 1985;37(5):495-501.
261. Zhao B, Moochhala SM, Lu J, et al. Determination of pyridostigmine bromide and its metabolites in biological samples. *J Pharm Pharm Sci*. 2006;9(1):71-81.
262. Gupta A, Goyal V, Srivastava AK, et al. Remission and relapse of myasthenia gravis on long-term azathioprine: an ambispective study. *Muscle Nerve*. 2016;54(3):405-412.
263. Lavrnic D, Vujic A, Rakocevic-Stojanovic V, et al. Cyclosporine in the treatment of myasthenia gravis. *Acta Neurol Scand*. 2005;111(4):247-252.
264. U.S. Food and Drug Administration. Prescribing information for Imuran. Accessed June 13, 2023. https://www.accessdata.fda.gov/drugsatfda_docs/label/2011/016324s034s035lbl.pdf
265. U.S. Food and Drug Administration. Prescribing information for Neoral. Accessed June 13, 2023. https://www.accessdata.fda.gov/drugsatfda_docs/label/2009/050715s027,050716s028lbl.pdf
266. Heatwole C, Ciafaloni E. Mycophenolate mofetil for myasthenia gravis: a clear and present controversy. *Neuropsychiatr Dis Treat*. 2008;4(6):1203-1209.
267. U.S. Food and Drug Administration. Prescribing information for CellCept. Accessed June 13, 2023. https://www.accessdata.fda.gov/drugsatfda_docs/label/2009/050722s021,050723s019,050758s019,050759s024lbl.pdf
268. U.S. Food and Drug Administration. Prescribing information for Firdapse. Accessed June 27, 2023. https://www.accessdata.fda.gov/drugsatfda_docs/label/2022/208078s008lbl.pdf
269. German CL, Baladi MG, McFadden LM, et al. Regulation of the dopamine and vesicular monoamine transporters: pharmacological targets and implications for disease. *Pharmacol Rev*. 2015;67(4):1005-1024.
270. Yao Z, Wei X, Wu X, et al. Preparation and evaluation of tetrabenazine enantiomers and all eight stereoisomers of dihydrotetrabenazine as VMAT2 inhibitors. *Eur J Med Chem*. 2011;46(5):1841-1848.
271. Mehvar R, Jamali F, Watson MW, et al. Pharmacokinetics of tetrabenazine and its major metabolite in man and rat. Bioavailability and dose dependency studies. *Drug Metab Dispos*. 1987;15(2):250-255.
272. Derangula VR, Pilli NR, Nadavala SK, et al. Liquid chromatography-tandem mass spectrometric assay for the determination of tetrabenazine and its active metabolites in human plasma: a pharmacokinetic study. *Biomed Chromatogr*. 2013;27(6):792-801.
273. U.S. Food and Drug Administration. Prescribing information for Ingrezza. Accessed June 13, 2023. https://www.accessdata.fda.gov/drugsatfda_docs/label/2017/209241lbl.pdf
274. Grigoriadis DE, Smith E, Hoare SRJ, et al. Pharmacologic characterization of valbenazine (NBI-98854) and its metabolites. *J Pharmacol Exp Ther*. 2017;361(3):454-461.
275. Adinolfi S, Iannuzzi C, Prischi F, et al. Bacterial frataxin CyaY is the gatekeeper of iron-sulfur cluster formation catalyzed by IscS. *Nat Struct Mol Biol*. 2009;16(4):390-396.
276. Lee A. Omaveloxolone: first approval. *Drugs*. 2023;83(8):725-729.
277. Abeti R, Baccaro A, Esteras N, et al. Novel Nrf2-inducer prevents mitochondrial defects and oxidative stress in Friedreich's ataxia models. *Front Cell Neurosci*. 2018;12:188.
278. U.S. Food and Drug Administration. Prescribing information for Skyclarys. Accessed June 20, 2023. https://www.accessdata.fda.gov/drugsatfda_docs/label/2023/216718Orig1s000lbl.pdf

Structure Challenge Answers

1a. D and E, 1b. D, 1c. Opicapone (D) is indicated for off-episodes of PD and is not contraindicated in patients with liver disease.
2a. A and G, 2b. G, 2c. Monomethyl fumarate (G) is not contraindicated in patients with risk or previous diagnosis of cancer, whereas cladribine (A) is.
3a. B and F, 3b. B, 3c. Metaxalone (B) is less likely to have drug-drug interactions with CYP2C19 inhibitors, such as esomeprazole, compared to carisoprodol (F), which is primarily metabolized by CYP2C19.
4a. C and H, 4b. H, 4c. Ropinirole (H) is primarily metabolized by CYPs and not cleared renally, whereas pramipexole (C) is primarily cleared via the kidneys.

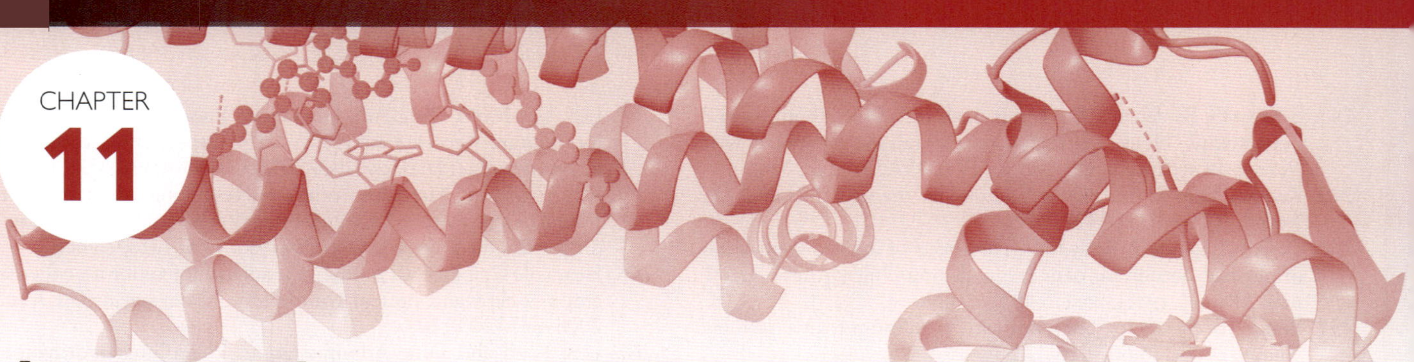

CHAPTER

11

Antipsychotic and Anxiolytic Drugs

Clinton E. Canal

Drugs covered in this chapter:

ANTIPSYCHOTIC DRUGS

PHENOTHIAZINES AND THIOXANTHENES
- Chlorpromazine
- Fluphenazine
- Perphenazine
- Prochlorperazine
- Thioridazine
- Thiothixene
- Trifluoperazine

BUTYROPHENONES
- Droperidol
- Haloperidol
- Lumateperone

DIPHENYLBUTYLPIPERIDINES
- Pimozide

DIARYLAZEPINES
- Asenapine
- Clozapine
- Loxapine
- Olanzapine
- Quetiapine

BENZISOXAZOLE/BENZISOTHIAZOLES
- Iloperidone
- Lurasidone
- Paliperidone
- Risperidone
- Ziprasidone

BENZAMIDES
- Amisulpride

PHENYLPIPERAZINES
- Aripiprazole
- Brexpiprazole
- Cariprazine

MISCELLANEOUS DRUGS
- Pimavanserin for Parkinson disease psychosis
- Tetrabenazines for tardive dyskinesia

ANXIOLYTIC DRUGS ACTING AT GABA RECEPTORS

MISCELLANEOUS DRUGS
- Baclofen

BENZODIAZEPINES
- Alprazolam
- Chlordiazepoxide
- Diazepam
- Flurazepam
- Lorazepam
- Midazolam
- Oxazepam

NONBENZODIAZEPINES
- Eszopiclone
- Zaleplon
- Zolpidem

NON-GABAERGICS
- Buspirone
- Gepirone

Abbreviations

ACh acetylcholine
AADC l-aromatic amino acid decarboxylase
α alpha
CNS central nervous system
COMT catechol-*O*-methyltransferase
CPZ chlorpromazine
CYP cytochrome P450
D, DA dopamine
DAT dopamine transporter
7-DHC 7-dehydrocholesterol
DOPAC dihydroxyphenylacetate
DSM-5 *Diagnostic and Statistical Manual of Mental Disorders of the American Psychiatric Association*
FDA U.S. Food and Drug Administration
FMRP Fragile X Messenger Ribonucleoprotein
GABA γ-aminobutyric acid
$GABA_A$ γ-aminobutyric acid receptor A
$GABA_B$ γ-aminobutyric acid receptor B
GPCR G protein–coupled receptor
HVA homovanillic acid
HPP^+ haloperidol pyridinium
HPTP haloperidol 1,2,3,6-tetrahydropyridine
5-HT serotonin
IC50 inhibitory concentration at 50%
M muscarinic acetylcholine receptor
MAO monoamide oxidase
MPP^+ 1-methyl-4-phenylpyridinium
NE norepinephrine
NMDA *N*-methyl-D-aspartate
PAM positive allosteric modulator
PANSS Positive and Negative Syndrome Scale
QT Q wave and T wave (on an electrocardiogram)
SNRIs serotonin/norepinephrine reuptake inhibitors
TOH tyrosine hydroxylase
VMAT vesicular monoamine transporter

SHORT TESTIMONIAL

In treating individuals with varying psychiatric disorders, a clinician must have a thorough understanding of all the variables that contribute to the selection and application of drug therapies explicitly tailored to the individual.

The pharmacology, pharmacodynamics, pharmacokinetics, and adverse effects of psychotropic drugs are widely variant and dependent on chemical structure, potency at receptors, and resultant physiological effects. Understanding medicinal chemistry is critical to understanding a drug's effectiveness and adverse effects. Learning about the pharmacodynamics of the highly effective antipsychotic clozapine drove, in part, the development of a newly FDA-approved combination agent, xanomeline/trospium (Cobenfy (TM), Karuna Therapeutics). Xanomeline, a centrally acting muscarinic receptor agonist, is combined with tropsium, a peripherally-restricted muscarinic antagonist, to blunt peripheral adverse effects of xanomeline. Cobenfy (TM) showed remarkable efficacy in clinical trials to treat positive and negative symptoms of schizophrenia. Focusing on the chemical structure and pharmacology of an already known agent, like clozapine, will aid in designing new agents with different mechanisms of action from current practice. It is how scientists and clinicians keep pushing innovation forward to overcome the challenge of treating negative symptoms of schizophrenia and other psychotic disorders.

The principles of medicinal chemistry are critical in applying the principles of pharmacotherapeutics. They are complementary sciences that, taken together, promote an in-depth scientific understanding of drug action that can inform rational decision-making in the care of patients with neuropsychiatric disorders.

Katelynn Mayberry, PharmD

Overview of Antipsychotic and Anxiolytic Medicines

Psychotherapeutic agents differ in their ability to treat unique psychiatric symptoms. Thus, an appropriate clinical diagnosis—currently founded on the presence of distinct clinical symptoms—is critical to selecting an efficacious drug. The definitive diagnostic criteria for psychiatric disorders in the United States are described in the *Diagnostic and Statistical Manual of Mental Disorders of the American Psychiatric Association* (*DSM-5*).[1] This chapter focuses on the medicinal chemistry of drugs that treat psychotic disorders and anxiety disorders.

Psychoses and Anxiety Disorders

Psychotic disorders are arguably the most severe mental illnesses and are characterized foremost by hallucinations and/or delusions, wherein consensus reality is distorted or has disintegrated in the patient. Defined psychotic disorders include schizophrenia, schizoaffective disorder, schizophreniform disorder, delusional disorder, postpartum psychosis, psychosis associated with bipolar disorder or depression, psychosis caused by a general medical disorder (eg, Parkinson disease psychosis), and substance-induced psychosis. Lifetime prevalence of psychotic disorders is about 0.75%,[2] and recent studies reveal that about 6% of otherwise healthy people report isolated psychotic experiences—reports of hallucinations are much more common than delusions.[3] Schizophrenia, the most common psychotic disorder, has a prevalence of about 0.64%.[2] Schizophrenia's economic burden is estimated to be as high as 1.65% of gross domestic product.[4]

In anxiety disorders, the ability to perceive and comprehend reality is retained, but cognition and mood problems can be disabling. Anxiety can be defined as a sense of apprehensive expectation. In reasonable amounts and at appropriate times, anxiety is helpful (eg, anxiety before an examination may motivate a student to initiate an appropriate study plan). Too much anxiety, however, can be deleterious. Anxiety can be considered pathological when it significantly interferes with activities of daily living or work. The estimates for lifetime morbid risk/12-month prevalence are 18%/12% for specific phobia, 13%/7% for social phobia, 9%/2% for generalized anxiety disorder, 7%/2% for panic disorder, and 4%/2% for agoraphobia,[5] though, during the COVID-19 pandemic, the Centers for Disease Control and Prevention reported significant fluctuations in these numbers in the United States.

Schizophrenia

A thorough description of schizophrenia was reported 100 years ago by the German psychiatrist Emil Kraepelin. Patients presented with a severe, progressive and chronic type of mental enfeeblement, which was not caused by known infections or brain injury. Kraepelin carefully annotated symptoms that included hallucinations (eg, hearing voices), delusions (eg, being persecuted), incoherence of thought and thought disturbances (eg, thoughts are "pushed" into the mind or do not belong to the patient), stereotyped thinking (persistence of single ideas) and behaviors (eg, echolalia), bizarre movements (eg, "waxy flexibility"), inattention, inappropriate emotions, intellectual and behavioral negativism (eg, knowingly responding incorrectly to questions or acting contrarily), blunted affect, avolition (eg, catatonia) and loss of will power, susceptibility to influence, social withdrawal (autistic-like), and language or speech problems (eg, paraphasia).[6] Kraepelin also described bodily symptoms, including sleep and appetite disturbances. Meanwhile, the Swiss psychiatrist Eugen Bleuler had coined this disorder "schizophrenia" as there was a perceived "schism" or splitting in mental functioning.[7]

The modern definition of schizophrenia as defined by the *DSM-5*[8] takes into account three major root characteristics: (1) chronicity and poor outcomes, as described by Kraepelin[6]; (2) dissociative and negative symptoms—diminished emotional expression or avolition—as described by Bleuler[7]; and (3) reality distortion or positive symptoms, as described by Schneider.[9] The diagnostic criterion for characteristic symptoms of schizophrenia, "Criterion A," requires two or more of the following to be present for a significant proportion of time during a 1-month period: (1) delusions, (2) hallucinations, (3) disorganized speech, (4) grossly disorganized or catatonic behavior, (5) negative symptoms. At least one of the characteristic symptoms must be delusions, hallucinations, or disorganized speech. In addition to Criterion A, there are two other criteria, "Criterion B" and "Criterion C." The former notes that "for a significant portion of the time since the onset of the disturbance, one or more major areas of functioning, such as work, interpersonal relations, or self-care, are markedly below the level achieved prior to the onset (or when the onset is in childhood or adolescence, failure to achieve expected level of interpersonal, academic, or occupational achievement)."[8] "Criterion C" states that continuous symptoms must persist for 6 months. Finally, before a diagnosis of schizophrenia is made, schizoaffective and mood disorders as well as psychotic symptoms caused by substances (eg, medications or illicit drugs) or other medical conditions must be ruled out. The *DSM-5* also introduced psychopathological dimensions—presence/absence of specific psychiatric symptoms and numerically categorized symptom severity—to improve the ability to describe the heterogeneity of schizophrenia in a valid and clinically useful manner.[10] *DSM-5* criteria for schizophrenia do not consider cognitive symptoms observed in schizophrenia, even though they are prominent and impair quality of life. These include deficits in working memory, attention, and verbal learning and memory. Most clinical trials evaluating the efficacy of antipsychotics use the Positive and Negative Syndrome Scale (PANSS).

Etiology of Schizophrenia

Schizophrenia is a neurodevelopmental disorder that often manifests during late adolescence. Although environmental factors influence the development of schizophrenia, heritability is about 80%.[11] Its genetic etiology involves numerous common alleles with small to moderate effect, and rare to ultrarare, but highly penetrant copy number variations.[12] A large (~150,000 subjects) genome-wide association study reported 108 schizophrenia-associated loci.[13] Genes within associated loci included *DRD2* (dopamine D_2 receptor), *CHRNA3*, *CHRNA5*, and *CHRNB4* (nicotinic acetylcholine receptors), as well as genes involved in glutamate (eg, *GRM3*, glutamate mGluR3 receptor) and GABA (eg, *IGSF9B*) neurotransmission, synaptic development and plasticity, and several others that encode mRNAs that interact with Fragile X Messenger Ribonucleoprotein (FMRP), the protein lost in fragile X syndrome (the most common monogenic cause of intellectual disability and autism).[12-14]

Many of the genes implicated in schizophrenia map to glutamatergic pyramidal cells and GABAergic interneurons in the cortex and to dopamine D_1- and D_2-containing medium spiny neurons in the striatum,[15] inferring alterations in excitatory-inhibitory homeostasis as well as dysregulation of dopamine neurotransmission. These observations support the predominant theories of schizophrenia etiology (described next). Most of the genetic polymorphisms observed across studies, however, do not change exonic sequences; in other words, schizophrenia-associated genes likely alter splicing, transcription, and noncoding RNAs.

A revealing development from several massive, genome-wide association studies is that alterations in common loci observed in schizophrenia are also observed in other psychiatric disorders, including bipolar disorder, clinical depression, autism spectrum disorder, attention deficit hyperactivity disorder, and posttraumatic stress disorder, pointing to common underlying and/or interconnected pathologies.[16-18] Also revealing, the personality trait "neuroticism" associates with almost every psychiatric disorder, including schizophrenia.[19] Despite clarifications regarding the genetics of schizophrenia, recent findings have not yet converged on any new, well-defined targets for medicinal chemistry drug discovery, with the exception of central muscarinic receptors.

Investigations of environmental influences have focused on prenatal and perinatal risk factors for abnormal brain development. Retrospective analyses show that schizophrenia is associated with influenza or other virus exposure and Rh factor incompatibility during prenatal development, and with obstetrical complications, such as asphyxia during childbirth. These environmental insults activate inflammatory processes including cytokines and brain microglia that likely contribute to gray matter loss in schizophrenia.[20] Research also reveals that schizophrenia (as well as bipolar depression and major depressive disorder) is associated with increased levels of certain blood cytokines, suggesting immune dysregulation. Genetic and environmental interactions—involving several common polymorphisms and a perturbed womb environment—may converge with precipitating factors such as psychosocial stress and synaptic pruning in the cortex during adolescence to cause schizophrenia.

Neuroanatomical changes associated with psychoses include loss of dendritic arbors and synaptic spines in cortical pyramidal neurons, thinning of cortical layers, decreased hippocampal CA1 volume, and enlargement of the brain's ventricular system. Also, neurochemical abnormalities, including changes in the central dopamine system, are well-documented in psychoses. Neuropathology in schizophrenia (eg, overt loss of nerve cells), however, is not as striking as neurodegenerative diseases such as Parkinson or Alzheimer disease.

Models of Schizophrenia Etiology

There are three interrelated models for studying schizophrenia etiology: (1) the neurodevelopmental model, (2) the excitation-inhibition imbalance model, and (3) the "dopamine hypothesis"[21] (now well-tested and verified to be a model). Alterations of dopaminergic neurotransmission in psychoses have been studied for more than 50 years; thus, there is substantially more knowledge surrounding the dopamine model (discussed in detail in the next section). The neurodevelopmental and the excitation-inhibition imbalance models have evolved more recently. Collectively, the models posit that schizophrenia is caused by disruptions in GABAergic and glutamatergic networks and perturbations in dopamine signaling in subcortical and cortical brain regions during critical periods of synaptic formation and rearrangement. The excitation-inhibition model of schizophrenia asserts that cortical pyramidal neurons are in a hyperexcited, disorganized state, creating neural noise that interferes with normal reality judgment. Cortical hyperexcitability results from a loss of inhibition from GABAergic interneurons. This model emerged in part from observations that glutamate *N*-methyl-D-aspartate (NMDA) receptor antagonists (eg, phencyclidine, PCP or "angel dust") can cause a psychotomimetic state that includes positive and negative symptoms. Blockade of glutamate NMDA receptors expressed on GABAergic interneurons inhibits GABA neurotransmission, subsequently enhancing glutamate neurotransmission.[22] Neuroimaging studies in patients with schizophrenia support this model,[23] but thus far, no compounds that directly modify glutamate neurotransmission have succeeded in clinical trials for schizophrenia.

Dopamine Model

According to the dopamine model of schizophrenia, psychosis symptoms result from aberrant dopamine neurotransmission—specifically, increased dopamine neurotransmission in the mesolimbic pathway (including the ventral striatum) and decreased dopamine neurotransmission in the mesocortical pathway (including the prefrontal cortex). The model arose initially from observations that the first effective antipsychotic drugs, the phenothiazines (eg, chlorpromazine), affected brain dopamine metabolism.[24] Further support emanated from observations of elevated psychostimulant-induced dopamine release in the striatum, but reduced release in the prefrontal cortex in persons with schizophrenia. Also, acutely psychotic patients, as well as patients prodromal for schizophrenia, display increased presynaptic striatal dopamine synthesis.[25] Increases in expression of dopamine D_2 receptors, as well as genetic polymorphisms at a locus that includes the D_2 gene, *DRD2*, have also been observed.[13]

Many antipsychotic medications bind to D_2 receptors with high affinity (K_i <10 nM) (Table 11.1), and their affinities for D_2 strongly correlate with their average therapeutic doses.[26] Binding to dopamine D_2 receptors in vivo also correlates with clinical efficacy[27]; neuroimaging studies suggest about 65% occupancy of dopamine D_2 receptors is required for efficacy of typical antipsychotics. Although most antipsychotics block D_2 receptors, functional interactions are complex, involving competitive antagonism, inverse agonism, and partial agonism. Moreover, it is now realized that G protein–coupled receptors (GPCRs), including D_2, can couple to multiple, distinct, intracellular signaling pathways, and drugs can possess a bias for activating or inactivating certain pathways.[28] In other words, based on the unique chemical interactions they have with the receptor, ligands can stabilize unique receptor conformations, resulting in unique cellular effects.[29-31] Thus, the biochemical effects and, by extension, clinical and side effects of antipsychotics are likely not due to simple blockade of endogenous agonist (dopamine) access to the D_2 receptor. More likely, they reduce dopamine neuron activity via unique actions at D_2 receptors. Antipsychotic drug discovery programs are exploring D_2-biased agonists that might maximize efficacy while minimizing side effects.[32]

Dopamine Receptors in Schizophrenia

There are five genetically encoded dopamine receptors (D_1, D_2 [with short and long splice variants], D_3, D_4, and D_5) and each is a GPCR. Historically, there were few medicinal chemical probes specific enough to distinguish between the five subtypes; thus, dopamine receptors often are classified as the D_1-type (includes D_5), which stimulates adenylyl cyclase, and the D_2-type (includes D_3 and D_4), which inhibits adenylyl cyclase. Several chemical probes are available that can distinguish between the general D_1-type and D_2-type receptor families (Fig. 11.1). The *R*-(+)-isomer of the benzazepine derivative, SKF 38393, is used for research as a selective D_1-type partial agonist. Meanwhile, the structurally related benzazepine derivative, *R*-(+)-SCH 23390, is used as a selective D_1-type receptor antagonist. Although not very selective for D_1-type over D_2-type receptors, the rigid benzophenanthridine derivative (+)-dihydrexidine is a useful research tool because it is a D_1-type full-efficacy agonist.[33] Although binding to dopamine D_1 receptors does not correlate with antipsychotic potencies, some studies suggest altered levels of cortical D_1 receptors in drug naïve patients with psychosis.[34] Since D_1 activation can improve cognitive function, such as working memory, which is impaired in schizophrenia, researchers are developing D_1-selective agonists to treat cognitive dysfunction in schizophrenia.[35] D_1 activation, however, is associated with nausea and vomiting.

D_2-type full agonists, such as the pyrazole derivative (−)-quinpirole, and D_2-type antagonists, such as (−)-sulpiride and raclopride, also are available to researchers, but these compounds do not distinguish D_2 and D_3 receptors well. The dopamine D_3 receptor has been of interest to neuropharmacologists and medicinal chemists since the early 1990s because of its preferential distribution in certain limbic regions of mammalian brain—notably in the nucleus accumbens (part of the ventral striatum), where it modulates glutamate and dopamine neurotransmission.[36] It was proposed that D_3-selective drugs might be developed as antipsychotic agents with preferential limbic antidopaminergic actions while sparing the extrapyramidal basal ganglia. Theoretically, this tactic would treat psychotic symptoms but prevent the neurological movement disorder side effects associated with antipsychotic drug therapy.

The D_3-preferring tetrahydronaphthalene, (+)-7-hydroxy-N,N-di-*n*-propyl-2-aminotetralin (7-OH-DPAT) helped elucidate the distribution of D_3 receptors in the brain ex vivo, though in vivo, under conditions of high extracellular NaCl conditions, 7-OH-DPAT does not adequately discriminate D_3 from D_2.[36] (+)-PD 128907, a congener of 7-OH-DPAT, remains one of the most selective D_3 agonists for experimental

Table 11.1 **Representative Food and Drug Administration–Approved Antipsychotics: Affinities at Receptor Targets Implicated in Therapeutic and Side Effects, Oral Doses and Half-Lives**

Drug / Target	5-HT_{1A}	5-HT_{2A}	5-HT_{2C}	5-HT_7	D_1	D_2	D_3	D_4	α_1	α_2	H_1	M_1	M_2	M_3	M_4	M_5	Oral Dose	Half-Life
Aripiprazole																	10	75
Asenapine																	10**	24
Brexpiprazole													*NA*	*NA*	*NA*	*NA*	2	91
Cariprazine					*NA*			*NA*				*NA*	*NA*	*NA*	*NA*	*NA*	1.5	72
Chlorpromazine																	500@	3@
Clozapine																	300	8
Haloperidol																	1	24
Iloperidone																	24	26
Loxapine																	60	3
Lurasidone*			*NA*		*NA*		*NA*										40	18
Olanzapine																	10	33
Paliperidone																	3	23@@
Perphenazine															*NA*	*NA*	12	11
Pimavanserin				*NA*			*NA*								*NA*	*NA*	34	57
Pimozide								*NA*				*NA*	*NA*		*NA*	*NA*	2	55
Quetiapine																	150	6
Risperidone																	4	20
Ziprasidone																	80	8

Black represents very high affinity (K_i < 1 nM). **Red** represents high affinity (K_i < 10 nM). **Grey** represents moderate affinity (K_i < 300 nM). **Light red** represents low affinity (K_i > 300 nM). *NA* denotes that data have not been reported. Values were culled from the PDSP website (Roth et al., 2000) in 2018, July or from the initial reported characterization of the drug and represent affinities at human cloned or human brain receptors, with the exception of * where some data are from rat or guinea pig brain tissue, as human data have not been reported. "Atypical" antipsychotics are emboldened. Half-life refers to approximate elimination half-life in hours, and oral dose is the lowest recommended target dose in mg/24 h for adults with schizophrenia, provided in prescribing information.

**Sublingual formulation.

@Not firmly established.

@@Extended-release formulation.

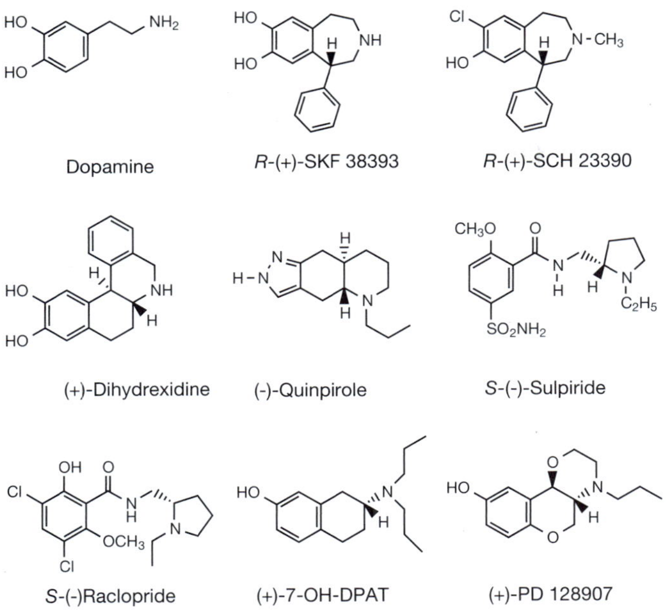

Figure 11.1 Structures of compounds useful for characterizing dopamine receptors.

purposes. Confirmatory results for targeting D_3 for schizophrenia were not observed until 2017, when F17464, a preferential D_3 antagonist, was shown to be efficacious in a placebo-controlled phase 2 study of patients with an acute exacerbation of schizophrenia.[37] The antipsychotics cariprazine, asenapine, and perphenazine bind D_3 with very high affinity (K_i <1 nM) (see Table 11.1), and there is some evidence that targeting D_3 may improve negative symptoms of schizophrenia, which are more difficult to treat than positive symptoms.

Enthusiasm for D_4 was sparked when it was found that the prototypical and highly effective second-generation antipsychotic, clozapine, had higher affinity at D_4 relative to all other dopamine receptors. D_4 ligands, however, failed in clinical trials for schizophrenia. Nevertheless, there remains a groundswell of interest in developing selective D_4 ligands as pharmacotherapies for Parkinson's disease, addiction, and other disorders.[38] A small number of human genetic studies have reported associations between the D_5 gene (DRD5) and schizophrenia, but there has been only limited interest from the medicinal chemistry community. An extremely high affinity (K_i <0.1 nM) D_5 antagonist has been reported,[39] but there are no others.

The dopamine D_1-type and D_2-type receptor families are differentially distributed in mammalian forebrain dopaminergic pathways. The extrapyramidal nigrostriatal pathway, which plays a key role in locomotor coordination, consists of neurons with cell bodies in the A9 pars compacta of the substantia nigra in the midbrain. These neurons project to the basal ganglia structures caudate nucleus and putamen (collectively referred to as the dorsal striatum) in the forebrain (Fig. 11.2). Degeneration of neurons in the nigrostriatal pathway is the hallmark pathologic feature of Parkinson disease, clinically manifested as bradykinesia, muscular rigidity, resting tremor, and impairment of postural balance.

The mesolimbic and mesocortical pathway, involved in integrating emotions and perceptions, motivated behaviors, and executive functions, consist of neurons with cell bodies in the A8 and A10 ventral tegmentum area. These neurons project to limbic forebrain structures, including the nucleus accumbens (ventral striatum) and the amygdala, and to higher levels of cerebral function, such as the frontal cortex (see Fig. 11.2). Reiterating, according to the dopamine model, increased dopaminergic neurotransmission in limbic pathways contributes to positive symptoms (eg, hallucinations and delusions), but negative symptoms (eg, catatonia) may be mediated by hypoactivity of dopaminergic signaling in the prefrontal cortex.

All antipsychotics, except pimavanserin, act in both extrapyramidal and limbic brain regions at D_2-type dopamine receptors that can be located postsynaptically (on cell bodies, dendrites, and nerve terminals of other neurons) as well as

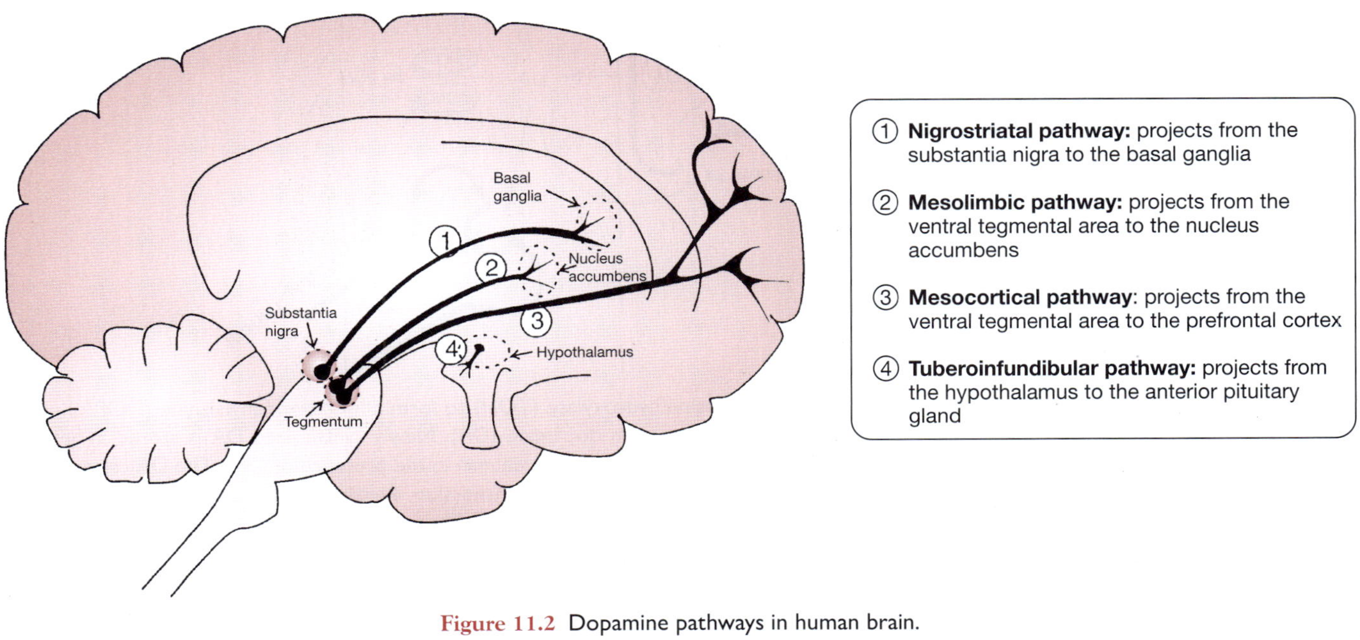

Figure 11.2 Dopamine pathways in human brain.

presynaptically on dopamine neurons. Dopamine receptors located presynaptically on dopamine cell bodies and nerve terminals are called autoreceptors—typically D_2 receptors—and act to decrease dopamine synthesis and release and to decrease neuronal firing probability (Fig. 11.3). Low concentrations of certain dopamine agonists can stereospecifically activate dopamine D_2-type autoreceptors to decrease dopamine synthesis and release,[40,41] thus reducing dopaminergic neurotransmission. Consistent with the dopamine model of schizophrenia, selective dopamine autoreceptor agonists could, theoretically, be pharmacotherapeutic agents in schizophrenia and related mental illnesses, and indeed newer antipsychotics, including aripiprazole, brexpiprazole, and cariprazine, possess D_2 autoreceptor agonist activity.

Pharmacotherapy of Schizophrenia and Related Psychoses

Antipsychotic drugs were historically called neuroleptics. This term suggested they "take hold" (*lepsis*) of the central nervous system (CNS) to suppress movement in addition to psychotic symptoms. While treating psychosis, classic neuroleptics, such as haloperidol, also cause debilitating extrapyramidal movement side effects. Indeed, the term "neuroleptic" is so synonymous with neurologic side effects that later developed antipsychotic drugs, with reduced risk of extrapyramidal effects, such as clozapine, were coined atypical neuroleptic drugs or second-generation antipsychotics. All new antipsychotics since clozapine are now simply called atypical antipsychotics. Though, likely forthcoming is an updated nomenclature based on a therapeutic continuum that considers: (1) efficacy to treat distinct psychiatric and cognitive symptoms and (2) specific side effects and side effect severity.

Chemical classes of typical antipsychotics include the phenothiazines, thioxanthenes, and butyrophenones. Atypical antipsychotic drug classes include the diarylazepines, benzisoxazoles, benzamides, and phenylpiperazines. In general, pharmacotherapy with either typical/first-generation or atypical/second-generation antipsychotics effectively treats positive symptoms of schizophrenia, whereas negative symptoms—which greatly impair quality of life—are not as appreciably affected despite concerted drug discovery efforts. There is some evidence that certain atypical antipsychotics, including clozapine, amisulpride, olanzapine, risperidone, and cariprazine, have better efficacy than the typical antipsychotic, haloperidol, in the treatment of negative symptoms. However, pivotal double-blind, randomized, clinical trials comparing a first-generation/typical antipsychotic (perphenazine) versus second-generation/atypical antipsychotics (olanzapine, quetiapine, risperidone, ziprasidone) revealed no substantial differences in overall efficacy. All medications were associated with high discontinuation rates due to intolerable side effects or inefficacy. Moreover, extrapyramidal side effects, unexpectedly, were not less frequent in patients treated with the atypical drugs. Clozapine was the most effective drug for individuals with a poor symptom response to previous antipsychotics.[42] Despite these findings, atypical

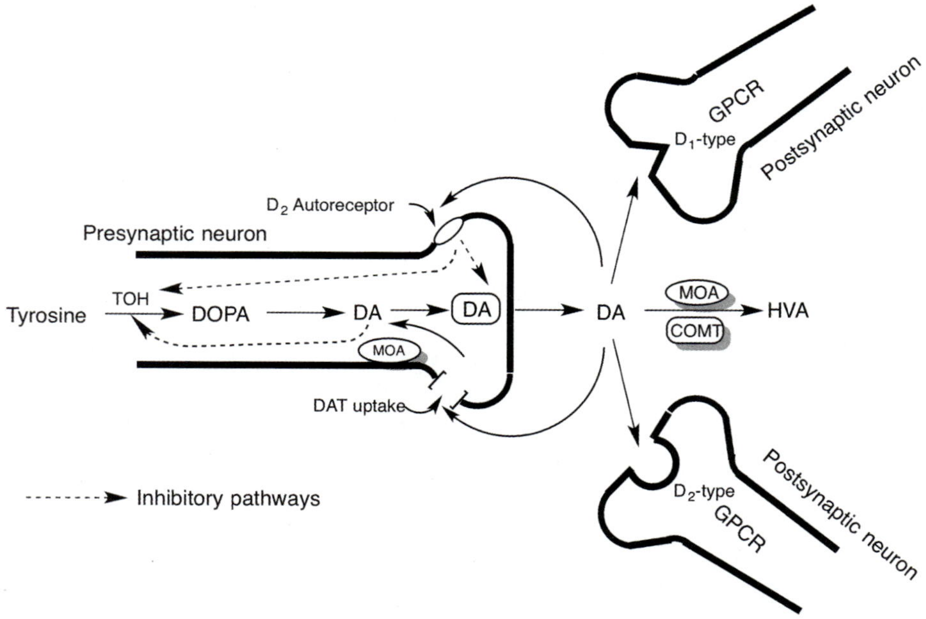

Figure 11.3 Tyrosine is hydroxylated in a rate-limiting step by tyrosine hydroxylase (TOH) to form dihydroxyphenylalanine (DOPA), which is decarboxylated by L-aromatic amino acid decarboxylase (AADC) to form dopamine (DA). Newly synthesized DA is stored in vesicles, from which release occurs into the synaptic cleft by depolarization of the presynaptic neuron in the presence of Ca^{2+}. The DA released into the synaptic cleft stimulates postsynaptic D_1- and D_2-type receptors enabling neurotransmission. Released DA also stimulates presynaptic D_2-type autoreceptors that modulate DA synthesis and release through negative feedback. The action of synaptic DA is inactivated largely via uptake into the presynaptic neuron by the DA transporter (DAT) located on the nerve terminal membrane. Cytoplasmic pools of DA may undergo metabolic deamination by monoamine oxidase (MAO), an enzyme bound to the outer membrane of mitochondria, to form dihydroxyphenylacetaldehyde, which oxides to dihydroxyphenylacetate (DOPAC). The DA or DOPAC may undergo methylation by catechol-*O*-methyltransferase (COMT), ultimately forming homovanillic acid (HVA), a metabolite excreted in urine.

antipsychotic prescriptions for new patients far exceed typical antipsychotic prescriptions.

A more recent and thorough meta-analysis showed superior efficacy of clozapine, amisulpride, olanzapine, and risperidone compared to several other antipsychotics, regardless of typical versus atypical designation. For example, clozapine and amisulpride (both atypicals) were more efficacious than lurasidone and iloperidone (both atypicals).[43] Differences between antipsychotic drugs are particularly evident in their side-effect profiles,[43,44] but again, they are not parsed by typical versus atypical categorization. We urge students, therefore, to pay close attention to chemical structures and unique receptor pharmacology and pharmacokinetic profiles to gain a clearer understanding of mechanisms and side effects of specific antipsychotics until further recategorization of antipsychotics occurs. Indeed, each antipsychotic, by nature of its structure, and hence engagement with targets (its affinity, on/off kinetics, receptor function biases), is unique.

Mechanism of Action of Antipsychotics

Given that the pathogenesis of schizophrenia and other psychotic disorders remains unclear—beyond burgeoning views involving neurocytoarchitecture development, synapse formation and pruning, coordination of excitation and inhibition processes, neuroinflammation, and alterations in dopamine function—it is perhaps naïve to describe how drugs act at the molecular level to relieve the symptoms of these disorders. Nevertheless, it generally is agreed that the mechanism of action of nearly all antipsychotics includes modulation of dopamine neurotransmission in the mesolimbic-mesocortical pathways via direct interaction with D_2 receptors. Though, all antipsychotics also have an affinity for $5\text{-}HT_{2A}$ receptors[45] (Table 11.1), which likely contributes to antipsychotic efficacy. Indeed, activation of $5\text{-}HT_{2A}$ receptors potentiates dopamine release and can disturb perception and cognition[46-48]—antipsychotics are $5\text{-}HT_{2A}$ inverse agonists[49,50] that block these effects. Most convincingly, pimavanserin selectively targets $5\text{-}HT_{2A}$ (and to a lesser extent $5\text{-}HT_{2C}$) receptors as an inverse agonist and effectively treats psychosis in Parkinson disease.[51]

Aside from affinity for D_2 and $5\text{-}HT_{2A}$, receptor-binding characteristics of different antipsychotics are unique (Table 11.1). Certain antipsychotics target other (non-D_2-type) dopamine receptors, serotonin $5\text{-}HT_{1A}$ and/or $5\text{-}HT_{2C}$, acetylcholine muscarinic, and/or histamine H_1 receptors, all of which are known to modulate dopamine synthesis and/or release in striatal and cortical systems, potentially contributing to efficacy.[52-55]

Furthermore, activation of $5\text{-}HT_{2C}$ receptors (converse to activation of $5\text{-}HT_{2A}$ receptors) produces antipsychotic-like effects in various rodent models of schizophrenia,[48,54,56] and aripiprazole possesses $5\text{-}HT_{2C}$ partial agonist activity. The most recent antipsychotics approved for schizophrenia (cariprazine and brexpiprazole—see later) include $5\text{-}HT_{1A}$ partial agonist activity, similar to several other atypical antipsychotics. $5\text{-}HT_{1A}$ receptors are expressed at much higher densities in the cortex, relative to the striatum, and activation of $5\text{-}HT_{1A}$ receptors increases dopamine release in the cortex, potentially contributing to antipsychotic efficacy, especially regarding negative and cognitive symptoms.[57]

Structure-Activity Relationships

GPCR targets of antipsychotics share a three-dimensional structure consisting of a bundle of seven transmembrane alpha helices, connected by alternating intracellular and extracellular loops, with the N-terminus in the extracellular domain and C-terminus in the intracellular domain. Antipsychotics bind to the orthosteric (endogenous ligand) pocket inside of GPCRs. This pocket is characterized by many hydrophobic side chains from residues in transmembranes two, three, five, six, and seven. There is a fair to high degree of amino acid sequence overlap within the transmembrane helices between different GPCRs, and even more overlap in the sequences that form the binding sites of endogenous ligands. This contributes to the polypharmacology of antipsychotics (ie, their high affinity for multiple GPCRs).

All extant antipsychotics possess a basic amine (a protonatable nitrogen atom) that forms a salt bridge with the side chain carboxylate of an aspartate residue in the third transmembrane, Asp3.32, present in all aminergic GPCRs. This interaction is crucial for binding.[58] Also, antipsychotics have hydrogen bond acceptors and donors, hydrophobic groups, and aromatic rings that form distinct interactions with GPCR residues. These interactions determine affinities and the functional activities of antipsychotics at GPCRs. The detailed molecular structure of the human dopamine D_3 receptor, in complex with eticlopride, a potent D_2/D_3 receptor antagonist, is resolved and illustrates: (1) how an antagonist binds to the receptor and (2) the shape of an inactive GPCR highly targeted by antipsychotics.[59] Canonical interactions include a disulfide bond bridging a cysteine in the second extracellular loop and a cysteine in transmembrane three (Cys3.25). Another interaction believed to be critical in stabilizing an inactive GPCR conformation is the ionic lock—a salt bridge between the charged Arg3.50 in the conserved "D[E]RY" (aspartic acid, [glutamic acid], arginine, tyrosine) motif and Asp6.30 (or Glu6.30) at the cytoplasmic side of transmembrane three and six.

Side Effects and U.S. Federal Drug Administration Drug Warnings

Up to two-thirds of patients with psychoses are nonadherent or cease taking their antipsychotic medications often because of obvious and serious side effects (including extrapyramidal symptoms, weight gain, sedation, lethargy, and emotional dampening) that interfere with activities of daily living and cause psychological distress. Though it is more apparent with some antipsychotics than others, sedation is a side effect of every antipsychotic agent. Since sedation can exacerbate negative symptoms of schizophrenia, such as avolition, it exemplifies a major challenge in treating both positive and negative symptoms.

Extrapyramidal side effects occur in up to 50% of patients taking antipsychotics. They tend to present within 8 weeks of initiating treatment, and despite the development of numerous atypical antipsychotics, they continue to be the greatest side-effect burden. Extrapyramidal side effects include akathisia, tardive dyskinesia, dystonia—such as facial grimacing, torticollis, and oculogyric crisis—and parkinsonian-type symptoms, such as bradykinesia, cogwheel rigidity, tremor, masked face, and shuffling gait. Akathisia, a feeling of inner restlessness or an urge to move, occurs in about 20% of patients on antipsychotics. Incidence in patients treated with haloperidol, aripiprazole, or quetiapine is about 60%, 18%, and 4%, respectively.[60] Tardive dyskinesia occurs in 20% to 30% of patients on antipsychotics and is characterized by stereotyped, involuntary, repetitive, choreiform movements of the face, eyelids, mouth (grimaces), tongue, extremities, and trunk. A new medicine was recently developed to treat tardive dyskinesia—valbenazine, a highly selective vesicular monoamine transporter 2 inhibitor that modulates the packaging and release of dopamine[61] (covered in Specific Drugs).

Extrapyramidal side effects are caused by prolonged blockade of dopamine binding to D_2 receptors in the nigrostriatal pathway. Similarly, hyperprolactinemia (elevation of blood levels of the lactation hormone, prolactin) is caused by D_2 blockade in the tuberoinfundibular (connecting the hypothalamus to the pituitary gland) pathway and is a common side effect of various antipsychotics. Closely titrating antipsychotic dose or switching to a different antipsychotic is necessary to reduce the likelihood or severity of these side effects. Certain antipsychotics (eg, clozapine, quetiapine) have a low incidence of extrapyramidal and hyperprolactinemia side effects; likely contributing factors include reduced affinity at D_2, and similarly, unique binding kinetics at D_2 receptors—namely unique association and dissociation rates.[62] An optimal kinetic profile for antipsychotics would permit endogenous dopamine to continue acting at the D_2 receptor, while also permitting the drug to sufficiently modulate the receptor's function. Insurmountable binding to D would completely block dopamine's ability to function, but slower on rates and faster off rates would allow time for dopamine to bind and function. This is notable, as, in general, antipsychotics that are more potent on a dose basis produce more side effects, suggesting tighter binding to D_2.

Additional side effects of antipsychotics such as sedation, hypotension, tachycardia, and other autonomic effects reflect blockade of histamine H_1 and adrenergic α_1/α_2 receptors. Antimuscarinic (M_{1-5} receptors) actions of certain antipsychotics account for other autonomic side effects, such as cardiac, ophthalmic, xerostomia, gastrointestinal, and genitourinary disturbances. On the other hand, it has been proposed that modulation of muscarinic cholinergic activity might be beneficial in controlling negative symptoms in patients with schizophrenia, and specifically targeting muscarinic receptors in the brain is coming to fruition with the success of KarXT (see "Short Testimonial") in phase 3 clinical trials. Also, the severity of extrapyramidal side effects increases with the ratio of antidopaminergic to anticholinergic potency, and anticholinergic medications can reverse some extrapyramidal side effects. Antimuscarinic alkaloids found in belladonna can be used in Parkinson disease therapy,[63] suggesting that selective antagonism of distinct muscarinic receptors may be favorable for preventing extrapyramidal symptoms.

Weight gain and general metabolic dysregulation that lead to type 2 diabetes and cardiovascular disease are problematic for many typical and atypical antipsychotic drugs. The mechanism for antipsychotic-induced weight gain and metabolic syndrome is not known for certain but might involve serotonin $5\text{-}HT_{2C}$ and histamine H_1 GPCR antagonism or inverse agonism.[64-66] It is notable that haloperidol and aripiprazole treatment is associated with relatively low incidence of weight gain[43]; haloperidol has no activity at $5\text{-}HT_{2C}$ receptors, whereas aripiprazole is a $5\text{-}HT_{2C}$ partial agonist. Meta-analyses consistently show that clozapine and olanzapine cause more weight gain and metabolic side effects,[43,67] and both are potent $5\text{-}HT_{2C}$ inverse agonists. Conversely, selective activation of $5\text{-}HT_{2C}$ receptors reduces food intake, and may improve metabolic function, as evidenced by the $5\text{-}HT_{2C}$ selective agonist, lorcaserin, which was approved for obesity.

Relatively common dermatologic reactions, such as, urticaria and photosensitivity, are observed especially with the phenothiazines. Antipsychotics also can prolong the heart's QT interval (measured from electrocardiograms), which potentiates the risk of serious ventricular arrhythmias. Antipsychotics are associated with increased risk of seizures, especially at high doses, and they carry a black box warning of increased risk of mortality in elderly patients with dementia-related psychosis. Deaths are typically attributed to cardiovascular events or infection. Antipsychotics also cause a 3-fold increase in the risk of stroke in older adults.

The FDA also revised the Pregnancy section of drug labels to warn about adverse effects to neonates of all antipsychotics taken during pregnancy. Babies born from mothers taking antipsychotics during the third trimester of pregnancy have an increased risk of abnormal muscle movements (ie, extrapyramidal symptoms) and withdrawal symptoms, including agitation, abnormal muscle tone, respiratory distress, tremor, somnolence, difficulty breathing, and trouble feeding. Medications to treat withdrawal include the γ-aminobutyric acid (GABA) potentiators phenobarbital and benzodiazepines.

Despite the vast number of approved antipsychotic medications, almost a third of patients with schizophrenia have an insufficient treatment response, and almost 10% are treatment-resistant (do not respond to at least two antipsychotic medications). These data illustrate the need for pharmacotherapies with novel mechanisms of action; see the "Short Testimonial" regarding KarXT—an M_1/M_4 preferring muscarinic agonist, xanomeline, combined with a peripherally restricted muscarinic receptor antagonist, trospium—that recently met primary endpoints in a phase III clinical trial for schizophrenia that can treat negative symptoms and likely will circumvent many of the adverse effects of extant antipsychotics that act at dopamine receptors.

First-Generation (Typical) Antipsychotic Drugs

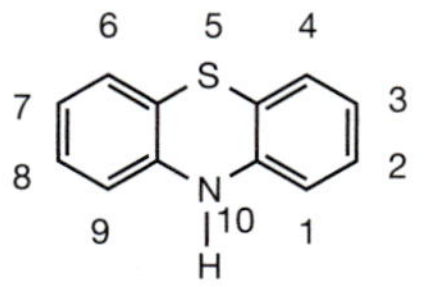

Phenothiazine

The phenothiazine nucleus was synthesized in 1883. It was used as an anthelmintic (antiparasitic) for many years, but it has no antipsychotic activity. The basic structure from which the phenothiazine antipsychotic drugs trace their origins is benzodioxane, and type I benzodioxanes are antihistamines (Fig. 11.4). In 1937, Bovet hypothesized that specific substances antagonizing histamine should exist, tried various compounds known to act on the autonomic nervous system, and was the first to recognize antihistamine activity with the discovery of piperoxan.[68] Starting with the benzodioxanes (Fig. 11.4 I), many molecular modifications were carried out in various laboratories in search of other types of antihistamines.

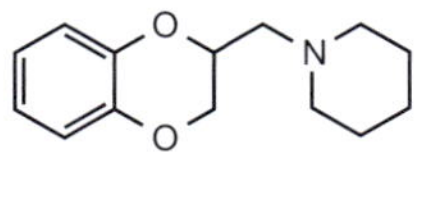

Piperoxan

The benzodioxanes led to ethers of ethanolamine (Fig. 11.4 II), which, after further modifications, led to the benzhydryl ethers that are characterized by the clinically useful antihistamine diphenhydramine (Fig. 11.4 III) or to ethylenediamine (Fig. 11.4 IV), which led to antihistamine drugs, such as tripelennamine (Fig. 11.4 V). Further modification of the ethylenediamine type of antihistamine resulted in the incorporation of one of the nitrogen atoms into a phenothiazine ring system, which produced phenothiazine, a compound found to have antihistamine properties

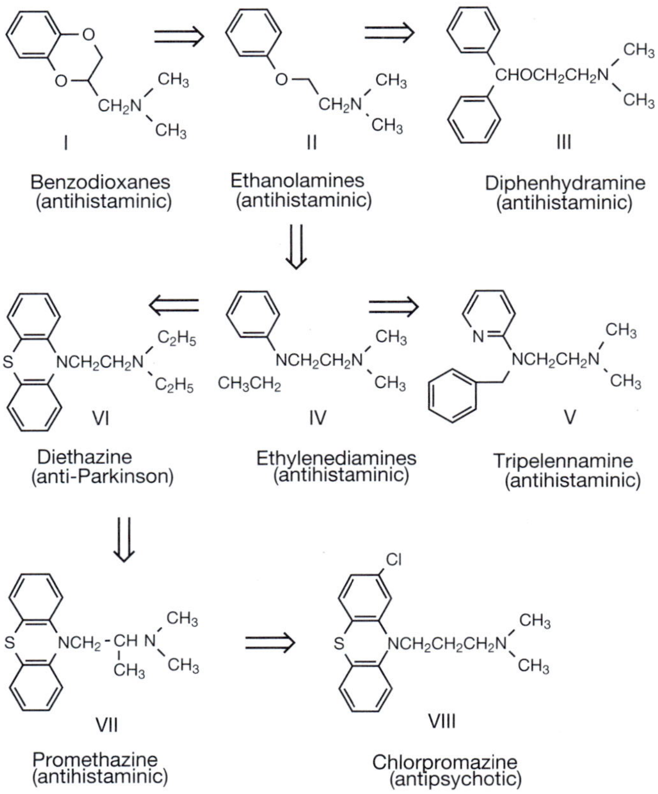

Figure 11.4 Development of phenothiazine-type antipsychotic drugs.

and, similar to many other antihistamines, a strong sedative effect. Diethazine (Fig. 11.4 VI) is more useful in the treatment of Parkinson disease (because of its potent antimuscarinic action) than in allergies, whereas promethazine (Fig. 11.4 VII) is clinically used as an antihistamine. After it was discovered that promethazine prolongs barbiturate-induced sleep in rodents, the drug was introduced into clinical anesthesia as a potentiating agent.

Chlorpromazine and Related Phenothiazines and Thioxanthenes

To enhance the sedative effects of such phenothiazines, Charpentier and Courvoisier synthesized and evaluated many analogs of promethazine. This research effort eventually led to the synthesis of chlorpromazine (Fig. 11.4 VIII) in 1950 at the Rhône-Poulenc Laboratories. Soon thereafter, the French surgeon Laborit and his coworkers described the ability of this compound to potentiate anesthetics and produce artificial hibernation.[69] They noted that chlorpromazine, by itself, did not cause a loss of consciousness but did produce a tendency to sleep and a marked disinterest in the surroundings. The first attempts to treat mental illness with chlorpromazine were made in Paris in 1951 and early 1952 by Paraire and Sigwald.

In 1952, Delay and Deniker began their important work with chlorpromazine.[70] They were convinced that chlorpromazine achieved more than symptomatic relief of agitation or anxiety, and that this drug had an ameliorative effect on psychosis. Thus, what initially involved minor molecular modifications of an antihistamine that produced sedative side effects resulted in the development of a major class of drugs that initiated a new era in drug therapy for the mentally ill—chlorpromazine spawned the "psychopharmacological revolution."[71] More than anything else in the history of psychiatry, the phenothiazines and related drugs have positively influenced the lives of schizophrenic patients, enabling them to assume a greatly improved role in society.

More than 24 phenothiazine and the related thioxanthene derivatives are used in medicine, with many of them used for treating psychosis, such as perphenazine, fluphenazine, trifluoperazine, prochlorperazine, thioridazine, and thiothixene. The structures, doses, and effects of those currently in use are listed in Table 11.2. Antipsychotics are also combined with antidepressants to treat moderate to severe anxiety, agitation, and depression. An example is perphenazine and amitriptyline, a tricyclic antidepressant (see Chapter 12). One phenothiazine, fluphenazine, is available in a long-acting injectable formulation, fluphenazine decanoate.

It is presumed that phenothiazine and thioxanthene antipsychotic drugs mediate their effects mainly through interactions at D_2-type dopamine receptors. Examination of the x-ray structures of dopamine (in the preferred *trans* α-rotamer conformation) and chlorpromazine shows that these two structures can be partly superimposed (Fig. 11.5).[72] In the preferred conformation of chlorpromazine, its side chain tilts away from the midline toward the chlorine-substituted ring.

Table 11.2 Phenothiazine- and Thioxanthene-Type Antipsychotic Drugs and Their Prominent Adverse Effects

	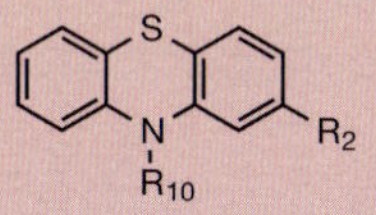		Adult Antipsychotic Oral Dose Range (mg/d)	Side Effects[a]			Other Effects
	R_{10}	R_2		Sedation	Extrapyramidal	Hypotension	
Phenothiazine Type							
Chlorpromazine	$(CH_2)_3N(CH_3)_2$	Cl	300-800	+++	++	Oral ++ IM +++	Antiemetic dose 10-25 mg every 4-6 h
Thioridazine	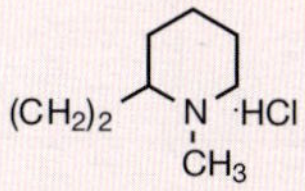	SCH_3	200-600	+++	+	++	Antiemetic dose 5-10 mg every 4-6 h
Perphenazine	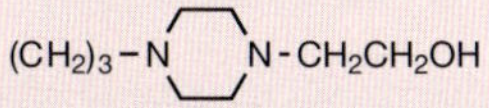	Cl	8-32	++	+++	+	
Prochlorperazine	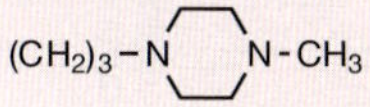	Cl	75-100	++	+++	+	
Fluphenazine	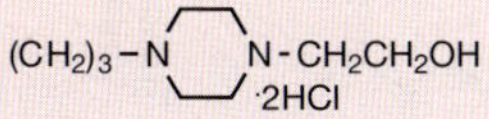	CF_3	1-20	+	+++	+	
Trifluoperazine	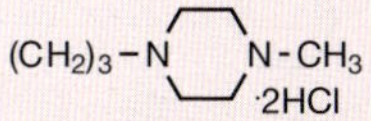	CF_3	6-20	+	+++	+	
Thioxanthene Type							
Thiothixene	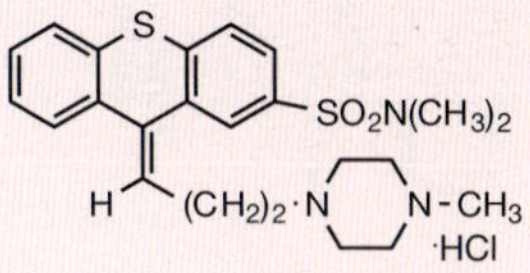		6-30	++	++	++	

[a]+++, high; ++, medium; +, low.

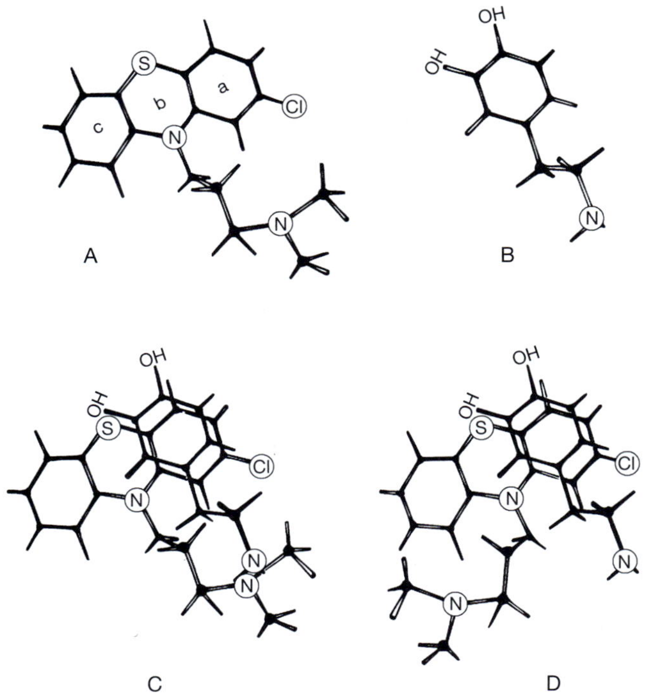

Figure 11.5 Conformations of chlorpromazine (A), dopamine (B), and their superposition (C) as determined by x-ray crystallographic analysis. The a, b, and c in (A) designate rings. Also shown (D) is another conformation in which the alkyl side chain of chlorpromazine is in the *trans* conformation (ring a and amino side chain), which is not superimposable onto dopamine. (Adapted from Horn AS, Snyder SH. Chlorpromazine and dopamine: conformational similarities that correlate with the antischizophrenic activity of phenothiazine drugs. *Proc Natl Acad Sci* USA. 1971;68:2325-2328, with permission.)

The electronegative chlorine atom on ring "a" is responsible for imparting asymmetry to this molecule, and the attraction of the amine side chain (protonated at physiologic pH) toward the ring containing the chlorine atom indicates an important structural feature of such molecules. Phenothiazine and related compounds lacking a chlorine atom in this position are, in most cases, inactive as antipsychotic drugs. In addition to the ring "a" substituent, another major requirement for therapeutic efficacy of phenothiazines is that the side-chain amine contains three carbons separating the two nitrogen atoms (Fig. 11.5). Phenothiazines with two carbon atoms separating the two nitrogen atoms lack antipsychotic efficacy. Compounds such as promethazine (Fig. 11.4 VII) are primarily antihistamines and are less likely to assume the preferred conformation.

When thioxanthene derivatives that contain an olefinic double bond between the tricyclic ring and the side chain are examined, it can be seen that such structures can exist in either the *cis* or *trans* isomeric configuration. The *cis* isomer of the antipsychotic thiothixene is several-fold more active than both the *trans* isomer and the compound obtained from saturation of the double bond. Structure D in Figure 11.5 shows that the active structure of dopamine does not superimpose with a *trans*-like conformer of chlorpromazine that would be predicted to be inactive.

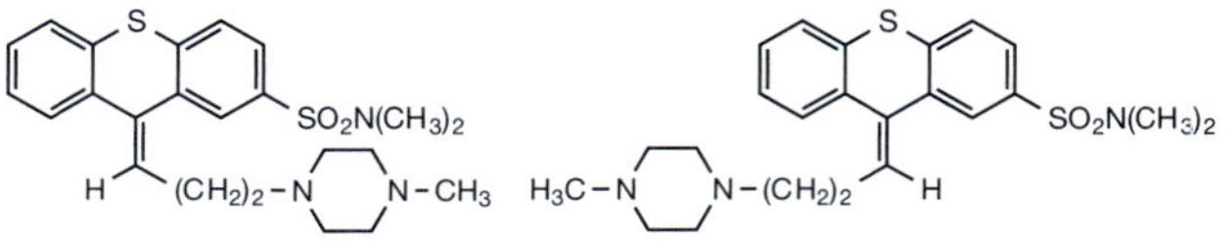

Cis isomer *Trans* isomer

Thiothixene

Some metabolic pathways for chlorpromazine are shown in Figure 11.6. It should be kept in mind that during metabolism, several processes can and do occur for the same molecule. For example, chlorpromazine can be demethylated, sulfoxidized, hydroxylated, and glucuronidated to yield 7-O-glu-nor-chlorpromazine-sulfoxide. The combination of such processes leads to more than 100 identified metabolites. Evidence indicates that the 7-hydroxylated derivatives and possibly other hydroxylated derivatives as well as the mono- and di-desmethylated products (nor_1-chlorpromazine, nor_2-chlorpromazine) are active in vivo and at dopamine D_2 receptors, whereas the sulfoxide (chlorpromazine-sulfoxide) is inactive. Although the thioxanthenes are closely related to the phenothiazines in their pharmacologic effects, there seems to be at least one major difference in metabolism—most of the thioxanthenes do not form ring-hydroxylated derivatives. Metabolic pathways for phenothiazines and thioxanthenes are significantly altered, both quantitatively and qualitatively, by a number of factors, including age, gender, interaction with other drugs, and route of administration.

Butyrophenone Antipsychotics

In the late 1950s, Janssen and coworkers synthesized the propiophenone and butyrophenone analogues of meperidine in an effort to increase its analgesic potency.[73] Both had greater analgesic potency than meperidine, but the butyrophenone analogue also displayed activity resembling that of chlorpromazine. The structure-activity results of Janssen and coworkers showed that it was possible to eliminate the analgesic activity and, simultaneously, enhance the chlorpromazine-like antipsychotic activity in the butyrophenone series.

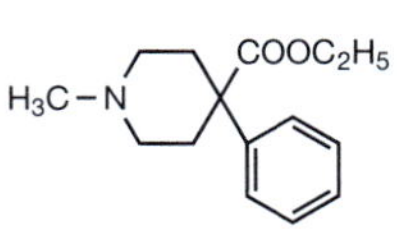

Meperidine

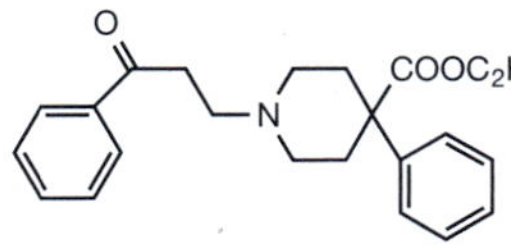

Propiophenone analog

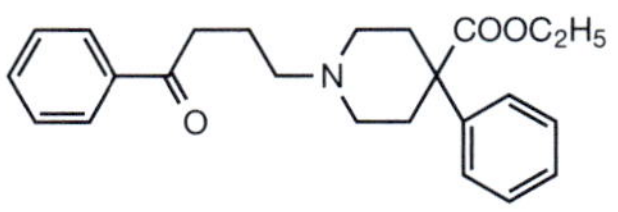

Butyrophenone analog

All butyrophenone derivatives displaying high antipsychotic potency, including haloperidol and droperidol, have the following general structure:

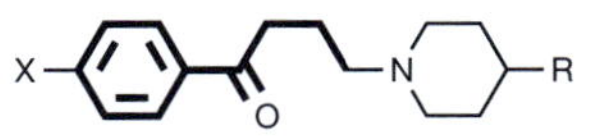

X = F or OCH_3

Scaffold of butyrophenone antipsychotics
The butyrophenone core is emboldened.

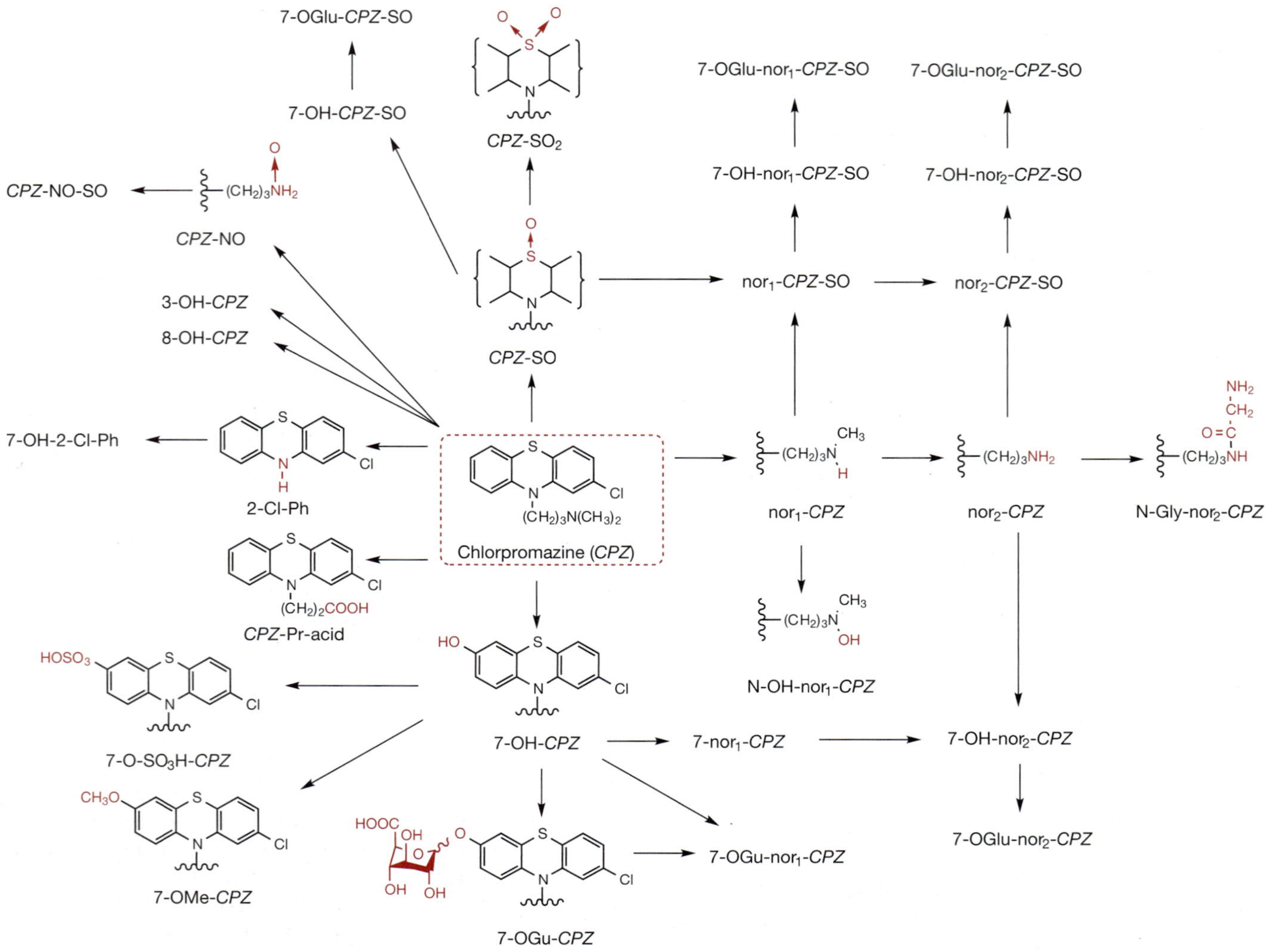

Figure 11.6 Metabolism of chlorpromazine. CPZ, chlorpromazine; NO, *N*-oxide; O-Glu, O-glucuronide; O-SO_3H, sulfate; Ph, phenothiazine; Pr-acid, propionic acid; SO, sulfoxide; SO_2, sulfone.

The attachment of a tertiary amino group to the fourth carbon of the butyrophenone skeleton is essential for antipsychotic activity; lengthening, shortening, or branching of the three-carbon propyl chain decreases antipsychotic potency. Replacement of the keto moiety (eg, with the thioketone group as in the butyrothienones, with olefinic or phenoxy groups, or reduction of the carbonyl group) decreases antipsychotic potency. In addition, most potent butyrophenone compounds have a fluorine substituent in the para position of the benzene ring. Variations are possible in the tertiary amino group without loss of antipsychotic potency; for example, the basic nitrogen usually is incorporated into a six-membered ring (piperidine, tetrahydropyridine, or piperazine) that is substituted in the para position.

In most respects, the pharmacological effects of butyrophenones differ in degree, but not in kind, from those of the piperazine phenothiazines. Consistent with its higher affinity for dopamine D_2 receptors, haloperidol—the prototypical butyrophenone antipsychotic—is more potent and produces a higher incidence of extrapyramidal reactions than chlorpromazine, but sedative effects in moderate doses are less than that observed with phenothiazines. Butyrophenones have less prominent autonomic effects, than the phenothiazine-type antipsychotic drugs, and only mild hypotension occurs. Also, haloperidol has less propensity to induce weight gain than chlorpromazine and most of the second-generation antipsychotic drugs.

Haloperidol (Haldol) was introduced for the treatment of psychoses in Europe in 1958 and in the United States in 1967. It is an effective alternative to phenothiazine antipsychotics and also is used for the manic phase of bipolar disorder. Haloperidol decanoate has been introduced as depot maintenance therapy. When injected every 4 to 6 weeks, the drug appears to be as effective as daily orally administered haloperidol. Other currently available (mostly in Europe) butyrophenones include the very potent spiperone (spiroperidol) as well as trifluperidol and droperidol (Inapsine) (Fig. 11.7). Droperidol, a short-acting butyrophenone, is used in anesthesia for antiemetic effects and sometimes—off-label—in psychiatric emergencies as a sedative antipsychotic. Droperidol is often administered in combination with the potent narcotic analgesic fentanyl for pre-anesthetic sedation and anesthesia. Caution should be exercised when administering droperidol due to its rapid induction of a prolongation of the QT interval.

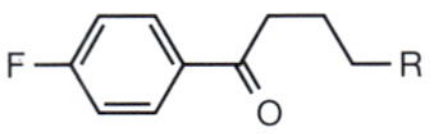

Generic names	Trade names	R
Haloperidol	Haldol	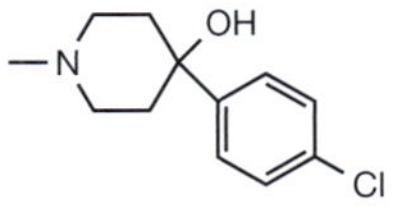
Haloperidol decanoate		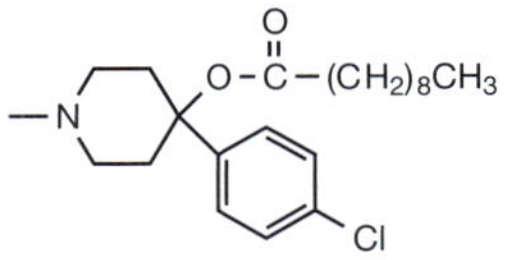
Droperidol	Inapsine	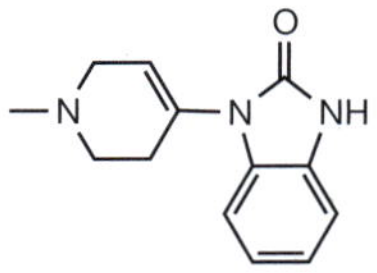

Figure 11.7 Haloperidol and its analogues.

Haloperidol is readily absorbed from the gastrointestinal tract. The drug is concentrated in the liver and CNS and is mostly bound to plasma proteins.[74] Peak plasma levels occur 2 to 6 hours after ingestion. Approximately 15% of a given dose is excreted in the bile, and approximately 40% is eliminated through the kidney. Figure 11.8 shows the typical oxidative metabolic pathway of butyrophenones as exemplified by haloperidol.

NEUROTOXICOLOGY OF HALOPERIDOL

As discussed in the section on Side Effects of antipsychotics, untoward extrapyramidal effects occur in up to 50% of patients receiving standard doses of typical antipsychotics. The severe and sometimes irreversible dyskinesias associated with haloperidol pharmacotherapy are hypothesized to result from neurotoxicity involving dopaminergic systems. In fact, the central and peripheral biochemical and resulting pathophysiological features of haloperidol-induced movement disorders are similar to the potent dopaminergic neurotoxicant and parkinsonian-producing agent, 1-methyl-4-phenyl-1,2,3,6-tetrahydropyridine (MPTP).

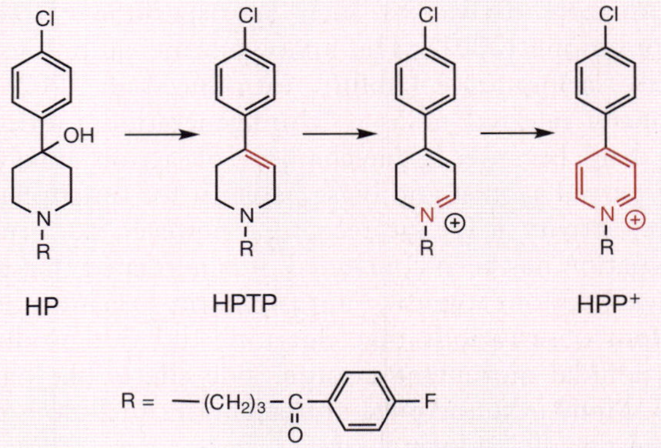

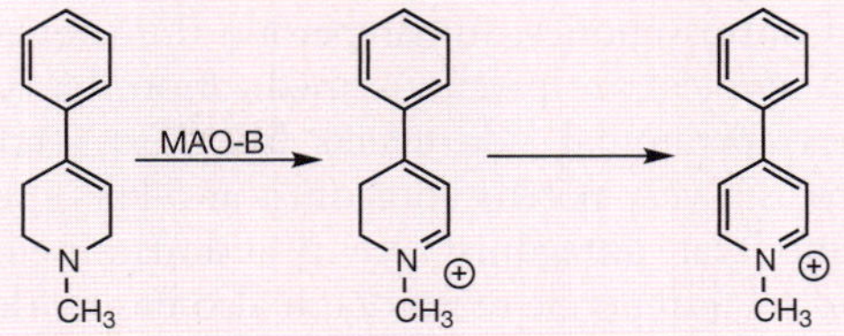

MPTP MPDP+ MPP+

Proposed neurotoxicological mechanisms for haloperidol-induced dyskinesias similar to that of dopaminergic toxicant MPTP.

Microsomal-catalyzed dehydration of haloperidol (HP) yields the corresponding haloperidol 1,2,3,6-tetrahydropyridine derivative (HPTP) that is a close analogue of the parkinsonian-inducing neurotoxicant MPTP. Long-term (58-week) administration of HPTP to nonhuman primates alters both presynaptic and postsynaptic dopaminergic neuronal function, which may contribute to the parkinsonian-type side effects and tardive dyskinesia that are relatively common with haloperidol pharmacotherapy.[75] In baboons treated chronically with HPTP, animals developed orofacial dyskinesia, and histopathological studies revealed volume loss in the basal forebrain and hypothalamus, along with other neuronal cell loss that may be relevant to the pathophysiology of tardive dyskinesia.[76] In humans and baboons, HPTP is oxidized in vivo to the corresponding haloperidol pyridinium species (HPP+) similar to the oxidation of MPTP to its ultimate neurotoxic species 1-methyl-4-phenylpyridinium (MPP+). HPP+ is neurotoxic to dopaminergic and, especially, serotonergic neurons in vivo in rats,[77] and HPP+ has been identified in the urine of humans treated with haloperidol.[78] Furthermore, in a study involving psychiatric patients who were treated chronically with haloperidol, the severity of tardive dyskinesia and parkinsonism was associated with an increased serum concentration ratio of HPP+ to haloperidol,[79] providing compelling clinical evidence for the neurotoxicity of HPP+. Investigations continue to determine if antipsychotic-induced pathology of the extrapyramidal motor system, such as that associated with tardive dyskinesia, may be related to production of MPP+/HPP+-type species in humans.

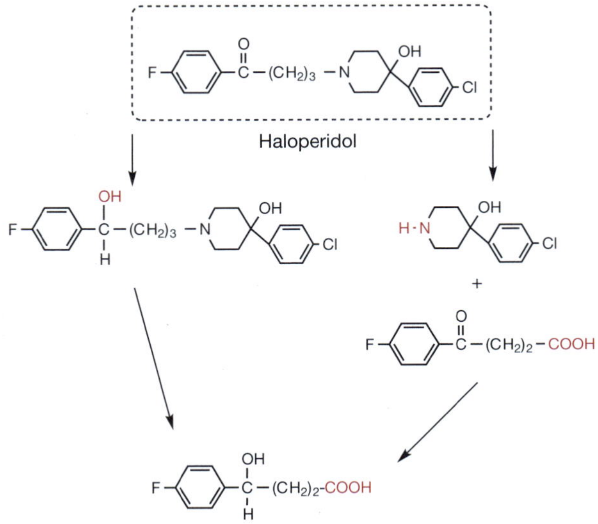

Figure 11.8 Metabolism of haloperidol.

Lumateperone (Caplyta). Although in the butyrophenone class of antipsychotics, lumateperone (lumateperone tosylate) is an atypical antipsychotic medication, based on its lack of extrapyramidal side effects (see next section). Lumateperone is a very potent antagonist at 5-HT_{2A} receptors and has moderate antagonist activity at dopamine D_2 as well as D_4 and α1-adrenergic receptors; it also has moderate inhibitory activity at the serotonin transporter, a primary pharmacodynamic property of first-line medications for depression (see Chapter 12). Uncommon amongst antipsychotics, lumateperone has partial agonist activity at presynaptic D_1 receptors, which can potentiate glutamate signaling via phosphorylation of the GluN2B subunit of the glutamate NMDA receptor.[80] The free base structure of lumateperone has a quinoxaline ring system that may confer its D_1 receptor activity. The antipsychotic asenapine also has high D_1 receptor affinity (Table 11.1), and has a core structure, oxepino[4,5-c]pyrrole, that is similar to lumateperones that may underlie its D_1 activity. Lumateperone has low activity at muscarinic and histamine receptors.

Lumateperone is a relatively new antipsychotic (approved in 2019) and is approved for the treatment of schizophrenia and bipolar I and II depression, as either monotherapy or adjunctive therapy (with lithium or valproate). Lumateperone is metabolized primarily by CYB3A4, and thus is not prescribed with medicines that induce CYB3A4; lower doses are prescribed for patients taking medicines that inhibit CYB3A4. It also is a substrate for several other metabolic enzymes, including but not limited to UGT1A, CYP2C8 and CYB1A2, which together produce >20 metabolites. The majority of lumateperone is excreted in the urine, followed by the feces. Lumateperone is highly bound to plasma proteins, and has a long elimination half-life (~18 hours). The most common side effect is somnolence or sedation, which is consistent with its principal pharmacology; 5-HT_{2A} antagonists cause sedation and were tested clinically to treat insomnia, and the antidepressant drug trazodone that has potent antagonist activity at 5-HT_{2A} receptors is prescribed off-label to treat insomnia. In clinical trials, lumateperone showed potential benefits for sleep maintenance.

In its phase 3 clinical trials, lumateperone's efficacy, scored by the PANSS, was compared to placebo and the positive control, risperidone. Secondary endpoints included Clinical Global Impression-Severity, and effects on social behavior and metabolic parameters. It significantly reduced positive symptoms of schizophrenia, and did not cause significant weight gain, metabolic disturbances, QTc prolongation, extrapyramidal symptoms or prolactin elevation, or sexual dysfunction. That it has a low risk of producing extrapyramidal symptoms and elevating prolactin is likely due to the observations that at its prescribed dose, 42 mg orally, it has high occupancy at cortical 5-HT_{2A} but relatively low occupancy at striatal D_2 receptors.[81] It also did not impair cognition, putatively owing to its glutamate-stimulating property.

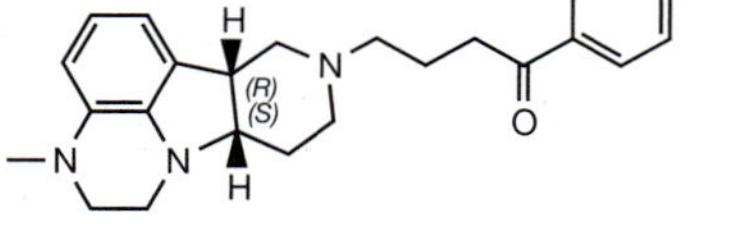

Lumateperone (Caplyta)

Diphenylbutylpiperidines

Replacement of the haloperidol butyrophenone side chain with a di-4-flourophenylmethane moiety results in diphenylbutylpiperidine antipsychotics, such as pimozide, penfluridol, and fluspirilene, which have a longer duration of action than the butyrophenone analogues. Penfluridol and fluspirilene are discontinued in the United States, and pimozide is now approved as a treatment for motor and phonic tics in patients with Tourette syndrome who have failed to respond to other treatments. Tourette syndrome is a movement disorder that is characterized by facial tics, grimaces, emitting of strange and uncontrollable sounds, and sometimes, involuntary shouting of obscenities. This disorder can be misdiagnosed by clinicians as schizophrenia. Typically, the onset of Tourette syndrome occurs at age 10, and standard treatment for Tourette syndrome has been antipsychotics. Chronic treatment of Tourette syndrome with pimozide and other typical antipsychotics carries the risk of producing tardive dyskinesia.

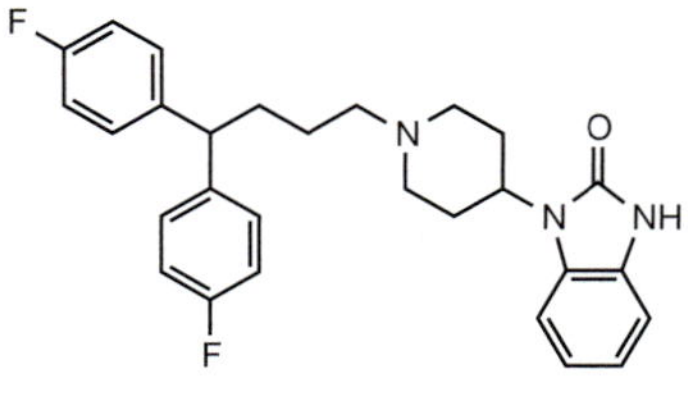

Pimozide

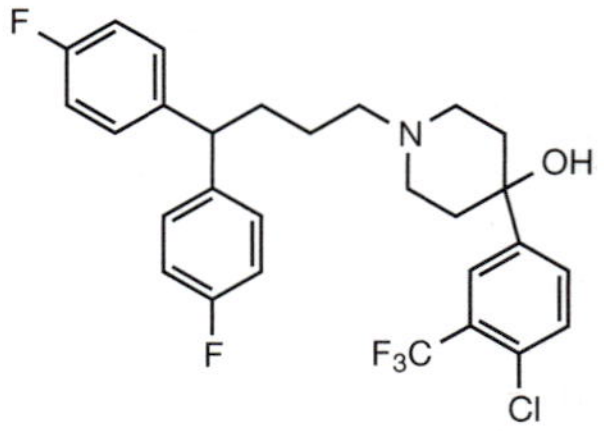

Penfluridol

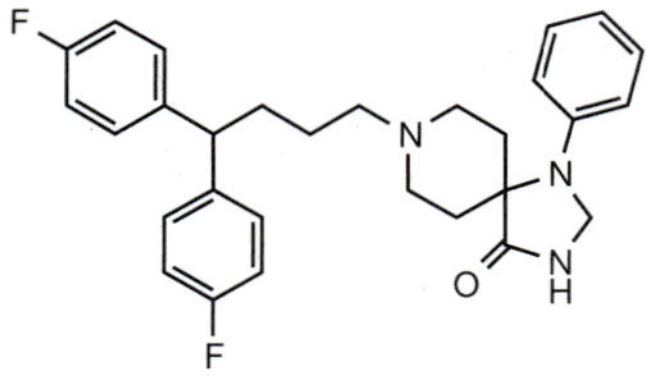

Fluspirilene

Second-Generation (Atypical) Antipsychotic Drugs

Atypical antipsychotic drugs first emerged with the introduction of the diarylazepine derivative, clozapine. This was followed by approval of the first benzisoxazole and benzisothiazole derivatives such as risperidone (1994) and ziprasidone (2001). The arylpiperazine quinolinone derivative, aripiprazole (Abilify, introduced in 2002) is occasionally referred to as a "third-generation" antipsychotic drug because its mechanism of action involves unique partial agonist and biased agonist (or functionally selective) activity at D_2 autoreceptors; however, no formal re-designation has been concluded. It is reiterated that the second-generation/atypical antipsychotic classification grew from observations that clozapine did not produce extrapyramidal movement disorder side effects like haloperidol. Many other atypical antipsychotics including risperidone and lurasidone, however, have a propensity to produce motor side effects, and akathisia is a common side effect of new antipsychotics, including the most recently approved medications, brexpiprazole, cariprazine, asenapine, and lurasidone. Other side effects, also, do not reliably define boundaries of classic, first-generation versus second-generation antipsychotics. Numerous investigators, therefore, suggest reclassification of antipsychotics.[82,83]

Diarylazepine and Related Analogues

The structures of the diarylazepine derivatives, clozapine, olanzapine, quetiapine, loxapine, amoxapine (an active metabolite of loxapine, indicated for symptoms of depression in patients with neurotic depressive disorders as well as psychotic depressions), and the related dibenzo-oxepine asenapine are shown in Figure 11.9.

Clozapine (Clozaril, Versacloz). Clozapine is the quintessential, atypical antipsychotic drug. It carries minimal extrapyramidal side effects and does not produce tardive dyskinesia with long-term use. It is believed this is due to its selective targeting of limbic rather than striatal dopamine receptors, its receptor binding kinetics, and/or its activity at muscarinic receptors. Clozapine maintains superiority to nearly all other antipsychotics, effectively alleviating both positive and negative symptoms of schizophrenia.[84] Furthermore, recent research suggests that clozapine has a protective effect on suicide. Serious drawbacks to the use of clozapine, however, are metabolic effects (weight gain, hyperglycemia, diabetes, dyslipidemia), and with rarer incidence, potentially fatal agranulocytosis (decreased white blood cell count). Agranulocytosis is reported to occur in ~0.7% of patients and may be related to a rare mutation, which also affects agranulocytosis susceptibility related to

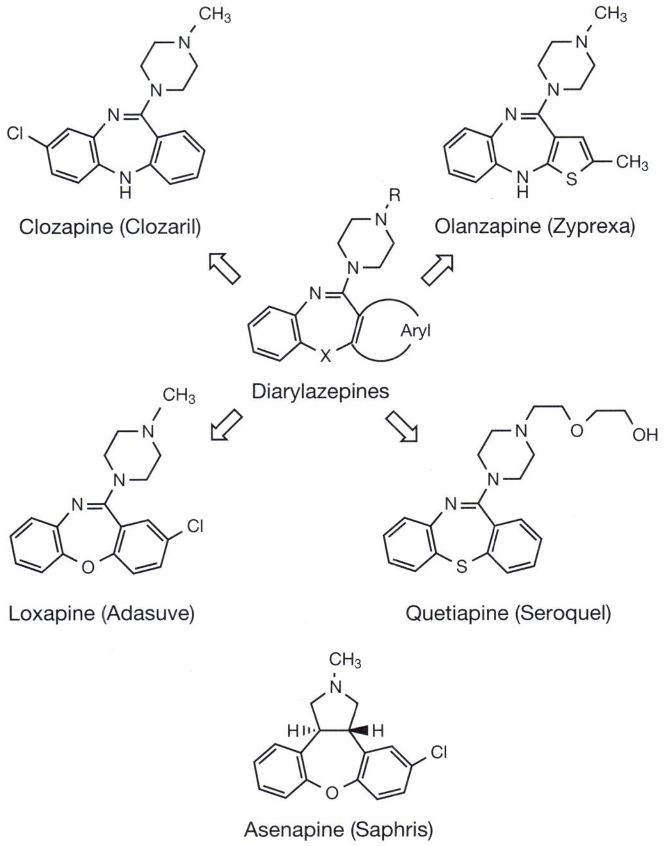

Figure 11.9 Metabolism of clozapine.

other medications.[85] Because of this risk, clozapine is reserved only for (1) use in the treatment of severely ill patients with schizophrenia who fail to respond adequately to other antipsychotics or (2) for reducing recurrent suicidal behavior in patients with schizophrenia or schizoaffective disorder. All patients treated with clozapine must have a baseline white blood cell count and absolute neutrophil count before and regularly during treatment and for at least 4 weeks after discontinuation. Clozapine can also cause constipation, and the FDA strengthened its warning that untreated constipation caused by clozapine can lead to bowel problems that can be fatal. This may be due to its activities at muscarinic receptors, as muscarinic receptors on smooth muscle cells in the intestine are critical for gastrointestinal motility.

The GPCR profile for clozapine is well characterized with respect to binding. In addition to D_2 and 5-HT_{2A}, clozapine has high to moderate affinity at dopamine D_1, D_3, D_4, D_5, serotonin 5-HT_{1A}, 5-HT_{2B}, 5-HT_{2C}, 5-HT_3, 5-HT_6, 5-HT_7, adrenergic α_{1A}, α_{1B}, α_{2A}, α_{2B}, α_{2C}, cholinergic $M_{1\text{-}5}$, histamine H_1 and H_2 GPCRs. It is notable that clozapine has high affinity at 5-HT_{2A} (K_i <10 nM) and only moderate affinity (K_i ~300 nM) at D_2, distinguishing it from most other antipsychotics that have high affinity at D_2. Clozapine's pharmacology with respect to function, which is necessary for understanding physiological effects, is not as well understood. Clozapine is generally considered an antagonist or inverse at most of its targets' canonical signaling pathways, but there are peculiar exceptions at noncanonical pathways and at targets for which it apparently has no affinity. Clozapine activates noncanonical 5-HT_{2A} signaling, leading to Akt phosphorylation, an effect blocked by a selective 5-HT_{2A} antagonist,[86] and although apparently not directly binding to them, clozapine modulates the function of $GABA_B$ receptors, as well as the glycine site on the NMDA receptor.[87,88] Furthermore, clozapine is a partial agonist at M_4, and its active metabolite, *N*-desmethylclozapine, is an agonist at muscarinic M_1 and M_4 GPCRs.[89,90] All of these pharmacologic properties may be relevant to its superior antipsychotic efficacy.

Clozapine is orally active and metabolized primarily by CYP1A2 with a smaller contribution from CYP3A4, although there is a high degree of between-subject and within-subject variability (Fig. 11.10).[91] It has a half-life of about 8 hours. The main products of metabolism are inactive

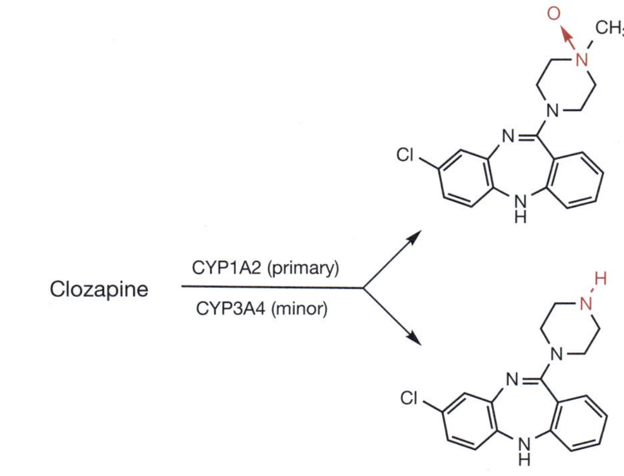

Figure 11.10 Diarylazepine derivatives.

hydroxyl and *N*-oxide derivatives. *N*-desmethylclozapine has a receptor binding profile similar to that of clozapine, although with higher affinity at 5-HT_{1A}. It is noted that caffeine is metabolized primarily by CYP1A2, and it has been observed that some patients who consume caffeine-containing beverages while taking clozapine show signs of increased arousal and extrapyramidal symptoms; removal of caffeine results in resolution of these problems,[92] suggesting a clinically relevant drug interaction. Also, cigarette smoking induces activity of CYP1A2, and patients who smoke while taking clozapine can have significantly lower serum levels of clozapine.[93,94]

OLANZAPINE (ZYPREXA). The thienobenzodiazepine olanzapine—available in several formulations—shares close structural resemblance to clozapine and has a similar receptor-binding profile, except it has higher affinity at dopamine D_2 and serotonin 5-HT_{2A} receptors but lower affinity at 5-HT_{1A} and α-adrenergic receptors. Olanzapine is effective at treating positive and negative symptoms. Its side-effect profile is similar to that of clozapine, with the exception of agranulocytosis that is not usually seen with olanzapine use. Also, olanzapine causes serious weight gain; prolonged use can cause some patients to gain 30 lbs. or more. Olanzapine is well absorbed after oral administration and is metabolized mainly by CYP1A2 to inactive metabolites similar to those seen with clozapine (*N*-oxide and N-demethylation) along with methyl oxidation and phase 2 glucuronidation (Fig. 11.11).[95,96] The drug has a variable half-life of approximately 20 to 50 hours. There is available a long-acting injectable formulation, olanzapine pamoate, Zyprexa Relprevv, and a combination therapy, Lybalvi, that contains olanzapine and samidorphan (an opioid antagonist) for schizophrenia and bipolar I disorder.

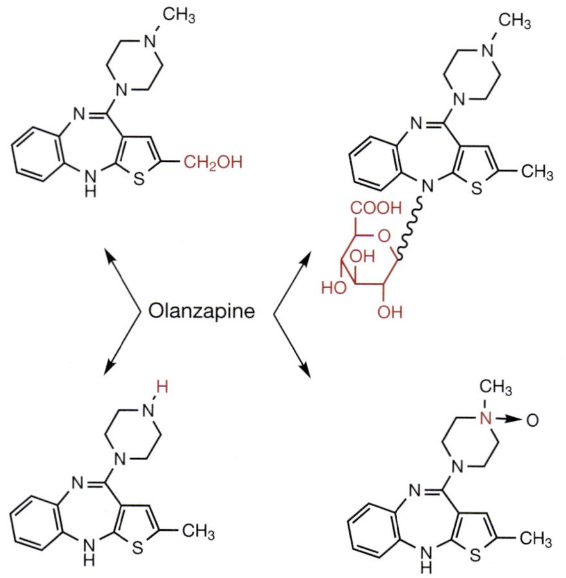

Figure 11.11 Metabolism of olanzapine.

QUETIAPINE (SEROQUEL). Quetiapine is a dibenzothiazepine that binds with high affinity at histamine H_1 GPCRs, but with low to moderate affinity at most other targets. Quetiapine is 100% bioavailable, but first-pass metabolism yields at least 20 metabolites, with the major metabolites shown in Figure 11.12. The major products are the sulfoxide (catalyzed by CYP3A4) and the carboxylic acid.[97] *N*-desalkylquetiapine has high affinity at several GPCRs, is a 5-HT_{1A} agonist, and potently inhibits the norepinephrine transporter, which may contribute to antidepressant activity.[98] It does not appear that CYP2D6 or CYP1A2 is involved in quetiapine metabolism, and cigarette smoking does not affect the pharmacokinetics of this drug. Relative to many other antipsychotics, but similar to clozapine, quetiapine has a short half-life, approximately 6 hours (Table 11.1). Also akin to clozapine, quetiapine carries a low incidence of extrapyramidal side effects, likely owing to its relatively low affinity at dopamine D_2 receptors.

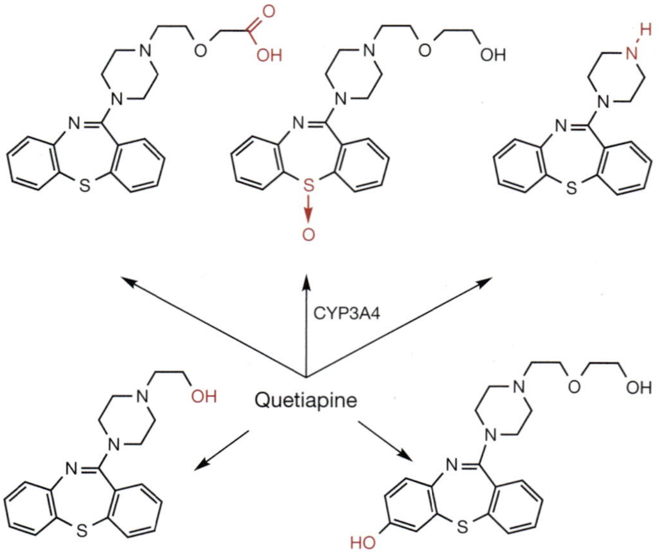

Figure 11.12 Major metabolic products of quetiapine.

LOXAPINE. The dibenzoxazepine loxapine has high affinity for dopamine D_2-type, serotonin 5-HT_2-type, and histamine H_1 GPCRs. It also has moderate affinity for 5-HT_6, 5-HT_7, α-adrenergic, M_1 and M_3 receptors. Loxapine has a short half-life of about 3 hours, undergoing phase I aromatic hydroxylation to yield several phenolic metabolites that have higher affinity for D_2-type receptors than the parent drug. Loxapine also undergoes N-desmethylation, via CYP1A2, to form amoxapine. Similarly, aromatic hydroxylation of amoxapine via CYP3A4 and CYP2D6 produces metabolites that have D_2 antagonist activity similar to haloperidol. Unlike loxapine, amoxapine has moderate affinity for serotonin, norepinephrine, and dopamine neurotransporters and blocks reuptake of these neurotransmitters; it is used clinically as an antidepressant.

ASENAPINE (SAPHRIS, SECUADO). Asenapine is a dibenzo-oxepino pyrrole that is unique in that it has very high to high affinity at several targets. These include 5-HT_{1A}, 5-HT_{1B}, 5-HT_{2A}, 5-HT_{2B}, 5-HT_{2C}, 5-HT_5, 5-HT_6, 5-HT_7, D_1, D_2, D_3, D_4, α_{1A}, α_{2A}, α_{2B}, α_{2C}, H_1, and H_2. It is reported that asenapine antagonizes all of its targets.[99] Also, in contrast to other diarylazepines asenapine, it has essentially no affinity (K_i >10 μM) for cholinergic muscarinic (M_1-M_5) GPCRs. Despite its unique polypharmacology, there does not appear to be any efficacy advantages for asenapine over other antipsychotic drugs (typical or atypical) for treating schizophrenia

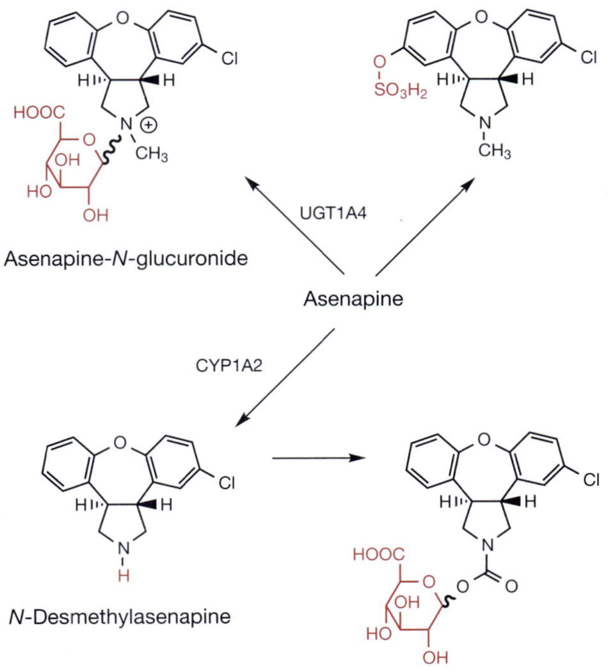

Figure 11.13 Major metabolic plasma products for asenapine.

or bipolar disorder.[43] Moreover, its side-effect profile is similar to that of other antipsychotics, except that it produces a lower incidence of extrapyramidal effects and prolactin secretion compared to haloperidol, and weight gain is less than with olanzapine. The most common adverse reactions are akathisia, oral hypoesthesia, and somnolence.

When given as a sublingual tablet, asenapine's bioavailability is about 35% (<2%, orally) with a half-life of 24 hours. The drug is extensively metabolized to compounds with little or no contributing activity. Elimination is primarily by direct glucuronidation by UGT1A4, yielding asenapine-N-glucuronide, and by N-demethylation and aromatic oxidation (primarily by CYP1A2) followed by conjugation (Fig. 11.13). Approximately 50% of the administered dose is lost via the kidney and 40% via the fecal route.

Benzisoxazole and Benzisothiazole Derivatives. Because certain diarylazepine type antipsychotic agents with high affinity for 5-HT_{2A} receptors produce low extrapyramidal and prolactinemia side effects (ie, clozapine), investigators predicted that combined, selective D_2 and 5-HT_{2A} receptor blockade would effectively treat schizophrenia without causing such adverse events. Linking the chemical features present in potent benzamide D_2 antagonists (eg, remoxipride, discussed below) with those of the benzothiazolyl piperazine 5-HT_{2A} antagonists (eg, tiospirone; Fig. 11.14) led to the development of the 3-(4-piperidinyl)-1,2-benzisoxazole nucleus present in risperidone and ziprasidone (Fig. 11.14). Post-marketing analyses of these medications have not supported the D_2 plus 5-HT_{2A} antagonist hypothesis for reduced extrapyramidal and prolactinemia side-effect risks.

Risperidone (Risperdal, Perseris) and Paliperidone (Invega). Risperidone—available in several formulations—is a benzisoxazole piperidine that has very high affinity at serotonin 5-HT_{2A} and high affinity at dopamine D_2 GPCRs, where it has been shown to act as an antagonist or inverse agonist. Despite this pharmacology, risperidone and its active 9-OH metabolite, marketed as paliperidone (see Fig. 11.14), demonstrate higher incidence of extrapyramidal side effects compared to clozapine and others, and no difference compared to amisulpride,[43] a benzamide discussed later that is a selective D_2-type antagonist with no activity at 5-HT_{2A}. Compared to haloperidol, extrapyramidal incidents are lower, but hyperprolactinemia incidents are higher with risperidone and paliperidone. Both produce significant weight gain on par with most other antipsychotics, excluding haloperidol, ziprasidone, and lurasidone which produce minimal weight gain. Other aspects of risperidone's and paliperidone's GPCR binding profile include high affinity at α_1- and α_2-type, and 5-HT_7 receptors, with moderate affinity at H_1, H_2, D_1, 5-HT_{2B}, and 5-HT_{2C} receptors.

Risperidone is well absorbed orally and undergoes hepatic CYP2D6- and CYP3A4-catalyzed N-dealkylation and 9-hydroxylation—paliperidone is the racemic version of the 9-hydroxy metabolite (see Fig. 11.14). Paliperidone

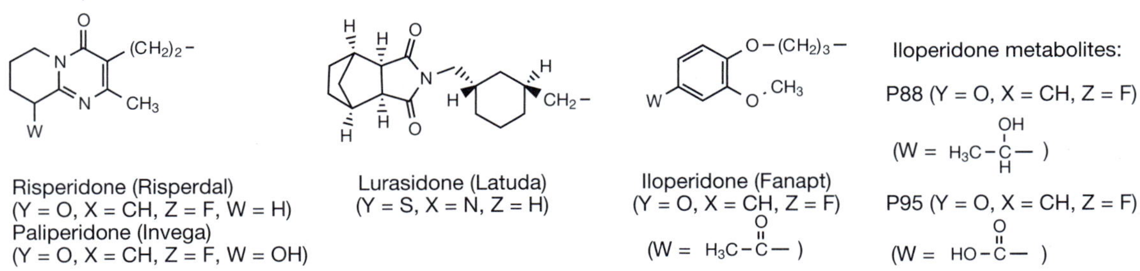

Figure 11.14 Benzisoxazole and benzisothiazole antipsychotic agents.

is not extensively metabolized by the liver and is excreted largely unchanged through the kidney. The half-lives of risperidone and paliperidone are approximately 23 hours. Patients differ regarding proportions of the (+)- and (−)-enantiomers of paliperidone produced in vivo, with the (+)-enantiomer arising from hydroxylation of risperidone by CYP2D6 and the (−)-enantiomer being formed mainly by action of CYP3A4.[100] There are no remarkable differences between risperidone and paliperidone regarding therapeutic activity, but reduced QTc prolongation with paliperidone compared to risperidone is a notable difference. Most clinical trials for both drugs were conducted versus placebo, but meta-analyses do not show superiority of these agents over other atypical antipsychotics.[43] Both drugs are available as long-acting injectable forms: risperidone in a physical complex with carbohydrate microspheres and paliperidone as the palmitate fatty acid ester.

Iloperidone (Fanapt). Like paliperidone, this benzisoxazole is very similar to risperidone regarding both its chemical structure and its GPCR binding profile—with the exception that iloperidone has additional moderate affinity for 5-HT_{1A} receptors. Iloperidone functions as an antagonist at all tested GPCRs. The affinities of the active metabolites P88 and P95 (see Fig. 11.14) are similar to that of the parent compound.[101] In the few studies where iloperidone was compared to other antipsychotic drugs (haloperidol, risperidone, ziprasidone), there was no difference in antipsychotic efficacy. Iloperidone produces significant weight gain, more than risperidone (2.1 vs 1.8 kg). Interestingly, iloperidone and risperidone have about the same affinity for serotonin 5-HT_{2C} and histamine H_1 receptors, which are thought to be responsible for antipsychotic-induced weight gain. Unlike risperidone and paliperidone, iloperidone is not associated with an increase in prolactin release. As is the case for risperidone, iloperidone is well absorbed orally and undergoes hepatic CYP2D6- and CYP3A4-catalyzed N-dealkylation. A majority of iloperidone is recovered unchanged in feces, indicating biliary excretion. Prescribing information reports that elimination half-lives for iloperidone, P88, and P95 in CYP2D6 extensive metabolizers are 18, 26, and 23 hours, respectively, whereas in poor metabolizers, half-lives are 33, 37, and 31 hours, respectively.

Ziprasidone (Geodon). Ziprasidone—available in several formulations—is chemically similar to risperidone, but with a substitution of piperazinyl and benzisothiazole for piperidinyl and benzisoxazole and with minor aromatic modifications (see Fig. 11.14) that impact its pharmacology and side effects. Like risperidone, ziprasidone has very high affinity at 5-HT_{2A}, but also at 5-HT_{2C}, receptors. It has high affinity at 5-HT_{1B}, 5-HT_{1D}, 5-HT_7, α_{1B}, D_2, D_3, and moderate affinity at 5-HT_{1A}, 5-HT_{2B}, 5-HT_5, 5-HT_6, α_{1A}, α_{2A}, α_{2B}, α_{2C}, D_1, D_4, and H_1 GPCRs. Ziprasidone also has moderate affinity at the serotonin transporter and the norepinephrine transporter. Moreover, ziprasidone can activate 5-HT_{1A} receptors that regulate dopaminergic neurotransmission in brain regions involved in critical cognitive functions.[102] Ziprasidone can cause hyperprolactinemia and extrapyramidal side effects, but incidents of hyperprolactinemia are low, relative to risperidone and paliperidone. Akathisia incidents are very low. Ziprasidone has a relatively low propensity for inducing weight gain despite its significant affinity at histamine H_1 and serotonin 5-HT_{2C} receptors. Ziprasidone oral bioavailability is approximately 60%, which can be enhanced in the presence of fatty foods. It is extensively metabolized (<5% excreted unchanged) by aldehyde oxidase, which results in reductive cleavage of the S–N bond, and then by S-methylation. Ziprasidone also can undergo CYP3A4-catalyzed N-dealkylation and S-oxidation. It has a half-life of about 8 hours.

Lurasidone (Latuda). Lurasidone is a benzoisothiazole piperazine structurally similar to ziprasidone. It has very high affinity at serotonin 5-HT_7 receptors; high affinity at 5-HT_{2A}, 5-HT_{1A}, and dopamine D_2; and moderate affinity at D_4, α_1- and α_2-type GPCRs. Lurasidone is an antagonist at these receptors, with the exception of 5-HT_{1A}, where it behaves as a partial agonist. Lurasidone has a low incidence of weight gain but can cause significant extrapyramidal side effects and prolactin increases. Lurasidone, like paliperidone, lumateperone, and aripiprazole (discussed below), is unique among many antipsychotics because it carries a low risk of QTc prolongation. Metabolism is reported as oxidative N-dealkylation, hydroxylation of the norbornane ring, and S-oxidation, mainly by CYP3A4. It has a half-life of 18 hours and is suitable for once-daily dosing.

Benzamide Derivatives

Analogues of the benzamide antiemetic and gastroparesis medication, metoclopramide, in which the side chain is incorporated into a pyrrolidine ring include S-(−)-sulpiride, S-(−)-remoxipride, and racemic amisulpride. Each is a potent D_2 receptor antagonist that displays antipsychotic properties.

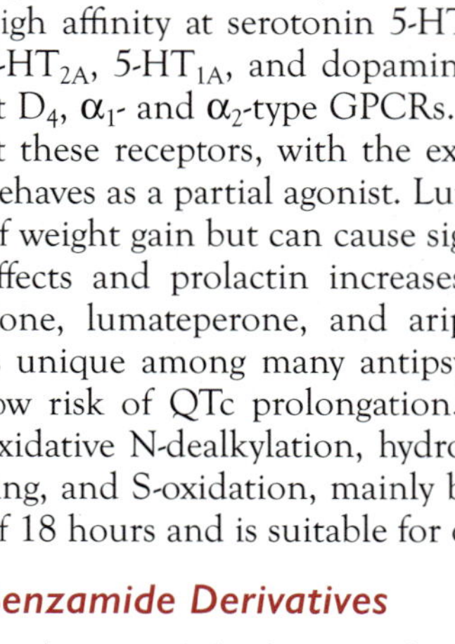

Metoclopramide (Reglan)

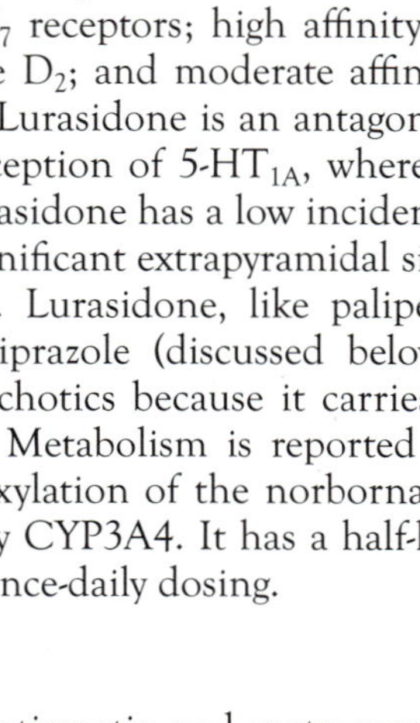

S-(-)-Sulpiride, R = H, R' = NH_2
Amisulpride, R = NH_2, R' = Et

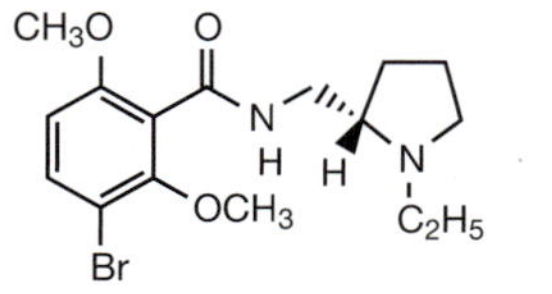

S-(-)-Remoxipride

Benzamide Derivatives

The hydrophilic properties of sulpiride might account for its poor oral absorption, limited penetration into the CNS and resulting low potency. Remoxipride was a promising antipsychotic that is comparable to haloperidol in potency and efficacy and has less incidence of extrapyramidal and autonomic side effects. Life-threatening aplastic anemia, however, was reported with remoxipride use, which prompted its withdrawal from the market.

AMISULPRIDE. The racemic para-amino congener of sulpiride, amisulpride, is used as an antipsychotic agent outside of the United States. [Within the United States, it is approved as a postoperative antiemetic under the brand name Barhemsys.] It is distinguished from other antipsychotics, because it has high affinity for dopamine D_2 and D_3 receptors, as well as $5\text{-}HT_{2B}$ and $5\text{-}HT_7$ receptors ($K_i <$ 15 nM); it has very low affinity (K_i = 1,000-10,000 nM) for all other common GPCR targets of antipsychotics, including $5\text{-}HT_{2A}$. A meta-analysis shows amisulpride to be the next most effective antipsychotic behind clozapine, and it can treat patients with predominant negative symptoms of schizophrenia.[43] Extrapyramidal effects, weight gain, sedation, and overall discontinuation rates are relatively low with amisulpride, especially at low doses that treat negative symptoms. Low extrapyramidal risk may be due to preferential blockade of mesolimbic compared to nigrostriatal D_2 and D_3 receptors, as shown in animal studies. QTc prolongation incidents with amisulpride treatment are high compared to most other antipsychotics. There are contraindications with citalopram and (S)-citalopram (escitalopram) because of increased risk of ventricular arrhythmia, particularly torsades de pointes. Amisulpride, like sulpiride, can also cause hyperprolactinemia.

Amisulpride bioavailability is 48%. It is poorly metabolized; two inactive metabolites account for only about 4% of the total amount of drug eliminated. Amisulpride is eliminated unchanged in the urine. Amisulpride does not accumulate, and its pharmacokinetics remain the same after repeated administration. The elimination half-life is approximately 12 hours after an oral dose.

Phenylpiperazines

ARIPIPRAZOLE (ABILIFY). Aripiprazole (Fig. 11.15)—available in several formulations—is an arylpiperazine quinolinone derivative that has received a lot of attention in the clinical and basic science literature. Aripiprazole has high affinity at $5\text{-}HT_{1A}$, $5\text{-}HT_{2A}$, and D_3 and very high affinity at D_2 receptors. Although its efficacy is not superior to other antipsychotic drugs, it has an improved side effect profile compared to that of many others. Aripiprazole does not prolong the QTc and causes relatively minimal weight gain.[43]

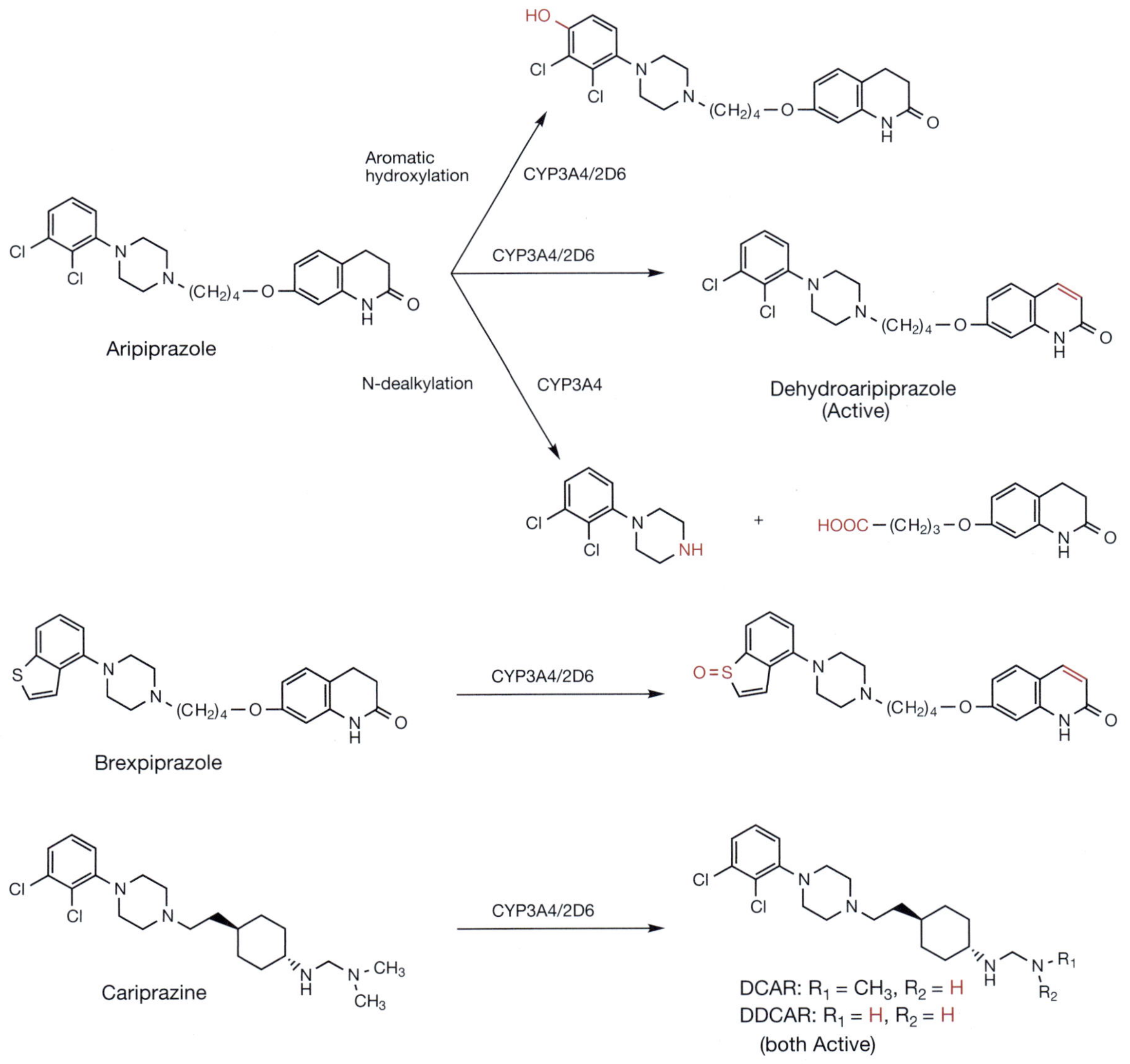

Figure 11.15 Structures and metabolism of aripiprazole, brexpiprazole, and cariprazine.

Also, despite its very high affinity at dopamine D_2, aripiprazole has a relatively low propensity to cause extrapyramidal symptoms, with the exception of akathisia (affecting ~10% of patients), and does not increase prolactin.[43,103] Partly, this may be explained by its GPCR functional profile.

Aripiprazole is a partial agonist at dopamine D_2, D_3, serotonin 5-HT_{1A}, and 5-HT_{2C} receptors—with efficacies depending on the cellular milieu—and is an antagonist at 5-HT_{2A} receptors.[57] Recall that prolonged D_2 blockade produces extrapyramidal and hyperprolactinemia side effects. As a D_2 receptor partial agonist with moderate intrinsic activity, aripiprazole may partially block D_2 receptor signaling in neural systems with high dopaminergic tone, that is, the striatal dopamine system of schizophrenic patients. Conversely, it may partially activate D_2 receptors in neural systems with low dopaminergic tone, that is, the mesocortical system in schizophrenic patients. This may account for its efficacy to treat psychoses.[80,104] Other proposed pharmacologic mechanisms focus on aripiprazole's full agonism at presynaptic D_2 autoreceptors in vivo in animal models.[57,80,104,105] D_2 autoreceptors modulate dopamine neurotransmission via a negative feedback mechanism. For example, at relatively high dopamine concentrations (or during phasic dopamine release), presynaptic D_2 autoreceptors are activated to decrease dopamine synthesis and release, and somatodendritic D_2 autoreceptors decrease neuronal firing rate. Striatal dopamine neurons express high levels of D_2 autoreceptors, whereas they are scantly expressed in the mesocortical dopamine pathway. Thus, aripiprazole, by acting as a D_2-autoreceptor agonist, may decrease dopaminergic tone selectively in the striatum. Combined with antagonist activity at postsynaptic D_2 receptors in vivo, this pharmacology may contribute to its unique clinical effects. Finally, aripiprazole's functional effects at the D_2 receptor vary depending on signaling pathway, cell type, and cellular context, providing evidence that it may be a biased agonist at the D_2 receptor in vivo. Aripiprazole's partial agonist activity at 5-HT_{1A} and 5-HT_{2C} receptors might also contribute to its efficacy for treating negative symptoms, and to its low propensity to induce weight gain, respectively.

Aripiprazole has high oral bioavailability (90%) with a half-life of approximately 75 hours. It undergoes hepatic CYP3A4- and CYP2D6-catalyzed N-dealkylation and hydroxylation as well as dehydrogenation to dehydroaripiprazole, which is an active metabolite with a half-life of about 90 hours. Recent preclinical data show that aripiprazole, as well as cariprazine (discussed later), and a common metabolite of each, 2,3-(dichlorophenyl) piperazine, inhibit cholesterol biosynthesis at the conversion of 7-dehydrocholesterol (7-DHC) to cholesterol.[106] The inhibition of this enzymatic step by mutations in the *DHCR7* gene leads to Smith-Lemli-Opitz syndrome, a severe developmental disorder that affects many parts of the body and causes intellectual and behavioral problems. Thus, risks associated with aripiprazole usage during pregnancy should be strongly considered.

BREXPIPRAZOLE (REXULTI). Brexpiprazole is a close analogue of aripiprazole and similarly, has been shown to be effective at treating positive and negative symptoms of schizophrenia, as measured by the PANSS. In addition to schizophrenia, brexpiprazole is also approved as an adjunctive treatment of major depressive disorder. Brexpiprazole has high affinity at many serotonin, α-adrenergic, and dopamine receptors. Brexpiprazole, compared to its predecessor aripiprazole, has at least 10-fold higher affinity at D_4, 5-HT_{1A}, 5-HT_{2A}, α_{1A}, α_{1B}, and α_{2C} and similar affinity at all other GPCRs tested.[107] Brexpiprazole exhibits D_2, D_3, 5-HT_{1A}, and 5-HT_{2C} partial agonism, similar to aripiprazole. However, brexpiprazole exhibits lower intrinsic activity at dopamine D_2 receptors relative to aripiprazole. Its functional activities at D_3 and 5-HT_{2C}, also, are very weak. It behaves as an antagonist at 5-HT_{2A}, 5-HT_{2B}, and α1- and α_2-type receptors. It also has inhibitory activity at the serotonin (IC_{50} = 29 nM) and norepinephrine (IC_{50} = 139 nM) transporters that is similar to fluoxetine.[107] This likely contributes to its antidepressant activity. Like aripiprazole, akathisia is a common adverse effect of brexpiprazole, but incidence is reportedly lower than aripiprazole, which might be due lower D_2 intrinsic activity. Other adverse events are comparable to placebo.

Brexpiprazole has high absolute bioavailability (95%), is highly bound to plasma protein (>99%), and undergoes CYP3A4 and CYP2D6 metabolic oxidation to the major inactive metabolite DM-3411, which apparently does not contribute to clinical effects. Various other oxidative metabolites have been reported. The terminal elimination half-lives of brexpiprazole and its major metabolite, DM-3411, are 91 hours and 86 hours, respectively.

CARIPRAZINE (VRAYLAR). Cariprazine is effective at treating both positive and negative symptoms of schizophrenia. A recent clinical trial reported superiority at treating negative symptoms compared to risperidone.[108] In addition to schizophrenia, cariprazine is also approved to treat manic or mixed episodes associated with bipolar I disorder in adults. Like its structurally similar counterparts, aripiprazole and brexpiprazole, cariprazine is a 5-HT_{1A}, dopamine D_2 and D_3 receptor partial agonist, with efficacies depending on cellular milieu. Cariprazine has very high affinity for both the D_2 and D_3 receptors, but is unique among antipsychotics for possessing higher selectivity for the dopamine D_3 receptor (D_3 K_i <0.1 nM; D_2 K_i <1 nM). This was corroborated in a clinical trial that showed preferential binding to D_3 in patients with schizophrenia when administered at low doses.[109] At doses 1.5 mg/d and higher, D_2 and D_3 receptor occupancy is at least 75%. In addition to the usual targets, cariprazine also shows moderate affinity for σ1 receptors. Long-term administration of cariprazine changes the expression of dopamine, serotonin, and glutamate receptor subtypes in multiple brain regions.[110,111]

Cariprazine is metabolized by CYP3A4 and to a lesser extent by CYP2D6 to two clinically active metabolites, desmethyl-cariprazine and didesmethyl-cariprazine, which are excreted in the urine with only a small amount of the unchanged parent drug. Cariprazine has a half-life of 2 to 4 days, and didesmethyl-cariprazine has a terminal half-life of 2 to 3 weeks. At high doses (>6 mg/d), there is increased incidence of extrapyramidal effects (akathisia and Parkinson disease symptoms) and hypertension.[112] Akathisia and other extrapyramidal symptoms were particularly high in patients treated with cariprazine—in some cases, 14% and 20% of patients reported these respective side effects (compared

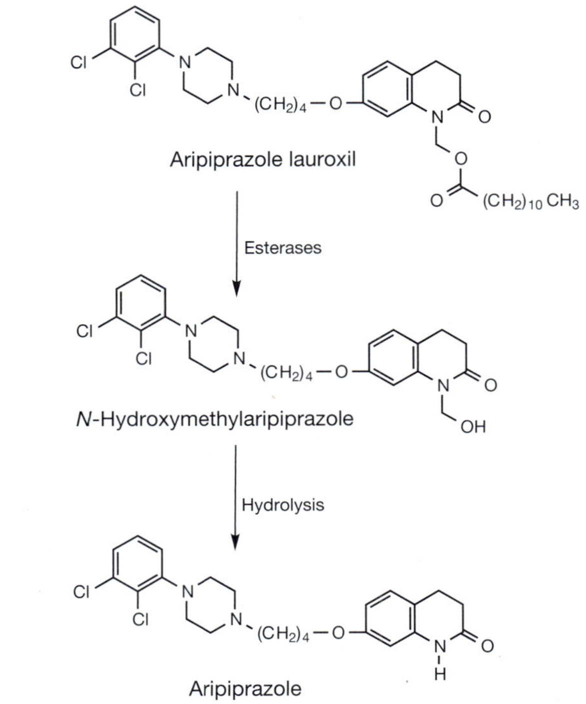

Figure 11.16 Hydrolysis of aripiprazole lauroxil to aripiprazole.

to 4% and 8% with placebo). Cariprazine (6 mg/d or less) showed no clinically relevant effects on QTc prolongation or prolactin elevation.

Long-Acting Antipsychotics

The duration of action of many of the antipsychotics with a free hydroxyl moiety can be considerably prolonged by the preparation of a long-chain fatty acid ester analogue. Fluphenazine decanoate and fluphenazine enanthate (the latter discontinued) were the first of such esters to appear in clinical use and are longer acting, with fewer side effects than the unesterified parent drug. The ability to treat patients with a single intramuscular injection every 1 to 2 weeks with the enanthate or every 2 to 3 weeks with the decanoate ester means that problems associated with patient compliance to the drug regimens and with drug malabsorption can be reduced.

Aripiprazole also is available in a long-acting form, aripiprazole lauroxil (Aristada). It is an intramuscular injectable formulation administered monthly, every 6 weeks, or every 2 months, depending on dose. Aripiprazole lauroxil undergoes esterase-catalyzed hydrolysis to *N*-hydroxymethyl aripiprazole, which is then hydrolyzed to aripiprazole (Fig. 11.16).[113]

Miscellaneous Medications

VALBENAZINE (INGREZZA) FOR TARDIVE DYSKINESIA. Tetrabenazine and its prodrug forms, deutetrabenazine and valbenazine (Fig. 11.17), are vesicular monoamine transporter 2 (VMAT2) inhibitors approved to treat tardive dyskinesia, a common extrapyramidal side effect of high-dose antipsychotics. Both tetrabenazine and deutetrabenazine also have been approved for treatment of chorea associated with Huntington

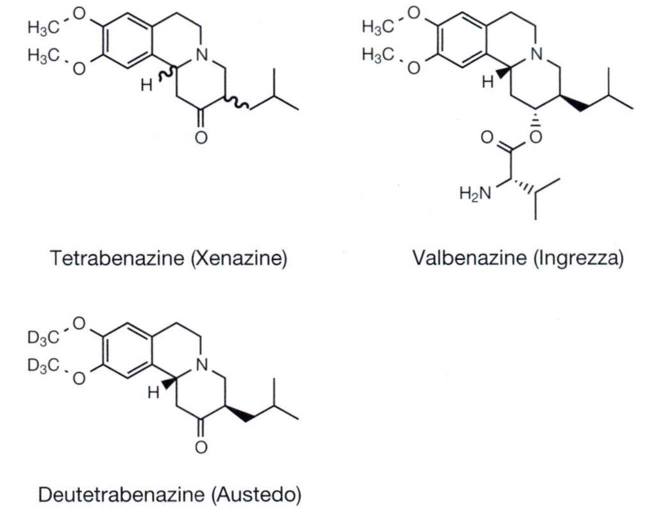

Figure 11.17 Structures of tetrabenazine and its prodrug forms valbenazine and deutetrabenazine.

disease. The keto moiety of tetrabenazine (an enantiomeric mixture) undergoes rapid and extensive hepatic metabolism by carbonyl reductase to an enantiomeric mixture of dihydrotetrabenazines (Fig. 11.18). Plasma concentrations of tetrabenazine are not detected after oral administration due to rapid metabolism to dihydrotetrabenazines. These then undergo oxidative demethylation by CYP2D6 to inactive metabolites that subsequently undergo phase II metabolism to sulfates and glucuronidates (Fig. 11.18). The half-life for tetrabenazine is 10 hours, whereas the half-life of the active drug metabolite, (*R*,*R*,*R*)-α-dihydrotetrabenazine, is 2 to 8 hours.

(*R*,*R*,*R*)-α-Dihydrotetrabenazine is active to inhibit VMAT2, an antiporter protein found within the membrane of dopamine vesicles. These vesicles regulate dopamine (and to a lesser extent serotonin and norepinephrine) uptake from the cytoplasm into synaptic vesicles, which stores neurotransmitters prior to their subsequent release

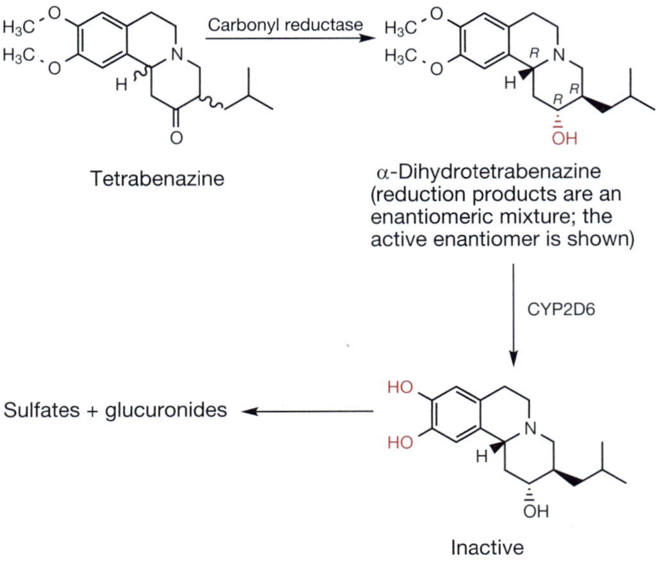

Figure 11.18 Metabolism of tetrabenazine.

into extracellular zones. Reversible binding of tetrabenazine to VMAT2 reduces storage and synaptic concentrations of dopamine. The reduction in synaptic dopamine levels is hypothesized to address the pathophysiology of tardive dyskinesia. Specifically, it is believed that prolonged antipsychotic drug blockade of dopamine receptors results in receptor hypersensitivity that leads to tardive dyskinesia. Reducing synaptic dopamine levels by VMAT2 inhibition decreases activity of dopamine receptors to alleviate tardive dyskinesia.

Valbenazine (see Fig. 11.17) is a single enantiomer prodrug form of tetrabenazine containing an L-valine ester moiety that is hydrolyzed in vivo to the single active enantiomer (*R*,*R*,*R*)-α-dihydrotetrabenazine.[114] The hydrolysis step occurs slowly; thus, valbenazine has a half-life of 15 hours. Deutetrabenazine[115] (see Fig. 11.17) is the first deuterated drug approved by the FDA (2017). Analogously to tetrabenazine, deutetrabenazine undergoes reduction to an enantiomeric mixture of deutdihydrotetrabenazines, with the active drug being the (*R*,*R*,*R*) enantiomer of α-deutdihydrotetrabenazine. The substitution of carbon-hydrogen with carbon-deuterium on the methoxy moiety of (*R*,*R*,*R*)-α-deutdihydrotetrabenazine is presumed to slow CYP2D6-catalyzed oxidative demethylation, resulting in a half-life of 9 hours for the active drug and a reduced dosing frequency for prodrug deutetrabenazine.

Sedation is the most common adverse effect of tetrabenazine and its analogues. The incidence of extrapyramidal symptoms is low and includes mainly dyskinesia, not akathisia. Tetrabenazine and its analogues carry a black box warning of the potential for depression and suicidality. Additionally, deutetrabenazine is contraindicated in patients with hepatic impairment, in patients taking monoamine oxidase inhibitors and in patients taking reserpine.

Pimavanserin (Nuplazid) for Parkinson Disease Psychosis.[50] Up to 60% of patients with Parkinson disease develop psychosis, which may be caused by dopamine agonist medications or may be related to pathology. Management often includes a reduction in dopaminergic medications or the introduction of an atypical antipsychotic medication, such as clozapine. The serious side effects associated with clozapine, such as metabolic syndrome, however, created an opportunity for new drug development that avoided direct targeting of dopamine receptors. Pimavanserin is a selective serotonin 5-HT_{2A} (and to a lesser extent 5-HT_{2C}) receptor inverse agonist approved for Parkinson disease psychosis in 2016. In a randomized, double-blind, placebo-controlled study, pimavanserin improved psychotic symptoms in patients with Parkinson disease, while also leading to improved sleep and decreased caregiver burden.[51] Pimavanserin is predominantly metabolized by CYP3A4 and CYP3A5; CYP3A4 is the major enzyme responsible for the formation of its major active metabolite. The half-life of pimavanserin is very long (54 hours), and it is recommended to reduce the dose by half if patients are also taking strong inhibitors of CYP3A4, such as ketoconazole.

Confusional state (6%), peripheral edema (7%), and hallucinations (7%, paradoxically) were reported side effects occurring in at least 5% of patients receiving pimavanserin that did not also occur at or above this frequency with placebo. There are no data on long-term efficacy and safety in patients with Parkinson disease, but it may prolong the QTc interval. Post-marketing side effects of pimavanserin reported include rash, urticaria, potential angioedema, and somnolence. Pimavanserin, like other antipsychotics, carries a black box warning of increased mortality in older adults with dementia-related psychosis. Pimavanserin is not currently approved for psychosis unrelated to Parkinson disease. However, in a phase 2, randomized, placebo-controlled, double-blind study, it was effective for Alzheimer disease psychosis after 6 weeks of treatment; effects did not endure to 12 weeks[116]; in 2022, the FDA responded they could not approve pimavanserin for Alzheimer disease psychosis, based on the current evidence submitted by Acadia, the drug maker.

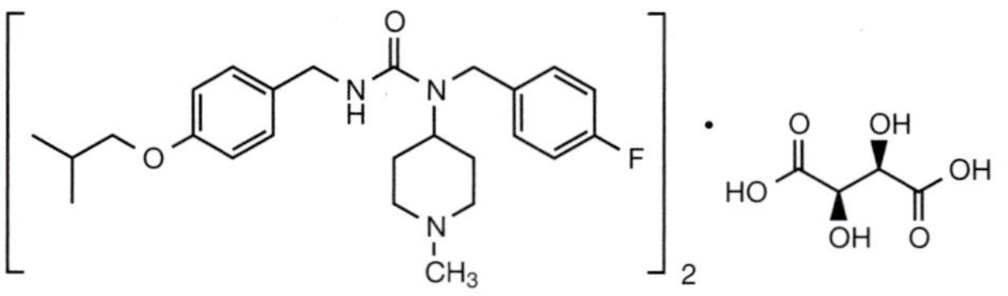

Pimavanserin tartrate (Nuplazid)

Anxiety Disorders

In the *DSM-5*, anxiety disorders include generalized anxiety disorder, separation anxiety disorder, social anxiety disorder (social phobia), specific phobia, panic disorder, agoraphobia, and selective mutism (a disorder in which a person normally capable of speech does not speak in specific situations or to certain people). Notably, anxiety disorders are considered separate from obsessive-compulsive disorders and trauma and stressor-related disorders (including posttraumatic stress disorder), albeit several of the drugs discussed in this chapter that target GABA receptors to treat anxiety disorders are often used to treat obsessive-compulsive disorder. To meet general *DSM-5* reference criteria, anxiety symptoms cannot be caused by an exogenous factor (eg, caffeine) or a medical condition (eg, hyperthyroidism), and at least three (one in children) of the following symptoms must occur more days than not for at least 6 months: restlessness, irritability, muscle tension, difficulty to concentrate, sleep disturbance, and fatigue. Moreover, an anxiety disorder diagnosis requires that the mental and/or physical symptoms impair social, occupational, and/or other important areas of functioning.

Etiology of Anxiety Disorders

Studies of patients with anxiety disorders have not revealed a general gross neuroanatomical lesion. In vivo functional imaging studies, however, show altered blood oxygen levels (as a manifestation of blood flow) or glucose utilization in specific brain areas in patients with anxiety conditions,[117,118] including panic disorder[119,120] and specific phobia,[121,122] mostly implicating the prefrontal cortex and limbic areas as being involved in pathologic anxiety. Although there is some evidence linking acid-sensitive channels and catechol-O-methyltransferase to panic disorder, genetic mechanisms underlying general symptoms of anxiety remain unclear. It is also important to note that there is a high degree of comorbidity for anxiety and major depressive disorder in both children and adults,[123,124] suggesting mechanistic overlap between the disorders. Indeed, first-line treatments for generalized anxiety disorder, panic disorder, and social anxiety disorder are the antidepressants selective serotonin reuptake inhibitors (SSRIs) and serotonin/norepinephrine reuptake inhibitors (SNRIs) (see Chapter 12).

A variety of neurotransmitters, neuromodulators (eg, adenosine), and neuropeptides (eg, cholecystokinin, corticotropin-releasing factor, and neuropeptide Y) are suggested to be involved in the pathophysiology of anxiety. Abundant evidence exists to document the involvement of the neurotransmitters GABA, glutamate, norepinephrine, serotonin, and dopamine in anxiety. Notably, most drugs effective for anxiety disorders affect one or several of these neurotransmitters. Anxiety disorders, however, are not simply a deficiency or excess of one neurotransmitter or another—research increasingly is revealing that these neurotransmitter systems have complex anatomical and functional interrelationships. Such complexity helps explain the unpredictable and sometimes paradoxical responses to medications.

GABA Receptors

The major inhibitory neurotransmitter in the mammalian CNS, GABA, is widespread with approximately one-third of all synapses in the CNS utilizing this neurochemical for intercellular communication. The two major classes of GABA receptors are inotropic $GABA_A$ and metabotropic $GABA_B$ receptors[125]. The so-called $\rho GABA_A$ receptor is the preferred term to describe a gene product that was identified, precloning, as a GABA receptor-like protein with pharmacology distinct from $GABA_A$ and $GABA_B$ receptors.[126] Based on primary sequence and function, $\rho GABA_A$ appears closely related to $GABA_A$ receptors, and it is currently recommended by the International Union of Pharmacology to not use the term "$GABA_C$" receptor to describe $\rho GABA_A$ receptors.[125]

$GABA_A$ Receptor

The $GABA_A$ receptor is a member of the gene superfamily of ligand-gated ion channels that is known as the "cys-loop" family because of the presence of a cysteine loop in their N-terminal domain. These receptors exist as heteropentameric subunits arranged around a central ion channel (Fig. 11.19A). Each of the five polypeptide subunits is composed of an extracellular region, four membrane-spanning α-helical cylinders, and a large intracellular cytoplasmic loop.

The second of the four membrane-spanning α-helical cylinders, from each of the five subunits, forms the $GABA_A$ ion channel, which conducts chloride to hyperpolarize the cell, for example, decreases the firing probability of a neuron. The first $GABA_A$ subunit was sequenced in 1987.[127] In humans, so far, 16 different genetically distinct subunits for the $GABA_A$ receptor have been isolated. These polypeptides are denoted as $\alpha_{1\text{-}6}$, $\beta_{1\text{-}3}$, $\gamma_{1\text{-}3}$, δ, ε, π, and θ. The subunits can combine in varied proportions and alternatively spliced variants are common. Thus, many possible receptor subtypes may exist. The major (60%) $GABA_A$ receptor isoform in the adult brain consists of two α_1 subunits, two β_2 subunits,

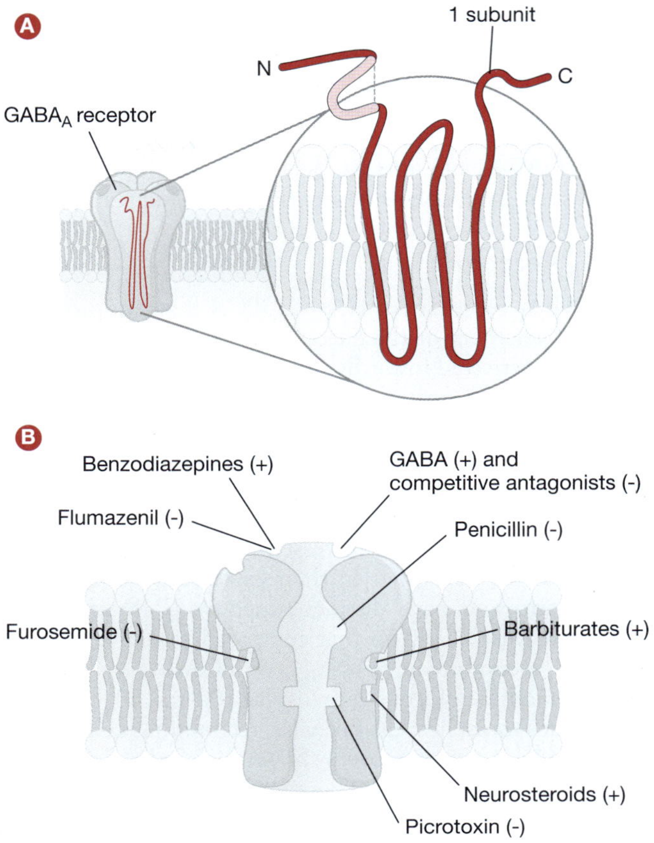

Figure 11.19 Schematic representation of the γ-aminobutyric $acid_A$ ($GABA_A$) receptor. A. $GABA_A$ receptors have a pentameric structure composed predominantly of α, β, and γ subunits arranged, in various proportions, around a central ion channel that conducts chloride (refer to text). Each subunit has four membrane-spanning regions and a cysteine loop in the extracellular *N*-terminal domain (dashed line). B. There are several unique ligand-binding sites on the $GABA_A$ receptor, where drugs can bind to impact $GABA_A$ receptor function. (From Chou J, Strichartz GR, Lo EA. Pharmacology of excitatory and inhibitory neurotransmission. In: Golan DE, ed. *Principles of Pharmacology*. Lippincott Williams & Wilkins; 2005:142; with permission.)

and one γ_2 subunit.[128] Recently, cryo-electron microscopy structures with overall resolution of 3.9 Å of the human $\alpha_1\beta_2\gamma_2$ $GABA_A$ receptor, bound to GABA and flumazenil (an antagonist of the site on the $GABA_A$ receptor where benzodiazepines bind, see below), were reported.[129] In contrast to $GABA_A$ receptors, ρ subunits alone can form functional homo- and heteropentameric $\rho GABA_A$ receptors. So far, three different human rho subunits ($\rho_{1\text{-}3}$) have been identified as structural components of the $\rho GABA_A$ receptor.

The $GABA_A$ receptor contains many distinct binding sites (Fig. 11.19B), including a site for GABA (orthosteric site) as well as sites where neuroactive drugs—for example, benzodiazepines, barbiturates, picrotoxin, ethanol, and neurosteroids (allosteric sites)—bind. The recently resolved $GABA_A$ crystal structure also revealed several additional binding sites that will likely aid in the design of novel $GABA_A$ targeting medication candidates. The orthosteric, GABA binding site is at the interface between α and β subunits, whereas the allosteric binding site for benzodiazepines, commonly prescribed as anxiolytic and sedative agents, is defined by the α and γ subunits. The distinct composition of α and γ subunits determines the affinity and efficacy of unique benzodiazepines, and specific positive allosteric modulation of distinct $GABA_A$ subunits (α, β, and γ) can produce distinct effects, such as anxiolysis or sedation (see Chapter 14).[130]

$GABA_B$ Receptors

The $GABA_B$ receptor is a class-C GPCR that can modulate (via $G\alpha_{i/o}$) activity of the effector proteins adenylyl cyclase, G protein–activated inwardly rectifying K^+ channels (GIRK) channels, and G protein–dependent neuronal Ca^{2+} channels. Like $GABA_A$, neurophysiological effects of $GABA_B$ signaling include hyperpolarization of neurons and inhibition of neurotransmitter release. The $GABA_B$ GPCR exists as two major subtypes, $GABA_{B(1)}$ and $GABA_{B(2)}$. The $GABA_{B(1)}$ subtype can be expressed as $GABA_{B(1a)}$ and $GABA_{B(1b)}$ isoforms that differ in their extracellular NH_2-terminal domains and have distinct functions.[131] Interestingly, it was discovered early on that compared to native $GABA_B$ receptors, recombinant $GABA_{B(1a)}$ and $GABA_{B(1b)}$ receptors expressed in heterologous cells display 100- to 150-fold lower affinity for agonist ligands. Likewise, recombinant $GABA_{B(1a)}$ and $GABA_{B(1b)}$ receptors were shown to couple inefficiently to their effector systems. These surprising pharmacologic findings were explained by the discovery that recombinant $GABA_{B(1a)}$ and $GABA_{B(1b)}$ receptors expressed in heterologous cells are retained in the endoplasmic reticulum. In fact, it turned out that $GABA_{B(1)}$ receptors do not traffic to the cell membrane surface in the absence of $GABA_{B(2)}$ receptors. This remarkable discovery that the $GABA_{B(2)}$ receptor co-expresses on the cell surface with the $GABA_{B(1a)}$ or $GABA_{B(1b)}$ receptor to form a functional heterodimeric GPCR was reported simultaneously by three research groups from the pharmaceutical industry in 1998.[132-134] $GABA_B$ receptors were the first GPCR shown to function not as a single protein but rather, as two distinct subunits, neither of which is functional by itself (Fig. 11.20). Recently, it was determined that the $GABA_B$ receptor is also expressed on the

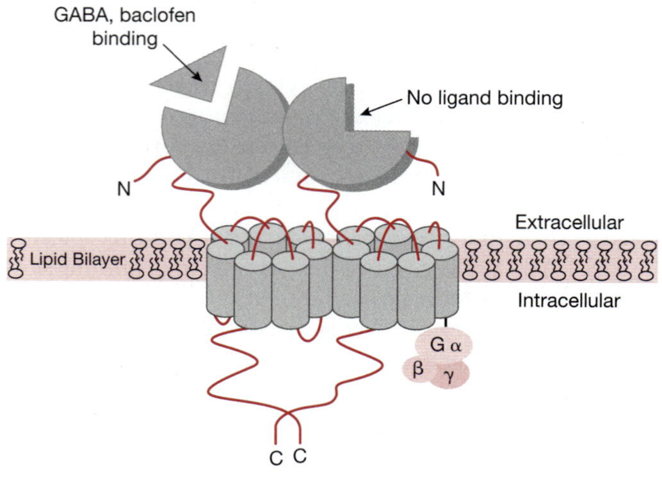

Figure 11.20 Schematic representation of the γ-aminobutyric $acid_B$ ($GABA_B$) receptor.

cell surface as a large oligomeric complex.[135] Homo- and/or heterodimerization, as well as oligomerization, has been documented for many GPCRs and may account for the diverse signaling functionality for this protein family.

The solved structure[136,137] of the extracellular orthosteric ligand-binding region of the heterodimeric $GABA_{B(1b)}$/$GABA_{B(2)}$ GPCR is very different and considerably more complex in comparison to other aminergic GPCRs that are able to function as monomers. In accordance with the Venus flytrap model for class-C GPCRs,[138] the extracellular domains of the $GABA_{B(1b)}$ and $GABA_{B(2)}$ subunits each are a pair of globular lobes, with a hinge region separating each lobe within the pair. Only the $GABA_{B(1b)}$ subunit binds orthosteric ligands, while the $GABA_{B(2)}$ unit couples with G protein. The $GABA_{B(2)}$ subunit also interacts with potassium channel tetramerization-domain proteins that modulate kinetic parameters of G protein signaling. Upon binding of an orthosteric agonist (eg, GABA or the clinical drug baclofen) to the $GABA_{B(1b)}$ subunit, the flytrap closes and the $GABA_B$ receptor is activated.[139] Binding of an antagonist ligand (usually containing a bulky chemical moiety) to the $GABA_{B(1b)}$ subunit sterically hinders flytrap closure and stabilizes an inactive conformation of receptor. The $GABA_{B(1a)}$ subunit is proposed to possess the same ligand-binding function within the heteromer as the $GABA_{B(1b)}$ subunit.

$GABA_B$ receptors are reported to play a role in the pathophysiology and perhaps pharmacotherapy of a variety of CNS diseases and disorders, including Alzheimer disease, addiction (especially ethanol), anxiety, autism spectrum disorder, fragile X syndrome, depression, epilepsy, Huntington disease, pain, Parkinson disease, schizophrenia, and stroke, as well as muscle spasticity disorders and gastroesophageal reflux. The only drug currently in clinical use that selectively interacts with the $GABA_B$ receptor is baclofen (β-*p*-chlorophenyl-GABA). Baclofen was first synthesized in 1962 and was shown to have potent muscle relaxant and analgesic activity. In 1972, the R/S racemate was marketed (Lioresal) to treat spasticity disorders. In 1980, the *R*-(−)-enantiomer of baclofen was shown to stereoselectively interact as an agonist with what is now known as the $GABA_B$ receptor. Currently, baclofen is indicated only for the relief of muscle spasticity in patients with multiple sclerosis and spinal cord injuries. It is proposed that baclofen inhibits spinal cord monosynaptic and polysynaptic reflexes via $GABA_B$ receptor–mediated opening of neuronal potassium channels that leads to hyperpolarization of primary afferent fiber terminals. In spinal motor neurons, baclofen suppresses excitability by reducing calcium persistent inward currents. Baclofen is used off-label to treat some of the many other conditions thought to involve $GABA_B$ receptors (as listed above), including anxiety, especially associated with alcohol withdrawal, albeit there currently is not compelling evidence $GABA_B$ receptors play a major role in the pathophysiology or pharmacotherapy of anxiety disorders. Although baclofen is rapidly absorbed after oral administration, absorption is mainly limited to the upper small intestine, and therapeutic concentrations in brain are difficult to achieve because it is transported out of the brain via the organic acid transporter. Baclofen also has a short duration of action (half-life 3-4 hours) and is rapidly cleared from circulation, largely eliminated unchanged, via renal excretion.

The investigational compound, arbaclofen placarbil, is a prodrug of (*R*)-baclofen developed to enhance oral absorption compared to the parent compound.[140] After oral administration, arbaclofen placarbil is efficiently absorbed and rapidly converted to *R*-baclofen. Although arbaclofen has been studied to treat symptoms of autism and fragile X syndrome, convincing efficacy has not been established and the prodrug has not been approved. Adverse effects with oral baclofen include muscle weakness, nausea, somnolence, and paresthesia. Rapid tolerance to its therapeutic effects occurs. Intrathecal baclofen can bypass the difficulty to obtain therapeutic CNS concentrations via oral administration, allowing for a minimized dose and perhaps minimized untoward effects.

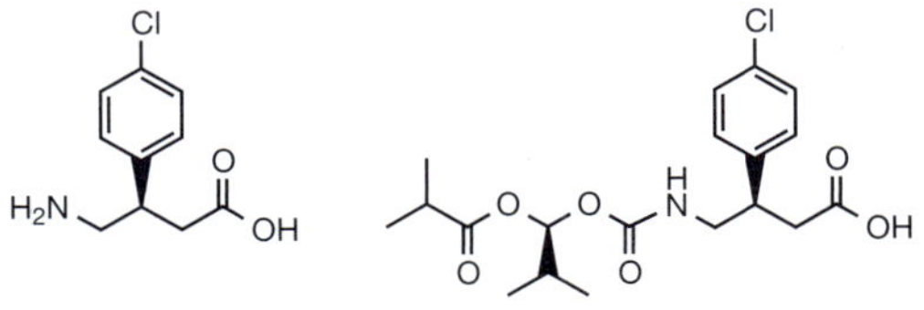

R-(-)-Baclofen Arbaclofen placarbil

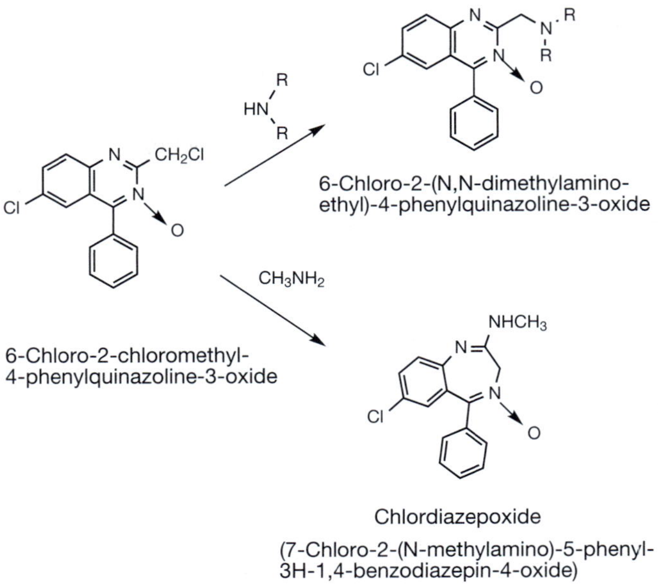

Figure 11.21 Synthesis of chlordiazepoxide.

Drugs Targeting $GABA_A$ Receptors for the Treatment of Anxiety

Benzodiazepines

Benzodiazepines are efficacious drugs for treating anxiety disorders, including generalized anxiety, social anxiety, and panic disorders. Some are also approved to treat seizures and alcohol withdrawal symptoms. Benzodiazepines are not first-line pharmacotherapies for anxiety disorders owing to rapid tolerance, dependency, abuse, and overdose liabilities. Furthermore, long-term use (beyond a few weeks) is not recommended, as discontinuation increases the risk of death. Benzodiazepines vary considerably in their pharmacokinetics and anxiolytic potencies, and several dose-equivalency conversion tools are easily accessible on the internet. Triazolam is the most potent approved benzodiazepine—1 mg, orally, is equivalent to 2-mg alprazolam (the second most potent) and 75 mg of chlordiazepoxide.

Chlordiazepoxide was the first benzodiazepine to be marketed for clinical use in 1960. Its effectiveness and safety margin were major advances over previously used drugs, such as barbiturates, that possess greater health risks. A variety of new benzodiazepines followed. The major factors to be considered when selecting a benzodiazepine include rate and extent of absorption, presence or absence of active metabolites, and degree of lipophilicity. These factors help determine how a benzodiazepine is marketed and used; for example, an agent that is rapidly absorbed and fast-acting, such as alprazolam, is approved to treat panic attacks, which often occur quickly and unexpectedly.

Development of Benzodiazepine Anxiolytics. In the 1950s, the medicinal chemist Sternbach noted that "basic groups frequently impart biological activity," and in accordance with this observation, he synthesized, at the New Jersey laboratories of Hoffman LaRoche, a series of compounds by treating various chloromethylquinazoline *N*-oxides with amines to produce what he hoped would be products with "tranquilizer" activity.[141,142] Studies by Sternbach included the reaction of 6-chloro-2-chloromethyl-4-phenylquinazoline-3-oxide with methylamine, which yielded the unexpected rearrangement product 7-chloro-2-(*N*-methylamino)-5-phenyl-3H-1, 4,-benzodiazepin-4-oxide (Fig. 11.21). This product was given the code name RO 50690 and screened for pharmacological activity in 1957. Subsequently, Randall et al[143,144] reported that RO 50690 was hypnotic and sedative and had anti-strychnine properties similar to the propanediol meprobamate, a sedative that has tranquilizer (anxiolytic) properties only at intoxicating doses. Renamed chlordiazepoxide, RO 50690 was marketed in 1960 as Librium, a safe and effective anxiolytic agent.

Chlordiazepoxide turned out to have rather remarkable pharmacological properties and tremendous potential as a pharmacotherapeutic agent, but it possessed a number of unacceptable physical chemical properties. In an effort to enhance its "pharmaceutical elegance," structural modifications of chlordiazepoxide were undertaken that eventually led to the synthesis of diazepam in 1959. In contrast to the maxim that basic groups impart biological activity, diazepam contains no basic nitrogen moiety. Diazepam, however, was found to be 3- to 10-fold more potent than chlordiazepoxide and was marketed in 1963 as the anxiolytic drug Valium. Subsequently, thousands of benzodiazepine derivatives were synthesized, and more than 10 benzodiazepines are in clinical use in the United States (Fig. 11.22).

A major advance in the benzodiazepine field was made in 1981 with the first report that the imidazobenzodiazepinone derivative, flumazenil, binds with high affinity to the benzodiazepine binding site and blocks the pharmacological effects of the classical benzodiazepines in vitro and in vivo.[149] Binding of [^{3}H]flumazenil to the benzodiazepine binding site is not affected by GABA and has no intrinsic activity of its own.[150] It is therefore a neutral antagonist. Flumazenil is used clinically to reverse benzodiazepine-induced sedation in overdose.

BENZODIAZEPINE BINDING-SITE LIGANDS

An endogenous ligand with affinity for the CNS benzodiazepine binding site of the $GABA_A$ receptor complex has not been identified conclusively. Several compounds of endogenous origin, however, that inhibit the binding of radiolabeled benzodiazepines to the benzodiazepine binding site have been reported. In 1980, Braestrup et al[145] reported the presence of β-carboline-3-carboxylic acid ethyl ester (βCCE) in normal human urine, which has very high affinity for the benzodiazepine binding site complex. It was subsequently shown, however, that βCCE formed as an artifact from Braestrup's extraction procedure, during which the urine extract was heated with ethanol at pH 1, a condition favoring formation of the ethyl ester from β-carboline-3-carboxylic acid, a tryptophan metabolite.

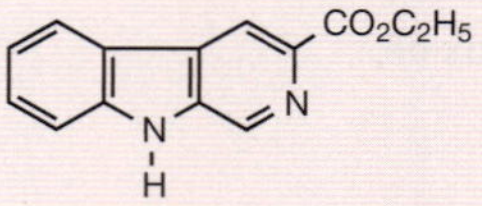

βCCE

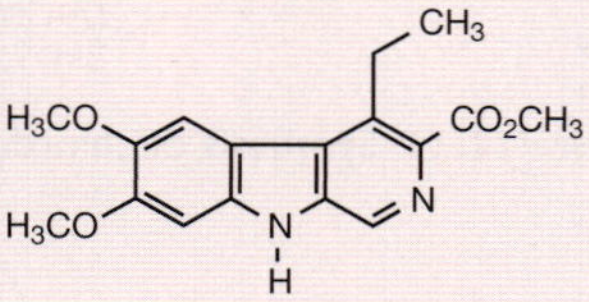

DMCM

Beta-carboline

Although βCCE actually was shown not to be of endogenous origin, its discovery as a high-affinity benzodiazepine binding site ligand stimulated research that led to the synthesis of a series of β-carboline derivatives with a variety of intrinsic activities, presumably mediated through the benzodiazepine binding site on the $GABA_A$ receptor. For example, although βCCE is considered to be a partial inverse agonist at this site, 6,7-dimethoxy-4-ethyl-β-carboline-3-carboxylic acid methyl ester (DMCM) appears to be a full inverse agonist.[146] In fact, βCCE blocks the convulsions produced by DMCM.[147] βCCE has approximately 10-fold higher affinity for the benzodiazepine binding site labeled by [^{3}H]diazepam than DMCM.[148] The β-carbolines currently are important research tools to probe the agonist, competitive antagonist, inverse agonist, and partial agonist/inverse agonist pharmacophores of the benzodiazepine binding site/on the $GABA_A$ receptor.

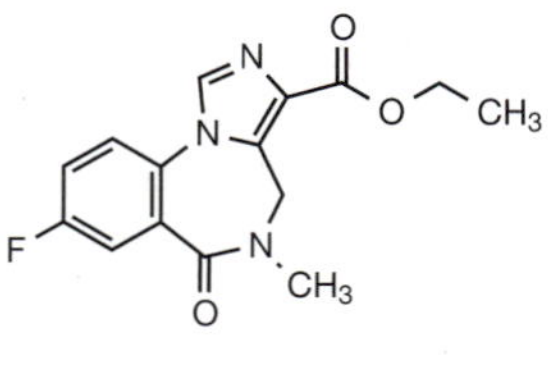

Flumazenil

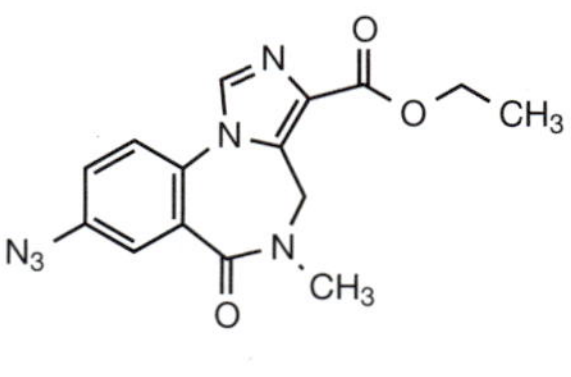

RO 15-4513

Mechanism of Action of Anxiolytic Benzodiazepines. A representation of the relationship between ligand interaction with the benzodiazepine binding site and intrinsic activity to modulate $GABA_A$ receptor function is shown in Figure 11.23. Anxiolytic benzodiazepines indirectly alter transmembrane chloride conduction to produce their anxiolytic effects; they are positive allosteric modulators (PAMs) of GABA binding to $GABA_A$. When an anxiolytic benzodiazepine binds to the benzodiazepine site, it greatly increases the affinity of GABA at $GABA_A$, which leads to a strong potentiation of chloride conductance through the channel and an increase in cell hyperpolarization (eg, decreases activity of a neuron). Neutral antagonist benzodiazepines, such as flumazenil, bind to the benzodiazepine site, but have no effect on the intrinsic activity of the $GABA_A$ receptor. That is, they do not affect chloride conductance. Neutral antagonists, however, block access of other drugs (eg, PAMs and negative allosteric modulators) to the site—for example, RO 15-4513. Negative allosteric modulators (or inverse agonists), such as RO 15-4513, bind to the benzodiazepine site and decrease GABA binding, which decreases chloride conductance through the channel, leading to cell depolarization (eg, increases activity of a neuron).

The benzodiazepine site can be rendered benzodiazepine-insensitive by a point mutation in the α subunit, replacing a critical histidine residue for arginine.[151] The affinity, intrinsic activity, and efficacy of benzodiazepines are determined by the nature of both the α and γ subunits. Different α and γ subunit compositions give rise to subtypes of the $GABA_A$ receptor that are pharmacologically distinct with regard to ligand affinity and intrinsic activity, providing a mechanistic basis for development of ligands that are anxioselective (ie, anxiolysis in the absence of sedation, muscle relaxation, amnesia, and ataxia). Thus, current drug discovery approaches target specific α and γ molecular subunits of the $GABA_A$ receptor in the quest for benzodiazepine and nonbenzodiazepine (see later) drugs that demonstrate anxioselectivity. In studies using nonhuman primates, it was suggested several decades ago that $GABA_A$ α_2, α_3, and α_5 subunits mediate anxiolytic and muscle relaxant effects of benzodiazepines, whereas α_1 receptors mediate the sedative effects.[152] Currently used benzodiazepines, however, are not selective for particular α subtypes. Several putative anxioselective benzodiazepines have reached the clinic; however, they have not exhibited the degree of anxioselectivity predicted from preclinical testing and, usually, have lower efficacy than standard benzodiazepines.

Structure-Activity Relationships. Thousands of benzodiazepine derivatives with a variety of substituents have been synthesized that interact with the benzodiazepine site, and structure-activity relationships for classical 5-phenyl-1,4-benzodiazepine-2-one anxiolytic agents are well known. Most pharmacophore models that describe ligand functional activity are based on binding activity at a single benzodiazepine site, and this approach is used here to summarize the structure-activity relationship for benzodiazepine derivatives.

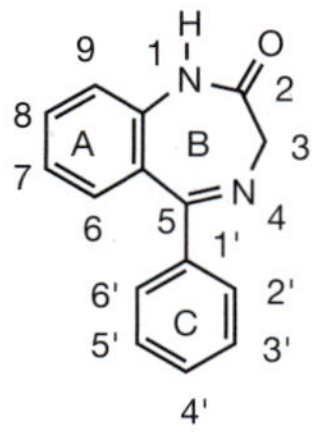

Benzodiazepine structure

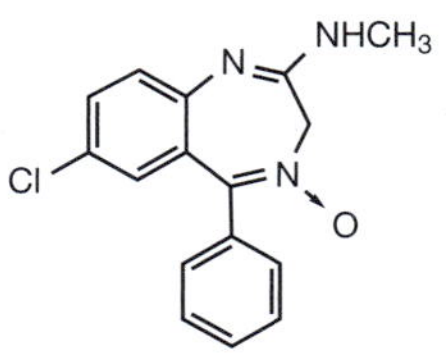

Chlordiazepoxide
(Librium)

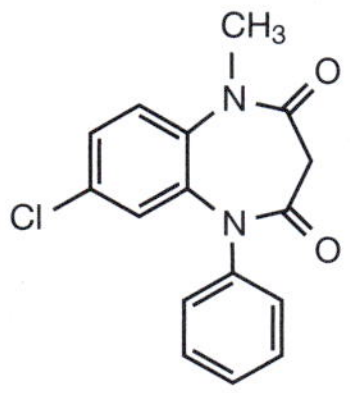

Clobazam
(Frisium)

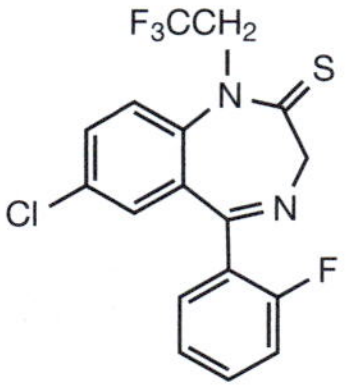

Quazepam
(Doral)

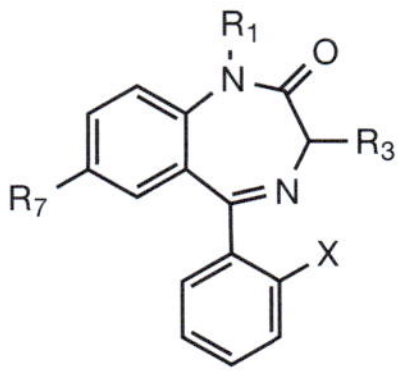

Class A
Benzodiazepines

Generic name	Trade name	R_1	R_3	R_7	X
Clonazepam	Klonopin	H	H	NO_2	Cl
Clorazepate	Tranxene	H	COOH	Cl	H
Diazepam	Valium	CH_3	H	Cl	H
Flurazepam	Generic	$(CH_2)_2NC_2H_5)_2$	H	Cl	F
Lorazepam	Ativan	H	OH	Cl	Cl
Oxazepam	Generic	H	OH	Cl	H
Temazepam	Restoril	CH_3	OH	Cl	H

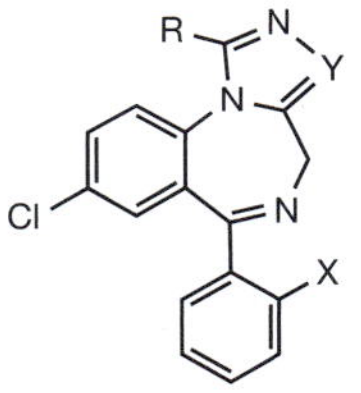

Class B
Benzodiazepines

Generic name	Trade name	R	X	Y
Alprazolam	Xanax	CH_3	H	N
Estazolam	ProSom	H	H	N
Midazolam	Versed	CH_3	F	CH
Triazolam	Halcion	CH_3	Cl	N

Figure 11.22 Structures of some commercially available anxiolytic benzodiazepines.

Ring A. In general, the minimum requirement for binding of 5-phenyl-1,4-benzodiazepin-2-one derivatives to the benzodiazepine site includes an aromatic or heteroaromatic ring (ring A), which is believed to participate in π-π stacking with aromatic amino acid residues of the receptor. Substituents on ring A have varied effects on binding of benzodiazepines to the benzodiazepine site, but such effects are not predictable on the basis of electronic or (within reasonable limits) steric properties. It is generally true, however, that an electronegative group (eg, halogen or nitro) substituted at the 7-position markedly increases functional anxiolytic activity, albeit effects on binding affinity in vitro are not as dramatic. On the other hand, substituents at positions 6, 8, or 9 generally decrease anxiolytic activity. Other 1,4-diazepine derivatives in which ring A is replaced by a heterocycle generally show weak binding affinity in vitro and even less pharmacological activity in vivo when compared to phenyl-substituted analogues.

Ring B. A proton-accepting group is believed to be a structural requirement of both benzodiazepine and nonbenzodiazepine ligand binding to the $GABA_A$ receptor, putatively for interactions with a histidine residue that serves as a proton source in the $GABA_A$ α_1 subunit. For the benzodiazepines, optimal affinity occurs when the proton-accepting group in the 2-position of ring B (ie, the carbonyl moiety) is in a coplanar spatial orientation with the

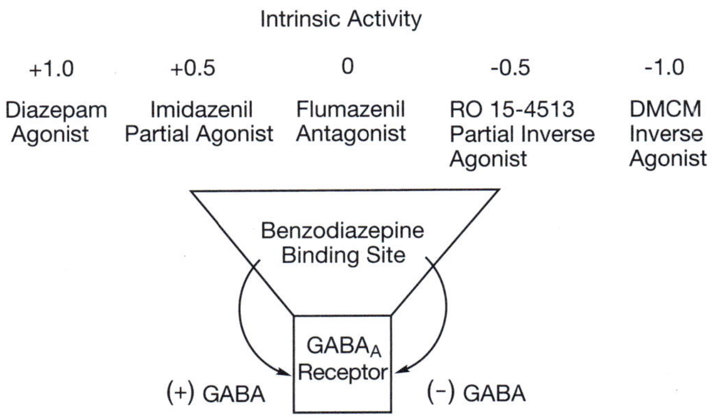

Figure 11.23 Ligand interaction with the γ-aminobutyric acid A ($GABA_A$) benzodiazepine binding site. Drugs with a range of different chemical structures, which produce different pharmacological activity, bind at the $GABA_A$ benzodiazepine binding site to modulate GABA binding at the $GABA_A$ receptor. Certain drugs (eg, flumazenil) can block the binding of other drugs to the benzodiazepine binding site.

aromatic ring A. Substitution of sulfur for oxygen at the 2-position may affect selectivity for binding to GABA receptors, but anxiolytic activity is maintained. Substitution of the methylene 3-position or the imine nitrogen is sterically unfavorable for antagonist activity but has no effect on PAM (ie, anxiolytic) activity. Derivatives substituted with a 3-hydroxy moiety have potency comparable to nonhydroxylated analogues and are excreted faster. Esterification of a 3-hydroxy moiety also is possible without loss of potency. Neither the 1-position amide nitrogen nor its substituent is required for in vitro binding to the benzodiazepine site, and many clinically used analogues are not N-alkylated (see Fig. 11.22). Although even relatively long *N*-alkyl side chains do not dramatically decrease affinity, sterically large substituents like tert-butyl drastically reduce receptor affinity and in vivo activity. Neither the 4,5-double bond nor the 4-position nitrogen (the 4,5-[methyleneimino] group) in ring B is required for in vivo anxiolytic activity, albeit in vitro affinity is decreased if the C=N bond is reduced to C–N. It is proposed that in vivo activity of such derivatives results from oxidation back to C=N. It follows that the 4-oxide moiety of chlordiazepoxide can be removed without loss of anxiolytic activity.

Ring C. Ring C (5-phenyl) is not required for binding to the benzodiazepine site in vitro. This accessory aromatic ring may contribute favorable hydrophobic or steric interactions to receptor binding, however, and its relationship to ring A planarity may be important. Substitution at the 4′-(para)-position of an appended 5-phenyl ring is unfavorable for PAM activity, but 2′-(ortho)-substituents are not detrimental, suggesting that limitations at the para position are steric, rather than electronic, in nature.

1,2-Annelation. Annelating the 1,2-bond of ring B with an additional "electron-rich" (ie, proton acceptor) ring, such as *S*-triazole or imidazole, also results in pharmacologically active benzodiazepine derivatives with high affinity for the benzodiazepine site. For example, the *S*-triazolobenzodiazepines triazolam, alprazolam, and estazolam and the imidazo-benzodiazepine midazolam are clinically effective anxiolytic agents (see Fig. 11.22).

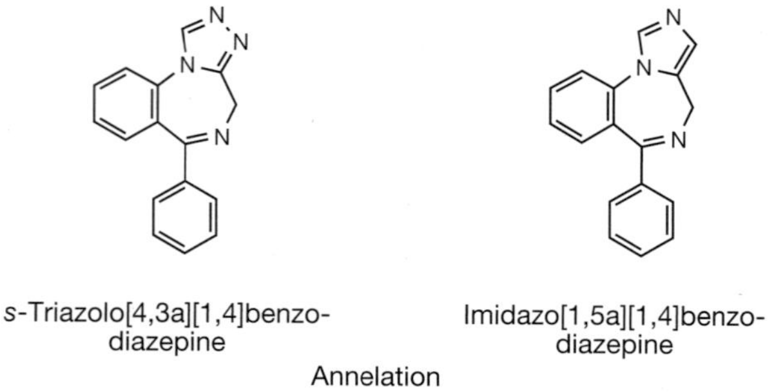

Annelation

STEREOCHEMISTRY. Most clinically useful benzodiazepines do not have a chiral center; however, the seven-membered ring B may adopt one of the two possible boat conformations, *a* and *b*, that are "enantiomeric" (mirror images) to each other. Nuclear magnetic resonance studies indicate that the two conformations can easily interconvert at room temperature, making it impossible to predict which conformation is active at the benzodiazepine site, a priori. Evidence for stereospecificity for binding to the benzodiazepine site was provided by introducing a 3-substituent into the benzodiazepine nucleus to provide a chiral center and enantiomeric pairs of derivatives. In vitro binding affinity and in vivo anxiolytic activity of several 3-methylated enantiomers were found to reside in the *S*-isomer. Moreover, the *S*-enantiomer of 3-methyldiazepam was shown to stabilize conformation *a* for ring B, whereas the *R*-enantiomer stabilizes conformation *b*. Also, the 3-S configuration and *a* conformation for ring B is present in both the crystalline state[153] and in solution[154] for 3-methyldiazepam. In spite of the enantioselectivity demonstrated for benzodiazepines, the commonly used 3-hydroxylated derivatives (eg, lorazepam and oxazepam) are commercially available only as racemic mixtures.

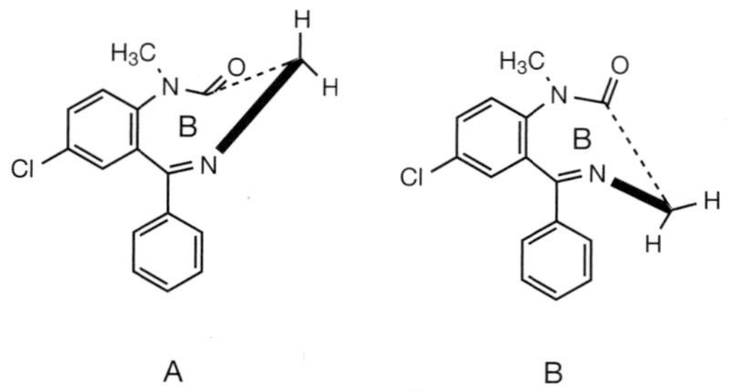

Stereochemistry

PHYSIOCHEMICAL AND PHARMACOKINETICS. The physiochemical and pharmacokinetic properties of the various benzodiazepines vary widely, and these properties have clinical implications. For example, depending on the nature of substituents, particularly with regard to electronegative substituents, the lipophilicity of the benzodiazepines may vary by more than three orders of magnitude, which affects absorption, distribution, and metabolism. In general, most benzodiazepines have relatively high lipid:water partition coefficients (Log *P* values) and are completely absorbed after oral administration and rapidly distributed to the brain and other highly perfused organs. A notable exception is clorazepate that is rapidly decarboxylated at the 3-position to *N*-desmethyldiazepam and, subsequently, quickly absorbed. Overall, clorazepate clinical and pharmacokinetic properties are similar to chlordiazepoxide and diazepam (see later).

Most benzodiazepines and their metabolites bind to plasma proteins. The degree of protein binding is dependent on lipophilicity of the compound and varies from approximately 70% for more polar benzodiazepines, such as alprazolam, to 99% for very lipophilic derivatives, such as diazepam. As shown in Figure 11.24, hepatic microsomal oxidation, including N-dealkylation and aliphatic hydroxylation by a wide variety of CYP enzymes, accounts for the major metabolic disposition of most benzodiazepines. Subsequent conjugation of microsomal metabolites by glucuronyl transferases yields polar glucuronides that are excreted in urine. In general, the rate and product of benzodiazepine metabolism varies, depending on route of administration and the individual drug.

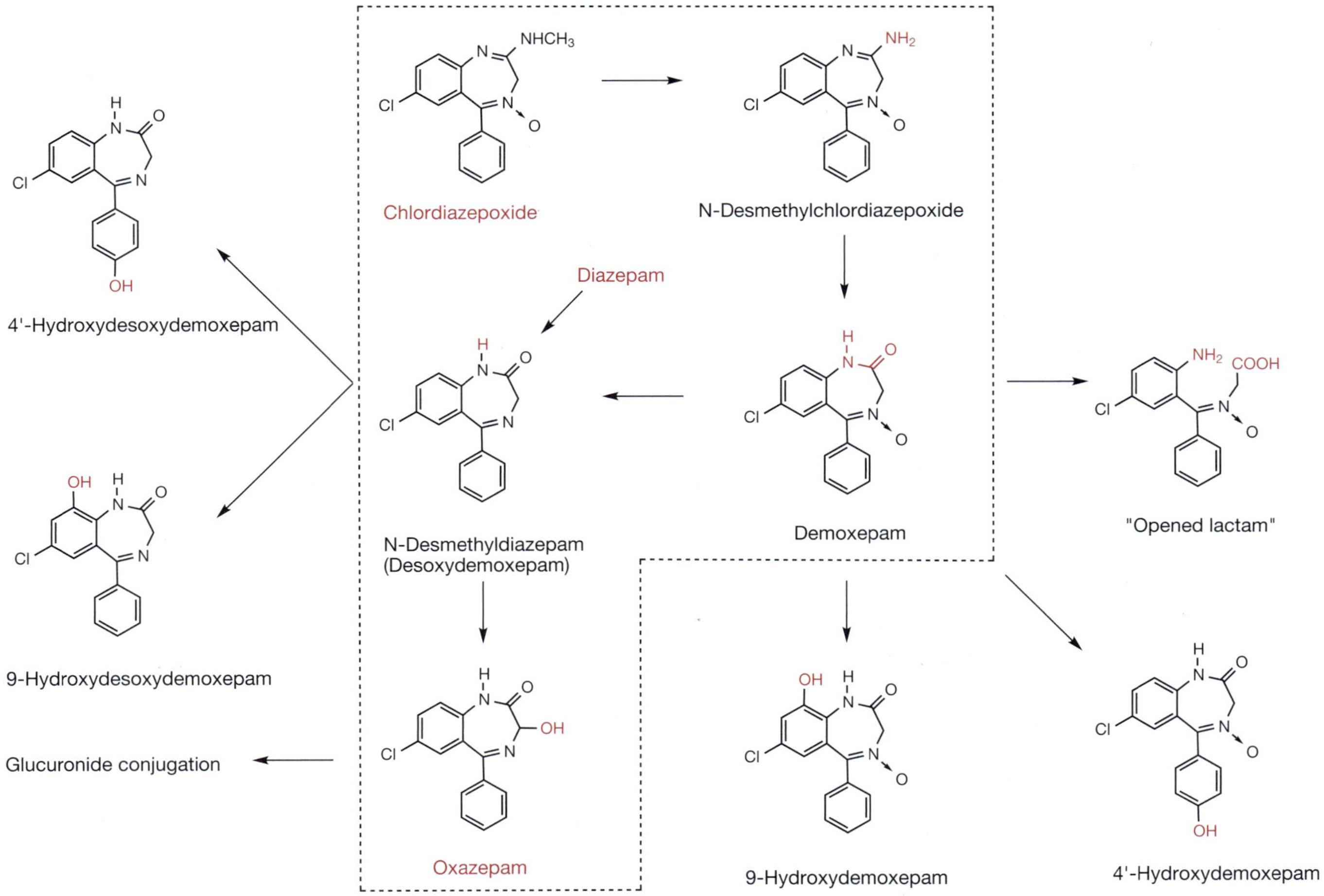

Figure 11.24 Metabolism of chlordiazepoxide and related benzodiazepines.

Specific Drugs

Alprazolam (Xanax). Alprazolam is a benzodiazepine approved to treat anxiety as well as panic disorders. Intriguingly, before the development of alprazolam, panic disorder was not a defined disorder in the DSM. Alprazolam is rapidly absorbed after oral administration and reaches peak plasma concentrations in 1 to 2 hours. Alprazolam's fast onset is why it is a preferred benzodiazepine for panic disorder, as panic attacks are severe and often occur unexpectedly. It has a volume of distribution of 0.8 to 1.3 L/kg and a plasma protein binding of 80%. It is extensively metabolized primarily to 4-hydroxyalprazolam and α-hydroxyalprazolam—which have less potency and activity than the parent drug—by CYP3A4. Thus, it is contraindicated in patients taking strong CYP3A4 inhibitors, except ritonavir. The elimination half-life of alprazolam is about 11.2 hours, but it can vary depending on age, hepatic function, and concomitant drug use. Like other benzodiazepines, alprazolam has a high potential for abuse, which can lead to overdose or death, especially when combined with alcohol or μ-opioid agonists. It can also cause withdrawal symptoms if discontinued abruptly.

Chlordiazepoxide. Chlordiazepoxide is well absorbed after oral administration, and peak blood concentration usually is reached in approximately 4 hours. Intramuscular absorption of chlordiazepoxide, however, is slower and erratic. The half-life of chlordiazepoxide is variable but usually quite long (6-30 hours). Hepatic metabolism is mainly by CYP3A4 to give the initial N-desmethylation product, N-desmethylchlordiazepoxide. This metabolite undergoes deamination to form the demoxepam (see Fig. 11.24), which is extensively metabolized, with less than 1% of a dose of chlordiazepoxide excreted as demoxepam. Demoxepam can undergo four different metabolic fates. Removal of the N-oxide moiety yields the active metabolite, N-desmethyldiazepam (desoxydemoxepam). This product is a metabolite of both chlordiazepoxide and diazepam and can be hydroxylated to yield oxazepam, another active metabolite that is rapidly glucuronidated and excreted in the urine. Another possibility for metabolism of demoxepam is hydrolysis to the "opened lactam," which is inactive (see Fig. 11.24). The two other metabolites of demoxepam are the products of ring A hydroxylation (9-hydroxydemoxepam) or ring C hydroxylation (4′-hydroxydemoxepam), both of which are inactive. The majority of a dose of chlordiazepoxide is excreted as glucuronide conjugates of oxazepam and other phenolic (9- or 4′-hydroxylated) metabolites. As with diazepam (see next), repeated administration of chlordiazepoxide can result in accumulation of parent drug and its active metabolites, which may have important clinical implications, including excessive sedation.

Diazepam. Diazepam is rapidly and completely absorbed after oral administration. (There are several other formulations, including in a rectal gel to treat seizures.) Maximum peak blood concentration after oral administration occurs in 2 hours, and elimination is slow, with a half-life of approximately 20 to 50 hours. As with chlordiazepoxide, the major metabolic product of diazepam, generated by CYP3A4, is *N*-desmethyldiazepam, which is pharmacologically active and undergoes even slower metabolism than its parent compound. Repeated administration of diazepam (or chlordiazepoxide) leads to accumulation of *N*-desmethyldiazepam, which can be detected in the blood for more than 1 week after discontinuation of the drug. Hydroxylation of *N*-desmethyldiazepam at the 3-position gives the active metabolite oxazepam (see Fig. 11.24).

FLURAZEPAM. Flurazepam, approved for insomnia, is administered orally as the dihydrochloride salt. It is rapidly N-dealkylated primarily by CYP3A4 to produce *N*1-desalkylflurazepam, and it subsequently follows the same metabolic pathways as chlordiazepoxide and diazepam (see Fig. 11.24). The half-life of flurazepam is relatively short (~2.3 hours).

LORAZEPAM (ATIVAN). Lorazepam, the 2′-chloro derivative of oxazepam (see Fig. 11.22), is approved to treat anxiety and status epilepticus (a type of seizure disorder), depending on the formulation, in tablets or solutions for oral administration compared to liquids for injection, respectively. Lorazepam is absorbed rapidly and completely after oral administration, with an absolute bioavailability of 90%. It reaches peak plasma concentrations in about 2 hours. Lorazepam is mainly metabolized in the liver by glucuronidation at the 3-hydroxy group, then excreted in the urine, and lorazepam does not accumulate in the plasma with repeated administration. Lorazepam has a mean plasma half-life of about 12 hours. Lorazepam is highly bound to plasma proteins, about 85%.

MIDAZOLAM. Midazolam has a pK_a of 6.2, making it one of the few benzodiazepines that is highly water soluble (pH <4) as well as highly lipid soluble (pH >4). It is the most commonly used benzodiazepine as a premedication for anesthesia, with a quick onset (1-2 minutes) and recovery (20 minutes) after a bolus injection.[155] The time to full alertness after midazolam premedication, however, is about 40 minutes, which is much longer than for nonbenzodiazepine agents such as propofol (10 minutes). The intravenously administered preparation is a dihydrochloride salt preparation that is buffered to pH 3—at this pH, acid-catalyzed diazepine ring opening at the 4,5-double bond occurs that assists water solubility but renders the compound inactive. The dihydrochloride salt preparation consists of about 80% to 85% of the ring-opened structure II and 15% to 20% of the ring-closed form Ia.[156] The diazepine ring completely reforms to the active midazolam compound (I) upon intravenous injection, that is, at pH 7.4. Midazolam undergoes hepatic metabolism mainly by CYP3A4 and CYP3A5 to yield primarily hydroxylated derivatives that likely do not contribute to pharmacological activity at usual doses; these are subsequently excreted as glucuronide conjugates.

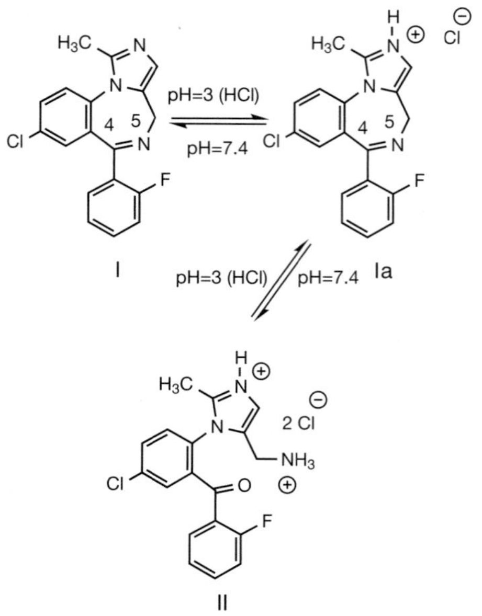

Midazolam

Oxazepam. Oxazepam is an active metabolite of both chlordiazepoxide and diazepam and is marketed separately, as a short-acting anxiolytic agent. Similar to lorazepam, oxazepam is rapidly inactivated to glucuronidated metabolites that are excreted in the urine (Fig. 11.24). The half-life of oxazepam is approximately 4 to 8 hours, and cumulative effects with chronic therapy are much less than with long-acting benzodiazepines, such as chlordiazepoxide and diazepam.

PHARMACOKINETICS OF BENZODIAZEPINES. Detailed pharmacokinetic analysis for most benzodiazepines is complex. Two-compartment models may be adequate to describe the disposition of most derivatives, but three-compartment models are necessary for highly lipophilic agents, such as diazepam. The distribution of such lipophilic drugs is further complicated by enterohepatic circulation. Thus, the usually stated elimination half-life of benzodiazepines may not adequately account for the pharmacodynamics of the distributive phase of the drug, which can be clinically important. For example, the distributive (α) half-life of diazepam is approximately 1 hour, whereas the elimination (β) half-life is approximately 1.5 days, acutely, and even longer after chronic dosing that results in accumulation of the drug. Furthermore, plasma concentration and clinical effectiveness of benzodiazepines is difficult to correlate, and only a 2-fold increase in clinically effective levels produces sedative side effects. Consequently, despite the long half-life of many benzodiazepines, they are not safe or effective when given as a once-daily dose and usually are divided into two to four doses per day for treatment of daytime anxiety. Both therapeutic and toxic effects may persist several days after discontinuation of chronically administered, long-acting benzodiazepines, such as chlordiazepoxide, clonazepam, and diazepam. Thus, short-acting benzodiazepines, such as oxazepam, alprazolam, and lorazepam, that are rapidly metabolized to inactive products should be considered in elderly or hepato-compromised patients.

Nonbenzodiazepine Agonists at the Benzodiazepine Site of the $GABA_A$ Receptor

Relatively few structural classes of nonbenzodiazepine compounds have clinically relevant affinity for the benzodiazepine site and show desired anxiolytic or other pharmacological activity in vivo. Representative drugs of these classes in current clinical use include the cyclopyrrolone eszopiclone, the pyrazolopyrimidine zaleplon, and the imidazopyridazine zolpidem, used for insomnia (see Chapter 14). These ligands show greater selectivity for $GABA_A$ receptors containing the α_1 subunit; however, it should be noted that the α_2, α_3, α_5, and γ subunits may be important in mediating anxiolytic effects.

Cyclopyrrolones. The cyclopyrrolone drug zopiclone is described as a "superagonist" of the benzodiazepine site with the subunit composition $\alpha_1\ \beta_2\ \gamma_2$ and $\alpha_1\ \beta_2\ \gamma_3$ because it potentiates the GABA-gated current more than the benzodiazepine (flunitrazepam) reference agonist.[157] Racemic zopiclone has been available in Europe since 1992 and the higher-affinity *S*-enantiomer (eszopiclone) was marketed in the United States in 2005. It is used primarily to treat insomnia because of its rapid onset and moderate duration (half-life, ~6 hours) of hypnotic-sedative effect.[158] Less than 10% of orally administered eszopiclone is excreted unchanged because it undergoes extensive CYP3A4- and CYP2E1-catalyzed oxidation and demethylation to metabolites excreted primarily in urine (see Chapter 12).

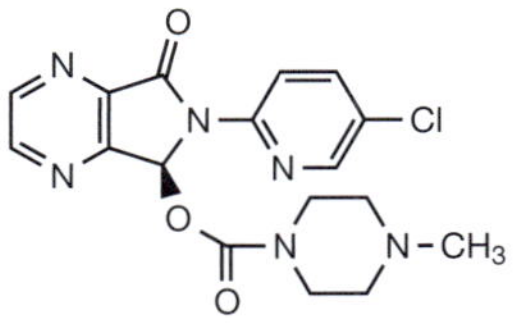

Eszopiclone

Pyrazolopyrimidines. The pyrazolopyrimidine zaleplon has selective high affinity for α_1-containing benzodiazepine sites but also produces effects at other $GABA_A$ binding sites. In patients with insomnia, zaleplon is effective to decrease sleep latency and does not appear to induce withdrawal symptoms or rebound insomnia on discontinuation. Zaleplon is absorbed rapidly and reaches peak plasma concentrations in approximately 1 hour, with a half-life of approximately 1 hour as well. Less than 1% of a dose of zaleplon is excreted unchanged because most is oxidized by aldehyde dehydrogenase and CYP3A4 to inactive metabolites, which are converted to glucuronides and eliminated in urine (see Chapter 12).

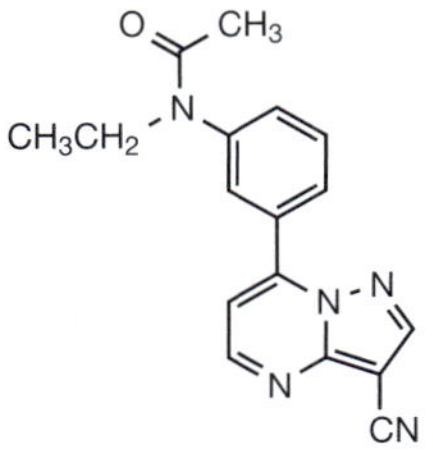

Zaleplon (Sonata)

Imidazopyridines. The imidazopyridines, zolpidem and alpidem, represent another example of α_1 subunit-selective ligands of the benzodiazepine that have clinical profiles different from those of typical benzodiazepines. For example, although the activating effects of zolpidem on $GABA_A$ receptors qualitatively resemble those of benzodiazepines, clinically it shows a weaker anticonvulsant effect and a stronger sedative effect. Zolpidem was marketed as a sedative-hypnotic in the United States in 1993 and is effective in shortening sleep latency and prolonging total sleep time, without affecting sleep stages, in patients with insomnia.[159] Zolpidem is readily absorbed from the gastrointestinal tract and is extensively metabolized by the liver to inactive oxidized products, with a half-life of approximately 2 hours (see Chapter 14).

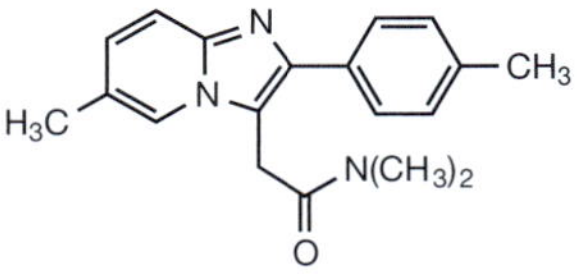

Zolpidem (Ambien)

$GABA_A$ Partial Positive Allosteric Modulators

Partial agonists (partial PAMs) of the benzodiazepine site offer some theoretical and practical advantages over full agonists, including less side effects (sedation and ataxia) and abuse potential. For example, imidazenil is an imidazobenzodiazepine carboxamide that has higher affinity than diazepam but is only about half as efficacious at potentiating GABA effects on chloride currents. Consistent with the general pharmacological principle that partial agonists may show antagonist functional effects in competition with a more efficacious agonist, imidazenil blocks the sedative and ataxic effects of diazepam.[160] Interestingly, however, imidazenil does not block the anticonvulsant effects of diazepam; accordingly, it has been proposed as a better alternative to flumazenil in the alleviation of benzodiazepine-induced withdrawal symptoms. In addition to imidazenil, several other structural classes of $GABA_A$ partial agonists have been evaluated; however, no $GABA_A$ partial agonist has reached the marketplace because data from clinical trials did not support promising preclinical results.[161]

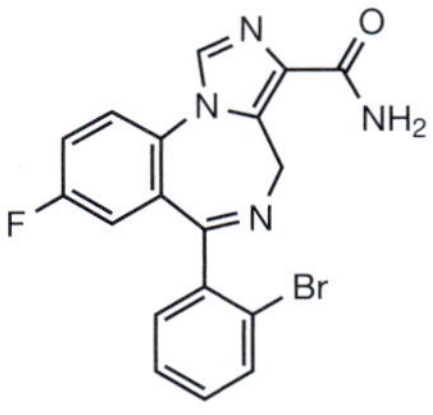

Imidazenil

Miscellaneous Medications

Buspirone (Buspar) and Gepirone (Exxua). Buspirone and gepirone are azapirones, a class of drugs that act as partial agonists of the $5\text{-}HT_{1A}$ receptor. They are approved to treat anxiety (buspirone) and depression (gepirone, approved in 2023). The chemical structures of buspirone and gepirone are very similar, except with gepirone having a dimethyl group in place of the cyclopentyl of buspirone. This makes gepirone more polar and less lipophilic than buspirone. The pharmacodynamics of buspirone and gepirone are similar, but they differ in their potency, selectivity, and efficacy. Buspirone is more potent than gepirone at 5-HT_{1A} and has off-targets including dopamine D_2, D_3, D_4, and α-adrenergic receptors. Gepirone has similar off-targets, though, it binds less potently at the dopamine receptors.[162] Gepirone has a higher efficacy at the 5-HT_{1A} receptor than buspirone. How this translates clinically in terms of clinical efficacy and safety is currently unknown. Historically, efficacious activation of 5-HT_{1A} was thought to cause serotonin syndrome, a potentially life-threatening condition with clinical symptoms, including agitation, several autonomic effects, such as increased heart rate and blood pressure, body temperature, and sweating, as well as changes in muscle tone, such as muscle rigidity and spasms. With the approval of gepirone, researchers and physicians are reevaluating the impact of 5-HT_{1A} receptor activation in serotonin syndrome. 5-HT_{1A} receptors are expressed both pre- and postsynaptically on neurons, and pre- and postsynaptic 5-HT_{1A} receptors have divergent physiological effects.[162] Though, concomitant use of gepirone and serotonergics increases serotonin syndrome risk, reinforcing that 5-HT_{1A} receptors have a role in serotonin syndrome.

The pharmacokinetics of buspirone and gepirone differ in terms of bioavailability, metabolism, and elimination. Buspirone has a low bioavailability of about 4%, while gepirone has a higher bioavailability of about 20%. Buspirone is extensively metabolized by the liver, mainly by the CYP3A4. One of its major metabolites—also a metabolite of gepirone—is 1-pyrimidinylpiperazine, which has similar activity at 5-HT_{1A} and α_{2A}-adrenergic receptors as the parent compounds. Buspirone has a half-life of 2.5 hours. Gepirone is also metabolized by liver CYP3A4 enzymes, and is contraindicated in patients taking strong CYB3A4 inhibitors (or inducers). Co-administration of ketoconazole (an antifungal medication) and verapamil (a calcium channel blocker used to treat hypertension), whose metabolism involves CYB3A4, significantly increase plasma concentrations of gepirone. In addition to 1-pyrimidinylpiperazine, its other major metabolites is 3′-OH-gepirone, which also has 5-HT_{1A} receptor activity. Gepirone has a half-life of 1.5 hours.

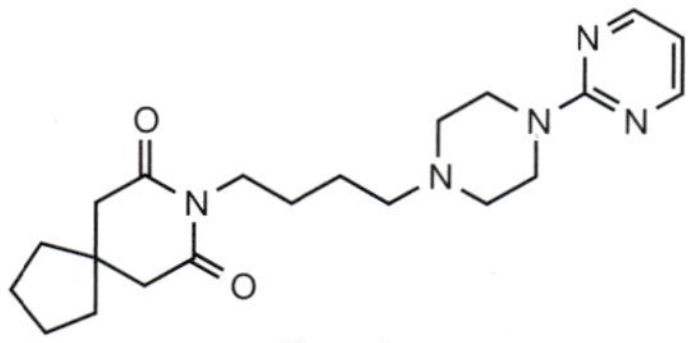

Buspirone

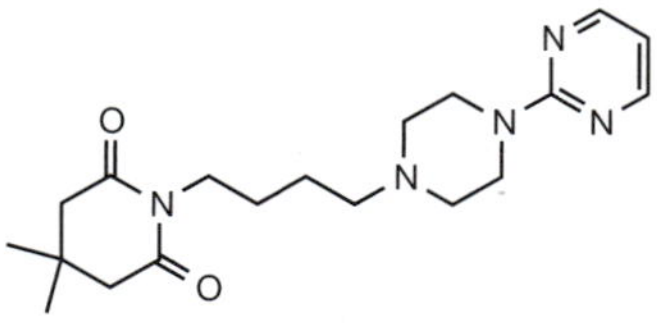

Gepirone

Structure Challenge

Below are the structures of six medicines from this chapter. Use your knowledge of drug chemistry, pharmacodynamics, and pharmacokinetics to identify the most appropriate recommendation for each patient described below.

1. A patient who exhibits anxiety attacks that occur rapidly and unexpectedly
2. A patient with schizophrenia and suicidality who has failed to respond to other antipsychotic pharmacotherapies
3. A patient with psychosis associated with Parkinson disease
4. A patient with generalized anxiety disorder and no history of a substance use disorder who has not responded to first-line pharmacotherapies (eg, SSRIs; see Chapter 12)
5. A patient with schizophrenia taking the antidepressant nefazodone, a potent CYP3A4 inhibitor
6. A patient with schizophrenia taking haloperidol who is developing clinical signs of tardive dyskinesia warranting a new pharmacotherapy to treat her schizophrenia

A.

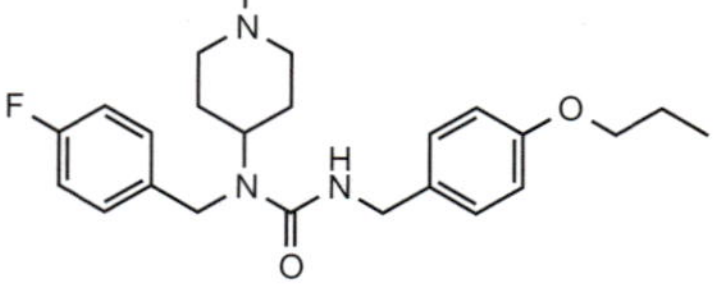

B.

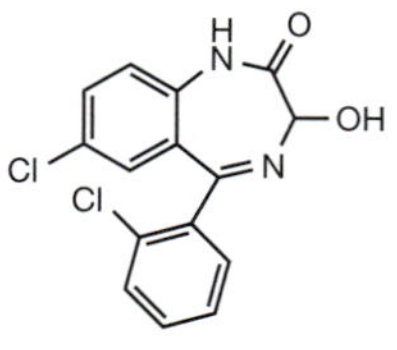

C.

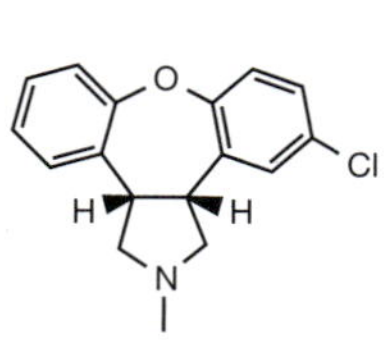

D.

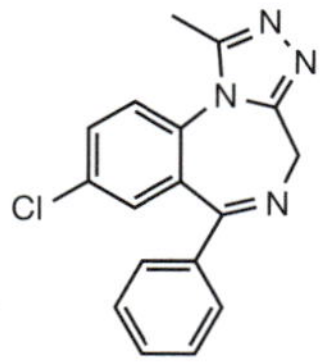

E.

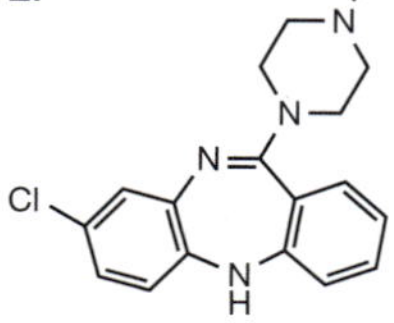

F.

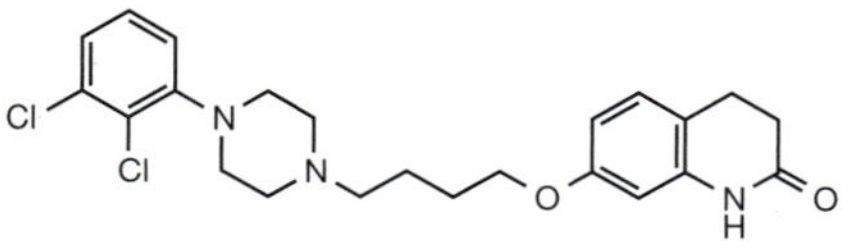

Structure Challenge answers found immediately after References.

REFERENCES

1. American Psychiatric Association; DSM-5 Task Force. *Diagnostic and Statistical Manual of Mental Disorders: DSM-5*. 5th ed. American Psychiatric Association; 2013.
2. Moreno-Kustner B, Martin C, Pastor L. Prevalence of psychotic disorders and its association with methodological issues. A systematic review and meta-analyses. *PLoS One*. 2018;13(4):e0195687.
3. McGrath JJ, Saha S, Al-Hamzawi A, et al. Psychotic experiences in the general population: a cross-national analysis based on 31,261 respondents from 18 countries. *JAMA Psychiatry*. 2015;72(7):697-705.
4. Chong HY, Teoh SL, Wu DB, Kotirum S, Chiou CF, Chaiyakunapruk N. Global economic burden of schizophrenia: a systematic review. *Neuropsychiatr Dis Treat*. 2016;12:357-373.
5. Kessler RC, Petukhova M, Sampson NA, Zaslavsky AM, Wittchen HU. Twelve-month and lifetime prevalence and lifetime morbid risk of anxiety and mood disorders in the United States. *Int J Methods Psychiatr Res*. 2012;21(3):169-184.
6. Kraepelin E, Barclay RM, Robertson GM. *Dementia Praecox and Paraphrenia*. E. & S. Livingstone; 1919.
7. Bleuler E. *Dementia Praecox*. International Universities Press; 1950.
8. Tandon R, Gaebel W, Barch DM, et al. Definition and description of schizophrenia in the DSM-5. *Schizophr Res*. 2013;150(1):3-10.
9. Schneider K. *Clinical Psychopathology*. Grune & Stratton; 1959.
10. Barch DM, Bustillo J, Gaebel W, et al. Logic and justification for dimensional assessment of symptoms and related clinical phenomena in psychosis: relevance to DSM-5. *Schizophr Res*. 2013;150(1):15-20.
11. Hilker R, Helenius D, Fagerlund B, et al. Heritability of schizophrenia and schizophrenia spectrum based on the Nationwide Danish twin register. *Biol Psychiatry*. 2018;83(6):492-498.
12. O'Tuathaigh CM, Desbonnet L, Moran PM, Waddington JL. Susceptibility genes for schizophrenia: mutant models, endophenotypes and psychobiology. *Curr Top Behav Neurosci*. 2012;12:209-250.
13. Schizophrenia Working Group of the Psychiatric Genomics Consortium. Biological insights from 108 schizophrenia-associated genetic loci. *Nature*. 2014;511(7510):421-427.
14. Genovese G, Fromer M, Stahl EA, et al. Increased burden of ultra-rare protein-altering variants among 4,877 individuals with schizophrenia. *Nat Neurosci*. 2016;19(11):1433-1441.
15. Skene NG, Bryois J, Bakken TE, et al. Genetic identification of brain cell types underlying schizophrenia. *Nat Genet*. 2018;50(6):825-833.
16. Wray NR, Ripke S, Mattheisen M, et al. Genome-wide association analyses identify 44 risk variants and refine the genetic architecture of major depression. *Nat Genet*. 2018;50(5):668-681.
17. Duncan LE, Ratanatharathorn A, Aiello AE, et al. Largest GWAS of PTSD (N=20 070) yields genetic overlap with schizophrenia and sex differences in heritability. *Mol Psychiatry*. 2018;23(3):666-673.
18. Cross-Disorder Group of the Psychiatric Genomics Consortium. Identification of risk loci with shared effects on five major psychiatric disorders: a genome-wide analysis. *Lancet*. 2013;381(9875):1371-1379.
19. Anttila V, Bulik-Sullivan B, Finucane HK, et al. Analysis of shared heritability in common disorders of the brain. *Science*. 2018;360(6395):eaap8757.
20. Howes OD, McCutcheon R. Inflammation and the neural diathesis-stress hypothesis of schizophrenia: a reconceptualization. *Transl Psychiatry*. 2017;7(2):e1024.
21. Howes OD, Kapur S. The dopamine hypothesis of schizophrenia: version III—the final common pathway. *Schizophr Bull*. 2009;35(3):549-562.
22. Moghaddam B, Javitt D. From revolution to evolution: the glutamate hypothesis of schizophrenia and its implication for treatment. *Neuropsychopharmacology*. 2012;37(1):4-15.
23. Poels EM, Kegeles LS, Kantrowitz JT, et al. Imaging glutamate in schizophrenia: review of findings and implications for drug discovery. *Mol Psychiatry*. 2014;19(1):20-29.
24. Carlsson A, Lindqvist M. Effect of chlorpromazine or haloperidol on formation of 3-methoxytyramine and normetanephrine in mouse brain. *Acta Pharmacol Toxicol (Copenh)*. 1963;20:140-144.
25. Howes O, Bose S, Turkheimer F, et al. Progressive increase in striatal dopamine synthesis capacity as patients develop psychosis: a PET study. *Mol Psychiatry*. 2011;16(9):885-886.
26. Snyder SH. *Drugs and the Brain*. Scientific American Books: Distributed by W.H. Freeman; 1986.
27. Heinz A, Knable MB, Weinberger DR. Dopamine D2 receptor imaging and neuroleptic drug response. *J Clin Psychiatry*. 1996;57(suppl 11):84-88; discussion 89-93.
28. Kenakin T, Christopoulos A. Measurements of ligand bias and functional affinity. *Nat Rev Drug Discov*. 2013;12(6):483.
29. Kenakin T. Inverse, protean, and ligand-selective agonism: matters of receptor conformation. *FASEB J*. 2001;15(3):598-611.
30. Liu Y, Canal CE, Cordova-Sintjago TC, Zhu W, Booth RG. Mutagenesis analysis reveals distinct amino acids of the human serotonin 5-HT2C receptor underlying the pharmacology of distinct ligands. *ACS Chem Neurosci*. 2017;8(1):28-39.
31. Mottola DM, Kilts JD, Lewis MM, et al. Functional selectivity of dopamine receptor agonists. I. Selective activation of postsynaptic dopamine D2 receptors linked to adenylate cyclase. *J Pharmacol Exp Ther*. 2002;301(3):1166-1178.
32. Chen X, McCorvy JD, Fischer MG, et al. Discovery of G protein-biased D2 dopamine receptor partial agonists. *J Med Chem*. 2016;59(23):10601-10618.
33. Lovenberg TW, Brewster WK, Mottola DM, et al. Dihydrexidine, a novel selective high potency full dopamine D-1 receptor agonist. *Eur J Pharmacol*. 1989;166(1):111-113.
34. Cervenka S. PET radioligands for the dopamine D1-receptor: application in psychiatric disorders. *Neurosci Lett*. 2019;691:26-34.
35. Arnsten AFT, Girgis RR, Gray DL, Mailman RB. Novel dopamine therapeutics for cognitive deficits in schizophrenia. *Biol Psychiatry*. 2017;81(1):67-77.
36. Sokoloff P, Le Foll B. The dopamine D3 receptor, a quarter century later. *Eur J Neurosci*. 2017;45(1):2-19.
37. Bitter I, Groc M, Delsol C, et al. Efficacy of F17464, a new preferential D3 antagonist in a placebo-controlled phase 2 study of patients with an acute exacerbation of schizophrenia. *Eur Psychiatry*. 2017;41:S387.
38. Lindsley CW, Hopkins CR. Return of D4 dopamine receptor antagonists in drug discovery. *J Med Chem*. 2017;60(17):7233-7243.
39. Mohr P, Decker M, Enzensperger C, Lehmann J. Dopamine/serotonin receptor ligands. 12(1): SAR studies on hexahydro-dibenz[d,g]azecines lead to 4-chloro-7-methyl-5,6,7,8,9,14-hexahydrodibenz[d,g]azecin-3-ol, the first picomolar D5-selective dopamine-receptor antagonist. *J Med Chem*. 2006;49(6):2110-2116.
40. Arbilla S, Langer SZ. Stereoselectivity of presynaptic autoreceptors modulating dopamine release. *Eur J Pharmacol*. 1981;76(4):345-351.
41. Booth RG, Baldessarini RJ, Kula NS, Gao Y, Zong R, Neumeyer JL. Presynaptic inhibition of dopamine synthesis in rat striatal tissue by enantiomeric mono- and dihydroxyaporphines. *Mol Pharmacol*. 1990;38(1):92-101.
42. Lieberman JA, Stroup TS. The NIMH-CATIE schizophrenia study: what did we learn? *Am J Psychiatry*. 2011;168(8):770-775.
43. Leucht S, Cipriani A, Spineli L, et al. Comparative efficacy and tolerability of 15 antipsychotic drugs in schizophrenia: a multiple-treatments meta-analysis. *Lancet*. 2013;382(9896):951-962.
44. Haddad PM, Das A, Keyhani S, Chaudhry IB. Antipsychotic drugs and extrapyramidal side effects in first episode psychosis: a systematic review of head-head comparisons. *J Psychopharmacol*. 2012;26(5 suppl):15-26.

45. Roth BL, Lopez E, Patel S, Kroeze WK. The multiplicity of serotonin receptors: uselessly diverse molecules or an embarrassment of riches? *Neuroscientist*. 2000;6(4):252-262.
46. Canal CE. Serotonergic psychedelics: experimental approaches for assessing mechanisms of action. *Handb Exp Pharmacol*. 2018;252:227-260.
47. Nichols DE. Psychedelics. *Pharmacol Rev*. 2016;68(2):264-355.
48. Canal CE, Murnane KS. The serotonin 5-HT2C receptor and the non-addictive nature of classic hallucinogens. *J Psychopharmacol*. 2017;31(1):127-143.
49. Weiner DM, Burstein ES, Nash N, et al. 5-hydroxytryptamine2A receptor inverse agonists as antipsychotics. *J Pharmacol Exp Ther*. 2001;299(1):268-276.
50. Vanover KE, Weiner DM, Makhay M, et al. Pharmacological and behavioral profile of *N*-(4-fluorophenylmethyl)-*N*-(1-methylpiperidin-4-yl)-*N'*-(4-(2-methylpropyloxy)phen ylmethyl) carbamide (2R,3R)-dihydroxybutanedioate (2:1) (ACP-103), a novel 5-hydroxytryptamine(2A) receptor inverse agonist. *J Pharmacol Exp Ther*. 2006;317(2):910-918.
51. Cummings J, Isaacson S, Mills R, et al. Pimavanserin for patients with Parkinson's disease psychosis: a randomised, placebo-controlled phase 3 trial. *Lancet*. 2014;383(9916):533-540.
52. Choksi NY, Nix WB, Wyrick SD, Booth RG. A novel phenylaminotetralin (PAT) recognizes histamine H1 receptors and stimulates dopamine synthesis in vivo in rat brain. *Brain Res*. 2000;852(1):151-160.
53. Johnson EA, Tsai CE, Shahan YH, Azzaro AJ. Serotonin 5-HT1A receptors mediate inhibition of tyrosine hydroxylation in rat striatum. *J Pharmacol Exp Ther*. 1993;266(1):133-141.
54. Pogorelov VM, Rodriguiz RM, Cheng J, et al. 5-HT2C agonists modulate schizophrenia-like behaviors in mice. *Neuropsychopharmacology*. 2017;42(11):2163-2177.
55. Perez XA, Bordia T, Quik M. The striatal cholinergic system in L-DOPA-induced dyskinesias. *J Neural Transm (Vienna)*. 2018;125(8):1251-1262.
56. Canal CE, Morgan D, Felsing D, et al. A novel aminotetralin-type serotonin (5-HT) 2C receptor-specific agonist and 5-HT2A competitive antagonist/5-HT2B inverse agonist with preclinical efficacy for psychoses. *J Pharmacol Exp Ther*. 2014;349(2):310-318.
57. Casey AB, Canal CE. Classics in chemical neuroscience: aripiprazole. *ACS Chem Neurosci*. 2017;8(6):1135-1146.
58. Katritch V, Cherezov V, Stevens RC. Structure-function of the G protein-coupled receptor superfamily. *Annu Rev Pharmacol Toxicol*. 2013;53:531-556.
59. Chien EY, Liu W, Zhao Q, et al. Structure of the human dopamine D3 receptor in complex with a D2/D3 selective antagonist. *Science*. 2010;330(6007):1091-1095.
60. Juncal-Ruiz M, Ramirez-Bonilla M, Gomez-Arnau J, et al. Incidence and risk factors of acute akathisia in 493 individuals with first episode non-affective psychosis: a 6-week randomised study of antipsychotic treatment. *Psychopharmacology*. 2017;234(17):2563-2570.
61. Hauser RA, Factor SA, Marder SR, et al. KINECT 3: a phase 3 randomized, double-blind, placebo-controlled trial of valbenazine for tardive dyskinesia. *Am J Psychiatry*. 2017;174(5): 476-484.
62. Sykes DA, Moore H, Stott L, et al. Extrapyramidal side effects of antipsychotics are linked to their association kinetics at dopamine D2 receptors. *Nat Commun*. 2017;8(1):763.
63. Snyder SH, Greenberg D, Yamumura HI. Antischizophrenic drugs: affinity for muscarinic cholinergic receptor sites in the brain predicts extrapyramidal effects. *J Psychiatr Res*. 1974;11:91-95.
64. Reynolds GP, Kirk SL. Metabolic side effects of antipsychotic drug treatment–pharmacological mechanisms. *Pharmacol Ther*. 2010;125(1):169-179.
65. Kroeze WK, Hufeisen SJ, Popadak BA, et al. H1-histamine receptor affinity predicts short-term weight gain for typical and atypical antipsychotic drugs. *Neuropsychopharmacology*. 2003;28(3): 519-526.
66. Lord CC, Wyler SC, Wan R, et al. The atypical antipsychotic olanzapine causes weight gain by targeting serotonin receptor 2C. *J Clin Invest*. 2017;127(9):3402-3406.
67. Zhang Y, Liu Y, Su Y, et al. The metabolic side effects of 12 antipsychotic drugs used for the treatment of schizophrenia on glucose: a network meta-analysis. *BMC Psychiatry*. 2017;17(1):373.
68. Ungar G, Parrot JL, Bovet D. The inhibition of the effects of histamine on the isolated intestine of the Guinea pig by some sympathicolytic and sympathicomimetic substances. *Cr Soc Biol*. 1937;124:445-446.
69. Laborit H, Huguenard P, Alluaume R. A new vegetative stabilizer; 4560 R.P. *Presse Med (1893)*. 1952;60(10):206-208.
70. Delay J, Deniker P, Harl J. Utilization therapeutique psychiatrique d'une phenothiazine d'action centrale elective. *Ann Med Psychol (Paris)*. 1952;110:112-117.
71. López-Muñoz F, Alamo C, Cuenca E, Shen WW, Clervoy P, Rubio G. History of the discovery and clinical introduction of chlorpromazine. *Ann Clin Psychiatry*. 2005;17(3):113-135.
72. Horn AS, Snyder SH. Chlorpromazine and dopamine: conformational similarities that correlate with the antischizophrenic activity of phenothiazine drugs. *Proc Natl Acad Sci U S A*. 1971;68(10):2325-2328.
73. Janssen PA. The evolution of the butyrophenones, haloperidol and trifluperidol, from meperidine-like 4-phenylpiperidines. *Int Rev Neurobiol*. 1965;8:221-263.
74. Murray M. Role of CYP pharmacogenetics and drug-drug interactions in the efficacy and safety of atypical and other antipsychotic agents. *J Pharm Pharmacol*. 2006;58(7):871-885.
75. Subramanyam B, Pond SM, Eyles DW, Whiteford HA, Fouda HG, Castagnoli N Jr. Identification of potentially neurotoxic pyridinium metabolite in the urine of schizophrenic patients treated with haloperidol. *Biochem Biophys Res Commun*. 1991;181(2):573-578.
76. Halliday GM, Pond SM, Cartwright H, McRitchie DA, Castagnoli N Jr, Van der Schyf CJ. Clinical and neuropathological abnormalities in baboons treated with HPTP, the tetrahydropyridine analog of haloperidol. *Exp Neurol*. 1999;158(1):155-163.
77. Igarashi K, Matsubara K, Kasuya F, Fukui M, Idzu T, Castagnoli N Jr. Effect of a pyridinium metabolite derived from haloperidol on the activities of striatal tyrosine hydroxylase in freely moving rats. *Neurosci Lett*. 1996;214(2-3):183-186.
78. Rollema H, Skolnik M, D'Engelbronner J, Igarashi K, Usuki E, Castagnoli N Jr. MPP(+)-like neurotoxicity of a pyridinium metabolite derived from haloperidol: in vivo microdialysis and in vitro mitochondrial studies. *J Pharmacol Exp Ther*. 1994;268(1):380-387.
79. Ulrich S, Sandmann U, Genz A. Serum concentrations of haloperidol pyridinium metabolites and the relationship with tardive dyskinesia and Parkinsonism: a cross-section study in psychiatric patients. *Pharmacopsychiatry*. 2005;38(4):171-177.
80. Snyder GL, Vanover KE, Zhu H, et al. Functional profile of a novel modulator of serotonin, dopamine, and glutamate neurotransmission. *Psychopharmacology*. 2015;232:605-621.
81. Davis RE, Vanover KE, Zhou Y, et al. ITI-007 demonstrates brain occupancy at serotonin 5-HT2A and dopamine D2 receptors and serotonin transporters using positron emission tomography in healthy volunteers. *Psychopharmacology (Berl)*. 2015;232(15):2863-2872.
82. Mailman RB, Murthy V. Third generation antipsychotic drugs: partial agonism or receptor functional selectivity? *Curr Pharm Des*. 2010;16(5):488-501.
83. Gründer G, Hippius H, Carlsson A. The "atypicality" of antipsychotics: a concept re-examined and re-defined. *Nat Rev Drug Discov*. 2009;8:197-202.
84. Wenthur CJ, Lindsley CW. Classics in chemical neuroscience: clozapine. *ACS Chem Neurosci*. 2013;4(7):1018-1025.

85. Goldstein JI, Jarskog LF, Hilliard C, et al. Clozapine-induced agranulocytosis is associated with rare HLA-DQB1 and HLA-B alleles. *Nat Commun*. 2014;5:4757.
86. Schmid CL, Streicher JM, Meltzer HY, Bohn LM. Clozapine acts as an agonist at serotonin 2A receptors to counter MK-801-induced behaviors through a betaarrestin2-independent activation of Akt. *Neuropsychopharmacology*. 2014;39(8):1902-1913.
87. Wu Y, Blichowski M, Daskalakis ZJ, et al. Evidence that clozapine directly interacts on the GABAB receptor. *Neuroreport*. 2011;22(13):637-641.
88. Schwieler L, Linderholm KR, Nilsson-Todd LK, Erhardt S, Engberg G. Clozapine interacts with the glycine site of the NMDA receptor: electrophysiological studies of dopamine neurons in the rat ventral tegmental area. *Life Sci*. 2008;83(5-6): 170-175.
89. Sur C, Mallorga PJ, Wittmann M, et al. N-desmethylclozapine, an allosteric agonist at muscarinic 1 receptor, potentiates N-methyl-D-aspartate receptor activity. *Proc Natl Acad Sci U S A*. 2003;100(23):13674-13679.
90. Gigout S, Wierschke S, Dehnicke C, Deisz RA. Different pharmacology of N-desmethylclozapine at human and rat M2 and M 4 mAChRs in neocortex. *Naunyn Schmiedebergs Arch Pharmacol*. 2015;388(5):487-496.
91. Raedler TJ, Hinkelmann K, Wiedemann K. Variability of the in vivo metabolism of clozapine. *Clin Neuropharmacol*. 2008;31(6):347-352.
92. Vainer JL, Chouinard G. Interaction between caffeine and clozapine. *J Clin Psychopharmacol*. 1994;14(4):284-285.
93. Desai HD, Seabolt J, Jann MW. Smoking in patients receiving psychotropic medications: a pharmacokinetic perspective. *CNS Drugs*. 2001;15(6):469-494.
94. Haring C, Meise U, Humpel C, Saria A, Fleischhacker WW, Hinterhuber H. Dose-related plasma levels of clozapine: influence of smoking behaviour, sex and age. *Psychopharmacology (Berl)*. 1989;99(suppl 1):S38-S40.
95. Urichuk L, Prior TI, Dursun S, Baker G. Metabolism of atypical antipsychotics: involvement of cytochrome p450 enzymes and relevance for drug-drug interactions. *Curr Drug Metab*. 2008;9(5):410-418.
96. Kassahun K, Mattiuz E, Nyhart E Jr, et al. Disposition and biotransformation of the antipsychotic agent olanzapine in humans. *Drug Metab Dispos*. 1997;25(1):81-93.
97. DeVane CL, Nemeroff CB. Clinical pharmacokinetics of quetiapine: an atypical antipsychotic. *Clin Pharmacokinet*. 2001;40(7):509-522.
98. Jensen NH, Rodriguiz RM, Caron MG, Wetsel WC, Rothman RB, Roth BL. N-desalkylquetiapine, a potent norepinephrine reuptake inhibitor and partial 5-HT1A agonist, as a putative mediator of quetiapine's antidepressant activity. *Neuropsychopharmacology*. 2008;33(10):2303-2312.
99. Shahid M, Walker GB, Zorn SH, Wong EHF. Asenapine: a novel psychopharmacologic agent with a unique human receptor signature. *J Psychopharmacol*. 2009;23(1):65-73.
100. Yasui-Furukori N, Hidestrand M, Spina E, Facciola G, Scordo MG, Tybring G. Different enantioselective 9-hydroxylation of risperidone by the two human CYP2D6 and CYP3A4 enzymes. *Drug Metab Dispos*. 2001;29(10):1263-1268.
101. Subramanian N, Kalkman HO. Receptor profile of P88-8991 and P95-12113, metabolites of the novel antipsychotic iloperidone. *Prog Neuropsychopharmacol Biol Psychiatry*. 2002;26(3): 553-560.
102. Newman-Tancredi A, Gavaudan S, Conte C, et al. Agonist and antagonist actions of antipsychotic agents at 5-HT1A receptors: a [35S]GTPgammaS binding study. *Eur J Pharmacol*. 1998;355(2-3):245-256.
103. Hirose T, Uwahodo Y, Yamada S, et al. Mechanism of action of aripiprazole predicts clinical efficacy and a favourable side-effect profile. *J Psychopharmacol*. 2004;18(3):375-383.
104. Shapiro DA, Renock S, Arrington E, et al. Aripiprazole, a novel atypical antipsychotic drug with a unique and robust pharmacology. *Neuropsychopharmacology*. 2003;28(8):1400-1411.
105. Lawler CP, Prioleau C, Lewis MM, et al. Interactions of the novel antipsychotic aripiprazole (OPC-14597) with dopamine and serotonin receptor subtypes. *Neuropsychopharmacology*. 1999;20(6):612-627.
106. Genaro-Mattos TC, Tallman KA, Allen LB, et al. Dichlorophenyl piperazines, including a recently-approved atypical antipsychotic, are potent inhibitors of DHCR7, the last enzyme in cholesterol biosynthesis. *Toxicol Appl Pharmacol*. 2018;349:21-28.
107. Maeda K, Sugino H, Akazawa H, et al. Brexpiprazole I: in vitro and in vivo characterization of a novel serotonin-dopamine activity modulator. *J Pharmacol Exp Ther*. 2014;350(3): 589-604.
108. Nemeth G, Laszlovszky I, Czobor P, et al. Cariprazine versus risperidone monotherapy for treatment of predominant negative symptoms in patients with schizophrenia: a randomised, double-blind, controlled trial. *Lancet*. 2017;389(10074): 1103-1113.
109. Girgis RR, Slifstein M, D'Souza D, et al. Preferential binding to dopamine D3 over D2 receptors by cariprazine in patients with schizophrenia using PET with the D3/D2 receptor ligand [(11)C]-(+)-PHNO. *Psychopharmacology (Berl)*. 2016;233(19-20):3503-3512.
110. Choi YK, Adham N, Kiss B, Gyertyán I, Tarazi FI. Long-term effects of cariprazine exposure on dopamine receptor subtypes. *CNS Spectr*. 2014;19(3):268-277.
111. Choi YK, Adham N, Kiss B, Gyertyán I, Tarazi FI. Long-term effects of aripiprazole exposure on monoaminergic and glutamatergic receptor subtypes: comparison with cariprazine. *CNS Spectr*. 2017;22(6):484-494.
112. Earley W, Durgam S, Lu K, Laszlovszky I, Debelle M, Kane JM. Safety and tolerability of cariprazine in patients with acute exacerbation of schizophrenia: a pooled analysis of four phase II/III randomized, double-blind, placebo-controlled studies. *Int Clin Psychopharmacol*. 2017;32(6):319-328.
113. Rohde M, Rk NM, Hakansson AE, et al. Biological conversion of aripiprazole lauroxil—an N-acyloxymethyl aripiprazole prodrug. *Results Pharma Sci*. 2014;4:19-25.
114. O'Brien CF, Jimenez R, Hauser RA, et al. NBI-98854, a selective monoamine transport inhibitor for the treatment of tardive dyskinesia: a randomized, double-blind, placebo-controlled study. *Mov Disord*. 2015;30(12):1681-1687.
115. Anderson KE, Stamler D, Davis MD, et al. Deutetrabenazine for treatment of involuntary movements in patients with tardive dyskinesia (AIM-TD): a double-blind, randomised, placebo-controlled, phase 3 trial. *Lancet Psychiatry*. 2017;4(8): 595-604.
116. Ballard C, Banister C, Khan Z, et al. Evaluation of the safety, tolerability, and efficacy of pimavanserin versus placebo in patients with Alzheimer's disease psychosis: a phase 2, randomised, placebo-controlled, double-blind study. *Lancet Neurol*. 2018;17(3):213-222.
117. Campbell-Sills L, Simmons AN, Lovero KL, Rochlin AA, Paulus MP, Stein MB. Functioning of neural systems supporting emotion regulation in anxiety-prone individuals. *Neuroimage*. 2011;54(1):689-696.
118. Martin EI, Ressler KJ, Binder E, Nemeroff CB. The neurobiology of anxiety disorders: brain imaging, genetics, and psychoneuroendocrinology. *Clin Lab Med*. 2010;30(4):865-891.
119. Nordahl TE, Semple WE, Gross M, et al. Cerebral glucose metabolic differences in patients with panic disorder. *Neuropsychopharmacology*. 1990;3(4):261-272.
120. Beutel ME, Stark R, Pan H, Silbersweig D, Dietrich S. Changes of brain activation pre- post short-term psychodynamic inpatient psychotherapy: an fMRI study of panic disorder patients. *Psychiatry Res*. 2010;184(2):96-104.

121. Rauch SL, Savage CR, Alpert NM, et al. A positron emission tomographic study of simple phobic symptom provocation. *Arch Gen Psychiatry*. 1995;52(1):20-28.
122. Caseras X, Mataix-Cols D, Trasovares MV, et al. Dynamics of brain responses to phobic-related stimulation in specific phobia subtypes. *Eur J Neurosci*. 2010;32(8):1414-1422.
123. Gershenfeld HK, Philibert RA, Boehm GW. Looking forward in geriatric anxiety and depression: implications of basic science for the future. *Am J Geriatr Psychiatry*. 2005;13(12): 1027-1040.
124. Cheung A, Mayes T, Levitt A, et al. Anxiety as a predictor of treatment outcome in children and adolescents with depression. *J Child Adolesc Psychopharmacol*. 2010;20(3):211-216.
125. Olsen RW, Sieghart W. International Union of Pharmacology. LXX. Subtypes of gamma-aminobutyric acid(A) receptors: classification on the basis of subunit composition, pharmacology, and function. Update. *Pharmacol Rev*. 2008;60(3): 243-260.
126. Cutting GR, Lu L, O'Hara BF, et al. Cloning of the gamma-aminobutyric acid (GABA) rho 1 cDNA: a GABA receptor subunit highly expressed in the retina. *Proc Natl Acad Sci U S A*. 1991;88(7):2673-2677.
127. Schofield PR, Darlison MG, Fujita N, et al. Sequence and functional expression of the GABA A receptor shows a ligand-gated receptor super-family. *Nature*. 1987;328(6127):221-227.
128. Wisden W, Laurie DJ, Monyer H, Seeburg PH. The distribution of 13 GABAA receptor subunit mRNAs in the rat brain. I. Telencephalon, diencephalon, mesencephalon. *J Neurosci*. 1992;12(3):1040-1062.
129. Zhu S, Noviello CM, Teng J, Walsh RM Jr, Kim JJ, Hibbs RE. Structure of a human synaptic GABAA receptor. *Nature*. 2018;559(7712):67-72.
130. Sieghart W. Anxioselective anxiolytics: additional perspective. *Trends Pharmacol Sci*. 2013;34(3):145-146.
131. Frangaj A, Fan QR. Structural biology of GABAB receptor. *Neuropharmacology*. 2018;136(pt A):68-79.
132. Kaupmann K, Malitschek B, Schuler V, et al. GABA(B)-receptor subtypes assemble into functional heteromeric complexes. *Nature*. 1998;396(6712):683-687.
133. Couve A, Filippov AK, Connolly CN, Bettler B, Brown DA, Moss SJ. Intracellular retention of recombinant GABA(B) receptors. *J Biol Chem*. 1998;273(41):26361-26367.
134. Jones KA, Borowsky B, Tamm JA, et al. GABA(B) receptors function as a heteromeric assembly of the subunits GABA(B)R1 and GABA(B)R2. *Nature*. 1998;396(6712):674-679.
135. White JH, Wise A, Main MJ, et al. Heterodimerization is required for the formation of a functional GABA(B) receptor. *Nature*. 1998;396(6712):679-682.
136. Stewart GD, Comps-Agrar L, Norskov-Lauritsen LB, Pin JP, Kniazeff J. Allosteric interactions between GABA(B1) subunits control orthosteric binding sites occupancy within GABA(B) oligomers. *Neuropharmacology*. 2018;136:92-101.
137. Geng Y, Bush M, Mosyak L, Wang F, Fan QR. Structural mechanism of ligand activation in human GABA(B) receptor. *Nature*. 2013;504(7479):254-259.
138. Pin JP, Galvez T, Prezeau L. Evolution, structure, and activation mechanism of family 3/C G-protein-coupled receptors. *Pharmacol Ther*. 2003;98(3):325-354.
139. Brown KM, Roy KK, Hockerman GH, Doerksen RJ, Colby DA. Activation of the gamma-aminobutyric acid type B (GABA(B)) receptor by agonists and positive allosteric modulators. *J Med Chem*. 2015;58(16):6336-6347.
140. Lal R, Sukbuntherng J, Tai EH, et al. Arbaclofen placarbil, a novel R-baclofen prodrug: improved absorption, distribution, metabolism, and elimination properties compared with R-baclofen. *J Pharmacol Exp Ther*. 2009;330(3):911-921.
141. Garattini S, Mussini E, Randall LO. *The Benzodiazepines*. Raven Press; 1973.
142. Sternbach LH. The benzodiazepine story. *J Med Chem*. 1979;22(1):1-7.
143. Randall LO, Schallek W, Heise GA, Keith EF, Bagdon RE. The psychosedative properties of methaminodiazepoxide. *J Pharmacol Exp Ther*. 1960;129:163-171.
144. Randall LO, Scheckel CL, Banziger RF. Pharmacology of the metabolites of chlordiazepoxide and diazepam. *Curr Ther Res Clin Exp*. *1965*;7(9):590-606.
145. Braestrup C, Nielsen M, Olsen CE. Urinary and brain beta-carboline-3-carboxylates as potent inhibitors of brain benzodiazepine receptors. *Proc Natl Acad Sci U S A*. 1980;77(4):2288-2292.
146. Cole BJ, Hillmann M, Seidelmann D, Klewer M, Jones GH. Effects of benzodiazepine receptor partial inverse agonists in the elevated plus-maze test of anxiety in the rat. *Psychopharmacology (Berl)*. 1995;121(1):118-126.
147. Braestrup C, Schmiechen R, Neef G, Nielsen M, Petersen EN. Interaction of convulsive ligands with benzodiazepine receptors. *Science*. 1982;216(4551):1241-1243.
148. Haefely W, Kyburz E, Gerecke M, et al. Recent advances in the molecular pharmacology of benzodiazepine receptors and the structure-activity relationships of these agonists and antagonists. In: *Advances in Drug Research. Vol* 14. Academic Press; 1985:166-322.
149. Hunkeler W, Mohler H, Pieri L, et al. Selective antagonists of benzodiazepines. *Nature*. 1981;290(5806):514-516.
150. Mohler H, Richards JG. Agonist and antagonist benzodiazepine receptor interaction in vitro. *Nature*. 1981;294(5843):763-765.
151. Wieland HA, Luddens H, Seeburg PH. A single histidine in GABA-A receptors is essential for benzodiazepine agonist binding. *J Biol Chem*. 1992;267(3):1426-1429.
152. Rowlett JK, Platt DM, Lelas S, Atack JR, Dawson GR. Different GABAA receptor subtypes mediate the anxiolytic, abuse-related, and motor effects of benzodiazepine-like drugs in primates. *Proc Natl Acad Sci U S A*. 2005;102(3):915-920.
153. Blount JF, Fryer RI, Gilman NW, Todaro LJ. Quinazolines and 1,4-benzodiazepines. 92. Conformational recognition of the receptor by 1,4-benzodiazepines. *Mol Pharmacol*. 1983;24(3):425-428.
154. Sunjic V, Lisini A, Sega A, Kovac T, Kajfez F, Ruscic B. Conformation of 7-chloro-5-phenyl-D5-3(S)-methyldihydro-1,4-benzodiazepin-2-one in solution. *J Heterocyclic Chem*. 1979;16(4):757-761.
155. Olkkola KT, Ahonen J. Midazolam and other benzodiazepines. In: Schüttler J, Schwilden H, eds. *Modern Anesthetics. Handbook of Experimental Pharmacology*. Vol 182. Springer; 2008.
156. Gerecke M. Chemical structure and properties of midazolam compared with other benzodiazepines. *Br J Clin Pharmacol*. 1983;16(suppl 1):11S-16S.
157. Davies M, Newell JG, Derry JM, Martin IL, Dunn SM. Characterization of the interaction of zopiclone with gamma-aminobutyric acid type A receptors. *Mol Pharmacol*. 2000;58(4): 756-762.
158. Rosenberg R, Caron J, Roth T, Amato D. An assessment of the efficacy and safety of eszopiclone in the treatment of transient insomnia in healthy adults. *Sleep Med*. 2005;6(1):15-22.
159. Herrmann WM, Kubicki ST, Boden S, Eich FX, Attali P, Coquelin JP. Pilot controlled double-blind study of the hypnotic effects of zolpidem in patients with chronic 'learned' insomnia: psychometric and polysomnographic evaluation. *J Int Med Res*. 1993;21(6):306-322.
160. Auta J, Costa E, Davis JM, Guidotti A. Imidazenil: an antagonist of the sedative but not the anticonvulsant action of diazepam. *Neuropharmacology*. 2005;49(3):425-429.
161. Basile AS, Lippa AS, Skolnick P. Anxioselective anxiolytics: can less be more? *Eur J Pharmacol*. 2004;500(1-3):441-451.
162. Newman-Tancredi A, Depoortère RY, Kleven MS, Kołaczkowski M, Zimmer L. Translating biased agonists from molecules to medications: Serotonin 5-HT1A receptor functional selectivity for CNS disorders. *Pharmacol Ther*. 2022 229:107937.

Structure Challenge Answers

1. **D.** Alprazolam (Xanax)
2. **E.** Clozapine (Clozaril)
3. **A.** Pimavanserin (Nuplazid)
4. **B.** Lorazepam (Ativan)
5. **C.** Asenapine (Saphris)
6. **F.** Aripiprazole (Abilify)

CHAPTER 12

Drugs Used to Treat Depression

David A. Williams

Drugs covered in this chapter:

Tricyclic tertiary amines
- Amitriptyline
- Clomipramine
- Doxepin
- Imipramine
- (+)-Trimipramine

Tricyclic secondary amines
- Amoxapine
- Desipramine
- Maprotiline
- Nortriptyline
- Protriptyline

Selective serotonin reuptake inhibitors
- (±)-Citalopram
- (+) Escitalopram (*S*-citalopram)
- (±)-Fluoxetine
- Fluvoxamine
- (−)-Paroxetine
- (+)-Sertraline

Atypical drugs
- (−)-Atomoxetine
- Bupropion
- Desvenlafaxine
- (−)-Duloxetine
- (±) Mirtazapine
- Trazodone
- Venlafaxine
- Vilazodone
- Vortioxetine

Neuroactive steroid
- Brexanolone (allopregnanolone)
- Zuranolone

Monoamine oxidase inhibitors
- Phenelzine
- Tranylcypromine

Mood stabilizers
- Lithium carbonate

***N*-methyl-D-aspartate receptor antagonists**
- Dextromethorphan/bupropion
- Ketamine
  - Ketamine spray
  - Esketamine spray

Abbreviations

5-HT serotonin (5-hydroxytryptamine)
5-MeO-DMT 5-methoxy-*N*,*N*-dimethyltryptamine
ACh acetylcholine
ACTH adrenocorticotropic hormone
ADH alcohol dehydrogenase
ADHD attention-deficit/hyperactivity disorder
ALDH aldehyde dehydrogenase
AMPAR α-amino-3-hydroxy-5-methyl-4-isoxazolepropionic acid receptor
AUC area under the curve
BBB blood-brain barrier
BDNF brain-derived neurotrophic factor
BHP British Herbal Pharmacopoeia
CA catecholamine
cAMP cyclic adenosine monophosphate
CDC U.S. Centers for Disease Control and Prevention
CNS central nervous system
CRF corticotropin-releasing factor
CSF cerebrospinal fluid
CT computed tomography
CYP cytochrome P450
DA dopamine
DAT dopamine reuptake transporter
DDI drug-drug interaction
DSM-5 Diagnostic and Statistical Manual of Mental Disorders, Fifth Edition
ECT electroconvulsive therapy
eGFR estimated glomerular filtration rate
ESCOP European Scientific Cooperative on Phytotherapy
FDA U.S. Food and Drug Administration
GABA γ-aminobutyric acid
GAD generalized anxiety disorder
GI gastrointestinal
GSK-3 glycogen synthase kinase-3
HLM human liver microsome
HNK hydroxynorketamine
HPA hypothalamic-pituitary-adrenal
IC50 half-maximal inhibitory concentration
iRs ionotropic receptors
IP_3 inositol 1,4,5-trisphosphate
IV intravenous
K_i inhibition constant
LSD lysergic acid diethylamide
LVM levomilnacipran
mAChRs muscarinic acetylcholine receptors
MADRS Montgomery-Asberg Depression Rating Scale
MAO monoamine oxidase

Abbreviations—continued

MAOIs monoamine oxidase inhibitors
m-CPP *m*-chlorophenylpiperazine
MDD major depressive disorder
mGlu metabotropic glutamate
mRs metabotropic receptors
nAChRs nicotinic acetylcholine receptors
NaSSAs noradrenergic and specific serotonergic antidepressants
NDA new drug application
NE norepinephrine
NET norepinephrine reuptake transporter
NMDA *N*-methyl-D-aspartate
NMDAR *N*-methyl-D-aspartate receptor
NSAID nonsteroidal anti-inflammatory drug
OCD obsessive-compulsive disorder
ODV *O*-desmethylvenlafaxine
OTC over the counter
PAM positive allosteric modulation
PCP phencyclidine
PMDD premenstrual dysphoric disorder
PMS premenstrual syndrome
PPD postpartum depression
PTSD posttraumatic stress disorder
REMS Risk Evaluation and Mitigation Strategy
SARIs serotonin receptor modulators (serotonin antagonist reuptake inhibitors)
SERT serotonin reuptake transporter
SMSs serotonin modulators and stimulants
SNRIs serotonin-norepinephrine reuptake inhibitors
SPARI 5-HT partial agonist-reuptake inhibitor
SSRIs selective serotonin reuptake inhibitors
STAR*D Sequenced Treatment Alternatives to Relieve Depression
TCAs tricyclic antidepressants
TM transmembrane domain
TRD treatment-resistant depression
UGT UDP-glucuronosyl-transferase
UV ultraviolet
WHO World Health Organization

CLINICAL SIGNIFICANCE

In patients with depression, it is important to match the correct medication to the patient's symptoms. The medications used to treat depression work on multiple complex pathways. Because of this, utilizing the inhibition constant (K_i) becomes important in understanding how strong a certain medication will bind to a receptor. For instance, venlafaxine, a serotonin-norepinephrine reuptake inhibitor (SNRI), demonstrates higher affinity for the serotonin or 5-hydroxytryptamine (5-HT) receptor at lower doses than the norepinephrine (NE) receptor, which means that if the patient requires more NE in their synapses higher doses of venlafaxine will need to be used. In contrast, duloxetine, also an SNRI, has much more potent affinity for both the 5-HT and NE receptors, which provides more flexible dosing to balance both NE and 5-HT levels at all doses.

Holly Lassila, DrPH, MSEd, RPh, LPC

Canst thou not minister to a mind diseas'd
Pluck from the memory a rooted sorrow,
Raze out the written troubles of the brain
And with some sweet oblivious antidote
Cleanse the stuff'd bosom of that perilous stuff
Which weighs upon the heart?

—William Shakespeare

Introduction

Depression is a common anxiety-mood disorder representing a social problem in the United States and worldwide, which is predicted to become the largest disease burden in 2030 by the World Health Organization (WHO).[1-4] Depression can be triggered by traumatic life events, hormone imbalance, medications, drug and alcohol use, lack of exercise, and several other factors. In contrast, a healthy lifestyle including consuming a nutritious diet and exercising regularly is an effective preventive and/or treatment strategy for depression. These triggers are known to cause or contribute to neurotransmitter imbalances. However, engaging in a healthy lifestyle may not be effective enough, and medication can help. The discovery of the first-generation antidepressants (ie, monoamine oxidase inhibitors [MAOIs], tricyclic antidepressants [TCAs], followed by selective serotonin reuptake inhibitors [SSRIs], mixed-acting serotonin-norepinephrine reuptake inhibitors [SNRIs], atypical antidepressants, and a few others) significantly improved the treatment and prognosis of depression, in addition to promoting the investigation of its possible biologic mechanisms.[5] However, the long latency of therapeutic effect and the presence of side effects and treatment resistance are still major problems with most antidepressant medications. For these reasons, the pharmacologic treatment of depression is still far from being satisfactory. Other mechanisms are being explored in the attempt to discover novel and effective antidepressants (see discussion regarding ketamine).

Depression is an ancient and prevalent mental condition that has been referenced throughout history in song, poetry, and literature.[6]

People do not know how to handle their depression. Depression isn't just a feeling and you can't just snap out of it. It's like a hatred that sucking inside of you and you have no happiness, no joy, and you do not know what to do next, you're lost.

-John Holcomb, Echoes of Gunfire, The Week, April 14, 2023

Clinical depression immobilizes a person, affecting both men and women, rich and poor, and young and old alike.[4,7] Depression symptoms include exhaustion, feelings of worthlessness and helplessness, and thoughts that lead to suicidal ideation. Depression affects appetite and sleep with normal day-to-day functioning. Clinical depression is not the same as a passing "blue" mood (temporary state of depression).[8,9] Without suitable treatment, depressive symptoms can last for weeks, months, or years. Appropriate treatment, however, can help most people who have depression. Negative thinking fades as treatment begins to take effect. Unfortunately, many people do not recognize that depression is a treatable illness. Much of this suffering is unnecessary, because depression is one of the most treatable mental illnesses.

Depression is the flaw in love. The meaninglessness of every enterprise and every emotion, the meaninglessness of life itself, becomes self-evident. The only feeling left in this loveless state is insignificance.

My depression had grown on me as that vine had conquered the oak; it had been a sucking thing that had wrapped itself around me, ugly and more alive than I. It had a life of its own that bit by bit asphyxiated all of my life out of me. My moods belonged to the depression as surely as the leaves on that oak tree's high branches belonged to the vine.

Drug therapy hacks through the vine. You can feel it happening, how the medication seems to be poisoning the parasite so that bit by bit it withers away. You feel the weight going, feel the way that the branches can recover much of their natural bent. But even with the vine gone, you may still have a few leaves and shallow roots and the rebuilding of yourself cannot be achieved with any drugs that now exist. Rebuilding of the self in and after depression requires love, insight and most of all, time.

—Andrew Solomon, The Noonday Demon: An Atlas of Depression

One in four women and 1 in 10 men can expect to develop depression during their lifetime.[7-9] In the United States alone, approximately 20 million adults are affected yearly with some type of depression, and at least 50% of these with major depressive disorder (MDD) will experience one or more repeated episodes during their lifetime. Depression affects at least 1 in 50 children under age 11 years and 1 in 20 teenagers, mostly girls. The increased rate of depression among adolescent girls is related more to physical changes that occur during puberty, suggestive of hormonal changes. Further evidence of hormonal involvement in depression is associated with premenstrual syndrome (PMS) and postpartum depression (PPD). Studies indicate that the majority of patients inadequately respond to monoamine antidepression therapy. Approximately 63% of patients failed to achieve remission after initial treatment with an SSRI. Of those patients who did not respond, 69% did not achieve remission upon switching to a second antidepressant. In patients who do achieve remission, residual symptoms, including insomnia, weight gain, and impaired concentration/decision-making, are common.

In a depressed state, a person feels hopeless and experiences an overwhelming sense of despair.[10] Depression immobilizes a person, making them feel exhausted, worthless, and helpless. It is an illness that involves the body, mood, and thoughts and affects the way the patient eats and sleeps, the way they feel about themself, and the way they think about things. It often interferes with normal functioning, causing pain and suffering not only to themselves but also to those around them. Depression can destroy family life as well as the life of the person who is ill.

About 11% of men and 16% of women will experience major depression in the course of their lives. Depression can limit quality of life, affect relationships, lead to lost time from work or school, and contribute to other chronic diseases.[11,12] Sometimes, it leads to suicidal ideation. Fortunately, for most people, MDD can be effectively treated with antidepressant drugs and psychotherapy. Everyone has periods of unhappiness in their lives, such as from the loss of a loved one or job dissatisfaction. Many people become temporarily down when things do not seem to be going well. These feelings are a normal part of life. Depressive episodes may appear at any age; however, MDD is most prevalent in adults (ages 18-64 years) with a median age of onset in their 20s. For example, adults are twice as likely to be diagnosed with MDD as compared to both adolescents (13-17 years) and older adults (65+ years). About half of all cases of depression go unrecognized and untreated, and approximately 10% to 15% of those with depression take their own lives yearly.

Depression in older adults (17%-35%) often is dismissed as a normal part of aging and may go undiagnosed and untreated, causing needless suffering for the family and for the individual who could otherwise live a fruitful life.[11] Often, the symptoms described usually are physical, and the older person is reluctant to discuss feelings of hopelessness, sadness, loss of interest in normally pleasurable activities, or extremely prolonged grief after a loss. Some symptoms may be the result of adverse (side) effects of medication that the older person is taking for other physical problems, or they may be caused by a concurrent illness. Improved recognition and treatment of depression will make life more enjoyable and fulfilling for the depressed older adult, the family, and the caretakers.[12]

The economic cost for depressive illnesses in the United States is estimated to be $210 billion per year, according to the newest data available from the U.S. Centers for Disease Control and Prevention (CDC) from 2014, but the cost in human suffering cannot be estimated. In 2016, antidepressant drugs (primarily TCAs, reuptake inhibitors of both norepinephrine [NE] and 5-hydroxytryptamine [5-HT], and SSRIs) ranked in the top 50 drugs dispensed, third in total prescriptions written, and third in total dollar prescription sales, at approximately $11.5 billion (~5% of total prescription drug sales).

Although there are several treatment options (both pharmacologic and nonpharmacologic) for depression, 34% to 46% of patients with MDD do not adequately respond to treatment. These patients are categorized as having treatment-resistant depression (TRD).

Clinicians have developed a strategic plan for TRD called Sequenced Treatment Alternatives to Relieve Depression (STAR*D).[12] STAR*D provides a four-step treatment plan, in which a patient proceeds to the next treatment step if they do not achieve full remission under the current treatment step. SSRIs are the first treatment step, and, as patients progress through the treatment steps, they will be introduced to new antidepressant drugs with different mechanism of actions (eg, bupropion, TCAs, etc). Patients that achieve full remission and tolerate treatment at a specific step are then placed on long-term treatment with that drug. The results from a large-scale long-term study found a cumulative remission rate of 67% (across all four treatment steps); however, those patients who progressed through more treatment steps had higher relapse rates as compared to those patients that achieved remission in the first treatment step. The annual suicide rate in the United States is 13 in 100,000.

Types of Depressive Disorders

Major Depressive Disorder

MDD (also called clinical depression) is the most serious type of depression that is manifested by a combination of symptoms that interfere with the ability to work, study, sleep, eat, and enjoy once-pleasurable activities and may reoccur multiple times during a lifetime.[3,10,12] Many people with MDD cannot continue to function normally. Major depression seems to run in families, suggesting that depressive illnesses can be inherited. The treatments for MDD are antidepressants, psychotherapy, and, in extreme cases, electroconvulsive therapy (ECT). MDD causes a persistent feeling of sadness and loss of interest. It affects how the person feels, thinks, and behaves and can lead to a variety of emotional and physical problems. They may have trouble doing normal day-to-day activities, and sometimes they may feel as if life is not worth living. More than just a bout of the blues, MDD is not a weakness, and the patient cannot simply "snap out" of it. Depression may require long-term treatment. Most people with MDD feel better with medication, psychotherapy, or both. Although major depression may occur only once, people typically have multiple episodes. During these episodes, symptoms occur most of the day, nearly every day, and may include[10,12,13]:

- Feelings of sadness, tearfulness, emptiness, or hopelessness
- Angry outbursts, irritability, and frustration, even over small matters
- Loss of interest or pleasure in most or all normal activities, such as sex, hobbies, and sports
- Sleep disturbances, including insomnia or sleeping too much
- Tiredness and lack of energy, so even small tasks take extra effort
- Reduced appetite and weight loss or increased cravings for food and weight gain
- Anxiety, agitation, and restlessness
- Slowed thinking, speaking, and body movements
- Feelings of worthlessness or guilt, fixating on past failures, and self-blame
- Trouble thinking, concentrating, making decisions, and remembering things
- Frequent or recurrent thoughts of death, suicidal thoughts, suicide attempts, and suicide
- Unexplained physical problems, such as back pain and headaches

For many people with depression, symptoms usually are severe enough to cause noticeable problems in day-to-day activities, such as work, school, social activities, and relationships with others. Some people may feel generally miserable or unhappy without really knowing why.

Common signs and symptoms of MDD in children and teenagers are similar to those of adults, but there can be some differences. In younger children, symptoms of depression may include sadness, irritability, clinginess, worry, aches and pains, refusing to go to school, and being underweight. In teens, symptoms may include sadness, irritability, feeling negative and worthless, anger, poor performance or poor attendance at school, feeling misunderstood and extremely sensitive, using recreational drugs or alcohol, eating or sleeping too much, self-harm, loss of interest in normal activities, and avoidance of social interaction.

Depression in older adults is not a normal part of growing older, and it should never be taken lightly.[11] Unfortunately, depression often goes undiagnosed and untreated in older adults, and they may feel reluctant to seek help. Symptoms of depression may be different or less obvious in older adults, such as memory difficulties or personality changes, physical aches or pain, fatigue, loss of appetite, sleep problems, and loss of interest in sex—not caused by a medical condition or medication, often wanting to stay at home, rather than going out to socialize or doing new things, and suicidal thinking or feelings, especially in older men.[13]

Persistent Depressive Disorder (Dysthymia)

This is a mild, chronic depression that lasts for 2 years (1 year for children and adolescents) or longer and is characterized by chronic symptoms that do not disable but keep the person from functioning well or from feeling good about themselves.[3] Many of those with dysthymia also experience major depressive episodes at some point in their lives. Most people may not realize that they are depressed and continue to function at work or school, but often with the feeling that they are "just going through the motions." Antidepressants or psychotherapy can help.

Other Types of Depressive Disorders

Seasonal Affective Disorder

Other, less common types of depression include seasonal affective disorder, a popular name that describes a type of depression that happens during particular seasons of the year (seasonal pattern) but is a Diagnostic and Statistical Manual of Mental Disorders, Fifth Edition (DSM-5) diagnosis.[3] This disorder involves symptoms of depression that occur during the fall and winter seasons, when the days are shorter, and there is less exposure to natural sunlight. When the spring and summer seasons begin, and there is greater exposure to longer hours of daylight, the symptoms of depression disappear. Adjustment disorder with depressed mood is a type of depression that results when a person has something bad happen that depresses them (eg, job loss can cause this type of depression). It generally fades as time passes, and the person gets over whatever it was that happened.[1] Additional factors involved in its onset include stresses at home, work, or school, and symptoms may persist for as long as 6 months.

Depression in Women

Contrary to popular belief, depression is not a "normal part of being a woman" nor is it a "female weakness."[7] Depression is a treatable medical illness that can occur in any woman, at any time, and for various reasons regardless of age, ethnicity, or income.[14,15] Approximately 11 million women in the United States experience depression each year. About one in every eight women can expect to develop depression during their lifetime. Depression occurs most frequently in women ages 25 to 44. Many factors may contribute to depression in women, such as developmental (puberty), reproductive, menstrual, genetic, and other biologic differences (eg, PMS, childbirth, infertility, and menopause).[14,15] Social factors may also lead to higher rates of depression among women, including stress from work, family responsibilities, the roles and expectations of women, increased rates of sexual abuse, and poverty. Women experience depression at roughly twice the rate of men. Girls ages 14 to 18 years have consistently higher rates of depression than boys in this age group. Around 20% to 40% of women may experience PMS, and an estimated 3% to 5% have symptoms severe enough to be classified as MDD.

Postpartum Depression

PPD is a common debilitating illness that affects 15% to 20% of women, who experience significant depressive symptoms after the birth of a child.[16-19] Of these, 5% to 10% experience severe depressive symptoms, meaning that about 1% of women develop severe depression after childbirth. PPD is associated with substantial morbidity, and improved pharmacologic treatment options are needed. The U.S. Food and Drug Administration (FDA) approved brexanolone (Zulresso, an intravenous [IV] infusion formulation of allopregnanolone) for treatment of moderate to severe PPD.[20,21] A 60-hour infusion of brexanolone temporarily returned the level of allopregnanolone to predelivery levels, thus allowing the brain to adjust to a more gradual decrease in this steroid's levels. The results at the end of the 60-hour infusion were dramatic. Women treated with the active drug had a marked response—full remission of symptoms—in comparison to 1 of 10 women who were treated with placebo. Importantly, the benefits of the drug were still apparent 30 days after the beginning of the infusion. The treatment was also well tolerated by all who achieved remission of depressive symptoms. Many believe it is normal for a mother to feel depressed for at least 2 weeks after giving birth.

ALLOPREGNANOLONE. Allopregnanolone (3α-hydroxy-5α-pregnan-20-one) is a neurosteroid and a metabolite of progesterone.[16] It is a positive allosteric modulator of γ-aminobutyric acid $(GABA)_A$ receptors for the treatment of moderate to severe PPD.[14] Allosteric modulation of a neurotransmitter receptor is known to cause different degrees of desired activity, instead of total activation or inhibition of the receptor. It has strong sedative and anxiolytic properties, and low endogenous levels have been associated with depressed mood.[17,22,23] Allopregnanolone is a potent $GABA_A$ receptor modulator and impacts central nervous system (CNS) activity through positive allosteric modulation (PAM) of the $GABA_A$ receptor (see Chapter 8) at synaptic or extrasynaptic $GABA_A$ receptors. It is ideally suited for parenteral administration due to its low oral bioavailability. PAMs are allosteric regulators or potentiators, thereby inducing the amplification of the effect of the $GABA_A$ receptor, much like tuning a radio. Most anxiolytic benzodiazepines act as PAMs at the $GABA_A$ receptor. Zuranolone is an oral derivative of brexanolone that is under development by Sage Therapeutics for the oral treatment of MDD, PPD, Parkinson disease, insomnia, and seizures.[24,25] It is a synthetic, orally effective, inhibitory pregnane neurosteroid of allopregnanolone, with a half-life of 16 to 23 hours, and acts as a PAM of the $GABA_A$ receptor. The drug was developed as an improvement over brexanolone with high oral bioavailability and a biologic half-life suitable for once-daily administration for MDD, PPD, and Parkinson disease and is in phase 3 clinical studies for insomnia and seizures.

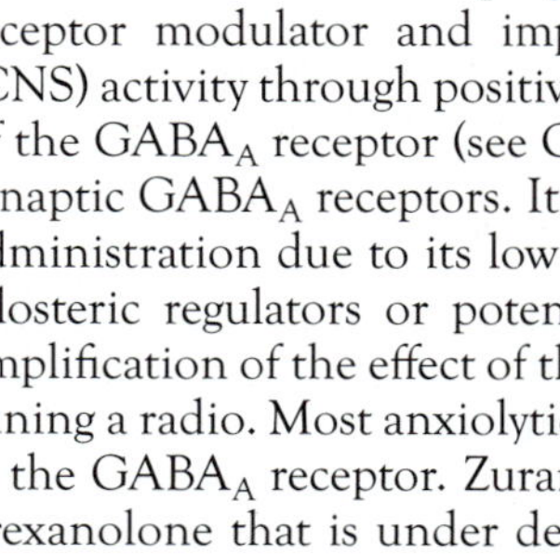

Allopregnanolone (Brexanolone)

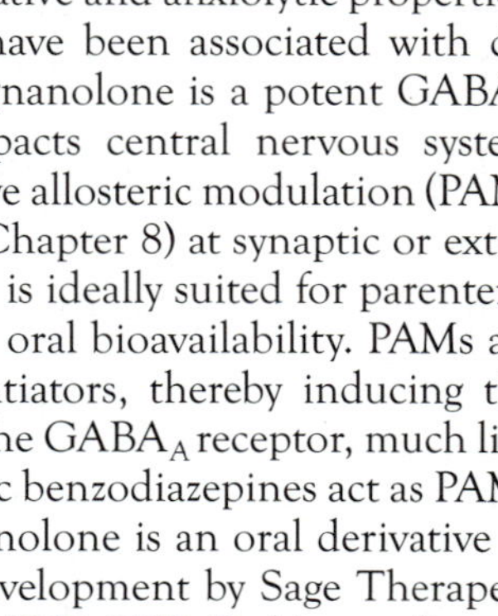

Zuranolone

As the primary inhibitory neurotransmitter in the CNS, GABA can influence a wide range of behavioral states, such as anxiety levels, seizures, sleep, vigilance, and memory.[26] $GABA_A$ receptors are the target for numerous clinically relevant drugs such as benzodiazepines, barbiturates, and anesthetics. Allopregnanolone allosterically enhances GABAergic signaling at $GABA_A$ receptors. Allopregnanolone is synthesized in the brain from progesterone, but the main sources of serum allopregnanolone in nonpregnant women are the corpus luteum and the adrenal cortex.[16] Low bioavailability and oxidation of the 3α-hydroxyl to a 3-ketone limit the therapeutic use of allopregnanolone. During the menstrual cycle, serum allopregnanolone concentrations vary between around 0.5 and 4 to 5 nmol/L. During pregnancy, fetoplacental synthesis causes the maternal serum concentrations of allopregnanolone to rise to reach more than 10 times the maximum menstrual cycle levels. After delivery, the allopregnanolone level rapidly drops to 2 nmol/L within a few days. When administered IV to nonpregnant women, pregnancy-like allopregnanolone serum concentrations are sedative, suggesting that a tolerance to allopregnanolone develops during pregnancy. Low levels of allopregnanolone have been implicated in the pathophysiology of mood disorders such as PPD. For example, successful treatment with SSRIs increases plasma and cerebrospinal fluid (CSF) levels of allopregnanolone in patients with MDD. However, increased serum allopregnanolone has also been observed after unsuccessful treatment with antidepressants. Furthermore, lowered allopregnanolone levels have been observed in women with depression compared to women with no history of depression.

However, lower allopregnanolone plasma levels after delivery have been found in women who develop postpartum blues, and, for this reason, postpartum blues have been suggested to be an effect of withdrawal from allopregnanolone.[22,23,27] Women with higher allopregnanolone concentrations during pregnancy may be protected against depressed mood during pregnancy and could be subject to a more marked drop after delivery, thus being more susceptible to depressive symptoms postpartum. Both progesterone and allopregnanolone levels change substantially during pregnancy, increasing up to 30-fold and then rapidly returning to normal levels at the time of delivery. Allopregnanolone is known to be anxiolytic, whereas prolonged administration or withdrawal from allopregnanolone may precipitate increased anxiety. Allopregnanolone is partly responsible for the decreased hypothalamic-pituitary-adrenal (HPA) response to stress seen in rats during pregnancy. Thus, higher levels of allopregnanolone during late pregnancy would be protective against concurrent symptoms of depressed mood and anxiety. It is also likely that allopregnanolone withdrawal following delivery has a larger influence during the first days following delivery than several weeks into the postpartum period. The results are relevant for generally healthy pregnant women who experience mood symptoms during pregnancy. When allopregnanolone levels drop dramatically after delivery, the nerve cells containing GABA take a while to adjust to the decrease. It is thought that this delay might trigger depressive symptoms in some women.

The new drug application (NDA) for zuranolone has been approved by the FDA as a rapid-acting, once-daily, 14-day, oral short-course treatment for MDD and PPD in women. Zuranolone is an oral neuroactive steroid $GABA_A$ receptor PAM for the treatment of MDD and PPD.[24] The $GABA_A$ system is the major inhibitory signaling pathway of the brain and CNS and contributes to regulating brain function. Altered neurotransmission of GABA has been implicated in the pathogenesis of depression. Zuranolone was developed as an oral improvement to brexanolone, approved for the treatment of PPD. Zuranolone has better bioavailability with a half-life of 10 to 23 hours and can be administered orally, whereas brexanolone is administered IV. According to data, zuranolone has demonstrated rapid and sustained improvement of depressive symptoms, a consistent safety profile, and generally good tolerability.

Previous studies have linked low levels of allopregnanolone to depression, anxiety, anorexia, obesity, and posttraumatic stress disorder (PTSD).[28,29] Women with anorexia nervosa and obesity having low levels of allopregnanolone add to the picture that the role of allopregnanolone is under-recognized in mood disorders. The results also suggest that those who presented with severe symptoms of MDD or anxiety had lower levels of allopregnanolone, concluding that there is a distinct correlation between the level of allopregnanolone and the severity of the mood disorders.

If someone with PTSD is going through an ongoing trauma, such as being in an abusive relationship, both of the problems need to be addressed. Other ongoing problems can include panic disorder, depression, substance abuse, and feeling suicidal.

The most studied type of medication for treating PTSD are antidepressants, which may help control PTSD symptoms such as sadness, worry, anger, and feeling numb inside. Other medications may be helpful for treating specific PTSD symptoms, such as sleep problems and nightmares. Clinicians and patients can work together to find the best medication or medication combination, as well as the right dose. Check the FDA website for the latest information on patient medication guides, warnings, and newly approved medications.

Psychotherapy (sometimes called "talk therapy") involves talking with a mental health professional to treat a mental illness. Psychotherapy can occur one-on-one or in a group. Talk therapy treatment for PTSD usually lasts 6 to 11 weeks, but it can last longer. Research shows that support from family and friends can be an important part of recovery. Talk therapies teach people helpful ways to react to the frightening events that trigger their PTSD symptoms.

Premenstrual Dysphoric Disorder

Premenstrual dysphoric disorder (PMDD) is diagnosed when a woman experiences severe symptoms of depression, tension, and irritability in the week prior to menstruation.[18,19] While it is not uncommon for most women to experience emotional and physical changes prior to menstruation, women who meet criteria for PMDD experience changes that impact their lives and include sudden mood swings, irritability, and anger; depressed mood and feelings of hopelessness, anxiety, tension, and being overwhelmed or out of control; decreased interest in usual activities; difficulty staying focused in attention or thinking; fatigue; change in appetite and food cravings; and trouble sleeping or sleeping too much. Physical symptoms include breast tenderness, joint or muscle pain, weight gain, and bloating. The distinction between PMDD and MDD is that symptoms begin a week prior to menstruation and end within the first few days post-menstruation. Treatment can include hormone treatment, psychotherapy, and antidepressants. With treatment, most women experience partial or full improvement in symptoms.

Married couples have a lower rate of depression than those living alone. However, unhappily married women have the highest rates of depression; happily married men have the lowest rates.[26] Approximately 10% to 15% of all new mothers get PPD, which most frequently occurs within the first months after the birth of a child. Also, research shows a strong relationship between eating disorders (anorexia and bulimia nervosa) and depression in women. About 90% to 95% of cases of anorexia occur in young females. Reported rates of bulimia nervosa vary from one to three out of 100 people. Although men are more likely than women to die by suicide, women report attempting suicide approximately twice as often as men. An estimated 15% of people hospitalized for depression eventually take their own lives. Depression in women is misdiagnosed approximately 30% to 50% of the time. Fewer than half of the women who experience clinical depression will ever seek care. Fortunately, clinical depression is a very treatable illness. More than 80% of people with depression can be treated successfully with medication, psychotherapy, or a combination of both. More than half of women believe it is "normal" for a woman to be depressed during menopause and that treatment is not necessary. More than half of women believe depression is a "normal part of aging."

Bipolar Disorder (Manic-Depressive Illness)

Bipolar disorder, formerly called manic depression, is a mental health condition that causes extreme mood swings (mania or hypomania) and lows (depression) including changes in thoughts, mood, and behavior.[3] A person with bipolar disorder may experience periods of mania, hypomania, and depressive episodes. When they become depressed, they may feel sad or hopeless and lose interest or pleasure in most activities. When their mood shifts to mania or hypomania (less extreme than mania), they may feel euphoric, full of energy, or unusually irritable. These mood swings can affect sleep, energy, activity, judgment, behavior, and the ability to think clearly. Episodes of mood swings may occur rarely or multiple times a year. While most people will experience some emotional symptoms between episodes, some may not experience any. Although bipolar disorder is a lifelong condition, mood swings and other symptoms can be managed by following a treatment plan. In most cases, bipolar disorder is treated with medications other than MDD drugs and psychological counseling (psychotherapy).

Bipolar disorder affects men and women in roughly equal numbers, but there are some gender differences. Women with bipolar disorder tend to have more depressive and fewer manic episodes, and are more likely to have bipolar II disorder and rapid cycling. Women's hormonal changes and reproductive factors can influence the onset, relapse, and treatment of the disorder. Women with bipolar disorder are more likely to experience depressive episodes than men. They may require hospitalization during these times to help manage symptoms and potential safety concerns.

Symptoms can cause unpredictable changes in mood and behavior, resulting in significant distress and difficulty in life. There are several types of bipolar and related disorders, including bipolar I disorder, bipolar II disorder, and cyclothymic disorder.

Bipolar I Disorder. Bipolar I disorder is a condition that causes periods of severe changes in mood, activity levels, energy, and ability to carry out everyday tasks. Bipolar I disorder can cause unpredictable high and low mood swings, also known as manic-depressive episodes. It is impossible to predict how long mood episodes may last. The patient might be severely depressed either for a brief or extended period of time before entering into a manic episode. Mania could last anywhere from a week to months. Patients may even experience manic and depressive symptoms at the same time, which is known as a mixed episode. Bipolar I diagnosis involves at least one manic or mixed episode lasting at least 1 week or resulting in hospitalization. The episode may come before or after a hypomanic or depressive episode. However, someone can have bipolar I without having a depressive episode. These changes are commonly called "mood episodes." Three million Americans are affected by bipolar I disorder each year. While anyone can develop bipolar I disorder, it often starts in the late teen or early adult years, and it lasts a lifetime. It can result from many factors, including an imbalance of certain neurochemicals in the brain, which may be too high or too low. Bipolar I disorder often runs in families.

Bipolar II Disorder. Diagnosis of bipolar II disorder involves a current or past major depressive episode lasting for at least 2 weeks. The person must also have had a current or past episode of hypomania.

Mania. Mania is a state of elevated mood. During manic episodes, a person may feel very high-spirited, energetic, and creative. They may also feel irritable or may engage in high-risk behaviors, such as substance misuse, increased sexual activity, spending money foolishly, making bad financial investments, or behaving in other reckless ways. Manic episodes can last for a week or longer. Patients may experience either visual or auditory hallucinations or delusions; these are referred to as "psychotic features."

Hypomania. Hypomania is a less severe form of mania. During hypomanic episodes, a patient may be in a state of elevated mood similar to those that occur with mania. These elevated moods are less intense than manic moods, though, and have less impact on one's ability to function. Women are more likely to develop hypomania than men.

Depression. People with bipolar disorder may experience depressive episodes, with intense sadness and a significant loss of energy. These episodes last at least 2 weeks, which can cause severe impairment. Women are more likely to experience depressive symptoms than men. A major depressive episode includes symptoms that can be severe enough to cause noticeable difficulty in day-to-day activities, such as work, school, social activities, and relationships. An episode includes five or more of these symptoms: depressed mood, such as feeling sad, empty, hopeless, or tearful (in children and teens, depressed mood can appear as irritability); marked loss of interest or feeling no pleasure in all—or almost all—activities; significant weight loss when not dieting, weight gain, or decrease or increase in appetite (in children, failure to gain weight as expected can be a sign of depression); insomnia or sleeping too much; restlessness or slowed behavior; fatigue or loss of energy; feelings of worthlessness or excessive or inappropriate guilt; decreased ability to think or concentrate or indecisiveness; and thinking about, planning, or attempting suicide.

Mixed Mania. In addition to separate manic and depressive episodes, people with bipolar disorder may also experience mixed mania. This is also known as a mixed episode. With a mixed episode, both manic and depressive symptoms may be experienced daily for a week or longer. Women are more likely to experience mixed episodes than men.

Rapid Cycling. Bipolar episodes can also be characterized by how quickly the episodes alternate. Rapid cycling is a pattern of bipolar disorder that occurs when there are at least four manic or depressive episodes within 1 year.

Cyclothymic Disorder. People with cyclothymic disorder may experience ongoing bipolar symptoms that do not meet the full criteria for a bipolar I or bipolar II diagnosis. Cyclothymic disorder is considered a less severe form of bipolar disorder. It involves the frequent recurrence of hypomanic and depressive symptoms that never become severe enough to be diagnosed as having bipolar II disorder. These symptoms generally persist for a 2-year period.

Bipolar Disorder in Children and Adolescents. Symptoms of bipolar disorder can be difficult to identify in children and teens. It is often hard to tell whether these are normal ups and downs, or signs of a mental health problem other than bipolar disorder. Symptoms of bipolar disorder in children include serious mood swings that differ from their usual mood swings. These happen often, can last a long time, and greatly affect the way a child acts, such as being very hyperactive, impulsive, and aggressive, which affects how a child acts socially and in other areas of life. They can have racing thoughts, sometimes shown by quickly and often changing subjects when talking. Risky and reckless behaviors that are out of character, such as having frequent casual sex with many partners, are common. Other examples include alcohol or drug misuse, wild spending sprees, and unable to sleep or greatly decreased need for sleep. During a depressive bout, depressed or irritable mood occurs most of the day, nearly every day. Suicidal thoughts or behaviors can occur. These symptoms occur more often in older children and teens. When a child or teen with bipolar disorder experiences symptoms, it is called an episode. Between these episodes, they can return to their usual behavior and mood. Making a diagnosis of bipolar disorder is complicated. It often involves several assessments, sessions, and sources of information. There are no laboratory, genetic, medical, or brain imaging tests that a health care provider can use to diagnose bipolar disorder. If a child has serious mood swings, depression, or behavior problems, the parent should seek help from a mental health provider who specializes in working with children and teens. Mood and behavior issues caused by bipolar disorder or other mental health conditions can lead to major problems. Early treatment can help prevent serious issues and decrease the effects of mental health problems as the child gets older. Children and teens may have distinct major depressive or manic or hypomanic episodes, but the pattern can vary from that of adults with bipolar disorder, and moods can rapidly shift during episodes. Some children may have periods without mood symptoms between episodes. The most prominent signs of bipolar disorder in children and teenagers may include severe mood swings that are different from their usual mood swings.

Bipolar disorder is most often identified in young adults, but it can also occur in teenagers. It is rare but possible in younger children. Emotional unrest and behaviors that disrupt others are common in the childhood and teen years. In most cases, these behaviors are not a sign of a mental health problem that needs to be treated. All kids go through rough periods, feeling down, irritable, angry, hyperactive, or impulsive at times. But if the child's symptoms are severe or ongoing or causing big problems, it may be more than just a phase.

Despite the mood extremes, people with bipolar disorder often do not recognize how much their emotional instability disrupts their lives and the lives of their loved ones and do not get the treatment they need. Some people with bipolar disorder may enjoy the feelings of euphoria and cycles of being more productive. However, this euphoria is always followed by an emotional crash that can leave them depressed; worn out; and perhaps in financial, legal, or relationship trouble. Bipolar disorder does not get better on its own. Getting treatment from a mental health professional with experience in bipolar disorder can help get symptoms under control. Suicidal thoughts and behavior are common among people with bipolar disorder. Depressive and manic episodes are often triggered by something. Being aware of triggers or warning signs can help manage mood episodes. Common triggers for bipolar I disorder may include: sleep deprivation, medications, seasonal changes, and substance misuse. Some triggers can be controlled or managed, while others may not. Treatments for MDD may not be effective for patients with bipolar I disorder, so it is important to get the right diagnosis. Lithium, carbamazepine, topiramate, and valproic acid are effective mood-stabilizing treatments for bipolar disorders.

Neurodevelopmental Disorders, Obsessive-Compulsive and Related Disorders, and Posttraumatic Stress Disorder

A discussion of these disorders[3] is included in this chapter because patients with these disorders are more likely to experience comorbid depression.

Neurodevelopmental disorders include:

- Autism spectrum disorder: a group of developmental disabilities that can cause significant social, communication, and behavioral challenges
- Attention-deficit/hyperactivity disorder (ADHD): one of the most common neurodevelopmental disorders of childhood, usually first diagnosed in childhood and often lasts into adulthood; children with ADHD may have trouble paying attention, controlling impulsive behaviors (may act without thinking about what the result will be), or be overly active
- Tic disorders: patients must have had ≥2 motor tics and ≥1 vocal tic for a year, with onset before age 18 years; a computed tomography (CT) scan is done to rule out other causes of the symptoms.

Obsessive-compulsive disorder (OCD) is a pattern of unwanted thoughts and fears (obsessions) that induce repetitive behaviors (compulsions).

PTSD is a mental and behavioral disorder that can develop because of exposure to a traumatic event, such as sexual assault, warfare, traffic collisions, child abuse, domestic violence, or other threats on a person's life.

Biologic Basis of Depression

Monoamine Hypothesis

It has been almost 50 years since the monoamine hypothesis of depression was first described.[30,31] The monoamine hypothesis proposes that patients with depression have depleted concentrations of 5-HT, NE, or dopamine (DA). Two primary lines of evidence led to the development of the monoamine hypothesis: (1) the effects of reserpine on 5-HT and catecholamines (CAs) and (2) the pharmacologic mechanisms of action of antidepressant drugs.

The classic antidepressants that modulate monoaminergic systems are not sufficiently effective and require long systematic application. Recent studies suggest that substances that modulate the glutamatergic system may produce an antidepressant effect that is not only faster but also more sustained. The intensive preclinical and clinical research on N-methyl-D-aspartate (NMDA) and metabotropic glutamate (mGlu) receptor ligands, which is currently ongoing, could contribute to the awaited breakthrough in the field of novel antidepressant drug discovery. This line of research may also lead to a new understanding of the biologic basis of depression.[32]

Reserpine, an alkaloid extracted from *Rauwolfia serpentina*, was utilized as a treatment for hypertensive disease in the 1950s; however, reserpine was found to precipitate depression in some patients.[30,31] The depression produced by reserpine was reversed after the treatment was terminated and following either rest or electric shock therapy. Additionally, reserpine was found to produce depressive-like effects in animals. Reserpine was found to inhibit the monoamine transporter and, as a result, depletes brain monoamines (ie, 5-HT and CAs), which provided evidence for the role of 5-HT, NE, or DA in depression. The second line of evidence was based on the underlying pharmacologic mechanisms of action of monoamine oxidase (MAO) inhibitors and TCAs. For example, antidepressant drugs primarily target the monoamine neurotransmitters (ie, 5-HT, NE, or DA) in an attempt to increase the presence of these monoamine neurotransmitters in the synaptic space to activate postsynaptic receptors.[32] The SSRIs, which were developed later, provided additional support for the monoamine hypothesis. More recent clinical studies have provided evidence suggesting that the monoamine hypothesis for MDD needs to be revised and is not as simple as depleted concentrations of 5-HT, NE, or DA leading to MDD. For example, monoamine depletion in healthy subjects does not produce depressive symptoms. Furthermore, monoamine or tryptophan depletion does not increase depressive symptoms in unmedicated patients with MDD.[33] Thus, the revised monoamine hypothesis suggests that monoamine depletion may play more of a modulatory role such that it influences other neurobiologic systems (eg, intracellular signaling, brain-derived neurotrophic factor [BDNF], or other neurotransmitter and neuropeptide systems) or must be present in the context of stressors. The development and description of the mechanisms of actions for each of the seven major antidepressant drug classes are presented.

Although the underlying pathophysiology of depression has not been clearly defined, preclinical and clinical evidence suggest disturbances in the neuroaminergic system, 5-HT, NE, or DA neurotransmission in the CNS.[32,33] Most all currently available antidepressants act on one or more of the following mechanisms: inhibition of reuptake of 5-HT or NE and DA, antagonism of inhibitory presynaptic 5-HT or NE receptors, or inhibition of MAO. All of these mechanisms enhance the neurotransmission of 5-HT and/or NE. Evidence for the involvement of NE in depression is abundant, and recent studies on neuronal pathways and symptoms highlight the specific role of NE in this disorder.[30,31] NE plays a role in regulating cognition, motivation, and intellect, which are fundamental in social relationships. NE-deficit depressions are associated with decreased concentration, low motivation, poor energy, inattention, poor self-care, and cognitive difficulties, whereas 5-HT-deficit depressions are associated with anxiety, suicidality, and appetite disturbances (Fig. 12.1).

The classic monoamine hypothesis of depression posits in an oversimplified manner that depression arises due to a deficiency in monoamine neurotransmitters.[30,31] Although direct evidence for the monoamine hypothesis is lacking, virtually all currently available antidepressants directly affect one or more monoamine neurotransmitter systems.

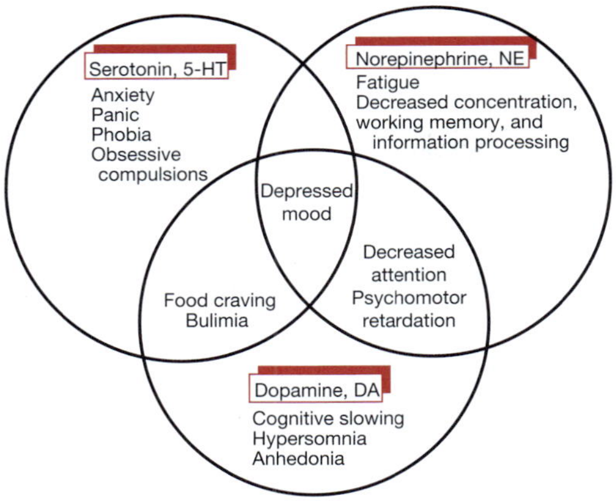

Figure 12.1 Neurotransmitter deficiency syndromes and their interactions.

However, despite the fact that such agents increase monoamine levels shortly after initiating treatment, the therapeutic benefits are often delayed by several weeks.

As a result, the focus has now shifted away from the neurotransmitters themselves to their receptors, transporters, and the downstream molecular events that these receptors trigger in order to explain the mechanism of action of antidepressants. Treatment with agents targeting the monoamine pathway, such as SSRIs, has been shown to increase neurogenesis formation of new neurons in the hippocampus. These effects may be mediated by activating the cyclic adenosine monophosphate (cAMP) response.[33]

The monoamine hypothesis is still driving clinical development of new antidepressants. Virtually all currently available antidepressants act on one or more mechanisms compatible with the monoamine hypothesis. The confirmation of the clinical activity of these antidepressants has done much to reinforce the monoamine hypothesis. Although the precise nature of depression is not fully understood at the level of the chemistry in the brain, several theories have been proposed to explain the role of NE, 5-HT, and glutamine in the causes of depression. Schildkraut et al[34] postulated that depression arises as a consequence of a deficiency of NE and that the effects caused by CA depletion can be reversed by the TCAs. Depression in animals following reserpine administration can be reversed by TCAs, suggesting that the stimulating effects of desipramine (a secondary amine TCA) and MAOIs were NE based.

During the late 1960s, Kielholz,[33] a Swiss psychiatrist, argued that different antidepressants did quite different things and that it was important to select the right antidepressant for the right patient. He differentiated the TCAs based on whether they possessed the ability to sedate (eg, trimipramine), to stimulate (eg, desipramine or nortriptyline), or to improve mood (eg, clomipramine). By the end of the 1960s, the broad consensus was that secondary amine TCAs (like desipramine or nortriptyline) inhibited the reuptake of NE into noradrenergic neurons and that blocking 5-HT reuptake by tertiary amine TCAs (such as clomipramine) explained the mood elevation of some antidepressants.

The CA hypothesis was then modified to include 5-HT in the etiology of depression.[32] Inhibition of 5-HT biosynthesis reverses the therapeutic effects of treatment with antidepressants that have predominantly 5-HT reuptake inhibitory activity (eg, fluoxetine) but less so with those that have predominantly NE reuptake inhibitory activity (eg, desipramine). Also, inhibition of 5-HT biosynthesis produced a relapse in patients who are depressed who had their depression successfully treated with imipramine or tranylcypromine, whereas inhibitors of DA or NE synthesis had no effect on these patients who are depressed. A depletion of CA reverses the therapeutic effects of desipramine more than that of fluoxetine or sertraline. These studies appear to confirm that the antidepressive action of antidepressants is, indeed, a function of their monoamine activity.

Kielholz further reasoned that because NE reuptake inhibitors (activating antidepressants) were likely to trigger suicide and 5-HT reuptake inhibitors would be less likely to lead to suicide, therefore, it would be worth developing drugs that selectively inhibited the reuptake of 5-HT, producing agents more useful for the treatment of depression. Genetic studies of NE function have indicated the multiple roles that NE plays in normal and pathologic states. Functional deletion (knockout) of the NE transporter in mice results in increased extracellular levels of NE.[34] This model functionally mimics the therapeutic effects of selective NE antidepressants. Studies in patients with depression who are in remission and no longer taking medication have shown that a drastic reduction of NE levels (by inhibition of the key synthetic enzyme, tyrosine hydroxylase, with α-methyl-*p*-tyrosine) results in a rapid reappearance of depressive symptoms. Interestingly, however, CA depletion in healthy control volunteers does not result in depressed mood. Analysis of the unresolved symptoms suggests that a specific set of symptoms related to decreased positive affect respond poorly to serotonergic antidepressants, namely loss of pleasure, interest, and energy and fatigue. There is evidence to suggest that antidepressants that enhance NE and DA activity offer a therapeutic advantage over 5-HT antidepressants in the treatment of symptoms associated with reduced positive affect.[34]

Although currently available antidepressants increase monoamine levels soon after the start of treatment, therapeutic benefits are often delayed by several weeks or months, and the majority of patients with MDD fail to achieve an adequate response (treatment resistance) to first- or second-line therapies targeting monoamines.[33] The recent approval of the NMDA antagonist esketamine (Spravato) given intranasally for TRD has reinforced the need for agents with rapid onset with alternate mechanisms of action. Dextromethorphan/bupropion (Auvelity), recently FDA approved, is one such candidate. The use of agents with more rapid onsets of action, such as ketamine, is restricted due to the need for monitoring, risk of serious side effects, and the potential for abuse/misuse.

Considerations for Major Depressive Disorder and Treatment-Resistant Depression

Research suggests that combination therapy with multimodal agents is more effective than antidepressant monotherapy.[35,36] While 25% of patients treated with an SSRI alone for 6 weeks achieved remission, 52% of those treated with an SSRI in combination with a noradrenergic and specific serotonergic antidepressant (NaSSA) and 46% of those treated with a NaSSA in combination with bupropion achieved remission, resulting in more rapid and robust decreases in depression rating scale scores than bupropion treatment alone. With its similar pharmacologic properties to ketamine, dextromethorphan/bupropion combination (Auvelity) represents a promising new investigational agent for depression. Spravato is the only FDA-approved nasal spray for TRD (see "Esketamine" section).[37]

Changes in NE and 5-HT levels do not affect mood in everyone.[36] Some evidence also suggests that for a subset of patients, DA plays a role in depression.[38] Dopaminergic substances have been used as antidepressants when other measures have failed. The DA hypothesis of schizophrenia and the emphasis on other neurotransmitters, most notably NE and 5-HT, in the pathogenesis of depression have focused attention away from DA and its role in affective disorders.[38,39] Recent clinical evidence suggests the involvement of DA in several subtypes of depression, psychomotor retardation, and diminished motivation and in seasonal mood disorder.[38,39] The biochemical evidence in patients with depression indicates diminished DA turnover. In addition, a considerable amount of pharmacologic evidence exists regarding the efficacy of antidepressants with dopaminergic effects in the treatment of depression. However, the role of DA in depression must be understood in the context of existing theories involving other neurotransmitters that may act independently and interact with DA and other neurochemicals to contribute to depression.

Thus, the clinical efficacy/toxicity produced by these antidepressants is due to a combination of inhibitory actions on different targets including reuptake transporters for the neurotransmitters 5-HT, NE, and DA; nicotinic acetylcholine receptors (nAChRs); histamine H_1 receptors; and α1-adrenergic receptors.[40,41]

Limitations of the Monoamine Hypothesis

While the monoamine deficiency hypothesis of depression has been commonly used for more than 60 years to explain the mechanism of actions of the antidepressant drugs, a growing body of evidence has been accumulating over the past two decades supporting alternative non-monoamine mechanisms of action: the hypercholinergic hypothesis of depression and NMDA antagonists and neurohormones.[33]

Drugs increasing the synaptic availability of 5-HT and NE (biogenic amine–based agents) have been used to treat depression for more than 50 years. However, significant symptom improvement requires 2 to 4 weeks of treatment, and a first course of therapy provides symptom relief to only 60% to 65% of patients. NMDA receptor (NMDAR) antagonists targeting the NR2B subtype for TRD are under development.[32,33] The NR2B receptor is an NMDAR class of ionotropic glutamate receptors. The NMDAR channel has been shown to be involved in long-term increase in the efficiency of synaptic transmission thought to underlie certain kinds of memory and learning. NMDAR channels are heterotetramers composed of two molecules of the key receptor subunit NMDAR1 and two drawn from one or more of the four NMDAR2 subunits: The NR2 subunit acts as the agonist-binding site for glutamine, one of the predominant excitatory neurotransmitter receptors in the mammalian brain. Its function has been associated with age- and visual experience–dependent plasticity in the neocortex of rats, where an increased NR2B correlates directly with the stronger excitatory in young animals. Glutamine-based therapies might represent an effective alternative to biogenic amine–based agents for depression and provide perspectives on the development of glutamine-based therapies.

Treatment of MDD including TRD remains a major unmet need. Although there are several classes of dissimilar antidepressant drugs approved for MDD, the monoaminergic drugs have either limited efficacy or are associated with undesirable side effects and withdrawal symptoms.[33] The efficacy and side effects of antidepressant drugs are mainly attributed to their actions on different monoamine neurotransmitters (5-HT, NE, and DA). Development of new antidepressants with novel targets beyond the monoamine pathways may fill the unmet need in treatment of MDD and TRD.[32,33] The recent approval of intranasal esketamine (a glutamatergic agent) in conjunction with an oral antidepressant for the treatment of adults with TRD was the first step toward expanding beyond the monoamine targets.[37] Several other glutamatergic and GABAergic (brexanolone, zuranolone) drugs have been FDA approved for MDD and TRD. The renaissance of psychedelic drugs and the emergence of preliminary positive clinical trial results with psilocybin, 5-methoxy-*N*,*N*-dimethyltryptamine (5-MeO-DMT), and lysergic acid diethylamide (LSD) may pave the way toward establishing glutamatergic drugs as a class of drugs that are effective therapies for MDD, TRD, and other neuropsychiatric disorders. Going beyond the monoamine targets appears to be an effective strategy to develop novel antidepressant drugs with superior efficacy, safety, and tolerability for the improved treatment of MDD and TRD.[37]

Cholinergic Hypothesis of Depression

More than 40 years ago, the cholinergic theory of depression and mania hypothesized a balance between cholinergic and adrenergic systems, suggesting that hyperactivity of the cholinergic system over the adrenergic system would lead to symptoms of depression, mediated through excessive neuronal nicotinic receptor activation.[42] Thus the therapeutic actions of many antidepressants may be, in part, mediated through inhibition of these nAChRs. On the other hand, hypocholinergic activity would lead to symptoms of mania. Consistent with this hypothesis, physostigmine (a cholinesterase inhibitor causing a hypercholinergic response), when administered to normal subjects, produces symptoms of depression including anxiety, irritability, aggressiveness, and hostility. When physostigmine was administered to patients with MDD, the depressive symptoms were more pronounced and longer lasting in these patients: physostigmine also induced depression in patients with acute mania. The hypercholinergic effects of physostigmine are mediated primarily through acetylcholine (ACh) activation of neuronal nAChRs, not muscarinic receptors.[42] Over the past 20 years, various groups have reported on the nAChR inhibitory actions of classic TCAs including imipramine, nortriptyline, amitriptyline, and desipramine and the serotonin reuptake inhibitors including fluoxetine, sertraline, paroxetine, and citalopram. The nAChRs modulate not only the release of monoamines, but also GABA, topiramate, and various neuropeptides. Perhaps one of the most interesting antidepressants to have nAChR inhibitory activity is the atypical antidepressant bupropion. Bupropion is unique because it is metabolized to hydroxybupropion, which is an SNRI and a reuptake inhibitor of DA, with little or no direct action on serotoninergic neurotransmission, used in nicotine cessation.

In addition, transdermal nicotine administration (patch) has been shown to substantially improve the depressive symptoms of patients with MDD, an effect believed to be due to nicotine's antagonist effects on nAChRs. These effects have been attributed primarily to inhibition of a high-affinity nAChR subtype ($\alpha4\beta2$) in the brain, representing the predominant mammalian brain nAChR subtype. Thus, cigarette smoking may exert antidepressant effects in MDD refractory to SSRI treatment,[42] supporting the view that people with depression who smoke self-medicate by smoking.

Thus, there is an increasing amount of evidence supporting a possible role of neuronal nAChRs in depression as well as in the clinical effectiveness of antidepressants and that the therapeutic action of many antidepressants may be mediated, at least partially, through inhibition of excessive neuronal nAChR activity.[42]

Yet, evidence for hypercholinergic mechanisms in depression and hypocholinergic mechanisms in mania has been building over the last several decades, especially the clinical relationships between tobacco use and depression, which suggest important effects of nicotine in MDD.[42] About 110 years ago, Willoughby (*Lancet*, 1889) first reported the use of pilocarpine (a cholinomimetic) to treat acute mania. During the 1970s, Janowski and others hypothesized that a cholinergic imbalance (ie, hypercholinergic tone) was a primary factor in depressive illnesses. Since that time, a number of key findings from both animal and human studies have supported this hypothesis, with focus specifically on central nicotinic cholinergic rather than muscarinic pathways. Further support for this hypothesis is the loss of high-affinity nicotinic cholinergic receptors in patients with Alzheimer's.[39] Most clinically prescribed antidepressants target NE and 5-HT neurotransmitter systems; however, many of the drugs that target these systems, such as SSRIs, SNRIs, and TCAs, also act as potent noncompetitive antagonists of nAChRs at clinically effective doses for the treatment of major depression. The rapid monoamine effects of the antidepressants and their delayed therapeutic onset of action have led to reconsideration of alternative hypotheses regarding the mechanism of action of antidepressants.

Animal treatments with the NMDA antagonist ketamine have consistently shown antidepressant effects within a few hours of its administration; thus, it produces its antidepressant response in a much shorter period of time than existing antidepressant medications. Understanding the molecular basis of the NMDA can lead to the development of improved antidepressant pharmacotherapy rather than simply furthering our knowledge of current standard antidepressants.

Hormonal Hypothesis

The hormonal hypothesis suggests that changes in the HPA can influence the levels of 5-HT, NE, and ACh released by nerve cells in the brain and, subsequently, their function.[38] In the event of stress, ACh stimulates the hypothalamus to produce a hormone locally in the brain called corticotropin-releasing factor (CRF), which, in turn, stimulates the pituitary gland to secrete adrenocorticotropic hormone (ACTH) into the blood, where it stimulates the adrenal glands to release hydrocortisone (cortisol), which prepares the body for dealing with stress. Stress also directly stimulates the adrenal gland to secrete epinephrine and NE. Hydrocortisone can cause depression, especially when released in higher-than-usual amounts. The release of hydrocortisone may push the individual over the edge into depression or contribute to the component of anxiety that so often accompanies depressive illnesses. Approximately 50% of those with MDD have elevated hydrocortisone levels as a result of increased CRF activity.

Moreover, one of the most replicated findings in biologic psychiatry is that large numbers of unmedicated patients who are depressed exhibit HPA hyperactivity. The available evidence suggests that nAChRs play important roles in mediating stress-related and possibly depression-inducing neuroendocrine effects of ACh. ACh (hypercholinergic activity), in response to stress, can stimulate the HPA through activation of nAChRs. Thus, antidepressants may reduce symptoms of depression, in part, through blockade of nAChRs involved with stress-induced activation of the HPA.[39,42]

Living organisms operate in a state of imbalance and the neural (autonomic) and endocrine systems have evolved to modify the rates of biochemical pathways to maintain homeostasis. One of the hallmarks of these regulatory systems is the short-lived nature of the nerve signals produced. The half-life of neurotransmitters is measured in seconds, whereas those of the circulating hormones may be in minutes or hours. A rationale for the short-lived nature of the neurotransmitters is to permit these signaling pathways to quickly reset themselves to meet the next challenge. Readjustments (ie, plasticity) in these systems include uncoupling of receptor responses from signaling events, degradation of receptors and up- and downregulation of signaling molecules that affect the primary signaling pathway. These hypotheses are not mutually exclusive, and in each it is assumed that the more extreme the event, the more severe the clinical outcome.

Neurotropic Hypothesis of Depression

Several theories of depression have been proposed, including the monoamine hypothesis, neuroendocrine mechanisms, hormone hypotheses, and the neurotrophic hypothesis of depression.[43,44] However, these theories have not been sufficient for completely explaining the pathology and treatment of MDD. Recent evidence supports the neurotropic hypothesis of depression in its prediction that BDNF is involved in depression. However, some key questions remain unanswered, including whether abnormalities in BDNF persist beyond the clinical state of depression, whether BDNF levels are related to the clinical features of depression, and whether distinct antidepressants affect BDNF levels equally. Neurotropic factors are critical regulators of the formation and plasticity of neuronal networks. The "neurotrophin hypothesis of depression" is based largely on correlations between stress or antidepressant treatment and down- or upregulation, respectively, of BDNF. Serum BDNF levels were low in antidepressant-free patients with depression relative to controls and elevated for patients with depression who were treated with an antidepressant. The antidepressant-associated upregulation of serum BDNF in patients with depression was confined to SSRIs and St John's wort.[45] Thus, BDNF may be a target of antidepressants but not the sole mediator of MDD. Advances in BDNF cell biology may provide new insights into its role in mood disorders.[46] The BDNF is abundant in the brain and periphery and is found in both serum and plasma. Animal studies have demonstrated that stress reduces BDNF expression, and that this reduction can be prevented by treatment with antidepressant drugs.[47,48] A similar change in BDNF activity occurs in the brain of patients with MDD. The hypothesis of MDD postulates that a loss of BDNF is directly involved in the pathophysiology of MDD, and that its restoration may underlie the therapeutic efficacy of antidepressant treatment.[48] While this theory has received considerable experimental support, an increasing number of studies have generated evidence that is not only inconsistent, but also directly contradicts the hypothesis. Numerous clinical and preclinical studies demonstrate the contrasting role of BDNF in regulating mood and antidepressant effects throughout the brain. Neuronal plasticity, or neuroplasticity, is the biologic process by which the brain reorganizes its synapses in response to environmental stimuli.[49] The brain always aims to optimize its functioning, and, because of this, biologic systems are in place that frequently enhance patterns of thinking, making relevant neural networks stronger and irrelevant ones weaker, supporting processes such as learning and memory.[49] Human and animal studies have investigated the association of a BDNF single-nucleotide polymorphism (Val66Met) with depression pathogenesis.

BDNF is an essential mechanism of MDD. Insufficient signaling by BDNF, an important role in neural plasticity, has been considered as a key factor for MDD and antidepressant responses.[48] Neural plasticity, a fundamental mechanism of neuronal adaptation, is disrupted in MDD.[49] The changes in neural plasticity induced by stress and other negative stimuli play a significant role in the onset and development of MDD. Antidepressant treatments have also been found to exert their antidepressant effects through regulatory effects on neural plasticity. However, the detailed mechanisms of neural plasticity in depression remain unclear.

The review of preclinical and clinical papers demonstrates that BDNF plays a role in the pathophysiology of MDD.[50] Experimental studies suggest that BDNF expression is induced by chronic antidepressant treatments, and that BDNF itself has antidepressant activity in animal models of depression. Antidepressant treatment for at least 4 weeks can restore the decreased BDNF function up to the normal value. Therefore, MDD is associated with impaired neuronal plasticity.[51] Suicidal behavior can be a consequence of severe impaired neuronal plasticity in the brain. Antidepressant treatment promotes increased BDNF activity.[52] BDNF is a protein found in the brain of humans that is encoded by the *BDNF* gene. BDNF is a member of the neurotrophin family of growth factors, which are found in the brain and the periphery. BDNF was first isolated from a pig brain in 1982. *BDNF* gene regulation has been linked to the pathophysiology of MDD. Patients with MDD show cognitive deficit (ability to think and reason). Taken together, these findings may pave the way for future progress in neural plasticity studies.

Stress and depression are associated with reduced synaptic connectivity in brain regions that contribute to depressive behaviors, and that antidepressant treatment can reverse these deficits. The serum BDNF level was found to be consistently lower in patients with depression compared to healthy controls. In antidepressant treatment trials, the BDNF levels were found to be higher posttreatment than pretreatment. Studies revealed that it was more likely that BDNF serum levels were lower as a result of depression than representing an etiologic factor for the illness.

The relationships between serum BDNF protein levels and patients with MDD and the effects of antidepressants on the serum BDNF protein levels demonstrated significantly lower serum BDNF protein levels in patients with depression than in healthy controls. Additionally, changes in serum BDNF protein levels were significantly increased in patients taking antidepressants during a period of 4 weeks. There were significantly increased changes in serum BDNF protein levels. These analytical results suggest that low serum BDNF may play an important role in MDD, and antidepressant treatment significantly increases serum BDNF. However, further studies of larger populations are necessary to confirm these results and elucidate the effects of different classes of antidepressants on serum BDNF protein levels.

These findings show that the neurotrophic hypothesis of depression is more complex than previously assumed. Animal studies have shown a correlation between stress, diminished BDNF expression in the brain, and depressive-like behavior. Studies in humans suggest that the decrease in serum BDNF is a consequence of the depression. Thus, BDNF may be a target of antidepressants but not the sole mediator of depression or anxiety. Advances in BDNF cell biology may provide new insights into its role in mood disorders.

The serum levels of BDNF in drug-naive patients with MDD were significantly decreased as compared with normal controls.[50] These findings suggest that low BDNF levels may play a pivotal role in the pathophysiology of MDD. In order to determine the precise mechanism underlying the relationship between reduced BDNF levels and the etiology of MDD under both genetic and environmental backgrounds, further detailed study will be necessary.

Glutaminergic System

Half a century after the first formulation of the monoamine hypothesis, compelling evidence implies that long-term changes in brain areas and circuits mediating complex cognitive-emotional behaviors represent the biologic underpinnings of mood/anxiety disorders.[53,54] A large number of clinical studies suggest that the pathophysiology of depression is associated with dysfunction of the glutamatergic system, malfunction in the mechanisms regulating clearance and metabolism of glutamine, and maladaptive changes in a number of brain areas mediating cognitive-emotional behaviors. A wealth of data from animal models have shown that different types of environmental stress enhance glutamine release/transmission in limbic/cortical areas and exert powerful structural effects, resembling those observed in patients with depression.[55] Because a vast majority of neurons use glutamine as neurotransmitter, it would be limiting to maintain that glutamine is in some way "involved" in mood/anxiety disorders.[56,57] It should be recognized that the glutaminergic system is a primary mediator of depressive disorders and the pathway for the therapeutic action of antidepressant agents. A paradigm shift from a monoamine hypothesis of depression to a hypothesis focused on glutamine may represent a substantial advancement in the working glutamine hypothesis that drives research for new drugs and therapies. Despite the availability of multiple classes of drugs with monoamine-based mechanisms of action, there remains a large percentage of patients who fail to achieve a sustained remission of depressive symptoms. The unmet need for improved pharmacotherapies for TRD means there is a large space for the development of new compounds with novel mechanisms of action such as glutamine transmission and related pathways.[54,57] MDD affects around 16% of the world's population at some point in their lives.

Drugs increasing the synaptic availability of 5-HT and NE (biogenic amine–based agents) have been used to treat depression for more than 50 years. However, significant symptom improvement requires at least 2 to 4 weeks of treatment, and a first course of therapy provides symptom relief to only 60% to 65% of patients.[56] There is evidence that glutamate-based therapies might represent an effective alternative to biogenic amine–based agents for depression and provide perspectives on the development of these agents.[54]

Ketamine, functioning as a channel blocker of the excitatory glutamine-gated NMDARs, displays fast-acting and sustained antidepressant effects for TRD.[53] Over the past decades, clinical and preclinical studies have implied that the pathology of depression is associated with dysfunction of glutamatergic transmission.[56] The discovery of antidepressant agents regulating NMDAR function (eg, Auvelity) has prompted breakthroughs for depression treatment compared with conventional antidepressants targeting the monoaminergic system.[57] The pathway of the ketamine-mediated antidepressant effects is based on the glutamine hypothesis of depression. This hypothesis postulates that ketamine antidepressant effects occur within different brain areas, including NMDAR antagonism on GABAergic interneurons, NMDAR-mediated antagonism, and ketamine blocking.[54] The structural basis of NMDAR channel blockers and NMDAR regulators has been reported to exert potential antidepressant effects in animal models or in clinical trials. Integrating the cutting-edge technologies of the next generation of first-in-class rapid antidepressants targeting NMDARs is an emerging direction for depression therapeutics.

In spite of intensive research, the problems of treating TRD still exist. Treatment of MDD usually takes weeks to months to achieve an adequate response; however, remission may be solved with esketamine nasal spray. The past decade has seen a steady accumulation of evidence supporting a role for the excitatory amino acid neurotransmitter glutamine and its mR1 and mR5 receptors in depression and antidepressant activity.[53] Glutamine plays an essential role as a neurotransmitter in many physiologic functions, and an increase in glutamine release can result in activation of the NMDAR, an underlying cause for depression and anxiety. Glutamine is the major excitatory neurotransmitter in the CNS and plays a central role in learning, cognition, and memory. A growing body of evidence suggests that the glutamine system, especially the abnormalities of the NMDAR, contribute to the pathophysiology of MDD.[57] An imbalance in glutamine neurotransmission may contribute to increased levels of NMDA agonism, thereby enhancing glutamine excitatory activity in most brain circuits involved in MDD. Most drugs acting at NMDARs showed biochemical effects indicative of antidepressant activity in both clinical and preclinical studies. Overall, NMDAR regulation may facilitate the release of neurotransmitters associated with treatment response to depression in humans. The glutamine system represents a target for effective intervention in MDD.[57] Specifically, those glutamine medications targeting NMDAR by inhibiting the release of neurotransmitters or regulating its postsynaptic responses may serve as molecular modulators with specific antidepressant properties. The brain possesses approximately 5 to 15 nmol/kg of glutamine, depending on the region, and only a small fraction of this total accumulates in the extracellular space.

Glutaminergic Antagonist

As mentioned earlier, glutamate is the major excitatory neurotransmitter in the CNS and plays a central role in synaptic plasticity (adaptability of brain to environmental changes), learning, cognition, and memory.[54] Glutamine can be synthesized from glucose through the Krebs/tricarboxylic acid cycle or through recycling of glutamine by the glutamine-glutamine cycle and packaged in calcium-dependent synaptic vesicles by vesicular glutamate transporters and soon after into the synaptic cleft, where it interacts with ionotropic (iRs) and metabotropic (mRs) receptors. The iRs are ion channels that selectively allow an influx of Ca^{2+} and Na^{+}, promoting depolarization of the neuron.[54] An imbalance in glutaminergic neurotransmission may contribute to increased levels of NMDA agonism, thereby enhancing glutamine excitatory activity in most brain circuits involved in MDD. Most drugs acting at NMDARs showed biochemical effects indicative of antidepressant activity in both clinical and preclinical studies.[55] Overall, NMDAR modulation may facilitate the release of neurotransmitters associated with treatment response to depression in humans. The glutamine system represents a target for effective intervention in MDD. Specifically, those glutamine medications targeting NMDARs by inhibiting the release of neurotransmitters or regulating its postsynaptic responses may serve as molecular regulators with specific antidepressant properties.[54]

N-Methyl-D-Aspartate Receptor Antagonists

NMDAR antagonists are a class of drugs that work to antagonize, or block the action of, the NMDAR. They are commonly used as anesthetics (ie, ketamine) for animals and humans. NMDAR antagonists were the first class of therapeutic agents for depression (ketamine) via ligand-gated receptors (NMDAR and α-amino-3-hydroxy-5-methyl-4-isoxazolepropionic acid receptors [AMPARs]). The complex structure of the NMDAR provides multiple sites for therapeutic inhibition.[54] Competitive NMDAR antagonists bind directly to the glutamine site of the NMDAR to inhibit the action of glutamine. Noncompetitive antagonists block the NMDAR-associated ion channel. Other sites on the NMDAR susceptible to antagonism are the glycine site and the polyamine site. Prototypes of these competitive and noncompetitive NMDAR antagonists (such as dextromethorphan; see Auvelity) have been studied in phase 3 clinical trials for the treatment of depression.[56] Recent evidence suggests that the glutamatergic system (see Chapter 8), especially the abnormalities of glutamine and NMDARs, contributes to the pathophysiology of MDD. An imbalance in glutamine neurotransmission may contribute to increased levels of NMDA agonism, thereby enhancing excitatory activity in most brain circuits involved in MDD. Although NMDAR antagonists have been demonstrated to possess antidepressant-like activity, the molecular changes in NMDAR underlying abnormal glutamine signaling remain poorly understood.[57,58]

The glutamine system represents a target for effective intervention in the treatment of MDD and resistant hypertension.[57] Specifically, those glutamine medications targeting NMDAR by inhibiting the release of neurotransmitters or modulating its postsynaptic responses may serve as molecule modulators with specific antidepressant properties. Ketamine, one of the most popular NMDAR antagonists, is an example.[56]

Targeting NMDARs using antagonists such as dextromethorphan and esketamine represents important alternative antidepressants options in treatment of MDD.[59] Antidepressant-like effects of NMDAR antagonists have shown antidepressant properties in preclinical studies, either alone or combined with traditional antidepressants, such as bupropion. The mechanism of action of bupropion in the treatment of MDD is unclear; however, it may be related to noradrenergic and/or dopaminergic mechanisms.

General Approaches to Treatment of Depression

Before 1950, there were no antidepressants—at least not as we know them today.[60] The two treatments for depressive illness were either amphetamine stimulants, which often were ineffective and had the general effect of increasing energy and activity, or ECT, which was effective but had the disadvantage of terrifying and often endangering the patient. Not until the late 1950s were the first generation of antidepressants discovered (TCAs and MAOIs), not by design but by chance. While searching for "chlorpromazine-like" compounds to treat schizophrenia, imipramine was recognized by Kuhn[40] for its antidepressant properties, thus becoming the forerunner for the tricyclic class of monoamine reuptake inhibitor antidepressants (ie, the TCAs). The second compound to be discovered was the antitubercular drug isoniazid, which proved to have powerful mood-enhancing properties, becoming the forerunner of the MAOIs. With the introduction of imipramine and isoniazid, the theory and treatment of depression changed.[41] These early studies still summarize much of our current knowledge regarding the therapeutic effects of antidepressant treatments.

Between 1960 and 1980, TCAs were the major pharmacologic treatment for depression.[37] The TCAs, however, have many other actions in addition to blocking monoamine reuptake and nicotinic receptors, including anticholinergic, antihistaminergic, and cardiotoxic side effects that are related to their affinity for muscarinic, H_1 and α_1-adrenergic receptors as well as their action on cardiac and CNS sodium channels in membranes (Table 12.1). The improved safety, tolerability, and reuptake selectivity of the newer antidepressants (ie, SSRIs, atypical SNRIs, serotonin modulators and stimulants [SMSs]) have resulted in displacement of the TCAs as the first choice for the treatment of MDD. The TCAs occupy a narrower—but still important—role in psychopharmacologic therapy.

The early MAOIs irreversibly inhibited the oxidative deamination of the neurotransmitter monoamines, the proposed mechanism of their antidepressant activity. The biggest liability for these MAOIs was their potential to cause life-threatening hypertensive reactions, resulting from the irreversible inhibition of both MAO-A and MAO-B, which decreases the gastrointestinal (GI) and hepatic degradation of dietary sources of tyramine.[41] The inhibition of MAO allows excessive amounts of dietary tyramine, a weak sympathomimetic vasoconstrictor, to be absorbed from food, resulting in increased blood pressure (refer to the section on MAOIs in this chapter for more details). Inhibition of MAOs also can alter the pharmacokinetics of monoamine over the counter (OTC) and prescription drugs, allowing them to accumulate in the blood and, thus, increasing their potential for causing adverse drug effects and drug-drug interactions (DDIs). Minimizing drug and food interactions of these early MAOIs inspired the development of a new generation of MAOIs that are both reversible and selective for MAO-A. The demise of the early MAOIs allowed the TCAs to become the gold standard for the treatment of depressive disorders.[41]

Discovery of Selective Serotonin Reuptake Inhibitor Antidepressants

The discovery that certain antihistaminic agents without the condensed aromatic ring systems are selective inhibitors of 5-HT reuptake with little affinity for the other neuroreceptors and almost devoid of cardiotoxicity questioned the need for the 10,11-ethylene bridge for the TCAs. Thus, the search for inhibitors that selectively blocked 5-HT reuptake without the seven-membered central ring of the TCAs resulted in the synthesis of the diarylpropylamine analogues of the TCAs (Fig. 12.2). Thus, during the late 1960s and early 1970s, antihistamine molecules were structurally manipulated in the search for compounds that selectively inhibited 5-HT reuptake with greater potency.[60-62] The initial

Table 12.1 Antidepressant Classes of Drugs, Generic, Trade Name, and Common Side Effects

Generic Name	Trade Name	Amine Effects	Seizures	Sedation	Hypotension	Anticholinergic Effects	GI Effects	Sexual Effects	Cardiac Effects
Tricyclic Tertiary Amines									
Amitriptyline	Elavil and generic	NE, 5-HT	2+	3+	3+	3+	+	2+	3+
Clomipramine	Anafranil	NE, 5-HT	3+	2+	2+	+	2+	3+	
Doxepin	Adapin, Sinequan	NE, 5-HT	2+	3+	2+	+	2+	3+	
Imipramine	Tofranil and generic	NE, 5-HT	2+	2+	2+	2+	+	2+	3+
(+)-Trimipramine	Surmontil	NE, 5-HT	2+	3+	2+	3+	+	2+	3+
Tricyclic Secondary Amines									
Amoxapine	Asendin	NE, DA	2+	+	2+	+	+	+	2+
Desipramine	Norpramin	NE	+	+	+	+	+	2+	2+
Maprotiline	Ludiomil	NE	3+	2	2	0	+	2+	2
Nortriptyline	Pamelor	NE	+	+	+	0	+	2+	2+
Protriptyline	Vivactil	NE	2+	0	+	0	+	2+	2+
Selective Serotonin Reuptake Inhibitors (SSRIs)									
(±)-Citalopram	Celexa	5-HT	0	0/+	0	0	3+	3+	0
(+)-Escitalopram	Lexapro	5-HT	0	0/+	0	0	3+	3+	0
(±)-Fluoxetine	Prozac	5-HT	+	0/+	0	0	3+	3+	0
Fluvoxamine	Luvox	5-HT	0	0/+	0	0	3+	3+	0
(−)-Paroxetine	Paxil	5-HT	0	0/+	0	0	3+	3+	0
(+)-Sertraline	Zoloft	5-HT	0	0/+	0	0	3+	3+	0
Serotonin-Norepinephrine Reuptake Inhibitors (SNRIs)									
(−)-Atomoxetine	Strattera	NE	0	0	0	0	0	0	0
(+)-Duloxetine	Cymbalta	NE, 5-HT	0/+	0/+	0/+	0	0/+	0/+	0/+
Levomilnacipran	Fetzima	5-HT, NE	0	4+	0	0	0	0	0
(±)-Mirtazapine	Remeron	5-HT, NE	0	4+	0	0	0	0	0
(±)-Venlafaxine	Effexor	5-HT	0	+	0	0	3+	3+	0
Desvenlafaxine	Pristiq	5-HT	0	+	0	0	3+	3+	0

(continued)

Table 12.1 Antidepressant Classes of Drugs, Generic, Trade Name, and Common Side Effects (*continued*)

Generic Name	Trade Name	Amine Effects	Seizures	Sedation	Hypotension	Anticholinergic Effects	GI Effects	Sexual Effects	Cardiac Effects
Serotonin Modulators and Stimulants (SMSs) and Serotonin Receptor Modulators (SARIs)									
Vilazodone	Viibryd	5-HT	0/+	+	0	0	3+	2+	1+
Vortioxetine	Brintellix	5-HT	0	0	0	2+	3+	3+	0
Trazodone	Desyrel	5-HT	0	0	3+	0	2+		
Norepinephrine-Dopamine Reuptake Inhibitors (NDRIs)									
Bupropion	Wellbutrin, Zyban, etc	NE, DA	3+	0	0	0/+	2+	0/+	0/+
Monoamine Oxidase Inhibitors (MAOIs)									
Phenelzine	Nardil	NE, 5-HT, DA	+	+	0	+	3+	0	
Tranylcypromine	Parnate	NE, 5-HT, DA	0	+	0	+	2+	0	

5-HT, serotonin; DA, dopamine; NE, norepinephrine.

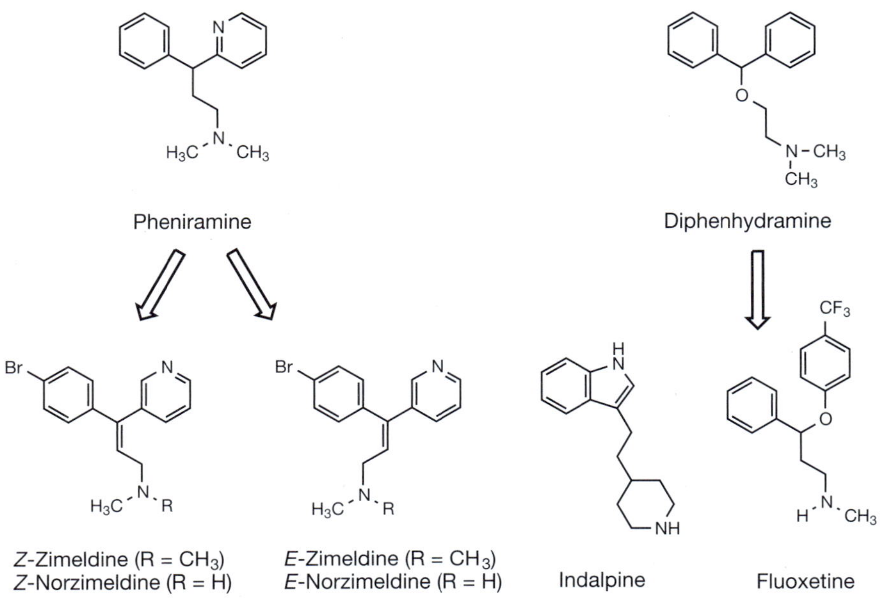

Figure 12.2 Structural relationship between antihistamines and antidepressants that block the reuptake of serotonin (5-HT).

breakthrough came with the synthesis of Z-zimeldine (the *cis*-isomer) (aka, zimelidine, patented in 1971), the first SSRI that selectively inhibited the presynaptic reuptake of 5-HT without the adverse events associated with the multireceptor activities of the TCAs.[61,62] Zimeldine was synthesized from the manipulation of the antihistamine pheniramine into a diaryl allylamine, the *cis*-isomer (rigid analogue) of the propylamine group (Fig. 12.2).[62]

Another structural change that enhanced its potency and selectivity for blocking 5-HT reuptake was moving the regional position of the 2-pyridyl ring of pheniramine to the 3-pyridyl position and substitution of a halogen into the 4-position of the phenyl ring (2-substitutions selectively block NE reuptake).[63] The secondary amine and primary metabolite, norzimeldine, was 15 times more potent than zimeldine for blocking 5-HT reuptake. On the other hand, (*E*)-zimeldine (the *trans*-isomer) is an inhibitor of both 5-HT and NE reuptake, whereas its corresponding secondary amine is a potent and selective inhibitor of NE reuptake. It is not unusual for geometric isomers to differ markedly from each other with regard to their receptor or transporter selectivity, affinity, and pharmacodynamic properties. Thus, zimeldine became the first SSRI to be marketed as an antidepressant, but unfortunately, several cases of Guillain-Barré syndrome (an autoimmune disorder attacking the peripheral nervous system) were associated with the use of this drug and led to its withdrawal from the market in 1983. During postmarketing clinical studies, zimeldine showed an increase in the number of suicide attempts than had been expected—this adverse event was to become a major issue with the SSRIs 20 years later.

The success of zimeldine as an SSRI, however, led to the discovery and marketing of several nontricyclic SSRIs from multiple pharmaceutical companies worldwide.[64] Another manipulation of the antihistamines produced indalpine (patented in 1977 by Rhône Poulenc) (see Fig. 12.2). It produced responses in patients who had not responded to the TCAs or MAOIs but then ran into trouble, because clinical trials suggested that it might cause agranulocytopenia (lowering of the white blood cell count). For the most part, this is not a serious problem, but in rare cases, if undetected, it can be fatal. It was removed from the European market in 1985 and was never marketed in the United States.

Other SSRIs developed during this period that have become household words include paroxetine (patented in 1975 by Ferrosan to SmithKline Beecham then to GlaxoKline), citalopram (patented in 1979 by Lindberg, licensed to Forest Labs), fluoxetine (patented in 1982 by Lilly), and sertraline (patented in 1985 to Pfizer).

Scientists at Lilly Research Laboratories synthesized more than 50 phenoxypropylamines derived from the antihistamine diphenhydramine (Benadryl) before discovering fluoxetine[64,65] (see Fig. 12.2). The first of these compounds was nisoxetine, a potent SNRI that was clinically developed but never marketed. Other derivatives that have since been marketed by Lilly include atomoxetine and duloxetine (atypical SNRIs).

Fluoxetine (Prozac) was heralded as the prototype for the next generation of SSRI antidepressants possessing fewer adverse effects and with a greater margin of safety when compared with the TCAs and also lacking the food-interaction toxicity of MAOIs.[64,65] Fluoxetine was marketed in 1987 and, within a few years, it boasted worldwide sales of nearly $1.2 billion a year. During the past 20 years, nontricyclic selective NE- or 5-HT reuptake inhibitors and TCA reuptake inhibitors of both NE and 5-HT as well as reversible selective MAOIs have been approved for use in depression. These newer additions allow exploration of the roles of NE versus 5-HT using treatments that are devoid of confounding receptor activities. Conscious targeting of more than one neurotransmitter activity (eg, of serotonergic and noradrenergic mechanisms or of NE and DA), while retaining specificity, is the target for the development of the next generation of antidepressants. The majority of TCAs in current use selectively inhibit the reuptake of 5-HT and NE.[63] Based on the previously neglected role proposed for DA in depression, it has been hypothesized that a "broad-spectrum" antidepressant will produce a more rapid onset and/or higher efficacy than agents inhibiting the selective reuptake of 5-HT and/or NE.[63] Broad-spectrum antidepressants are compounds that inhibit the reuptake of NE, 5-HT, and DA, the three biogenic amines most closely linked to depression.

Traditionally, antidepressants have been classified according to their structure (ie, secondary or tertiary amine TCAs) or their principal mechanism of action.[63] With the appearance of increasing numbers of second- and third-generation antidepressants, however, a better way of classifying and describing the antidepressants was necessary. For the purposes of this chapter, the antidepressants are organized into seven classes (see Table 12.1) and discussed according to their distinct and different mechanisms of action (Fig. 12.3). Considerable overlap exists in their mechanism of actions and uses, but these different classes of antidepressants work by distinct mechanisms, have different side-effect profiles, and may be favored for different types of depressive illnesses.

A key step that determines the intensity and duration of monoamine signaling at synapses is the reuptake of the released neurotransmitter into nerve terminals through high-affinity plasma membrane transporters.[66] Reuptake is the process of rapidly removing the monoamine neurotransmitters from the synaptic cleft and allowing most of the released neurotransmitter to be recycled for further use. The advantage of reuptake is that it is faster than passive diffusion through the membrane. Any monoamine neurotransmitter remaining in the synaptic cleft is then absorbed and metabolized into inactive metabolites. The monoamine reuptake transporter protein binds the released neurotransmitter in the extracellular fluid and transports the monoamine across the presynaptic plasma membrane back into the intracellular fluid of the presynaptic neuron (Fig. 12.4). Monoamine transporters (Fig. 12.5 and sidebar for more detail) are embedded in the plasma membrane of the nerve terminals (perisynaptically) of dopaminergic, noradrenergic, and serotonergic neurons rather than intrasynaptically (along the portion of the nerve terminal forming the synapse).[67] They are members of a larger sodium-dependent transporter family and represent a major mechanism terminating the action of released monoamine neurotransmitters in the synaptic cleft. These transporters are important targets for many antidepressive drugs and substances of abuse (ie, cocaine). Transporter proteins are specific to their respective neurotransmitter: serotonin reuptake transporter (SERT), NE reuptake transporter (NET), and dopamine reuptake transporter (DAT).[67] None of the reuptake antidepressants exhibit significant affinity for DA transporters, which may be related to their ineffectiveness in types of depression that is resistant to the SNRIs and SSRIs. The TCAs and nontricyclic SNRIs block the reuptake transporters for both NE and 5-HT, and the SSRIs selectively block SERT. The antidepressant reuptake inhibitors also may contribute to relief of depression by decreasing the expression of their respective transporter proteins.

Figure 12.6 illustrates the selectivity of the reuptake inhibitors for their respective transporters.[68,69] The selectivity ratios for inhibiting SERT (ratio, >1) are obtained by dividing the affinity of the inhibitor (K_i) for inhibiting SERT with its affinity (K_i) for inhibiting NET, whereas the selectivity ratio for inhibiting NET (ratio <1) is obtained by dividing its affinity (K_i) for inhibiting NET with the affinity (K_i) for inhibiting SERT. For example, a value of approximately 1 for amitriptyline means that amitriptyline will inhibit both NET and SERT at the same concentration (ie, no selectivity with regard to their mechanism of antidepressant activity). The value of ~30 for desipramine means that desipramine is 30 times more potent at inhibiting the NET than the SERT, although the SSRIs with selectivity ratio values of greater than 100 are more than 100 times more potent at inhibiting the SERT than the NET. Furthermore, because the

TRANSPORTER PROTEINS

The monoamine transporter protein (molecular weights, 60-80 kDa) is a string of amino acids that weaves in and out of the presynaptic membrane 11 times (see Fig. 12.4)—that is, 11 transmembrane domains (TMs) with a large extracellular loop between TM3 and TM4. Both the N- and C-termini of the transporters are located within the cytoplasm. There are six potential sites of phosphorylation by protein kinase A and protein kinase C, which regulate the transporters. The large extracellular loop and the cytoplasmic parts of the N- and C-termini do not appear to be the target sites for the transporter inhibitors (ie, antidepressants). Rather, the areas important for selective monoamine affinity appear to be localized within TM1 to TM3 and TM8 to TM11 that project into the synapse, and these areas of the transporters have a common binding site for the monoamine and many of its inhibitors (see Fig. 12.4). To transport protonated 5-HT (5-HT$^+$), SERT cotransports one sodium ion (Na^+) and one chloride ion (Cl^-) while countertransporting a potassium ion (K^+) (see Fig. 12.5). The SERT then flips inside the cell, releasing the 5-HT$^+$ and the Na^+ and Cl^- into the cytoplasm of the neuron. On releasing the 5-HT$^+$ and the Na^+ and Cl^-, SERT flips back out, with the unoccupied binding site exposed to the synaptic cleft, ready to receive and transport another 5-HT$^+$ molecule. To transport protonated NE (NE$^+$), NET also cotransports Na^+ and Cl^- with intracellular K^+ stimulation and no K^+ efflux. The initial complex of the monoamine, Na^+ and Cl^-, with the transporter protein creates a conformational change in the transporter protein. The driving force (electrical potential) for the energetically unfavorable transport of the monoamine is the Na^+ concentration gradient. The Na^+/K^+ transporter (Na^+/K^+-ATPase) maintains the extracellular Na^+ concentration as well as the intracellular K^+ concentration. The Na^+/K^+-ATPase transport three Na^+ ions for each two K^+ ions pumped into the cell. Unlike channels that stay open or closed, transporters undergo conformational changes (changes in their three-dimensional shape) and move one monoamine molecule in each cycle.

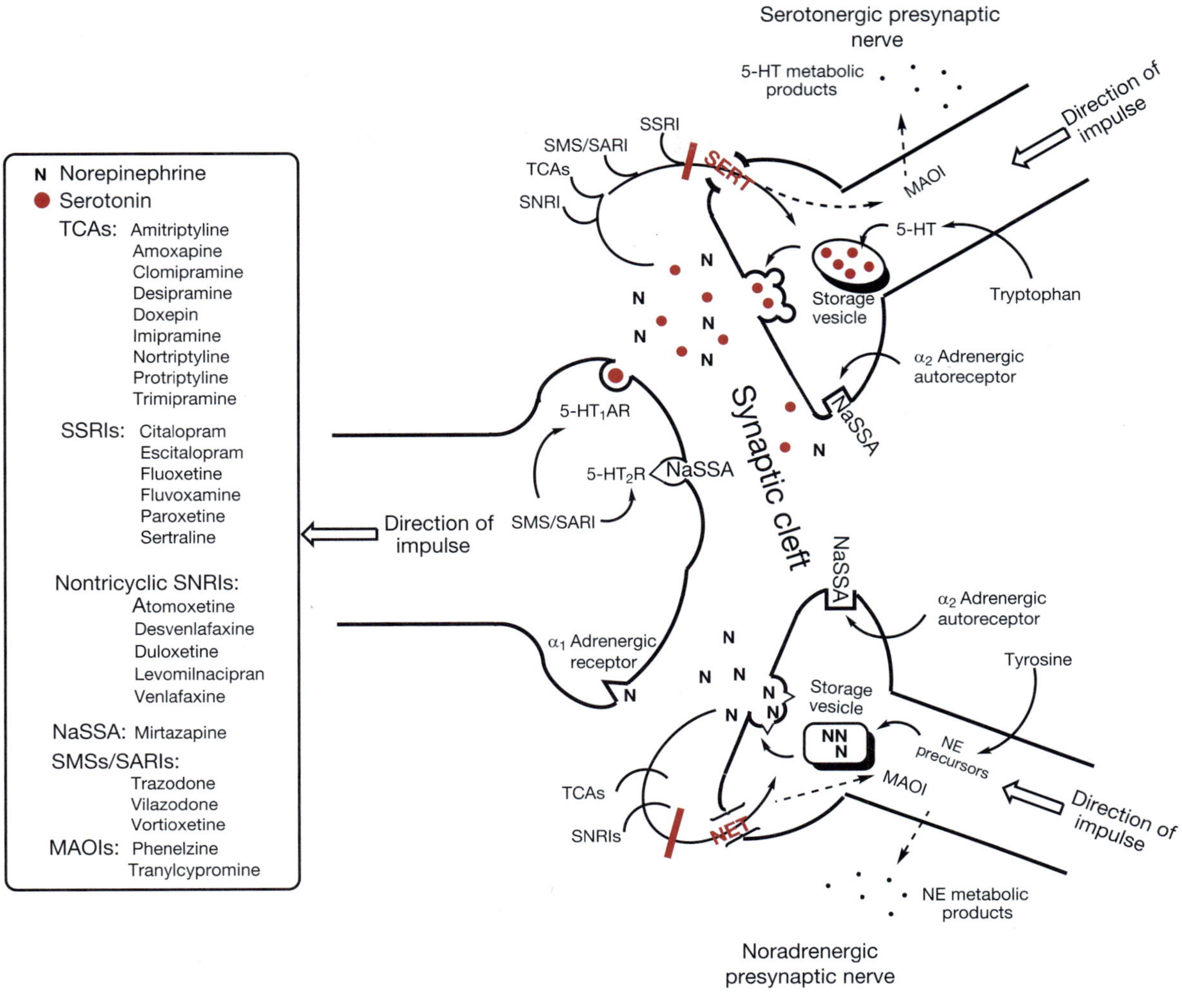

Figure 12.3 Sites of action of the antidepressants.

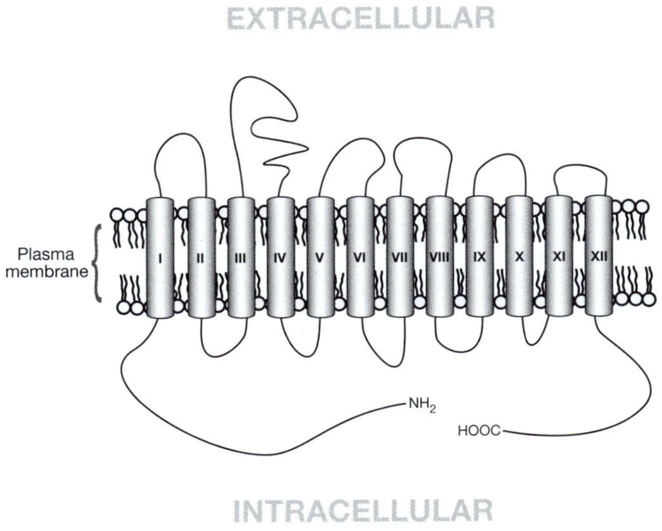

Figure 12.4 Monoamine reuptake transporter.

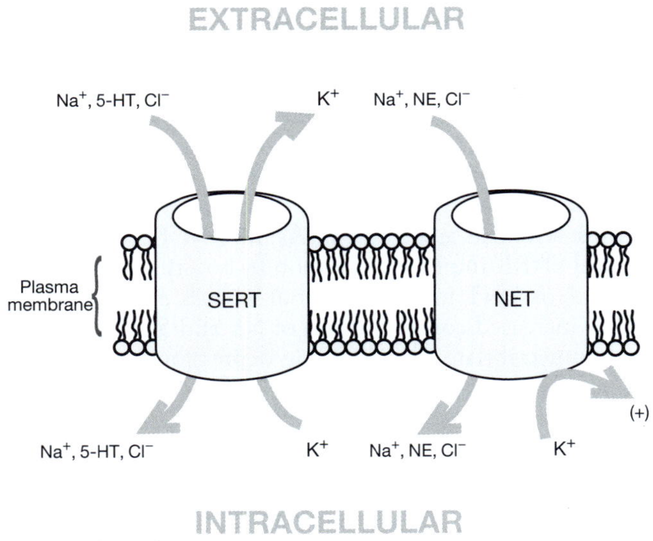

Figure 12.5 Model of the NET and SERT and the ion-coupled NE and 5-HT reuptake. Reuptake of 5-HT is dependent on the cotransport of Na^+ and Cl^- and countertransport of K^+. Reuptake of NE is dependent on the cotransport of Na^+ and Cl^- with intracellular K^+ stimulation but without K^+ efflux.

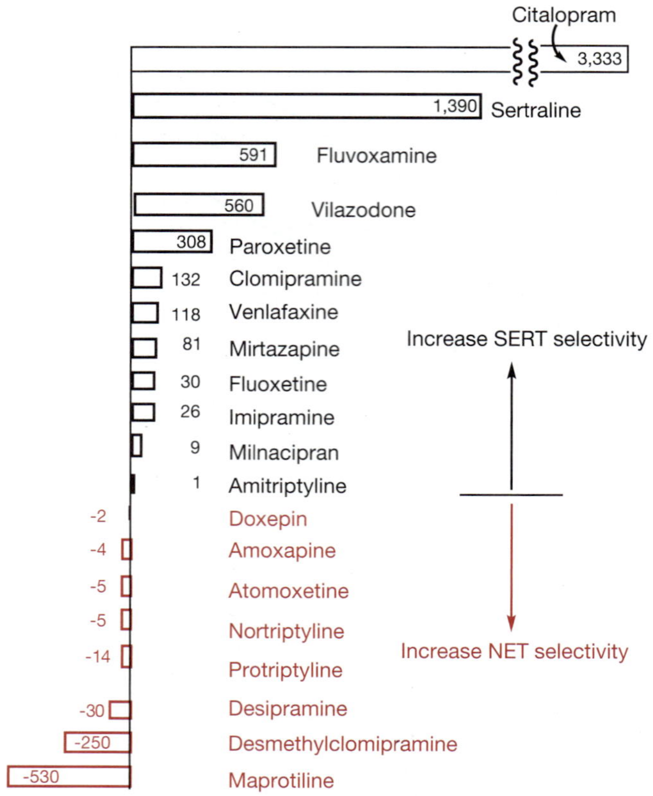

Figure 12.6 In vitro selectivity ratios for reuptake inhibitors. NET, norepinephrine reuptake transporter; SERT, serotonin reuptake transporter;

selectivity ratio for most SSRIs is more than 100, a plasma concentration of any SSRI that will produce inhibition of the SERT will produce no physiologically meaningful inhibition of NET. The converse will be true regarding selectivity for the NET. Clinically, such selectivity ratios of greater than 100 translate into being able to produce all the physiologic effects mediated by inhibiting one transporter without causing any effects that will be produced by inhibiting the other uptake transporter. When the selectivity ratio is less than 30, such as with fluoxetine, the difference is small enough that inhibition of both reuptake transporters may occur under therapeutic doses and, thus, can contribute to the broad antidepressant activity of the drug.

Most scientists agree that TCAs, MAOIs, SSRIs, and the atypical SNRIs improve depression by boosting the levels of NE and/or 5-HT in the brain, but what is not established is how increased concentrations of NE and 5-HT and their synergism translate into reducing depression.[70] One problem with the original monoamine model was that, whereas plasma concentrations of the antidepressant and binding to the monoamine transporter occur almost immediately, chronic administration of antidepressants is needed before clinical efficacy is attained.[69] The therapeutic effect of an antidepressant is almost always observed after a period of 3 to 6 weeks of treatment. This suggests that certain adaptive changes are occurring with chronic administration of these drugs that may be important for their antidepressant action. Over the years, mechanisms such as downregulation of β-adrenergic receptors, desensitization of presynaptic α_2-adrenoceptors, increased postsynaptic 5-HT receptor sensitivity, downregulation of 5-HT_2 receptors, and desensitization of presynaptic 5-HT_{1A} receptors have been cited either as the final common pathway or as one of many possible final common pathways.

It should be remembered that the neurotransmitter and downregulation hypotheses are incomplete explanations for how antidepressants work. Antidepressants most likely set off an intricate chain of reactions that occur between the time the patient first takes them and the following few weeks, when they finally produce their effect.[69] What the neurotransmitter and downregulation hypotheses do provide are useful—if simplistic—models for comprehending at least some of the basic biochemical processes triggered by antidepressants.

ANTIDEPRESSANTS IN PSYCHOTHERAPY

Depression is a common condition, affecting an estimated 1 in 10 adults at some point in their lives. Antidepressants are widely prescribed in primary and secondary care, along with psychological interventions such as cognitive behavioral or interpersonal therapy. Comparative efficacy and acceptability of 21 antidepressant drugs for the acute treatment of adults with MDD has been recently reported in a systematic review and network meta-analysis.[70]

The most effective antidepressants for adults revealed in a major review of 522 antidepressant trials by Cipriani et al[69] found that all of the 21 antidepressant drugs studied performed better than placebo in short-term trials measuring response to treatment. However, effectiveness varied widely, and the researchers ranked drugs by effectiveness and acceptability after 8 weeks of treatment. Five antidepressants appear more effective and better tolerated than others and include escitalopram, paroxetine, sertraline, agomelatine (not available in the United States), and mirtazapine. The most effective antidepressant compared to placebo was the TCA amitriptyline, which increased the chances of treatment response more than 2-fold. The least effective was reboxetine (available in the UK), which is a selective NE inhibitor. People were 30% more likely to stop taking the tricyclic clomipramine than placebo or the SSRI fluoxetine. There has been uncertainty in recent years about the effectiveness of antidepressants. Their mode of action is poorly understood, and improvement in mood tends to be modest. A 2008 meta-analysis suggested that antidepressants gave little benefit over placebo for mild-to-moderate depression. However, it did not assess antidepressants compared to other treatments such as cognitive behavioral therapy or treatments in combination.

The introduction of the second-generation classes of antidepressants in the 1980s and 1990s (SSRIs, atypical SRNIs, SMSs, serotonin antagonist/reuptake inhibitors [SARIs], and NaSSAs; see Table 12.1 and Fig. 12.3) has been regarded as the major pharmacologic advance in the treatment of depression since the appearance of the TCAs and MAOIs. The SSRIs and atypical SNRIs have proven to be effective for a broad range of depressive illnesses, dysthymia, several anxiety disorders, and bulimia. The SSRIs are the most widely prescribed antidepressant drugs and rank in the top 50 drugs in terms of total US sales for 2022. In addition to being the usual first-line treatments for major depression, the SSRIs also are first-line treatments for panic disorder, OCD, social phobia, PTSD, and bulimia. They also may be the best medications for treatment of dysthymia and generalized anxiety disorder (GAD).

Differences in general tolerability of the different classes of antidepressants and in their side-effect profiles are well known and generally accepted. Compared with the TCAs, the SSRIs cause significantly more nausea, diarrhea, agitation, sexual dysfunction, anorexia, insomnia, nervousness, and anxiety, whereas the TCAs cause more cardiotoxicity, dry mouth, constipation, dizziness, sweating, and blurred vision.[71] Although the SSRIs and SNRIs possess improved safety margins and fewer cardiovascular adverse effects than tertiary TCAs and utility for treating other non-depressive disorders, they offer no real gain in efficacy than the first-generation TCAs. Despite pharmacologic differences in their mechanisms of actions, the general view has been that all antidepressants are of equal efficacy. Only within the last 10 years has this general assumption come under serious challenge from comparisons of antidepressants with dual mechanisms of action, which can be acting in a complementary and perhaps synergistic manner to improve depression versus those with a single mechanism of action.[70] Often, a variety of antidepressants will be prescribed and the dosage adjusted before the most effective antidepressant or combination of antidepressants is found. Although some improvements may be seen during the first few weeks, the antidepressants must be taken regularly for 3 to 4 weeks (and, in some cases, for as many as 8 weeks) before the full therapeutic effect occurs. Patient compliance can become an issue, because they often are tempted to stop medication too soon as a result of feeling better and, thus, thinking they no longer need the medication. Additionally, they may have problems with the adverse effects, or they may think the medication is not helping at all. It is important for the patient to keep taking the antidepressant until it has a chance to work, although side effects often appear before antidepressant activity does. Once the individual is feeling better, it is important to continue the medication for at least 4 to 9 months (or longer) to prevent a recurrence of the depression. Antidepressants alter the brain chemistry; therefore, they must be stopped gradually to give the brain time to adjust. For some individuals with bipolar disorder or chronic major depression, antidepressant therapy may need to be maintained indefinitely.[71] All patients who are prescribed antidepressants should be informed that discontinuation/withdrawal symptoms may occur on stopping; on missing doses; or, occasionally, on reducing the dose of the drug. These symptoms usually are mild and self-limiting, but they can sometimes be severe, particularly if the drug is stopped abruptly. Symptoms of antidepressant withdrawal include nausea, vomiting, anorexia, headache, restlessness, agitation, "chills," and insomnia as well as, sometimes, hypomania, panic-anxiety and extreme motor restlessness, especially if an antidepressant (particularly an MAOI) is stopped suddenly after regular administration for 8 weeks or more.

In addition to the wide use of antidepressants to treat depression, chronic neuropathic pain disorders, which include fibromyalgia and diabetic and other peripheral neuropathic syndromes, have responded at least partly to treatment with tertiary TCAs and the SNRIs duloxetine, milnacipran, and venlafaxine. The SNRIs appear to be superior to the SSRIs.[69]

Effect of Physicochemical Properties and Stereochemistry on Antidepressant Efficacy

Small substituent changes in molecular structure can affect the pharmacokinetic and pharmacodynamic (clinical) properties of antidepressant drug molecules, resulting in profound differences between their transporter selectivity and their antidepressant effect—for example, a difference of a 2-chloro group between the structurally related antidepressants imipramine and clomipramine or the *o*- versus *p*-substituents between duloxetine and atomoxetine (SNRIs) (Fig. 12.7).[72] Furthermore, a seemingly simple isosteric

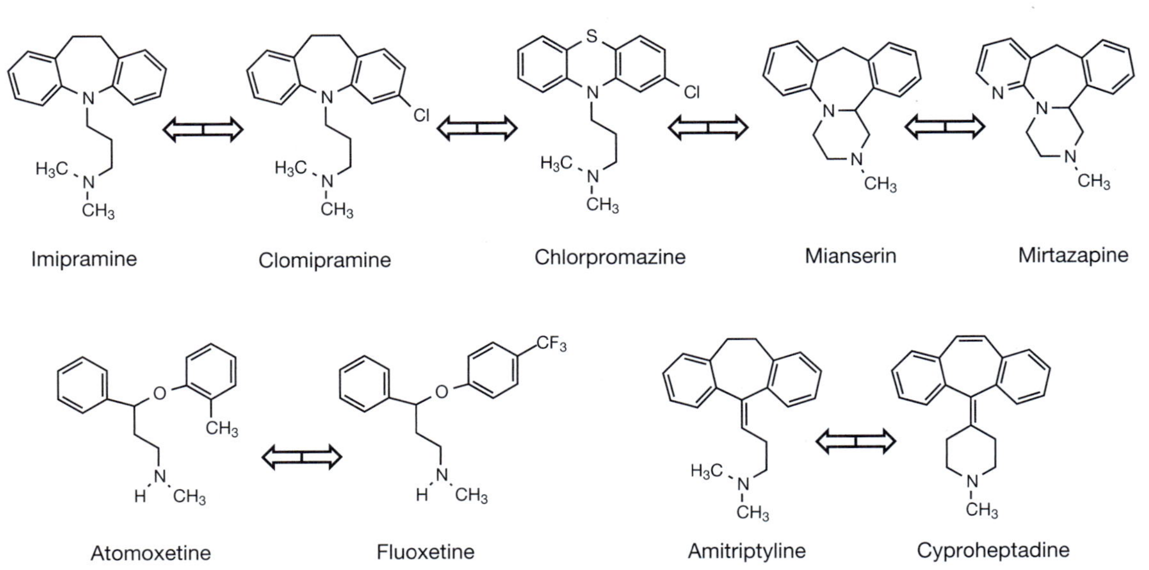

Figure 12.7 Structural relationship between selected molecular structures.

replacement of a sulfur atom in the central ring of chlorpromazine with an ethylene group to give a seven-membered azepine ring (clomipramine) or the replacement of the methylpiperidylidene at the 5-position for the antihistamine/5-HT antagonist cyproheptadine with a dimethylaminopropylidene for the antidepressant reuptake inhibitor amitriptyline has profound effects on the physicochemical properties, pharmacokinetics, mechanisms of action, and therapeutic activities (see Fig. 12.7).[73] On the other hand, the physicochemical differences can translate into differences in in vitro and in vivo pharmacologic and clinical properties, as exemplified between mianserin and mirtazapine (see Fig. 12.7).[73] The isosteric replacement of a benzene ring (mianserin) with a pyridine (mirtazapine) resulted in significant changes in their dipole moments, lipophilicity (log P), pK_a values, and electronegativity, resulting in different mechanisms of action and regioselectivity in the formation of hydroxylated metabolites.

Many antidepressants are stereoisomers and contain either a chiral center or a center of unsaturation by which chiral metabolites could result.[72,73] Often, such chiral drugs are marketed as a mixture of the resultant enantiomers (racemates) or of geometric isomers (eg, levomilnacipran [LVM], *1S,2R*, and *1R,2S*). These enantiomers or geometric isomers may differ markedly from each other with regard to their pharmacodynamic and/or pharmacokinetic properties.[73,74] Increased knowledge about the molecular structure of specific drug targets and an awareness of several possible advantages to using single enantiomers rather than racemic mixtures of drugs have led to an increased emphasis on understanding the role of chirality in drug development of antidepressant drugs. Several notable examples of antidepressants (the SSRIs) currently are available in which the individual enantiomers or geometric isomers differ considerably with regard to factors such as binding to SERTs and NETs, interactions with receptors and metabolizing enzymes, and clearance rates from the body. Examples of the effects of chiral centers or geometric centers on such properties include racemic mixtures, such as (±)-fluoxetine, (±)-citalopram, (±)-bupropion, and (±)-trimipramine; single enantiomers, such as (+)-sertraline, (−)-paroxetine, (−)-escitalopram, and (−)-atomoxetine; and geometric isomers, such as 1*S*,2*R*-*cis*-levomilnacipran, *Z*-zimeldine, *Z*-doxepin, and *E*-fluvoxamine. Recent developments in analytical and preparative resolution of racemic and geometric drug mixtures as well as increased interest in developing new drugs that interact with specific targets, which have been described in detail at the molecular level, have resulted in increased emphasis on stereochemistry in antidepressant drug development.[74,75]

Structure-Activity Relationship of the Tricyclic Antidepressants

The tricyclic ring structure can be found in a variety of different drugs and, for the most part, represents a method for medicinal chemists to restrict the conformational mobility of two phenyl rings attached to a common carbon or hetero atom.[74] The tricyclic ring structure is formed by joining the two phenyl rings into 6-6-6 or 6-7-6 ring systems, in which the central ring is either a six-membered or a seven-membered carbocyclic or heterocyclic ring, respectively. Small molecular changes, such as ring flexibility, substituents or heteroatoms in the tricyclic ring structure, can bring about significant changes in physicochemical, electronegativity (dipole moments), and pharmacodynamic properties (eg, anticholinergics [antimuscarinic], cholinesterase inhibitors, antihistamine, antipsychotics, and antidepressants). This suggests that the tricyclic structure is not associated with affinity for any particular receptor but, rather, contributes to a range of multiple CNS pharmacodynamic (adverse) effects because of increased lipophilicity. The most common tricyclic ring found in drugs is the near-planar phenothiazine ring common to most of the antipsychotic drugs (Fig. 12.8).[74] The TCAs are classified as such because they contain a 6-7-6 ring arrangement in which the central seven-membered ring is either carbocyclic or heterocyclic, saturated or unsaturated, which is fused to two phenyl rings (see Figs. 12.9 and 12.10 for tertiary and secondary TCAs, respectively). The side chain may be attached to any one of the atoms in the central seven-membered ring, but

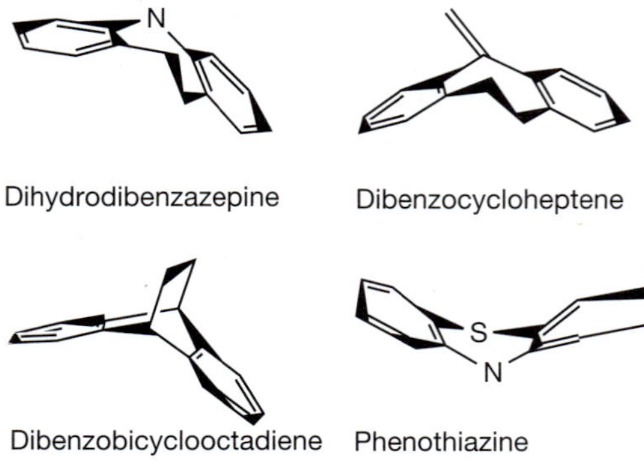

Figure 12.8 Three-dimensional models of the tricyclic and tetracyclic ring systems.

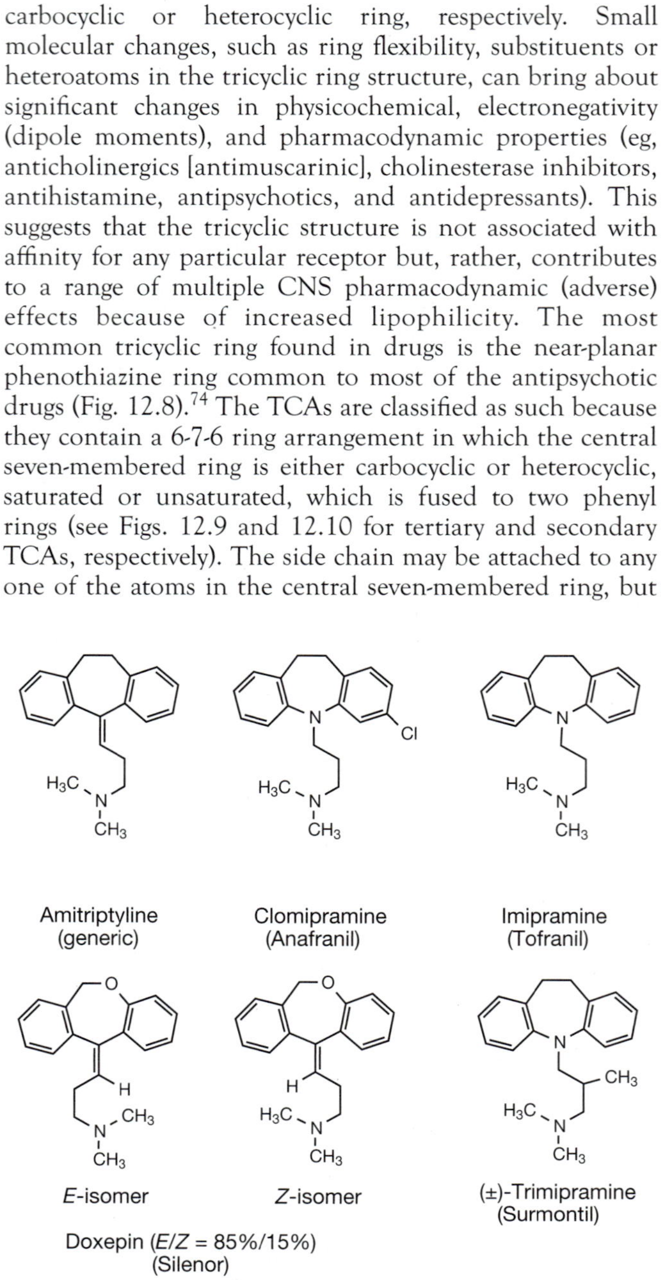

Figure 12.9 Tertiary amine tricyclic antidepressants.

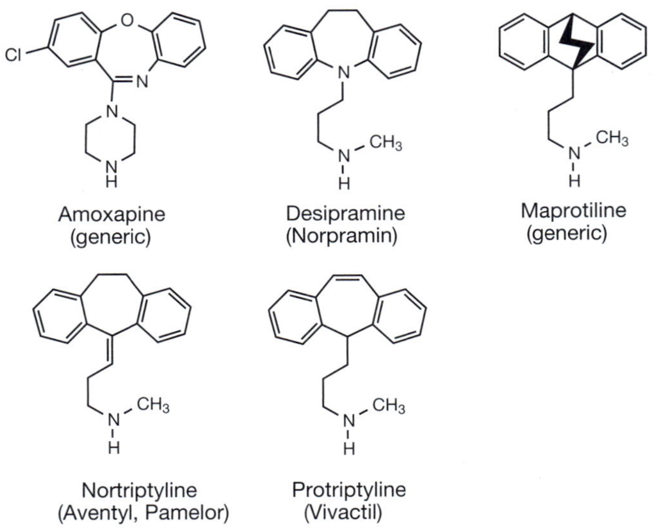

Figure 12.10 Secondary amine tricyclic antidepressants.

it must be three carbon atoms, either saturated (propyl) or unsaturated (propylidene) and have a terminal amine group (secondary or tertiary). The TCAs differ structurally from the antipsychotic phenothiazines in that the two phenyl (aromatic) rings are connected by a 2-carbon link to form a central seven-membered ring instead of a sulfur bridge.

The TCAs are subdivided into a dihydrodibenzazepine ring (aka, iminodibenzyl, from which the name imipramine is derived), a dibenzocycloheptene ring whereby the ring nitrogen of imipramine is replaced by an exocyclic olefinic group (eg, amitriptyline), a dibenzoxazepine ring as a bioisosteric modification of imipramine (eg, doxepin), a dibenzocycloheptene ring that replaces the dihydroethylene group of imipramine with an olefinic ethylene group (eg, protriptyline), or a tetracyclic (bicyclic ring, eg, maprotiline) derivative. The tricyclic ring system has little significance regarding selectivity for inhibiting the NET or SERT, but it appears to be important for DA transporter inhibition.[75]

The secondary and tertiary amine TCAs differ markedly with regard to their selectivity ratios (see Fig. 12.6) and their pharmacodynamic and/or pharmacokinetic properties (Tables 12.2 and 12.3). Substituting a halogen (ie, chlorine; clomipramine) or cyano group into the 3-position of the dihydrodibenzazepine ring enhances preferential affinity for SERT.[75,76] 3-Cyanoimipramine was investigated as a potent SSRI but was never marketed as an antidepressant agent. It is used as a research probe for studying 5-HT transporters. Branching the propyl side chain with a 2-methyl group (as in trimipramine) significantly reduces the affinity (~100 times) of imipramine for both the SERT and NET. The Z (*cis*) geometry for the propylidene group in chiral TCAs appears to be important for transporter selectivity and affinity (eg, doxepin).

Studies correlating the binding of the TCAs with the SSRIs found that the TCAs and SSRIs bind to different sites on the transporter and that the TCAs may act as a modulator of monoamine reuptake by producing conformational changes in the transporter, affecting affinity for the monoamine neurotransmitter.[75]

Table 12.2 Pharmacokinetics of the Tricyclic Tertiary Amine Antidepressants

Parameters	Amitriptyline	Clomipramine	Doxepin	Imipramine	Trimipramine
Oral bioavailability (%)	31-61	~50	13-45	29-77	44
Lipophilicity (Log $D_{7.4}$)	2.96	3.31	2.50	2.68	3.04
Protein binding (%)	95	96-98	ND	89-95	95
Volume of distribution (L/kg)	11-18	17 (9-25)	11-28	23 (15-31)	~31
Elimination half-life (hours)	10-26	32 (19-37)	11-16	11-25	9-11
Cytochrome P450 major isoform	2D6	2D6	2D6 and 2C19	2D6 and 2C19	2D6 and 2C19
Major active metabolites	Nortriptyline	Desmethylclomipramine (54-77 h)	Nordoxepin (~30 h)	Desipramine	Desmethyltrimipramine (30 h)
Peak plasma concentration (hours)	2-11	2-6 (4.7)	<2	1-2	<2
Excretion (%)	Urine 25-50	Urine 51-60 (14 d)	Renal ~50	Urine ~40 (24 h)	Feces 80-90
	Feces minor	Feces 24-32	Feces minor	Feces minor	Urine <5
Plasma half-life (hours)	21 (10-46)	34 (22-84)	8-24	18 (9-24)	9
Time to steady-state concentration	—	1-2 wk	ND	ND	ND

ND, not determined.

Table 12.3 Pharmacokinetics of the Tricyclic Secondary Amine Antidepressants

Parameters	Desipramine	Nortriptyline	Amoxapine	Protriptyline	Maprotiline
Oral bioavailability (%)	60-70	32-79	ND	77-93	66-75
Lipophilicity (Log $D_{7.4}$) Protein binding (%)	1.58 91	2.28 92	1.70 92	1.85 92	2.10 88
Volume of distribution (L/kg)	17-42	14-22	ND	22	15-28
Elimination half-life (hours)	30 (11-30)	30 (18-44)	8 (8-30)	67-89	43 (27-58)
Major active metabolites	None	10-E-hydroxy	8-OH (30 h) 7-OH (6.5 h)	None	(60-90 h)
Peak plasma concentration (hours)	4-6	7-9	90 min	24-30	8-24
Excretion (%)	Urine	Urine 40	Urine 60 (6 d)	Urine 50 (16 d)	Urine 65 (21 d)
	Feces	Feces minor	Feces 7-18	Feces minor	Feces 30
Plasma half-life (hours)	14-62	18-93	8	54-198	21-52
Time to steady-state concentration	ND	ND	ND		7 d

ND, not determined.

Although similar in a two-dimensional plane to the antipsychotic (neuroleptic) phenothiazines, the ethylene bridge linking the two phenyl rings of the TCAs causes the two phenyl rings to be twisted out of the plane, leading to a less rigid and more conformationally mobile molecular structures than the phenothiazines (Fig. 12.8). The conformational mobility for the TCAs, including ring inversion of the tricyclic ring system, flexing of the CH_2-X bridge (X= CH_2, O, N, or S) in the central seven-membered ring, and flexibility of the alkyl side chain, can result in substantial changes in the overall shape of the molecules. This, in turn, can affect transporter affinity and selectivity, diverse neuroreceptor affinity, and the drug's physicochemical properties. The rate of ring flexibility seems to be correlated with their differences in clinical potency. A dibenzazepine ring system exhibits a greater degree of conformational ring flexing, whereas the dibenzocycloheptene ring system and inserting heteroatoms into the benzylic position reduce the rate of ring flexing in TCAs and their potency.[74,75] Thus, the differences in the pharmacologic activity between these TCAs allows selective binding to their respective transporter proteins. The angle between the two aromatic rings ranges from 106° to 110° for the TCAs and the large lipophilic ring enhances the affinity of TCA to block the CNS muscarinic, H_1-, and α_1-adrenergic receptors and to block sodium channels, contributing to its multiple pharmacodynamic effects.

Drug Metabolism and Drug-Drug Interactions

Antidepressant treatment carries increased risks of adverse drug events because of age-related physiologic changes, polypharmacotherapy, and individual variability in drug metabolism (eg, genetic factors, concurrent disease, diet, and eating habits).[77] Pharmacokinetic DDIs occur when one medication (the precipitant drug) significantly affects the plasma concentration, half-life, or both of another medication (the object drug) by altering its absorption, distribution, metabolism, or elimination. For object drugs with narrow therapeutic indices, even small elevations in plasma drug concentration can cause potentially serious adverse reactions. Pharmacodynamic DDIs occur when the precipitant drug affects the ability of the object drug to bind with its therapeutic target (eg, transporter protein) or receptor. Some compounds compete directly for binding to a receptor; others indirectly affect the ability of an object drug to interact with its site of action. Many medications can bind to multiple receptor types (eg, first-generation TCAs), causing diverse adverse reactions. Thus, before adding a new drug to an existing antidepressant regimen, it is wise to determine whether any medications can be eliminated. Reduction of total drug burden, adjustment of dose levels, and careful selection of an appropriate agent are important steps toward avoiding adverse drug interactions. In addition, the documented and potential drug interactions of the various classes of antidepressants—and of the specific drugs within each class—should be considered. Each patient should be treated individually and monitored carefully during the initiation and maintenance of antidepressant therapy.

The infamous DDIs between mibefradil (Propulsid) and terfenadine (Seldane) and other drugs metabolized by cytochrome P450 (CYP) 3A4 resulted in these drugs being withdrawn from the market, which placed a spotlight on hepatic drug metabolism as a significant participant in DDIs. Nearly all the antidepressants are metabolized by at least one CYP isoform, and these drugs and their metabolites may be substrates or inhibitors for the CYPs (Table 12.4).

Table 12.4 Cytochrome P450 Metabolism

Antidepressant	Major CYP	Minor CYP	Metabolism Pathway	CYP Inhibitor
Amitriptyline	2D6	3A4, 2C19, 2C9, 1A2, and 2B6	2D6, 3A4, 2C19, and 1A2 *N*-demethylation 2D6 and 2B6 E-10-hydroxylation	2D6, 2C19, 1A2, and 2C9[a]
Clomipramine	2D6	3A4, 2C19, 1A2, and 2C9	2D6, 3A4, 2C19, 2C9, and 1A2 *N*-demethylation 2D6 2- and 8-hydroxylation	2D6
Desipramine	2D6	1A2 and 2C19	1A2 and 2C19 *N*-demethylation	2D6 and 2C19[a]
			2D6 and 2C19 2-hydroxylation	
E-Doxepin	2D6 and 2C9	3A4, 1A2, and 2C19	2D6 and 2C9 hydroxylation	
			3A4 and 1A2 *N*-demethylation	
Z-Doxepin	2C19	2C9, 3A4, and 1A2	2C19 and 2C9 *N*-demethylation	
			3A4 and 1A2 *N*-demethylation	
Imipramine	2D6	3A4, 2C19, 1A2, 2B6, and 2C9	1A2 and 2C19 *N*-demethylation 2D6, 1A2, 3A4, and 2C19 2- and 10-hydroxylation	1A2, 2D6, and 2C19
Maprotiline	2D6	1A2	2D6 and 1A2 *N*-demethylation	
Nortriptyline	2D6	3A4, 2C19, and 1A2	2D6, 3A4, 2C19, and 1A2 *N*-demethylation 2D6 *E*-10-hydroxylation	2D6 and 2C19[a]
Trimipramine	2D6	2C9 and 2C19	2-hydroxyl, 10-hydroxyl, and *N*-demethylation	2D6
(±)-Citalopram	2C19	3A4, 2D6	2C19, 3A4, *N*-demethylation 2D6 *N*-oxidation	1A2[a] and 2D6[a]
Escitalopram	2D6	1A2 and 2C19	2D6, 2C19, and 3A4 *N*-demethylation	
			2D6 *N*-oxidation	
(±)-Fluoxetine	2D6	3A4, 2C9, 2C19, and 1A2	2D6 and 2C19 *N*-dealkylation	2D6 (*S*-fluoxetine)
			1A2 and 2C9 *O*-dealkylation	1A2,[a] 2C19,[a] 3A4,[a] 2C9,[a] and 2D6[a]
Sertraline	3A4	2D6 and 2C19	3A4, 2C19, 2D6, and 2C9	2C19,[a] 3A4,[a] and 2D6[a]
			N-demethylation	
Fluvoxamine	1A2	3A4, 2C19, and 2D6	2D6 and 1A2 *O*-dealkylation	2C19, 1A2,[a] and 3A4[a]
Paroxetine	2D6	3A4, 1A2, and 2C9	2D6 cleavage methylene dioxy	2D6,[b] 2C19,[a] and 3A4[a]
Venlafaxine	2D6	3A4, 2C19, and 2C9	2D6, 2C19, and 2C9 *O*-demethylation	2D6[a]
			2C19, 2C9, and 3A4 *N*-demethylation	
Atomoxetine	2D6	3A4, 2C19, and 1A2	2D6, 1A2, 2B6, and 2C19 4-hydroxylation	
			2C19, 3A4, and 2B6 *N*-demethylation	
Duloxetine	2D6	1A2	4- and 6-hydroxylation	2D6
Mirtazapine	2D6	3A4 and 1A2	2D6 and 1A2 8-hydroxylation	3A4[a] and 2D6[a]
			3A4 *N*-demethylation	
			3A4 and 1A2 *N*-oxidation	

Table 12.4 Cytochrome P450 Metabolism (*continued*)

Antidepressant	Major CYP	Minor CYP	Metabolism Pathway	CYP Inhibitor
Vilazodone	3A4/5	2C19, 2D6	6-aromatic hydroxylation of indole ring	
Vortioxetine	2D6	2C9, 2C19, 3A4	2D6 and 2C19 methyl hydroxylation 2D6 and 2C9 aromatic hydroxylation 3A4 *N*- and *S*-oxidation	2D6
Bupropion	2B6	2E1, 3A4, and 2D6	Hydroxylation *t*-butyl group	2D6[a]
Trazodone	3A4	2D6	*N*-dealkylation to chlorophenylpiperazine	
			Aromatic ring hydroxylation	
Tranylcypromine		3A4, 2A6, 2D6, 2C19, and 2C9	Aromatic ring hydroxylation	2A6[b]
Levomilnacipran	3A4		*N*-deethylation and *p*-hydroxylation	

CYP, cytochrome.
[a]Weak CYP inhibitor.
[b]Mechanism-based inhibition.
Rendic S. Summary of information on human CYP enzymes: human P450 metabolism data. *Drug Metab Rev.* 2002;34(1-2):83-448. doi: 10.1081/dmr-120001392

When an antidepressant is metabolized by more than one CYP isoform in parallel, the antidepressant is unlikely to be affected by drug interactions or genetic polymorphisms and to cause clinically significant drug interactions via CYP isoform inhibition.[77,78] However, if the drug is metabolized (depending upon enzyme kinetics) primarily by CYP3A4 or the polymorphic CYP2C18 or CYP2D6 isoforms, the potential for DDIs increases. Therefore, knowledge regarding the metabolic pathways of antidepressants as well as knowledge about substrates and inhibitors of the CYP isoforms can assist in the selection of a proper drug and its dose, thus minimizing the risks of DDIs.[77,78]

Drug Safety

Clinical trials have concluded that two or three of every 100 children and teenagers treated with antidepressants might be at higher risk of suicidal behavior. Data regarding suicidal behavior vary among the antidepressants, which leads to the conclusion that no antidepressant is free from risk at this time. Most of the suicides have occurred with the SSRIs, especially paroxetine (Paxil) and fluoxetine (Prozac); only fluoxetine has been proven to be effective and is approved for treating pediatric depression. Approximately 7% of antidepressant prescriptions are written for children. Thus, the FDA in 2007 approved that "black box labeling" be included on antidepressant product packaging, alerting physicians to avoid prescribing antidepressants to children because of possible risks of suicidal behavior and to watch for signs of worsening depression or suicidal thoughts in children who are taking any antidepressant. In 2018, the FDA directed manufacturers of all antidepressant drugs to revise the labeling for their products to include a black box warning and expanded warning statements that alert health care providers to an increased risk of suicidality (suicidal thinking and behavior) in children and adolescents being treated with these antidepressants, and to include additional information about the results of pediatric studies. The FDA also informed these manufacturers that it has determined that a patient medication guide (medguide), which will be given to patients receiving the drugs to advise them of the risks and precautions that can be taken, is appropriate for these drug products. The risk of suicidality for these antidepressant drugs was identified in a combined analysis of short-term (up to 4 months) placebo-controlled trials of nine antidepressant drugs, including the SSRIs, SNRIs, and atypical others, in children and adolescents with MDD, OCD, and other affective disorders. The analysis showed a greater risk of suicidality during the first few months of treatment in those receiving antidepressants. The average risk of such events was 4%, twice the placebo risk of 2%. Among the antidepressants, only Prozac is approved for use in treating MDD in pediatric patients. Fluoxetine, sertraline, fluvoxamine, and clomipramine are approved for OCD in pediatric patients. Pediatric patients being treated with antidepressants for any indication should be closely observed for clinical worsening as well as agitation, irritability, suicidality, and unusual changes in behavior, especially during the initial few months of a course of drug therapy, or at times of dose changes, either increases or decreases. In addition to the boxed warning and other information in professional labeling on antidepressants, medguides are being prepared for all of the antidepressants to provide information about the risk of suicidality in children and adolescents directly to patients and their families and caregivers. Medguides are intended to be distributed by the pharmacist with each prescription or refill of a medication. SSRIs are safer than the TCAs for older people because they do not disturb heart rhythms and rarely cause dizziness that results in falls, but liver function is less efficient in older people, so there is a greater risk of drug interactions involving the CYP450 system (see Table 12.4). For this reason, older people do best with rapidly metabolized SSRIs like sertraline.

Specific Drugs

Tricyclic Tertiary Amine Antidepressants

Despite the current popularity of the SSRIs for the treatment of depression, the noradrenergic neurons should not be overlooked, because they also influence the depressed mood.[73] The noradrenergic system appears to be associated with NE-deficit depressions with decreased concentration, low motivation, poor energy, inattention, poor self-care, and cognitive difficulties, whereas 5-HT-deficit depressions are associated with changes in mood, anxiety, suicidality, and appetite disturbances (see Fig. 12.1). Thus, the different symptoms of depression may benefit from drugs acting mainly on one or the other of the neurotransmitter systems. The secondary amine TCAs (see Fig. 12.10) seem to be at least as effective as the SSRIs in the treatment of depressive illness by acting specifically at noradrenergic sites. Thus, the SSRIs and secondary amine TCAs influence depression by parallel, independent pathways. The secondary amine TCAs have a role in the treatment of depression, either alone or as adjunct therapy. The secondary amine TCAs are well tolerated but possess different adverse-event profiles.

The selectivity ratios (see Fig. 12.6) show that the TCAs, as a group, are potent inhibitors of the SERT and NET, and that the secondary amine TCAs are substantially more potent with regard to their inhibition of NE reuptake in comparison to the SSRIs. Their in vitro affinity for inhibiting the NET essentially mirrors more or less their clinical efficacy as antidepressants: desipramine > protriptyline > amitriptyline = nortriptyline > maprotiline > amoxapine > imipramine. The secondary amine TCAs are primarily NE reuptake inhibitors, with no clinically relevant 5-HT reuptake except where large doses are used, and include protriptyline, nortriptyline, and desipramine as examples.

The tricyclic tertiary amines (see Fig. 12.9) have a relatively low bioavailability, suggesting first-pass metabolism (*N*-demethylation) to their secondary amine active metabolites (nor- or desmethyl metabolites) and aromatic ring hydroxylation (see Table 12.2). Despite the fact that steady-state serum plasma levels are reached within 1 to 2 days, their onset of antidepressant action typically is at least 2 to 3 weeks or longer. Their volume of distribution is very high, suggesting distribution into the CNS and protein binding (see Table 12.2). Excretion is primarily as metabolites via renal elimination. Renal and liver function can affect the elimination and metabolism of the parent TCA and its metabolites, leading to increased potential for adverse effects, especially in those patients (ie, older adults) with renal disease (see Table 12.2).

Meaningful differences between the TCA tertiary amines are largely related to their pharmacokinetics, metabolism to active metabolites, inhibition of CYP isoforms, potential for DDIs, and half-lives.

Mechanisms of Action Common to Tricyclic Tertiary Amine Antidepressants

The exact mechanism of action for the tertiary amine TCAs is unclear, but it is known that the parent tertiary amine TCA exhibits mixed inhibition of the NET and SERT. The result is an increase in both NE and 5-HT concentrations in the synaptic cleft. The in vivo antidepressant activity for these TCAs is more complex, however, because of the formation of secondary amine TCA metabolites, which, in many cases, annuls the 5-HT affinity of the parent TCA, leading to NET selectivity. The plasma concentrations for the secondary amine metabolites usually are higher than that of their parent tertiary amine TCA because of rapid *N*-demethylation metabolism. Note that none of the tertiary amine TCAs have any significant affinity for the DA transporter. During chronic therapy with the tertiary amine TCAs, downregulation of the noradrenergic and serotonergic receptors occurs, which is a result of neurotransmitter hypersensitivity caused by the continued high concentrations of NE and 5-HT at the postsynaptic receptor. The TCA tertiary amines are less potent inhibitors than the SSRIs for SERT.

Therapeutic Uses Common to Tricyclic Tertiary Amine Antidepressants

For the most part, the therapeutic uses for the tertiary amine TCAs are very similar as a group, but these TCAs may be used in different cases of depression because of their variability in their dual mechanism of action as inhibitors of NE and 5-HT reuptake and the adverse effects. Their efficacy in treating depression suggests that mixed inhibition of NET and SERT influences depression by parallel and independent pathways. The tertiary TCAs may offer an option in the treatment of major depression for patients who have failed treatment with or who do not tolerate atypical SNRIs or SSRIs.

Adverse Effects Common to Tricyclic Tertiary Amine Antidepressants

Because of their potent and multiple pharmacodynamic effects at H_1, muscarinic, and α_1-adrenergic receptors, the tertiary amine TCAs exhibit greater anticholinergic, antihistaminic, and hypotensive adverse effects than the secondary amine TCAs (see Table 12.5). Increased cardiotoxicity or frequency of seizures is higher for the tertiary amine TCAs than for the secondary amine TCAs, because they are potent inhibitors of sodium channels, leading to changes in nerve conduction. Cardiotoxicity can occur at plasma concentrations approximately 5 to 10 times higher than therapeutic blood levels. These concentrations can occur in individuals who take an overdose of a tertiary amine TCA or who are slow metabolizers and develop higher plasma concentrations on what usually are therapeutic doses.

Drug-Drug Interactions Common to Tricyclic Tertiary Amine Antidepressants

For the most part, DDIs for the tertiary amine TCAs are very similar to those for the secondary amine TCAs. These interactions, however, may be more pronounced. The concurrent use of tertiary amine TCAs with SSRIs and other serotonergic drugs may result in 5-HT syndrome (see the discussion of drug interactions of SSRIs). Coadministration of a tertiary amine TCA with a MAOI is potentially hazardous and may result in severe adverse effects associated with 5-HT syndrome.

Because protein binding of the tertiary amine TCAs is high, displacement interactions with other highly

Table 12.5 Patient Information and Recommendations for Tricyclic Secondary Amine Antidepressants

Patient Information	Recommendations
Potential drug-drug and drug-health interactions	Share medical conditions, other medicines (including over-the-counter and herbal medicines), allergies to tricyclic antidepressants (TCAs), fertility status, or breastfeeding with pharmacist.
Seizures, breathing difficulties, fever and sweating, loss of bladder control, muscle stiffness, unusual weakness or tiredness	Discontinue therapy and consult physician (TCAs may increase risk of seizures).
Course of therapy	Complete full course of therapy.
Discontinuance of therapy	Consult physician; abrupt discontinuance not recommended, because it may cause nausea, headache, and malaise.
Alcohol use	Avoid alcohol.
Central nervous system depressants	May exacerbate TCAs.
Drowsiness, dizziness, blurred vision	Avoid driving or performing tasks requiring alertness and coordination.
Sun/sunlamp exposure	Avoid prolonged exposure because of photosensitivity.

protein-bound drugs and drugs with narrow therapeutic indices, although not fully evaluated, may be important. Concurrent use of tertiary amine TCAs with anticholinergic drugs requires close supervision and careful adjustment of the dosage because of potential additive anticholinergic effects (ie, spastic colon). An additional disadvantage of the tertiary amine TCAs is their toxicity from overdosage, especially in those who are being treated for depression having suicidal thoughts.

The plasma concentrations of tertiary amine TCAs usually are lower and plasma concentrations of their secondary amine metabolites higher, as a result of CYP1A induction.

Patient Information Common to Tricyclic Tertiary Amine Antidepressants

Common patient information and recommendations are similar to those given to patients who are prescribed secondary amine TCAs (Table 12.5).

Unique Properties of Specific Tricyclic Tertiary Amine Antidepressants

AMITRIPTYLINE. Amitriptyline is a tricyclic tertiary amine dibenzocycloheptadiene TCA with a propylidene side chain extending from the central carbocyclic ring (see Fig. 12.9). The diarylpropylideneamine moiety for amitriptyline makes it sensitive to photo-oxidation; therefore, its hydrochloride solutions should be protected from light to avoid ketone formation and precipitation.

Pharmacokinetics. Amitriptyline is rapidly absorbed from the GI tract and from parenteral sites. Its pharmacokinetics are shown in Table 12.2. Amitriptyline and its active metabolite, nortriptyline, are distributed into breast milk. Amitriptyline is primarily (65%) metabolized by *N*-demethylation by CYP2D6 to nortriptyline and hydroxylation to its *E*-10-hydroxy metabolite. Nortriptyline is pharmacologically active as a secondary amine TCA. Amitriptyline shows approximately equal affinity for 5-HT and NE transporters.

IMIPRAMINE. Imipramine is a 10,11-dihydrodibenzazepine tricyclic tertiary amine TCA (see Fig. 12.9) that is marketed as hydrochloride and pamoate salts, both of which are administered orally. Although the hydrochloride salt may be administered in divided daily doses, imipramine's long duration of action suggests that the entire oral daily dose may be administered at one time. On the other hand, imipramine pamoate usually is administered as a single daily oral dose. Imipramine preferentially inhibits 5-HT reuptake over NE; however, the formation of its *N*-desmethyl metabolite removes whatever 5-HT activity imipramine had, with the net result of enhanced noradrenergic activity from inhibition of NE reuptake at the presynaptic neuronal membrane. Imipramine shares the pharmacologic and adverse-effect profile of the other tertiary TCAs.

The pharmacokinetics for imipramine are shown in Table 12.2. Imipramine is completely absorbed from the GI tract. Imipramine is primarily metabolized by CYP2D6 to its 2- and 10-hydroxylated metabolites and *N*-demethylated via CYP2C11 and CYP1A2 to desipramine, its *N*-monodemethylated metabolite.

Therapeutic Uses. Besides being used in the clinical treatment of depression, imipramine also has been used for the treatment of functional enuresis in children who are at least 6 years old (25 mg daily administered 1 hour before bedtime, not to exceed 2.5 mg/kg daily).

DOXEPIN. Doxepin is a tricyclic tertiary amine dibenzoxazepine derivative with an oxygen replacing one of the ethylene carbons in the bridge. The oxygen introduces asymmetry into the tricyclic ring system, resulting in the formation of two geometric isomers: *E* (*trans*) and *Z* (*cis*) (see Fig. 12.9). No commercial attempt was made to separate the isomers; thus, doxepin is administered as an 85:15 mixture of *E*- and *Z*-stereoisomers, with the *Z*-isomer being the more active stereoisomer for inhibiting the reuptake of 5-HT.[79] The *E*-isomer inhibits the reuptake of NE.[40] Unless otherwise specified, the reported in vitro and in vivo studies with doxepin were done with the 85:15 geometric mixture.

Mechanism of Action. Because doxepin is administered as an 85:15 mixture of geometric isomers, its mechanism of action and antidepressant properties reflect this ratio. Therefore, doxepin's selectivity for inhibiting presynaptic NE reuptake is most likely caused by the 85% presence of the *E*-isomer in the geometric mixture. Its antidepressant activity is similar to amitriptyline. Data suggest NE reuptake inhibitory potency comparable to imipramine and clomipramine; the fact that doxepin is an 85:15 mixture of *E*- and *Z*-geometric isomers clouds its true efficacy for SERT or NET. The formation of *N*-desmethyldoxepin results in inhibition of NE reuptake with enhanced noradrenergic activity. As a result of these mixed effects on the 5-HT and NE transporters, doxepin shares the pharmacologic and adverse-effect profile of the other TCAs.

The pharmacokinetics for oral doxepin are described in Table 12.2. After oral dosing, no significant difference was found between the bioavailability of the *E*- and *Z*-isomers. The plasma concentrations of the doxepin isomers remained roughly those of the administered drug, whereas the ratio for the metabolites *E*-*N*-desmethyldoxepin and *Z*-*N*-desmethyldoxepin was approximately 1:1.[78,79] This similarity in ratios of metabolites is attributed to *E*-doxepin being primarily metabolized in parallel by CYP2D6 and CYP2C19, whereas *Z*-doxepin is primarily metabolized only by CYP2C19 and not at all by CYP2D6 (see Table 12.2). Its *Z*-*N*-demethylated metabolite is pharmacologically more active than its *E*-metabolite as an inhibitor of 5-HT and NE reuptake. Both isomers of doxepin showed large volumes of distribution and relatively short half-lives in plasma, suggestive of extensive distribution and/or tissue binding. Renal clearances did not differ for the isomers.[79]

CLOMIPRAMINE. Clomipramine is considered to be the most powerful antidepressant ever made. This tricyclic tertiary dihydrodibenzazepine TCA, with actions on both the NE and 5-HT transporters, was the last of the major TCAs to come to market. Initially, the FDA regarded it as another "me-too" drug, and, accordingly, they did not license it. Subsequently, however, it was licensed for the treatment of OCD. Clomipramine differs from imipramine only by the addition of a 3-chloro group (see Fig. 12.9).

Mechanism of Action. Clomipramine is different from the other tertiary amine TCAs, exhibiting preferential selectivity for inhibiting the reuptake of 5-HT at the presynaptic neuronal membrane. Its antidepressant mechanism of action as an inhibitor of the 5-HT transporter is reduced in vivo, however, because of the formation of its active metabolite, *N*-desmethylclomipramine, which inhibits the reuptake of NE. As a result of its common structure with the other TCAs, clomipramine shares the pharmacologic and adverse-effect profile of the other TCAs.

The efficacy of clomipramine relative to the other TCAs in the treatment of OCD may be related to its potency in blocking 5-HT reuptake at the presynaptic neuronal membrane, suggesting a dysregulation of 5-HT for the pathogenesis of OCD. Clomipramine appears to decrease the turnover of 5-HT in the CNS, probably because of a decrease in the release and/or synthesis of 5-HT.

Although in vitro studies suggest that clomipramine is approximately 4 times more potent than fluoxetine as a 5-HT reuptake inhibitor, in vivo studies suggest the opposite. This difference has been attributed to the relatively long elimination half-lives for fluoxetine and its principal serotonergic metabolite norfluoxetine. In addition, metabolism of clomipramine to its *N*-desmethyl secondary amine metabolite decreases the potency and selectivity of 5-HT reuptake inhibition of clomipramine, but not fluoxetine.

Pharmacokinetics. Clomipramine appears to be well absorbed from the GI tract following oral administration, with an oral bioavailability of approximately 50%, suggesting some first-pass metabolism (see Table 12.2). Food does not appear to substantially affect its bioavailability. Clomipramine and its active metabolite, *N*-desmethylclomipramine, exhibit nonlinear pharmacokinetics at 25 to 150 mg daily. At dosages exceeding 150 mg daily, their elimination half-lives may be considerably prolonged, allowing plasma concentrations to accumulate, which may increase the incidence of plasma concentration–dependent adverse effects, particularly seizures. Because of the relatively long elimination half-lives of clomipramine and *N*-desmethylclomipramine, their steady-state plasma concentrations generally are achieved within approximately 1 to 2 weeks. Plasma concentration of *N*-desmethylclomipramine generally is greater than that for clomipramine at steady-state conditions. Clomipramine crosses the placenta and is distributed into breast milk.

Clomipramine is primarily metabolized by CYP2D6 *N*-dealkylation to its pharmacologically active metabolite (*N*-desmethylclomipramine), the 2- and 8-hydroxylated metabolites and their glucuronides and clomipramine *N*-oxide (Fig. 12.11). *N*-dealkylation also involves CYP3A4, CYP2C19, CYP2C9, and CYP1A2. Like all the other secondary amine TCAs, *N*-desmethylclomipramine is significantly more potent as an inhibitor of NE reuptake than clomipramine. Although *N*-desmethylclomipramine

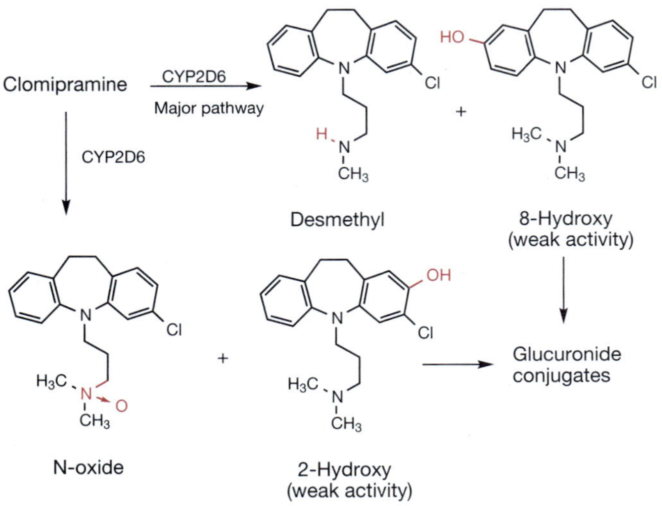

Figure 12.11 Metabolism of clomipramine.

is pharmacologically active, its efficacy in OCD is not known. 8-Hydroxyclomipramine and 8-hydroxydesmethylclomipramine also are pharmacologically active, but their clinical importance remains unknown. The hydroxylation and *N*-demethylation of clomipramine highlight CYP2D6 polymorphism in healthy adults who were phenotyped as either extensive metabolizers or poor metabolizers of clomipramine. Interindividual variation in plasma concentrations may be caused by genetic differences in the metabolism of the drug. In addition, CYP1A2 ring hydroxylates clomipramine. Less than 1% of an oral dose of clomipramine was excreted unmetabolized into the urine, with 8-hydroxyclomipramine glucuronide as the principal metabolite found in the urine. The effects of renal clearance suggest that clomipramine and desmethylclomipramine should be decreased in patients with renal impairment.

Pharmacogenetic differences in the metabolism of clomipramine after a single oral dose are apparent as increased plasma clomipramine concentrations in patients of Indian and Pakistani origin compared with patients of White origin. In patients of Japanese origin, substantial interindividual variation in demethylation and hydroxylation of clomipramine was observed, although the prevalence of poor demethylators and poor hydroxylators of clomipramine has been estimated to be less than 1%.

If inhibition of SERT is critical to the desired clinical effect for clomipramine, then a patient may fail to respond, because of higher levels of *N*-desmethylclomipramine as opposed to the parent drug. On the other hand, if a patient who had responded well and was stabilized to a dose of clomipramine is exposed to an environmental agent that is capable of inducing CYP1A or CYP3A4, the drug might lose efficacy.

Adverse Effects. Male patients taking clomipramine should be informed of sexual dysfunction as a side effect associated with antidepressants having significant serotonergic activity. Sexual dysfunction in men appears as ejaculatory incompetence, ejaculatory retardation, decreased libido, or inability to obtain or maintain an erection. Sexual dysfunction is dose-related and may be treated by simply lowering the drug dose.

TRIMIPRAMINE. Trimipramine is also a tertiary amine dihydrodibenzazepine TCA that differs structurally from imipramine in that the 5-propyl side chain is branched by a methyl group creating a chiral center (see Fig. 12.9). Trimipramine is marketed as a racemic mixture.[80] No data are available regarding the activity of the enantiomers. Apparently, branching the propyl side chain reduces affinity by 100 times for both 5-HT and NE transporters, but the selectivity ratio favors the 5-HT transporter.[81] Although trimipramine has the weakest binding affinity for the monoamine transporters, it shares the pharmacologic and toxicity actions of the other TCAs and is used primarily in the treatment of depression.

The pharmacokinetics for trimipramine are shown in Table 12.2. Trimipramine is rapidly absorbed. Trimipramine demonstrates stereoselectivity in its metabolism to its three major metabolites. (−)-Trimipramine is primarily metabolized via CY2D6 hydroxylation to 2-hydroxytrimipramine, whereas (+)-trimipramine is preferentially metabolized by CYP2C19 *N*-demethylation to desmethyltrimipramine. Desmethyltrimipramine is further hydroxylated to 2-hydroxydesmethyltrimipramine. (−)-Trimipramine is metabolized by CYP3A4/5 to an unknown metabolite.[80,81] Most of the oral dose is excreted in urine in 72 hours, primarily as *N*-demethylated or hydroxylated and conjugated metabolites. The pharmacokinetics of trimipramine in geriatric individuals (age ≥65 years) do not differ substantially from those in younger adults.

Trimipramine is one of the TCA antidepressants with the most pronounced differences in pharmacokinetics caused by the CYP2D6 genetic polymorphism.[80,81] Its bioavailability and systemic clearance depend significantly on the CYP2D6 isoform with a linear dose relationship. Its mean bioavailability was 44% in individuals without CYP2D6 (poor metabolizers) but 16% and 11% in those individuals with two and three active genes of CYP2D6 (fast and ultrafast metabolizers), respectively. Consequently, the mean total clearances of the oral dose were 27, 151, and 253 L/h in poor, extensive, and ultrarapid metabolizers, respectively. The 44% bioavailability combined with low systemic clearance of trimipramine in poor metabolizers of CYP2D6 substrates results in a very high exposure to trimipramine with the risk of adverse drug reactions. On the other hand, the presystemic elimination may result in subtherapeutic drug concentrations in carriers of CYP2D6 gene duplications with a high risk of poor therapeutic response.

Tricyclic Secondary Amine Antidepressants

Pharmacokinetics Common to Secondary Amine Tricyclic Antidepressants

The secondary amine TCAs are rapidly and well absorbed following oral administration. Although the pharmacokinetics are approximately similar within the tertiary and secondary amine groups, the pharmacokinetics are different between the two groups (see Tables 12.2 and 12.3). The secondary amine TCAs have relatively high bioavailability. Their primary routes of hepatic metabolism are *N*-demethylation to inactive primary amine metabolites and aromatic ring hydroxylation (see Table 12.3). Despite the fact that serum plasma levels are reached within 1 to 2 days, their onset of antidepressant action typically is at least 2 to 3 weeks or longer. Their volume of distribution is very high, suggesting distribution into the CNS and protein binding. Elimination is primarily as metabolites and their conjugates via renal elimination. Renal and liver function can affect the elimination and metabolism of the parent secondary amine TCA and its metabolites, leading to increased potential for adverse effects, especially in those patients (ie, older adults) with renal disease.

Mechanisms of Action Common to Secondary Amine Tricyclic Antidepressants

The exact mechanism of action for the secondary TCAs is unclear, but the secondary amine TCAs exhibit substantially more affinity than the SSRIs and the tertiary TCAs for inhibiting the NET. None of the secondary TCAs has significant affinity for the DAT. Blocking the reuptake of

NE increases its concentration in the synaptic cleft and its ability to interact with synaptic NE receptors. When drugs are selective for a transporter, differences in potency become clinically irrelevant, because the plasma concentration can be dose-adjusted to achieve inhibition of the desired transporter without affecting the other transporters. During chronic therapy with the TCAs, adaptive changes at the noradrenergic receptor occur (ie, downregulation) as a result of neurotransmitter hypersensitivity from low concentrations of NE at the postsynaptic receptor. These changes involve the α_1-adrenergic receptor. The antidepressant action of the NE selective secondary amine TCAs such as desipramine and nortriptyline suggests a major involvement of NE neurotransmission in depression, although these compounds or their metabolites also have some action on the 5-HT system. The selective NE reuptake inhibitor, reboxetine, has demonstrated equivalent efficacy to TCAs in some studies.

Drug-Drug Interactions Common to the Secondary Amine Tricyclic Antidepressants

The secondary amine TCAs were once first-line therapy for depression because of their efficacy in a broad range of depressive disorders. Today, however, these agents generally are reserved for second-line treatment because of their narrow therapeutic-to-toxicity ratios and troublesome adverse-effect profiles. Even the better-tolerated nortriptyline is fatal in overdose and may have significant adverse effects at therapeutic dose levels. Most TCAs are metabolized by multiple CYP enzymes and, thus, are likely to be object drugs for many common medications. Because these TCAs have narrow therapeutic indices, any interference with their metabolism can lead to serious adverse reactions resulting from increased plasma concentrations (eg, arrhythmias, seizures, and confusion). Such reactions are both more common and more likely to be life threatening in older adult patients because of age-related pharmacokinetic alterations. Therefore, although specific secondary amine TCAs are useful for some conditions (eg, major depression), coadministration with other drugs should be done cautiously.

Concurrent administration of these TCAs and MAOIs is contraindicated, and at least 2 weeks should elapse between discontinuance of TCA therapy and initiation of MAOI therapy and vice versa, to allow washout. Coadministration of SNRIs, TCAs, and MAOIs is potentially hazardous and may result in severe adverse effects associated with hypertension.

Because protein binding of secondary amine TCAs is high, displacement interactions with other highly protein-bound drugs with narrow therapeutic indices, although not yet fully evaluated, may be important. Concurrent use of the secondary amine TCAs with anticholinergics requires close supervision and careful adjustment of the dosage because of potential additive anticholinergic effects (ie, spastic colon) and increased blood pressure and heart rate. An additional disadvantage of these TCAs is their toxicity from overdosage, especially in those being treated for depression who may have suicidal thoughts.

In addition, the secondary amine TCAs are inhibitors of sodium channels and, thus, can slow ventricular conduction at therapeutic doses. If the patient overdoses or drug interactions result in increased plasma concentration of the TCA, severe conduction block contributing to cardiotoxicity may result in ventricular arrhythmias. Also, changes in CNS conduction can result in seizures. Patients who are sensitive to one TCA may be sensitive to other TCAs.

The effect of smoking on the activity of CYP1A2 does not appear to have an effect on the plasma concentrations of the secondary TCAs. This is because CYP1A2 is not involved with the *N*-dealkylation to their primary amine metabolites. For common patient information and recommendations, see Table 12.5.

Unique Properties for Specific Secondary Amine Tricyclic Antidepressants

DESIPRAMINE. Desipramine is a dihydrodibenzazepine secondary amine TCA that is also the active metabolite of imipramine (see Fig. 12.10). Desipramine appears to have a bioavailability comparable to the other secondary TCAs (see Table 12.3). Desipramine is distributed into milk in concentrations similar to those present at steady state in maternal plasma. This drug is metabolized primarily by CYP2D6 to its 2-hydroxy metabolite and by CYP1A2 and CYP2C19 to its *N*-demethylated (primary amine) metabolite (see Table 12.4).

Desipramine exhibits a greater potency and selectivity for the NET than the other secondary TCAs do (see Fig. 12.6). Its antidepressant effect results from increases in the level of NE in CNS synapses and long-term administration causes a downregulation of α_1-adrenoceptors and desensitization of presynaptic α_2-receptors, equilibrating the noradrenergic system and, thus, correcting the dysregulated output of patients who are depressed. The SSRIs do not produce this effect. Desipramine also downregulates NET, but not SERT. Substantial loss of NET binding sites takes 15 days to occur and is accompanied by a marked reduction of NET function in vivo. Desipramine has weak effects on 5-HT reuptake.

NORTRIPTYLINE. Nortriptyline is a secondary amine dibenzocycloheptene TCA (see Fig. 12.10) as well as the major metabolite of amitriptyline. Similar to desipramine, nortriptyline appears in breast milk and is metabolized by CYP2D6 to the primary amine and by ring hydroxylation to its *E*-10-hydroxy metabolite (see Table 12.3). Approximately a third of a dose of nortriptyline is excreted in urine as metabolites within 24 hours and small amounts are excreted in feces via biliary elimination.

AMOXAPINE. Amoxapine is a dibenzoxazepine TCA (see Fig. 12.10) with antidepressant and antipsychotic effects that have shown therapeutic effectiveness in patients with delusional depression. Additionally, it is the *N*-desmethyl metabolite of the antipsychotic loxapine. Amoxapine differs structurally from the other secondary TCAs in that it has both a nitrogen and an oxygen atom in its seven-membered central ring and a piperazinyl ring rather than a propylamino side chain attached to the central ring.

Amoxapine is a less potent inhibitor of neuronal NE reuptake compared with the other secondary TCAs, with a mechanism of action similar to that of desipramine. Amoxapine shares the toxic potentials of the TCAs, and the usual precautions of TCA administration should be observed. Amoxapine resembles the atypical antipsychotic drugs in its affinity as an antagonist of DA_2 and of 5-HT_2 receptors.

Amoxapine is rapidly and almost completely absorbed from the GI tract. Its pharmacokinetics are shown in Table 12.3. Amoxapine and its 8-hydroxyamoxapine metabolite have been detected in human milk at concentrations below steady-state therapeutic concentrations. Amoxapine has the shortest elimination time (~8 hours) of the secondary TCAs. It is metabolized in the liver principally to 8-hydroxyamoxapine and to 7-hydroxyamoxapine. Both of these metabolites are pharmacologically active and have half-lives of 30 and 6.5 hours, respectively. The hydroxylation of amoxapine is inhibited by ketoconazole, suggesting the involvement of CYP3A4.

Protriptyline. Protriptyline is a dibenzocycloheptriene TCA that differs from the other tricyclics by having an unsaturated ethylene bridge joining the two aromatic rings and a secondary aminopropyl side chain (see Fig. 12.10). Protriptyline is completely absorbed from the GI tract and slowly eliminated. Its pharmacokinetic data are shown in Table 12.3. Metabolism data are limited for protriptyline, but it is most likely metabolized via the same pathways as the other TCAs are (see Table 12.4). Very little drug is excreted in the feces via bile.

Protriptyline exhibits high selectivity for the NET, but with less potency than desipramine (see Fig. 12.10). Its mechanism of action is similar to that of desipramine. Minimal effect on 5-HT reuptake has been observed.

Maprotiline. Maprotiline is a tetracyclic secondary amine dibenzobicyclooctadiene that differs structurally from the TCAs by having an ethylene bridge in its central ring, resulting in a rigid bicyclo-molecular skeleton (see Figs. 12.8 and 12.10). The tetracyclics have diverse pharmacology and differ from TCAs in a number of ways. They do not inhibit the reuptake of 5-HT, but do inhibit the reuptake of NE. They block the 5-HT_2 receptors similarly to TCAs. Besides mirtazapine, they also block the α_1-adrenergic receptor. The tetracyclics also block the histamine H_1 receptor similarly to the TCAs, but tend to be even stronger antihistamines than TCAs. On the other hand, in contrast to almost all TCAs, they have only low affinity for the neuronal muscarinic (m) AChRs and, for this reason, are associated with few or no anticholinergic side effects.

Maprotiline exhibits the highest affinity and selectivity for the NE transporter (see Fig. 12.6). Its antidepressant mechanism of action is similar to that of desipramine, with an onset of action of up to 2 to 3 weeks.

Maprotiline is slowly but completely absorbed from the GI tract, and, like the other TCAs, it is metabolized by CYP2D6 and CYP2C19 isoforms in the liver, primarily to pharmacologically active *N*-desmethylmaprotiline and to maprotiline-*N*-oxide. Its pharmacokinetics are shown in Table 12.3. Maprotiline is distributed into breast milk at concentrations similar to those found at steady state in maternal blood. The elimination half-life of maprotiline averages 43 hours (60-90 hours for its *N*-desmethyl metabolite).

Maprotiline shares the toxic potentials of the secondary TCAs, and the usual precautions of TCA administration should be observed. Although most of the TCAs have been reported to induce seizures, it is generally recognized that maprotiline may be associated with a higher incidence of dose-dependent seizures compared with the other secondary TCAs. Maprotiline has been reported to produce sedation in patients who are depressed and to reduce aggressive behavior in animals. Maprotiline also shares the anticholinergic and cardiovascular effects of the secondary TCAs and may cause electrocardiographic changes, tachycardia, and postural hypotension.

Therapeutic Uses Common to All Tricyclic Antidepressants

The efficacy of the secondary and tertiary amine TCAs in the clinical treatment of depressive illness is recommended for various conditions, including major depressive episodes, dysthymia, panic disorder, social phobia, bulimia, narcolepsy, attention-deficit disorder with or without hyperactivity, migraine headache and various other chronic pain syndromes, enuresis in children, and OCD (clomipramine). The TCAs possibly are useful as well for a broader range of depressive conditions described as dysthymia or depressive neurosis and even for prolonged or pathologic mourning, agoraphobia without panic attacks, and some of the symptoms (eg, nightmares) in PTSD.

Adverse Effects Common to All Tricyclic Antidepressants

The family of TCAs has many undesirable side effects and behaves like "five drugs wrapped into one." They not only block the reuptake of NE and 5-HT but also block muscarinic receptors (anticholinergic), α_1-adrenergic receptors (hypotension), H_1-receptors (antihistamine), and sodium channels. The common adverse effects and appropriate responses are given in Table 12.6.

Table 12.6 Common Adverse Effects With Tricyclic Antidepressants and Recommendations

Side Effect	Treatment Recommendations
Dry mouth	Drink sips of water; chew sugarless gum; clean teeth daily
Constipation	Diet rich in bran cereals, prunes, fruit, and vegetables
Bladder complaints (weak urine stream, emptying difficulty, painful urination)	Consult physician
Sexual problems	Consult physician
Blurred vision	Commonly will pass with time
Dizziness	Rise slowly from the bed or chair
Daytime drowsiness	Do not drive; take medication at bedtime; commonly will pass with time

Selective Serotonin Reuptake Inhibitors

Serotonin Hypothesis of Depression

5-HT is a major player in depressive illness, and serotonergic pathways are closely related to mood disorders, especially depression (see Fig. 12.1).[82,83] Thus, drugs affecting the 5-HT levels in the neural synapse and serotonergic pathways may lead to effective therapy of depression.

5-HT is synthesized from tryptophan, packaged into vesicles, and released into the synaptic cleft following an action potential. Once in the synaptic cleft, 5-HT interacts with both the pre- and postsynaptic serotonergic receptors.[84] Evidence implicating multiple abnormalities in serotonergic pathways as a cause of depression includes:

1. Low urinary concentrations of 5-HT's major metabolite, 5-hydroxyindoleacetic acid
2. Low density of brain and platelet 5-HT transporters in individuals who are depressed
3. High density of brain and platelet 5-HT-binding sites
4. Low synaptic concentration of tryptophan, which is used in 5-HT synthesis

Of these, the low level of SERTs in patients who are depressed has received the most attention in the development and synthesis of the SSRIs. The precise antidepressant mechanism of action for the SSRIs eludes neuroscientists, but the SSRIs have been shown to alleviate depression and are the most commonly used drugs in the therapy for depression.[82] Claims of decreased adverse effects (adverse drug reactions) and less toxicity in overdose than both the MAOIs and the TCAs, together with increased safety, have led to their extensive use and several are ranked in the top 50 prescription drugs dispensed in the United States during 2022.

The SSRIs are proven treatments for depression, OCD, and panic disorder and are helpful in a variety of other conditions as well. The most substantial benefit to the SSRIs compared with the TCAs is their reduced adverse-effect profile and the fact that they are better tolerated. Although the SSRIs have become the most commonly prescribed drugs for depression, there are clinical situations in which TCAs may be more appropriate (eg, melancholic depression).[84] Meaningful differences between the individual SSRIs are largely related to their pharmacokinetics, metabolism to active metabolites, inhibition of CYP isoforms, effect of DDIs, and the half-life of the individual SSRI.

The SSRIs are expensive, and it has been common to have nonadherent patients (especially older adults) relapse because they cannot afford their medications. Persuading the patient to take their medication as prescribed is extremely important for potentially suicidal patients with depression. Because of this, it is exceedingly important that patients receive the lowest effective (and, thereby, the most cost-effective) dose of any drug they are prescribed. Also, the SSRIs have a history of increased risk of suicide for reasons that are not clearly understood.

Discovery of Selective Serotonin Reuptake Inhibitors

Although the TCAs, as a group, are effective antidepressants, their adverse-event profile and high potential for toxicity have limited their use. The early antidepressants indicated that 5-HT might play a significant role in depression. Therefore, medicinal chemists set out in search of the ideal SSRI with the goal of developing drugs with[84]:

- High affinity and selectivity for the 5-HT uptake transporter
- Ability to slow or inhibit the transporter when bound to it
- Low affinity for the multiple neuroreceptors known to be responsible for many of the adverse effects of the TCAs (eg, ACh, histamine, and adrenergic receptors)
- No inhibition of the fast sodium channels that cause the cardiotoxicity problems associated with TCAs

Initial success occurred with the synthesis of zimeldine, in which the central ring of amitriptyline was opened to form a diphenylpropylidene analogue. *Z*-zimeldine displayed selective inhibition of 5-HT reuptake, with minimal inhibition of NE reuptake. Most importantly, zimeldine was without the adverse-event profile exhibited by the TCAs. Thus, zimeldine became the template for the second-generation SSRIs shown in Figures 12.2, 12.12, and 12.13.

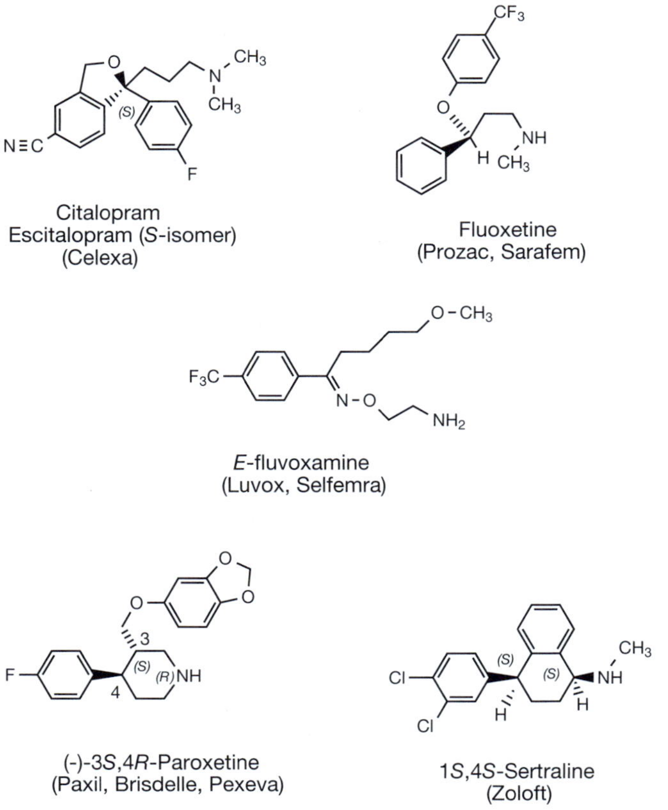

Figure 12.12 Selective serotonin reuptake inhibitors (SSRIs).

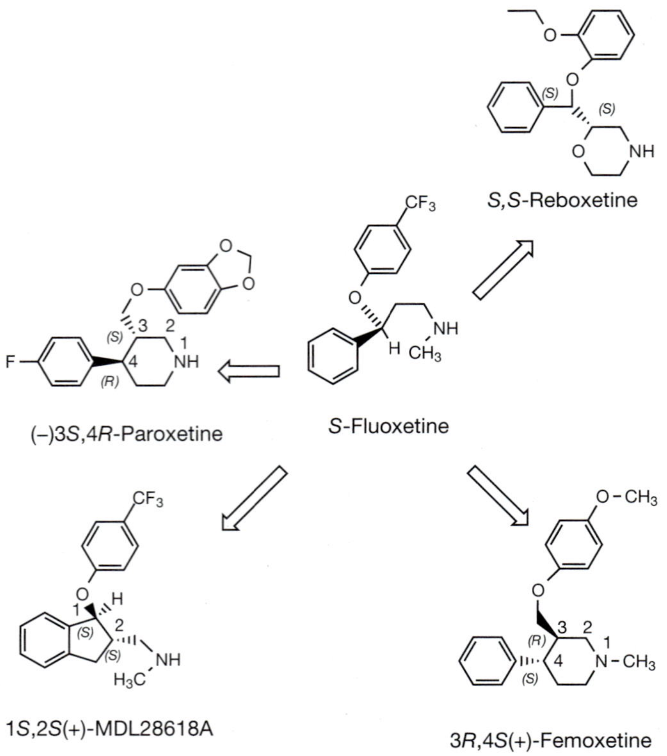

Figure 12.13 Structural relationships for the phenoxyphenylalkylamines.

Mechanisms of Action Common to the Selective Serotonin Reuptake Inhibitors

The SSRIs preferentially act to inhibit SERT (the reuptake transporter for 5-HT) with minimal or no affinity for NET and DAT.[84] These drugs have a high and selective affinity for SERT (see Fig. 12.6) and, therefore, block 5-HT from binding to SERT and being absorbed into presynaptic cells (see Fig. 12.3). The excess 5-HT in the synaptic cleft means overactivation of the postsynaptic receptors. Over an extended period of time, this causes downregulation of pre- and postsynaptic receptors, a reduction in the amount of 5-HT produced in the CNS, and a reduction in the number of SERTs expressed. Long-term administration of SSRIs causes downregulation of the SERT, but not the NET. Substantial loss of SERT binding sites takes 15 days to occur and is accompanied by a marked reduction of SERT function in vivo. These compensatory responses at receptors and transporters are thought to produce the antidepressant effects of SSRIs. This onset delay may, in part, explain the delayed onset of action of SSRIs in the treatment of depression.[83,85] Similar to the binding of 5-HT, SSRIs likely bind to SERT at the same site as 5-HT does, although it has not been determined conclusively. Although not as selective as the SSRIs, drugs of abuse, such as cocaine, fenfluramine, and 3,4-methylenedioxymethamphetamine ("Ecstasy"), are inhibitors of SERT.

The affinity data for the SSRIs show that the SSRIs, as a group, are very potent and selective inhibitors for SERT compared with their affinity for NET and DAT (see Fig. 12.6) and are more potent inhibitors of 5-HT reuptake than are the tertiary amine TCAs.[82,84] None of the SSRIs has substantial effect on NET or DAT. Of the SSRIs, sertraline exhibits the most potent inhibition of DAT, although it is still 100 times less potent in terms of inhibiting DAT versus SERT. Therefore, the plasma concentration of sertraline would have to be increased by as much as 100 times to inhibit DAT. When drugs are this selective for the reuptake transporters, differences in potency become clinically irrelevant, because the plasma concentration can be dose-adjusted to achieve inhibition of the desired transporter without affecting the other transporters. Clomipramine displays less affinity for SERT than citalopram, fluvoxamine, paroxetine, or sertraline does and is more potent than fluoxetine. In terms of the ability to inhibit the NET, the SSRIs are 2 to 3 times less potent than the SNRI TCA desipramine.

Their in vitro potency for selectively inhibiting the SERT more or less mirrors their clinical efficacy as SSRIs[86]: paroxetine > sertraline > clomipramine > fluoxetine > citalopram > fluvoxamine > imipramine > amitriptyline > reboxetine > venlafaxine = milnacipran > desipramine. Clinically, however, all the SSRIs are equally effective over time, suggesting that these variations in potency do not affect efficacy or adverse effects.[87] The SSRIs have less affinity for α_1, α_2, H_1, and muscarinic receptors, which may explain the adverse-effect profile differences between TCAs and SSRIs.

The results in Table 12.7 show the therapeutic doses that produce approximately 60% to 80% inhibition of the SERT.[85,87] The inhibition of SERT is relevant to the antidepressant efficacy of the SSRIs and suggests that approximately 70% to 80% inhibition of this transporter usually is necessary to produce an antidepressant effect. Higher doses of these drugs do not produce a greater antidepressant response on average (ie, a flat dose-response curve for antidepressant efficacy) but do increase the incidence and severity of adverse effects mediated by excessive 5-HT reuptake inhibition. Obviously, the results shown in Table 12.7 pertain to the average patient. A patient who has a rapid clearance of the SSRI may need a higher-than-average dose to achieve an effective concentration, whereas a patient who has a slow clearance may do better in terms of the ratio of efficacy to adverse effects on a minimum dose.

The β-adrenergic blocker pindolol blocks the presynaptic 5-HT_{1A} receptors, thereby increasing 5-HT neuronal transmission. The 5-HT_{1A} receptors do not require prolonged exposure (several weeks) to excessive amounts of 5-HT to promote downregulation. This results in augmentation and acceleration of the antidepressant effect of the SSRIs when combined with a 5-HT_{1A} inhibitor. Bordet et al[88] demonstrated the accelerated antidepressant response of pindolol with paroxetine.

Table 12.7 Relationship Between Dose, Plasma Level, Potency, and Serotonin Uptake

SSRI	Dose (mg/d)	Plasma Level	In Vitro Potency (IC50)	Inhibition of Serotonin Transporter (%)
Citalopram	40	85 ng/mL (260 nM)	1.8	60
Fluoxetine	20	200 ng/mL (300 nM)[a]	3.8	70
Fluvoxamine	150	100 ng/mL (300 nM)	3.8	70
Paroxetine	20	40 ng/mL (130 nM)	0.29	80
Sertraline	50	25 ng/mL (65 nM)	0.19	80

SERT, serotonin reuptake transporter; SSRI, selective serotonin reuptake inhibitor.
[a]Plasma level for fluoxetine represents the total of fluoxetine plus norfluoxetine given comparable effects on SERT; parent SSRI alone shown for all others. Also, plasma levels are a total of both enantiomers for citalopram and fluoxetine. Values for the parent drug and for the respective major metabolite are in parentheses.

Pharmacokinetics Common to the Selective Serotonin Reuptake Inhibitors

The SSRIs share a number of pharmacokinetic characteristics (Table 12.8).[85,88] They are well absorbed orally, although the presence of food in the stomach may alter the absorption of some SSRIs. Food, however, does not affect the area under the curve (AUC) and does not appear to affect clinical efficacy. The SSRIs are highly lipophilic and are highly plasma protein bound.

Current SSRIs tend to be characterized by high volumes of distribution, which results in relatively long plasma

Table 12.8 Pharmacokinetics of the Selective Serotonin Reuptake Inhibitors

Parameters	(±)-Fluoxetine	(−)-Sertraline	(−)-Paroxetine	E-Fluvoxamine	(±)-Citalopram ([+]-Escitalopram)
Oral bioavailability (%)	70	20-36	50	>50	80 (51-93)
Lipophilicity (log $D_{7.4}$)	1.75	3.14	1.46	1.08	1.27
Protein binding (%)	95	96-98	95	77	~56 (70-80)
Volume of distribution (L/kg)	11-18	17 (9-25)	25 (11-28)	15-31	11-16
Elimination half-life (hours)	50	24 (19-37)	22	15-20	36 (27-32) Older adult ~48
Cytochrome P450 major isoform	2D6	3A4	2D6	2D6	2C19, 2D6, and 3A4
Major active metabolites	*O*-desmethylfluoxetine (240 h)	*N*-desmethyl (62-104 h)	None	None	Desmethylcitalopram (30 h)
	Norfluoxetine (96-364 h)				
Peak plasma concentration (hours)	6-8	4-8	2-8	3-8	4 (1-6)
Excretion (%)	Urine 25-50	Urine 51-60	Renal ~50%	Urine ~40% (24 h)	Feces 80%-90%
	Feces minor	Feces 24-32	Feces minor	Feces minor	Urine <5%
Plasma half-life (hours)	1-4 d (norfluoxetine 7-15 d)	22-35	24	7-63	36 (23-75)
Time to steady-state concentration (days)	~4 wk	7-10 d older adults 2-3 wk	7-14 d	10 d	7 d

concentrations (typically 4-8 hours). The SSRIs display a range of elimination half-life values for the parent drugs, from half-life values of approximately 20 hours for paroxetine and fluvoxamine to 2 days for fluoxetine. Only sertraline and citalopram exhibit linear pharmacokinetics, whereas fluvoxamine, fluoxetine, and paroxetine exhibit nonlinear pharmacokinetics (ie, changes in plasma concentration are not proportional to dose) as a result of their longer plasma half-lives within the usual therapeutic ranges (see Table 12.8). Sertraline stands out as having the best effects on depression among all antidepressants. Fluoxetine and fluvoxamine are least likely to penetrate into breast milk. Thus, the SSRI antidepressants best suited for pharmacokinetic optimization of therapy are the following: sertraline, fluvoxamine, and citalopram.[87] All the SSRIs are extensively metabolized by CYP isoforms to pharmacologically active *N*-demethylated metabolites, which are then excreted in urine and feces. Except for sertraline, the drugs fluoxetine, paroxetine, and fluvoxamine are metabolized by polymorphic CYP isoforms, a matter of concern for poor and extensive metabolizers who may need dose adjustments. Citalopram is metabolized almost equally by CYP2C19, CYP2D6, and CYP3A4 (see Table 12.8). Peak plasma levels usually are reached in approximately 6 to 8 hours and steady-state plasma levels in approximately 7 to 10 days except for fluoxetine (~4 weeks). The half-lives are variable depending on the specific SSRI and the presence and plasma concentration of an active metabolite, but the half-lives tend to be prolonged. No evidence indicates that serum drug monitoring of SSRIs is a useful strategy to predict response. The SSRIs in general exhibit a flat, dose-independent antidepressant response curve (ie, the antidepressant activity does not improve with increasing dose, only side effects increase).[88]

Some of the key differences among the SSRIs are the result of differences in their pharmacokinetic properties and metabolism to active metabolites (see Table 12.8). Fluoxetine is unique because of its long half-life and the long half-life of its active metabolite norfluoxetine.[52] Although sertraline also has an active metabolite, it is 10 times less potent than sertraline and probably is not clinically relevant. Fluvoxamine and paroxetine have no active metabolites. Because of the differences in half-lives and activities of metabolites, a much longer washout period is necessary when switching from fluoxetine (a long-acting SSRI) to another SSRI or MAOI. These differences can cause considerable therapeutic delays in the treatment of refractory cases.

Adverse Effects Common to the Selective Serotonin Reuptake Inhibitors

The SSRIs are reported to have fewer side effects than the TCAs, which have strong anticholinergic and cardiotoxic properties.[86,87] Among the SSRIs, there are few differences in adverse effects. The adverse effects observed for the SSRIs include dry mouth, nausea, headaches, nervousness, restlessness, trouble sleeping, sexual dysfunction, and anxiety. Fewer patients have discontinued SSRIs than TCAs (amitriptyline and imipramine and not nortriptyline, desipramine, doxepin, and clomipramine).

Sexual dysfunction is reported in both men and women, such as decreased libido, anorgasmia, ejaculatory incompetence, ejaculatory retardation, and inability to obtain or maintain an erection. The basic pharmacologic similarities among the SSRIs suggest that the effects on sexual function should be similar for each drug and that no one SSRI was more likely to cause the reported sexual adverse effects than another. Moreover, evidence suggests that SSRI-induced sexual dysfunction may be dose-related and may be treated by simply lowering its dose. In patients who cannot have their SSRI dosage reduced, another option is simply to wait and reassess sexual function after several months. If the above measures are ineffective in managing SSRI-induced sexual dysfunction, the next step is to consider an alternative antidepressant without serotonergic activity (eg, bupropion). Orgasm difficulties and impotence occurred more frequently with paroxetine as compared with sertraline and fluoxetine. The addition of amantadine, cyproheptadine, yohimbine, or sildenafil has been reported to be effective in some patients with SSRI-induced sexual dysfunction.

Drug Interactions Common to the Selective Serotonin Reuptake Inhibitors

The most serious DDI for the SSRIs is their potential to produce the "serotonin syndrome" (ie, hyperserotonergic effect), which typically develops within hours or days following the addition of another serotonergic agent to a drug regimen that already includes serotonergic-enhancing drugs.[87] Symptoms of the 5-HT syndrome include agitation, diaphoresis, diarrhea, fever, hyperreflexia, incoordination, confusion, myoclonus, shivering, and tremor.

The 5-HT syndrome interaction between MAOIs and SSRIs is the most important drug interaction for the SSRIs, necessitating a washout ranging from 2 to 5 weeks depending on the plasma half-life of the SSRI. These differences in washout times for the SSRIs when switching to an MAOI are key differences between SSRIs and should be remembered if an MAOI is planned as a possible subsequent treatment in the event of SSRI failure. The differences among SSRIs are not important, when a patient is switched from an MAOI to an SSRI. However, in this case, a 10- to 14-day washout for the MAOI is necessary, regardless of which SSRI is used, to allow regeneration of MAO. The drug interaction between TCAs and SSRIs is of particular importance because of the potential for the development of toxic TCA concentrations, 5-HT syndrome, and subsequent adverse effects.[85]

Coadministration of the antihistamine cyproheptadine or other 5-HT antagonists with SSRIs might be expected to result in a pharmacodynamic interaction (ie, reduced effectiveness for the SSRI). Cyproheptadine acts to block postsynaptic 5-HT. Lack of antidepressant efficacy has been reported when cyproheptadine was given concurrently with fluoxetine and paroxetine.

Clinically, the potency of the SSRIs to inhibit CYP2D6 decreases from paroxetine to fluoxetine to norfluoxetine and then to fluvoxamine, with sertraline and citalopram being metabolized by CYP3A4 and CYP2C19, respectively, explaining the extent of differences in pharmacokinetic interactions between the SSRIs and other CYP2D6 substrates.[89] Fluvoxamine is associated with drug interactions from its inhibition of CYP1A2, CYP2C9, CYP2C19, and CYP3A4. Because all the SSRIs are extensively metabolized in the liver, it is possible that other drugs that inhibit or induce hepatic CYP microsomal enzyme systems may alter SSRI plasma concentrations (AUCs) (see Table 12.8). The SSRIs may inhibit or interfere with the metabolism of other frequently prescribed drugs that are CYP hepatically metabolized, increasing the potential for DDIs (see Table 12.4). Although similar drug interactions are possible with other SSRIs, there is considerable variability among the drugs in the extent to which they inhibit CYP2D6. Fluoxetine and paroxetine appear to be more potent in this regard than sertraline.[89] The extent to which this potential interaction may become clinically important depends on the extent of inhibition of CYP2D6 by the SSRI and the therapeutic index of the concurrently administered drug. The drugs for which this potential interaction is of greatest concern are those that are metabolized principally by CYP2D6 and have a narrow therapeutic index. Caution should be exercised whenever concurrent therapy with fluoxetine and other drugs metabolized by CYP2D6 is considered.[90] The clinical significance of these possible interactions with the CYP isoforms is questionable, however, because there is no known correlation between plasma concentration and therapeutic response for any of the SSRIs.[90] If an interaction is suspected, the patient's SSRI dosage can be easily adjusted.

The SSRIs are highly protein bound and may affect the pharmacodynamic effect of other protein-bound drugs with narrow therapeutic indices (eg, warfarin). The changes appear to be clinically significant, however, only for fluoxetine, fluvoxamine, and paroxetine.[90] Close monitoring of prothrombin time and international normalized ratio is necessary if these drugs are used together.

The SSRIs have a high toxic to therapeutic ratio and, therefore, are safer than the TCAs or MAOIs in acute overdose. The SSRI overdoses can result in drowsiness, tremor, nausea and vomiting, seizures, electrocardiographic changes, and coma. Fatalities are uncommon with pure SSRI overdoses.

Therapeutic Uses Common to the Selective Serotonin Reuptake Inhibitors

The primary uses for the SSRIs include MDD and bipolar depression (fluoxetine, paroxetine, sertraline, and citalopram), "atypical" depression (ie, patients who are depressed with unusual symptoms, such as hypersomnia, weight gain, and interpersonal rejection sensitivity; fluoxetine, paroxetine, sertraline, and citalopram), anxiety disorders, panic disorder (sertraline and paroxetine), dysthymia, PMS, PPD, dysphoria, bulimia nervosa (fluoxetine), obesity, borderline personality disorder, OCD (fluvoxamine, fluoxetine, paroxetine, and sertraline), alcohol use disorder, rheumatic pain, and migraine headache. Among the SSRIs, there are more similarities than differences; however, the differences between the SSRIs could be clinically significant.[87]

The SSRIs, such as paroxetine and fluoxetine, need stronger pediatric use warnings because of the possible risks of suicidal thoughts and behavior in some children and teenagers. Such risks may be unrelated to any specific SSRI. Recent clinical trials have concluded that two or three of every 100 young people treated with antidepressants might be at higher risk of suicidal behavior. Only fluoxetine has been proven to be effective and is approved for the treatment of pediatric depression.

Phenoxyphenylalkylamine Selective Serotonin Reuptake Inhibitors

(±)-FLUOXETINE

Structure-Activity Relationship. Fluoxetine is a 3-phenoxy-3-phenylpropylamine that exhibits selectivity and high affinity for human SERT and low affinity for NET (see Fig. 12.10).[89,90] It is marketed as a racemic mixture of *R*- and *S*-fluoxetine. Its selectivity for SERT inhibition depends on the position of the substituent in the phenoxy ring (Table 12.9). Mono-substitution in the 4-(*para*) position of the phenoxy group (with an electron-withdrawing group, eg, trifluoromethyl group, as in fluoxetine) results in selective inhibition of 5-HT reuptake. Disubstitution (2,4- or 3,4-disubstitution) results in loss of SERT selectivity. Constraining fluoxetine into semirigid analogues, such as MDL28618A or a phenylpiperidine (ie, femoxetine), maintains selectivity for SERT, but both have approximately 10% of the affinity of fluoxetine for SERT (Fig. 12.13).[90] The *trans*-(1*S*,2*S*)-MDL28618A stereoisomer is approximately 10 times more potent than the *cis*-(−)enantiomer.[89,90] The *trans*-(3*R*,4*S*)-(+)-enantiomer of femoxetine has approximately 10% the affinity of fluoxetine for SERT.[53] *N*-demethylation of femoxetine to its secondary amine enhances affinity for SERT by 10 times (comparable to fluoxetine). Femoxetine is not only an analogue of fluoxetine and paroxetine but also the (3*R*,4*S*)-diastereomer of a paroxetine analogue.

Mechanism of Action. Fluoxetine is a potent and selective inhibitor of 5-HT reuptake, but not of NE or DA uptake in the CNS. Its mechanism of action is common to the SSRIs.[89] Fluoxetine does not interact directly with postsynaptic 5-HT receptors and has weak affinity for the other neuroreceptors. Both enantiomers of fluoxetine display similar affinities for human SERT. The NE/5-HT selectivity ratio, however, indicates that the *S*-enantiomer is approximately 100 times more selective for SERT inhibition than the *R*-enantiomer. The *R*-(+)-stereoisomer is approximately 8 times more potent an inhibitor of SERT together with a longer duration of action than the *S*-(−)-isomer. However, the *S*-(−)-norfluoxetine metabolite is 7 times more potent as an inhibitor of the 5-HT transporter than the *R*-(+)-metabolite, with a selectivity ratio approximately equivalent to that of *S*-fluoxetine.[89,90]

Pharmacokinetics. The pharmacokinetics of fluoxetine fit the general characteristics of the SSRIs (see Table 12.8). Of particular importance is its long half-life contributing to its nonlinear pharmacokinetics. In vitro studies show that fluoxetine and norfluoxetine are potent inhibitors of CYP2D6 and CYP3A4 and less potent inhibitors of

Table 12.9 Structure-Activity Relationships for Atypical Phenoxyphenylpropylamines

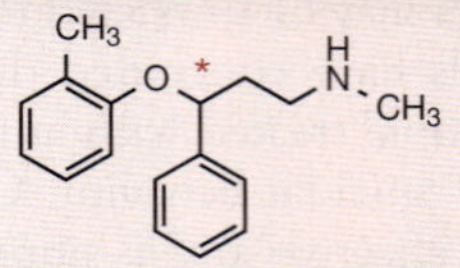

R (drug)	Inhibition of Reuptake (K_i nM) (28)	
	5-HT	NE
H	102	200
2-OCH_3 (nisoxetine)	1,371	2.4
2-SCH_3 (thionisoxetine)	130	0.2
2-CH_3 (atomoxetine)	390	3.4
2-F	898	5.3
2-I	25	0.4
2-CF_3	1,489	4,467
3-CF_3	16	1,328
4-CF_3 (fluoxetine)	17	2,703
4-CF_3 (norfluoxetine, NH_2)	17	2,176
4-CH_3	95	570
4-OCH_3	71	1,107
4-Cl	142	568
4-F	638	1,176

5-HT, serotonin; NE, norepinephrine.

CYP2C9, CYP2C19, and CYP1A2.[89] Fluoxetine is metabolized primarily by CYP2D6 *N*-demethylation to its active metabolite norfluoxetine and, to a lesser extent, *O*-dealkylation to form the inactive metabolite *p*-trifluoromethylphenol.[89] Following oral administration, fluoxetine and its metabolites are excreted principally in urine, with approximately 73% as unidentified metabolites, 10% as norfluoxetine, 10% as norfluoxetine glucuronide, 5% as fluoxetine *N*-glucuronide, and 2% as unmetabolized drug.

Both *R*- and *S*-norfluoxetine were less potent than the corresponding enantiomers of fluoxetine as inhibitors of NE uptake. Inhibition of 5-HT uptake in the cerebral cortex persisted for more than 24 hours after administration of *S*-norfluoxetine similar to fluoxetine. Thus, *S*-norfluoxetine is the active *N*-demethylated metabolite responsible for the persistently potent and selective inhibition of 5-HT uptake in vivo.[90]

The pharmacokinetics of fluoxetine in healthy geriatric individuals do not differ substantially from those in younger adults. Because of its relatively long half-life and nonlinear pharmacokinetics, the possibility of altered pharmacokinetics in geriatric individuals could exist, particularly those with systemic disease and/or in those receiving multiple medications concurrently. The elimination half-lives of fluoxetine and norfluoxetine do not appear to be altered substantially in patients with renal or hepatic impairment.

Drug Interactions. Fluoxetine and its norfluoxetine metabolite, like many other drugs metabolized by CYP2D6, inhibit the activity of CYP2D6 and, potentially, may increase plasma concentrations of concurrently administered drugs that also are metabolized by this enzyme.[90] Fluoxetine may make normal CYP2D6 metabolizers resemble poor metabolizers. Fluoxetine can inhibit its own CYP2D6 metabolism, resulting in higher-than-expected plasma concentrations during upward dose adjustments. Therefore, switching from fluoxetine to another SSRI or other serotonergic antidepressant requires a washout period of at least 5 weeks or a lower-than-recommended initial dose with monitoring for adverse events.

Fluoxetine is highly protein bound and may affect the free plasma concentration and, thus, the pharmacologic effect of other highly protein-bound drugs (eg, warfarin sodium).

(−)-Paroxetine

Structure-Activity Relationship. Paroxetine is a constrained analogue of fluoxetine in which the linear phenylpropylamine group has been folded into a piperidine ring (Fig. 12.14). Paroxetine contains two chiral centers, with the possibility of four stereoisomers. One of these stereoisomers, the (3*S*,4*R*)-(−)-enantiomer, is marketed as paroxetine. Paroxetine is a potent and selective inhibitor of SERT and displays high affinity for human SERT and little affinity for NE and DA transporters (see Fig. 12.5).[91] Converting the secondary amine of the piperidine ring into a tertiary amine with a methyl group reduces affinity for SERT by 100 times (Fig. 12.14). Substituting the 4-fluoro with either a hydrogen or methyl reduces affinity for human SERT by approximately 10 times; replacing the 3,4-methylenedioxy group with a 4-methoxy group in the phenoxy ring also reduces affinity by a factor of 10. Stereochemical factors affect affinity of the paroxetine molecule for SERT. Therefore, substitution into the 2-(*ortho*) position of either aromatic ring decreases affinity for rat SERT by as much as 10 to 100 times, with the greatest loss

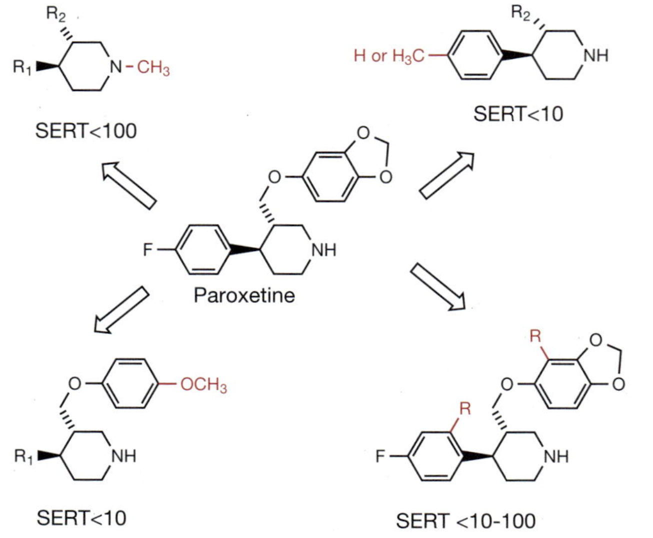

Figure 12.14 Structural changes to paroxetine and effects on serotonin reuptake transporter (SERT) affinity.

occurring in the phenoxy ring. In vitro binding studies suggest that paroxetine is a more selective and potent inhibitor of 5-HT reuptake than fluoxetine. The drug essentially has no effect on NE or DA reuptake, nor does it show affinity for other neuroreceptors. Its onset of action is 1 to 4 weeks.

Pharmacokinetics. Paroxetine appears to be slowly but well absorbed from the GI tract following oral administration with an oral bioavailability of approximately 50%, suggesting first-pass metabolism (see Table 12.8), reaching peak plasma concentrations in 2 to 8 hours.[91,92] Food does not substantially affect the absorption of paroxetine. Paroxetine is distributed into breast milk. Approximately 80% of an oral dose of paroxetine is oxidized by CYP2D6 to a catechol intermediate, which is then either O-methylated or O-glucuronidated. These conjugates are then eliminated in the urine.

Paroxetine exhibits a preincubation-dependent increase in inhibitory potency of CYP2D6 consistent with a mechanism-based inhibition of CYP2D6.[92,93] The inactivation of CYP2D6 occurs via the formation of an *o*-quinonoid reactive metabolite.

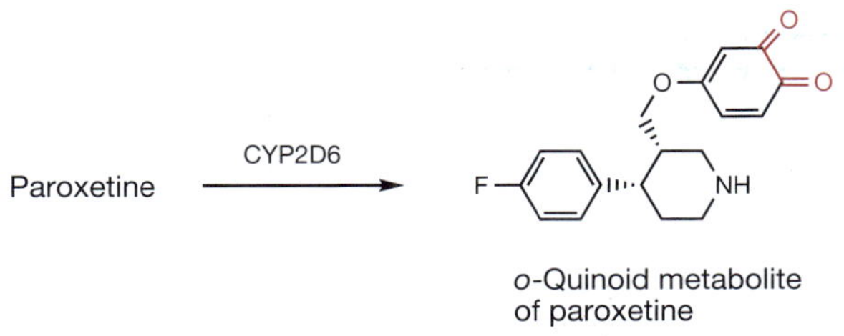

Paroxetine

The methylenedioxy has been associated with mechanism-based inactivation of other CYP isoforms.[92,93] In contrast, fluoxetine, a potent inhibitor of CYP2D6 activity, did not exhibit a mechanism-based inhibition of CYP2D6. As a result of mechanism-based inhibition, saturation of CYP2D6 at clinical doses appears to account for its nonlinear pharmacokinetics observed with increasing dose and duration of paroxetine treatment, which results in increased plasma concentrations of paroxetine at low doses. Older adults may be more susceptible to changes in doses and, therefore, should be started off at lower doses. Following oral administration, paroxetine and its metabolites are excreted in both urine and feces.

Oral administration of a single dose resulted in unmetabolized paroxetine accounting for 2% and metabolites accounting for 62% of the excretion products. The effect of age on the elimination of paroxetine suggests that hepatic clearance of paroxetine can be reduced, leading to an increase in elimination half-life (eg, to ~36 hours) and increased plasma concentrations. The metabolites of paroxetine have been shown to possess no more than 2% of the potency of the parent compound as inhibitors of 5-HT reuptake; therefore, they are essentially inactive (see Fig. 12.14).

Because paroxetine is a potent mechanism-based inhibitor of CYP2D6, this type of inhibition yields nonlinear and long-term effects on drug pharmacokinetics, because the inactivated or complexed CYP2D6 must be replaced by newly synthesized CYP2D6 protein.[92,93] Thus, coadministration of paroxetine with CYP2D6-metabolized medications should be closely monitored or, in certain cases, avoided, as should upward dose adjustment of paroxetine itself.

(±)-Citalopram. In trying to create a new antidepressant to inhibit NE reuptake, Lundbeck chemists accidentally synthesized two new compounds (talopram and talsupram) having the phenylspiro-isobenzofuran nucleus (Fig. 12.15). These compounds were potent SNRIs, but considering that a number of suicide attempts were reported during clinical studies with these compounds, Lundbeck discontinued the studies. Undeterred, the chemists subsequently modified talopram by addition of a 5-cyano to the isobenzofuran ring and a 4-fluoro to the benzene ring in the formation of citalopram. Therapeutic activity for (±)-citalopram resides in the *S*-(+)-isomer. Isosteric substitution of the isobenzofuran ring in citalopram with an isobenzothiophene yields talsupram, which changes selectivity from an inhibitor of SERT to a potent inhibitor of NET (Fig. 12.15). Citalopram was marketed in the United States in 1996 as the most selective SSRI and, therefore, is the least likely to cause the adverse effects observed with most of the other antidepressants (see Fig. 12.6). It is used to treat depression, anxiety, eating disorders, and OCD among other mood disorders.

Mechanism of Action. Citalopram, primarily through its *S*-enantiomer, selectively blocks 5-HT reuptake, leading to potentiation of serotonergic activity in the CNS.[94,95] Citalopram exhibits the greatest in vitro selectivity for 5-HT reuptake inhibition compared with the other SSRIs (see Fig. 12.6). The drug essentially has no effect on NE or DA reuptake, nor does it show affinity for other neuroreceptors.

Pharmacokinetics. The pharmacokinetics of citalopram are shown in Table 12.8. Unlike several of the other

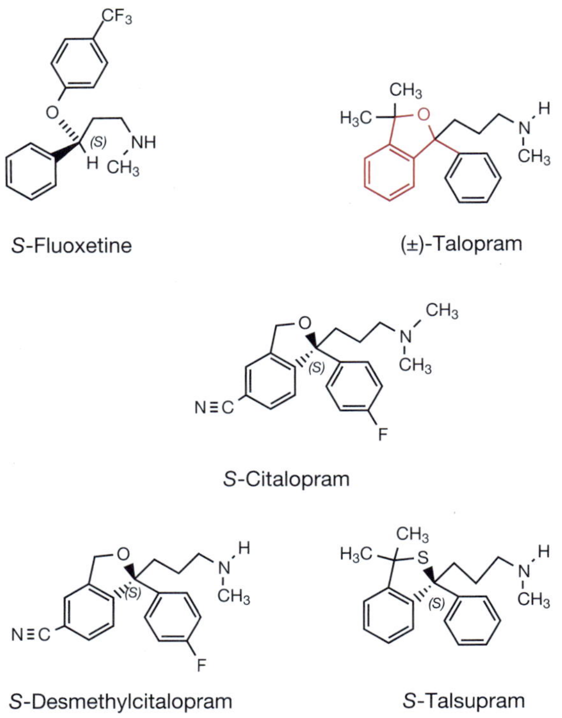

Figure 12.15 Structural relationships for citalopram selective serotonin reuptake inhibitors (SSRIs).

SSRIs, citalopram does not undergo first-pass metabolism; it has an oral bioavailability of approximately 80%. Food does not affect absorption. Citalopram is highly lipophilic and widely distributed throughout the body, including the blood-brain barrier (BBB). However, its metabolite, desmethylcitalopram does not cross the BBB well. The drug is metabolized via hepatic *N*-demethylation to its major metabolite, *N*-desmethylcitalopram, almost equally by CYP2C19, CYP2D6, and CYP3A4 (see Table 12.4). The major metabolite exhibits approximately 50% of the potency of citalopram as an inhibitor of 5-HT reuptake.[95] Because the metabolite concentration in the plasma is lower than that of citalopram, it should not add significantly to citalopram's antidepressant effects. Citalopram exhibits dose-proportional linear pharmacokinetics in a dosage range of 10 to 60 mg/d; plasma levels increase proportionately with each increasing dose. Approximately 11% to 23% of an oral dose was recovered in the urine as unmetabolized drug and 10% in feces. The clearance of orally administered citalopram was reduced by 37% and 17% in patients with hepatic and renal function impairment, respectively.

Citalopram and its desmethyl metabolite are weak inhibitors of the CYP isoforms, suggesting a low potential for drug interactions. Although no relevant in vivo interactions between citalopram and CYP2D6-metabolized medications have been reported, caution is advised when coadministering citalopram with potential object drugs, especially those having narrow therapeutic indices, in older adults. Because citalopram is metabolized in parallel by CYP2C19, CYP2D6, and CYP3A4, it would have little inhibitory effect on the metabolism of other drugs metabolized by these isoenzymes. Citalopram is less highly protein bound than the other SSRIs, reducing the potential for drug interactions with protein-bound drugs having narrow therapeutic indices.

ESCITALOPRAM. Escitalopram is the *S*-enantiomer of citalopram that binds with high affinity and selectivity to the human SERT equivalent to (±)-citalopram.[94] It has been reported that nearly all the activity resides in the *S*-enantiomer and that *R*-citalopram actually counteracts the action of the *S*-enantiomer.[94,95] Studies show that escitalopram exhibits twice the activity of citalopram and is at least 27 times more potent than the *R*-enantiomer. The *R*-enantiomer inhibits the *S*-enantiomer at the transporter.[95] Escitalopram's mechanism of action is common to the SSRIs.

The pharmacokinetics for escitalopram do not exhibit stereoisomer selectivity and, therefore, are similar to that for citalopram (see Table 12.8). Likewise, it exhibits linear pharmacokinetics so that plasma levels increase proportionately and predictably with increased doses, and its half-life of 27 to 32 hours is consistent with once-daily dosing. It also has been found that *R*-citalopram is cleared more slowly than the *S*-enantiomer. Therefore, when the drug is used as a racemic mixture (citalopram), the inactive isomer predominates at steady state. This is an added incentive for use of the enantiomerically pure escitalopram. Escitalopram has negligible effects on CYP isoforms, suggesting a low potential for DDIs. Escitalopram is indicated for patients with MDD, GAD, panic disorder, and social anxiety disorder.

Escitalopram is metabolized to *S*-desmethylcitalopram by CYP2C19 (37%), CYP2D6 (28%), and CYP3A4 (35%) and to *S*-didesmethylcitalopram (only by CYP2D6) in human liver microsomes (HLMs) and in expressed cytochromes. Escitalopram and its desmethyl metabolite were negligible inhibitors of CYP1A2, CYP2C9, CYP2C19, CYP2E1, and CYP3A and were weakly inhibited by CYP2D6. *R*-citalopram and its metabolites had properties very similar to those of the corresponding *S*-enantiomers. Because escitalopram is biotransformed by three CYP isoforms in parallel, escitalopram is unlikely to be affected by drug interactions or genetic polymorphisms and is unlikely to cause clinically important drug interactions via CYP inhibition.

Phenylalkylamine Selective Serotonin Reuptake Inhibitors

SERTRALINE. Although sertraline appears to differ structurally from the other SSRIs, it is a phenylaminotetralin, in which the diphenylbutylamine nucleus is constrained into a rigid bicyclic ring system (Fig. 12.16). In the early work with the discovery of SSRIs at Pfizer, tametraline was initially synthesized in 1978. Animal studies showed it to be a stimulant and to block NE and DA uptake, a use that Pfizer was not interested in pursuing. Subsequently, one or two chlorine atoms were introduced into tametraline to produce new molecules that were potent inhibitors of 5-HT reuptake in the CNS. One of the dichloro compounds was to become known as sertraline.

Sertraline contains two chiral centers and only the *S*,*S*-(+)-diastereomer is marketed. The *R*,*R*-, *R*,*S*-, and *S*,*R*-diastereomers are significantly weaker as inhibitors of 5-HT reuptake. Sertraline was marketed in the United States in 1992, emphasizing its pharmacokinetic differences from the other SSRIs.

Mechanism of Action. Sertraline is a potent and selective inhibitor of the neuronal reuptake 5-HT transporter. In vitro binding studies suggest that sertraline has a substantially higher selectivity for inhibiting 5-HT reuptake than other SSRIs or tertiary TCAs, including clomipramine (see Fig. 12.6). It has only weak effects on neuronal uptake of NE and DA. Its mechanism of action is common to the SSRIs. Sertraline is very selective, lacking affinity for other neuroreceptors at therapeutic concentrations.

Pharmacokinetics. Sertraline appears to be well absorbed from the GI tract following oral administration with an oral bioavailability in humans from 20% to 36% (see Table 12.8), suggesting extensive first-pass metabolism to its *N*-desmethylated metabolite.[95] Food enhances its oral absorption, decreasing the time to achieve peak plasma

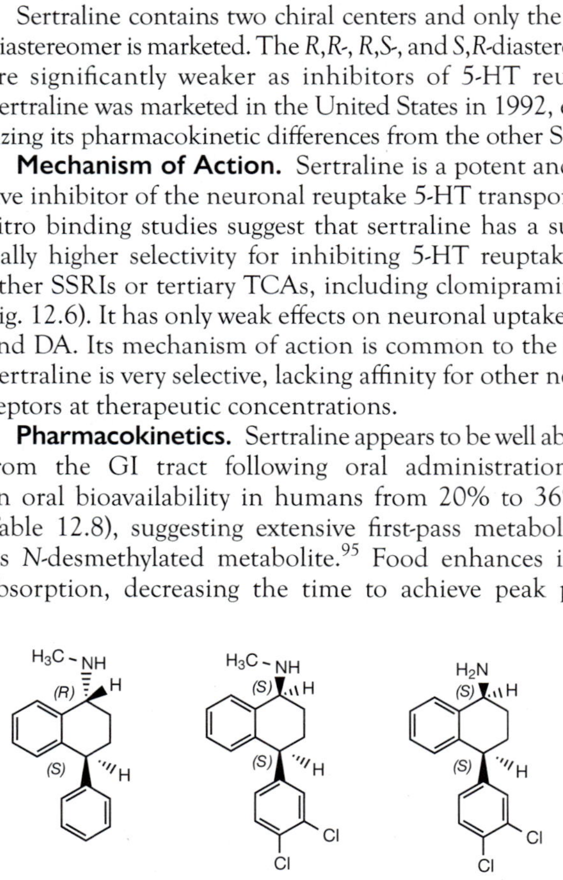

Figure 12.16 Structural relationships for the phenylalkylamine selective serotonin reuptake inhibitors (SSRIs).

concentrations from approximately 8 to 6 hours. Following multiple dosing, steady-state plasma sertraline concentrations are proportional and linearly related to dose (half-life: single dose, 24 hours; multiple doses, 24 hours). *N*-desmethylsertraline, sertraline's principal metabolite, exhibits dose-dependent pharmacokinetics. Sertraline and *N*-desmethylsertraline are distributed into breast milk. Protein binding is approximately 98%, although, in older adults, the elimination half-life is increased to approximately 36 hours. This effect does not appear to be clinically important and does not warrant dosing alterations. Sertraline is primarily metabolized to *N*-desmethylsertraline through the action of CYP2B6[96] and to a minor extent by CYP2C9, CYP2C19, CYP2D6, and CYP3A4 (Fig. 12.17). *N*-desmethylsertraline is approximately 5 to 10 times less potent as an inhibitor of 5-HT reuptake than sertraline. The formation of sertraline ketone can occur either through the action of CYP or MAO, but studies have not been reported to indicate the role of either or both. The formation of sertraline *N*-carbamoyl glucuronide is a unique product that was shown to form in vitro through the action primarily by UGT2B7. The involvement of multiple enzymes in the metabolism of sertraline suggests that no single drug could significantly alter sertraline pharmacokinetics and produce any DDIs. Sertraline and *N*-desmethylsertraline undergo further metabolism via oxidative deamination and ring hydroxylation and glucuronide conjugation. *N*-desmethylsertraline has an elimination half-life approximately 2.5 times that of sertraline. Following oral administration, sertraline and its conjugated metabolites are excreted in both urine and feces and unmetabolized sertraline accounts for less than 5% of the oral dose. Plasma clearance of sertraline was approximately 40% lower in geriatric patients. The elimination half-life of sertraline in patients with hepatic disease was prolonged to a mean of 52 hours, compared with 22 hours in individuals without hepatic disease.

Drug Interactions. Sertraline is not a potent inhibitor of CYP3A4 and because CYP2D6 metabolism is a minor pathway for sertraline, DDIs with these isoforms are unlikely to be of clinical importance. Sertraline is metabolized by more than one CYP isoform in parallel; therefore, drug interactions or genetic polymorphisms are unlikely to cause clinically significant drug interaction via CYP isoform inhibition. Caution is advised, however, when coadministering sertraline with potential object drugs, especially those with narrow therapeutic indices in older adults. For example, sertraline has been shown to reduce the clearance of desipramine and imipramine as a result of CYP2D6 inhibition.

Because sertraline is highly protein bound, patients receiving it concurrently with any highly protein-bound drug should be observed for potential adverse effects associated with combined therapy.

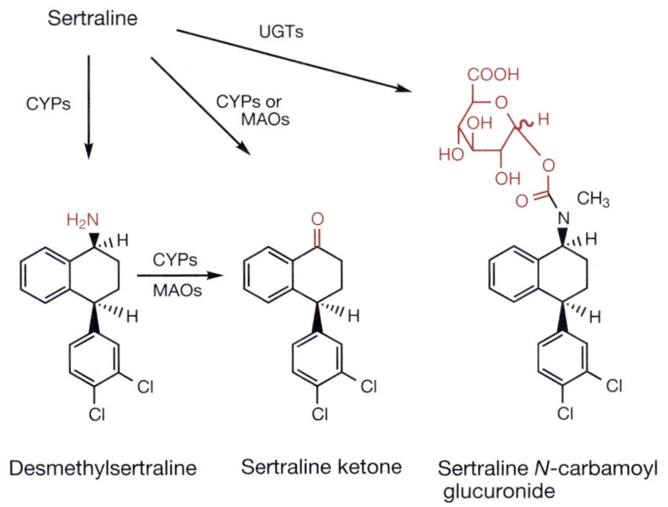

Figure 12.17 Metabolic products formed from sertraline metabolism.

Aralkylketone Selective Serotonin Reuptake Inhibitor

FLUVOXAMINE. Fluvoxamine is a nontricyclic SERT inhibitor that is structurally unique among the SSRIs by being the (*E*)-isomer of a 2-aminoethyl oxime ether of an aralkylketone (see Fig. 12.18). The C=N double bond is isosteric with the propylidene group in amitriptyline and, thus, imparts geometric *E* or *Z* stereoisomerism to fluvoxamine. The oxime ether is found in a previously marketed analogue of amitriptyline called noxiptiline (1966 by Bayer AG [Germany]). Thus, fluvoxamine may be considered to be an open-chain analogue of the tricyclic noxiptiline. The 4-trifluoromethyl group or other electronegative group is essential for SERT affinity and selectivity. The C=N double bond also enhances the susceptibility of fluvoxamine to photoisomerization by ultraviolet (UV)-B light (290-320 nm). When fluvoxamine solutions were exposed to UV-B light, photoisomerization to the pharmacologically inactive *Z*-isomer occurred. Thus, fluvoxamine solutions should be protected from sunlight to prevent loss of antidepressant efficacy. No studies have been reported regarding its solid-state stability to UV-B light.

Mechanism of Action. Fluvoxamine is a highly selective inhibitor of 5-HT reuptake at the presynaptic membrane.[97] Potency data from in vitro affinity studies suggest that fluvoxamine is less potent than the other SSRIs (eg, paroxetine, sertraline, and citalopram). Its mechanism of action is similar to that of the other SSRIs. Fluvoxamine appears to have little or no effect on the reuptake of NE or DA. In vitro studies have demonstrated that fluvoxamine possesses virtually no affinity for other neuroreceptors. Its

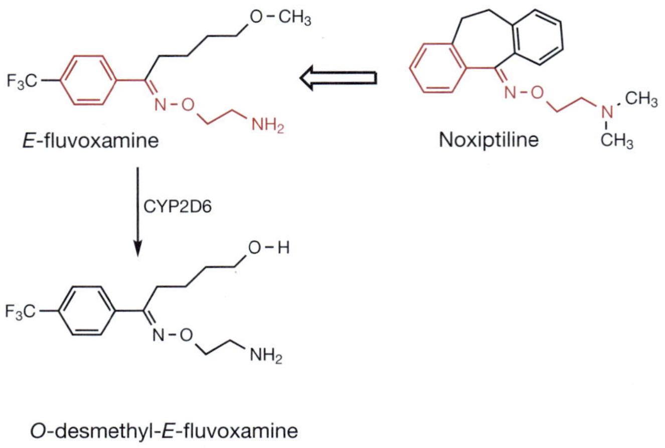

Figure 12.18 Structural relationships for fluvoxamine and its metabolism.

onset of action is similar to the other SSRIs (2-4 weeks). It is also used to treat symptoms of OCD in adults and children.

Pharmacokinetics. Fluvoxamine is well absorbed, with a bioavailability of approximately 50%, because of first-pass metabolism (Table 12.8). At steady-state doses, fluvoxamine demonstrates nonlinear pharmacokinetics over a dosage range of 100 to 300 mg/d, which results in higher plasma concentrations at higher doses than would be predicted by lower-dose kinetics (single dose, 15 hours; multiple dosing, 22 hours). Food does not significantly affect oral bioavailability. The mean apparent volume of distribution for fluvoxamine reflects its lipophilic nature, extensive tissue distribution, and protein binding. Fluvoxamine is distributed into breast milk. Fluvoxamine is preferentially metabolized by CYP2D6 by O-demethylation to its alcohol metabolite, which is subsequently oxidized to a carboxylic acid and on to a O-glucuronide. Oxidative deamination and nine other metabolites have been identified, none of which shows significant pharmacologic activity.

Adverse Effects. The adverse effects for fluvoxamine include symptoms of drowsiness, nausea or vomiting, abdominal pain, tremors, sinus bradycardia, and mild anticholinergic symptoms. Toxic doses could produce seizures and severe bradycardia.

Drug Interactions. In vitro studies have shown fluvoxamine to be a potent inhibitor of CYP1A2, to inhibit CYP3A4 and CYP2C19, and to weakly inhibit CYP2D6. The bioavailability of fluvoxamine is significantly decreased in those who smoke compared with nonsmokers, possibly because of induction of CYP1A2 metabolism of fluvoxamine. Therefore, interactions with drugs that inhibit CYP1A2 also should be considered (eg, theophylline and caffeine).

Therapeutic Uses. Fluvoxamine is approved for use in OCD.

Atypical Antidepressants

The atypical antidepressants are distinct from other classes of antidepressants that include SSRIs, TCAs, SMSs, SARIs, and MAOIs.[97] Atypical antidepressants are frequently used in patients with major depression who have inadequate responses or intolerable side effects during first-line treatment with SSRIs. However, atypical antidepressants are often first-line treatment if the drug has a desirable characteristic (eg, sexual side effects and weight gain occur less often with bupropion than SSRIs). Examples of atypical antidepressants include mirtazapine, bupropion, trazodone, vilazodone, and vortioxetine. Atypical antidepressants are unlike the SSRIs, TCAs, and MAOIs and act mainly as SNRIs, SMSs, and SARIs.[97]

Nontricyclic Serotonin-Norepinephrine Reuptake Inhibitors

Clinical studies suggest that compounds that increase the synaptic availability of both NE and 5-HT have greater efficacy than single-acting drugs such as SSRIs in the treatment of MDD.[97] Thus began the efforts to design a drug that combined the properties of SSRIs and SNRIs that only blocked SERTs and NETs and without the unwanted adverse effects of TCAs.[97] Currently, the nontricyclic mixed inhibitors of 5-HT and NE uptake are venlafaxine, desvenlafaxine, LVM, atomoxetine, and duloxetine (Fig. 12.19).

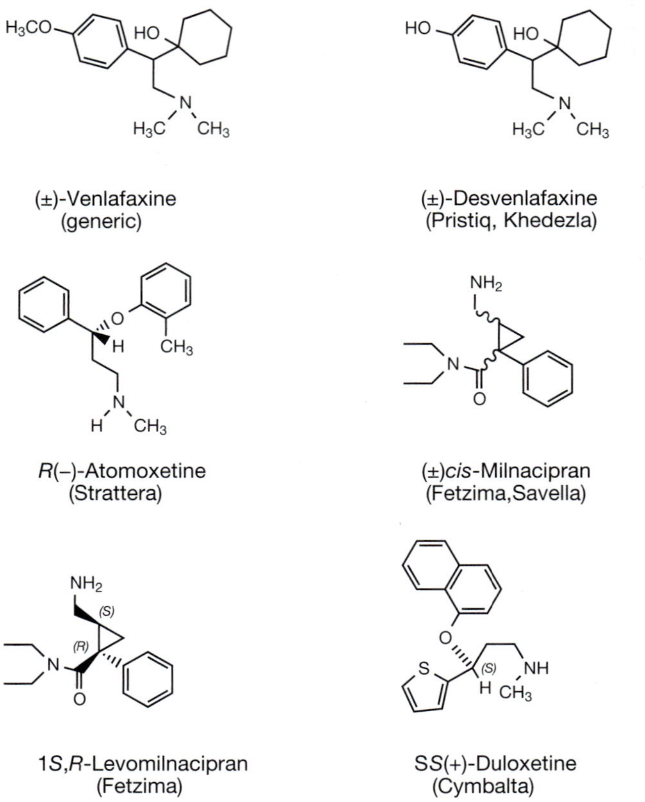

Figure 12.19 Nontricyclic serotonin-norepinephrine reuptake inhibitors (SNRIs).

Based on preclinical studies, venlafaxine, desvenlafaxine, LVM, milnacipran, atomoxetine, and duloxetine inhibit the reuptake of 5-HT and NE both in vitro and in vivo in the following order of decreasing potency: duloxetine > LVM > venlafaxine > desvenlafaxine. All the mixed reuptake inhibitors exhibit low affinity at neuronal receptors of the other neurotransmitters, suggesting a low side-effect potential. Desvenlafaxine, LVM, atomoxetine, and duloxetine have repeatedly shown to be as efficacious as TCA drugs in treating MDD. These non-TCAs are reported to produce a faster and greater antidepressant response than an SSRI alone, suggesting that these mixed mechanisms of action can be synergistic in terms of mediating antidepressant efficacy. Meaningful differences between the nontricyclic SNRIs are largely related to their pharmacokinetics, metabolism to active metabolites, inhibition of CYP isoforms, effect of DDIs, and the half-life of the nontricyclic SNRIs.[97]

VENLAFAXINE. Venlafaxine is a methoxyphenylethylamine antidepressant that resembles an open TCA with one of the aromatic rings replaced by a cyclohexanol ring and a dimethylaminomethyl group rather than a dimethylaminopropyl chain (Fig. 12.19).

Venlafaxine and its active metabolite, O-desmethylvenlafaxine (ODV), have mixed mechanisms of action, with preferential affinity for 5-HT reuptake and weak inhibition of NE and DA reuptake. Venlafaxine is approximately 30 times more potent as an inhibitor of SERT than of NET. Because of the 30-fold difference in transporter affinities, increasing the dose of venlafaxine from 75 to 375 mg/d can sequentially inhibit both SERT and NET. Thus, venlafaxine displays an

Table 12.10 Pharmacokinetics of the Nontricyclic Serotonin-Norepinephrine Reuptake Inhibitors

Parameters	Venlafaxine	Desvenlafaxine	Levomilnacipran	Duloxetine	Atomoxetine
Oral bioavailability (%)	45	45	92	>90	70
Lipophilicity (cLog $D_{pH7.4}$)	1.93	1.93	−1.09	ND	1.06
Protein binding	27	30	22	>90	>97
Volume of distribution (L/kg)	7.5±3.7	5.7±1.8	387-473	1,640	93-328 (250)
Elimination half-life (hours)	5	11	11	11	4 (3-6) (EM) 17-21 (PM)
Major active metabolites	Desvenlafaxine (ODV)	None	None	None	None
Peak plasma concentration (hours)	2	7.5	32-48	6-10	3
Excretion (%)	Urine 87	Urine 30	Urine 58	Urine 70 Feces 20	Urine >80 Feces <17
Plasma half-life (hours)		30	32-48	6	5 (EM) 22 (PM)
Time to steady-state concentration (days)	3	ND	6-8	3	5 (EM) 22 (PM)

ND, not determined; ODV, *O*-desmethylvenlafaxine; EM, extensive metabolizers and PM, poor metabolizers.

ascending dose-dependent antidepressant response in contrast to the flat dose-antidepressant response curve observed with the SSRIs. This sequential action for venlafaxine also is consistent with its dose-dependent adverse-effect profile. Its mechanism of action is similar to imipramine.

Venlafaxine is rapidly and well absorbed, but with a bioavailability of 45%, which has been attributed to first-pass metabolism (see Table 12.10). Food delays its absorption but does not impair the extent of absorption. Venlafaxine is distributed into breast milk. Venlafaxine is primarily metabolized in the liver by CYP2D6 to its primary metabolite, ODV, which is approximately equivalent in pharmacologic activity and potency to venlafaxine. In vitro studies indicate that CYP3A4 also is involved in the metabolism of venlafaxine to its minor and less active metabolite, *N*-desmethylvenlafaxine (Fig. 12.20). Protein binding for venlafaxine and ODV is low and is not a problem for drug interactions. In patients with hepatic impairment, elimination half-lives were increased by approximately 30% for venlafaxine and

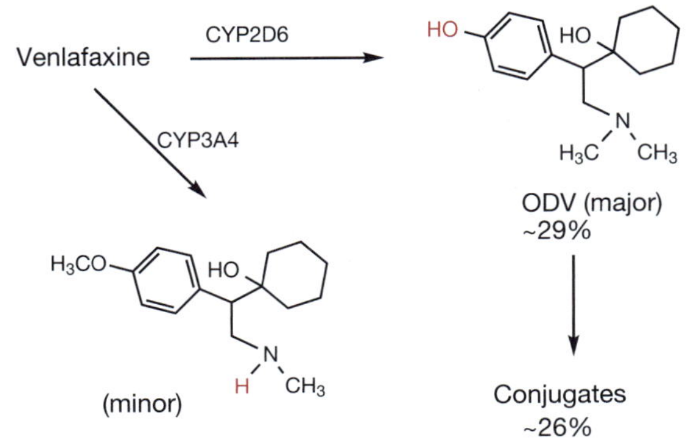

Figure 12.20 Metabolism of venlafaxine.

approximately 60% for ODV (Table 12.10). In patients with renal function impairment, elimination half-lives were increased by approximately 40% to 50% for venlafaxine and for ODV. At steady-state doses, venlafaxine and ODV exhibit dose-proportional linear pharmacokinetics over the dose range of 75 to 450 mg/d. Steady-state concentrations of venlafaxine and ODV are attained within 3 days with regular oral dosing. Venlafaxine and its metabolites are excreted primarily in the urine (87%).

The potential for cardiotoxicity with venlafaxine during normal use and for various toxicities in overdose situations is a key concern. Venlafaxine displays minimal in vitro affinity for the other neural neurotransmitter receptors and, thus, a low probability for adverse effects. To minimize GI upset (eg, nausea), venlafaxine can be taken with food without affecting its GI absorption. Venlafaxine should be administered as a single daily dose with food at approximately the same time each day. The extended-release capsules should be swallowed whole with fluid and should not be divided, crushed, chewed, or placed in water.

Whenever venlafaxine is being discontinued after more than 1 week of therapy, it generally is recommended that the patient be closely monitored, and the dosage of the drug be tapered gradually to reduce the risk of withdrawal symptoms.

Although venlafaxine is a weak inhibitor of CYP2D6, variability has been observed in the pharmacokinetic parameters of venlafaxine in patients with hepatic or renal function impairment. As a precaution, older adults taking venlafaxine concurrently with a drug that has a narrow therapeutic index and also is metabolized by CYP2D6 should be carefully monitored. Concurrent use of CYP3A4 inhibitors with venlafaxine has been shown to interfere with its metabolism and clearance. Similar to the other antidepressants that block 5-HT reuptake, venlafaxine may interact pharmacodynamically to cause toxic levels of 5-HT to accumulate, leading to the 5-HT syndrome.

DESVENLAFAXINE. ODV, as previously described, is the main active CYP2D6 metabolite of venlafaxine (Figs. 12.19 and 12.20). Similar to venlafaxine, ODV is an SNRI and has been approved for use in the United States and Canada as an antidepressant but is not approved for use in the European market. Non-FDA-approved (off-label) use is as a non-hormonal-based vasomotor (hot flashes) treatment for menopause. The European Union has not approved ODV for any indication because, in relation to its parent, venlafaxine, desvenlafaxine seemed to be less effective with no advantages in terms of safety and tolerability. Since venlafaxine is already approved for the treatment of MDD and is almost entirely transformed into ODV, it would be expected that efficacy and safety of ODV in the treatment of MDD would be very similar to that of venlafaxine. ODV is approximately 10-fold more potent at inhibiting 5-HT reuptake than NE reuptake. When most normal metabolizers take venlafaxine, ~70% of the parent drug is metabolized into ODV, so the effects are very similar. Side effects for ODV include nausea (most common 30%-50% vs placebo 9%-11%) and is the most common reason for discontinuation. Other adverse reactions were dizziness, insomnia, sweating, constipation, somnolence, decreased appetite, priapism, night terrors, anxiety, and delayed ejaculation, which are consistent with those of other SNRIs. Suicidal risk was significant in some patients in each study.

Structure-Activity Relationships for the Phenoxyphenylpropylamines

(±)-NISOXETINE. Nisoxetine (see Fig. 12.21) was the initial phenoxyphenylpropylamine synthesized in the Lilly Research Laboratories during the early 1970s from the rearrangement of an oxygen atom in diphenhydramine, a diphenylmethoxyethylamine, to a phenoxyphenylpropylamine (see Fig. 12.2). Nisoxetine was discovered to be a potent and very selective SNRI, with little affinity for other receptors. It underwent clinical studies as an alternative to Lilly's best-selling antidepressant, nortriptyline, but without the adverse effects associated with the tricyclic secondary amines. It was never marketed, however, because of a greater interest in developing its 4-trifluoromethyl analogue, fluoxetine, an SSRI.

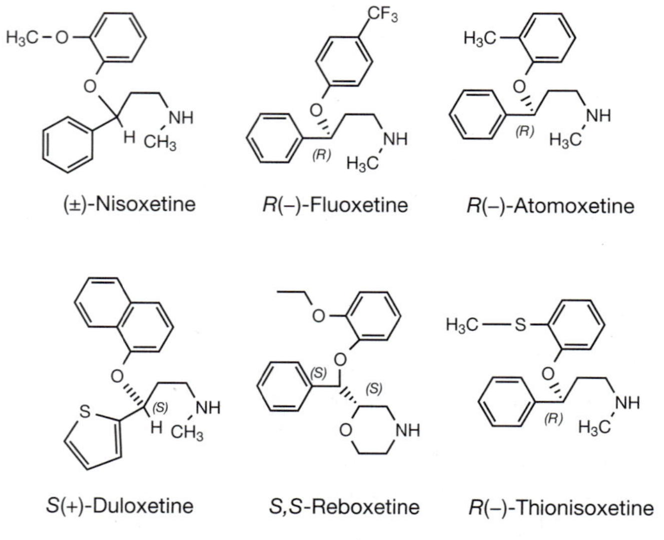

Figure 12.21 Structural relationships for the nontricyclic serotonin-norepinephrine reuptake inhibitors (SNRIs).

The type and position of the ring substitution plays a critical role in the mechanism of action for these phenoxyphenylpropyamines (see Table 12.9 for structure-activity relationships of the phenoxypropylamines). The unsubstituted molecule is a weak SSRI. However, 2-substitution into the phenoxy ring (except for the 2-trifluoromethyl) yields compounds with high potency and selectivity for blocking NE reuptake, whereas the 4-substitution results in compounds having potent SSRI activity, with the 4-trifluoromethyl group (fluoxetine) being the most potent and selective for SERT.[98] The substantial changes in transporter selectivity for NET and SERT, and the differences in affinity, are more likely attributed to the bulky 2-(*ortho*)-substituted groups, which restricts the flexibility of the aromatic rings, thereby enhancing alignment of the hydrogen-bond acceptor group (the methoxy) with a donor group on the binding site on the NET for NE that is not available for the 5-HT binding site. The *R*-isomer of nisoxetine has 20 times greater affinity than its *S*-isomer for NET. The NET K_i for nisoxetine is 0.8 nM and is 40 times more selective for NET than for SERT. Its tertiary amine is approximately 100 times less effective at inhibiting NET. Increasing the size of the methylamino with ethyl or larger alkyl groups eliminates all activity. The 2- and 4-analogues exhibited weak effects on neuronal uptake of DA and lack affinity for other neuroreceptors at therapeutic concentrations. Substituting the 2-methoxy with the isosteric 2-methylthio (thionisoxetine) produced a more potent SNRI (K_i 0.2 nM for the *R*-enantiomer) and 600 times more selective for NET than for SERT. Thionisoxetine is approximately 10 times more potent than nisoxetine at inhibiting NET and, unlike nisoxetine, it reduces food consumption in rodents and has been studied for the treatment of obesity and eating disorders. Substitution of the phenoxy group with a naphthyloxy group and the phenyl ring with the isosteric thienyl (thiophene) group results in a drug with mixed inhibition of NE and 5-HT reuptake (ie, duloxetine) (see Fig. 12.19).

R(−)-ATOMOXETINE. *R*(−)-Atomoxetine, 2-methylphenoxyphenylpropylamine, was marketed in 2003 as a "nonstimulant" treatment for ADHD in both adults and children and for treatment of adult depression.[99] The 2-methyl substitution (cf, nisoxetine) (see Figs. 12.19 and 12.21) confers selectivity for inhibiting NE reuptake (see Fig. 12.6).[100] The *R*-enantiomer is 10 times more potent than the *S*-enantiomer as a NET reuptake inhibitor. Atomoxetine has a low propensity for anticholinergic and adverse cardiovascular effects.

Pharmacokinetics. Atomoxetine is well absorbed from the GI tract and cleared primarily by metabolism, with the majority of the dose being excreted into the urine. Atomoxetine is metabolized primarily by CYP2D6 to its major active metabolite, 4-hydroxyatomoxetine, which is eliminated as its glucuronide (see Fig. 12.22).[100] Peak plasma concentrations of atomoxetine occur 1 to 2 hours after oral administration. Significant differences are seen in the elimination half-life between normal metabolizers, extensive metabolizers, and

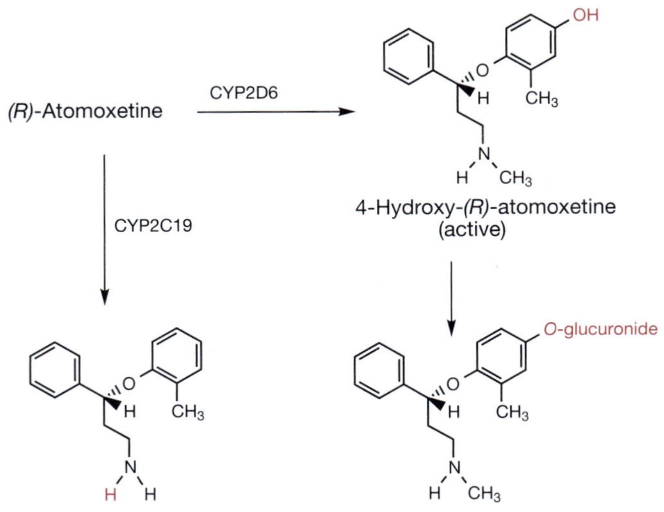

Figure 12.22 Atomoxetine metabolism.

poor metabolizers (see Table 12.4). Atomoxetine exhibited an elimination half-life of 3 to 6 hours for normal and extensive metabolizers and 17 to 21 hours for poor metabolizers. CYP2C19 is the other enzyme primarily responsible for the formation of its minor metabolite *N*-desmethylatomoxetine.

Adverse Effects. At therapeutic doses, no serious drug-related adverse effects have been encountered. Adverse effects have included modest increases in diastolic blood pressure and heart rate, anorexia, weight loss, somnolence, dizziness, GI effects (nausea), dry mouth, and skin rash.

Therapeutic Uses. Atomoxetine is used as a safe and well-tolerated "nonstimulant" treatment of ADHD in both adults and children and of depression. Among children and adolescents ages 8 to 18 years, atomoxetine was superior to placebo in reducing symptoms of ADHD and in improving social and family functioning symptoms. Oral atomoxetine is promoted as an alternative to conventional ADHD therapy with methylphenidate, dextroamphetamine, and pemoline. It also can be a replacement for bupropion or for TCAs. Onset of action is approximately 7 days.

MILNACIPRAN. (±)-Milnacipran is the *cis*-aminomethyl derivative of phenylcyclopropanecarboxamide (see Fig. 12.19) that acts as an SNRI. It is structurally different from the other SNRIs and currently is only available in Europe as a racemic mixture, with both enantiomers exhibiting antidepressant activity. It is marketed in the United States as 1S,2*R*-levomilnacipran. Substituting the aminomethyl group of LVM with an aminopropyl gives a milnacipran homologue (*cis*-1-Phenyl-2-[1-aminopropyl]-*N*,*N*-diethylcyclopropanecarboxamide) that exhibits antidepressant activity as a potent NMDAR antagonist. A glutamate hypothesis is being investigated as an alternative mechanism of depression (see the subsection on NMDA antagonists).

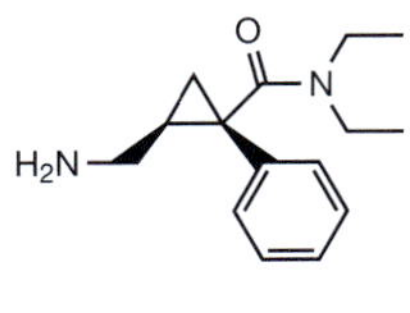

cis-Milnacipran
(Fetzima, Savella)

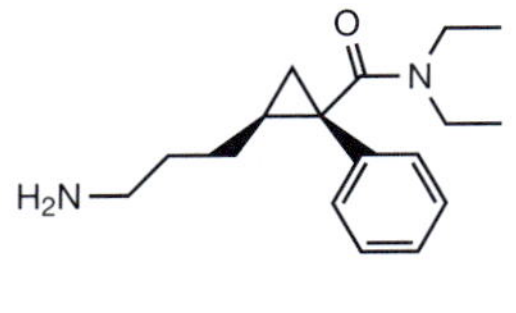

cis-1-Phenyl-2-[1-aminopropyl]-
N,*N*-diethylcyclopropanecarboxamide

Levomilnacipran. Recently, LVM (*1S*, *2R*-milnacipran) was approved by the FDA for the treatment of MDD.[101,102] It is the *levo* enantiomer of the racemic drug, milnacipran, which is approved for the treatment of MDD in Europe and Japan and for fibromyalgia in the United States. LVM has been developed solely as a sustained-release formulation (once per day). Preclinical studies have found that LVM is a more potent inhibitor of NE and 5-HT (50 and 13 times, respectively) than the less active enantiomer (*1R*, *2S*).[64] Furthermore, it has a better pharmacokinetic profile than its enantiomer, having a longer elimination half-life with a higher maximal concentration (see Table 12.10). LVM binds with high affinity to human 5-HT and NE transporters (K_i 11 and 91 nM, respectively). It inhibits 5-HT and NE reuptake (IC50 16-19 and 11 nM, respectively). LVM does not bind to any other receptors, ion channels, or transporters, including serotonergic (5-HT_{1-7}), α- and β-adrenergic, muscarinic, or histaminergic receptors and Ca^{2+}, Na^+, K^+, or Cl^- channels to a significant degree. LVM does not inhibit MAO. Thus, LVM is a dual neurotransmitter reuptake inhibitor of NE and 5-HT. It is unique among other dual neurotransmitter reuptake inhibitors in that it predominantly potentiates NE over 5-HT; it has over a 15-fold higher selectivity for NE versus 5-HT reuptake inhibition compared with duloxetine, desvenlafaxine, or venlafaxine. Interestingly, both in vitro and in vivo animal studies suggest that, at higher doses, serotonergic activity increases so that inhibition of NE reuptake approaches that of inhibition of 5-HT reuptake. LVM lacks affinity for other receptors, including the dopaminergic, adrenergic, histaminic, muscarinic, and opioid receptors.

In contrast with other selective SNRIs, including duloxetine and desvenlafaxine, LVM has greater selectivity for inhibiting NE reuptake than 5-HT reuptake. In short-term studies, LVM was found to be more effective than placebo in reducing depression, whereas long-term studies found LVM was not significantly superior to placebo. LVM is fairly well tolerated, with the most common adverse events being nausea, headache, dry mouth, and constipation. Adverse events were not dose-related except for urinary hesitancy and erectile dysfunction. LVM was not toxic to the liver, and did not cause clinically significant QTc prolongation. LVM is a relatively safe alternative antidepressant treatment with minimal DDIs. In addition, LVM might be effective in NE-deficit depression, atypical depression, or seasonal depression.

Pharmacokinetics. The pharmacokinetics of LVM follow linear dynamics with a half-life of approximately 11 hours, and a time to peak concentration of 32 to 48 hours.[103] Absorption is not affected by food intake, and the drug is 22% bound to protein. Metabolism is primarily through CYP3A4, which can contribute to potential DDIs if the concomitant drug is a strong inhibitor of cytochrome 3A4, such as ketoconazole, clarithromycin, or ritonavir.[104] Therefore, in these situations, a dose adjustment is recommended. Excretion of LVM is predominantly via the kidney. LVM should not be used in patients with end-stage renal disease.

Relative to other SNRIs, LVM as well as milnacipran differ in that they are much more balanced reuptake inhibitors of 5-HT and NE. To demonstrate, the 5-HT/NE ratios of SNRIs are as follows: venlafaxine, 30/1; duloxetine, 10/1; desvenlafaxine, 14/1; and LVM, 1/2.[103] The clinical implications of more balanced elevations of 5-HT and NE are unclear, but may include improved effectiveness, though also increased side effects.[104]

LVM is a selective SNRI, lacking significant affinity for other target sites. LVM is an NMDAR antagonist at high concentrations. It has a high oral bioavailability of 92% and a low plasma protein binding of 22%. It is metabolized in the liver by the CYP3A4 by *N*-deethylation to norlevomilnacipran, thereby making the medication susceptible to grapefruit-drug interactions. The drug has an elimination half-life of approximately 11 hours, allowing for once-daily administration. LVM is excreted in the urine.

DULOXETINE. Duloxetine (see Figs. 12.19 and 12.21) has been approved for the treatment of depression and diabetic peripheral neuropathic pain, but not for stress urinary incontinence or fibromyalgia.[103-105] It is manufactured and marketed by Eli Lilly and Company. It is another analogue in the line of fluoxetine-based products from Lilly, in which the phenyl and phenoxy groups of fluoxetine have been respectively replaced with the benzene isostere thiophene and a naphthyloxy group (previously described under fluoxetine). Duloxetine exhibits dual inhibition with high affinity for the SERTs (K_i 0.8 nM) and NETs (K_i 7.5 nM), with a 9-fold preferential inhibition of the SERT.[106] Duloxetine appears to be a more potent in vitro blocker of SERTs and NETs than venlafaxine. In humans, duloxetine has a low affinity for the other neuroreceptors, suggesting low incidence of unwanted adverse effects.

Duloxetine appears to be fairly well absorbed after oral doses, with peak plasma levels in 6 to 10 hours and linear pharmacokinetics (see Table 12.10).[106] The drug is extensively metabolized in the liver to active metabolites, with 72% of an oral dose primarily excreted in the urine as conjugated metabolites and up to 15% appearing in the feces. Its elimination half-life, time to steady-state blood levels, and mean volume of distribution are shown in Table 12.10.

N-Demethylation to an active metabolite (CYP2D6) and hydroxylation of the naphthyl ring (CYP1A2) at either the 4-, 5-, or 6-positions are the main metabolic pathways for duloxetine. Its metabolites are primarily excreted into the urine as glucuronide, sulfate, and *O*-methylated conjugation products (Fig. 12.23). The major metabolites found

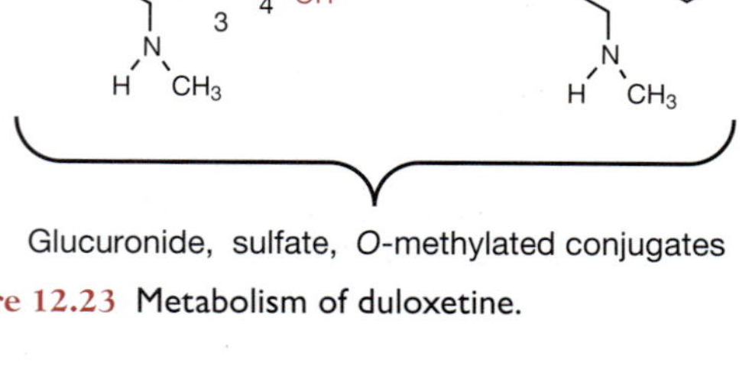

Figure 12.23 Metabolism of duloxetine.

in plasma also were found in the urine. Preclinical data for 4-hydroxyduloxetine suggest it has a similar pharmacologic profile to duloxetine, with selective inhibition of SERT but less activity at NET.

Adverse effects have included insomnia, somnolence, headache, nausea, diarrhea, and dry mouth. Mild withdrawal symptoms on abrupt discontinuation have been described in studies with healthy subjects.[107]

Duloxetine is a moderately potent CYP2D6 inhibitor (intermediate between paroxetine and sertraline). Thus, duloxetine should be used with caution when CYP2D6 substrates and inhibitors are coadministered.

Dopamine-Norepinephrine Reuptake Inhibitor

BUPROPION. Bupropion is an arylisopropylaminoketone that is structurally related to the phenylisopropylamine CNS stimulant methamphetamine, the phenylisopropylaminoketone cathinone (a constituent in khat), and the anorexiant diethylpropion (see Fig. 12.24). Although structurally similar to the CNS stimulants, bupropion exhibits distinctively different pharmacologic and therapeutic effects mostly because of its metabolites. The absence of the tricyclic ring system in bupropion results in a better adverse-effect profile than with the TCAs. The tertiary butyl group in bupropion prevents its *N*-dealkylation to metabolites that could possess sympathomimetic and/or anorexigenic properties.

Wellbutrin and Zyban (an aid in smoking cessation treatment) are trade name products for bupropion.[108] Therefore, the potential exists for an overdose toxicity in a patient receiving multiple brand name and generic prescriptions containing bupropion for the treatment of depression, smoking cessation, and other off-label uses.

Mechanism of Action. The mechanism of antidepressant action for bupropion is more complex because of its metabolism to its three principal metabolites (see Fig. 12.24), which contribute to its antidepressant mechanism of action because their accumulated plasma concentrations are higher than those of bupropion, with a longer duration of action.[109,110] Bupropion appears to be a selective inhibitor of DA reuptake at the DA presynaptic neuronal membrane and an SNRI (see Table 12.11) as well as inducing the release of DA and NE. An additional mechanism of action for bupropion is a noncompetitive antagonist of several neuronal nAChRs. Thus, the mixed antidepressant and anti-nicotinic activity of bupropion is mediated by its stimulatory action on the DA and NE systems and inhibition of the neuronal nAChRs. The neuronal nAChRs are ligand-gated ion channels of the CNS that regulate synaptic activity from both pre- and postsynaptic sites. Bupropion blocks noncompetitively the activation of $\alpha_3\beta_2$, $\alpha_4\beta_2$, and α_7 neuronal nAChRs and is approximately 5 and 11 times more effective blocking $\alpha_3\beta_2$ and $\alpha_4\beta_2$ (the brain nicotine-binding site) than α_7 receptors. Bupropion at high concentration failed to displace nicotine from the $\alpha_4\beta_2$ receptors. Bupropion inhibition of $\alpha_3\beta_2$ and $\alpha_4\beta_2$ ion channel receptors on neuronal nAChRs involves initial binding to the ion channels in the resting state, decreasing the probability of the ion channels opening and further interaction with a binding domain in the ion channel shared with the TCAs.[108] Bupropion does not exhibit clinically

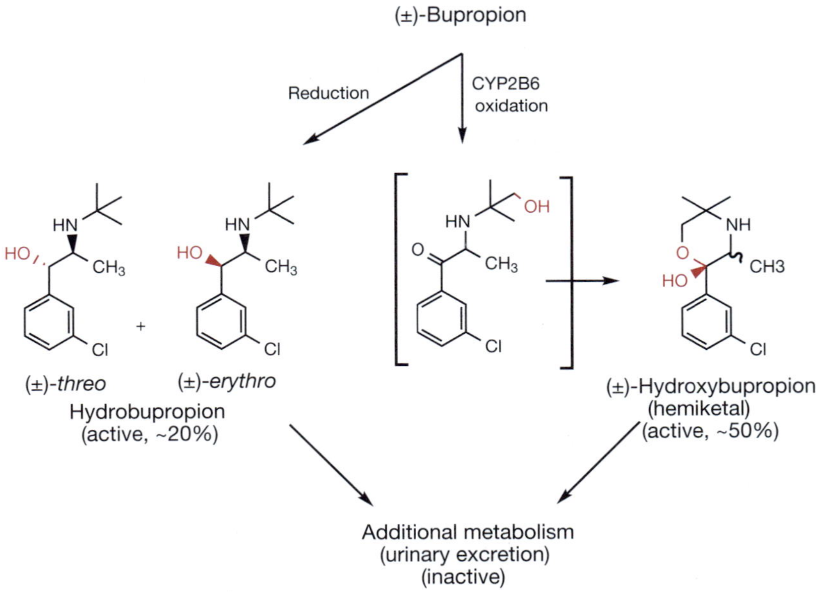

Figure 12.24 Bupropion, related derivatives and metabolites.

significant anticholinergic, antihistaminic, or α_1-adrenergic blocking activity or MAO inhibition.

Bupropion is also effective in nicotine dependence by blocking nicotine's pharmacologic effects, suggesting that bupropion possesses some selectivity for neuronal nAChRs underlying various nicotinic effects. In addition, bupropion blocks noncompetitively the activation of $\alpha_3\beta_2$, $\alpha_4\beta_2$, and α_7 neuronal nAChRs. It was approximately 50 and 11 times more effective blocking $\alpha_3\beta_2$ and $\alpha_4\beta_2$ than α_7 receptors.[110] Bupropion at high concentration failed to displace nicotine from brain nicotine-binding sites, a site largely composed of $\alpha_4\beta_2$ receptors. The inhibition of $\alpha_3\beta_2$ and $\alpha_4\beta_2$ receptors suggests bupropion may not be acting as an open channel blocker.

Bupropion reduces the discomfort and craving associated with smoking cessation, which suggests that the principal mode of action by bupropion as an aid in smoking cessation is on the withdrawal symptoms following smoking cessation.[108] The efficacy of bupropion in smoking cessation does not appear to depend on the presence of depression. The current presumed mechanism of action of bupropion involves modulation of dopaminergic and noradrenergic systems that have been implicated in addiction, by increasing extracellular CNS DA concentrations, most likely as a result of its inhibition of DA and noradrenaline reuptake transporters (see Table 12.1).[108] As nicotine CNS concentrations drop with smoking cessation, the firing rates of noradrenergic neurons increase, which may be the basis for the withdrawal symptoms. Thus, during withdrawal, bupropion and its active metabolite hydroxybupropion reduce the firing rates of these noradrenergic neurons in a dose-dependent manner, attenuating the symptoms of smoking cessation. Furthermore, its ability to block the nicotinic receptors also may prevent relapse by attenuating the reinforcing properties of nicotine but probably cannot acutely reduce smoking.[108]

Bupropion is extensively metabolized in humans with its three major hydroxylated metabolites reaching plasma levels higher than those of bupropion itself. These hydroxylated metabolites share many of the pharmacologic properties of bupropion, so they can play a greater role in attenuating the withdrawal and relapse by which bupropion exerts its activity in smoking cessation.[109,110]

Pharmacokinetics. Bupropion is absorbed from the GI tract, with a low oral bioavailability as a result of first-pass metabolism. The pharmacokinetic properties of bupropion are shown in Table 12.11. Food does not appear to substantially affect its peak plasma concentration or AUC. Following oral administration, peak plasma concentrations usually are achieved within 2 hours for bupropion and 3 hours for sustained-released bupropion products, followed by a biphasic decline for bupropion. Plasma concentrations are dose-proportional (linear pharmacokinetics) following single doses of 100 to 250 mg/d. The fraction of a dose excreted unmetabolized was less than 1%.

Bupropion hydroxylation of the *tert*-butyl group to hydroxypropion intermediate, which cyclizes to a phenylmorpholinol metabolite, is mediated exclusively by CYP2B6.[110] Other metabolites include reduction of the aminoketone to the amino-alcohol isomers *threo*-hydrobupropion and *erythro*-hydrobupropion (see Fig. 12.24). Further oxidation of the bupropion side chain results in the formation of *m*-chlorobenzoic acid, which is eliminated in the urine as its glycine conjugate. Hydroxybupropion is approximately 50% as potent as bupropion, whereas *threo*-hydrobupropion and *erythro*-hydrobupropion have 20% of the potency of bupropion. Peak plasma concentrations for hydroxybupropion are approximately 20 times the peak level of the parent drug at steady state, with an elimination half-life of approximately 20 hours. Thus, CYP2B6-catalyzed bupropion hydroxylation is a clinically important bioactivation and elimination pathway. The times to peak concentrations for the *erythro*-hydrobupropion and *threo*-hydrobupropion metabolites are similar to that of the hydroxybupropion metabolite. The plasma levels of the *erythro*-hydrobupropion correlate

Table 12.11 Pharmacokinetics of the Norepinephrine/Dopamine Reuptake Inhibitors and Serotonin Receptor Modulators

Parameters	Bupropion	Trazodone	Mirtazapine	Levomilnacipran	Vilazodone	Vortioxetine
Oral bioavailability (%)	5-20	65 (60-70)	~50	92	72	75
Lipophilicity (Log $D_{7.4}$)	2.88	2.59	2.40	−1.09	ND	3.37
Protein binding (%)	80	90-95	85	22	98	98
Volume of distribution (L/kg)	19-21	0.84 (0.5-1.2)	107	387-473		2,600
Elimination half-life (hours)	21 (14-24) ~20 (*S,S*)-hydroxy	7 (4-9)	16-40	11	25	66
Cytochrome P450 major isoform	2B6	3A4	3A4 and 2D6	3A4	3A4	2D6, 3A4/5
Major active metabolites	(*S,S*)-Hydroxyl	*m*-chlorophenyl piperazine	None	None	None	None
Peak plasma concentration (hours)	2-3 8 (*S,S*)-hydroxy	1-2	2	6-8	4-5	7-11
Excretion (%)	Urine 87	Urine 70-75	Urine 75	Urine 58	Urine >90	Urine 60
	Feces 10	Feces 25-30	Feces 15		Feces 2	
Plasma half-life (hours)	3-4 20 (*S,S*)-hydroxy	6 (4-8)	2			
Time to steady-state concentration (days)	5-8 (*S,S*)-hydroxy	3-7	5			

ND, not determined.

with several side effects, such as insomnia and dry mouth. Their elimination half-lives, however, are longer (~33 and 37 hours, respectively) and steady-state AUCs are 1.5 and 7.0 times that of bupropion, respectively. The hepatic clearance in patients with liver disease was increased from 19 to 29 hours. The median observed T_{max} was 19 hours for hydroxybupropion and 31 hours for *threo-/erythro*-hydrobupropion. The mean half-lives for hydroxybupropion and *threo-/erythro*-hydrobupropion were increased by 5 and 2 times, respectively, in patients with severe hepatic cirrhosis compared with healthy volunteers. Bupropion and its metabolites are distributed into breast milk.[109,110]

In geriatric patients, the apparent half-life of hydroxybupropion averaged approximately 34 hours. Reduction in renal or hepatic function may affect elimination of the major metabolites, because these compounds are moderately polar and are likely to be metabolized further or conjugated in the liver before urinary excretion.

The pharmacokinetic parameters for bupropion and hydroxybupropion did not differ between smokers and nonsmokers, but adolescent females exhibited increased AUCs and volume of distribution (normalized to body weight) and a longer elimination half-life than males. No differences in clearance between males and females, however, were observed.[110]

Drug Interactions. Inhibition studies with the SSRIs and bupropion suggest that bupropion is a potent CYP2D6 inhibitor. Bupropion hydroxylation was strongly inhibited by, in the following order, paroxetine > fluvoxamine > sertraline > desmethylsertraline > norfluoxetine > fluoxetine and only weakly inhibited by venlafaxine, ODV, citalopram, and desmethylcitalopram. The inhibition of bupropion hydroxylation in vitro by SSRIs suggests the potential for clinical drug interactions. Therefore, coadministration of drugs that inhibit CYP2D6 warrants careful monitoring. Because of its selective inhibition of DA reuptake, pharmacodynamic interactions with DA agonists (eg, levodopa) and antagonists should be anticipated. Coadministration of bupropion with drugs that lower the seizure threshold should be avoided because of the risk of serious seizures. Drugs that affect metabolism by CYP2B6 (eg, methadone, nicotine, and cyclophosphamide) also have the potential to interact with bupropion.

Therapeutic Uses. Besides being used to treat depression, bupropion is a non-nicotine aid in the cessation of smoking. The efficacy of bupropion in smoking cessation is comparable to that of nicotine replacement therapy and should be considered as a second-line treatment in smoking cessation.[108] It possesses a broad spectrum of infrequent adverse effects, however, with potential drug metabolism interactions with TCAs, β-adrenergic blocking drugs, and class IC antiarrhythmics.

Serotonin Receptor Modulators and Stimulators

SMSs, sometimes referred to more simply as 5-HT modulators (regulators), have multiple pharmacologic modes of action at receptor sites specific to the 5-HT neurotransmitter system. SMSs simultaneously regulate one or more 5-HT receptors and inhibit the reuptake of 5-HT.

SMSs are a distinct class of atypical antidepressants used to treat MDD. SMSs have several modes of interaction with the various 5-HT receptors in the brain and simultaneously modulate one or more 5-HT receptors and inhibit the reuptake of 5-HT.[111] There are many different subtypes of 5-HT receptors (at least 15 in total are currently known); however, not all of these receptors appear to be involved in the antidepressant effects of SSRIs. A drug that combines the actions of SSRI, 5-HT_{1A} partial agonism, and 5-HT_7 receptor antagonism could prove more effective than pure SSRIs, improving tolerability. They were developed to address problems with 5-HT uptake related to depression and the increasing numbers of 5-HT receptors. An alternative term is 5-HT partial agonist-reuptake inhibitor (SPARI), which can be applied only to vilazodone.

SMS describes the mechanism of action of the serotonergic antidepressant vortioxetine, which acts as an SSRI, agonist at the 5-HT_{1A} receptor, and antagonist at the 5-HT_3 and 5-HT_7 receptors. Drugs in this class of antidepressants include trazodone, mirtazapine, vilazodone, and vortioxetine. A serious adverse effect of SMSs is hepatic failure, and they should be used with precaution in patients with cardiac abnormalities. Patients should be monitored for suicidal thinking and behavior. There is also the risk of hypotension and of abnormal bleeding.[111]

General Mechanism of Action. SMSs are a class of antidepressants, the function of which is to modulate the concentration of 5-HT in the brain. A neuromodulator functions as a "volume control in the brain and nervous system," regulating the other neurotransmitters through its receptors in the brain in response to external stimuli. The serotonergic system modulates a large number of physiologic events, such as temperature regulation, sleep, learning and memory, behavior, sexual function, hormonal secretions, and immune activity and is implicated in stress, anxiety, aggressiveness, and depression disorders. Of the various types of 5-HT receptors mediating serotonergic activity, the 5-HT_{1B} receptors play an important role in modulating the serotonergic system. The 5-HT_{1B} receptors are autoreceptors localized on serotonergic presynaptic nerve terminals, where they inhibit the release of 5-HT and its biosynthesis; they also inhibit the release of other neurotransmitters, such as ACh, GABA, and NE. Excessive amounts of 5-HT in the brain may cause relaxation, sedation, and a decrease in sexual drive; inadequate amounts of 5-HT can lead to psychiatric disorders. Therefore, the SMSs exert their antidepressant effects by mechanisms that enhance noradrenergic or serotonergic transmission by acting as dual 5-HT antagonists/5-HT reuptake inhibitors ([SARIs] trazodone and vilazodone), α_2-adrenergic antagonists, and 5-HT_2 and 5-HT_3 antagonists ([NaSSAs] mirtazapine). Chronic antidepressant treatment with SARIs and NaSSAs modulates 5-HT receptor expression and, in turn, 5-HT function.

Arylpiperazine Antidepressants. In order to avoid benzodiazepine's undesirable side effects, a third-generation anxiolytic agent, buspirone, the focus of the arylpiperazine group of anti-anxiety agents, has been introduced recently as a new class of antidepressant agent. Arylpiperazine derivatives work as 5-HT_{1A} receptor partial agonists and are known as 5-HT modulators and inhibitors of 5-HT uptake. Recent developments in the pharmacology of arylpiperazine antidepressant drugs have focused on compounds that enhance the neurotransmission of 5-HT, such as 5-HT uptake inhibitors and 5-HT_{1A} receptor agonists and 5-HT antagonists. Clinical and preclinical studies support the efficacy of 5-HT_{1A} receptor partial agonists as antidepressants. The antidepressant activity of the arylpiperazines may be due to the activation of postsynaptic 5-HT_{1A} receptors, although 5-HT_{1A} receptor agonists also activate autoreceptors that diminish the release of 5-HT. Evidence also does not support the involvement of buspirone in the antidepressant activity of 5-HT_{1A} receptor–selective azapirones. The arylpiperazine derivatives have no sedative and muscle relaxant effects, but they have a rather weak anxiolytic action and a slow onset of action.

The 5-HT_{1A} receptors are located presynaptically, where they act as autoreceptors to inhibit the firing rate of 5-HT neurons. Most 5-HT_{1A} agonists are readily absorbed but are also rapidly eliminated, thereby often producing either suboptimal therapeutic responses at low doses or cumbersome adverse effects at higher doses. Extended-release formulations allow once-daily dosing regimens, thus avoiding sharp peak plasma concentrations. This improves adherence and permits the use of higher dosages, which may be associated with enhanced efficacy and better tolerability relative to the immediate-release formulations. In conclusion, 5-HT_{1A} receptor agonists represent a valuable and efficacious therapeutic approach to major depression.

Trazodone. Trazodone is a phenylpiperazine-triazolopyridine antidepressant that is structurally unrelated to most of the other antidepressant classes (see Fig. 12.25). It acts as a mixed 5-HT agonist and 5-HT reuptake inhibitor (also known as SARIs).[111]

Mechanism of Action. Although the exact mechanism of action is unknown, trazodone acts as an antagonist at 5-HT_{2A} receptors and is a weak inhibitor of 5-HT reuptake at the presynaptic neuronal membrane, potentiating the

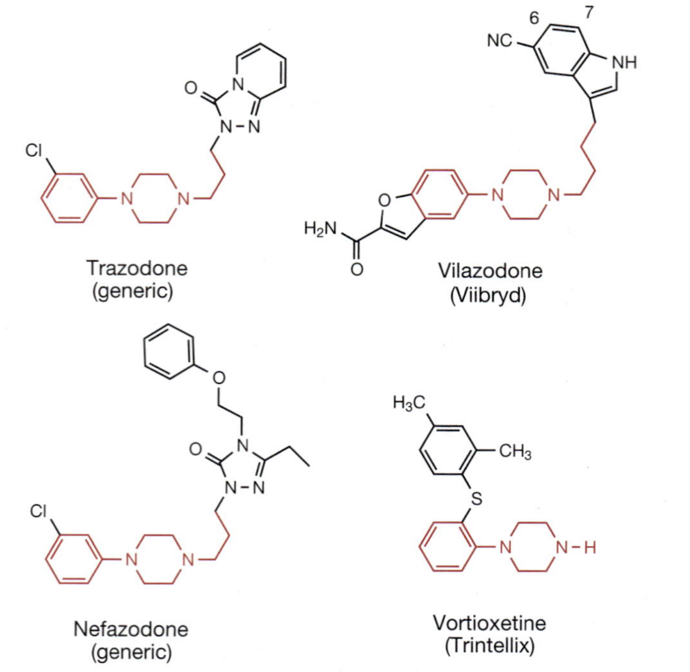

Figure 12.25 Serotonin receptor modulators.

synaptic effects of 5-HT. Its mechanism of action is complicated by the presence of its metabolite, *m*-chlorophenylpiperazine (*m*-CPP) (Fig. 12.26), which is a 5-HT_{2C} agonist.[112] At therapeutic dosages, trazodone does not appear to affect the reuptake of DA or NE within the CNS. It has little anticholinergic activity and is relatively devoid of toxic cardiovascular effects. The increase in serotonergic activity with long-term administration of trazodone decreases the number of postsynaptic serotonergic (ie, 5-HT_2) and β-adrenergic binding sites in the brains of animals, decreasing the sensitivity of adenylyl cyclase to stimulation by β-adrenergic agonists. It has been suggested that postsynaptic serotonergic receptor modification is mainly responsible for the antidepressant action observed during long-term administration of trazodone.[113] Trazodone does not inhibit MAO and, unlike amphetamine-like drugs, does not stimulate the CNS.

Trazodone is rapidly and almost completely absorbed from the GI tract following oral administration, with an oral bioavailability of approximately 65% (see Table 12.11).[114] Peak plasma concentrations of trazodone occur approximately 1 hour after oral administration when taken on an empty stomach or 2 hours when taken with food. At steady state, its plasma concentrations exhibit wide interpatient variation.

Trazodone is extensively metabolized in the liver by *N*-dealkylation to its primary circulating active metabolite *m*-CPP, which subsequently undergoes aromatic hydroxylation to *p*-hydroxy-*m*-CPP (see Fig. 12.26).[115] In vitro studies indicate that CYP3A4 is the major isoform involved in the production of *m*-CPP from trazodone (and CYP2D6 to a lesser extent). 4′-Hydroxy-*m*-CPP and triazolopyridinonepropionic acid (the major metabolite excreted in urine) are conjugated with glucuronic acid. Less than 1% of a dose is excreted unmetabolized. *m*-CPP is 4′-hydroxylated by CYP2D6. *m*-CPP is of significant interest because of its 5-HT_{2C} agonist and 5-HT_{2A} antagonist activities that may contribute to trazodone antidepressant action.[114]

Trazodone therapy has been associated with several cases of idiosyncratic hepatotoxicity. Although the mechanism of hepatotoxicity remains unknown, the generation of an iminoquinone, an epoxide reactive metabolite, or both may play a role in the initiation of trazodone-mediated hepatotoxicity (see Fig. 12.26).[115,116] Studies have shown that the bioactivation of trazodone involves, first, aromatic hydroxylation of the 3-chlorophenyl ring, followed by its oxidation to a reactive iminoquinone intermediate, which then reacts with glutathione or oxidation of the triazolopyridinone ring to an electrophilic

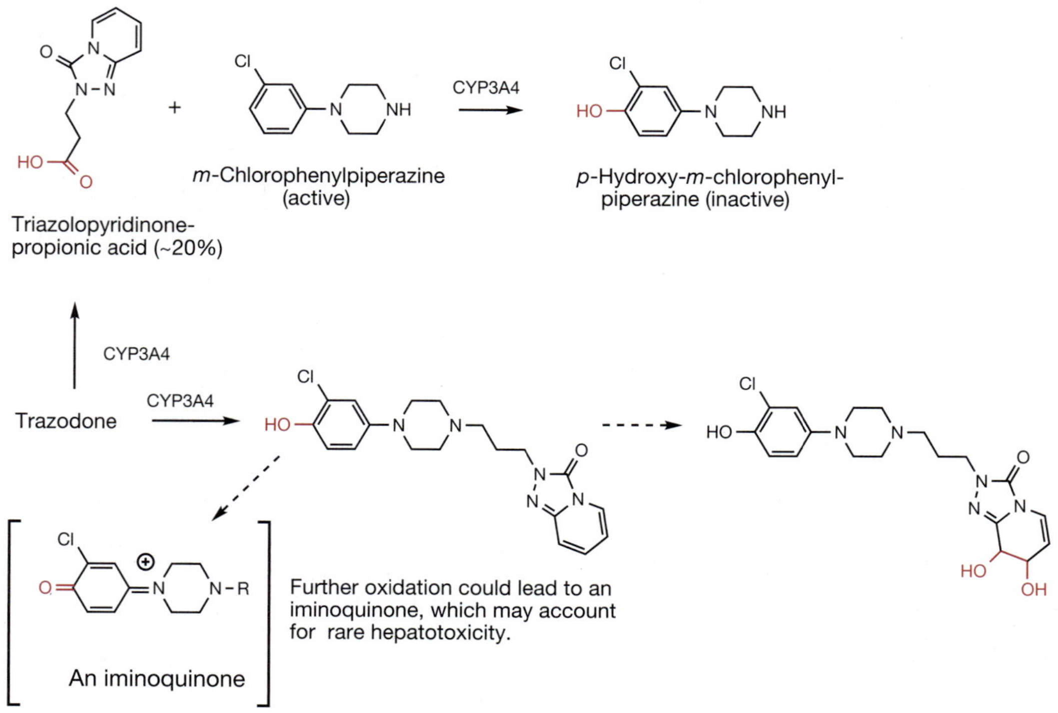

Figure 12.26 Metabolism of trazodone.

epoxide and ring opening by either a nucleophile or to generate the corresponding hydrated trazodone-nucleophile conjugate or the stable diol metabolite, respectively.[114,115] The pathway involving trazodone bioactivation to the iminoquinone also has been observed with many para-hydroxyanilines (eg, acetaminophen). The reactive intermediates consume the available glutathione, allowing the reactive intermediate to react with hepatic tissue leading to liver damage.

Unlike the TCAs, trazodone does not block the fast sodium channels and, thus, does not have significant arrhythmic activity. Compared with the SSRIs, it has a lesser tendency to cause drug-induced male sexual dysfunction as a side effect. Although trazodone displays α_1-adrenergic blocking activity, hypotension is relatively uncommon. Signs of overdose toxicity include nausea, vomiting, and decreased level of consciousness. Trazodone produces a significant amount of sedation in patients who are normal and mentally depressed (principally from its central α_1-adrenergic blocking activity and antihistaminic action).

Drug Interactions. Trazodone possesses serotonergic activity; therefore, the possibility of developing 5-HT syndrome should be considered in patients who are receiving trazodone and other SSRIs or serotonergic drugs concurrently. When trazodone is used concurrently with drugs metabolized by CYP3A4, caution should be used to avoid excessive sedation. Trazodone can cause hypotension, including orthostatic hypotension and syncope; concomitant administration of antihypertensive therapy may require a reduction in dosage of the antihypertensive agent. The possibility of DDIs with trazodone and other substrates, inducers, and/or inhibitors of CYP3A4 exists.[113]

Therapeutic Uses. Trazodone is used primarily in the treatment of insomnia, depression, and depression/anxiety disorders. The drug also has shown some efficacy in the treatment of benzodiazepine or alcohol dependence, diabetic neuropathy, and panic disorders.

NEFAZODONE

Nefazodone is an arylpiperazine antidepressant structurally related to trazodone, but it differs pharmacologically from trazodone, the SSRIs, the MAOIs, and the TCAs (see Fig. 12.25). When compared with trazodone, nefazodone displays approximately twice the affinity potency for SERT. Nefazodone therapy, however, was associated with life-threatening cases of idiosyncratic hepatotoxicity and as a result, nefazodone was withdrawn from both the North American and European market in 2003. The mechanism of hepatotoxicity remains unknown, but nefazodone, being structurally similar to trazodone (see Fig. 12.24), is metabolized to *p*-hydroxynefazodone, *m*-CPP, and phenoxyethyltriazoledione. In turn, *p*-hydroxynefazodone is thought to be oxidized to an iminoquinone and/or an epoxide reactive metabolite, which may play a role in the initiation of nefazodone-mediated hepatotoxicity.

Vilazodone. Vilazodone is an arylpiperazine-2-benzofurancarboxamide antidepressant that is structurally related to trazodone (see Fig. 12.25). It acts as a dual 5-HT receptor partial agonist and 5-HT reuptake inhibitor.[117]

Mechanism of Action. The mechanism of the antidepressant effect of vilazodone is not fully understood but could be related to its enhancement of CNS serotonergic activity through selective inhibition of 5-HT reuptake.[118] In addition, vilazodone is also a partial agonist at 5-HT_{1A} receptors. Vilazodone binds with high affinity to the 5-HT reuptake site (K_i 0.1 nM), but not to the NE (K_i 56 nM) or DA (K_i 37 nM) reuptake sites. Vilazodone is a potent and selective inhibitor of 5-HT reuptake (IC50 1.6 nM) (see Fig. 12.6). As a 5-HT_{1A} receptor partial agonist, it binds selectively with high affinity to 5-HT_{1A} receptors (IC50 2.1 nM). Vilazodone does not prolong the QTc interval as do the TCAs and is below the threshold for clinical concern. Clinical trials of vilazodone showed significant antidepressant efficacy with an onset of effect in 1 week, unlike other antidepressants. The 1-week onset of its antidepressant action has been linked to its partial agonist action at the 5-HT_{1A} receptor.[118,119]

Pharmacokinetics. The antidepressant activity for vilazodone activity is due primarily to the parent drug. Vilazodone exhibits dose-proportional linear pharmacokinetics and steady state is achieved in about 3 days.[120] Elimination of vilazodone is primarily by hepatic metabolism with a terminal half-life of approximately 25 hours (see Table 12.11). Peak plasma concentrations (T_{max}) occur 4 to 5 hours after oral administration. The absolute bioavailability of vilazodone is 72% with food. The C_{max} of vilazodone with food (high fat or light meal) increases oral bioavailability by approximately 147% to 160%, and AUC increases by approximately 64% to 85%. Vilazodone is widely distributed and approximately 96% to 99% protein bound. Vilazodone is extensively metabolized by CYP3A4 to 6-hydroxyvilazodone (inactive metabolite) with minor contributions from CYP2C19 and CYP2D6.[120-122] Only 1% of the oral dose is recovered in the urine and 2% recovered in the feces as unchanged vilazodone. In vitro studies indicate that vilazodone is unlikely to inhibit or induce the metabolism of other CYP (except for CYP2C8) substrates and did not alter the pharmacokinetics of CYP2C19, 2D6, and 3A4 substrates.[121] Renal impairment or mild or moderate hepatic impairment did not affect the clearance of vilazodone, thus no dose adjustment is required.[121,122] Coadministration of vilazodone with ethanol or with a proton pump inhibitor (eg, pantoprazole) did not affect the rate or extent of vilazodone absorption. Vilazodone is excreted into the milk of lactating rats, and the effect on lactation and nursing in humans is unknown. Breastfeeding in women treated with vilazodone should be considered only if the potential benefit outweighs the potential risk to the child. A pharmacokinetic study in older adults (age >65 years) versus young (24- to 55-year-old) subjects demonstrated that the pharmacokinetics were generally similar between the two age groups. No dose adjustment is recommended on the basis of age. Greater sensitivity of some older individuals to vilazodone cannot be ruled out. After adjustment for body weight, the systemic exposures between males and females are similar.[120,122]

Adverse Effects. The most commonly observed adverse reactions in vilazodone-treated MDD with an incidence greater than 5% were diarrhea, nausea, vomiting, and insomnia. Sexual dysfunction was minimal with vilazodone. As with all antidepressants, use vilazodone cautiously in patients with a history or family history of bipolar disorder, mania, or hypomania. Vilazodone has safety risks associated with the induction of suicidal thoughts in young adults, adolescents, and children (a black box warning).

Drug Interactions. The risk of using vilazodone in combination with other CNS-active drugs has not been evaluated. Because of potential interactions with MAOIs, vilazodone should not be prescribed concomitantly with an MAOI or within 14 days of discontinuing or starting an MAOI. Based on the drugs' mechanism of action and the potential for 5-HT toxicity (serotonin syndrome), caution is advised when coadministered with other drugs that may affect the serotonergic neurotransmitter systems (eg, MAOI, SSRIs, SNRIs, triptans, buspirone, tramadol, tryptophan products, etc). Because 5-HT release by platelets plays an important role in hemostasis, concurrent use of a nonsteroidal anti-inflammatory drug (NSAID) or aspirin with vilazodone may potentiate the risk of abnormal bleeding. Altered anticoagulant effects, including increased bleeding, have been reported when SSRIs and SNRIs are coadministered with warfarin. Thus, patients receiving warfarin therapy should be carefully monitored when vilazodone is initiated or discontinued. Concomitant use of vilazodone and strong/moderate inhibitors of CYP3A4 (eg, ketoconazole) can increase vilazodone plasma concentrations by approximately 50%, requiring a dosage adjustment. No dose adjustment is recommended when coadministered with mild inhibitors of CYP3A4 (eg, cimetidine). Concomitant use of vilazodone with inducers of CYP3A4 has the potential to reduce vilazodone plasma levels. Concomitant administration of vilazodone with inhibitors of CYP2C19 and CYP2D6 is not expected to alter its plasma concentration. These isoforms are minor elimination pathways in the metabolism of vilazodone. Coadministration of vilazodone with substrates for CYP1A2, CYP2C9, CYP3A4, or CYP2D6 is unlikely to result in clinically significant changes in the concentrations of the CYP substrates. Vilazodone coadministration with mephenytoin resulted in a small (11%) increase in mephenytoin biotransformation, suggestive of a minor induction of CYP2C19. In vitro studies have shown that vilazodone is a moderate inhibitor of CYP2C19 and CYP2D6. In vitro studies suggest that vilazodone may inhibit the biotransformation of substrates of CYP2C8, thus coadministration of vilazodone with a CYP2C8 substrate may lead to an increase in the plasma concentration of the CYP2C8 substrate. Chronic administration of vilazodone is unlikely to induce the metabolism of drugs metabolized by CYP1A1, 1A2, 2A6, 2B6, 2C9, 2C19, 2D6, 2E1, or 3A4/5. Because vilazodone is highly bound to plasma protein, administration to a patient taking another drug that is highly protein bound may cause increased free concentrations of the other drug.[121,122]

Vortioxetine. Vortioxetine was FDA approved in 2013 for the treatment of adults with MDD. Vortioxetine is classified as an SMS as it has a multimodal mechanism of action toward the 5-HT neurotransmitter system, whereby it simultaneously modulates one or more 5-HT receptors and inhibits the reuptake of 5-HT (Fig. 12.25). Vortioxetine is an arylpiperazine that also acts as a partial agonist of the 5-HT_{1B} receptor; an agonist of 5-HT_{1A}; and antagonist of the 5-HT_3, 5-HT_{1D}, and 5-HT_7 receptors.[123] It reduces depressive symptoms for treatment of MDD and to maintain an antidepressant response.

Mechanism of Action. Its mechanism of action is not fully understood, but it binds with high affinity to the SERT (K_i 1.6 nM) in the CNS inhibition of 5-HT reuptake but not to the NE (K_i 113 nM) or DA (K_i >1,000 nM) transporters. Vortioxetine potently and selectively inhibits reuptake of 5-HT by inhibition of the SERT (IC50 5.4 nM). Vortioxetine displays binding affinity to 5HT_3 (K_i 3.7 nM), 5HT_{1A} (K_i 15 nM), 5HT_7 (K_i 19 nM), 5HT_{1D} (K_i 54 nM), and 5HT_{1B} (K_i 33 nM) receptors and is a 5HT_3, 5HT_{1D}, and 5HT_7 receptor antagonist; 5HT_{1B} receptor partial agonist; and 5HT_{1A} receptor agonist.[124] Vortioxetine's binding affinity is dose-proportional. Based on its receptor binding affinities, vortioxetine displays reuptake blockade of the SERT and acts as an agonist at the 5-HT_{1A} receptor and a partial agonist at the 5-HT_{1B} receptor, both of which function as presynaptic autoreceptors for serotonergic neurotransmission. It also displays antagonism at the 5-HT_{1D}, 5-HT_7, and 5-HT_3 receptors. Agonist and partial agonist activity at the 5-HT_{1A} and 5-HT_{1B} receptors can lead to further 5-HT release and could theoretically cause additional antidepressant activity. Antagonistic activity at the 5-HT_7 receptor potentiates the effects of SERT inhibition by additional release of 5-HT through downstream mechanisms.[125] Animal studies suggest that vortioxetine increases extracellular levels of all five neurotransmitters in major regions of the brain associated with depression, including the prefrontal cortex and hippocampus, and that this multimodal action produces an additional clinical benefit. Vortioxetine can be discontinued 1 week before complete discontinuation.[124,126]

Drug Interactions. Since vortioxetine is an agonist and antagonist of multiple 5-HT receptors, potential interactions may occur with other medications that alter the serotonergic pathways. There is an increased risk of the serotonin syndrome when vortioxetine is used in combination with other serotonergic agents. Medications that should be avoided because of the increased risk of serotonin syndrome when combined with vortioxetine include SNRIs, SSRIs, TCAs, triptans, MAOIs, lithium, and antipsychotic agents. St John's wort and dextromethorphan, common OTC medications, should also be avoided because of their serotonergic effects. Vortioxetine has been known to cause abnormal bleeding with NSAIDs, warfarin, and aspirin, and patients should watch for signs and symptoms of abnormal bleeding.[126]

Pharmacokinetics. Vortioxetine is extensively metabolized by CYP2D6, with minor CYP3A4/5, CYP2C19, and CYP2C9 metabolism and subsequent glucuronic acid conjugation (see Fig. 12.27 and Table 12.11). CYP2D6 hydroxylates vortioxetine into its phenolic inactive metabolite and hydroxylates the arylmethyl group to hydroxymethyl and alcohol dehydrogenase (ADH)/aldehyde dehydrogenase (ALDH) oxidation to the carboxylic acid metabolite. Since vortioxetine primarily goes through CYP2D6, the probability of interactions with CYP2D6 inhibitors and inducers affecting its concentration is high. The half-life of vortioxetine is approximately 66 hours, and it is primarily eliminated in urine (59%) and feces (26%), with a negligible amount of unchanged vortioxetine in the urine. Drug interactions involve inhibitors and inducers of CYP2D6. The dose of vortioxetine should be reduced by half when it is combined with strong CYP2D6 inhibitors, and the dose of vortioxetine should be increased if strong CYP2D6 inducers are used for 14 days or longer (up to 3 times the maximum

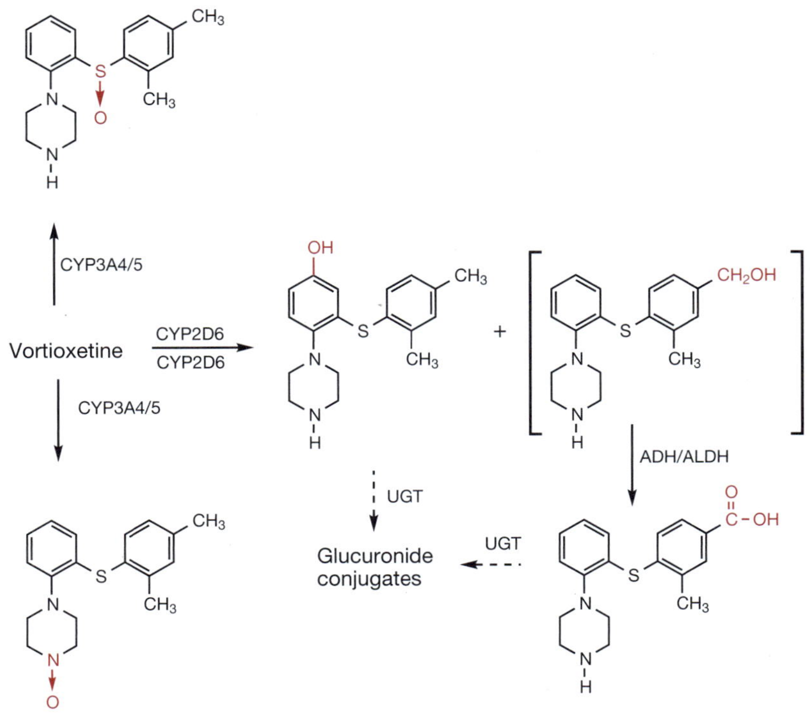

Figure 12.27 Metabolism of vortioxetine.

recommended dose can be used with strong CYP2D6 inducers). After oral administration, vortioxetine is absorbed from the GI tract and exhibits peak plasma concentrations in about 7 to 11 hours. Its oral bioavailability is 75%. Consumption of food does not affect the bioavailability, and taking vortioxetine with food has not been shown to increase its C_{max}. The steady-state concentration is achieved in about 2 weeks. Vortioxetine has a linear and dose-proportional pharmacokinetic profile with single daily dosing of 2.5 to 60 mg.[124]

Therapeutic Effects. There was a statistically significant short-term reduction at week 8 for the 10-mg vortioxetine group compared with placebo. All doses of vortioxetine showed reductions in antidepressant scores by weeks 2 and 8, but 10 mg demonstrated better efficacy, suggesting a potential dose effect. In addition, all doses were statistically superior to placebo in regard to response rates, as well as remission rates.

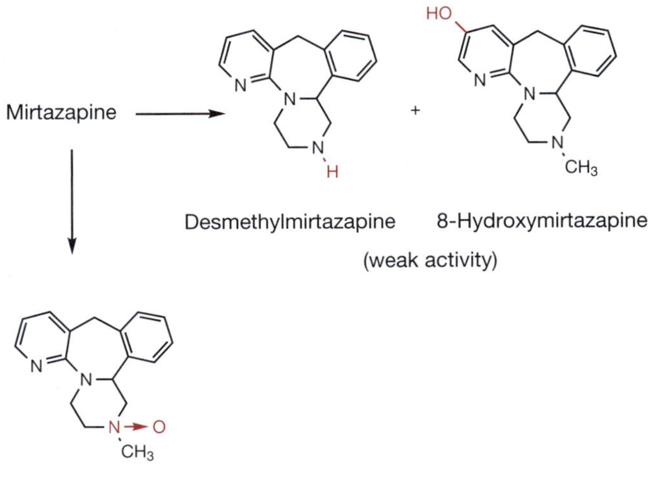

Figure 12.28 Metabolism of mirtazapine.

MIRTAZAPINE. Mirtazapine is a pyrazinopyridobenazepine antidepressant that is an isostere of the antidepressant mianserin (Fig. 12.28).[127] A seemingly simple isosteric replacement of an aromatic methine group (CH) in mianserin with a nitrogen to give a pyridine ring (mirtazapine) has profound effects on the physicochemical properties, pharmacokinetics, mechanisms of action, and antidepressant activities (Table 12.12). Profound differences between receptor affinity and transporter affinity, pharmacokinetics, regioselectivity in the formation of metabolites, and toxicity are observed for mianserin and mirtazapine and their antidepressant mechanisms of action.[127] The pyridine ring increases the polarity of the molecule and decreases the measured partition coefficient and the basicity. Mianserin is a potent inhibitor of NET, whereas mirtazapine has negligible effects on the inhibition of NET and SERT (K_i >4,600 and >10,000 nM respectively).

Mianserin is currently marketed in Europe as an antidepressant. Mianserin has not been approved by the FDA for

Table 12.12 Physicochemical Properties of Mirtazapine and Mianserin

Properties	Mirtazapine	Mianserin
pK_a	7.1	7.4
Lipophilicity (log $D_{7.4}$)	2.72	3.17
Polarity	2.63 debye	0.82 debye
NET affinity (pK_i)	5.8	7.1
5-HT release	Yes	No

5-HT, serotonin; NET, norepinephrine reuptake transporter.

use in the United States because of its serious adverse effects of agranulocytosis and leukopenia. Mirtazapine has not exhibited this adverse effect.

Mechanism of Action. Mirtazapine demonstrates a dual mode of action as an NaSSA and is an antagonist of central presynaptic α_2-adrenergic autoreceptors (K_i 20 nM)[128] and α_2-adrenergic heteroreceptors on both NE and 5-HT presynaptic axons, plus it is a potent antagonist of postsynaptic 5-HT_2 and 5-HT_3 receptors (K_i 6.3 and 8 nM) (see Fig. 12.3). It shows no significant affinity for 5-HT_{1A} or 5-HT_{1B} receptors (K_i >4,000 nM). Blocking these receptors inhibits the negative feedback loop, which increases the release of NE into the synapse. It enhances the release of NE and 5-HT_{1A}-mediated serotonergic transmission. This dual mode of action may conceivably be responsible for mirtazapine's rapid onset of action. The net outcome of these effects is increased noradrenergic activity together with increased serotonergic activity, especially at 5-HT_{1A} receptors.[128] This mechanism of action minimizes many of the adverse effects common to both TCAs and SSRIs. Mirtazapine has an onset of clinical effect in 2 to 4 weeks, similar to other antidepressants. Mirtazapine is extensively metabolized in the liver. CYP1A2, CYP2D6, and CYP3A4 are mainly responsible for its metabolism.[129] Steady-state concentrations are reached after 4 days in adults and 6 days in older adults. In vitro studies suggest that mirtazapine is unlikely to cause clinically significant DDIs. Dry mouth, sedation, and increases in appetite and body weight are the most common adverse effects. In contrast to the SSRIs, mirtazapine has no sexual side effects. In major depression, its efficacy is comparable to that of amitriptyline, clomipramine, doxepin, fluoxetine, paroxetine, citalopram, and venlafaxine. It seems to be safe and effective during long-term use. It displays some anticholinergic properties, and it produces sedative effects because of potent histamine H_1-receptor antagonism and orthostatic hypotension (because of moderate antagonism at peripheral α_1-adrenergic receptors). Its antidepressant effect is comparable to the TCAs and may be better than some SSRIs, especially in patients with depression of the melancholic type, but, at higher doses, it may cause drowsiness and weight gain. The drug generally is well tolerated, producing no more adverse events than the SSRIs and fewer adverse events than the TCAs.[129]

The pharmacokinetics for mirtazapine are shown in Table 12.11. Mirtazapine absorption is rapid and complete, with a bioavailability of approximately 50% as a result of first-pass metabolism.[129] The rate and extent of mirtazapine absorption are minimally affected by food. Dose and plasma levels are linearly related over a dose range of 15 to 80 mg. The elimination half-life of the (−)-enantiomer is approximately twice that of the (+)-enantiomer. In females of all ages, the elimination half-life is significantly longer than in males (mean half-life 37 vs 26 hours).[129]

Following oral administration, mirtazapine undergoes first-pass metabolism by *N*-demethylation and ring hydroxylation to its 8-hydroxy metabolite, followed by O-glucuronide conjugation.[129] In vitro studies indicate that CYP2D6 and CYP1A2 are involved in the formation of the 8-hydroxy metabolite and that CYP3A4 is responsible for the formation of the *N*-desmethyl and *N*-oxide metabolites (see Fig. 12.28). The 8-hydroxy and *N*-desmethyl metabolites possess weak pharmacologic activity, but their plasma levels are very low and thus are unlikely to contribute to the antidepressant action of mirtazapine. Clearance for mirtazapine may decrease in patients with hepatic or renal impairment, increasing its plasma concentrations. Therefore, it should be used with caution in these patients. In vitro studies have shown mirtazapine to be a weak inhibitor of CYP1A2, CYP2D6, and CYP3A4.

Esmirtazapine had been under development by Organon/Merck for the treatment of insomnia and vasomotor symptoms (eg, hot flashes) associated with menopause and as a potential antidepressant, but Merck terminated its clinical development in March 2010. Esmirtazapine is the (*S*)-(+)-enantiomer of mirtazapine and possesses similar overall pharmacologic activity to (±)-mirtazapine, enhancing the release of NE and 5-HT through blockage of presynaptic α_2-adrenergic receptors. It also blocks both 5-HT_2 and 5-HT_3 receptors and is a potent histamine H_1-receptor antagonist.

Gepirone. The FDA recently (September 2023) approved gepirone extended release (gepirone ER; EXXUA) for oral use for the treatment of MDD in adults. Gepirone is an azapirone compound related to the anxiolytic buspirone (see Chapter 11 for a more complete discussion of these compounds). Gepirone acts as a full agonist at serotonin 5-HT_{1A} autoreceptors as well as a partial agonist at postsynaptic serotonin 5-HT_{1A} receptors. The recommended starting dose is 18.2 mg once a day with food. Depending on clinical response, the dose may be titrated to as high as 72.6 mg daily over 7 days. For patients with compromised kidney function (<50 mL/min clearance), the starting dose of 18.2 mg daily may be increased to a maximum of 36.3 mg daily. Gepirone is primarily metabolized by CYP3A4 and excreted via the kidneys (~81%) as well as in the feces (~13%). Dosage should be adjusted if gepirone is given concomitantly with strong and moderate CYP3A4 inhibitors (eg, ketoconazole or verapamil).

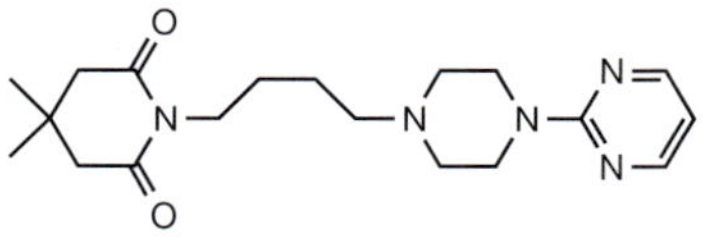

Gepirone

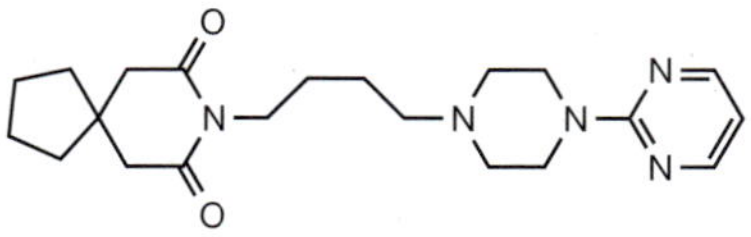

Buspirone

Monoamine Oxidase Inhibitors

The discovery of MAOIs resulted from a search for derivatives of isoniazid (isonicotinic acid hydrazide) (see Fig. 12.29) with antitubercular activity. During clinical trials with this hydrazine derivative, a rather consistent beneficial effect of mood elevation was noted in patients with tuberculosis who are depressed.[130] Although no longer used clinically, iproniazid (see Fig. 12.29), the first derivative to be synthesized, was found to be hepatotoxic at dosage levels required for

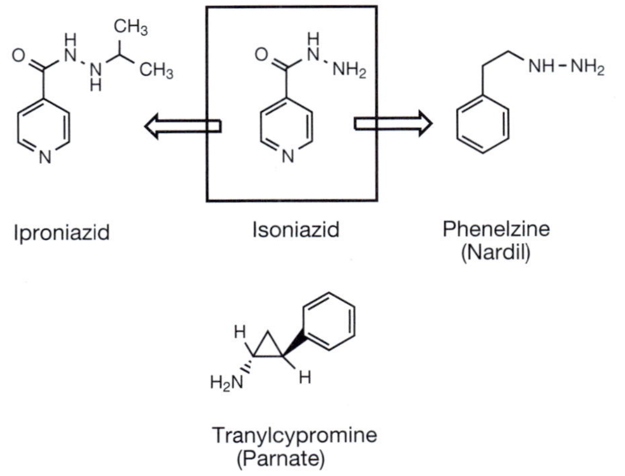

Figure 12.29 Monoamine oxidase inhibitor (MAOI) antidepressants.

antitubercular and antidepressant activity. The antidepressant activity of iproniazid, however, prompted a search for other MAOIs, which resulted in the synthesis of hydrazine and nonhydrazine MAOIs that were relatively less toxic than iproniazid.

The MAOIs can be classified as hydrazines (eg, phenelzine) and nonhydrazines (eg, tranylcypromine), which can block the oxidative deamination of naturally occurring monoamines.[131] MAOIs can also be classified according to their ability to selectively or inhibit MAO-A or MAO-B (nonselective inhibitors). The currently available MAOI antidepressants (phenelzine and tranylcypromine) (see Fig. 12.29) are considered to be irreversible inhibitors of both MAO-A and MAO-B.[130] The mechanism of antidepressant action of the MAOIs suggests that an increase in free 5-HT and NE and/or alterations in other amine concentrations within the CNS are mainly responsible for their antidepressant effect.

Mechanisms of Action Common to Monoamine Oxidase Inhibitors

An enzyme found mainly in nerve tissue and in the liver and lungs, MAO catalyzes the oxidative deamination of various amines, including epinephrine, NE, DA, and 5-HT. At least two isoforms of MAO exist, MAO-A and MAO-B, with differences in substrate preference, inhibitor specificity, and tissue distribution. The MAO-A substrates include 5-HT, and the MAO-B substrates include phenylethylamine. Tyramine, epinephrine, NE, and DA are substrates for both MAO-A and MAO-B. The cloning of MAO-A and MAO-B has demonstrated unequivocally that these enzymes consist of different amino acid sequences and also has provided insight regarding their structure, regulation, and function.[130] Both MAO-A and -B knockout mice exhibit distinct differences in neurotransmitter metabolism and behavior. The MAO-A knockout mice have elevated brain levels of 5-HT, NE, and DA, and they manifest aggressive behavior similar to human males with a deletion of MAO-A. In contrast, MAO-B knockout mice do not exhibit aggression, and only levels of phenylethylamine are increased. Both MAO-A and -B knockout mice show increased reactivity to stress.[131] These knockout mice are valuable models for investigating the role of monoamines in psychoses and in neurodegenerative- and stress-related disorders.

The pharmacologic effects of MAOIs are cumulative. A latent period of a few days to several months may occur before the onset of the antidepressant action, and effects may persist for up to 3 weeks following discontinuance of therapy.[131]

Adverse Effects Common to Monoamine Oxidase Inhibitors

Common side effects for the nonselective MAOIs include difficulty getting to sleep and broken sleep, daytime insomnia, agitation, dizziness on standing that results in fainting (orthostatic hypotension), dry mouth, tremor (slight shake of muscles of arms and hands), syncope, palpitations, tachycardia, dizziness, headache, confusion, weakness, overstimulation including increased anxiety, constipation, GI disturbances, edema, dry mouth, weight gain, and sexual disturbances.

Drug Interactions Common to Monoamine Oxidase Inhibitors

The most significant drug interaction limiting the efficacy of the nonselective MAOIs is with certain foods that have the potential to cause hypertensive crisis because of the release and potentiation of CAs. The severity and consequences of such interactions vary among individuals from only minor increases in blood pressure to substantial and rapid increases in blood pressure within 20 minutes. These patients may experience symptoms associated with brain hemorrhage or cardiac failure (Table 12.13).

Hypertensive crises with MAOIs have occurred in some patients following ingestion of foods containing large amounts of tyramine or tryptophan. In general, patients taking MAOIs should avoid protein foods that have undergone protein breakdown by aging, fermentation, pickling, smoking, or bacterial contamination. Some of the common foods to avoid are shown in Table 12.13. Patients should be warned against eating foods with a high tyramine content, because hypertensive crisis may result. Excessive amounts of caffeine also reportedly may precipitate hypertensive crisis.

The MAOIs interfere with the hepatic metabolism of many prescription and OTC drugs and may potentiate the actions of their pharmacologic effects (ie, cold decongestants, sympathomimetic amines, general anesthetics, barbiturates, and morphine).

Therapeutic Uses Common to Monoamine Oxidase Inhibitors

The MAOIs are indicated in patients with atypical (exogenous) depression and in some patients who are unresponsive to other antidepressive therapy. They rarely are a drug of first choice. Unlabeled uses have included bulimia (having characteristics of atypical depression), treatment of cocaine addiction (phenelzine), night terrors, PTSD, some migraines resistant to other therapies, seasonal affective disorder (30 mg/d), and treatment of some panic disorders. A list of information that should be transmitted to the patient concerning use of MAOIs is shown in Table 12.14.

Table 12.13 Foods to Be Avoided Due to Potential Monoamine Oxidase Inhibitor–Food Interactions

Cheeses	**Cheddar**	**Meats**	**Chicken Livers**
	Camembert		Genoa salami
	Stilton		Hard salami
	Processed cheese		Pepperoni
	Sour cream		Lebanon bologna
Spirits	Chianti	**Fruit**	Figs (overripe/canned)
	Champagne		Raisins
	Alcohol-free/reduced wines		Overripe bananas
Fish	Pickled herring	**Dairy product**	Yogurt
	Anchovies	**Vegetable products**	Yeast extract
	Caviar		Pods, broad beans
Miscellaneous	Shrimp paste		Bean curd
	Chocolate		Soy sauce
	Meat tenderizers (papaya)		Avocado

Table 12.14 Common Information for Patients Taking Monoamine Oxidase Inhibitors

Patient Information	Recommendation
Discontinuance of therapy or dose adjustment	Consult physician.
Adding medication (prescription/over the counter)	Consult physician.
Tyramine-containing foods and over-the-counter products	Avoid.
Drowsiness, blurred vision	Avoid driving or performing tasks requiring alertness or coordination.
Dizziness, weakness, fainting	Arise from sitting position slowly.
Alcohol use	Avoid alcohol.
Onset of action	Effects may be delayed for a few weeks.
Severe headache, palpitation, tachycardia, sense of constriction in throat or chest, sweating, stiff neck, nausea or vomiting	Consult physician.
New physician or dentist	Inform practitioner of use.

Nonselective Monoamine Oxidase Inhibitor Antidepressants

PHENELZINE. Phenelzine is a hydrazine MAOI (see Fig. 12.29). Its mechanism of action is the prolonged, nonselective irreversible inhibition of MAO-A and MAO-B.[131] Phenelzine has been used with some success in the management of bulimia nervosa. The MAOIs, however, are potentially dangerous in patients with binge eating and purging behaviors, and the American Psychiatric Association states that MAOIs should be used with caution in the management of bulimia nervosa.

Limited information is available regarding MAOI pharmacokinetics of phenelzine (Table 12.15). Phenelzine appears

Table 12.15 Pharmacokinetics of Monoamine Oxidase Inhibitors

Parameters	Phenelzine (Nardil)	Tranylcypromine (Parnate)
Oral bioavailability (%)	NA	~50
Lipophilicity (Log $D_{7.4}$)	0.51	0.46
Protein binding (%)		NA
Volume of distribution (L/kg)	NA	1.1-5.7
Elimination half-life (hours)	NA	79
Peak plasma concentration (hours)	2-3	1.5 (0.7-3.5)
Excretion route	Urine	Urine 62
		Feces

NA, not available.

to be well absorbed following oral administration; however, maximal inhibition of MAO occurs within 5 to 10 days. Acetylation of phenelzine to its inactive acetylated metabolite appears to be a minor metabolic pathway. Phenelzine is a substrate as well as an inhibitor of MAO, and major identified metabolites of phenelzine include phenylacetic acid and *p*-hydroxyphenylacetic acid. Phenelzine also elevates brain GABA levels, probably via its β-phenylethylamine metabolite. The clinical effects of phenelzine may continue for up to 2 weeks after discontinuation of therapy. Phenelzine is excreted in the urine mostly as its *N*-acetyl metabolite. Interindividual variability in plasma concentrations has been observed among patients who are either slow or fast acetylators. Slow acetylators of hydrazine MAOIs may yield exaggerated adverse effects after standard dosing. If adverse neurologic reactions occur during phenelzine therapy, phenelzine-induced pyridoxine deficiency should be considered. Pyridoxine supplementation can correct the deficiency while allowing continuance of phenelzine therapy.

TRANYLCYPROMINE. Tranylcypromine is a nonhydrazine, irreversible MAOI antidepressant agent that was designed as the cyclopropyl analogue of amphetamine (Fig. 12.29). Instead of exhibiting amphetamine-like stimulation, its mechanism of action is nonselective, irreversible inhibition of MAO. Its onset of antidepressant action is more rapid than for phenelzine. Tranylcypromine is well absorbed following oral administration (Table 12.15). Metabolism occurs via aromatic ring hydroxylation and *N*-acetylation. It is a competitive inhibitor of CYP2C19 and CYP2D6 and a noncompetitive inhibitor of CYP2C9.[131] Most metabolism studies suggest that tranylcypromine is not metabolized to amphetamine, contrary to debate. Maximal MAO inhibition, however, occurs within 5 to 10 days. The GI absorption of the tranylcypromine shows interindividual variation and may be biphasic in some individuals, achieving an initial peak within approximately 1 hour and a secondary peak within 2 to 3 hours. It has been suggested that this apparent biphasic absorption in some individuals may represent different absorption rates. Following discontinuance of tranylcypromine, the drug is excreted within 24 hours. On withdrawal of tranylcypromine, MAO activity is recovered in 3 to 5 days (possibly in up to 10 days). Concentrations of urinary tryptamine, an indicator of MAO-A inhibition, return to normal within 72 to 110 hours.

Mood Stabilizers

Bipolar disorder is a prevalent mental disorder with a global impact. Mood stabilizers have acute and long-term effects and, at a minimum, are prophylactic for manic or depressive disorders.[132] Lithium is the classic mood stabilizer and exhibits significant effects on mania and depression but may be augmented or substituted by some antiepileptic drugs. The biochemical basis for mood stabilizer therapies or the molecular origins of bipolar disorder is unknown. Lithium ion directly inhibits two signal transduction pathways. It suppresses inositol 1,4,5-trisphosphate (IP_3) signaling through depletion of intracellular inositol and inhibits glycogen synthase kinase-3 (GSK-3), a multifunctional protein kinase. A number of GSK-3 substrates are involved in neuronal function and organization and, therefore, present plausible targets for manic depression. Despite these intriguing observations, it remains unclear how changes in IP_3 signaling underlie the origins of bipolar disorder.[132]

Inositol (myo-inositol), a naturally occurring isomer of glucose, is a key intermediate of the phosphatidylinositol signaling pathway, a second-messenger system used by noradrenergic, serotonergic, and cholinergic receptors. The suggestion that lithium might treat mania via its reduction of inositol levels led to experiments showing that oral doses of inositol reverse the behavioral effects of lithium in animals and the side effects of lithium in humans. CSF levels of inositol are low in individuals who are depressed.[133] The effectiveness of inositol in treating manic depression was shown in a double-blind trial that large doses of inositol (11 g) increased inositol concentrations in human CSF by 70% and led to improvement in patients who are depressed compared to placebo.[133] Valproic acid and carbamazepine are antiepileptic drugs with mood-stabilizing properties that also inhibit IP_3 signaling through the inositol-depletion mechanism.

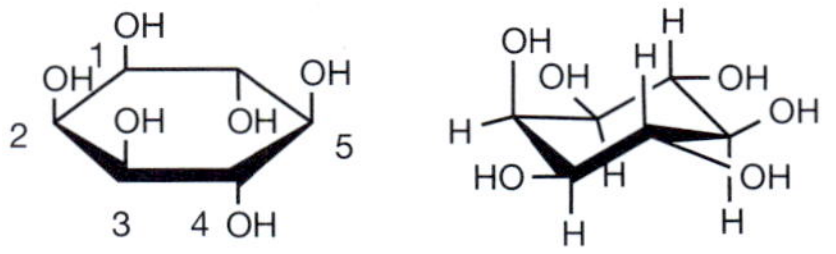

myo-Inositol

Inositol significantly reduced the number of panic attacks per week in patients as compared to fluvoxamine and without the nausea and tiredness that are common with fluvoxamine. Inositol has few known side effects, thus making it attractive for administration to patients with manic depression who are ambivalent about taking other antidepressant drugs.

Lithium

Lithium (from the Greek word *lithos*, meaning "stone") is a monovalent cation that competes with sodium, potassium, calcium, and magnesium ions at intracellular binding sites, sugar phosphatases, protein surfaces, carrier binding sites, and transport sites. Because of its small ionic size, lithium ion (Li^+) readily passes through sodium channels of cellular membranes, and high concentrations can block the narrow potassium channels during impulse conduction. In the 1870s, claims for the healthful effects of Li^+ fueled the market for products such as Lithia Beer and Lithia Springs Mineral Water (in 1887, analysis of Lithia Springs Mineral Water proved the water to be rich not only in Li^+ but also in potassium, calcium, magnesium, fluoride and other essential trace minerals). In 1890, the Lithia Springs Sanatorium (Georgia) was established, using natural lithium water to treat alcohol and opium addiction and compulsive behavior, even though manic depression had not been identified as a form of mental illness until the early 1900s.

Lithium's mood-stabilizing properties were revitalized in the 1940s when Australian physician John Cade hypothesized that a toxin in the blood was responsible for bipolar illness.[133] Believing that uric acid would protect individuals from this toxin, he began studying the effects of a mixture of uric acid and Li^+ in rats. Lithium carbonate was used to dissolve the uric acid. He observed a calming effect of this combination on the rats and subsequently determined that the Li^+, rather than the uric acid, was responsible for this calming effect. He then speculated that lithium might be useful in humans as a mood attenuator, subsequently administered lithium to a sample of patients with bipolar disorder, and discovered that Li^+ not only decreased the symptoms of mania but also prevented the recurrence of both depression and mania when taken regularly by these patients. After a decade of clinical trials, the FDA approved lithium for treatment of mania in 1970.[133,134]

Lithium carbonate (Eskalith) is the most commonly used salt of lithium to treat manic depression. Lithium carbonate dosage forms are labeled in mg and mEq/dosage unit, and lithium citrate (Lithobid) is labeled as mg equivalent to lithium carbonate and mEq/dosage unit. Lithium is effectively used to control and prevent manic episodes in 70% to 80% of those with bipolar disorder as well as to treat other forms of depression. Those who respond to lithium for depression often are those who have not responded to TCAs after several weeks of treatment. When taking lithium in addition to their antidepressants, some of these people have shown significant improvement.

Mechanism of Action. Lithium therapy for disorders is believed to be effective because of its ability to reduce signal transduction through the phosphatidylinositol signaling pathway (Fig. 12.30).[133,134] In this pathway, the second messengers diacylglycerol and IP_3 are produced from the enzymatic hydrolysis of phosphatidylinositol-4,5-bisphosphate (a membrane phospholipid) by the receptor-mediated activation of the membrane-bound, phosphatidylinositol-specific phospholipase C. The second-messenger activity for IP_3 is terminated by its hydrolysis in three steps by inositol monophosphatases to inactive inositol, thus completing the signaling pathway. To recharge the signaling pathway, inositol must be recycled back to phosphatidylinositol bisphosphate by inositol phospholipid–synthesizing enzymes in the CNS, because inositol is unable to cross the BBB into the CNS in sufficient concentrations to maintain the signaling pathway. By uncompetitive inhibition of inositol phosphatases in the signaling pathway, the therapeutic plasma concentrations of lithium ion deplete the pool of inositol available for the resynthesis of phosphatidylinositol-4,5-bisphosphate, ultimately decreasing its cellular levels and, thereby, reducing the enzymatic formation of the second messengers.[133] Thus, Li^+ restores the balance among aberrant signaling pathways in critical regions of the brain.

The effects of Li^+ on disorders are surprisingly specific because of the inability of inositol to cross the BBB and replenish depleted inositol levels. Li^+ exerts its greatest influence on this signaling pathway when the Li^+ concentration is at saturation conditions.

The clinical efficacy of lithium in the prophylaxis of recurrent affective episodes in bipolar disorder is characterized by a lag in onset and remains for weeks to months after

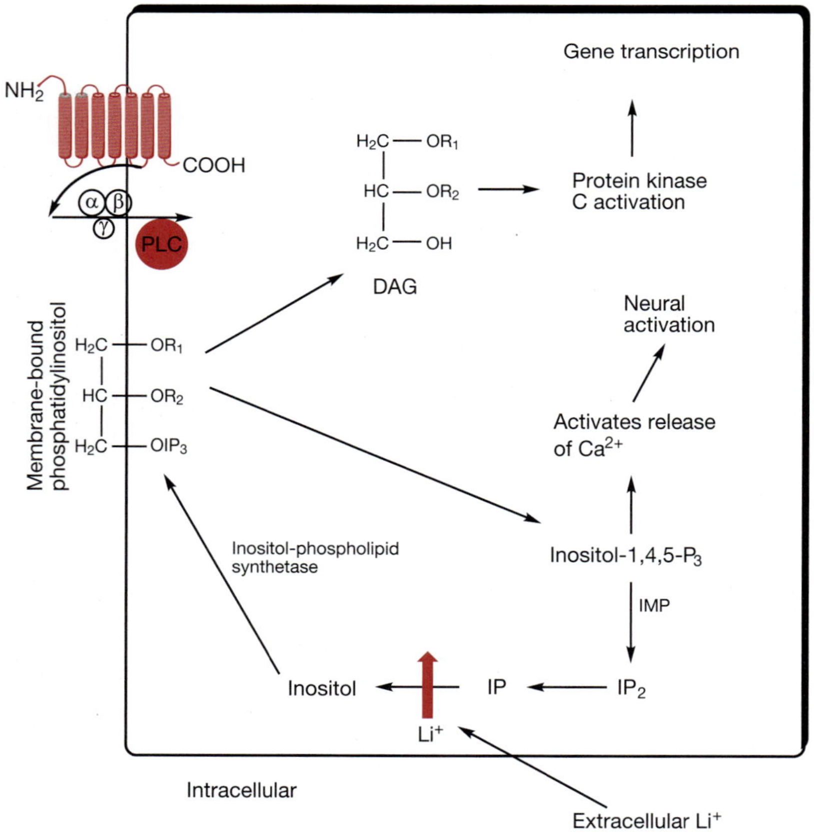

Figure 12.30 Intracellular phosphatidylinositol signaling pathway and site of action for lithium. Phospholipase (PLC) is a membrane-bound enzyme. DAG, diacylglyceride; IMP, inositol monophosphatase; IP, inositol phosphate; IP_2, inositol bisphosphate.

discontinuation. Thus, the long-term therapeutic effect of lithium likely requires reprogramming of gene expression. Protein kinase C and GSK-3 signal transduction pathways are perturbed by chronic lithium at therapeutically relevant concentrations and have been implicated in modulating synaptic function in nerve terminals.[134]

Pharmacokinetics. The absorption of Li^+ is rapid and complete within 6 to 8 hours. The absorption rate of slow-release capsules is slower, and the total amount of Li^+ absorbed lower than with other dosage forms. Li^+ is not protein bound. The elimination half-life for older adults (39 hours) is longer than that for adult patients (24 hours), which, in turn, is longer than that for adolescent patients (18 hours). The time to peak serum concentration for lithium carbonate is dependent on the dosage form (tablets, 1-3 hours; extended tab, 4 hours; slow release, 3 hours). Steady-state serum concentrations are reached in 4 days, with the desirable dose targeted to give a maintenance Li^+ plasma concentration range of 0.6 to 1.2 mEq/L, with a level of 0.5 mEq/L for older adults.[134] The risk of bipolar recurrence was approximately 3-fold greater for patients with Li^+ dosages that gave plasma concentrations of 0.4 to 0.6 mEq/L. Adverse reactions are frequent at therapeutic doses, and adherence is a big problem. Toxic reactions are rare at serum Li^+ levels of less than 1.5 mEq/L. Mild-to-moderate toxic reactions may occur at levels from 1.5 to 2.5 mEq/L, and severe reactions may be seen at levels from 2.0 to 2.5 mEq/L, depending on individual response. The onset of therapeutic action for clinical improvement is 1 to 3 weeks. Renal elimination of Li^+ is 95%, with 80% actively reabsorbed in the proximal tubule. The rate of Li^+ urinary excretion decreases with age. Fecal elimination is less than 1%.

Drug Interactions. Lithium pharmacokinetics may be influenced by a number of factors, including age. Older adults require lower doses of Li^+ to achieve serum concentrations similar to those observed in younger adults as a result of reduced volume of distribution and reduced renal clearance. Li^+ clearance decreases as the glomerular filtration rate decreases with increasing age. Reduced Li^+ clearance is expected in patients with hypertension, congestive heart failure, or renal dysfunction. Larger Li^+ maintenance doses are required in patients who are obese compared with those who are nonobese. The most clinically significant pharmacokinetic drug interactions associated with lithium involve drugs that are commonly used in older adults and that can increase serum Li^+ concentrations. People who are taking lithium should consult their physician before taking the following drugs: acetazolamide, antihypertensives, angiotensin-converting enzyme inhibitors, NSAIDs, calcium channel blockers, carbamazepine, thiazide diuretics, hydroxyzine, muscle relaxants, neuroleptics, table salt, baking powder, tetracycline, TCAs, MAOIs, and caffeine. The tolerability of lithium is lower in older adult patients. Lithium toxicity can occur in older adults at concentrations considered to be "therapeutic" in the general adult populations. Serum concentrations of Li^+ ion need to be markedly reduced in the older adult population—and particularly so in the very old and frail.[134]

Adverse Effects. Common side effects of Li^+ include nausea, loss of appetite, and mild diarrhea, which usually taper off within the first few weeks. Dizziness and hand tremors also have been reported. Increased production of urine and excessive thirst are two common side effects that usually are not serious problems, but patients with kidney disease should not be given Li^+. Taking the day's dosage of Li^+ at bedtime also seems to help with the problem of increased urination. Other side effects of Li^+ include weight gain, hypothyroidism, increased white blood cell count, skin rashes, and birth defects.[133,134]

While on Li^+, a patient's blood level must be closely monitored. If the blood level of Li^+ is too low, the patient's symptoms will not be relieved. If the blood level of lithium ion is too high, there is a danger of a toxic reaction.

Therapeutic Uses. For many years, lithium has been the treatment of choice for bipolar disorder, because it can be effective in smoothing out the mood swings common to this condition. Its use must be carefully monitored, however, because the range between an effective and a toxic dose is small.

Non-Monoaminergic Antidepressants

N-Methyl-D-Aspartate Receptor Antagonists

NMDARs have received much attention over the last few decades, due to their role in many types of neural plasticity on the one hand, and their involvement in excitotoxicity on the other hand.[54,55] There is great interest in developing clinically relevant NMDAR antagonists that would block NMDAR activation, without interfering with NMDAR function needed for normal synaptic transmission and plasticity.[54] Current understanding of the structure of NMDARs, the mechanisms of NMDAR activation and modulation, and data describing the properties of various types of NMDAR inhibition provide information for the development of NMDAR inhibitors with desirable antidepressant properties. These compounds show voltage-independent block that is predicted to preferentially target excessive tonic NMDAR activation. These antidepressants are also all compatible and display minimal disruption of normal synaptic transmission. Thus, NMDAR inhibitors are a promising class of antidepressants that may lead to the development of neuroprotective drugs with optimal therapeutic profiles.[56] The past decade has seen a steady accumulation of evidence supporting a role for the excitatory amino acid neurotransmitter, glutamine, and its mGluR1 and mGluR5 receptors in depression and antidepressant activity.[56] Glutamine plays an essential role as a neurotransmitter in many physiologic functions, and an increase in glutamine release can result in activation of NMDARs, an underlying cause for depression and anxiety. The NMDAR is a ligand-gated ion channel that mediates excitatory synaptic transmission in the CNS (see Chapter 8). This channel opening and receptor activation are triggered by synaptically released glutamine and require the binding of glycine, which is a coagonist. NMDAR antagonists of mGluR1 and mGluR5 receptors, as well as positive modulators of AMPARs, have antidepressant-like activity in a variety of preclinical models. Furthermore, evidence implicates disturbances in glutamine metabolism, NMDA, and mGluR1/5 receptors in depression and suicidality.[57]

cis-1-Phenyl-2-[1-aminopropyl]-*N*,*N*-diethylcarboxamide, an NMDAR antagonist and homologue of milnacipran, produces sustained relief from depressive symptoms. Several studies have shown that chronic antidepressant treatment can modulate NMDAR expression and function. Preclinical studies with this and other NMDAR antagonists have demonstrated their potential antidepressant properties.[54,57-59]

KETAMINE. Ketamine, a nonselective NMDAR antagonist, is used widely in medicine as an anesthetic agent. However, ketamine's mechanisms of action lead to widespread physiologic effects, some of which are now coming to the forefront of research for the treatment of diverse medical disorders, including the treatment of depression; pain syndromes including acute pain, chronic pain, and headache; neurologic applications including neuroprotection and seizures; and alcohol and substance use disorders.[135] Ketamine has a potential role in the treatment of all of these conditions. A single subanesthetic dose of ketamine produces rapid (within hours) and long-lasting antidepressant effects in patients who are resistant to other antidepressants. Ketamine is a racemic mixture of *S*- and *R*-ketamine enantiomers, with the *S*-ketamine isomer being the more active antidepressant.[136] However, research in this area is still in its early stages, and larger studies are required to evaluate ketamine's efficacy for non-anesthetic purposes in the general population.

The electron microscope structures of human GluN1-GluN2A and GluN1-GluN2B NMDARs in complex with *S*-ketamine, glycine, and glutamate show that the binding pocket for *S*-ketamine is between the channel gate and binding pocket.[136] Molecular dynamics simulation showed that *S*-ketamine moves between two distinct locations within the binding pocket. Two amino acids, leucine 642 on GluN2A (homologous to leucine 643 on GluN2B) and asparagine 616 on GluN1, were identified as key residues that form hydrophobic and hydrogen-bond interactions with ketamine, and mutations at these residues reduced the potency of ketamine in blocking NMDAR channel activity. These findings show structurally how ketamine binds to and acts on human NMDARs, and pave the way for the future development of ketamine-based antidepressants.[135] Ketamine acts by modulating glutamine, one of the brain's key neurotransmitters, an amino acid found in 80% of neurons. Glutamine is the most plentiful of all the neurotransmitters, and it influences the formation of, and the number of, brain synapses—the vital connections between neurons. Glutamine also acts with another important neurotransmitter, GABA, to maintain a healthy and well-functioning nervous system. An imbalance between GABA and glutamine can cause problems, including anxiety, difficulty sleeping, overstimulation, and other mental conditions. Evidence suggests ketamine helps rebalance the glutamine system by acting as an NMDAR antagonist, and this increase in glutamine is believed to be one key factor in enabling the antidepressant effect of ketamine.

For the past 20 years, researchers at top scientific institutions and universities have researched the efficacy of ketamine in the treatment of mental health disorders and shown positive results.[54] Despite the availability of numerous monoaminergic-based antidepressants, most patients require several weeks, if not months, to respond to these treatments, and many patients never attain sustained remission of their symptoms. The noncompetitive, glutamatergic NMDAR antagonist (*R,S*)-ketamine exerts rapid and sustained antidepressant effects after a single dose in patients with depression, but its use is associated with undesirable side effects.[135] The metabolism of (*R,S*)-ketamine to (2*S*,6*S*;2*R*,6*R*)-hydroxynorketamine (HNK) is essential for its antidepressant effects, and that the (2*R*,6*R*)-HNK enantiomer exerts behavioral and antidepressant-related actions in humans.[137] These antidepressant actions are independent of NMDAR inhibition but involve early and sustained activation of AMPARs (see Chapter 8).

Several preclinical studies in the 1990s revealed an important role for NMDAR antagonists in the mechanism of action of antidepressants and has generated considerable interest in NMDAR as a target for new antidepressant therapies.[136] Recent human studies have shown that the noncompetitive NMDAR antagonist ketamine leads to rapid and sustained antidepressant effects in patients with TRD.[136] These findings have given rise to the hypothesis that the NMDA antagonist ketamine (an anesthetic) might have potential as an antidepressant, which has been validated in drug-free patients with MDD. A significant reduction in depression was observed 3 hours after a single infusion of ketamine, and this effect was sustained for at least 72 hours.[138] This rapid antidepressant effect of ketamine has been replicated using larger sample sizes and patients with TRD. This rapid effect has a high therapeutic value in patients with depression who are suicidal who might benefit from such a rapid and marked effect, as their acute mortality risk is not considerably diminished with conventional antidepressants owing to their long delay in onset of action (usually 2-3 weeks). Suicidal thoughts were reduced 24 hours after a single ketamine infusion.[138] Ketamine therapy could be extended to other disorders in which NMDARs are implicated, such as bipolar disorder and addiction.

Thus, the therapeutic effects of monoaminergic antidepressants, ketamine, and other NMDA antagonists may be mediated by increased AMPA-to-NMDA glutamine receptor throughput in critical neuronal circuits, and ketamine directly mediates this throughput.[139] Since the monoaminergic antidepressants work indirectly and gradually, this may explain, in part, the lag of onset of several weeks to months that is observed with traditional antidepressants.[140] These studies suggest that an intimate relationship exists between regulation of monoaminergic and excitatory amino acid neurotransmission and antidepressant effects.

ESKETAMINE. Esketamine, also known as (*S*+)-ketamine, is the *S*-enantiomer of ketamine, a dissociative hallucinogen drug used as a general anesthetic and as an antidepressant.[141] Esketamine acts primarily as a noncompetitive NMDAR antagonist and also as a DAT. It works differently by acting on a glutamine pathway in the brain. The exact way esketamine works is not fully understood. It shows properties of being a rapid-acting antidepressant. Esketamine was introduced for medical use as an anesthetic in Germany in 1997 and was subsequently marketed in other countries. Esketamine was approved as a Schedule III drug by the FDA as the first rapid-acting therapy for MDD and TRD in 2018. Esketamine is the only Schedule III FDA-approved nasal spray for adult patients with MDD who have had an inadequate response to two or more oral antidepressants (TRD). Esketamine is not for use to prevent or relieve pain (anesthetic). It is not known if esketamine is safe or effective as an anesthetic medicine and in preventing suicide or in reducing suicidal thoughts or actions. It is not known if esketamine is safe and effective in children.

Esketamine, *S*(+)-ketamine (Spravato nasal spray) enantiomer is a general anesthetic and a dissociative hallucinogen.[137] It is given by IV infusion or spray. Esketamine is approximately twice as potent as an anesthetic as (±)-ketamine.[137] It is eliminated from the human body more quickly than arketamine *R*(−)-ketamine or (±)-ketamine. In mice studies, the rapid antidepressant effect of arketamine was greater and lasted longer than that of esketamine or 2*R*,6*R*-HNK, a major metabolite of *R*-ketamine.[142] Esketamine inhibits DAT 8 times more than arketamine, thus increasing DA activity in the brain. Patients also generally recover mental function more quickly after being treated with pure esketamine, because it is cleared from the system more quickly.[142]

Esketamine has an affinity for the PCP-binding site of the NMDAR 3 to 4 times greater than that of arketamine. Esketamine generally has a more dissociative or hallucinogenic effect, while arketamine is reportedly more relaxing.

Esketamine nasal spray could provide the first new mechanism of action in 30 years to treat MDD and TRD. It can be self-administered by patients under the supervision of health care professionals for TRD. It can also be used to treat MDD in patients with imminent risk for suicide.[138]

Arketamine. Arketamine, also (*R*)-(−)-ketamine, is the (*R*)-(−)-enantiomer of ketamine. Similarly to (±)-ketamine and esketamine, arketamine is biologically active; however, it is less potent as an NMDAR antagonist and anesthetic and thus has never been approved or marketed for clinical use as an enantiopure drug. Relative to esketamine, arketamine possesses 4 to 5 times less affinity for the phencyclidine (PCP) site of the NMDAR. It is significantly less potent than (±)-ketamine and especially esketamine in terms of anesthetic, analgesic, and sedative-hypnotic effects. It has been suggested that arketamine may play a role in the hallucinogenic effects of racemic ketamine and that it may be responsible for the lowering of the seizure threshold seen with (±)-ketamine. Esketamine inhibits the DAT 8 times more potently as a DA reuptake inhibitor. Arketamine and esketamine possess similar potency for interaction with the muscarinic AChRs. Thus, arketamine appears to be more effective as a rapid-acting antidepressant than esketamine.

A study conducted in mice found that ketamine's antidepressant activity is not caused by ketamine inhibiting the NMDAR, but rather by sustained activation of a different glutamine receptor, the AMPAR, by a metabolite, (2*R*,6*R*)-HNK.[139] Arketamine is an AMPAR agonist. Arketamine shows greater and longer-lasting rapid antidepressant effects in animal models of depression relative to esketamine. It has been suggested that this activity may be due to affinity at α_7-nicotinic receptor, as norketamine and HNK are potent antagonists of this receptor and markers of potential rapid antidepressant effects.

The currently available antidepressant medications that work through optimizing the monoaminergic system are often limited by their lack of efficacy or their adverse effects. There is increasing evidence that some neuropeptides, including substance P, CRF, neuropeptide Y, vasopressin, and galanin, may have relevance in both depression and anxiety. Modulation of monoaminergic transmission is the most likely mechanism by which neuropeptides may work in these disorders. These neuropeptides and their receptors may serve not only as potential therapeutic targets for treatment of depression and anxiety, but may also help enhance our understanding of the psychopathology of these two major psychiatric disorders.

Ketamine Pharmacokinetics. (*R*,*S*)-Ketamine is extensively metabolized involving enantioselective *N*-demethylation to (*R*,*S*)-norketamine by HLMs and confirmed by expressed CYPs (Fig. 12.31).[137,142] The *N*-demethylation of (*S*)-ketamine to (*S*)-norketamine is greater than that of (*R*)-ketamine to (*R*)-norketamine. The CYPs associated with the metabolic *N*-demethylation of (*R*,*S*)-ketamine to (*R*,*S*)-norketamine was primarily 2B6 with some contribution of CYP2A6 and CYP3A4/5.[142] Expressed studies with (*S*)-ketamine and (*R*)-ketamine suggest that CYP3A4/5 plays a greater role in the metabolic clearance of (*R*)-ketamine than (*S*)-ketamine.

In addition to *N*-demethylation, (*R*,*S*)-norketamine is further transformed regio- and enantioselectively into a series of diastereomeric HNK metabolites arising from hydroxylation of the cyclohexanone ring at the C6, C5, and C4 positions, with (*S*)-hydroxylation being preferred at these positions. (*R*,*S*)-Norketamine hydroxylation is enantioselective and regioselective with (*S*)-norketamine preferentially converted to (2*S*,6*S*)- and (2*S*,6*R*)-HNK (2a) and to (2*R*,6*S*)-and (2*R*,6*R*)-HNK diastereomer (2b).[142] The CYP isoforms associated with the regio- and enantioselective 6-hydroxylation of (*R*,*S*)-norketamine have demonstrated that the *S*-hydroxylation is mediated primarily by CYP2B6 and CYP2A6.

The enantioselective hydroxylation of (*S*)-ketamine predominates relative to (*R*)-ketamine.[137] Thus, the primary hydroxyketamine (HK) diastereomeric metabolite from the HLM incubation of (*R*,*S*)-ketamine is (2*S*,6*S*)-HK and (2*R*,6*S*)-HK, respectively (1a,1b). With expressed enzymes, (*R*)- and (*S*)-ketamine were hydroxylated into the HK diastereomers with the formation of (2*R*,6*S*)-HK diastereomer (1b) slightly favored relative to the (2*S*,6*R*)-HK diastereomer (1a).[142] The expressed CYP isoforms associated with the regio- and enantioselective 6-hydroxylation of (*R*,*S*)-ketamine have demonstrated that the 6*S*-hydroxylation is primarily mediated by CYP2B6 and CYP2A6, with minor contribution from CYP3A4/5. Regio-hydroxylation at the 6-position is the preferred site of hydroxylation because of C-H activation by the adjacent 1-ketone group. The HK diastereomers are further transformed by *N*-demethylation into the corresponding HNK diastereomers, 2a and 2b. The 4- and 5-HNK diastereomers are found in minor amounts. Recent results indicate that the incubation of (*R*,*S*)-ketamine with HLMs also produced phenolic metabolites.

The rates of formation of 1a and 1b diastereomers with expressed CYP3A4/5 suggest their greater role in the metabolic clearance of (*R*)-ketamine than (*S*)-ketamine. The

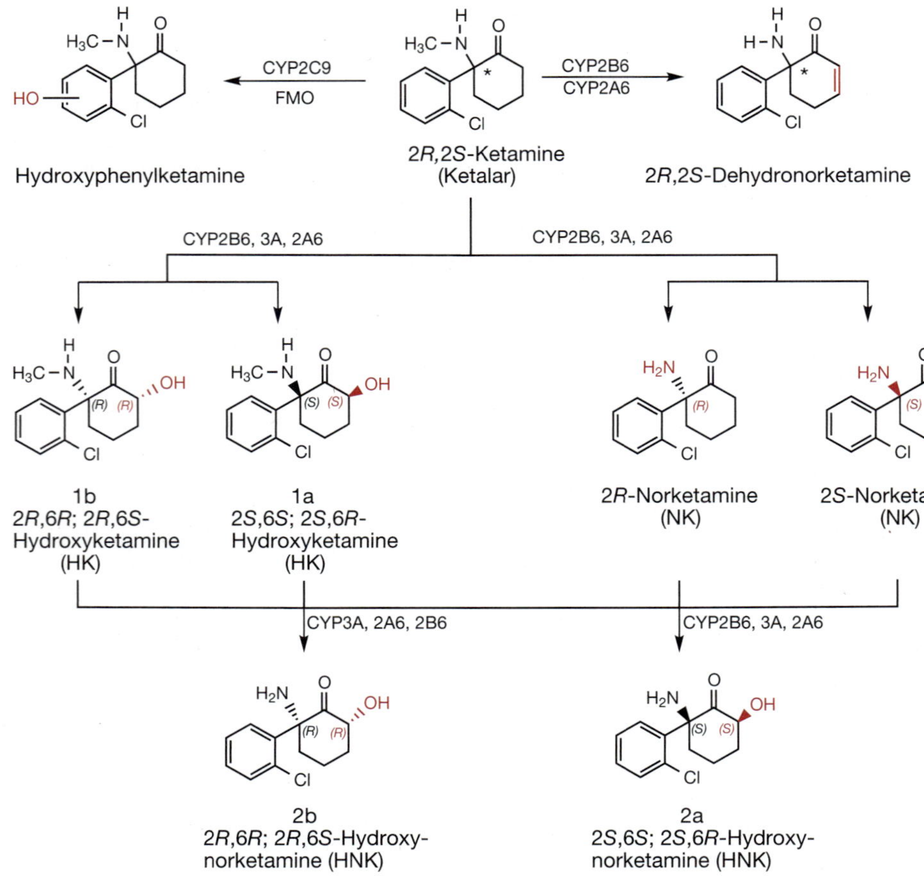

Figure 12.31 Metabolism of ketamine.

formation of 1a,1b is enantioselective with the hydroxylation of (*S*)-ketamine predominating relative to (*R*)-ketamine, and the reaction is enantiospecific producing primarily a *S*-configuration at the C6 carbinol.[142] Thus, the primary HK metabolite from the expressed incubation of (*S*)-ketamine with CYP2B6 is (2*S*,6*S*)-HK. (*R*,*S*)-Ketamine was hydroxylated into the HK diastereomers, 2a and 2b, with the formation of (2*R*,6*S*)-HK slightly favored relative to the (2*S*,6*R*)-HK diastereomer.

(*R*,*S*)-Ketamine is also transformed into the enantiomeric 5,6-dehydronorketamine ((*R*,*S*)-DHNK), and the expressed results suggest that DHNK is derived from 5-HNK produced by CYP2B6-mediated hydroxylation at the C5-position on the cyclohexanone ring of norketamine.[142] The primary isoform associated with the formation of the phenolic metabolite from (*R*,*S*)-ketamine was CYP2C9, while flavin monooxygenase (FMO) enzymes appeared to be the major factor in the formation of this metabolite from (*S*)-ketamine.[142]

The metabolic transformations observed in the in vitro HLM studies are consistent with the metabolism and disposition of (*R*,*S*)-ketamine determined in clinical studies. (*R*,*S*)-Ketamine, (*R*,*S*)-norketamine, and (*R*,*S*)-DHNK were identified in plasma samples obtained from patients receiving (*R*,*S*)-ketamine, and all of the major metabolites of (*R*,*S*)-ketamine were identified in urine samples from a single 50-mg oral dose of (*R*,*S*)-ketamine.[142]

The most typical route of administration is via IV infusion, which rapidly attains maximum plasma concentrations 5 to 30 minutes after administration. Oral bioavailability of (*R*,*S*)-ketamine is 16% to 29%, with peak concentration levels of the drug occurring within 20 to 110 minutes because of extensive first-pass hepatic metabolism. Oral bioavailability of (*S*)-ketamine is 8% to 11% with greater first-pass metabolism. Intranasal bioavailability is 45% to 50%. Intranasal administration is considered an attractive alternative to the IV administration of (*R*,*S*)-ketamine because it is less invasive, results in rapid systemic absorption, and is not subject to first-pass hepatic metabolism. Oral bioavailability of (2*S*,6*S*)-HNK was estimated to be 46.3% in rats and mice, and the oral bioavailability of (2*R*,6*R*)-HNK is estimated to be approximately 50%.

(*R*,*S*)-Ketamine is rapidly distributed into the brain, resulting in a large steady-state volume of distribution (V_d = 3-5 L/kg). A single IV bolus administration of an anesthetic dose of (*R*,*S*)-ketamine in humans (2 mg/kg) leads to equal plasma concentrations of (*S*)-ketamine and (*R*)-ketamine 1 minute post-administration. Although plasma levels of (*R*,*S*)-ketamine are below detectable limits within 1 day following an IV antidepressant dose (40-minute infusion), circulating levels of 2*R*,6*R*;2*S*,6*S*-HNK were observed for up to 3 days after (±)-ketamine infusion in patients diagnosed with bipolar depression. Norketamine and ketamine were detectable for up to 14 and 11 days, respectively, in the urine of children.[141]

A short elimination half-life (155-158 minutes) was demonstrated for both (*S*)-ketamine and (*R*)-ketamine.

Elimination of (*R,S*)-ketamine is primarily performed by the kidneys. The majority of the drug (80%) is excreted as glucuronide conjugates of HK and HNK in urine and bile. In adult humans, the IV terminal plasma half-life was 186 minutes, and the intramuscular half-life was 155 minutes. In humans, (*S*)-ketamine has a slightly longer elimination half-life than racemic ketamine: 1.5 hours for (*S*)-ketamine versus 2 to 4 hours for racemic ketamine. This may suggest an inhibition of (*S*)-ketamine's clearance by the (*R*)-ketamine enantiomer when the racemic mixture is administered.

Utility of Ketamine's Hydroxynorketamine Metabolites as Drug Treatments[106,110]. It has been reported that the metabolism of ketamine is necessary for its full antidepressant action in mice. Specific metabolites, (2*S*,6*S*)-HNK and (2*R*,6*R*)-HNK, derived from the metabolism of (*S*)-ketamine and (*R*)-ketamine, respectively, do not bind to or inhibit the NMDAR at antidepressant-relevant concentrations but do exert antidepressant behavioral effects similar to those observed following administration of ketamine itself.[141] These findings further challenge the NMDAR inhibition hypothesis of ketamine's antidepressant actions. In addition, (2*R*,6*R*)-HNK exerts antidepressant effects without the sensory dissociation, ataxia, and abuse liability of ketamine in animal tests. Indeed, the psychoactive side effects of ketamine, including dissociation and changes in sensory perception, as well as its abuse potential, have been attributed to the NMDAR *R*-enantiomer effects of ketamine.

The recent findings that ketamine metabolites are involved in the antidepressant actions of ketamine suggest the possible use of these metabolites in the treatment of depression and open new paths for investigating their role in other brain disorders.[141] HNK metabolites may contribute to the clinical effects of subanesthetic doses of ketamine, perhaps due to their direct actions on nAChRs, which may provide a framework for a novel ketamine metabolite paradigm, which posits clinically relevant effects dependent on metabolic conversion of ketamine, but it does not involve NMDAR inhibition. Nevertheless, future preclinical studies are needed to support the contention that NMDAR inhibition is not required for the effectiveness of ketamine's metabolites as fast-acting antidepressants and to identify the underlying mechanism of action of these metabolites.

Esketamine Nasal Spray for Depression (Spravato). Ketamine nasal spray (Schedule III) (as alternative to esketamine) is being used for both pain and as an alternative therapy for MDD. This dosage method is not FDA approved but may provide quick relief for depression. Ketamine nasal spray is prepared by a commercial compounding pharmacy and can be provided in any strength, but the drug's solubility is limited at 200 mg/mL. It is important to keep this strength at room temperature, to prevent the drug from precipitating from solution. The administration schedule is 2 to 3 times a week. Preserved water is used in the formulation, so the risk of bacterial contamination is minimal. Most common is a 100 mg/mL concentration. Dosages vary widely, but each pump of the spray bottle is 0.1 mL, so each pump will deliver 10 mg of ketamine. Many times, one dose will provide a remarkable turnaround.

The nasal spray is a convenient dosage mechanism for bypassing oral delivery. The nose has nerve fibers within its cavity that directly connects to the brainstem, thus bypassing the BBB. The tight cell junctions of the nasal cavity stop most drugs delivered via the bloodstream from entering the brain. This system also prevents harmful pathogens as a protective mechanism. However, delivering the drug via the nasal cavity has proven to be a dependable method for administering many useful drugs, including ketamine, oxytocin, fentanyl, flumazenil, vitamin B12, and many other large peptide analogs.

The FDA has recently approved esketamine nasal spray (Spravato) for depression and TRD. Because of its potential for abuse and misuse, the FDA will restrict availability and monitor use tightly.

In addition to its fast action, Spravato provides a number of benefits over other antidepressants. Esketamine nasal spray seems to have a very safe profile with few side effects, while many other antidepressants cause a number of side effects. Many patients appreciate the convenient dosing schedule of the spray, which is usually 2 to 3 times a week, rather than daily. The nasal spray delivery makes it discreet and easy to use. The safe, effective, and speedy relief from depression that esketamine nasal spray provides can change the lives of people with this mood disorder. After treatment, many patients are able to return to work, take care of their families, and enjoy their favorite hobbies. Most go on to lead happy, productive lives.

Spravato is a nasal spray that is often used together with oral antidepressant medication to treat adults with TRD.[141,143] Spravato is only available to adults through a restricted program called the Spravato Risk Evaluation and Mitigation Strategy (REMS) Program. This medicine can only be administered at a health care setting certified in the REMS Program and to patients enrolled in the program.[47,144] This medicine cannot be used at home. Spravato is used only in a health care setting where patients can be watched closely for at least 2 hours after each dose. The patient will need someone to drive them home after using it. They must be registered in the program and understand the risks and benefits of this medicine.

Warnings. Spravato can cause severe drowsiness or feelings of being disconnected from the body or thoughts or surroundings. Some people have thoughts about suicide while taking esketamine. The patient should stay alert to changes in their mood or symptoms and report any new or worsening symptoms to their health care provider. There is a risk for abuse and dependence with esketamine treatment. The health care provider should check for signs of abuse and dependence before and during treatment with this medicine. The patient should tell their health care provider if they have ever misused or been dependent on alcohol, prescription medicines, or street drugs because of the risks for sedation, dissociation, and abuse and misuse.

Spravato may cause worsening of depression and suicidal thoughts and behaviors, especially during the first few months of treatment and when the dose is changed. The patient should tell their health care provider right away if they have any new or sudden changes in mood, behavior, thoughts, or feelings.

To make sure Spravato is safe, the patient should tell their health care provider if they have heart problems, such as chest pain, heart failure, or a heart valve disorder; slow heartbeats that have caused them to faint; high blood pressure; a heart attack or stroke; a brain injury or increased pressure in their brain; mental illness or psychosis; suicidal thoughts or actions; a family history of depression; alcohol or drug addiction; or liver disease.

Some people have thoughts about suicide when first using an antidepressant. The health care provider should check the patient's progress at regular visits. The family or other caregivers should also be alert to changes in mood or symptoms. Esketamine is contraindicated if the patient is pregnant, as it may harm a fetus. Breastfeeding while using esketamine is contraindicated.

Spravato is usually given twice per week at first (induction phase) and then once every 1 to 2 weeks.[145] The health care provider will tell the patient how often they need to use the medicine. The usual adult dose for weeks 1 to 4 is 56 mg intranasally once, then subsequent doses of 56 to 84 mg intranasally twice a week. The maintenance phase for weeks 5 to 8 is 56 to 84 mg intranasally once a week. For weeks 9 and after, the dose is 56 to 84 mg intranasally every 2 weeks or once a week. Treatment sessions should be directly supervised by a health care provider; treatment sessions should include nasal administration of the dose and post-administration observation. Patients who require nasal corticosteroids/decongestants should use the agent(s) at least 1 hour before using this drug. Patients should be advised to avoid eating foods for at least 2 hours before treatment and to avoid drinking liquids for at least 30 minutes before administration. After the induction phase, evidence of therapeutic benefit should be evaluated to determine the need for continued treatment. After week 8, the dosing frequency should be individualized to the least frequent dosing to maintain remission. After 4 weeks, evidence of therapeutic benefit should be evaluated to determine the need for continued treatment. The dosage may be decreased to 56 mg intranasally 2 times a week if intolerable symptoms occur.

Antidepressant medicines may increase suicidal thoughts and actions in some people ages 24 years and younger, especially within the first few months of treatment or when the dose is changed. Esketamine is not for use in children.

Common Side Effects of Spravato. A temporary increase in blood pressure may last for about 4 hours after taking a dose. Check blood pressure before taking Spravato and for at least 2 hours after. Tell the health care provider right away if chest pain, shortness of breath, sudden severe headache, change in vision, or seizures occur after taking esketamine.

Other side effects include bladder problems, such as trouble urinating, a frequent or urgent need to urinate, pain when urinating, or urinating frequently at night; feeling disconnected, dizzy, nauseous, sleepy, anxious, drunk, very happy or excited; experiencing a spinning sensation, decreased sensitivity (numbness), or a lack of energy; and vomiting. If these common side effects occur, they usually happen right after taking Spravato and go away the same day.

Dextromethorphan/Bupropion (Auvelity)

Current antidepressant therapies exhibit low therapeutic efficiency and delayed onset of antidepressant action of about 4 to 6 weeks.[145,146] Thus, the search for better-acting oral agents is a continuous process. One of the primary targets for the development of new antidepressant drugs are the noncompetitive antagonists of the NMDAR (see Chapter 6). Auvelity is an orally acting combination of dextromethorphan and bupropion and was recently approved by the FDA for the oral treatment of MDD in adults. Auvelity is the first and only rapid-acting oral medication approved for MDD with labeling of statistically significant antidepressant efficacy compared to placebo starting at 1 week (Fig. 12.32).

Auvelity uses the first new oral mechanism of action for MDD developed in more than 60 years. It works on the NMDAR, an ionotropic glutamate receptor, and on the σ-1 receptor in the brain via its dextromethorphan component. The bupropion component is an aminoketone, which increases blood levels of dextromethorphan by competitively inhibiting CYP2D6, which is the major biotransformation pathway for dextromethorphan. Given the debilitating nature of depression, the efficacy of Auvelity observed at 1 week and sustained thereafter may have a significant impact on the current treatment paradigm for this condition. The efficacy of Auvelity for MDD was demonstrated in a placebo-controlled study, and confirmatory evidence was established comparing Auvelity to bupropion sustained-release tablets.

According to study findings, Auvelity showed statistically significant superiority to placebo in improvement of depressive symptoms as measured by the trial's primary endpoint, change in the Montgomery-Asberg Depression Rating Scale (MADRS) total score at week 6. To evaluate the speed of onset of action, the changes in MADRS total score from baseline to week 1 and from baseline to week 2 were prespecified secondary efficacy endpoints. The difference between Auvelity and placebo in change from baseline in MADRS total score was statistically significant at weeks 1 and 2.

Auvelity is a combination of dextromethorphan and bupropion. Bupropion increases plasma levels of dextromethorphan by competitively inhibiting CYP2D6, which catalyzes a major biotransformation pathway for dextromethorphan. Bupropion is a relatively weak inhibitor of the neuronal reuptake of NE and DA and does not inhibit MAO or the reuptake of 5-HT. Dextromethorphan when coadministered with bupropion displays nonlinear pharmacokinetics at steady state, with greater-than-dose-proportional changes in AUC and C_{max} for varying doses of dextromethorphan (60-120 mg times the maximum recommended dose of Auvelity) and less-than-dose-proportional changes for varying doses of bupropion (150-300 mg times the maximum recommended dose of

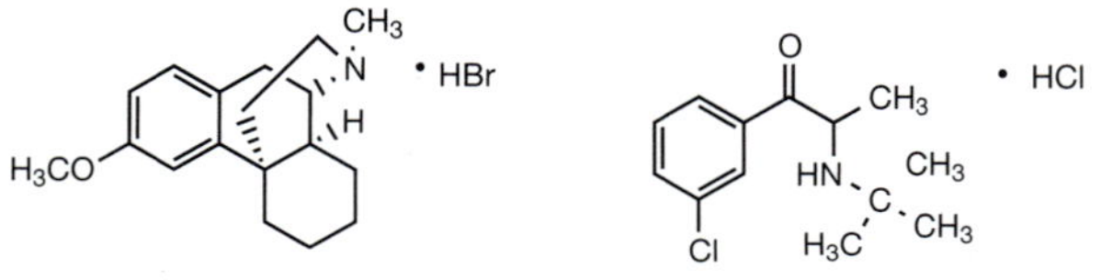

Dextromethorphan hydrobromide + Bupropion hydrochloride (Auvelity)

Figure 12.32 Auvelity.

Auvelity). Steady-state plasma concentrations of dextromethorphan and bupropion when given as Auvelity are achieved within 8 days. The accumulation ratios for dextromethorphan at steady state when given as Auvelity are 20 and 32, respectively, based on C_{max} and $AUC_{0\text{-}12}$, compared to 1.3 and 1.4, respectively, for dextromethorphan given without bupropion. The accumulation ratios for bupropion at steady state are 1.1 and 1.5, respectively, based on C_{max} and $AUC_{0\text{-}11}$. The median T_{max} of dextromethorphan and bupropion when given as Auvelity was 3 and 2 hours, respectively.

The multimodal pharmacologic activity of Auvelity therapy also contributes to more rapid efficacy than traditional antidepressant monotherapy. Patients with a confirmed diagnosis of moderate to severe MDD were randomized to receive Auvelity. Each tablet contains 32.98 mg of dextromethorphan base in an immediate-release formulation and 91.14 mg bupropion base in an extended-release formulation (Auvelity) or extended release of bupropion (105 mg) twice daily for 6 weeks. Treatment with Auvelity resulted in significantly lower depression rating total scores by week 2 as compared to bupropion monotherapy. In addition, 26% of patients treated with Auvelity had achieved remission by week 2 versus 3% of those receiving bupropion monotherapy. Notably, no NMDA dissociative/psychotomimetic events were observed in the trial. The formulation achieves pharmacologic synergy by simultaneously targeting monoamines, NMDARs, and σ-1 receptors.

Dextromethorphan. Dextromethorphan is a noncompetitive NMDAR, σ-1 receptor agonist, and nAChR as a negative allosteric modulator, among other actions, whereas bupropion acts as an NE/DA reuptake inhibitor and nAChR negative allosteric modulator. Dextromethorphan is a prodrug of dextrorphan, which is the actual mediator of most of its antidepressant effects through acting as a more potent noncompetitive NMDAR antagonist and a σ-1 receptor agonist. Auvelity is a combination of dextromethorphan and bupropion, a weak NE and DA inhibitor, and strong CYP2D6 inhibitor (see previous discussion for a full description of bupropion).

Dextromethorphan shares pharmacologic properties in common with antidepressants and, in particular, ketamine, a drug with demonstrated rapid-acting antidepressant activity. Pharmacodynamic similarities include actions on NMDA, σ-1 receptor, calcium channel, 5-HT transporter, and muscarinic sites. Additional unique properties potentially contributory to an antidepressant effect include actions at β, α-2, and 5-HT1b/d receptors. Therefore, dextromethorphan may have antidepressant efficacy in bipolar, MDD, and TRD depressive disorders, and may display a rapid onset of antidepressant response. The clinical utility of dextromethorphan is limited by its extensive CYP2D6 metabolism. Auvelity is formulated with bupropion to increase the bioavailability and half-life of dextromethorphan through CYP2D6 inhibition of its metabolism by bupropion.

Tabuteau and colleagues concluded that Auvelity showed rapid and statistically significant antidepressant efficacy compared to bupropion as the active comparator on multiple clinician- and patient-reported measures of depression severity.[145] Study limitations include exclusion of patients with lower levels of symptom severity and other psychiatric or medical comorbidities. This study demonstrated that the dextromethorphan/bupropion combination significantly improves depressive symptoms compared to bupropion alone and was generally well tolerated.[47] On average, patients taking Auvelity had a rapid improvement in their depressive symptom scores versus placebo at 1 week. More people taking Auvelity reached remission at 2 weeks than those taking placebo.

Auvelity is associated with significantly greater reduction in MDD scores versus bupropion with statistically significant differences beginning at week 2. Response and remission at week 6 were significantly more likely in the Auvelity study and was also associated with greater improvement. The prevalence of adverse events was 73% in the Auvelity group and 65% in the bupropion group. The most common adverse events were dizziness, nausea, dry mouth, decreased appetite, and anxiety. There were no serious adverse events in the trial. Auvelity was not associated with psychotomimetic effects, weight gain, sexual dysfunction, increased suicidality, or significant changes in laboratory parameters and vital signs.

Bupropion. The bupropion component of Auvelity is a potent CYP2D6 inhibitor that serves to increase and prolong the blood levels of dextromethorphan (see previous discussion for more details on bupropion).

Dextromethorphan is alternatively used for temporary relief of coughs by certain infections of the air passages such as sinusitis and the common cold.

Dextromethorphan Pharmacokinetics. The mechanism of dextromethorphan in the treatment of MDD is unclear. Following oral administration, dextromethorphan is rapidly absorbed from the GI tract, where it enters the bloodstream and crosses the BBB. At therapeutic doses, dextromethorphan acts centrally. It is rapidly absorbed from the GI tract and converted into its active metabolite dextrorphan in the liver by CYP2D6. Dextromethorphan has an elimination half-life of approximately 4 hours in individuals who are extensive CYP2D6 metabolizers and is increased to approximately 13 hours when dextromethorphan is given in combination with a CYP2D6 inhibitor (ie, bupropion). Around 1 in 10 of the Caucasian population has little or no CYP2D6 enzyme activity, leading to long-lived high drug levels of dextromethorphan.

The main metabolic pathways of dextromethorphan metabolism are catalyzed by CYP3A4 and CYP2D6 and UDP-glucuronosyl-transferase (UGT). The first pass through the hepatic portal vein results in some of the drug being metabolized by CYP2D6 *O*-demethylation into an active metabolite called dextrorphan. The antidepressant activity of dextromethorphan is believed to be caused by both the drug and its metabolite. Dextromethorphan also undergoes *N*-demethylation by CYP3A4 to 3-methoxymorphinan and partial conjugation with glucuronic acid and sulfate ions. Hours after dextromethorphan therapy, (in humans) the metabolite dextrorphan and traces of the unchanged drug are detectable in the urine. *O*-demethylation of dextromethorphan to dextrorphan contributes to at least 80% of the dextrorphan formed during dextromethorphan metabolism.

CYP2D6 is a major metabolic pathway in the O-demethylation of dextromethorphan. The duration of action and effects of dextromethorphan can be increased by as much as 3 times in poor CYP2D6 metabolizers. In one study on 252 Americans, 84% were found to be "fast" (extensive) metabolizers, 7% "intermediate" metabolizers, and 9% "slow" metabolizers of dextromethorphan. A number of alleles for CYP2D6 are known, including several completely inactive variants. The distribution of alleles is uneven among ethnic groups. *N*-demethylation is primarily accomplished by CYP3A4, contributing to at least 90% of the primary metabolite of nordextromethorphan.

A large number of drugs are potent inhibitors of CYP2D6, which include certain SSRIs and TCAs, some antipsychotics, and the antihistamine diphenhydramine. Therefore, the potential for DDIs exists between dextromethorphan and medications that inhibit CYP2D6, particularly in slow metabolizers.

Auvelity can be taken with or without food. Dextromethorphan C_{max} and $AUC_{0\text{-}12}$ were unchanged and decreased by 14%, respectively, and bupropion C_{max} and $AUC_{0\text{-}12}$ were increased by 3% and 6%, respectively, when Auvelity was administered with food. The plasma protein binding of dextromethorphan is approximately 60% to 70%, and bupropion is 84%. The extent of protein binding of the hydroxybupropion metabolite is similar to that for bupropion, whereas the extent of protein binding of the *threo*-hydroxybupropion metabolite is about half that seen with bupropion (see Fig. 12.24).

Following 8 days of administration of Auvelity in extensive metabolizers, the mean elimination half-life of dextromethorphan was increased approximately 3-fold to 22 hours, as compared to dextromethorphan given without bupropion. The mean elimination half-life of dextromethorphan and bupropion was 22 and 15 hours, respectively. In CYP2D6 extensive metabolizers, approximately 37% to 52% of the orally administered dose of dextromethorphan is recovered in the urine. Less than 2% of the administered dose is excreted as unchanged parent drug in the urine. In CYP2D6 poor metabolizers, approximately 45% to 83% of the administered dose is recovered in the urine. Approximately 26% of the administered dose is excreted as unchanged parent drug in the urine. Following oral administration of 200 mg of 14C-bupropion in humans, 87% and 10% of the radioactive dose were recovered in the urine and feces, respectively. Only 0.5% of the oral dose was excreted as unchanged bupropion.

Adverse Effects. Auvelity may cause serious adverse effects. There is a risk of seizures during treatment with Auvelity. The risk is higher at higher doses, in patients that have certain medical problems, and when taking Auvelity with certain other medicines. If a seizure occurs during treatment, Auvelity should be discontinued and not restarted. Some people may get high blood pressure during treatment with Auvelity. Check blood pressure before taking and during treatment with Auvelity. The pharmacokinetics of Auvelity have not been studied in patients 65 years and older. The pharmacokinetics of Auvelity in pediatric patients have not been studied. No significant pharmacokinetic differences based on sex and ethnicity have been observed for Auvelity.

Dosage and Administration. Starting dosage is one tablet once daily in the morning. After 3 days, increase to the maximum recommended dosage of one tablet twice daily, separated by at least 8 hours. Do not exceed two doses within the same day.

Contraindications. Auvelity should not be used in the setting of a current or prior diagnosis of bulimia or anorexia nervosa. Auvelity should not be used within 14 days of discontinuing an MAOI.

Warnings and Precautions. Seizure risk is dose-related. Discontinue if seizure occurs. Auvelity can increase blood pressure and cause hypertension. Blood pressure should be assessed before initiating treatment and monitored periodically during treatment.

Patients should be screened for bipolar disorder. Auvelity with SSRIs or TCAs increases the risk of bipolar disorder. Discontinue if this occurs. Advise pregnant females of the potential risk to a fetus. Discontinue treatment in pregnant females and use alternative treatment for females who are planning to become pregnant.

Adverse Reactions. Most common adverse reactions (≥5% and more than twice as frequently as placebo) include dizziness, headache, diarrhea, somnolence, dry mouth, sexual dysfunction, and hyperhidrosis.

Drug Interactions. For strong CYP2D6 inhibitors, the recommended dosage is one tablet by mouth once daily in the morning. For strong CYP2B6 inducers, avoid use of CYP2D6 substrates; Auvelity increases the exposures of drugs that are substrates of CYP2D6. For drugs that lower the seizure threshold, coadministration may increase risk of seizure.

Renal Impairment. Dosage adjustment of Auvelity is recommended in patients with moderate renal impairment (estimated glomerular filtration rate [eGFR] 30-59 mL/min/1.73 m^2). The pharmacokinetics of Auvelity have not been evaluated in patients with severe renal impairment. Auvelity is not recommended in patients with severe renal impairment (eGFR 15-29 mL/min/1.73 m^2).

Hepatic Impairment. No dose adjustment of Auvelity is recommended in patients with mild or moderate hepatic impairment. The pharmacokinetics of Auvelity have not been evaluated and are not recommended in patients with severe hepatic impairment.

CYP2D6 Poor Metabolizers. Dosage adjustment is recommended in patients known to be poor CYP2D6 metabolizers because these patients have higher dextromethorphan concentrations than extensive/intermediate CYP2D6 metabolizers.

Herbal Therapy

In the past few years, much interest has been generated regarding the use of herbs in the treatment of both depression and anxiety.[147-149] Recent studies, however, have revealed potentially fatal interactions between herbal remedies and traditional drugs. Numerous natural herbs have been clinically and traditionally proven to reduce depression symptoms and increase the quality of life. Just like with all supplemental changes, consult a medical practitioner if consider altering a standard health care routine.

Ten Best Herbs for Depression

The following are the best research-backed herbs for mild depression, not for MDD.[150] These herbal antidepressants have been shown to support mental health through a variety of different mechanisms.[149,151]

St John's Wort (*Hypericum perforatum*)

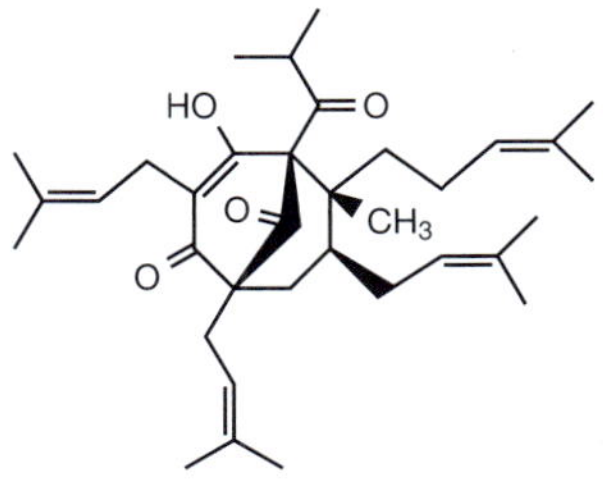

Hyperforin

Numerous studies have shown that St John's wort is a safe and effective natural herb for depression. It is typically used for moderate depression. The active drug in St John's wort is hyperforin.[150] A 2017 review article summarizing in a participant pool of SSRIs found that St John's wort was as effective as SSRIs in alleviating depressive symptoms. In a double-blind study, St John's wort extract was compared to fluoxetine (an SSRI) in a group of older adults with mild-to-moderate depression. Researchers found that St John's wort was just as effective as fluoxetine and elicited no adverse effects on cognitive performance. Another clinical trial comparing St John's wort extract to imipramine (a TCA) found that both treatments were effective in improving the quality of life in subjects with depression. Although they were comparable, St John's wort was found to be better tolerated among participants. Two different types of St John's wort extract were examined in another double-blind study. Researchers discovered that the content level of hyperforin was responsible for the effectiveness of the extract. The higher the hyperforin content, the more effective the extract was found to be. In a trial observing those with depression, St John's wort extract was found to be effective for treating mild-to-moderate forms of depression. However, the extract was found not helpful for those with MDD. The Commission E, a German government health agency, mentions that St John's wort is appropriate to use in cases of depressive moods, anxiety, and nervous unrest. The European Scientific Cooperative on Phytotherapy (ESCOP) also reports that St John's wort is useful for mild-to-moderate depressive states, restlessness, anxiety, and irritability.

Lemon Balm (*Melissa officinalis*)

Lemon balm is known to be one of the best herbs for PPD. As such, it is especially helpful for pregnant or nursing mothers. In a clinical trial, 60 women who underwent cesarean sections were observed for PPD. Lemon balm was administered at 500 mg, 3 times a day for 10 days. The lemon balm was shown to significantly reduce the occurrence of PPD. An 8-week study found that lemon balm was helpful for reducing symptoms of depression in participants with sleeping issues and anxiety. The results also showed improved sleep quality as well as a reduction in stress and anxiety levels. In another trial, lemon balm tea, when taken twice a day, was found to ease anxiety and depression in hospitalized burn patients. The tea was also able to improve sleep quality. A combination study of lemon balm and Persian lavender had the ability to improve depression and anxiety symptoms in those with severe insomnia.

Bacopa (*Bacopa monnieri*)

Bacopa is generally well known for its cognition-enhancing abilities, but clinical studies have found that bacopa may also be a beneficial herb for depression, anxiety, and mood. In one comparative clinical study, participants with lack of pleasure were either treated with a common antidepressant citalopram or a combination of citalopram and 300 mg of bacopa. The citalopram/bacopa combination treatment group displayed significant improvements in both depression and anhedonia when compared to the group only treated with citalopram. In a placebo-controlled trial, 48 older adults were treated with either a placebo or 300 mg of bacopa extract every day for 12 weeks. The group treated with *Bacopa monnieri* extract experienced lower levels of depression and anxiety when compared to the group treated with a placebo, who, interestingly, saw increases in depression and anxiety. In one clinical trial involving 100 individuals experiencing poor sleep, it was found that participants treated with a standardized bacopa extract had significantly better well-being, mood, and overall health when compared to the group given a placebo. It should be noted, however, that neither group experienced significant increases in sleep quality. In one stress-induced animal model of depression, administration of bacopa extract in rats seemed to lower stress and have antidepressant actions, much like common antidepressant medications. Finally, in an animal study conducted on mice exposed to chronic stress, it was found that supplementation with bacopaside, a beneficial constituent in bacopa, lowered cortisol levels and increased BDNF, an important compound for overall brain function that is often reduced in individuals with depression.

Chamomile (*Matricaria chamomilla*)

Chamomile is considered one of the best herbs for depression as it is highly supportive of the CNS. An exploratory study found that chamomile was able to significantly reduce depression scores in subjects with only depression, only anxiety, or both. These effects were seen in all subjects. A double-blind, placebo-controlled trial found that 1,500 mg of chamomile extract daily had an antidepressant and anxiolytic effect on those with GAD and depression. Researchers believe this effect may be due to chamomile's ability to regulate the body's stress response. The flavonoid apigenin is thought to be the phytochemical behind chamomile's natural antidepressant effects. This constituent is known to reduce anxiety, so researchers believe there may be a tie to depression symptoms as well.

Ashwagandha (Withania somnifera)

Ashwagandha is an herb that is highly revered for both depression and anxiety. Research shows that ashwagandha may be useful as a natural remedy for depression due to its ability to support stress management. In a clinical study, ashwagandha proved to be promising for treating depression symptoms in individuals with schizophrenia. The participants' depression and anxiety scores improved significantly after taking 1,000 mg daily for 3 months. In a published research review, researchers mention that ashwagandha was able to alleviate depression and insomnia symptoms in both humans and animals. They also noted that they believe this was a result of ashwagandha's ability to regulate the HPA axis (the body's stress command center).

Lavender (Lavandula angustifolia)

Lavender has been clinically proven to be a supportive herb for depression and anxiety.

A study involving 93 participants with high levels of stress and anxiety discovered that lavender aromatherapy was able to improve mood and reduce anxiety. While the short-term anxiolytic effects were significant, these effects went away after the aromatherapy stopped. In a pilot study, researchers found that the lavender essential oil blend administered via aromatherapy was supportive for women with PPD and anxiety. The essential oil was administered in 15 minutes/session (twice weekly for 4 weeks) and helped to lower both depression and anxiety scores.

Hops (Humulus lupulus)

Hops is an herb known as a natural mood booster for mental health issues. A study observing healthy young adults with mild depression, anxiety, and stress discovered that hops extract was able to reduce symptoms after 1 month. Those taking the hops extract saw a significant reduction in depression scores. Hops has also been used as a traditional herb for depression and anxiety. It is popular in the United States and Germany for its anxiolytic properties.

Passionflower (Passiflora incarnata)

Passionflower is an herb historically known to reduce insomnia, a common symptom of depression. This makes passionflower a very powerful natural sleep aid. A placebo-controlled study observing subjects with insomnia found that passionflower extract was able to improve sleep efficiency as well as decrease depression, anxiety, and stress levels. This research shows that passionflower extract may have a positive effect on depression through its ability to improve sleep. Another trial found that passionflower tea was able to improve sleep quality in participants with insomnia. Due to the relationship between depression and poor sleep quality, passionflower tea may help those with depression-induced insomnia. The European Medicines Agency mentions that passionflower is safe and effective for those with mild anxiety and/or insomnia. A review of passionflower notes that passionflower has therapeutic properties that help reduce and regulate stress and therefore may be helpful for the treatment of depression, insomnia, and anxiety.

American Skullcap (Scutellaria lateriflora)

Skullcap is a natural herbal remedy for depression that is well known for its ability to promote sleep and reduce anxiety. A placebo-controlled study discovered that skullcap extract has the ability to improve mood in those with mild anxiety. Researchers believe that the extract may be helpful for enhancing mood in those with anxiety and comorbid depression since there was no reduction in energy or cognition (a common side effect of antidepressant drugs). An in vivo study of skullcap extract found that its antioxidant properties may be helpful for those with stress-induced depression. Skullcap is able to reduce oxidative stress, which may have a powerful effect on the body's stress response. The British Herbal Pharmacopoeia (BHP) notes that skullcap is certified to support against stress and insomnia that may be stemming from depression.

Blue Vervain (Verbena hastata)

Blue vervain is an herb traditionally known as a natural antidepressant that is helpful for alleviating depression and can act as a gentle anxiolytic. Blue vervain combined with ashwagandha, St John's wort, licorice (*Glycyrrhiza glabra*), and Asian ginseng (*Panax ginseng*) was beneficial for PPD and irritability.

Electroconvulsive Therapy

ECT has been in use since the late 1930s to treat a variety of severe mental illnesses, most notably major depression.[152] Use of ECT is beneficial particularly for individuals whose depression is severe or life threatening or who cannot take antidepressant medication. Often, ECT is effective in cases in which antidepressant drugs do not provide sufficient relief of symptoms.

ECT remains the "gold standard" for the treatment of major depression and a variety of other psychiatric and neurologic disorders.[152] Because of the effectiveness and resurgence of ECT, more patients are considered to be good candidates for this treatment option. Overall, these patients are medication refractory and older adults and, thus, are more sensitive to polypharmacy. Additionally, these patients tend to have more coexisting medical problems.

In recent years, ECT has been much improved. A muscle relaxant is given before treatment, which is done under brief anesthesia. Electrodes are placed at precise locations on the head to deliver electrical impulses. The stimulation causes a brief (~30 seconds) seizure within the brain. The person receiving ECT does not consciously experience the electrical stimulus. For full therapeutic benefit, at least several sessions of ECT, typically given at the rate of three per week, are required. ECT appears to increase the sensitivity of postsynaptic 5-HT receptors and upregulation of 5-HT_{1A} postsynaptic receptors.

Side effects may result from the anesthesia, the ECT treatment, or both. Common side effects include temporary short-term memory loss, nausea, muscle aches, and headache. Some people may have longer-lasting problems with memory after ECT. Sometimes, a person's blood pressure or heart rhythm changes. If these changes occur, they are carefully watched during the ECT treatments and are immediately treated.

Structure Challenge

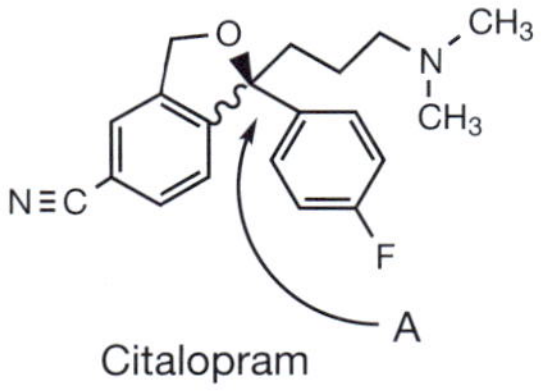

Citalopram

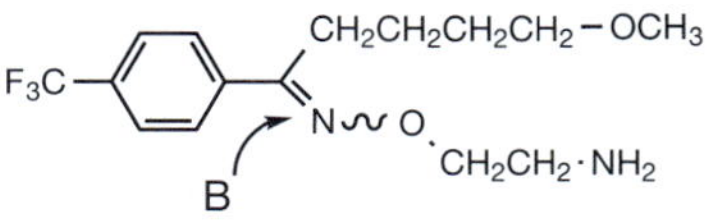

Fluvoxamine

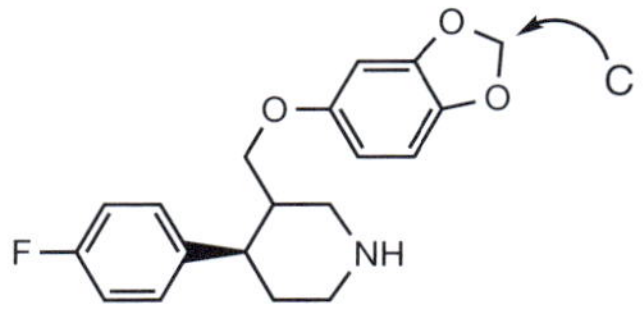

Paroxetine

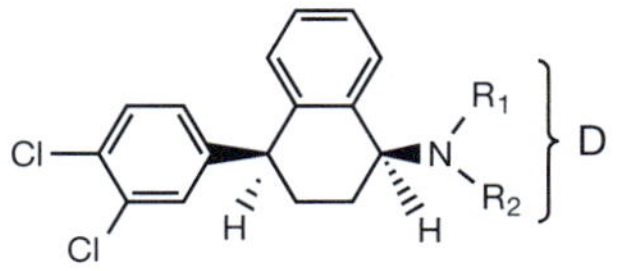

Sertraline

Which of the following statements is correct for the drugs shown?

A. Stereochemistry at site A is extremely important in promoting antidepressant effects.
B. Stereochemistry at site B is unimportant.
C. Paroxetine is a prodrug that requires removal of the methylene (C) for activation.
D. Primary, secondary, or tertiary amine at D all exhibit equal activity as an SSRI.

Structure Challenge answers found immediately after References.

REFERENCES

1. National Institute of Mental Health. (2015). *Depression: What You Need to Know* (NIH Publication No. 15-3561). U.S. Government Printing Office.
2. Zhang Y, Jia XJ, Yang Y, et al. Change in the global burden of depression from 1990-2019 and its prediction for 2030. *J Psych Res.* 2024;178:16-22.
3. American Psychiatric Association. *Diagnostic and Statistical Manual of Mental Disorders (DSM-5).* 5th ed. American Psychiatric Association; 2013.
4. Monroe SM, Harkness KL. Major depression and its recurrences: life course matters. *Annu Rev Clin Psychol.* 2022;18:329-357.
5. Wang HQ, Wang ZZ, Chen NH. The receptor hypothesis and the pathogenesis of depression: genetic bases and biological correlates. *Pharmacol Res.* 2021;167:105542.
6. Kendler KS. The origin of our modern concept of depression—the history of melancholia from 1780-1880: a review. *JAMA Psychiatry.* 2020;77:863-868.
7. Brandis M. A feminist analysis of the theories of etiology of depression in women. *Nurs Leadersh Forum.* 1998;3:18-23.
8. Paris J. The mistreatment of major depressive disorder. *Can J Psychiatry.* 2014;59(3):148-151.
9. Dwyer JB, Aftab A, Radhakrishnan R, et al. Hormonal treatments for major depressive disorder: state of the art. *Am J Psychiatry.* 2020;1778:686-705.
10. Bain N, Abdijerdid S. Major depressive disorder. In *StatPearls* [Internet]. StatPearls Publishing; 2023.
11. Reynolds CF 3rd, Lenze E, Mulsant BH. Assessment and treatment of major depression in older adults. *Handb Clin Neurol.* 2019;167:429-435.
12. Cuijpers P, Quero S, Dowrick C, Arroll B. Psychological treatment of depression in primary care: recent developments. *Curr Psychiatry Rep.* 2019;21:129.
13. Manji HK, Lenox RH. Signaling: cellular insights into the pathophysiology of bipolar disorder. *Biol Psychiatry.* 2000;48:518-530.
14. Schüle C, Nothdurfter C, Rupprecht R. The role of allopregnanolone in depression and anxiety. *Prog Neurobiol.* 2014;113:79-87.

15. Osborne LM, Gispen F, Sanyal A, et al. Lower allopregnanolone during pregnancy predicts postpartum depression: an exploratory study. *Psychoneuroendocrinology*. 2017;79:116-111.
16. Bäckström T, Bixo M, Johansson M, et al. Allopregnanolone and mood disorders. *Prog Neurobiol*. 2014;113:88-94.
17. O'Hara MW, McCabe JE. Postpartum depression: current status and future directions. *Annu Rev Clin Psychol*. 2013;9:379-407.
18. Pearlstein T, Howard M, Salisbury A, Zlotnick C. Postpartum depression. *Am J Obstet Gynecol*. 2009;200:357-364.
19. Kroska EB, Stowe ZN. Postpartum depression: identification and treatment in the clinic setting. *Obstet Gynecol Clin North Am*. 2020;47:409-419.
20. Kanes S, Colquhoun H, Gunduz-Bruce H, et al. Brexanolone (SAGE-547 injection) in post-partum depression: a randomised controlled trial. *Lancet*. 2017;390:480-489.
21. Meltzer-Brody S, Colquhoun H, Riesenberg R, et al. Brexanolone injection in post-partum depression: two multicentre, double-blind, randomised, placebo-controlled, phase 3 trials. *Lancet*. 2018;392:1058-1070.
22. Hellgren C, Åkerud H, Skalkidou A, et al. Low serum allopregnanolone is associated with symptoms of depression in late pregnancy. *Neuropsychobiology*. 2014;69(3):147-153.
23. Stewart DE, Vigod SN. Postpartum depression: pathophysiology, treatment, and emerging therapeutics. *Annu Rev Med*. 2019;70:183-196.
24. Deligiannidis KM, Meltzer-Brody S, Gunduz-Bruce H, et al. Effect of zuranolone vs placebo in postpartum depression: a randomized clinical trial. *JAMA Psychiatry*. 2021;78:959.
25. Ali M, Ullah I, Diwan MN, et al. Zuranolone and its role in treating major depressive disorder: a narrative review. *Horm Mol Biol Clin Investig*. 2023;44(2):229-236.
26. Schiller CE, Schmidt PJ, Rubinow DR. Allopregnanolone as a mediator of affective switching in reproductive mood disorders. *Psychopharmacology (Berl)*. 2014;231:3557-3567.
27. Payne JL, Maguire J. Pathophysiological mechanisms implicated in postpartum depression. *Front Neuroendocrinol*. 2019;52:165-180.
28. Brummelte S, Galea LA. Postpartum depression: etiology, treatment and consequences for maternal care. *Horm Behav*. 2016;77:153-166.
29. Sockol LE, Epperson CN, Barber JP. Preventing postpartum depression: a meta-analytic review. *Clin Psychol Rev*. 2013;33:1205-1217.
30. Moret C, Briley M. The importance of norepinephrine in depression. *Neuropsychiatr Dis Treat*. 2011;7(suppl 1):9-13.
31. Delgado PL, Moreno FA. Role of norepinephrine in depression. *J Clin Psychiatry*. 2000;61(suppl 1):5-11.
32. Duman RS, Heninger GR, Nestler EJ. A molecular and cellular theory of depression. *Arch Gen Psychiatry*. 1997;54:597-606.
33. Kielholz P. The classification of depressions and the activity profile of the antidepressants. *Prog Neuropsychopharmacol*. 1979;3(1-3):59-63.
34. Schildkraut JJ, Klerman GL, Hammond R, et al. Excretion of 3-methoxy-mandelic acid (VMA) in depressed patients treated with antidepressant drugs. *J Psychiatr Res*. 1965;2:257-266.
35. van Praag HK, Korf J. Endogenous depressions with and without disturbances in the 5-hydroxytryptamine metabolism: a biochemical classification? *Psychopharmacology*. 1971;19:148-152.
36. Coppen A, Prange AJ Jr, Whybrow PC, et al. Abnormalities of indoleamines in affective disorders. *Arch Gen Psychiat*. 1972;26:474-478.
37. Lenox RH, Frazer A. Mechanism of action of antidepressants and mood stabilizers. In: Davis KL, Charney D, Coyle JT, et al, eds. *Neuropsychopharmacology: The Fifth Generation of Progress*. Lippincott Williams & Wilkins; 2002:1139-1164.
38. Brown AS, Gershon S. DA and depression. *J Neural Transm*. 1993;91:75-109.
39. Shytle RD, Silver AA, Lukas RJ, et al. Nicotinic acetylcholine receptors as targets for antidepressants. *Mol Psychiatry*. 2002;7:525-535.
40. Kuhn R. Uber die behandlung depressives zustande mit einem iminobenzylderivat (G 22,355). *Schweiz Med Wschr*. 1957;87:1135-1140.
41. Loomer HP, Saunders JC, Kline NS. A clinical and pharmacodynamic evaluation of iproniazid as a psychic energizer. *Psychiatr Res Rep Am Psychiatr Assoc*. 1957;8:119-141.
42. Janowsky DS, Davis JM. Adrenergic-cholinergic balance in affective disorders. *Psychopharmacol Bull*. 1978;14(4):58-60.
43. Zhang JC, Yao W, Hashimoto K. Brain-derived neurotrophic factor (BDNF)-TrkB signaling in inflammation-related depression and potential therapeutic targets. *Curr Neuropharmacol*. 2016;14:721-731.
44. Gelle T, Samey RA, Plansont B, et al. BDNF and pro-BDNF in serum and exosomes in major depression: evolution after antidepressant treatment. *Prog Neuropsychopharmacol Biol Psychiatry*. 2021;109:110229.
45. Carniel BP, da Rocha NS. Brain-derived neurotrophic factor (BDNF) and inflammatory markers: perspectives for the management of depression. *Prog Neuropsychopharmacol Biol Psychiatry*. 2021;108:110151.
46. Caviedes A, Lafourcade C, Soto C, Wyneken U. BDNF/NF-κB signaling in the neurobiology of depression. *Curr Pharm Des*. 2017;23:3154-3163.
47. Keam SJ. Dextromethorphan/bupropion: first approval. *CNS Drugs*. 2022;36:1229-1238.
48. Wang JQ, Mao L. The ERK pathway: molecular mechanisms and treatment of depression. *Mol Neurobiol*. 2019;56:6197-6205.
49. Rana T, Behl T, Sehgal A, et al. Unfolding the role of BDNF as a biomarker for treatment of depression. *Mol Neurosci*. 2021;71:2008-2021.
50. Mondal AC, Fatima M. Direct and indirect evidences of BDNF and NGF as key modulators in depression: role of antidepressants treatment. *Int J Neurosci*. 2019;129(3):283-296.
51. Carboni E, Carta AR. BDNF alterations in brain areas and the neurocircuitry involved in the antidepressant effects of ketamine in animal models, suggest the existence of a primary circuit of depression. *J Integr Neurosci*. 2022;21(5):144.
52. Kojima M, Matsui K, Mizui T. BDNF pro-peptide: physiological mechanisms and implications for depression. *Cell Tissue Res*. 2019;377:73-79.
53. Katz EG, Hough D, Doherty T, et al. Benefit-risk assessment of esketamine nasal spray vs. placebo in treatment-resistant depression. *Clin Pharmacol Ther*. 2021;109(2):536-546.
54. Skolnick P, Popik P, Trullas R. Glutamate-based antidepressants: 20 years on. *Trends Pharmacol Sci*. 2009;30:563-569.
55. Ono S, Ogawa K, Yamashita K, et al. Conformational analysis of the NMDA receptor antagonist (1*S*,2*R*)-1-phenyl-2-[*S*-1-aminopropyl]-*N*,*N*-diethylcyclopropanecarboxamide (PPDC) designed by a novel conformational restriction method based on the structural feature of cyclopropane ring. *Chem Pharm Bull (Tokyo)*. 2002;50:966-968.
56. Gonda X, Dome P, Neill JC, Tarazi FI. Novel antidepressant drugs: beyond monoamine targets. *CNS Spectr*. 2023;28(1):6-15.
57. Pałucha-Poniewiera A, Pilc A. Glutamate-based drug discovery for novel antidepressants. *Expert Opin Drug Discov*. 2016;11:873-883.
58. Garay R, Zarate CA Jr, Cavero I, et al. The development of glutamate-based antidepressants is taking longer than expected. *Drug Discov Today*. 2018;23:1689-1692.
59. Chaki S, Fukumoto K. Potential of glutamate-based drug discovery for next generation antidepressants. *Pharmaceuticals (Basel)*. 2015;8(3):590-606.
60. Baldessarini RJ. Drug therapy of depression and anxiety disorders. In: Brunton LL, Lazo JS, Parker KL eds. *Goodman & Gilman's the Pharmacological Basis of Therapeutics*. 11th ed. McGraw-Hill; 2006:429-460.

61. Hogberg T, Ulff B, Renyi AL, et al. Synthesis of pyridylallylamines related to zimelidine and their inhibition of neuronal monoamine uptake. *J Med Chem.* 1981;24:1499-1507.
62. Ogren SO, Ross SB, Hall H, et al. The pharmacology of zimelidine: a 5-HT selective reuptake inhibitor. *Acta Psychiatr Scand Suppl.* 1981;290:117-151.
63. Skolnick P, Popik P, Janowsky A, et al. "Broad spectrum" antidepressants: is more better for the treatment of depression? *Life Sci.* 2003;73:3175-3179.
64. Wong DT, Bymaster FP, Horng JS, et al. A new selective inhibitor for uptake of serotonin into synaptosomes of rat brain: 3-(p-trifluoromethylphenoxy). *N*-methyl-3-phenylpropylamine. *J Pharmacol Exp Ther.* 1975;193:804-811.
65. Wong DT, Bymaster FP, Engleman EA. Prozac (fluoxetine, lilly 110140), the first selective serotonin uptake inhibitor and an antidepressant drug: twenty years since its first publication. *Life Sci.* 1995;57:411-441.
66. Torres GE, Gainetdinov RR, Caron MG. Plasma membrane monoamine transporters: structure, regulation and function. *Nat Rev Neurosci.* 2003;4:13-25.
67. Owens MJ, Morgan WN, Plott SJ, et al. Neurotransmitter receptor and transporter binding profile of antidepressants and their metabolites. *J Pharmacol Exp Ther.* 1997;283:1305-1322.
68. Sanchez C, Hyttel J. Comparison of the effects of antidepressants and their metabolites on reuptake of biogenic amines and on receptor binding. *Cell Mol Neurobiol.* 1999;19:467-489.
69. Cipriani A, Furukawa TA, Salanti G, et al. Comparative efficacy and acceptability of 21 antidepressant drugs for the acute treatment of adults with major depressive disorder: a systematic review and network meta-analysis. *Lancet.* 2018;391:1357-1366.
70. Brunello N, Mendlewicz J, Kasper S, et al. The role of noradrenaline and selective noradrenaline reuptake inhibition in depression. *Eur Neuropsychopharmacol.* 2002;11:461-475.
71. Mandrioli R, Protti M, Mercolini L. New-generation, non-SSRI antidepressants: therapeutic drug monitoring and pharmacological interactions. Part 1: SNRIs, SMSs, SARIs. *Curr Med Chem.* 2018;25:772-792.
72. Kelder J, Funke C, De Boer T, et al. A comparison of the physicochemical and biological properties of mirtazapine and mianserin. *J Pharm Pharmacol.* 1997;49:403-411.
73. Baker GB, Prior TI. Stereochemistry and drug efficacy and development: relevance of chirality to antidepressant and antipsychotic drugs. *Ann Med.* 2002;34:537-543.
74. Budău M, Hancu G, Rusu A, et al. Chirality of modern antidepressants: an overview. *Adv Pharm Bull.* 2017;7:495-500.
75. Norregaard L, Gether U. The monoamine neurotransmitter transporters: structure, conformational changes and molecular gating. *Curr Opin Drug Discov Dev.* 2001;4:591-601.
76. Casarotto MG, Craik DJ. Ring flexibility within tricyclic antidepressant drugs. *J Pharm Sci.* 2001;90:713-719.
77. Venkatakrishnan K, Von Moltke LL, Greenblatt DJ. Human drug metabolism and the cytochromes P450: application and relevance of in vitro models. *J Clin Pharmacol.* 2001;41:1149-1179.
78. Haritos VS, Ghabrial H, Ahokas JT, et al. Role of cytochrome P450 2D6 (CYP2D6) in the stereospecific metabolism of *E*- and *Z*-doxepin. *Pharmacogenetics.* 2000;10:591-603.
79. Yan JH, Hubbard JW, McKay G, et al. Absolute bioavailability and stereoselective pharmacokinetics of doxepin. *Xenobiotica.* 2002;32:615-623.
80. Eap CB, Bender S, Gastpar M, et al. Steady-state plasma levels of the enantiomers of trimipramine and of its metabolites in CYP2D6-, CYP2C19- and CYP3A4/5-phenotyped patients. *Ther Drug Monit.* 2000;22:209-214.
81. Kirchheiner J, Muller G, Meineke I, et al. Effects of polymorphisms in CYP2D6, CYP2C9 and CYP2C19 on trimipramine pharmacokinetics. *J Clin Psychopharmacol.* 2003;23:459-466.
82. Eriksson E. Antidepressant drugs: does it matter if they inhibit the reuptake of noradrenaline or serotonin? *Acta Psychiatr Scand Suppl.* 2000;402:11-17.
83. Cowen PJ. Serotonin hypothesis. In: Feighner JP, Boyer WR, eds. *Selective Serotonin Re-uptake Inhibitors.* 2nd ed. Wiley-Blackwell; 1996:63-86.
84. Olivier B, Soudjin W, van Wijngaarden I. Serotonin, DA and norepinephrine transporters in the CNS and their inhibitors. In: Jucker E, ed. *Progress in Drug Research.* Vol 54. Birkhäuser-Verlag; 2000:59-110.
85. Preskorn SH. *Clinical pharmacology of SSRIs.* Accessed December 8, 2018. http://www.preskorn.com
86. Preskorn SH. Clinically relevant pharmacology of selective serotonin reuptake inhibitors. An overview with emphasis on pharmacokinetics and effects on oxidative drug metabolism. *Clin Pharmacokinet.* 1997;32(suppl 1):1-19.
87. Hyttel J. Pharmacological characterization of selective serotonin reuptake inhibitors (SSRIs). *Int Clin Psychopharmacol.* 1994;9(suppl 1):19-26.
88. Bordet R, Thomas P, Dupuis B. Effect of pindolol on onset of action of paroxetine in the treatment of major depression: intermediate analysis of a double-blind, placebo-controlled trial. Reseau de Recherche et d'Experimentation Psychopharmacologique. *Am J Psychiatr.* 1998;155:1346-1351.
89. Wong DT, Threlkeld PG, Robertson DW. Affinities of fluoxetine, its enantiomers and other inhibitors of serotonin uptake for subtypes of serotonin receptors. *Neuropsychopharmacology.* 1991;5:43-47.
90. Wong DT, Bymaster FP, Reid LR, et al. Norfluoxetine enantiomers as inhibitors of serotonin uptake in rat brain. *Neuropsychopharmacology.* 1993;8:337-344.
91. Bertelsen KM, Venkatakrishnan K, Von Moltke LL, et al. Apparent mechanism-based inhibition of human CYP2D6 in vitro by paroxetine: comparison with fluoxetine and quinidine. *Drug Metab Dispos.* 2003;31:289-293.
92. Nakajima M, Suzuki M, Yamaji R, et al. Isoform selective inhibition and inactivation of human cytochrome P450s by methylenedioxyphenyl compounds. *Xenobiotica.* 1999;29:1191-1102.
93. Bolton JL, Acay NM, Vukomanovic V. Evidence that 4-allyl-*o*-quinones spontaneously rearrange to their more electrophilic quinone methides: potential bioactivation mechanism for the procarcinogen safrole. *Chem Res Toxicol.* 1994;7:443-450.
94. Sanchez C, Bogeso KP, Ebert B, et al. Escitalopram versus citalopram: the surprising role of the *R*-enantiomer. *Psychopharmacology.* 2004;174:163-176.
95. Owens MJ, Knight DL, Nemeroff CB. Second-generation SSRIs: human monoamine transporter binding profile of escitalopram and *R*-fluoxetine. *Biol Psychiatry.* 2001;50:345-350.
96. Obach RS, Cox LM, Tremaine LM. Sertraline is metabolized by multiple cytochrome P450 enzymes, monoamine oxidases and glucuronyl transferase in human; an in vitro study. *Drug Met Disposition.* 2005;33:262-270.
97. Wong DT, Bymaster FP. Dual serotonin and noradrenaline uptake inhibitor class of antidepressants potential for greater efficacy or just hype? *Prog Drug Res.* 2002;58:169-222.
98. Bymaster FP, Dreshfield-Ahmad LJ, Threlkeld PG, et al. Comparative affinity of duloxetine and venlafaxine for serotonin and norepinephrine transporters in vitro and in vivo, human serotonin receptor subtypes and other neuronal receptors. *Neuropsychopharmacology.* 2001;25:871-880.
99. Zerbe RL, Rowe H, Enas GG, et al. Clinical pharmacology of atomoxetine, a potential antidepressant. *J Pharmacol Exp Ther.* 1985;232:139-143.
100. Sauer JM, Ponsler GD, Mattiuz EL, et al. Disposition and metabolic fate of atomoxetine hydrochloride: the role of CYP2D6 in human disposition and metabolism. *Drug Metab Dispos.* 2003;31:98-107.

101. Asnis GM, Henderson MA. Levomilnacipran for the treatment of major depressive disorder: a review. *Neuropsychiatr Dis Treat.* 2015;11:115-135.
102. Vaishnavi SN, Nemeroff CB, Plott SJ, et al. Milnacipran: a comparative analysis of human monoamine uptake and transporter binding affinity. *Biol Psychiatry.* 2004;55:320-322.
103. Chen L, Greenberg WM, Gommoll C, et al. Levomilnacipran pharmacokinetics in healthy volunteers versus patients with major depressive disorder and implications for norepinephrine and serotonin reuptake inhibition. *Clin Ther.* 2015;37(9):2059-2070.
104. Iozzo C, Panconi E, Deprez D. Pharmacology and pharmacokinetics of milnacipran. *Int Clin Psychopharmacol.* 2002;17(suppl 1):S25-S35.
105. Brunner V, Maynadier B, Chen L, et al. Disposition and metabolism of [14C]-levomilnacipran, a serotonin and norepinephrine reuptake inhibitor, in humans, monkeys, and rats. *Drug Des Devel Ther.* 2015;9:3199-3215
106. Lantz RJ, Gillespie TA, Rash TJ, et al. Metabolism, excretion and pharmacokinetics of duloxetine in healthy human subjects. *Drug Metab Dispos.* 2003;31:1142-1150.
107. Jensen TS, Madsen CS, Finnerup NB. Pharmacology and treatment of neuropathic pains. *Curr Opin Neurol.* 2009;22:467-474.
108. Warner C, Shoaib M. How does bupropion work as a smoking cessation aid? *Addict Biol.* 2005;10:219-231.
109. Coles R, Kharasch ED. Stereoselective metabolism of bupropion by cytochrome P4502B6 (CYP2B6) and human liver microsomes. *Pharm Res.* 2008;25:1405-1411.
110. Hesse LM, Venkatakrishnan K, Court MH, et al. CYP2B6 mediates the in vitro hydroxylation of bupropion: potential drug interactions with other antidepressants. *Drug Metab Dispos.* 2000;28:1176-1183.
111. Bryant SG, Ereshefsky L. Antidepressant properties of trazodone. *Clin Pharm.* 1982;15:406-417.
112. Stahl SM. Mechanism of action of trazodone: a multifunctional drug. *CNS Spectr.* 2009;14:536-546.
113. Karhu D, Gossen ER, Mostert A, Cronjé T, Fradette C. Safety, tolerability, and pharmacokinetics of once-daily trazodone extended-release caplets in healthy subjects. *Int J Clin Pharmacol Ther.* 2011;49:730-743.
114. Wen B, Ma L, Rodrigues AD, Zhu M. Detection of novel reactive metabolites of trazodone: evidence for CYP2D6-mediated bioactivation of *m*-chlorophenylpiperazine. *J Chromatogr B Analyt Technol Biomed Life Sci.* 2008;871:44-54.
115. Boulton DW, Miller LF, Miller RL. Pharmacokinetics of trazodone and its major metabolite *m*-chlorophenylpiperazine in plasma and brain of rats. *Drug Metab Dispos.* 2008;36:841-850.
116. Rotzinger S, Fang J, Baker GB. Trazodone is metabolized to *m*-chlorophenylpiperazine by CYP3A4 from human sources. *Drug Metab Dispos.* 1998;26:572-575.
117. Iranikhah M, Wensel TM, Thomason AR. Vilazodone for the treatment of major depressive disorder. *Pharmacotherapy.* 2011;32(10):958-965.
118. Reinhold JA, Mandos LA, Lohoff FW, Rickels K. Evidence for the use of vilazodone in the treatment of major depressive disorder. *Expert Opin Pharmacother.* 2011;13:2215-2224.
119. McCormack PL. Vilazodone: a review in major depressive disorder in adults. *Drugs.* 2015;75(16):1915-1923.
120. El-Bagary R, Hashem H, Fouad M, Tarek S. UPLC-MS-MS method for the determination of vilazodone in human plasma: application to a pharmacokinetic study. *J Chromatogr Sci.* 2016;54:1365-1372.
121. Shi L, Wang J, Xu S, Lu Y. Efficacy and tolerability of vilazodone for major depressive disorder: evidence from phase III/IV randomized controlled trials. *Drug Des Devel Ther.* 2016;10:3899-3907.
122. Stuivenga M, Giltay EJ, Cools O, et al. Evaluation of vilazodone for the treatment of depressive and anxiety disorders. *Expert Opin Pharmacother.* 2018;26:1-10.
123. Connolly KR, Thase ME. Vortioxetine: a new treatment for major depressive disorder. *Expert Opin Pharmacother.* 2016;17:421-431.
124. Chen G, Højer AM, Areberg J, Nomikos G. Vortioxetine: clinical pharmacokinetics and drug interactions. *Clin Pharmacokinet.* 2018;57:673-686.
125. Chen G, Nomikos GG, Affinito J, et al. Effects of intrinsic factors on the clinical pharmacokinetics of vortioxetine. *Clin Pharmacol Drug Dev.* 2018;7:880-888.
126. Greenblatt DJ, Harmatz JS, Chow CR. Vortioxetine disposition in obesity: potential implications for patient safety. *J Clin Psychopharmacol.* 2018;38:172-179.
127. Benjamin S1, Doraiswamy PM. Review of the use of mirtazapine in the treatment of depression. *Expert Opin Pharmacother.* 2011;11:1623-1632.
128. Thompson C. Mirtazapine versus selective serotonin reuptake inhibitors. *J Clin Psychiatry.* 1999;60(suppl 17):18-22.
129. Stormer E, von Moltke LL, Shader RI, et al. Metabolism of the antidepressant mirtazapine in vitro: contribution of cytochromes P-450 1A2, 2D6 and 3A4. *Drug Metab Dispos.* 2000;28:1168-1175.
130. Shih JC, Chen K, Ridd MJ. MAO: from genes to behavior. *Annu Rev Neurosci.* 1999;22:197-217.
131. Baker GB, Urichuk LJ, McKenna KF, et al. Metabolism of monoamine oxidase inhibitors. *Cell Mol Neurobiol.* 1999;19:411-426.
132. Harwood AJ. Neurodevelopment and mood stabilizers. *Curr Mol Med.* 2003;3:472-482.
133. Berridge MJ. The Albert Lasker Medical Awards. Inositol trisphosphate, calcium, lithium and cell signaling. *JAMA.* 1989;262:1834-1841.
134. Lenox RH, Wang L. Molecular basis of lithium action: integration of lithium-responsive signaling and gene expression networks. *Mol Psychiatry.* 2003;8:135-144.
135. Machado-Vieira R, Salvadore G, Diazgranados N, Zarate CA. Ketamine and the next generation of antidepressants with a rapid onset of action. *Pharmacol Ther.* 2009;113:143-150.
136. Aan het Rot M, Collins KA, Murrough JW, et al. Safety and efficacy of repeated-dose intravenous ketamine for treatment-resistant depression. *Biol Psychiatry.* 2010;67:139-145.
137. Zanos P, Moaddel R, Morris PJ, et al. Ketamine and ketamine metabolite pharmacology: insights into therapeutic mechanisms. *Pharmacol Rev.* 2018;70:621-660.
138. Hasselmann HWW. Ketamine as antidepressant? Current state and future perspectives. *Curr Neuropharmacol.* 2014;11:57-70.
139. Zanos P, Gould TD. Mechanisms of ketamine action as an antidepressant. *Mol Psychiatry.* 2018;23:801-811.
140. Zanos P, Thompson SM, Duman RS, et al. Convergent mechanisms underlying rapid antidepressant action. *CNS Drugs.* 2018;32:197-227.
141. Zanos P, Gould TD. Intracellular signaling pathways involved in (*S*)- and (*R*)-ketamine antidepressant actions. *Biol Psychiatry.* 2018;83:2-4.
142. Desta Z, Moaddel R, Ogburn ET, et al. Stereoselective and regiospecific hydroxylation of ketamine and norketamine. *Xenobiotica.* 2011;42:1076-1087.
143. Abuzoor A, El-Alfy AT, Busse K. Auvelity (dextromethorphan/bupropion). *WMJ.* 2023;122:P4.
144. Dextromethorphan/bupropion (Auvelity) for depression. *Med Lett Drugs Ther.* 2022;26:201-203.
145. Khabir Y, Hashmi MR, Ali Asghar A. Rapid-acting oral drug (Auvelity) for major depressive disorder. *Ann Med Surg (Lond).* 2022;82:104629.
146. Chaki S, Watanabe M. Collection antidepressants in the post-ketamine Era: pharmacological approaches targeting the glutamatergic system. *Neuropharmacology.* 2023;223:109348.
147. Aschenbrenner DS. New combination drug for depression. *Am J Nurs.* 2023;123:24-25.

148. Ioannides C. Pharmacokinetic interactions between herbal remedies and medicinal drugs. *Xenobiotica*. 2002;32:451-478.
149. British Herbal Medicine Association. *British Herbal Pharmacopoeia*. British Herbal Medicine Association; 1983.
150. Muller WE, Singer A, Wonnemann M. Hyperforin—antidepressant activity by a novel mechanism of action. *Pharmacopsychiatry*. 2001;34(suppl 1):S98-S102.
151. Parker, J. (2020) 10 Best Medicinal Herbs and Their Health Benefits. Accessed May, 2025. https://motherofhealth.com/best-medicinal-herbs
152. Christopher EJ. Electroconvulsive therapy in the medically ill. *Curr Psychiatry Rep*. 2003;5:225-230.

Structure Challenge Answers

A

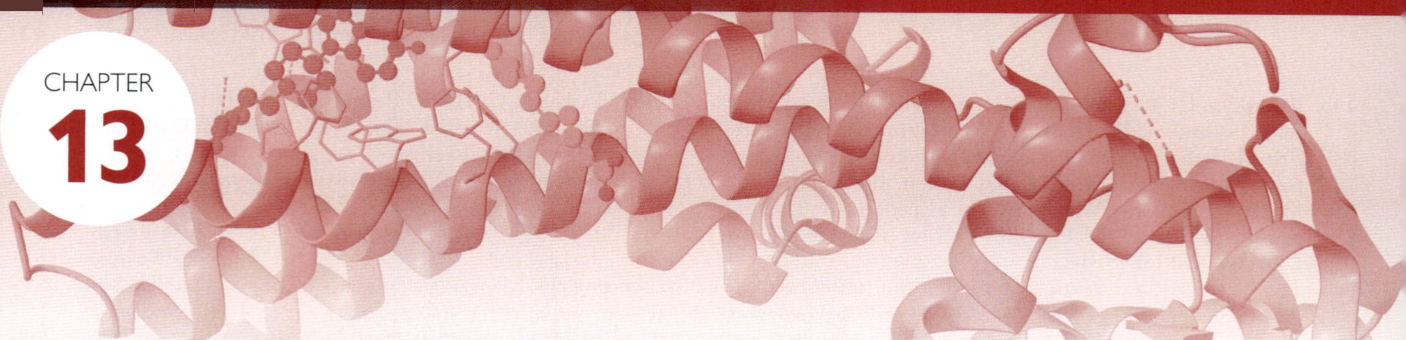

CHAPTER 13

Drugs Used to Treat Alzheimer Disease and Attention-Deficit/Hyperactivity Disorder

Patrick T. Flaherty

Drugs covered in this chapter:

ALZHEIMER DISEASE DRUGS

CHOLINESTERASE INHIBITORS
- Donepezil
- Galantamine
- Rivastigmine

NMDA-RECEPTOR ANTAGONISTS
- Memantine

BIOLOGICS
- Aducanumab
- Donanemab-azbt
- Lecanemab

ATTENTION-DEFICIT/HYPERACTIVITY DISORDER DRUGS

NONSTIMULANTS
- Atomoxetine
- Bupropion
- Clonidine
- Guanfacine
- Imipramine

STIMULANTS
- Dexmethylphenidate
- Dextroamphetamine
- Lisdexamphetamine
- Methylphenidate

Abbreviations

Aβ amyloid-beta peptide
ACh acetylcholine
AChE acetylcholinesterase
AD Alzheimer disease
ADAS-cog14 14-item cognitive subscale of the Alzheimer's Disease Assessment Scale
ADCOMS Alzheimer's Disease Composite Score
ADCS-ADL Alzheimer's Disease Cooperative Study–Instrumental Activities of Daily Living Inventory
ADHD attention-deficit/hyperactivity disorder
APO apolipoprotein
APOE ε4 apolipoprotein E ε4
APP/sAPP amyloid precursor protein/soluble amyloid precursor protein
ARIA amyloid-related imaging abnormality
BACE β-amyloid cleaving enzyme
BuChE butyrylcholinesterase
CAA cerebral β-amyloid angiopathy
C_{max} maximum serum concentration
CNS central nervous system
CSF cerebrospinal fluid
CYP cytochrome P450
DA dopamine
DAT dopamine transporter
DMT disease-modifying therapy
DSM-5 *Diagnostic and Statistical Manual of Mental Disorders* of the American Psychiatric Association
FAD familial Alzheimer disease
FDA U.S. Food and Drug Administration
GFAP glial fibrillary acidic protein
5-HT serotonin
iADRS Integrated Alzheimer Disease Rating Scale
mAb monoclonal antibody
MCI mild cognitive impairment
MMSE Mini-Mental State Examination
NAP 3-[1-(*N*,*N*-dimethylamino)ethyl] phenol
NE norepinephrine
NET norepinephrine transporter
NFT neurofibrillary tangles
NIA/NIH National Institute on Aging/National Institutes of Health
NMDA *N*-methyl-D-aspartate
NP neuritic plaques
p-tau phosphorylated tau
QC glutaminyl cyclase
SAD sporadic Alzheimer's disease
SERT serotonin transporter
$t_{1/2}$ half-life
T_{max} time to maximum serum concentration
VMAT vesicular monoamine transporter

CLINICAL SIGNIFICANCE

Alzheimer disease (AD), the most common and most costly dementia, requires informed clinicians to optimize patient outcomes. Cognition enhancement via blockade of acetylcholinesterase and/or blockade of N-methyl-D-aspartate receptors requires a delicate balance of symptom control while recognizing and managing side effects. For example, initiation of an acetylcholinesterase inhibitor may result in gastrointestinal disturbances or incontinence; quick recognition of these new symptoms as side effects may prevent unnecessary treatment and polypharmacy in older adults. U.S. Food and Drug Administration (FDA)-approved monoclonal antibody therapy against Aβ carries potential for disease-modification but requires consideration of cost, modest cognitive and functional outcomes, and significant amyloid-related imaging abnormality side effects to optimize outcomes for patients with AD.

Christine K. O'Neil, PharmD, BCPS, BCGP

Drugs Used to Treat Alzheimer Disease

I have–so to say–lost myself.

Augusta D., first patient diagnosed with Alzheimer disease.

Introduction

Alzheimer disease (AD) was first described by Alois Alzheimer as pre-senile dementia in 1906.[1] His patient, 51-year-old Augusta D., presented with disorientation in familiar locations, decreased knowledge of prior skills, an increased inability to recognize persons with whom she was familiar, and increased fearfulness and disorientation. Alzheimer, a trained histologist as well as physician, conducted a postmortem brain histologic study with silver stain and identified unusual extra-neuronal protein amyloid deposits and intraneuronal neurofibrils that had formed tangles. According to the Alzheimer's Association,[2] in 2024, almost 6.9 million U.S. citizens over 65 years old were living with this diagnosis and being cared for by an estimated 11 million unpaid providers. AD is the sixth leading cause of death in the United States and, in 2024, is projected to burden the health care system with an estimated annual cost of $360 billion. It is calculated that 25% of cost is "out-of-pocket" expense, with 64% of the total cost supported by Medicare and Medicaid. Even after demographic adjustment for COVID-19, prevalence of AD for persons 65 and older by 2060 is projected to be 13.8 million and reach an annual cost of $1 trillion by 2025.

Etiology

Increasingly, AD is seen as the most prevalent form of related dementias[3] characterized by functional loss correlated with anatomically characterized progressive neuronal cell death. Categorization of dementia type is based on both anatomical location and spread of neuronal cell death, as well as aberrantly processed protein deposition.[4] AD accounts for 60% to 80% of all dementia,[5,6] with the vast majority of these cases being sporadic (SAD) versus the 1% to 2% caused by genetic mutation.[7] While SAD can involve predisposing genetic factors (specifically one or more apolipoprotein E ε4 alleles), genetic-driven AD is most often associated with genetic variations in the sequence of amyloid precursor protein (APP) or proteases that process APP such as presenilin (PS1 or PS2).[7] Known as familial Alzheimer disease (FAD), this aggressive form of the disease commonly presents earlier in life and progresses more rapidly than SAD.

All forms of AD can be characterized by the location and progressive deposition of extracellular amyloid plaques and soluble oligomers composed of amyloid-beta peptide (Aβ), intracellular neurofibrillary tangles (NFTs) and extra-neuronal neuritic plaques (NPs). Both NFTs and NPs are composed of hyperphosphorylated tau, a microtubule-associated protein that normally stabilizes the cytoskeletal structure of axonal projections.[4,5,7] Phosphorylated tau (p-tau)[8] found in NFTs and NPs is uniquely hyperphosphorylated at multiple sites, including p-tau181, p-tau217, and p-tau231. These forms of p-tau self-associate and precipitate as NFTs and NPs.

In healthy individuals, soluble amyloid precursor protein (sAPP) undergoes peptide hydrolysis by α- or β-secretases to generate soluble peptide products. In contrast, AD patients produce insoluble Aβ through sequential cleavage of APP by β- then γ-secretase to produce insoluble proteins that misfold into a hairpin structure, then stack into insoluble neurotoxic β-sheet oligomers. Two variations of Aβ (Aβ40 and Aβ42) are associated with acetylcholinergic cell death. These Aβ oligomers are neurotoxic, promote additional self-association, accelerate subsequent neurotoxicity, and drive neuronal death.[9] Aβ40 is more prone to self-associate, oligomerize, deposit Aβ plaques, and is more neurotoxic than Aβ42. Despite intense research, development of γ-secretase inhibitors as an anti-AD therapeutic strategy has been problematic. Promising clinical candidates with good intrinsic γ-secretase inhibitory activity and appropriate pharmacokinetic properties failed in clinical trials due to collateral off-target NOTCH inhibition that drove melanoma development.[7]

The primacy of Aβ pathology versus the primacy of tau hyperphosphorylation, although not resolved at the current time, is increasingly better understood. A biphasic process for Aβ mediated toxicity is currently proposed.[10] In the initial stage, early deposited Aβ oligomers are proposed as priming events that drive inflammatory processes, which vary from individual to individual. Proposed inflammatory processes include activation of glia, conversion of astrocytes into a neurotoxic phenotype, and alteration of tau phosphorylation patterns due to neuronal cytoskeletal instability. As the initial stage progresses to the second stage of Aβ toxicity, clinically observable symptoms, including loss of spatial orientation and memory, become apparent. The second stage of Aβ-mediated toxicity is at least partially independent of increased Aβ production and deposition. In this later stage, hyperphosphorylation of tau drives formation of intracellular NFTs and NPs; these deposits can increase the inflammatory response, including increased Aβ production and Aβ deposition. This biphasic response recommends therapeutic strategies that can attenuate Aβ deposition in the presymptomatic phase of AD prior to disease conversion to the second phase, which is less susceptible to Aβ reduction therapeutic strategies. An awareness of a biphasic contribution from Aβ aggregation to AD progression argues strongly for development of early bioassays, which can facilitate development of disease-modifying therapeutic approaches and serve as clinically determined criteria for initiation of disease-modifying therapy (DMT) in responsive individuals.

Sustained neuronal cytosolic Ca^{2+} signaling can drive increased Aβ plaque and p-tau tangle production and has been proposed as a contributory factor for AD development.[7] Ca^{2+} dyshomeostasis within lysosomes, mitochondria, and endoplasmic reticulum may be the most impactful to AD pathogenesis, although much research remains to be conducted before a clear understanding of clinical relevance is gained.

Pathology and Approaches to Treatment

The preclinical or asymptomatic phase of AD can be as long as 20 years, during which cognitive changes are nonexistent or mild (prodromal AD). The first overt symptoms generally arise from loss of acetylcholinergic activity in the subiculum, entorhinal cortex, and hippocampal regions of the brain. Early neuronal loss matches deposition of Aβ, NFTs, and NPs, driving loss of function dependent on neural processing in these areas of the brain. This results in loss of orientation in place and time; loss of short-term memory; and an inability to recall familiar names, places, and events. Later, a depressed or flattened affect is presented. Decreased attention and concentration is noted, and skills related to planning, problem-solving, and completing complex tasks are impaired. Other symptoms include language problems, including difficulty recalling words, reduced vocabulary, and decreased complexity in speech and writing. Correct affective discernment becomes impaired consistent with increased impairment of the hippocampus and amygdala. Patients may withdraw from social engagements and begin to display more profound cognitive and communicative impairments, such as confusion and/or a presumption of external aggression by others. Patients may ultimately lose the ability to walk and/or swallow.[11] A total of seven drugs have received FDA approval to treat AD. This includes three monoclonal antibodies (mAbs) for treating AD recently approved by the FDA: aducanumab (Aduhelm), lecanemab (Leqembi), and donanemab-azbt (Kisunla).

Without a defined path to cure, AD management is aimed primarily at attenuating symptoms and slowing progression of its hallmark outcome (dementia), with much effort focused on prevention.[5] Primary prevention strategies seek to minimize disease acquisition risk as we currently understand it through healthy diet and lifestyle choices, fostering cardiovascular health and encouraging ongoing educational enrichment and mental stimulation. Secondary prevention seeks to forestall disease progression before significant loss of cognitive function; strategies including nutritional guidance, exercise, social and mental engagement, and cardiovascular risk factor management are being studied.

Recent initiatives by the National Institute on Aging (NIA)/National Institutes of Health (NIH) have emphasized several key areas for research that have the potential to drive significant advances in understanding and treating AD. Development of bioassays to determine the state of disease progression, as well as providing a basis for assessing the utility of novel treatment strategies, is actively being examined. A better understanding of early events that could tip the homeostatic balance from neuroprotection toward neurodegeneration and/or identification of yet uncharacterized processes driving subsequent neurotoxicity are also actively under examination. The larger goal is to understand AD and associated neurodegenerative processes at a fundamental level to enable therapeutic interventions that prevent neuronal death, prevent functional loss, and enable a more durable presence of the patient.[12]

Pharmacotherapy

Figure 13.1 provides the structures of the four small molecule anti-AD drugs currently marketed in the United States, three structurally distinct acetylcholinesterase (AChE) inhibitors (donepezil, galantamine, rivastigmine), and one *N*-methyl-D-aspartate (NMDA) receptor allosteric antagonist (memantine).

The neurotransmitter acetylcholine (ACh) is critical to cognition, and diminished levels of cholinergic neurons in the basal forebrain of AD patients result in diminished function for the patient.[13,14] ACh is rapidly hydrolyzed to inactive acetate and choline by the enzyme AChE. Inhibition of AChE increases the intraneuronal levels of ACh and its neurotransmission. AChE inhibitors are generally recommended in the early stages of the disease when patients are exhibiting mild-to-moderate symptoms.[7,14] Other approaches to augmenting ACh in cognitively impaired brains have been tried (specifically ACh precursors and synthetic muscarinic agonists) but they were not successful, primarily due to challenging pharmacokinetic and/or adverse effect profiles.[14] As the disease progresses, patients are subject to neuronal destruction via the overstimulation of NMDA receptors by the excitatory neurotransmitter glutamate. NMDA receptors are intimately involved in learning and memory. Memantine is an allosteric blocker of the NMDA receptor at the inter-channel magnesium ion binding site. This allosteric antagonism reduces the glutamate firing frequency in a use-dependent manner, reducing glutamate excitotoxicity in patients with moderate-to-severe disease.[7,13]

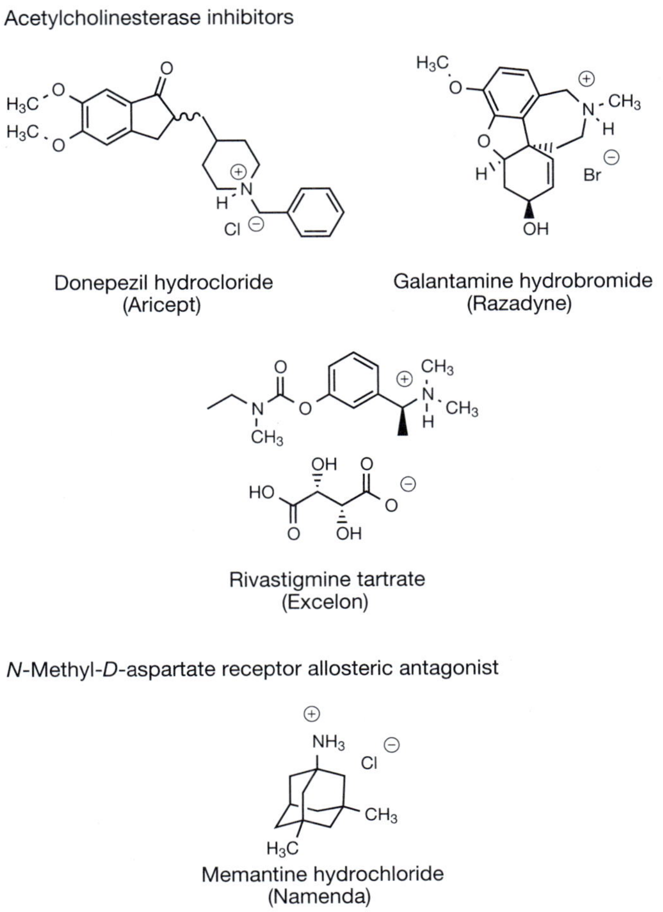

Figure 13.1 Small molecule drugs available to treat Alzheimer disease.

Selected pharmacokinetic parameters of these four agents are provided in Table 13.1.[15] All are administered orally in immediate- or extended-release formulations, and the AChE inhibitors donezepil and rivastigmine are also available in a transdermal patch dosage form.

Acetylcholinesterase Inhibitors

AChE's catalytic site contains a Ser203 residue activated for nucleophilic attack at ACh's electrophilic carbonyl carbon through an intramolecular association with a His447 and Glu334 (residue numbers for the human enzyme).[16,17] Although contained within a deeply recessed active site, this catalytic triad is a powerful hydrolyzing "machine," cleaving up to 25,000 ACh molecules per second.[16] Other domains that appropriately orient and hold ACh in place include: (1) an anionic domain that, despite its name, has only aromatic residues that anchor the onium head of ACh through cation-π interactions, (2) an acyl pocket containing sterically restricting Phe residues that ensure no choline esters larger than ACh can enter, and (3) an oxyanion hole with Gly and Ala residues and one structured water molecule that facilitates enzyme-substrate binding, as well as the tetrahedral hydrolytic transition state.[17]

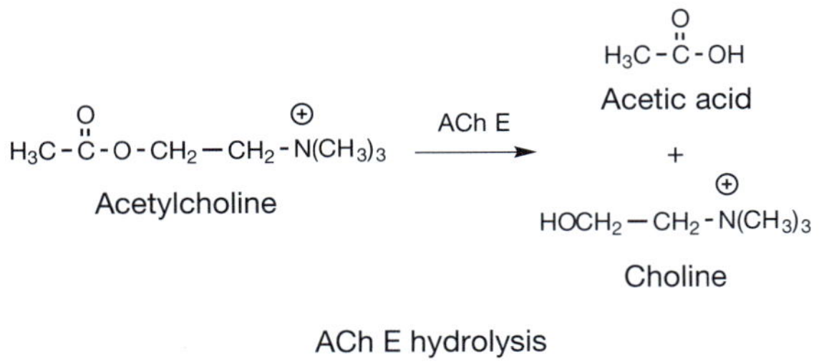

Tacrine was the first cholinesterase inhibitor to be marketed in the United States but was discontinued due to reversible hepatotoxicity as safer options became available. In addition to elevating central levels of ACh, AChE inhibitors also block the cytotoxicity-promoting action of AChE on Aβ aggregation and p-tau hyperphosphorylation, thus decreasing the formation of destructive plaques and neurofibrillary tangles.[13] AChE inhibitors can modestly improve cognition and the ability to engage in the activities of daily living (ADLs), but only about 30% to 40% of patients respond, and the duration of therapeutic benefit is generally limited to 2 years or less.[14] While there is currently no

Table 13.1 Selected Pharmacokinetic Parameters of Anti-Alzheimer Drugs

Drug	$t_{1/2}$ (h)	T_{max} (h)	Protein Binding (%)	Metabolism	Renal Excretion (%)
Donepezil	70	3-8 (dose dependent)	96	CYP2D6, CYP3A4, glucuronidation	57
Galantamine	7	1 (IR); 4.5-5 (ER)	18	O-demethylation (CYP2D6), N-oxidation (CYP3A4)	20
Rivastigmine	1.5; 3 (TD)	1; 8-16 (TD)	40	Hydrolysis, N-demethylation, sulfonation (non-CYP)	97
Memantine	60-80	3-7 (IR); 9-12 (ER)	45	Hepatic (non-CYP)	74

Orally administered unless otherwise noted.

clearly defined way to identify responders prior to therapy, apolipoprotein E ε4 (APOE ε4) carrier status has been associated with a lack of responsiveness, as this allele appears to thwart compensatory hippocampal cholinergic sprouting in lesion-induced mammalian brain damage designed to mimic early AD.[14]

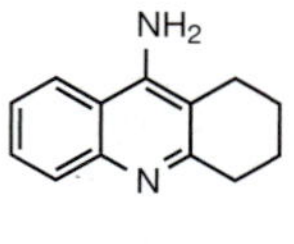

Tacrine (Cognex)

Cholinergic augmentation through AChE inhibition is proposed to have an important place at the therapeutic table due to its neuroprotective and compensatory neuronal plasticity benefits.[14] Research into the development of new inhibitors is ongoing, and four goals have been recommended to advance therapeutic efficacy: (1) ability to bind to both the catalytic and peripheral sites of the esterase, (2) ability to inhibit both synaptic, membrane-bound AChE and the more ubiquitous, nonspecific and glial-based butyrylcholinesterase (BuChE), which may take over for AChE when the latter enzyme is specifically inhibited, (3) targeted delivery to/activity in the basal forebrain, and (4) attention to the impact/timing of ACh release on presynaptic autoreceptor stimulation (which inhibits further release) and the ability to respond to postsynaptic phasic cholinergic signaling.[14] Combination therapies that couple AChE inhibitors with anti-amyloid, antioxidant, and/or anti-inflammatory agents (among others) are also being actively explored, as is the development of highly selective and centrally active M_1 muscarinic receptor agonists that could serve as DMTs.

Specific Drugs

Donepezil Hydrochloride. Donepezil was the second AChE inhibitor approved for use in AD and is currently the oldest such drug clinically available.[16] It is chemically classified as a 2-benzylpiperidine-indenone, and structure-activity studies have confirmed that both the basic benzylpiperidine moiety and the indenone C_1 carbonyl are essential. Expansion of the cyclopentenone component of the indenone ring to six- or seven-membered systems diminished activity. The aromatic methoxy groups at indenone C_5 and C_6 increase activity over 25-fold compared to the unsubstituted derivative, and the activity provided by the methylene spacer between rings is second only to propylene. While marketed as the racemic mixture, AChE inhibiting activity resides exclusively in the *R* isomer.[16]

Donepezil binding to the AChE active site is reversible, highly selective (minimal BuChE inhibition occurs), and predominantly noncompetitive. Key interactions with AChE isolated from *Torpedo californica* (electric eel) are shown in Figure 13.2. The essential cationic piperidine nitrogen anchors to Asp72, as well as to Phe330 and Tyr121, the latter bridged through a water molecule. Trp residues engage in affinity-enhancing π-π interactions with both aromatic systems, and another molecule of water links the two methoxy oxygen atoms to anionic Glu185. The carbonyl oxygen serves an orientation function to permit edge-on π-π stacking

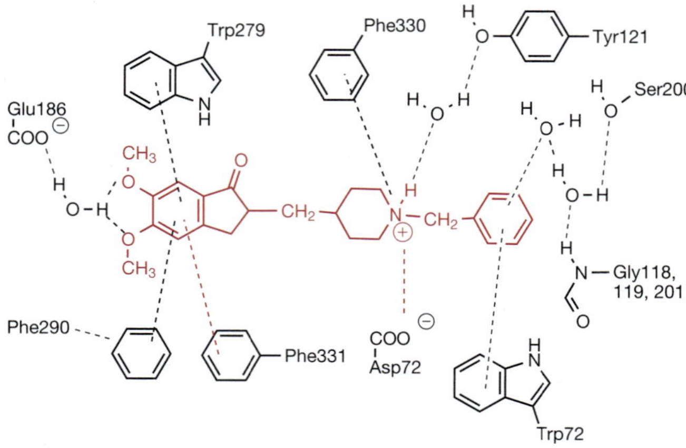

Figure 13.2 Binding interactions between *Torpedo californica* acetylcholinesterase and donepezil.

with Phe331 and Phe290. Three Gly residues and Ser200, again working through water molecules, interface with the aromatic segment of the benzyl moiety.[16] The bound drug is believed to inhibit both the formation of the endogenous enzyme-substrate (ACh) complex and the hydrolysis of any neurotransmitter that finds its way into the catalytic pocket.

In addition to binding at the enzyme's active site, donepezil also interacts within a peripheral anionic site adjacent to the recessed catalytic gorge, which inhibits other nonhydrolytic enzyme functions.[17,18] Aβ is known to bind to this peripheral site, and inhibiting its association with the enzyme protects cholinergic neurons from complex-induced cytotoxicity, as well as minimizes AChE-induced fibrillation of the Aβ protein. Some have postulated neuroprotective effects for donepezil independent of AChE inhibition (including protection against Aβ- and glutamate-induced cell destruction, ischemia, and hippocampal atrophy) that might qualify it as a DMT.[18] A systemic review of donepezil, rivastigmine, and galantamine[19] on the potentially multifaceted clinical mechanism of donepezil in early to late-stage AD is ongoing.[20,21]

As noted in Table 13.2, donepezil is vulnerable to CYP-catalyzed metabolism and is excreted primarily via the kidneys. Only about 15% of the dose found in the urine is in parent drug form. CYP2D6 and CYP3A4 are both involved in donepezil biotransformation, and blood levels can be significantly impacted by 2D6 phenotype. The active *R* isomer is metabolized more readily than the inactive *S* enantiomer,[16] but clinically relevant interactions with co-administered drugs are fairly rare due to the generally slow rate of metabolic transformation. However, strong CYP3A4 inhibitors, such as conazole antifungal agents, can significantly elevate serum levels of the drug.

The most prevalent donepezil metabolite (M1) is the 6-phenol (11% of the administered dose), which is essentially equally active with donepezil.[16,17] A minor *p*-hydroxybenzyl metabolite[22] (M3) also exhibits activity on a par with the parent drug. The most common phase 1 metabolic reactions, or those that produce an active metabolite, are shown in Figure 13.3.[16,23] Glucuronidation (M1, M2) or sulfonation (M3) of phenolic metabolites is known to occur prior to excretion.[16]

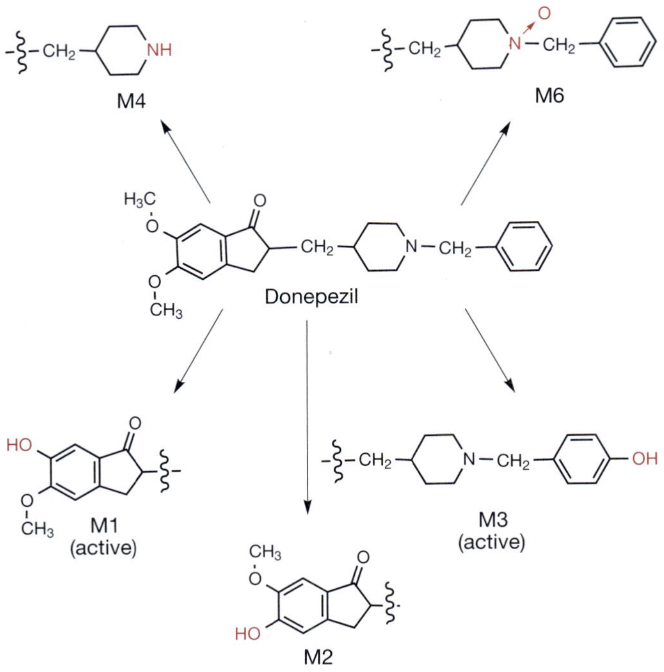

Figure 13.3 Major CYP2D6- and CYP3A4-catalyzed phase 1 metabolism of donepezil.

Donepezil is marketed as 5-, 10-, and 23-mg tablets. The two lower doses are also available in a disintegrating tablet formulation that may be particularly helpful in patients who are losing the ability to swallow safely, and the 23-mg tablet is film coated. The 5- and 10-mg doses are reserved for patients with mild-to-moderate cognitive symptoms, and inhibition of AChE runs between 20% and 40%.[16] The 23-mg dose provides a significantly increased C_{max} and more persistently high serum levels, making it useful in more advanced disease. The therapeutic value of the 23-mg dose was initially questioned, as disease severity as measured by several markers (including the Mini-Mental State Examination [MMSE]) was not noticeably improved over the lower doses. Interestingly, the actions of the 23-mg dose cannot be duplicated by simply taking more doses of the 5- or 10-mg tablets.

Patients should be slowly and carefully titrated to their optimum dosage, and it is recommended that the 23-mg dose not be started until the patient has shown success on lower doses for 3 to 4 months. The most commonly observed adverse effects are those associated with elevated cholinergic activity, including bradycardia, nausea, vomiting, and diarrhea as well as muscle cramping and vertigo.[16] Adverse effects are dose-dependent,[24] and providers and caregivers should work collaboratively when assessing relative risks and benefits of ongoing therapy.

Donepezil is also available as once-weekly transdermal patches in two dosage forms: the equivalent of 5 or 10 mg/d.[25,26] This improves on prior transdermal patches with rivastigmine that required daily patch application. The primary advantage over orally administered donepezil is ease of administration in an institutional setting and avoiding difficulties in swallowing; side effects and drug interactions are similar to those of solid-dosage forms. Donepezil patches require storage under refrigeration, then normalization to room temperature prior to application. Skin irritation in healthy subjects with non- or lightly-pigmented skin (median age 54 years) was determined with the patch on days 1, 2, and 3 and after removal of the patch at days 8, 15, and 22 days, with a combined skin irritation prevalence score of 2% contrasted to 0% for placebo.[25]

Galantamine Hydrobromide. Galantamine, an alkaloid found in bulbs and flowers of plants of the genus *Galanthus* used in traditional medicine for over 2000 years, has enjoyed current therapeutic use in several neuromuscular-related pathologies, including myasthenia gravis and residual poliomyelitis.[17] Its ability to concentrate in the central nervous system (CNS) and impact cholinergic systems made it a natural for investigation in the treatment of AD, and it received FDA approval in 2001 for use in mild-to-moderate disease.

Galantamine's selective, competitive, and reversible binding to AChE involves the catalytic and acyl pockets as well as the adjacent peripheral anionic site (Fig. 13.4). Hydrogen and hydrophobic interactions predominate, but an important cation-π bond between the protonated amine and Tyr337 mimics the interaction of the onium head of endogenous ACh with the enzyme. Molecular docking studies performed with *N*-aralkyl-modified analogs document that affinity for the peripheral anionic site increases significantly due to π-π stacking interactions with Tyr341 (not shown).[17] Studies in animal models have demonstrated the ability of galantamine to promote Aβ clearance and microglial phagocytosis.[27] The drug is known to uniquely modulate nicotinic cholinergic receptors through allosteric binding, leading to increased intracellular Ca^{2+}, augmented release of ACh and norepinephrine (NE) from central synapses, and potentially enhanced cognition.[24,27] Despite this, the clinical relevance of nicotinic receptor involvement[28,12] in anticholinergic AD drug action is being revaluated.[14]

Galantamine absorption is complete and minimally impacted by food. The majority of galantamine is metabolized by CYP2D6 and CYP3A4, which generates

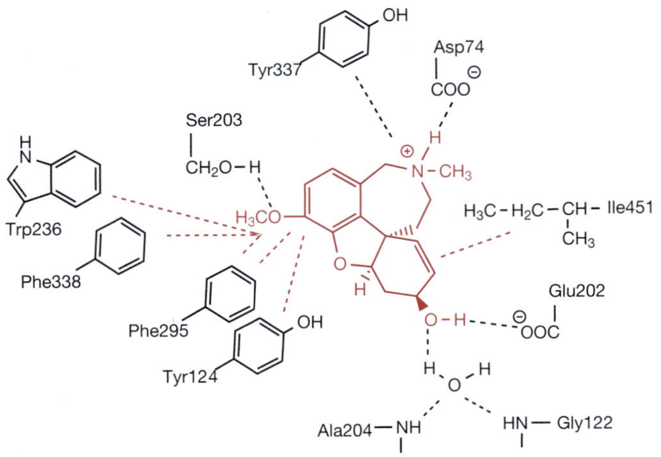

Figure 13.4 Binding interactions between human acetylcholinesterase and galantamine. Hydrophobic interactions are shown in red.

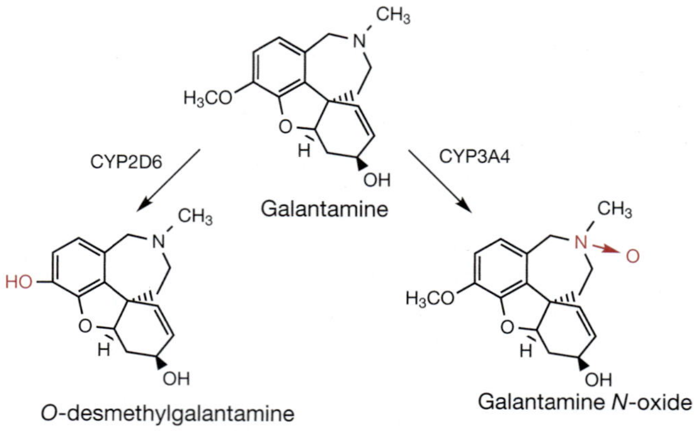

Figure 13.5 CYP2D6- and CYP3A4-catalyzed phase 1 metabolism of galantamine.

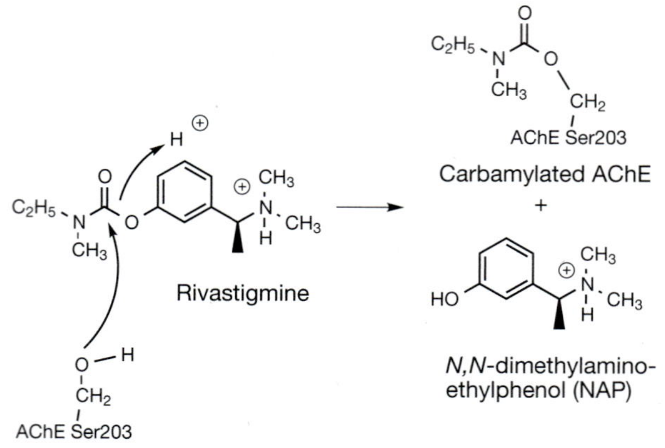

Figure 13.6 Rivastigmine carbamoylation of acetylcholinesterase.

O-dealkylated phenol and *N*-oxide metabolites, respectively (Fig. 13.5).[27,29] Unlike donepezil, neither metabolite retains therapeutic activity. Approximately 75% of a dose will be biotransformed, and both the parent drug and metabolites can undergo glucuronidation prior to renal excretion. CYP2D6 phenotype impacts the rate of O-desmethyl metabolite generation; however, dosage adjustments for poor 2D6 metabolizers are not required.[27] Likewise, drug-drug interactions (DDIs) based on metabolic vulnerabilities are of only minor clinical concern, although strong inhibitors of these isoforms should be used with appropriate caution.[15,27]

A meta-analysis of galantamine efficacy in AD showed cognition enhancement when compared to placebo and, with long-term use, improvement in performance of ADL.[30] It has been shown to be an acceptable alternative for mild-moderate AD patients who are nonresponsive to donepezil therapy[31] and is available in tablet, extended-release capsule, and oral solution dosage forms. The daily maintenance dose ranges from 16 to 24 mg administered once (extended-release) or in two divided doses (immediate-release) in a 24-hour period, most commonly with meals. Initial doses are half the lower maintenance dose, and 4 weeks should elapse between dose escalations. Adverse effects that can prompt drug discontinuation are primarily gastrointestinal in nature (nausea, vomiting, diarrhea), vertigo, and urinary tract infection.[27,30] More serious adverse effects include dermatological toxicity, including Stevens-Johnson syndrome, and arrhythmia (bradycardia, AV block). Additive effects with co-administered drugs that prolong the QT interval can lead to potentially fatal arrhythmia, including Torsade de Pointes.

Rivastigmine Tartrate. Unlike the other cholinesterase inhibitors used in AD, *S*(−)-rivastigmine stereoselectively inhibits both AChE and BuChE in the CNS, which is advantageous in patients experiencing disease-associated loss of AChE.[32] Rivastigmine acts through the covalent carbamoylation of the catalytic site Ser hydroxyl residue of both cholinesterases, destroying their ability to act as a hydrolytic nucleophile on endogenous ACh.[33] The carbamoylation reaction with hAChE Ser203 is shown in Figure 13.6; the reaction with BuChE is analogous, although this enzyme is known to have a less-constrained active site cavity.[33] After carbamoylation, the normal interaction of the other two catalytic triad residues, His and Glu, is sterically disrupted by rivastigmine's *N*-ethyl moiety and/or the displaced 3-[1-(*N,N*-dimethylamino)ethyl]phenol (NAP). This hinders the positioning of the water molecule needed to liberate the carbamoylated esterase,[33,34] with the result being a prolonged "pseudoirreversible" or slowly reversible covalent inhibition of the enzyme that persists for 10 hours or longer. Enzyme inhibition is enhanced by the displaced NAP, as it is believed to be captured within the anionic domain of the esterase.

Imaging studies have demonstrated that patients responding to rivastigmine show enhanced hippocampal metabolism and metabolic activity in memory-related areas of the brain compared to nonresponders. In patients with likely AD, BuChE inhibition in cerebral spinal fluid was associated with improvement in attentiveness and memory more so than AChE inhibition, and these clinical benefits persisted for up to 6 months of therapy.[35] BuChE with the A539T mutation (known as a K-variant) shows a 30% decrease in hydrolytic efficacy compared to the wild-type enzyme. Patients expressing this polymorph experience less aggressive disease progression and respond less vigorously to rivastigmine.[35] Meta-analyses on the relative value of rivastigmine in AD compared to donepezil and galantamine are mixed, but the risk of gastrointestinal adverse effects is generally highest for oral rivastigmine.[36]

Rivastigmine metabolism is straightforward and involves hydrolytic cleavage of the carbamate with possible N-demethylation and/or phase 2 sulfonation of the resultant NAP metabolite (Fig. 13.7).[37] The relative lack of CYP involvement in biotransformation, along with a low affinity for serum protein, translates to a decreased risk of DDIs in a highly vulnerable population.[38] Oral absorption from the capsule formulation is rapid and complete within an hour. The initial dose is 1.5 mg administered twice daily with meals and can be gradually increased up to a maximum of 12 mg daily as long as there is a 2-week interval between dosing elevations.

As noted, gastrointestinal distress, coupled with difficulty swallowing and/or challenges in achieving optimal

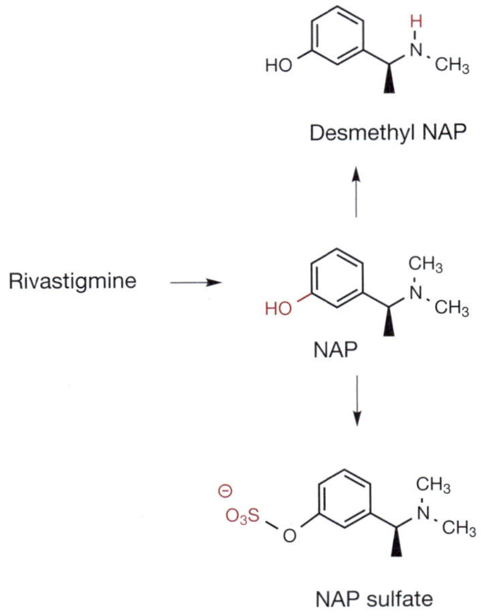

Figure 13.7 Metabolism of rivastigmine.

plasma concentrations, can compromise patient well-being and may result in drug discontinuation. This therapeutic reality prompted the development of a transdermal patch formulation of rivastigmine.[38,39] Drug release is controlled through an acrylic polymer mixture, and the silicone matrix against the skin optimizes patch adherence while minimizing trauma on removal (important in the often fragile skin of older adults).[39] Rivastigmine patches can deliver 4.6, 9.5, or 13.3 mg of drug per 24 hours. The 9.5 mg daily dose has been shown to lower the maximum serum concentration (C_{max}) while prolonging time to achieve C_{max} (T_{max}) compared to the maximum oral dose (6 mg capsules taken twice daily) without compromising overall drug exposure, thus improving pharmacokinetic stability and overall tolerability.[39,40] Efficacy is dose dependent, with the 13.3 mg transdermal dose providing greater therapeutic benefit than the 4.6 mg daily dose relative to cognition, ADLs, and overall function.[35] A minimum of 4 weeks on a lower dose should precede dose escalation. The adverse effect profile (including weight loss) is significantly decreased compared to the capsule formulation, with some studies showing gastrointestinal distress with the 9.5 mg/d dose on par with placebo.[39,40] The short 3-hour elimination half-life ($t_{1/2}$) ensures that serum levels will fall quickly if the patch must be removed in an emergency.[40]

Rivastigmine bioavailability from the patch formulation is highest when applied to the upper or lower back, upper arm, or chest.[39,40] While skin reactions are possible, they can be minimized by site rotation and do not generally result in therapy discontinuation.[39,40] Convenience/compliance advantages for the patch include simplified once-daily administration without regard to meals and readily visible confirmation of medication adherence for caregivers.[39]

Rivastigmine is the only anti-AD cholinesterase inhibitor approved for use in Parkinson disease–related dementia. It has also shown value in the symptomatic treatment of dementia resulting from subcortical vascular insufficiency.[39]

N-Methyl-D-Aspartate Antagonists

The fact that augmentation of central cholinergic activity does not, in and of itself, permanently halt the progression of AD exemplifies the multifaceted pathology of this disease. Glutamate is another neurotransmitter linked to neurophysiologic health and cognition, which has provided a novel avenue for dementia drug development, as levels of glutamate are known to be elevated in AD.[41]

NMDA Receptors, Excitotoxicity, and Uncompetitive Receptor Antagonism. NMDA receptors are ligand-gated calcium ion channels (Chapter 8). When stimulated by the endogenous excitatory neurotransmitter glutamate or an exogenous agonist, NMDA receptors depolarize, liberate a bound regulatory Mg^{2+} ion, and open a channel permitting influx of Ca^{2+} and Na^{+} ions into the postsynaptic neuron. The liberation of Mg^{2+} and the short-term opening of the channel is associated with synaptic plasticity in the hippocampus (the central seat of episodic memory) and improves the ability to learn, think, and remember.[13,41] Overstimulation of NMDA receptors by moderately (but chronically) elevated levels of glutamate or neuronal insult from Aβ results in excitotoxicity. Excitotoxicity damages neurons secondary to excessively high levels of intracellular Ca^{2+} by generating free radicals and other neurotoxins.[41,42] Overexcited neurons become highly depolarized with an excessive intraneuronal positive charge that repels Mg^{2+} ions and inhibits normal inhibition of NMDA channels by Mg^{2+}. This generates a persistently open ion channel that negatively impacts cognition.[42] NMDA hyperactivity also stimulates the hyperphosphorylation of tau to increase NFT formation. The interconnectedness of glutamate, NMDA receptors, Aβ (particularly soluble oligomers of the Aβ protein), and p-tau has been described in the literature.[43]

Uncompetitive blockade of NMDA receptors by compounds like memantine at the Mg^{2+} site antagonizes excessive overstimulation by glutamate, leaving homeostatic stimulation unaffected. It does this through low-affinity binding to the receptor-associated Ca^{2+} channel in its open state, with minimal retention in the channel during its closed state after hyperpolarization. This keeps Ca^{2+} concentrations in check and improves cognition in moderate-to-advanced disease without the risk of adverse effects that a complete and total receptor block could induce (eg, dissociation, excessive sedation, hallucinations).[42]

An important distinction between uncompetitive and noncompetitive receptor antagonism is the former's requirement for a receptor activated by an agonist. An uncompetitive NMDA-receptor antagonist must gain access to the ion channel after it is opened by glutamate, and this requires that the channel stay open long enough for it to enter (longer than homeostatic opening). This is why the antagonist shows greater efficacy when levels of glutamate are high (pathologic) as opposed to low (homeostatic). The antagonist should not bind too tightly or work too aggressively when the receptor is only minimally activated, but it should spend a longer time in the channel than the endogenous Mg^{2+} gatekeeper.[42] To paraphrase a famous line in a familiar children's story, to achieve therapeutic efficacy, the "dwell time" in the channel should not be too long (homeostatic antagonism) or too short (ineffective excitotoxicity blockade), but "just right."

Memantine Hydrochloride. Memantine blocks glutamate-induced excitotoxicity by binding close to the Mg^{2+} site within the NMDA-associated ion channel. It gains access to this site through its monocationic protonated amine. Two bridgehead CH_3 groups and large hydrophobic bridged structure help retain it in situ for the appropriate amount of time. Memantine blocks neurodegeneration driven by glutamate overstimulation of NMDA receptors, resulting in neuroprotection and, therefore, has characteristics of DMT.[41,42]

Randomized controlled trials on efficacy and therapeutic value have produced conflicting results: safe and effective versus a high risk for adverse effects. However, a meta-analysis with well-defined inclusion criteria published in 2015 found evidence of significant benefits to cognition, ADL, mental state, and the clinician's global impression of status, primarily due to memantine's ability to retard mental and functional decline in patients with moderate-to-severe disease.[44] Approximately 4,100 patients with AD from 13 double-blinded placebo-controlled trials were included in the analysis, and the investigators determined that the only troublesome or serious adverse effect more likely with memantine compared to placebo was somnolence. These outcomes were confirmed in a 2017 meta-analysis conducted by others.[45]

Memantine is available in immediate-release tablets and extended-release capsules. Memantine is extensively plasma bound with a long $t_{1/2} = 60$ hours enabling once a day dosing. The immediate-release medication is started at 5 mg daily and slowly titrated upward on a weekly basis in 5-mg increments to a maximum of 20 mg/d. The same approach is taken with the extended-release formulation, only the starting and maximum doses are 7 and 28 mg/d, respectively. An oral 2 mg/mL solution is also commercially available. Absorption of memantine is complete and food independent. Patients with alkaline urine may show higher than normal serum levels of drug and should be monitored for adverse effects. In addition to drowsiness, dizziness may be a problem for some patients; however, discontinuation rates are comparable to placebo.[46] Metabolism is CYP-independent and none of the four primary metabolites are active (Fig. 13.8).

Memantine/Donepezil Combination Therapy. Combination NMDA/AChE antagonist therapy has been proposed to be beneficial, as glutamatergic terminal reorganization occurs in brain regions that exhibit cholinergic plasticity.[14] Additional evidence of the interconnectedness of these two neurotransmitter systems has been documented.[47] Specifically, glutamatergic neurons interact directly with cholinergic neurons in several areas of the brain, including the hippocampus, and it has been proposed that

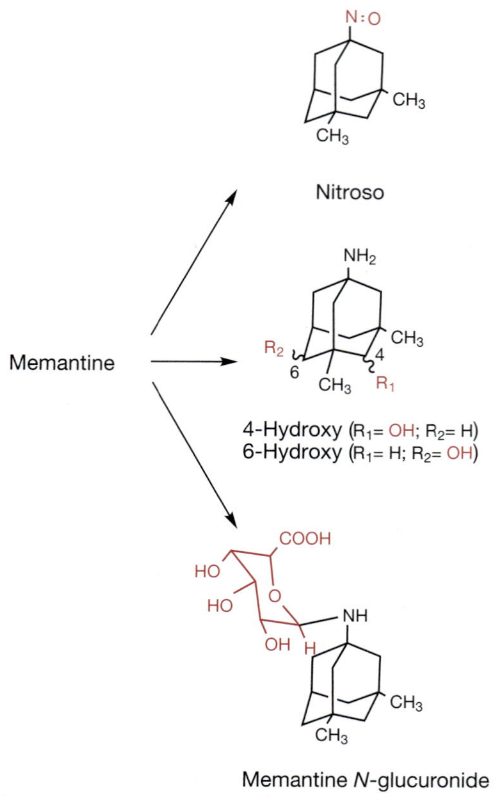

Figure 13.8 Metabolism of memantine.

NMDA-receptor activation stimulates the release of ACh from neurons in the basal forebrain. Glutamate-induced excitotoxicity and accompanying neuronal cell death takes a toll on cholinergic neurons in the cerebral cortex, and inhibition of that destructive process can protect cholinergic receptors and synaptic AChE.

In short, both cholinergic and NMDA-related dysfunction underpin AD pathology, with distinct mechanisms of action that are complementary for additive positive impact on learning, memory, cognitive function, and emotional well-being. NMDA antagonists may have the benefit of reducing agitation and delusional thinking while AChE inhibitors can more positively impact anxious and depressive behaviors and apathetic affect, so combining the two can allow for a broader approach to therapeutic intervention. Preclinical studies have documented the value of combination NMDA/AChE antagonist therapy over monotherapy with either agent alone.[47]

A memantine/donepezil combination product is marketed as Namzaric and intended for use in patients with moderate-to-severe AD previously stabilized on 10 mg donepezil.[48] The extended-release capsules contain 10 mg of donepezil hydrochloride and 7, 14, 21, or 28 mg of memantine hydrochloride. While the combination product is more costly than monotherapy ($535 per month vs $16 per month for both generic drugs administered separately in 2022), it has been reported that the overall economic savings are higher with the combination product due to a 4-month delay in admission to a skilled care facility.[48] A pharmacoeconomic study of AD therapy options (including memantine/donepezil combination therapy) that evaluated 38 articles containing economic models was published in 2018, but several limitations, including the prevalence of industry-funded studies in the data set, compromised data evaluation.[49]

Importantly, combining memantine and donepezil into a single dosage form does not significantly alter the efficacy of either drug, nor the adverse effect profile or discontinuation rate compared to monotherapy with either agent.[46-48] There are several potential advantages to the combination product, including: (1) improved adherence to therapeutic regimens, (2) decreased caregiver burden related to medication administration, and (3) the ability to sprinkle the contents of the capsule on applesauce for safer consumption in patients with swallowing difficulties.[48] In the opinion of some, the combination product represents first-line therapy for moderate-severe AD, with memantine monotherapy as the second-line approach.[46]

Monoclonal Antibody Therapy: Aducanumab, Lecanemab, and Donanemab-azbt

At the time of this writing, three biologic agents for treating AD have been approved by the FDA, with the first two being aducanumab (Aduhelm) in 2021 and lecanemab (Leqembi) in 2023.[50-52] Aducanumab recognizes the sequence EFRHD (residues 3-7) of Aβ42, while lecanemab recognizes the sequence DAEFRHDSGYEVHHQK (residues 1-16). Both peptide sequences remain solvent-exposed in the precipitated Aβ plaque.[53] Aducanumab and lecanemab were approved under an accelerated drug-development process due to significant need for DMTs for AD and related dementias (Chapter 38). All are human immunoglobulin (Ig)G1 monoclonal antibodies (mAbs) raised against, and therefore targeting, Aβ.[53]

The development of these biologic agents is founded on the Aβ hypothesis, and clinical trials were conducted on patients with late-stage AD versus age and sex-matched controls with AD. Because these clinical trials were conducted over a multi-year period based upon the multi-year progression of AD, they lagged several years behind leading edge understanding of the neurodegenerative cascade present in AD. Biomarkers used in the clinical trials were based upon a diagnosis of AD using Pittsburgh compound B[54] and Aβ aggregation profiles in cerebrospinal fluid (CSF). To meet clinical trial qualifying criteria, patients would have progressed into the partially independent phase two of Aβ-driven neurotoxicity. Antibody therapies were approved on the basis of a positive biomarker response and less cognitive decline than for control patients.

Cognitive response was determined using the 14-item cognitive subscale of the Alzheimer's Disease Assessment Scale (ADAS-cog14), the Alzheimer's Disease Composite Score (ADCOMS), and the score on the Alzheimer's Disease Cooperative Study–Activities of Daily Living Scale for Mild Cognitive Impairment (ADCS-ADL MCI). In the 1,795 patents enrolled in the lecanemab phase 3 clinical trial; there was a modest reduction in cognitive loss compared to placebo controls after 18 months of treatment.[52] In clinical trials with 3,285 participants with AD, aducanumab also displayed modest reduction in cognitive loss compared to placebo controls during the same time period,[51] but at about 50% of the reduction level seen with lecanemab.

Significant side effects of both FDA-approved antibody therapies include cerebral edema, microhemorrhages, and superficial siderosis. These vascular adverse effects were observed using MRI imaging and are therefore termed amyloid-related imaging abnormality (ARIA) events. Increased ARIA events with lecanemab were seen in 12.6% of the treated patients versus 1.7% for patients receiving placebo.[52] Aducanumab was associated with a 35.2% prevalence of ARIA events versus 2.7% for placebo.[51] ARIA events presented clinically primarily as dizziness and resolved within 18 months after discontinuation of treatment. Additionally, 26.4% of patients administered either lecanemab or aducanumab experienced mild-to-moderate infusion-related reactions contrasted to 7.4% for placebo. ARIA events for either lecanemab or aducanumab increased for patients with a better cognitive response, with APOE4 homozygosity, and with increased antibody dose, consistent with a drug-induced side effect driven by primary pharmacological action. These ARIA events are also consistent with alteration of glial and astrocyte function and alteration of mechanical integrity of vascular tissues and correlated with histological determination of cerebral β-amyloid angiopathy (CAA). CAA occurs in phase 2 of Aβ toxicity and argues against use of antibody therapy with blood thinning (antiplatelet) agents. Use of platelet aggregation inhibitors has been fatal in patents with CAA.[53]

An additional consideration for use of mAbs for AD therapy[55] is the significant cost for these therapies. Lecanemab is dosed biweekly, while aducanumab is administered every 4 weeks. Yearly direct drug cost is estimated to be $27,000 to $56,000 for biweekly administration, with the final cost doubled when administration cost is included. Based on significant cost, marginal therapeutic improvement, and the high incidence of side effects, the Centers for Medicare and Medicaid Services (CMS) restricts coverage of lecanemab and aducanumab to clinical trials only.

In July 2024, the third biologic therapy for AD, donanemab-azbt (Kisunla), received FDA approval for early disease patients with mild cognitive impairment. Donanemab-azbt is a 145 kDA humanized IgG1 mAb raised against the pyroglutamate (pE) capped N-terminal truncated Aβ42 sequence, $A\beta_{pE3\text{-}x}$, where the Aβ42 (DAEFRHDSGY EVHHQKLVFF AEDVGSNKGA IIGLMVGGVV IA) is replaced by $A\beta_{pE3\text{-}x}$ (pEFRHDSGY EVHHQKLVFF AEDVGSNKGA IIGLMVGGVV IA). $A\beta_{pE3\text{-}x}$ is a more stable and more lipophilic peptide than Aβ and was originally identified as a component in the core of Aβ plaques by Mori in 1992.[56] It is currently proposed that $A\beta_{pE3\text{-}x}$ is present in neurotoxic protofibrils, uniquely identified in Aβ deposits of patients with AD versus healthy controls. In vivo generation of $A\beta_{pE3\text{-}x}$ arises from sAPP cleavage by the endoprotease β-amyloid cleaving enzyme (BACE) or the metalloprotease meprin-β, followed by N-terminal exoprotease cleavage of aspartate by aminopeptidase A (APA), N-terminal exoprotease cleavage of alanine by either meprin-β or DPP4, with final cyclodehydration catalyzed by glutaminyl cyclase (QC). All of these processing enzymes are therapeutic targets of current drug design programs. End-capping the N-termini of proteins is an established strategy to increase the stability of cytokines, suggesting an inflammatory component to $A\beta_{pE3\text{-}x}$ generation. Subsequent analysis of humanized IgG1 mAbs raised against $A\beta_{pE3\text{-}x}$ formed the basis of the TRAILBLAZER-ALZ clinical trial[57-59] that led to the development of donanemab-azbt. The TRAILBLAZER-ALZ trial examined 273 patients with early symptomatic AD (median age 74 years old) with a 71.8% and 74.4% completion rate for treatment and placebo arms.

The primary outcome of the TRAILBLAZER-ALZ trial was a change in the Integrated Alzheimer Disease Rating Scale (iADRS: 0-144). Lower scores indicate greater functional and cognitive impairment. The PET emitters florbetapir or flortaucipir, which bind to amyloid and tau proteins, respectively, were employed in the imaging bioassay to determine changes in amyloid deposits. Secondary outcomes were determined with the ADCS-ADL and the MMSE. Decrease of amyloid plaque burden by 65% by week 21 with a maximal reduction to 80% was achieved by week 76. Tau load was only modestly affected. Functional and cognitive impairment determined with either ADCS-ADL or the MMSE indicated better retention of abilities than placebo after 24 weeks of treatment: decrease was slower by 22% to 35% for patients who were treated than for patients receiving placebo.[59]

The most common adverse effects associated with donanemab were headache and ARIA with ARIA-E (characterized by vasogenic edema and/or sulcal effusions) occurring in 27% of all patients and ARIA-H (characterized by superficial siderosis, microhemorrhages, and macrohemorrhages) occurring in 30% of patients. The incidence of ARIA-E was nearly double (40%) with the ApoE ε4/ε4 phenotype. Consequently, ApoE ε4 phenotype assessment is recommended prior to initiating therapy. Reviews of aducanumab, lecanemab, and donanemab described comparable modest cognitive and functional outcomes[60,61] with significant ARIA side effects remaining a concern.[60-63]

Emerging Biomarker Assays

Significant advancements have been made in the development of AD biomarkers. Aβ40 and Aβ42 can be differentially determined with tandem mass spectrometry (MS/MS) on blood,[64] tears, or CSF. This bioassay is marketed direct to consumers as an over-the-counter test employing tear fluid as the testing medium; this test is not FDA approved. In the clinic, the test is usually conducted on a blood draw with immunoprecipitation, followed by liquid chromatography (LC)-MS/MS analysis of the Aβ42/40 ratio. A low ratio (<0.107) is alleged to correlate with lower cognitive scores after 5 years. However, independent studies by the FDA indicated there is no evidence that it can reliably be used to predict who will develop AD.

Determination of NFT-associated p-tau[12], including p-tau181, p-tau217, and p-tau231 variations, can be determined with a similar immunoprecipitation followed by LC-MS/MS analysis. Determination of glia reactivity and astrocyte activation can be assayed through determination of triggering receptors expressed on myeloid cells 2 (Trem2)[65] and glial fibrillary acidic protein (GFAP)[66], respectively. In presymptomatic AD, the trajectories of these biomarkers closely parallel those of phase 1 Aβ-deposition. CSF levels of neurofilament light chain (NEFL) increase after half-maximal Aβ deposition and could be used as an indicator of progression from phase 1 to phase 2 Aβ toxicity.[53]

Drugs Used to Treat Attention-Deficit/Hyperactivity Disorder

Introduction

Children, adolescents, and adults who demonstrate a pattern of inattention, impulsivity, and hyperactivity may be diagnosed with attention-deficit/hyperactivity disorder (ADHD). ADHD is considered a neurodevelopmental disorder that often significantly impairs functioning and places children at an elevated risk for a variety of adverse outcomes. The *Diagnostic and Statistical Manual of Mental Disorders*, Fifth Edition (*DSM-5*)[67] identifies diagnostic criteria for ADHD within two main subtypes: (1) inattention and (2) hyperactivity/impulsivity. It allows for combined criteria, along with the stipulation that several symptoms must have been present prior to age 12.[67-70] International prevalence of ADHD varies significantly from one country to the next, driven by differences between *DSM-5* versus International Classification of Mental and Behavioral Disorders (ICD)[71] criteria for ADHD diagnosis, specialist training, and cultural perspectives.[72] Although ADHD is most often a disorder of children and adolescents that commonly manifests in a learning environment, there is now a body of evidence that suggests it is also a relevant diagnosis in adults.[73]

ADHD patients exhibit deficits in attention to detail, do not readily follow instructions, can show poor organization, and may make careless mistakes at or fail to complete work. Children with ADHD can show inattention while playing because they are easily sidetracked and may have difficulty listening to others. Hyperactivity-impulsivity symptoms include a general increase in psychomotor behavior. People with ADHD often fidget and can have difficulty sitting still. Excessive talking and interrupting are also common.

An accurate prevalence of ADHD is difficult to determine, as there remains debate in the medical literature about whether the disorder is overdiagnosed.[53,72-74] In 2012, the prevalence of ADHD in children and adolescents aged 4 to 17 years was reported to be 11% (6.4 million), with the inattentive subtype predominating.[75] The prevalence of diagnosed ADHD in children increased 28% from 2007 to 2011, and, by 2016, 5.2% of all children ages 2 to 17 years in the United States were taking ADHD medication. There is a higher incidence in males, with the male/female ratio ranging from 2:1 to 9:1.[74-77]

Although environmental factors can play a significant role in the etiology, it is generally believed that ADHD might be an inherited disorder.[78-80] Numerous studies have identified several genes associated with ADHD, including dopamine 4/5 receptor genes (*DRD4*, *DRD5*), the dopamine transporter gene (*DAT1*), the dopamine β-hydroxylase gene (*DBH*), and the noradrenergic adrenoceptor α2 gene (*ADRA2A*).[76,81] A great deal more research is needed to identify and confirm the link between genetics and ADHD.

Treatment of Attention-Deficit/Hyperactivity Disorder

Therapy for ADHD generally requires a combination of pharmacological and nonpharmacological behavioral therapeutic approaches. Nonpharmacological treatment, often referred to as psychosocial intervention, consists of family therapy and cognitive behavioral therapy. The key to success with this therapy is to educate against the stigma of ADHD, enhance academic organization, modify behavior in the classroom and at home, and develop social skills. A healthy balanced diet is always recommended, although diet is not directly related to ADHD behaviors.[82]

Pharmacologic Treatment of Attention-Deficit/Hyperactivity Disorder

In 1937, Charles Bradley, a Rhode Island pediatrician, treated what were then mistakenly called "problem children" with benzedrine (amphetamine sulfate) for headaches and discovered that this CNS stimulant had a profound positive effect on their behavior.[83] Ever since, the phenylethylamine stimulants amphetamine, methylphenidate, and their analogs have been the drugs of choice for ADHD treatment.[84] These stimulants work by mimicking the structures of dopamine (DA) and NE and modulate their release, reuptake, and signaling within the brain. This leads to an increased concentration of DA and NE within the synaptic cleft and has led to the theory that ADHD is a disorder of DA and NE release in the striatal and prefrontal cerebral areas.[85] This theory is perhaps an oversimplification, since ADHD may present with comorbidities such as anxiety disorder, major depression, autism spectrum disorder, or Tourette disorder, which implies a more complicated etiology.[86] The overall objective of therapy is to realize meaningful improvement in core ADHD symptoms of inattention, hyperactivity, and impulsivity. Although psychosocial therapy is recommended along with medication, studies have not shown significant improvements of outcomes over medication alone.[82]

In addition to CNS stimulants, the second-line drugs used in ADHD treatment are discussed in Chapters 12 and 19 and are listed in Table 13.2. They include the serotonin/norepinephrine-reuptake inhibitor (SNRI) atomoxetine, α-adrenergic agonist antihypertensives (eg, clonidine and guanfacine), and several antidepressants (eg, the TCA imipramine and bupropion).

Stimulants

Amphetamine Salts. The stimulant mechanism of amphetamine derives from its structural similarity to the neurotransmitters DA, NE, and (to a lesser extent) serotonin (5-HT), since it has the arylethylamine moiety in common with all of these endogenous molecules. It competes for reuptake via their transporters (dopamine transporter [DAT]), (norepinephrine transporter [NET]), and 5-HT transporter [SERT]) in the striatum and prefrontal cortex. In addition, amphetamine inhibits translocation of DA and NE from the cytosol into storage vesicles in the neuron by inhibiting the vesicular monoamine transporter 2 (VMAT2). Through this type of competition, amphetamine actually overloads the transporters and causes a reversal of their action, pumping DA and NE out of the neurons into the synapse.[87,88]

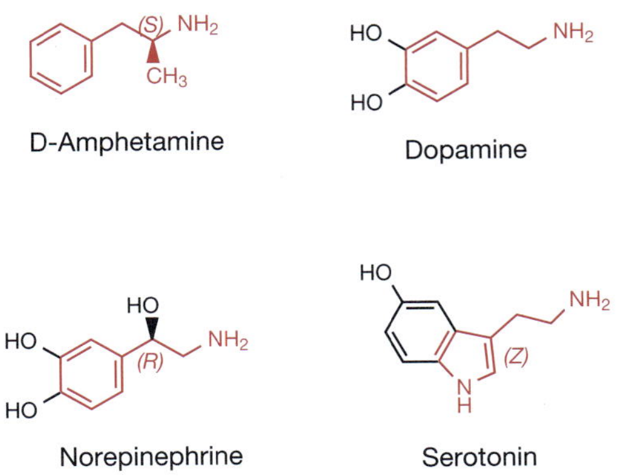

Relationship of amphetamine (shown in red) to endogenous neurotransmitters.

Since amphetamine has a single chiral center, it is optically active and exists in enantiomeric forms (Fig. 13.9). While chirality is now preferably noted using *R* (rectus, or right) and *S* (sinister, or left) designations that describe three-dimensional structure, the D (dextro) and L (levo) terminology (which describes optical rotation) is still in use in designating amphetamine stereoisomerism. D-Amphetamine is the more potent isomer (~4X L-amphetamine) and has been marketed in isomerically pure form since the early 1940s. It has subsequently been determined that both enantiomers are effective in treating ADHD, but the only current use of L-amphetamine is in the mixed enantiomeric salt product Adderall (Table 13.3), which consists of a 3:1 mixture of D and L isomers. D-Amphetamine is a more potent stimulant of DA release; however, L-amphetamine is equal to, or more potent than, its enantiomer in promoting the release of NE. In addition, the L-isomer in the 3:1 mixture appears to prolong the efflux of DA, presumably due to modulation of the ability of the D-isomer to competitively bind to DAT, resulting in transporter overload, as described.[88]

Amphetamine is metabolized by oxidative deamination to benzoic acid via a pathway that involves CYP2C isoforms. A common 4-hydroxynorephedrine metabolite is generated via two pathways that require CYP2D6 and dopamine β-hydroxylase (Fig. 13.10). The benzoic acid metabolite is excreted in the urine as the hippuric acid conjugate (a product of glutathione metabolism), and 4-hydroxynorephedrine is excreted as either the glucuronide or sulfate conjugate of the phenolic hydroxy. Amphetamine is 30% to 40% excreted unchanged,

Table 13.2 Nonstimulant Drugs for Attention-Deficit/Hyperactivity Disorder Treatment

Drug	Structure	Mechanism of Action	Indication	Detailed Discussion Chapter
Atomoxetine	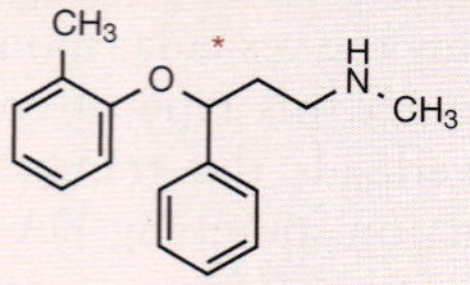	SNRI	ADHD +/− enuresis, tic disorder, anxiety, oppositionality + ADHD	12
Bupropion	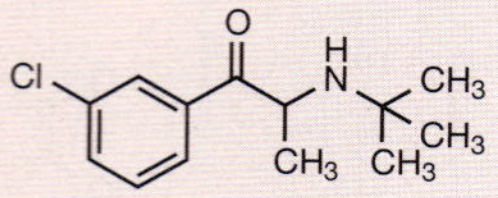	Antidepressant DNRI	ADHD +/− depression Anxiety disorder, obsessive compulsive disorder (OCD)	12
Clonidine	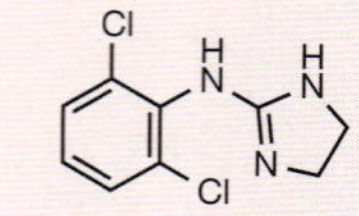	Antihypertensive Central α_2-agonist	Tourette syndrome, aggression, self-abuse, oppositionality + ADHD	19
Guanfacine	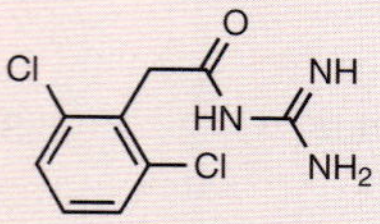	Antihypertensive Central α_2-agonist	Tourette syndrome, aggression, self-abuse, oppositionality + ADHD	19
Imipramine	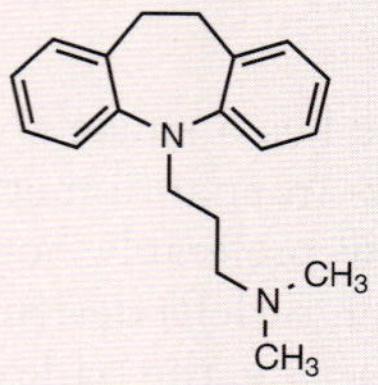	Tricyclic Antidepressant (TCA)	ADHD +/− enuresis, TIC disorder, anxiety disorder, oppositionality + ADHD	12

DNRI, dopamine/norepinephrine-reuptake inhibitor; SNRI, selective norepinephrine-reuptake inhibitor.

and the pH of the urine has an effect on its elimination. Alkaline urine promotes the unionized amine conjugate, decreasing water solubility and promoting renal tubular reabsorption over elimination. In contrast, acidic urine promotes the protonated (cationic) amine conjugate, increasing water solubility and retention in urine for subsequent elimination.[89]

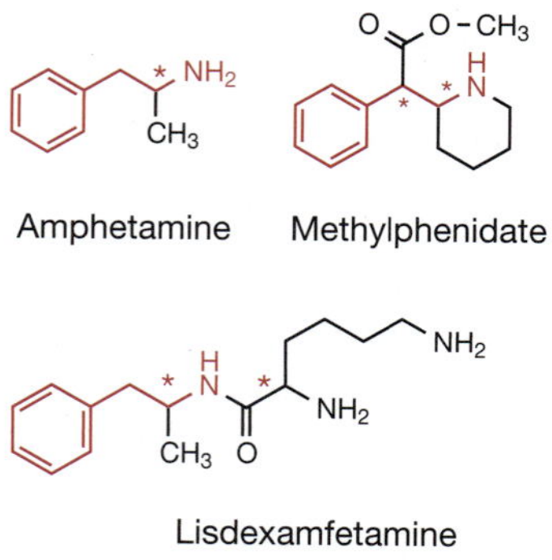

Figure 13.9 Structures of stimulant drugs used to treat attention-deficit/hyperactivity disorder. Common phenylethylamine moiety is shown in red.

There are multiple pharmacologic dosage forms for amphetamine salts that modify release and, consequently, duration of action. This permits dosing regimens designed to achieve a duration of action compatible with patient needs in a typical school setting. Amphetamine is available in immediate-release tablets, as well as a number of extended-release formulations (see Table 13.3). Orally administered intermediate-release amphetamine is rapidly absorbed and has high bioavailability. These fast-acting formulations demonstrate dose-proportional pharmacokinetics with a T_{max} of 2 to 3 hours and age-dependent $t_{1/2}$ ranging from 7 to 10 hours. Body weight has an inverse effect on amphetamine's C_{max} and systemic exposure. Extended-release formulations typically have a T_{max} of 8 to 12 hours. As body weight decreases, volume of distribution, clearance, and $t_{1/2}$ all increase.[90]

Amphetamine has a high abuse potential, and all marketed products come with a boxed warning to that effect. The common adverse effects include decreased appetite, weight loss, insomnia, headache, and irritability, and jitteriness. The less common adverse effects[69] can be noted with prolonged use and include dysphoria, hypertension

Table 13.3 Stimulant Medications for the Treatment of Attention-Deficit/Hyperactivity Disorder

Medication	Product Name	Formulation	DOA (h)	Recommended Dose
Methylphenidate	Ritalin	Short-acting tablet	3-5	5-10 mg/bid to tid
	Ritalin-SR	Intermediate/WM	8	20-30 mg/bid
	Ritalin LA	Long-acting/SODAS	8-12	10-60 mg/qdam
	Concerta	Long-acting/OROS	12	18-36 mg/qdam
	Metadate ER	Intermediate-acting/WM	8	10-20 mg/bid to tid
	Metadate CD	Long-acting/CD	12	20-60 mg/qdam
	Methylin	Short-acting tablet	3-4	5-60 mg/bid
	Methylin CT	Short-acting chewable	3-4	5-60 mg/bid
	Daytrana Patch	Transdermal	12	10-30 mg/qdam
	Equasym XL	Long-acting/CD/DC	8	
	QuilliChew ER	Short-acting chewable	3-4	20-60 mg/qdam
	Quillivant XR	Oral suspension	8-12	20-60 mg/qdam
	Aptensio XR	Long-acting/SRB	3-12	10-60 mg/qdam
Dexmethylphenidate	Focalin	Short-acting tablet	3-4	2.5-10 mg/bid to tid
	Focalin XR	Intermediate-acting/MSRP	6-8	5-20 mg/qdam
Dextroamphetamine (D-amphetamine)	Dexedrine	Intermediate-acting Spansules	8	5-40 mg/bid
*D:L*amphetamine 1:1	Evekeo	Short acting	3-4	2.5-40 mg/bid to tid
*D:L*amphetamine 3.2:1	Dyanavel XR	Long-acting oral suspension	12	5-20 mg/qdam
*D:L*amphetamine 3:1	Adzenys XR-ODT	Long-acting/ODT	10-12	3.1-18.8 mg/qdam
Lisdexamfetamine	Vyvanse	Long-acting amphetamine prodrug	12	30-70 mg/qdam
Dextroamphetamine 3:1D/L amphetamine salts	Adderall	Intermediate-acting	4-6	5 mg bid Increase to 40 mg max
	Adderall XR	Long-acting/SRB	12	5-30 mg/qdam

bid, twice a day; CD, controlled delivery; DC, diffucaps; ODT, oral disintegrating tablet; OROS, osmotic release oral system; qdam, once a day in the morning; SODAS, spheroidal oral drug absorption system; SRB, sustained release beads; tid, three times a day; WM, wax matrix.

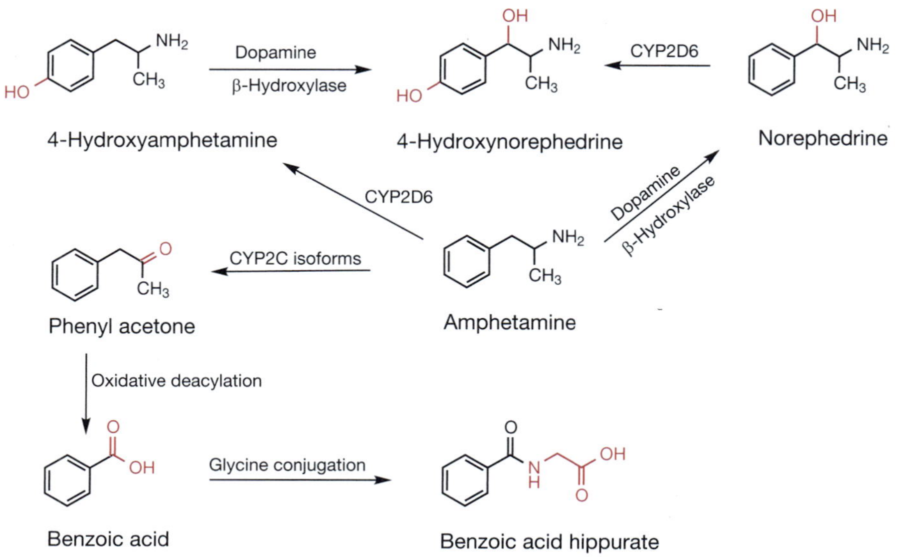

Figure 13.10 Metabolism of amphetamine.

(<2.0 mm Hg in healthy individuals), and psychosis. Dose adjustment usually attenuates these toxicities.[68,91]

Lisdexamfetamine (Vyvanse) is the first amphetamine prodrug approved for ADHD treatment. Structurally, it is the lysine amide derivative of D-amphetamine (see Fig. 13.9) and is unlikely to cross the blood-brain barrier. Lisdexamphetamine is metabolized in red blood cells to D-amphetamine by amide hydrolysis. The hydrolysis is a rate-limited process, and the release of D-amphetamine is slowed compared with the immediate-release formulation. The area under the curve (AUC) values are comparable, but the C_{max} of the prodrug was lower by 50%, and the T_{max} was doubled. This pharmacokinetic effect produces a gradual and sustained increase of striatal DA and a much slower decline as compared to immediate-release D-amphetamine, resulting in a longer duration of action (8-14 hours). Lisdexamfetamine is eliminated via the urine, 42% as amphetamine metabolites, 2% as unchanged lisdexamfetamine, and 25% as the hippuric acid conjugate.[88,92] As a D-amphetamine prodrug, lisdexamfetamine has the same boxed warning for potential abuse and adverse effect profile as amphetamine. In 2016, the dimesylate salt of lisdexamfetamine was approved by the FDA to treat binge-eating disorder.

METHYLPHENIDATE. Methylphenidate was the leading stimulant for ADHD treatment since its marketing (as Ritalin) in 1955, but the use of enantiomeric amphetamine salts (Adderall) has advanced to nearly equal to the use of Ritalin since its introduction in 1996. Methylphenidate is an amphetamine analog that contains the phenylethylamine pharmacophore incorporated into its methyl 2-phenyl-2-piperidin-2-ylacetate structure (see Fig. 13.9). Its mechanism of action is similar to that of amphetamine in that it increases DA and NE by inhibition of DAT, NET, and redistribution of VMAT2 in the striatum and prefrontal cortex.[93] Methylphenidate has little effect on SERT but does have low (micromolar) affinity and agonist activity at both the 5-HT_{1A} and α_2-adenergic receptors, resulting in a procognitive effect. The clinical importance of this is not clearly understood.[81,93]

Methylphenidate has two chiral centers and, therefore, there are four possible stereoisomers (two enantiomeric pairs): D/L-*threo* and D/L-*erythro*-methylphenidate. Only the racemic mixture of D/L-*threo*-methylphenidate is used clinically since the D/L-*erythro* pair has a greater adverse effect profile. The clinical effect of D/L-*threo*-methylphenidate is attributed to the D-enantiomer since the L-enantiomer has no stimulant effect when administered alone. Subsequently, a pure D-*threo*-methylphenidate formulation has become available (see Table 13.3).[94,95]

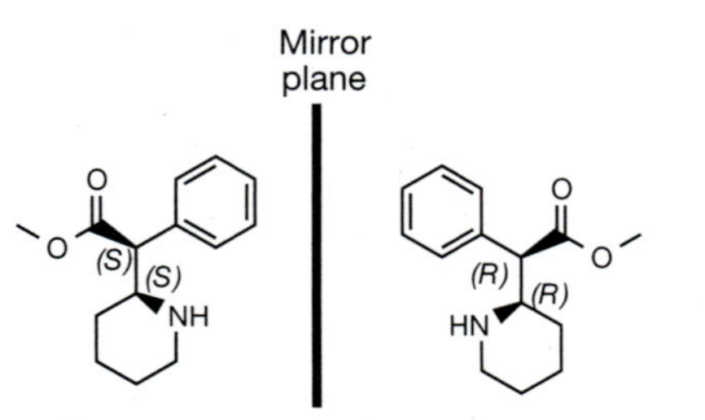

The absolute oral bioavailability of methylphenidate is only about 30% due to presystemic metabolism. Studies have shown that racemic *threo*-methylphenidate is metabolized by ester hydrolysis by carboxylesterase 1A1 and that the hydrolysis is stereoselective. This enzyme is present in the stomach and liver and shows a preference for L-*threo*-methylphenidate. Consequently, after an oral dose of the racemic mixture, plasma concentration of the D-*threo* isomer is higher than that of its enantiomer. The product of methylphenidate hydrolysis is racemic ritalinic acid (2-phenyl-2-piperidin-2-ylacetic acid).[96]

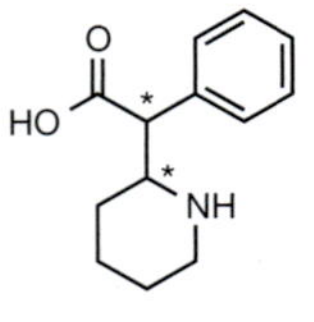

Ritalinic acid

Methylphenidate is well absorbed orally and, after extensive first-pass metabolism, peak plasma levels from the immediate-release formulation occur within 2 hours of administration.[97] Protein binding is low (10%-30%) and the apparent distribution volume after IV dosing is about 6 L/kg. Excretion is via the kidneys, with 78% to 97% of the dose being excreted as metabolites (primarily ritalinic acid). Only minor amounts of unchanged methylphenidate appear in the urine or feces. The excretion $t_{1/2}$ varies from 2.5 to 7 hours depending on the formulation.[84]

The adverse effects of methylphenidate are analogous to those seen with amphetamine: overstimulation of the CNS, including insomnia, night terrors, nervousness, restlessness, euphoria, and irritability.[93] Often these effects can be followed by fatigue and depression. Other potentially use-limiting effects include dry mouth, anorexia, gastrointestinal disturbances (eg, abdominal cramps), headache, dizziness, and sweats. Additionally, tachycardia, myocardial infarction, and altered libido have been identified as less common side effects. Like amphetamine, there is an abuse potential associated with methylphenidate, and the FDA has issued a boxed warning to that effect.[98] Methylphenidate is the preferred medication in adult populations for treatment of ADHD. However, interplay of comorbid psychiatric conditions, either as independent or as consequential conditions, complicates interpertation.[93]

Future Directions in Attention-Deficit/Hyperactivity Disorder Research and Therapy

Emerging opportunities for ADHD treatment can be categorized into the broad areas of diagnosis,[77,99,100] resolving the contributions of immediate versus adaptive pharmacological mechanisms to optimize patient outcomes,[69,98,101] and the role of ADHD diagnosis and treatment in adult populations.[93]

Structure Challenge

The following structures are used in the treatment of Alzheimer disease or attention-deficit/hyperactivity disorder (ADHD). Demonstrate your ability to apply structure-activity analysis to answer the questions below.

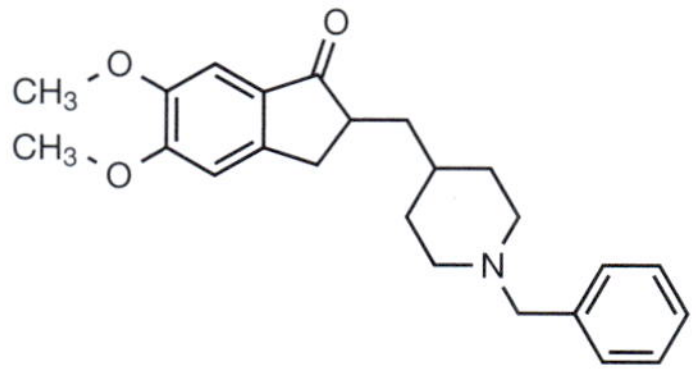

A

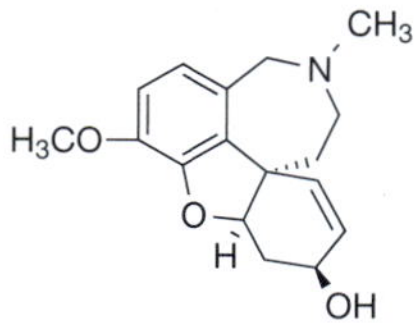

B

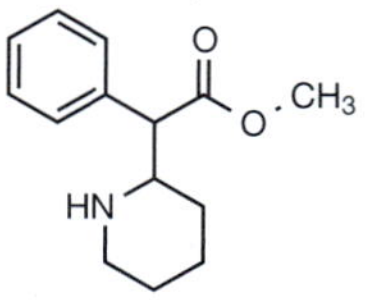

C

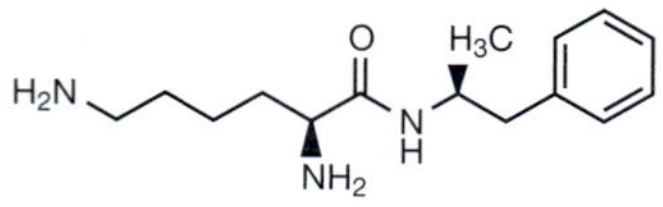

D

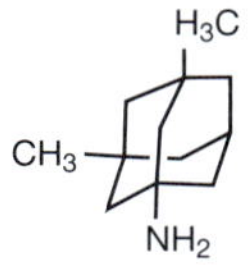

E

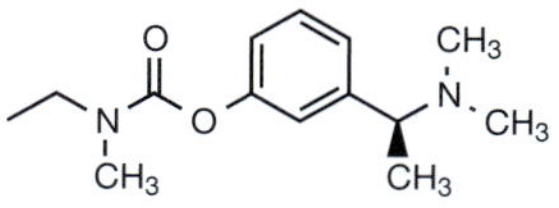

F

1. Which of these drugs would increase the amount of the neurotransmitter acetylcholine in central neurons? Select all that apply.
2. Which of these drugs is a prodrug that is devoid of activity until converted through phase 1 metabolism into the active therapeutic agent?
3. Which of these drugs can be used to treat ADHD? Select all that apply.
4. Which of these drugs exert its primary pharmacology at the NMDA receptor?
5. Which drug inactivates butyrylcholinesterase through carbamoylation of the enzyme?

Structure Challenge answers found immediately after References.

ACKNOWLEDGMENT

The author wishes to acknowledge the work of Victoria F. Roche, PhD, and S. William Zito, PhD, who authored content used within this chapter in a previous edition of this text.

REFERENCES

1. Dahm R. Alzheimer's discovery. *Curr Biol.* 2006;16(21):R906-R910.
2. Alzheimer's Association. 2024 Alzheimer's disease facts and figures. Accessed July 28, 2024. https://www.alz.org/alzheimers-dementia/facts-figures
3. Ali F, Baringer SL, Neal A, et al. Parvalbumin-positive neuron loss and amyloid-β deposits in the frontal cortex of Alzheimer's disease-related mice. *J Alzheimers Dis.* 2019;72(4):1323-1339.
4. Montine TJ, Phelps CH, Beach TG, et al. National Institute on Aging–Alzheimer's Association guidelines for the neuropathologic assessment of Alzheimer's disease: a practical approach. *Acta Neuropathol.* 2012;123(1):1-11.
5. Crous-Bou M, Miguillon C, Gramunt N, Molinuevo JL. Alzheimer's disease prevention: from risk factors to early intervention. *Alzheimers Res Ther.* 2017;9:71.
6. Gustavsson A, Green C, Jones RW, et al. Current issues and future research priorities for health economic modelling across the full continuum of Alzheimer's disease. *Alzheimers Dement.* 2017;13:312-321.
7. Tong BC-K, Wu AJ, Li M, et al. Calcium signaling in Alzheimer's disease and therapies. *Biochim Biophys Acta Mol Cell Res.* 2018;1865:1745-1760.
8. Ashton NJ, Janelidze S, Mattsson-Carlgren N, et al. Differential roles of Aβ42/40, p-tau231 and p-tau217 for Alzheimer's trial selection and disease monitoring. *Nat Med.* 2022;28(12):2555-2562.
9. Lee JH, Oh I-H, Lim HK. Stem cell therapy: a prospective treatment for Alzheimer's disease. *Psychiatry Investig.* 2016;13:583-589.
10. Jucker M, Walker LC. Alzheimer's disease: from immunotherapy to immunoprevention. *Cell.* 2023;186(20):4260-4270.
11. *Alzheimer's Association. 2018 Alzheimer's disease facts and figures.* Accessed July 28, 2018. https://www.alz.org/media/HomeOffice/Facts%20and%20Figures/facts-and-figures.pdf
12. Srivastava S, Ahmad R, Khare SK. Alzheimer's disease and its treatment by different approaches: a review. *Eur J Med Chem.* 2021;216:113320.
13. Anand A, Patience AA, Sharma N, et al. The present and future of pharmacotherapy of Alzheimer's disease: a comprehensive review. *Eur J Pharmacol.* 2017;815:365-375.
14. Douchamps F, Mathis C. A second wind for the cholinergic system in Alzheimer's therapy. *Behav Pharmacol.* 2017;28:112-123.
15. Facts & Comparisons [database online]. St. Louis, MO: Wolters Kluwer Health, Inc.; March, 2005.
16. Brewster JT II, Dell'Acqua S, Thach DQ, Sessler JL. Classics in chemical neuroscience: donepezil. *ACS Chem Neurosci.* 2019;10:155-167.
17. Atanasova M, Yordanov N, Dimitrov I, et al. Molecular docking study on galantamine derivatives as cholinesterase inhibitors. *Mol Inform.* 2015;34:394-403.
18. Kim SH, Kandiah N, Hsu JL, Suthisisang C, Udommongkol C, Dash A. Beyond symptomatic effects: potential of donepezil as a neuroprotective agent and disease modifier in Alzheimer's disease. *Br J Pharmacol.* 2017;174:4224-4232.
19. Li DD, Zhang YH, Zhang W, Zhao P. Meta-analysis of randomized controlled trials on the efficacy and safety of donepezil,

galantamine, rivastigmine, and memantine for the treatment of Alzheimer's disease. *Front Neurosci.* 2019;13:472.
20. Pardo-Moreno T, Gonzalez-Acedo A, Rivas-Dominguez A, et al. Therapeutic approach to Alzheimer's disease: current treatments and new perspectives. *Pharmaceutics.* 2022;14:1117.
21. Vecchio I, Sorrentino L, Paoletti A, Marra R, Arbitrio M. The state of the art on acetylcholinesterase inhibitors in the treatment of Alzheimer's disease. *J Cent Nerv Syst Dis.* 2021;13:1-13.
22. Matsui K, Mashima M, Nagai Y, *Yuzuriha T, Yoshimura T*. Absorption, distribution, metabolism and excretion of donepezil (Aricept) after a single oral administration to rat. *Drug Metab Dispos.* 1999;27:1406-1414.
23. Meier-Davis SR, Murgasova R, Toole C, et al. Comparison of metabolism of donepezil in rat, mini-pig, and human, following oral and transdermal administration, and in an in vitro model of human epidermis. *J Drug Metab Toxicol.* 2012;3(5):129.
24. Adlimoghaddam A, Neuendorff M, Roy B, et al. A review of clinical treatment considerations of donepezil in severe Alzheimer's disease. *CNS Neurosci Ther.* 2018;24:876-888.
25. Sabbagh MN, Mathew P, Blau, A. A randomized double-blind study to assess the skin irritation and sensitization potential of a once-weekly donepezil transdermal delivery system in healthy volunteers. *Alzheimer Dis Assoc Disord.* 2023;37(4):290-295.
26. Tariot PN, Braeckman R, Oh C. Comparison of steady-state pharmacokinetics of donepezil transdermal delivery system with oral donepezil. *J Alzheimers Dis.* 2022;90:161-172.
27. Farlow MR. Clinical pharmacokinetics of galantamine. *Clin Pharmacokinet.* 2003;42:1383-1392.
28. Fontana IC, Kumar A, Nordberg A. The role of astrocytic α7 nicotinic acetylcholine receptors in Alzheimer disease. *Nat Rev Neurol.* 2023;19(5):278-288.
29. Mannens GS, Snel CA, Hendrickx J, et al. The metabolism and excretion of galantamine in rats, dogs, and humans. *Drug Metab Dispos.* 2002;30(5):553-563.
30. Jiang D, Yang X, Li M, et al. Efficacy and safety of galantamine treatment for patients with Alzheimer's disease: a meta-analysis of randomized controlled trials. *J Neural Transm.* 2015;122:1157-1166.
31. Hwang T-Y, Ahn I-S, Kim S, et al. Efficacy of galantamine on cognition in mild-to-moderate Alzheimer's dementia after failure to respond to donepezil. *Psychiatry Investig.* 2016;13:341-348.
32. Wang L, Wang Y, Tian Y, et al. Design, synthesis, biological evaluation, and molecular modeling studies of chalcone-rivastigmine hybrids as cholinesterase inhibitors. *Biorg Med Chem.* 2017;25:360-371.
33. Bar-On P, Millard CB, Harel M, et al. Kinetic and structural studies on the interaction of cholinesterases with the anti-Alzheimer's drug rivastigmine. *Biochem.* 2002;41:3555-3564.
34. Bolognesi ML, Bartolini M, Cavalli A, et al. Design, synthesis, and biological evaluation of conformationally restricted rivastigmine analogues. *J Med Chem.* 2004;47:5945-5952.
35. Kandiah N, Pai M-C, Senanarong V, et al. Rivastigmine: the advantage of dual inhibition of acetylcholinesterase and butyrylcholinesterase and its role in subcortical vascular dementia and Parkinson's disease dementia. *Clin Interv Aging.* 2017;12:697-707.
36. Hansen RA, Gartlehner G, Webb AP, et al. Efficacy and safety of donepezil, galantamine, and rivastigmine for the treatment of Alzheimer's disease: a systematic review and meta-analysis. *Clin Interv Aging.* 2008;3:211-225.
37. Williams BR, Nazarians A, Gill MA. A review of rivastigmine: a reversible cholinesterase inhibitor. *Clin Ther.* 2003;25:1634-1653.
38. Sadowsky CH, Micca JL, Grossberg GT, et al. Rivastigmine from capsule to patch: therapeutic advances in the management of Alzheimer's disease and Parkinson's disease dementia. *Prim Care Companion CNS Disord.* 2014;16(5):10.4088/PCC.14r01654.
39. Emre M, Bernabei R, Blesa R, et al. Drug profile: transdermal rivastigmine patch in the treatment of Alzheimer disease. *CNS Neurosci Ther.* 2010;16:246-253.
40. Kurz A, Farlow M, Lefevre G. Pharmacokinetics of a novel transdermal rivastigmine patch for the treatment of Alzheimer's disease: a review. *Int J Clin Pract.* 2009;63:799-805.
41. Molinuevo JL, Llado A, Rami L. Memantine: targeting glutamate excitotoxicity in Alzheimer's disease and other dementias. *Am J Alzheimers Dis Other Demen.* 2005;20:77-85.
42. Lipton SA. The molecular basis of memantine action in Alzheimer's disease and other neurologic disorders: low-affinity, uncompetitive antagonism. *Curr Alzheimer Res.* 2005;2:155-165.
43. Danysz W, Parsons CG. Alzheimer's disease, β-amyloid, glutamate, NMDA receptors and memantine—searching for the connections. *Br J Pharmacol.* 2012;167:324-352.
44. Jiang J, Jiang H. Efficacy and adverse effects of memantine treatment for Alzheimer's disease from randomized controlled trials. *Neurol Sci.* 2015;36:1633-1641.
45. Kishi T, Matsunaga S, Oya K, et al. Memantine for Alzheimer's disease: an updated systematic review and meta-analysis. *J Alzheimers Dis.* 2017;60:401-425.
46. Matsunaga S, Kishi T, Normura I, et al. The efficacy and safety of memantine for the treatment of Alzheimer's disease. *Expert Opin Drug Saf.* 2018;17:1053-1061.
47. Parsons CG, Danysz W, Dekundy A, et al. Memantine and cholinesterase inhibitors: complementary mechanisms in the treatment of Alzheimer's disease. *Neurotox Res.* 2013;24:358-369.
48. Calhoun A, King C, Khoury R, et al. An evaluation of memantine ER + donepezil for the treatment of Alzheimer's disease. *Expert Opin Pharmacother.* 2018;15:1711-1717.
49. Ebrahem AS, Oremus M. A pharmacoeconomic evaluation of cholinesterase inhibitors and memantine in the treatment of Alzheimer's disease. *Expert Opin Pharmacother.* 2018;19:1245-1259.
50. Wu W, Ji Y, Wang Z, et al. The FDA-approved anti-amyloid-β monoclonal antibodies for the treatment of Alzheimer's disease: a systematic review and meta-analysis of randomized controlled trials. *Eur J Med Res.* 2023;28(1):544.
51. Salloway S, Chalkias S, Barkhof F, et al. Amyloid-related imaging abnormalities in 2 phase 3 studies evaluating aducanumab in patients with early Alzheimer disease. *JAMA Neurol.* 2022;79(1):13-21.
52. van Dyck CH, Swanson CJ, Aisen P, et al. Lecanemab in early Alzheimer's disease. *N Engl J Med.* 2023;388(1):9-21.
53. van Langen MJM, van Hulst BM, Durston S. Hidden in plain sight: how individual ADHD stakeholders have conflicting ideas about ADHD but do not address their own ambivalence. *Eur Child Adolesc Psychiatry.* 2024;33(6):1921-1933.
54. Ikonomovic MD, Abrahamson EE, Price JC, et al. Early AD pathology in a [C-11]PiB-negative case: a PiB-amyloid imaging, biochemical, and immunohistochemical study. *Acta Neuropathol.* 2012;123(3):433-447.
55. Lecanemab (Leqembi) for Alzheimer's disease. *Med Lett Drugs Ther.* 2023;65(1669):17-18.
56. Bayer TA. Pyroglutamate Aβ cascade as drug target in Alzheimer's disease. *Mol Psychiatry.* 2022;27(4):1880-1885.
57. Mintun MA, Wessels AM, Sims JR. Donanemab in early Alzheimer's disease. Reply. *N Engl J Med.* 2021;385(7):667.
58. Mintun MA, Lo AC, Evans CD, et al. Donanemab in early Alzheimer's disease. *N Engl J Med.* 2021;384(18):1691-1704.
59. Klein EG, Schroeder K, Wessels AM, et al. How donanemab data address the coverage with evidence development questions. *Alzheimers Dement.* 2024;20(4):3127-3140.
60. Terao I, Kodama W. Comparative efficacy, tolerability and acceptability of donanemab, lecanemab, aducanumab and lithium on cognitive function in mild cognitive impairment and Alzheimer's disease: a systematic review and network meta-analysis. *Ageing Res Rev.* 2024;94:102203.
61. Angioni D, Delrieu J, Coley N, et al. Drugs for Alzheimer's disease: where are we coming from? Where are we going? *Sci Bull.* 2024:69(10):1369-1374.

62. Hoeilund-Carlsen PF, Alavi A, Barrio JR, et al. Donanemab, another anti-Alzheimer's drug with risk and uncertain benefit. *Ageing Res Rev.* 2024;99:102348.
63. Couzin-Frankel J. New Alzheimer's drug clears FDA advisory vote despite unknowns. *Science.* 2024;384(6701):1164-1165.
64. Teunissen CE, Verberk IMW, Thijssen EH, et al. Blood-based biomarkers for Alzheimer's disease: towards clinical implementation. *Lancet Neurol.* 2022;21(1):66-77.
65. Morenas-Rodriguez E, Li Y, Nuscher B, et al. Soluble TREM2 in CSF and its association with other biomarkers and cognition in autosomal-dominant Alzheimer's disease: a longitudinal observational study. *Lancet Neurol.* 2022;21(4):329-341.
66. Pereira JB, Janelidze S, Smith R, et al. Plasma GFAP is an early marker of amyloid-β but not tau pathology in Alzheimer's disease. *Brain.* 2021;144(11):3505-3516.
67. American Psychiatric Association; DSM-5 Task Force. *Diagnostic and Statistical Manual of Mental Disorders: DSM-5.* 5th ed. American Psychiatric Association; 2013.
68. Sparrow EP, Erhardt D. *Essentials of ADHD Assessment for Children and Adolescents.* John Wiley & Sons; 2014.
69. Cortese S. Pharmacologic treatment of attention deficit-hyperactivity disorder. *N Engl J Med.* 2020;383(11):1050-1056.
70. Drugs for ADHD. *Med Lett Drugs Ther.* 2020; 62(1590):9-15.
71. Conrad P, Bergey MR. The impending globalization of ADHD: notes on the expansion and growth of a medicalized disorder. *Soc Sci Med.* 2014;122:31-43.
72. Te Meerman S, Freedman JE, Batstra L. ADHD and reification: four ways a psychiatric construct is portrayed as a disease. *Front Psychiatry.* 2022;13:1055328.
73. Surman C, Biederman J, Spencer T, et al. Understanding deficient emotional self-regulation in adults with attention deficit hyperactivity disorder: a controlled study. *Atten Defic Hyperact Disord.* 2013;5:273-281.
74. Batstra L, Nieweg EH, Hadders-Algra M. Exploring five common assumptions on Attention Deficit Hyperactivity Disorder. *Acta Paediatr.* 2014:103(7):696-700.
75. Willcutt EG. The prevalence of DSM-IV attention-deficit/hyperactivity disorder: a meta-analytic review. *Neurotherapeutics.* 2012;9:490-499.
76. Visser SN, Danielson ML, Bitsko RH, et al. Trends in the parent-report of health care provider-diagnosed and medicated attention-deficit/hyperactivity disorder: United States, 2003–2011. *J Am Acad Child Adolesc Psychiatry.* 2014;53:34-46.e2.
77. Kazda L, Bell K, Thomas R, et al. Overdiagnosis of attention-deficit/hyperactivity disorder in children and adolescents: a systematic scoping review. *JAMA Netw Open.* 2021;4(4):e215335.
78. Sciberras E, Mulraney M, Silva D, et al. Prenatal risk factors and the etiology of ADHD-review of existing evidence. *Curr Psychiatry Rep.* 2017;19:1.
79. Gallo EF, Posner J. Moving towards causality in attention-deficit hyperactivity disorder: overview of neural and genetic mechanisms. *Lancet Psychiatry.* 2016;3:555-567.
80. Faraone SV, Larsson H. Genetics of attention deficit hyperactivity disorder. *Mol Psychiatry.* 2019;24(4):562-575.
81. Faraone SV. The pharmacology of amphetamine and methylphenidate: relevance to the neurobiology of attention-deficit/hyperactivity disorder and other psychiatric comorbidities. *Neurosci Biobehav Rev.* 2018;87:255-270.
82. Pelsser LM, Frankena K, Toorman J, Rodrigues Pereira R. Diet and ADHD, Reviewing the Evidence: A Systematic Review of Meta-Analyses of Double-Blind Placebo-Controlled Trials Evaluating the Efficacy of Diet Interventions on the Behavior of Children with ADHD. *PLoS One.* 2017;12(1):e0169277. Published 2017 Jan 25. doi:10.1371/journal.pone.0169277
83. Strohl MP. Bradley's Benzedrine studies on children with behavioral disorders. *Yale J Biol Med.* 2011;84:27-33.
84. Sharma A, Couture J. A review of the pathophysiology, etiology, and treatment of attention-deficit hyperactivity disorder (ADHD). *Ann Pharmacother.* 2014;48:209-225.
85. Levy F, Swanson JM. Timing, space and ADHD: the dopamine theory revisited. *Aust N Z J Psychiatry.* 2001;35:504-511.
86. Austerman J. ADHD and behavioral disorders: assessment, management, and an update from DSM-5. *Cleve Clin J Med.* 2015;82:S2-S7.
87. Wang KH, Penmatsa A, Gouaux E. Neurotransmitter and psychostimulant recognition by the dopamine transporter. *Nature.* 2015;521:322-327.
88. Heal DJ, Smith SL, Gosden J, et al. Amphetamine, past and present—a pharmacological and clinical perspective. *J Psychopharmacol.* 2013;27:479-496.
89. Yamada H, Shiiyama S, Soejima-Ohkuma T, et al. Deamination of amphetamines by cytochromes P450: studies on substrate specificity and regioselectivity with microsomes and purified CYP2C subfamily isozymes. *J Toxicol Sci.* 1997;22:65-73.
90. Markowitz JS, Patrick KS. The clinical pharmacokinetics of amphetamines utilized in the treatment of attention-deficit/hyperactivity disorder. *J Child Adolesc Psychopharmacol.* 2017;27:678-689.
91. Cortese S, Holtmann M, Banaschewski T, et al. Practitioner review: current best practice in the management of adverse events during treatment with ADHD medications in children and adolescents: practitioner review: management of AEs with ADHD medications. *J Child Psychol Psychiatry.* 2013;54:227-246.
92. Dopheide JA, Pliszka SR. Attention-deficit-hyperactivity disorder: an update. *Pharmacotherapy.* 2009;29:656-679.
93. Jaeschke RR Sujkowska E, Sowa-Kucma M. Methylphenidate for attention-deficit/hyperactivity disorder in adults: a narrative review. *Psychopharmacology (Berl).* 2021;238(10):2667-2691.
94. Markowitz JS, Straughn AB, Patrick KS. Advances in the pharmacotherapy of attention-deficit-hyperactivity disorder: focus on methylphenidate formulations. *Pharmacotherapy.* 2003;23:1281-1299.
95. Markowitz JS, Patrick KS. Differential pharmacokinetics and pharmacodynamics of methylphenidate enantiomers: does chirality matter? *J Clin Psychopharmacol.* 2008;28:S54-S61.
96. Sun Z, Murry DJ, Sanghani SP, et al. Methylphenidate is stereoselectively hydrolyzed by human carboxylesterase CES1A1. *J Pharmacol Exp Ther.* 2004;310:469-476.
97. Cortese S, D'Acunto G, Konofal E, et al. New formulations of methylphenidate for the treatment of attention-deficit/hyperactivity disorder: pharmacokinetics, efficacy, and tolerability. *CNS Drugs.* 2017;31:149-160.
98. Golmirzaei J, Mahboobi H, Yazdanparast M, et al. Psychopharmacology of attention-deficit hyperactivity disorder: effects and side effects. *Curr Pharm Des.* 2016;22:590-594.
99. Koutsoklenis A, Honkasilta J. ADHD in the DSM-5-TR: what has changed and what has not. *Front Psychiatry.* 2022;13:1064141.
100. Faraone SV, Banaschewski T, Coghill D, et al. The World Federation of ADHD International Consensus Statement: 208 evidence-based conclusions about the disorder. *Neurosci Biobehav Rev.* 2021;128:789-818.
101. Drechsler R, Brem S, Brandeis D, et al. ADHD: current concepts and treatments in children and adolescents. *Neuropediatrics.* 2020;51(5):315-335.

Structure Challenge Answers

1-A, B, F; 2-D; 3-D, C; 4-E; 5-F.

CHAPTER 14

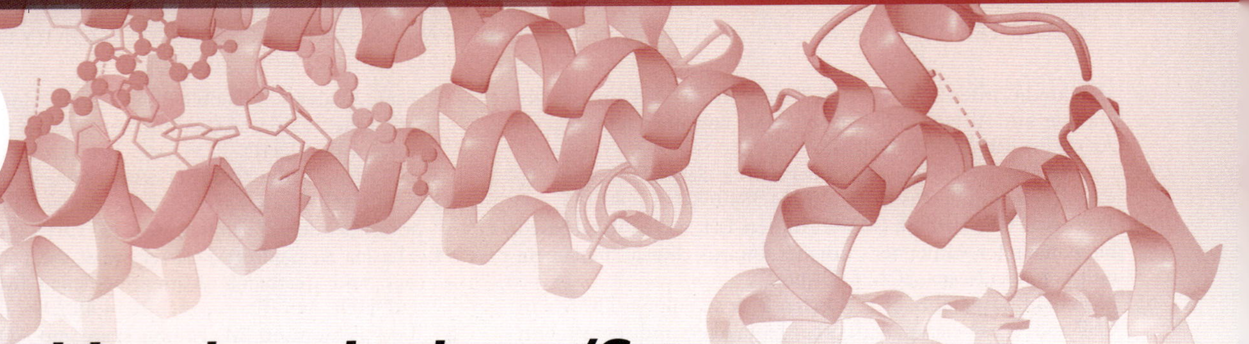

Drugs Used to Induce/Support Sedation or Anesthesia

Nader H. Moniri

Drugs covered in this chapter:

AGENTS THAT INDUCE OR PROMOTE SEDATION AND SLEEP

BARBITURATES
- Amobarbital
- Butabarbital
- Pentobarbital
- Phenobarbital
- Secobarbital

BENZODIAZEPINE SEDATIVE HYPNOTICS
- Estazolam
- Flurazepam
- Quazepam
- Remimazolam
- Temazepam
- Triazolam

NONBENZODIAZEPINE SEDATIVE HYPNOTICS
- Eszopiclone
- Zaleplon
- Zolpidem

MELATONIN RECEPTOR AGONISTS
- Ramelteon
- Tasimelteon

OREXIN RECEPTOR ANTAGONISTS
- Daridorexant
- Lemborexant
- Suvorexant

HISTAMINE H1 RECEPTOR ANTAGONISTS
- Diphenhydramine
- Doxepin
- Doxylamine

AGENTS THAT INDUCE OR PROMOTE GENERAL ANESTHESIA

THIOBARBITURATES
- Thiamylal
- Thiopental

INHALED ANESTHETICS
- Desflurane
- Isoflurane
- Nitrous oxide
- Sevoflurane

INTRAVENOUS ANESTHETICS
- Etomidate
- Ketamine
- Propofol

NEUROMUSCULAR JUNCTION–BLOCKING AGENTS
- Atracurium
- Cisatracurium
- *d*-Tubocurarine
- Pancuronium
- Rocuronium
- Succinylcholine
- Vecuronium

Abbreviations

ACh acetylcholine
ACTH adrenocorticotropic hormone
AMP adenosine monophosphate
AMPA α-amino-3-hydroxy-5-methyl-4-isoxazolepropionic acid
APR antiplanar region
ARAS ascending reticular activating system
BZ benzodiazepine
BZ1R BZ1 receptor
BZ2R BZ2 receptor
CHO Chinese hamster ovary cells
CNS central nervous system
CYP cytochrome P-450
DEA US Drug Enforcement Agency
DORA dual orexin receptor antagonist
EEG electroencephalograph
ERR electron-rich region
FDA US Food and Drug Administration
FRAR freely rotating aromatic ring region
GA general anesthetic
$GABA_A$ γ-aminobutyric acid-A receptor
GPCR G protein–coupled receptor
IC_{50} inhibitory concentration 50%
IM intramuscular
IV intravenous
MACs minimum alveolar concentrations
MT melatonin
MT1R melatonin1 receptor
MT2R melatonin2 receptor
nAChR nicotinic acetylcholine receptor
NE norepinephrine
NMDA-R *N*-methyl-*D*-aspartate receptor
NMJ neuromuscular junction
OTC over-the-counter
OXR orexin receptor
OX1R $orexin_1$ receptor
OX2R $orexin_2$ receptor
PKA cAMP-dependent protein kinase
P-gp P-glycoprotein
REM rapid eye movement
SAR structure-activity relationship
SCN suprachiasmatic nucleus
SORA single orexin receptor antagonist
TMH transmembrane helix
TMN tuberomammillary nucleus
U.S. United States

CLINICAL SIGNIFICANCE

The medicinal chemistry of the agents used to treat insomnia plays an especially important role in allowing the clinician to understand the molecular interactions of the agent with the specific central nervous system (CNS) target responsible for inducing sedation and sleep. Knowledge of structure-activity relationships (SARs) and medicinal chemistry allows the clinician to predict metabolism of the agents in order to minimize drug-drug interactions and residual next-day side effects that may result from improper metabolic breakdown of sleep-inducing drugs. Taken together, mechanism of action, pharmacokinetics, and metabolism can all be informed by drug chemistry and SARs and are factors that should be considered in order to appropriately optimize each unique patient's drug regimen.

Susan W. Miller, PharmD

Agents That Induce or Promote Sedation and Sleep

Neurobiology of Sleep

Sleep is a reversible process typified by sensory and motor inactivity as well as reduced cortical responses to external stimuli. This process is distinct from complete states of unconsciousness (eg, general anesthesia or coma), in which decreased cortical activity is unresponsive to all external stimuli. In human physiology, sleep/wake cycles are regulated to a large degree by endogenous circadian rhythms as well as homeostatic mechanisms, which in turn are governed by a myriad of neuronal pathways. Critical experiments performed in felines in the late 1940s demonstrated that impairment of the reticular formation within the brainstem triggered behavioral and electroencephalographic (EEG) activity consistent with comalike states, suggesting that this area of the brain was involved in regulating sleep and wakefulness.[1] This was contrary to observations that showed that felines with lesions of ascending sensory neurons distal to the reticular formation displayed no impairment to wakefulness or sleep, indicating that sleep/wake regulation by the reticular formation was not dependent on sensory neurons that leave it.[2] Further experiments showed that the reticular formation contained a high density of afferent input and that direct stimulation of the reticular formation facilitated wakefulness.[3] Taken together, these key observations suggested that sleep and wakefulness were likely controlled by factors within the reticular formation and that this structure behaves as a relay center that transmits afferent input to the cortex.

These and other pioneering studies led to the ascending reticular activating system (ARAS) hypothesis of sleep/wake regulation and subsequent identification of ARAS function as being critical in modification of sleep/wake transitions. Many decades of ensuing research on sleep/wake responses of the ARAS have revealed that projections to and from various nuclei within the brainstem can modulate ARAS activity in order to facilitate wakefulness and sleep. These include serotonergic neurons of the raphe nucleus within the reticular formation itself; cholinergic neurons of the pedunculopontine tegmentum and noradrenergic neurons of the locus coeruleus, within the pons; as well as dopaminergic neurons of the substantia nigra and ventral tegmental areas of the midbrain. These structures themselves are regulated in a highly orchestrated manner primarily by the excitatory neurotransmitter glutamate and the inhibitory neurotransmitter γ-aminobutyric acid (GABA) to regulate their respective activities.

In addition to the cell structures that make up the brainstem ARAS, there are additional populations of highly specialized cells that modulate sleep/wakefulness, either independently or in concert with cells of the ARAS. For example, stimulation of the tuberomammillary nucleus (TMN) within the posterior hypothalamus facilitates wakefulness and arousal, and these cells are predominantly active only during wakeful periods.[4] TMN-mediated regulation of wakefulness is dependent on histaminergic neurons that densely project into the cortex as well as other wake-promoting structures within the brainstem.[5] The firing rate of these cortical projecting histaminergic TMN neurons decreases upon sleep and increases upon arousal, while lesioning of histaminergic neurons within the TMN promotes sleep.[6-8] Biochemically, the release of histamine from these neurons is increased upon and during wakefulness and is under the control of glutaminergic-stimulatory and GABAergic-inhibitory circuits.[9,10] Studies with histamine receptor knockout mice as well as in vivo pharmacological studies have established that the TMN effects of histamine on wakefulness and sleep are mediated primarily by histamine H_1 G protein–coupled receptors (GPCRs; see Chapter 6).

While the posterior hypothalamic TMN is involved in regulating arousal, the anterior hypothalamus, specifically the suprachiasmatic nucleus (SCN), is involved in induction of sleep. Studies have shown that lesions of the posterior hypothalamus (eg, TMN) induce sleepfulness, while lesions of the anterior hypothalamus are associated with wakefulness.[11] Decades of further work have established that the SCN is critical for the maintenance of circadian rhythms, in essence, behaving as the brain's endogenous master clock, thereby regulating sleep/wake cycles and synchronizing circadian phase timings with other brain structures. Importantly, the SCN receives visual input from the retina via the retinohypothalamic tract, and this key connection serves to synchronize circadian rhythms to daylight.[12] The firing rate of SCN neurons is strongly correlated with day/night cycles, which serve to establish an approximate 24-hour circadian rhythm. While the SCN is largely under the control of glutaminergic and GABAergic neurons, which originate in the preoptic nucleus, it also works in concert with the pineal gland to regulate circadian rhythms.[13] As such, inhibitory GABAergic outflow from SCN neurons to the pineal is enhanced during the daylight hours and declines proportionally to decreases in daylight. Light-sensitive neurons from the SCN project to the hypothalamic paraventricular nuclei and through the lateral horn of the spinal cord primarily by way of vasopressin and GABAergic neurons. The signal is then relayed to the pineal gland through noradrenergic ganglionic sympathetic fibers that directly innervate the pineal gland. Hence, during periods of light, GABA output is elevated, which inhibits the release of norepinephrine (NE) at the pineal gland. In contrast, during periods of darkness the inhibitory GABAergic outflow from the SCN is reduced, resulting in increased levels of NE released at the level of the pineal gland.[12] Here, NE acts primarily through pineal β_1- and α_{1B}-adrenergic receptors to stimulate a rapid and profound (~10-fold) synthesis and release of melatonin, another key regulator of circadian rhythms and the sleep/wake cycle, into the bloodstream.[14]

The synthesis of melatonin occurs within the pineal gland, where the amino acid *l*-tryptophan is converted to serotonin, which is subsequently acetylated to yield *N*-acetylserotonin by the enzyme arylalkylamine *N*-acetyltransferase (AA-NAT). *N*-acetylserotonin is converted to melatonin by the enzyme hydroxyindole O-methyltransferase (HIOMT) (Fig. 14.1). The activity of AA-NAT is greatly influenced by β_1-adrenergic receptors that are activated upon the release of NE via the SCN circuit described earlier.

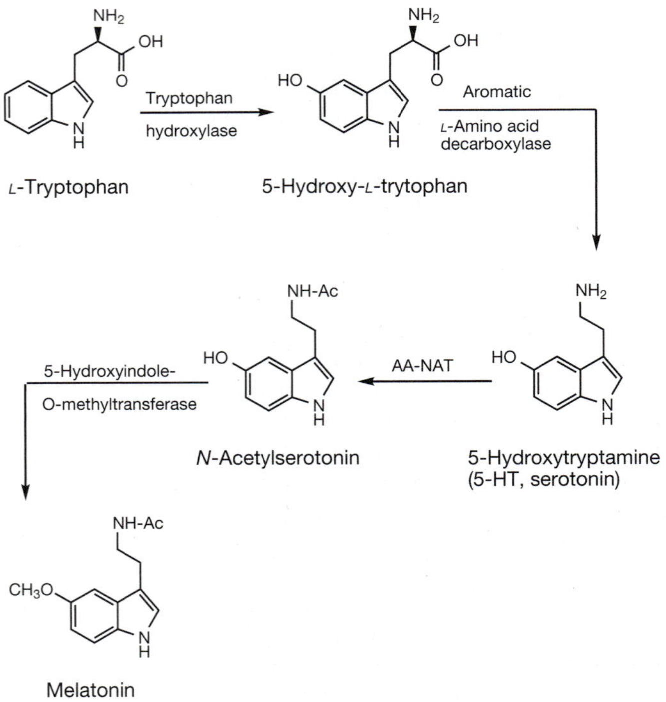

Figure 14.1 Biosynthesis of melatonin. AA-NAT, arylalkylamine *N*-acetyltransferase.

β_1-Receptor-mediated increases in intracellular cyclic AMP stimulate AA-NAT expression, and it also increases PKA-mediated phosphorylation of AA-NAT, which stabilizes and activates the enzyme.[15] The rhythm of AA-NAT activity is thus correspondingly coupled to light exposure, as increases in light lead to decreases in AA-NAT activity. Activity of AA-NAT can also be effectively abolished by lesions of the SCN, further demonstrating that melatonin synthesis is dependent on retinohypothalamic input.[16] Once synthesized, melatonin diffuses into capillary blood vessels and rapidly reaches all tissues of the body, where it can agonize its cognate GPCRs, melatonin receptor-1 (MT1R), and melatonin receptor-2 (MT2R), leading to various physiologic responses. With specific regard to sleep, melatonin has profound effects on the SCN, where it agonizes MT1R to mediate the acute inhibition of SCN neurons, thereby promoting sleep. Additionally, agonism of MT2R in the SCN is associated with the phase-shifting effects on circadian rhythms.

In addition, orexinergic neurons within the lateral hypothalamus receive an abundance of afferent input from emotional, physiological, and environmental stimuli that regulate the synthesis and secretion of the excitatory neuropeptides orexin-A and orexin-B, also referred to as hypocretins.[17-19] In turn, these orexinergic neuronal projections innervate all of the brain regions noted to promote wakefulness and arousal, including the dorsal raphe nucleus, locus coeruleus, TMN, and cortex.[20] Release of the orexins into synapses at these sites activates two separate GPCRs, orexin receptor-1 (OX1R) and orexin receptor-2 (OX2R), which together modulate the activities of the orexin neuropeptides.[19] Specifically, agonism of postsynaptic OX1R/OX2R by orexins facilitates depolarization and subsequent activity of postsynaptic neurons that promote wakefulness and arousal via excitatory neurotransmission toward the complement of wake-promoting brain regions.[21]

Human Sleep Cycles

The EEG has afforded researchers the ability to assess the electrical activity of the brain during the course of sleep, and these findings have revealed the presence of distinct EEG activity, which correlates to five stages of sleep. These stages, which cycle throughout the night, include four non-REM (rapid eye movement) stages, often referred to as "quiet sleep," as well a single stage of REM sleep, referred to as "active sleep." Non-REM sleep stages correlate to periods of low metabolic rate and low neuronal activity; hence brain activity and EEG events are "quiet." In non-REM sleep, heart rate and blood pressure are also reduced due to an increase in parasympathetic nervous system activity coupled with a decrease in sympathetic outflow. As a result of these autonomic reflexes, non-REM sleep also causes pupillary constriction, which diminishes the amount of light that is allowed to enter the retina.[22]

The initial period of sleep is stage 1, which lasts only a brief period of time (5-15 minutes) and represents the period of transitioning from wakefulness to sleep. While EEG activity in awake humans mainly consists of high-frequency (15-25 Hz) α-wave events, the progression to stage 1 sleep results in the emergence of slower θ waves with lower frequency (4-10 Hz) as the individual progresses to the light or drowsy sleep characterized by stage 1. In stage 2 sleep, which often lasts 15 to 20 minutes, background θ waves continue but are periodically interrupted by characteristic sleep spindles, which are short bursts of higher frequency (12-15 Hz) EEG events. Stage 2 of the sleep cycle is still considered a light sleep; however, skeletal muscle activity is decreased in this stage compared to the transitionary stage 1. Stages 3 and 4, often referred to as slow-wave sleep, are characterized by the appearance of higher amplitude, slower frequency (0.5-4 Hz) δ waves that occur less often in stage 3 and more often in stage 4. Both of these stages represent deep sleep, as the characteristic δ-activity is least similar to arousal state α-activity. If awakened in this stage of sleep, an individual will likely be confused and disoriented.[23]

The fifth stage of sleep is referred to as REM sleep and is characterized by increases in eye movement, respiration rate, and brain activity. EEG changes in REM sleep include high-voltage firing spikes that originate in the pons, lateral geniculate nucleus, and occipital cortex, and these spikes are correlated with bursts of REMs associated with this stage of sleep.[24] The increased brain activity in REM sleep is consistent with an increase in dreaming as well as an increase in metabolic rate, thus the naming convention "active sleep." However, given that REM sleep effectively paralyzes skeletal muscle, this stage of sleep is inversely proportional to skeletal muscle tonicity.

The sleep stages are normally cycled every 90 to 100 minutes throughout the night, and it is important to note that sleep does not necessarily advance sequentially through the five stages. Healthy adults typically enter sleep through a progression through the stages, with the first REM stage occurring after 75 to 90 minutes of non-REM sleep and a typical return to stage 2 or 3 sleep thereafter. As sleep progresses over the course of a night, the amount of time spent in REM sleep increases such that, over a typical 8-hour sleep cycle, approximately 55% to 60% of sleep time is spent in stages 1 to 2 (light sleep), 20% in stages 3 to 4 (deep sleep), and 20% to 25% in stage 5 (REM sleep).

Pharmacologic Targets of Sedative Hypnotic Agents

As described, many physiologic and biochemical factors can influence the various stages of sleep, and as such, numerous targets for pharmacological intervention have arisen. In fact, nearly every neurotransmitter system in the mammalian brain, including adenosinergic, serotonergic, dopaminergic, adrenergic, histaminergic, and cholinergic systems, has at one time or another been associated with induction of sleep or wakefulness. Despite this wide breadth of potential biochemical targets, the development of sedative hypnotic agents has primarily focused on (1) agents that cause CNS depression via agonism of $GABA_A$ receptors and (2) agents that modulate hypothalamic histaminergic, melatonergic, or orexinergic systems, which, as described, regulate sleep and arousal. This section will focus on chemical perspectives toward SARs, pharmacodynamics, and pharmacokinetics of these agents, including barbiturates, benzodiazepines (BZs), and nonbenzodiazepine $GABA_A$ agonists, as well as melatonin receptor agonists and histamine H1 and OXR antagonists.

$GABA_A$ Receptors

γ-Aminobutyric acid (GABA) is the major inhibitory neurotransmitter in the mammalian CNS and is critical in balancing neuronal excitation. GABA is widely distributed throughout the CNS and can be in found at concentrations up to 1,000-fold (high μM to low mM) greater than that of monoaminergic neurotransmitters in various CNS nuclei. GABA-induced physiological functions are mediated by at least two distinct classes of membrane-bound receptors: ionotropic $GABA_A$ receptors and metabotropic $GABA_B$ receptors. $GABA_B$ receptors belong to the second messenger–linked GPCR superfamily and share homology with metabotropic glutamate receptors. Meanwhile, $GABA_A$ receptors are ligand-gated ion channels that modulate conductance of chloride ions (Cl^-) through the cell membrane upon binding of GABA. The activation of $GABA_A$ receptors on excitable neurons leads to membrane hyperpolarization, facilitating an increase in the firing threshold potential and consequently reducing the likelihood of generating a neuronal action potential. Hence, agonism of $GABA_A$ receptors leads to neuronal inhibition and CNS depression. Not surprisingly, $GABA_A$ receptors are important targets for treatment of a variety of CNS disorders in which CNS depression provides a therapeutic benefit, including anxiety (see Chapter 11), convulsions and seizures (see Chapter 15), sleep disorders, and anesthesia. In this regard, drugs that increase $GABA_A$-mediated Cl^- flux (eg, $GABA_A$ agonists) provide anxiolytic, anticonvulsant, sedative hypnotic, and anesthetic activity, while agents that block the Cl^- channel (eg, picrotoxin) can lead to convulsions and heightened states of awareness and arousal.

The $GABA_A$ receptor-channel complex is related to the nicotinic acetylcholine receptor (nAChR) superfamily, which also includes the strychnine-sensitive glycine receptors and serotonin $5\text{-}HT_3$ receptors. In the human brain, $GABA_A$ complexes are formed by oligomerization of individual subunits that produce heteropentomeric complexes consisting of α, β, γ, δ, ε, or ρ subunits that assemble a ligand-gated channel with a central pore that allows for the conductance of Cl^- (Fig. 14.2).[25] Moreover, the α, β, and γ subunits of $GABA_A$ receptors are expressed as distinct alternatively spliced variants (eg, $\alpha_{[1\text{-}6]}$, $\beta_{[1\text{-}3]}$, $\gamma_{[1\text{-}3]}$). Functional channels typically require multiple α and β subunits in combination with another subunit, allowing for tremendous diversity in the makeup of the channels (Fig. 14.2). The distribution of various $GABA_A$ receptors varies according to the subtype combinations. The $\alpha_1\beta_2\gamma_2$, $\alpha_2\beta_3\gamma_2$, and $\alpha_3\beta_3\gamma_2$ subtypes are the most abundant receptors, accounting for nearly 80% of $GABA_A$ receptors in the mammalian brain.[25] The α_1 subunit is the most widely expressed, while α_4, α_5, and α_6 subunits are restricted to localized neuronal populations.[25] Two distinct GABA binding sites are formed at the two α and β subunit interfaces, while the binding sites for GABA-modulating drugs such as barbiturates and BZs are at allosteric sites (Fig. 14.2). Upon binding of barbiturates or BZs

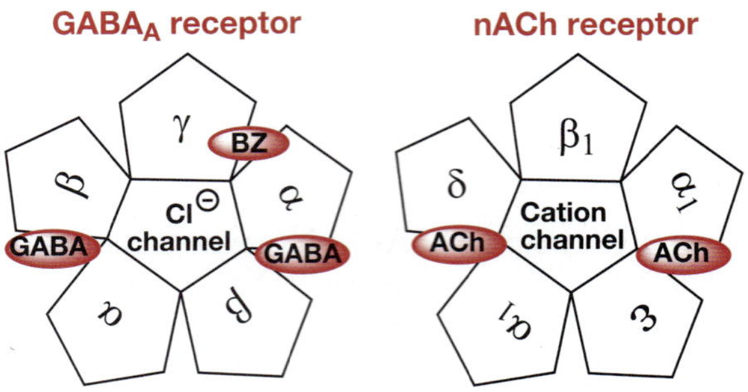

Figure 14.2 Pentameric assembly of γ-aminobutyric acid-A (GABA$_A$) receptors (left) and neuromuscular αβδε nicotinic acetylcholine receptors (nAChR) (right), whose monomers assemble to form the ion channel at the center. The GABA and benzodiazepine (BZ) binding sites of a distinct αβγ-type GABA$_A$ receptor are noted (left). The two acetylcholine (ACh) binding sites on the αβδε nAChR are noted (right).

to their respective allosteric sites on the GABA$_A$ receptor, alterations in the conductance of Cl^- occur, as described for each class of agent next.

Barbiturates. Barbiturates are potent CNS depressants with sedative hypnotic, anesthetic, and anticonvulsant activity and were widely considered sedative hypnotic agents of choice until the marketing of BZs in the late 1960s. Barbiturates played a crucial role in our understanding of GABA$_A$ receptor function, and while there are special instances, which call for barbiturate use, they have largely been replaced as sedative hypnotic agents by other agents due to safety concerns, including tolerance, dependence, potential for abuse, as well as a relatively low toxicity threshold that can lead to overdosage and poisoning. Historically, five barbiturates have been approved at one time or another by the US Food and Drug Administration (FDA) for use as sedative hypnotics: amobarbital, butabarbital, pentobarbital, phenobarbital, and secobarbital. While all of these are covered in this chapter since they are all available for research use, it is important to note that currently, only phenobarbital and pentobarbital are available for clinical use. Similarly, two thiobarbiturate derivatives, thiamylal and thiopental, are currently available only for research use as general anesthetics, based on their ultra-short–acting properties, and will be discussed in the "general anesthetics" section.

Barbiturate Mechanism of Action. Upon binding of GABA to the GABA$_A$ receptor, the Cl^- conductance channel opens in bursts of approximately 1, 5, and 10 ms of duration, followed by brief periods of closure. Channel opening increases in frequency and duration upon increases in GABA concentrations. Binding of barbiturates to their GABA$_A$ binding site causes an increase in the binding of GABA to the receptor, enhancing the actions of GABA and leading to prolongation of the longest-duration open state.[26] While the exact site of barbiturate binding on GABA$_A$ receptors remains elusive, the barbiturate binding site does not seem to require specific subunits, and it is distinct from both of the better characterized GABA and BZ binding sites. Indeed, using related bacterial receptor orthologs, it was recently shown that barbiturates bind deep within the central ion channel pore.[27] Higher therapeutic concentrations of barbiturates can also enhance the binding of BZs, while supratherapeutic concentrations of barbiturates can cause opening of the channel independently of GABA, although the clinical importance of this response has not been widely studied.[28] Notably, in addition to their augmentation of GABA$_A$ responses, the physiological effects of higher concentrations of barbiturates can also be mediated by kainite-sensitive AMPA glutamate receptors, as well as voltage-gated Na^+ and Ca^{2+} channels.

Pharmacologic Effects of Barbiturates. Barbiturates act as reversible inhibitors of virtually all excitable neurons and can produce dose-dependent CNS depression that ranges in effect from weak sedation to general anesthesia. With regard to their effects on sleep, barbiturates significantly decrease the time it takes to fall asleep, known as sleep latency, increase the total time of sleep, and decrease occurrences of nighttime awakenings. Because of these effects, barbiturates significantly impair psychomotor abilities and also decrease memory as well as cognitive performance. Additionally, barbiturates can cause physical dependence, and sudden withdrawal of these agents can lead to serious neuropsychiatric symptoms as well as convulsions of excitable tissue, an effect that can facilitate seizures and respiratory spasms. Long-term use of barbiturates has also been shown to lead to tolerance, in which higher doses of the agent are needed to achieve the same therapeutic endpoints (eg, sleep) previously obtained with a lower dose. Since these agents have relatively narrow safety margins, higher doses due to tolerance can lead to toxicity. Due to these concerns, the use of barbiturates in treatment of insomnia has been virtually discontinued, and when these agents are used for treatment of insomnia, they are used in special cases and/or restricted to only short-term use.

Structure-Activity Relationships of Barbiturates. Barbiturates are derivatives of a cyclized ureide of malonic acid, commonly referred to as barbituric acid (2,4,6-trioxyhexahydropyrimidine) (Fig. 14.3), which is itself devoid of sedative **hypnotic, anesthetic, anxiolytic, and anticonvulsant activity. As shown in Figure 14.3, barbituric** acid can undergo pH-dependent keto-enol tautomerization through transfer of either an imino hydrogen or methylene hydrogen to a carbonyl oxygen. This tautomerization is based on a fairly acidic enol (pK_a ~4) at the 2-position that is stabilized in either molecular form based on the acidity

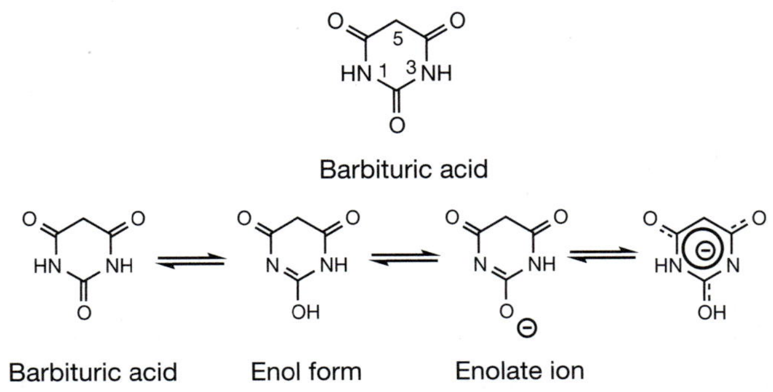

Figure 14.3 Structure of barbituric acid (top) and tautomerization of barbituric acid (bottom).

of the solution. Empirical and computational studies have demonstrated that the tricarbonyl form is the most stable in aqueous solutions, while the 4,6-dialcohol tautomeric forms are the least stable.[29,30] While barbituric acid itself lacks pharmacological activity, addition of 5,5-disubstituents to the barbituric backbone yields compounds with potent sedative hypnotic, anesthetic, anxiolytic, and anticonvulsant activity. Termed barbiturates, the 5,5-disubstituted barbituric acids all possess a high degree of lipophilicity and, as weak acids, can be easily converted to sodium salts by treatment with sodium hydroxide.

Despite the fact that thousands of barbiturate-like compounds have been synthesized, the 5,5-disubstituted barbituric acid backbone is the primary pharmacophore required for sedative hypnotic and anesthetic activity, and efforts to further derivatize this backbone lead to a general loss in these activities. These efforts show that amide formation at either of the 1,3-diazine nitrogen atoms decreases hypnotic activity. While substitution of these nitrogens with aliphatic carbons retained anticonvulsant effects, it led to only weak hypnotic activity for *N*-methylated substituents, and this activity was lost upon increases in chain length and/or bulk.[31,32] Likewise, esterification of the 5-position substituents (eg, 5-phenyl, 5-methylester) yielded agents with analgesic activity but only weak hypnotic effects.[33] While an early work on barbiturate derivatization demonstrated the importance of the 5-position substitutions on CNS depressant activity, the inclusion of polar functional groups at C_5 resulted in compounds that were fully devoid of sedative hypnotic, anesthetic, or anticonvulsant activity.[34]

As noted, only phenobarbital and pentobarbital are available for clinical use in the United States, while amobarbital, secobarbital, and butabarbital are available and readily used in research settings, prompting their discussion in this chapter (Fig. 14.4). Structurally, pharmacological activity is imparted to all five compounds due to the lipophilic disubstitutions at the 5-position (eg, 5^a and 5^b, Table 14.1). The first commercially marketed barbiturate, barbital, contained identical 5,5-diethyl substituents, and as such, a plane of symmetry. However, many clinically useful barbiturates

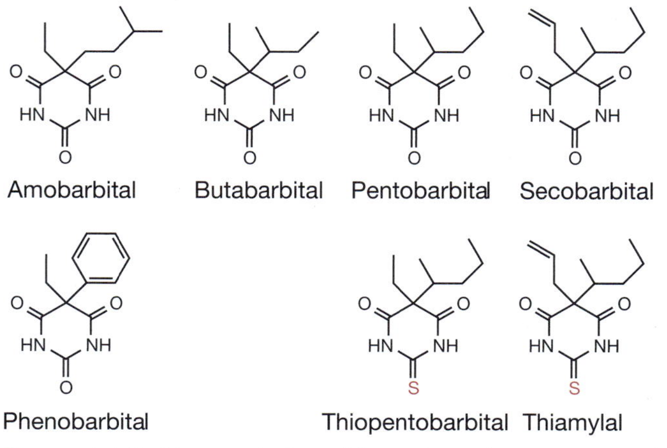

Figure 14.4 Barbiturates indicated for sedative hypnotic use and the anesthetic-acting thiobarbiturates underneath their respective oxybarbiturate congeners.

contain distinct 5,5-disubstitutions and substituted nitrogens that form an asymmetric chiral center at C_5 and/or within one of the 5-position alkyl chains. While barbiturates are dispensed as racemic mixtures, *l*-stereoisomers typically have twice the potency of the respective *d*-stereoisomers, consistent with observations that demonstrate stereoselectivity of GABAA receptors. With the exception of secobarbital, which contains an allylic group at 5^a, the remaining agents contain ethyl substitutions at this position (Fig. 14.4; Table 14.1). Differences in these sedative hypnotic barbiturates occur at the 5^b position, where substitutions can affect the potency, rate of onset, and duration of action of the various congeners.

The activity of these agents is strongly influenced by the lipophilicity of both substituents at the 5-position. As the number of carbon atoms at the 5^b position increases, the lipophilicity of the barbiturate will also increase such that comparative predictions on activity and time to onset can be made. For example, pentobarbital is more potent and has faster onset compared to butabarbital, which contains one less methylene group and is thus less lipophilic (Fig. 14.4, Table 14.1). Although the lipophilicity of the molecule greatly influences its ability to cross the blood-brain barrier, leading to potency and effecting the time of onset (see "Pharmacokinetics and Metabolism of Barbiturates" section), too high a degree of lipophilicity will offset the required hydrophilicity that is necessary for dissolution and solubility of the compound in aqueous fluids. Hence, a limit to lipophilicity is reached and pharmacological activity will begin to decrease if this threshold is surpassed. A somewhat paradoxical situation exists in the case of phenobarbital (Fig. 14.4; Table 14.1), which contains a 5^b-phenyl substitution that, on first look, appears to increase lipophilicity of the molecule, due to the six carbons and increased π-electron density afforded by the aromatic ring. However, the high electron density of phenobarbital stabilizes the formation of the more hydrophilic enolate anion due to the tautomerization process described. Because of this electronic effect, phenobarbital exhibits a higher degree of hydrophilicity compared to the other barbiturates, as demonstrated by its lower log P (Table 14.1). The consequence of this is lower sedative hypnotic potency and a longer time of onset.

A final note regarding the SAR of barbiturates is more critical in the role of this class as anesthetic agents. Specifically, modification of the C_2 oxygen of the barbiturate backbone with the larger sulfur atom yields thiobarbiturate derivatives with increased lipophilicity, faster time of onset, and shorter duration of action compared to the oxy-derivatives. For example, thiobarbital and thiamylal, which are no longer available for clinical use in the United States but are used heavily in research settings, have much faster onset and shorter durations than their respective oxy-congeners, pentobarbital and secobarbital, respectively (Fig. 14.4). Thus, thiobarbiturates have specialized roles as anesthetics, as described in further details in the "general anesthetics" section.

Pharmacokinetics and Metabolism of Barbiturates. The barbiturate salts are rapidly and completely absorbed following oral ingestion, in contrast to the free acids, which are absorbed at a much slower rate. The time of onset and

Table 14.1 Pharmacokinetic Parameters of Barbiturates Approved for Sedative Hypnotic Use

Barbiturate	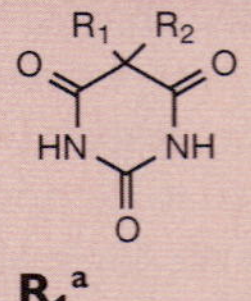 R_1[a]	R_2[b]	Log P	Onset Time (min)[c]	Duration of Action (h)[c]	Classification
Pentobarbital	C_2H_5	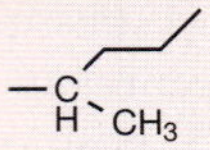	2.10[a]	10-15	3-4	Short acting
Secobarbital	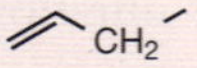	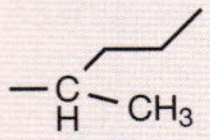	2.36[b]	10-15	3-4	Short acting
Amobarbital	C_2H_5	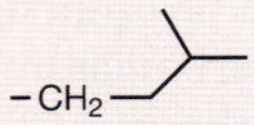	2.07[d]	45-60	6-8	Intermediate acting
Butabarbital	C_2H_5	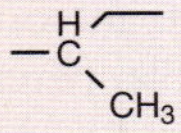	1.60[b]	45-60	6-8	Intermediate acting
Phenobarbital	C_2H_5	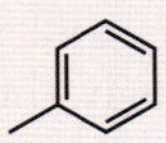	1.46[b]	30-60	10-16	Long acting

[a]From Freese IE, Levin BC, Pearce R, et al. Correlation between the growth inhibitory effects, partition coefficients and teratogenic effects of lipophilic acids. *Teratology*. 1979;20:413-444.
[b]Average determinations from Slater B, McCormack A, Avdeef A, et al. Comparison of partition coefficients determined by HPLC and potentiometric methods to literature values. *J Pharm Sci*. 1994;83:1280-1283, with permission from Elsevier.
[c]On oral administration.
[d]From Kakemi K, Arita T, Hori R, Konishi R. Absorption and excretion of drugs. XXXI. On the relationship between partition coefficients and chemical structures of barbituric acid derivatives. *Chem Pharm Bull*. 1967;15:1705-1712.

duration of action are also significantly influenced by the lipophilicity of the individual agent as well as the route of administration. The barbiturates described here are all highly lipophilic, with corresponding log *P* values above 1.4 compared to barbital, which has a log *P* of 0.65 (Table 14.1).[35] Given the high proportion of cardiac output that is directed toward the brain, more lipophilic barbiturates are more rapidly distributed to the CNS and will have a faster time of onset. As with other CNS-acting agents, the time of onset is also dependent on the route of administration, with intravenous (IV) administration being the fastest and having near immediate effects, followed by intramuscular (IM) administration, which leads to faster brain distribution than the 10 to 60 minutes typical of orally administered sedative hypnotics (Table 14.1).

While the lipophilic nature of barbiturates coupled with the high cardiac output to the brain dictates a rapid CNS distribution leading to fast time of onset, lipophilicity also facilitates the relatively short duration of action of these agents due to redistribution from the brain to other body compartments upon equilibration. This redistribution (eg, to muscle or adipose tissue) is the major mechanism that contributes to the loss of sedative hypnotic and anesthetic activity of these agents. Durations of 3 to 8 hours define the short- and intermediate acting agents, while phenobarbital, due to the electronic influence described, has the lowest lipophilicity and, therefore, the longest (10-16 hours) duration of action (Table 14.1). Since lipophilicity and route of administration can affect both time to onset and duration of action of barbiturates, these factors will influence a particular barbiturate's place in therapy. The anticonvulsant barbiturates are typically less lipophilic (eg, phenobarbital) and correspondingly have slow onset and long durations upon oral dosing, while the sedative hypnotic agents described here are typically administered orally to achieve an optimum balance between achievement of sleep onset and duration. In contrast, anesthesia-inducing barbiturates such as thiamylal are termed ultra-short acting due to their extremely high lipophilicity (log $P > 3$), which confers immediate onset and very short durations upon IV injection.

While loss of barbiturate sedative hypnotic activity occurs primarily due to redistribution, the agents are also metabolically transformed. Metabolism of barbiturates is dependent on their individual degrees of lipid solubility: the more lipophilic compounds generally have greater hepatic penetration and, hence, undergo greater metabolic transformation. It is important to understand that metabolism of barbiturates leads to metabolites that lack a high degree of lipophilicity, and as a result, lack sedative hypnotic activity. To achieve loss of lipophilicity, barbiturates are typically converted to phase 2 glucuronide or sulfate conjugates that are strongly ionized and, therefore, hydrophilic and will allow for renal excretion of the agents. The most important pathway of barbiturate metabolism is oxidation or removal

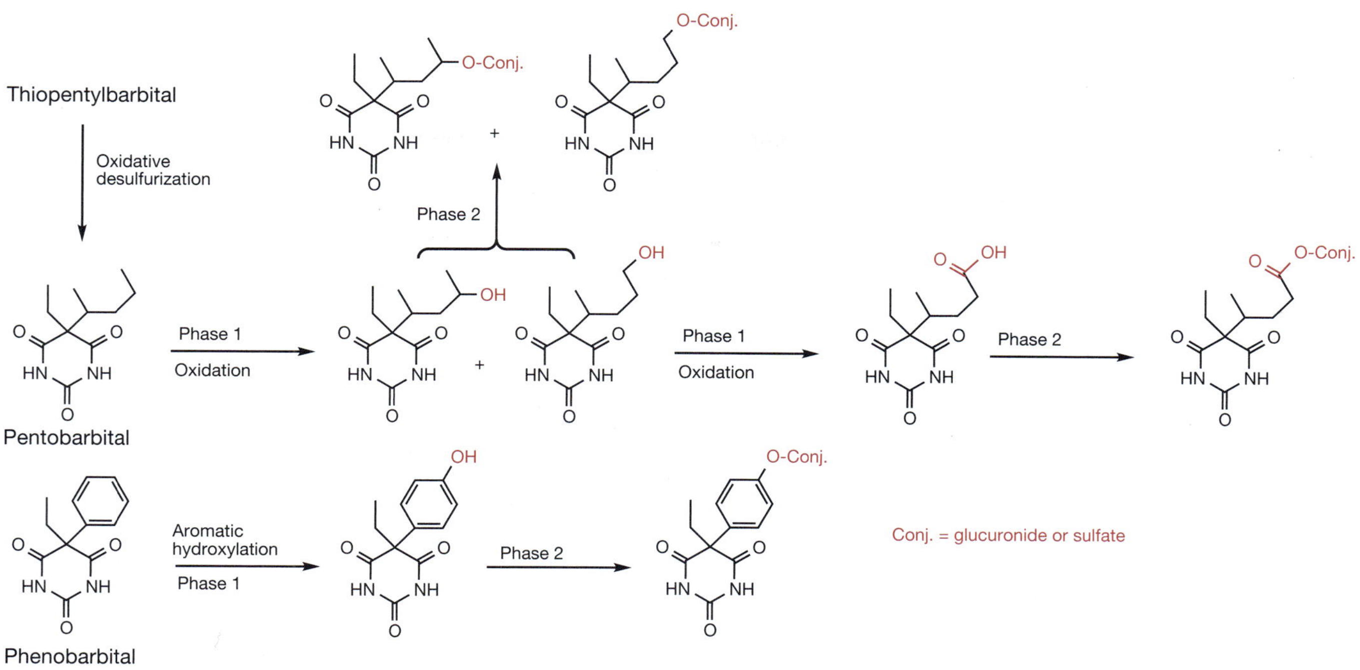

Figure 14.5 Major routes of metabolism of barbiturates. Thiobarbital and pentobarbital are used as examples to describe metabolism of alkyl thio- and oxybarbiturates, while phenobarbital is used as an example to describe metabolism of aromatic barbiturates.

of the substituents at the 5-position (Fig. 14.5). These phase 1 oxidation transformants are typically alcohols or phenols in the case of phenobarbital, which can appear in the urine as either free or conjugated metabolites, the latter as a result of further phase 2 reactions with glucuronic acid or sulfate. The alcohols formed can also be further oxidized to yield ketones or carboxylic acid metabolites, which can be excreted freely or also conjugated (Fig. 14.5). Although not as significant as the route described, oxidative desulfuration of thiobarbiturates can also occur, leading to more hydrophilic oxybarbiturates. Oxybarbiturate metabolites of thiamylal and thiobarbital are subsequently oxidized by the phase 1 and phase 2 reactions as described (Fig. 14.5).

Benzodiazepines. As with the barbiturates, BZs modulate the function of $GABA_A$ receptors, leading to neuronal hyperpolarization and CNS depressant effects. In contrast to the barbiturate binding site of $GABA_A$ receptors, the benzodiazepine binding site has been well characterized and is known to be formed by the interface of α and γ subunits. Not surprisingly, $GABA_A$ receptors lacking the γ subunit (eg, $\alpha_6\beta\delta$) are completely insensitive to all BZs. Additionally, it has been shown that isoforms of the α subunit have differential BZ binding affinities, with the α_1 subunit–containing receptors (often termed Bz_1 receptors) having high benzodiazepine affinity and the α_2, α_3, and α_5 subunit–containing receptors (often termed Bz_2 receptors) having moderate affinity. Furthermore, some combinations that include α_4 or α_6 subunits are completely insensitive to benzodiazepine agonists, even in the presence of an appropriate γ subunit.[25]

Binding of BZs to the allosteric BZ binding site produces agonist or partial agonist physiological responses, leading to CNS depressant activity. For this reason, BZ agonists are used clinically as sedative hypnotic agents as well as for anesthesia. Moreover, BZs have a prominent role in the treatment of anxiety and convulsant disorders, in accordance with their ability to allosterically augment GABA-mediated inhibitory Cl^- conductance through the $GABA_A$ channel. Specifically, binding of BZs to the BZ site leads to increases in the binding on-rate and affinity of one GABA molecule to the first GABA binding site of the receptor.[33] The increased affinity and rate of binding of GABA correlate with an increase in the frequency of the open channel bursts.[33] It is important to distinguish that BZs increase the frequency of channel opening, while barbiturates increase the duration of the open channel, and, as such, the two classes of agents have distinct molecular effects on the $GABA_A$ receptor. Furthermore, unlike barbiturates, BZs lack any effects in the absence of GABA. Refer to Chapter 11 for more detailed descriptions of benzodiazepine receptor binding and function.

Pharmacologic Effects of Benzodiazepines. All BZs are capable of producing sedative hypnotic effects; however, currently only five shorter-acting benzodiazepine agents are approved by the FDA for use as sedative hypnotics: estazolam, flurazepam, quazepam, temazepam, and triazolam. Moreover, remimazolam has recently been approved for induction and maintenance of sedation for procedures lasting 30 minutes or less. Residual hypnosis as well as psychomotor and cognitive inhibition are common side effects associated with their use. All of these agents are agonists of the BZ site of $GABA_A$ receptors containing α and γ subunits. Physiologically, they significantly reduce sleep latency and the number and duration of nighttime awakenings, resulting in an increase in total sleep time. The clinical use of these agents as sedative hypnotics is not free from adverse effects, which are primarily manifested as excessive residual next-day sleepiness, tolerance upon long-term use, and withdrawal upon discontinuation. Another clinically important effect is the ability of BZs to produce a high degree of anterograde amnesia, in which recent events are not transferred to long-term memory.[36]

Structure-Activity Relationships of Benzodiazepines. The SAR of BZs are described in detail in Chapter 11. There are five BZs approved for sedative hypnotic use and two that are approved for use in procedural sedation, that are described in more detail within this chapter (Fig. 14.6). All seven agents contain the 5-phenyl-1,4-benzodiazepine-2-one backbone required for $GABA_A$ activity, and all include an electronegative 7-position halogen substitution on ring A (see Chapter 11 and Fig. 14.6). Similarly, all contain a pendant 5-phenyl ring (ring C), which is required for in vivo agonism and can be substituted with *o*-electronegative halogens to increase lipophilicity, as is the case with flurazepam, quazepam, temazepam, triazolam, and midazolam. Importantly, *p*-substitution on ring C leads to inactive BZs, suggesting that steric restrictions are important at this site. Of note, several BZs, including estazolam, are metabolized at the C-ring *p* (4′) position, leading to inactivation of the agent. The major structural differences, which impart distinct pharmacokinetic properties to the sedative hypnotic BZs, are located within ring B, the major site of metabolic transformation of these agents. The structural features of ring B that contribute to metabolic vulnerability are discussed later.

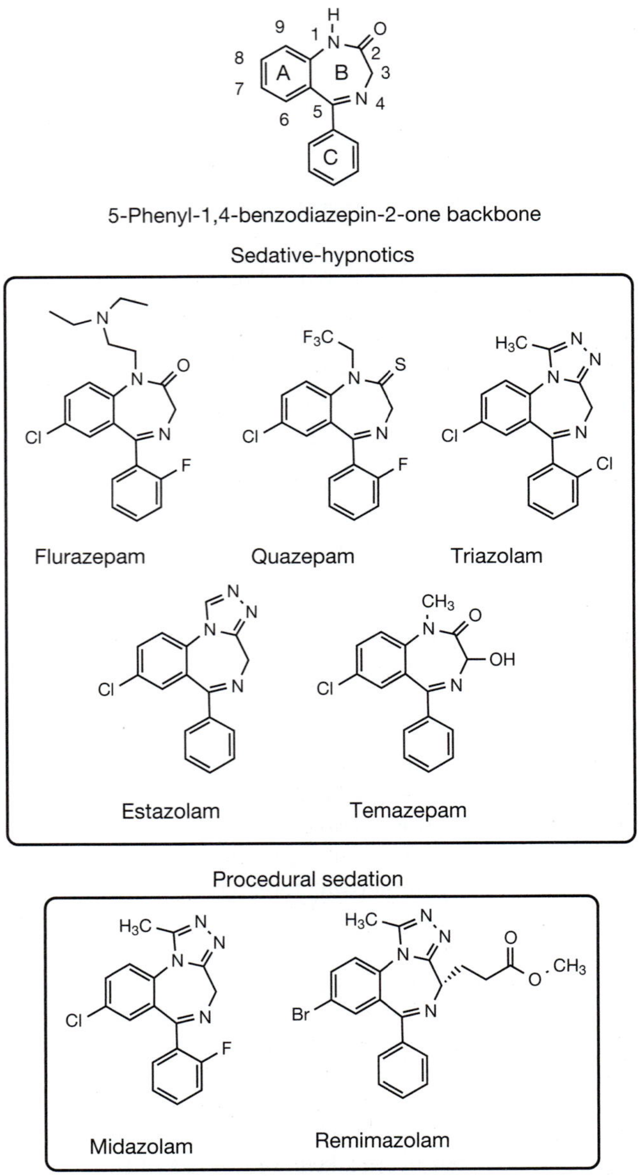

Figure 14.6 Benzodiazepine backbone and the benzodiazepines indicated for use as sedative hypnotics (top) and procedural sedation (bottom).

Pharmacokinetics and Metabolism of Benzodiazepines. Benzodiazepine agents, like the barbiturates, are lipophilic and can be easily absorbed upon oral ingestion and rapidly distributed to the brain. Among the oral benzodiazepine formulations specifically indicated for the treatment of insomnia, flurazepam is absorbed most rapidly, achieving mean peak plasma concentrations within 0.5 to 1.0 hours. Temazepam and triazolam reach mean peak plasma concentrations within 0.5 to 2.0 hours, while estazolam and quazepam take longer (Table 14.2).

The sedative hypnotic duration and side effect potential of BZs are greatly influenced by metabolism of the parent agent and the activity of resulting metabolites. Flurazepam has an elimination half-life of approximately 2 hours and is primarily metabolized by cytochrome P450-3A4 mediated *N*-dealkylation and hydroxylation, yielding active N1-desethyl and N1-hydroxyethyl metabolites with elimination half-lives of 47-100 and 2-4 hours, respectively (Fig. 14.7; Table 14.2).[37] Following a single 30-mg dose, the N1-hydroxyethyl metabolite is undetectable in the plasma after 24 hours. On the contrary, levels of N1-desethylflurazepam are 5- to 6-fold higher after 7 days of administration than they are following 24 hours, suggesting buildup of this active metabolite. Conjugation of N1-hydroxyethylflurazepam in phase 2 reactions allows for urinary excretion, and this conjugate is the major urinary metabolite, accounting for up to 55% of a single dose (Fig. 14.7). The long half-life of these metabolites explains the clinical findings that flurazepam exhibits faster sleep latency and decreases in total wake time following several days of use and also why it is still efficacious for one to two nights following discontinuation of the parent drug. These observations are especially important in older adult populations, in whom the elimination half-life of N1-desethylflurazepam is significantly higher, upward of 160 hours.

Quazepam is metabolized by CYP3A4 to yield 2-oxoquazepam, which is subsequently *N*-dealkylated to *N*-desalkyl-2-oxoquazepam (Fig. 14.7).[38] Both of these metabolites are pharmacologically active and have long durations, with mean plasma elimination half-lives of 40 and 73 hours, respectively (Table 14.2).[38] Both 2-oxoquazepam and *N*-desalkyl-2-oxoquazepam can be further hydroxylated at the 3-position, yielding 3-hydroxy-2-oxoquazepam and 3-hydroxy-*N*-desalkyl-2-oxoquazepam, respectively. These hydroxylated metabolites are subsequently *O*-glucuronidated and excreted readily in the urine (Fig. 14.7). As a consequence of the slow elimination of multiple active metabolites of both flurazepam and quazepam, residual hypnotic

Table 14.2 Pharmacokinetic Parameters of Benzodiazepines Approved for Sedative hypnotic Use

	Flurazepam	Quazepam	Estazolam	Triazolam	Temazepam
Log P[a]	2.35	4.03	3.51	2.42	2.19
Time to peak concentration (h)	0.5-1.0	~2	0.5-6.0	<2	1.2-1.6
Parent elimination half-life (h)	~2	39	10-24	1.5-5.5	0.4-0.6
Major metabolites (half-life, h)	N1-desethyl- (47-100, active) N1-hydroxyethy- (2-4, active)	2-Oxo-(40, active) *N*-desalkyl-(73, active)	4-Hydroxy- 4′-Hydroxy- 1-Oxo (all inactive)	α-hydroxy- (50%-100% active) 4-hydroxy-(inactive)	*O*-Glucuronides (Major) Oxazepam (Minor)
Predominant CYP isoforms involved	3A4	3A4/2C9	3A4	3A4	

[a]Data from Sangster Research Laboratories LOGKOW database.

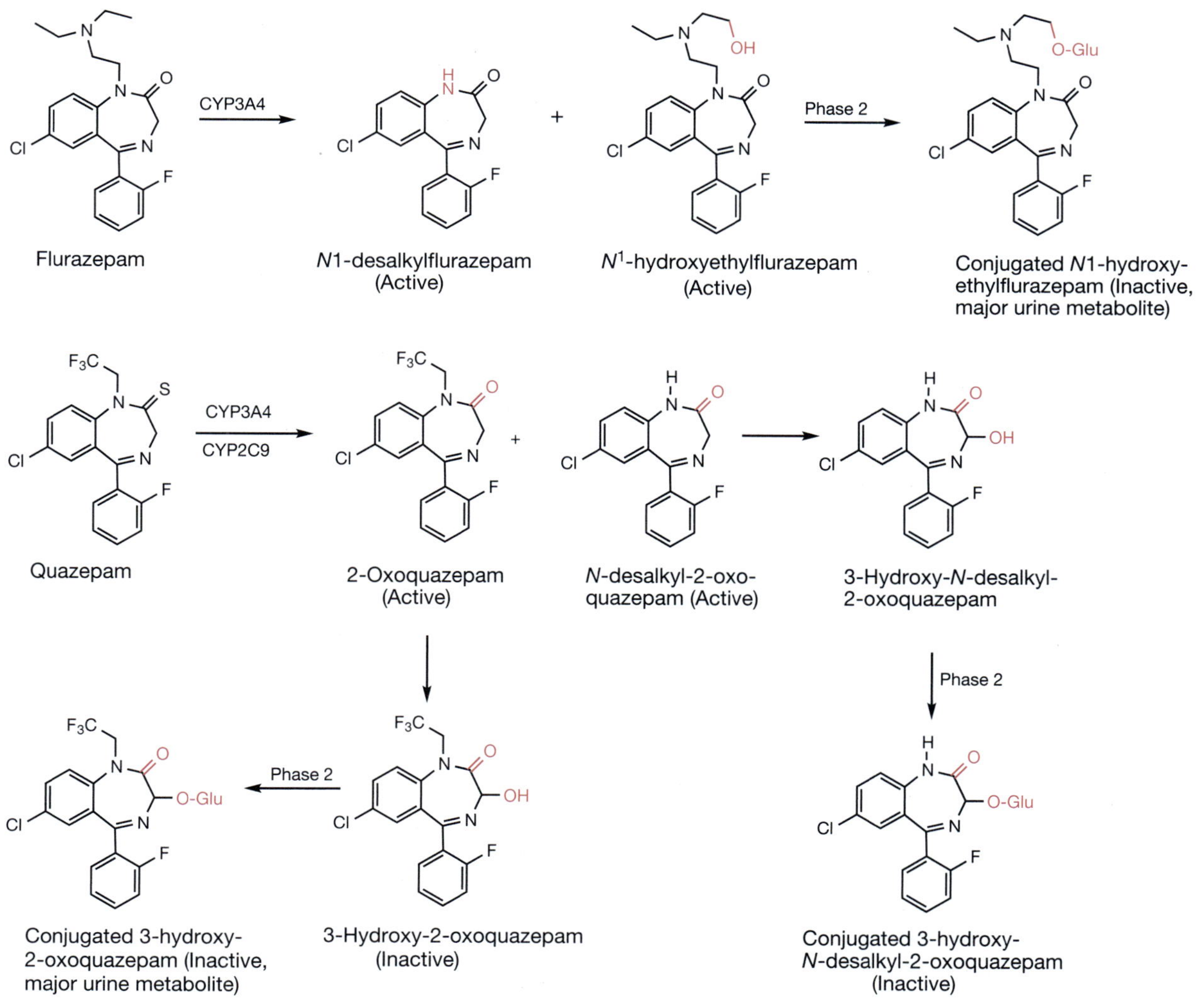

Figure 14.7 Metabolism of flurazepam and quazepam leads to formation of multiple long-acting active metabolites.

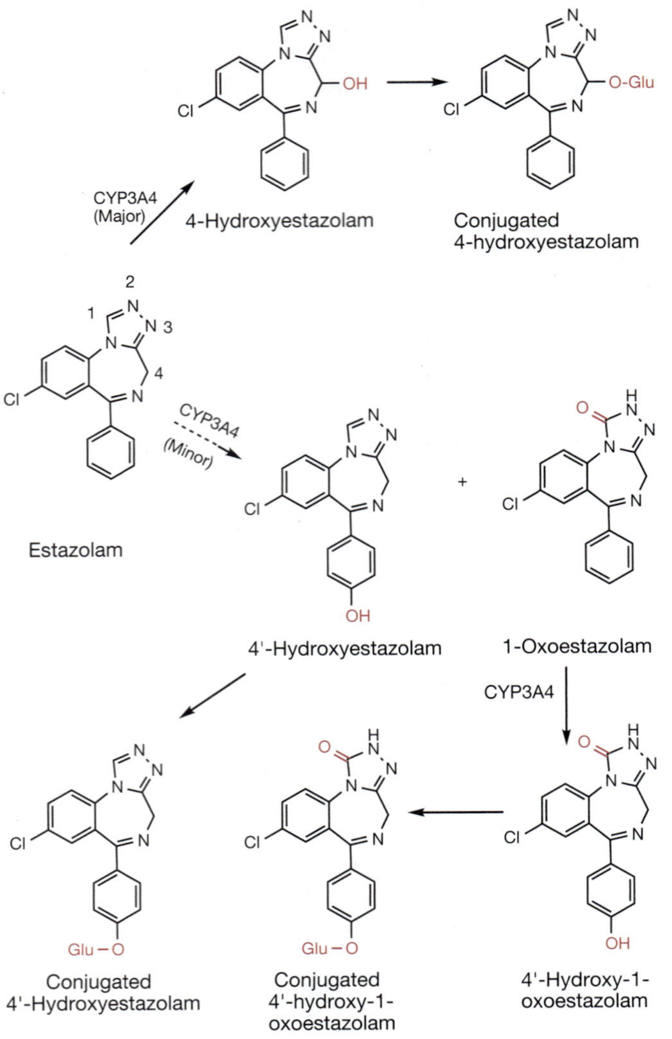

Figure 14.8 Metabolism of estazolam.

effects, including excessive daytime drowsiness and over-sedation as well as cognitive decline and confusion, are common and clinically relevant adverse effects.

These problems led to the development of newer triazolobenzodiazepines, such as estazolam and triazolam, with high $GABA_A$ receptor affinity and relatively shorter durations. The 1,4-triazolo ring of these congeners prevents oxidative metabolism typical of the BZs, which in the case of flurazepam and quazepam results in formation of active metabolites with long elimination half-lives. The presence of the fused fourth ring of these agents also changes the numbering convention, such that numbering priority proceeds around the triazole ring (Fig. 14.8). Estazolam has a longer elimination half-life (10-24 hours) compared to flurazepam, but this agent is primarily metabolized by CYP3A4, yielding 4-hydroxyestazolam as a major metabolite, which accounts for 70% of the biotransformation. Two minor metabolites 4′-hydroxyestazolam and 1-oxoestazolam, account for 23% and 7%, respectively (Fig. 14.8, Table 14.2).[39] While these metabolites have weak pharmacologic activity, three important factors prevent them from contributing to any significant sedative hypnotic effects. The first is the low affinities of the metabolites for the $GABA_A$ receptor. In particular, 4′-hydroxestazolam is sterically hindered from optimal $GABA_A$ binding, consistent with SAR findings described earlier showing that *p*-substitutions of ring C lead to decreased potency. The second factor that impedes the activity of estazolam metabolites is their decreased lipophilicity compared to the parent drug. This decrease facilitates the final factor, which is that the circulating metabolites are found in low concentrations due to direct excretion of the hydrophilic free metabolites or their rapid O-glucuronidation to highly ionized and readily excreted conjugates (Fig. 14.8).

Triazolam has a short duration of approximately 4 hours and is metabolized in humans to six metabolites, one of which, α-hydroxytriazolam, has been shown to retain 50% to 100% of the potency of the parent compound. While only small amounts of the parent drug are found in the urine, glucuronides of α-hydroxytriazolam as well as 4-hydroxytriazolam are the principal metabolites found in the urine, and these account for approximately 80% of triazolam excretion (Fig. 14.9).[40] There is no evidence of accumulation of triazolam metabolites, and the clinical effects of the active α-hydroxytriazolam are unclear, as this metabolite has been detected in the plasma primarily in its glucuronidated form. Taken together, the relatively short half-life of the parent, coupled with the urinary excretion of glucuronidated metabolites, affords triazolam a relatively short duration of action compared with other BZs.

Temazepam is unique among the sedative hypnotic BZs in that it contains a 3-hydroxy group and, as such, the agent circumvents phase 1 oxidation reactions prior to conjugation and excretion. The O-glucuronide of temazepam accounts for more than 90% of all metabolites recovered in man, and this feature affords a 0.4 to 0.6 hour elimination half-life and rapid excretion of the parent, while also providing the additional benefit of bypassing oxidative hepatic metabolism (Fig. 14.9).[41] In a secondary pathway, temazepam can also be *N*-demethylated to *N*-desmethyltemazepam, which itself is marketed as oxazepam. Oxazepam is further metabolized by phase 2 conjugation, yielding the O-glucuronide of oxazepam or *N*-desmethyltemazepam (Fig. 14.9).[41] Importantly, these metabolites are also formed independent of CYP450 isoforms and are rapidly excreted in the urine, with half-lives of approximately 2 hours.[41] Due to the rapid excretion of the phase 2 conjugates of temazepam, the metabolism of the parent drug serves as the rate-limiting step in the termination of the sedative hypnotic effect.

On the contrary to these, remimazolam was developed as a rapid onset, short duration agent and is considered an ultra-short–acting BZ. The basis of its development was modeled after the ultra-short–acting μ-opioid analgesic agent remifentanil that takes advantage of an active carboxylic acid ester, which, when hydrolyzed by tissue esterases, leads to an inactive agent. Similar to this model, remimazolam contains a 3-position (S)-oriented carboxylic ester that exists as the active BZ receptor agonist with very high affinity (~30 nM) for the BZ binding site.[42] The 7-chloro-substituent present on other highly hypnotic BZs was replaced with a

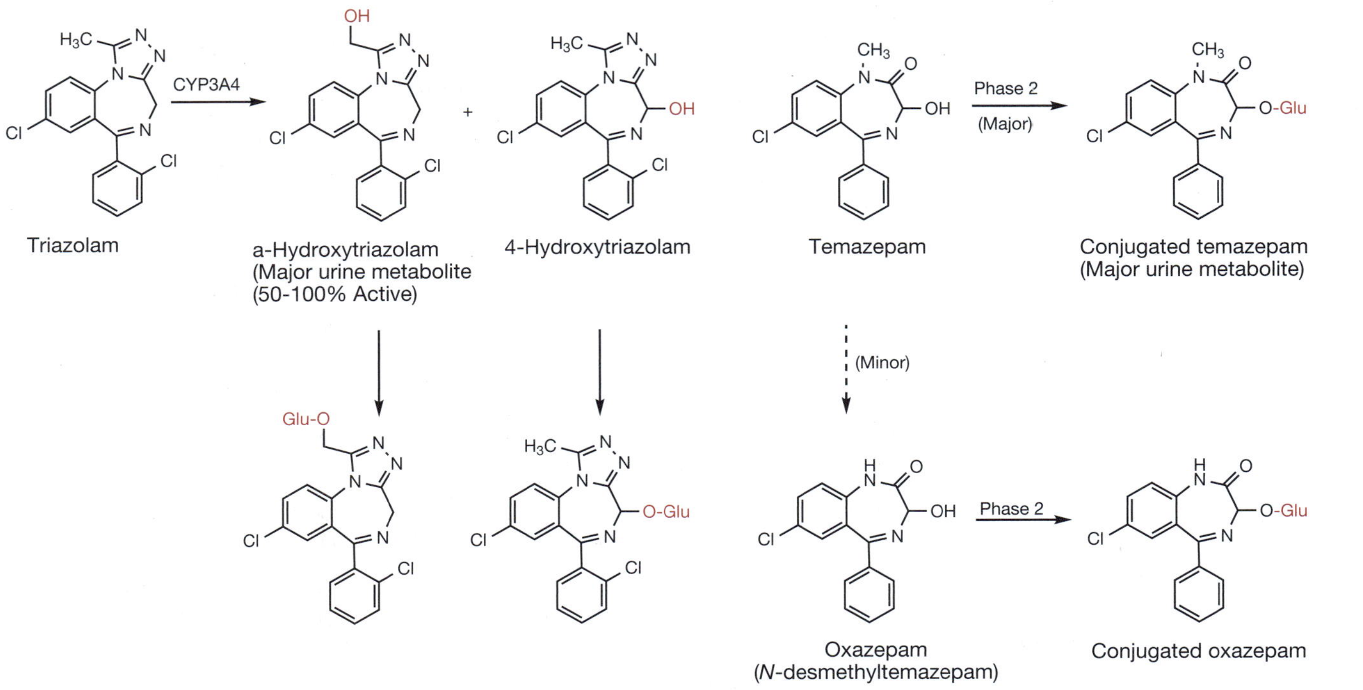

Figure 14.9 Metabolism of triazolam and temazepam.

similarly lipophilic bromo-substituent in this agent. The potency of remimazolam is greater than midazolam, an agent that is also commonly used for procedural anesthesia, at a variety of common GABA-R subtypes, including $\alpha1\beta2\gamma2$, $\alpha2\beta2\gamma2$, $\alpha3\beta2\gamma2$, and $\alpha5\beta2\gamma2$, and the efficacy of inducing GABA currents was greater for remimazolam at $\alpha1$- and $\alpha5$-containing GABA-R, compared to midazolam.[42] Importantly, remimazolam is rapidly inactivated by nonspecific tissue esterases to yield the carboxylic acid (Fig. 14.10), which has poor (~13 μM) affinity for the BZ site, facilitating deactivation of the anesthetic effectiveness. Four hours after IV administration, 98.63% of remimazolam is present in the urine as the inactive carboxylic acid metabolite (M01) (Fig. 14.10). Another 1% consisted of two oxidation products of M01, one of which was identified as oxidation of the imidazoline methyl group (Fig. 14.10), while the other was detected as oxidation via mass spectrometry, but whose site was not localized.[43] Finally, 0.36% of the dose was detected as glucuronide conjugates of these oxidized produces and 0.27% remained as the active parent (Fig. 14.10).[43] In the plasma, only remimazolam (0.33%) and the inactive M01 metabolite (99.67%) are present, consistent with the role of ester-mediated hydrolysis.[43]

In clinical trials, remimazolam yielded dose-dependent effects with the mean duration of sedation and loss of consciousness increasing with the dose.[44] The systemic clearance of the agent was rapid with linear kinetics across the dose range studied, while the clearance of the inactive carboxylic acid metabolite was slower than the active parent.[44] Compared to midazolam, patients on remimazolam recover from the hypnotic effect more rapidly, owing to the residence time of 0.5 hours compared to 3.56 hours for midazolam, which contributes to 3-fold faster clearance of remimazolam compared to midazolam.

Adverse Effects of Benzodiazepines. BZs are used as sedative hypnotic agents, as well as general muscle relaxants, anxiolytics, and anticonvulsants; however, as mentioned previously, their use can be confounded by presentation of undesirable side effects. While death by benzodiazepine overdose is rare and typically only results as a consequence of concomitant use with other CNS depressants, these agents are not free from adverse side effects and toxicities. Nearly all BZs have been reported to cause dose-dependent alterations in behavior, specifically, bizarre uninhibited and confused behaviors. The propensity of BZs to cause tolerance and

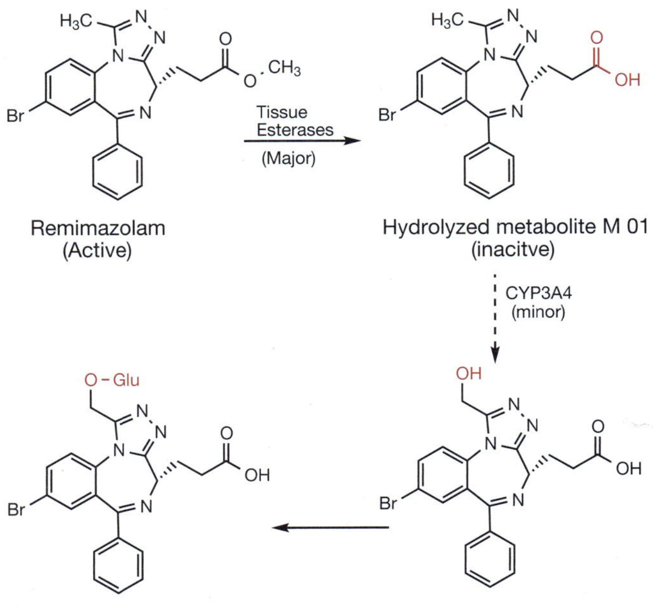

Figure 14.10 Inactivation of remimazolam by ester hydrolysis and subsequent metabolism.

their potential for physical dependence and abuse also limits their use. Additionally, misuse of rapid onset hypnotic BZs such as flunitrazepam (Rohypnol) has had profound social and medicolegal implications due to their use as "date-rape" or "robbery" drugs. This illicit use is based on the ability to produce rapid hypnosis in combination with anterograde amnesia. In addition to cognitive effects, BZs may also exhibit respiratory depressant effects depending on the dose and the duration, and as such, they are contraindicated in patients with pulmonary conditions or sleep apnea. These factors contributed to the development of nonbenzodiazepine sedative hypnotics devoid of many of the adverse effects induced by classical BZs.

Nonbenzodiazepine $GABA_A$ Agonists. Due to advances in molecular biology, genetics, and pharmacology in the late 1980s to early 1990s, numerous lines of evidence demonstrated that different $GABA_A$ receptor subtypes may bring about distinct functions depending on their localization in the brain. Future work revealed that α_2, α_3, and α_5 subtype–containing $GABA_A$ receptors (Bz_2) play critical roles in the anxiolytic, anticonvulsant, muscle relaxant, and cognitive impairment properties of classical BZs, while modulation of the α_1-containing $GABA_A$ receptor subtypes (Bz_1) was shown to be the key to benzodiazepine-induced sedation and hypnosis.[45-49] Importantly, these findings revealed that it could be feasible to design functionally selective drugs that act as selective agonists at specific $GABA_A$ subtypes to yield the appropriate pharmacotherapeutic outcomes. For example, selective α_2- or α_3-acting agents could have anxiolytic properties while being devoid of sedative effects, whereas selective α_1-acting agents would behave specifically as sedative hypnotic agents. While classical BZs described here and in Chapter 11 are nonselective and demonstrate sedative hypnotic as well as anxiolytic and other effects, the discovery of novel nonbenzodiazepine compounds with a high degree of selectivity for α_1 subtype–expressing $GABA_A$ receptors allowed for the specific use of these agents as sedative hypnotics. Currently, three structurally distinct non-BZs, zolpidem, eszopiclone, and zaleplon, which are often referred to as the Z-drugs, are approved in the United States for treatment of insomnia, and several other investigational agents are in various stages of clinical trials.

Zolpidem

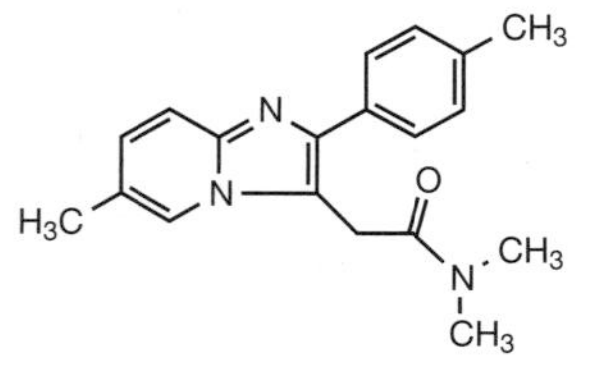

Zolpidem is an imidazopyridine that is a highly selective agonist of the α_1 subunit-expressing $GABA_A$ receptors (Bz_1), demonstrating 5- and 10-fold greater affinity for α_1 versus α_2 and α_3 subtypes, respectively.[50] Similar to the BZs, zolpidem lacks appreciable affinity for α_4 and α_5 receptors.[50] Of the three marketed nonbenzodiazepine drugs, zolpidem also has the greatest functional potency at potentiating GABA currents.[51] The hypnotic effects of zolpidem parallel those seen for temazepam and triazolam, but based on its selective pharmacological profile, zolpidem demonstrates weaker anxiolytic, anticonvulsant, and muscle relaxant effects compared to the classical BZs. Zolpidem has been shown to significantly improve sleep latency and prolong the duration of sleep in healthy volunteers as well as in patients with insomnia. Studies that compare the sleep outcomes of zolpidem with those of BZs have generally revealed comparable onset and sleep durations, while also showing that zolpidem leads to significantly fewer nighttime awakenings and, at the same time, being free from residual morning sedation, confusion, or memory impairment.[51-55] Further studies demonstrated that zolpidem exhibits significant improvements with regard to sleep latency as well as subjective accounts of sleep quality compared to BZs. Extensive review of trial data, which compare sleep outcomes of zolpidem to various BZs, shows that zolpidem is comparable or superior to various BZs with respect to sleep outcomes.[56-58]

Zolpidem is currently available in the United States in multiple formulations including immediate or controlled release oral tablets as well as sublingual tablets and an oral spray. Oral administration leads to bioavailability of approximately 70% and peak maximal plasma concentrations within 1.6 hours, while the sublingual formulation peaks at 35 to 75 minutes (Table 14.3). While plasma concentrations of zolpidem begin to decrease at approximately 2 hours following administration of the immediate release formulation, the extended-release formulation produces a more sustained peak plasma concentration that results in higher plasma concentrations over an 8-hour period. Direct comparison of the two formulations shows that plasma concentration profiles are generally identical for 2 hours following administration, after which decreases in blood levels are seen with the immediate release formulation. The controlled release formulation allows for this peak blood level to be extended for approximately 1 to 2 additional hours, allowing for correspondingly sustained blood levels throughout the night. Administration of the agent with food doubles the time required to reach peak and lowers the peak concentration by 30%. Accumulation of zolpidem does not seem to occur upon repeated exposure, regardless of the formulation. In addition, an available zolpidem oral spray formulation is distinguished by the fact that it allows for significantly faster time of onset of approximately 15 minutes (Table 14.3) and, as such, is clinically useful for patients with difficulties in achieving sleep initiation.

Structure-Activity Relationships of Zolpidem. There have been a great deal of medicinal-chemical efforts to define the SARs of zolpidem and to characterize interaction of the agent with the Bz_1 receptor. Anzini and colleagues have integrated these models using the structurally similar, but non-α_1-selective, imidazopyridine anxiolytic agent alpidem.[59] Based on these results, they have described a freely rotating aromatic ring region (FRAR), an electron-rich region (ERR), an antiplanar region (APR), and a planar aromatic region (PAR) (Fig. 14.11), which contribute to the binding of alpidem to benzodiazepine receptors. Studies on each of these regions have demonstrated that the replacement of alpidem's electronegative

Table 14.3 Pharmacokinetic Parameters of Nonbenzodiazepines Approved for Sedative Hypnotic Use

	Zolpidem	Eszopiclone	Zaleplon
Log P	2.31	−0.34	1.23
Time to peak concentration (h)	Immediate release—1.6[a]/1.6[b] Controlled release—1.5[c] Oral spray—0.25 Sublingual—0.5-1.0	1	1
Parent elimination half-life (mean, h)	Immediate release—2.5[a]/2.6[b] Controlled release—2.6[c]	6.5	1
Major metabolites (half-life, h)	None active	*N*-oxide (inactive) *N*-desmethyl (active, lower affinity)	None active
Predominant CYP isoforms involved	3A4 (major) 2C9, 1A2, and 2D6 (minor)	3A4, 2E1, 2C8	3A4 (minor)

[a]5 mg tablets.
[b]10 mg tablets.
[c]12.5 mg tablets.

chloro groups at both the FRAR and PAR with methyl groups, as in zolpidem, does not affect receptor binding affinity, but significantly increases the selectivity for α_1-subtype receptors.[60]

Further studies on the ERR have shown that conversion of either of imidazopyridine's H-bond–accepting imidazole nitrogen atoms to a hydrogen donor (ie, indole nitrogen) leads to complete loss of selectivity for α_1-subtype $GABA_A$ receptors, suggesting an interaction of this H-bonding H-acceptor with the $GABA_A$ receptor.[59] The importance of the ERR is also demonstrated by studies that convert the imidazole of zolpidem to its azaisostere congener. This simple change does not affect binding to α_1 subtype receptors

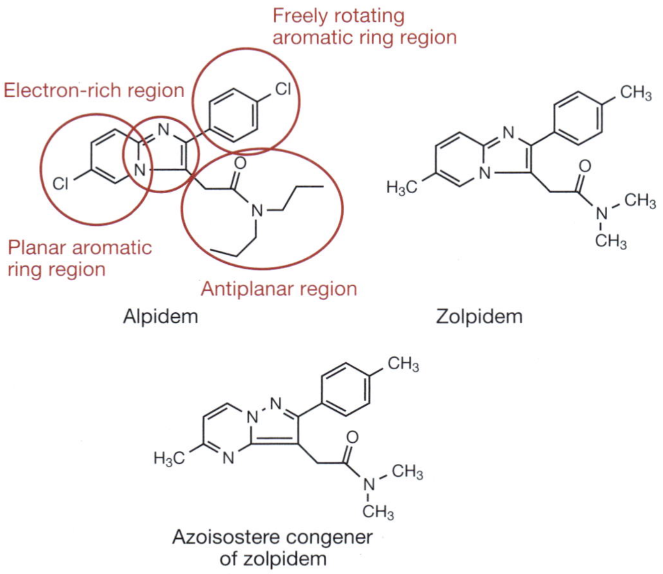

Figure 14.11 Structures of alpidem, zolpidem, and an azaisostere of zolpidem.

but decreases binding to α_2 and α_3 such that potency at these subtypes is negligible, similar to that seen for the α_5 subtype.[61]

The APR has also been shown to be critical in facilitating binding to $GABA_A$ receptors by allowing for hydrogen bonding interactions. Molecular modeling studies have shown that the APR carbonyl group of zolpidem can hydrogen bond to Ser204 or near Thr206/Gly207 within the backbone of loop C of α_1 subunits, as well as to Arg194 within loop F of γ_2 subunits, which form $\alpha_1\gamma_2$ complexes.[62] Finally, the APR also contributes to binding selectivity and affinity, as sterically hindered bulky amide nitrogen substitutions show decreased binding to α_1-subtype receptors. This study also identifies three additional α_1 and three additional γ_2 residues that are within 5 Å of zolpidem upon molecular docking simulations, suggesting that other hydrogen bonding or salt bridge interactions can occur within the ligand-binding domain.

Metabolism of Zolpidem. Zolpidem is rapidly eliminated with a mean half-life of approximately 2.5 hours (Table 14.3). Repeated doses do not seem to accumulate, and elimination of the parent is achieved through extensive metabolism, with only trace amounts of unchanged drug being found in urine or feces.[63] In humans, zolpidem can be oxidatively metabolized to yield four metabolites, MII, MIV, MX, and MXI, all of which lack pharmacological activity. As shown in Figure 14.12, the major metabolite is formed by CYP3A4-mediated hydroxylation of the *p*-tolyl methyl group yielding MIII, which is subsequently oxidized to the corresponding carboxylic acid, MI, by alcohol dehydrogenase.[64] The MI metabolite is the principal metabolite found in human urine, accounting for approximately 70% to 85% of the administered dose. CYP1A2, CYP2C9, and CYP2D6 can also metabolize a minor proportion of zolpidem to the MIII metabolite (Fig. 14.12).[64,65]

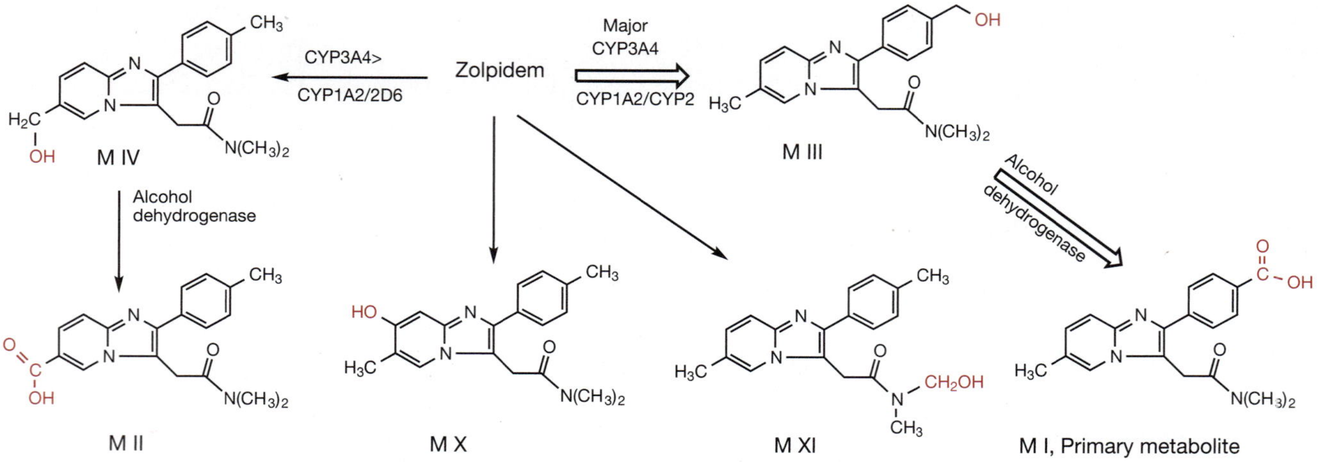

Figure 14.12 Metabolism of zolpidem.

Similarly, microsomal enzyme-mediated hydroxylation of the *p*-methyl substituent on the imidazopyridine backbone can also occur, leading to formation of metabolite MIV. As with formation of MIII, this occurs primarily via CYP3A4, with more minor contributions through either CYP1A2 or CYP2 isoforms. The MIV metabolite can be further oxidized to the corresponding carboxylic acid MII, accounting for approximately 10% of the administered dose.[64,65] Since expression of CYP1A2 and CYP2D6 in human liver is generally significantly less than that of CYP3A4, the clinical contribution of these enzymes in transformation of zolpidem to MIII and MIV is expected to be minor, and it is now well accepted that CYP3A4 plays the clinically more significant role.

More recent studies have confirmed these suspicions and demonstrated that the contribution of CYP enzymes to zolpidem metabolism is greatest for CYP3A4 (61%), followed by CYP2C9 (22%), CYP1A2 (14%), and less than 3% for CYP2D6.[65] Since MIII and MIV are not detectable in human urine or feces, but rather, the respective carboxylic acids MI and MII are, it was proposed that rapid formation of these secondary metabolites occurs. Indeed, studies in rodents have demonstrated that the conversion of the alcohol metabolites to their corresponding acids occurs very rapidly and requires a nonmicrosomal enzyme, perhaps alcohol dehydrogenase.[66] Finally, as shown in Figure 14.12, CYP3A4-mediated aromatic and side chain oxidation of zolpidem can lead to formation of the minor metabolites MX and MXI, respectively.

In older adult populations, dose adjustments must be made to account for the 50% increase in elimination half-life of the drug.[67] Similarly, in patients with hepatic dysfunction, the plasma concentration of zolpidem doubles, with an increase in elimination half-life to a mean of 10 hours. There has been recent interest in the likelihood of differential gender-based metabolism of zolpidem based on the ability of circulating free testosterone to increase CYP3A4 activity.[67,68] Given this correlation, women are likely to have higher plasma concentrations of zolpidem and, as such, may be more likely to have higher degrees of zolpidem-mediated adverse effects.[69] For this reason, the dose given to women is 50% of that given to men.

Eszopiclone

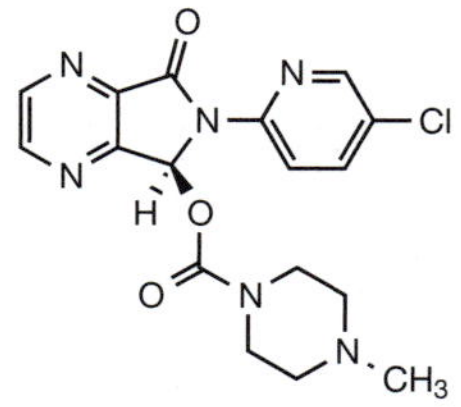

Eszopiclone, a pyrrolopyrazine derivative of the cyclopyrrolone class, is the active (*S*)-enantiomer of zopiclone, a racemic mixture that is no longer marketed in the United States. Compared to zopiclone, eszopiclone significantly improves sleep latency and sleep maintenance and increases the time spent in stage III and IV sleep. It is distinguished by the fact that its approval is not limited to short-term utilization and that it has no potential for development of tolerance or abuse. Several trials have demonstrated that hypnotic efficacy is maintained and eszopiclone is well tolerated upon chronic dosing up to 12 months.[70] In contrast to the racemic zopiclone, eszopiclone is devoid of substantial residual next-day sedative and cognitive effects. Unlike zolpidem, eszopiclone is not subtype selective. However, despite this lack of selectivity, it does not behave as a classical benzodiazepine with respect to its pharmacodynamics and pharmacological activity (see "Structure-Activity Relationships of Benzodiazepines" section). Eszopiclone binds with higher affinity to α_1-subtype-containing receptors but also has appreciable affinity for α_3 subunits and thus has hypnotic as well as other CNS activities. The affinity for α_1-subtype receptors is less than the other marketed nonbenzodiazepine agonists.

Eszopiclone is rapidly absorbed following oral administration, and peak plasma concentrations are reached within 1 hour. The elimination half-life of 6.5 hours is the longest of the nonbenzodiazepine hypnotics (Table 14.3). Similar to zolpidem, eszopiclone does not accumulate following repeated administration, and administration after a high-fat meal delays the time to peak plasma concentration by 1 hour and decreases this concentration by over 20%.[71] Eszopiclone dosing in older adults must also be adjusted to account for 41% greater drug levels and a significantly longer half-life of 9 hours. Similar dose adjustments must be made in patients with liver dysfunction, as total exposure to eszopiclone increases 2-fold at the 2-mg dose, although the time to peak concentration and the concentration itself were unaffected.[71]

Structure-Activity Relationships of Eszopiclone. Eszopiclone exhibits 50-fold greater binding affinity for $GABA_A$ receptors than does the (*R*)-enantiomer. This leads to significant improvement in GABA agonist potency, but more importantly, enantiomeric separation of the (*S*)-enantiomer seems to reduce adverse effects such as residual sedation seen with racemic zopiclone, despite the fact that the racemic mixture has a shorter half-life (5.0 vs 6.5 hours). Racemization of one enantiomer to the other does not occur in mammals in vivo.

While SAR studies for cyclopyrrolones have not been performed to a great degree, it is known that this subclass recognizes a distinct site of the $GABA_A$ receptor complex that is allosteric to the recognition site for classical BZs.[72] The regional distribution and specificity of sites labeled by radiolabeled cyclopyrrolones are similar to those labeled by classical benzodiazepine ligands, suggesting that the cyclopyrrolone binding site resides on the BZ site of the $GABA_A$ complex.[72] However, unlike classical benzodiazepine agonists, binding of cyclopyrrolones is not affected by GABA or barbiturates. Furthermore, radioreceptor displacement binding studies revealed a noncompetitive interaction of cyclopyrrolones at sites labeled by classical BZs, whereas displacement of radiolabeled cyclopyrrolones by classical BZs occurred competitively, validating that cyclopyrrolones recognize a site on the BZ receptor complex that is allosteric to the recognition site of classical BZs.[72] Others have suggested that perhaps cyclopyrrolones can interact with one of the multiple BZ binding sites on the $GABA_A$ receptor and, in doing so, cause allosteric changes in ligand affinity at the remaining sites. In this manner, eszopiclone could be thought to act in a positive cooperative binding manner with respect to itself.

With regard to binding within the ligand recognition site, molecular modeling and mutagenesis studies have shown that eszopiclone is within 4 Å of many amino acid residues within the GABA-BZ complex binding pocket, and such proximity allows anchoring and stabilization by multiple hydrogen bonding interactions with Arg144, Tyr209, Tyr159, and various other residues.[62] These studies also revealed that the structural requirements for eszopiclone binding are different than that for zolpidem, and these differences may account for the lack of selectivity of eszopiclone.[62]

Metabolism of Eszopiclone. Eszopiclone is metabolized extensively by CYP3A4 and CYP2E1 isozymes that yield the primary metabolites (*S*)-*N*-desmethylzopiclone and (*S*)-*N*-oxidezopiclone, respectively, in addition to a variety of minor metabolites (Fig. 14.13).[73] The racemic parent zopiclone was also noted to be extensively metabolized by CYP2C8, making it possible that this isoform also metabolizes the (*S*)-enantiomer.[74] The *N*-oxide metabolite is inactive, while *N*-desmethyleszopiclone exhibits lower potency and affinity at $GABA_A$ receptors and therefore has only very weak hypnotic activity compared to the parent (Fig. 14.13).

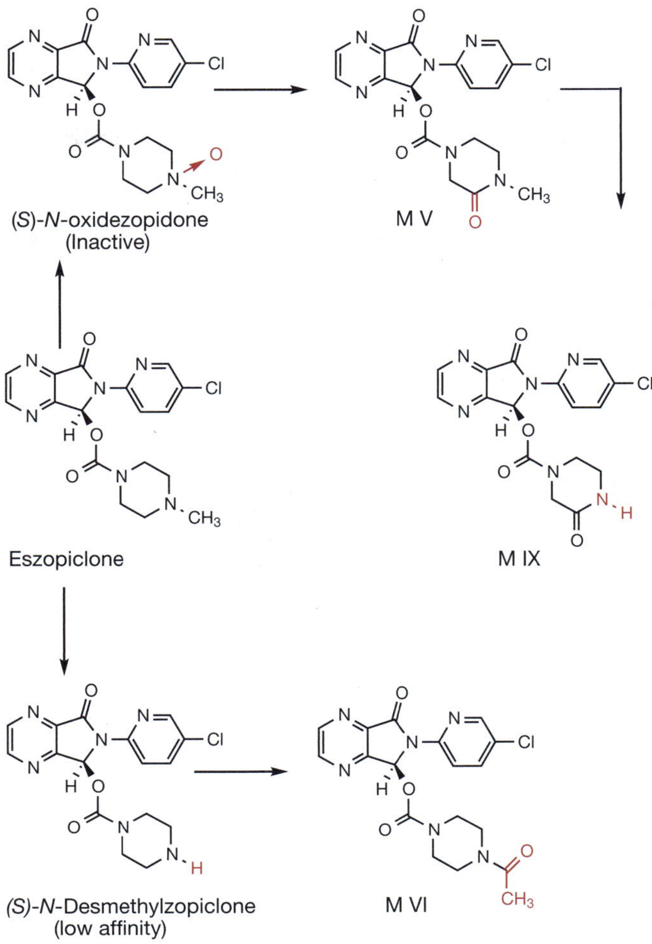

Figure 14.13 Metabolism of eszopiclone.

Interestingly, due to its lower affinity and lack of subtype selectivity, together with its weak sedative effects, this metabolite has been investigated as a novel anxiolytic agent. Only small amounts (<7%) of unchanged eszopiclone are excreted in the urine, and more than 75% of a dose is excreted via this route as inactive transformants of the two primary metabolites. In this regard, (*S*)-*N*-oxidezopiclone is further oxidized at a methylene of the piperazine group to yield the ketopiperazine metabolite MV, which can be further demethylated to form MIX, while (*S*)-*N*-desmethylzopiclone can be further oxidized to the amide derivative MVI (Fig. 14.13).[73]

Zaleplon

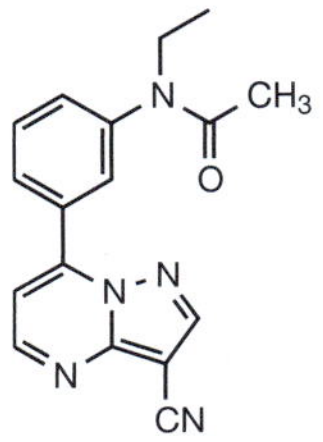

Zaleplon, a pyrazolopyrimidine, is a hypnotic agent that has a pharmacological profile similar to that of zolpidem but is primarily distinguished by its extremely rapid onset and short half-life. Similar to zolpidem, zaleplon has greater affinity at the α_1- versus α_2- and α_3-containing receptors, albeit with one-third to one-half the potency of zolpidem.[75] Unlike zolpidem, which does not recognize α_5-containing receptors with any appreciable affinity, zaleplon is able to potentiate the effects of GABA at α_5-containing receptors; however, its affinity for these receptors is approximately 15-fold less than that for α_1-containing receptors.[75] Thus, zaleplon is considered an α_1-selective GABA modulator, which lacks the classical benzodiazepine effects on non–sleep-related physiology.

The distinguishing features that afford zaleplon a unique place in the therapy of insomnia are its rapid rate of onset combined with its relatively fast rate of excretion. Oral administration of zaleplon leads to a peak plasma concentration in less than 1 hour, regardless of dose, the fastest of the non-BZs.[76] While zaleplon is completely absorbed following oral administration, it is subject to first-pass metabolism, leading to an absolute bioavailability of 30% (Table 14.3).[76] As with zolpidem and eszopiclone, administration with heavy meals, particularly high-fat foods, delays the time to peak plasma concentration to 3 hours and reduces the peak plasma concentration by 35%.[77,78] Following oral administration, zaleplon is rapidly eliminated with a mean elimination half-life of 1 hour, an effect that is delayed significantly in patients with hepatic dysfunction. Taken together, these pharmacokinetic properties facilitate the rapid onset and short duration hypnotic effects.[77,78]

Clinically, zaleplon is distinguished by its ability to significantly reduce sleep latency for up to 5 weeks compared to placebo, an effect that can be contributed to its rapid onset.[78,79] However, numerous clinical trials have failed to consistently show that a 5- or 10-mg nightly dose of zaleplon significantly improves sleep duration, decreases the number of awakenings, or improves overall sleep quality compared with placebo. This is likely due to the short half-life of the agent, which precludes hypnotic effects throughout the night. Higher nightly doses of zaleplon (20 mg) do significantly improve both sleep latency and duration, but effects on total sleep quality and number of awakenings compared to placebo have been inconsistent in clinical trials at this dose.[78] Tolerance and withdrawal effects have not been reported during short-term treatment (up to 5 weeks), and the agent also seems to be free from rebound insomnia and residual next-day sedative effects, similar to other nonbenzodiazepine hypnotics.[79] As a result of these effects, zaleplon is approved only for patients with difficulties falling asleep; however, an extended-release formulation, which could improve sleep maintenance and duration, has been under development for some time.

Structure-Activity Relationships of Zaleplon. Unlike zolpidem and eszopiclone, extensive studies that examine the SARs of zaleplon with regard to binding potency and interaction within the binding pocket have not been conducted. However, there have been numerous studies comparing the binding and function of zaleplon to the closely related compound indiplon (Fig. 14.14), allowing for deduction of SAR from pharmacological results. These studies show that zaleplon exhibits approximately 7- and 10-fold greater selectivity for α_1- over α_3- and α_5-containing $GABA_A$ receptors, respectively, whereas indiplon demonstrates only 1.6- and 4-fold selectivity.[80] Importantly, indiplon has 3-, 12-, and 7-fold higher affinity at α_1-, α_3-, and α_5-containing receptors, respectively, than does zaleplon. Further work has demonstrated that indiplon is 100-fold more potent than zaleplon at potentiating GABA currents through α_1-containing receptors but is also 46- and 25-fold more potent at doing so through α_3- and α_5-containing receptors, respectively.[51,80] This work suggests that the thiophene-2-carbonyl moiety of indiplon (Fig. 14.14) drives higher binding affinity and thus potency, but decreases overall selectivity for one subtype

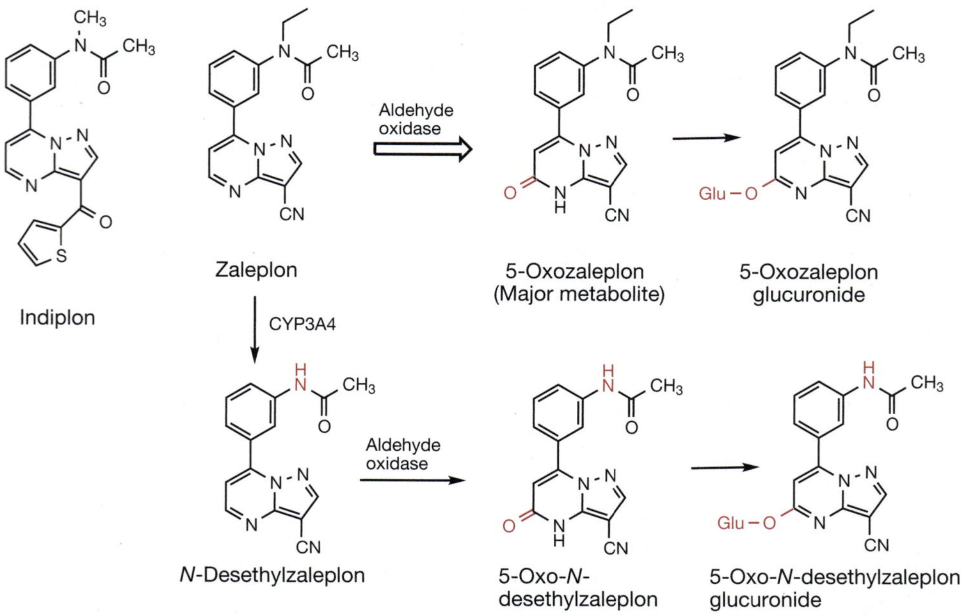

Figure 14.14 Structural relationship of zaleplon to indiplon and metabolism of zaleplon.

over another. Meanwhile, zaleplon contains only a cyano group at this position, suggesting that electronic rather than steric factors influence selectivity.

Metabolism of Zaleplon. As described, zaleplon is subject to significant first-pass metabolism that accounts for its low oral bioavailability. Following oral administration of the agent in humans, less than 0.1% of the drug is recovered unchanged in the urine. Animal studies have demonstrated distinct interspecies variability in the metabolism of orally administered zaleplon due to differences in the activity of hepatic aldehyde oxidase, which is the principle metabolic enzyme responsible for the transformation of zaleplon.[81] In rodents and canines, which have decreased expression and activity of aldehyde oxidase, zaleplon is predominantly metabolized by CYP3A4 to *N*-desethylzaleplon, with only minor oxidation by aldehyde oxidase to yield 5-oxozaleplon. In humans, these metabolic routes are interchanged due to greater activity of aldehyde oxidase, and as a result, the major metabolite is 5-oxozaleplon, while CYP3A4-mediated transformation, yielding *N*-desethylzaleplon, is a minor route (Fig. 14.14). Both primary metabolites are inactive and, once formed, can either be directly eliminated in the urine or oxidized further and excreted as a glucuronide conjugate. In addition, the *N*-desethylzaleplon metabolite can be rapidly converted, presumably also via aldehyde oxidase, to 5-oxo-*N*-desethylzaleplon (Fig. 14.14).[77] Following oral administration of radiolabeled zaleplon to healthy volunteers, 70% of the dose was recovered in the urine within 2 days, almost exclusively as the two primary metabolites or their *O*-glucuronide conjugates (Fig. 14.14).[77] The 5-oxozaleplon metabolite also predominates in the feces, where over 15% of an administered dose can be found within 6 days.[77]

The non-BZs represent major advancements in treatment of insomnia. They are highly effective hypnotic agents with negligible residual daytime drowsiness and are generally free from the psychomotor and cognitive side effects of classical BZs. Despite their primary use at nighttime and their relatively short half-lives, these agents are also not completely devoid of adverse side effects. There are reported occurrences of nonbenzodiazepine-induced sleepwalking and associated amnesic sleep-related complex sleep behaviors such as sleep driving, sleep eating, sleep cooking, sleep talking, and sleep sex.[82-90] These effects have been reported at therapeutic as well as supratherapeutic doses and are potentiated by alcohol consumption. Importantly, patients do not have any recall or memory of these events. While these unintended effects are rare, they are potentially very serious, as they can affect social, emotional, and physical health and pose risks for fatal incidents.

MELATONIN RECEPTOR AGONISTS. As described, melatonin is a neurohormone that is primarily synthesized in the pineal gland from its precursor, serotonin (Fig. 14.1). Since melatonin synthesis is concurrent with sleep, the increase in endogenous nighttime melatonin levels correlates with the onset of sleepiness. The sleep-promoting and circadian effects of melatonin are due to agonism of both MT_1 and MT_2 receptors (MT1R, MT2R), both of which are present in very high density (~ 4 fmol/mg protein) within the SCN.[91] Agonism of SCN MT1R directly facilitates inhibition of SCN neuron firing, promoting sleep, while activation of SCN MT2R effects the circadian rhythm settings related to the central clock.[92,93]

Melatonin itself is a poor chemotherapeutic agent due to its poor absorption and low oral bioavailability of less than 10% as well as its ubiquitous effects on sleep and circadian rhythms. Moreover, because melatonin is a supplement that is unregulated by the FDA, preparations vary in their purity and concentration and, as a result, poor sleep outcomes are often encountered. The significant effects of MT receptor agonism on sleep, coupled with the relatively poor nature of melatonin as a drug, prompted intense medicinal-chemical efforts to develop novel small molecule congeners of melatonin that behave as potent agonists of MT receptors. These efforts led to the successful launch of the first-in-class melatonin receptor agonist (*S*)-ramelteon, which has an excellent sleep and safety profile. Similarly, tasimelteon selectively agonizes MT1 and MT2 receptors and is approved for treatment of non–24-hour sleep-wake disorder.

Structure-Activity Relationships of Melatonin Receptor Agonists. SARs for melatonin and its congeners have been reviewed at length.[94-99] Early studies demonstrated that the indole backbone of melatonin was not required for activity as long as it was replaced by an aromatic isostere as in ramelteon (which contains an indane) or as in other MTR agonists such as tasimelteon and agomelatine (Fig. 14.15).[97] It has been proposed that the importance of the aromatic ring system is to offer an optimum distance between the amide side chain at position-3 and the 5-methoxy substituent.[98,99] The aromatic moiety has also been suggested to interact with aromatic receptor residues within the binding pocket through π-π stacking.[98,99] While the aromatic portion contributes to spacing and likely π-π-interactions, the 3-position amide and the 5-methoxy side chains are responsible for binding and functional activation of the receptors by interacting with two proposed binding pockets.

The amide group is critical for agonist activity at both MT receptors and is thought to interact with key serine (Ser110 and Ser114) and asparagine (Asn175) residues in transmembrane helix (TMH) III of MT_1 and TMH IV of TM2, respectively.[100] Meanwhile, the 5-methoxy moiety is critical for functional effects. It has been proposed that the methoxy

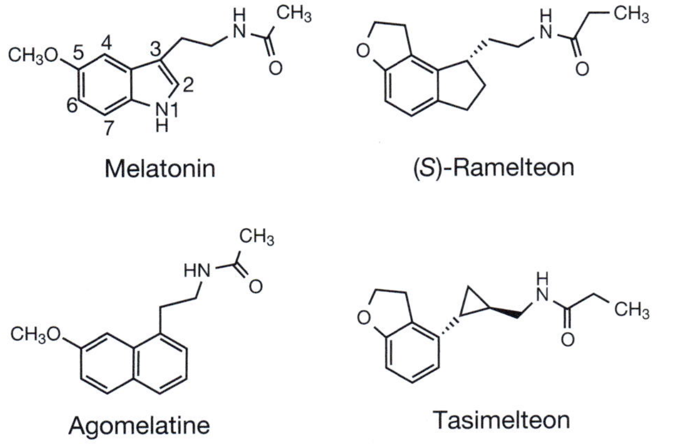

Figure 14.15 Structures of melatonin and the melatonin receptor agonists (*S*)-ramelteon, agomelatine, and tasimelteon.

oxygen interacts with His195 and His208 within TMH VI of MT1R and MT2R, respectively.[99,101] Movement of the methoxy group to the 4-, 6-, or 7-positions significantly decreases functional activity, suggesting that distance to these conserved histidine residues is critical in maintaining binding affinity and functional activity.[95] Additionally, Val192, which is located nearly one turn above His195 within the ligand-binding domain, has been shown to be involved in binding the methyl component of the methoxy group.[99]

Finally, the binding pocket of MTRs is highly stereoselective, an important feature that must be considered for drug design. As a consequence of the three-dimensional requirements of binding to MT receptors, ramelteon (discussed next) is dispensed as the enantiomerically pure (*S*)-enantiomer, which has 500-fold greater affinity for MT1R than does (*R*)-ramelteon.

Ramelteon

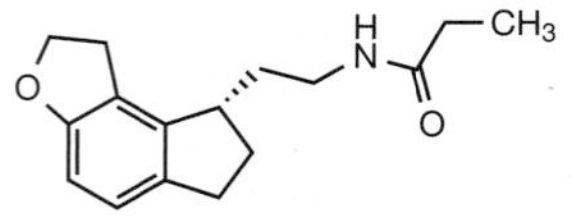

(*S*)-Ramelteon selectively binds to both MT1R and MT2R, recognizing the human receptors with extremely high affinity of 14 and 112 pM (picomolar), respectively. This represents an 8- to 10-fold greater affinity for MT1R compared to MT2R, and 6-fold greater affinity than melatonin for MT1R.[102] The high potency and slight preference for MT1R correlate to the ability of the drug to primarily reduce sleep latency, as opposed to influencing regulation of phase—circadian rhythms, which is primarily mediated by MT2R.

With regard to functional pharmacology, in Chinese hamster ovary (CHO) cells ectopically expressing the human MT1R and MT2R, ramelteon was 4- and 17-fold more potent at inhibiting cyclic AMP production compared to melatonin, respectively, consistent with observations that demonstrate coupling of MT receptors to $G\alpha_{i/o}$ proteins.[102] Moreover, ramelteon does not have any appreciable affinity for a third physiologically relevant melatonin-binding site known as MT3R, which is a melatonin-sensitive quinine reductase not involved in sleep/wake functions.[103,104] Taken together, the absence of binding to brain receptors other than MT1R/MT2R, along with its potent activity at these melatonin receptors, makes ramelteon an efficacious sleep-inducing agent that is free from many of the CNS side effects common to other sedative hypnotics.

Animal studies demonstrate that ramelteon significantly decreases wakefulness and increases both short wave and REM sleep compared with placebo.[103-105] In clinical trials, no effects on short wave sleep have been noted, but the agent leads to significant decreases in sleep latency and increases in total sleep duration over a 5-week period compared to placebo.[106-108] Importantly, ramelteon, consistent with its melatonin receptor–related mechanism which is free of endogenous GABAergic signaling, does not produce residual next-day sedation or decreases in psychomotor function.[107] Likewise, due to its unique mechanism, ramelteon does not hinder learning, cognition, and memory like the benzodiazepine agents do. It also lacks the potential for abuse, does not lead to tolerance, and poses no risk of withdrawal or rebound insomnia upon discontinuation.[107-109] One potential adverse effect, which can be predicted for melatonin receptor agonists, is based on the ability of melatonin to influence prolactin and testosterone levels via agonism of MT1R and MT2R located within endocrine and reproductive tissue. Similarly, ramelteon has been reported to affect mean free and total testosterone levels.[103] Further studies are necessary to gauge the clinical consequences, if any, that exogenous melatonin receptor agonists have on endocrine and reproductive function. In summary, from a sleep-therapy standpoint, melatonin receptor agonists such as ramelteon have highly efficacious hypnotic effects while being free of many of the cognitive and residual effects common to $GABA_A$-modulating agents.

Metabolism of Ramelteon. (*S*)-Ramelteon is rapidly absorbed following oral administration and mean peak plasma concentrations are achieved at 0.75 hours. In a study on healthy volunteers who were administered radiolabeled ramelteon, 84% of recovered radioactivity was found in the urine and 4% in the feces, suggesting that at least 84% of the drug was absorbed. However, ramelteon is subject to extensive first-pass metabolism, leading to an absolute oral bioavailability of only approximately 2%.[110] Ramelteon has a short elimination half-life of 1 to 2.5 hours, and once-nightly dosing does not lead to accumulation of the drug. The time to peak plasma concentration was delayed by 45 minutes upon administration with food, and the peak plasma concentrations were decreased by 22% in this case.[110]

Ramelteon is primarily metabolized by oxidation in phase 1 reactions, with secondary metabolites being excreted as glucuronide conjugates.[111] Hepatic CYP1A2 is the major isoform responsible for transformation (49%), while CYP2C19 (42%) and CYP3A4 (8.6%) isoforms are also contributors to ramelteon metabolism in the liver. In contrast, in the intestines, only CYP3A4 contributes to transformation.[112] The major metabolite of ramelteon in humans is the hydroxylated propionamide MII metabolite (Fig. 14.16), which is active, has a 2- to 5-hour half-life, and has 20- to 100-fold greater systemic exposure than the parent, suggesting slower removal from the circulation.[110,111] Moreover, this metabolite has 1/5 to 1/10 the binding affinity of the parent for human MT_1 and MT_2 receptors and shows potent hypnotic effects in animals, suggesting that it may contribute to the sedative hypnotic effects of ramelteon.[109-112] In addition to the MII metabolite, ramelteon can be oxidized to the ring-opened MI metabolite or transformed to a carboxy-metabolite, MIII (Fig. 14.16), both of which are inactive. Biotransformation of the MII and MIII metabolites by sequential oxidation can lead to formation of MIV. The rank order of prevalence of the four metabolites in human serum is MII, MIV, MI, and MIII, and all three of the hydroxylated metabolites can be excreted as glucuronide conjugates (Fig. 14.16).

Importantly, ramelteon is also subject to significant drug interactions upon coadministration with the antidepressant fluvoxamine, the fluoroquinolone antibiotic ciprofloxin, or the over-the-counter (OTC) H_2-antagonist cimetidine, which are all relatively strong CYP1A2 inhibitors. Coadministration of any of these agents with ramelteon significantly

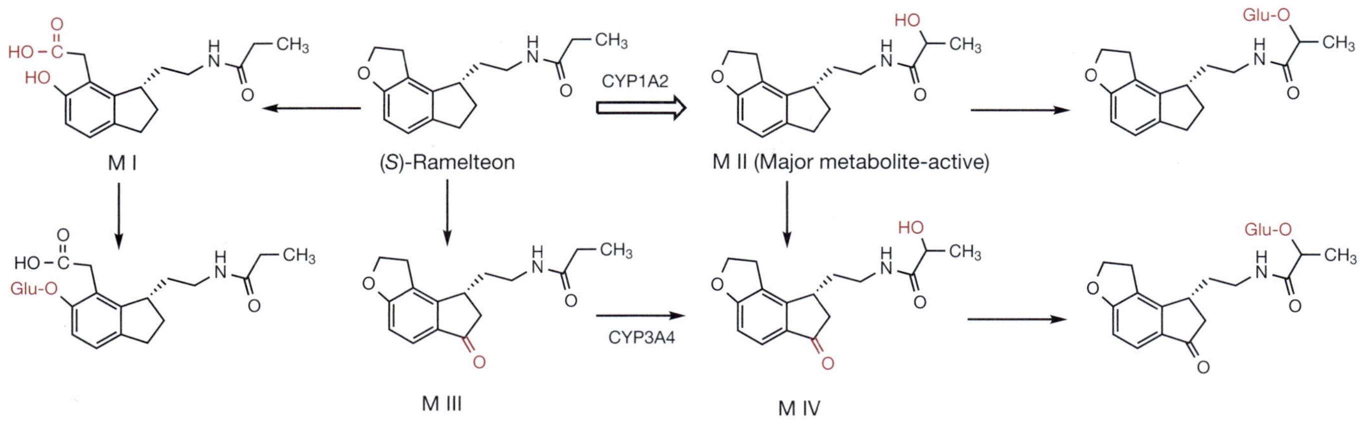

Figure 14.16 Metabolism of (*S*)-ramelteon.

increases the total systemic exposure of ramelteon (>100-fold in the case of fluvoxamine) and should be avoided.

Tasimelteon. Tasimelteon exhibits strong subnanomolar affinity and full agonist activity at both MT1R (Ki = 300-350 pM) and MT2R (Ki = 69-170 pM), with only 2- to 4-fold greater affinity for the MT2 subtype.[113] Given the prominent role of MT2R in regulating circadian rhythm and the hypothalamic master clock as discussed, the somewhat enhanced potency of tasimelteon at MT2R dictates the agent's therapeutic usefulness in treatment of sleep-wake disorders such as non–24-hour circadian disorder. This is in distinct contrast to ramelteon, which has 8- to 10-fold greater affinity for the MT1 subtype versus MT2. Similar to ramelteon, tasimelteon has a highly favorable on-target selectivity, lacking any appreciable affinity toward over 160 receptors and enzymes.[113]

Metabolism of Tasimelteon. Oral administration of tasimelteon reaches maximal plasma levels rapidly (T_{max}, 0.5 hours), with an absolute bioavailability of 38% and elimination half-life of approximately 1 hour, similar to that seen with ramelteon and the nonbenzodiazapine Z-drugs.[114] The bioavailability of tasimelteon is greater than that of both melatonin and ramelteon, and the low overall bioavailability of all is attributed to significant first-pass oxidative metabolism. Interestingly, among the three, tasimelteon is unique in that 80% of radiolabeled drug is recovered as parent or metabolites in the urine, suggesting that although the agent is subjected to first-pass metabolism, a significant proportion of this occurs after systemic exposure rather than prior to it.[114] Given this, it is unsurprising that tasimelteon is heavily metabolized by CYP1A1, CYP1A2, CYP2D6, CYP2C9, and CYP3A4 with at least nine distinct metabolites identified in humans.[115,116] No metabolism of the parent drug is seen in the presence of CYP2A6, 2B6, 2C8, 2C19, or 2E1 isoforms (Fig. 14.17).[115,116] The proposed metabolic route of transformation of tasimelteon yields the phenolic carboxylic acid M9 (19.8% of plasma AUC), the 7-hydroxylated M13 (14.6%), the 8-hydroxy M14 (7.1%), the 8-hydrox M12 (3.9%), and the diol M11 (3.6%) as the major primary metabolites (Fig. 14.17). The phase 2 glucuronidated products M1, M2, and M3 combine to comprise an additional 14.5% of the plasma drug exposure (Fig. 14.17).[115-117] All of the metabolites of tasimelteon had 13-fold or less activity at MT1 and MT2 receptors compared to parent agent.[115-117]

Orexin Receptor Antagonists. As described, the hypothalamic neuropeptides orexin-A and orexin-B activate their cognate GPCRs, OX1R, and OX2R, to depolarize and excite downstream neurons in order to promote arousal and alertness. Hypothalamic orexin neurons are highly active during wakefulness and quiesce during all stages of sleep, which correlates with heightened levels of orexin-A during wake periods that fall significantly during sleep.[118-120] The discovery that disturbances in orexinergic function are linked to the pathophysiology of narcolepsy, coupled with evidence linking loss of function mutations of OX2R to heritable narcolepsy in animals, demonstrates the critical role of OXRs in regulating vigilance and arousal.[121,122]

Consistent with these observations, exogenous administration of orexins in mammals increases wakefulness, decreases REM and non-REM sleep, and increases locomotor activity.[123,124] On the contrary, antagonism of the orexin GPCRs facilitates hyperpolarization of postsynaptic neurons, which promotes drowsiness and somnolence. Using genetic knockout models coupled to approaches that utilize selective single- or dual-OXR antagonists (ie, SORA and DORA, respectively), it has become evident that arousal is principally regulated by the OX2R, while both OXRs are involved in modulating vigilance states within the sleep/wake architecture.[125] In addition, dual-OXR knockout animals exhibit the most pronounced sleep phenotype compared to single OXR knockouts, and when compared to SORA, DORA provide enhanced in vivo and clinical sleep efficacy. Consequently, recent drug discovery efforts have led to development of DORA for clinical therapy of insomnia.

Almorexant (structure shown at the end of the section) was one of the first DORA to be assessed clinically for the treatment of insomnia and proved to be effective at increasing total sleep time and decreasing sleep latency, including time to induction of REM sleep. This is consistent with its reported low nanomolar affinity for both OXR (inhibitory concentration 50% (IC_{50}) of 13 and 8 nM for OX1R and OX2R, respectively).[126-128] Unlike zolpidem, almorexant lacked sedative hypnotic effects in OX1R/OX2R knockout mice and had no effects on next-day motor function

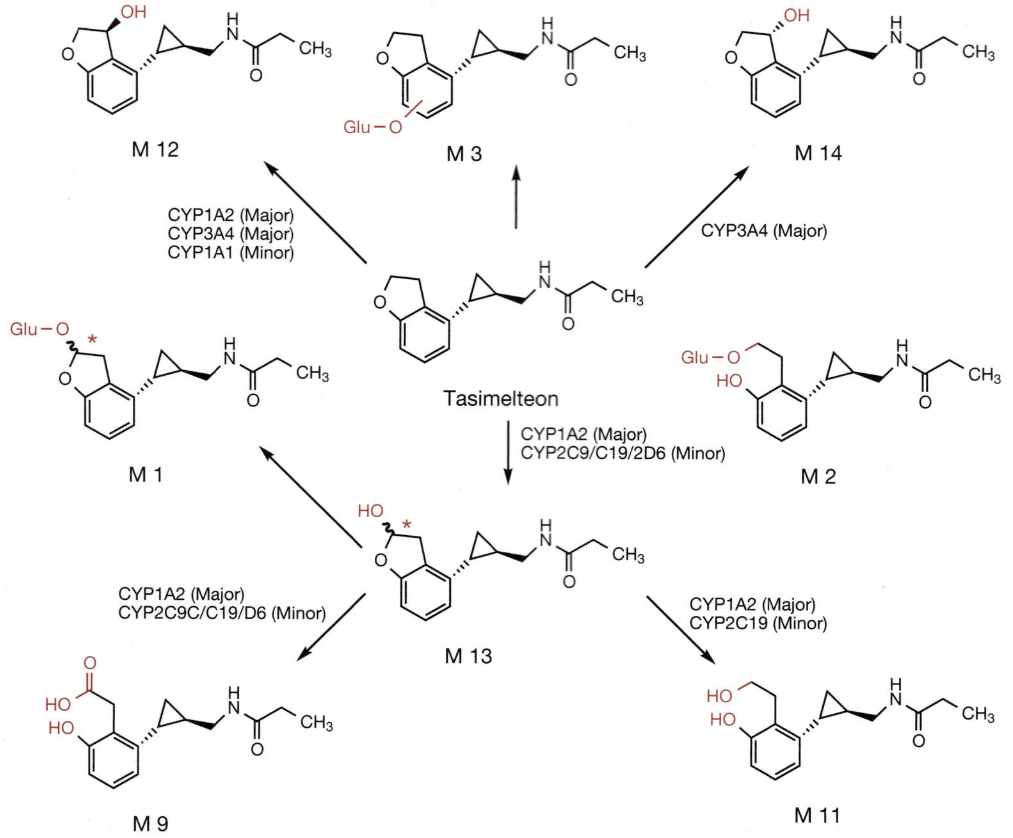

Figure 14.17 Proposed metabolic transformation of tasimelteon. * denotes a chiral center with both enantiomers produced.

or muscle relaxation.[126,129] In clinical trials, almorexant improved measures of sleep efficiency and showed minimal residual next-day impairments to motor function or cognition in insomniac patients; however, development of this agent was halted in late 2011 due to undisclosed reasons.

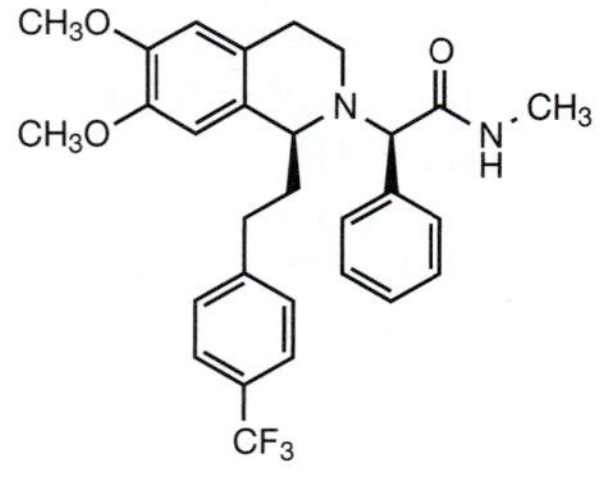

Suvorexant. Suvorexant, developed by Merck & Co. as MK-4305, was the first DORA approved for the treatment of insomnia. Suvorexant has high binding affinity of 0.55 and 0.35 nM for OX1R and OX2R, respectively. This translates to 50 and 56 nM functional potency, as determined by the ability to inhibit orexin-mediated Ca^{2+}-mobilization in clonal CHO expression systems.[130] In an off-target screen of 170 enzymes, receptors, and ion channels, suvorexant displays a noteworthy more than 10,000-fold selectivity for the OXR, an effect that alleviates concerns regarding ancillary target profiles.[130]

Pharmacokinetically, suvorexant has moderate passive brain permeability owing to a high degree of lipophilicity (log P = 3.6) and is not a substrate for *P*-glycoprotein (P-gp) efflux from the brain.[130] In animals, suvorexant significantly increased REM sleep and δ-stage activity (stage 4 sleep) and induced corresponding decreases in wake time, with analogous receptor occupancy of more than 90%.[130]

In human clinical trials of durations ranging from 1 month to more than 1 year, suvorexant was dose-dependently superior to placebo in regard to time to sleep onset and time to onset of REM sleep.[131-134] Furthermore, suvorexant increased total sleep time and decreased number and time of awakenings compared to placebo.[131-134] It was also demonstrated to be effective in reducing time to sleep onset and total sleep time in older adults with insomnia.[134,135] Together, these clinical data demonstrate that suvorexant is effective for both latency and maintenance of sleep.

In clinical trials, as would be expected given the indicated use of the agent, the most common adverse effect of suvorexant was somnolence, which was dose dependent.[136] Interestingly, the incidence of somnolence was significantly higher in women (8%) than in men (3%), suggesting that gender-based metabolism plays a role in metabolic breakdown of suvorexant. Gender-specific metabolism was also seen with zolpidem. Residual somnolence, drowsiness, and general CNS depressant effects may persist for several days following discontinuation of suvorexant. Of note, this effect led to a clinically meaningful next-morning impaired driving performance, and consequently, patients on suvorexant should be warned about residual next-day impairments to mental alertness. Given its unique mechanism of action, suvorexant would be predicted to have a distinct adverse effect profile compared to other sedative hypnotic agents. After somnolence, the next most frequently occurring adverse effects were headache, abnormal dreams, and dry mouth, which while occurring in a dose-dependent manner in suvorexant-treated patients[128] are common to many CNS-acting agents. Mechanistically curious adverse effects noted in clinical trials included a significant dose-dependent increase in serum cholesterol, which became apparent after 4 weeks of treatment, as well as a dose-dependent increase in suicidal ideation.[136] Overall, the adverse effects in older adults were consistent with those observed in younger patients, and the long-term (ie, up to 1 year) adverse effects were consistent with those observed in the first 3 months of suvorexant treatment.

Finally, although there was no evidence for physical dependence or withdrawal symptoms after discontinuation, an abuse liability study in a small sampling of recreational drug users showed that suvorexant was similar to zolpidem in producing subjective drug-desirableness, lending to its categorization as a DEA Schedule IV controlled substance.

Structure-Activity Relationships of Suvorexant. Suvorexant (Fig. 14.18) was derived from high-throughput screening efforts that identified diazepane-based compounds as novel high affinity antagonists of both OXRs and which promoted sleep in rodents.[130] The early diazepane derivatives contained chloro-benzisothiazole or quinazoline ring substituents relative to the central 1,4-diazepane ring; however, compounds with these substituents yielded poor in vivo bioavailabilities in rats and canines as a consequence of first-pass metabolism and heightened clearance rates.[130] Assessment of these metabolites revealed oxidation of both the central diazepane ring and the quinazoline substituent, prompting synthetic efforts to modify the quinazoline ring in order to prevent rapid oxidation and clearance. Halogenation of the 6-position of the quinazoline ring improved OX1R/OX2R affinities and also reduced clearance of the agent, leading to enhanced bioavailability. Replacement of the entire quinazoline ring with a 5-chloro-benzoxazole ring, as seen with suvorexant, resulted in additional decreases in clearance, increasing bioavailability and preserving affinity for both OXRs.[130] Suvorexant is dispensed as the enantiomerically resolved (7*R*)-isomer (as shown in Fig. 14.18), which has 10- to 20-fold greater functional potency at both OXRs compared to the (*S*)-enantiomer.[130]

The crystal structure of the human OX2 receptor bound to suvorexant was resolved to a resolution of 2.5 Å and sheds a great degree of insight into the atomic interactions of the antagonist with the receptor.[137] As shown in Figure 14.19A, suvorexant is accessible to the OX2R binding pocket via a solvent accessible channel that is enclosed by amino acid residues from TMH II, VI, VI, and VII, as well as a β-hairpin turn from extracellular loop 2.[137] As shown by early SAR studies,[130] the early 1,4-disubstituted diazepane OX1R/OX2R antagonists, including suvorexant, exhibited hindered rotations about the C-N bond between the central diazepane and the quinazoline rings, a structural feature that facilitates U-shaped, or horseshoelike, conformations of the outer heterocyclic ring systems. This allows for an unusual intramolecular π-π stacking between the aromatic *p*-toluene and benzoxazole moieties.[130] These early observations were

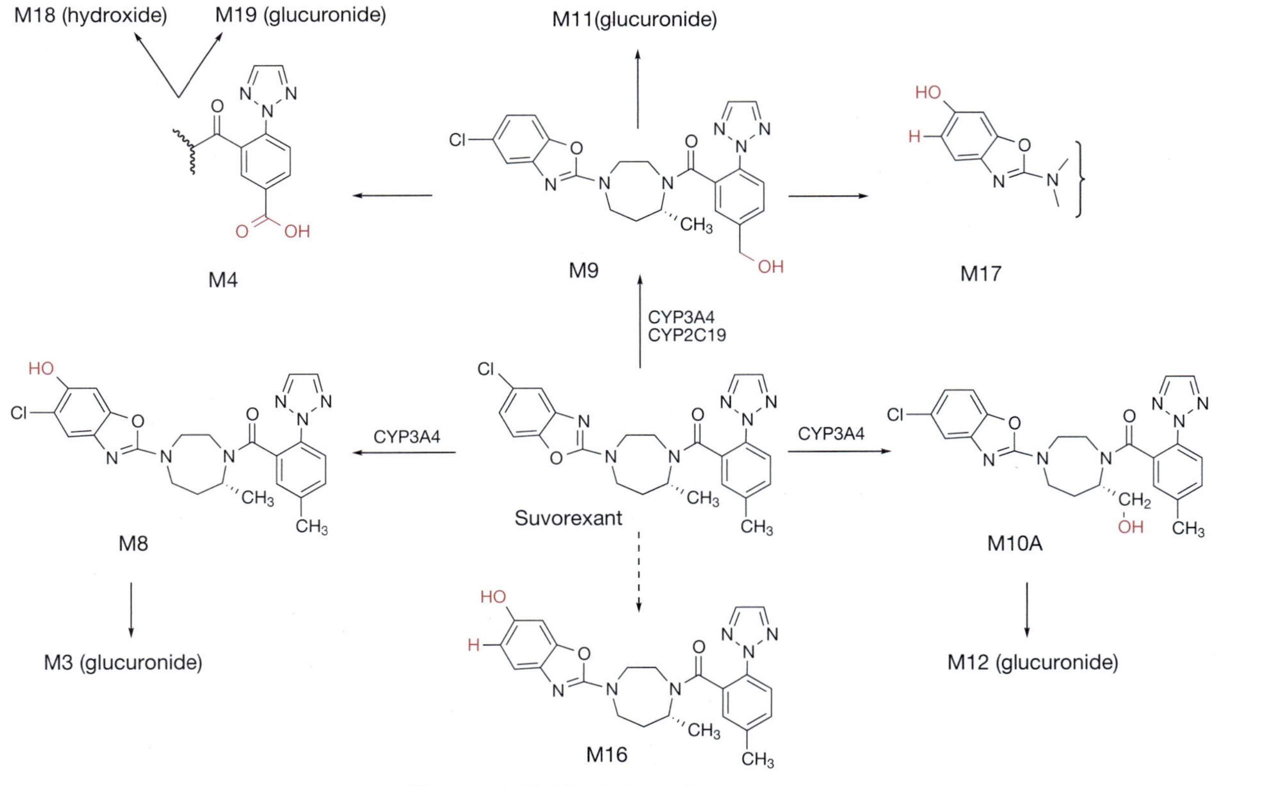

Figure 14.18 Metabolism of suvorexant.

confirmed in the crystal structure, revealing that suvorexant rests in the ligand-binding pocket of OX2R in a horseshoe configuration (Fig. 14.19C), due to a boat conformation of the diazepane ring and intramolecular π-π stacking of the aromatic benzoxazole and *p*-toluamide functional groups.

As shown in Figure 14.19B, C, suvorexant makes contact with all OX2R TMH except for TMH I. A hydrogen bond exists between Asn324 in TMH VI and the carbonyl group of the suvorexant amide, while a water molecule that is centrally located 2.85 Å from the amide and 2.92 Å from His350 in TMH VII coordinates additional hydrogen bond interactions; and together, these form a water bridge between these polar functional groups to the agent (Fig. 14.19). The aromatic functionality of His350 is also responsible to contributing to π-π stacking with the aromatic *p*-toluene moiety of suvorexant, while neighboring Tyr317 contributes to π-π stacking with the triazole moiety (Fig. 14.19). Additionally, van der Waals interactions occur between Phe227 and the I-oriented methyldiazepane ring, which is itself in boat conformation due to the horseshoe orientation noted. Meanwhile, the chlorobenzoxazole moiety is stabilized via interactions with Ile130 and Pro131 in TMH III and Ala110 and Thr111 in TMH II (Fig. 14.19).[137]

Metabolism and Pharmacokinetics of Suvorexant. Maximal suvorexant plasma concentrations are obtained within 2 hours after oral administration under fasting conditions, an effect that is delayed to 3.5 hours if administered with a high-fat meal.[136] Given a mean elimination half-life of 12.3 hours (range of 9-15 hours), it is reasonable to expect some residual next-day drowsiness.[138] Indeed, in phase III trials, patients on the 40-mg dose had 12-hour plasma concentrations equivalent to the T_{max} observed in patients taking the 20-mg dose. Therefore, the nightly dose should not exceed 20 mg.

As shown in Figure 14.18, suvorexant is metabolized in humans primarily by CYP3A4 with an additional minor contribution from CYP2C19.[138] Following single oral dose administration of radioactive suvorexant to healthy human volunteers, 66% of the dose is recovered in the feces while 23% is recovered in the urine, with the majority (82%) of the dose being excreted in 6 days.[138] The major proposed metabolites of suvorexant found in the urine include the carboxylic acid M4 and its glucuronide conjugate M19, which account for 4.1% and 5.3% of the administered dose, respectively (Fig. 14.18).[138] Glucuronide conjugates of metabolites M8, M10A, and M9, yielding M3, M12, and M11, respectively, accounted for the remaining urinary metabolites. These phase 2 conjugates were respectively responsible for 3.8%, 2.7%, and 1.4% of the total dose. No other metabolites nor the parent drug was localized to the urine. As seen in the urine, the major metabolite accounted for in the feces was the carboxylic acid M4, which accounted for 17% of the total dose. Further oxidation of M4 to M18 represented 10.6%, while oxidation of the *p*-toluene to the alcohol M9 and oxidation of the methyldiazepan to the alcohol M10A each represented 9% of the dose. Given the

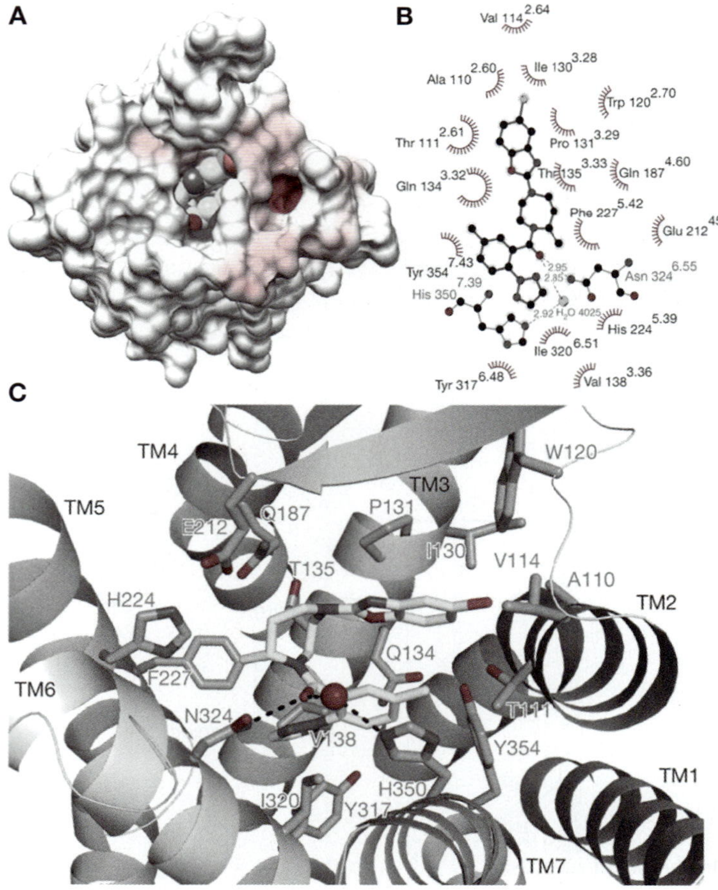

Figure 14.19 Crystallographic interactions of suvorexant with the human orexin-2 receptor. A. Accessibility of suvorexant to the OX2R binding pocket via a solvent accessible channel. B and C. Suvorexant interactions with amino acids in TMH II-VII of the OX2R binding pocket. (Reprinted by permission from Springer *Nature*: From GmbH. Yin J, Mobarec JC, Kolb P, et al. Crystal structure of the human OX2 orexin receptor bound to the insomnia drug suvorexant. *Nature*. 2015;519:247-250. License date May 10, 2023.)

role of CYP3A4 and CYP2C19 on suvorexant metabolism, analysis of CYP inhibitory properties revealed that the agent weakly inhibits both P450 enzymes, with IC50's of 4.0 and 4.0 μM, respectively.[138]

Daridorexant. Daridorexant is a recently approved dual orexin receptor antagonist (DORA) that was selected for development in part via physiologic-based pharmacodynamic/pharmacokinetic modeling used within the preclinical progression of candidate DORAs. The agent has sub-nanomolar antagonistic potency at both OX1R (620 pM) and OX2R (820 pM), with optimal PK/PD profile among the series of agents investigated.[139] In clinical studies, 25- and 50-mg doses significantly reduced wake time after sleep onset and sleep latency compared to placebo and patients had significantly improved self-reported total sleep at 1- and 3-month intervals. The higher dose also improved daytime function in patients with insomnia disorder.[140] To date, no structure-activity relationship studies have been performed for the agent; however, it is likely that it takes advantage of similar binding sites as those described for suvorexant (Fig. 14.19).

Metabolism and Pharmacokinetics of Daridorexant. Maximal daridorexant plasma concentrations are reached 1 to 2 hours after oral administration, with lower doses achieved faster T_{max}, and steady-state achieved after 3 days with no accumulation of the drug. The elimination half-life of the agent is also dose dependent and ranges from 5.9 to 9.2 hours for the 10-, 25-, and 75-mg doses on day 1 and was not different after day 5.[141] This PK profile facilitates fast onset of sedation, within 1 hour, which correlates to a maximal plasma concentration peak achieved within 0.8 to 2.8 hours, and a mean terminal half-life of 5.9 to 8.8 hours for doses ranging from 5 to 200 mg.[142] Using a radioactive daridorexant microtracer, it was found that fecal excretion accounts for 56.6% of an oral dose, while 27.9% was excreted in the urine. Daridorexant is extensively metabolized in humans, primarily via CYP3A4, with a total of 77 reported metabolites identified, of which 30 were found to exist in the plasma (Fig. 14.20).[143] Metabolic transformation in humans is primarily mediated via CYP3A4 isozymes (~90%), while CYP2D6, CYP2C19, CYP1A2, CYP2C8, and CYP2C9 play minor additional roles.[144,145] As shown in Figure 14.20, the majority of the metabolites existing in the plasma were formed via four primary reactions, including demethylation of the methoxy (M4); oxidation of the benzyl to form an alcohol (M3) and subsequent oxidation to an aldehyde (M1) and acid (M2); cleavage of the pyrrolidine ring forming an aldehyde and cyclization with the benzimidazole ring (M5); or oxidation of the triazolyl-phenyl group at a variety of positions, the exact site of which remains uncharacterized (M11, A7). A variety of other metabolites that contained various combinations of these were also reported (eg, M10); however, the exact order of sequence that these were formed was not deduced.[143-145] In addition, 12 phase 2 glucuronide conjugates were identified in the plasma, including derivatives of M5 (conjugate M29), M3 (conjugate M30), M11 (conjugate M6), and A7 (conjugate M8) (Fig. 14.20), as well as others derived from various combinations of the four primary reactions.[143-145] In addition to these, two metabolites were formed via different reactions

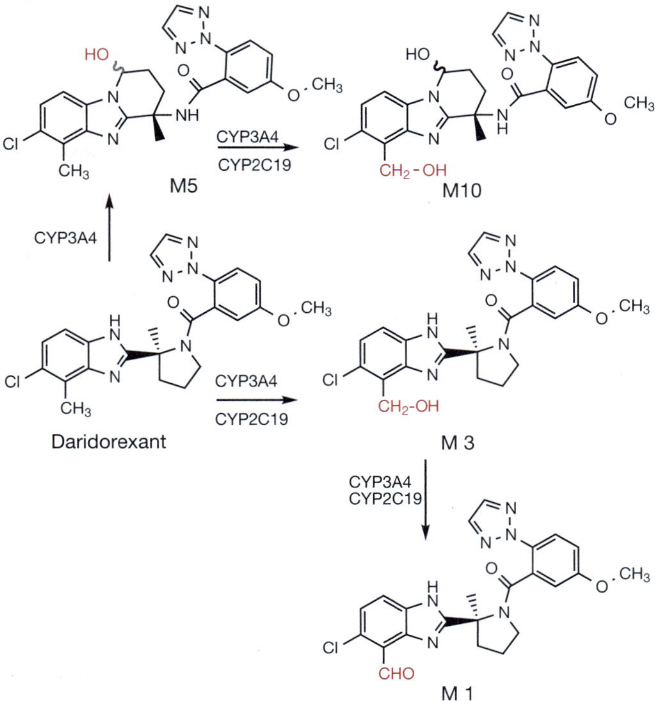

Figure 14.20 Metabolism of daridorexant.

that these four with A8 being formed upon oxidation of the chloro, and A9, which is speculated to exist as a consequence of degradation of the acidic triazol-phenyl moiety (Fig. 14.20).[143-145] Following a radioactive dose of daridorexant, 21% of the total radioactivity in the plasma represented the unchanged parent drug, while 29% represented M3, 13% represented M1, and 9% represented M10. In addition to the 30 metabolites identified in the plasma, 28 metabolites were found in the urine, five of which were not found in the plasma, and 60 metabolites were identified in the feces, 43 of which were not detected in either plasma or urine, suggesting extensive first-pass or microbiota-mediated metabolism of the agent, which generates these later metabolites prior to their systemic exposure.[143-145]

Lemborexant. Lemborexant is another recently approved DORA derived from a series of cyclopropane core structures with low nanomolar affinity of 6 nM and 2.6 nM toward OX1R and OX2R, respectively.[146] Like the other DORAs, lemborexant displayed high selectivity for OXRs, as it lacks any appreciable affinity for more than 80 other receptors, transporters, and ion channels, although it did interact in vitro as an antagonist with MT1R at only the highest concentrations used (30 μM).[146] In clinical trials, treatment with 5- or 10-mg doses of lemborexant resulted in significantly decreased time to sleep latency compared to both placebo and extended-release formulations of zolpidem on nights 1 and 2, as well as on nights 29 and 30 of use. Subjective measures of sleep quality and latency were also significantly improved compared to placebo, but where not different compared to zolpidem.[147] Longer term studies over a 6- and 12-month period of use have also demonstrated significant improvement in time to sleep latency and subjective sleep onset latency.[148]

Structure-Activity Relationships of Lemborexant. SAR and modeling studies on lemborexant reveal that the agent binds the same π-electron stacked horseshoe conformation within the OXR-receptor binding pocket as described for suvorexant, and which are presumed to occur with daridorexant.[139,149] Here, the π-stacking is upheld by interaction of the 2,4-dimethylpyrimidine ring (ring A, Fig. 14.21) with the 5-fluoropyridine ring (ring B) in a "face-to-face" manner. In the OXR2 binding pocket, ring A was predicted to also form another π-π interaction with His350 in TM VII and upholds a water bridge to both Thr111 and Tyr354, the former of which is similar to suvorexant.[139,149] Meanwhile, the amide-linked B-ring forms a hydrogen bond with Gln134, while the 3-fluorophenyl C-ring is surrounded by a variety of hydrophobic residues, predicting additional π-electron or electrostatic interactions with these.[146] Modeling of the binding of lemborexant in the OXR1 binding pocket was identical, with only slight differences in the placement of the interacting histidine, glutamine, and threonine residues due to differences in the amino acid sequences between the two OXR.[146]

Modifications to the A-ring of the backbone greatly influence activity given the importance of this pharmacophore in upholding both the intramolecular horseshoe π-stacking and the π-stacking with the respective OXR residues. While pyrazole-based or ethyl or methoxy-substituted A-rings demonstrated high OXR binding affinity, these agents exhibited poor solubility or undesired P-gp or CYP3A4 affinity and results of ASRs demonstrated that a dimethyl pyrimidine containing group provided ideal balance between OXR affinity, solubility, and CYP3A4 inhibition (Fig. 14.21).[149] SAR studies with 2-, 3-, or 4-pyridine B-rings showed that 3- and 4-pyridine rings exhibited greater P-gp effects; hence, the 2-pyridine backbone for this ring was selected. B-ring para-substitutions resulted in markedly improved affinity compared to the meta-substitutions, while in general halogens exhibited stronger binding affinity than methyl substitutions (Fig. 14.21).[149] Interestingly, incorporation of a *p*-F and an *m*-CH_3 on the B-ring profoundly increased receptor affinity, but also significantly decreased solubility. Based on the identification of an optimal backbone containing a dimethyl pyrimidine A-ring with the *p*-halogen substituted 2-pyridine B-ring, modification of the C-ring using a fluorine scan found that the *m*-F substitution yielded optimal binding affinity and CYP3A4/P-gp parameters, compared to the respective *o*-F and *p*-F-substituted or di-F substituted congener.[149]

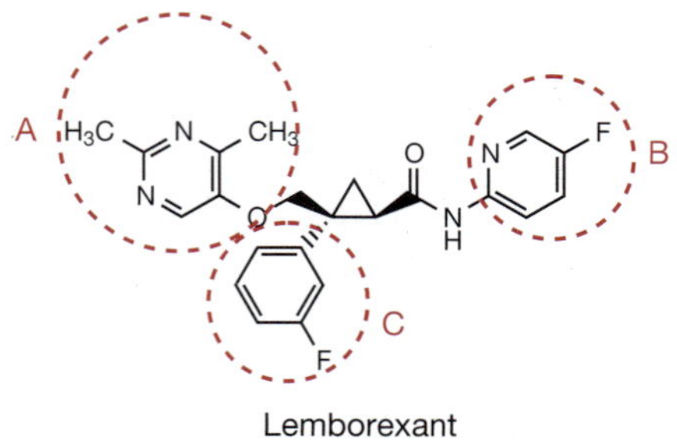

Figure 14.21 Structure of lemborexant depicting the A, B, and C rings.

Metabolism and Pharmacokinetics of Lemborexant. After a single oral administration of 10 mg of radiolabeled lemborexant, both plasma lemborexant concentrations and total plasma radioactivity peaked at 1 hour following the dose and declined with elimination half-life of 43.6 hours for lemborexant and 45.2 hours for all radioactivity.[150] The primary route of excretion of radioactive lemborexant was via feces (57.4%), while urinary excretion accounted for 29.1% and only 90% of radioactivity was recovered in urine and feces after 20 days.[150] Lemborexant is heavily metabolized via hydrolysis, oxidation, reduction, methylation, and phase 2-glucuronidation and sulfation reactions forming a total of 41 unique metabolites after a single dose, which range from 1% to 12.5% of the total drug exposure in the plasma (Fig. 14.22).[150] The primary route of metabolism is via oxidation to mono-oxidized metabolites, with further oxidation to dioxy or carboxylated derivatives, some of whose structures remain unresolved (Fig. 14.22) as well as the glucuronidated or sulfated phase 2 products. A more minor role for amide hydrolysis is also described that leads to another glucuronide conjugate (Fig. 14.22).[150] The primary mono-oxy metabolites of lemborexant exhibit peak concentrations 2 to 4 hours following the dose and their elimination half-lives (27-36 hours) are shorter than those of the parent. The affinity of these mono-oxy metabolites is of equal potency to that of lemborexant, suggesting a strong contribution of these congeners to the overall clinical effect.[150] Following mono-oxidation, the agents are all metabolized further via subsequent oxidations, methylation, amide hydrolysis and phase 2 conjugation reactions, all of which would be expected to significantly deactivate further receptor activity. The major metabolic enzyme responsible for lemborexant is CYP3A4, while CYP3A5 also plays a role.

Histamine H1 Receptor Antagonists. The first generation of ethanolamine ether histamine H_1 receptor antagonists (ie, antihistamines) that cross the blood-brain barrier are used for acute insomnia due to their sedation-promoting side effects. In particular, diphenhydramine and doxylamine,

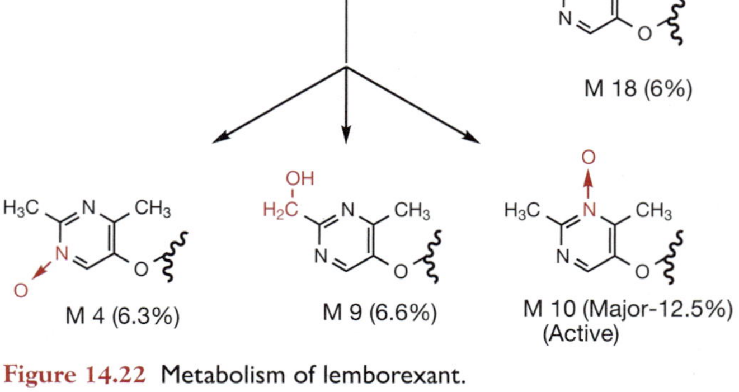

Figure 14.22 Metabolism of lemborexant.

both high affinity (low nanomolar) H_1 receptor antagonists, are sold as OTC sleep aids. The tricyclic antidepressant doxepin, a potent subnanomolar-affinity H_1 antagonist, has also been approved for treatment of insomnia at lower doses than that used for depression (Silenor). The benefit of these agents for treatment of insomnia comes from H_1 receptor antagonism within the TMN of the posterior hypothalamus, where the normal release of histamine during the day causes arousal, and its decreased release at night reduces arousal responses. Antagonism of H_1 receptors within the TMN promotes sedation and drowsiness by inhibiting TMN outflow to other brain structures such as the dorsal raphe nucleus, paraventricular nucleus, and locus coeruleus.

Overall, antihistamines bring about increased drowsiness and sedation with marginal beneficial effects on sleep latency and total sleep time. There is very little in the way of rigorous clinical trial data that support their sedative hypnotic efficacy, and to the contrary, some results reveal that these agents disrupt sleep architecture by delaying the onset to, and duration of, REM sleep. Regardless, these drugs are utilized heavily as sedative hypnotics, and in the case of diphenhydramine and doxylamine, patients are able to readily self-medicate due to the ease in their availability.

While diphenhydramine, doxylamine, and doxepin also exhibit antimuscarinic activity, leading to corresponding side effects such as dry mouth, urinary retention, and blurred vision, a major side effect of these agents is excessive daytime drowsiness and residual next-day sedation. These next-day effects can lead to impaired cognition and performance and are attributed to their relatively long half-lives. Finally, nightly use of first-generation antihistamines as sleep aids has been associated with tolerance to the hypnotic effect with long-term use.

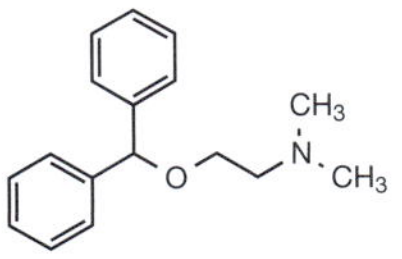

Diphenhydramine

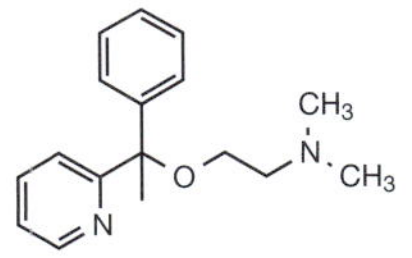

Doxylamine

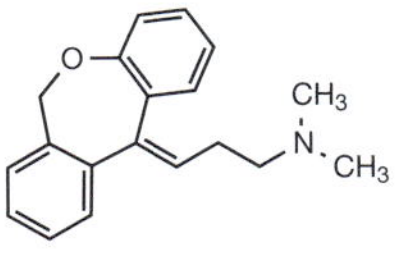

Doxepin

Agents that Induce or Maintain General Anesthesia

Historic records document the use of a myriad of natural products, including a variety of herbs, as well as wines, vapors, and the opium poppy for use in anesthesia. In the early 1500s, the first use of ether was documented to provide a robust anesthetic effect in animals, while in the late 1700s, the discovery of nitrous oxide (N_2O), commonly referred to as "laughing gas," led to observations that it could "destroy physical pain." Based on these and similar observations, in the mid-1800s, Georgia physician and pharmacist Crawford Long pioneered the use of inhaled sulfuric ether as an anesthetic, which gave rise to efforts to investigate novel anesthetics such as diethyl ether, chloroform, and cocaine going into the 20th century. While the theoretical considerations and kinetic principles of anesthesia have been covered in depth in prior editions of this text, the aim of the current section is to provide the reader with the neurochemical basis for understanding anesthesia as well as an in depth discussion of the chemical perspectives regarding SAR, pharmacodynamics, and pharmacokinetics of agents used for general anesthesia.

Neurobiology of Anesthesia

Anesthesia is defined as the loss of feeling or sensation, and can (but does not necessarily have to) be coupled to concurrent loss of consciousness. Drug-induced anesthesia typically refers to either the systemic administration of agents that promote loss of sensation and consciousness through CNS depression (ie, general anesthesia) or, alternatively, regional administration of agents that promote loss of sensation by inhibiting local sensory neurotransmission in a given tissue (ie, local anesthesia). In addition, sedative hypnotics, analgesics, and neuromuscular blocking agents can induce or potentiate anesthesia and are routinely utilized clinically for such use.

While sleep is characterized by diminished consciousness that is responsive to external stimuli, general anesthesia is typified by the complete loss of consciousness that is not responsive to external stimuli. Importantly, induction of general anesthesia is also characterized by amnesia, analgesia, and temporary paralysis of muscles, allowing for its utility in clinical diagnostic procedures as well as surgical and operative procedures. Based on current understanding of the effects of anesthetics in consciousness, the induction of general anesthesia and the emergence from it back toward conscious states are driven primarily by acetylcholine (ACh) neurons within the thalamus. The same glutamatergic, GABAergic, and orexinergic neurons within the reticular formation, thalamus, and hypothalamus noted as being responsible for sedative/hypnotic effects are also involved. Upon induction of anesthesia with certain agents, cerebral blood flow and brain glucose metabolism are drastically affected within the thalamus,[151-153] suggesting that this region of the brain is greatly influenced by GAs. Certain anesthetics have also been shown to influence brain metabolism in a manner that is directly proportional to density of GABA receptor expression within a given brain region, such that higher levels of GABA receptors in the thalamus may be responsible for the reduced metabolism seen in that region upon induction. Since the thalamus behaves as a relay center for ascending and descending processing to and from the cortex, the thalamocortical axis is a major regulator of anesthetic-induced unconsciousness.[154,155] Indeed, it is typically well accepted that GAs induce unconsciousness by inhibiting the high-frequency pulses of arousal sensing information through the thalamocortical and reticulo-thalamocortical ascending arousal structures.[156-158] Mechanistically, this is thought to occur primarily via four pharmacological targets, modulation of which facilitates hyperpolarization of neurons that are responsible for arousal, awareness, and conscious states. These four targets include (1) $GABA_A$ receptors, activation of which enhances inhibitory neurotransmission; (2) *N*-methyl-D-aspartate receptor receptors (NMDA-R), antagonism of which inhibits excitatory neurotransmission; (3) nicotinic ACh receptors (nAChR), antagonism of which inhibits excitatory neurotransmission; and (4) two-pore–domain K^+ channels (eg, K2P channels) that modulate background K^+ currents, agonism of which directly hyperpolarizes neurons. As will be described here, GAs will function through one or more of these routes to inactivate brain regions, resulting in CNS depression and loss of consciousness.

In contrast to GA, where loss of sensory perception is coupled with unconsciousness, local anesthesia causes a reversible loss of sensory perception with no effect on central arousal state. These agents are administered topically or by injection directly into localized areas. The local administration of these agents causes the loss of propagation of the action potential in peripheral nerve fibers, thereby blocking nerve conductance that transmits sensory and nociceptive information from the localized area to the brain. Local anesthetics, which are discussed in detail in Chapter 17, block nerve conductance by binding to specific sites on voltage-gated Na+ channels on excitable nerves, thereby preventing the passage of Na+ and interfering with the action potential that is required for excitability.

Stages of General Anesthesia

The early works that characterized the inhaled effects of diethyl ether led to Arthur Guedel's classification of the stages of anesthesia in the late 1930s. In the first stage, referred to as *analgesia*, the patient experiences mild thalamocortical depression leading to pain relief without amnesia. In the second stage, referred to as *excitement*, CNS depression deepens, particularly within reticulothalamic centers, and the patient may appear excitable or even delirious but is fully amnesic. Here, respiration, cardiac chronotropy, and blood pressure may increase, and involuntary muscle activity could occur. The ideal anesthetic agent should produce very little time in the first two stages, and increased concentrations of the GA can shorten time in these stages. Stage III, referred to as *surgical anesthesia*, begins with normalization of unconscious respiration and chronotropy and extends to four distinct planes as the depth of anesthesia increases. These planes include cessation of ocular activity, paralysis of the intercostal muscles, dilation of pupils, and the loss of muscle tone. If the depth of anesthesia is allowed to increase, the paralysis of the diaphragm and respiratory function, known as *apnea*, ensues in stage IV, which is indicative of severe depression of vasomotor medullary activity in the brainstem. Under the careful observation of the anesthesiologist, stages I to II should occur as rapidly as possible, while stage IV should never occur.

General Anesthetics

Clinically Useful Inhalation Agents

The gaseous GA agents include the volatile fluorinated hydrocarbons isoflurane, sevoflurane, and desflurane, which, along with the nonvolatile gas nitrous oxide (N_2O), make up the family of clinically useful inhalation agents that are administered under the care of the anesthesiologist

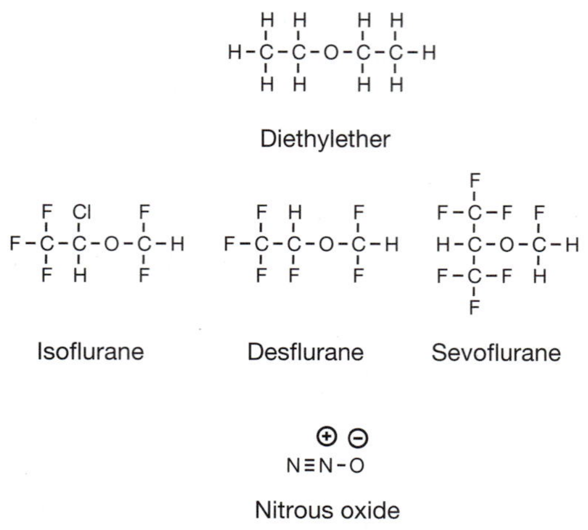

Figure 14.23 Structures of inhaled general anesthetics.

(Fig. 14.23). The concentration of inhaled anesthetics is carefully controlled by the anesthesiologist in order to maximize the anesthetic effect while ensuring proper emergence from it. The volatile anesthetics are vaporized prior to inhalation with O_2, whereas N_2O can be inhaled directly as a gas mixed with O_2. Upon inhalation, the concentration of anesthetic in the bronchiolar alveoli reaches equilibrium with that in the inspired gas mixture. Transfer from the alveolar space to the blood proceeds quickly, as the partial pressure (tension) in the alveoli is in equilibrium with the blood. Subsequent passage to the brain and other tissue moves toward equilibrium of the partial pressures in each compartment based on the solubility and physiochemical characteristics of each individual agent (Table 14.4). Since the partial pressure of the inhaled anesthetic equilibrates throughout the body in this manner, the alveolar concentration of the agent is reflective of the amount in the brain.

Solubility of the inhaled anesthetics is defined by the partition coefficient, the ratio of the concentration of the dissolved gas in the blood or tissue to the concentration in the gaseous phase at equilibrium (ie, blood/gas or blood/tissue partition coefficient, respectively) (Table 14.4). Due to lipophilicity, the solubility of the anesthetic in the blood will differ from that in the tissue, and the partition coefficient plays an essential role of the kinetics of these agents. While the fluorinated agents, all derived from diethyl ether (Fig. 14.23), all have high degrees of lipophilicity, before significant amounts of the anesthetic enter the brain from the blood, the latter must be saturated with the anesthetic. The blood-tissue/gas partition coefficients explain the ability of the agent to partition within a given target at equilibrium, when the partial pressures of the agent will be the same. For example, the blood/gas partition coefficient of isoflurane is 1.4, and at equilibrium, the concentration in the blood will be 1.4-fold the concentration in the alveolar space. Therefore, the blood/gas partition coefficient and the brain/blood partition coefficient play meaningful roles in anesthetic effects. Practically, this implies that agents that have higher blood/gas coefficients will have longer times to saturate the blood compartment before the partial pressure rises enough to induce anesthesia in the brain. As a consequence, these agents have longer anesthesia induction onset

Table 14.4 Partition Coefficients, Minimum Alveolar Concentrations (MACs), and Ion Channel Modulation of Clinically Utilized Inhaled Anesthetics[a]

Anesthetic	Blood/Gas Partition Coefficient	MAC[b] (Vol %)		Ion Channel Modulation[c]							
		$-N_2O$	$+N_2O$	$GABA_A$	Glycine	nAChR	$5\text{-}HT_3$	NMDA	AMPA	K+	Na+
Isoflurane	1.4	1.15	0.50	+++	+++	−−−	−	−−	−−	++	−
Sevoflurane	0.63	1.71	0.66	+++	+++	−−−	−	−−	−−	++	−
Desflurane	0.42	6.0	2.83	+++	+++	−−−	−	−−	−−	++	−
Nitrous oxide	0.47	104	–	Weak	Weak	−−	Weak	−−	None	+	None

[a]Adapted from Refs.[146-161]
[b]Minimum alveolar concentration.
[c]Modulatory activity is indicated by "+" for agonism and "−" for antagonism. The number of symbols correlates to the degree of either activity at the given site of action.

times. In general, agents with higher partition coefficients have higher lipophilicity and higher blood solubility, meaning that more anesthetic will need to be dissolved to saturate the blood in order to reach the brain, yielding a slower induction.

Given that the rate of inhaled anesthetic induction is not dependent on absorption of the drug, but rather, primarily on the relative partial pressure in each compartment, the rate of emergence from anesthesia is correlated to the induction rate, such that agents with high blood solubility and slow induction will also exhibit slow recovery and emergence from anesthesia. In contrast, agents with low blood solubility and lower blood/gas partition coefficients will quickly saturate the blood and then rapidly enter the brain for a quick inductive effect, as well as faster emergence and recovery from the anesthetic effect. In addition to this important physiochemical characteristic, induction of anesthesia can be modulated by other factors, including concentration, ventilation, and cardiac output, the latter of which is inversely correlated to induction. Greater levels of cardiac output will remove more anesthetic from the gas phase via the greater blood flow to the lungs.

Blood/gas partition coefficients for the inhaled anesthetics are in the rank order of isoflurane > sevoflurane > nitrous oxide ≥ desflurane, as shown in Table 14.4.[159] Since the initial alveolar concentration of inhaled agent drives blood and brain permeation, the potency of inhaled anesthetics is measured as the minimum alveolar concentration (MAC). MAC is defined as the concentration of vapor (as a percentage of 1 atmosphere in the alveoli) required to prevent motor responses in 50% of adult patients subjected to a standardized surgical stimulus. Importantly, MAC values assume that equilibrium between the gas/alveoli/blood/brain compartments has been reached, and a variety of patient factors, including body temperature, acidosis, blood pressure, pregnancy, and age, can alter MAC. Nonetheless, a lower MAC value denotes a more potent anesthetic effect. The rank order of potencies for the anesthetics discussed here in 100% oxygen, as MAC_{50}, is isoflurane> sevoflurane> desflurane> nitrous oxide (Table 14.4).[159] Additionally, the coadministration of nitrous oxide with a volatile anesthetic is additive; in general, a 1% increase in nitrous oxide allows for a similar percentage reduction in the MAC of the volatile anesthetic.[160,161]

Mechanism of Action of Inhaled Anesthetics. In the early 1900s, Meyer and subsequently Overton noted a strong correlation between the potency of volatile anesthetics and their lipophilicity and, based on this, theorized that these agents act nonspecifically on protein targets or on lipid components of CNS cells.[162] However, other highly lipophilic agents, lipid disruptors, and membrane modulators lack anesthetic capabilities, suggesting that other mechanisms are at play. The pharmacological characterization of the effects of the agents on a variety of CNS-acting ion channels, along with the structural diversity of the different types of inhaled anesthetics that have been used over the years, now supports the concept that myriad mechanisms are utilized by inhaled GAs to promote anesthesia. Indeed, the now-accepted mechanism of these agents is based on their ability to modulate a diverse assortment of CNS ion channels, including all of the "cysteine loop" neurotransmitter receptors, which include $GABA_A$, nACh, $5\text{-}HT_3$, and glycine receptors, as well as the excitatory glutaminergic NMDA and AMPA receptors.[163-165] The known in vitro and in vivo pharmacologic effects of the halogenated agents and nitrous oxide on these receptors are summarized in Table 14.4. The volatile agents are known to inhibit voltage-gated Na^+ channels in addition to nAChR, NMDA, AMPA, and $5\text{-}HT_3$ receptors, while at the same time enhancing the activity of $GABA_A$, two-pore–domain K^+ channels, and glycine receptors.[166-180] Modulation of these ion channels facilitates membrane hyperpolarization and decreases synaptic neuronal excitability. On the contrary, nitrous oxide has only weak activity at potentiating $GABA_A$ and glycine receptor currents but can activate two-pore K^+ channels and also inhibits nAChR and NMDA-R flux.

Chemical Considerations and Structure-Activity Relationships of Inhaled Anesthetics. The volatile inhaled anesthetics are derived from the structure of diethyl ether (Fig. 14.23). Replacement of diethyl ether's hydrogen groups with fluorine atoms preserves the steric features of the small hydrogen atom while greatly enhancing lipophilicity of the fluorinated congeners. This effect also lowers the boiling point, decreases flammability and toxicity, and increases stability. Halothane, an older agent described in previous editions of this text, is a halogenated alkane; however, this structural backbone was associated with cardiac arrhythmias. On the contrary, an ether backbone reduces the likelihood of this effect 4-fold, and hence the clinically useful agents of today are based on the halogenated methyl ethyl ether backbone.

Given these considerations, one would speculate that SARs for this family of anesthetics would be easily concluded. On the contrary, no definitive SAR exists for these agents that allow for accurate predictions of anesthetic activity, other than that at least one hydrogen is necessary for anesthetic effect. In this regard, full halogenation of the agents shown in Figure 14.23 results in loss of anesthetic effect and promotes convulsant effects, suggesting that the role of electron-withdrawing groups, coupled with heightened lipophilicity, mediate vastly different effects on excitatory versus inhibitory neurotransmission.[181] All of the clinically useful fluorinated anesthetics contain a chiral carbon and, hence, exist as (+) and (−) enantiomers, although all of the commercially available formulations contain racemic mixtures. Early works with enantiomerically resolved isoflurane showed that (+)-isoflurane was more effective at inducing anesthesia compared to the (−) enantiomer. This observation correlated with in vitro studies showing that the (+) enantiomer has 2-fold the efficacy of the (−) enantiomer in potentiating K^+-efflux and inhibiting nAChR.[182-185] Similarly, (+)-isoflurane is significantly more potent that (−)-isoflurane in potentiating effects at $GABA_A$ receptors.[165,166] Such results argue further against the Meyer and Overton theory and, given the known stereoselective requirements of ion channels and receptors, further support modulation of these channels by inhaled anesthetics as part of their mechanisms of action.

Properties and Metabolism of Individual Inhaled Anesthetic Agents.

Isoflurane. Isoflurane, 1-chloro-2,2,2-trifluoroethyl difluoromethyl ether, has a blood/gas partition coefficient that is intermediate compared to the highly insoluble sevoflurane and desflurane. Given this property, 3% isoflurane induction time is in the 7- to 12-minutes range, and single dose recovery times are within the 10- to 20-minutes range. Since isoflurane has a pungent odor, too rapid rates of inhalation administration may produce unpleasant or adverse effects such as cough, laryngospasm, or inadvertent breath-holding. Greater than 99% of inhaled isoflurane is expired unchanged from the lungs. Isoflurane is unique compared to sevoflurane, given that it is fairly resistant to human metabolism, with less than 0.5% of the agent being biotransformed by the liver to yield trifluoroacetic acid and F^- (Fig. 14.24).[186]

Sevoflurane. Sevoflurane, fluoromethyl 2,2,2-trifluoro-1-(trifluoromethyl) ethyl ether, is an isopropyl ether with a significantly lower blood/gas partition coefficient (0.63) compared to isoflurane, allowing for rapid induction of anesthesia and rapid recovery following discontinuation from inhalation. Inhalation anesthesia induction times are achieved in 1 to 2 minutes, and single dose emergence is slightly shorter than that of isoflurane, ranging from 4 to 10 minutes.[187,188] Based on this profile as well as its more pleasant sweet odor and less propensity to irritate the airway, sevoflurane is widely used in outpatient surgical and pediatric care settings. Approximately 40% of inhaled sevoflurane is excreted unchanged in expired air, while hepatic CYP2E1 is responsible for oxidative defluorination of 3% to 5% of the inspired agent. The remainder is likely metabolized by unknown extrahepatic mechanisms, yielding hexafluoroisopropanol and F^- (Fig. 14.24).[189-191] As blood concentrations of sevoflurane approach 0.6 mM, F^- levels that result from this biotransformation can exceed 50 μM, which is potentially nephrotoxic. However, this is greatly dose and time dependent, and serum levels of fluoride rapidly decrease following discontinuation. For example, 3% sevoflurane exposure for 1 hour causes a peak of 22 μM of F^- load in blood, decreasing to 4 μM after 24 hours.[189-191]

Desflurane. Desflurane, 1,2,2,2-tetrafluoroethyl-difluoromethyl ether, differs from isoflurane by a single atom fluoro- for chloro- substitution. However, this effect is significant, as it decreases blood solubility substantially (blood/gas partition coefficient of 1.4 for isoflurane vs 0.42 for desflurane),

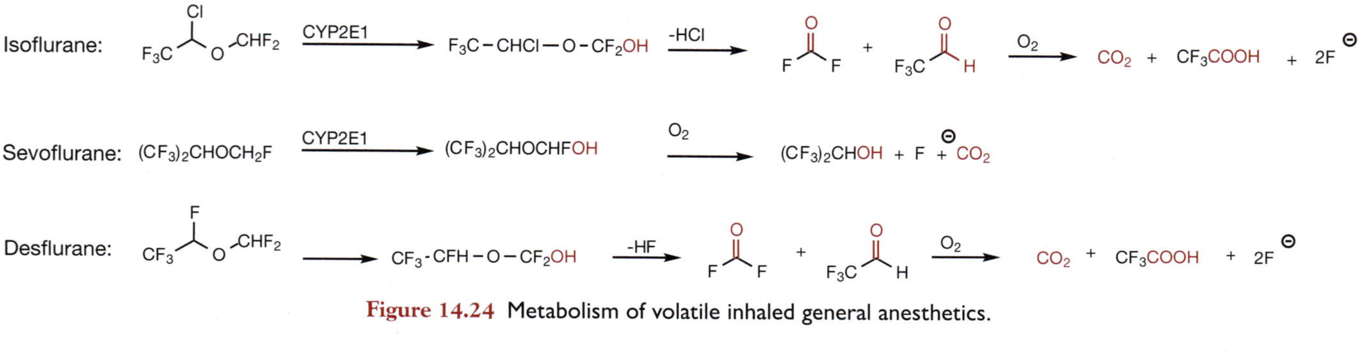

Figure 14.24 Metabolism of volatile inhaled general anesthetics.

distinguishing desflurane as the least soluble of the volatile GAs. This single atom change also significantly decreases the boiling point (48.5 °C for isoflurane and 22.8 °C for desflurane), while greatly increasing the room temperature vapor pressure of desflurane (669 mm Hg) compared to isoflurane (238 mm Hg). These physical properties make desflurane incompatible with conventional vaporizers at room temperatures, as inconceivable gas flow would be required to deliver clinically meaningful doses. As a consequence, desflurane is delivered via specially designed vaporizers that can be heated to 39 °C to facilitate vaporization. Nonetheless, due to its low blood solubility, desflurane is characterized by very rapid induction and emergence compared to the other volatile GAs. Inhalation anesthesia induction times are achieved in 1 to 2 minutes, and single dose emergence occurs within 5 to 6 minutes.[192,193] However, similar to isoflurane, desflurane also has a pungent odor and can also cause airway irritation and laryngospasm, decreasing its clinical utility in inducing anesthesia. For these reasons, desflurane is better suited for use in maintenance of anesthesia. Also similar to isoflurane, desflurane is resistant to human biotransformation, with more than 99% being recoverable from expired air. Less than 0.02% of the dose is converted, presumably via hepatic oxidation like isoflurane, to F^- and trifluoroacetic acid, neither of which are readily detectible in urine (Fig. 14.24).[194,195]

Nitrous Oxide. Historically referred to as "laughing gas," nitrous oxide (N_2O) has very a low blood/gas partition coefficient (0.47), allowing for rapid induction. However, with an MAC of 105%, it is incapable of producing surgical anesthesia when used alone. Hence, when used as monotherapy, it is most efficacious in instances where full surgical anesthesia is not necessary, for example, in dental procedures or as an adjuvant to local anesthesia. The relatively low anesthetic potency of nitrous oxide monotherapy may be ancillary to its strong analgesic and weak muscle relaxant properties. Most commonly, nitrous oxide is used in combination with other GAs, where it synergizes the anesthetic effects, allowing for reductions in the concentration of the other agent required to produce the desired anesthetic response.

Although the exact mechanism of nitrous oxide–mediated analgesia remains elusive, in vivo positron emission tomography (PET) imaging reveals decreases in pain-induced activation of thalamocortical brain regions as described, suggesting that the effects of nitrous oxide may be similar to that of the volatile GAs. Pharmacologically, nitrous oxide has been postulated to exert its effects through blockade of nAChR and NMDA channels, as well as via activation of two-pore K^+ channels. However, it is very likely that other mechanisms are also involved.[168-178]

Nitrous oxide is rapidly and nearly fully eliminated unchanged from expired air, with minor excretion from the skin. Major toxicities associated with nitrous oxide use include cardiac arrhythmia and the N_2O-induced irreversible oxidation of the cobalt atom of vitamin B_{12}. In the latter case, the gas converts the monovalent cobalt form of vitamin B_{12} (Co^+) to the divalent form that is incapable of acting as a cofactor for the enzyme methionine synthetase, which is itself critical for nucleic acid synthesis and neurotransmission and specifically for the synthesis of myelin. Methionine synthetase activity is reduced in a small percentage of patients after acute inhalation of N_2O and can be restored only upon de novo translation of the enzyme. This effect has possible consequences related to vitamin B_{12}–dependent effects such as erythropoiesis, anemia, and myelosuppression.

Clinically Useful Parenteral Agents

The clinically useful parenteral agents are small molecules characterized by high lipophilicity, allowing for a high degree of partitioning into the well-perfused tissue (such as the brain) within a single cycle of blood circulation following IV administration. As described with the highly lipophilic barbiturate agents, time-dependent redistribution from the CNS to less well-perfused or less lipophilic tissues greatly influences the kinetics of these agents. The IV agents discussed here, which include the barbiturates thiopental and thiamylal, as well as propofol, ketamine, and etomidate, have a faster rate of anesthetic action than the inhaled GAs and, as a consequence, are utilized greatly in the induction of anesthesia.

Thiopental and Thiamylal

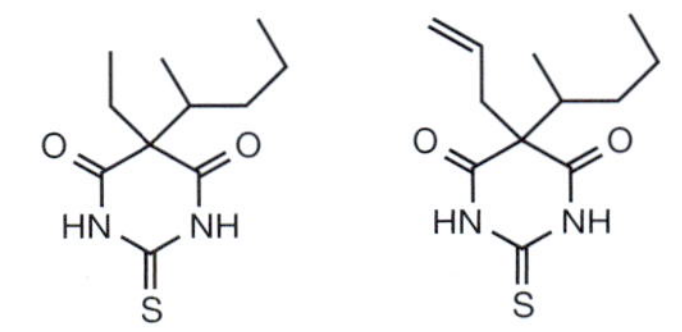

Thiopentobarbital Thiamylal

Although the thiobarbiturates are no longer available for clinical use in the United States, they are still heavily used in animal procedures for research use. As described in the sedative hypnotic section, the oxybarbiturates thiopental (thiopentylbarbital) and thiamylal contain 2-position sulfur atoms within the barbiturate backbone. This increases lipophilicity and allows for ultrarapid anesthetic effects compared to their 2-oxy congeners, due to rapid penetration to the brain, which typically occurs within 10 to 20 seconds. The effects are rapidly lost within 5 to 7 minutes of a bolus dose due to redistribution from the CNS into the muscle, adipose, and other less lipophilic tissues. While the effects of single bolus dose thiobarbiturates are short acting, continuous infusion or multiple administrations can lead to long-lasting unconsciousness because of a change from first-order to zero-order kinetics with slow biotransformation and elimination (Fig. 14.5). This may be particularly problematic in hepatic and renal dysfunction and in pregnancy.[196,197] In this regard, the approximate 1.5 to 3.0 mL/kg/min clearance rate of thiopental is the slowest among the injectable GAs and can cause prolonged unconsciousness if not used acutely.[198,199] Thiobarbiturate mechanisms of action, SARs, and metabolism are described with sedative hypnotic agents.

Similarly, adverse effects of thiobarbitals mimic those seen with their oxy-congeners and can include hypotension, decreases in cardiac inotropy, and respiratory depression. As described, since barbiturates tautomerize and are active in the enolate form (Fig. 14.3), they are formulated in alkaline solutions. Mixing these agents with other drugs in more acidic solutions inhibits tautomerization and shifts the equilibrium, stabilizing the inactive barbituric acid form. Hence, when used for anesthesia, barbiturates are administered first and should clear the tubing prior to administration of other IV agents.

Propofol

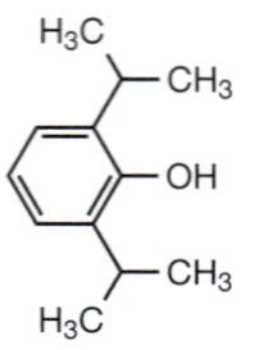

Propofol (2,6-diisopropylphenol) is a very popular GA that is commonly used in surgical and diagnostic procedures. Propofol exerts its anesthetic action via modulation of neuronal $GABA_A$ receptors. Specifically, propofol significantly decreases the dissociation rate of the endogenous neurotransmitter from the receptor, thereby enhancing GABA binding. This effect facilitates Cl^- flux, postsynaptic hyperpolarization, and CNS depression, similar to that described for other GABAergic agents. Propofol has synergistic effects with other GABAergics (eg, BZs and barbiturates), enhancing their effects. In addition, propofol inhibits presynaptic GABA uptake and may also influence GABA release in addition to modulation of glycine, nACh, and NMDA receptors.[200]

Structure-Activity Relationships of Propofol. SARs of early 2,6-dialkylphenols revealed that the anesthetic potencies and kinetics are strongly correlated to the lipophilicity and steric bulk/localization of the substitutions.[201] As a class, mono-*o*-substituted alkyl phenols showed only moderate hypnotic/anesthetic effects with poor therapeutic ratios, while mono-*p*-substituted phenols, like the parent phenol compound, proved to be toxic, yielding high degrees of respiratory depression. Similarly, compounds with *m*-alkyl substitutions or di-, tri-, or tetrasubstitutions that included a *m*-position alkyl displayed poor anesthetic properties.

Meanwhile, propofol-like 2,6-disubstituted alkyl derivatives with linear ethyl, *n*-propyl, or *n*-butyl groups displayed moderate anesthetic properties with slow induction and increased durations as the chain lengths increased. A further series of 2-*n*-alkyl, 6-*sec*-alkyl substitutions further increased anesthetic potency until the total number of carbons in the substituents reached 8, while cyclohexyl substitution decreased potency. Interestingly, 2,6-di-sec substituted alkyl congeners yielded highest anesthetic potencies as long as the total number of carbons did not exceed six and the substitutions were acyclic. Similarly, anesthetic kinetics were rapid and sleep times were short when the total carbons were less than seven, while induction became slow and recovery prolonged when the total number of carbons in the substituents surpassed eight. Of congeners within the 2,6-di-sec substituted alkyl series, 2,6-diisopropyl (ie, propofol) was noted to have exceptional characteristics denoted by a smooth and rapid induction and recovery, as well as a short but useful duration.[201]

Pharmacokinetics and Metabolism of Propofol. Propofol has pharmacokinetic properties that are similar to those of thiobarbitals and, yet, has distinct and important differences. Like the thiobarbitals, it is a highly lipophilic agent that produces rapid CNS effects with a fast blood-brain equilibrium half-life of 3 minutes and rapid redistribution from the CNS after a single bolus dose.[198] This property allows for onset within a single circulation time and recovery periods of 3 to 8 minutes, depending on the dose.[199] However, unlike thiobarbitals, propofol has a very high rate of clearance of 25 to 50 mL/kg/min, a roughly 10-fold faster rate than thiopental, and this characteristic allows for much faster recovery when administered in multiple doses or upon infusion.[202]

Propofol is metabolized rapidly via hepatic CYP2B6-mediated biotransformation to 4-hydroxy propofol (2,6-diisopropyl-1,4-hydroquinone) followed by conjugation of either the 1- or 4-position hydroxy with glucuronic acid or sulfate, accounting for approximately 60% of the urinary detectible dose. Direct phase 2 conjugation of the parent accounts for the remainder of the major metabolites found in the urine (Fig. 14.25).[203-205] Less than 0.3% of the parent drug is recovered unchanged in the urine, and the recovery

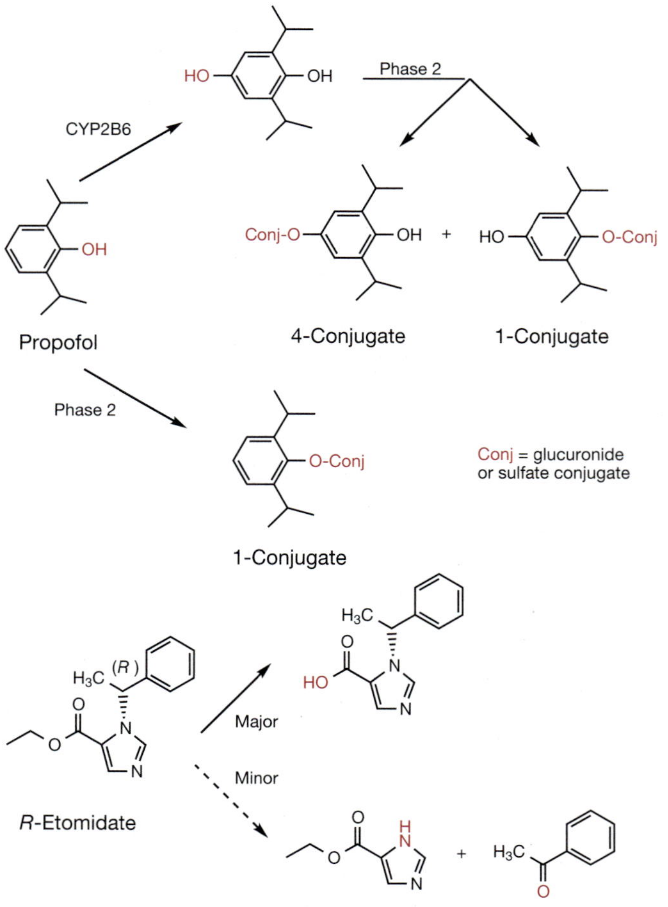

Figure 14.25 Metabolism of propofol and etomidate.

of metabolites is comparable in male and female patients, consistent with the observation that clinical pharmacokinetics of propofol exhibit no gender-based differences. Due to its very poor water solubility, propofol is formulated in a 10 mg/mL emulsion with 10% (w/v) soybean oil, 1.2% egg phosphatide, and 2.25% glycerol, a formulation that can support bacterial growth and, as such, requires the use of strict aseptic technique.

Adverse Effects of Propofol. Propofol can reduce blood pressure and respiration to a greater degree than the thiobarbiturates and can also cause bradycardia and decreased cardiac output. The effects on blood pressure are mediated by vasodilation and decreased peripheral resistance secondary to reductions in sympathetic nervous system tone. More than 60% of patients report pain at the injection site.

Etomidate

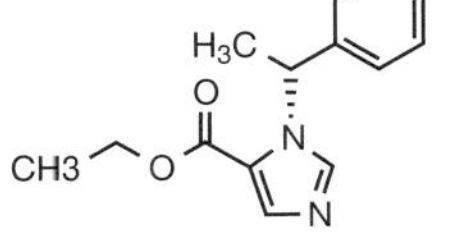

Etomidate, ethyl 3-(1-phenylethyl)imidazole-4-carboxylate, is a phenyl-substituted carboxylated imidazole that was initially developed as part of a novel series of antifungal agents and is primarily used as an induction anesthetic owing to its ultrarapid hypnotic onset and short duration of action. Distinct from propofol, etomidate seems to exert its hypnotic and anesthetic effects exclusively via modulation of $GABA_A$ receptors and, more specifically, $GABA_A$ receptors that contain the β_2 or β_3 subunits.[206] At clinically relevant concentrations of etomidate, the agent potentiates the binding of GABA to $GABA_A$ receptors, an effect that causes postsynaptic hyperpolarization. At higher concentrations, etomidate directly and allosterically agonizes $GABA_A$ receptors in the absence of GABA.[207]

Structure-Activity Relationships of Etomidate. Stereoselectivity is a critical aspect of etomidate's ability to either potentiate the binding of GABA to the $GABA_A$ receptor or directly stimulate the receptor. The *R*-(+)-enantiomer is 10- to 20-fold more potent at modulating these activities compared to the *l*-(-)-enantiomer, and as such, the clinically used agent contains the resolved *R*-(+)-enantiomer (Fig. 14.25). SARs of the series of 1-(1-substituted)-imidazole-5-carboxylic acid esters showed that these agents exhibited extremely potent hypnotic effects with short durations.[208] The nature of the imidazole nitrogen substituent is critical to hypnotic/anesthetic effect, and a one-carbon distance between the aryl substitution and nitrogen affords greatest hypnotic/anesthetic effects. Branching at the opposite end of the α-carbon also affected potency, with alkyl substituents having the greatest activity, especially smaller methyl substitutions.[208] Anesthetic activity was completely lost if the side chain was lengthened to two carbons, if the α-carbon was unbranched, or if the aryl group was directly attached to the imidazole nitrogen.[208] An ester moiety at the 4-position was essential for anesthetic effects, as corresponding carboxylic acids lacked activity. However, the absolute nature of the ester substitution allowed for variability, as methyl, ethyl, *n*-propyl, or isopropyl substituents all provided high activity. Of the series, etomidate, which contains an ethyl ester and phenylethyl-imidazole substitution, provided the ideal safety ratio, which takes into account the hypnotic activity and toxicity.

Pharmacokinetics and Metabolism of Etomidate. After a single IV injection, (*R*)-etomidate induces anesthesia with an onset time on the order of 10 to 20 seconds and emergence from anesthesia in 2 to 10 minutes, depending on the dose used.[209,210] While the duration of anesthetic action is somewhat limited by redistribution of the agent out of the brain into other compartments, biotransformation of etomidate occurs rapidly due to plasma and hepatic hydrolysis of the ester, which is the primary driver of the limited duration. As noted, the SAR requirement for an ester group to retain anesthetic activity signifies that the carboxylic acid metabolite formed upon hydrolysis of the ester is inactive (Fig. 14.25). Oxidative metabolism of etomidate can also produce benzoic acid, and together, these metabolites account for the urinary (75%) and biliary (25%) excretion of etomidate (Fig. 14.25).[211,212] Etomidate also provides effective anesthesia upon rectal administration, although the onset of action is significantly delayed (~5 minutes).

Adverse Effects of Etomidate. Although a major advantage of etomidate compared to other agents is the decreased incidence of cardiovascular and respiratory adverse effects, etomidate does precipitate other adverse activities. Nearly 40% of patients exhibit pain at the site of injection, and over 25% demonstrate involuntary movements that are directly due to GABAergic disinhibition within the basal ganglia. Consistent with its initial envisioned use as an antifungal agent intended to disrupt fungal steroidogenesis, etomidate also has high inhibitory affinity for the adrenocortical enzyme 11β-hydroxylase, which is intricately involved in adrenal cortisol synthesis. As a consequence, prolonged use of etomidate strongly inhibits adrenal gland function and profoundly suppresses cortisol in a manner that is unresponsive to Adrenocorticotropic hormone (ACTH), an effect that occurs at the level of the adrenal cortex itself.

Ketamine

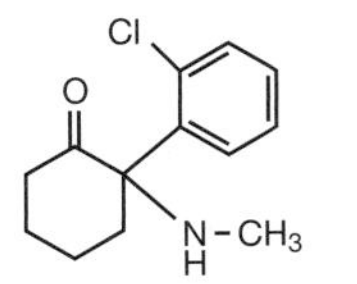

Ketamine, 2-(*o*-chlorophenyl)-2-methylaminocyclohexanone, is a structural derivative of the abused dissociative drug phencyclidine (ie, PCP or "angel dust"). Phencyclidine was initially used as an anesthetic; however, patients often emerged into lengthy states of delirium, prompting efforts to modify the structure to optimize anesthetic effects with a lesser degree of psychogenic disturbances. These efforts led to the discovery of ketamine, an agent with pronounced anesthetic and analgesic effects and a lower propensity to induce psychiatric effects compared to phencyclidine. As a consequence of its similarities to phencyclidine, ketamine is the only IV GA that produces dissociative anesthesia, which is characterized by analgesia, catatonia, catalepsy, and amnesia. This is distinct from other GAs, as the patient's eyes could remain open, and they may breathe spontaneously.

As opposed to the GABAergic acting agents that disrupt thalamocortical and reticulothalamo-cortical brain activity, the resulting anesthesia is thought to be due to thalamoneocortical and limbic system disruption secondary to direct antagonism of excitatory glutamate NMDA receptors. Other results suggest that ketamine may also function indirectly by modulation of opioid, norepinephrine, serotonin, and ACh neurotransmission. Together, these activities prevent ascending brain pathways from perceiving pain or auditory/visual sensations, producing a disconnected cataleptic state with amnesia and analgesia, with minimal depression of respiration.[213] Based on this unique dissociative mechanism, emergence from analgesia can be accompanied by reactions that include confused mental state, hallucination, dreamlike states, and delirium, which typically can last a few hours.

Structure-Activity Relationships of Ketamine. A chiral center within the cyclohexanone ring affords two optical isomers of ketamine, *R*-(-)- and *S*-(+)-, both of which are included in the commercial preparation of the agent. However, in animals, *S*-(+)-ketamine has a significantly greater therapeutic index than the racemate or the *R*-(-)-enantiomer, and exhibits 3- and 1.5-fold more analgesic and hypnotic potency as the *R*-(-)-enantiomer.[214] These observations extend to human studies where *S*-(+)-ketamine produces more effective anesthesia than the racemate or *R*-(-)-ketamine, and also produced less of the ketamine-emergence reactions described. Moreover, patients anesthetized with *R*-(-)-ketamine were more agitated that those induced with the racemate or *S*-(+)-ketamine. When compared to phencyclidine, ketamine has a lower calculated log P and only a slightly lower affinity for human recombinant NMDA receptors. Heterocyclic substitution of the cyclohexanone ring results in a significant loss of antagonistic activity and lipophilicity, while substitution of the second *o*-position of this ring also lowers activity.[215] Previous SAR studies on phencyclidine derivatives have shown that agents with electron-withdrawing substituents on the aromatic ring, such as the halogen on ketamine, decrease psychotropic effects, while *N*-alkyl substitution increases the hypnotic potency.

Pharmacokinetics and Metabolism of Ketamine. The analgesic effects of ketamine occur at much lower doses than those required for anesthesia (40-200 ng/mL vs 1,500 to >2,000 ng/mL). A single IV injection of ketamine in this range induces anesthesia within 30 to 40 seconds, while an IM dose provides a slower onset time of 3 to 4 minutes.[216] Ketamine is also clinically useful following oral, nasal, rectal, or epidural administration. The duration of action following a single IV dose is 5 to 10 minutes, with longer recovery times upon IM (12-25 minutes), nasal (45-60 minutes), or epidural (>240 minutes) administration.[217,218] Like the other agents described here, duration is limited by the redistribution of ketamine from the brain to the muscle and peripheral tissues over time.[218]

The activity of ketamine is also regulated by its extensive hepatic metabolism, which is thought to play an important role in its therapeutic utilization. Oral ketamine is subject to significant first-pass metabolism leading to 15% bioavailability. As shown in Figure 14.26, CYP2B6 is the primary enzyme required for in vitro and clinically meaningful biotransformation of ketamine enantiomers, with the 2A6, 3A4, and 3A5 isoforms also playing minor roles.[219-224] Both *R*-(-)- and *S*-(+)-ketamine are *N*-demethylated to the primary major metabolite *R*-(-)- and *S*-(+)-norketamine, respectively. Norketamine is an active circulating metabolite with approximately one-third the analgesic and anesthetic potency of the respective parent enantiomer and is the primary basis for the use of oral ketamine to provide analgesia and anesthesia. Peak concentrations of norketamine appear in 60 and 75 minutes following an oral or IM dose, respectively.[217] The primary norketamine metabolites can be further biotransformed to the respective enantiomers of dehydronorketamine or to three pairs of hydroxylated norketamine diastereomers via *o*-, *m*-, or *p*-hydroxylation to 4-, 5-, or 6-hydroxynorketamine, respectively (Fig. 14.26). Ketamine can also be metabolized to hydroxyketamine, which is not abundant in human circulation, as it is further *N*-demethylated to 6-hydroxynorketamine (Fig. 14.26). After IV administration of ketamine, the major circulating human metabolites are *R*-(-)- and *S*-(+)-norketamine, (2*S*,6*S*;2*R*,6*R*)-6-hydroxynorketamine, (2*S*,5*R*;2*R*,5*S*)- 5-hydroxynorketamine, and *R*-(-)- and *S*-(+)-dehydronorketamine.[219-224] The majority of the dose is excreted by the kidneys as either the hydroxylated metabolites or their conjugates, while less than 4% is excreted unchanged or as norketamine.[213]

Adverse Effects of Ketamine. As a dissociative anesthetic, ketamine has unique properties and induces adverse effects that are distinct from other IV anesthetics. In this regard, ketamine exhibits sympathomimetic activity that increase both blood pressure and cardiac chronotropy and output. This effect can also produce heightened salivation and elevated muscle tone. Similarly, it can increase cerebral blood flow, cerebral metabolic rate, and intracranial pressure. Taken together, these effects are precisely in opposition to those seen with the other IV agents. Due to its unique mechanism, psychiatric effects upon emergence from anesthesia (ie, emergence delirium), which are characterized by vivid and unpleasant dreams, out-of-body experiences, hallucinations, confusion, and agitation, occur in a high percentage of patients (12%-50%).

Neuromuscular Junction–Blocking Agents

Neuromuscular blocking agents promote muscle relaxation, and as a result, their primary therapeutic utility is as an adjuvant to GA. The muscle relaxant effects of these agents afford reductions in the depth requirement for GAs and allows for optimization of induction and recovery times. This allows for intracavitary operative procedures such as abdominal or thoracic surgeries, as well as placement of devices into muscle-laden organs—for example, tracheal intubation or insertion of ventilation tubes within the airway.

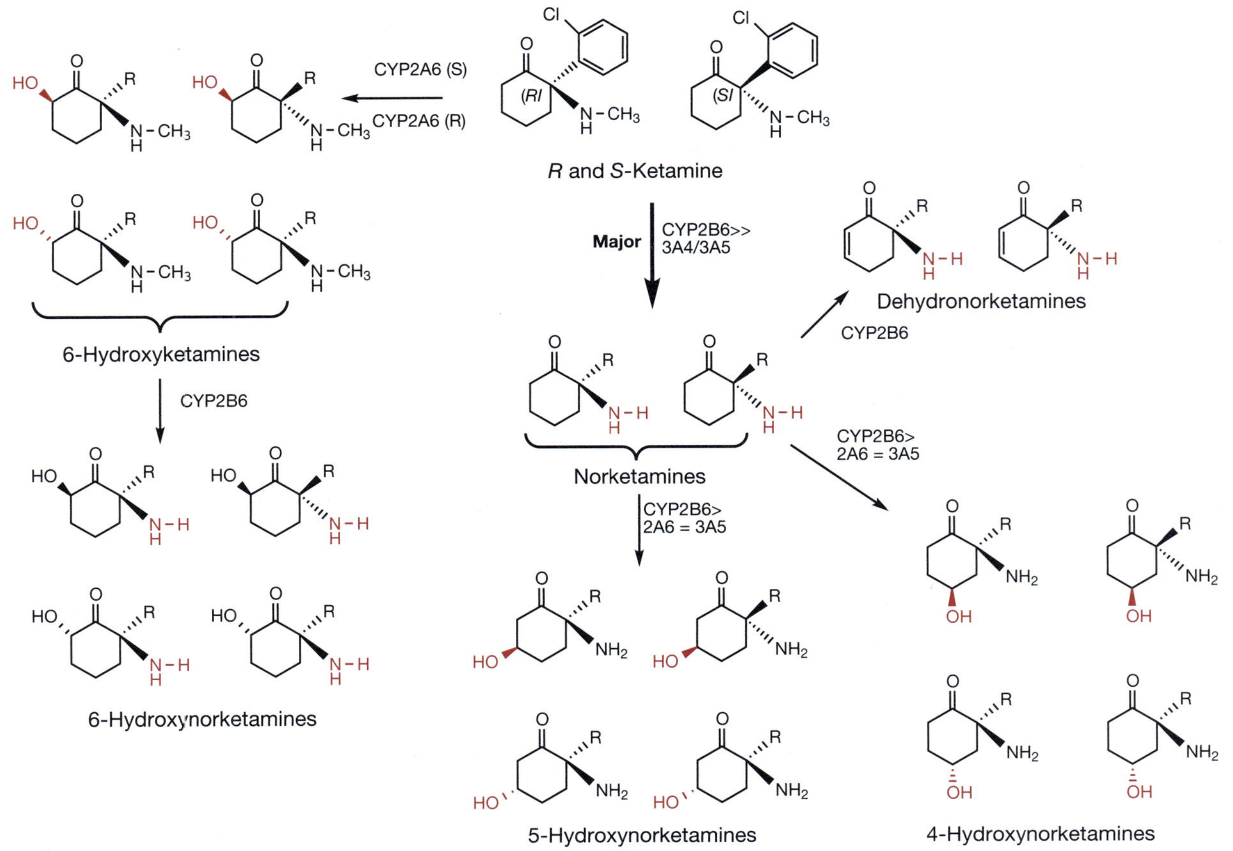

Figure 14.26 Metabolism of ketamine.

When used systemically, the fast-twitching smaller muscles (eg, ocular and facial muscles) are affected first, followed by the muscles of the neck, abdomen, and limbs, and finally, the larger intercostal muscles and diaphragm. The recovery from paralysis typically occurs in the reverse order.

Mechanism of Action of Neuromuscular Blocking Agents

All neuromuscular blockers act via inhibition of propagation of the action potential at the neuromuscular junction (NMJ), which serves as a distinct synapse that allows for the transmission of electrical impulses from nerves to muscle cells at the motor end plate. At this site, the depolarization of "presynaptic" parasympathetic neurons at the NMJ facilitates the voltage- and Ca^{2+}-dependent release of ACh into the synaptic cleft. Within this synapse, ACh rapidly binds to and stimulates postsynaptic nicotinic ACh receptors (nAChR) on the muscle cell end plate. Once activated by ACh, these ligand-gated nAChR modulate the robust influx of Na^+ and smaller relative efflux of K^+, within the muscle cells of the end plate, leading to a muscle action potential.

The nACh receptors (Fig. 14.2) are similar to the heteropentameric $GABA_A$ receptors previously described. Human adult motor end plates specifically express high levels of postsynaptic nAChRs that contain $\alpha_1\beta_1\varepsilon\delta$ subunits that assemble in a 2:1:1:1 ratio to give rise to the postsynaptic ligand-gated cation channel (see Fig. 14.2). Also, similar to $GABA_A$ receptors, postsynaptic $\alpha_1\beta_1\varepsilon\delta$-containing nAChR are composed of two distinct clusters of anionic amino acids that form two separate ACh binding sites: a high affinity site formed by one $\alpha_1\delta$ interface and a low-affinity site formed by another $\alpha_1\varepsilon$ interface. Upon binding of ACh to the high affinity site, conformational changes allow for positive cooperative binding of another ACh molecule to the low-affinity site, and together, these drive further conformational changes that allow for Na^+/K^+ antitransport through the pore. In addition to these postsynaptic receptors, neuronal nAChR consisting of $\alpha_3\beta_2$ subunits act as presynaptic ACh autoreceptors that further promote the release of ACh in a positive feedback manner, thereby further increasing release of the neurotransmitter into the NMJ.

Upon neuronal release of ACh and subsequent agonism of $\alpha_1\beta_1\varepsilon\delta$ nAChRs, the resulting Na^+ influx and K^+ efflux in the postsynaptic muscle cells cause the local motor end plate membrane potential to change. This change is directly correlated to the magnitude of nAChR activity and leads to activation and opening of voltage-gated Na^+ channels on the motor end plate. The high density of Na^+ channels here amplifies the membrane potential signal and produces the electrical gradient that facilitates an action potential and subsequent generation of muscle contraction. The effects of ACh within the NMJ are tightly regulated by acetylcholinesterase (AChE), which rapidly degrades the neurotransmitter and resets the motor end plate.

The neuromuscular blocking agents can be divided into two subclasses, depolarizing and nondepolarizing, based on their differing abilities to modulate this normal NMJ transmission. The only depolarizing NMJ blocking agents used clinically is succinylcholine (Fig. 14.27), which consists of two molecules of ACh linked endwise. In this paradoxical mechanism, succinylcholine binds to postsynaptic nAChRs to profoundly depolarize the motor end plate, as ACh itself does. Since the succinylcholine molecule is intrinsically more resistant to hydrolysis than ACh, the effects are prolonged and more intensified, leading to repeated muscle contractions manifesting as fasciculations due to the vast activation of nAChRs. As a consequence of this overexcitation of the motor end plate, the requirement for repolarization of the membrane that must exist to elicit the next contraction does not occur and the muscle tone effectively becomes flaccidly paralyzed. This phenomenon is referred to as phase I depolarizing block, and inhibition of AChE at this stage in the process further promotes succinylcholine-mediated paralysis. Upon continued activity of succinylcholine at the NMJ, the nAChR become desensitized and refractory to the effects of the agent, while at the same time, repolarization is occurring as normal primarily due to end plate Na^+/K^+-ATPase activity. Despite the repolarization, upon desensitization of nAChRs, Na^+ channels on the NMJ become inactivated through mechanisms that remain elusive, and this combination of inhibited Na^+ flux effectively paralyzes the muscle cells. This is referred to as phase II depolarizing block, and these effects can be reversed by inhibition of AChE, which allows ACh to compete with the succinylcholine for the nAChR.

In contrast to this depolarizing mechanism, the second subclass of NMJ blocking agents, which include all other FDA-approved agents, behave as nondepolarizing competitive antagonists of ACh binding for both pre- and postsynaptic nAChRs. Unlike succinylcholine, these agents do not possess intrinsic receptor modulating activity; rather, they inhibit muscle contraction by directly competing with ACh

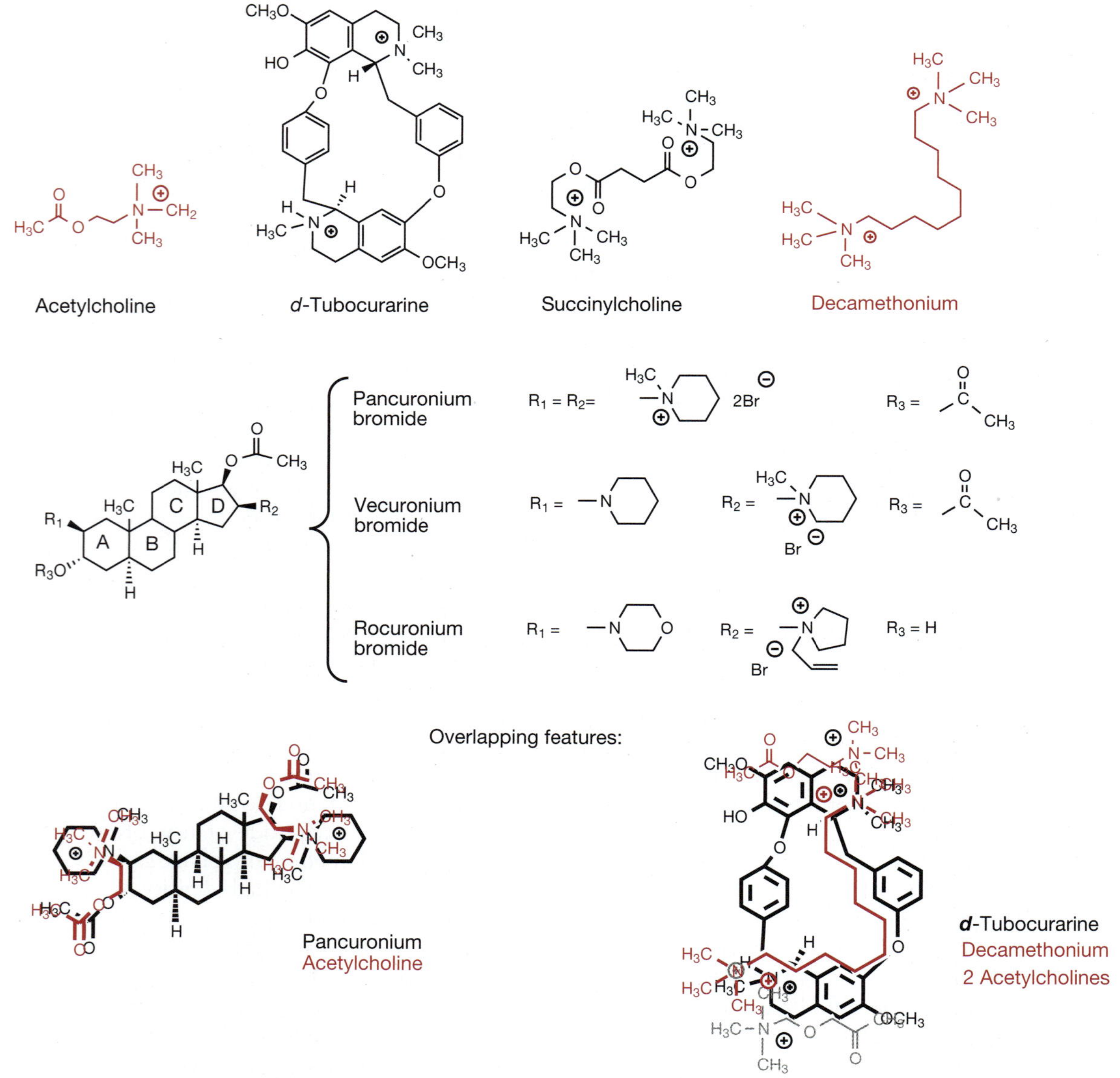

Figure 14.27 Structures of acetylcholine, succinylcholine, *d*-tubocurarine, and the aminosteroid neuromuscular blocking agents. Overlapping features are shown for pancuronium/acetylcholine and *d*-tubocurarine, acetylcholine, and decamethonium.

for the dianionic receptor binding sites. As a consequence of this mechanism, it can be inferred that structurally, these agents will possess dicationic pharmacophores (see later). Inhibition of binding of ACh to postsynaptic nAChR by these agents facilitates flaccid paralysis of musculature without producing depolarization of the motor end plate and lessens the amount of anesthetic required for surgical procedures. Nondepolarizing NMJ blocking agents also inhibit ACh binding to neuronal nAChR, thereby inhibiting the positive feedback role of the autoreceptor. This effectively decreases additional synaptic ACh release and further promotes NMJ blockade.

Structure-Activity Relationships of Neuromuscular Blocking Agents

The historical use of NMJ blocking agents can be dated to the 1500s, where South American natives utilized crude extracts of the climbing vine *Chondrodendron tomentosum* to construct "poisoned" arrows with which they hunted animals. These poisoned arrows, termed "ourare" (ie, curare) by the indigenous population, effectively asphyxiated the prey once injected into the animal, yet ingestion of the meat of the animal did no harm. Pioneering experiments by Claude Bernard in the 1850s led to the recognition that these extracts acted at a site between a nerve and the skeletal muscle, now known as the NMJ. In the late 1800s, curare extracts were found to contain a variety of quaternary ammonium–containing alkaloids, and in the 1930s, Henry Dale demonstrated that ACh acted at the NMJ and that curare blocked this activity. In 1935, Harold King was the first to isolate and publish the chemical structure of one of the active curare alkaloids, which he called tubocurarine. Importantly, in this published work, King[225] described that the structure of the active *d*-tubocurarine contained two quaternary nitrogen functional groups (ie, bisquaternary amine), and this discovery prompted development of derivatives of *d*-tubocurarine, such as decamethonium, as novel NMJ blockers based on the requirement for bisquaternary ammonium nitrogens.

It was not until 35 years after King's initial report that it was found that the structure of *d*-tubocurarine actually contained a single quaternary ammonium functional group in addition to a tertiary amine functional group (Fig. 14.27). At physiological pH, the tertiary nitrogen is primarily ionized, so overall, King's assessment of two positively charged centers holds true to form. Nonetheless, the bisquaternary ammonium–based structure served as the basis for development of many of the agents used clinically today. Since these agents all contain bis-ionizable nitrogen groups, they are poorly permeable through cell membranes and are hence not orally available, requiring direct IV or IM injection. This structural feature also explains why animals that were injected with curare arrows could be eaten with no harm to the consumer.

In addition to activation of nAChRs, acetylcholine nonselectively stimulates muscarinic GPCRs (mAChR), and previous studies have demonstrated that the distance from the center of the quaternary nitrogen to the van der Waals radius of the carbonyl oxygen of ACh is critical to selectivity for agonism of mAChR versus nAChR. In this regard, an N-O distance of 4.4 Å was proposed to yield muscarinic selectivity, while a distance of 5.9 Å would yield nicotinic activity.[226] This difference implies that nAChRs are receptive to larger agents with greater distance between the ionized amine and H-bond donor oxy groups.

The depolarizing agents such as decamethonium and succinylcholine provided much of the acquired knowledge of NMJ blocking agent SAR. As shown in Figure 14.27, these two agents typify the family of bismethonium-containing compounds that contain two bulky nitrogen-containing heads separated by a distinct number of atoms. The positively charged dicationic nitrogen groups play critical roles by binding to the two anionic ACh binding sites of the nAChRs. The bismethonium NMJ blocking agents contain the general structure of $(H_3C)_3N^+\text{-}(CH_2)_n\text{-}N^+(CH_3)_3$ and display nicotinic agonistic activity when n is equal to either 5 to 12 or 18 carbons. The optimal depolarizing neuromuscular blockade occurs when $n = 10$, which approximates to the 5.9 Å optimal distance for nAChR agonism by ACh. Bismethonium agents with five to six carbons are also effective as ACh ganglionic blockers, while agents with long carbon chains (eg, 18 or longer) regain neuromuscular blocking activity but become nondepolarizing.[227] While the SAR requirements of succinylcholine and decamethonium are in agreement with those of the nondepolarizing agent *d*-tubocurarine, which also has 10 atoms that span between the two cationic nitrogens (Fig. 14.27 overlay), it is well accepted that, like ACh, a single succinylcholine molecule exists in its lowest energy conformation in a bent arrangement (as shown in Fig. 14.27), which cannot span both anionic sites of the nAChR. Rather, two molecules of succinylcholine act individually on each anionic site of a single nAChR to modulate channel activity.[228] In contrast, the nondepolarizing agents such as *d*-tubocurarine that contain bis-nitrogen groups allow for simultaneous engagement of both anionic ACh binding sites of a single nAChR by each individual molecule, which spans the channel.[228]

In addition to *d*-tubocurarine, aminosteroid-, and tetrahydroisoquinoline-based agents function as competitive antagonists of nAChRs with a greater degree of clinical utility as highly efficacious nondepolarizing NMJ blocking agents. The clinically useful agents that make up the aminosteroid subfamily discussed here include pancuronium, vecuronium, and rocuronium, while tetrahydroisoqunolines are typified by atracurium and cisatracurium. The androstane-derived aminosteroids that contained monoquaternary ammonium salts were first noted to possess weak NMJ blocking activity in the 1960s. These early derivatives included ACh-likeness in the form of A-ring acetyl esters linked to the monoquaternary ammonium group (Fig. 14.27). Addition of a similar D-ring ACh mimic, as in pancuronium, facilitated markedly enhanced NMJ blocking activity (Fig. 14.27). As shown in Figure 14.27, pancuronium contains identical bisquaternary piperidinium substitutions (R_1 and R_2) and bisacetyloxy moieties that overlay identically with that of the structure of ACh. Meanwhile, the androstane backbone provides a rigid and bulky structural base to uphold a critical three-dimensional geometry.

In this regard, the A-ring ACh mimic is maintained in a *trans*-orientation, with the ionized ammonium in an upward β-position in reference to the plane of the androstane backbone, while the acetoxy moiety is oriented in a downward α-position (Fig. 14.27). Single crystal x-ray diffraction studies on pancuronium demonstrate that the A-ring is held in a twisted-boat orientation that mimics the binding of ACh to the high affinity anionic binding site of the nAChR.[229] On the eastern face of the molecule, the D-ring has a cis-orientation with both the quaternary ammonium and the acetoxy groups facing in the upward β-position relative to the androstane backbone (Fig. 14.27). Due to the critical role of the ionized nitrogen groups in binding to nAChR, SAR studies show that the highest potency steroid-based NMJ blocking agents have at least one quaternary ammonium, which, in addition to a second tertiary nitrogen, is capable of being ionized on the D-ring. Abiding to the structural mimicry of ACh, diacetate ester substitutions have greater potency than dipropionate esters, which were more potent than dipivalate or dibenzoate esters. Finally, *N*-alkyl substitution on the heterocyclic rings (R_1 and R_2, Fig. 14.27) affects potency with methyl providing optimal potency, followed by allyl substituents.[230]

In comparison to pancuronium, vecuronium contains a nonmethylated (nor) A-ring piperidine substitution (Fig. 14.27), hence the initial marketing under the brand name Norcuron. This tertiary amine substitution preserves potency but markedly alters the pharmacokinetics and side effect potential as described later and, perhaps more significantly, provides structural insight that the quaternary substitution at the D-ring is likely more important than that of the A-ring. Similar to vecuronium, rocuronium loses the quaternary functional group at the R_1 position of the A-ring but also loses the acetoxy ester moiety at R_3, in essence, losing its ACh-likeness on the western face (ie, A-ring) of the molecule (Fig. 14.27). As can be expected, this change imparts nearly 10-fold less potency to rocuronium compared to the other two steroid-based agents but produces a favorable pharmacokinetic profile, as discussed later.

The final grouping of NMJ blocking agents discussed here are the tetrahydroisoquinolines, of which, atracurium and cisatracurium are utilized clinically to a high degree. These compounds were rationally designed to be nonsteroidal, nondepolarizing NMJ blocking agents that could be biodegraded in vivo in a manner independent of hepatic or renal transformation. The structural similarity of atracurium to ACh is readily apparent, with the former having a long and flexible diester-containing chain that connects two quaternary onium heads, (Fig. 14.28), both of which engage the two anionic ACh binding sites of the nAChR. Importantly, the ester linkage of atracurium is reversed from that of ACh. This two atom separation between the quaternary nitrogen and the ester carbonyl readily allows for pH- and temperature-dependent elimination of the α-β carbons from the quaternary nitrogen in a process termed Hofmann elimination, which, along with ester hydrolysis, provides the basis for organ-independent breakdown of these agents (see "Pharmacokinetics and Metabolism of Neuromuscular Blocking Agents" section). Atracurium contains four chiral centers (denoted by asterisks in Fig. 14.28) that give rise to

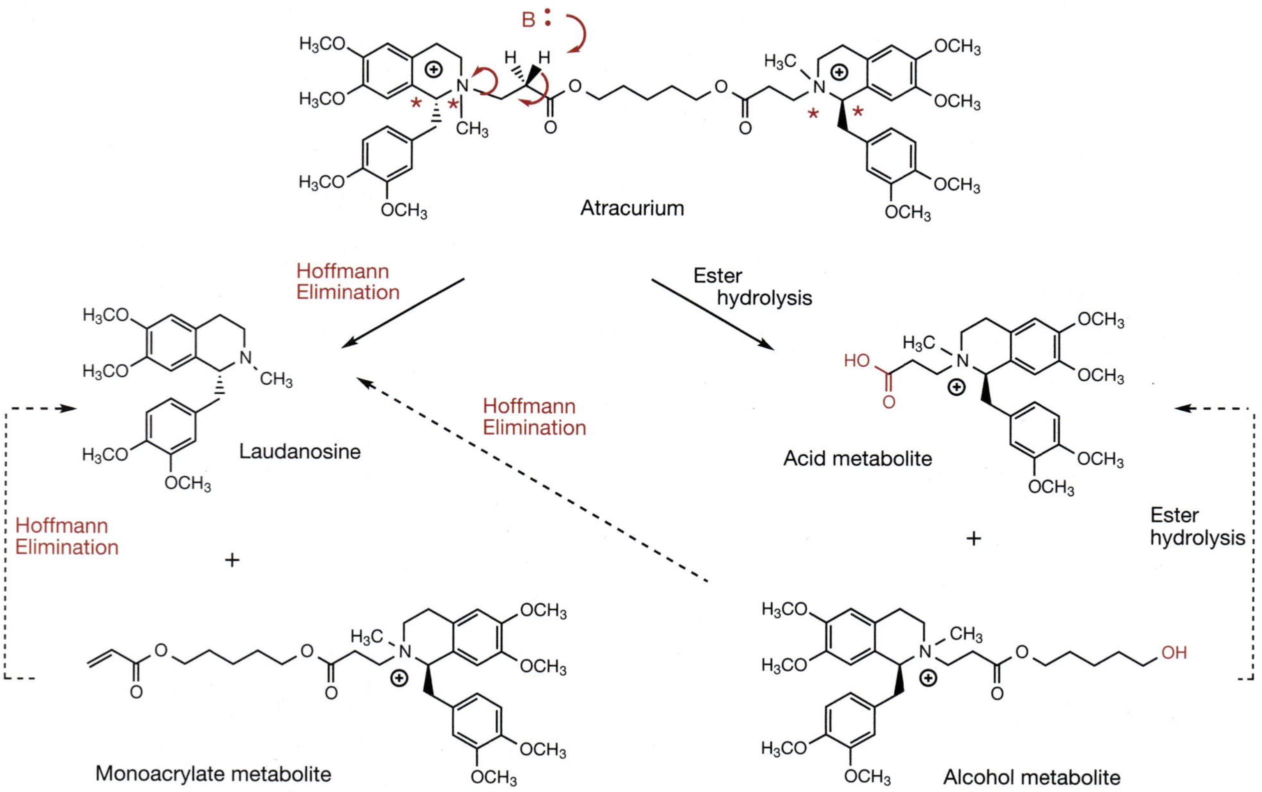

Figure 14.28 Structure of atracurium and organ-independent metabolism of atracurium.

16 enantiomers. However, since a plane of symmetry exists between the two ester moieties, the commercial product contains six meso structures and 10 optically distinct active enantiomers. Only six of the 10 stereoisomers have NMJ blocking activity, and of these, the *cis*-(1*R*, 2*R*, 1′*R*, 2′*R*) absolute isomer, which is commercialized as cisatracurium, is approximately 4-fold more potent than atracurium and is devoid of atracurium's side effects.

Adverse Effects of Neuromuscular Blocking Agents

Many of the adverse effects of NMJ blocking agents are outcomes directly related to their mechanism or durations of actions—for example, prolonged muscle relaxation, paralysis, or myalgia. However, other serious reactions can occur, including apnea due to paralysis of respiratory muscles and cardiovascular effects due to direct ganglionic blockade or secondary to histamine release. Succinylcholine, atracurium, and especially *d*-tubocurarine, but not so much the steroid-based agents or cisatracurium, can directly stimulate mast cells to facilitate the release of histamine, which can cause clinically manifested complications such as hypotension, bronchospasm, and hypersecretion. The depolarizing agents, prototyped by succinylcholine, can also release K^+, leading to hyperkalemia and cardiovascular and muscular issues, including rhabdomyolysis. Pancuronium can produce vagolytic effects, putatively via blockage of cardiovascular mAChRs, which can give rise to serious cardiovascular effects, including hypertension, tachycardia, and increased cardiac output. The newer steroid-based agents, including vecuronium and rocuronium, provide a greater degree of cardiostability and are relatively free from these effects. Atracurium is associated with hypotension, tachycardia, and flushing, while cisatracurium is relatively free from these adverse reactions.

Pharmacokinetics and Metabolism of Neuromuscular Blocking Agents

The pharmacokinetic profiles of the NMJ blocking agents are summarized in Table 14.5. Succinylcholine produces neuromuscular blockade within 30 to 60 seconds of IV administration and within 1 to 4 minutes of IM administration. The duration of action for these routes is 6 to 10 minutes and 15 to 20 minutes, respectively.[231] Unlike ACh, succinylcholine is fairly resistant to break down by AChE but is readily hydrolyzed by plasma pseudocholinesterases,

Table 14.5 Classification and Pharmacokinetics of Neuromuscular Junction–Blocking Agents

Agent	Structural Classification	Mechanism	Time to Peak (min)	Single Dose Duration of Action (min)	Elimination	Distinct Effects
Succinylcholine	Diacetylcholine ester	Depolarizing Ultra-short acting	0.5-1 (IV) 1-4 (IM)	6-10 (IV) 15-20 (IM)	Hydrolysis by plasma pseudocholinesterases	Histamine release K^+ release
d-Tubocurarine	Isoquinoline alkaloid	Nondepolarizing Long acting	1-2 (IV) 10-25 (IM)	20-120	Renal (88%-90%) Biliary (10%-12%)	Histamine release CV effects
Pancuronium	Androstane—amino-steroid	Nondepolarizing Long acting	2-3 (IV)	45-60 (IV)	Renal (69%) Hepatic (25%)	CV effects Hepatic effects
Vecuronium	Androstane—amino-steroid	Nondepolarizing Intermediate acting	2-5 (IV)	30-40 (IV)	Renal (15%) Biliary (50%) Hepatic (33%)	Cardioselective, lacks CV effects of others
Rocuronium	Androstane—amino-steroid	Nondepolarizing Intermediate acting	0.8-2 (IV)	22-40 (IV)	Renal (33%) Biliary (67%)	Cardioselective, lacks CV effects of others
Atracurium	Tetrahydroisoquinoline	Nondepolarizing Intermediate acting	2-3 (IV)	60-70 (IV)	Hofmann elimination Ester hydrolysis	Flushing, hypotension
Cisatracurium	Tetrahydroisoquinoline	Nondepolarizing Intermediate acting	2-8 (IM)	42-90 (IV)	Hofmann elimination Ester hydrolysis	

CV, cardiovascular; IM, intramuscular; IV, intravenous.

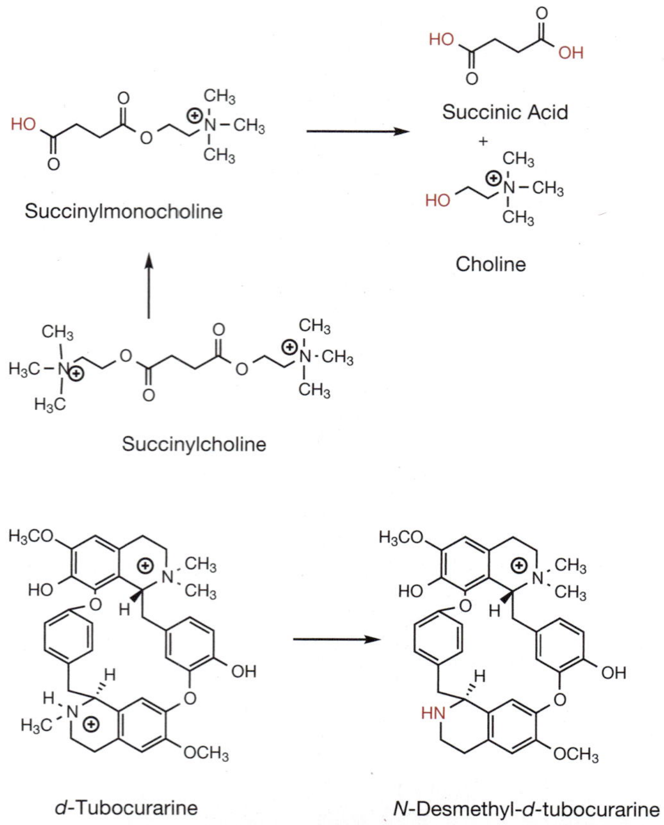

Figure 14.29 Metabolism of succinylcholine and *d*-tubocurarine.

including butyrylcholinesterase, yielding succinylmonocholine, which is itself 20- to 50-fold less active as an NMJ blocker than the parent drug.[232] About 70% of a bolus dose of succinylcholine is degraded to succinylmonocholine within 1 minute, and the metabolite is then further degraded to succinic acid and choline (Fig. 14.29).

Tubocurarine provides NMJ blockade within 2 minutes of an IV dose and within 10 to 25 minutes of an IM dose. Following a single IV dose, paralysis usually lasts 20 to 30 minutes, but the duration of blockade depends on the number of doses used and the overall depth of anesthesia, often lasting 60 to 120 minutes. Most of the drug is excreted unchanged by the kidneys within 24 hours, while 10% to 12% can be excreted in the bile, which also contains a small percentage (~1%) of *N*-demethylated metabolite (Fig. 14.29).[233]

For the steroid-based agents, peak blockade for pancuronium, vecuronium, and rocuronium occurs within 2 to 3, 2 to 5, and 0.8 to 2 minutes, respectively. The duration of action of a single IV dose of each agent is 45 to 60, 30 to 40, and 22 to 40 minutes, respectively. Notably, the loss of the quaternizing methyl in vecuronium is directly responsible for reduction of the duration by a third of that seen with pancuronium. Similarly, the loss of ACh-likeness at the A-ring of rocuronium decreases the time to onset and the duration of action of this agent compared to the androstane-steroid agents.

The majority of a pancuronium dose (69%) is excreted unchanged in the urine after 24 hours, while 25% is hepatically metabolized to an active 3-desacetyl (3-OH-containing) metabolite that is excreted in the urine. The remainder appears in the urine as 17-desacetyl or 3,17-desacetyl metabolites (Fig. 14.30).[234] For vecuronium, approximately 15% of an administered dose is recovered unchanged in the urine, while nearly 50% is excreted in the bile and 33% is metabolized hepatically to 3-desacetyl-, 17-desacetyl-, or 3,17-descetylvecuronium metabolites, all of which have activity as NMJ blocking agents (Fig. 14.30). Accumulation of the 3-desacetylvecuronium metabolite in critically ill patients may be associated with prolonged neuromuscular blockade in those receiving long-term therapies.[235-237] The major route of elimination of rocuronium is via biliary excretion, with approximately one-third of a dose also being excreted unchanged in the urine. Hepatic metabolism accounts for the formation of an inactive 17-desacetyl metabolite with no clinical relevance (Fig. 14.30).[238,239]

Atracurium and cisatracurium are fast-onset NMJ blocking agents, with peak blockade occurring within 2 to 3 and 2 to 8 minutes of IV injection, respectively. Single dose durations via this route are 60 to 70 and 42 to 90 minutes, respectively. These agents are not metabolized by organ-based transformation, but rather, as discussed in the SAR section, via Hofmann elimination and ester hydrolysis in the blood. The base-catalyzed Hofmann elimination of atracurium coupled with ester hydrolysis is illustrated in Figure 14.28 and leads to formation of laudanosine, a quaternary monoacrylate, a monoquaternary carboxylic acid, and a dialcohol, all of which are inactive. At physiological temperature and pH, base-mediated abstraction of one of the α-hydrogens respective to the ester carbonyl facilitates bond movements that, together with the ionized nitrogen, weakens its adjacent bonds, allows for the fissure of the molecule at the β-carbon respective to the ester carbonyl (Fig. 14.28). This forms laudanosine and the monoacrylate metabolite, which itself can undergo Hofmann elimination to yield laudanosine (Fig. 14.28). At the same time, ester hydrolysis of atracurium in plasma can lead to the formation of the acid and the alcohol metabolites, the latter of which can undergo further ester hydrolysis to the acid metabolite or Hofmann

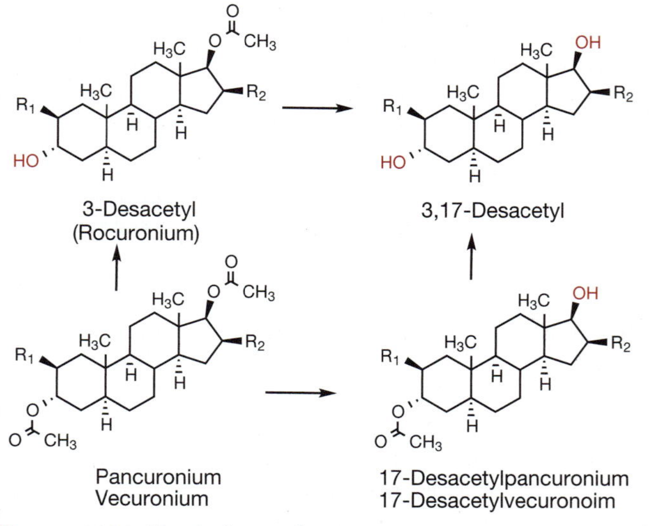

Figure 14.30 Metabolism of pancuronium, vecuronium, and rocuronium.

elimination to yield laudanosine.[240,241] This biodegradative pathway also holds true for cisatracurium and together, due to their independence from hepatic or renal biotransformation, atracurium and cisatracurium, are useful especially in patients with liver or kidney dysfunction.

REFERENCES

1. Moruzzi G, Magoun HW. Brain stem reticular formation and activation of the EEG. *Electroencephalogr Clin Neurophysiol.* 1949;1:455-473.
2. Lindsley DB, Schreiner LH, Knowles WB, Magoun HW. Behavioral and EEG changes following chronic brain stem lesions in the cat. *Electroencephalogr Clin Neurophysiol.* 1950;2:483-498.
3. Maghoun HW. Caudal and cephalic influences of the brain stem reticular formation. *Physiol Rev.* 1950;30:459-474.
4. Lu J, Greco MA. Sleep circuitry and the hypnotic mechanism of GABAA drugs. *J Clin Sleep Med.* 2006;2:S19-S26.
5. Panula P, Pirvola U, Auvinen S, Airaksinen MS. Histamine immunoreactive nerve fibers in the rat brain. *Neuroscience.* 1989;28:585-610.
6. Takahashi K, Lin JS, Sakai K. Neuronal activity of histaminergic tuberomammillary neurons during wake-sleep states in the mouse. *J Neurosci.* 2006;26:10292-10298.
7. Reiner PB, McGeer EG. Electrophysiological properties of cortically projecting histamine neurons of the rat hypothalamus. *Neurosci Lett.* 1987;73:43-47.
8. Lin JS, Sakai K, Jouvet M. Evidence for histaminergic arousal mechanisms in the hypothalamus of cat. *Neuropharmacology.* 1988;27:111-122.
9. Mochizuki T, Yamatodani A, Okakura K, Horii A, Inagaki N, Wada H. Circadian rhythm of histamine release from the hypothalamus of freely moving rats. *Physiol Behav.* 1992;51:391-394.
10. Lin JS, Sakai K, Vanni-Mercier G, Jouvet M. A critical role of the posterior hypothalamus in the mechanisms of wakefulness determined by microinjection of muscimol in freely moving cats. *Brain Res.* 1989;479:225-240.
11. Nauta WH. Hypothalamic regulation of sleep in rats. *J Neurophysiol.* 1946;9:285-316.
12. Moore RY. Retinohypothalamic projection in mammals: a comparative study. *Brain Res.* 1973;49:403-409.
13. Kalsbeek A, Cutrera RA, Van Heerikhuize JJ, Van Der Vliet J, Buijs RM. GABA release from suprachiasmatic nucleus terminals is necessary for the light-induced inhibition of nocturnal melatonin release in the rat. *Neuroscience.* 1999;91:453-461.
14. Roseboom PH, Coon SL, Baler R, McCune SK, Weller JL, Klein DC. Melatonin synthesis: analysis of the more than 150-fold nocturnal increase in serotonin N-acetyltransferase messenger ribonucleic acid in the rat pineal gland. *Endocrinology.* 1996;137:3033-3045.
15. Ganguly S, Weller JL, Ho A, Chemineau P, Malpaux B, Klein DC. Melatonin synthesis: 14-3-3-dependent activation and inhibition of arylalkylamine N-acetyltransferase mediated by phosphoserine-205. *Proc Natl Acad Sci U S A.* 2005;102:1222-1227.
16. Klein DC, Moore RY. Pineal N-acetyltransferase and hydroxyindole-O-methyltransferase: control by the retinohypothalamic tract and the suprachiasmatic nucleus. *Brain Res.* 1979;174:245-262.
17. Yoshida K, McCormack S, España RA, Crocker A, Scammell TE. Afferents to the orexin neurons of the rat brain. *J Comp Neurol.* 2006;494:845-61.
18. de Lecea L, Kilduff TS, Peyron C, et al. The hypocretins: hypothalamus-specific peptides with neuroexcitatory activity. *Proc Natl Acad Sci U S A.* 1998;95:322-327.
19. Sakurai T, Amemiya A, Ishii M, et al. Orexins and orexin receptors: a family of hypothalamic neuropeptides and G protein-coupled receptors that regulate feeding behavior. *Cell.* 1998;92:573-585.
20. Saper CB, Scammell TE, Lu J. Hypothalamic regulation of sleep and circadian rhythms. *Nature.* 2005;437:1257-1263.
21. van den Pol AN, Gao XB, Obrietan K, Kilduff TS, Belousov AB. Presynaptic and postsynaptic actions and modulation of neuroendocrine neurons by a new hypothalamic peptide, hypocretin/orexin. *J Neurosci.* 1998;18:7962-7971.
22. Steriade M. Acetylcholine systems and rhythmic activities during the waking-sleep cycle. *Prog Brain Res.* 2004;145:179-196.
23. Datta S. Cellular and chemical neuroscience of mammalian sleep. *Sleep Med.* 2010;11:431-440.
24. Datta S. Cellular basis of pontine ponto-geniculo-occipital wave generation and modulation. *Cell Mol Neurobiol.* 1997;17: 341-365.
25. McKernan RM, Whiting PJ. Which GABAA-receptor subtypes really occur in the brain? *Trends Neurosci.* 1996;19:139-143.
26. Macdonald RL, Rogers CJ, Twyman RE. Barbiturate regulation of kinetic properties of the GABAA receptor channel of mouse spinal neurones in culture. *J Physiol.* 1989;417:483-500.
27. Fourati Z, Ruza RR, Laverty D, et al. Barbiturates bind in the GLIC ion channel pore and cause inhibition by stabilizing a closed state. *J Biol Chem.* 2017;292:1550-1558.
28. Akaike N, Maruyama T, Tokutomi N. Kinetic properties of the pentobarbitone-gated chloride current in frog sensory neurones. *J Physiol.* 1987;394:85-98.
29. Vida JA, Hooker ML, Samour CM. Anticonvulsants. 4. Metharbital and phenobarbital derivatives. *J Med Chem.* 1973;16:1378-1381.
30. Vida JA, Samour CM, O'Dea MH, et al. Analgesics. 2. Selected 5-substituted 5-(1-phenylethyl)barbituric acids. *J Med Chem.* 1974;17:1194-1197.
31. Blicke FH, Cox RH, eds. *Medicinal Chemistry.* Vol 4. Wiley; 1959.
32. Basak SC, Harriss DK, Magnuson VR. Comparative study of lipophilicity versus topological molecular descriptors in biological correlations. *J Pharm Sci.* 1984;73:429-437.
33. Lavoie AM, Twyman RE. Direct evidence for diazepam modulation of GABAA receptor microscopic affinity. *Neuropharmacology.* 1996;35:1383-1392.
34. Twyman RE, Rogers CJ, Macdonald RL. Differential regulation of gammaaminobutyric acid receptor channels by diazepam and phenobarbital. *Ann Neurol.* 1989;25:213-220.
35. Windholz M, ed. *The Merck Index.* 9th ed. Merck & Co.; 1976.
36. Mejo SL. Anterograde amnesia linked to benzodiazepines. *Nurse Pract.* 1992;17:49-50.
37. Clatworthy AJ, Jones LV, Whitehouse MJ. The gas chromatography mass spectrometry of the major metabolites of flurazepam. *Biomed Mass Spectrom.* 1977;4:248-254.
38. Zampaglione N, Hilbert JM, Ning J, *Chung M, Gural R, Symchowicz S.* Disposition and metabolic fate of 14C-quazepam in man. *Drug Metab Dispos.* 1985;13:25-29.
39. Miura M, Otani K, Ohkubo T. Identification of human cytochrome P450 enzymes involved in the formation of 4-hydroxyestazolam from estazolam. *Xenobiotica.* 2005;35:455-465.
40. Eberts FS Jr, Philopoulos Y, Reineke LM, *Vliek RW.* Triazolam disposition. *Clin Pharmacol Ther.* 1981;29:81-93.
41. Schwarz HJ. Pharmacokinetics and metabolism of temazepam in man and several animal species. *Br J Clin Pharmacol.* 1979;8:23S-29S.
42. Kilpatrick GJ, McIntyre MS, Cox RF, et al. CNS 7056: a novel ultra-short-acting Benzodiazepine. *Anesthesiology.* 2007;107(1):60-66.
43. Zhou Y, Hu P, Jiang J. Metabolite characterization of a novel sedative drug, remimazolam in human plasma and urine using ultra high-performance liquid chromatography coupled with synapt high-definition mass spectrometry. *J Pharm Biomed Anal.* 2017;137:78-83.
44. Antonik LJ, Goldwater DR, Kilpatrick GJ, Tilbrook GS, Borkett KM. A placebo- and midazolam-controlled phase I single ascending-dose study evaluating the safety, pharmacokinetics, and pharmacodynamics of remimazolam (CNS 7056): Part

I. Safety, efficacy, and basic pharmacokinetics. *Anesth Analg.* 2012;115(2):274-283.
45. Sanger DJ, Benavides J, Perrault G, et al. Recent developments in the behavioral pharmacology of benzodiazepine (omega) receptors: evidence for the functional significance of receptor subtypes. *Neurosci Biobehav Rev.* 1994;18:355-372.
46. McKernan RM, Rosahl TW, Reynolds DS, et al. Sedative but not anxiolytic properties of benzodiazepines are mediated by the GABA(A) receptor alpha1 subtype. *Nat Neurosci.* 2000;3:587-592.
47. Löw K, Crestani F, Keist R, et al. Molecular and neuronal substrate for the selective attenuation of anxiety. *Science.* 2000;290:131-134.
48. Collinson N, Kuenzi FM, Jarolimek W, et al. Enhanced learning and memory and altered GABAergic synaptic transmission in mice lacking the alpha 5 subunit of the GABAA receptor. *J Neurosci.* 2002;22:5572-5580.
49. Crestani F, Keist R, Fritschy JM, et al. Trace fear conditioning involves hippocampal alpha5 GABA(A) receptors. *Proc Natl Acad Sci U S A.* 2002;99:8980-8985.
50. Smith AJ, Alder L, Silk J, et al. Effect of alpha subunit on allosteric modulation of ion channel function in stably expressed human recombinant gamma-aminobutyric acid(A) receptors determined using (36)Cl ion flux. *Mol Pharmacol.* 2001;59:1108-1118.
51. Petroski RE, Pomeroy JE, Das R, et al. Indiplon is a high-affinity positive allosteric modulator with selectivity for alpha1 subunit-containing GABAA receptors. *J Pharmacol Exp Ther.* 2006;317:369-377.
52. Frattola L, Maggioni M, Cesana B, et al. Double blind comparison of zolpidem 20 mg versus flunitrazepam 2 mg in insomniac in-patients. *Drugs Exp Clin Res.* 1990;16:371-376.
53. Bensimon G, Foret J, Warot D, et al. Daytime wakefulness following a bedtime oral dose of zolpidem 20 mg, flunitrazepam 2 mg and placebo. *Br J Clin Pharmacol.* 1990;30:463-469.
54. Declerck AC, Ruwe F, O'Hanlon JF, Vermeeren A, Wauquier A. Effects of zolpidem and flunitrazepam on nocturnal sleep of women subjectively complaining of insomnia. *Psychopharmacology.* 1992;106:497-501.
55. Roger M, Attali P, Coquelin JP. Multicenter, double-blind, controlled comparison of zolpidem and triazolam in elderly patients with insomnia. *Clin Ther.* 1993;15:127-136.
56. Priest R, Terzano M, Parrino L, Boyer P. Efficacy of zolpidem in insomnia. *Eur Psychiatry.* 1997;12(suppl 1):5-14.
57. Kerkhof G, Van Vianen BG, Kamphuisen HC. A comparison of zolpidem and temazepam in psychophysiological insomniacs. *Eur Neuropsychopharmacol.* 1996;6:155-156.
58. Holm KJ, Goa KL. Zolpidem: an update of its pharmacology, therapeutic efficacy and tolerability in the treatment of insomnia. *Drugs.* 2000;59:865-889.
59. Anzini M, Cappelli A, Vomero S, et al. Molecular basis of peripheral vs central benzodiazepine receptor selectivity in a new class of peripheral benzodiazepine receptor ligands related to alpidem. *J Med Chem.* 1996;39:4275-4284.
60. Trapani G, Franco M, Ricciardi L, et al. Synthesis and binding affinity of 2-phenylimidazo[1,2-alpha]pyridine derivatives for both central and peripheral benzodiazepine receptors. A new series of high-affinity and selective ligands for the peripheral type. *J Med Chem.* 1997;40:3109-3118.
61. Selleri S, Bruni F, Costagli C, et al. A novel selective GABA(A) alpha1 receptor agonist displaying sedative and anxiolytic-like properties in rodents. *J Med Chem.* 2005;48:6756-6760.
62. Hanson SM, Morlock EV, Satyshur KA, Czajkowski C. Structural requirements for eszopiclone and zolpidem binding to the gamma-aminobutyric acid type-A (GABAA) receptor are different. *J Med Chem.* 2008;51:7243-7252.
63. Sauvantet JP, Langer SZ, Morselli PL, eds. *Imidazopyridines in Sleep Disorders.* Raven Press; 1988.
64. Pichard L, Gillet G, Bonfils C, et al. Oxidative metabolism of zolpidem by human liver cytochrome P450S. *Drug Metab Dispos.* 1995;23:1253-1262.
65. Von Moltke LL, Greenblatt DJ, Granda BW, et al. Zolpidem metabolism in vitro: responsible cytochromes, chemical inhibitors, and in vivo correlations. *Br J Clin Pharmacol.* 1999;48:89-97.
66. Gillet G, Thénot JP, Morselli PL. *In vitro and in vivo metabolism of zolpidem in three animal species and in man.* Paper presented at: Proceedings *of the* 3rd Intl ISSX Meeting, *Amsterdam,* The *Netherlands;* 1991:153.
67. Olubodun JO, Ochs HR, von Moltke LL, et al. Pharmacokinetic properties of zolpidem in elderly and young adults: possible modulation by testosterone in men. *Br J Clin Pharmacol.* 2003;56:297-304.
68. Nakamura H, Nakasa H, Ishii I, et al. Effects of endogenous steroids on CYP3A4-mediated drug metabolism by human liver microsomes. *Drug Metab Dispos.* 2002;30:534-540.
69. Cubala WJ, Landowski J, Wichowicz HM. Zolpidem abuse, dependence and withdrawal syndrome: sex as susceptibility factor for adverse effects. *Br J Clin Pharmacol.* 2008;65:444-445.
70. Hair PI, McCormack PL, Curran MP. Eszopiclone: a review of its use in the treatment of insomnia. *Drugs.* 2008;68:1415-1434.
71. U.S. Food and Drug Administration. Prescribing information: Lunesta (eszopiclone) tablets 1 mg, 2 mg, 3 mg. Sepracor, Inc; 2009. https://dailymed.nlm.nih.gov/dailymed/drugInfo.cfm?setid=3821f4b7-a3c8-4920-ba80-18aa96532c09.
72. Trifiletti RR, Snyder SH. Anxiolytic cyclopyrrolones zopiclone and suriclone bind to a novel site linked allosterically to benzodiazepine receptors. *Mol Pharmacol.* 1984;26:458-469.
73. Gaillot J, Heusse D, Hougton GW, Marc Aurele J, Dreyfus JF. Pharmacokinetics and metabolism of zopiclone. *Pharmacology.* 1983;27(suppl 2):76-91.
74. Becquemont L, Mouajjah S, Escaffre O, Beaune P, Funck-Brentano C, Jaillon P. Cytochrome P-450 3A4 and 2C8 are involved in zopiclone metabolism. *Drug Metab Dispos.* 1999;27(9):1068-1073.
75. Sanna E, Busonero F, Talani G, et al. Comparison of the effects of zaleplon, zolpidem, and triazolam at various GABA(A) receptor subtypes. *Eur J Pharmacol.* 2002;451:103-110.
76. Rosen AS, Fournié P, Darwish M, et al. Zaleplon pharmacokinetics and absolute bioavailability. *Biopharm Drug Dispos.* 1999;20:171-175.
77. U.S. Food and Drug Administration. Prescribing information: Sonata (zaleplon) capsules 5 mg, 10 mg. King Pharmaceuticals, Inc; 2006. https://labeling.pfizer.com/ShowLabeling.aspx?id=710.
78. Dooley M, Plosker GL. Zaleplon: a review of its use in the treatment of insomnia. *Drugs.* 2000;60:413-445.
79. Walsh JK, Vogel GW, Scharf M, et al. A five week, polysomnographic assessment of zaleplon 10 mg for the treatment of primary insomnia. *Sleep Med.* 2000;1:41-49.
80. Wegner F, Deuther-Conrad W, Scheunemann M, et al. GABAA receptor pharmacology of fluorinated derivatives of the novel sedative-hypnotic pyrazolopyrimidine indiplon. *Eur J Pharmacol.* 2008;580:1-11.
81. Kawashima K, Hosoi K, Naruke T, *Shiba T, Kitamura M, Watabe T.* Aldehyde oxidase-dependent marked species difference in hepatic metabolism of the sedative-hypnotic, zaleplon, between monkeys and rats. *Drug Metab Dispos.* 1999;27:422-428.
82. Dolder CR, Nelson MH. Hypnosedative-induced complex behaviours: incidence, mechanisms and management. *CNS Drugs.* 2008;22:1021-1036.
83. Hoque R, Chesson AL Jr. Zolpidem-induced sleepwalking, sleep related eating disorder, and sleep-driving: fluorine-18-flourodeoxyglucose positron emission tomography analysis, and a literature review of other unexpected clinical effects of zolpidem. *J Clin Sleep Med.* 2009;5:471-476.
84. Tsai JH, Yang P, Chen CC, et al. Zolpidem-induced amnesia and somnambulism: rare occurrences? *Eur Neuropsychopharmacol.* 2009;19:74-76.
85. Siddiqui F, Osuna E, Chokroverty S. Writing emails as part of sleepwalking after increase in zolpidem. *Sleep Med.* 2009;10:262-264.
86. Doane JA, Dalpiaz AS. Zolpidem-induced sleep-driving. *Am J Med.* 2008;121:e5.
87. Sansone RA, Sansone LA. Zolpidem, somnambulism, and nocturnal eating. *Gen Hosp Psychiatry.* 2008;30:90-91.

88. Iruela LM. Zolpidem and sleepwalking. *J Clin Psychopharmacol.* 1995;15:223.
89. Ferentinos P, Paparrigopoulos T. Zopiclone and sleepwalking. *Int J Neuropsychopharmacol.* 2009;12:141-142.
90. Liskow B, Pikalov A. Zaleplon overdose associated with sleepwalking and complex behavior. *J Am Acad Child Adolesc Psychiatry.* 2004;43:927-928.
91. Gauer F, Masson-Pevet M, Stehle J, Pevet P. Daily variations in melatonin receptor density of rat pars tuberalis and suprachiasmatic nuclei are distinctly regulated. *Brain Res.* 1994;641: 92-98.
92. Liu C, Weaver DR, Jin X, et al. Molecular dissection of two distinct actions of melatonin on the suprachiasmatic circadian clock. *Neuron.* 1997;19:91-102.
93. Dubocovich ML, Yun K, Al-Ghoul WM, Benloucif S, Masana MI. Selective MT2 melatonin receptor antagonists block melatonin-mediated phase advances of circadian rhythms. *FASEB J.* 1998;12:1211-1220.
94. Mor M, Plazzi PV, Spadoni G, Tarzia G. Melatonin. *Curr Med Chem.* 1999;6:501-518.
95. Spadoni G, Mor M, Tarzia G. Structure-affinity relationships of indole-based melatonin analogs. *Biol Signals Recept.* 1999;8:15-23.
96. Rivara S, Mor M, Bedini A, et al. Melatonin receptor agonists: SAR and applications to the treatment of sleep-wake disorders. *Curr Top Med Chem.* 2008;8:954-968.
97. Yous S, Andrieux J, Howell HE, et al. Novel naphthalenic ligands with high affinity for the melatonin receptor. *J Med Chem.* 1992;35:1484-1486.
98. Sugden D, Davidson K, Hough KA, *Teh MT.* Melatonin, melatonin receptors and melanophores: a moving story. *Pigment Cell Res.* 2004;17:454-460.
99. Dubocovich ML, Delagrange P, Krause DN, Sugden D, Cardinali DP, Olcese J. International union of basic and clinical pharmacology. LXXV. Nomenclature, classification, and pharmacology of G protein-coupled melatonin receptors. *Pharmacol Rev.* 2010;62:343-380.
100. Farce A, Chugunov AO, Logé C, et al. Homology modeling of MT1 and MT2 receptors. *Eur J Med Chem.* 2008;43:1926-1944.
101. Gerdin MJ, Mseeh F, Dubocovich ML. Mutagenesis studies of the human MT2 melatonin receptor. *Biochem Pharmacol.* 2003;66:315-320.
102. Kato K, Hirai K, Nishiyama K, et al. Neurochemical properties of ramelteon (TAK-375), a selective MT1/MT2 receptor agonist. *Neuropharmacology.* 2005;48:301-310.
103. Miyamoto M, Nishikawa H, Doken Y, et al. The sleep-promoting action of ramelteon (TAK-375) in freely moving cats. *Sleep.* 2004;27:1319-1325.
104. Nosjean O, Ferro M, Coge F, et al. Identification of the melatonin-binding site MT3 as the quinone reductase 2. *J Biol Chem.* 2000;275: 31311-31317.
105. Yukuhiro N, Kimura H, Nishikawa H, *Ohkawa* S, Yoshikubo S, Miyamoto M. Effects of ramelteon (TAK-375) on nocturnal sleep in freely moving monkeys. *Brain Res.* 2004;1027:59-66.
106. Mini L, Wang-Weigand S, Zhang J. Ramelteon 8 mg/d versus placebo in patients with chronic insomnia: post hoc analysis of a 5-week trial using 50% or greater reduction in latency to persistent sleep as a measure of treatment effect. *Clin Ther.* 2008;30:1316-1323.
107. Roth T, Stubbs C, Walsh JK. Ramelteon (TAK-375), a selective MT1/MT2-receptor agonist, reduces latency to persistent sleep in a model of transient insomnia related to a novel sleep environment. *Sleep.* 2005;28:303-307.
108. Erman M, Seiden D, Zammit G, *Sainati S, Zhang J.* An efficacy, safety, and dose-response study of Ramelteon in patients with chronic primary insomnia. *Sleep Med.* 2006;7:17-24.
109. Griffiths RR, Johnson MW. Relative abuse liability of hypnotic drugs: a conceptual framework and algorithm for differentiating among compounds. *J Clin Psychiatry.* 2005;66:31-41.
110. U.S. Food and Drug Administration. Prescribing information: Rozerem (ramelteon) tablets 8 mg. Takeda Pharmaceuticals America, Inc; 2008. https://content.takeda.com/?contenttype=PI&product=ROZ&language=ENG&country=GBL&documentnumber=1
111. Karim A, Tolbert D, Cao C. Disposition kinetics and tolerance of escalating single doses of ramelteon, a high-affinity MT1 and MT2 melatonin receptor agonist indicated for treatment of insomnia. *J Clin Pharmacol.* 2006;46:140-148.
112. Obach RS, Ryder TF. Metabolism of ramelteon in human liver microsomes and correlation with the effect of fluvoxamine on ramelteon pharmacokinetics. *Drug Metab Dispos.* 2010;38:1381-1391.
113. Lavedan C, Forsberg M, Gentile AJ. Tasimelteon: a selective and unique receptor binding profile. *Neuropharmacology.* 2015;91:142-147.
114. Torres R, Dressman MA, Kramer WG, Baroldi P. Absolute bioavailability of Tasimelteon. *Am J Ther.* 2015;22(5):355-360.
115. Vachharajani NN, Yeleswaram K, Boulton DW. Preclinical pharmacokinetics and metabolism of BMS-214778, a novel melatonin receptor agonist. *J Pharm Sci.* 2003;92(4):760-772.
116. U.S. Food and Drug Administration. Prescribing information: ETLIOZ (tasimelteon) capsules 20 mg. Vanda Pharmaceuticals Inc; 2020. https://hetlioz.com/assets/HetliozPI-20a5211da72736c030cecdefae6e021b0588589715dae78082a0776052b2d6ba.pdf
117. Center for Drug Evaluation and Research. HETLIOZ (tasimelteon): clinical pharmacology review—new drug application 205-677. Vanda Pharmaceuticals Inc; 2013. https://www.accessdata.fda.gov/drugsatfda_docs/nda/2014/205677Orig1s000PharmR.pdf
118. Lee MG, Hassani OK, Jones BE. Discharge of identified orexin/hypocretin neurons across the sleep-waking cycle. *J Neurosci.* 2005, 25:6716-6720.
119. Takahashi K, Lin JS, Sakai K. Neuronal activity of orexin and non-orexin waking-active neurons during wake-sleep states in the mouse. *Neuroscience.* 2008, 153:860-870.
120. Mileykovskiy BY, Kiyashchenko LI, Siegel JM. Behavioral correlates of activity in identified hypocretin/orexin neurons. *Neuron.* 2005;46:787-798.
121. Lin L, Faraco J, Li R, Kadotani H, et al. The sleep disorder canine narcolepsy is caused by a mutation in the hypocretin (orexin) receptor 2 gene. *Cell.* 1999; 98:365-376.
122. Aldrich MS, Reynolds PR. Narcolepsy and the hypocretin receptor 2 gene. *Neuron.* 1999;23:625-626.
123. Hagan JJ, Leslie RA, Patel S, et al. Orexin A activates locus coeruleus cell firing and increases arousal in the rat. *Proc Natl Acad Sci U S A.* 1999;96:10911-10916.
124. España RA, Plahn S, Berridge CW. Circadian-dependent and circadian-independent behavioral actions of hypocretin/orexin. *Brain Res.* 2002, 943:224-236.
125. Gotter AL, Webber AL, Coleman PJ, Renger JJ, Winrow CJ. International union of basic and clinical pharmacology. LXXXVI. Orexin receptor function, nomenclature and pharmacology. *Pharmacol Rev.* 2012;64:389-420.
126. Mang GM, Dürst T, Bürki H, et al. The dual orexin receptor antagonist almorexant induces sleep and decreases orexin-induced locomotion by blocking orexin 2 receptors. *Sleep. 2012*;35: 1625-1635.
127. Hoever P, de Haas SL, Dorffner G, *Chiossi E, van Gerven JM, Dingemanse J.* Orexin receptor antagonism: an ascending multiple-dose study with almorexant. *J Psychopharmacol.* 2012;26: 1071-1080.
128. Brisbare-Roch C, Dingemanse J, Koberstein R, et al. Promotion of sleep by targeting the orexin system in rats, dogs and humans. *Nat Med.* 2007;13:150-155.
129. Steiner MA, Lecourt H, Strasser DS, et al. Differential effects of the dual orexin receptor antagonist almorexant and the GABA(A)-α1 receptor modulator zolpidem, alone or combined with ethanol, on motor performance in the rat. *Neuropsychopharmacology.* 2011; 36:848-856.
130. Cox CD, Breslin MJ, Whitman DB, et al. Discovery of the dual orexin receptor antagonist [(7R)-4-(5-chloro-1,3-benzoxazol-2-yl)-7-methyl-1,4-diazepan-1-yl][5-methyl-2-(2H-1,2,3-triazol-2-yl)phenyl]methanone (MK-4305) for the treatment of insomnia. *J Med Chem.* 2010;53:5320-5332.

131. Michelson D, Snyder E, Paradis E, et al. Safety and efficacy of suvorexant during 1-year treatment of insomnia with subsequent abrupt treatment discontinuation: a phase 3 randomised, double-blind, placebo-controlled trial. *Lancet Neurol.* 2014;13:461-471.
132. Herring WJ, Snyder E, Budd K, et al. Orexin receptor antagonism for treatment of insomnia: a randomized clinical trial of suvorexant. *Neurology.* 2012;79:2265-2274.
133. Herring WJ, Connor KM, Ivgy-May N, et al. Suvorexant in patients with insomnia: results from two 3-month randomized controlled clinical trials. *Biol Psychiatry.* 2016; 79:136-148.
134. Herring WJ, Connor KM, Snyder E, et al. Suvorexant in elderly patients with insomnia: pooled analyses of data from phase III randomized controlled clinical trials. *Am J Geriatr Psychiatry.* 2017;25:791-802.
135. Herring WJ, Connor KM, Snyder E, et al. Suvorexant in patients with insomnia: pooled analyses of three-month data from phase-3 randomized controlled clinical trials. *J Clin Sleep Med.* 2016;12:1215-1225.
136. U.S. Food and Drug Administration. Prescribing information: Belsomra® (suvorexant) tablets 10 mg, 20 mg, 40 mg. Merck & Co, Inc; 2016. https://www.merck.com/product/usa/pi_circulars/b/belsomra/belsomra_pi.pdf.
137. Yin J, Mobarec JC, Kolb P, Rosenbaum DM. Crystal structure of the human OX2 orexin receptor bound to the insomnia drug suvorexant. *Nature.* 2015;519:247-250.
138. Cui D, Cabalu T, Yee KL, et al. In vitro and in vivo characterisation of the metabolism and disposition of suvorexant in humans. *Xenobiotica.* 2016;46:882-895.
139. Treiber A, de Kanter R, Roch C, et al. The use of physiology-based pharmacokinetic and pharmacodynamic modeling in the discovery of the dual orexin receptor antagonist ACT-541468. *J Pharmacol Exp Ther.* 2017;362(3):489-503.
140. Mignot E, Mayleben D, Fietze I, et al. Safety and efficacy of daridorexant in patients with insomnia disorder: results from two multicentre, randomised, double-blind, placebo-controlled, phase 3 trials. *Lancet Neurol.* 2022;21(2):125-139.
141. Muehlan C, Brooks S, Zuiker R, van Gerven J, Dingemanse J. Multiple-dose clinical pharmacology of ACT-541468, a novel dual orexin receptor antagonist, following repeated-dose morning and evening administration. *Eur Neuropsychopharmacol.* 2019;29(7):847-857.
142. Muehlan C, Heuberger J, Juif PE, Croft M, van Gerven J, Dingemanse J. Accelerated development of the dual orexin receptor antagonist ACT-541468: integration of a microtracer in a first-in-human study. *Clin Pharmacol Ther.* 2018;104(5):1022-1029.
143. Muehlan C, Fischer H, Zimmer D, et al. Metabolism of the dual orexin receptor antagonist ACT-541468, based on microtracer/accelerator mass spectrometry. *Curr Drug Metab.* 2019;20(4):254-265.
144. Treiber A, Delahaye S, Weigel A, Aeänismaa P, Gatfield J, Seeland S. The metabolism of the dual orexin receptor antagonist daridorexant. *Xenobiotica.* 2023;11:1-11.
145. Treiber A, Aissaoui H, Delahaye S, et al. CYP3A4 catalyzes the rearrangement of the dual orexin receptor antagonist daridorexant to 4-hydroxypiperidinol metabolites. *ChemMedChem.* 2023;18(10):e202300030.
146. Beuckmann CT, Suzuki M, Ueno T, Nagaoka K, Arai T, Higashiyama H. In vitro and in silico characterization of lemborexant (E2006), a novel dual orexin receptor antagonist. *J Pharmacol Exp Ther.* 2017;362(2):287-295.
147. Rosenberg R, Murphy P, Zammit G, et al. Comparison of lemborexant with placebo and zolpidem tartrate extended release for the treatment of older adults with insomnia disorder: a phase 3 randomized clinical trial. *JAMA Netw Open.* 2019;2(12):e1918254.
148. Yardley J, Kärppä M, Inoue Y, et al. Long-term effectiveness and safety of lemborexant in adults with insomnia disorder: results from a phase 3 randomized clinical trial. *Sleep Med.* 2021;80:333-342.
149. Yoshida Y, Naoe Y, Terauchi T, et al. Discovery of (1R,2S)-2-{[(2,4-dimethylpyrimidin-5-yl)oxy]methyl}-2-(3-fluorophenyl)-N-(5-fluoropyridin-2-yl)cyclopropanecarboxamide (E2006): a potent and efficacious oral orexin receptor antagonist. *J Med Chem.* 2015;58(11):4648-4664.
150. Ueno T, Ishida T, Aluri J, et al. Disposition and metabolism of [14C]lemborexant in healthy human subjects and characterization of its circulating metabolites. *Drug Metab Dispos.* 2021;49(1):31-38.
151. Alkire MT, Miller J. General anesthesia and the neural correlates of consciousness. *Prog Brain Res.* 2005;150:229-244.
152. Heinke W, Schwarzbauer C. In vivo imaging of anaesthetic action in humans: approaches with positron emission tomography (PET) and functional magnetic resonance imaging (fMRI). *Br J Anaesth.* 2002;89:112-122.
153. Alkire MT, Haier RJ. Correlating in vivo anaesthetic effects with ex vivo receptor density data supports a GABAergic mechanism of action for propofol, but not for isoflurane. *Br J Anaesth.* 2001;86:618-626.
154. Alkire MT, Haier RJ, Fallon JH. Toward a unified theory of narcosis: brain imaging evidence for a thalamocortical switch as the neurophysiologic basis of anesthetic-induced unconsciousness. *Conscious Cogn.* 2000;9:370-386.
155. Hentschke H, Schwarz C, Antkowiak B. Neocortex is the major target of sedative concentrations of volatile anaesthetics: strong depression of firing rates and increase of GABAA receptor-mediated inhibition. *Eur J Neurosci.* 2005;21:93-102.
156. French JD, Livingston RB, Hernandez-Peon R. Cortical influences upon the arousal mechanism. *Trans Am Neurol Assoc.* 1953;3:57-58.
157. Nicoll RA, Madison DV. General anesthetics hyperpolarize neurons in the vertebrate central nervous system. *Science.* 1982;217:1055-1057.
158. Dringenberg HC, Olmstead MC. Integrated contributions of basal forebrain and thalamus to neocortical activation elicited by pedunculopontine tegmental stimulation in urethane-anesthetized rats. *Neuroscience.* 2003;119:839-853.
159. Torri G. Inhalation anesthetics: a review. *Minerva Anestesiol.* 2010;76:215-228.
160. Di Fazio CA, Brown RE, Ball CG, Heckel CG, Kennedy SS. Additive effects of anesthetics and theories of anesthesia. *Anesthesiology.* 1972;36:57-63.
161. Torri G, Damia G, Fabiani ML. Effect of nitrous oxide on the anaesthetic requirement of enflurane. *Br J Anaesth.* 1974;46:468-72.
162. Meyer H. Zur Theorie der Alkoholnarkose. *Arch Exp Pathol Pharmakol.* 1899;42:109-118.
163. Mennerick S, Jevtovic-Todorovic V, Todorovic SM, Shen W, Olney JW, Zorumski CF. Effect of nitrous oxide on excitatory and inhibitory synaptic transmission in hippocampal cultures. *J Neurosci.* 1998;18:9716-9726.
164. Narahashi T, Aistrup GL, Lindstrom JM, et al. Ion channel modulation as the basis for general anesthesia. *Toxicol Lett.* 1998;100:185-191.
165. Franks NP, Lieb WR. Which molecular targets are most relevant to general anaesthesia? *Toxicol Lett.* 1998;100:1-8.
166. Olsen RW. The molecular mechanism of action of general anesthetics: structural aspects of interactions with GABAA receptors. *Toxicol Lett.* 1998;100:193-201.
167. Harrison NL, Kugler JL, Jones MV, Greenblatt EP, Pritchett DB. Positive modulation of human gamma-aminobutyric acid type A and glycine receptors by the inhalation anesthetic isoflurane. *Mol Pharmacol.* 1993;44:628-632.
168. Flood P, Role LW. Neuronal nicotinic acetylcholine receptor modulation by general anesthetics. *Toxicol Lett.* 1998;100:149-153.
169. Mascia MP, Machu TK, Harris RA. Enhancement of homomeric glycine receptor function by long-chain alcohols and anaesthetics. *Br J Pharmacol.* 1996;119:1331-1336.
170. Violet JM, Downie DL, Nakisa RC, Lieb WR, Franks NP. Differential sensitivities of mammalian neuronal and muscle nicotinic acetylcholine receptors to general anesthetics. *Anesthesiology.* 1997; 86:866-874.

171. Dilger JP, Vidal AM, Mody HI, Liu Y. Evidence for direct actions of general anesthetics on an ion channel protein: a new look at a unified mechanism of action. *Anesthesiology*. 1994; 81: 431-442.
172. Raines DE, Claycomb RJ, Scheller M, Forman SA. Nonhalogenated alkane anesthetics fail to potentiate agonist actions on two ligand-gated ion channels. *Anesthesiology*. 2001; 95:470-477.
173. Kendig JJ. In vitro networks: subcortical mechanisms of anaesthetic action. *Br J Anaesth*. 2002;89:91-101.
174. Jenkins A, Franks NP, Lieb WR. Actions of general anaesthetics on 5-HT3 receptors in N1E-115 neuroblastoma cells. *Br J Pharmacol*. 1996;117:1507-1515.
175. Perouansky M, Baranov D, Salman M, Yaari Y. Effects of halothane on glutamate receptor-mediated excitatory postsynaptic currents: a patch-clamp study in adult mouse hippocampal slices. *Anesthesiology*. 1995;83:109-119.
176. Lin LH, Chen LL, Harris RA. Enflurane inhibits NMDA, AMPA, and kainate-induced currents in Xenopus oocytes expressing mouse and human brain mRNA. *FASEB J*. 1993; 7:479-485.
177. Kohro S, Hogan QH, Nakae Y, Yamakage M, Bosnjak ZJ. Anesthetic effects on mitochondrial ATP-sensitive K channel. *Anesthesiology*. 2001;95:1435-1440.
178. Huneke R, Jungling E, Skasa M, et al. Effects of the anesthetic gases xenon, halothane, and isoflurane on calcium and potassium currents in human atrial cardiomyocytes. *Anesthesiology*. 2001;95:999-1006.
179. Yost CS. Potassium channels: basic aspects, functional roles, and medical significance. *Anesthesiology*. 1999;90:1186-1203.
180. Patel AJ, Honore E, Lesage F, Fink M, Romey G, Lazdunski M. Inhalational anesthetics activate two-pore-domain background K+ channels. *Nat Neurosci*. 1999;2:422-426.
181. Terrell RC. The invention and development of enflurane, isoflurane, sevoflurane and desflurane. *Anesthesiology*. 2008;108:531-533.
182. Lysko GS, Robinson JL, Casto R, Ferrone RA. The stereospecific effects of isoflurane isomers in vivo. *Eur J Pharmacol*. 1994;263: 25-29.
183. Franks NP, Lieb WR.What is the molecular nature of general anaesthetic target sights. *Trends Pharmacol Sci*. 1987;8: 169-174.
184. Moody EJ, Harris BD, Skolnick P. Stereospecific actions of the inhalation anesthetic isoflurane at the GABAA receptor complex. *Brain Res*. 1993;615:101-106.
185. Harris B, Moody EJ, Basile T, Skolnick P. Volatile anesthetics bidirectionally and stereospecifically modulate ligand binding to GABA receptors. *Eur J Pharmacol*. 1994;267:269-274.
186. Holaday DA, Fiserova-Bergerova V, Latto IP, Zumbiel MA. Resistance of isoflurane to biotransformation in man. *Anesthesiology*. 1975;43:325-332.
187. Quinn AC, Newman PJ, Hall GM, Grounds RM. Sevoflurane anaesthesia for major intra-abdominal surgery. *Anaesthesia*. 1994 49:567-571.
188. Frink EJ Jr, Malan P, Atlas M, Dominguez LM, DiNardo JA, Brown BR Jr. Clinical comparison of sevoflurane and isoflurane in healthy patients. *Anesth Analg*. 1992;74:241-245.
189. Kharasch ED, Thummel KE. Identification of cytochrome P450 2E1 as the predominant enzyme catalyzing human liver microsomal defluorination of sevoflurane, isoflurane, and methoxyflurane. *Anesthesiology*. 1993;79:795-807.
190. Van Obbergh LJ, Verbeeck RK, Michel I, et al. Extrahepatic metabolism of sevoflurane in children undergoing orthoptic liver transplantation. *Anesthesiology*. 2000;92:683-686.
191. Jiaxiang NI, Sato N, Fujii K, Yuge O. Urinary excretion of hexafluoroisopropanol glucuronide and fluoride in patients after sevoflurane anaesthesia. *J Pharm Pharmacol*. 1993; 45:67-69.
192. Van Hemelrijck J, Smith I, White PF. Use of desflurane for outpatient anesthesia: a comparison with propofol and nitrous oxide. *Anesthesiology*. 1991;75:197-203.
193. Wrigley SR, Fairfield JE, Jones RM, Black AE. Induction and recovery characteristics of desflurane in day case patients: a comparison with propofol. *Anaesthesia*. 1991;46:615-622.
194. Smiley RM, Ornstein E, Pantuck EJ, Pantuck CB, Matteo RS. Metabolism of desflurane and isoflurane to fluoride ion in surgical patients. *Can J Anaesth*. 1991;38:965-968.
195. Jones RM, Koblin DD, Cashman JN, Eger EI 2nd, Johnson BH, Damask MC. Biotransformation and hepato-renal function in volunteers after exposure to desflurane (I-653). *Br J Anaesth*. 1990;64:482-487.
196. White PF. Clinical uses of intravenous anesthetic and analgesic infusions. *Anesth Analg*. 1989;68:161-171.
197. Swerdlow BN, Holley FO. Intravenous anaesthetic agents: pharmacokinetic-pharmacodynamic relationships. *Clin Pharmacokinet*. 1987;12:79-110.
198. Schuttler J, Schwilden H, Stoeckel H. Pharmacokinetic-dynamic modelling of diprivan. *Anesthesiology*. 1986;65:A549.
199. Adam HK, Kay B, Douglas EJ. Blood disoprofol levels in anaesthetised patients. *Anaesthesia*. 1982;37:536-540.
200. Trapani G, Altomare C, Liso G, Sanna E, Biggio G. Propofol in anesthesia. Mechanism of action, structure-activity relationships, and drug delivery. *Curr Med Chem*. 2000;7: 249-271.
201. James R, Glen JB. Synthesis, biological evaluation, and preliminary structure-activity considerations of a series of alkylphenols as intravenous anesthetic agents. *J Med Chem*. 1980;23:1350-1357.
202. Diprivan(R), propofol US prescribing information. Fresenius Kabi USA, LLC. 2014. https://www.diprivan-us.com/wp-content/uploads/US-PH-Diprivan_FK-AU451575A_Jan_2020_Austria-PI.pdf
203. Oda Y, Hamaoka N, Hiroi T, et al. Involvement of human liver cytochrome P4502B6 in the metabolism of propofol. *Br J Clin Pharmacol*. 2001;51:281-285.
204. Sneyd JR, Simons PJ, Wright B. Use of proton NMR spectroscopy to measure propofol metabolites in the urine of the female Caucasian patient. *Xenobiotica*. 1994;24:1021-1028.
205. Simons PJ, Cockshott ID, Douglas EJ, Gordon EA, Hopkins K, Rowland M. Disposition in male volunteers of a subanaesthetic intravenous dose of an oil in water emulsion of 14C-propofol. *Xenobiotica*. 1988;18:429-440.
206. Sanna E, Murgia A, Casula A, Biggio G. Differential subunit dependence of the actions of the general anesthetics alphaxalone and etomidate at gamma-aminobutyric acid type A receptors expressed in Xenopus laevis oocytes. *Mol Pharmacol*. 1997;51:484-490.
207. Rüsch D, Zhong H, Forman SA. Gating allosterism at a single class of etomidate sites on alpha1beta2gamma2L GABA A receptors accounts for both direct activation and agonist modulation. *J Biol Chem*. 2004;279:20982-20989.
208. Godefroi EF, Janssen PAJ, Van der Eycken CAM, Vanheertum AH, Niemegeers CJ. DL-(1-arylalkyl)imidazole-5-carboxylate esters. A novel type of hypnotic agents. *J Med Chem*. 1965;56:220-223.
209. Tornetta FJ, Song S, Smoyer AD. Etomidate: a pharmacologic profile of a new hypnotic. *J Am Assoc Nurse Anesthetists*. 1980;48:517-525.
210. Morgan M, Lumley J, Whitwam JG. Etomidate, a new water-soluble nonbarbiturate intravenous induction agent. *Lancet*. 1975;1:955-956.
211. Fragen RJ, Caldwell N, Brunner EA. Clinical use of etomidate for anesthesia induction: a preliminary report. *Anesth Analg*. 1976;55:730-733.
212. Gooding JM, Corssen G: Etomidate: an ultrashort-acting nonbarbiturate agent for anesthesia induction. *Anesth Analg*. 1976;55: 286-288.
213. White PF, Way WL, Trevor AJ. Ketamine—its pharmacology and therapeutic uses. *Anesthesiology*. 1982;56:119-136.
214. Marietta MP, Way WL, Castagnoli N Jr, Trevor AJ. On the pharmacology of the ketamine enantiomorphs in the rat. *J Pharmacol Exp Ther*. 1977;202:157-165.

215. Zarantonello P, Bettini E, Paio A, Simoncelli C, Terreni S, Cardullo F. Novel analogues of ketamine and phencyclidine as NMDA receptor antagonists. *Bioorg Med Chem Lett.* 2011;21:2059-2063.
216. Ketalar(R), ketamine hydrochloride. US prescribing information. Monarch Pharmaceuticals, Inc. 1998. https://labeling.pfizer.com/ShowLabeling.aspx?id=14017
217. Grant IS, Nimmo WS, Clements JA. Pharmacokinetics and analgesic effects of IM and oral ketamine. *Br J Anaesth.* 1981;53:805-810.
218. Kreter B. Ketamine as an anesthetic agent for interventional radiology. *Semin Intervent Radiol.* 1987;4:183-188.
219. Desta Z, Moaddel R, Ogburn ET, et al. Stereoselective and regiospecific hydroxylation of ketamine and norketamine. *Xenobiotica.* 2012;42:1076-1087.
220. Kharasch ED, Herrmann S, Labroo R. Ketamine as a probe for medetomidine stereoisomer inhibition of human liver microsomal drug metabolism. *Anesthesiology.* 1992;77: 1208-1214.
221. Yanagihara Y, Kariya S, Ohtani M, et al. Involvement of CYP2B6 in N-demethylation of ketamine in human liver microsomes. *Drug Metab Dispos.* 2001;29:887-890.
222. Portmann S, Kwan HY, Theurillat R, Schmitz A, Mevissen M, Thormann W. Enantioselective capillary electrophoresis for identification and characterization of human cytochrome P450 enzymes which metabolize ketamine and norketamine in vitro. *J Chromatogr A.* 2010;1217:7942-7948.
223. Hijazi Y, Boulieu R. Contribution of CYP3A4, CYP2B6, and CYP2C9 isoforms to N-demethylation of ketamine in human liver microsomes. *Drug Metab Dispos.* 2002;30:853-858.
224. Li Y, Coller JK, Hutchinson MR, et al. The CYP2B6*6 allele significantly alters the N-demethylation of ketamine enantiomers in vitro. *Drug Metab Dispos.* 2013;41:1264-1272.
225. King H. Curare alkaloids. Part 1: tubocurarine. *J Chem Soc.* 1935;5:1381-1389.
226. Beers WH, Reich E. Structure and activity of acetylcholine. *Nature.* 1970;22: 917-922.
227. Paton WDM, Zaimis EJ. The pharmacological actions of polymethylene bistrimethylammonium salts. *Br J Pharmacol.* 1949;4381-4400.
228. Lee C. Structure, conformation, and action of neuromuscular blocking drugs. *Br J Anaesth.* 2001;87:755-769.
229. Savage DS, Cameron AF, Ferguson G, Hannaway C, Mackay IR. Molecular structure of pancuronium bromide (3α,17β-diacetoxy-2β,16β-dipiperidino-5α-androstane dimethobromide), a neuromuscular blocking agent. Crystal and molecular structure of the water: methylene chloride solvate. *J Chem Soc B.* 1971;410-415.
230. Buckett WR, Hewett CL, Savage DS. Pancuronium bromide and other steroidal neuromuscular blocking agents containing acetylcholine fragments. *J Med Chem.* 1973;16:1116-1124.
231. Donati F, Bevan JC, Devan DR. Neuromuscular blocking drugs in anaesthesia. *Can Anaesth Soc J.* 1984;31:324-335.
232. Thompson MA. Muscle relaxant drugs. *Br J Hosp Med.* 1980;23:164-179.
233. Ramzan MI, Somogyi AA, Walker JS, Shanks CA, Triggs EJ. Clinical pharmacokinetics of the nondepolarizing muscle relaxants. *Clin Pharmacokinet.* 1981;6:25-60.
234. Agoston S, Vermeer GA, Kertsten UW, Meijer DK. The fate of pancuronium bromide in man. *Acta Anaesthesiol Scand.* 1973;17:267-275.
235. Hilgenberg JC. Comparison of the pharmacology of vecuronium and atracurium with that of other currently available muscle relaxants. *Anesth Analg.* 1983;62:524-531.
236. Segredo V, Matthay MA, Sharma ML, Gruenke LD, Caldwell JE, Miller RD. Prolonged neuromuscular blockade after long-term administration of vecuronium in two critically ill patients. *Anesthesiology.* 1990;72:566-570.
237. Watling SM, Dasta JF. Prolonged paralysis in intensive care unit patients after the use of neuromuscular blocking agents: a review of the literature. *Crit Car Med.* 1994;22:884-893.
238. Wierda JMKH, Kleef UW, Lambalk LM, Kloppenburg WD, Agoston S. The pharmacodynamics and pharmacokinetics of Org 9426, a new non-depolarizing neuromuscular blocking agent, in patients anaesthetized with nitrous oxide, halothane and fentanyl. *Can J Anaesth.* 1991;38:430-435.
239. Agoston S, Vandenbrom RHG, Wierda JMKH. Clinical pharmacokinetics of neuromuscular blocking drugs. *Clin Pharmacokinet.* 1992;22:94-115.
240. Basta SJ, Ali HH, Savarese JJ, et al. Clinical pharmacology of atracurium besylate (BW 33A): a new non-depolarizing muscle relaxant. *Anesth Analg.* 1982; 61:723-729.
241. Stenlake JB, Waigh RD, Urwin J, Dewar GH, Coker GG. Atracurium: conception and inception. *Br J Anaesth.* 1983;55: 3S-10S.

Clinical Scenario

ANESTHESIA AND SEDATIVE HYPNOTICS

Susan W. Miller, PharmD and Nader H. Moniri, PhD

BR, a 72-year-old White woman underwent surgery to repair a fracture of her right hip at 7:30 AM. The anesthesiologist used propofol as the anesthetic for the procedure. BR's medical problems (and medications) include type 2 diabetes (glipizide 5 mg orally every day), hypertension (metoprolol tartrate 50 mg and hydrochlorothiazide 25 mg orally every day), osteoporosis (alendronate 70 mg orally once weekly, calcium citrate 200 mg/vitamin D 250 IU 2 tabs orally twice a day), and chronic insomnia (ramelteon 8 mg orally as needed at bedtime). BR's medical problems are under control and stable, with a hemoglobin A1C at 6.8%, and a blood pressure at 126/78 mm Hg. BR took all of her medications as prescribed on the day prior to surgery and was *nil per os* starting at 11:00 PM the night prior to the surgery, except for her metoprolol/hydrochlorothiazide dose that she took at 6:00 am on the morning of the surgery with a sip of water. BR's 150-minute (2 ½ hour) surgery was successful and she was transferred to recovery about 10:00 AM. In the waiting room, BR's daughter is very concerned that her mom should get a good night's sleep and asks if there is an order for the ramelteon that she usually takes about 9:00 PM every night. Should BR receive the 8-mg dose of ramelteon at 9:00 PM? Are there additional concerns regarding BR's chronic medications and the propofol used for anesthesia during the surgical procedure?

CHEMICAL ANALYSIS

Propofol: Propofol induces anesthesia by decreasing the dissociation GABA binding from the GABAA receptor, thereby promoting the effects of endogenous GABA at the receptor, which includes neuronal hyperpolarization and CNS depression.

Clinical Scenario (continued)

Based on its mechanism, propofol potentiates the effects of other GABAergic acting agents, including benzodiazepines, Z-drugs, and barbiturates. Propofol is highly lipophilic and produces rapid effects due to fast blood-brain equilibration, followed by rapid redistribution from the CNS, which directly influences its duration. Propofol also exhibits a rapid clearance rate, roughly 10-fold faster than thiobarbiturates, allowing for fast recovery from the anesthetic effects. Additionally, propofol is rapidly metabolized rapidly via direct 1-position conjugation or phase I oxidation via CYP2B6, which is followed by 4- or 1-position conjugation to hydrophilic and readily excreted metabolites:

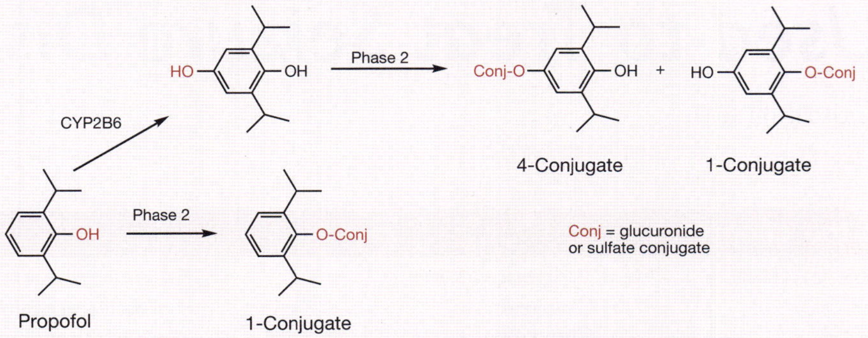

Ramelteon: Ramelteon induces sedative hypnotic effects independently of GABA-acting systems, via activation of MT1 and MT2 melatonin receptors in the hypothalamus. Ramelteon exhibits nearly 10-fold selectivity toward MT1, consistent with its greater effects in sleep rather than circadian rhythm regulation. Ramelteon has an elimination half-life of 1 to 2.5 hours and is primarily excreted via phase I metabolism and phase II conjugation; however, the major metabolite (MII) is active at MT1R/MT2R, and exhibits a 2- to 5-hour half-life and slower removal from circulation:

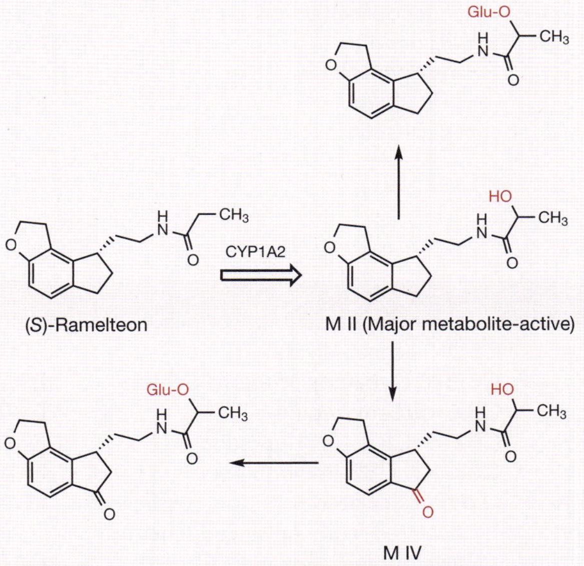

While propofol and ramelteon affect distinct sleep-promoting pathways and the latter is free from GABAergic modulation, they are both classified as CNS depressants that facilitate similar clinical outcomes related to the range of sedation, hypnosis, and anesthesia. Important considerations include the half-lives of propofol, ramelteon, and its active MII metabolite, as well as any drug interactions that may interfere with proper metabolism of either agent.

Furthermore, the health care provider should monitor the clinical status of the patient related to sedation and sleep in order to determine if ramelteon can be administered safely the night of the surgery. *If the clinical status of BR is stable at 9:00 pm, the ramelteon dose may be administered.*

Moreover, BR is on metoprolol and hydrochlorothiazide for blood pressure, and propofol can further reduce blood pressure by inducing vasodilation and decreased peripheral resistance due to altered sympathetic tone. In addition, metoprolol, hydrochlorothiazide, and propofol can also cause bradycardia and decreased cardiac output, necessitating the health care provider to monitor this potential effect. An additional postoperative consideration, particularly in older adults and those with a history of insomnia or sleep-wake disturbance, is postoperative delirium, which is another factor that should be monitored. *The care team should closely monitor the postoperative clinical status of BR, particularly in regard to the cardiac status and mental status and adjust therapy as necessary.*

CHAPTER

15

Drugs Used to Treat Seizure Disorders

Christopher W. Cunningham

Drugs covered in this chapter:

VOLTAGE-GATED SODIUM CHANNEL BLOCKERS:
- Carbamazepine
- Eslicarbazepine acetate
- Fosphenytoin
- Lacosamide
- Lamotrigine
- Oxcarbazepine
- Phenytoin
- Rufinamide

VOLTAGE-GATED CALCIUM CHANNEL BLOCKERS:
- Ethosuximide
- Gabapentin
- Pregabalin

GABA MODULATORS:
- Clobazam
- Clonazepam
- Clorazepate
- Diazepam
- Ganaxolone
- Lorazepam
- Midazolam
- Phenobarbital
- Primidone
- Stiripentol
- Tiagabine
- Vigabatrin

GLUTAMATE ANTAGONISTS:
- Brivaracetam
- Levetiracetam
- Perampanel

MULTIMODAL ANTISEIZURE MEDICATIONS:
- Cannabidiol
- Cenobamate
- Felbamate
- Fenfluramine
- Topiramate
- Valproic acid
- Zonisamide

Abbreviations

ADH alcohol dehydrogenase
AKR aldo-keto reductase
ALT alanine transaminase
AMPA α-amino-3-hydroxy-5-methyl-4-isoxazolepropionic acid
AMPAR α-amino-3-hydroxy-5-methyl-4-isoxazolepropionic acid receptor
ASM antiseizure medication
AUC area under the (dose-response) curve
BBB blood-brain barrier
BCS Biopharmaceutics Classification System
BDNF brain-derived neurotrophic factor
BZR benzodiazepine receptor
CA carbonic anhydrase
Ca_v voltage-gated calcium channels
CB1R cannabinoid receptor 1
CB2R cannabinoid receptor 2
CBD cannabidiol
CBDQ cannabidiolquinone
CBDV cannabidivarin
CBMA carbamoylpropionaldehyde
CBZ carbamazepine
CBZ-E CBZ-10,11-epoxide
CBZ-IQ CBZ-iminoquinone
cLogP calculated partition coefficient calculated from Advanced Chemical Development, Toronto, Canada, 2018
CNS central nervous system
CRMP2 collapsin response mediator protein 2
DDI drug-drug interaction
DEA Drug Enforcement Administration
DHFR dihydrofolate reductase
DMT *N*,*N*-dimethyltryptamine
DRESS drug reaction with eosinophilia and systemic symptoms
EAAC-1 excitatory amino acid carrier-1
ECSS endocannabinoid signaling system
EEG electroencephalography
ESL eslicarbazepine acetate
EWG electron-withdrawing group
FAAH fatty acid amide hydrolase
FABP fatty acid–binding protein
FDA U.S. Food and Drug Administration
GABA γ-aminobutyric acid
GABA-AT GABA aminotransferase
GABA-T GABA transaminase
GAD glutamate decarboxylase
GAT1 GABA transporter 1
$GEFS_+$ generalized epilepsy with febrile seizures plus
GIT gastrointestinal tract
GVG γ-vinyl-GABA
HBA hydrogen bond acceptor
hCE human carboxyesterase
HPPH 5-(4′-hydroxyphenyl)-5-phenylhydantoin
3α-HSD 3α-hydroxysteroid dehydrogenase

Abbreviations—continued

5-HT_2 type-2 serotonin receptors
HVA high voltage–activated
ILAE International League Against Epilepsy
IM intramuscular
I_{NaP} persistent sodium current
I_{NaT} transient sodium current
IR immediate release
IV intravenous
KR kainate receptor
LAT system L amino acid transporter
MAOIs monoamine oxidase inhibitors
MDMA methylenedioxymethamphetamine
MHD monohydroxyderivatives
MOA mechanism of action
mTOR mammalian target of rapamycin
MZD midazolam
Na_v voltage-gated sodium channels
NDA New Drug Application
NDMC *N*-desmethylclobazam
NIH National Institutes of Health
NMDAR *N*-methyl-D-aspartate receptor
OXC oxcarbazepine
PAM positive allosteric modulator
PAP pyridoxamine-5′-phosphate
PEMA phenylethylmalonamide
P-gp P-glycoprotein
PK pharmacokinetics
PKU phenylketonuria
PLP pyridoxal-5′-phosphate
REMS Risk Evaluation and Mitigation Strategy
SAR structure-activity relationship
SERT serotonin transporter
SHARE Support, Help, and Resources for Epilepsy Program
SJS Stevens-Johnson syndrome
SNRIs serotonin/norepinephrine reuptake inhibitors
SRA serotonin-releasing agent
SSAH succinic semialdehyde
SSRIs selective serotonin reuptake inhibitors
SV2 synaptic vesicle 2
TEN toxic epidermal necrosis
Δ^9-THC Δ^9 -tetrahydrocannabinol
TPSA topological polar surface area
TRP transient receptor potential
TSC tuberous sclerosis complex
UGT UDP-glucuronosyltransferase
UV ultravoilet
V_d volume of distribution
VFD visual field defects
VPA valproic acid
WHO World Health Organization

CLINICAL SIGNIFICANCE

Antiepileptic/anticonvulsant medications often represent the pinnacle of the clinician decision-making conundrum in medicine: risk versus benefit, therapeutic versus toxic, and desirable versus undesirable effects for patients. Many of these medications are impacted by protein binding, plagued by a narrow therapeutic index, and are associated with unique adverse effects. This creates challenges not only in seizure management, but also in the patient experience. For clinicians, an understanding of the wide scope of medicinal chemistry and pharmacology is necessary to managing this fine balance and the dose-response relationship. Understanding the significance of the pharmacology of voltage-gated channel blockade informs agent selection and monitoring for seizure prevention and management. Distinguishing the structure and binding behavior of the γ-aminobutyric acid (GABA)-A modulators permits clinician drug selection to halt existing seizure activity and represents a critical tool for those responding to toxicity-induced seizures. Recognizing that many epilepsy patients require multimodal therapy, knowledge of unique mechanisms of medications like levetiracetam, zonisamide, cannabidiol, and others is vital for creating an effective therapy plan for patients.

Elizabeth A. Laubach, PharmD, DABAT

Overview of Seizure Disorders

Epileptic seizures were documented over 4,000 years ago in early Babylonian and Hebrew writings. The work of Hippocrates, *On the Sacred Disease* (400 BC), was the first to characterize epileptic seizures as a treatable medical disorder and not a product of spiritual origin. To this point, seizure disorders were seen as a divine affliction handed down by the gods; the remedies include avoiding "unwholesome" foods and shunning black robes that are "expressive of death." However, Hippocrates proposed that seizures are a result of a hereditary dysregulation of the patient's brain. This is largely seen as a turning point in medicine: if seizures are due to an affliction in the brain, then they might be treatable with the proper medication.[1]

A seminal publication on the modern treatments of seizure disorders was released by British epileptologist William Aldren Turner in 1907. His book, *Epilepsy–A Study of the Idiopathic Disease*, outlined a patient-centered approach to treating epileptic seizures that focused on the use of medications to stop active seizures and prophylactic treatments, control of diet, stress management, and also surgery to prevent future seizures. Turner considered bromide salts, first reported in the mid-1800s in London,[2] as the treatment of choice for patients with uncontrolled epilepsy. His studies concluded that bromide therapy was effective in 50% of his patients, with long-term remission in 23.5%; however, use of chronic, high-dose bromides resulted in "bromism," which, he remarked, "is characterized by a blunting of the intellectual faculties, impairment of the memory, and the production of a dull and apathetic state."[3] The use of bromides continued into the early 20th century when small molecule antiepileptic drugs, phenobarbital (phenobarbitone) and phenytoin, emerged as rivals with improved outcomes, in the 1920s to 1930s.

The period between 1938 and 1958 saw the approval of 14 antiseizure medications (ASMs) by the U.S. Food and Drug Administration (FDA). The first-in-class medications were discovered largely through serendipitous findings in animal seizure models, and combinations of these medications were often more effective at preventing seizures, than one drug alone. More effective second-generation ASMs were developed in the 1950s to 1970s, which operate simultaneously through multiple mechanisms of action (MOA) and can be used as monotherapy. The third-generation ASMs were developed using modern drug discovery and medicinal chemistry techniques to avoid the side effects of first- and second-generation agents. Despite the many advances made, modern ASM therapy still suffers from some of the same side effects that Dr Turner observed in his bromide-treated patients: somnolence, memory impairment, and cognitive slowing, hindering patient satisfaction and compliance. Newer medications that operate through novel, nonion channel inhibitory mechanisms may provide therapeutic benefits without these adverse cognitive effects.

Epilepsy affects 2.2 to 3 million Americans and more than 65 million people worldwide. An estimated one in 26 people in the United States will develop epilepsy at some point in their lives, making it the fourth most common neurological disorder. Recent estimates put the costs of treating seizure disorders around US$15.5 billion. This figure does not include the intangible adverse impact of seizure disorders on patients' quality of life.[4]

What Are Seizures?

Definitions of epileptic seizures and epilepsy are available from the International League Against Epilepsy (ILAE). An epileptic seizure is "a transient occurrence of signs and/or symptoms due to abnormal excessive or synchronous neuronal activity in the brain."[5] A hallmark of this abnormal neuronal activity is the rapid firing of electrical impulses caused by uncontrolled ion-channel gating. These electrical impulses are monitored using electroencephalography (EEG). EEG measures the fluctuation of electric current throughout the brain using noninvasive electrodes attached to the skin. Analysis of EEG readouts helps clinicians diagnose epilepsy and seizure disorders: for example, diagnosis of Lennox-Gastaut syndrome is aided by EEGs that show a definitive pattern of slow, sharp waves and paroxysmal fast activity.[6] When a patient experiences a single seizure for 5 or more minutes, or two seizures within 5 minutes, they are said to be experiencing status epilepticus.

The ILAE defines epilepsy as "a disorder of the brain characterized by an enduring predisposition to generate epileptic seizures and by the neurobiologic, cognitive, psychologic, and societal consequences of this condition."[5] These definitions clarify that a patient must experience at least one epileptic seizure in order to be diagnosed with epilepsy. Seizures may be either symptomatic—meaning the underlying cause for the seizure is known—or idiopathic. For example, symptomatic seizures may result from brain lesions, cortical malformations, or tumors, whereas the mechanisms causing idiopathic seizures are unknown. Distinguishing between classifications of seizures and epilepsy disorders is critical to providing optimal patient care. For example, patients with Dravet syndrome—a symptomatic seizure disorder—should not be administered lamotrigine and carbamazepine, as these the ASMs may exacerbate seizures in these patients.[7,8]

Types of Seizures

Seizure types are classified based on three key parameters: (1) onset of action, (2) the level of consciousness in the patient, and (3) whether motor symptoms are observed. The ILAE has published guidelines that clarify these seizure types (Table 15.1).[9] These guidelines were developed, in part, to be easier to understand and to aid in classification of previously difficult-to-classify seizure types. These guidelines may also permit targeted selection of the appropriate medications to treat different disease states. Throughout this section, we will refer to historically used terms; their modern counterparts can also be found in Table 15.1.

Table 15.1 Classification of Seizure Types

Onset (ILAE 2017)[a]	Examples
Partial Onset (Focal)	
Simple (aware)	
Complex (impaired awareness)	
Motor onset	Automatisms, atonic, clonic, epileptic spasms, hyperkinetic, myoclonic, tonic
Nonmotor onset	Autonomic, behavior arrest, cognitive, emotional, sensory
Generalized Onset	
Motor onset	Tonic-clonic or grand mal seizures, myoclonic, atonic, epileptic spasms
Nonmotor onset	Absence or petit mal seizures, myoclonic
Unknown Onset	
Motor onset	Epileptic spasms, tonic-clonic
Nonmotor onset	Behavior arrest

Seizures are first classified by their region of onset, if it is known. Partial seizures are then classified according to the level of consciousness of the patient. All seizures are classified according to whether abnormal motor function is present (motor onset) or absent (nonmotor onset).

[a]Modern terms proposed by the ILAE in 2017.

Adapted from Fisher RS, Cross JH, French JA, et al. Operational classification of seizure types by the International League Against epilepsy: position paper of the ILAE Commission for classification and terminology. *Epilepsia*. 2017;58(4):522-530.

Seizures are first classified by the degree of localization of onset in the brain. Seizures that are generalized originate simultaneously throughout the cortex in two or more of the frontal, temporal, parietal, and occipital lobes. Focal seizures (partial seizures) are those that are localized initially in a single region. A distinguishing factor between generalized and partial seizures is whether patients experience physical responses throughout the whole body as opposed to only a single region. For example, a patient experiencing visual disturbances without cognitive impairment may be experiencing a seizure localized within the occipital lobe. Seizures where the region of onset was missed or is obscured would be considered unknown onset seizures.

Partial or focal seizures can be further subdivided by the patient's level of awareness during the event. A seizure is considered simple or aware when a patient is conscious and maintains memory during the seizure; conversely, a seizure is classified as complex or impaired awareness if any of these features is lost at any point during the event. The new terminology for a simple partial seizure is "focal aware seizure," and a complex partial seizure can be considered a "focal impaired awareness seizure." Simple partial seizures are the most common form of seizure in adults. When describing a seizure event, the patient's level of awareness may not be communicated, particularly if it is either not known or not applicable. For example, impaired awareness may not be able to be communicated explicitly in a patient experiencing a generalized seizure.

Seizures can be further categorized as motor or nonmotor onset based on the most prominent observed effects. A motor seizure is the one that causes the patient to experience motor disturbances, whereas a seizure that does not cause motor disturbances is considered a nonmotor or absence seizure. Tonic motor seizures cause an increase in muscle tone, which results in sudden muscle stiffening. The affected muscles are related to the localization of the seizure: for example, a seizure that results in sudden stiffening of only a single region of the body would be considered a partial or focal tonic seizure, whereas seizures that affect the whole body tonus would be considered a generalized tonic seizure. A clonic seizure is the one that causes the patient's muscles to contract and relax rapidly (a "clonus"). As with tonic seizures, clonic seizures can be either generalized or partial. A patient who experiences tonic effects followed by clonic effects is experiencing a tonic-clonic seizure, sometimes referred to as grand mal. The duration of the clonus in a tonic-clonic seizure can be several minutes. Myoclonic seizures are those that affect a single muscle or a group of muscles and result in brief spasms that last on the order of seconds. Myoclonic seizures typically affect both sides of the body simultaneously. Absence seizures were previously called petit mal seizures, and are characterized by a brief loss of consciousness and return to normal function without subsequent lethargy.

Epilepsy Syndromes

The ILAE defines an epilepsy syndrome as "a group of clinical entities that are reliably identified by a cluster of electroclinical characteristics."[10] Epilepsy syndromes are classified by the type of seizures experienced, their frequency, and the patient population affected. Not all epilepsy syndromes may be treated using ASMs; for example, seizures from benign rolandic epilepsy generally remit spontaneously before adulthood, and ASMs may not provide much added benefit.[11]

Dravet syndrome in infants younger than age 1 often begins as severe febrile seizures, which are seizures precipitated by hyperthermia. These seizures progress to myoclonic or tonic-clonic seizures and may precipitate developmental delay. In 70% to 85% of cases, Dravet syndrome is associated with a missense mutation in the *SNC1A* gene encoding the voltage-gated sodium channel 1α subunit ($Na_V1.1$) that causes a loss-of-function phenotype.[12,13] Patients with Dravet syndrome should not be treated with Na_V channel blockers, which may exacerbate the pathology inherent in this phenotype.

Lennox-Gastaut syndrome is a childhood-onset epilepsy syndrome characterized by (1) tonic, atonic, and atypical absence seizures, (2) cognitive and behavioral abnormalities, (3) EEGs with generalized or diffuse slow spikes and waves, and generalized paroxysmal fast activity. Comorbidities, such as autism, cognitive, and behavioral delays, are common. Treatment of Lennox-Gastaut syndrome is challenging: over 90% of children with Lennox-Gastaut syndrome have drug-resistant epilepsy, and patients may experience additive side effects from the use of multiple medications.[14] When traditional pharmacologic treatments are ineffective, patients may experience benefits from a ketogenic diet.[15] Surgical options include the use of vagal nerve stimulation and corpus callostomy, wherein the corpus callosum is severed to block the spread of generalized seizures from one brain hemisphere to the other.[16]

West syndrome, more generally termed epileptic spasms or infantile spasms, is a rare seizure disorder in infants and young children that is characterized by three symptoms: (1) myoclonic convulsions ("lightning attacks") that affect the whole body, (2) sudden convulsions of neck muscles that cause the chin to jerk toward the chest ("nodding attacks"), (3) sudden flexor spasms of the trunk and contraction of the legs and arms ("jackknife or Salaam attacks"). Most cases of West syndrome are symptomatic, rather than idiopathic. The most common cause of West syndrome is tuberous sclerosis complex (TSC), a genetic condition associated with benign tumors that precipitate seizures. Targeted therapies to treat TSC, and possibly West syndrome, are in development.

Physiologic Mechanisms Involved in Seizures

Seizures are the result of uncontrolled, asynchronous neuronal firing. Although the source(s) of this uncontrolled signaling can differ between seizure disorders and epileptic syndromes, all pharmacologic treatments modulate excitatory and inhibitory neurotransmission. Most classes of ASMs block seizures through one of the three general mechanisms: (1) direct modulation of ion channels involved in neuronal depolarization, (2) inhibition of excitatory neurotransmission, and (3) enhancement of inhibitory neurotransmission. A visual representation of the pharmacologic targets of ASMs can be found in Figure 15.1.

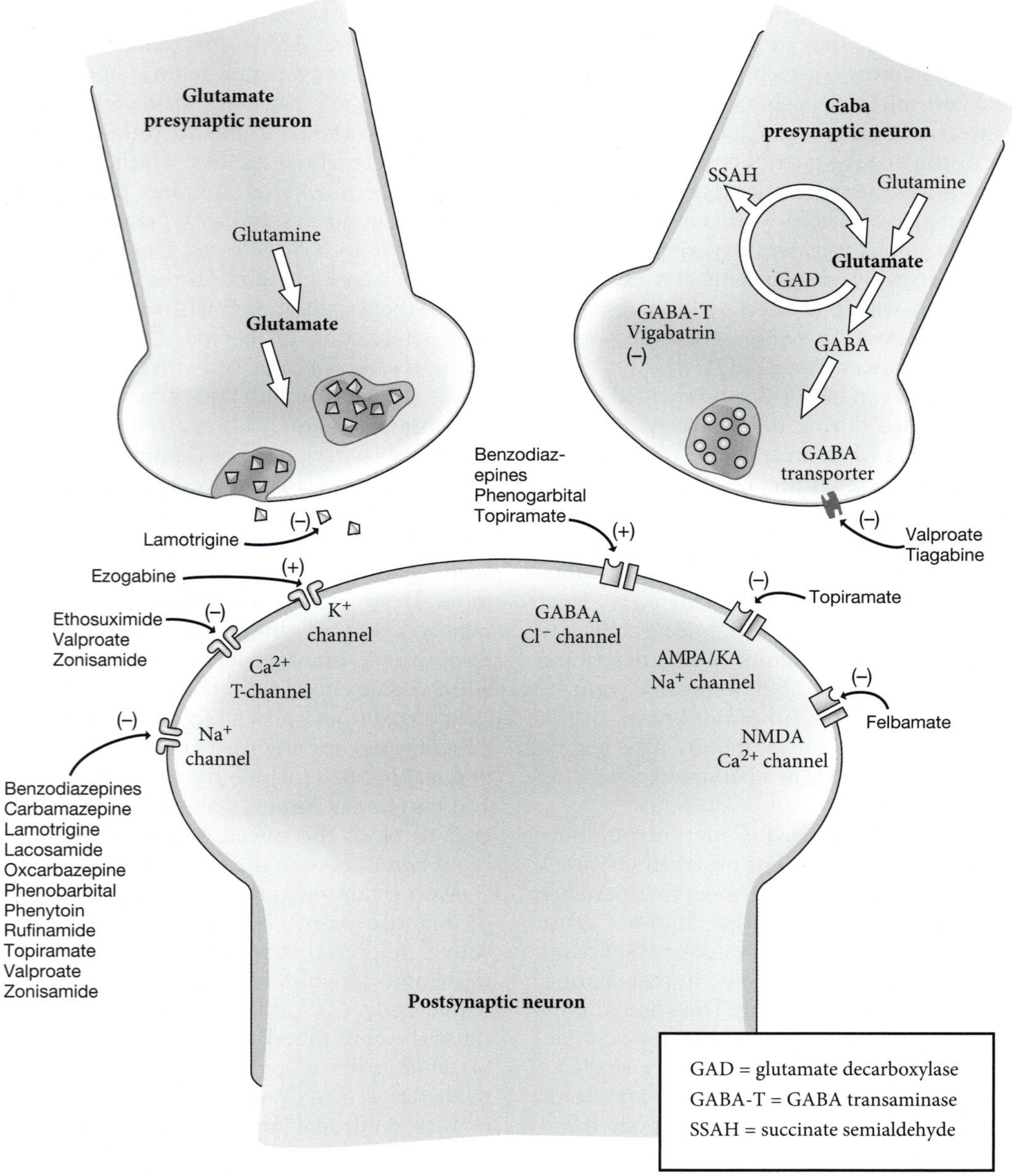

Figure 15.1 Summary of the sites of action for the antiepileptic drugs. (Adapted from Taylor CP. Mechanisms of new antiepileptic drugs. In: Delgado-Escueta AV, Wilson WA, Olsen RW, Olsen RW, Delgado-Escueta AV, eds. *Jasper's Basic Mechanisms of the Epilepsies.* 3rd ed. Advances in Neurology, Vol 79. Lippincott Williams & Wilkins; 1999:1012-1027, with permission.)

As described in more detail in Chapter 8, neurons maintain a resting potential of −70 mV. This polarized state is normally maintained by ion channels that regulate the movement of anions and cations across the cellular membrane. Channel opening that permits the influx of positively charged metal ions—sodium (Na^+), potassium (K^+), calcium (Ca^{2+})—causes cellular depolarization. Once the membrane potential is approximately −55 mV, it is said to have reached the threshold potential. Reaching the threshold potential triggers a rapid depolarization phase, which initiates an action potential at approximately +40 mV. After depolarization, a repolarization phase occurs, returning the membrane potential to a hyperpolarized state below −70 mV (approximately −80 mV). Hyperpolarization is reached when ion channels open to permit efflux of Na^+ or K^+ or influx of chloride (Cl^-) ions.

Ion channels activated by neurotransmitters are considered ligand-gated ion channels. Once released to the synapse, excitatory neurotransmitters like glutamate and aspartate activate ion channels such as α-amino-3-hydroxy-5-methyl-4-isoxazolepropionic acid receptors (AMPARs), *N*-methyl-D-aspartate receptors (NMDARs), and kainate receptors (KRs). These channels facilitate the influx of Na^+ and Ca^{2+} ions, which leads to cellular depolarization. Thus, AMPAR, NMDAR, and KR blockers are able to attenuate uncontrolled neuronal firing associated with epilepsy. Following ion-channel activation, excess glutamate and aspartate is taken up into presynaptic cells by excitatory amino acid transporters (EAACs), notably EAAC-1. In contrast, binding of the inhibitory neurotransmitter γ-aminobutyric acid (GABA) to the $GABA_A$ ion channel causes a conformational change, which permits influx of Cl^-. This causes cellular hyperpolarization, which makes the neuron less capable of firing. Positive allosteric modulators (PAMs) of $GABA_A$ channels block seizures by lowering the membrane potential of the cell.

Ion channels that are responsive to changes in membrane potential and not activated by neurotransmitters are called voltage-gated ion channels. A voltage-gated channel that senses a threshold potential will change conformation from a closed, resting state to an open, active state that is permeable to small metal ions (eg, Na^+, K^+, Ca^{2+}). Once the action potential has been reached, these channels adopt an inactive state conformation that is unresponsive to a stimulus. This is different from a resting state in that a channel in a resting state can respond to a suitable electric potential.

Voltage-gated ion channels are classified based on ionic permeability: for example, voltage-gated sodium (Na_v) channels are exclusively permeable to Na^+ ions. Because they respond quickly to membrane potentials, voltage-gated ion channels are involved in the rapid depolarization and repolarization phases of the action potential. Once the threshold potential is reached, postsynaptic Na_v channels open to permit the influx of Na^+ ions, causing neuronal depolarization. Reaching the action potential triggers two events: first, Na_v channels close, adopting an inactive state that limits Na^+ influx and depolarization. Then, postsynaptic voltage-gated potassium channels open, permitting the influx of K^+ ions into the cell. These two events combine to form the rapid repolarization phase of the action potential.

Voltage-gated calcium (Ca_v) channels mediate the release of excitatory neurotransmitters from presynaptic vesicles. The Ca_v channels consist of pore-forming α1 subunits, an extracellular glycoprotein dimer of α2δ subunits, and an intracellular β subunit.[17] Although dozens of Ca_v channels are expressed throughout the body, the most relevant to epileptic disorders are the P/Q-type ("Purkinje") channels and N-type ("neural") channels. These channels are expressed throughout the brain, with P/Q-type channels located in high concentrations on Purkinje neurons in the cerebellum. These channels are members of the high voltage–activated (HVA) family of voltage-gated ion channels. A critical role of HVA Ca_v channels is to mediate the release of glutamate from presynaptic vesicles in response to a high-voltage action potential, thereby propagating a signal. Thus, agents that inhibit glutamate release would decrease neuronal signaling by reducing excitatory neurotransmission. Low voltage–activated Ca_v channels are also known as T-type ("transient") or Ca_v3. T-type Ca_v channels can open at lower membrane potential and have smaller, shorter conductance. Hyperfunction of Ca_v3 channels contributes specifically to absence seizures.

Presynaptic vesicles respond to intracellular Ca^{2+} by releasing excitatory neurotransmitters. The synaptic vesicle 2 (SV2) family of membrane glycoproteins consists of three isoforms (SV2A, SV2B, SV2C) that are expressed on vesicular membranes throughout the brain. Of these, SV2A is the most widely expressed on glutamatergic and GABAergic vesicles. SV2A regulates the response of vesicles to an increase in intracellular Ca^{2+} mediated by presynaptic Ca^{2+} ion channels. Because SV2A is expressed on both excitatory and inhibitory vesicles, regulation of protein expression and function is critical to maintaining proper neuronal excitability. For example, both genetic knockout animals and overexpressing SV2A animals show a proconvulsant phenotype, perhaps due to decreased inhibitory neurotransmission and increased excitatory neurotransmission, respectively.[18,19] Animal studies also suggest an increase in SV2A expression in response to seizure kindling[20]; therefore, agents that control SV2A function regulate the neuronal hyperactivity during seizures. "Kindling" here refers to the process by which an animal seizure model is generated by repeated electrical stimulation, resulting in a permanent epilepsy state.

Inherited genetic mutations that affect ion-channel function are called channelopathies.[21] The most common channelopathies associated with seizure disorders affect Na^+ and K^+ channels that are involved in the fast depolarization and repolarization phases, respectively. In generalized epilepsy with febrile seizures plus (GEFS+), mutations in the *SCN1A* gene result in modifications of the pore-forming α-subunit of $Na_V1.1$, which can lead to hyperexcitability. Mutation of the *SCN1B* gene impairs the ability of β-subunits to inactivate $Na_V\beta1$ channels, causing an extended depolarization phase.[22,23] Mutations to voltage-gated potassium-channel genes *KCNQ2* and *KCNQ3* are associated with benign neonatal epilepsy disorders.[22-27] Genetic disruption of GABAergic signaling is associated with human idiopathic epilepsies. Mutations to the *GABRA1* and *GABRG2* genes result in impaired $GABA_A$-channel function due to modifications of α1 and γ2 subunits, respectively.[28-30]

Augmenting inhibitory neurotransmission dampens neuronal hyperexcitability. Glutamate is converted to the inhibitory GABA by glutamate decarboxylase (GAD; Fig. 15.2) and stored in presynaptic vesicles. In response to a stimulus, vesicular GABA is transported to the axonal membrane, where it is drawn into the synapse to interact with $GABA_A$ channels. Synaptic GABA is then taken up into presynaptic cells by GABA transporters (GATs), such as GAT1.[31] Degradation of GABA by GABA-transaminase (GABA-T) results in succinic semialdehyde, which no longer binds $GABA_A$ channels. Inhibitors of GABA-T block this process, thereby increasing synaptic GABA concentrations and inhibitory neurotransmission. Blocking GAT1 and preventing cellular uptake is another mechanism for increasing synaptic GABA.

Polypharmacy and polypharmacology are important topics when discussing ASMs. Polypharmacy is the concomitant use of multiple medications, generally agreed to be approximately five or more. In treating patients with seizures, particularly those with seizures that are refractory to ASM monotherapy, many patients will be prescribed

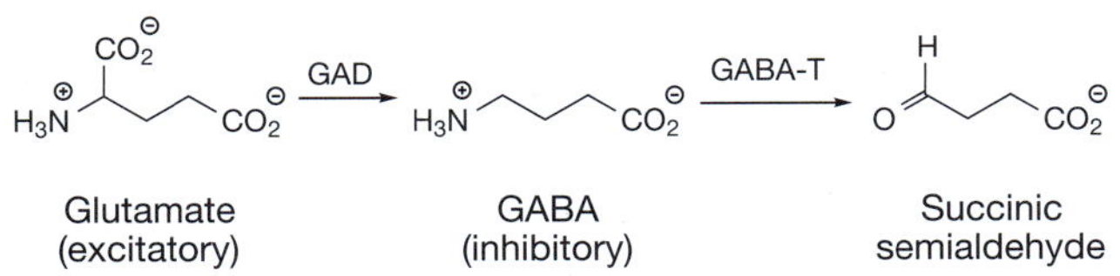

Figure 15.2 Regulation of glutamate and GABA. GAD, glutamate decarboxylase; GABA-T, GABA-transaminase.

multiple ASMs. Polypharmacology describes the situation where a single agent operates through multiple MOA. For example, valproic acid produces anticonvulsant actions through binding to glutamatergic, GABAergic, and even monoamine neurotransmitter targets (eg, dopamine, serotonin). Although a single "magic bullet" medication may be the most desirable from a patient compliance and tolerance perspective, in many cases, a rational polytherapeutic approach may lead to optimal outcomes. In this approach, two ASMs with complementary, synergistic MOA may be used in combination to best control seizures.[32]

Chemistry of Commonly Used Antiepileptic Drugs

Over 20 ASMs are available to treat seizure disorders, and the most commonly used ASMs covered in this chapter are described in Table 15.2. Health care providers may rationally combine medications that operate through synergistic MOA to afford optimal outcomes. A visual representation of the therapeutic applications of ASMs can be found in Figure 15.3.

Table 15.2 Mechanisms of Action (MOA) of Antiseizure Medications

Generic Name	Trade Name[a]	Approval (Year)[b]	Generation	Pharmacologic Targets[c]
Voltage-Gated Sodium Channel Blockers				
Phenytoin sodium	Dilantin	1953	First	Na_V
Carbamazepine	Tegretol	1968	First	Na_V
Oxcarbazepine	Trileptal	1990	Second	Na_V
Lamotrigine	Lamictal	1994	Second	Na_V, Ca_V1-3, DHFR
Fosphenytoin sodium	Cerebyx	1996	Second	Na_V
Lacosamide	Vimpat	2008	Third	Na_V(slow), CRMP2
Rufinamide	Banzel	2008	Third	Na_V1.1, Na_V1.6
Eslicarbazepine acetate	Aptiom	2013	Third	Na_V
Voltage-Gated Calcium Channel Blockers				
Ethosuximide	Zarontin	1958	First	Ca_V3
Gabapentin	Neurontin	1993	Second	$Ca_v(\alpha2\delta)$
Pregabalin	Lyrica	2005	Third	$Ca_V(\alpha2\delta)$
GABA Modulators				
Phenobarbital	Luminal	1912	First	$GABA_A$-PAM
Primidone	Mysoline	1954	First	$GABA_A$-PAM
Diazepam	Valium	1963	First	$GABA_A$-BZR
Clonazepam	Klonopin	1964	First	$GABA_A$-BZR
Midazolam	Versed	1976	First	$GABA_A$-BZR
Lorazepam	Ativan	1977	First	$GABA_A$-BZR
Clorazepate	Tranxene	1987	Second	$GABA_A$-BZR
Tiagabine	Gabitril	1997	Second	GAT-1
Vigabatrin	Sabril	2009	Third	GABA-T
Clobazam	Onfi	2011	Third	$GABA_A$-BZR
Stiripentol	Diacomit	2018	Third	$GABA_A$-PAM
Ganaxolone	Ztalmy	2022	Third	$GABA_A$-PAM

Table 15.2 Mechanisms of Action (MOA) of Antiseizure Medications (*continued*)

Generic Name	Trade Name[a]	Approval (Year)[b]	Generation	Pharmacologic Targets[c]
Glutamate Antagonists				
Levetiracetam	Keppra	1999	Second	SV2A
Brivaracetam	Briviact	2016	Third	SV2A
Perampanel	Fycompa	2016	Third	AMPAR
Antiseizure Medications with Multiple MOA				
Valproic acid	Depakene, Depakote, Depacon	1976	First	GABA-T, Na_v, NMDAR, DA, 5-HT
Felbamate	Felbatol	1993	Second	$GABA_A$, Na_v, NMDAR
Topiramate	Topamax	1996	Second	Na_v, Ca_v, GABA, AMPAR, CA-II, CA-IV
Zonisamide	Zonegran	2000	Second	Na_v, Ca_V3, DA, EAAC, GAT-1, CA
Cannabidiol	Epidiolex	2018	Third	CB1R-NAM, 5-HT1AR, GPR55, others
Cenobamate	Xcopri	2019	Third	Na_v, GABA release
Fenfluramine	Fintepla	2020	Third	5-HT release, 5-HT2R, σ1

[a]FDA-approved trade name.
[b]Year of FDA approval.
[c]See abbreviations section at the beginning of this chapter.

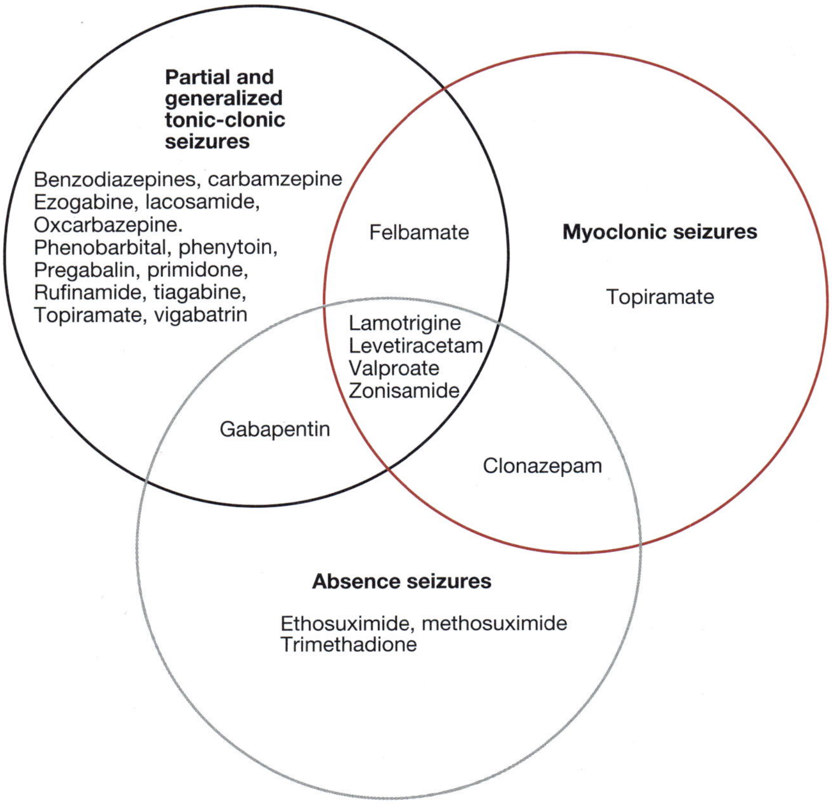

Figure 15.3 Antiseizure drugs used in treatment of the various seizures.

Many ASMs are enzyme inducers, which can lead to clinically relevant drug-drug interactions (DDIs) by inducing the transcription of cytochromes P450 (CYP450s) and UDP-glucuronosyltransferases (UGTs) that are involved in metabolism and clearance of ASMs and non-ASMs. Because ASMs are frequently given in combination, it is important to understand how inducing and noninducing ASMs interact across drug classes.

Voltage-Gated Sodium Channel Blockers

Iminostilbenes

One of the oldest and most widely used classes of antiepileptic drugs is iminostilbenes. Since the approval of carbamazepine (CBZ) in 1968, two additional iminostilbenes have reached the market, namely oxcarbazepine (OXC) and (S)-(+)-licarbazepine (eslicarbazepine) (Fig. 15.4).

Receptor Binding/Mechanism of Action. Iminostilbenes bind to the intracellular surface of the inactive state of Na_v channels, preventing transition to the resting state. The inactive state is therefore unable to respond when the hyperactive neuron reaches threshold. By preferentially stabilizing the inactive state of Na_v, iminostilbenes have some selectivity for hyperfunctioning neurons compared to normal neuronal signaling; however, this selectivity is lost at higher doses of the older drugs, CBZ and OXC. These agents have a slow onset and long duration of anticonvulsant action.

Structure-Activity Relationship. Iminostilbenes consist of a dibenzazepine core functional moiety that resembles the tricyclic pharmacophore of chlorpromazine and other tricyclic antidepressants (see Chapter 11). In fact, CBZ produces similar anticholinergic side effects as these medications do. The drug retains activity when the ethylene group connecting the two aromatic rings is metabolically oxidized (Fig. 15.5). The dibenzazepine nitrogen is functionalized by a terminal urea group. This urea must be unsubstituted: alkylation here leads to a dramatic loss of anticonvulsant activity.

Physicochemical and pharmacokinetic properties of iminostilbene antiseizure agents are provided in Table 15.3.

Carbamazepine (Tegretol). CBZ was one of the first ASMs discovered and developed entirely by the pharmaceutical industry. Initially designed as an antidepressant and

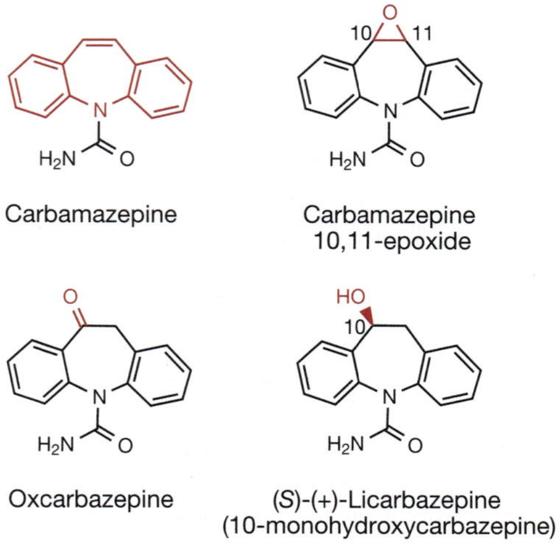

Figure 15.4 Iminostilbenes.

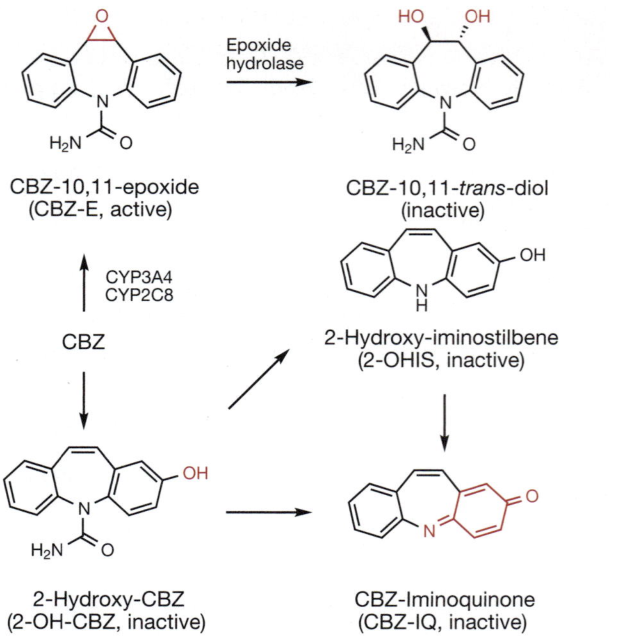

Figure 15.5 Bioactivation pathways for carbamazepine. Reactive portions of intermediates shown in red.

antipsychotic, CBZ is one of the most commonly prescribed ASMs and is considered the gold standard against which new ASM medications are compared. CBZ is indicated for complex partial and generalized tonic-clonic seizures, but is inactive against absence seizures. CBZ is on the World Health Organization's (WHO) 20th List of Essential Medicines.

Metabolism. The major route of metabolism of CBZ is CYP3A4 and CYP2C8 oxidation of the stilbene to the active metabolite, CBZ-10,11-epoxide (CBZ-E), followed by hydrolytic cleavage to the *trans*-diol by epoxide hydrolase (Fig. 15.5). A minor route of biotransformation is oxidation of the 2-position to produce 2-hydroxy-CBZ (2-OH-CBZ). Secondary oxidation of 2-OH-CBZ removes the urea to produce the pharmacologically inactive 2-hydroxyiminostilbene (2-OHIS), which can be converted to the iminoquinone (CBZ-IQ). CBZ-IQ may also be produced directly from 2-OH-CBZ. Some intermediates are reactive and can cause toxicities at high concentrations: for example, CBZ-E and CBZ-IQ form covalent adducts with CYP3A4 and other nucleophiles in vivo. The iminoquinone of CBZ-IQ consists of two Michael acceptors that are highly electrophilic and reactive with cell nucleophiles. The epoxide has been associated with ataxic gait in certain patients, and both reactive products may contribute to idiosyncratic toxicities.[33-35]

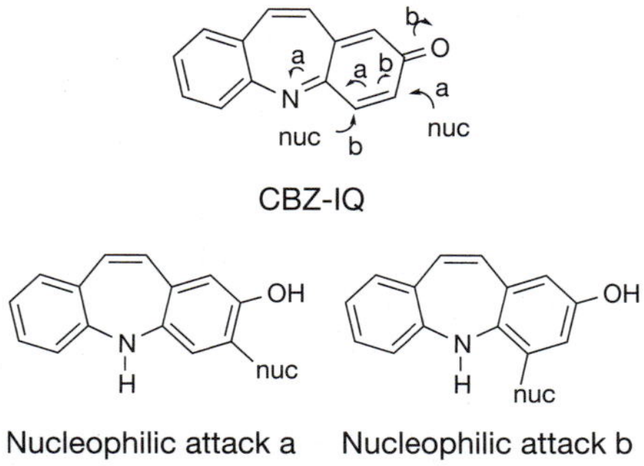

Table 15.3 Physicochemical and Pharmacokinetic Properties of Iminostilbenes

	CBZ	OXC	ESL[a]
cLogP	2.67	1.44	0.93
Solubility (mg/mL)	0.018	0.16	0.11
TPSA (Å²)	43.33	63.4	72.63
f (%)[b]	85-90	>95	>95
$t_{1/2}$ (h)	26.2[b] 12.3[c] 8.2[d]	1-5[e] 7-20[f]	9
t_{max} (h)	3-8	1-3	1-4
Protein binding (%)	75	37-40	30
V_d (L/kg)	0.79-1.86	0.3-0.8	0.65-0.85
Metabolized by:	CYP3A4 CYP2C8	AKR UGT	Esterases AKR
Inducer of:	CYP1A2 CYP2B6 CYP2C9 CYP3A4 UGTs P-gp	CYP3A4 CYP3A5	CYP3A4
Inhibitor of:	none	CYP2C19	CYP2C19

AKR, aldo-keto reductase; CBZ, carbamazepine; ESL, eslicarbazepine acetate; f, oral bioavailability; OXC, oxcarbazepine; TPSA, topologic polar surface area; UGT, UDP-glucuronosyltransferase; V_d, volume of distribution.
[a]Active (*S*)-licarbazepine metabolite.
[b]After a single dose.
[c]After repeated doses.
[d]When taken with other ASMs.
[e]Parent drug.
[f]Active monohydroxy derivative (MHD) metabolite.

The inductive effect of CBZ on CYP3A4 stimulates its own metabolism (ie, metabolic autoinduction). Because CBZ is metabolized by CYP3A4 and induces its metabolic activity, repeated administration of CBZ results in increasingly faster clearance. In practice, this means that the dose of CBZ must be increased in patients over time to maintain therapeutic plasma levels.

Physicochemical Properties. The clogP of CBZ is approximately 2.67, and the topological polar surface area (TPSA) is 46.33 Å. CBZ contains no ionizable functional groups and, as a result, is practically insoluble in water (17.7 μg/mL).

Pharmacokinetics. Tablet, capsule, and suspension formulations of CBZ are available in the United States. Dissolution of CBZ from tablets is slow; therefore, absorption is unpredictable. Absorption of CBZ from the suspension is faster than that of the immediate release (IR) tablet; thus, when substituting the suspension for the IR tablet, the dosing interval should be shortened without changing the daily dose. The IR tablet formulation has high apparent bioavailability (f_{app} = 85%-90%) and the t_{max} is 3 to 8 hours. Plasma protein binding is approximately 75%, and volume of distribution (V_d) is 0.79 to 1.86 L/kg.[36] Approximately 97% of CBZ is metabolized, leaving little parent drug excreted unchanged. Elimination of CBZ and metabolites is largely renal (~70%). A pharmacokinetics study in 1985 found that the single dose $t_{1/2}$ is 26.2 hours; this was much lower in patients on CBZ monotherapy ($t_{1/2}$ 12.3 hours) and in patients taking CBZ concomitantly with other ASMs ($t_{1/2}$ 8.2 hours). Enhanced CBZ elimination means lower circulating plasma levels in these patients.[37] CBZ is a possible P-glycoprotein (P-gp) substrate.[38]

Specific Adverse Events and Drug-Drug Interactions. Toxic epidermal necrosis (TEN) and Stevens-Johnson syndrome (SJS) are rare, but serious, side effects of CBZ. The incidence is greater in patients with the *HLA-B*1502* gene variant, found almost exclusively in patients of Chinese ancestry. The risk of aplastic anemia and agranulocytosis is low, although patients should be monitored for cardiac and hepatic toxicities.[39] When coadministered with valproic acid, plasma protein binding of CBZ is reduced, causing increased free plasma fractions.[40] CBZ is an inducer of CYP1A2, CYP2B6, CYP2C9, and CYP3A4, the latter of which is the primary enzyme responsible for CBZ metabolism. Thus, coadministration of CBZ with antiepileptic drugs metabolized by these enzymes will enhance their metabolism and increase clearance. Metabolism of CBZ is also impacted by other enzyme-inducing ASMs, including phenytoin and phenobarbital: these drugs increase CBZ-E/CBZ ratio when coadministered.[41]

During pregnancy, CBZ-E/CBZ ratio is increased, and CBZ and CBZ-diol plasma levels are decreased. This is a result of CYP upregulation and epoxide hydrolase downregulation. CBZ and CBZ-E cross the placental barrier and are found in breast milk; daily exposure is approximately 2 to 5 mg, doses sufficiently low to minimize concern when breastfeeding.[42] CBZ significantly decreases areas under the curve (AUCs) of the oral contraceptives norethisterone and ethinylestradiol by approximately 50%, increasing the risk of unplanned pregnancy unless other contraceptive methods are employed.

Oxcarbazepine (Trileptal). Originally developed alongside CBZ in the 1960s, OXC was approved for clinical use as monotherapy or adjunctive therapy for partial seizures in adults and children in 1990. This makes OXC a second-generation ASM. Though OXC and CBZ are structurally similar and act through similar mechanisms of action (MOAs), the safety and tolerability profile of OXC offers some clinical advantages over CBZ.

Metabolism. OXC is rapidly oxidized into a mixture of (*R*)- and (*S*)-monohydroxy derivatives (MHDs, also known as licarbazepine) by hepatic aldo-keto reductase (AKR) (Fig. 15.6). This is largely a stereoselective reduction, as the ratio of (*S*)- to (*R*)-MHD is approximately 80:20. In healthy volunteers, it was found that circulating levels of the active MHD metabolites were approximately 6-fold higher than

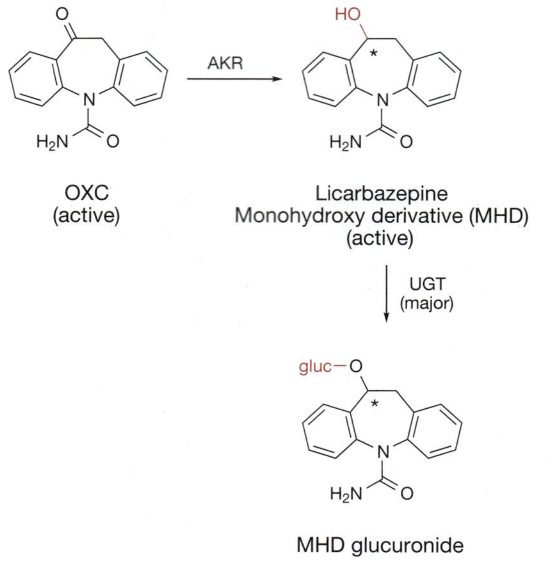

Figure 15.6 Metabolism of OXC (* = chiral center). AKR, aldo-keto reductase; UGT, UDP-glucuronosyltransferase.

those of OXC.[43] Glucuronidation of the resulting alcohols is the major phase 2 metabolic pathway. Unlike CBZ, OXC is not metabolized into CBZ-E and CBZ-10,11-*trans*-diol metabolites, the entities responsible for CBZ-induced neurotoxicities[44] and hepatic enzyme induction,[45] respectively.

Physicochemical Properties. Like CBZ, OXC contains no ionizable functional groups and is practically insoluble in water. cLogP is 1.44, and TPSA is 63.4. Compared to CBZ, OXC is slightly more hydrophilic and polar than CBZ due to the ketone at C5. Though OXC is more hydrophilic and polar than CBZ, aqueous solubility remains low due to a lack of ionizable functional groups.

Pharmacokinetics. OXC is rapidly and completely absorbed, reaching peak concentrations within 1 to 3 hours. The mixture of active MHD metabolites reaches peak concentration within 2 to 4 hours post dose at steady state.[45] Though the AUC and C_{max} for OXC were increased when taken with food, this has negligible impact on therapeutic dosing. Calculation of the V_d of OXC is difficult because OXC is rapidly and completely metabolized. The apparent V_d of the MHD metabolites is 0.3 to 0.8 L/kg, with low plasma protein binding (37%-40%).[46] OXC exhibits first-order linear kinetics: $t_{1/2}$ of OXC is 1 to 5 hours, and $t_{1/2}$ for MHD is between 7 and 20 hours on oral administration. Elimination of oral OXC is mostly renal (96%), with an OXC/MHD/MHD-glucuronide ratio of approximately <1%:27%:49%.[45] Several studies estimated that renal clearance in healthy volunteers is approximately 21 mL/min, which increases in older adult patients with impaired renal function. OXC is a P-gp substrate.[38]

Specific Adverse Events and Drug-Drug Interactions. Because OXC is not a CYP substrate and, therefore, is not biotransformed to the same reactive metabolites as CBZ, tolerability of OXC is generally improved. Specifically, fewer allergic reactions and psychomotor impairments have been reported.[47] Pharmacokinetic DDIs are less pronounced for OXC compared to CBZ.[46] Only CYP3A4 and CYP3A5 are induced by OXC, compared to the pan-induction by CBZ. This is clinically relevant in that metabolic autoinduction does not occur, meaning that therapeutic dose does not need to be increased with long-term use. Coadministration with hormonal contraceptives still causes plasma levels of ethinylestradiol and progrestins to decrease. OXC is an inhibitor of CYP2C19, suggesting that DDIs are possible when high doses of OXC are coadministered with ASMs phenytoin and phenobarbital, both of which are substrates of this isoform.[46]

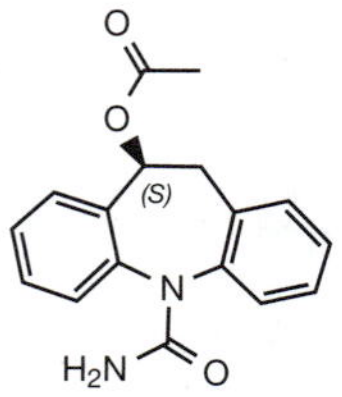

Eslicarbazepine acetate
(Aptiom)

Eslicarbazepine Acetate (Aptiom). Eslicarbazepine acetate (ESL) is a third-generation ASM approved in 2013 as an add-on medication for the treatment of partial seizures. The activity of ESL is similar to other iminostilbenes in that they are structurally related and operate through the same MOS, yet ESL possesses fewer toxic side effects due to a unique receptor binding profile. ESL derives its name as the acetate ester of the (*S*)-enantiomer of licarbazepine, which, as noted above, is another name for the OXC monohydroxy derivative metabolites (MHDs).

Receptor Binding/Mechanism of Action. Like CBZ and OXC, ESL and its active metabolites stabilize the inactivated state of Na_v channels, thereby preventing transition to the resting state. Unlike CBZ and OXC, ESL has lower affinity for the resting state of Na_v channels; thus, ESL is expected to be more selective for rapidly firing neurons over those firing at normal, baseline levels. This means ESL is expected to produce less toxic side effects compared to other agents in this class.[48]

Structure-Activity Relationship. ESL was designed to be a prodrug of (*S*)-licarbazepine, an active MHD product of OXC metabolism (Fig. 15.6). A series of racemic aliphatic and aromatic O-esters were synthesized and evaluated for neuroprotection in a rat seizure model and a rotarod test to determine motor toxicity.[49] The greatest neuroprotection occurred with the O-acetate. Extending the ester alkyl chain to ethyl and propyl led to progressively lower antiepileptic potency. When tested for neurotoxicity, ESL was found to be 2 to 3 times less toxic than CBZ and OXC when given by intraperitoneal injection, resulting in a wider therapeutic window.

Metabolism. ESL is rapidly metabolized by hepatic esterases to the active metabolite, (*S*)-licarbazepine. This is the (*S*)-enantiomer of the same active MHD metabolite discussed earlier for OXC; thus, the metabolic fate of ESL metabolites is the same for these two agents. A minor redox biotransformation is catalyzed by AKR, which oxidatively converts (*S*)-licarbazepine to OXC and then, OXC is reduced back to enantiomeric licarbazepine, as shown in Figure 15.6.

Physicochemical Properties. Like other iminostilbenes, ESL contains no ionizable functional groups at physiologic pH. ESL is moderately more hydrophilic than OXC, with cLogP of 0.93. The polar ester functional group affords ESL a TPSA of 72.63. Less than 1 mg/mL is soluble in water.

Pharmacokinetics. ESL is readily absorbed following oral administration and undergoes rapid first-pass hydrolytic metabolism to the active (S)-licarbazepine by liver esterases. Food does not affect absorption. The drug is bound to plasma protein (~30%) and blood cells (~46%). Most (92%) of the administered ESL is eliminated in the urine as (S)-licarbazepine (67%) and (S)-licarbazepine-O-glucuronide (33%), along with other metabolites (8%). The half-life for (S)-licarbazepine is approximately 9 hours.[50] ESL is a probable P-gp substrate.[38]

Specific Adverse Events and Drug-Drug Interactions. Adverse effects are generally mild and consist of somnolence, vomiting, diplopia, headaches, and dizziness. Adverse effects are dose related. Increased doses may augment the risk of depression, and suicidal thoughts and behavior are occasionally seen with antiepileptic drugs in general. The extent of CYP induction is considerably lower compared to CBZ. The parent drug ESL does not induce major CYP isoforms, although the (S)-licarbazepine MHD metabolite does induce CYP3A4. This can reduce plasma levels of ethinylestradiol and progestin hormonal contraceptives. Both ESL and MHD are inhibitors of CYP2C19 and enhance blood plasma levels of phenytoin and phenobarbital.[51]

Hydantoins

The hydantoins have been used as ASMs since the mid-1950s. The antiepileptic efficacy of the first hydantoin to be discovered, phenytoin (Fig. 15.7), resulted from a rational search of structurally related analogues of phenobarbital that do not cause sedation. Several hydantoin analogues have been developed since, including fosphenytoin, mephenytoin, and ethotoin.

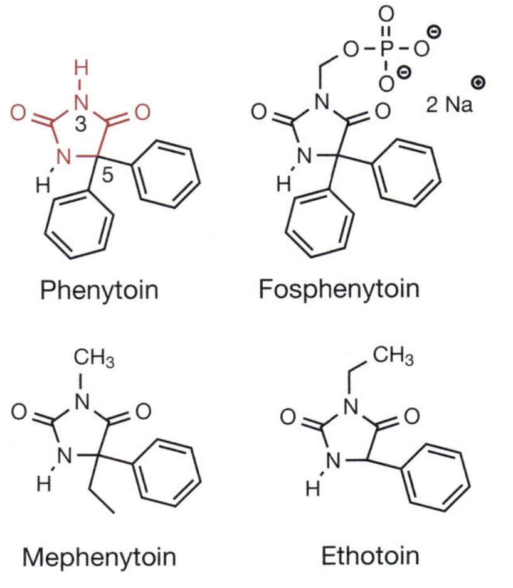

Figure 15.7 Hydantoins. The pharmacophore is shown in red.

RECEPTOR BINDING/MECHANISM OF ACTION. Like iminostilbenes, hydantoins inhibit Na_v channels. Since the pharmacologic actions of hydantoins—slow onset and long duration of action—so closely resemble those of other Na_v blockers, it is proposed that they all share a similar molecular mechanism of action.[52] As shown in Figure 15.8, the two aromatic rings of phenytoin occupy a similar chemical space as the two aromatic rings of the Na^+-channel blockers CBZ and lamotrigine. Molecular modeling using a Na_v homology model suggests that hydantoins, like iminostilbenes and lamotrigine, are capable of binding to a lipophilic domain containing Tyr1771 and Phe1764.[53] In this model, the imide NH of phenytoin (bolded in Fig. 15.8) engages in a unique hydrogen bond with the π-electrons of the Phe side chain.

STRUCTURE-ACTIVITY RELATIONSHIP. Hydantoins contain a common five-membered core called a ureide. The term "ureide" is derived from the functional groups "urea" and "imide." The imide nitrogen (position 3, Fig. 15.7) of phenytoin bears a weakly acidic proton with a pK_a of approximately 8 to 9. The conjugate base form is resonance-stabilized by the two adjacent carbonyl groups. The acidic character of the imide is nonessential, as the imide nitrogen can also be alkylated (mephenytoin, ethotoin) and retain activity. Another critical element to the hydantoin pharmacophore is the presence of one to two unsubstituted phenyl rings on position 5. Substitution on even one phenyl ring, such as addition of a *p*-fluorine, results in a substantial loss of activity.[54,55]

Physicochemical and pharmacokinetic properties of Na_v antiseizure agents, including hydantoins, are provided in Table 15.4.

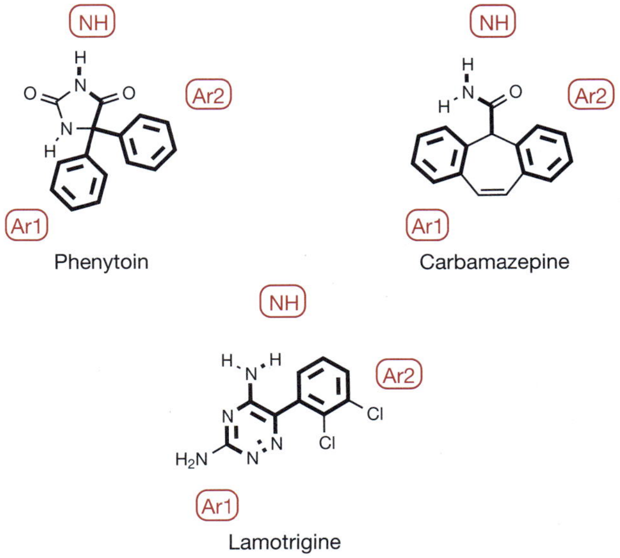

Figure 15.8 Proposed common binding mode within the Na_v channel for phenytoin, carbazepine, and lamotrigine. Ar1 and Ar2 on each agent may interact with F978, L1465, I1469, and Y1771, and the bolded NH is proposed to engage in an orthogonal π-dipole interaction with F1771. Ar1, aromatic ring 1; Ar2, aromatic ring 2.

Table 15.4 Physicochemical and Pharmacokinetic Properties of Na_V Blockers

	PHT	FPHT	LTG	LAC	RFM
cLogP	2.52	0.47	−0.19	0.90	0.05
Solubility (mg/mL)	0.02 (free acid) 3 (Na^+ salt)	142	0.17	20.1	0.03
TPSA (Å^2)	58.2	116.17	89.12	67.43	73.8
f (%)	70-100	100[a]	>98	100	80-85
$t_{1/2}$ (h)	15-22	<0.2	25-30	12-16	6-10
t_{max} (h)	1.5-3	3	1.4-4.8	0.5-4	4-6
Protein binding (%)	95	95-99	55	<15	26-34
V_d (L/kg)	0.7-0.8	0.04-0.13	0.9-1.3	0.6	0.8-1.2
Metabolized by:	CYP2C9 CYP2C19	Phosphatases	UGT1A4	CYP2C19	CEs
Inducer of:	CYP3A4 CYP2C9	CYP3A4[b] CYP2C9	None	None	CYP3A4
Inhibitor of:	None	None	None	None	None

CE, carboxyesterase; f, oral bioavailability; FPHT, fosphenytoin; LAC, lacosamide; LTG, lamotrigine; PHT, phenytoin; RFM, rufinamide; TPSA, topologic polar surface area; V_d, volume of distribution.

[a]Bioavailability of phenytoin after biotransformation.

[b]Based on conversion to phenytoin.

Phenytoin Sodium (Dilantin). Phenytoin was the first hydantoin discovered that effectively suppresses electrically induced convulsions in animals.[56,57] In fact, the name "phenytoin" is derived from the common name of its chemical structure, which is a 5,5-diphenylhydantoin. An analogue of phenobarbital, an ASM with potent sedative/hypnotic activity, phenytoin was found to be anticonvulsant absent sedative effects.[58] At the time of its discovery, phenytoin was the most potent, nonsedating anticonvulsant available. Oral dosage forms of phenytoin are approved to treat tonic-clonic and focal seizures, and fast-acting injectable formulations of phenytoin sodium are available to treat status epilepticus. Phenytoin is on the WHO 20th List of Essential Medicines.

Metabolism. Phenytoin is metabolized extensively (>95%) by CYP2C9 and CYP2C19 to the *p*-phenol metabolite, 5-(4′-hydroxyphenyl)-5-phenylhydantoin (HPPH), and to a lesser extent to the corresponding catechol (Fig. 15.9). The first step in oxidation occurs through the formation of an arene oxide intermediate. This epoxide is highly reactive to proteins, including the CYP enzymes responsible

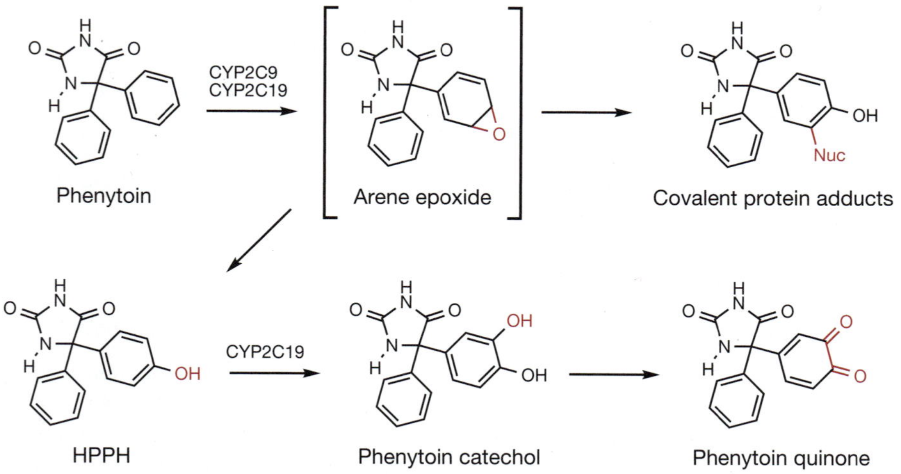

Figure 15.9 Phase 1 metabolism of phenytoin. Nuc, nucleophile.

for its formation. Formation of covalent protein adducts is one possible mechanism underlying phenytoin toxicity.[59] Further oxidation of HPPH to the phenytoin catechol can be catalyzed by a number of CYP isoforms, with CYP2C19 potentially playing a key role. The catechol is subjected to further oxidation to the *o*-quinone, which is capable of direct oxidation of DNA.[60] This second mechanism of oxidative toxicity may also contribute to the toxicologic profile of phenytoin.[61,62] Conversion of phenytoin and HPPH into innocuous metabolites by UGTs is a protective mechanism against toxicity.[63]

Physicochemical Properties. Phenytoin is weakly acidic (pK_a 8.3). With a cLogP of 2.52, it is lipophilic and poorly water soluble (20-30 μg/mL).[64] While the sodium salt is substantially more soluble in water (3 mg/mL), it is still considered to be of low aqueous solubility. The polar surface area is 58.2 Å and is readily able to enter the brain.

Pharmacokinetics. Oral capsule, tablet, and suspensions of phenytoin show high bioavailability (70%-100%) and high plasma protein binding (90%). In adults, V_d is approximately 0.7 to 0.8 L/kg, and C_{max} is reached between 1.5 and 3 hours. The elimination $t_{1/2}$ of phenytoin ranges from 15 to 22 hours following repeated dosing of a standard 300-mg oral dose. Phenytoin is a substrate for P-gp.[38]

Phenytoin demonstrates nonlinear pharmacokinetics. From a therapeutic perspective, this means that higher doses cause saturation of metabolizing enzymes and a decrease in elimination rate. Once metabolic saturation has been reached, a small increase in phenytoin dose can cause a large increase in drug plasma levels. Furthermore, there is wide interpatient variability in phenytoin metabolism and elimination, as discussed above. For these reasons, phenytoin therapeutic drug monitoring is clinically important, especially so in patients with hepatic or renal dysfunction.

Specific Adverse Events and Drug-Drug Interactions. Severe toxicities associated with unintentional phenytoin poisoning include SJS and TEN, both of which can be life-threatening. A rare disorder called purple glove syndrome can occur in older adult patients taking high doses of phenytoin. This is characterized by localized pain, swelling, and a blue-purple discoloration of the skin proximal to the injection of intravenous (IV) phenytoin. In extreme cases, the skin will become necrotic and may require excision. Fetal hydantoin syndrome is the collection of teratogenic effects in children of mothers administered phenytoin during pregnancy. Children are born with microcephaly as well as limb and cardiac birth defects, and often experience cognitive and developmental delays. Due to poor solubility in aqueous solution, injectable phenytoin formulations contain propylene glycol and ethanol, which may contribute to cardiac toxicities. These toxicities are rare with ingested phenytoin.

Phenytoin has a narrow therapeutic window; thus, coadministration with other agents that enhance absorption and distribution, or inhibit metabolism and elimination, will potentially cause an increase in toxicities. Because phenytoin has high plasma protein binding (90%), coadministration with other highly bound agents, or in patients with renal impairment, free (unbound) drug levels will be enhanced to potentially toxic levels. Enzyme-inducing ASMs, such as CBZ and OXC, enhance phenytoin metabolism, shortening duration. Phenytoin induces CYP2C9 and CYP3A4. This can significantly impact the clearance of coadministered agents, including certain ASMs and hormonal contraceptives.

Other Important Aspects of Drug Chemistry. *Although phenytoin sodium is available as an injectable formulation to treat status epilepticus, significant issues arise on injection. As discussed earlier, phenytoin and phenytoin sodium are poorly aqueous-soluble. Phenytoin sodium is formulated in pH 12 buffer containing 40% propylene glycol/10% ethanol to facilitate solubility and dissolution. Precipitation of active drug following IV administration can cause significant soft tissue pain and irritation to the local venous environment. Intramuscular (IM) injection also produces intense pain due to precipitation of the drug in muscle. Furthermore, rapid injection of phenytoin sodium can result in severe, life-threatening hypotension.*

FOSPHENYTOIN SODIUM (CEREBYX)

Due to the clinical success of phenytoin in treating seizures, and the significant adverse effect profile associated with the injectable formulation, development began in the early 1980s to develop an aqueous-soluble prodrug of phenytoin. The result of a decade of research was fosphenytoin sodium (Cerebyx) (Fig. 15.7), a second-generation ASM approved in 1996 to treat convulsive status epilepticus.

Metabolism. Fosphenytoin sodium is rapidly and completely metabolized by phosphatases to 3-hydroxymethylphenytoin. This 3-hydroxymethyl intermediate is chemically unstable and rapidly degrades to release the active phenytoin and a formaldehyde byproduct. The rate of metabolic conversion to phenytoin is on the order of 8 to 10 minutes. Unchanged fosphenytoin is not detected in urine samples. Metabolism of phenytoin then occurs as described earlier (Fig. 15.9).

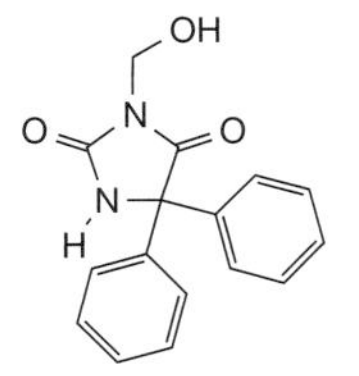

3-Hydroxymethylphenytoin

Physicochemical Properties. Fosphenytoin sodium is more than 4,400 times more aqueous-soluble than phenytoin (142 mg/mL vs 0.02 mg/mL).[64] The phosphate ester prodrug has two acidic pK_a values (1.46 and ~6.4) and is formulated as the disodium salt. The polar surface area of the prodrug is 116.17 Å, which would suggest poor central bioavailability; however, rapid bioactivation produces phenytoin, which, with a polar surface area of only 58.2 Å, can readily be able to cross the blood-brain barrier (BBB).

Pharmacokinetics. The bioavailability of fosphenytoin's active metabolite, phenytoin, is nearly 100% following IM injection based on the AUC of IV phenytoin.[65] When given orally, the phenytoin AUC for fosphenytoin sodium solution is indistinguishable from oral phenytoin.[66] Compared to IV phenytoin, administration of IM fosphenytoin sodium results in a lower C_{max} (8.92 ± 0.35 vs 5.68 ± 0.20 μg/mL, respectively) and higher t_{max} (0.32 ± 0.03 vs

3.13 ± 0.23 hour, respectively).[67] This may be due to the poor aqueous solubility of phenytoin suspension interfering with bioavailability.[66] Due to high polarity and plasma protein binding, fosphenytoin has an apparent V_d of approximately 0.04 to 0.13 L/kg.[68] Fosphenytoin clearance ranges from 12.9 to 22.8 L/h as a function of dose and infusion rate, with higher doses leading to higher unbound fraction and enhanced clearance.[68]

Specific Adverse Events and Drug-Drug Interactions. The adverse event profile of fosphenytoin is similar to that of phenytoin. A statistically relevant observation in clinical trials is that fewer patients experience injection-site pain with fosphenytoin sodium (6%) than with phenytoin sodium (25%).[69]

Miscellaneous Na_v Channel Blockers

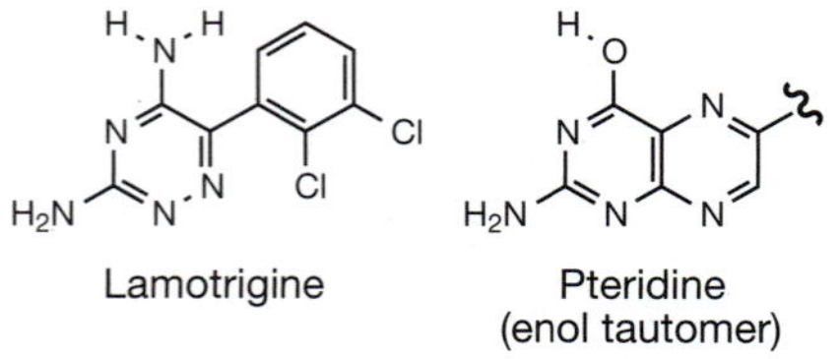

LAMOTRIGINE (LAMICTAL). Lamotrigine was approved in 1994 as adjunctive therapy for partial seizures, Lennox-Gastaut syndrome, and primary generalized tonic-clonic seizures in adults and pediatric patients older than age 2. Lamotrigine is also approved for conversion to monotherapy for adults with partial seizures who are receiving another single ASM.

Receptor Binding/Mechanism of Action. Lamotrigine works similarly to CBZ and phenytoin, as an inhibitor of presynaptic fast Na_v channels. Evidence supports additional anticonvulsant mechanisms, including blockade of L-, N-, and P/Q/R-type Ca_v channels, which may lead to a broader spectrum of anticonvulsant activity. Lamotrigine is an inhibitor of dihydrofolate reductase. This does not impact anticonvulsant activity but may contribute to a unique adverse effect profile.

Structure-Activity Relationship. Lamotrigine is a 1,2,4-triazine, the only approved ASM with this structural core. The central hypothesis that led to the discovery of lamotrigine was that, because other ASMs known in the 1960s (phenytoin and phenobarbital) caused folate deficiency, perhaps anticonvulsant activity was directly related to folate antagonism. Wellcome Research Laboratories studied several series of *N*-heterocycles that mimic the pteridine ring system of folic acid and found that BW430C, later known as lamotrigine, produced strong anticonvulsant effects with weak antifolate activity.[70]

Metabolism. Lamotrigine is extensively metabolized to pharmacologically inactive products. The major metabolite is the N_2-glucuronide (LMG-N2-G; Fig. 15.10), which accounts for 75% to 90% of the dose. A minor route of metabolism results in generation of an arene epoxide intermediate that is highly reactive to biologic nucleophiles such as reduced glutathione (GSH). Reaction of GSH with this arene oxide may result in a lamotrigine-GSH adduct, which could be responsible for the ASM hypersensitivity reactions seen in some patients.[71]

Physicochemical Properties. The 1-amino substituent of lamotrigine is weakly basic, with $pK_a = 5.87$. This means that over 90% of the drug will be in the uncharged conjugate base state at physiologic pH. Lamotrigine is very slightly soluble in water (0.17 mg/mL). The physicochemical properties of lamotrigine tend to be more polar and hydrophilic than one might expect for a centrally acting drug (cLogP = −0.19, TPSA = 89.12 Å); nevertheless, lamotrigine is effective at reaching the brain and preventing seizures.

Pharmacokinetics. Lamotrigine is rapidly and completely absorbed on oral administration (absolute bioavailability >98%) with negligible first-pass metabolism. Food does not impact absorption, and t_{max} is reached between 1.4 and 4.8 hours. The estimated V_d range is 0.9 to 1.3 L/kg and is not altered in patients with epilepsy compared to healthy volunteers. Lamotrigine is not extensively bound to plasma proteins (55%). The major route of inactivation is through N_2-glucuronidation (Fig. 15.10). Elimination is largely renal (94%) and consists of 10% unchanged drug, 85% glucuronides, and around 5% other minor metabolites (eg, GSH conjugate). The elimination $t_{1/2}$ in patients taking only lamotrigine ranges from 25 to 30 hours over single and multiple doses. Apparent plasma clearance is 0.44 to 0.58 mL/min/kg. Patients with renal and hepatic insufficiency have significantly increased $t_{1/2}$ and lowered plasma clearance. Lamotrigine is a P-gp substrate.[38]

Specific Adverse Events and Drug-Drug Interactions. Serious adverse events related to ASM hypersensitivity syndrome may be seen, especially when coadministered with valproic acid. The development of myoclonus after 2 to 3 years of treatment has also been reported.[72] Other common side effects include somnolence, headache, dizziness, diplopia, ataxia, and nausea. Concomitantly administered ASMs that induce UGT enzymes cause a significant decrease in blood plasma levels of lamotrigine. Valproate significantly reduces lamotrigine clearance by inhibiting UGT; thus, the dose of lamotrigine should be reduced to avoid toxicities.

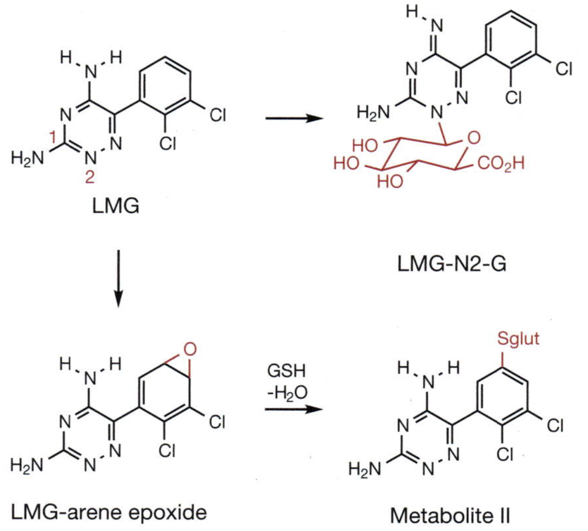

Figure 15.10 Metabolism of lamotrigine (LMG). GSH, glutathione; glut, glutathione.

Coadministration with the oral contraceptive ethinylestradiol doubled apparent clearance of lamotrigine, but the ASM did not impact ethinylestradiol pharmacokinetics.[73] In contrast to estrogens, progestins have no effect on lamotrigine pharmacokinetics. While lamotrigine itself has no effect on the plasma levels of coadministered ethinylestradiol, it does impact the clearance of progestins.

LACOSAMIDE (VIMPAT). Lacosamide is a third-generation ASM approved by the FDA in 2008 as an adjuvant for partial onset seizures in adults. The deceptively simple amino acid structure of lacosamide belies a complex mechanism of action that remains incompletely understood. Lacosamide has an improved safety profile over older Na_v channel blockers, with minimal DDIs or induction of metabolic enzymes.

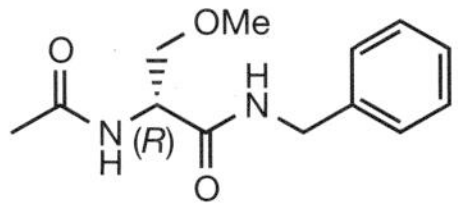

(*R*)-Lacosamide
(Motpoly XR, Vimpat)

Receptor Binding/Mechanism of Action. Lacosamide has a multimodal mechanism of action. First, lacosamide inhibits hyperexcitability through enhanced slow inactivation of Na_v channels. This is different from CBZ and phenytoin, which modify fast inactivation of Na_v channels. This distinct mechanism of Na_v blockade suggests that lacosamide may potentially be effective as an adjuvant for patients with drug-resistant epilepsy.[74,75]

A second lacosamide mechanism that may contribute to its antiepileptic effects involves the intracellular phosphoprotein collapsin responsemediator protein 2 (CRMP2).[76] CRMP2 is involved in neuronal differentiation and axonal outgrowth induced by brain-derived neurotrophic factor (BDNF). Since CRMP2 function is dysregulated in treatment-resistant epilepsy patients compared to controls,[77] there is a potentially unique neuroprotective mechanism of lacosamide in treating refractory epilepsy disorders.[78]

Structure-Activity Relationship. Lacosamide can be considered a "functionalized amino acid" because of a simple substituted amino acid backbone. Since the discovery that *N*-acetyl-D, L-alanine benzyl amide was effective in animal models of epilepsy, extensive SAR studies showed several key trends that led to the development of lacosamide. First, there is a stereochemical preference for (*R*)- over (*S*)-enantiomers, with a eudismic (*R*)/(*S*) ratio of approximately 10. Second, there is a preference for heteroatoms separated from the amino acid backbone by a single carbon atom; in lacosamide, the methyl ether assumes this role. Substitution of this side chain with heteroaromatic groups—particularly 2-furyl, 2-pyrrolyl, or 2-pyridinyl that possesses the properly spaced heteroatom—also maintains activity. The *N*-acetamide can be replaced by a *t*-butyl amide with a modest loss of potency, but other modifications are not tolerated. The benzyl group is also required for activity and is modestly sensitive to substitution.[79,80]

Metabolism. Compared to Na^+-channel blockers described previously, lacosamide is stable to metabolism. Approximately 40% of the parent drug is excreted unchanged, and 30% is eliminated as the inactive *O*-desmethyl metabolite. The rest of the dose is excreted as presently unidentified polar metabolites. The enzyme primarily responsible for this metabolism is CYP2C19.

Physicochemical Properties. Lacosamide solubility in phosphate-buffered saline at pH 7.5 is 20.1 mg/mL.[78] As an amino acid derivative, lacosamide is modestly polar with a cLogP of approximately 0.90. The TPSA of lacosamide is 67.43 Å, which is appropriate for high central bioavailability.

Pharmacokinetics. Lacosamide displays linear pharmacokinetics. The drug is rapidly and completely absorbed (100%) following oral administration, with a t_{max} of 0.5 to 4 hours after dose. Peak plasma concentrations (C_{max}) rise proportionately with increasing dose: in a phase I trial in healthy volunteers, C_{max} following a single 400 mg dose was 8.7 ± 1.8 μg/mL and 14.3 ± 2.3 μg/mL after a 600 mg dose.[81] Lacosamide has low (<15%) plasma protein binding, and the V_d is 0.6 L/kg.[82] The elimination $t_{1/2}$ is approximately 3 hours in otherwise healthy patients, which increases with severe renal impairment. Renal excretion accounts for around 95% of lacosamide elimination, which should also be monitored in renally impaired patients.[81] An intravenous form of lacosamide is available for refractory status epilepticus.[83]

Specific Adverse Events and Drug-Drug Interactions. Compared to other ASMs, lacosamide is generally well-tolerated with few serious adverse effects. In preclinical animal studies, ataxia and reduced motility were mild and dose limiting. A particular advantage of lacosamide over other ASMs like phenytoin, valproate, and zonisamide is the lack of teratogenic effects.[78] Emerging evidence suggests patients with cardiac risk factors should be monitored when taking lacosamide because of its effect on modulating slow inactivation of Na^+ channels in cardiac cells.[84]

Preclinical evaluation of lacosamide revealed no induction of five CYP isoforms (1A2, 2B6, 2C9, 2C19, 3A4) in human hepatocytes, and only weak inhibition of a panel of 10 CYPs at concentrations 30-fold higher than therapeutic plasma levels.[78] Thus, there are few clinically relevant DDIs to consider with lacosamide.

Other Important Aspects of Drug Chemistry. Like many ASMs, lacosamide is also effective in certain pain conditions—for example, neuropathic pain.[85] Lacosamide is a Drug Enforcement Administration (DEA) Schedule V drug.

RUFINAMIDE (BANZEL). Rufinamide was FDA-approved in 2008 as an adjuvant agent to treat children older than 4 years and adults with Lennox-Gastaut syndrome. More recent evidence suggests that rufinamide may also be effective as an add-on for treating refractory partial seizures.[86] As a third-generation ASM, rufinamide operates through a unique mechanism of action that may aid in treating refractory seizures, and its pharmacokinetic properties suggest enhanced safety and tolerability compared to older agents.

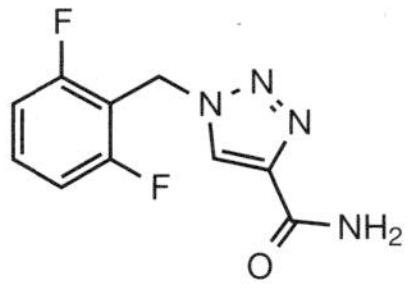

Rufinamide
(Banzel)

Receptor Binding/Mechanism of Action. Like the ASMs described earlier, the mechanism of action of rufinamide includes inhibition of Na_v channels. Unlike other Na_v inhibitors, however, rufinamide appears to selectively alter $Na_V1.1$- and $Na_V1.6$-channel activation. Rufinamide prolongs Na_V channel time in the inactive state by slowing the recovery from inactivation.

Structure-Activity Relationship. Rufinamide is the sole member of a class of N-benzyltriazole-based ASMs. Little is definitively understood about the SAR of this class. The benzyl ring is substituted at the 2,6 (*ortho*) positions with fluorines. These fluorine atoms are not hard-and-fast requirements, however, as defluorinated analogues maintain inhibitory efficacy at $Na_V1.1$ channels.[87] The central triazole core is substituted at the 4-position by a terminal carboxamide group. This amide group appears to be essential for activity, as the carboxylic acid metabolite (Fig. 15.11) and a synthetic alcohol derivative are both inactive at Na_V channels.

Metabolism. Rufinamide is biotransformed into an inactive carboxylic acid metabolite by human carboxyesterase-1 (hCE-1; Fig. 15.11). Other minor metabolites found in the urine appear to be acyl glucuronides of this acid metabolite.[88]

Physicochemical Properties. Rufinamide is a chemically neutral small molecule, with a cLogP of 0.05 and TPSA of 73.8 Å. Rufinamide is practically insoluble in aqueous solution (31 μg/mL) and is very slightly soluble in ethanol (440 μg/mL).[89]

Pharmacokinetics. Oral bioavailability of rufinamide is 80% to 85%, which is enhanced when taken with food. Rufinamide has low (26%-34%) plasma protein binding, and t_{max} 4 to 6 hours. The V_d is 0.8 to 1.2 L/kg. The $t_{1/2}$ for rufinamide is 6 to 10 hours, which is not altered by renal impairment. Only ~2% of parent drug is excreted in urine. Elimination of rufinamide follows nonlinear Michaelis-Menten kinetics.

Specific Adverse Events and Drug-Drug Interactions. Rufinamide is generally well tolerated in children and adults. An analysis from clinical trials found that the most common side effects in children were somnolence, vomiting, and headache, which can be limited by slowing the increase in dose. [90] Another trial found that rufinamide causes no cognitive impairment over a range of therapeutic doses.[91] Children can also experience a higher incidence of rash and ASM hypersensitivity syndrome, both of which subside on discontinuation.[92]

Though rufinamide does not inhibit major CYP isoforms at therapeutic doses, significant DDIs are possible, particularly in younger patients. Induction of CYP3A4 may be responsible for the observed increase in metabolism of midazolam, ethinylestradiol, and progestins that are metabolized by this isoform. Rufinamide has no effect on the plasma concentrations of valproate, topiramate, or olanzapine, and may decrease plasma levels of CBZ and lamotrigine and increase levels of phenobarbital and phenytoin. Valproate increases plasma concentrations of rufinamide, possibly through inhibition of hCE-1. Phenobarbital, primidone, and phenytoin modestly decrease plasma levels of rufinamide through unknown mechanisms.[93]

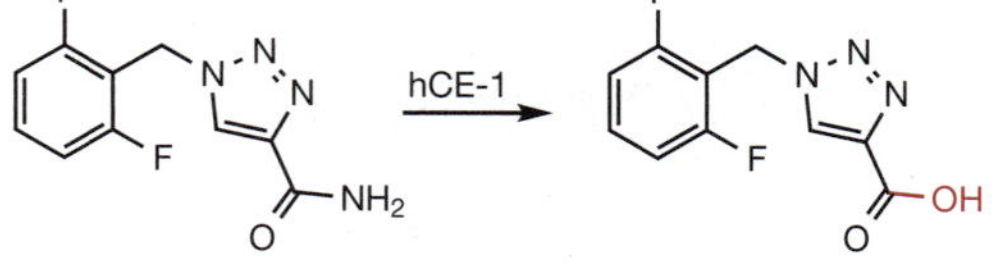

CGP 47,292

Rufinamide
(CGP 33,101)

Figure 15.11 Rufinamide (CGP 33,101) and its inactive carboxylic acid metabolite. hCE-1, human carboxyesterase-1.

Voltage-Gated Calcium Channel Blockers

Gabapentinoids

The most successful class of Ca_v-channel modulators are actually structural analogues of GABA, known as gabapentinoids (Fig. 15.12). Owing to the serendipity of drug discovery, both agents were initially designed to mimic GABA binding to GABAergic targets: in the case of gabapentin, the idea was to develop a more lipophilic and bioavailable $GABA_A$ receptor agonist, and pregabalin was designed as a GABA-T inhibitor. Instead, both compounds are potent blockers of HVA Ca_v channels.

Receptor Binding/Mechanism of Action. The gabapentinoids bind to the α2δ subunit of Ca_v channels. The α2δ subunit is a membrane glycoprotein with a large extracellular domain that binds to Ca_v α1 pore-forming subunits.[94] In the absence of a cocrystal structure, site-directed mutagenesis studies suggest that gabapentin and pregabalin bind to a conserved Arg217 of α2δ-1 and α2δ-2 isoforms, presumably through an ionic bond with the carboxylic acid group.[95,96] Both gabapentin and pregabalin modulate HVA Ca_v-channel gating, causing a net reduction in glutamate release.[97] By attenuating the release of this excitatory neurotransmitter, gabapentinoids reduce excessive hyperactivity associated with seizures.

A second critical target of gabapentinoids is the system L-amino acid transporter (LAT). As amino acids,

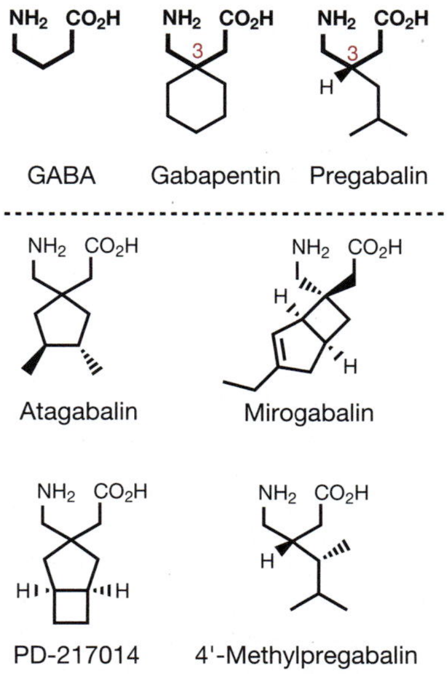

Figure 15.12 Structures of gabapentinoid Ca_v channel blockers. The GABA backbone is shown in bold.

gabapentinoids are poorly permeable by passive diffusion and must be taken up by a facilitated transport mechanism. The LAT family recognizes dietary amino acids like leucine, isoleucine, valine, and phenylalanine. The close structural similarity between the gabapentinoids and dietary amino acids is responsible for active uptake by LAT.

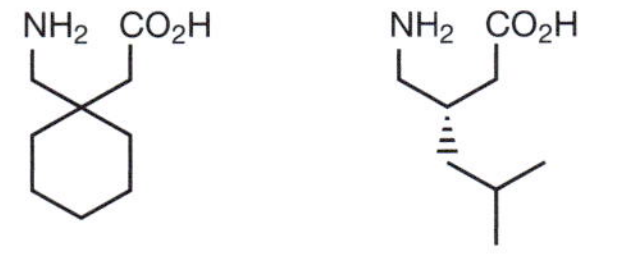

Gabapentin Pregabalin

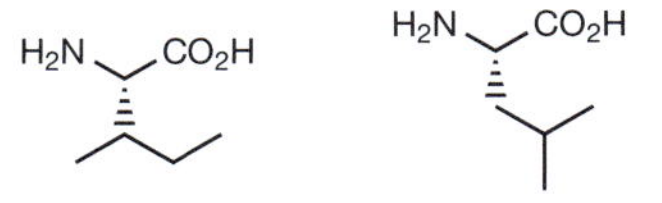

L-Ile L-Leu

Structure-Activity Relationship. Gabapentin and pregabalin contain a GABA amino acid core (Fig. 15.12). The pharmacophore for this class of ASMs consists of (1) a weakly acidic carboxylic acid or bioisostere, (2) cyclic or acyclic hydrocarbons attached to the 3-position, (3) a weakly basic primary amine. For gabapentin, the 3-position alkyl modification is a cyclohexane ring: careful inspection of the structure shows that this is a molecule of GABA modified by the addition of five carbons to form the cyclohexane moiety. This is the basis for the name "gabapentin." Alternate cycloalkyl analogues have been shown to produce even more potent antiepileptic activity in vitro than the parent and are currently under development. For example, atagabalin (a "gababutin") demonstrates more potent α2δ inhibitory effects in vitro, though LAT-mediated transport limits its clinical efficacy in vivo.

Physicochemical and pharmacokinetic properties of Ca_v blockers are provided in Table 15.5.

Metabolism. Gabapentin and pregabalin are not appreciably metabolized. This means no meaningful DDIs are expected, and dose adjustments from metabolically compromised patients are likewise unnecessary.

Gabapentin (Neurontin). Gabapentin was FDA-approved in 1993 as adjunctive treatment of partial seizures and is also approved to treat postherpetic neuralgia. Gabapentin is available in the form of capsules, tablets, and oral solution.

Physicochemical Properties. Gabapentin has both weakly acidic and weakly basic functional groups, making it a zwitterionic compound. The pK_a of the carboxylic acid is 3.7, and the pK_a of the primary amine is 10.7, meaning gabapentin predominately exists in a charged, zwitterionic state at pH 7. Gabapentin is highly water soluble (>100 mg/mL) with a cLogP (n-octanol/0.05 M phosphate buffer) of −1.25 at pH 7.4.[98]

Pharmacokinetics. The zwitterionic nature of gabapentin suggests poor passive permeability across cell membranes. As introduced earlier, LAT type 1 (LAT-1) contributes to the high systemic bioavailability of gabapentin. At high doses, gabapentin overwhelms LAT-1, resulting in dose-limited absorption.[99] This corresponds to a sizable difference in oral bioavailability between low doses (80%, 100 mg every 8 hour) and high doses (27%, 1,600 mg every 8 hour).[100]

Table 15.5 Physicochemical and Pharmacokinetic Properties of Ca_v Blockers

	GBP	PGB	ETX
cLogP	1.19	1.12	0.38
Solubility (mg/mL)	10	>30	39.2
TPSA (Å^2)	63.32	63.32	46.17
f (%)	80	>90	90-95
$t_{1/2}$ (h)	5-7	6.3	30-40 (children) 40-60 (adults)
t_{max} (h)	3.3-3.5	0.6 (fasted) 2-3 (with food)	1-4
Protein binding (%)	None	None	None
V_d (L/kg)	0.8	0.5	0.7
Metabolized by:	None	None	CYP3A
Inducer of:	None	None	None
Inhibitor of:	None	None	None

ETX, ethosuximide; f, oral bioavailability; GBP, gabapentin; PGB, pregabalin; TPSA, topologic polar surface area; V_d, volume of distribution.

Peak plasma concentrations (C_{max}) of approximately 3 to 3.5 μg/mL occur at a t_{max} of 3.3 to 3.5 hours. There is a modest effect of food, which causes ~10% increase in C_{max} and AUC.[101] Due to high aqueous solubility, hydrophilicity, and low plasma protein binding, gabapentin has a V_d of 0.8 L/kg, similar to total body water. Gabapentin $t_{1/2}$ ranges from 5 to 7 hours. Gabapentin is renally excreted, and doses must be monitored in renally compromised patients accordingly. Gabapentin is a possible P-gp substrate.[38]

Specific Adverse Events and Drug-Drug Interactions. Gabapentin, at therapeutic concentrations, neither inhibits nor induces major CYP isoforms, which is suggestive of a safer DDI profile compared to other ASMs. Dizziness and somnolence are the most frequent adverse effects, which are dose-dependent and reversible.[102]

Due to an active uptake mechanism within the gastrointestinal tract (GIT), agents that prolong gastric transit time may enhance gabapentin bioavailability. For example, coadministration with the mu opioid receptor agonist morphine causes a 50% increase in bioavailability of a 600 mg dose of gabapentin.[103] Cimetidine, which is also excreted through a renal elimination route, reduces gabapentin clearance by approximately 12%.[104]

Pregabalin (Lyrica). Pregabalin was approved in 2005 as adjunctive treatment of partial onset seizures. Pregabalin is also approved to treat neuropathic pain, generalized anxiety disorder, and fibromyalgia. Pregabalin is available as oral capsule and suspension formulations. A controlled-release formulation, Lyrica-CR, is approved to treat diabetic peripheral neuropathy and postherpetic neuralgia; however, it has not been tested in seizure disorders.

Physicochemical Properties. Pregabalin is a zwitterionic GABA analogue with weakly acidic and basic functional groups. The pK_a of the carboxylic acid is 4.2, and the pK_a of the basic amine is 10.6. Pregabalin is highly soluble in water (>30 mg/mL).

Pharmacokinetics. Like gabapentin, the zwitterionic pregabalin is actively transported by LAT transporters. A key difference between the absorption of these two agents is that pregabalin is a substrate of multiple LAT transporters, not just LAT-1. This means the absorption of pregabalin is linear and approximately 3-fold greater than gabapentin. Peak plasma concentrations for a single dose during a fasted state are reached within an hour (t_{max} = 0.6 hour), which can rise to 2 to 3 hours with food.[100] Pregabalin is not plasma protein bound and has a V_d of 0.5 L/kg. The $t_{1/2}$ of pregabalin in healthy patients is 6.3 hours. A population pharmacokinetic study showed that patients with creatinine clearance of 100 mL/min had pregabalin clearance of 70 mL/min, indicative of renal resorption.[100]

Specific Adverse Events and Drug-Drug Interactions. Pregabalin has few adverse events or clinically relevant DDIs. Dizziness and somnolence are common side effects and are dose-limited. Pregabalin does not induce or inhibit major CYP isoforms. Pregabalin is a Schedule V drug.

Succinimides and Oxazolidinediones

Older classes of Ca_v blockers that are structurally related to the ureides are the succinimides and oxazolidinediones (Fig. 15.13). Following the success of phenytoin, these agents were originally developed in the 1940s and 1950s to be safer seizure-reducing analogues of phenobarbital. The oxazolidinediones trimethadione and paramethadione were the first of this series to show efficacy at treating absence seizures, although severe toxicities, including hemeralopia and agranulocytosis, limited their therapeutic use. As a serendipitous discovery, the succinimide ethosuximide (Zarontin) emerged in 1958 with an alternate mechanism of action and a better safety profile when compared to both phenobarbital and phenytoin. As such, ethosuximide is clinically effective at treating absence seizures, whereas these other ASMs are not.

RECEPTOR BINDING/MECHANISM OF ACTION. In contrast to α2δ subunits of HVA currents that modulate neurotransmitter release, T-type Ca_v channels (Ca_v 3) are responsible for "low-threshold Ca^{2+} spikes." These channels are located in the thalamus and cause bursting and intrinsic oscillations, which are hallmarks of generalized absence seizures. Succinimides block firing of several Ca_v3-channel types, including α1G (Ca_v3.1), α1H (Ca_v3.2), and α1I (Ca_v3.3). The mechanism of Ca_v3-channel blockade appears to include both blockade of the open (activated) state of the channel and preferential blockade of inactivated channels.[105]

STRUCTURE-ACTIVITY RELATIONSHIP. Like phenytoin, oxazolidinediones and succinimides share a similar pharmacophore: (1) a five-membered heterocyclic ring system containing an imide and (2) an sp^3-hybridized carbon containing up to

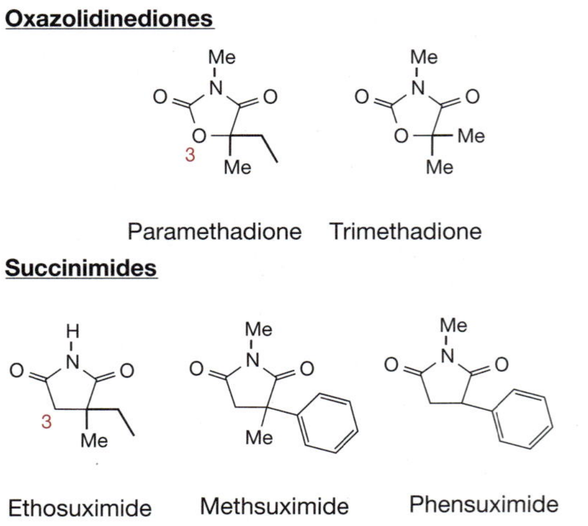

Figure 15.13 Oxazolidinediones and succinimides.

two hydrocarbon groups, of which only one may be aromatic (Fig. 15.13). A key difference in the pharmacophore responsible for the divergent pharmacodynamics of these classes is the lack of a *gem*-diphenyl substituent that is posited to be required for Na_v blockade (Fig. 15.8). The Ca_v-selective oxazolidinediones and succinimides do not have this group and are, thus, inactive at Na_v channels. Another point of differentiation between the classes can be found at position 3. The hydantoins have a nitrogen atom at this position, which is exchanged for an oxygen (oxazolidinediones) or a carbon (succinimides) atom. Although this modification has little impact on pharmacodynamics, there are modest differences in pharmacokinetics between these classes. Both *N*-methyl and *N*-desmethyl succinimide metabolites are pharmacologically active.

ETHOSUXIMIDE (ZARONTIN)

Metabolism. Ethosuximide is metabolized by both phase 1 and phase 2 mechanisms to inactive metabolites. As shown in Figure 15.14, the major route of elimination is ω-1 oxidation of the 2-ethyl group (40%-60% of the administered dose). Since ethosuximide is administered as a racemic mixture of (2*R*) and (2*S*) isomers, the resulting 2-(1-hydroxyethyl) metabolites are generated as a mixture of four diastereomeric products. The same is true when the ring itself is oxidized at the 3-position (3-hydroxylation, 7%-8%). This metabolic route is not possible in the hydantoin series. A minor route of metabolism is oxidation of the terminal carbon of the 2-ethyl substituent to give 2-(2-hydroxyethyl) succinimide. This product can be oxidized further to the terminal carboxylic acid metabolite. These phase 1 metabolic pathways are mediated selectively by CYP3A isoforms. Glucuronidation of these hydroxylated metabolites is a major metabolic route, accounting for 20% to 40% of the administered dose of ethosuximide.[106,107]

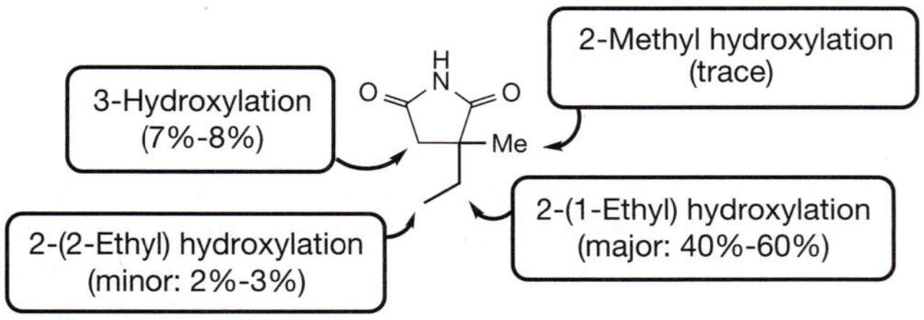

Figure 15.14 Sites of metabolic inactivation of ethosuximide.

Physicochemical Properties. The *gem*-dialkyl-substituted carbon of ethosuximide is a chiral center. No significant differences in pharmacologic activity have been reported for (*R*)- and (*S*)-enantiomers, and ethosuximide is administered as the racemate. Like phenytoin, the imide of ethosuximide is weakly acidic, with a pK_a of 9.3. Ethosuximide is more hydrophilic than phenytoin (cLogP 0.38 compared to 2.52) and is also more water soluble (39.2 mg/mL). The TPSA is 46.17 Å and is freely centrally bioavailable.

Pharmacokinetics. Ethosuximide has high oral bioavailability (90%-95%), reaching maximum concentration at t_{max} of 1 to 3 hours. The syrup formulation is absorbed faster than capsules, though the AUCs are similar. Ethosuximide is not bound to plasma proteins and has V_d of 0.7 L/kg. This suggests few DDIs when coadministered with plasma-bound ASMs. The $t_{1/2}$ is approximately 40 to 60 hours in adults and 30 to 40 hours in children, meaning once-daily dosing is appropriate. In light of the substantial effect of CYP3A metabolism on the pharmacokinetic profile of ethosuximide, $t_{1/2}$ may increase in patients with hepatic impairment. Elimination follows first-order kinetics. Clearance is 0.01 L/kg/h in adults and 0.016 to 0.013 L/kg/h in children.[108-110] Ethosuximide is unlikely to be a P-gp substrate.[38]

Specific Adverse Events and Drug-Drug Interactions. Like other ASMs, ethosuximide can cause somnolence, headache, and dizziness. Confusion, sleep disturbances, depression, and aggression can be behavioral consequences of ethosuximide use.[111] Episodes of psychotic behavior have been reported that are resolved on discontinuation.[112]

Unlike other first-generation ASMs, ethosuximide does not induce CYPs or UGT enzymes. One report showed a significant decrease in serum concentration of valproic acid.[113] Due to extensive hepatic metabolism by CYP3A enzymes, there is a significant decrease in ethosuximide plasma concentrations when coadministered with CYP-inducing ASMs—for example, carbamazepine, phenytoin, and phenobarbital.[114] Likewise, care should be taken when administering ethosuximide with other CYP3A inhibitors, which may increase drug plasma levels.

Modulators of GABA Signaling

The first clinically used ASMs, the barbiturates, produce potent sedative/hypnotic effects through inhibitory mechanisms. We now understand that GABA is the predominant inhibitory neurotransmitter system in the brain, and extensive research into the mechanisms behind GABAergic signaling has revealed many therapeutic targets for treating epilepsy disorders.

Barbiturates

The discovery of the anticonvulsant properties of the sedative hypnotic phenobarbital arguably began the era of development of pharmacotherapies to treat seizure disorders. Attempts to separate the anticonvulsant properties from sedation, hypnosis, and abuse potential of phenobarbital resulted in the hydantoins, succinimides, and oxazolidinediones. The sedative hypnotic effects of barbiturates are discussed in more detail in Chapter 14; here, we will focus on the properties of barbiturates that afford anticonvulsant activity.

Receptor Binding/Mechanism of Action. At clinically relevant doses, barbiturates (Fig. 15.15) are PAMs of $GABA_A$ channels. Barbiturates increase the amount of time the channel stays open when bound by GABA but have no effect on the frequency of channel opening. At high doses, barbiturates can act as $GABA_A$ agonists in the absence of GABA. Barbiturates also inhibit α-amino-3-hydroxy-5-methyl-4-isoxazolepropionic acid (AMPA) and kainate receptors (KRs) (glutamate receptors), nicotinic receptors, and at higher doses, P/Q-type Ca_v channels and glutamate release. The exact binding site for barbiturates on $GABA_A$ channels is not fully understood, though evidence suggests β subunits are involved.[115]

Structure-Activity Relationship. Barbiturates are characterized by their barbituric acid core, a six-membered ring system consisting of alternating imide carbonyl and nitrogen atoms (Fig. 15.16, R1=R2=H). To be pharmacologically active, barbituric acid must be *gem*-disubstituted at position 5 (R1=R2=alkyl or aryl). Most barbiturates are substituted with an ethyl group (R1=ethyl), and the nature of R2 substitution determines the onset and duration of action, and consequently the indication. For example, when R2=phenyl (phenobarbital), the low lipophilicity (cLogP = 1.67) means less drug is distributed to peripheral tissues than more lipophilic drugs such as the ultra-short-acting thiopental, which is no longer marketed in the United States (R2 = *sec*-pentyl, cLogP 2.99). Long-acting hydrophilic barbiturates are useful as ASMs due to infrequent dosing. Alkylation of the imide nitrogen atoms is a prodrug strategy for enhancing duration of action and avoiding reinforcing effects that can cause abuse. To be fully-active ASMs, both imides must be secondary, which requires dealkylation of tertiary imide prodrugs. This was the rationale behind the design of nonmarketed drugs, mephobarbital, metharbital, eterobarb, and

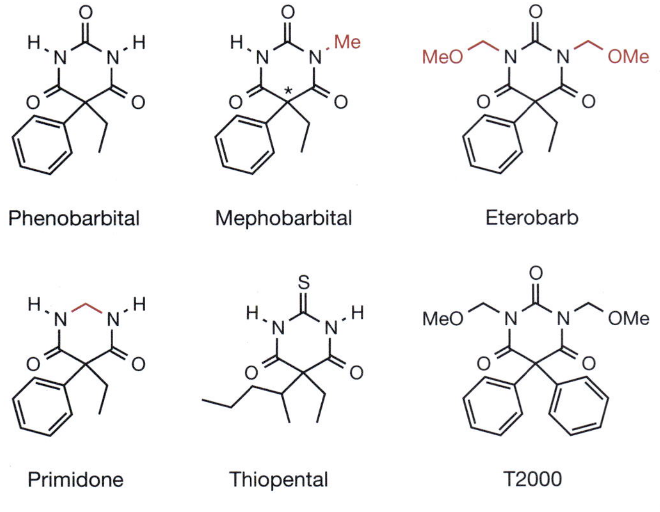

Figure 15.15 Anticonvulsant barbiturates. Labile portions of analogues that are metabolized to phenobarbital are shown in red (* = chiral center).

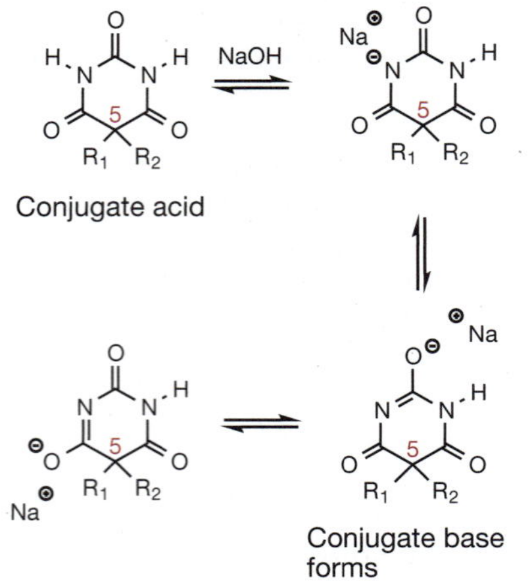

Figure 15.16 Conjugate acid and base forms of barbiturates.

the investigational drug T2000: the delayed onset of action reduces the rapid rewarding effects.

Physicochemical Properties. Barbituric acids are weakly acidic (pK_a 7.4). In the presence of weak base such as sodium hydroxide, the imide is deprotonated to one of the three conjugate base forms (Fig. 15.16). The sodium salt of the conjugate base is much more water soluble than the protonated free conjugate acid form and is therefore available for parenteral injection. Long-acting anticonvulsant barbiturates are generally more hydrophilic (cLogP approximately 0.5) than shorter-acting derivatives used for anesthetic and sedative hypnotic purposes. Double-prodrugs like eterobarb and T2000 are neutral until metabolized into their active barbituric acid–derived products.

Physicochemical and pharmacokinetic properties of barbiturate antiseizure agents are provided in Table 15.6.

Table 15.6 Physicochemical and Pharmacokinetic Properties of Barbiturates and Benzodiazepines

	PBT	PRM	CLB	CLO	CZM	DZP	LZP	MDZ
cLogP	1.67	0.40	1.69	2.90	2.34	2.91	2.47	3.93
Solubility (mg/mL)	1[a] 1,000[b]	0.6	0.18	0.02	0.01	0.005	0.08	>5 (HCl salt)
TPSA (Å^2)	75.27	58.20	40.62	78.76	87.28	32.67	61.69	27.96
f (%)	>90	100	87	90	>95	>90	100 (IM)	>90 (IM) 75-80 (oromucosal)
$t_{1/2}$ (h)	>48[c] >120[d]	10	24	30-100	17-56	48[e] ~100[f]	14	3-4
t_{max} (h)	0.5-4	1.5-3	0.5-2	1-3	1-4	0.5-1	3	0.5-1
Protein binding (%)	50	20-30	90	98	85	98	>90	98
V_d (L/kg)	0.7	0.4-1.0	1.31	0.8-1.0	1.5-4.4	0.8-1.0	1.3	5.3
Metabolized by:	CYP2C9 CYP2C19	CYPs[g]	CYP2C19 CYP3A4	CYP3A4[h]	CYP3A4	CYP2C19 CYP3A4	UGTs	CYP3A4
Inducer of:	CYP2C9 CYP2C19 CYP3A4	CYP2C9 CYP2C19 CYP3A4 UGTs	CYP3A4	None	None	None	None	None
Inhibitor of:	None	None	CYP2D6 CYP2C19[i] UGTs[i]	None	None	None		None

CLB, clobazam; CLO, clorazepate; CZM, clonazepam; DZP, diazepam; f, oral bioavailability; IM, intramuscular; LZP, lorazepam; MZD, midazolam; PBT, phenobarbital; PRM, primidone; TPSA, topologic polar surface area; V_d, volume of distribution.

[a]Free acid.

[b]Na^+ salt.

[c]In children.

[d]In adults.

[e]Initial distribution phase.

[f]Active metabolite, nordiazepam.

[g]Isoform(s) unknown.

[h]Clorazepate is chemically unstable to acid and converted to nordiazepam, which is metabolized by CYP3A4.

[i]NDMC metabolite.

PHENOBARBITAL (LUMINAL). Phenobarbital is one of the first clinically used anticonvulsants, and its use has been consistent through the past century. Its high effectiveness and low cost make phenobarbital a reasonable treatment option in situations where alternatives are cost-prohibitive. Its common modern use is in tonic-clonic and partial seizures. Originally developed and approved in 1912 as a sedative/hypnotic, its anticonvulsant activity was discovered serendipitously by Alfred Hauptmann to help his epileptic patients—and therefore himself—sleep through the night. He found that one dose of Luminal blocked their seizures in addition to helping them sleep. This discovery led to phenobarbital usurping bromides as the treatment of choice for seizures, causing a revolution in ASM treatment.[3] Phenobarbital is on the World Health Organization (WHO) 20th List of Essential Medicines.

Physicochemical Properties. Phenobarbital has a cLogP of 1.67 and TPSA of 75.27 Å. The free acid is only slightly soluble in water (1 mg/mL), whereas the sodium salt is highly water soluble (1,000 mg/mL).

Metabolism. The phenyl ring of phenobarbital is oxidized to the arene oxide intermediate II (Fig. 15.17), which undergoes an National Institutes of Health (NIH) shift to the inactive *p*-phenol. The particular isoform(s) responsible for this transformation remain unexplored, but the reaction may be catalyzed in part by CYP2C9.[116]

Pharmacokinetics. Phenobarbital bioavailability is greater than 90% when given orally in tablet or elixir form. The low cLogP of phenobarbital (1.67) contributes to low plasma protein binding of approximately 50%. Thus, clinically relevant DDIs due to plasma protein binding are not anticipated. The V_d of phenobarbital is 0.7 L/kg. Approximately 20% of phenobarbital dose is eliminated unchanged in the urine through a first-order process. Clearance in children (Cl = 4 mL/kg/h) is faster when compared to that in adults (Cl = 4 mL/kg/h) and older adults (3 mL/kg/h). Consequently, the $t_{1/2}$ in children (2.5 d) and adults (5 d) permits once-daily dosing.[117] Therapeutic drug monitoring should be undertaken for patients with renal and kidney disease. Phenobarbital is a substrate and inducer of CYP2C9 and has autoinducing properties. Phenobarbital is a P-gp substrate.[38]

Specific Adverse Events and Drug-Drug Interactions. As a sedative/hypnotic, phenobarbital causes severe somnolence at higher doses as well as disrupts memory and cognition. Maternal use of phenobarbital during pregnancy and exposure to phenobarbital during the first 3 years of life are associated with increased risk of cognitive and intelligence deficits.[118,119]

Phenobarbital is an inducer of CYP2C9, CYP2C19, CYP3A4, and UGT enzymes, which is responsible for many DDIs with other ASMs and non-anticonvulsants, such as hormonal contraceptives. Thus, care should be taken when using phenobarbital with other CYP substrates in polydrug therapy. Additionally, the use of other enzyme-inducing ASMs impacts phenobarbital clearance, underscoring the point that therapeutic drug monitoring is critical when using this agent.[120] Phenobarbital is a Schedule IV controlled substance.

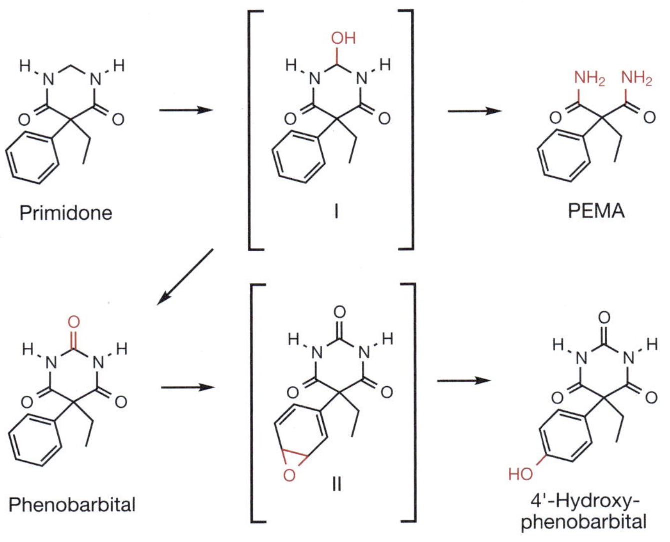

Figure 15.17 Metabolism of primidone and phenobarbital. PEMA, phenylethylmalonamide.

PRIMIDONE (MYSOLINE). Primidone was FDA approved in 1954 and is used to treat generalized seizures. Primidone is a prodrug of phenobarbital and is not entirely understood whether the anticonvulsant properties of primidone are due exclusively to metabolism to phenobarbital in vivo, or whether the parent drug contributes to the pharmacologic profile.

Metabolism. Primidone is metabolized to phenobarbital through an oxidized intermediate I (Fig.15.17). This step is CYP-dependent, although the identities of the responsible isoforms are unknown. Intermediate I can also undergo hydrolysis to phenylethylmalonamide (PEMA). Whether PEMA contributes to the anticonvulsant effects of primidone is controversial, although evidence suggests it does not. The ratio of phenobarbital/PEMA is approximately 1:2.5.

Physicochemical Properties. Primidone is technically not a barbituric acid derivative, although it is a prodrug of phenobarbital. Instead of a barbituric acid core, primidone contains two uncharged amides within a six-membered ring. Primidone is poorly water soluble (0.6 mg/mL) and, unlike barbiturates, is not weakly acidic and, therefore, cannot be formulated as the sodium salt. Primidone has a cLogP of 1.12 and a TPSA of 58.2 Å.

Pharmacokinetics. It is important to consider that primidone is metabolized to phenobarbital; thus, phenobarbital contributes to the observed clinical effects of primidone. Primidone is nearly completely absorbed on oral administration, with t_{max} occurring within 1.5 to 3 hours. The V_d is approximately 0.4 to 1 L/kg, and plasma protein binding is low (20%-30%). Hepatic metabolism accounts for approximately 60% of the elimination of primidone, with the remaining 40% of the unchanged parent drug found in the urine. Around 25% of the dose is excreted as PEMA. Phenobarbital (2%) and *p*-OH-phenobarbital (2%) are minor metabolites, as are *p*-OH-phenobarbital conjugates. Clearance of PEMA is significantly lower in older adults owing to the renal elimination of this metabolite.[121]

Specific Adverse Events and Drug-Drug Interactions. Side effects of primidone are similar to other barbiturates, though generally milder. Like phenobarbital and phenytoin, primidone is associated with osteoporosis and osteopenia. Primidone, like its phenobarbital metabolite, is a CYP and UGT inducer, thereby impacting the clearance of coadministered CYP and UGT substrates. Though primidone is metabolized to phenobarbital in vivo, it is not a scheduled substance.

Benzodiazepines

The serendipitous discovery by Leo Sternbach in the 1950s that the benzodiazepine, chlordiazepoxide, is active against seizures and anxiety disorders quickly proved to be revolutionary. This important class of agents is discussed in greater detail in Chapters 11 and 14; this section will focus on the features of benzodiazepines that are important for their antiepileptic MOA (Fig. 15.18). The benzodiazepines most frequently used to treat epilepsy disorders are clonazepam (Klonopin), diazepam (Valium, Diastat), chlorazepate (Tranxene), lorazepam (Ativan), midazolam (Versed), and clobazam (Onfi). Midazolam (buccal, oromucosal solution) and diazepam (rectal gel) are special formulations that can be used in emergency situations to treat status epilepticus. Diazepam, lorazepam, and midazolam are on the WHO 20th List of Essential Medicines.

Receptor Binding/Mechanism of Action. Like barbiturates, benzodiazepines augment $GABA_A$-channel signaling through an allosteric mechanism; however, benzodiazepines bind $GABA_A$ via a different binding site that increases the frequency of channel opening when bound by GABA. The allosteric binding sites are flanked by α and γ subunits on pentameric $GABA_A$ ion channels. When bound by ligands, these "benzodiazepine receptors" (BZRs) permit a conformational change in the channel that promotes enhanced channel opening in the presence of GABA. It should be noted that the BZR is not a receptor in itself, but rather is a specific binding site on $GABA_A$ channels. Of the six cloned and characterized α subunits, only α4 and α6 are insensitive to classical benzodiazepines and, thus, are not responsible for their antiepileptic mechanism. All currently available benzodiazepines are nonselective PAMs of α1 to α3 and α5. Reported $GABA_A$ channelopathies contribute to seizure disorders through mutations of γ2 subunits that reduce channel signaling.[29,30]

Structure-Activity Relationship. Figure 15.19 shows the SAR of benzodiazepines in the "azepam" (Series A) and "azolam" (Series B) series. In Series A, short-chain *N*-alkyl groups are tolerated at position 1 (R1), as is the nonalkylated 2° amide. Position 2 must have a hydrogen bond–accepting carbonyl or bioisostere. Position 3 can be unsubstituted or oxidized to a secondary alcohol. Chlorazepate, which has an exocyclic carboxylate group at the 3-position, is a prodrug that is converted to the active metabolite through decarboxylation. Most benzodiazepines have an imine in the 4,5-position, though the newest anticonvulsant benzodiazepine, clobazam, has an amide. The role of this structural region is to maintain rigidity in the diazepine ring. Electron-withdrawing groups at position 7 enhance antiepileptic activity, as well as sedative and hypnotic effects. Halogens at the 2′ position are also tolerated and add to the sedative actions of the molecule.

Metabolism. Clonazepam, diazepam, and clorazepate are N-dealkylated by CYP3A4 into active *N*-desmethyl metabolites II (Fig. 15.20). Clorazepate is chemically unstable in acid and is converted to *N*-desmethyldiazepam (II, R1 = H, R7 = Cl, R2′ = H) in the acidic environment of the stomach. Intermediates of type II can be oxidized further at position 3 into active 3-hydroxy metabolites (III) by CYP3A4, or inactivated to 9-hydroxy (IV) or 4′-hydroxy (V) metabolites. Oxidized metabolites III to V can be glucuronidated by UGT enzymes prior to elimination.

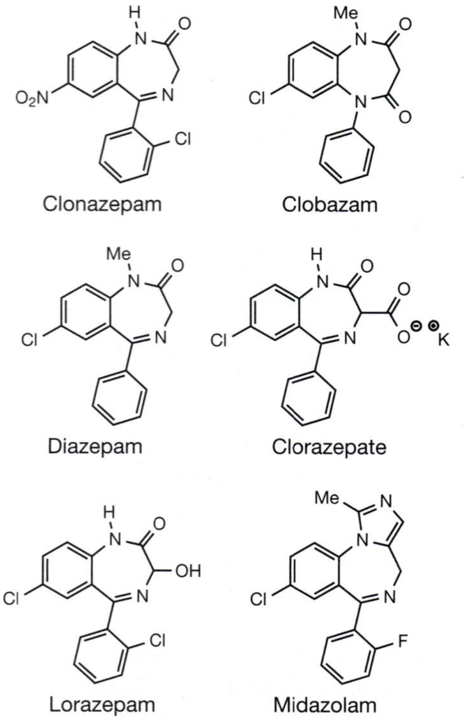

Figure 15.18 Benzodiazepines used to treat seizures.

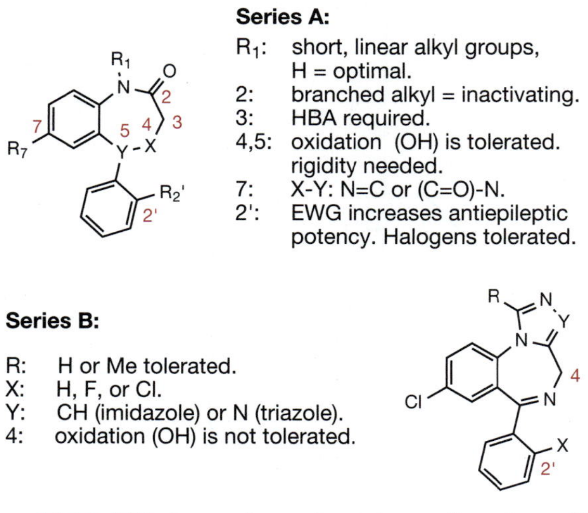

Figure 15.19 SAR for anticonvulsant benzodiazepines. EWG, electron-withdrawing group; HBA, hydrogen bond acceptor.

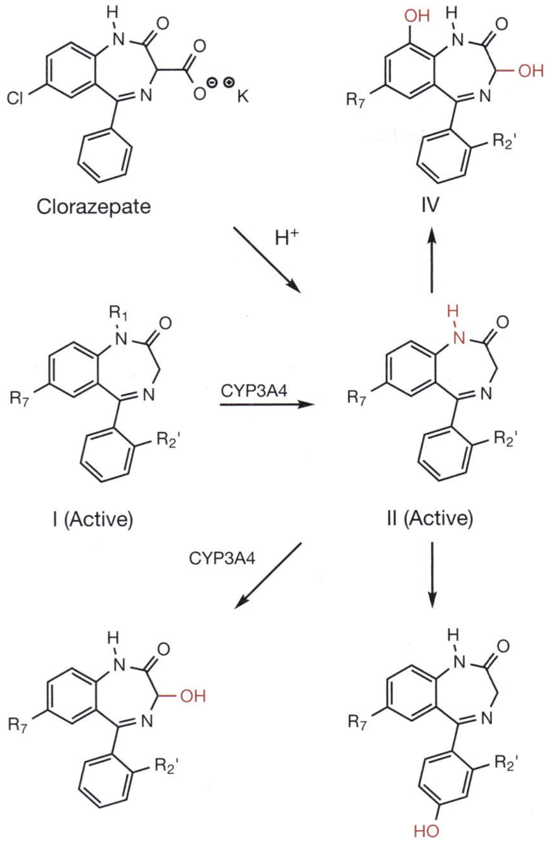

Figure 15.20 Metabolism of clonazepam, diazepam, and clorazepate. Clonazepam: R_1 = H, R_7 = NO_2, R_2' = Cl. Diazepam: R_1 = Me, R_7 = Cl, R_2' = H. Site of metabolism shown in red. Oxidized metabolites III-V can be metabolized further into inactive glucuronide conjugates.

PHYSICOCHEMICAL PROPERTIES. Benzodiazepines of the "azepam" class generally have poor aqueous solubility (<1 mg/mL) and can be given orally or by injection. Injection of aqueous-insoluble benzodiazepines requires the use of propylene glycol, which can cause local pain. Clorazepate is an exception: the chemically unstable carboxylic acid prodrug is formulated as the disodium salt. Benzodiazepines are modestly lipophilic, with cLogP values ranging from 1.69 (clobazam) to 2.91 (diazepam). The TPSA of benzodiazepines ranges from 32.67 Å (diazepam) to 93.27 Å (clonazepam). The 7-nitro substituent of clonazepam likely contributes to this higher value.

Physicochemical and pharmacokinetic properties of benzodiazepine antiseizure agents are provided in Table 15.6.

SPECIFIC ADVERSE EVENTS AND DRUG-DRUG INTERACTIONS. Tolerance to benzodiazepines can develop quickly, leading to decreased effectiveness with continued use. Abrupt discontinuation of benzodiazepines can lower seizure threshold, leading to increased risk of convulsions. Benzodiazepines are sedative-hypnotics; thus, sedation and memory impairment are common side effects that may be undesirable when treating seizure disorders. Benzodiazepines used as ASMs can cause life-threatening respiratory events and excessive sedation, so their use should be monitored in emergency settings. Respiratory depression is exacerbated by opioids, meaning that benzodiazepine doses should be lowered when given concomitantly. Benzodiazepines carry abuse and dependence potential and are, thus, on the Schedule IV list.

LORAZEPAM (ATIVAN). Lorazepam is a first-generation ASM that has sedative hypnotic and antiepileptic properties. Though tablet formulations are prescribed to treat anxiety and sleeping disorders, injectable formulations of lorazepam are available as treatments for status epilepticus. Lorazepam is on the WHO List of Essential Medicines.

Metabolism. The 3-hydroxyl group of lorazepam is extensively metabolized through phase 2 processes by UGT enzymes from the UGT1A and UGT2B subfamilies. The resulting lorazepam-3-O-glucuronide is pharmacologically inactive. This is in contrast to the metabolites of other "azepams" used as ASMs that can be biotransformed through phase 1 mechanisms to pharmacologically active products.

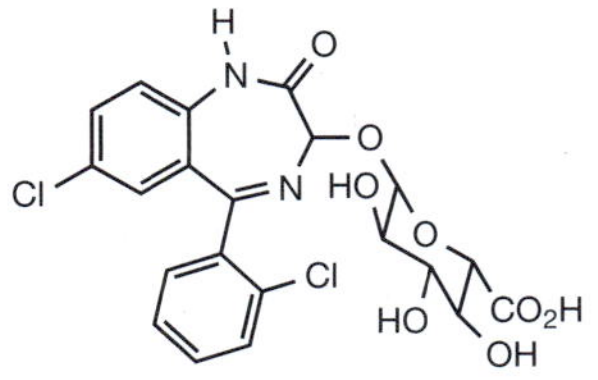

Lorazepam-3-*O*-glucuronide

Pharmacokinetics. Pharmacokinetic parameters are similar for IV or IM administration of lorazepam. Bioavailability is high (100%) on IM administration. Maximal concentrations are slightly lower for IM (C_{max} = 48 ng/mL) compared to IV (C_{max} = 90 ng/mL). Lorazepam is lipophilic (cLogP = 2.47) and plasma protein bound (90%). Maximal concentrations are reached within 3 hours, similar to other "azepam" benzodiazepines; the terminal half-life of lorazepam is shorter than that of clonazepam and diazepam ($t_{1/2}$ = 14 h). The V_d (1.3 L/kg) and Cl (1.1 ± 0.4 mL/min/kg) are similar to other benzodiazepines. The hepatic metabolite lorazepam-3-O-glucuronide undergoes enterohepatic recycling and is eliminated by the kidneys. Renal impairment significantly impacts half-life and clearance: patients with renal dysfunction or under hemodialysis experience 55% to 125% increase in $t_{1/2}$ and 75% to 90% decrease in clearance compared to healthy controls.[122]

Specific Adverse Events and Drug-Drug Interactions. Lorazepam should not be used in pregnant patients in the first trimester except for in life-threatening situations due to the potential to produce fetal abnormalities. Both lorazepam and lorazepam-3-O-glucuronide have been found in umbilical cord blood. Poor aqueous solubility (<0.1 mg/mL) requires formulation in benzyl alcohol that can cause hypotension and other toxicities in neonates and preterm infants. Use of lorazepam in these patients should be minimized.

Coadministration of lorazepam with valproic acid causes a significant decrease in formation of the 3-O-glucuronide metabolite due to competition with UGT enzymes. The dose of lorazepam should be lowered in patients taking valproic acid as a prophylactic treatment for seizures. Women on hormonal contraception experience a significant increase in metabolic clearance of lorazepam; doses of lorazepam need to be increased in these patients. Lorazepam is unlikely to be a P-gp substrate.

Clobazam (Onfi). Clobazam is a structurally unique benzodiazepine in that it contains a 1,5-diazepine ring instead of a 1,4-diazepine. Originally developed in the 1970s as an anxiolytic, clobazam was FDA-approved in 2011 for the adjunctive treatment of Lennox-Gastaut syndrome in patients older than age 2. It is also used as an adjuvant to treat refractory seizures. Clobazam is available in tablet and suspension forms.

Metabolism. Hepatic metabolism of clobazam is afforded through CYP3A4 and CYP2C19. Both enzymes are implicated in the generation of the active metabolite, *N*-desmethylclobazam (NDMC; Fig. 15.21), although the higher expression of CYP3A4 in the liver suggests this isoform is the most clinically relevant. Conversion of NDMC to the inactive 4′-OH-NDMC is mediated by CYP2C19. Though NDMC has preferential affinity for α2-containing $GABA_A$ channels, this does not impact its antiepileptic profile.[123]

Pharmacokinetics. Clobazam is rapidly and extensively absorbed when given orally. Peak concentrations are reached between 0.5 and 2 hours after a single dose, which increases on multiple dosing. Food has no effect on C_{max}, AUC, or t_{max}. The apparent V_d of clobazam is approximately 1.31 L/kg. Clobazam and NDMC are highly protein bound (89%-90% and 70%, respectively). Elimination is primarily renal, although only approximately 2% of clobazam is recovered unchanged in the urine. The most prevalent urinary metabolites are NDMC and its conjugates (94%). Circulating concentrations of NDMC are 3 to 5 times higher than those of the parent drug. The elimination $t_{1/2}$ is 24 hours. Clearance of clobazam is significantly impaired in older adult patients, although renal and hepatic impairment has a small effect on pharmacokinetics.[124]

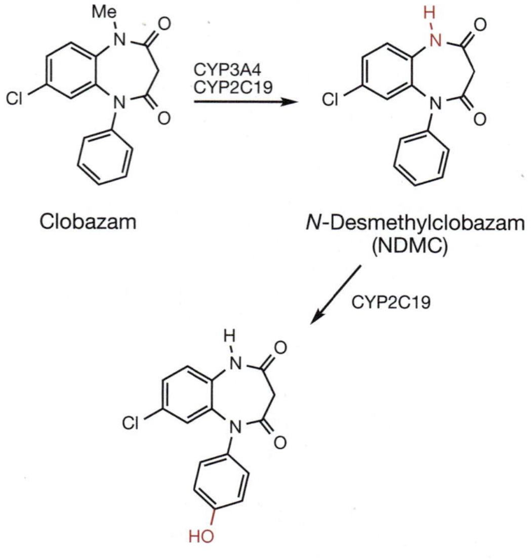

Figure 15.21 Metabolism of clobazam.

Specific Adverse Events and Drug-Drug Interactions. Like all benzodiazepines, excessive somnolence and lethargy are frequent side effects. Patients who are poor metabolizers of CYP2C19 may have trouble clearing NDMC, leading to artificially high plasma levels of active drug. Coadministration of clobazam with CYP-inducing ASMs accelerates clobazam metabolism to NDMC and 4′-OH-NDMC. Furthermore, coadministration with a CYP2C19 inhibitor like felbamate inhibits the clearance of NDMC, causing an increase in plasma concentrations of this active metabolite. Such combinations may cause toxicities.[125,126] Clobazam is a weak CYP3A4 inducer and CYP2D6 inhibitor. NDMC is a weak inhibitor of CYP2C9 and several UGT isoforms.[124] The CYP3A4-inducing effect of clobazam may contribute to a loss of contraceptive efficacy.

Midazolam (Versed). Midazolam plays an important role in treating seizure disorders as an emergency medication to treat status epilepticus. The unique chemical and pharmacokinetic properties of midazolam are perfect for oromucosal absorption, effective distribution, and rapid metabolism. In this way, emergency personnel may treat patients who are unable to receive intravenous injections, and the sedative effects will subside in a relatively short order.

Physicochemical Properties. As an "azolam" benzodiazepine, the physicochemical properties of midazolam are quite different from classical, "azepam" benzodiazepines. The two-position of the fused imidazole is weakly basic, with a pK_a of 6.15. This means midazolam may be formulated as the hydrochloride salt (Fig. 15.22), which has higher aqueous solubility (>5 mg/mL). In acidic solutions (pH 3.3), the diazepine ring is in equilibrium between ring-closed states (80%-85%) and hydrolyzed

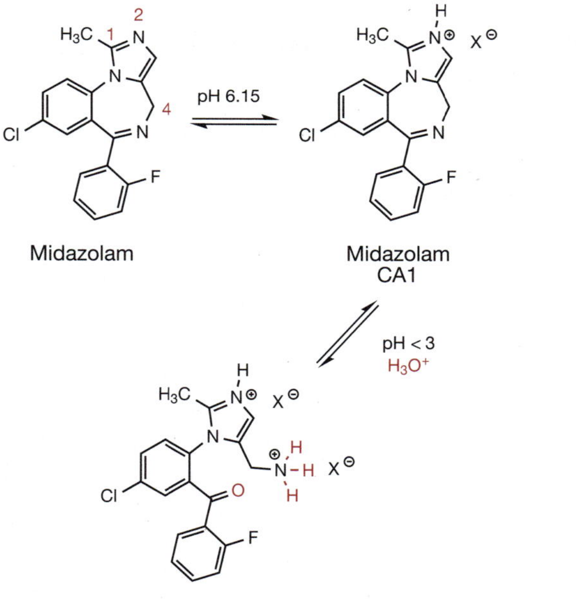

Figure 15.22 Equilibrium between charged conjugate acid (CA) states of midazolam. In aqueous buffer (pH 3.3), the CA1/CA2 ratio is approximately 80:20.

ring-open states (15%-20%). This means midazolam has two conjugate acid forms (CA1, CA2; Fig. 15.22). In the bloodstream (pH 7.4), the dihydrochloride (CA2) shifts its equilibrium back to the ring-closed free base state, which has a cLogP of 3.93 and TPSA of 27.96 Å. These properties make midazolam highly BBB-penetrating, with a fast onset of antiepileptic action.[127]

Metabolism. Midazolam is rapidly metabolized to inactive products. The major route of inactivation is CYP3A4-mediated oxidation of the α-carbon on position 1 of the imidazole ring (Fig. 15.23). This is responsible for the short duration of antiepileptic and sedative action. The α-OH-midazolam metabolite is conjugated and eliminated as the glucuronide. A minor route of metabolism is oxidation at the 4-position, analogous to the 3-position of classical "azepams." Unlike 3-hydroxylated azepam metabolites, 4-OH-midazolam is inactive.[127]

Pharmacokinetics. Approximately 75% to 80% of oromucosal midazolam hydrochloride is absorbed with a t_{max} within 30 minutes in children. Midazolam is lipophilic, highly protein bound (98%), and extensively distributed (V_d 5.3 L/kg). Midazolam is 60% metabolized by hepatic oxidation (CYP3A4) to inactive metabolites. The major metabolite is α-hydroxymidazolam and its glucuronide conjugate. This metabolite is more prevalent in children than in adults. Plasma clearance in children is 30 mL/kg/min, which is increased in hepatically impaired patients. The elimination $t_{1/2}$ of oromucosal midazolam is around 200 minutes. Renal impairment does not impact clearance.

Specific Adverse Events and Drug-Drug Interactions. Midazolam can cause life-threatening respiratory depression and arrest in adults, children, and neonates. Thus, patients should be monitored for labored breathing when given midazolam and other benzodiazepines. Reversal of benzodiazepine overdose is achieved with the $GABA_A$ antagonist, flumazenil. Importantly, flumazenil will only reverse the effects of benzodiazepines, and not other concomitantly administered ASMs. Midazolam can cross the placental barrier and enter human milk.

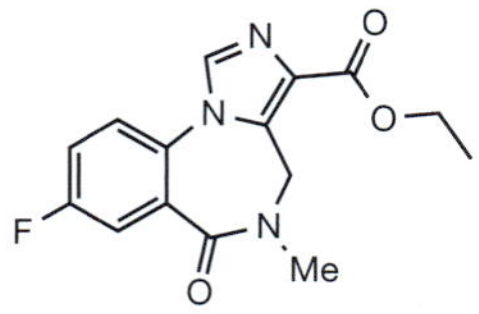

Flumazenil

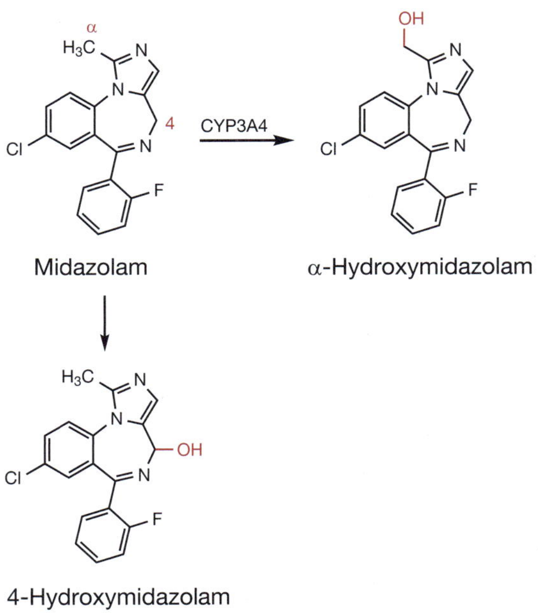

Figure 15.23 Metabolism of midazolam.

Miscellaneous $GABA_A$ Potentiators

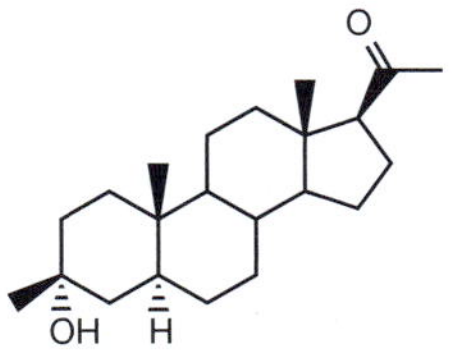

Ganaxolone
(Ztalmy)

GANAXOLONE (ZTALMY). Ganaxolone was approved in March 2022 to treat seizures associated with cyclin-dependent kinase-like five deficiency disorder (CDD) in patients aged 2 years and older. It is the first and, so far, only medication specifically approved to treat CDD.

Receptor Binding/Mechanism of Action. Like the other $GABA_A$ potentiators mentioned in this section, ganaxolone is an allosteric potentiator (positive allosteric modulator, PAM) of $GABA_A$ channels. Unlike these other agents, ganaxolone is a derivative of a class of neurosteroids and binds to an allosteric site that is not shared by benzodiazepines or barbiturates. Another unique feature of ganaxolone is that it is active against both synaptic $GABA_A$ receptors that contain α, β, and γ subunits, and extrasynaptic $GABA_A$ channels that contain α, β, and δ subunits. This gives ganaxolone an enhanced neuronal suppression against seizures. Like the barbiturates, ganaxolone appears to increase the frequency of receptor firing to GABA.

Structure-Activity Relationship. Ganaxolone is a semisynthetic derivative of the neurosteroid allopregnanolone. The key difference between ganaxolone and allopregnanolone is the presence of a β-methyl group at position 3. This turns the 3-OH group from secondary in allopregnanolone to tertiary and prevents oxidation by 3α-hydroxysteroid dehydrogenase (3α-HSD) to the progestin 5α-dihydroprogesterone. This increases duration of action and prevents activation of progesterone receptors.

Metabolism. Ganaxolone is metabolized extensively by CYP3A4/5, CYP2B6, CYP2C19, and CYP2D6 into dozens of metabolites. The 20-position ketone can be reduced to the secondary alcohol, which can then undergo phase-II conjugation. All of the metabolites of ganaxolone are inactive.

Physicochemical Properties. Ganaxolone does not contain any functional groups that would be ionizable under physiologically relevant pH. The LogP is predicted to be 4.37, and the TPSA is 37.3 Å^2. As a steroid, ganaxolone has negligible solubility in water.

Pharmacokinetics. Ganaxolone is administered as an oral suspension and reaches t_{max} between 2 and 3 hours. As a lipophilic compound, taking ganaxolone with a high-fat meal will significantly increase AUC. The oral bioavailability in the fed state is low (approximately 10%). Ganaxolone is widely distributed and has a tissue-to-plasma level of more than 5:1. The apparent $t_{1/2}$ is over 20 hours. Elimination is predominately through the feces (as metabolites), though approximately 20% of the metabolites are eliminated via the urine.[128]

Specific Adverse Effects and Drug-Drug Interactions. When compared to other ASMs, the side effect profile of ganaxolone is relatively marginal. As a $GABA_A$-PAM, ganaxolone has abuse and dependence liability; however, the risk is low, and ganaxolone is placed in Schedule V. Somnolence and sedation are the most commonly observed side effects. As with all ASMs, ganaxolone comes with a warning to monitor for suicidal thoughts and ideation, though the risk of ganaxolone specifically is unclear.

Ganaxolone is neither an inducer nor inhibitor of any major phase I or phase II enzymes at clinically relevant concentrations, and is neither a substrate nor inhibitor of any major transport proteins. Coadministration with CYP3A4 inducers and inhibitors will significantly lower and raise plasma concentrations of ganaxolone, respectively.

Stiripentol (Diacomit). Stiripentol has a long history of use in the world as an ASM, having been first approved by the European Medicines Agency for the treatment of Dravet syndrome in 2001. The FDA-approved stiripentol as an add-on therapy with clobazam, and is also frequently coadministered with valproic acid-based therapeutics. Once thought to only be effective as an inhibitor of the metabolism of coadministered ASMs, emerging evidence suggests that stiripentol has ASM activity of its own.

Receptor Binding/Mechanism of Action. Stiripentol exerts its ASM activity via direct binding to $GABA_A$ channels and potentiation of GABAergic signaling. Targeted studies suggest that stiripentol binds to the same site as barbiturates and, like barbiturates, increases the duration of channel opening when bound. Some studies suggest that stiripentol also increases synaptic GABA via inhibition of GABA transporters (eg, GAT-1); however, this is not a fully accepted mechanism.[129] Stiripentol contains a chiral center and is administered as a racemate. The aromatic ring contains a methylenedioxy group that is readily metabolized (see next section).

Metabolism. Stiripentol undergoes extensive hepatic metabolism by CYP1A2, CYP2C19, and CYP3A4 via a proposed pathway shown in Figure 15.24. Oxidation of the methylenedioxy ring removes the connecting carbon, revealing the catechol. Either phenolic OH group can be methylated, leaving the para-OH (P-OH) or meta-OH (M-OH) metabolites. Of these, P-OH is an active metabolite and M-OH is inactive. All metabolites can be conjugated in a phase-II process and eliminated.[130]

Physicochemical Properties. Stiripentol does not contain ionizable functional groups and will have no charge in the body. The LogP is 3.01 and TPSA is 38.69 Å^2. Stiripentol has negligible solubility in water.

Pharmacokinetics. Stiripentol is administered either as oral capsules or as a powder to make an oral suspension. Peak plasma concentrations are reached at t_{max} between

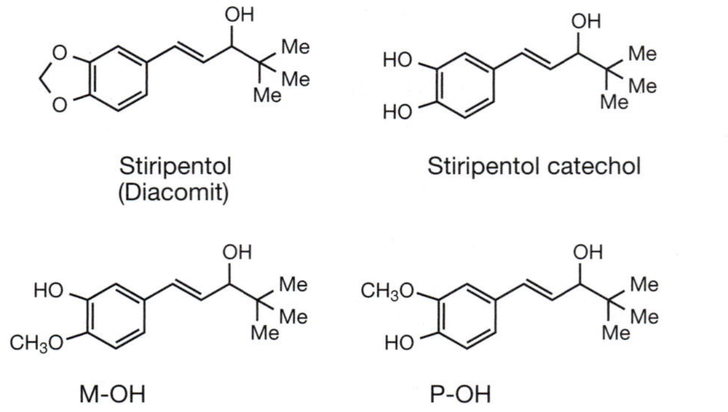

Figure 15.24 Structures of stiripentol and its major metabolites. Only the P-OH metabolite is active.

1 and 3 hours when taken with food; absolute bioavailability is unknown, as is the impact of food. Stiripentol exhibits nonlinear pharmacokinetics. The apparent V_d at steady-state ranges between 32 and 192 L as body weight increases from 10 to 60 kg. The elimination $t_{1/2}$ is between 4.5 and 13 hours, increasing with dose. Metabolites are eliminated primarily in the urine (73% of dose), and the parent drug is eliminated in the feces (13%-24%).[131] Because elimination is largely renal, patients with renal impairment should be advised against taking stiripentol.

Specific Adverse Effects and Drug-Drug Interactions. As a $GABA_A$-PAM, stiripentol carries a risk of causing somnolence by itself and when in combination with other central nervous system (CNS) depressants (eg, clobazam). If the patient is experiencing excessive drowsiness, consider decreasing the dose of other coadministered, sedating ASMs. Furthermore, patients should not immediately discontinue stiripentol due to a potential to put the patient at risk of seizures. Decreased appetite and body weight are other important considerations. Decreased neutrophil and platelet counts are possible when taking stiripentol. For this reason, hematologic testing should be obtained before taking stiripentol and during therapy (every 6 months).

Patients with phenylketonuria (PKU) need to know that the Diacomit suspension—but not the capsule formulation—contains phenylalanine. PKU is a rare disorder that prevents patients from being able to break down phenylalanine from their diet and other sources such as aspartame. Each 500-mg packet of Diacomit suspension contains 2.80 mg of phenylalanine. For patients with PKU, this needs to be factored into their daily intake levels. All ASMs carry a risk of increased suicidal behavior.

Stiripentol is both an inducer and inhibitor of many CYP enzymes, including CYP1A2, CYP2B6, CYP3A4, CYP2C8, and CYP2C19. The inhibitory effect means that doses of concomitantly administered CYP substrates should be decreased. Particularly relevant is the impact of stiripentol with the $GABA_A$-PAM, clobazam. CYP3A4 and CYP2C19 are responsible for metabolizing clobazam into its active metabolite (NDMC) and further into the inactive 4′-OH-NDMC. Inhibition of this metabolism causes a buildup of the parent drug and active metabolite. While this would be a desired outcome in CYP2C19 and CYP3A4 fast metabolizers, stiripentol can cause levels of clobazam and NDMC to build up to unsafe levels in some patients. Because stiripentol is metabolized by many CYPs into inactive metabolites, its use with CYP-inducing ASMs should be avoided.

Inhibitors of GABA Uptake and Metabolism

Physicochemical and pharmacokinetic properties of GABA modulators are provided in Table 15.7.

TIAGABINE (GABITRIL). Tiagabine is a structurally unique ASM that was FDA-approved in 1997 as an adjunctive agent to treat partial seizures in patients over age 12. Tiagabine is the first agent approved that inhibits GABA uptake as its primary mechanism of action.

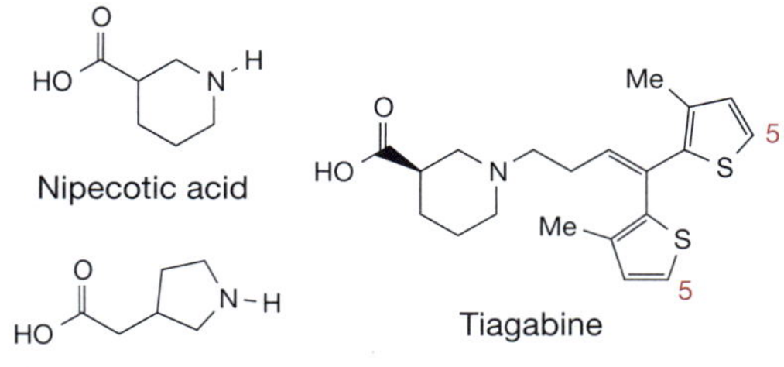

Nipecotic acid

Tiagabine

Homo-β-proline

Receptor Binding/Mechanism of Action. Tiagabine is a selective inhibitor of GAT-1, the most abundant isoform of the GAT family. Little is known definitively about the molecular mechanisms by which tiagabine binds GAT-1. Homology modeling suggests that the carboxylate anion engages a sodium ion in the GAT-1 active site, and the protonated amine engages in an ion/dipole bond with the backbone carbonyl of Phe294. The diaryl tail group engages a hydrophobic cleft stabilized by π-stacking with Tyr140.[132]

Structure-Activity Relationship. Tiagabine emerged from the observation that two conformationally constrained GABA analogues, nipecotic acid and homo-β-proline, were GABA uptake inhibitors in vitro that were BBB-impermeable in vivo. The BBB permeability of the lead nipecotic acid was improved by enhancing the lipophilicity, ultimately resulting in tiagabine.[133] The basic amine and carboxylic acid are required for GAT-1 binding (see previous section), and the lipophilic tail enhances GAT-1 affinity and CNS bioavailability.

Metabolism. Tiagabine is extensively metabolized by CYP3A oxidation. The primary sites of oxidation are the equivalent 5-positions on the thiophene rings. These 5-oxo-thiophene metabolites are pharmacologically inert.

Table 15.7 Physicochemical and Pharmacokinetic Properties of Glutamate and GABA Modulators

	TGB	VGB	LEV	BRV	PER	GNX	STP
cLogP	5.69	−0.10	−0.67	0.88	3.70	4.37	3.01
Solubility (mg/mL)	11	55.1	>40	>40	<0.01	<0.01	<0.01
TPSA (Å²)	40.54	63.32	63.40	63.40	56.46	37.30	38.69
f (%)[a]	95	>90	99	100	100	10	
$t_{1/2}$ (h)	7-9		6-8	7-8	105	>20	4-13
t_{max} (h)	0.75[b] 2[a]	0.5-1.0[b] 2[a]	1.3	1.0	1.0	2-3	1-3
Protein binding (%)	96	None	None	17	95	99	99
V_d (L/kg)	1.0	1.0-1.1	0.5-0.7	0.5	0.6-0.7		1.03
Metabolized by:	CYP3A4,5	None	Hydrolysis	CYP2C8	CYP3A4	CYP3A4/5 CYP2B6 CYP2C19 CYP2D6	CYP1A2 CYP2C19 CYP3A4
Inducer of:	None	None	None	None	None	None	CYP1A2 CYP2B6 CYP3A4 CYP2C8 CYP2C19
Inhibitor of:	None	None	None	EH	CYP2C8	None	CYP1A2 CYP2B6 CYP3A4 CYP2C8 CYP2C19

BRV, brivaracetam; EH, epoxide hydrolase; *f*, oral bioavailability; GNX, ganaxolone; LEV, levetiracetam; PER, perampanel; STP, stiripentol; TGB, tiagabine; TPSA, topologic polar surface area; V_d, volume of distribution; VGB, vigabatrin.

[a]With high-fat meal.

[b]Fasting.

Glucuronide conjugates are also common, though their exact structures remain to be determined.[134]

Physicochemical Properties. Tiagabine possesses both weakly acidic (pK_a 4.14) and basic (pK_a 9.26) functional groups. Thus, tiagabine carries a molecular charge across the pH scale. The hydrochloride salt is sparingly soluble in water (11 mg/mL), and the TPSA is 40.54 Å.

Pharmacokinetics. Tiagabine is rapidly and nearly completely absorbed (95%), exhibiting a linear pharmacokinetic profile. The t_{max} occurs around 45 minutes, which is extended to 2.5 hours when given with a high-fat meal. The extent of absorption (AUC) is not affected by food. Two peaks can be found in the plasma profile curve of tiagabine, suggestive of enterohepatic recycling. Tiagabine is highly bound to plasma proteins (96%) and has a V_d of 1 L/kg. Tiagabine is heavily metabolized, with only 2% of the parent drug eliminated unchanged. Elimination of metabolites occurs in the urine (25%) and feces (63%). Tiagabine $t_{1/2}$ (7-9 hours) and clearance (109 mL/min) is impacted by concomitantly administered CYP-inducing ASMs. No dose adjustments are needed for patients with renal impairment, though those with hepatic insufficiency should see dose reductions.[134]

Specific Adverse Events and Drug-Drug Interactions. Nonepileptic patients may experience new-onset seizures and status epilepticus while taking tiagabine. Since tiagabine is frequently given as an adjuvant with enzyme-inducing drugs, the dose should be decreased if given alone or in noninduced patients. Enzyme-inducing ASMs increase clearance by about 60% and valproate reduces plasma protein binding by approximately 2%, leading to a 40% increase in blood plasma levels of tiagabine. Tiagabine is not an inducer of CYP or UGT enzymes.

VIGABATRIN (SABRIL). Vigabatrin was approved by the FDA in 2009 as monotherapy in the treatment of infantile spasms, spasms due to West syndrome, and generalized tonic-clonic seizures. It is approved to treat refractory complex partial seizures in adults over age 10. It is a mechanism-based "suicide-inhibitor," and perhaps the first ASM that was rationally designed.

Receptor Binding/Mechanism of Action. Vigabatrin is a first-in-class inhibitor of GABA-transaminase (GABA-T), an enzyme that catalyzes the breakdown of GABA into inactive succinic semialdehyde (Fig. 15.24). The mechanism by which GABA-T converts the primary amine into an aldehyde is shown in Figure 15.25A. In the first step, GABA reacts with pyridoxal-5′-phosphate (PLP) to form Schiff base I. An active site lysine (Lys329) within GABA-T removes a proton α to the iminium ion, forming a second unstable aldimine intermediate II. Hydrolysis of II forms pyridoxamine-5′-phosphate (PAP) and releases succinic semialdehyde (SSA). PAP can then be converted back to PLP by converting α-ketoglutarate to glutamate. The action of vigabatrin is shown in Figure 15.25B. Like GABA, vigabatrin reacts with PAP to form aldimine III, and then Lys329 removes the α-proton, forming enimine IV. Regeneration of the conjugate base of Lys329 affords imine V. Here, the vinyl group is susceptible to nucleophilic Michael attack by Lys329, resulting in product VI that has covalently bound the substrate, enzyme, and cofactor, permanently inactivating GABA-T.[135]

Structure-Activity Relationship. Vigabatrin is also known as γ-vinyl-GABA (GVG). In fact, the name "vigabatrin" arises from the fact that it is a vinyl GABA-transaminase inhibitor. The simple addition of a vinyl group to the γ-carbon is key to the mechanism of covalent binding (see earlier text). If this alkene were not exactly one carbon removed from the γ-amine, vigabatrin would not covalently bind GABA-T. Conformationally constrained GVG analogues are in development, which orient this double bond toward the lysine. Such agents are designed to be much more potent irreversible GABA-T inhibitors.

Metabolism. Like other GABA analogues, vigabatrin is not extensively metabolized.

Physicochemical Properties. Vigabatrin contains both acidic (pK_a 4.61) and basic (pK_a 9.91) functional groups. An amino acid, vigabatrin is zwitterionic and soluble in aqueous solution (55.1 mg/mL) and can be administered as an oral solution or tablet. Vigabatrin is hydrophilic, with cLogP −0.10.

Pharmacokinetics. Vigabatrin displays linear pharmacokinetics over single and repeated doses between 0.5 and 4 g. Vigabatrin is fully absorbed following oral administration, with t_{max} reached within 0.5 to 1 hours. The effect of food is a 33% decrease in C_{max} and an increase of $t_{1/2}$ to approximately 2 hours, with no significant change in AUC. Vigabatrin is not bound to plasma proteins and has V_d = 1.0 to 1.1 L/kg. Elimination is renal and age-dependent: $t_{1/2}$(infants, 0.5-2 years) = 5.7 hours, $t_{1/2}$(children, 10-16 years) = 9.5 hours, $t_{1/2}$(adults) = 10.5 hours. This translates to substantial differences in clearance: Cl(infants) = 2.4 L/h, Cl(children) = 5.8 L/h, Cl(adults) = 7 L/h. Dose adjustment in renally impaired patients should be taken into consideration, as the AUC increases substantially in these patients and may cause toxicities.[136] Unlike gabapentin and pregabalin, vigabatrin is not known to be transported by LAT-1; however, evidence suggests alternate amino acid transporters contribute to oral bioavailability.[137] Vigabatrin is unlikely to be a P-gp substrate.[38]

Specific Adverse Events and Drug-Drug Interactions. The potential for producing severe, permanent visual field defects (VFDs) led to a Black Box warning for vigabatrin. The estimated prevalence of vigabatrin-induced VFD is 15% to 31% in infants, 15% in children, and 25% to 50% in adults. ASM-induced VFD is specific to vigabatrin, although the exact mechanism is unknown.[138] Due to this severe side effect, vigabatrin is only available through the Support, Help and Resources for Epilepsy (SHARE) program. As part of SHARE, patients are routinely tested for evidence of vision loss and potential markers for future toxicities.

Vigabatrin is a selective inducer of CYP2C9. This does not require dose adjustments with other coadministered ASMs, although clearance of non-ASM CYP2C9 substrates may be impacted.

Other Important Aspects of Drug Chemistry. Initial studies performed in rats[139] and human subjects[140] support the efficacy of vigabatrin in treating cocaine and methamphetamine addiction disorders, although subsequent clinical trials were less impressive.

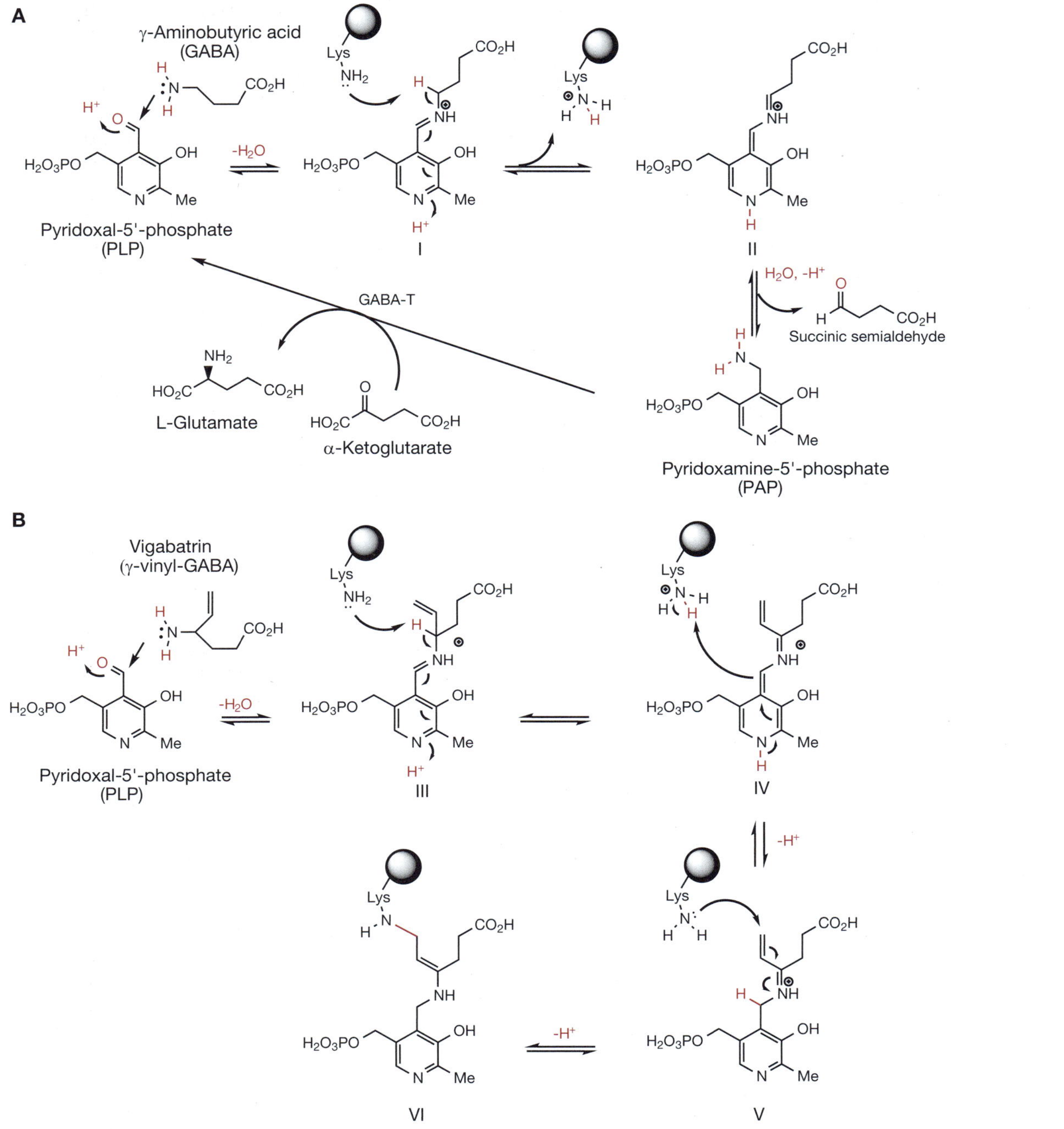

Figure 15.25 Mechanism of covalent inhibition of GABA-T. A. Mechanism of GABA-T metabolism of GABA. B. The role of the vinyl group of vigabatrin in covalent alkylation of the active site lysine.

Inhibitors of Glutamate Signaling

Physicochemical and pharmacokinetic properties of glutamate modulators are provided in Table 15.7.

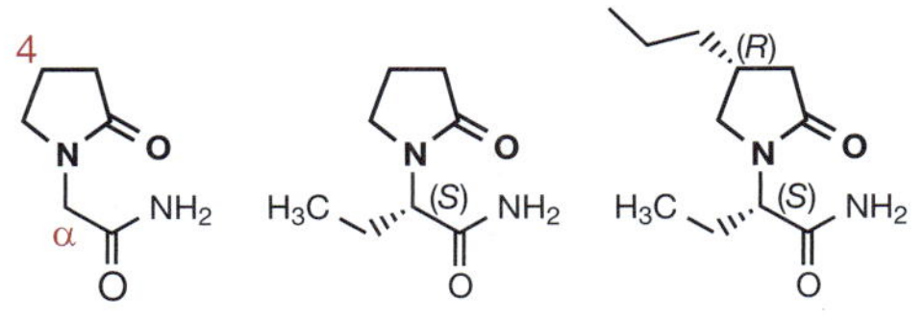

Piracetam | Levetiracetam (Keppra) | Brivaracetam (Briviact)

BRIVARACETAM (BRIVIACT) AND LEVETIRACETAM (KEPPRA). Brivaracetam has been approved by the FDA as an adjunct for the treatment of partial onset seizures. Brivaracetam and the structurally related levetiracetam are members of the racetam class characterized by an *N*-substituted pyrrolidinone core. Animal studies suggest that brivaracetam is more potent and has a broader spectrum of activity when compared to levetiracetam.

Receptor Binding/Mechanism of Action. Brivaracetam and levetiracetam are ligands for the synaptic vesicle protein SV2A, which appears to account for antiseizure activity by protecting against epileptiform responses.

Brivaracetam binds SV2A with an affinity approximately 10× that of levetiracetam. In addition, brivaracetam inhibits voltage-gated sodium currents and reversibly blocks the effects of inhibitory GABA and glycine receptors on currents.

Structure-Activity Relationship. Piracetam is a nootropic that was shown to produce modest anticonvulsant effects in animal models. Addition of an ethyl group to the α-carbon of piracetam (etiracetam) enhanced this activity, and isolation of the enantiomers showed that the (*S*)-*levo* isomer (levetiracetam) is over 1,000 times more potent than the (*R*)-*dextro* isomer. An unsubstituted carboxamide group is required for activity, as is a cyclic pyrrolidinone. Addition of unbranched alkyl groups to position 4 is also tolerated, with *n*-propyl (brivaracetam) being the most potent.

Metabolism. Brivaracetam was the main product identified in the plasma, while metabolites M9, M1b, and M4b accounted for 34.2%, 15.9%, and 15.2% of the administered dose, respectively (Fig. 15.26). Approximately 8.6% of the parent drug was recovered in the urine. The hydrolysis products M9 and M4b are associated with amide hydrolases, while the major oxidizing enzyme is CYP2C8.[141] Unlike brivaracetam, levetiracetam is not extensively metabolized.[142] Approximately 34% of the dose is metabolized, with the major inactive metabolite (LO57) generated by a hydrolytic mechanism.

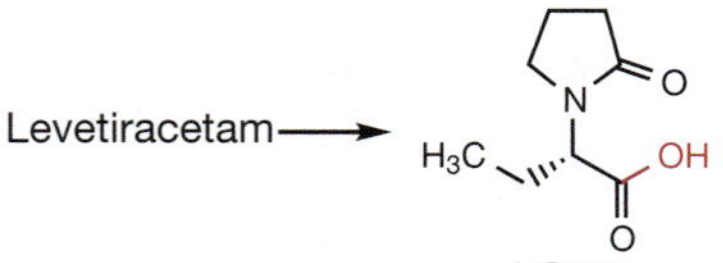

LO57

Physicochemical Properties. Brivaracetam and levetiracetam contain two amide functional groups and are net neutral molecules. Racetams are relatively hydrophilic molecules, with log $D_{pH7.4}$ in the range of −0.64 (levetiracetam) to 1.04 (brivaracetam).[143] Levetiracetam and brivaracetam are therefore highly soluble in aqueous solutions and are considered BCS class I substances. The TPSA for both agents is 63.4 Å, which is well within ranges suggestive of high brain permeability.[144]

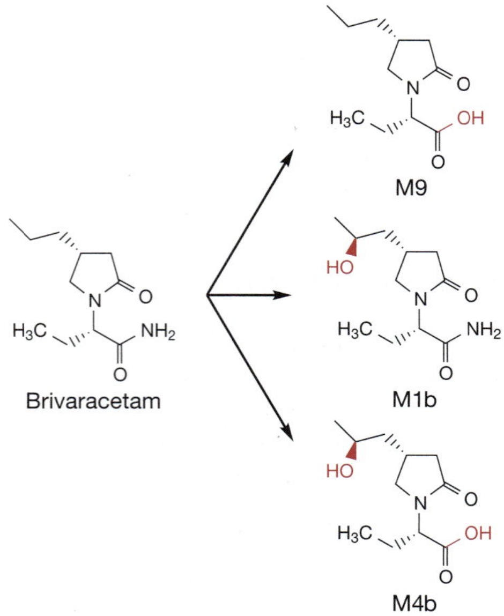

Figure 15.26 Metabolism of brivaracetam.

Pharmacokinetics. Brivaracetam is rapidly absorbed and has an elimination $t_{1/2}$ of 7 to 8 hours. The drug is poorly bound to plasma protein (~17%). Brivaracetam and its metabolites are excreted primarily in the urine. Absorption of levetiracetam is rapid (t_{max} 1.3 hours) and not impacted by food. Levetiracetam is not bound to plasma proteins and has a V_d of 0.5 to 0.7 L/kg. Elimination is primarily renal; thus, older adult patients and those with compromised creatinine clearance may need dosage adjustment. Levetiracetam is a probable P-gp substrate.[38]

Specific Adverse Events and Drug-Drug Interactions. The most common adverse effects consist of nausea, vomiting, dizziness, and drowsiness. Brivaracetam has no effect on plasma levels of CBZ; however, plasma levels of the reactive epoxide metabolite, CBZ-E, are increased due to inhibition of epoxide hydrolase by brivaracetam. Enzyme induction by CBZ enhances clearance of brivaracetam.[145] Brivaracetam is on the Schedule V list, and levetiracetam is not scheduled.

Miscellaneous Glutamate Antagonists

Perampanel (Fycompa)

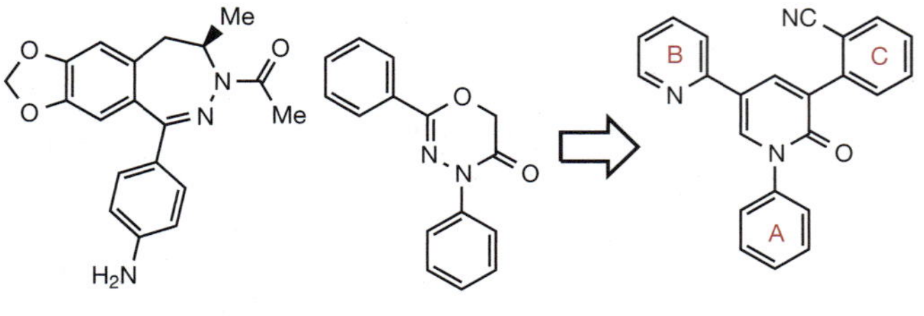

Talampanel HTS hit Perampanel

Perampanel is the only approved ASM that works through an AMPAR-blocking mechanism. It is approved as adjunctive treatment for partial onset seizures, with or without secondarily generalized seizures, in patients aged 12 years and older. Compared to talampanel, an earlier AMPAR blocker in development, perampanel has a long duration of action that permits once-daily dosing.

Receptor Binding/Mechanism of Action. Perampanel is a selective, noncompetitive antagonist of AMPARs. As a noncompetitive agonist, it is expected that perampanel will produce less sedation compared to competitive antagonists.

Structure-Activity Relationship. Four aromatic rings are required for potent noncompetitive AMPAR binding. Introduction of basic groups is tolerated by rings B and C. Electron-withdrawing substitutions on ring A at the *o*-position enhance affinity 5-fold. Bioisosteres for the aromatic phenyl rings (eg, thiophene) are generally not tolerated. The AMPAR binding site is generally not tolerant of charged or sterically demanding functional groups.[146]

Metabolism. Over 15 metabolites of perampanel have been isolated in urine and feces. More than 60% of the dose is metabolized to oxidized products on rings A and

C (M7, M13, M14). Metabolite M7 arises from hydrolytic ring-opening of arene oxide intermediate M19 (Fig. 15.27). The pyridine ring-opened metabolite M2 is generated by a ring-contraction/rearrangement (M6). Metabolism is mediated primarily by CYP3A4 and CYP3A5.[147]

Physicochemical Properties. Perampanel is a sparingly soluble triaryl pyridone. The pyridine is weakly basic, with pK_a of 4.0. The calculated cLogP is 3.70, and TPSA is 56.46 Å.

Pharmacokinetics. Perampanel follows linear kinetics. Perampanel is readily absorbed from the GIT (~100%), with no significant first-pass metabolism. The t_{max} is approximately 1 hour, which is delayed by a high-fat meal (2-3 hours). Though C_{max} is also lowered by 28% to 40%, food does not affect AUC. Perampanel is highly protein bound (95%) to both albumin and α-1-acid glycoprotein. Perampanel is metabolized 90% by liver enzymes of the CYP3A family; patients with hepatic impairment will have substantially increased AUC and elimination $t_{1/2}$ compared to healthy cohorts. Clearance is approximately 0.6 to 0.7 L/h, which is not affected by age. The elimination $t_{1/2}$ is highly variable among patients, with a mean of 105 hours. No dose adjustments are required for patients with mild-to-moderate renal impairment.

Specific Adverse Events and Drug-Drug Interactions. Perampanel carries a Black Box warning indicating that severe behavioral reactions, such as aggression, hostility, irritability, and homicidal ideation, should be monitored. Like other ASMs, drowsiness and somnolence are frequent side effects. Perampanel is a weak inhibitor of CYP2C8 at high concentrations (30 μmol/L) and a substrate of CYP3A4. Perampanel does not induce CYP or UGT isoforms and has few clinically relevant DDIs with other ASMs. Coadministration with enzyme-inducing ASMs (CBZ, OXC, phenytoin) decreases perampanel AUC by 50%. Ketoconazole, a significant CYP3A4 inhibitor, was found to increase perampanel AUC values by approximately 20%.

Other Important Aspects of Drug Chemistry. Perampanel is a C-III-controlled substance. Subjective assessments in phase III clinical trials reported that some patients (<1%) reported feeling drunk and euphoric while taking perampanel. A recent study comparing perampanel with alprazolam and ketamine reports similar subjective, "drug liking" effects for all three agents at supratherapeutic doses.[148]

Multimodal Antiseizure Medications

Physicochemical and pharmacokinetic properties of multimodal ASMs are provided in Table 15.8.

Cannabidiol (Epidiolex)

Promising research findings and shifting trends toward societal acceptance have led to intense research into the anticonvulsant potential of phytocannabinoids isolated from *Cannabis sativa* and *Cannabis indica*. Reports of cannabis use to treat convulsive disorders originate as far back as 2900 BC in Sumerian and Arabic texts. Following a medical trip to India, British surgeon William O'Shaughnessy wrote in 1843 about the efficacy of cannabis in treating epilepsy. In the years since, unsupervised use of medical cannabis preparations has been documented in many anecdotal reports regarding safety and efficacy in treating rare and severe epilepsies in children and adults. Reviews conducted by the American Academy of Neurology and Cochrane Database conclude that medical cannabis is of "unknown efficacy" to treat epilepsy[149,150]; nonetheless, clinical trials of

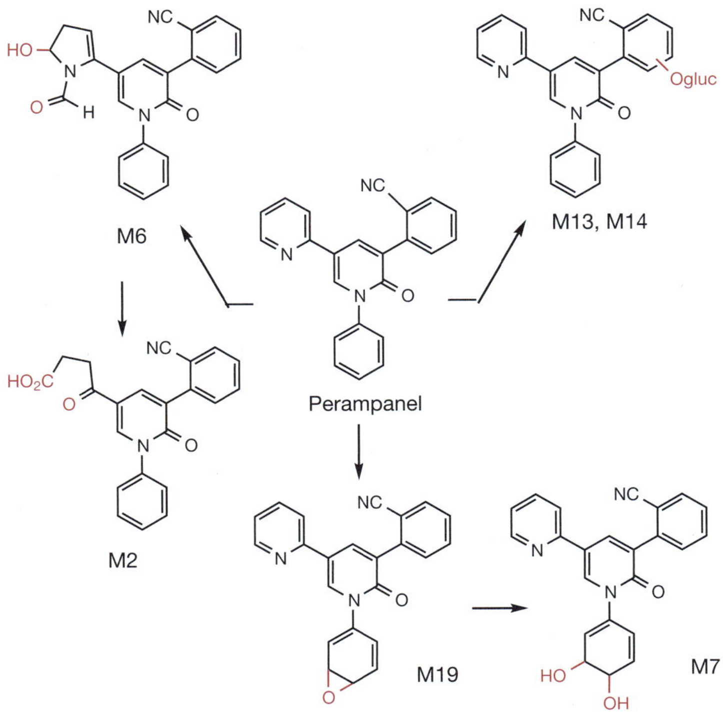

Figure 15.27 Metabolic profile of perampanel.

Table 15.8 Physicochemical and Pharmacokinetic Properties of Multimodal ASMs

	CBD	FBM	FFA	TPM	VPA	ZNS
cLogP	6.10	1.20	3.30	2.97	2.72	−0.16
Solubility (mg/mL)	<0.1	0.7	412	9.8	1.3 (free acid) 50 (Na^+ salt)	0.8
TPSA (Å^2)	40.46	104.64	12.03	115.54	37.3	81.75
f (%)[a]	13-19	>90	70	80	100	100
$t_{1/2}$ (h)	56-61	20-23	20	21	9-18	63[b] 105[a]
t_{max} (h)	3.0	3-5	3-5	1-2	2-3 (IR) 5-10 (SR)	2-6
Protein binding (%)	>94	<25	50	15-41	>90	40
V_d (L/kg)		0.8	11.9	0.8-0.55[c]	0.13-0.19	1.45
Metabolized by:	CYP3A4 CYP2C19	Esterases ADH CYP3A4 CYP2E1	CYP1A2 CYP2B6 CYP2D6 CYP3A4/5	CYP3A4	UGTs CYP2C9 CYP2A6 CYP2B6	CYP3A4
Inducer of:	None	None	None	CYP3A4	None	None
Inhibitor of:	CYP2C8 CYP2C9 CYP2C19 UGT1A9 UGT2B7	CYP2C19	CYP2D6	CYP2C19	Epoxide hydrolase	None

CBD, cannabidiol; f, oral bioavailability; FBM, felbamate; FFA, fenfluramine; IR, immediate release; SR, sustained release; TPM, topiramate; TPSA, topologic polar surface area; UGT, UDP-glucuronosyltransferase; V_d, volume of distribution; VPA, valproic acid; ZNS, zonisamide.
[a]In erythrocytes.
[b]In plasma.
[c]V_d is inversely related to dose.

phytocannabinoids—agents of plant-based origin that engage cannabinoid receptors, CB1R and CB2R—were undertaken to clarify these unknowns.[151]

While Δ^9-tetrahydrocannabinol (Δ^9-THC, Fig. 15.28) is perhaps the most well-known of the phytocannabinoids, its cousin cannabidiol (CBD) has proven to be a much more clinically viable ASM. That is not to say that Δ^9-THC is without efficacy at reducing convulsions: preclinical studies demonstrated that Δ^9-THC produced an anticonvulsive effect in over 60% of animal seizure model studies. In this study, another 32% showed no significant effect, and Δ^9-THC is primarily responsible for the psychomotor and reinforcing

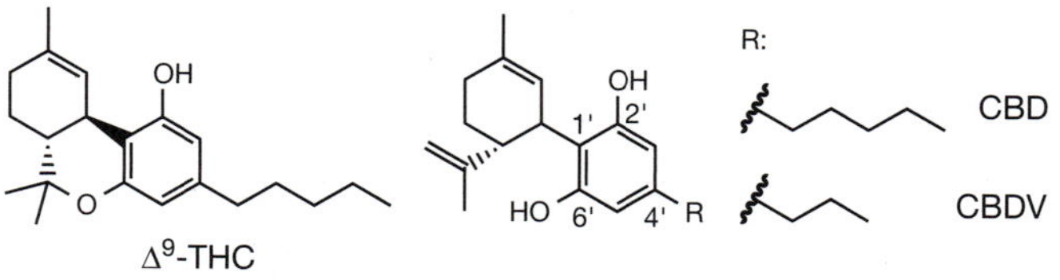

Figure 15.28 Phytocannabinoids with ASM activity: Δ^9-THC, CBD, CBDV.

effects of cannabis. Comparatively, the non-psychoactive phytocannabinoids CBD and the related cannabidivarin (CBDV) were effective in 80% of 41 animal seizure model studies.[151] Also advantageous to ASM development, these lesser-known phytocannabinoids have thus far proven to be a much more viable option to treating seizure disorders. The efficacy of CBD was recently demonstrated in a clinical trial of 214 children with drug-resistant Dravet syndrome,[152] and in 2017 a New Drug Application (NDA) was submitted to the FDA for CBD (Epidiolex, GW Pharmaceuticals) for the treatment of Dravet and Lennox-Gastaut syndromes. On June 25, 2018, Epidiolex was approved by the FDA to treat seizures associated with these severe diseases. This is significant because Epidiolex is the first FDA-approved medication containing a purified agent from cannabis plant material and is also the first approved drug for the treatment of patients with Dravet syndrome.

Receptor Binding/Mechanism of Action. The pharmacologic targets of CBD are numerous and include transient receptor potential (TRP) channels, 5-HT_{1A} receptors, T-type Ca_v channels, and GPR55. Like Δ^9-THC, CBD is a modulator of the endocannabinoid signaling system

(ECSS), a "master regulator" that is ubiquitously expressed throughout the central and peripheral nervous systems. Unlike Δ^9-THC, however, CBD is not an agonist at type-1 and type-2 cannabinoid receptors (CB1R or CB2R); in fact, recent studies suggest CBD may act as a CB1R negative allosteric modulator.[153] Other ECSS targets of CBD include fatty acid amide hydrolase (FAAH), the enzyme that breaks down the endocannabinoid, anandamide, and fatty acid–binding proteins (FABPs). Inhibition of FAAH and FABPs results in an increase in anandamide levels, thereby indirectly activating the ECSS and regulating neuronal activity.[154] Taken together, the pharmacologic activity of CBD is a true exercise in polypharmacology.

Structure-Activity Relationship. CBD is considered a phytocannabinoid, or a compound isolated from *Cannabis sativa* and contains a chemical structure that resembles Δ^9-THC. The structure of CBD consists of a central aromatic core group that contains two phenolic hydroxyl groups in a *meta*-orientation to each other (positions 2′ and 6′, Fig. 15.28). This functional group is called resorcinol, which is present in many natural products. Attached between these hydroxyl groups at position 1′ is a substituted cyclohexene. This group is free to rotate and even adopt an orthogonal orientation to the resorcinol ring. Oxidation of this group is tolerated, though only in specific ways as discussed more in the next section. At resorcinol position 4′ is an *n*-pentyl chain. This group has considerable conformational flexibility and is believed to occupy a lipophilic region within the cannabinoid receptor CB1R.

Metabolism. The major metabolites of CBD are found in Figure 15.29. The only major active metabolite of CBD is 7-OH-CBD. This metabolite is produced by CYP3A4 and CYP2C19 and is an example of an allyl oxidation process. 7-OH-CBD can be oxidized further into 7-COOH-CBD, which is inactive. Other oxidation pathways, particularly concerning the lipophilic tail at position 4′, are possible, but are minor and inactive. Phase-II glucuronidation of one of the resorcinol phenols results in an inactive metabolite.

At clinically relevant concentrations, CBD inhibits phase I enzymes, CYP2C8, CYP2C9, and CYP2C19, and phase II enzymes UGT1A9 and UGT2B7. CBD and 7-OH-CBD do not inhibit drug transporters (P-gp, BCRP), but 7-COOH-CBD does inhibit BCRP.

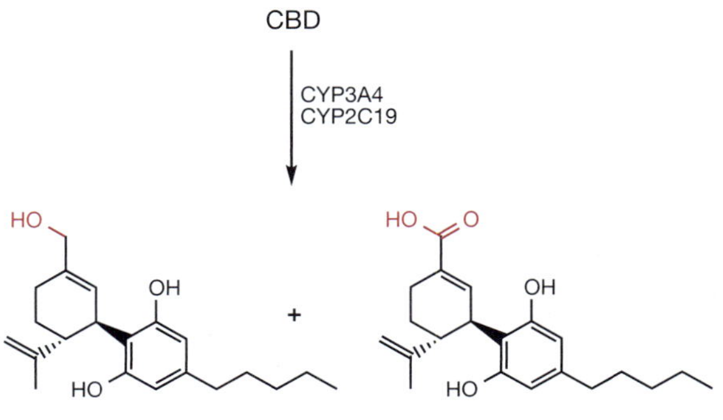

7-OH-CBD
(active)

7-COOH-CBD
(inactive)

Figure 15.29 Oxidized products of CBD. 7-OH-CBD (active) and 7-COOH-CBD (inactive) are major metabolites. Cannabidiolquinone (CBDQ) is an oxidized degradation product that results from exposure to air and sunlight.

Physicochemical Properties. CBD is very lipophilic (LogP 6.1) and is practically insoluble in water (<0.1 mg/mL). Thus, oral CBD is formulated as a solution in sesame oil. The resorcinol of CBD has two weakly acidic phenol groups, the most acidic phenol having a pK_a of 9.13. The TPSA of CBD is 40.46Å^2, which indicates CBD is likely to have high central bioavailability once it reaches systemic circulation.

Pharmacokinetics. The clinical pharmacokinetics of CBD was reviewed in 2018.[155] Epidiolex is formulated as an oral solution and is dosed using a 1- or 5-mL calibrated syringe. The oral bioavailability of CBD is low, approximately 13% to 19%, and is increased when taken with a high-fat meal. This impact of food is to be expected for such a lipophilic drug. The V_d is very high (>20,000 L) and heavily protein bound (>94%). The $t_{1/2}$ is 56 to 61 hours after twice-daily dosing for 7 days. Plasma clearance from a single dose (1,500 mg) is 1,111 L/h. CBD is eliminated primarily through the feces.

Specific Adverse Effects and Drug-Drug Interactions. There is a risk of hepatocellular injury (elevation in serum transaminases alanine transaminase (ALT)) when using CBD. The risk of such injury is highest when patients are taking valproate and clobazam concomitantly. For these reasons, ALT, and bilirubin levels should be obtained prior to initiation on CBD. Clinicians should consider discontinuing valproic acid and clobazam if transaminase levels rise while taking CBD.

Somnolence and sedation are common (>30% of patients) and dose-related side effects when taking CBD. Excessive sedation may occur if coadministered with other CNS depressants. Fatigue, malaise, and asthenia were other CNS adverse effects observed in clinical trials. Decreased appetite and diarrhea were among the observed gastrointestinal adverse effects.

The prescribing information for Epidiolex[156] describes an increased risk of suicide as a broad statement regarding all ASM medications; however, there is little evidence that CBD specifically increases suicide risk and/or suicidal ideation. The need for more research in this space is warranted.[157]

Care should be taken when co-administering CBD with strong inducers or inhibitors of CYP3A4 and CYP2C19, as these will increase and reduce metabolism of CBD, respectively. CBD can inhibit the metabolism of other CYP2C8, CYP2C9, and CYP2C19 substrates.

Other Important Aspects of Drug Chemistry. Like other phytocannabinoids, CBD has low stability when exposed to air and sunlight; for these reasons, Epidiolex is stored in an amber bottle (to protect against ultraviolet (UV) light) and should be discarded after 12 weeks of opening. Oxidation of CBD to the degradation product cannabidiolquinone (CBDQ, Fig. 15.29) results in a red-purple color.[158]

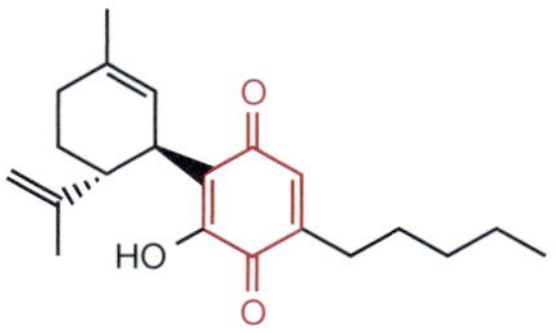

CBDQ

CENOBAMATE (XCOPRI). Cenobamate is one of the newest ASMs to be approved by the FDA, receiving approval for the treatment of partial onset (focal) seizures in adults in November 2019.

Receptor Binding/Mechanism of Action. Cenobamate was originally developed as a Na_v blocker. Unlike other Na_v blockers described earlier, which block the transient sodium current (I_{NaT}) as their primary MOA, cenobamate preferentially blocks the persistent sodium current (I_{NaP}). The I_{NaT} refers to the rapid flow of sodium ions through the channel during the open (activated) state; this occurs during the depolarization phase of neuronal firing and ends when the receptor pore is closed (closed or inactivated state). In contrast, the I_{NaP} persists, and can result in augmented receptor firing during epilepsy.[159] How these differences in modulating sodium channel conduction contribute to therapeutic and adverse effect profiles of Na_v blockers is an area of much ongoing research.[160]

A second mechanism of action of cenobamate is enhancement of $GABA_A$ signaling via binding to a nonbenzodiazepine binding site.[161]

Structure-Activity Relationship. Details recounting the path from discovery to development of cenobamate are lacking. Cenobamate is a member of the structural class of ASMs that contains a primary carbamate ($H_2NCO_2^-$) functional group; this class can be easily remembered by their generic names containing the suffix "-bamate." The drug is administered as the (*R*)-enantiomer, though it is unclear how this contributes to its activity. Another key feature is the tetrazole, which contains four nitrogen atoms that likely influence its physicochemical properties.

Metabolism. Cenobamate undergoes extensive metabolism, with only 6.8% of an oral dose eliminated unchanged. The primary route of metabolism is via phase-II glucuronidation. The glucuronide is attached to the carbamate nitrogen primarily by UGT2B7. Other minor oxidative metabolites are produced by CYP2E1, CYP2A6, and CYP2B.

Physicochemical Properties. Cenobamate does not contain any readily ionizable functional groups at any relevant physiologic pH. The predicted LogP is 1.98, and the TPSA is 95.92 $Å^2$. Cenobamate has high aqueous solubility (1.7 mg/mL) and is administered via a tablet formulation.

Pharmacokinetics. Oral cenobamate is almost completely absorbed via the gut (88%). The V_d is 40 to 50 L, and plasma protein binding (albumin) is 60%. The time to reach peak plasma concentrations (t_{max}) is 1 to 4 hours and is not impacted by food. Metabolism is near-complete, with only 6.8% of an oral dose eliminated unchanged in the urine. The apparent half-life is 50 to 60 hours, and oral clearance is 0.45 to 0.63 L/h over doses ranging 100 to 400 mg/d. Elimination is predominately renal (88% eliminated in the urine), though fecal elimination also occurs (5%). Patients with hepatic and/or renal impairment would be expected to have higher plasma levels of cenobamate. Indeed, patients with mild-to-moderate hepatic impairment have AUC approximately 2-fold higher than patients with normal liver function.[162]

Specific Adverse Events and Drug-Drug Interactions. Severe adverse effects are possible when taking cenobamate, including shortening of the QT interval, suicidal thoughts and depression, and severe multiorgan hypersensitivities. These adverse effects are not common, but should be considered when making prescribing or dose decisions with vulnerable populations (eg, patients with familial short QT syndrome, patients taking medications that shorten QT interval, patients with depression). Otherwise, cenobamate is generally well-tolerated and adverse effects are typically mild and dose related. Results from two phase-II clinical trials found that somnolence, dizziness, headache, fatigue, and diplopia (double-vision) were observed in at least 10% of patients.

In early clinical trials of cenobamate, three cases of drug reaction with eosinophilia and systemic symptoms (DRESS) were observed. DRESS is a severe idiosyncratic drug reaction that is similar in severity and presentation as SJS and TEN. In subsequent trials to determine strategies that would mitigate the potential for cenobamate to cause DRESS, clinicians observed no instances of DRESS when they used a "start low/go slow" titration approach beginning at 12.5 mg/d.[163]

Cenobamate is an inhibitor of CYP2C19 and an inducer of CYP2B6 and CYP3A4. Consequently, cenobamate will be expected to decrease plasma concentrations of carbamazepine, lamotrigine, and midazolam, and increase concentrations of phenytoin and phenobarbital.[162] Among non-ASMs, cenobamate decreased plasma concentrations of bupropion (CYP2B6 substrate) and increased concentrations of omeprazole (CYP2C19 substrate). Due to CYP induction, women who are taking oral contraceptives should be advised to use additional or nonhormonal birth control when taking cenobamate due to the potential increase in metabolism and elimination.[164] Cenobamate is neither a substrate nor inhibitor of P-gp. Cenobamate is a Schedule V controlled substance in the United States.

FELBAMATE (FELBATOL). Felbamate was approved in 1993 to treat refractory partial seizures and Lennox-Gastaut syndrome, and is available in tablet and oral suspension dosage forms. Despite excellent efficacy in treating difficult disease states, the severe idiosyncratic toxicity profile led to a Black Box warning and massive drop in its use.

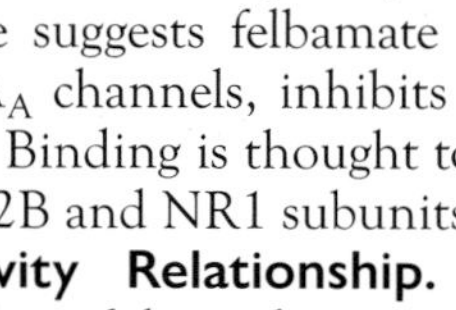

Felbamate

Receptor Binding/Mechanism of Action. The mechanism of action of felbamate is poorly understood and controversial. Evidence suggests felbamate potentiates GABA currents via $GABA_A$ channels, inhibits Na_v channels, and inhibits NMDARs. Binding is thought to occur through interactions with NR2B and NR1 subunits of NMDARs.[165]

Structure-Activity Relationship. Like cenobamate, felbamate is a member of the carbamate class of ASMs; however, unlike cenobamate, felbamate contains two primary carbamate groups and is therefore considered a biscarbamate. The biscarbamate possess skeletal muscle relaxant effects in addition to antiseizure activity. A comprehensive SAR study showed that the 2-position (Fig. 15.30) is tolerant of diverse alkyl substitutions to maintain antiseizure activity. Disubstitution at this position—for example, with two alkyl or aromatic groups—generally enhances muscle relaxant activity. The most potent anticonvulsant effects were found with the mono-phenyl substitution (felbamate). Importantly, the EC_{50} for anticonvulsant activity is over 40-fold lower than the EC_{50} for muscle relaxant effects. Anticonvulsant potency is reduced, and muscle relaxant activity increased on carbamate hydrolysis (monocarbamoyl felbamate, MCF; Fig. 15.30).

Metabolism. Felbamate metabolism is shown in Figure 15.30. Esterase hydrolysis of one carbamate produces MCF. The resulting alcohol is a substrate for alcohol dehydrogenase (ADH), which oxidizes the alcohol to an aldehyde (carbamoylpropionaldehyde, CBMA). Chemical instability of CBMA results in the loss of carbamic acid and the formation of atropaldehyde, a highly reactive product that has acrolein-like toxicity in vivo. The analogue 2-fluorofelbamate was designed as a safer alternative that is a weak ADH substrate and, therefore, is not metabolized to atropaldehyde.[166] The 2′- and 4′-positions of felbamate are also prone to oxidation by CYP3A4 and CYP2E1 to the alcohol or phenol, respectively.

Physicochemical Properties. Felbamate is available in tablet, capsule, and suspension formulations. The structure consists of a 1,3-propanediol core with a single phenyl substitution at position 2. The terminal alcohols are modified as unsubstituted carbamates. Felbamate is uncharged under normal physiologic conditions and has no ionizable functional groups. The cLogP is approximately 1.20 and the TPSA is 104.64 Å. Despite this high polar surface area, felbamate readily penetrates into the CNS. Felbamate has poor aqueous solubility (<1 mg/mL).

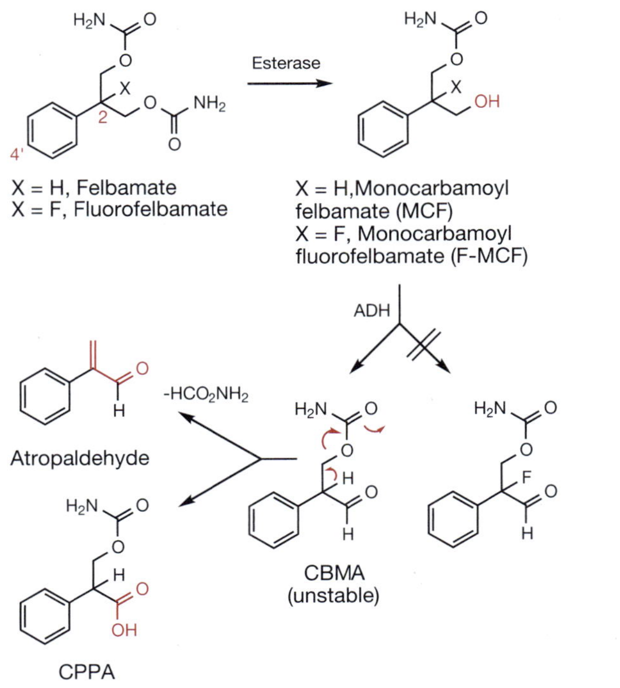

Figure 15.30 Metabolism of felbamate that leads to the generation of toxic metabolite atropaldehyde. Fluorofelbamate is not converted to atropaldehyde. ADH, alcohol dehydrogenase; CBMA, carbamoylpropionaldehyde; CPPA, 3-carbamoyl-2-phenylpropionic acid; MCF, mono-carbamoyl felbamate.

Pharmacokinetics. Felbamate follows linear pharmacokinetics. More than 90% is absorbed on oral administration, and the absorption is not impacted by food. Felbamate shows weak plasma protein binding (<25% to albumin) and a V_d of 0.8 L/kg. The brain/plasma ratio is approximately 1.8:1, meaning high penetration into the CNS. The terminal $t_{1/2}$ is 20 to 23 hours, and clearance is 26 to 30 mL/h/kg in healthy patients. Renally impaired patients show a 40% to 50% reduction in total body clearance and an increase in $t_{1/2}$ of 9 to 15 hours. Approximately 50% of the parent drug is eliminated unchanged, and 10% is eliminated as the 2′- or 4′-hydroxy metabolites. The carboxylic acid metabolite, 3-carbamoyl-2-phenylpropionic acid (CPPA), accounts for roughly 10% of the metabolites isolated in the urine. The remainder (30%) is excreted as glucuronide conjugates.[167] Felbamate is a possible P-gp substrate.[38]

Specific Adverse Events and Drug-Drug Interactions. Idiosyncratic toxicities are common in patients taking felbamate, particularly aplastic anemia and hepatotoxicity. These are likely due to generation of the highly reactive atropaldehyde in vivo.[168] Felbamate is an inhibitor of CYP2C19, which influences phenytoin clearance but is not an inducer of any enzyme. Enzyme-inducing ASMs increase felbamate clearance.

FENFLURAMINE (FINTEPLA). The path from discovery to development to approval of fenfluramine as an ASM was a long and difficult one. Originally developed and approved as an appetite suppressant in combination with phentermine ("fen-phen"), the amphetamine analog was withdrawn in the United States in 1997 due to the occurrence of valvular heart disease. After clinical trials demonstrated its effectiveness in treating Lennox-Gastaut and Dravet syndromes,[169,170] fenfluramine (Fintepla) was approved by the FDA in June 2020.

Receptor Binding/Mechanism of Action. Fenfluramine has long been known to increase levels of synaptic serotonin and is thus considered a serotonin-releasing agent (SRA). This activity is shared by other amphetamines (eg, methylenedioxymethamphetamine, MDMA) and tryptamines (eg, *N,N*-dimethyltryptamine, DMT). The increased release of serotonin is thought to occur via a reversal of transporter flux via the serotonin transporter (SERT). Not all SRAs or SERT blockers are effective at blocking seizures; an emerging hypothesis is that fenfluramine reduces seizures via a second mechanism of action, namely potentiation of sigma-1 receptor activity.[171] Fenfluramine has weak direct agonist activity at type-2 serotonin receptors ($5\text{-}HT_{2A,2B,2C}$), though it is not clear that this contributes to its therapeutic effects.

Structure-Activity Relationship. Fenfluramine is a substituted amphetamine. Details of the SAR of amphetamines can be found in Chapter 13. Briefly, substitutions to the aromatic ring generally decrease "amphetamine-like" activity, thus fenfluramine has low abuse potential. The α-methyl group enhances SERT affinity; like amphetamine, the dextrorotary D-enantiomer has higher SRA activity than the levorotary L-enantiomer. A secondary amine is not a requirement for SRA activity, as the *N*-desethyl derivative norfenfluramine is also active; however, a basic amine is required at a position that is two carbons removed from the aromatic ring.

Metabolism. The primary route of metabolism is N-dealkylation to the active metabolite norfenfluramine (Fig. 15.31). Norfenfluramine can be oxidized further to ketone metabolites that have the basic amine removed. Only norfenfluramine is pharmacologically active. This route of metabolism is similar to that of other primary monoamines. Metabolism is primarily mediated by CYP1A2, CYP2B6, and CYP2D6. A minor, but still potentially impactful, route of metabolism is mediated by CYP3A4/5.

Physicochemical Properties. As a secondary monoamine, fenfluramine is weakly basic with a pK_a of 10.2. It is formulated as the hydrochloride salt in an aqueous solution. The LogP is 3.3, and TPSA is 12.03 Å^2. It has high aqueous solubility (412 mg/L) owing to its salt form.

Pharmacokinetics. Fenfluramine oral solution is administered via syringe. Oral bioavailability is high (~70%) and is not impacted by food. The t_{max} at steady state is approximately 3 to 5 hours. Fenfluramine has a moderate V_d (11.9 L/kg) following oral administration and is 50% protein bound. Elimination $t_{1/2}$ of fenfluramine is 20 hours, and clearance is 24.8 L/h in healthy volunteers. Metabolism is extensive and metabolites are predominately eliminated in the urine.

Specific Adverse Effects and Drug-Drug Interactions. The severe cardiac toxicity liability of fenfluramine is well established. The mechanism by which fenfluramine causes this toxicity is unknown, but is likely associated with its weak agonism at 5-HT$_{2B}$ receptors. For this reason, patients must be screened (echocardiogram) for valvular heart disease and pulmonary arterial hypertension prior to, and during, treatment with fenfluramine. Access to fenfluramine is restricted under the Fintepla Risk Evaluation and Mitigation Strategy (REMS). Fenfluramine can cause decreases in appetite and body weight; this should be expected based on its history as a weight loss aid. Pediatric patients should be monitored carefully for signs of weight loss and doses should be modified accordingly.[172] Other serious adverse effects that have been observed with fenfluramine include hypertension and mydriasis. Patients with a family history of hypertension should be monitored regularly, and the drug should be discontinued if feelings of ocular pain or visual disturbances are noticed. All ASMs have a warning to monitor for increased suicidal ideation.

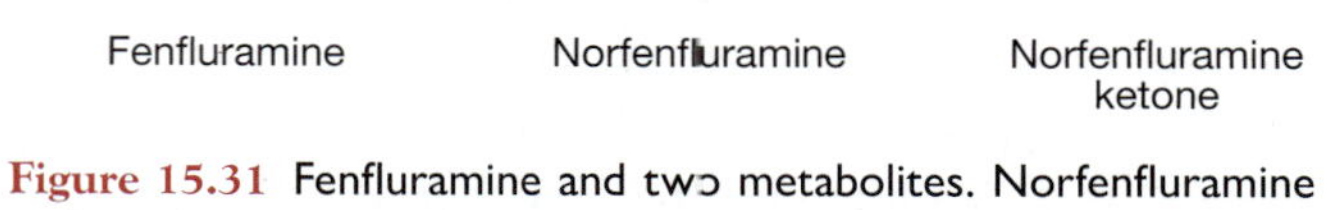

Figure 15.31 Fenfluramine and two metabolites. Norfenfluramine is the only active metabolite.

Strong inhibitors of CYP1A2, CYP2B6, CYP2D6, and CYP3A4/5 will increase fenfluramine concentrations. Coadministration with stiripentol and clobazam increases fenfluramine concentrations. In these cases, the maximum daily dose of fenfluramine should be reduced to avoid life-threatening cardiac toxicity. Strong inducers of these enzymes will enhance fenfluramine clearance and lower ASM efficacy. A specific interaction to consider with fenfluramine involves its activity on the serotonergic system. As a serotonin releaser, fenfluramine increases the risk of developing serotonin syndrome if coadministered with other drugs that increase synaptic serotonin—for example, selective serotonin reuptake inhibitors (SSRIs), serotonin/norepinephrine reuptake inhibitors (SNRIs), and monoamine oxidase inhibitors (MAOIs).

TOPIRAMATE (TOPAMAX). Topiramate was originally designed as an antidiabetic drug, although its powerful anticonvulsant activity was seen as much more promising. Topiramate was FDA-approved in 1996 as monotherapy or adjunctive therapy in patients older than age 2 with partial-onset or primary generalized tonic-clonic seizures, and as adjunctive therapy in treating Lennox-Gastaut syndrome. It can also be used as prophylactic treatment of migraines. Topiramate is available as a tablet or sprinkle capsules. It was heralded for its powerful antiepileptic effects, but a poor side effect profile remains a considerable drawback.

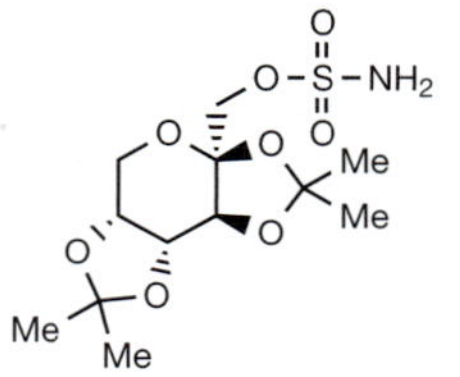

Topiramate
(Topamax)

Receptor Binding/Mechanism of Action. Topiramate produces antiepileptic effects through multiple mechanisms: (1) blockade of voltage-gated Na$_v$ channels and HVA Ca$_v$ channels, (2) augmentation of GABA$_A$-channel activity, (3) inhibition of AMPA/KRs, (4) inhibition of carbonic anhydrase isoforms II and IV (CA-II, CA-IV). It is thought that the broad efficacy of topiramate in treating seizures and its considerable side-effect profile are related to its multiple MOA.

Structure-Activity Relationship. Topiramate is a unique pharmacologic agent: the core of the molecule is a simple sugar, fructose, which is modified at the 1-position by a sulfamate functional group. The hydroxyl groups attached to the central pyran ring are connected by acetonide ethers (2,3- and 4,5-acetonide). Extensive SAR studies indicated a eudismic ratio of 1.5 in favor of the (*S*)-enantiomer found in topiramate. The unmodified sulfamate group is required for activity, as is a linking group between the oxygen atoms at the 4,5-position. Replacement of the 4,5-acetonide with a sulfate is approximately as active as the parent.[173]

Metabolism. Topiramate is not extensively metabolized. The major metabolites arise from hydrolysis of the 2,3- and 4,5-acetonide groups and result in inactive products. A second route of oxidative metabolism is ω-oxidation at the acetonide carbons at positions 9 and 10 (Fig. 15.32). The CYP

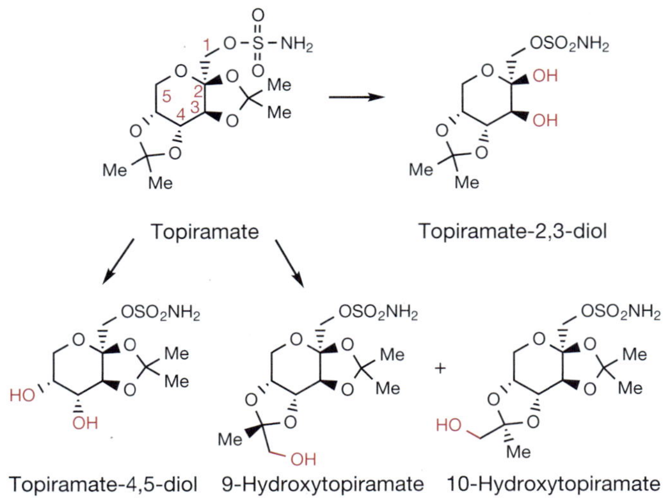

Figure 15.32 Metabolism of topiramate.

isoforms responsible for the oxidation of topiramate are unknown, although CYP3A4 may be involved (see "Specific Adverse Events and Drug-Drug Interactions" section). Some glucuronide metabolites have also been observed.

Physicochemical Properties. The sulfamate group is weakly acidic, $pK_a = 8.66$. Topiramate is relatively hydrophilic and polar compared to other ASMs, with cLogP = 2.97 and TPSA = 115.54 Å. These values are outside of typically accepted ranges for agents with high passive CNS permeability. Topiramate is soluble in water (9.8 mg/mL).

Pharmacokinetics. Topiramate is rapidly and completely absorbed with $t_{max} = 2$ hours, following an oral dose. Pharmacokinetics is linear over a therapeutic dose range. The V_d is inversely related to dose: 0.8 to 0.55 L/kg between 100 and 1,200 mg. V_d for female patients is approximately 50% of the values found in men. The mean plasma elimination $t_{1/2}$ is 21 hours, meaning steady state concentration is reached within 4 days. Topiramate is modestly protein bound (15%-41%). Coadministration with valproate decreased topiramate protein binding by 13% to 23%. Approximately 70% of the oral dose is eliminated unchanged in the urine, and only 5% of the administered dose is excreted as one of the six oxidized and conjugated metabolites. Oral plasma clearance is approximately 23 to 30 mL/min. Animal studies suggest renal tubule reabsorption is possible with topiramate. Dose reduction may be necessary in older adult patients or those with renal impairment.[174] Topiramate is a possible P-gp substrate.[38]

SPECIFIC ADVERSE EVENTS AND DRUG-DRUG INTERACTIONS. Cases of metabolic acidosis have been reported for topiramate. This is likely caused by inhibition of CA-II and CA-IV. Other significant adverse events include paresthesia, weight loss, difficulty with concentration and memory, and depression. The severity of adverse events is responsible for nearly one-third of patients discontinuing treatment.[174] Coadministration with enzyme-inducing ASMs (phenytoin, carbamazepine, phenobarbital) has a significant enhancing effect on topiramate clearance. Coadministration with valproate causes a modest, clinically insignificant decrease in topiramate clearance. Lamotrigine and topiramate can be coadministered without incident.[175] When given in high doses, topiramate is an inducer of CYP3A4, which may be responsible for increased clearance of ethinylestradiol and other CYP3A4 substrates.[176]

VALPROIC ACID. Valproic acid (VPA; Depakene), divalproex sodium (Depakote), and valproate sodium (Depacon) are indicated for monotherapy and adjunctive therapy of complex partial seizures and simple and complex absence seizures. In 1976, valproate was initially approved only for treatment of absence seizures. Divalproex sodium is a mixture of valproate sodium and its conjugate acid, VPA. It is available in many dosage forms, including tablets and capsules, syrup, and intravenous injection. VPA was discovered serendipitously in France in 1962: it was being used as a delivery solvent for a series of experimental tranquilizers when it was discovered that the solvent itself had exceptional anticonvulsant action.[177] VPA is on the WHO 20th List of Essential Medicines.

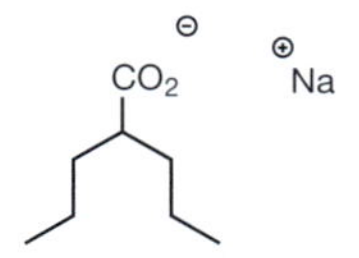

Sodium valproate
(Depakote, Dyzantil, Epilim)

Receptor Binding/Mechanism of Action. Although the molecular mechanism or mechanisms are unknown, VPA produces anticonvulsant effects through inhibitory and excitatory mechanisms: enhancement of GABA synthesis and release and inhibition of the release of β-hydroxybutyric acid, an excitatory neurotransmitter. The enhanced levels of synaptic GABA may be due to inhibition of GABA-T. VPA may also block NMDAR signaling and Na_v channels. Dopaminergic and serotonergic neurotransmission is also altered by VPA, though the exact mechanisms are unknown.[178]

Structure-Activity Relationship. When administered as the sodium salt, the drug dissipates rapidly in weakly acidic solution, generating the uncharged conjugate acid (VPA). A carboxylic acid or amide bioisostere and two alkyl chains are required for activity. Anticonvulsant activity is directly associated with lipophilicity, with increasing alkyl chain length and branching generally resulting in more potent agents. Adding rigidity to the chains, for example, through introducing a double bond, modestly lowers activity.

Metabolism. VPA is extensively metabolized by phase 1 and phase 2 mechanisms (Fig. 15.33). The principal metabolite (50%) is the carboxylic acid conjugate VPA glucuronide. This is mediated by several UGT isoforms. Oxidation occurs primarily at the 3- and 5-positions to produce the respective alcohols. This occurs primarily in the mitochondria (~40%) by several CYP isoforms (~10%).[179] Dehydration of these intermediates results in Δ^2- and Δ^4-VPA, respectively. Conjugation of Δ^4-VPA by coenzyme A produces the intermediate Δ^4-VPA-SCoA, which is rapidly metabolized to $\Delta^{2,4}$-VPA-SCoA. The α,β,γ,δ-unsaturated carbonyl group is extremely reactive to Michael attack by endogenous nucleophiles, including plasma proteins, enzymes, and glutathione.[180] This is likely responsible for the toxicity profile of VPA.

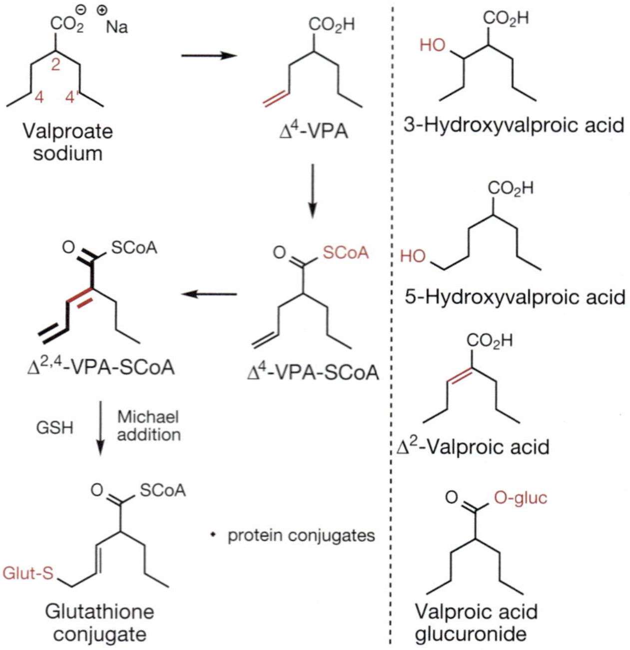

Figure 15.33 Metabolism of valproate. Left: mechanism by which ω-oxidation to Δ^4-valproate-SCoA (Δ^4-VPA-S-coenzyme A) leads to hepatotoxic metabolites. The electrophilic α,β,γ,δ-unsaturated Michael acceptor portion of $\Delta^{2,4}$-valproate-SCoA ($\Delta^{2,4}$-VPA-S-coenzyme A) is shown in bold. Right: Nontoxic phase 1 and phase 2 metabolites. GSH, glutathione.

Physicochemical Properties. VPA is an amphiphilic, branched, short-chain fatty acid derivative. The cLogP is 2.72, and the TPSA is 37.3 Å. VPA is slightly soluble in water in its free acid form ($pK_a = 4.8$, solubility = 1.3 mg/mL), which is greatly enhanced by formulation as the sodium salt (valproate sodium solubility = 50 mg/mL).

Pharmacokinetics. VPA dose/concentration relationships are nonlinear due to saturable plasma protein binding. VPA is almost completely bioavailable on oral administration, although formulation and route of delivery play a role in t_{max}. The t_{max} for non-enteric–coated or immediate release (IR) formulations is reached within 2 to 3 hours; this rises to 5 to 10 hours for sustained-release formulations. VPA is more than 90% albumin-bound, with V_d between 0.13 and 0.19 L/kg and brain/plasma ratio between 0.1 and 0.5. Active transport mechanisms, specifically anion exchange uptake transporters in the BBB, aid central bioavailability. Due to impaired plasma protein binding, older adult patients may need a reduction in dose. The $t_{1/2}$ of valproic acid is between 9 and 18 hours, which drops to 5 to 12 when taken with enzyme-inducing ASMs. VPA is extensively metabolized by multiple CYP isoforms, including CYP2C9, CYP2A6, and CYP2C19, and less than 3% is excreted unchanged in urine. Mean clearance for multiple day dosing ranges from 6.67 to 8.20 mL/h/kg to 500 to 1,500 mg/d.[181] VPA is a possible P-gp substrate.[38]

Specific Adverse Events and Drug-Drug Interactions. Hepatotoxicity and pancreatitis due to the generation of a toxic metabolite are severe and can be life-threatening. According to the Black Box warning for VPA, "children under the age of 2 years are at a considerably increased risk of developing fatal hepatotoxicity, especially those on multiple anticonvulsants, those with congenital metabolic disorders, those with severe seizure disorders accompanied by mental retardation, and those with organic brain disease."[182] VPA can also cause birth defects, and this should be considered when given to females of childbearing age. Platelet counts should be monitored for thrombocytopenia. As with many ASMs, suicidal ideation and somnolence are possible and should be monitored.[182]

Enzyme-inducing ASMs (iminostilbenes, hydantoins, barbiturates) significantly enhance VPA metabolism and clearance. VPA is not an enzyme-inducer, though clinically important increases in plasma concentrations of phenobarbital and lamotrigine are known to occur. Inhibition of epoxide hydrolase may increase CBZ-mediated toxicities by blocking metabolism of the intermediate CBZ-10,11-epoxide (Fig. 15.5). Other plasma protein-bound ASMs may be displaced by valproate—for example, phenytoin.[178]

ZONISAMIDE (ZONEGRAN). Like lamotrigine, zonisamide produces antiepileptic effects through inhibition of voltage-gated ion channels, Na_v and Ca_v. In contrast to lamotrigine, evidence suggests zonisamide has effects on multiple neurotransmitter systems that may contribute to a wider spectrum of anticonvulsant activity. Zonisamide capsules are indicated as adjunctive therapy in treating partial seizures in adults, and the drug is effective in treating complex partial seizures, generalized tonic-clonic seizures, myoclonic seizures, and Lennox-Gastaut syndrome. Used in Japan and Korea since 1990, zonisamide was first approved in the United States in 2000.

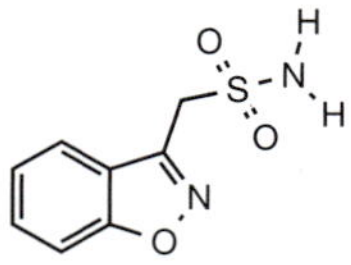

Zonisamide
(Zonegran, Zonisade)

Receptor Binding/Mechanism of Action. Available evidence indicates that zonisamide binds and stabilizes inactivated Na_v channels, slowing recovery from inactivation. Zonisamide also inhibits T-type $Ca_v3.2$ channels and glutamate release, though the magnitude of this effect suggests that it only partially contributes to the anticonvulsant mechanism of action. Zonisamide modulates dopaminergic signaling and may also affect free radical scavenging. Evidence shows that chronic zonisamide causes upregulation of excitatory amino acid carrier-1 (EAAC-1) and downregulation of GAT-1. This is expected to decrease synaptic glutamate levels and increase synaptic GABA availability.[183] Although zonisamide contains a sulfonamide function that resembles the sulfonamide class of CA inhibitors, zonisamide is a very weak CA inhibitor.

Structure-Activity Relationship. Detailed SAR of zonisamide at multiple targets is lacking. An early SAR study showed that sulfonamide N-alkylation by one or two short-chain (eg, methyl, ethyl) groups was tolerated, although longer chain derivatives were inactive. The fact that N,N-dialkylation was tolerated suggests that an acidic group is not a rigid requirement in this region. Halogen substitution of the aromatic ring enhances anticonvulsant and neurotoxic potency, resulting in a net drop in therapeutic index.

Metabolism. Zonisamide is subject to extensive CYP-mediated oxidation, reduction, and acetylation (Fig. 15.34). The major route of metabolism is reduction of the benzisoxazole heterocyclic ring to a short-lived, ring-opened imine intermediate that rapidly decomposes to 2-(sulfamoylacetyl)-phenol (2-SMAP). This is catalyzed by CYP3A4. Glucuronide conjugation produces metabolite M3 (12.6%). Acetylation (M8, 7.7%) and conjugation (M6, 7.6%) are minor metabolic pathways.[184]

Physicochemical Properties. Zonisamide is the only ASM with a benzisoxazole core. Like other CA inhibitors, zonisamide has a weakly acidic primary sulfonamide group ($pK_a = 10.2$). Zonisamide is relatively hydrophilic, with calculated cLogP = −0.16, and it has a modestly high TPSA (81.75 Å). In spite of this, zonisamide has high central bioavailability. Zonisamide is only slightly soluble in aqueous solution (0.80 mg/mL).

Pharmacokinetics. Zonisamide is rapidly and completely absorbed, with peak plasma concentrations reached in 2 to 6 hours. Food modestly delays t_{max} (4-6 hours), but AUC is unaffected. Zonisamide is extensively concentrated in plasma erythrocytes, likely due to the affinity of zonisamide for CA enzymes. Absorption is linear until high concentrations (800 mg) saturate erythrocyte binding. Apparent V_d is 1.45 L/kg, and plasma protein binding is modest at around 40%. Approximately 60% of the oral dose is found unchanged in the urine, and major metabolites are glucuronide conjugates of 2-SMAP (metabolite M3; Fig. 15.30). Plasma $t_{1/2}$ is 63 hours, and the elimination $t_{1/2}$ in red blood cells is approximately 105 hours. Plasma clearance during monotherapy is 0.30 to 0.35 mL/min/kg, which is increased to 0.50 mL/min/kg when taken with enzyme-inducing ASMs. In patients with renal damage (CrCl <20 mL/min), renal clearance dropped from 3.5 to 2.23 mL/min and AUC rose to 35%. Doses should be decreased in these patients. There is no effect of age on zonisamide pharmacokinetics. Zonisamide is unlikely to be a P-gp substrate.[38]

Specific Adverse Events and Drug-Drug Interactions. Zonisamide is a sulfonamide and should not be given to patients with sulfonamide allergies, as this could lead to life-threatening reactions (eg, SJS, TEN). Thus, discontinuation of zonisamide should be considered if a rash is observed. Oligohidrosis (deficient sweat production) and hyperthermia in pediatric patients are also potentially life-threatening side effects of zonisamide therapy. Women of childbearing age should be aware of teratogenic effects and fetal abnormalities when taking zonisamide. Psychiatric (depression, psychosis) and psychomotor slowing (difficulty concentrating, speech and language problems) are cognitive adverse events. Somnolence and fatigue are also common.[185]

Zonisamide does not induce metabolic enzymes. When taken with enzyme-inducing ASMs, the $t_{1/2}$ falls to 27 hours (phenytoin), 38 hours (phenobarbital, CBZ), and 46 hours (valproate). Plasma protein binding is not affected by other ASMs.

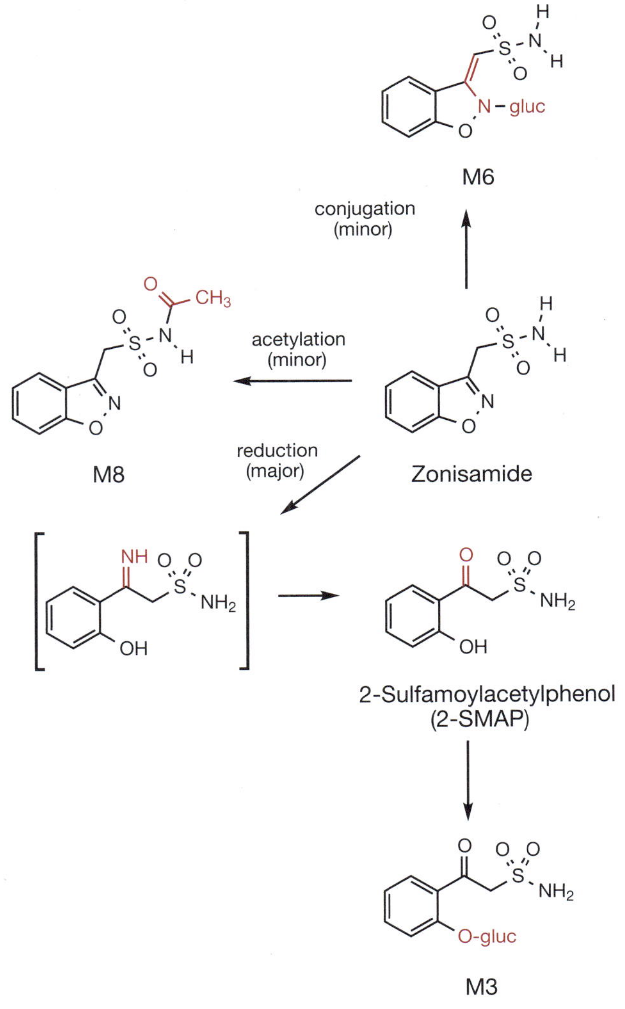

Figure 15.34 Metabolism of zonisamide.

Antiseizure Medications in the Pipeline

The quest continues for the discovery of efficacious ASMs with an optimal adverse effect profile. The current pipeline of ASM drug development is shown in Table 15.9.[186] Some general takeaways can be made regarding how epilepsy disorders may be treated in the future. First, there are no candidates that are currently in late-stage (phase 3) clinical trials, so the next generation of ASMs will take some time to develop. Next, we see that the "tried-and-true" neurotransmitter targets—GABA, glutamate, potassium/sodium/calcium channels, multimodal mechanisms—are still here, though the mechanisms by which these systems are targeted are different. For example, CVL-865 targets $GABA_A$ channels bearing α2,3 subunits, whereas currently available $GABA_A$-PAMs bind α1 subunits. OV329 GABA aminotransferase (GABA-AT) and E2730 (GAT1) are thought to enhance synaptic GABA by inhibiting its degradation

Table 15.9 Antiepileptic drug candidates in the clinical pipeline. Candidates are organized by broad mechanism of action and development phase

	Preclinical	Phase I	Phase II
Glutamate, GABA modulators	OV329	SAGE 324 JNJ-55511118 E2730	JNJ-40411813 CVL-865 Selurampanel
Potassium-channel modulators	KB-3061		XEN1101
Sodium channel modulators	TD561, TD562	XEN901	
Calcium channel modulators	FV-137	ACT-709478	CX-8998
Anti-inflammatory	GAO-3-02	VX-765	
Serotonin modulator			EPX-100 Lorcaserin
Multimodal	FV-082		Carisbamate Naluzotan Padsevonil
Other mechanisms	2-deoxy-D-glucose PQR530, PQR620, PQR626	Huperzine A	soticlestat

and uptake, respectively. The success of fenfluramine (serotonin-releasing agent) has fueled additional research in repurposing serotonergic modulators. EPX-100 (the antihistamine clemazole) and lorcaserin (Belviq, currently withdrawn treatment for obesity) are two such examples. As our understanding of the neuroinflammatory contributions to epilepsy continue to develop, so too are therapies targeting neuronal inflammation. Finally, natural products, such as huperzine A, isolated from the Chinese moss *Huperzia serrata*, are also under development as potential new leads.

Status Epilepticus Case Study

You are on an emergency medicine rotation in an urban underserved clinic. Due to your close proximity to this marginalized community, many of your patients come to your clinic for emergency prescriptions. Your preceptor tells you about a patient that came to the clinic late on Friday worried that her son's antiseizure medication ran out and she is not able to get a new one from her primary care physician until Monday. The ideal medication for her son will provide long-acting, once-daily prophylaxis against seizures.

To assess your knowledge of SAR, your preceptor asks you to identify the drug structure from the options below that would be best suited to help this patient. Conduct a structural analysis: to which drug class do these options belong? What is the mechanism of action of each? How does metabolism and SAR contribute to their duration of action? With this information, choose the ideal compound to help control the patient's son's seizures.

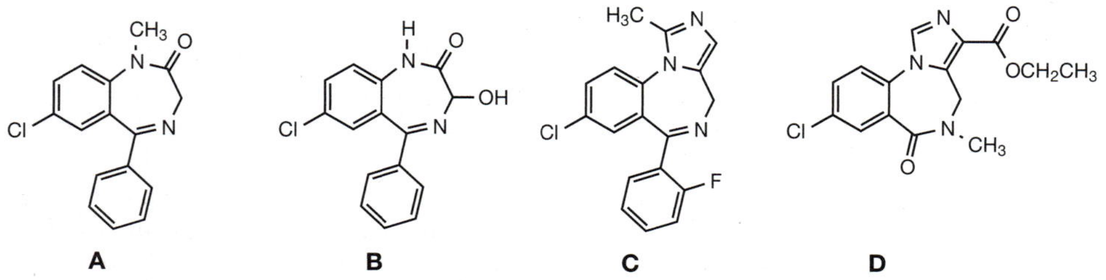

REFERENCES

1. Stevenson DC. Hippocrates: on the sacred disease. The Internet Classics Archive. Accessed December 27, 2017. http://classics.mit.edu/Hippocrates/sacred.html
2. Friedlander WJ. *History of Modern Epilepsy: The Beginning, 1865-1914*. Greenwood Press; 2001.
3. Shorvon SD. Drug treatment of epilepsy in the century of the ILAE: the first 50 years, 1909-1958. *Epilepsia*. 2009;50:69-92.
4. Institute of Medicine. *Epilepsy Across the Spectrum: Promoting Health and Understanding*. The National Academies Press; 2012.
5. Fisher RS, van Emde Boas W, Blume W, et al. Epileptic seizures and epilepsy: definitions proposed by the International League Against Epilepsy (ILAE) and the International Bureau for Epilepsy (IBE). *Epilepsia*. 2005;46:470-472.
6. Liang JG, Lee D, Youn SE, Kim HD, Kim NY. Electroencephalography network effects of corpus callosotomy in patients with Lennox-Gastaut syndrome. *Front Neurol*. 2017;8:456.
7. Genton P. When antiepileptic drugs aggravate epilepsy. *Brain Dev*. 2000;22:75-80.
8. Ceulemans B, Boel M, Claes L, et al. Severe myoclonic epilepsy in infancy: toward an optimal treatment. *J Child Neurol*. 2004;19:516-521.
9. Fisher RS, Cross JH, French JA, et al. Operational classification of seizure types by the International League Against Epilepsy: position paper of the ILAE commission for classification and terminology. *Epilepsia*. 2017;58:522-530.
10. Berg AT, Berkovic SF, Brodie MJ, et al. Revised terminology and concepts for organization of seizures and epilepsies: report of the ILAE commission on classification and terminology, 2005-2009. *Epilepsia*. 2010;51:676-685.
11. Guerrini R, Pellacani S. Benign childhood focal epilepsies. *Epilepsia*. 2012;53:9-18.
12. Wu YW, Sullivan J, McDaniel SS, et al. Incidence of Dravet syndrome in a US population. *Pediatrics*. 2015;136:e1310-e1315.
13. Yu FH, Mantegazza M, Westenbroek RE, et al. Reduced sodium current in GABAergic interneurons in a mouse model of severe myoclonic epilepsy in infancy. *Nat Neurosci*. 2006;9:1142-1149.
14. Ostendorf AP, Ng YT. Treatment-resistant Lennox-Gastaut syndrome: therapeutic trends, challenges and future directions. *Neuropsychiatr Dis Treat*. 2017;13:1131-1140.
15. Hartman AL, Gasior M, Vining EP, Rogawski MA. The neuropharmacology of the ketogenic diet. *Pediatr Neurol*. 2007;36:281-292.
16. Lancman G, Virk M, Shao H, et al. Vagus nerve stimulation vs. corpus callosotomy in the treatment of Lennox-Gastaut syndrome: a meta-analysis. *Seizure*. 2013;22:3-8.
17. Catterall WA. Voltage-gated calcium channels. *Cold Spring Harb Perspect Biol*. 2011;3:a003947.
18. Venkatesan K, Alix P, Marquet A, et al. Altered balance between excitatory and inhibitory inputs onto CA1 pyramidal neurons from SV2A-deficient but not SV2B-deficient mice. *J Neurosci Res*. 2012;90:2317-2327.
19. Nowack A, Malarkey EB, Yao J, Bleckert A, Hill J, Bajjalieh SM. Levetiracetam reverses synaptic deficits produced by overexpression of SV2A. *PLoS One*. 2011;6:e29560.
20. Winden KD, Karsten SL, Bragin A, et al. A systems level, functional genomics analysis of chronic epilepsy. *PLoS One*. 2011;6:e20763.
21. Hess EJ. Migraines in mice? *Cell*. 1996;87:1149-1151.
22. Wallace RH, Wang DW, Singh R, et al. Febrile seizures and generalized epilepsy associated with a mutation in the Na^+-channel beta1 subunit gene SCN1B. *Nat Genet*. 1998;19:366-370.
23. Sugawara T, Mazaki-Miyazaki E, Ito M, et al. Nav1.1 mutations cause febrile seizures associated with afebrile partial seizures. *Neurology*. 2001;57:703-705.
24. Biervert C, Schroeder BC, Kubisch C, et al. A potassium channel mutation in neonatal human epilepsy. *Science*. 1998;279:403-406.
25. Singh NA, Charlier C, Stauffer D, et al. A novel potassium channel gene, KCNQ2, is mutated in an inherited epilepsy of newborns. *Nat Genet*. 1998;18:25-29.
26. Charlier C, Singh NA, Ryan SG, et al. A pore mutation in a novel KQT-like potassium channel gene in an idiopathic epilepsy family. *Nat Genet*. 1998;18:53-55.
27. Dedek K, Kunath B, Kananura C, Reuner U, Jentsch TJ, Steinlein OK. Myokymia and neonatal epilepsy caused by a mutation in the voltage sensor of the KCNQ2 K^+ channel. *Proc Natl Acad Sci U S A*. 2001;98:12272-12277.
28. Cossette P, Liu L, Brisebois K, et al. Mutation of GABRA1 in an autosomal dominant form of juvenile myoclonic epilepsy. *Nat Genet*. 2002;31:184-189.
29. Wallace RH, Marini C, Petrou S, et al. Mutant GABA(A) receptor gamma2-subunit in childhood absence epilepsy and febrile seizures. *Nat Genet*. 2001;28:49-52.
30. Baulac S, Huberfeld G, Gourfinkel-An I, et al. First genetic evidence of GABA(A) receptor dysfunction in epilepsy: a mutation in the gamma2-subunit gene. *Nat Genet*. 2001;28:46-48.
31. Sarup A, Larsson OM, Schousboe A. GABA transporters and GABA-transaminase as drug targets. *Curr Drug Targets CNS Neurol Disord*. 2003;2:269-277.
32. Brodie MJ, Sills GJ. Combining antiepileptic drugs–rational polytherapy? *Seizure*. 2011;20:369-375.
33. Pearce RE, Uetrecht JP, Leeder JS. Pathways of carbamazepine bioactivation in vitro: II. The role of human cytochrome P450 enzymes in the formation of 2-hydroxyiminostilbene. *Drug Metab Dispos*. 2005;33:1819-1826.
34. Pearce RE, Lu W, Wang Y, Uetrecht JP, Correia MA, Leeder JS. Pathways of carbamazepine bioactivation in vitro. III. The role of human cytochrome P450 enzymes in the formation of 2,3-dihydroxycarbamazepine. *Drug Metab Dispos*. 2008;36:1637-1649.
35. Lu W, Uetrecht JP. Peroxidase-mediated bioactivation of hydroxylated metabolites of carbamazepine and phenytoin. *Drug Metab Dispos*. 2008;36:1624-1636.
36. Bertilsson L. Clinical pharmacokinetics of carbamazepine. *Clin Pharmacokinet*. 1978;3:128-143.
37. Eichelbaum M, Tomson T, Tybring G, Bertilsson L. Carbamazepine metabolism in man. Induction and pharmacogenetic aspects. *Clin Pharmacokinet*. 1985;10:80-90.
38. Zhang C, Kwan P, Zuo Z, Baum L. The transport of antiepileptic drugs by P-glycoprotein. *Adv Drug Deliv Rev*. 2012;64:930-942.
39. U.S. Food and Drug Administration. Prescribing information for Tegretol. Accessed November 16, 2017. https://www.accessdata.fda.gov/drugsatfda_docs/label/2009/016608s101,018281s048lbl.pdf
40. Mattson GF, Mattson RH, Cramer JA. Interaction between valproic acid and carbamazepine: an in vitro study of protein binding. *Ther Drug Monit*. 1982;4:181-184.
41. Bertilsson L, Tomson T. Clinical pharmacokinetics and pharmacological effects of carbamazepine and carbamazepine-10,11-epoxide: an update. *Clin Pharmacokinet*. 1986;11:177-198.
42. Froescher W, Eichelbaum M, Niesen M, Dietrich K, Rausch P. Carbamazepine levels in breast milk. *Ther Drug Monit*. 1984;6:266-271.
43. Larkin JG, McKee PJ, Forrest G, et al. Lack of enzyme induction with oxcarbazepine (600 mg daily) in healthy subjects. *Br J Clin Pharmacol*. 1991;31:65-71.
44. Patsalos PN, Stephenson TJ, Krishna S, Elyas AA, Lascelles PT, Wiles CM. Side-effects induced by carbamazepine-10,11-epoxide. *Lancet*. 1985;2:496.
45. Lloyd P, Flesch G, Dieterle W. Clinical pharmacology and pharmacokinetics of oxcarbazepine. *Epilepsia*. 1994;35:S10-S13.
46. May TW, Korn-Merker E, Rambeck B. Clinical pharmacokinetics of oxcarbazepine. *Clin Pharmacokinet*. 2003;42:1023-1042.
47. Dam M, Ekberg R, Loyning Y, Waltimo O, Jakobsen K. A double-blind study comparing oxcarbazepine and carbamazepine in patients with newly diagnosed, previously untreated epilepsy. *Epilepsy Res*. 1989;3:70-76.
48. Almeida L, Soares-da-Silva P. Eslicarbazepine acetate (BIA 2-093). *Neurotherapeutics*. 2007;4:88-96.

49. Benes J, Parada A, Figueiredo AA, et al. Anticonvulsant and sodium channel-blocking properties of novel 10,11-dihydro-5H-dibenz[b,f]azepine-5-carboxamide derivatives. *J Med Chem.* 1999;42:2582-2587.
50. Bialer M, Soares-da-Silva P. Pharmacokinetics and drug interactions of eslicarbazepine acetate. *Epilepsia.* 2012;53:935-946.
51. Brown ME, El-Mallakh RS. Role of eslicarbazepine in the treatment of epilepsy in adult patients with partial-onset seizures. *Ther Clin Risk Manag.* 2010;6:103-109.
52. Kuo CC. A common anticonvulsant binding site for phenytoin, carbamazepine, and lamotrigine in neuronal Na^+ channels. *Mol Pharmacol.* 1998;54:712-721.
53. Lipkind GM, Fozzard HA. Molecular model of anticonvulsant drug binding to the voltage-gated sodium channel inner pore. *Mol Pharmacol.* 2010;78:631-638.
54. Poupaert JH, Adline J, Claesen MH, Laey PD, Dumont PA. Stereochemical aspects of the metabolism of 5-(4′-fluorophenyl)-5-phenylhydantoin in the rat. *J Med Chem.* 1979;22:1140-1142.
55. Nelson WL, Kwon YG, Marshall GL, Hoover JL, Pfeffer GT. Fluorinated phenytoin anticonvulsant analogs. *J Pharm Sci.* 1979;68:115-117.
56. Friedlander WJ. Putnam, Merritt, and the discovery of Dilantin. *Epilepsia.* 1986;27:S1-S20.
57. Glazko AJ. Addendum to "Putnam, Merritt, and the discovery of Dilantin". *Epilepsia.* 1987;28:87-88.
58. Putnam TJ, Merritt HH. Experimental determination of the anticonvulsant properties of some phenyl derivatives. *Science.* 1937;85:525-526.
59. Spielberg SP, Gordon GB, Blake DA, Goldstein DA, Herlong HF. Predisposition to phenytoin hepatotoxicity assessed in vitro. *N Engl J Med.* 1981;305:722-727.
60. Winn LM, Wells PG. Phenytoin-initiated DNA oxidation in murine embryo culture, and embryo protection by the antioxidative enzymes superoxide dismutase and catalase: evidence for reactive oxygen species-mediated DNA oxidation in the molecular mechanism of phenytoin teratogenicity. *Mol Pharmacol.* 1995;48:112-120.
61. Munns AJ, De Voss JJ, Hooper WD, Dickinson RG, Gillam EM. Bioactivation of phenytoin by human cytochrome P450: characterization of the mechanism and targets of covalent adduct formation. *Chem Res Toxicol.* 1997;10:1049-1058.
62. Cuttle L, Munns AJ, Hogg NA, et al. Phenytoin metabolism by human cytochrome P450: involvement of P450 3A and 2C forms in secondary metabolism and drug-protein adduct formation. *Drug Metab Dispos.* 2000;28:945-950.
63. Kim PM, Winn LM, Parman T, Wells PG. UDP-glucuronosyltransferase-mediated protection against in vitro DNA oxidation and micronucleus formation initiated by phenytoin and its embryotoxic metabolite 5-(p-hydroxyphenyl)-5-phenylhydantoin. *J Pharmacol Exp Ther.* 1997;280:200-209.
64. Varia SA, Schuller S, Sloan KB, Stella VJ. Phenytoin prodrugs III: water-soluble prodrugs for oral and/or parenteral use. *J Pharm Sci.* 1984;73:1068-1073.
65. Browne TR, Davoudi H, Donn KH, et al. Bioavailability of ACC-9653 (phenytoin prodrug). *Epilepsia.* 1989;30:S27-S32.
66. Burstein AH, Cox DS, Mistry B, Eddington ND. Phenytoin pharmacokinetics following oral administration of phenytoin suspension and fosphenytoin solution to rats. *Epilepsy Res.* 1999;34:129-133.
67. Boucher BA. Fosphenytoin: a novel phenytoin prodrug. *Pharmacotherapy.* 1996;16:777-791.
68. Fischer JH, Patel TV, Fischer PA. Fosphenytoin: clinical pharmacokinetics and comparative advantages in the acute treatment of seizures. *Clin Pharmacokinet.* 2003;42:33-58.
69. Boucher BA, Feler CA, Dean JC, et al. The safety, tolerability, and pharmacokinetics of fosphenytoin after intramuscular and intravenous administration in neurosurgery patients. *Pharmacotherapy.* 1996;16:638-645.
70. Cohen AF, Ashby L, Crowley D, Land G, Peck AW, Miller AA. Lamotrigine (BW430C), a potential anticonvulsant. Effects on the central nervous system in comparison with phenytoin and diazepam. *Br J Clin Pharmacol.* 1985;20:619-629.
71. Maggs JL, Naisbitt DJ, Tettey JN, Pirmohamed M, Park BK. Metabolism of lamotrigine to a reactive arene oxide intermediate. *Chem Res Toxicol.* 2000;13:1075-1081.
72. Janszky J, Rasonyi G, Halasz P, et al. Disabling erratic myoclonus during lamotrigine therapy with high serum level–report of two cases. *Clin Neuropharmacol.* 2000;23:86-89.
73. U.S. Food and Drug Administration. Prescribing information for Lamictal. Accessed December 29, 2017. https://www.accessdata.fda.gov/drugsatfda_docs/label/2006/020241s10s21s25s26s27,020764s3s14s18s19s20lbl.pdf
74. Chung SS. Lacosamide: new adjunctive treatment option for partial-onset seizures. *Expert Opin Pharmacother.* 2010;11:1595-1602.
75. Casas-Fernandez C, Martinez-Bermejo A, Rufo-Campos M, et al. Efficacy and tolerability of lacosamide in the concomitant treatment of 130 patients under 16 years of age with refractory epilepsy: a prospective, open-label, observational, multicenter study in Spain. *Drugs R D.* 2012;12:187-197.
76. Wilson SM, Khanna R. Specific binding of lacosamide to collapsin response mediator protein 2 (CRMP2) and direct impairment of its canonical function: implications for the therapeutic potential of lacosamide. *Mol Neurobiol.* 2015;51:599-609.
77. Czech T, Yang JW, Csaszar E, Kappler J, Baumgartner C, Lubec G. Reduction of hippocampal collapsin response mediated protein-2 in patients with mesial temporal lobe epilepsy. *Neurochem Res.* 2004;29:2189-2196.
78. Beyreuther BK, Freitag J, Heers C, Krebsfänger N, Scharfenecker U, Stöhr T. Lacosamide: a review of preclinical properties. *CNS Drug Rev.* 2007;13:21-42.
79. Conley JD, Kohn H. Functionalized DL-amino acid derivatives. Potent new agents for the treatment of epilepsy. *J Med Chem.* 1987;30:567-574.
80. Kohn H, Sawhney KN, LeGall P, Conley JD, Robertson DW, Leander JD. Preparation and anticonvulsant activity of a series of functionalized alpha-aromatic and alpha-heteroaromatic amino acids. *J Med Chem.* 1990;33:919-926.
81. Cawello W, Fuhr U, Hering U, Maatouk H, Halabi A. Impact of impaired renal function on the pharmacokinetics of the antiepileptic drug lacosamide. *Clin Pharmacokinet.* 2013;52:897-906.
82. U.S. Food and Drug Administration. Prescribing information for Vimpat. Accessed December 22, 2017. https://www.accessdata.fda.gov/drugsatfda_docs/label/2013/022253s024,022254s018,022255s010lbl.pdf
83. Tilz C, Resch R, Hofer T, Eggers C. Successful treatment for refractory convulsive status epilepticus by non-parenteral lacosamide. *Epilepsia.* 2010;51:316-317.
84. DeGiorgio AC, Desso TE, Lee L, DeGiorgio CM. Ventricular tachycardia associated with lacosamide co-medication in drug-resistant epilepsy. *Epilepsy Behav Case Rep.* 2013;1:26-28.
85. McCleane G, Koch B, Rauschkolb C. Does SPM 927 have an analgesic effect in human neuropathic pain? An open label study. *Neurosci Lett.* 2003;352:117-120.
86. Brodie MJ, Rosenfeld WE, Vazquez B, et al. Rufinamide for the adjunctive treatment of partial seizures in adults and adolescents: a randomized placebo-controlled trial. *Epilepsia.* 2009;50(8):1899-1909.
87. Gilchrist J, Dutton S, Diaz-Bustamante M, et al. Nav1.1 modulation by a novel triazole compound attenuates epileptic seizures in rodents. *ACS Chem Biol.* 2014;9:1204-1212.
88. U.S. Food and Drug Administration. Prescribing information for Banzel. Accessed December 22, 2017. https://www.accessdata.fda.gov/drugsatfda_docs/label/2008/021911lbl.pdf
89. U.S. Food and Drug Administration. Center for drug evaluation research: application number 21-911: environmental assessment. Accessed December 22, 2017. https://www.accessdata.fda.gov/drugsatfda_docs/nda/2008/021911s000_EA.pdf

90. Wheless JW, Conry J, Krauss G, Mann A, LoPresti A, Narurkar M. Safety and tolerability of rufinamide in children with epilepsy: a pooled analysis of 7 clinical studies. *J Child Neurol.* 2009;24:1520-1525.
91. Aldenkamp AP, Alpherts WC. The effect of the new antiepileptic drug rufinamide on cognitive functions. *Epilepsia.* 2006;47:1153-1159.
92. Chu-Shore CJ, Thiele EA. New drugs for pediatric epilepsy. *Semin Pediatr Neurol.* 2010;17:214-223.
93. Perucca E, Cloyd J, Critchley D, Fuseau E. Rufinamide: clinical pharmacokinetics and concentration-response relationships in patients with epilepsy. *Epilepsia.* 2008;49:1123-1141.
94. Dolphin AC. The alpha2δ subunits of voltage-gated calcium channels. *Biochim Biophys Acta.* 2013;1828:1541-1549.
95. Wang M, Offord J, Oxender DL, Su TZ. Structural requirement of the calcium-channel subunit alpha2delta for gabapentin binding. *Biochem J.* 1999;342:313-320.
96. Bian F, Li Z, Offord J, et al. Calcium channel alpha2-delta type 1 subunit is the major binding protein for pregabalin in neocortex, hippocampus, amygdala, and spinal cord: an ex vivo autoradiographic study in alpha2-delta type 1 genetically modified mice. *Brain Res.* 2006;1075:68-80.
97. Dooley DJ, Mieske CA, Borosky SA. Inhibition of K(+)-evoked glutamate release from rat neocortical and hippocampal slices by gabapentin. *Neurosci Lett.* 2000;280:107-110.
98. U.S. Food and Drug Administration. Prescribing Information for Neurontin. Accessed December 27, 2023. https://www.accessdata.fda.gov/drugsatfda_docs/label/2017/020235s064_020882s047_021129s046lbl.pdf
99. Stewart BH, Kugler AR, Thompson PR, Bockbrader HN. A saturable transport mechanism in the intestinal absorption of gabapentin is the underlying cause of the lack of proportionality between increasing dose and drug levels in plasma. *Pharm Res.* 1993;10:276-281.
100. Bockbrader HN, Wesche D, Miller R, Chapel S, Janiczek N, Burger P. A comparison of the pharmacokinetics and pharmacodynamics of pregabalin and gabapentin. *Clin Pharmacokinet.* 2010;49:661-669.
101. Bockbrader HN, Radulovic LL, Posvar EL, et al. Clinical pharmacokinetics of pregabalin in healthy volunteers. *J Clin Pharmacol.* 2010;50:941-950.
102. Eisenberg E, River Y, Shifrin A, Krivoy N. Antiepileptic drugs in the treatment of neuropathic pain. *Drugs.* 2007;67:1265-1289.
103. Eckhardt K, Ammon S, Hofmann U, Riebe A, Gugeler N, Mikus G. Gabapentin enhances the analgesic effect of morphine in healthy volunteers. *Anesth Analg.* 2000;91:185-191.
104. Radulovic LL, Turck D, von Hodenberg A, et al. Disposition of gabapentin (neurontin) in mice, rats, dogs, and monkeys. *Drug Metab Dispos.* 1995;23:441-448.
105. Gomora JC, Daud AN, Weiergraber M, Perez-Reyes E. Block of cloned human T-type calcium channels by succinimide antiepileptic drugs. *Mol Pharmacol.* 2001;60:1121-1132.
106. Horning MG, Stratton C, Nowlin J, Harvey DJ, Hill RM. Metabolism of 2-ethyl-2-methylsuccinimide (ethosuximide) in the rat and human. *Drug Metab Dispos.* 1973;1:569-576.
107. Sarver JG, Bachmann KA, Zhu D, Klis WA. Ethosuximide is primarily metabolized by CYP3A when incubated with isolated rat liver microsomes. *Drug Metab Dispos.* 1998;26:78-82.
108. Eadie MJ, Tyrer JH, Smith GA, McKauge L. Pharmacokinetics of drugs used for petit mal 'absence' epilepsy. *Clin Exp Neurol.* 1977;14:172-183.
109. Vajda FJ, Eadie MJ. The clinical pharmacology of traditional antiepileptic drugs. *Epileptic Disord.* 2014;16:395-408.
110. Buchanan RA, Fernandez L, Kinkel AW. Absorption and elimination of ethosuximide in children. *J Clin Pharmacol J New Drugs.* 1969;9:393-398.
111. Nadkarni S, Devinsky O. Psychotropic effects of antiepileptic drugs. *Epilepsy Curr.* 2005;5:176-181.
112. Landolt H. Serial electroencephalographic investigations during psychotic episodes in epileptic patients and during schizophrenic attacks. In: de Haas L, ed. *Lectures on Epilepsy.* Vol 3. Elsevier; 1958: 91-133.
113. Salke-Kellermann RA, May T, Boenigk HE. Influence of ethosuximide on valproic acid serum concentrations. *Epilepsy Res.* 1997;26:345-349.
114. Warren JW, Benmaman JD, Wannamaker BB, Levy RH. Kinetics of a carbamazepine-ethosuximide interaction. *Clin Pharmacol Ther.* 1980;28:646-651.
115. Greenfield LJ. Molecular mechanisms of antiseizure drug activity at GABAA receptors. *Seizure.* 2013;22:589-600.
116. Pacifici GM. Clinical pharmacology of phenobarbital in neonates: effects, metabolism and pharmacokinetics. *Curr Pediatr Rev.* 2016;12:48-54.
117. Messina S, Battino D, Croci D, Mamoli D, Ratti S, Perucca E. Phenobarbital pharmacokinetics in old age: a case-matched evaluation based on therapeutic drug monitoring data. *Epilepsia.* 2005;46:372-377.
118. Reinisch JM, Sanders SA, Mortensen EL, Rubin DB. In utero exposure to phenobarbital and intelligence deficits in adult men. *JAMA.* 1995;274:1518-1525.
119. Farwell JR, Lee YJ, Hirtz DG, Sulzbacher SI, Ellenberg JH, Nelson KB. Phenobarbital for febrile seizures–effects on intelligence and on seizure recurrence. *N Engl J Med.* 1990;322:364-369.
120. Lambie DG, Johnson RH. The effects of phenytoin on phenobarbitone and primidone metabolism. *J Neurol Neurosurg Psychiatry.* 1981;44:148-151.
121. Martines C, Gatti G, Sasso E, Calzetti S, Perucca E. The disposition of primidone in elderly patients. *Br J Clin Pharmacol.* 1990;30:607-611.
122. U.S. Food and Drug Administration. Prescribing information for Ativan. Accessed April 21, 2018. https://www.accessdata.fda.gov/drugsatfda_docs/label/2017/018140s041s042lbl.pdf
123. Ralvenius WT, Acuna MA, Benke D, et al. The clobazam metabolite *N*-desmethyl clobazam is an α2 preferring benzodiazepine with an improved therapeutic window for antihyperalgesia. *Neuropharmacology.* 2016;109:366-375.
124. U.S. Food and Drug Administration. Prescribing information for Onfi. Accessed December 29, 2017. https://www.accessdata.fda.gov/drugsatfda_docs/label/2016/203993s005lbl.pdf
125. Contin M, Riva R, Albani F, Baruzzi AA. Effect of felbamate on clobazam and its metabolite kinetics in patients with epilepsy. *Ther Drug Monit.* 1999;21:604-608.
126. Giraud C, Tran A, Rey E, Vincent J, Tréluyer J-M, Pons G. In vitro characterization of clobazam metabolism by recombinant cytochrome P450 enzymes: importance of CYP2C19. *Drug Metab Dispos.* 2004;32:1279-1286.
127. Gerecke M. Chemical structure and properties of midazolam compared with other benzodiazepines. *Br J Clin Pharmacol.* 1983;16:11S-16S.
128. Nohria V, Giller E. Ganaxolone. *Neurotherapeutics.* 2007;4:102-105.
129. Quilchini PP, Chiron C, Ben-Ari Y, Gozlan H. Stiripentol, a putative antiepileptic drug, enhances the duration of opening of GABA-A receptor channels. *Epilepsia.* 2006;47:704-716.
130. Levy RH, Lin H-S, Blehaut HM, Tor JA. Pharmacokinetics of stiripentol in normal man: evidence of non-linearity. *J Clin Pharmacol.* 1983;23:523-533.
131. U.S. Food and Drug Administration. Clinical pharmacology and biopharmaceutics review(s). NDA #206709. Accessed May 20, 2023. https://www.accessdata.fda.gov/drugsatfda_docs/nda/2018/206709Orig1s000,207223Orig1s000ClinPharmR.pdf
132. Jurik A, Zdrazil B, Holy M, Stockner T, Sitte HH, Ecker GF. A binding mode hypothesis of tiagabine confirms liothyronine effect on γ-aminobutyric acid transporter 1 (GAT1). *J Med Chem.* 2015;58:2149-2158.
133. Andersen KE, Braestrup C, Gronwald FC, et al. The synthesis of novel GABA uptake inhibitors. 1. Elucidation of the structure-activity studies leading to the choice of

(R)-1-[4,4-bis(3-methyl-2-thienyl)-3-butenyl]-3-piperidinecarboxylic acid (tiagabine) as an anticonvulsant drug candidate. *J Med Chem*. 1993;36:1716-1725.
134. U.S. Food and Drug Administration. Prescribing information for Gabitril. Accessed December 29, 2017. https://www.accessdata.fda.gov/drugsatfda_docs/label/2009/020646s016lbl.pdf
135. Nanavati SM, Silverman RB. Mechanisms of inactivation of gamma-aminobutyric acid aminotransferase by the antiepilepsy drug gamma-vinyl GABA (vigabatrin). *J Am Chem Soc*. 1991;113:9341-9349.
136. U.S. Food and Drug Administration. Prescribing information for Vigabatrin. Accessed December 30, 2017. https://www.accessdata.fda.gov/drugsatfda_docs/label/2013/020427s010s011s012,022006s011s012s013lbl.pdf
137. Abbot EL, Grenade DS, Kennedy DJ, Gatfield KM, Thwaites DT. Vigabatrin transport across the human intestinal epithelial (Caco-2) brush-border membrane is via the H^+ -coupled amino-acid transporter hPAT1. *Br J Pharmacol*. 2006;147:298-306.
138. Hawker MJ, Astbury NJ. The ocular side effects of vigabatrin (Sabril): information and guidance for screening. *Eye (Lond)*. 2008;22:1097-1098.
139. Kushner SA, Dewey SL, Kornetsky C. The irreversible gamma-aminobutyric acid (GABA) transaminase inhibitor gamma-vinyl-GABA blocks cocaine self-administration in rats. *J Pharmacol Exp Ther*. 1999;290:797-802.
140. Brodie JD, Case BG, Figueroa E, et al. Randomized, double-blind, placebo-controlled trial of vigabatrin for the treatment of cocaine dependence in Mexican parolees. *Am J Psychiatry*. 2009;166:1269-1277.
141. Sargentini-Maier ML, Espie P, Coquette A, Stockis A. Pharmacokinetics and metabolism of 14C-brivaracetam, a novel SV2A ligand, in healthy subjects. *Drug Metab Dispos*. 2008;36:36-45.
142. Patsalos PN. Clinical pharmacokinetics of levetiracetam. *Clin Pharmacokinet*. 2004;43:707-724.
143. Nicolas JM, Hannestad J, Holden D, et al. Brivaracetam, a selective high-affinity synaptic vesicle protein 2A (SV2A) ligand with preclinical evidence of high brain permeability and fast onset of action. *Epilepsia*. 2016;57:201-209.
144. Rankovic Z. CNS drug design: balancing physicochemical properties for optimal brain exposure. *J Med Chem*. 2015;58:2584-2608.
145. Stockis A, Chanteux H, Rosa M, Rolan P. Brivaracetam and carbamazepine interaction in healthy subjects and in vitro. *Epilepsy Res*. 2015;113:19-27.
146. Hibi S, Ueno K, Nagato S, et al. Discovery of 2-(2-oxo-1-phenyl-5-pyridin-2-yl-1,2-dihydropyridin-3-yl)benzonitrile (perampanel): a novel, noncompetitive α-amino-3-hydroxy-5-methyl-4-isoxazolepropanoic acid (AMPA) receptor antagonist. *J Med Chem*. 2012;55:10584-10600.
147. Patsalos PN. The clinical pharmacology profile of the new antiepileptic drug perampanel: a novel noncompetitive AMPA receptor antagonist. *Epilepsia*. 2015;56:12-27.
148. Hawkins KL, Gidal BE. When adverse effects are seen as desirable: abuse potential of the newer generation antiepileptic drugs. *Epilepsy Behav*. 2017;77:62-72.
149. Koppel BS, Brust JC, Fife T, et al. Systematic review: efficacy and safety of medical marijuana in selected neurologic disorders: report of the Guideline Development Subcommittee of the American Academy of Neurology. *Neurology*. 2014;82:1556-1563.
150. Gloss D, Vickrey B. Cannabinoids for epilepsy. *Cochrane Database Syst Rev*. 2014;2014(3):CD009270.
151. Rosenberg EC, Tsien RW, Whalley BJ, Devinsky O. Cannabinoids and epilepsy. *Neurotherapeutics*. 2015;12:747-768.
152. Devinsky O, Cross JH, Laux L, et al. Trail of cannabidiol for drug-resistant seizures in the Dravet syndrome. *N Engl J Med*. 2017;376:2011-2020.
153. Laprairie RB, Bagher AM, Kelly ME, Denovan-Wright EM. Cannabidiol is a negative allosteric modulator of the cannabinoid CB1 receptor. *Br J Pharmacol*. 2015;172:4790-4805.
154. Deutsch DG. A personal retrospective: elevating anandamide (AEA) by targeting fatty acid amide hydrolase (FAAH) and the fatty acid binding proteins (FABPs). *Front Pharmacol*. 2016;7:370.
155. Millar SA, Stone NL, Yates AS, O'Sullivan SE. A systematic review on the pharmacokinetics of cannabidiol in humans. *Front Pharmacol*. 2018;9:1365.
156. U.S. Food and Drug Administration. Prescribing information for Cannabidiol. Accessed May 21, 2023. https://www.accessdata.fda.gov/drugsatfda_docs/label/2018/210365lbl.pdf
157. Moazen-Zadeh E, Galynker II. Suicidality and cannabidiol: opportunities and challenges. *Curr Neuropharmacol*. 2021;19:733-735.
158. Caprioglio D, Mattoteja D, Pollastro F, et al. The oxidation of phytocannabinoids to cannabinoquinoids. *J Nat Prod*. 2020;83:1171-1175.
159. Stafstrom CE. Persistent sodium current and its role in epilepsy. *Epilepsy Curr*. 2007;7:15-22.
160. Guignet M, Campbell A, White HS. Cenobamate (XCOPRI): can preclinical and clinical evidence provide insight into its mechanism of action? *Epilepsia*. 2020;61:2329-2339.
161. Sharma R, Nakamura M, Neupane C, et al. Positive allosteric modulation of $GABA_A$ receptors by a novel antiepileptic drug cenobamate. *Eur J Pharmacol*. 2020;879:173117.
162. Specchio N, Pietrafusa N, Vigevano F. Is cenobamate the breakthrough we have been wishing for? *Int J Mol Sci*. 2021;22:9339.
163. Sperling MR, Klein P, Aboumatar S, et al. Cenobamate (YKP3089) as adjunctive treatment for uncontrolled focal seizures in a large, phase 3, multicenter, open-label safety study. *Epilepsia*. 2020;61:1099-1108.
164. U.S. Food and Drug Administration. Prescribing information for Cenobamate. Accessed June 3, 2023. https://www.accessdata.fda.gov/drugsatfda_docs/label/2019/212839s000lbl.pdf
165. Chang HR, Kuo CC. Molecular determinants of the anticonvulsant felbamate binding site in the N-methyl-D-aspartate receptor. *J Med Chem*. 2008;51:1534-1545.
166. Parker RJ, Hartman NR, Roecklein BA, et al. Stability and comparative metabolism of selected felbamate metabolites and postulated fluorofelbamate metabolites by postmitochondrial suspensions. *Chem Res Toxicol*. 2005;18:1842-1848.
167. Dieckhaus CM, Thompson CD, Roller SG, Macdonald TL. Mechanisms of idiosyncratic drug reactions: the case of felbamate. *Chem Biol Interact*. 2002;142:99-117.
168. Popovic M, Nierkens S, Pieters R, Uetrecht J. Investigating the role of 2-phenylpropenal in felbamate-induced idiosyncratic drug reactions. *Chem Res Toxicol*. 2004;17:1568-1576.
169. Lagae L, Sullivan J, Knupp K, et al. Fenfluramine hydrochloride for the treatment of seizures in Dravet syndrome: a randomized, double-blind, placebo-controlled trial. *Lancet*. 2019;394:2243-2254.
170. Knupp K, Scheffer IE, Ceulemans B, et al. Efficacy and safety of fenfluramine for the treatment of seizures associated with Lennox-Gastaut syndrome: a randomized clinical trial. *JAMA Neurol*. 2022;79:554-564.
171. Martin P, de Witte PAM, Maurice T, Gammaitoni A, Farfel G, Galer B. Fenfluramine acts as a positive modulator of sigma-1 receptors. *Epilepsy Behav*. 2020;105:106989.
172. U.S. Food and Drug Administration. Prescribing information for Fenfliramine. Accessed May 30, 2023. https://www.ucb-usa.com/fintepla-prescribing-information.pdf
173. Maryanoff BE, Costanzo MJ, Nortey SO, et al. Structure-activity studies on anticonvulsant sugar sulfamates related to topiramate. Enhanced potency with cyclic sulfate derivatives. *J Med Chem*. 1998;41:1315-1343.
174. U.S. Food and Drug Administration. Prescribing information for Topamax. Accessed December 29, 2017. https://www.accessdata.fda.gov/drugsatfda_docs/label/2009/020505s038s039,020844s032s034lbl.pdf

175. Britzi M, Perucca E, Soback S, et al. Pharmacokinetic and metabolic investigation of topiramate disposition in healthy subjects in the absence and in the presence of enzyme induction by carbamazepine. *Epilepsia*. 2005;46:378-384.
176. Nallani SC, Glauser TA, Hariparsad N, et al. Dose-dependent induction of cytochrome P450 (CYP) 3A4 and activation of pregnane X receptor by topiramate. *Epilepsia*. 2003;44:1521-1528.
177. Shorvon SD. Drug treatment of epilepsy in the century of the ILAE: the second 50 years, 1959-2009. *Epilepsia*. 2009;50:93-130.
178. Perucca E. Pharmacological and therapeutic properties of valproate: a summary after 35 years of clinical experience. *CNS Drugs*. 2002;16:695-714.
179. Ghodke-Puranik Y, Thorn CF, Lamba JK, et al. Valproic acid pathway: pharmacokinetics and pharmacodynamics. *Pharmacogenet Genomics*. 2013;23:236-241.
180. Kassahun K, Farrell K, Abbott F. Identification and characterization of the glutathione and N-acetylcysteine conjugates of (E)-2-propyl-2,4-pentadienoic acid, a toxic metabolite of valproic acid, in rats and humans. *Drug Metab Dispos*. 1991;19:525-535.
181. Bowdle AT, Patel IH, Levy RH, Wilensky AJ. Valproic acid dosage and plasma protein binding and clearance. *Clin Pharmacol Ther*. 1980;28:486-492.
182. U.S. Food and Drug Administration. Prescribing information for Depakote. Accessed December 29, 2017. https://www.accessdata.fda.gov/drugsatfda_docs/label/2011/018723s037lbl.pdf
183. Ueda Y, Doi T, Tokumaru J, Willmore LJ. Effect of zonisamide on molecular regulation of glutamate and GABA transporter proteins during epileptogenesis in rats with hippocampal seizures. *Brain Res*. 2003;116:1-6.
184. Stiff DD, Zemaitis MA. Metabolism of the anticonvulsant agent zonisamide in the rat. *Drug Metab Dispos*. 1990;18:888-894.
185. U.S. Food and Drug Administration. Prescribing information for Zonegran. Accessed December 27, 2017. https://www.accessdata.fda.gov/drugsatfda_docs/label/2003/20789scm001_zonegran_lbl.pdf
186. Löscher W, Klein P. The pharmacology and clinical efficacy of antiseizure medications: from bromide salts to cenobamate and beyond. *CNS Drugs*. 2021;35:935-963.

Case Study Answer

All four of the compounds your preceptor showed you are benzodiazepines. You can tell this by the benzene ring ("benzo") fused to a seven-membered ring containing two nitrogen atoms ("diazepine"). All benzodiazepines bind to a benzodiazepine binding site on $GABA_A$ ion channels called a "benzodiazepine receptor" (BZR) site. This is an allosteric binding site that can either increase or decrease the activity of the receptor when GABA is bound. When GABA binds GABAA channels, the channel opens to allow chloride anions into the cell, causing hyperpolarization and a decrease in neuronal activity. Whether the compound increases or decreases the activity of GABA depends on the presence of an extra benzene ring attached to the benzodiazepine core. Inspection of A-C shows that an extra benzene is attached to A-C and is not present in D. Thus, A-C are all positive allosteric modulators (PAMs) and D is a negative allosteric modulator (NAM). This means that A-C will lead to more hyperpolarization and better control of seizures, and compound D might actually increase neuronal activity during a seizure.

To determine which of A-C would be most appropriate, you need to understand how each drug is metabolized and whether any of those metabolites would be active. Compound A is an "-azepam," which means N-demethylation at position 1 is tolerated, as is oxidation at position 3. This means there are three possible active metabolites: the *N*-demethylated product (A-1), the 3-hydroxylated product (A-2), and the product that has both N-demethylation and 3-hydroxylation (A-3). Compound 2 does not have any active metabolites: there is nothing to remove at position 1, and position 3 is already oxidized. Oxidation to any other position on the molecule leads to inactive metabolites, so there are no predicted active metabolites. Compound C is an "-azolam." You can tell by the fact that there is an imidazole fused to positions 1 and 2. The SAR of "-azolams" are different from those of "-azepams" in that all oxidized metabolites are inactive. Because compound A has three active metabolites and compounds B and C have none, the duration of action of A is expected to be the longest. This drug (which is diazepam) is the most appropriate for this patient.

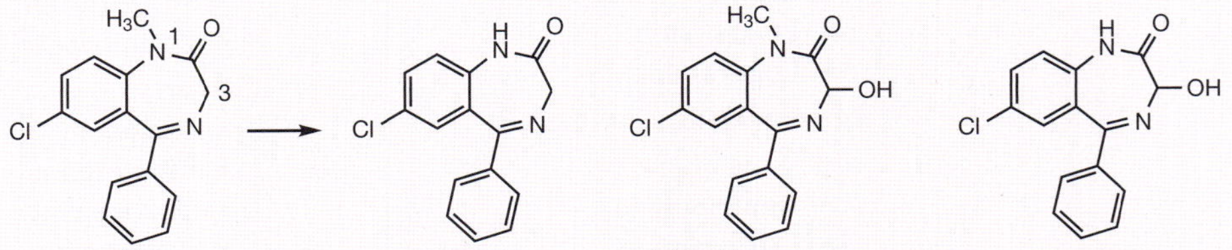

A A-1 A-2 A-3

SECTION 2

Drugs Impacting Pain Perception

CHAPTER

16

Drugs Used to Treat Pain: Centrally Acting Agents

Christopher W. Cunningham and Victoria F. Roche

Drugs covered in this chapter:

OPIOID ANALGESICS

PHENANTHRENE-BASED RIGID M AGONISTS

- Buprenorphine
- Codeine
- Hydrocodone
- Hydromorphone
- Levorphanol
- Morphine
- Oxycodone
- Oxymorphone

PHENANTHRENE-BASED RIGID κ AGONISTS/μ ANTAGONISTS

- Butorphanol
- Nalbuphine
- Pentazocine

FLEXIBLE μ AGONISTS

- Alfentanil
- Fentanyl
- Meperidine
- Methadone
- Remifentanil
- Sufentanil
- Tapentadol (dual action)
- Tramadol (dual action)

OPIOID ANTAGONISTS

- Methylnaltrexone bromide
- Naldemedine
- Nalmefene
- Naloxegol
- Naloxone
- Naltrexone

PERIPHERALLY SELECTIVE OPIOID-BASED ANTIDIARRHEALS

- Difenoxin
- Diphenoxylate
- Eluxadoline
- Loperamide

NEUROPATHIC ANALGESICS

FIRST-LINE AGENTS

- Amitriptyline
- Desipramine
- Duloxetine
- Gabapentin
- Nortriptyline
- Pregabalin

SECOND-LINE AGENTS

- Capsaicin
- Lidocaine

ANTIMIGRAINE DRUGS

TRIPTANS

- Almotriptan
- Eletriptan
- Frovatriptan
- Naratriptan
- Rizatriptan
- Sumatriptan
- Zolmitriptan

GEPANTS

- Atogepant
- Rimegepant
- Ubrogepant
- Zavegepant

Abbreviations

5-HT serotonin
AC adenylyl cyclase
ACE angiotensin-converting enzyme
ADF abuse-deterrent formulation
AMPA α-amino-3-hydroxy-5-methyl-4-isoxazolepropionic acid
APPE advanced pharmacy practice experience
ATP adenosine triphosphate
β-arr2 β-arrestin2
BBB blood-brain barrier
cAMP cyclic adenosine monophosphate
CGRP calcitonin gene–related peptide

Abbreviations—continued

CNS central nervous system
CRLR calcitonin receptor–like receptor
DAT dopamine transporter
DEA US Drug Enforcement Agency
EASE Entereg Access Support Education
EDDP 2-ethylene-1,5-dimethyl-3,3-diphenylpyrrolidine
EDMP 2-ethylene-5-methyl-3,3-diphenyl-1-pyrrolidine
FDA US Food and Drug Administration
FMO flavin monooxygenase
FRS fentanyl-related substances
GABA γ-aminobutyric acid
GI gastrointestinal
GPCR G-protein–coupled receptor
HBA hydrogen-bond acceptor
HBD hydrogen-bond donor
IM intramuscular
IMs intermediate metabolizers
IV intravenous
LDN low-dose naltrexone
MAO monoamine oxidase
MAT medication-assisted treatment
MCT-1 monocarboxylate transporter-1
MEGX monoethylglycine xylidide
MPP+ phenylpyridine
NET norepinephrine transporter
NE norepinephrine
NMDA *N*-methyl-D-aspartate
NSAIDs nonsteroidal anti-inflammatory drugs
OIC opioid-induced constipation
ORL 1 opioid receptor–like 1
OTC over the counter
PAMORAs peripherally acting μ opioid–receptor antagonists
PCPs primary care physicians
PEG polyethylene glycol
PKA protein kinase A
P-gp P-glycoprotein
PMs poor metabolizers
RAMP receptor activity–modifying protein
RCP receptor-component protein
REMS Risk Evaluation and Mitigation Strategy
Rx prescription
SAMHSA Substance Abuse and Mental Health Services Administration
SAR structure-activity relationship
SNP single-nucleotide polymorphism
SSRI selective serotonin-reuptake inhibitor
TCA tricyclic antidepressant
TIRF transmucosal immediate-release fentanyl
TMH transmembrane helix
TPSA topologic polar surface area
TRPV1 transient receptor potential vanilloid 1
UGT UDP-glucuronosyltransferase
WCS wooden chest syndrome
UMs ultrarapid metabolizers

CLINICAL SIGNIFICANCE

Pain management practice is heavily influenced by the medicinal chemistry of analgesic pharmacotherapy. Clinicians are required to have a strong understanding of the metabolism pathways of frequently used μ-opioid analgesics, especially when assessing urine drug screening outcomes often used to identify aberrant behaviors such as diversion, polysubstance use, and nonadherence. Misinterpretation of drug screening results, including erroneous assumptions of illicit morphine-based drug administration in patients prescribed codeine-based analgesics, can lead to negative patient outcomes, including abrupt discontinuation with subsequent withdrawal symptoms and, in some cases, patient abandonment. Recognition of lipophilicity differences in fentanyl-based opioids can help clinicians select agents with the proper onset/duration parameters to meet therapeutic needs.

Jordan L. Wulz, PharmD, MPH, BC-ADM

PAIN

"The greatest evil is physical pain"

St. Augustine

While not everyone would agree with St. Augustine's sweeping characterization, most people will go to great lengths to avoid physical pain. Pain is defined as an unpleasant sensory and emotional experience associated with actual or potential tissue damage, or described in terms of such damage.[1,2] Pain is part of the body's defense system, is designed to protect against more serious injury (ie, a "necessary evil"), and usually resolves once the offensive stimulus is removed and healing is complete. However, some pain persists well after offending injuries have healed and/or arises in the absence of any detectable stimulus.[3]

Regardless of how it presents, serious pain can be disabling, demoralizing, and destructive to a person's quality of life. Reflecting this importance to well-being, in 1995 the President of the American Pain Society, Dr James Campbell, proposed that pain be considered the fifth vital sign to raise awareness among health care providers on the need to adequately treat it.[4] However, some have questioned whether pain management has advanced as a result of this characterization.[5] Although supporting the goal of pain assessment in all patients, the fifth vital sign concept was never formally endorsed by the Joint Commission.[6] In 2016, the American Medical Association House of Delegates voted that it be eliminated from professional standards based on concerns related, at least in part, to reimbursement.[7] A possible link between the fifth vital sign view and increases in opioid prescribing has been raised in the literature, as has the critical need for expanded medical education on pain assessment and management.[8,9]

The intensity, character, and tolerability of each person's pain are subjective and challenging to assess objectively. Differences in pain prevalence, perception, tolerance thresholds, and/or management are associated with, among other factors, age, economic status, race/ethnicity, genetics, and gender. To account for variability in perception, standardized pain scales, such as the Wong-Baker FACES Pain Rating Scale,[10] are commonly used to clue providers on patients' pain intensity. They are also used to evaluate the effectiveness of therapy, although some would criticize these scales for their simplicity. Differences and/or disparities in pain perception, coping, and treatment based on a patient's race/ethnicity are claimed to have psychosocial components. Research and professional education designed to address current inequities in quality pain care have been advocated.[11]

In 2011, the economic toll of pain in the United States, including the cost of treatment and the impact of lost productivity, was estimated at $634 billion.[8,12] Additionally, the economic burden associated with opioid analgesic misuse contributed an estimated $78.5 billion in 2013 when the cost of criminal justice system involvement was considered.[13] In 2017, a 13-year retrospective study on pain prevalence in a US population of more than 6.5 million adults documented that a mean of 2.68 distinct pain diagnoses commonly occur in individual patients.[12] Back pain was cited as the most prevalent diagnosis, and more than half (58%) of the pain patients in the study population were women.

More recently, Yong et al have confirmed that chronic pain continues to exact a heavy toll on quality of life and economic well-being in the United States.[14] Based on the results of a 2019 National Health Interview Survey study, the authors estimate that 20% of the US adult population (50.2 million people) experience chronic pain that occurs "most days" or daily, most commonly in the lower extremities and back. Approximately half are classified as having "high-impact" pain, which is sufficiently frequent/intense to restrict the ability to work, play and/or engage independently in activities of daily living. Using the same data set, Zelaya et al confirmed that chronic pain, (including high-impact pain) was higher in women and those aged 65 years and older.[15] Yong and collaborators estimate that, in 2019, close to $80 billion in lost wages and $300 billion in lost productivity could be attributed to the disabling effects of chronic pain.[14]

Pathophysiology of Pain

Pain is categorized based on its pathophysiology as nociceptive, neuropathic, or due to sensory hypersensitivity.

Nociceptive Pain

Nociceptive pain is due to trauma, inflammation, or other injury occurring in nonneural tissue. It is mediated through nociceptors located in the skin, bone, connective tissue, muscle, and viscera.[16] Nociceptive pain is often described with adjectives such as tender, dull, aching, throbbing, or cramping[3] and usually responds to nonsteroidal anti-inflammatory drugs (NSAIDs) and opioids.

The nociceptive pain mechanism is highly complex.[2,16] Tissue damage in the periphery depolarizes neuronal membranes and releases chemical mediators such as prostaglandins, bradykinin, serotonin, substance P, and histamine, which stimulate nociceptors. The ensuing action potential travels along afferent neurons, designated as C fibers and Aδ fibers, to receptors at the dorsal horn of the spinal cord. There, the excitatory amino acid glutamate is released and stimulates α-amino-3-hydroxy-5-methyl-4-isoxazolepropionic acid (AMPA) receptors on secondary neurons. A surge of released glutamate allows activation of *N*-methyl-D-aspartate (NMDA) receptors normally inhibited by Mg^{2+}, leading to central sensitization. Pain perception is due to the transmission of the nociceptive message from the thalamus to the somatosensory cortex, parietal lobe, frontal lobe, and limbic system.

Aδ fibers are thinly myelinated and transmit the action potentials more rapidly (~20 m/s) than unmyelinated C fibers (~2 m/s). Aδ axons associated with acute pain mediate the reflex process that results in avoidance of the noxious stimuli (eg, pulling away from a hot surface or sharp implement). The more slowly conducting C fibers are responsible for the longer-lasting pain that follows acute injury.

Neuropathic Pain

Neuropathic pain involves damage to peripheral or central neurons. Peripheral neuropathic pain is commonly associated with diseases such as diabetes, polio, herpes zoster virus (shingles), cancer, and some cancer chemotherapies. Central neuropathic pain can be experienced by patients who have suffered a stroke or spinal cord injury.[3]

Excitatory impulses are repeatedly transmitted in neuropathic pain, leading to sensitization of peripheral nociceptors, hyperexcitability of central neurons, and ultimately to structural and/or functional changes in these neurons. The result can be recurrent or continuous abnormal responses to painful stimuli, including hyperalgesia (excessive response), hypoalgesia (attenuated response), and/or paresthesia or dysesthesia (annoying or more intensely unpleasant sensations, respectively).[16,17]

Adjectives commonly used to describe neuropathic pain include tingling, shock-like, pins and needles, burning, and stabbing.[3] Patients living with neuropathic pain are also at higher risk for anxiety, depression, and sleep disturbances compared to the general population and are known to have a lower health-related quality of life.[17]

Sensory Hypersensitivity

Sensory hypersensitivity can be thought of as neuropathic pain without identifiable nerve damage.[3,17] Sustained functional disruption of central neurons is believed to result in lowered pain thresholds and an augmentation of pain impulses. Generalized hypersensitivity of central neurons can also lead to exaggerated responses to other environmental stimuli, such as light, sounds, and/or smells. The pathophysiologic mechanisms of these two categories of pain are believed to be very similar, and they respond to similar therapeutic interventions (eg, α2δ ligands, tricyclic antidepressants [TCAs], and serotonin [5-HT]- or norepinephrine

[NE]-reuptake inhibitors). Opioids, of use primarily in nociceptive pain, are third-line therapy in neuropathic pain and contraindicated in sensory hypersensitivity.

Fibromyalgia, chronic fatigue syndrome, and restless leg syndrome are examples of disorders resulting in sensory hypersensitivity-related pain. Patients can present with complaints of widely disseminated pain, hyperalgesia, allodynia (pain in response to nonpainful stimuli), fatigue, and disorders in cognition and/or mood.

Acute Pain

Acute pain is defined as the normal and predictable physiologic response to an identifiable noxious stimulus, such as surgery, trauma, inflammation, or short-term illness.[1,8] Acute pain results from nociceptor activation at the site of tissue damage and is viewed as adaptive since it attenuates activities that would exacerbate the pain-inducing pathology and/or jeopardize healing.[18] Acute pain is typically self-limiting and resolves over days to weeks, but it can persist for months or longer as healing occurs. It can also be episodic, as in the case of migraine headaches or dysmenorrhea, and is classified "breakthrough" when it manifests during a period of otherwise controlled pain.

Approaches to therapeutic management of acute pain often involve an "analgesic ladder" of drugs known to be effective in nociceptive pain. Peripheral agents such as local anesthetics, NSAIDS, and/or acetaminophen are considered first-line therapy, with central analgesics (opioids) of increasing potency added if pain intensifies or persists.[19] An overview of systematic reviews of the efficacy of nonprescription pain medications in treating acute postoperative pain was published in 2015.[20] Physical pain can be complicated by psychological, emotional, social, cultural, and spiritual elements,[18,19] which reinforces the wisdom of introducing nonpharmacological approaches to pain management, as appropriate.

While often viewed as straightforward and "simpler" than chronic pain, Radnovich et al[18] argue that acute pain is complex, dynamic, and highly variable in its manifestations. There is significant potential for negative patient care outcomes if acute pain is inadequately treated, including longer hospitalizations; compromised cardiac, pulmonary, and immunological functioning; and the risk of progression to chronic pain situations. Therefore, acute pain warrants comprehensive and multidimensional assessments to guide holistic therapy and minimize risk of inadequate management due to patient-provider miscommunications or assumptions.[18,21]

Chronic Pain

Chronic pain persists at least 3 to 6 months after an initiating stimulus has resolved. Chronic pain can be related to degenerative disease such as rheumatoid arthritis, and it can be a lifelong phenomenon. It has been referred to as maladaptive since it has no protective purpose and serves no recognizably useful function.[18] The US Centers for Disease Control and Prevention reported that the prevalence of chronic pain among US adults in 2021 was estimated at 20.9%, or 51.6 million people. Another 6.9% (17.1 million) experienced high-impact chronic pain.[22] It carries a significant public health and economic burden.[3,23]

Chronic pain is commonly caused by mixed pathophysiologic mechanisms (nociceptive, neuropathic, sensory hypersensitivity) with approximately 20% arising from neuropathic origins.[24] While the literature often distinguishes chronic malignant pain from noncancer-related chronic pain due to the complexity of cancer's etiology, pathology, and level of patient care, the underlying physiologic processes may be the same.[3,25]

Chronic pain that is predominantly nociceptive is routinely treated with peripheral and/or central analgesics. As with acute pain, a therapeutic ladder is recommended that initiates pharmacotherapy with peripheral agents (NSAIDs, acetaminophen) and moves to opioids only if/when truly warranted.[3] As noted earlier, chronic pain with a significant neuropathic component is commonly treated with antiepileptic $\alpha 2\delta$ ligands (gabapentin, pregabalin), antidepressants (venlafaxine, imipramine), local anesthetics (lidocaine), or central analgesics (tramadol, tapentadol), but only 40% to 60% of patients may see significant benefits.[24] Surgical or other invasive procedures, such as deep brain stimulation, may be employed if indicated by the etiology and/or if noninvasive pain control strategies prove insufficient. Enzymes that regulate neuronal function and impact glial activation are currently being investigated as potential targets for the development of novel therapies to treat chronic pain.[24,26,27]

In addition to conventional pharmacologic therapies, patients living with chronic pain often seek alternative treatments such as chiropractic adjustments, acupuncture, traditional Chinese medicine, cognitive behavior therapy (eg, relaxation, hypnosis), massage, and, more recently, virtual reality therapy.[28] Chronic pain induces pathophysiologic changes in the central nervous system (CNS) that negatively impact body, mind, and spirit,[29] and it can rob patients of a sense of control over their well-being. Delgado et al[30] suggest that the use of alternative therapies may allow patients to play a proactive and empowering role in their own holistic healing. Stanos et al[3] reinforce the importance of individualized treatment that incorporates nonpharmacologic therapies deemed appropriate after a rigorous physiologic and psychosocial assessment. They also emphasize the importance of an interprofessional team approach (including pharmacists) to the treatment of chronic pain.

Similarly, Peppin et al[31] have commented on the traditionally linear approach to chronic pain therapy that adopts an opioid-focused model of care delivered, in large measure, by primary care physicians (PCPs). They advocate for a nonlinear "complexity model" of personalized collaborative care involving PCPs and pain specialists, who stratify patient care needs after an extensive and multifaceted pain evaluation that includes things such as medical comorbidities, body mass index, history of sleep disorders/head trauma/tobacco use, education/employment status, social support, and risk for medication abuse/diversion.

Opioid Analgesics and Antagonists

"Oh! just, subtle, and mighty opium! That to the hearts of poor and rich alike, for the wounds that will never heal, and for 'the pangs that tempt the spirit to rebel,' bringest an assuaging balm"

Thomas de Quincey, Confessions of an English Opium Eater

The juice (*opium* in Greek) or latex from the unripe seed pods of the poppy *Papaver somniferum* is among the oldest recorded medication used by humans and may have been used as a tonic as early as 3500 BC. In 1803, the German pharmacist Friedrich Surtürner isolated an alkaloid from opium he named morphine, after Morpheus, the Greek god of dreams. Later, other valuable alkaloids were isolated from opium, namely codeine and thebaine. Collectively, these three compounds are considered *opiates* because they are alkaloids isolated from opium. As will be discussed, all other related synthetic and semisynthetic analgesics are called *opioids*. The discovery of morphine revolutionized pain management and greatly altered the course of human history, being the subject of geopolitical battles (the "Opium wars" and the ongoing Opioid Public Health Crisis in the United States).[32] Morphine is considered the "gold standard" treatment for chronic, severe pain and has been used to characterize the endogenous opioid neurotransmitter system, which is a target for analgesics, alcohol deterrents, and antidiarrheals. For all of these reasons, discovery by Sertürner was invaluable to modern medicine.

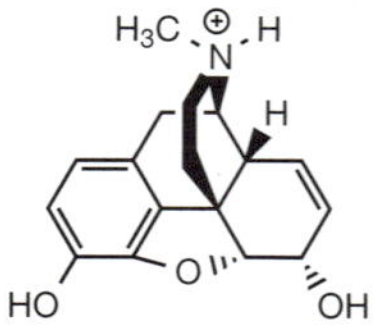

Morphine

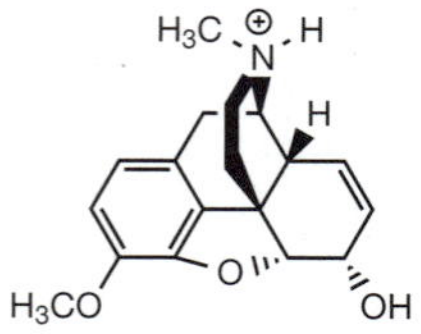

Codeine

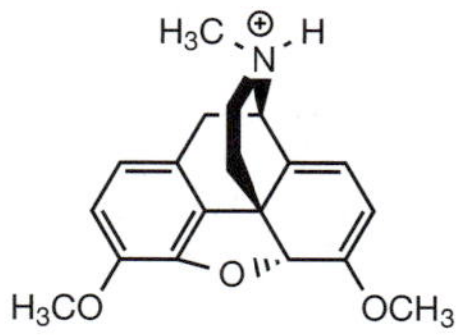

Thebaine

Opioid Receptors

The primary targets of morphine and related opioids are opioid receptors. There are three types of opioid peptide receptors, namely μ (mu, μOP, MOP), κ (kappa, κOP, KOP), and δ (delta, δOP, DOP). All of these are class A G-protein–coupled receptors (GPCRs), and each produces unique pharmacologic responses when agonized. These are summarized in Table 16.1. The strongest analgesic effects of opioids are mediated through activation of μ and κ receptors. The psychiatric adverse effect profile of μ and κ agonists differ: whereas μ receptor agonists cause rewarding euphoric effects, κ receptor agonists cause dysphoria and hallucinations. Although δ receptor agonism also produces analgesic effects, it is widely accepted that the magnitude of pain control is lower for δ receptor agonism as compared to μ and κ receptor activation. Agonists of δ receptors also have therapeutic potential as antidepressants. Early research supported the hypothesis that δ receptor agonism results in a pro-convulsant effect; however, subsequent investigation reveals not all δ receptor ligands produce convulsions; thus, certain δ receptor agonists may be viable therapeutic leads.[33]

Centrally, μ receptors are found in abundance in the arcuate nucleus, periaqueductal gray, and thalamic areas of the brain, while κ receptor density is highest in the dorsal horn and substantia gelatinosa of the spinal cord. The δ receptors are expressed in highest levels in the basal ganglia and neocortical regions in the brain and in the superficial dorsal horn of the spinal cord.[33]

Table 16.1 Effects of Opioid Agonists

μ Agonists	κ Agonists	δ Agonists
Analgesia	Analgesia	Analgesia (weaker than μ or κ)
Sedation	Sedation	Mood-elevating/ antidepressant
Nausea and vomiting	Dysphoria	Anxiolytic
Constipation[a]	Diuresis	Convulsions
Miosis[a]	Increase in cardiac workload (excluding nalbuphine)	
Respiratory depression	Respiratory depression	
Euphoria		
Tolerance and dependence		

[a]No tolerance to these adverse reactions.

Opioid receptors are also found in the periphery. Activation of μ opioid receptors expressed in the gastrointestinal (GI) tract results in decreased intestinal motility. This is the mechanism by which many μ agonist–based analgesics cause opioid-induced constipation (OIC) during opioid pain management. The presence of κ receptors in cardiac tissue is a likely mechanism by which κ agonists can induce cardiopulmonary toxicity.[34] Opioids acting at peripheral κ receptors may have value in attenuating inflammatory visceral pain.[35] Antagonism of δ opioid receptors in the intestine attenuates the slowed GI effects of μ agonists and blocks the development of constipation.

Opioid receptors signal through various intracellular signaling pathways. Opioid receptors are coupled to inhibitory $G_{i/o}$ proteins (see Chapter 6, G Protein–Coupled Receptors) and mediate analgesia through the activation of adenosine triphosphate (ATP)-gated K^+ channels and the inhibition of voltage-gated Ca^{2+} channels, leading to decreases in intracellular Ca^{2+} and cyclic adenosine monophosphate (cAMP).[36] A second key protein is the regulatory protein β-arrestin2 (β-arr2). Certain agonists cause a conformational change in the receptor that allows phosphorylation at Ser375, which recruits β-arr2. When β-arr2 binds to the μ receptor, it uncouples the G protein from the receptor and initiates receptor internalization. Both steps result in a termination of agonist response. Not all μ agonists are capable of recruiting β-arr2. Those that only stimulate G-protein–mediated signaling events and do not recruit β-arr2 are termed *biased agonists* and may produce therapeutic benefits with limited adverse effects like constipation[37]; however, the biased agonists produced to date still have significant liabilities (nausea, tolerance, dependence), meaning their benefits over other μ agonists are still limited.

Of potential clinical interest is the fact that individuals with the single-nucleotide polymorphism (SNP) A118G in the gene coding for the μ receptor have reduced expression of this protein and, as a result, higher μ agonist dosing requirements. While this has been claimed to be of questionable importance in the general population, many Asian populations carry this modified gene with a frequency significantly higher than that of Whites (40%-50% vs 10%). Some hypothesize the A118G SNP to be the biggest contributing factor to the attenuated response to opioids observed in some patients of Asian ancestry.[38]

Endogenous Opioid Peptides

The three opioid receptors are activated by endogenous peptides, collectively termed *endorphins*, which is a portmanteau of "endogenous morphine." Examples of endorphins are Met- and Leu-enkephalin, β-endorphin, endomorphin-1 and -2, and dynorphin.[39] The endogenous opioid peptides are agonists of their respective opioid receptor types. β-Endorphin is the peptide with the highest affinity for μ receptors, dynorphin for κ receptors, and the enkephalins for δ receptors. β-Endorphin and the enkephalins are considered nonselective agonists of μ and δ receptors.

All opioid peptides share the same N-terminal sequence: Tyr-Gly-Gly-Phe. The protonated amine, aromatic ring, and phenolic hydroxyl group of the Tyr residue, along with the aromatic ring of the Phe moiety, are important in holding these peptides to opioid receptors. The Tyr residue is also found in the structure of morphine, signifying that the two classes share a molecular mechanism of action of binding opioid receptors. Other parts of larger peptides can confer target selectivity. Dynorphin contains two basic Arg residues at positions 6 and 7 that are believed to interact with weakly acidic regions of the κ receptor.

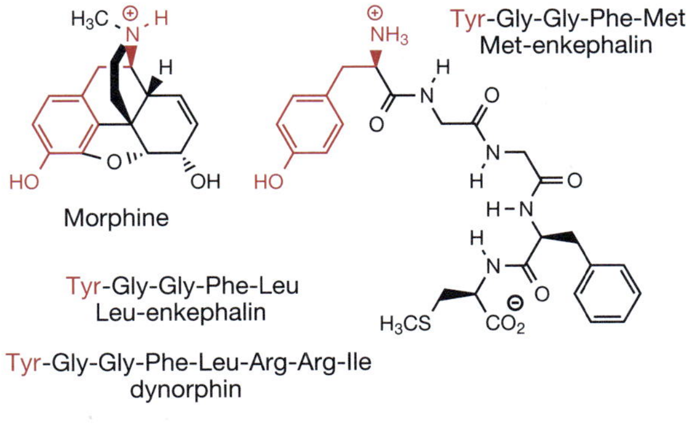

Tolerance and Dependence

Tolerance is the phenomenon where increasingly larger doses of drug are required to produce the same degree of biologic response that had previously been obtained with a lower dose. There are several ways that tolerance to opioid analgesia can occur. As discussed earlier, receptor desensitization can occur if G proteins are unable to bind μ receptors due to β-arr2 or if their downstream effector pathways are uncoupled. As noted earlier, β-arr2 can also promote receptor internalization in some cases, and receptor downregulation can also occur. Other global mechanisms of tolerance have also been explored, including an increase in opioid metabolism or an increase in active efflux from target cells. These are both areas of ongoing research.

Dependence is distinct from tolerance. Physiologic dependence occurs when withdrawal symptoms are experienced when drug use is abruptly ceased. Examples of symptoms associated with opioid withdrawal include nausea and vomiting, hallucinations, and diarrhea. Dependence can occur as a result of compensatory upregulation of adenylyl cyclase (AC), a downstream effector target of $G\alpha_{i/o}$. Prolonged inhibition of AC causes neurons to increase the expression of the enzyme. When the agonist used on a chronic basis is suddenly withdrawn, the inhibition of AC abruptly stops, and all enzymes begin producing cAMP. The significantly elevated cAMP concentrations are believed to be responsible for the physiologic symptoms of opioid withdrawal.

Opioid Addiction

Although frequently used as a synonym for dependence, addiction is a distinct phenomenon that must be addressed differently. Addiction is defined by the National Institute on Drug Abuse as a "chronic, relapsing disorder characterized by compulsive drug seeking and use despite adverse consequences."[40] This is different from dependence. A patient can be physiologically dependent on a medication without being addicted. An important distinction is that addiction has a strong psychosocial and genetic component, leading to drug-craving and drug-seeking behavior in the absence of pain, destructive behavior patterns, and compulsive use in the face of negative mental and/or social consequences. The risk of addiction in patients with chronic pain on opioids has been estimated at 3.3%, with genetic predisposition possibly accounting for 40% to 60% of that risk,[41] but some claim that data corresponding to addiction risk in patients with chronic pain are inconsistent.[42]

Prescription opioids are a major source of the drugs misused, abused, and diverted in the United States.[43] More than 259 million opioid prescriptions were written in 2012, representing a significant increase from 1999. Although opioid prescribing rates have since declined due to intense professional attention to the connection between prescribing practices and the ongoing opioid epidemic, a recent publication[44] cited a 2017 article stating that the opioid prescribing rate remained higher in the United States than in other high-income countries. Additionally, a 2013 study claimed that approximately one-quarter of patients prescribed opioids engaged in misuse/abuse. Similarly, a 2020 multicenter study of postsurgical opioid prescribing found that, compared to their international counterparts, US physicians: (1) prescribed an "alarmingly large amount" of opioids, (2) exhibited a wider variation in prescribing patterns, and (3) authorized more opioid prescription refills despite refills seldom being required.[45] Given this, it might not be surprising that 92% of pain patients are prescribed more opioids than required to manage their postoperative pain, and 77% admitted to not storing or disposing of surplus opioids appropriately, leaving the diversion door wide open.[45] The economic burden of opioid abuse and misuse, born extensively by payers, has been documented by many.[13,42,46,48]

In 2016, the National Safety Council determined that 80% of those abusing heroin started their addiction journey with prescription opioids.[49] A 2017 study found that opioid overdose claimed approximately one US life every 36 minutes,[50] and, 1 year later, that estimate had increased to 115 lives per day.[44] Zhou et al[51] noted that the rise in opioid-induced mortality coincidentally corresponded with the increase in opioid prescribing secondary to more relaxed views on the use of opioids to treat chronic nonmalignant pain, along with widespread marketing efforts by opioid manufacturers. In response, some states have enacted legislation to limit the number of opioids, the length of initial treatment, and/or the doses physicians can prescribe. In early 2018, the makers of controlled-release OxyContin, an oxycodone product with a high misuse/abuse potential, voluntarily cut their sales force by more than half and halted the active marketing of the analgesic to physicians.

Changes to federal prescribing guidelines have also positively impacted the opioid crisis in the United States. In 2016, the US Centers for Disease Control and Prevention (CDC) issued new evidence-based guidelines for prescribing opioids for chronic pain. Included among these changes were recommendations to increase communications between prescribers and patients to discuss the risks and benefits of opioid therapy. To measure the effectiveness of these changes, a 2023 report used dispensing data from the Xponent database (IQVIA) to monitor rates of opioid prescribing among US states. The authors found that rates of opioid prescribing went down between 2012 and 2018 and that these prescribing/dispensing decreases accelerated following the new 2016 CDC guidelines.[52]

Overdose deaths from prescription opioids have leveled off since 2011, as deaths from fatal administrations of heroin and illicitly produced fentanyl and its more potent analogs (eg, carfentanil) have risen.[53] The number of opioid overdose deaths quadrupled between 1999 and 2013[51] and continues to escalate: more than 100,000 drug-involved overdose deaths occurred in 2021, including 70,601 overdose deaths involving synthetic opioids other than methadone.[54] For context, this is up from less than 10,000 in 2015. The reasons behind the massive increase in fentanyl-related overdose deaths are multifaceted and complex. Beyond the high potency and unique adverse effect profile that will be discussed later, fentanyl is relatively simple to synthesize in clandestine laboratories using commercially available starting materials. As an extension, fentanyl analogs, termed *fentanyl-related substances* (*FRS*), are also easily made and can avoid detection by law enforcement.[55] Many FRS have not been rigorously tested for safety or efficacy, and users of these substances put themselves and others at great risk of overdose or unintended toxicity. In response to the proliferation of FRS, the US Drug Enforcement Administration (DEA) enacted a class-wide ban on FRS in 2018 by temporarily placing them on the Schedule I controlled substances list. While helpful from a prosecutorial perspective, this move is controversial, as it limits the ability for many scholars to conduct research with FRS.[56]

Some states are now making the rapid-acting opioid antagonist naloxone (autoinjector and nasal spray) available to law enforcement, librarians, high school staff, and/or family and caregivers of addicted individuals. Naloxone administered by intramuscular (IM), subcutaneous, or intranasal routes reverses life-threatening overdose within minutes. Pharmacists have a vital role to play in educating these first responders and the public at large on the safe and effective use of this life-saving drug.

The US opioid epidemic was officially declared a national public health emergency in October 2017, which stopped short of the national emergency status that would have deployed additional federal resources to combat it. Those interested in reading more about the national approach to the US opioid crisis are directed to the references cited.[57-60]

Euphoria and Dysphoria

The ability of μ agonists to induce profound euphoria is well known. The agonist-induced decrease in cAMP inhibits the release of the inhibitory neurotransmitter γ-aminobutyric acid (GABA) from the ventral tegmental area, which is upstream of the nucleus accumbens. The nucleus accumbens is the brain's self-reward or pleasure center and is activated by dopamine. GABA normally inhibits dopamine release from this cerebral "candy land," so the decrease in GABA levels induced by μ-receptor stimulation enhances dopamine release from these terminals. The subsequent elevation in dopamine receptor stimulation in the nucleus accumbens is perceived as a feeling of intense well-being or euphoria. Euphoria is the psychological driver behind opioid addiction.

In contrast, κ agonists have the potential to induce dysphoria, a feeling of intense discomfort. Stimulation of κ receptors in the nucleus accumbens results in a direct inhibitory effect on presynaptic dopaminergic neurons, resulting in a decrease in dopamine and an attenuation of pleasure-related responses that translates as dysphoria.

Clinical Use

Opioid analgesics are the therapeutic mainstay in the treatment of moderate to severe pain, and there is no question that they are effective.

A study published in 2017 examined beliefs and attitudes on opioid analgesic use among a small sample of PCPs in the United States (high use) and Japan (low use) and found that differences in health systems, regulations, provider education, and cultural mindsets likely impacted the 26-fold prescribing difference for six high-potency opioids.[50] The drive to alleviate suffering and to secure patient satisfaction with their care plan impacted opioid prescribing patterns in both physician cohorts. A more robust retrospective study of 377,345 Medicare patients treated in (and discharged from) US emergency rooms between 2008 and 2011 identified a wide variability in opioid prescribing patterns among emergency care physicians, with patients treated by "high-intensity prescribers" significantly more likely to remain on long-term opioid therapy.[61] A 2017 retrospective study of opioid use in US pediatric care settings over the course of 1 year found that 43.5% of more than 8,000 inpatients 18 years or younger were prescribed an opioid, and that 75% of these were treated for less than 5 days (ie, acute therapy).[62] Cancer, followed by cardiac disorders, was the most common diagnosis in pediatric patients receiving opioids for longer than 1 month.

The relationship between legitimate chronic opioid use and abuse is a significant public health concern. Using a system dynamics approach, Schmidt et al[63] identified 12 data gaps that must be bridged to better understand the use and potential misuse of prescribed opioids, including incidence/diagnosis rate/opioid use in treating nonmalignant chronic pain, the fraction of opioid prescriptions diverted for nonmedical use, and the "thwart rate" of prescription forgery and "doctor shopping" to secure multiple prescriptions for opioids of choice. Recommendations for expanding current data collection efforts to address these knowledge gaps were provided. In 2016, Kattan et al[64] described the positive impact of an opioid public health detailing initiative to health care providers in Staten Island, NY, based on the knowledge of sound opioid prescribing practices and prescribing rate. They recommended their successful approach be expanded to other communities and jurisdictions. Given that people who are opioid-dependent can also experience painful illnesses or surgical interventions requiring potent analgesia, Raub and Vettese[65] offered an evidence-based review and clinician's guide on the use of opioids in this patient population.

Clearly, while the aforementioned studies advocated for the reality-based and evidence-focused education of providers and patients alike on the risks and benefits of opioid use, there is a continuing need for a scientific approach to the use of these powerful molecules—one that mitigates risk while allowing patients in significant pain access to provider-monitored pharmacotherapy that can give them a better quality of life. The importance of a collaborative patient-provider partnership in assuring the appropriate use of opioid analgesics cannot be overstated.

Opioid Chemistry

When making a clinical decision over which opioid ligand is appropriate for a patient, one needs to know: (1) the receptors that are targeted by the drug; (2) the location of the receptors; and (3) whether the drug is an agonist or antagonist. Once this is known, it is critical to understand whether the drug is active when administered or bioactivated into an active metabolite. As will be seen, some opioids are prodrugs that are activated by metabolism, others are inactivated by metabolism, and some change their pharmacodynamic profile once metabolized.

Opioid Receptor Binding and the "Opioid Pharmacophore"

It was initially understood that all opioid receptor ligands contained a consensus "opioid pharmacophore" that was required for tight binding to the μ opioid receptor. This consensus was built through rigorous investigation of the structure-activity relationships (SARs) of morphine. The opioid pharmacophore consists of a tertiary, basic amine, a two to three carbon–linking group, and an aromatic ring that contains a phenol group. As discussed earlier, this pharmacophore essentially mimics the terminal Tyr residue that is present in all endogenous opioid peptides. Thus, opioid receptor ligands that share this pharmacophore bind in a similar manner as the endogenous neurotransmitters. However, not all opioid receptor ligands contain this pharmacophore or follow the same SAR rules. For example, fentanyl and meperidine do not contain a phenol group, and their aromatic rings do not occupy the same chemical space (Fig. 16.1). Furthermore, the requirement for a basic amine is also challenged by the finding that the nonnitrogenous neoclerodane diterpenes, salvinorin A, and herkinorin are potent κ and μ agonists, respectively.[66] This means that different structural classes bind to opioid receptors via different molecular interactions, and thus there is not a single pharmacophore that unites all opioid receptor ligands.

Three-dimensional structures of ligand-bound μ, κ, and δ receptors have been solved based on x-ray crystallography and cyro-EM electron microscopy. These structures can be observed online at the Protein DataBank (rcsb.org). The commercially available μ opioid receptor agonists and antagonists all contain weakly basic amine groups that are protonated at physiologic pH. These basic amines engage in an ionic bonding interaction with a conserved Asp147 that is located near the top of transmembrane helix 3 (TMH3). The opioids that contain the opioid pharmacophore are further "anchored" by an adjacent Tyr148 that participates

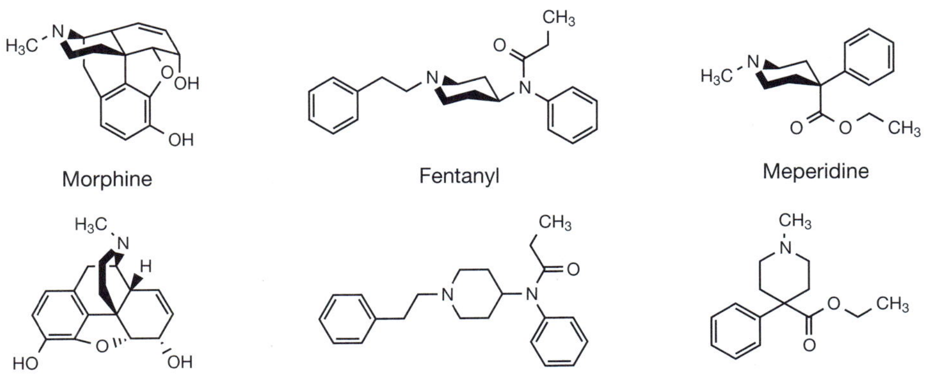

Figure 16.1 Structures of μ opioid–receptor ligands drawn from the side (top) and in a typical "flat" view. These opioid receptor ligands share a central piperidine core function.

in a hydrogen bond with the 4,5-epoxy group oxygen. The phenol is then positioned to form a hydrogen bond with Lys233. This binding is facilitated by a water molecule. The weakly basic μ ligands that do not contain the opioid pharmacophore also engage with Asp147 but form distinct interactions with other active site residues. For example, Tyr326 stabilizes fentanyl binding by forming a π-stacking interaction with the anilido aryl group. Maps of ligand-receptor binding can be found in Figure 16.2.

Opioid Structure-Activity Relationships and the "Message-Address Concept"

The natural opiates morphine and codeine are members of a phenanthrene-type pentacyclic scaffold. Members of this class are most properly called 4,5-epoxymorphinans, though they can also be generally referred to as morphine analogs. During the course of determining SARs of 4,5-epoxymorphinans, the rings A through E (Fig. 16.3) were systematically removed to determine whether each was strictly necessary for activity. Many of the resulting scaffolds retained affinity for opioid receptors and became new structural classes. For example, removal of ring E resulted in a new class called morphinans, and removal of ring C resulted in benzomorphans. Certain structures that retain only piperidine ring D are active as opioid receptor ligands, and in certain cases, removing all scaffolding rings results in fully flexible ligands. Finally, rings can be added to the 4,5-epoxymorphinan scaffold. The orvinols are an important example of 4,5-epoxymorphinans that has an additional ring. Each of these structural classes has its own SAR; the SAR for 4,5-epoxymorphinans often overlap with other structural classes, though sometimes they can differ substantially.

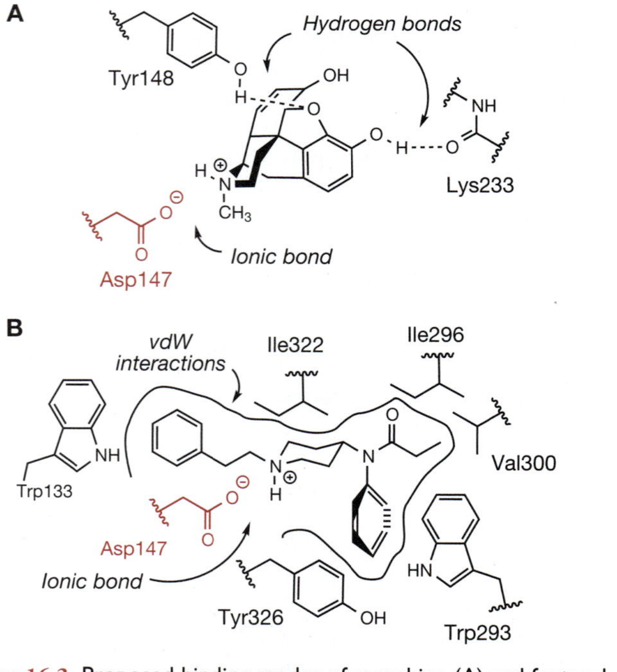

Figure 16.2 Proposed binding modes of morphine (A) and fentanyl (B) at the μ opioid receptor. Ionic bonds and hydrogen bonds are highlighted for morphine, and van der Waals (vdW) interactions are shown for fentanyl.

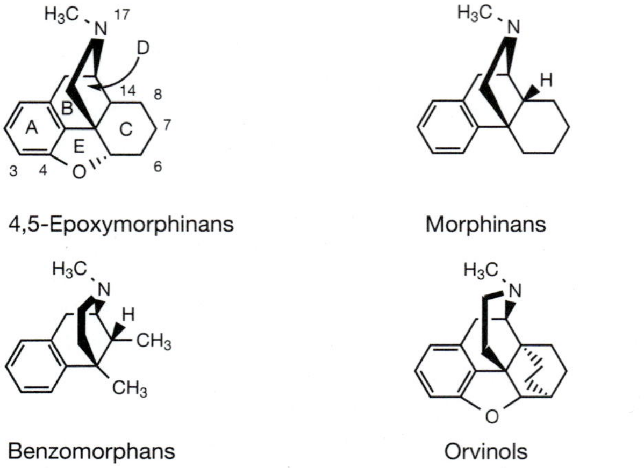

Figure 16.3 Skeletons of the phenanthrene-based rigid opioid classes. The ring system designations (A-E) and key carbon numbers are shown.

One approach that has been used to rationalize 4,5-epoxymorphinan SAR is called the *"message-address concept."* This concept, which was first applied to opioid SARs by Portoghese,[67] proposes that there are some regions of a molecular structure that strongly influence receptor binding affinity and selectivity (the "address") and others that have a greater impact on efficacy upon binding those receptors (the "message"). As will be discussed in the next section, the rigid 4,5-epoxymorphinan core imparts a high level of selectivity for opioid receptors over other neurotransmitter receptors (the "address"); the N-substituent largely governs whether a ligand will be an agonist or antagonist when it binds those receptors (the "message").

4,5-Epoxymorphinans. The 4,5-epoxymorphinan core is a pentacyclic structure with at least four contiguous stereocenters. The rings are commonly designated by letters A to E, and each position in the scaffold carries a number (see Fig. 16.3). Naturally occurring levorotatory (−)-morphine has the 5*R*,6*S*,9*R*,13*S*,14*R* absolute configuration, which is the most active isomeric form at μ opioid receptors. The dextrorotary enantiomer, (+)-morphine, has negligible affinity for opioid receptors, yet certain (+)-4,5-epoxymorphinans have activity at non-opioid targets. Rings B and C are connected via a *cis*-ring fusion, giving the 4,5-epoxymorphinan structure a distinct T shape. This can be observed in the "side-view" orientation that is shown in Figure 16.1. This view also shows that ring A occupies an axial orientation relative to piperidine ring D. This locks ring A into an orientation relative to the basic amine that perfectly overlaps with the N-terminal Tyr of the endorphins. The phenol acts as a hydrogen-bond donor (HBD) with the active site. A recent cryo-EM structure suggests that the hydrogen-donating phenol points toward the backbone carbonyl of Lys233, which serves as the hydrogen-bond acceptor (HBA).[68] This interaction is conserved with the endorphin N-terminal Tyr, which also has a phenol.

Though medicinal chemists have thoroughly investigated the entire 4,5-epoxymorphinan scaffold, only modifications to carbon positions 3, 6, 14, and N-17 contribute substantially to activity in opioid receptor ligands approved by the

US Food and Drug Administration (FDA). Certain modifications to ring C can also influence opioid receptor binding and will be discussed briefly. In general, modifications to the carbon positions influence opioid receptor binding (the "address"), and modifications to the basic amine group influence efficacy (the "message"). Structures of clinically used 4,5-epoxymorphinans are shown in Figure 16.4.

Structure-Activity Relationship of Ring A: Position 3. Modifications to position 3 most strongly influence opioid receptor binding affinity. Highest affinity ligands will have a hydrogen bond–donating group at this position to form the critical H-bond, with the H-accepting Lys233. In most cases, this will be a phenolic hydroxyl group; however, carboxamide groups are also tolerated here. Removing this hydrogen bond–donating group will lower affinity. Functional groups that can be metabolized to reveal a phenol are considered prodrugs. For example, codeine, the 3-O-methyl ether derivative of morphine, has a much lower μ opioid receptor affinity as compared to morphine. Phase I-mediated O-demethylation converts codeine into morphine, which has much higher affinity. Similarly, heroin contains a 3-O-acetate that is rapidly metabolized by esterases to reveal the more active phenol. Phenols are frequent targets of Phase II conjugation reactions, including glucuronidation and sulfonation. Glucuronide conjugation requires UDP-glucuronosyltransferase (UGT) enzymes. Conjugation at position 3 results in inactive metabolites. Phenols also undergo in vitro oxidation to therapeutically inactive quinones. Phenolic drugs, including active opioids, should always be protected from light, base, and oxygen in the air or, over time, they can decompose. Removing the 3-substituent entirely has a strongly negative impact on opioid receptor binding.

Structure-Activity Relationship of Ring C: Positions 6, 7 and 8, and 14. Position 6 can be modified in ways that influence opioid receptor binding affinity ("address"). The naturally occurring opiates, morphine and codeine, have a α-hydroxyl group at position 6. This group does not contribute substantially to target binding; however, structural modifications at this position enhance the overall lipophilicity of the compound and improve potency. In most FDA-approved opioids, this is achieved by oxidation to a ketone. Hydromorphone and hydrocodone are two examples of 6-keto-substituted 4,5-epoxymorphinans. Oxidation in this way removes a hydrogen bond–donating group and makes the molecule less polar. Other ways to reduce hydrogen bonding potential include making alkyl ethers or esters. Heroin, which has a 6-O-acetate group, is a relevant example here, too. Removing all substitutions entirely results in desomorphine, a high-potency recreational product that has substantial abuse liability. Desomorphine is also known as "krokodil" in Russia for its potential to cause injection site skin necrosis that resembles the scaly skin of a crocodile.

The 6α-OH group of morphine and codeine is associated with mast cell degranulation and histamine release, which can lead to an allergic-like response involving hypotension, intense pruritus, and rash.[69] The mechanism involves activation of protein kinase A and inositol triphosphate kinase, which not only releases histamine but also stimulates the production of proinflammatory chemokines in mast cells.[70] Pruritus induced via this mechanism is not reversed by opioid antagonists.[70,71] A μ receptor–linked pruritus mechanism, which can be reversed with low-dose antagonists, has also been proposed. The pruritus associated with opioids increases significantly with intravenous (IV) and/or epidural administration. This adverse effect is particularly intense

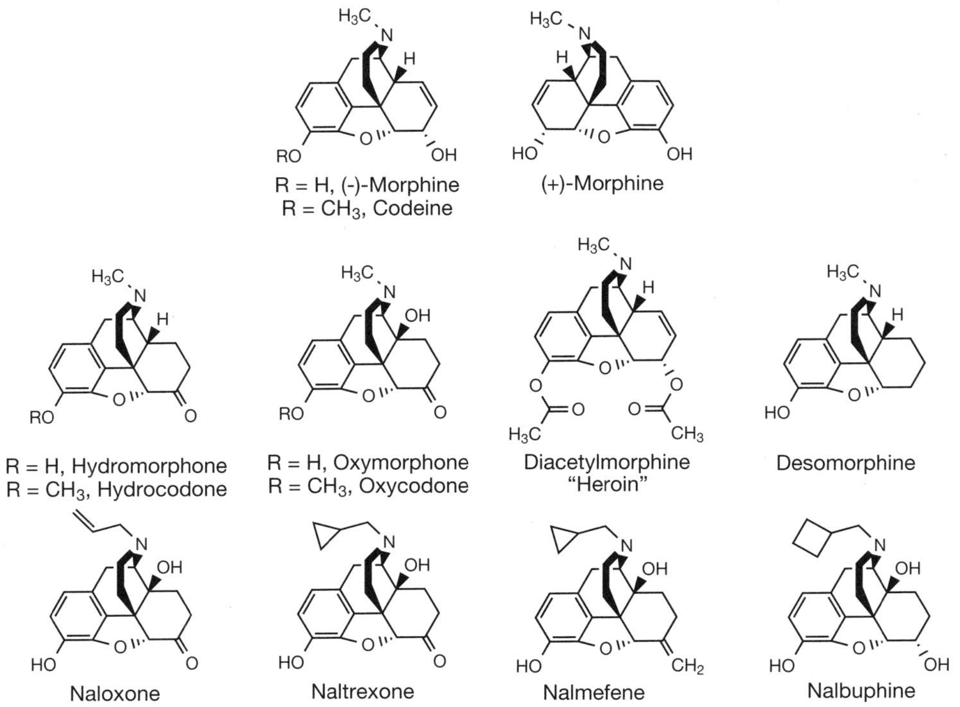

Figure 16.4 Rigid 4,5-epoxymorphinan–based opioid receptor agonists and antagonists.

with codeine, and as a result, parenteral administration of this analgesic is generally not recommended. Pruritus and hypotension are not generally observed with 6-keto or 6-desoxy opioids,[71,72] and the risk of nausea may also be lowered. The κ agonists that have μ antagonist action do not induce pruritus.[71]

Positions 7 and 8 in the natural opiates are connected by a double bond, which makes ring C occupy a "pseudo-boat" conformation. Reduction of this olefin causes a modest increase in opioid activity, again through making ring C more lipophilic. The 6,7-olefin is most often reduced in this way when the 6-position is oxidized into a ketone: a double bond next to a ketone (known as an α,β-unsaturated ketone) can act as a Michael acceptor (electrophile) and cause nonspecific toxicities secondary to alkylation of cell nucleophiles. Adding rigid aromatic groups to position 7 is an approach to introducing affinity and selectivity for δ opioid receptors: the 6,7-fused indole, naltrindole, is a δ-selective antagonist that is used in research.

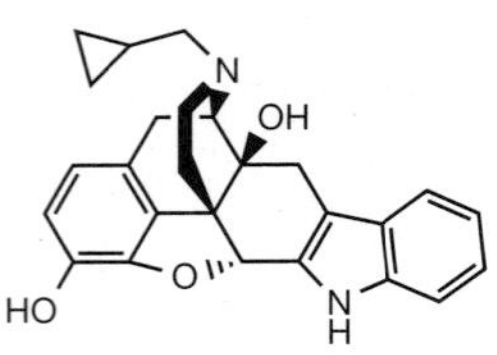

Naltrindole

Position 14 typically contains either a β-H or β-hydroxyl group. Though this amounts to a modification that adds a polar functional group, which would be expected to reduce potency, hydroxylation here generally increases potency. One potential explanation for this is that the OH group forms an additional hydrogen bonding interaction with the receptor. Another explanation could be that this OH group engages in either an intramolecular ion-dipole bond with the protonated basic amine N-17 or a hydrogen bond with the 6-ketone (14 β-OH as a hydrogen bond-donor). Examples of 14-hydroxylated 4,5-epoxymorphinans include oxymorphone and oxycodone.

Structure-Activity Relationship of Ring D: Position N-17. A basic amine is an essential feature of all 4,5-epoxymorphinan opioids because, in its cationic conjugate acid form, it forms an essential electrostatic bond with an Asp residue conserved in TMH3. The N-17 substituent plays a key role in the "message" of 4,5-epoxymorphinans and generally dictates whether the efficacy at μ-opioid receptors will be high or low. The "agonist message" group here is most frequently methyl, but *N*-phenethyl groups can also be μ agonists. No *N*-phenethyl-4,5-epoxymorphinans are marketed currently.

The "antagonist message" is seen with *N*-allyl and *N*-cyclopropylmethyl groups, such as those seen in naloxone and naltrexone, respectively. The allyl double bond and cyclopropyl ring are electron-rich compared to methyl, and both occupy a narrow, primarily hydrophobic cleft formed between the side chains of Asp, Met, Tyr, Ile, and Gly residues.[73] Tyr326 and Trp293 have also been suggested as antagonist substituent-binding residues.[74] Some authors caution that ligand-induced conformational changes in receptor proteins can obscure or otherwise complicate the binding specifics.[75] Another *N*-cyclopropylmethyl μ receptor antagonist of note is nalmefene. Nalmefene differs from naltrexone in that the 6-position ketone is replaced by a methylene. Though these groups occupy similar chemical space, this small change significantly impacts opioid receptor pharmacodynamics: nalmefene is a bifunctional μ antagonist/κ partial agonist. It is not known why this modification influences activity at κ receptors. If the ring strain of the cyclopropylmethyl group is eased to a cyclobutylmethyl group, κ agonism (analgesia) becomes the therapeutically predominant action. A relevant example is nalbuphine. Nalbuphine is a mixed low-efficacy μ partial agonist/high-efficacy κ partial agonist.

Morphinans and Benzomorphans. Morphinans are related to the 4,5-epoxymorphinans in that they contain rings A through D, but are missing the 4,5-ether bridge that creates ring E (Fig. 16.5). Many of the SARs that describe 4,5-epoxymorphinan activity also hold for the morphinans. For example, the tyrosine portion of the opioid pharmacophore–basic amine, 2 carbon linker, phenol–must be present for morphinans to be active as opioids. The SAR of the 3-position phenol holds as well: phenols here have the highest opioid receptor affinity, and methyl ethers are modestly lower affinity prodrugs. The stereochemical requirements hold as well: the levorotary (−)-enantiomers bind opioid receptors and the dextrorotary (+)-enantiomers do not. Notable examples here are levomethorphan (μ agonist, analgesic) and dextromethorphan (NMDA receptor antagonist, antitussive). N-substituent SARs

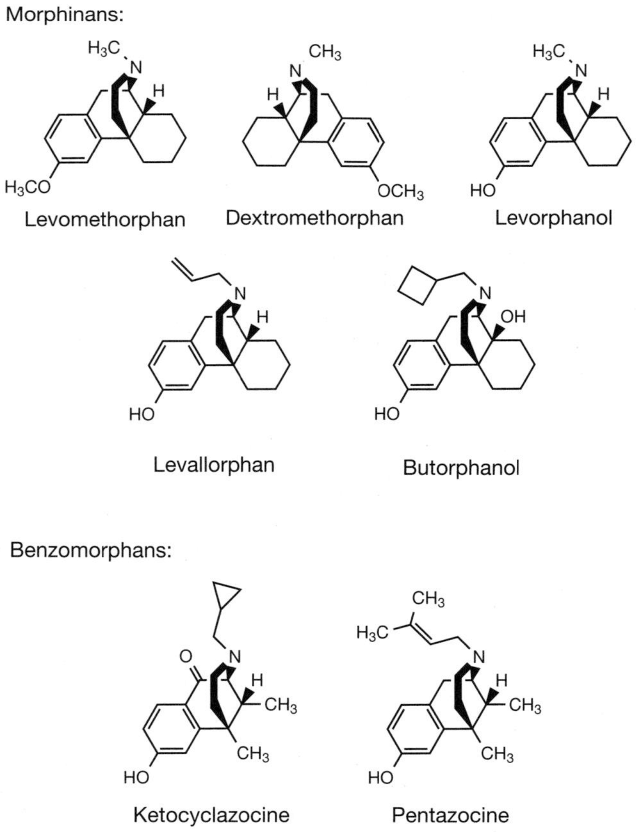

Figure 16.5 Morphinans and benzomorphans.

also hold at μ-opioid receptors: N-methyl substitution results in agonists (eg, levorphanol, a clinically available analgesic), while N-allyl and N-cyclopropylmethyl groups reduce efficacy at μ receptors. A key divergence point is seen at κ receptors. These electron-rich groups typically maintain high-efficacy κ agonism, resulting in "mixed-efficacy" κ-agonist/μ-antagonist analgesics and anesthetics. As κ agonists, morphinans are expected to cause hallucinations and dysphoria, and thus they are not widely used. For example, the *N*-methyl morphinan, levorphanol, is a mixed agonist at μ and κ receptors, and the *N*-allyl derivative levallorphan is a μ antagonist and κ agonist. Both levorphanol and levallorphan, due to κ agonism, have the potential to cause hallucinations.

There are only a few benzomorphans in clinical use, though their persistence as drugs of abuse merits discussion. Lacking rings C and E, the benzomorphans contain the "opioid pharmacophore" and thus are likely to bind opioid receptors in a similar way as the endorphins. As a class, the benzomorphans have highest affinity for κ receptors over μ and δ receptors. As κ agonist–based analgesics, the benzomorphans are capable of producing strong analgesia with limited respiratory depression and potential to cause reward; however, hallucinations and dysphoria are significant adverse effects. Notable examples of benzomorphans include ketocyclazocine (ketazocine) and pentazocine. Pentazocine, in combination with the opioid antagonist naloxone, is the only benzomorphan left on the US market. Ketocyclazocine is notable because it was used to characterize the κ receptor and, thus, this receptor was given the Greek letter κ.

Orvinols. The orvinols, as a therapeutic class, were discovered serendipitously in the laboratories of Bentley and Hardy (Fig. 16.6). As an exercise in basic organic chemistry, the C ring of thebaine contains an electron-rich diene system; such systems are poised to react well with electron-poor dienophiles under conditions that would promote a Diels-Alder–type cyclization. Reacting thebaine with methyl vinyl ketone results in thevinone, a product that itself has weak opioid receptor binding. The ketone group of thevinone is primed to react with alkyl magnesium bromides under Grignard conditions to give tertiary alcohols. The resulting orvinols are among the most potent opioid receptor ligands discovered to date. The discovery that orvinols are therapeutically valuable was a completely serendipitous finding.

Like all opioids discussed thus far, the orvinols contain the "opioid pharmacophore" and are thought to bind opioid receptors in the same way as endorphins. Unlike the 4,5-epoxymorphinans, the orvinols possess an additional ring system that occupies an allosteric region of opioid receptors. Being able to form additional contacts with opioid receptors is one hypothesis as to why orvinols are so potent. Another factor influencing potency is lipophilicity. Etorphine (logP 3.29) and buprenorphine (logP 4.53) are both substantially more lipophilic than morphine (logP 0.99) and thus are more likely to be centrally bioavailable.

Minor differences exist between the SAR of orvinols and 4,5-epoxymorphinans. Notably, the N-substituent does not control efficacy as neatly as seen with 4,5-epoxymorphinans. For example, the *N*-methyl-substituted etorphine is a μ-/κ-/δ-receptor agonist; however, buprenorphine (*N*-cyclopropylmethyl) is a mixed-efficacy μ partial agonist/κ and δ antagonist.

Flexible Opioids: Anilidopiperidines. The anilidopiperidine analgesics, commonly known as the fentanyls, are the only class of flexible opioids with more than two members (Fig. 16.7). The crystal structure of fentanyl has confirmed a chair conformation of the piperidine ring and the equatorial conformation of the 4-phenylpropanamide moiety.[73] In that conformation, the phenyl ring may interact with the μ receptor residue that normally binds Phe4 of enkephalin, and no phenolic OH group is incorporated into their structures. The anilidopiperidine opioids bind opioid receptors via different binding modes and, thus, they do not share the same pharmacophore and SAR as the rigid 4,5-epoxymorphinans. Anilidopiperidine opioids are highly lipophilic molecules that distribute rapidly across the blood-brain barrier (BBB), resulting in a fast and potent, albeit short-lived, analgesic response.[76] As discussed earlier, the emergence of FRS has confounded law enforcement in the United States. Understanding the SAR of 4-anilidopiperidines is critical to stopping the proliferation of these dangerous drugs.

Structure-Activity Relationship of the N-Substituent. There are similarities and differences between SARs of anilidopiperidines and 4,5-epoxymorphinans. First, while

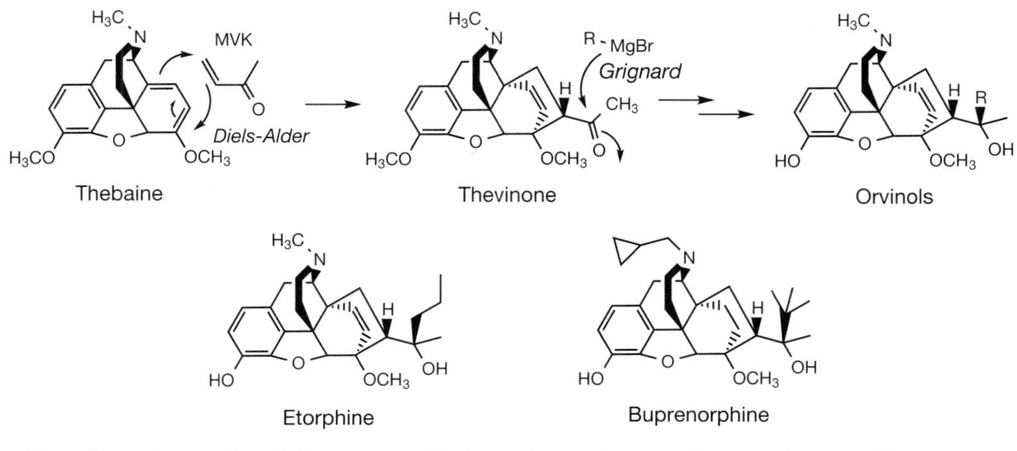

Figure 16.6 Clinically used orvinols and their structural relationship to the natural opiate, thebaine. MVK, methyl vinyl ketone.

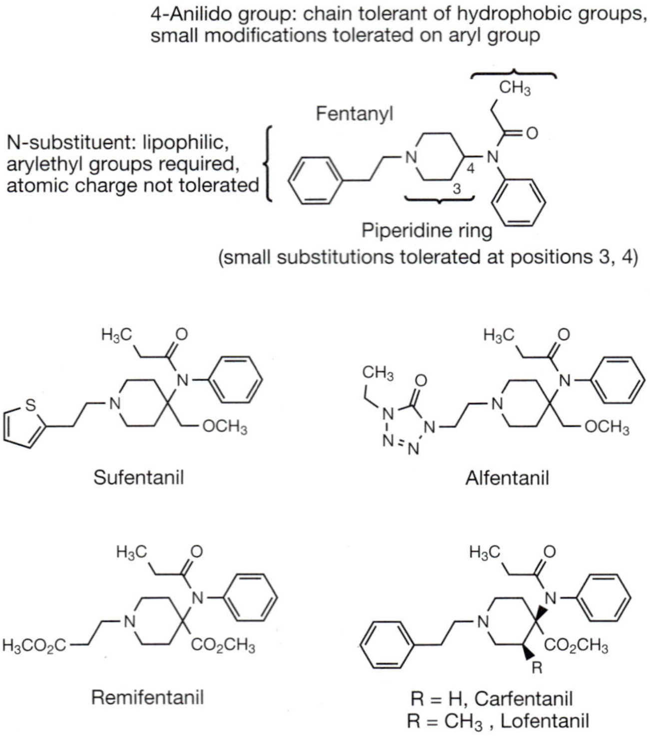

Figure 16.7 Summary of the structure-activity relationship of anilidopiperidine analgesics (top) and notable members of the class (bottom).

phenethyl groups result in high-affinity agonists in both classes, N-methyl substituents are inactive in the anilidopiperidines. The group attached to the nitrogen must be lipophilic to be active, and various lipophilic groups are tolerated here. An arylethyl moiety is the most common N-substituent in anilidopiperidines and FRS. These groups—phenethyl and thienylethyl of fentanyl and sufentanil, respectively—promote a very fast penetration of the BBB and a very high affinity at μ receptors through hydrophobic and π-stacking interactions. This results in an analgesic activity that runs between 80- and 800-fold greater than that of morphine. The substantial lipophilicity of these aralkyl substituents contributes to the very high calculated/experimental logP values of fentanyl (4.12/4.05) and sufentanil (3.4/3.95).[77]

Replacing the lipophilic aryl ring with the polar tetrazolinone system found in alfentanil (calculated/experimental log P = 2.2/2.16)[77] produces some complex but predictable changes in in vivo drug behavior. One might logically expect the decrease in molecular lipophilicity to translate to a more sluggish journey across the BBB. However, this strongly electron-withdrawing ring system decreases the pK_a of the piperidino nitrogen atom to 6.5 compared to 8.4 for fentanyl's basic nitrogen atom,[78] which significantly decreases the ratio of ionized to unionized conjugate forms in the bloodstream. Contrary to what would be expected from a simple comparison of logP values, the lower pK_a of alfentanil allows for a faster penetration of the BBB. However, this depressed ionized/unionized ratio is maintained at the receptor surface, which means less cationic drug is available for essential ion-ion anchoring with the μ receptor Asp147. Therefore, despite a positive CNS distribution profile, the potency of alfentanil decreases to 25-fold that of morphine because of a lower μ-receptor affinity.

The nitrogen substituent of remifentanil looks very different than those described so far. First, as with alfentanil, the electron-withdrawing ester lowers the amine pK_a to 7.1, increasing the fraction of unionized drug in the bloodstream and facilitating rapid penetration into the CNS. The fact that the amine pK_a is higher than alfentanil translates to a higher percentage of cationic drug at the receptor surface (33% vs 11%) and augmented receptor affinity. A second important aspect of drug chemistry concerns the rate of metabolism of this methyl ester. Esterase-mediated hydrolysis is rapid and leaves behind a carboxylic acid; this group is now hydrophilic and is not tolerated in this lipophilic region of the μ-opioid receptor. This means that the duration of action of remifentanil is very short (3-10 minutes) and appropriate for the induction or maintenance of anesthesia.

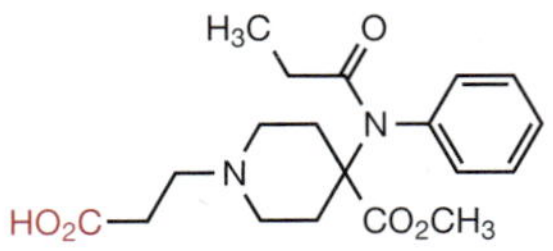

Remifentanil acid metabolite
(inactive)

Unlike the SAR of the N-substituent of 4,5-epoxymorphinans, N-allyl and N-cyclopropylmethyl groups do not result in μ antagonists. This is rationalized by the fact that the N-groups of fentanyl and morphine are oriented toward different pockets of the receptor and thus contribute differently to opioid binding and efficacy.

Structure-Activity Relationship of the 4-Anilido Group. At the 4-position of the piperidine ring is a functional group called an *anilide*. The term comes from the combination of aniline and amide. An aniline is an amine that is directly attached to an aromatic phenyl ring. The anilide group is not charged at any pH. All of the commercially available fentanyl analogs share the same anilido group: an aniline conjugated with a propionic acid to generate a propionamide. The phenyl ring and amide are both tolerant of diverse substitutions, however. Many FRS that have been identified in illicit drug seizures have structural modifications in these regions. Examples of FRS can be found in a recent review.[55] The reagents used to make these types of analogs are inexpensive and widely commercially available. The fact that these regions are so tolerant to diverse substitutions makes it very difficult to control their synthesis and proliferation.

Structure-Activity Relationship of the Piperidine Ring. While no 3-substituted anilidopiperine analgesics are currently marketed, it bears mentioning that a methyl group at position 3 increases μ receptor affinity and analgesic activity. Stereochemistry is critical, with the *cis* isomers being 6 to 8 times as active as the *trans*, and the *cis* (+) isomer being approximately 120-fold more potent than its (−) enantiomer.[76] The synthesis of myriad fentanyl analogs has added significantly to our understanding of anilidopiperidine SARs.[79]

The 4-position is tolerant of substitutions adjacent to the anilido group. The axial methoxymethyl moiety at C_4 of the piperidine ring of sufentanil and alfentanil is lipophilic and contributes to their rapid distribution to central sites of action. It also promotes high-affinity binding at the μ-receptor surface. A similar spike in μ affinity is realized with a 4-methylcarboxylate moiety (eg, carfentanil, lofentanil). Ester modifications to the 4-position are shielded from esterase-mediated hydrolysis by the large anilido group, and are thus metabolically stable.

Flexible Opioids: Dual-Action Agents. Inhibiting central monoamine reuptake in descending nociceptive pathways has been shown to alleviate chronic pain. While both NE and 5-HT have a mechanistic role to play,[80] NE-reuptake inhibition appears to provide the stronger analgetic response.[81] Structurally, many of the multimodal acting analgesics are less rigid and more flexible than the 4,5-epoxymorphinans that have high affinity for opioid receptor targets. This can be rationalized by observing that highly flexible, simple molecules can more easily rotate into conformations that permit binding to alternate receptor targets than conformationally rigid compounds can. Examples of multimodal opioids include meperidine, tapentadol, tramadol, and methadone (Fig. 16.8).

Meperidine is a relatively weak μ opioid receptor agonist and is less effective at controlling severe pain than morphine. The mechanism of action of meperidine includes μ opioid receptor agonism and dopamine transporter (DAT) and norepinephrine transporter (NET) inhibition. Like fentanyl, meperidine contains a piperidine core function; however, the SAR of meperidine and fentanyl are very different. As with other opioids discussed so far, meperidine requires a weakly basic, tertiary amine to be active. Substitutions beyond *N*-methyl that make this group more lipophilic will increase potency, though allyl and cyclopropylmethyl groups will not result in antagonists. Metabolism of the N-methyl group reveals a secondary amine product (normeperidine) that is inactive as a μ agonist and produces convulsions. The phenyl ring is tolerant to substitutions, including addition of a phenol as in ketobemidone. The ethyl ester group in meperidine is also modified to a bioisosteric ketone in ketobemidone, demonstrating that this region is also tolerant to modifications. An "inversed ester" derivative of meperidine showed up in illicit batches of "bathtub meperidine" in the 1970s. Though also a μ opioid receptor agonist, this inversed ester was subject to esterase hydrolysis and reveals a chemically unstable tertiary alcohol. Further conversion of this metabolite reveals a product called *N*-methyl-4-phenylpyridine (MPP+), a potent neurotoxin.

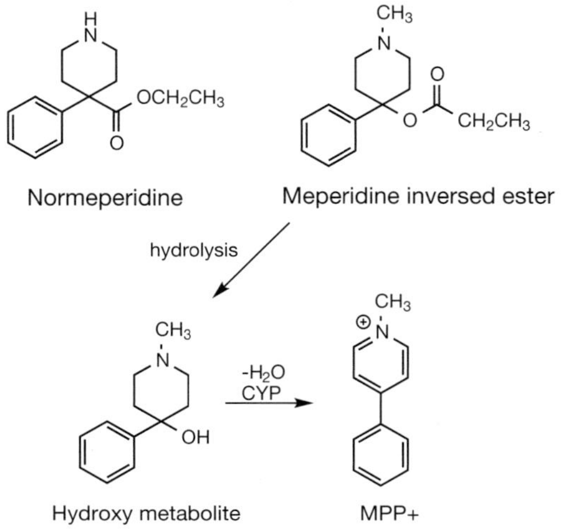

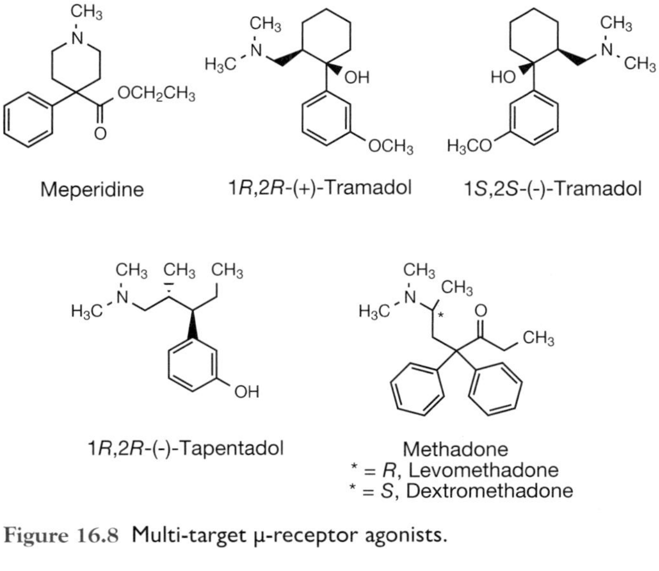

Figure 16.8 Multi-target μ-receptor agonists.

Tapentadol and tramadol (see Fig. 16.8) both inhibit central NE reuptake to about the same extent, but the former drug, administered as the pure 1*R*,2*R*-(−) isomer, does so selectively. Complicating its therapeutic activity profile, tramadol is marketed as a racemic mixture of *cis* isomers, each of which targets a different neurotransmitter. 1*S*,2*S*-(−)-Tramadol inhibits the reuptake of NE, while the 1*R*,2*R*-(+) enantiomer blocks 5-HT reuptake.[82]

Both tapentadol and tramadol also elicit analgesia through μ-receptor agonism that synergizes with the pain relief gained through inhibition of neurotransmitter reuptake. Phenolic (−)-tapentadol, a rationally designed drug that is the more potent analgesic of the two, is active intact. Similar to codeine-based analgesics, tramadol's aromatic methoxy group must be O-dealkylated by CYP2D6 before significant μ-receptor binding can occur, and only the (+) isomer generates a clinically active μ agonist. CYP3A4 may play a secondary role in tramadol O-dealkylation.[82] Since neurotransmitter-reuptake activity resides primarily in the parent tramadol structure, the mechanism by which this drug provides analgesia shifts as O-dealkylation progresses.[81] In addition to selective NE reuptake, the time-independent mechanism of tapentadol's analgetic action is viewed as a distinct therapeutic advantage. The chemical and mechanistic distinctions of tramadol and tapentadol are summarized in Table 16.2.

The dimethylamino moiety is an essential feature for both analgetic mechanisms of tramadol and tapentadol. While the binding affinity of tapentadol to the human μ receptor is almost 50-fold less than the (+)-phenol metabolite of tramadol, the opioid agonist potency of tapentadol is higher due to a more favorable CNS distribution profile.[82]

Table 16.2 Chemical and Mechanistic Properties of Tramadol and Tapentadol

	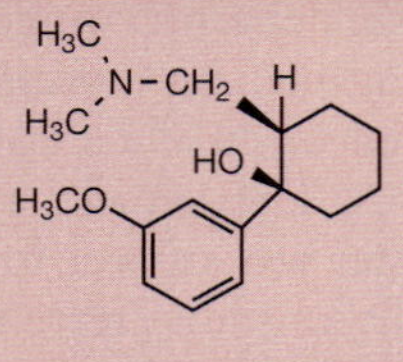 1*R*,2*R*-(+)-Tramadol	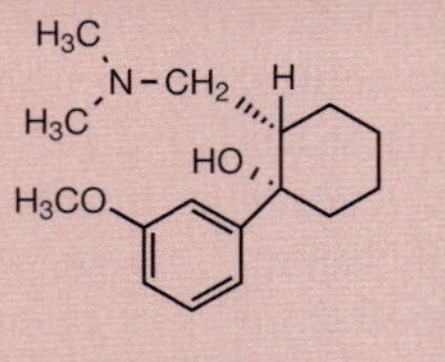 1*S*,2*S*-(-)-Tramadol	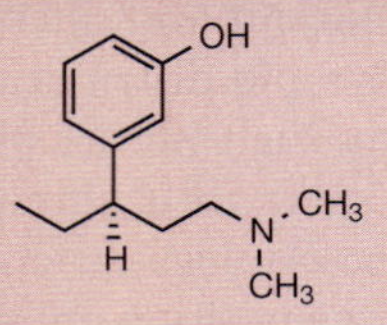 1*R*,2*R*(-)-Tapentadol
Aliphatic structure	Cyclic		Open chain
Marketed as	Racemic mixture of *cis* isomers		Single isomer
Neurotransmitter-reuptake profile	Serotonin and norepinephrine (1*S*,2*S*)		Norepinephrine
Prodrug opioid?	Yes: activated by CYP2D6-catalyzed O-dealkylation		No: active intact
μ-Agonist isomer	Dextrorotatory		Levorotatory
μ-Agonist potency	Weak		Weak-moderate (1.5-4 times tramadol)
Analgesic mechanism	Time dependent: neurotransmitter reuptake (parent drug) decreases as μ agonism ([+]-phenol metabolite) increases		Time independent: neurotransmitter reuptake and μ agonism provided by parent drug
Inactivating metabolism	CYP3A4/CYP2B6-catalyzed *N*-dealkylation; glucuronic acid or sulfate conjugation		CYP2C-catalyzed *N*-dealkylation (13%), glucuronic acid (55%) or sulfate (15%) conjugation
Abuse potential	C-IV		C-II

Its μ-agonist activity is commonly compared against morphine or oxycodone.

Shen et al[83] have confirmed that the active phenolic metabolite of (+)-tramadol binds to the μ receptor in a manner similar to morphine. Molecular docking studies indicate that ion-ion anchoring to Asp147, hydrophobic bonding of N-substituents with Trp293 and Tyr326, and H-bonding of the phenolic OH with Lys233 occur with both structures.

Methadone is one of the most conformationally flexible μ-receptor agonists in clinical use. Of note, there is no molecular "scaffolding" (ie, rings) connecting the basic amine to the other parts of the molecule. Like the other flexible, multi-target analgesics discussed in this section, there is a *N*-propyl-phenyl linkage present in methadone. Methadone is administered as the racemic mixture of (*R*)- and (*S*)-enantiomers. Both enantiomers have high affinity and selectivity for μ over κ and δ receptors and also inhibit the monoamine serotonin and norepinephrine transporters serotonin transport protein (SERT) and norepinephrine transport protein (NET), respectively. Monoamine transport blockade may contribute to the therapeutic and adverse effects of methadone.

Common Metabolic Reactions

The common metabolic pathways of opioids are predictable from their structure. Many μ agonists have an N-methyl group that can be dealkylated by CYP3A4.[84] From a therapeutic standpoint, the resulting nor-metabolites have limited clinical relevance due to a decrease in distribution-enhancing lipophilicity and the loss of an agonist-promoting hydrophobic interaction with the receptor.

In contrast, CYP2D6-mediated O-dealkylation of the aryl methoxy group of codeine analogs (Fig. 16.9) and tramadol are required to generate the phenolic OH group essential for μ opioid–receptor binding. As noted, patients deficient in this activating enzyme may show an attenuated response to these prodrug analgesics. Within the United States, the incidence of CYP2D6 poor metabolizer (PM) phenotype has been estimated at approximately 10%.[85] Although the *CYP2D6*3* and *CYP2D6*4* alleles common in White PMs are present in only 1% or less of persons of Asian ancestry, the *CYP2D6*10* allele associated with reduced CYP2D6 catalytic capability (intermediate metabolizer [IM] phenotype) is found in up to 50% of Asians.[86-88] Approximately 1% to 2% of the US population is of the ultrarapid metabolizer (UM) phenotype, but the incidence rises to up to 28% in individuals of Arab, Ethiopian, and North African descent.[85,89]

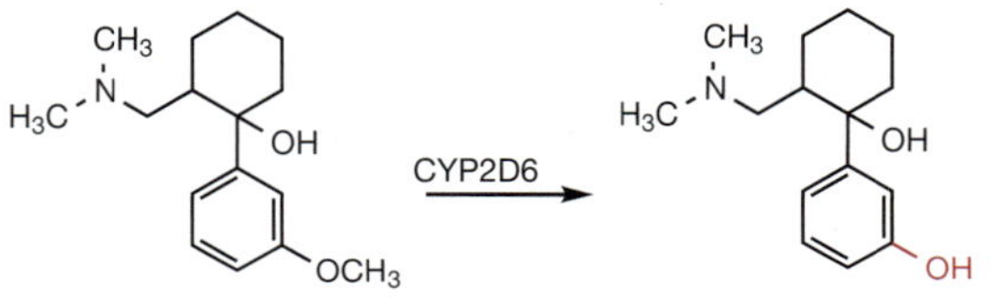

Tramadol (inactive) — *O*-Desmethyltramadol (active)

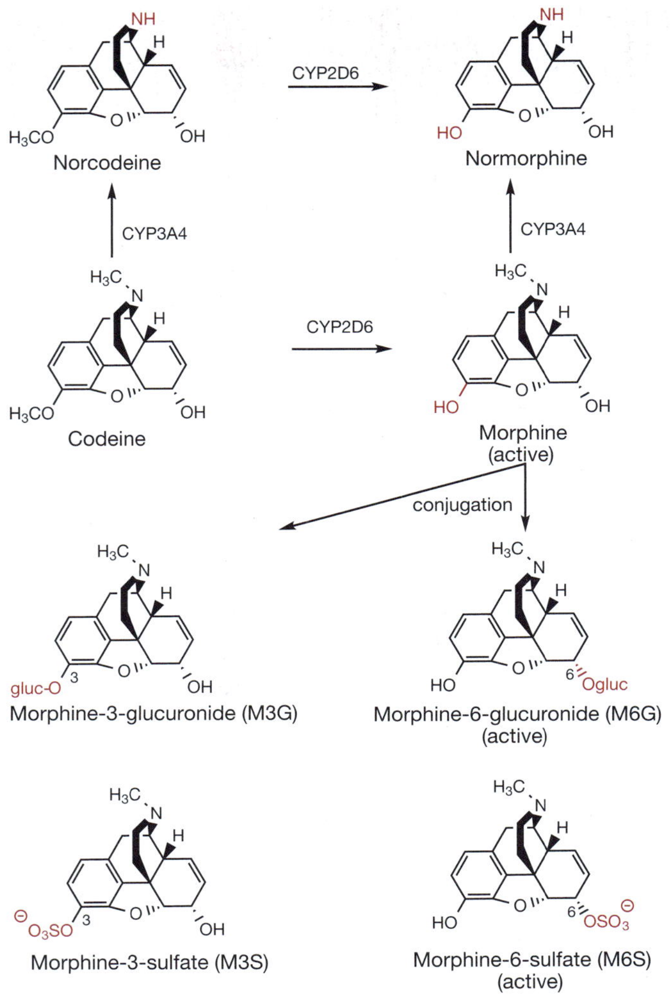

Figure 16.9 Common metabolic reactions of morphine and codeine. Active metabolites are shown in red.

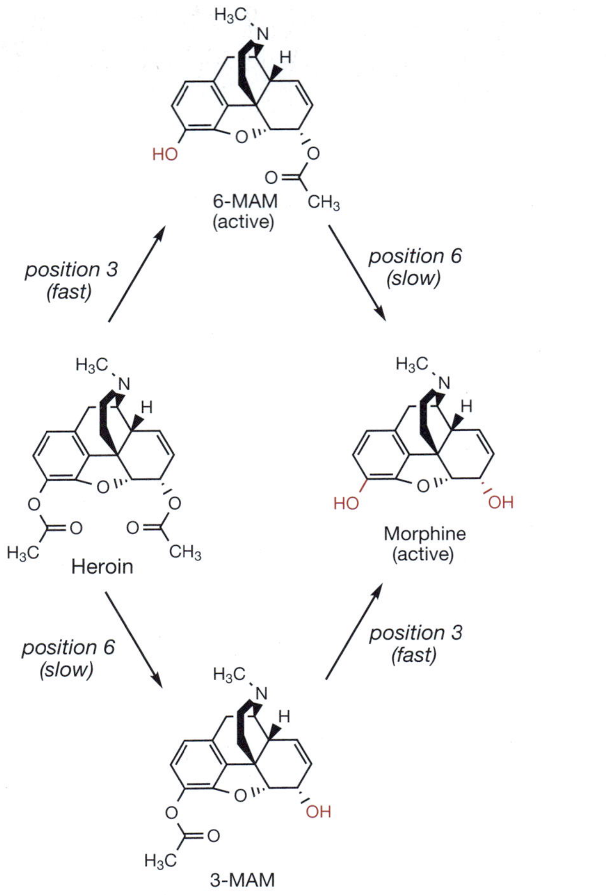

Figure 16.10 Hydrolysis of heroin into metabolites 3-monoacetylmorphine (3-MAM), 6-monoacetylmorphine (6-MAM), and morphine. Active metabolites are shown in red.

While no clinically marketed opioid analgesic has a C_3-ester, the need for metabolic liberation of the phenol would still hold true. For example, the 3-acetate ester of heroin is readily hydrolyzed in the CNS to generate the μ agonist, 6-monoacetylmorphine (6-MAM), which contributes to the strong reinforcing effects of heroin (Fig. 16.10). 6-MAM is more lipophilic than morphine by virtue of the fact that the hydroxyl group has been replaced by a lipophilic ester; thus, 6-MAM penetrates into the brain faster, and the metabolite is highly rewarding. The 6-acetate ester is slower to cleave because it is more sterically hindered by the 4,5-epoxymorphinan ring C, but it will eventually succumb to hydrolysis to produce morphine.

Opioids are also subject to phase II metabolism prior to excretion. The opioids that have the highest potential for forming phase II conjugates are those possessing phenols or secondary alcohols. Glucuronide and sulfate conjugates are found in the urine of patients taking most opioids. One must consider the SAR of the structural class to determine if these metabolites are active. For example, morphine contains two alcohol groups that can form conjugates: the 3-phenol and the 6-α-hydroxyl. Conjugates that are found in the urine include morphine-3-glucuronide (M-3-G), morphine-6-glucuronide (M-6-G), morphine-3-sulfate (M-3-S), and morphine-6-sulfate (M-6-S). According to SAR of the 3-position, M-3-G and M-3-S are likely to be inactive because the hydrogen bond–donating phenol has been replaced. On the other hand, because the 6-position does not engage in beneficial binding interactions and is tolerant of diverse substitutions, it is possible that M-6-G and M-6-S would be active metabolites. Indeed, M-6-G and M-6-S have high affinity for μ opioid receptors and likely contribute to the observed analgesic effects of morphine.[84,90] Phase II conjugation in the GI tract impacts the oral bioavailability of many phenolic opioids (Table 16.3). Those administered by mouth must be given in doses higher than one would administer parenterally, and/or they are formulated to promote rapid absorption and limit exposure to intestinal transferase enzymes. Glucuronidation at both C_3 and C_6 is catalyzed by UGT2B7.

The metabolic pathway of codeine (see Fig. 16.9) is illuminating in that it contains essentially all the aforementioned biotransformations and includes reactions that are analgetically activating, inactivating, attenuating, and augmenting.

Table 16.3 Selected Physicochemical and Pharmacokinetics Properties of Opioid Analgesics and Antagonists

Opioid Analgesic: Rigid Phenanthrene-Based	Log P (Calc)	Oral Bioavailability (%)	Extended-Release Dosage Form Available?	Protein Binding (%)
Buprenorphine	4.53	NA 31 (sl)	No	96
Butorphanol	3.65	5-17 60-70 (nas)	No	80
Codeine	1.2	90	Yes	7-25
Hydrocodone	2.13	–	Yes	19-45
Hydromorphone	1.69	24	Yes	19
Levorphanol	3.29	Low	No	40
Morphine	0.99	30	Yes	30-40
Oxycodone	1.04	60-87	Yes	45
Oxymorphone	1.26	10	Yes	8-19
Nalbuphine	2.0	NA 81-83 (im) 76-79 (sc)	No	Little appreciable binding
Pentazocine	4.44	Low	No	
Opioid Analgesic: Flexible				
Alfentanil	2.2	NA	No	92
Fentanyl	4.12	50 (buccal) 92 (td)	No	80-85
Meperidine	2.9	50-60	No	60-80
Methadone	4.14	36-100	No	85-90
Remifentanil	1.75	NA	No	70
Sufentanil	3.4	NA	No	91-93
Tapentadol	3.47	32	Yes	20
Tramadol	2.71	75	Yes	20
Opioid Antagonist				
Naloxone	1.47	NA	No	10
Naltrexone	2.07	5-40	Yes	21
Methylnaltrexone bromide	0.59	Low (approx. 2%)	No	11-15
Naloxegol	1.73	–	No	4.2
Alvimopan	3.25	<7%	No	80-90%
Naldemedine	3.14	–	No	93-94%

Table 16.3 Selected Physicochemical and Pharmacokinetics Properties of Opioid Analgesics and Antagonists (*continued*)

Opioid Analgesic: Rigid Phenanthrene-Based	Onset (min) of Analgesia (po unless noted)	$T_{1/2}$ (h)	Duration of Action (h)	Excretion (%)	T_{max} (h) (po unless noted)
Buprenorphine	15 (im)	2.2 (iv) 37 (sl)	≥6 (im)	10-30 renal 70 fecal	0.67-3.5 (sl) 1 (im) 72 (td)
Butorphanol	≤15	18	3-4 (im, iv) 4-5 (nas)	70-80 renal 15 fecal	0.5-1 (im, iv) 1-2 (nas)
Codeine	30-60	2.5-3.5	4-6	90 renal	1-1.5
Hydrocodone	60	1.5-3	3-4	26 renal	2
Hydromorphone	15-30	2-3	3-4	Primarily renal	0.5-1
Levorphanol	10-60	11-16	≤8	Primarily renal	1
Morphine	30 5-10 (iv)	2-4	3-5	90 renal 7-10 fecal	0.5
Oxycodone	10-15	2-4	3-6	80 renal	0.5-1
Oxymorphone	5-10 (im, sc, iv)	7-9 (po)	3-6 (im, sc, iv)	49 renal	–
Nalbuphine	2-3 (iv) <15 (sc, im)	5	3-6	Primarily fecal 7 renal	1 (sc, im)
Pentazocine	15-30 (sc, im)	2-3	4-6	Primarily renal	0.25-1 (sc, im)
Opioid Analgesic: Flexible					
Alfentanil	2-3 iv	1.5-2	0.5-1	Primarily renal	15 min (im)
Fentanyl	<1 iv 7-8 (im) 6 h (td) 5-15 (buc, sl, nas)	2-4 (iv) 20-27 (td)	72 (td) 0.5-1 (iv) 1-2 (im)	75 renal 9 fecal	0.25-8 (buc, sl, nas) 20-72 (td)
Meperidine	10-15 (im, sc)	2.5-4	2-4 (po, sc, im) 2-3 (iv)	Primarily renal	2 1 (im, sc)
Methadone	30-60 10-20 (im, sc, iv)	8-59	4-8	Primarily renal	1-2 (im, sc) 3-5 d (continuous po)
Remifentanil	1-3 (iv)	<0.33	0.05-0.17 (iv)	Primarily renal	<0.080 (iv)
Sufentanil	1-3 iv	2.7	0.5 (iv) 1.7 (epidural)	Primarily renal	
Tapentadol	32	4	4-6	99 renal	1.25
Tramadol	60-75	6-8	4-6	90 renal 10 fecal	2
Opioid Antagonist					
Naloxone	2-5 (im, sc, nas)	0.5-1.5 (im, sc, iv) 2 (nas)	0.5-2	40 renal (<6 h)	0.25 (im, sc) 0.33-0.5 (nas)

(continued)

Table 16.3 Selected Physicochemical and Pharmacokinetics Properties of Opioid Analgesics and Antagonists (*continued*)

Opioid Analgesic: Rigid Phenanthrene-Based	Onset (min) of Analgesia (po unless noted)	$T_{1/2}$ (h)	Duration of Action (h)	Excretion (%)	T_{max} (h) (po unless noted)
Naltrexone	–	4 5-10 d (im)	24-72 4 wk (im)	53-79 renal 5-10 fecal	1 2 (im, 1st phase) 48-72 (im, second phase)
Methylnaltrexone bromide	–	15 (po)	–	44-45 renal 17 fecal	1.5 (po) 0.5 (sc)
Naloxegol	–	6-11	–	16 renal 68 fecal	<2 h

buc, buccal; im, intramuscular; iv, intravenous; nas, intranasal; po, oral; sc, subcutaneous; sl, sublingual; $T_{1/2}$, elimination half-life; td, transdermal; T_{max}, time to peak plasma concentration.

Data from Drug Bank. Accessed September 30, 2017. https://www.drugbank.ca/; *Drug Facts and Comparisons. Facts & Comparisons* [Database Online]. In: Louis S, ed. Wolters Kluwer Health, Inc; 2005; Lexicomp Online Lexi-drugs Hudson. Lexi-Comp, Inc.

Physicochemical and Pharmacokinetic Properties

As GPCR ligands, opioids have a tertiary amine that will be predominantly cationic at pH 7.4. Amine pK_a values range from 6.5 (alfentanil) to 9.4 (tramadol). Phenolic opioids are sensitive to in vitro oxidation and must be protected from light, air, and elevated pH. As drugs with a central mechanism of action, opioid agonists and antagonists are generally highly lipophilic structures capable of penetrating the BBB. Only morphine, the most polar opioid, has a predicted log P value less than 1.0. As noted earlier, the analgetic action of chiral opioids is highly stereoselective, with the (–) isomer being the clinically active form for all but tramadol.

Many opioid pharmaceuticals are administered only by parenteral, buccal, sublingual, or transdermal routes due to inactivating prehepatic or first pass metabolism. Those that could be given orally are usually given in doses higher than would be administered by injection. Extended duration dosage forms are available for many agents, although concerns about their potential for abuse and fatal misuse have prompted the removal of some from the marketplace (eg, Opana ER).

Key physicochemical and pharmacokinetic properties of marketed opioid agonists and antagonists are provided in Table 16.3.[77,91,92]

Phenanthrene-Based Rigid μ Agonists

The opioid agonists discussed next are those that currently enjoy the most widespread clinical use as analgesics. One can easily name these drugs by looking at the key structural positions discussed at length earlier (see Fig. 16.4). First, look at positions 6, 7, and 8: if there is an OH at 6 and an alk*ene* between 7 and 8, the drug name will end in "-ine." If there is a ket*one* at position 6, then the drug name will end in "-one." Next, look at position 3: a phenol will have the prefix "morph" because morphine has a 3-phenol, and a methyl ether will have the prefix "cod" because codeine has a methyl ether. Finally, for the 6-ketones, look to position 14: if there is a *hydro*gen here, the prefix "hydro" is used, and if there is an oxygen (OH), the prefix "oxy" is used.

MORPHINE SULFATE. Morphine is the prototypical opioid agonist, and all synthetic multicyclic analgesics are based on the morphine nucleus to some degree. The presence of the N-CH_3 substituent, phenolic hydroxyl, and B/C *cis* configuration assure potent and selective μ agonism. Despite being well absorbed from the GI tract, morphine has very poor oral bioavailability due to extensive prehepatic and first-pass metabolism to inactive 3-glucuronide and 3-sulfate conjugates. The C_3 glucuronide undergoes extensive enterohepatic cycling, so if oral administration is required, large initial doses must be given followed by lower maintenance doses. At 0.99, morphine's logP is low, and opioids of higher lipophilicity exhibit better oral bioavailability, as well as a faster onset of analgesic action (see Table 16.3). Polar and metabolically vulnerable morphine is generally considered 3- to 6-fold more active by parenteral routes than by the oral route.

Approximately 5% of a dose of morphine is metabolized by CYP3A4-mediated N-dealkylation to normorphine[93] (see Fig. 16.9) which, at 1/20 the activity of the parent drug, is not clinically relevant. Inactivation is primarily a result of C_3 glucuronidation by UGT2B7 (57%), with sulfonation taking on a minor conjugating role. Glucuronidation of the C_6-OH (5%-10%) by the same UGT isoform provides a highly active metabolite, M-6-G.[94,95] The potency ratio between morphine and M-6-G in humans has been estimated between 1:2 and 1:3,[95,96] and the metabolite is believed to account for up to 85% of morphine's analgesic action.[97] Polar morphine-6-glucuronide has a log P of 0.13,[77] and it passively crosses the BBB with some difficulty. Along with morphine, it is a substrate for central P-glycoprotein (P-gp) efflux proteins.[93,98] To facilitate entry into the CNS, the molecule can hide its polar groups through folding,[95] and active transport mechanisms are being investigated, but more work is needed to fully elucidate how these powerful analgesics reach central receptors.[98] The M-6-G metabolite can accumulate in patients with renal failure or poor renal function (eg, older adults),[94,95] increasing the risk of inadvertent overdose. A small study found that M-6-G did not induce the pruritus associated with the free 6α-OH group of morphine and codeine.[99] Phase II clinical trials have demonstrated efficacy of M-6-G in the treatment of postoperative pain. Compared to morphine, M-6-G provides long-lasting (12-24 hours) analgesia with a significantly slower onset of action and fewer and/or less severe adverse effects.[95,96]

Morphine is one of the safest opioids to use to treat the pain of myocardial infarction, unstable angina, and other ischemic disorders because of its positive hemodynamic effects.[100] Its negative chronotropic effect and venous and arterial vasodilation result in a decrease in myocardial oxygen demand. Morphine decreases blood pressure secondary to histamine release, an activity linked to the 6α-OH group and must be used with caution in patients with hypovolemia.

Extreme caution is advised with the use of all opioids in patients with head trauma because opioids can increase intracranial pressure, which in turn can exacerbate respiratory depression. Inhibition of cough reflex, however, is a valuable action in this situation because it helps keep intracranial pressure within defined limits. Morphine lacks the 14β-OH group that attenuates cough suppression and, along with fentanyl, it is the opioid most commonly used to treat pain in patients with head injury.[101] On a precautionary note, inflammation associated with head injury may downregulate efflux proteins such as P-gp and multidrug-resistant protein, resulting in an accumulation of morphine and the active 6-glucuronide in cerebral tissue.[102]

Morphine is available in a variety of dosage forms, including solution for injection, oral solution, tablets, extended-release tablets, suppositories, and patient-controlled intramuscular (IM) administration devices. Oral dosage forms must be swallowed whole and not chewed, crushed, or dissolved in liquid.

Extended-release morphine sulfate is marketed as MS Contin. All extended-release opioids are for use only when continuous long-term analgesia requiring "around the clock" opioid agonist therapy is warranted. Patients taking this and all extended-release products must not be opioid-naïve, or potentially fatal respiratory depression could result. The consumption of alcohol while on opioid agonists is never advised, but it could prove fatal when taking extended-release capsules because alcohol can promote rapid capsule dissolution in the GI tract. Consuming alcohol and/or other CNS depressants (eg, benzodiazepines) with opioids, regardless of formulation, can increase the risk of respiratory depression, excessive sedation, coma, and death. Some patients will experience an allergic-like reaction to morphine (attributed to the free 6α-OH) while others may be hypersensitive to the phenanthrene structural moiety.[103] Hypersensitive patients may react to all rigid opioid agonists, regardless of whether they contain a 6α-OH group.

Hydromorphone Hydrochloride and Oxymorphone Hydrochloride. Hydromorphone differs in structure from morphine only in the area of ring C. The 7,8-dihydro-6-1 structural motif adds flexibility to the system and increases lipophilicity. The increase in analgesic action arising from these modifications has been estimated at 4- to 7-fold by the oral route.[104] As μ receptor–elicited analgesia and side effects such as respiratory depression and constipation go hand in hand, the risk of toxicity with hydromorphone as compared to morphine also increases. Hydromorphone is metabolized primarily by C_3 glucuronidation, but a small amount undergoes reduction of the 6-keto group to isomeric alcohols (morphols), both of which are active.[105]

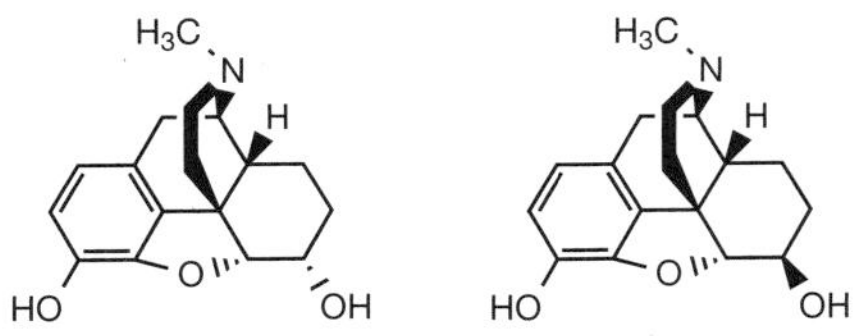

6α-hydromorphol 6β-hydromorphol

A 2016 Cochrane Review of the use of hydromorphone in cancer pain, including pain that disrupts sleep, revealed efficacy similar to other μ agonists like morphine and oxycodone but concluded that more comprehensive studies were needed to positively document relative value in this patient population.[106] A 2017 retrospective study on inpatient deaths due to hydromorphone or morphine underscores the importance of vigilance against errors in prescribing, dispensing, administration, and monitoring.[107]

Hydromorphone hydrochloride is available as a solution for IM or IV injection, rectal suppositories, tablets, liquid for oral administration, and extended-release tablets, with the latter reserved for use in patients tolerant to and dependent on μ agonists who require high-potency pain management on a chronic basis. As with morphine, boxed warnings caution patients and providers on hydromorphone's potential for abuse/addiction, profound respiratory depression, and life-threating interactions if coadministered with other CNS depressants.

Oxymorphone's 14β-OH group increases analgesic action approximately 3- to 4-fold over hydromorphone due to an increase in μ-receptor affinity. It is considered approximately 10 times more potent than morphine,[108,109] and its metabolic pathway mirrors that of hydromorphone. Since only a small amount is reduced to the isomeric 6-oxymorphol metabolites, it can be used in patients sensitive to the histamine-releasing action of the 6α-OH opioids codeine and morphine.[109] As oxymorphone is not metabolized by CYP enzymes, there is essentially no risk for CYP-related drug-drug interactions.

Oxymorphone is commercially available as tablets and a solution for injection. Abuse-deterrent extended-release tablets were marketed for a time as Opana ER and the abuse-deterrent formulation (ADF) chemical strategy for this potent opioid was claimed to be the same as that used for an ADF of oxycodone (OxyContin). However, a study involving more than 12,000 individuals with an opioid abuse disorder showed that, while abuse via insufflation (snorting) decreased with both ADF drugs, abuse by IV injection decreased only for oxycodone, while a trend toward increased oxymorphone misuse was observed.[110] In mid-2017, the FDA recommended that sales of Opana ER be suspended due to "dangerous unintended consequences" as a result of its high potential for misuse/abuse. Within a month, the manufacturer voluntarily withdrew the product from the market.

Codeine Sulfate, Hydrocodone Bitartrate, and Oxycodone Hydrochloride. Codeine, hydrocodone, and oxycodone are the 3-methoxy analogs of morphine, hydromorphone, and oxymorphone, respectively, and they have the same potency relationship to one another, as their parent structures demonstrated. All are prodrugs that must undergo CYP2D6-mediated activation to the phenol required for high-affinity binding to μ receptors.

Unlike morphine, CYP3A4-mediated N-dealkylation plays a major role in oxycodone metabolism. Noroxycodone represents 23% of oxycodone urinary metabolites, while CYP2D6-generated oxymorphone represents only 11%.[111] Although N-dealkylation is not as prominent, these two reactions are also the major phase I biotransformation processes for hydrocodone and, to a lesser extent, codeine.[91,112] In contrast to hydrocodone and oxycodone, glucuronidation comprises a major component (70%) of codeine metabolism. The phase I metabolic pathways of oxycodone are shown in Figure 16.11.

A clinical guideline on the use of codeine in patients of varying CYP2D6 phenotypes has been published,[113] and hydrocodone analgesia has also been assumed to be linked to this genetic profile.[112] Interestingly, CYP2D6 genotype is reported to be relatively unimportant to the analgesic response to oxycodone, despite having the predicted impact on the extent of O-dealkylation.[111,114] The risk of drug-drug interactions involving oxycodone is also claimed to be less significant with CYP2D6 inducers and inhibitors than with modifiers of CYP3A4 activity. Codeine's diminished risk of CYP-related interactions (particularly CYP3A4) is related to its strong metabolic reliance on glucuronidation, although CYP3A4 inhibition can complicate the codeine response picture when coupled with other factors, such as CYP2D6 genotype.[113]

All three drugs are available as single-agent products. Although the potency of each is about 10- to 12-fold lower than its phenolic counterpart, oral bioavailability is greatly enhanced (Table 16.3). They are efficacious analgesics that

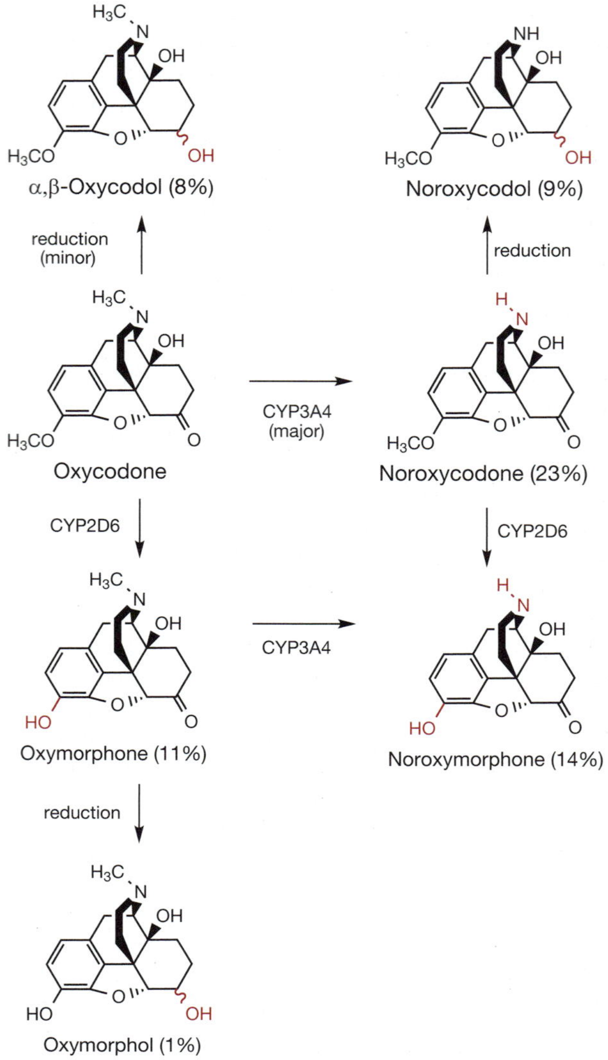

Figure 16.11 Oxidative and reductive metabolism of oxycodone. All metabolites have some level of pharmacologic activity. Conjugation at the 3-position (eg, 3-*O*-glucuronides of oxymorphone, noroxymorphone, and oxymorphol) are essentially inactive.

are generally well tolerated. Codeine and oxycodone are available as immediate-release tablets and as a solution for injection. As previously noted, the risk of a severe pseudoallergic reaction to parenterally administered codeine phosphate is high due to the presence of the 6α-OH group. Very little reduction to 6-OH metabolites occurs with hydrocodone (3%)[90] or oxycodone (10%),[111] so the risk of significant histamine release is slight.

All three codeine-based opioids are also formulated with peripheral analgesics acetaminophen, ibuprofen, or aspirin. These combination analgesics attack pain on both central and peripheral mechanistic fronts and allow lower doses of each potentially toxic drug to be utilized. Codeine and hydrocodone are found in combination with a variety of antihistamines, adrenergic agonist decongestants, and expectorants for use in treating cold symptoms that include serious cough. The attenuating impact of the 14β-OH group of oxycodone on cough suppression, along with the fact that protracted cough requiring opioid therapy is best treated with lower-potency agents, explains the lack of similar oxycodone-containing combination products.

Oxycodone was one of the first μ agonist analgesics to be made available in controlled-release tablet form (OxyContin). There was much focus in the literature and lay press on the potential for misuse/abuse of this drug when it was first released, leading to the development of the ADFs in use today. Abuse-deterrent extended-release tablets and capsules are the only single-agent hydrocodone dosage forms available, and they too generated controversy at the national level before they came to market. The risk-benefit of extended-release hydrocodone (misuse:abuse liability vs long-acting analgesia without fear of acetaminophen-induced hepatoxicity with chronic use), along with the pros and cons of various extended-release formulations, has been described in the literature.[112]

In April 2017, the FDA issued a special safety alert cautioning against administering codeine (and tramadol) to children younger than 12 years due to a high risk of excessive sedation and respiratory depression leading to death.[115] In 2010, codeine or oxycodone use in older adults for longer than 6 months was reported to increase the risk of serious or fatal cardiovascular events and to increase all-cause mortality when used for more than 30 days.[116] While this observation has been questioned by others, the call for additional research into this potentially serious and relatively unique cardiovascular health risk is clearly warranted.[117]

Buprenorphine Hydrochloride. Buprenorphine is a member of the orvinol class of highly potent opioids that has an equally unique and interesting SAR.[118,119] Despite the presence of the N-cyclopropylmethyl group that normally imposes μ antagonist action, buprenorphine is a very potent partial μ agonist. As a partial agonist, its intrinsic activity at μ receptors is less than maximal, and pharmacological actions eventually hit a ceiling as doses are increased. This significantly limits toxicity, including respiratory depression, physical dependence, and abuse potential.[120]

Estimates of buprenorphine's analgesic potency in comparison to morphine have ranged between 30:1 and 115:1, depending on the route of administration.[121,122] Buprenorphine's superior potency is attributed to high lipophilicity that facilitates concentration in the CNS and a very high affinity for μ receptors secondary to additional hydrophobic and hydrogen bonding capabilities of the C_7 side chain. Buprenorphine also antagonizes κ receptors[123] and stimulates the opioid receptor–like 1 (ORL 1) protein, which some claim may help minimize hyperalgesia, dysphoria, and the development of tolerance.[121,122]

The μ-receptor binding of buprenorphine is strong enough to be classified as pseudoirreversible,[123] which provides an exceptionally long half-life of 37 hours and permits once-daily dosing. Slow dissociation from μ receptors minimizes withdrawal symptoms even if the drug is abruptly discontinued.[121,124] Any discomfort a patient experiences after abrupt withdrawal of buprenorphine normally occurs 5 to 14 days after the last dose. The downside of pseudoirreversible binding is that it is difficult to reverse receptor-mediated side effects, such as respiratory depression.[125] While less common or severe than that induced by full μ agonists, this adverse effect can be clinically significant, and it can take up to 10-fold the normal dose of naloxone to reverse. Buprenorphine-induced respiratory depression can outlast naloxone's duration of action, and a regimen of 2 to 3 mg of naloxone followed by a 4-mg/h continuous infusion has been shown to restore normal breathing in respiratory-depressed patients within an hour. Kinetic models to explain this clinical observation have been published.[123] As with all opioids, the risk of potentially fatal respiratory depression increases significantly if other CNS depressants, including alcohol, are coadministered.

Buprenorphine undergoes significant first-pass metabolism. The CYP3A4-generated *N*-dealkylated metabolite norbuprenorphine retains analgesic activity, albeit 40-fold lower than the parent drug. Both buprenorphine and its nor metabolite are glucuronidated at the C_3 position prior to fecal excretion.[122,126] The buprenorphine parent structure can be hepatotoxic in high doses secondary to inhibition of mitochondrial respiration and subsequent adenosine triphosphate depletion,[127] and the nor metabolite is believed to be responsible for buprenorphine-related respiratory depression.[122] Blood levels of norbuprenorphine are normally less than 10% of the parent drug,[122] but the buprenorphine dose may need to be adjusted if coadministered with CYP3A4 substrates or inhibitors.

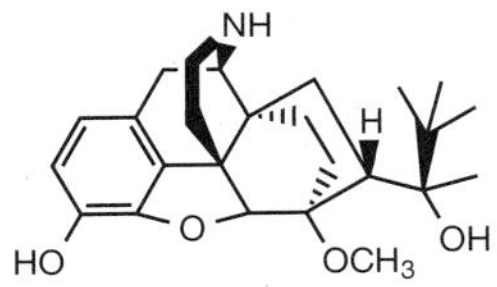

Norbuprenorphine

While pharmacologically classified as a partial μ agonist, buprenorphine has demonstrated full clinical efficacy in a large number of clinical trials evaluating relief of postoperative and cancer-related pain.[128] It is also viewed as effective in treating chronic noncancer pain[129] and, while additional studies are needed, it may have value in neuropathic pain.[122,130,131] Buprenorphine's relatively low risk of respiratory depression, constipation, and tolerance are considered therapeutic positives.[121] Additional reasons some have advocated for its use as a "frontline analgesic" include relative safety in older adults and patients with renal failure, minimal impact on gonadal function, and lack of significant cardiotoxicity and immunosuppression.[122]

Buprenorphine is commonly administered sublingually, buccally (75-900 μg film) or via injection to avoid inactivating conjugation in the gut and on first pass. The relative bioavailability of the sublingual and buccal formulations is 30% to 50% and 28%, respectively.[122] Plasma levels of buprenorphine peak in 1.5 (sublingual) and 3 (buccal) hours, and consumption of liquids can lower blood levels from the buccal film by up to 37%. A transdermal patch formulation of buprenorphine (Butrans) is available in strengths ranging from 5 to 20 μg/h. Steady-state concentrations are achieved in 72 hours, and patches are changed weekly. The previously described precaution on using extended-release opioids only in opioid-tolerant patients also applies to transdermal buprenorphine. In addition, patients must avoid exposing the applied patch to heat, as the release of drug from the patch matrix is temperature dependent and exposure to active drug can increase up to 55%.[91]

In addition to its use as an analgesic, buprenorphine is also employed in opioid addiction recovery. In 2-mg doses, buprenorphine blocks the euphoric effects of μ opioid-receptor agonists. It has been shown to be as active as 30 mg of methadone in addiction treatment programs and is considered a safer alternative due to lower risks of overdose,[132] cardiovascular toxicity,[123] and drug-drug interactions.[110] Treatment programs generally range from 6 months to over 2 years. Patients initiating replacement therapy with buprenorphine must be opioid-free for at least 12 hours.[110] Either under the direct supervision of their physician or at home, the patient enters the preliminary phase of opioid withdrawal before the first dose of buprenorphine is administered. The partial μ agonism will suppress withdrawal symptoms, but it would have precipitated active withdrawal if the patient had been under the influence of opioids at the time of buprenorphine induction.

Buprenorphine induction is followed by the stabilization (dose optimization) and maintenance phases of therapy. If recovering patients relapse (common in the first years of abstinence) and increase the buprenorphine dose in an attempt to achieve euphoria, they will hit the partial agonist activity plateau and the attempt to abuse will be thwarted. When the time comes, the patient can be withdrawn from buprenorphine with few, if any, withdrawal symptoms due to its slow dissociation from the receptors and slow disappearance from the body. The patient's receptors essentially wean themselves off of the drug.[133]

Several formulations are available to deliver buprenorphine to patients in addiction recovery programs. As noted earlier, buprenorphine alone is marketed in 2- and 8-mg sublingual tablets.[90,120] In November 2017, the FDA approved a once-monthly injectable extended-release formulation of buprenorphine (Sublocade) for patients previously treated with transmucosally delivered drug for a minimum of 7 days. Sublocade utilizes the Atrigel Delivery System and is provided in prefilled syringes. After subcutaneous administration by health care providers, the delivery system forms a solid depot under the skin which releases active buprenorphine as the depot degrades. If the drug were to be injected IV, the mass formed would likely occlude vessels or form a mobile embolus, either of which could prove fatal. While the drug will not be dispensed directly to patients, the need for patient education is clear.

While buprenorphine's partial μ agonism attenuates abuse liability, diversion and misuse can still occur.[134] Dosage forms combining buprenorphine with the opioid antagonist naloxone, most commonly in a 4:1 mg ratio, were designed to block euphoria if drug is extracted from the sublingual tablets or buccal film and injected IV. Naloxone has limited activity by the transmucosal route and does not interfere with buprenorphine actions when the combination product is used as prescribed.

The addition of buprenorphine to opioid addiction recovery therapeutic options is significant in that it allows recovering patients to receive care from the hands of their own physicians and pharmacists, environments that can be less emotionally stressful than a methadone clinic.[135] Once appropriately trained through the Substance Abuse and Mental Health Services Administration (SAMHSA), physicians may dispense a small supply of buprenorphine (with or without naloxone) to patients in their office. Pharmacists can then dispense the combination product for long-term treatment. Patients in the maintenance phase of therapy require weekly-monthly monitoring, providing opportunities for interprofessional physician-pharmacist collaboration to promote positive patient care outcomes over the duration of recovery.[136] While buprenorphine is more expensive than methadone, the economic and quality-of-life costs to patients over the prolonged time course of recovery may actually be less due to, among other things, fewer office visits.[130,137] Expansion of buprenorphine use in addiction recovery will require greater patient access to SAMHSA-waivered physicians (especially problematic in rural areas), supportive insurance plans and reimbursement rates, interprofessional collaboration (including addiction specialists and counselors), and provider/patient education.[135]

ETORPHINE AND DIPRENORPHINE

Predictably, replacing the N-cyclopropylmethyl substituent of buprenorphine with a methyl group provides a full μ agonist, as seen with etorphine. In addition to an N-methyl group, etorphine's structural differences include the presence of a *n*-propyl chain instead of a *t*-butyl group and a double bond in the *endo*-alkyl group (*endo*-etheno vs buprenorphine's *endo*-ethano bridge). Etorphine is approximately 10,000 to 30,000 times more potent than morphine with an LD50 of 3 μg in humans. This extreme potency makes etorphine too dangerous for use in humans, though it has been widely used in veterinary medicine and as an immobilizer to permit the safe capture and/or handling of zoo animals and large game. Marketed alone or in combination with the sedative antiemetic acetylpromazine, etorphine has enjoyed the descriptive trade names of Captivon and Immobilon, respectively. Buprenorphine can also be converted into a potent and pure opioid antagonist (diprenorphine) simply by replacing the *t*-butyl moiety on the C_7 side chain with methyl group. Under the equally descriptive trade name Revivon, diprenorphine is the specific antidote to etorphine and other extremely potent agonists like carfentanil due to its own high-potency antagonist effects. Nonetheless, diprenorphine is also not safe for use in humans because its weak μ partial agonist effects could exacerbate an overdose. Only a "silent antagonist" like naloxone should be used, even in cases of etorphine or carfentanil overdose.

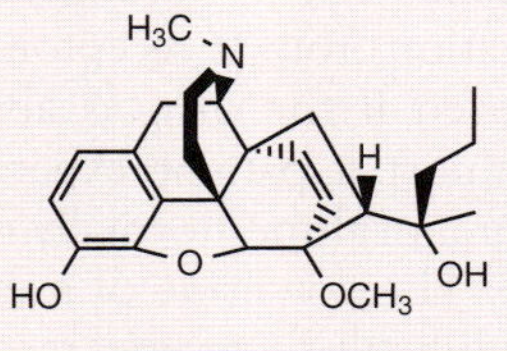

Etorphine

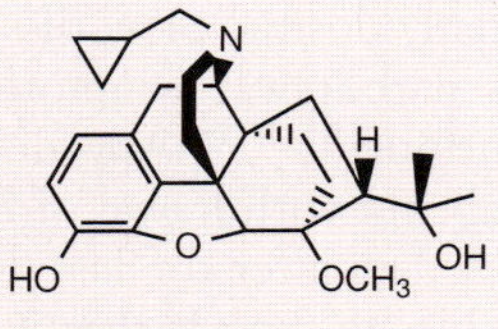

Diprenorphine

Phenanthrene-Based Rigid κ Agonists

NALBUPHINE HYDROCHLORIDE, BUTORPHANOL TARTRATE, AND PENTAZOCINE LACTATE. Replacing μ agonist–directing amine substituents with cyclobutylmethyl (nalbuphine, butorphanol) or dimethylallyl (pentazocine) groups results in clinically useful κ receptor–mediated analgesia (see Figs. 16.4 and 16.5). In analgesic doses, these structures also exhibit partial μ agonism (butorphanol, pentazocine) or partial μ antagonism (nalbuphine), and all will precipitate a withdrawal episode if administered to patients dependent on full μ agonists. They are less commonly utilized for pain control than the rigid μ agonists discussed earlier, possibly because of the risk of drug-induced dysphoria, particularly with pentazocine and butorphanol. Other κ-associated adverse effects include diuresis and sedation, but the risk of respiratory depression, constipation, euphoria, and addiction is lower than for μ agonists. Kappa agonist analgesics are generally more effective and/or longer acting in women, particularly when used in dental pain, and some studies have demonstrated an anti-analgesic effect in men.[138-140]

All three κ analgesics undergo significant first-pass metabolism, and only pentazocine is available in an oral dosage form. Pentazocine tablets contain naloxone in a 100:1 mg ratio to discourage misuse/abuse by drug extraction and IV injection. The major phase I metabolites of each κ agonist are shown in the upcoming sections, and clinically relevant information is provided in Table 16.4.

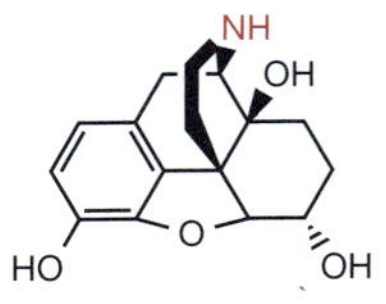

Nornalbuphine

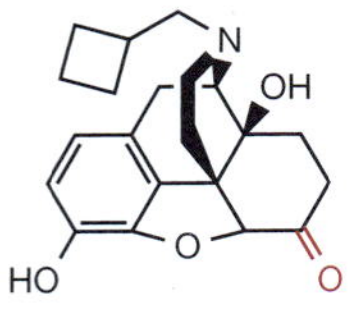

6-Ketonalbuphine

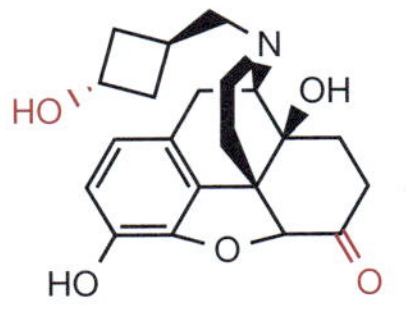

trans-3'-Hydroxybutorphanol

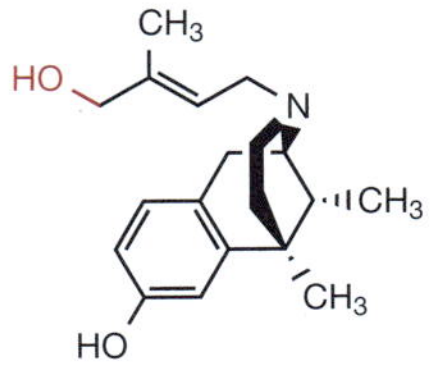

Hydroxypentazocine

Flexible Opioid Agonists

The flexible opioids, including the dual-action agents, are all μ agonists (see Fig. 16.7). The anilidopiperine analgesics fentanyl and alfentanil, along with the dual-action analgesic tramadol, enjoy the most widespread use within this major structural class for the treatment of pain and/or as adjuncts to anesthesia. Methadone is used predominantly in opioid addiction recovery.

Meperidine has fallen out of favor due to its serious adverse effect profile, which includes histamine release, serotonin syndrome, and neurotoxicity, leading to seizures, with the latter attributed to the N-demethylated metabolite, normeperidine. As noted previously, tapentadol has several mechanistic advantages over tramadol, but is not

Table 16.4 Clinically Important Information on Less Commonly Prescribed Opioids

Opioid	Pharmacodynamics	Analgesic Potency (× Morphine)	Dosage Forms	Schedule	Precipitate Withdrawal in μ Agonist–Dependent Patient?
Levorphanol	Mixed μ/κ agonist	4-8	Tab	C-II	No
Nalbuphine	κ agonist/partial μ agonist	0.5-1	Sol for inj	Rx	Yes
Butorphanol	κ agonist/partial μ agonist	5-7	Sol for inj, nas	C-IV	Yes
Pentazocine	κ agonist/partial μ agonist	0.16-0.33	Sol for inj, tab (with naloxone)	C-IV	Yes
Meperidine	Full μ agonist	0.1	Tab, sol for inj, po sol	C-II	No
Sufentanil	Full μ agonist	600-900	Sol for inj	C-II	No
Remifentanil	Full μ agonist	≥80	Sol for inj	C-II	No
Tapentadol	Full μ agonist	0.4-1	Tab, ER tab	C-II	No

ER, extended-release; inj, injection; nas, intranasal; po, oral; Rx, prescription; sol, solution; tab, tablets.

as commonly employed in the clinic. Meperidine and tapentadol, along with sufentanil (a more lipophilic, faster/shorter-acting adjunct to anesthesia than the parent fentanyl), are included in Table 16.4.

FENTANYL BASE AND FENTANYL CITRATE SALT. Fentanyl is a very sedative and euphoria-inducing analgesic with a potency approximately 75 to 100 times that of morphine. The high activity of anilidopiperidines is due, in part, to their very high lipophilicity, which allows them to quickly penetrate the BBB and concentrate in the CNS. Because they also leave the brain quickly, their duration of analgesic action is short (30-60 minutes for fentanyl). Fentanyl citrate and its analogs are commonly administered IV as adjuncts to anesthesia, but all formulations carry the risk of potentially fatal respiratory depression and other common μ-opioid adverse effects.

Transdermal and transmucosal formulations of fentanyl are available to treat chronic pain, including the pain of cancer.[141,142] The transdermal patch formulation releases fentanyl free base to maintain therapeutic blood levels for 72 hours, providing a convenient and reliable mechanism for patients with chronic pain to achieve analgesia at home. Strengths ranging from 12.5 to 100 μg/h are available. Great care must be taken when disposing of used patches so that opioid-naïve individuals do not accidently come in contact with residual drug. Serious toxicity or death can result, with children at particularly high risk. As with transdermal formulations of other high-potency opioids, exposure of fentanyl patches to external heat accelerates drug release and absorption and can have fatal consequences.

Transmucosal formulations of fentanyl in a wide range of strengths are often used to treat chronic and/or breakthrough pain in patients with opioid tolerance and in pediatric burn patients undergoing painful cleansings and dressing changes. While many dosage forms have been discontinued in the United States in recent years, a buccal lozenge "lollipop" of generic fentanyl citrate is marketed in strengths (expressed as free base) ranging from 200 to 1,600 μg. Effervescent buccal tablets (Fentora) containing fentanyl citrate, citric acid, sodium bicarbonate, and sodium carbonate are also available in 100 to 800-μg strengths (expressed as free base). When placed at the back of the mouth between the cheek and gum, the citric acid drops salivary pH to a minimum of 5.0, producing soluble protonated fentanyl. The tablet generally dissolves within 15 to 25 minutes. The dissolved citric acid reacts with sodium bicarbonate and sodium carbonate to generate sodium citrate and carbonic acid (H_2CO_3), which dissociates to CO_2 and H_2O. As CO_2 is expired, citric acid is consumed, and salivary pH rises to 9 to 10. This shifts the fentanyl equilibrium to favor lipophilic fentanyl free base, which is readily absorbed across buccal membranes.[143] The absolute bioavailability is 65%, which represents a 30% greater fentanyl exposure compared to the buccal lozenge. If there is a need to switch a patient from the lozenge to the effervescent tablet, the dose should be cut by 25% to 50% to avoid life-threatening toxicity. This explains why Fentora is marketed in strengths that are half that of the buccal lollipop formulation.

The FDA requires transmucosal immediate-release fentanyl (TIRF) products be prescribed only by practitioners enrolled in and certified by the Risk Evaluation and Mitigation Strategy (TIRF REMS) program. This program carries strict responsibilities for provider education, patient and/or caregiver counseling, and the establishment of formal care agreements with each patient being treated. Prescribers must re-enroll in the TIRF REMS program on a biannual basis. All transdermal and transmucosal dosage forms carry a boxed warning related to unintentional overdose, toxicity, and intentional abuse.

A toxic adverse effect observed in the high-potency μ agonists is a phenomenon called "wooden chest syndrome" (WCS). The effects of WCS are reversed by naloxone, suggesting an opioid receptor–mediated mechanism of action. It is believed that WCS is caused by a release of adrenaline that causes episodic "breath-holding spells," and that cholinergic mechanisms may also contribute. Practitioners should be careful when using naloxone to reverse the effects of WCS, as high doses may put the patient into withdrawal.

Fentanyl is extensively biotransformed via CYP3A4-mediated N-dealkylation to an inactive metabolite, norfentanyl, and practitioners must be alert to the risk for potency-enhancing (CYP3A4 inhibitors or competitors) or attenuating (CYP3A4 inducers) interactions. Anilidopiperidines do not release histamine like meperidine and 6α-hydroxylated phenanthrenes do, and there is no risk of histamine-mediated allergic responses when fentanyl is administered IV. The fentanyl adverse reaction of greatest concern is respiratory depression. This potentially fatal reaction is persistent and can outlast the action of antagonists used to reverse it. The risk is significantly lower with sufentanil and alfentanil, as respiratory depression generally occurs only at doses higher than those needed to relieve pain or support anesthesia.

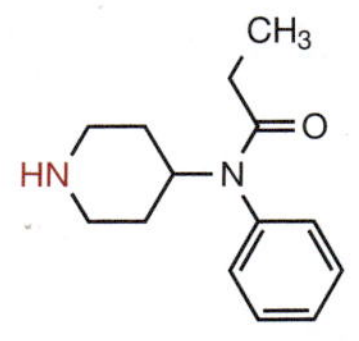

Norfentanyl

ALFENTANIL HYDROCHLORIDE. Alfentanil is the least potent of the currently marketed anilidopiperidine opioids, but it distributes and redistributes across the BBB more rapidly than either fentanyl or sufentanil. Analgesic action begins within 5 minutes of IV administration and lasts between 0.5 to 1 hour. It is commonly administered to patients undergoing very short surgical or medical procedures requiring anesthesia/sedation (eg, colonoscopy). More recently, it has found use in attenuating pain during bedside burn dressing changes in patients with uncompromised respiration.[144]

REMIFENTANIL. Remifentanil hydrochloride (Ultiva) is typically administered to adults as a 0.5- to 1.0-μg/kg/min continuous IV infusion. The shortest-acting of the μ opioid–receptor agonists, remifentanil has a metabolic half-life of 3 to 6 minutes, and recovery occurs within 5 to 10 minutes. The short duration of action is due to the presence of a strategic methyl ester attached to the pyridine N-substituent: this group is rapidly metabolized by plasma and tissue esterases to the corresponding carboxylic acid, which is inactive. This approach of adding a metabolically labile functional group in the hopes that it will shorten duration of effect is called a *soft drug strategy*.

METHADONE HYDROCHLORIDE. Methadone is one of only three marketed opioid analgesics that do not contain a piperidine ring. The N-methyl substituent accurately predicts its μ agonist-activity profile, and the activity-attenuating impact of ketone reduction supports a receptor binding role for the C_3 carbonyl oxygen. There is some evidence to suggest that methadone may function as a β-arrestin-biased μ agonist.[145] While most commonly associated with use in addiction recovery (methadone maintenance), its use as an analgesic is on the rise.[146,147] Despite its complex pharmacological and pharmacokinetic profile, it may be of value in patients who are nonresponsive to other opioids. The hydrochloride salt is marketed as an injectable solution and in a variety of oral dosage forms.

Methadone contains a chiral center and is marketed as the racemic mixture. The *R*(−) isomer is responsible for opioid analgesic action and the *S*(+) enantiomer antagonizes the NMDA receptor.[148] Though NMDA antagonism may be beneficial in neuropathic and opioid-resistant pain, this may contribute to potentially serious cardiovascular toxicities such as a prolonged QT interval and torsades de pointes.[149] The analgesic activity of methadone is shorter than its 1- to 2-day elimination half-life would suggest, and it can induce respiratory depression that outlasts the analgesic phase. Methadone's naturally long half-life is due in part to the generation of several active metabolites (Fig. 16.12), and it can be significantly increased in basified urine. Deaths from cardiac arrhythmia and respiratory depression have been noted, particularly as the drug is being introduced and/or the dose titrated. Dosing more frequently than once daily can allow drug accumulation, which sets the stage for serious and/or potentially fatal toxicity.

A review of methadone metabolism and transport has called into question the long-held belief in the pivotal role of CYP3A4 in methadone N-demethylation. Kharasch[148] summarized studies that demonstrated no impact of this isoform on single-dose methadone metabolism and clearance, and stated that methadone is not a CYP3A4 substrate. Rather, evidence was provided that identified CYP2B6 as the preferential methadone dealkylating isoform and confirmed previous understanding of its stereoselective action [*S*(+) > *R*(−)]. Evaluation of methadone plasma levels in patients of varying CYP2B6 genotype documented elevated concentrations in PMs (*CYP2B6*6*) compared to EMs (*CYP2B6*1*), with the lowest concentrations of parent drug coming from ultrarapid metabolizers (UMs) (*CYP2B6*4*). The metabolic autoinduction known to occur over the first weeks of methadone therapy was attributed to CYP2B6 upregulation. Kharasch referred to the continued reference to CYP3A4-catalyzed methadone metabolism in literature and tertiary drug information resources as "CYP3A inertia." Because of the risk of serious/fatal cardiac and respiratory toxicity, pharmacists should be vigilant with regard to

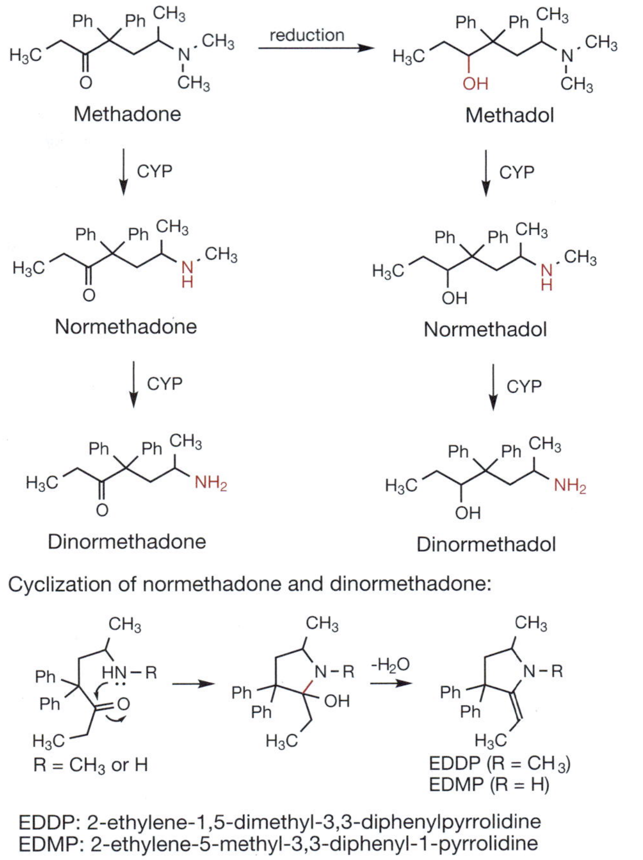

Figure 16.12 Methadone metabolism. The N-dealkylated and reduced alcohol derivatives at the top are all active. Cyclization of normethadone and dinormethadone results in inactive products EDDP (2-ethylene-1,5-dimethyl-3,3-diphenylpyrrolidine) and EDMP (2-ethylene-5-methyl-3,3-diphenyl-1-pyrrolidine).

monitoring for metabolism-related interactions with CYP competitors, inhibitors, and inducers.

The *N*-dealkylated metabolites of methadone (but not methadol) can cyclize to form inactive pyrrolidine-based structures that are found in the urine of patients on methadone (see Fig. 16.12). These compounds are commonly known as EDDP (2-ethylene-1,5-dimethyl-3,3-diphenylpyrrolidine) and EDMP (2-ethylene-5-methyl-3,3-diphenyl-1-pyrrolidine), which are acronyms for their chemical names. The parent drug is incapable of generating a cyclic pyrrolidine metabolite because the N,N-dimethyl substitution pattern of the parent drug provides steric hindrance to nucleophilic attack by the unionized amine at the electrophilic carbonyl carbon. EDDP, and to a lesser extent EDMP, has recently been shown to be mechanism-based inhibitors of CYP2C19.[150] EDDP has an elimination half-life of 40 to 48 hours.

As noted, methadone has found its greatest use in addiction recovery programs. Its high oral bioavailability, long duration of action, daily dosing regimen, slow tolerance development, and relative lack of physical dependence are beneficial advantages in its use in medication-assisted treatment (MAT). Unlike buprenorphine, methadone used in addiction recovery is administered in strictly regulated federal- and state-licensed methadone clinics, commonly under direct supervision. The drug is administered in water or an acidic juice to ensure solubility and avoid unintended buccal absorption of unionized drug. If buccal absorption is required (eg, patients with swallowing disorders), a basified solution can be held in the mouth for 2.5 minutes before expectorating.

Patients receiving methadone maintenance therapy are titrated upward from an initial 20- to 30-mg daily dose to a maintenance daily dose that is most commonly 80 to 120 mg.[133] Therapy usually continues over 1 to 2 (or more) years. Compliance can be tracked by quantifying urinary levels of EDDP and calculating the EDDP/urine creatinine ratio. This analytical technique provides results related to the consumed quantity of methadone that are independent of patient hydration status and resistant to attempts to adulterate the sample with agents like soap, bleach, or methadone itself.[151] When the time is right to discontinue methadone, any withdrawal symptoms experienced will generally be mild due to the prolonged duration of action of the drug and the presence of multiple active metabolites. However, the patient will still be both tolerant to, and dependent on, methadone, which, unlike buprenorphine, is not a pseudoirreversible μ agonist. Therefore, the protocol for medically supervised drug discontinuation involves a "stair-step" dose-attenuation process, with reductions of less than 10% of the maintenance dose taking place no sooner than every 10 to 14 days.

TRAMADOL HYDROCHLORIDE. The dual mechanism of tramadol's analgesic action is complex and time-dependent.[152] Over time, as the parent isomers are O-dealkylated to phenolic metabolites, the μ receptor–agonist component of activity increases, while the monoamine reuptake–inhibition mechanism decreases. The μ-receptor affinity of the (+) phenol is 300 times that of the parent drug and is the clinically relevant opioid entity. As in codeine analogs, CYP2D6 catalyzes the O-dealkylation reaction, and patients deficient in this isoform will either not experience the μ-agonist component of tramadol's action or require dosage increases of up to 30%. Inactivating glucuronide or sulfate conjugation of the phenol will occur prior to urinary excretion. CYP3A4 and CYP2B6 catalyze inactivating N-dealkylation to secondary and primary amine metabolites.[108]

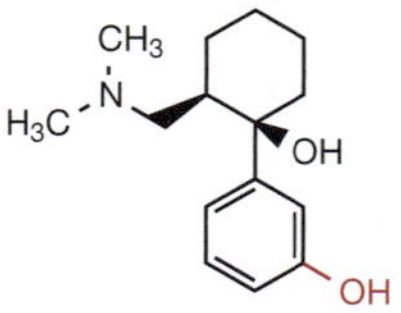

1*R*,2*R*-(+)-*O*-Desmethyltramadol (μ agonist)

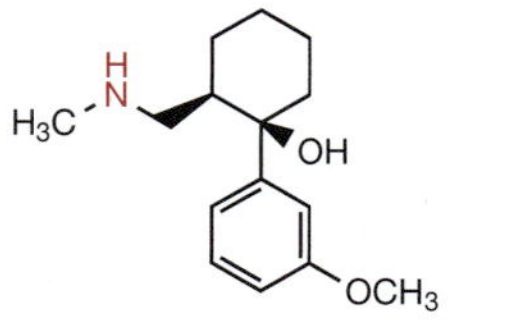

1*R*,2*R*-(+)-Nortramadol (inactive)

Since the (+) 1*R*,2*R* isomer of tramadol inhibits 5-HT reuptake, it has the potential to induce or exacerbate serotonin syndrome, a potentially life-threatening condition.[153] The symptoms of serotonin syndrome include neuromuscular hyperactivity with loss of coordination, cardiovascular and pulmonary distress, and cognitive dysfunction. Patients at greatest risk include those of advanced age and/or on high-dose therapy, coadministration of selective serotonin-reuptake inhibitor (SSRI) antidepressants or CYP2D6 inhibitors, and CYD2D6 PM phenotype.[153-155] Tramadol is not recommended in suicidal patients due to the elevation of central 5-HT.

Tramadol also carries a risk of seizure, especially in patients taking drugs that increase central levels of monoamines or whose seizure threshold is otherwise reduced. Seizures have been documented in doses as low as 200 mg (which is close to the maintenance dose of 50-100 mg) and generally occur within 6 hours of drug ingestion. Tramadol generally induces less respiratory depression, constipation, and abuse liability than other opioids, but withdrawal symptoms have been noted upon abrupt discontinuation. Life-threatening respiratory depression risk is increased in patients of CYP2D6 UM phenotype[156] and in children younger than age 12 years. As a result, the FDA issued a safety alert in April 2017 restricting tramadol use in preteen patients. GI distress and sedation are the most commonly reported adverse effects.[108]

Tramadol is available in immediate-release tablets, administered every 4 to 6 hours, and extended-release tablets and capsules (ConZip), administered once daily. An oral solution (Qdolo) and kits for compounding tramadol into a suspension (Synapryn FusePaq) or a cream (EnovaRx) formulation are also marketed. Tramadol has demonstrated efficacy in chronic pain of moderate intensity, including low back pain and the pain of rheumatoid arthritis. Although further studies are needed, the drug may have a place in the treatment of premature ejaculation.[157]

Biased μ Opioid–Receptor Agonists

OLICERIDINE (OLINVYK). Oliceridine is a first-in-class medication that is a G-protein–biased μ opioid–receptor agonist. As discussed, a "biased agonist" is one that stabilizes a GPCR in a conformation that only allows signaling through a single intracellular signaling pathway. In this case, oliceridine biases the μ receptor toward $G_{\alpha i}$ signaling and away from β-arrestin signaling. The theory is that β-arrestin signaling specifically contributes toward the adverse effects of μ agonists, namely respiratory depression and constipation, whereas the therapeutic analgesic effects of μ agonism are associated with $G_{\alpha i}$. As the theory goes, the $G_{\alpha i}$-biased oliceridine would have a diminished impact on these adverse events. In practice, however, oliceridine shares a qualitatively similar adverse effect profile as canonical μ agonists, including drug reward. For these reasons, the US DEA placed oliceridine under Schedule II of the Controlled Substances Act. Oliceridine is only available as an IV injection due to poor oral bioavailability, though other analogs, such as TRV734, are currently in clinical trials as orally available biased μ agonists. The promise of biased μ agonists has not yet lived up to the hype, fueling questions about their past and future: perhaps the currently available pharmacologic techniques are not yet capable of truly measuring bias, or whether in vitro measures can be translated into living systems.

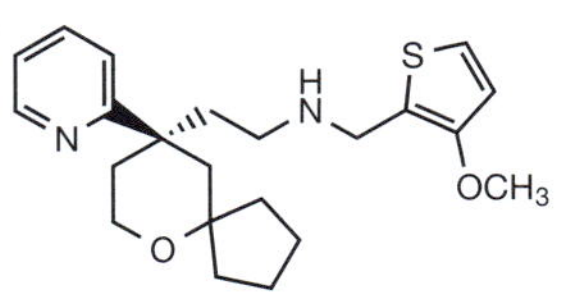

Oliceridine

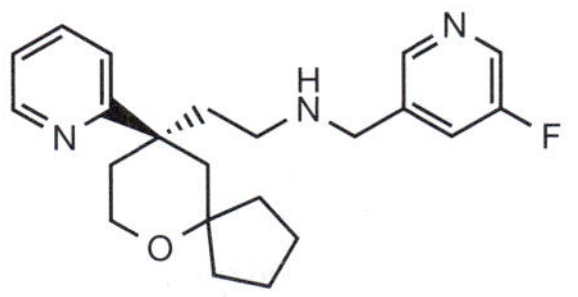

TRV734

NOTABLE NATURAL PRODUCTS: SALVIA AND KRATOM

Many plant-based natural products have been tested over the years for analgesic activity in the hopes of finding analgesics with an improved adverse effect profile as compared to existing agents. Two examples are worth discussing due to their complex opioid pharmacology. Salvia divinorum, also known as ska maria pastora, diviner's sage, or simply "salvia," is a member of the mint family that grows in Oaxaca, Mexico and has been used by Mazatec shamans for centuries in divination rituals. The hallucinogenic principle, salvinorin A, was discovered in 2002 to be a potent, selective κ opioid receptor agonist.[158] Salvinorin A is a unique opioid ligand in that it does not contain a basic amine group, and thus binds receptors by different mechanisms. An analog, named herkinorin, was discovered to be a high-potency, high-affinity μ opioid–receptor biased agonist, one of the first biased μ agonists reported.[159] Another notable plant is a member of the coffee family, *Mitragynine speciosa*, also known as kratom. *M. speciosa* grows naturally in Southeast Asia and has two uses by the local population: at low doses, kratom tea produces mild psychostimulant effects, and at higher doses kratom produces mild opioid-like analgesic actions. The main psychoactive principle, mitragynine, has an indole alkaloid structure that shares little structural similarity to other known opioid ligands. Extensive research into the psychoactivity profile of mitragynine and its metabolite, 7-hydroxymitragynine, suggests that the mechanisms of action of these secondary metabolites are complex, and include activity at opioid receptors, adrenergic receptors, and 5-HT receptors.[160] Kratom products are increasingly available in the United States, and, like any alternative or natural medicine, pharmacists and healthcare providers should be aware that they are not regulated for content or purity in the same way as FDA-approved medications.

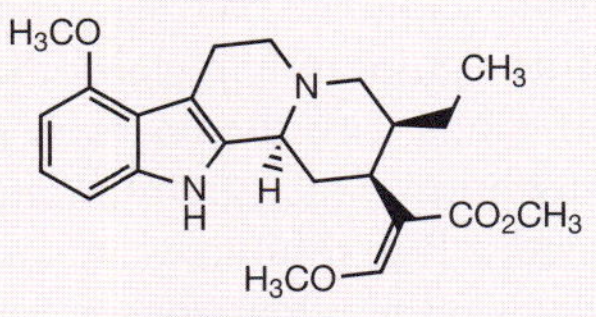

Mitragynine

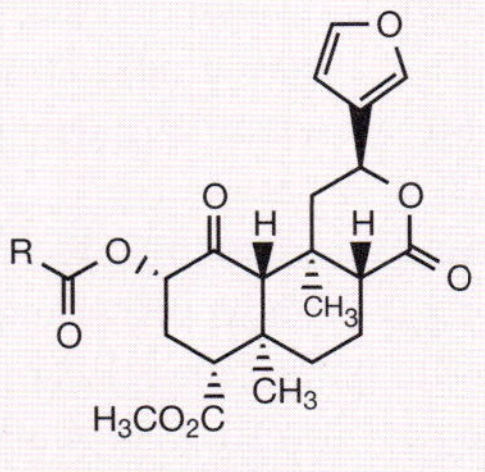

R = CH_3, Salvinorin A
R = C_6H_5, Herkinorin

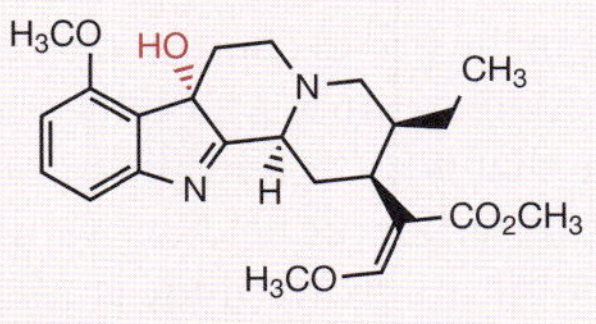

7-Hydroxymitragynine

Opioid Antagonists

NALOXONE HYDROCHLORIDE AND NALTREXONE HYDROCHLORIDE. Two pure opioid antagonists are marketed to reverse the central actions of opioid agonists, although they antagonize peripheral opioid receptors with equal ease. They both have a classic antagonist-directing amine substituent on a pentacyclic scaffold and contain the requisite 14β-OH and the 7,8-dihydro-6-one C ring (see Fig. 16.5). With a four-carbon *N*-cyclopropylmethyl substituent, naltrexone is twice as potent as the allyl-substituted naloxone, presumably due to enhanced distribution to central sites of action (see Fig. 16.4).

As noted earlier, each antagonist is incorporated into selected oral dosage forms of potent μ agonists to thwart misuse and abuse by agonist extraction and IV or intranasal administration. Either antagonist can rescue patients from life-threatening opioid overdose, but only naloxone carries that indication. Naloxone undergoes extensive glucuronide conjugation in the gut and liver and, therefore, is useful as a deterrent in combination products that are not administered parenterally. In selected states, naloxone hydrochloride autoinjector (Evzio) and nasal spray (Narcan) formulations are being made available to first responders, teachers, family, and others likely to come into contact with individuals experiencing life-threatening overdose ("buddy-administration"), as well as to opioid-dependent persons for self-injection. More recently, it has been made available from community pharmacies; in most states no prescription is needed. Naloxone is also marketed in solution for IV or IM administration in the clinical setting.

In contrast, naltrexone has sufficient bioavailability (5%-40%) for oral administration, which enhances its utility in outpatient opioid dependence and alcoholism recovery programs. Naltrexone is effective in patients with alcohol use disorder because it blocks the activity of μ-agonist endorphins that are released when a patient consumes ethanol. It is available in 50-mg tablets and as a suspension for IM injection. Patients should be opioid-free for 7 to 10 days prior to initiating relapse prophylaxis therapy. Naltrexone's major metabolite is 6β-naltrexol, which is produced by dehydrogenase-mediated reduction. Naltrexone is not readily metabolized by CYP enzymes.

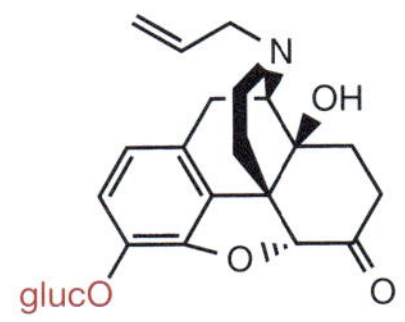

Naloxone-3-glucuronide

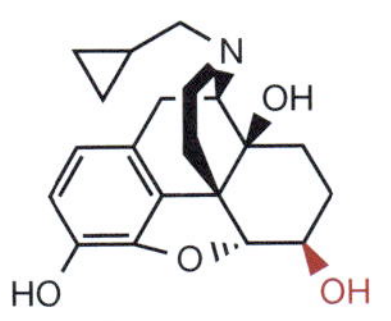

6β-*N*altrexol

In synergistic combination with a sustained-release formulation of the atypical antidepressant bupropion, sustained-release naltrexone was approved for use in the treatment of obesity in adult populations in 2014. A review of clinical efficacy and safety data for this combination product (Contrave), along with a summary of pharmacodynamic and kinetic profiles of each agent, has been published.[161] Preliminary data also indicate a potential role for low-dose naltrexone (LDN, 4.5 mg/d) in inducing remission in Crohn disease, possibly by stimulating production of Met-enkephalin, which attenuates cell proliferation through a receptor-mediated process.[162,163] The mechanisms by which LDN is effective at treating pain—for example, in cases of autoimmune disease and multiple sclerosis, are incompletely understood.

Peripherally Restricted μ Antagonists: Methylnaltrexone Bromide, Naloxegol Oxalate, Naldemedine Tosylate, and Alvimopan. Unlike centrally acting naloxone and naltrexone, methylnaltrexone bromide (Relistor), naloxegol (PEGylated naloxol, Movantik), naldemedine (Symproic), and Alvimopan (Entereg) were designed to work as prokinetic agents in the gut to reverse the intractable constipation that is a hallmark of long-term μ opioid use (Fig. 16.13). OIC impacts up to 40% of patients on chronic opioid therapy (some sources claim up to 90%), with older adults and patients with cancer at higher risk. Tolerance to this adverse effect does not develop. OIC has a very negative impact on quality of life and can limit the dose of opioid prescribed to manage pain.[164] These peripherally selective antagonists will displace agonist from intestinal μ receptors and restore GI motility and bowel tone. Since none of these drugs penetrates the BBB to any significant extent,[165] they will not precipitate a withdrawal episode in opioid-dependent patients suffering from OIC. Review articles on the action, efficacy, and safety of peripherally acting μ opioid–receptor antagonists (PAMORAs) have been published.[165,166]

The molecular mechanisms that keep these agents from entering the CNS are related to their physicochemical properties, namely drug polarity and charge: methylnaltrexone bromide is a quaternary ammonium salt; the polyethylene glycol (PEG) group present at the 6 position of naloxegol adds significant polarity and molecular size; naldemedine has a high polar surface area (141.18 Å^2); and alvimopan has weakly acidic and basic groups that are both charged at physiologic pH. Because these compounds are peripherally restricted due to physicochemical properties and not active efflux mechanisms, there is no concern that they will become centrally bioavailable, for example due to a drug-drug or drug-herb interaction.

Opioid antagonist therapy for OIC is recommended when dietary and activity-related modifications and maintenance laxatives have been less than optimally effective in restoring bowel function. Abdominal pain is the most common adverse effect, and patients with bowel obstructions should not receive these drugs until the blockage has been fully resolved. Laxatives should be discontinued for at least 3 days while antagonist therapy is established. They can then be reintroduced if the antagonist does not produce satisfactory results.

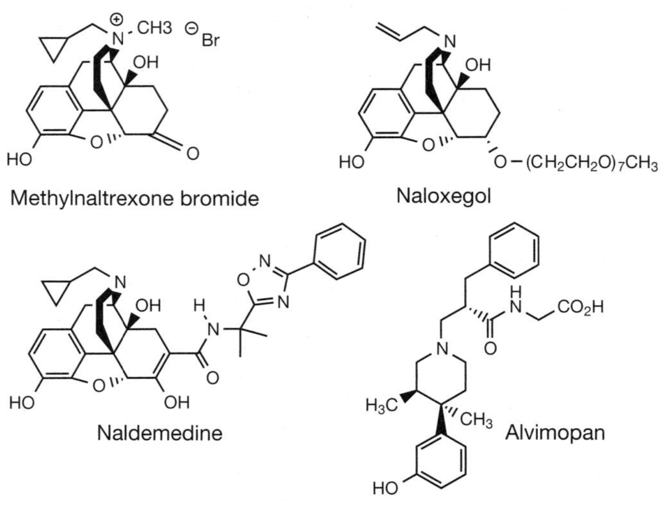

Figure 16.13 Peripherally restricted μ antagonists.

Methylnaltrexone bromide[166,167] is administered orally (450 mg daily) or by subcutaneous injection. In seriously ill patients, the subcutaneous dose is based on patient weight and initiated on an every-other-day schedule. If warranted, the frequency can be increased to a maximum of once daily. OIC associated with chronic noncancer pain is often treated orally or with a daily 12-mg injection. The permanently water-soluble drug is excreted in the urine and feces primarily unchanged. The biotransformation that does occur involves reduction of the 6-keto group to isomeric alcohols and phenol sulfonation, so CYP-related drug-drug interactions are of little concern.

Naloxegol is dosed at 25 mg once daily, although 12.5 mg daily can be administered to patients with significant renal dysfunction or who do not tolerate the higher dose. The drug should be taken 1 to 2 hours before the morning meal to ensure an empty stomach. As naloxegol is N- and O-dealkylated by CYP3A4 prior to predominantly fecal elimination, coadministration with CYP substrates, inducers, or inhibitors (including grapefruit juice) should be avoided or undertaken with care. For example, removal of the 6-O-PEG group would result in 6α-naloxol, which would be a centrally bioavailable μ antagonist. Naloxegol is also a substrate for P-gp, suggesting that coadministration with strong P-gp inhibitors could increase central bioavailability and block the effects of μ agonists[165]; however, passive permeability of naloxegol is low, and this interaction is not believed to be clinically relevant.[168,169]

Naldemedine is structurally related to naltrexone, where a 7-position functionalized amide group increases molecular size and polarity. Naldemedine[170] has many properties in common with naloxegol, including CYP3A4-catalyzed N-dealkylation to an active secondary amine metabolite. Coadministration of CYP3A4 competitors or inhibitors can increase the risk of adverse effects, and grapefruit juice should be avoided. C_3-glucuronidation is minor, but a significant fraction undergoes amide hydrolysis in the gut to produce naldemedine carboxylic acid. Like naloxegol, naldemedine has affinity for P-gp, but its significantly higher binding to serum proteins (94% vs 4%), along with the relatively polar C_7 side chain, limits BBB penetration. Still, careful monitoring for adverse effects is warranted if P-gp inhibitors are coadministered. Unlike naloxegol, there is no requirement for administration on an empty stomach, and the drug and its metabolites are excreted primarily in the urine (57%) compared to feces (35%).

Alvimopan is an orally administered benzazocine derivative that is hydrolyzed by the action of gut flora to provide an active carboxylic acid derivative. Both the parent and this metabolite are zwitterionic at physiologic pH, limiting bioavailability (6%) and permeability across the BBB. There is minimal hepatic metabolism, and the drug is excreted primarily by secretion into the bile.[171] This PAMORA is administered exclusively in the inpatient setting to treat postsurgical ileus. Institutions providing the drug must be registered with the Entereg Access Support Education (EASE) program, which assures that providers are appropriately instructed on its actions and use restrictions. Patients receive one dose prior to surgery and up to 14 additional doses administered twice daily for a maximum of 7 days. The use of alvimopan accelerates bowel function recovery without antagonizing opioid analgesia and can result in shorter hospital stays.[172]

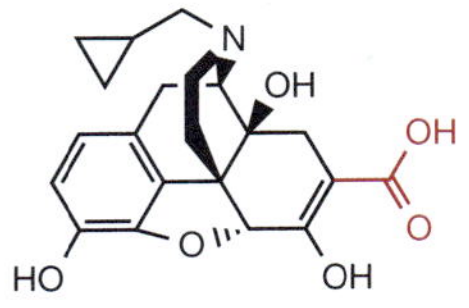

Naldemedine carboxylic acid

Alvimopan carboxylic acid

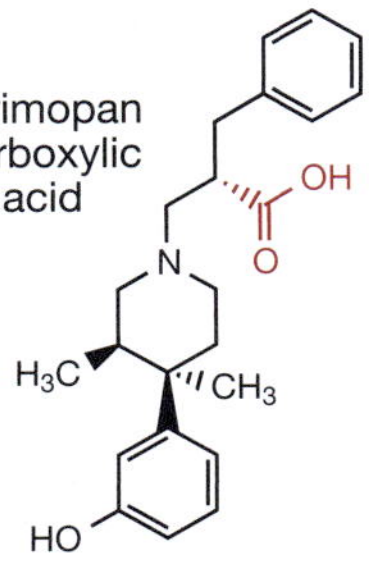

Peripherally Restricted μ Agonists: Antidiarrheals

"You've probably been asked to care about things like HIV/AIDS or TB or measles, but diarrhea kills more children than all those three things put together. It's a very potent weapon of mass destruction."

Rose George

As previously discussed, OIC is one of the most discomforting and, at times, serious complications of opioid analgesic use. However, medicinal chemists, following the old adage "When life hands you lemons, make lemonade," have modified the structure of the flexible μ agonist meperidine to limit BBB penetration without compromising GI mobility inhibition.[173] Two orally administered peripherally selective μ agonists, diphenoxylate and loperamide (Fig. 16.14), have enjoyed significant therapeutic use as antidiarrheals for years. A newer medication, eluxadoline, was approved in 2015.

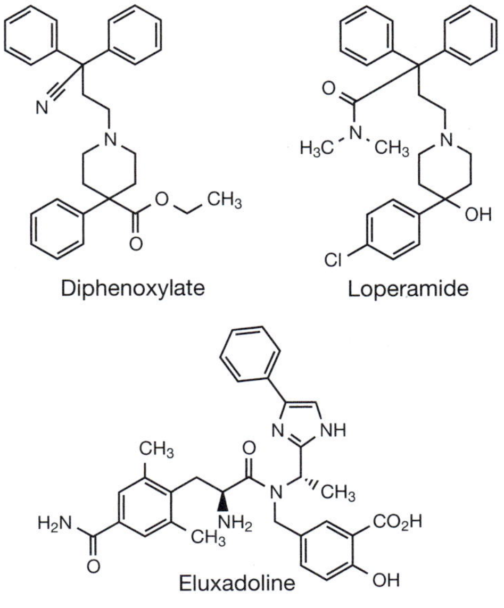

Figure 16.14 Peripherally restricted μ agonists.

Diphenoxylate Hydrochloride

Diphenoxylate (Lomotil) bears a close resemblance to the parent meperidine structure (see Fig. 16.8). The only chemical difference between the two compounds is the nature of the amine substituent; meperidine has the prototypical μ agonist-directing methyl group while diphenoxylate has a more complex 3,3,-diphenyl-3-cyanopropyl functional group. The ethylcarboxylate ester is readily cleaved by plasma esterases, yielding a carboxylic acid metabolite that is approximately 5 times as active as diphenoxylate as an antidiarrheal. The zwitterionic metabolite, which is marketed as difenoxin, does not readily distribute into the CNS in therapeutic doses. In higher doses, the chemical reluctance to cross the BBB is overcome, and central μ receptors can be stimulated.

For reasons both therapeutic (anticholinergic) and abuse related, diphenoxylate and difenoxin are only available in combination with atropine sulfate. If a potential abuser attempts to extract the antidiarrheal agent with the intent to inject and abuse, the atropine will also be extracted and injected, leading to nausea, weakness, sedation, and annoying peripheral effects such as dry mouth, blurred vision, and urinary retention. The diphenoxylate combination product is a Schedule V drug, indicating that there is a slight potential for abuse and/or addiction, whereas the difenoxin combination product is classified as Schedule IV (a medically useful drug with a low potential for abuse and/or addiction). If used alone, these antidiarrheals would be classified as Schedule II agents, indicating that they have a significant potential for abuse and/or addiction without the atropine "safety net."

Loperamide Hydrochloride

Loperamide (Imodium) is a nonhydrolyzable amide analog of meperidine that is available over the counter (OTC) for the treatment of diarrhea. Meperidine's ethylcarboxylate ester has been replaced by a tertiary hydroxyl group, and the phenyl ring has been chlorinated at the *para* position. The amine substituent is reminiscent of that incorporated into diphenoxylate, although a dimethylamide moiety has replaced the nitrile. While the highly lipophilic drug (Log P_{calc} 4.44) acts as a full μ-receptor agonist in the gut, it lacks central μ agonist action due to very low oral bioavailability and extensive P-gp-mediated exclusion from the CNS.[174,175] In contrast to diphenoxylate, which is not a P-gp substrate,[176] loperamide was assumed to have no potential for abuse, which allowed it to be available without a prescription.[177] In addition to and/or in concert with its μ agonist action, loperamide's GI motility inhibition has been linked to the μ agonist-mediated release of 5-HT[178] and calcium-channel antagonism.[179]

N-Demethylation of loperamide's tertiary amide is catalyzed by CYP3A4 and CYP2C8.[180] While few interactions with CYP3A4 substrates have been reported, clinically relevant interactions are known to occur with P-gp inducers (decreased serum concentrations) and inhibitors (increased serum concentrations). Significant first-pass metabolism minimizes oral bioavailability. Desmethylloperamide, the major metabolite, does not bind to μ receptors and is inactive as an antidiarrheal.

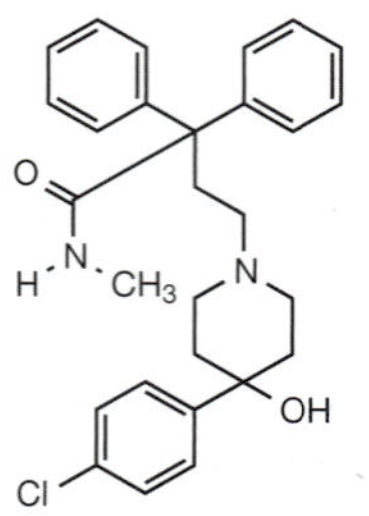

N-Desmethylloperamide

Loperamide has been compared favorably to diphenoxylate with regard to potency, duration and specificity of action, and safety margin.[173] However, the misuse/abuse of this drug, termed the "poor man's methadone" because of its ready availability and low cost, is currently on the rise. Data collected from the National Poison Data System show a consistent uptick in intentional misuse of loperamde from around 100 cases reported in 2009 to nearly 400 in 2017.[181] When taken in doses 40 to 100 times, the recommended maximum dose of 8 (OTC) to 16 (Rx) mg per day, loperamide can saturate P-gp, cross the BBB, and induce euphoria or attenuate withdrawal symptoms.[175] The drug is cardiotoxic when taken chronically at these high doses. Prolonged QTc interval, widened QRS complex, ventricular tachycardia, torsades de pointes, heart block, and sudden cardiac death have all been documented. Interference with myocardial Na^+/K^+-channel conductivity, including blockade of the hERG K^+ channel, has been proposed as a possible arrhythmogenic mechanism.[175,182] Symptoms can persist for as long as 4 to 5 days, and treatment sometimes requires an overdrive pacemaker in addition to drugs like lidocaine, amiodarone, isoproterenol, and metoprolol. In 2016, the FDA issued a warning about the risk of potentially fatal cardiotoxicity due to loperamide misuse/abuse.

Eluxadoline

While not currently as commonly used as diphenoxylate and loperamide, eluxadoline (Viberzi) is indicated for use in irritable bowel syndrome with diarrhea. Eluxadoline has a complex opioid receptor profile, with μ- and κ-agonist and δ-antagonist actions, and it acts directly in the GI tract to inhibit motility and ease discomfort. The δ-antagonist effects of eluxadoline are thought to attenuate the development of constipation that is sometimes observed when patients take loperamide or diphenoxylate for long periods of time. Nonetheless, constipation was noted in phase 3 clinical trials.[183] Administration with food decreases T_{max} from 2 to 1.5 hours, although a high-fat meal cuts C_{max} in half.[91] The standard dose is 75 to 100 mg twice daily. Eluxadoline is a substrate and an inhibitor of the hepatic OATP1B1 carrier protein, and the lower dose is used if coadministered with other drugs also known to inhibit this transporter.

Eluxadoline is 81% protein bound and excreted primarily in feces. The complete metabolic pathway has not been determined, but glucuronic acid conjugation of the carboxylic acid moiety is believed to occur. Adverse effects are predominantly GI-related and include nausea, abdominal pain, and constipation. Therapy should be discontinued if severe constipation develops.

Drugs Used to Treat Neuropathic Pain

"We may not look sick, but turn our bodies inside out and they would tell different stories."

—Wade Sutherland

It has been estimated that 25% of the US population suffers from neuropathic pain, which represents an enormous public health burden.[184] Most of this pain is peripheral in origin, arising from injury, trauma (including surgical trauma), or disease such as diabetes or polio, with the remainder arising from CNS disorders such as Parkinson disease, multiple sclerosis, and phantom limb pain. Individual differences in pain perception, along with mechanism-related complexity and varied concurrent pain sensations, complicate the diagnosis of this pervasive type of pain despite the availability of a variety of validated screening and assessment tools.[17,185,186] However, an accurate diagnosis is critical, since many OTC analgesics that patients might independently gravitate to from past experience in treating nociceptive pain are ineffective in neuropathic pain.

The Neuropathic Pain Special Interest Group of the International Association for the Study of Pain has developed evidence-based guidelines to assist practitioners in approaching therapy,[187] and a review of neuropathic pain management from etiology to contemporary approaches to treatment has been published.[17] Treatment options include pharmacotherapy and procedures such as spinal cord stimulation, radiotherapy, nerve block, and neurofeedback. Levels of proinflammatory cytokines are known to be elevated during times of pain flare and may potentially serve as biomarkers to assist in the evaluation of various therapeutic interventions.[184]

A number of drugs and natural products have been tested in neuropathic pain, including μ opioid–receptor agonists, cannabinoids, angiotensin-receptor blockers, dynorphin A, Botulinum toxin A, and ziconotide. Currently, only a few selected anticonvulsants (pregabalin, gabapentin), 5-HT- and/or NE-reuptake inhibitors (duloxetine), and antidepressants (amitriptyline, nortriptyline, desipramine) are considered first-line therapy.[17,188] The topically applied local anesthetic lidocaine and the chili pepper extract capsaicin are second-line drugs for this indication (Fig. 16.15).[17,188-190]

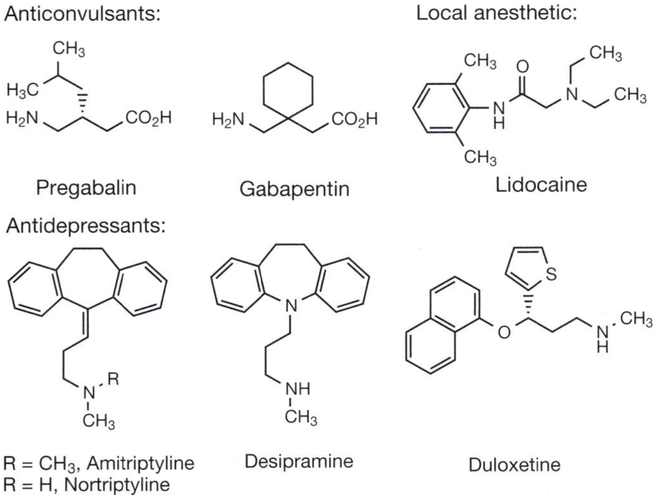

Figure 16.15 Medications most commonly used to treat neuropathic pain.

DRUGS LESS COMMONLY USED TO TREAT NEUROPATHIC PAIN

- Carbamazepine
- Lacosamide
- Oxcarbazepine
- Tramadol
- Venlafaxine
- Metanex

Pregabalin and Gabapentin

Pregabalin (Lyrica) and gabapentin (Neurontin) are anticonvulsant ligands of the α_2-δ subunit of central voltage-gated calcium channels, and they inhibit the release of several excitatory neurotransmitters, including glutamate and substance P. Immediate-release formations are dosed twice (pregabalin) or 3 times (gabapentin) daily, with the standard daily dose of gabapentin between 3 and 6 times that of pregabalin.

Pregabalin has demonstrated efficacy in a wide variety of peripheral and central neuropathic pathologies, including fibromyalgia, diabetic peripheral neuropathy, postherpetic neuralgia, and pain resulting from neuromas and spinal cord injury. It is well absorbed orally and follows linear pharmacokinetics. Its metabolism in humans is negligible, leading to 90% being recovered in the urine as unchanged zwitterionic drug. The N-methylated derivative, the major metabolite, accounts for only 0.9% of the dose. The lack of interaction with metabolizing enzymes and the absence of protein binding leads to essentially no drug-drug interactions. However, synergism with other CNS depressants may be noted. Among the more concerning adverse effects are suicidal ideation, angio- and peripheral edema, thrombocytopenia, vision disturbances, and myopathy secondary to elevated creatine kinase.[91]

Similar to pregabalin, zwitterionic gabapentin has negligible protein binding (<3%) and is metabolism-resistant. The entire dose is renally excreted as unchanged drug. Unlike pregabalin, its use is restricted to postherpetic neuralgia, and the pharmacokinetics of the immediate-release formulation are nonlinear. Due to a saturable L-amino acid transport-facilitated absorption process, there is a "ceiling effect" limiting bioavailability at high doses. Gabapentin enacarbil is an extended-release prodrug preparation marketed as Horizant and is also actively absorbed via monocarboxylate transporter-1 (MCT-1). Hydrolysis to the active gabapentin metabolite is predominantly intestinal, and the time to peak serum concentrations is essentially twice that of the immediate-release formulation (3 vs 6 hours). Gabapentin tablets (immediate and extended release), capsules, and oral solutions are marketed. Suspensions and cream formulations can also be extemporaneously compounded. Adverse effects shared with pregabalin include sedation, vertigo, vision disturbances, impaired thinking, and edema leading to weight gain.

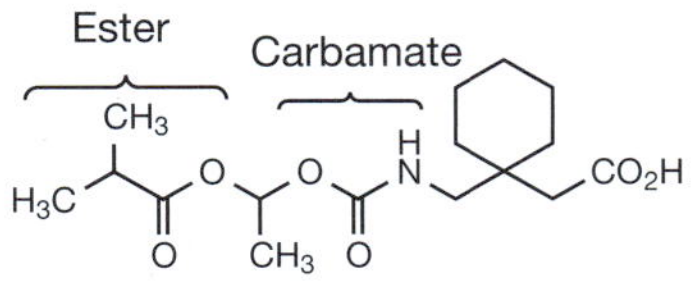

Gabapentin enacarbil

Duloxetine Hydrochloride

Duloxetine hydrochloride (Cymbalta) is dosed at 60 mg once daily in diabetic neuropathy and titrated to no more than 60 mg daily after a 7-day initial regimen of 30 mg daily in fibromyalgia. Gradual dose increases can also be employed in patients with diabetic peripheral neuropathy if tolerance is an issue. Its relatively early onset of pain relief (typically within the first week) is in contrast to the 2 to 3 weeks it may take to elicit a sustained antidepressant effect. However, the dual action is viewed as particularly beneficial in patients with these comorbidities.[190]

Duloxetine is over 90% protein bound and extensively metabolized by the highly polymorphic CYP2D6 (N-demethylation) and CYP1A2 (aromatic hydroxylation), leading to a high risk of drug-drug interactions. CYP1A2 is induced by cigarette smoke, and smokers experience a 33% decrease in duloxetine bioavailability.[91] Nausea, sedation, and constipation are among the most common adverse effects. Morning administration may help attenuate any negative impact on sleep quality.[17,190]

Tricyclic Antidepressants

The secondary TCAs desipramine and nortriptyline selectively inhibit NE reuptake, while tertiary TCAs (eg, amitriptyline) inhibit the reuptake of 5-HT in parent form, and NE once N-dealkylated by CYP2D6. Numerous studies have confirmed the efficacy of TCAs in the treatment of neuropathic pain, particularly diabetic peripheral neuropathy and postherpetic neuralgia, although it can take up to 8 weeks for the maximum benefit to be realized.[189] TCA-induced analgesia is independent of the antidepressant effect but, as with duloxetine, these agents are frequently used in depressed patients suffering with neuropathic pain. The marked anticholinergic actions associated with tertiary TCAs, including their cardiovascular adverse effects, have led to a preference for the secondary amine derivatives. This is particularly true in older adults at risk for falls and fractures, mental confusion or hallucinations, vision impairment, heart block, and/or sedation. While daily doses of 25 to 150 mg are allowed, the risk of sudden death is minimized if doses are kept to less than 100 mg/d.[189]

Lidocaine and Capsaicin

The local anesthetic lidocaine (Lidoderm) and the transient receptor potential vanilloid 1 (TRPV1) agonist capsaicin (Qutenza) are topical agents available in patch form for the treatment of localized peripheral neuropathic pain.[17,188,191] While the body of evidence for the efficacy of 8% capsaicin is stronger than for 5% lidocaine, the higher safety margin of the latter has kept it in the second-line therapeutic category.

Lidocaine inhibits nerve conduction by blocking voltage-gated sodium channels and it is used in postherpetic neuralgia. Up to three patches (the maximum daily dose) may be applied to painful intact skin and left in place for 12 hours. Approximately 3% of the dose reaches the general circulation. A study of lidocaine metabolism in healthy human skin documents the formation of the monoethylglycine xylidide (MEGX) metabolite in quantities less than 12.8% of the amount of drug found in skin after a 2 hour exposure to 5 mg/cm² of 5% lidocaine.[192]

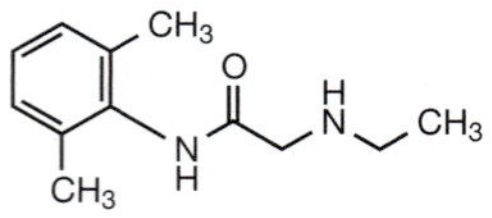

Monoethylglycine xylidide (MEGX)

The capsaicin patch is indicated in general neuropathic pain and is thought to work by calming ("defunctionalizing") hyperactive cutaneous nerve endings. Up to four patches can be applied to intact skin at the most painful sites and left on for up to an hour. The head and face should be avoided, and 3 months should elapse between applications. The major adverse effect is burning at the site of application, but pretreatment with a topical anesthetic can ease the discomfort. Patients taking angiotensin-converting enzyme (ACE) inhibitors may notice an increase in drug-induced cough.[190] A 0.075%-cream formulation is available for off-label use in painful diabetic peripheral neuropathy and, to be effective, should be applied 4 times daily on a chronic basis.

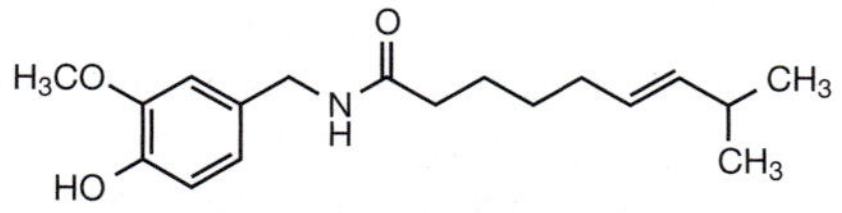

Capsaicin

Antimigraine Drugs

"Migraines...the only time when taking a hammer to your own skull seems like an appropriate solution."

—CoyoteRed

Migraine impacts more than 14% of the US population, approximately 35 million people, with women suffering from the disorder more commonly than men.[193,194] Presentation includes throbbing headache (which is often unilateral and can last from hours to days), environmental sensitivity (eg, light, sound, odors, activity), and nausea and/or vomiting.[195] In approximately 20% to 30% of migraine sufferers (called migraineurs), headache is preceded by an aura (most commonly lines and shapes in the visual field, but also sensory tingling and numbness) that persists for up to an hour. Between 10% and 20% of patients experience a 1- to 2-day prodrome phase characterized by specific behaviors (eg, irritability), feelings (eg, depression), or conditions (eg, constipation). In addition to symptoms, the frequency of migraine "attacks" also informs the diagnosis; headache on at least half the days in a month for 3 months, with at least 8 of those days being "migraine-like," warrants a diagnosis of chronic migraine.[195] The chronically episodic and often incapacitating symptoms of migraine interfere with school, employment, and social engagement. Migraine presents a serious economic and public health burden and is considered one of the 40 most disabling conditions in the world.[196-198]

Migraine Pathology

The pathology of migraine headache is complex, genetically rooted, and believed to involve dysfunction in the trigeminal innervation of cranial vasculature impacting parasympathetic outflow.[196] Activation of central and peripheral trigeminal nociceptive pathways is also evident. As intracranial extracerebral vessels dilate, blood volume increases with each heartbeat, leading to pulsating pain. Inflammatory neuropeptides such as calcitonin gene–related peptide (CGRP) and substance P are released, augmenting pain and stimulating hallmark symptoms of nausea/vomiting and aversion to light. Nitric oxide may also play a role in pain induction.

Migraine Prophylaxis

Prevention of migraine headaches often involves dietary/activity/sleep-related lifestyle modifications, headache trigger management, and nonpharmacologic interventions such as deep breathing, biofeedback, and cognitive behavior modification. If needed, certain nonselective/selective β_1-receptor blockers or antiseizure agents can be prescribed, but side effects can be use-limiting (Fig. 16.16). Interestingly, central accumulation is not required for β-blocker therapeutic efficacy.[196] OnabotulinumtoxinA (Botox) is a better-tolerated approach to migraine prophylaxis despite the need for administration by multiple facial IM injections. Newer strategies under investigation to prevent or

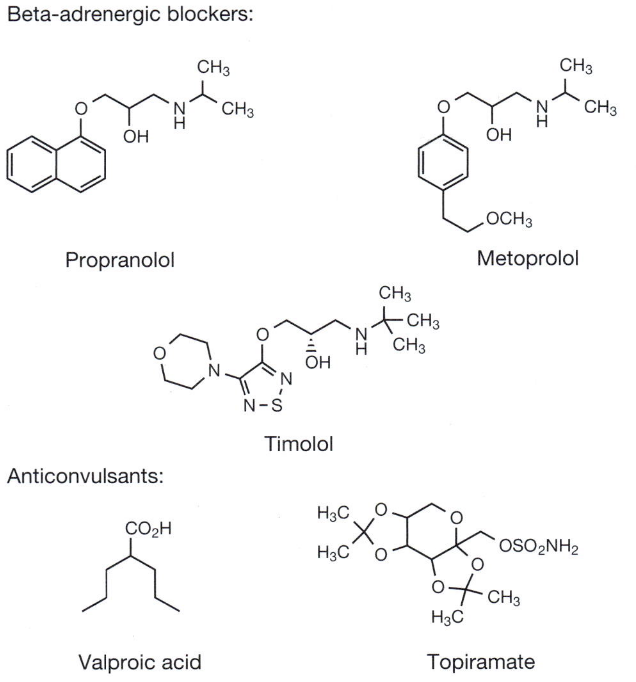

Figure 16.16 Medications used to prevent migraines.

abort migraine headaches include antagonism of CGRP and glutamate receptors, stimulation of adenosine A_1 and nociception ORL 1 receptors, inhibition of nitric oxide synthase, and transcranial magnetic and/or vagal nerve stimulation.[195,197,199,200]

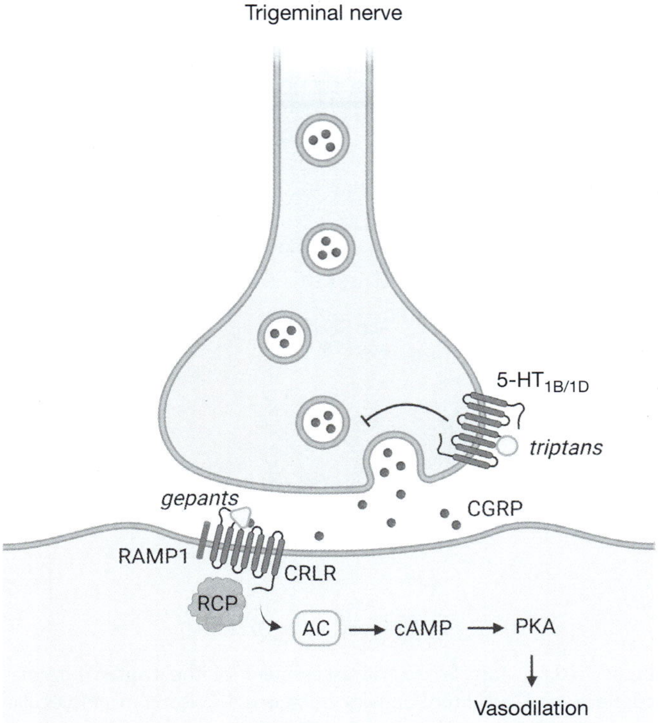

Figure 16.17 Schematic of the calcitonin gene–related peptide (CGRP) pathway. Agonists of 5-HT1B/1D (triptans) and antagonists of the calcitonin receptor–like receptor (CRLR, gepants) block the vasodilating effects of CGRP. AC, adenylyl cyclase; PKA, protein kinase A; RAMP1, receptor activity-modifying protein 1; RCP, receptor component protein. Image created using BioRender.

Pharmacotherapy of Active Migraine

When a migraine headache begins, the release of CGRP in the trigeminal nerve activates a CGRP receptor that consists of three subunits: the calcitonin receptor–like receptor (CRLR), receptor activity-modifying protein 1 (RAMP1), and receptor-component protein (RCP). Activation of CRLR stimulates $G\alpha_s$, which activates AC, increases intracellular cAMP, and activates protein kinase A (PKA), ultimately leading to vasodilation and the experience of migraine pain.

Many receptor types and subtypes have been associated with migraine pathology and pharmacotherapy, but the $5\text{-HT}_{1B/1D}$ target has received the most focused drug development attention. When stimulated, these two closely related subtypes induce constriction of cranial vessels (5-HT_{1B}) and inhibit trigeminal vascular activity, inflammatory neuropeptide release (CGRP), and nociception (5-HT_{1D}) (Fig. 16.17).[196,201] Ergotamine and dihydroergotamine were among the first nonselective $5\text{-HT}_{1B/1D}$ agonists used in the treatment of acute migraine. Ergotamine is a natural product that is isolated from the ergot fungus, *Claviceps purpurea*, and dihydroergotamine is a semisynthetic derivative. While still commercially available, they are considered second-line agents since the development of the more selective and efficacious triptans. If ergotamines are used, patients must be cautioned about nausea and vomiting, and prescribers need to know that nonselective 5-HT_{2B} receptor agonism of these compounds could cause cardiac-specific adverse effects.

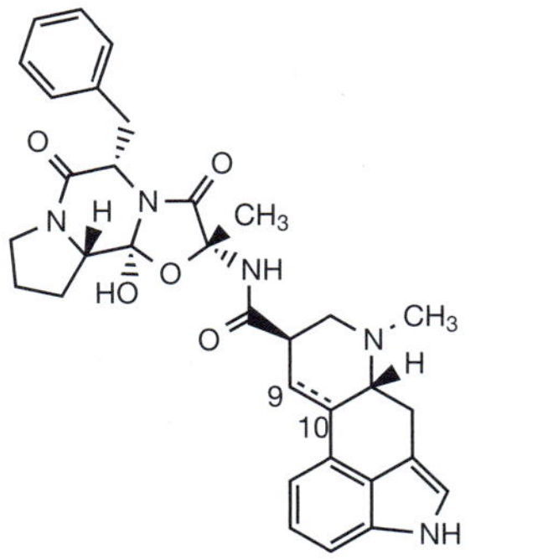

$\Delta^{9,10}$ = double bond, Ergotamine
$\Delta^{9,10}$ = single bond, Dihydroergotamine

Triptans

The success of ergotamines demonstrated the value that 5-HT-receptor agonism has on aborting an active migraine; however, this class is not subtype-selective and therefore produces a constellation of adverse side effects. The challenge thus becomes designing a selective 5-HT receptor agonist. The class of centrally active $5\text{-HT}_{1B/1D}$ receptor agonists known collectively as triptans was created by modifying the structure of 5-HT (Figs. 16.18 and 16.19). Opioids are not used to treat migraine pain and can actually accelerate the progression from episodic to chronic migraine.[202]

Triptans have been in clinical use for over 25 years, and they have a well-recognized effect on pain relief and function,

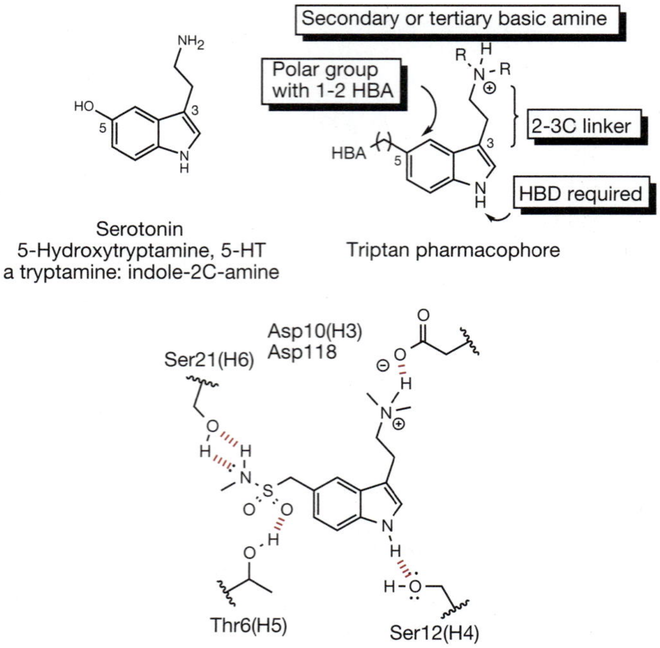

Figure 16.18 Top: Structural assessment of the triptan pharmacophore and structure-activity relationship. Bottom: Molecular mechanism of triptan binding 5-HT1B/1D predicted using computational modeling. Key hydrogen bonding interactions shown in red. HBA, hydrogen-bond acceptor; HBD, hydrogen-bond donor.

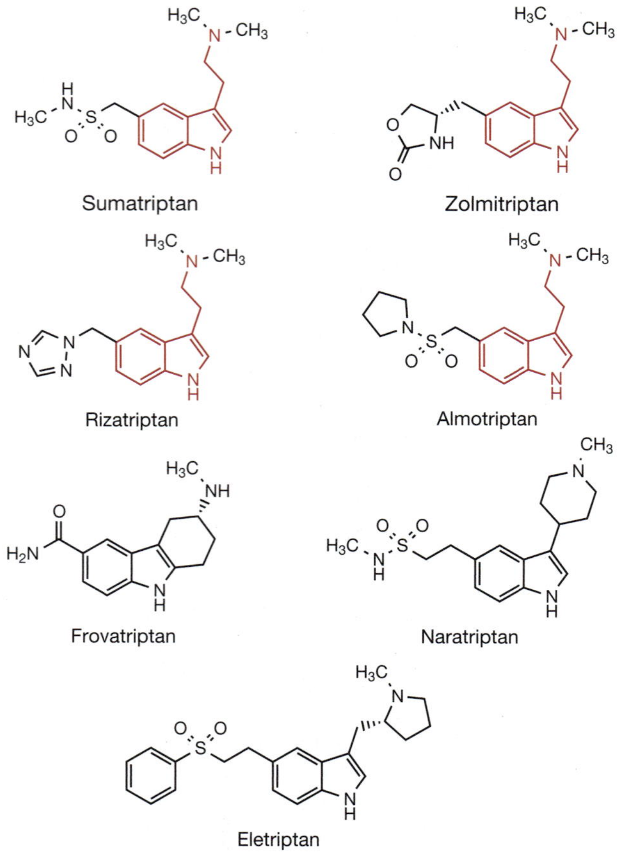

Figure 16.19 Members of the triptan class of antimigraine agents. Top two rows: triptans that contain a tryptamine pharmacophore (shown in red). Bottom row: triptans that do not contain a tryptamine pharmacophore. FMO, flavin monooxygenase; MAO-A, monoamine oxidase-A.

and thus on patient quality of life. However, some studies have shown that an initial incomplete or inconsistent response to a prescribed triptan, coupled with problematic adverse effects, can cause up to 60% of patients to not refill their medication. Up to 9% switch immediately to a different triptan, rather than persisting with the original drug for the recommended number of trials.[203] The importance of detailed and descriptive medical and pain histories, along with patient-provider discussion of preferred dosage forms and education on clinical expectations, is paramount to arriving expediently at the optimal therapeutic approach for each patient having migraine.

Mechanism and Pharmacokinetics. All seven marketed triptans act by constricting intracranial extracerebral vessels, attenuating neuroinflammation, and inhibiting the release of neurotransmitters at trigeminal nociceptive terminals. While their mechanism is identical, they differ significantly in their pharmacokinetic properties (Table 16.5).[198,201] The triptans have calculated logP values ranging from 1.17 (sumatriptan) to 3.84 (eletriptan). Oral bioavailability also varies widely, and nasal spray formulations are available for some products on the lower end of the scale. Gastric emptying slows during active migraine attacks, which can delay drug absorption. Therapeutic action generally begins within 2 hours of oral administration, and elimination half-lives are commonly in the 2- to 4-hour range. Serum levels can be elevated in patients with significant hepatic or renal dysfunction.

In general, the higher the bioavailability and the faster the penetration of the BBB, the more beneficial the therapeutic action. However, patients nonresponsive to one triptan might be robust responders to another, depending on the individual patient's constellation of symptoms and the pharmacokinetic advantages of the effective agent.[204] Treatment should begin when pain intensity is low, and doses titrated until efficacy is achieved or the maximum allowed dose is reached. If therapy is delayed until central trigeminal sensitization has occurred (signaled by cutaneous allodynia), triptan therapy can become ineffective.[198] Approximately 25% to 35% of migraineurs get no relief from triptans, and 60% of those who do not respond to NSAIDs fall into the triptan-resistant category. Although in the early stages, pharmacogenomics studies hope to eventually identify genes related to disease susceptibility and etiology so that more rational and individualized approaches to pharmacotherapy can be implemented.[205]

Chemistry. The first triptans were designed based on 5-HT and thus share a tryptamine core group that consists of an indole and basic amine separated by an ethyl group at position 3 of the indole ring. Subsequent agents replaced the flexible ethyl spacer with various ring systems that maintain this ethyl spacer: for example, frovatriptan has constrained the ethyl group into a cyclohexyl group, and eletriptan has the amine constrained as a pyrrolidine (see Fig. 16.19). In naratriptan, three carbons separate the indole ring from the terminal amine, but the distance is shortened by incorporating the amine into a piperidine ring. All triptans are tertiary amines except frovatriptan, which is secondary. Amine substituents are limited in size to methyl, presumably to restrict steric hindrance to electrostatic interaction

Table 16.5 Triptan Pharmacokinetics

Parameters	Sumatriptan	Zolmitriptan	Naratriptan	Rizatriptan	Almotriptan	Frovatriptan	Eletriptan
Trade name	Imitrex	Zomig	Amerge	Maxalt	Axert	Frova	Relpax
Log P (calc)	1.17	2.25	2.16	1.67	2.04	1.2	3.84
Oral Bioavailability (%)	15 17-19 (nas) 97 (sc)	40 102 (nas compared to po)	74	45	70	20-30[a]	50
Protein binding (%)	14-21	25	28-31	14	35	15	85
Volume of distribution (po unless noted)	2.7 L/kg 50 L (sc)	7 L/kg 8.4 L/kg (nas)	170 L	110-140 L[a]	180-200 L	3-4.2 L/kg	138 L
$T_{1/2}$ (h) (po unless noted)	2 1.8 (nas) 2 (sc)	3 3 (nas)	6	2-3	3-5	26-30	4
Major phase I metabolites (%)	Indoleacetic acid	*N*-Desmethyl (act)	Hepatic: 50%	Indole acetic acid	Indole acetic acid	*N*-Desmethyl (act)	*N*-Desmethyl (act)
		Indole ethyl alcohol		*N*-Desmethyl (act)	GABA	*N*-Ac-desmethyl	
		Indole acetic acid		6-OH	*N*-Desmethyl		
Metabolizing enzymes	MAO-A	CYP1A2	CYP3A4 and other isoforms	MAO-A	CYP3A4/CYP2D6	CYP1A2	CYP3A4
		MAO-A	MAO-A		MAO-A		
Excretion (%)	60 renal 40 fecal (3-22 unchanged drug)	60 renal 30 fecal (8 unchanged drug)	30 renal 15 fecal (50 unchanged drug)	82 renal 12 fecal (14 unchanged drug)	75 renal 13 fecal (~53 unchanged drug)	32 renal 62 fecal	90 renal <10 fecal (<20 unchanged drug)
T_{max} (h) (po unless noted)	2-2.5 0.75-1.5 (nas) 0.2 (sc)	1.5[b] 3 (dt) 3 (nas)	2-3[b]	1-1.5 1.6-2.5 (dt)	1-3	2-4	1.5-2[b]
C_{max} (mg/L) (po)	54	10[a]	12.6[a]	19.8[a]	49.5	4.2-7.0[a]	246[b]

(continued)

Table 16.5 Triptan Pharmacokinetics (*continued*)

Parameters	Sumatriptan	Zolmitriptan	Naratriptan	Rizatriptan	Almotriptan	Frovatriptan	Eletriptan
% Pain relief[c] at 2 h (at 4 h) (po unless noted)	56-67 (71) 72-74 (nas) 80 (sc)	62-65 (70-75)	40 (60-68)	67-77	70	38 (68)	77
Initial dosage range (mg) (po unless noted)	25-100 5-20 (nas) 6 (sc)	1.25-5 2.5 (nas)	1-2.5	5-10	6.25-12.5	2.5-5	20-40
Maximum p.o. dose (mg/24 h)	200	10	5	30	25	7.5	80

act, active; C_{max}, peak plasma concentration after po administration; dt, disintegrating tablets; nas, intranasal; po, oral; sc, subcutaneous; $T_{1/2}$, elimination half-life; T_{max}, time to peak plasma concentration.

[a]Gender dependent (women > men).

[b]Increased during active migraine.

[c]Compared to placebo.

Data from Drug Bank. Accessed September 30, 2017. https://www.drugbank.ca/; *Drug Facts and Comparisons. Facts & Comparisons* [Database Online]. In: Louis S, ed. Wolters Kluwer Health, Inc.; 2005; Burch R, Loder S, Loder E, et al. The prevalence and burden of migraine and severe headache in the United States: updated statistics from government health surveillance studies. *Headache*. 2015;55:21-34; Weatherall M. The diagnosis and treatment of chronic migraine. *Ther Adv Chronic Dis*. 2015;6:115-123.

of the protonated amine at G-protein-coupled 5-$HT_{1B/1D}$ receptors.

The 5-phenol of the serotonin moiety is replaced by a more metabolically stable polar functional group such as an amide (frovatriptan), secondary or tertiary sulfonamide (sumatriptan, almotriptan, naratriptan), sulfone (eletriptan), or heterocyclic ring (zolmitriptan, rizatriptan). In all cases but frovatriptan, the polar moiety is separated from the indole ring by one to two carbon atoms. The polar group must have at least one HBA group that is separated from the indole by at least one to three atoms. This group is hypothesized to accept a hydrogen from a serine or threonine (HBD) in the active sites of 5-$HT_{1B/1D}$, and likely the strongest contributor to 5-HT receptor–subtype selectivity.[206]

METABOLISM.[207-213] Organizing the triptans into two groups, triptans that contain a tryptamine and those that do not, simplifies understanding of how they are metabolized (Fig. 16.20). All triptans can be N-demethylated to give the corresponding desmethyl metabolite. For most triptans, this results in a secondary amine. Frovatriptan is N-demethylated to the primary amine metabolite. Those that contain a tryptamine core can be transformed in another way: like 5-HT, the tryptamine-based triptans can have their amine removed entirely by monoamine oxidase-A (MAO-A), resulting in the corresponding indole-3-acetic acid metabolites. Because the trypamine-based triptans closely resemble 5-HT, the enzyme metabolizes them in the same manner. The cyclic rings in frovatriptan, naratriptan, and eletriptan are too sterically hindered to allow oxidation by MAO-A. Rizatriptan and almotriptan are oxidized by flavin monooxygenase (FMO) to inactive N-oxides. Some triptans are subjected to minor metabolic pathways that oxidize the 6- or 7-position of the indole core (6-hydroxyrizatriptan, 1-hydroxyfrovatriptan), rendering them inactive. Finally, the pyrrolidine ring of almotriptan can undergo CYP3A4 or CYP2D6 oxidation to an unstable hydroxyl intermediate, which breaks down into a γ-aminobutyric acid metabolite.

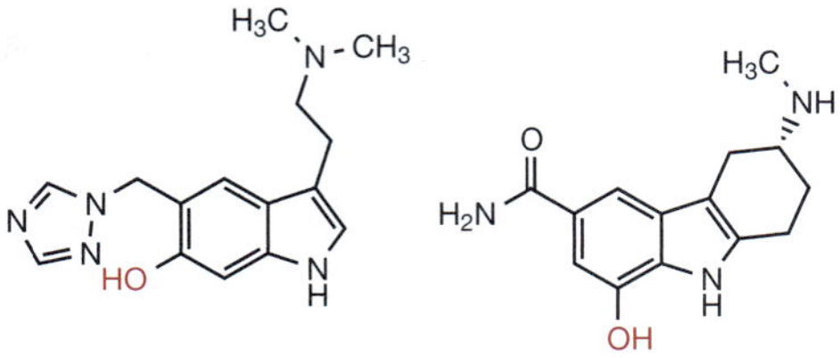

6-Hydroxyrizatriptan Hydroxyfrovatriptan

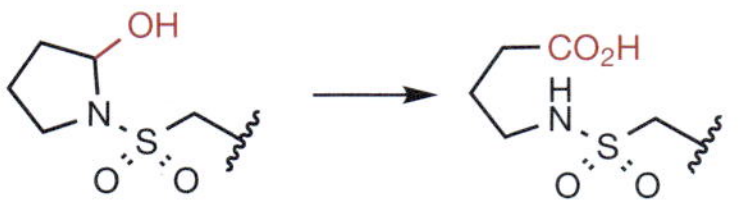

Hydroxyalmotriptan Gamma-aminobutyric (acid metabolite)

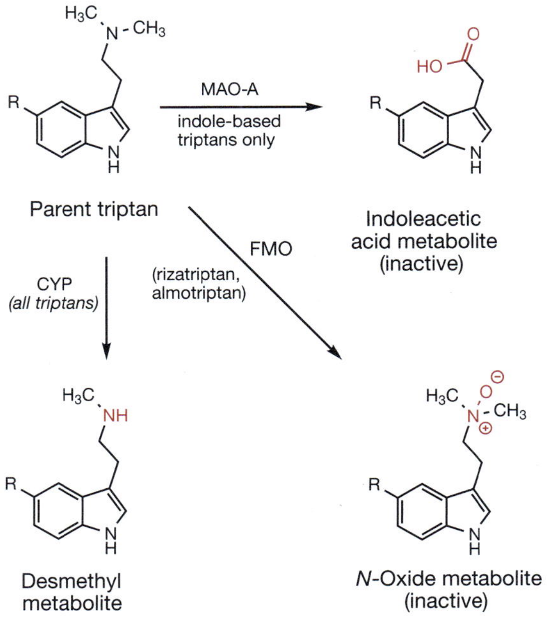

Figure 16.20 Common metabolic pathways of triptans.

The isoforms involved in CYP-vulnerable triptan metabolism vary and include 2D6 (almotriptan), 1A2 (frovatriptan, zolmitriptan), and 3A4 (naratriptan, almotriptan, and eletriptan). The desmethyl metabolites of rizatriptan, zolmitriptan, eletriptan, and frovatripan are active. Desmethylrizatriptan is approximately equipotent with rizatriptan, and desmethylzolmitriptan's activity is between 2 and 6 times that of the parent drug. The 50% longer half-life of desmethylzolmitriptan likely contributes to its augmented potency.[198,211] Desmethyleletriptan has a half-life and time to maximum plasma concentration (T_{max}) similar to its parent drug, but the peak concentrations are about 3-fold lower. Desmethylfrovatriptan binds to target receptors with approximately one-third the affinity of its parent, but has a 3-fold longer half-life.[198] Sumatriptan, almotriptan, and naratriptan have no active metabolites, which is one proposed reason for their lower incidence of central adverse effects. The metabolites that no longer have a basic amine–the indoleacetic acids and N-oxides–are all inactive.

ADVERSE EFFECTS. While they have no affinity for 5-HT_{2A} receptors that mediate the majority of 5-HT-linked coronary vasoconstriction, triptans can bind to the small 5-HT_{1B} subtype reserve in that tissue and have the potential to constrict coronary vessels.[214] While serious cardiac events are uncommon, triptans should be avoided in patients with known or suspected ischemic or vasoactive coronary artery disease. To minimize the risk of synergistic vasoconstriction, patients should be restricted to a single triptan, and triptans and ergot derivatives should not be coadministered in the same 24-hour period.[215]

Molecular lipophilicity of triptans and their active metabolites has been positively correlated with risk of CNS adverse effects, including drowsiness, dizziness, and cognition or sensory disturbances. This is of clinical importance since the fear of CNS toxicity is known to prompt decisions to delay therapy, leading to prolonged pain and patient disengagement from social or work- related activities.[198] Nausea and dry mouth can also occur with triptan use.

TRIPTAN DRUG-DRUG INTERACTIONS

- Ergot derivatives
  - Augmented ergot-induced vasoconstriction
- 5-HT_3 antagonist antiemetics
  - Serotonin syndrome
- Opioid analgesics
  - Serotonin syndrome[216]
- Antipsychotic drugs
  - Serotonin syndrome and/or neuroleptic malignant syndrome
- Metoclopramide
  - Serotonin syndrome and/or neuroleptic malignant syndrome
- Droxidopa
  - Augmented droxidopa-induced hypertension
- CYP3A4 inhibitors
  - Strong: Elevated eletriptan and almotriptan serum levels
  - Moderate: Elevated eletriptan serum levels
- MAO inhibitors
  - Elevated sumatriptan, zolmitriptan, rizatriptan, and almotriptan serum levels

Specific Drugs

Sumatriptan Succinate. Sumatriptan (Imitrex) was the first triptan to be marketed, and it stands alone in the "first generation" class of triptan antimigraine drugs. It has one of the lowest lipophilicities of the triptans, and its activity is predominantly peripheral.[201] It is marketed in a variety of dosage forms, including tablets, nasal solution, nasal exhaler powder (Onzetra Xsail), solution for subcutaneous injection, and subcutaneous autoinjector (Imitrex StatDose, Zembrace SymTouch). A combination product with the NSAID naproxen sodium is marketed in tablet form as Treximet.

Subcutaneous administration provides faster and more efficacious pain-relieving action than tablets and is useful in patients whose pain is escalating or who are nauseated. However, the injection formulation is associated with an elevated risk of usually short-lived adverse effects such as dizziness, sensory disturbances, chest/throat tightness, and shortness of breath. Likewise, the nasal spray relieves pain more quickly than the tablets, but patients can experience recurrent headache at the 2-hour pain relief benchmark, as well as an unpleasant taste.[215] Regardless of formulation, the dose can be repeated no sooner than 2 hours (oral, nasal) or 1 hour (injection) after the initial dose, and the maximum allowed dose should not be exceeded (see Table 16.5).

Zolmitriptan. Zolmitriptan was designed to improve upon sumatriptan's fairly low oral bioavailability. Its higher lipophilicity promotes absorption from the GI tract and penetration of the BBB, although clinical efficacy of the two triptans is essentially equivalent. The ability of a second dose of zolmitriptan to address unresolved headache pain 2 hours post-administration led to the establishment of a secondary (4-hour) endpoint for evaluating clinical efficacy, and it is uniquely effective when a second dose is taken for persistent headache.[215] As noted previously, the N-desmethyl metabolite has an activity between 2 and 6 times that of the parent drug with a 50% longer half-life. Women may show higher mean serum concentrations of zolmitriptan compared to men.[91] The use of oral contraceptives increases maximum serum concentrations by 30% while delaying time to peak concentrations by 30 minutes.[201]

Zolmitriptan (Zomig) is one of two triptans available in a disintegrating tablet formulation (rizatriptan is the other). Absorption is intestinal (not buccal), but patients with nausea may appreciate not having to swallow the tablet formulation, plus it can be taken when water is not immediately at hand. The nasal spray formulation has similar advantages and disadvantages as sumatriptan's intranasal dosage form.[215]

Naratriptan Hydrochloride. Naratriptan's relative low incidence of adverse effects has caused it to be termed the "gentle triptan" by some.[215] Available only in tablet form (Amerge), it has the highest oral bioavailability of any marketed triptan and a longer half-life than all but frovatriptan. Still, its single-dose efficacy is among the lowest of the triptan antimigraine drugs, but the risk of recurrent headache is also lower compared to zolmitriptan or sumatriptan. The time to peak serum concentration is delayed to 3 to 4 hours during acute migraine episodes, leading to enhanced pain relief at 4 hours (60%-68%) versus 2 hours (40%). Similar to zolmitriptan, serum levels are about 1.5 times higher in women, and oral contraceptive use contributes to this by decreasing clearance by 26%. The fact that smoking increases clearance by 30% lends support to the concept of CYP1A2 being involved in naratriptan metabolism.[201]

Rizatriptan Benzoate. As noted, rizatriptan (Maxalt) is available in oral disintegrating tablets as well as traditional tablets. Its onset of action is among the fastest, and elimination half-life among the shortest, of currently marketed triptans. It has the highest 2-hour clinical efficacy and is able to sustain a pain-free state up through 24 hours. The low (45%) bioavailability is due to significant first-pass metabolism, with the equally active desmethyl metabolite being formed to a relatively minor extent (14%). Serum levels of both the parent drug and active metabolite increase dramatically in the presence of MAO inhibitors and substrates, requiring dose reductions when coadministration cannot be avoided.[201]

While the drug is known to accumulate in rodent breast milk, rizatriptan has been assigned a Briggs category rating of Probably Compatible, indicating that available data suggest no significant risk to nursing infants. All other triptans received the same rating with the exception of sumatriptan, which was classified as Compatible (safe) despite being excreted into human milk.[217] Still, given the low protein-binding potential of triptans, coupled with their moderate half-lives and fairly low molecular weights, care and counseling is warranted when prescribing these drugs for breastfeeding patients.

Almotriptan Malate. Almotriptan is lipophilic and rapidly absorbed from the GI tract. Marketed only in tablet form, two-thirds of the dose is delivered to the bloodstream within 1 hour post-administration, and patients can begin to experience relief within 30 minutes.[201,215] It is well tolerated, but drug-drug interactions are possible with agents that impact the availability and activity of CYP3A4 and CYP2D6 (especially strong CYP3A4 inhibitors) and MAO-A. The adverse effect profile is mild, with dizziness and drowsiness being the most commonly observed effects.

Frovatriptan Succinate. Frovatriptan, marketed only as tablets (Frova), has a lipophilicity, oral bioavailability, and protein binding profile very similar to sumatriptan. While its onset of action is relatively sluggish, its half-life is extended approximately 15-fold compared to sumatriptan, regardless of dose or route of administration. This allows it to have its major impact on pain relief at the 4-hour (vs 2-hour) efficacy benchmark. Frovatriptan has the highest affinity for 5-HT_{1B} receptors of all triptans and demonstrates selectivity for cerebral, as opposed to coronary, vessels, making it safer to use in patients with coronary artery disease.[201] Appropriate caution, counseling, and monitoring, however, is always warranted.

Like eletriptan, frovatriptan is not metabolized by MAO-A and can be more safely administered with drugs that are MAO-A substrates or inhibitors. It is a recommended agent for the treatment of migraine headaches triggered by menstruation.[195]

Eletriptan Hydrobromide. Eletriptan is a cyclized *N*-methylpyrrolidine analog of sumatriptan. In this constrained conformation, affinity for 5-HT_{1D} receptors rises to the highest level of all triptans, and its affinity for the 5-HT_{1B} subtype is second only to frovatriptan.[201] It is the most lipophilic triptan and rapidly reaches peak plasma concentrations that are higher by severalfold than any other drug in the class (see Table 16.5). Like frovatriptan, it is effective in treating menstruation-related migraine, and its efficacy is not impacted by the concomitant use of oral contraceptives.[201]

Eletriptan is marketed only in tablet form (Relpax). The adverse effect risk appears to be dose-related and includes nausea, dizziness, drowsiness, and general weakness. It carries the highest risk of toxicity when coadministered with CYP3A4 substrates or inhibitors, although some studies have shown the adverse effect profile insignificantly impacted by CYP3A4 activity modulators.[215]

Gepants

Though the triptans have been the mainstay of migraine prophylaxis and pharmacotherapy for decades, there are significant drawbacks to their use, including weight gain, migraine recurrence, and an increased progression from episodic migraine to chronic migraine with triptan overuse. Significantly, triptans are contraindicated in patients with uncontrolled hypertension due to their vasoconstrictive actions. A newer class of antimigraine agents, called gepants, avoid many of these risks—in particular, the cerebrovascular adverse effects. As of the end of 2023, three gepants are FDA approved for acute treatment of migraine: ubrogepant (Ubrelvy, 2019), rimegepant (Nurtec ODT, 2020), and zavegepant (Zavzpret, 2023). Additionally, two gepants are approved for migraine prevention: rimegepant and atogepant (Qulipta, 2021). Finally, atogepant was approved in 2023 for the prevention of chronic migraine.[219]

Mechanism and Pharmacokinetics. The gepants are small molecule antagonists of the CGRP receptor known as CRLR. The gepant binding site can be found at the interface between CRLR and RAMP1, also known as CRLR/RAMP1. Inhibiting CRLR/RAMP1 at the level of the trigeminal nerve blocks the meningeal vasodilatory actions of CGRP. Intracellularly, CRLR blockade reverses the increased cAMP that is caused by AC activation. The pharmacokinetic parameters of the gepants vary wildly among the members of the class (Table 16.6). This can be rationalized by the fact that the gepants are structurally distinct from each other and do not share a consensus "gepant pharmacophore" (Fig. 16.21). Most gepants are strong P-gp substrates and are thus readily cleared from the brain. This is not a detriment to antimigraine action, however, as blocking

Table 16.6 Clinical Pharmacokinetic Properties of the Gepant Antimigraine Drugs

Parameters	Atogepant	Rimegepant	Ubrogepant	Zavegepant
Trade name	Qulipta	Nurtec ODT	Ubrelvy	Zavzpret
Route of administration	Oral (tablet)	Oral disintegrating tablet	Oral (tablet)	Intranasal
Predicted Log P	3.62	2.68	3.07	2.85
Aqueous solubility	Insoluble	Slightly soluble	Insoluble	Freely soluble
Bioavailability	unknown	64%	unknown	5%
T_{max}	2-3 h	1.5 h[a]	0.7-1.5 h[a]	0.5 h
Protein binding	95%	96%	87%	90%
Volume of distribution	292 L	120 L	350 L	1,774 L
$T_{1/2}$	11 h	11 h	5-7 h	6.5 h
Metabolism (% unchanged)	Moderate (47%)	Minor (77%)	Major	Minor (90%)
Metabolized by	CYP3A4, UGT	CYP3A4, CYP2C9	CYP3A4, UGT	CYP3A4
Route of elimination	Fecal	Fecal > urine	Fecal	Fecal

[a]Taking with a high-fat meal causes an increase in T_{max} and a decrease in C_{max}.
Data from Drug Bank. Accessed October 10, 2023. https://www.drugbank.ca/

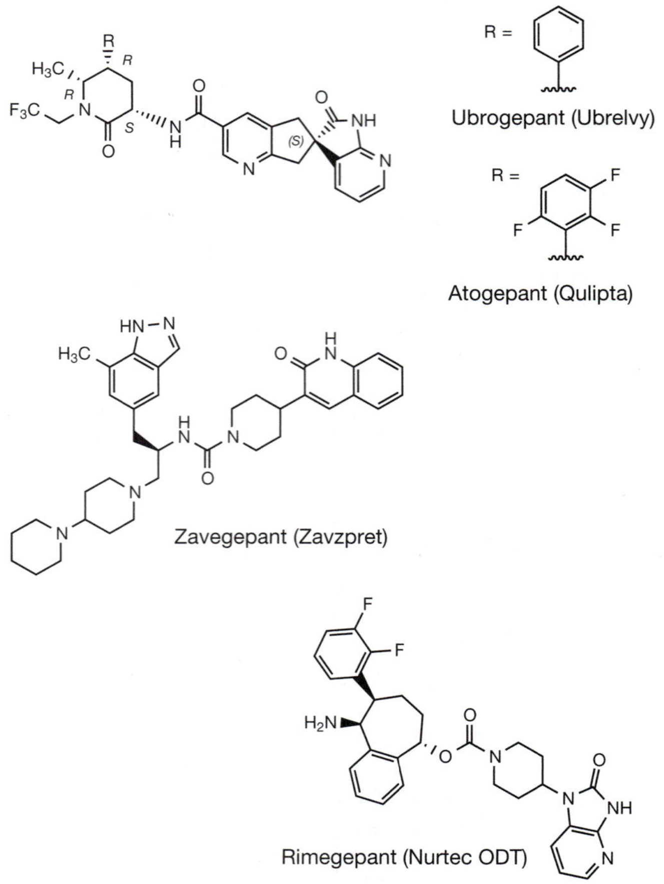

Figure 16.21 Gepant class of antimigraine agents.

GRLR/RAMP1 at the level of the trigeminal nerve does not require transport across the BBB. All gepants are available as oral formulations, with the exception of zavegepant, which is an intranasal spray.

Chemistry and Metabolism. Unlike other medications classes discussed in this chapter, the gepants arose from hit-to-lead development campaigns beginning from hits discovered via high-throughput screening of small molecule libraries. Because different pharmaceutical companies started from different hits, the final products all look different; hence, there is no "gepant pharmacophore." Notably, ubrogepant and atogepant are structurally similar because they were both developed by Merck. Nonetheless, all of the gepant drugs inhibit CRLR/RAMP1 via a consensus binding site that mimics CGRP binding.[219] As a class, the gepants are generally large (MW >500 Da) and have high topologic polar surface area (TPSA). With the exception of zavegepant, the gepants are nonionizable at physiologic pH: zavegepant has two tertiary, basic amine functional groups that enhance aqueous solubility and permit formulation as an intranasal spray.

Few details are presently available regarding the specific metabolic fates of the gepants. Rimegepant and zavegepant are not heavily metabolized (77% and 90% of the dose is eliminated unchanged, respectively), although oxidized metabolites produced by CYP3A4 have been detected. Atogepant and ubrogepant are metabolized by CYP3A4 and eliminated as glucuronide conjugates. The specific structures of these metabolites have not been disclosed.

Adverse Effects. In general, the gepant drugs are well-tolerated. No severe adverse drug reactions have been reported, though, as stated, these are relatively "new" medications, and some have not yet reached the market. Nonetheless, pharmacists should be sure to report any potential adverse effects as part of post-marketing surveillance. The most common adverse drug reactions are nausea and fatigue.

Acknowledgment

The authors wish to acknowledge the work of Edward B. Roche, PhD, who authored content used within this chapter in a previous edition of this text.

Learning Activity
Central Pain Case Study

As a senior pharmacy student, you have elected an advanced pharmacy practice experience (APPE) hospital rotation in a rural community. Your service-minded preceptor volunteers with the local fire department and is preparing an in-service for firefighters and paramedics on the medication they use to resuscitate people at risk of dying from respiratory depression secondary to opioid overdose, most commonly heroin and fentanyl.

To assess your knowledge of SARs, she asks you to identify the drug structure from the four shown below that would be effective in saving these lives, explaining the structural basis for why your selected agent would be appropriate and the others would not. How do you respond? How do the structures of heroin and fentanyl tell you that these are high-efficacy μ opioid–receptor agonists?

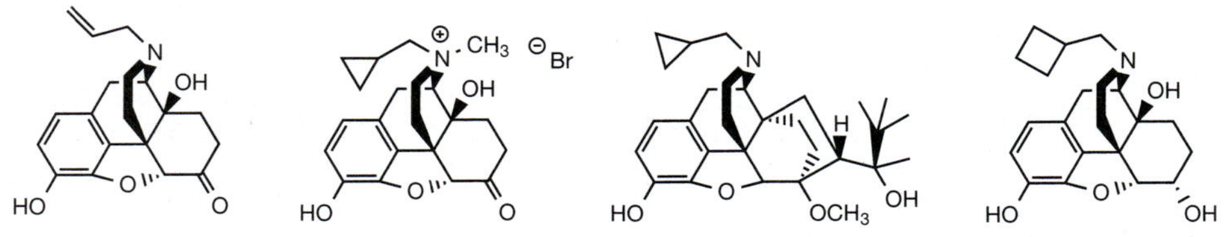

A B C D

REFERENCES

1. Merskey H, Bogduk N. *Classification of Chronic Pain*. 2nd ed. International Association for the Study of Pain Press; 2004:209-214.
2. Griffen RS, Woolf CJ. Pharmacology of analgesia. In: Golan DE, Armstrong EJ, Armstrong AW, eds. *Principles of Pharmacology: The Pathophysiologic Basis of Drug Therapy*. 4th ed. Wolters Kluwer; 2016:288-307.
3. Stanos S, Brodsky M, Argoff C, et al. Rethinking chronic pain in a primary care setting. *Postgrad Med*. 2016;128:502-515.
4. Campbell J. APS presidential address. *J Pain*. 1996;5:85-88.
5. Mularski R, White-Chu F, Overbay D, et al. Measuring pain as the 5th vital sign does not improve quality of pain management. *J Gen Int Med*. 2006;21:607-612.
6. Joint Commission Statement on Pain Management. Accessed July 30, 2017. https://www.jointcommission.org/joint_commission_statement_on_pain_management/
7. Stanos SP. The AMA and AAPM. A historical partnership now advocating for the "Future of Pain Medicine". *Pain Med*. 2017;18(8): 1411-1412. Accessed January 20, 2025. https://academic.oup.com/painmedicine/article/18/8/1411/3988392
8. Institute of Medicine. *Relieving Pain in America; a Blueprint for Transforming Prevention, Care, Education and Research*. The National Academies Press (US); 2011.
9. Morone N, Weiner D. Pain as the 5th vital sign: exposing the vital need for pain education. *Clin Ther*. 2013;35:1728-1732.
10. Wong-Baker FACES Foundation. Accessed July 30, 2017. http://wongbakerfaces.org
11. Tait R, Chibnall T. Racial/ethnic disparities in the assessment and treatment of pain. *Am Psychologist*. 2014;69:131-141.
12. Murphy K, Han J, Yang S, et al. Prevalence of specific types of pain diagnoses in a sample of United States adults. *Pain Phys*. 2017;20: E247-E268.
13. Abd-Elsayed A, Fischer M, Dimbert J, et al. Prescription drugs and the US workforce: results from a National Safety Council survey. *Pain Phys*. 2020:23;1-16.
14. Yong RJ, Mullins PM, Bhattacharyya N. Prevalence of chronic pain among adults in the United States. *Pain*. 2022;163(2):e328-e332.
15. Zelaya CE, Dahlhamer JM, Lucas JW, et al. *Chronic Pain and High-Impact Chronic Pain Among U.S. Adults, 2019. NCHS Data Brief, No 390*. National Center for Health Statistics; 2020.
16. Fornasari D. Pain mechanisms in patients with chronic pain. *Clin Drug Invest*. 2012;32:45-52.
17. McCarberg B, D'Arcy Y, Parsons B, et al. Neuropathic pain: a narrative review of etiology, assessment, diagnosis and treatment for primary care providers. *Curr Med Res Opin*. 2017;33:1361-1369 (and references therein).
18. Radnovich R, Chapman C, Gudin J, et al. Acute pain: effective management requires comprehensive assessment. *Postgrad Med*. 2014;126:59-72.
19. Tawfic Q, Faris A. Acute pain service: past present and future. *Pain Manag*. 2015;5:47-58.
20. Moore R, Wiffen P, Derry S, et al. Non-prescription (OTC) oral analgesics for acute pain – an overview of Cochrane reviews. *Cochrane Database Syst Rev*. 2015;11:1-30.
21. Gordon D. Acute pain assessment tools: let us move beyond simple pain ratings. *Curr Opin*. 2015;28:565-569.
22. Rikard S, Strahan A, Schmit K, et al. Chronic pain among adults—United States, 2019-2021. *MMWR Morb Mortal Wkly Rep*. 2023;72:379-385.
23. Zidarov D, Visca R, Gogovor A, et al. Performance and quality indicators for the management of non-cancer chronic pain: a scoping review protocol. *BMJ Open*. 2016;6:e010487.
24. Lisi L, Aceto P, Navarra P, et al. mTOR kinase: a possible pharmacological target in the management of chronic pain. *Biomed Res Int*. 2015;2015:394257.
25. Turk D. Remember the distinction between malignant and benign pain? Well forget it. *Clin J Pain*. 2002;18:75-76.
26. Sun R, Zhang W, Bo J, et al. Spinal activation of alpha7-nicotinic acetylcholine receptor attenuates posttraumatic stress disorder chronic pain via suppression of glial activation. *Neuroscience*. 2016;344:243-254.
27. Loo L, Wright B, Zylka M. Lipid kinases as therapeutic targets for chronic pain. *Pain*. 2015;156(suppl 1):S2-S10.
28. Jones T, Moore T, Choo J. The impact of virtual reality on chronic pain. *PLoS One*. 2016;11:e0167523.
29. Pain Management Task Force Final Report: Providing a standardized DoD and VHA vision and approach to pain management to optimize the care for warriors and their families. Accessed August 1, 2017. https://permanent.access.gpo.gov/gpo60064/Pain-Management-Task-Force.pdf
30. Delgado R, York A, Lee C, et al. Assessing the quality, efficacy and effectiveness of the current evidence base of active self-care complementary and integrative medicine therapies for the management of chronic pain: a rapid evidence assessment of the literature. *Pain Med*. 2014;15:S9-S20.
31. Peppin J, Cheatle M, Kirsh K, et al. The complexity model: a novel approach to improve chronic pain care. *Pain Med*. 2015; 16:653-666.
32. Devereaux A, Mercer S, Cunningham C. DARK classics in chemical neuroscience: morphine. *ACS Chem Neurosci*. 2018;9: 2395-2407.
33. Peppin J, Raffa R. Delta opioid agonists: a concise update on potential therapeutic applications. *J Clin Pharmacol Ther*. 2015;40: 155-166.
34. Lendeckel U, Muller C, Rocken C, et al. Expression of opioid subtypes and their ligands in fibrillating human atria. *PACE*. 2005; 28:S275-S279.
35. Riviere P-M. Peripheral kappa opioid agonists for visceral pain. *Br J Pharmacol*. 2004;141:1331-1334.
36. DeWire S, Yamashita D, Rominger D, et al. A G protein-biased ligand at the mu opioid receptor is potently analgesic with reduced gastrointestinal and respiratory dysfunction compared with morphine. *J Pharmacol Exp Ther*. 2013;344:708-717.
37. Bohn L, Gainetdinov P, Lin F-T, et al. Mu opioid receptor desensitization by beta-arrestin-2 determines morphine tolerance but not dependence. *Nature*. 2000;408:720-723.
38. Somogyi A, Coller J, Barratt D. Pharmacogenetics of opioid response. *Clin Pharmacol Ther*. 2015;97:125-127.
39. Hughes J, Smith T, Kosterlitz H, et al. Identification of two related pentapeptides from the brain with potent opiate agonist activity. *Nature*. 1975;258:577-579.
40. National Institute on Drug Abuse. Drugs, brains, and behavior: the science of addiction. Drug misuse and addiction. Accessed September 12, 2023. https://nida.nih.gov/publications/drugs-brains-behavior-science-addiction/drug-misuse-addiction
41. Jan S. Introduction: landscape of opioid dependence. *J Manag Care Pharm*. 2010;16:S4-S8.
42. Lipman A, Webster L. The economic impact of opioid use in the management of chronic nonmalignant pain. *J Manag Care Spec Pharm*. 2015;21:891-899.
43. Center for Behavioral Health Statistics and Quality. 2015 National Survey on Drug Use and Health: detailed tables. Substance Abuse and Mental Health Services Administration. Accessed August 12, 2017. https://www.samhsa.gov/data/sites/default/files/NSDUH-DetTabs-2015/NSDUH-DetTabs-2015/NSDUH-DetTabs-2015.pdf
44. Rowe S, Zagales I, Fanfan D, et al. Postoperative opioid prescribing practices in US adult trauma patients: a systematic review. *J Trauma Acute Care Surg*. 2022;92(2):456-463.
45. Kaafarani HMA, Han K, Moheb ME, et al. Opioids after surgery in the United States versus the rest of the world. *Ann Surg*. 2020;272(6):879-886.
46. Oderda G, Lake J, Rudell K, et al. Economic burden of prescription opioid misuse and abuse: a systematic review. *J Pain Palliat Care Pharmacother*. 2015;29:388-400.
47. Kirson N, Scarpati L, Enloe C, et al. The economic burden of opioid abuse: updated findings. *J Manag Care Spec Pharm*. 2017;23: 427-445.
48. Sanyal C. Economic burden of opioid crisis and the role of pharmacist-led interventions. *J Am Pharm Assoc*. 2021;61:e70-e74.

49. National Safety Council. Prescription nation 2016: addressing America's drug epidemic. Accessed January 20, 2025. https://dpbh.nv.gov/uploadedFiles/dpbh.nv.gov/content/Programs/ClinicalSAPTA/Meetings/National%20Safety%20Council%20Report.pdf
50. Onishi E, Kobayashi T, Dexter E, et al. Comparison of opioid prescribing patterns in the United States and Japan: primary care physicians' attitudes and perceptions. *J Am Board Fam Med.* 2017;30:248-254.
51. Zhou C, Florence C, Dowell D. Payments for opioids shifted substantially to public and private insurers while consumer spending on these medications declined, 1999-2012. *Health Aff.* 2016;35:824-831.
52. Lyu X, Guy G, Baldwin G, et al. State-to-state variation in opioid dispensing changes following the release of the 2016 CDC Guideline for Prescribing Opioids for Chronic Pain. *JAMA Network Open.* 2023;6:e2332507.
53. Garnett MF, Miniño AM. *Drug Overdose Deaths in the United States, 2003-2023.* NCHS Data Brief, No 522. National Center for Health Statistics; 2024. Accessed January 20, 2025. https://www.cdc.gov/nchs/products/databriefs/db522.htm
54. National Institute on Drug Abuse. Drug overdose death rates. Accessed September 12, 2023. https://nida.nih.gov/research-topics/trends-statistics/overdose-death-rates
55. Burns S, Cunningham C, Mercer S. DARK Classics in chemical neuroscience: Fentanyl. *ACS Chem Neurosci.* 2018;9:2428-2437.
56. Comer S, Pravetoni M, Coop A, et al. Potential unintended consequences of class-wide drug scheduling based on chemical structure: a cautionary tale for fentanyl-related compounds. *Drug Alcohol Depend.* 2021;221:108530. doi:10.1016/j.drugalcdep.2021.108530
57. Volkow N, Collins F. The role of science in addressing the opioid crisis. *New Eng J Med.* 2017;377:391-394.
58. Volkow N. NIH's efforts to reduce the opioid epidemic. Accessed August 15, 2017. https://acd.od.nih.gov/documents/presentations/06092017Volkow.pdf
59. Secretary Price announces HHS strategy for fighting opioid crisis. Accessed August 15, 2017. https://www.hhs.gov/about/leadership/secretary/speeches/2017-speeches/secretary-price-announces-hhs-strategy-for-fighting-opioid-crisis/index.html
60. Opioid crisis. Accessed August 15, 2017. https://www.drugabuse.gov/drugs-abuse/opioids/opioid-crisis
61. Barnett M, Olenski A, Jena A. Opioid-prescribing patterns of emergency physicians and risk of long term use. *New Eng J Med.* 2017;376:663-673.
62. Walco G, Gove N, Phillips J, et al. Opioid analgesics administered for pain in the inpatient pediatric setting. *J Pain.* 2017;18:1270-1276.
63. Schmidt T, Haddox J, Nielsen A, et al. Key data gaps regarding the public health issues associated with opioid analgesics. *J Behav Health Serv Res.* 2015;42:540-553.
64. Kattan J, Tuazon E, Paone D, et al. Public health detailing—a successful strategy to promote judicious opioid analgesic prescribing. *Am J Pub Health.* 2016;106:1430-1438.
65. Raub J, Vettese T. Acute pain management in hospitalized adult patients with opioid dependence: a narrative review and guide for clinicians. *J Hosp Med.* 2017;12:371-379.
66. Cunningham C, Rothman R, Prisinzano T. Neuropharmacology of the naturally occurring kappa opioid hallucinogen salvinorin A. *Pharmacol Rev.* 2011;63:316-347.
67. Portoghese P, Sultana M, Nagase H, et al. Application of the message-address concept in the design of highly potent and selective non-peptide delta opioid receptor antagonists. *J Med Chem.* 1988;31:281-282.
68. Zhuang Y, Wang Y, He B, et al. Molecular recognition of morphine and fentanyl by the human μ-opioid receptor. *Cell.* 2022;185:4361-4375.
69. Voorhorst R, Sparreboom S. Four cases of recurrent pseudo-scarlet fever caused by phenathrene alkaloids with a 6-hydroxy group (codeine and morphine). *Ann Allergy.* 1980;44:116-120.
70. Sheen C, Schleimer R, Kulka M. Codeine induces mast cell chemokine and cytokine production: involvement of G-protein activation. *Allergy.* 2007;62:532-538.
71. Golembiewski J. Opioid-induced pruritus. *J Perianesth Nurs.* 2013;28:247-249.
72. Katcher J, Walsh D. Opioid-induced itching: morphine sulfate and hydromorphone hydrochloride. *J Pain Symptom Manage.* 1999;17:70-72.
73. Pogozheva I, Lomize A, Mosberg H. Opioid receptor three-dimensional structures from distance geometry calculations with hydrogen bonding constraints. *Biophys J.* 1998;75:612-634.
74. Manglik A, Kruse A, Kobilka T, et al. Crystal structure of the mu opioid receptor bound to a morphinan antagonist. *Nature.* 2012;485:321-326.
75. Cui X, Yeliseev A, Liu R. Ligand interaction, binding site and G-protein activation of the mu opioid receptor. *Eur J Pharmacol.* 2013;702:309-315.
76. Vuckovic S, Prostran M, Ivanovic M, et al. Fentanyl analogs: structure-activity relationship study. *Curr Med Chem.* 2009;16:2468-2474.
77. Drug Bank. Accessed September 30, 2017. https://www.drugbank.ca/
78. Williams D. p*K*a values for some drugs and miscellaneous organic acids and bases. In: Lemke T, Williams D, Roche V, et al, eds. *Foye's Principles of Medicinal Chemistry.* 7th ed. Lippincott Williams & Wilkin; 2103:1469-1477.
79. Vardanyan R, Hruby V. Fentanyl-related compounds and derivatives: current status and future prospects for pharmaceutical applications. *Future Med Chem.* 2014;6:385-412.
80. Nossaman V, Ramadhyani U, Kadowitz P, et al. Advances in perioperative pain: use of medications with dual analgesic mechanisms, tramadol and taptentadol. *Anesthesiol Clin.* 2010;28:647-666.
81. Guay D. Is tapentadol an advantage on tramadol? *Consult Pharm.* 2009;24:833-840.
82. Raffa R, Buschmann H, Christoph T, et al. Mechanistic and functional differentiation of tapentadol and tramadol. *Expert Opin Pharmacother.* 2012;13:1437-1449.
83. Shen Q, Qian Y, Xu X, et al. Design, synthesis and biological evaluation of N-phenylalkyl-substituted tramadol derivatives as novel mu opioid receptor ligands. *Acta Pharmacol Sin.* 2015;36:887-894.
84. Coller JK, Christrup LL, Somogyi AA. Role of active metabolites in the use of opioids. *Eur J Clin Pharmacol.* 2009;65:121-139.
85. Gammal R, Crews K, Haidar C, et al. Pharmacogenetics for safe codeine use in Sickle Cell disease. *Pediatrics.* 2016;138:e20153479.
86. Bernard S, Neville K, Nguyen A, et al. Interethnic differences in genetic polymorphisms of CYP2D6 in the U.S. population: clinical implications. *Oncologist.* 2006;11:126-135.
87. Matsui A, Azuma J, Witcher J, et al. Pharmacokinetics, safety and tolerability of atomoxetine and effect of CYP2D6*10/*10 genotype in healthy Japanese men. *J Clin Pharmacol.* 2012;52:388-403.
88. Zhou S-F. Polymorphism of human cytochrome P450 2D6 and its clinical significance. Part 1. *Clin Pharmacokinet.* 2009;48:689-723.
89. Hudak M. Codeine pharmacogenetics as a proof of concept for pediatric precision medicine. *Pediatrics.* 2016;138:e320161359.
90. Mazák K, Noszál B, Hosztafi S. Physicochemical and pharmacological characterization of permanently charged opioids. *Curr Med Chem.* 2017;24:3633-3648.
91. Drug Facts and Comparisons. Facts & Comparisons [Database Online]. In: Louis S, ed. Wolters Kluwer Health, Inc.; 2005.
92. Lexicomp Online® Lexi-drugs® Hudson. Lexi-Comp, Inc. Accessed January 20, 2025. https://www.wolterskluwer.com/en/solutions/uptodate/enterprise/lexidrug-facts-and-comparisons
93. Sverrisdottir E, Lund T, Olesen A, et al. A review of morphine and morphine-6-glucuronide's pharmacokinetic-pharmacodynamic relationships in experimental and clinical pain. *Eur J Pharm Sci.* 2015;74:45-62.
94. Klimas R, Milus G. Morphine-6-glucuronide is responsible for the analgesic effect after morphine administration: a quantitative review of morphine, morphine-6-glucuronide, and morphine-3-glucuronide. *Br J Anaesth.* 2014;113:935-944.
95. van Dorp E, Morariu A, Dahan A. Morphine-6-glucuronide: potency and safety compared with morphine. *Exp Opin Pharmacother.* 2008;9:1955-1961.
96. van Dorp E, Romberg R, Sarton E, et al. Morphine-6-glucuronide: morphine's successor for postoperative pain relief? *Anesth Analg.* 2006;102:1789-1797.

97. Hand C, Blunnie W, Claffey LP, et al. Potential analgesic contribution from morphine-6-glucuronide in CSF. *Lancet.* 1987;2:1207-1208.
98. De Gregori S, De Gregori M, Ranzani G, et al. Morphine metabolism, transport and brain disposition. *Metab Brain Dis.* 2012;27:1-5.
99. Hannah M, Peat S, Knibb A, et al. Disposition of morphine-6-glucuronide and morphine in healthy volunteers. *Br J Anaesth.* 1991;66:103-107.
100. Kou V, Nassisi D. Unstable angina and non-ST segment myocardial infarction: an evidence-based approach to management. *Mt Sinai J Med.* 2006;73:449-468.
101. Hocker S, Fogelson J, Rabinstein A. Refractory intracranial hypertension due to fentanyl administration following closed head injury. *Front Neurol.* 2013;4:3.
102. Roberts D, Goralski K, Renton K, et al. Effect of acute inflammatory brain injury on the accumulation of morphine and morphine 3- and 6-glucuronide in the human brain. *Crit Care Med.* 2009;37:2767-2774.
103. Saljoughian M. Opioids: allergy vs. pseudoallergy. *US Pharm.* 2006;7:HS-5-HS-9.
104. Stanford School of Medicine. Palliative care: opioid conversion/equivalency table. Accessed Octobor 18, 2017. https://palliative.stanford.edu/opioid-conversion/equivalency-table/
105. Cone E, Darwin W, Buchwald W, et al. Oxymorphone metabolism and urinary excretion in human, rat, Guinea pig, rabbit and dog. *Drug Metab Dispos.* 1983;11:446-450.
106. Bao Y, Hou W, Kong X, et al. Hydromorphone for cancer pain. *Cochrane Database Syst Rev.* 2016;10:1-45.
107. Lowe A, Hamilton M, Greenall J, et al. Fatal overdoses involving hydromorphone and morphine among inpatients: a case series. *CMAJ Open.* 2017;5:E184-E189.
108. Vadivelu N, Chang D, Helander E, et al. Ketorolac, oxymorphone, tapentadol and tramadol: a comprehensive review. *Anesthesiol Clin.* 2017;35:e1-e20.
109. Vadivelu N, Maria M, Jolly S, et al. Clinical applications of oxymorphone. *J Opioid Manag.* 2103;9:439-452.
110. Cicero T, Ellis M, Kasper Z. A tale of 2 ADFs: differences in the effectiveness of abuse-deterrent formations of oxymorphone and oxycodone extended-release drugs. *Pain.* 2016;157;1232-1238.
111. Olkkola K, Kontinen V, Saari T. Does the pharmacology of oxycodone justify its increasing use as an analgesic? *Trends Pharmacol Sci.* 2013;23:206-214.
112. Krashin D, Murinova N, Trescot A. Extended-release hydrocodone—gift or curse? *J Pain Res.* 2013;6:53-57.
113. Madadi P, Amstutz U, Rieder M, et al. Clinical practice guideline: CYP2D6 genotyping for safe and efficacious codeine therapy. *J Popul Ther Clin Pharmacol.* 2013;20:e369-396.
114. Andreassen T, Eftedal I, Kelpstad P, et al. Do CYP2D6 genotypes reflect oxycodone requirements for cancer patients treated for cancer apin? A cross-sectional multi-centre study. *Eur J Clin Pharmacol.* 2012;68:55-64.
115. Gardiner S, Chang A, Marchant J, et al. Codeine versus placebo in chronic cough in children. *Cochrane Database Syst Rev.* 2016;7:1-23.
116. Soloman D, Rassen J, Glynn R, et al. The comparative safety of opioids of nonmalignant pain in older adults. *Arch Intern Med.* 2010;170:1979-1986.
117. Becker W, O'Connor P. The safety concerns of opioid analgesics in the elderly: new data raise new concerns. *Arch Intern Med.* 2010;170:1986-1988.
118. Heel R, Brogden R, Speight T, et al. Buprenorphine: a review of its pharmacological properties and therapeutic efficacy. *Drugs Aging.* 1979;17:81-110.
119. Jasinski D, Pevnick J, Griffith J. Human pharmacology and abuse potential of the analgesic bupenorphine. *Arch Gen Psych.* 1978;35:501-516.
120. Barnwal P, Das S, Mondal S, et al. Probuphine (buprenorphine implant): a promising candidate in opioid dependence. *Ther Adv Psychopharmacol.* 2017;7:119-134.
121. Cote J, Montgomery L. Sublingual buprenorphine as an analgesic in chronic pain: a systematic review. *Pain Med.* 2014;15:1171-1178.
122. Davis M. Twelve reasons for considering buprenorphine as a frontline analgesic in the management of pain. *J Support Oncol.* 2012;10:209-219.
123. Dahan A, Aarts L, Smith T. Incidence, reversal and prevention of opioid-induced respiratory depression. *Anesthesiology.* 2010;112:226-238.
124. Fudala P, Jaffe J, Dax E, et al. Use of buprenorphine in the treatment of opioid addiction II. Physiologic and behavior effects of daily and alternate day administration and abrupt withdrawal. *Clin Pharmacol Ther.* 1990;47:525-534.
125. Gal T. Naloxone reversal of buprenorphine-induced respiratory depression. *Clin Pharmacol Ther.* 1989;45:66-71.
126. Kobayashi K, Yamamoto T, Chiba K, et al. Human buprenorphine N-dealkylation is catalyzed by cytochrome P450 3A4. *Drug Metab Dispos.* 1998;26:818-821.
127. Berson A, Fau D, Fornacciari R, et al. Mechanisms for experimental buprenorphine hepatotoxicity: major role of mitochondria dysfunction versus metabolic activation. *J Hepatol.* 2001;34:261-269.
128. Raffa R, Haidery M, Huang H-M, et al. The clinical analgesic efficacy of buprenorphine. *J Clin Pharm Ther.* 2014;39:577-583.
129. Buprenorphine for chronic pain: a review of the clinical effectiveness [Internet]. Canadian Agency for Drugs and Technologies in Health; 2017:1-22.
130. Wiffin P, Derry S, Moore T, et al. Buprenorphine for neuropathic pain in adults. *Cochrane Database of Syst Rev.* 2015;9:1-2.
131. Hans G. Buprenorphine—a review of its role in neuropathic pain. *J Opioid Manag.* 2007;3:195-206.
132. Kahan M, Srivastava A, Ordean A, et al. Buprenophine: new treatment of opioid addiction in primary care. *Can Fam Phys.* 2011;57:281-289.
133. Nicholls L, Bragaw L, Ruetsch C. Opioid dependence: treatment and guidelines. *J Manag Care Pharm.* 2010;16:S14-S21.
134. Lofwall M, Walsh S. A review of buprenorphine diversion and misuse: the current evidence base and experiences from around the world. *J Addict Med.* 2014;8:315-326.
135. Murphy S, Fishman P, McPherson S, et al. Determinants of buprenorphine treatment for opioid dependence. *J Subst Abuse Treat.* 2014;46:315-319.
136. DiPaula B, Menachery E. Physician-pharmacist collaborative care model for buprenorphine-maintained opioid-dependent patients. *J Am Pharm Assoc.* 2015;55:187-192.
137. Barnett P. Comparison of costs and utilization among buprenorphine and methadone patients. *Addiction.* 2009;104:982-992.
138. Rasakham K, Liu-Chen L-Y. Sex difference in kappa opioid pharmacology. *Life Sci.* 2011;88:2-16.
139. Vijay A, Wang S, Worhunsky P, et al. PET imaging reveals sex differences in kappa opioid receptor availability in humans, in vivo. *Am J Nucl Med Mol Imaging.* 2016;6:205-214.
140. Gear R, Miaskowski C, Gordon N, et al. Kappa-opioids produce significantly greater analgesia in women than in men. *Nat Med.* 1996;2:1248-1250.
141. Prommer E, Thompson L. Intranasal fentanyl for pain control: current status with a focus on patient considerations. *Patient Prefer Adherence.* 2011;5:157-164.
142. Rodriguez D, Urrutia G, Escobar Y, et al. Efficacy and safety of oral or nasal fentanyl for treatment of breakthrough pain in cancer patients: a systematic review. *J Pain Palliat Care Pharmacother.* 2015;29:228-246.
143. Durfee S, Messina J, Khankari R. Fentanyl effervescent buccal tablets: enhanced buccal absorption. *Am J Drug Deliv.* 2006;4:1-5.
144. Fontaine M, Latarjet J, Payre J, et al. Feasibility of monomodal analgesia with IV alfentanil during burn dressing changes at bedside (in spontaneously breathing non-intubated patients). *Burns.* 2017;43:337-342.
145. Doi S, Tomohisa M, Uzawa N, et al. Characterization of methadone as a beta-arrestin-biased mu-opoioid receptor agonist. *Mol Pain.* 2016;12:1-9.
146. Kharasch E. Current concepts in methadone metabolism and transport. *Clin Phamacol Drug Dev.* 2017;6:125-134.

147. Kreutzwiser D, Tawfic Q. Methadone for pain management: a pharmacotherapeutic review. *CNS Drugs*. 2020;34:827-839.
148. Moryl N, Tamasdan C, Tarcatu D, et al. A phase I study of D-methadone in patients with chronic pain. *J Opioid Manag*. 2016;12:47-55.
149. Romero J, Baldinger S, Goodman-Meza D, et al. Drug-induced torsades de pointes in an underserved urban population. Methadone: is there therapeutic equipoise. *J Interv Card Electrophysiol*. 2016;45:37-45.
150. Wenjie J, Bies R, Kamden L, et al. Methadone: a substrate and mechanism-based inhibitor of CYP2C19 (Aromatase). *Drug Metab Dispos*. 2010;38:1308-1313.
151. Larson M, Richards T. Quantification of a methadone metabolite (EDDP) in urine: assessment of compliance. *Clin Med Res*. 2009;7:134-141.
152. Grond S, Sablotzki A. Clinical pharmacology of tramadol. *J Pharmacol Exp Ther*. 2004;43:879-923.
153. Beakley B, Kaye A, Kaye A. Tramadol pharmacology, side efects, and serotonin syndrome: a review. *Pain Phys*. 2015;18:395-400.
154. Park S, Wackernah R, Stimmel G. Serotonin syndrome: is it a reason to avoid the use of tramadol with antidepressants? *J Pharm Pract*. 2014;27:71-78.
155. Miotto K, Cho A, Khali M, et al. Trends in tramadol: pharmacology, metabolism and misuse. *Anesth Clin Pharmacol*. 2017; 124:44-51.
156. "Weak" opioid analgesics codeine, dihydrocodeine and tramadol: no less risky than morphine. *Prescrire Intern*. 2016;25:45-51.
157. Kirby E, Carson C, Coward R. Tramadol for the management of premature ejaculation: a timely systematic review. *Int J Impot Res*. 2015;27:121-127.
158. Roth B, Baner K, Westkaemper R, et al. Salvinorin A: a potent naturally occurring nonnitrogenous κ opioid selective agonist. *Proc Natl Acad Sci U S A*. 2002;99:11934-11939.
159. Groer C, Tidgewell K, Moyer R, et al. An opioid agonist that does not induce mu-opioid receptor-arrestin interactions or receptor internalization. *Mol Pharmacol*. 2007;71:549-557.
160. Hiranita T, Obeng S, Sharma A, et al. In vitro and in vivo pharmacology of kratom. *Adv Pharmacol*. 2022; 93:35-76.
161. Saunders K, Igel L, Aronne L. An update on naltrexone/bupropion extended release in the treatment of obesity. *Expert Opin Pharmacother*. 2016;17:2235-2242.
162. Segal D, Macdonald J, Chande N. Low dose naltrexone for induction of remission in Crohn's disease. *Cochrane Database Syst Rev*. 2014;21:1-21.
163. Ludwig M, Zagon I, McLaughlin P. Serum [Met5]-enkephalin levels are reduced in multiple sclerosis and restored by low-dose naltrexone. *Exp Biol Med*. 2017;242:1524-1533.
164. Prichard D, Norton C, Bharucha A. Management of opioid-induced constipation. *Br J Nurs*. 2016;25:S4-S11.
165. Garnock-Jones K. Naloxegol: a review of its use in patients with opioid-induced constipation. *Drugs*. 2015;75:419-425.
166. Siemens W, Becker G. Methylnaltrexone for opioid-induced constipation: review and meta-analysis for objective plus subjective efficacy and safety outcomes. *Ther Clin Risk Manag*. 2016;12: 401-412.
167. Bader S, Jaroslawski K, Blum H, et al. Opioid-induced constipation in advanced illness: safety and efficacy of methylnaltrexone bromide. *Clin Med Insights Oncol*. 2011;5:201-211.
168. Bui K, She F, Zhou D, et al. The effect of quinidine, a strong P-glycoprotein inhibitor, on the pharmacokinetics and central nervous system distribution of naloxegol. *J Clin Pharmacol*. 2016;56:497-505.
169. Floettmann E, Bui K, Sostek M, et al. Pharmacologic profile of naloxegol, a peripherally acting μ-opioid receptor antagonist, for the treatment of opioid-induced constipation. *J Pharmacol Exp Ther*. 2017;361:280-291.
170. Baker D. Formulary drug review: naldemedine. *Hosp Pharm*. 2017;52:464-468.
171. Erowele G. Alvimopan (Entereg), a peripherally acting mu-opioid receptor antagonist for postoperative ileus. *Pharm Therap*. 2008;33:574-583.
172. Xu L-L, Zhou X-Q, Yi P-S, et al. Alvimopan combined with enhanced recovery strategy for managing postoperative ileus after open abdominal surgery: a systematic review and meta-analysis. *J Surg Res*. 2016;203:211-221.
173. Niemegeers C, McGuire JL, Heykants J, et al. Dissociation between opiate-like and antidiarrheal activities of antidiarrheal drugs. *J Pharmacol Exp Ther*. 1979;210:327-333.
174. Sadeque A, Wandel C, He H, et al. Increased drug delivery to the brain by P-glycoprotein inhibition. *Clin Pharmacol Ther*. 2000;68:231-237.
175. Akel T, Bekheit S. Loperamide toxicity: "A brief review". *Ann Noninvasive Electrocardiol*. 2017;e12505:1-4.
176. Crowe A, Wong P. Potential roles of P-gp and calcium channels in loperamide and diphenoxylate transport. *Toxicol Appl Pharmacol*. 2003;193:127-137.
177. Baker D. Loperamide: a pharmacological review. *Rev Gastroenterol Disord*. 2007;7(suppl 3):S11-S18.
178. De Luca A, Coupar I. Difenoxin and loperamide: studies on possible mechanisms of intestinal antisecretory action. *Naunyn-Schmiedebergs Arch Pharmacol*. 1993;347:231-237.
179. Reynolds I, Gould R, Snyder S. Loperamide: blockade of calcium channels as a mechanism for antidiarrheal effects. *J Pharmacol Exp Ther*. 1984;231:628-632.
180. Kim K-A, Chung J, Jung D-H, et al. Identification of cytochrome P450 isoforms involved in the metabolism of loperamide in human liver microsomes. *Eur J Clin Pharmacol*. 2004;60:575-581.
181. Powell J, Presnell S. Loperamide as a potential drug of abuse and misuse: fatal overdoses at the Medical University of South Carolina. *J Forensic Sci*. 2019;64:1726-1730.
182. Salama A, Levin Y, Jha P, et al. Ventricular fibrillation due to overdose of loperamide, the "poor man's methadone". *J Community Hosp Intern Med Perspect*. 2017;7:222-226.
183. Lembo A, Lacy B, Zuckerman M, et al. Eluxadoline for irritable bowel syndrome with diarrhea. *N Engl J Med*. 2016;374:242-253.
184. Nwagwu C, Sarris C, Tao Y-X, et al. Biomarkers for chronic neuropathic pain and their potential application in spinal cord stimulatin: a review. *Transl Perioper Pain Med*. 2016;1:33-38.
185. Diagnostic methods for neuropathic pain: a review of diagnostic accuracy [Internet]. Canadian Agency for Drugs and Technologies in Health. 2015:1-11.
186. Morgan K, Anghelescu D. A review of adult and pediatric neuropathic pain assessment tools. *Clin J Pain*. 2017;33:844-452.
187. O'Connor A, Dworkin R. Treatment of neuropathic pain: an overview of recent guidelines. *Am J Med*. 2009;122:S22-S32.
188. Finnerup N, Attal N, Haroutounian S, et al. Pharmacotherapy for neuropathic pain in adults: a systematic review and meta-analysis. *Lancet Neurol*. 2015;14:162-173.
189. Kerstman E, Ahn S, Battu S, et al. Neuopathic pain. In: Barnes M, Good D, eds. *Handbook of Clinical Neurology*. Vol 110. Elsevier BV; 2013:175-187.
190. Mendlik M, Uritsky T. Treatment of neuropathic pain. *Curr Treat Options Neurol*. 2015;17:50.
191. Binder A, Baron R. The pharmacological therapy of chronic neuropathic pain. *Dtsch Arztebl Int*. 2016;113:616-626.
192. Rolsted K, Benfeldt E, Kissmeyer A-M, et al. Cutaneous in vivo metabolism of topical lidocaine formulation in human skin. *Skin Pharmacol Physiol*. 2009;22:124-127.
193. Stewart W, Lipton R, Celentano D, et al. Prevalence of migrane headache in the United States. Relation to age, income, race, and other sociodemographic factors. *J Am Med Assoc*. 1992; 267:64-69.
194. Burch R, Loder S, Loder E, et al. The prevalence and burden of migraine and severe headache in the United States: updated statistics from government health surveillance studies. *Headache*. 2015;55:21-34.
195. Antonaci F, Ghiotto N, Wu S, et al. Recent advances in migraine therapy. *Springerplus*. 2016;5:673-686.
196. Mehrotra S, Gupta S, Chan K, et al. Current and prospective pharmacological targets in relation to antimigraine action. *Naunyn Schmiedelbergs Arch Pharmacol*. 2008;378:371-394.

197. Weatherall M. The diagnosis and treatment of chronic migraine. *Ther Adv Chronic Dis.* 2015;6:115-123.
198. Dodick D, Martin V. Triptans and CNS side effects: pharmacokinetic and metabolic mechanisms. *Cephalalgia.* 2004;24:417-424.
199. Goadsby P. Post-triptan era for the treatment of acute migraine. *Curr Pain Headache Rep.* 2004;8:393-398.
200. Rapoport A, Bigal M. Migraine preventative therapy: current and emerging treatment options. *Neurol Sci.* 2005;26:S111-S120.
201. Jhee S, Shiovitz T, Crawford A, et al. Pharmacokinetics and pharmacodynamics of the triptan antimigraine agents. *Clin Pharmacokinet.* 2001;40:189-205.
202. Bigal M, Ferrari M, Silberstein S, et al. Migraine in the triptan era: lessons from epidemiology, pathophysiology and clinical sciences. *Headache.* 2009;49:S21-S33.
203. Messali A, Yang M, Gillard P, et al. Treatment persistence and switching in triptan users: a systematic literature review. *Headache.* 2014;54:1120-1130.
204. Rapoport A, Tepper S, Sheftell F, et al. Which triptan for which patient? *Neurol Sci.* 2006;27:S123-S129.
205. Johnson M, Fernandez F, Colson N, et al. A pharmacogenomic evaluation of migraine therapy. *Exp Opin Pharmacother.* 2007;8:1821-1835.
206. Bremner D, Ringan N, Wishart G. Modeling the agonist binding site of serotonin human 5-HT1A, 5-HT1Dα and 5-HT1Dβ receptors. *Eur J Med Chem.* 1997;32:59-69.
207. Vyas K, Halpin R, Geer L. Disposition and pharmacokinetics of the antimigraine drug, rizatriptan, in humans. *Drug Metab Dispos.* 2000;28:89-95.
208. Buchan P, Keywood C, Wade A, et al. Clinical pharmacokinetics of frovatriptan. *Headache.* 2002;42(suppl 2):S54-S62.
209. Wild M, McKillop D, Butters C. Determination of the human cytochrome P450 isoforms involved in the metabolism of zolmitriptan. *Xenobiotica.* 1999;29:847-857.
210. Dixon C, Park G, Tarbit M. Characterization of the enzyme responsible for the metabolism of sumtriptan in human liver. *Biochem Pharmacol.* 1994;47:1253-1257.
211. Yu A-M. Indolealkylamines: biotransformations and potential drug-drug interactions. *AAPS J.* 2008;10:242-253.
212. Evans D, O'Connor D, Lake B, et al. Eletriptan metabolism by human hepatic CYP450 enzymes and transport by human P-glycoprotein. *Drug Metab Dispos.* 2003;31:861-869.
213. Salva M, Jansat J, Martinez-Tobed A, et al. Identification of human liver enzymes involved in the metabolism of the antimigraine agent almotriptan. *Drug Metab Dispos.* 2003;31:404-411.
214. Bigal M, Krymchantowski A, Ho T. Migraine in the tripan era. *Arq Neuropsiquiatr.* 2009;67:559-569.
215. Rapoport A, Tepper S, Bigal M, et al. The triptan formulations: how to match patients and products. *CNS Drugs.* 2003;17:431-447.
216. Baldo B. Opioid analgesic drugs and serotonin toxicity (syndrome): mechanisms, animal models, and links to clinical effects. *Arch Toxicol.* 2018;92:2457-2473.
217. Hutchingson S, Marmura M, Calhoun A, et al. Use of common migraine treatments in breast-feeding women: a summary of recommendations. *Headache.* 2013;53:614-627.
218. Li D, Abreu J, Tepper S. A brief review of gepants. *Curr Pain Headache Rep.* 2023;27:479-488.
219. Dubowchik G, Conway C, Xin A. Blocking the CGRP pathway for acute and preventive treatment of migraine: the evolution of success. *J Med Chem.* 2023;63:6600-6623.

Learning Activity Answers
Central Pain Case Study Answer

Heroin and fentanyl are opioids with an N-methyl and N-phenethyl substituent, respectively, making them both μ-agonist analgesics. Their individual chemistry gives them high affinity for μ receptors and they pose a very high risk for adverse effects such as respiratory depression leading to death. To reverse their potentially lethal effects requires potent and fast-acting μ-receptor antagonism.

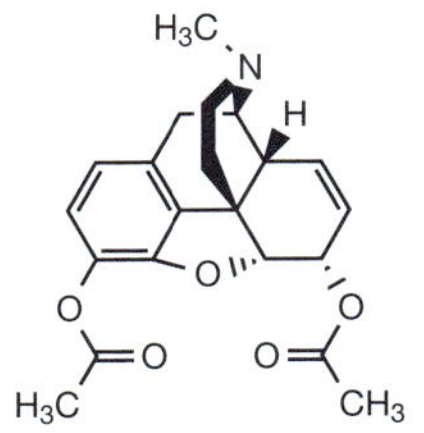

Heroin

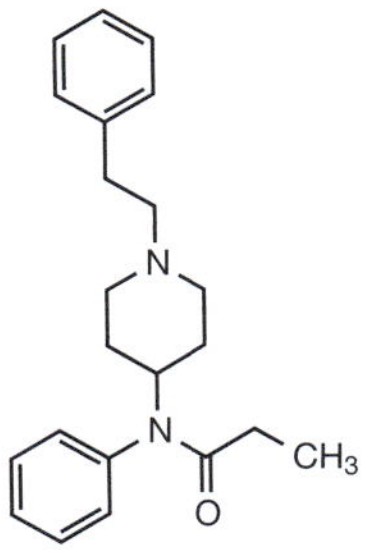

Fentanyl

As shown, all of the therapeutic candidates form water-soluble salts for injection or formulation into an aqueous-based nasal spray, which are the fast-acting dosage forms needed in this clinical situation. All contain the epoxymorphinan structural framework common in opioid ligands, and all have the essential 3-phenolic hydroxyl group. Most also have an affinity-enhancing 14β-OH group. However, evaluation of their remaining structural features quickly leads to the elimination of three candidates.

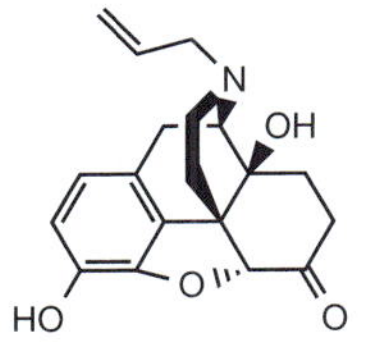

A

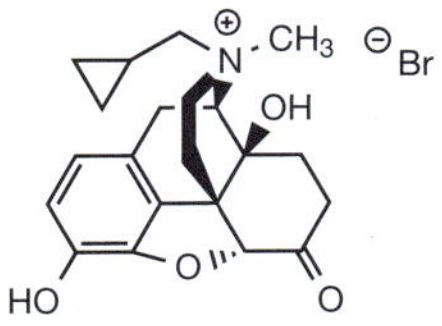

B

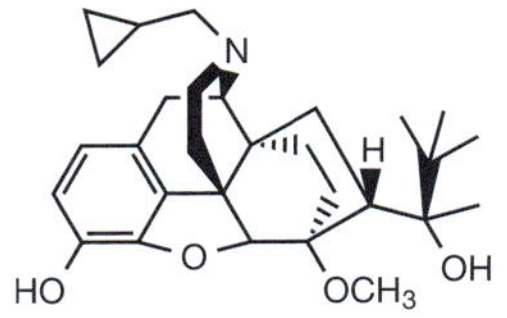

C

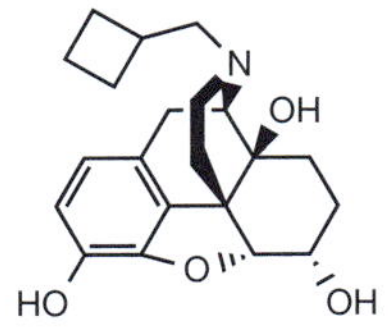

D

(continued)

Learning Activity Answers
Central Pain Case Study Answer (continued)

Candidate B: While this drug has the cyclopropylmethyl N-substituent associated with μ-antagonist action, it also has a N-CH_3 substituent that makes the amine quaternary and charged at all pH values. Since it will be fully charged in the bloodstream, it will not be able to penetrate the BBB to reach central sites of action. Therefore, it will not be able to reverse respiratory depression, a central adverse effect. This peripherally restricted antagonist (naltrexone methylbromide) is used clinically to reverse the constipating effect of μ agonists in the gut.

Candidate C: This tertiary amine drug can penetrate the BBB and it also has the cyclopropylmethyl nitrogen substituent, which generally confers μ-antagonist action. However, its unique structure that incorporates a C-ring *endo*-ethano bridge and a large hydrophobic substituent at C_7 changes its μ-receptor binding characteristics to provide partial μ agonism of an affinity sufficiently high to be considered pseudoirreversible. This drug's bicyclic C ring allows it to be structurally classified as an orvinol, rather than a true epoxymorphinan. As a μ agonist, this drug (buprenorphine) can induce respiratory depression and its high receptor affinity means it is very hard to reverse. It would exacerbate the clinical problem these overdosed patients are experiencing, rather than reverse it.

Candidate D: This centrally acting tertiary opioid has an N-substituent reminiscent of the cyclopropylmethyl group of Candidates B and C, but the ring has been expanded by one carbon (cyclobutylmethyl). This is enough to shift its primary pharmacologic action from μ antagonist to κ agonist. This drug (nalbuphine) is used clinically as an analgesic, although its κ-agonist action makes use-limiting dysphoria a potential adverse effect. Furthermore, the cyclobutylmethyl group makes candidate D a weak μ receptor partial agonist; like candidate C, this could exacerbate an overdose due to the partial agonist effect. In patients who are at risk of losing their life to μ agonist–induced respiratory depression, a pure and potent μ antagonist is needed.

Candidate A: This drug (naloxone) provides everything required to save lives from μ agonist overdose. The *N*-allyl substituent is electron-rich and confers μ antagonist action, and the pentacyclic structure with the requisite 3-OH, affinity-enhancing 14β-OH, and molecular flexibility provided by the 7,8-dihydro C ring` makes that antagonist action pure. There is no agonist action at any receptor at any dose and, as a tertiary amine, it can readily penetrate the BBB and reverse respiratory depression. In water-soluble hydrochloride salt form, this potent μ antagonist can be delivered intranasally or by injection for almost immediate action.

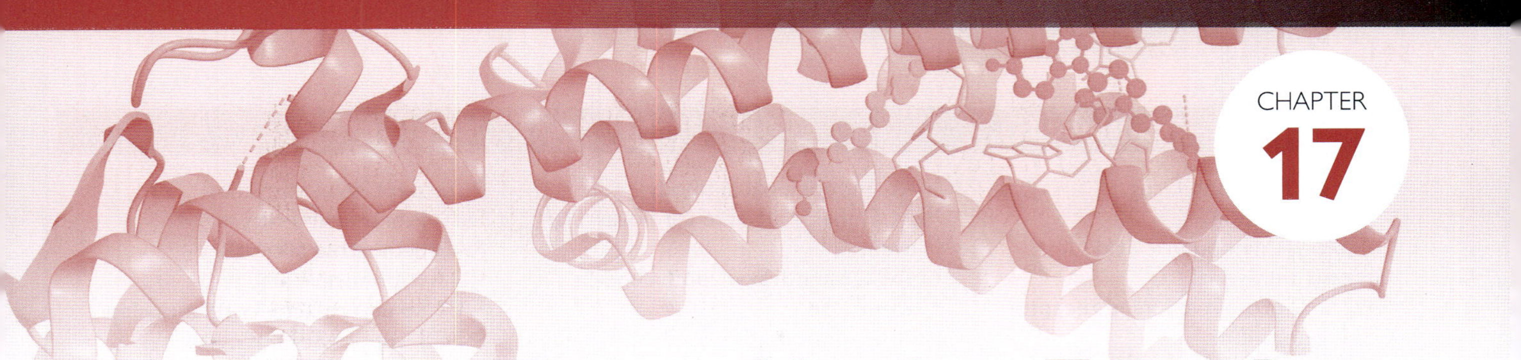

CHAPTER
17

Drugs Used to Treat Pain: Peripherally Acting Agents

Dave Weldon and Abby Weldon

Drugs covered in this chapter:

Antipyretic Analgesics
- Acetaminophen

Anti-inflammatory Analgesics
- Aspirin and other salicylates
- Bromfenac
- Diclofenac
- Diflunisal
- Etodolac
- Fenoprofen
- Flurbiprofen
- Ibuprofen
- Indomethacin
- Ketoprofen
- Ketorolac
- Meclofenamic acid
- Mefenamic acid
- Meloxicam
- Nabumetone
- Naproxen
- Nepafenac
- Oxaprozin
- Piroxicam
- Sulindac
- Tolmetin

COX-2 Inhibitors
- Celecoxib

Monoclonal Antibodies for Rheumatoid Arthritis
- Adalimumab
- Certolizumab
- Golimumab
- Infliximab
- Rituximab
- Secukinumab
- Siltuximab
- Tocilizumab

Disease-modifying Drugs for Rheumatoid Arthritis
- Abatacept
- Anakinra
- Apremilast
- Baricitinib
- Etanercept
- Gold salts
- Hydroxychloroquine
- Leflunomide
- Methotrexate
- Sulfasalazine
- Tofacitinib
- Upadacitinib

Drugs for the Treatment of Gout
- Allopurinol
- Colchicine
- Febuxostat
- Lesinurad
- Pegloticase
- Probenecid

Local Anesthetics
- Articaine
- Benzocaine
- Bupivacaine
- Chloroprocaine
- Dibucaine
- Lidocaine
- Mepivacaine
- Prilocaine
- Procaine
- Ropivacaine
- Tetracaine

Abbreviations

ACR American College of Rheumatology
APC antigen-presenting cell
Apo apolipoprotein
5-ASA 5-aminosalicylic acid
AUC area under the (plasma concentration) curve
cAMP cyclic adenosine monophosphate
CDC Centers for Disease Control
CHO Chinese hamster ovary
C_{max} maximum plasma concentration
C_{min} minimum plasma concentration
CNS central nervous system
CoASH coenzyme A
COVID-19 coronavirus disease 2019
COX cyclooxygenase
CTLA-4 cytotoxic T-lymphocyte antigen-4
CXCL chemokines
CYP cytochrome P450
DAG diacylglycerol
DHODH dihydroorotate dehydrogenase
DMARD disease-modifying antirheumatic drug
DNA deoxyribonucleic acid
EMLA eutectic mixture of a local anesthetic

Abbreviations—continued

FDA US Food and Drug Administration
GABA γ-aminobutyric acid
GI gastrointestinal
GPCR G protein–coupled receptor
GSH glutathione
HDL high-density lipoprotein
hOAT3 human organic anion transporter
HPETE hydroperoxy-eicosatetraenoic acid
IC_{50} 50% of maximal inhibitory concentration
IFNγ interferon-γ
IL-1Rα IL-1 receptor antagonist
IL-1R1 IL-1 type 1 receptor
Ig immunoglobulin
IL interleukin
IM intramuscular
IV intravenous
JAK Janus-activated kinase
JAKis Janus-activated kinase inhibitors
LDL low-density lipoprotein
LT leukotriene
LTB_4 leukotriene B_4
MAb monoclonal antibody
MACE major adverse cardiovascular event
6MNA 6-methoxynaphthalene-2-acetic acid
mPEG monomethoxypoly(ethylene glycol)
NAPQI *N*-acetyl-*p*-benzoquinoneimine
NF nuclear factor
NMDA *N*-methyl-D-aspartate
NO nitric oxide
NSAID nonsteroidal anti-inflammatory drug
OA osteoarthritis
OATP organic anion transporting polypeptide
OTC over the counter
PABA *p*-aminobenzoic acid
PDE phosphodiesterase
PEG polyethylene glycol
P-gp P-glycoprotein
PG prostaglandin
PIAS protein inhibitors of activated STAT
PLTs peptidoleukotrienes
PsA psoriatic arthritis
RA rheumatoid arthritis
RNA ribonucleic acid
SAR structure-activity relationship
SOCS suppressors of cytokine signaling
SRS-A slow-reacting substance of anaphylaxis
STAT signal transducer and activator of transcription
TC total cholesterol
T_{max} time to maximum serum concentration
TNF tumor necrosis factor
TNFR tumor necrosis factor receptor
TLR4 toll-like receptor 4
TYK tyrosine kinase
TX thromboxane
TXA2 thromboxane A2
URAT1 urate anion transporter
USAN US Adopted Names
VEGF vascular endothelial growth factor
VTE venous thromboembolism

CLINICAL SIGNIFICANCE

The nonsteroidal anti-inflammatory drugs (NSAIDs) are one of the oldest and most widely utilized classes of medications. Both prescription and over-the-counter NSAIDs are commercially available and are frequently used in the treatment of pain, fever, and inflammation. While NSAIDs are a chemically heterogeneous class of drugs, they share a similar mechanism of action by inhibiting the cyclooxygenase (COX) enzymes responsible for prostaglandin (PG) synthesis in the arachidonic acid pathway. Most NSAIDs are nonselective and inhibit varying degrees of COX-1 and COX-2. However, many newer NSAIDs predominantly inhibit the COX-2 isoform, with celecoxib being the only commercially available COX-2 selective inhibitor.

Although NSAIDs are commonly prescribed medications, as a class, they are associated with serious adverse effects, including gastrointestinal bleeding, cardiovascular events, and nephrotoxicity, specifically with high doses, long duration of use, or the combination thereof.

NSAIDs will continue to remain an important class of drugs in the management of pain, fever, and inflammation. An understanding of the chemical features underlying the pharmacokinetic and pharmacodynamic variability of these drugs will allow clinicians to select the best NSAID for the patient.

Amy M. Pick, PharmD, BCOP

INTRODUCTION

Pain management is an essential part of a health care team's responsibility for patient well-being in operative, postoperative, emergency, and acute and chronic disease situations. This chapter will focus on drugs that elicit pain relief in the periphery. These drugs include antipyretic analgesics, NSAIDs, small molecule and monoclonal antibody (MAb) therapies for rheumatoid arthritis (RA), and local anesthetic agents.

INFLAMMATION

Inflammation is a normal and essential response to any noxious stimulus that threatens the host and can vary from a localized to a generalized response.[1] One of the primary mechanisms for an inflammatory event is the release of proinflammatory chemical mediators (eg, histamine, serotonin, leucokinins, slow-reacting substance of anaphylaxis [SRS-A], lysosomal enzymes, lymphokinins, and PGs). The most common sources of these chemical mediators include neutrophils, basophils, mast cells, platelets, macrophages, and lymphocytes. Currently available drugs relieve the painful symptoms of the disease but are not considered curative.

The anti-inflammatory drugs discussed in this chapter act by modulating any one of several mechanisms, including immunologic processes, activation of complement system, cellular activities such as phagocytosis, interference with the formation and release of the chemical mediators of inflammation, or stabilization of lysosomal membranes. In 1971, J.R. Vane published a classic paper in which he reported that some NSAIDs, including aspirin, inhibited the biosynthesis of PGs from arachidonic acid.[2] This theory has become the most widely accepted mechanism of action of NSAIDs.

Mediators of Inflammation

Prostaglandins, Thromboxanes, Prostacyclin, and Leukotrienes

PROSTAGLANDINS. PGs are eicosanoids, which are a group of autocoids that also include thromboxanes (TX), prostacyclin, and leukotrienes (LT). PGs are naturally occurring products produced in mammalian tissue. They are found throughout the body and, through the activation of specific G protein–coupled receptors (GPCRs), possess many pharmacological properties impacting the cardiovascular system, platelets, inflammation, smooth muscle, central nervous system, and endocrine system. The inhibition of PG biosynthesis is the primary mechanism of NSAID-mediated anti-inflammatory activity.

Prostaglandin Structure. PGs are 20-carbon cyclopentanofatty acid derivatives produced from polyunsaturated fatty acids. The general structure of the PGs is shown in Figure 17.1. All naturally occurring PGs have a 15α-hydroxy group and a *trans* double bond at C13. The chain containing the carboxylic acid group is the α-chain, and the chain substituted with the 15α-hydroxyl group is labeled the β-chain. The PGs are classified by the capital letters A, B, C, D, E, F, G, H, and I (eg, PGA, PGB, PGC) depending on the nature and stereochemistry of oxygen substituents at the 9- and 11-positions. For example, members of the PGE series possess a keto function at C9 and an α-hydroxy group at C11, whereas members of the PGF series possess α-hydroxy groups at both of these positions. The number of double bonds in the side chains connected to the cyclopentane ring is designated by subscripts 1, 2, or 3. The subscript 2 indicates an additional *cis* double bond between C5 and C6, and the subscript 3 indicates a third double bond (C17-18) of *cis* stereochemistry. Members of the PGG and PGH series are cycloendoperoxide intermediates in the biosynthesis of PGs and contain a peroxide group bridging the C9 and C11 carbons, as depicted in Figure 17.2.

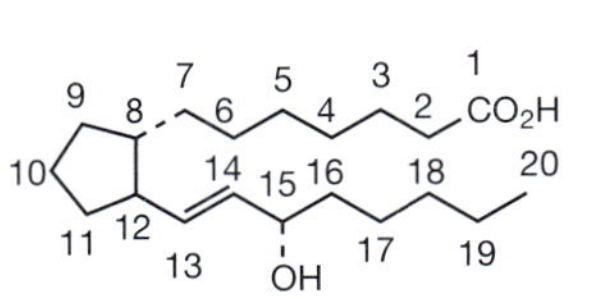

Figure 17.1 General structure of the prostaglandins.

Prostaglandin Biosynthesis. PGs are derived biosynthetically from unsaturated fatty acid precursors (see Fig. 17.2). The number of double bonds contained in the naturally occurring PGs reflects the nature of the biosynthetic precursors. The most common of these fatty acids in humans is arachidonic acid, which is derived from dietary linoleic acid or is ingested from the diet and esterified to phospholipids (primarily phosphatidylethanolamine or phosphatidylcholine) in cell membranes.[3]

The primary source of arachidonic acid is stored as acyl chains in membrane glycerophospholipids. Liberation of free arachidonic acid can occur through a variety of enzymatic reactions (see Fig. 17.2). When activated by various initiating factors that interact with membrane receptors coupled to guanine nucleotide–binding regulatory proteins (G proteins; see Chapter 6), phospholipase A2 catalyzes the hydrolysis of the two acyl chains from the glycerol backbone of the phospholipid. Other phospholipases (eg, phospholipase C [PLC]) also play a role. PLC hydrolyzes the phosphodiester bond, forming 1,2-diacylglycerides from phospholipids with the subsequent release of arachidonic acid by the actions of mono- and diacylglyceride lipases.[4] An inflammation-mediating polypeptide produced by leukocytes, interleukin-1, increases phospholipase activity and, thus, arachidonic acid release.

Once arachidonic acid is released, arachidonic acid cyclooxygenase (PG endoperoxide synthase, COX) produces PGs, along with thromboxanes and prostacyclin. Alternatively, arachidonic acid is susceptible to lipoxygenase activity to produce leukotrienes.

Cyclooxygenases. COX, in the presence of oxygen and heme, first produces the cyclic endoperoxide PGG_2 from arachidonic acid, and then, through its peroxidase activity, PGH_2. Both PGG_2 and PGH_2 are chemically unstable due to the reactive peroxide group and decompose rapidly (half-life of 5 minutes) to generate more persistent PGs (see Fig. 17.2). PGE_2 is a proinflammatory PG formed by the action of PGE isomerase and PGD_2 by the actions of isomerases or glutathione-S-transferase on PGH_2, whereas proinflammatory $PGF_2\alpha$ is formed from PGH_2 via an endoperoxide reductase system (see Fig. 17.2). Interestingly, PGE_1 is a reduced form of PGE_2 and possesses GI cytoprotective properties (discussed next in the "Prostaglandin Effects on the Gastrointestinal Tract" section). The biologic target for NSAIDs is COX, where they inhibit PG biosynthesis to prevent inflammation.

Three isoforms of COX have been identified: COX-1, COX-2, and COX-3. COX was first purified in 1976.[5] Interestingly, COX-2 expression is inducible by cytokines and growth factors.[6-10] Attenuated COX-1 proteins have been identified; however, their clinical impact is yet to be determined.[11] The primary mechanism by which NSAIDS are believed to produce their pharmacologic effects is attributed to inhibition of the COX-1 and COX-2 enzymes. Both isoforms carry out the same two reactions in the PG biosynthetic pathway: the double dioxygenation of arachidonic acid to PGG_2 at the cyclooxygenase active site and the subsequent reduction to PGH_2 at the peroxidase site.[12] Analgesic/antipyretic drugs selectively target COX-3; thus,

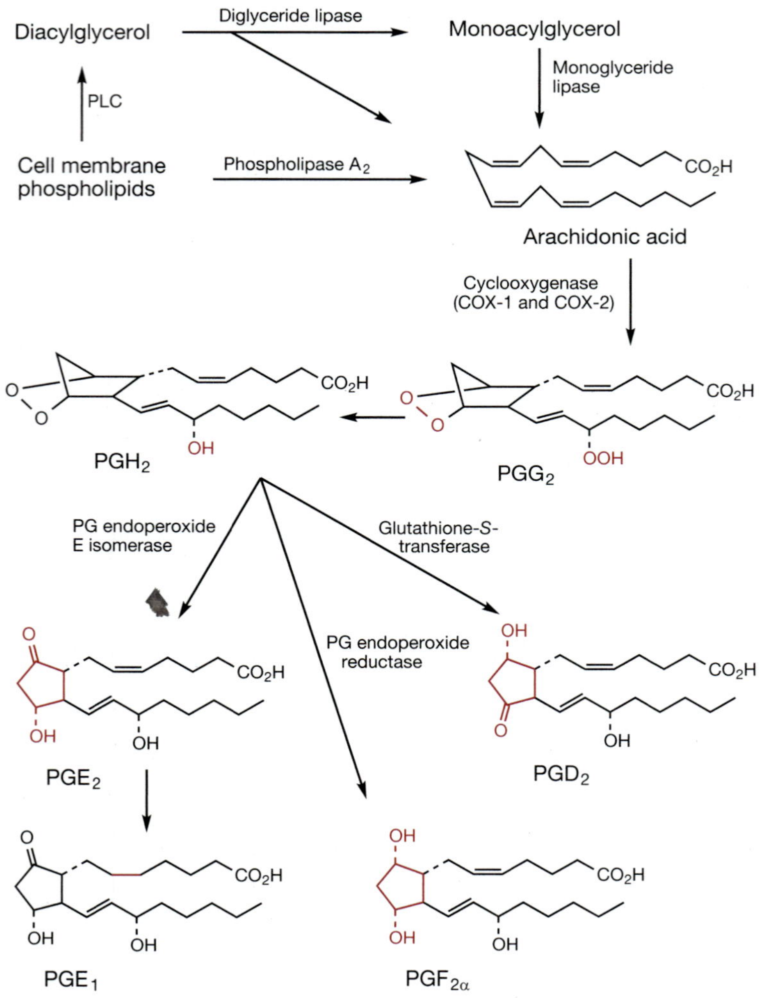

Figure 17.2 Biosynthesis of prostaglandins from arachidonic acid.

inhibition of COX-3 can represent a primary mechanism by which acetaminophen decreases pain and fever.[14]

Both human COX-1 and COX-2 are quite similar in structure (60% homology) and almost identical in length, varying from 599 (COX-1) to 604 (COX-2) amino acids.[13-16] The active site cavities of COX-1 and COX-2 are illustrated in Figure 17.3.[14] Residues that form the substrate binding and catalytic sites, and residues immediately adjacent to those sites, are essentially identical with two minor, however important, exceptions. The Ile at positions 434 and 523 in COX-1 is exchanged for Val in COX-2. The smaller size of Val434 and Val523 in COX-2 allows inhibitor access to an allosteric pocket adjacent to the active site, whereas the longer side chain of Ile in COX-1 sterically blocks inhibitor access. The available space in the binding pocket of COX-2 is 20% to 25% larger than that of the COX-1 binding site because of the replacement of the smaller Val434 and Val523 residues in COX-2 for the larger Ile434 and Ile523 residues in COX-1 and, thus, is the basis for COX-2 selectivity. Large inhibitors that utilize this extra space are essentially too big to fit in the COX-1 site, making them COX-2 selective.

From a therapeutic standpoint, the major difference between COX-1 and COX-2 lies in physiologic function rather than in structure. The concentration of COX-1 is quite high in resting cells as compared to COX-2, which is minimally present in resting cells. However, COX-2 can be induced at sites of inflammation by cytokines in vascular smooth muscle, fibroblasts, and epithelial cells. COX-1 functions to produce PGs that are involved in normal homeostatic cellular activity, and COX-2 produces PGs at inflammatory sites.[17] Inducible COX-2 linked to inflammatory cell types and tissues is believed to be the target enzyme in the treatment of inflammatory disorders by NSAIDs. Most NSAIDs inhibit both COX-1 and COX-2, with varying degrees of selectivity, and are termed "nonselective." Selective COX-2 inhibitors can attenuate (but not eliminate) COX-1–related adverse effects commonly associated with NSAIDs, such as gastric and renal effects.

Prostaglandin Effects on the Gastrointestinal Tract. One of the primary adverse effects of nonselective NSAIDs primarily targeting COX-1 is GI disturbances, which is due to the reduction of specific PGs in the GI tract. Specifically, PGE_1 exerts a protective effect on gastroduodenal mucosa by stimulating secretion of an alkaline mucus and bicarbonate ion and by maintaining or increasing mucosal blood flow. Thus, inhibition of PG biosynthesis in the GI tract is unfavorable because it can cause disruption of mucosal integrity, resulting in GI distress, including peptic ulcer disease that is commonly associated with the use of NSAIDs.

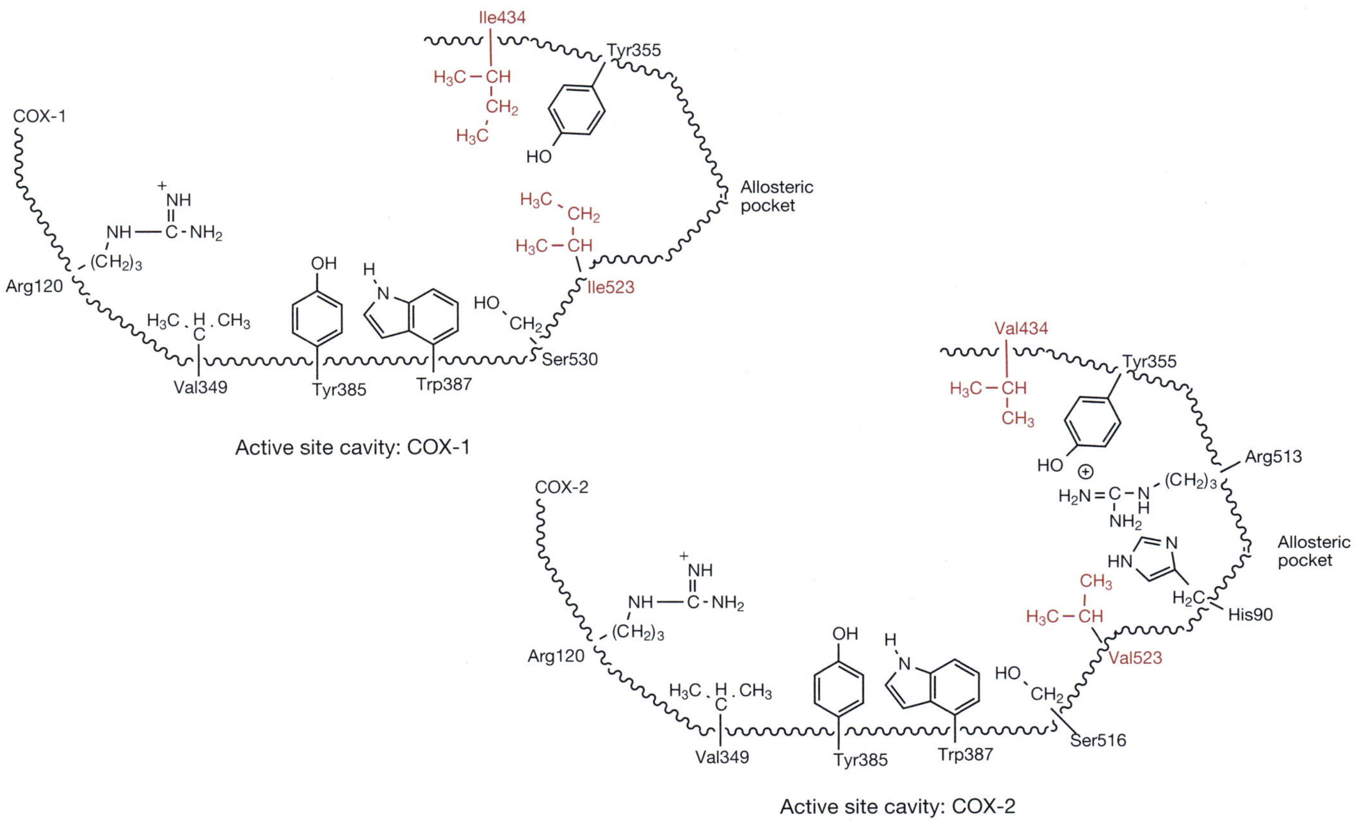

Figure 17.3 Representations of COX-1 and COX-2 active sites. (Reprinted from Roche VF. A receptor-grounded approach to teaching nonsteroidal anti-inflammatory drug chemistry and structure-activity relationships. *Am J Pharm Educ.* 2009;73(8):143, with permission.)

NONPROSTANOID PRODUCTS OF THE ARACHIDONIC ACID PATHWAY

Thromboxane and Prostacyclin. In addition to forming the various PGs, nonprostanoids can also be formed from PGH_2, as illustrated in Figure 17.4. Thromboxane synthase acts on PGH_2 to produce thromboxane A_2 (TXA_2), whereas prostacyclin synthase converts PGH_2 to prostacyclin (PGI_2), both of which possess short biologic half-lives. A potent vasoconstrictor and inducer of platelet aggregation, TXA_2 has a biologic half-life of approximately 30 seconds, being rapidly and nonenzymatically converted to the more stable, but inactive, TXB_2. Prostacyclin, a potent hypotensive and inhibitor of platelet aggregation, has a half-life of approximately 3 minutes and is nonenzymatically converted to 6-keto-$PGF_1\alpha$. Platelets contain primarily thromboxane synthase, whereas endothelial cells contain primarily prostacyclin synthase. Considerable research efforts are being expended in the development of stable prostacyclin analogues and thromboxane antagonists as cardiovascular drugs. The pharmacologic effects of some PGs, TXA_2, and prostacyclin are summarized in Table 17.1.

Leukotrienes. With NSAID therapy, in which COX enzymes are inhibited, arachidonic acid is now forced to be metabolized by lipoxygenase enzymes. Lipoxygenases are a group of enzymes that oxidize polyunsaturated fatty acids possessing two *cis* double bonds separated by a methylene group to produce lipid hydroperoxides.[18] Arachidonic acid is thus metabolized by lipoxygenase enzymes to a number of hydroperoxy-eicosatetraenoic acid (HPETE) derivatives. Lipoxygenases differ in the position at which they peroxidize arachidonic acid and in their tissue specificity. For example, platelets possess only a 12-lipoxygenase, whereas leukocytes possess both a 12-lipoxygenase and a 5-lipoxygenase.[19] Leukotrienes are products of the 5-lipoxygenase pathway and are divided into two major classes: hydroxylated eicosatetraenoic acids (LTs), represented by leukotriene B_4 (LTB_4), and peptidoleukotrienes (pLTs), such as LTC_4, LTD_4, and LTE_4. 5-Lipoxygenase will produce leukotrienes from 5-HPETE, as shown in Figure 17.5.

LTA synthase converts 5-HPETE to an unstable epoxide called LTA4, which can be converted by LTA hydrolase to the leukotriene LTB_4 or by glutathione-*S*-transferase to LTC_4. Other cysteinyl leukotrienes (eg, LTD_4, LTE_4, and LTF_4) can then be formed from LTC_4 by the removal of glutamic acid and glycine and then reconjugated with glutamic acid. The cysteinyl leukotrienes produce airway edema, smooth muscle constriction, and altered cellular activity associated with the inflammatory process, all of which are associated with the pathophysiology of asthma. Cysteinyl leukotrienes activate at least two receptors, designated as CysLT1 and CysLT2. A long-recognized mediator of inflammation, SRS-A, is primarily a mixture of leukotrienes LTC_4 and LTD_4.

The physiologic role of LTB_4 is a potent chemotactic agent for polymorphonuclear leukocytes, causing the accumulation of leukocytes at inflammation sites.[20] Both LTC_4

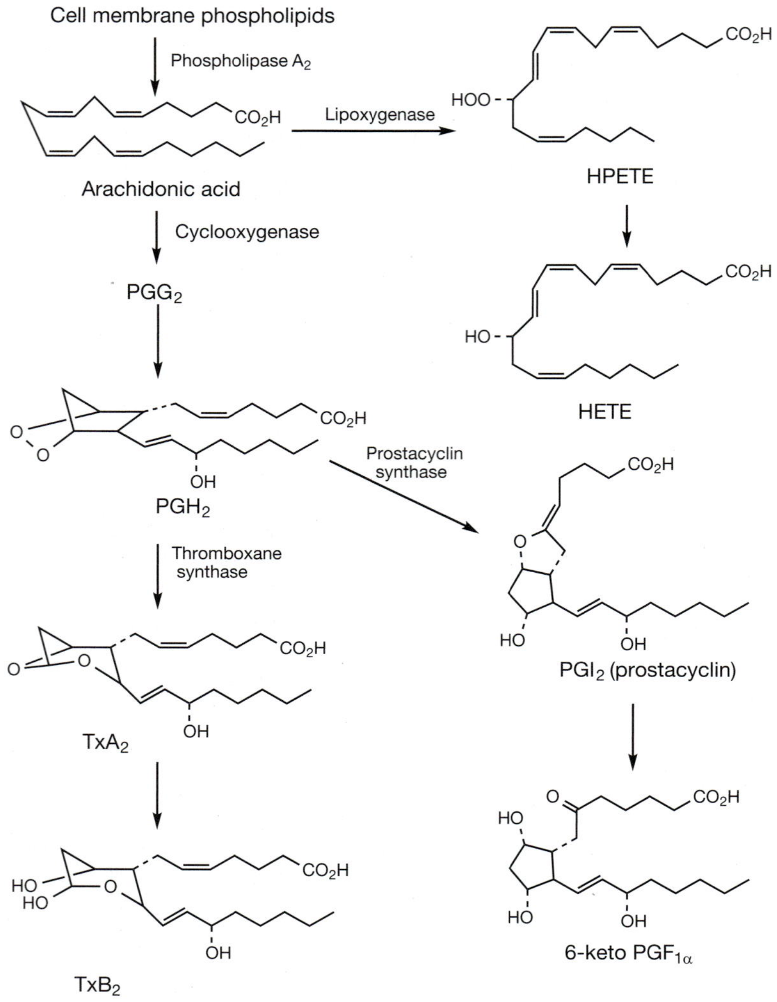

Figure 17.4 Biosynthesis of thromboxanes, prostacyclin, and leukotrienes.

and LTD_4 are potent hypotensives and bronchoconstrictors and are the leukotrienes responsible for NSAID-induced asthmatic responses.

General Gastrointestinal Considerations for Nonsteroidal Anti-inflammatory Drug Therapy

NSAIDs do have some use-limiting adverse effects, including GI, renal, and cardiovascular toxicities. However, GI toxicity remains the most common adverse effect observed with chronic NSAID users. GI toxicities include dyspepsia, abdominal pain, heartburn, gastric erosion leading to wall perforation, peptic ulcer formation, bleeding, and diarrhea. These gastric ailments are attributed to one or two arms of the dual insult mechanism (Fig. 17.6). Nearly all NSAIDs are weak acids, with pK_a values of approximately 3, making them poorly soluble in gastric fluid, which has a pH of ~1.5. The primary insult is committed when pieces of insoluble NSAID lodge in gastric mucosa, resulting in direct tissue damage. The secondary insult is committed through reduction in cytoprotective PG concentrations in the GI tract, which is primarily mediated through COX-1 inhibition. The secondary insult is a significant reason for the development

Table 17.1 Pharmacologic Properties of Prostaglandins, Thromboxane, and Prostacyclin

	PGE_2	PGF_2^{α}	PGI_2	TXA_2
Uterus	Oxytocic dilation	Oxytocic constriction		
Bronchi	Dilation	Constriction		Constriction
Platelets			Pro-aggregatory	Anti-aggregatory
Blood vessels	Dilation	Constriction	Dilation	Constriction

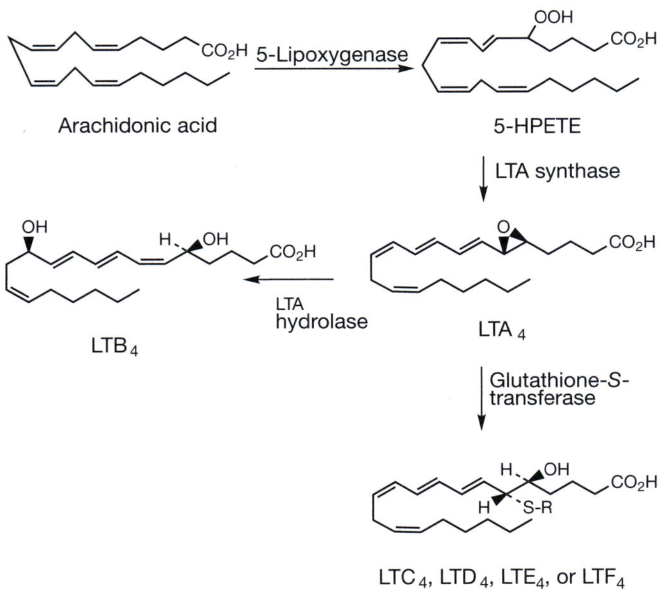

Figure 17.5 Biosynthesis of leukotrienes.

of COX-2 selective inhibitors; however, they are accompanied by significant cardiotoxic liabilities (discussed later).

Therapeutic Classifications

Antipyretic Analgesics

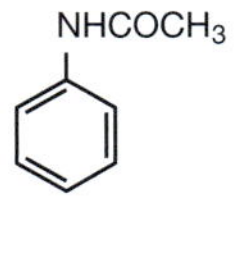

Acetanilide

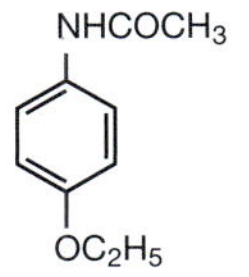

Phenacetin

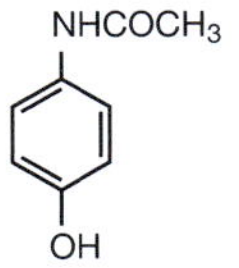

Acetaminophen

Mechanism of Action

Drugs included in this class possess analgesic and antipyretic actions, but lack anti-inflammatory effects. Antipyretics interfere with pyrogenic factors that produce fever, but they do not appear to lower body temperature in afebrile subjects. It had been historically accepted that the antipyretics exert their actions within the central nervous system (CNS), primarily at the hypothalamic thermoregulatory center. Endogenous leukocytic pyrogens can be released from cells that have been activated by various stimuli, and antipyretics can act by (1) inhibiting the activation of these cells by an exogenous pyrogen or (2) by inhibiting the release of endogenous leukocytic pyrogens from the cells once they have been activated by the exogenous pyrogen. Substantial evidence exists suggesting a central antipyretic mechanism, an antagonism that can result from either a direct competition of a pyrogen and the antipyretic agent at CNS receptors or an inhibition of PG synthesis in the CNS.[21,22]

Despite the extensive use of acetaminophen, the mechanism of action is not fully clear.[23] Acetaminophen can inhibit pain impulses by exerting a depressant effect on peripheral receptors, and an antagonistic effect on the actions of bradykinin can also play a role. The antipyretic effects might not result from inhibition of release of endogenous pyrogen from leukocytes but, rather, from inhibiting its action on hypothalamic thermoregulatory centers. As noted earlier, the fact that acetaminophen is an effective antipyretic/analgesic, but an ineffective anti-inflammatory agent, may be explained by its greater inhibition of PG biosynthesis via inhibition of the COX-3 isoform (a splice variant of COX-1) in the CNS compared with that in the periphery.

The ability of selected analgesic/antipyretic drugs to inhibit COX-1, COX-2, and COX-3 is shown in Table 17.2.[11]

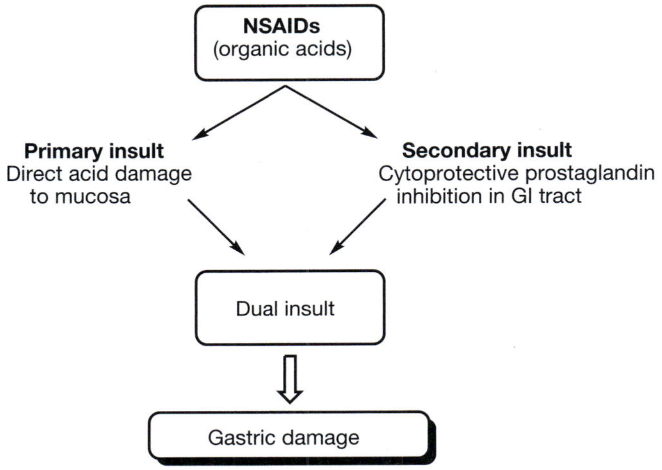

Figure 17.6 NSAID-induced production of gastric damage by a dual-insult mechanism.

Structure-Activity Relationships

The structure-activity relationships of *p*-aminophenol derivatives have been widely studied. Based on the comparative toxicity of acetanilide and acetaminophen, aminophenols are less toxic than the corresponding aniline derivatives, although *p*-aminophenol itself is too toxic for therapeutic purposes. Etherification of the phenolic function with methyl or propyl groups produces derivatives with more side effects than ethyl groups. Substituents on the nitrogen atom that reduce basicity reduce activity unless that substituent is metabolically labile (eg, acetyl). Amides derived from aromatic acids (eg, *N*-phenylbenzamide) are less active or inactive.

Table 17.2 Potency (IC_{50}, μM) of Selected Nonsteroidal Anti-inflammatory Drugs for the COX Enzymes

Drug	COX-1	COX-2	COX-3
Acetaminophen	>1,000	>1,000	460
Phenacetin	>1,000	>1,000	102
Aspirin	10	>1,000	3.1
Diclofenac	0.035	0.041	0.008
Ibuprofen	2.4	5.7	0.24
Indomethacin	0.010	0.66	0.016

Acetaminophen

Acetaminophen is indicated for use as an antipyretic/analgesic and may be particularly useful in individuals displaying an allergy or sensitivity to aspirin. It is weakly acidic (phenolic $pK_a = 9.51$) and not extensively bound to plasma proteins (18%-25%).[24] It does not possess anti-inflammatory activity; however, it will produce analgesia in a wide variety of arthritic and musculoskeletal disorders. It is available in various formulations, including suppositories, tablets, capsules, granules, and solutions. The usual adult dose is 325 to 650 mg every 4 to 6 hours. Doses greater than 2.6 g/d are not recommended for long-term therapy because of potential hepatotoxicity. Acetaminophen, unlike aspirin, is stable in aqueous solution, making liquid formulations readily available, which is particularly advantageous in pediatric patients. Because acetaminophen is water insoluble, liquid formulations are prepared with solvents such as propylene glycol to keep acetaminophen in solution; otherwise, the formulation is administered as a suspension.

METABOLISM AND TOXICITY. The metabolism of acetaminophen is illustrated in Figure 17.7.[25] Both acetanilide and phenacetin are metabolized to acetaminophen. Additionally, both undergo hydrolysis to yield aniline derivatives that produce significant methemoglobinemia and hemolytic anemia (either directly or through conversion to hydroxylamines), which resulted in their removal from the US market. Acetaminophen undergoes rapid first-pass metabolism in the GI tract primarily by conjugation reactions, with the *O*-sulfate being the primary metabolite in children and the *O*-glucuronide being the primary metabolite in adults.

It has been known for more than 40 years that cytochrome P450 (CYP450)–mediated metabolism is responsible for the hepatotoxicity of acetaminophen.[26] A minor, but significant, product of acetaminophen is *N*-hydroxyamide produced by CYP2E1 and CYP3A4.[27] CYP2E1 is the rate-limiting enzyme that initiates the cascade of events leading to acetaminophen hepatotoxicity; in the absence of this enzyme, toxicity will only be apparent at high concentrations.[27] The *N*-hydroxyamide metabolite is converted to a reactive toxic metabolite, an acetimidoquinone (*N*-acetyl-*p*-benzoquinoneimine, or NAPQI) that has been suggested to produce the nephrotoxicity and hepatotoxicity associated with acetaminophen and phenacetin.[28,29] Normally, this iminoquinone is detoxified by conjugation with hepatic glutathione. In cases of ingestion of large doses or overdoses of acetaminophen, however, hepatic stores of glutathione can be depleted by more than 70%, allowing the electrophilic quinone to react with nearby nucleophilic functional groups, primarily thiol (-SH) groups, on hepatic proteins, resulting

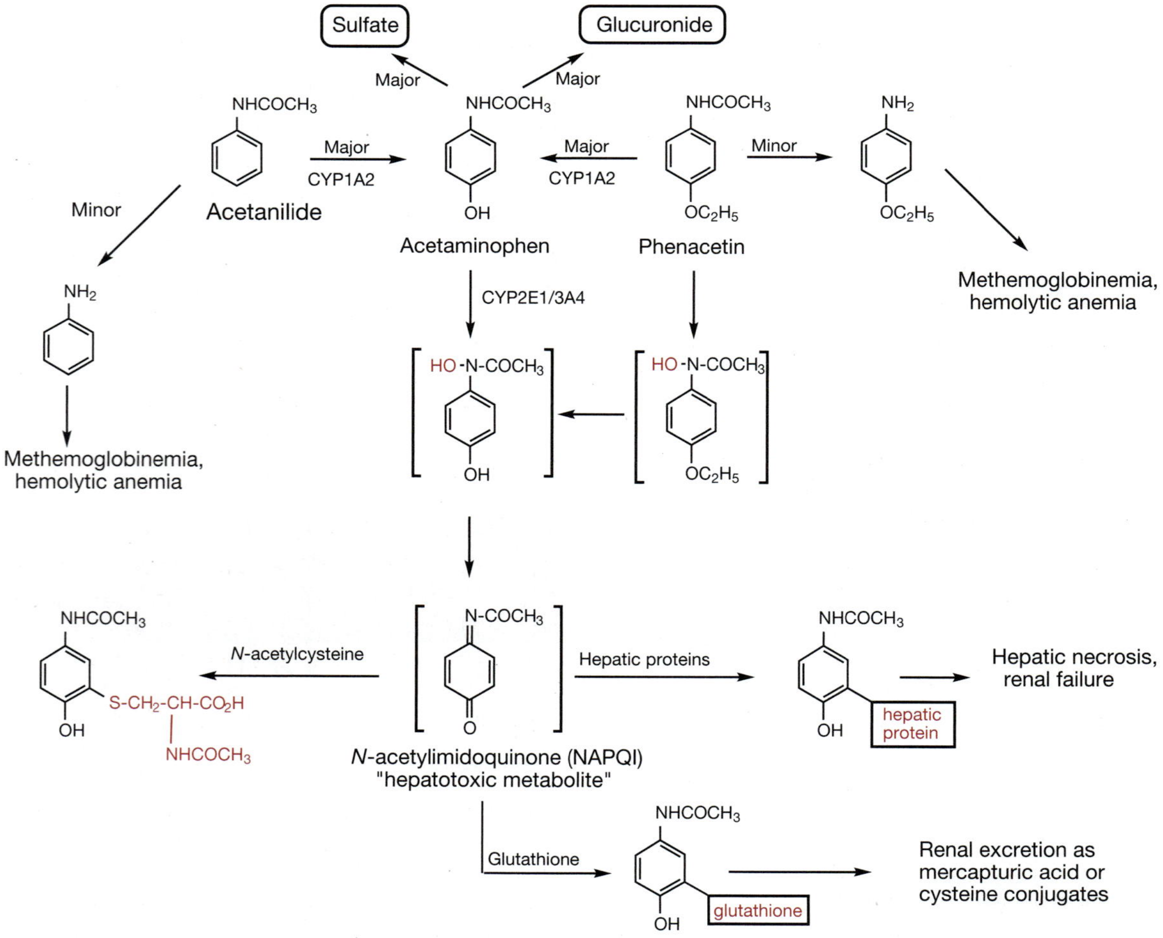

Figure 17.7 Metabolism of acetaminophen.

in the formation of covalent adducts that produce hepatic necrosis. Both CYP2E1 and CYP3A4 are induced by the ingestion of alcohol, accounting for the increase in acetaminophen toxicity, especially among alcoholics, observed upon the concomitant consumption of alcoholic beverages and acetaminophen.[30]

Various sulfhydryl-containing compounds were found to be useful as antidotes to acetaminophen overdose. The most useful is *N*-acetylcysteine (Mucomyst, Acetadote), a thiol-containing reagent that serves as a substitute for the endogenous and depleted glutathione and competes with hepatic protein thiols for reaction with the electrophilic and toxic NAPQI. *N*-acetylcysteine is also a cysteine prodrug, thereby enhancing hepatic glutathione stores.[31,32]

Drug Interactions. Hepatic necrosis develops at much lower doses of acetaminophen in people who chronically consume large amounts of ethanol, potentially because of the induction of the CYP2E1 system, depletion of glutathione stores, aberrations in the primary sulfate and glucuronide conjugation pathways, or a combination of all three.[25] Acetaminophen is weakly bound to plasma proteins and can also interfere with the enzymes involved in vitamin K–dependent coagulation factor synthesis. Chemical incompatibilities have also been reported based on hydrolysis by strong acids or bases or by phenolic oxidation in the presence of oxidizing agents. Acetaminophen forms "sticky" mixtures with diphenhydramine HCl and discolors under humid conditions in the presence of caffeine or codeine phosphate, two drugs with which it is commonly used in combination.

Anti-inflammatory Drugs

Salicylate-based Therapeutics

Salicylates are one of the oldest classes of drugs in history. Their use dates back to 5 BC, where Hippocrates prescribed chewing willow bark, a natural source for salicylic acid, for pain relief. Salicylates have many therapeutic actions, including antipyretic, analgesic, and anti-inflammatory properties. The most prevalent and widely used salicylate is aspirin, and its medical use began in 1899 and continues to gain therapeutic utility today. For example, recent studies have shown aspirin's ability to help prevent cardiovascular disease[33] and colorectal cancer.[34] However, the salicylates target COX-1 preferentially; thus, many undesirable side effects stem from GI disturbances. There are many marketed salicylate products; however, many of them have reduced clinical use.

Mechanism of Action. Salicylate-based NSAIDs exhibit their pain relief primarily through the inhibition of COX enzymes, thereby blocking PG biosynthesis. This class is generally more active against COX-1 over COX-2, as exemplified in Table 17.2 for aspirin. The salicylate-based NSAIDs, except for aspirin, are competitive inhibitors, blocking COX-mediated oxidation of arachidonic acid. Aspirin is a suicide-, irreversible, or mechanism-based COX inhibitor, meaning it reacts with and covalently modifies the enzyme by acetylating Ser530 in COX-1 and Ser516 in COX-2 (Fig. 17.8). Acetylation of COX-1 renders it inactive; however, acetylation of COX-2 converts it to more of

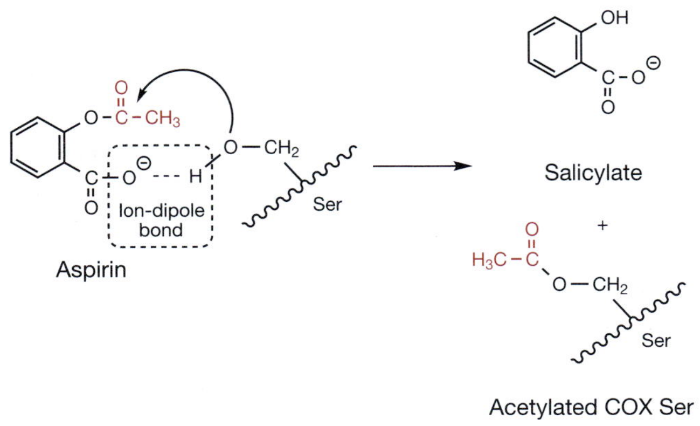

Figure 17.8 Acetylation of COX Ser by aspirin.

a lipoxygenase, where it can still produce the monooxygenated product 15(*R*)-hydroxyeicosatetraenoic acid.[15]

Structure-Activity Relationships

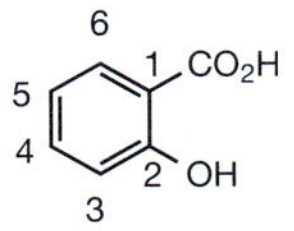

Salicylic acid

Salicylic acid is a 2-hydroxybenzoic acid and comprises the core requirements for all salicylate analogues. The carboxylic acid functional group at position 1 has a pK_a ~3; thus, at physiological pH, it is highly ionized. This is important, as the resultant carboxylate anion (except for aspirin) makes a key ion-ion bond with Arg120 in COX active sites. For aspirin, the carboxylate's role is to reduce the pK_a of the active site Ser residue, resulting in its increased nucleophilicity for attack on the acetoxy carbonyl carbon (see Fig. 17.8). The phenolic hydroxy group at the 2-position, whether free or acetylated, is also important for anti-inflammatory activity as hydroxy substitutions at the 3- and 4-positions are inactive. The addition of a second conjugated aromatic ring to the salicylate phenyl ring increases anti-inflammatory activity, as the resultant analogue makes more effective van der Waals and hydrophobic interactions with Tyr348, Val349, Tyr385, and Trp387.

Absorption and Metabolism. Most salicylates are rapidly and effectively absorbed after oral administration. The rate of absorption and the extent of oral bioavailability are dependent on a number of factors, including formulation, gastric pH, food in the stomach, gastric emptying time, the presence of buffering agents or antacids, and particle size.[35] Salicylates are weak acids (aspirin pK_a = 3.5) and highly unionized in the stomach; thus, solubility in gastric fluid is poor. This is one of the primary reasons for GI distress of the salicylates. Absorption takes place primarily from the small intestine because of better drug dissolution, where unionized molecules can passively diffuse across the gut wall.

The major metabolic routes of salicylic acid are illustrated in Figure 17.9 and have been extensively reviewed.[36]

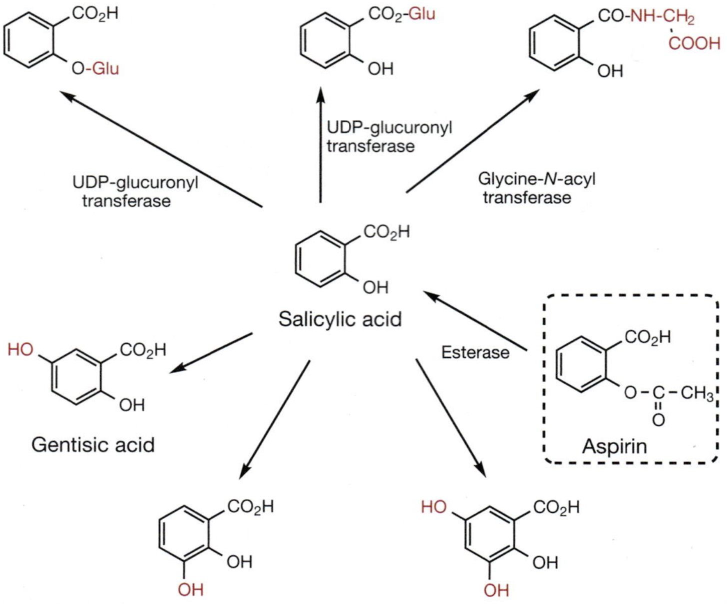

Figure 17.9 Metabolism of salicylic acid derivatives (Glu = glucuronide conjugate).

The initial route of metabolism for aspirin is conversion to salicylic acid, which can be excreted in the urine as the free acid (10%) or undergo conjugation with glycine or glucuronic acid.[37] The major metabolite is the glycine conjugate (75%), with glucuronide ethers and esters accounting for 15% of metabolites.[37] In addition, microsomal aromatic hydroxylation of salicylic acid also occurs, albeit to a limited extent.

Adverse Effects. Although the rate of salicylate poisoning has declined, salicylates still account for a significant percentage of all accidental poisonings in the United States.[38] The most commonly observed side effects associated with the use of salicylates relate to disturbances of the GI tract, including nausea, vomiting, epigastric discomfort, aggravation of peptic ulcers, gastric ulcerations, erosive gastritis, and GI hemorrhage. These adverse effects typically occur in individuals on high doses of aspirin. The incidence of these side effects is rarer at low doses, but a single dose of aspirin can cause GI distress in 5% of individuals. Salicylate-induced GI distress is typically mediated by the dual insult (see Fig. 17.6) and/or inhibition of platelet aggregation, which promotes bleeding.

Reye syndrome is an acute and potentially fatal condition that can follow influenza and chickenpox infections in children from infancy to their late teens, with the majority of cases occurring between ages 5 and 14.[39] It is characterized by symptoms including sudden vomiting, violent headaches, and unusual behavior in children who appear to be recovering from a viral infection. Reye syndrome is a rare disease, and incidence rates are largely unknown, since reporting to the Centers for Disease Control (CDC) is not mandated; however, two or fewer cases per year have been reported since 1994.[39] The vast majority (>90%) of children diagnosed with Reye syndrome were on aspirin therapy while afflicted with their viral infection. Based on these statistics, the FDA has mandated that aspirin and other salicylates be labeled with a warning against their use in children younger than 16 years with influenza, chickenpox, or other flu-like illnesses. Acetaminophen is suggested to be the drug of choice in children with these conditions.

Commonly Used Salicylate-based Therapeutics. The structures of the commonly used salicylate-based therapeutics are presented in Figure 17.10. The physicochemical and pharmacokinetic properties of all NSAIDs, including aspirin, are provided in Table 17.3.

Aspirin. Acetylsalicylic acid, or aspirin, is indicated for the relief of minor aches and mild to moderate pain, arthritis, and related arthritic conditions, to reduce the risk of transient ischemic attacks, myocardial infarction prophylaxis, and as a platelet aggregation inhibitor. Aspirin contains the acetoxy functional group; therefore, it is able to irreversibly acetylate the COX active site Ser residue. This is especially important for aspirin's action as a platelet aggregation inhibitor. Platelets utilize COX-1 to produce TXA_2 (a pro-aggregatory prostanoid), and since platelets cannot produce new COX-1 protein because they do not have any deoxyribonucleic acid (DNA) biosynthetic machinery, acetylation of COX-1 Ser leads to prolonged inhibitory action. Patients should take care not to take another nonselective NSAID for pain concurrently with low-dose "heart healthy" aspirin, as the other NSAID would compete for COX-1 active site residues, leading to ineffective COX-1 inhibition in platelets. The acetoxy

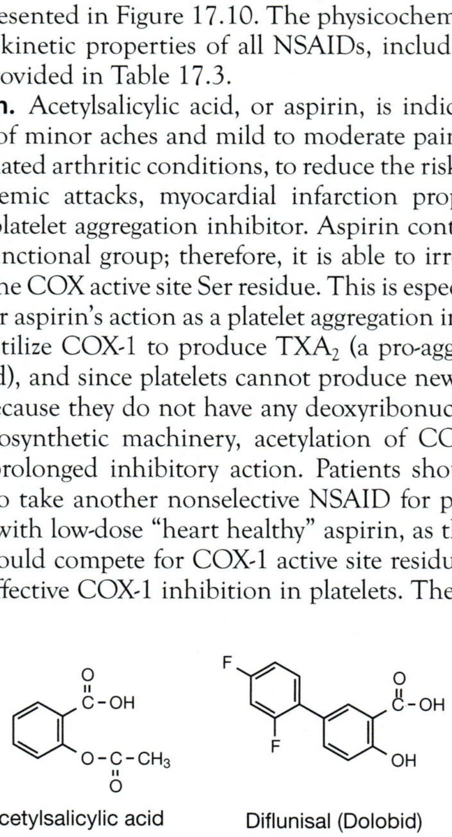

Figure 17.10 Commonly used salicylate-based NSAIDs.

Table 17.3 Pharmacokinetic and Physicochemical Properties of Nonsteroidal Anti-inflammatory Drugs

Drug	Anti-Inflammatory Dose (mg)	Onset (Duration) of Action	Peak Plasma Levels (h)	Protein Binding (%)	Biotrans-formation	Elimination Half-Life (h)	p*K*a
Aspirin	3,200-6,000	ND	2	90	Plasma hydrolysis and hepatic	<30 min	3.5
Diclofenac (Voltaren)	100-200	30 min (~8 h)	1.5-2.5	99	Hepatic; first-pass metabolism: 3A4	1-2	4.0
Diflunisal (Dolobid)	500-1,000	1 h (8-12 h)	2-3	99	Hepatic	8-12	3.3
Etodolac (Lodine)	800-1,200	30 min (4-6 h)	1-2	99	Hepatic: 2C9	6-7	4.7
Fenoprofen calcium (Nalfon)	1,200-2,400	NR	2	99	Hepatic: 2C9	3	4.5
Flurbiprofen (Ansaid)	200-300	NR	1.5	99	Hepatic: 2C9	6 (2-12)	4.2
Ibuprofen (Motrin, Advil)	1,200-3,200	30 min (4-6 h)	2	99	Hepatic; first-pass metabolism: 2C9, 2C19	~2	4.4
Indomethacin (Indocin)	75-150	2-4 h (2-3 d)	2-3	97	Hepatic: 2C9	5 (3-11)	4.5
Ketoprofen (Orudis)	150-300	NR	0.5-2	99	Hepatic: 2C9, 3A4	~2	5.9
Meclofenamate sodium (Meclomen)	200-400	1 h (4-6 h)	4.0	99	Hepatic: 2C9	2-3	NR
Mefenamic acid (Ponstel)	1,000	NR	2-4	79	Hepatic: 2C9	2	4.2
Meloxicam (Mobic)	7.5-15	NR	4-5	99	Hepatic 2C9	15-20	1.1, 4.2
Nabumetone[a] (Relafen)	1,500-2,000	NR	2.5 ($^{1-8}$) 6MNA	99[b]	Hepatic; first-pass metabolism to 6MNA	6MNA, 23	Neutral
Naproxen (Naprosyn, Anaprox)	500-1,000	NR	2-4	99	Hepatic: 3A4, 1A2	13	4.2
Oxaprozin (Daypro)	1,200	NR	3-5	99	Hepatic: 2C9	25	4.3
Piroxicam (Feldene)	20	2-4 h (24 h)	2	99	Hepatic: 2C9	50	1.8, 5.1

(continued)

Table 17.3 Pharmacokinetic and Physicochemical Properties of Nonsteroidal Anti-inflammatory Drugs (*Continued*)

Drug	Anti-Inflammatory Dose (mg)	Onset (Duration) of Action	Peak Plasma Levels (h)	Protein Binding (%)	Biotransformation	Elimination Half-Life (h)	pKa
Sulindac[a] (Clinoril)	400	NR	2-4	93	Hepatic; sulfide metabolite active	50	4.5
Tolmetin (Tolectin)	1,200	NR	<1	99	Hepatic	5	3.5

6MNA, 6-methoxynaphthalene-2-acetic acid; ND, not determined; NR, not reported.
[a]Prodrug.
[b]Protein binding data is for the active 6-MNA metabolite.

group is responsible for aspirin's short duration of action, since it is susceptible to plasma esterase–catalyzed hydrolysis. Aspirin is stable in a dry environment; however, it can be hydrolyzed to salicylic acid and acetic acid under humid or moist conditions or when exposed to basic media. Salicylic acid contains a typically light-sensitive phenol functional group, which commonly degrade to provide inactive colored quinones. Thus, if an aspirin medication smells like vinegar (acetic acid; CH_3COOH) or has discolored, it has degraded and should be discarded. Aspirin is available in a large number of dosage forms and strengths as tablets, suppositories, capsules, enteric-coated tablets, and buffered tablets.

Drug Interactions. Aspirin is highly bound to plasma proteins (see Table 17.3)[40] and can compete with other drugs, leading to drug interaction concerns. The interaction of salicylates with oral anticoagulants (eg, warfarin) represents one of the most widely documented and clinically significant drug interactions reported to date.[41] The plasma concentration of free anticoagulant increases in the presence of salicylates through one of the following two mechanisms: (1) the salicylate may simply block expected anticoagulant plasma protein binding or (2) the salicylate may displace bound anticoagulant. These pharmacokinetic implications may require a reduced dose of anticoagulant. These interactions are also evident with other nonsalicylated NSAIDs, and coadministration can increase the incidence and severity of GI distress. Ingestion of alcohol also exacerbates salicylate-induced gastric bleeding.[42]

Diflunisal (Dolobid). Diflunisal is indicated for mild to moderate pain, RA, and osteoarthritis (OA). Diflunisal lacks the reactive acetoxy group seen in aspirin; therefore, it is a competitive and reversible inhibitor of the COX enzymes. It is more potent than aspirin because of the second conjugated phenyl ring on the 5-position of the salicylic acid moiety that can make more effective van der Waals and hydrophobic interactions with COX aromatic and hydrophobic residues. It is rapidly and completely absorbed on oral administration.[43] The *p*-fluorine atom increases duration of action because it blocks phase 1 oxidative metabolism. The metabolism of diflunisal occurs primarily through phase 2 conjugation, and it is excreted in the urine primarily as glucuronide ester and ether conjugates.[44] The most frequently reported side effects include disturbances of the GI system (eg, nausea, dyspepsia, and diarrhea), dermatologic reactions, and CNS effects (eg, dizziness and headache). Lastly, it does not have any effect on platelet aggregation.

Arylalkanoic Acids

General Structure-Activity Relationships

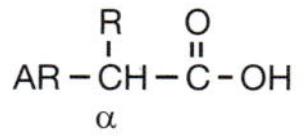

R = H, CH_3 or alkyl
AR = aryl or heteroaryl

Arylalkanoic acid

The general structure-activity relationships (SARs) that apply to all arylalkanoic acids will be discussed here, and specific SAR or exceptions to these general rules will be presented with each drug or drug class.

The arylalkanoic acid class of NSAIDs structurally comprises aromatic rings attached to carboxylic acid groups primarily through a one- or two-saturated carbon chain. The bridging carbon is termed "the α-carbon" and can accommodate a methyl group substituent. If there is no substituent (ie, R = H), then the compounds are identified as the arylacetic acid class. When the α-carbon is substituted with a methyl group, the resulting α-methyl acetic acid, or arylpropionic acid, analogues have been given the class name "profens" by the US Adopted Names (USAN) Council. If all other structural features are identical, the arylpropionic acid class has improved activity over the arylacetic acid class.

Introduction of a methyl group makes the α-carbon a chiral center. For chiral NSAIDs, the *S* enantiomer is the active isomer. Activity increases with the addition of a second conjugated aromatic ring. Introduction of aromatic substituents that increase non-coplanarity of the two rings also enhances activity by optimizing the van der Waals and hydrophobic interactions with COX aromatic and aliphatic residues.

Aryl- and Heteroarylacetic Acids. The structures of the aryl- and heteroarylacetic acid derivatives ("fenacs") and the aryl- and heteroarylpropionic acids ("profens") clinically available are presented in Figure 17.11.

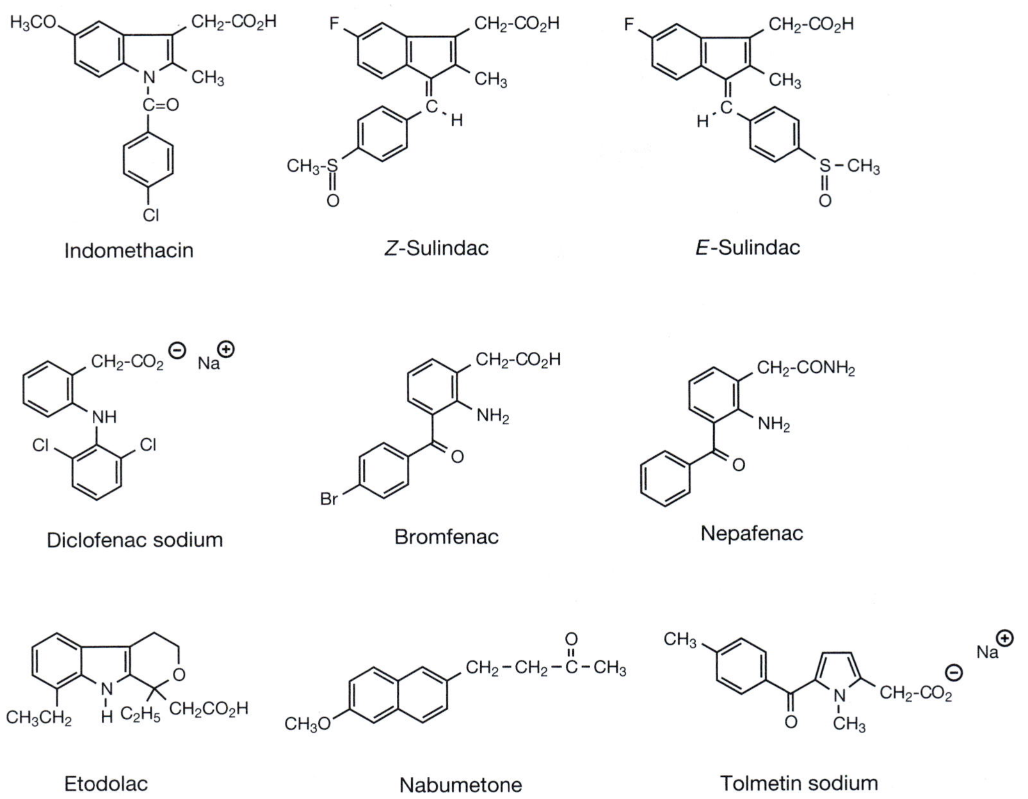

Figure 17.11 Aryl- and heteroarylacetic acid derivatives.

Diclofenac (Cataflam, Volataren). Diclofenac is one of the most widely used NSAID globally and is indicated for the treatment of RA, OA, ankylosing spondylitis, and mild to moderate pain. In addition, diclofenac is often administered to patients with tuberculosis for inflammation and has been shown to synergize with streptomycin against *Mycobacterium tuberculosis*, the causative pathogen for tuberculosis.[45] Diclofenac is a phenylacetic acid substituted at the 2-position with a 2,6-dichloroanilino group and displays anti-inflammatory, analgesic, and antipyretic properties. It is twice as potent as indomethacin as an anti-inflammatory agent and 450 times as potent as aspirin. As an analgesic, it is 6 times more potent than indomethacin and 40 times as potent as aspirin. As an antipyretic, it is twice as potent as indomethacin and more than 350 times as potent as aspirin. Diclofenac is unique among NSAIDs in that it possesses three putative mechanisms of action: (1) inhibition of the COX system, resulting in a decreased production of PGs and thromboxanes; (2) inhibition of the lipoxygenase pathway, resulting in decreased production of leukotrienes, particularly the proinflammatory LKB4; and (3) inhibition of arachidonic acid release and stimulation of its reuptake, resulting in a reduction of arachidonic acid availability.[46]

Structure-Activity Relationships. Diclofenac is a bioisostere of salicylic acid where the 2-hydroxyl group on salicylic acid has been replaced with an -NH- group. This nitrogen atom adopts an sp2 hybridization, which maintains conjugation between the two aromatic rings. The two *o*-chloro groups are significant potency boosters, which is a primary reason for its high anti-inflammatory potency (estimated at 3-1,000 times as that of most other NSAIDs). The two *o*-chloro groups sterically hinder the C3-hydrogen and the carboxylic acid group on the phenylacetic acid moiety, forcing a non-coplanar conformation between the halogenated phenyl ring and the phenyl acetic acid portion, thus optimizing binding to the active site of the COX.[47] They also add to the lipophilicity of the compound, which promotes passive penetration into inflamed tissue.

Absorption and Metabolism. Diclofenac is rapidly and completely absorbed on oral administration.[48] The free acid ($pK_a = 4.0$) is highly bound to serum proteins.[49] Only 50% to 60% of an oral dose is bioavailable due to extensive hepatic metabolism (Fig. 17.12). This is primarily due to the high lipophilicity and open *p*-positions. The major CYP3A4-catalyzed metabolite is the 4′-hydroxy derivative and accounts for 20%-30% of the excreted dose, whereas the 5-hydroxy, 3′-hydroxy, and 4′,5-dihydroxy metabolites are catalyzed by CYP2C9 and account for 10% to 20% of the excreted dose.[50] Phase 2 conjugation yields sulfate conjugates, which is unusual because most other NSAIDs are excreted as a glucuronide conjugate.

Diclofenac can also produce a hepatotoxic quinoneimine metabolite similar to that reported in the metabolism of acetaminophen.[51] The formation and reactivity of the quinoneimine metabolite is shown in Figure 17.13. The 4′-hydroxy metabolite formed under normal CYP3A4 oxidation can undergo further oxidation to the reactive and toxic quinoneimine metabolite. The carbons on the quinoneimine at the 3′- and 5′-positions are highly electrophilic (δ+) and will nonspecifically react with nearby nucleophiles.

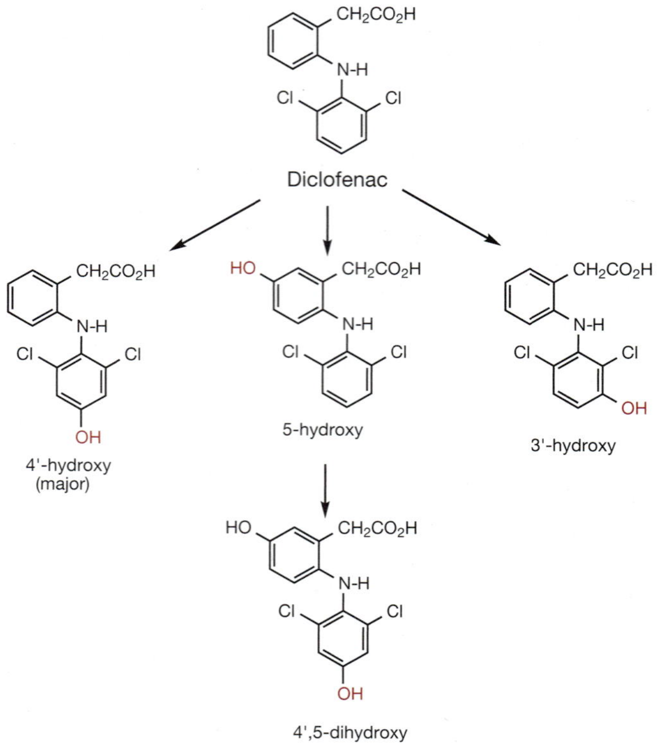

Figure 17.12 Metabolism of diclofenac.

The quinoneimine is normally inactivated via conjugation with glutathione but, if glutathione (GSH) levels are depleted, can induce chemically predictable hepatotoxicity. Nucleophilic Cys residues on liver hepatocytes will attack the electrophilic quinoneimine metabolite, leaving them irreversibly alkylated. This is particularly important because diclofenac is currently the only NSAID capable of active transport into the liver mediated through the OATP1B3 transporter protein.[52] Therefore, it is important that patients taking diclofenac have their liver function monitored regularly.

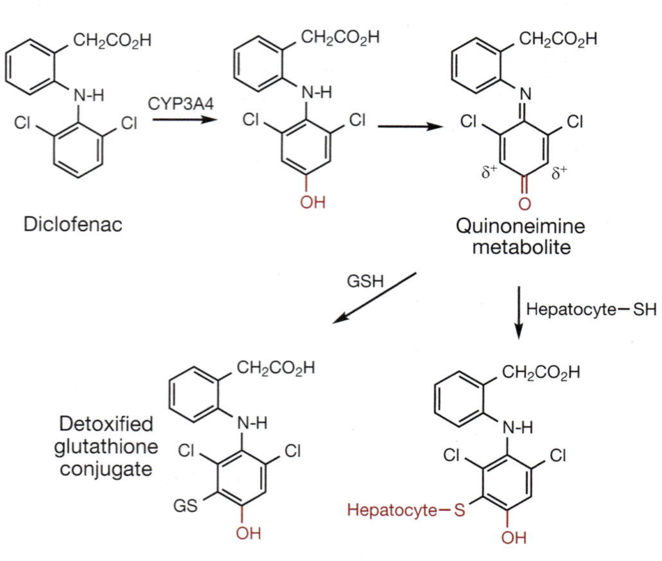

Figure 17.13 Formation of diclofenac's quinoneimine metabolite and reactions with GSH and hepatocyte Cys.

Nabumetone (Relafen). Nabumetone is indicated for the acute and chronic treatment of OA and RA. However, studies have linked nabumetone use to an increased risk of acute pancreatitis.[53] Nabumetone is a nonacidic prodrug, making it quite a unique NSAID. It is rapidly metabolized after absorption to form a major active metabolite, 6-methoxynaphthaleneacetic acid (6MNA) (Fig. 17.13). Since nabumetone is nonacidic, it does not induce the primary insult (direct GI mucosal damage). An additional benefit to nabumetone's action is that it is not metabolized to the active metabolite until after absorption; therefore, nabumetone does not engage in the secondary insult (COX-1 inhibition in GI tract). The net result is that gastric side effects of nabumetone are reduced. Once the parent drug enters the circulatory system, however, it is metabolized to the active 6MNA metabolite, which is an effective inhibitor of COX enzymes.

Structure-Activity Relationships. Alkylation of the butanone side chain with either methyl or ethyl groups reduced anti-inflammatory activity. Removal of the methoxy group at the 6-position reduced activity, but replacement of the methoxy with a methyl or chloro group resulted in active compounds.[54] In contrast, replacement of the methoxy with hydroxy, acetoxy, or *N*-methylcarbamoyl, or positional isomers of the methoxy group at the 2- or 4-positions reduced activity.[54] 6MNA is closely related to naproxen structurally (discussion on naproxen below), differing only by the lack of an α-methyl group. Interestingly, the ketone precursor 4-(6-methoxy-2-naphthyl)pentan-2-one that would be expected to produce naproxen as a metabolite via a metabolic mechanism similar to that which produces 6-MNA was inactive in chronic models of inflammation.

Absorption and Metabolism. Nabumetone is absorbed primarily from the duodenum. Milk and food increase the rate of absorption and the bioavailability of the active metabolite.[55] Higher plasma levels of the active metabolite were seen in older adults.[56] Nabumetone undergoes rapid and extensive metabolism in the liver, with a mean absolute bioavailability of the active metabolite of 38% (Fig. 17.14). The 6-MNA metabolite is formed via β-oxidase catalysis. O-dealkylation of the 6-methoxy group is mediated through CYP2C9. However, this reaction is sluggish; thus, nabumetone's duration of action is extended over most other NSAIDs, affording once-a-day dosing. Metabolites where the carbonyl has been reduced to the secondary alcohol are inactive.

ARYL- AND HETEROARYLPROPIONIC ACIDS. Members of this class represent the most widely used NSAIDs because several members of the class are available over the counter (OTC). The introduction of the α-methyl group in the carboxylic acid side chain results in a chiral carbon atom and thus, the existence of enantiomers, with oxaprozin being the sole exception. The structures of aryl- and heteroarylpropionic acid derivatives are shown in Figure 17.15.

Ibuprofen (Advil, Motrin). Ibuprofen is available as a nonprescription (OTC) and prescription drug and is indicated for the relief of the signs and symptoms of RA and OA, the relief of mild to moderate pain, the reduction of fever, and the treatment of dysmenorrhea. It is marketed as the racemic mixture, although biologic activity resides almost exclusively in the S-(+)-isomer. Ibuprofen is more potent than aspirin, but less potent than indomethacin in

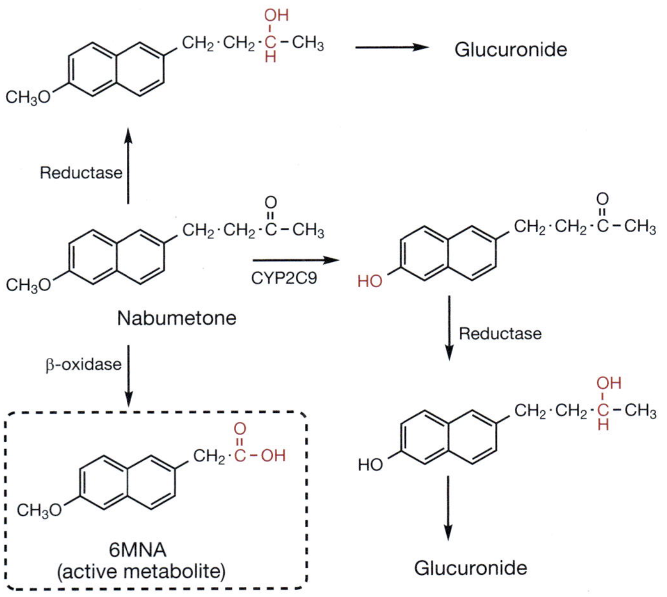

Figure 17.14 Metabolism of nabumetone.

anti-inflammatory and PG biosynthesis inhibition assays, and it produces moderate degrees of gastric irritation. Ibuprofen has been linked to cardiovascular toxicities, and caution should be taken when administering to patients with existing cardiovascular disease or risk factors, including hypertension.[57-59]

Structure-Activity Relationships. Ibuprofen has only one aromatic ring; thus, its potency and anti-inflammatory activity is lower than that of other NSAIDs that contain two conjugated aromatic moieties. The 4-isobutyl group is hydrophobic and compensates, to some extent, for the lack of the second conjugated aromatic ring. The substitution of an α-methyl group on the alkanoic acid portion of arylacetic acid NSAIDs enhances anti-inflammatory actions and reduces many side effects.[60] The α-methyl group creates a chiral center and, as with many other chiral NSAIDs that are marketed as a racemic mixture, the *S*-(+)-enantiomer of ibuprofen possesses greater anti-inflammatory activity than the *R*-(−)-isomer.

Absorption and Metabolism. Ibuprofen is rapidly absorbed on oral administration.[61] As with most acidic NSAIDs, ibuprofen is extensively bound to plasma proteins; however, displacement interactions do not seem to be clinically significant.[62,63] Ibuprofen is metabolized rapidly to many inactive metabolites, explaining why it has a short duration of action requiring dosing every 4 to 6 hours. Ibuprofen is nearly completely excreted in the urine as either unchanged drug or oxidative metabolites within 24 hours after administration (Fig. 17.16).[63]

Metabolism by CYP2C9 (90%) and CYP2C19 (10%) involves primarily ω-1 and ω-oxidation of the *p*-isobutyl side chain, followed by oxidation of the primary alcohol via sequential reactions with alcohol dehydrogenase and aldehyde dehydrogenase to the corresponding carboxylic acid.[64] When ibuprofen is administered as the individual enantiomers, the major metabolite isolated is the *S*-(+)-enantiomer, regardless of the configuration of the starting enantiomer. The inactive *R*-(−)-enantiomer is completely inverted to the active *S*-(+)-enantiomer in vivo via a reaction also requiring coenzyme A (CoASH), accounting for the observation that the two enantiomers are bioequivalent.[65] This is a metabolic phenomenon that has also been observed for other arylpropionic acids, such as ketoprofen, benoxaprofen, fenoprofen, and naproxen.[66]

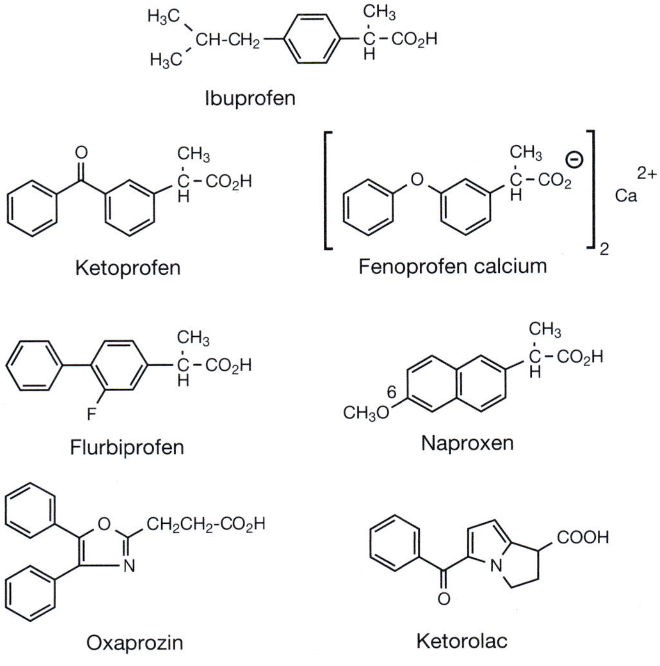

Figure 17.15 Aryl- and heteroarylpropionic acid derivatives.

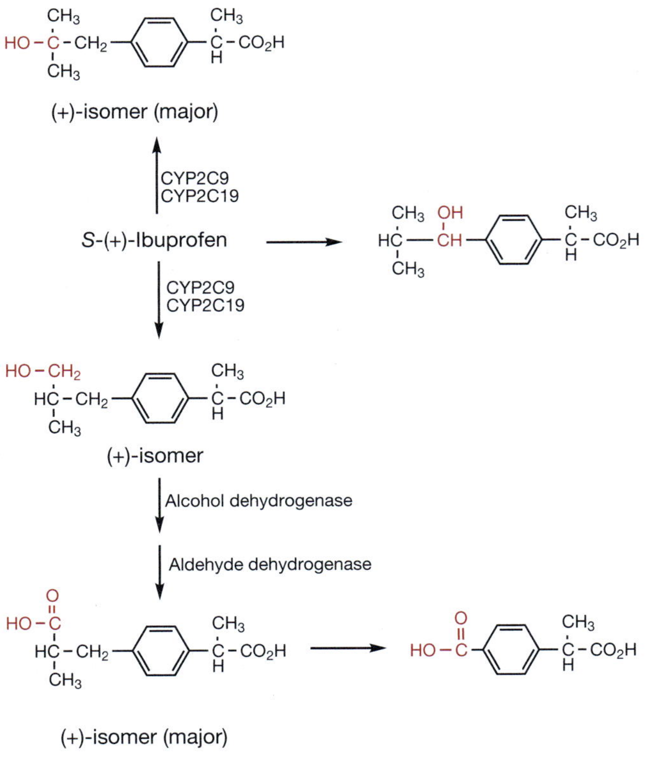

Figure 17.16 Metabolism of ibuprofen.

Naproxen (Aleve, Naprosyn). Naproxen is available as a nonprescription (OTC) and prescription drug and is indicated for the treatment of RA, OA, juvenile arthritis, ankylosing spondylitis, tendinitis, bursitis, acute gout, and primary dysmenorrhea and for the relief of mild to moderate pain. It is marketed as the pure S-(+)-enantiomer. Naproxen contains two fused benzene rings (naphthalene), which is considered a single aromatic moiety; therefore, naproxen's potency is relatively low compared to other NSAIDs that have two distinct conjugated aromatic rings.

Structure-Activity Relationships. In a series of substituted 2-naphthylacetic acids, substitution in the 6-position led to maximum anti-inflammatory activity. Small lipophilic groups such as chloro, methylsulfide, and difluoromethoxy were active analogues, with methoxy being the most potent.[67] Larger groups were found to be less active.[67] Removal of the α-methyl group from the acetic acid side chain reduced activity. Prodrug mimics of naproxen that replaced the carboxylic acid group with functional groups capable of being metabolized to the carboxylic acid function (eg, methyl ester, aldehyde, or hydroxymethyl) led to retention of activity. Not surprising, the S-(+)-isomer is the most potent enantiomer. Naproxen is the only arylalkanoic acid NSAID currently marketed as the optically pure S enantiomer.

Absorption and Metabolism. Naproxen is almost completely absorbed following oral administration.[68] Like most of the acidic NSAIDs, it is highly bound to plasma proteins. Approximately 70% of an administered dose is eliminated as either unchanged drug (60%) or conjugates of unchanged drug (10%).[69] The remainder is slowly O-dealkylated to the 6-O-desmethyl metabolite by either CYP2C9 or CYP1A2. Similar to nabumetone, this slow inactivating metabolic reaction accounts for naproxen's extended duration of action, allowing for twice-a-day dosing. Phase 2 glucuronide conjugation of the demethylated metabolite occurs.[70] Like most of the arylalkanoic acids, the most common side effects associated with the use of naproxen are irritation to the GI tract and CNS disturbances.

N-ARYLANTHRANILIC ACIDS (FENAMIC ACIDS). The anthranilic acid class of NSAIDs are bioisosteres of the salicylic acid class, where an –NH– has replaced the -OH of salicylic acid. Additionally, they could be considered structural analogues of the phenylacetic acid derivative, diclofenac (Fig. 17.11). The fenamic acids possess little advantage over the salicylates with respect to their anti-inflammatory and analgesic properties, and this has diminished interest in their large-scale development relative to the arylalkanoic acids. The structures of the fenamic acids are shown in Figure 17.17.

The fenamic acids share a number of pharmacologic properties with the other NSAIDs. They were shown to block PG biosynthesis primarily through the inhibition of COX enzymes, which is their primary mechanism of therapeutic action.[71,72] Interestingly, fenamic acid NSAIDs, including mefenamic acid, have shown promise for Alzheimer disease in animal models through a mechanism of action independent of COX inhibition.[73] Side effects are those primarily associated with GI disturbances, some CNS effects, skin rashes, and transient hepatic and renal abnormalities.

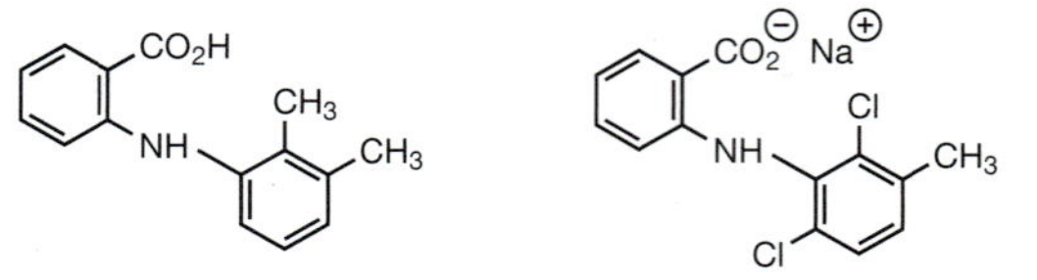

Figure 17.17 *N*-arylanthranilic acids (fenamic acids).

General Structure-Activity Relationships

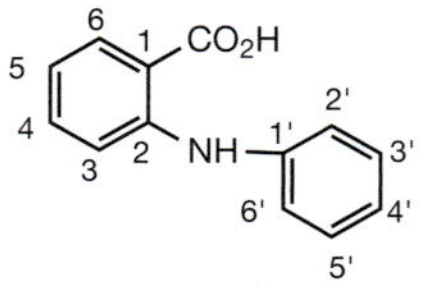

Fenamate numbering

The benzoic acid portion of the fenamic acid structure is essential for activity, as the carboxylic acid group makes an essential ion-ion bond with the COX active site Arg120. Replacement of the carboxylic acid function with the isosteric tetrazole moiety has little effect on activity. The *o*-anilino group increases COX's binding capabilities, as the second conjugated ring makes more effective van der Waals and hydrophobic interactions in the COX active sites. Substituents on the anilino ring that promote non-coplanarity with the benzoic acid ring enhance binding at this site and, thus, activity. This can account for the enhanced anti-inflammatory activity of meclofenamic acid, which has two large *o*-substituents forcing this ring out of the plane of the anthranilic acid ring. Meclofenamic acid (conjugate acid of meclofenamate sodium) possesses 25 times greater anti-inflammatory activity than mefenamic acid, likely attributable to both steric and lipophilicity-related parameters of the aromatic chloro substituents of the former. The NH-moiety of anthranilic acid appears to be essential for activity, as replacement of the NH function with oxygen, methylene (CH_2), sulfur, sulfone (SO_2), N-CH_3, or acetamide (N-$COCH_3$) functionalities significantly reduces activity.[74] The *o*-substituted anilino group is critical for activity, as *m*- and *p*- substitutions are inactive.

Drug Interactions. The fenamic acid class of acidic NSAIDs are highly plasma protein bound, and significant drug interactions can occur with other highly plasma protein bound drugs. The most common interactions reported are those of mefenamic acid and meclofenamic acid with oral anticoagulants, potentially requiring a reduction in anticoagulant dose.[75]

OXICAMS. The enolic acid class of NSAIDs has been termed "oxicams" by the USAN Council to describe the series of 4-hydroxy-1,2-benzothiazine carboxamides that possess anti-inflammatory and analgesic properties.

General Structure-Activity Relationships. Given the general structure shown in the following image, the cyclic sulfonamide must be tertiary and optimum activity was observed when R_1 was methyl. The carboxamide substituent, R, is optimal with an aryl or heteroaryl substituent. Alkyl substituents for R are less active.

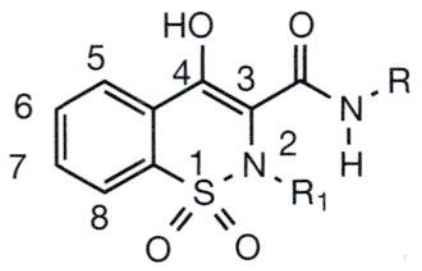

Oxicam

Oxicams have an acidic enol functional group with pK_a values in the range of 4 to 6. The acidic nature of the enol is attributed to stabilization of the enolate anion (conjugate base of enolic acid) by (1) an intramolecular ion-dipole bond (shown in structure A) and (2) extended resonance, as illustrated in the figure at the top of the next page in resonance hybrid A and hybrid B.[76] This explains the observation that secondary carboxamides are more potent than the corresponding tertiary derivatives, because no N–H bond would be available to enhance the stabilization of the enolate anion in the latter.

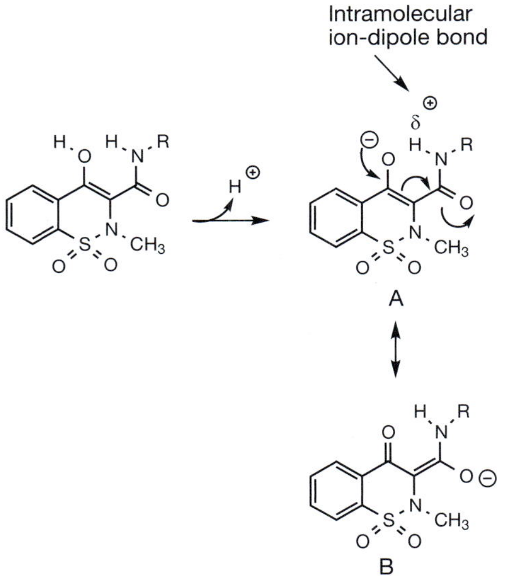

Piroxicam enolate stabilization

The optimal substituents on the secondary carboxamide group are heteroaromatics such as 2-pyridyl (piroxicam), 2-thiazolyl (meloxicam), or 3-(5-methyl) isoxazolyl ring system substituents. In addition to possessing anti-inflammatory activity equal to or greater than indomethacin, the heteroaryl carboxamides also possess longer plasma half-lives, providing less frequent dosing regimens.

Drug Interactions. A number of reports of therapeutically significant interactions of oxicams with other drugs have appeared. Concurrent administration of aspirin has been shown to reduce oxicam plasma levels by approximately 20%, whereas anticoagulant effects can be potentiated, presumably as a result of plasma protein displacement.[77,78]

Specific Drugs

Meloxicam (Mobic). Meloxicam is indicated for the treatment of OA. Meloxicam is an analogue of piroxicam where the 2-pyridyl ring has been replaced with a 5-methylthiazolyl ring. Despite having such similar structural features to piroxicam, meloxicam is a COX-2 preferential inhibitor having approximately 2 times more COX-2 inhibitory activity over other non-COX-2 selective NSAIDs.[79,80] Due to meloxicam being COX-2 preferential, it carries a lower risk of GI disturbances. Meloxicam is readily absorbed when administered orally and is highly bound to plasma proteins.[81]

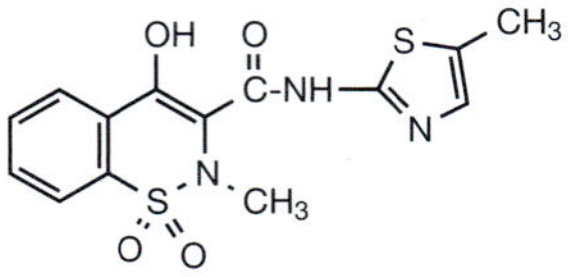

Meloxicam

Metabolism. Meloxicam is extensively metabolized in the liver, primarily by CYP2C9 and, to a lesser extent, by CYP3A4.[82] The 5-methyl group on the thiazole ring is akin to a benzylic carbon and is highly susceptible to CYP oxidation. Oxidation of the thiazole methyl to the primary alcohol is catalyzed by CYP2C9/CYP3A4. The primary alcohol metabolite then undergoes subsequent oxidation reactions to the carboxylic acid.[82] All metabolites are inactive.[82] The metabolism of meloxicam is shown in Figure 17.18.

Selective COX-2 Inhibitors

Since COX-2 is inducible in inflammatory events, and COX-1 is homeostatic and produces cytoprotective PGs, a COX-2 selective inhibitor would, in theory, be an active anti-inflammatory agent with significantly reduced GI toxicity. Selectivity for COX-2 over COX-1 can be achieved through structures that are large enough to be rejected by the sterically restricted COX-1 active site, but which can still bind within the allosteric binding pocket that serves as a secondary site of enzyme inhibition. The allosteric domain in COX-2 is accessible because it has two Val gatekeeper residues flanking the active site cavity that are smaller than the corresponding Ile residues found on COX-1.

Several selective COX-2 inhibitors reached the US market (celecoxib, rofecoxib, lumiracoxib, and valdecoxib), but safety risks and cardiovascular side effects led to the voluntary removal of all except celecoxib (the first to be marketed and the least COX-2 selective of them all). The development of other selective COX-2 inhibitors, such as parecoxib and etoricoxib, has been halted (Fig. 17.19). To explain why the least COX-2 selective agent was the only one to survive, it is important to note that, while COX-1 is found in platelets and is involved in the biosynthesis of the vasoconstrictive and pro-aggregatory

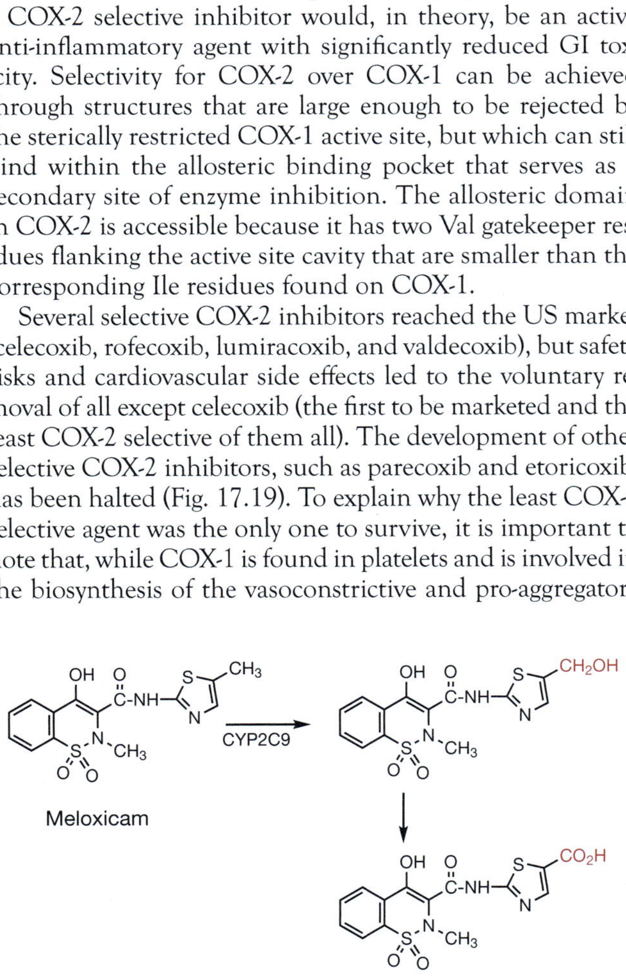

Figure 17.18 Metabolism of meloxicam.

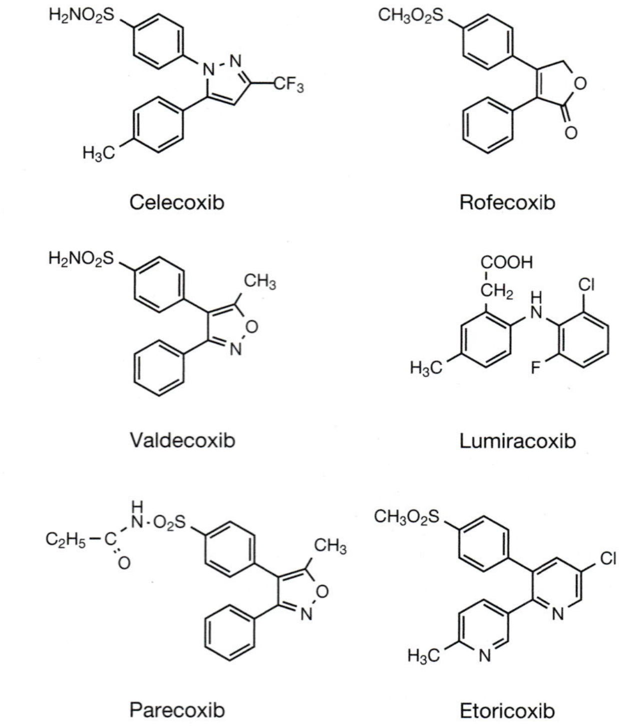

Figure 17.19 Selective COX-2 inhibitors.

thromboxane A_2, COX-2 is the enzyme that catalyzes the biosynthesis of the vasodilating and anti-aggregatory prostacyclin (PGI_2) in the vessel wall. Therefore, the more COX-2 selective an inhibitor, the higher the TXA_2/PGI_2 ratio and the greater the risk for platelet aggregation–facilitated cardiovascular damage. Rofecoxib was the first COX-2 selective NSAID pulled from the US market (soon followed by valdecoxib and, later, lumiracoxib) due to the very real risk of potentially fatal myocardial infarction, stroke, and other serious cardiovascular pathologies.[83] Patients with underlying cardiovascular disease are most vulnerable to these toxicities, and older adults are at increased risk for all serious NSAID adverse events, including those induced by COX-2 selective inhibitors. An excellent review of the various chemical classes of selective COX-2 inhibitors has been published.[83]

Perhaps as interesting as the role that COX-2 selective inhibitors have played in reducing the incidence of GI side effects caused by NSAIDs are the reports of other potential therapeutic uses for this new class of drugs, including in Alzheimer disease and carcinomas of various types. Epidemiologic studies suggest a significant reduction in the risk for colon cancer in patients regularly taking aspirin.[34] Additionally, NSAIDs have been reported to reduce the growth rate of polyps in the colon of humans, as well as the incidence of colonic tumors in animals. The expression of COX-2 appears to be significantly upregulated in carcinoma of the colon. The effectiveness of NSAIDs in the prevention and treatment of other cancers, such as prostate cancer and mammary carcinoma, has been reported as well.[84] This effectiveness is more noticeable among COX-2 selective drugs, as this is the isoform upregulated in pathological conditions; however, the potential for this drug class is not certain, as clinical trials have yielded mixed results.[85,86]

Specific Drugs

Celecoxib (Celebrex). Celecoxib was the first NSAID to be marketed as a truly selective COX-2 inhibitor. Celecoxib is indicated for the relief of OA and RA and to reduce the number of adenomatous colorectal polyps in familial adenomatous polyposis as an adjunct to usual care. Celecoxib is well absorbed from the GI tract, with peak plasma concentrations normally being attained within 3 hours of administration.[87] Celecoxib is excreted in the urine and feces primarily as inactive metabolites, with less than 3% of an administered dose being excreted as unchanged drug.[88] Metabolism occurs primarily in the liver by CYP2C9 and involves hydroxylation of the benzylic 4-methyl group to the primary alcohol, which is subsequently oxidized to the corresponding inactive carboxylic acid, the major metabolite (73% of the administered dose) (Fig. 17.20).[89] The carboxylic acid can conjugate with glucuronic acid to form a minor phase 2 metabolite. None of the metabolites are active. Drug interactions are a concern for other drugs metabolized by CYP2D6, as celecoxib inhibits this isoform.

Celecoxib is at least as effective as naproxen in the symptomatic management of OA, and at least as effective as naproxen and diclofenac in the symptomatic treatment of RA, while being less likely to cause adverse GI effects. Unlike aspirin, celecoxib does not exhibit antiplatelet activity (a COX-1–mediated activity), but concomitant administration of aspirin and celecoxib in an effort to secure the cardiovascular benefits of nonselective COX inhibitors can increase the incidence of GI side effects. Another notable potential drug interaction with celecoxib is its ability to reduce the blood pressure response to angiotensin-converting enzyme inhibitors, an effect it shares with other NSAIDs. A more detailed discussion of the chemical, pharmacologic, pharmacokinetic, and clinical aspects of celecoxib is available.[90]

Gastroenteropathy Induced by Nonselective COX-Inhibiting Nonsteroidal Anti-inflammatory Drugs

The effectiveness and popularity of the NSAIDs make this one of the most commonly used classes of therapeutic entities. As emphasized several times in this chapter, most

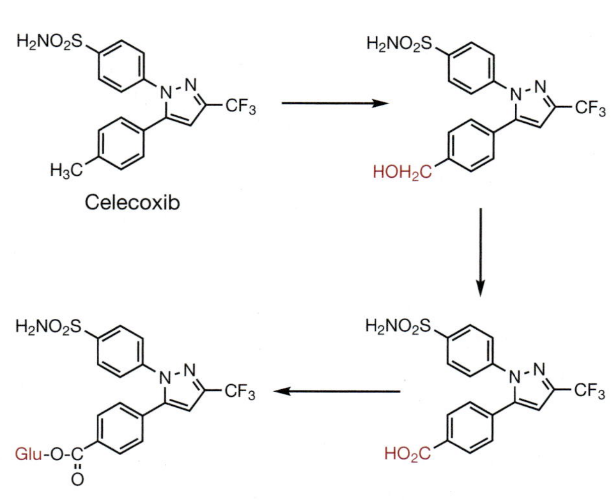

Figure 17.20 Metabolism of celecoxib.

NSAIDs are nonselective COX-1 and COX-2 inhibitors and may exhibit damaging effects to gastric and intestinal mucosa, resulting in erosion, ulcers, and GI bleeding, and these represent the major adverse reactions to the use of NSAIDs.[91]

Normally, the stomach protects itself from the harmful effects of hydrochloric acid and pepsin by a number of protective mechanisms referred to as the gastric mucosal barrier, which consists of epithelial cells, the mucous and bicarbonate layer, and mucosal blood flow. Gastric mucosa is actually a gel consisting of polymers of glycoprotein, which limit the diffusion of hydrogen ions. These polymers reduce the rate at which hydrogen ions (produced in the lumen) and bicarbonate ions (secreted by the mucosa) mix; thus, a pH gradient is created across the mucus layer. Normally, gastric mucosal cells are rapidly repaired when they are damaged by factors such as food, ethanol, or acute ingestion of NSAIDs. Among the cytoprotective mechanisms is the ability of PGs of the PGE series, particularly PGE_1, to increase the secretion of bicarbonate ion and mucus and to maintain mucosal blood flow. The PGs also decrease acid secretion, permitting the gastric mucosal barrier to remain intact.

The use of exogenously administered PGE_1 to reduce NSAID-induced gastric damage is limited by the fact that it is ineffective orally and degrades rapidly on parenteral administration, primarily by oxidation of the secondary 15-hydroxy group. To overcome these limitations, Misoprostol (Cytotec) was introduced as a PG prodrug analogue in which oral activity was achieved by administering the drug as the methyl ester. The methyl ester must be hydrolyzed by esterases before misoprostol is active. In comparison to PGE_1, the hydroxy group has been moved from C15 to C16. The 16-hydroxy group is now tertiary, which prevents it from being oxidized to the inactive ketone.

Misoprostol was introduced in 1989 as a mixture of C16-stereoisomers for the prevention of NSAID-induced gastric ulcers (but not duodenal ulcers) in patients at high risk of complications from a gastric ulcer, particularly older adults and patients with concomitant debilitating disease and in individuals with a history of gastric ulcers. However, misoprostol should be used with caution, as it is an abortifacient and should not be given to pregnant patients who want to remain pregnant. Another approach to preventing GI distress is the administration of proton pump inhibitors, which stop the active secretion of acid into the gastric lumen in combination with an NSAID.[92]

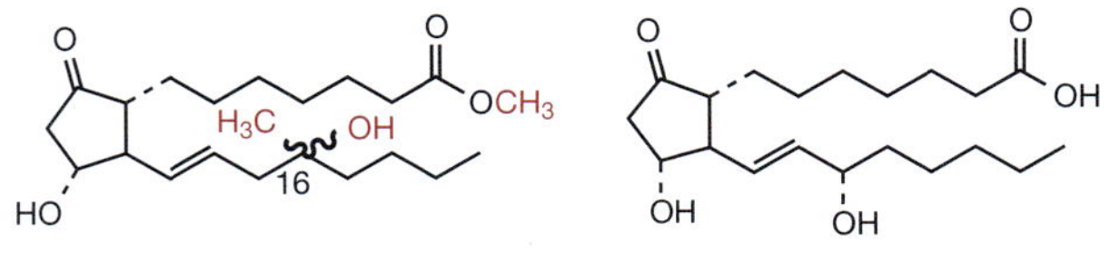

Misoprostol PGE$_1$

Disease-Modifying Antirheumatic Drugs

Disease-modifying antirheumatic drugs (DMARDs) differ from the previously discussed NSAIDs in that they retard or halt the underlying disease progression, limiting the amount of joint damage that occurs in RA while lacking the anti-inflammatory and analgesic effects observed with NSAIDs. Although both NSAIDs and DMARDs improve symptoms of active RA, only DMARDs have been shown to alter the disease course. DMARDs should be considered for chronic rheumatic disease and are generally slow acting, taking as long as 3 months to experience a therapeutic benefit. Therefore, DMARDs are routinely used with an NSAID or a corticosteroid, as the latter improves the immediate symptoms and limits inflammation while the DMARD affects the disease itself. Interestingly, taking DMARDs at early stages in the development of RA has been shown to be especially important to slow the disease and to save the joints and other tissues from permanent damage.[93,94]

The DMARDS can be divided into two general categories: synthetic DMARDS, which can be taken orally, and biologic DMARDS, which are given by intravenous (IV) infusion or subcutaneously. Both classes target and inactivate cell proteins (cytokines) and T lymphocytes (T cells) from causing irreversible joint inflammation.

Synthetic Disease-Modifying Antirheumatic Drugs

Gold Compounds

Mechanism of Action. The biochemical and pharmacologic properties shared by gold compounds are quite diverse. The mechanism by which they produce their antirheumatic actions has not been totally determined. Several hypotheses were advanced, and ultimately discarded or fell out of favor. Specifically:

- *Antimicrobial activity*—Gold compounds do not consistently inhibit microbial growth in vitro while inhibiting the arthritic process independent of microbial origins.
- *Immunosuppression*—While enzymatic proinflammatory mediators released as a result of the immune response can be inhibited, no direct effect on either immediate or delayed cellular responses is evident to suggest any immunosuppressive mechanism.
- *Macroglobulin aggregation*—Gold compounds may inhibit the aggregation of macroglobulins, leading to immune complex formation, thus slowing connective tissue degradation; however, this has not been widely accepted as the primary mechanism of action.
- *Collagen reactivity reduction*—Interaction with collagen fibrils and, thus, reduction of collagen reactivity that alters the course of the arthritic process has been also postulated, but not yet fully accepted.

The most widely accepted mechanism of antiarthritic action for gold compounds is inhibition of lysosomal enzymes, the release of which promotes the inflammatory response. The lysosomal enzymes glucuronidase, acid phosphatase, collagenase, and acid hydrolases are inhibited by these agents, putatively through stable and reversible gold–thiol interactions.

Specific mechanistic observations have been made relative to specific gold compounds. Gold sodium thiosulfate is a potent uncoupler of oxidative phosphorylation. Gold sodium thiomalate is a fairly effective inhibitor of PG biosynthesis in vitro, but the relationship of this effect to the antiarthritic actions of gold compounds has not been clarified. More recent studies suggest that auranofin suppressed the toll-like receptor 4 (TLR4)–mediated activation of the transcription factors by nuclear factor-κB (NF-κB) and IRF3, thus preventing the expression of cytokines and COX-2.[95] Previously it was shown that zinc is a necessary component of NF-κB for DNA binding and that gold ion can block this binding by oxidizing Cys residues associated with zinc.[96] Auranofin has also been shown to decrease tumor necrosis factor (TNF)-α–induced NF-κB activation, suggesting that effective inhibitors of NF-κB can be useful immunosuppressive and anti-inflammatory agents.[97]

Adverse Effects. Toxic side effects have been associated with the use of gold compounds, with the incidence of reported adverse reactions in patients on chrysotherapy (aurotherapy or treatment with gold salts) being as high as 55%. Serious toxicity occurs in 5% to 10% of reported cases. The most common adverse reactions include dermatitis (eg, erythema, papular, vesicular, and exfoliative dermatitis), mouth lesions (eg, stomatitis preceded by a metallic taste and gingivitis), pulmonary disorders (eg, interstitial pneumonitis), nephritis (eg, albuminuria and glomerulitis), and hematologic disorders (eg, thrombocytopenic purpura, hypoplastic and/or aplastic anemia, and eosinophilia; blood dyscrasias are rare in incidence but can be severe). Less commonly reported reactions are GI disturbances (eg, nausea, anorexia, and diarrhea), ocular toxicity (eg, keratitis with inflammation and ulceration of the cornea and subepithelial deposition of gold in the cornea), and hepatitis. In those cases in which severe toxicity occurs, excretion of gold can be markedly enhanced by the administration of chelating agents, the two most common of which are dimercaprol (British Anti-Lewisite) and penicillamine. Glucocorticoids also suppress the symptoms of gold toxicity, and the concomitant administration of dimercaprol and corticosteroids has been recommended in cases of severe gold intoxication.

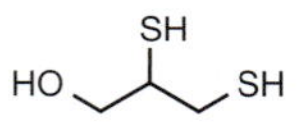

Dimercaprol

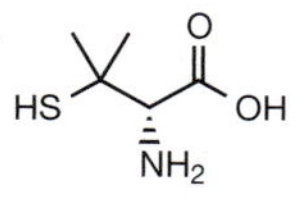

Penicillamine

General Structure-Activity Relationships. Despite the longevity that gold compounds have enjoyed over the last century, the SAR of gold compounds is limited. Monovalent gold (aurous ion [Au+]) is more effective than trivalent gold (auric ion [Au3+]). Only compounds with aurous ions attached to a sulfur-containing ligand are active (Fig. 17.21). Substituents attached to the aurous ion are typically polar and designed to enhance water solubility and primarily impact tissue distribution and excretion. Aurous ion is short-lived in solution, being rapidly converted to metallic gold or auric ion. Aqueous solutions decompose on standing at room temperature, posing a stability problem for gold compounds formulated as injections (aurothioglucose and gold sodium thiomalate).

In order to increase solution-phase aurous ion stability, complexation of Au+ with phosphine ligands, such as triethylphosphine (Fig. 17.21), has been employed.

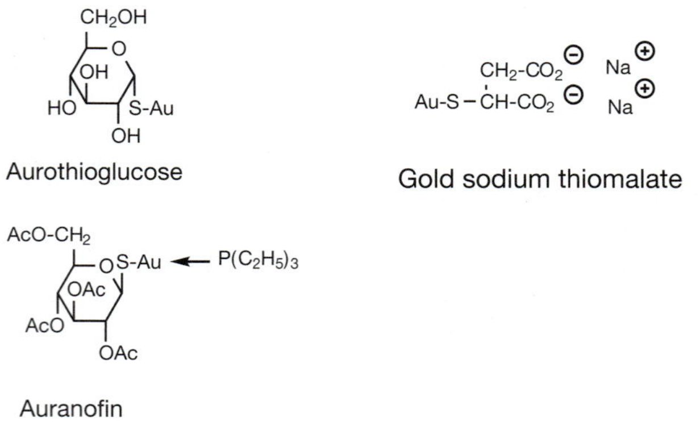

Figure 17.21 Gold compounds as disease-modifying antirheumatic drugs (DMARDs).

Triethylphosphine stabilizes the reduced valence state and results in both nonionic complexes that are soluble in organic solvents and enhanced oral bioavailability. Phosphine compounds lacking an aurous ion are ineffective in arthritic assays; however, compared to other groups bound to gold, the phosphine ligand in the gold coordination complexes appears to play a role in promoting antiarthritic activity. The structures of the three therapeutically available gold compounds in the United States are shown in Figure 17.21.

Absorption and Metabolism. Gold compounds are rapidly absorbed following IM injection, and the gold is widely distributed in the body. The highest concentrations are found in the reticuloendothelial system and in adrenal and renal cortices. They are also highly bound to plasma proteins.[98] Binding of gold from orally administered agents to red blood cells is higher than that of injectable gold.[99] Gold accumulates in inflamed joints, where high levels persist for at least 20 days after injection. Although gold is excreted primarily in the urine, the bulk of injected gold is retained. Gold can be found in the urine months after therapy has been discontinued.

Drug Interactions. The only significant drug interactions reported for gold compounds are concurrent administration of drugs that decrease excretion of gold compounds, leading to blood dyscrasias (most notably the antimalarial and immunosuppressive drugs).

Specific Drugs

Gold Sodium Thiomalate. Gold sodium thiomalate is indicated as an anti-inflammatory agent in the treatment of RA. Gold thiomalate inhibits glucosamine-6-phosphate synthase, a rate-limiting step involved in the mucopolysaccharide biosynthetic pathway. Gold sodium thiomalate (actually a mixture of mono- and disodium salts of gold thiomalic acid) is highly water soluble and is available as a light-sensitive aqueous solution of pH 5.8 to 6.5. The gold content is approximately 50%. It is administered as an IM injection and is not orally bioavailable.

Aurothioglucose. Aurothioglucose is indicated for the adjunctive treatment of adult and juvenile RA when other anti-inflammatory agents have been ineffective. It is a glucose analogue where the α-hydroxy group at the 1-position is substituted with an aurothio group, making it highly water soluble. However, aqueous solutions are unstable and decompose;

therefore, it is available as a suspension in sesame oil for IM injection. The gold content is approximately 50%. It is highly bound to plasma proteins (95%), and peak plasma levels are achieved within 2 to 6 hours. The half-life ranges from 3 to 27 days, but following successive weekly doses, the half-life increases to 14 to 40 days after the third dose. The therapeutic effect does not correlate with serum plasma gold levels but appears to depend on total accumulated gold.

Auranofin. Auranofin is indicated for use in adults with active RA who have not responded sufficiently to one or more NSAIDs. It is an analogue of aurothioglucose in which all the hydroxy groups have been acetylated and the aurothio group at the 1-position has been epimerized to the β-configuration. The increased lipophilicity of auranofin makes it orally effective, and it is the first orally bioavailable gold compound used to treat RA. Auranofin contains approximately 29% gold. Daily oral doses produce a rapid increase in kidney and blood gold levels for the first 3 days of treatment, with a more gradual increase on subsequent administration. Oral absorption is not complete, as plasma gold levels after oral administration are lower than those attained with parenteral gold compounds. The major route of excretion is via the urine. Auranofin can produce fewer adverse reactions than parenteral gold compounds, but its therapeutic efficacy can also be less.

Aminoquinolines

HYDROXYCHLOROQUINE SULFATE. Hydroxychloroquine sulfate, a 4-aminoquinoline, is indicated for the treatment of RA, systemic lupus erythematosus, and malaria. While the nonhydroxylated analogue chloroquine was discontinued for use in the treatment of RA due to corneal and renal toxicities, hydroxychloroquine, being less toxic, is still indicated for this use. The mechanism of antirheumatic action is currently unknown; however, it is largely accepted that it accumulates in and stabilizes lysosomes.

Hydroxychloroquine sulfate is highly water soluble and is readily absorbed on oral administration, reaching peak plasma levels within 1 to 3 hours. It concentrates in organs such as the liver, spleen, kidneys, heart, lung, and brain, thereby prolonging elimination. Hydroxychloroquine is metabolized by N-dealkylation of the tertiary amine, followed by oxidative deamination of the resulting primary amine to the carboxylic acid derivative. In addition to possessing mild corneal and renal toxicity, hydroxychloroquine can also cause CNS, neuromuscular, GI, and hematologic side effects.

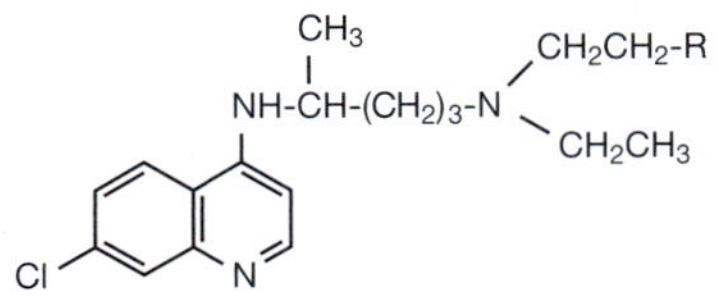

Chloroquine (R = H)
Hydroxychloroquine (R = OH)

Immunosuppressants

Several substances that suppress the immune system have been explored as antirheumatic drugs because the etiology of RA can involve a destructive immune response. Thus, unlike drugs previously discussed, immunosuppressive drugs can act at the steps involved in the pathogenesis of the inflammatory disorders. As a group, however, these drugs (shown in Fig. 17.22) are cytotoxic, as evidenced by their initial development as anticancer agents.

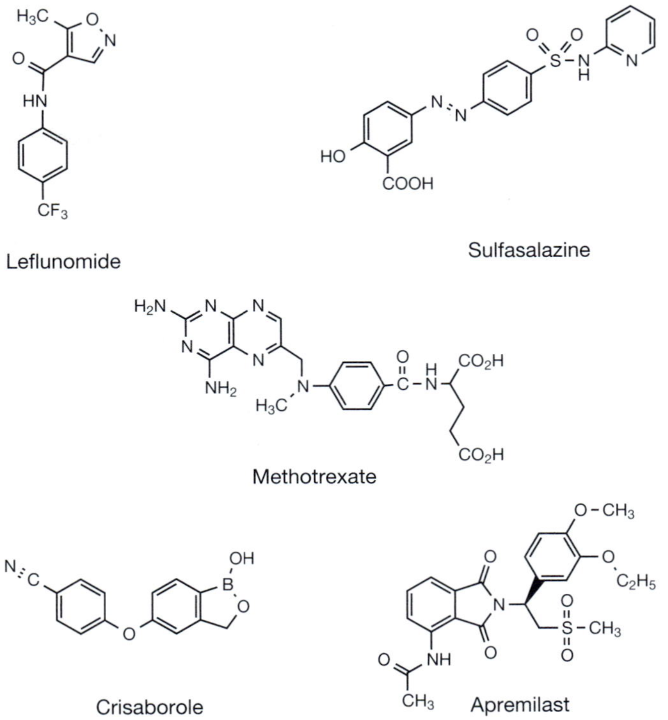

Figure 17.22 Disease-modifying antirheumatic immunosuppressants.

SPECIFIC DRUGS

Leflunomide. Leflunomide is a DMARD used for the management of RA. It retards structural damage associated with arthritis in adults who have moderate to severe active RA.

Leflunomide is a prodrug that is rapidly and almost completely metabolized (half-life <60 min) after oral administration.

The mechanism of action of leflunomide is through teriflunomide's ability to inhibit the pyrimidine biosynthetic pathway, specifically inhibiting dihydroorotate dehydrogenase. Inhibition of the pyrimidine biosynthetic pathway results in decreasing DNA and ribonucleic acid (RNA) nitrogen-containing bases and arresting the B-cell and T-cell proliferation cycles and production of antibodies (Fig. 17.23). It is the reduction of B-cell concentrations that downregulates the immune process.

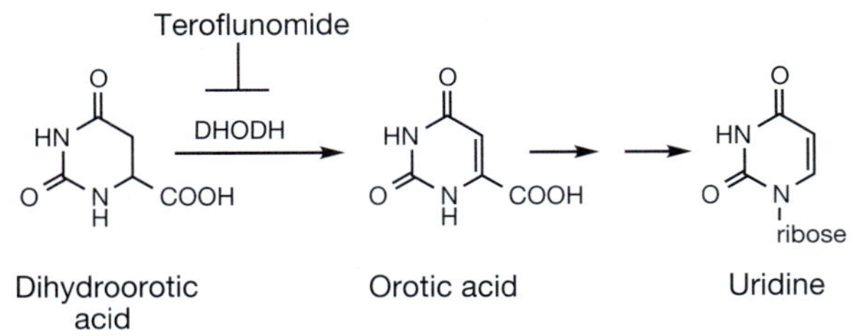

Figure 17.23 Dihydroorotate dehydrogenase (DHODH) pathway.

At high therapeutic doses, leflunomide inhibits protein tyrosine kinases. Leflunomide is administered orally as a single daily dose without regard to meals. Therapy can be initiated with a loading dosage given for 3 days, followed by the usual maintenance dose. It undergoes primarily enterohepatic circulation, extending its duration of action.

Methotrexate. Methotrexate (Fig. 17.22) is an antifolate approved for the treatment of severe active RA in adults who are intolerant to, or have had an insufficient response to, first-line therapy. There are many putative mechanisms of action for the antirheumatic activity of methotrexate.[100] Similar to leflunomide, methotrexate blocks the pyrimidine biosynthetic pathway and the proliferation of B cells by interfering with DNA synthesis, repair, and replication. It accomplishes this by pseudoirreversibly inhibiting dihydrofolate reductase. An additional action implicated in methotrexate's antirheumatic activity is the inhibition of the production of polyamines that can be responsible for inducing tissue damage and the activation of NF-κB. Methotrexate is well absorbed after oral administration, and oral bioavailability is approximately 60%, where food can delay absorption and reduce peak serum concentrations. Methotrexate is approximately 50% bound to plasma proteins.

Approximately 10% to 20% of a dose of methotrexate is metabolized to active polyglutamated and 7-hydroxylated metabolites.[101] Some prehepatic metabolism occurs in the GI tract after oral administration. Methotrexate is actively transported by the human organic anion transporter (hOAT3) into the urine and is excreted primarily unchanged. Its elimination half-life is 3 to 10 hours.

Life-threatening drug interactions are known to occur between methotrexate and NSAIDs, probenecid, and penicillin G. These drugs inhibit hOAT3-mediated active transport of methotrexate into the urine. Thus, patients with RA should not take NSAIDs while taking methotrexate. Methotrexate therapy requires monitoring of liver enzymes and is contraindicated in those with hepatic disease and in patients who are pregnant or considering pregnancy.

Sulfasalazine (Azulfidine). Sulfasalazine is used for the treatment of mild to moderate ulcerative colitis, as adjunct therapy in the treatment of severe ulcerative colitis, for the treatment of Crohn disease, and for the treatment of RA or ankylosing spondylitis. Sulfasalazine is a prodrug that is hydrolyzed by colonic bacteria into 5-aminosalicylic acid (5-ASA; mesalamine) and sulfapyridine (Fig. 17.24). Some controversy exists regarding which of these two products is responsible for the activity of sulfasalazine. 5-ASA, like aspirin, is an inhibitor of PG biosynthesis and is known to have therapeutic benefit. However, it is not clear whether sulfapyridine adds any further benefit, since it is the metabolite that is more extensively absorbed. It was shown to inhibit purine biosynthesis by inhibiting 5-aminoimidazole-4-carboxamisoribonucleotide transformylase and to enhance adenosine release, enhancing the ability of adenosine to decrease inflammation by binding to A2 adenosine receptors on inflammatory cells.[102] Sulfasalazine and/or its metabolites have been shown to inhibit the release of inflammatory cytokines and TNFα. In the colon, the products created by the breakdown of sulfasalazine work as anti-inflammatory

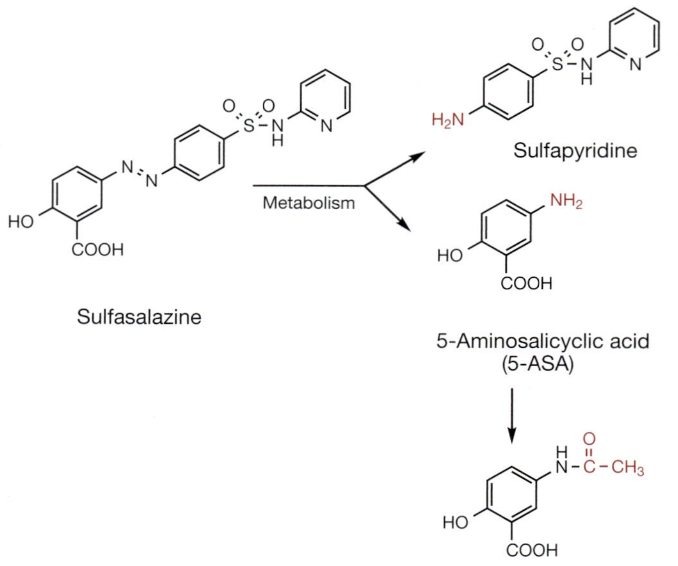

Figure 17.24 Metabolism of sulfasalazine.

agents for treating colon inflammation. The beneficial effect of sulfasalazine is believed to result from a local effect on the bowel, although there can also be a beneficial systemic immunosuppressant effect.

Apremilast (Otezla). Apremilast (Fig. 17.22) is a phthalimide analogue approved for treatment of active psoriatic arthritis or plaque psoriasis, and is being tested for a number of additional inflammatory conditions such as ankylosing spondylitis, Behcet disease, and RA.[103,104] The treatment of psoriatic arthritis (PsA) normally calls for the use of costly biologicals, which are administered via injection. The advent of an orally active low molecular weight drug is highly desirable.

A variety of inflammatory mediators are associated with the onset of psoriasis. These include TNF, a number of interleukins (ILs), interferon-γ (IFNγ), vascular endothelial growth factor (VEGF), and several chemokines (CXCL). The most recent therapeutic approach to attenuating the inflammatory impact of these mediators has been to inhibit the hydrolysis of cyclic adenosine monophosphate (cAMP). The concentration of cAMP is regulated by adenylyl cyclases (synthesis) and phosphodiesterase (PDE) (degradation); therefore, inhibition of cAMP hydrolysis translates to inhibition of PDE.

Apremilast is an orally active PDE4 inhibitory drug, which does not show selectivity for any particular PDE4 receptor subclass.[105] Among the PDEs, the PDE4 isoforms are found within immune cells such as lymphocytes, granulocytes, and cells of the monocyte/macrophage system. Important PDEs within immune cells are PDE4A, B, and D. Unfortunately, nonspecific inhibitors of PDE4 cause significant adverse events, including diarrhea by binding to intestinal ion channels and stimulating chloride ion secretion into the small intestine, and emesis. Headache, a runny and/or stuffy nose, upper respiratory tract infections, and abdominal pain may also be experienced.

Apremilast is rapidly absorbed following oral administration and exhibits a long half-life (~8 hours). The T_{max}

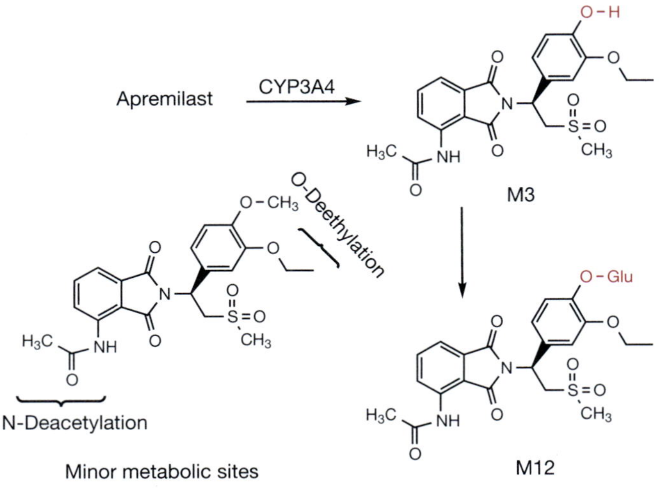

Figure 17.25 Metabolism of apremilast.

occurs at approximately 2.5 hours. Apremilast is extensively metabolized to a wide variety of products, and only 7% of the drug is excreted unchanged. It is primarily inactivated through CYP3A4-mediated O-dealkylation of the methoxy group, forming metabolite M3, followed by glucuronide conjugation to give M12 (Fig. 17.25).[106] Apremilast should not be administered to patients taking CYP3A4 inducers, as this results in significantly reduced serum concentrations. The addition of ketoconazole to the regimen results in a significant increase in the AUC, also suggesting CYP3A4/5 as the metabolizing enzyme. Minor metabolites include those generated through O-deethylation, N-deacetylation, and additional aromatic hydroxylation reactions. The majority of the metabolites are found in the urine, and all are inactive.

Crisaborole (Eucrisa). Crisaborole is an immunosuppressant approved for the treatment of atopic dermatitis and has also completed phase 2 clinical trials for the treatment of psoriasis.[107] Atopic dermatitis is commonly associated with an increased level of phosphodiesterase 4B activity, which, in turn, leads to increased levels of TNFα, IL-12, and IL-23. The disease is characterized by the symptoms of severe pruritus and skin barrier disruption. Crisaborole contains a boron atom, which is typically not seen in pharmaceuticals; however, it is essential for its activity and also promotes skin penetration. Crisaborole is structurally similar to the topical antifungal agent, tavaborole. The most common adverse effect consists of pain at the site of application.

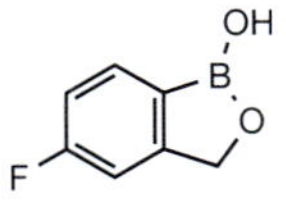

Tavaborole

Crisaborole is an inhibitor of PDE4 and, as such, results in decreased levels of TNFα and various ILs (Fig. 17.26).[108] As with apremilast, inhibition of PDE4 by crisaborole leads to increased levels of cAMP[108] but, unlike apremilast, it has been shown to exhibit selectivity toward isoforms A and B of the PDE4 enzyme. More specifically, the boron atom binds

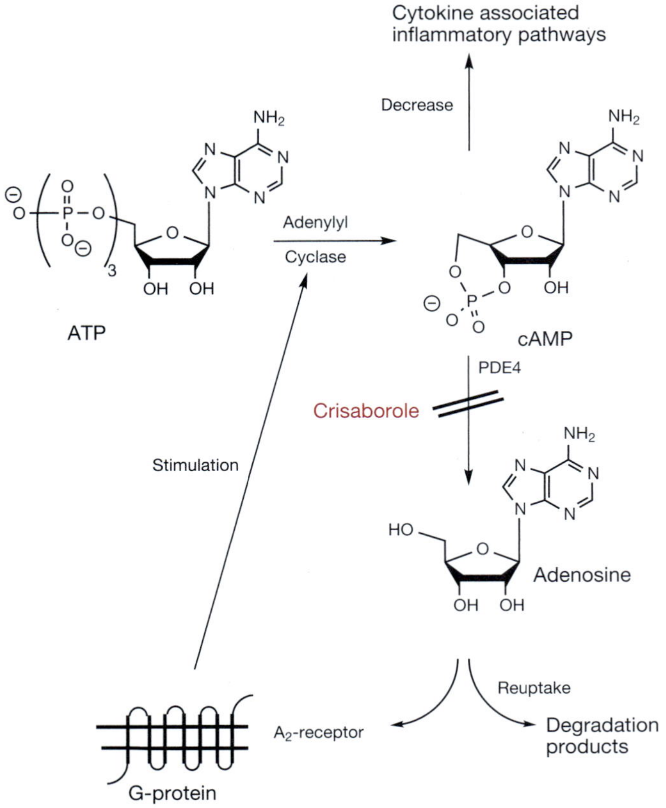

Figure 17.26 Mechanism of action for crisaborole.

in a tetrahedral configuration to bimetal ions in the catalytic site of the PDE4B enzyme.[109] In so doing, crisaborole, through the hydrated boron atom, appears to be taking the normal binding site that the phosphate in cAMP would occupy, which spares the cyclic nucleotide from hydrolytic destruction.[109]

Crisaborole is available as a 2% ointment and is used topically. The drug is absorbed following topical administration (~25%), extensively metabolized to inactive metabolites (Fig. 17.27), and excreted via the urine. The major CYP3A4- and 1A1/2-generated metabolite results from oxidative deboronation followed by hydrolysis of crisaborole, yielding 5-(4-cyanophenoxy)-2-hydroxyl benzyl alcohol. The primary alcohol is then further oxidized to the carboxylic acid. The drug is highly bound to plasma protein.

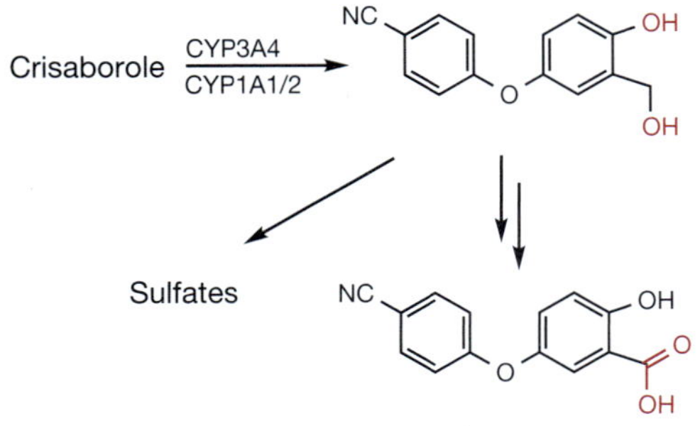

Figure 17.27 Metabolism of crisaborole.

Biologic Disease-Modifying Antirheumatic Drugs

Interleukin-1 Receptor Antagonist

ANAKINRA (KINERET). Anakinra is approved for use in adults with moderate to severe active RA and in whom conventional DMARD therapy was ineffective, and it can be used in combination with methotrexate.[110] Anakinra is a recombinant, nonglycosylated form of the human IL-1 receptor antagonist (IL-1Rα) that neutralizes the inflammatory activity of the proinflammatory IL-1 cytokine by competing with IL-1 for binding to its IL-1 type 1 receptor (IL-1R1). IL-1R1 activation leads to increases in the formation of nitric oxide (NO), PGE_2, and collagenase in synovial cells, resulting in cartilage degradation and stimulation of bone resorption. IL-1R1 receptor activity is regulated by the endogenous antagonist IL-1Rα. Synovial fluid has increased concentrations of IL-1 in rheumatoid synovium, resulting in imbalance between IL-1 and IL-1Rα leading to rheumatic progression. The levels of the naturally occurring IL-lRα in synovium and synovial fluid from patients with rheumatoid are insufficient to compete with the elevated amount of locally produced IL-1; therefore exogenous anakinra (IL-1Rα analogue) can be administered to effectively neutralize the proinflammatory activity of IL-1 through competitive inhibition of IL-1RI.

Anakinra consists of 153 amino acids and has a molecular weight of 17.3 kDa. It is produced by recombinant DNA technology using an *Escherichia coli* bacterial expression system and differs from native human IL-1Rα by the addition of a single Met residue at its amino terminus.

Anakinra is administered subcutaneously on a once-daily basis, and its elimination half-life ranges from 4 to 6 hours. Some potential side effects include injection site reactions, decreased white blood cell counts, headache, and an increase in upper respiratory infections. There can be a slightly higher rate of respiratory infections in people who have asthma or chronic obstructive pulmonary disease. Persons with an active infection are advised not to use anakinra.

Interleukin-6 Receptor Antagonist

TOCILIZUMAB (ACTEMRA). Tocilizumab is approved for use in adults with moderate to severe active RA, cytokine release syndromes, and giant cell arteritis. It can be used in combination with methotrexate and is an alternative therapy for rheumatic patients not responding to TNFα blockers (discussed later). Tocilizumab is a recombinant humanized antihuman monoclonal antibody that binds to and inhibits solubilized and membrane-bound IL-6 receptors.[111] IL-6 is the endogenous proinflammatory agonist for the IL-6 receptors. Tocilizumab is a member of the IgG1κ subclass with a typical H2L2 (two heavy and two light chains) polypeptide structure. Each light chain consists of 214 amino acids, whereas the heavy chain contains 448 residues. The four polypeptide chains are linked by disulfide bonds both intra- and intermolecularly. It has a molecular weight of approximately 148 kDa.

Tocilizumab's dosing regimen is either 4 or 8 mg/kg IV every 4 weeks. Steady-state is reached following the first administration for C_{max} and AUC, respectively, and after 16 weeks for C_{min}. The half-life is concentration dependent and is 11 days for the 4 mg/kg dose and 13 days for the 8 mg/kg dose. The total dose should not exceed 800 mg per infusion. The most frequently observed adverse effects are upper respiratory tract infection, headache, hypertension, increased alanine transaminase activity, and nasopharyngitis.

Costimulation Modulators

Two signals are required to activate a T-cell response to an antigen, and the process is referred to as costimulation. Costimulation activation is shown in Figure 17.28. The two signals for the costimulation process are:

1. An unactivated antigen-presenting cell (APC) "presents" an antigen complex that is recognized by the T-cell receptor
2. A costimulatory ligand, such as B7, that interacts with CD28 on the T-cell surface to form a B7-CD28 complex and that is also presented by the APC

If only process 1 happens, the T cell does not respond and becomes unreactive and nonresponsive to any further antigenic stimuli. If both processes occur, T-cell proliferation and differentiation in response to the antigenic stimulus is initiated and T cell binding proinflammatory cytokines are released, further enhancing its activation. T-cell costimulation activation is regulated by T-lymphocyte antigen 4

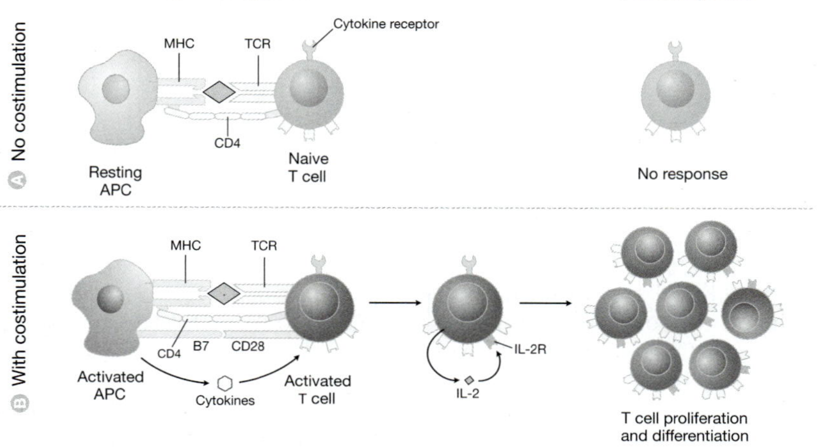

Figure 17.28 Costimulation in the T-cell activation pathway.

(CTLA-4), which is also expressed on the T-cell surface and is upregulated on T-cell activation. B7 ligands on the surface of APCs now have a choice on where to bind on the surface of T cells, CD28 or CTLA-4. The B7 ligands bind with a greater affinity to CTLA-4 than to CD28, preventing delivery of the costimulatory signal. This built-in limit prevents T-cell activation from spiraling out of control.

Abatacept (Orencia). As described, the costimulatory process ends with a B7-CD28 complex between the APC and the T-cell, resulting in T-cell activation and the subsequent proliferation and release of proinflammatory cytokines. Abatacept, a costimulation modulator acting through reduced T-cell activation, was designed to inhibit this process and is an alternative for rheumatic patients who have failed on TNF blockers (discussed later).[112] Abatacept is a novel chimeric CTLA-4–IgG1 fused protein created from the fusion of the extracellular domain of the mouse CTLA-4 with the modified heavy-chain constant region of human IgG1. It acts like an antibody, where the extracellular portion binds with high affinity to B7 ligands and prevents them from interacting with CD28 on activated T-cells. This inhibits the costimulatory process, suppresses T-cell proliferation and release of proinflammatory cytokines, and slows bone and cartilage damages while relieving rheumatic symptoms.

Abatacept is available for subcutaneous administration weekly or by IV infusion monthly and side effects can include headache, nausea, and mild infections such as upper respiratory tract infections. Serious infections, such as pneumonia, can occur. There is some concern that blocking of the suppressive signal from B7 to CTLA-4 can have a negative effect on regulatory T cells and thus, eventually, promote autoimmunity.

Cytokine Inhibitors

T cells are activated as described, and therefore, they multiply and release cytokines that promote the destruction of tissues surrounding the joints and cause the signs and symptoms of RA.[113] This section describes antirheumatic therapeutics that act downstream from T-cell activation, inhibiting cytokine activity.

Tumor Necrosis–Factor Blockers. Upon T-cell activation, the expression of the cytokines, IL-1, IL-6, and TNFα by the rheumatoid synovium is upregulated leading to RA disease progression. More specifically, TNFα is a proinflammatory cytokine that has a major role in the pathological inflammatory process of RA. As TNFα concentrations increase in joints, it leads to joint inflammation and ultimately, joint destruction. Therefore, rendering TNFα inactive has become an effective therapy for RA, as well as ankylosing spondylitis and psoriatic arthritis.[102]

Two effective approaches have been developed to decrease TNFα activity.

1. Soluble TNF receptor (TNFR) decoys that bind present TNFα (etanercept)
2. Anti-TNFα antibodies that bind to TNFα, preventing it from activating TNFRs (infliximab, adalimumab, golimumab, certolizumab)

These actions help reduce pain, morning stiffness, and tender or swollen joints, usually within 1 or 2 weeks after treatment begins. TNF blockers work synergistically with methotrexate, and the two drugs are often coadministered. Common adverse effects include blood disorders, lymphoma, demyelinating diseases, and increased risk of infection. Because TNF is also important for host defense against infections, the effects of long-term use on toxicity may be problematic.

Structural illustrations of the anti-TNF agents etanercept, infliximab, adalimumab, golimumab, and certolizumab are provided in Figure 17.29. For a comprehensive review of biologic DMARD drug, see the recent publication by Combe et al.[114]

Etanercept (Enbrel). Etanercept is used for the treatment of RA in patients who have not adequately responded to one or more of the synthetic DMARDs. It can also be used in psoriatic arthritis and ankylosing spondylitis.

Etanercept is a dimeric soluble form of p75 TNFR and acts as a decoy receptor capable of binding to two TNFα molecules in the circulation, rendering them unavailable for binding to the TNFR. It consists of the extracellular ligand binding portion of the 75-kDa human TNFR fused to the Fc portion of human immunoglobulin (Ig) G1. The Fc component of etanercept contains the CH_2 domain, the CH_3 domain, and the hinge region, but not the CH_1 domain of IgG1. It consists of 934 amino acids and has an apparent molecular weight of approximately 150 kDa, requiring specific disulfide bridging for optimal activity.[115] Etanercept

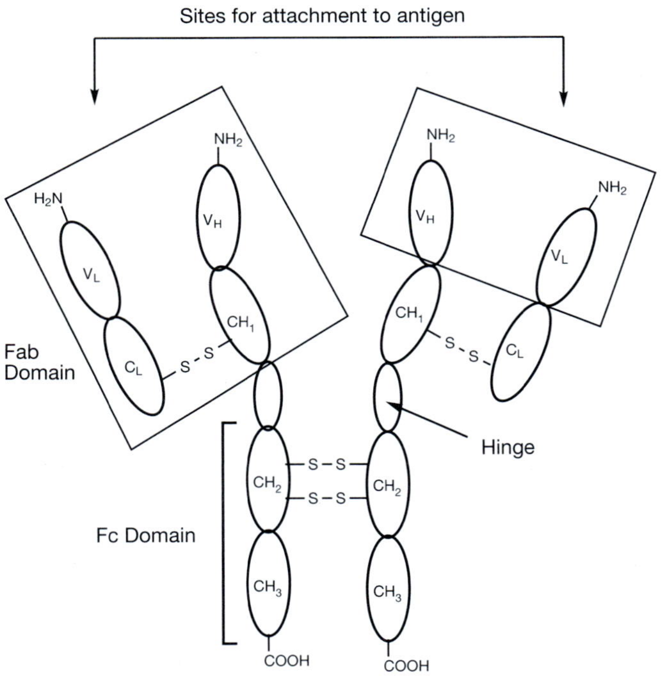

Figure 17.29 Anti-tumor necrosis factor (TNF) agents. Etanercept is the extracellular portion of the human TNF receptor fused to the Fc domain of human immunoglobulin (Ig) G1. Infliximab is a partially humanized monoclonal antibody against TNFα. The Fv domains are derived from mouse antihuman sequences, whereas the Fc domain is composed of human IgG1 sequence. Adalimumab is fully humanized antibody to human TNFα (Fv and Fc derived from human sequences). Golimumab is a fully humanized antibody. Certolizumab has a human Fab domain and no Fc domain. The Fc domain for certolizumab is replaced with PEG.

also binds TNFβ. Some concern exists because of reports that etanercept can cause serious infections and could have contributed to the deaths of several patients using the drug. A review of the clinical utility of etanercept is available.[116]

Etanercept is available as a powder to be reconstituted for injection. Dosing can be once (50 mg/dose) or twice (25 mg/dose) a week. Patients may experience irritation at the injection site.

Infliximab (Remicade). Infliximab is indicated for the treatment of RA in combination with methotrexate and to induce remission in patients with moderate to severe Crohn disease who have not responded to conventional therapy. It can also be used to treat psoriatic arthritis and ulcerative colitis. Infliximab is a chimeric IgG1κ monoclonal antibody to human TNFα, blocking its ability to bind TNFRs. The Fv domain of the mouse antibody responsible for recognizing TNFα is combined with a human Fc domain of IgG1 (IgG1κ). This fused protein has been "humanized" and has increased immunostability with a lower risk of degradation by the host's immune system. Infliximab has an approximate molecular weight of 149 kDa. It blocks TNFα activity by binding both the transmembrane and soluble forms of TNFα. It does not bind to TNFβ (lymphotoxin A), a related cytokine that uses the same receptors as TNFα and, thus, is more specific in its action than etanercept. Cells expressing transmembrane TNFα bound by infliximab can be lysed.

Infliximab is supplied as a lyophilized powder to be formulated for IV infusion in sterile water. The solution should be used immediately after reconstitution, as the product does not contain antibacterial preservatives. The volume of distribution at steady-state is independent of dose. The terminal half-life of infliximab is 8.0 to 9.5 days, which is sufficiently long enough to allow dosing every 6 to 8 weeks. No systemic accumulation of infliximab occurred on continued repeated treatment at 4- or 8-week intervals.

Long-term use can be associated with the development of anti-infliximab antibodies, an effect that does not appear when it is used in combination with methotrexate. Warnings associated with the use of infliximab include risks of autoimmunity, infections, hypersensitivity reactions, and worsening congestive heart failure. Reviews and reports of the properties and use of infliximab are available.[117,118]

Adalimumab (Humira). Adalimumab is a recombinant human IgG1 monoclonal antibody targeted for human TNFα. It is fully humanized and comprises human-derived, heavy- and light-chain variable regions (Fab) and human IgG1κ constant regions. It consists of 1330 amino acids and has a molecular weight of approximately 148 kDa. Adalimumab has the same mechanism of action as infliximab; however, since it is a fully humanized IgG1 monoclonal antibody, there is increased immune-stability and lessened chance for degradation by the immune system. In addition, similar to infliximab, adalimumab does not bind or inactivate TNFβ. It is supplied in single-use, prefilled, glass syringes as a sterile, preservative-free, colorless solution for biweekly subcutaneous administration. Irritation at the site of injection may occur. The pharmacokinetics of adalimumab are linear over the dose range of 0.5 to 10.0 mg/kg following a single IV dose. The mean elimination half-life is approximately 2 weeks.

Golimumab (Symponi). Golimumab is a human IgG1k monoclonal antibody specific for human TNFα. It is an alternative to etanercept, adalimumab, and infliximab for the treatment of RA. Golimumab weighs approximately 150 to 151 kDa[119] and binds to both the soluble and transmembrane forms of human TNFα, with high affinity.[112] The advantage golimumab possesses over other anti-TNFα agents is the once-monthly subcutaneous dosing.

The average terminal half-life of golimumab is 2 weeks. Subcutaneous dosing every 4 weeks leads to steady-state serum concentrations by week 12. Its metabolic pathway is unknown. The most frequent adverse effects are upper respiratory tract infection, sore throat, and nasopharyngitis. Serious infections can occur, along with lymphomas and other malignancies. Labeling includes a boxed warning that alerts patients to the risk of tuberculosis and invasive fungal infections.

Certolizumab Pegol (Cimzia). Certolizumab is a monoclonal antibody directed against TNFα.[120] It selectively inhibits TNFα over lymphotoxin A (TNFβ). Certolizumab is composed of a humanized anti-TNFα antibody Fab' fragment, which is linked to polyethylene glycol (PEG). The purpose of linking the antibody to PEG (pegolate) is to (1) reduce the immunogenicity of the antibody, (2) increase the circulating half-life of the antibody, which expands the dosing range to once every 4 weeks, rather than the every-2-week regimen common with non-pegylated MAbs, and (3) enhance TNFα targeting. The Fab' fragment is composed of a light chain with 214 amino acid residues and a heavy chain with 229 amino acids. The antibody lacks an Fc portion and thus binds to only TNFα without having to bind to the cell surface receptors for antibodies. One of the major advantages of certolizumab over the other monoclonal antibodies directed against TNFα is its lower cost.

Subcutaneous and single IV dosing studies of certolizumab demonstrate predictable and linear dose-related plasma concentrations. Metabolism of the Fab' fragment is unknown, whereas the PEG moiety is excreted in the urine. The major adverse effects are mild and include rash and upper respiratory and urinary tract infections.

B-Lymphocyte Blocker

Rituximab (Rituxan). Rituximab, in combination with methotrexate, can reduce signs and symptoms of RA in adult patients with moderate to severe disease who have had an inadequate response to one or more TNF blockers. Rituximab is a genetically engineered, fused mouse/human anti-CD20 MAb that targets B lymphocytes by binding specifically to the CD20 antigen, a protein found on the surface of B cells at certain stages in the life cycle. Rituximab is composed of two heavy chains of 451 amino acids and two light chains of 213 amino acids with an approximate molecular weight of 145 kDa. Its binding affinity for the CD20 antigen is approximately 8.0 nM. The mouse light- and heavy-chain Fab domains of rituximab, which bind to the CD20 antigen on B cells, are linked to the human Fc domains of IgG1κ. Once the rituximab molecule attaches to the B cells, it initiates B-cell lysis, inducing rapid and profound depletion of peripheral B cells, with patients showing near-complete B-cell depletion within 2 weeks after receiving the first dose of rituximab.

Rituximab is a sterile, clear, colorless, preservative-free, liquid concentrate formulated for IV administration. It is given as two 1,000-mg IV infusions separated by 2 weeks. Adverse effects include hypersensitivity and flu-like symptoms such as fever, chills, and nausea. Patients experiencing significant hypersensitivity can show bronchospasm, hypotension, myocardial infarction, and ventricular fibrillation that can be fatal. Interested readers are referred to published reviews on the clinical applications of rituximab.[121,122]

Janus Kinase Inhibitors

Janus-activated kinase (JAK) inhibitors (JAKis) are oral synthetic DMARDs used to treat a variety of chronic inflammatory disorders, such as RA, PsA, ulcerative colitis, and atopic dermatitis, which may involve continuous or increased activation of the JAK/signal transducer and activator of transcription (STAT) signaling pathway.[123] JAKs are dimerized enzyme-linked receptors that transmit extracellular signals intracellularly through phosphorylation and dimerization of STATs to induce gene transcription pathways. This leads to the production of cytokines, chemokines, and growth factors that are involved in coordinating the function of immune cells.[124] JAK/STAT signaling is complex due to multiple JAK and tyrosine kinase (TYK) receptor combinations (eg, JAK1/JAK2, JAK1/JAK3, and JAK2/TYK2). The JAK-STAT pathway is activated by cytokines (eg, IL-2, IL-6, IL-10, and interferon-gamma) binding to these extracellular receptors.[125] Normally, suppressors of cytokine signaling (SOCS) and protein inhibitors of activated STAT (PIAS) proteins impede JAK/STAT signaling.[123] However, these regulators are dysfunctional in RA.[123] Elevated levels of IL-6 and IL-10, cytokines generated from the activation of the JAK/STAT pathway, are implicated in dyslipidemia in chronic inflammatory disorders.[125] Inhibiting the JAK/STAT signaling pathway improves therapeutic outcomes partly by reducing disease activity; however, whether selective inhibition of the JAK/STAT pathway reduces adverse effects is still being evaluated.[126]

JAKi class effects include increased infection risk, cytopenia, and lipid abnormalities. In addition, JAKis should be used with caution in patients with a history of diverticulitis or NSAID use due to an increased risk of gastrointestinal perforations.[126] Other common adverse effects include upper respiratory infections, urinary tract infections, nasopharyngitis, nausea, headaches, and occasional diarrhea. Although these side effects are well-tolerated, black box warnings indicate an increased risk for serious events, such as serious infections, neoplasms, major adverse cardiovascular event (MACE), thrombosis, and death.[127] Specifically, JAKi use strongly correlates with lipid abnormalities, resulting in increased levels of total cholesterol (TC), low-density lipoprotein (LDL), high-density lipoprotein (HDL), apolipoprotein (Apo)AI, and ApoB. These aberrant lipid levels are typically observed within the first 4 weeks and, ultimately, stabilize by 12 weeks of treatment.[128] The underlying mechanism partly involves dysfunctional cholesterol ester metabolism and impaired antioxidant capacity despite elevated HDL levels.[129] JAKis may also reverse the lipid paradox, thereby restoring or increasing lipid levels within RA patients.[130] Given that RA patients are susceptible to adverse cardiovascular events, these JAKi-induced phenomena further contribute to the development of MACE and venous thromboembolism (VTE).[131,132] While European RA guidelines reflect this risk by recommending JAKis be reserved for patients refractory to first-line DMARDs who have been screened for associated risk factors, the American College of Rheumatology (ACR) guidelines currently do not distinguish between preference for biologic DMARD or targeted synthetic DMARD.[133,134]

Tofacitinib (Xeljanz). Tofacitinib was the first JAKi to be FDA approved for the treatment of RA in 2012. In subsequent years, it was also approved for four additional autoimmune-based disease states: PsA, ulcerative colitis, polyarticular course juvenile idiopathic arthritis, and ankylosing spondylitis. For RA, tofacitinib is formulated as an immediate-release tablet (5 mg twice daily) or an extended-release tablet (11 mg once daily). It is noted that patients may see the inert tablet shell in the feces because it is not absorbable; however, the active medication has been absorbed by the time it fully passes through the gut. Tofacitinib has an absolute bioavailability of 74%, with an elimination half-life of approximately 3 hours. It is metabolized via CYP3A4 primarily and can have potential drug interactions with other CYP3A4 inhibitors/inducers.[135-137]

Baricitinib (Olumiant). Baricitinib was the second JAKi to be FDA approved for the treatment of RA in 2018. In 2022, it was also approved for coronavirus disease 2019 (COVID-19) in certain hospitalized adults and severe alopecia areata. For RA, tofacitinib is formulated as a 2-mg tablet, while a 4-mg tablet is indicated for COVID-19 and alopecia areata. Baricitinib has an absolute bioavailability of 97%, with an elimination half-life of approximately 12 hours.[138]

Upadacitinib (Rinvoq). Upadacitinib is the most recent JAKi to be FDA approved for the treatment of RA in 2019. It is also approved for PsA (2021), atopic dermatitis (2022), ulcerative colitis (2022), ankylosing spondylitis (2022), spondylarthritis (2022), and Crohn disease (2023). For RA, upadacitinib is formulated as 30-mg, 45-mg, and 60-mg extended-release tablets.[139,140]

Drugs Used to Treat Gout

Pathophysiology

Gout is an acute or chronic form of inflammatory arthritis characterized by significant joint pain, tenderness, redness, and swelling. It is the most common inflammatory arthritis in men, with the incidence in Black men almost twice that of White men. The major factors that can precipitate gout include lifestyle, genetics, and medications. Lifestyle factors include high meat and seafood diet, emotional stress, physical trauma, and excessive alcohol intake. Medications such as diuretics, β-blockers, and even aspirin have also been attributed to gout attacks. Gout is also associated with an increased risk of kidney stones.[141]

Gout results from elevated levels of uric acid in the blood with subsequent accumulation of needle-like crystals of monosodium urate monohydrate within the joints, synovial fluid, and periarticular tissue. The formation of uric acid from adenine and guanine is illustrated in Figure 17.30. Xanthine is a common metabolic product formed from

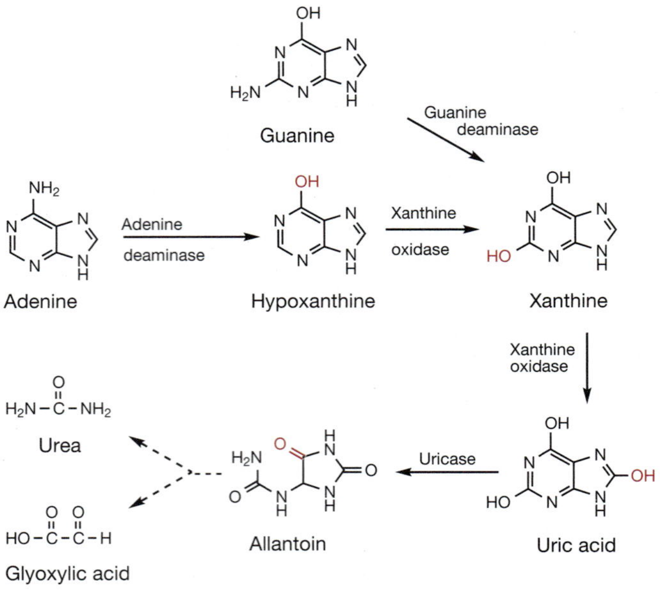

Figure 17.30 Formation of uric acid, urea, and glyoxylic acid from purines.

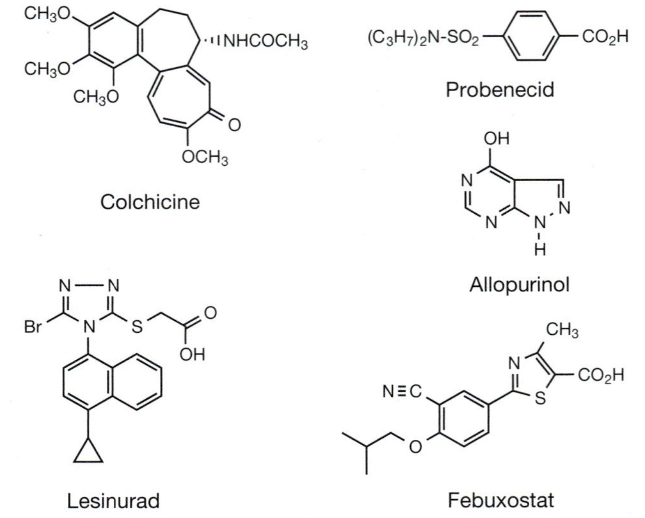

Figure 17.31 Agents used to control gout.

either adenine or guanine. Adenine deaminase converts the 6-amino group of adenine to a 6-hydroxy group, forming hypoxanthine. Xanthine oxidase then oxidizes hypoxanthine at the 2-position, yielding xanthine. Uric acid is subsequently formed by the oxidation of xanthine by the enzyme xanthine oxidase. Finally, uric acid is metabolized by uricase, forming allantoin with subsequent hydrolysis to provide urea and glyoxylic acid.

Uric acid is a weak acid with two pK_a values (5.7 and 10.3), and at physiologic pH, it exists primarily as the urate monoanion. Uric acid has low water solubility (~6 mg/100 mL); however, the urate monoanion is approximately 50 times more soluble in aqueous media. When levels of uric acid in the body increase, the solubility limits of urate monoanion are exceeded, and precipitation of sodium urate from the resulting supersaturated solution causes deposits of urate crystals. It is the formation of these urate crystals in joints and connective tissue that initiate attacks of gouty arthritis.

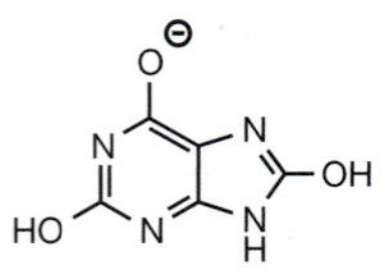

Urate monoanion

Blood levels of urate monoanion are maintained by a careful balance between its formation and excretion. The kidney has a dominant role in urate elimination, excreting about 70% of the daily urate production. Excretion of urate requires the urate anion transporter (URAT1) located in renal proximal tubule cells, which also has a central role in urate homeostasis. The URAT1 is targeted by uricosuric and antiuricosuric agents that affect urate excretion.

The structures of the drugs used to treat gout are shown in Figure 17.31.

Treatment of Acute Gout

The management of gout has been approached with the following therapeutic strategies: (1) control of acute attacks with drugs that reduce inflammation caused by the deposition of urate crystals and (2) control of chronic gout by increasing the rate of uric acid excretion and halting the biosynthesis of uric acid by inhibiting the enzyme xanthine oxidase. Treatment of acute gout includes NSAIDs such as indomethacin or naproxen (see previous NSAID discussion), colchicine, and glucocorticoids. The choice of an NSAID is usually based on the side effect profile.

Colchicine

Colchicine is a natural product obtained from various species of *Colchicum*, primarily *Colchicum autumnale* L, and is used in the prophylaxis and treatment of acute gout. It darkens on exposure to light and possesses moderate water solubility.

Colchicine does not alter serum levels of uric acid; however, it does appear to retard the inflammation attributed to the deposition of urate crystals. Colchicine's mechanism of action is multifaceted and essentially reduces proinflammatory mechanisms while increasing anti-inflammatory chemical mediators. A comprehensive review of colchicine's mechanism of action as it relates to the treatment of gout has been published.[142] The FDA approved the first single-ingredient oral colchicine formulation, Colcrys, for the treatment of acute gout flares in 2010. The drug is also approved for the treatment of familial Mediterranean fever.[143] Because colchicine does not lower serum urate levels, it is beneficial to combine it with a uricosuric agent, most commonly probenecid.

Absorption and Metabolism. Colchicine is absorbed on oral administration, with peak plasma levels being attained within 0.5 to 2 hours after dosing. Plasma protein binding is only 31%. It concentrates primarily in the GI tract, liver, kidney, and spleen, and is excreted primarily in the feces, with only 20% of an oral dose being excreted in the urine.

It is retained in the body for considerable periods of time, being detected in the urine and leukocytes for 9 to 10 days following a single dose. This is partially attributed to colchicine being recycled in the bile through enterohepatic circulation. Metabolism occurs in the liver via demethylation by CYP3A4, with the major metabolites being 2-O-demethylcolchicine and 3-O-demethylcolchine.

Adverse Effects. Colchicine can produce bone marrow depression, with long-term therapy resulting in thrombocytopenia or aplastic anemia. At maximum dose levels, GI disturbances (eg, nausea, diarrhea, and abdominal pain) can occur. Acute toxicity is characterized by GI distress, including severe diarrhea resulting in excessive fluid loss, respiratory depression, and kidney damage. Treatment normally involves measures that prevent shock, as well as morphine and atropine administration to diminish abdominal pain. A number of drug interactions have been reported. In general, the actions of colchicine are potentiated by alkalinizing substances and inhibited by acidifying agents, consistent with its mechanism of action of increasing the pH of synovial fluid. Responses to CNS depressants and to sympathomimetic drugs appear to be enhanced. Clinical tests can be affected; most notably, elevated alkaline phosphatase and serum glutamate oxaloacetate transaminase values, and decreased thrombocyte values. Because colchicine is a P-glycoprotein (P-gp) and CYP3A4 substrate, life-threatening drug interactions have been reported as a result of significant increases in colchicine plasma levels in patients treated with P-gp and strong CYP3A4 inhibitors.

Treatment of Chronic Gout

Drugs That Increase Uric Acid Secretion

Probenecid. Probenecid is insoluble in water and acidic solutions, but is soluble in alkaline solutions buffered to pH 7.4. Probenecid promotes the excretion of uric acid by inhibiting the URAT1 transporter, which decreases the reabsorption of uric acid in the proximal tubules and promoting its excretion. With the increase in uric acid excretion, blood concentrations decrease, leading urate depositions to decrease due to enhanced solubilization. Probenecid is an N-dialkylsulfamoyl benzoate, and increased uric acid excretion occurs with smaller N-alkyl substituents.

Probenecid is essentially completely absorbed from the GI tract on oral administration, with peak plasma levels observed within 2 to 4 hours. Like most acidic compounds that are highly ionized at physiologic pH, probenecid ($pK_a = 3.4$) is extensively plasma protein bound (93%-99%). It is extensively metabolized, with only 5% to 10% excreted unchanged. The metabolic reactions of probenecid are shown in Figure 17.32. The primary phase 1 metabolites result from N-dealkylation and ω-oxidation of the *n*-propyl side chain, followed by subsequent oxidation of the resulting primary alcohol to the carboxylic acid via sequential alcohol dehydrogenase and aldehyde dehydrogenase enzymatic reactions. Phase 2 reactions include glycine conjugation with the carboxylic acids. All metabolites retain uricosuric activity. The primary route of elimination of probenecid and its metabolites is the urine.

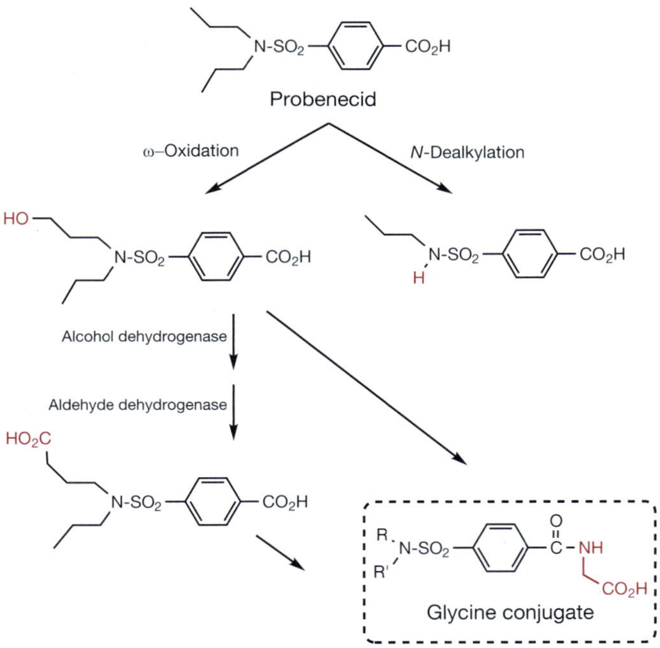

Figure 17.32 Metabolism of probenecid.

Probenecid is well tolerated with few adverse reactions. The primary side effects are mild GI irritation and hypersensitivity reactions. Despite the high degree of plasma protein binding, displacement interactions with other drugs bound to plasma proteins do not appear to occur to any significant extent, although other drug interactions have been reported. For example, salicylates can block the uricosuric effects of probenecid. Probenecid can block the tubular secretion of penicillin, aminosalicylic acid, methotrexate, sulfonamides, dapsone, sulfonylureas, naproxen, indomethacin, rifampin, and sulfinpyrazone, yielding higher plasma concentrations for these drugs.

Drugs That Decrease Uric Acid Formation

Allopurinol (Zyloprim, Lopurin)

Mechanism of Action. Allopurinol is effective for chronic gout and acts through inhibition of the uric acid biosynthetic pathway. Specifically, allopurinol is a xanthine mimic and a competitive inhibitor of xanthine oxidase. It is a purine analogue where the pyrimidine ring is fused to a pyrazole ring instead of imidazole, and the 6-position has been oxidized. Allopurinol has an affinity for xanthine oxidase that is 15 to 20 times higher than that of the endogenous substrate xanthine. Therefore, when allopurinol is administered, xanthine and hypoxanthine are elevated in the urine, and uric acid levels decrease. When this happens, plasma urate monoanion concentrations decrease and urate crystal deposits dissolve, eliminating the primary cause of gout.

Absorption and Metabolism. Allopurinol is well absorbed on oral administration, with peak plasma concentrations appearing within 1 hour. Decreases in uric acid plasma levels can be observed within 24 to 48 hours. Allopurinol is metabolized via C2 oxidation (Fig. 17.33). The major oxidative metabolite, alloxanthine or oxypurinol, has a much longer half-life than the parent drug (18-30 vs 2-3 hours) and

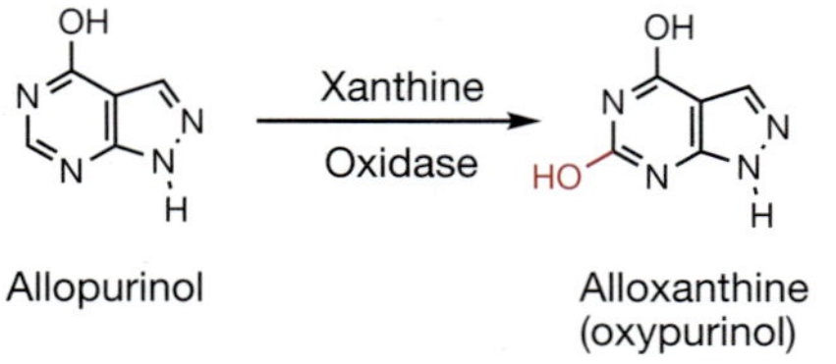

Figure 17.33 Metabolism of allopurinol.

is also an inhibitor of xanthine oxidase. Thus, the extended plasma half-life of alloxanthine leads to once-a-day dosing. Allopurinol and alloxanthine are not bound to plasma proteins. Their excretion occurs primarily in the urine, with approximately 20% of a dose being excreted in the feces.

Adverse Effects. The primary adverse effects of allopurinol are GI distress (nausea, vomiting, and diarrhea) and dermatologic allergic reactions (typically skin rash). Luckily, these symptoms tend to disappear when the medication is discontinued. Allopurinol can also initiate attacks of acute gouty arthritis during the early stages of therapy due to the release of tissue uric acid, requiring the concomitant administration of colchicine and an NSAID. Drug interactions can occur with xanthine oxidase competitors, some of which are therapeutically beneficial. For example, the oxidation of 6-mercaptopurine, an antineoplastic agent used to treat acute lymphoblastic anemia, is inhibited, permitting a reduction in the therapeutic dose of the toxic anticancer agent. Allopurinol also has an inhibitory effect on hepatic microsomal enzymes and can prolong the half-lives of vulnerable drugs that normally are metabolized and inactivated by these enzymes. As might be anticipated, this effect is quite variable. The incidence of ampicillin-related skin rashes increases with the concurrent administration of allopurinol.

Allopurinol is indicated for the treatment of primary and secondary gout and for the treatment of patients with recurrent calcium oxalate calculi. Recently, a fixed combination of lesinurad and allopurinol (Duzallo) has been approved for the treatment of hyperuricemia in gout patients.

FEBUXOSTAT (ULORIC). Febuxostat is the first nonpurine selective inhibitor of xanthine oxidase. It is indicated for the chronic management of hyperuricemia in patients with gout and for patients who cannot tolerate allopurinol. Febuxostat is a noncompetitive inhibitor of both the oxidized and reduced forms of xanthine oxidase, thereby inhibiting the oxidation of the endogenous substrates hypoxanthine and xanthine.[144,145] Therefore, similar to allopurinol, plasma uric acid levels are attenuated. Since febuxostat is a nonpurine analogue, it does not inhibit enzymes involved in purine (or pyrimidine) metabolism, resulting in fewer adverse events compared to allopurinol.

Absorption and Metabolism. Febuxostat is well absorbed on oral administration, with peak plasma concentrations appearing within 1.5 hours and a half-life of 5 to 8 hours. Phase 1 oxidative metabolism of febuxostat is primarily mediated by CYP1A1, generating the O-dealkylated and ω-1 hydroxy products (Fig. 17.34).[146] CYP2C9 is responsible for oxidation of the ω carbon of the isobutyl group. Phase 2 metabolic reactions are catalyzed by glucuronosyltransferase enzymes, including UGT1A1, UGT1A3, UGT1A9, and UGT2B7, forming the glucuronide ester through either carboxylic acid.[146,147] Excretion of febuxostat, as various metabolites and their conjugates, occurs primarily in the urine (49%) and feces (45%). From an administered dose, only 3% and 12% are recovered as unchanged drug in the urine and feces, respectively.

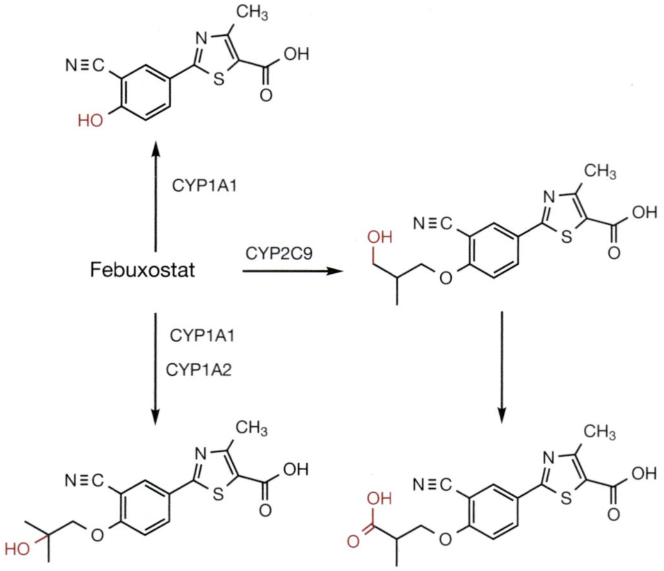

Figure 17.34 Metabolism of febuxostat.

Adverse Effects. The major adverse effects of febuxostat include GI distress, liver function abnormalities, and headache. Cardiovascular safety is concurrently monitored, as there is evidence of increased myocardial infarction and stroke.[148] Similar to allopurinol, initial dosing can initiate gout flares and may require the concomitant administration of an NSAID or colchicine. Drug interactions include those drugs that are also metabolized by xanthine oxidase, such as azathioprine, mercaptopurine, and theophylline. A review of the clinical properties of febuxostat as a treatment option for chronic gout has been published.[149]

Drugs Acting by Enhancing the Degradation of Uric Acid

PEGLOTICASE. Pegloticase is indicated for the treatment of chronic gout in patients in whom traditional small-molecule therapy has failed. Pegloticase is a recombinant porcine-like uricase that enhances the elimination of uric acid by converting it to allantoin (see Fig. 17.30). Pegloticase is a uric acid–specific enzyme that consists of recombinant modified mammalian uricase produced by a genetically modified strain of *E. coli* and then covalently joined to monomethoxypoly(ethylene glycol) (mPEG). The cDNA coding for uricase was derived from mammalian sequences, and each uricase subunit is approximately 34 kDa. The average molecular weight of pegloticase (tetrameric enzyme conjugated to mPEG) is approximately 540 kDa.

Adverse Effects. The recommended dose of pegloticase is 8 mg administered IV every 2 weeks. After administration, common adverse effects are GI distress, allergic reaction (sore throat, runny nose, hives), and new gout flares. Prior to beginning the infusion, premedication with antihistamines and corticosteroids is recommended to prevent infusion reactions and possible anaphylaxis, which are thought to result from cytokine release. To counter new gout flares that can occur, NSAIDs and/or colchicine should be started at least 1 week prior to pegloticase therapy.

LOCAL ANESTHETICS

Anesthesia is a medically and chemically induced loss of sensation with or without loss of consciousness. There are generally three accepted forms of anesthetics, including general, sedation, and local. Although various mechanisms of action are attributed to anesthetics, they all produce their action by inhibiting neurons.

Local anesthetic agents are drugs that, when given either topically or administered directly into a localized area, produce a state of local anesthesia by reversibly blocking nerve conductance that transmits the sensations of pain from this localized area to the brain. Conductance occurs when sodium ions (Na+) pass through the pores of Na+ ion channels. Local anesthetics bind to specific sites on the Na+ ion channel and inhibit its function. The anesthesia produced by local anesthetics is without loss of consciousness or impairment of vital central cardiorespiratory functions.

Discovery of Local Anesthetics

As with many drugs in the era of rational drug design, the initial leads for the design of clinically useful local anesthetics originated from natural sources. In 1860, A. Niemann obtained a crystalline alkaloid from coca leaves to which he gave the name cocaine, and who noted the anesthetic effect on the tongue (Fig. 17.35). In 1884, the first successful surgical use of cocaine was performed by C. Koller, and this discovery led to the rapid development of new local anesthetic agents and anesthetic techniques.[150]

Cocaine dependence (or addiction) is psychological dependency on the regular use of cocaine.

Although the structure of cocaine was not known until 1924, many attempts were made to prepare new analogues that lacked its addicting liability and other therapeutic shortcomings, such as allergic reactions, tissue irritations, and poor stability in aqueous solution. For example, cocaine is easily decomposed to hydrolysis products ecgonine and benzoic acid, when the solution is sterilized (Fig. 17.35).

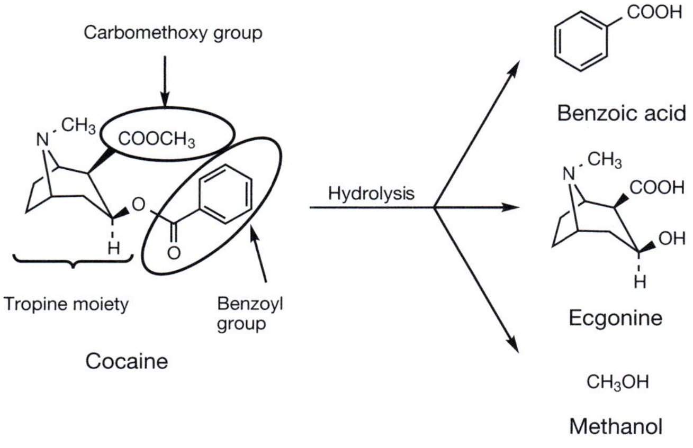

Figure 17.35 Cocaine and its hydrolysis products.

When the chemical structure of ecgonine became known, the preparation of active compounds containing the ecgonine nucleus accelerated. It was soon realized that a variety of benzoyl esters of amino alcohols, including benzoyltropine, exhibited strong local anesthetic properties without any of cocaine's addiction liability. Thus, removal of the methyl ester group at the 2-position from cocaine abolished its addiction liability. This discovery eventually led to the discovery of procaine, which then became the local anesthetic prototype for nearly half a century, due to its lower toxicity.

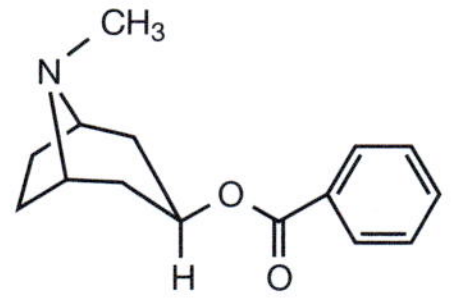

Benzoyltropine

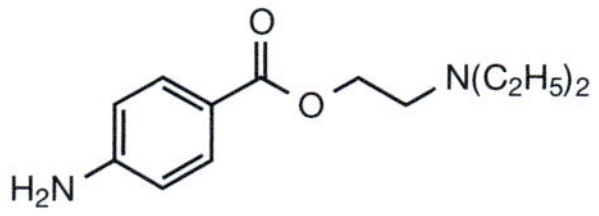

Procaine

Although procaine did enjoy many years of first-line local anesthetic use, it did have some liabilities, including low potency and a short duration. To address these therapeutic shortcomings, tetracaine was discovered and remains the most potent, long-acting, ester-type local anesthetic agent, which is used by injection in spinal anesthesia and also found in some topical combination products.

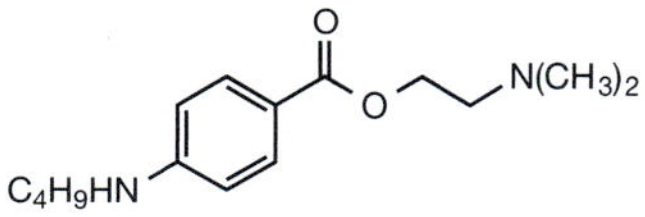

Tetracaine

The serendipitous discovery of the local anesthetic activity of another natural alkaloidal product, isogramine, in 1935 by H. von Euler and H. Erdtman was the next major turning point in the development of clinically useful local anesthetic agents. This observation led to the synthesis of lidocaine (Xylocaine) by N. Löfgren in 1946; lidocaine was the first nonirritating, amide-type local anesthetic agent with good local anesthetic properties, yet less prone to allergenic reactions than procaine analogues, and was found to be stable in aqueous solution due to its amide functionality. Structurally, lidocaine can be viewed as an open-chain bioisosteric analogue of isogramine.

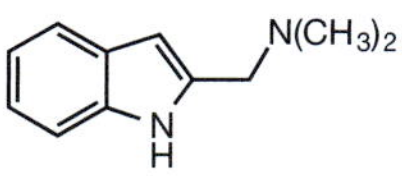

Isogramine

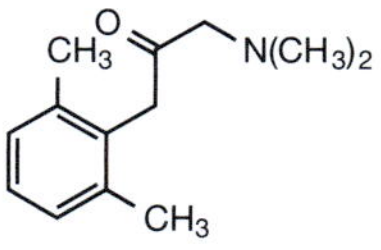

Lidocaine

Characteristics of an Ideal Local Anesthetic

The ideal local anesthetic should produce reversible blockade of sensory neurons, with a minimal effect on the motor neurons. It also should possess a rapid onset, have a sufficient duration of action for the completion of surgical procedures without any systemic toxicity, and be easily sterilized and not inordinately expensive (Table 17.4). There is opportunity for an improved local anesthetic with regard to its selective actions on the Na+ ion channels. Additional leads for the design of ideal local anesthetics could also come from a more systematic metabolic and toxicity study of currently available agents.

Therapeutic Considerations for Using Local Anesthetic Drugs

Since the discovery of cocaine in 1880 as a surgical local anesthetic, several thousand new compounds have been tested and found to produce anesthesia by blocking nerve conductance. Among these agents, approximately 20 are currently clinically available in the United States as local anesthetic preparations (Table 17.5). Figure 17.36 provides the chemical structures of the agents in common use.

Pharmaceutical Preparations

Local anesthetic agents generally are prepared in various dosage forms: aqueous solutions for parenteral injection, and creams and ointments for topical applications. Thus, chemical stability and aqueous solubility become primary factors in the preparations of suitable pharmaceutical dosage forms. Compounds containing an amide linkage are ideal, as they have greater chemical hydrolytic stability than do the esters. In this regard, an aqueous solution of an amino ester–type local anesthetic is more likely to hydrolyze under normal conditions of use and cannot withstand heat sterilization as a result of base-catalyzed hydrolysis of the ester.

Table 17.4 Characteristics of the Ideal Local Anesthetic Agent

Produces a reversible blockade
Selective for sensory neurons with no effect on motor neurons
Rapid onset
Sufficient duration of action
Chemically stable when sterilized
No systemic toxicity
Wide margin of safety
Compatible with other coadministered drugs
Absence of adverse effects
Inexpensive

Table 17.5 Clinically Available Local Anesthetics

Generic Name	Trade Name	Recommended Application
Articaine	Septocaine, Septanest	Parenteral (dental)
Benzocaine	Americaine, Anbesol, Benzodent, Orajel, Oratect, Rid-A-Pain, Hurricaine	Topical
Bupivacaine	Marcaine, Sensorcaine	Parenteral
Chloroprocaine	Nesacaine	Parenteral
Cocaine	Cocaine Topical	Topical
Dibucaine	Nupercainal, Cinchocaine	Topical
Lidocaine	Xylocaine, l-Caine, DermaFlex, Dolocaine, Lidoject, Lignocaine, Octocaine	Parenteral, topical
Mepivacaine	Carbocaine, Polocaine, Isocaine	Parenteral, topical
Prilocaine	Citanest	Parenteral, topical
Procaine	Novocain	Parenteral
Proparacaine	Proxymetacaine	Topical
Ropivacaine	Naropin	Parenteral
Tetracaine	Pontocaine, Amethocaine, Prax	Parenteral, topical

Local anesthetic activity usually increases with increasing lipid solubility, although this is inversely related to water solubility and suitable parenteral dosage forms may not be possible. For this reason, a suitable parenteral dosage form might not be available for these agents because of poor water solubility under acceptable conditions. For example, benzocaine, which contains an anilino amine and is not basic enough for salt formation, is insoluble in water at pH values used in parenteral dosage forms. Protonation of the anilino amine in benzocaine results in a conjugate acid with a pK_a of 2.78, which is far too acidic for use by injection. For this reason, benzocaine is used mostly in creams or ointments to provide topical anesthesia.

The only commonly accepted organic additives to local anesthetics are vasoconstrictors, such as epinephrine and levonordefrin (α-methylnorepinephrine). These compounds

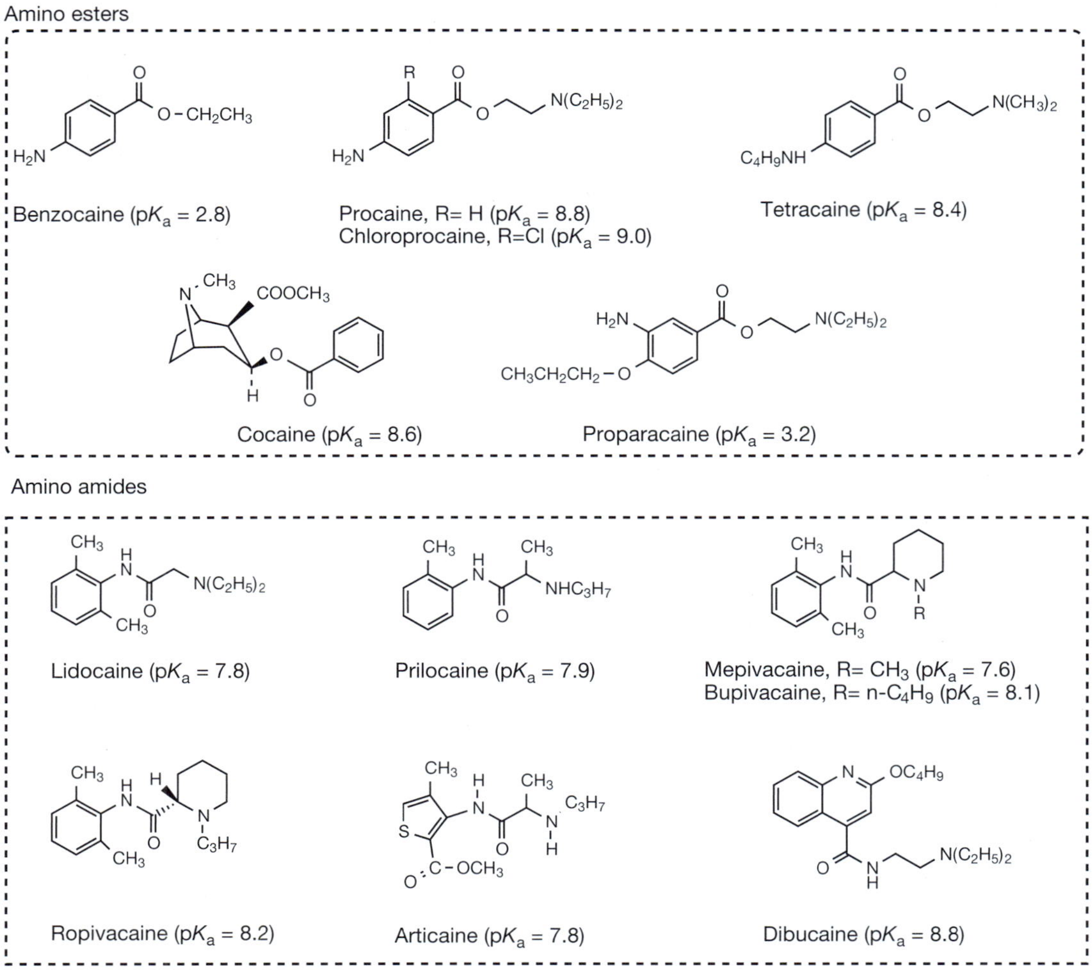

Figure 17.36 Commonly used local anesthetics.

often increase the frequency of successful anesthesia and, to a limited degree, increase the duration of activity by reducing the rate of drug loss from the injection site by constricting arterioles that supply blood to the area of the injection. The effect of these vasoconstrictors is less pronounced if they are injected in an area that has profuse venous drainage, but is remote from an arterial supply.

Administration of a local anesthetic in a carbonic acid–carbon dioxide aqueous solution, rather than the usual solution of a hydrochloride salt, appreciably improves the time to onset and the duration of action without causing increased local or systemic toxicity. Carbon dioxide is believed to potentiate the action of local anesthetics by initial indirect depression of the axon, followed by diffusion trapping of the active form of the local anesthetic within the nerve.

A eutectic mixture of a local anesthetic (EMLA) cream containing 2.5% lidocaine and 2.5% prilocaine (or etidocaine) is used for the topical application through the keratinized layer of the intact skin to provide dermal or epidermal analgesia. This mode of administration allows the use of higher concentrations of local anesthetic with minimal local irritation and lower systemic toxicity. The use of EMLA creams, especially those containing prilocaine, on mucous membranes is not recommended, however, because of the faster absorption of the drugs and, therefore, the increasing risk of systemic toxicity, such as methemoglobinemia.[150]

Toxicity and Adverse Effects

The toxicity of local anesthetics seems to be related to their actions on other excitable membrane proteins, such as in the Na+ and K+ channels in the heart, the nicotinic acetylcholine receptors in the neuromuscular junctions, and the nerve cells in the CNS. In general, neuromuscular junctions and the CNS are more susceptible than the cardiovascular system to the toxic effects of local anesthetics. The actions on skeletal muscles tend to be transient and reversible, whereas the CNS side effects can be more deleterious. The primary effect of the toxicity seems to be convulsions, followed by severe CNS depression, particularly of the respiratory and cardiovascular centers. This can be related to an initial depression of inhibitory neurons, such as GABAergic systems, causing convulsions, followed by depression of other neurons, leading to general depression of the CNS.

The amino amide–type local anesthetics (lidocaine derivatives) are, in general, more likely to produce CNS side effects than the amino ester–type compounds (procaine analogue). However, it should be noted that the toxic effects observed depend heavily on the route and site of administration, as well as on the lipid solubility and metabolic stability of a given local anesthetic molecule. For example, most amide-type local anesthetics are first degraded via N-dealkylation by hepatic enzymes (discussed later). Unlike lidocaine, however, the initial metabolic degradation of prilocaine in humans is hydrolysis of the amide linkage to give *o*-toluidine and N-propylalanine. Formation of *o*-toluidine and its metabolites can cause methemoglobinemia in some patients.[151]

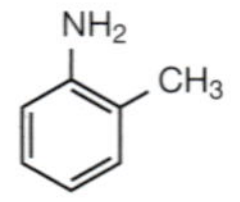

o-Toluidine

Allergic reactions to local anesthetics, although rare, are known to occur exclusively with *p*-aminobenzoic acid (PABA) ester–type local anesthetics.[152] This may be attributed to increased concentrations of PABA, since it is formed upon ester hydrolysis. However, the preservatives, such as methylparaben, used in the preparation of amide-type local anesthetics are metabolized to the PABA analogue *p*-hydroxybenzoic acid. Thus, patients who are allergic to amino ester–type local anesthetics should be treated with a preservative-free amino amide–type local anesthetic.

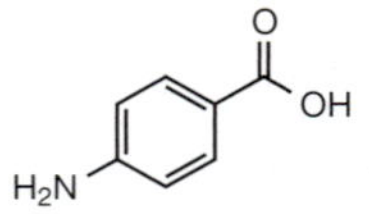

PABA

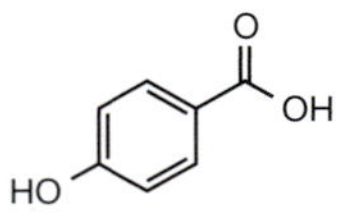

p-Hydroxy benzoic acid

Amide-type local anesthetics (eg, procainamide and lidocaine) also possess antiarrhythmic activity when given parenterally and at subanesthetic doses. Although this action is likely an extension of their effects on Na+ channels in cardiac tissues, some evidence suggests an alternative mechanism of action with respect to the modulation of channel receptors' binding sites for these compounds.[153,154]

Chemical and Pharmacodynamic Aspects of Local Anesthetics

Mechanism of Action

Local anesthetics act by decreasing the excitability of nerve cells without affecting the resting potential. Because the action potential, or the ability of nerve cells to be excited, is associated with the movement of Na+ across the nerve membranes, anything that interferes with the movement of these ions will interfere with cell excitability. For this reason, many hypotheses have been suggested to explain how local anesthetics regulate the changes in Na+ permeability that underlie the nerve impulse. These hypotheses include direct action on ion channels that interfere with ionic fluxes and interaction with phospholipids and calcium that reduces membrane flexibility and responsiveness to changes in electrical fields. The nonspecific membrane actions of local anesthetics can be easily ruled out because most clinically useful agents, in contrast to general anesthetics, possess a defined SAR. At much higher drug concentrations, local anesthetics also bind and block K+ channels.

Structure-Activity Relationships

Figure 17.36 shows the two major classes of marketed local anesthetics: amino esters (procaine analogues) and amino amides (lidocaine analogues). Most of the clinically useful local anesthetics are basic tertiary amines with pK_a values of 7.0 to 9.0. Thus, under physiologic conditions, both protonated forms (cationic) and the molecular (unionized) forms are available for binding to the channel proteins. The ratio between the protonated [HB+] and the unionized molecules [B] can be easily calculated based on the pH of the medium and the pK_a of the drug molecule by the Henderson-Hasselbalch equation: $pH - pK_a = \log [B]/[HB+]$. The effect of pH changes on the potency of local anesthetics has been extensively investigated.[155]

It is the protonated conjugate [HB+] capable of selective binding to and inhibiting Na+ channels. For this reason, any structural modifications that significantly alter the lipid solubility, pK_a, and rate/extent of metabolic inactivation have a pronounced effect on the ability of a drug molecule to reach or interact with the hypothetical binding sites, thus modifying its local anesthetic properties.

Lipophilic Portion. The lipophilic portion of the molecule is essential for local anesthetic activity. For most of the clinically useful local anesthetics, this portion of the molecule consists of an aromatic group directly attached to either a carbonyl function (the amino ester series) or through an –NH– group (the amino amide series) (Fig. 17.37). Lipophilic aromatic rings incorporated into the amino ester series that have *o*- or *p*- (or both) electron donating groups typically as amino or alkoxy groups increase potency. The aromatic rings incorporated into the amino amide series are routinely

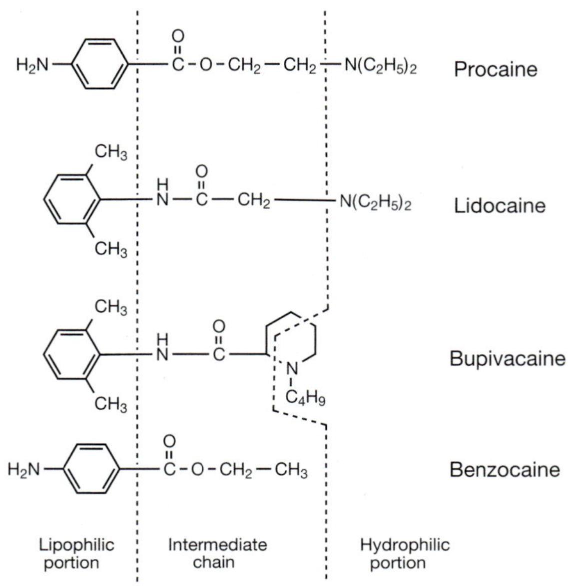

Figure 17.37 Structure-activity relationship comparison of local anesthetics.

disubstituted at the *o*-position with methyl groups but may be monosubstituted. The lipophilic aromatic rings appear to play an important role in the binding of local anesthetics to the channel proteins.

As illustrated in Figure 17.38, resonance is expected to give rise to a zwitterionic resonance hybrid. Neither drawn resonance hybrid of procaine in Figure 17.38 can accurately represent the structure of procaine, as the actual structure is a combination of all resonance hybrids whether protonated or not. This is also true for procaine when it interacts with the local anesthetic binding site; however, the greater the resemblance to the zwitterionic form, the greater the affinity for the binding site. Thus, addition of any aromatic substitution that can enhance the formation of the zwitterionic form through electron donation will produce more potent local anesthetic agents. Electron-withdrawing groups, such as nitro ($-NO_2$), hinder the formation of the zwitterion and, thus, reduce the local anesthetic activity.

Insertion of a methylene group between the aromatic moiety and the carbonyl function, as shown below in the procaine analogue, blocks extended electron delocalization and prohibits the formation of the zwitterionic form with a resonance hybrid where the negative charge localizes on the carbonyl oxygen. Therefore, this procaine analogue has greatly reduced anesthetic potency. When an amino or an alkoxy group is attached to the *m*-position of the aromatic ring, no resonance delocalization of their electrons can localize at the carbonyl oxygen. The addition of this function only increases (alkoxy group) or decreases (amino group) the lipophilicity of the molecule, where increased lipophilicity increases potency.

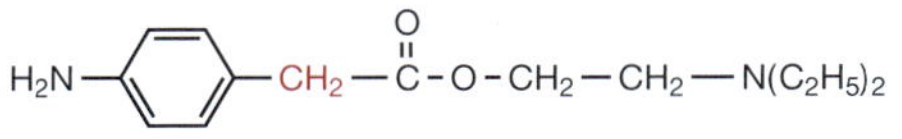

Procaine analogue

Tetracaine is approximately 50-fold more potent than procaine. Experimentally, this increase in potency cannot be correlated solely with the 2,500-fold increase of lipid solubility by the *n*-butyl group (Log $D_{pH\ 7.4} = 2.73$ vs procaine Log $D_{pH\ 7.4} = -0.32$). Perhaps part of this activity potentiation can be attributed to the electron-releasing property of the *n*-butyl group via the positive inductive effect, which indirectly enhances the electron density of the *p*-amino group. This, in turn, increases electron donation through resonance to the carbonyl oxygen, promoting the formation of zwitterion for optimal interaction with the binding site proteins.

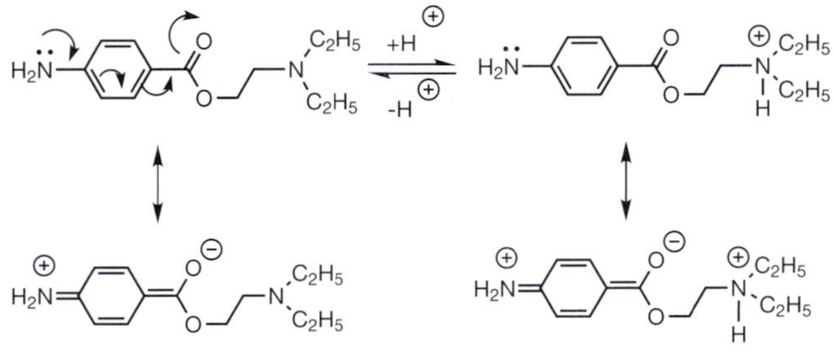

Figure 17.38 Resonance hybrid structures of procaine.

In the amino amides (lidocaine analogues), the *o,o*-dimethyl groups offer steric and electronic (positive induction) protection from amide hydrolysis, increasing duration of action. The shorter duration of action, however, observed with chloroprocaine when compared with that of procaine can be explained by the negative inductive effect of the *o*-chloro group, which pulls the electron density away from the carbonyl function, thus making it more susceptible to nucleophilic attack by the plasma esterases.

Intermediate Chain. The intermediate chain almost always contains a short alkyl segment of one to three carbons linked to the aromatic ring via several possible functional groups. The nature of this intermediate chain determines the chemical stability of the drug, which directly influences the duration of action and relative toxicity. In general, amino amides are more resistant to metabolic hydrolysis than the amino esters and, thus, have a longer duration of action. The placement of small alkyl groups (ie, branching), especially around the ester function or the amide function, also hinders esterase- or amidase-catalyzed hydrolysis, prolonging the duration of action. It should be mentioned, however, that prolonging the duration of action of a compound usually increases its systemic toxicities unless it is more selective toward the voltage-gated Na+ channel, as in the case of the levorotatory isomer of bupivacaine (levobupivacaine).[156,157]

Hydrophilic Portion. Most clinically useful local anesthetics have a tertiary alkylamine, which readily forms water-soluble salts with organic and inorganic acids, and this portion is commonly considered to be the hydrophilic portion of the molecule (Fig. 17.37). The necessity of this portion of the molecule for amino ester–type local anesthetics remains a matter of debate. The strongest opposition for requiring a basic amino group for local anesthetic action comes from the observation that benzocaine, which lacks the basic aliphatic amine function, has potent local anesthetic activity. For this reason, it is often suggested that the tertiary amine function in procaine analogues is needed only for the formation of water-soluble salts suitable for pharmaceutical preparations. With the understanding of the voltage-activated Na+ channel, it is logical that the cations produced by protonation of the tertiary amine group are also required for binding in the voltage-gated Na+ channels.

The hydrophilic group in most of the clinically useful drugs can be in the form of a secondary or tertiary alkylamine or part of a nitrogen heterocycle (see Fig. 17.37). As mentioned, most of the clinically useful local anesthetics have pK_a values of 7.0 to 9.0. The effects of an alkyl substituent on the pK_a depend on the size, length, and hydrophobicity of the group; and thus, it is difficult to see a clear SAR among these structures. It is generally accepted that local anesthetics with higher lipid solubility and lower pK_a values appear to exhibit more rapid onset of action through more effective tissue penetration and lower toxicity.

Stereochemistry

A number of clinically used local anesthetics contain a chiral center (ie, bupivacaine, mepivacaine, and prilocaine); however, the effect of optically pure isomers on isolated nerve preparations revealed a lack of stereospecificity. In a few cases (eg, prilocaine, bupivacaine), however, small differences in the total pharmacologic profile of optical isomers have been noted when administered in vivo.[158-160]

The stereochemistry of the local anesthetics, however, plays an important role in their observed toxicity and pharmacokinetic properties. For example, ropivacaine, the only optically active local anesthetic currently being marketed, has considerably lower cardiac toxicities than its closest structural analogue, bupivacaine.[161] Since ropivacaine is marketed as the pure *S*-(−) isomer, the observed cardiac toxicity of racemic bupivacaine has been attributed to the *R*-(+)-bupivacaine enantiomer.[158-160] Furthermore, the degree of separation between motor and sensory blockade is more apparent with ropivacaine relative to bupivacaine at a lower end of the dosage scale.[162]

Metabolism of Local Anesthetics

The amino ester–type local anesthetics are rapidly hydrolyzed by plasma esterase, which is widely distributed in body tissues. Compounds that either inhibit or compete with local anesthetics for access to esterase will prolong local anesthetic activity and/or toxicity. Another potential drug interaction with clinical significance is between benzocaine and sulfonamides because benzocaine is hydrolyzed to PABA, which can antagonize the antibacterial activity of sulfonamides.

The amino amide–type local anesthetics, however, are metabolized primarily in the liver, involving CYP1A2 isozymes.[163] A general metabolic scheme for lidocaine is shown in Figure 17.39.

Lidocaine is N-dealkylated via CYP1A2 to the monoethylglycinexylidide metabolite. This reaction occurs again, leading to the primary amine (glycinexylidide). In addition, the monoethylglycinexylidide can also undergo amide hydrolysis, forming 2,6-xylidine. The metabolite 2,6-xylidine can then undergo aromatic or benzylic oxidation ending with either phenol- or carboxylic acid–based metabolites. These are then susceptible to phase 2 metabolic conjugation reactions. Although the exact mechanism for the CNS toxicity of lidocaine remains unclear, the metabolic studies of lidocaine provide some insight for future studies. Of all the metabolites of lidocaine, only monoethylglycinexylidide (and not glycinexylidide) contributes to some of the CNS side effects of lidocaine.

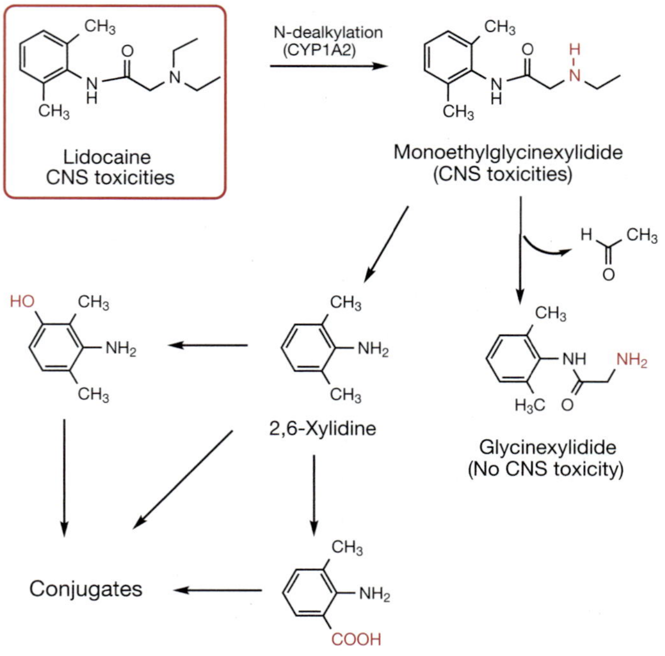

Figure 17.39 Metabolic scheme for lidocaine.

Common Agents Used for Local Anesthesia

Local anesthetics are widely used in many primary care settings. Techniques for their administration in these settings include topical application, local infiltration, field block, and peripheral nerve block. Their use can be maximized by an understanding of their potencies, durations of action, routes of administration, and pharmacokinetic and side effect profiles. The generic name, trade name, and recommended application are given in Table 17.5, and the chemical structures of these agents can be found in Figure 17.36.

Articaine

Articaine has been widely used in dentistry due to its quick onset and short duration of action. The structure differs from the structures of all other amino amide–type local anesthetics in that it contains a thiophene ring instead of a benzene ring and a unique methyl ester group. Both of these groups make articaine more lipophilic and, thus, makes it easier to cross membranes to reach sodium channel binding sites.

Articaine's local anesthetic potency is approximately 1.5-fold that of lidocaine, which can primarily be attributed to the increase in lipophilicity and plasma protein binding (76%) properties. The carbomethoxy ester is hydrolyzed primarily by plasma esterases and, therefore, articaine has a much shorter duration of action than lidocaine (ie, only approximately one-fourth that of lidocaine). The hydrolysis product, articainic acid, is eliminated either unchanged (75%) or as its glucuronides (25%). Compared with other short-acting, amino amide–type local anesthetics, such as mepivacaine, lidocaine, or prilocaine, articaine is said to be a much safer drug for regional anesthesia.[164,165]

Articaine hydrolysis

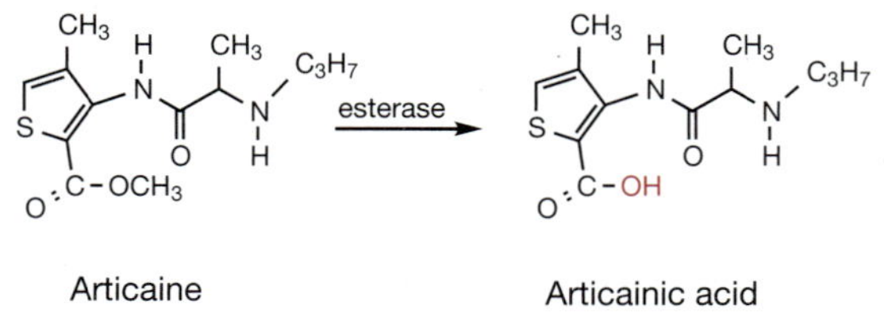

Benzocaine

Benzocaine is used topically alone or in combination with menthol or phenol in nonprescription dosage forms such as gels, creams, ointments, lotions, aerosols, and lozenges to relieve pain or irritation caused by such conditions as sunburn, insect bites, toothache, teething, cold sores or canker sores in or around the mouth, and fever blisters. Benzocaine is a lipophilic local anesthetic agent with a short duration of action.

Like most amino ester–type local anesthetics, it is easily hydrolyzed by plasma esterase. Benzocaine has a low pK_a and is primarily unionized at physiological pH. Therefore, when administered topically to abraded skin, it can easily cross membranes into the systemic circulation to cause systemic toxicities. Furthermore, being a PABA derivative, it has similar allergenic properties to procaine and is contraindicated with sulfonamide antibacterial agents.

Bupivacaine

Bupivacaine hydrochloride is a racemic mixture of the *S*-(−)- and *R*-(+)-enantiomers. Bupivacaine has higher lipid solubility ($\log D_{pH\ 7.4} = 2.54$) and a much decreased rate of hepatic degradation compared with lidocaine, leading to an extended duration of action. For this reason, bupivacaine has significantly greater tendency than lidocaine to produce cardiotoxicity. Because of its greater affinity for voltage-gated Na+ channels, the *R*-(+)-enantiomer confers greater cardiotoxicity than racemic bupivacaine.

Possible pathways for metabolism of bupivacaine include CYP1A2 aromatic 3-hydroxylation, CYP3A4 N-dealkylation, and to a minor extent, the amide hydrolysis (Fig. 17.40). Only the N-dealkylated product, however, has been identified in the urine after epidural or spinal anesthesia.

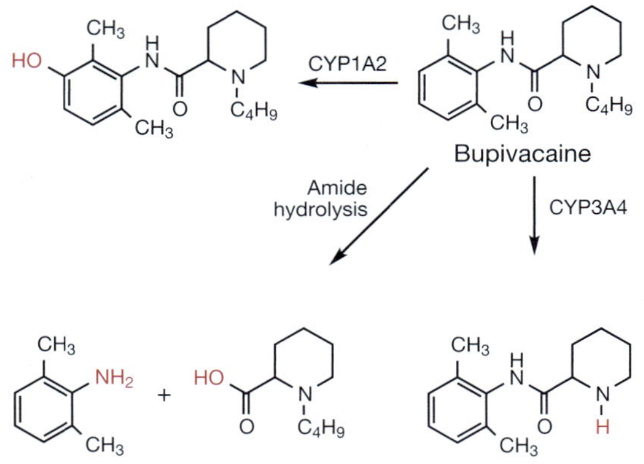

Figure 17.40 Metabolism of bupivacaine.

Chloroprocaine

Chloroprocaine is a very short-acting, amino ester–type local anesthetic used to provide regional anesthesia by infiltration as well as by peripheral and central nerve block, including lumbar and caudal epidural blocks.[166,167] The presence of a chlorine atom ortho to the carbonyl of the ester function increases its lipophilicity. Its rate of hydrolysis by plasma esterase is at least 3-fold that of procaine and benzocaine due to an enhancement of the electrophilic character of the carbonyl carbon. Like PABA, the hydrolysis product of chloroprocaine is 4-amino-2-chlorobenzoic acid, which also inhibits the action of sulfonamides. Therefore, its use with sulfonamides should be avoided.

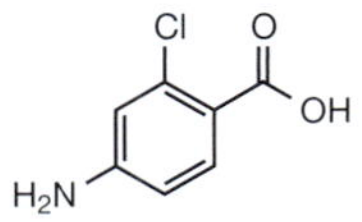
4-Amino-2-chlorobenzoic acid

Lidocaine

Lidocaine is the most commonly used amino amide–type local anesthetic. Lidocaine is very lipid soluble ($\log D_{pH\ 7.4} = 2.26$) and, thus, has a more rapid onset and a longer duration of action than most amino ester–type local anesthetics, such as procaine and tetracaine. It can be administered parenterally (with or without epinephrine) or topically either alone or in combination with prilocaine as a eutectic mixture that is very popular with pediatric patients.

Adverse effects of the CNS are the most frequently observed systemic toxicities of lidocaine. The initial manifestations are restlessness, vertigo, tinnitus, and slurred speech. Eventually, seizures, followed by CNS depression with a cessation of convulsions and the onset of unconsciousness and respiratory depression or cardiac arrest, can occur. This biphasic effect occurs because local anesthetics initially block the inhibitory GABAergic pathways, resulting in stimulation, and eventually block both inhibitory and excitatory pathways (ie, block the Na+ channels associated with the NMDA receptors, resulting in overall CNS inhibition).[168]

Lidocaine is extensively metabolized in the liver by CYP3A4 N-dealkylation and aromatic hydroxylation catalyzed by CYP1A2 (see Fig. 17.39). Lidocaine also possesses a weak inhibitory activity toward the CYP1A2 isozymes and, therefore, can interfere with metabolism of other medications.[169]

Mepivacaine

Mepivacaine hydrochloride is an amino amide–type local anesthetic agent widely used to provide regional analgesia and anesthesia by local infiltration, peripheral nerve block, and epidural and caudal blocks. The pharmacologic and toxicologic profile of mepivacaine is quite similar to that of lidocaine, except that mepivacaine is less lipophilic ($\log D_{pH\ 7.4} = 1.95$), has a slightly longer duration of action, and lacks the vasodilator activity of lidocaine. For this reason, it serves as an alternate choice for lidocaine when addition of epinephrine is not recommended (eg, in patients with hypertensive vascular disease).

Mepivacaine undergoes extensive hepatic metabolism similar to bupivacaine. Phase 1 metabolism of mepivacaine is catalyzed by CYP3A4 and CYP1A2, with only a small percentage of the administered dosage (<10%) being excreted unchanged in the urine. The major metabolic biotransformations of mepivacaine are N-dealkylation (to give the N-demethylated compound 2′,6′-pipecoloxylidide) and aromatic hydroxylations. These metabolites are excreted as their corresponding glucuronides.

Ropivacaine

S(−)-Ropivacaine hydrochloride is the first optically active, amino amide–type local anesthetic marketed. It combines the anesthetic potency and long duration of action of racemic bupivacaine with a side effect profile intermediate

Structure Challenge

NSAID and gout structure challenge. Evaluate the NSAID/gout structures drawn below and answer the questions.

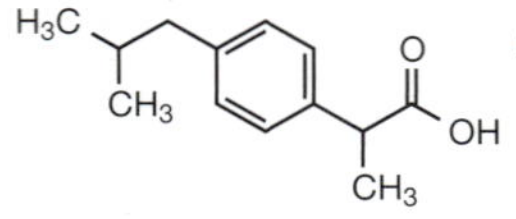

A.

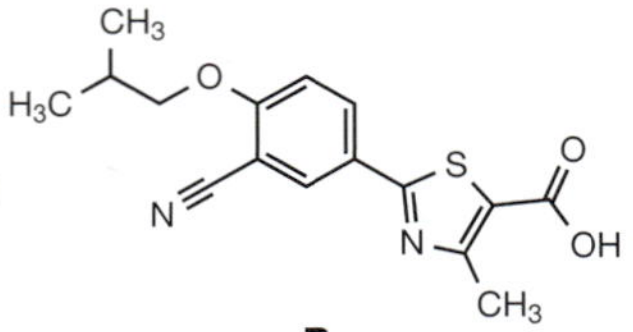

B.

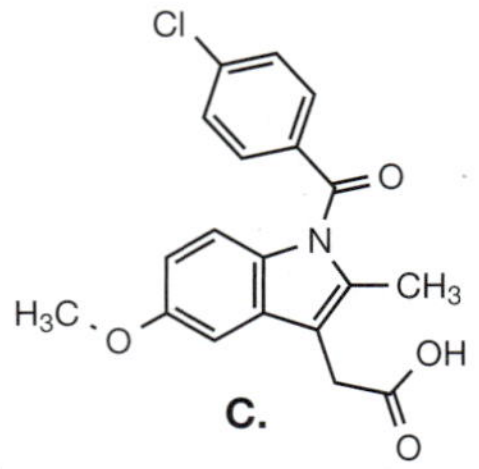

C.

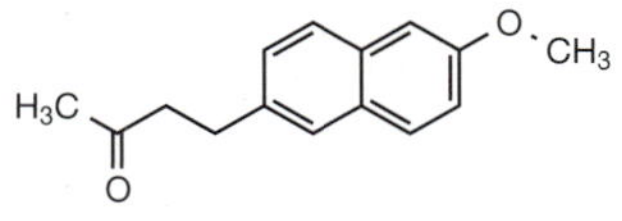

D.

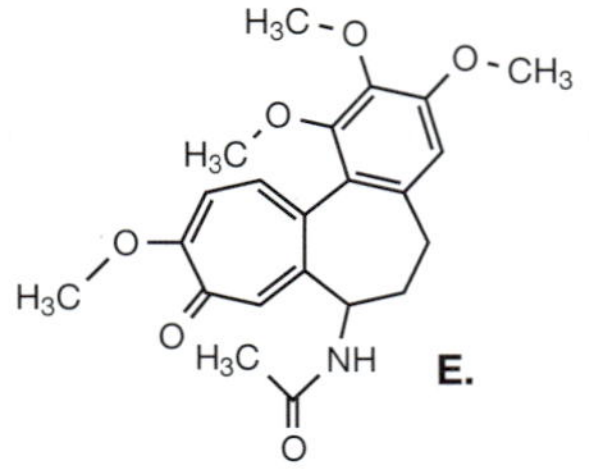

E.

1. Which of the structures is the first nonpurine medication for gout?
2. Which of the structures for peripheral pain possess acidic functional groups, including those structures that are prodrugs?
3. Which of the structures is a natural product and what is the primary indication?
4. Which of the structures would you expect to be the NSAID with the lowest incidence of GI disturbance and stomach irritation as a side effect?

Structure Challenge answers found immediately after References.

between those of bupivacaine and lidocaine. Although ropivacaine has a pK_a nearly identical to that of bupivacaine, it is 2- to 3-fold less lipid soluble and has a smaller volume of distribution, a greater clearance, and a shorter elimination half-life than bupivacaine in humans.

The metabolism of ropivacaine in humans is mediated by hepatic CYP1A2 and, to a minor extent, by CYP3A4.[169] The major metabolite is 3-hydroxyropivacaine, and the minor metabolite is *S*-2′,6′-pipecoloxylidide (an N-dealkylated product).

ACKNOWLEDGMENTS

The authors wish to acknowledge the work of the late Ronald Borne, PhD, Mark Levi, PhD, Timothy J. Maher, PhD, Norman Wilson, PhD, and E. Jeffrey North, PhD who authored a significant component of the content used within this chapter in previous editions of this text.

REFERENCES

1. Hamor GH. Non-steroidal anti-inflammatory drugs. In: Foye WO, ed. *Principles of Medicinal Chemistry*. 3rd ed. Lea & Febiger; 1989:503-530.
2. Gund P, Shen TY. A model for the prostaglandin synthetase cyclooxygenation site and its inhibition by antiinflammatory arylacetic acids. *J Med Chem*. 1977;20(9):1146-1152.
3. von Euler US. On the specific vaso-dilating and plain muscle stimulating substances from accessory genital glands in man and certain animals (prostaglandin and vesiglandin). *J Physiol*. 1936;88(2):213-234.
4. Miyamoto T, Ogino N, Yamamoto S, Hayaishi O. Purification of prostaglandin endoperoxide synthetase from bovine vesicular gland microsomes. *J Biol Chem*. 1976;251(9):2629-2636.
5. Hla T, Neilson K. Human cyclooxygenase-2 cDNA. *Proc Natl Acad Sci U S A*. 1992;89(16):7384-7388.
6. Jones DA, Carlton DP, McIntyre TM, Zimmerman GA, Prescott SM. Molecular cloning of human prostaglandin endoperoxide synthase type II and demonstration of expression in response to cytokines. *J Biol Chem*. 1993;268(12):9049-9054.
7. Kennedy BP, Chan CC, Culp SA, Cromlish WA. Cloning and expression of rat prostaglandin endoperoxide synthase (cyclooxygenase)-2 cDNA. *Biochem Biophys Res Commun*. 1993;197(2):494-500.
8. Kujubu DA, Fletcher BS, Varnum BC, Lim RW, Herschman HR. TIS10, a phorbol ester tumor promoter-inducible mRNA from Swiss 3T3 cells, encodes a novel prostaglandin synthase/cyclooxygenase homologue. *J Biol Chem*. 1991;266(20):12866-12872.
9. Xie WL, Chipman JG, Robertson DL, Erikson RL, Simmons DL. Expression of a mitogen-responsive gene encoding prostaglandin synthase is regulated by mRNA splicing. *Proc Natl Acad Sci U S A*. 1991;88(7):2692-2696.
10. Chandrasekharan NV, Dai H, Roos KL, et al. COX-3, a cyclooxygenase-1 variant inhibited by acetaminophen and other analgesic/antipyretic drugs: cloning, structure, and expression. *Proc Natl Acad Sci U S A*. 2002;99(21):13926-13931.
11. Blobaum AL, Marnett LJ. Structural and functional basis of cyclooxygenase inhibition. *J Med Chem*. 2007;50(7):1425-1441.
12. Flower RJ. The development of COX2 inhibitors. *Nat Rev Drug Discov*. 2003;2:179-191.

13. Roche VF. A receptor-grounded approach to teaching nonsteroidal antiinflammatory drug chemistry and structure-activity relationships. *Am J Pharm Educ.* 2009;73(8):143.
14. Chang HW, Jahng Y. Selective cyclooxygenase-2 inhibitors as anti-inflammatory agents. *Eur J Med Chem.* 1998;8:48-79.
15. Vane JR, Bakhle YS, Botting YM. Cyclooxygenases 1 and 2. *Annu Rev Pharmacol Toxicol.* 1998;38:97–120.
16. Botting JH. Nonsteroidal anti-inflammatory agents. *Drugs Today.* 1999;35:225-235.
17. Hata AN, Breyer RM. Pharmacology and signaling of prostaglandin receptors: multiple roles in inflammation and immune modulation. *Pharmacol Ther.* 2004;103(2):147-166.
18. Okazaki T, Sagawa N, Okita JR, Bleasdale JE, MacDonald PC, Johnston JM. Diacylglycerol metabolism and arachidonic acid release in human fetal membranes and decidua vera. *J Biol Chem.* 1981;256(14):7316-7321.
19. Rubin P, Mollison KW. Pharmacotherapy of diseases mediated by 5-lipoxygenase pathway eicosanoids. *Prostaglandins Other Lipid Mediat.* 2007;83(3):188-197.
20. Clark WG. Mechanisms of antipyretic action. *Gen Pharmacol.* 1979;10(2):71-77.
21. Aronoff DM, Neilson EG. Antipyretics: mechanisms of action and clinical use in fever suppression. *Am J Med.* 2001;111(4):304-315.
22. Graham GC, Scott RF. Mechanism of action of paracetamol. *Am J Ther.* 2005;12:46-55.
23. Forrest JA, Clements JA, Prescott LF. Clinical pharmacokinetics of paracetamol. *Clin Pharmacokinet.* 1982;7(2):93-107.
24. Kunkel DB. *Emergency Medicine.* Geigy Pharmaceuticals; 1985.
25. Mitchell JR, Jollow DJ, Potter WZ, Davis DC, Gillette JR, Brodie BB. Acetaminophen-induced hepatic necrosis. I. Role of drug metabolism. *J Pharmacol Exp Ther.* 1973;187(1):185-194.
26. McGill MR, Jaeschke H. Metabolism and disposition of acetaminophen: recent advances in relation to hepatotoxicity and diagnosis. *Pharm Res.* 2013;30(9):2174-2187.
27. Calder IC, Creek MJ, Williams PJ, et al. N-hydroxylation of p-acetophenetidide as a factor in nephrotoxicity. *J Med Chem.* 1973;16(5):499-502.
28. Yan M, Huo Y, Yin S, Hu H. Mechanisms of acetaminophen-induced liver injury and its implications for therapeutic interventions. *Redox Biol.* 2018;17:274-283.
29. Sinclair J, Jeffery E, Wrighton S, et al. Alcohol-mediated increases in acetaminophen hepatotoxicity: role of CYP2E and CYP3A. *Biochem Pharmacol.* 1998;55(10):1557-1565.
30. Buckpitt AR, Rollins DE, Mitchell JR. Varying effects of sulfhydryl nucleophiles on acetaminophen oxidation and sulfhydryl adduct formation. *Biochem Pharmacol.* 1979;28(19):2941-2946.
31. Atkuri KR, Mantovani JJ, Herzenberg LA, Herzenberg LA. N-Acetylcysteine—a safe antidote for cysteine/glutathione deficiency. *Curr Opin Pharmacol.* 2007;7(4):355-359.
32. Capodanno D, Angiolillo DJ. Aspirin for primary prevention of cardiovascular disease. *Lancet.* 2018;392(10152):988-990.
33. Garcia-Albeniz X, Chan AT. Aspirin for the prevention of colorectal cancer. *Best Pract Res Clin Gastroenterol.* 2011;25(4-5):461-472.
34. Verbeeck RK, Blackburn JL, Loewen GR. Clinical pharmacokinetics of non-steroidal anti-inflammatory drugs. *Clin Pharmacokinet.* 1983;8(4):297-331.
35. Davison C. Salicylate metabolism in man. *Ann N Y Acad Sci.* 1971;179:249-268.
36. Hutt AJ, Caldwell J, Smith RL. The metabolism of aspirin in man: a population study. *Xenobiotica.* 1986;16(3):239-249.
37. Gummin DD, Mowry JB, Spyker DA, et al. 2016 annual report of the American Association of Poison Control Centers' National Poison Data System (NPDS): 34th annual report. *Clin Toxicol (Phila).* 2017;55(10):1072-1252.
38. Chapman J, Arnold JK. *Reye Syndrome.* StatsPearls Publishing; 2018. Accessed December 20, 2018. https://www.ncbi.nlm.nih.gov/books/NBK526101/
39. Ghahramani P, Rowland-Yeo K, Yeo WW, Jackson PR, Ramsay LE. Protein binding of aspirin and salicylate measured by in vivo ultrafiltration. *Clin Pharmacol Ther.* 1998;63(3):285-295.
40. Chan TY. Adverse interactions between warfarin and nonsteroidal antiinflammatory drugs: mechanisms, clinical significance, and avoidance. *Ann Pharmacother.* 1995;29(12):1274-1283.
41. Goulston K, Cooke AR. Alcohol, aspirin, and gastrointestinal bleeding. *Br Med J.* 1968;4(5632):664-665.
42. Jayamani E, Tharmalingam N, Rajamuthiah R, et al. Characterization of a *Francisella tularensis-Caenorhabditis elegans* pathosystem for the evaluation of therapeutic compounds. *Antimicrob Agents Chemother.* 2017;61(9):e00310-17.
43. Verbeeck R, Tjandramaga TB, Mullie A, Verbesselt R, Verberckmoes R, de Schepper PJ. Biotransformation of diflunisal and renal excretion of its glucuronides in renal insufficiency. *Br J Clin Pharmacol.* 1979;7(3):273-282.
44. Sylvia L. The pharmacology of indomethacin. *Headache.* 2016;56(2):436-446.
45. Gan TJ. Diclofenac: an update on its mechanism of action and safety profile. *Curr Med Res Opin.* 2010;26(7):1715-1731.
46. Moser P, Sallmann A, Wiesenberg I. Synthesis and quantitative structure-activity relationships of diclofenac analogues. *J Med Chem.* 1990;33(9):2358-2368.
47. Davies NM, Anderson KE. Clinical pharmacokinetics of diclofenac. Therapeutic insights and pitfalls. *Clin Pharmacokinet.* 1997;33(3):184-213.
48. Chan KK, Vyas KH, Brandt KD. In vitro protein binding of diclofenac sodium in plasma and synovial fluid. *J Pharm Sci.* 1987;76(2):105-108.
49. Tang W. The metabolism of diclofenac—enzymology and toxicology perspectives. *Curr Drug Metab.* 2003;4(4):319-329.
50. Poon GK, Chen Q, Teffera Y, et al. Bioactivation of diclofenac via benzoquinone imine intermediates—identification of urinary mercapturic acid derivatives in rats and humans. *Drug Metab Dispos.* 2001;29(12):1608-1613.
51. Kindla J, Muller F, Mieth M, Fromm MF, König J. Influence of non-steroidal anti-inflammatory drugs on organic anion transporting polypeptide (OATP) 1B1- and OATP1B3-mediated drug transport. *Drug Metab Dispos.* 2011;39(6):1047-1053.
52. Hunter EB, Johnston PE, Tanner G, Pinson CW, Awad JA. Bromfenac (Duract)-associated hepatic failure requiring liver transplantation. *Am J Gastroenterol.* 1999;94(8):2299-2301.
53. Goudie AC, Gaster LM, Lake AW, et al. 4-(6-Methoxy-2-naphthyl) butan-2-one and related analogues, a novel structural class of antiinflammatory compounds. *J Med Chem.* 1978;21(12):1260-1264.
54. Hyneck ML. An overview of the clinical pharmacokinetics of nabumetone. *J Rheumatol Suppl.* 1992;36:20-24.
55. Davies NM. Clinical pharmacokinetics of nabumetone. The dawn of selective cyclo-oxygenase-2 inhibition? *Clin Pharmacokinet.* 1997;33(6):404-416.
56. Arfe A, Scotti L, Varas-Lorenzo C, et al. Non-steroidal anti-inflammatory drugs and risk of heart failure in four European countries: nested case-control study. *BMJ.* 2016;354:i4857.
57. Wen YC, Hsiao FY, Chan KA, Lin ZF, Shen LJ, Fang CC. Acute respiratory infection and use of nonsteroidal anti-inflammatory drugs on risk of acute myocardial infarction: a nationwide case-crossover study. *J Infect Dis.* 2017;215(4):503-509.
58. Bally M, Dendukuri N, Rich B, et al. Risk of acute myocardial infarction with NSAIDs in real world use: Bayesian meta-analysis of individual patient data. *BMJ.* 2017;357:j1909.
59. Goldkind L, Laine L. A systematic review of NSAIDs withdrawn from the market due to hepatotoxicity: lessons learned from the bromfenac experience. *Pharmacoepidemiol Drug Saf.* 2006;15(4):213-220.
60. Davies NM. Clinical pharmacokinetics of ibuprofen. The first 30 years. *Clin Pharmacokinet.* 1998;34(2):101-154.
61. Aarons L, Grennan DM, Siddiqui M. The binding of ibuprofen to plasma proteins. *Eur J Clin Pharmacol.* 1983;25(6):815-818.

62. Bushra R, Aslam N. An overview of clinical pharmacology of ibuprofen. *Oman Med J.* 2010;25(3):155-1661.
63. Kepp DR, Sidelmann UG, Hansen SH. Isolation and characterization of major phase I and II metabolites of ibuprofen. *Pharm Res.* 1997;14(5):676-680.
64. Rudy AC, Knight PM, Brater DC, Hall SD. Stereoselective metabolism of ibuprofen in humans: administration of R-, S- and racemic ibuprofen. *J Pharmacol Exp Ther.* 1991;259(3):1133-1139.
65. Hutt AJ, Caldwell J. The metabolic chiral inversion of 2-arylpropionic acids—a novel route with pharmacological consequences. *J Pharm Pharmacol.* 1983;35(11):693-704.
66. Nash JF, Bechtol LD, Bunde CA, et al. Linear pharmacokinetics of orally administered fenoprofen calcium. *J Pharm Sci.* 1979;68(9):1087-1090.
67. Davies NM, Anderson KE. Clinical pharmacokinetics of naproxen. *Clin Pharmacokinet.* 1997;32(4):268-293.
68. Segre EJ. Naproxen metabolism in man. *J Clin Pharmacol.* 1975;15(4 pt 2):316-323.
69. Miners JO, Coulter S, Tukey RH, Veronese ME, Birkett DJ. Cytochromes P450, 1A2, and 2C9 are responsible for the human hepatic O-demethylation of R- and S-naproxen. *Biochem Pharmacol.* 1996;51(8):1003-1008.
70. Geisslinger G, Lötsch J, Menzel S, Kobal G, Brune K. Stereoselective disposition of flurbiprofen in healthy subjects following administration of the single enantiomers. *Br J Clin Pharmacol.* 1994;37(4):392-394.
71. Scherrer RA. Aryl- and heteroarylcarboxylic acids. In: Scherrer RA, Whitehouse MW, eds. *Anti-inflammatory Agents.* Vol 1. Academic Press; 1974:56-74.
72. Daniels MJD, Rivers-Auty J, Schilling T, et al. Fenamate NSAIDs inhibit the NLRP3 inflammasome and protect against Alzheimer's disease in rodent models. *Nat Commun.* 2016;7:12504.
73. Brannigan LH, Hodge RB, Field L. Biologically oriented organic sulfur chemistry. 14. Antiinflammatory properties of some aryl sulfides, sulfoxides, and sulfones. *J Med Chem.* 1976;19(6):798-802.
74. Diana FJ, Veronich K, Kapoor AL. Binding of nonsteroidal anti-inflammatory agents and their effect on binding of racemic warfarin and its enantiomers to human serum albumin. *J Pharm Sci.* 1989;78(3):195-199.
75. Sato J, Yamane Y, Ito K, et al. Structures of mefenamic acid metabolites from human urine. *Biol Pharm Bull.* 1993;16(8):811-812.
76. Wells PS, Holbrook AM, Crowther NR, Hirsh J. Interactions of warfarin with drugs and food. *Ann Intern Med.* 1994;121(9):676-683.
77. Olkkola KT, Brunetto AV, Mattila MJ. Pharmacokinetics of oxicam nonsteroidal anti-inflammatory agents. *Clin Pharmacokinet.* 1994;26(2):107-120.
78. Verbeeck RK, Richardson CJ, Blocka KL. Clinical pharmacokinetics of piroxicam. *J Rheumatol.* 1986;13(4):789-796.
79. Fleischmann R, Iqbal I, Slobodin G. Meloxicam. *Expert Opin Pharmacother.* 2002;3(10):1501-1512.
80. Turck D, Roth W, Busch U. A review of the clinical pharmacokinetics of meloxicam. *Br J Rheumatol.* 1996;35(suppl 1):13-16.
81. Chesné C, Guyomard C, Guillouzo A, Schmid J, Ludwig E, Sauter T. Metabolism of meloxicam in human liver involves cytochromes P4502C9 and 3A4. *Xenobiotica.* 1998;28(1):1-13.
82. Laine L. The gastrointestinal effects of nonselective NSAIDs and COX-2-selective inhibitors. *Semin Arthritis Rheum.* 2002;32(3 suppl 1):25-32.
83. Zhao X, Xu Z, Li H. NSAIDs use and reduced metastasis in cancer patients: results from a meta-analysis. *Sci Rep.* 2017;7(1):1875.
84. Dai P, Li J, Ma XP, Huang J, Meng JJ, Gong P. Efficacy and safety of COX-2 inhibitors for advanced non-small-cell lung cancer with chemotherapy: a meta-analysis. *OncoTargets Ther.* 2018;11:721-730.
85. Liu B, Qu L, Yan S. Cyclooxygenase-2 promotes tumor growth and suppresses tumor immunity. *Cancer Cell Int.* 2015;15:106.
86. Davies NM, McLachlan AJ, Day RO, Williams KM. Clinical pharmacokinetics and pharmacodynamics of celecoxib: a selective cyclo-oxygenase-2 inhibitor. *Clin Pharmacokinet.* 2000;38(3):225-242.
87. Gong L, Thorn CF, Bertagnolli MM, Grosser T, Altman RB, Klein TE. Celecoxib pathways: pharmacokinetics and pharmacodynamics. *Pharmacogenet Genomics.* 2012;22(4):310-318.
88. Sandberg M, Yasar U, Strömberg P, Höög JO, Eliasson E. Oxidation of celecoxib by polymorphic cytochrome P450 2C9 and alcohol dehydrogenase. *Br J Clin Pharmacol.* 2002;54(4):423-429.
89. Penning TD, Talley JJ, Bertenshaw SR, et al. Synthesis and biological evaluation of the 1,5-diarylpyrazole class of cyclooxygenase-2 inhibitors: identification of 4-[5-(4-methylphenyl)-3-(trifluoromethyl)-1H-pyrazol-1-yl]benze nesulfonamide (SC-58635, celecoxib). *J Med Chem.* 1997;40(9):1347-1365.
90. Demoruelle MK, Deane KD. Treatment strategies in early rheumatoid arthritis and prevention of rheumatoid arthritis. *Curr Rheumatol Rep. 2012*;14(5):472-480.
91. Yuan JQ, Tsoi KK, Yang M, et al. Systematic review with network meta-analysis: comparative effectiveness and safety of strategies for preventing NSAID-associated gastrointestinal toxicity. *Aliment Pharmacol Ther.* 2016;43(12):1262-1275.
92. Zarghi A, Arfaei S. Selective COX-2 inhibitors: a review of their structure-activity relationships. *Iran J Pharm Res.* 2011;10(4):655-683.
93. McEvoy GK. American Hospital Formulary Service Drug Information 2011. Published 2017. Accessed November 2, 2017.
94. Korpela M, Laasonen L, Hannonen P, et al. Retardation of joint damage in patients with early rheumatoid arthritis by initial aggressive treatment with disease-modifying antirheumatic drugs: five-year experience from the FIN-RACo study. *Arthritis Rheum.* 2004;50(7):2072-2081. https://acrjournals.onlinelibrary.wiley.com/doi/epdf/10.1002/art.20351
95. Youn HS, Lee JY, Saitoh SI, Miyake K, Hwang DH. Auranofin, as an anti-rheumatic gold compound, suppresses LPS-induced homodimerization of TLR4. *Biochem Biophys Res Commun.* 2006;350(4):866-871.
96. Yang JP, Merin JP, Nakano T, Kato T, Kitade Y, Okamoto T. Inhibition of the DNA-binding activity of NF-kappa B by gold compounds in vitro. *Febs Lett.* 1995;361(1):89-96.
97. Blocka KL, Paulus HE, Furst DE. Clinical pharmacokinetics of oral and injectable gold compounds. *Clin Pharmacokinet.* 1986;11(2):133-143.
98. Capparelli EV, Bricker-Ford R, Rogers MJ, McKerrow JH, Reed SL. Phase I clinical trial results of auranofin, a novel antiparasitic agent. *Antimicrob Agents Chemother.* 2017;61(1):e01947-16.
99. Brown PM, Pratt AG, Isaacs JD. Mechanism of action of methotrexate in rheumatoid arthritis, and the search for biomarkers. *Nat Rev Rheumatol.* 2016;12(12):731-742.
100. Kremer JM, Galivan J, Streckfuss A, Kamen B. Methotrexate metabolism analysis in blood and liver of rheumatoid arthritis patients. Association with hepatic folate deficiency and formation of polyglutamates. *Arthritis Rheum.* 1986;29(7):832-835.
101. Flanagan ME, Blumenkopf TA, Brissette WH, et al. Discovery of CP-690,550: a potent and selective Janus kinase (JAK) inhibitor for the treatment of autoimmune diseases and organ transplant rejection. *J Med Chem.* 2010;53(24):8468-8484.
102. Palfreeman AC, McNamee KE, McCann FE. New developments in the management of psoriasis and psoriatic arthritis: a focus on apremilast. *Drug Des Devel Ther.* 2013;7:201-210.
103. Wittmann M, Helliwell PS. Phosphodiesterase 4 inhibition in the treatment of psoriasis, psoriatic arthritis and other chronic inflammatory diseases. *Dermatol Ther.* 2013;3(1):1-15.
104. Schafer P. Apremilast mechanism of action and application to psoriasis and psoriatic arthritis. *Biochem Pharmacol.* 2012;83(12):1583-1590.
105. Hoffmann M, Kumar G, Schafer P, et al. Disposition, metabolism and mass balance of [(14)C]apremilast following oral administration. *Xenobiotica.* 2011;41(12):1063-1075.

106. Zane LT, Chanda S, Jarnagin K, Nelson DB, Spelman L, Gold LS. Crisaborole and its potential role in treating atopic dermatitis: overview of early clinical studies. *Immunotherapy*. 2016;8(8):853-866.
107. Moustafa F, Feldman SR. A review of phosphodiesterase-inhibition and the potential role for phosphodiesterase 4-inhibitors in clinical dermatology. *Dermatol Online J*. 2014;20(5):22608.
108. Freund YR, Akama T, Alley MR, et al. Boron-based phosphodiesterase inhibitors show novel binding of boron to PDE4 bimetal center. *Febs Lett*. 2012;586(19):3410-3414.
109. Singh JA, Hossain A, Tanjong Ghogomu E, et al. Biologics or tofacitinib for rheumatoid arthritis in incomplete responders to methotrexate or other traditional disease-modifying antirheumatic drugs: a systematic review and network meta-analysis. *Cochrane Database Syst Rev*. 2016;2016(5):CD012183.
110. Oldfield V, Dhillon S, Plosker GL. Tocilizumab: a review of its use in the management of rheumatoid arthritis. *Drugs*. 2009;69(5):609-632.
111. Shealy DJ, Cai A, Staquet K, et al. Characterization of golimumab, a human monoclonal antibody specific for human tumor necrosis factor alpha. *MAbs*. 2010;2(4):428-439.
112. Gadangi P, Longaker M, Naime D, et al. The anti-inflammatory mechanism of sulfasalazine is related to adenosine release at inflamed sites. *J Immunol*. 1996;156(5):1937-1941.
113. Combe B, Lula S, Boone C, Durez P. Effects of biologic disease-modifying anti-rheumatic drugs on the radiographic progression of rheumatoid arthritis: a systematic literature review. *Clin Exp Rheumatol*. 2018;36(4):658-667.
114. Lamanna WC, Mayer RE, Rupprechter A, et al. The structure-function relationship of disulfide bonds in etanercept. *Sci Rep. 2017*;7(1):3951.
115. Scott LJ. Etanercept: a review of its use in autoimmune inflammatory diseases. *Drugs*. 2014;74(12):1379-1410.
116. Naguwa SM. Tumor necrosis factor inhibitor therapy for rheumatoid arthritis. *Ann N Y Acad Sci*. 2005;1051:709-715.
117. Perdriger A. Infliximab in the treatment of rheumatoid arthritis. *Biologics*. 2009;3:183-191.
118. McCluggage LK, Scholtz JM. Golimumab: a tumor necrosis factor alpha inhibitor for the treatment of rheumatoid arthritis. *Ann Pharmacother*. 2010;44(1):135-144.
119. Kaushik VV, Moots RJ. CDP-870 (certolizumab) in rheumatoid arthritis. *Expert Opin Biol Ther*. 2005;5(4):601-606.
120. King KM, Younes A. Rituximab: review and clinical applications focusing on non-Hodgkin's lymphoma. *Expert Opin Biol Ther*. 2001;1(2):177-186.
121. Schioppo T, Ingegnoli F. Current perspective on rituximab in rheumatic diseases. *Drug Des Devel Ther*. 2017;11:2891-2904.
122. Ferrari P, Bonny O. [Diagnosis and prevention of uric acid stones]. *Ther Umsch*. 2004;61(9):571-574.
123. Malemud CJ. The role of the JAK/STAT signal pathway in rheumatoid arthritis. *Ther Adv Musculoskelet Dis*. 2018;10(5-6):117-127. doi:10.1177/1759720X18776224
124. Morinobu A. JAK inhibitors for the treatment of rheumatoid arthritis. *Immunol Med*. 2020;43(4):148-155. doi:10.1080/25785826.2020.1770948
125. Hu X, Li J, Fu M, Zhao X, Wang W. The JAK/STAT signaling pathway: from bench to clinic. *Signal Transduct Target Ther*. 2021;6(1):402. doi:10.1038/s41392-021-00791-1
126. U.S. Food and Drug Administration. MedWatch: the FDA safety information and adverse event reporting program. Accessed December 1, 2023. www.fda.gov/medwatch
127. Ytterberg SR, Bhatt DL, Mikuls TR, et al. Cardiovascular and cancer risk with tofacitinib in rheumatoid arthritis. *N Engl J Med*. 2022;386(4):316-326. doi:10.1056/NEJMOA2109927
128. Czókolyová M, Hamar A, Pusztai A, et al. Effects of one-year tofacitinib therapy on lipids and adipokines in association with vascular pathophysiology in rheumatoid arthritis. *Biomolecules*. 2022;12(10):1483. doi:10.3390/biom12101483
129. Yan J, Yang S, Han L, et al. Dyslipidemia in rheumatoid arthritis: the possible mechanisms. *Front Immunol*. 2023; 14:1254753. doi:10.3389/fimmu.2023.1254753
130. Myasoedova E, Crowson CS, Kremers HM, et al. Lipid paradox in rheumatoid arthritis: the impact of serum lipid measures and systemic inflammation on the risk of cardiovascular disease. *Ann Rheum Dis*. 2011;70(3):482-487. doi:10.1136/ard.2010.135871
131. Linton MF, Yancey PG, Davies SS, et al. The role of lipids and lipoproteins in atherosclerosis. In: Feingold KR, Anawalt B, Blackman MR, et al, eds. *Endotext* [Internet]. MDText.com, Inc.; 2000.
132. Charles-Schoeman C, Fleischmann R, Davignon J, et al. Potential mechanisms leading to the abnormal lipid profile in patients with rheumatoid arthritis versus healthy volunteers and reversal by tofacitinib. *Arthritis Rheumatol*. 2015;67(3):616-625. doi:10.1002/art.38974
133. Fraenkel L, Bathon JM, England BR, et al. 2021 American College of Rheumatology guideline for the treatment of rheumatoid arthritis. *Arthritis Care Res (Hoboken)*. 2021;73(7):924-939. doi:10.1002/acr.24596
134. Smolen JS, Landewé RBM, Bergstra SA, et al. EULAR recommendations for the management of rheumatoid arthritis with synthetic and biological disease-modifying antirheumatic drugs: 2022 update. *Ann Rheum Dis*. 2023;82(1):3-18. doi:10.1136/ard-2022-223356
135. Riese RJ, Krishnaswami S, Kremer J. Inhibition of JAK kinases in patients with rheumatoid arthritis: scientific rationale and clinical outcomes. *Best Pract Res Clin Rheumatol*. 2010;24(4):513-526.
136. Prakash C, Lin J, Chan G, Boy M. Metabolism, pharmacokinetics and excretion of a Janus kinase-3 inhibitor, CP-690,550, in healthy male volunteers. *AAPS J*. 2008;10:2492.
137. Lawendy N, Krishnaswami S, Wang R, et al. Effect of CP-690,550, an orally active Janus kinase inhibitor, on renal function in healthy adult volunteers. *J Clin Pharmacol*. 2009;49(4):423-429.
138. Shi JG, Chen X, Lee F, et al. The pharmacokinetics, pharmacodynamics, and safety of baricitinib, an oral JAK 1/2 inhibitor, in healthy volunteers. *J Clin Pharmacol*. 2014;54(12):1354-1361.
139. Mohamed MF, Klünder B, Othman AA. Clinical pharmacokinetics of upadacitinib: review of data relevant to the rheumatoid arthritis indication. *Clin Pharmacokinet*. 2020;59(5):531-544. doi:10.1007/s40262-019-00855-0
140. Mohamed MF, Zeng J, Marroum PJ, Song IH, Othman AA. Pharmacokinetics of upadacitinib with the clinical regimens of the extended-release formulation utilized in rheumatoid arthritis phase 3 trials. *Clin Pharmacol Drug Dev*. 2019;8(2):208-216. doi:10.1002/cpdd.462
141. Leung YY, Yao Hui LL, Kraus VB. Colchicine—Update on mechanisms of action and therapeutic uses. *Semin Arthritis Rheum*. 2015;45(3):341-350.
142. Portincasa P. Colchicine, biologic agents and more for the treatment of familial Mediterranean fever. The old, the new, and the rare. *Curr Med Chem*. 2016;23(1):60-86.
143. Bruce SP. Febuxostat: a selective xanthine oxidase inhibitor for the treatment of hyperuricemia and gout. *Ann Pharmacother*. 2006;40(12):2187-2194.
144. Stamp LK, O'Donnell JL, Chapman PT. Emerging therapies in the long-term management of hyperuricaemia and gout. *Intern Med J*. 2007;37(4):258-266.
145. Grabowski BA, Khosravan R, Vernillet L, Mulford DJ. Metabolism and excretion of [14C] febuxostat, a novel nonpurine selective inhibitor of xanthine oxidase, in healthy male subjects. *J Clin Pharmacol*. 2011;51(2):189-201.
146. Mukoyoshi M, Nishimura S, Hoshide S, et al. In vitro drug-drug interaction studies with febuxostat, a novel non-purine selective inhibitor of xanthine oxidase: plasma protein binding, identification of metabolic enzymes and cytochrome P450 inhibition. *Xenobiotica*. 2008;38(5):496-510.
147. White WB, Saag KG, Becker MA, et al. Cardiovascular safety of febuxostat or allopurinol in patients with gout. *N Engl J Med*. 2018;378(13):1200-1210.

148. Frampton JE. Febuxostat: a review of its use in the treatment of hyperuricaemia in patients with gout. *Drugs*. 2015;75(4):427-438.
149. Liljestrand G. The historical development of local anesthesia in local anesthetics. In: Lechat P, ed. *International Encyclopedia of Pharmacology and Therapeutics*. Pergamon Press; 1971:1-38.
150. Arthur GR. Pharmacokinetics of local anesthetics. In: Strichartz GR, ed. *Local Anesthetics Handbook of Experimental Pharmacology*. Vol 81. Springer; 1987:165-186.
151. Eggleston ST, Lush LW. Understanding allergic reactions to local anesthetics. *Ann Pharmacother*. 1996;30(7-8):851-857.
152. Bean BP, Cohen CJ, Tsien RW. Lidocaine block of cardiac sodium channels. *J Gen Physiol*. 1983;81(5):613-642.
153. Makielski JC, Sheets MF, Hanck DA, January CT, Fozzard HA. Sodium current in voltage clamped internally perfused canine cardiac Purkinje cells. *Biophys J*. 1987;52(1):1-11.
154. Narahashi T, Frazier DT. Site of action and active form of local anesthetics. *Neurosci Res*. 1971;4:65-99.
155. Mather LE, Chang DH. Cardiotoxicity with modern local anaesthetics: is there a safer choice? *Drugs*. 2001;61(3):333-342.
156. Rood JP, Coulthard P, Snowdon AT, et al. Safety and efficacy of levobupivacaine for postoperative pain relief after the surgical removal of impacted third molars: a comparison with lignocaine and adrenaline. *Br J Oral Maxillofac Surg*. 2002;40(6):491-496.
157. Rutten AJ, Mather LE, McLean CF. Cardiovascular effects and regional clearances of i.v. bupivacaine in sheep: enantiomeric analysis. *Br J Anaesth*. 1991;67(3):247-256.
158. Denson DD, Behbehani MM, Gregg RV. Enantiomer-specific effects of an intravenously administered arrhythmogenic dose of bupivacaine on neurons of the nucleus tractus solitarius and the cardiovascular system in the anesthetized rat. *Reg Anesth*. 1992;17(6):311-316.
159. Rutten AJ, Mather LE, McLean CF, et al. Tissue distribution of bupivacaine enantiomers in sheep. *Chirality*. 1993;5(7):485-491.
160. McClure JH. Ropivacaine. *Br J Anaesth*. 1996;76(2):300-307.
161. Markham A, Faulds D. Ropivacaine. A review of its pharmacology and therapeutic use in regional anaesthesia. *Drugs*. 1996;52(3):429-449.
162. Imaoka S, Enomoto K, Oda Y, et al. Lidocaine metabolism by human cytochrome P-450s purified from hepatic microsomes: comparison of those with rat hepatic cytochrome P-450s. *J Pharmacol Exp Ther*. 1990;255(3):1385-1391.
163. Shirvani A, Shamszadeh S, Eghbal MJ, et al. Effect of preoperative oral analgesics on pulpal anesthesia in patients with irreversible pulpitis-a systematic review and meta-analysis. *Clin Oral Investig*. 2017;21(1):43-52.
164. Tong HJ, Alzahrani FS, Sim YF, et al. Anaesthetic efficacy of articaine versus lidocaine in children's dentistry: a systematic review and meta-analysis. *Int J Paediatr Dent*. 2018;28(4):347-360.
165. Goldblum E, Atchabahian A. The use of 2-chloroprocaine for spinal anaesthesia. *Acta Anaesthesiol Scand*. 2013;57(5):545-552.
166. Forster JG, Rosenberg PH, Harilainen A, et al. Chloroprocaine 40 mg produces shorter spinal block than articaine 40 mg in day-case knee arthroscopy patients. *Acta Anaesthesiol Scand*. 2013;57(7):911-919.
167. Castañeda-Castellanos DR, Nikonorov I, Kallen RG, Recio-Pinto E. Lidocaine stabilizes the open state of CNS voltage-dependent sodium channels. *Brain Res Mol Brain Res*. 2002;99(2):102-113.
168. Wei X, Dai R, Zhai S, Thummel KE, Friedman FK, Vestal RE. Inhibition of human liver cytochrome P-450 1A2 by the class IB antiarrhythmics mexiletine, lidocaine, and tocainide. *J Pharmacol Exp Ther*. 1999;289(2):853-858.
169. Arlander E, Ekstrom G, Alm C, et al. Metabolism of ropivacaine in humans is mediated by CYP1A2 and to a minor extent by CYP3A4: an interaction study with fluvoxamine and ketoconazole as in vivo inhibitors. *Clin Pharmacol Ther*. 1998;64(5):484-491.

Structure Challenge Answers

1. Answer: B (Febuxostat)
2. Answer: A (Ibuprofen-Carboxylic acid), C (Indomethacin-Carboxylic acid), and D (Nabumetone is a prodrug-Carboxylic acid)
3. Answer: E. Colchicine is a natural product that is indicated for the treatment of acute gout.
4. Answer: D. Nabumetone will have a lower incidence of GI side effects because it is a non-acidic prodrug and is not converted to a carboxylic acid until it is in the plasma.

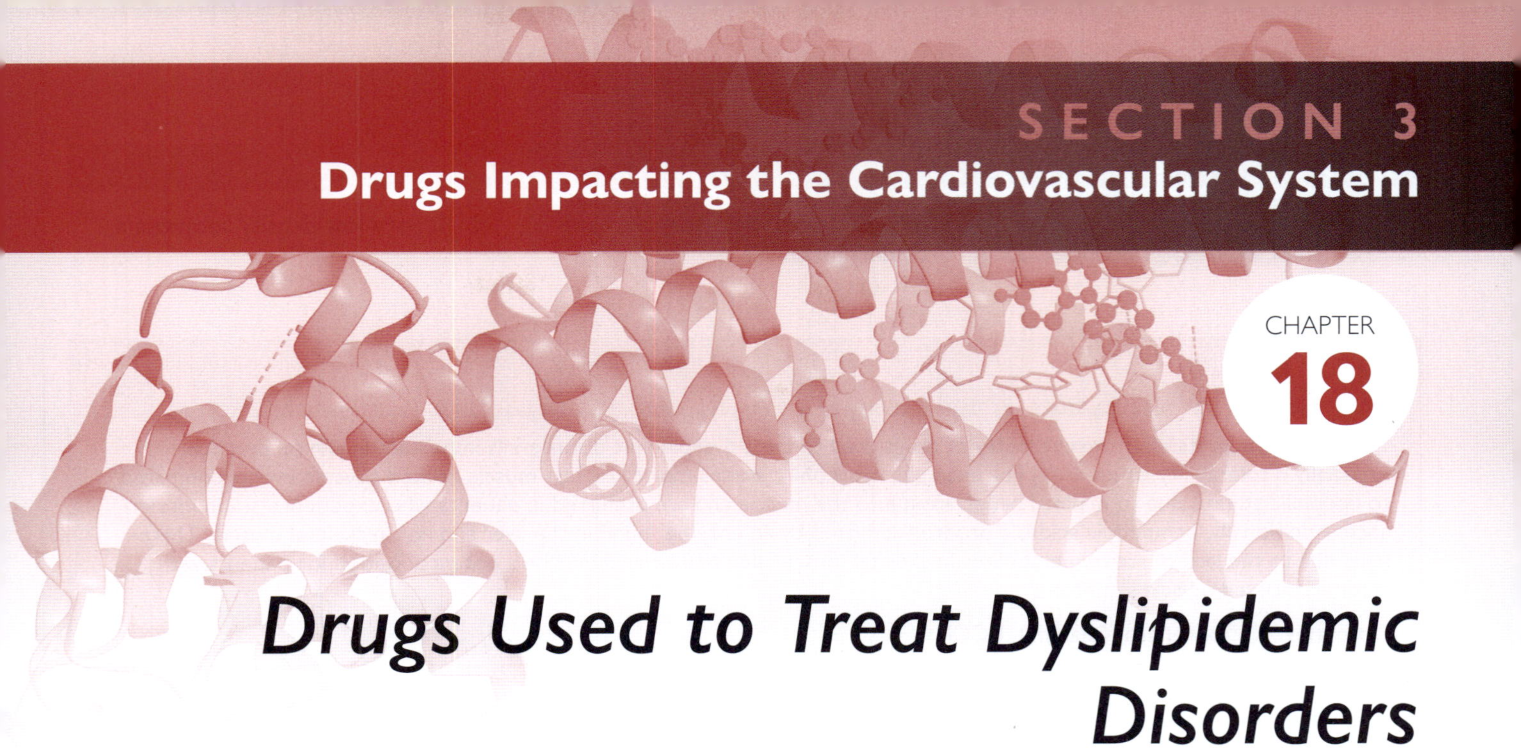

SECTION 3
Drugs Impacting the Cardiovascular System

CHAPTER 18

Drugs Used to Treat Dyslipidemic Disorders

Marc W. Harrold

Drugs covered in this chapter:

- Alirocumab
- Atorvastatin
- Bempedoic acid
- Cholestyramine
- Clofibrate
- Colesevelam
- Colestipol
- Docosahexaenoic acid (DPA)
- Eicosapentaenoic acid (EPA)
- Evinacumab
- Evolocumab
- Ezetimibe
- Fenofibric acid
- Fluvastatin
- Gemfibrozil
- Inclisiran
- Lomitapide
- Lovastatin
- Mipomersen
- Nicotinic acid/niacin
- Pitavastatin
- Pravastatin
- Rosuvastatin
- Simvastatin

Abbreviations

ACAT acyl CoA-cholesterol acyltransferase
ACL ATP-citrate lyase
ACSVL1 very-long-chain acyl CoA synthetase-1
aka also known as
ALT alanine transaminase
Apo apolipoprotein
ASCVD atherosclerotic cardiovascular disease
ASGPR asialoglycoprotein receptor
AST aspartate transaminase
BCRP breast cancer resistance protein
CETP cholesteryl ester transfer protein
CHD coronary heart disease
CoA coenzyme A
Fab fragment antigen binding
FC free unesterified cholesterol
FDA U.S. Food and Drug Administration
FFA free fatty acids
GalNAc *N*-acetylgalactosamine
GERD gastroesophageal reflux disorder
GI gastrointestinal
HDL high-density lipoprotein
HeFH heterozygous familial hypercholesterolemia
HMG-CoA 3-hydroxy-3-methylglutaryl coenzyme A
HMGR HMG-CoA reductase
HMGRIs HMG-CoA reductase inhibitors
HoFH homozygous familial hypercholesterolemia
LCAT lecithin-cholesterol acyltransferase
IDL intermediate-density lipoprotein
IgG immunoglobulin G
LDL low-density lipoprotein
LDL-C low-density lipoprotein cholesterol
MI myocardial infarction
mRNA messenger RNA
MTTP microsomal triglyceride transport protein
NAD^+ nicotinamide adenine dinucleotide
$NADP^+$ nicotinamide adenine dinucleotide phosphate
NPC1L1 Niemann-Pick C1-like 1
OATPs organic anion transporter polypeptides
PCSK9 proprotein convertase subtilisin kexin type 9
P-gp permeability glycoprotein (aka multidrug resistance protein 1; MDR1)
PPARs peroxisome proliferator-activated receptors
RCT reverse cholesterol transport
RISC RNA-induced silencing complex
SAR structure-activity relationship

Abbreviations—continued

SC subcutaneous
siRNA small, interfering ribonucleic acid
SREBP-2 sterol regulatory element–binding protein-2
VLDL very-low-density lipoprotein

CLINICAL SIGNIFICANCE

Understanding the chemistry of drugs used to treat dyslipidemic disorders is important in clinical practice, especially if tolerability issues arise. For example, hydrophilic statins may cause less muscle-related adverse events compared to lipophilic statins, due to minimal penetration into the muscle and are preferred in patients who experience statin intolerance. Additionally, bempedoic acid is a prodrug activated by an enzyme found in the liver and not in skeletal muscle. Therefore, due to the lack of active metabolites in skeletal muscle, bempedoic acid may be a potential option for patients with statin-associated muscle symptoms.

Courtney A. Montepara, PharmD, BCCP

Chemistry and Biochemistry of Plasma Lipids

The major lipids found in the bloodstream are cholesterol, cholesterol esters, triglycerides, and phospholipids. An abnormal concentration of one or more of these endogenous compounds is known as dyslipidemia. Since most abnormalities cause an increase in these endogenous lipids, the term "hyperlipidemia" is often used. Dyslipidemia/hyperlipidemia has been strongly associated with atherosclerotic lesions and coronary heart disease (CHD).[1,2] Prior to discussing lipoproteins, their role in cardiovascular disease, and drugs to decrease their concentrations, it is essential to review the biochemistry and normal physiologic functions of cholesterol, triglycerides, and phospholipids.

Synthesis and Degradation of Cholesterol

Cholesterol is a C_{27} steroid that serves as an important component of all cell membranes and is the precursor for androgens, estrogens, progesterone, and adrenocorticoids (Fig. 18.1). It is synthesized from acetyl coenzyme A (CoA), as shown in Figure 18.2.[3,4] The first stage of the biosynthesis is the formation of isopentenyl pyrophosphate from three acetyl-CoA molecules.

The conversion of 3-hydroxy-3-methylglutaryl (HMG)-CoA to mevalonic acid is especially important because it is a primary control site for cholesterol biosynthesis. This reaction is catalyzed by HMG-CoA reductase and reduces the thioester of HMG-CoA to a primary hydroxyl group. The second stage involves the coupling of six isopentenyl pyrophosphate molecules to form squalene. Initially, three isopentenyl pyrophosphate molecules are condensed to form farnesyl pyrophosphate, a C_{15} intermediate. Two farnesyl pyrophosphate molecules are then combined using a similar type of reaction. The next stage involves the cyclization of squalene to lanosterol. This process involves an initial epoxidation of squalene, followed by a subsequent cyclization requiring a concerted flow of four pairs of electrons and the migration of two methyl groups. The final stage involves the conversion of lanosterol to cholesterol. This process removes three methyl groups from lanosterol, reduces the side-chain double bond, moves the other double bond within the ring structure, and requires approximately 20 steps.[3,4]

Cholesterol is enzymatically transformed by two different pathways. As illustrated in Figure 18.1, cholesterol can be oxidatively cleaved by the enzyme desmolase (aka side chain–cleaving enzyme). The resulting compound, pregnenolone, serves as the common intermediate for the biosynthesis of all other endogenous steroids. Cholesterol can also be converted to bile acids and bile salts (Fig. 18.3). This pathway represents the most important mechanism for cholesterol catabolism. 7α-hydroxylase catalyzes the initial, rate-limiting step in this metabolic pathway and, thus, is the key control enzyme for this pathway. Cholic acid and its derivatives are primarily (99%) conjugated with either glycine (75%) or taurine (24%). Bile salts, such as glycocholate, are surface active agents that act as anionic detergents.[5,6]

The bile salts are synthesized in the liver, stored in the gallbladder, and released into the small intestine, where they emulsify dietary lipids and fat-soluble vitamins. This solubilization promotes the absorption of these dietary compounds through the intestinal mucosa. Bile salts are predominantly reabsorbed through enterohepatic circulation and returned to the liver, where they exert a negative feedback control on 7α-hydroxylase and, thus, regulate any subsequent conversion of cholesterol.[3,5,7]

The terms "bile acid" and "bile salt" refer to the unionized and ionized forms, respectively, of these compounds. For illustrative purposes only, Figure 18.3 shows cholic acid as an unionized bile acid and glycocholate as an ionized sodium bile salt. At physiologic and intestinal pH values, both compounds would exist almost exclusively in their ionized forms.

Overview of Triglycerides

Triglycerides (or, more appropriately, triacylglycerols) are highly concentrated stores of metabolic energy. They are formed from glycerol-3-phosphate and acylated CoA (Fig. 18.4) and accumulate primarily in the cytosol of adipose cells. When required for energy production, triglycerides are hydrolyzed by lipase enzymes to liberate free fatty acids, which are then subjected to β-oxidation, the citric acid cycle, and oxidative phosphorylation.[3,4]

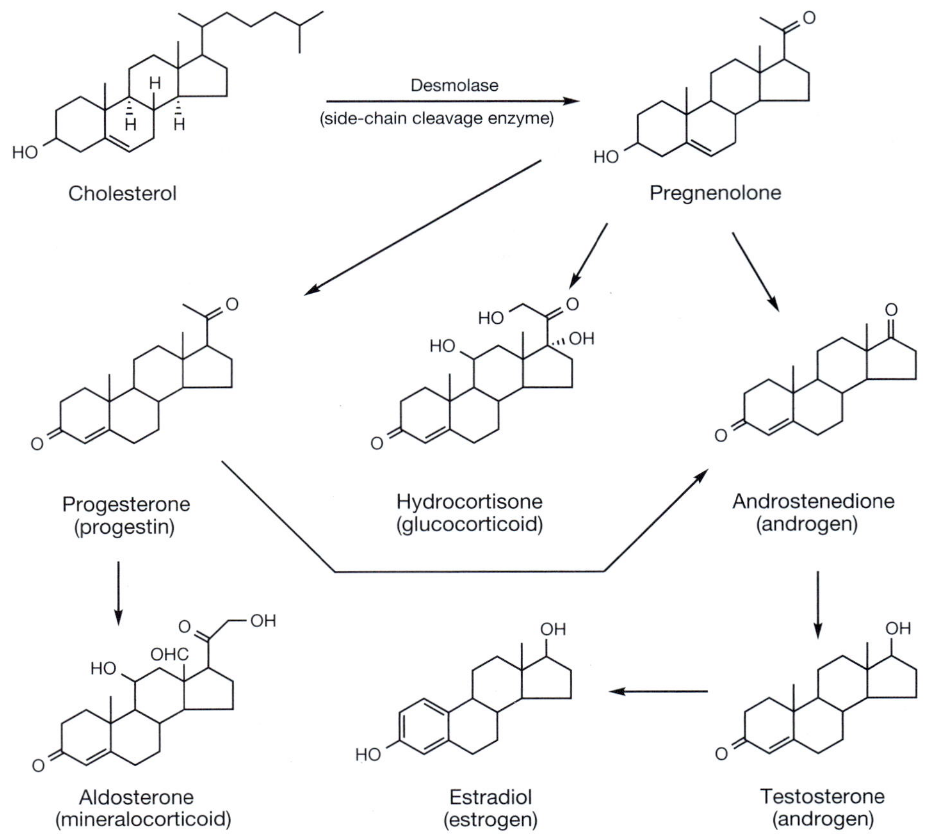

Figure 18.1 Cholesterol's role as a key intermediate in the biosynthesis of endogenous steroids.

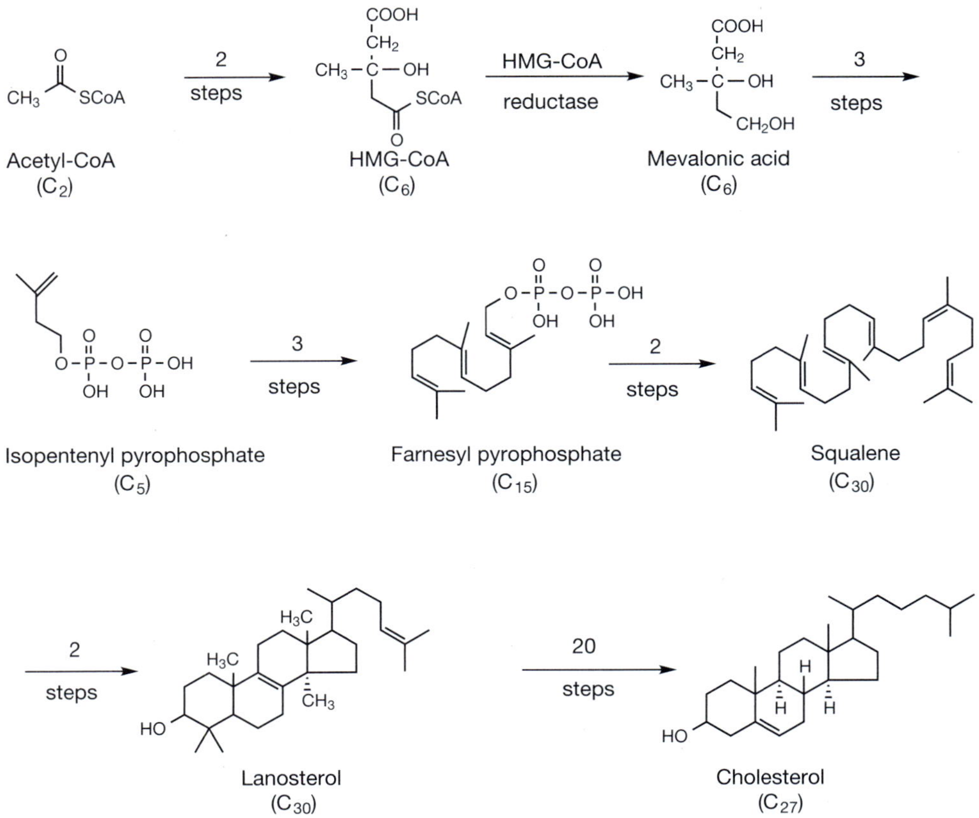

Figure 18.2 Biosynthesis of cholesterol.

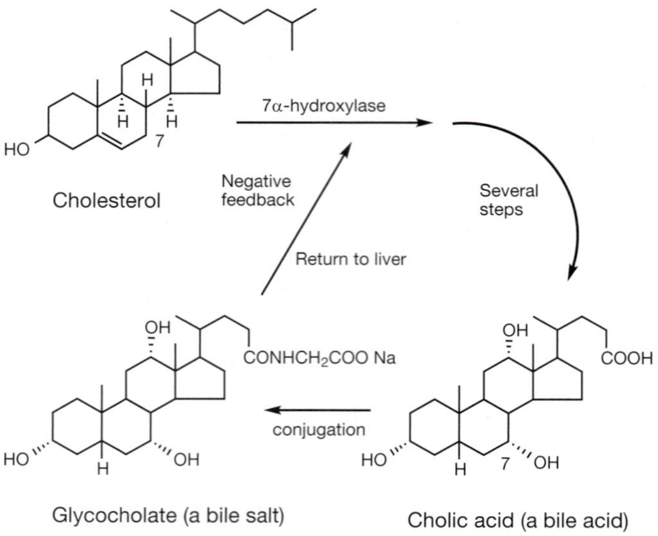

Figure 18.3 Conversion of cholesterol to bile acids and bile salts.

Lipoproteins and Transport of Cholesterol and Triglycerides

Cholesterol and triglycerides are freely soluble in organic solvents, such as isopropanol, chloroform, and diethyl ether, but are relatively insoluble in aqueous physiologic fluids. To be transported within the blood, these lipids are solubilized through association with macromolecular aggregates known as lipoproteins. Each lipoprotein is associated with additional proteins, known as apolipoproteins, on their outer surface. These apolipoproteins provide structural support and stability, bind to cellular receptors, and act as cofactors for enzymes involved in lipoprotein metabolism. The compositions and primary functions of the six major lipoproteins are listed in Table 18.1.[7-9]

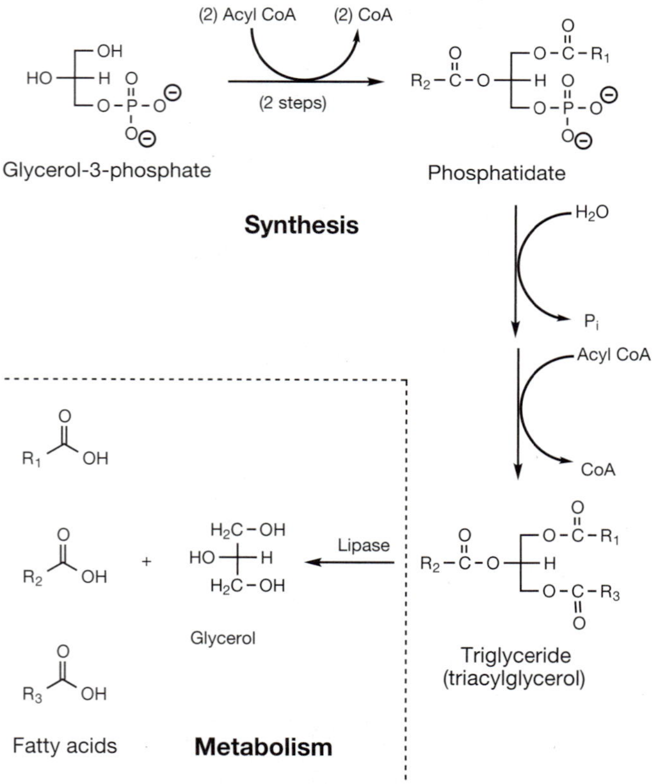

Figure 18.4 Biosynthesis and metabolism of triglycerides.

Lipoprotein nomenclature is based on the mode of separation. When preparative ultracentrifugation is used, lipoproteins are separated according to their density and identified as very-low-density lipoproteins (VLDLs), intermediate-density lipoproteins (IDLs), low-density lipoproteins (LDLs), and high-density lipoproteins (HDLs). When electrophoresis is used in the separation, lipoproteins are designated as pre-β, β, and α. The IDLs are mainly found in the pre-β fraction as a second electrophoretic band and are currently believed to be an intermediate lipoprotein in the catabolism of VLDL to LDL. Chylomicron remnants and IDLs may show similar electrophoretic and ultracentrifugation separation characteristics. In general, VLDL, LDL, and HDL correspond to pre-β, β, and α lipoprotein, respectively.

The interrelationship among the lipoproteins is shown in Figure 18.5.[8-10] As illustrated, the pathway can be divided into exogenous (dietary intake) and endogenous (synthetic) components. The exogenous pathway begins after the ingestion of a fat-containing meal or snack. Dietary lipids are absorbed in the form of cholesterol and fatty acids, with fatty acids being the predominant lipid. The fatty acids are then re-esterified within the intestinal mucosal cells and, along with the cholesterol, are incorporated into chylomicrons, the largest lipoprotein. During circulation, chylomicrons are degraded into remnants by the action of lipoprotein lipase, a plasma membrane enzyme located on capillary endothelial cells in adipose and muscle tissue. The interaction of chylomicrons with lipoprotein lipase requires apolipoprotein (apo) C-II. The absence of either the enzyme or the apolipoprotein can lead to hypertriglyceridemia and pancreatitis. The liberated free acids are then available for either storage or energy generation by these tissues. The remnants are predominantly cleared from the plasma by liver parenchymal cells via recognition of the apoE portion of the carrier.

The endogenous pathway begins in the liver with the formation of VLDL. Similar to chylomicrons, triglycerides are present in a higher concentration than either cholesterol or cholesterol esters; however, the concentration difference between these lipids is much less than that seen in chylomicrons. Also, the metabolism of VLDL is similar to that of chylomicrons in that lipoprotein lipase decreases the triglyceride content of VLDL and increases the availability of free fatty acids to the muscle and adipose tissue. The resulting lipoprotein, IDL, can be further metabolized to LDL, or it can be transported to the liver for receptor-mediated endocytosis. This latter effect involves an interaction of the LDL receptor with the apolipoproteins apoB-100 and apoE on IDL. The amount of IDL delivered to the liver is approximately the same as that converted to LDL. The half-life of IDL is relatively short when compared to that of LDL and, thus, accounts for only a small portion of total plasma cholesterol. In contrast, LDL accounts for approximately two-thirds of total plasma cholesterol and serves as the primary source of cholesterol for both hepatic and extrahepatic cells. As with IDL, the uptake of LDL by these cells is mediated by a receptor interaction with the apoB-100 on LDL.

Table 18.1 Classification and Characteristics of Major Plasma Lipoproteins

Classification	Composition	Major Apolipoproteins	Primary Function(s)
Chylomicrons	Triglycerides 80%-95%, free cholesterol 1%-3%, cholesterol esters 2%-4%, phospholipids 3%-9%, apoproteins 1%-2%	apoA-I, apoA-IV, apoB-48, apoC-I, apoC-II, apoC-III	Transport dietary triglycerides to adipose tissue and muscle for hydrolysis by lipoprotein lipase
Chylomicron remnants	Primarily composed of dietary cholesterol esters	apoB-48, apoE	Transport dietary cholesterol to liver for receptor-mediated endocytosis
VLDL	Triglycerides 50%-65%, free cholesterol 4%-8%, cholesterol esters 16%-22%, phospholipids 15%-20%, apoproteins 6%-10%	apoB-100, apoE, apoC-I, apoC-II, apoC-III	Transport endogenous triglycerides to adipose tissue and muscle for hydrolysis by lipoprotein lipase
IDL	Intermediate between VLDL and LDL	apoB-100, apoE, apoC-II, apoC-III	Transport endogenous cholesterol for either conversion to LDL or receptor-mediated endocytosis by the liver
LDL	Triglycerides 4%-8%, free cholesterol 6%-8%, cholesterol esters 45%-50%, phospholipids 18%-24%, apoproteins 18%-22%	apoB-100	Transport endogenous cholesterol for receptor-mediated endocytosis by either the liver or extrahepatic tissues
HDL	Triglycerides 2%-7%, free cholesterol 3%-5%, cholesterol esters 15%-20%, phospholipids 26%-32%, apoproteins 45%-55%	apoA-I, apoA-II, apoE, apoC-I, apoC-II, apoC-III	Removal of cholesterol from extrahepatic tissues via transfer of cholesterol esters to IDL and LDL

apo, apolipoprotein; HDL, high-density lipoprotein; IDL, intermediate-density lipoprotein; LDL, low-density lipoprotein; VLDL, very-low-density lipoprotein.

There is a direct correlation between the number of LDL receptors on the cell surface, the cholesterol content within the cell, and the regulation of cellular LDL uptake. It has been shown that high plasma LDL levels are associated with a low number of LDL receptors, and that low plasma LDL levels are associated with a high number of LDL receptors. Cells requiring increased amounts of cholesterol will increase the biosynthesis of LDL receptors. Conversely, it has been demonstrated that increased hepatic concentrations of cholesterol will inhibit both HMG-CoA reductase and the production of LDL receptors. A decrease in cellular cholesterol levels triggers the transport of sterol regulatory element–binding protein-2 (SREBP-2) from the endoplasmic reticulum to the Golgi. The cleavage and activation of SREBP by protease enzymes then allows SREBP-2 to migrate to the nucleus and activate genes involved in the formation of LDL receptors. In contrast, an increase in cellular cholesterol blocks the transport and activation of SREBP-2, resulting in a decrease in the formation of LDL receptors. The regulation of LDL receptors is also mediated by proprotein convertase subtilisin kexin type 9 (PCSK9), a protein that binds to LDL receptors on the surface of hepatocytes and promotes their degradation. Further regulation of cellular cholesterol is mediated by the conversion of hepatic cholesterol to bile acids and bile salts and their enterohepatic circulation.[9,11,12]

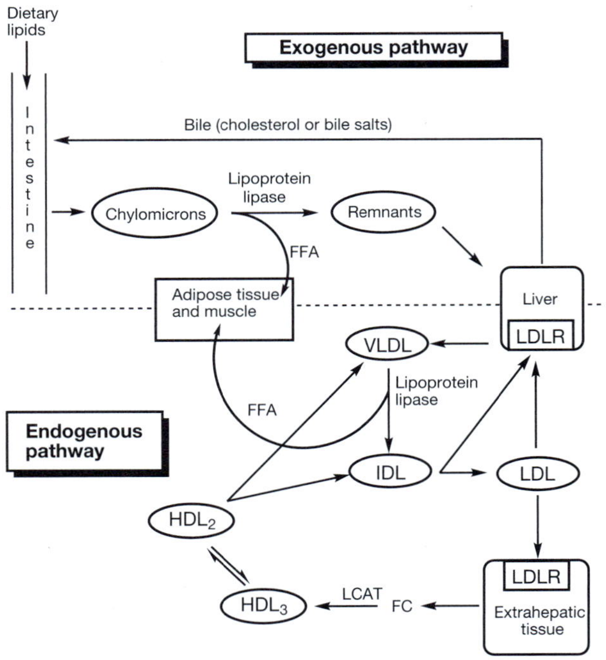

Figure 18.5 Endogenous and exogenous pathways for lipid transport and metabolism. FC, free unesterified cholesterol; FFA, free fatty acids; LCAT, lecithin-cholesterol acyltransferase; LDLR, low-density lipoprotein receptor.

Synthesized in the liver and intestine, HDL initially exists as a dense, phospholipid disk composed primarily of apoA-I. The primary function of HDL is to act as a scavenger to remove cholesterol from extrahepatic cells and to facilitate its transport back to the liver. Nascent HDL accepts free, unesterified cholesterol. A plasma enzyme, lecithin-cholesterol acyltransferase, then esterifies the cholesterol. This process allows the resulting cholesterol esters to move from the surface to the core and results in the production of spherical HDL_3 particles. As cholesterol content is added, HDL_3 is converted to HDL_2, which is larger and less dense than HDL_3. The ultimate return of cholesterol from HDL_2 to the liver is known as reverse cholesterol transport (RCT) and is accomplished via an intermediate transfer of cholesterol esters from HDL_2 to either VLDL or IDL. This process regenerates spherical HDL_3 molecules that can recirculate and acquire excess cholesterol from other tissues. In this manner, HDL serves to prevent the accumulation of cholesterol in arterial cell walls and other tissue, and may serve as the basis for its cardioprotective properties.[7-9]

Therapeutic Overview

Diseases and Disorders Caused by Hyperlipidemias

Atherosclerosis, which is named from the Greek terms for "gruel" (*athere*) and "hardening" (*sclerosis*), is the underlying cause of CHD. It is a gradual process in which an initial accumulation of lipids in the arterial intima leads to thickening of the arterial wall, plaque formation, thrombosis, and occlusion.[13-15] The involvement of LDL cholesterol in this process is shown in Figure 18.6. Within the extracellular space of the intima, LDL is more susceptible to oxidative metabolism because it is no longer protected by plasma antioxidants. This metabolism alters the properties of LDL such that it is readily scavenged by macrophages. Unlike normal LDL, the uptake of oxidized LDL is not regulated; thus, macrophage cells can readily become engorged with oxidized LDL. Subsequent metabolism produces free cholesterol, which can either be released into the plasma or be reesterified by the enzyme acyl CoA-cholesterol acyltransferase (ACAT). Cholesterol released into plasma can be scavenged by HDL_3 and returned to the liver, thus preventing any accumulation or damage. In this manner, HDL acts as a cardioprotective agent because high concentrations of reesterified cholesterol can morphologically change macrophages into foam cells. Accumulation of lipid-engorged foam cells in the arterial intima results in the formation of fatty streaks, the initial lesion of atherosclerosis. Later, the deposition of lipoproteins, cholesterol, and phospholipids causes the formation of softer, larger plaques. Associated with this lipid deposition is the proliferation of arterial smooth muscle cells into the intima and the laying down of collagen, elastin, and glycosaminoglycans, leading to fibrous plaques. Ultimately, the surface of the plaque deteriorates, and an atheromatous ulcer is formed, with a fibrous matrix, accumulation of necrotic tissue, and appearance of cholesterol and cholesterol ester crystals. A complicated lesion also

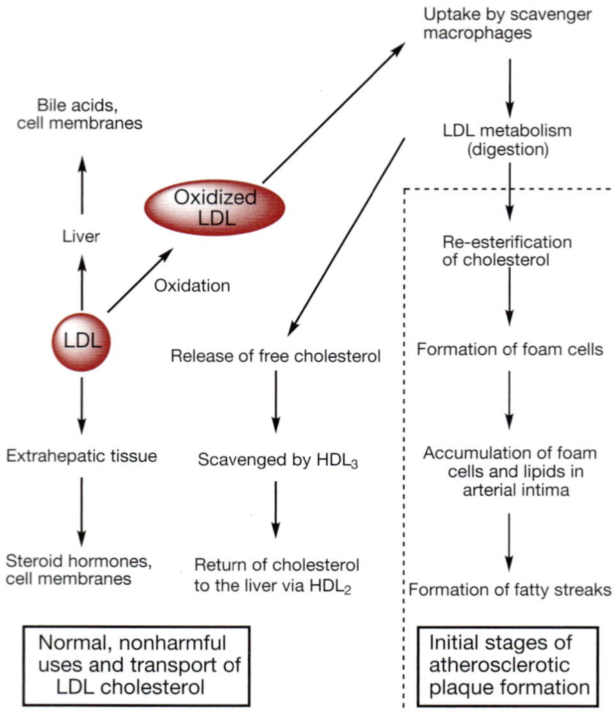

Figure 18.6 Role of LDL cholesterol in the development of atherosclerotic plaques and the cardioprotective role of HDL. The oxidation of LDL occurs within the extracellular space of the intima.

shows calcification and hemorrhage with the formation of organized mural thrombi. Thrombosis results from changes in the arterial walls and in the blood-clotting mechanism.

Elevated plasma triglyceride levels can contribute to atherosclerosis and CHD in mixed hyperlipoproteinemias, whereas pure hypertriglyceridemias are primarily associated with pancreatitis and show little to no relationship to CHD.[7,8]

Classification of Hyperlipoproteinemias

Hyperlipoproteinemia can be divided into primary and secondary disorders. Primary disorders are the result of genetic deficiencies or mutations, whereas secondary disorders are the result of other conditions or diseases. Secondary hyperlipoproteinemia has been associated with diabetes, hypothyroidism, renal disease, liver disease, alcoholism, and certain drugs.[7,8,13]

In 1967, Fredrickson et al[10] classified primary hyperlipoproteinemias into six phenotypes (I, IIa, IIb, III, IV, and V), based on which lipoproteins and lipids were elevated. Current literature and practice, however, appear to favor the more descriptive classifications and subclassifications listed in Table 18.2. Primary disorders are currently classified as those that primarily cause hypercholesterolemia, those that primarily cause hypertriglyceridemia, and those that cause a mixed elevation of both cholesterol and triglycerides. Subclassifications are based on the specific biochemical defect responsible for the disorder. Classifications developed by Fredrickson have been included in Table 18.2 under the heading *Previous Classification* for comparative and reference purposes.

Table 18.2 Characteristics of the Major Primary Hyperlipoproteinemias

Current Classification	Biochemical Defect	Elevated Lipoproteins	Previous Classification
Hypercholesterolemias			
Familial hypercholesterolemia	Deficiency of LDL receptors	LDL	IIa
Familial defective apoB-100	Mutant apoB-100	LDL	IIa
Polygenic hypercholesterolemia	Unknown	LDL	IIa
Hypertriglyceridemias			
Familial hypertriglyceridemia	Unknown	VLDL	IV
Familial lipoprotein lipase deficiency	Deficiency of lipoprotein lipase	Chylomicrons, VLDL	I (chylomicron elevation only), V
Familial apoC-II deficiency	Deficiency of apoC-II	Chylomicrons, VLDL	I (chylomicron elevation only), V
Mixed hypercholesterolemia and hypertriglyceridemia			
Familial combined hyperlipidemia	Unknown	VLDL, LDL	IIb
Dysbetalipoproteinemia	Presence of $apoE_2$ isoforms	VLDL, IDL	III

apo, apolipoprotein; IDL, intermediate-density lipoprotein; LDL, low-density lipoprotein; VLDL, very-low-density lipoprotein.

As shown in Table 18.2, some disorders are well characterized, whereas others are not.[7,10,13] Familial hypercholesterolemia is caused by a deficiency of LDL receptors. This results in a decreased uptake of IDL and LDL by hepatic and extrahepatic tissues and an elevation in plasma LDL levels. The homozygous form of this disorder is rare, but results in extremely high LDL levels as well as early morbidity and mortality because of the total lack of LDL receptors. A related disorder, familial defective apoB-100, also results in elevated LDL levels, but is caused by a genetic mutation rather than by a deficiency. Alteration of apoB-100 decreases the affinity of LDL for the LDL receptor and, thus, hinders normal uptake and metabolism. Elevations in chylomicron levels can result from a deficiency of either lipoprotein lipase or apoC-II. These deficiencies cause decreased or impaired triglyceride hydrolysis, and result in a massive accumulation of chylomicrons in the plasma. Dysbetalipoproteinemia results from the presence of an altered form of apoE and is the only mixed hyperlipoproteinemia with a known cause. Proper catabolism of chylomicron and VLDL remnants requires apoE. The presence of a binding-defective form of apoE, known as $apoE_2$, results in elevated levels of VLDL and IDL triglyceride and cholesterol levels.

Prevalence and Public Health Burden of Coronary Heart Disease

According to a 2023 report, CHD, which includes acute myocardial infarction (MI), ischemic heart disease, and angina pectoris, affects approximately 20.5 million Americans who are aged 20 years or more, and is the leading cause of mortality in the United States.[16] The overall prevalence of CHD in this age group is 7.1%, with the prevalence being higher for men (8.7%) than for women (5.8%). On the basis of the Framingham Heart Study, more than 50% of all cardiovascular events occurring in patients aged 75 years or less are due to CHD. In 2020, CHD was responsible for slightly less than 382,850 deaths and an underlying cause of one in every seven deaths. The CHD age-adjusted death rates were higher in men than in women, with non-Hispanic Black men having the highest incidence per 10,000 individuals (153.6), followed by non-Hispanic White men (128.5), Hispanic men (102.2), non-Hispanic Black women (85.9), non-Hispanic White men (63.8), and Hispanic women (54). From a positive perspective, the percentage of US adults with a 10-year predicted atherosclerotic cardiovascular disease (ASCVD) greater than 20% has decreased from 13% in 1999 to 2000 to 9.4% in 2011 to 2012. Risk factors associated with CHD include hypertension, cigarette smoking, elevated plasma cholesterol levels, physical inactivity, diabetes, and obesity.[17]

Economic Impact of Therapy

Recent studies have estimated that the annual cost of cardiovascular disease (CVD) in the United States is over $400 billion, when both direct and indirect costs are considered. This cost includes over $250 billion in expenditures, including the cost of physicians, other health professionals, hospital services, and prescribed medications. In 2018 and 2019, CVD was responsible for approximately 12% of the total US health expenditures, a figure that was higher than any other major diagnostic group.[18] As such, the selection of appropriate therapy based on desired patient outcomes plays a key role in the pharmacotherapy of treating risk factors such as dyslipidemia.

Studies have been conducted for the cost-effectiveness of two major classes of drugs used to treat dyslipidemia: HMG-CoA reductase inhibitions (HMGRIs) (commonly known as statins) and PCSK9 inhibitors. A study published in 2022 examined the cost-effectiveness of the preventive use of statins over a 10-year risk period. Results of the study indicated that the availability of generic pricing and patient eligibility increased the use of statins and reduced the risk of CVD in a cost-effective manner.[19] Current clinical guidelines from the American College of Cardiology/American

Heart Association (ACC/AHA) recognize both the benefits and economic impact of PCSK9 inhibitors. Simulation models have been used to assess both the cost-effectiveness and economic value for the use of this class of drugs. These models predict that, in order for PCSK9 inhibitors to be cost-effective, the cost needs to be reduced by up to 70%. The models have also shown that the economic value of PCSK9 inhibitors would be improved by restricting use to patients who have a very high-risk of ASCVD, as defined by current guidelines.[20]

Drugs Used to Treat Dyslipidemia

Current guidelines for lowering plasma LDL cholesterol (LDL-C) focus on the use of HMGRIs, and other dietary and pharmacologic/chemical classes of drugs commonly known as nonstatin therapy.[20,21] These guidelines define four patient population groups that would benefit from the use of statins as well as other factors that need to be considered. These include adherence, lifestyle, the control of other risk factors, the balance between risks and benefits of using a statin, the patient's preference for one medication over another, the total LDL reduction that is set as the patient's goal, and patient monitoring. Current drug options beyond statin therapy include ezetimibe (an inhibitor of dietary cholesterol absorption), PCSK9 inhibitors, bempedoic acid (an inhibitor of cholesterol biosynthesis acting upstream of the statins), bile acid sequestrants, mipomersen (a microsomal triglyceride transfer protein inhibitor), evinacumab (an angiopoietin-like protein 3 inhibitor), and lomitapide (an apoB-100 protein translation inhibitor). Additionally, niacin, fibrates, and the ω-3 fish oils have been found to be useful for lowering triglyceride levels and reducing the risk of pancreatitis. Low plasma HDL levels, defined as less than 40 mg/dL for men and less than 50 mg/dL for women, are known risk factors for CVD.[20] Both niacin and the fibrates have been shown to increase HDL levels and favorably decrease this risk factor.[22,23]

The discussion of drugs in this chapter is organized based on the current treatment guidelines. HMGRIs are discussed first, followed by nonstatin therapy, to treat patients with primary or secondary hypercholesterolemia. For most patients, nonstatin therapy includes ezetimibe, PCSK9 inhibitors, bempedoic acid, and bile acid sequestrants; however, for patients with homozygous familial hypercholesterolemia (HoFH), lomitapide, mipomersen, and evinacumab are available options. The chapter concludes with discussions of niacin, fibrates, and ω-3 fatty acids, drugs used in the treatment of hypertriglyceridemias and mixed dyslipidemias.

HMG-CoA Reductase Inhibitors

The development and use of HMGRIs began in 1976 with the discovery of mevastatin, a lactone-containing prodrug. Originally named compactin, this fungal metabolite was isolated from two different species of *Penicillium*. Its hydrolyzed metabolite demonstrated potent, competitive inhibition of HMG-CoA reductase, with an affinity that was 10,000-fold greater than that of the substrate HMG-CoA.[24] Several years later, a structurally similar compound known as mevinolin was isolated from *Monascus ruber* and *Aspergillus terreus*. Mevinolin was later renamed lovastatin, and its hydrolyzed metabolite was shown to be more than 2-fold more potent than mevastatin (Fig. 18.7). The top portions of these structures contain a 3,5-dihydroxy acid that mimics the intermediate that is formed by HMG-CoA reductase (HMGR). Clinical trials of mevastatin were halted after reports of altered intestinal morphology in dogs[25]; however, lovastatin received approval by the U.S. Food and Drug Administration (FDA) in 1987, representing the first HMGRI to be available in the United States for therapeutic use.

All HMGRIs are approved for the treatment of primary hypercholesterolemia and mixed dyslipidemia (Fig. 18.8). Additional indications for this class of drugs include primary dysbetalipoproteinemia, hypertriglyceridemia, homozygous familial hyperlipidemia, and primary and secondary prevention of cardiovascular events (eg, MI, stroke). Specific indications for each drug can be found in their respective product literature or online resources.[26,27] At their highest approved doses, atorvastatin and rosuvastatin have been shown to be the most effective drugs at lowering LDL cholesterol levels.[23]

Mechanism of Action

Inhibitors of HMG-CoA reductase lower plasma cholesterol levels by three related mechanisms: inhibition of cholesterol biosynthesis, enhancement of receptor-mediated LDL uptake, and reduction of VLDL precursors.[7,8,26] HMG-CoA reductase catalyzes the rate-limiting step in cholesterol biosynthesis. Competitive inhibition of this enzyme causes an initial decrease in hepatic cholesterol. As previously discussed, this decrease in cellular cholesterol levels triggers the activation of SREBP and an increase in the formation of LDL receptors.[9,11] While not beneficial, compensatory

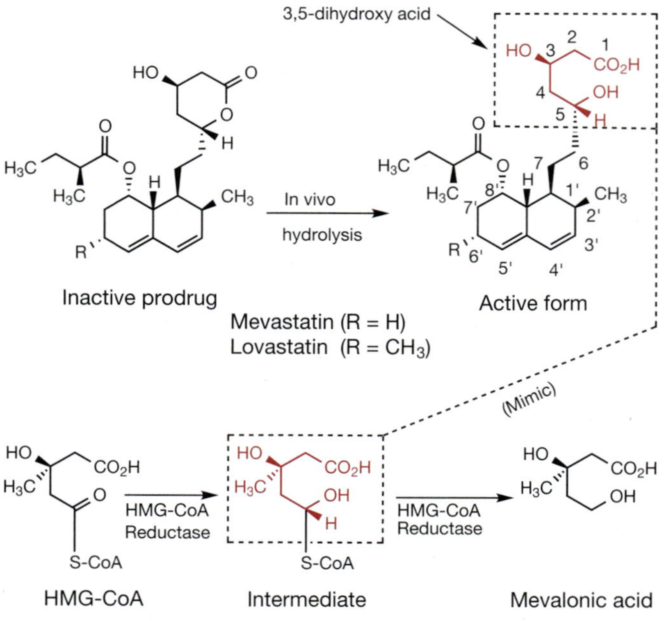

Figure 18.7 Mechanism of action of mevastatin and lovastatin. Hydrolysis of these prodrugs produces a 3,5-dihydroxy acid that mimics the tetrahedral intermediate produced by HMG-CoA reductase.

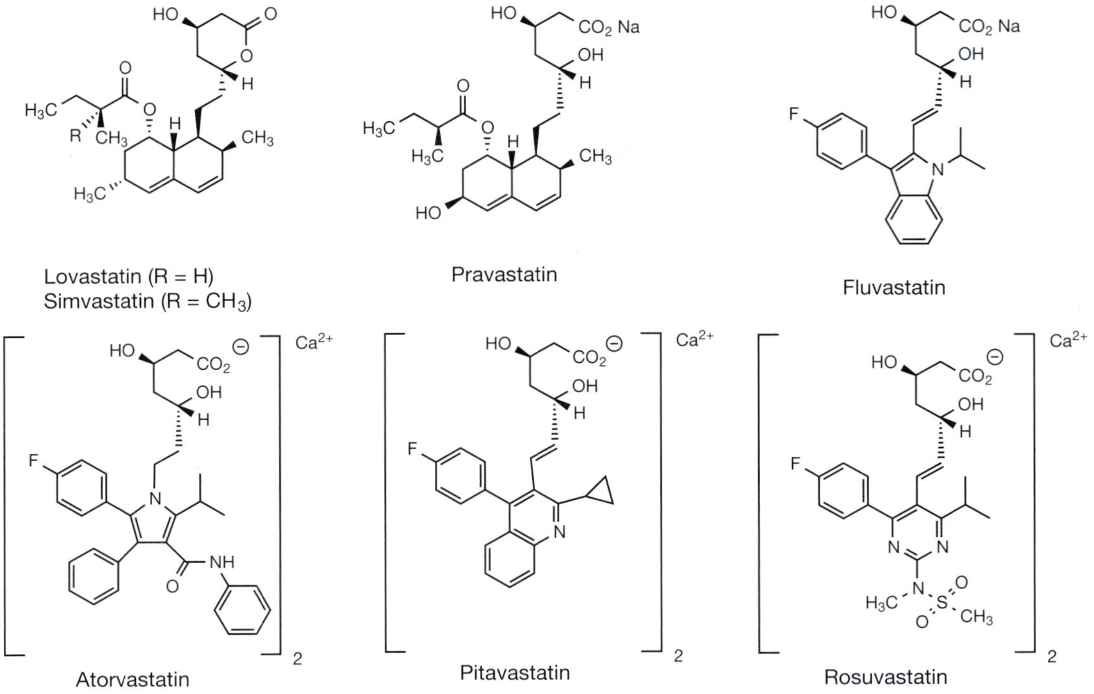

Figure 18.8 Commercially available HMG-CoA reductase inhibitors.

mechanisms also result in an enhanced expression of HMG-CoA reductase. The net result of all these effects is a slight to modest decrease in cholesterol biosynthesis, a significant increase in receptor-mediated LDL uptake, and an overall lowering of plasma LDL levels. Evidence to support the theory that enhanced LDL receptor expression is the primary mechanism for lowering LDL levels comes from the fact that most statins do not lower LDL levels in patients who are unable to produce LDL receptors (ie, HoFH). The increased number of LDL receptors may also increase the direct removal of VLDL and IDL. Because these lipoproteins are precursors to LDL, this action may contribute to the overall lowering of plasma LDL cholesterol. Finally, all HMGRIs can produce a modest (6%-12%) increase in HDL.[7,8]

Atorvastatin, rosuvastatin, and simvastatin appear to have some effects beyond those seen with the other HMGRIs. These drugs have been shown to decrease plasma LDL levels in patients with HoFH, an effect that is proposed to result from their ability to produce a more significant decrease in the hepatic production of LDL cholesterol. Additionally, atorvastatin and rosuvastatin can produce a significant lowering of plasma triglycerides. In the case of atorvastatin, this effect has been attributed to its ability to produce an enhanced removal of triglyceride-rich VLDL.[7,28-30]

A number of additional cardioprotective effects, other than lowering LDL cholesterol, are thought to be associated with HMGRIs. HMGRIs cause an upregulation of nitric oxide synthase expression, resulting in vasodilation and improved endothelial function, and they have been postulated to stabilize plaques, provide an anti-inflammatory effect, reduce the susceptibility of LDL to oxidation, and reduce platelet aggregation.[30]

Role of Organic Anion Transporter Polypeptides on HMGRIs

In general, organic anion transporter polypeptides (OATPs) facilitate the transport of amphipathic organic drugs and biomolecules across gastrointestinal (GI) and cellular membranes. The HMGRIs are amphipathic drugs in that they contain both polar and nonpolar regions in their structures. There are a number of OATP isoforms, with OATP1B1 and OATP2B1 being the most important for HMGRI therapy. OATP2B1 is relatively ubiquitous and is present in the intestine, liver, heart, and skeletal muscles. OATP2B1 has been shown to be important for the GI absorption of HMGRIs. The effects of OATP2B1 are pH dependent with enhanced activity at a more acidic pH. OATP1B1 is primarily expressed in human liver cells and plays a significant role in hepatic uptake and clearance of HMGRIs. Genetic polymorphism of OATP1B1 at specific locations produces an allele (ie, variant) with a reduced activity. The presence of this variant results in a decreased concentration of the HMGRI in hepatocytes, an increased concentration of the HMGRI in the plasma concentration, and an increased risk of statin-induced myopathy. Studies evaluating the effects of OATB1B1 variant found that the above effects are not the same for all HMGRIs. In the presence of the variant, the plasma concentrations of atorvastatin, lovastatin, pitavastatin, and simvastatin were increased by approximately 3.4-fold, while the plasma concentrations of the two most water-soluble HMGRIs were increased by approximately 1.8-fold. Interestingly, the plasma concentrations of fluvastatin were not significantly altered when the variant was present.[31-34]

Common Adverse Effects

The most prevalent or significant side effects of HMGRIs are highlighted in the box titled "Adverse Effects of HMGRIs."[7,26] In general, this class of drugs is well tolerated. GI disturbances are the most common side effect; however, these and other adverse reactions tend to be mild and transient. Elevations in hepatic transaminase levels can occur with all HMGRIs. These increases usually occur shortly after the initiation of therapy and resolve after the discontinuation of medication. In a small percentage of patients, these levels can increase to more than 3-fold the upper limit of normal. Current guidelines require that liver function tests be performed prior to starting HMGRI therapy and, if there is a clinical indication during therapy. Routine monitoring is not required or recommended based on the facts that serious hepatic injury is rare, and that routine monitoring has not been shown to detect or prevent hepatic injury. Approximately 5% to 10% of patients will experience mild increases in creatine phosphokinase levels; however, only 1% to 2% will develop symptoms of myalgia and myopathy. Symptoms of statin-induced myopathy include fever, fatigue, muscle aches, muscle tenderness, muscle cramps, and unusual tiredness or weakness. Tests for creatine phosphokinase levels should be performed in patients reporting muscle complaints. Rhabdomyolysis (ie, massive muscle necrosis with secondary acute renal failure) has occurred, but this is rare.

The incidence of statin-induced myopathy is related to the lipophilic nature of the drug. Atorvastatin, lovastatin, and simvastatin are more prone to induce myopathy than are the relatively more hydrophilic statins, fluvastatin, pravastatin, and rosuvastatin. Lipophilic drugs can more easily penetrate passively (ie, do not require OATPs) into muscle cells and tissue and, thus, have an increased potential to cause myopathy.[35,36]

Common Interactions

With the exception of rosuvastatin and pravastatin, all other HMGRIs are metabolized by CYP3A4 (primarily) and CYP2C9; therefore, other drugs that inhibit or induce these isozymes will increase or decrease the levels of HMGRIs, respectively. Inhibition of CYP3A4 may increase the risk of myopathy and rhabdomyolysis; therefore, specific dosage reductions are suggested whenever an HMGRI is used in combination with a strong CYP3A4 inhibitor. Statin transport out of the gut, into the liver, and within the systemic circulation depends upon OATPs, P-glycoprotein (P-gp), and breast cancer resistance protein (BCRP). Drugs that affect the actions of these proteins may increase or decrease statin levels. Concurrent use of cyclosporine (CYP3A4 inhibitor) or gemfibrozil (OATP inhibitor and competitor of statin phase 2 metabolizing enzymes) will increase the plasma concentrations of all statins and will increase the risk of rhabdomyolysis. Rhabdomyolysis involves the breakdown of damaged muscle, the release of muscle cell proteins and electrolytes into the blood, and potential organ damage. The use of high-dose niacin with statins has been associated with an increased risk of myopathy and rhabdomyolysis. If used in combination with strongly cationic bile acid sequestrants, anionic HMGRIs should be administered at least 1 hour prior to, or 4-6 hours after, the bile acid sequestrant, to avoid decreased absorption. Inhibitors of HMG-CoA reductase are contraindicated in pregnancy. Fetal development requires cholesterol as a precursor for the synthesis of steroids and cell membranes; thus, inhibition of its synthesis may cause fetal harm. Additionally, HMGRIs are excreted in breast milk and should not be used by nursing mothers.[7,8,23,26]

ADVERSE EFFECTS OF HMGRIs

Cardiovascular: Chest pain
Central nervous system: Headache
GI: Abdominal pain, constipation, diarrhea, dyspepsia, flatulence, nausea, vomiting
Metabolic: Elevated hepatic enzymes
Musculoskeletal: Arthralgia, muscle cramps, myalgia, myopathy, rhabdomyolysis
Pulmonary: Rhinitis, sinusitis

Drug Development, Receptor Binding, and Structure-Activity Relationships

Drug Development

Mevastatin and lovastatin served as lead compounds in the development of additional HMGRIs. The only structural difference between lovastatin and mevastatin was the presence of a methyl group at the 6′ position of the bicyclic decalin ring of lovastatin. As illustrated in Figure 18.7, mevastatin and lovastatin can bind very tightly with HMG-CoA reductase because their hydrolyzed lactones mimic the tetrahedral intermediate produced by the reductase enzyme.[7] Studies published in 1985 confirmed this theory and established that the decalin portion of these compounds bind to the CoA site of the enzyme.[37]

Initial research published by Merck Pharmaceuticals examined alterations of the lactone and decalin ring system as well as the ethylene bridge between them. The results demonstrated that the lactone ring must be hydrolyzed in vivo to a carboxylic acid and a C_5-hydroxyl group, the stereochemistry at the C_3 and C_5 positions must mimic that of the intermediate shown in Figure 18.7, and that the two-carbon length of the bridge connecting the two ring systems is optimal. Additionally, it was found that the decalin ring system of mevastatin and lovastatin could be replaced with other lipophilic rings, and that the size and shape of these other ring systems were important to the overall activity of the compounds.[38]

Minor modifications of the decalin ring system and side-chain ester of lovastatin produced simvastatin and pravastatin (Fig. 18.8). Pravastatin, a ring-opened dihydroxy acid with a 6′α-hydroxyl group, is much more hydrophilic than either lovastatin or simvastatin. Proposed advantages of this enhanced hydrophilicity are minimal penetration into the lipophilic membranes of peripheral cells, better selectivity for hepatic tissues, and a reduction in the incidence of myopathy and other side effects seen with lovastatin and simvastatin.[39,40]

The replacement of the decalin ring system of lovastatin with various substituted aromatic ring systems led to the development of atorvastatin, fluvastatin, pitavastatin, and rosuvastatin (Fig. 18.8). The initial rationale centered on a desire to simplify the structures of mevastatin and lovastatin. The 2,4-dichlorophenyl analogue (compound A) was one of the first compounds to demonstrate that this type of substitution was possible; however, compound A was considerably less potent than mevastatin. Subsequent research investigated a variety of aromatic substitutions and heterocyclic ring systems to optimize HMGRI activity. The substituted pyrrole (compound B) retained 30% of the activity of mevastatin[41] and was a key intermediate in the development of atorvastatin. The 4-fluorophenyl and isopropyl (or cyclopropane) substitutions found in compound B are also seen in the indole, quinoline, and pyrimidine ring systems of fluvastatin, pitavastatin, and rosuvastatin, respectively, and most likely represent the optimum substitutions at their respective positions. The design of all four of these compounds included the ring-opened dihydroxy acid functionality first seen in pravastatin.

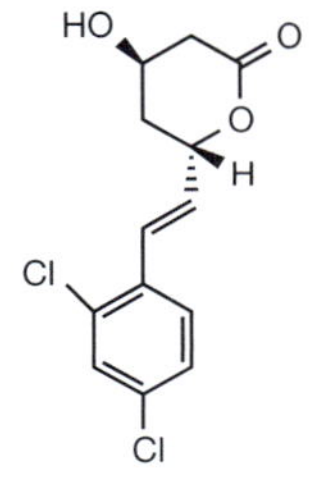

Compound A

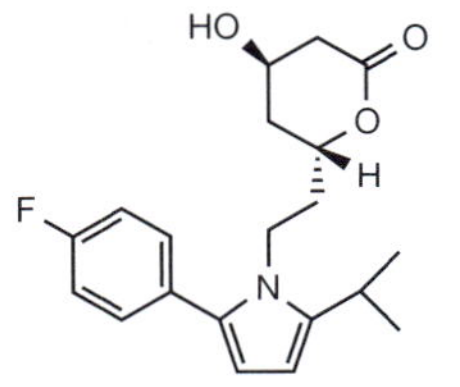

Compound B

Receptor Binding

Molecular modeling studies reported key binding interactions between the statins and HMGR.[42,43] An example illustrating the results of these studies is shown in Figure 18.9, with the binding of rosuvastatin. The 7-substituted-3,5-dihydroxyheptanoic acid is an essential structural feature for all statins. The carboxylic acid can form ionic bonds with Lys692, Arg702, and/or Lys735. The C_3-hydroxyl group can participate in an ion-dipole bond with Arg702, and the C_5-hydroxyl group can participate in an ion-dipole bond with Lys691. Other amino acids may also interact with these two hydroxyl groups, including Ser684 and Asp690 (not shown in Fig. 18.9). The hydrophobic regions of the statins participate in van der Waals interactions with Leu562, Val683, Leu853, Ala856, and Leu857. These interactions vary due to the structural differences in the individual ring systems. The *p*-fluoro group present with the heterocyclic rings of atorvastatin, fluvastatin, pitavastatin, and rosuvastatin has been shown to interact with Arg590. Additionally, these modeling studies have shown that the *p*-fluoro–substituted aromatic ring must be approximately perpendicular to the heterocyclic ring for effective receptor binding. Structural alterations that prevent rotation and cause the *p*-fluoro ring to be coplanar with the heterocyclic ring are inactive.

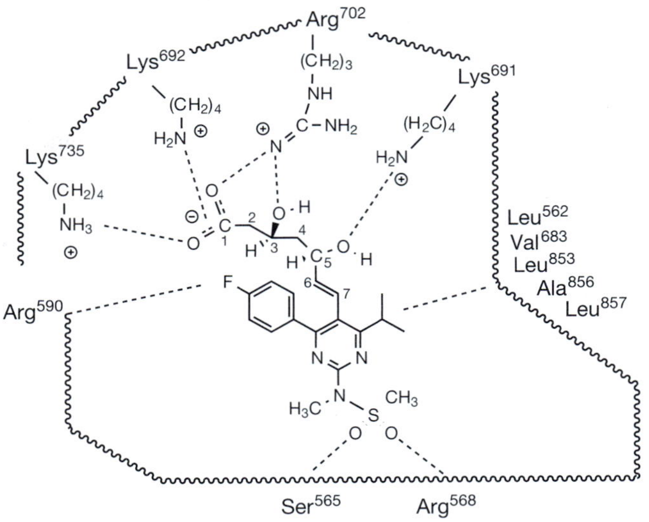

Figure 18.9 Binding interactions of rosuvastatin with HMG-CoA reductase.

Atorvastatin and rosuvastatin have additional binding interactions with Ser565 and Arg568 due to the presence of the electron-rich *N*-methyl sulfonamide of rosuvastatin and the amide of atorvastatin. As a result of these additional binding interactions, atorvastatin and rosuvastatin have the strongest overall interactions with HMG-CoA.[42,43] The enhanced binding interactions of atorvastatin and rosuvastatin correlates with their overall efficiency in lowering LDL levels. Current guidelines classify statins as either high-intensity statins, moderate-intensity statins, or low-intensity statins based on their relative abilities to lower LDL-C at prescribed doses. As seen in Table 18.3, atorvastatin and rosuvastatin can lower a patient's LDL-C by over 50% when used at their highest doses.[7,8,20]

Table 18.3 Classification of Statins by LDL-C Reduction and Dose

High-Intensity Statins *Lower LDL-C by >50%*	Moderate-Intensity Statins *Lower LDL-C by 30% to <50%*	Low-Intensity Statins *Lower LDL-C by <30%*
Atorvastatin 40-80 mg Rosuvastatin 20-40 mg	Atorvastatin 10-20 mg Fluvastatin 40 mg twice daily Fluvastatin XL 80 mg Lovastatin 40 mg Pitavastatin 2-4 mg Pravastatin 40-80 mg Rosuvastatin 5-10 mg Simvastatin 20-40 mg	Fluvastatin 20-40 mg Lovastatin 20 mg Pitavastatin 1 mg Pravastatin 10-20 mg Simvastatin 10 mg

All doses are once daily unless noted.

Statin Structure-Activity Relationships

A summary of the structure-activity relationships (SARs) for HMGRIs is presented in Table 18.4. The structures of all HMGRIs contain a 7-substituted-3,5-dihydroxyheptanoic acid, which is required for activity. Additionally, this class of drugs can be subclassified based on the nature of the C_7 ring substituent. Drugs related to the natural products mevastatin and lovastatin have structural features common to those of ring A, whereas those that are completely synthetic have structural features common to those of ring B.[38,40,41,44-50]

Physicochemical Properties

In their active forms, all HMGRIs contain a carboxylic acid. This functional group is required for inhibitory activity, has a pK_a in the range of 2.5 to 3.5, and will be primarily ionized at physiologic pH. Lovastatin and simvastatin are neutral lactone prodrugs and should be classified as nonelectrolytes. Pravastatin, fluvastatin, and atorvastatin can be classified as acidic drugs. The nitrogen atoms in the indole and pyrrole rings of fluvastatin and atorvastatin, respectively, are aromatic nitrogen atoms that are not ionizable. This is because the lone pair electrons of these atoms are involved in maintaining the aromaticity of their respective rings and are not available to bind protons. Pitavastatin and rosuvastatin are amphoteric compounds; however, their quinoline and pyrimidine rings are weakly basic and will be primarily unionized at physiologic pH.

The calculated log *P* values for the HMGRIs are shown in Table 18.5.[51,52] Although some variations exist among the values for lovastatin, pravastatin, and simvastatin, the general trends are the same, regardless of what program was used to calculate the values. Atorvastatin, fluvastatin, pitavastatin, and the prodrugs lovastatin and simvastatin have a much higher lipid solubility than either pravastatin or rosuvastatin. Hydrolysis of the lactone ring for the two prodrugs produces a 3,5-dihydroxycarboxylate, which significantly improves water solubility.

The HMG-CoA reductase enzyme is stereoselective. The 3*R*, 5*R* stereochemistry seen in the active forms of mevastatin and lovastatin (see Fig. 18.7) is required for inhibitory activity and is present in all other HMGRIs. The stereochemistry of substituents on the decalin ring system of lovastatin, simvastatin, and pravastatin is less crucial to activity, as described in Table 18.4.

Table 18.4 Structure-Activity Relationship of HMG-CoA Reductase Inhibitors

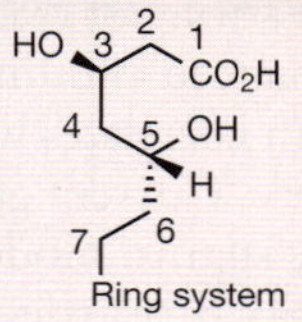

7-Substituted-3,5-dihydroxyheptanoic acid

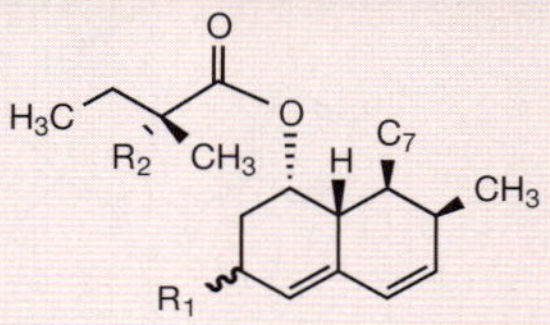

Ring A

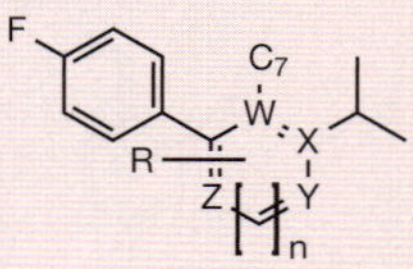

Ring B

Common for all HGMIs	1. The 3,5-dihydroxycarboxylate is essential for inhibitory activity. Drugs containing a lactone are prodrugs requiring in vivo hydrolysis. 2. The absolute stereochemistry of the 3- and 5-hydroxyl groups must be the same as that found in mevastatin and lovastatin. 3. Altering the two-carbon distance between C_5 and the ring system diminishes, or fails to improve, activity. 4. A double bond between C_6 and C_7 can either increase or decrease activity. The ethyl group provides optimal activity for compounds containing ring A and some heterocyclic rings (eg, pyrrole ring of atorvastatin). The ethenyl group is optimal for compounds with other ring systems, including the indole, quinoline, and pyrimidine rings seen in fluvastatin, pitavastatin, and rosuvastatin, respectively.
Ring A subclass	1. The decalin ring is essential for anchoring the drug to the enzyme active site. Replacement with a cyclohexane ring resulted in a 10,000-fold decrease in activity. 2. Stereochemistry of the ester side chain is not important for activity; however, conversion of this ester to an ether results in a decrease in activity. 3. Methyl substitution at the R_2 position increases activity (ie, simvastatin is more potent than lovastatin). 4. β-Hydroxyl group substitution at the R_1 position enhances hydrophilicity and may provide some cellular specificity.
Ring B subclass	1. Substituents W, X, Y, and Z can be either carbon or nitrogen; n is equal to either zero or one (ie, five- or six-member heterocyclic). 2. The *p*-fluorophenyl cannot be coplanar with the central aromatic ring. (Structural restraints to cause coplanarity have resulted in a loss of activity.) 3. R substitution with aryl groups, hydrocarbon chains, amides, or sulfonamides enhances lipophilicity and inhibitory activity.

Table 18.5 Pharmacokinetic Parameters of HMG-CoA Reductase Inhibitors

Drug	Calculated log P[a]	Oral Bioavailability (%)	Active Metabolite(s)	Protein Binding (%)	Time to Peak Concentration (h)	Elimination Half-Life (h)	Major Route(s) of Elimination
Atorvastatin	4.13	12-14	*o*- and *p*-hydroxylated	98	1-2	14-19	Biliary/fecal (>90%) Renal (<2%)
Fluvastatin	3.62	20-30	None	98	0.5-1.0	1	Biliary/fecal (95%) Renal (5%)
Lovastatin	4.07 (4.04)[b]	5	3,5-Dihydroxy acid	>95	2	3-4	Fecal (83%) Renal (10%)
Pravastatin	1.44 (0.5)[b]	17	None	43-55	1.0-1.5	2-3	Fecal (70%) Renal (20%)
Pitavastatin	3.45	51	None	>99	1	12	Fecal (79%) Renal (15%)
Rosuvastatin	0.42	20	*N*-Desmethyl	88	3-5	19-20	Fecal (90%) Renal (10%)
Simvastatin	4.42 (4.2)[b]	5	3,5-Dihydroxy acid	95	4	3	Fecal (60%) Renal (13%)

[a]A commercial program was used for calculated values.[47]
[b]Calculated using the CLOG program.[48]

Metabolism

Lovastatin and simvastatin are inactive prodrugs that must undergo in vivo hydrolysis to produce their effects (see Fig. 18.7). The active forms of these two drugs as well as most HMGRIs undergo extensive first-pass metabolism.[26-29,53] The CYP3A4 isozyme is responsible for the oxidative metabolism of atorvastatin, lovastatin, and simvastatin. In the case of atorvastatin, the *o*- and *p*-hydroxylated metabolites are equiactive with the parent compound and contribute significantly to the overall activity of the drug (Table 18.5). Rosuvastatin is metabolized to a limited extent by CYP2C9 to form an N-desmethyl metabolite that can contribute to activity but is 7-fold less potent. Approximately 90% of rosuvastatin is excreted unchanged. In contrast, the activity of lovastatin and simvastatin resides primarily in the initial hydrolysis product. Further oxidation decreases activity. Fluvastatin is metabolized by the CYP2C9 and CYP3A4 isozymes to active hydroxylated metabolites; however, these metabolites do not circulate systemically and do not contribute to the overall activity. Pravastatin also undergoes oxidative metabolism, but the resulting metabolites retain only minimal activity and are not significant. Neither pitavastatin, pravastatin, nor rosuvastatin is metabolized by CYP3A4; therefore, these drugs are potentially advantageous for patients who must take concurrent medication that alters the activity of this isozyme. Pitavastatin is primarily metabolized by glucuronide conjugation, with oxidative metabolism by CYP2C9 and CYP2C8 representing a minor metabolic pathway. As shown in Figure 8.10, the initial glucuronide conjugate undergoes reversible lactonization to regenerate the active drug. This metabolic process contributes to the enhanced duration of pitavastatin's action.[54,55]

Pharmacokinetic Properties

The pharmacokinetic parameters and dosing information for HMGRIs are summarized in Tables 18.5 and 18.6,[7,8,23,26-29,52,53] respectively. With a few exceptions, these drugs have similar onsets of action, durations of action, dosing intervals, and plasma protein binding.

Despite the ability to attain a peak plasma concentration in 1 to 4 hours, HMGRIs require approximately 2 weeks to demonstrate an initial lowering of plasma cholesterol. Peak reductions of plasma cholesterol occur after 4 to 6 weeks of therapy for most compounds. Studies with atorvastatin, however, indicate that it may only need 2 weeks to produce its peak reduction. Atorvastatin, rosuvastatin, and pitavastatin are also unique in that they have much longer durations of action than the other compounds. With the exception of pravastatin, which is one of the more hydrophilic drugs in this class, most HMGRIs bind extensively to plasma proteins.

Because of first-pass metabolism, the oral bioavailability of this class of drugs generally is low and does not reflect the actual absorption of the individual drugs. For example, 60% to 80% of a dose of simvastatin is orally absorbed, but only 5% is available to produce an effect. The same is true with fluvastatin, pravastatin, and lovastatin, which have oral absorptions of 90%, 34%, and 35%, respectively, but have much lower bioavailability. Pitavastatin has the highest oral bioavailability in this class of compounds (see Table 18.5). With the exception of lovastatin, the concurrent administration of food does

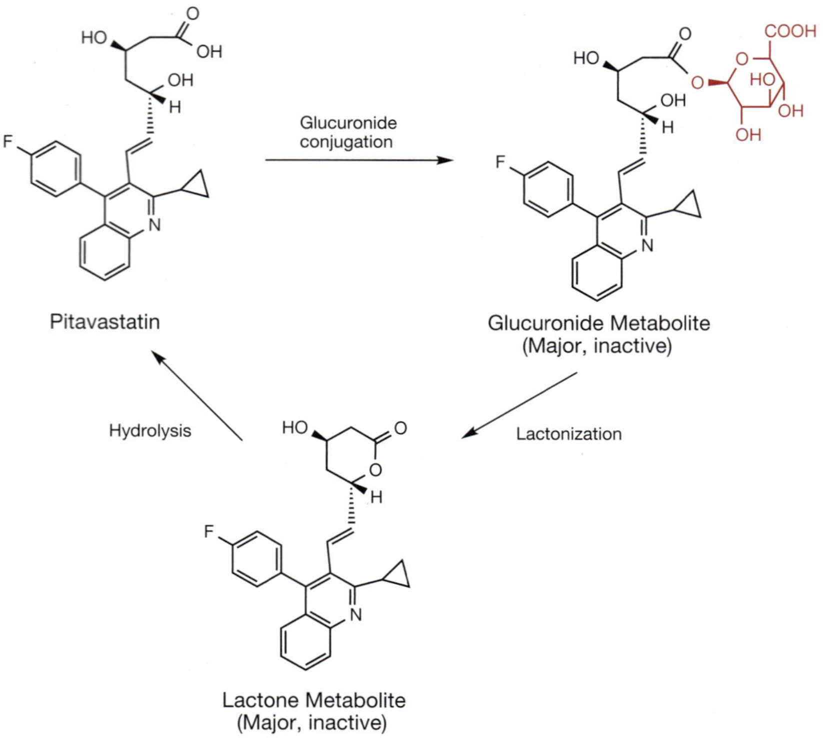

Figure 18.10 Metabolism and reversible lactonization of pitavastatin.

Table 18.6 Dosing Information for HMG-CoA Reductase Inhibitors

Generic Name	Brand Name(s)[a]	Dosing Range	Maximum Daily Dose	Dose Reduction with Renal Dysfunction	Tablet Strengths (mg)
Atorvastatin	Lipitor Atorvaliq	10-80 mg once daily	80 mg	No	10, 20, 40, 80 (oral suspension: 20 mg/5 mL)
Fluvastatin	Lescol XL	20-80 mg once daily or b.i.d.	80 mg	Caution in severe impairment	20, 40, 80 (XR)
Lovastatin	Altoprev	20-80 mg once daily	80 mg (60 mg if XR)	Only with severe impairment	10, 20, 40, 20 (XR), 40 (XR), 60 (XR)
Pitavastatin	Livalo Zypitamag	1-4 mg once daily	4 mg	Yes	1, 2, 4
Pravastatin	Pravachol	10-80 mg once daily	80 mg	Yes	10, 20, 40, 80
Rosuvastatin	Crestor Ezallor Sprinkle	5-40 mg once daily	40 mg (10 mg with fibrate)	Only with severe impairment	5, 10, 20, 40
Simvastatin	Zocor FloLipid	5-40 mg once daily	80 mg	Only with severe impairment	5, 10, 20, 40, 80 (Oral suspension: 20 mg/5 mL; 40 mg/5 mL)

b.i.d., twice a day; XR, extended release.
[a]Brand names are USA only.

not affect the overall therapeutic effects of HMGRIs. Lovastatin should always be administered with food to maximize oral bioavailability. Failure to do this results in a 33% decrease in plasma concentrations. In general, HMGRIs should be administered in the evening or at bedtime to counteract the peak cholesterol synthesis, which occurs in the early morning hours. Exceptions to this are atorvastatin, rosuvastatin, and pitavastatin, which, because of their long half-lives, are equally effective regardless of when they are administered. The primary route of elimination of these compounds is through the feces. Because of extensive hepatic transformation and the ability to elevate hepatic enzymes, HMGRIs are contraindicated in patients with active hepatic disease or unexplained persistent elevations in serum aminotransferase concentrations. Dosage reductions in patients with renal dysfunction depend on the individual drug. Atorvastatin, which has minimal renal excretion, requires no dosage reduction and may be the best agent for patients with renal disorders. Fluvastatin, rosuvastatin, and simvastatin require dosage reductions only in cases of severe renal impairment and are better choices than lovastatin, pitavastatin, and pravastatin, which require dosage reductions in mild or moderate impairment.

Cholesterol Absorption Inhibitor

Mechanism of Action

Ezetimibe (Zetia), currently the only drug to act via this mechanism, lowers plasma cholesterol levels by inhibiting the absorption of cholesterol at the brush border of the small intestine.[7,55,56] Specifically, ezetimibe binds to the sterol transporter, Niemann-Pick C1-like 1 (NPC1L1). This transporter is located in the epithelial cells of small intestine and is required for the intestinal uptake of cholesterol and phytosterols. Ezetimibe appears to be selective in its actions in that it does not interfere with the absorption of triglycerides, lipid-soluble vitamins, or other nutrients. The decreased absorption of cholesterol eventually leads to enhanced receptor-mediated LDL uptake similar to that seen with HMGRIs. When used as monotherapy, the decreased absorption of cholesterol causes a compensatory increase in cholesterol biosynthesis; however, it is insufficient to override the overall LDL-lowering effects of ezetimibe. Overall, ezetimibe has been shown to reduce LDL-C levels by 15% to 20% and can be used in combination with statin therapy.[7,8]

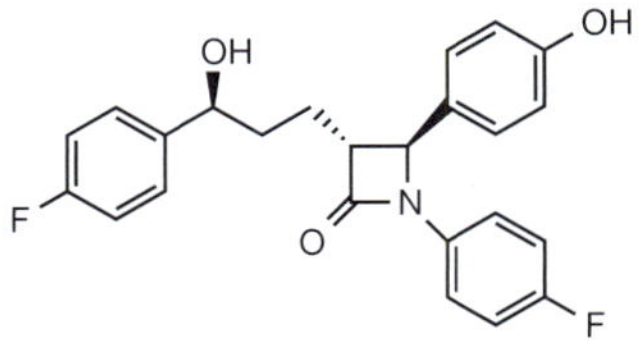

Ezetimibe

Common Adverse Effects and Drug Interactions

Ezetimibe generally is well tolerated. The most common adverse effects are abdominal pain, diarrhea, back pain, cough, pharyngitis, sinusitis, fatigue, and viral infection. More serious adverse effects, such as rhabdomyolysis, hepatitis, pancreatitis, and thrombocytopenia, have been reported, but causal relationships have not been established. In one clinical study, the incidence of adverse effects when used in combination with an HMGRI was similar to that seen with HMGRI monotherapy.[23,26,57]

Drug interactions for ezetimibe are listed in Table 18.7.

Receptor Binding and Structure-Activity Relationship

The 1,4-diaryl-β-lactam ring is essential for the binding of ezetimibe to NPC1L1. Hydrolysis of the β-lactam ring or the use of larger lactam rings produce inactive compounds. It has been proposed that this ring primarily serves as a scaffold to orient the two aromatic rings and the aliphatic chain for optimum receptor affinity. The phenolic and aliphatic hydroxyl groups enhance activity, although a *p*-methoxy group has also been shown to be active. The hydrophilic nature of these two functional groups is important for helping ezetimibe localize in the small intestine. The *p*-fluoro group prevents aromatic oxidation and thus prolongs the duration of action.[58,59]

Physicochemical Properties

Ezetimibe is a crystalline powder that is practically insoluble in water but is freely soluble in ethanol and other organic solvents. Its calculated log P value is 3.50.[52] The phenol present in ezetimibe allows this compound to be classified as acidic; however, the phenol has a pK_a of 9.72 and is predominantly unionized at physiologic pH.

Metabolism

After oral administration, ezetimibe is rapidly and extensively metabolized in the intestinal wall and the liver via conjugation to a phenolic glucuronide (Fig. 18.11). Both ezetimibe and its glucuronide conjugate are active, with the conjugated metabolite comprising 80% to 90% of the plasma drug levels. The glucuronide metabolite is excreted in the bile back to

Table 18.7 Drug Interactions for Ezetimibe

Drug	Result of Interaction
Bile acid sequestrants	Decreased bioavailability of ezetimibe if administration is not adequately spaced
Cyclosporine	Increased ezetimibe plasma concentration
Fibrates	Increased ezetimibe plasma concentration and possible increased risk of cholelithiasis. With the exception of fenofibrate, concomitant use is not recommended
Inhibitors of OATP1B1/1B3	May increase the ezetimibe plasma concentration

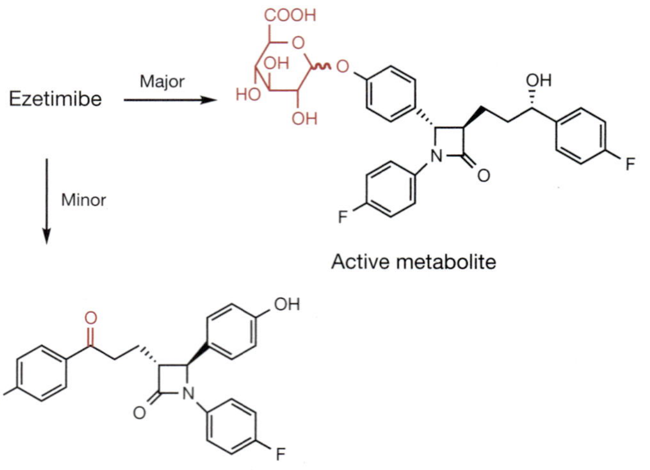

Figure 18.11 Metabolism of ezetimibe to its active and inactive metabolites.

its active site. A small amount (<5%) of ezetimibe undergoes oxidation to convert the benzylic hydroxyl group to a ketone; however, ezetimibe does not appear to exert any significant effect on the activity of CYP450 enzymes.[26,53,56]

Pharmacokinetic Properties

Ezetimibe is administered orally; however, its absolute bioavailability cannot be determined because of its aqueous insolubility and the lack of an injectable formulation. Based on its area under the curve values, the oral absorption ranges from 35% to 60%. Mean peak concentrations of the active glucuronide metabolite are reached within 1 to 2 hours. Both ezetimibe and its glucuronide conjugate are extensively bound (>90%) to plasma proteins. The relative plasma concentrations of ezetimibe and its glucuronide conjugate range from 10% to 20% and from 80% to 90%, respectively. Both compounds have a long half-life of approximately 22 hours. The coadministration of food with ezetimibe has no effect on the extent of absorption. The normal dose of ezetimibe is 10 mg once daily. Dosage reduction for patients with renal impairment, intermittent hemodialysis, or mild hepatic impairment is not necessary. Because of insufficient data, the use of ezetimibe is not recommended in patients with moderate to severe hepatic impairment.[7,26,53]

Proprotein Convertase Subtilisin/Kexin Type 9 Inhibitors

The hepatic enzyme PCSK9 is involved in cholesterol homeostasis. The binding of this enzyme to LDL receptors leads to their degradation and an overall increase in plasma LDL-C levels.[7,60] Inhibition of this enzyme can be accomplished by using monoclonal antibodies or small, interfering ribonucleic acid (siRNA).

Monoclonal Antibodies

Alirocumab (Praluent) and evolocumab (Repatha) are human monoclonal immunoglobulin G (IgG) antibodies that bind to PCSK9 and inhibits its action. Both drugs have been approved for treatment of hypercholesterolemia in individuals with severe forms of hereditary high cholesterol who cannot tolerate or who do not exhibit sufficient LDL lowering by HMGRIs.

Mechanism of Action

The normal function of circulating PCSK9 is to bind to LDL receptors located on the surface of hepatocytes. Internalization of the resulting complex leads to LDL receptor destruction and the inability of the liver to remove LDL from the plasma. This in turn increases plasma LDL cholesterol. While this regulatory function is crucial for maintaining normal plasma LDL levels in healthy patients, it can contribute to hypercholesterolemia in other patients. Both alirocumab and evolocumab inhibit the binding of PCSK9 to LDL receptors, thus increasing the number of functional LDL receptors available to clear plasma LDL and lower LDL-C.[7,23,61]

Common Adverse Effects and Drug Interactions

Alirocumab and evolocumab are well tolerated but can cause injection site reactions, muscle aches, rash, and itching. Flu-like symptoms, nasopharyngitis, allergic skin reactions, and cognitive effects (ie, confusion, dementia, and memory impairment) may also occur. To date, there are no reported drug interactions with either alirocumab or evolocumab.[7,26,62,63]

Receptor Binding and Structure-Activity Relationship

Similar to other antibodies, alirocumab and evolocumab are proteins composed of two heavy chains linked through disulfide bonds to two light chains. The two heavy chains are also linked together through a disulfide bond. The fragment antigen binding (Fab) regions on both of these drugs have complementary binding areas, which allow the antibodies to bind to a specific site on PCSK9 and, thus, prevent it from binding to LDL receptors.[62,63]

Physicochemical and Pharmacokinetic Properties

Both alirocumab and evolocumab are human monoclonal antibodies, a specialized type of proteins. The molecular weights of these drugs are approximately 146 and 144 kDa, respectively. Neither of these drugs is orally active and they must be administered as a subcutaneous (SC) injection. They require approximately 3 to 7 days to achieve peak serum concentrations.[62,63]

Due to their peptidic nature, metabolism occurs via degradation to smaller peptides and amino acids.

Small, Interfering Ribonucleic Acid

Inclisiran (Leqvio) is the first siRNA to be approved by the FDA. The normal function of an siRNA is to target and cleave a specific messenger RNA (mRNA).[64] Inclisiran (Fig. 18.12) is a synthetic siRNA that selectively targets the mRNA of PCSK9, resulting in a decreased production of the enzyme, a decrease in the degradation of LDL receptors, and an

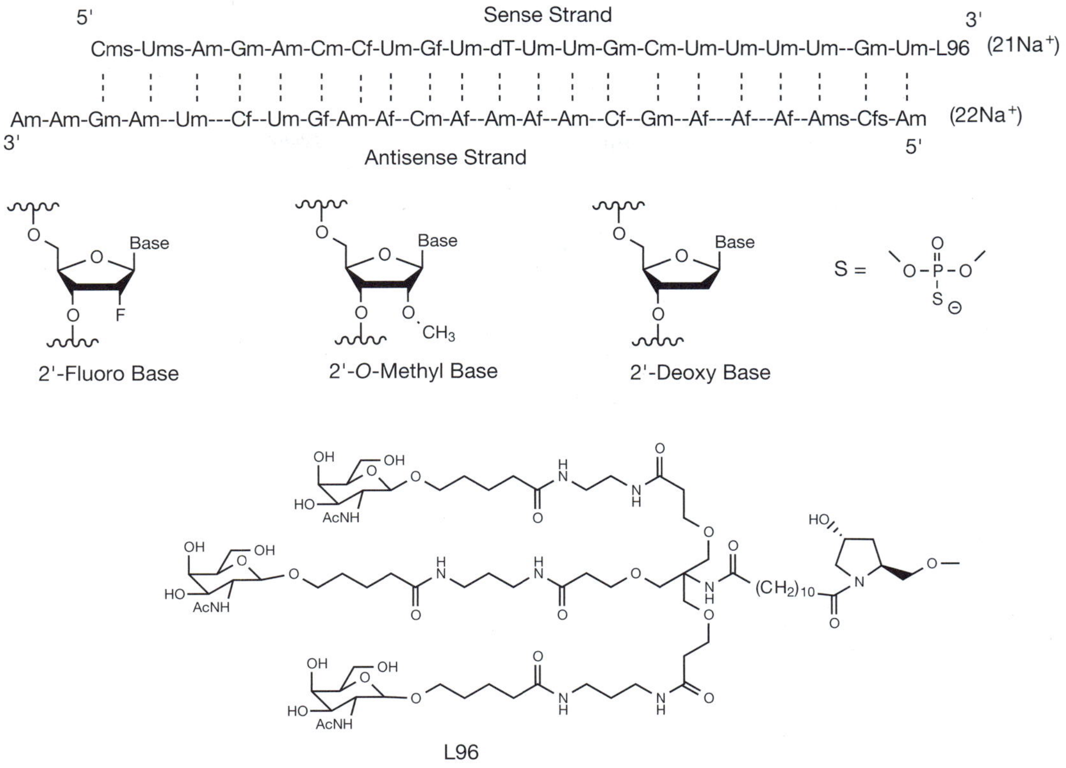

Figure 18.12 Structure of inclisiran. The f, m, and s designations next to the nucleotides indicate the presence of a 2′-F sugar, a 2′-*O*-methyl sugar, and a phosphorothiolate linker, respectively.

overall decrease in plasma LDL-C.[65,66] Inclisiran is approved as an adjunct to diet and statin therapy for the treatment of adults with heterozygous familial hypercholesterolemia (HeFH) who require additional lowering of LDL-C.[26]

Mechanism of Action

The synthetically modified double-stranded siRNA allows it to selectively target hepatocytes and degrade PCSK9 mRNA. This mechanism is illustrated in Figure 18.13 and involves six steps. The sense strand of inclisiran is conjugated to a triantennary *N*-acetylgalactosamine (GalNAc) ligand, identified as L96 (Fig. 18.12). The initial step in this mechanism involves the binding of the GalNAc ligand to the asialoglycoprotein receptor (ASGPR), a receptor that is expressed primarily on hepatocytes. Once bound, the siRNA-GalNAc complex enters the hepatocyte through endocytosis (step 2). Within the endosome, the GalNAc portion of the complex is removed and degraded, and the ASGPR is recycled,

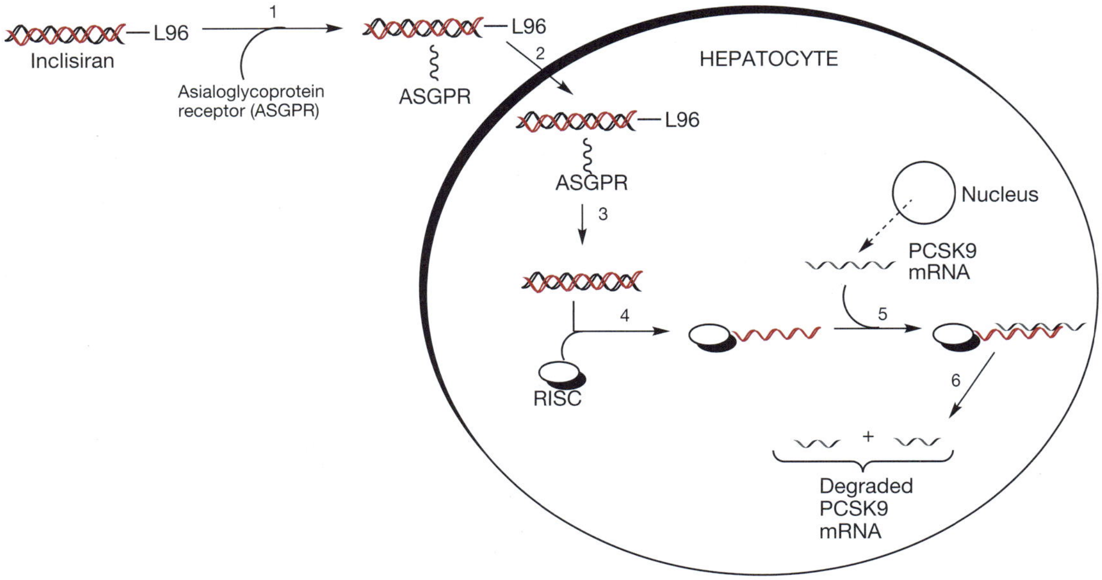

Figure 18.13 Mechanism of action of inclisiran.

leaving only the siRNA portion of inclisiran (step 3). The siRNA is slowly released to the cytoplasm of the hepatocyte and binds to the RNA-induced silencing complex (RISC). Once bound to the RISC, the sense strand of inclisiran is degraded, leaving only a single antisense strand (step 4). Using this antisense strand, the RISC scans the cytoplasm for the complementary mRNA for PCSK9. The mRNA for PCSK9 then binds with the antisense strand of inclisiran (step 5), and the RISC degrades it (step 6). The overall effect of these actions is a decrease in the amount of the PCSK9 enzyme, a decrease in the degradation of LDL-C receptors, and an increased ability of the hepatocyte to remove LDL-C from the plasma.[66,67]

Common Adverse Effects and Drug Interactions

Inclisiran is generally well tolerated. The most common adverse effects are injection site reactions, which can include erythema, pain, or a rash. Other adverse effects are arthralgia, antibody development, and bronchitis. There are no known drug interactions.[26,67]

Receptor Binding and Structure-Activity Relationship

As discussed in the mechanism of action section, the tri-antennary GalNAc ligand (L96) is essential for the binding of inclisiran to ASGPR and its ability to selectively enter the hepatocyte. The structure of inclisiran is composed of 44 nucleotides, one with a normal deoxyribose sugar, 11 with a modified 2′-fluoro sugar, and 32 with a modified 2′-O-methyl sugar. Additionally, six phosphodiester bonds are modified to phosphorothiolate bonds. These structural modifications were made to decrease the degradation of the RNA by nucleases. These types of modifications are a known chemical strategy to enhance the duration of action of nucleotide-based drugs.[66-68]

Physicochemical and Pharmacokinetic Properties

Inclisiran is a modified nucleotide and contains 43 acidic phosphate or thiophosphate functional groups that are formulated as their respective sodium salts. Due to its size and hydrophilicity, inclisiran is not orally active and is administered as a subcutaneous injection. Once inclisiran enters the hepatic cells, it has a long duration of action due to its slow release from endosomes and its binding to RISC. The half-life of a single dose of inclisiran is approximately 9 hours; however, its long duration allows it to be initially dosed every 3 months and then once every 6 months. Inclisiran is 87% plasma protein bound, and is metabolized by nucleases to form smaller nucleotides of varying lengths.[26,49,69]

Bempedoic Acid

Bempedoic acid (Nexletol) provides adjunct therapy in adult patients with HeFH who are on maximally tolerated statin therapy and require additional lowering of LDL-C. Bempedoic acid is available either as a single agent or in combination with ezetimibe.

Mechanism of Action

Bempedoic acid is a prodrug that is activated by the addition of coenzyme A, as shown in Figure 18.14. The enzyme responsible for this activation is known as very-long-chain acyl CoA synthetase-1 (ACSVL1). This enzyme is primarily expressed in the liver and is absent in adipose tissue and muscles. The active metabolite, bempedoyl-CoA, inhibits ATP-citrate lyase (ACL), an enzyme upstream of HMG-CoA reductase in the cholesterol biosynthesis pathway. Specifically, ACL catalyzes the cleavage of citrate to acetyl-CoA and oxaloacetate, and links carbohydrate metabolism in the liver to the synthetic pathways for cholesterol and fatty acids. The inhibition of ACL by bempedoic acid decreases cholesterol and fatty acid synthesis, resulting in the upregulation of LDL-C receptors, increased uptake of LDL-C by the liver, and reduced blood LDL-C levels. The end point of this mechanism, the upregulation of LDL-C receptors, is the same as that seen with the HMGRIs.[70,71]

Common Adverse Effects and Drug Interactions

Bempedoic acid appears to be well tolerated. The most common adverse effects, in order of frequency, are upper respiratory tract infection, muscle spasms, hyperuricemia, back pain, abdominal pain or discomfort, bronchitis, pain in extremity, anemia, and elevated liver enzymes. The ability of bempedoic acid to inhibit renal tubular OATP2 and increase serum uric acid levels is responsible for hyperuricemia. Bempedoic acid has also been associated with an increased risk of benign prostatic hyperplasia and tendon rupture; however, instances of these effects are seen in less than 1% of patients.

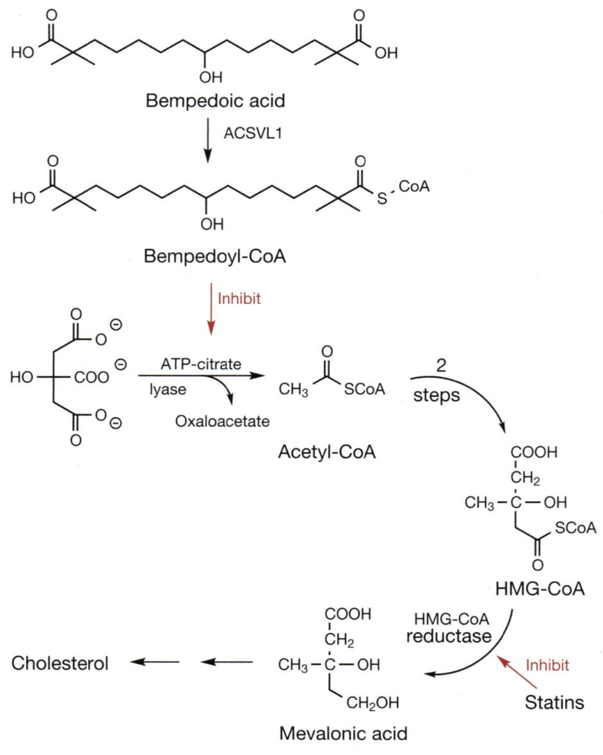

Figure 18.14 Mechanism of action of bempedoic acid and its comparison to the statins in inhibiting cholesterol biosynthesis.

Bempedoic acid and its glucuronide metabolite weakly inhibit OATP1B1 and have the potential to causes drug interactions with HMGRIs. Studies examining the coadministration of bempedoic acid with simvastatin, pravastatin, atorvastatin, and rosuvastatin found that bempedoic acid increased the plasma concentrations of simvastatin and pravastatin, but not atorvastatin or rosuvastatin. Specific dosing parameters have been established for simvastatin and rosuvastatin when taken in combination with bempedoic acid.[23,26,27]

Since the activation of bempedoic acid by ACSVL1 occurs in the liver and is absent in skeletal muscle cells, bempedoic acid may be a potential option for patients with statin-associated muscle symptoms.

Receptor Binding and Structure-Activity Relationship

As shown in Figure 18.14, bempedoic acid is a symmetrical fatty acid. Activation of one of these carboxylic acids with ACSVL1 allows it to mimic an intermediate in the mechanism of ATP-citrate lyase and cause inhibition.[72,73] Similar to citric acid, the structure of bempedoic acid contains two terminal carboxylic acids and a hydroxyl group in the center of molecule. While bempedoic acid is much larger than citric acid, it is flexible and can bind to its target enzyme, causing inhibition. The dimethyl groups adjacent to both carboxylic acids prevent the active CoA form of bempedoic acid from undergoing β-oxidation.

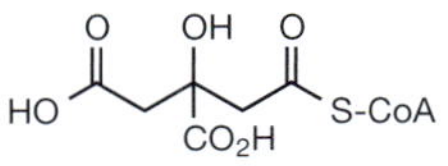

Intermediate in ATP-citrate lyase mechanism

Physicochemical and Pharmacokinetic Properties

Bempedoic acid is an acidic drug. The approximate pK_a values for the carboxylic acid functional groups are 4.4. It also contains a significant amount of lipid solubility due to the hydrocarbon chain and the methyl groups. The log P value is 3.65, and it is greater than 99% plasma protein bound. Bempedoic acid is administered orally, with the maximum concentration reached after 3.5 hours and a duration that allows once daily dosing. Bempedoic acid is reversibly converted to an active ketone metabolite (ESP15228), and both the parent drug and the ketone metabolite undergo glucuronide conjugation to inactive metabolites. Glucuronide conjugation sites highlighted in red below.[26,69]

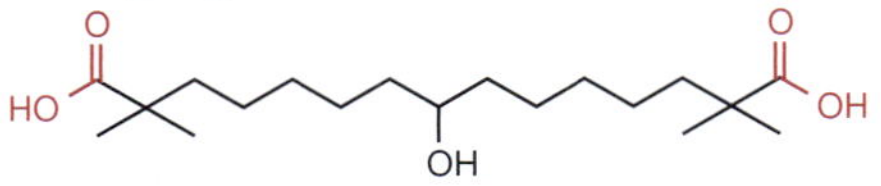

Bempedoic acid

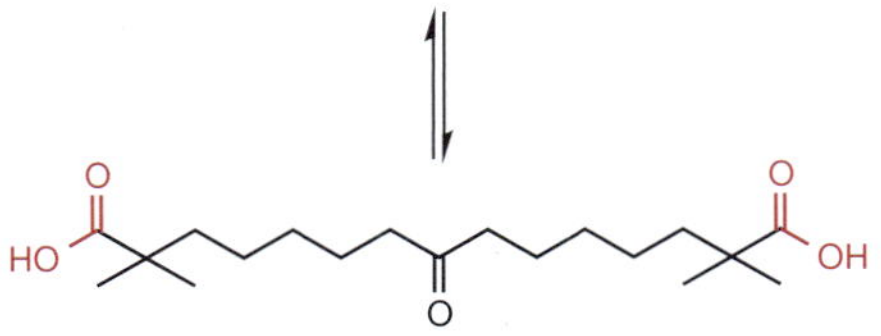

ESP15228

Bile Acid Sequestrants

Cholestyramine (Questran, Prevalite) was originally developed in the 1960s to treat pruritus secondary to elevated plasma concentrations of bile acids in patients with cholestasis. Its ability to bind (ie, to hold or to sequester) bile acids and to increase their fecal elimination was subsequently shown to produce beneficial effects in lowering serum cholesterol levels.

Mechanism of Action

Cholestyramine, colestipol (Colestid), and colesevelam (Welchol) lower plasma LDL levels by indirectly increasing the rate at which LDL is cleared from the bloodstream. Under normal circumstances, approximately 97% of bile acids are reabsorbed into the enterohepatic circulation. As previously discussed, bile acids are returned to the liver where they regulate their own production. Bile acid sequestrants are not orally absorbed but act locally within the gastrointestinal tract to interrupt this process. They bind the two major bile acids, glycocholic acid and taurocholic acid, and greatly increase their fecal excretion. As a result, decreased concentrations of these compounds are returned to the liver. This removes the feedback inhibition of 7α-hydroxylase and increases the hepatic conversion of cholesterol to bile acids (see Fig. 18.3). The decrease in hepatic cholesterol concentrations causes an increased expression of LDL receptors and an increased hepatic uptake of plasma LDL similar to that previously described for HMGRIs, ezetimibe, and bempedoic acid. Compensatory responses also lead to the induction of HMG-CoA reductase and increased biosynthesis of cholesterol; however, similar to ezetimibe, these effects are insufficient to counteract the decrease in plasma LDL. The combination use of a bile acid sequestrant with an HMGRI will counter this compensatory response and provide and additive effect in lowering LDL cholesterol.[7,26,74,75]

The decreased return of bile acids to the liver will also produce an increase in triglyceride synthesis and a transient rise in VLDL levels; however, the increased expression of LDL receptors will eventually return VLDL levels to originally observed levels. One exception to this is seen in patients with preexisting hypertriglyceridemia. For these patients, the increase in LDL receptors is inadequate to counter the rise in VLDL levels.[7]

Common Adverse Effects

Because bile acid sequestrants are not orally absorbed, they produce minimal systemic side effects and, thus, are one of the safest drugs to use for hypercholesterolemia. Constipation is by far the most frequent patient concern. Increasing dietary fiber or using bulk-producing laxatives, such as psyllium, often can minimize this adverse effect. Other GI symptoms include bloating, heartburn, nausea, eructation, and abdominal discomfort. These adverse effects usually dissipate with continued use; however, the possibility of fecal impaction requires that extreme caution be used in patients with preexisting constipation.[23,26]

Common Drug Interactions

Because of their mechanism of action, bile acid sequestrants can potentially bind with and decrease the oral absorption of almost any other drug. Because these drugs contain numerous positive charges, they are much more likely to bind to acidic compounds (which have anionic conjugate bases) than to basic compounds or nonelectrolytes. This is not an absolute, however, because cholestyramine and colestipol have been reported to decrease the oral absorption of propranolol (a basic drug with a cationic conjugate acid) and the lipid-soluble vitamins A, D, E, and K (nonelectrolytes). As a result, the current recommendation is that all other oral medication should be administered at least 1 hour before or 4 hours after cholestyramine and colestipol. Colesevelam seems to be less likely to interfere with the absorption of concurrently administered drugs; however, drugs that have not been studied in combination with colesevelam should be spaced similar to cholestyramine and colestipol.[7,23,26]

Receptor Binding and Structure-Activity Relationship

Cholestyramine, colestipol, and colesevelam (Fig. 18.15) do not bind to specific receptors but rather to negatively charged atoms or functional groups present on drug molecules or biomolecules. Since they can selectively bind and exchange negatively charged atoms and molecules, they are chemically classified as anion-exchange resins. The selectivity comes from the fact that these positively charged resins do not bind equally to all anions. For example, the chloride ion of cholestyramine can be displaced by, or exchanged with, other anions (eg, bile acids) that have a greater affinity for the positively charged functional groups on the resin.

All three of these drugs are large polycationic polymers. Cholestyramine is a copolymer consisting primarily of polystyrene, divinylbenzene, and approximately 4 mEq of fixed quaternary ammonium groups per gram of dry resin. Colestipol is a copolymer of tetraethylenepentamine and epichlorohydrin, and is commercially marked as its hydrochloride salt. The key functional groups on colestipol are the basic secondary and tertiary amines.

Colesevelam is a more diverse polymer containing four different basic and/or quaternary fragments; however, similar to colestipol, epichlorohydrin acts to cross-link these fragments. The key structural feature of all three of these polymers is the presence of multiple basic (and, therefore, potentially cationic at gastrointestinal pH) or quaternary functional groups that can bind to negatively charged atoms or functional groups.[7,26,27]

Physicochemical Properties

All bile acid sequestrants are large, hygroscopic, water-insoluble resins. The molecular weight of cholestyramine is reported to be greater than 1,000,000 Da; however,

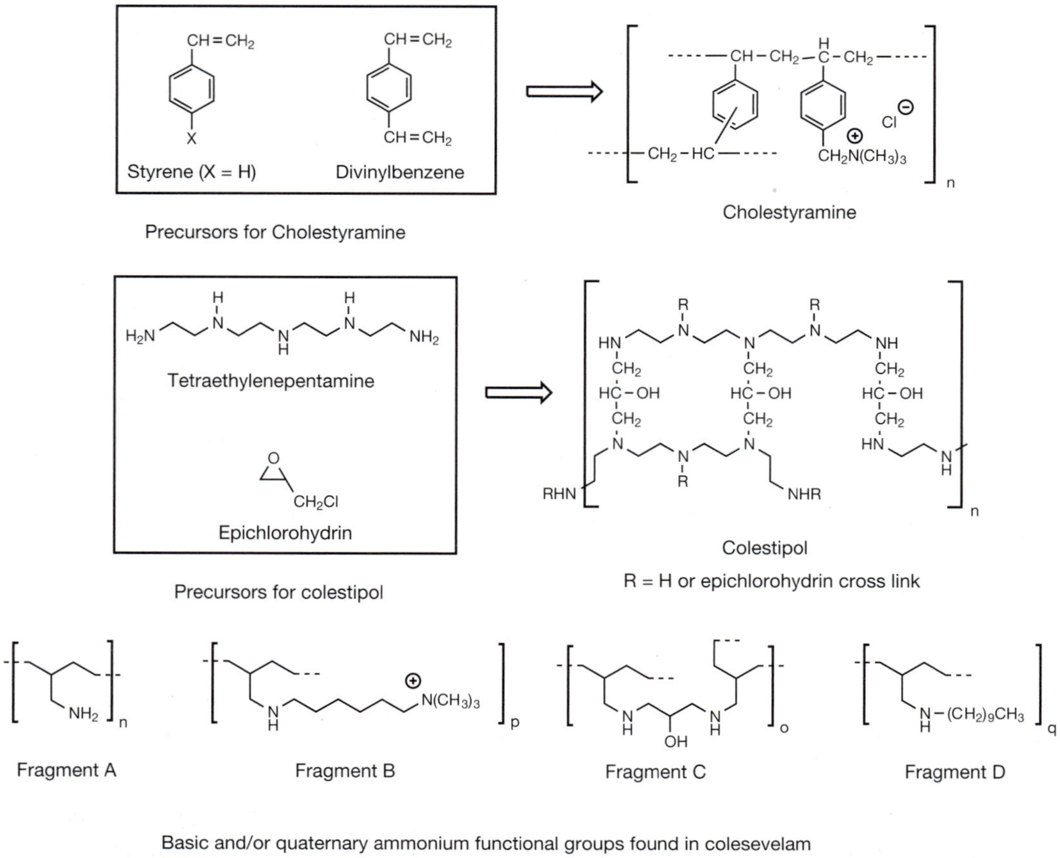

Figure 18.15 Structures of cholestyramine, colestipol, and precursors for these polymeric resins. Also included are the basic and quaternary functional groups found on colesevelam. Note that cholestyramine will contain a fraction of unsubstituted aromatic rings (ie, those that are neither cross-linked nor contain a quaternary ammonium group).

no specific molecular weight has been assigned to either colestipol or colesevelam. Cholestyramine contains a large number of quaternary ammonium groups and has multiple permanent positive charges. Colestipol contains a large number of secondary and tertiary amines, whereas colesevelam contains quaternary ammonium groups as well as primary and secondary amines. Normal pKa values for the amines range from 9.0 to 10.5; thus, all of these functional groups should be primarily ionized and positively charged at intestinal pH.

Metabolism and Pharmacokinetic Properties

Cholestyramine, colestipol, and colesevelam are not orally absorbed and are not metabolized by gastrointestinal enzymes. They are excreted in the feces as an insoluble complex with bile acids. Their onset of action occurs within 24 to 48 hours; however, it may take up to 1 month to achieve peak response.[7,26,53] Cholestyramine is available as a powder that is mixed with water, juice, or other noncarbonated beverages to create a slurry to drink. Colestipol is available as either granules or 1-g tablets. The granules should be taken in a manner similar to that described for the cholestyramine powder. Colesevelam is available as a 625-mg tablet and a 3.75-g powder for suspension. Both formulations should be taken with a meal.

ORPHAN DRUGS FOR THE TREATMENT OF HOMOZYGOUS FAMILIAL HYPERCHOLESTEROLEMIA

Homozygous familial hypercholesterolemia (HoFH) results from genetic mutations of the LDL receptor in both parents. Patients with HoFH can develop severe hypercholesterolemia within the first two decades of life and can develop accelerated atherosclerosis and CHD. The overall prevalence of HoFH is one case in a million individuals. In comparison, the overall prevalence of HeFH is one case in 500 individuals.[76]

Lomitapide, mipomersen, and evinacumab have been approved for the treatment of this rare genetic disorder. According to current therapeutic guidelines, these drugs are indicated for patients with HoFH who have a baseline LDL-C of at least 190 mg/dL and who have had an inadequate response to statins with or without ezetimibe and PCSK9 inhibitors.[20]

Lomitapide

Mechanism of Action

Lomitapide (Juxtapid) exerts its mechanism of action by inhibiting the microsomal triglyceride transport protein (MTTP) located in the lumen of the endoplasmic reticulum. This prevents the assembly of apoB-containing lipoproteins (ie, VLDL and LDL) in both hepatocytes and enterocytes. The overall result of these actions is an initial decrease in the synthesis of chylomicrons and VLDL and an ultimate reduction in plasma LDL cholesterol.[7,23,26]

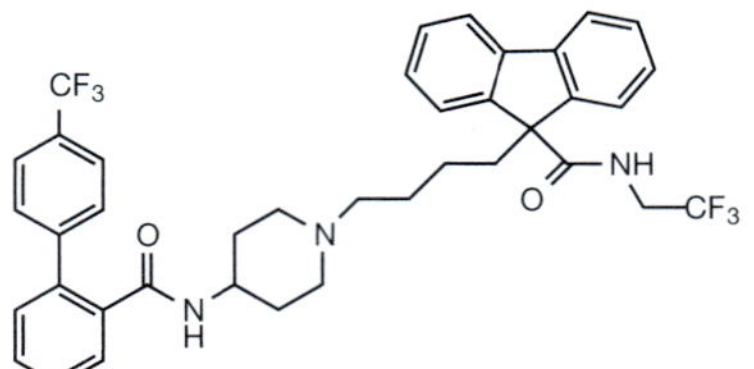

Lomitapide

Common Adverse Effects and Drug Interactions

The most commonly seen adverse effects of lomitapide involve the GI tract and include abdominal discomfort, abdominal distension, abdominal pain, constipation, diarrhea, flatulence, gastroenteritis, gastroesophageal reflux disorder (GERD), nausea, and vomiting. The most serious adverse effect is an increased risk of hepatotoxicity.

Lomitapide normally undergoes oxidative metabolism by CYP3A4. Inhibitors of this isozyme will increase the plasma concentrations of lomitapide. Because of this, concurrent use of lomitapide with strong or moderate inhibitors of CYP3A4 is contraindicated. A 50% dosage reduction is required if lomitapide is used in combination with a weak CYP3A4 inhibitor. Patients taking this drug should also avoid grapefruit juice.[7,23,26]

Physicochemical Properties

The structure of lomitapide contains a basic tertiary amine that will be primarily ionized at all physiologic environments. Overall, lomitapide is highly lipid soluble and over 99% is bound to plasma proteins.

Metabolism and Pharmacokinetic Properties

Due to its high lipid solubility, lomitapide is extensively metabolized in the liver via a variety of oxidations followed by glucuronide conjugation. The primary metabolic route is N-dealkylation of the piperidine ring (Fig. 18.16). This essentially breaks the molecule in half and renders the drug inactive. Lomitapide is administered orally; however, it has a very low bioavailability (~7%) due to its high lipid solubility. While it can easily pass through lipid-soluble membranes, it has a lower ability to initially dissolve in the GI tract.[26,27]

Mipomersen

Mechanism of Action

Mipomersen (Kynamro) is a stable oligonucleotide that contains a modified DNA sequence that is complementary to the coding region of the mRNA for apoB-100. This complementary, or antisense, nature allows it to bind to the mRNA and create a 20-nucleotide hybrid DNA/mRNA sequence. This results in RNase-H-mediated degradation of the mRNA and an inhibition of the production of the apoB-100 protein required for the synthesis of both LDL and VLDL.[26,27]

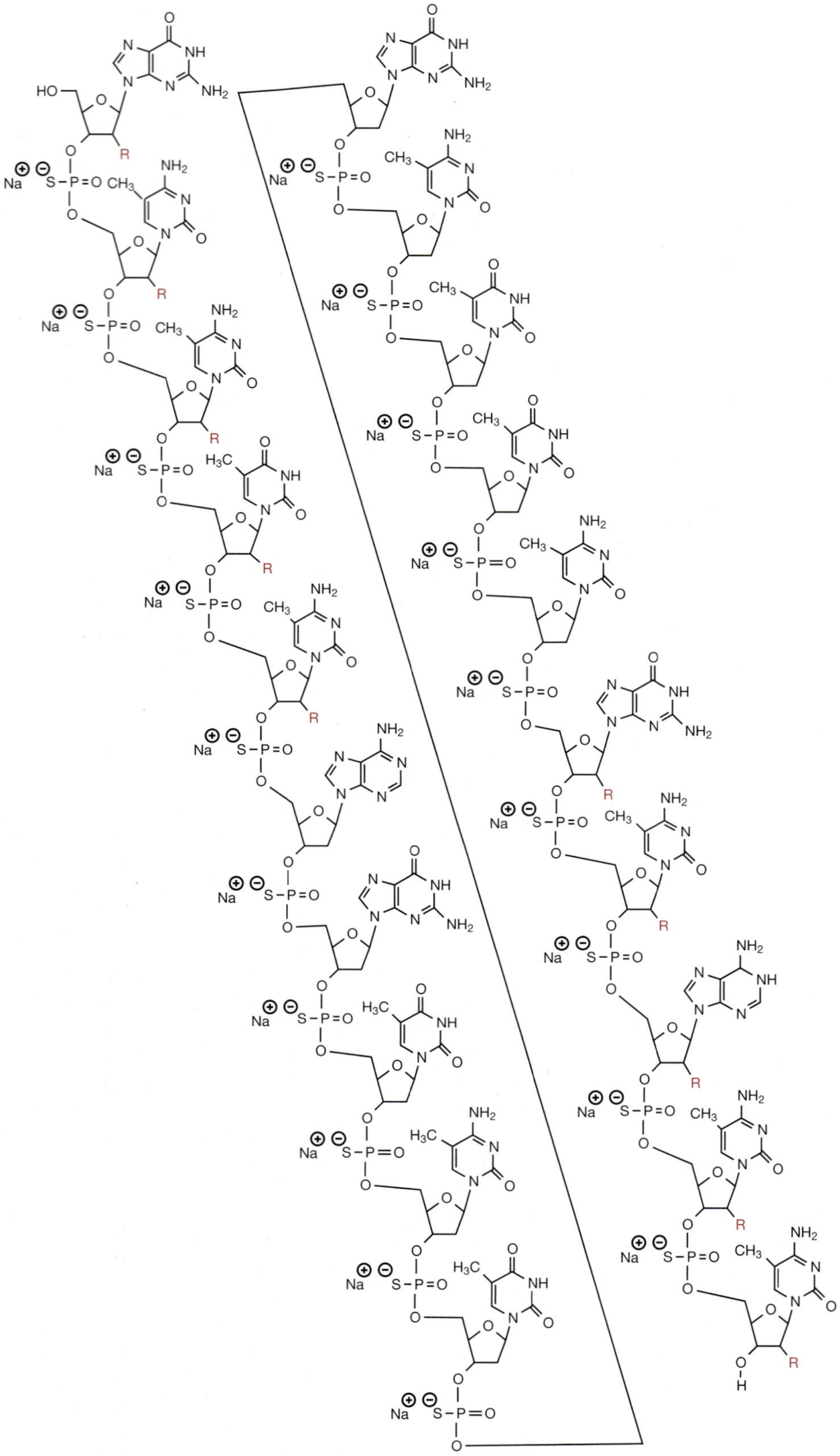

Mipomersen sodium

R = 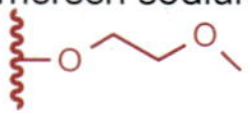

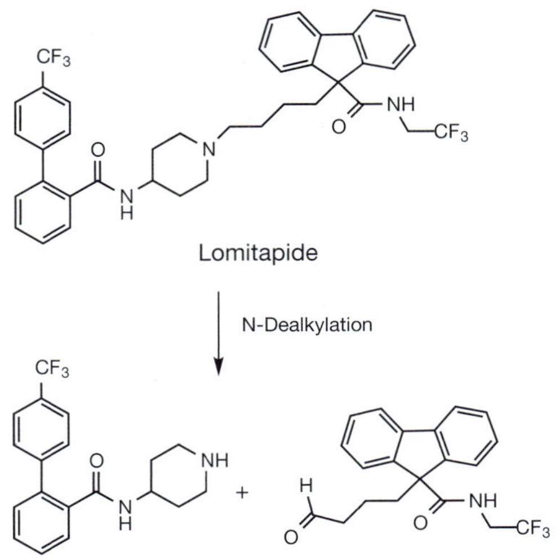

Figure 18.16 Metabolism of lomitapide.

Common Adverse Effects and Drug Interactions

Injection site reactions (including erythema, pain, hematoma, pruritus, swelling, discoloration, and rash) are the most common adverse effects seen with mipomersen. Approximately 85% of patients will experience one or more of these reactions. Other common adverse effects include elevations in serum alanine transaminase (ALT) levels, flu-like symptoms, headache, and nausea. The most serious adverse effect is an increased risk of hepatotoxicity. To date, no clinically relevant drug interactions have been reported; however, caution should be exercised when using mipomersen in combination with other medications known to have potential for hepatotoxicity.[26,27]

Receptor Binding and Structure-Activity Relationship

The 20 nucleotides present within the structure of mipomersen form hydrogen bonds consistent with Watson-Crick pairing with a specific, complementary sequence in the mRNA of apoB-100. The isosteric replacement of phosphate oxygen atoms with sulfur atoms increases the chemical stability of the oligonucleotide, while the 2′-O-(2-methoxyethyl) groups present on the terminal five nucleotides at the 5′ and 3′ ends inhibit nuclease action. These two chemical alterations enhance the duration of action.[27]

Metabolism and Physicochemical and Pharmacokinetic Properties

The phosphorothioate groups that link the nucleotides are acidic in nature and allow for the formation of sodium salts. Mipomersen is administered once weekly as a SC injection. The estimated bioavailability ranges from 54% to 78%, and the elimination half-life is 1 to 2 months. It is greater than 90% plasma protein bound. Metabolism of mipomersen involves endonuclease activity to produce shorter oligonucleotides that are further metabolized by exonucleases. Additionally, mipomersen is eliminated renally.[26,27]

Evinacumab

Mechanism of Action

Evinacumab (Evkeeza) is an angiopoietin-like protein 3 (ANGPTL3) inhibitor. ANGPTL3 is primarily expressed in the liver, where its normal function is to regulate lipid metabolism by inhibiting lipoprotein lipase and endothelial lipase. These actions increase the plasma levels of triglycerides, LDL-C, and HDL. Thus, inhibition of ANGPTL3 with evinacumab lowers the plasma levels of all of these lipids. The actions of evinacumab on LDL-C are independent of low-density lipoprotein receptor (LDLR), and are the result of promoting VLDL processing and clearance upstream of LDL formation. The dependence of LDL synthesis on VLDL was previously discussed and shown in Figure 18.5. The actions of evinacumab on triglycerides and HDL are due to removal of the inhibition of lipoprotein lipase and endothelial lipase, respectively.[7,26,77] The actions of endothelial lipase have been shown to have an inverse relationship with HDL levels (ie, increased endothelial lipase expression leads to decreased HDL levels).[78]

Common Adverse Effects and Drug Interactions

The most common adverse effect seen with evinacumab is nasopharyngitis. Other adverse effects include abdominal pain, constipation, nausea, hypersensitivity reactions, asthenia, dizziness, pain in the extremities, flu-like symptoms, nasal congestion, rhinorrhea, upper respiratory tract infection, and infusion-related reactions. To date, no clinically relevant drug interactions have been reported.[26,27]

Receptor Binding and Structure-Activity Relationship

Evinacumab is a recombinant human IgG4 monoclonal antibody that was genetically engineered to bind and inhibit circulating ANGPTL3. Evinacumab consists of two disulfide-linked heavy chains and light chains. The heavy chains are also covalently linked to the light chains by disulfide bonds. Similar to other monoclonal antibodies, the key binding interactions occur between the Fab regions of evinacumab and specific complementary sites on ANGPTL3.[72]

Metabolism and Physicochemical Properties

Evinacumab is not orally active and is administered via an intravenous (IV) infusion over 60 minutes once monthly. Due to its peptide nature, it is metabolized by endo- and exopeptidases to form smaller, inactive peptides. These metabolic pathways are similar to the known catabolic pathways for endogenous IgG antibodies and can produce amino acids that can be recycled for protein synthesis or further metabolized for other purposes. Because of their molecular size, monoclonal antibodies are not generally excreted into the urine. The elimination $t_{1/2}$ for evinacumab is not a constant but is a function of the serum concentration.[7,26,77]

POTENTIAL DRUG TARGETS

Despite the success of current therapy in decreasing plasma LDL-C, investigators continue to look for potential drug targets that will help optimize patient outcomes. Over the past two decades, there have been three specific targets that have received a significant amount of attention; however, due to problems with efficacy and adverse effects, they have not yet been used to produce a viable therapeutic drug. Since these targets may ultimately produce alternatives to currently available therapy, a brief overview of each of these targets is provided here.

Potential Target 1: Squalene synthase is an enzyme responsible for catalyzing the two-step conversion of two molecules of farnesyl pyrophosphate to squalene. Squalene synthase catalyzes the first committed step in sterol biosynthesis and offers some potential advantages over HMG-CoA reductase as a drug target. The latter group of drugs inhibits cholesterol synthesis at an early stage of the pathway and, thus, lacks specificity. Mevalonic acid, the immediate product of HMG-CoA reductase, is a common intermediate in the biosynthesis of other isoprenoids, such as ubiquinone (an electron carrier in oxidative phosphorylation), dolichol (a compound involved in oligosaccharide synthesis), and farnesylated proteins (the farnesyl portion targets the protein to cell membrane, as opposed to the cytosol). Inhibitors of squalene synthase target an enzyme involved in a later stage of cholesterol biosynthesis and could potentially accomplish the same desired outcomes as currently available agents without interfering with the biosynthesis of other essential, nonsteroidal compounds. An additional advantage of squalene synthase inhibitors is that they do not cause the myopathies seen with the statins. While squalene synthase inhibitors have reached phase 2 and phase 3 clinical trials, adverse effects, specifically hepatotoxicity, have halted their approval.[79,80]

Potential Target 2: Inhibitors of ACAT have been investigated as cholesterol-lowering or antiatherosclerotic agents. In addition to its role in foam cell formation, ACAT is also required for esterification of cholesterol in intestinal mucosal cells and for synthesis of cholesterol esters in hepatic VLDL formation. Thus, ACAT inhibitors have the potential of providing three beneficial effects in patients with hypercholesterolemia: decreased cholesterol absorption, decreased hepatic VLDL synthesis, and decreased foam cell formation. To date, the development of ACAT inhibitors has been hampered by toxicity profiles and the inability to provide effective cholesterol reduction in human patients. Interestingly, the most effective compound in these studies turned out to be an azetidinone derivative that blocked cholesterol absorption through binding to the sterol transporter NPC1L1 instead of ACAT. Further structural modification of this lead compound produced ezetimibe.[81,82]

Potential Target 3: Cholesteryl ester transfer protein (CETP) interacts with HDL, LDL, and VLDL to mediate the transfer of cholesterol esters from HDL (primarily HDL_2) to LDL and VLDL while balancing this exchange in a 1:1 fashion with a transfer of triglycerides from LDL and VLDL to HDL. The end result of this process is a higher concentration of LDL cholesterol and a lower concentration of HDL cholesterol. It has been postulated that CETP inhibitors would produce a therapeutic benefit due to their ability to prevent these transfers and favorably increase HDL cholesterol and lower LDL cholesterol. The initial development of potent CETP inhibitors proved to be challenging due to the nonenzymatic nature of a transport protein, the lack of a transition state and/or tightly bound intermediates, and the lack of potent natural and synthetic inhibitors. A number of chemical classes of compounds have been investigated over the years; however, despite some success in clinical trials, no drug has been approved yet. Key factors preventing approval at the current time are adverse effects and the inability to show superiority in secondary end points.[82-84]

NICOTINIC ACID (NIACIN)

Nicotinic acid, also known as niacin, is a vitamin that is an essential structural component of nicotinamide adenine dinucleotide (NAD^+) and nicotinamide adenine dinucleotide phosphate ($NADP^+$), two cofactors involved in electron transport and intermediary metabolism.[85] In 1955, Altschul et al[86] observed that high doses of nicotinic acid lowered cholesterol levels in humans, an activity unrelated to its properties as a vitamin. While nicotinic acid shows favorable effects in lowering both triglycerides and LDL-C, it is primarily used in adjunctive therapy for severe hypertriglyceridemia in adults at risk of pancreatitis. Studies have shown that addition of niacin to statin therapy does not significantly improve cardiac outcomes.[23]

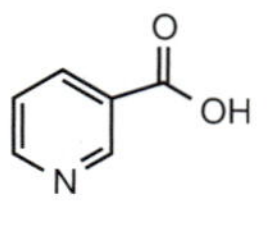

Nicotinic acid

Mechanism of Action

Nicotinic acid exerts a variety of effects on lipoprotein metabolism.[7,74,87] One of its most important actions is the inhibition of lipolysis in adipose tissue. Impaired lipolysis decreases the mobilization of free fatty acids, thus reducing their plasma levels and their delivery to the liver. In turn, this decreases hepatic triglyceride synthesis and results in a decreased production of VLDL. Enhanced clearance of VLDL through stimulation of lipoprotein lipase has also been proposed to contribute to the reduction of plasma VLDL levels. Because LDL is derived from VLDL (see Fig. 18.5), the decreased production of VLDL ultimately leads to a decrease in LDL levels. The sequential nature of this process has been clinically demonstrated. The reduction in triglyceride levels occurs within several hours after initiation of nicotinic acid therapy, whereas the reduction in cholesterol does not occur until after several days of therapy.

Nicotinic acid also inhibits diacylglycerol acyltransferase-2 in hepatic cells. This enzyme catalyzes the final step in hepatic triglyceride synthesis and limits the availability of triglycerides for the formation of VLDL.[69,88]

Nicotinic acid favorably increases HDL levels due to a reduction in the clearance of apoA-I, an essential component of HDL. Nicotinic acid does not have any effects on cholesterol catabolism or biosynthesis.

Common Adverse Effects and Drug Interactions

The most common (and often, dose-limiting) side effects of nicotinic acid are cutaneous vasodilation (flushing and pruritus) and gastrointestinal intolerance, which may occur in 20% to 50% of treated patients. Flushing and pruritus are prostaglandin-mediated effects and may be prevented by taking aspirin, indomethacin, or another nonsteroidal anti-inflammatory drug prior to nicotinic acid. GI side effects, such as flatulence, nausea, vomiting, and diarrhea, can be minimized if nicotinic acid is taken either with or immediately after meals. All of these effects can be minimized by slowly titrating the dose of nicotinic acid. Hepatic dysfunction is one of the more serious complications of high-dose nicotinic acid. Plasma aspartate transaminase (AST), ALT, lactate dehydrogenase, and alkaline phosphatase levels are often elevated but usually return to normalcy when therapy is either adjusted or discontinued.[7,8,26]

Drug interactions for nicotinic acid are listed in Table 18.8.

Receptor Binding and Structure-Activity Relationship

The actions of nicotinic acid on lipolysis have been suggested to be due to its ability to bind to a G protein–coupled receptor. The carboxylic acid is essential in providing either an ionic bond or an ion-dipole bond. Conversion of the carboxylic acid to an amide, as seen with nicotinamide, results in an inactive compound. The pyridine ring can interact with the receptor through hydrogen bond formation (as the acceptor), van der Waals interactions, and charge-transfer interactions. Structural changes to nicotinic acid result in loss of activity.[89,90]

Table 18.8 Drug Interactions for Nicotinic Acid

Drug	Result of Interaction
Antidiabetic drugs	Nicotinic acid can induce insulin resistance, requiring alteration of the dosing of antidiabetic drugs
Bile acid sequestrants	Decreased bioavailability of nicotinic acid if administration is not adequately spaced
Ethanol	Potential enhanced hepatotoxicity and excessive peripheral or cutaneous vasodilation
HMG-CoA reductase inhibitors	Increased risk of myopathy and rhabdomyolysis

Physicochemical Properties

Nicotinic acid (niacin) is a stable, nonhygroscopic, white, crystalline powder. Its carboxylic acid has a pK_a of 4.76 and, thus, is predominantly ionized at physiologic pH. The pyridine nitrogen is a very weak base (pK_a = 2.0) and, therefore, primarily exists in the unionized form. Nicotinic acid is freely soluble in alkaline solutions and has a measured log P of −0.20 at pH 6.0.[69]

Metabolism

Nicotinic acid is a B-complex vitamin that is converted to nicotinamide, NAD^+, and $NADP^+$. The latter two biomolecules are coenzymes and are required for oxidation/reduction reactions in a variety of biochemical pathways. Additionally, nicotinic acid is metabolized to a number of inactive compounds, including nicotinuric acid and N-methylated derivatives. Normal biochemical regulation and feedback prevent large doses of nicotinic acid from producing excess quantities of NAD^+ and $NADP^+$. Thus, small doses of nicotinic acid, such as those used for dietary supplementation, will be primarily excreted as metabolites, whereas large doses, such as those used for the treatment of hyperlipoproteinemia, will be primarily excreted unchanged by the kidney.[7,26,69]

Pharmacokinetic Properties

Nicotinic acid is readily absorbed. Peripheral vasodilation is seen within 20 minutes, and peak plasma concentrations occur within 45 minutes. The half-life of the drug is approximately 1 hour, thus necessitating frequent dosing or an extended-release formulation. Extended-release tablets produce peripheral vasodilation within 1 hour, reach peak plasma concentrations within 4 to 5 hours, and have a duration of 8 to 10 hours.

Dosing of nicotinic acid should be titrated to minimize adverse effects. An initial dose of 50 to 100 mg 3 times a day is often used with immediate-release tablets. The dose then is gradually increased by 50 to 100 mg every 3 to 14 days, up to a maximum of 6 g/d, as tolerated. Therapeutic monitoring to assess efficacy and prevent toxicity is essential until a stable and effective dose is reached. Similar dosing escalations are available for extended-release products, with doses normally starting at 500 mg once daily at bedtime to minimize patient awareness of vasodilation-mediated adverse effects.[7,26,53]

FIBRATES

The use of this class of drugs to treat hyperlipoproteinemias can be traced back to 1962 and, thus, predates the use of most of the other drugs in this chapter. The name of this class of drugs is an acronym for ethyl *p*-chloro<u>ph</u>enox<u>y</u>iso<u>b</u>uty<u>rate</u>, the chemical name of clofibrate (Fig. 18.17). Clofibrate was approved for therapeutic use in 1967 and was initially a widely prescribed drug. Results from a 1978 World Health Organization trial changed the acceptance of clofibrate and dramatically decreased its use. These trials indicated that despite a 9% lowering of cholesterol, patients taking clofibrate showed no reduction of cardiovascular events and actually had an increase in overall mortality.[91] Although clofibrate is no longer available in the United States, it has served as the prototype for the design of safer and more effective fibrates. Structural modifications, focused primarily on ring substitutions and the addition of spacer groups, have produced gemfibrozil and fenofibrate (Fig. 18.17).

Mechanism of Action

Overall, fibrates decrease plasma triglyceride levels much more dramatically than they decrease plasma cholesterol levels. They significantly decrease VLDL levels, cause a moderate increase in HDL levels, and have variable effects on LDL concentrations. As an example of this latter point, gemfibrozil will raise LDL levels in patients with hypertriglyceridemia but will lower LDL levels in patients with normal triglyceride levels. The exact mechanisms for these actions have not been fully elucidated; however, studies have shown that this class of compounds can produce a variety of beneficial effects on lipoprotein metabolism. It has been proposed that these effects are mediated through the activation of peroxisome proliferator-activated receptors (PPARs) and an alteration of gene expression. Specifically, fibrates bind to PPARα.[7,23,26,91]

Decreases in plasma VLDL levels primarily result from the ability of these drugs to stimulate the activity of lipoprotein lipase, the enzyme responsible for removing triglycerides from plasma VLDL (see Fig. 18.5). Additionally, fibrates can lower VLDL levels through PPARα-mediated stimulation of fatty acid oxidation, inhibition of triglyceride synthesis, and reduced expression of apoC-III. This latter effect enhances the action of lipoprotein lipase because apoC-III normally serves as an inhibitor of this enzyme. Favorable effects on HDL levels appear to be related to increased transcription of apoA-I and apoA-II as well as a decreased activity of CETP.

All fibrates accelerate the turnover and removal of cholesterol from the liver. This increases the biliary secretion of cholesterol, enhances its fecal excretion, and may cause cholelithiasis (ie, gallstone formation).

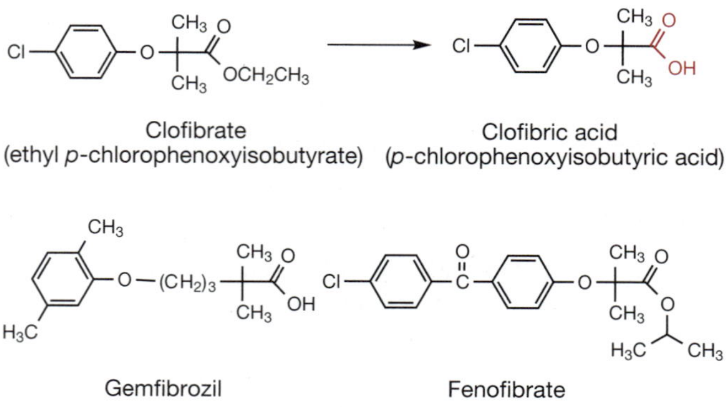

Figure 18.17 Bioactivation of clofibrate and chemical structures of other fibrates.

Common Adverse Effects and Drug Interactions

The most prevalent or significant side effects caused by the fibrates are highlighted in the box titled "Adverse Effects of Fibrates."[7,8,23,26] Overall, fibrates are usually well tolerated. GI issues are the most common but do not usually cause discontinuation of therapy. The combination of gemfibrozil with higher doses of statins has been shown to increase the incidence of myopathies. This increase is due to the ability of gemfibrozil to inhibit the hepatic uptake of statins by OATP1B1 and elevate the plasma level of the statins. The combination of statins with fenofibrate is less likely to cause myopathy than combination therapy with gemfibrozil. Fibrates also cause increases in plasma AST, ALT, and creatine phosphokinase levels.

Drug interactions for fibrates are listed in Table 18.9.

Table 18.9 Drug Interactions for Fibrates

Drug	Fibrate	Result of Interaction
Antidiabetic agents	All	Increased hypoglycemic effect through increased sensitivity and decreased glucagon secretion
Bexarotene	Gemfibrozil	Increased bexarotene plasma concentrations
Bile acid sequestrants	All	Decreased bioavailability of fibrate if administration is not adequately spaced
Colchicine	All	Increased potential for myopathy
Cyclosporine	Fenofibrate	Increased potential for nephrotoxicity
Drugs requiring CYP2C8 or OATP1B1	Gemfibrozil	Gemfibrozil may increase the plasma concentrations of drugs requiring this enzyme or transporter
Ezetimibe	All	Increased ezetimibe plasma concentrations and possible increased risk of cholelithiasis; concomitant use is not recommended
HMG-CoA reductase inhibitors	All	Increased risk of severe myopathy or rhabdomyolysis
Oral anticoagulants	All	Increased hypoprothrombinemic effect
Repaglinide	Gemfibrozil	Increased repaglinide plasma concentrations

ADVERSE EFFECTS OF FIBRATES

Central nervous system: Dizziness, drowsiness, headache, mental depression
GI: Abdominal pain, constipation, diarrhea, dyspepsia, flatulence, nausea, vomiting
Hematologic: Anemia, eosinophilia leukopenia
Hepatic: Cholelithiasis, cholestasis, jaundice, pancreatitis
Musculoskeletal: Myopathy, myositis, rhabdomyolysis
Skin: Pruritus, rash
Urogenital: Impotence, decreased libido
Vision: Blurred vision

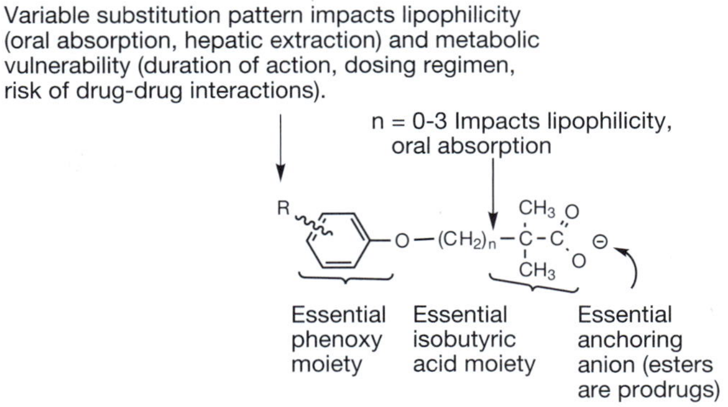

Figure 18.18 Fibrate pharmacophore and summary of SAR.

Receptor Binding and Structure-Activity Relationship

All fibrates are analogues of phenoxyisobutyric acid. A structure of this pharmacophore, as well as a summary of the SAR for this class of drugs, is shown in Figure 18.18. Fibrates bind to PPARα via an ion-dipole bond with a tyrosine residue. Fenofibrate, which contains an ester, is a prodrug and requires in vivo hydrolysis in order to be active. The isobutyric acid group is essential for activity; however, PPARα has some flexibility and will accommodate a spacer up to three carbon atoms between the isobutyric acid and the phenoxy ring, as seen with gemfibrozil. This spacer enhances lipid solubility and allows gemfibrozil to be absorbed through the gastrointestinal membrane without the need of an ester prodrug. Substitution at the *p* position of the aromatic ring with a chloro group or a chlorine-containing cyclopropyl ring produces compounds with significantly longer half-lives.[92]

Physicochemical Properties

As noted, a carboxylic acid is a required structural feature for fibrate binding and activity. The pK_a of the carboxylic acid of gemfibrozil is reported to be 4.4, and thus, it will be primarily ionized at physiologic pH.[69] The pK_a and ionization of the active metabolite of fenofibrate can reasonably be assumed to be similar. Fenofibrate is a neutral, ester prodrug and can be classified as nonelectrolyte, while gemfibrozil can be classified as an acidic drug. The calculated log P values for fenofibrate and gemfibrozil are shown in Table 18.10.[69] Both drugs are highly lipid soluble; however, a structural analysis provides an explanation as to why fenofibrate has a higher log *P* value than gemfibrozil. The structure of fenofibrate contains a nonionizable isopropyl ester and two aromatic rings, while the structure of gemfibrozil contains an ionizable carboxylic acid and a single aromatic ring. Despite the presence of an ionizable carboxylic acid, gemfibrozil still contains significant lipid character due to two structural features. Its 2,5-dimethyl aromatic ring is predicted to be slightly more hydrophobic than the 4-chloro ring of fenofibrate, and the propyl bridge between the isobutyric acid and the aromatic ring adds additional lipid solubility.[93] All currently available fibrates are achiral molecules and not subject to stereochemical concerns.

Metabolism

The metabolic pathways of gemfibrozil and fenofibrate are shown in Figure 18.19. Oxidation of the aromatic methyl groups of gemfibrozil by CYP3A4, alcohol dehydrogenase, and aldehyde dehydrogenase produces inactive hydroxymethyl and carboxylic acid metabolites. These functional groups can be further metabolized by conjugation with glucuronic acid. Fenofibrate is a prodrug that undergoes rapid hydrolysis to produce fenofibric acid. This active metabolite can then be conjugated with glucuronic acid, similar to gemfibrozil. The *p*-chloro group of fenofibric acid deactivates the ring from aromatic oxidation. Both drugs are primarily excreted as glucuronide conjugates in the

Table 18.10 Pharmacokinetic Parameters of Fibrates

Drug	Calculated log P	Oral Bioavailability (%)	Active Metabolite	Protein Binding (%)	Time to Peak Concentration (h)	Elimination Half-Life (h)	Major Route(s) of Elimination
Fenofibrate	5.24	60-90	Fenofibric acid	99	4-8	20-22	Renal (60%-90%) Fecal (5%-25%)
Gemfibrozil	3.9	>90	None	99	1-2	1.5	Renal (70%) Fecal (6%)

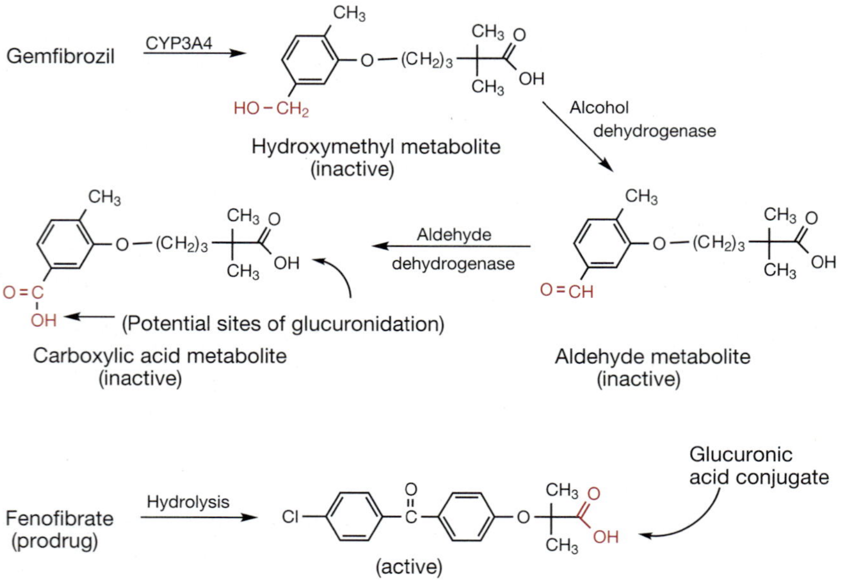

Figure 18.19 Metabolic pathways for gemfibrozil and fenofibrate.

urine. While oxidation of gemfibrozil requires the CYP3A4 isozyme, it can be conjugated and eliminated either with or without oxidation. As such, drug interactions with gemfibrozil and other drugs affecting the CYP3A4 system are less important here than with other drug classes.

Pharmacokinetic Properties

The pharmacokinetic properties for fenofibrate and gemfibrozil are summarized in Table 18.10.[7,26,27,53,69] The prodrug, fenofibrate, requires a longer time to reach peak concentrations compared with gemfibrozil. Because of differences in aromatic substitution, fenofibrate also has a much longer half-life than gemfibrozil. The 2,5-dimethyl substitution in gemfibrozil is much more susceptible to oxidative metabolism than the terminal *p*-chloro-substituted aromatic ring of fenofibrate. Changes in lipid levels are not seen immediately, and up to 2 months may be required to reach maximal clinical effects and to determine the overall clinical efficacy. Fenofibrate and gemfibrozil have excellent bioavailability and are extensively bound to plasma proteins. Because food can significantly enhance their oral absorption, these drugs should be taken either with or just before meals. Renal elimination is the primary route through which these drugs are excreted from the body. Patients with mild renal dysfunction often can be managed with minor dosage adjustments, whereas those with severe impairment or renal failure may have to discontinue its use.

ω-3 Fatty Acids

ω-3 Fatty acids are essential to the human diet because human cells do not possess the enzymes required to add double bonds at the ω-3 and the ω-6 positions on fatty acids. The three main ω-3 fatty acids are α-linolenic acid (ACA), eicosapentaenoic acid (EPA), and docosahexaenoic acid (DPA) (Fig 18.20). ACA is found in plant oils such as soybean and canola oils, while EPA and DPA are found in fish oils. Studies have shown that EPA and DPA can reduce triglyceride levels by 20% to 50%; however, the ability of these drugs to decrease the risk of ASCVD has not been firmly established.[23,94-96] Both of these drugs are available as adjunct therapy to treat hypertriglyceridemia and cardiovascular risk reduction in patients with hypertriglyceridemia. Vegetable oils, such as ACA, can be converted to EPA and DPA; however, this conversion is limited due to other available biochemical pathways. Thus, vegetable oils are not viable alternatives to fish oils. The current dosage recommendations for EPA or the combination of EPA and DPA is 4 g, taken once or twice daily.

Mechanism of Action

ω-3 fatty acids EPA and DPA inhibit the enzyme acyl CoA:1,2-diacylglycerol *O*-acyltransferase. This enzyme catalyzes the formation of triglycerides by transferring an activated fatty acid (ie, acyl CoA) to diacylglycerol. Both EPA and DPA have a high affinity for this enzyme; however, they are poor substrates and result in an inhibition of triglyceride

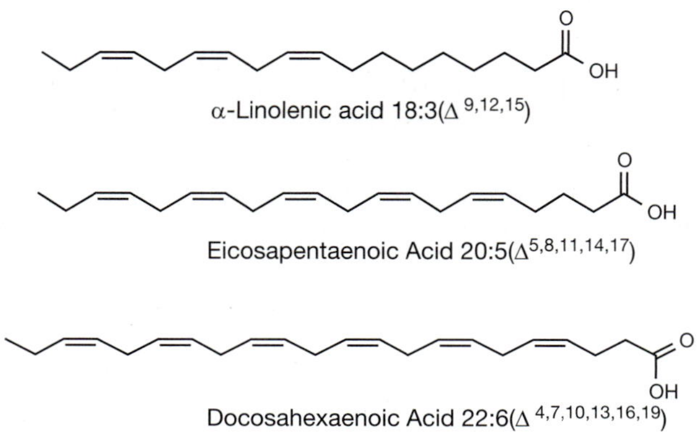

Figure 18.20 ω-3 fatty acids.

synthesis. Due to the decrease in triglyceride synthesis, the hepatic production of VLDL is subsequently decreased. The decrease in VLDL production is also due to enhanced degradation of apolipoprotein B in the liver, thus preventing its assembly and secretion. The ability of both EPA and DPA to induce lipoprotein lipase results in the clearance of triglycerides from both chylomicrons and VLDL. Additional beneficial effects that have been reported include a decrease in platelet aggregation and a slight reduction in blood pressure.[23,94,95]

Common Adverse Effects and Drug Interactions

The most common adverse effects of EPA and DPA are eructation (ie, belching), dyspepsia, arthralgia, unpleasant aftertaste, and rash. Higher doses have been reported to alter glycemic control in patients with diabetes. Due to their effects on platelet aggregation, EPA and DPA can increase the risk of bleeding if used in combination with other anticoagulants or antiplatelet drugs.[7,23,26,94]

Structure Challenge

1. Shown here are the structures of atorvastatin, pitavastatin, and rosuvastatin. Evaluate their structures and answer the following questions.
   a. Provide a chemical explanation why atorvastatin and rosuvastatin have a higher binding affinity for HMGR as compared to pitavastatin.
   b. If a patient is currently taking other medications that interfere with both CYP3A4 and the enzymes required for glucuronide conjugation, which one of these three drugs would be preferred, and why?

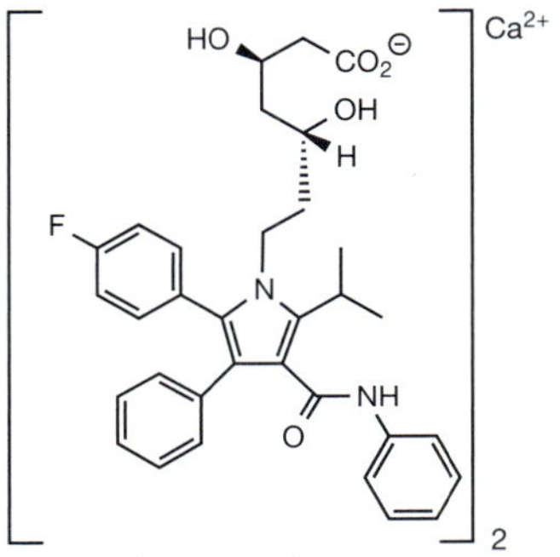

Atorvastatin

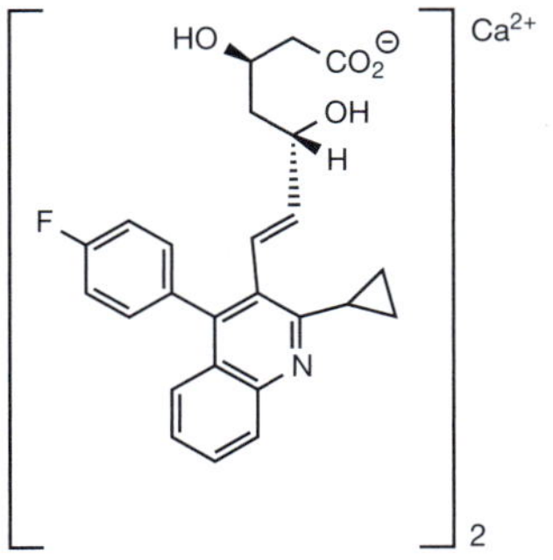

Pitavastatin

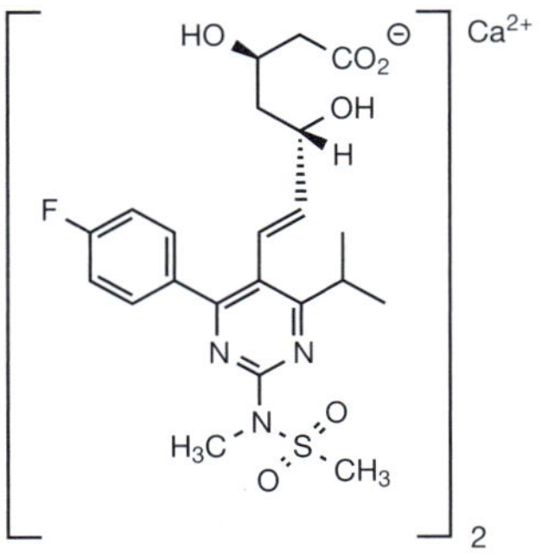

Rosuvastatin

2. Shown here is the structure of atorvastatin and two potential analogues. For each potential analogue, indicate if it would be expected to enhance the binding to HMGR or decrease the binding. Provide a rationale for your responses.

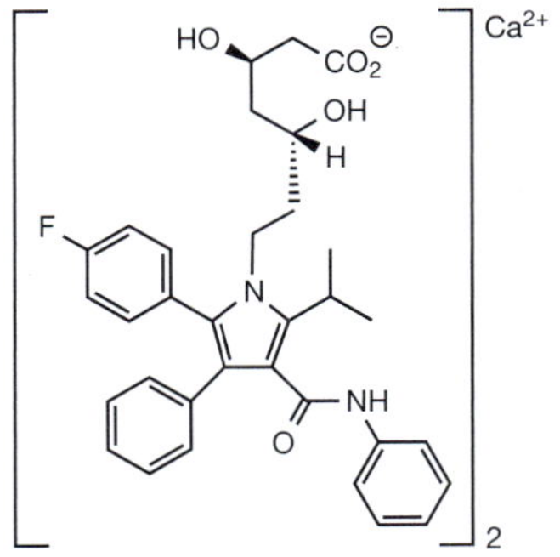

Atorvastatin

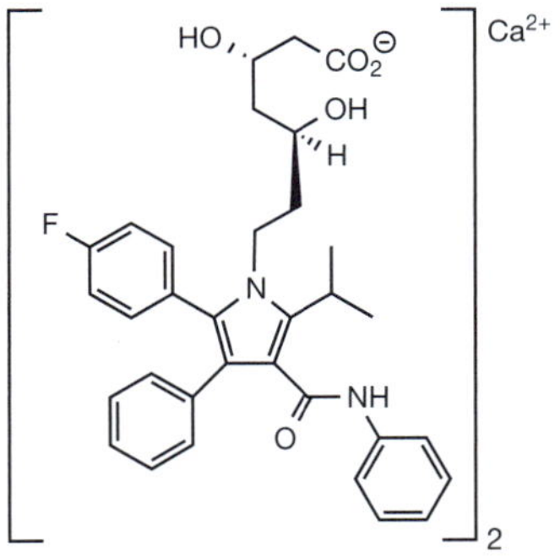

Analogue A

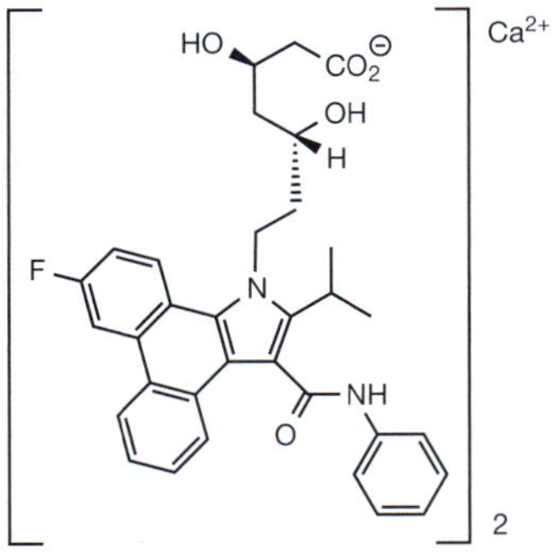

Analogue B

3. The following questions pertain to the structure of cholestyramine.
   a. Why does cholestyramine produce minimal systemic adverse effects?
   b. Why must other medications be taken 1 hour before or 4 hours after cholestyramine, and what would happen if this dosing guideline was ignored?

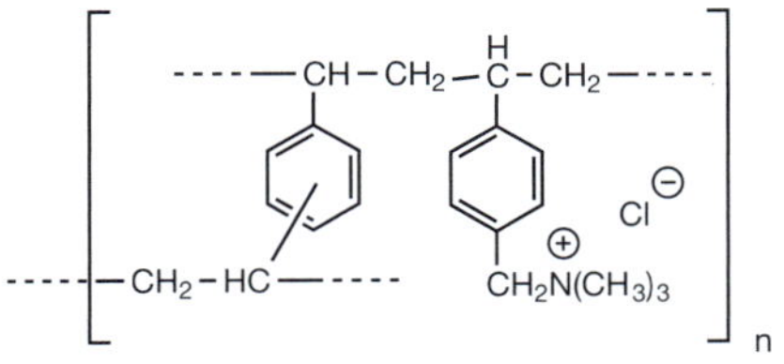

Cholestyramine

Structure Challenge answers found immediately after References.

Receptor Binding and Structure-Activity Relationship

In order for fatty acids to be added to glycerol, monoacylglycerol, or diacylglycerol, they must be at least 16 carbon atoms long and can be either saturated, monounsaturated, or polyunsaturated. Both EPA and DPA meet these structural requirements. Similar to all other fatty acids, EPA and DPA must first be activated via the addition of coenzyme A to form a thioester acyl CoA. As mentioned, the activated acyl CoA intermediates of EPA and DPA have a high affinity for acyl CoA:1,2-acylglycerol O-acyltransferase. Since these fatty acids are not normally present in triglycerides, they are not good substrates, but act as inhibitors for this enzyme.[4,26,94]

Physicochemical Properties, Metabolism, and Pharmacokinetic Properties

Both EPA and DPA are highly lipophilic and are administered as ethyl ester prodrugs. They are hydrolyzed in the small intestine and absorbed as their active carboxylic acid metabolites. Similar to other fatty acids, EPA and DPA are incorporated into chylomicrons with phospholipids, cholesterol, and triglycerides. As free fatty acids, both EPA and DPA are greater than 99% plasma protein bound. They are metabolized by β-oxidation similar to other fatty acids. The elimination $t_{½}$ is approximately 50 to 80 hours.[7,26,69]

REFERENCES

1. Gaziano TA, Gaziano JM. Epidemiology of cardiovascular disease. In: Loscalzo J, Fauci A, Kasper D, *Hauser S, Longo D, Jameson J*, eds. *Harrison's Principles of Internal Medicine*. 21st ed. McGraw Hill; 2022.
2. Arnett DK, Blumenthal RS, Albert MA, et al. ACC/AHA guideline on the primary prevention of cardiovascular disease: executive summary: a report of the American College of Cardiology/American Heart Association Task Force on Clinical Practice Guidelines. *Circulation*. 2019;140:e563-e595.
3. Berg JM, Tymoczko JL, Gatto GJ, Stryer, L. *Biochemistry*. 8th ed. Freeman & Company; 2015:767-800.
4. Nelson DL, Cox MM. *Lehninger Principles of Biochemistry*. 8th ed. Macmillan Learning; 2021:744-793.
5. Javitt NB. Bile acid synthesis from cholesterol: regulatory and auxiliary pathways. *FASEB J*. 1994;8(15):1308-1311.
6. Šarenac TM, Mikov M. Bile acid synthesis: from nature to the chemical modification and synthesis and their applications as drugs and nutrients. *Front Pharmacol*. 2018;9:939.
7. Ruiz-Negrón N, Blumenthal DK. Drug therapy for dyslipidemias. In: Brunton L, Knollman B, eds. *Goodman & Gilman's the Pharmacological Basis of Therapeutics*. 14th ed. McGraw Hill; 2023:729-746.
8. Dixon DL, Riche DM. Dyslipidemia. In: Dipiro JT, Yee GC, Posey LM, *Haines* ST, *Nolin* TD, *Ellingrod* V, eds. *Pharmacotherapy: A Pathophysiologic Approach*. 11th ed. McGraw Hill; 2020:117-136.
9. Feingold KR. Introduction to lipids and lipoproteins. In: Feingold KR, Anawalt B, Blackman MR, et al, eds. *Endotext*. MDText.com, Inc.; 2000. Updated January 19, 2021. Accessed May 5, 2023. https://www.ncbi.nlm.nih.gov/books/NBK305896
10. Fredrickson DS, Levy RI, Lees RS. Fat transport in lipoproteins—an integrated approach to mechanisms and disorders. *N Engl J Med*. 1967;276:34-42.
11. Goldstein JL, DeBose-Boyd RA, Brown MS. Protein sensors for membrane sterols. *Cell*. 2006;124:35-46.
12. Bayly GR. Lipids and disorders of lipoprotein metabolism. In: Marshall WJ, Lapsley M, Day AP, *Ayling R*, eds. *Clinical Biochemistry: Metabolic and Clinical Aspects*. 3rd ed. Churchill Livingstone; 2014:702-736.
13. Ginsberg HN, Goldberg IJ. Disorders of lipoprotein metabolism. In: Fauci AS, Braunwald E, Isselbacher KJ, et al, eds. *Harrison's Principles of Internal Medicine*. 14th ed. McGraw Hill; 1998:2138-2149.
14. Libby P. Atherosclerosis. In: Fauci AS, Braunwald E, Isselbacher KJ, et al, eds. *Harrison's Principles of Internal Medicine*. 14th ed. McGraw Hill; 1998:1345-1352.
15. Sliskovic DR, White AD. Therapeutic potential of ACAT inhibitors as lipid lowering and antiatherosclerotic agents. *Trends Pharmacol Sci*. 1991;12:194-199.
16. Tsao CW, Aday AW, Almarzooq ZI, et al. Heart disease and stroke statistics—2023 update: a report from the American Heart Association. *Circulation*. 2023;147:e93-e621.
17. Ford ES, Will JC, Mercado CI, Loustalot F. Trends in predicted risk for atherosclerotic cardiovascular disease using the pooled cohort risk equations among US adults from 1999 to 2012. *JAMA Intern Med*. 2015;175:299-302.
18. Agency for Healthcare Research and Quality. Medical Expenditure Panel Survey (MEPS): household component summary tables: medical conditions, United States. Accessed April 5, 2023. https://meps.ahrq.gov/mepsweb/
19. Kohli-Lynch CN, Lewsey J, Boyd KA, et al. Beyond 10-year risk: a cost-effectiveness analysis of statins for the primary prevention of cardiovascular disease. *Circulation*. 2022;145:1312-1323.
20. Grundy SM, Stone NJ, Bailey AL, et al. 2018 AHA/ACC/AACVPR/AAPA/ABC/ACPM/ADA/AGS/APhA/ASPC/NLA/PCNA guideline on the management of blood cholesterol: a report of the American College of Cardiology/American Heart Association Task Force on Clinical Practice Guidelines. *Circulation*. 2019;139:e1082-e1143.
21. Lloyd-Jones DM, Morris PB, Ballantyne CM, et al. 2017 Focused update of the 2016 ACC expert consensus decision pathway on the role of non-statin therapies for LDL-cholesterol lowering in the management of atherosclerotic cardiovascular disease risk. *J Am Coll Cardiol*. 2017;70(14):1785-1822.
22. Skulas-Ray AC, Wilson PWF, Harris WS, et al; American Heart Association Council on Arteriosclerosis, Thrombosis and Vascular Biology; Council on Lifestyle and Cardiometabolic Health; Council on Cardiovascular Disease in the Young; Council on Cardiovascular and Stroke Nursing; Council on Clinical Cardiology. Omega-3 fatty acids for the management of hypertriglyceridemia: a science advisory from the American Heart Association. *Circulation*. 2019;140:e673-e691.
23. Lipid-lowering drugs. *Med Lett Drugs Ther*. 2022;64:145-152.
24. Heathcock CH, Hadley CR, Rosen T, Theisen PD, Hecker SJ. Total synthesis and biological evaluation of structural analogues of compactin and dihydromevinolin. *J Med Chem*. 1987;30:1858-1873.
25. Cutler SJ, Cocolas GH. Cardiovascular agents. In: Block JH, Beale JM, eds. *Wilson and Gisvold's Textbook of Organic Medicinal and Pharmaceutical Chemistry*. 11th ed. Lippincott Williams & Wilkins; 2004:657-663.
26. Lexicomp. UpToDate Lexidrug: evidence-based drug referential content for teams. Wolters Kluwer. Accessed May 2023. https://www.wolterskluwer.com/en/solutions/lexicomp
27. U.S. Food and Drug Administration. Drugs@FDA: FDA-approved drugs. U.S. Food and Drug Administration. Accessed May 2023. https://www.accessdata.fda.gov/scripts/cder/daf/
28. Atorvastatin—a new lipid-lowering drug. *Med Lett Drugs Ther*. 1997;39:29-31.
29. Rosuvastatin—a new lipid-lowering drug. *Med Lett Drugs Ther*. 2003;45:81-83.
30. Cutler SJ, Cocolas GH. Cardiovascular agents. In: Block JH, Beale JM, eds. *Wilson and Gisvold's Textbook of Organic Medicinal and Pharmaceutical Chemistry*. 11th ed. Lippincott Williams & Wilkins; 2004:657-663.
31. du Souich P, Roederer G, Dufour R. Myotoxicity of statins: mechanism of action. *Pharmacol Ther*. 2017;175:1-16.

32. Nwobodo NN. Effects of organic anion transporting polypeptide (OATP1B1/SLCO1B1) genetic polymorphism on statin therapy. *Biomed J.* 2013;6:429-433.
33. Varma MV, Rotter CJ, Chupka J, et al. pH-Sensitive interaction of HMG-CoA reductase inhibitors (statins) with organic anion transporting polypeptide 2B1. *Mol Pharm.* 2011;8:1303-1313.
34. Rodrigues AC. Efflux and uptake transporters as determinants of statin response. *Expert Opin Drug Metab Toxicol.* 2010;6:621-632.
35. Sathasivam S, Lecky B. Statin induced myopathy. *BMJ.* 2008;337:a2286.
36. Rosenson RS. Current overview of statin-induced myopathy. *Am J Med.* 2004;116:408-416.
37. Adams JL, Metcalf BW. Therapeutic consequences of the inhibition of sterol metabolism. In: Hansch C, Sammes PG, Taylor JB, eds. *Comprehensive Medicinal Chemistry.* Vol 2. Pergamon Press; 1990:333-363.
38. Stokker GE, Hoffman WF, Alberts AW, et al. 3-Hydroxy-3-methylglutaryl–coenzyme A reductase inhibitors. 1. Structural modification of 5-substituted 3,5-dihydroxypentanoic acids and their lactone derivatives. *J Med Chem.* 1985;28:347-358.
39. Sliskovic DR, Blankley CJ, Krause BR, et al. Inhibitors of cholesterol biosynthesis. 6. trans-6-[2-(2-N-heteroaryl-3,5-disubstituted-pyrazol-4-yl)ethyl/ethenyl]tetrahydro-4-hydroxy-2H- pyran-2-ones. *J Med Chem.* 1992;35:2095-2103.
40. Bone EA, Davidson AH, Lewis CN, Todd RS. Synthesis and biological evaluation of dihydroeptastatin, a novel inhibitor of 3-hydroxy-3-methylglutaryl–coenzyme A reductase. *J Med Chem.* 1992;35:3388-3393.
41. Roth BD, Ortwine DF, Hoefle ML, et al. Inhibitors of cholesterol biosynthesis. 1. trans-6-(2-pyrrol-1-ylethyl)-4-hydroxypyran-2-ones, a novel series of HMG-CoA reductase inhibitors. 1. Effects of structural modifications at the 2- and 5-positions of the pyrrole nucleus. *J Med Chem.* 1990;33:21-31.
42. Istvan ES, Deisenhofer J. Structural mechanism for statin inhibition of HMG-CoA reductase. *Science.* 2001;292:1160-1164.
43. da Costa RF, Freire VN, Bezerra EM. Explaining statin inhibition effectiveness of HMG-CoA reductase by quantum biochemistry computations. *Phys Chem Chem Phys.* 2012;14:1389-1398.
44. Hoffman WF, Alberts AW, Cragoe EJ Jr, et al. 3-Hydroxy-3-methylglutaryl–coenzyme A reductase inhibitors. 2. Structural modification of 7-(substituted aryl)-3,5-dihydroxy-6-heptenoic acids and their lactone derivatives. *J Med Chem.* 1986;29:159-169.
45. Stokker GE, Alberts AW, Anderson PS, et al. 3-Hydroxy-3-methylglutaryl-coenzyme A reductase inhibitors. 3. 7-(3,5-Disubstituted [1,1′-biphenyl]-2-yl)-3,5-dihydroxy-6-heptenoic acids and their lactone derivatives. *J Med Chem.* 1986;29:170-181.
46. Heathcock CH, Davis BR, Hadley CR. Synthesis and biological evaluation of a monocyclic, fully functional analogue of compactin. *J Med Chem.* 1989;32:197-202.
47. Lee TJ, Holtz WJ, Smith RL, Alberts AW, Gilfillan JL. 3-Hydroxy-3-methylglutaryl–coenzyme A reductase inhibitors. 8. Side chain ether analogues of lovastatin. *J Med Chem.* 1991;34:2474-2477.
48. Hoffman WF, Alberts AW, Anderson PS, Chen JS, Smith RL, Willard AK. 3-Hydroxy-3-methylglutaryl-coenzyme A reductase inhibitors. 4. Side chain ester derivatives of mevinolin. *J Med Chem.* 1986;29:849-852.
49. Stokker GE, Alberts AW, Gilfillan JL, Huff JW, Smith RL. 3-Hydroxy-3-methylglutaryl–coenzyme A reductase inhibitors. 5. 6-(Fluoren-9-yl)- and 6-(fluoren-9-ylidenyl)-3,5-dihydroxyhexanoic acids and their lactone derivatives. *J Med Chem.* 1986;29:852-855.
50. Procopiou PA, Draper CD, Hutson JL, Inglis GG, Ross BC, Watson NS. Inhibitors of cholesterol biosynthesis. 2. 3,5- dihydroxy-7-(*N*-pyrrolyl)-6-heptenoates, a novel series of HMG-CoA reductase inhibitors. *J Med Chem.* 1993;36:3658-3662.
51. *Advanced Chemistry Development, Inc.* Values calculated by author using ACD/ChemSketch. Version12.01. 2010. Obtained from Advanced Chemistry Development, Inc. Accessed May 2023. http://www.acdlabs.com
52. Craig PN. Drug compendium. In: Hansch C, Sammes PG, Taylor JB, eds. *Comprehensive Medicinal Chemistry.* Vol 6. Pergamon Press; 1990:237-991.
53. Micromedex. Solutions. Merative US L.P. Accessed May 2023. https://www.merative.com/clinical-decision-support
54. Mukhtar RYA, Reid J, Reckless JPD. Pitavastatin. *Int J Clin Pract.* 2005;59:239-252.
55. Phan BA, Dayspring TD, Toth PP. Ezetimibe therapy: mechanism of action and clinical update. *Vasc Health Risk Manag.* 2012;8:415-427.
56. Kosoglou T, Statkevich P, Johnson-Levonas AO, Paolini JF, Bergman AJ, Alton KB. Ezetimibe: a review of its metabolism, pharmacokinetics, and drug interactions. *Clin Pharmacokinet.* 2005;44:467-494.
57. Cannon CP, Blazing MA, Giugliano RP, et al. Ezetimibe added to statin therapy after acute coronary syndromes. *N Engl J Med.* 2015;372:2387.
58. Clader JW, Burnett DA, Caplen MA, et al. 2-Azetidinone cholesterol absorption inhibitor: structure-activity relationship on the heterocyclic nucleus. *J Med Chem.* 1996;39:3684-3693.
59. Rosenblum SB, Huynh T, Afonso A, et al. Discovery of 1-(4-fluorophenyl)-(3P)-[3-(4- fluorophenyl)-(35)-hydroxypropyl]-(45) -(4-hydroxyphenyl)-2-azetidinone (SCH 58235): a designed, potent, orally active inhibitor of cholesterol absorption. *J Med Chem.* 1998;41:973-980.
60. Peterson AS, Fong LG, Young SG. PCSK9 function and physiology. *J Lipid Res.* 2008;49(6):1152-1156.
61. Rosenson R, Hegele R, Fazio S, Cannon CP. The evolving future of PCSK9 inhibitors. *J Am Coll Cardiol.* 2018;72(3):314-329.
62. Praluent (Alirocumab). Prescribing information. Regeneron Pharmaceuticals, Inc. 2022. Accessed May 2023. https://www.praluent.com
63. Repatha (Evolocumab). Prescribing information. Amgen Inc. 2023. Accessed May 2023. https://www.repathahcp.com
64. Dana H, Chalbatani GM, Mahmoodzadeh H, et al. Molecular mechanisms and biological functions of siRNA. *Int J Biomed Sci.* 2017;13(2):48-57.
65. Handelsman Y, Lepor NE. PCSK9 inhibitors in lipid management of patients with diabetes mellitus and high cardiovascular risk: a review. *J Am Heart Assoc.* 2018;7:e008953.
66. Soffer D, Stoekenbroek R, Plakogiannis R. Small interfering ribonucleic acid for cholesterol lowering—inclisiran: inclisiran for cholesterol lowering. *J Clin Lipidol.* 2022;16:574-582.
67. Migliorati JM, Jin J, Zhong X. siRNA drug Leqvio (inclisiran) to lower cholesterol. *Trends Pharmacol Sci.* 2022;43:455-456.
68. Bege M, Borbás A. The medicinal chemistry of artificial nucleic acids and therapeutic oligonucleotides. *Pharmaceuticals (Basel).* 2022;15:909-948.
69. DrugBank Online. Version 5.1.10. Published 2023. Accessed May 2023. https://go.drugbank.com/drugs
70. Markham A. Bempedoic acid: first approval. *Drugs.* 2020;80:747-753.
71. Agarwala A, Quispe R, Goldberg AC, Michos ED. Bempedoic acid for heterozygous familial hypercholesterolemia: from bench to bedside. *Drug Des Devel Ther.* 2021;15:1955-1963.
72. Granchi C. ATP citrate lyase (ACLY) inhibitors: an anti-cancer strategy at the crossroads of glucose and lipid metabolism. *Eur J Med Chem.* 2018;157:1276-1291.
73. Bilen O, Ballantyne CM. Bempedoic acid (ETC-1002): an investigational inhibitor of ATP citrate lyase. *Curr Atheroscler Rep.* 2016;18:61.
74. Cendella RJ. Cholesterol and hypocholesterolemic drugs. In: Craig CR, Stitzel RE, eds. *Modern Pharmacology with Clinical Applications.* 5th ed. Little, Brown & Co; 1997:279-289.
75. Brown MS, Goldstein JL. A receptor-mediated pathway for cholesterol homeostasis. *Science.* 1986;232:34-47.
76. Raal FJ, Santos RD. Homozygous familial hypercholesterolemia: current perspectives on diagnosis and treatment. *Atherosclerosis.* 2012;223:262-268.

77. Sosnowska B, Adach W, Surma S, Rosenson RS, Banach M. Evinacumab, an ANGPTL3 inhibitor, in the treatment of dyslipidemia. *J Clin Med.* 2022;12:168.
78. Ishida T, Choi S, Kundu RK, et al. Endothelial lipase is a major determinant of HDL level. *J Clin Invest.* 2003;111:347-355.
79. Kourounakis AP, Charitos C, Rekka EA, Kourounakis PN. Lipid-lowering (hetero)aromatic tetrahydro-1,4-oxazine derivatives with antioxidant and squalene synthase inhibitory activity. *J Med Chem.* 2008;51:5861-5865.
80. Liao JK. Squalene synthase inhibitor lapaquistat acetate: could anything be better than statins? *Circulation.* 2011;123:1925-1928.
81. Roth B. ACAT inhibitors: evolution from cholesterol-absorption inhibitors to antiatherosclerotic agents. *Drug Discov Today.* 1998;3:19-25.
82. Edmondson SE, Weber AE, Elliot J. Cardiovascular and metabolic diseases: 50 years of progress. In: Desai MC, ed. *2015 Medicinal Chemistry Reviews.* Vol 50. American Chemical Society; 2015:83-116.
83. Sikorski JA. Oral cholesteryl ester transfer protein (CETP) inhibitors: a potential new approach for treating coronary artery disease. *J Med Chem.* 2006;49:1-22.
84. Cannon CP, Shah S, Dansky HM, et al. Safety of anacetrapib in patients with or at high risk for coronary heart disease. *N Engl J Med.* 2010;363:2406-2415.
85. Xiao W, Wang RS, Handy DE, Loscalzo J. NAD(H) and NADP(H) redox couples and cellular energy metabolism. *Antioxid Redox Signal.* 2018;28:251-272.
86. Altschul R, Hoffer A, Stephen JD. Influence of nicotinic acid on serum cholesterol in man. *Arch Biochem Biophys.* 1955;54:558-559.
87. Drood JM, Zimetbaum PJ, Frishman WH. Nicotinic acid for the treatment of hyperlipoproteinemia. *J Clin Pharmacol.* 1991;31:641-650.
88. Kamanna VS, Kashyap ML. Mechanism of action of niacin. *J Am Coll Cardiol.* 2008;101(8):S20-S26.
89. Zhang Y, Schmidt RJ, Foxworthy P, et al. Niacin mediates lipolysis in adipose tissue through its G-protein coupled receptor HM74A. *Biochem Biophys Res Commun.* 2005;334:729-732.
90. DiPalma J, Thayer WS. Use of niacin as a drug. *Annu Rev Nutr.* 1991;11:169-187.
91. Bersot TP. Drug therapy for hypercholesterolemia and dyslipidemia. In: Brunton L, Chabner B, Knollman B, eds. *Goodman & Gilman's the Pharmacological Basis of Therapeutics.* 12th ed. McGraw Hill; 2011:877-908.
92. Balendiran GK, Verma M, Perry E. Chemistry of fibrates. *Curr Chem Biol.* 2007;1(3):311-316.
93. Hansch C, Leo A. *Substituent Constants for Correlation Analysis in Chemistry and Biology.* Wiley; 1979:49-54.
94. Koski RR. Omega-3-acid ethyl ester (Lovaza) for severe hypertriglyceridemia. *P T.* 2008;33:271-281.
95. Weitz D, Weintraub H, Fisher E, *Schwartzbard* AZ. Fish oil for the treatment of cardiovascular disease. *Cardiol Rev.* 2010;18:258-263.
96. Bhatt DL, Steg PG, Miller M, et al. Cardiovascular risk reduction with icosapent ethyl for hypertriglyceridemia. *N Engl J Med.* 2019;380:11-22.

Structure Challenge Answers

1. ***Part a.*** All three of these drugs contain similar structural features: a carboxylic acid, two hydroxyl groups at the C_3 and C_5 positions, a heterocyclic ring, a *p*-substituted aromatic ring, and either an isopropyl or a cyclopropyl group. The primary structural difference among these drugs is the presence of a hydrogen bonding group in both atorvastatin and rosuvastatin. These functional groups, an amide in atorvastatin and a sulfonamide in rosuvastatin, allow these drugs to form additional binding interactions with HMGR, which allows for a higher binding affinity. These binding interactions are not possible for pitavastatin nor for any of the other HMGRIs.

   Part b. Rosuvastatin would be the best choice in the scenario provided. Atorvastatin and pitavastatin are much more lipid soluble than rosuvastatin and undergo significant hepatic metabolism. Atorvastatin is primarily inactivated by oxidative pathways requiring CYP3A4, and pitavastatin is primarily inactivated by glucuronide conjugation. The *N*-methyl sulfonamide attached to the pyrimidine ring of rosuvastatin provides significant water solubility as compared to hydrophobic aromatic rings present in the structures of atorvastatin and pitavastatin. As a result, rosuvastatin undergoes minimal hepatic metabolism by CYP2C9, is primarily excreted unchanged, and would be unaffected by the other medications that the patient is currently taking.

2. Performing a structural analysis of atorvastatin and Analogue A reveals that the only difference between these structures is the stereochemistry at the C_3-OH group. As described with the SAR of the statins, the 3,5-dihydroxyheptanoic acid portion of HMGRIs mimics the substrate, product, and/or transition state intermediate of the enzymatic reaction. Alteration of the stereochemistry at the C_3-OH position decreases the ability of Analogue A to mimic the natural substrate and would be expected to decrease binding.

   Performing a structural analysis of atorvastatin and Analogue B reveals that the only difference between these structures is that the *p*-fluoro ring has been fused with the adjacent phenyl ring to form a flat, rigid, and coplanar ring system. In order for any drug to bind to its receptor, it must be able to meet the steric requirements and be able to "fit" into the binding site. Thus, in order for Analogue B to bind to HMGR, the enzyme would need to have a similar large, flat area within its binding site. Studies have shown that this binding feature is not present within HMGR and that the *p*-fluoro ring must be able to freely rotate in order to fit into the enzyme binding site. As a result, Analogue B would not be expected to properly bind to HMGR and would most likely be inactive.

3. ***Part a:*** While the questions specifically pertained to cholestyramine, the concepts provided in the answers below are also applicable to colestipol and colesevelam. Cholestyramine contains multiple quaternary nitrogen atoms and permanently positive charges within its structure. Additionally, cholestyramine is a large polymer with a molecular weight reported to be greater than 1,000,000 Da. Extremely large molecules with multiple positive charges are not able to penetrate the GI membrane; therefore, cholestyramine would not be expected to be absorbed systemically and would not be expected to produce systemic adverse effects. Its main adverse effect is constipation due to a local effect within the GI tract.

Structure Challenge Answers (continued)

Part b: Cholestyramine is a large molecule with multiple positive charges. Its mechanism of action involves the binding and elimination of negatively charged bile acids. The actions of cholestyramine on bile acids is not specific; therefore, it is possible for cholestyramine to bind and eliminate other drugs that are administered at the same time as cholestyramine, thus decreasing their absorption and activity. While acidic drugs would be expected to be more susceptible to this drug interaction since they can become anionic at intestinal pH, it has been shown that this can also occur with basic drugs, amphoteric drugs, and drugs that are nonelectrolytes.

If this guideline was ignored, the primary effect would be a decrease in the absorption of the drug that is administered with cholestyramine. In comparing the relative doses of cholestyramine (4-16 g once or twice daily) to those of many other drugs (10-200 mg), it should be apparent that cholestyramine alters the absorption and affects other drugs much more than other drugs that affect cholestyramine.

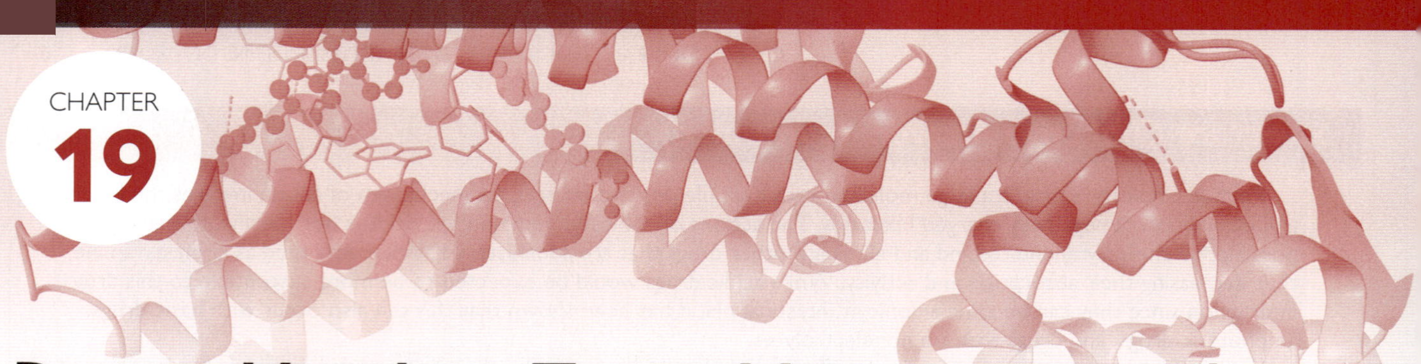

CHAPTER

19

Drugs Used to Treat Hypertensive/Hypotensive Disorders

Peter J. Harvison and Rami A. Al-Horani

Drugs covered in this chapter[a]:

Osmotic Diuretics
- Mannitol
- Sorbitol

Carbonic Anhydrase Inhibitors
- Acetazolamide
- Brinzolamide/dorzolamide
- Methazolamide

Thiazide Diuretics
- Bendroflumethiazide
- Chlorothiazide
- Hydrochlorothiazide
- Hydroflumethiazide
- Methyclothiazide

Thiazide-Like Diuretics
- Chlorthalidone
- Indapamide
- Metolazone

Loop Diuretics
- Bumetanide
- Ethacrynic acid
- Furosemide
- Torsemide

Aldosterone Antagonists (Mineralocorticoid Receptor Antagonists)
- Eplerenone
- Finerenone
- Spironolactone

Potassium-Sparing Diuretics
- Amiloride
- Triamterene

Angiotensin-Converting Enzyme Inhibitors
- Benazepril
- Captopril
- *Cilazapril*
- Enalapril
- Fosinopril
- Lisinopril
- Moexipril
- Perindopril
- Quinapril
- Ramipril
- *Spirapril*
- Trandolapril

Angiotensin II Receptor Blockers
- Azilsartan
- Candesartan
- Eprosartan
- *Fimasartan*
- Irbesartan
- Losartan
- Olmesartan
- Sparsentan
- Telmisartan
- Valsartan

Renin Inhibitor
- Aliskiren

Calcium Channel Blockers
- Amlodipine
- Clevidipine
- Diltiazem
- Felodipine
- Isradipine
- Nicardipine
- Nifedipine
- Nimodipine
- Nisoldipine
- Verapamil

β-Nonselective Blockers
- Carteolol
- Levobunolol
- Nadolol
- Penbutolol
- Pindolol
- Propranolol
- Timolol

β_1-Selective Blockers
- Acebutolol
- Atenolol
- Betaxolol
- Bisoprolol
- Esmolol
- Metoprolol
- Nebivolol

α_1-Blockers
- Doxazosin
- Prazosin
- Terazosin

Mixed α-/β-Blockers
- Carvedilol
- Labetalol

α_2-Agonists
- Clonidine
- Guanabenz
- Guanfacine
- Methyldopa
- Moxonidine
- Rilmenidine

α_1-Agonists
- Metaraminol
- Methoxamine
- Phenylephrine

Vasodilators
- Diazoxide
- Hydralazine
- Minoxidil

Nitrodilator
- Sodium nitroprusside

[a] *Drugs listed include those that are available inside and outside the United States; drugs available outside the United States are shown in italics.*

Abbreviations

ACE angiotensin-converting enzyme
ACEI angiotensin-converting enzyme inhibitor
ADH antidiuretic hormone, vasopressin
ADHD attention-deficit/hyperactivity disorder
AR androgen receptor
ARB angiotensin receptor blocker
AT_1 angiotensin II type 1 receptor
AT_2 angiotensin II type 2 receptor
AT-II angiotensin II
ATP adenosine triphosphate
AUC area under the curve
AV atrioventricular
BB β-blocker
CAD, coronary artery disease
CaM calmodulin
cAMP cyclic adenosine monophosphate
CCB calcium channel blocker
cGMP cyclic guanosine monophosphate
CNS central nervous system
COMT catechol-*O*-methyltransferase
COX-2 cyclooxygenase-2
CS chronic stable angina
DAG diacylglycerol
DCT distal convoluted tubule
DLH descending limb of the Loop of Henle
1,4-DHPs 1,4-dihydropyridines
ENaC epithelial sodium channel
eNOS endothelial nitric oxide synthase
ER extended release
ET endothelin
FDA U.S. Food and Drug Administration
GFR glomerular filtration rate
GPCRs G-protein–coupled receptors
GI gastrointestinal
GR glucocorticoid receptor
HVA high-voltage activated
IC_{50} half maximal inhibitory concentration
IgA immunoglobulin A
iNOS inducible nitric oxide synthase
IP3 inositol triphosphate
ISA intrinsic sympathomimetic activity
IV intravenous
JNC8 Eighth Joint National Committee
L-DOPA L-dihydroxyphenylalanine
LVA low-voltage activated
MAO monoamine oxidase
MAP mitogen-activated protein
MI myocardial infarction
MLCK myosin light-chain kinase
MR mineralocorticoid receptor
MRA mineralocorticoid receptor antagonist
NDMA *N*-nitroso-*N*-dimethylamine
NMDA *N*-methyl-D-aspartate
nNOS neuronal nitric oxide synthase
NADH nicotinamide adenine dinucleotide hydrogen
NADPH nicotinamide adenine dinucleotide phosphate hydrogen
NO nitric oxide
NOS nitric oxide synthase
PCT proximal convoluted tubule
PDC potential-dependent Ca^{2+} channels
PIP_2 phosphatidylinositol
PKC protein kinase C
PLC phospholipase C
PR progesterone receptor
PST proximal straight tubule
PSVT paroxysmal supraventricular tachycardia
PVD peripheral vascular disease
ROC receptor-operated Ca^{2+} channels
SAR structure-activity relationship
SLE systemic lupus erythematosus
SR sarcoplasmic reticulum
TALH thick ascending limb of the loop of Henle
VSM vascular smooth muscle

CLINICAL SIGNIFICANCE

Hypertension is a risk factor for cardiovascular diseases and stroke. There are over 80 antihypertensive agents belonging to 18 pharmacological mechanistic classes and subclasses. The abundance of antihypertensive agents is largely attributed to the application of medicinal chemistry concepts to continuously develop new agents and improve existing ones. Rationale structural design has led to the development of novel antihypertensive agents that serve specific clinical purposes. The application of structure-activity relationship (SAR) studies and prodrug preparation strategies have enabled the optimization of efficacy, potency, specificity, oral bioavailability, duration of action, and metabolic stability. Health care providers with knowledge of the medicinal chemistry and history of antihypertensive drugs will be able to improve patient outcomes by enhancing compliance, reducing adverse effects, and maintaining healthy blood pressures.

Ahlam Ayyad, PharmD

Cardiovascular Hypertension

Overview

Hypertension is the most common cardiovascular disease and is the major risk factor for coronary artery disease, heart failure, stroke, and renal failure. According to the 2023 American Heart Association statistics (period from 2017 to 2020)[1], approximately 122.4 million adult (age ≥20 years) Americans (59.6 million women and 62.8 million men) have a systolic or diastolic blood pressure at least 130/80 mm Hg, and the incidence of this disease increases with age in both sexes.[1] The highest prevalence is observed in Black men and women.[1]

The importance of controlling blood pressure is well documented,[1] although the rates of awareness, treatment, and control of hypertension have not risen as expected in the National Health and Nutrition Examination Survey.[2] This survey showed that 68% of Americans are aware that they have high blood pressure but that only 53% are receiving treatment and only 27% have their blood pressure under control. Since 1976, there has been a significant improvement in the rates of awareness, treatment, and control of hypertension; however, since 1990, whatever progress had been achieved has now reached a plateau.[2] Although the age-adjusted death rates from stroke and coronary heart disease during this period have fallen by 59% and 53%, respectively, their rates of decline also appear to have reached a plateau.[2] These troubling trends should awaken clinicians to be more aggressive in the treatment of patients with hypertension.

When the decision to initiate hypertensive therapy is made, physicians often are presented with the dilemma of which of more than 80 antihypertensive products, representing more than 18 different mechanistic drug classes, to use in their patients (Table 19.1).[1,3] The factors that can affect the outcomes from the treatment of hypertension, including potential adverse effects, clinically significant drug-drug interactions (especially when so many different drug classes are involved), patient adherence, affordability, risk/benefit ratios, and dosing frequency, must be considered.[3] Having considered these factors, the health care provider (clinician or pharmacist) arrives at an appropriate choice of antihypertensive drug.[3] Once the patient is stabilized with an antihypertensive medication, some of these issues need to be reevaluated. Patients should be continually asked about side effects because many of the antihypertensive drugs possess side effects that the patient cannot tolerate.[1] This problem and the cost of drug therapy can affect compliance to drug therapy especially for older adults and those on fixed incomes.[4]

Table 19.1 Classification of Antihypertensive Activity According to Mechanism of Action

Drug Class	Drug Subclass
Diuretics	1. Osmotic diuretics 2. Carbonic anhydrase inhibitors 3. Thiazide diuretics 4. Thiazide-like diuretics 5. Loop diuretics 6. Aldosterone antagonists 7. Potassium-sparing diuretics
Angiotensin-converting enzyme inhibitors	
Angiotensin II receptor blockers	
Renin inhibitor	
Calcium channel blockers	
Sympatholytic drugs	1. β-Adrenergic receptor blockers 2. α_1-Adrenergic receptor blockers 3. Mixed α-/β-adrenergic receptor blockers 4. α_1-Adrenergic receptor agonists 5. α_2-Adrenergic receptor agonists
Vasodilators	1. Arterial 2. Arterial and venous

Drug therapy in the management of hypertension must be individualized and adjusted based on coexisting risk factors, including the degree of blood pressure elevation, severity of the disease (eg, presence of target organ damage), presence of underlying cardiovascular or other risk factors, response to therapy (single or multiple drugs), and tolerance to drug-induced adverse effects.[1,3] Antihypertensive therapy is generally reserved for patients who fail to respond to nondrug therapies along with lifestyle modifications, such as diet (including sodium restriction and adequate potassium intake), regular aerobic physical activity, moderation of alcohol consumption, and weight reduction.[3]

It is not surprising that compliance with antihypertensive therapy can be as low as 40% when one considers that the patient, if he or she has other chronic diseases, can be taking as many as 10 different drugs and up to 40 tablets or capsules per day.[4] To achieve better compliance requires educating the patient and simplifying the drug regimen by reducing the number of drugs being taken.

Hypertension in pregnancy presents a formidable therapeutic challenge and requires comprehensive management with close monitoring for both maternal and fetal welfare.[5] Mechanisms involved with pregnancy-related hypertension include a hyperadrenergic state, plasma volume reduction, reduction in uteroplacental perfusion, hormonal control of vascular reactivity, and prostacyclin deficiency and can result from or activate the mechanisms that elevate blood pressure. Effective blood pressure control for pregnancy-related hypertension can often be achieved with methyldopa (recommended), β-blockers (BBs), or mixed α-/β-blockers (dual combination of α- and β-blocker activity). The vasodilating agent hydralazine is used to treat hypertensive emergencies associated with eclampsia.[1,6] The presence or development of proteinuria (preeclampsia) in a hypertensive pregnant woman implies a major increase in risk to the fetus and warrants immediate admission to a hospital for specialist management.[5]

Patients with diabetes have a much higher rate of hypertension than would be expected in the general population. Regardless of the antihypertensive agent used, a reduction in blood pressure helps prevent or reduce diabetic microvascular and macrovascular complications, such as blindness and kidney failure. Angiotensin-converting enzyme (ACE) inhibitors (ACEIs) and angiotensin receptor blockers (ARBs) are considered first-line therapy in patients with diabetes and hypertension because of their well-established renal protective effects. Most patients with diabetes having hypertension require combination therapy with low-dose diuretics and BBs to achieve optimal blood pressure goals.

Combination Antihypertensive Therapy

It is well documented that monotherapy adequately controls hypertension only in approximately 50% of patients.[7,8] Therefore, a large percentage of patients will require at least a combination of two drugs to control their blood pressure

Table 19.2 Initial Drug Choices (JNC8)

Without Compelling Risk Factors		With Compelling Risk Factors
Blood pressure goal, <120/80 mm Hg		Blood pressure goal, <130/80 mm Hg
Stage 1 hypertension	Stage 2 hypertension	Compelling risk factors include
SBP 130-139 or DBP 80-89 mm Hg	SBP ≥140 or DBP ≥90 mm Hg	Heart failure After myocardial infarction High coronary disease risk Diabetes Chronic kidney disease Recurrent stroke prevention
Monotherapy with first-line drugs (thiazide-type diuretics, ACEIs, ARBs, or CCBs) or combinations to achieve blood pressure goal	Two first-line drugs (thiazide-type diuretics, ACEIs, ARBs, or CCBs) in different classes	Drugs for compelling indications: Stage 1 drugs and other antihypertensive drugs
Not at Blood Pressure Goal		
Optimize stage 2 drug treatment, or add additional classes of antihypertensive drugs until blood pressure goal is achieved		

ACEI, angiotensin-converting enzyme inhibitor; ARB, angiotensin receptor blocker; CCB, calcium channel blocker; DBP, diastolic blood pressure; SBP, systolic blood pressure.

and symptoms of hypertension. By combining different antihypertensive drug classes in low doses, their different mechanisms of action result in synergistic blood pressure lowering as well as in minimizing the adverse effects and improving compliance issues.[1,8] For example, the addition of a low-dose thiazide diuretic dramatically increases the rates of response to methyldopa, ACEIs, and BBs without producing the undesirable side effects. In the latest guidelines for treatment of hypertension, the Joint National Committee for Prevention, Detection, Evaluation, and Treatment of High Blood Pressure (JNC8), clinicians are encouraged to begin initially with thiazide-type diuretics, ACEIs, ARBs, or calcium channel blockers (CCBs) in hypertensive patients without compelling risk factors (Table 19.2). These drug classes have been shown to decrease morbidity and mortality in long-term clinical trials.[2] Other antihypertensive drugs (including stage 1 agents) are considered in patients with compelling risk factors, such as heart disease, clinical manifestations of cardiovascular diseases or diabetes (Table 19.2). In patients with compelling risk factors for cardiovascular disease, treatment should be more aggressive, with the goal of reducing blood pressure to less than 130/80 mm Hg (Table 19.3). These recommendations reflect the current awareness of the importance of addressing other cardiovascular conditions aside from just lowering the blood pressure.

Diuretics

Overview

Diuretics are chemicals that increase the rate of urine formation.[9] Diuretic usage leads to increased excretion of electrolytes (especially sodium and chloride ions) and water from the body by increasing the urine flow rate, without affecting protein, vitamin, glucose, or amino acid reabsorption. These pharmacological properties have led to the use of diuretics in the treatment of edematous conditions resulting from a variety of causes (eg, congestive heart failure, nephrotic syndrome, and chronic liver disease) and in the management of hypertension. Diuretic drugs also are useful as the sole agent or as adjunct therapy in the treatment of a wide range of other clinical conditions, including hypercalcemia, diabetes insipidus, acute mountain sickness, primary hyperaldosteronism, and glaucoma.

The primary target organ for diuretics is the kidney, where these drugs interfere with the reabsorption of sodium and other ions from the lumina of the nephrons, which are the functional units of the kidney. The amount of ions and

Table 19.3 Risk Factors for Cardiovascular Disease

Correctable	Noncorrectable
Cigarette smoking	Age >60 y
Hypertension	Sex (men and postmenopausal women)
Elevated cholesterol	Family history of cardiovascular disease or stroke (women <65 y, men <55 y)
Reduced HDL (high-density lipoprotein) cholesterol	Target organ damage
Diabetes	
Obesity	
HDL	

accompanying water that are excreted as urine following administration of a diuretic, however, is determined by many factors, including the chemical structure of the diuretic, the site or sites of action of the agent, the salt intake of the patient, and the amount of extracellular fluid present. In addition to having a direct effect in impairing solute and water reabsorption from the nephron, diuretics can also trigger compensatory physiologic events that impact either the magnitude or the duration of the diuretic response. Thus, it is important to be aware of the normal mechanisms of urine formation and renal control mechanisms to understand clearly the ability of chemicals to induce diuresis.

Normal Physiology of Urine Formation

Two important functions of the kidney are (1) to maintain a homeostatic balance of electrolytes and water and (2) to excrete water-soluble end products of metabolism. The kidney accomplishes these functions through the formation of urine by the nephrons (Fig. 19.1). Each kidney contains approximately one million nephrons and is capable of forming urine independently. The nephrons are composed of a specialized capillary bed called the glomerulus and a long tubule divided anatomically and functionally into the proximal tubule, loop of Henle, and distal tubule. Each component of the nephron contributes to the normal functioning of the kidney in a unique manner; thus, all are targets for different classes of diuretic agents.

Urine formation begins with the filtration of blood at the glomerulus. Approximately 1,200 mL of blood per minute flows through both kidneys and reaches the nephron by way of afferent arterioles. About 20% of the blood entering the glomerulus is filtered into Bowman capsule to form the glomerular filtrate. The glomerular filtrate is composed of blood components with a molecular weight less than that of albumin (~69,000 Da) and not bound to plasma proteins. The glomerular filtration rate (GFR) averages 125 mL/min in humans but can vary widely even in normal functional states.

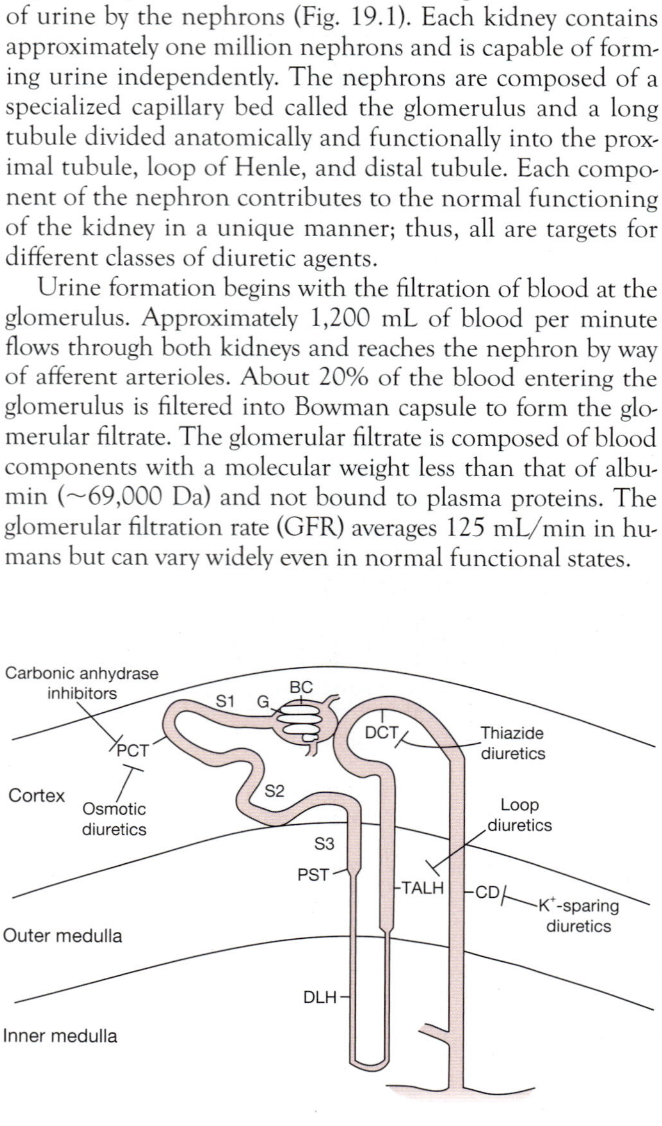

Figure 19.1 Nephron. BC, Bowman capsule; CD, collecting duct; DCT, distal convoluted tubule; DLH, descending limb of the Loop of Henle; G, glomerulus; PCT, proximal convoluted tubule; PST, proximal straight tubule; TALH, thick ascending limb of the loop of Henle.

The glomerular filtrate leaves the Bowman capsule and enters the proximal convoluted tubule (S1, S2 segments, Fig. 19.1), where the majority (50%-60%) of filtered sodium is reabsorbed osmotically. Sodium reabsorption is coupled electrogenetically with the reabsorption of glucose, phosphate, and amino acids and nonelectrogenetically with bicarbonate reabsorption. Glucose and amino acids are completely reabsorbed in this portion of the nephron, whereas phosphate reabsorption is between 80% and 90% complete. The early proximal convoluted tubule also is the primary site of bicarbonate reabsorption (80%-90%), a process that is mainly sodium dependent and coupled to hydrogen ion secretion. The reabsorption of sodium and bicarbonate is facilitated by the enzyme carbonic anhydrase, which is present in proximal tubular cells and catalyzes the formation of carbonic acid from water and carbon dioxide. The carbonic acid provides the hydrogen ion, which drives the reabsorption of sodium bicarbonate. Chloride ions are reabsorbed passively in the proximal tubule, where they follow actively transported sodium ions into tubular cells.

The reabsorption of electrolytes and water also occurs isosmotically in the proximal straight tubule or pars recta (S3 segment, Fig. 19.1). By the end of the straight segment, between 65% and 70% of water and sodium, chloride, and calcium ions; 80% to 90% of bicarbonate and phosphate; and essentially 100% of glucose, amino acids, vitamins, and protein have been reabsorbed from the glomerular filtrate. The proximal tubule also is the site for active secretion of weakly acidic and weakly basic organic compounds. Thus, many of the diuretics can enter luminal fluid not only by filtration at the glomerulus but also by active secretion.

The descending limb of the loop of Henle is impermeable to ions, but water can freely move from the luminal fluid into the surrounding medullary interstitium, where the higher osmolality draws water into the interstitial space and concentrates luminal fluid. Luminal fluid continues to concentrate as it descends to the deepest portion of the loop of Henle, where the fluid becomes the most concentrated. The hypertonic luminal fluid next enters the water-impermeable, thick ascending limb of the loop of Henle. In this segment of the nephron, approximately 20% to 25% of the filtered sodium and chloride ions are reabsorbed via a cotransport system ($Na^+/K^+/2Cl^-$) on the luminal membrane. Reabsorption of sodium and chloride in the medullary portion of the thick ascending limb is important for maintaining the medullary interstitial concentration gradient. Reabsorption of sodium chloride in the cortical component of the thick ascending limb of the loop of Henle and the early distal convoluted tubule contributes to urinary dilution, and as a result, these two nephron sections sometimes are called the cortical diluting segment of the nephron.

Luminal fluid leaving the early distal tubule next passes through the late distal tubule and cortical collecting tubule (collecting duct), where sodium is reabsorbed in exchange for hydrogen and potassium ions. This process is partially controlled by the primary mineralocorticoid, aldosterone, and accounts for the reabsorption of between 2% and 3% of filtered sodium ions. Although the reabsorption of sodium ions from these segments of the nephron is not large, this sodium/potassium/hydrogen ion exchange system determines the final acidity and potassium content of urine. Several factors, however, can influence the activity of this exchange system, including the amount of sodium ions delivered to these segments, the status of the acid-base balance in the body, and the levels of circulating aldosterone.

The urine formed during this process represents only approximately 1% to 2% of the original glomerular filtrate, with more than 98% of electrolytes and water filtered at the glomerulus being reabsorbed during passage through the nephron. Thus, a change in urine output of only 1% to 2% could double urine volume. Urine leaves the kidney through the ureters and travels to the bladder, where it is stored until urination removes it from the body.

Normal Regulation of Urine Formation

The body contains several control mechanisms that regulate the volume and contents of urine. These systems are activated by changes in solute or water content of the body, by changes in systemic or renal blood pressure, and by a variety of other stimuli. Activation of one or more of these systems by diuretics can modify the effectiveness of these drugs to produce their therapeutic response and may require additional therapeutic measures to ensure a maximal response.

The kidney can respond to changes in the GFR through the action of specialized distal tubular epithelial cells called the macula densa. These cells are in close contact with the glomerular apparatus of the same nephron and detect changes in the rate of urine flow and luminal sodium chloride concentration. An increase in the urine flow rate at this site (as can occur with the use of some diuretics) activates the macula densa cells to communicate with the granular cells and vascular segments of the juxtaglomerular apparatus. Stimulation of the juxtaglomerular apparatus causes renin to be released, which leads to the formation of angiotensin II and subsequent renal vasoconstriction. Renal vasoconstriction leads to a decrease in GFR and, possibly, a decrease in the effectiveness of the diuretic. Renin release also can be stimulated by factors other than diuretics, including decreased renal perfusion pressure, increased sympathetic tone, and decreased blood volume.

Another important regulatory mechanism for urine formation is antidiuretic hormone (ADH), also known as vasopressin, which is released from the posterior pituitary in response to reduced blood pressure and elevated plasma osmolality. In the kidney, ADH acts on the collecting tubule to increase water permeability and reabsorption via increased aquaporin (water channel) expression. As a result, the urine becomes more concentrated, and water is conserved in the presence of ADH.

Role of Fluid Volume in Hypertension and Other Cardiovascular Disorders

The diuretic drugs are used primarily to treat two medically important conditions, edema and hypertension.[10-13] Both conditions are common, although some patients exhibit refractory disease states that require additional modification of the drug regimen to include alternative diuretics or the addition of nondiuretic drugs. Edema (excessive extracellular fluid) normally results from disease of the heart, kidney, or liver. Decreased cardiac function (eg, congestive heart disease) can result in decreased perfusion of all organs (eg, kidney) and limbs and an accumulation of edema fluid in the extremities, particularly around the ankles and in the hands. Left-sided heart failure can lead to the development of acute pulmonary edema, which is a medical emergency. Right-sided heart failure shifts extracellular fluid volume from the arterial circulation to the venous circulation, which leads to general edema formation.

Kidney dysfunction can lead to edema because of decreased formation of urine and the subsequent imbalance of water and electrolyte (eg, sodium ion) homeostasis. Retention of salt and water results in an expansion of the extracellular fluid volume and edema. Thus, when salt intake exceeds salt excretion, edema can form. Edema is also associated with deceased protein levels in blood, as seen in nephrotic syndrome and liver disease. Cirrhosis of the liver leads to increased lymph in the space of Disse. Eventually, the increased lymph volume results in movement of fluid into the peritoneal cavity and ascites develops.

Patients with hypertension are at increased risk for developing cardiovascular disease. One key element in controlling blood pressure is the sodium ion concentration, and early antihypertensive effects of diuretics are related to increased salt and water excretion. Additionally, however, diuretics have long-term effects, resulting in decreased vascular resistance that contribute to blood pressure control. Although effects on vascular calcium-activated potassium channels have been proposed as contributing to the chronic antihypertensive effects of thiazide diuretics, the exact mechanisms of long-term effects remain to be determined.

Diuretics also are useful in treating a number of other conditions, including increased cranial (trauma or surgery) or intraocular (glaucoma) pressure (eg, osmotic diuretics), diabetes insipidus (eg, thiazides), hypercalcemia (eg, loop diuretics), acute mountain sickness (eg, carbonic anhydrase inhibitors), primary hyperaldosteronism (eg, aldosterone antagonists), and osteoporosis (eg, thiazides).

General Therapeutic Approaches

Diuretic drugs may be administered acutely or chronically to treat edematous states. When immediate action to reduce edema (eg, acute pulmonary edema) is needed, intravenous administration of a loop diuretic is often the approach of choice. Thiazide or loop diuretics normally are administered orally to treat nonemergency edematous states. The magnitude of the diuretic response is directly proportional to the amount of edema fluid that is present. As the volume of edema decreases, so does the magnitude of the diuretic response with each dose. If concern exists about the development of diuretic-induced hypokalemia, then a potassium supplement or potassium-sparing diuretic may be added to the drug regimen. The development of hypokalemia is particularly important for patients with congestive heart failure who also are taking cardiac glycosides, such as digoxin.

Digoxin has a narrow therapeutic index, and developing hypokalemia can potentiate digitalis-induced cardiac effects with potentially fatal results.

Diuretic drugs are typically administered orally to help control blood pressure in the treatment of hypertension. Diuretics often are the first drugs used to treat hypertension, and they also may be added to other drug therapies used to control blood pressure with beneficial effects.

Diuretics have also been used illicitly by some athletes for "sport doping"[14] because of the drugs' ability to quickly produce weight loss (via increased excretion of water) and masking of urine contents (via dilution of other drugs or metabolites that might be present in the urine). Furosemide, triamterene, and hydrochlorothiazide are the most commonly used diuretics for sport doping, as they are eliminated rapidly and are therefore more difficult to detect in urine samples taken at later time points after use. Another consideration is that some diuretics can degrade in urine samples; for example, thiazides may hydrolyze to aminobenzenedisulfonamide derivatives.[15] Use of diuretics by athletes without a documented therapeutic need has been banned since 1988, and routine monitoring for these drugs and their degradation products is commonplace. A list of banned drugs, including diuretics, is maintained and updated by the International Olympic Committee and the World Anti-Doping Agency.

Diuretic Drug Classes

History

Compounds that increase the urine flow rate have been known for centuries. One of the earliest substances known to induce diuresis is water, an inhibitor of ADH release. Calomel (mercurous chloride) was used as early as the 16th century as a diuretic, but because of poor absorption from the gastrointestinal tract and toxicity, calomel was replaced clinically by the organomercurials (eg, chlormerodrin). The organomercurials represented the first group of highly efficacious diuretics available for clinical use. The need to administer these drugs parenterally, the possibility of tolerance, and their potential toxicity, however, soon led to the search for newer, less toxic diuretics. Today, the organomercurials are no longer used as diuretics, but their discovery began the search for many of the diuretics used today. Other compounds previously used as diuretics include the acid-forming salts (eg, ammonium chloride) and methylxanthines (eg, theophylline).

Diuretic Classification

Diuretics are classified (Table 19.4) by their chemical class (thiazides), mechanism of action (carbonic anhydrase inhibitors and osmotics), site of action (loop diuretics), or effects on urine contents (potassium-sparing diuretics). These drugs vary widely in their efficacy (ie, their ability to increase the rate of urine formation) and their site of action within the nephron. Efficacy often is measured as the ability of the diuretic to increase the excretion of sodium ions filtered at the glomerulus (ie, the filtered load of sodium) and should not be confused with potency, which is the amount of the diuretic required to produce a specific diuretic response.

Efficacy is determined, in part, by the site of action of the diuretic. Drugs (eg, carbonic anhydrase inhibitors) that act primarily on the proximal convoluted tubule to induce diuresis are weak diuretics because of the ability of the nephron to reabsorb a significant portion of the luminal contents at downstream sites. Likewise, drugs (potassium-sparing diuretics) that act at the more distal segments of the nephron are weak diuretics because most of the glomerular filtrate

Table 19.4 Diuretics: Sites and Mechanisms of Action

Diuretic Class	Site of Action	Mechanism of Action
Osmotics	Proximal tubule	Osmotic effects decrease sodium and water reabsorption
	Loop of Henle	Increases medullary blood flow to decrease medullary hypertonicity and reduce sodium and water reabsorption
	Collecting tubule	Sodium and water reabsorption decreases because of reduced medullary hypertonicity and elevated urinary flow rate
Carbonic anhydrase inhibitors	Proximal convoluted tubule	Inhibition of renal carbonic anhydrase decreases sodium bicarbonate reabsorption
Thiazides and thiazide-like	Cortical portion of the thick ascending limb of loop of Henle and distal tubule	Inhibition of Na^+/Cl^- symporter
Loop or high ceiling	Thick ascending limb of the loop of Henle	Inhibition of the luminal $Na^+/K^+/2Cl^-$ transport system
Potassium sparing	Distal tubule and collecting duct	Inhibition of sodium and water reabsorption by competitive inhibition of aldosterone (eplerenone, finerenone, and spironolactone) or blockade of sodium channel at the luminal membrane (triamterene and amiloride)

has already been reabsorbed in the proximal tubule and ascending limb of the loop of Henle before reaching the distal tubule. Thus, the most efficacious diuretics discovered so far, the high-ceiling or loop diuretics, interfere with sodium chloride reabsorption at the ascending limb of the loop of Henle, which is situated after the proximal tubule but before the distal portions of the nephron and collecting tubule (Fig. 19.1).

Osmotic Diuretics

Therapeutic Role of Osmotic Diuretics

Osmotic diuretics are not frequently used in medicine today except in the prophylaxis of acute renal failure, in which these drugs inhibit water reabsorption and maintain urine flow. They may also be helpful in maintaining urine flow in cases where urinary output is diminished because of severe bleeding or traumatic surgical experiences. The osmotic diuretics have also been used to acutely reduce increased intracranial or intraocular pressure.

Mannitol is the most commonly used osmotic diuretic and is administered intravenously in solutions of 5% to 50% at a rate of administration that is adjusted to maintain the urinary output at 30 to 50 mL/h.[16] Sorbitol, a close structural analog of mannitol (see later), is used as a hyperosmotic laxative for the treatment of constipation.

Pharmacology Overview of Osmotic Diuretics

Mechanism of Action. Osmotic diuretics are low-molecular-weight compounds that are freely filtered through the Bowman capsule.[16] Once in the renal tubule, osmotic diuretics have limited reabsorption because of their high-water solubility. When administered as a hypertonic (hyperosmolar) solution, these agents increase intraluminal osmotic pressure, causing water to pass from the body into the tubule. As the osmotic agent and associated water are not reabsorbed from the nephron, a diuretic effect is observed. Osmotic diuretics increase the volume of urine and the excretion of water and almost all electrolytes.

Common Adverse Effects. Osmotic diuretics induce few adverse effects, but expansion of the extracellular fluid volume can occur, which limits their use in treating ordinary edemas. Alteration of blood sodium levels can be seen, and these drugs should not be used in anuric or unresponsive patients. If cranial bleeding is present, mannitol should not be used.

Common Interactions. Mannitol may interfere with lithium therapy by increasing urinary elimination of that drug.

Medicinal Chemistry of Osmotic Diuretics

Receptor Binding, Structure-Activity Relationships, and Physicochemical Properties. These drugs do not interact with a receptor and exert their diuretic or laxative activity via an osmotic effect. Mannitol and sorbitol are highly water-soluble sugar alcohols and differ from each other only in the stereochemical orientation of the hydroxyl group on carbon atom 2.

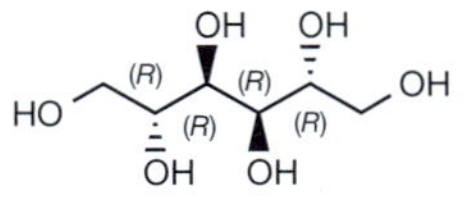

Mannitol

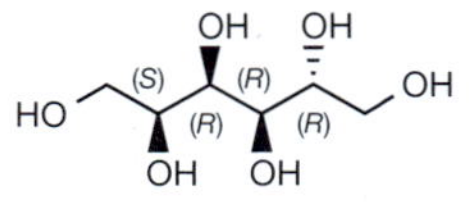

Sorbitol

Pharmacokinetic Properties and Metabolism. Due to their polarity, mannitol and sorbitol have poor oral bioavailability and are administered intravenously or rectally. They undergo limited hepatic metabolism and are excreted mostly as unchanged parent drugs (see Table 19.5 for pharmacokinetic properties of mannitol). Sorbitol is metabolized by intestinal bacteria.

Carbonic Anhydrase Inhibitors

Therapeutic Role of Carbonic Anhydrase Inhibitors

Carbonic anhydrase inhibitors are not currently used in the management of hypertension. Their most common therapeutic role is in the treatment of glaucoma, in which they inhibit carbonic anhydrase in the eye, reduce the rate of aqueous humor formation, and consequently reduce intraocular pressure.[17] These compounds have also found some limited use in the treatment of absence seizures, to alkalinize the urine, to treat familial periodic paralysis, to reduce metabolic alkalosis, and, prophylactically, to reduce acute mountain sickness.

With prolonged use of carbonic anhydrase inhibitors, the urine becomes more alkaline, and the blood becomes more acidic. When acidosis occurs, the carbonic anhydrase inhibitors lose their effectiveness as diuretics. They remain ineffective until normal acid-base balance in the body has been regained.

Acetazolamide, a thiadiazole derivative, was the first carbonic anhydrase inhibitors to be used as an orally effective diuretic, with a therapeutic effect that lasts ca. 8 to 12 hours (Table 19.5).

Pharmacology Overview of Carbonic Anhydrase Inhibitors

Mechanism of Action. In 1937, it was proposed that the normal acidification of urine was caused by secretion of hydrogen ions by the tubular cells of the kidney. These ions were provided by the action of the enzyme carbonic anhydrase, which catalyzes the formation of carbonic acid (H_2CO_3) from carbon dioxide and water.

$$CO_2 + H_2O \xrightarrow{\text{carbonic anhydrase}} H_2CO_3 \rightleftharpoons H^{\oplus} + HCO_3^{\ominus}$$

It was also observed that sulfanilamide rendered the urine of dogs alkaline because of the inhibition of carbonic anhydrase. This inhibition of carbonic anhydrase resulted in a lesser exchange of hydrogen ions for sodium ions in the kidney tubule. Sodium ions, along with bicarbonate ions, and associated water molecules were then excreted, and a diuretic effect was noted.

Carbonic anhydrase inhibitors induce diuresis by inhibiting the formation of carbonic acid within proximal

Table 19.5 Pharmacologic and Pharmacokinetic Properties of the Nonthiazide Diuretics

Drug	Trade Name	Relative Potency	Oral Absorption (%)	Peak Plasma	Half-Life	Duration of Effect	Elimination
Osmotic Diuretics							
Mannitol			<20	1-3 h IV	0.5-1.5 h	6-8 h	Urine, as parent drug
Carbonic Anhydrase Inhibitors							
Acetazolamide	Diamox		>90	1-3 h	6-9 h	8-12 h	Urine (major), as parent drug (70%-100%)
Methazolamide	Neptazane		>90	NA	~14 h	10-18 h	Urine, as parent drug (~25%) and metabolites
Brinzolamide	Azopt		topical use only (eye)	NA	~111 d[a]	8-12 h	Urine, as parent drug (major)
Dorzolamide	Trusopt		topical use only (eye)	NA	4 mo[a]	8-12 h	Urine, as parent drug (major)
Loop Diuretics							
Furosemide	Lasix	1	11-90[b]	4-5 h	0.5-4 h (>3 h)[c]	6-8 h	Urine/feces, as parent drug (60%-70%) and metabolites
Bumetamide	Bumex	40	80-100	<2 h	1-1.5 h (>3 h)[c]	5-6 h	Urine (major), as parent drug (~50%) and ~5 metabolites
Torsemide	Demadex	3	80-100	1-2 h	0.8-4 h	6-8 h	Urine/feces (2:8), as parent drug
Ethacrynic acid	Edecrin	0.7	>90	2 h	0.5-1 h	6-8 h	Urine/feces, as parent drug (30%-60%) and mercapturic acid
Mineralocorticoid Receptor Antagonists							
Spironolactone	Aldactone	20-40	>90[d]	1-2 h	1-3 h (parent drug)	2-3 d	Urine/feces, as active metabolite(s)
Eplerenone	Inspra	1	70	1.5 h	4-6 h	NA	Urine/feces (2:1), as metabolites (>95%)
Potassium-Sparing Diuretics							
Amiloride	Midamor	1	~50[b]	3-4 h	6-9 h normal (21 h)[c]	24 h	Urine/feces (5:4), as parent drug
Triamterene	Dyrenium	0.1	>70	2-4 h	2-3 h	Can be ≥24 h	Urine, as parent drug and metabolites

NA, data not available.
[a]Strongly bound to red blood cells.
[b]Food affects bioavailability.
[c]In patients with renal insufficiency.
[d]Formulation affects bioavailability.

Data from AHFS Drug Information (2010), American Society of Health-System Pharmacists (available at: www.tetondata.com/titles#|q=ahfs); *Lexicomp Online* (2011), Lexicomp (available at: www.wolterskluwer.com/en/solutions/uptodate/enterprise/lexidrug); *Facts and Comparisons* (2010), Wolters Kluwer Health (available at: www.wolterskluwer.com/en/solutions/uptodate/enterprise/lexidrug-facts-and-comparisons).

(proximal convoluted tubule; S2 segment) and distal tubular cells to limit the number of hydrogen ions available to promote sodium reabsorption. For a diuretic response to be observed, more than 99% of the carbonic anhydrase enzymes must be inhibited. Although carbonic anhydrase activity in the proximal tubule regulates the reabsorption of approximately 20% to 25% of the filtered load of sodium, the carbonic anhydrase inhibitors are not highly efficacious diuretics. An increased excretion of only 2% to 5% of the filtered load of sodium is seen with carbonic anhydrase inhibitors because of increased reabsorption of sodium ions by the ascending limb of the loop of Henle and more distal nephron segments.

Common Adverse Effects. The carbonic anhydrase inhibitors generally do not produce serious side effects. However, monitoring for electrolyte disturbances may be necessary. Symptoms resulting from adverse effects on the gastrointestinal tract (nausea, vomiting, etc), nervous system (sedation, headache, etc), and kidneys (formation of stones) have been reported. Although they contain sulfonamide groups, hypersensitivity reactions with other sulfonamide-containing drugs are not common. As noted above, these drugs can produce metabolic acidosis.

Common Interactions. Carbonic anhydrase inhibitors may increase the elimination of lithium and consequently decrease the therapeutic activity of this drug.

As they alkalinize urine, carbonic anhydrase inhibitors may decrease the elimination of basic drugs. This occurs because the higher pH shifts the equilibrium to the nonionized base, which is more extensively reabsorbed from the renal tubular fluid than the ionized conjugate acid.

Medicinal Chemistry of Carbonic Anhydrase Inhibitors

Receptor Binding, Structure-Activity Relationships, and Physicochemical Properties. Sulfanilamide inhibits carbonic anhydrase; however, the large doses required for inhibition and the side effects associated with this compound prompted a search for more effective carbonic anhydrase inhibitors as diuretics. This led to the discovery that the sulfonamide portion of an active diuretic molecule could not be monosubstituted or disubstituted.[18,19] As a result, it was reasoned that a more acidic sulfonamide would bind more tightly to the carbonic anhydrase enzyme. Synthesis of more highly acidic sulfonamides produced compounds with activities greater than 2,500-fold that of sulfanilamide. Acetazolamide was introduced in 1953 as an orally effective diuretic drug. Methazolamide is a close structural analog of acetazolamide in which one of the active hydrogens in the thiadiazole ring has been replaced by a methyl group. This decreases polarity of the compound and permits a greater penetration into the ocular fluid, where it acts as a carbonic anhydrase inhibitor, reducing intraocular pressure.

Brinzolamide and dorzolamide contain ionizable amino groups and are the result of efforts to develop water-soluble compounds that retain sufficient lipophilicity to penetrate the cornea.[11] They are indicated only for topical eye administration in glaucoma patients.

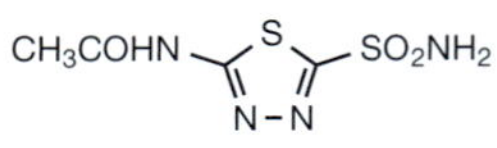

Acetazolamide

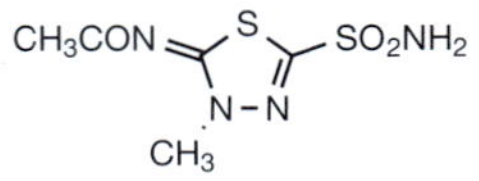

Methazolamide

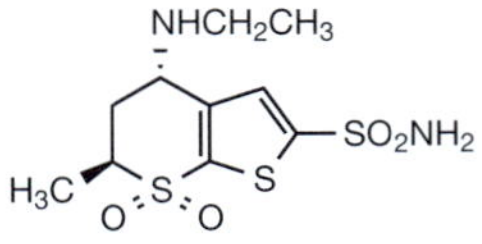

Dorzolamide

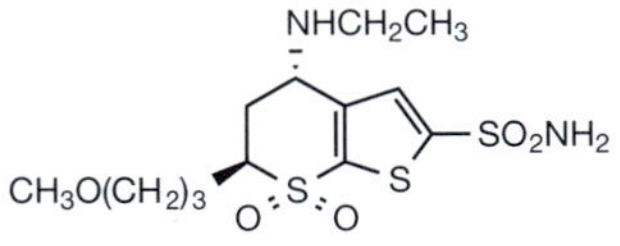

Brinzolamide

Pharmacokinetic Properties and Metabolism. The pharmacokinetic properties of the carbonic anhydrase inhibitors are summarized in Table 19.5. These drugs are administered orally or topically to the cornea (for ocular use) and are eliminated in urine predominantly as unchanged parent compounds.

Thiazide Diuretics

Therapeutic Role of Thiazide Diuretics

Thiazide and thiazide-like (see next section) diuretics are a mainstay in the treatment of hypertension.[20,21] Interestingly, increasing doses of thiazides correlates with an increase in adverse effects, but not in diuretic activity. Consequently, the doses currently used are lower than when these drugs first came into clinical use. They are also used to treat edemas caused by cardiac decompensation as well as in hepatic or renal disease. Their effect may be attributed to a reduction in blood volume and a direct relaxation of vascular smooth muscle. The thiazide diuretics are administered once a day or in divided daily doses. Some have a duration of action that permits administration of a dose every other day. They are used in monotherapy and in combination with other antihypertensive drugs, including ACE inhibitors, ARBs, and β-blockers.[21] The specific structures for the thiazide diuretics, relative activities, and inhibitory potencies are summarized in Table 19.6.

Pharmacology Overview of Thiazide Diuretics

Mechanism of Action. Further study of the benzene disulfonamide derivatives was undertaken to find more efficacious carbonic anhydrase inhibitors. These studies provided some compounds with a high degree of diuretic activity. Chloro and amino substitution gave compounds with increased activity, but these compounds were weak carbonic anhydrase inhibitors. When the amino group was acylated, an unexpected ring closure took place. These compounds possessed a diuretic activity independent of the carbonic anhydrase inhibitory activity, and a new series of diuretics called the benzothiadiazines (thiazides) was discovered.[20]

These diuretics are actively secreted in the proximal tubule and are carried to the loop of Henle and to the distal tubule. The major site of action of these compounds is in the distal convoluted tubule, where these drugs compete for the chloride binding site of the Na^+/Cl^- symporter and inhibit the reabsorption of sodium and chloride ions. For this reason, they are referred to as saluretics. They also inhibit the reabsorption of potassium and bicarbonate ions, but to a lesser degree.

Table 19.6 Pharmacologic and Pharmacokinetic Properties of the Thiazide Diuretics

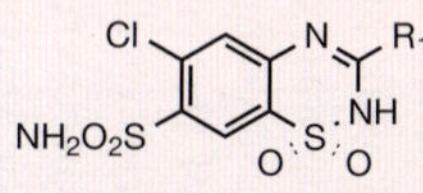

Thiazides: Structure I

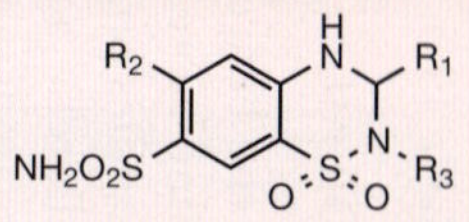

Thiazides: Structure II

Generic Name	Trade Name	Structure	Relative Potency[a]	Carbonic Anhydrase Inhibition[b]	Bioavailability	Peak Plasma	Half-Life	Duration of Effect	Elimination
Bendroflumethiazide	Naturetin	Structure II: R_1 = benzyl; R_2 = CF_3; R_3 = H	1.8	3×10^{-4} M	>90%	4 h	8.5 h	6-12 h	Urine, as parent drug
Chlorothiazide	Diuril	Structure I: R_1 = H	0.8	2×10^{-6} M	<25%	4 h	0.75-2 h	12-16 h	Urine, as parent drug
Hydrochlorothiazide	HydroDiuril Esidrix	Structure II: R_1 = H; R_2 = Cl; R_3 = H	1.4	2×10^{-5} M	>80%	4-6 h	6-15 h	12-16 h	Urine, as parent drug
Hydroflumethiazide	Saluron Diucardin	Structure II: R_1 = H; R_2 = CF_3; R_3 = H	1.3	2×10^{-4} M	Inc	3-4 h	17 h	18-24 h	Urine, as parent drug and metabolites
Methyclothiazide	Aquatensen	Structure II: R_1 = CH_2Cl; R2 = Cl; R3 = CH_3	1.8		Var	6 h	NA	>24 h	Urine, as parent drug

Inc, incomplete absorption; NA, data not available; Var, variables absorption.

[a]The numerical values refer to potency ratios (in humans) with the natriuretic response to that of a standard dose of meralluride, which is given a value of one.

[b]50% inhibition of carbonic anhydrase in vitro.

Data from AHFS Drug Information (2010), American Society of Health-System Pharmacists; Lexicomp Online (2011), Lexicomp; Facts and Comparisons (2010), Wolters Kluwer Health.

COMMON ADVERSE EFFECTS. Thiazide diuretics may induce several adverse effects, including hypersensitivity reactions, gastric irritation, nausea, and electrolyte imbalances, such as hyponatremia, hypokalemia, hypomagnesemia, hypochloremic alkalosis, hypercalcemia, and hyperuricemia. Individuals who exhibit hypersensitivity reactions to one thiazide are likely to have a hypersensitivity reaction to other thiazides and sulfamoyl-containing diuretics (eg, thiazide-like and some high-ceiling diuretics). Potassium and magnesium supplements may be administered to treat hypokalemia or hypomagnesemia, but their use is not always indicated. These supplements usually are administered as potassium chloride, potassium gluconate, potassium citrate, magnesium oxide, or magnesium lactate. The salts are administered as solutions, tablets, or timed-release tablets. Potassium-sparing diuretics (eg, triamterene or amiloride) may also be used to prevent hypokalemia. Combination preparations of hydrochlorothiazide and a potassium-sparing diuretic are available.

Long-term use of thiazide diuretics may also result in decreased glucose tolerance and increased blood lipid (low-density lipoprotein cholesterol, total cholesterol, and total triglyceride) content.

COMMON INTERACTIONS. As noted earlier, the thiazides may be used in combination with ACE inhibitors or ARBs to achieve an enhanced antihypertensive effect. However, it may be necessary to monitor blood pressure or adjust doses to avoid hypotension.[21] Potentiation of antihypertensive activity can also be seen with other drugs, such as barbiturates, MAO inhibitors, and tricyclic antidepressants.

Nonsteroidal anti-inflammatory drugs (NSAIDs) can cause retention of sodium ions, which may antagonize the therapeutic effects of the thiazides.[12,21] Glucocorticoid-induced hyperkalemia can also exert an antagonistic effect. Oral thiazides should be taken 1 hour before or 4 hours after cholestyramine or colestipol (bile acid sequestrants) to avoid a decrease in absorption and consequent reduction in diuretic activity.

Thiazides can enhance toxicity of other drugs,[21] including digitalis (increased risk of cardiac arrhythmias and ventricular tachycardia), lithium (decreased renal excretion of lithium resulting in increased toxicity), and allopurinol (increased allergic response).

Medicinal Chemistry of Thiazide Diuretics

RECEPTOR BINDING, STRUCTURE-ACTIVITY RELATIONSHIPS, AND PHYSICOCHEMICAL PROPERTIES. Although these compounds inhibit carbonic anhydrase (Table 19.6), there is no correlation of this activity with their saluretic effect. In fact, their diuretic activity is due to an effect on the Na^+/Cl^- symporter in the distal convoluted tubule.

Thiazide diuretics are weakly acidic compounds, with a common benzothiadiazine 1,1-dioxide nucleus.

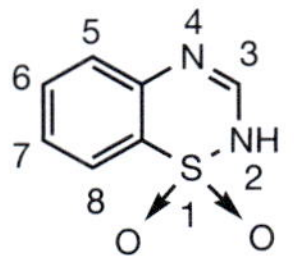

Chlorothiazide is the simplest member of this series, with pK_a values of 6.7 and 9.5. The hydrogen atom at the N_2 position is the most acidic because of the electron-withdrawing effects of the neighboring sulfone group. The sulfonamide group that is substituted at the C_7 position provides an additional point of acidity in the molecule but is less acidic than the N_2 proton. These acidic protons make possible the formation of a water-soluble sodium salt that can be used for intravenous administration of the diuretics.

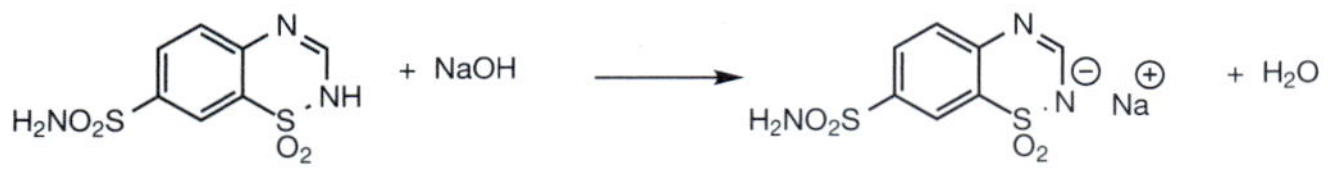

An electron-withdrawing group is necessary at position 6 for diuretic activity. Little diuretic activity is seen with a hydrogen atom at position 6, whereas compounds with either chloro (eg, chlorothiazide, hydrochlorothiazide, and methyclothiazide) or trifluoromethyl (eg, bendroflumethiazide and hydroflumethiazide) substituents are highly active.[19-21] The trifluoromethyl-substituted diuretics are more lipid soluble and have a longer duration of action than their chloro-substituted analogs. When electron-releasing groups, such as methyl or methoxyl, are placed at position 6, the diuretic activity is markedly reduced.

Replacement or removal of the sulfonamide group at position 7 yields compounds with little or no diuretic activity. Saturation of the double bond to give a 3,4-dihydro derivative (cf. chlorothiazide and hydrochlorothiazide) produces a diuretic that is 10-fold more active than the unsaturated derivative. Substitution with a lipophilic group at position 3 gives a marked increase in the diuretic potency. Haloalkyl, aralkyl, or thioether substitution increases the lipid solubility of the molecule and yields compounds with a longer duration of action. Alkyl substitution on the 2-*N* position also decreases the polarity and increases the duration of diuretic action (Table 19.6).

PHARMACOKINETIC PROPERTIES AND METABOLISM. The pharmacokinetic properties of the thiazide diuretics are summarized in Table 19.6. Several of these compounds are rapidly absorbed orally and can show their diuretic effect within an hour. These drugs are highly bound to plasma proteins and therefore are primarily cleared from the circulation via renal tubular secretion.[21] Thiazides are not extensively metabolized and are primarily excreted unchanged in the urine.

Thiazide-Like Diuretics

Therapeutic Role of Thiazide-Like Diuretics

This is a structurally diverse group of sulfonamide-containing compounds that are derivatives of quinazolin-4-one, phthalimidine, or indoline. In spite of their dissimilar structures and lack of a benzothiadiazine ring, these drugs have the same mechanism of action and similar therapeutic activities and adverse effects as the thiazide diuretics.[21]

However, in contrast to thiazide diuretics, metolazone (2.5-20 mg given as a single oral dose) may be effective as a diuretic when the GFR falls below 40 mL/min. In addition, chlorthalidone has a long duration of action (48-72 hours). For example, although metolazone is administered daily, chlorthalidone may be administered in doses of 25 to 100 mg 3 times a week. Uses of indapamide include the treatment of essential hypertension and edema resulting from congestive heart failure. Like metolazone, indapamide is an effective diuretic drug when the GFR is below 40 mL/min. The duration of action is approximately 24 hours, with the normal oral adult dosage starting at 2.5 mg given each morning. The dose may be increased to 5.0 mg/d, but doses beyond this level do not appear to provide additional results.

Pharmacology Overview of Thiazide-Like Diuretics

Mechanism of Action. These drugs have the same mechanism of action as the thiazide diuretics.

Common Adverse Effects. Side effects for the thiazide-like diuretics are similar to those of the thiazides.

Common Interactions. These drugs have the same interactions as the thiazide diuretics.

Medicinal Chemistry of Thiazide-Like Diuretics

Receptor Binding, Structure-Activity Relationships, and Physicochemical Properties. The quinazolin-4-one molecule has been structurally modified in a manner similar to the modification of the thiazide diuretics. Metolazone ($pK_a = 9.7$) is an example of this class of drug (Table 19.7). The structural difference between the quinazolinone and thiazide diuretics is the replacement of the 4-sulfone group ($-SO_2-$) in the former with a 4-keto group (–CO–) in the latter. Because of their similar structures, it is not surprising that the quinazolin-4-ones have a diuretic effect similar to that of the thiazides.

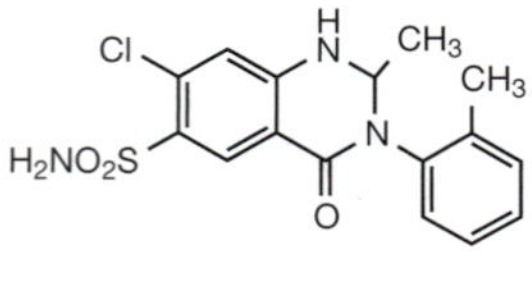

Metolazone

Chlorthalidone ($pK_a = 9.4$) is an example of a diuretic in this class of compounds that bears a structural analogy to the quinazolin-4-ones (Table 19.7). This compound may be named as a 1-oxo-isoindoline or a phthalimidine. Although the molecule exists primarily in the phthalimidine form, the ring may be opened to form a benzophenone derivative. The benzophenone form illustrates the relationship to the quinazolin-4-one series of diuretics.

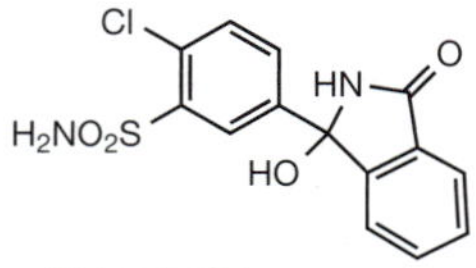

Chlorthalidone
(Thalitone)

The prototypic indoline diuretic is indapamide, which was reported as a diuretic in 1984. Indapamide contains a polar chlorobenzamide moiety and a nonpolar lipophilic methylindoline group. In contrast to the thiazides, indapamide does not contain a thiazide ring, and only one sulfonamide group is present within the molecular structure of this drug ($pK_a = 8.8$).

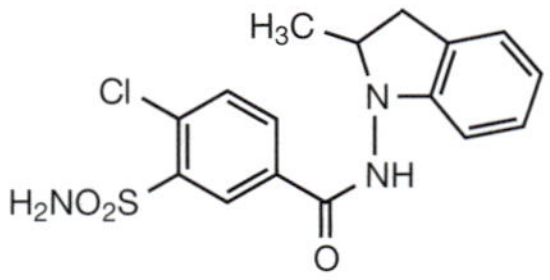

Indapamide

Pharmacokinetic Properties and Metabolism. The pharmacokinetic properties for the thiazide-like diuretics are listed in Table 19.7.

Chlorthalidone binds extensively to plasma proteins, as well as carbonic anhydrase in erythrocytes, and consequently has a long duration of action, up to 72 hours.[21] When chlorthalidone is formulated with the excipient povidone, the product has greater bioavailability (>90%) and reaches peak plasma concentrations in a shorter time.

Like chlorthalidone, metolazone binds to plasma proteins and carbonic anhydrase in erythrocytes and has a long

Table 19.7 Pharmacokinetic Properties for the Thiazide-Like Diuretics

Generic Name	Trade Name	Bioavailability	Peak Plasma	Half-Life	Duration	Elimination
Chlorthalidone	Hygroton Thalitone[a]	Var/Inc	4 h	35-50 h[b]	48-72 h	Urine, as parent drug (50%-65%)
Indapamide	Lozol	>90%	2-3 h	14-18 h	24-36 h	Urine/feces (6:2), as parent drug (70%) and metabolites
Metolazone	Zaroxolyn	<65%	8-12 h	14 h	12-24 h	Urine/feces (8:2), as parent drug (>70%)

Inc, incomplete absorption; NA, data not available; *Var*, variable absorption.

[a]Not interchangeable with a similar drug.

[b]Strongly bound to red blood cells.

Data from AHFS Drug Information (2010), American Society of Health-System Pharmacists; Lexicomp Online (2011), Lexicomp; Facts and Comparisons (2010), Wolters Kluwer Health.

duration of action, 12 to 24 hours.[21] Metolazone has a bioavailability of 65% (Zaroxolyn) and a prolonged onset to reach peak plasma concentrations of action ranging from 8 to 12 hours.

Indapamide is rapidly and completely absorbed from the gastrointestinal tract and reaches its peak plasma level in 2 to 3 hours, with a duration of action of up to 36 hours.[21] This prolonged effect is associated with its extensive binding to carbonic anhydrase in the erythrocytes. It exhibits biphasic kinetics, with a half-life of 14 to 18 hours and an elimination half-life of 24 hours. Indapamide is extensively metabolized (60%-70%), with several of the metabolites being shown in Figure 19.2.[22,23] In vitro studies support aromatic hydroxylation as a metabolic route. Less than 10% of the drug is excreted unchanged, while the remaining 20% to 30% is eliminated via enterohepatic recycling.

High-Ceiling or Loop Diuretics

Therapeutic Role of High-Ceiling or Loop Diuretics

This class of drugs is characterized more by its pharmacological similarities than by its chemical similarities.[24,25] Examples include furosemide, bumetanide, torsemide, and ethacrynic acid. These drugs produce a peak diuresis much greater than that observed with the other commonly used diuretics, hence the name high-ceiling diuretics. Their diuretic effect appears in approximately 30 minutes and lasts for approximately 6 hours. However, the loop diuretics are less effective in treating hypertension than thiazide diuretics. As they have a different mechanism of action, they may be used in combination with other diuretics for improved antihypertensive effects.

Furosemide has a saluretic effect 8- to 10-fold that of the thiazide diuretics; however, it has a shorter duration of action (~6-8 hour). It can cause a marked excretion of sodium, chloride, potassium, calcium, magnesium, and bicarbonate

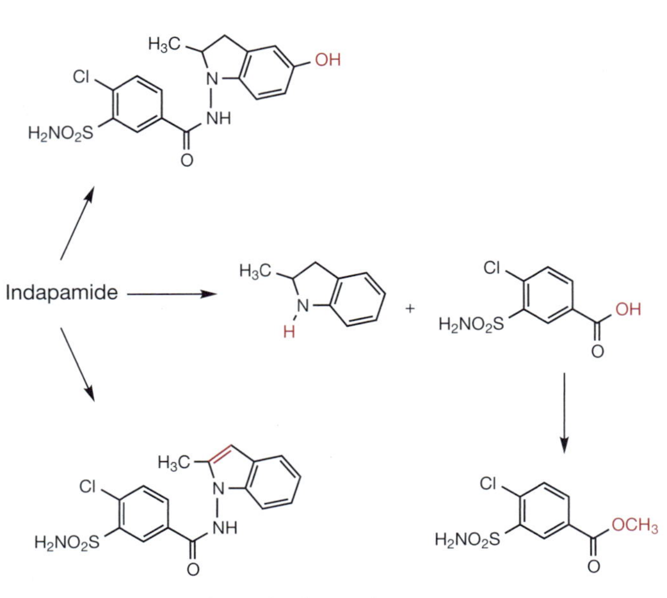

Figure 19.2 Metabolism of indapamide.

ions, with as much as 25% of the filtered load of sodium excreted in response to initial treatment. It is effective for the treatment of edemas connected with cardiac, hepatic, and renal sites.

Bumetanide has a duration of action of approximately 4 hours. The dose of bumetanide is 0.5 to 2 mg/d given as a single dose. Like other high-ceiling diuretics, torsemide exerts its effect in the ascending limb of the loop of Henle to promote the excretion of sodium, potassium, chloride, calcium, and magnesium ions and water. An additional effect on the peritubular side at chloride channels may enhance the luminal effects of torsemide. In contrast to furosemide and bumetanide, however, torsemide does not act at the proximal tubule and, therefore, does not increase phosphate or bicarbonate excretion.

Another major class of high-ceiling diuretics are the phenoxyacetic acid derivatives, of which ethacrynic acid is the prototypical agent. These compounds were developed at about the same time as furosemide but were designed to act mechanistically like the organomercurials (ie, via inhibition of sulfhydryl-containing enzymes involved in solute reabsorption). Ethacrynic acid is the only loop diuretic that is not a sulfonamide derivative and may be useful in patients who are allergic to sulfonamides.

Pharmacology Overview of High-Ceiling or Loop Diuretics

Mechanism of Action. The main site of action for the high-ceiling (loop) diuretics is believed to be on the thick ascending limb of the loop of Henle, where they inhibit the luminal $Na^+/K^+/2Cl^-$ symporter. Additional effects on the proximal and distal tubules are also possible. High-ceiling diuretics are characterized by a quick onset and short duration of activity.[24,25]

The mechanism of action of ethacrynic acid appears to be more complex than the simple Michael addition of the α,β-unsubstituted ketone of the drug to enzyme sulfhydryl groups. When the double bond of ethacrynic acid is reduced, the resulting compound is still active, although the diuretic activity is diminished. The sulfhydryl groups of the enzyme would not be expected to add to the drug molecule in the absence of the α,β-unsaturated ketone.

Common Adverse Effects. Clinical toxicity of furosemide and other loop diuretics primarily involves abnormalities of fluid and electrolyte balance. As with the thiazide diuretics, hypokalemia is an important adverse effect that can be prevented or treated with potassium supplements or coadministration of potassium-sparing diuretics. Increased calcium ion excretion can be a problem for postmenopausal osteopenic women, and furosemide generally should not be used in these individuals. Hyperuricemia, glucose intolerance, increased serum lipid levels, ototoxicity, and gastrointestinal side effects might be observed as well. Hypersensitivity reactions are also possible with furosemide (a sulfonamide-based drug), and cross-reactivity with other sulfonamide-containing drugs is possible. The adverse effects of bumetanide and torsemide are similar to those induced by furosemide. In patients with cirrhosis and ascites, torsemide should be used with caution.

Toxicity induced by ethacrynic acid is similar to that induced by furosemide and bumetanide. Ethacrynic acid is not widely used as a diuretic because it also induces a greater incidence of ototoxicity and more serious gastrointestinal effects than furosemide or bumetanide.

Common Interactions. The loop diuretics exhibit many of the same interactions with other drugs as occurs with the thiazides.[25] For example, hypotension may result when they are used in combination with ACE inhibitors or ARBs, and their activity may be antagonized by NSAIDs and glucocorticoids.

Loop diuretics may alter the pharmacokinetics of the anticoagulant warfarin by displacing this highly protein-bound drug from its binding sites on serum albumin; this interaction may necessitate a dosage reduction for warfarin.[25]

Kidney damage may be increased when the loop diuretics are used together with other nephrotoxic drugs, including aminoglycosides and NSAIDs. The combination of a loop diuretic and the anticancer drug cisplatin may increase the risk of nephrotoxicity and ototoxicity in patients receiving both drugs.[25]

Medicinal Chemistry of High-Ceiling or Loop Diuretics

Receptor Binding, Structure-Activity Relationships, and Physicochemical Properties. High-ceiling diuretics exert their diuretic effects via inhibition of $Na^+/K^+/2Cl^-$ symporter in the thick ascending limb of the loop of Henle.

Research on 5-sulfamoylanthranilic acids at the Hoechst Laboratories in Germany showed them to be effective diuretics.[19] The most active of a series of variously substituted derivatives was furosemide.

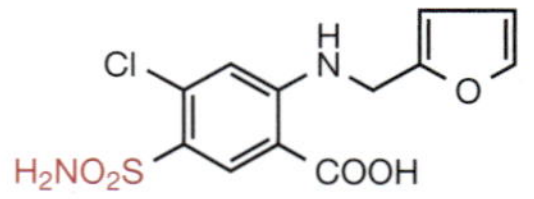

Furosemide

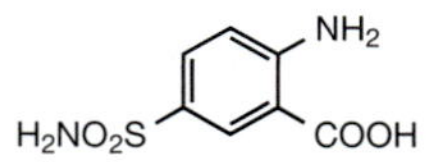

5-Sulfamoyl-anthranilic acid

Chlorine and sulfonamide substituents are also found in other diuretics. Because the molecule possesses a free carboxyl group, furosemide is a stronger acid than the thiazide diuretics ($pK_a = 3.9$). This drug is excreted primarily unchanged.[26] A small amount of metabolism, however, can take place on the furan ring, which is substituted on the aromatic amino group. See Table 19.5 for its other pharmacokinetic properties.

In bumetanide, a phenoxy group has replaced the customary chloro or trifluoromethyl substituents seen in other diuretic molecules.[27] The phenoxy group is an electron-withdrawing group similar to the chloro or trifluoromethyl substituents. The amine group customarily seen at position 6 has been moved to position 5. These minor variations from furosemide produced a compound with a mode of action similar to that of furosemide, but with a marked increase in diuretic potency. The short duration of activity is similar, but the compound is approximately 50-fold more potent. Replacement of the phenoxy group at position 4 with a C_6H_5NH- or C_6H_5S- group also gives compounds with a favorable activity. When the butyl group on the C_5 amine is replaced with a furanylmethyl group, such as in furosemide, however, the results are not favorable.

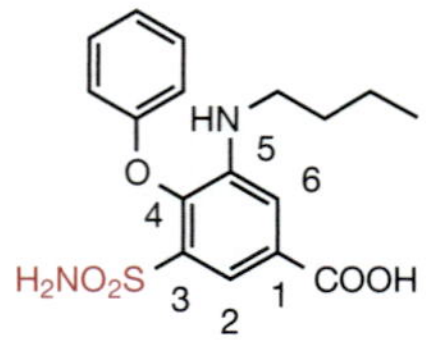

Bumetanide

Further modification of furosemide-like structures led to the development of torsemide.[28] Instead of the sulfonamide group found in furosemide and bumetanide, torsemide contains a sulfonylurea moiety.

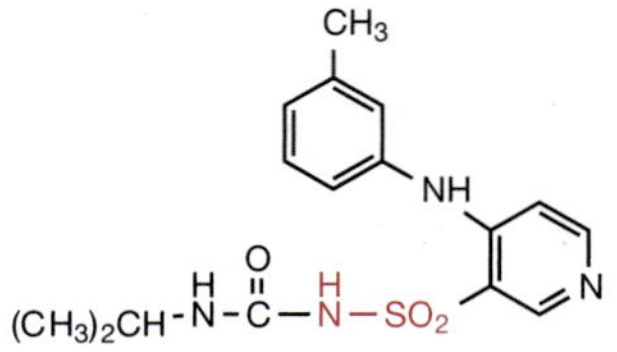

Torsemide

Optimal diuretic activity was obtained when an oxyacetic acid group was positioned para to an α,β-unsaturated carbonyl (or other sulfhydryl-reactive group) and chloro or methyl groups were placed at the 2- or 3-position of the phenyl ring.[29] In addition, hydrogen atoms on the terminal alkene carbon also provided maximum reactivity. Thus, a molecule with a weakly acidic group to direct the drug to the kidney and an alkylating moiety to react with sulfhydryl groups and lipophilic groups seemed to provide the best combination for a diuretic in this class. These features led to the development of ethacrynic acid as the prototypic agent in this class.

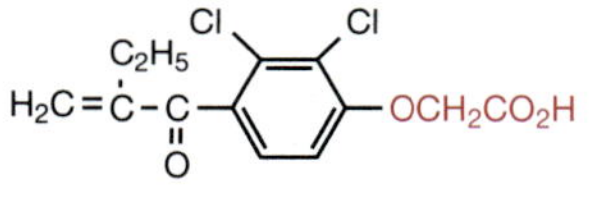

Ethacrynic acid

Pharmacokinetic Properties and Metabolism. The pharmacokinetic properties for the loop diuretics are listed in Table 19.5. Furosemide is orally effective but may be used parenterally when a prompter diuretic effect is desired, such as in the treatment of acute pulmonary edema. The dosage of furosemide, 20 to 80 mg/d, may be given in divided doses because of the short duration of action of the drug and carefully increased up to a maximum of 600 mg/d. Bumetanide exhibits similar pharmacokinetics to furosemide. Both drugs are eliminated in urine and feces (furosemide) as a mixture of parent compounds and metabolites.

The oral bioavailability of torsemide is very good (~80%), and absorption is not affected by the presence of food in the gastrointestinal tract.[28] Peak diuresis is observed 1 to 2 hours following oral or intravenous administration, with a duration of action of approximately 6 hours (Table 19.5). Torsemide is indicated for the treatment of edema resulting from congestive heart failure and for the treatment of hypertension. In contrast to furosemide and bumetanide, torsemide is eliminated predominantly as unmetabolized parent drug.

Oral administration of ethacrynic acid results in diuresis within 1 hour and a duration of action of 6 to 8 hours. This drug is eliminated renally and hepatically as parent compound and metabolites, including a mercapturic acid derivative.

Mineralocorticoid Receptor Antagonists

Therapeutic Role of Mineralocorticoid Receptor Antagonists

The adrenal cortex secretes a potent mineralocorticoid called aldosterone, which promotes salt and water retention and potassium and hydrogen ion excretion. Aldosterone exerts its biological effects through binding to the mineralocorticoid receptor (MR), a nuclear transcription factor.[30]

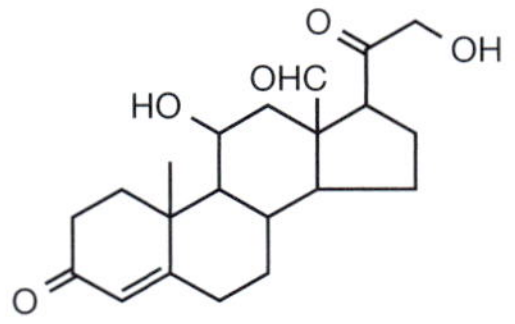

Aldosterone
(aldol from)

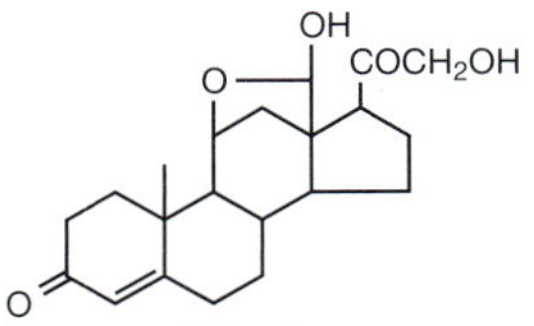

Aldosterone
(hemiacetal form)

Other mineralocorticoids influence the electrolytic balance of the body, but aldosterone is the most potent. Its ability to cause increased reabsorption of sodium and chloride ion and increased potassium ion excretion is approximately 3,000-fold that of hydrocortisone. A substance that antagonizes the effects of aldosterone could conceivably be a good diuretic drug. Spironolactone and eplerenone are examples of such mineralocorticoid receptor antagonists (MRAs). These drugs are also classified as potassium-sparing diuretics. The pharmacological properties of spironolactone and eplerenone are summarized in Table 19.5.

Spironolactone (first generation MRA) is useful in treating edema resulting from primary hyperaldosteronism and refractory edema associated with secondary hyperaldosteronism. Spironolactone is the drug of choice for treating edema resulting from cirrhosis of the liver. The dose of spironolactone is 100 mg/d given in single or divided doses. Another use of spironolactone is coadministration with a potassium-depleting diuretic (eg, a thiazide or loop diuretic) to prevent or treat diuretic-induced hypokalemia. However, it should not be combined with potassium-sparing diuretics (eg, triamterene or amiloride). Spironolactone can be administered in a fixed-dose combination with hydrochlorothiazide for this purpose, but optimal individualization of the dose of each drug is recommended.

Eplerenone (second-generation MRA) came out of efforts to develop spironolactone analogs with reduced adverse effects.[31,32] Like spironolactone, eplerenone is used alone or with other diuretics for the treatment of hypertension or left ventricular systolic dysfunction and congestive heart failure after myocardial infarction (MI). Single daily oral doses are 25 to 50 mg.

Pharmacology Overview of Mineralocorticoid Receptor Antagonists

Mechanism of Action. Spironolactone and eplerenone competitively inhibit aldosterone binding to the MR,[30] thereby interfering with reabsorption of sodium and chloride ions and the associated water. The most important renal site of the MRs, and hence the primary site of action of spironolactone and eplerenone, is in the late distal convoluted tubule and collecting system (collecting duct).

Common Adverse Effects. The primary concern with the use of spironolactone is the development of hyperkalemia, which can be fatal. Spironolactone may cause hypersensitivity reactions, gastrointestinal disturbances, and peptic ulcer. Sexual side effects (ie, gynecomastia, decreased libido, and impotence) can also occur and are due to nonselective binding of spironolactone to the androgen receptor (AR), glucocorticoid receptor (GR), or progesterone receptor (PR). It has also been implicated in tumor production during chronic toxicity studies in rats, but human risk has not been documented.

Hyperkalemia is also a serious and potentially fatal side effect with eplerenone. However; in contrast to spironolactone, eplerenone has limited or no inhibitory effects on AR, GR, and PR and is therefore a more selective aldosterone antagonist.[31,32] Consequently, it has fewer sexual side effects.

Common Interactions. The MRAs can produce additive effects when combined with other antihypertensive drugs.[25] As seen with other diuretics, NSAIDs and glucocorticoids may exert antagonistic effects. Hyperkalemia may result if MRAs are used in combination with other drugs (eg, ACE inhibitors, ARBs, and BBs) that elevate blood potassium levels.

Eplerenone is extensively metabolized by CYP3A4. Combination with inhibitors (eg, ketoconazole or erythromycin) of this CYP isozyme may therefore alter eplerenone metabolism and pharmacokinetics.[25]

Medicinal Chemistry of Mineralocorticoid Receptor Antagonists

Receptor Binding, Structure-Activity Relationships, and Physicochemical Properties. MRA activity is dependent on the presence of a γ-lactone ring on the C_{17} atom and a substituent on the C_7 atom that is present in spironolactone and structurally related compounds.[33,34] Interaction of C_7-unsubstituted agonists, such as aldosterone, with a methionine residue in the MR ligand binding domain is important for receptor activation and subsequent transcription. However, this interaction is sterically hindered by the C_7 substituents on aldosterone antagonists, thereby leaving MR in an inactive conformation.[33,34]

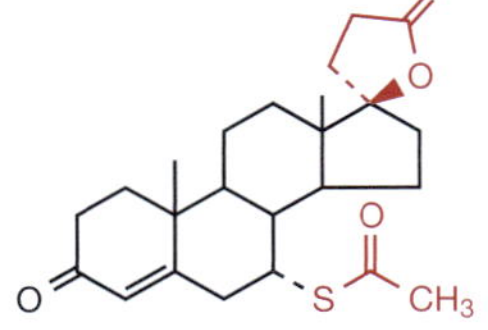

Spironolactone

In addition to the lactone ring and the C_7 substituent (in this case an acetyl group) that are important for MR antagonism, eplerenone has a 9α,11α-epoxy group as part of its structure. Like spironolactone, it binds to the MR and is an aldosterone antagonist. However, it has a 20- to 40-fold lower affinity for the MR than spironolactone (see Table 19.5).[31] This reduced binding is believed to be due to the epoxy group.[35,36] Nevertheless, eplerenone is an effective diuretic and has certain therapeutic advantages over spironolactone.

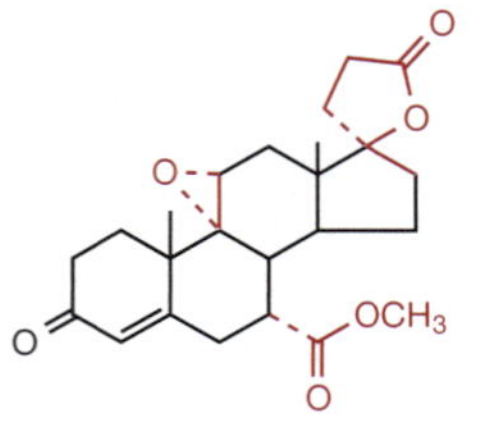

Pharmacokinetic Properties and Metabolism. The pharmacokinetic properties of spironolactone and eplerenone are summarized in Table 19.5. On oral administration, approximately 90% of the dose of spironolactone is absorbed and is significantly metabolized during its first passage through the liver to its major active metabolite, canrenone, which is interconvertible with its canrenoate anion (Fig. 19.3).[37,38] Canrenone is an antagonist to aldosterone and exists in equilibrium with its ring-opened form, canrenoate.

The canrenoate anion is not therapeutically active but acts as an aldosterone antagonist because of its conversion back to canrenone, which exists in the lactone form. Canrenone has been suggested to be the active form of spironolactone as an aldosterone antagonist. The formation of canrenone, however, cannot fully account for the total activity of spironolactone.[37,38] Both canrenone and potassium canrenoate are used as diuretics in other countries, but they are not available in the United States.

Eplerenone has good (~70%) oral bioavailability and, unlike spironolactone, only undergoes limited first-pass

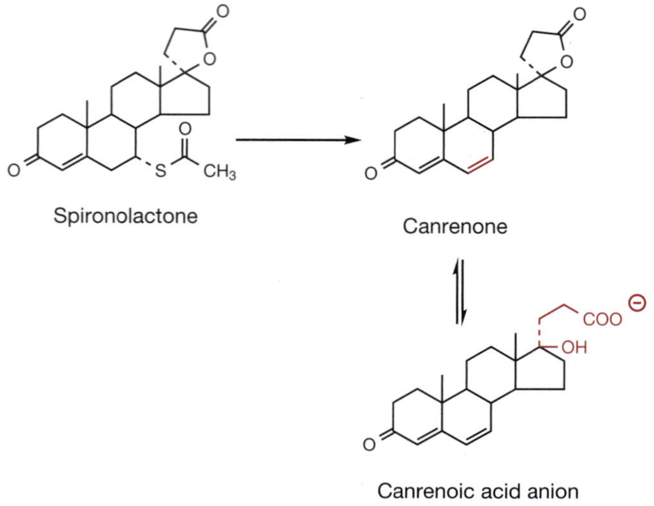

Figure 19.3 Metabolic conversion of spironolactone to canrenone.

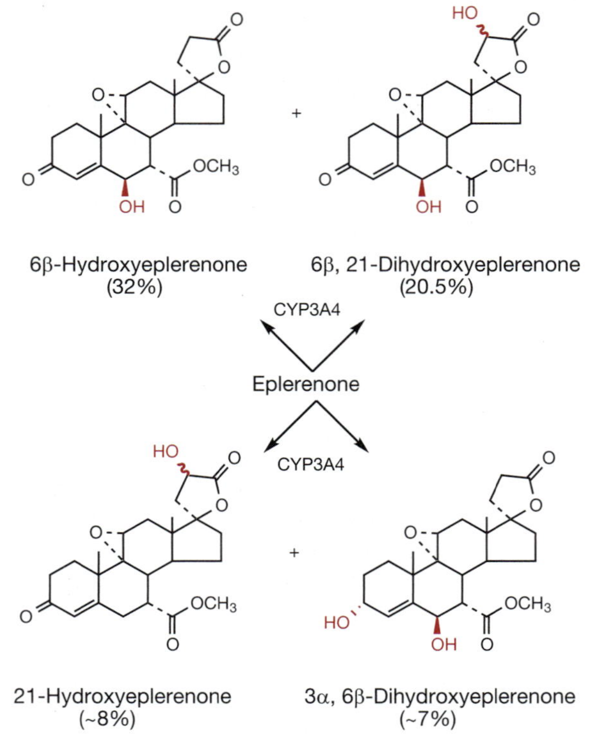

Figure 19.4 Major metabolic products formed from eplerenone.

metabolism (Table 19.5). Absorption is not affected by the presence of food in the GI tract. In plasma, it is about 50% bound to plasma α_1-acid glycoprotein. Eplerenone has a half-life of approximately 5 hours and undergoes extensive metabolism by hepatic CYP3A4 to inactive metabolites (Fig. 19.4).[39] Elimination occurs in the urine and feces.

THIRD-GENERATION MINERALOCORTICOID RECEPTOR ANTAGONISTS

The need for more efficacious MRAs with fewer adverse effects led to the development of third-generation drugs, such as finerenone, which was approved by the U.S. Food and Drug Administration (FDA) in 2021.[40,41] Finerenone is indicated for the treatment of cardiovascular conditions that are associated with chronic kidney disease in patients with type 2 diabetes. Unlike spironolactone and eplerenone, finerenone has a more limited effect on blood pressure.[41] Although it targets the same receptor as the flat, steroidal MRAs, finerenone is a bulky, nonsteroidal molecule. Binding of finerenone to the MR results in an unstable drug-receptor complex that cannot recruit co-regulators needed for transcription.[41,42] Finerenone is a 1,4-dihydropyridine derivative and is a more selective and potent antagonist (IC_{50} = 17.8 nM) at the MR than spironolactone (IC_{50} = 24 nM) or eplerenone (IC_{50} = 990 nM).[41]

THIRD-GENERATION MINERALOCORTICOID RECEPTOR ANTAGONISTS (*continued*)

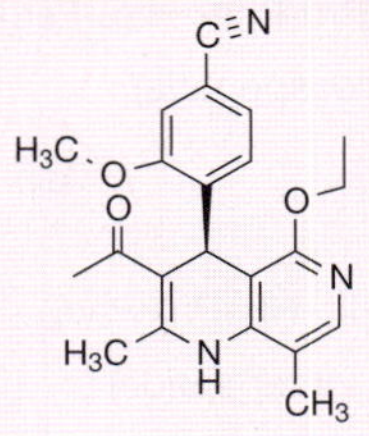

Finerenone

It has no affinity for other nuclear receptors, such as AR, GR, and PR.[40] The lack of finerenone binding to AR, GR, and PR reduces the incidence of sexual side effects (eg, gynecomastia, reduced libido). In contrast to spironolactone and eplerenone, which exhibit greater penetration into the kidneys than cardiac tissue, the distribution of finerenone into these tissue sites in rats is comparable, this may help explain its reduced potential to cause hyperkalemia in patients.[40,41] Due to its lower lipophilicity than the steroidal MRAs, finerenone does not cross the blood-brain barrier. Finerenone is a substrate for the CYP3A4 isozyme and is extensively converted into inactive metabolites. Less than 1% of the dose is excreted as the parent drug in urine (major) and feces (minor).[43] The half-life of finerenone (2-3 hour) is shorter than that of eplerenone (3-6 hour) or spironolactone (>12 hour).[42]

Potassium-Sparing Diuretics

Therapeutic Role of Potassium-Sparing Diuretics

Two drugs in this class of diuretics are triamterene and amiloride (Table 19.5), which are derivatives of pteridine and aminopyrazine, respectively. Individually, amiloride and triamterene exert a mild diuretic effect and are usually used in combination with other diuretic agents.

Triamterene is useful in combination with a thiazide or loop diuretic in the treatment of edema or hypertension. Liddle syndrome, which is due to an inherited mutation in the epithelial sodium channel (ENaC) leading to increased activity of the receptor, may also be treated with a sodium channel blocking drug, such as triamterene or amiloride. Triamterene is administered initially in doses of 100 mg twice a day. A maintenance dose for each patient should be individually determined. This dose may vary from 100 mg a day to as low as 100 mg every other day.

Like triamterene, amiloride combined with a thiazide or loop diuretic is used to treat edema or hypertension. Aerosolized amiloride has shown some benefit in improving mucociliary clearance in patients with cystic fibrosis.

Pharmacology Overview of Potassium-Sparing Diuretics

Mechanism of Action. In vitro experiments have shown that triamterene and amiloride exert a diuretic effect by blocking an ENaC in principal cells of the late distal convoluted tubule and collecting duct.[44,45] Both drugs are weak organic bases and inhibit ENaC in a voltage- and pH-dependent manner. Inhibition occurs because amiloride and triamterene bind to negatively charged regions of the sodium channel in the ENaC. The greater potency (approximately 100-fold in vitro) of amiloride is probably due to the fact that it is a stronger base ($pK_a = 8.7$) and is therefore more extensively protonated at physiological pH than triamterene ($pK_a = 6.2$). Sodium channel inhibitors block the reabsorption of sodium ion and inhibit the secretion of potassium ion. The net result is increased sodium and chloride ion excretion in the urine and almost no potassium excretion. Consequently, amiloride and triamterene can be used to offset the effect of other diuretics that result in loss of potassium.

Common Adverse Effects. The most serious side effect associated with the use of triamterene is hyperkalemia. For this reason, potassium supplements are contraindicated, and serum potassium levels should be checked regularly. Triamterene is also used in combination with hydrochlorothiazide. Here, the hypokalemic effect of the hydrochlorothiazide counters the hyperkalemic effect of the triamterene. Other side effects that are seen with the use of triamterene are nausea, vomiting, and headache. Amiloride can produce similar side effects as triamterene, including hyperkalemia.

Common Interactions. Hypotension can result if amiloride or triamterene are used in combination with other diuretics and other antihypertensive agents.[25]

Medicinal Chemistry of the Potassium-Sparing Diuretics

Receptor Binding, Structure-Activity Relationships, and Physicochemical Properties. Pteridine ring–containing compounds have a marked potential for influencing biological processes. Early screening of pteridine derivatives revealed that 2,4-diamino-6,7-dimethylpteridine had diuretic activity.

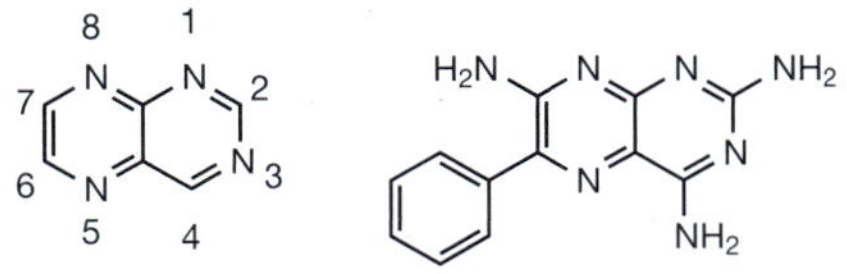

Pteridine Triamterene

Structural modifications of the pteridine nucleus led to the development of triamterene. Further alterations of the triamterene structure are not usually beneficial in terms of diuretic activity. Activity is retained if an amine group is replaced with a lower alkylamine group. Introduction of a para-methyl group on the phenyl ring decreases the activity by approximately half. Introduction of a para-hydroxyl group on the phenyl ring yields a compound that is essentially inactive as a diuretic.

Amiloride is an aminopyrazine structurally related to triamterene as an open-chain analog.

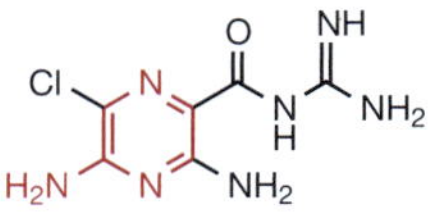

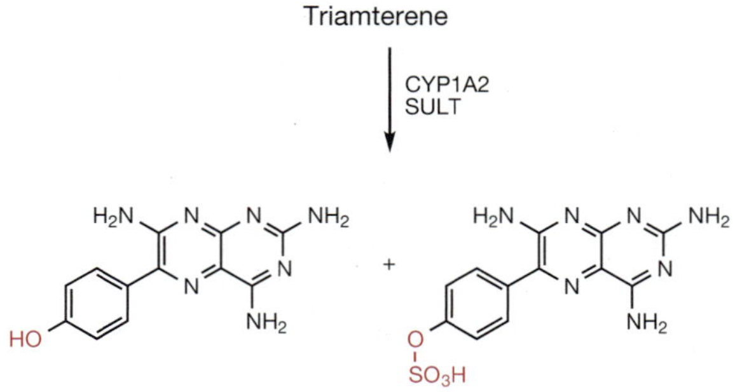

Figure 19.5 Metabolism of triamterene. Coloration indicates site of metabolism.

Pharmacokinetic Properties and Metabolism. Triamterene is more than 70% absorbed on oral administration (see Table 19.5 for its other pharmacokinetic properties). The diuretic effect occurs rapidly (~30 minutes) and reaches a peak plasma concentration in 2 to 4 hours, with a duration of action of more than 24 hours. This drug is extensively metabolized to 4′-hydroxytriamterene, which subsequently undergoes sulfation (Fig. 19.5). Both metabolites are still active as diuretics and, along with the parent drug triamterene, are excreted in the urine.[46]

Oral amiloride is approximately 50% absorbed (see Table 19.5 for its other pharmacokinetic properties), with a duration of action of up to about 24 hours, which is slightly shorter than that of triamterene. Although triamterene is extensively metabolized, approximately 50% of amiloride is excreted unchanged. Renal impairment can increase its elimination half-life. The dose of amiloride is 5 to 10 mg/d. Amiloride is also combined with hydrochlorothiazide in a fixed-dose combination.

Renin-Angiotensin Pathway

Overview

The renin-angiotensin system plays a vital role in maintaining blood volume, electrolyte balance, and arterial blood pressure through a sophisticated and tightly controlled pathway. This pathway involves two key enzymes, renin and angiotensin-converting enzyme (ACE), which work together to generate angiotensin II from its endogenous precursor, angiotensinogen (Fig. 19.6). Angiotensin II is a potent vasoconstrictor that affects peripheral resistance, renal function, and cardiovascular structure.[47] Angiotensin II also promotes the release of another hormone called aldosterone from the adrenal cortex. Aldosterone promotes salt and water retention in the kidneys.

In 1898, Tiegerstedt and Bergman made a significant discovery by demonstrating the presence of a pressor substance in raw kidney extracts, marking the initial recognition of the renin-angiotensin system. It took approximately four decades for two separate research groups to independently reveal that this pressor substance, initially known as renin, was actually an enzyme, and that the true pressor substance was a peptide produced through the catalytic action of renin. Initially, this peptide pressor substance received two different names, angiotonin and hypertensin. However, these names were eventually merged to form the current term, angiotensin. During the 1950s, a significant breakthrough occurred when it was discovered that angiotensin exists in two forms: an inactive decapeptide called angiotensin I and an active octapeptide known as angiotensin II. Furthermore, it was discovered that the conversion of angiotensin I to II is facilitated by an enzyme different from renin.[48]

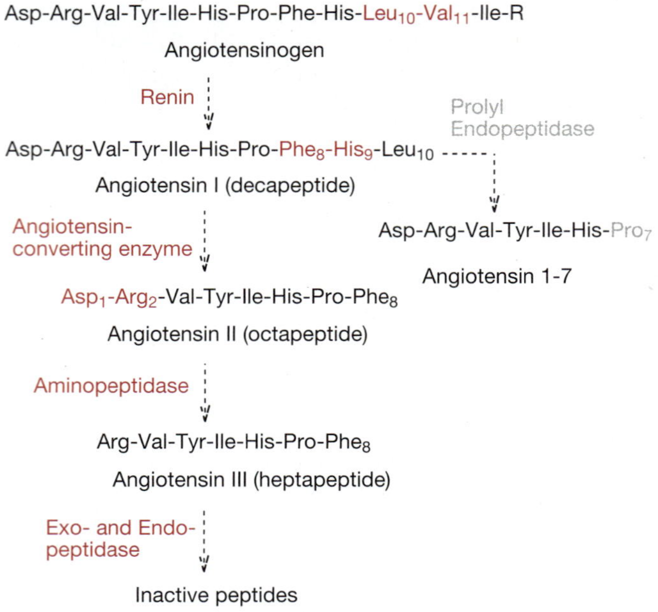

Figure 19.6 Schematic representation of the renin-angiotensin pathway. The labile peptide bonds of angiotensinogen, angiotensin I, and angiotensin II are highlighted.

Angiotensinogen, a plasma protein, is an α_2-globulin with a molecular weight ranging from 58 to 61 kDa. It consists of 452 amino acids and is primarily synthesized and released by the liver. Its production is influenced by various hormones such as glucocorticoids, thyroid hormone, and angiotensin II. The most important portion of this biomolecule is the N-terminus, specifically the Leu10-Val11 bond. This bond is cleaved by renin and produces the decapeptide angiotensin I. The Phe8-His9 peptide bond of angiotensin I is then cleaved by ACE to produce the octapeptide angiotensin II. Aminopeptidase can further convert angiotensin II to the active heptapeptide angiotensin III by removing the N-terminal aspartic acid residue. Further actions of carboxypeptidases, aminopeptidases, and endopeptidases result in the formation of inactive peptide fragments. An additional peptide can be formed by the action of a prolyl-endopeptidase on angiotensin I. Cleavage of the Pro7-Phe8 bond of angiotensin I produces a heptapeptide known as angiotensin 1-7.[48]

Physiologic Actions of the Renin-Angiotensin Pathway

Renin, an aspartyl protease, plays a crucial role in regulating the production of angiotensin II and exhibits a higher level of specificity compared to ACE. Its main function involves cleaving the leucine-valine bond located at residues 10 and 11 of angiotensinogen. The release of renin is tightly controlled by a combination of hemodynamic, neurogenic, and humoral signals (Fig. 19.7). The renal juxtaglomerular cells play a crucial role in hemodynamic signaling. These cells are responsive to the stretch of the afferent glomerular arteriole, which reflects changes in blood pressure. When there is an increase in the stretch, indicating elevated blood pressure, renin release is reduced. Conversely, a decrease in the stretch leads to an increase in renin secretion. Furthermore, these cells are also sensitive to the flux of NaCl across the neighboring macula densa. An increase in NaCl flux inhibits renin release, while a decrease in flux stimulates its release. Neurogenic factors also contribute to the enhancement of renin release, achieved through the activation of β_1-receptors. Additionally, the release of renin is influenced by various hormonal signals. Somatostatin, atrial natriuretic factor, and angiotensin II inhibit renin release, whereas vasoactive intestinal peptide, parathyroid hormone, and glucagon stimulate its release.[49]

In contrast to renin, ACE, also referred to as kininase II, is a zinc protease that operates with minimal physiological regulation. It does not serve as a rate-limiting factor in the production of angiotensin II. Instead, ACE acts as a relatively nonspecific dipeptidyl carboxypeptidase, requiring only a tripeptide sequence as a substrate. The sole structural requirement for ACE is that the penultimate amino acid of the peptide substrate cannot be proline. For this reason, angiotensin II, which contains a proline in the penultimate position, is not further metabolized by ACE. ACE's lack of specificity and control contributes to its involvement in the bradykinin pathway, as illustrated in Figure 19.8. Bradykinin, a nonapeptide, exerts local effects such as pain generation, vasodilation, increased vascular permeability, stimulation of prostaglandin synthesis, and bronchoconstriction. Similar to angiotensin II, bradykinin is generated through proteolytic cleavage of a precursor peptide. The protease kallikrein cleaves kininogens, producing a decapeptide

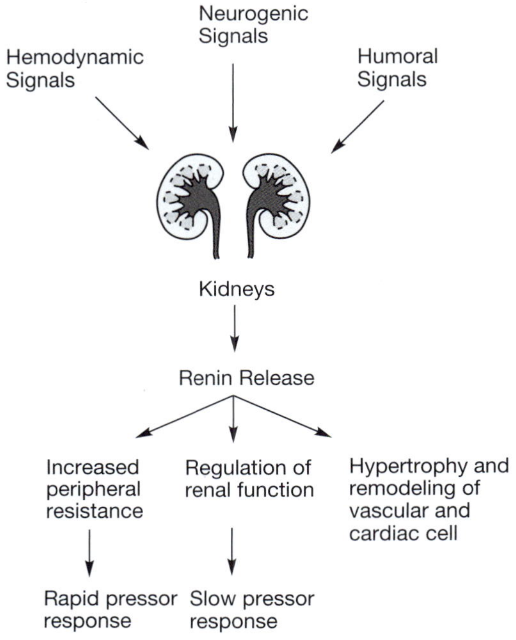

Figure 19.7 Summary of the factors involved in renin release and the effects mediated by angiotensin II.

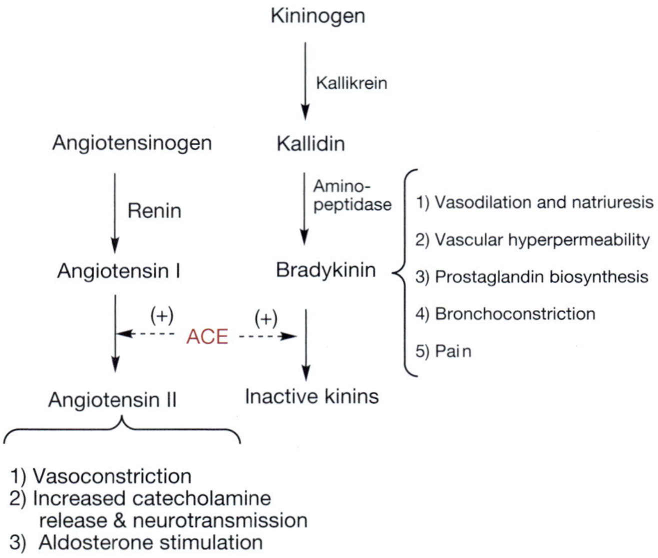

Figure 19.8 Schematic representation of the bradykinin pathway and its relationship to angiotensin-converting enzyme (ACE) and the renin-angiotensin pathway.

referred to as either kallidin or lysyl-bradykinin. Subsequent cleavage of the N-terminal lysine by aminopeptidase results in the formation of bradykinin. ACE plays a role in the degradation of bradykinin into inactive peptides. Thus, in addition to producing a potent vasoconstrictor, angiotensin II, ACE also deactivates a potent vasodilator, bradykinin.[47,49,50]

Angiotensin II, the primary peptide produced in the renin-angiotensin pathway (see Fig. 19.7), holds a dominant role. It acts as a potent vasoconstrictor, contributing to an increase in total peripheral resistance through multiple mechanisms. These mechanisms include direct vasoconstriction, stimulation of catecholamine release and neurotransmission within the peripheral nervous system, as well as heightened sympathetic discharge. Collectively, these actions swiftly lead to a pressor response. Furthermore, angiotensin II elicits a slow pressor response that helps in the long-term stabilization of arterial blood pressure. This effect is achieved by regulating renal function. Angiotensin II directly enhances sodium reabsorption in the proximal tubule, influences renal hemodynamics, and prompts the release of aldosterone from the adrenal cortex. Moreover, angiotensin II induces hypertrophy and remodeling of both vascular and cardiac cells through a combination of hemodynamic and nonhemodynamic effects. These effects contribute to the structural changes observed in these cells over time.[47]

The secondary peptides, angiotensin III and angiotensin 1-7, can contribute to the overall effects of the renin-angiotensin pathway. Angiotensin III demonstrates potency comparable to that of angiotensin II in stimulating aldosterone secretion; however, it is only 10% to 25% as effective in increasing blood pressure. On the other hand, angiotensin 1-7 does not induce aldosterone secretion or vasoconstriction. Nevertheless, it possesses potent effects that differ from those of angiotensin II. Similar to angiotensin II, angiotensin 1-7 can cause neuronal excitation and release of vasopressin. Additionally, it enhances the production of prostaglandins through a receptor-mediated process that does not involve an elevation in intracellular calcium levels. It has been proposed that angiotensin 1-7 plays an important role in modulating cell-to-cell interactions within cardiovascular and neural tissues.[51]

Role of Renin-Angiotensin Pathway in Hypertension and Other Cardiovascular Disorders

Dysfunctions within the renin-angiotensin pathway, such as excessive renin release and overproduction of angiotensin II, can contribute to hypertension by triggering both the rapid and slow pressor responses mentioned earlier. Additionally, elevated levels of angiotensin II can lead to the development or worsening of heart failure, a condition characterized by the heart's inability to adequately supply blood to meet the body's demands. Similar to hypertension, heart failure can arise through various mechanisms. Any pathophysiological event that impairs systolic or diastolic function can result in heart failure. Systolic dysfunction, which involves reduced contractility, may be caused by conditions like dilated cardiomyopathies, ventricular hypertrophy, or a decrease in muscle mass. On the other hand, diastolic dysfunction, characterized by limitations in ventricular filling, can occur due to increased ventricular stiffness, stenosis of the mitral or tricuspid valves, or pericardial disease. Both ventricular hypertrophy and myocardial ischemia can contribute to increased ventricular stiffness.

The actions of angiotensin II contribute to the onset and progression of heart failure through several mechanisms. It increases systemic vascular resistance, leading to heightened workload on the heart. Additionally, it promotes the retention of sodium, stimulates the release of aldosterone, and induces ventricular hypertrophy and remodeling. These combined effects of angiotensin II contribute to the development and worsening of heart failure. Heart failure is a prevalent condition, affecting around 6 million Americans, and it represents the most common reason for hospital discharge among individuals over the age of 65 years. From an economic perspective, the annual expenses associated with heart failure reach or surpass approximately $40 billion dollars.[52] Without improvements to the cost of care by the year 2030, costs are predicted to reach $69.8 billion.[53]

Development of Drugs to Block the Actions of the Renin-Angiotensin Pathway

Development of Angiotensin-Converting Enzyme Inhibitors

Cushman et al. developed a hypothetical model of the binding site of ACE that led to the development of captopril, the first FDA-approved ACE inhibitor.[54-57] Their model was based upon the enzymatic actions of ACE, the actions of several naturally occurring peptides, and the similarities between ACE and pancreatic carboxypeptidases. The original peptides were isolated from the venom of the South American pit viper *Bothrops jararaca*, and contained a proline residue at their carboxylate terminus.[58,59] These peptides, represented by teprotide (L-pyroglutamyl-L-tryptophyl-L-prolyl-L-arginyl-L-prolyl-L-glutaminyl-L-isoleucyl-L-prolyl-L-proline), were shown to inhibit ACE and potentiate the actions of bradykinin.

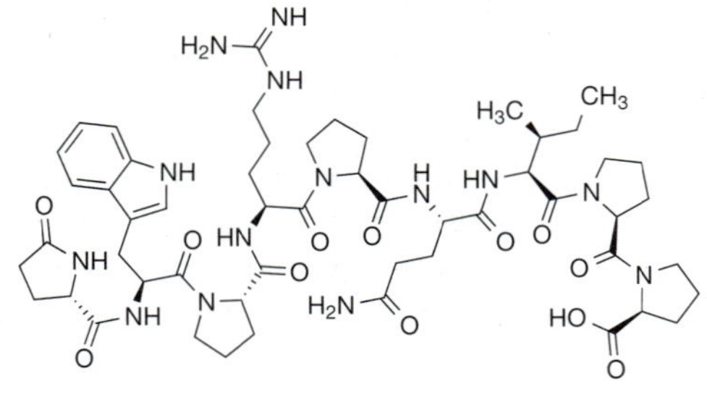

Teprotide

Similar to ACE, carboxypeptidase A is an exopeptidase that contains zinc ion. When a substrate binds to carboxypeptidase A, it involves three significant interactions, as depicted in Figure 19.9A. These interactions include: (1) an ionic interaction between the negatively charged carboxylate terminus of the substrate and the positively charged Arg145 on the enzyme, (2) van der Waals interactions between a hydrophobic pocket within the enzyme and the side chains of C-terminal aromatic or nonpolar residues of the substrate, and (3) a complexation between a zinc ion and the carbonyl of the labile peptide bond. The zinc ion helps polarize the carbonyl bond and stabilize the resulting negatively charged tetrahedral intermediate.[60] The binding of substrates to ACE was proposed to involve similar interactions with three specific differences (Fig. 19.9B). First, because ACE cleaves dipeptides instead of single amino acids, the position of the zinc ion was assumed to be located two amino acids away from the cationic center for it to be adjacent to the labile peptide bond. Second, ACE does not show specificity for C-terminal hydrophobic amino acids; however, it was proposed that the side chains, R_1 and R_2, of ACE substrates could contribute to the overall binding affinity. Finally, as the C-terminal peptide bond is nonlabile

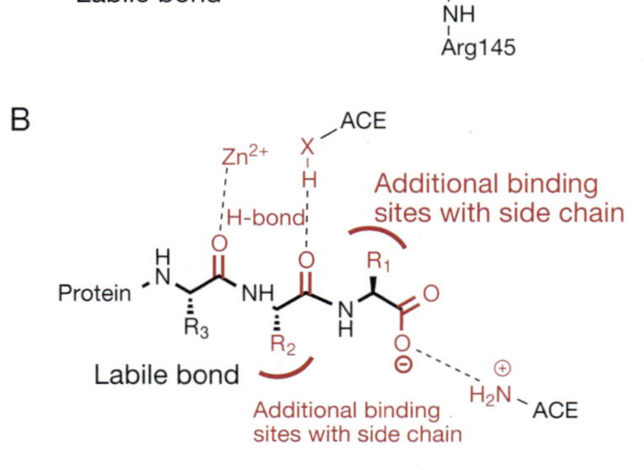

Figure 19.9 Model of substrate binding to carboxypeptidase A (A) and ACE (B). ACE substrate binding sites are highlighted in red.

(ie, not cleaved), it was assumed to provide hydrogen bonding between the substrate and ACE.

Using this model and the knowledge that D-2-benzylsuccinic acid was an extremely potent inhibitor of carboxypeptidase A, Cushman et al. sequentially examined succinyl L-proline analogs (Fig. 19.10). Given that proline was present as the C-terminal amino acid in teprotide, it was used instead of leucine, the C-terminal amino acid present in angiotensin I. One of the most important alterations to succinyl-L-proline was the replacement of the succinyl carboxylate with a sulfhydryl group. The further addition of a methyl group yielded captopril. Captopril is a dipeptide mimic and a competitive inhibitor of ACE. It has a K_i value of 1.7 nM and was the first ACE inhibitor to be marketed.

The presence of the sulfhydryl group in captopril played a significant role not only in its potent inhibitory activity but also in causing two frequently encountered side effects: skin rashes and taste disturbances, such as metallic taste and loss of taste. Typically, these side effects diminish upon reducing the dosage or discontinuing captopril. The sulfhydryl group was identified as the source of these effects, as similar reactions had been observed with penicillamine, another agent containing a sulfhydryl group that is used in the treatment of Wilson disease and rheumatoid arthritis.[61,62]

Researchers at Merck[63] sought to develop drugs that lacked the sulfhydryl group of captopril yet maintained the same ability to chelate zinc ion. Their investigations lead to the development of carboxylate-containing tripeptide inhibitors that have the general structure shown below.

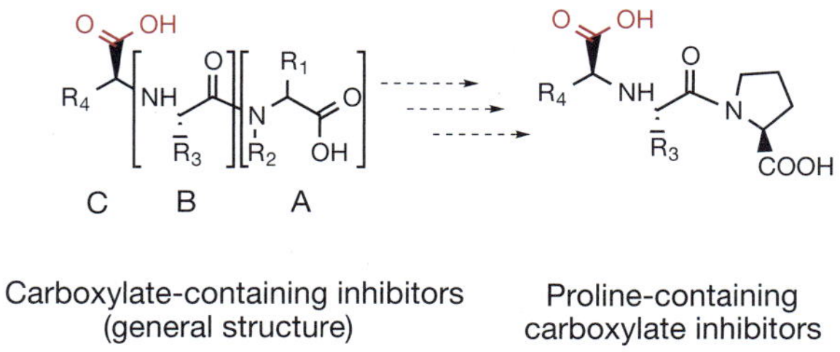

These tripeptide substrate analogs maintain the C-terminal (A) and penultimate (B) amino acids while isosterically replacing the third amino acid with a substituted *N*-carboxymethyl group (C). Similar to the findings in the development of captopril,

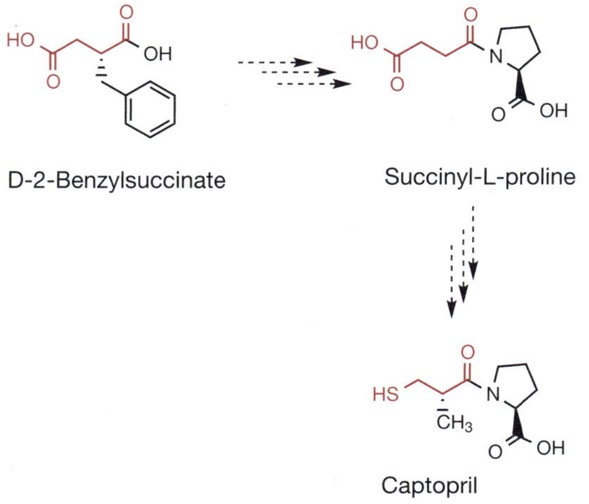

Figure 19.10 Development of captopril from D-2-benzylsuccinate.

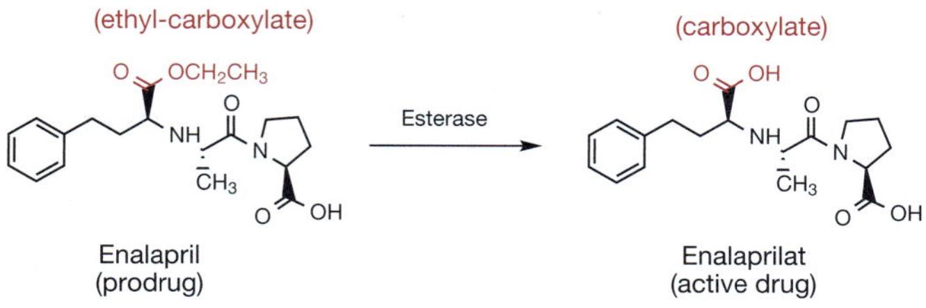

Figure 19.11 Bioactivation of enalapril to enalaprilat.

analogs with a C-terminal proline demonstrated optimal activity. Specifically, the incorporation of a methyl group at R_3 (B = Ala) and a phenylethyl group at R_4 resulted in the creation of enalaprilat. Comparing the activity of captopril and enalaprilat revealed that enalaprilat, with a K_i value of 0.2 nM, exhibited approximately 10-fold greater potency than captopril. However, enalaprilat had poor oral bioavailability despite its remarkable intravenous (IV) activity. To address this issue, esterification of enalaprilat was performed, leading to the development of enalapril, a drug with significantly improved oral bioavailability (Fig. 19.11). The success of both enalapril and enalaprilat paved the way for the subsequent development of eight additional carboxylate-containing inhibitors.

The search for ACE inhibitors that lacked the sulfhydryl group also led to the investigation of phosphorous-containing compounds.[64] The phosphinic acid shown in Figure 19.12 is capable of binding to ACE in a manner similar to that of enalaprilat. The interaction between the zinc ion and the phosphinic acid resembled that observed with the sulfhydryl and carboxylate groups. Moreover, this compound was capable of forming ionic, hydrogen, and hydrophobic bonds similar to those seen with enalaprilat and other analogs containing carboxylate groups. Further modification of the proline ring led to the development of fosinoprilat, a drug that exhibited higher inhibitory activity than captopril.

Development of Angiotensin II Receptor Blockers

From an historical perspective, the angiotensin II receptor was the initial target for developing drugs that could inhibit the renin-angiotensin pathway. The pursuit of angiotensin II receptor antagonists commenced in the early 1970s, primarily focusing on peptide-based analogs of the endogenous agonist. Although these peptide analogs demonstrated the ability to lower blood pressure, they faced limitations in terms of oral bioavailability and exhibited undesired partial agonist activity. To overcome these challenges, researchers

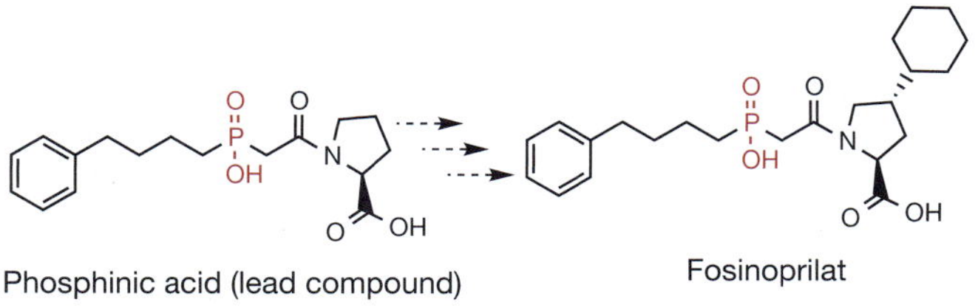

Figure 19.12 Structures of a phosphinic acid lead compound and fosinoprilat.

turned to peptide mimetics as an alternative approach. This shift in strategy eventually led to the creation of losartan, the first nonpeptide angiotensin II receptor blocker (ARB). Unlike the peptide analogs, losartan offered improved oral bioavailability and lacked partial agonist activity, making it a significant milestone in the development of ARBs.[47,65]

In 1982, two patent publications described the antihypertensive effects of a series of imidazole-5-acetic acid analogs. Exemplified by S-8038 (Fig. 19.13), these analogs were found to selectively block the angiotensin II receptor without producing any unwanted agonist activity. A computerized molecular modeling overlap of angiotensin II with the structure of S-8308 revealed three common structural features: The ionized carboxylate of S-8308 correlated with the C-terminal carboxylate of angiotensin II, the imidazole ring of S-8308 correlated with the imidazole side chain of the His6 residue, and the *n*-butyl group of S-8308 correlated with the hydrocarbon side chain of the Ile5 residue (Fig. 19.13). The benzyl group of S-8308 was proposed to lie in the direction of the N-terminus of angiotensin II; however, it was not believed to have any significant receptor interactions.

By considering S-8308, a number of molecular modifications were carried out in an attempt to improve receptor binding and lipid solubility, with the latter being important to assure adequate oral absorption. These changes resulted in losartan, a drug with high receptor affinity (IC_{50} = 19 nM) and oral activity (Fig. 19.14). Several additional ARBs have been subsequently approved for therapeutic use.

Development of Renin Inhibitors

In 1957, Skeggs et al. reported the activities of a purified amino acid sequence that could function as a renin substrate and proposed that the inhibition of renin would be beneficial in the treatment of hypertension.[66] Renin is a very specific enzyme that recognizes the Pro7-Phe8-His9-Leu10-Val11-Ile12-His13-Asn14 octapeptide sequence of angiotensinogen. Initial attempts to design renin inhibitors focused upon peptide analogs designed to mimic portions

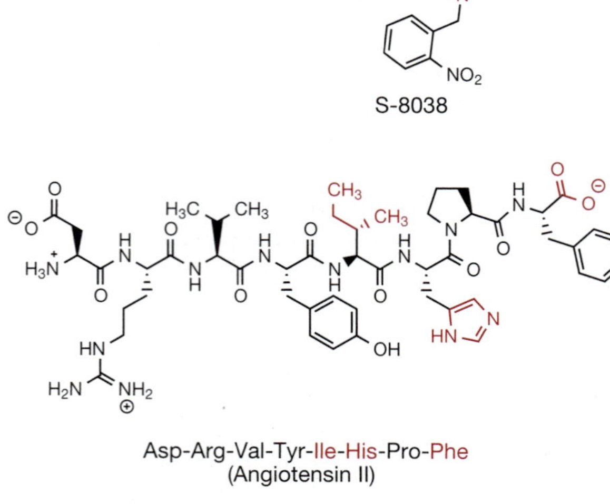

Figure 19.13 Structural comparison of S-8308, an imidazole-5-acetic acid analog, with angiotensin II.

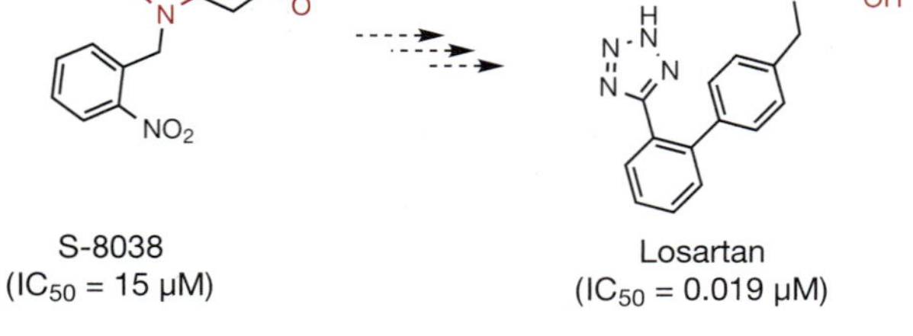

S-8038
(IC_{50} = 15 μM)

Losartan
(IC_{50} = 0.019 μM)

Figure 19.14 Development of losartan from S-8308.

or all of this sequence. Many of these analogs, exemplified by CGP29287 in Figure 19.15, showed effective inhibition of renin; however, susceptibility to proteolytic cleavage, poor or absent oral bioavailability, and short durations of action limited the therapeutic utility of these peptidic agents. Sequential structural modifications produced peptide-based compounds with the ability to mimic the transition state of angiotensinogen cleavage. Compounds such as zankiren and CGP38 560 (Fig. 19.15) possessed improved potency, favorable lipid solubility, and better oral bioavailability as compared to their predecessors. Unfortunately, the cost of synthetic preparation coupled with the success of newly approved ARBs temporarily curtailed commercial interest in this area. Success was finally obtained when the peptide backbone was abandoned and replaced with a nonpeptidic template. This template was used in the development of aliskiren (*Tekturna*) (Fig. 19.15), the first nonpeptide, low-molecular-weight, orally active, transition-state renin inhibitor.[67-69] Essential in the structure of aliskiren is the α,β-aminol moiety, which makes ion-dipole contacts with the key Asp32 and Asp215 residues in the active site of renin. Aliskiren is generally used in combination with thiazide diuretics such as hydrochlorothiazide or calcium channel blockers such as amlodipine, to treat hypertension.[70]

Therapeutic Role of Drugs That Block the Renin-Angiotensin Pathway

All ACE inhibitors, ARBs, and aliskiren are approved for the treatment of hypertension. In addition, specific ACE inhibitors and ARBs have also been approved for the treatment and management of coronary syndromes, stable coronary artery disease, heart failure with reduced ejection fraction, post-MI heart failure, left ventricular dysfunction, stroke, primary aldosteronism, post-transplant erythrocytosis in kidney transplant recipients, and diabetic and nondiabetic proteinuric chronic kidney disease. Very recently, sparsentan was shown to significantly reduce proteinuria in patients with primary immunoglobulin A nephropathy and, thus, was approved in the United States by the FDA for this indication following the accelerated approval procedure. It is worth mentioning that sparsentan is a dual endothelin and angiotensin II receptor antagonist.[71] Although all ACE inhibitors and ARBs block the action of angiotensin II, the approved indications differ among the currently available drugs.[72,73] These drugs can be used either individually or in combination with other classes of drugs. Drugs that are

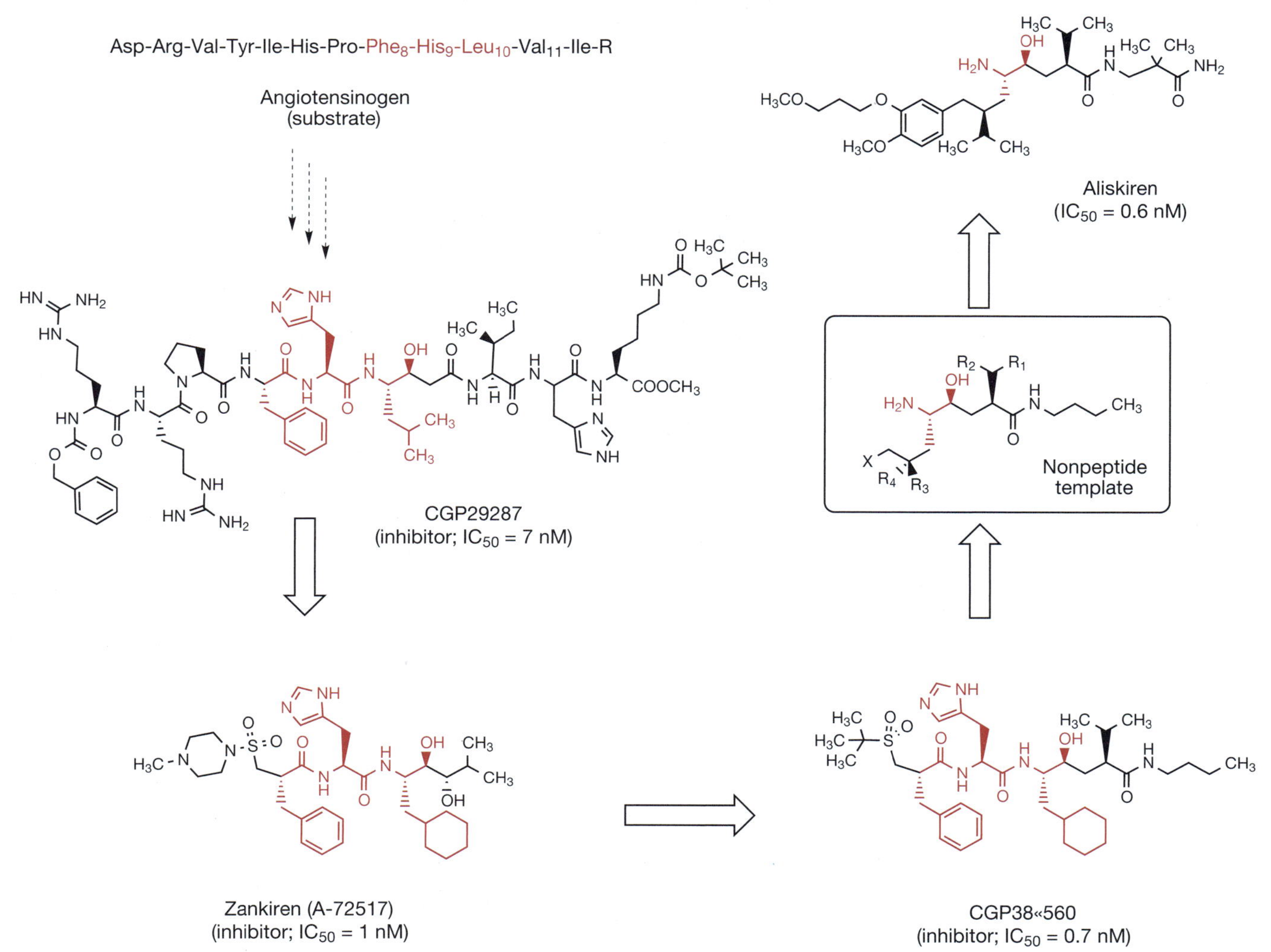

Figure 19.15 Aliskiren and predecessor renin inhibitors.

approved in other countries are the ACEIs cilazapril and spirapril, and the ARB fimasartan.

According to the 2014 report from the Eighth Joint National Committee (JNC8), ACE inhibitors and ARBs, along with thiazide-type diuretics and calcium channel blockers, are recommended for the treatment of hypertension in the general non-Black population. Additionally, ACE inhibitors and ARBs are recommended as either initial or add-on therapy for hypertension in patients with chronic kidney disease aged 18 years or older.[74] Arterial and venous dilation seen with ACE inhibitors not only lowers blood pressure but also has favorable effects on both preload and afterload in patients with heart failure. According to the American College of Cardiology/American Heart Association Task Force on Clinical Practice Guidelines, ACE inhibitors and ARBs are among the medications recommended for patients with chronic heart failure with reduced ejection fraction.[75] The ability of ACE inhibitors to cause regression of left ventricular hypertrophy has been demonstrated to reduce the incidence of further heart disease in patients with hypertension. The use of ACE inhibitors and ARBs in patients with MI is based on their ability to decrease mortality by preventing postinfarction left ventricular hypertrophy and heart failure. Both ACE inhibitors and ARBs are beneficial to patients with impaired left ventricular systolic impairment regardless of the presence of observable symptoms due to their ability to block the vascular and cardiac hypertrophy and remodeling caused by angiotensin II. Finally, ACE inhibitors and ARBs have also been reported to slow the progression of diabetic nephropathy and, thus, are preferred agents in the treatment of hypertension in patients with diabetes.[47,76,77]

UNLABELED USES OF DRUGS THAT BLOCK THE RENIN-ANGIOTENSIN PATHWAY

ACEIs and ARBs can also be used for hypertensive crises, renovascular hypertension, neonatal and childhood hypertension, stroke prevention, HIV-associated nephropathy, Marfan syndrome with aortic aneurysm, migraine prevention, nondiabetic nephropathy, chronic kidney disease, scleroderma renal crisis, Raynaud phenomenon, and Bartter syndrome.[69,70,72,73,78-80]

Pharmacology Overview of Drugs That Block the Renin-Angiotensin Pathway

Mechanisms of Action

Angiotensin-Converting Enzyme Inhibitors. The ACE inhibitors decrease the effects of the renin-angiotensin system by inhibiting the conversion of angiotensin I to II (Fig. 19.6). Inhibition of angiotensin II production lowers blood pressure and increases natriuresis. They also inhibit the conversion of angiotensin I to III; however, this action appears to have only a minor role in the overall cardiovascular effects of these drugs. They are selective in that they do not directly interfere with any other components of the renin-angiotensin system; however, they do cause other effects that are unrelated to the decrease in angiotensin II concentration. Since ACE has many physiologic substrates, its inhibition has multiple outcomes, including inhibition of bradykinin degradation, which has useful antihypertensive and protective effects (Fig. 19.8). Furthermore, ACE inhibitors also increase renin release and the rate of angiotensin I conversion by interfering with negative feedback on renin release. Accumulation of angiotensin I directs its metabolic fate into alternative routes, resulting in enhanced production of angiotensin 1-7 and other vasodilatory peptides. ACE inhibitors also increase the circulating levels of the stem cell regulator Ac-SDKP, which may contribute to their cardioprotective effects.[47]

Angiotensin II Receptor Blockers. The angiotensin II receptor exists in at least two subtypes: type 1 (AT_1) and type 2 (AT2), both of which are G-protein–coupled receptors (GPCRs). The AT_1 receptors are located in the brain, neuronal, vascular, renal, hepatic, adrenal, and myocardial tissues and mediate the hypertensive, renal, hypertrophic, and central nervous system (CNS) effects of angiotensin II. AT_1 receptors are associated with several signal transduction systems, producing effects that vary with the cell type. In most cells, AT_1 receptors are coupled to $G_{q/11}$ to activate the phospholipase C (PLC)/β-IP_3-Ca^{2+} pathway. Secondary responses to $G_{q/11}$ activation include activation of eicosanoid production, protein kinase C, phospholipase A_2, and phospholipase D, Ca^{2+}-dependent and mitogen-activated protein (MAP) kinases, and Ca^{2+}-calmodulin–dependent activation of nitric oxide synthase. Eventually, angiotensin II influences the expression of several genes, particularly genes that regulate cell growth and production of extracellular matrix components. Interaction of angiotensin II with AT_1 also stimulates the activity of a membrane-bound NADH/NADPH (nicotinamide adenine dinucleotide hydrogen/nicotinamide adenine dinucleotide phosphate hydrogen) oxidase that generates reactive oxygen species, to which many detrimental effects are attributed.

On the other hand, activation of the AT_2 receptors counteracts the effects of the AT_1 receptors that are activated by the same endogenous ligand. These effects are antihypertensive, anti-inflammatory, antiproliferative, vasodilatory, and natriuretic effects. The AT_2 receptors are more widely distributed in fetal tissues than in adults, and thus, they have been proposed to mediate a variety of growth, development, and differentiation processes. The AT_2 receptor signaling is mediated by G protein–independent and G protein–dependent ($G_i\alpha_2$ and $G_i\alpha_3$) pathways. Specific effects of AT_2 receptor activation include inhibition of Ca^{2+} channel functions; activation of phosphotyrosine phosphatases; and increasing the production of nitric oxide, cGMP, and bradykinin. Interestingly, AT_2 receptors can bind, antagonize, and reduce the expression of AT_1 receptors.[47]

All currently available ARBs are 10,000 to 30,000-fold more selective for the AT_1 receptor subtype and primarily act as competitive antagonists at this site, although some can be noncompetitive antagonists. Considering their relative affinity, azilsartan, candesartan, and olmesartan have the greatest affinity for AT_1 receptors; irbesartan and eprosartan have a somewhat modest affinity; and telmisartan, valsartan, and losartan have the lowest affinity. All ARBs inhibit most biological effects of angiotensin II, including the rapid and slow pressor responses, vascular smooth muscle (VSM) contraction, the release of vasopressin and adrenal catecholamines, the secretion of aldosterone, the increases in sympathetic tone, the enhancement of noradrenergic neurotransmission, changes in renal function, and cellular hypertrophy and hyperplasia.[81,82]

Renin Inhibitors. Aliskiren is currently the only FDA-approved renin inhibitor. It directly inhibits renin, thereby preventing the formation of angiotensins I and II. As previously mentioned, renin is the rate-limiting step in the formation of angiotensin II. Renin is secreted by the granular cells within the juxtaglomerular apparatus. The secretion of renin is regulated by the macula densa, intrarenal baroreceptors, and β_1-adrenergic receptors. Studies have shown that there are two potential advantages of inhibiting this enzyme when compared to inhibiting ACE or using an ARB. Inhibiting the renin-angiotensin pathway through the use of ACE inhibitors or ARBs has been shown to cause a compensatory increase in renin concentration, which is not seen with the renin inhibitor aliskiren. Furthermore, alternate pathways, such as the chymostatin-sensitive pathway present in the heart, can convert angiotensin I to angiotensin II. While this alternate pathway could affect the efficacy of ACE inhibitors, it would not alter the effects of direct renin inhibition.[66-69,83]

Common Adverse Effects

The most prevalent or significant adverse effects of drugs affecting the renin-angiotensin pathway have been well reported.[47,72,73,81-84] While some adverse effects can be directly related to the mechanism of action of this class of drugs, others can be attributed to specific functional groups within individual agents.

Angiotensin-Converting Enzyme Inhibitors. Common adverse effects of all drugs affecting the renin-angiotensin pathway are hypotension and hyperkalemia. Hypotension results from an extension of the desired physiological effect, whereas hyperkalemia results from a decrease in aldosterone secretion secondary to a decrease in angiotensin II production. Hyperkalemia is particularly seen in patients with renal insufficiency or diabetes or if used with potassium supplements, potassium-sparing diuretics, β-receptor blockers, or NSAIDs.

ACE inhibitors can induce a bothersome, dry cough. It is seen in 5% to 20% of patients, usually is not dose-dependent, and apparently results from the lack of selectivity of this class of drugs. As previously discussed, ACE inhibitors prevent the breakdown of bradykinin (Fig. 19.8), and because bradykinin stimulates prostaglandin synthesis, prostaglandin levels also increase. The increased levels of bradykinin, prostaglandins, and in some cases substance P, in the lungs have been proposed to be responsible for the cough.[84] Bradykinin accumulation has also been linked to angioedema manifested as rapid swelling in the nose, throat, mouth, glottis, larynx, lips, and/or tongue. This adverse drug reaction is rare (0.1%-0.5%) and occurs at a higher incidence in Black patients than in non-Black patients. ACE inhibitors should be immediately discontinued if angioedema occurs. The dry cough and angioedema are notably absent with ARBs and aliskiren. This is because these drugs are more specific in their action and do not affect the levels of bradykinin or prostaglandins.[47]

The ACE inhibitors can also cause maculopapular rashes, sometimes with itch, which may spontaneously resolve or can be treated with antihistamines. The higher incidence of maculopapular rashes and taste disturbances observed among patients using captopril have been linked to the presence of the sulfhydryl group. Other rare adverse effects include acute renal insufficiency, hepatotoxicity, anemia, neutropenia, and glycosuria. ACE inhibitors and ARBs have also been associated with renal developmental defects when administered in the third trimester of pregnancy, and potentially earlier, owing to fetal hypotension. Fortunately, ACE inhibitors do not affect plasma concentrations of uric acid or calcium, and in fact, they may improve glucose tolerance and insulin sensitivity in patients with insulin resistance. They may also decrease lipoprotein (a) and cholesterol levels in proteinuric renal disease.[47,72]

Angiotensin II Receptor Blockers. The occurrence of cough and angioedema with ARBs is less than with ACE inhibitors. ARBs can cause hypotension, oliguria, progressive azotemia, or acute renal failure. ARBs are potentially teratogenic and should be discontinued in pregnancy. Other rare effects include anaphylaxis, hepatotoxicity, vasculitis, agranulocytosis, neutropenia, leukopenia, hyponatremia, pruritus, urticaria, and alopecia.[47]

Aliskiren. Adverse events are generally mild and include gastrointestinal symptoms (abdominal pain, dyspepsia, gastroesophageal reflux, and diarrhea), dizziness, fatigue, headache, upper respiratory tract infection, and back pain. Cough and angioedema are much less common than ACEIs. Other adverse effects include rash, hyperkalemia, hypotension, elevated uric acid, gout, and renal stones. Aliskiren is contraindicated in pregnancy. Concomitant use with ACEIs and ARBs in patients with diabetes is also contraindicated.[47]

Drug Interactions

Angiotensin-Converting Enzyme Inhibitors. Coadministration of other drugs may complicate the use of ACE inhibitors by affecting their pharmacokinetics and/or pharmacodynamics. In fact, some can also worsen their adverse effects. Pharmacokinetically, antacids and the phosphate-binding agent lanthanum carbonate (Fosrenol) may decrease the bioavailability of ACE inhibitors. ACE inhibitors may increase plasma concentrations of lithium and digoxin and hypersensitivity reactions to allopurinol and other drugs. Probenecid decreases the clearance of captopril and increases its blood level. Rifampin (CYP3A4 inducer) decreases the plasma level of enalapril. Iron salts can also reduce captopril levels unless administration is separated by at least 2 hours. Quinapril may reduce the absorption of tetracycline, potentially because of the high magnesium content of quinapril tablets.

Pharmacodynamically, NSAIDs, including aspirin, may decrease the antihypertensive response to ACE inhibitors because they decrease the biosynthesis of prostaglandins. Studies have shown that indomethacin, naproxen, and piroxicam have a greater tendency for causing this interaction. In contrast, phenothiazines may increase the pharmacological effects of ACE inhibitors. Diuretics may also result in excessive reduction in blood pressure. Potassium supplements and potassium-sparing diuretics or drospirenone, a birth control drug, may exacerbate ACEI-induced hyperkalemia. Coadministration of pregabalin, alteplase, everolimus, and dipeptidyl peptidase-IV inhibitors such as sitagliptin may also increase the risk of developing angioedema. Lastly, capsaicin may worsen ACEI-induced cough.[47] It is worth mentioning that the consequences of interactions with potassium supplements, potassium-sparing diuretics, drospirenone, NSAIDs, and lithium are the same among all drugs affecting the renin-angiotensin pathway.

Angiotensin II Receptor Blockers. Many drug interactions are similar to those of ACEIs. For example, rifampin, CYP3A4 inducer, can decrease the plasma levels of losartan and its active metabolite, EXP-3174. ARBs may also impair the excretion of digoxin, and thus, increase its plasma concentration.

Aliskiren. While aliskiren shares similar drug interactions with ACEIs and ARBs, there are a few that are unique. Aliskiren plasma levels are increased by drugs that inhibit P-glycoprotein, such as atorvastatin, cyclosporine, and ketoconazole. Aliskiren decreases the absorption of furosemide by 50%, and irbesartan reduces the maximum plasma concentration of aliskiren by 50%.[47]

Medicinal Chemistry of Angiotensin-Converting Enzyme Inhibitors

General Structure and Classification

With the exception of benazepril, clinically used ACE inhibitors can be represented by the general structure given in Figure 19.16. These ACE inhibitors possess a central domain, which is generally known as the zinc-binding domain. This domain is terminal in captopril, the smallest ACE inhibitor. The zinc-binding domain is composed of an essential structural moiety that mimics the endogenous transition state in the catalytic mechanism of ACE. It also binds with the zinc ion in the enzyme's active site, resulting in the enzyme inhibition. Because of this, ACE inhibitors are mechanistically classified as transition-state mimetic, competitive enzyme inhibitors. Considering

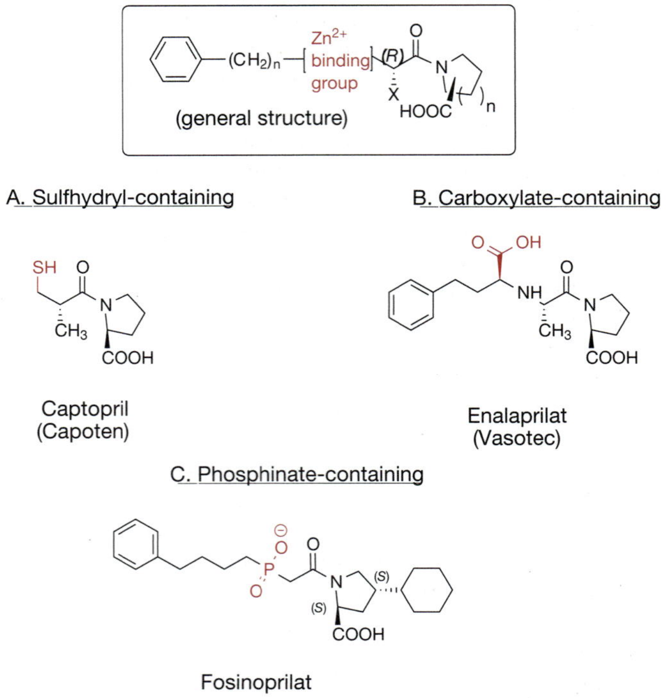

Figure 19.16 General structure of ACEIs.

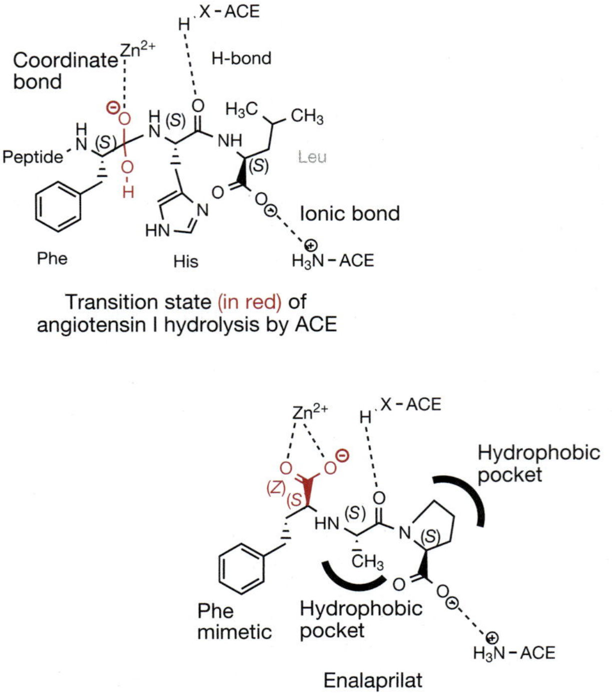

Figure 19.17 Comparison of enalaprilat and the transition state of angiotensin I hydrolysis by ACE.

the zinc-binding domain, ACE inhibitors are classified as either sulfhydryl-containing (only captopril), carboxylate-containing (several including enalaprilat), or phosphinate-containing (only fosinoprilat) ACE inhibitors.

Receptor Binding and Structure-Activity Relationship

With the exception of captopril, all ACE inhibitors mimic the Phe8-His9-Leu10 tripeptide sequence at the C-terminus of angiotensin I (see Fig. 19.6). As ACE is a relatively nonspecific dipeptidyl carboxypeptidase, the side chains of His9 and Leu10 are replaced by Ala and either Pro or Pro analogs, respectively. A comparison of the transition state of angiotensin I hydrolysis by ACE and the binding of enalaprilat is shown in Figure 19.17. The structure of enalaprilat and all carboxylate-containing ACE inhibitors have a tetrahedral carbon atom in place of the labile peptide. Moreover, the carboxylic acid attached to this tetrahedral carbon atom can chelate with the enzyme-bound zinc ion. Enalaprilat and other carboxylate-containing ACE inhibitors possess a second carboxylic acid that is located at the C-terminal proline or proline analog. These drugs are occasionally referred to as dicarboxylate-containing ACEIs. This second carboxylic acid can form an ionic bond with either a lysine or arginine residue in the active site of ACE. The nonlabile peptide bond between the alanine and proline analog can form a hydrogen bond with ACE, while the phenylethyl group mimics the hydrophobic side chain of Phe_8 that is present in angiotensin I. All of these binding interactions closely resemble the binding of angiotensin I-transition state to ACE.

Captopril and fosinoprilat demonstrate similar binding to ACE with a few structural changes (Fig. 19.18). Captopril is more of a dipeptide mimetic, whereas fosinopril, similar to enalaprilat, is a tripeptide mimetic. The structure of captopril does not contain the tetrahedral carbon atom or the phenylethyl group seen in enalaprilat; however, the sulfhydryl group is superior to the carboxylic acid in binding to the zinc ion. Fosinoprilat binds to ACE in a manner similar to that of enalaprilat. The interaction of the zinc ion with the phosphinic acid is similar to that seen with sulfhydryl group of captopril and carboxylate group of enalaprilat. The phosphinic acid is able to truly mimic the ionized, tetrahedral intermediate of peptide hydrolysis. Although the

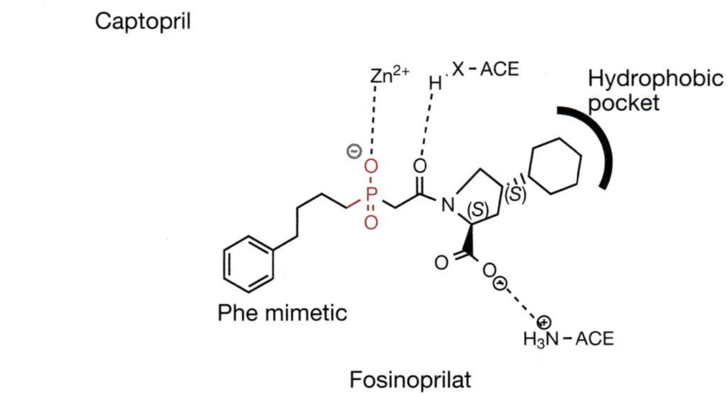

Figure 19.18 Binding of captopril and fosinoprilat to ACE.

spatial orientation of the functional groups in fosinoprilat is slightly different from enalaprilat, it still is able to occupy the same space of the side chains of Phe8 and Leu10.

While the carboxylic acid of enalaprilat is required to bind to the zinc ion, the overall oral bioavailability of the drug is poor. The two carboxylate groups and the secondary amine will be primarily ionized under the physiological pH of the gastrointestinal (GI) tract, which will impede its absorption and limit its bioavailability. As depicted in Figure 19.11, masking the zinc-binding carboxylic acid in the form of ethyl ester produced enalapril, a prodrug with superior oral bioavailability. Interestingly, the ester prodrug has a significant effect on the pK_a of the adjacent secondary amine. The ester group forms a hydrogen bond with the adjacent secondary amine and decreases its pK_a to 5.49. Thus, the secondary amine will be primarily unionized in the gastrointestinal tract, and zwitterion formation with the proline carboxylic acid will be unlikely. This adds to the overall enhanced lipid solubility and absorbability of enalapril.[85,86] Bioactivation by hepatic esterases (Fig. 19.11) has been suggested as the most probable mechanism for the conversion of the prodrug enalapril to the active drug enalaprilat.[87,88]

Similar to the carboxylic acid group in enalaprilat, the ionization of the phosphinic acid group in the structure of fosinoprilat significantly reduces its gastrointestinal absorption following oral administration. The prodrug fosinopril contains an (acyloxy)alkyl group, which prevents the phosphinic acid from ionization in the gastrointestinal environment, and thus, allows better lipid solubility and improved bioavailability.[64] Bioactivation via esterase activity in the intestinal wall and liver produces fosinopril (Fig. 19.19).

Nine other carboxylate-containing ACE inhibitors (Fig. 19.20) have been approved in the United States and other countries for various therapeutic indications. All of the carboxylate-containing ACEIs are ethyl ester prodrugs (Fig. 19.20A-C) that require esterase-mediated bioactivation, except lisinopril (Figure 19.20D). Lisinopril is chemically different in two respects. First, it contains the basic amino acid lysine side chain (-$CH_2CH_2CH_2CH_2NH_2$) instead of the standard nonpolar side chain of alanine (-CH_3). Second, it is an active drug on its own and does not require bioactivation, because neither of its two carboxylic acids (the zinc-binding acidic group and the terminal acidic group) is esterified. Lisinopril was developed at the same time as enalapril. Despite the addition of another ionizable group, the oral absorption of lisinopril was found to be better than that of enalaprilat but less than that of enalapril. In vitro studies indicated that lisinopril is slightly more potent than enalaprilat.[87,88]

The major structural difference among the remaining carboxylate-containing ACE inhibitors is in the ring of the C-terminal amino acid. As previously mentioned, proline was the C-terminal amino acid in the naturally occurring snake venom peptides used to develop ACE inhibitors. Attempts to replace it with other amino acids were unsuccessful. Nevertheless, structural variations of proline with larger hydrophobic ring systems enhanced binding and potency as compared to enalapril and lisinopril, the two original drugs from this subclass. The larger hydrophobic ring systems include proline-containing bicyclic systems present in the structures of ramipril, spirapril, trandolapril, and perindopril; a tetrahydroisoquinoline-3-carboxylic acid system present in the structures of quinapril and moexipril; and an azepane-containing bicyclic systems present in the structures of cilazapril and benazepril. The larger hydrophobic ring systems also led to differences in the following pharmacokinetic parameters among these drugs: absorption, plasma protein binding, elimination, onset of action, duration of action, and dosing.

A summary of the SAR for ACE inhibitors is provided in Table 19.8. ACE is a stereoselective enzyme. Because all currently available ACE inhibitors are either di- or tripeptide substrate analogs, they must contain a stereochemistry that is consistent with the L-amino acids present in ACE's endogenous substrates. This was demonstrated very early in the development of ACE inhibitors when compounds with C-terminal D-amino acids were discovered to be very poor inhibitors.[89] The stereochemical requirement was subsequently reinforced by the work of Patchett et al.[63] They reported a 100- to 1,000-fold loss in inhibitor activity when the configuration of either the zinc-binding carboxylate or the X substituent (L-alanine or L-Lysine) (Table 19.8) was changed. The *S,S,S*-configuration seen in enalapril and other carboxylate inhibitors meets the stereochemical requirement, resulting in an optimal enzyme inhibition activity.

Physicochemical Properties

Captopril and fosinopril are acidic drugs, but all other ACE inhibitors are amphoteric (ie, possess acidic and basic functional groups). The carboxylic acid attached to the *N*-ring

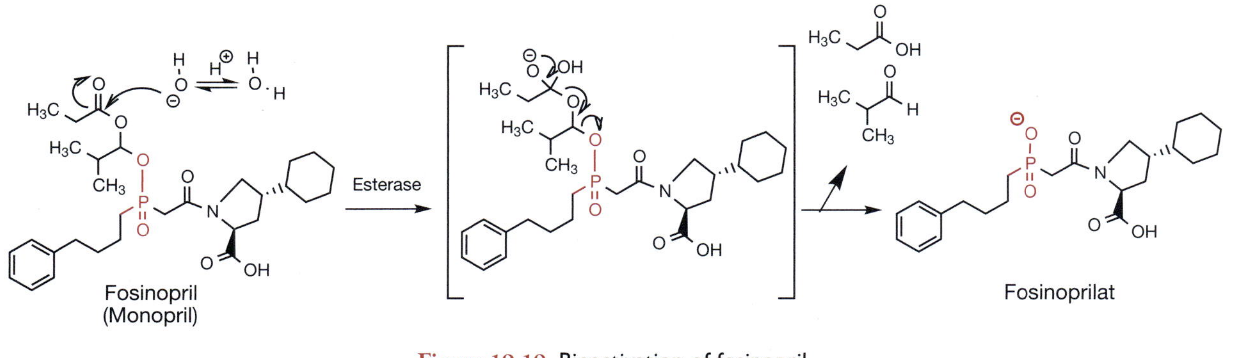

Figure 19.19 Bioactivation of fosinopril.

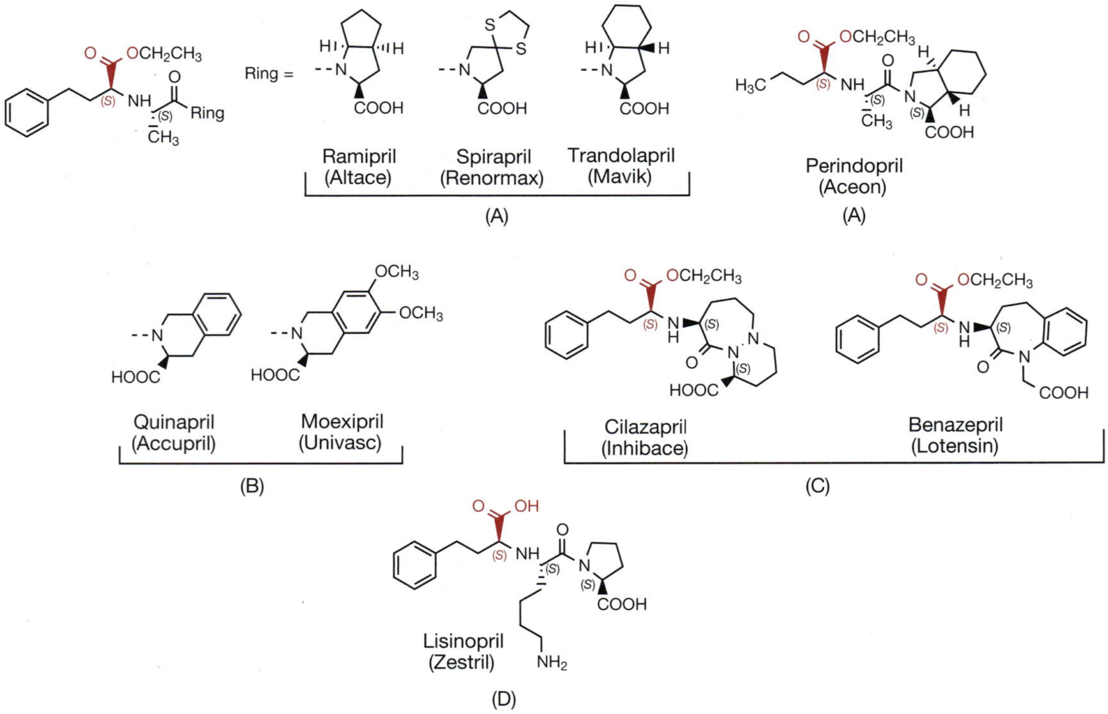

Figure 19.20 Chemical structures of carboxylate-containing ACEIs. Variations are primarily attributed to the nature of the ring system, which can be proline-based (A), tetrahydroisoquinoline-3-carboxylic acid-based (B), or azepane-based (C); and to the active drug versus prodrug status. Drugs in (A), (B), and (C) are all prodrugs, whereas lisinopril (D) is an active drug.

is a common structural feature in all ACE inhibitors with a pK_a value in the range of 2.5 to 3.5. It will be primarily ionized at physiological pH. In the carboxylate series, the pK_a and the ionization of the secondary amine depend on whether the adjacent functional group is in the prodrug or active form. In the prodrug form, the amine is adjacent to an ester, is less basic, and is primarily unioinized at physiological pH. Following bioactivation, the amine is adjacent to an ionized carboxylic acid that enhances both the basicity (pK_a = 8.02) and the ionization of the amine. Similarly, the basic nitrogen enhances the acidity of the adjacent carboxylic acid such that it usually has a lower pK_a than the carboxylic acid attached to the *N*-ring. As an example, the pK_a values of the two carboxylic acids in enalaprilat are

Table 19.8 Structure-Activity Relationships of Angiotensin-Converting Enzyme Inhibitors

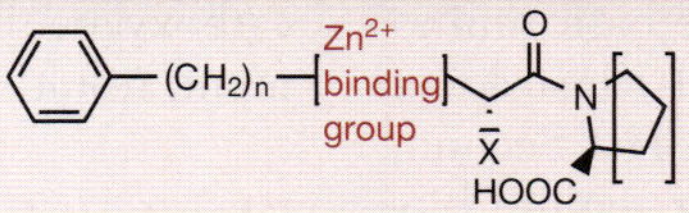

a. The zinc-binding group can be either sulfhydryl, a carboxylic acid, or a phosphinic acid. Esterification of the carboxylate or phosphinate produces an orally bioavailable prodrug.

b. The sulfhydryl group shows superior binding to zinc (the side chain mimicking the Phe in carboxylate and phosphinic acid inhibitors partially compensates for the lack of a sulfhydryl group).

c. Inhibitors that bind to zinc through either a carboxylate or phosphinate mimic the peptide hydrolysis transition state and enhance binding.

d. X is usually methyl to mimic the side chain of alanine. Within the carboxylate series, when X equals *n*-butylamine (lysine side chain), this produces a compound that does not require prodrug for oral activity.

e. The *N*-ring must contain a carboxylic acid to mimic the C-terminal carboxylate of ACE substrates.

f. Large hydrophobic heterocyclic rings increase potency and alter pharmacokinetic parameters.

g. The X group and the *N*-ring can be fused as in cilazapril and benazepril.

h. Optimal activity occurs when the stereochemistry of the inhibitor is consistent with L-amino acid stereochemistry present in endogenous substrates.

i. Owing to the sulfhydryl group, captopril has shorter duration of action because of dimerization and disulfide formation and is associated with a high incidence of skin rash and taste disturbances.

2.30 and 3.39. These values correspond to the carboxylic acid adjacent to the amine and the carboxylic acid on the *N*-ring, respectively. The analogous values for these functional groups in lisinopril are 1.7 and 3.3.[86]

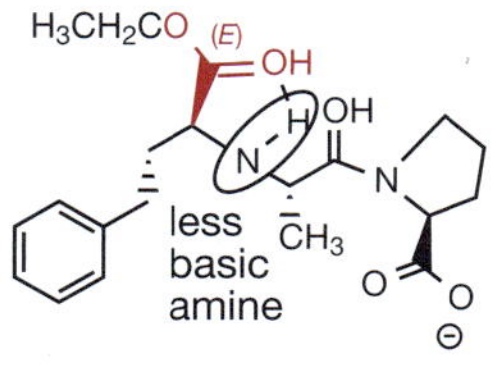

Enalapril [prodrug]
(more lipophilic)

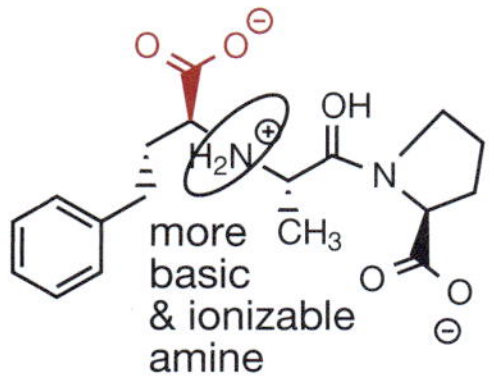

Enalaprilat [active drug]
(less lipophilic)

The calculated log P values[86] along with other pharmacokinetic parameters for the ACE inhibitors are shown in Table 19.9. With three notable exceptions (captopril, enalaprilat, and lisinopril), all of the drugs possess good lipid solubility. Generally, ACEIs that contain bicyclic ring systems are more lipid soluble than those that contain proline. A comparison of the log P values of benazepril, fosinopril, moexipril, perindopril, quinapril, ramipril, spirapril, and trandolapril to those of captopril and enalapril illustrates this fact. An exception to this is seen in cilazapril. While it has a bicyclic ring system, this ring system is saturated, contains a tertiary amine, and is much less lipid soluble. As previously discussed, enalaprilat is much more hydrophilic than its ester prodrug and is currently the only ACE inhibitor marked for IV administration. In terms of solubility, lisinopril is an interesting drug in that it is the most hydrophilic inhibitor, yet unlike enalaprilat, it is orally active. One plausible justification for this phenomenon is that in the duodenum, lisinopril will exist as a di-zwitterion in which the ionized groups can internally bind to one another. Therefore, lisinopril may be able to pass through the lipid bilayer with an overall net neutral charge.

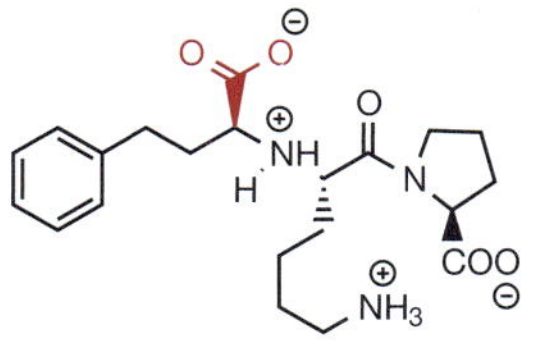

The di-zwitterion
form of lisinopril

Pharmacokinetic Properties

The pharmacokinetic parameters and dosing information for ACE inhibitors are summarized in Tables 19.9 and 19.10, respectively.[47,72,86,90] The oral bioavailability of this class of drugs ranges from 13% to 95%. Variations in lipid solubility and first-pass metabolism susceptibility account for this wide variation. Both parameters should be considered when comparing any two or more drugs. With the exceptions of enalapril and lisinopril, the concurrent administration with food adversely affects the oral absorption of ACE inhibitors. For captopril and moexipril, the literature specifically instructs that the former should be taken 1 hour before meals and that the latter should be taken in the fasting state. Similar instructions may potentially benefit patients taking an ACE inhibitor whose absorption is affected by food.

The extent of protein binding also exhibits wide variability among different drugs. The data suggest that this variation might correlate with the calculated log P values for the drugs (Table 19.9). Three of the more lipophilic drugs—fosinopril, quinapril, and benazepril—exhibit protein binding of greater than 90%, whereas three of the least lipophilic drugs—lisinopril, enalapril, and captopril—exhibit much lower protein binding. Another way to predict the potential for plasma protein binding is to consider the nature of the ring systems. Inhibitors with a monocyclic ring system—lisinopril, enalapril, and captopril—are most likely to demonstrate less than 50% potential to bind to plasma proteins, whereas drugs with multicyclic ring systems are most likely to exhibit more than 50% plasma protein binding. This can be attributed to the potential of nonspecific hydrophobic interactions between these rings and cyclic amino acids in plasma proteins.

Renal elimination is the primary route of elimination for most ACE inhibitors. With the exceptions of fosinopril and spirapril, altered renal function significantly reduces the plasma clearance of ACE inhibitors. Thus, the dosage of most ACE inhibitors should be reduced in patients with renal impairment.[47]

All orally administered ACE inhibitors have a similar onset of action (~1 hour), duration of action (~24 hours), and dosing interval (once or twice daily), except for captopril. The smallest drug among all ACEIs, captopril, has a more rapid onset of action (~0.25 hour) and a shorter duration (6-12 hours). Its short duration of action can be attributed to its ability to self-dimerize or cross-dimerize to form a disulfide bond with itself or with other endogenous molecules containing sulfhydryl group, respectively. Thus, the maximum dose of captopril (450 mg) is larger than any of the other ACEIs and is administered more frequently than any of the other ACEIs (3 times a day). When oral dosing is inappropriate, enalaprilat can be used IV. The normal dose administered to hypertensive patients is 0.625 to 1.25 mg every 6 hours. The dose is usually administered over 5 minutes and may be titrated up to 5 mg IV every 6 hours.

Metabolism

Lisinopril and enalaprilat are excreted unchanged, whereas all other ACE inhibitors undergo variable levels of metabolic biotransformation.[47,72,86,90] As illustrated in Figures 19.11 and 19.19, all carboxylate and phosphinate prodrugs must undergo bioactivation via hepatic esterases. Additionally, based on their structural features, specific drugs can undergo metabolic inactivation via various pathways (Fig. 19.21). Because of its sulfhydryl group, captopril is subject to oxidative dimerization or conjugation. Approximately 40% to 50% of a dose of captopril is excreted unchanged, whereas the remainder is excreted as either a disulfide dimer or a captopril-cysteine disulfide. Glucuronide conjugation has been reported for benazepril, fosinopril, quinapril, and ramipril. This conjugation can occur either with the parent prodrug or with the activated drug. Benazepril, with the *N*-substituted glycine, is especially susceptible to this reaction because of the limited steric hindrance. For all ACE inhibitors, except benazepril, the terminal carboxylic

Table 19.9 Pharmacokinetic Parameters of Angiotensin-Converting Enzyme Inhibitors

Drug	Calculated Log P	Oral Bioavailability (%)	Effect of Food on Absorption	Active Metabolite	Protein Binding (%)	Onset of Action (h)	Duration of Action (h)	Major Route(s) of Elimination
Benazepril	5.50	37	Slows absorption	Benazeprilat	>95	1	24	Renal (primary) Biliary (secondary)
Captopril	0.27	60-75	Reduced	NA	25-30	0.25-0.50	6-12	Renal
Cilazapril	0.73	60	Slows absorption to a minor extent (therapeutically irrelevant)	Cilazaprilat	—	1	24	Renal
Enalapril	2.43	60	None	Enalaprilat	50-60	1	24	Renal/fecal
Enalaprilat	1.54	NA	NA	NA	—	0.25	6	Renal
Fosinopril	6.09	36	Slows absorption	Fosinoprilat	95	1	24	Renal (50%) Hepatic (50%)
Lisinopril	1.19	25-30	None	NA	25	1	24	Renal
Moexipril	4.06	13	Reduced	Moexiprilat	50	1	24	Fecal (primary) Renal (secondary)
Perindopril	3.36	65-95	Reduced	Perindoprilat	60-80	1	24	Renal
Quinapril	4.32	60	Reduced	Quinaprilat	97	1	24	Renal
Ramipril	3.41	50-60	Slows absorption	Ramiprilat	73	1-2	24	Renal (60%) Fecal (40%)
Spirapril	3.16	50	—	Spiraprilat	—	1	24	Renal (50%) Hepatic (50%)
Trandolapril	3.97	70	Slows absorption	Trandolaprilat	80	0.5-1.0	24	Fecal (primary) Renal (secondary)

—, data not available; NA, not applicable.

Table 19.10 Dosing Information for Orally Available Angiotensin-Converting Enzyme Inhibitors

Generic Name	Trade Name(s)	Approved Indications	Dosing Range (Treatment of Hypertension)	Maximum Daily Dose	Dose Reduction With Renal Dysfunction	Available Tablet Strengths (mg)
Benazepril	Lotensin	Hypertension	40 mg once daily or b.i.d.	80 mg	Yes	5, 10, 20, 40
Captopril	Capoten	Hypertension, hypertensive crisis, heart failure, left ventricular dysfunction (post-MI), diabetic nephropathy	25-150 mg b.i.d. or t.i.d.	450 mg	Yes	12.5, 25, 50, 100
Enalapril	Vasotec	Hypertension, heart failure, left ventricular cardiac dysfunction, asymptomatic (ejection fraction ≤35%)	2.5-40 mg once daily or b.i.d.	40 mg	Yes	2.5, 5, 10, 20
Fosinopril	Monopril	Hypertension, heart failure	10-40 mg once daily	80 mg	No	10, 20, 40
Lisinopril	Prinivil, Zestril	Hypertension, heart failure, improve survival post-MI	10-40 mg once daily	80 mg	Yes	2.5, 5, 10, 20, 30, 40
Moexipril	Univasc	Hypertension	7.5-30 mg once daily or b.i.d.	30 mg	Yes	7.5, 15
Perindopril	Aceon	Hypertension, stable CAD	4-8 mg once daily or b.i.d.	16 mg	Yes	2, 4, 8
Quinapril	Accupril	Hypertension, heart failure	10-80 mg once daily or b.i.d.	80 mg	Yes	5, 10, 20, 40
Ramipril	Altace	Hypertension, heart failure (post-MI), reduce risk of MI, stroke, and death from cardiovascular causes	2.5-20 mg once daily or b.i.d.	20 mg	Yes	1.25, 2.5, 5, 10
Trandolapril	Mavik	Hypertension, heart failure (post-MI), left ventricular dysfunction (post-MI)	1-4 mg once daily	8 mg	Yes	1, 2, 4

b.i.d., twice a day; CAD, coronary artery disease; MI, myocardial infarction; t.i.d., three times a day.

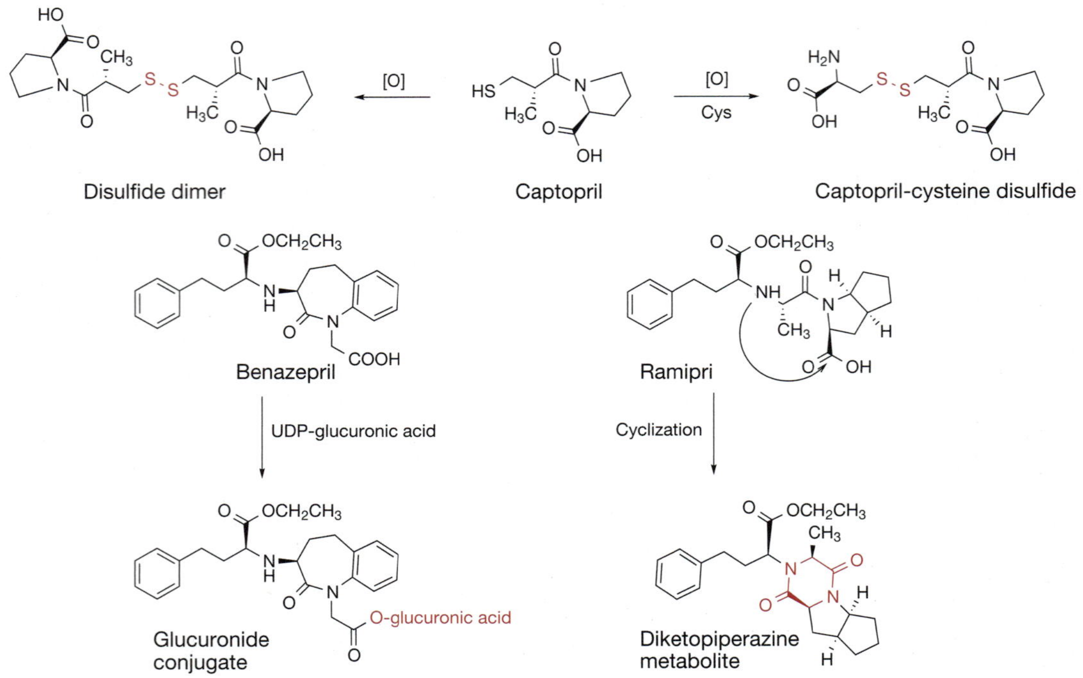

Figure 19.21 Metabolic routes of ACE inhibitors.

acid is substituted on the ring system, which creates some steric hindrance to conjugation. However, the same terminal carboxylic group in benazepril extends relatively farther from the rings system, given the unsubstituted methylene bridge. Thus, this terminal carboxylic group now exists in a relatively less sterically hindered chemical environment and is more accessible, thus facilitating conjugation. Moexipril, perindopril, and ramipril can undergo cyclization to produce diketopiperazines. This cyclization can occur with either the parent or active forms of the drugs.

Medicinal Chemistry of Angiotensin II Receptor Blockers

Receptor Binding and Structure-Activity Relationships

Angiotensin II receptor blockers have structural features that mimic the side chains of certain amino acids present within the structure of angiotensin II, as illustrated with losartan in Figure 19.22. All other ARBs, with the exception of eprosartan, are biphenyl analogs of losartan, and they share similar structural features and binding abilities (Fig. 19.23). Azilsartan medoxomil, candesartan cilexetil, and olmesartan medoxomil are prodrugs that are rapidly and completely hydrolyzed to the corresponding carboxylic acids.

In terms of SAR, all commercially available ARBs are analogs of the following general structure:

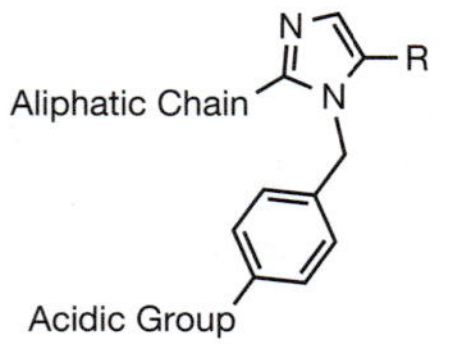

1. The "acidic group" is thought to mimic either the Tyr4 phenol or the Asp1 carboxylate of angiotensin II. Groups capable of such a role include a phenyl tetrazole (as seen in losartan, olmesartan, valsartan, irbesartan, fimasartan, and candesartan), a benzoic acid (as seen in telmisartan), a phenyl oxadiazole moiety (as seen in azilsartan), a benzene-sulfonamide moiety (as seen in sparsentan), and a carboxylic acid (as seen in eprosartan).
2. In the biphenyl series, the tetrazole, carboxylate, oxadiazole, and sulfonamide groups must be in the ortho position for optimal activity. Relative to the carboxylic acid, the other groups appear to be superior in terms of metabolic stability, lipophilicity, and oral bioavailability.
3. The "aliphatic chain" mimics the side chain of Ile5 of angiotensin II and it supports hydrophobic binding to the angiotensin II receptor. It can be an *n*-butyl group, an *n*-propyl, or an ethylether, suggesting that this substituent should be a 3- to 4-atom extended chain.
4. The imidazole ring or its isosteric equivalent is required to mimic the His6 side chain of angiotensin II.
5. Substitution can vary at the "R" position. The most frequent R group is the carboxylic acid, which can be masked in the form of a carbonate-containing ester to improve oral bioavailability. Other R groups present in currently available ARBs include a hydroxymethyl group (losartan), a ketone group (irbesartan, sparsentan, and fimasartan), or a benzimidazole ring (telmisartan). The R group is thought to interact with the AT_1 receptor through either ionic, ion-dipole, or dipole-dipole bonds. The thienyl ring present within the structure of eprosartan isosterically mimics the Phe8 phenyl ring of angiotensin II.

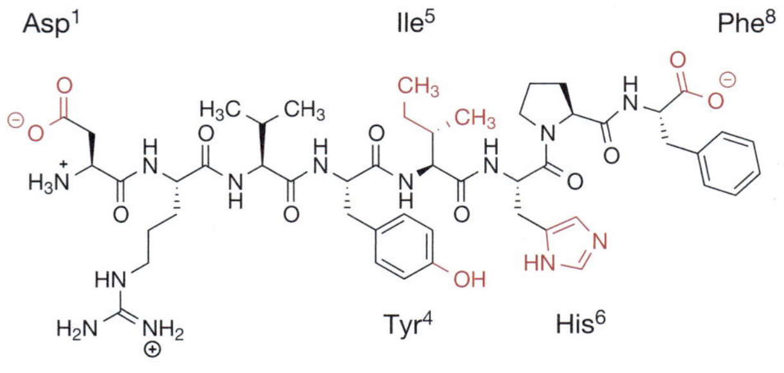

Asp-Arg-Val-Tyr-Ile-His-Pro-Phe
(Angiotensin II)

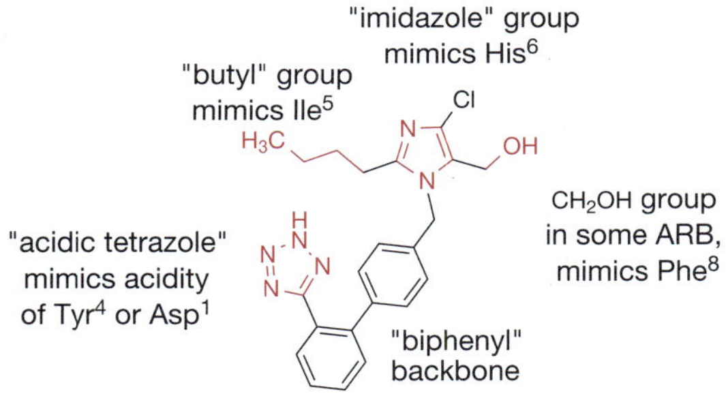

Losartan
(Competitive ARB)

Figure 19.22 Structural similarities between angiotensin II and losartan.

Physicochemical Properties

All ARBs contain acidic functional groups. The tetrazole ring present within the structures of losartan, olmesartan, valsartan, irbesartan, fimasartan, and candesartan, and has a pK_a of approximately 6 and will be at least 90% ionized at physiological pH. The 5-oxo-1,2,4-oxadiazole ring present in azilsartan is a tetrazole isostere and has a similar pK_a value. The carboxylic acids found on valsartan, candesartan, olmesartan, telmisartan, azilsartan, and eprosartan have pK_a values in the range of 3 to 4 and will also be primarily ionized. The sulfonamide group in sparsentan has a pK_a value of about 5.7 and will also be primarily ionized under physiological pH. Currently, available agents have adequate, but not excellent, lipid solubility. As previously mentioned, the tetrazole group is more lipophilic than a carboxylic acid. Additionally, the four nitrogen atoms present in the tetrazole ring can create a greater charge distribution than that available for a carboxylic acid. These properties have been proposed to be responsible for the enhanced binding and bioavailability of the tetrazole-containing drugs.[91] Similar to ACE inhibitors, the stereochemistry of valsartan is consistent with the L-amino acids in the endogenous agonist.

Pharmacokinetic Properties

The pharmacokinetic parameters and dosing information for ARBs are summarized in Tables 19.11 and 19.12, respectively.[73,90,92-95] With the exception of azilsartan medoxomil (60%), irbesartan (60%-80%) and, possibly, telmisartan (42%-58%), all of these drugs have low, but adequate, oral bioavailability (15%-33%). Given the fact that most of the drugs are excreted unchanged, the most probable reasons for the low bioavailability are poor lipid solubility and incomplete absorption. The effect of food on the absorption of ARBs has been generally deemed to be clinically insignificant; thus, these drugs can be taken either with or without food. All ARBs have similar onsets of action, are highly plasma protein bound, have elimination half-lives that enable once- or twice-daily dosing, and with the exception of olmesartan, are primarily eliminated via the fecal route. Candesartan, telmisartan, and sparsentan appear to require a slightly longer time to reach peak plasma concentrations.

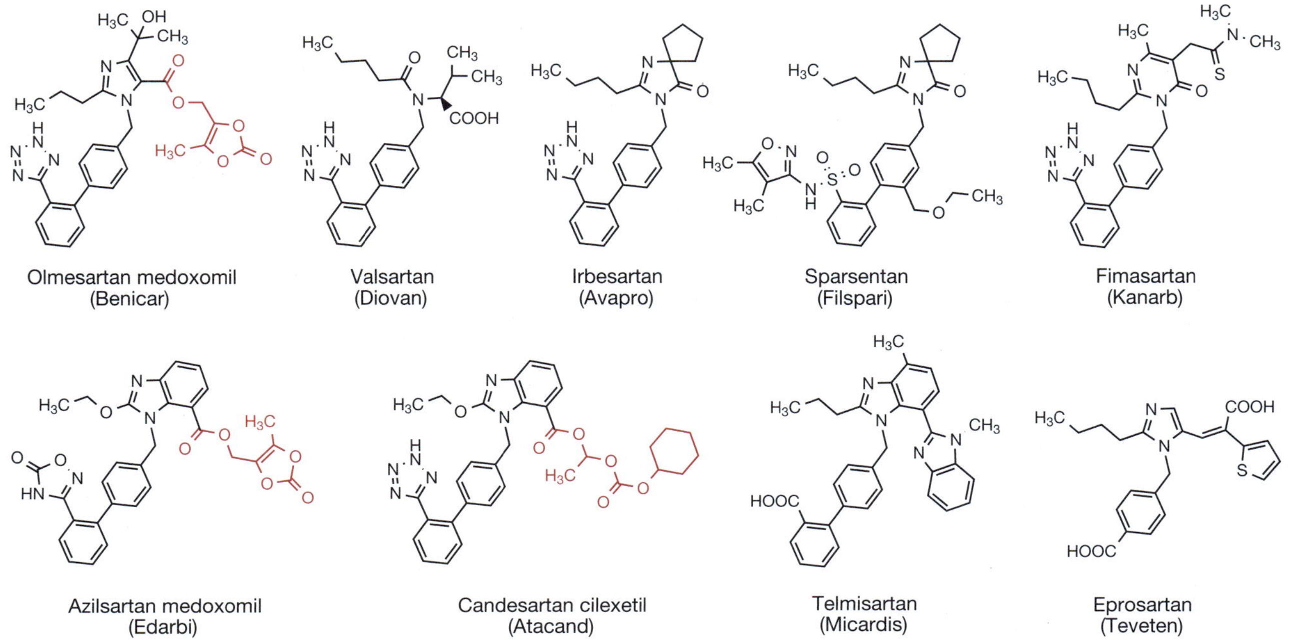

Figure 19.23 Structures of ARBs. The highlighted portions of candesartan cilexetil, olmesartan medoxomil, and azilsartan medoxomil are hydrolyzed via esterases to produce their respective active carboxylate metabolites.

Table 19.11 Pharmacokinetic Parameters of Angiotensin II Receptor Blockers

Drug	Oral Bioavailability (%)	Active Metabolite	Protein Binding (%)	Time to Peak Plasma Concentration (h)	Elimination Half-Life (h)	Major Route(s) of Elimination
Azilsartan Medoxomil	60	Azilsartan	99	1.5-3.0	11	Fecal (55%) Renal (42%)
Candesartan Cilexetil	15	Candesartan	99	3-4	9	Fecal (67%) Renal (33%)
Eprosartan	15	None	98	1-2	5-9	Fecal (90%) Renal (10%)
Fimasartan	19	Desulfo-metabolite	9	0.5-3.0	5-16	Fecal (>90%)
Irbesartan	60-80	None	90	1.5-2.0	11-15	Fecal (80%) Renal (20%)
Losartan	33	EXP-3174	98.7 (losartan)	1 (losartan)	1.5-2.0 (losartan)	Fecal (60%)
			99.8 (EXP-3174)	3-4 (EXP-3174)	6-9 (EXP-3174)	Renal (35%)
Olmesartan Medoxomil	26	Olmesartan	99	1.5-3.0	10-15	Fecal (35%-50%) Renal (50%-65%)
Sparsentan	Dose-dependent	None	>99	2-8	9.6	Fecal (80%; 9% unchanged) Renal (2%)
Telmisartan	42-58	None	100	5	24	Fecal (97%)
Valsartan	25	None	95	2-4	6	Fecal (83%) Renal (13%)

Table 19.12 Dosing Information for Angiotensin II Receptor Blockers

Generic Name	Trade Name(s)	Approved Indications	Dosing Range (Treatment of Hypertension)	Maximum Daily Dose	Initial Dose Reduction With Hepatic Dysfunction	Dose Reduction With Renal Dysfunction	Available Tablet Strengths (mg)
Azilsartan Medoxomil	Edarbi	Hypertension	40-80 mg once daily	80 mg	No	No	40, 80
Candesartan Cilexetil	Atacand	Hypertension, heart failure	8-32 mg once daily	32 mg	No	Only with severe impairment	4, 8, 16, 32
Eprosartan	Teveten	Hypertension	400-800 mg once daily or b.i.d.	900 mg	No	Decrease maximum daily dose to 600 mg	600

Table 19.12 Dosing Information for Angiotensin II Receptor Blockers (*continued*)

Generic Name	Trade Name(s)	Approved Indications	Dosing Range (Treatment of Hypertension)	Maximum Daily Dose	Initial Dose Reduction With Hepatic Dysfunction	Dose Reduction With Renal Dysfunction	Available Tablet Strengths (mg)
Fimasartan	Kanarb	Hypertension and heart failure	60-120 mg	120 mg	The drug is not recommended in moderate to severe hepatic impairment	No dose adjustment required in mild to moderate renal impairment, but <30 mL/min creatinine clearance starting dose is 30 mg	30, 60, 120
Irbesartan	Avapro	Hypertension, nephropathy in type 2 diabetics	150-300 mg once daily	300 mg	No	No	75, 150, 300
Losartan	Cozaar	Hypertension, nephropathy in type 2 diabetics, stroke prevention in hypertensive patients with left ventricular hypertrophy	25-100 mg once daily or b.i.d.	100 mg	Yes (reduce to 25 mg once daily)	Adults, no Children, yes	25, 50, 100
Olmesartan Medoxomil	Benicar	Hypertension	20-40 mg once daily	40 mg	No	No	5, 20, 40
Sparsentan	Filspari	Primary IgA nephropathy	200-400 mg once daily	400	Contraindicated	No	200, 400
Telmisartan	Micardis	Hypertension, cardiovascular risk reduction of MI and stroke	40-80 mg once daily	80 mg	Yes (reduce to 20 mg once daily)	No	20, 40, 80
Valsartan	Diovan	Hypertension, heart failure, post-MI in patients with left ventricular failure or dysfunction	80-320 mg once daily	320 mg	No	No	40, 80, 160, 320

b.i.d., *twice a day;* IgA, *immunoglobulin A;* MI, *myocardial infarction*

Metabolism

Approximately 14% of a dose of losartan is oxidized by the isozymes CYP2C9 and CYP3A4 to produce EXP-3174, a noncompetitive AT_1 receptor antagonist that is 10- to 40-fold more potent than losartan (Fig. 19.24). The overall cardiovascular effects seen with losartan result from the combined actions of the parent drug and the active metabolite. Therefore, losartan is not considered as a prodrug.[47] As previously mentioned, azilsartan medoxomil, candesartan cilexetil, and olmesartan medoxomil are prodrugs that are rapidly and completely hydrolyzed to azilsartan, candesartan, and olmesartan, respectively, in the intestinal wall. These active metabolites have the

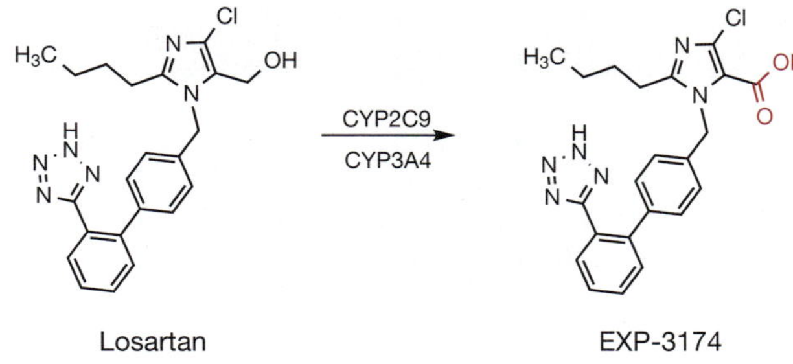

Figure 19.24 Metabolic conversion of losartan to EXP-3174 by cytochrome P450 isozymes.

highest renal elimination within this drug class given the added aqueous solubility attributed to the newly exposed carboxylic group.

Regarding metabolism, approximately 20% of valsartan is metabolized to inactive compounds via mechanisms that do not appear to involve the CYP450 system. The primary circulating metabolites for irbesartan, telmisartan, and eprosartan are inactive glucuronide conjugates. A small amount of irbesartan is oxidized by CYP2C9; however, irbesartan does not substantially induce or inhibit the CYP450 enzymes normally involved in drug metabolism.[47,73,90,92-95] Azilsartan is primarily metabolized by CYP2C9 to an inactive O-dealkylated metabolite. Animal studies also indicated that fimasartan is extensively metabolized to provide de-*N*-dimethyl-fimasartan acid, oxygenated pyrimidinone metabolite, *N*-glucuronide, desulfo-metabolite (active), and hydroxy-*n*-butyl metabolite.[96] Likewise, in vitro studies indicated that sparsentan is a substrate, inhibitor, and inducer of CYP3A, and an inducer of CYP2B6, CYP2C9, and CYP2C19.[97] Given the metabolic and excretion profiles of ARBs, losartan and telmisartan require initial dose reductions in patients with hepatic impairment. Because of significantly increased plasma concentration, patients with impaired hepatic function or biliary obstructive disorders should avoid the use of telmisartan. Fimasartan is not recommended in patients with moderate to severe hepatic impairment; however, no dose adjustment is required in mild to moderate renal impairment. Patients with a creatinine clearance less than 30 mL/min should have their starting dose of fimasartan reduced to 30 mg. Sparsentan appears to be contraindicated in patients with hepatic dysfunction.

In 2019, there was a massive recall of the generic versions of tetrazole-containing ARBs, particularly losartan, valsartan, and irbesartan from the world market. It appears that the generic manufacturer(s) changed the manufacturing process of tetrazole-containing ARBs to use *N,N*-dimethyl-formamide (DMF) as a processing solvent in the making of the tetrazole intermediate. At elevated temperatures, DMF decomposes to carbon monoxide and dimethylamine, which subsequently reacts with another reagent in the synthesis process to form *N*-nitroso-*N*-dimethylamine (NDMA). Nitrosamines such as NDMA are potential carcinogens and mutagens. More recently, more possible contaminants were revealed including nitrosodiethylamine (NDEA), nitrosomethylaminobutyric acid (NMBA) and azidomethyl biphenyl tetrazole (AZBT).[98]

Medicinal Chemistry of Aliskiren

Receptor Binding and Structure-Activity Relationships

Renin is an aspartyl protease that uses two aspartic acid residues to cleave angiotensinogen between the Leu10 and Val11 peptide bond. As shown in Figure 19.25, the structure of aliskiren contains two isopropyl groups that are capable of mimicking the side chains of these two amino acids, while the secondary hydroxyl group is able to mimic the transition state of peptide hydrolysis. An additional interaction can occur between the α,β-aminol moiety and the Asp32 and Asp215 residues. The spacing of the two isopropyl groups is longer than the endogenous substrate; however, it has been proposed that these two groups occupy the S_1 and S_1' sites of the enzyme. Additionally, the ether side chain has been proposed to occupy an S_3 subpocket of the enzyme. The drug's flexible nature has been proposed to enhance binding through hydrogen bonds (oxygen atom) and van der Waals interactions (carbon atoms).[99,100]

Physicochemical Properties

Aliskiren is a basic drug and is marketed as its hemifumarate salt. The calculated log P value for the unionized form of aliskiren is 4.32[86]; however, its salt form is highly water soluble. Aliskiren contains four chiral centers and is marketed as the pure 2S, 4S, 5S, 7S enantiomer.[90]

Pharmacokinetic Properties

Aliskiren is poorly absorbed and has a bioavailability of approximately 2.5%. Following oral administration, peak plasma concentrations are achieved within 1 to 3 hours, and steady-state blood concentration is attained within 7 to 8 days. Its volume of distribution is 135 L, and it moderately binds to plasma protein (47%-51%). The terminal elimination half-life of aliskiren is about 40 hours (range: 34-41 hours). The normal, initial dose of aliskiren is 150 mg once daily. This may be increased to 300 mg once daily in patients whose blood pressure is not adequately controlled. The antihypertensive effects are usually attained within 2 weeks. High-fat meals have been shown to significantly decrease absorption, and patients are encouraged to establish a fixed/routine time to take aliskiren. No adjustment in dose is required for older adults or those with mild renal impairment or hepatic insufficiency. It should be cautiously used in patients with severe renal impairment.[71,83,90]

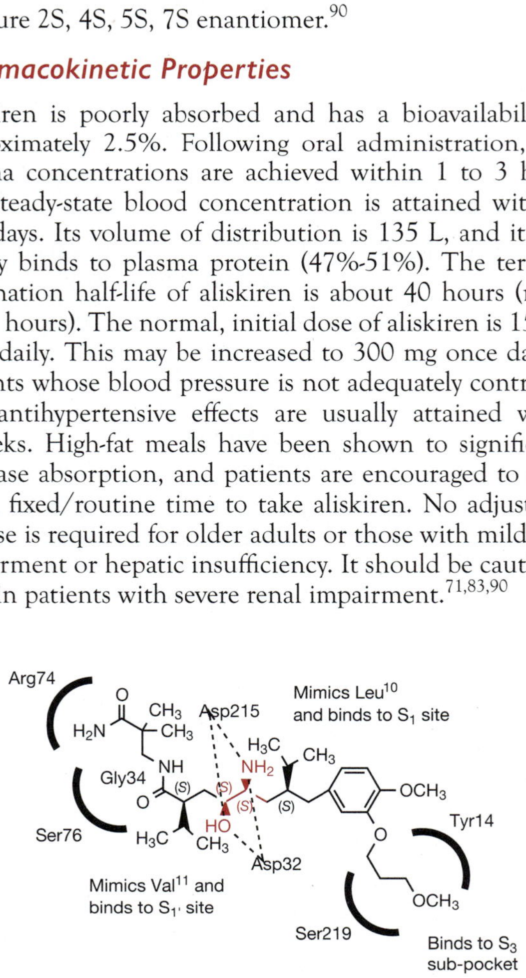

Figure 19.25 Binding interactions of aliskiren with renin.

Metabolism

Approximately 90% of aliskiren is eliminated unchanged in the feces. Given its poor bioavailability, the extent of systemic metabolism is unclear; however, clearance through the hepatobiliary tract appears to be the primary route of elimination. While metabolism is a minor pathway, the two major metabolites of aliskiren are an O-demethylated alcohol derivative and a carboxylic acid derivative. It is unknown how much of the absorbed dose is metabolized. Approximately 25% of the absorbed dose appears in the urine as unchanged drug. In vitro studies indicate that the major enzyme responsible for aliskiren metabolism is CYP3A4. Aliskiren does not inhibit the CYP450 isoenzymes.[71,83,90]

Calcium Channel Blockers

Calcium and Muscles

Calcium ions play a significant role in the regulation of many cellular processes, including neurotransmission and muscle contraction. The role of calcium in these processes is to serve either as a second messenger or as a biochemical regulator to regulate, for example, the functions of enzymes and ion channels. The importance of calcium ions to physiological functions was first realized by Ringer, who observed the role of the calcium ion in cardiac contractility in 1883.[101]

Within the cardiovascular system, calcium ions are key components of the excitation-contraction coupling process. Increased cytosolic calcium concentration results in its binding to a regulatory protein, either calmodulin in vascular smooth muscles or troponin C in cardiac and skeletal muscles. This initial binding of calcium exposes myosin binding sites on the actin molecule, and subsequent interactions between actin and myosin result in muscle contraction. If the cytosolic concentration of calcium drops, all above events retreat. In this situation, calcium binding to calmodulin or troponin C is reduced or removed, myosin binding sites are masked, actin and myosin can no longer interact, and muscle contraction ceases.[102]

Calcium Movement and Storage

Calcium is essentially important as a messenger, linking cellular excitation to cellular response. This role has been made possible by the existence of calcium-specific influx, efflux, and sequestering mechanisms (Fig. 19.26), in addition to the existence of specific, intracellular high affinity calcium-binding proteins (calmodulin and troponin) as well as the significant inwardly directed calcium concentration and electrochemical gradients.[103]

The influx of calcium can occur through the Na^+/Ca^{2+} exchange process (site 1), receptor-operated channels (site 2), potential-dependent channels (site 3), and "leak" pathways (site 4). The Na^+/Ca^{2+} exchange process can promote either influx or efflux because the direction of Ca^{2+} movement depends on the relative intracellular and extracellular ratios of Na^+ and Ca^{2+}. Influx via either receptor-operated or potential-dependent channels has been proposed to be the major entry pathway for Ca^{2+}. In principle, receptor-operated

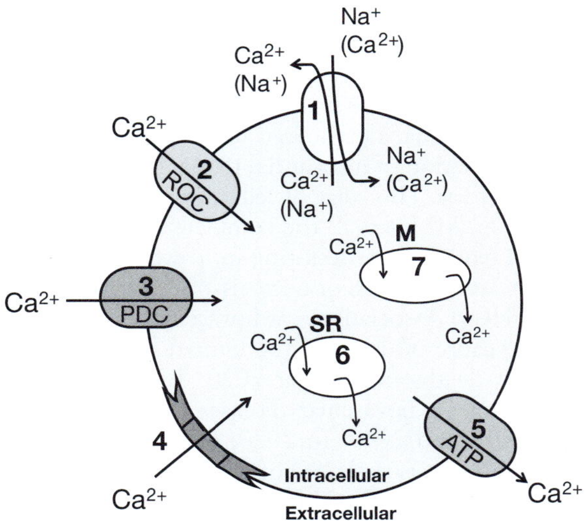

Figure 19.26 Cellular mechanisms for the influx, efflux, and sequestering of Ca^{2+}. *M*, mitochondria; PDC, potential-dependent Ca^{2+} channels; ROC, receptor-operated Ca^{2+} channels; SR, sarcoplasmic reticulum.

channels are associated with cellular membrane receptors and activated by specific agonist-receptor interactions. In contrast, potential-dependent channels, also known as voltage or voltage-gated calcium channels, are channels activated by membrane depolarization. The "leak" pathways, which include unstimulated Ca^{2+} entry as well as entry during the fast inward Na^+ phase of an action potential, play only a minor role in calcium influx.

Efflux can occur through either an ATP-driven membrane pump (site 5) or via the Na^+/Ca^{2+} exchange process (site 1). In addition to these influx and efflux mechanisms, the sarcoplasmic reticulum (site 6) and the mitochondria (site 7) serve as internal storage and release sites. These sites work in harmony with the influx and efflux processes to maintain cytosolic calcium levels adequate for cellular processes. While influx and release processes are essential for excitation-contraction coupling, efflux and sequestering processes are equally important for terminating the contractile process as well as for protecting the cell from the detrimental effects of calcium overload.[103,104]

Potential-Dependent Calcium Channels in Hypertension and Other Cardiovascular Disorders

Given the role of calcium in excitation-contraction coupling process, vascular tone and muscular contraction are primarily determined by the availability of calcium from intracellular or extracellular sources. Potential-dependent calcium channels regulate the influx of calcium, and thus, regulate blood pressure through their effects on vasoconstriction and vasodilation. Inhibition of calcium flow through these channels results in both vasodilation and decreased cellular response to contractile stimuli. Coronary and cerebral arterial vessels are more sensitive to the action of these channels than other arterial beds, which are subsequently more sensitive than venous smooth muscle.[105] Given that Ca^{2+}-channel antagonists relax arterial smooth muscle, they decrease arterial resistance, blood pressure, and cardiac afterload, all of which are very beneficial in treating hypertension.

Ischemic heart disease includes pathologies that result in myocardial ischemia, a pathological reduction in blood supply and oxygenation of myocardial tissue. Its main symptom is angina pectoris. This stage of cell injury is generally reversible. However, MI refers to the complete blockage of blood supply and oxygenation, resulting in irreversible cell injury, which indicates cell death or necrosis.[106,107] According to the American Heart Association, cardiovascular disease remains the leading cause of death in the United States, accounted for 928,741 deaths in the year 2020. Total direct and indirect costs of cardiovascular diseases were $407.3 billion between 2018 and 2019. In 2020, coronary heart disease was the leading cause (41.2%) of deaths attributable to cardiovascular disease in the United States, followed by stroke (17.3%), other cardiovascular diseases (16.8%), high blood pressure (12.9%), heart failure (9.2%), and diseases of the arteries (2.6%).[108]

Myocardial ischemia leads to angina pectoris, a chest pain behind the sternum. Myocardial ischemia occurs because of an imbalance in the myocardial oxygen supply and demand relationship. This imbalance can be attributed to an increase in myocardial oxygen demand, or by a decrease in myocardial oxygen supply, or sometimes by both. Typical angina is felt as a heavy, pressing substernal discomfort, often radiating to the left shoulder, the flexor of the left arm, jaw, or epigastrium. Angina pectoris is common and affects approximately 8 million Americans. Angina pectoris may occur in a stable pattern over many years or may become unstable, increasing in severity or frequency, and even occurring at rest. In typical stable angina (exercise-induced angina), the pathologic reason is a fixed atherosclerotic narrowing of an epicardial coronary artery. In variant angina, focal or diffuse coronary vasospasm episodically reduces coronary flow. In most patients with unstable angina, a local platelet deposition at an atherosclerotic plaque decreases coronary blood flow.[106-108] Given that Ca^{2+}-channel antagonists relax coronary artery smooth muscle, they increase the blood flow and blood oxygen supply, which is beneficial in treating some types of angina pectoris.

Excitation-contraction coupling in the heart is different from that in vascular smooth muscle in that a portion of the inward current is carried by Na^+ through the fast channel. Nevertheless, depolarization depends primarily on the movement of Ca^{2+} through the slow channel in the sinoatrial and atrioventricular (AV) nodes. Attenuation of this Ca^{2+} movement produces a negative inotropic effect and decreased conduction through the AV node. This latter effect is especially useful in treating paroxysmal supraventricular tachycardia (PSVT), an arrhythmia primarily caused by AV nodal reentry and AV reentry.[105-108]

Development of Calcium Channel Blockers

Several CCBs are approved for clinical use. They are structurally diverse and include numerous dihydropyridines (1,4-DHPs represented by nifedipine), the phenylalkylamine verapamil, and the benzothiazepine diltiazem (Fig. 19.27).

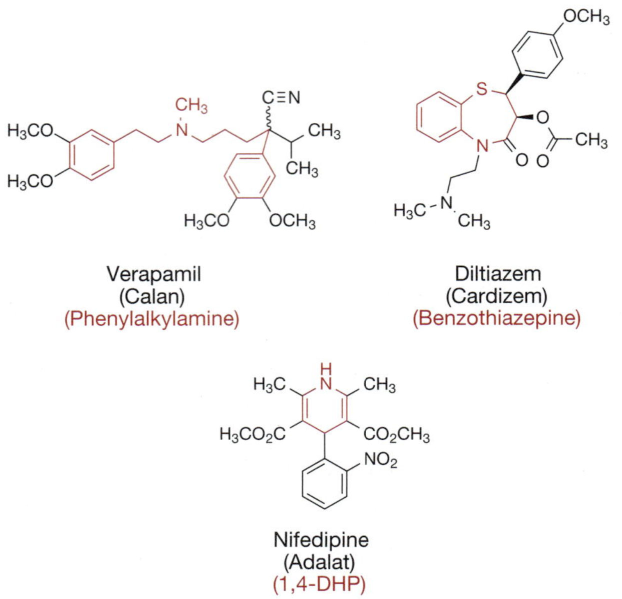

Figure 19.27 Chemical classes of CCBs.

Although these drugs are commonly classified together as CCBs, there are fundamental differences among them with respect to pharmacokinetics, pharmacodynamics, drug interactions, and toxicities.

Identification of drugs that block the inward movement of Ca^{2+} through slow cardiac channels occurred during 1960s. Verapamil and other phenylalkylamines were shown to possess negative inotropic and chronotropic effects that were distinct from other coronary vasodilators. In 1967, Fleckenstein suggested that the negative inotropic effect resulted from the inhibition of excitation-contraction coupling and that the mechanism involved reduced movement of Ca^{2+} into cardiac myocytes. Verapamil was the first clinically available calcium channel blocker. Subsequently, derivatives of verapamil, as well as other chemical classes of drugs (including the benzothiazepine, diltiazem), were shown to competitively block Ca^{2+} movement through the slow channel and, thus, alter the cardiac action potential. Thus, CCBs are also known as slow channel blockers, calcium entry blockers, and calcium antagonists.[103-106]

The development of 1,4-DHPs can be traced back to an 1882 article in which Hantzsch described their utility as intermediates in the synthesis of substituted pyridines. Subsequently, it was discovered that a 1,4-DHP ring was responsible for the "hydrogen-transfer" properties of the coenzyme NADH. Numerous biochemical studies followed this discovery; however, it was not until the early 1970s that the pharmacologic properties of 1,4-DHPs were fully investigated. As shown in Figure 19.28, the Hantzsch multicomponent reaction is composed of ammonia, aldehyde,

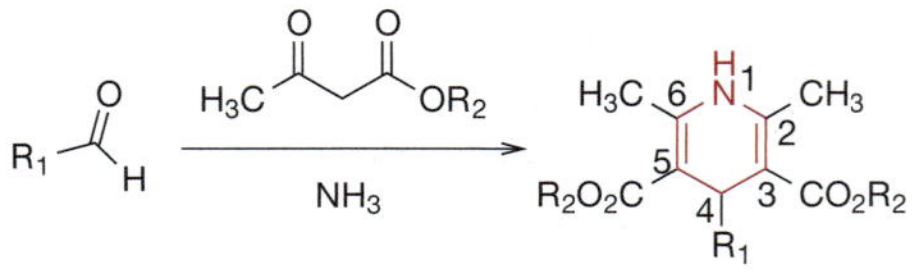

Figure 19.28 Synthesis of 1,4-DHPs using the Hantzsch reaction.

and acetylacetate. It produced a symmetrical compound, in which both the esters (ie, CO_2R_2) and the C_2 and C_6 substituents (ie, CH_3) are identical with each other. Structural requirements necessary for activity were identified by sequentially modifying the C_4 substituent (ie, the R_1 group), the C_3- and C_5-esters (ie, the R_2 groups), the C_2- and C_6-alkyl groups, and the N_1-H substituent. Nifedipine was the first 1,4-DHP to be approved for therapeutic use.[109-113]

Therapeutic Role of Calcium Channel Blockers

The CCBs have been investigated for a wide range of clinical applications. They have been approved for the treatment of hypertension, angina pectoris, subarachnoid hemorrhage, and specific types of arrhythmias. All CCBs cause vasodilation and decrease peripheral resistance. With the exception of nimodipine, which is approved for subarachnoid hemorrhage, all are approved to treat hypertension. According to the 2014 report from the JNC8, CCBs are recommended as the first-line treatment of hypertension in general populations. Because they have a well-documented effect on cardiovascular end points and total mortality, the CCBs are among the preferred drugs for the treatment of hypertension, both as monotherapy and in combination with other antihypertensives. The combination of the ACE inhibitor, perindopril, and the CCB, amlodipine, proved superior to the combination of the β-blocker, atenolol, and the diuretic, hydrochlorothiazide. Amlodipine demonstrated better therapeutic outcomes than hydrochlorothiazide when combined with the ACE inhibitor benazepril. Importantly, CCBs do not have significant effects on the release of renin or cause long-term changes in glucose or lipid metabolism.[90,101,105,109] Studies have indicated that immediate-release formulations of short-acting CCBs, especially nifedipine, can cause an abrupt vasodilation that can result in MI. As a result, only the sustained-release formulations of nifedipine and diltiazem are used in the treatment of essential hypertension.[114] Due to its short duration of action, clevidipine is approved for the parenteral treatments of perioperative hypertension as well as hypertensive urgency or emergency.

Verapamil, diltiazem, nifedipine, amlodipine, and nicardipine are approved for the treatment of angina pectoris. Verapamil is the most versatile agent in that it is indicated for all three types of angina: stable, unstable, and variant. Amlodipine and nifedipine are indicated for both chronic stable and variant angina, whereas diltiazem and nicardipine are indicated only for chronic stable angina. Nimodipine is unique in that it has a greater effect on cerebral arteries than on other arteries. As a result, nimodipine is approved to improve the neurologic deficits caused by spasm following subarachnoid hemorrhage from ruptured congenital intracranial aneurysms. Verapamil and diltiazem are pharmacologically different from the 1,4-DHPs in that they block sinus and AV nodal conduction. As a result, verapamil and diltiazem are parenterally indicated for the management of PSVT, atrial fibrillation, and atrial flutter. Verapamil also can be used orally, either alone (for prophylaxis of repetitive PSVT) or in combination with digoxin (for atrial flutter or atrial fibrillation).

Besides their approved indications, CCBs are used off-label for a number of other conditions (Table 19.13).[90,115]

Table 19.13 Unlabeled Uses of Calcium Channel Blockers

Calcium Channel Blocker	Unlabeled Use
Verapamil	Prophylaxis for cluster headache Coronary arteriosclerosis Electroconvulsive therapy Hypertrophic cardiomyopathy Keloid scar Kidney disease Subarachnoid hemorrhage Supraventricular tachycardia
Diltiazem	Coronary artery bypass graft Disorder related to transplantation Pulmonary hypertension Unstable and variant angina
Nifedipine	Chilblains Diffuse spasm of esophagus Disorder of anus; disorder of rectum Pregnancy and transplantation hypertension Preterm labor; short-term to allow for administration of antenatal steroids Raynaud's phenomenon Renovascular hypertension High-altitude pulmonary edema
Nicardipine	Electroconvulsive therapy Hypertension due to acute stroke Hypotension; induction and maintenance Malignant hypertension Migraine Subarachnoid hemorrhage Variant angina
Amlodipine	Diabetic nephropathy Disorder related to transplantation Left ventricular hypertrophy Pulmonary hypertension Raynaud phenomenon Silent myocardial ischemia Systolic hypertension
Nisoldipine	Renovascular hypertension
Felodipine	Angina pectoris Chronic cyclosporin A nephrotoxicity
Isradipine	Angina pectoris

Unlabeled uses are from Micromedex Solutions. Merative US LP 1973. 2023. Accessed July 2023. https://www.micromedexsolutions.com/home/dispatch; and Lexicomp. UpToDate Lexidrug: evidence-based drug referential content for teams. Wolters Kluwer Health. Accessed June 4, 2023. https://www.wolterskluwer.com/en/solutions/lexicomp.

Pharmacology of Calcium Channel Blockers

Mechanisms of Action

CCBs exert their effects through interaction with potential-dependent channels. Six functional subclasses, or types, of potential-dependent calcium channels have been identified: T, L, N, P, Q, and R, differing in their electrophysiological and pharmacological characteristics. They can be divided into two major groups: low-voltage activated (LVA) channels and high-voltage activated (HVA) channels. Only the T (transient, tiny) channel is designated as LVA channel because it can be rapidly activated and inactivated, with small changes in the cell membrane potential. The T channel is most commonly found in neurons (cells having pacemaker activity) and osteocytes. All other channels require a larger depolarization and are thus designated as HVA channels. The L (long-lasting, large) channel is the site of action for currently available CCBs and, therefore, has been extensively studied. It is located in skeletal, cardiac, and smooth muscle and, thus, is highly important for the cardiovascular system. The N channel is found in neuronal tissue (central and peripheral tissue) and exhibits kinetics and inhibitory sensitivity distinct from both L and T channels. The P channel has been named for its presence in the Purkinje cells, whereas the Q and R (Residual) channels have been characterized by their abilities to bind to certain polypeptide toxins, and they may be involved in neurotransmitter release, dendritic calcium transients, and hormone release.[116-118]

The L channel is a pentameric complex consisting of α_1, α_2, β, γ, and δ polypeptides (Fig. 19.29).[118] The α_1 subunit is a transmembrane-spanning protein, consisting of four domains (I-IV) that functions as the pore-forming subunit. The α_1 subunit also contains binding sites for all currently available CCBs. The other four subunits surround the α_1 portion of the channel and contribute to the overall channel hydrophobicity of the pentamer, which allows it to be embedded in the cell membrane. The α_2 and β subunits appear to be on the extracellular and the intracellular sides, respectively. The α_2, δ, and β subunits also modulate the function of α_1 subunit. Other types of potential-dependent channels are similar to the L channel. They all have a central α_1 subunit; however, molecular cloning studies have revealed that there are at least six α_1 *genes:* α_{1S}, α_{1A}, α_{1B}, α_{1C}, α_{1D}, and α_{1E}. Some differences were noted among the L channels located in different organs and tissues. The L channels of skeletal muscles result from the α_{1S} gene; those in the heart, aorta, lung, and fibroblast result from the α_{1C} gene; and those in endocrine tissue result from the α_{1D} gene. Both α_{1C} and α_{1D} are used for L channels in the brain. Furthermore, differences in α_1 genes and differences among the other subunits are responsible for the variations seen among the other five types of potential-dependent calcium channels.[116,119]

CCBs do not occlude the channel but bind to specific binding sites located within the central α_1 subunit of L-type calcium channels and prevent the influx of calcium into the cell. Three distinct, but allosterically linked, binding sites

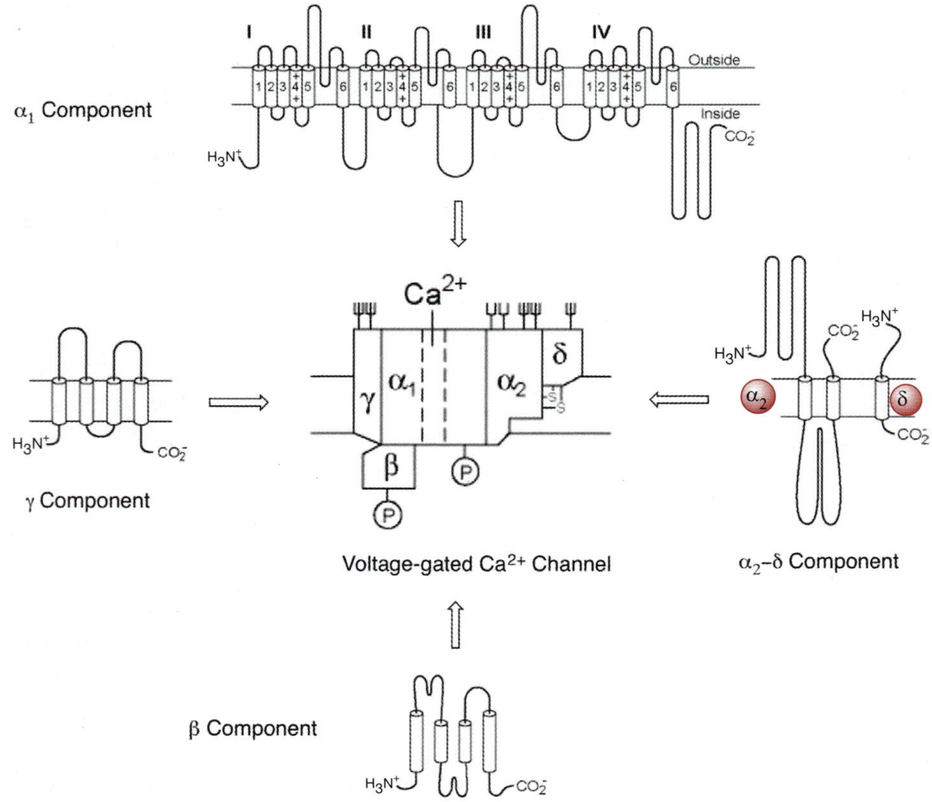

Figure 19.29 Representation of the structure of the voltage-gated Ca^{2+} channel (L channel) composed of several subunits—α_1, α_2-δ, β, γ—organized as depicted in the central area.[161]

Table 19.14 Actions of Calcium Channel Blockers and Interactions Among Their Receptor Sites

Calcium Channel Blocker	Effect on Ca^{2+} Channel	Allosteric Effect on the Binding of		
		Verapamil	*Diltiazem*	*1,4-DHPs*
Verapamil	Antagonist; blocks channel	NA	Inhibits	Inhibits
Diltiazem	Antagonist; blocks channel	Inhibits	NA	Enhances
1,4-DHPs	Antagonist/agonist; can either block or open channel	Inhibits	Enhances	NA

NA, not applicable.

have been identified for verapamil, diltiazem, and the 1,4-DHPs. As shown in Table 19.14, the binding of verapamil to its binding site inhibits the binding of both diltiazem and the 1,4-DHPs to their respective binding sites. Likewise, the binding of either diltiazem or the 1,4-DHPs inhibits the binding of verapamil. In contrast, diltiazem and the 1,4-DHPs mutually enhance the binding of each other.[110]

Potential-dependent calcium channels can exist in one of three conformations: (1) a resting state, which can be stimulated by membrane depolarization; (2) an open state, which allows the Ca^{2+} to enter; and (3) an inactive state, which is refractory to further depolarization. CCBs are shown to be more effective with increasing frequency or intensity and duration of membrane depolarization. This suggests that these drugs preferentially interact with their binding sites when the Ca^{2+} channel is either open or inactivated. This state dependence is not identical for all classes of CCBs and, in combination with the different binding sites, allostery, and solubility, may be responsible for the pharmacological differences among the different classes. A summary of these differences is provided in Table 19.15. Verapamil and diltiazem are vasodilators and cardiodepressants, whereas the 1,4-DHPs are primarily vasodilators. The increased heart rate seen with the 1,4-DHPs results from a baroreceptor reflex mechanism that attempts to overcome the vasodilation and subsequent drop in blood pressure caused by these drugs. In contrast, the compensatory mechanism does not occur to the same extent with verapamil or diltiazem because they block the AV nodal conductance. Ultimately, these pharmacological differences are reflected in their clinical uses.[104,109,110]

Table 19.15 Similarities and Differences Among Verapamil, Diltiazem, and 1,4-DHPs

Cardiovascular Effect	Verapamil and Diltiazem	1,4-DHPs
Peripheral vasodilation	Increase	Increase
Blood pressure	Decrease	Decrease
Heart rate	Decrease or no effect	Increase
Atrioventricular node conduction	Decrease	No effect
Contractility	Decrease	No effect or moderate increase

Common Adverse Effects

The most frequent or significant side effects of CCBs are listed in the box below.[90,101-106,109,115] In most cases, these side effects do not cause long-term complications, and they often resolve with time or dosage adjustments. Many of these effects are extensions of the pharmacological effects of this class of drugs. Excessive vasodilation results in edema, flushing, hypotension, nasal congestion, headache, and dizziness. Subclass-specific side effects also occur and include the palpitations, chest pain, and tachycardia seen with 1,4-DHPs, which are the result of sympathetic responses to the vasodilatory effects of this class. In this case, a β-blocker with a 1,4-DHP can minimize the compensatory effects and can be very useful in treating hypertension. Subclass-specific side effects also include bradycardia and AV block seen with verapamil and diltiazem because of their ability to depress AV nodal conduction. Because of risks associated with additive cardiodepressive effects, they should not be used in combination with β-blockers. Clevidipine is formulated as an oil-in-water emulsion that contains soybean oil, glycerin, and purified egg yolk phospholipids. Therefore, clevidipine in the current formulation is contraindicated in patients with egg hypersensitivity or soya lecithin hypersensitivity. The emulsion used in this formulation can also aggravate preexisting disorders of lipid metabolism.

Common Interactions

Drug interactions for CCBs[90,101-106,109,115] are listed in Table 19.16.

ADVERSE EFFECTS OF CALCIUM CHANNEL BLOCKERS

Edema, flushing, hypotension, nasal congestion, palpitations, chest pain, tachycardia, headache, fatigue, dizziness, rash, nausea, abdominal pain, constipation, diarrhea, vomiting, shortness of breath, weakness, bradycardia, and AV block are side effects of CCBs.

Table 19.16 Drug Interactions for Calcium Channel Blockers

Drug	Calcium Channel Blocker(s)	Result of Interaction
Pharmacokinetic interactions		
Azole antifungals	Felodipine, isradipine, nifedipine, nisoldipine	Increased serum concentrations of the calcium channel blockers
α_1-Blockers (prazosin, terazosin)	Verapamil	Increased prazosin and terazosin levels
Buspirone	Diltiazem, verapamil	Increase buspirone levels
Carbamazepine, oxcarbazepine	Felodipine, diltiazem, verapamil	Carbamazepine and oxcarbazepine decrease felodipine levels; verapamil and diltiazem increase carbamazepine levels
Cimetidine	All	Increased 1,4-DHP levels
Cyclosporine	Felodipine, nicardipine, nifedipine, diltiazem, verapamil	Increased cyclosporine levels when used with all of these except for nifedipine; cyclosporine increases felodipine and nifedipine levels
CYP3A4 inhibitors	All	Potentially can increase the plasma levels of calcium channel blockers
Digoxin	Nifedipine, diltiazem, verapamil	Increased digoxin levels
Dofetilide	Verapamil	Increased dofetilide levels
Doxorubicin	Verapamil	Increased doxorubicin levels
Erythromycin, clarithromycin	All	Increased 1,4-DHP levels and increased toxicity
HMG-CoA reductase inhibitors	Diltiazem, verapamil	Increase levels of HMG-CoA reductase inhibitor
Imipramine	Diltiazem, verapamil	Increased imipramine levels
Lithium	Diltiazem, verapamil	Decreased lithium levels with verapamil; neurotoxicity with diltiazem
Methylprednisolone	Diltiazem, verapamil	Increased methylprednisolone levels
Moricizine	Diltiazem	Increased moricizine levels; decreased diltiazem levels
Phenobarbital	All	Decreased bioavailability of calcium channel blocker
Rifampin	Diltiazem, isradipine, nicardipine, nifedipine, verapamil	Decreased levels of calcium channel blocker
Sirolimus, tacrolimus	Diltiazem, nifedipine, verapamil	Increased sirolimus and tacrolimus levels
Theophylline	Diltiazem, verapamil	Increased theophylline levels and toxicity
Valproic acid	Nimodipine	Increased nimodipine levels
Vecuronium	Verapamil	Increased vecuronium levels
Vincristine	Nifedipine	Increased vincristine levels
St John wort	Nifedipine	Decreased nifedipine levels (St John wort most likely increases the metabolism of all calcium channel blockers)

Table 19.16 Drug Interactions for Calcium Channel Blockers (*continued*)

Drug	Calcium Channel Blocker(s)	Result of Interaction
Pharmacodynamic interactions		
Amiodarone	Diltiazem, verapamil	Increased bradycardia and cardiotoxicity; decreased cardiac output
Aspirin	Verapamil	Increased incidence of bruising
β-Blockers	All	Coadministration may cause additive or synergistic effects; increased cardiodepressant effects (more extensive with verapamil and diltiazem); inhibition of β-blocker metabolism by diltiazem, isradipine, nicardipine, nifedipine, and verapamil
Barbiturates	Felodipine, nifedipine, verapamil	Decreased pharmacologic effects of the calcium channel blockers
Disopyramide, flecainide	Verapamil	Additive cardiodepressant effects
Fentanyl	All	Severe hypotension and/or bradycardia
General anesthetics	All	Potentiation of the cardiac effects and vascular dilation associated with anesthetics
Lovastatin	Isradipine	Decreased effects of lovastatin
Melatonin	All	Decreased therapeutic effects of calcium channel blockers
Midazolam, triazolam	Diltiazem, verapamil	Increased effects of these benzodiazepines
Phenytoin	All	Decreased effectiveness of calcium channel blocker due to induction of metabolism
Quinidine	Diltiazem, nifedipine, nisoldipine, verapamil	Variable responses: quinidine decreases AUC of nisoldipine but increases actions of nifedipine; diltiazem and verapamil increase the effects of quinidine; nifedipine decreases quinidine levels and actions

AUC, area under the curve; 1,4-DHP, 1,4-dihydropyridine; HMG-*CoA*, 3-hydroxy-3-methyl-glutaryl-coenzyme A.

Medicinal Chemistry of Calcium Channel Blockers

Receptor Binding and Structure-Activity Relationships

The specific structures of the 1,4-DHPs are described in Figure 19.30. The following is a concise summary of the most relevant SAR studies.

1. A substituted phenyl ring at the C_4 position optimizes activity. Heteroaromatic rings, such as pyridine, produce similar therapeutic effects but are not used because of observed animal toxicity. C_4 substitution with a small nonplanar alkyl or cycloalkyl group decreases or abolishes the vasodilatory activity.
2. The steric nature and the position of the phenyl substituent at the C_4-position are more important for the vasodilatory activity than its electronic properties. Drugs with *ortho*- or *meta*-substituents possess optimal activity, whereas those that are substituted at the *para*-position or even unsubstituted demonstrate a significantly decreased activity. Although all commercially available 1,4-DHPs have electron-withdrawing *ortho*- and/or *meta*-substituents, drugs with electron-donating groups at these same positions have also demonstrated good activity. The importance of the *ortho*- and *meta*- substituents is to provide sufficient bulk to "lock" the conformation of the 1,4-DHP such that it is perpendicular to the C_4 aromatic ring (Fig. 19.31). This perpendicular conformation has been proposed to be essential for the activity of the 1,4-DHPs.
3. The 1,4-DHP ring is essential for activity. Substitution at the N_1-position or the use of reduced (pyridine) or fully oxidized (piperidine) ring systems greatly decreases or abolishes activity.
4. Ester groups at the C_3 and C_5 positions optimize activity. Other electron-withdrawing groups exhibit

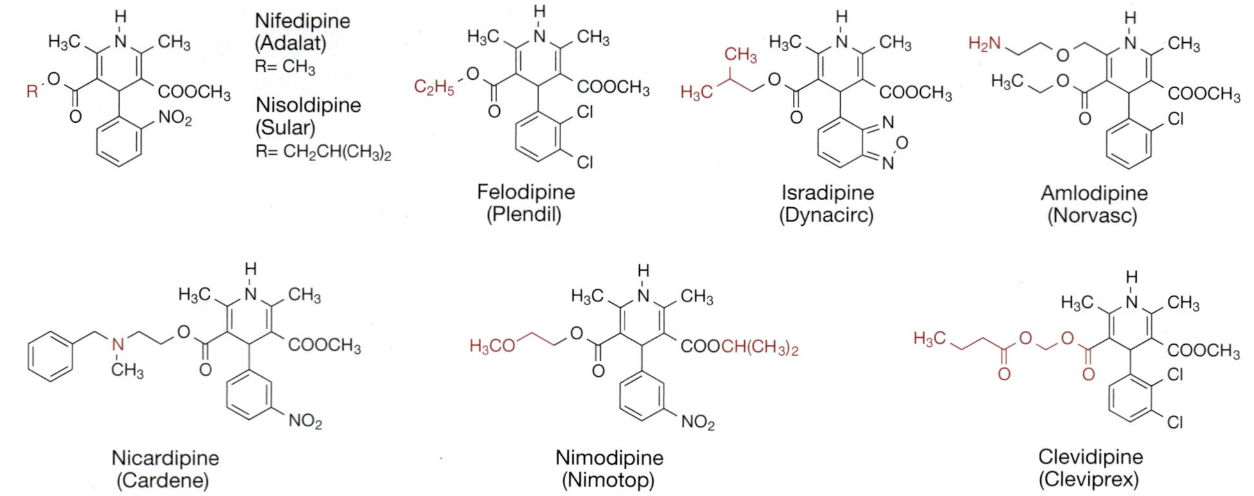

Figure 19.30 Chemical structures of clinically used CCBs. Highlighted in red are functional groups important to distinguish among the depicted drugs.

reduced antagonist activity and may even show agonist activity. For example, the replacement of the C_3 ester of isradipine with a nitro group produces a calcium channel activator or agonist, suggesting the term "calcium channel modulators" to be more appropriate for the classification of the 1,4-DHPs.

5. Stereoselectivity comes into play when the esters at C_3 and C_5 are nonidentical, creating a chiral center at the C_4-position. Evidence suggests that the C_3 and C_5 positions of the DHP ring are not necessarily equivalent. Crystal structures of nifedipine, a symmetrical 1,4-DHP, have shown that the C_3 carbonyl is synperiplanar to the C_2-C_3 bond but that the C_5 carbonyl is antiperiplanar to the C_5-C_6 bond (Fig. 19.32). Asymmetrical drugs have shown enhanced selectivity for specific blood vessels and were preferentially developed. Nifedipine is the first and the only symmetrical 1,4-DHP to be marketed in this chemical class.
6. All 1,4-DHPs, except amlodipine, have methyl groups at C_2 and C_6-positions. The enhanced potency of amlodipine compared with nifedipine potentially indicates that the 1,4-DHP binding site on the L-type potential-dependent calcium channel can accept larger substituents at these positions and that an enhanced activity can be obtained by altering these groups.

In addition to the 1,4-DHPs provided in Figure 19.30, there are a number of others that meet the described SAR and that are used around the world. Some examples are provided in Figure 19.33. Since verapamil and diltiazem are the sole molecules in their chemical classes, their SARs will not be discussed here.

Physicochemical Properties

The chemical structures of verapamil and diltiazem both contain tertiary amines, with pK_a values of 8.9 and 7.7,[86] respectively, which makes them basic in nature. They are generally prepared as hydrochloride salts for administration. However, the 1,4-DHPs are considerably less basic than verapamil and diltiazem. The nitrogen atom of the 1,4-DHP ring is part of a conjugated carbamate. Its electrons are involved in resonance delocalization and are much less available for protonation. Thus, verapamil and diltiazem are primarily ionized at physiological pH, whereas the 1,4-DHPs are primarily unionized, except for amlodipine and nicardipine. The former contains a primary amine, whereas the latter possesses a tertiary amine. The basic amine groups are part of the side chains connected to the 1,4-DHP ring. Although the 1,4-DHP ring of these drugs is unionized, the side-chain amines of amlodipine and nicardipine will be primarily ionized at physiological pH. Due to their basicity,

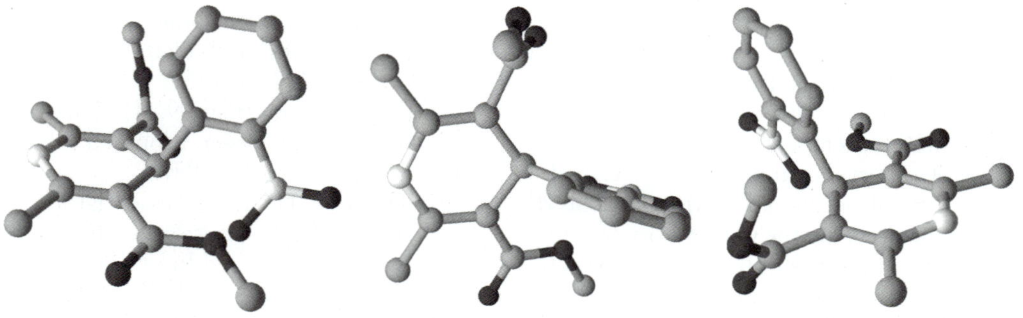

Figure 19.31 Molecular models of nifedipine. The ortho-nitro group of nifedipine provides steric bulk and ensures that the required perpendicular nature of the phenyl and dihydropyridine rings is maintained.[120]

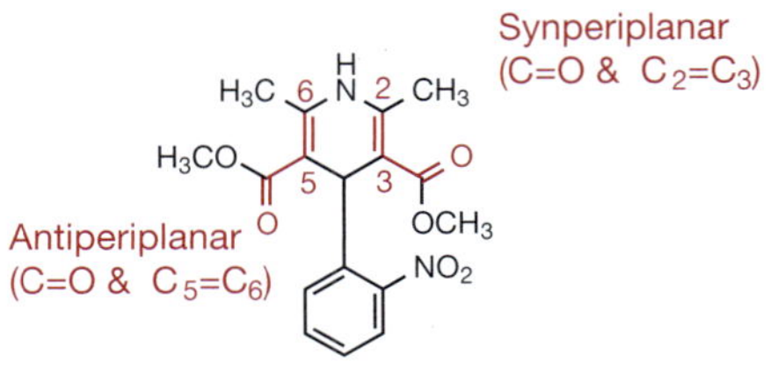

Nifedipine

Figure 19.32 Conformation of the C_3 and C_5 esters of nifedipine. The C_3 carbonyl is synperiplanar to the C_2-C_3 bond, and the C_5 carbonyl is antiperiplanar to the C_5-C_6 bond.

they are pharmaceutically available as besylate and hydrochloride salts, respectively. Because an ionic attraction often is the initial interaction between a drug and its receptor, the differences in basicity between the 1,4-DHP ring and the tertiary amines of verapamil and diltiazem are consistent with the fact that the binding sites for verapamil and diltiazem are distinct from that for the 1,4-DHPs.

The calculated log P values for the CCBs are listed in Table 19.17.[86] As indicated by their calculated log P values (2.4–4.7), all of these drugs possess good lipid solubility and, hence, excellent oral absorption. Within the 1,4-DHP class, enhanced lipid solubility occurs in drugs that contain either larger ester groups or disubstituted phenyl rings. A comparison of the log P values of nifedipine and nisoldipine illustrates this fact. It should be noted that the calculated log P values listed in Table 19.17 are for the unionized forms. These values significantly decrease for the ionized forms of amlodipine, nicardipine, verapamil, and diltiazem such that the latter three agents possess sufficient water solubility to be used both parenterally as well as orally.

All CCBs, with the exception of nifedipine (because of its symmetry), contain at least one chiral center; however, they are all marketed in their racemic mixtures. The *S*-(-)-enantiomers of verapamil and other phenylalkylamines are more potent than the *R*-(+)-enantiomers. Furthermore, very few SAR studies are available for diltiazem; however,

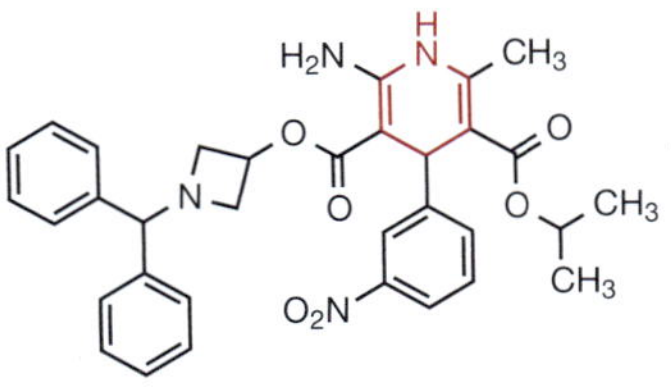

Azelnidipine

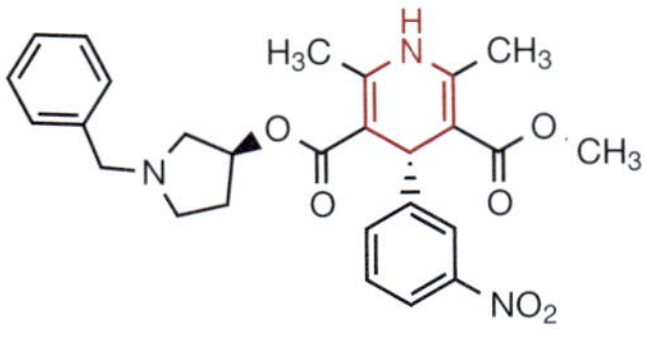

Barnidipine

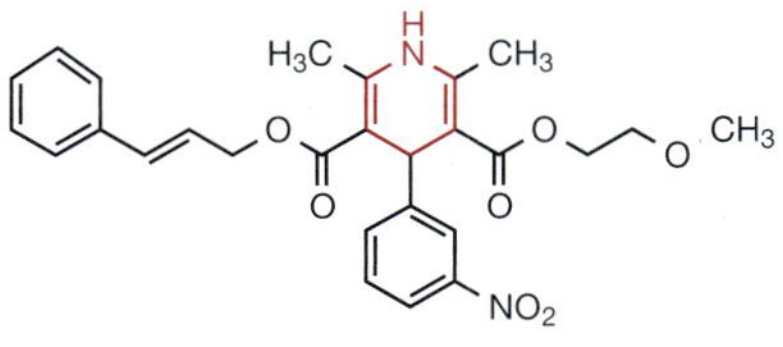

Cilnidipine

Figure 19.33 Chemical structures of other CCBs used worldwide. The chemical structures are consistent with the SAR described in the summary.

the *cis*-arrangement of the acetyl ester and the substituted phenyl ring is required for activity.[110] As previously mentioned, 1,4-DHPs with asymmetrically substituted esters exhibit stereoselectivity between the enantiomers.

Pharmacokinetic Properties

The pharmacokinetic parameters and oral dosing information for CCBs are summarized in Tables 19.17 and 19.18, respectively.[90,115] The primary differences among the drugs are their oral bioavailability, onsets of action, and half-lives. Although all CCBs have excellent oral absorption, their oral bioavailability is considerably variable depending on the extent of first-pass metabolism in the liver. Furthermore, CCBs are highly plasma protein bound and primarily eliminated as inactive metabolites in the urine. Because of extensive hepatic transformation, CCBs should be used cautiously in patients with hepatic disease. Recommendations for these patients include dosage reductions, monitoring, and titrations. Diltiazem and verapamil are both metabolized to active metabolites that are renally eliminated and, hence, they also require dosage adjustments in patients with renal dysfunction because that can significantly increase the concentrations of their active metabolites. Dosage adjustments usually are not required for the 1,4-DHPs because they are metabolized to inactive metabolites, or in the case of nisoldipine to significantly weak active metabolites.

Immediate-release and sustained-release formulations vary from one drug to another and are described in Table 19.18. Unlike immediate-release solid dosage forms, sustained-release formulations cannot be crushed or chewed because this may lead to an immediate release of the medication, producing an overdose and subsequent toxicities in the patient. Clevidipine, nicardipine, verapamil, and diltiazem are also available as parenteral preparations. Nicardipine is incompatible with lactated Ringer solution (an isotonic, crystalloid fluid classified as a balanced or buffered solution used for fluid replacement), and verapamil will precipitate in solutions having a pH greater than or equal to 6. Moreover, parenteral preparations of nicardipine and verapamil are incompatible with IV solutions containing sodium bicarbonate because it increases the pH of the solution, resulting in the precipitation of the CCB. Given its basicity, it is reasonable to assume that a similar interaction may occur for diltiazem.[90,115]

Metabolism

With the exception of clevidipine, all CCBs are substrates for the CYP3A4 isozyme in the liver and undergo extensive first-pass metabolism.[90,115] Several of these drugs can also inhibit CYP3A4, suggesting significant drug-drug interaction profiles. Clevidipine was designed to have an ultra-short duration of action. The "double ester" prodrug design enables an enzyme-mediated hydrolysis of the remote "exposed" ester followed by spontaneous hydrolysis of the resulting internal "hidden" ester. Upon IV infusion, clevidipine exerts its antihypertensive actions within 2 to 4 minutes. Rapid hydrolysis of the double ester moiety (Fig. 19.34) inactivates the drug and allows it to be used in patients with either renal or hepatic dysfunction without any dosage adjustments.

Table 19.17 Pharmacokinetic Parameters of Calcium Channel Blockers

Drug	Calculated Log P	Oral Bioavailability (%)	Effect of Food on Absorption	Active Metabolite	Protein Binding (%)	T_{max} (h)	Elimination Half-Life (h)	Major Route(s) of Elimination
1,4-Dihydropyridines								
Amlodipine	2.76	64-90	None	None	93-97	6-12	35-50	Renal (60%) Fecal (20%-25%)
Clevidipine	2.96	NA	NA	None	>99	2-4 (min)	0.15	Renal (63%-74%) Fecal (7%-22%)
Felodipine	4.69	10-25	Increase	None	>99	2.5-5.0	11-16	Renal (70%) Fecal (10%)
Isradipine	3.19	15-24	Reduced rate, same extent	None	95	7-18 (CR)	8	Renal (60%-65%) Fecal (25%-30%)
Nicardipine	4.27	35	Reduced	None	>95	0.5-2.0 (IR) 1-4 (SR)	2-4	Renal (60%) Fecal (35%)
Nifedipine	2.40	45-70 86 (SR)	None	None	92-98	0.5 (IR) 6 (SR)	2-5 (IR) 7 (SR)	Renal (60%-80%) Biliary/fecal (15%)
Nimodipine	3.14	13	Reduced	None	>95	1	8-9	Renal
Nisoldipine	3.86	5	High-fat meal increases immediate release but lowers overall amount	Hydroxylated analog	>99	6-12	7-12	Renal (70%-75%) Fecal (6%-12%)
Phenylalkylamines								
Verapamil	3.53	20-35	Reduced (SR form only)	Norverapamil	90	1-2 (IR) 7-11 (SR) 0.1-0.2 (IV)	3-7 (IR) 12 (SR)	Renal (70%) Fecal (16%)
Benzothiazepines								
Diltiazem	3.55	40-60	None	Deacetyldilti-azem	70-80	2-4 (IR) 6-14 (SR)	3.0-4.5 (IR) 4.0-9.5 (SR) 3.4 (IV)	Renal (35%) Fecal (60%-65%)

CR, controlled-release product; IR, immediate-release product; IV, intravenous administration; NA, not applicable; SR, sustained-release product; T_{max}, time to maximum blood concentration.

Table 19.18 Oral Dosing Information for Calcium Channel Blockers

Generic Name	Brand Name(s)	Approved Indications	Normal Dosing Range	Maximum Daily Dose	Precautions With Hepatic Dysfunction	Available Tablet or Capsule Strengths (mg)
1,4-Dihydropyridines						
Amlodipine	Norvasc	Angina (V, CS), hypertension	5-10 mg once daily	10 mg	Reduce dosage	2.5, 5, 10
Clevidipine	Cleviprex	Hypertension	4-6 mg/h IV	32 mg/h IV	None	25 mg/50 mL emulsified suspension
Felodipine	Plendil	Hypertension	2.5-10.0 mg once daily	10 mg	Reduce dosage	ER: 2.5, 5, 10
Isradipine	DynaCirc	Hypertension	2.5-10.0 mg b.i.d.	20 mg	Titrate dosage	2.5, 5
Nicardipine	Cardene, Cardene IV	Angina (CS), hypertension	20-40 mg t.i.d. (SR: 30-60 mg b.i.d.) (IV: 5-15 mg/h)	120 mg	Titrate dosage	20, 30 (ER: 30, 45) (IV: 2.5 mg/mL)
Nifedipine	Procardia, Adalat	Angina (V, CS), hypertension	10-20 mg t.i.d. (SR: 30-60 mg once a day)	180 mg (SR: 90 mg)	Reduce dosage	10, 20 (ER: 30, 60, 90)
Nimodipine	Nimotop	Subarachnoid hemorrhage	60 mg every 4 h for 21 d	360 mg	Reduce dosage	30 (30 mg/10 mL oral suspension)
Nisoldipine	Sular	Hypertension	17-34 mg once daily	34 mg	Closely monitor blood pressure	ER: 8.5, 17, 20, 25.5, 30, 34, 40
Phenylalkylamines						
Verapamil	Calan, Isoptin, Verelan	Angina (V, CS, U), hypertension, atrial fibrillation/flutter, PSVT	80-120 mg t.i.d. or q.i.d. (SR: 180-480 mg once daily or b.i.d.)	480 mg	Reduce dosage	40, 80, 120 (SR: 100, 120, 180, 200, 240, 300, 360) (IV: 2.5 mg/mL)
Benzothiazepines						
Diltiazem	Cardizem, Cartia, Dilt-CD, Dilt-XR, Diltzac, Matzim, Taztia, Tiazac	Angina (V, CS), hypertension, atrial fibrillation/flutter, PSVT	30-120 mg t.i.d. or q.i.d. (SR: 120-480 mg once daily)	480 mg (SR: 540 mg)	Reduce dosage	30, 60, 90, 120 (SR: 60, 90,120,180, 240, 300, 360, 420) (IV: 5 mg/mL)

b.i.d., twice a day; CR, controlled release; CS, chronic stable angina; ER, extended release; IV, intravenous; PSVT, paroxysmal supraventricular tachycardia; q.i.d., four times a day; SR, sustained release; t.i.d., three times a day; U, unstable angina; V, vasospastic angina.

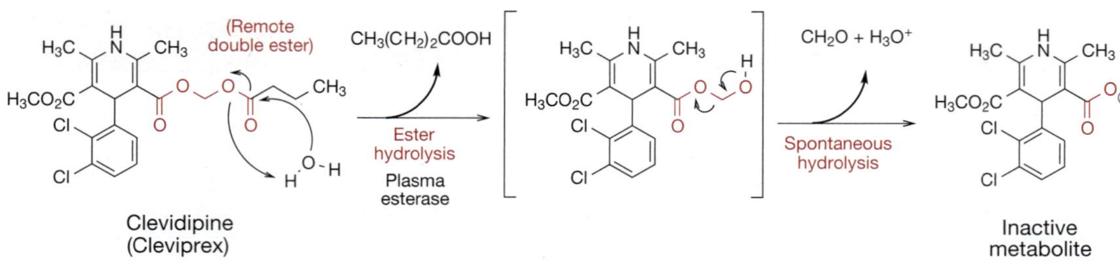

Figure 19.34 In vivo metabolic hydrolysis of clevidipine to an inactive metabolite.

All other 1,4-DHPs are oxidatively metabolized to a variety of inactive compounds. In many cases, the dihydropyridine ring is initially oxidized to an inactive pyridine analog (Fig. 19.35). The lack of activity of the pyridine analog is likely attributed to the loss of the essential perpendicular shape of the parent compound (Fig. 19.36). These initial metabolites are further metabolized by hydrolysis, conjugation, and additional oxidation pathways. Nisoldipine is also subject to these processes; however, it is the only 1,4-DHP that is associated with an active metabolite. Hydroxylation of the isobutyl ester moiety of nisoldipine produces a metabolite that retains 10% of the activity of the parent compound. In addition to the drug-drug interactions listed in Table 19.16, an interesting drug-food interaction occurs with the 1,4-DHPs and grapefruit juice.[121] Coadministration of 1,4-DHPs with grapefruit juice increases the systemic concentration of the 1,4-DHPs. The mechanism of this interaction appears to result from the inhibition of intestinal CYP450 by flavonoids and furanocoumarins specifically found in grapefruit juice. Limiting the daily grapefruit intake to either an 8-oz. glass of juice or half of a grapefruit would likely eliminate the risk of significant drug interactions not only with 1,4-DHPs, but also with most CYP3A4-metabolized drugs.[122]

Verapamil is primarily converted to the corresponding *N*-demethylated metabolite, norverapamil, which retains about 20% of the pharmacologic activity of verapamil and can reach or exceed the steady-state plasma levels of verapamil. Unexpectedly, the more active *S*-(-)-isomer undergoes more extensive first-pass hepatic metabolism than does the less active *R*-(+)-isomer. This is important because when given IV, verapamil prolongs the PR interval of the electrocardiogram to a greater extent than when it is given orally.[123] This is because the parenteral administration limits the metabolism prospect of the more active stereoisomer.

Diltiazem is primarily hydrolyzed to deacetyldiltiazem. This metabolite retains 25% to 50% of the coronary vasodilatory effects of diltiazem and is present in the plasma at levels of 10% to 45% of the parent compound. Both verapamil and diltiazem undergo other less important oxidative O- or N-demethylation, resulting in weakly active or nonactive metabolites (Fig. 19.37).

Central and Peripheral Sympatholytics and Vasodilators

Background

Arterial pressure is the product of cardiac output and peripheral vascular resistance and, therefore, can be lowered by decreasing or inhibiting either or both of these physiologic responses.[105,106,124] This section will discuss antihypertensives that are classified as either sympatholytics (ie, having a central or peripheral mechanism of action) or vasodilators. These classes of drugs are less commonly used today because of the higher incidence of side effects associated with inhibition of the sympathetic nervous system (sympathoinhibition) or vasodilation. In many instances, they have been replaced because of availability of newer and more effective antihypertensive drugs with fewer side effects, such as ACEIs and ARBs.

Overview of Vascular Tone

Before beginning the discussion of the sympatholytics and vasodilators, it is important to review the nature of vascular tone. The term "vascular tone" refers to the degree of constriction experienced by a blood vessel relative to its

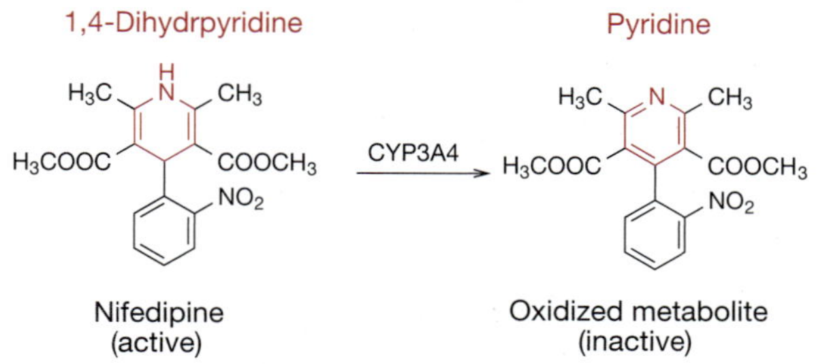

Figure 19.35 Oxidation of the 1,4-dihydropyridine ring of nifedipine.

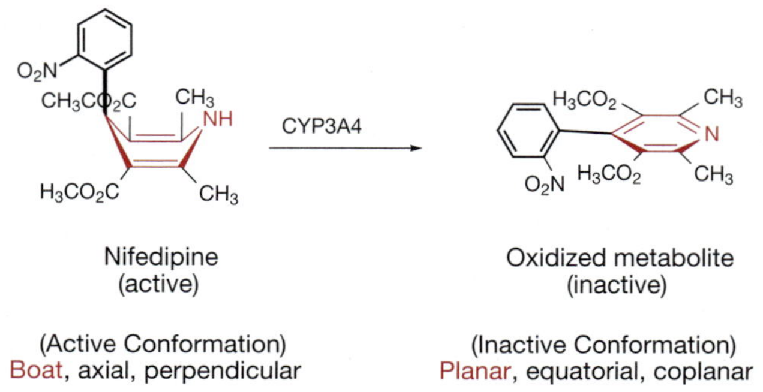

Figure 19.36 Change in conformation upon the oxidation of the dihydropyridine ring of nifedipine.

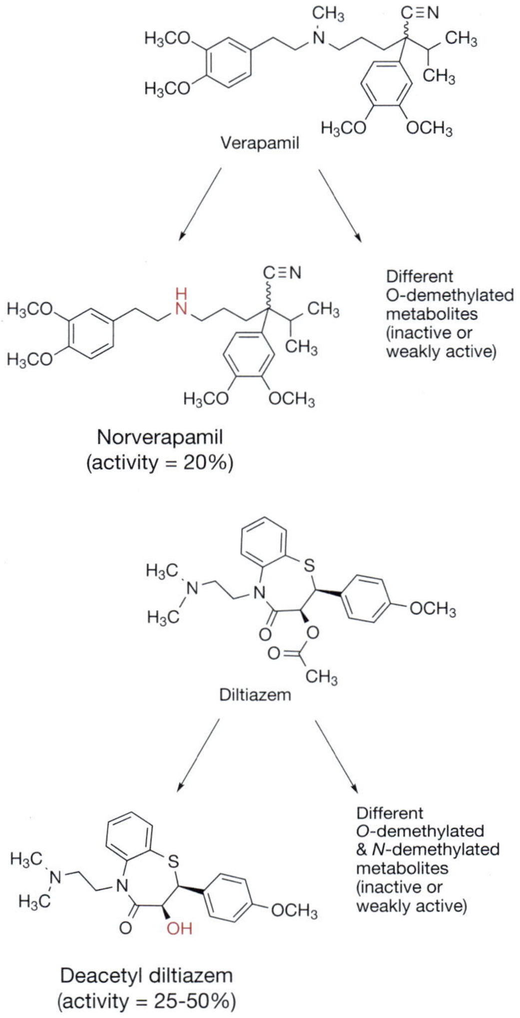

Figure 19.37 Metabolism of verapamil and diltiazem.

maximally dilated state. All resistance (arteries) and capacitance (venous) vessels under basal conditions exhibit some degree of smooth muscle contraction, which determines the diameter and, hence, the tone of the vessel.[124]

Basal vascular tone varies among organs. Those organs having a large vasodilatory capacity (eg, myocardium, skeletal muscle, skin, and splanchnic circulation) have high vascular tone, whereas organs having relatively low vasodilatory capacity (eg, cerebral and renal circulations) have low vascular tone. Vascular tone is determined by many different competing vasoconstrictor and vasodilator influences acting on the blood vessel. Influences such as sympathetic nerves and circulating angiotensin II regulate arterial blood pressure by increasing vascular tone (ie, vasoconstriction). On the other hand, mechanisms for local blood flow regulation within an organ include endothelial factors (eg, nitric oxide [NO] and endothelin [ET]) or local hormones/chemical substances (eg, prostanoids, thromboxanes, histamine, and bradykinin) that can either increase or decrease tone. The mechanisms by which the above influences either constrict or relax blood vessels involve a variety of signal transduction mechanisms that, ultimately, influence the interaction between actin and myosin in the smooth muscle.

Overview of the Regulation of Vascular Smooth Muscle Contraction and Relaxation

The contractile characteristics and the mechanisms that cause contraction of vascular smooth muscle (VSM) are very different from those of cardiac muscle.[124] The VSM undergoes slow, sustained, tonic contractions, whereas cardiac muscle contractions are rapid and of relatively short duration (a few hundred milliseconds). Although VSM contains actin and myosin, it does not have the regulatory protein troponin, as is found in the heart. Furthermore, the arrangement of actin and myosin in VSM is not organized into distinct bands, as it is in cardiac muscle. This is not to imply that the contractile proteins of VSM are disorganized and not well developed. Actually, they are highly organized and well suited for their role in maintaining tonic contractions and reducing lumen diameter.

Contraction of the VSM can be initiated by mechanical, electrical, and chemical stimuli. Passive stretching of VSM can cause contraction that originates from the smooth muscle itself and, therefore, is termed a "myogenic response." Electrical depolarization of the VSM cell membrane also elicits contraction, most likely by opening voltage-dependent calcium channels (L-type calcium channels) and causing an influx (increase) in the intracellular concentration of calcium ion. Finally, a number of chemical stimuli, such as norepinephrine, angiotensin II, vasopressin, endothelin-1, and thromboxane A_2, can cause contraction. Each of these substances binds to specific receptors on the VSM cell (or to receptors on the endothelium adjacent to the VSM), which then leads to VSM contraction. The mechanism of contraction involves different signal transduction pathways, all of which converge to increase intracellular Ca^{2+}.

The mechanism by which an increase in intracellular Ca^{2+} stimulates VSM contraction is illustrated in the left panel of Figure 19.38.

An increase in free intracellular Ca^{2+} results from either increased flux of Ca^{2+} into the VSM cell through calcium channels or by release of Ca^{2+} from intracellular stores of the sarcoplasmic reticulum (SR). The SR is an internal membrane system within the VSM that functions as the major regulator of Ca^{2+} for managing VSM contractility and relaxation. The SR releases Ca^{2+} during contraction, and the released free intracellular Ca^{2+} binds to a special calcium-binding protein called calmodulin (CaM), which in turn activates myosin light-chain kinase (MLCK), an enzyme that phosphorylates the myosin light chains by means of adenosine triphosphate (ATP). Phosphorylation of the myosin light chain leads to actin-myosin cross-bridge formation between the myosin heads and the actin filaments and, hence, VSM contraction. Dephosphorylation of the phosphorylated myosin light chain by myosin light-chain phosphorylase yields myosin light chain, which results in relaxation of the VSM. The concentration of intracellular Ca^{2+} depends on the balance between the Ca^{2+} that enters the VSM cells, the Ca^{2+} released by the SR, and the removal of Ca^{2+} either transported by an ATP-dependent calcium pump back into SR, where the Ca^{2+} is resequestered or removed from the VSM cell to the external environment by an ATP-dependent calcium pump or by the sodium/calcium exchanger.

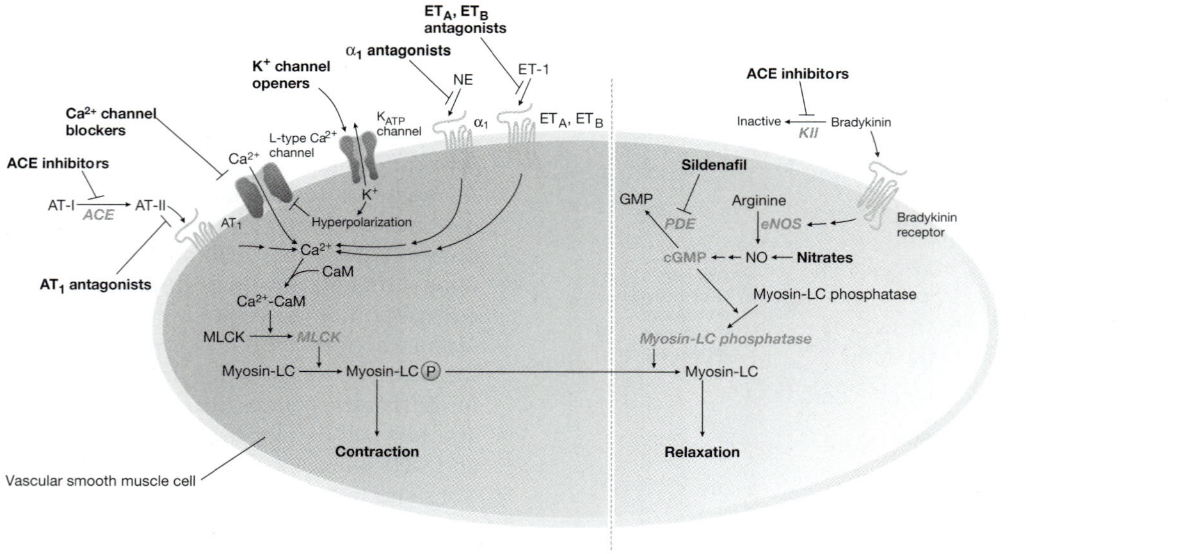

Figure 19.38 Calcium second messenger mechanism of vascular smooth muscle contraction and relaxation and sites of action of the peripheral and centrally acting sympatholytics and vasodilators. ACE, angiotensin-converting enzyme; AT, angiotensin; CaM, calmodulin; ET-1, endothelin peptide; *eNOS*, endothelial nitric oxide synthase; ET$_A$ and ET$_B$, endothelin receptors; KII, kininase II or ACE; MLCK, myosin light-chain kinase; PDE, phosphodiesterase. (From Yeh DC, Michel T. Pharmacology of vascular tone. In: Golan DE, Tashjian A, Armstrong E, et al, eds. *Principles of Pharmacology: The Pathophysiologic Basis of Drug Therapy*. 2nd ed. Wolters Kluwer/Lippincott Williams & Wilkins; 2008:367-385, with permission.)

The activation of the calcium second messenger system by hormones, neurotransmitters, local mediators, and sensory stimuli is very important in regulating VSM contraction. Several signal transduction mechanisms modulate intracellular calcium concentration and, therefore, the state of vascular tone. These calcium second messenger systems are the phosphatidylinositol (PIP$_2$)/G$_q$ protein–coupled pathway, the cyclic adenosine monophosphate (cAMP)/G$_s$ protein–coupled pathway, and the NO/cyclic guanosine monophosphate (cGMP) pathway.

The PIP$_2$ pathway in VSM is similar to that found in the heart (Fig. 19.39). The VSM membrane is lined with specific receptors for norepinephrine (α_1-adrenoceptors), angiotensin II (AT-II), or endothelin-1 (ET-1, which binds one of two receptors ET$_A$ or ET$_B$), that stimulate G$_q$ protein, activating phospholipase C (PLC) and resulting in the formation of inositol triphosphate (IP3) from PIP$_2$ in the membrane. Then, IP$_3$ stimulates the SR to release calcium, which in turn activates the phosphorylation of myosin light chain, causing contraction. The formation of diacylglycerol (DAG) activates protein kinase C (PKC), which also contributes to VSM contraction via protein phosphorylation.

The cAMP/G$_s$ protein–coupled pathway stimulates adenylyl cyclase, which catalyzes the formation of cAMP (Fig. 19.39). In VSM, unlike the heart, an increase in intracellular cAMP concentrations stimulated by a β_2-adrenoceptor agonist, such as epinephrine or isoproterenol, binding to the β-receptor inhibits myosin light-chain phosphorylation, causing VSM relaxation. Therefore, drugs that increase cAMP (eg, β_2-adrenoceptor agonists, PDE3 phosphodiesterase inhibitors) cause vasodilation. On the other hand, stimulation of G$_i$ protein inhibits adenylyl cyclase.

A third mechanism that is also very important in regulating VSM tone is the NO/cGMP pathway (Fig. 19.38, right panel). The formation of NO in the endothelium activates guanylyl cyclase, which causes increased formation of cGMP and vasodilation. The precise mechanisms by which cGMP relaxes VSM is unclear; however, cGMP can activate a cGMP-dependent PKC, inhibit calcium entry into the VSM, activate K$^+$ channels, and decrease IP$_3$.

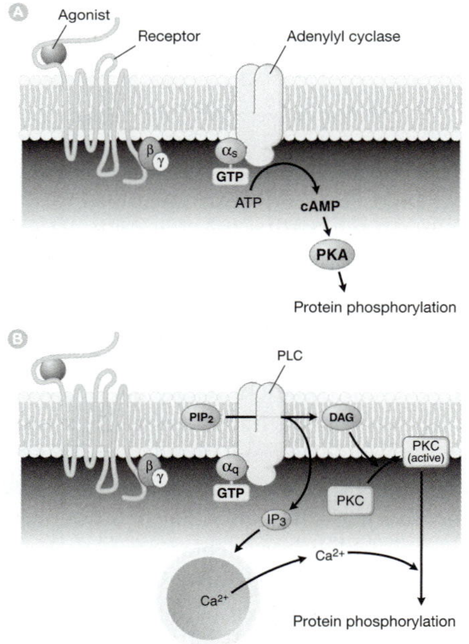

Figure 19.39 Mechanism of activation of the cyclic adenosine monophosphate (cAMP)/G$_s$ protein–coupled pathway and the phospholipase C/phosphatidylinositol (PIP$_2$) pathway in vascular smooth muscle. DAG, diacylglycerol; IP$_3$, inositol triphosphate; PKA, protein kinase A. (From Cairo CW, Simon JB, Golan, DE. Drug-receptor interactions. In: Golan DE, Tashjian A, Armstrong E, et al, eds. *Principles of Pharmacology: The Pathophysiologic Basis of Drug Therapy*. 2nd ed. Wolters Kluwer/Lippincott Williams & Wilkins; 2008:3-18, with permission).

Sympatholytics

Adrenergic Drugs

Adrenergic drugs are a broad class of agents employed in the treatment of disorders of widely varying severity. Adrenergic drugs include popular prescription drugs, such as albuterol for asthma and atenolol for hypertension, as well as many common over-the-counter cold remedies, such as the nasal decongestant pseudoephedrine.

Adrenergic drugs act on effector cells through adrenoceptors that normally are activated by the neurotransmitter norepinephrine (noradrenaline), or they can act on the neurons that release the neurotransmitter. The term "adrenergic" stems from the discovery early in the 20th century that administration of the hormone adrenaline (epinephrine) had specific effects on selected organs and tissues similar to the effects produced by stimulation of the sympathetic (adrenergic) nervous system. For a number of years, adrenaline was thought to be the neurotransmitter in the sympathetic nervous system, but it was also recognized that the effects of administered epinephrine were not quite identical to those of sympathetic stimulation. Finally, in the 1940s, norepinephrine was identified as the true neurotransmitter at the terminus of the sympathetic nervous system.[125,126] Adrenoceptors are widely located in various organs and tissues as well as on neurons of both the peripheral nervous system and central nervous system (CNS).

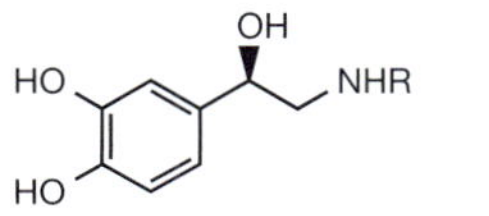

Norepinephrins, R = H
Epinephrine, R = CH_3

Norepinephrine and epinephrine are members of a class of pharmacologically active substances known as catecholamines because they contain within their structures both an amine and an *ortho*-dihydroxybenzene moiety, which is known by the common chemical name of catechol.

Neurons at the terminus of an adrenergic neuron fiber release norepinephrine to influence the target tissue through binding to receptors on cells of the tissue or organ. The cells bearing the receptors are called effector cells because they produce the effect seen by adrenergic stimulation.

Norepinephrine has limited clinical application because of the nonselective nature of its action, which causes both vasoconstriction and cardiac stimulation. In addition, it must be given intravenously because it has no oral activity (poor oral bioavailability) due to its rapid metabolism by intestinal and liver catechol O-methyltransferase (COMT) and monoamine oxidase (MAO), 3′-O-glucuronidation/sulfation in the intestine, and low lipophilicity. Rapid metabolism by MAO and COMT limits its duration of action to only 1 or 2 minutes, even when given by infusion. The drug is used to counteract various hypotensive crises because its α-activity raises blood pressure, and as an adjunct treatment in cardiac arrest, where its β-activity stimulates the heart.

Epinephrine is far more widely used clinically than norepinephrine, although it also lacks oral activity for the same reasons as norepinephrine. Epinephrine, like norepinephrine, is used to treat hypotensive crises and, because of its greater β-activity, to stimulate the heart in cardiac arrest. The β_2-activity of epinephrine leads to its administration intravenously and in inhalers to relieve bronchoconstriction in asthma and to its application in inhibiting uterine contractions. Because it has significant α-activity, epinephrine has been used in nasal decongestants. Constriction of dilated blood vessels in mucous membranes shrinks the membranes and reduces nasal congestion, although significant rebound congestion can limit its utility.

Characterization of Adrenergic Receptor Subtypes

The discovery of subclasses of adrenergic receptors and the ability of relatively small-molecule drugs to stimulate differentially or block these receptors represented a major advance in several areas of pharmacotherapeutics. Adrenergic receptors were subclassified by Ahlquist[127] in 1948 into α- and β-adrenoreceptor classes, according to their responses to different adrenergic receptor agonists, principally norepinephrine, epinephrine, and isoproterenol. These catecholamines can stimulate α-adrenoceptors in the following descending order of potency: epinephrine > norepinephrine > isoproterenol. In contrast, β-adrenoceptors are stimulated in the following descending order of potency: isoproterenol > epinephrine > norepinephrine.

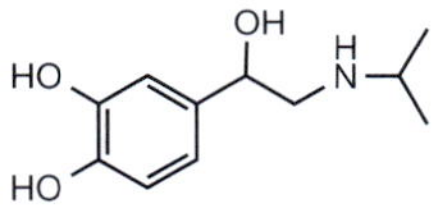

Isoproterenol

In the years since Ahlquist original classification, additional small-molecule agonists and antagonists have been used to allow further subclassification of α- and β-receptors into the α_1 and α_2 subtypes of α-receptors and the β_1, β_2, and β_3 subtypes of β-adrenoceptors. The powerful tools of molecular biology have been used to clone, sequence, and identify even more subtypes of α-receptors for a total of six. Currently, three types of α_1-adrenoceptors, called α_{1A}, α_{1B}, and α_{1D}, are known (there is no α_{1C} because identification of this supposed subtype was found to be incorrect). Three subtypes of α_2, known as α_{2A}, α_{2B}, and α_{2C}, are also known.[128] The data derived from molecular biology provide a wealth of information on the structures and biochemical properties of both α- and β-receptors. Intensive research continues in this area, and the coming years can provide evidence of additional subtypes of both α- and β-receptors. At this time, however, only the α_1-, α_2-, β_1-, and β_2-receptor subtypes are sufficiently well differentiated by their small-molecule binding characteristics to be clinically significant in pharmacotherapeutics, although therapeutic agents acting selectively on β_3-adrenoceptors to induce fat catabolism could become available in the near future.[129]

Therapeutic Relevance of Adrenergic Receptor Subtypes

The clinical utility of receptor-selective drugs becomes obvious when one considers the adrenoreceptor subtypes and effector responses of only a few organs and tissues innervated by the sympathetic nervous system. The major adrenoceptor subtypes are listed in Table 19.19. For example, the predominant response to adrenergic stimulation of smooth muscle of the peripheral vasculature is constriction, causing a rise in blood pressure. Because this response is mediated through α_1-receptors, an α_1-antagonist would be expected to cause relaxation of the blood vessels and a drop in blood pressure with clear implications for treating hypertension. The presence of α_1-adrenoceptors in the prostate gland also leads to the use of α_1-antagonists in treating benign prostatic hyperplasia. The principal therapeutic uses of adrenergic agonists and antagonists are shown in Table 19.20. A smaller number of β_2-receptors on VSM mediate arterial dilation, particularly to skeletal muscle, and a few antihypertensives act through stimulation of these β_2-receptors. Adrenergic stimulation of the lungs causes smooth muscle relaxation and bronchodilation mediated through β_2-receptors. Drugs acting as β_2-agonists are useful for alleviating respiratory distress in persons with asthma or other obstructive pulmonary diseases. Activation of β_2-receptors in the uterus also causes muscle relaxation, and so some β_2-agonists are used to inhibit uterine contractions in premature labor. Adrenergic stimulation of the heart causes an increase in rate and force of contraction, which is mediated primarily by β_1-receptors. Drugs with β_1-blocking activity slow the heart rate and decrease the force of contraction. These drugs have utility in treating hypertension, angina, and certain cardiac arrhythmias.

Table 19.19 Selected Tissue Responses to Stimulation of Adrenoceptor Subtypes

Organ or Tissue	Major Receptor Type	Response
Arterioles, vascular bed	α_1, α_2	Constriction
Skeletal muscle	β_2	Dilation
Eye (radial muscle)	α_1	Contraction (papillary dilation)
Heart	β_1	Increased rate and force
Lungs	β_2	Relaxation (bronchodilation)
Liver	α_1, β_2	Increased gluconeogenesis and glycogenolysis
Fat cells	α_1, β_3	Lipolysis
Uterus (pregnant)	α_1	Contraction
	β_2	Relaxation
Intestine	α_1, β_2	Decreased motility

Table 19.20 Principal Therapeutic Uses of Adrenergic Agonists and Antagonists

Adrenoceptor	Drug Action	Therapeutic Uses
α_1	Agonists	Shock, hypotension (to raise blood pressure)
		Nasal decongestants
	Antagonists	Antihypertensives
		Benign prostatic hyperplasia
α_2	Agonists	Antihypertensives
		Glaucoma
		Analgesia
		Sedatives
β_1	Antagonists	Antihypertensives
		Antiarrhythmics
β_2	Agonists	Bronchodilators (asthma and chronic obstructive pulmonary disease)
		Glaucoma
β_3	Agonists	Weight loss (investigational drugs)

Peripherally Acting Sympatholytics

β-Adrenergic Receptor Blockers

Therapeutic Overview of β-Adrenergic Receptor Blockers. β-Blockers (BBs) decrease arterial blood pressure by reducing cardiac output.[6,124,130] Many forms of hypertension are associated with an increase in blood volume and cardiac output. Therefore, reducing cardiac output by β-blockade can be an effective treatment for hypertension, especially when used in conjunction with a diuretic. Hypertension in some patients is caused by emotional stress, which causes enhanced sympathetic activity. BBs are very effective in these patients and are especially useful in treating hypertension caused by a pheochromocytoma, which results in elevated circulating catecholamines. BBs have an additional benefit as a treatment for hypertension in that they inhibit the release of renin by the kidneys (the release of which is partly regulated by β_1-adrenoceptors in the kidney). Decreasing circulating plasma renin leads to a decrease in angiotensin II and aldosterone, which enhances renal loss of sodium and water and further diminishes arterial pressure. Acute treatment with a BB is not very effective in reducing arterial pressure because of a compensatory increase in systemic vascular resistance. This can occur because of the baroreceptor reflexes working in conjunction with the removal of β_2 vasodilatory influences that normally offset, to a small degree, α-adrenergic–mediated vascular tone. Chronic treatment with a BB lowers arterial pressure more than acute treatment possibly because of reduced renin release and effects of β-blockade on central and peripheral nervous systems.

Several of the nonselective BBs are also used to reduce intraocular pressure in the treatment of glaucoma. These include carteolol, levobunolol, and timolol.

The selection of oral BBs as monotherapy for stage 1 or 2 hypertension without compelling risk factors (see Table 19.2) is based on several factors, including their cardioselectivity and preexisting conditions, ISA, lipophilicity, metabolism, and adverse effects (exception is esmolol) (Table 19.21). Esmolol is a very short-acting cardioselective β_1-blocker administered by infusion because of its rapid hydrolysis by plasma esterases to a rapidly excreted zwitterionic metabolite (plasma half-life, 9 minutes). After the discontinuation of esmolol infusion, blood pressure returns to preexisting conditions in approximately 30 minutes. The older adult with hypertension (age, ≥65 years) cannot tolerate or respond to these drugs because of their mechanism of lowering cardiac output and increasing systemic vascular resistance.[131]

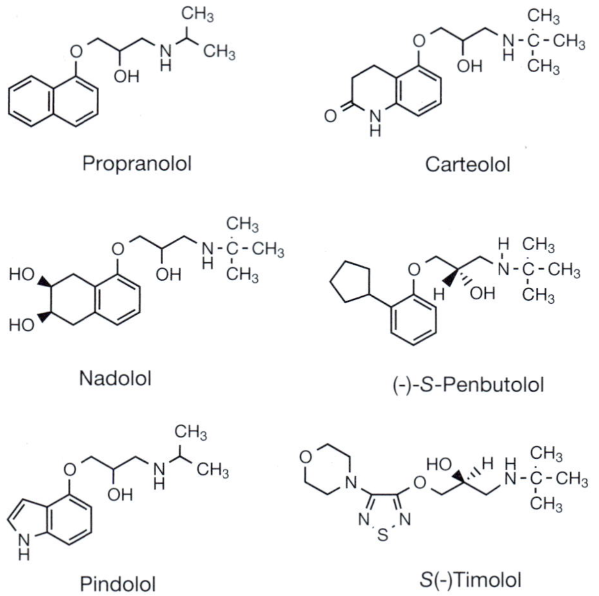

Figure 19.40 Nonselective β-adrenergic blockers.

Pharmacology Overview of β-Adrenergic Receptor Blockers

Mechanism of Action. The VSMs are lined with β_2-adrenoceptors that normally are activated by norepinephrine released from sympathetic adrenergic nerves or by circulating epinephrine. These receptors, like those in the heart, are coupled to a G_s protein, which stimulates the formation of cAMP. Although increased cAMP enhances cardiac contraction, with VSM an increase in cAMP leads to smooth muscle relaxation (Fig. 19.39). Therefore, increases in intracellular cAMP caused by β_2-agonists inhibit MLCK, thereby producing less contractile force (ie, promoting relaxation). Inhibition of cardiac β_1- and β_2-adrenoceptors reduces the contractility of the myocardium (negative inotropic), decreasing heart rate (negative chronotropic), blocking sympathetic outflow from the central nervous system (CNS), and suppressing renin release.[105,106]

BBs are drugs that bind to β-adrenoceptors and, thereby, block the binding of norepinephrine and epinephrine to these receptors, causing inhibition of normal sympathetic effects. Therefore, BBs are sympatholytic drugs. Some BBs, when they bind to the β-adrenoceptor, partially activate the receptor while preventing norepinephrine from binding to the receptor. These partial agonists therefore provide some "background" of sympathetic activity while preventing normal and enhanced sympathetic activity. These particular BBs (partial agonists) are said to possess intrinsic sympathomimetic activity (ISA). Some BBs also possess what is referred to as membrane-stabilizing activity. This effect is similar to the membrane-stabilizing activity of sodium channel blockers that represent class I antiarrhythmics.

The first generation of BBs were nonselective, meaning that they blocked both β_1- and β_2-adrenoceptors (Fig. 19.40). Second-generation BBs are more cardioselective because they are relatively selective for β_1-adrenoceptors (Fig. 19.41). Note that this relative selectivity can be lost at higher drug doses. Finally, the third-generation BBs are drugs that also possess vasodilator actions through blockade of vascular α-adrenoceptors (mixed α_1-/β_1-adrenergic blockers) (see Fig. 19.42). Their structure-activity relationship, pharmacokinetics, and metabolism are presented in Table 19.21. In addition to uncomplicated hypertension, they can also be used as monotherapy in the treatment of angina, arrhythmias, mitral valve prolapse, myocardial infarction, migraine headaches, performance anxiety, excessive sympathetic tone, or "thyroid storm" in hyperthyroidism.[6]

Common Adverse Effects. Common adverse effects for the BBs include decreased exercise tolerance, cold extremities, depression, sleep disturbance, and impotence, although these side effects can be less severe with the β_1-selective blockers, such as metoprolol, atenolol, or bisoprolol.[132] The use of lipid-soluble BBs, such as propranolol (Table 19.21), has been associated with more CNS side effects, such as dizziness, confusion, or depression.[6,124] These side effects can be avoided, however, with the use of hydrophilic drugs, such as nadolol or atenolol. The use of β_1-selective drugs also helps minimize adverse effects associated with β_2-blockade, including suppression of insulin release and increasing the chances for bronchospasms (asthma).[6,124] It is important to emphasize that none of the BBs, including the cardioselective ones, are cardiospecific. At high doses, these cardioselective BBs can still adversely affect asthma, peripheral vascular disease, and diabetes.[6,124] Nonselective BB are contraindicated in patients with bronchospastic disease (asthma), and β_1-selective blockers should be used with caution in these patients. BBs with ISA, such as acebutolol, pindolol, carteolol, or penbutolol (Table 19.21), partially stimulate the β-receptor while also blocking it.[133] The proposed advantages of BBs with ISA over those without ISA include less cardiodepression and resting bradycardia as well as neutral effects on lipid and glucose metabolism. Neither cardioselectivity nor ISA, however, influences the efficacy of BBs in lowering blood pressure.[6]

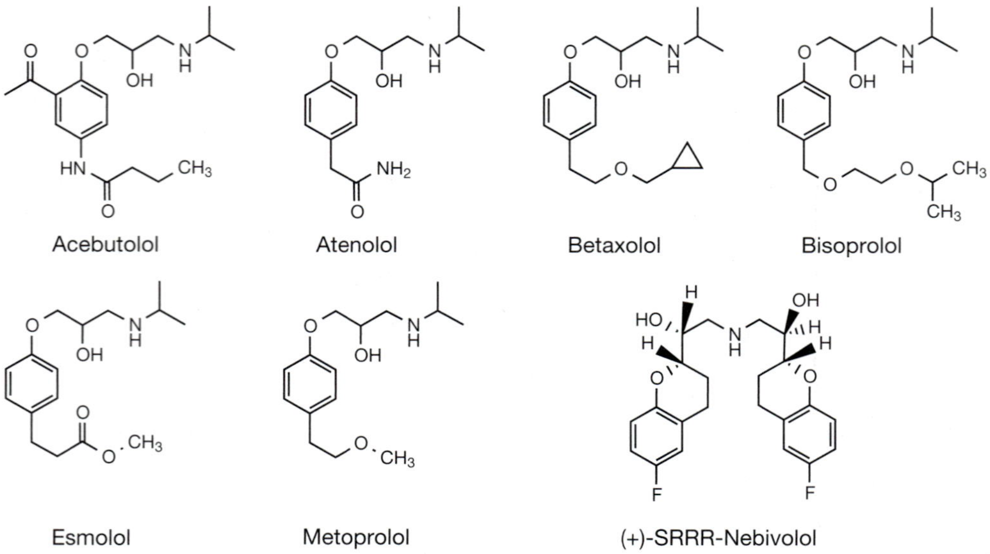

Figure 19.41 β_1-Selective–adrenergic blockers.

Common Interactions. Table 19.22 summarizes common drug-drug interactions for the β-adrenergic receptor blockers.

Medicinal Chemistry of β-Adrenergic Receptor Blockers

Receptor Binding, Structure-Activity Relationships, and Physicochemical Properties. In the 1950s, dichloroisoproterenol, a derivative of isoproterenol in which the catechol hydroxyl groups had been replaced by chlorine atoms, was discovered to be a β-antagonist that blocked the effects of sympathomimetic amines on bronchodilation, uterine relaxation, and heart stimulation.[134] Although dichloroisoproterenol had no clinical utility, replacement of the 3,4-dichloro substituents with a carbon bridge to form a naphthylethanolamine derivative did afford a clinical candidate, pronethalol, which was introduced in 1962 only to be withdrawn in 1963 because of tumor induction in animal tests.

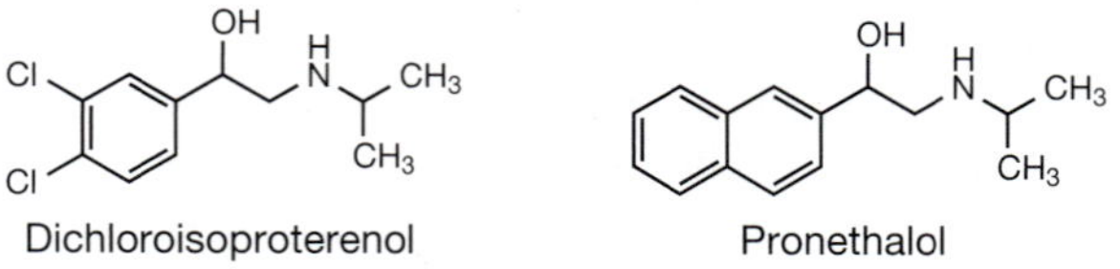

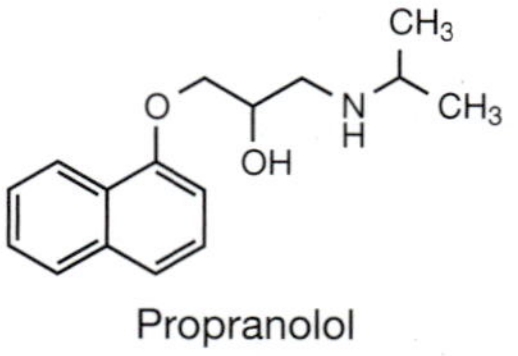

Shortly thereafter, a major innovation in drug development for the β-adrenergic antagonists was introduced when it was discovered that an oxymethylene bridge, OCH_2, could be inserted into the arylethanolamine structure of pronethalol to afford propranolol, an aryloxypropanolamine and the first clinically successful β-blocker. Note that along with the introduction of the oxymethylene bridge, the side chain was moved from C_2 of the naphthyl group to the C_1 position. In general, the aryloxypropanolamines are more potent β-blockers than the corresponding arylethanolamines, and most of the β-blockers currently being used clinically are aryloxypropanolamines. β-Blockers have found wide use in treating hypertension and certain types of glaucoma.

Initially, it might appear that lengthening the side chain would prevent appropriate binding of the required functional groups to the same receptor site. Molecular models, however, show that the side chains of aryloxypropanolamines can adopt a conformation that places the hydroxyl and amine groups into approximately the same position in space (Fig. 19.43). Although the simple two-dimensional drawing in Figure 19.43 exaggerates the true degree of overlap, elaborate molecular modeling studies confirm that the aryloxypropanolamine side chain can adopt a low-energy conformation that permits close overlap with the arylethanolamine side chain.[135]

A factor that sometimes causes confusion when comparing the structures of arylethanolamines with aryloxypropanolamines is the stereochemical nomenclature of the side-chain carbon bearing the hydroxyl group. For maximum effectiveness in receptor binding, the hydroxy group

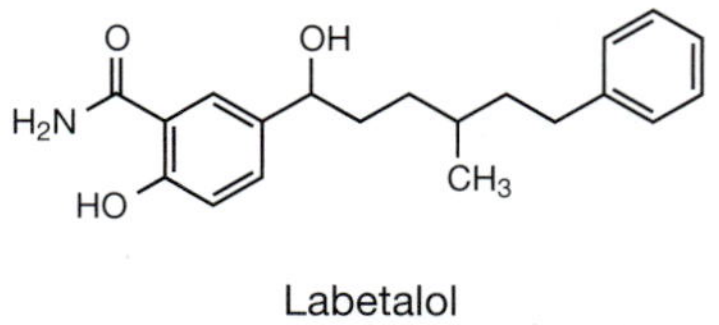

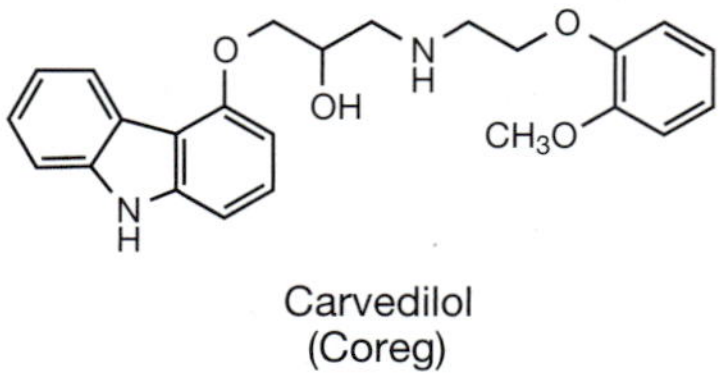

Figure 19.42 Mixed α-/β-selective–adrenergic blockers.

Table 19.21 Pharmacologic/Pharmacokinetic Properties of Antihypertensive β-Adrenergic Blocking Agents

Drug	Adrenergic Receptor Blocking Activity	Membrane-Stabilizing Activity	Intrinsic Sympathomimetic Activity	Lipophilicity[a] (cLog D at pH 7.4)	Extent of Absorption (%)	Absolute Oral Bioavailability (%)	Half-Life (h)	Protein Binding (%)	Metabolism/Excretion
Acebutolol (Sectral)	β_1[b]	+	+	−0.38	90	20-60	3-4	26	Hepatic; renal excretion 30%-40%, nonrenal excretion 50%-60% (bile)
Atenolol (Tenormin)	β_1[b]	0	0	−1.85	50	50-60	6-9	5-16	~50% excreted unchanged in feces
Betaxolol (Kerlone)	β_1[b]	0	0	0.76	~100	89	14-22	50	Hepatic; >80% recovered in urine, 15% unchanged
Bisoprolol (Zebeta)	β_1[b]	0	0	0.12	≥0	80	9-12	30	~50% excreted unchanged in urine, remainder as inactive metabolites; <2% excreted in feces
Esmolol (Brevibloc)	β_1[b]	0	0	−0.08	NA	NA	0.15	55	Rapid metabolism by esterases in cytosol of red blood cells
Metoprolol (Lopressor)	β_1[b]	0[c]	0	−0.25	95	40-50	3-7	12	Hepatic; renal excretion, <5% unchanged
Metoprolol, LA			—	—	77	—			
Nebivolol (Bystolic)	β_1[b]	0	0	2.36	NA	12-fast metabolizers 96-poor metabolizers	12-19	98	Hepatic; glucuronidation, N-dealkylation and oxidation by CYP2D6 Renal: 38%-67%; <1% renal unchanged; fecal 13%-44%
Carteolol (Cartrol, Ocupress)	β_1 β_2	0	++	−0.24	80	85	6	23-30	50%-70% excreted unchanged in urine
Levobunolol (Betagan)	β_1 β_2	0	0	0.50	NA	NA	NA	NA	Ophthalmic

(continued)

Table 19.21 Pharmacologic/Pharmacokinetic Properties of Antihypertensive β-Adrenergic Blocking Agents (*continued*)

Drug	Adrenergic Receptor Blocking Activity	Membrane-Stabilizing Activity	Intrinsic Sympathomimetic Activity	Lipophilicity[a] (cLog D at pH 7.4)	Extent of Absorption (%)	Absolute Oral Bioavailability (%)	Half-Life (h)	Protein Binding (%)	Metabolism/Excretion
Nadolol (Corgard)	β_1 β_2	0	0	−0.86	30	30-50	20-24	30	Urine, unchanged
Penbutolol (Levatol)	β_1 β_2	0	+	1.80	~100	>90	5	80-98	Hepatic (conjugation, oxidation); renal excretion of metabolites (17% as conjugate)
Pindolol (Visken)	β_1 β_2	+	+++	−0.32	95	>90	3-4[d]	40	Urinary excretion of metabolites (60%-65%) and unchanged drug (35%-40%)
Propranolol (Inderal)	β_1 β_2	++	0	1.15	90	30	3-5	90	Hepatic; <1% excreted unchanged in urine
Propranolol, LA						9-18	8-11		
Timolol (Blocadren, Timoptic)	β_1 β_2	0	0	−0.35	90	75	4	10	Hepatic; urinary excretion of metabolites and unchanged drug
Labetalol[e] (Normodyne)	β_1 β_2 α_1	0	0	0.85	100	30-40	5.5-8.0	50	55%-60% excreted in urine as conjugates or unchanged drug
Carvedilol (Coreg)	β_1 β_2 α_1	0	0	3.04	>90	25-35	7-10	98	

NA, not applicable (available as intravenous only); 0, none; +, low; ++, moderate; +++, high.
[a]Calculated c Log D values at pH 7.4 from Appendix A.
[b]Inhibits β_2-receptors (bronchial and vascular) at higher doses.
[c]Detectable only at doses much greater than required for β-blockade.
[d]In older adults with hypertension with normal renal function; half-life variable, 7 to 15 hour.
[e]Not labetalol monograph.
Data from *Drug Facts and Comparisons* (2024), Wolters Kluwer Health (available at: www.wolterskluwer.com/en/solutions/uptodate/enterprise/lexidrug-facts-and-comparisons).

Table 19.22 Common Drug Interactions for Adrenergic Drugs

Drug Class	Interactions
β-Adrenergic receptor blockers	Other antihypertensive agents may produce additive effects Nonsteroidal anti-inflammatory drugs (NSAIDs) may reduce antihypertensive activity Use with some cardiovascular agents may adversely impact atrioventricular (AV) or sinoatrial (SA) node conduction Activity of metoprolol and other β-blockers that are metabolized by CYP2D6 may be altered by inhibitors of this isozyme
α-/β-Adrenergic receptor blockers	Other antihypertensive agents may produce additive effects Activity of carvedilol and other α-/β-blockers that are metabolized by CYP2D6 may be altered by inhibitors of this isozyme
α_1-Adrenergic receptor blockers	Other antihypertensive agents may produce additive effects Displacement of prazosin from plasma proteins by other drugs is possible
α_2-Adrenergic receptor agonists	Other antihypertensive agents may produce additive effects Levodopa may enhance the antihypertensive activity of methyldopa Oral iron (ferrous salts) may reduce absorption of methyldopa from the gastrointestinal tract Tricyclic antidepressants may antagonize antihypertensive activity of clonidine Metabolism of guanfacine may be increased by microsomal enzyme inducers
α_1-Adrenergic receptor agonists	Possible increase in activity when phenylephrine is used with monoamine oxidase (MAO) inhibitors
Vasodilators	Other antihypertensive agents may produce additive effects Diazoxide may displace other drugs that are highly bound to plasma proteins

Data from *AHFS Drug Information* (2018), American Society of Health-System Pharmacists (available at: www.tetondata.com/titles#|q=ahfs).

must occupy the same region in space as it does for the phenylethanolamine agonists in the *R* absolute configuration. Because of the insertion of an oxygen atom in the side chain of the aryloxypropanolamines, the Cahn-Ingold-Prelog priority of the substituents around the asymmetric carbon changes, and the isomer with the required special arrangement now has the *S* absolute configuration. This is an effect of the nomenclature rules; the groups still have the same spatial arrangements (Fig. 19.44).

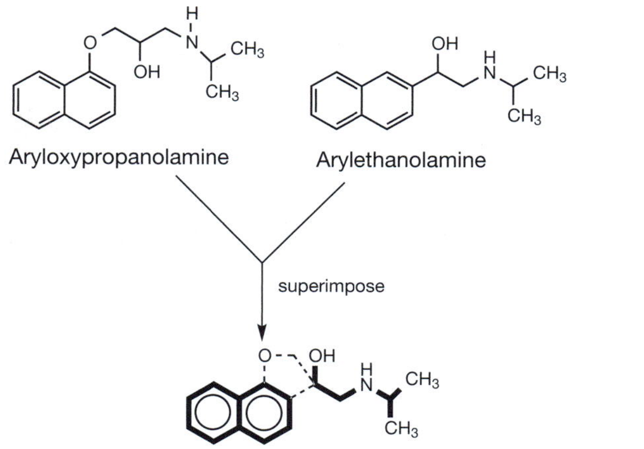

Figure 19.43 Overlap of aryloxypropanolamines and arylethanolamines. The structures of prototype β-antagonists propranolol and pronethalol can be superimposed, so the critical functional groups occupy the same approximate regions in space, as indicated by the bold lines in the superimposed drawings. The dotted lines are those parts that do not overlap but are not necessary to receptor binding.

Unlike the conventional cardioselective β_1-receptor blockers, nebivolol, a third-generation BB, also exhibits an NO-potentiating vasodilatory effect for the treatment of hypertension. Although nebivolol has four chiral centers with 16 possible stereoisomers, only 10 distinct stereoisomers exist due to the symmetrical nature of the molecule. Two of the stereoisomers are active. Clinically, this drug is used as a racemic mixture consisting of (+)-nebivolol ([+]-SRRR nebivolol) and (−)-nebivolol ([−]-RSSS nebivolol) that differ chemically and pharmacologically from other BBs. The selective β_1-blocking effect is due almost exclusively to the (+)-stereoisomer. In contrast, (−)-nebivolol is primarily responsible for the vasodilatory activity. The combination of (+)-nebivolol and (−)-nebivolol therefore acts synergistically to produce a cardiovascular profile that differs noticeably from that of conventional BBs with respect to enhanced blood pressure reduction at lower doses. This drug is highly selective for β_1-receptors at low doses (≤10 mg), but at higher doses, it loses its cardioselectivity and blocks both β_1- and β_2-receptors. (-)-Nebivolol exerts its activity through a unique β_3-adrenergic receptor-mediated stimulation of endothelial nitric oxide synthase (eNOS). The product of this reaction, nitric oxide (NO), produces vasodilation, which

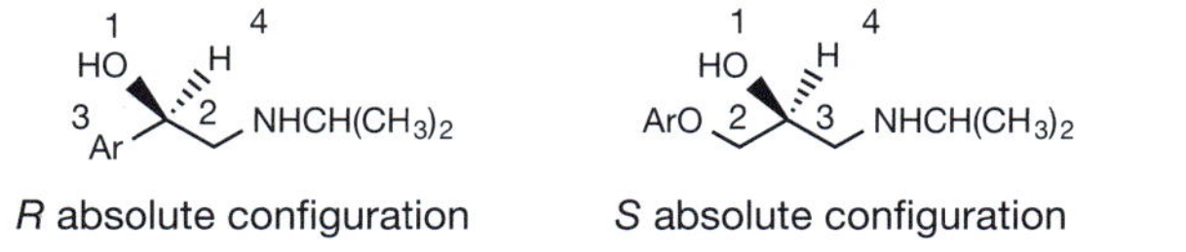

Figure 19.44 Stereochemical nomenclature for arylethanolamines versus aryloxypropanolamines. The relative positions in space of the four functional groups are the same in the two structures; however, one is designated *R* and the other *S*. This is because the introduction of an oxygen atom into the side chain of the aryloxypropanolamine changes the priority of two of the groups used in the nomenclature assignment.

reduces peripheral vascular resistance and blood pressure. Neither nebivolol nor its stereoisomers show any intrinsic sympathomimetic activity, without the undesirable BB effects, such as a decrease in cardiac output.

Pharmacokinetic Properties and Metabolism. Details about the pharmacokinetic parameters and metabolism of the β-blockers are provided in Table 19.21. Esmolol is the methyl ester of a carboxylic acid, which makes it susceptible to hydrolysis by serum esterases. The acid metabolite generated by hydrolysis is essentially inactive and readily excreted as its zwitterion. For this reason, esmolol has a half-life of approximately 8 minutes and is used to control supraventricular tachycardia during surgery when a short-acting β_1-adrenergic antagonist is desirable.

Another physicochemical parameter with some clinical correlation is the relative lipophilicity of different agents. Propranolol is by far the most lipophilic of the available β-blockers, and it enters the CNS far better than the less lipophilic agents, such as atenolol or nadolol. Lipophilicity as measured by octanol-water partitioning also correlates with the primary site of clearance, as seen in Table 19.21. The more lipophilic drugs are primarily cleared by the liver, whereas the more hydrophilic agents are cleared by the kidney. This could influence the choice of agents in cases of renal failure or liver disease. Several of the β-blockers must be dose adjusted in patients with impaired renal function.

Nebivolol undergoes biotransformation via glucuronidation and CYP2D6-mediated hydroxylation. Areas under the curve (AUCs) and half-lives are higher in CYP2D6 poor metabolizers than in CYP2D6 extensive (normal) metabolizers. However, the metabolites exhibit BB activity and contribute to the therapeutic effects of the parent compound. As a result, dosage adjustments do not appear to be necessary, regardless of an individual's CYP2D6 phenotype.

α_1-Adrenergic Receptor Blockers

Therapeutic Overview of α_1-Adrenergic Receptor Blockers.

α_1-Blockers are effective agents for the initial management of hypertension and are especially advantageous for older men who also suffer from symptomatic benign prostatic hyperplasia.[6,136] Prazosin, the first known selective α_1-blocker, was discovered in the late 1960s[137] and is now one of a small group of selective α_1-antagonists that includes other quinoxaline antihypertensives such as terazosin and doxazosin. They have been shown to be as effective as other major classes of antihypertensives in lowering blood pressure in equivalent doses. α_1-Blockers possess a characteristic "first-dose" effect, which means that orthostatic hypotension frequently occurs with the first few doses of the drug. This side effect can be minimized by slowly increasing the dose and by administering the first few doses at bedtime.

Pharmacology Overview of α_1-Adrenergic Receptor Blockers

Mechanism of Action. These drugs block the effect of sympathetic nerves on blood vessels by selectively binding to α_1-adrenoceptors located on the VSM (Fig. 19.38), which then stimulate the G_q protein, activating smooth muscle contraction through the IP_3 signal transduction pathway. Most of these drugs act as competitive antagonists by competing with the binding of norepinephrine to α_1-adrenergic receptors on VSM. Some α-blockers are noncompetitive (eg, phenoxybenzamine), which greatly prolongs their action. Prejunctional α_2-adrenoceptors located on the sympathetic nerve terminals serve as a negative feedback mechanism for norepinephrine release.

α-Blockers dilate both arteries and veins because both vessel types are innervated by sympathetic adrenergic nerves. The vasodilator effect is more pronounced, however, in the arterial resistance vessels. Because most blood vessels have some degree of sympathetic tone under basal conditions, these drugs are effective dilators. They are even more effective under conditions of elevated sympathetic activity (eg, during stress) or during pathologic increases in circulating catecholamines caused by an adrenal gland tumor (pheochromocytoma).[105,106] α_2-Adrenoceptors are also abundant in the smooth muscle of the bladder neck and prostate and, when inhibited, cause relaxation of the bladder muscle, increasing urinary flow rates and the relief of benign prostatic hyperplasia.

Common Adverse Effects. The most common side effects are related directly to α_1-adrenoceptor blockade. These side effects include dizziness, orthostatic hypotension (because of loss of reflex vasoconstriction on standing), nasal congestion (because of dilation of nasal mucosal arterioles), headache, and reflex tachycardia (especially with nonselective α-blockers). Fluid retention is also a problem that can be rectified by use of a diuretic in conjunction with the α_1-blocker. α-Blockers have not been shown to be beneficial in heart failure or angina and should not be used in these conditions.

Common Interactions. Common drug-drug interactions for the α_1-adrenergic receptor blockers are summarized in Table 19.22.

Medicinal Chemistry of α_1-Adrenergic Receptor Blockers

Receptor Binding, SAR, and Physicochemical Properties. The structures for the available α_1-receptor blockers are shown in Figure 19.45. These include prazosin ($\log D_{7.4} = 1.70$), doxazosin ($\log D_{7.4} = 1.97$), and terazosin ($\log D_{7.4} = 2.13$). Prazosin, doxazosin, and terazosin contain a 4-amino-6,7-dimethoxyquinazoline ring system attached to a piperazine ring.

Pharmacokinetic Properties and Metabolism. Important structural differences between these drugs are the heterocyclic acyl groups attached to the second nitrogen of the piperazine or the propyl chain. The differences in

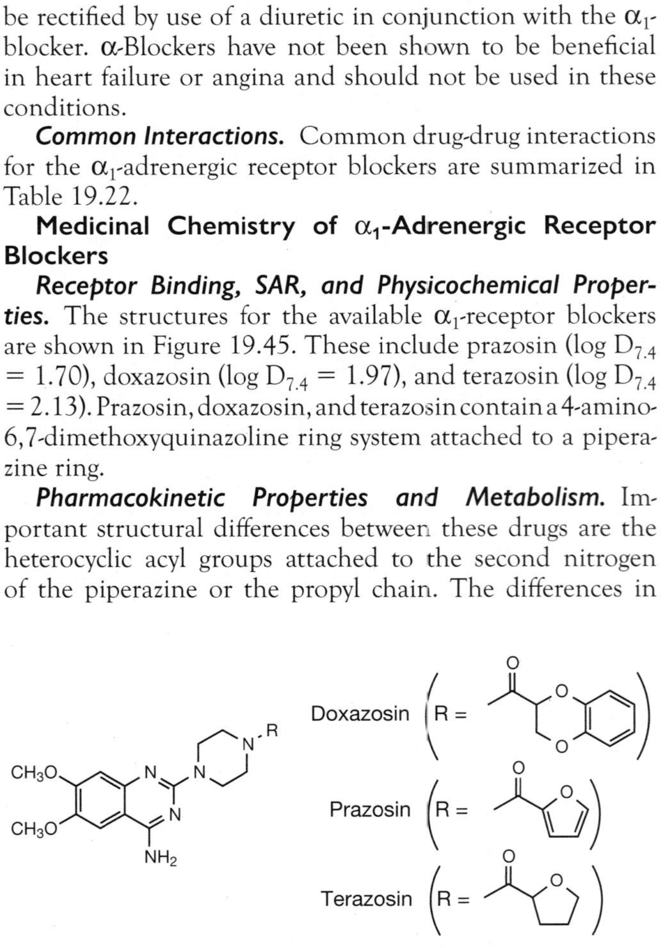

Figure 19.45 α_1-Selective–adrenergic blockers.

these groups afford dramatic differences in some of the pharmacokinetic properties of these agents (Table 19.23). For example, reduction of the furan ring for prazosin to the tetrahydrofuran ring of terazosin increases its duration of action by altering its rate of metabolism. Some of the important clinical parameters of the quinazolines are shown in Table 19.23.

MIXED α-/β-ADRENERGIC RECEPTOR BLOCKERS

Therapeutic Overview of Mixed α-/β-Adrenergic Receptor Blockers. Monotherapy with carvedilol or labetalol, mixed-acting α-/β-receptor blockers, reduces blood pressure as effectively as other major antihypertensives and their combinations.[138-140] Selection of mixed α-/β-blockers is recommended for management of hypertension when the stage 2 family of drugs cannot be used alone or when a compelling indication (Table 19.2) is present that requires the use of a specific drug. Both drugs effectively lower blood pressure in essential and renal hypertension. Carvedilol is also effective in ischemic heart disease.

Pharmacology Overview of Mixed α-/β-Adrenergic Receptor Blockers

Mechanism of Action. The mixed α-/β-receptor blocking properties in the same molecule confer some advantages in the lowering of blood pressure. Vasodilation via α_1-blockade lowers peripheral vascular resistance to maintain cardiac output, thus preventing bradycardia more effectively when compared to pure BBs.[140] β-Blockade helps avoid the reflex tachycardia sometimes observed with the other vasodilators listed later in this chapter.

Common Adverse Effects. Any adverse effects are usually related to β_1- or α_1-blockade. The β effects are usually less bothersome because the α_1-blockade reduces the effects of β-blockade.

Common Interactions. Table 19.22 summarizes common drug-drug interactions for the mixed α-/β-adrenergic receptor blockers.

Medicinal Chemistry of Mixed α-/β-Adrenergic Receptor Blockers

Receptor Binding, Structure-Activity Relationships, and Physicochemical Properties. Carvedilol[138] and labetalol[139] are the currently available mixed α-/β-receptor blockers (Fig. 19.42). The α-methyl substituent attached to the N-arylalkyl group appears to be responsible for the α-adrenergic blocking effect. Carvedilol is administered as its racemate; its *S*-(−)-enantiomer is both an α- and nonselective β-blocker, whereas its *R*-(+)-enantiomer is an α_1-blocker. Labetalol possesses two chiral centers and, therefore, is administered as a mixture of four stereoisomers, of which $R(CH_3),R(OH)$ is the active β-blocker diastereomer with minimal α_1-blocking activity and the $S(CH_3),R(OH)$ diastereomer is predominantly an α_1-blocker. The *R,R*-diastereomer is also known as dilevalol, which was not approved by the FDA because of hepatotoxicity. The $S(CH_3),S(OH)$ and $R(CH_3),S(OH)$ diastereomers are both inactive. The comparative potency for labetalol reflects the fact that 25% of the diastereomeric mixture is the active *R,R*-diastereomer. The β-blocking activity of labetalol is approximately 1.5-fold that of its α_1-blocking activity. Carvedilol has an estimated β-blocking activity 10- to 100-fold its α_1-blocking activity.

Pharmacokinetic Properties and Metabolism. The pharmacokinetic properties and metabolism of carvedilol and labetalol are summarized in Table 19.21.

α_1-ADRENERGIC RECEPTOR AGONISTS

Therapeutic Overview of α_1-Adrenergic Receptor Agonists. Examples of drugs in this class include metaraminol, methoxamine, and phenylephrine. Their α_1-agonist activity makes them strong vasoconstrictors, and their primary systemic use is limited to treating hypotension during surgery or severe hypotension accompanying shock.

Pharmacology Overview of α_1-Adrenergic Receptor Agonists

Mechanism of Action. Metaraminol, methoxamine, and phenylephrine are selective agonists for α_1-receptors in the peripheral vasculature and have minimal cardiac stimulatory properties.

Common Adverse Effects. Table 19.24 lists common adverse effects for the α_1-adrenergic receptor agonist phenylephrine.

Common Interactions. Common drug-drug interactions for the α_1-adrenergic receptor agonists are summarized in Table 19.22.

Medicinal Chemistry of α_1-Adrenergic Receptor Agonists

Receptor Binding, Structure-Activity Relationships, and Physicochemical Properties. The aromatic ring substitution pattern in phenylethanolamines is an important structural factor in adrenergic receptor selectivity. In compounds with only 3′-OH substituents, such as phenylephrine and metaraminol, activity is reduced at α_1 sites but almost eliminated at β sites, thus affording selective α_1-agonists. Indication that α_1 sites have a wide range of substituent tolerance for agonist activity is shown by the 2′,5′-dimethoxy substitution pattern of methoxamine.

Table 19.23 Selected Clinical Parameters of α_1-Adrenergic Antagonists

Drug	Trade Name	c Log P/log D_{pH} 7.0	Half-Life (h)	Duration of Action (h)	Bioavailability (%)
Prazosin	Minipress	−1.1/−1.3[a]	2-3	4-6	45-65
Terazosin	Hytrin	−1.0/−1.0[a]	12	>18	90
Doxazosin	Cardura	0.7/0.5[a]	22	18-36	65

[a]Chemical Abstracts, American Chemical Society, calculated using Advanced Chemistry Development (ACD/Labs) Software V8.19 for Solaris (1994-2011 ACD/Labs).

Table 19.24 Common Adverse Effects of α_1-Agonists, Direct Vasodilators, and Potassium Channel Openers

Drug Class	Interactions
α_1-Adrenergic receptor agonists	Systemic use of phenylephrine can be associated with a number of side effects impacting the cardiovascular system (eg, bradycardia, vasoconstriction that may decrease blood flow to tissues) and the central nervous system (eg, dizziness and anxiety) Sensitive patients may exhibit allergic reactions (potentially severe) to sodium metabisulfite, a preservative that is added to some parenteral preparations of phenylephrine
Vasodilators (direct-acting)	Common sites for adverse effects associated with hydralazine include the cardiovascular system (eg, tachycardia) and the central nervous system (CNS) (eg, headache) An autoimmune syndrome resembling systemic lupus erythematosus (SLE) has been reported in patients using hydralazine. This is characterized by the presence of antinuclear antibodies in the circulation and can negatively impact multiple organs in the body. The incidence of this condition is more common with higher doses of the drug and may correlate with a patient's acetylator status (see upcoming sections) Hydralazine has been shown to be mutagenic in bacterial assays, carcinogenic in mice, and teratogenic in some laboratory animal species
Vasodilators (potassium channel openers)	Heart palpitations and increased heart rate can occur in patients who are taking diazoxide Chronic use of diazoxide has been associated with CNS effects (extrapyramidal effects), an hyperglycemia, which may be severe Diazoxide has been shown to be teratogenic in rabbits Retention of water and sodium has been shown to occur with both diazoxide and minoxidil Minoxidil is commonly associated with tachycardia in patients. Severe cardiac effects have also been noted, and patients receiving this drug should be closely monitored Increased hair growth has been observed with minoxidil, and the drug has been marketed for this purpose to treat hair loss under the trade name Rogaine

Data from AHFS Drug Information (2018), American Society of Health-System Pharmacists.

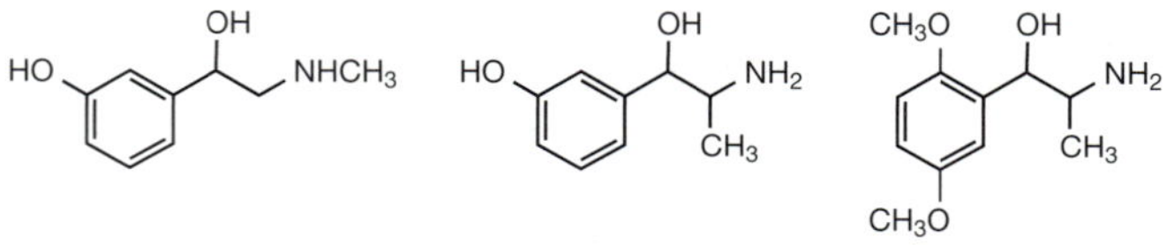

Phenylephrine Metaraminol Methoxamine

Pharmacokinetics and Metabolism. Because they are not substrates for catechol-O-methyltransferase (COMT), the duration of action for the α_1-agonists is significantly longer than that of norepinephrine. Methoxamine is bioactivated by 5′-O-demethylation to an active 5′-phenolic metabolite. The β-blocking activity of methoxamine, which is seen at high concentrations, affords some use in treating tachycardia. Phenylephrine, which is also a selective α_1-agonist, is used similarly to metaraminol and methoxamine for hypotension. It is widely used as a nonprescription nasal decongestant in both oral and topical preparations. However, its oral bioavailability is less than 10% because of its hydrophilic properties and intestinal 3′-O-glucuronidation/sulfation.

Centrally Acting Sympatholytics

α_2-Adrenergic Receptor Agonists

Therapeutic Overview of α_2-Adrenergic Receptor Agonists. The sympathetic adrenergic nervous system plays a major role in the regulation of arterial pressure. Activation of these nerves to the heart increases the heart rate (positive chronotropy), contractility (positive inotropy), and velocity of electrical impulse conduction (positive chronotropy). Within the medulla are located preganglionic sympathetic excitatory neurons, which travel from the spinal cord to the ganglia. They have significant basal activity, which generates a level of sympathetic tone to the heart and vasculature even under basal conditions. The sympathetic neurons within the medulla receive input from other neurons within the medulla, and together, these neuronal systems regulate sympathetic (and parasympathetic) outflow to the heart and vasculature. Sympatholytic drugs can block this sympathetic adrenergic system on three different levels. First, peripheral sympatholytic drugs, such as α-adrenoceptor and β-adrenoceptor antagonists, block the influence of norepinephrine at the effector organ (heart or blood vessel). Second, there are ganglionic blockers that block impulse transmission at the sympathetic ganglia. Third, centrally acting sympatholytic drugs block sympathetic activity within the brain. Centrally acting sympatholytics block sympathetic activity by binding to and activating α_2-adrenoceptors, which reduces sympathetic outflow to the heart, thereby decreasing cardiac output by decreasing heart rate and contractility. Reduced sympathetic output to the vasculature decreases sympathetic vascular tone, which causes vasodilation and reduced systemic vascular resistance, which in turn decreases arterial pressure.

Methyldopa is used in the management of moderate to severe hypertension and is reserved for patients who fail to achieve blood pressure goals with stage 2 drugs.[6,124] Methyldopa is also coadministered with diuretics and other classes of antihypertensive drugs, permitting a reduction in the dosage of each drug and minimizing adverse effects while maintaining blood pressure control. Methyldopa has been used in the management of hypertension during pregnancy without apparent substantial adverse effects on the fetus and also for the management of pregnancy-induced hypertension (ie, preeclampsia).[5] Intravenous methyldopate can be used for the management of hypertension when parenteral hypotensive therapy is necessary. Because of its slow onset of action; however, other agents, such as sodium nitroprusside, are preferred when a parenteral hypotensive agent is employed for hypertensive emergencies.

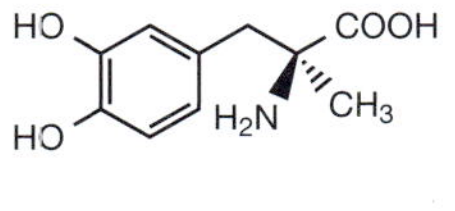

Methyldopa

Clonidine, guanabenz, and guanfacine (Fig. 19.46) are used in the management of mild to moderate hypertension or when stage 2 drugs have been ineffective in achieving blood pressure goals.[6,101] They have been used as monotherapy or to achieve lower dosages in combination with other classes of antihypertensive agents. The centrally acting sympatholytics are generally reserved for patients who fail to respond to therapy with a stage 1 drug (eg, diuretics, β-adrenergic blocking agents, ACEIs, or ARBs). Clonidine, guanabenz, and guanfacine can be used in combination with diuretics and other stage 1 hypotensive agents, permitting a reduction in the dosage of each drug, which minimizes adverse effects while maintaining blood pressure control. Geriatric patients, however, cannot tolerate the adverse cognitive effects of these sympatholytics. All three drugs reduce blood pressure to essentially the same extent in both supine and standing patients; thus, orthostatic effects are mild and infrequently encountered. Exercise does not appear to affect the blood pressure response to guanabenz and guanfacine in patients with hypertension. Plasma renin activity can be unchanged or reduced during long-term therapy with these drugs.

Clonidine is administered twice a day for the management of mild to moderate hypertension in those patients not achieving the blood pressure goal with stage 2 drugs.[6]

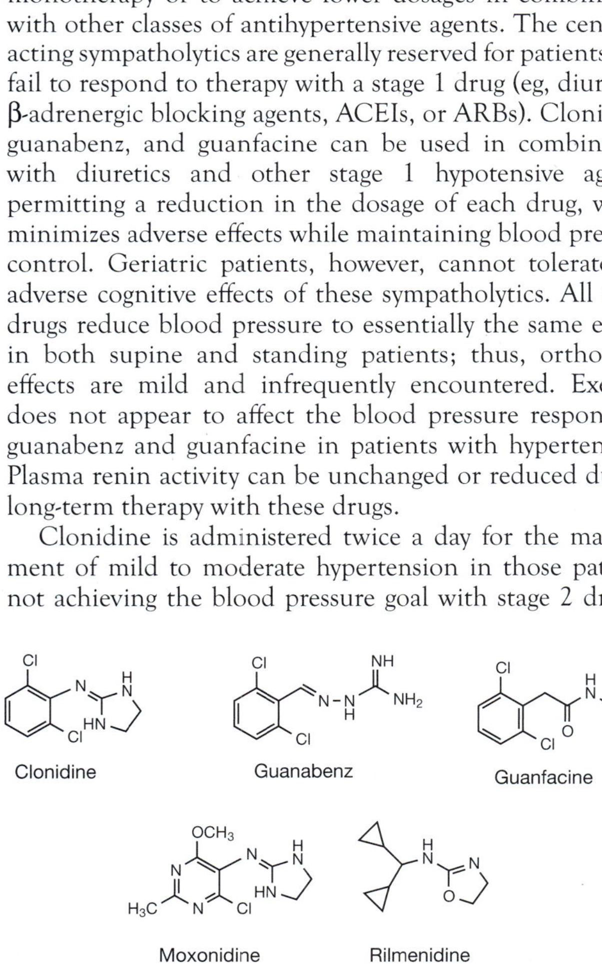

Figure 19.46 Centrally acting sympatholytics.

Transdermal clonidine has also been successfully substituted for oral clonidine in some patients with mild to moderate hypertension whose compliance with a daily dosing regimen can be a problem.[141] When administered by epidural infusion, clonidine is used as adjunct therapy in combination with opiates for the management of severe cancer pain not relieved by opiate analgesics alone. Other nonhypertensive uses for clonidine include the prophylaxis of migraine headaches, the treatment of severe dysmenorrhea, menopausal flushing, and rapid detoxification in the management of opiate withdrawal in opiate-dependent individuals. Additionally, in conjunction with benzodiazepines, clonidine is used for the management of alcohol withdrawal, and for the treatment of tremors associated with the adverse effects of methylphenidate in patients with attention-deficit/hyperactivity disorder (ADHD). Clonidine has been used to reduce intraocular pressure in the treatment of open-angle and secondary glaucoma. Clonidine, a nonstimulant drug, is also used in reducing the symptoms of ADHD and bipolar disorders, whose mechanism of action is thought to regulate norepinephrine release from the locus ceruleus, part of the brain stem involved with physiologic responses to stress and panic. Clonidine can also reduce symptoms of aggression as with patients with bipolar disorders and reduce the insomnia associated with CNS stimulants such as methylphenidate. Once stabilized, children on larger doses can be switched to the transdermal clonidine patch.

The therapeutic applications for guanabenz are similar to those of clonidine and other α_2-adrenergic agonists. One advantage for guanabenz is its once-a-day dosing schedule. Guanabenz has been used in diabetic patients with hypertension without adverse effects in the control of or therapy for diabetes, and it has been effective in hypertensive patients with chronic obstructive pulmonary disease, including asthma, chronic bronchitis, or emphysema. Guanabenz has been used alone or in combination with naltrexone in the management of opiate withdrawal in patients physically dependent on opiates and undergoing detoxification. Guanabenz has also been used as an analgesic in a limited number of patients with chronic pain.

The therapeutic applications for guanfacine are similar to those of the other centrally acting α_2-adrenergic agonists and methyldopa.[6,142] It has been effective as monotherapy in the treatment of patients with mild to moderate hypertension. One advantage for guanfacine is its once-a-day dosing schedule. The use of diuretics to prevent accumulation of fluid can allow a reduction in the dosage for guanfacine. Somnolence and sedation were commonly reported adverse events in clinical trials. The most common adverse events associated with guanfacine treatment include somnolence/sedation, abdominal pain, dizziness, hypotension/decreased blood pressure, dry mouth, and constipation.

Guanfacine extended-release tablets have been FDA approved for the nonstimulant treatment of ADHD in children and adolescents in the ages of 6 to 17 years. Although the mechanism of action for treatment of ADHD is unknown, guanfacine is thought to directly bind to postsynaptic α_2-adrenoceptors in the prefrontal cortex of the brain, an area of the brain that has been linked to ADHD. Stimulation of these adrenoceptors is theorized to strengthen working memory, reduce susceptibility to distraction, improve attention regulation, improve behavioral inhibition, and enhance impulse control. Guanfacine treatment can cause decreases in blood pressure and heart rate, which can lead to syncope. This drug should be used with caution in patients with ADHD having a history of hypotension, heart block, bradycardia, cardiovascular disease, syncope, orthostatic hypotension, or dehydration and should be used with caution in patients being treated concomitantly with antihypertensive agents or other drugs that reduce blood pressure or heart rate or increase the risk of syncope. Guanfacine extended-release tablets should not be crushed, chewed, or broken before they are swallowed and not substituted for immediate-release tablets. Patients with ADHD should be reevaluated periodically for the long-term usefulness of this drug. When ADHD therapy with guanfacine is discontinued, the dose should be tapered over a period of 7 days.

Pharmacology Overview of α_2-Adrenergic Receptor Agonists

Mechanism of Action. The central mechanism for the antihypertensive activity of the prodrug methyldopa is not caused by its inhibition of norepinephrine biosynthesis but, rather, by its metabolism in the CNS to α-methylnorepinephrine, an α_2-adrenergic agonist (Fig. 19.47).[105,106] Other more powerful inhibitors of aromatic l-amino acid decarboxylase (eg, carbidopa) have proven to be clinically useful, but not as antihypertensives. Rather, these agents are used to inhibit the metabolism of exogenous L-DOPA administered in the treatment of Parkinson disease.

The mechanism of the central hypotensive action for methyldopa is attributed to its transport into the CNS via an aromatic amino acid transport mechanism, where it is decarboxylated and hydroxylated into α-methylnorepinephrine (Fig. 19.47).[105,106] This active metabolite of methyldopa decreases total peripheral resistance, with little change in

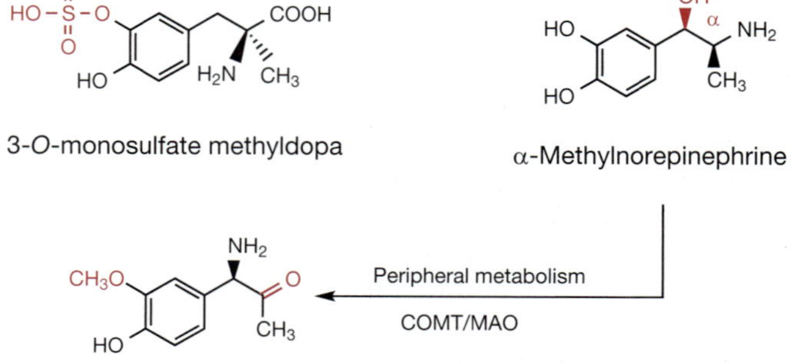

Figure 19.47 Metabolism of methyldopa. COMT, catechol-*O*-methyltransferase; MAO, monoamine oxidase.

cardiac output and heart rate, through its stimulation of central inhibitory α_2-adrenoceptors. A reduction of plasma renin activity can also contribute to the hypotensive action of methyldopa. Postural hypotension and sodium and water retention are also effects related to a reduction in blood pressure. If a diuretic is not administered concurrently with methyldopa, tolerance to the antihypertensive effect of the methyldopa during prolonged therapy can result.

The overall mechanism of action for the centrally active sympatholytics, clonidine, guanabenz, and guanfacine, appears to be stimulation of α_2-adrenoceptors and specific binding to nonadrenergic imidazoline I_1 receptors in the CNS (mainly in the medulla oblongata), causing inhibition of sympathetic output (sympathoinhibition).[143,144] This effect results in reduced peripheral and renovascular resistance and leads to a decrease in systolic and diastolic blood pressure. Through the use of imidazoline and α_2-adrenergic antagonists, specific I_1 receptors have recently been characterized in CNS control of blood pressure.[145] The I_1 receptors are pharmacologically distinct from α_2-receptors because they are not activated by catecholamines but characterized by their high affinity for 2-iminoimidazolines (or 2-aminoimidazolines) and low affinity for guanidines.[145] Thus, the central hypotensive action for clonidine, other 2-aminoimidazolines, and structurally related compounds needs both the I_1 and α_2-adrenoceptors to produce their central sympatholytic response.[144] Because of this discovery, a new generation of centrally acting antihypertensive agents selective for the I_1 receptor has been developed and includes moxonidine (a pyrimidinyl aminoimidazoline) and rilmenidine (an alkylaminooxazoline) (Fig. 17.40). Rilmenidine and moxonidine are both highly selective for the I_1 receptor while having low affinity for α_2-adrenoceptors, and both control blood pressure effectively without the adverse effects associated with binding to α_2-receptors (eg, sedation, bradycardia, and mental depression).[144] Clonidine appears to be more selective for α_2-adrenoceptors than for I_1 receptors.

In addition to its central stimulation of I_1 receptors and α_2-adrenoceptors,[144,145] clonidine (as well as other α_2-adrenergic agonists), when administered epidurally, produces analgesia by stimulation of spinal α_2-adrenoceptors, inhibiting sympathetically mediated pain pathways that are activated by nociceptive stimuli, thus preventing transmission of pain signals to the brain.[105,106] The administration of clonidine, while blocking opiate withdrawal, causes sympathetic inhibition and reduction in arterial pressure. The actions of clonidine on morphine pain response and withdrawal are most likely mediated by its ability to block *N*-methyl-D-aspartate (NMDA) receptor channels. Analgesia resulting from clonidine therapy is not antagonized by opiate antagonists. Activation of α_2-adrenoceptors also apparently stimulates acetylcholine release and inhibits the release of substance P, an inflammatory neuropeptide.

Common Adverse Effects. The most common adverse effect for methyldopa is drowsiness, which occurs within the first 48 to 72 hours of therapy and can disappear with continued administration of the drug.[6] Sedation commonly recurs when its dosage is increased. A decrease in mental acuity, including impaired ability to concentrate, lapses of memory, and difficulty in performing simple calculations, can occur and usually necessitates withdrawal of the drug. Patients should be warned that methyldopa can impair their ability to perform activities requiring mental alertness or physical coordination (eg, operating machinery or driving a motor vehicle). Nightmares, mental depression, orthostatic hypotension, and symptoms of cerebrovascular insufficiency can occur during methyldopa therapy and are indications for dosage reduction. Orthostatic hypotension can be less pronounced with methyldopa than with guanethidine but can be more severe than with reserpine, clonidine, hydralazine, propranolol, or thiazide diuretics. Nasal congestion commonly occurs in patients receiving methyldopa. Positive direct antiglobulin (Coombs) test results have been reported in approximately 10% to 20% of patients receiving methyldopa, usually after 6 to 12 months of therapy. This phenomenon is dose related. Methyldopa should be used with caution in patients with a history of previous liver disease or dysfunction, and it should be stopped if unexplained drug-induced fever and jaundice occur. These effects commonly occur within 3 weeks after initiation of treatment.

Dosage forms of methyldopa and methyldopate can contain sulfites, which can cause allergic-type reactions, including anaphylaxis and life-threatening or less severe asthmatic episodes. These allergic reactions are observed more frequently in asthmatic than in nonasthmatic individuals. Methyldopa is contraindicated in patients receiving MAO inhibitors.

Overall, the frequency of adverse effects produced by clonidine, guanabenz, and guanfacine are similar and appear to be dose related.[6] Drowsiness, tiredness, dizziness, weakness, bradycardia, headache, and dry mouth are common adverse effects for patients receiving clonidine, guanabenz, and guanfacine. The sedative effect for these centrally acting sympatholytics can result from their central α_2-agonist activity. The dry mouth induced by these drugs can result from a combination of central and peripheral α_2-adrenoceptor mechanisms, and the decreased salivation can involve inhibition of cholinergic transmission via stimulation of peripheral α_2-adrenoceptors. Orthostatic hypotension does not appear to be a significant problem with these drugs because there appears to be little difference between supine and standing systolic and diastolic blood pressures in most patients. Other adverse effects include increased urinary frequency (nocturia), urinary retention, sexual dysfunction (eg, decreased libido, erectile dysfunction, and impotence), nasal congestion, tinnitus, blurred vision, and dry eyes. These symptoms most often occur within the first few weeks of therapy and tend to diminish with continued therapy, or they can be relieved by a reduction in dosage. Although adverse effects of these drugs are generally not severe, discontinuance of therapy has been necessary in some patients because of intolerable sedation or dry mouth. Sodium and fluid retention can be avoided or relieved by administration of a diuretic.

Adverse effects occurring with transdermal clonidine generally appear to be similar to those occurring with oral therapy.[141,146] They have been mild and have tended to diminish with continued treatment. Hypotension has occurred in patients receiving clonidine by epidural infusion as adjunct therapy with epidural morphine for the treatment of cancer pain. With the transdermal system, localized skin reactions, such as erythema and pruritus, have occurred in some patients. The use of clonidine and methylphenidate in combination for managing ADHD can adversely affect cardiac conduction and increase risk for arrhythmias. Patients with ADHD need to be closely monitored and screened for a patient or family history of rhythm disturbances, and periodic monitoring of blood pressure, heart rate, and rhythm is recommended. Within 2 to 3 hours following the abrupt withdrawal of oral clonidine therapy, a rapid increase in systolic and diastolic blood pressures occurs, and blood pressures can exceed pretreatment levels. Associated with the clonidine withdrawal syndrome, the symptoms observed include nervousness, agitation, restlessness, anxiety, insomnia, headache, sweating, palpitations, increased heart rate, tremor, and increased salivation. The exact mechanism of the withdrawal syndrome following discontinuance of α_2-adrenergic agonists has not been determined but can involve increased concentrations of circulating catecholamines, increased sensitivity of adrenoceptors, enhanced renin-angiotensin system activity, decreased vagal function, failure of autoregulation of cerebral blood flow, and failure of central α_2-adrenoceptor mechanisms to regulate sympathetic outflow from the CNS.[6] The clonidine withdrawal syndrome is more pronounced after abrupt cessation of long-term therapy and with administration of high oral dosages (>1.2 mg daily). Withdrawal symptoms have been reported following discontinuance of transdermal therapy or when absorption of the drug is impaired because of dermatologic changes (eg, contact dermatitis) under the transdermal system. Epidural clonidine can prolong the duration of the pharmacologic effects, including both sensory and motor blockade, of epidural local anesthetics.

Overall, the frequency of adverse effects produced by guanabenz is similar to that produced by clonidine and the other α_2-adrenergic agonists, but the incidence is lower.[6,147] As with the other centrally active sympatholytics (eg, clonidine), abrupt withdrawal of guanabenz can result in rebound hypertension, but the withdrawal syndrome symptoms appear to be less severe.

Although the frequency of troublesome adverse effects produced by guanfacine is similar to that produced by clonidine and the other centrally acting sympatholytics, their incidence and severity are lower with guanfacine.[6,142] Unlike clonidine, abrupt discontinuation of guanfacine rarely results in rebound hypertension. When a withdrawal syndrome has occurred, its onset was slower and its symptoms are less severe than the syndrome observed with clonidine.

Common Interactions. Table 19.22 summarizes common drug-drug interactions for the α_2-adrenergic receptor agonists. More detailed information follows.

A pharmacokinetic-based interaction occurs where oral iron preparations (ferrous salts) interfere with the absorption of methyldopa from the gastrointestinal tract, reducing its systemic bioavailability.

The hypotensive actions for clonidine, guanabenz, and guanfacine can be additive with, or can potentiate the action of, other CNS depressants, such as opiates or other analgesics, barbiturates or other sedatives, anesthetics, or alcohol.[6] Coadministration of opiate analgesics with clonidine can also potentiate the hypotensive effects of clonidine. Tricyclic antidepressants (ie, imipramine and desipramine) have reportedly inhibited the hypotensive effect of clonidine, guanabenz, and guanfacine, and increase in blood pressure usually occurs during the second week of tricyclic antidepressant therapy. Dosage should be increased to adequately control hypertension if necessary. Sudden withdrawal of clonidine, guanabenz, and guanfacine can result in an excess of circulating catecholamines; therefore, caution should be exercised in concomitant use of drugs that affect the metabolism or tissue uptake of these amines (MAO inhibitors or tricyclic antidepressants, respectively). Because clonidine, guanabenz, and guanfacine can produce bradycardia, the possibility of additive effects should be considered if these drugs are given concomitantly with other drugs, such as hypotensive drugs or cardiac glycosides.

Medicinal Chemistry of α_2-Adrenergic Receptor Agonists

Receptor Binding, Structure-Activity Relationships, and Physicochemical Properties. Methyldopa is structurally and chemically related to L-dihydroxyphenylalanine (L-DOPA) and the catecholamines. To increase its water solubility for parenteral administration, the zwitterion methyldopa is esterified and converted to its hydrochloride salt, methyldopate ethyl ester hydrochloride (referred to as methyldopate). Methyldopate ester hydrochloride is used to prepare parenteral solutions of methyldopa, having a pH in the range of 3.5 to 6.0. Methyldopa is unstable in the presence of oxidizing agents (ie, air), alkaline pH, and light. Being related to the catecholamines, which are subject to air oxidation, metabisulfite/sulfite can be added to dosage formulations to prevent oxidation. Some patients, especially those with asthma, can exhibit sulfite-related hypersensitivity reactions. Methyldopate hydrochloride injection has been reported to be physically incompatible with drugs that are poorly soluble in an acidic medium (eg, sodium salts of barbiturates and sulfonamides) and with drugs that are acid labile. Incompatibility depends on several factors (eg, concentrations of the drugs, specific diluents used, resulting pH, and temperature).

Clonidine is an aryl-2-aminoimidazoline (Fig. 19.46) that is more selective for α_2-adrenoceptors than for I_1 receptors in producing its hypotensive effect. It is available as oral tablets, injection, or a transdermal system. Clonidine was originally synthesized as a vasoconstricting nasal decongestant but, in early clinical trials, was found to have dramatic hypotensive effects—in contrast to all expectations for a vasoconstrictor.[148] Subsequent pharmacologic investigations showed that clonidine not only has some α_1-agonist (vasoconstrictive) properties in the periphery but also is a powerful α_2-adrenergic agonist and exhibits specific binding to nonadrenergic imidazoline binding sites in the CNS (mainly in the medulla oblongata), causing inhibition of sympathetic output (sympathoinhibition). Because of its peripheral activity on extraneuronal vascular postsynaptic α_{2B}-receptors,[149] initial doses of clonidine can produce a transient vasoconstriction and an increase in blood pressure that is soon overcome by vasodilation as clonidine penetrates the blood-brain barrier and interacts with CNS α_{2A}-receptors.

Clonidine has lipophilic ortho-dichloro substituents on the phenyl ring, and the uncharged form of clonidine exists as a pair of tautomers as shown.

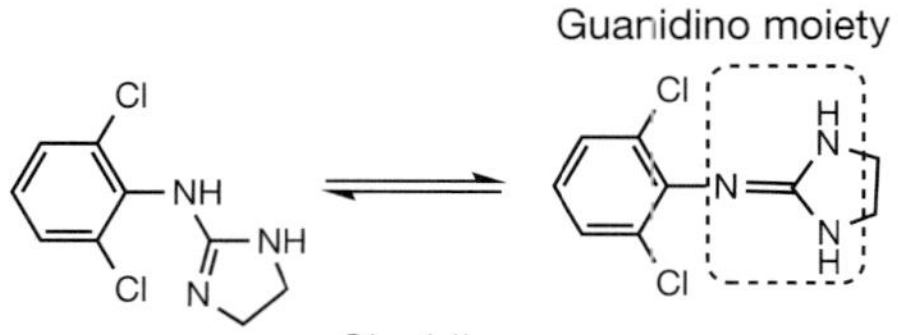

Clonidine

The pK_a of clonidine is 8.3 and it is approximately 80% ionized at physiologic pH. Its experimental log $D_{pH\ 7.4}$ = 1.03. The positive charge is shared through resonance by all three nitrogens of the guanidino group. Steric crowding by the bulky ortho-chlorine groups does not permit a coplanar conformation of the two rings, as shown.

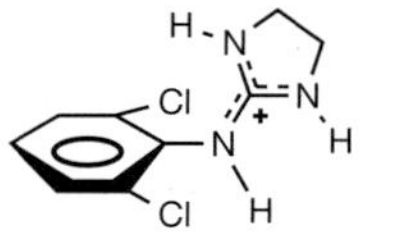

Protonated clonidine

After the discovery of clonidine, extensive research into the SAR of central α_2-agonists showed that the imidazoline ring was not necessary for activity in this class but that the phenyl ring required at least one ortho chlorine or methyl group. Two clinically useful antihypertensive agents resulting from this effort are guanabenz and guanfacine.

Guanabenz, a centrally active hypotensive agent, is pharmacologically related to clonidine but differs structurally from clonidine by the presence of an aminoguanidine side chain rather than an aminoimidazoline ring (Fig. 19.46). Guanabenz (pK_a = 8.1; log $D_{7.4}$ = 2.42) occurs largely (~80%) in the nonionized, lipid-soluble base form. Guanabenz can be given as a single daily dose administered at bedtime to minimize adverse effects.

Guanfacine, a phenylacetyl guanidine derivative (pK_a = 7.1; log $D_{7.4}$ = 1.52) (Fig. 19.46) is a centrally acting sympatholytic that is more selective for α_2-adrenoceptors than is clonidine. Its mechanism of action is similar to clonidine and is an effective alternative to that of the other centrally acting antihypertensive drugs. Although guanfacine is 5- to 20-fold less potent than clonidine on a weight basis, comparable blood pressure–lowering effects have been achieved when the two drugs were given in equipotent dosages. Its relatively long elimination half-life permits a once-a-day dosing schedule. Guanfacine activates peripheral α_2-adrenoceptors because a transient increase in blood pressure is observed in normotensive, but not in hypertensive, patients.

Pharmacokinetics and Metabolism. Methyldopa is an α_2-agonist acting in the CNS via its active metabolite, α-methylnorepinephrine (Fig. 19.47).[150] Methyldopa is transported across the blood-brain barrier, where it is decarboxylated by aromatic L-amino acid decarboxylase in the brain to α-methyldopamine, which is then stereospecifically hydroxylated to 1*R*,2*S*-α-methylnorepinephrine. This stereoisomer is a selective α_2-agonist and acts as an antihypertensive agent much like clonidine to inhibit sympathetic neural output from the CNS, thus lowering blood pressure. α-Methylnorepinephrine and α-methyldopamine do not cross the blood-brain barrier because of their hydrophilicity.

Originally synthesized as a norepinephrine biosynthesis inhibitor, methyldopa was thought to act through a combination of inhibition of norepinephrine biosynthesis through DOPA decarboxylase inhibition and metabolic decarboxylation to generate α-methylnorepinephrine. The latter was thought to replace norepinephrine in the nerve terminal and, when released, to have less intrinsic activity than the natural neurotransmitter. This latter mechanism is an example of the concept of a false neurotransmitter.

The oral bioavailability of methyldopa ranges from 20% to 50% and varies among individuals. Optimum blood pressure response occurs in 12 to 24 hours in most patients. After withdrawal of the drug, blood pressure returns to pretreatment levels within 24 to 48 hours. Methyldopa and its metabolites are weakly bound to plasma proteins. Although 95% of a dose of methyldopa is eliminated in hypertensive patients with normal renal function, with a plasma half-life of approximately 2 hours, in patients with impaired renal function, the half-life is doubled to approximately 3 to 4 hours, with about 50% of it excreted. Orally administered methyldopa undergoes presystemic first-pass metabolism in the GI tract to its 3-O-monosulfate metabolite (Fig. 19.47). Sulfate conjugation occurs to a greater extent when the drug is given orally rather than intravenously. Its rate of sulfate conjugation is decreased in patients with renal insufficiency. Methyldopa is excreted in urine as its mono-O-sulfate conjugate. Any peripherally decarboxylated α-methylnorepinephrine is metabolized by COMT and MAO (Fig. 19.47).

Methyldopate is slowly hydrolyzed in the body to form methyldopa. The hypotensive effect of IV methyldopate begins in 4 to 6 hours and lasts 10 to 16 hours.

Clonidine has an oral bioavailability of more than 90%, with a log $D_{7.4}$ of 1.82. It is well absorbed topically when applied to the eye, and percutaneously following application of a transdermal system to the arm or chest.[141,146,151] Following the application of a clonidine transdermal patch, therapeutic plasma concentrations are attained within 2 to 3 days. Studies have indicated that release of clonidine from the patch averages from 50% to 70% after 7 days of wear. Plasma clonidine concentrations attained with the transdermal systems are generally similar to twice-daily oral dosing regimens of the drug. Percutaneous absorption of the drug from the upper arm or chest is similar, but less drug is absorbed from the thigh.[146] Replacement of the transdermal system at a different site at weekly intervals continuously maintains therapeutic plasma clonidine concentrations. After discontinuance of transdermal therapy, therapeutic plasma drug concentrations persist for approximately 8 hours and then decline slowly over several days; over this time period, blood pressure returns gradually to pretreatment levels.

Blood pressure begins to decrease within 30 to 60 minutes after an oral dose of clonidine, with the maximum decrease in approximately 2 to 4 hours.[6] The hypotensive effect lasts up to 8 hours. Following epidural administration of a single bolus dose of clonidine, it is rapidly absorbed into the systemic circulation and into cerebrospinal fluid (CSF), with maximal analgesia within 30 to 60 minutes. Although the CSF is not the presumed site of action of clonidine-mediated analgesia, the drug appears to diffuse rapidly from the CSF to the dorsal horn of the spinal cord. After oral administration, clonidine appears to be well distributed throughout the body, with the lowest concentration in the brain. Clonidine is approximately 20% to 40% bound to plasma proteins, and it crosses the placenta. The plasma half-life of clonidine is 6 to 20 hours in patients with normal renal function and 18 to 41 hours in patients with impaired renal function. Clonidine is metabolized in the liver to its inactive major metabolite 4-hydroxyclonidine and its glucuronide and sulfate conjugates (10%-20%) (Fig. 19.48). In humans, 40% to 60% of an oral or IV dose of clonidine is excreted in the urine as unchanged drug within 24 hours. Approximately 85% of a single dose is excreted within 72 hours, with 20% of the dose excreted in the feces, probably via enterohepatic circulation.

The effective oral dose range for rilmenidine is 1 to 3 mg, with a dose-dependent duration of action of 10 to 20 hours. Moxonidine is administered once a day at a dose range of 0.2 to 0.4 mg. The oral bioavailability of moxonidine in humans is greater than 90%, with approximately 40% to 50% of the oral dose excreted unmetabolized in the urine.[152,153] The principal route of metabolism for moxonidine is oxidation of the 2-methyl group in the pyrimidine ring to 2-hydroxymethyl and 2-carboxylic acid derivative as well as the formation of corresponding glucuronides. After an oral dose of moxonidine, peak hypotensive effects occur within 2 hours, with an elimination half-life of greater than 8 hours.[153,154] Rilmenidine is readily absorbed from the GI tract, with an oral bioavailability greater than 95%. It is poorly metabolized and is excreted unchanged in the urine, with an elimination half-life of 8 hours.[155,156] After IV or oral administration of these

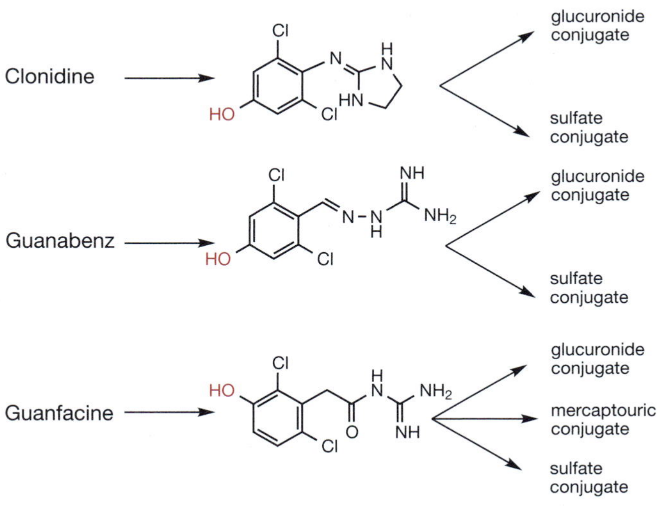

Figure 19.48 Metabolites formed from clonidine, guanabenz, and guanfacine.

drugs in normotensive patients, an initial hypertensive response to the drug occurs that is caused by activation of the peripheral α_2-adrenoceptors and the resulting vasoconstriction. This response is not observed, however, in patients with hypertension.

The oral bioavailability of guanabenz is 70% to 80%. After an oral dose, the hypotensive effect of guanabenz begins within 1 hour, peaks within 2 to 7 hours, and is diminished within 6 to 8 hours. It has an elimination half-life averaging 4 to 14 hours. The blood pressure response can persist for at least 12 hours. After IV dosing, guanabenz is distributed into the CNS, with brain concentrations 3 to 70 times higher than concurrent plasma concentrations. Guanabenz is approximately 90% bound to plasma proteins. In patients with hepatic or renal impairment, its elimination half-life can be prolonged.

Guanabenz is metabolized principally by hydroxylation to its inactive metabolite, 4-hydroxyguanabenz, which is eliminated in the urine as its glucuronide (major) and sulfate conjugates (Fig. 19.48). Guanabenz and its inactive metabolites are excreted principally in the urine, with approximately 70% to 80% of its oral dose excreted in the urine within 24 hours and approximately 10% to 30% excreted in the feces via enterohepatic cycling. Approximately 40% of an oral dose of guanabenz is excreted in the urine as 4-hydroxyguanabenz and its glucuronide, and less than 5% is excreted unchanged. The remainder is excreted as unidentified metabolites and their conjugates.

The pharmacokinetic properties of guanfacine differ from those of clonidine, guanabenz, and α-methyldopa.[142,157,158] At pH 7.4, guanfacine is predominantly (67%) in the nonionized, lipid-soluble base form, which accounts for its high oral bioavailability (>80%). Following an oral dose, peak plasma concentrations occur in 1 to 4 hours, with a relatively long elimination half-life of 14 to 23 hours. The maximum blood pressure response occurs in 8 to 12 hours after oral administration and is maintained up to 36 hours after its discontinuation. After IV dosing, guanfacine achieves the highest concentrations in the liver and kidney, with low concentrations in the brain. Guanfacine is 64% bound to plasma proteins. In patients with hepatic or renal impairment, its elimination half-life can be prolonged.

Guanfacine is metabolized principally by hepatic hydroxylation to its inactive metabolite, 3-hydroxyguanfacine (20%), which is eliminated in the urine as its glucuronide (30%), sulfate (8%), or mercapturic acid conjugate (10%), and 24% to 37% is excreted as unchanged guanfacine (Fig. 19.48). Its nearly complete bioavailability suggests no evidence of any first-pass effect. Guanfacine and its inactive metabolites are excreted principally in the urine, with approximately 80% of its oral dose excreted in the urine within 48 hours.

Vasodilators

Overview

Vasodilator drugs relax the smooth muscle in blood vessels, which causes the vessels to dilate.[124] Dilation of arterial vessels leads to a reduction in systemic vascular resistance, which leads to a fall in arterial blood pressure. Dilation of venous vessels decreases venous blood pressure.

Arterial dilator drugs are used to treat systemic and pulmonary hypertension, heart failure, and angina. They reduce arterial pressure by decreasing systemic vascular resistance, thereby reducing the afterload on the left ventricle and enhancing stroke volume and cardiac output. They also decrease the oxygen demand of the heart and, thereby, improve the oxygen supply/demand ratio. The primary functions of venous dilators in treating cardiovascular hypertension include reduction in venous pressure, thus reducing preload on the heart and decreasing cardiac output and capillary fluid filtration and edema formation (a decrease in capillary hydrostatic pressure). Therefore, venous dilators sometimes are used in the treatment of heart failure along with other drugs because they help reduce pulmonary and/or systemic edema resulting from heart failure.

There are three potential drawbacks in the use of vasodilators: First, vasodilators can lead to a baroreceptor-mediated reflex stimulation of the heart (increased heart rate and inotropy) from systemic vasodilation and arterial pressure reduction. Second, they can impair the normal baroreceptor-mediated reflex vasoconstriction when a person stands up, which can lead to orthostatic hypotension and syncope on standing. Third, they can lead to renal retention of sodium and water, increasing blood volume and cardiac output.

Vasodilator drugs are classified either based on their site of action (arterial vs venous) or, more commonly, by their primary mechanism of action.

Direct-Acting Vasodilators

THERAPEUTIC OVERVIEW OF DIRECT-ACTING VASODILATORS. Hydralazine, the only drug in this class, is used in the management of moderate to severe hypertension.[6] It is reserved for patients with compelling indications and for those who fail to respond adequately to a stage 2 antihypertensive regimen. This drug is recommended for use in conjunction with cardiac glycosides and other vasodilators for the short-term treatment of severe congestive heart failure. Patients who engage in potentially hazardous activities, such as operating machinery or driving motor vehicles, should be warned about possible faintness, dizziness, or weakness. Hydralazine should be used with caution in patients with cerebrovascular accidents or with severe renal damage.

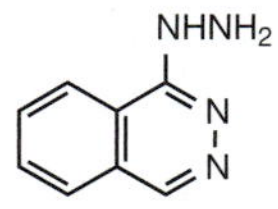

Hydralazine

Parenteral hydralazine can be used for the management of severe hypertension when the drug cannot be given orally or when blood pressure must be lowered immediately. Other agents (eg, sodium nitroprusside) are preferred for the management of severe hypertension or hypersensitive emergencies when a parenteral hypotensive agent is used.

PHARMACOLOGY OF DIRECT-ACTING VASODILATORS

Mechanism of Action. Hydralazine does not fit neatly into the other mechanistic classes of vasodilators, in part, because its mechanism of action is not entirely clear. It seems to have multiple, direct effects on the VSM. First, it causes smooth muscle hyperpolarization, quite likely through the opening of K^+ channels. Activation, therefore, increases the efflux of potassium ions from the cells, causing hyperpolarization of VSM cells and, thus, prolonging the opening of the potassium channel and sustaining a greater vasodilation on arterioles than on veins.[105,106] It can also inhibit the second messenger, IP_3-induced release of calcium from the smooth muscle SR (the PIP_2 signal transduction pathway) (Fig. 19.39). Finally, hydralazine stimulates the formation of NO by the vascular endothelium, leading to cGMP-mediated vasodilation (Fig. 19.38). The arterial vasodilator action of hydralazine reduces systemic vascular resistance and arterial pressure. Diastolic blood pressure is usually decreased more than systolic pressure. The hydralazine-induced decrease in blood pressure and peripheral resistance causes a reflex response, which is accompanied by increased heart rate, cardiac output, and stroke volume and an increase in plasma renin activity. It has no direct effect on the heart.[6] This reflex response could offset the hypotensive effect of arteriolar dilation, limiting its antihypertensive effectiveness. Hydralazine also causes sodium and water retention and expansion of plasma volume, which could develop tolerance to its antihypertensive effect after prolonged therapy. Thus, coadministration of a diuretic improves the therapeutic outcome.

Common Adverse Effects. Examples of adverse effects associated with the use of hydralazine are summarized in Table 19.24.

Common Interactions. The coadministration of hydralazine with diuretics and other hypotensive drugs can have a synergistic effect, resulting in a marked decrease in blood pressure.

MEDICINAL CHEMISTRY OF DIRECT-ACTING VASODILATORS

Receptor Binding, Structure-Activity Relationships and Physicochemical Properties. Hydralazine, a phthalazine-substituted hydrazine antihypertensive drug with a pK_a of 7.3 and log $D_{7.4}$ of 0.52, is highly specific for arterial vessels, producing its vasodilation by a couple of different mechanisms.

Pharmacokinetic Properties and Metabolism. Hydralazine is well absorbed from the GI tract and is metabolized in the GI mucosa (prehepatic systemic metabolism) and in the liver by acetylation, hydroxylation, and conjugation with glucuronic acid (Fig. 19.49).[6,105,106] Little of the hydralazine dose is excreted unchanged while most of the dose appears as metabolites in the urine, which are without significant therapeutic activity. A small amount of hydralazine is reportedly converted to a hydrazone, most likely with vitamin B_6 (pyridoxine), which can be responsible for some

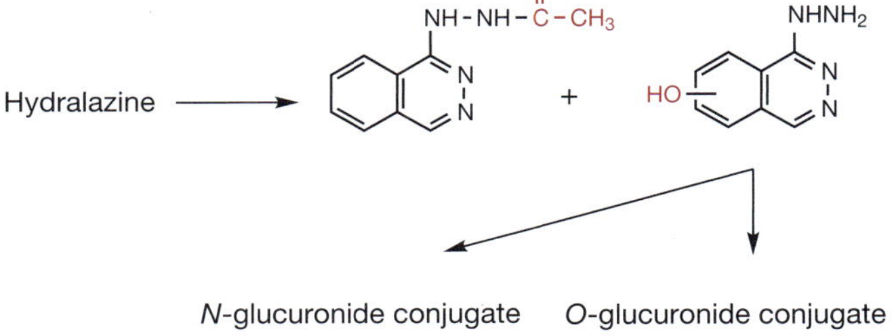

Figure 19.49 Metabolism of hydralazine.

its neurotoxic effects. Following the oral administration of hydralazine, its antihypertensive effect begins in 20 to 30 minutes and lasts 2 to 4 hours. The plasma half-life of hydralazine is generally 2 to 4 hours but can be up to 8 hours in some patients (ie, slow acetylators). In slow acetylator patients or in those with impaired renal function, the plasma concentrations for hydralazine are increased and, possibly, prolonged. Approximately 85% of hydralazine in the blood is bound to plasma proteins following administration of usual doses.

First-pass acetylation in the GI mucosa and liver is related to genetic acetylator phenotype. Acetylation phenotype is an important determinant of the plasma concentrations of hydralazine when the same dose of hydralazine is administered orally. Slow acetylators have an autosomal recessive trait that results in a relative deficiency of the hepatic enzyme *N*-acetyl transferase, thus prolonging the elimination half-life of hydralazine. This population of hypertensive patients will require an adjustment in dose to reduce the increased overactive response. Approximately 50% of African American and White as well as the majority of Native American and Asian populations are rapid acetylators of hydralazine. These patients will have subtherapeutic plasma concentrations of hydralazine because of its rapid metabolism to inactive metabolites and shorter elimination times. Patients with hydralazine-induced systemic lupus erythematosus frequently are slow acetylators.[105,106]

Potassium Channel Openers

THERAPEUTIC OVERVIEW OF POTASSIUM CHANNEL OPENERS. The two drugs in this class are minoxidil and diazoxide. Being effective arterial dilators, potassium channel openers are used in the treatment of hypertension. However, these drugs are not first-line therapy for hypertension because of their side effects; therefore, they are relegated to treating refractory, severe hypertension. They are generally used in conjunction with a BB and a diuretic to attenuate the reflex tachycardia and retention of sodium and fluid, respectively.

Minoxidil is used in the management of severe hypertension. It is reserved for resistant cases of hypertension that have not been managed with maximal therapeutic dosages of a diuretic and two other hypotensive drugs or for patients who have failed to respond adequately with hydralazine. To minimize sodium retention and increased plasma volume, minoxidil must be used in conjunction with a diuretic. A BB must be given before beginning minoxidil therapy and should be continued during minoxidil therapy to minimize minoxidil-induced tachycardia and increased myocardial workload. Minoxidil is also used topically to stimulate regrowth of hair in patients with androgenic alopecia (male pattern alopecia, hereditary alopecia, or common male baldness) or alopecia areata.

Intravenous diazoxide has been used in hypertensive crises for emergency lowering of blood pressure when a prompt and urgent decrease in diastolic pressure is required in adults with severe nonmalignant and malignant hypertension and in children with acute severe hypertension.[6] However, other IV hypotensive agents are preferred for the management of hypertensive crises. Diazoxide is intended for short-term use in hospitalized patients only. Although diazoxide has also been administered orally for the management of hypertension, its hyperglycemic and sodium-retaining effects make it unsuitable for chronic therapy. Diazoxide is also administered orally in the management of hypoglycemia caused by hyperinsulinism associated with inoperable islet cell adenoma or carcinoma or extrapancreatic malignancy in adults.

Pharmacology Overview of Potassium Channel Openers

Mechanism of Action. Potassium channel openers are drugs that activate (ie, open) ATP-sensitive K^+ channels in the VSM (Fig. 19.38).[159] By opening these potassium channels, there is increased efflux of potassium ions from the cells, causing hyperpolarization of VSM, which closes the voltage-gated calcium channels and, thereby, decreases intracellular calcium. With less calcium available to combine with calmodulin, there is less activation of MLCK and phosphorylation of myosin light chains. This leads to relaxation and vasodilation. Because small arteries and arterioles normally have a high degree of smooth muscle tone, these drugs are particularly effective in dilating these resistance vessels, decreasing systemic vascular resistance, and lowering arterial pressure. The fall in arterial pressure leads to reflex cardiac stimulation (baroreceptor-mediated tachycardia).

Minoxidil, as its active metabolite minoxidil O-sulfate, prolongs the opening of the potassium channel, sustaining greater vasodilation on arterioles than on veins. The drug decreases blood pressure in both the supine and standing positions, and there is no orthostatic hypotension. Associated with the decrease in peripheral resistance and blood pressure is a reflex response that is accompanied by increased heart rate, cardiac output, and stroke volume, which can be attenuated by the coadministration of a BB.[6] Along with this decrease in peripheral resistance is increased plasma renin activity and sodium and water retention, which can result in expansion of fluid volume, edema, and congestive heart failure. The sodium- and water-retaining effects of minoxidil can be reversed by coadministration of a diuretic. When minoxidil is used in conjunction with a β-adrenergic blocker, pulmonary artery pressure remains essentially unchanged.

Diazoxide reduces peripheral vascular resistance and blood pressure by a direct vasodilating effect on the VSM with a mechanism similar to that described for minoxidil by activating (opening) the ATP-modulated potassium channel.[160] Thus, diazoxide prolongs the opening of the potassium channel, sustaining greater vasodilation on arterioles than on veins.[105,106] The greatest hypotensive effect is observed in patients with malignant hypertension. Although oral or slow IV administration of diazoxide can produce a sustained fall in blood pressure, rapid IV administration is required for maximum hypotensive effects, especially in patients with malignant hypertension.[6] Diazoxide-induced decreases in blood pressure and peripheral vascular resistance are accompanied by a reflex response, resulting in an increased heart rate, cardiac output, and left ventricular ejection rate. In contrast to the thiazide diuretics, diazoxide causes sodium and water retention and decreased urinary output, which can result in expansion of plasma and extracellular fluid volume, edema, and congestive heart failure, especially during prolonged administration.

Diazoxide increases blood glucose concentration (diazoxide-induced hyperglycemia) by several different mechanisms: inhibition of pancreatic insulin secretion, stimulating the release of catecholamines, and/or increasing the hepatic release of glucose.[6,105,106] The precise mechanism of inhibition of insulin release has not been elucidated but, possibly, can result from an effect of diazoxide on cell membrane potassium channels and calcium flux.

Common Adverse Effects. Common adverse effects for the potassium channel openers, diazoxide and minoxidil, are listed in Table 19.24.

Common Interactions. When minoxidil is administered with diuretics or other hypotensive drugs, the hypotensive effect of minoxidil increases, and concurrent use can cause profound orthostatic hypotensive effects.

Medicinal Chemistry of Potassium Channel Openers

Receptor Binding, Structure-Activity Relationships, and Physicochemical Properties. Minoxidil is the *N*-oxide of a piperidinopyrimidine hypotensive agent with a pK_a 4.6 and log $D_{7.4}$ of 0.62. Diazoxide is a nondiuretic hypotensive and hyperglycemic agent that is structurally related to the thiazide diuretics. Being a sulfonamide with a pK_a of 8.5 and log $D_{7.4}$ of 1.28, it can be solubilized in alkaline solutions (pH of injection is 11.6). Solutions or oral suspension of diazoxide are unstable to light and will darken when exposed to light. Such dosage forms should be protected from light, heat, and freezing. Darkened solutions can be subpotent and should not be used.

Pharmacokinetic Properties and Metabolism. Minoxidil is not an active hypotensive drug until it is metabolized by hepatic thermolabile phenol sulfotransferase (SULT1A1) to minoxidil *N*-O-sulfate.[105,106] Plasma concentrations for minoxidil sulfate peak within 1 hour and then decline rapidly. Following an oral dose of minoxidil, its hypotensive effect begins in 30 minutes, is maximal in 2 to 8 hours, and persists for approximately 2 to 5 days. The delayed onset of the hypotensive effect for minoxidil is attributed to its metabolism to its active metabolite. The drug is not bound to plasma proteins. The major metabolite for minoxidil is its *N*-O-glucuronide, which unlike the sulfate metabolite, is inactive as a hypotensive agent. Approximately 10% to 20% of an oral dose of minoxidil is metabolized to its active metabolite, minoxidil O-sulfate, and approximately 20% of minoxidil is excreted unchanged.

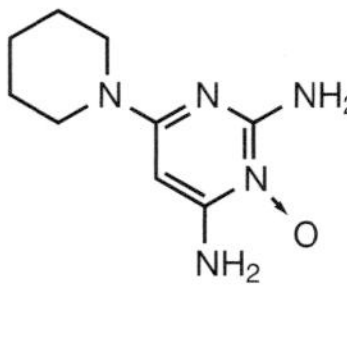

Minoxidil

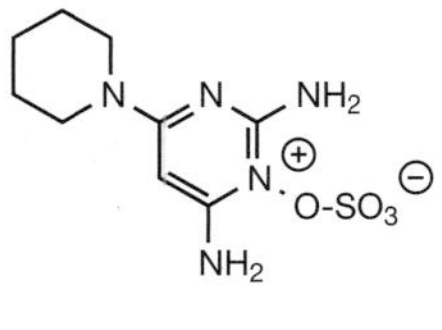

Minoxidil *N-O*-sulfate

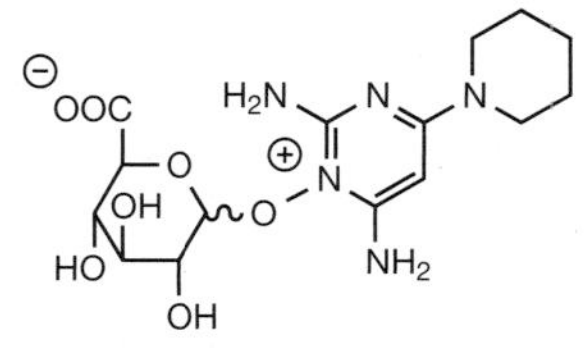

Minoxidil *N-O*-glucuronide

After rapid IV administration, diazoxide produces a prompt reduction in blood pressure, with maximum hypotensive effects occurring within 5 minutes.[6] The duration of its hypotensive effect varies from 3 to 12 hours, but ranges from 30 minutes to 72 hours have been observed. The elimination half-life of diazoxide following a single oral or IV dose has been reported to range from 21 to 45 hours in adults with normal renal function. In patients with renal impairment, the half-life is prolonged. Approximately 90% of the diazoxide in the blood is bound to plasma proteins. Approximately 20% to 50% of diazoxide is eliminated unchanged in the urine, along with its major metabolites, resulting from the oxidation of the 3-methyl group to its 3-hydroxymethyl- and 3-carboxyl-metabolites.

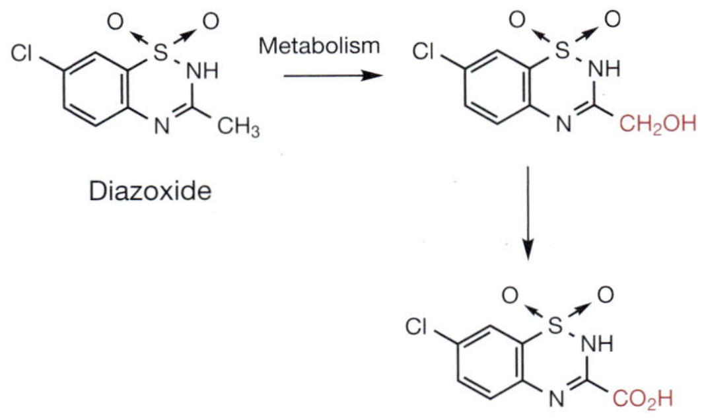

Nitrodilators

THERAPEUTIC OVERVIEW OF NITRODILATORS. Intravenous sodium nitroprusside is used as an infusion for hypertensive crises and emergencies.[6] The drug is consistently effective in the management of hypertensive emergencies, irrespective of etiology, and can be useful even when other drugs have failed. It can be used in the management of acute congestive heart failure.

PHARMACOLOGY OF NITRODILATORS

Mechanism of Action. Nitric oxide (NO), a molecule produced by many cells in the body, has several important actions. NO is a highly reactive gas that participates in many chemical reactions. It is one of the nitrogen oxides ("NOx") in automobile exhaust and plays a major role in the formation of photochemical smog, but NO also has many physiologic functions. It is synthesized within cells by an enzyme NO synthase (NOS). There are three isoenzymes: neuronal NOS (nNOS or NOS-1), inducible NOS (iNOS or NOS-2)—found in macrophages, and endothelial NOS (eNOS or NOS-3)—found in the endothelial cells that line the lumen of blood vessels. Whereas the levels of nNOS and eNOS are relatively steady, expression of iNOS genes awaits an appropriate stimulus. All types of NOS produce NO from arginine with the aid of molecular oxygen and NADPH. Because NO diffuses freely across cell membranes, there are many other molecules with which it can interact, and NO is quickly consumed close to where it is synthesized. Thus, NO affects only cells adjacent to its point of synthesis. NO relaxes the smooth muscle in the walls of the arterioles. At each systole, the endothelial cells that line the blood vessels release a puff of NO, which diffuses into the underlying smooth muscle cells, causing them to relax and, thus, to permit the surge of blood to pass through easily. The signaling functions of NO begin with its binding to protein receptors on or in the cell, triggering the formation of cGMP from soluble guanylyl cyclase (Fig. 19.38). Mice in which the genes for the NOS found in endothelial cells (eNOS) have been "knocked out" suffer from hypertension. Nitroglycerin, which is often prescribed to reduce the pain of angina, does so by generating NO, which relaxes venous walls and arterioles, improving the oxygen supply/demand ratio (see Chapter 20). NO also inhibits the aggregation of platelets and, thus, keeps inappropriate clotting from interfering with blood flow. Other actions on smooth muscle include penile erection and peristalsis aided by the relaxing effect of NO on the smooth muscle in intestinal walls. NO also inhibits the contractility of the smooth muscle wall of the uterus, but at birth, the production of NO decreases, allowing contractions to occur. Nitroglycerin has helped some women who were at risk of giving birth prematurely to carry their baby to full term. The NO from iNOS inhibits inflammation in blood vessels by blocking the release of mediators of inflammation from the endothelial cells, macrophages, and T lymphocytes. NO produced by iNOS has also been shown to S-nitrosylate cyclooxygenase-2 (COX-2), increasing its activity, and drugs that prevent this interaction could work synergistically with the nonsteroidal anti-inflammatory drugs inhibiting COX-2. NO affects hormonal secretion from several endocrine glands. Hemoglobin transports NO at the same time that it carries oxygen, and when it unloads oxygen in the tissues, it also unloads NO.

Since the dawn of recorded human history, nitrates have been used to preserve meat from bacterial spoilage. Harmless bacteria in our throat convert nitrates in our food into nitrites. When the nitrites reach the stomach, the acidic gastric juice (pH ~1.4) generates NO from these nitrites, killing almost all the bacteria that have been swallowed in our food.

In the cardiovascular system, NO is produced primarily by vascular endothelial cells. This endothelial-derived NO has several important functions, including relaxing VSM (vasodilation), inhibiting platelet aggregation (antithrombotic), and inhibiting leukocyte-endothelial interactions (anti-inflammatory). These actions involve NO-stimulated formation of cGMP (Fig. 19.38). Nitrodilator are drugs that mimic the actions of endogenous NO by releasing NO or forming NO within tissues. These drugs act directly on the VSM to cause relaxation and, therefore, serve as endothelial-independent vasodilators.

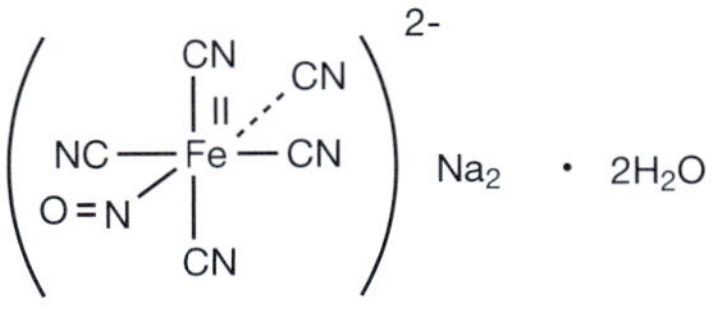

Sodium nitroprusside

There are two basic types of nitrodilators: those that release NO spontaneously (eg, sodium nitroprusside) and those that require an enzyme activation to form NO (organic nitrates). Sodium nitroprusside is a direct-acting vasodilator on VSM, producing its vasodilation by the release of NO. Since 1929, it has been known as a rapidly acting hypotensive agent when administered as an infusion. It is chemically and structurally unrelated to other available hypotensive agents.

Common Adverse Effects. The most clinically important adverse effects of sodium nitroprusside are profound hypotension and the accumulation of cyanide and thiocyanate.[6] Thiocyanate can accumulate in the blood of patients receiving sodium nitroprusside therapy, especially in those with impaired renal function. Thiocyanate is mildly neurotoxic at serum concentrations of 60 μg/mL and can be life-threatening at concentrations of 200 μg/mL. Other adverse effects of thiocyanate include inhibition of both the uptake and binding of iodine, producing symptoms of hypothyroidism.

Sodium nitroprusside can bind to vitamin B_{12}, interfering with its distribution and metabolism, and it should be used with caution in patients having low plasma vitamin B_{12} concentrations. Use of this drug can result in the formation of methemoglobin (which contains ferric iron in its heme groups), an oxidized form of hemoglobin that cannot bind or transport oxygen, in erythrocytes.

Common Interactions. The hypotensive effect of sodium nitroprusside is augmented by concomitant use of other hypotensive agents and is not blocked by adrenergic blocking agents. It has no direct effect on the myocardium, but it can exert a direct coronary vasodilator effect on VSM. When sodium nitroprusside is administered to hypertensive patients, a slight increase in heart rate commonly occurs, and cardiac output is usually decreased slightly. Moderate doses of sodium nitroprusside in patients with hypertension produce renal vasodilation without an appreciable increase in renal blood flow or decrease in glomerular filtration.[6]

MEDICINAL CHEMISTRY OF NITRODILATORS

Receptor Binding, Structure-Activity Relationships and Physicochemical Properties. The potency of sodium nitroprusside is expressed in terms of the dihydrated drug. When reconstituted with 5% dextrose injection, sodium nitroprusside solutions are reddish-brown in color, with a pH of 3.5 to 6.0. Its crystals and solutions are sensitive and unstable to light and should be protected from extremes of light and heat. The exposure of sodium nitroprusside solutions to light causes deterioration, which can be evidenced by a change from a reddish-brown to a green

Structure Challenge

The structures of several antihypertensive agents discussed in this chapter are shown below.

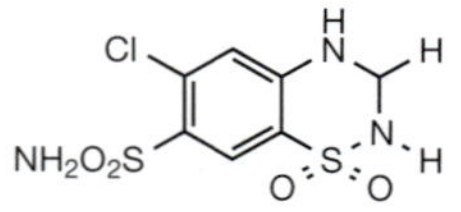

Hydrochlorothiazide

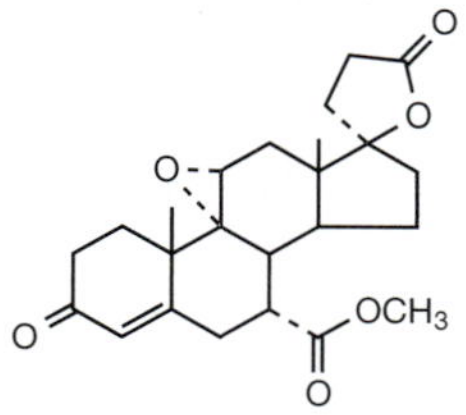

Eplerenone

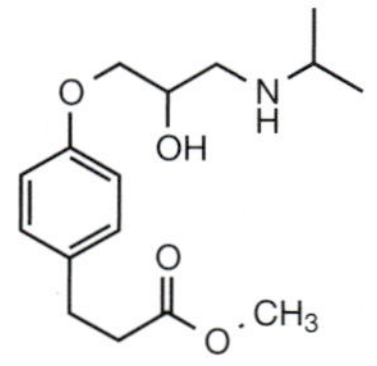

Esmolol

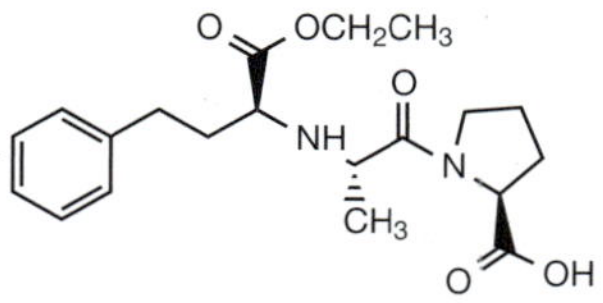

Enalapril

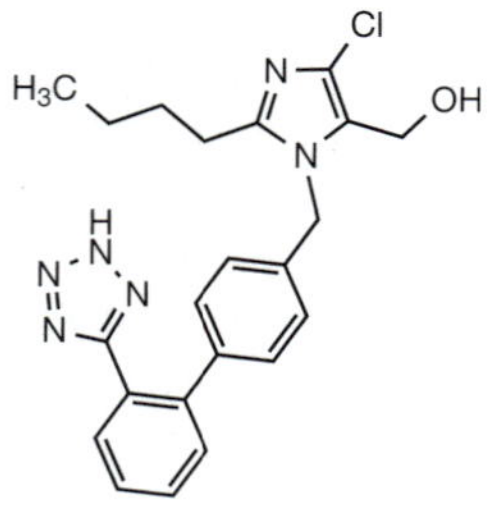

Losartan

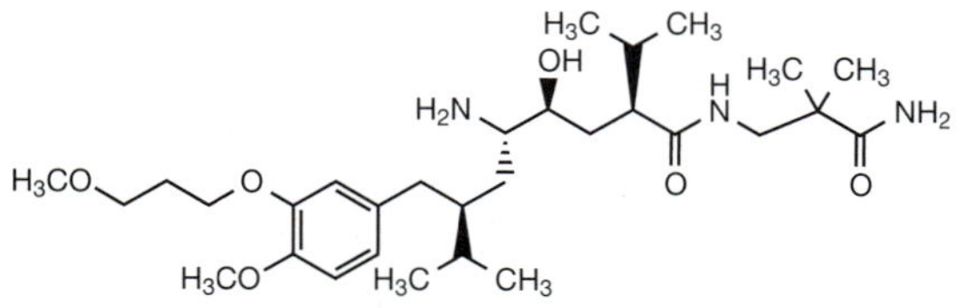

Aliskiren

For each drug provide the following information:

1. Mechanism of action.
2. Important structural features that are required for its mechanism of action.
3. Effect of drug metabolism on its therapeutic activity and how the drug and/or its metabolite(s) are eliminated from the body.

Structure Challenge answers found immediately after References.

to a blue color, indicating a rearrangement of the nitroso to the inactive isonitro form. Sodium nitroprusside solutions in glass bottles undergo approximately 20% degradation within 4 hours when exposed to fluorescent light and even more rapid degradation in plastic bags. Sodium nitroprusside solutions should be protected from light by wrapping the container with aluminum foil or other opaque material. When adequately protected from light, reconstituted solutions are stable for 24 hours. Trace metals, such as iron and copper, can catalyze the degradation of nitroprusside solutions, releasing cyanide. Any change in color for the nitroprusside solutions is an indication of degradation, and the solution should be discarded. No other drug or preservative should be added to stabilize sodium nitroprusside infusions.

Pharmacokinetic Properties and Metabolism. Intravenous infusion of sodium nitroprusside produces an almost immediate reduction in blood pressure. Blood pressure begins to rise immediately when the infusion is slowed or stopped and returns to pretreatment levels within 1 to 10 minutes.

Sodium nitroprusside is not an active hypotensive drug until metabolized to its active metabolite, NO, the mechanism of action of which has been previously described (Fig. 19.38). Studies with sodium nitroprusside suggest that it releases NO by its interaction with glutathione or with sulfhydryl groups in the erythrocytes and tissues to form an S-nitrosothiol intermediate, which spontaneously produces NO, which in turn freely diffuses into the VSM, thereby increasing intracellular cGMP concentration.[6,105,106] NO also activates K^+ channels, which leads to hyperpolarization and relaxation.

Sodium nitroprusside undergoes a redox reaction that releases cyanide.[6,105,106] The cyanide that is produced is rapidly converted into thiocyanate in the liver by the enzyme thiosulfate sulfurtransferase (rhodanese) and is excreted in the urine.[6,105,106] The rate-limiting step in the conversion of cyanide to thiocyanate is the availability of sulfur donors, especially thiosulfate. Toxic symptoms of thiocyanate begin to appear at plasma thiocyanate concentrations of 50 to 100 μg/mL. The elimination half-life of thiocyanate is 2.7 to 7.0 days when renal function is normal but longer in patients with impaired renal function.

ACKNOWLEDGMENTS

The authors wish to acknowledge the work of Marc W. Harrold who authored content used within this chapter in previous editions of this text.

REFERENCES

1. Tsao CW, Aday AW, Amarzooq ZI, et al. Heart disease and stroke statistics—2023 update: a report from the American Heart Association. *Circulation*. 2023;147:e93-e621.
2. Weibert RT. Hypertension. In: Herfindal ET, Gourley DR, eds. *Textbook of Therapeutics: Drug and Disease Management*. 7th ed. Lippincott Williams & Wilkins; 2000:795-824.
3. James PA, Oparil S, Carter BL, et al. evidence-based guideline for the management of high blood pressure in adults: report from the panel members appointed to the Eighth Joint National Committee (JNC 8). *JAMA*. 2014;311(5):507-520.
4. Brown MJ, Haydock S. Pathoetiology, epidemiology and diagnosis of hypertension. *Drugs*. 2000;59(suppl 2):1-12.
5. Sibai B. Treatment of hypertension in pregnant women. *N Engl J Med*. 1996;335:257-265.
6. McEvoy GK, ed. *AHFS 2000 Drug Information*. American Society of Health-System Pharmacists; 2000:1658-1726.
7. Kaplan NM. Combination therapy for systemic hypertension. *Am J Cardiol*. 1995;76:595-597.
8. Abernethy DR. Pharmacological properties of combination therapies for hypertension. *Am J Hypertens*. 1997;10:13S-16S.
9. Reilly RF, Jackson EK. Regulation of renal function and vascular volume. In: Brunton LL, Chabner BA, Knollmann BC, eds. *Goodman and Gilman's the Pharmacological Basis of Therapeutics*. 12th ed. McGraw Hill; 2011:671-719.
10. Padilla MCA, Armas-Hernandez MJ, Hernandez RH, et al. Update of diuretics in the treatment of hypertension. *Am J Ther*. 2007;14:154-160.
11. Supuran CT. Diuretics: from classical carbonic anhydrase inhibitors to novel applications of the sulfonamides. *Curr Pharm Des*. 2008;14:641-648.
12. Ernst ME, Moser M. Use of diuretics in patients with hypertension. *N Engl J Med*. 2009;361:2153-2164.
13. Ernst ME, Gordon JA. Diuretic therapy: key aspects in hypertension and renal disease. *J Nephrol*. 2010;23:487-493.
14. Cadwallader AB, de la Torre X, Tieri A, et al. The abuse of diuretics as performance-enhancing drugs and masking agents in sport doping: pharmacology, toxicology and analysis. *Brit J Pharmacol*. 2010;161:1-16.
15. Deventer K, Baele G, Van Eenoo P, et al. Stability of selected chlorinated thiazide diuretics. *J Pharm Biomed Anal*. 2009;49: 519-524.
16. Nissenson AR, Weston RE, Kleeman CR. Mannitol. *West J Med*. 1979;131:277-284.
17. Mincione F, Menabuoni L, Supuran CT. Clinical applications of carbonic anhydrase inhibitors in ophthalmology. In: Supuran CT, Scozzafava A, Conway J, eds. *Carbonic Anhydrase Its Inhibitors and Activators*. CRC Press; 2004:243-254.
18. Sprague JM. The chemistry of diuretics. *Ann NY Acad Sci*. 1958;71:328-342.
19. Maren TH. Relations between structure and biological activity of sulfonamides. *Annu Rev Pharmacol Toxicol*. 1976;16:309-327.
20. Fitzgerald D. Trails of discovery: a cornerstone of cardiovascular therapy: the thiazide diuretics. *Dialogues Cardiovasc Med*. 2005;10:175-182.
21. Tamargo J, Segura J, Ruilope LM. Diuretics in the treatment of hypertension. Part 1: thiazide and thiazide-like diuretics. *Expert Opin Pharmacother*. 2014;15:527-547.
22. Campbell DB, Taylor AR, Hopkins YW, et al. Pharmacokinetics and metabolism of indapamide: a review. *Curr Med Res Opin*. 1977;5(suppl S1):13-24.
23. Sun H, Moore C, Dansette PM, et al. Dehydrogenation of the indoline-containing drug 4-chloro-*N*-(2-methyl-1-indolinyl)-3-sulfamoylbenzamide (Indapamide) by CYP3A4: correlation with in silico predictions. *Drug Metab Dispos*. 2009;37:672-684.
24. Wargo KA, Banta WM. A comprehensive review of the loop diuretics: should furosemide be first line? *Ann Pharmacother*. 2009;43:1836-1847.
25. Tamargo J, Segura J, Ruilope LM. Diuretics in the treatment of hypertension. Part 2: loop diuretics and potassium-sparing agents. *Expert Opin Pharmacother*. 2014;15:605-621.
26. Beermann B, Dalen E, Lindstrom B, et al. On the fate of furosemide in man. *Eur J Clin Pharmacol*. 1975;9:57-61.
27. Feit PW. Bumetanide—the way to its chemical structure. *J Clin Pharmacol*. 1981;21:531-536.
28. Blose JS, Adams KF, Patterson JH. Torsemide: a pyridine-sulfonylurea loop diuretic. *Ann Pharmacother*. 1995;29:396-402.

29. Koechel DA. Ethacrynic acid and related diuretics: relationship of structure to beneficial and detrimental actions. *Annu Rev Pharmacol Toxicol.* 1981;21:265-293.
30. Fogerson FM, Brennan FE, Fuller PJ. Mineralocorticoid receptor binding, structure and function. *Mol Cell Endocrinol.* 2004;217:203-212.
31. Garthwaite SM, McMahon EG. The evolution of aldosterone antagonists. *Mol Cell Endocrinol.* 2004;217:27-31.
32. Craft J. Eplerenone (Inspra), a new aldosterone antagonist for the treatment of systemic hypertension and heart failure. *Proc (Bayl Univ Med Cent).* 2004;17:217-220.
33. Fagart J, Seguin C, Pinon GM, et al. The Met852 residue is a key organizer of the ligand-binding cavity of the human mineralocorticoid receptor. *Mol Pharmacol.* 2005;67:1714-1722.
34. Huyet J, Pinon GM, Fay MR, et al. Structural basis of spironolactone recognition by the mineralocorticoid receptor. *Mol Pharmacol.* 2007;72:563-571.
35. de Gasparo M, Joss U, Ramjoue HP, et al. Three new epoxy-spironolactone derivatives: characterization in vivo and in vitro. *J Pharmacol Exp Ther.* 1987;240:650-656.
36. Rogerson FM, Yao Y, Smith BJ, et al. Differences in the determinants of eplerenone, spironolactone and aldosterone binding to the mineralocorticoid receptor. *Clin Exp Pharmacol Physiol.* 2004;31:704-709.
37. Ramsay L, Shelton J, Harrison I, et al. Spironolactone and potassium canrenoate in normal man. *Clin Pharmacol Ther.* 1976;20:167-177.
38. Overdiek HW, Merkus FW. The metabolism and biopharmaceutics of spironolactone in man. *Drug Metab Drug Interact.* 1987;5:273-302.
39. Cook CS, Berry LM, Bible RH, et al. Pharmacokinetics and metabolism of [14C]eplerenone after oral administration to humans. *Drug Metab Dispos.* 2003;31:1448-1455.
40. Singh AK, Singh A, Singh R, et al. Finerenone in diabetic kidney disease: a systematic review and critical appraisal. *Diabetes Metab Syndr.* 2022;16:102638.
41. Di Lullo L, Lavalle C, Scatena A, et al. Finerenone: questions and answers- the four fundamental arguments on the new-born promising non-steroidal mineralocorticoid receptor antagonist. *J Clin Med.* 2023;12:3992.
42. Barrera-Chimal J, Kolkhof P, Lima-Posada I, et al. Differentiation between emerging non-steroidal and established steroidal mineralocorticoid receptor antagonists: head-to-head comparisons of pharmacological and clinical characteristics. *Expert Opin Investig Drugs.* 2021;30:1141-1157.
43. Lerma EV, Wilson DJ. Finerenone: a mineralocorticoid receptor antagonist for the treatment of chronic kidney disease associated with type 2 diabetes. *Expert Rev Clin Pharmacol.* 2022;15:501-513.
44. Canessa CM, Schild L, Buell G, et al. Amiloride-sensitive epithelial Na^+ channel is made of three homologous subunits. *Nature.* 1994;367:463-467.
45. Busch AE, Suessbrich H, Kunzelmann K, et al. Blockade of epithelial Na^+ channels by triamterenes—underlying mechanisms and molecular basis. *Pflugers Arch Eur J Physiol.* 1996;432:760-766.
46. Fuhr U, Kober S, Zaigler M, et al. Rate-limiting biotransformation of triamterene is mediated by CYP1A2. *Int J Clin Pharmacol Ther.* 2005;43:327-334.
47. Sriram K, Insel PA. Renin and angiotensin. In: Brunton LL, Knollmann BC, eds. *Goodman & Gilman's: The Pharmacological Basis of Therapeutics.* 14th ed. McGraw Hill; 2023.
48. Skeggs L. Historical overview of the renin-angiotensin system. In: Doyle AE, Bearn AG, eds. *Hypertension and the Angiotensin System: Therapeutic Approaches.* Raven Press; 1984:31-45.
49. Vallotton MB. The renin-angiotensin system. *Trends Pharmacol Sci.* 1987;8:69-74.
50. Skidgel RA, Kaplan AP, Erdos EG. Histamine, bradykinin, and their antagonists. In: Brunton LL, Chabner BA, Knollman BC, eds. *Goodman & Gilman's the Pharmacological Basis of Therapeutics.* 12th ed. McGraw Hill; 2011:911-935.
51. Ferrario CM, Brosnihan KB, Diz DI, et al. Angiotensin-(1–7): a new hormone of the angiotensin system. *Hypertension.* 1991;18(5 suppl):126-133.
52. Agarwal SK, Chambless LE, Ballantyne CM, et al. Prediction of incident heart failure in general practice: the Atherosclerosis Risk in Communities (ARIC) study. *Circ Heart Fail.* 2012;5:422-429.
53. Patel J. Heart failure population health considerations. *Am J Manag Care.* 2021;27(9 suppl):S191-S195.
54. Harvison PJ, Harrold MW. Drugs used to treat hypertensive/hypotensive disorders. In: Lemke TL, Williams DA, Roche VF, et al, eds. *Foye's Principles of Medicinal Chemistry.* 8th ed. Wolters Kluwer/Lippincott Williams & Wilkins; 2019:694-721.
55. Ondetti MA, Rubin B, Cushman DW. Design of specific inhibitors of angiotensin-converting enzyme: new class of orally active antihypertensive agents. *Science.* 1977;196:441-444.
56. Cushman DW, Cheung HS, Sabo EF, et al. Design of potent competitive inhibitors of angiotensin-converting enzyme. Carboxyalkanoyl and mercaptoalkanoyl amino acids. *Biochemistry.* 1977;16:5484-5491.
57. Ondetti MA, Cushman DW. Enzymes of the renin-angiotensin system and their inhibitors. *Annu Rev Biochem.* 1982;51:283-308.
58. Ferreira SH, Bartelt DC, Lewis LJ. Isolation of bradykinin-potentiating peptides from Bothrops jararaca venom. *Biochemistry.* 1970;9:2583-2593.
59. Bakhle YS. Conversion of angiotensin I to angiotensin II by cell-free extracts of dog lung. *Nature.* 1968;220:919-921.
60. Stryer L. *Biochemistry.* 4th ed. Freeman and Company; 1995:218-222.
61. Klaassen CD. Heavy metals and heavy-metal antagonists. In: Brunton L, Lazo J, Parker K, et al, eds. *Goodman & Gilman's the Pharmacological Basis of Therapeutics.* 11th ed. McGraw Hill; 2006:1753-1775.
62. Atkinson AB, Robertson JIS. Captopril in the treatment of clinical hypertension and cardiac failure. *Lancet.* 1979;2:836-839.
63. Patchett AA, Harris E, Tristram EW, et al. A new class of angiotensin-converting enzyme inhibitors. *Nature.* 1980;288:280-283.
64. Krapcho J, Turk C, Cushman DW, et al. Angiotensin-converting enzyme inhibitors. Mercaptan, carboxyalkyl dipeptide, and phosphinic acid inhibitors incorporating 4-substituted prolines. *J Med Chem.* 1988;31:1148-1160.
65. Timmermans PB, Wong PC, Chiu AT, et al. Angiotensin II receptors and angiotensin II receptor antagonists. *Pharmacol Rev.* 1993;45:205-213.
66. Skeggs L, Kahn JR, Lentz K, et al. Preparation, purification and amino acid sequence of a polypeptide renin substrate. *J Exp Med.* 1957;106:439-453.
67. Sepehrdad R, Frishman WH, Steier C, et al. Direct inhibition of renin as a cardiovascular pharmacotherapy: focus on aliskiren. *Cardiol Rev.* 2007;15:242-256.
68. Maibaum J, Stutz S, Goschke R, et al. Structural modification of the P2' position of 2,7-dialkyl-substituted 5(S)-amino-4(S)-hydroxy-8-phenyl-octanecarboxamides: the discovery of aliskiren, a potent nonpeptide human renin inhibitor active after once daily dosing in marmosets. *J Med Chem.* 2007;50:4832-4844.
69. Fisher NDL, Hollenberg NK. Renin inhibition: what are the therapeutic opportunities? *J Am Soc Nephrol.* 2005;16:592-599.
70. Vaidyanathan S, Jarugula V, Dieterich HA, et al. Clinical pharmacokinetics and pharmacodynamics of aliskiren. *Clin Pharmacokinet.* 2008;47(8):515-531.
71. Heerspink HJL, Radhakrishnan J, Alpers CE, et al. Sparsentan in patients with IgA nephropathy: a prespecified interim analysis from a randomised, double-blind, active-controlled clinical trial. *Lancet.* 2023;401(10388):1584-1594.
72. Goyal A, Cusick AS, Thielemier B. ACE inhibitors. In: *StatPearls* [Internet]. StatPearls Publishing; 2023. Updated July 12, 2022. Accessed June 29, 2023. https://www.ncbi.nlm.nih.gov/books/NBK430896/

73. Hill RD, Vaidya PN. Angiotensin II receptor blockers (ARB). In: *StatPearls* [Internet]. StatPearls Publishing; 2023. Updated March 27, 2023. Accessed June 29, 2023. https://www.ncbi.nlm.nih.gov/books/NBK537027/
74. James PA, Oparil S, Carter BL, et al. 2014 evidence-based guideline for the management of high blood pressure in adults. *JAMA*. 2014;311(5):507-520.
75. Heidenreich PA, Bozkurt B, Aguilar D, et al. 2022 AHA/ACC/HFSA guideline for the management of heart failure: executive summary: a report of the American College of Cardiology/American Heart Association Joint Committee on Clinical Practice Guidelines. *J Am Coll Cardiol*. 2022;79(17):1757-1780.
76. Parker RB, Nappi JM, Cavallari LH. Chronic heart failure. In: Dipiro JT, Talbert RL, Yee GC, et al, eds. *Pharmacotherapy: A Pathophysiologic Approach*. 9th ed. McGraw Hill; 2014:85-122.
77. Saseen JJ, MacLaughlin EJ. Hypertension. In: Dipiro JT, Talbert RL, Yee GC, et al, eds. *Pharmacotherapy: A Pathophysiologic Approach*. 9th ed. McGraw Hill; 2014:49-84.
78. Bokhari SRA, Zulfiqar H, Mansur A. Bartter syndrome. In: *StatPearls* [Internet]. StatPearls Publishing; 2023. Updated December 24, 2022. Accessed June 29, 2023. https://www.ncbi.nlm.nih.gov/books/NBK442019/
79. Pitcher A, Spata E, Emberson J, et al. Angiotensin receptor blockers and β blockers in Marfan syndrome: an individual patient data meta-analysis of randomised trials. *Lancet*. 2022;400(10355):822-831.
80. Dziadzio M, Denton CP, Smith R, et al. Losartan therapy for Raynaud's phenomenon and scleroderma: clinical and biochemical findings in a fifteen-week, randomized, parallel-group, controlled trial. *Arthritis Rheum*. 1999;42(12):2646-2655.
81. Bauer JH, Reams GP. The angiotensin II type 1 receptor antagonists: a new class of antihypertensive drugs. *Arch Intern Med*. 1995;155:1361-1368.
82. Miura S, Karnik SS, Saku K. Review: angiotensin II type 1 receptor blockers: class effects versus molecular effects. *J Renin Angiotensin Aldosterone Syst*. 2011;12(1):1-7.
83. Aliskiren (Tekturna) for hypertension. *Med Lett Drugs Ther*. 2007;49:29-31.
84. Lacourciere Y, Brunner H, Irwin R, et al. Effects of modulators of the renin-angiotensin-aldosterone system on cough. Losartan Cough Study Group. *J Hypertens*. 1994;12:1387-1393.
85. Gringauz A. *Introduction to Medicinal Chemistry*. Wiley; 1997:450-461.
86. ChemSketch (Freeware), version 2022.2.3 (File Version C45E41, Build 130928, December 16, 2022). Advanced Chemistry Development. Available at: https://www.acdlabs.com/resources/free-chemistry-software-apps/chemsketch-freeware/.
87. Gross DM, Sweet CS, Ulm EH, et al. Effect of *N*-[(*S*)-1-carboxy-3-phenylpropyl]-L-Ala-L-Pro and its ethyl ester (MK-421) on angiotensin converting enzyme in vitro and angiotensin I pressor responses in vivo. *J Pharmacol Exp Ther*. 1981;216:552-557.
88. Ulm EH, Hichens M, Gomez HJ, et al. Enalapril maleate and a lysine analogue (MK-521): disposition in man. *Br J Clin Pharmacol*. 1982;14:357-362.
89. Oparil S, Koerner T, Tregear GW, et al. Substrate requirements for angiotensin I conversion in vivo and in vitro. *Circ Res*. 1973;32:415-423.
90. Khan MOF, Murphy K. Drugs affecting renin-angiotensin system. In: *Medicinal Chemistry of Drugs Affecting Cardiovascular and Endocrine Systems*. Medicinal Chemistry for Pharmacy Students. 2024;3:1-39. doi:10.2174/9789815179729124030004.
91. Carini DJ, Duncia JV, Aldrich PE, et al. Nonpeptide angiotensin II receptor antagonists: the discovery of a series of *N*-(biphenylylmethyl)imidazoles as potent, orally active antihypertensives. *J Med Chem*. 1991;35:2525-2547.
92. Pradhan A, Gupta V, Sethi R. Fimasartan: a new armament to fight hypertension. *J Family Med Prim Care*. 2019;8(7):2184-2188.
93. Angeli F, Verdecchia P, Trapasso M, et al. PK/PD evaluation of fimasartan for the treatment of hypertension current evidences and future perspectives. *Expert Opin Drug Metab Toxicol*. 2018;14(5):533-541.
94. Kim JH, Lee JH, Paik SH, et al. Fimasartan, a novel angiotensin II receptor antagonist. *Arch Pharm Res*. 2012;35(7):1123-1126.
95. Komers R, Gipson DS, Nelson P, et al. Efficacy and safety of sparsentan compared with irbesartan in patients with primary focal segmental glomerulosclerosis: randomized, controlled trial design (DUET). *Kidney Int Rep*. 2017;2(4):654-664.
96. Kim TH, Shin S, Bashir M, et al. Pharmacokinetics and metabolite profiling of fimasartan, a novel antihypertensive agent, in rats. *Xenobiotica*. 2014;44(10):913-925.
97. Syed YY. Sparsentan: first approval [published correction appears in *Drugs*. 2023;83(10):955]. *Drugs*. 2023;83(6):563-568.
98. Salim H, Jones AM. Angiotensin II receptor blockers (ARBs) and manufacturing contamination: a retrospective National Register Study into suspected associated adverse drug reactions. *Br J Clin Pharmacol*. 2022;88(11):4812-4827.
99. Lunney EA, Hamilton HW, Hodges JC, et al. Analyses of ligand binding in five endothiapepsin crystal complexes and their use in the design and evaluation of novel renin inhibitors. *J Med Chem*. 1993;36:3809-3820.
100. Matter H, Scheiper B, Steinhagen H, et al. Structure-based design and optimization of potent renin inhibitors on 5- or 7-azaindole-scaffolds. *Bio Med Chem Lett*. 2011;21:5487-5492.
101. Cutler SJ, Cocolas GH. Cardiovascular agents. In: Block JH, Beale JM, eds. *Wilson and Gisvold's Textbook of Organic Medicinal and Pharmaceutical Chemistry*. 11th ed. Lippincott Williams & Wilkins; 2004:622-675.
102. Silverthorn DU. *Human Physiology: An Integrated Approach*. 4th ed. Benjamin Cummings; 2006:397-432.
103. Janis RA, Triggle DJ. New developments in Ca^{2+} channel antagonists. *J Med Chem*. 1983;26:775-785.
104. Swamy VC, Triggle DJ. Calcium channel blockers. In: Craig CR, Stitzel RE, eds. *Modern Pharmacology with Clinical Applications*. 6th ed. Lippincott Williams & Wilkins; 2003:218-224.
105. Eschenhagen T. Treatment of hypertension. In: Brunton LL, Hilal-Dandan R, Knollmann BC, eds. *Goodman & Gilman's: The Pharmacological Basis of Therapeutics*. 13th ed. McGraw Hill; 2017.
106. Eschenhagen T. Treatment of ischemic heart disease. In: Brunton LL, Knollmann BC, eds. *Goodman & Gilman's: The Pharmacological Basis of Therapeutics*. 14th ed. McGraw Hill; 2023.
107. Oakes SC. Cell injury, cell death, and adaptations. In: Kumar V, Abbas AK, Aster JC, eds. *Robbins & Cotran Pathologic Basis of Disease*. 10th ed. Elsevier; 2021:33-35.
108. Tsao CW, Aday AW, Almarzooq ZI, et al. Heart disease and stroke statistics-2023 update: a report from the American Heart Association [published correction appears in *Circulation*. 2023;147(8):e622]. *Circulation*. 2023;147(8):e93-e621.
109. Vaghy PL. Calcium antagonists. In: Brody TM, Larner J, Minneman KP, et al, eds. *Human Pharmacology: Molecular to Clinical*. 2nd ed. Mosby; 1994:203-213.
110. Triggle DJ. Drugs acting on ion channels and membranes. In: Hansch C, Sammes PG, Taylor JB, eds. *Comprehensive Medicinal Chemistry*. Vol 3. Pergamon Press; 1990:1047-1099.
111. Loev B, Ehrreich SJ, Tedeschi RE. Dihydropyridines with potent hypotensive activity prepared by the Hantzsch reaction. *J Pharm Pharmacol*. 1972;24:917-918.
112. Loev B, Goodman MM, Snader KM, et al. "Hantzsch-type" dihydropyridine hypotensive agents. *J Med Chem*. 1974;17:956-965.
113. Triggle AM, Shefter E, Triggle DJ. Crystal structures of calcium channel antagonists: 2,6-dimethyl-3,5-dicarbomethoxy-4-[2-nitro, 3-cyano-, 4-(dimethylamino)-, and 2,3,4,5,6-pentafluorophenyl]-1,4-dihydropyridine. *J Med Chem*. 1980;23:1442-1445.
114. Safety of calcium-channel blockers. *Med Lett Drugs Ther*. 1997;39:13-14.

115. Lexicomp. UpToDate Lexidrug: evidence-based drug referential content for teams. Wolters Kluwer Health. Accessed June 4, 2023. https://www.wolterskluwer.com/en/solutions/lexicomp
116. Varadi G, Mori Y, Mikala G, et al. Molecular determinants of Ca^{2+} channel function and drug action. *Trends Pharmacol Sci.* 1995;16:43-49.
117. Gilmore J, Dell C, Bowman D, et al. Neuronal calcium channels. *Annu Rep Med Chem.* 1995;30:51-60.
118. Zamponi GW, Striessnig J, Koschak A, et al. The physiology, pathology, and pharmacology of voltage-gated calcium channels and their future therapeutic potential. *Pharmacol Rev.* 2015;67(4):821-870.
119. Catterall WA, Perez-Reyes E, Snutch TP, et al. International Union of Pharmacology. XLVIII. Nomenclature and structure-function relationships of voltage-gated calcium channels. *Pharmacol Rev.* 2005;57(4):411-425.
120. Calculated using ChemBioDraw Ultra Software V12.0 (1986–2009). CambridgeSoft. Available at: https://revvitysignals.com/products/research/chemdraw.
121. Bailey DG, Arnold JMO, Spence JD. Grapefruit juice and drugs: how significant is the interaction? *Clin Pharmacokinet.* 1994;26:91-98.
122. Drug interactions with grapefruit juice. *Med Lett Drugs Ther.* 2004;46:2-4.
123. Sampson KJ, Kass RS. Anti-arrhythmic drugs. In: Brunton LL, Chabner BA, Knollman BC, eds. *Goodman & Gilman's the Pharmacological Basis of Therapeutics.* 12th ed. McGraw Hill; 2011:815-848.
124. Yeh D, Michel T. Pharmacology of vascular tone. In: Goan DE, Tashjian A, Armstrong E, et al, eds. *Principles of Pharmacology: The Pathophysiologic Basis of Drug Therapy.* Lippincott Williams & Wilkins; 2004:317-330.
125. Von Euler US. Synthesis, uptake, and storage of catecholamines in adrenergic nerves: the effect of drugs. In: Blaschko H, Marshall E, eds. *Catecholamines.* Springer; 1972:186-230.
126. Griffith RK. Adrenergics and adrenergic-blocking drugs. In: Abraham DJ, ed. *Burger's Medicinal Chemistry and Drug Discovery.* John Wiley and Sons; 2003:1-37.
127. Ahlquist RP. A study of the adrenotropic receptors. *Am J Physiol.* 1948;153:586-600.
128. Harrison JK, Pearson WR, Lynch KR. Molecular characterization of α1- and α2-adrenoceptors. *Trends Pharmacol Sci.* 1991;12:62-67.
129. De Souza CJ, Burkey BF. β3-Adrenoceptor agonists as anti-diabetic and antiobesity drugs in humans. *Curr Pharm Des.* 2001;7:1433-1449.
130. Robertson JIS. State-of-the-art review: β-blockade and the treatment of hypertension. *Drugs.* 1983;25(suppl 2):5-11.
131. Freis ED, Papademetriou V. Current drug treatment and treatment patterns with antihypertensive drugs. *Drugs.* 1996;52:1-16.
132. Husserl FE, Messerli FH. Adverse effects of antihypertensive drugs. *Drugs.* 1981;22:188-210.
133. Goldberg M, Fenster PE. Clinical significance of intrinsic sympathomimetic activity of beta blockers. In: *Drug Therapy.* 1991;21:35-43.
134. Moran NC. New adrenergic blocking drugs: their pharmacological, biochemical, and clinical actions. *Ann NY Acad Sci.* 1967;139:545-548.
135. Jen T, Frazee JS, Schwartz MS, et al. Adrenergic agents. 8. Synthesis and β-adrenergic agonist activity of some 3-tert-butylamino-2-(substituted phenyl)-1-propanols. *J Med Chem.* 1977;20:1263-1268.
136. Cauffield JS, Gums JG, Curry RW. Alpha blockers: a reassessment of their role in therapy. *Am Fam Physician.* 1996;54:263-270.
137. Scriabine A, Constantine JW, Hess HJ, et al. Pharmacological studies with some new antihypertensive aminoquinazolines. *Experientia.* 1968;24:1150-1151.
138. Dunn CJ, Lea AP, Wagstaff AJ. Carvedilol: a reappraisal of its pharmacological properties and therapeutic use in cardiovascular disorders. *Drugs.* 1997;54:161-185.
139. Goa KL, Benfield P, Sorkin EM. Labetalol: a reappraisal of its pharmacology, pharmacokinetics and therapeutic use in hypertension and ischemic heart disease. *Drugs.* 1989;37:583-627.
140. Van Zwieten PA. An overview of the pharmacodynamic properties and therapeutic potential of combined α- and β-adrenoreceptor antagonists. *Drugs.* 1993;45:509-517.
141. Fujimura A, Ebihara A, Ohashi K-I, et al. Comparison of the pharmacokinetics, pharmacodynamics and safety of oral (Catapres) and transdermal (M-5041T) clonidine in healthy subjects. *J Clin Pharmacol.* 1994;34:260-265.
142. Cornish LA. Guanfacine hydrochloride: a centrally acting antihypertensive agent. *Clin Pharm.* 1988;7:187-197.
143. Bousquet P, Feldman J. Drugs acting on imidazoline receptors: a review of their pharmacology, their use in blood pressure control and their potential interest in cardioprotection. *Drugs.* 1999;58:799-812.
144. Piletz JE, Regunathan S, Ernsberger P. Agmatine and imidazolines: their novel receptors and enzymes. *Ann NY Acad Sci.* 2003;1009:xv-xvi.
145. Dardonville C, Rozas I. Imidazoline binding sites and their ligands: an overview of the different chemical structures. *Med Res Rev.* 2004;24:639-661.
146. Ebihara A, Fujimura A, Ohashi K-I, et al. Influence of application site of a new transdermal clonidine M-5041T on its pharmacokinetics and pharmacodynamics in healthy subjects. *J Clin Pharmacol.* 1993;33:1188-1191.
147. Holmes B, Brogden RN, Heel RC, et al. Guanabenz: a review of its pharmacodynamic properties and therapeutic efficacy in hypertension. *Drugs.* 1983;26:212-225.
148. Kobinger W. Central α-adrenergic systems as targets for hypotensive drugs. *Rev Physiol Biochem Pharmacol.* 1978;81:39-100.
149. Kanagy NL. α2-Adrenergic receptor signaling in hypertension. *Clin Sci (Lond).* 2005;109:431-437.
150. Skerjanec A, Campbell NRC, Robertson S, et al. Pharmacokinetics and presystemic gut metabolism of methyldopa in healthy human subjects. *J Clin Pharmacol.* 1995;35:275-280.
151. Langley MS, Heel RC. Transdermal clonidine: a preliminary review of its pharmacodynamic properties and therapeutic efficacy. *Drugs.* 1988;35:123-142.
152. Ziegler D, Haxhiu MA, Kaan EC, et al. Pharmacology of moxonidine, an I1–imidazoline receptor agonist. *J Cardiovascular Pharmacol.* 1996;27(suppl 3):S26-S37.
153. Theodor R, Weimann HJ, Weber W, et al. Absolute bioavailability of moxonidine. *Eur J Drug Metab Pharmacokinet.* 1991;16:153-159.
154. Chrisp P, Faulds D. Moxonidine: a review of its pharmacology and therapeutic use in essential hypertension. *Drugs.* 1992;44:993-1012.
155. Genissel P, Bromet N, Fourtillan JB, et al. Pharmacokinetics of rilmenidine in healthy subjects. *Am J Cardiol.* 1988;61:47D-53D.
156. Genissel P, Bromet N. Pharmacokinetics of rilmenidine. *Am J Med.* 1989;87:8S-23S.
157. Sorkin EM, Heel RC. Guanfacine: a review of its pharmacodynamic and pharmacokinetic properties and therapeutic efficacy in the treatment of hypertension. *Drugs.* 1986;31:301-336.
158. Carchman SH, Crowe JT, Wright GJ. The bioavailability and pharmacokinetics of guanfacine after oral and intravenous administration to healthy volunteers. *J Clin Pharmacol.* 1987;27:762-767.
159. Duty S, Weston AH. Potassium channel openers: pharmacological effects and future uses. *Drugs.* 1990;40:785-791.
160. Campese VM. Minoxidil: a review of its pharmacological properties and therapeutic use. *Drugs.* 1981;22:257-278.
161. Catterall WA, Few AP. Calcium channel regulation and presynaptic plasticity. *Neuron.* 2008;59(6):882-901.

Structure Challenge Answers

1. Mechanism of Action
   A. Hydrochlorothiazide inhibits the Na^+/Cl^- symporter in the distal convoluted tubule of the nephron and therefore blocks reabsorption of Na^+, Cl^-, and H_2O.
   B. Eplerenone is an MR antagonist and inhibits binding of aldosterone to the receptor.
   C. Esmolol is a selective β_1-adrenergic receptor antagonist (β-blocker, BB).
   D. Enalapril is metabolized to enalaprilat, which is an ACE inhibitor.
   E. Losartan is an ARB.
   F. Aliskiren is a direct renin inhibitor and blocks conversion of the precursor angiotensinogen to angiotensin I.
2. Important Structural Features
   A. Hydrochlorothiazide is a member of the thiazide group of diuretics in which the sulfonamide group is necessary for diuretic activity.
   B. Eplerenone contains a steroid nucleus; the γ-lactone ring on C_{17} and substituent at C_7 are also important for its antidiuretic activity. The epoxy group in eplerenone results in a lower affinity for the MR than spironolactone.
   C. Esmolol is an aryloxypropanolamine that contains structural resemblance to norepinephrine.
   D. Enalaprilat, the active metabolite of enalapril, is a structural mimic of a three amino acid sequence (Phe_8-His_9-Leu_{10}) at the carboxy end of ACE; the carboxylic acid is required for binding to an enzyme-bound Zn^{2+} ion.
   E. Losartan has a biphenyl backbone; the tetrazole ring, pyrazole ring, and the n-butyl side-chain mimic amino acids in the structure of angiotensin II.
   F. The structure of aliskiren contains two isopropyl groups that mimic the side chains of two Asp amino acid residues in renin, a hydroxy group that mimics the transition state, and an ether side chain that occupies a subpocket in the enzyme.
3. Metabolism/Elimination
   A. Hydrochlorothiazide does not undergo extensive metabolism and is eliminated in the urine primarily as the parent drug.
   B. Eplerenone is converted to inactive metabolites by CYP3A4, which are eliminated in the urine and feces.
   C. Esmolol undergoes metabolism by esterases to an inactive metabolite, which is eliminated in the urine.
   D. Enalapril is a prodrug and must be metabolized by esterases to the active drug, enalaprilat, which is eliminated in the urine.
   E. Losartan is metabolized (14%) by CYP2C9 and CYP3A4 to the active metabolite EXP-3174; elimination of parent drug and metabolite, occur via the feces (predominant) and urine.
   F. Aliskiren is eliminated in the feces primarily (90%) as the parent drug.

CHAPTER

20

Drugs Used to Treat Ischemic Heart Disease, Heart Failure, and Arrhythmias

Raghunandan Yendapally and Helmut B. Gottlieb

Drugs covered in this chapter:

ANTIANGINAL AGENTS

NITRATES AND NITRITES
- Amyl nitrite
- Isosorbide dinitrate and mononitrate
- Nitroglycerin
- Pentaerythritol tetranitrate

CALCIUM CHANNEL BLOCKERS
- Amlodipine
- Diltiazem
- Nicardipine
- Nifedipine
- Verapamil

β-BLOCKERS
- Atenolol
- Bisoprolol
- Carvedilol
- Esmolol
- Metoprolol
- Propranolol

SODIUM-CHANNEL BLOCKER
- Ranolazine

I_F INHIBITOR
- Ivabradine

DRUGS USED TO TREAT HEART FAILURE

CARDIAC GLYCOSIDES POSITIVE INOTROPIC AGENTS
- Digoxin
- Digitoxin

NONGLYCOSIDIC POSITIVE INOTROPIC AGENTS
- Dobutamine
- Dopamine
- Inamrinone
- Milrinone

NITRATE VASODILATORS
- Isosorbide dinitrate and mononitrate
- Isosorbide dinitrate in combination with hydralazine
- Nitroglycerin

NEPRILYSIN INHIBITOR/ANGIOTENSIN II–RECEPTOR BLOCKER
- Sacubitril/valsartan

SOLUBLE GUANYLYL CYCLASE STIMULATOR
- Vericiguat

TRANSTHYRETIN TETRAMERS STABILIZER
- Tafamidis

ANTI-ARRHYTHMIC AGENTS

CLASS IA
- Disopyramide
- Procainamide
- Quinidine

CLASS IB
- Lidocaine
- Mexiletine
- Phenytoin

CLASS IC
- Flecainide
- Propafenone

CLASS II
- Esmolol

CLASS III
- Amiodarone
- Dofetilide
- Dronedarone
- Ibutilide
- Sotalol

CLASS IV
- Diltiazem
- Verapamil

MISCELLANEOUS AGENTS
- Adenosine
- Magnesium sulfate

Abbreviations

ACC American College of Cardiology
ACE angiotensin-converting enzyme
AHA American Heart Association
ANP atrium natriuretic peptide
AP action potential
ARB angiotensin II-receptor blocker
ATP adenosine triphosphate
ATPase adenosine triphosphatase
ATTR-CM Transthyretin amyloid cardiomyopathy
AT1 angiotensin type I receptor
AUC area under the curve
AV atrioventricular
BBB blood-brain barrier
BCRP breast cancer resistance protein
CAD coronary artery disease
cAMP cyclic adenosine monophosphate
CCB calcium channel blocker
cGMP cyclic guanosine 3′,5′-monophosphate
CHF congestive heart failure
CNS central nervous system
COMT catechol-*O*-methyltransferase
CYP cytochrome P450
DCI dichloroisoproterenol
DDI drug-drug interaction
DHP dihydropyridine
1,4-DHPs 1,4-dihydropyridines
DOPAC 3,4-dihydroxyphenylacetic acid
DOPAL 3,4-dihydroxyphenylacetal-dehyde
DOPET 3,4-dihydroxyphenylethanol
ECG electrocardiogram
FDA US Food and Drug Administration
FS Frank-Starling
1,2-GDN 1,2-glyceryl dinitrate
1,3-GDN 1,3-glyceryl dinitrate
GFR glomerular filtration rate
GI gastrointestinal
Gs stimulatory guanine nucleotide binding proteins
HF heart failure
HFrEF heart failure with reduced ejection fraction
HH hydralazine hydrazone
IBW ideal body weight
IHD ischemic heart disease
IV intravenous
MAO monoamine oxidase
MEGX monoethylglycinexylidide
MI myocardial infarction
mtALDH mitochondrial aldehyde dehydrogenase
NAcHPZ *N*-acetylhydrazinophthalazinone
Non-DHP non-dihydropyridine
NEP neprilysin endopeptidase
NO nitric oxide
NTG nitroglycerin
NYHA New York Heart Association
PDE phosphodiesterase
PDE3 phosphodiesterase-3
PDE4 phosphodiesterase-4
PDE5 phosphodiesterase-5
PEDN pentaerythrityl dinitrate
PEMN pentaerythrityl mononitrate
PETN/PENT/PENTA/TEN pentaerythrityl tetranitrate
PETriN pentaerithrityl trinitrate
PNS parasympathetic nervous system
PZ phthalazinone
ROS reactive oxygen species
SA sinoatrial
sGC soluble guanylyl cyclase
SNO *S*-nitrosothiol
SNS sympathetic nervous system
TP triazolophthalazine
TTR transthyretin

CLINICAL SIGNIFICANCE

The agents described in this chapter are used to treat one or more cardiovascular diseases, including ischemic heart disease (IHD), heart failure (HF), and arrhythmias. Many of these agents are the most prescribed medications, so understanding the medicinal and pharmacokinetic properties of these drugs is important. Physicochemical properties such as lipophilicity and hydrophilicity affect drug distribution. Additionally, structural differences can influence the selectivity, with metoprolol succinate having a lesser impact on blood pressure than carvedilol. Chemical structures also play an important role in potential drug toxicities. For example, the iodine moiety of amiodarone's chemical structure results in an extensive adverse effect profile, including amiodarone-induced thyrotoxicosis. A thorough grasp of medicinal chemistry ensures that these medications are used safely and effectively.

Kathleen A. Lusk, PharmD, BCPS, BCCP

Drugs for the Treatment of Angina

Ischemic Heart Disease

According to the US Centers for Disease Control and Prevention, cardiovascular disease is the #1 cause of death in the United States. Cardiovascular disease encompasses several heart and blood vessel diseases and includes atrial fibrillation, HF, coronary heart disease, hypertension, and stroke. The American Heart Association (AHA) estimates that by 2035, nearly half of the United States population will have some form of cardiovascular disease. It also projects that the estimated US economic burden is about to increase from $555 billion in 2016 to more than $1 trillion by 2035.[1] More than half of the deaths are caused by heart disease, and coronary artery disease (CAD) is the most frequent type of heart disease. Because of its prevalence, CAD is one of the costliest chronic diseases. With the aging of the "Baby Boom" population, it is predicted that the health care cost, mortality, and morbidity rate associated with CAD will continue to rise. Although our understanding and treatment of CAD has improved over the last few years, these efforts have been insufficient to slow down or reverse the epidemic trend.

One of the most common manifestations of CAD is ischemic heart disease (IHD), which is also known as angina pectoris. IHD is manifested as asymptomatic (silent IHD) or symptomatic chest pain.[2] In both cases, it is caused by the buildup of atherosclerotic plaques in the coronary arteries, or by the disruption and rupture of atherosclerotic plaque's protective fibrous cap. An increase in plaque buildup leads to a reduction in the coronary artery lumen radius, which results in a decrease of blood flow to certain areas of the heart. In contrast, rupture of the plaque's cap leads to thrombosis, which can completely occlude the coronary blood vessel. A thrombus can also be dislodged and travel within the blood vessels, which is known as an embolus. Eventually an embolus can lodge within a small blood vessel and completely block the blood supply, resulting in an embolism. Thus, if an embolism occurs in the coronary arteries, it can deprive the myocardium of essential blood flow, which is essential for the maintenance of healthy tissue and results in a myocardial infarction (MI). As such, angina pectoris occurs when there is an imbalance between the amount of oxygenated blood being delivered to the heart (supply) versus the amount of blood required by the heart to maintain its required metabolic needs (demand).[3] It is widely accepted that decreased blood delivery, either by partial or total occlusion, to coronary arteries will lead to myocardial ischemia with consequent damage or death of the myocardial tissue. This ultimately leads to an increased mortality and morbidity, as well as the development of other cardiovascular diseases discussed in this chapter (HF and arrhythmias). IHD is typically divided into three major classes.[2,4,5]

1. Stable IHD is caused by the partial blockade or narrowing of the coronary artery. In these patients, exertion typically causes an increase in demand with no significant change in the supply of oxygenated blood. Resting and drug therapy typically resolve chest pain within a few minutes. Drug therapy for most patients includes agents that decrease the workload of the heart and thus decrease the frequency of angina attacks. Drugs that cause vasodilation to increase the delivery of blood to the ischemic site may also be utilized. Finally, drugs such as statins and aspirin are useful in maintaining the supply of blood flow and are indicated for patients with other comorbidities.
2. Unstable IHD is caused by the rupture of atherosclerotic plaques, which lead to thrombosis and embolism. In this case, aggressive drug therapy and surgical procedures may be required to resolve and prevent further damage to the myocardium. Prophylactic therapy is aimed at reducing clot formations or increasing plaque cap stability.
3. Coronary artery vasospasm (a.k.a. Prinzmetal or variant angina) is triggered by the quivering of the coronary smooth muscle and can occur in both atherosclerotic and nonatherosclerotic coronary arteries. However, patients with variant angina are typically younger and do not have many IHD risk factors. Drug therapy is aimed at producing vasodilation at the coronary artery and restoring blood flow.

There are several factors that can affect the myocardial oxygen demand. The primary site of action is the heart itself, which is modulated by the parasympathetic nervous system (PNS) and sympathetic nervous system (SNS).[6] Under exercise conditions, the SNS, via the release of norepinephrine, activates β-adrenergic receptors. Activation of these receptors produces an increase in heart rate and strength of myocardial contraction and decreased diastolic filling time. These responses lead to an increase in cardiac output and the demand for oxygen. In addition, an increase in intramyocardial wall tension can also increase the need for oxygen. Among the factors that can change wall tension are the preload, afterload, and wall thickness.[7] Preload, also known as diastolic pressure, is directly related to the volume of blood in the left ventricle at the end of diastole. Preload is typically affected by venous smooth muscle tension and urine output. The higher the preload is, the harder the ventricles must work to pump blood forward. Afterload, also known as systolic pressure, is determined by the arterial smooth muscle resistance against which the heart must pump to open the valves and eject blood into the main circulation. Similar to the preload, the higher the afterload, the higher the oxygen demand. Finally, the ventricular wall thickness can also play a role. The thicker the ventricular wall is, the more oxygen it will require to maintain normal function. In contrast, myocardial oxygen supply can be affected by perfusion pressure, hemoglobin-dependent oxygen carrying capacity, and coronary blood flow. In patients with advanced atherosclerotic plaque buildup or who have experienced myocardium ischemia, there is development or growth of new blood vessels. This phenomenon is known as collateral blood flow, which is a compensatory mechanism designed to bypass the narrowed coronary blood vessel and reestablish blood flow.[8] The severity or extent of CAD can be determined by several tests, including electrocardiogram (ECG), cardiac stress test, and angiography. In patients who are experiencing severe chest pain, emergency physicians may check laboratory biomarkers to differentiate between stable and unstable IHD. The most common biomarkers are cardiac troponin, creatine kinase, creatine kinase-MB, and lactate dehydrogenase.

As such, drugs used to treat CAD and IHD diseases are designed to decrease the workload of the heart, thus decreasing the oxygen demand (Table 20.1). Alternatively, drugs that increase the supply of blood by inducing coronary vasodilation may also be used (Table 20.1). Drugs that decrease the progression of atherosclerotic plaque buildup or thrombus formation may be beneficial a well.

Mechanism of Action of Antianginal Agents

Organic Nitrates. Nitroglycerin (NTG), isosorbide dinitrate, and isosorbide mononitrate are the three most commonly used drugs in this class. These drugs have several

Table 20.1 Pharmacologic Summary of Drugs Used to Treat Ischemic Heart Disease

Drug Class		Drug Name	Mechanism of Action	Primary Site of Action	Pharmacological Effect	IHD Effect
Organic Nitrates		Nitroglycerin, isosorbide dinitrate, isosorbide mononitrate	NO donor	Arteries, veins, and coronary arteries	Decrease preload and afterload	Decrease workload and increase blood supply
CCBs	Dihydropyridine CCBs	Amlodipine, nifedipine, nicardipine, etc	L-type Ca^{2+} channel	Arteries and coronary arteries	Decrease afterload	Decrease workload and increase blood supply
	Non-dihydropyridine CCBs	Verapamil, diltiazem	L-type Ca^{2+} channel	Arteries, heart, and coronary arteries	Decreases heart rate and afterload	Decrease workload and increase blood supply
β-blockers	Selective β_1-blockers	Metoprolol, atenolol, etc	Selective β_1-adrenergic receptor antagonist	Heart	Decreases heart rate and myocardial contractile force	Decrease workload
	Nonselective β-blockers	Propranolol, etc	Nonselective β_1- and β_2-adrenergic receptor antagonist	Heart	Decreases heart rate and myocardial contractile force	Decrease workload
	Mixed α- and β-blockers	Carvedilol labetalol	Nonselective β_1-, β_2-, and α_1-adrenergic receptor antagonist	Heart, arteries, and veins	Decreases heart rate, myocardial contractile force, afterload, and preload	Decrease workload
Late Na^+ channel blocker		Ranolazine	Late Na^+ channel blocker	Heart	Prevents Ca^{2+} overload	Prevents worsening of ischemic effects
I_f channel antagonist		Ivabradine	I_f channel antagonist	Heart	Bradycardia	Decrease workload

CCBs, calcium-channel blockers; IHD, ischemic heart disease; NO, nitric oxide.

routes of administration and can be used in combination with other drug classes to decrease the demand and, in some cases, to increase the supply of blood to the ischemic heart. Organic nitrates have very similar pharmacodynamic properties, which is the release of nitric oxide (NO) upon metabolism. NO easily dissolves across bilayer membranes and works in the cytoplasm of smooth muscles of blood vessels. It couples with soluble guanylate cyclase and activates the enzyme, leading to an increased production of cyclic guanosine 3′,5′-monophosphate (cGMP), which is a second messenger that is responsible for the dephosphorylation of myosin light chain kinase and smooth muscle relaxation.[9] At lower doses, the primary site of action of organic nitrates is the venous smooth muscle and coronary arteries (Table 20.1). By increasing the levels of cGMP in these tissues, drugs such as NTG can decrease preload and consequently, decrease ventricular wall tension. These two effects ultimately lead to a decreased workload of the heart. By producing vasodilation in the coronary arteries, it may also increase coronary blood flow and thus, increases the supply of oxygenated blood.[10] In patients with variant angina, NTG via its vasodilatory properties can also relieve the coronary vasospasm. At higher doses, it becomes less site-specific, and it can also vasodilate arterial smooth muscle. These drugs have a quick onset of action and may cause a marked decrease in arterial pressure. This sudden decrease in afterload will decrease the baroreceptor tone and increase SNS output to the heart, which may be counterproductive since activation of β-adrenergic receptors in the heart increases the workload of the heart. This is typically not a problem since β-blockers are first line drug therapy for IHD, and it would prevent this baroreceptor-mediated reflex tachycardia.

Calcium-Channel Blockers. Calcium channel blockers (CCBs) are used to treat several cardiovascular diseases, including hypertension, IHD, and arrhythmias. CCBs are broadly divided into two groups—that is, dihydropyridines (DHPs) and non-dihydropyridines (non-DHPs).[11] The DHPs are composed of several drugs, including amlodipine, nifedipine, nicardipine, and others. Non-DHP analogs include verapamil and diltiazem. Both groups of drugs have an affinity for the L-type Ca^{2+} channels that are present in the arterial smooth muscle, and they block/prevent the influx of Ca^{2+} into the smooth muscle.[12] Therefore, CCBs decrease afterload and, consequently, the workload of the heart. These drugs are also believed to produce coronary vasodilation, which may increase the supply of oxygenated blood or decrease the quivering associated with variant angina. Among the CCBs, it is accepted that drugs belonging to the DHP class are more potent than non-DHPs with respect to their vasodilatory effects but have little to no net effect on the heart. In addition to their effects on the arterial and coronary smooth muscle, verapamil and diltiazem can also bind to voltage dependent L-type Ca^{2+} channels in the atrioventricular (AV) node and decrease the slope of phase 0.[13] This results in a slowing down of AV node conduction, which is reflected as a prolongation of the PR interval on the ECG (see corresponding subsection in antiarrhythmic drugs).[14] As a result, heart rate is reduced, which in turn reduces the myocardial oxygen requirement. When comparing the effects that CCBs evoke in the myocardium, verapamil and diltiazem produce the greatest reduction in the heart rate when compared to the DHP drugs but are weaker vasodilators.

β-Blockers. β-Blockers are one of the oldest and most widely prescribed medications used to treat several types of cardiovascular diseases.[15] There are several β-blockers available in the United States, and their pharmacological response is dependent on the drug-receptor affinity and selectivity.[16] At normal therapeutic doses, cardioselective β-blockers such as atenolol, metoprolol, bisoprolol, and nebivolol are more selective toward the β_1-adrenergic receptor subtype. Other drugs like propranolol antagonize both β_1- and β_2-adrenergic receptors. Drugs like carvedilol and labetalol are mixed adrenergic antagonists that not only block β_1- and β_2-receptors, but also block α_1-adrenergic receptors.[17] In addition, some research suggests that certain β-blockers can produce antioxidant effects, improve NO release, and act as partial agonists at the β_2-adrenergic receptors.[18] β_1-Receptors are one of the major receptors expressed in the heart that are involved in its function. Because all β-blockers have an affinity for the β_1-receptor, this class of drugs inhibits the binding of norepinephrine and epinephrine, which slows heart rate and decreases myocardium contractile force and myocardium rate of relaxation. As such, β-blockers are utilized in IHD to decrease the workload of the heart. β_1-receptors are also present in the juxtaglomerular cells of the kidney, and activation of these receptors can produce an increase in renin secretion.[19] Renin is the rate-limiting enzyme involved in the production of angiotensin II, a powerful vasoconstrictor. Thus, β-blockers may decrease the secretion of renin, which would decrease plasma levels of angiotensin II and potentially decrease preload and afterload. Although β_2 appears to be the predominant receptor subtype in the central nervous system (CNS), β_1-selective drugs can also produce CNS side effects. Activation of β-adrenergic receptors in the brain has been associated with increased sympathetic activity. Thus, β-blockers may produce additional beneficial effects via a decrease in SNS tone to the heart and vasculature. α_1-Adrenergic receptors are primarily expressed in the eye, brain, and arterial and venous blood vessels. Activation of the α_1-receptors by the SNS is one of the major pathways in which the body controls blood pressure. Certain β-blockers such as carvedilol and labetalol can also antagonize α_1-adrenergic receptors, which reduces the workload of the heart by decreasing the preload and afterload.[20]

Ranolazine. Ranolazine's anti-ischemic mechanism of action is primarily associated with its ability to block the late inward sodium channel.[21] Under normal physiological conditions, these late sodium channels are mostly closed. The Na^+/K^+-ATPase (adenosine triphosphatase) and Na^+/Ca^{2+} exchangers are involved in the reestablishment of ion balance homeostasis, which promotes relaxation of the left ventricle.[22] During hypoxic/ischemic events, there is an increase in the production of metabolites and reactive oxygen species (ROS) by the myocytes that triggers an increase in the opening of late inward sodium channels. This increase in intracellular sodium concentration causes a reversal of the Na^+/Ca^{2+} exchanger and consequently increases intracellular Ca^{2+} overload in an attempt to restore blood flow to the ischemic site. Unfortunately, an increase in Ca^{2+} binding to contractile elements aggravates the ischemia by increasing left ventricle wall tension, adenosine triphosphate (ATP) consumption, and diastolic contractile dysfunction. At optimum therapeutic dose, ranolazine prevents cardiac overload by preventing myocardial Ca^{2+} overload during ischemia without major changes in heart rate or blood pressure.[21] In animal models, ranolazine has also been shown to block the delayed rectifier potassium channels and inhibit fatty acid oxidation.[23] Although these alternative mechanisms of action may provide additional pathways to decrease ischemia angina, its effect in humans is still not determined.

Ivabradine. Ivabradine decreases the workload of the heart by decreasing heart rate, which increases diastolic perfusion time. It is an antagonist at the I_f channel, which is the primary channel responsible for spontaneous diastolic depolarization, and is also known as the pacemaker current.[22] This channel was first named as the "funny current."[24] It allows sodium influx, which increases the slope of the sinoatrial node, which then makes the membrane potential less negative and allows for the opening of voltage-gated ion channels. I_f channels are one of the major determinants of automaticity and heart rate. Ivabradine decreases the heart rate by dose-dependent selective inhibition of the I_f channel, which decreases the slope of depolarization, and produces a prolongation of sinus node recovery time. It is a novel approach to decrease the heart rate and differs from β-blockers by not affecting the myocardial contractile force or AV conduction. In addition to being used for angina, ivabradine has also been approved by the US Food and Drug Administration (FDA) for use in patients with HF.

Chemistry of Nitrates and Nitrites

NTG or glyceryl trinitrate (Fig. 20.1) is a synthetic molecule that was discovered by an Italian scientist Ascanio Sobrero in 1846 by reacting glycerol with the classical nitration mixture (nitric and sulfuric acid).[25] He not only observed its uncontrolled explosive properties, but when tasted in small quantities, he noted its headache causing properties.[26] An important invention of the era was made by Alfred Nobel by combining nitroglycerin with kieselguhr and developed dynamite, which is explosive under controlled conditions.[25] This has led to the success of the Nobel family, and eventually much of his wealth was used in the establishment of the renowned Nobel Prize that has been awarded since 1901.[26,27]

The medicinal properties of amyl nitrite (Fig. 20.1) for the treatment of angina were documented in 1867 by British Physician, Thomas Lauder Brunton.[28] In the following decade, it was largely replaced by nitroglycerin because of the ease of administration and long duration of action.[29] In fact, in 1890, Alfred Nobel's physician prescribed him nitroglycerin for the treatment of his heart disease.[30]

NTG is a prodrug (Fig. 20.2).[31] It is primarily bioactivated in smooth muscles by undergoing complex metabolic reactions and is converted to nitric oxide (NO) or a related compound S-nitrosothiol (SNO) intermediate.[32] Recently, a few scientists have questioned whether nitroglycerin's effect on smooth muscle relaxation is dependent on the generation of free nitric oxide or not.[33] There are several hypotheses that have been put forward regarding the activation of nitroglycerin including enzymatic (eg, glutathione S-transferase, cytochrome P450 [CYP]-related enzymes) and nonenzymatic (eg, cellular thiol compounds) activation.[10] NTG metabolic activation primarily takes place by the enzyme mitochondrial aldehyde dehydrogenase (mtALDH), a novel reductase mechanism.[32] Human mtALDH contains two cysteine thiols in the active site and nitroglycerin serves as a substrate and is converted to 1,2-glyceryl dinitrate (1,2-GDN).[34]

Pentaerythritol tetranitrate (PETN) (Fig. 20.1) is similar to NTG and is synthesized by nitration of the polyalcohol pentaerythritol instead of glycerol.[35] PETN appears more spherical in shape than the glycerol backbone of NTG.[36]

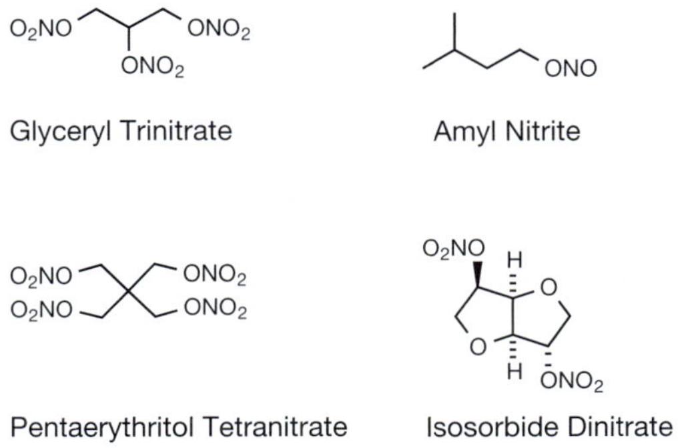

Figure 20.1 Organic nitrates and nitrites.

PETN contains a central carbon, which, in turn, is attached to four $-CH_2$-ONO_2 groups.[36] PETN is not frequently used in the United States but is widely used in Europe.[37] Pentaerythritol tetranitrate is abbreviated as PETN but is also referred to as PENT, PENTA, and TEN. It is also used as an explosive for military purposes.[36]

Isosorbide (see Fig. 20.1) is a bicyclic sugar derivative that is prepared by the dehydration of sorbitol. Chemically, isosorbide mono- and dinitrate are nitrate ester derivatives of isosorbide.[36] The nitrate attached to the sugar largely reduces the explosive properties, which makes it a more stable compound.[36] The difference in the number of nitrate groups (mono- and dinitrate) results in pharmacokinetic differences.

Pharmaceutical Preparations. NTG is available in various formulations. It is administered orally in the form of extended-release capsules, translingual spray, sublingual powder, and tablets; topically in the form of ointment, transdermal patch; and parenterally in the form of intravenous (IV) infusion. Isosorbide mono- and dinitrate are available as oral immediate- and extended-release formulations. Isosorbide dinitrate is also available as a sublingual formulation. PETN is available as an oral formulation.

Pharmacokinetics. The onset of action of NTG varies depending on its formulation and route of administration. The onset of action of an IV NTG formulation is immediate, and the onset is rapid when sublingual tablets or a translingual spray (2 minutes) is administered. The onset of action is slower for topical administration (15-30 minutes), extended-release capsules (60 minutes), and transdermal patches (about 30 minutes).[38] Therefore, for acute anginal attacks, IV or sublingual formulations are appropriate choices of treatment when compared to other routes.

The duration of action of an IV nitroglycerin formulation is about 3 to 5 minutes, and a sublingual tablet is about 25 minutes, whereas an extended-release capsule (4-8 hours), a transdermal patch (10-12 hours), and topical preparations (about 7 hours) have a longer duration of action, making these formulations suitable for a sustained effect.[38]

The plasma kinetics of NTG is highly variable due to intra- and inter-individual differences.[39] When administered by IV infusion, NTG was shown to have a high apparent volume of distribution of approximately 3 L/kg and a short plasma half-life of about 3 minutes.[39]

NTG is metabolized in systemic vasculature, liver, lungs, kidneys, and erythrocytes. The amount and extent of metabolites formed is also dependent on the route of administration. For example, the IV, sublingual, and transdermal routes of administration avoid first-pass metabolism and have higher bioavailability than orally administered capsules. Irrespective of the route of administration, the amount of metabolites formed far exceeds the intact NTG, indicating extensive metabolism.[40] NTG is metabolized to 1,2-GDN, 1,3-glyceryl dinitrate (1,3-GDN), NO, and SNO.[32] The NO that is generated via an obligate intermediate nitrite ion leads to vascular smooth muscle relaxation (see Fig. 20.2).[32] Dinitrates of NTG can further be metabolized by denitration into 1-glyceryl mononitrate, 2-glyceryl mononitrate, and subsequently to glycerol.[40] Dinitrate and mononitrate

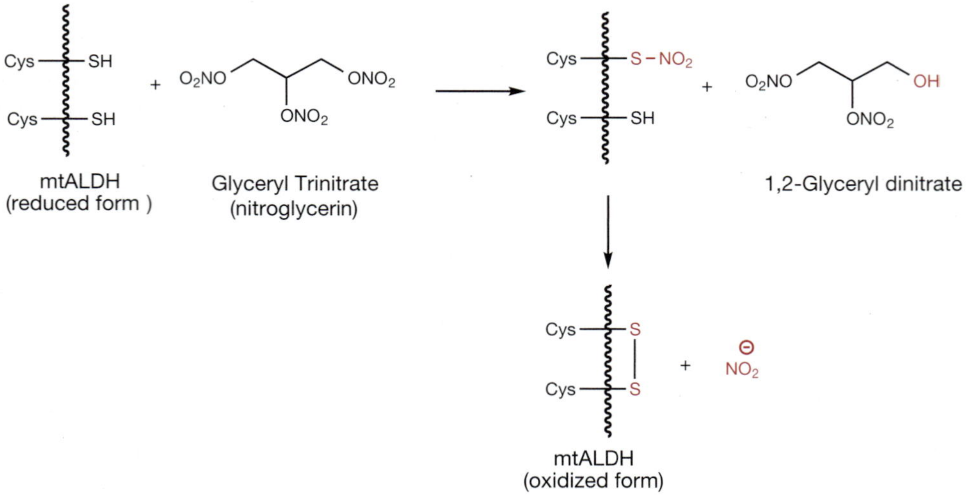

Figure 20.2 Activation of glyceryl trinitrate.

NTG may also undergo glucuronide conjugation.[41] Pharmacokinetics of pentaerythrityl tetranitrate is different from nitroglycerin. When administered orally, PETN is metabolized to pentaerythrityl dinitrate (PEDN), pentaerythrityl mononitrate (PEMN), and not much of pentaerithrityl trinitrate (PETriN) is observed. The PEDN and PEMN metabolites are less effective than the PETN.[36,42]

When administered orally, isosorbide dinitrate is rapidly absorbed. It has only about 30% bioavailability because of extensive first-pass metabolism in the liver.[43,44] Isosorbide dinitrate is distributed rapidly and primarily metabolized by denitration to 2-isosorbide mononitrate (~25%) and 5-isosorbide mononitrate (~75%).[43,44] The half-life elimination of oral, sublingual, and IV isosorbide dinitrate is about 30 minutes, 5 minutes, and 9 minutes, respectively.[43,44] To the contrary, its metabolites 2-isosorbide mononitrate and 5-isosorbide mononitrate have longer elimination half-lives of about 2 hours and 5 hours, respectively.[43,44] Majority of isosorbide metabolites are eliminated in the urine.

The orally administered isosorbide mononitrate is rapidly and completely absorbed, with a bioavailability close to 100%.[43] It is metabolized by conjugation and denitration to inactive metabolites isosorbide and sorbitol, which are predominantly eliminated renally.

Adverse Effects. Headache due to the vasodilation of blood vessels in the brain is the most common side effect associated with NTG, especially with the longer duration of action formulations. Other side effects include hypotension associated with syncope, nausea, and vomiting.

Nitrate Tolerance. The major limitation of chronic administration of organic nitrates is tolerance, which results in decreased antianginal efficacy because of desensitization of blood vessels.[32] NTG tolerance is partly due to the impaired bioactivation and the loss of mtALDH function.[32] NTG tolerance is also attributed to its ability to generate free radical reactive oxygen species (ROS) by the endothelium, which are capable of oxidizing membrane lipids.[37] On the contrary, PETN is not associated with an increase in ROS and does not cause tolerance.[37]

Drug-Drug Interactions. Organic nitrates may have significant drug interactions and have profound hypotensive effects with other vasodilators. Riociguat and phosphodiesterase-5 (PDE5) inhibitors must be avoided in combination with organic nitrates. Riociguat used for the treatment of pulmonary hypertension is a direct activator of the soluble guanylate cyclase (sGC) enzyme.[45] In addition, it can also sensitize the sGC to the endogenous nitric oxide, which is produced by the activation of the NO synthase enzyme. In contrast, PDE5 inhibitors such as sildenafil block the PDE5 enzyme, which is involved in the breakdown of cGMP.[46] Concurrent use of NTG with either one of these drugs may lead to a marked increase in cGMP and a severe drop in blood pressure. On the contrary, concurrent administration of vasoconstricting agents, such as ergot alkaloids (eg, ergotamine), may lead to a decreased antianginal efficacy of NTG.

Chemistry of Calcium Channel Blockers

The clinically available DHPs and non-DHP CCBs act on L-type or long-lasting channels; however, the structural diversity of these compounds emphasizes the importance of their specificities in cardiac tissues and arteriolar vasculature.[47] Since clinically available DHPs contain hydrogen atoms at 1 and 4 positions on the DHP ring, they are specifically referred to as 1,4-dihydropyridines (1,4-DHPs). Several 1,4-DHPs are also effective in the treatment of hypertension.[48] The 1,4-DHPs that are primarily used in the management of angina include amlodipine, nifedipine, and nicardipine (Fig. 20.3). The non-DHPs can further be divided into a phenylalkylamine derivative (verapamil), a benzothiazepine derivative (diltiazem), and a diaminopropanol ether derivative (bepridil). Currently, verapamil and diltiazem are the only non-DHPs that are clinically available in the United States (Fig. 20.4). Verapamil is the first calcium channel blocker that was discovered based on the structure of papaverine, one of the important constituents of opium poppy alkaloids.[49] Verapamil was first synthesized as D365 (Iproveratril) by Dr Ferdinand Dengel at the German pharmaceutical company Knoll AG, and in the early 1960s, its coronary vasodilatory properties and anti-arrhythmic properties were discovered.[49,50]

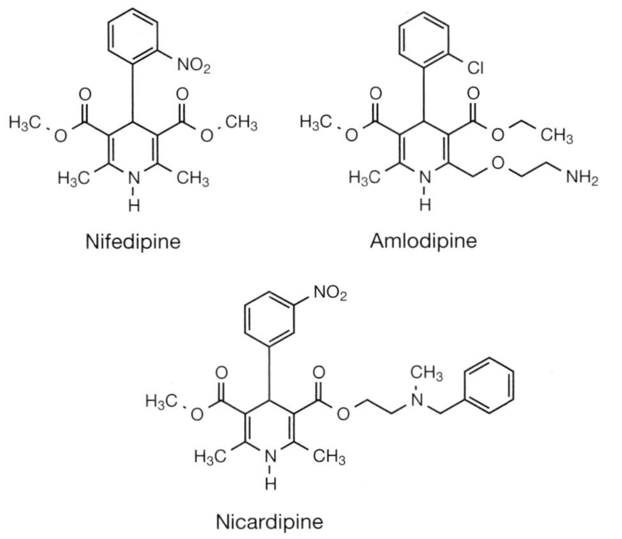

Figure 20.3 1,4-Dihydropyridine calcium channel blockers.

1,4-DIHYDROPYRIDINES. Nifedipine is the prototype molecule in the 1,4-DHP class of CCBs and was discovered in the early 1970s.[51] Nifedipine is a symmetrical 1,4-DHP, in which both esters (methyl ester) at the C_3 and C_5 positions, as well as substitutions at the C_2 and C_6 positions (methyl group) are identical. Nifedipine is light sensitive and undergoes decomposition into a pyridine analog and a nitroso pyridine analog.[52]

The replacement of the 1,4-DHP ring with other rings leads to compounds with reduced or loss of activity, indicating the importance of the ring for optimal activity.[53] The 1,4-DHP ring adopts a boat confirmation.[53] The hydrogen atom attached to the nitrogen atom in the 1,4 DHP ring forms hydrogen bonding with tyrosine in the receptor.[53] Replacement of the hydrogen atom with other groups and oxidation of the nitrogen are detrimental to its activity.[53] The presence of C_3 and C_5 ester groups on the 1,4-DHP ring is required for optimal activity. The C_4 atom is attached to an *ortho* and/or *meta* electron-withdrawing phenyl ring.[53] The *ortho* and/or *meta* derivatives are considered to be critical for activity because they lock the phenyl ring perpendicular to the 1,4-DHP ring.[53] Nifedipine contains an *ortho*-nitrophenyl group, amlodipine contains an *ortho*-chlorophenyl group, and nicardipine contains a *meta*-nitrophenyl group (see Fig. 20.3).

Nicardipine and amlodipine have distinguishable physiochemical properties among the 1,4-DHP derivatives.[54]

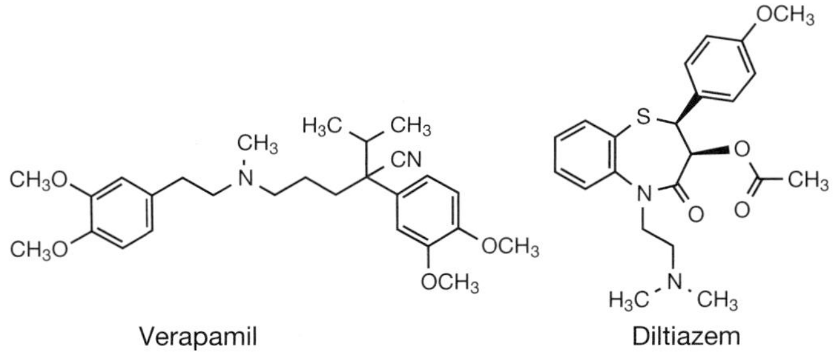

Figure 20.4 Non-dihydropyridine calcium channel blockers.

Amlodipine besylate and nifedipine hydrochloride salt forms have good aqueous solubility. Amlodipine has an amino-ethoxy methyl side chain, and nicardipine has an *N*-benzyl-*N*-methylamino side chain (see Fig. 20.3). Therefore, at physiological pH, they exist as ionized forms, which have higher hydrophilicity than their unionized forms.[54]

NON-DIHYDROPYRIDINES. Verapamil contains a basic tertiary nitrogen and is marketed as a hydrochloride salt. It contains one chiral center, but it is administered as a racemic mixture of the *R*- and *S*-enantiomers. The *S*(-)-isomer of verapamil is about 10 to 20 times more potent than the *R*(+)-isomer as a vasodilator.[55] However, the *R*-isomer is less cardiotoxic than the *S* isomer.[55] The clinically available diltiazem is a (+)-*cis* isomer and has two chiral centers with a 2*S*, 3*S* configuration.[56] The (-)-*cis* enantiomer, with a 2*R*, 3*R* configuration, does not have vasodilatory properties. The *trans* diastereomers (2*R*, 3*S* and 2*S*, 3*R*) have weak activity.[56] Therefore, stereochemistry has an absolute impact on the pharmacological activity of diltiazem.[56]

PHARMACEUTICAL PREPARATIONS. Amlodipine is available as oral tablets, solution, and suspension. Nifedipine is available as oral capsules and extended-release tablets,[57] whereas nicardipine is available both in oral and IV formulations.[57] The oral formulations of verapamil and diltiazem are used in the treatment of angina, and IV formulations are used in supraventricular tachycardias.[57]

PHARMACOKINETICS. The bioavailability of orally administered nifedipine is about 45% to 70%.[58] Nifedipine is highly protein bound (>95%), primarily to albumin.[59] Nifedipine undergoes significant first-pass metabolism in the liver and intestine.[58] It is primarily oxidized by CYP3A4 to a pyridine ring, which is further metabolized into acid metabolites by ester hydrolysis.[58,60] Nifedipine immediate-release formulation has a half-life elimination of 2 hours, and it reaches the maximum blood concentration in about 30 minutes,[61] whereas the controlled-release formulation of nifedipine has a half-life elimination of 7 hours and the time to reach the maximum blood concentration is 1.6 to 4 hours.[61] About 60% to 80% of orally administered nifedipine is eliminated in the urine, predominantly as metabolites with the remaining drug eliminated in the feces.[62] In patients with liver cirrhosis, there is an increased bioavailability and reduced systemic clearance of nifedipine, necessitating the need for adjustment of doses.[63] Nifedipine pharmacokinetic parameters may be affected by genetic differences. For example, South Asian people have a lower systemic clearance than White people, and, as a result, the half-life of nifedipine is significantly higher in the South Asian population.[58]

Nicardipine is completely and rapidly absorbed after oral administration.[64] The bioavailability is moderately low (35%) because of extensive first-pass metabolism.[64] The bioavailability of nicardipine is further decreased when food is consumed before or along with nicardipine.[64] The bioavailability is further dependent on the dose because of the saturable pre-systemic effect.[64] Nicardipine undergoes extensive serum protein binding (>95%).[65] It binds to albumin, lipoproteins, and erythrocytes.[65] Nicardipine has a half-life elimination of 1 to 4 hours, and the maximum blood concentration is achieved in 0.5 to 2 hours.[61] It is predominantly metabolized in the liver.[64] Apart from the oxidation of the 1,4-DHP ring to a pyridine ring, the *N*-benzyl side chain also undergoes debenzylation, which is further metabolized.[64] Glucuronide conjugates are also identified in the urine.[64] About 60% (primarily in the form of metabolites) of nicardipine is eliminated in the urine, and 25% is eliminated in the feces.[66]

Amlodipine has unique pharmacokinetic properties because of its high degree of ionization.[54] Food does not have an effect on the bioavailability of amlodipine, and the estimated bioavailability is about 64% to 90%.[67] Amlodipine has a large volume of distribution of about 21 L/kg and a high degree of protein binding of about 98%.[54] Amongst 1,4-DHP's, amlodipine has the highest elimination half-life, 35 to 50 hours, and the duration it takes to reach the maximum blood concentration is 6 to 12 hours.[61] Amlodipine once-daily dosing is effective for the treatment of angina pectoris owing to its slow clearance.[61] Amlodipine does not undergo extensive first-pass metabolism; however, it does undergo significant metabolism in the liver.[54] CYP3A4 plays a major role in metabolizing the 1,4-DHP ring of amlodipine to its oxidized pyridine metabolite.[68] It can further undergo metabolism via O-demethylation, O-dealkylation, and oxidative deamination.[68] The elimination half-life of amlodipine is significantly prolonged in patients with hepatic cirrhosis ($t_{1/2}$ is ~60 hours), leading to a greater accumulation.[69] About 60% of the administered amlodipine is eliminated in the urine predominantly in the form of metabolites.[70] In older adults, amlodipine has a prolonged elimination half-life because of decreased clearance and may require adjustment of doses.[69]

Verapamil is well absorbed orally.[71] However, the bioavailability is only 10%-35% because of extensive hepatic first-pass metabolism.[71,72] Verapamil is extensively bound to proteins (about 90%).[73] Verapamil undergoes stereoselective metabolism, and the *S*-enantiomer is metabolized at a faster rate than the *R*-enantiomer.[74,75] Verapamil undergoes N-demethylation catalyzed extensively by CYP3A4 and CYP3A5 to norverapamil.[75] Verapamil and norverapamil further undergo O-demethylation by CYP2C8.[75] Norverapamil has about 20% cardiovascular activity when compared to verapamil. The immediate-release formulation of verapamil has an elimination half-life of about 3 to 10 hours, but is extended up to 17 hours during chronic administration.[76] Norverapamil has a longer elimination half-life than verapamil.[76] About 70% of the administered verapamil is eliminated in the urine and 16% is eliminated in feces primarily as metabolites.

The absolute bioavailability of diltiazem is 40% to 50%.[77] The volume of distribution of diltiazem is 8 to 14 L/kg.[77] About 80% of the diltiazem is protein bound with significant inter-individual differences.[78] It is primarily bound to lipoproteins and α_1-acid glycoprotein.[78] Diltiazem undergoes extensive metabolism, and less than 5% of the drug is eliminated unchanged.[79] Diltiazem primarily undergoes O-deacetylation by esterases to desacetyl diltiazem and N-demethylation by CYP3A4 to *N*-monodesmethyl diltiazem.[79,80] Diltiazem also undergoes O-demethylation by CYP2D6.[81] The desacetyl diltiazem and *N*-monodesmethyl diltiazem are pharmacologically active vasodilators; therefore, the activity is due to the intact drug and its active metabolites.[79] Diltiazem and its *N*-monodesmethyl and *N,N*-didesmethyl metabolites are CYP3A4 inhibitors.[80] The half-life elimination of immediate- and extended-release formulations are 3 to 4.5 and 4 to 9 hours, respectively.[57,78] During chronic oral administration, *N*-monodesmethyl diltiazem accumulates to a greater extent than desacetyl diltiazem.[82] During chronic therapy, the accumulation of diltiazem metabolites leads to the decreased elimination of diltiazem.[80]

ADVERSE EFFECTS. The most common side effects of CCBs are related to their vasodilatory abilities on smooth muscle vasculature. As such, patients may complain of dizziness, fatigue, headache, constipation, and flushing. Because of their potency, some patients may experience peripheral edema and palpitations with dihydropyridines. This is most likely caused by the baroreceptor-mediated increase in sympathetic tone to the venous system and heart. Gastrointestinal (GI) side effects are also observed. Verapamil frequently produces gingival hyperplasia and constipation.

DRUG-DRUG INTERACTIONS. CCBs are contraindicated in patients with HF because of the risk of developing pulmonary edema. Because β-blockers are first line therapy for most patients with HF, concurrent administration of β-blockers with verapamil or diltiazem may lead to severe bradycardia and potential heart block.

Simvastatin, used in the treatment of hypercholesterolemia, is predominantly metabolized by the CYP3A4 enzyme. Amlodipine co-administration may increase the plasma concentrations of simvastatin, but it is a safer option than verapamil and diltiazem.[83] Verapamil is a potent CYP3A4 inhibitor, and co-administration of verapamil with other drugs that are metabolized by CYP3A4 may lead to altered drug concentrations.[84] For instance, verapamil is shown to increase the plasma concentrations of simvastatin by about 3-fold and increase the adverse effects of statins such as rhabdomyolysis.[84] Therefore, simvastatin doses should be adjusted and appropriately monitored when combined with verapamil.[84]

Rifamycin, a potent CY3A4 inducer, may increase the metabolism and systemic elimination of CCBs, thereby diminishing their therapeutic effects.[85] To the contrary, some azole antifungal agents, such as itraconazole, are potent CYP3A4 inhibitors and may decrease the metabolism and enhance the plasma concentrations of CCBs.[86] Itraconazole may further potentiate negative inotropic effects associated with verapamil and diltiazem.[57] Grapefruit juice is a known CYP3A4 and CYP3A5 inhibitor.[87] It predominantly inhibits the CYPs in the intestine, with a minor effect on hepatic CYP enzymes.[87] Amongst DHPs, amlodipine and nifedipine are less affected by grapefruit juice because their oral bioavailability is greater than other DHPs.[87] However, the blood levels of these two drugs may still be increased by about 15% to 30% when coadministered with grapefruit juice.[87] Therefore, caution and monitoring are essential when CCBs are coadministered with grapefruit juice.

Verapamil is a substrate and inhibitor of P-glycoprotein.[88] Co-administration of verapamil with digoxin, a P-glycoprotein substrate, may decrease renal tubular elimination and increase plasma concentrations of digoxin.[89] Since this can lead to deleterious effects of digoxin, the dose of digoxin should be reduced when given in combination with verapamil.[90] Verapamil may inhibit the P-glycoprotein in the blood-brain barrier (BBB) and thereby preventing the efflux of drugs.[91] This could have either beneficial or deleterious effects. A beneficial effect is seen with the antiepileptic drug, carbamazepine. Verapamil can limit the P-glycoprotein efflux in the BBB of carbamazepine and thereby increase the intracellular concentrations of carbamazepine in the brain and potentially provide an advantage in patients with seizures.[91] On the contrary, it may be a disadvantage and may lead to unwanted toxic drug-drug interactions (DDIs) in some other cases. For instance, verapamil being a P-glycoprotein inhibitor may have the potential to increase antidiarrheal loperamide (P-glycoprotein substrate) concentrations in the BBB, which may lead to loperamide unwanted opioid CNS side effects such as respiratory depression.[92] Verapamil and diltiazem may also precipitate the neurotoxic side effects associated with anticonvulsants such as carbamazepine and phenytoin.[93,94] Therefore, the combination should either be avoided or patients must carefully be monitored.

Chemistry and Development of β-Blockers

Catecholamines such as norepinephrine and epinephrine are synthesized from the amino acid L-tyrosine.[95] Tyrosine is in turn obtained from the diet and biosynthesized from the amino acid L-phenylalanine via catalysis by the enzyme tyrosine hydroxylase.[95] Catecholamines bind and intrinsically activate G protein–coupled α- and β-adrenergic receptors.

Isoproterenol, a synthetic catecholamine, is a potent β-adrenergic agonist. In the 1950s, the 3,4-dihydroxy groups in isoproterenol were replaced with the dichloro group to afford dichloroisoprenaline or dichloroisoproterenol (DCI) (Fig. 20.5).[96] DCI was shown to inhibit the adrenergic effects of epinephrine and isoproterenol[96]; however, DCI was not clinically useful as a β-blocker because of its potent intrinsic sympathomimetic activity.[97] In 1962, Sir James Black et al. noted that the development of β-blockers free of intrinsic sympathomimetic activity could potentially be valuable for the treatment of angina and tachycardias.[97] The 3,4-dichlorophenyl ring in DCI was replaced with the naphthyl ring to afford pronethalol (Fig. 20.5)[97]; however, pronethalol has serious unpleasant side effects.[98] In mice, pronethalol induced malignant tumors, primarily thymic and lymphosarcomata.[98] Pronethalol also has intrinsic sympathomimetic activity, albeit not as potent as DCI.[98] Sir Black et al continued further research to discover newer drug molecules with decreased toxicity. An important breakthrough was achieved by introducing the oxymethylene (-OCH_2) group between the aryl (naphthyl) ring and ethanolamine to yield aryloxypropanolamine.[98] This modification resulted in the discovery of propranolol (Fig. 20.5), a prototype β-blocker that was devoid of carcinogenic properties and the intrinsic sympathomimetic activity possessed by pronethalol.[98] In 1988, Sir Black received the Nobel Prize in Physiology or Medicine for his contribution to the "important principles for drug treatment."[99]

The classification of β-receptors into β_1 and β_2 was first reported in 1967 by Lands et al.[100] This has paved the way for the classification of β-blockers into nonselective β-blockers, antagonizing both β_1- and β_2-receptors and cardioselective β-blockers that specifically antagonize β_1-receptors at low doses.[101] Selective β_1-blockers may have a better safety profile in patients with bronchospasm than nonselective β-blockers.[101] Practolol (Fig. 20.6) was the first clinically available selective β_1-blocker, but was later withdrawn from clinical use because of adverse oculomucocutaneous syndrome characterized by vision loss, fibrous or plastic peritonitis, mucosal and nasal ulceration, otitis media, and rashes.[101,102] Practolol is a phenyloxypropanolamine containing *N*-acetamide (-$NHCOCH_3$) at the *para* position (see Fig. 20.5). It possibly undergoes deacetylation to yield an aromatic amine, which may be responsible for its untoward side effects.[103] Replacement of the acetamide -$NHCOCH_3$ with -CH_2CONH_2 at the *para* position led to the discovery of atenolol (see Fig. 20.5). Unlike practolol, atenolol did not possess severe oculomucocutaneous side effects.[102]

Today, several selective and nonselective β-blockers are available worldwide for the treatment of hypertension (clinical use of β-blockers to treat hypertensive disorders is discussed in Chapter 19), angina, HF, arrhythmias, and glaucoma. All clinically available β-blockers end with the suffix -lol; nonselective β-blockers include carteolol, nadolol, penbutolol, pindolol, propranolol, sotalol, and timolol (Fig. 20.7). Selective β_1-blockers include acebutolol, atenolol, betaxolol, bisoprolol, esmolol, metoprolol, and nebivolol (Fig. 20.8). Labetalol and carvedilol are mixed adrenergic antagonists blocking both α_1- and β-adrenergic receptors (Fig. 20.7).[101]

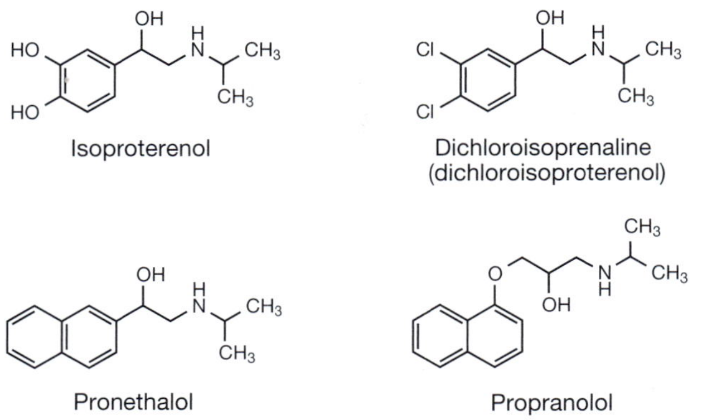

Figure 20.5 Development of β-adrenergic antagonists.

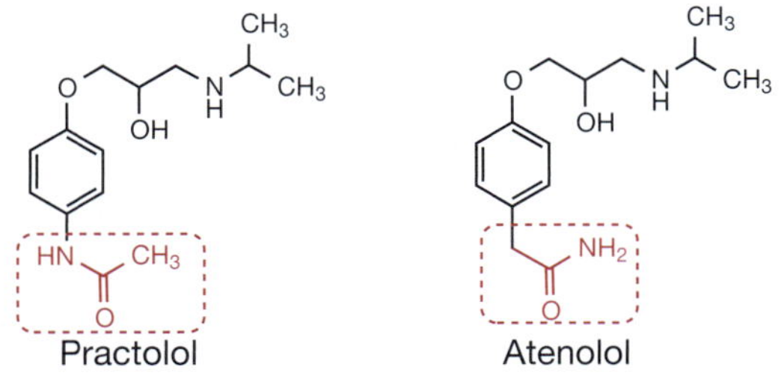

Figure 20.6 Development of selective β_1 adrenergic antagonists.

Structural Properties of β-Blockers. The chemical features of clinically available β-blockers are listed below.[104]

1. All β-blockers have at least one aromatic and/or heteroaromatic ring system.[104] They are devoid of catechol functional groups.
2. The aromatic/heteroaromatic ring is in turn attached to an alkyl side chain containing a chiral secondary hydroxyl group and an amine.[104] The amine group is either attached to an isopropyl or a tertiary butyl group with few exceptions.
3. Most β-blockers are aryloxypropanolamine derivatives with two exceptions. Sotalol is an arylethanolamine derivative containing a sulfonamide group at the *para* position, and labetalol lacks the oxymethylene group.
4. The majority of the clinically available selective β_1-blockers are phenyloxypropanolamine derivatives containing substitutions at the *para* position.
5. Due to the presence of the oxymethylene (-OCH_2) group in aryloxypropanolamine, the *S*- enantiomer of aryloxypropanolamine side chain occupy similar space in the β-receptor as the *R*-enantiomer side chain of arylethanolamine. In general, in β-blockers with one chiral center, the *S*(-)-enantiomer has better β-receptor binding affinity than the *R*(+)-enantiomer.[104]
6. The majority of β-blockers are clinically administered as a racemic mixture. Exceptions include timolol, which is only available as *S*(-)-timolol.[104]

β-blockers, based on their partition coefficient, can be classified into lipophilic and hydrophilic β-blockers. This may account for the pharmacokinetic differences between β-blockers. For example, a lipophilic β-blocker such as propranolol has a higher partition coefficient (LogP = 2.65; CLogP = 2.75)[105] because of the hydrocarbon naphthyl ring system, and as a result, it has a greater ability to penetrate the BBB. On the contrary, hydrophilic β-blockers such as atenolol containing a polar acetamide group (LogP = 0.5; CLogP = -0.1)[105] are less likely to cross the CNS.[106] Lipophilic β-blockers undergo extensive hepatic metabolism, leading to shorter half-lives than the hydrophilic β-blockers, which are minimally metabolized by the liver.[107]

The commonly used β-blockers for the treatment of angina are propranolol, atenolol, metoprolol, bisoprolol, and carvedilol.

Propranolol. Propranolol (Fig. 20.7), a lipophilic nonselective β-blocker, is almost completely absorbed after oral administration.[108] However, the bioavailability is poor (about 25%) because of extensive hepatic metabolism.[109] Protein-rich food may increase its bioavailability.[110] The S(-)-propranolol is about 100 times more potent than the *R*(+)-propranolol.[111] It is well distributed to various tissues, and about 90% of the drug is protein bound.[108] The volume of distribution of propranolol is about 6 L/kg.[109] The naphthyl ring in propranolol is hydroxylated at the 4 and 5 positions predominantly by CYP2D6 and undergoes N-desisopropylation by CYP1A2.[112] The 4-hydroxy propranolol metabolite possesses potent β-blocking properties similar to propanol and is also a weak CYP2D6 inhibitor.[113] Propranolol is also metabolized by glucuronidation.[111] Propranolol is predominantly excreted in the urine as metabolites, and only <1% is eliminated as the intact drug.[114] Since propranolol crosses the BBB it may cause depression.[115] However, its CNS effects may be beneficial in patients with anxiety.[116] Propranolol is also used as a prophylactic agent in migraine.[117]

Propranolol is available as oral conventional propranolol hydrochloride and extended-release capsules. The extended-release formulation takes a longer time for dissolution and

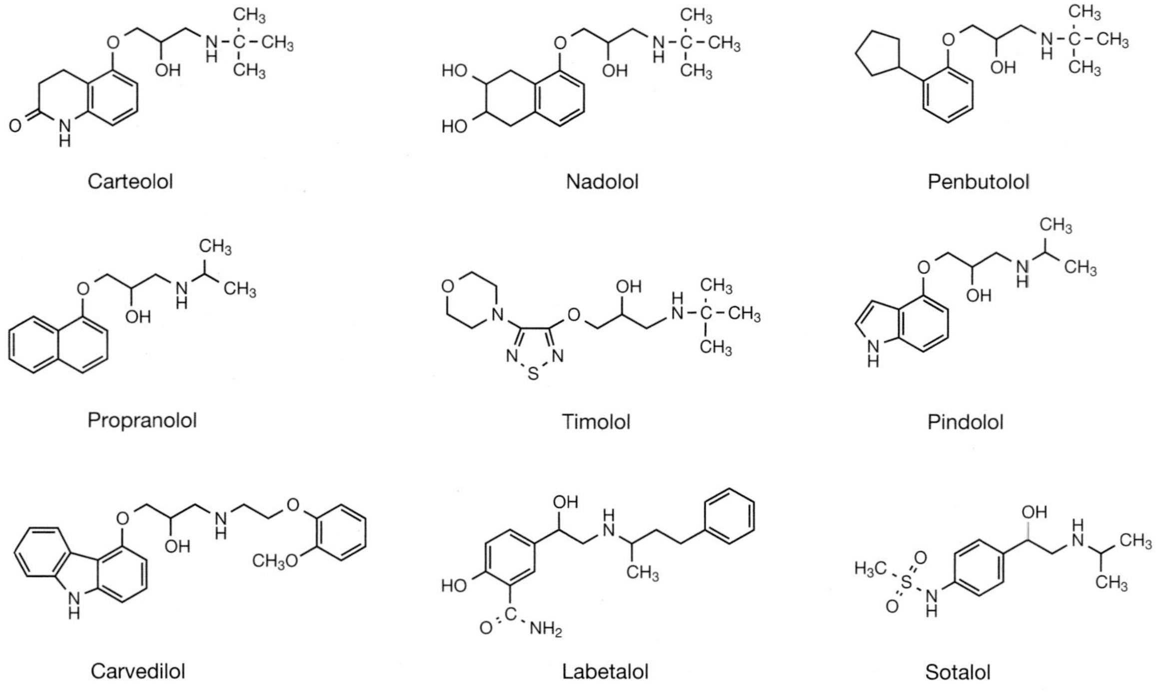

Figure 20.7 Nonselective β-adrenergic antagonists.

releases the drug in a controlled and predictable manner when compared to the conventional formulation.[118] In extended-release formulation the bioavailability is lower, the time to attain peak plasma levels is longer, and the peak plasma levels are lower than the conventional formulation.[118,119] The elimination half-life of conventional propranolol is about 3 to 6 hours and requires multiple dosing,[108] whereas the elimination half-life of the extended-release formulation is significantly longer (8-11 hours).[119] The extended-release capsule constantly maintains the plasma concentrations for 24 hours, which allows for once-daily dosing and thereby improves patient compliance.[119]

Atenolol. Atenolol (Fig. 20.8) is a hydrophilic selective β_1-blocker and is incompletely absorbed after oral administration.[120] The oral bioavailability is about 50%, and the peak plasma levels are attained in 2 to 4 hours.[120] Atenolol is not significantly bound to plasma proteins (3%-5%).[121] While the majority of β-blockers undergo metabolism, atenolol is not significantly metabolized.[122] Only 5% to 10% of the drug is metabolized in the liver.[120] About 50% of the orally administered drug is eliminated unchanged by the kidneys, and the remaining percentage in feces.[122] After IV administration, about 85% of atenolol is eliminated unchanged in the urine.[123] The elimination half-life is about 6 to 9 hours and is increased in patients with renal impairment.[120]

Metoprolol Tartrate and Succinate. Metoprolol is a moderately lipophilic (LogP = 1.72; CLogP = 1.48)[105] selective β_1-blocker. Chemically, it is a phenyloxypropanolamine containing methyloxyethyl substitution (ether moiety) at the *para* position (Fig. 20.8). It is sold as the tartrate and succinate dicarboxylate salt forms. Metoprolol tartrate (Fig. 20.8) is an immediate-release and a short-acting formulation dosed twice daily.[124] Metoprolol succinate (Fig. 20.8) is an extended-release formulation that provides consistent β-blocking properties for over 24 hours, allowing once-daily administration.[125] Metoprolol succinate was shown to reduce the relative risk of mortality and provides substantial morbidity benefits in patients with HF.[125] Orally administered metoprolol is well absorbed in the intestine, but the bioavailability is only about 50% because it undergoes extensive first-pass hepatic metabolism.[126] The bioavailability may be enhanced when taken with food and during chronic administration.[126] In patients with hepatic cirrhosis, bioavailability may be increased because of decreased first-pass metabolism.[126] Approximately 15% of metoprolol is bound to plasma proteins.[127] Metoprolol is metabolized via hydroxylation to α-hydroxymetoprolol and O-dealkylation to yield a primary alcohol, which is further oxidized to the carboxylic acid metabolite.[128,129] Metoprolol is predominantly metabolized by CYP2D6 and exhibits genetic polymorphism.[130] The elimination half-life of metoprolol in extensive and poor CYP2D6 metabolizers is about 3.1 hours and 7.2 hours, respectively.[131] The peak plasma concentrations of metoprolol is about 3-fold higher in poor CYP2D6 metabolizers than extensive metabolizers.[131] Consequently, poor CYP2D6 individuals may be associated with a greater risk of metoprolol adverse effects.[132] It is predominantly excreted as metabolites in the urine.[126] In patients with impaired renal function, metabolites may accumulate in the body for a longer time.[126]

Bisoprolol. Bisoprolol is a moderately lipophilic (LogP = 1.94; CLogP = 1.79)[105] selective β_1-blocker containing an

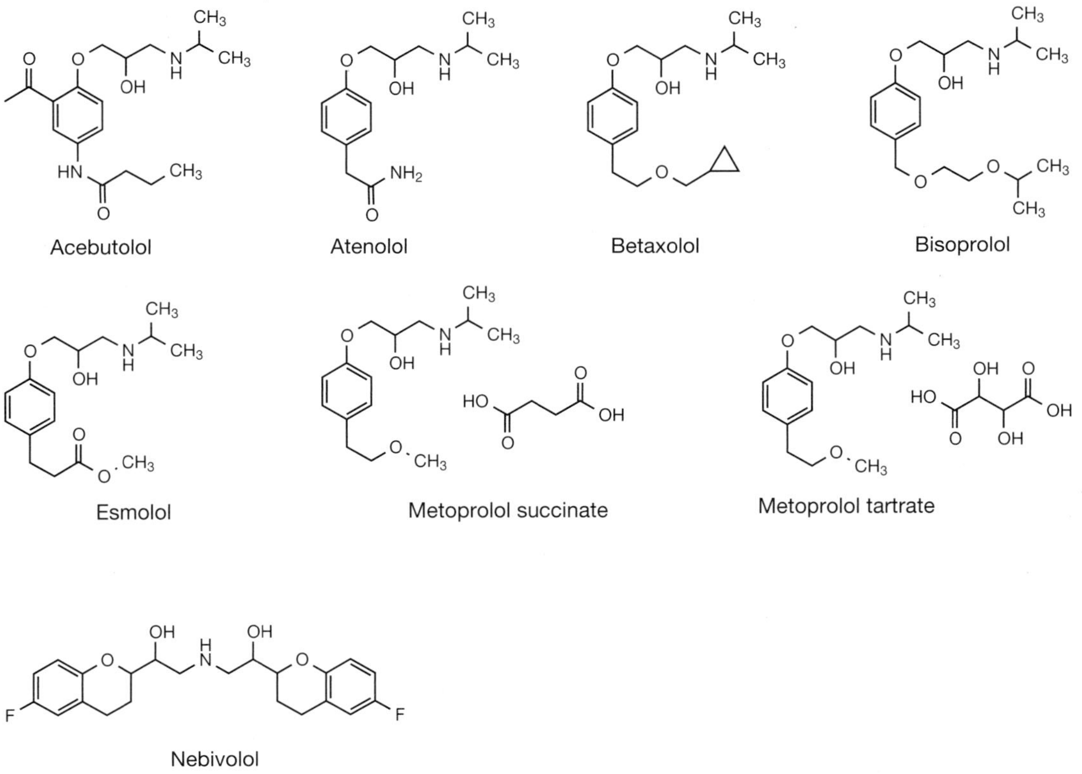

Figure 20.8 Selective β_1 adrenergic antagonists.

ether substitution (Fig. 20.8). It is sold as its fumarate salt. It exhibits relatively small inter- and intra-individual variability with predictable pharmacokinetics.[133] Orally administered bisoprolol is well absorbed, and the bioavailability is about 90%.[133] About 30% of the drug is protein bound. It undergoes moderate first-pass metabolism and is primarily metabolized by CYP3A4 and CYP2D6 to inactive metabolites.[133,134] The plasma half-life is relatively long (~10-11 hours), allowing for once-daily dosing.[133] Bisoprolol is eliminated renally and hepatically in similar proportions.[133]

Carvedilol. Carvedilol is a weakly basic (pKa = 7.8) lipophilic (LogP = 2.68; CLogP = 3.28)[105] blocker antagonizing α_1-, β_1-, and β_2-receptors (Fig. 20.7).[135,136] Carvedilol prevents reflex tachycardia by acting as a potent competitive antagonist at β_1- and β_2-receptors.[137] Carvedilol vasodilatory properties are due to α_1-adrenoceptor blockade.[137] At high concentrations, carvedilol acts as a calcium channel antagonist, and in cutaneous circulation, it increases blood flow.[137] It contains one chiral center, but it is marketed as a racemic mixture consisting of the *S*(-)-enantiomer and *R*(+)-enantiomer.[138,139] Carvedilol contains a unique tricyclic heterocyclic ring system known as carbazole. Carbazole contains a central five-membered heteroaromatic ring system, which is in turn fused to two phenyl rings on either side. The β-blocking properties of carvedilol is about 10 times more potent than the α-blocking properties.[138] The *S*(-)-enantiomer is almost exclusively responsible for its β-blocking properties; whereas, both *S*(-)- and *R*(+)-enantiomers equally block α_1-receptors.[138]

After oral administration, carvedilol is rapidly absorbed and undergoes extensive hepatic first-pass metabolism.[138] The absolute oral bioavailability is about 25%.[140] The peak plasma concentration is achieved in about 1 to 2 hours.[138,140] The absorption is delayed when taken with food.[138] It undergoes extensive protein binding (>98%) and is primarily bound to albumin.[135] The volume of distribution is about 115 L.[135] Carvedilol undergoes both phase-I and phase II metabolic reactions.[140] Carvedilol phase-I reactions involve aromatic ring hydroxylation and side chain cleavage.[140] The hydroxylated and demethylated carvedilol also have activity.[135] Specifically, the 4′-hydroxyphenyl metabolite of carvedilol is about 13-fold more potent β-blocker than carvedilol.[135] Phase II metabolism occurs predominantly by glucuronidation.[140] Carvedilol displays stereoselective drug disposition.[139] In poor CYP2D6 metabolizers, the plasma concentrations of *R*-carvedilol is significantly greater than extensive metabolizers.[139] However, the plasma concentrations of *S*-carvedilol is similar in both poor and extensive metabolizers. Therefore, poor CYP2D6 metabolizers may have significant α-blockade.[139] Other CYP enzymes that are involved in the metabolism of carvedilol include CYP2C9, CYP1A2, and CYP3A4.[141] The majority of carvedilol is eliminated as metabolites. About 60% is eliminated in feces.[140] Only 2% of the intact drug and 16% as metabolites are eliminated in the urine.[142]

DRUG INTERACTIONS. The drug interactions associated with β-blockers are pharmacodynamic or pharmacokinetic interactions.[143] Pharmacodynamic interactions are attributed to the mechanism of action of administered drugs, while pharmacokinetic interactions are attributed to alterations of drug metabolizing enzymes such as CYP enzymes and transporters such as MDR1 (P-glycoprotein).[143] Diphenhydramine, a first-generation antihistamine, inhibits CYP2D6 metabolism of metoprolol in extensive metabolizers.[144] This will potentiate the adverse effects of metoprolol such as prolonged negative chronotropic and inotropic effects.[144] Therefore, CYP2D6 inhibitors (eg, quinidine, paroxetine, fluoxetine) may increase the plasma concentrations of CYP2D6 β-blocker substrates.[145,146] Carvedilol is a potent inhibitor of P-glycoprotein and increases plasma digoxin levels.[90,147] Bisoprolol also significantly inhibits P-glycoprotein, whereas, atenolol, metoprolol, and sotalol are not P-glycoprotein inhibitors.[90,148] Carvedilol is also a P-glycoprotein substrate, and co-administration with rifampin leads to significantly decreased carvedilol serum concentrations.[149]

ADVERSE EFFECTS. The side effects associated with β-blockers include AV blockade, bradycardia, hypotension, gastrointestinal disturbances, and pruritic rash.[150] Pulmonary side effects such as bronchitis and bronchospasm are associated with all β-blockers; however, cardiovascular selectivity may be achieved with small doses of selective β_1-blockers.[150] Nonselective β-blockers are contraindicated in patients with a history of reactive airway disease (eg, asthma). Lipophilic β-blockers have a greater ability to cause CNS disturbances such as insomnia, dreams, hallucinations, and depression.[150] Some of the β-blockers may cause a rare oculomucocutaneous reaction.[150] β_2-Adrenergic receptors play a significant role in insulin release and gluconeogenesis. Nonselective β-blockers are also contraindicated in patients with insulin-dependent (type 1) diabetes. Nonselective β-blockers can slow down the recovery of insulin-induced hypoglycemia and block/mask most of these signs of hypoglycemia with the exception of sweating. Patients should also avoid sudden discontinuation of β-blockers because of the risk for hypertensive crises caused by the receptor up-regulation.

Chemistry of Ranolazine

Ranolazine was approved by the US FDA in 2006.[151] Chemically, it is *N*-(2,6-dimethylphenyl)-2-(4-(2-hydroxy-3-(2-methoxyphenoxy)propyl)piperazin-1-yl)acetamide.[151] It contains a chiral center, but is synthesized and sold as a racemic mixture.[152] Ranolazine immediate-release capsule and oral solution have a short elimination half-life, which had subsequently led to the development of an extended-release formulation, which allows for twice daily dosing.[152]

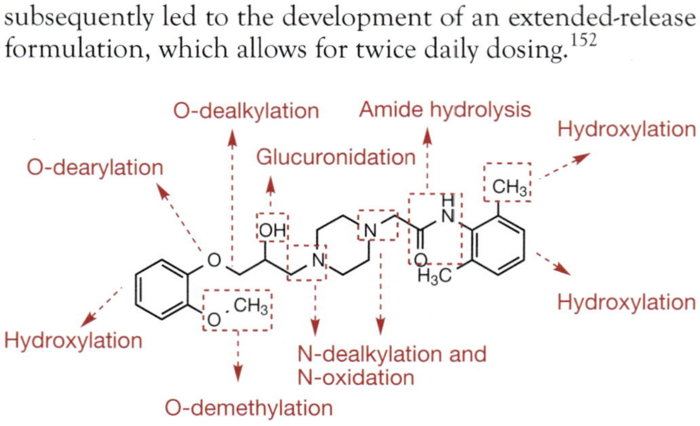

Metabolic sites of ranolazine

Pharmacokinetics. Ranolazine has an absolute oral bioavailability of 35% to 50%. The amount and extent of ranolazine absorption from an extended-release formulation is not significantly affected by food.[152] Approximately 60% of the drug is protein bound.[152] Ranolazine is extensively metabolized in the liver by CYP3A4 and is a minor substrate for CYP2D6.[152] Ranolazine undergoes methyl group hydroxylation and aromatic hydroxylation.[153] The amide group attached to the aromatic ring undergoes amide hydrolysis to yield a piperazine carboxylic acid metabolite and 2,6-dimethyl aniline.[153] It undergoes N-dealkylation metabolic reactions at the either side of the piperazine ring system.[153] It is metabolized by O-dearylation and O-demethylation at the methoxy phenoxy end. Nitrogen atoms on the piperazine ring can directly undergo N-oxidation.[153] Ranolazine also directly undergoes glucuronidation, and several of its metabolites are further metabolized by glucuronidation and sulfation.[153,154] The half-life elimination of immediate- and extended-release ranolazine is about 2 and 7 hours, respectively.[152] Approximately 75% of ranolazine and its metabolites are excreted in the urine, and less than 5% of the intact drug is excreted unchanged.[152] The plasma concentration of ranolazine is increased in patients with renal impairment.[152] HF and diabetes do not significantly alter pharmacokinetic parameters of ranolazine.[152] Ranolazine peak plasma concentration is increased in patients with cirrhosis. Therefore, ranolazine is contraindicated in patients with liver cirrhosis.

Drug-Drug Interactions. Ranolazine is a weak CYP3A4 inhibitor and increases simvastatin plasma concentrations by about 2-fold.[152] Ranolazine is a P-glycoprotein inhibitor and increases plasma digoxin concentrations.[152] Concurrent administration of other CYP3A4 inhibitors such as ketoconazole increases ranolazine concentration by about 4-fold and verapamil increases ranolazine concentration by about 2-fold.[152] Since ranolazine is only a minor substrate for CYP2D6, concurrent administration of other drugs that are CYP2D6 inhibitors or inducers have a minor effect on ranolazine plasma concentrations.[152]

Adverse Effects. The most common adverse effects associated with ranolazine include nausea, dizziness, headache, and constipation.[155] Ranolazine prolongs the QT interval and may potentially contribute to torsades de pointes, a unique form of polymorphic ventricular tachycardia.[156]

Chemistry of Ivabradine

Scientists at the Servier Research Institute screened various compounds to reduce the heart rate.[157] In that screen, they identified two potent classes of molecules, benzocyclobutane and indane derivatives.[157] Indane derivatives prolonged the action potential (AP) duration; however, success was found with ivabradine, an optically pure *S* isomer of a benzocyclobutane analog (Fig. 20.9).[157]

Pharmacokinetics. Ivabradine is completely absorbed, but the absolute oral bioavailability is about 40% due to extensive intestinal and hepatic first-pass metabolism by CYP3A4.[158] The peak plasma levels are achieved in about 1 hour after the oral administration under fasting conditions.[158] Even though

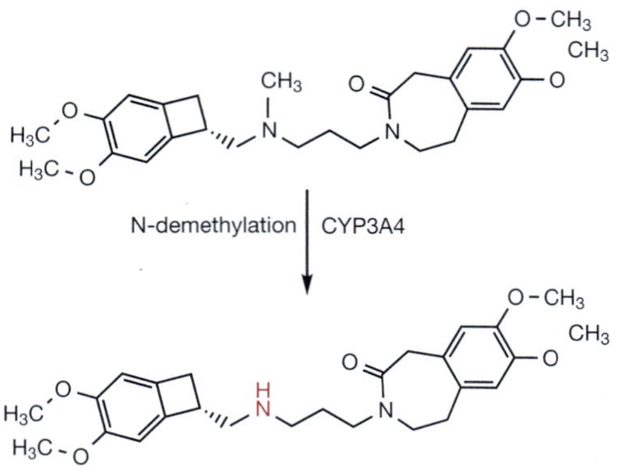

Figure 20.9 Metabolism of ivabradine.

food delays the absorption of ivabradine, it enhances the plasma level by about 20% to 40%.[158] Ivabradine is about 70% bound to plasm proteins. Ivabradine undergoes N-demethylation by CYP3A4 to form desmethyl ivabradine, which may further be metabolized (see Fig. 20.9).[158] Both ivabradine and desmethyl metabolite have equal potency.[158] The half-life elimination of ivabradine is about 6 hours. Ivabradine is excreted in feces and urine.[158]

Drug-Drug Interactions. Since ivabradine is metabolized by CYP3A4, DDIs may occur with CYP3A4 inhibitors and inducers.[159] Carbamazepine, which is an anticonvulsant drug and a CYP3A4 inducer, increases the first-pass metabolism of ivabradine and decreases plasma concentrations and the area under the curve (AUC) by about 5-fold.[160] Phenytoin, used in the treatment of epilepsy, is a potent CYP3A4 inducer, which significantly decreases the plasma concentrations and bioavailability of ivabradine.[159] Therefore, coadministration of ivabradine with CYP3A4 inducers may lead to reduced biological response. Potent CYP3A4 inhibitors such as itraconazole and clarithromycin may increase the plasma concentrations of ivabradine, leading to increased toxic side effects.[158]

Toxic Effects. Even though toxic effects are extremely rare, ivabradine has the potential to cause sinus bradycardia. Ivabradine should be avoided in patients with sick sinus syndrome because it acts on the sinus node.[161] Ivabradine can prolong the QT interval, but by itself may not cause torsades de pointes.[161] Ivabradine should not be coadministered with other agents that can cause the QT prolongation and/or agents that lower the heart rate.[161] Ivabradine binds to the I_h channels in the eye, and at high doses, it leads to changes in the electroretinogram.[161] In about 15% patients, it resulted in mild to moderate visual disturbances.[161]

Drugs for the Treatment of Heart Failure

Heart Failure

According to the AHA, it is estimated that HF affects over 6.5 million adult Americans (2011-2014) and is projected to increase to 46% between 2012 and 2030. Projections show that heart failure costs will increase by 127% from 2012 to 2030.[162] Congestive heart failure (CHF) is a debilitating disease with a high rate of morbidity and mortality. The 5-year prognosis for patients with CHF is either a heart transplant or mortality of 50%. CHF is a complex disease that involves several neuronal and humoral pathways. It is characterized by the body's inability to maintain its normal metabolic needs, which is caused by the functional or structural loss of viable myocardial cells. This can occur over a long (chronic) or short (acute) period. There are several comorbidities that cause CHF, but the most common causes are IHD, hypertension, MI, and diabetes. In addition, improvements in diagnostic techniques have established that a mutation in the transthyretin (TTR) protein has been associated with misfolding of TTR and aggregation into amyloid fibrils in the heart. The deposition of amyloid in the extracellular space leads to amyloidosis and HF.[163,164] HF is classified by the New York Heart Association (NYHA) into four classes: I, II, III, and IV. Patients in class I are the least severe and do not present any limitations or symptoms. Classes II and III are described as patients who are comfortable at rest but demonstrate symptoms at different degrees of physical activity. In contrast, patients in class IV are the most severe with symptoms at rest and are unable to carry out any physical activities without symptoms. In addition to the NYHA, the American College of Cardiology (ACC) and the AHA have developed a system that focuses on the progression of the disease. In this system, patients are classified by stages A through D. Stage A indicates that patients are at risk for HF (eg, previous medical history of chronic hypertension) but do not yet have symptoms or structural or functional heart disease. Stage B indicates that patients are without current or previous symptoms of HF but with either structural heart disease or other risk factors. Stage C indicates that patients with current or previous symptoms of HF but are well controlled. Stage D indicates that patients have HF symptoms that interfere with daily life functions or lead to repeated hospitalizations.[165]

From a physiologic standpoint, HF can be divided into left ventricle HF or right ventricle HF. It can also be further divided into diastolic HF (the heart cannot relax and fill the ventricle properly) or systolic heart failure (cannot contract and eject blood properly). The major purpose of the circulation is to move blood forward and perfuse organs and tissues. However, if the heart cannot relax or contract properly, blood starts to accumulate in the ventricles and/or move backward. This backward movement of blood will lead to accumulation of fluids and edema. Right ventricle failure typically leads to peripheral edema, as observed by swelling of the ankles. Left ventricle failure produces accumulation of fluid in the lungs. As a result of fluid overload, patients will present with signs and symptoms that are usually characterized by shortness of breath, increased fatigue, edema, nausea, lack of appetite, and arrhythmias.[166]

Under normal physiologic tone, the cardiac output (4-8 L/min) is defined as the product of heart rate times stroke volume. Stroke volume is directly affected by three factors: myocyte contractile force, preload (left ventricle end-diastolic pressure), and afterload (systolic pressure).

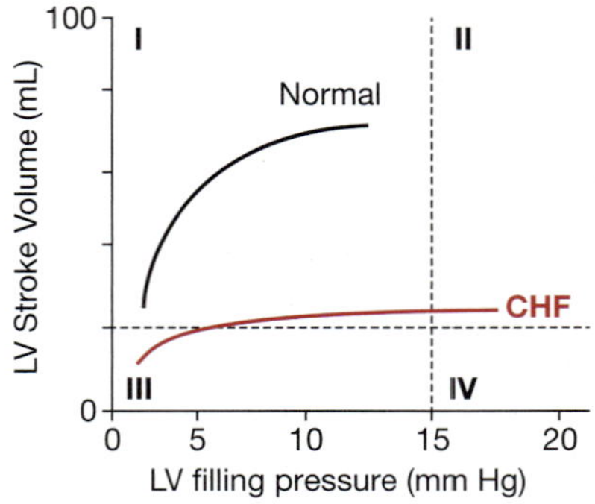

Figure 20.10 Frank-Starling curve.

The relationship between the stroke volume and left-ventricle filling pressure (LVFP) is represented by the Frank-Starling (FS) curve (Fig. 20.10).[167] Under normal physiologic conditions, the stroke volume is directly proportional to LVFP and/or the myocardium contractile force. As a result, the stroke volume increases as the LVFP and/or the myocardium contractile force increases. In contrast, the stroke volume is indirectly proportional to afterload. Stroke volume decreases as systemic vascular resistance increases because it requires greater workload for the heart to compensate for this increase in arterial pressure.[168] The FS curve relationship can be subdivided into four quadrants. The FS curve in healthy individuals is typically in quadrant I with enough room for compensation. If the preload is further increased, the LVFP would exceed the normal range (10-15 mm Hg), and the stroke volume would plateau and extend into quadrant II. In this case, patients would become congested and show symptoms of edema. If contractile force is markedly reduced or the afterload is too high, patients may fall under quadrant III. This would lead to poor organ perfusion and possible organ damage. Patients who fall into quadrant IV are decompensated and would demonstrate symptoms of both poor organ perfusion and congestion. This FS curve reflects severe stage IV CHF. In these patients, the FS curve plateaus much faster at a lower volume. Drugs used in the treatment of CHF are designed to modify preload, afterload and contractility as a therapeutic approach to increase stroke volume, decrease edema, and perfuse organs.[169]

Mechanism of Action of Drugs Used to Treat Heart Failure

Glycosidic Positive Inotropic Agents

Digoxin and digitoxin are potent and selective antagonists at the Na^+/K^+-ATPase pump.[170] The Na^+/K^+-ATPase is one of the major pumps involved in the reestablishment of ion homeostasis in the myocyte.[171] Digoxin binds to the Na^+/K^+-ATPase pump and blocks its ability to efficiently move Na^+ out and K^+ into the cell, leading to an increase in intracellular Na^+ concentrations. This in turn causes the reversal of the Na^+/Ca^{2+} exchanger, leading to an increase in intracellular Ca^{2+} levels, which contributes to an increase in contractile force and consequently stroke volume. Digoxin has not been shown to decrease mortality, but it improves the quality of life.[172]

Nonglycosidic Positive Inotropic Agents

Phosphodiesterase Inhibitors. PDEs are a group of intracellular enzymes that catalyze the breakdown of cyclic adenosine monophosphate (cAMP) and cyclic guanosine monophosphate (cGMP), and are distributed ubiquitously throughout the human body.[173,174] Eleven different isoenzymes (PDE 1-11) have been identified.[174] The PDE3 (phosphodiesterase-3) isoenzyme is mainly responsible for cleaving cAMP to AMP.[175] Inhibition of PDE3 leads to a decreased degradation and increased intracellular cAMP, and thereby increases the myocardium contraction.[175] Therefore, PDE3 inhibitors are therapeutically used for the short-term treatment of CHF.[173] PDE4 (phosphodiesterase-4) inhibitors are being investigated for their use in inflammatory airway diseases.[173] PDE5 inhibitors such as sildenafil citrate are used in the treatment of erectile dysfunction.[173]

Milrinone is a PDE3 antagonist with a lower affinity for other PDE isoenzyme subtypes. Its major sites of action are the heart and vasculature. By blocking the PDE3 in the heart, milrinone increases intracellular levels of cAMP, resulting in a Ca^{2+} mediated increase in inotropic contractile force.[176] Although the benefit of increased contractile force appears to be useful in the short-term, milrinone increases the workload of the heart and the risk for arrhythmias in the long term, which may increase mortality. In addition to its effects in the heart, milrinone also increases the levels of cAMP in the vasculature. An increase of cAMP in the arteries and veins leads to a reduction in afterload and preload, respectively. These two effects are believed to be beneficial since it decreases the myocardium oxygen demand. This class of drugs can be used for the short-term support of critically ill patients with chronic HF.[177] However, patients who have ischemia appear to present with prolonged hospitalization and have an increase in mortality compared to patients without ischemia.[178]

Dopamine and Dobutamine. Both dopamine and dobutamine increase myocardium contractile force by activating β_1-adrenergic receptors.[179,180] These receptors are coupled to a Gs (stimulatory guanine nucleotide binding proteins) G-protein. Activation leads to increased levels of cAMP, and consequently Ca^{2+} ions. Dobutamine not only increases the force of contraction (inotropic), but also the speed of contraction (chronotropic). At low to moderate therapeutic doses, the effects on the heart are predominant, with the effects on β_2 (vasodilator) offsetting the effects of the α_1-receptors (vasoconstriction). At higher infusion doses, dobutamine's effect on the α_1-receptors start to predominate over its β_2 effect, which leads to an increase in blood pressure. The chronotropic effects also become more predominant and increase the risk for arrhythmias and angina pectoris. In contrast to dobutamine, dopamine at lower doses has higher affinity for the D_1- and D_2 dopamine receptors.[181] Activation of D_1 evokes primarily renal and mesenteric vasodilation via an increase in cAMP. The effects on the renal vasculature may increase the glomerular filtration rate (GFR) and benefit certain patients. At moderate doses, dopamine begins to bind and activate β_1-adrenergic receptors in the heart and produces an increase in the contractile force and heart rate. This effect is in addition to its renal effects. At higher doses, it becomes less selective and begins to bind and activate α_1-adrenergic receptors, which causes an increase in systemic vascular resistance. The increase in blood pressure will increase afterload and oxygen demand.

Nitrate Vasodilators

Refer to the "antianginal agents" section for the mechanism of action of organic nitrates.

Isosorbide Dinitrate in Combination with Hydralazine. The specific mechanism of action by which hydralazine produces its effect is not clear. However, it has been established that hydralazine is a potent vasodilator of arterial smooth muscle and decreases the afterload.[182] It is not usually used as monotherapy because of the compensatory effects it can evoke, including baroreflex-mediated tachycardia and water retention. In HF, hydralazine is used in combination with isosorbide dinitrate, resulting in a better outcome than with either drug alone.[183] This is due to the fact that hydralazine decreases the work load of the heart by decreasing afterload, while low doses of nitrates favor vasodilation of the venous system, thus decreasing preload. As a result, the stroke volume is improved and has also been shown to be more beneficial to African Americans who are resistant to angiotensin-converting enzyme (ACE) inhibitors.[183] Depending on the patients' genetics, sex, dose, and race, there is a risk for the development of drug-induced lupus syndrome and other autoimmune reactions.[184]

Other Vasodilators

The three β-blockers approved by the FDA for the treatment of CHF includes metoprolol succinate, bisoprolol, and carvedilol. All three have been shown to decrease mortality and morbidity. At therapeutic doses, bisoprolol and metoprolol are selective to the β_1-adrenergic receptors. In contrast, carvedilol is a nonselective β_1, β_2, and α_1-adrenergic receptor antagonist. Patients who are starting on these drugs should begin with the lowest doses and titrate their way up. Initial therapy with β-blockers in patients with HF causes a major decrease in cardiac output. However, by blocking the β_1-adrenergic receptor in the heart over the long term, patients not only improve their ejection fraction, but also decrease mortality.

In addition to β-blockers, drugs affecting the renin-angiotensin-aldosterone system have also been shown to be beneficial in patients with HF. Both ACE inhibitors and angiotensin II–receptor blockers (ARBs) decrease preload and afterload. ACE inhibitors block the conversion of angiotensin I into angiotensin II, and consequently decrease the activation of angiotensin type I receptor (AT1) by angiotensin II.[185] In addition, ACE inhibitors also decrease the breakdown of bradykinin. The increase in bradykinin plasma levels has been associated with the vasodilatory properties of ACE inhibitors. It is also accepted that by blocking the conversion of angiotensin I into angiotensin II, ACE inhibitors redirect the pathway and increase the production of angiotensin 1-7, which has been proposed to oppose the effects of angiotensin II. In contrast to ACE inhibitors, ARBs have a high affinity for the angiotensin AT1 receptor. Both ACE inhibitors and ARBs decrease cardiovascular remodeling and mortality. The specific drugs in these two classes, detailed mechanism of action, and side effects are further discussed in Chapter 19. However, both ACE inhibitors and ARBs cause similar side effects, including hypotension, hyperkalemia, increase in serum creatinine, and potential fetus damage.

Diuretics, in particular loop diuretics, have also been shown to decrease volume overload in patients with CHF. Furosemide is a prototypical drug, and it decreases preload by blocking the $Na^+/K^+/2Cl^-$transporter in the ascending loop of Henle. Although these drugs do not decrease mortality, they can decrease the symptoms associated with hypervolemia and decrease edema. Providers should be careful using these drugs since they may cause electrolyte imbalance and dehydration. See Chapter 19 for a full description of all loop diuretics.

Neprilysin Inhibitor/Angiotensin II–Receptor Blocker: Sacubitril/Valsartan

Sacubitril is the first drug in its class and is used in combination with valsartan.[186] Valsartan is an ARB that acts primarily by blocking the activation of AT1 receptors. Valsartan is approved as part of CHF therapy by the FDA for patients who cannot tolerate ACE inhibitors. Sacubitril is rapidly metabolized to sacubitrilat, a neprilysin endopeptidase (NEP) antagonist. NEP is involved in the breakdown of atrium natriuretic peptide (ANP), which belongs to a family of peptides that are released by the atria in response to an increase in preload and consequently atrial pressure via stretch-sensitive ion channels.[187] Once in the circulation, this peptide has natriuretic, diuretic, and vasodilatory properties. However, it has a short half-life and is readily metabolized in the liver, lung, and kidneys by the NEP enzyme. By blocking the NEP enzyme, sacubitril prolongs the half-life of ANP and increases its circulating plasma levels. When combined with valsartan, it further decreases preload and afterload in patients with HF.

Soluble Guanylate Cyclase Activator: Vericiguat

Vericiguat is a soluble guanylate cyclase (sGC) activator approved for the treatment of HF with reduced ejection fraction. It has a similar mechanism of action to riociguat, an FDA drug approved for the treatment of pulmonary hypertension.[45,188] Activation of the sGC increases the production of cGMP, which is a second messenger involved in smooth muscle vasodilation.[189] As such, activation of sGC independent of nitric oxide produces a decrease in preload and afterload. Clinical trials established that vericiguat was dose-dependently associated with an increase in left-ventricle ejection fraction and a reduction in clinical events.[190] Vericiguat appears to be relatively safe and most side effects, hypotension and syncope, are produced by the relaxation of arterial and venous arteries, respectively. Similar to nitric oxide donors, it should be avoided with drugs that also increase intracellular levels of cGMP, such as PDE 5 inhibitors.[191]

Transthyretin Tetramers Stabilizer: Tafamidis

Tafamidis is a small molecule that selectively binds and stabilizes the TTR tetramers proteins by binding to unoccupied T_4 binding sites.[192] TTR is a protein secreted from the liver, choroid plexus, and retinal epithelial cells.[193] It contains predominantly four β-sheets that circulate as a tetramer and acts as a carrier for thyroxine.[193] Mutations in the TTR gene are generally associated with the destabilizing of the tetramers and an acceleration of their dissociation and a promotion of amyloidogenesis.[194] The dissociation of transthyretin tetramers into monomers is the rate-limiting step in the amyloidogenic process.[194] Tafamidis is approved for the treatment of the cardiomyopathy of wild-type or hereditary transthyretin-mediated amyloidosis (ATTR-CM) in adults.[195] Tafamidis was reported to reduce all-cause mortality and cardiovascular-related hospitalizations as compared to placebo.[196] Although tafamidis does not directly affect cardiac function, it appears to slow down the progression of the disease. Tafamidis appears to be safe, with only post-market GI side effects.[195]

Chemistry, Physicochemical Properties, Adverse Effects, and Drug Interactions of Drugs Used to Treat Heart Failure

Chemistry of the Cardiac Glycosides

In ancient times, cardiac glycosides were applied to arrows and were used as poisons in human warfare.[197] In 1785, William Withering, a physician and botanist, described the medical uses of the foxglove plant (*Digitalis purpurea*) in "*An account of the foxglove, and some of its medical uses: with practical remarks on dropsy, and other diseases.*"[198] Reports indicate that even though the foxglove plant was used for many centuries for various purposes, it was Withering who paved the way for the standard use of cardiac glycosides in modern practice.[199] Sydney Smith in 1930 isolated the active ingredient digoxin from *Digitalis lanata*.[200] Cardiac glycosides are composed of carbohydrates and steroids. The steroid portion is commonly referred to as an aglycone or genin, and the carbohydrate portion is commonly referred to as a glycone.[201] The carbohydrate units are linked to one another as well as to the steroid template by glycosidic bonds.

Aglycones. The steroid template contains fused A, B, C, and D rings which in turn are fused to an unsaturated lactone ring at C_{17} in a β configuration.[197] Cardiac glycosides can be classified into cardenolides and bufadienolides, based on the aglycone portion.[197] Cardenolides contain a five-membered α, β unsaturated lactone (butyrolactone), and the steroid template (including the lactone ring) is composed of 23 carbon atoms.[202] In contrast, bufadienolides contain a six-membered unsaturated lactone (α-pyrone) ring, and the steroid template (including the lactone ring) is composed of 24 carbon atoms.[202] The cardiac glycosides commonly occur in plants, and the sources of important cardiac glycosides include the leaves of *Digitalis purpurea* and *Digitalis lanata*, and the seeds of *Stropanthus kombe* and *Stropanthus gratus*.[202] The major aglycones in *Digitalis* species include digitoxigenin, gitoxigenin, digoxigenin, and gitaligenin, whereas *Stropanthus* species include stropanthidin and ouabagenin (Fig 20.11).[202] The therapeutically used cardiac glycoside preparations are primarily obtained from

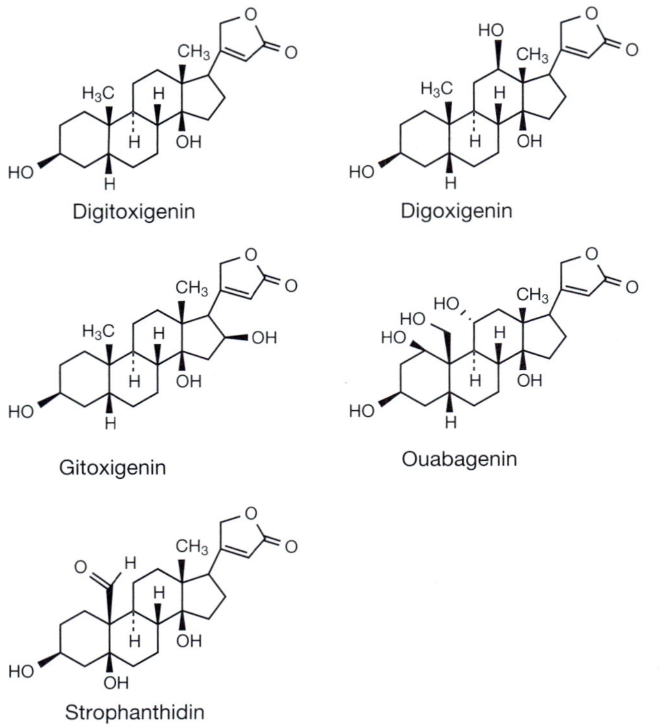

Figure 20.11 Cardenolide aglycones.

the *Digitalis* species. In nature, some animals also contain cardiac glycosides, such as the venom glands in the skin of toads contain bufadienolides.[202]

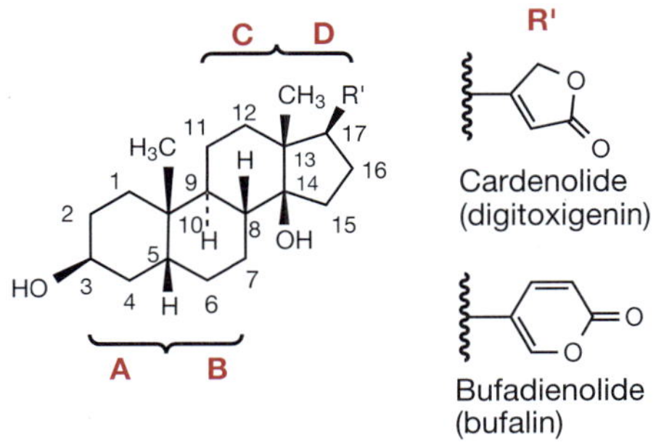

Cardenolide and bufadienolide aglycones

Glycones. The sugar portion of the cardiac glycoside contains one or more units typically attached at the 3-position of the steroid. The commonly occurring sugars in *Digitalis* species include glucose, 3-acteyl digitoxose, and/or digitoxose, whereas *Stropanthus* species include glucose, cymarose, and/or rhamnose (Fig. 20.12). The presence of side chains such as the 3-acetyl groups effects the physicochemical and pharmacokinetic properties of molecules. The sugars are predominantly linked to one another by the β (1 → 4) glycosidic bonds.

The two commonly used cardiac glycoside preparations are digoxin and digitoxin. In the United States, digoxin is the only cardiac glycoside approved for therapeutic use. The structure of digoxin contains the aglycone digoxigenin and three digitoxose sugars, whereas the structure of digitoxin contains the aglycone digitoxigenin and three digitoxose

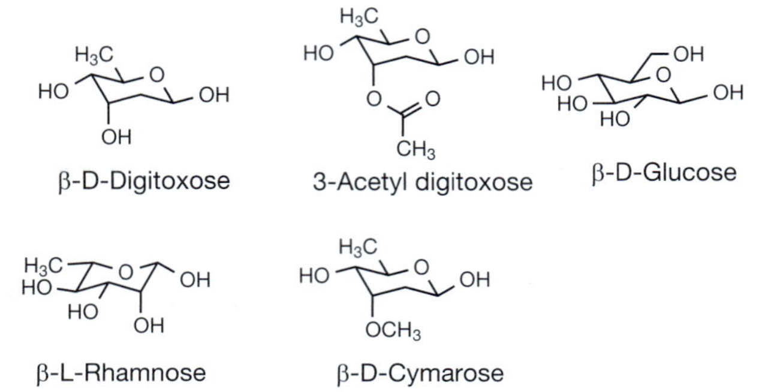

Figure 20.12 Selected sugars found in naturally occurring cardiac glycosides.

sugars.[202] In digoxigenin, digitoxigenin, and stropanthidin-based cardenolides, rings A-B, B-C, and C-D have *cis*, *trans*, and *cis* configurations (Fig 20.11). Because of this specific fusion of rings, the steroid template acquires a characteristic bent shape, as opposed to a flat shape.[197]

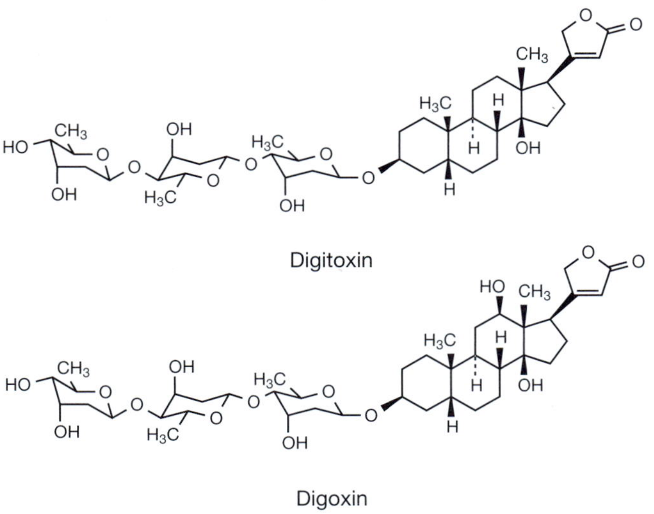

Structural Requirements for Cardiotonic Activity. The Na^+/K^+-ATPase contains both α and β subunits; the α subunit exists in α_1, α_2, α_3, and α_4 isoforms, and the β subunit exists in β_1, β_2, and β_3 isoforms.[203] The α_2 isoform is primarily present in skeletal, smooth, and cardiac muscle and is believed to be an important target of the cardiac glycosides.[204]

Importance of Sugars. The number of sugars attached to the steroid template appears to play a key role in its cardiotonic properties.[204,205] Tridigitoxosyl digoxigenin (digoxin) is more active than didigitoxosyl digoxigenin, which in turn is more active than monodigitoxosyl digoxigenin. On the contrary, tetradigitoxosyl digoxigenin is less active than digoxin. This indicates that the three sugars present in the structure of digoxin are optimal for its cardiotonic activity, and the hydrophilic pocket present in the enzyme can accommodate three sugars. Four sugars are sterically detrimental for the inhibitory activity.[170] Although the sugar portion of the glycoside is not absolutely essential, it is required for optimal cardiotonic activity.[204,205] Digoxigenin (only the steroid component of digoxin) has some cardiotonic properties, but its activity is significantly lower than monodigitoxosyl digoxigenin.[204,205]

Importance of the Steroid Nucleus. The specific fusion of the steroid rings seems to be very critical for the activity. For example, digitoxigenin, which has an A-B *cis* configuration, has 35 times higher binding affinity than Uzarigenin, which has an A-B *trans* configuration.[205] Introduction of polar head groups on the steroid template, such as the hydroxyl group, may reduce the activity.[205] For example, 16-hydroxy digitoxin (gitoxin) has about a 7-fold lower binding affinity than digitoxin.[205] Furthermore, it was recently shown that digoxin's steroid concave surface (α-surface) interacts with the hydrophobic surface by non-polar interactions.[170] Digoxin and digitoxin are both potent molecules. Digoxin has a hydroxy group at the 12-position on the steroid nucleus, making it slightly more hydrophilic than digitoxin, which is also one of the primary reasons for their pharmacokinetic differences.

Importance of the Lactone. The unsaturated lactone ring is optimal for activity. If the carbon-carbon double bond is reduced in the lactone ring, the binding affinity is tremendously diminished.[205] The lactone ring fits into the hydrophobic pocket, which most likely leads to the cationic-binding site occupied by Mg^{2+} or K^{+}.[170] The lack of the lactone ring may lead to compounds with some cardiotonic properties. For example, investigations of synthetic compounds in which the C-17 β lactone ring has been replaced with basic moieties such as guanylhydrazone and O-aminoalkyloximes androstane diol derivatives led to compounds with Na^+/K^+-ATPase inhibitory activity.[206,207] Overall, the cardiotonic properties of the cardiac glycosides are affected by the degree/type of glycosylation, the type of substituents/configuration of the steroid rings, and the size and degree of unsaturation of the lactone ring.[170]

Pharmacokinetics of the Cardiac Glycosides

Orally administered digoxin is primarily absorbed in the small intestine.[208] The amount of digoxin absorption is dependent on the type of oral formulation. Approximately 70% is absorbed when given in the form of tablets, and 80% absorbed in the form of elixir.[209] The discontinued *Lanoxicaps* capsules of digoxin had an oral bioavailability up to 100%.[210] Digoxin reaches a steady state concentration in about 5 to 7 days.[211] It has a high volume of distribution (7 L/kg)[208] and is highly bound to skeletal muscles, heart, and kidneys.[208] Only about 20% to 30% of digoxin is bound to serum albumin.[208] Digoxin is similarly distributed in normal and obese individuals when the ideal body weight (IBW) is considered.[212] Therefore, in obese individuals, digoxin dosages should be calculated based on the IBW rather than the total body weight, which includes the adipose tissue.[212] From the structural perspective, since the sugar portion of the digoxin contributes to its hydrophilic nature, it is not well distributed into lipophilic adipose tissue.[213] The volume of distribution is decreased in patients with impaired renal function, requiring dose reduction.[214] The apparent volume of distribution in infants is higher than in adults.[215] Digoxin, when administered to pregnant women, rapidly crosses the placental barrier and is equally distributed in maternal and fetal blood.[216]

Digoxin is primarily eliminated by the kidneys (~70%), predominantly as the unchanged drug. Approximately 25% to 30% of digoxin is eliminated by the hepatic and biliary routes, but the enterohepatic circulation is of less significance.[208,209] In the body, digoxin is hydrolyzed to digoxigenin bisdigitoxoside, digoxigenin monodigitoxoside, and digoxigenin. In about 10% of the patient population, the lactone ring on digoxin is reduced by gastrointestinal bacteria to dihydrodigoxin, a cardio inactive metabolite.[217] Further, administration of antibiotics such as tetracycline or erythromycin to individuals taking digoxin leads to an increased serum digoxin concentration, which indicates that any alteration of the gut flora may affect the absorption of digitalis.[217] The half-life elimination of digoxin in healthy volunteers is approximately 40 hours.[208] The major route of elimination is by glomerular filtration and, to a lesser extent, by tubular secretion and tubular reabsorption.[208] P-glycoprotein is involved in the tubular secretion of digoxin.[218] In older adults, digoxin has a longer half-life and increased blood concentration, which can be attributed to reduced body size and decreased urinary elimination.[219] Thus, the dosage of digoxin needs to be appropriately adjusted. It was observed that in patients with hypothyroidism, serum digoxin concentrations were at higher levels and in patients with hyperthyroidism, serum digoxin concentrations were at lower levels, which correlated with changes in the GFR and digoxin serum half-life.[220] Patients with hyperthyroidism also have higher digoxin clearances.[221]

Digitoxin has a long plasma half-life ranging from 5 to 7 days and requires 35 days to attain a plateau.[211] Digitoxin is less dependent on renal function than digoxin and about 50% of digitoxin is eliminated renally.[211,222] Digitoxin is metabolized by hydrolysis to digitoxigenin bisdigitoxoside, digitoxigenin monodigitoxoside, and digitoxigenin.[223,224] Digitoxin minimally undergoes hydroxylation at the C_{12} carbon of the aglycone to form digoxin.[223]

Toxicity of Cardiac Glycosides

Digoxin and other cardiac glycosides have a narrow therapeutic window. Within this window, they are therapeutically effective; however, variations in blood concentrations may lead to either toxic concentrations or subtherapeutic concentrations.[225] Increased digoxin serum levels more than 2 ng/mL is commonly associated with its toxicity.[226] Therefore, patients need to be carefully monitored for acute and chronic toxicity.[227] Digoxin toxicity includes gastrointestinal disturbances such as nausea, vomiting, anorexia, abdominal pain, and diarrhea; neuropsychiatric symptoms such as headache, delirium, hallucinations, convulsions, and drowsiness; yellow or green vision disturbances; cardiac disorders such as dysrhythmias and ventricular tachycardia.[227,228] Digoxin binding to Na^+/K^+-ATPase is inhibited by high levels of potassium. Therefore, hyperkalemia decreases digoxin activity and hypokalemia increases its toxicity.[229]

Drug Interactions of Cardiac Glycosides

Several drugs alter digoxin absorption, distribution, and elimination.[230] Digoxin is a well-known substrate for intestinal and renal P-glycoprotein.[231] Since P-glycoprotein is a multidrug efflux transporter, medications that are P-glycoprotein inhibitors can reduce the efflux of digoxin in the intestine and/or decrease the elimination of digoxin by the kidneys leading to increased plasma digoxin levels causing digoxin toxicity.[231,232] In contrast, P-glycoprotein inducers decrease plasma digoxin levels by an opposing mechanism, and as a result, digoxin may not reach therapeutic levels.[231,232] In vitro studies show that quinidine is a substrate for P-glycoprotein and a strong inhibitor of digoxin transport.[233] Co-administration of quinidine with digoxin increases digoxin's rate and extent of absorption, resulting in a 2-fold rise in its serum concentration.[234] Furthermore, the renal clearance of digoxin is reduced by 51% with an increase in its mean elimination half-life (up to 72 hours).[235,236] Concomitant administration of verapamil, a P-glycoprotein inhibitor, leads to non-competitive inhibition of digoxin's transport.[237] Verapamil reduces the total clearance of digoxin by 35% and increases its half-life by about 30%.[238,239] The anti-arrhythmic agent amiodarone, a P-glycoprotein inhibitor, increases the plasma concentration and AUC of digoxin.[240] This interaction may be sustained for several months potentiating its toxicity.[240] Cyclosporine inhibits renal tubular secretion and thereby increases digoxin's serum concentration by 50%.[241]

Rifampin, an intestinal P-glycoprotein inducer, decreases digoxin's oral bioavailability by about 30% and plasma levels up to 58%.[242] However, administration of rifampin does not significantly affect renal clearance and terminal half-life of digoxin.[242] Cholestyramine, a bile acid-binding sequestering resin used in reducing cholesterol levels, decreases digoxin's serum concentration and half-life probably by interfering with enterohepatic recycling and thereby leading to enhanced elimination of digoxin.[243] Antacids, such as magnesium carbonate and magnesium trisilicate, decrease the absorption of digoxin.[244] Macrolide antibiotics, especially clarithromycin, are associated with a high risk of digoxin toxicity.[232]

Drugs that decrease or increase potassium plasma levels should be avoided or used with caution. Loop (eg, furosemide) and thiazide (eg, hydrochlorothiazide) diuretics can cause hypokalemia, which may lead to an increased distribution of digoxin to its target receptor site resulting in an increased risk of toxicity. In contrast, potassium-sparing diuretics such as spironolactone can cause hyperkalemia, which may lead to a diminished therapeutic effect of digoxin.

Digoxin-Immune Fab

In acute and chronic digoxin poisoning, digoxin-specific antibody fragments is the effective choice of treatment.[245] Digoxin-immune Fab has a stronger affinity to digoxin than the affinity of digoxin toward its target receptor and biological membranes.[246] The administration of Digoxin-immune Fab results in the binding of free digoxin molecules to form a complex, and this shifts the equilibrium of digoxin bound to receptors.[246] Eventually, these complexes are eliminated, resulting in reduced digoxin levels in the body and decreased toxic effects.[246,247] Digoxin-immune Fab has an elimination half-life of about 16 to 20 hours, and its clearance can be reduced up to 75% in patients with renal failure.[247]

Nonglycosidic Positive Inotropic Agents

PHOSPHODIESTERASE 3 INHIBITORS: INAMRINONE AND MILRINONE. Milrinone and inamrinone are bipyridine derivatives (Fig. 20.13). Inamrinone was the first PDE3 bipyridine derivative approved for the treatment of CHF.[248] It was initially referred to as amrinone, but its name was later changed to inamrinone. The elimination half-life of IV inamrinone is up to 4 hours in healthy individuals.[249] In 2011, production of the inamrinone lactate injection in the United States was discontinued by its manufacturer, Bedford laboratories. Inamrinone has been replaced with milrinone, a less-toxic and more specific PDE3 inhibitor.[248] Milrinone has direct vasodilatory properties and is about 10 to 75 times more potent than inamrinone.[250]

An oral preparation of milrinone is not available in the United Sates. The prolonged administration of oral milrinone led to increased morbidity and mortality in patients with severe chronic HF, limiting its use.[251] Milrinone is only administered by IV in the form of its water-soluble lactate salt.[252] Milrinone has a quick onset of action of about 15 minutes, and approximately 70% of the drug is protein bound.[175] In adults, milrinone has an apparent volume of distribution 0.4 to 0.5 L/kg.[253] The half-life elimination of milrinone is about 2 hours. However, the half-life elimination can be extended up to 20 hours in patients undergoing continuous veno-venous hemofiltration.[254] The majority of milrinone (about 83%) is excreted unchanged renally. Metabolism of milrinone includes glucuronide conjugation. Milrinone doses should be adjusted in patients with moderate or severe kidney disease.[255]

Inamrinone may be associated with the increased risk of thrombocytopenia, which is usually not the case with milrinone.[248] Patients who are taking milrinone or inamrinone should be monitored for hepatic and renal functions.[248] Overdoses of PDE3 inhibitors may lead to hypotension and reflex tachycardia.[248] Since milrinone and other PDE3 inhibitors are associated with an increased risk of mortality and cardiovascular side effects in patients with chronic HF, long-term treatment of PDE3 inhibitors should be avoided.[256] Milrinone is chemically incompatible with the loop diuretic furosemide, and combining these two in admixture formulations results in precipitation.[257] Therefore, they should be administered separately.[257]

DOPAMINE. Dopamine (see Fig. 20.13) is an endogenous catecholamine that is biosynthesized from the amino acid L-tyrosine. Dopamine affects both the renal and

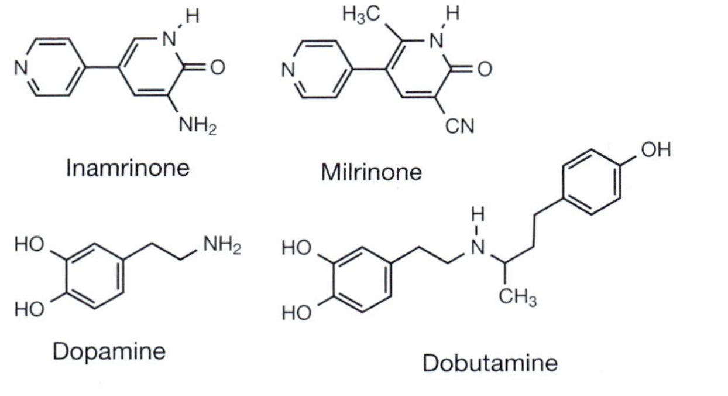

Figure 20.13 Nonglycosidic positive inotropic agents.

cardiovascular functions but only has a limited utility in the cardiogenic circulatory failure.[258] Dopamine plasma concentration, distribution, and metabolism is highly variable because of intra- and inter-individual differences.[259] Unlike PDE3 inhibitors, half-life elimination of catecholamines dopamine and dobutamine are in minutes.[175] When dopamine is administered exogenously, its agonistic activity at various receptors is dose and concentration dependent.[258] Dopamine metabolism is complex and undergoes both phase I and phase II metabolic reactions. Since dopamine undergoes quick metabolism, it is only administered through IV infusion. The free base dopamine is formulated in the form of water-soluble hydrochloride salt for IV infusion. The primary amine group in dopamine is oxidized by monoamine oxidase (MAO) to 3,4-dihydroxyphenylacetaldehyde (DOPAL). DOPAL further undergoes oxidation by aldehyde dehydrogenase to a carboxylic acid metabolite (3,4-Dihydroxyphenylacetic acid [DOPAC]) and reduction by alcohol dehydrogenase to an alcohol (3,4-dihydroxyphenylethanol [DOPET]).[260] Furthermore, catechol-O-methyltransferase (COMT) catalyzes 3-O-methylation of DOPAC to form homovanillic acid (HVA).[260] Dopamine is also directly metabolized by COMT to 3-methoxy tyramine, which is subsequently metabolized by MAO to 3-methoxy-4-hydroxyphenyl acetaldehyde.[260] The aldehyde metabolite further undergoes oxidation to the carboxylic acid metabolite HVA.[260] Dopamine also undergoes sulfation and glucuronidation.[260] The major excretion products of dopamine include dopamine conjugates, its metabolites HVA, DOPAC, and their glucuronide and sulfate conjugates.[260]

DOBUTAMINE. Dobutamine is a catecholamine that is synthetically produced in the laboratory. Dobutamine contains a secondary amine and a *sec*-butyl side chain that in turn is attached to a phenol (see Fig. 20.13). Dobutamine was developed in the early 1970s as part of structure-activity relationship studies of isoproterenol and dopamine.[261] Dobutamine contains a chiral center, but is clinically sold as a racemic mixture (±). The (+) enantiomer of dopamine is a potent α_1-adrenergic antagonist and the (–) enantiomer is a potent α_1-adrenergic agonist.[262] Both isomers are β-adrenergic agonists, but the (+)-isomer is much more potent than the (–) isomer.[262]

Like dopamine, dobutamine is administered by IV infusion and undergoes rapid metabolism. Dobutamine is formulated as the water-soluble hydrochloride salt and contains an antioxidant, sodium metabisulfite. Since it contains a sulfite in its formulation, it may trigger hypersensitive reactions such as rash and eosinophilia.[263] Dobutamine has a quick onset of action. Steady state concentration is achieved within 10 minutes, and the half-life elimination is about 2 minutes.[264] Dobutamine is predominantly metabolized by COMT to 3-O-methyldobutamine.[265] Dobutamine is excreted as dobutamine sulfate, 3-O-methyldobutamine, and 3-O-methyldobutamine sulfate conjugates.[265] Unlike dopamine, dobutamine appears not to be a substrate of MAO.[266] Its resistance to MAO metabolism is probably due to the bulky sec-butyl phenolic ring attached to the amine side chain. Dopamine is associated with increased urinary outflow and irregular heartbeat.[267] Dobutamine is associated with increased heart rate, increased systolic blood pressure, and premature ventricular beats.[268]

Nitrate Vasodilators

Nitroglycerin, isosorbide dinitrate, and mononitrate are used in the treatment of HF (refer to the section on drugs for the treatment of angina). In addition, the fixed dose of isosorbide dinitrate in combination with hydralazine is used as an adjunct therapy in patients with HF.[269] Hydralazine is also used as an antihypertensive agent. Chemically, hydralazine is a hydrazine derivative containing a phthalazine ring (Fig. 20.14).[270] The bioavailability of hydralazine in patients with HF for a single dose is about 10% to 26%.[271] Patients who are slow acetylators tend to have a higher percentage of bioavailability than fast acetylators probably due to lower first-pass metabolism. Increasing the dose and repeated administration of hydralazine increases its plasma concentration due to saturable first-pass metabolism.[271] Hydralazine reaches peak plasma concentration in 1 hour and the elimination half-life is about 4 hours, but is longer in slow acetylators.[271] Hydralazine undergoes extensive metabolism and several metabolites, including *N*-acetylhydrazinophthalazinone (NAcHPZ), triazolophthalazine (TP), phthalazinone (PZ), and hydralazine hydrazone (HH), are eliminated in the urine (Fig. 20.14).[272] The patient's acetylator phenotype influences hydralazine metabolism.[272] Slow acetylators are more prone to lupus syndrome than the rapid acetylators due to greater accumulation of non-acetylated metabolites.[272] Slow acetylators eliminate lower amounts of NAcHPZ and TP, but more of PZ and HH than the rapid acetylators.[272] The common side effects of this combination include headache, dizziness, nausea, and hypotension.[271]

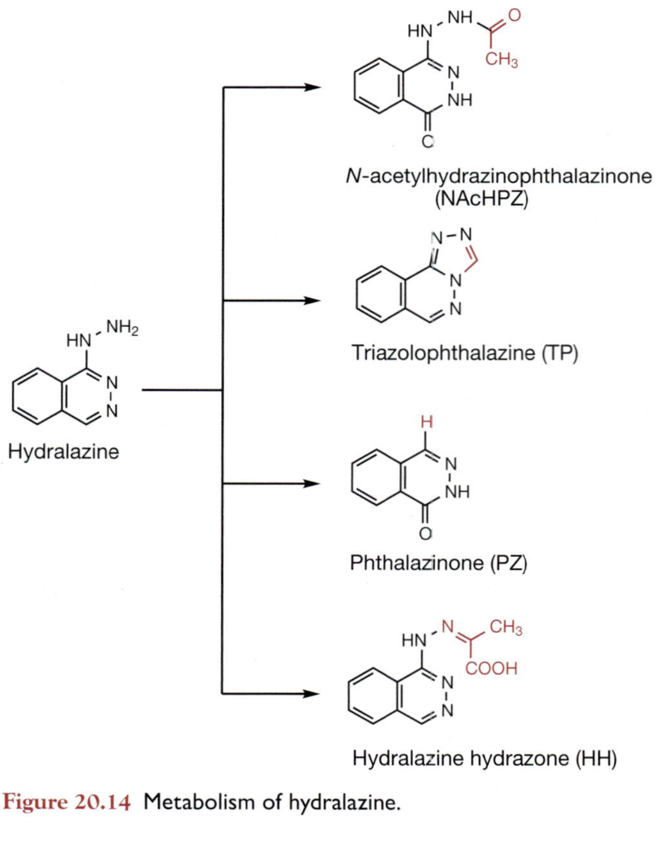

Figure 20.14 Metabolism of hydralazine.

Neprilysin Inhibitor/Angiotensin II–Receptor Blocker: Sacubitril/Valsartan

The combination of sacubitril and valsartan was approved by the FDA in 2015.[273] It was reviewed under the FDA's priority review program and was granted the fast track designation to reduce the risk associated with heart failure.[273] Sacubitril and valsartan are present in equal ratios in *Entresto*. Sacubitril is an ethyl ester prodrug, which undergoes rapid enzymatic hydrolysis to yield an active dicarboxylic metabolite (sacubitrilat or LBQ657) (Fig. 20.15).[274] Sacubitril and its metabolite (LBQ 657) are biphenyl derivatives containing two chiral centers. The most active form is the *R*, *S* isomer. Its enantiomer (*S*, *R*) and diastereomers (*S*, *S* and *R*, *R*) are less active, indicating the importance of stereospecificity on its biological activity.[275] Researchers at the Novartis Institutes for BioMedical Research Inc. studied the crystal structure of LBQ 657 with NEP, a zinc-dependent peptidase.[276] LBQ 657 interacts by reversible non-covalent interactions with NEP.[276] This study reveals several key interactions (Fig. 20.16)[276]:

1. The negatively charged oxygen on the carboxylate interacts with the zinc ion by ionic interactions.
2. The second carboxylate interacts with the Arg102 and Arg110 side chains by ionic interactions.
3. The amide backbone interacts with the side chains of Asn542 and Arg717 via hydrogen bonding.
4. The biphenyl ring and the methyl group fit into the hydrophobic binding pockets.

Chemically, valsartan contains a biphenyl ring and two acidic functional groups: a tetrazole ring (p*K*a = 4.73) and a carboxylic acid (p*K*a = 3.9).[277] Valsartan at physiological pH exists predominantly in its ionized form.[277] It is a unique ARB (refer to Chapter 19) containing an acylated valine amino acid.[278] It has one chiral center and is marketed as its (*S*)-isomer. Unlike sacubitril, valsartan does not require bioactivation and undergoes minimal metabolism to hydroxy valsartan.[279]

The sacubitril/valsartan combination has good aqueous solubility (>100 mg/mL).[280] Sacubitril has high permeability, and the bioavailability is predicted to be about 60%.[281] Although the absorption of valsartan is decreased with the food, it is not clinically significant. Therefore, this combination can be administered with or without food.[279] The peak plasma concentrations of sacubitril, LBQ657, and valsartan are achieved in 0.5, 2.5, and 2 hours, respectively.[282] Sacubitril, LBQ 657, and valsartan have high plasma protein binding (94%-97%).[279,281] Hepatic carboxylesterase-1 rapidly metabolizes oral sacubitril to

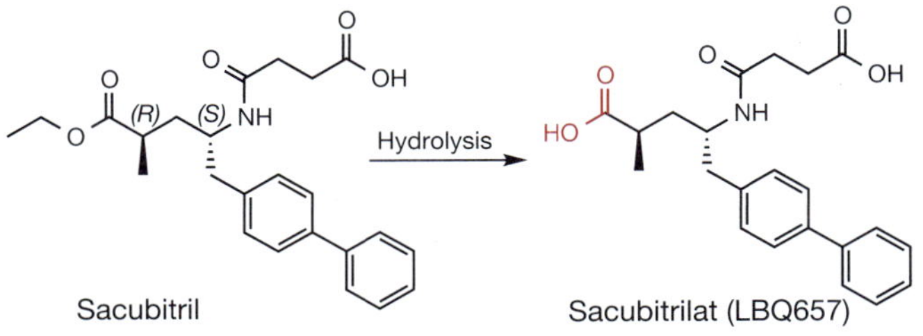

Figure 20.15 Metabolism of sacubitril.

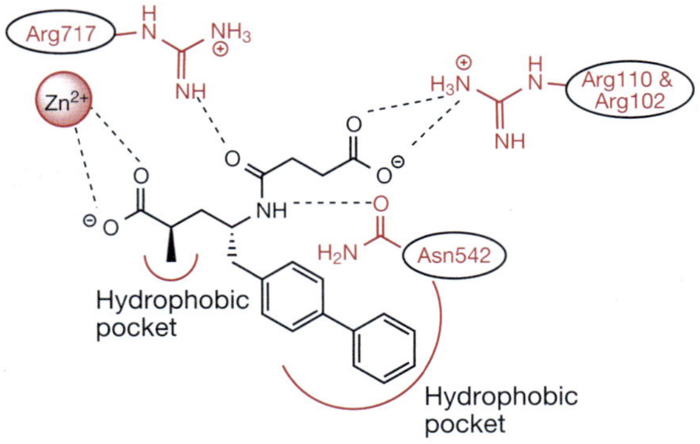

Figure 20.16 Sacubitrilat (LBQ657) binding to neprilysin.

LBQ 657.[283,284] Inter-individual variability in metabolic activation of sacubitril is attributed to genetic variants in carboxylesterase-1.[284] The plasma half-lives are about 4, 18, and 14 hours for sacubitril, LBQ657, and valsartan, respectively.[282] About 86% of sacubitril is eliminated as LBQ657 in the urine and feces.[283] About 86% of valsartan and its metabolites are eliminated in the feces.[279] In patients with moderate and severe renal impairment, the AUC of sacubitril is increased. Therefore, doses should be adjusted accordingly.[281] Sacubitril/valsartan should not be combined with nonsteroidal anti-inflammatory drugs because of the increased risk of renal failure.[279] In vitro studies indicate that sacubitril and LBQ 657 may not significantly inhibit or induce CYP enzymes to potentially cause clinically relevant CYP-mediated DDIs.[283] The use of sacubitril/valsartan is contraindicated in patients with a previous history of angioedema related to the use of ARB or ACE inhibitors.[279] Concomitant use with potassium-sparing diuretics is contraindicated because it may lead to increased potassium levels.[279] The common side effects include hypotension, hyperkalemia, cough, dizziness, elevated creatinine levels, and renal failure.[186,279]

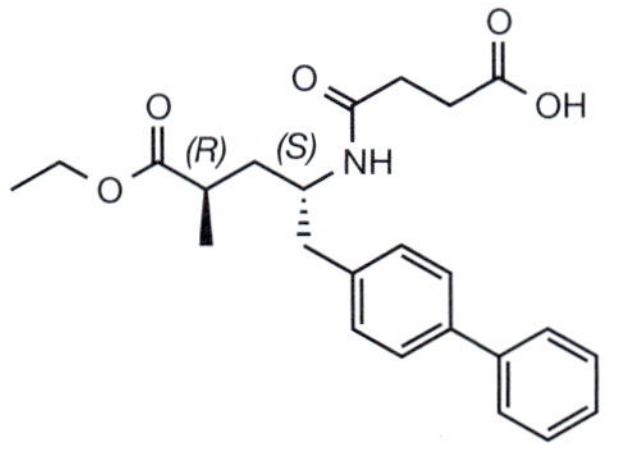

Sacubitril

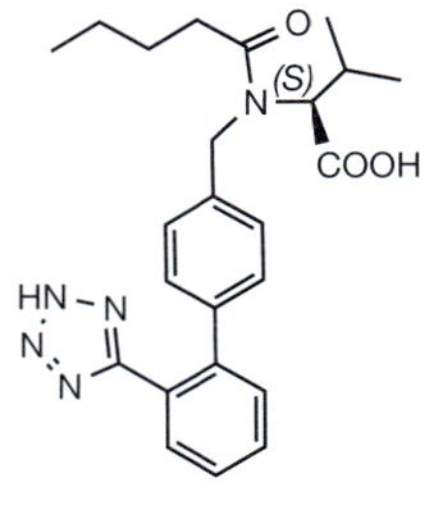

Valsartan

Soluble Guanylyl Cyclase Stimulator: Vericiguat

The suffix "ciguat" refers to all compounds that enhance the activity of sGC.[285] Vericiguat is a stimulator of sGC-cGMP and was the first drug approved for the treatment of symptomatic patients with chronic HF with reduced ejection fraction (HFrEF).[285] Riociguat is a sGC stimulator that was approved for the treatment of pulmonary arterial hypertension and chronic thromboembolic pulmonary hypertension.[286] However, riociguat has a short half-life. The structural modification of riociguat to reduce the clearance and increase the half-life led to the discovery of vericiguat.[285] Both vericiguat and riociguat contain a pyrazolo pyridine ring, but vericiguat contains an additional fluorine. Vericiguat and riociguat also differ in their carbamate functional groups. The carbamate nitrogen atom of vericiguat is unsubstituted, while the carbamate nitrogen atom of riociguat is attached to the methyl group. It is also important to have a terminal methyl group attached to the oxygen for prolonged metabolism.[285]

The absolute oral bioavailability of vericiguat is 93% when taken with food.[191] It is highly protein bound (98%), primarily to serum albumin. The half-life elimination in patients with HF is about 30 hours. Vericiguat is primarily metabolized by phase II glucuronidation.[285] It undergoes N-glucuronidation on the amino group on the pyrimidine ring. About 53% of vericiguat is eliminated renally (primarily as inactive metabolite) and 45% in feces as unchanged drug. The most common adverse effects of vericiguat are hypotension and anemia.[191]

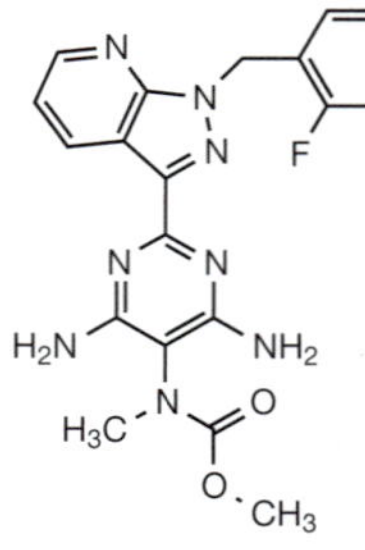

Riociguat

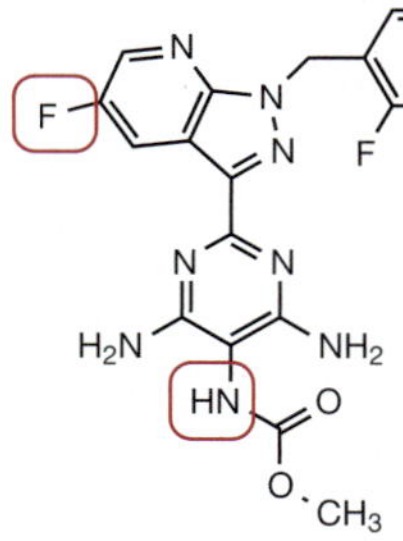

Vericiguat

Transthyretin Tetramers Stabilizer: Tafamidis

Tafamidis is a soft gelatinous capsule administered orally in its base form or as a meglumine salt.[195] Chemically, it is a benzoxazole carboxylic acid derivative. It binds to the thyroxine binding sites, thereby stabilizing the TTR by slowing the dissociation of tetramers into monomers.[195] It reaches the peak plasma concentrations within 4 hours and is highly protein bound (>99%). The half-life elimination is about 49 hours. Interestingly, the accumulation of tafamidis is 2.5 times higher after repeated dosing than that of a single dose. After a single dose administration of 20 mg tafamidis meglumine, approximately 59% of the drug is eliminated in the feces (predominantly unchanged) and 22% in the urine as a glucuronide metabolite. In vitro studies show that tafamidis induces CYP2B6 and CYP3A4. Tafamidis induces breast cancer resistance protein (BCRP), and it is observed that it increases the level of rosuvastatin, a BCRP substrate. The adverse effects associated with tafamidis include gastrointestinal disturbances such as diarrhea.[195]

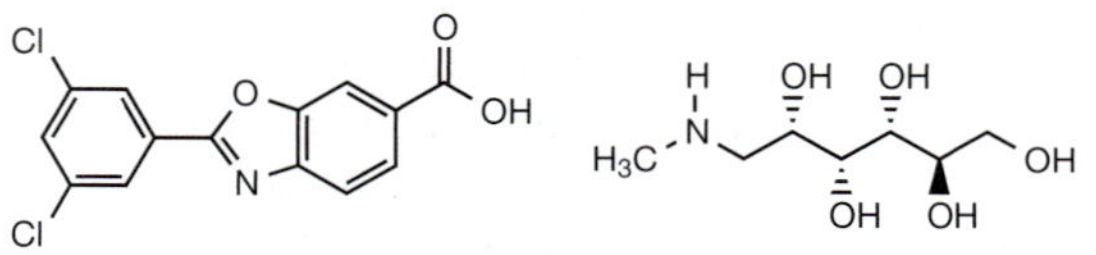

Tafamidis meglumine

Drugs for the Treatment of Cardiac Arrhythmia

Arrhythmias

Arrhythmia is a broad term used to describe a change, or the creation of an abnormal rate and/or rhythm, related to an AP propagation in the heart.[287] Drugs described in this section modulate the function of receptors involved in electrical impulses and/or myocyte contractile function. In order for the heart to function properly, an AP is generated and transmitted through the myocytes throughout the myocardial conduction system. This occurs by a coordinated and synchronized opening and closing of unique ion channels, which allows certain positive ions to influx or outflow from the cells.[288] These APs are repeated during every heart beat (normal range; 60-100 beats/min), in which cardiac cells undergo depolarization and repolarization. The type of ion channel and the direction of ion flow determine the shape and speed of the AP. Under normal situations, an AP starts in the sinoatrial node (SA node), which is the automatic focus or "pace maker" of the heart. The SA node's AP is spread through the atrial myocytes rejoining at the AV node, and then conducting down through the ventricles via the bundle of His, the left and right bundle branch system, and the Purkinje fibers. When all these APs are measured together, the electrical impulse on the ECG is generated. Because the ECG reflects the time required for an AP to travel over an area of the heart, only atrial (P wave), ventricle depolarization (QRS complex), and ventricular repolarization (T wave) are observed (Fig. 20.17).[289] The SA and AV nodes are too small to register in the ECG. However, the automaticity of these nodes can be determined by measuring how often a P wave occurs and how long it takes to go from the P wave to the QRS (PR interval). The smaller these intervals are, the faster the heart rate will occur.[290] For simplicity, the AP occurring in the SA node and ventricle will be discussed.

The SA and AV nodes express I_f channels, which passively open and are modulated by the autonomic nervous system.[291] Although the SA node can depolarize spontaneously, it is typically under the influence of the sympathetic and parasympathetic nervous systems. Thus, the autonomic nervous system can speed up or slow down the rate of depolarization, increasing or decreasing heart rate. I_f channels

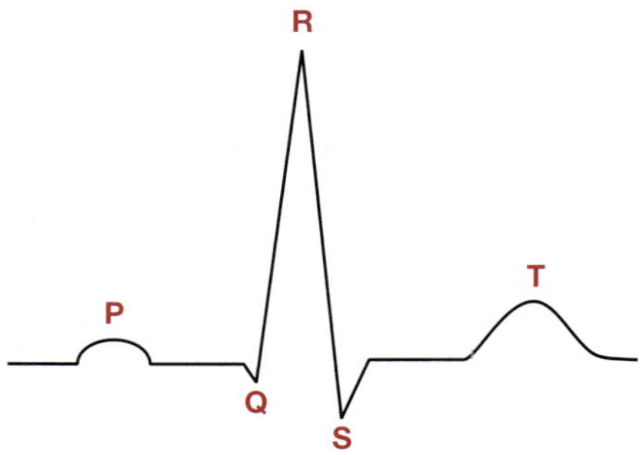

Figure 20.17 Depiction of electrocardiography recording.

allow Na^+, which is high outside of the cells, to follow its electrochemical gradient and move inside the cell. The influx of Na^+ makes the cell membrane potential more positive and eventually causes the opening of voltage-gated T-type Ca^{2+} channels, which leads to the influx of Ca^{2+} into the myocyte until it reaches the threshold (phase 4). At this point, voltage-gated L-type Ca^{2+} channels open and the SA node depolarizes (phase 0) (Fig. 20.18). Calcium is the depolarizing ion in the SA and AV node, but this Ca^{2+} current and the slope it creates are slower. Since it takes a little longer to depolarize, the SA and AV nodes are commonly referred to as slow AP. As it starts to reach its peak, voltage-gated potassium channels start to open and allow the movement of K^+ from inside of the cell to the outside. This is the beginning of the repolarization process (phases 2 and 3). It is important to note that I_f channels are not selective Na^+ channels and they also allow other ions to cross, but the function of these channels determines the rate of depolarization. From the SA node, the AP travels to the atrial myocytes producing the depolarization and contraction of the atrium. The AP reaches the AV node, which follows a very similar pattern of depolarization and repolarization as the SA node. Once the AP travels through the AV node and other fast AP tissues, it reaches the ventricular myocytes.

In the ventricles, Na^+ is the major depolarizing ion (phase 0; Fig. 20.19). As the tissue reaches the threshold, Na^+ channels move from the resting (closed) state to the active (open) state. The opening of these channels allows the influx of Na^+, which is responsible for the upstroke. During phase 1, Na^+ channels change their conformational state into the inactive mode, and Na^+ no longer can enter the cells. During phases 1 and 2, Ca^{2+} channels open and the entry of Ca^{2+} produces ventricle contraction, and the blood is pumped out of the ventricle into the main circulation. During phases 1, 2, and 3, K^+ channels open and that is the beginning of the repolarization process.[289] During these phases, Na^+ channels move from the inactive state into the resting state. The conformational state of the Na^+ channels define the refractory period, which can be characterized into two groups, absolute and relative refractory periods. During the absolute refractory period, an AP cannot be created because the majority of Na^+ channels are present in the inactive state. In contrast, during the relative refractory period

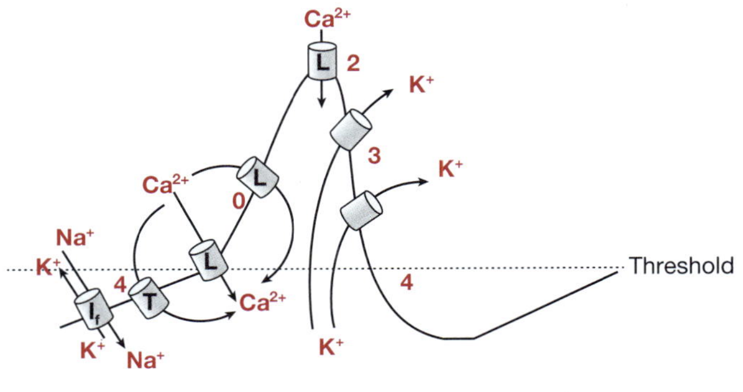

Figure 20.18 Depiction of cardiac action potential from a sinoatrial node.

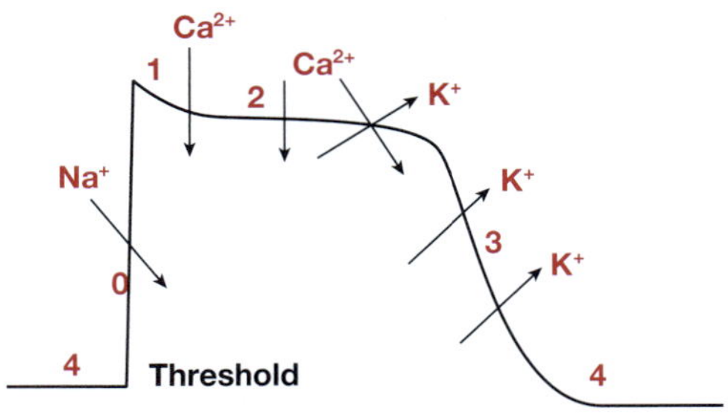

Figure 20.19 Depiction of cardiac action potential from a ventricle.

(which typically begins during phase 3), a smaller AP may be elicited depending how many Na^+ channels are present in the resting state. During phase 4, most of the sodium channels are restored to the resting states.

As described, arrhythmias occur when there is a perturbation in ion channel function that affects either the creation and/or propagation of the AP. This can result from high sympathetic input, myocardium infarction, and congenital defects.[292] Drugs in this class are used to either change the rate or the rhythm by altering the flow of specific ions.[185] Anti-arrhythmic drugs are classified based on the Vaughan-Williams classification.[293]

Class I: Sodium-channel blockers
Class II: β-Adrenergic blockers
Class III: Potassium channel blockers
Class IV: Calcium channel blockers
Miscellaneous Agents

Mechanism of Action of Anti-arrhythmic Drugs

Class I Anti-arrhythmic Drugs: Sodium-Channel Blockers

All drugs in this class have affinity for the Na^+ channels present in the fast AP tissue and decrease the influx of Na^+.[294] However, they differ in their selectivity, onset, and offset times.

Class IA Anti-arrhythmic Drugs. Drugs belonging to Class IA have an intermediate onset and offset binding, which can affect the myocardium AP during resting and arrhythmic states.[295] Procainamide, by blocking Na^+ channels, decreases the speed of conduction through the fast AP tissues (eg, ventricle) and increases the threshold. This can be observed on the ECG as a widening of the QRS complex. In addition, by also blocking the K^+ channels, there is a prolongation of the AP duration and an increase in the refractory period. This is observed by a prolongation of the QT interval.[296] The next drug in this class is quinidine, which has a more complex pharmacologic profile. In addition to blocking Na^+ channels, it can also bind and antagonize K^+ channels and α_1-adrenergic receptors. At higher doses, it may also block L-type Ca^{2+} channels. It produces greater hypotensive effects than procainamide due to the blockade of α_1-receptors, with a variable effect on the heart rate. Because it lacks receptor selectivity, quinidine produces a wide spectrum of side effects. The most concerning side effect is the marked prolongation of the QT interval. Disopyramide is another drug in this class, and it has affinity for the Na^+ channels. The (S)-enantiomer can also bind and block K^+ channels. One of the major differences between disopyramide and other drugs in this class is its pronounced antimuscarinic effects. In a similar fashion to the other two, it widens the QRS and prolongs the QT intervals. By blocking the muscarinic (M_2) receptor in the heart, it will increase the heart rate, as reflected by the shortening of the PR interval. It may also cause dry mouth and constipation associated with the blockade of the muscarinic system.

Class IB Anti-arrhythmic Drugs. Lidocaine, mexiletine, and phenytoin belong to class IB, and they have fast onset and fast offset kinetics. These drugs produce most of their effects when the heart is undergoing an arrhythmia or ischemic event. These selective Na^+ channel blockers primarily widen the QRS complex, with little to no significant effect on the PR and QT intervals. Lidocaine's preferred route of administration is intravenous, and mexiletine can be given orally.[297]

Class IC Anti-arrhythmic Drugs. Class IC drugs have slow onset/offset kinetics. Flecainide and propafenone are the two drugs in this class. These drugs have a high affinity for the Na^+ channels and will produce marked tonic blockade, which will lead to a decrease in automaticity, widening of the QRS, and an increase in AP durations. Flecainide also blocks K^+ channels, which is reflected as a prolongation of the QT interval and refractory period.[298] In addition, flecainide also blocks Ca^{2+} channels, thus decreasing the heart rate and prolonging the PR interval. Propafenone lacks affinity for the K^+ and Ca^{2+} channels, but it antagonizes β_1-adrenergic receptors. This results in a decrease of SA node automaticity and slowing down of the heart rate that is reflected as a prolongation of the PR interval.[299]

Class II Anti-arrhythmic Drugs: β-Adrenergic Blockers

Class II drugs are composed of β-blockers.[293] β_1-Adrenergic receptors are one of the most prominent receptors in the heart and are directly modulated by the SNS. By blocking the ability of norepinephrine from binding and activating β_1-receptors, these drugs produce a significant decrease in SA and AV nodes automaticity, which is reflected as a prolongation of the PR interval. The drugs in this class differ primarily on their selectivity (eg, metoprolol is a β_1-selective antagonist, and propranolol is a nonselective β_1- and β_2-antagonist).

Class III Anti-arrhythmic Drugs: Potassium Channel Blockers

Class III drugs are primarily K^+ channel antagonists. The drugs in this class include amiodarone, dronedarone, sotalol, dofetilide, and ibutilide.[300] Because all these drugs block the outflow of K^+, they tend to prolong the refractory period and AP duration. This is observed as a prolongation of the QT interval. Although there are K^+ channels on the SA and AV node, these drugs have affinity directed toward the K^+ channels present on the fast AP tissues.

Amiodarone is one of the most commonly used drugs in this class. In addition to blocking K^+ channels, it can also block Na^+ (widening of the QRS), Ca^{2+} (prolongation of the PR interval), α_1 (hypotension), and β_1-adrenergic receptors (sinus bradycardia).[301] Amiodarone has serious side effects, which increase with time. Dronedarone was developed to circumvent these side effects. In vitro studies suggest that dronedarone can bind and antagonize Na^+, K^+, and Ca^{2+} channels. It also has affinity for the α_1 and β_1-adrenergic receptors. However, clinical studies do not support improved efficacy for dronedarone when compared to amiodarone.

Sotalol is a K^+-channel blocker with affinity for the β-receptors.[302] As such, it prolongs both the QT and PR intervals. Ibutilide and dofetilide are selective K^+-channel antagonists, and these drugs will prolong the QT interval, with minimal effect on the PR or QRS complex.

Class IV Anti-arrhythmic Drugs: Calcium Channel Blockers

Class IV drugs belong to the class of non-DHP CCBs verapamil and diltiazem.[11] These drugs have the greatest affinity for the L-type CCBs present on the SA and AV nodes. By decreasing the influx of Ca^{2+}, these two drugs decrease the slope of phase 0 and prolong the refractory period of the SA and AV nodes.[303] This is reflected by a decrease in the heart rate and prolongation of the PR interval, thus taking longer for the AP to travel from the atrial myocardium to the ventricle.

Miscellaneous Agents

In addition to the drugs described, digoxin, adenosine, and magnesium may be used in the inpatient setting. Magnesium has been shown to be useful in terminating an ongoing torsades de pointes, but the exact mechanism of action is not fully understood.[304] Digoxin, in addition to its inotropic effects, enhances parasympathetic tone. This vagotonic effect decreases the heart rate, which is observed as a prolongation of the PR interval. This appears to be an indirect effect of digoxin that is not associated with the blockade of Na^+/K^+-ATPase. Adenosine is an endogenous nucleoside that binds to adenosine receptors. It works in a similar fashion to acetylcholine and appears to slow AP currents in the SA and AV nodes.

Physicochemical Properties, Pharmacokinetics, Drug Interactions, and Adverse Effects of Anti-arrhythmic Drugs

Class I Anti-arrhythmic Drugs: Sodium-Channel Blockers

Class IA Anti-arrhythmic Drugs

Quinidine. Quinidine (dextrorotatory [+]) and quinine (levorotatory [-]) are naturally occurring alkaloids that are isolated from the bark of the cinchona tree.[305] Quinidine (Fig. 20.20) is therapeutically used as an anti-arrhythmic agent, whereas quinine is used an antimalarial agent.[305] Quinidine and quinine each contain four chiral centers, and are diastereomers of one another. Chemically, quinidine contains a bicyclic amine known as quinuclidine and a methoxyquinoline ring. The quinoline and quinuclidine rings are linked by a hydroxy methylene group. Quinuclidine is further connected to a vinyl group. The quinuclidine tertiary aliphatic nitrogen atom is more basic (p*K*a = 8.4) than the quinoline aromatic nitrogen atom (p*K*a = 4.2).[306] As a result, quinidine can be converted into water-soluble salts by reacting it with acids. Commercially, quinidine is available as its sulfate and gluconate salt forms, and as immediate- and extended-release oral formulations. Quinidine gluconate is also available in an IV formulation. Quinidine sulfate and gluconate have 83% and 62% of quinidine base, respectively.[307] Since the two salt forms have different quinidine percentages, they are not directly interchangeable.[307] Quinidine formulations may contain dihydroquinidine as a common impurity.[308]

Oral quinidine is rapidly absorbed. It is moderately metabolized by hepatic first-pass metabolism and has a bioavailability of about 70% to 80%.[309] The apparent volume of distribution is about 2.4 L/kg.[310] Quinidine has high protein binding (70%-95%). It primarily binds to α_1-acid glycoprotein and serum albumin.[311] About 60% to 85% of quinidine is metabolized in the liver.[311] It is primarily metabolized by CYP3A4 into an active metabolite (3*S*)-3-hydroxy-quinidine.[312] Other metabolites of quinidine include quinidine *N*-oxide and dihydroquinidine.[312] About 15% to 40% of intact quinidine is excreted renally.[311] Quinidine has an elimination half-life of about 7 hours.[311] Age and disease states affect the clearance of quinidine. In older adults, quinidine clearance is reduced, and the half-life elimination is prolonged (~10 hours), which can lead to toxic side effects unless doses are adjusted accordingly.[310] The amount of serum albumin and α_1-acid glycoprotein is lower in patients with liver failure, resulting in an increase in unbound quinidine fraction and volume of distribution.[313] In patients with hepatic cirrhosis, the half-life elimination is significantly increased (~9 hours).[310] In patients with CHF, the volume of distribution of quinidine is decreased because of elevated levels of plasma proteins, and the total drug clearance is also reduced because of reduced unbound concentrations.[307,314] However, the average half-life of quinidine in patients with CHF is similar to normal individuals.[314]

Quinidine is a substrate and a strong inhibitor of P-glycoprotein.[233] P-glycoprotein-mediated inhibition by quinidine leads to decreased digoxin elimination and increased plasma levels.[233] Quinidine is also a potent inhibitor of CYP2D6.[315] Concurrent administration of quinidine with CYP2D6 substrates, such as metoprolol may lead to a significant increase in metoprolol concentrations and half-life.[145] Quinidine and its metabolites can cause QT prolongation leading to toxic torsades de pointes in about 1% to 3% of patients.[316] The combination of amiodarone and quinidine can have cumulative toxic side effects by enhancing the QT interval.[317] The adverse effects associated with quinidine include gastrointestinal disturbances, fever, hepatic dysfunction, leukopenia, cinchonism, hemolytic anemia, and cardiac arrhythmias.[318] Quinidine can also cause hypokalemia and decreased heart rate.[316]

Procainamide. Procainamide (see Fig. 20.20) is a bioisostere of procaine. Procaine, a local anesthetic agent, was used by cardiologists as an alternative to quinidine during World War II.[319] However, the clinical application of procaine as a cardiovascular agent is limited due to its rapid metabolism by esterases and high incidence of CNS side effects.[319] The ester group of procaine was later replaced with an amide functionality to produce procainamide, which is more resistant to hydrolysis by esterases. Procainamide, because of its lower lipophilicity, has fewer incidences of CNS side effects.[319]

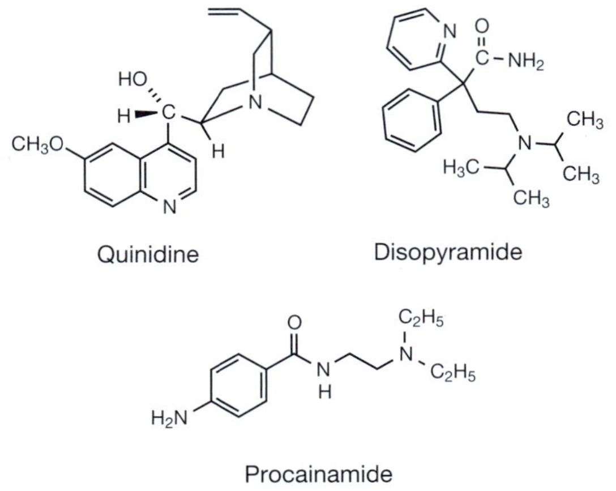

Figure 20.20 Class IA anti-arrhythmic agents.

Procainamide is rapidly and completely absorbed after oral administration. The oral bioavailability is about 75% to 95%.[320] It reaches peak plasma concentrations in about 1 to 2 hours.[320] The oral form of procainamide is not available in the United States, and it is only administered intravenously. Procainamide's volume of distribution is about 2 L/kg, and only 15% is bound to plasma proteins.[320] The half-life elimination of procainamide is about 3 hours and is longer in patients with the renal impairment.[320] Procainamide undergoes hepatic metabolism through *N*-acetyltransferase-II to *N*-acetylprocainamide, a major metabolite with similar pharmacological effects comparable to those of procainamide.[320] The acetylation metabolism of procainamide is genetically determined, and is dependent on the rapid or slow acetylation phenotypes.[321] Chronic oral administration of procainamide is associated with systemic lupus-like syndrome.[322] In slow acetylators, the rate at which procainamide induces antinuclear antibodies and lupus syndrome is much faster and more frequent than rapid acetylators, indicating the unacetylated procainamide is responsible for its side effect.[322] The *para*-amino group on procainamide undergoes oxidation to hydroxylamine and nitro derivatives, which are responsible for hypersensitive reactions.[323] Procainamide is also metabolized to *N*-hydroxyprocainamide by CYP2D6.[324] Ethnic background may play an important role in determining the dose and systemic lupus-like side effect.[325] In Caucasian and African American populations, about 50% are rapid acetylators; in Japanese and Alaska Native populations about 80% to 90% are rapid acetylators, and in Egyptian and certain Jewish populations, 20% or fewer are rapid acetylators.[325] About 50% of the intact procainamide and the majority of its metabolites are eliminated renally by glomerular filtration and active tubular secretion.[320] The plasma concentration of procainamide and *N*-acetylprocainamide is significantly increased in patients with impaired renal function because of reduced elimination.[326]

Drugs interfering with the tubular secretion of procainamide may potentially have significant DDIs.[325] Fluoroquinolone antibacterials, such as ciprofloxacin and levofloxacin, significantly decrease the renal clearance of procainamide and *N*-acetylprocainamide.[327] Cimetidine, a histamine H_2 receptor antagonist, is shown to decrease the clearance, increase the plasma levels, and enhance adverse effects of procainamide. Therefore, either of these combinations should be avoided, or doses should be adjusted accordingly and side effects carefully monitored.[328]

The adverse effects associated with procainamide include gastrointestinal upset, fever, bradycardia, and hypotension.[329] Procainamide increases the risk of developing torsades de pointes.

Disopyramide. Disopyramide (see Fig. 20.20) is a unique molecule containing a chiral carbon atom that is linked to a pyridine ring, phenyl ring, an amide, and an alky diisopropyl amine. It is commercially sold as a racemic mixture. The tertiary amine is converted into salts, such as phosphate, to improve water solubility.

Disopyramide is available as immediate- and controlled-release formulations.[330] The controlled-release formulation of disopyramide provides more constant pharmacological effects and lower interdose variation in unbound drug levels than the immediate-release formulation.[330] The oral bioavailability of disopyramide is about 85%.[331] It reaches peak plasma concentrations in about 0.5 to 3 hours.[332] Disopyramide has a unique and complex protein binding pattern that is dependent on the concentration of the drug and exhibits stereoselectivity. The *S*(+)-disopyramide is more highly protein bound than the *R*(–)-disopyramide.[333] Disopyramide is primarily bound (70%) to α_1-acid glycoprotein with high affinity.[334,335] About 5% of disopyramide is bound to albumin with low affinity.[334] Disopyramide when administered orally does not undergo significant first-pass metabolism.[332] About 55% of the drug is excreted unchanged primarily by the kidneys.[335] Disopyramide is metabolized in the liver by CYP3A4 N-dealkylation to mono-*N*-desisopropyldisopyramide, which is pharmacologically active.[335,336] Disopyramide has an elimination half-life of about 7 hours.[332] In patients with renal impairment, the levels of disopyramide and mono-*N*-desisopropyldisopyramide are increased.[337]

Concurrent administration of disopyramide with CYP3A4 inhibitors, such as macrolide antibiotics, can significantly enhance the plasma levels of disopyramide and could potentially cause ventricular tachycardia.[338,339] Disopyramide can cause anticholinergic side effects such as nausea, dry mouth (xerostomia), abdominal discomfort, constipation, and urinary urgency and retention.[340] Disopyramide, in combination with other anticholinergic agents such as ipratropium and tiotropium, should be avoided. Disopyramide can have negative inotropic actions and may reduce the contractions of the heart.[341]

CLASS IB ANTI-ARRHYTHMIC DRUGS

Lidocaine. Lidocaine (Fig. 20.21) was synthesized in the early 1940's.[342] Over the years, lidocaine has been used as a local anesthetic agent similar to procaine. Its anti-arrhythmic activity effect was first reported in 1950.[342] Lidocaine is widely used in the treatment of ventricular arrhythmias. Structurally, lidocaine contains a 2,6-dimethylphenyl ring attached to an *N*-acetamide that is linked to a diethylamine functional group (Fig. 20.21).[342] The tertiary amine is weakly basic (p*K*a = 8).[342]

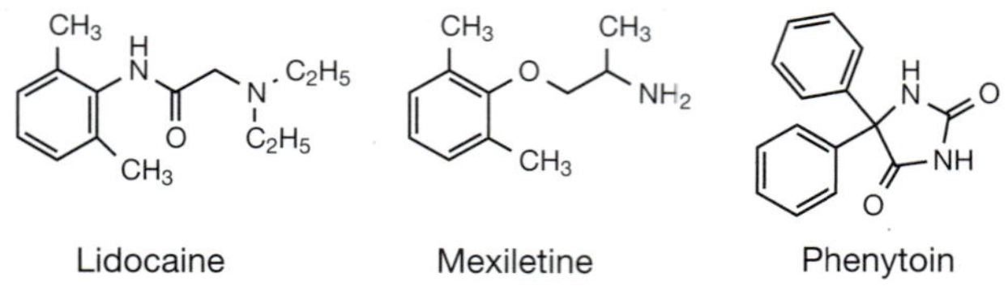

Figure 20.21 Class IB anti-arrhythmic agents.

The oral bioavailability is about 35%.[343] When administered orally, lidocaine undergoes extensive hepatic first-pass metabolism and does not attain sufficient plasma levels to have anti-arrhythmic effects.[343] Therefore, lidocaine is administered intravenously for its anti-arrhythmic effects.[343] Lidocaine is highly protein bound (60%-80%) to α_1-acid glycoprotein, and alteration of this glycoprotein concentration results in either decreased or increased protein binding.[344] Lidocaine's protein binding is variable and is dependent on inter- and intra-individual differences.[344] The volume of distribution is about 1.5 L/kg.[343,345] The liver is the primary site of metabolism, and the hepatic blood flow is very important for clearance of lidocaine because of its high hepatic extraction ratio.[342] The major metabolic pathway of lidocaine is by *N*-deethylation to yield monoethylglycinexylidide (MEGX), a pharmacologically active metabolite.[342] CYP1A2 and CYP3A4 are the two important isoforms that are responsible for the metabolism of lidocaine.[346] The amide moiety in MEGX undergoes hydrolysis to yield 2,6-xylidine (2,6-dimethyl aniline) and *N*-ethylglycine (amino acid).[342] Up to 10% of lidocaine is excreted unchanged in the urine.[342] Since lidocaine is a weak base, alkalization of the urine may decrease its clearance, and acidification of the urine may increase its clearance.[342] Lidocaine has a plasma half-life of about 1.5 hours.[343] Older adults may have a prolonged half-life when compared to young individuals.[347] In patients with hepatic failure, lidocaine metabolism is impaired, resulting in reduced plasma clearance and increased half-life (≥5 hours).[348] In patients with HF, lidocaine's clearance and volume of distribution are significantly reduced and doses must be reduced accordingly.[348] The side effects of lidocaine and its metabolites are concentration dependent.[349] Common side effects are CNS effects, which include dizziness, drowsiness, and euphoria.[349] At therapeutic levels, it can cause seizures, confusion, agitation, and psychosis.[349] At higher concentrations, it can cause cardiovascular side effects such as hypotension, AV block, and circulatory collapse.[349]

The concurrent administration of antidepressant fluvoxamine, a strong CYP1A2 inhibitor, significantly reduces the metabolism of lidocaine in patients with normal liver function.[350] Therefore, caution must be taken when lidocaine is administered with other CYP1A2 inhibitors. Erythromycin, a CYP3A4 inhibitor, is shown to modestly decrease the clearance of lidocaine and increase the levels of MEGX possibly by inhibiting its further metabolism.[351] Amiodarone, another CYP3A4 inhibitor, decreases the systemic clearance and increases the plasma levels of lidocaine.[352] Concurrent administration of cimetidine may decrease the clearance of lidocaine and may increase its plasma levels because of a decreased hepatic blood flow.[353]

Mexiletine. Mexiletine (see Fig. 20.21) was originally developed as an anticonvulsant agent, but its cardiac properties were quickly observed, and thereafter it was clinically used as an anti-arrhythmic agent.[354] The amide bond in lidocaine is replaced with the ether functional group to make it metabolically more resistant to hydrolysis (see Fig. 20.21). Mexiletine contains a chiral center and is sold as a racemic mixture.

Mexiletine is weakly basic (p*K*a = 8.5) and primarily exists in the ionized state (hydrophilic form) in the stomach; however, its ionization is significantly reduced in the intestines.[354] Therefore, most of the absorption takes place in the small intestine.[354] Orally administered mexiletine is rapidly and almost completely absorbed, with a bioavailability of about 80% to 90%.[297] It undergoes minimal first-pass hepatic metabolism.[297] About 70% of mexiletine is bound to plasma proteins (albumin and α_1-acid glycoprotein).[354] The volume of distribution ranges from 5 to 9 L/kg, and the distribution is to the heart, liver, and brain.[354] Mexiletine undergoes extensive metabolism in the liver into several metabolites.[354] The primary metabolic routes of mexiletine are hydroxylation of the primary amine to *N*-hydroxy-mexiletine, *para* or *meta* aromatic hydroxylation, hydroxylation of the methyl group on the aromatic ring to hydroxymethylmexiletine, and glucuronide conjugation.[354] CYP1A2 catalyzes the formation of *N*-hydroxymexiletine, and CYP2D6 predominantly catalyzes the formation of hydroxymethylmexiletine and *para/meta* hydroxymexiletine.[354] Genetic polymorphisms of CYP2D6 influence the metabolism of mexiletine, based on whether the individual is a poor or extensive metabolizer.[354] The clearance of hydroxymethylmexiletine and *para* and *meta* hydroxymexiletine is decreased in poor metabolizers as compared to extensive metabolizers.[354,355] The elimination half-life of mexiletine is about 10 hours and is prolonged in patients with hepatic failure, CHF, and MI.[356] The plasma concentration of mexiletine varies significantly with pH, and extreme pH values may lead to either decreased efficacy or increased risk of adverse effects.[357] An acidic urinary pH would significantly favor the elimination of mexiletine, resulting in decreased plasma concentrations.[357] In contrast, an increase in the urinary pH would decrease its elimination.[357]

Atropine decreases and metoclopramide enhances the rate of mexiletine absorption.[358] The time to reach the maximum plasma concentration of mexiletine is slightly increased by concurrent administration with antacids due to a delay in gastric emptying.[359] Concurrent administration of mexiletine with theophylline, a CYP1A2 substrate, increases the serum concentration of theophylline by about 2-fold, but mexiletine serum concentration is unaffected.[360] H_2-receptor antagonists, such as cimetidine, may slightly prolong the absorption and decrease the plasma concentration of mexiletine.[361] Strong CYP2D6 inhibitors (eg, quinidine) and CYP1A2 inhibitors may decrease the metabolism of mexiletine.[354,362] The common side effects associated with mexiletine include GI disturbances and CNS side effects such as dizziness, nervousness, and insomnia.[356]

Phenytoin. Chemically, phenytoin (see Fig. 20.21) is 5,5-diphenylhydantoin. It was discovered in 1936, and its clinical efficacy was established in 1937.[363] Since then, it is widely used as an antiepileptic drug. The use of phenytoin as an anti-arrhythmic drug is not officially approved. Phenytoin is a weakly acidic drug and has poor solubility. Therefore, it is usually administered as a sodium salt.[364] Phenytoin is administered either orally or intravenously.[365] Approximately 90% of phenytoin is bound to plasma proteins.[364] However, in patients with chronic kidney disease, phenytoin protein binding is significantly reduced, which may lead to increased free (unbound) concentrations of the drug.[366] Drugs that displace phenytoin from plasma protein binding sites, such as valproic acid, may increase the unbound fraction of phenytoin.[367]

Phenytoin is predominantly metabolized via hydroxylation by various CYP enzymes to a 5-hydroxylated metabolite.[368] CYP2C19 is the major metabolizing enzyme of phenytoin. Phenytoin metabolism is nonlinear, and metabolizing enzymes are saturated at therapeutic doses, leading to an increase in phenytoin concentrations and toxicity.[369] The mean elimination half-life is about 22 hours.[370] Phenytoin and its metabolites are excreted into bile and undergo reabsorption from the GI tract, and are eventually eliminated renally by glomerular filtration and tubular secretion.[370]

Co-administration of phenytoin with CYP2C19 inhibitors leads to an increased phenytoin plasma level and toxicity.[371] Poor CYP2C9 metabolizers are associated with reduced clearance and an increased phenytoin level in the body and serious adverse effects.[372] Phenytoin may cause hyperglycemia, skin rashes, and increase the risk of suicidal thoughts.[370]

Class IC Anti-arrhythmic Drugs

Flecainide. Flecainide (Fig. 20.22) is therapeutically used in maintaining the sinus rhythm in patients with atrial flutter.[373] Flecainide has a local anesthetic effect and is drastically different from Class IA or IB agents.[373] Flecainide is a bis-trifluoroethoxy benzamide derivative and sold as an acetate salt. It is well absorbed orally, and the bioavailability is about 70%.[374] Food does not significantly affect the rate and extent of absorption.[374] Only about 40% of flecainide is bound to plasma proteins, and the volume of distribution is 5 to 6 L/kg.[375] The plasma half-life of flecainide is 13 to 16 hours.[375] Flecainide is predominantly metabolized by CYP2D6 into two major metabolites, *meta*-O-dealkylated flecainide and *meta*-O-dealkylated lactam.[376] Flecainide metabolites do not have significant activity.[375] Pharmacokinetics of flecainide are influenced by genetic differences.[377] Poor and intermediate CYP2D6 metabolizers have reduced flecainide clearance.[377] About 86% of flecainide and its metabolites are eliminated

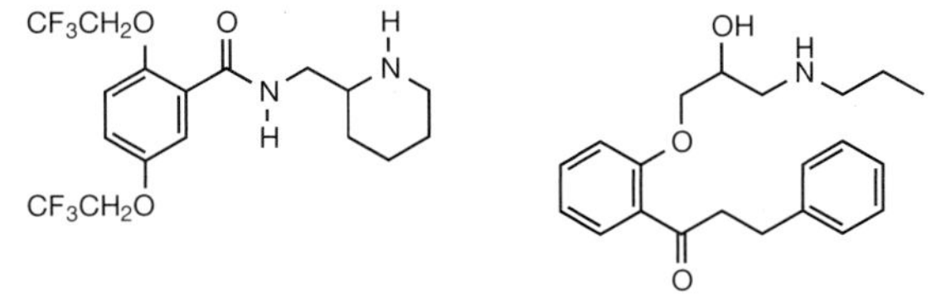

Flecainide Propafenone

Figure 20.22 Class IC anti-arrhythmic agents.

renally, and only about 5% are eliminated in the feces.[375] Renal elimination of flecainide is by both glomerular filtration and tubular secretion.[374] Flecainide's rate of elimination is possibly reduced with age.[375] Flecainide has a good safety profile, but it has proarrhythmic effects and may cause supraventricular proarrhythmia.[373] The less serious side effects of flecainide include headache, diarrhea, and nausea.[373] Concurrent administration of flecainide with digoxin or propranolol significantly prolongs the ECG PR interval.[378]

Propafenone. Propafenone contains a chiral center and is administered as a racemic mixture of *S*(+)- and *R*(−)-propafenone (Fig. 20.22).[379] Both enantiomers of propafenone have an equal anti-arrhythmic effect as sodium channel blockers, but the *S*(+)-isomer is primarily responsible for its β_1-blocking properties.[380] It contains a phenyloxypropanolamine group, which is structurally similar to some of the β_1-adrenergic antagonists.[380] Since it contains a weakly basic secondary amine, it is converted to the hydrochloride salt for improved water solubility.

More than 90% of propafenone is absorbed after oral administration.[379] Propafenone undergoes extensive first-pass metabolism, and the bioavailability varies from 5% to 50%.[379] Food may increase its bioavailability.[381] Peak plasma concentrations are reached in about 2 hours, and the amount of the drug that reaches the systemic circulation is dependent on the concentration.[379,382] The majority of propafenone is bound to α_1-acid glycoprotein.[383] Propafenone is distributed to the heart, liver, and lungs, and the apparent volume of distribution is 2.5 to 4 L/kg.[384] *R*(−)-propafenone (92.4%) is slightly less protein bound than the *S*(+) propafenone (95.1%).[385] The two major metabolic pathways of propafenone are CYP2D6-catalyzed hydroxylation to 5-hydroxypropafenone, and CYP3A4-catalyzed N-dealkylation to *N*-depropylpropafenone.[386,387] Both hydroxylated and *N*-dealkylated metabolites have anti-arrhythmic properties.[388] The metabolism of propafenone is influenced by genetic polymorphisms.[389] Individuals who are extensive metabolizers rapidly metabolize propafenone to 5-hydroxypropafenone when compared to poor metabolizers.[390] Approximately, 10% of Caucasians are poor metabolizers.[379] At high doses, both extensive and poor metabolizers are prone to β-blocking properties, but at low doses, poor metabolizers are more prone to its β-blocking properties than extensive metabolizers because of the greater accumulation of propafenone in the body.[389] Propafenone also undergoes phase II metabolism by glucuronidation.[391] The mean half-life of propafenone is about 6 hours and is subject to inter-individual variability.[392] In extensive metabolizers, the half-life elimination is 3.4 to 7.6 hours, and in poor metabolizers, it is 9 to 25 hours.[393] Propafenone exhibits stereoselectivity in elimination. Long-term administration of propafenone results in enhanced β-blocking properties and increased *S*(+)-propafenone concentrations due to faster rate elimination of the *R*(−)-isomer.[394]

Concurrent administration of propafenone with digoxin significantly increases digoxin's plasma concentrations and reduces digoxin's clearance.[395] Propafenone impairs warfarin's metabolism and increases its plasma concentration by about 38%, and this may lead to an enhanced anticoagulant effect.[396] Propafenone, when administered along with the CY2D6 substrate metoprolol, enhances metoprolol concentrations 2- to 5-fold.[397] In extensive metabolizers, the co-administration of quinidine, a potent CYP2D6 inhibitor, increases propafenone plasma concentrations more than 2 times and decreases its clearance and metabolism to 5-hydroxypropafenone.[398]

The most common adverse effects of propafenone include cardiovascular side effects such as aggravation of arrhythmia, induction or worsening of CHF, conduction abnormalities, gastrointestinal disturbances, and CNS side effects. The side effects are commonly observed during chronic therapy and at high doses (≥900 mg/d).[399]

Class II Anti-arrhythmic Drugs: β-Adrenergic Blockers

Refer to the antianginal section for chemical structures and other properties of β-blockers.

ESMOLOL. Esmolol is an ultrashort-acting selective β-blocker (Fig. 20.23), making it an effective agent for acute critical care settings.[400] It is only administered by the IV route. The *para* ester substituent is required for its β-blocking activity.[400] The onset of action is attained in about 2 minutes, and in 5 minutes, about 90% of the steady state β-blockade is achieved.[401] The ester group is rapidly hydrolyzed by esterases present in red blood cells into a carboxylic acid metabolite and methanol.[400,401] The carboxylic acid metabolite is essentially inactive, and methanol levels are in the normal endogenous range.[401] The elimination half-life is about 10 minutes.[402] The therapeutic effect of esmolol quickly dissipates in 30 minutes after its discontinuation.[402] The major side effects of esmolol includes hypotension and diaphoresis.[401]

Class III Anti-arrhythmic Drugs: Potassium Channel Blockers

SOTALOL. Sotalol (Fig. 20.24) is a phenyl-hydroxyethyl-isopropylamine *para*-methane sulfonamide.[403] Sotalol contains a chiral center and is sold as a racemic mixture of *d*(+)-sotalol and *l*(−)-sotalol.[404] Both enantiomers have potassium channel blocking (class III) properties.[404] In addition, the *l*(−) sotalol is 30 to 60 times more potent as a β-blocker (class II) than *d*(+)-sotalol.[404]

Sotalol is administered by oral and IV routes. It is rapidly and completely absorbed after oral administration.[405] The bioavailability is 90% to 100%, indicating minimal or no fast-pass metabolism.[405] The bioavailability is reduced by about 20% in the presence of food.[405] The peak plasma

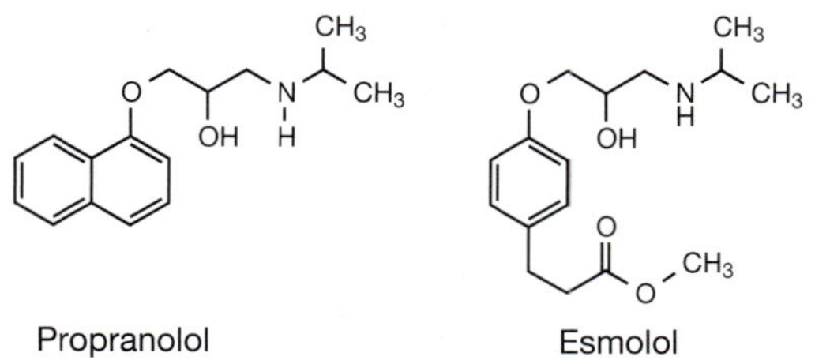

Figure 20.23 Class II anti-arrhythmic agents.

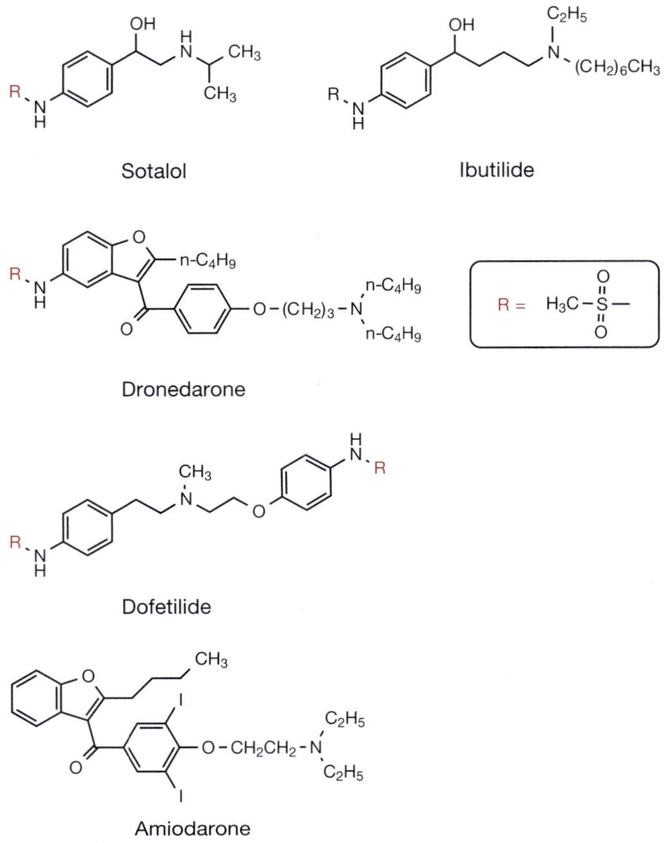

Figure 20.24 Class III anti-arrhythmic agents.

concentrations are attained rapidly in about 2 to 4 hours.[405] Sotalol is not significantly bound to plasma proteins and is well distributed to the lungs, liver, and kidneys, with an apparent volume of distribution of 1.2 to 2.4 L/kg.[404,405] It is hydrophilic in nature and not well distributed to the CNS.[405] Sotalol's metabolism is insignificant, and about 80% to 90% of the unchanged drug is eliminated in the urine.[404,405] In patients with renal impairment, sotalol doses should be adjusted accordingly.[404] Both *d*(+)- and *l*(−)-sotalol are eliminated equally in the urine.[405] The elimination half-life is in the range of 10 to 20 hours.[405]

Since sotalol does not undergo any significant metabolism, drug interactions associated with CYP inducers or inhibitors appear to be less likely.[406] However, several pharmacodynamic drug-drug interactions can occur.[406] Concurrent administration of sotalol with antacids such as magnesium hydroxide decreases sotalol's oral absorption and plasma levels, and this interaction can be avoided by administering the drugs at 2-hour intervals.[407] Sotalol may prolong the QT interval, and can cause syncope and ventricular tachycardia.[408] Concurrent administration with other Class IA or III anti-arrhythmic agents have a combined effect on QT prolongation, potentiating the possibility of torsades de pointes.[406] Sotalol may worsen bradycardia associated with digoxin when given in combination.[409] Sotalol should be used with caution with diuretics that cause hypokalemia since hypokalemia is a risk factor for prolonged QT interval.[408]

AMIODARONE. Amiodarone (see Fig. 20.24) is a highly lipophilic (LogP: 7.78) diiodinated benzofuran derivative.[410] The iodine content is 39.3% in amiodarone free base.[410] Amiodarone is a weakly basic molecule (p*K*a is 7.0)[411] and is converted into its hydrochloride salt to improve water solubility.

The oral absorption of amiodarone is erratic and incomplete, and the bioavailability is 22% to 86%.[410] Because of its high lipophilicity, it is sequestered in many body parts, including adipose tissue, liver, lungs, skin, and skeletal muscle.[410,412] Amiodarone has a high volume of distribution (66 L/kg), and about 96% of the drug is protein bound.[410,412] Orally administered amiodarone has a slow onset and offset of action.[412] The plasma half-life of a single oral dose of amiodarone is about 3 to 80 hours, but after withdrawal of chronic administration, the half-life can be as long as 100 days.[410] The onset of action after a single IV administration is within 30 minutes.[410] However, after oral administration, there is a delay of about 2 to 21 days to observe its complete therapeutic effects.[410] The duration of action could last up to 1 month even after withdrawing amiodarone.[410] The majority of the drug undergoes metabolism, and only about 1% of the drug is eliminated unchanged in the urine.[410] Amiodarone is hepatically metabolized by CYP3A4-catalyzed N-deethylation to desethylamiodarone, a major metabolite.[413] Desethylamiodarone is pharmacologically active and has a similar elimination half-life as amiodarone.[412] Minor metabolites include bis-*N*-desethylamiodarone and deiodinated metabolites.[412] Since amiodarone undergoes negligible renal elimination, dosage need not be reduced in patients with renal impairment.[412]

Amiodarone and its metabolite, desethylamiodarone, are CYP2C9, CYP2D6, and CYP3A4 inhibitors.[414] Amiodarone inhibits the metabolism of warfarin and thereby, increases its plasma levels and anticoagulant effect.[410] Concurrent administration of cholestyramine, a bile acid sequestrant, with amiodarone decreases the enterohepatic circulation of amiodarone and enhances its elimination.[415] Amiodarone also has calcium channel blocking properties and when combined with CCBs, it may have additive effects.[406,416] Amiodarone, when combined with diltiazem, could lead to sinus arrest and hypotension.[417] Amiodarone decreases cyclosporine clearance by more than 50% probably by inhibiting CYP3A4 in the GI mucosa.[406,418]

The common adverse effects of amiodarone are GI side effects, most commonly constipation; ocular disturbances related to the formation of corneal microdeposits; neuromotor effects in the form of tremor, ataxia, and sleeplessness; and photosensitivity in the form of sunburn, erythema, and swelling.[419,420] Amiodarone may cause a rise in hepatic enzymes, hypothyroidism, and hyperthyroidism.[419] It also has the potential to cause pulmonary fibrosis.[419] Side effects are dose dependent and chronic administration may increase its propensity to cause adverse reactions.[419,420]

DRONEDARONE. Dronedarone (see Fig. 20.24) is a nonidodinated benzofuran derivative of amiodarone that was approved by the FDA in 2009.[421] It was designed to reduce the toxic side effects associated with chronic amiodarone therapy.[422] The lack of the iodine atoms and the addition of the methanesulfonyl group makes dronedarone (LogP: 5.2) more hydrophilic in nature than amiodarone (LogP: 7.78).[422]

Orally administered dronedarone is well absorbed (70%-94%). However, it has poor bioavailability (15%) because it undergoes extensive first-pass metabolism primarily by hepatic CYP3A4.[423,424] Food increases its bioavailability 2- to 3-fold and a high fat meal can increase the bioavailability to 3- to 4.5-fold.[424] Relatively, dronedarone has a lower tissue distribution and a shorter half-life than amiodarone.[422] Dronedarone is well tolerated, and side effects include bradycardia, QT interval prolongation; gastrointestinal disturbances such as nausea, diarrhea, and vomiting; skin related events such as rash; and may increase serum creatinine.[422,425] Unlike amiodarone, dronedarone has a better side effect profile and does not significantly increase thyroid abnormalities and pulmonary disorders.[425]

IBUTILIDE. Ibutilide (see Fig. 20.24) is structurally similar to sotalol and is another methanesulfonamide derivative.[426] It contains hydroxy butyl and heptyl side chains.[427] Ibutilide is more effective than sotalol in terminating atrial fibrillation or atrial flutter.[428] Ibutilide is sold as its fumarate salt and has good water solubility (>100 mg/mL) at a pH less than 7.[427,429] Although ibutilide has a chiral center, it is sold as a racemic mixture since both the enantiomers have similar pharmacokinetic properties.[427] Ibutilide undergoes extensive first-pass metabolism, making it unsuitable for long-term oral administration.[426] Therefore, ibutilide is administered via intravenous infusion.[426] About 40% of the administered ibutilide is bound to plasma proteins.[429] Ibutilide is extensively distributed with a large volume of distribution of about 11 L/kg, and patients have high inter-individual variability.[427,429] Ibutilide is metabolized by hepatic enzymes into eight metabolites.[429] The heptyl side chain undergoes omega-oxidation and subsequently β-oxidation.[429] The metabolites are inactive, except the omega-hydroxyl metabolite, which showed in vitro activity in the rabbit myocardium model.[429] However, this metabolite is only 10% of the circulating plasma levels, indicating the activity is largely from the intact ibutilide and not from its metabolites.[429] It has high systemic plasma clearance and is also rapidly cleared from the body.[427] The average half-life elimination is about 6 hours.[427,429] About 82% of ibutilide is excreted in the urine and 18% in feces.[427,429]

Since ibutilide is not metabolized by CYP3A4 and CYP2D6, agents affecting these enzymes do not have DDIs.[429] Other cardiovascular drug such as CCBs, β-blockers or digoxin do not affect the safety and efficacy of ibutilide.[429] Ibutilide is associated with the risk of polymorphic ventricular tachycardia.[430] Ibutilide may prolong the QT interval and torsades de pointes.[430] Therefore, it should not be used with other drugs that significantly prolong the QT interval.

DOFETILIDE. Dofetilide is a bis-methanesulfonamide (see Fig. 20.24) derivative and is a highly selective potassium channel blocker when compared to sotalol and amiodarone.[431] Dofetilide is well absorbed with an absolute oral bioavailability more than 90%.[432] After oral administration, the time to reach maximum plasma concentrations is about 2 to 3 hours.[432,433] About 60% to 70% of dofetilide is protein bound, and the volume of distribution is about 3 L/kg. In vitro studies show that dofetilide is metabolized by CYP3A4. It predominantly undergoes N-demethylation to form the N-desmethyl metabolite.[434] It is also metabolized by N-oxidation to form the *N*-oxide, which has weak class I anti-arrhythmic properties.[434] Its biological response is largely due to unchanged dofetilide, and metabolites are either inactive or do not have significant activity.[434] The elimination half-life is approximately 10 hours.[435] Dofetilide is primarily eliminated renally (80%), and the majority of the drug is eliminated unchanged. Concurrent administration with other drugs that significantly interfere with renal elimination should be avoided.[435,436] For example, hydrochlorothiazide and triamterene significantly increase the plasma concentrations of dofetilide and must be avoided.[435] Co-administration of dofetilide with verapamil or organic cation transporter inhibitors such as cimetidine must also be avoided because they increase dofetilide plasma concentrations.[435]

Dofetilide prolongs the QT interval duration and is proportional to the plasma concentration of the drug.[432] Torsade de pointes ventricular tachycardia is the significant adverse side effect associated with dofetilide.[436] Patients with renal impairment and decreased creatinine clearance will experience an increased plasma concentration of dofetilide. Therefore, the dose must be adjusted according to the creatinine clearance and must be avoided in patients with severe renal impairment (creatinine clearance <20 mL/min).[435]

Class IV Anti-arrhythmic Drugs: Calcium Channel Blockers

The non-DHP CCBs verapamil and diltiazem comprise the class IV agents (see Fig. 20.4). Refer to the antianginal section for chemical structures and other properties.

Miscellaneous Agents

Adenosine is a naturally occurring purine nucleoside composed of an adenine base and a ribose sugar. Adenosine monophosphate is metabolized by dephosphorylation to adenine and inorganic phosphate. Adenosine is used as a drug in treating supraventricular tachycardias.[437] Adenosine is administered by rapid intravenous bolus and is quickly metabolized by erythrocytes and vascular endothelium.[437] The clinical effects of adenosine last for about 20 seconds, and it has an ultrashort-acting half-life up to 10 seconds.[437] After administration, the effectiveness is typically observed between 10 and 20 seconds, and is dependent on the dose, cardiac output, and speed of administration.[437] Dipyridamole, a PDE3 enzyme inhibitor, decreases the metabolism and increases adenosine concentrations and thereby, potentiates its effects.[438] Therefore, the adenosine dose should be lowered when administered with dipyridamole and should be used with extreme caution.[437] Methylxanthines such as theophylline and caffeine act as adenosine receptor antagonists primarily at the A_1 receptors.[439,440] Thus, in the presence of methylxanthine derivatives, adenosine may have reduced pharmacologic effect.[437] The most common side effects with adenosine include flushing due to coronary vasodilation, acute dyspnea due to transient bronchoconstriction, and

Structure Challenge

Heart failure and anti-arrhythmic structures challenge: Evaluate the structures drawn below and match the correct description associated with each of the drugs.

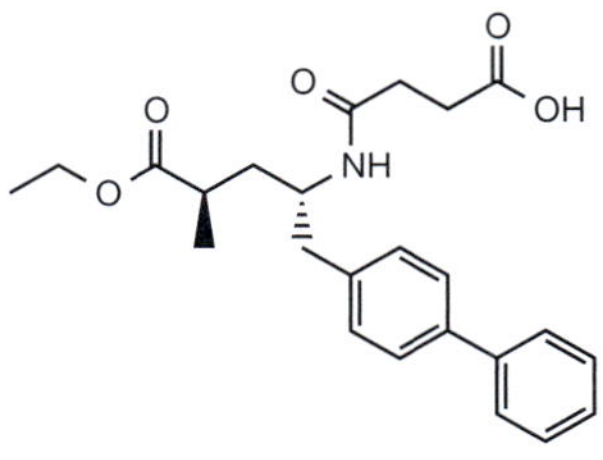

a

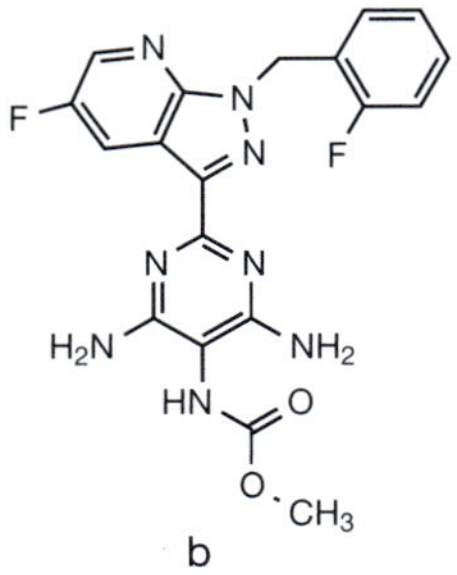

b

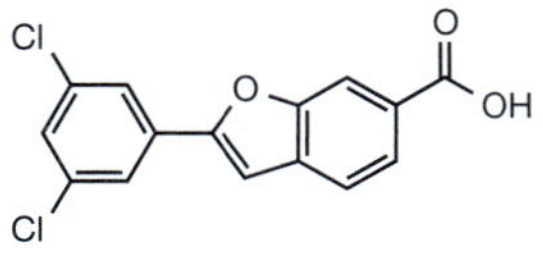

c

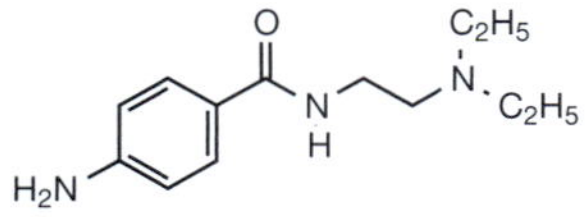

d

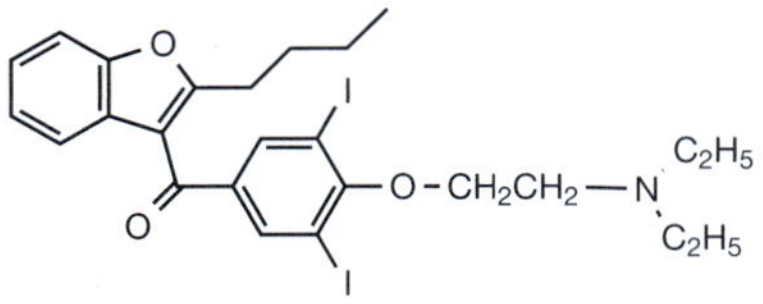

e

1. Highly lipophilic molecule that has the potential to cause hypo or hyperthyroidism
2. Prodrug that prevents the breakdown of the natriuretic peptide
3. Benzoxazole carboxylic acid derivative that stabilizes the TTR
4. Soluble guanylyl cyclase stimulator
5. Slow acetylators are more prone to lupus syndrome

Structure Challenge answers found immediately after References.

carotid body chemoreceptor activation.[437] Although rare, adenosine has significant proarrhythmic effects.[437]

Magnesium sulfate may be indicated in the treatment of torsades de pointes.[441] However, oral magnesium preparations do not have any effect as an anti-arrhythmic agent.[441]

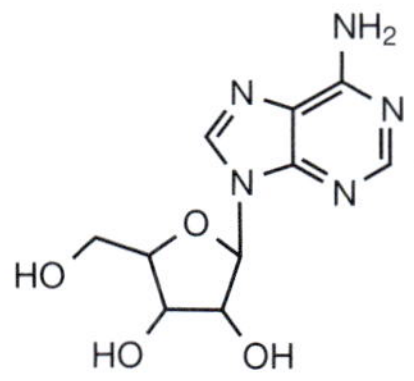

Adenosine

REFERENCES

1. The American Heart Association. Cardiovascular disease: a costly burden for America—projections through 2035. https://www.heart.org/-/media/Files/About-Us/Policy-Research/Fact-Sheets/Public-Health-Advocacy-and-Research/CVD-A-Costly-Burden-for-America-Projections-Through-2035.pdf
2. Ford TJ, Corcoran D, Berry C. Stable coronary syndromes: pathophysiology, diagnostic advances and therapeutic need. *Heart.* 2018;104:284-292.
3. Radico F, Cicchitti V, Zimarino M, et al. Angina pectoris and myocardial ischemia in the absence of obstructive coronary artery disease: practical considerations for diagnostic tests. *JACC Cardiovasc Interv.* 2014;7:453-463.
4. Braunwald E, Morrow DA. Unstable angina: is it time for a requiem? *Circulation.* 2013;127:2452-2457.
5. Ong P, Aziz A, Hansen HS, et al. Structural and functional coronary artery abnormalities in patients with vasospastic angina pectoris. *Circ J.* 2015;79:1431-1438.
6. Meyrelles SS, Mill JG, Cabral AM, et al. Cardiac baroreflex properties in myocardial infarcted rats. *J Auton Nerv Syst.* 1996;60:163-168.
7. Norton JM. Toward consistent definitions for preload and afterload. *Adv Physiol Educ.* 2001;25:53-61.
8. Ginsberg MD. Expanding the concept of neuroprotection for acute ischemic stroke: the pivotal roles of reperfusion and the collateral circulation. *Prog Neurobiol.* 2016;145-146:46-77.
9. Ferreira JC, Mochly-Rosen D. Nitroglycerin use in myocardial infarction patients. *Circ J.* 2012;76:15-21.
10. Mayer B, Beretta M. The enigma of nitroglycerin bioactivation and nitrate tolerance: news, views and troubles. *Br J Pharmacol.* 2008;155:170-184.
11. Godfraind T. Discovery and development of calcium channel blockers. *Front Pharmacol.* 2017;8:286.
12. Godfraind T. Calcium channel blockers in cardiovascular pharmacotherapy. *J Cardiovasc Pharmacol Ther.* 2014;19:501-515.
13. Diness JG, Bentzen BH, Sorensen US, et al. Role of calcium-activated potassium channels in atrial fibrillation pathophysiology and therapy. *J Cardiovasc Pharmacol.* 2015;66:441-448.
14. Elliott WJ, Ram CV. Calcium channel blockers. *J Clin Hypertens (Greenwich).* 2011;13:687-689.
15. Wallukat G. The beta-adrenergic receptors. *Herz.* 2002;27:683-690.
16. Smith C, Teitler M. Beta-blocker selectivity at cloned human beta 1- and beta 2-adrenergic receptors. *Cardiovasc Drugs Ther.* 1999;13:123-126.
17. Prichard BN, Richards DA. Comparison of labetalol with other anti-hypertensive drugs. *Br J Clin Pharmacol.* 1982;13:41S-47S.
18. Gupta S, Wright HM. Nebivolol: a highly selective beta1-adrenergic receptor blocker that causes vasodilation by increasing nitric oxide. *Cardiovasc Ther.* 2008;26:189-202.

19. Blumenfeld JD, Sealey JE, Mann SJ, et al. Beta-adrenergic receptor blockade as a therapeutic approach for suppressing the renin-angiotensin-aldosterone system in normotensive and hypertensive subjects. *Am J Hypertens.* 1999;12:451-459.
20. Schnabel P, Maack C, Mies F, et al. Binding properties of beta-blockers at recombinant beta1-, beta2-, and beta3-adrenoceptors. *J Cardiovasc Pharmacol.* 2000;36:466-471.
21. Wimmer NJ, Stone PH. Anti-anginal and anti-ischemic effects of late sodium current inhibition. *Cardiovasc Drugs Ther.* 2013;7:69-77.
22. Mason PK, DiMarco JP. New pharmacological agents for arrhythmias. *Circ Arrhythm Electrophysiol.* 2009;2:588-597.
23. Schram G, Zhang L, Derakhchan K, et al. Ranolazine: ion-channel-blocking actions and in vivo electrophysiological effects. *Br J Pharmacol.* 2004;142:1300-1308.
24. DiFrancesco D. The role of the funny current in pacemaker activity. *Circ Res.* 2010;106:434-446.
25. The Nobel Prize. Nitroglycerine and dynamite. http://www.nobelprize.org/alfred_nobel/biographical/articles/life-work/nitrodyn.html
26. Marsh N, Marsh A. A short history of nitroglycerine and nitric oxide in pharmacology and physiology. *Clin Exp Pharmacol Physiol.* 2000;27:313-319.
27. The Nobel Prize. Alfred Nobel's will. https://www.nobelprize.org/alfred-nobel/alfred-nobels-will/
28. Brunton TL. On the use of nitrite of amyl in angina pectoris. *Lancet.* 1867;2:97-98.
29. Nossaman VE, Nossaman BD, Kadowitz PJ. Nitrates and nitrites in the treatment of ischemic cardiac disease. *Cardiol Rev.* 2010;18:190-197.
30. The Nobel Prize. Alfred Nobel's health and his interest in medicine by Nils Ringertz. http://www.nobelprize.org/alfred_nobel/biographical/articles/ringertz/
31. Elkayam U, Bitar F, Akhter MW, et al. Intravenous nitroglycerin in the treatment of decompensated heart failure: potential benefits and limitations. *J Cardiovasc Pharmacol Ther.* 2004;9:227-241.
32. Chen Z, Zhang J, Stamler JS. Identification of the enzymatic mechanism of nitroglycerin bioactivation. *Proc Natl Acad Sci U S A.* 2002;99:8306-8311.
33. Kleschyov AL, Oelze M, Daiber A, et al. Does nitric oxide mediate the vasodilator activity of nitroglycerin? *Circ Res.* 2003;93:e104-e112.
34. Klemenska E, Beresewicz A. Bioactivation of organic nitrates and the mechanism of nitrate tolerance. *Cardiol J.* 2009;16:11-19.
35. Munzel T, Meinertz T, Tebbe U, et al. Efficacy of the long-acting nitro vasodilator pentaerithrityl tetranitrate in patients with chronic stable angina pectoris receiving anti-anginal background therapy with beta-blockers: a 12-week, randomized, double-blind, placebo-controlled trial. *Eur Heart J.* 2014;35:895-903.
36. Daiber A, Munzel T. Organic nitrate therapy, nitrate tolerance, and nitrate-induced endothelial dysfunction: emphasis on redox biology and oxidative stress. *Antioxid Redox Signal.* 2015;23:899-942.
37. Jurt U, Gori T, Ravandi A, et al. Differential effects of pentaerythritol tetranitrate and nitroglycerin on the development of tolerance and evidence of lipid peroxidation: a human in vivo study. *J Am Coll Cardiol.* 2001;38:854-859.
38. Lexidrug. Lexicomp. https://online.lexi.com/lco/action/search?q=nitroglycerin&t=name&acs=false&acq=nitroglycerin
39. McNiff EF, Yacobi A, Young-Chang FM, et al. Nitroglycerin pharmacokinetics after intravenous infusion in normal subjects. *J Pharm Sci.* 1981;70:1054-1058.
40. Hashimoto S, Kobayashi A. Clinical pharmacokinetics and pharmacodynamics of glyceryl trinitrate and its metabolites. *Clin Pharmacokinet.* 2003;42:205-221.
41. Hodgson JR, Lee CC. Trinitroglycerol metabolism: denitration and glucuronide formation in the rat. *Toxicol Appl Pharmacol.* 1975;34:449-455.
42. Neurath GB, Dunger M. Blood levels of the metabolites of glyceryl trinitrate and pentaerythritol tetranitrate after administration of a two-step preparation. *Arzneimittelforschung.* 1977;27:416-419.
43. Straehl P, Galeazzi RL. Isosorbide dinitrate bioavailability, kinetics, and metabolism. *Clin Pharmacol Ther.* 1985;38:140-149.
44. Sporl-Radun S, Betzien G, Kaufmann B, et al. Effects and pharmacokinetics of isosorbide dinitrate in normal man. *Eur J Clin Pharmacol.* 1980;18:237-244.
45. Ghofrani HA, Humbert M, Langleben D, et al. Riociguat: mode of action and clinical development in pulmonary hypertension. *Chest.* 2017;151:468-480.
46. Kloner RA. Novel phosphodiesterase type 5 inhibitors: assessing hemodynamic effects and safety parameters. *Clin Cardiol.* 2004;27:I20-I25.
47. Triggle DJ. Calcium-channel drugs: structure-function relationships and selectivity of action. *J Cardiovasc Pharmacol.* 1991;18 suppl 10:S1-S6.
48. Scholz H. Pharmacological aspects of calcium channel blockers. *Cardiovasc Drugs Ther.* 1997;10 suppl 3:869-872.
49. Davies MK, Hollman A. The opium poppy, morphine, and verapamil. *Heart.* 2002;88:3.
50. Melville KI, Shister HE, Huq S. Iproveratril: experimental data on coronary dilatation and antiarrhythmic action. *Can Med Assoc J.* 1964;90:761-770.
51. Vater W, Kroneberg G, Hoffmeister F, et al. [Pharmacology of 4-(2′-nitrophenyl)-2,6-dimethyl-1,4-dihydropyridine-3,5-dicarboxylic acid dimethyl ester (Nifedipine, BAY a 1040)]. *Arzneimittelforschung.* 1972;22:1-14.
52. Shamsipur M, Hemmateenejad B, Akhond M, et al. A study of the photo-degradation kinetics of nifedipine by multivariate curve resolution analysis. *J Pharm Biomed Anal.* 2003;31:1013-1019.
53. Shaldam MA, Elhamamsy MH, Esmat EA, El-Moselhy TF. 1,4-dihydropyridine calcium channel blockers: homology modeling of the receptor and assessment of structure activity relationship. *ISRN Med Chem.* 2014;1:1-14.
54. Meredith PA, Elliott HL. Clinical pharmacokinetics of amlodipine. *Clin Pharmacokinet.* 1992;22:22-31.
55. Nguyen LA, He H, Pham-Huy C. Chiral drugs: an overview. *Int J Biomed Sci.* 2006;2:85-100.
56. Ishii K, Minato K, Nakai H, Sato T. Simultaneous assay of four stereoisomers of diltiazem hydrochloride. Application to in vitro chiral inversion studies. *Chromatographia.* 1995;41:450-454.
57. Lexidrug. Lexicomp. https://online.lexi.com
58. Rashid TJ, Martin U, Clarke H, et al. Factors affecting the absolute bioavailability of nifedipine. *Br J Clin Pharmacol.* 1995;40:51-58.
59. Otto J, Lesko LJ. Protein binding of nifedipine. *J Pharm Pharmacol.* 1986;38:399-400.
60. Renwick AG, Robertson DR, Macklin B, et al. The pharmacokinetics of oral nifedipine—a population study. *Br J Clin Pharmacol.* 1988;25:701-708.
61. Wang JG, Kario K, Lau T, et al. Use of dihydropyridine calcium channel blockers in the management of hypertension in Eastern Asians: a scientific statement from the Asian Pacific Heart Association. *Hypertens Res.* 2011;34:423-430.
62. Food and Drug Administration. Adalat® CC. https://www.accessdata.fda.gov/drugsatfda_docs/label/2011/020198s023lbl.pdf
63. Kleinbloesem CH, van Harten J, Wilson JP, et al. Nifedipine: kinetics and hemodynamic effects in patients with liver cirrhosis after intravenous and oral administration. *Clin Pharmacol Ther.* 1986;40:21-28.
64. Graham DJ, Dow RJ, Hall DJ, et al. The metabolism and pharmacokinetics of nicardipine hydrochloride in man. *Br J Clin Pharmacol.* 1985;20 suppl 1:23S-28S.
65. Urien S, Albengres E, Comte A, et al. Plasma protein binding and erythrocyte partitioning of nicardipine in vitro. *J Cardiovasc Pharmacol.* 1985;7:891-898.

66. Food and Drug Administration. Cardene® SR. https://www.accessdata.fda.gov/drugsatfda_docs/label/2016/020005s014lbl.pdf
67. Judd E, Jaimes EA. Aliskiren, amlodipine and hydrochlorothiazide triple combination for hypertension. *Expert Rev Cardiovasc Ther.* 2012;10:293-303.
68. Zhu Y, Wang F, Li Q, et al. Amlodipine metabolism in human liver microsomes and roles of CYP3A4/5 in the dihydropyridine dehydrogenation. *Drug Metab Dispos.* 2014;42:245-249.
69. Abernethy DR. The pharmacokinetic profile of amlodipine. *Am Heart J.* 1989;118:1100-1103.
70. Beresford AP, McGibney D, Humphrey MJ, et al. Metabolism and kinetics of amlodipine in man. *Xenobiotica.* 1988;18:245-254.
71. Echizen H, Eichelbaum M. Clinical pharmacokinetics of verapamil, nifedipine and diltiazem. *Clin Pharmacokinet.* 1986;11:425-449.
72. Eichelbaum M, Ende M, Remberg G, et al. The metabolism of DL-[14C]verapamil in man. *Drug Metab Dispos.* 1979;7:145-148.
73. Keefe DL, Yee YG, Kates RE. Verapamil protein binding in patients and in normal subjects. *Clin Pharmacol Ther.* 1981;29:21-26.
74. Vogelgesang B, Echizen H, Schmidt E, et al. Stereoselective first-pass metabolism of highly cleared drugs: studies of the bioavailability of L- and D-verapamil examined with a stable isotope technique. *Br J Clin Pharmacol.* 1984;18:733-740.
75. Tracy TS, Korzekwa KR, Gonzalez FJ, et al. Cytochrome P450 isoforms involved in metabolism of the enantiomers of verapamil and norverapamil. *Br J Clin Pharmacol.* 1999;47:545-552.
76. Schwartz JB, Keefe DL, Kirsten E, et al. Prolongation of verapamil elimination kinetics during chronic oral administration. *Am Heart J.* 1982;104:198-203.
77. Ochs HR, Knuchel M. Pharmacokinetics and absolute bioavailability of diltiazem in humans. *Klin Wochenschr.* 1984;62:303-306.
78. Hermann P, Rodger SD, Remones G, et al. Pharmacokinetics of diltiazem after intravenous and oral administration. *Eur J Clin Pharmacol.* 1983;24:349-352.
79. Yeung PK, Prescott C, Haddad C, et al. Pharmacokinetics and metabolism of diltiazem in healthy males and females following a single oral dose. *Eur J Drug Metab Pharmacokinet.* 1993;18:199-206.
80. Sutton D, Butler AM, Nadin L, et al. Role of CYP3A4 in human hepatic diltiazem N-demethylation: inhibition of CYP3A4 activity by oxidized diltiazem metabolites. *J Pharmacol Exp Ther.* 1997;282:294-300.
81. Molden E, Johansen PW, Boe GH, et al. Pharmacokinetics of diltiazem and its metabolites in relation to CYP2D6 genotype. *Clin Pharmacol Ther.* 2002;72:333-342.
82. Montamat SC, Abernethy DR. N-monodesmethyldiltiazem is the predominant metabolite of diltiazem in the plasma of young and elderly hypertensives. *Br J Clin Pharmacol.* 1987;24:185-189.
83. Nishio S, Watanabe H, Kosuge K, et al. Interaction between amlodipine and simvastatin in patients with hypercholesterolemia and hypertension. *Hypertens Res.* 2005;28:223-227.
84. Kantola T, Kivisto KT, Neuvonen PJ. Erythromycin and verapamil considerably increase serum simvastatin and simvastatin acid concentrations. *Clin Pharmacol Ther.* 1998;64:177-182.
85. Yoshimoto H, Takahashi M, Saima S. [Influence of rifampicin on antihypertensive effects of dihydropiridine calcium-channel blockers in four elderly patients]. *Nihon Ronen Igakkai Zasshi.* 1996;33:692-696.
86. Jalava KM, Olkkola KT, Neuvonen PJ. Itraconazole greatly increases plasma concentrations and effects of felodipine. *Clin Pharmacol Ther.* 1997;61:410-415.
87. Sica DA. Interaction of grapefruit juice and calcium channel blockers. *Am J Hypertens.* 2006;19:768-773.
88. Kim RB. Drugs as P-glycoprotein substrates, inhibitors, and inducers. *Drug Metab Rev.* 2002;34:47-54.
89. Verschraagen M, Koks CH, Schellens JH, et al. P-glycoprotein system as a determinant of drug interactions: the case of digoxin-verapamil. *Pharmacol Res.* 1999;40:301-306.
90. Wessler JD, Grip LT, Mendell J, et al. The P-glycoprotein transport system and cardiovascular drugs. *J Am Coll Cardiol.* 2013;61:2495-2502.
91. Summers MA, Moore JL, McAuley JW. Use of verapamil as a potential P-glycoprotein inhibitor in a patient with refractory epilepsy. *Ann Pharmacother.* 2004;38:1631-1634.
92. Sadeque AJ, Wandel C, He H, et al. Increased drug delivery to the brain by P-glycoprotein inhibition. *Clin Pharmacol Ther.* 2000;68:231-237.
93. Bahls FH, Ozuna J, Ritchie DE. Interactions between calcium channel blockers and the anticonvulsants carbamazepine and phenytoin. *Neurology.* 1991;41:740-742.
94. Brodie MJ, MacPhee GJ. Carbamazepine neurotoxicity precipitated by diltiazem. *Br Med J (Clin Res Ed).* 1986;292:1170-1171.
95. Flatmark T. Catecholamine biosynthesis and physiological regulation in neuroendocrine cells. *Acta Physiol Scand.* 2000;168:1-17.
96. Powell CE, Slater IH. Blocking of inhibitory adrenergic receptors by a dichloro analog of isoproterenol. *J Pharmacol Exp Ther.* 1958;122:480-488.
97. Black JW, Stephenson JS. Pharmacology of a new adrenergic beta-receptor-blocking compound (Nethalide). *Lancet.* 1962;2:311-314.
98. Black JW, Duncan WA, Shanks RG. Comparison of some properties of pronethalol and propranolol. *Br J Pharmacol Chemother.* 1965;25:577-591.
99. The Nobel Prize. The Nobel Prize in Physiology or Medicine 1988. https://www.nobelprize.org/nobel_prizes/medicine/laureates/1988/press.html
100. Lands AM, Arnold A, McAuliff JP, et al. Differentiation of receptor systems activated by sympathomimetic amines. *Nature.* 1967;214:597-598.
101. Frishman WH. A historical perspective on the development of β-adrenergic blockers. *J Clin Hypertens.* 2007;9:19-27.
102. Wright P. Untoward effects associated with practolol administration: oculomucocutaneous syndrome. *Br Med J.* 1975;1:595-598.
103. Wall-Manning HJ. Problems with practolol. *Drugs.* 1975;10:336-341.
104. Mehvar R, Brocks DR. Stereospecific pharmacokinetics and pharmacodynamics of beta-adrenergic blockers in humans. *J Pharm Pharm Sci.* 2001;4:185-200.
105. LogP and CLogP reported using PerkinElmer ChemDraw 16.0.
106. McAinsh J, Cruickshank JM. Beta-blockers and central nervous system side effects. *Pharmacol Ther.* 1990;46:163-197.
107. Poirier L, Tobe SW. Contemporary use of beta-blockers: clinical relevance of subclassification. *Can J Cardiol.* 2014;30:S9-S15.
108. Shand DG. Pharmacokinetics of propranolol: a review. *Postgrad Med J.* 1976;52 suppl 4:22-25.
109. Borgström L, Johansson C-G, Larsson H, et al. Pharmacokinetics of propranolol. *J Pharmacokinet Biopharm.* 1981;9:419-429.
110. Liedholm H, Wahlin-Boll E, Melander A. Mechanisms and variations in the food effect on propranolol bioavailability. *Eur J Clin Pharmacol.* 1990;38:469-475.
111. Silber B, Riegelman S. Stereospecific assay for (-)- and (+)-propranolol in human and dog plasma. *J Pharmacol Exp Ther.* 1980;215:643-648.
112. Masubuchi Y, Hosokawa S, Horie T, et al. Cytochrome P450 isozymes involved in propranolol metabolism in human liver microsomes. The role of CYP2D6 as ring-hydroxylase and CYP1A2 as *N*-desisopropylase. *Drug Metab Dispos.* 1994;22:909-915.
113. Rowland K, Yeo WW, Ellis SW, et al. Inhibition of CYP2D6 activity by treatment with propranolol and the role of 4-hydroxy propranolol. *Br J Clin Pharmacol.* 1994;38:9-14.
114. Food and Drug Administration. Inderal®. https://www.accessdata.fda.gov/drugsatfda_docs/label/2011/016418s080,016762s017,017683s008lbl.pdf
115. Patten SB. Propranolol and depression: evidence from the antihypertensive trials. *Can J Psychiatry.* 1990;35:257-259.
116. Suzman MM. Propranolol in the treatment of anxiety. *Postgrad Med J.* 1976;52 suppl 4:168-174.

117. Garza I, Swanson JW. Prophylaxis of migraine. *Neuropsychiatr Dis Treat.* 2006;2:281-291.
118. McAinsh J, Baber NS, Smith R, et al. Pharmacokinetic and pharmacodynamic studies with long-acting propranolol. *Br J Clin Pharmacol.* 1978;6:115-121.
119. Nace GS, Wood AJ. Pharmacokinetics of long acting propranolol. Implications for therapeutic use. *Clin Pharmacokinet.* 1987;13:51-64.
120. Kirch W, Gorg KG. Clinical pharmacokinetics of atenolol—a review. *Eur J Drug Metab Pharmacokinet.* 1982;7:81-91.
121. Barber HE, Hawksworth GM, Kitteringham NR, et al. Protein binding of atenolol and propranolol to human serum albumin and in human plasma [proceedings]. *Br J Clin Pharmacol.* 1978;6:446P-447P.
122. Reeves PR, McAinsh J, McIntosh DA, et al. Metabolism of atenolol in man. *Xenobiotica.* 1978;8:313-320.
123. Food and Drug Administration. Tenormin®. https://www.accessdata.fda.gov/drugsatfda_docs/label/2011/018240s031lbl.pdf
124. Kukin ML, Mannino MM, Freudenberger RS, et al. Hemodynamic comparison of twice daily metoprolol tartrate with once daily metoprolol succinate in congestive heart failure. *J Am Coll Cardiol.* 2000;35:45-50.
125. Tangeman HJ, Patterson JH. Extended-release metoprolol succinate in chronic heart failure. *Ann Pharmacother.* 2003;37:701-710.
126. Regårdh CG, Johnsson G. Clinical pharmacokinetics of metoprolol. *Clin Pharmacokinet.* 1980;5:557-569.
127. Rigby JW, Scott AK, Hawksworth GM, et al. A comparison of the pharmacokinetics of atenolol, metoprolol, oxprenolol and propranolol in elderly hypertensive and young healthy subjects. *Br J Clin Pharmacol.* 1985;20:327-331.
128. McGourty JC, Silas JH, Lennard MS, et al. Metoprolol metabolism and debrisoquine oxidation polymorphism—population and family studies. *Br J Clin Pharmacol.* 1985;20:555-566.
129. Quarterman CP, Kendall MJ, Jack DB. The effect of age on the pharmacokinetics of metoprolol and its metabolites. *Br J Clin Pharmacol.* 1981;11:287-294.
130. Rau T, Heide R, Bergmann K, et al. Effect of the CYP2D6 genotype on metoprolol metabolism persists during long-term treatment. *Pharmacogenetics.* 2002;12:465-472.
131. Blake CM, Kharasch ED, Schwab M, et al. A meta-analysis of CYP2D6 metabolizer phenotype and metoprolol pharmacokinetics. *Clin Pharmacol Ther.* 2013;94:394-399.
132. Wuttke H, Rau T, Heide R, et al. Increased frequency of cytochrome P450 2D6 poor metabolizers among patients with metoprolol-associated adverse effects. *Clin Pharmacol Ther.* 2002;72:429-437.
133. Leopold G. Balanced pharmacokinetics and metabolism of bisoprolol. *J Cardiovasc Pharmacol.* 1986;8 suppl 11:S16-S20.
134. Zisaki A, Miskovic L, Hatzimanikatis V. Antihypertensive drugs metabolism: an update to pharmacokinetic profiles and computational approaches. *Curr Pharm Des.* 2015;21:806-822.
135. Food and Drug Administration. Coreg®. https://www.accessdata.fda.gov/drugsatfda_docs/label/2005/020297s013lbl.pdf
136. Hamed R, Awadallah A, Sunoqrot S, et al. pH-dependent solubility and dissolution behavior of carvedilol—case example of a weakly basic BCS class II drug. *AAPS PharmSciTech.* 2016;17:418-426.
137. Ruffolo RR Jr, Gellai M, Hieble JP, et al. The pharmacology of carvedilol. *Eur J Clin Pharmacol.* 1990;38 suppl 2:S82-S88.
138. Morgan T. Clinical pharmacokinetics and pharmacodynamics of carvedilol. *Clin Pharmacokinet.* 1994;26:335-346.
139. Zhou HH, Wood AJ. Stereoselective disposition of carvedilol is determined by CYP2D6. *Clin Pharmacol Ther.* 1995;57:518-524.
140. Neugebauer G, Akpan W, von Mollendorff E, et al. Pharmacokinetics and disposition of carvedilol in humans. *J Cardiovasc Pharmacol.* 1987;10 suppl 11:S85-S88.
141. Oldham HG, Clarke SE. In vitro identification of the human cytochrome P450 enzymes involved in the metabolism of *R*(+)- and *S*(-)-carvedilol. *Drug Metab Dispos.* 1997;25:970-977.
142. Gehr TW, Tenero DM, Boyle DA, et al. The pharmacokinetics of carvedilol and its metabolites after single and multiple dose oral administration in patients with hypertension and renal insufficiency. *Eur J Clin Pharmacol.* 1999;55:269-277.
143. Brodde OE, Kroemer HK. Drug-drug interactions of beta-adrenoceptor blockers. *Arzneimittelforschung.* 2003;53:814-822.
144. Hamelin BA, Bouayad A, Methot J, et al. Significant interaction between the nonprescription antihistamine diphenhydramine and the CYP2D6 substrate metoprolol in healthy men with high or low CYP2D6 activity. *Clin Pharmacol Ther.* 2000;67:466-477.
145. Johnson JA, Burlew BS. Metoprolol metabolism via cytochrome P4502D6 in ethnic populations. *Drug Metab Dispos.* 1996;24:350-355.
146. Molden E, Spigset O. [Interactions between metoprolol and antidepressants]. *Tidsskr Nor Laegeforen.* 2011;131:1777-1779.
147. Kakumoto M, Sakaeda T, Takara K, et al. Effects of carvedilol on MDR1-mediated multidrug resistance: comparison with verapamil. *Cancer Sci.* 2003;94:81-86.
148. Bachmakov I, Werner U, Endress B, et al. Characterization of beta-adrenoceptor antagonists as substrates and inhibitors of the drug transporter P-glycoprotein. *Fundam Clin Pharmacol.* 2006;20:273-282.
149. Giessmann T, Modess C, Hecker U, et al. CYP2D6 genotype and induction of intestinal drug transporters by rifampin predict presystemic clearance of carvedilol in healthy subjects. *Clin Pharmacol Ther.* 2004;75:213-222.
150. Frishman WH. Beta-adrenergic receptor blockers. Adverse effects and drug interactions. *Hypertension.* 1988;11:II21–II29.
151. Abrams J, Jones CA, Kirkpatrick P. Ranolazine. *Nat Rev Drug Discov.* 2006;5:453-454.
152. Jerling M. Clinical pharmacokinetics of ranolazine. *Clin Pharmacokinet.* 2006;45:469-491.
153. Jerling M, Huan BL, Leung K, et al. Studies to investigate the pharmacokinetic interactions between ranolazine and ketoconazole, diltiazem, or simvastatin during combined administration in healthy subjects. *J Clin Pharmacol.* 2005;45:422-433.
154. Penman AD, Eadie J, Herron WJ, et al. The characterization of the metabolites of ranolazine in man by liquid chromatography mass spectrometry. *Rapid Commun Mass Spectrom.* 1995;9:1418-1430.
155. Morrow DA, Scirica BM, Karwatowska-Prokopczuk E, et al. Effects of ranolazine on recurrent cardiovascular events in patients with non-ST-elevation acute coronary syndromes: the MERLIN-TIMI 36 randomized trial. *JAMA.* 2007;297:1775-1783.
156. Liu Z, Williams RB, Rosen BD. The potential contribution of ranolazine to Torsade de Pointe. *J Cardiovasc Dis Res.* 2013;4:187-190.
157. Vilaine JP. The discovery of the selective I(f) current inhibitor ivabradine. A new therapeutic approach to ischemic heart disease. *Pharmacol Res.* 2006;53:424-434.
158. Amgen Inc. Corlanor (ivabradine) prescribing information. http://pi.amgen.com/~/media/amgen/repositorysites/pi-amgen-com/corlanor/corlanor_pi.pdf
159. Vlase L, Popa A, Neag M, et al. Pharmacokinetic interaction between ivabradine and phenytoin in healthy subjects. *Clin Drug Investig.* 2012;32:533-538.
160. Vlase L, Neag M, Popa A, et al. Pharmacokinetic interaction between ivabradine and carbamazepine in healthy volunteers. *J Clin Pharm Ther.* 2011;36:225-229.
161. Savelieva I, Camm AJ. Novel If current inhibitor ivabradine: safety considerations. *Adv Cardiol.* 2006;43:79-96.
162. Benjamin EJ, Blaha MJ, Chiuve SE, et al. Heart disease and stroke statistics—2017 update: a report from the American Heart Association. *Circulation.* 2017;135:e146-e603.
163. Koike H, Katsuno M. Transthyretin amyloidosis: update on the clinical spectrum, pathogenesis, and disease-modifying therapies. *Neurol Ther.* 2020;9:317-333.

164. Manganelli F, Fabrizi GM, Luigetti M, et al. Hereditary transthyretin amyloidosis overview. *Neurol Sci.* 2022;43:595-604.
165. 100 Years. Classes and stages of heart failure. https://www.heart.org/en/health-topics/heart-failure/what-is-heart-failure/classes-of-heart-failure
166. Toschi-Dias E, Rondon M, Cogliati C, et al. Contribution of autonomic reflexes to the hyperadrenergic state in heart failure. *Front Neurosci.* 2017;11:162.
167. Kobirumaki-Shimozawa F, Inoue T, Shintani SA, et al. Cardiac thin filament regulation and the Frank-Starling mechanism. *J Physiol Sci.* 2014;64:221-232.
168. Sequeira V, van der Velden J. Historical perspective on heart function: the Frank-Starling Law. *Biophys Rev.* 2015;7:421-447.
169. LaCombe P, Lappin SL. *Physiology, Cardiovascular, Starling Relationships*. StatPearls Publishing; 2018.
170. Laursen M, Gregersen JL, Yatime L, et al. Structures and characterization of digoxin- and bufalin-bound Na+, K+-ATPase compared with the ouabain-bound complex. *Proc Natl Acad Sci U S A.* 2015;112:1755-1760.
171. Tian J, Xie ZJ. The Na-K-ATPase and calcium-signaling microdomains. *Physiology (Bethesda).* 2008;23:205-211.
172. Konstantinou DM, Karvounis H, Giannakoulas G. Digoxin in heart failure with a reduced ejection fraction: a risk factor or a risk marker. *Cardiology.* 2016;134:311-319.
173. Boswell-Smith V, Spina D, Page CP. Phosphodiesterase inhibitors. *Br J Pharmacol.* 2006;147 suppl 1:S252-S257.
174. Lugnier C. Cyclic nucleotide phosphodiesterase (PDE) superfamily: a new target for the development of specific therapeutic agents. *Pharmacol Ther.* 2006;109:366-398.
175. Lehtonen LA, Antila S, Pentikainen PJ. Pharmacokinetics and pharmacodynamics of intravenous inotropic agents. *Clin Pharmacokinet.* 2004;43:187-203.
176. Teerlink JR. A novel approach to improve cardiac performance: cardiac myosin activators. *Heart Fail Rev.* 2009;14:289-298.
177. Koster G, Bekema HJ, Wetterslev J, et al. Milrinone for cardiac dysfunction in critically ill adult patients: a systematic review of randomised clinical trials with meta-analysis and trial sequential analysis. *Intensive Care Med.* 2016;42:1322-1335.
178. Felker GM, Benza RL, Chandler AB, et al. Heart failure etiology and response to milrinone in decompensated heart failure: results from the OPTIME-CHF study. *J Am Coll Cardiol.* 2003;41:997-1003.
179. Tuttle RR, Hillmann CC, Toomey RE. Differential beta adrenergic sensitivity of atrial and ventricular tissue assessed by chronotropic, inotropic, and cyclic AMP responses to isoprenaline and dobutamine. *Cardiovasc Res.* 1976;10:452-458.
180. Ruffolo RR, Jr. The pharmacology of dobutamine. *Am J Med Sci.* 1987;294:244-248.
181. Clark D, Hjorth S, Carlsson A. Dopamine-receptor agonists: mechanisms underlying autoreceptor selectivity. I. Review of the evidence. *J Neural Transm.* 1985;62:1-52.
182. Gerber JG, Freed CR, Nies AS. Antihypertensive pharmacology. *West J Med.* 1980;132:430-439.
183. Cole RT, Kalogeropoulos AP, Georgiopoulou VV, et al. Hydralazine and isosorbide dinitrate in heart failure: historical perspective, mechanisms, and future directions. *Circulation.* 2011;123:2414-2422.
184. Ramsay LE, Cameron HA. The lupus syndrome induced by hydralazine. *Br Med J (Clin Res Ed).* 1984;289:1310-1311.
185. Roden DM. Antiarrhythmic drugs: from mechanisms to clinical practice. *Heart.* 2000;84:339-346.
186. Fala L. Entresto (sacubitril/valsartan): first-in-class angiotensin receptor neprilysin inhibitor FDA approved for patients with heart failure. *Am Health Drug Benefits.* 2015;8:330-334.
187. Volpe M, Carnovali M, Mastromarino V. The natriuretic peptides system in the pathophysiology of heart failure: from molecular basis to treatment. *Clin Sci (Lond).* 2016;130:57-77.
188. Gonzalez-Juanatey JR, Anguita-Sanchez M, Bayes-Genis A, et al. Vericiguat in heart failure: from scientific evidence to clinical practice. *Rev Clin Esp (Barc).* 2022;222:359-369.
189. Friebe A, Sandner P, Schmidtko A. cGMP: a unique 2nd messenger molecule—recent developments in cGMP research and development. *Naunyn Schmiedebergs Arch Pharmacol.* 2020;393:287-302.
190. Greenberg B. Novel therapies for heart failure—where do they stand? *Circ J.* 2016;80:1882-1891.
191. Food and Drug Administration. https://www.accessdata.fda.gov/drugsatfda_docs/label/2021/214377s000lbl.pdf
192. Obici L, Adams D. Acquired and inherited amyloidosis: knowledge driving patients' care. *J Peripher Nerv Syst.* 2020;25:85-101.
193. Hafeez AS, Bavry AA. Diagnosis of transthyretin amyloid cardiomyopathy. *Cardiol Ther.* 2020;9:85-95.
194. Coelho T, Merlini G, Bulawa CE, et al. Mechanism of action and clinical application of tafamidis in hereditary transthyretin amyloidosis. *Neurol Ther.* 2016;5:1-25.
195. Pfizer Labs. Vyndaqel (tafamidis meglumine) and Vyndamax (tafamidis) capsules prescribing information. https://labeling.pfizer.com/ShowLabeling.aspx?id=11685
196. Maurer MS, Schwartz JH, Gundapaneni B, et al. Tafamidis treatment for patients with transthyretin amyloid cardiomyopathy. *N Engl J Med.* 2018;379:1007-1016.
197. Agrawal AA, Petschenka G, Bingham RA, et al. Toxic cardenolides: chemical ecology and coevolution of specialized plant-herbivore interactions. *New Phytol.* 2012;194:28-45.
198. Withering W. *An Account of the Foxglove and Some of Its Medical Uses with Practical Remarks on Dropsy and Other Diseases.* G.G.J. and J. Robinson; 1785.
199. Wilkins MR, Kendall MJ, Wade OL. William Withering and digitalis, 1785 to 1985. *Br Med J.* 1985;290:7-8.
200. Smith S. Digoxin, a new digitalis glycoside. *J Chem Soc.* 1930:508-510.
201. Patel S. Plant-derived cardiac glycosides: role in heart ailments and cancer management. *Biomed Pharmacother.* 2016;84:1036-1041.
202. Hollman A. Plants and cardiac glycosides. *Br Heart J.* 1985;54:258-261.
203. Blanco G, Mercer RW. Isozymes of the Na-K-ATPase: heterogeneity in structure, diversity in function. *Am J Physiol.* 1998;275:F633–F650.
204. Katz A, Lifshitz Y, Bab-Dinitz E, et al. Selectivity of digitalis glycosides for isoforms of human Na,K-ATPase. *J Biol Chem.* 2010;285:19582-19592.
205. Erdmann E. Influence of cardiac glycosides on their receptor. In: Greef K, ed. *Cardiac Glycosides: Part I: Experimental Pharmacology.* Vol 56. Springer-Verlag; 1981:337-380.
206. Cerri A, Serra F, Ferrari P, et al. Synthesis, cardiotonic activity, and structure-activity relationships of 17 beta-guanylhydrazone derivatives of 5 beta-androstane-3 beta, 14 beta-diol acting on the Na+, K(+)-ATPase receptor. *J Med Chem.* 1997;40:3484-3488.
207. Cerri A, Almirante N, Barassi P, et al. 17beta-O-Aminoalkyloximes of 5beta-androstane-3beta,14beta-diol with digitalis-like activity: synthesis, cardiotonic activity, structure-activity relationships, and molecular modeling of the Na(+), K(+)-ATPase receptor. *J Med Chem.* 2000;43:2332-2349.
208. Iisalo E. Clinical pharmacokinetics of digoxin. *Clin Pharmacokinet.* 1977;2:1-16.
209. Aronson JK. Clinical pharmacokinetics of digoxin 1980. *Clin Pharmacokinet.* 1980;5:137-149.
210. Food and Drug Administration. Drugs@FDA: FDA-approved drugs. https://www.accessdata.fda.gov/scripts/cder/daf/index.cfm?event=overview.process&ApplNo=018118
211. Marcus FI. Digitalis pharmacokinetics and metabolism. *Am J Med.* 1975;58:452-459.
212. Abernethy DR, Greenblatt DJ, Smith TW. Digoxin disposition in obesity: clinical pharmacokinetic investigation. *Am Heart J.* 1981;102:740-744.
213. Noviasky J, Darko W, Akajabor D, et al. Digoxin. In: Cohen H, ed. *Casebook in Clinical Pharmacokinetics and Drug Dosing.* McGraw-Hill Education; 2015.

214. Cheng JW, Charland SL, Shaw LM, et al. Is the volume of distribution of digoxin reduced in patients with renal dysfunction? Determining digoxin pharmacokinetics by fluorescence polarization immunoassay. *Pharmacotherapy.* 1997;17:584-590.
215. Bendayan R, McKenzie MW. Digoxin pharmacokinetics and dosage requirements in pediatric patients. *Clin Pharm.* 1983;2:224-235.
216. Soyka LF. Digoxin: placental transfer, effects on the fetus, and therapeutic use in the newborn. *Clin Perinatol.* 1975;2:23-35.
217. Lindenbaum J, Rund DG, Butler VP Jr, et al. Inactivation of digoxin by the gut flora: reversal by antibiotic therapy. *N Engl J Med.* 1981;305:789-794.
218. Ito S, Woodland C, Harper PA, et al. P-glycoprotein-mediated renal tubular secretion of digoxin: the toxicological significance of the urine-blood barrier model. *Life Sci.* 1993;53:PL25-PL31.
219. Ewy GA, Kapadia GG, Yao L, et al. Digoxin metabolism in the elderly. *Circulation.* 1969;39:449-453.
220. Croxson MS, Ibbertson HK. Serum digoxin in patients with thyroid disease. *Br Med J.* 1975;3:566-568.
221. Bauer LA. Digoxin. In: Bauer LA, ed. *Applied Clinical Pharmacokinetics.* 3rd ed. McGraw-Hill Medical, 2015.
222. Kramer P. Digitalis pharmacokinetics and therapy with respect to impaired renal function. *Klin Wochenschr.* 1977;55:1-11.
223. Santos SR, Kirch W, Ohnhaus EE. Simultaneous analysis of digitoxin and its clinically relevant metabolites using high-performance liquid chromatography and radioimmunoassay. *J Chromatogr.* 1987;419:155-164.
224. Nokhodian A, Santos SR, Kirch W. Digitoxin and its metabolites in patients with liver cirrhosis. *Eur J Drug Metab Pharmacokinet.* 1993;18:207-213.
225. Currie GM, Wheat JM, Kiat H. Pharmacokinetic considerations for digoxin in older people. *Open Cardiovasc Med J.* 2011;5:130-135.
226. Dec GW. Digoxin remains useful in the management of chronic heart failure. *Med Clin North Am.* 2003;87:317-337.
227. Ehle M, Patel C, Giugliano RP. Digoxin: clinical highlights: a review of digoxin and its use in contemporary medicine. *Crit Pathw Cardiol.* 2011;10:93-98.
228. MacLeod-Glover N, Mink M, Yarema M, et al. Digoxin toxicity: case for retiring its use in elderly patients? *Can Fam Physician.* 2016;62:223-228.
229. Dawson AH, Buckley NA. Digoxin. *Medicine.* 2016;44:158-159.
230. Hooymans PM, Merkus FW. Current status of cardiac glycoside drug interactions. *Clin Pharm.* 1985;4:404-413.
231. de Lannoy IA, Silverman M. The MDR1 gene product, P-glycoprotein, mediates the transport of the cardiac glycoside, digoxin. *Biochem Biophys Res Commun.* 1992;189:551-557.
232. Gomes T, Mamdani MM, Juurlink DN. Macrolide-induced digoxin toxicity: a population-based study. *Clin Pharmacol Ther.* 2009;86:383-386.
233. Fromm MF, Kim RB, Stein CM, et al. Inhibition of P-glycoprotein-mediated drug transport: a unifying mechanism to explain the interaction between digoxin and quinidine [see comments]. *Circulation.* 1999;99:552-557.
234. Bigger JT Jr, Leahey EB Jr. Quinidine and digoxin. An important interaction. *Drugs.* 1982;24:229-239.
235. Schenck-Gustafsson K, Dahlqvist R. Pharmacokinetics of digoxin in patients subjected to the quinidine-digoxin interaction. *Br J Clin Pharmacol.* 1981;11:181-186.
236. Pedersen KE, Christiansen BD, Klitgaard NA, et al. Effect of quinidine on digoxin bioavailability. *Eur J Clin Pharmacol.* 1983;24:41-47.
237. Ledwitch KV, Barnes RW, Roberts AG. Unravelling the complex drug-drug interactions of the cardiovascular drugs, verapamil and digoxin, with P-glycoprotein. *Biosci Rep. 2016*;36:e00309.
238. Ledwitch KV, Roberts AG. Cardiovascular ion channel inhibitor drug-drug interactions with P-glycoprotein. *AAPS J.* 2017;19:409-420.
239. Pedersen KE, Dorph-Pedersen A, Hvidt S, et al. Digoxin-verapamil interaction. *Clin Pharmacol Ther.* 1981;30:311-316.
240. Robinson K, Johnston A, Walker S, et al. The digoxin-amiodarone interaction. *Cardiovasc Drugs Ther.* 1989;3:25-28.
241. Okamura N, Hirai M, Tanigawara Y, et al. Digoxin-cyclosporin A interaction: modulation of the multidrug transporter P-glycoprotein in the kidney. *J Pharmacol Exp Ther.* 1993;266:1614-1619.
242. Greiner B, Eichelbaum M, Fritz P, et al. The role of intestinal P-glycoprotein in the interaction of digoxin and rifampin. *J Clin Invest.* 1999;104:147-153.
243. Hall WH, Shappell SD, Doherty JE. Effect of cholestyramine on digoxin absorption and excretion in man. *Am J Cardiol.* 1977;39:213-216.
244. McElnay JC, Harron DW, D'Arcy PF, et al. Interaction of digoxin with antacid constituents. *Br Med J.* 1978;1:1554.
245. Chan BS, Buckley NA. Digoxin-specific antibody fragments in the treatment of digoxin toxicity. *Clin Toxicol (Phila).* 2014;52:824-836.
246. DIGIFab.health. Digifab prescribing information. http://www.digifab.us/download/DigiFab_Package_Insert.pdf
247. Ujhelyi MR, Robert S. Pharmacokinetic aspects of digoxin-specific Fab therapy in the management of digitalis toxicity. *Clin Pharmacokinet.* 1995;28:483-493.
248. Erdman R. A. Phosphodiesterase Inhibitors. In: Dart CR, ed. *Medical Toxicology.* 3rd ed. Lippincott Williams & Wilkins; 2004:706-710.
249. Levy JH, Bailey JM. Amrinone: pharmacokinetics and pharmacodynamics. *J Cardiothorac Anesth.* 1989;3:10-14.
250. Young RA, Ward A. Milrinone. A preliminary review of its pharmacological properties and therapeutic use. *Drugs.* 1988;36:158-192.
251. Packer M, Carver JR, Rodeheffer RJ, et al. Effect of oral milrinone on mortality in severe chronic heart failure. The PROMISE Study Research Group. *N Engl J Med.* 1991;325:1468-1475.
252. Shipley JB, Tolman D, Hastillo A, et al. Milrinone: basic and clinical pharmacology and acute and chronic management. *Am J Med Sci.* 1996;311:286-291.
253. Edelson J, Stroshane R, Benziger DP, et al. Pharmacokinetics of the bipyridines amrinone and milrinone. *Circulation.* 1986;73:III145-III152.
254. Taniguchi T, Shibata K, Saito S, et al. Pharmacokinetics of milrinone in patients with congestive heart failure during continuous venovenous hemofiltration. *Intensive Care Med.* 2000;26:1089-1093.
255. Woolfrey SG, Hegbrant J, Thysell H, et al. Dose regimen adjustment for milrinone in congestive heart failure patients with moderate and severe renal failure. *J Pharm Pharmacol.* 1995;47:651-655.
256. Amsallem E, Kasparian C, Haddour G, et al. Phosphodiesterase III inhibitors for heart failure. *Cochrane Database Syst Rev.* 2005;2005:CD002230.
257. Riley CM. Stability of milrinone and digoxin, furosemide, procainamide hydrochloride, propranolol hydrochloride, quinidine gluconate, or verapamil hydrochloride in 5% dextrose injection. *Am J Hosp Pharm.* 1988;45:2079-2091.
258. Maron BA, Rocco TP. Pharmacotherapy of Congestive Heart Failure. In: Brunton LL, Chabner BA, Knollmann BC, eds. *Goodman & Gilman's: The Pharmacological Basis of Therapeutics.* 12th ed. McGraw-Hill Education; 2011.
259. MacGregor DA, Smith TE, Prielipp RC, et al. Pharmacokinetics of dopamine in healthy male subjects. *Anesthesiology.* 2000;92:338-346.
260. Meiser J, Weindl D, Hiller K. Complexity of dopamine metabolism. *Cell Commun Signal.* 2013;11:34.
261. Tuttle RR, Mills J. Dobutamine: development of a new catecholamine to selectively increase cardiac contractility. *Circ Res.* 1975;36:185-196.
262. Ruffolo RR Jr, Spradlin TA, Pollock GD, et al. Alpha and beta adrenergic effects of the stereoisomers of dobutamine. *J Pharmacol Exp Ther.* 1981;219:447-452.

263. Kang SY, Lee JW, Park DE, et al. Hypereosinophilia with rash to dobutamine infusion; sulfite hypersensitivity diagnosed by in vitro stimulation assays. *Allergol Int.* 2016;65:477-480.
264. Hilal-Dandan R, Brunton LL. Adrenergic agonists and antagonists. In: Brunton L, Parker K, Blumenthal D, Buxton I, eds. *Goodman and Gilman's Manual of Pharmacology and Therapeutics.* 2nd ed. McGraw-Hill Education; 2016.
265. Yan M, Webster LT Jr, Blumer JL. 3-O-methyldobutamine, a major metabolite of dobutamine in humans. *Drug Metab Dispos.* 2002;30:519-524.
266. Yan M, Webster LT, Jr., Blumer JL. Kinetic interactions of dopamine and dobutamine with human catechol-O-methyltransferase and monoamine oxidase in vitro. *J Pharmacol Exp Ther.* 2002;301:315-321.
267. Sonne J, Goyal A, Lopez-Ojeda W. *Dopamine*. StatPearls Publishing; 2023. Updated July 3, 2023. https://www.ncbi.nlm.nih.gov/books/NBK535451/
268. Ashkar H, Adnan G, Makaryus AN. *Dobutamine*. [Updated 2023 Jan 19]. *StatPearls Publishing*. 2023. https://www.ncbi.nlm.nih.gov/books/NBK470431/.
269. Taylor AL, Ziesche S, Yancy C, et al. Combination of isosorbide dinitrate and hydralazine in blacks with heart failure. *N Engl J Med.* 2004;351:2049-2057.
270. Reece PA. Hydralazine and related compounds: chemistry, metabolism, and mode of action. *Med Res Rev.* 1981;1:73-96.
271. Arbor Pharmaceuticals, LLC. BIDIL (isosorbide dinitrate and hydralazine hydrochloride) tablet prescribing information. https://www.accessdata.fda.gov/drugsatfda_docs/label/2015/020727s005lbl.pdf
272. Facchini V, Timbrell JA. Further evidence for an acetylator phenotype difference in the metabolism of hydralazine in man. *Br J Clin Pharmacol.* 1981;11:345-351.
273. Food and Drug Administration. https://www.accessdata.fda.gov/drugsatfda_docs/nda/2015/207620Orig1s000OtherR.pdf
274. Gu J, Noe A, Chandra P, et al. Pharmacokinetics and pharmacodynamics of LCZ696, a novel dual-acting angiotensin receptor-neprilysin inhibitor (ARNi). *J Clin Pharmacol.* 2010;50:401-414.
275. Ksander GM, Ghai RD, deJesus R, et al. Dicarboxylic acid dipeptide neutral endopeptidase inhibitors. *J Med Chem.* 1995;38:1689-1700.
276. Schiering N, D'Arcy A, Villard F, et al. Structure of neprilysin in complex with the active metabolite of sacubitril. *Sci Rep. 2016*;6:27909.
277. Flesch G, Muller P, Lloyd P. Absolute bioavailability and pharmacokinetics of valsartan, an angiotensin II receptor antagonist, in man. *Eur J Clin Pharmacol.* 1997;52:115-120.
278. Criscione L, de Gasparo M, Buhlmayer P, et al. Pharmacological profile of valsartan: a potent, orally active, nonpeptide antagonist of the angiotensin II AT1-receptor subtype. *Br J Pharmacol.* 1993;110:761-771.
279. Novartis Pharmaceuticals Corporation. Entresto (sacubitril and valsartan) prescribing information. https://www.pharma.us.novartis.com/sites/www.pharma.us.novartis.com/files/entresto.pdf
280. Feng L, Karpinski PH, Sutton P, et al. LCZ696: a dual-acting sodium supramolecular complex. *Tetrahedron Lett.* 2012; 53(3):275-276.
281. Ayalasomayajula S, Langenickel T, Pal P, et al. Clinical pharmacokinetics of sacubitril/valsartan (LCZ696): a novel angiotensin receptor-neprilysin inhibitor. *Clin Pharmacokinet.* 2017;56(12):1461-1478.
282. Kobalava Z, Kotovskaya Y, Averkov O, et al. Pharmacodynamic and pharmacokinetic profiles of sacubitril/valsartan (LCZ696) in patients with heart failure and reduced ejection fraction. *Cardiovasc Ther.* 2016;34:191-198.
283. Flarakos J, Du Y, Bedman T, et al. Disposition and metabolism of [(14)C] sacubitril/valsartan (formerly LCZ696) an angiotensin receptor neprilysin inhibitor, in healthy subjects. *Xenobiotica.* 2016;46:986-1000.
284. Shi J, Wang X, Nguyen J, et al. Sacubitril is selectively activated by carboxylesterase 1 (CES1) in the liver and the activation is affected by CES1 genetic variation. *Drug Metab Dispos.* 2016;44:554-559.
285. Xia J, Hui N, Tian L, et al. Development of vericiguat: the first soluble guanylate cyclase (sGC) stimulator launched for heart failure with reduced ejection fraction (HFrEF). *Biomed Pharmacother.* 2022;149:112894.
286. Armstrong PW, Roessig L, Patel MJ, et al. A multicenter, randomized, double-blind, placebo-controlled trial of the efficacy and safety of the oral soluble guanylate cyclase stimulator: The VICTORIA Trial. *JACC Heart Fail.* 2018;6:96-104.
287. Antzelevitch C, Burashnikov A. Overview of basic mechanisms of cardiac arrhythmia. *Card Electrophysiol Clin.* 2011;3:23-45.
288. Klabunde RE. Cardiac electrophysiology: normal and ischemic ionic currents and the ECG. *Adv Physiol Educ.* 2017;41:29-37.
289. Glitsch HG. Electrophysiology of the sodium-potassium-ATPase in cardiac cells. *Physiol Rev.* 2001;81:1791-1826.
290. Wright SH. Generation of resting membrane potential. *Adv Physiol Educ.* 2004;28:139-142.
291. Bartos DC, Grandi E, Ripplinger CM. Ion channels in the heart. *Compr Physiol.* 2015;5:1423-1464.
292. Schmitt N, Grunnet M, Olesen SP. Cardiac potassium channel subtypes: new roles in repolarization and arrhythmia. *Physiol Rev.* 2014;94:609-653.
293. King GS, McGuigan JJ. *Antiarrhythmic Medications*. StatPearls Publishing LLC; 2018.
294. Grant AO, Starmer CF, Strauss HC. Antiarrhythmic drug action. Blockade of the inward sodium current. *Circ Res.* 1984;55:427-439.
295. Sheets MF, Fozzard HA, Lipkind GM, et al. Sodium channel molecular conformations and antiarrhythmic drug affinity. *Trends Cardiovasc Med.* 2010;20:16-21.
296. Cubeddu LX. QT prolongation and fatal arrhythmias: a review of clinical implications and effects of drugs. *Am J Ther.* 2003;10:452-457.
297. Manolis AS, Deering TF, Cameron J, et al. Mexiletine: pharmacology and therapeutic use. *Clin Cardiol.* 1990;13:349-359.
298. Salvage SC, Chandrasekharan KH, Jeevaratnam K, et al. Multiple targets for flecainide action: implications for cardiac arrhythmogenesis. *Br J Pharmacol.* 2018;175(8):1260-1278.
299. Bryson HM, Palmer KJ, Langtry HD, et al. Propafenone. A reappraisal of its pharmacology, pharmacokinetics and therapeutic use in cardiac arrhythmias. *Drugs.* 1993;45:85-130.
300. Naccarelli GV, Wolbrette DL, Khan M, et al. Old and new antiarrhythmic drugs for converting and maintaining sinus rhythm in atrial fibrillation: comparative efficacy and results of trials. *Am J Cardiol.* 2003;91:15D-26D.
301. Singh BN. Antiarrhythmic actions of amiodarone: a profile of a paradoxical agent. *Am J Cardiol.* 1996;78:41-53.
302. Anderson JL, Prystowsky EN. Sotalol: an important new antiarrhythmic. *Am Heart J.* 1999;137:388-409.
303. Singh B. A fourth class of anti-dysrhythmic action? Effect of verapamil and ouabain toxicity, on atrial and ventricular intracellular potentials, and on other features of cardiac function. *Cardiovasc Res.* 2000;45:39-42.
304. Thomas SH, Behr ER. Pharmacological treatment of acquired QT prolongation and torsades de pointes. *Br J Clin Pharmacol.* 2016;81:420-427.
305. Weinreb SM. Chemistry. Synthetic lessons from quinine. *Nature.* 2001;411:429, 431.
306. Warhurst DC, Craig JC, Adagu IS, et al. The relationship of physico-chemical properties and structure to the differential antiplasmodial activity of the cinchona alkaloids. *Malar J.* 2003;2:26.
307. Bauer LA. Quinidine. In: Bauer LA, ed. *Applied Clinical Pharmacokinetics.* 3rd ed. McGraw-Hill Medical; 2015.
308. Ueda CT, Williamson BJ, Dzindzio BS. Disposition kinetics of dihydroquinidine following quinidine administration. *Res Commun Chem Pathol Pharmacol.* 1976;14:215-225.

309. Ueda CT, Williamson BJ, Dzindzio BS. Absolute quinidine bioavailability. *Clin Pharmacol Ther.* 1976;20:260-265.
310. Ochs HR, Greenblatt DJ, Woo E, et al. Reduced quinidine clearance in elderly persons. *Am J Cardiol.* 1978;42:481-485.
311. Ochs HR, Greenblatt DJ, Woo E. Clinical pharmacokinetics of quinidine. *Clin Pharmacokinet.* 1980;5:150-168.
312. Nielsen F, Nielsen KK, Brosen K. Determination of quinidine, dihydroquinidine, (3S)-3-hydroxyquinidine and quinidine N-oxide in plasma and urine by high-performance liquid chromatography. *J Chromatogr B Biomed Appl.* 1994;660:103-110.
313. Mihaly GW, Ching MS, Klejn MB, et al. Differences in the binding of quinine and quinidine to plasma proteins. *Br J Clin Pharmacol.* 1987;24:769-774.
314. Ueda CT, Dzindzio BS. Quinidine kinetics in congestive heart failure. *Clin Pharmacol Ther.* 1978;23:158-164.
315. McLaughlin LA, Paine MJ, Kemp CA, et al. Why is quinidine an inhibitor of cytochrome P450 2D6? The role of key active-site residues in quinidine binding. *J Biol Chem.* 2005;280:38617-38624.
316. Roden DM, Thompson KA, Hoffman BF, et al. Clinical features and basic mechanisms of quinidine-induced arrhythmias. *J Am Coll Cardiol.* 1986;8:73A-78A.
317. Tartini R, Kappenberger L, Steinbrunn W, et al. Dangerous interaction between amiodarone and quinidine. *Lancet.* 1982;1:1327-1329.
318. Cohen IS, Jick H, Cohen SI. Adverse reactions to quinidine in hospitalized patients: findings based on data from the Boston Collaborative Drug Surveillance Program. *Prog Cardiovasc Dis.* 1977;20:151-163.
319. Sneader W. *Drug Discovery: A History.* John Wiley and Sons, Ltd.; 2005.
320. Karlsson E. Clinical pharmacokinetics of procainamide. *Clin Pharmacokinet.* 1978;3:97-107.
321. Giardina EG. Procainamide: clinical pharmacology and efficacy against ventricular arrhythmias. *Ann N Y Acad Sci.* 1984;432:177-188.
322. Woosley RL, Drayer DE, Reidenberg MM, et al. Effect of acetylator phenotype on the rate at which procainamide induces antinuclear antibodies and the lupus syndrome. *N Engl J Med.* 1978;298:1157-1159.
323. Uetrecht JP, Sweetman BJ, Woosley RL, et al. Metabolism of procainamide to a hydroxylamine by rat and human hepatic microsomes. *Drug Metab Dispos.* 1984;12:77-81.
324. Lessard E, Fortin A, Belanger PM, et al. Role of CYP2D6 in the N-hydroxylation of procainamide. *Pharmacogenetics.* 1997;7:381-390.
325. Bauer LA. Procainamide/N-acetyl procainamide. In: Bauer LA, ed. *Applied Clinical Pharmacokinetics.* 3rd ed. McGraw-Hill Medical; 2015.
326. Drayer DE, Lowenthal DT, Woosley RL, et al. Cumulation of N-acetylprocainamide, an active metabolite of procainamide, in patients with impaired renal function. *Clin Pharmacol Ther.* 1977;22:63-69.
327. Bauer LA, Black DJ, Lill JS, et al. Levofloxacin and ciprofloxacin decrease procainamide and N-acetylprocainamide renal clearances. *Antimicrob Agents Chemother.* 2005;49:1649-1651.
328. Bauer LA, Black D, Gensler A. Procainamide-cimetidine drug interaction in elderly male patients. *J Am Geriatr Soc.* 1990;38:467-469.
329. Lawson DH, Jick H. Adverse reactions to procainamide. *Br J Clin Pharmacol.* 1977;4:507-511.
330. Davies RF, Siddoway LA, Shaw L, et al. Immediate- versus controlled-release disopyramide: importance of saturable binding. *Clin Pharmacol Ther.* 1993;54:16-22.
331. Lima JJ, Haughey DB, Leier CV. Disopyramide pharmacokinetics and bioavailability following the simultaneous administration of disopyramide and 14C-disopyramide. *J Pharmacokinet Biopharm.* 1984;12:289-313.
332. Siddoway LA, Woosley RL. Clinical pharmacokinetics of disopyramide. *Clin Pharmacokinet.* 1986;11:214-222.
333. Lima JJ, Boudoulas H, Shields BJ. Stereoselective pharmacokinetics of disopyramide enantiomers in man. *Drug Metab Dispos.* 1985;13:572-577.
334. Lima JJ, Boudoulas H, Blanford M. Concentration-dependence of disopyramide binding to plasma protein and its influence on kinetics and dynamics. *J Pharmacol Exp Ther.* 1981;219:741-747.
335. Bredesen JE, Kierulf P. Relationship between alpha 1-acid glycoprotein and plasma binding of disopyramide and mono-N-dealkyldisopyramide. *Br J Clin Pharmacol.* 1984;18:779-784.
336. Echizen H, Tanizaki M, Tatsuno J, et al. Identification of CYP3A4 as the enzyme involved in the mono-N-dealkylation of disopyramide enantiomers in humans. *Drug Metab Dispos.* 2000;28:937-944.
337. Aitio ML. Plasma concentrations and protein binding of disopyramide and mono-N-dealkyldisopyramide during chronic oral disopyramide therapy. *Br J Clin Pharmacol.* 1981;11:369-375.
338. Granowitz EV, Tabor KJ, Kirchhoffer JB. Potentially fatal interaction between azithromycin and disopyramide. *Pacing Clin Electrophysiol.* 2000;23:1433-1435.
339. Hayashi Y, Ikeda U, Hashimoto T, et al. Torsades de pointes ventricular tachycardia induced by clarithromycin and disopyramide in the presence of hypokalemia. *Pacing Clin Electrophysiol.* 1999;22:672-674.
340. Teichman S. The anticholinergic side effects of disopyramide and controlled-release disopyramide. *Angiology.* 1985;36:767-771.
341. Di Bianco R, Gottdiener JS, Singh SN, et al. A review of the effects of disopyramide phosphate on left ventricular function and the peripheral circulation. *Angiology.* 1987;38:174-183.
342. Collinsworth KA, Kalman SM, Harrison DC. The clinical pharmacology of lidocaine as an antiarrhythymic drug. *Circulation.* 1974;50:1217-1230.
343. Boyes RN, Scott DB, Jebson PJ, et al. Pharmacokinetics of lidocaine in man. *Clin Pharmacol Ther.* 1971;12:105-116.
344. Routledge PA, Barchowsky A, Bjornsson TD, et al. Lidocaine plasma protein binding. *Clin Pharmacol Ther.* 1980;27:347-351.
345. Abernethy DR, Greenblatt DJ. Lidocaine disposition in obesity. *Am J Cardiol.* 1984;53:1183-1186.
346. Wang JS, Backman JT, Taavitsainen P, et al. Involvement of CYP1A2 and CYP3A4 in lidocaine N-deethylation and 3-hydroxylation in humans. *Drug Metab Dispos.* 2000;28:959-965.
347. Nation RL, Triggs EJ, Selig M. Lignocaine kinetics in cardiac patients and aged subjects. *Br J Clin Pharmacol.* 1977;4:439-448.
348. Thomson PD, Melmon KL, Richardson JA, et al. Lidocaine pharmacokinetics in advanced heart failure, liver disease, and renal failure in humans. *Ann Intern Med.* 1973;78:499-508.
349. Bauer LA. Lidocaine. In: Bauer LA, ed. *Applied Clinical Pharmacokinetics.* 2nd ed. McGraw-Hill; 2008.
350. Orlando R, Piccoli P, De Martin S, et al. Cytochrome P450 1A2 is a major determinant of lidocaine metabolism in vivo: effects of liver function. *Clin Pharmacol Ther.* 2004;75:80-88.
351. Orlando R, Piccoli P, De Martin S, et al. Effect of the CYP3A4 inhibitor erythromycin on the pharmacokinetics of lignocaine and its pharmacologically active metabolites in subjects with normal and impaired liver function. *Br J Clin Pharmacol.* 2003;55:86-93.
352. Ha HR, Candinas R, Stieger B, et al. Interaction between amiodarone and lidocaine. *J Cardiovasc Pharmacol.* 1996;28:533-539.
353. Knapp AB, Maguire W, Keren G, et al. The cimetidine-lidocaine interaction. *Ann Intern Med.* 1983;98:174-177.
354. Labbe L, Turgeon J. Clinical pharmacokinetics of mexiletine. *Clin Pharmacokinet.* 1999;37:361-384.
355. Turgeon J, Fiset C, Giguere R, et al. Influence of debrisoquine phenotype and of quinidine on mexiletine disposition in man. *J Pharmacol Exp Ther.* 1991;259:789-798.
356. Fenster PE, Comess KA. Pharmacology and clinical use of mexiletine. *Pharmacotherapy.* 1986;6:1-9.
357. Johnston A, Burgess CD, Warrington SJ, et al. The effect of spontaneous changes in urinary pH on mexiletine plasma concentrations and excretion during chronic administration to healthy volunteers. *Br J Clin Pharmacol.* 1979;8:349-352.

358. Wing LM, Meffin PJ, Grygiel JJ, et al. The effect of metoclopramide and atropine on the absorption of orally administered mexiletine. *Br J Clin Pharmacol.* 1980;9:505-509.
359. Herzog P, Holtermuller KH, Kasper W, et al. Absorption of mexiletine after treatment with gastric antacids. *Br J Clin Pharmacol.* 1982;14:746-747.
360. Ueno K, Miyai K, Seki T, et al. Interaction between theophylline and mexiletine. *DICP.* 1990;24:471-472.
361. Klein A, Sami M, Selinger K. Mexiletine kinetics in healthy subjects taking cimetidine. *Clin Pharmacol Ther.* 1985;37:669-673.
362. Broly F, Vandamme N, Caron J, et al. Single-dose quinidine treatment inhibits mexiletine oxidation in extensive metabolizers of debrisoquine. *Life Sci.* 1991;48:PL123-PL128.
363. Anderson RJ. The little compound that could: how phenytoin changed drug discovery and development. *Mol Interv.* 2009;9:208-214.
364. Richens A. Clinical pharmacokinetics of phenytoin. *Clin Pharmacokinet.* 1979;4:153-169.
365. Eddy JD, Singh SP. Treatment of cardiac arrhythmias with phenytoin. *Br Med J.* 1969;4:270-273.
366. Vanholder R, Van Landschoot N, De Smet R, et al. Drug protein binding in chronic renal failure: evaluation of nine drugs. *Kidney Int.* 1988;33:996-1004.
367. Perucca E, Hebdige S, Frigo GM, et al. Interaction between phenytoin and valproic acid: plasma protein binding and metabolic effects. *Clin Pharmacol Ther.* 1980;28:779-789.
368. Cuttle L, Munns AJ, Hogg NA, et al. Phenytoin metabolism by human cytochrome P450: involvement of P450 3A and 2C forms in secondary metabolism and drug-protein adduct formation. *Drug Metab Dispos.* 2000;28:945-950.
369. Aronson JK, Hardman M, Reynolds DJ. ABC of monitoring drug therapy. Phenytoin. *BMJ.* 1992;305:1215-1218.
370. Food and Drug Administration. Dilantin. https://www.accessdata.fda.gov/drugsatfda_docs/label/2009/084349s060lbl.pdf
371. Desta Z, Zhao X, Shin JG, et al. Clinical significance of the cytochrome P450 2C19 genetic polymorphism. *Clin Pharmacokinet.* 2002;41:913-958.
372. Franco V, Perucca E. CYP2C9 polymorphisms and phenytoin metabolism: implications for adverse effects. *Expert Opin Drug Metab Toxicol.* 2015;11:1269-1279.
373. Aliot E, Capucci A, Crijns HJ, et al. Twenty-five years in the making: flecainide is safe and effective for the management of atrial fibrillation. *Europace.* 2011;13:161-173.
374. Tjandra-Maga TB, Verbesselt R, Van Hecken A, et al. Flecainide: single and multiple oral dose kinetics, absolute bioavailability and effect of food and antacid in man. *Br J Clin Pharmacol.* 1986;22:309-316.
375. Conard GJ, Ober RE. Metabolism of flecainide. *Am J Cardiol.* 1984;53:41B-51B.
376. McQuinn RL, Quarfoth GJ, Johnson JD, et al. Biotransformation and elimination of 14C-flecainide acetate in humans. *Drug Metab Dispos.* 1984;12:414-420.
377. Doki K, Homma M, Kuga K, et al. Effect of CYP2D6 genotype on flecainide pharmacokinetics in Japanese patients with supraventricular tachyarrhythmia. *Eur J Clin Pharmacol.* 2006;62:919-926.
378. Lewis GP, Holtzman JL. Interaction of flecainide with digoxin and propranolol. *Am J Cardiol.* 1984;53:52B-57B.
379. Hii JT, Duff HJ, Burgess ED. Clinical pharmacokinetics of propafenone. *Clin Pharmacokinet.* 1991;21:1-10.
380. Stoschitzky K, Klein W, Stark G, et al. Different stereoselective effects of (*R*)- and (*S*)-propafenone: clinical pharmacologic, electrophysiologic, and radioligand binding studies. *Clin Pharmacol Ther.* 1990;47:740-746.
381. Axelson JE, Chan GL, Kirsten EB, et al. Food increases the bioavailability of propafenone. *Br J Clin Pharmacol.* 1987;23:735-741.
382. Hollmann M, Brode E, Hotz D, et al. Investigations on the pharmacokinetics of propafenone in man. *Arzneimittelforschung.* 1983; 33: 763–770.
383. Oravcova J, Lindner W, Szalay P, et al. Interaction of propafenone enantiomers with human alpha 1-acid glycoprotein. *Chirality.* 1991;3:30-34.
384. Funck-Brentano C, Kroemer HK, Lee JT, et al. Propafenone. *N Engl J Med.* 1990;322:518-525.
385. Brode E, Muller-Peltzer H, Hollmann M. Comparative pharmacokinetics and clinical pharmacology of propafenone enantiomers after oral administration to man. *Methods Find Exp Clin Pharmacol.* 1988;10:717-727.
386. Cai WM, Chen B, Cai MH, et al. The influence of CYP2D6 activity on the kinetics of propafenone enantiomers in Chinese subjects. *Br J Clin Pharmacol.* 1999;47:553-556.
387. Jazwinska-Tarnawska E, Orzechowska-Juzwenko K, Niewinski P, et al. The influence of CYP2D6 polymorphism on the antiarrhythmic efficacy of propafenone in patients with paroxysmal atrial fibrillation during 3 months propafenone prophylactic treatment. *Int J Clin Pharmacol Ther.* 2001;39:288-292.
388. Thompson KA, Iansmith DH, Siddoway LA, et al. Potent electrophysiologic effects of the major metabolites of propafenone in canine Purkinje fibers. *J Pharmacol Exp Ther.* 1988;244:950-955.
389. Lee JT, Kroemer HK, Silberstein DJ, et al. The role of genetically determined polymorphic drug metabolism in the beta-blockade produced by propafenone. *N Engl J Med.* 1990;322:1764-1768.
390. Kroemer HK, Mikus G, Kronbach T, et al. In vitro characterization of the human cytochrome P-450 involved in polymorphic oxidation of propafenone. *Clin Pharmacol Ther.* 1989;45:28-33.
391. Fromm MF, Botsch S, Heinkele G, et al. Influence of renal function on the steady-state pharmacokinetics of the antiarrhythmic propafenone and its phase I and phase II metabolites. *Eur J Clin Pharmacol.* 1995;48:279-283.
392. Connolly SJ, Kates RE, Lebsack CS, et al. Clinical pharmacology of propafenone. *Circulation.* 1983;68:589-596.
393. Siddoway LA, Thompson KA, McAllister CB, et al. Polymorphism of propafenone metabolism and disposition in man: clinical and pharmacokinetic consequences. *Circulation.* 1987;75:785-791.
394. Kroemer HK, Funck-Brentano C, Silberstein DJ, et al. Stereoselective disposition and pharmacologic activity of propafenone enantiomers. *Circulation.* 1989;79:1068-1076.
395. Calvo MV, Martin-Suarez A, Martin Luengo C, et al. Interaction between digoxin and propafenone. *Ther Drug Monit.* 1989;11:10-15.
396. Kates RE, Yee YG, Kirsten EB. Interaction between warfarin and propafenone in healthy volunteer subjects. *Clin Pharmacol Ther.* 1987;42:305-311.
397. Wagner F, Kalusche D, Trenk D, et al. Drug interaction between propafenone and metoprolol. *Br J Clin Pharmacol.* 1987;24:213-220.
398. Funck-Brentano C, Kroemer HK, Pavlou H, et al. Genetically-determined interaction between propafenone and low dose quinidine: role of active metabolites in modulating net drug effect. *Br J Clin Pharmacol.* 1989;27:435-444.
399. Ravid S, Podrid PJ, Novrit B. Safety of long-term propafenone therapy for cardiac arrhythmia—experience with 774 patients. *J Electrophysiol.* 1987;1:580-590.
400. Reynolds RD, Gorczynski RJ, Quon CY. Pharmacology and pharmacokinetics of esmolol. *J Clin Pharmacol.* 1986; 26(S1): A3-A14.
401. Wiest D. Esmolol. A review of its therapeutic efficacy and pharmacokinetic characteristics. *Clin Pharmacokinet.* 1995;28:190-202.
402. Turlapaty P, Laddu A, Murthy VS, et al. Esmolol: a titratable short-acting intravenous beta blocker for acute critical care settings. *Am Heart J.* 1987;114:866-885.
403. Lish PM, Weikel JH, Dungan KW. Pharmacological and toxicological properties of two new beta-adrenergic receptor antagonists. *J Pharmacol Exp Ther.* 1965;149:161-173.
404. Funck-Brentano C. Pharmacokinetic and pharmacodynamic profiles of d-sotalol and d,l-sotalol. *Eur Heart J.* 1993; 14 Suppl H: 30–35.

405. Hanyok JJ. Clinical pharmacokinetics of sotalol. *Am J Cardiol.* 1993;72:19A-26A.
406. Yamreudeewong W, DeBisschop M, Martin LG, et al. Potentially significant drug interactions of class III antiarrhythmic drugs. *Drug Saf.* 2003;26:421-438.
407. Laer S, Neumann J, Scholz H. Interaction between sotalol and an antacid preparation. *Br J Clin Pharmacol.* 1997;43:269-272.
408. McKibbin JK, Pocock WA, Barlow JB, et al. Sotalol, hypokalaemia, syncope, and torsades de pointes. *Br Heart J* 1984;51:157-162.
409. Singh S, Saini RK, DiMarco J, et al. Efficacy and safety of sotalol in digitalized patients with chronic atrial fibrillation. The Sotalol Study Group. *Am J Cardiol.* 1991;68:1227-1230.
410. Latini R, Tognoni G, Kates RE. Clinical pharmacokinetics of amiodarone. *Clin Pharmacokinet.* 1984;9:136-156.
411. Bonati M, Gaspari F, D'Aranno V, et al. Physicochemical and analytical characteristics of amiodarone. *J Pharm Sci.* 1984;73:829-831.
412. Singh BN. Amiodarone: the expanding antiarrhythmic role and how to follow a patient on chronic therapy. *Clin Cardiol.* 1997;20:608-618.
413. Trivier JM, Libersa C, Belloc C, et al. Amiodarone N-deethylation in human liver microsomes: involvement of cytochrome P450 3A enzymes (first report). *Life Sci.* 1993;52:PL91-PL96.
414. Ohyama K, Nakajima M, Suzuki M, et al. Inhibitory effects of amiodarone and its N-deethylated metabolite on human cytochrome P450 activities: prediction of in vivo drug interactions. *Br J Clin Pharmacol.* 2000;49:244-253.
415. Nitsch J, Luderitz B. [Acceleration of amiodarone elimination by cholestyramine]. *Dtsch Med Wochenschr.* 1986;111:1241-1244.
416. Wagner JA, Weisman HF, Levine JH, et al. Differential effects of amiodarone and desethylamiodarone on calcium antagonist receptors. *J Cardiovasc Pharmacol.* 1990;15:501-507.
417. Lee TH, Friedman PL, Goldman L, et al. Sinus arrest and hypotension with combined amiodarone-diltiazem therapy. *Am Heart J.* 1985;109:163-164.
418. Nicolau DP, Uber WE, Crumbley AJ 3rd, et al. Amiodarone-cyclosporine interaction in a heart transplant patient. *J Heart Lung Transplant.* 1992;11:564-568.
419. Harris L, McKenna WJ, Rowland E, et al. Side effects and possible contraindications of amiodarone use. *Am Heart J.* 1983;106:916-923.
420. Greene HL, Graham EL, Werner JA, et al. Toxic and therapeutic effects of amiodarone in the treatment of cardiac arrhythmias. *J Am Coll Cardiol.* 1983;2:1114-1128.
421. Baroletti S, Catella J, Ehle M, et al. Dronedarone: a review of characteristics and clinical data. *Crit Pathw Cardiol.* 2010;9:94-101.
422. Garcia D, Cheng-Lai A. Dronedarone: a new antiarrhythmic agent for the treatment of atrial fibrillation. *Cardiol Rev.* 2009;17:230-234.
423. Patel C, Yan GX, Kowey PR. Dronedarone. *Circulation.* 2009;120:636-644.
424. Dorian P. Clinical pharmacology of dronedarone: implications for the therapy of atrial fibrillation. *J Cardiovasc Pharmacol Ther.* 2010;15:15S-18S.
425. Hohnloser SH, Crijns HJ, van Eickels M, et al. Effect of dronedarone on cardiovascular events in atrial fibrillation. *N Engl J Med.* 2009;360:668-678.
426. Murray KT. Ibutilide. *Circulation.* 1998;97:493-497.
427. Pharmacia and Upjohn Company LLC. Corvert (ibutilide fumarate injection) prescribing information. http://labeling.pfizer.com/showlabeling.aspx?format=PDF&id=673
428. Vos MA, Golitsyn SR, Stangl K, et al. Superiority of ibutilide (a new class III agent) over DL-sotalol in converting atrial flutter and atrial fibrillation. The Ibutilide/Sotalol Comparator Study Group. *Heart.* 1998;79:568-575.
429. Cropp JS, Antal EG, Talbert RL. Ibutilide: a new class III antiarrhythmic agent. *Pharmacotherapy.* 1997;17:1-9.
430. Stambler BS, Wood MA, Ellenbogen KA, et al. Efficacy and safety of repeated intravenous doses of ibutilide for rapid conversion of atrial flutter or fibrillation. Ibutilide Repeat Dose Study Investigators. *Circulation.* 1996;94:1613-1621.
431. Gwilt M, Arrowsmith JE, Blackburn KJ, et al. UK-68,798: a novel, potent and highly selective class III antiarrhythmic agent which blocks potassium channels in cardiac cells. *J Pharmacol Exp Ther.* 1991;256:318-324.
432. Le Coz F, Funck-Brentano C, Morell T, et al. Pharmacokinetic and pharmacodynamic modeling of the effects of oral and intravenous administrations of dofetilide on ventricular repolarization. *Clin Pharmacol Ther.* 1995;57:533-542.
433. Allen MJ, Nichols DJ, Oliver SD. The pharmacokinetics and pharmacodynamics of oral dofetilide after twice daily and three times daily dosing. *Br J Clin Pharmacol.* 2000;50:247-253.
434. Walker DK, Alabaster CT, Congrave GS, et al. Significance of metabolism in the disposition and action of the antidysrhythmic drug, dofetilide. In vitro studies and correlation with in vivo data. *Drug Metab Dispos.* 1996;24:447-455.
435. Pfizer Inc. Tikosyn (dofetilide capsule) prescribing information. http://labeling.pfizer.com/ShowLabeling.aspx?id=639, http://labeling.pfizer.com/ShowLabeling.aspx?format=PDF&id=639
436. Torp-Pedersen C, Brendorp B, Kober L. Dofetilide: a class III anti-arrhythmic drug for the treatment of atrial fibrillation. *Expert Opin Investig Drugs.* 2000;9:2695-2704.
437. Wilbur SL, Marchlinski FE. Adenosine as an antiarrhythmic agent. *Am J Cardiol.* 1997;79:30-37.
438. Stafford A. Potentiation of adenosine and the adenine nucleotides by dipyridamole. *Br J Pharmacol Chemother.* 1966;28:218-227.
439. Biaggioni I, Paul S, Puckett A, et al. Caffeine and theophylline as adenosine receptor antagonists in humans. *J Pharmacol Exp Ther.* 1991;258:588-593.
440. Bertolet BD, Belardinelli L, Avasarala K, et al. Differential antagonism of cardiac actions of adenosine by theophylline. *Cardiovasc Res.* 1996;32:839-845.
441. Brugada P. Magnesium: an antiarrhythmic drug, but only against very specific arrhythmias. *Eur Heart J.* 2000;21:1116.

Structure Challenge Answers

1-E, 2-A, 3-C, 4-B, 5-D

CHAPTER

21

Drugs Used to Treat Thrombotic Disorders

Kimberly Beck

Drugs covered in this chapter:

ANTIPLATELET DRUGS

CYCLOOXYGENASE INHIBITOR
- Aspirin

$P2Y_{12}$-RECEPTOR ANTAGONISTS

THIENOPYRIDINES
- Clopidogrel
- Prasugrel

NUCLEOTIDE/NUCLEOSIDE ANALOGS
- Cangrelor
- Ticagrelor

THROMBIN PROTEASE–ACTIVATED RECEPTOR-1 ANTAGONIST
- Vorapaxar

GPIIB/IIIA INHIBITORS
- Eptifibatide
- Tirofiban

PHOSPHODIESTERASE 3 INHIBITOR
- Cilostazol

ANTICOAGULANTS

HEPARINS
- Dalteparin
- Enoxaparin
- Unfractionated heparin

ANTIDOTE TO HEPARIN TOXICITY
- Protamine sulfate

FACTOR XA INHIBITORS

INDIRECT FACTOR XA INHIBITOR
- Fondaparinux

DIRECT FACTOR XA INHIBITORS
- Apixaban
- Edoxaban
- Rivaroxaban

REVERSAL AGENT FOR RIVAROXABAN AND APIXABAN
- Andexanet alfa

DIRECT THROMBIN INHIBITORS
- Argatroban
- Bivalirudin
- Dabigatran etexilate

DABIGATRAN-REVERSAL AGENT
- Idarucizumab

VITAMIN K ANTAGONIST
- Warfarin

ANTIDOTE TO VITAMIN K–ANTAGONIST TOXICITY
- Vitamin K

ANTITHROMBOTIC/PROFIBRINOLYTIC OLIGONUCLEOTIDE
- Defibrotide

FIBRINOLYTIC DRUGS
- Alteplase
- Reteplase
- Tenecteplase

THROMBOPOIETIN-RECEPTOR AGONISTS
- Avatrombopag
- Eltrombopag
- Lusutrombopag
- Romiplostim

SPLEEN TYROSINE-KINASE INHIBITOR
- Fostamatinib

FIBRINOLYSIS INHIBITORS
- ε-Aminocaproic acid
- Tranexamic acid

Abbreviations

AA arachidonic acid
ACS acute coronary syndrome
ACT activated clotting time
ADP adenosine diphosphate
AF atrial fibrillation
AIS acute ischemic stroke
AMI acute myocardial infarction
APC activated protein C
aPTT activated partial thromboplastin time
ASA acetylsalicylic acid
ASCVD atherosclerotic cardiovascular disease
ATIII antithrombin III
ATP adenosine triphosphate
BCR B-cell receptor
BCRP breast cancer–resistance protein
CAD coronary artery disease
cAMP cyclic adenosine monophosphate
CLD chronic liver disease
COX cyclooxygenase
CPIC the Clinical Pharmacogenetics Implementation Consortium
CrCl creatinine clearance
DALY disability-adjusted life-year
DAPT dual antiplatelet therapy
DNA deoxyribonucleic acid

Abbreviations—continued

DOAC direct oral anticoagulant
DVT deep vein thrombosis
EACA ε-aminocaproic acid
FcγR Fc gamma receptors
FDA US Food and Drug Administration
GBD Global Burden of Disease
GI gastrointestinal
GPIIb/IIIa glycoprotein IIb/IIIa
hCE human carboxylesterase
HIT heparin-induced thrombocytopenia
HITT heparin-induced thrombocytopenia with thrombosis
HSCT hematopoietic stem-cell transplantation
IHD ischemic heart disease
INR international normalized ratio
ITP immune thrombocytopenia
IV intravenous
K kringle
LBSs lysine-binding sites
LDL low-density lipoproteins
LMWH low-molecular-weight heparin
M-CSF macrophage colony-stimulating factor
MACE major adverse cardiovascular events
MI myocardial infarction
MIDAS metal ion–dependent adhesion site
Mpl myeloproliferative leukemia virus receptors
MW molecular weight
MWavg average molecular weight
NET neutrophil extracellular trap
NO nitric oxide
NSAIDs nonsteroidal anti-inflammatory drugs
NSTE-ACS non-ST-elevation acute coronary syndromes
PAN plasminogen-apple-nematode
4PCC 4 factor prothrombin complex combination
P-gp P-glycoprotein
PAD peripheral artery disease
PAI-1 plasminogen activator inhibitor-1
PAR-1 protease-activated receptor-1
PCI percutaneous coronary intervention
PDE3 phosphodiesterase 3
PE pulmonary embolism
PF4 platelet factor 4
PGH_2 prostaglandin H_2
PGI_2 prostaglandin I_2, prostacyclin
PLATO Platelet Inhibition and Patient Outcomes
PPI proton-pump inhibitor
PT prothrombin time
RBCs red blood cells
RNA ribonucleic acid
SC subcutaneous
STEMI ST-elevation myocardial infarction
Syk spleen tyrosine kinase
TF tissue factor
TFPI tissue factor pathway inhibitor
TM transmembrane helices
TNK tenecteplase
tPA tissue plasminogen activator
TPO thrombopoietin
TPO-R thrombopoietin receptors
TPO-RA thrombopoietin receptor agonist
TXA tranexamic acid
TXA_2 thromboxane A_2
UA unstable angina
US United States
UFH unfractionated heparin
ULMWH ultra-low-molecular-weight heparin
USP United States Pharmacopeia
USPSTF US Preventive Services Task Force
V_d volume of distribution
VEGFR vascular endothelial growth factor
VKA vitamin K antagonist
VKOR vitamin K epoxide reductase
VOD/SOS veno-occlusive disease/sinusoidal obstruction syndrome
VTE venous thromboembolism
vWF von Willebrand factor
WAC wholesale acquisition cost

CLINICAL SIGNIFICANCE

As a clinician, it is often important to think about the chemistry of a drug when applying its use to specific patient situations. In the case of anticoagulation, this can be of utmost importance. When a patient is actively bleeding or at risk of bleeding due to an upcoming surgical procedure, clinicians must be able to accurately assess many variables relating to the drug's action to make an appropriate clinical plan. Does the drug have reversible or irreversible binding? How can the drug be monitored? Is there a reversal agent for the anticoagulant, and what is its mechanism? When could we expect to see efficacy when initiating a reversal agent? What is the half-life of the drug; how long will it be in the patient's system? These can help make a clinical plan for how long we may need to hold an anticoagulant dose or when we may be able to expect a change in bleeding.

In the clinical setting related to anticoagulation, the relationship between medicinal chemistry and clinical outcomes is also important in tailoring patient dose monitoring. Certain patients may respond differently to anticoagulants based on specific characteristics, and better knowledge of the activity of the drug may help guide usage in special populations. How is the drug metabolized? Will hepatic dysfunction, renal dysfunction, or drug-drug interactions affect drug action? Clinicians must have a thorough understanding of the medicinal chemistry, as well as the clinical outcomes of a drug, in order to make the best decisions for patients.

Lauren Czosnowski, PharmD, BCPS

Thrombosis is the inappropriate formation of blood clots and can occur anywhere in the body in both the arterial system and the venous system. A thrombus may partially or completely occlude blood flow in the affected vessel, ultimately leading to organ damage. A fragment(s) may dislodge from the original clot, forming an embolus, which travels and impedes blood flow in another vessel. Thrombosis is a component of multiple disease states. Disease states involving thrombus formation include many of the manifestations of atherosclerotic cardiovascular disease (ASCVD). Within ASCVD, thrombosis is a characteristic of acute coronary syndromes (ACS), such as type 1 myocardial infarction (MI) or unstable angina (UA), peripheral artery disease (PAD),[1] and acute ischemic stroke (AIS). Causes of AIS include thrombosis of an atherosclerotic lesion in a cerebral artery, cardioembolism due to atrial fibrillation (AF),[2] valvular disease or heart failure, and paradoxical embolism. Venous thromboembolism (VTE) includes deep vein thrombosis (DVT) and its sequelae pulmonary embolism (PE).[3,4] An increased risk of VTE is associated with multiple disease states, including cancer,[5] hospitalization for acute illness, including infection with COVID-19,[6-9] lower limb orthopedic surgery, pregnancy,[10] and patients with factor V Leiden mutation.

Epidemiology and Economic Impact of Thrombotic Diseases

Disorders involving thrombosis are associated with high morbidity and mortality. The number of patients worldwide affected by disease states involving thrombosis is enormous. The Global Burden of Disease (GBD) Study 2019 showed that ischemic heart disease (IHD) and stroke were the leading contributors to disease burden, ranking first and second, respectively, in the 50- to 74-year and the 75-years-and-older age groups, as measured in disability-adjusted life-years (DALYs).[11] DALYs combine the years of health lost due to the disability of the disease and the years of life prematurely lost due to the disease.[12] One DALY is the loss of 1 year of full health. IHD in the GBD 2019 study included MI and UA, and stable angina. The total number of DALYs caused by IHD globally in 2019 was 182 million. IHD caused 9.14 million deaths worldwide in 2019 with a prevalence of 197 million cases.[11,13] IHD is the leading cause of death in the United States, causing 558,100 deaths in 2019.[14] Stroke in the GBD 2019 study included ischemic stroke, intracerebral hemorrhage, and subarachnoid hemorrhage. Isolating ischemic stroke only, ischemic stroke was the cause of 63.5 million DALYs, 3.29 million deaths, and had a prevalence of 77.2 million cases globally in 2019.[11] Data from the GBD Study 2020 show the global prevalence of ischemic stroke to be 68.16 million cases.[14] In the United States, of all strokes, 87% are estimated to be ischemic strokes, whereas globally ischemic strokes represent 62.4% of all new strokes in 2019.[14] Ischemic stroke caused 109,000 deaths in the United States in 2019.[14]

In 2019, there was an estimated 643,000 cases of DVT and 393,000 cases of PE, for a total of 1,036,000 cases of VTE in the United States.[14] Globally, in 2019, the prevalence of PAD was 113 million cases causing 74,100 deaths.[11,13] The above numbers represent only a portion of all disease states in which thrombosis plays a role. This demonstrates that many people worldwide are affected by thrombosis.

Healthcare costs for treatment of diseases associated with thrombosis are expensive. An analysis of 154 health conditions in the United States found that IHD was the fourth highest in health care spending in 2016, at an estimated $89.3 billion.[15] It was estimated that the majority, 56.9%, of health care spending for IHD was for patients aged 65 years and older, although a significant portion, 42.7%, is estimated for patients 20 to 64 years old.

In a Medicare fee-for-service population in the United States, the median episode cost for ischemic stroke was found to be $9,973 in 2019.[16] Treatment with endovascular thrombectomy was associated with $24,631 in higher cost, and intravenous (IV) thrombolysis was associated with an increased cost of $5,474, although most patients in this population received neither therapy.[16]

In the United States, based on an estimate of 375,000 to 425,000 new cases of VTE each year, the annual health care costs associated with VTE are estimated to be $7 billion to $10 billion.[17] Treatment of acute VTE is associated with $12,000 to $15,000 (in 2014) per case among first-year survivors. Additional costs of $18,000 to $23,000 are estimated for subsequent complications, including adverse drug events from anticoagulation therapy. An analysis of a nationwide US population-based database found the median costs per admission for PAD to be over $15,000, and annual healthcare costs associated with PAD hospitalization are estimated to exceed $6 billion annually.[18]

Physiology of Hemostasis

Hemostasis is the cessation of bleeding at a site of injury. There are three steps in hemostasis: (1) vasoconstriction at the site of injury to impede blood loss, (2) formation of a platelet plug (primary hemostasis), and (3) coagulation (secondary hemostasis). In primary hemostasis, platelets bind to collagen exposed in the subendothelial layer of damaged endothelium via the plasma protein von Willebrand factor (vWF) and glycoprotein Ib receptors located on both platelets and collagen. Additionally, platelets bind to subendothelial collagen via platelet glycoprotein VI. Upon adhesion to the site of endothelial damage, platelets undergo activation. Platelet activation induces the release of platelet granular contents, including adenosine diphosphate (ADP), Ca^{2+}, serotonin, thromboxane A_2 (TXA_2), coagulation factors V and VIII, and polyphosphate.[19] Platelet activation also causes characteristic shape changes. Both granular content secretion and shape change lead to platelet aggregation, in which platelets are recruited to the site of injury and adhere to each other, forming a platelet plug that stops bleeding at the site of vascular injury. In addition, activated platelets provide a surface for coagulation factor activation.

Secondary hemostasis involves the activation of the coagulation cascade (Fig. 21.1). The coagulation cascade is composed of coagulation factors, which are proteins synthesized in the liver and circulate in the plasma in their

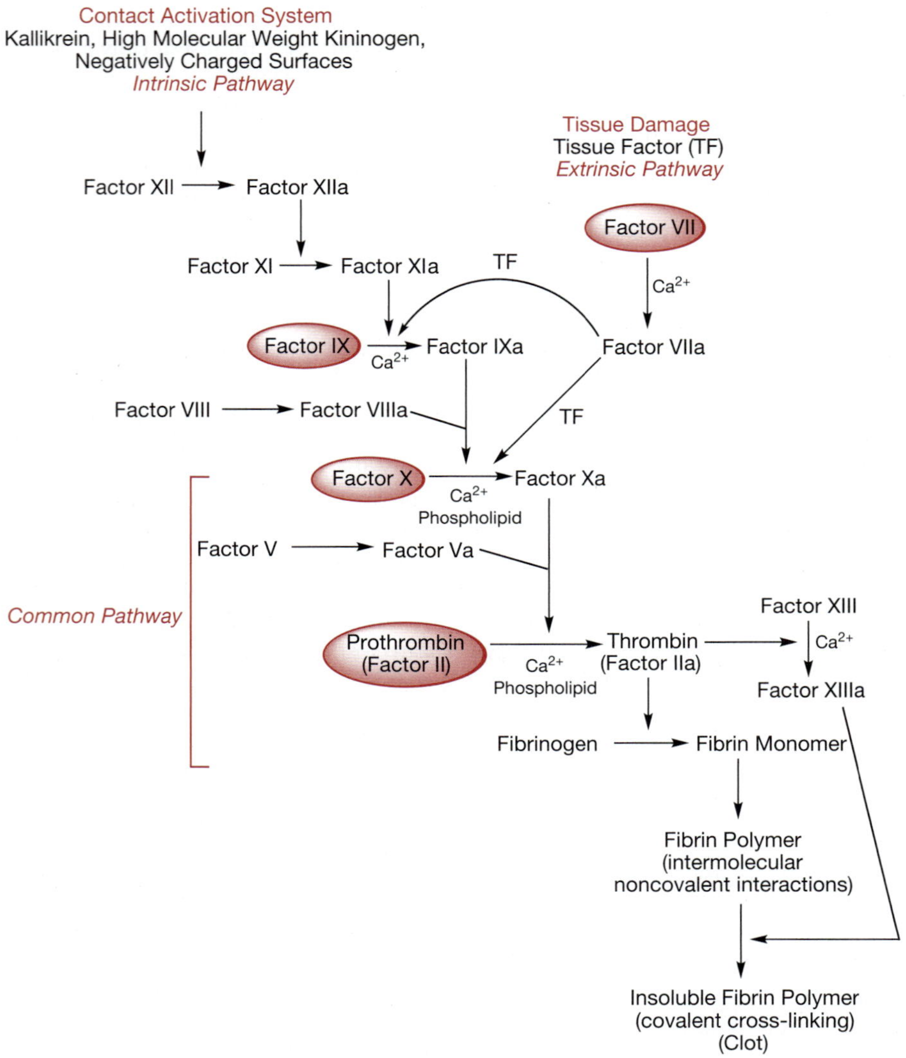

Figure 21.1 Coagulation cascade. Coagulation factors highlighted in red ovals are vitamin K–dependent. TF, tissue factor.

inactive precursor form (zymogen). Historically divided into the intrinsic pathway, extrinsic pathway, and the common pathway, the coagulation cascade involves the sequential proteolytic activation of coagulation factors, which catalyze subsequent coagulation factor activation in the cascade. In hemostasis, the coagulation cascade is triggered via the extrinsic pathway when tissue factor (TF), exposed at the site of vascular injury, binds and activates factor VII to form factor VIIa, or binds to circulating factor VIIa. The TF–factor VIIa complex activates factor IX from the intrinsic pathway and factor X of the common pathway. The intrinsic pathway begins by triggering the activation of factor XII and also leads to activation of factor X via the formation of the tenase complex, which includes factor IXa and factor VIIIa. Within the common pathway, the prothrombinase complex, including factors Va and Xa, activates prothrombin to thrombin (factor IIa). Thrombin catalyzes the conversion of fibrinogen to fibrin monomers and activates the transglutaminase factor XIIIa. Factor XIIIa catalyzes the formation of the crosslinked insoluble fibrin mesh, which traps red blood cells (RBCs) and platelets. This is the blood clot. Furthermore, thrombin amplifies platelet aggregation and the activation of factors V, VII, VIIII, and XI of the coagulation cascade.

Hemostasis is tightly regulated, and even as the blood clot forms, substances are secreted to limit clot growth and digest existing clot, as shown in Figure 21.2. Prostacyclin (PGI_2) and nitric oxide (NO) are secreted by endothelial cells, causing inhibition of platelet aggregation and vasodilation. Vasodilation increases blood flow and permits dilution of coagulation factors. Natural anticoagulants protein C and protein S are vitamin K–dependent glycoproteins synthesized in the liver.[20-23] Proteolytic cleavage of protein C by the thrombin-thrombomodulin complex bound to endothelial cells forms the serine protease activated protein C (APC). Protein S is a cofactor to APC, and together, they inactivate factor Va and factor VIIIa. By degrading factors Va and VIIIa, APC/protein S decreases thrombin generation. Tissue factor pathway inhibitors (TFPIs), another type of anticoagulation proteins, exist as two isoforms: TFPIα and TFPIβ.[24] TFPIα circulates in the plasma and is released from activated platelets. TFPIα binds to protein S to elicit its anticoagulant activity.[23,24] TFPIβ is anchored to the surface

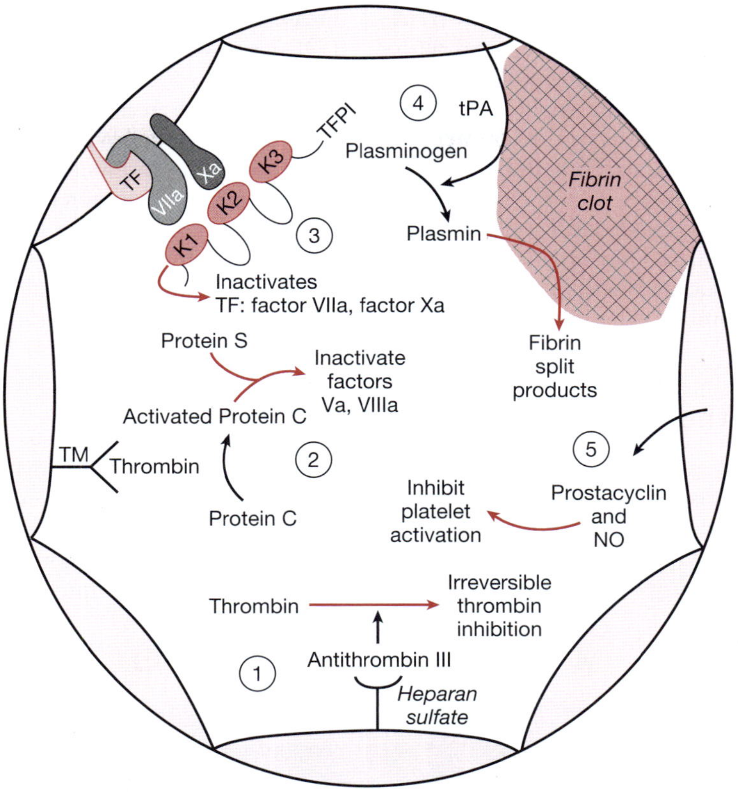

Figure 21.2 Endogenous protective mechanisms against thrombosis and vessel occlusion. (1) Inactivation of thrombin by antithrombin III (ATIII), the effectiveness that is enhanced by binding of ATIII to heparan sulfate. (2) Inactivation of clotting factors Va and VIIIa by activated protein C, an action that is enhanced by protein S. Protein C is activated by the thrombomodulin (TM)-thrombin complex. (3) Inactivation of tissue factor (TF):factor VIIa complex and factor Xa by tissue factor pathway inhibitor (TFPI). TFPI binds to factors VIIa and Xa at Kringle 1 (K1) and Kringle 2 (K2), respectively. TFPIα binds to protein S at Kringle 3 (K3). (4) Lysis of fibrin clots by tissue plasminogen activator (tPA). (5) Inhibition of platelet activation by prostacyclin (prostaglandin I_2, [PGI_2]) and nitric oxide (NO). (Modified from Berg DD, Sabatine MS, Lilly LS. Acute coronary syndromes. In: Lilly LS, ed. *Pathophysiology of Heart Disease: An Introduction to Cardiovascular Medicine.* 7th ed. Wolters-Kluwer; 2021:174, with permission.)

of endothelial cells and monocytes.[24] TFPIs inhibit the TF-factor VIIa complex and factor Xa. Antithrombin III (ATIII) is a serine protease inhibitor that circulates in the plasma and is capable of inactivating most of the coagulation factors, predominantly thrombin and factor Xa.[25] The activity of ATIII is increased by the binding of heparan sulfate present on the endothelial surface. Tissue plasminogen activator (tPA), secreted by the endothelium, catalyzes the proteolytic cleavage of plasminogen to plasmin. Plasmin causes fibrinolysis by cleaving fibrin into fibrin degradation products.

Pathophysiology of Thrombus Formation

Unlike hemostasis, where the goal is to stop bleeding at a site of damaged endothelium yet allow unperturbed blood flow through the vessel, thrombosis impedes or occludes blood flow through the vessel. Whereas the extrinsic pathway is the main driver of secondary hemostasis, the intrinsic pathway plays an important role in thrombus formation.[26-30] The three conditions predisposing a patient to thromboembolism are abnormal blood flow due to turbulence or stasis, hypercoagulability, and vascular endothelial dysfunction. Collectively, these three factors are known as the Virchow triad. Venous thrombi frequently form in the valve pockets of large veins in the lower limbs, with the veins of the calf being the most common site of DVT.[3,4] The valve pockets of deep veins are sites of blood stasis.[3,4] Blood stasis causes endothelial dysfunction and triggers the expression of surface adhesion molecules, including P-selectin and vWF, on endothelial cells creating a prothrombotic state.[3,4,31] Upon binding to the vascular endothelium, recruited platelets, leukocytes, and microparticles are activated. Platelet activation leads leukocytes, mostly neutrophils, to release neutrophil extracellular traps (NETs).[3,4,31] Via activation of factor XII and TF, NETs stimulate both the intrinsic and extrinsic pathway. Activated microparticles, along with monocytes recruited to the site of endothelial dysfunction, express TF. Collectively, platelet aggregation and coagulation ensue, creating a hypercoagulable state. DVT from the calf can propagate to behind the knee in the popliteal vein and in the thigh in the femoral vein.[4] When the DVT is more proximal, pieces of the thrombus are more likely to break off and travel to the pulmonary arteries, causing PE. PE is associated with a high risk of mortality.

Although originally proposed for VTE, the Virchow triad may also be applied to thromboembolism associated with AF. AF is associated with a high risk of thromboembolism and, ultimately, to ischemic stroke. The inefficient atrial contraction in AF results in blood stasis in the left atrium, causing thrombus formation, particularly in the left atrial appendage. In addition to blood stasis, endothelial damage to the atrial wall, inflammatory processes, and abnormalities in platelet function, coagulation, and fibrinolysis contribute to the prothrombotic state associated with AF.[32] An embolus from an AF-induced thrombus can travel to the brain and cause an ischemic stroke.

Pathophysiology of Atherothrombosis

Atherothrombosis of a coronary artery is the primary contributor to IHD. Coronary artery disease (CAD) is used to describe a syndrome in which atherosclerotic plaque builds up within the walls of coronary arteries. As shown in Figure 21.3, atherosclerotic plaque formation is a progressive chronic inflammatory disease. It begins with the diffusion of low-density lipoproteins (LDLs) into vessel walls in areas of intimal thickening where proteoglycan is found in the extracellular matrix.[33] LDLs are retained in these areas due to ionic bonding between negatively charged sugar groups in proteoglycan and a cluster of positively charged arginine and lysine residues on the apolipoprotein B (apoB) portion of lipoproteins.[33] Proteoglycan-bound LDLs in the intima are more prone to oxidation, and oxidized LDLs trigger an inflammatory response.[33]

Inflammation of the endothelial lining of the cardiac vessel lumen causes increased permeability. Typically, the endothelial cells of an arterial vessel do not interact with leukocytes. The inflammatory response, however, activates endothelial cells to express leukocyte adhesion molecules, chemoattractant cytokines (chemokines), and macrophage colony-stimulating factor (M-CSF).[34-37] The chemokines secreted by the activated endothelial cells attract mostly monocytes, which adhere to the adhesion molecules now expressed on the endothelial luminal surface. This allows these leukocytes to migrate into the intimal layer of a coronary

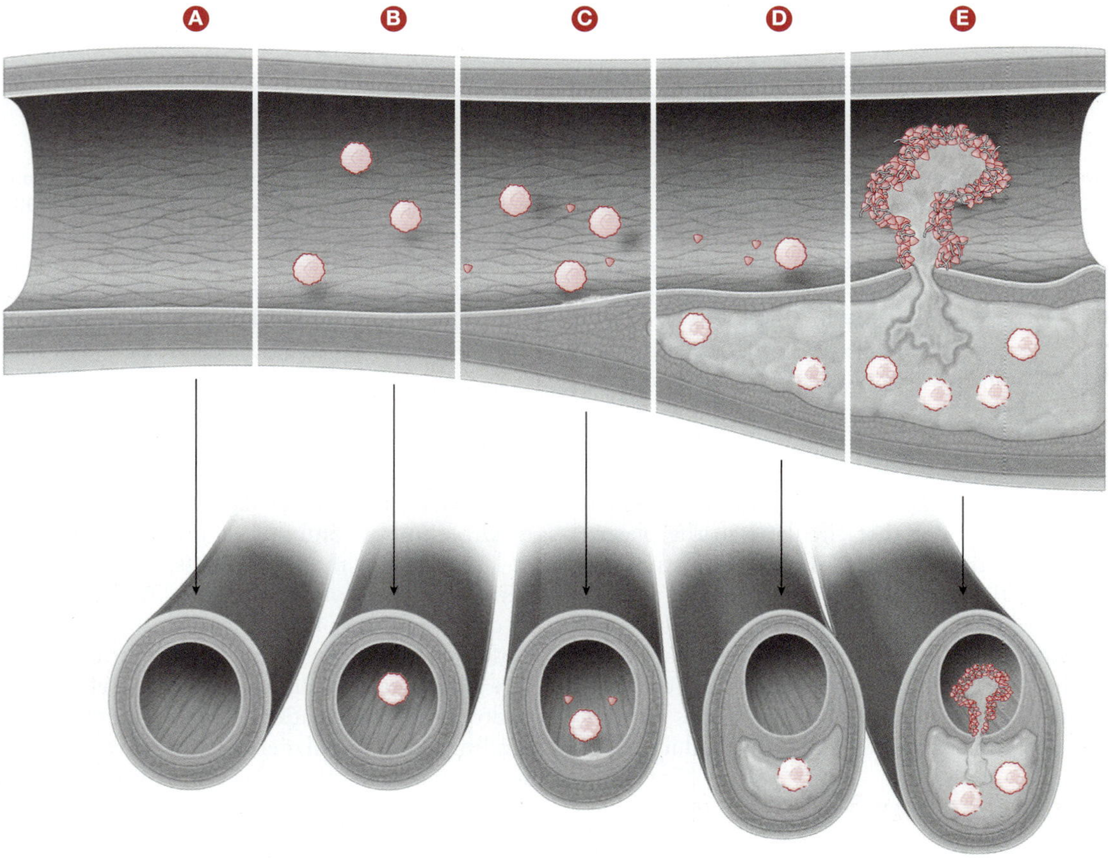

Figure 21.3 Pathogenesis of atherosclerosis in a coronary artery. A. A normal coronary artery has an intact endothelium surrounded by smooth muscle cells. B. Endothelial cell activation or injury recruit monocytes and T lymphocytes to the site of injury, leading to development of a fatty streak. C. Continued oxidative stress within a fatty streak leads to development of an atherosclerotic plaque. D. Macrophage apoptosis and continued cholesterol deposition cause further plaque organization and may induce the expression of additional inflammatory proteins and matrix metalloproteinases. At this stage, the cap of the fibroatheroma remains intact. E. Continued inflammation within an atherosclerotic plaque leads to thinning of the fibrous cap and, eventually, to plaque rupture or erosion. Exposure of plaque constituents to the bloodstream activates platelets and the coagulation cascade, with resulting coronary artery occlusion. (From McCabe JM, Armstrong EJ. Integrative cardiovascular pharmacology: hypertension, ischemic heart disease, and heart failure. In: Golan DE, Armstrong EJ, Armstrong AW, eds. *Principles of Pharmacology: The Pathophysiologic Basis of Drug Therapy*. 4th ed. Wolters Kluwer; 2017:482, with permission.)

artery, triggering the immune response. Once in the intima, monocytes differentiate into macrophages and proliferate under the influence of M-CSF. Some of these macrophages exhibit a proinflammatory phenotype and secrete proinflammatory/proatherogenic cytokines, such as interleukin 1β (IL-1β), IL-1β–induced IL-6, and IL-18.[38-41] Macrophages, within the intima, engulf lipids and change into foam cells. These lipid-filled foam cells cause fatty streaks within the lumen of a coronary artery, the first visible sign of atherosclerosis. Cholesterol continues to build up at the site of the atherosclerotic plaque, forming a lipid core. A detailed discussion regarding the role of lipids in the formation of atherosclerotic plaques can be found in Chapter 18.

Cytokines and growth factors produced by foam cells, activated platelets, and endothelial cells within the atherosclerotic plaque stimulate vascular smooth muscle cells from the media of the vessel wall to infiltrate the atherosclerotic plaque and proliferate. These smooth muscle cells produce collagen, elastin, and proteoglycans to form an extracellular matrix that gives structural integrity to the growing plaque and forms a collagen-rich fibrous cap over the surface that contains the atherosclerotic plaque.[35]

The accumulating macrophages and foam cells within the lipid core undergo apoptosis (cell death), and typically the resultant debris is cleared by phagocytes in a process called efferocytosis. In an advancing atherosclerotic plaque, efferocytosis is impaired such that the lipid core evolves into a necrotic core due to the necrosis of the sequestered apoptotic foam cells and smooth muscle cells.[35,38] Proinflammatory macrophages and foam cells within the lipid rich necrotic core secrete matrix metalloproteinases and other proteolytic enzymes that degrade collagen fibrils and other structures, which thins the fibrous cap.[41-43] Thin cap fibroatheromas are vulnerable atherosclerotic plaques prone to rupture.[41,43] Upon rupture, thrombogenic mediators within the necrotic core, such as TF, come in contact with the bloodstream and may trigger the formation of a thrombus that partially or completely occludes a coronary artery. Approximately 60% of coronary atherothrombosis is due to plaque rupture, leading to MI and cardiac death.[43,44] Plaque erosion, wherein the fibrous cap remains intact and thrombus formation is the result of endothelial damage exposing subendothelium to the blood, is the cause of approximately one-third of coronary thrombus formation.[41,43,44]

Coronary thrombosis due to plaque erosion is proposed to begin with disturbed blood flow at the site of the atherosclerotic plaque. As a result, endothelial cells are dislodged from the lumen of the coronary artery, triggering platelet and neutrophil activation. Neutrophil activation leads to NET formation, releasing a host of chemical mediators, including TF, which activates coagulation. NETs are also capable of entrapping platelets and fibrin. Ultimately, a platelet-rich thrombus is formed over the atherosclerotic lesion in the coronary artery. A summary of the mechanisms leading to thrombus formation in coronary arteries is shown in Figure 21.4. Figure 21.5 summarizes the consequences of coronary thrombosis.

Thrombosis Associated With Peripheral Artery Disease and Ischemic Stroke

Whereas atherothrombosis is a key component of the majority of IHD events, it is unclear that it is the primary contributor to thrombosis in PAD.[1,45] In a pathologic

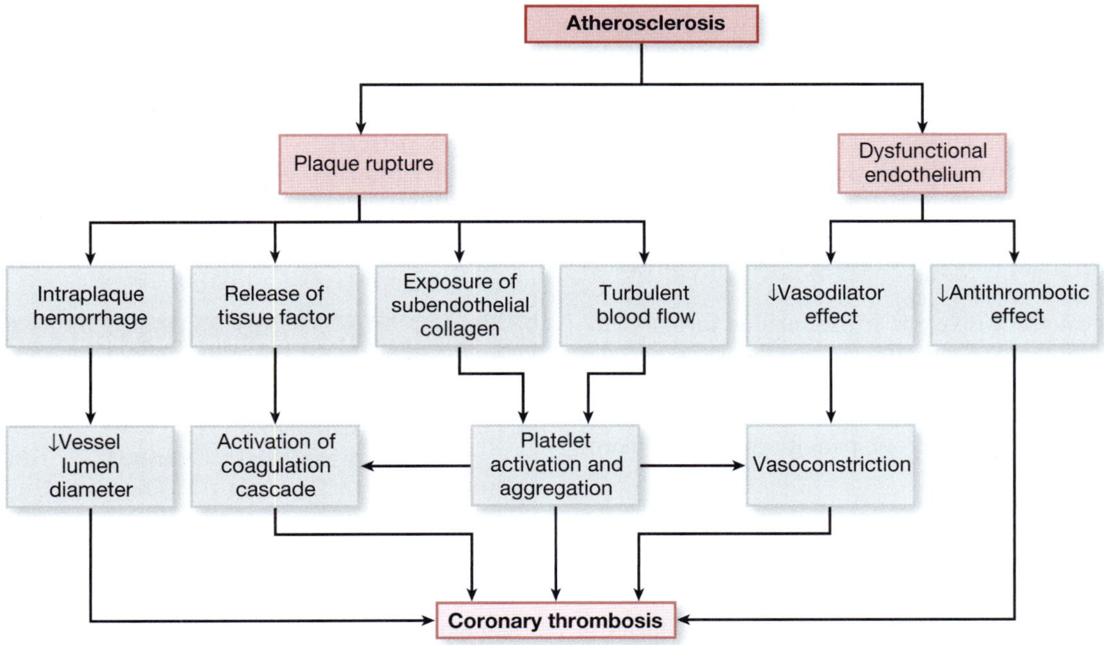

Figure 21.4 Mechanisms of coronary thrombus formation. Factors that contribute to this process include plaque disruption (eg, rupture or erosion) and inappropriate vasoconstriction and loss of normal antithrombotic defenses because of dysfunctional endothelium. (From Berg DD, Sabatine MS, Lilly LS. Acute coronary syndromes. In: Lilly LS, ed. *Pathophysiology of Heart Disease: An Introduction to Cardiovascular Medicine*. 7th ed. Wolters-Kluwer; 2021:175, with permission.)

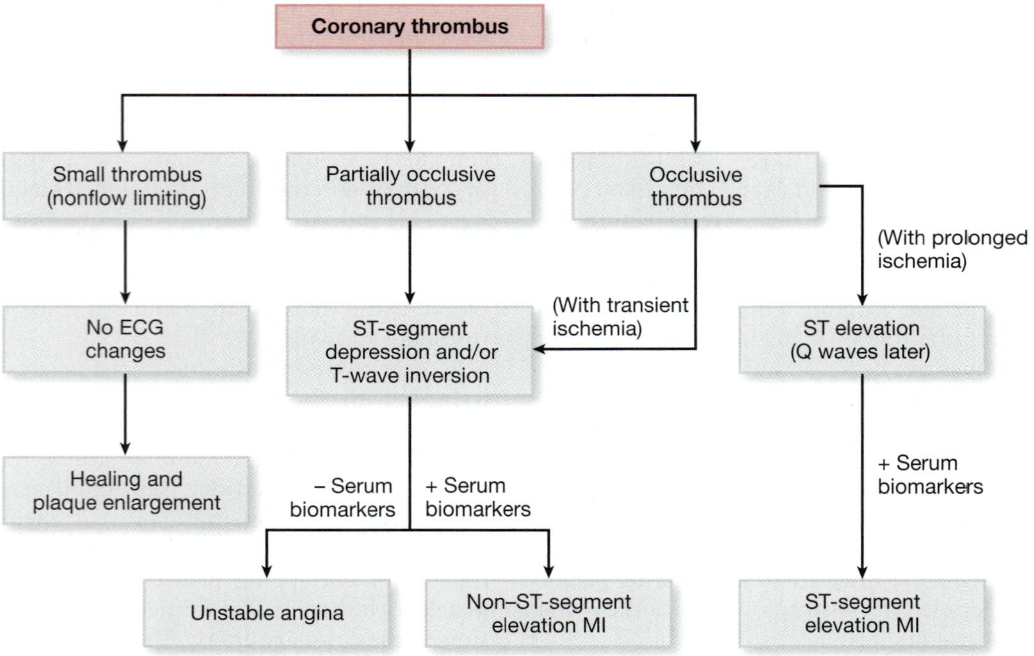

Figure 21.5 Consequences of coronary thrombosis. A small thrombus formed on superficial plaque rupture may not result in symptoms or electrocardiogram (ECG) abnormalities, but healing and fibrous organization may incorporate the thrombus into the plaque, causing the atherosclerotic lesion to enlarge. A partially occlusive thrombus narrows the arterial lumen, restricts blood flow, and can cause unstable angina or a non–ST-elevation MI, either of which may result in ST-segment depression and/or T-wave inversion on the ECG. A totally occlusive thrombus with prolonged ischemia is the most common cause of ST-elevation MI, in which the ECG initially shows ST-segment elevation, followed by Q-wave development if early reperfusion is not achieved. An occlusive thrombus that recanalizes, or one that develops in a region served by adequate collateral blood flow, may result in less prolonged ischemia and a non–ST-elevation MI instead. Serum biomarkers of myocardial necrosis include cardiac-specific troponins I and T. MI, myocardial infarction. (From Berg DD, Sabatine MS, Lilly LS. Acute coronary syndromes. In: Lilly LS, ed. *Pathophysiology of Heart Disease: An Introduction to Cardiovascular Medicine.* 7th ed. Wolters-Kluwer; 2021:177, with permission.)

analysis of PAD in 75 patients with above the knee or below the knee amputations due to critical limb ischemia, only a third of stenotic arteries associated with thrombi was linked to atherosclerosis.[46] Thrombotic luminal occlusion of the other two-thirds of lower limb vessels was associated with insignificant atherosclerosis. This suggests that mechanisms of thromboembolism other than atherosclerotic plaque rupture/erosion play a significant role in PAD.

Common causes of ischemic stroke include thromboembolism from large vessel atherosclerotic disease, especially in the internal carotid arteries, and cardioembolism due to AF.[47] One type of cerebral small vessel disease is thromboembolism from an atherosclerotic parent artery. This manifests as a lacunar stroke.

Composition of Thrombi

Venous thrombi are referred to as "red clots" as they are rich in RBCs. Consequently, as fragments of a deep vein thrombus, pulmonary emboli are also rich in RBCs. Arterial thrombi are referred to as "white clots," as they are rich in platelets. A study of arterial and venous thrombi and pulmonary emboli supports these generalizations (Table 21.1).[48] This is in contrast to the composition of stroke thrombi. Histologic analysis of 177 thrombi, retrieved by thrombectomy, from patients with AIS revealed that cerebral thrombi exhibit a typical heterogeneous pattern.[49] Ischemic stroke thrombi are composed of RBC-rich/platelet-poor areas and RBC-poor/platelet-rich areas. The composition of the thrombi can inform the appropriate antithrombotic medication therapy.

Table 21.1 Composition of Arterial and Venous Thrombi and Pulmonary Emboli

Component	Coronary Arterial Thrombi	Venous Thrombi	Pulmonary Emboli
Fibrin	43.3	35.0	41.2
Platelets	31.3	0.4	0.8
Red Blood Cells	17.1	63.4	48.6

Average volume fraction (%) of the overall thrombus composition.
Modified from Chernysh IN, Nagaswami C, Kosolapova S, et al. The distinctive structure and composition of arterial and venous thrombi and pulmonary emboli. *Sci Rep.* 2020;10:5112.

Antiplatelet Drugs

Platelet activation and aggregation are core components of coronary artery plaque formation and occlusion. Antiplatelet therapy is a cornerstone of the treatment of patients with ACS because it improves outcomes. Currently, aspirin and $P2Y_{12}$-receptor antagonists are the most frequently used antiplatelet agents in patients with ACS. Although used for decades, glycoprotein IIb/IIIa inhibitors are now used less frequently due to improved efficacy of the $P2Y_{12}$-receptor antagonists; however, they still have their role in certain scenarios. PAR-1 antagonism is another mechanism to achieve antiplatelet activity as seen with vorapaxar. Antiplatelet drugs are also used in the treatment of PAD and to prevent MI and stroke in patients at risk. All antiplatelet drugs are associated with a risk of bleeding, which needs to be considered when prescribed for patients.

Cyclooxygenase Inhibitor

Aspirin

An immediate loading dose (162-325 mg) of non–enteric-coated chewable aspirin (acetylsalicylic acid [ASA]) is first-line therapy for patients with non-ST-elevation acute coronary syndrome (NSTE-ACS).[50] Subsequently, a maintenance dose of aspirin (81-162 mg/d) is recommended indefinitely, for patients without contraindications because it decreases the incidence of death, recurrent MI, and stroke in patients with NSTE-ACS. In a recent study, there was no significant difference in efficacy between 81 mg of aspirin daily and 325 mg in the secondary prevention of cardiovascular events.[51] Aspirin administration is recommended within 24 to 48 hours after onset of AIS.[52]

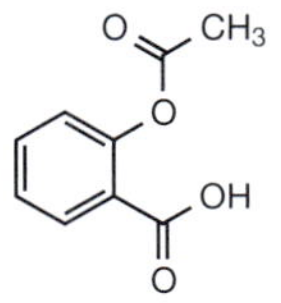

Aspirin
(Acetylsalicylic acid, ASA)

Mechanism of Antiplatelet Activity. Platelet aggregation plays a key role in the pathogenesis of atherosclerotic plaque and coronary artery thrombosis. Aspirin has antiplatelet activity by selectively and irreversibly inhibiting cyclooxygenase-1 (COX-1) at low doses (81-162 mg/d). The antiplatelet effect of aspirin occurs at doses that are more than 10- to 50-fold lower than doses required for analgesic, antipyretic, or anti-inflammatory activity.[53]

In platelets, COX-1 converts arachidonic acid (AA) to prostaglandin H_2 (PGH_2), which is further converted to TXA_2, a potent stimulator of platelet aggregation and inducer of vasoconstriction (Fig. 21.6). The mechanism by which TXA_2 causes platelet aggregation involves binding to discrete G protein–coupled TXA_2 receptors on the surface of platelets and is illustrated in Figure 21.7. Ultimately, the action of TXA_2 results in the activation of glycoprotein IIb/IIIa (GPIIb/IIIa) receptors on the surface of activated

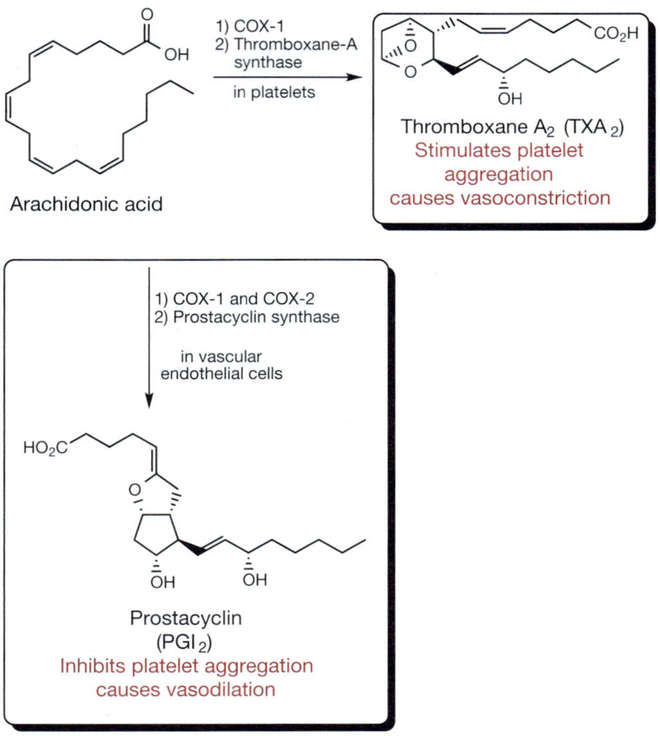

Figure 21.6 Biosynthesis of thromboxane A_2 and prostacyclin from arachidonic acid. Thromboxane A_2 and prostacyclin are synthesized predominately in platelets and vascular endothelium, respectively.

platelets. Each end of fibrinogen binds to GPIIb/IIIa receptors on neighboring platelets, linking platelets together and thereby causing platelet aggregation.

The active site of the COX enzymes is composed of a long hydrophobic channel that accommodates AA for the ultimate conversion to PGH_2.[54] The substrate binding site within the hydrophobic channel anchors AA in place via an ionic bond between the carboxylate of AA and the guanidinium side chain of Arg120. This ionic bond is reinforced with an electrostatic interaction between the same carboxylate and Tyr355. (The amino acid sequence numbering of COX enzymes typically refers to the ovine sequence.) Aspirin takes advantage of Arg120 and Tyr355 and binds in a similar manner as AA. This situates the acetyl group in close proximity to a serine residue at position 529 in human COX-1 (Fig. 21.8).[54] Tyr385 forms a hydrogen bond to the carbonyl oxygen of the acetyl group on aspirin. It is suggested that Tyr385 stabilizes the resultant tetrahedral intermediate formed in the process of acetylating the serine hydroxyl at position 529.[55] By hydrogen bonding to the phenolic hydroxyl of Tyr385, Tyr348 increases the hydrogen bonding capacity of Tyr385 to the acetyl group on aspirin.[55] The formation of the acetylated serine hydroxyl at position 529 of human COX-1 (serine 516 in human COX-2) irreversibly inhibits the enzyme. This serine residue is not critical for the catalytic function of COX-1. Instead, the acetylated serine residue sterically impedes the entrance of AA to its binding site on the COX enzyme, thereby inhibiting the conversion of AA to PGH_2 and ultimately prostaglandins and TXA_2.[56]

Mature platelets contain only COX-1, and as platelets are fragments of megakaryocytes and lack a nucleus, they

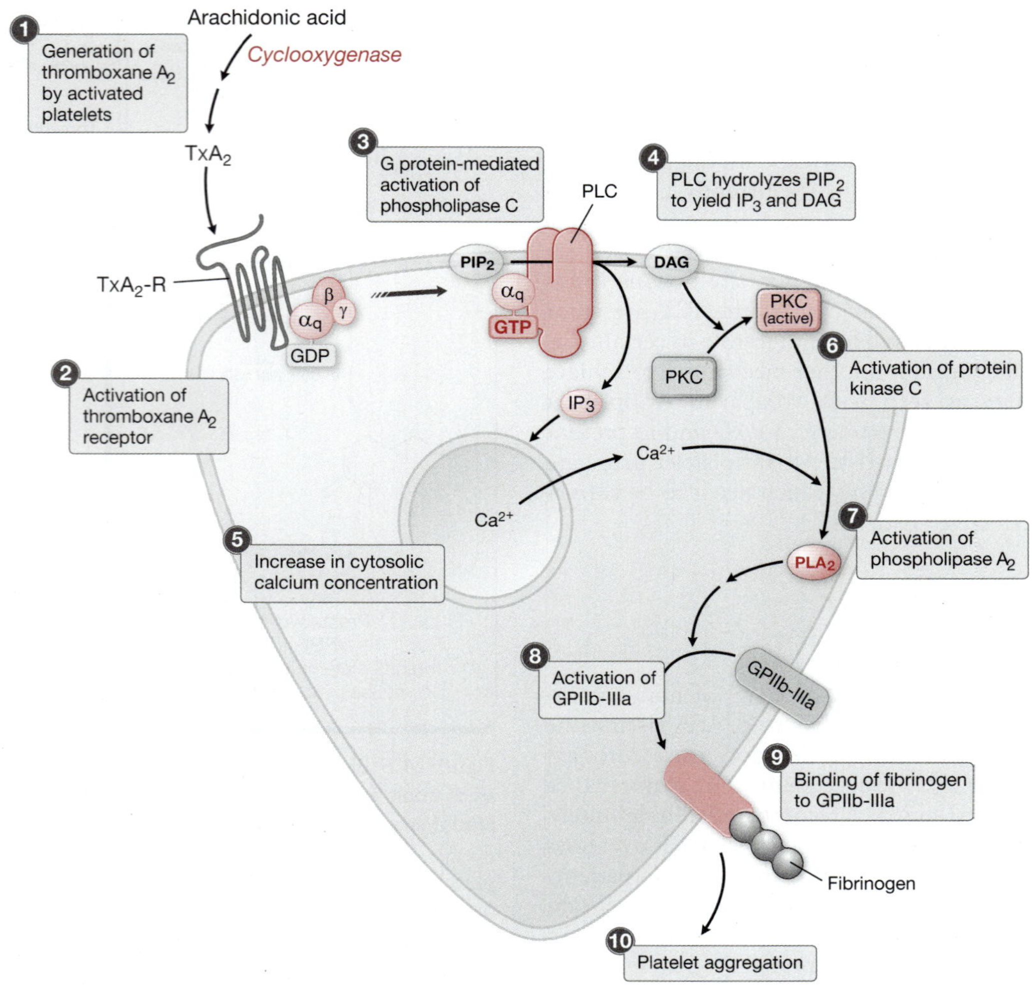

Figure 21.7 Platelet activation by thromboxane A_2. **1.** Thromboxane A_2 (TxA_2) is generated from arachidonic acid in activated platelets; cyclooxygenase catalyzes the committed step in this process. **2.** Secreted TxA_2 binds to the cell surface TxA_2 receptor (TxA_2-R), a G protein–coupled receptor. **3.** The Gα isoform of Gαq activates phospholipase C (PLC). **4.** PLC hydrolyzes phosphatidylinositol 4,5-biphosphate (PIP_2) to yield inositol 1,4,5-trisphosphate (IP_3) and diacylglycerol (DAG). **5.** IP_3 increases the cytosolic Ca^{2+} concentration by promoting vesicular release of Ca^{2+} into the cytosol. **6.** DAG activates protein kinase C (PKC). **7.** PKC activates phospholipase A_2 (PLA_2). **8.** Through an incompletely understood mechanism, activation of PLA_2 leads to the activation of glycoprotein (GP) IIb-IIIa. **9.** Activated GPIIb-IIIa binds to fibrinogen. **10.** Fibrinogen cross-links platelets by binding to GPIIb-IIIa receptors on other platelets. This cross-linking leads to platelet aggregation and formation of a primary hemostatic plug. GDP, guanosine diphosphate; GTP, guanosine triphosphate. (From Armstrong EJ, Golan DE. Pharmacology of hemostasis and thrombosis. In: Golan DE, Armstrong EJ, Armstrong AW, eds. *Principles of Pharmacology: The Pathophysiologic Basis of Drug Therapy*. 4th ed. Wolters-Kluwer; 2017:407, with permission.)

are unable to synthesize additional COX-1. Consequently, when platelet COX-1 is irreversibly inhibited by aspirin, TXA_2 synthesis is inhibited for the life of the platelet (8-10 days). In contrast, both COX-1 and COX-2 are present in vascular endothelial cells, where PGI_2 is ultimately synthesized from AA predominantly by COX-2. PGI_2 causes vasodilation and inhibits platelet aggregation. Aspirin is 10 to 100 times more potent at inhibiting COX-1 than COX-2, and at low doses of aspirin, COX-2 remains functional.[54,57] Furthermore, vascular endothelial cells are capable of synthesizing COX-2. Therefore, with low-dose aspirin therapy, while TXA_2 activity is inhibited, PGI_2 activity remains such that the overall balance is an antiplatelet effect (Table 21.2).

Pharmacokinetics. Aspirin is absorbed in the stomach and the small intestine. It is hydrolyzed via esterases in the gastrointestinal (GI) mucosa, liver, and plasma to salicylic acid. Lacking the critical acetyl group, salicylic acid does not have antiplatelet activity.

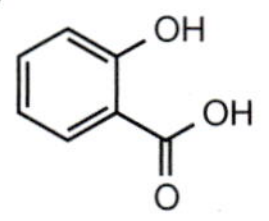

Salicylic acid

Evidence suggests that most of the COX-1 inhibition by aspirin occurs in platelets in the portal system (the presystemic circulation) before aspirin is deacetylated in the liver and before it gets into the systemic circulation.[58] Conversely, inhibition of PGI_2 formation in vascular endothelial cells occurs by aspirin in the systemic circulation.[58] The oral bioavailability of regular immediate release aspirin tablets is

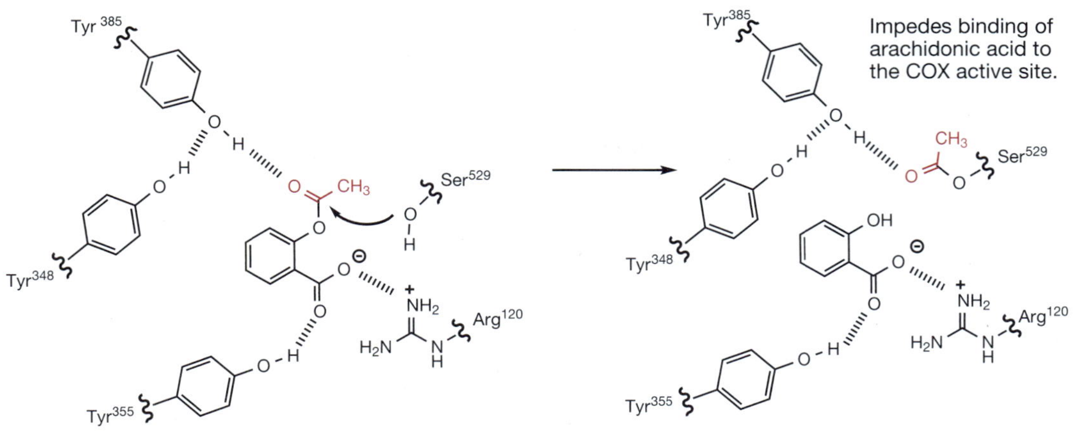

Figure 21.8 Model of irreversible acetylation of COX-1 by aspirin.[53-55] Important amino acid residues within COX-1 are noted and numbered according to the ovine sequence except for the serine residue. The serine hydroxyl that is acetylated by aspirin is at position 529 in human COX-1 (it is serine 530 in the ovine sequence). The acetylated serine residue sterically impedes binding of arachidonic acid to its binding site on COX. COX, cyclooxygenase.

40% to 50%, and peak plasma levels are achieved 30 to 40 minutes after oral ingestion.[57] The oral bioavailability of enteric formulations of aspirin is reduced, which may reduce the antiplatelet effect.[58-60] Furthermore, peak plasma levels of aspirin may not be achieved with enteric formulations until after 4 hours, rendering this formulation inappropriate for the treatment of ACS.[59,60]

Greater than 95% of TXA_2 activity must be inhibited to achieve an antiplatelet effect. While doses of aspirin as low as 30 mg/d completely suppress platelet TXA_2 production within a week by cumulative acetylation of platelet COX-1, a general maintenance dose of 75 mg to 100 mg/d is recommended.

Table 21.2 Cyclooxygenase Activity and Thrombosis

Characteristic	Platelets	Vascular Endothelial Cells
COX isoform	COX-1	COX-1 and COX-2
Ability to synthesize COX	No	Yes
AA metabolite	TXA_2	PGI_2
Activity of AA metabolite	• Stimulates platelet aggregation • Induces vasoconstriction	• Inhibits platelet aggregation • Induces vasodilation
With low-dose aspirin therapy	TXA_2 synthesis is inhibited; antiplatelet activity results	PGI_2 synthesis and inhibition of platelet aggregation activity remains

AA, arachidonic acid; COX, cyclooxygenase; PGI_2, prostacyclin; TXA_2, thromboxane A_2.

In the United States, low-dose aspirin chewable tablets are available as 81 mg. In patients with ACS, who were not previously taking aspirin, a rapid and complete inhibition of TXA_2 stimulated platelet aggregation can be achieved with a loading dose of 162 to 325 mg.[57] With the normal turnover of platelets, platelet function fully returns by about 3 days after the last dose of aspirin; therefore, patient compliance with daily aspirin is required for antithrombotic effects.

Adverse Effects. Even at low doses, inactivation of COX-1 by aspirin increases the risk of bleeding complications such as GI bleeds and hemorrhagic strokes.[61] These bleeding complications are the result of inhibition of TXA_2-induced platelet aggregation and decreased synthesis of COX-1–derived prostaglandin E_2 and PGI_2, which have cytoprotective effects on the gastric mucosa. The incidence of adverse effects of aspirin is dose related and increases at higher doses. Furthermore, at higher doses, aspirin loses COX-1 selectivity and also inhibits COX-2. Due to the small net benefit and the risk of bleeding, in 2022, the US Preventive Services Task Force (USPSTF) recommended that low-dose aspirin use for primary prevention of cardiovascular disease events in adults 40 to 59 years old who have a 10% or greater 10-year cardiovascular disease risk be considered only in patients not at increased risk for bleeding.[62] The USPSTF recommends against low-dose aspirin use for primary prevention of cardiovascular disease in adults 60 years or older because there is no net benefit.

Drug Interactions. Traditional nonsteroidal anti-inflammatory drugs (NSAIDs), such as ibuprofen or naproxen, reversibly bind to COX-1 with higher affinity than aspirin, thereby preventing the irreversible inhibition of aspirin.[63,64] NSAIDs also inhibit COX-2. Therefore, when given concomitantly, NSAIDs circumvent the antiplatelet effects of aspirin at low doses.

$P2Y_{12}$-Receptor Antagonists

Independent of TXA_2, platelet aggregation can be induced by ADP. Platelets possess two types of ADP receptors (also called purinergic receptors), $P2Y_1$ and $P2Y_{12}$, but currently available therapeutic agents are only able to antagonize ADP at $P2Y_{12}$ receptors. Upon ADP binding to the Gi-protein-coupled $P2Y_{12}$ receptors on the surface of platelets, adenylyl cyclase activity is inhibited, resulting in a decrease in the concentration of cyclic adenosine monophosphate (cAMP), which leads to platelet shape change and expression of GPIIb/IIIa, resulting in platelet aggregation (Fig. 21.9). ADP is released by activated platelets, thereby recruiting additional platelets to aggregate contributing to the thrombosis associated with CAD. Inhibiting the binding of ADP to $P2Y_{12}$ receptors and, consequently, inhibiting platelet aggregation, plays an important role in the treatment of ACS and as an adjunct to percutaneous coronary intervention (PCI).[50,65,66]

Treatment with the combination of low-dose aspirin (81 mg) and an oral $P2Y_{12}$ antagonist, termed dual antiplatelet therapy (DAPT), is established as standard therapy following an ACS or stent placement for the secondary prevention of ischemic events,[65,66] in treatment after some types of ischemic stroke,[52] and in other thrombotic disorders. DAPT inhibits platelet aggregation stimulated by two different mediators, intervening in the TXA_2 and the ADP pathways. $P2Y_{12}$ receptor antagonists to date, used in the treatment of ACS, are represented by two general types, the thienopyridine prodrugs and the nucleotide/nucleoside analogs. Table 21.3 is a comparison of $P2Y_{12}$ receptor antagonists with regard to their mode of binding and key clinical attributes.

Thienopyridines

The thienopyridines, clopidogrel and prasugrel, are irreversible antagonists of the $P2Y_{12}$ receptor.

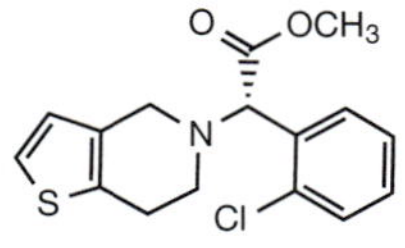

Clopidogrel
(Plavix)

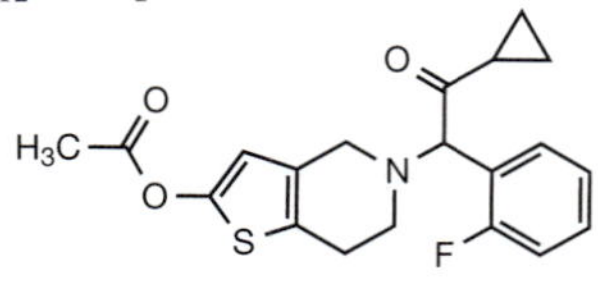

Prasugrel
(Effient)

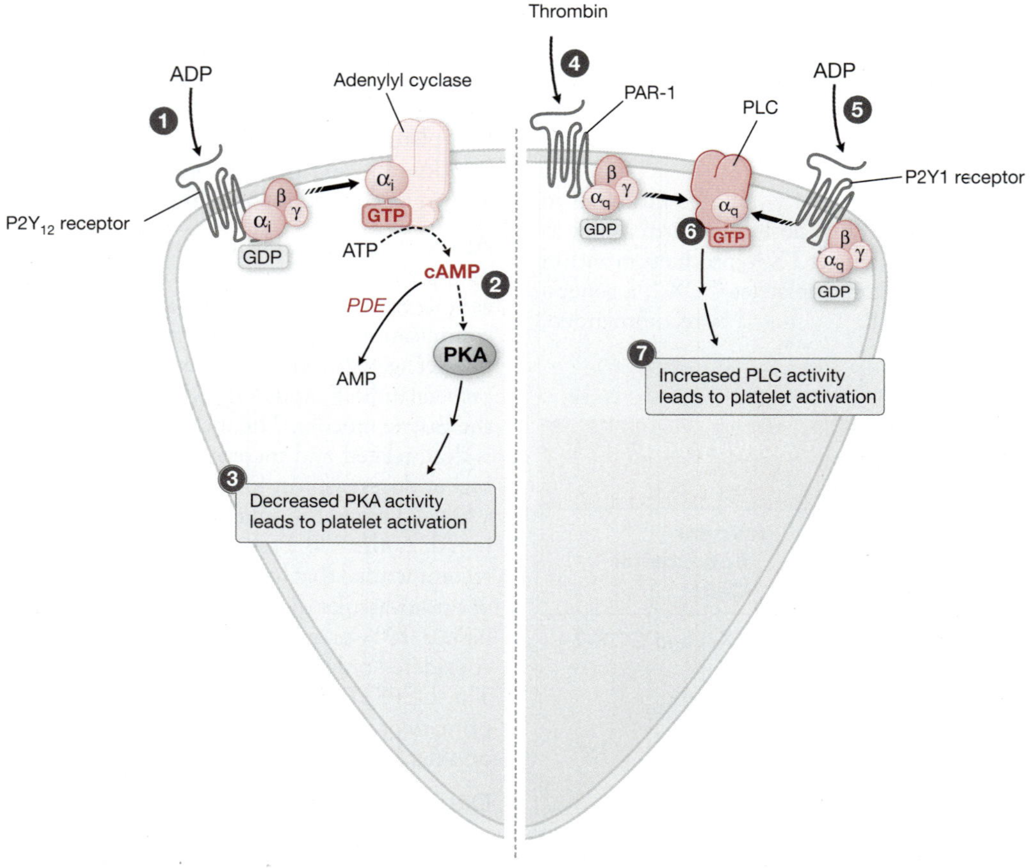

Figure 21.9 Platelet activation by ADP and thrombin. **Left panel: 1.** Binding of ADP to the $P2Y_{12}$ receptor activates a Gi protein, which inhibits adenylyl cyclase. **2.** Inhibition of adenylyl cyclase decreases the synthesis of cAMP and hence decreases protein kinase A (PKA) activation (dashed arrow). cAMP is metabolized to AMP by phosphodiesterase (PDE). **3.** PKA inhibits platelet activation through a series of incompletely understood steps. Therefore, the decreased PKA activation that results from ADP binding to the $P2Y_{12}$ receptor causes platelet activation. **Right panel: 4.** Thrombin proteolytically cleaves the extracellular domain of protease-activated receptor 1 (PAR-1). This cleavage creates a new N-terminus, which binds to an activation site on PAR-1 to activate a Gq protein. **5.** ADP also activates Gq by binding to the P2Y1 receptor. **6.** Gq activation (by either thrombin or ADP) activates phospholipase C (PLC). **7.** PLC activation leads to platelet activation, as shown in Figure21.7. Note that ADP can activate platelets by binding to either the $P2Y_{12}$ receptor or the P2Y1 receptor, although evidence suggests that full platelet activation requires the participation of both receptors. ADP, adenosine diphosphate; ATP, adenosine triphosphate;cAMP, cyclic adenosine monophosphate; GDP, guanosine diphosphate; GTP, guanosine triphosphate. (From Armstrong EJ, Golan DE. Pharmacology of hemostasis and thrombosis. In: Golan DE, Armstrong EJ, Armstrong AW, eds. *Principles of Pharmacology: The Pathophysiologic Basis of Drug Therapy*. 4th ed. Wolters-Kluwer; 2017:408, with permission.)

Table 21.3 Comparison of $P2Y_{12}$-Receptor Antagonists

Characteristics	Clopidogrel	Prasugrel	Ticagrelor	Cangrelor
Tradename	Plavix	Effient	Brilinta	Kengreal
Prodrug	Yes	Yes	No	No
Route of administration	Oral	Oral	Oral	IV
Mode of binding to target	Irreversible	Irreversible	Reversible	Reversible
Dosing frequency	Once a day	Once a day	Twice a day	Bolus followed by continuous infusion
Onset of inhibition of platelet aggregation	2-6 h	30 min to 4 h	30 min to 2 h	Within 2 min of infusion
Return of platelet function after discontinuing drug (time of withdrawal before CABG)	5 d	7 d	5 d	Within 1 h

CABG, coronary artery bypass graft surgery; IV, intravenous.
Modified from Golwala H, Bhatt DL. The timing of P2Y12 inhibitor initiation in the treatment of ACS? Does the evidence exist in this era? *Prog Cardiovasc Dis.* 2018;60:471-477.

Mechanism of Irreversible $P2Y_{12}$-Receptor Antagonism. Clopidogrel and prasugrel are oral prodrugs and require activation in vivo (Fig. 21.10). The main route of metabolism (~85%) of clopidogrel is hydrolysis of the methyl ester by human carboxylesterase 1 (hCE1) in the liver to the inactive carboxylic acid metabolite.[67] Activation of clopidogrel requires a two-step oxidation process involving multiple CYP enzymes in the liver.[68] The active thiol metabolite of clopidogrel forms a disulfide bond with a cysteine residue (cysteine 97 or cysteine 175) of the $P2Y_{12}$ receptor, irreversibly antagonizing platelet aggregation for the life of the platelet.[69,70] Activation of prasugrel requires ester hydrolysis predominantly via human carboxylesterase 2 (hCE2) in the small intestine and, to a limited degree, by hepatic hCE1 (Fig. 21.10).[71] The second step of prasugrel activation is CYP mediated, and generates the active thiol metabolite, which, like clopidogrel, forms an irreversible disulfide bond to a cysteine residue (cysteine 97 or cysteine 175) of the $P2Y_{12}$ receptor.[70] Overall, the metabolic activation of prasugrel is less reliant on hepatic oxidative metabolism than clopidogrel.

CYP2C19 Genetic Polymorphism and Clopidogrel Activity. CYP2C19 is genetically polymorphic. Patients who possess one loss of function allele, most frequently *CYP2C19*2* and to a lesser extent *CYP2C19*3* among others, have a decreased metabolizing phenotype and are defined as intermediate metabolizers. Patients with two loss of function *CYP2C19* alleles are considered poor metabolizers.

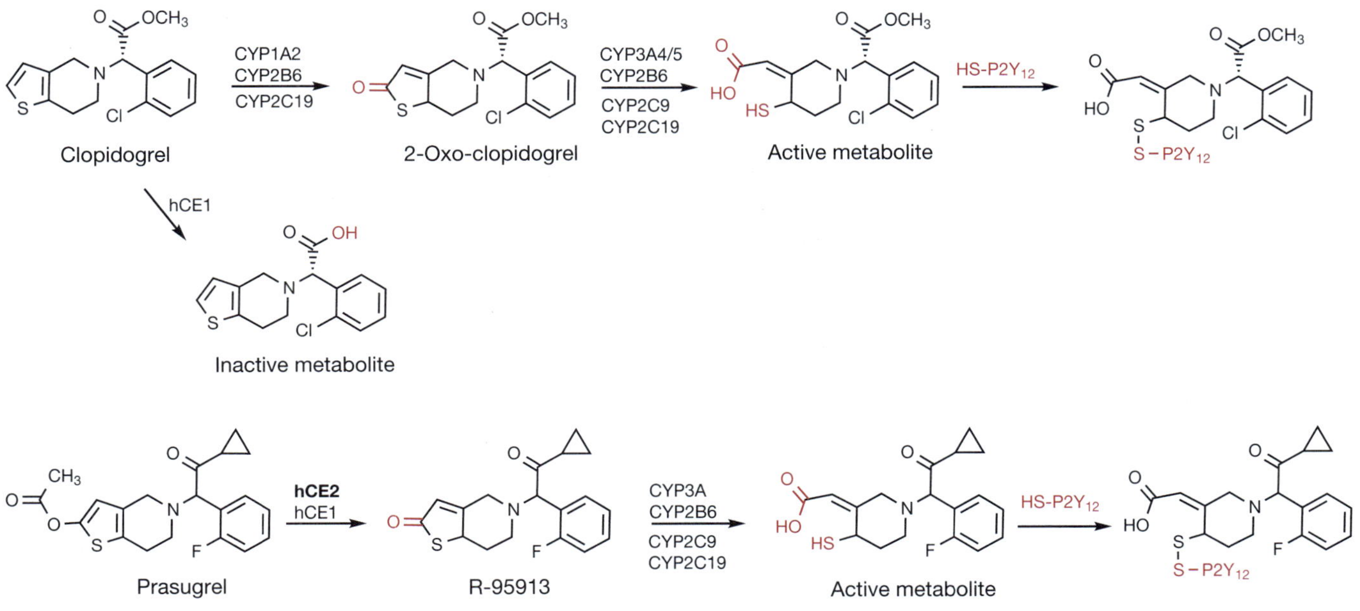

Figure 21.10 In vivo activation of clopidogrel and prasugrel. hCE1, human carboxylesterase 1; hCE2, human carboxylesterase 2; HS-$P2Y_{12}$, the thiol group of the cysteine residue at position 97 or 175 of the platelet surface $P2Y_{12}$ receptor.

Both steps necessary to produce the active metabolite of clopidogrel occur to a significant extent via CYP2C19. Studies have shown that patients with loss of function alleles exhibit decreased activation of clopidogrel, resulting in decreased $P2Y_{12}$ antagonist activity, thereby diminishing the platelet antiaggregatory effect.[72] Consequently, patients possessing at least one loss of function *CYP2C19* allele would be expected to have an increase in major adverse cardiovascular events (MACE), defined as death from cardiovascular causes, MI, and stroke, when taking clopidogrel in the treatment or prevention of ACS. This has been observed in some studies, but has not been a universal finding, thus making the role of CYP2C19 testing unclear.[72-75]

The current American Heart Association/American College of Cardiology guidelines do not include testing for CYP2C19 genotype for clopidogrel. However, the Clinical Pharmacogenetics Implementation Consortium (CPIC) does include guidelines for CYP2C19 testing and clopidogrel dosing.[76] Additionally, the US Food and Drug Administration (FDA) has issued a boxed warning in the clopidogrel package insert indicating that patients who are CYP2C19 poor metabolizers (those patients who have two loss of function alleles) will form less of the active metabolite of clopidogrel at recommended doses.[77] The recommendation is that another $P2Y_{12}$ antagonist should be used in CYP2C19 poor metabolizers. Conversely, *CYP2C19*17* is a gain of function allele, and a patient possessing at least one *CYP2C19*17* allele exhibits an ultrarapid metabolizing phenotype. CYP2C19 ultrarapid metabolizers would be expected to produce higher than normal amounts of clopidogrel active metabolite, with a normal dose increasing their risk of bleeding. A recent meta-analysis of 19 randomized controlled trials with 69,746 patients examined the risk of bleeding and ischemic events of unguided de-escalation of DAPT compared with personalized guided selection of DAPT.[78] The unguided de-escalation strategy included aspirin and a fixed-dose of a $P2Y_{12}$ antagonist and then changing potent $P2Y_{12}$ antagonists (prasugrel or ticagrelor) to less potent (clopidogrel) or reduced-dose (low-dose prasugrel) $P2Y_{12}$ antagonists 1 month after ACS. Unguided de-escalation of DAPT was associated with decreased risk of bleeding events without an increased risk of adverse cardiac events compared to either personalized guided DAPT strategies, which included aspirin and any $P2Y_{12}$ antagonist based on platelet function or genotype. Prasugrel activation is not affected by CYP2C19 genetic polymorphism.

DRUG INTERACTIONS. To reduce the risk of GI bleeding, a proton-pump inhibitor (PPI) is recommended for patients on DAPT with a history of GI bleeding or at increased risk of GI bleeding.[66] PPIs that strongly inhibit CYP2C19, most notably omeprazole and esomeprazole, inhibit the formation of the active thiol metabolite of clopidogrel and decrease its antiplatelet effect.[79,80] Whether or not this is clinically significant is unclear.[81] Several studies have shown no association between PPI use and risk of MACE with clopidogrel treatment.[81-83] The FDA-approved product information states that concomitant use of omeprazole with clopidogrel affects the formation of the active metabolite of clopidogrel the most, and deslanzoprazolehas the least effect on the antiplatelet activity of clopidogrel.[77] Prasugrel is not associated with a clinically relevant interaction with PPIs.

Coadministration of morphine with oral $P2Y^{12}$ receptor antagonists, including clopidogrel and prasugrel, delays absorption of the $P2Y^{12}$ receptor antagonist, decreases the plasma concentrations of the active metabolite and delays the onset of platelet inhibition.[84,85] Decreased GI motility caused by morphine is the proposed mechanism by which it decreases absorption of the oral $P2Y^{12}$ receptor antagonists. The effect of morphine is much more pronounced with clopidogrel than with prasugrel.

PRASUGREL CONTRAINDICATIONS. Prasugrel has a more rapid onset of antiplatelet activity and is a more potent inhibitor of ADP-induced platelet aggregation than clopidogrel.[86] Currently, the indication for prasugrel is for ACS patients undergoing PCI. In this patient population, the increased potency of prasugrel has been shown to decrease the rate of ischemic events, most notably MI, to a greater extent than clopidogrel. Prasugrel is also associated with a higher incidence of major bleeding, including fatal bleeding, compared to clopidogrel.[87] Consequently, prasugrel has a boxed warning and is contraindicated in patients with a history of stroke or transient ischemic attack, where the risk of harm outweighs any benefit.[88] Additionally, prasugrel should be avoided in patients at high risk of bleeding, such as patients aged 75 years or older and patients with a body weight of less than 60 kg.

Nucleotide/Nucleoside Analogs

Adenosine triphosphate (ATP) is a weak competitive antagonist of the $P2Y_{12}$ receptor, although it is not selective for $P2Y_{12}$ receptors. Cangrelor and ticagrelor were both designed based on the structure of ATP (Fig. 21.11), and they are both highly selective $P2Y_{12}$ antagonists that do not require bioactivation unlike the thienopyridines. They are direct and reversible inhibitors of ADP binding to the $P2Y_{12}$ receptor, resulting in platelet antiaggregatory activity. In addition to increasing the risk of bleeding, both cangrelor and ticagrelor are associated with an increased incidence of dyspnea.[89,90] The dyspnea appears to be dose-dependent and resolves upon discontinuation of the drug. The mechanism is unclear.[91]

CANGRELOR. Cangrelor is a nucleotide analog of ATP that is administered IV (Fig. 21.11). The triphosphate chain of ATP is sequentially dephosphorylated via ectonucleotidases, with the first dephosphorylation reaction liberating ADP, the potent inducer of platelet aggregation, via binding to the $P2Y_{12}$ receptor on the surface of platelets. The terminal phosphate anhydride oxygen of ATP was replaced with a dichloro-methylene group in cangrelor to prevent the hydrolysis to the proaggregatory diphosphate product.[92] Furthermore, the dichloro groups on the methylene bridge render the pK_a values within the triphosphate chain similar to those of ATP such that, like ATP, cangrelor exists as a tetraanion at physiological pH. The tetraanion is critical for high affinity to the $P2Y_{12}$ receptor and is important for conferring antagonist activity within the nucleotide template. The combination of the nonpolar trifluoromethyl thiopropyl group at position 2 of adenine and monoalkylation of the nitrogen at position 6 with a lipophilic methylthioethyl

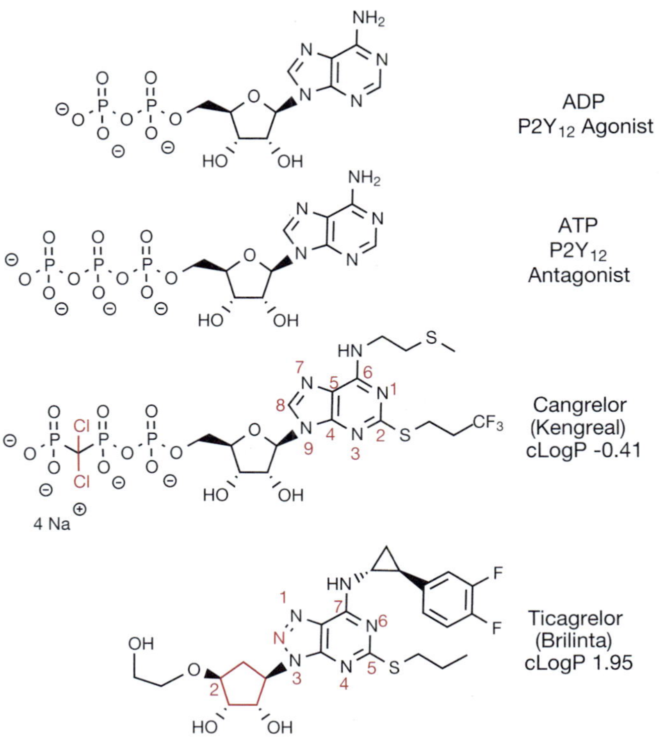

Figure 21.11 Nucleoside/nucleotide analogs as reversible $P2Y_{12}$ receptor antagonists. ADP, adenosine diphosphate; ATP, adenosine triphosphate. (Modified from Dobesh PP, Oestreich JH. Ticagrelor: pharmacokinetics, pharmacodynamics, clinical efficacy, and safety. *Pharmacotherapy*. 2014;34:1077-1090.)

group led to cangrelor, which has both high potency and a short half-life, allowing rapid recovery of platelet aggregation capability.[92]

Pharmacokinetics. The most rapid acting of all the $P2Y_{12}$ antagonists (Table 21.3), cangrelor is administered as a bolus followed by infusion and inhibits platelet aggregation within 2 minutes. Cangrelor is rapidly dephosphorylated in vivo by ectonucleotidases to an inactive nucleoside metabolite and has a plasma half-life of 3 to 6 minutes (Fig. 21.12).[93] Upon discontinuing the infusion of cangrelor, platelet function returns to normal within an hour. The rapid onset/offset characteristics of cangrelor make it suitable for antiplatelet therapy just before and during PCI, where it was found to decrease death, MI, ischemia-driven revascularization, and stent thrombosis at 48 hours more than clopidogrel without an increase in bleeding.[90]

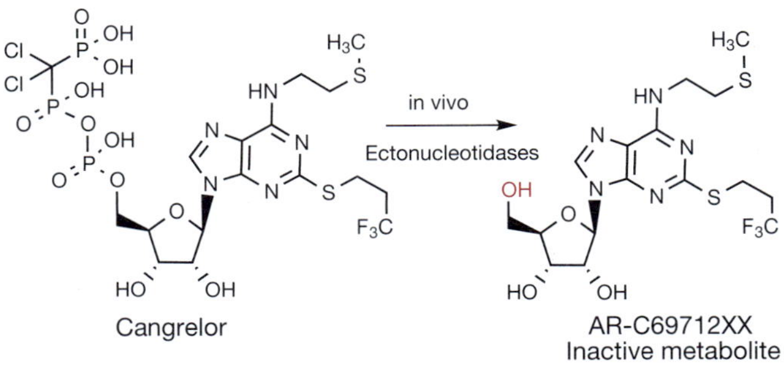

Figure 21.12 Metabolism of cangrelor.

Cangrelor has been found to block the irreversible binding of the thienopyridine active metabolites to the $P2Y_{12}$ receptor.[94] Therefore, when patients are transitioned from IV cangrelor to oral clopidogrel or prasugrel for continued antiplatelet therapy post-PCI, the thienopyridine must not be started until after the discontinuation of cangrelor infusion to insure effective antiplatelet activity.

Ticagrelor. Ticagrelor was designed to be an oral antiplatelet drug.[95] Before the design of ticagrelor, cangrelor had already been designed based on the structure of ATP as a short-acting water-soluble solution for injection. For oral activity, the compound would need to be longer acting and more lipid soluble. Similar to the nucleoside portion of cangrelor, the design of ticagrelor started with a 5,7-substituted purine derivative. The triazolopyrimidine ring is a bioisosteric replacement for the purine ring. Replacing the ribose sugar with a dihydroxycyclopentane bioisostere maintained potency and eliminated the potentially labile glycosidic bond. From more than 6,000 analogs, the thiopropyl group at position 5 and the 1*R*,2*S*-*trans*-phenylcyclopropylamine at position 7 of the triazolopyrimidine ring were found to have optimal potency and metabolic stability. The affinity to the $P2Y_{12}$ receptor and metabolic stability were enhanced with the addition of 3,4 difluoro substituents on the phenyl ring of the substituent at position 7. The triphosphate chain in ATP and the modified phosphate chain in cangrelor would not be suitable for oral bioavailability because these side chains are highly ionized, which precludes oral absorption, and they are metabolized rapidly via ectonucleotidases. The hydroxyethoxy group at the 2-position was found to be resistant to glucuronidation and had good oral bioavailability. Ticagrelor (cLogP = 1.95) is much more lipophilic than cangrelor (cLogP = −0.41), which makes it amenable to oral absorption.[96] Lacking phosphate groups, ticagrelor is a nucleoside analog of ATP. Ticagrelor is also referred to as a cyclopentyltriazolopyrimidine. Ticagrelor has a fast onset similar to prasugrel and is dosed twice a day (Table 21.3).

Contraindication and Aspirin Coadministration. Ticagrelor is a more potent inhibitor of platelet aggregation than clopidogrel.[97] As part of DAPT in patients with ACS, ticagrelor was shown to be more effective than clopidogrel in decreasing MACE in the international Platelet Inhibition and Patient Outcomes (PLATO) study, but was associated with a higher rate of non-coronary artery bypass graft major bleeding, including fatal intracranial bleeding.[98] Consequently, ticagrelor is contraindicated in patients with a history of intracranial bleeding.

A subgroup analysis of the data from the PLATO study showed that in the United States, ticagrelor showed a trend toward worse outcomes than clopidogrel.[99] One rationale for this regional difference is that more patients in the United States took a higher dose (≥300 mg/d) of aspirin than patients in the rest of the world. With ticagrelor, the lowest event rates were observed with low-dose (<300 mg/d) aspirin. Therefore, ticagrelor was initially FDA approved in 2011 with a boxed warning that maintenance doses of aspirin of more than 100 mg/d decrease the effectiveness of ticagrelor. As of March 2024, this information is no longer in a box warning, but is located throughout the most recent package insert.[100]

Metabolism. Oxidative metabolism, via CYP3A4 and CYP3A5, plays an important role in ticagrelor metabolism

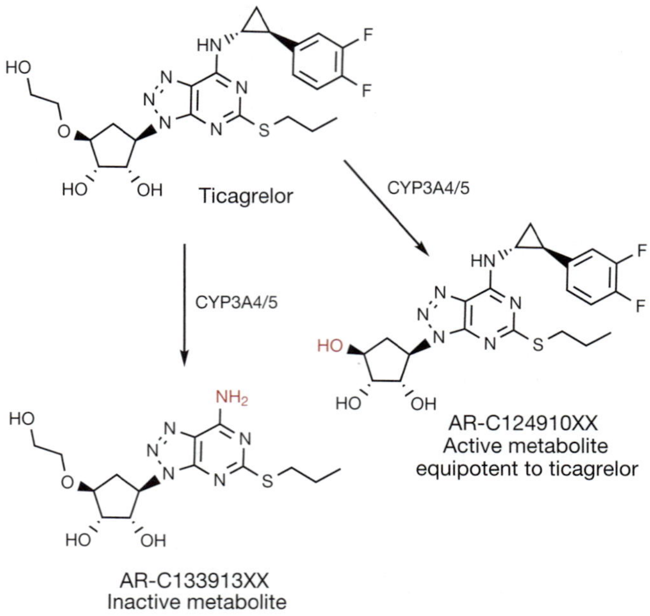

Figure 21.13 Metabolism of ticagrelor to active metabolite.

(Fig. 21.13).[101] The major plasma metabolite, AR-C124910XX is the result of CYP3A4/5-mediated O-dealkylation of the hydroxyethoxy group of ticagrelor. AR-C124910XX is equipotent to ticagrelor, and represents 30% to 40% of the exposure to ticagrelor.[100,101] AR-C133913XX, the product of CYP3A4/5 mediated N-dealkylation of ticagrelor, and its glucuronide are the major urinary metabolites.[101] AR-C133913XX is inactive. Coadministration of strong inducers or inhibitors of CYP3A with ticagrelor may result in decreased efficacy or increased risk of bleeding, respectively, and should be avoided.[100]

Drug Interaction. Like the other oral $P2Y_{12}$ receptor antagonists, morphine decreases the plasma levels and delays the platelet inhibitory activity of ticagrelor.[102] While decreased absorption is proposed as a reason for morphine's ability to decrease plasma levels and delay activity of oral $P2Y_{12}$ antagonists, administering methylnaltrexone, a peripherally restricted mu opioid receptor antagonist that circumvents the reduced GI motility associated with opioid use, along with morphine and ticagrelor, does not improve plasma levels of ticagrelor nor decrease time to platelet inhibition.[103,104]

Thrombin Protease–Activated Receptor-1 (PAR-1) Antagonist

In addition to being a key component of coagulation, thrombin is a potent inducer of platelet aggregation by binding predominantly to the PAR-1 receptor on the surface of platelets (see Fig. 21.9). Thrombin is a serine protease that cleaves the N-terminus of the PAR-1 receptor when bound to it. The resultant new N-terminus bears a sequence that acts as a tethered ligand and activates the Gq protein–coupled PAR-1 receptor.[110] Activation of the Gq protein stimulates phospholipase C, which leads to platelet aggregation.

Vorapaxar

Vorapaxar is an oral selective and competitive PAR-1 antagonist and the only marketed compound in this class, to date. It is indicated, in addition to aspirin and/or clopidogrel, for the secondary prevention of cardiovascular thrombotic events in patients with a history of MI and/or PAD.[111-113] Vorapaxar blocks thrombin-induced platelet aggregation. It was designed based on a lead structure discovered in a high-throughput screening program of analogs of the natural product (+)-himbacine

REVERSIBLE $P2Y_{12}$-RECEPTOR ANTAGONIST UNDER INVESTIGATION AS SUBCUTANEOUS INJECTION

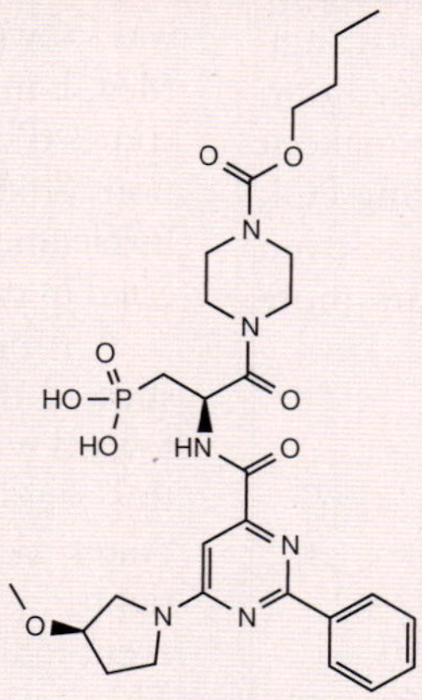

Selatogrel

Selatogrel, a reversible $P2Y_{12}$ receptor antagonist, is being developed as a subcutaneous (SC) autoinjector for the prehospital treatment of acute myocardial infarction (AMI) for patients with a recent history of AMI.[105]

Merging a scaffold derived from the structure of ticagrelor and the core template of a series of compounds with $P2Y_{12}$-receptor antagonist activity synthesized by Berlix Biosciences formed the starting 2-phenylpyrimidine-4-carboxamide structure that led to selatogrel.[106,107]

REVERSIBLE $P2Y_{12}$-RECEPTOR ANTAGONIST UNDER INVESTIGATION AS SUBCUTANEOUS INJECTION (*continued*)

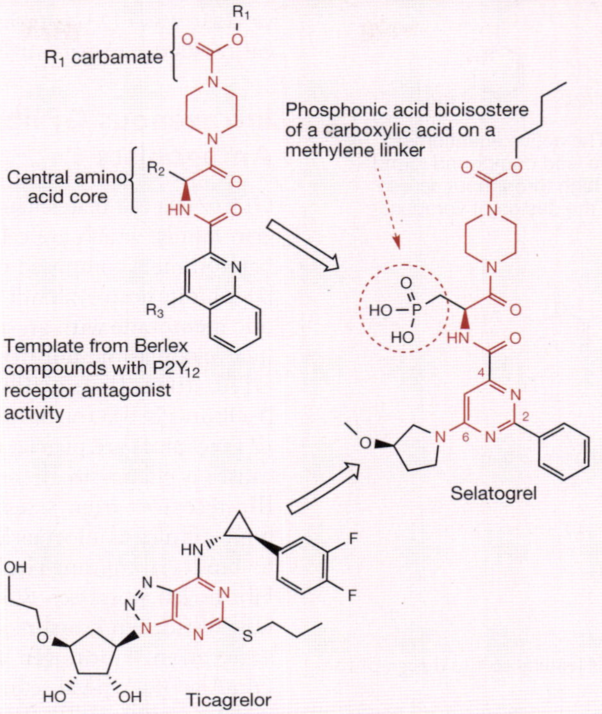

In structure-activity relationship studies, substitution of the 2-phenyl ring did not lead to improved activity and the 3-methoxypyrrolidin-1-yl group at position 6 of the pyrimidine ring conferred high affinity and activity.[106] Within the 4-carboxamide group, an acidic group was necessary at the amino acid core for high potency. Replacement of an L-glutamic acid residue with a phosphonic acid bioisostere of a carboxylic acid on a methylene linker had excellent potency and low metabolic clearance.[107] Modification of the piperazine ring was not tolerated. Extending the R_1 group on the carbamate from ethyl to *n*-butyl improved biological activity.

Selatogrel has poor oral bioavailability at about 1%. This is expected due to its large size (molecular weight [MW] 618), low lipid solubility ($LogD_7 = -0.3$),[108] and the phosphonate will be predominantly ionized in the small intestine with pK_a values of 1.38 and 7.39.[107] Selatogrel is mostly excreted unchanged in the urine and feces. About 8.5% of dose circulates as the major metabolite, a glucuronide metabolite, M21.[108] Whereas the oral $P2Y_{12}$ receptor antagonists require a minimum of 30 minutes to several hours to begin inhibition of platelet aggregation, the onset of antiplatelet action of selatogrel is reported to be 15 to 30 minutes when administered subcutaneously.[109] In the treatment of ACS, early inhibition of platelet aggregation can abruptly stop thrombus formation and lead to better outcomes. While cangrelor has a rapid onset within 2 minutes of infusion, it requires IV administration by a healthcare professional and has a half-life of 3 to 6 minutes. The half-life of selatogrel is 4 to 7.2 hours.[109]

(Fig. 21.14).[114,115] Vorapaxar has high affinity and a long dissociation half-life from the PAR-1 receptor of approximately 20 hours, which is critical, as it is competing with a tethered ligand.[115]

Pharmacokinetics. Vorapaxar is rapidly absorbed and has high oral bioavailability (<90%).[116,117] Vorapaxar completely inhibits (>80%) platelet aggregation stimulated by a thrombin receptor activating peptide within 1 week of initiating daily dosing. It has no effect on ADP-induced platelet aggregation. With a mean half-life of approximately of 173 to 269 hours, the antiplatelet effect of vorapaxar is essentially irreversible. Upon discontinuing daily dosing of vorapaxar, it takes 4 to 8 weeks to recover normal platelet function.[116] Vorapaxar specifically inhibits the platelet aggregatory effects of thrombin via PAR-1 antagonism and does not antagonize the effects of thrombin on the coagulation cascade. Therefore, vorapaxar has no effect on coagulation tests.[115,116]

Metabolism. Vorapaxar undergoes slow and extensive metabolism via CYP3A4 and CYP2J2 (Fig. 21.15).[117] Less than 2% of an oral dose of vorapaxar is excreted unchanged in the feces, and none is excreted unchanged in the urine. Vorapaxar does not require dose adjustment in patients with renal dysfunction. After a single dose, the main circulating metabolite is amine M19, primarily by CYP3A4 metabolism. The proposed mechanism of M19 formation is CYP-mediated hydroxylation of the secondary carbon of the ethyl group on the carbamate, followed by loss of acetaldehyde and CO_2.[117] After multiple doses, the omega hydroxylation product M20 is the main circulating metabolite at about 23% of the parent drug. M20 is an active metabolite and equipotent to vorapaxar. Concomitant administration of strong CYP3A4 inhibitors and inducers should be avoided when taking vorapaxar.[117]

Boxed Warning. In patients who have had an MI, when added to standard therapy of aspirin or DAPT, vorapaxar

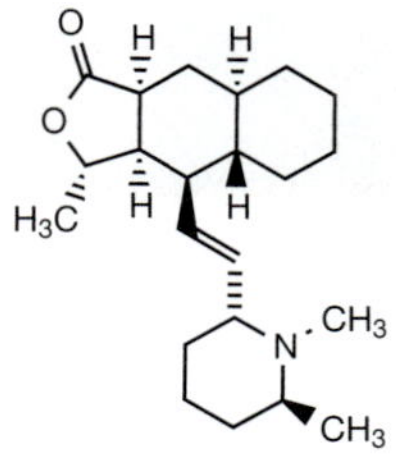

(+)-Himbacine
Natural product
(PAR-1 inactive)

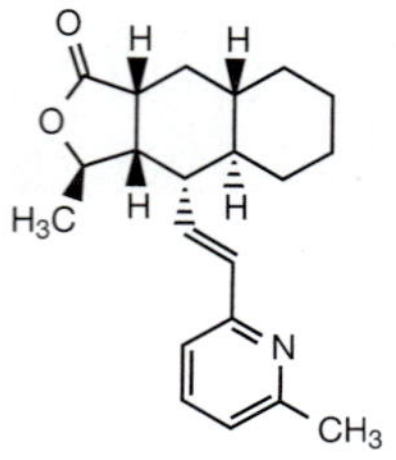

The active enantiomer
of a lead compound found
in high throughput screen
for the design of vorapaxar

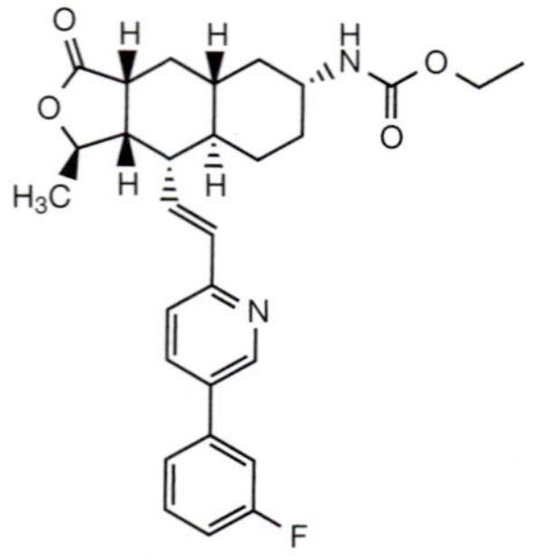

Vorapaxar
(Zontivity)

Figure 21.14 Structures of compounds leading to the design of the PAR-1 receptor antagonist vorapaxar.

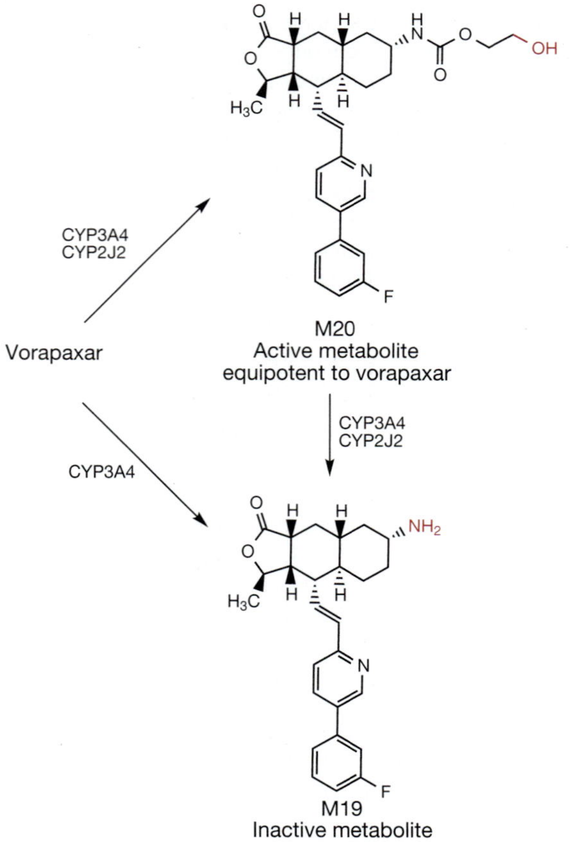

Figure 21.15 Metabolism of vorapaxar.

has been shown to decrease the rate of MACE, but there is an increase in bleeding, including intracranial bleeding.[112] Patients with a history of stroke had a significantly higher rate of intracranial bleeding with vorapaxar. As a result, vorapaxar was FDA approved with a box warning contraindicating its use in patients with a history of stroke.[111]

Intravenous GPIIb/IIIa-Receptor Antagonists

GPIIb/IIIa is a platelet surface membrane protein of the integrin family, which are cell adhesion molecules. Integrins are heterodimers composed of two subunits, an α subunit and a β subunit, noncovalently linked, which traverse the cytoplasmic membrane with an extracellular domain and an intracellular cytoplasmic tail from each subunit. The α subunit of GPIIb/IIIa is IIb (or αIIb in integrin nomenclature), and the β subunit is IIIa (or β3 in integrin nomenclature).[118] GPIIb/IIIa receptors are platelet αIIbβ3 integrins. Platelet activation causes a change in the extracellular domain of the GPIIb/IIIa receptors from a resting low affinity conformation to a high affinity conformation, which allows adhesive ligands to bind via arginine-glycine-aspartic acid (RGD) sequences. Fibrinogen possesses RGD sequences on each end. In this way, fibrinogen crosslinks activated platelets, causing platelet aggregation. Fibrinogen also binds to GPIIb/IIIa via a Lys-Gln-Ala-Gly-Asp-Val sequence at the carboxy terminus of the γ chains.[118,119] GPIIb/IIIa antagonists block the binding of fibrinogen, thereby inhibiting platelet aggregation, independent of the mediator of platelet activation, resulting in an antithrombotic effect.

Eptifibatide and Tirofiban

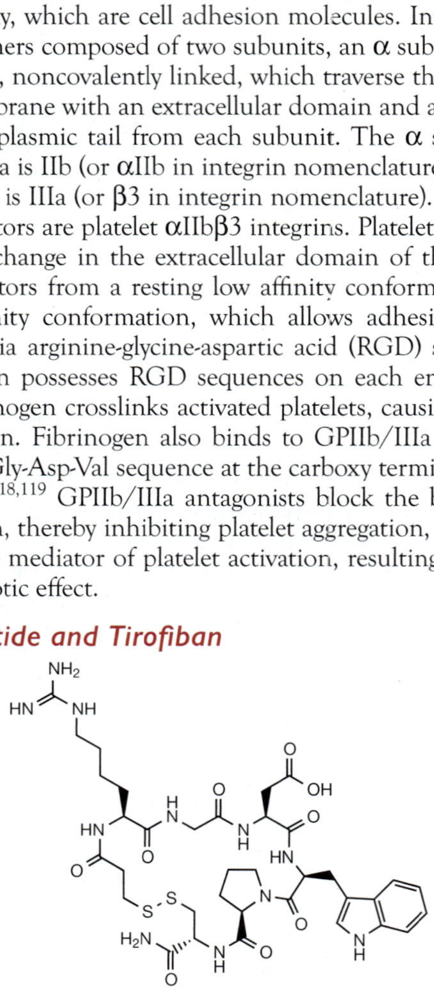

Eptifibatide
(Integrilin)

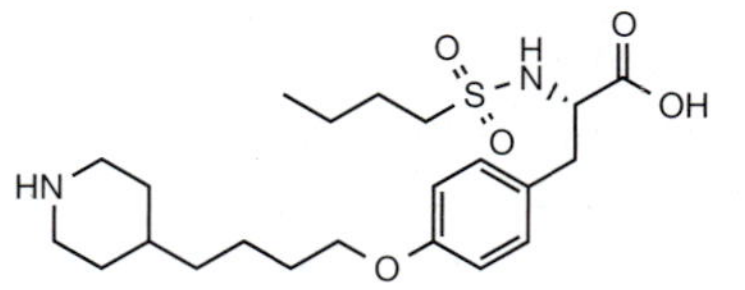

Tirofiban
(Aggrastat)

Currently, there are two commercially available GPIIb/IIIa antagonists, which were FDA approved in the 1990s. They vary widely in structure, and both are administered IV. They include a cyclic heptapeptide eptifibatide and a nonpeptide small-molecule tirofiban. Eptifibatide and tirofiban bind to

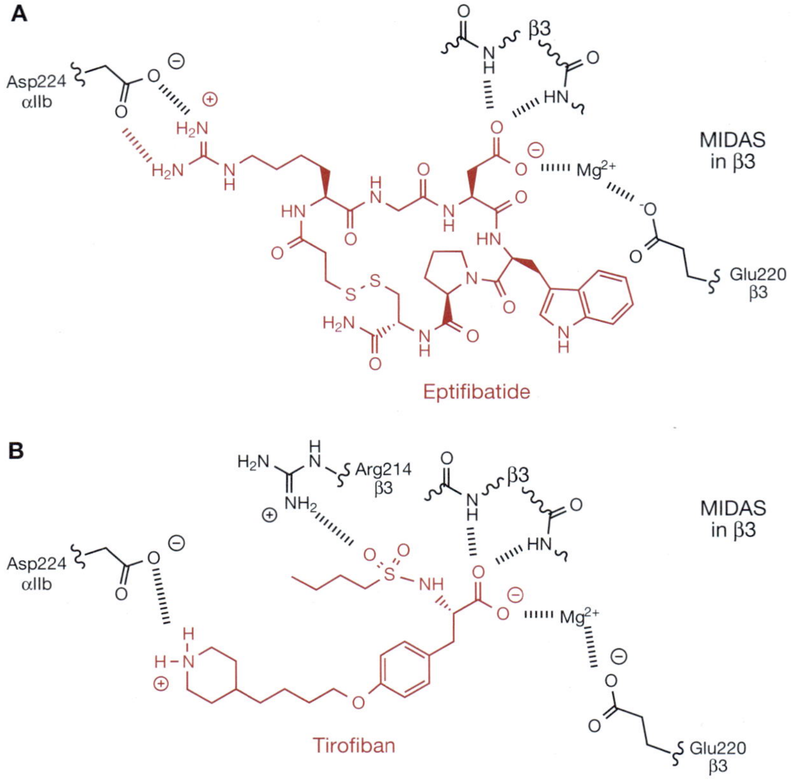

Figure 21.16 Important GPIIb/IIIa binding interactions with **(A)** eptifibatide and **(B)** tirofiban. Key amino acid residues within the GPIIb/IIIa binding site which interact with eptifibatide and tirofiban are shown in black. MIDAS, metal ion–dependent adhesion site.

GPIIb/IIIa in a drug-binding pocket located at the interface of the α and β subunits, and they are both specific for GPIIb/IIIa (Fig. 21.16).[120]

Structure-Activity Relationship. The design of eptifibatide is based on a Lys-Gly-Asp (KGD) sequence found in the 73 amino acid snake venom peptide barbourin.[121] Barbourin inhibits the binding of adhesive proteins, such as fibrinogen, specifically to GPIIb/IIIa receptors. A KGD containing cyclic heptapeptide, with potent GPIIb/IIIa antagonist activity was optimized to form eptifibatide. Modifying the ε-amino group of lysine to a guanidino group to form a homoarginine residue increased potency 5- to 10-fold and increased the specificity for GPIIb/IIIa over other integrins (Fig. 21.17).[121] In this way, eptifibatide is mimicking the RGD sequence of the natural ligands of GPIIb/IIIa. The large hydrophobic tryptophan residue next to the aspartic acid residue further increased affinity. The proline residue of eptifibatide restrains conformational flexibility of the heptapeptide ring to optimally position the homoarginine, aspartic acid, and tryptophan residues within the drug-binding pocket.[121] Removing the amino group of the N-terminus cysteine further improved potency.

Tirofiban, an L-tyrosine analog, was designed as a nonpeptide drug that maintains the distance between the basic moiety and the carboxylic acid similar to that in the RGD sequence (Fig. 21.17).[122] It possesses a basic piperidine nitrogen that mimics the arginine in RGD or the lysine in the additional fibrinogen binding sequence. The basic homoarginine residue of eptifibatide and the basic piperidine nitrogen of tirofiban

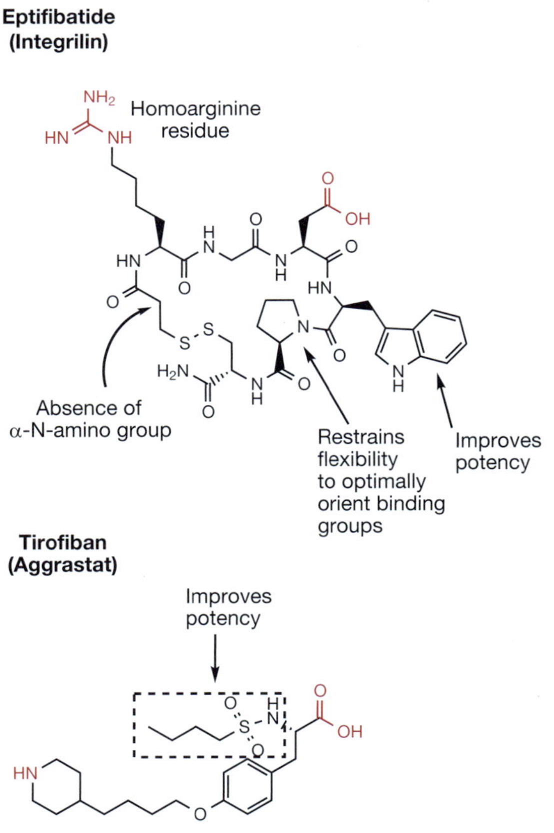

Figure 21.17 Structure-activity relationship of eptifibatide and tirofiban.

Table 21.4 Comparison of GPIIb/IIIa-Receptor Antagonists

Characteristics	Eptifibatide	Tirofiban
Tradename	Integrilin	Aggrastat
Molecular description	Cyclic heptapeptide	Nonpeptide small molecule
Molecular weight (Da)	832	495
Mechanism of action	Mimics RGD-binding sequence of natural ligands	Mimics RGD-binding sequence of natural ligands
Affinity for $\alpha IIb\beta 3$ (K_D)	120 nM	15 nM
Mode of binding to target	Reversible	Reversible
Selectivity for GPIIb/IIIa	Yes	Yes
Plasma $t_{1/2}$	~2.5 h	~2.0 h
Platelet-bound $t_{1/2}$	Seconds	Seconds
Excretion	Renal	Renal and biliary
Return of platelet function after discontinuing drug	4-8 h	4-8 h
Route of administration	IV	IV

IV, intravenous; K_D, dissociation constant; RGD, arginine-glycine-aspartic acid sequence.

each form an ionic bond with Asp224 of the αIIb subunit.[120] The carboxylic acid group in both eptifibatide and tirofiban coordinates with an Mg^{2+} ion in the metal ion–dependent adhesion site (MIDAS) located in the β3 subunit.[120,123] The binding of the Mg^{2+} ion in the MIDAS involves the assistance of Glu220 in the β3 subunit and induces a conformational change to the GPIIb/IIIa receptor. The *N*-α-sulfonamide group of tirofiban is critical to its potent activity.

Table 21.4 is a comparison of the two GPIIb/IIIa antagonists.[118,124] While GPIIb/IIIa antagonists continue to be used during PCI, their use in the noninvasive treatment of NSTE-ACS has been supplanted by oral $P2Y_{12}$ antagonists.

Metabolism. Eptifibatide does not undergo significant hepatic metabolism and is primarily eliminated by the kidneys.[125] Unchanged eptifibatide comprises 34% of the dose excreted in the urine, along with 19% of deamidated eptifibatide and 13% of various polar metabolites. The structures of the metabolites have not been published.

Tirofiban has not been shown to be metabolized by the liver and appears to be predominantly excreted unchanged.[126] Approximately 65% of tirofiban is excreted by the kidneys unchanged, and 25% is eliminated in feces.[127]

Adverse Effects. The GPIIb/IIIa antagonists are associated with bleeding and thrombocytopenia.[128-131] Thrombocytopenia associated with eptifibatide and tirofiban occurs in approximately 0.2% and 0.5% of patients, respectively.[132,133] Binding of eptifibatide or tirofiban to GPIIb/IIIa causes a conformational change in the β3 subunit that exposes epitopes, called ligand-induced binding sites (LIBS).[134,135] Some patients have innate antibodies that recognize these LIBS causing platelet destruction leading to acute thrombocytopenia.[134] Due to the risk of thrombocytopenia, the platelet count needs to be monitored in patients on IV GPIIb/IIIa antagonists.

Phosphodiesterase 3 Inhibitor

Cilostazol

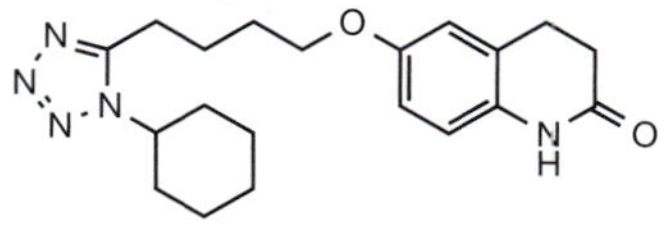

Cilostazol
(Pletal)

Cilostazol is a quinolinone derivative that inhibits platelet aggregation by inhibiting phosphodiesterase 3 (PDE3) in platelets, which increases the concentration of cAMP.[137] An increase in cAMP increases activation of protein kinase A, causing inhibition of platelet aggregation. Cilostazol also inhibits PDE3 in vascular smooth muscle, causing vascular smooth muscle relaxation, which leads to vasodilation. Cilostazol inhibits adenosine uptake, and that may also play a role in its ability to inhibit platelet aggregation.[137] Cilostazol is indicated in the treatment of intermittent claudication, a manifestation of PAD.[138]

Metabolism. Cilostazol is extensively metabolized by the liver to 11 metabolites. The two main metabolites of cilostazol are 3,4-dehydrocilostazol, formed via CYP3A4, and 4′-trans-hydroxycilostazol, formed predominantly via

NON–RGD-MIMETIC ANTAGONIST OF GPIIb/IIIa ON THE HORIZON

Clinical studies of oral GPIIb/IIIa antagonists that contained an RGD mimic as part of their structure revealed that these compounds caused an increase in mortality and a risk of bleeding and thrombocytopenia.[118,131] One theory for the increase in mortality is that RGD-mimetic GPIIb/IIIa antagonists activate the GPIIb/IIIa receptor by inducing a high affinity conformation that facilitates fibrinogen binding.[131,133] Thus when plasma concentrations of the oral GPIIb/IIIa antagonists are subtherapeutic, patients are left in a prothrombotic state. This phenomenon is commonly referred to as "priming" the GPIIb/IIIa receptor for fibrinogen binding. The same conformational change is associated with causing thrombocytopenia. A key aspect of this conformational change is binding of Mg^{2+} in the MIDAS of GPIIb/IIIa by RGD-mimetic inhibitors.[123,134,135] Zalunfiban (RUC-4) is a non–RGD-mimetic antagonist of GPIIb/IIIa that does not bind to the Mg^{2+} in the MIDAS and, therefore, does not induce the above conformational change.[134,135]

NON–RGD-MIMETIC ANTAGONIST OF GPIIB/IIIA ON THE HORIZON (*continued*)

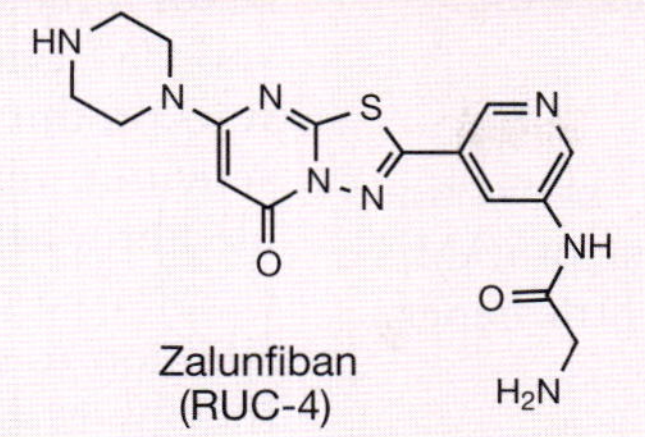

Zalunfiban
(RUC-4)

Shown below is the structure of zalunfiban in red, interacting with key amino acid residues in the GPIIb/IIIa binding site shown in black. Zalunfiban possesses a basic piperazine nitrogen and, like eptifibatide and tirofiban, forms an ionic bond with Asp224 of the αIIb subunit. The structure of zalunfiban lacks a carboxylic acid, but it possesses a primary amine that competes with Mg^{2+} and forms an ionic bond with Glu220 in the β3 subunit, which is reinforced by a hydrogen bond between the charged nitrogen and a backbone carbonyl oxygen. In this way, zalunfiban displaces the Mg^{2+} ion from the MIDAS on the β3 subunit and holds the GPIIb/IIIa receptor in an inactive conformation that does not prime the receptor for fibrinogen binding and does not expose neoepitopes.[134,135] Zalunfiban is under clinical investigation as a SC injection for prehospital administration in patients with ST-elevation myocardial infarction (STEMI).[136]

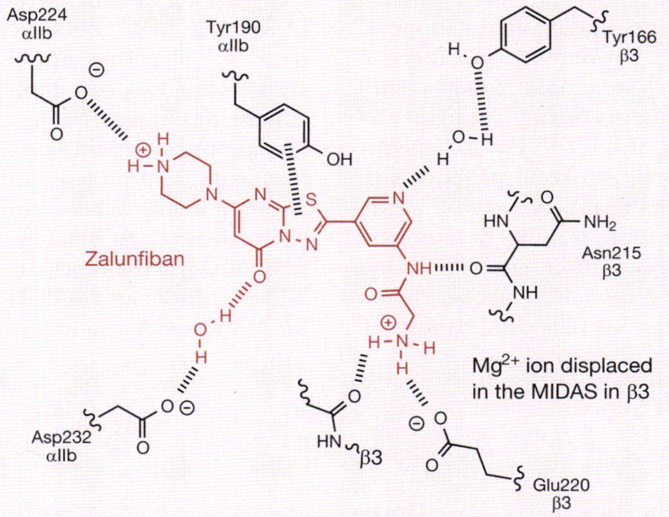

CYP3A5 and CYP2C19 (Fig. 21.18).[139,140] 3,4-Dehydrocilostazol represents 15% of the plasma levels after a single dose and is reported to be approximately 5 times as potent as cilostazol.[137] While active, the 4′-trans-hydroxylcilostazol metabolite is much weaker, with reportedly about 20% the activity of the parent cilostazol.[138] Furthermore, 4′-trans-hydroxycilostazol represents only 4% of the plasma levels.

Contraindication and Boxed Warning. Use of oral milrinone, a PDE3 inhibitor, in the treatment of heart failure has shown an increase in morbidity and mortality.[137,141] Cilostazol and its main metabolites have PDE3 inhibitory activity. Therefore, the clinical studies of cilostazol excluded patients with heart failure.[137] Cilostazol has a boxed warning in the package insert that it is contraindicated in patients with heart failure.[138]

Drug Interactions. Moderate and strong inhibitors of CYP3A4 increase the plasma concentration of cilostazol.[142] Moderate and strong inhibitors of CYP2C19 increase the plasma concentrations of cilostazol and the active metabolite 3,4-dehydrocilostazol.[143] When coadministering

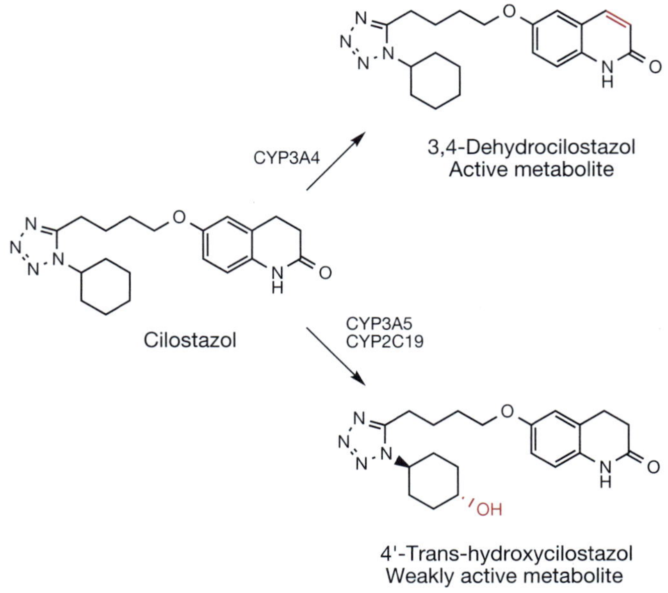

Figure 21.18 Metabolism of cilostazol to active metabolites.

cilostazol with strong or moderate inhibitors of CYP3A4 or CYP2C19, the package insert advises to reduce the dose of cilostazol from 100 mg twice a day to 50 mg twice a day.[138]

Dipyridamole

Dipyridamole, like cilostazol, inhibits cyclic nucleotide PDE3, thereby increasing cellular concentrations of cAMP. It also blocks adenosine uptake. The drug offers little benefit in the treatment of thrombotic conditions.

ANTICOAGULANTS

General Considerations

Anticoagulants are used to prevent a thrombus from forming, anywhere in the body, when a hypercoagulable state exists or to prevent the extension of an existing thrombus. For example, anticoagulants are used to prevent VTE in patients at high risk, this includes patients undergoing orthopedic surgery of the hip or knee,[144,145] patients with cancer,[146] critically ill patients (such as hospitalized patients with COVID19[147]), and in some patients during pregnancy.[148] They are used in the treatment of DVT.[149] Anticoagulants are used to prevent cardioembolic stroke in patients with AF[150] and in patients with mechanical heart values.[151] Atherosclerotic plaque rupture/erosion leading to coronary artery occlusion involves not only platelet aggregation, but also activation of the coagulation cascade. The coagulation cascade is triggered by the release of cells that express TF from the necrotic core of the ruptured plaque and by TF exposed on damaged endothelial cells. TF complexed with factor VIIa activates factor X. A complex of factors Xa, Va, and Ca^{2+} on anionic phospholipid membrane surfaces converts prothrombin to thrombin (factor IIa). Among its many activities, thrombin converts soluble fibrinogen to insoluble fibrin and activates factor XIII which converts fibrin to crosslinked polymers forming the fibrin clot. Therefore, in addition to antiplatelet therapy, parenteral anticoagulation therapy is recommended for all patients with NSTE-ACS to inhibit thrombus propagation.[50] Current anticoagulants target the indirect and direct inactivation of factor Xa and thrombin (factor IIa) and the synthesis of the vitamin K-dependent clotting factors. All anticoagulants currently marketed have a risk of bleeding as an adverse effect.

Heparins

Heparins are mixtures of acidic polymeric sugar fragments, of varying MW, obtained from porcine intestinal mucosa.[152,153] Heparin synthesis occurs in mast cells, where they are attached to a core protein, forming large proteoglycans. Commercial preparations of unfractionated heparin employ proprietary methods to digest and purify the heparin fragments from proteoglycan from the porcine source. The resultant highly sulfated polysaccharide chains, of the glycosaminoglycan (GAG) family, are 1,4-glycosidically linked patterns of D-glucosamine (GlcN), α-L-iduronic acid (IdoA), and β-D-glucuronic acid (GlcA) residues (Fig. 21.19).[152,153] The IdoA and GlcA residues can be sulfated at the 2-position.

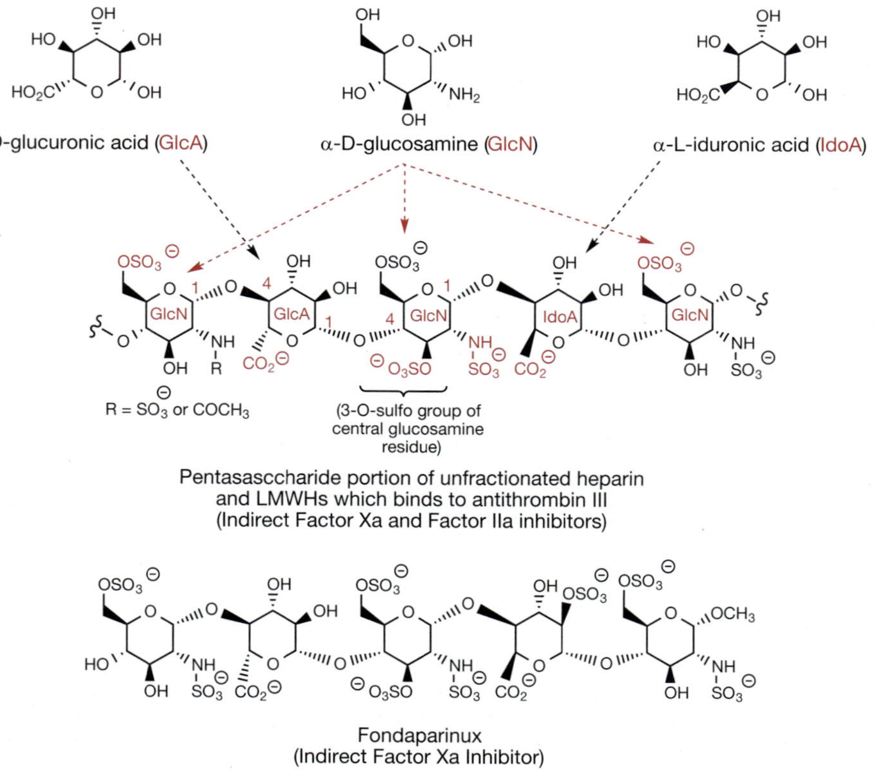

Figure 21.19 Essential pentasaccharide sequence in heparins necessary to bind to antithrombin III and the structure of fondaparinux. The **red bolded anionic groups** are critical for antithrombin III binding, particularly the 3-*O*-sulfo group in the central glucosamine residue. LMWHs, low-molecular-weight heparins.

The GlcN residues can form 3-O-sulfates and/or 6-O-sulfates. The 4-amino group of GlcN can be sulfonated or acetylated.

Unfractionated Heparin

Unfractionated heparin (UFH) is a heterogeneous mixture of fragments with an average MW (MWavg) between 15 and 19 kDa.[153] A MW of 15 kDa is approximately 45 monosaccharide chains.[154] UFH is formulated as standardized activity units measured as United States Pharmacopeia (USP) units/mL.

Mechanism of Action. Heparins indirectly elicit their anticoagulant activity by greatly potentiating the catalytic activity of the serine protease inhibitor ATIII to inactivate factor Xa and factor IIa. Via a specific pentasaccharide sequence (Fig. 21.19), the negative charges on heparin form ionic bonds to positively charged arginine and lysine residues on ATIII.[155] The heparin-ATIII complex produces a conformational change exposing the site on ATIII that interacts primarily with factor Xa and factor IIa, resulting in their inactivation (Fig. 21.20). To a lesser extent, the heparin-ATIII complex also inhibits factors IXa, XIa, and XIIa. The size of the heparin fragment dictates the action the fragment will exhibit. Anti-factor Xa activity requires fragments of at least the essential pentasaccharide unit to bind to ATIII. Heparin fragments of at least 18 saccharide units are required for anti-factor IIa activity. This includes the required pentasaccharide sequence to bind to ATIII along with an additional 13 saccharide units required to bind to thrombin (factor IIa), forming a ternary complex for inactivation.[156] Approximately one-third of the UFH fragments contain the required pentasaccharide sequence and virtually all of these fragments are capable of inactivating factor Xa or factor IIa, resulting in a 1:1 ratio of anti-factor Xa to anti-factor IIa activity. The remaining two-thirds of the dose has minimal anticoagulant activity and contributes to nonspecific binding.

Pharmacokinetics. Due to the large size of its heparin fragments, highly ionized nature, and glycosidic bonds, UFH has poor oral bioavailability and, consequently, it is administered IV and SC. Intramuscular injection of UFH may form

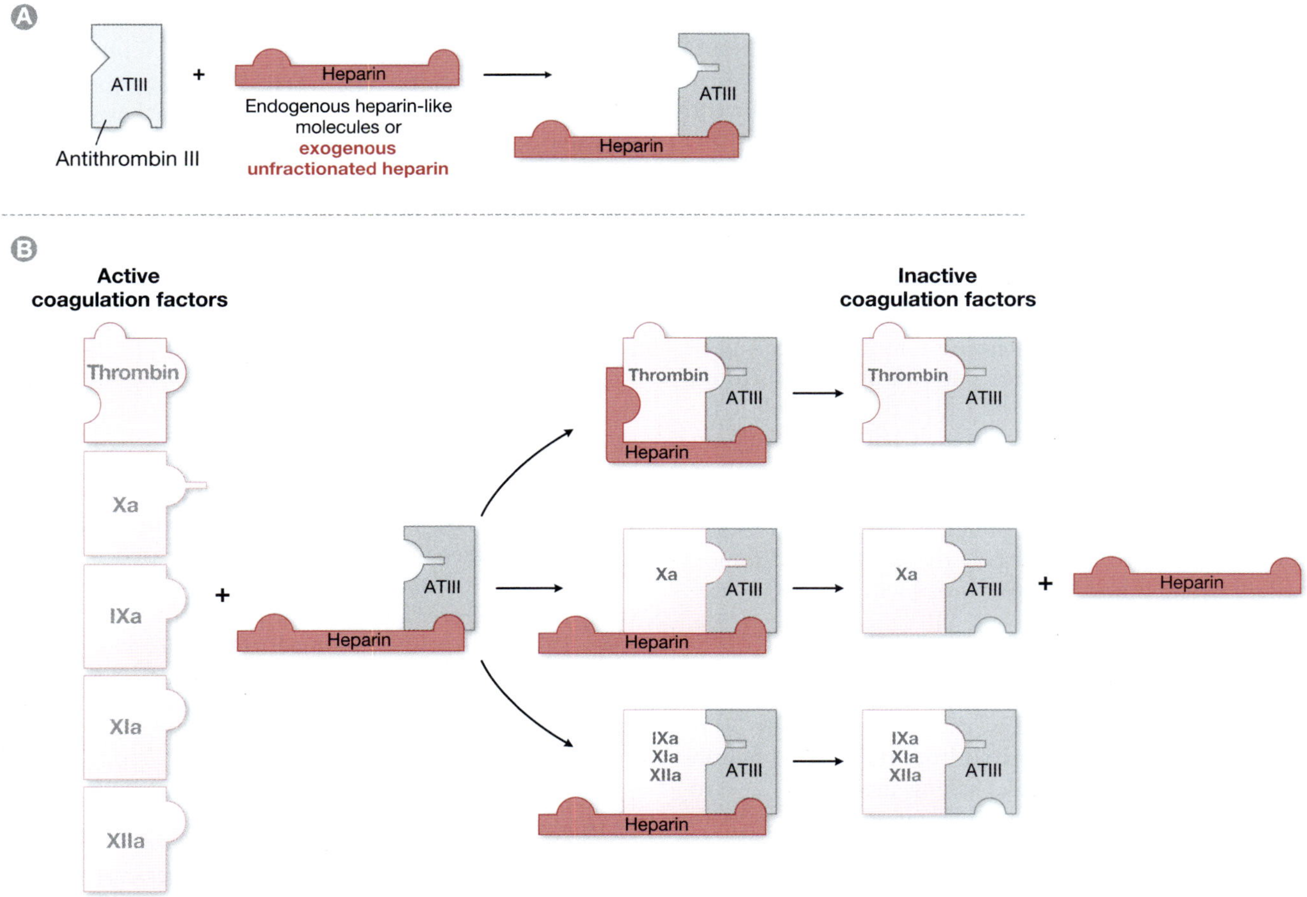

Figure 21.20 Mechanism of action of heparins. Antithrombin III (ATIII) inactivates thrombin and factors IXa, Xa, XIa, and XIIa by forming a stoichiometric complex with these coagulation factors. These reactions are catalyzed physiologically by heparin-like molecules expressed on healthy endothelial cells; sites of vascular injury do not express heparin-like molecules because the endothelium is denuded or damaged. Pharmacologically, these reactions are catalyzed by exogenously administered heparin. In more detail, the binding of heparin to ATIII induces a conformational change at ATIII (A) that allows ATIII to bind thrombin or coagulation factors IXa, Xa, XIa, or XIIa. The stoichiometric complex between ATIII and the coagulation factor is highly stable, allowing heparin to dissociate without breaking up the complex (B). (From Armstrong EJ, Golan DE. Pharmacology of hemostasis and thrombosis. In: Golan DE, Armstrong EJ, Armstrong AW, eds. *Principles of Pharmacology: The Pathophysiological Basis of Drug Therapy*. 4th ed. Wolters-Kluwer; 2017:411, with permission.)

hematoma and should be avoided. When administered SC, the onset of anticoagulation begins at approximately 1 hour and reaches its peak plasma level at approximately 3 hours.[154] For immediate anticoagulant activity, UFH is administered IV. UFH is highly plasma protein bound to a wide variety of plasma proteins, which decreases its bioavailability and contributes to variability in dose response. Longer chain heparins, as in UFH, can even bind to the spike proteins of SARS-CoV-2.[157] The dose-dependent half-life of IV UFH as a continuous infusion varies from 30 to 90 minutes.[158] Clearance of UFH involves two mechanisms. A rapid saturable hepatic uptake mechanism, thought to be due to binding to endothelial cells and macrophages, predominates at therapeutic doses. When UFH binds to endothelial cells and macrophages, it is internalized, depolymerized, and desulfated, respectively.[154,158] The slower nonsaturable mechanism involves renal clearance.[154]

As there is variability in dose response, UFH is monitored using the activated partial thromboplastin time (aPTT) or the anti-factor-Xa (anti-Xa) assay. UFH does not cross the placenta.

Adverse Effects. After bleeding, heparin-induced thrombocytopenia (HIT) is the most important adverse effect associated with UFH. HIT, which is associated with a mortality rate of 20% to 30%, has a prevalence of 0.1% to 5% in patients receiving heparin.[159,160] HIT involves a decline in platelet count after heparin exposure. The longer fragments of UFH participate in nonspecific binding. The mechanism of HIT involves the binding of polyanionic heparin fragments to the cationic platelet factor 4 (PF4) protein released from activated platelets. The formation of the heparin-PF4 complex causes conformational changes, exposing neoepitopes recognized by immunoglobulin G (IgG) antibodies.[159,160] The immune response to the heparin-PF4 complex leads to thrombocytopenia with or without thrombosis. HIT with thrombosis (HITT) is the result of activation of monocytes and platelets, which generates thrombin, platelet-fibrin thrombi, and other procoagulant mediators.

A decline in bone density is also associated with UFH. UFH suppresses osteoblast formation, which leads to activation of osteoclasts.[159] Together, these activities promote bone loss and may lead to osteoporosis with long-term use.

Antidote to heparin toxicity. The highly acidic anionic nature of UFH permits antidotal therapy with protamine sulfate. Protamine sulfate is a mixture of strongly basic arginine-rich cationic peptides, each approximately 30 to 32 amino acids in length, derived from the sperm of chum salmon harvested in Japanese fishing grounds.[161,162] Protamine forms a complex with UFH, via ionic bonds, completely neutralizing its anticoagulant effects by rendering it unable to complex with ATIII.

Protamine sulfate is administered by IV bolus and neutralizes the effects of UFH within 5 minutes after IV injection. The dose of protamine depends on the setting. Empiric dosing is 1 mg of protamine per 100 units of UFH, based on the UFH dose administered in the prior 2 to 3 hours.[162] Excess protamine is to be avoided due to an increased risk of bleeding and transfusions with higher protamine doses and risk of other adverse effects. Adverse effects of protamine include hypotension, pulmonary hypertension, bronchospasm, and anaphylaxis.

Low-Molecular-Weight Heparins

Low-molecular-weight heparin (LMWH) products are obtained from UFH by controlled enzymatic or chemical depolymerization processes. Currently, there are two LMWH products commercially available in the United States: dalteparin and enoxaparin. Dalteparin is produced by a nitrous oxide depolymerization process.[153,163] Enoxaparin is produced by initially forming heparin benzyl ester, followed by an alkaline depolymerization process.[153] Depolymerization processes produce mixtures composed of fragments with an MWavg of about 5,000, approximately a third the MWavg of UFH.[153,163] A comparison of the heparin products is shown in Table 21.5.

Mechanism of action. Due to the smaller fragments, LMWH has fewer fragments that possess the requisite 18 saccharides necessary to elicit anti-factor IIa activity. Only 25% to 50% of LMWH contain fragments with 18 or more saccharide units. Consequently, compared to UFH, LMWH is more selective for anti-factor Xa activity, with dalteparin and enoxaparin exhibiting a 2.7:1 and 3.8:1 ratio of anti-factor Xa to anti-factor IIa activity, respectively.[163] LMWH is administered SC.

Pharmacokinetics. Due to the difference in depolymerization methods, the LMWH products have different pharmacokinetic and pharmacodynamic characteristics. Therefore, LMWH products are not equivalent and are not interchangeable. Due to smaller fragments and less nonspecific binding to plasma proteins than UFH, LMWH is greater than 90% bioavailable upon SC injection and the anticoagulant response is predictable. The half-life of LMWH is 3 to 6 hours after SC administration.[163] This allows fixed doses of LMWH, and it does not require monitoring by coagulation tests. Due to decreased binding to macrophages, LMWH are renally cleared and may require dose reduction in patients with renal dysfunction.

Adverse effects. LMWH is associated with an increased incidence of bleeding. LMWH has decreased binding to PF4 and is associated with a decreased incidence of HIT compared to UFH. LMWH can complex with PF4; therefore, LMWH should be avoided in patients with HIT due to cross-reactivity with HIT antibodies. Also, LMWH has decreased binding to osteoblasts and is associated with less effect on lowering bone density. LMWH does not cross the placenta and is favored over UFH as an anticoagulant in pregnancy due to its predictable response, fewer adverse effects, and overall better safety profile.

Antidote to low-molecular-weight heparin toxicity. The interaction of protamine and heparin is affected by the MW of the heparin fragment. Protamine only partially reverses the anticoagulant effects of LMWH, as protamine does not bind to the smaller heparin fragments within LMWH because they lack a sufficient number of anionic sulfate groups.[159,162] Protamine neutralizes the antithrombin activity of LMWH (larger fragment of at least 18 saccharide units), but only approximately 60% of the anti-factor Xa activity of LMWH.

Table 21.5 Comparison of Heparin Derivatives[153,159,160,163,164]

Characteristics	UFH	Dalteparin	Enoxaparin	Fondaparinux
Tradename	Generic	Fragmin	Lovenox	Arixtra
Method of Preparation	Degradation and purification of porcine intestinal mucosa	Nitrous oxide depolymerization of UFH	Benzyl ester formation, followed by alkaline depolymerization of UFH	Chemical synthesis
MWavg (Da)	15,000	6,000	4,200	1,508—free acid
Route of administration	IV, SC	SC	SC	SC
Ratio anti-FXa/ anti-FIIa activity	1	2.7	3.8	Anti-FXa only
$t_{1/2}$	60-90 min (dose dependent)	3-6 h	3-6 h	17 h
Excretion	Reticuloendothelial system	Renal	Renal	Renal
Monitoring	aPTT, anti-Factor Xa assay, ACT during PCI	NA	NA	NA
Antidote	Complete reversal with protamine sulfate	Partial reversal with protamine sulfate	Partial reversal with protamine sulfate	None
Incidence of HIT	<5%	<1%	<1%	No

ACT, activated clotting time; anti-FXa, anti-factor Xa; anti-FIIa, anti-factor IIa; aPTT, activated partial thromboplastin time; HIT, heparin-induced thrombocytopenia; IV, intravenous; MWavg, molecular weight average; PCI, percutaneous coronary intervention; SC, subcutaneous, UFH, unfractionated heparin.

Factor Xa Inhibitors

Indirect Factor Xa Inhibitor

FONDAPARINUX. Fondaparinux (Fig. 21.19) is a synthetic analog modeled on the pentasaccharide sequence in heparin responsible for binding to ATIII. It is categorized as an ultra-low-molecular-weight heparin (ULMWH). As it has the required ATIII-binding pentasaccharide sequence only, it is too short to have anti-factor IIa activity (Table 21.5). Therefore, fondaparinux exclusively elicits anti-factor Xa activity. Like the heparins, fondaparinux indirectly inhibits factor Xa by binding to ATIII and increasing the catalytic activity of ATIII to inactivate factor Xa.

Pharmacokinetics. The pentasaccharide sequence of fondaparinux avoids nonspecific binding to plasma proteins and is more potent than UFH because it has a higher affinity for ATIII. Fondaparinux is 94% bound to plasma ATIII.[164] It is administered SC and has a $t_{1/2}$ of 17 hours, allowing once daily dosing. The dose response is predictable, and laboratory coagulation monitoring is not required with fondaparinux. Fondaparinux is excreted by the kidneys unchanged. Therefore, it is contraindicated in patients with a glomerular filtration rate less than 30 mL/h.

Adverse effects. The primary adverse effect of fondaparinux is bleeding. Due to exclusive renal clearance, the risk of bleeding increases with renal dysfunction. There are very few cases of HIT associated with fondaparinux. Protamine has no effect on fondaparinux, due to the small size of the pentasaccharide sequence.[162]

Direct Factor Xa Inhibitors

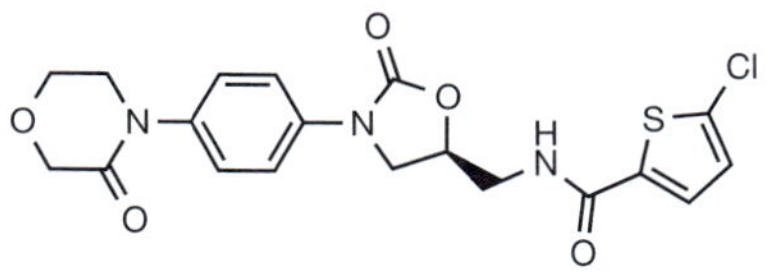

Rivaroxaban (Xarelto)

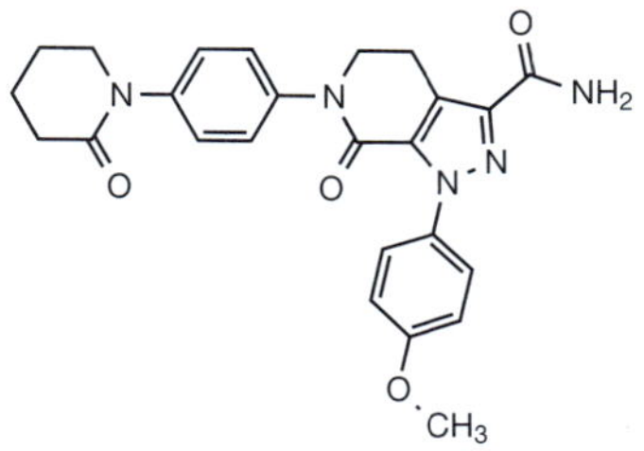

Apixaban (Eliquis)

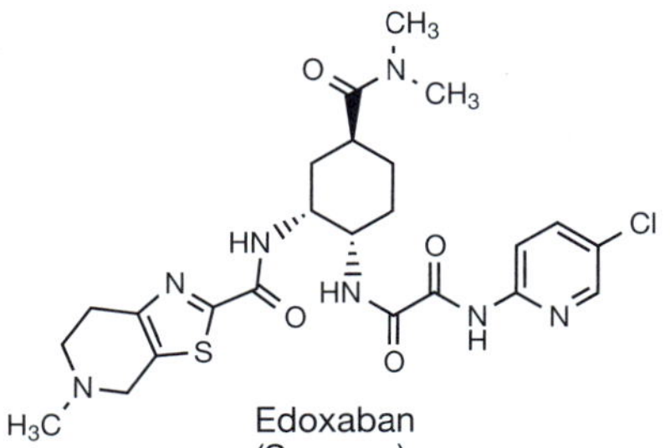

Edoxaban (Savaysa)

The direct factor Xa inhibitors currently marketed are rivaroxaban, apixaban, and edoxaban. The direct factor Xa inhibitors are oral drugs included in a classification called direct oral anticoagulants (DOACs).

Factor Xa is a trypsin-like serine protease. Within the prothrombinase complex of phospholipids, calcium ions and factor Va as the cofactor, factor Xa cleaves prothrombin at two sites, Arg320 and Arg271, to liberate thrombin. Nomenclature for a protease enzyme active site, such as in factor Xa, follows a convention initially described by Schechter and Berger.[165] It assumes that there are complementary binding sites within the protease active site that match the salient amino acid residues flanking each side of the peptide bond, which will be hydrolyzed in the natural substrate (Fig. 21.21). The amino acid residues from the labile peptide bond of the substrate are indicated by P1, P2, P3, P4, etc. going toward the amino-terminus, and P1′, P2′, P3′, P4′, etc. going toward the carboxy terminus of the natural substrate. Each amino acid side chain flanking the peptide bond to be cleaved is assumed to bind to a matching subsite within the catalytic site of the protease. The subsites are labeled S1, S2, S3, S4 and S1′, S2′, S3′, S4′ to match their counterpart amino acid on the substrate.

All three direct factor Xa inhibitors have been designed to accommodate the S1 and S4 pockets of the factor Xa active site.

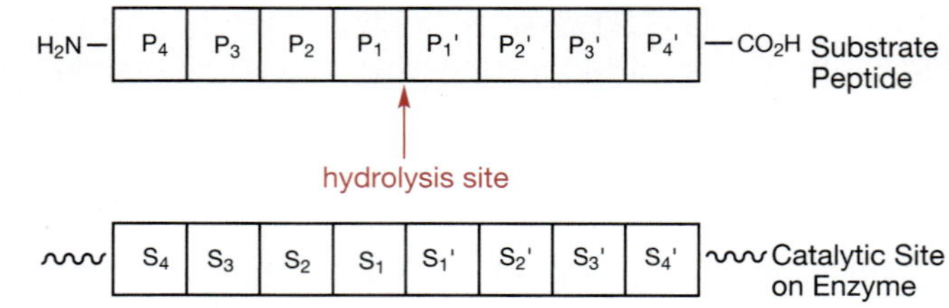

Figure 21.21 Nomenclature for peptide substrate binding to protease active site.

STRUCTURE-ACTIVITY RELATIONSHIP. The S1 pocket of factor Xa is predominantly hydrophobic.[166] The side chain of Tyr228, within the S1 pocket, is important for binding to the factor Xa inhibitors. The S4 pocket is a hydrophobic channel. The key amino acid residues in the S4 pocket important for factor Xa inhibitor binding include Tyr99, Phe174, and Trp215. In general, the factor Xa inhibitors possess a central scaffold ring system that orients functional groups into the S1 and S4 pockets (Fig. 21.22).

Rivaroxaban. Rivaroxaban was the first oral direct factor Xa inhibitor to be FDA approved. As shown in Figure 21.22, the central oxazolidinone ring of rivaroxaban forms a hydrogen bond between the carbonyl group of the oxazolidine ring and amino group of Gly219.[167] The *S*-enantiomer of the oxazolidinone ring is critical, as it allows the carbonyl oxygen of Gly219 to form a second hydrogen bond with the nitrogen of the amide within the S1 arm of rivaroxaban. This situates the chlorothiophene ring into the S1 pocket, where the chloro substituent interacts with the Tyr228 side chain. This interaction is key in conferring oral bioavailability to rivaroxaban.[168]

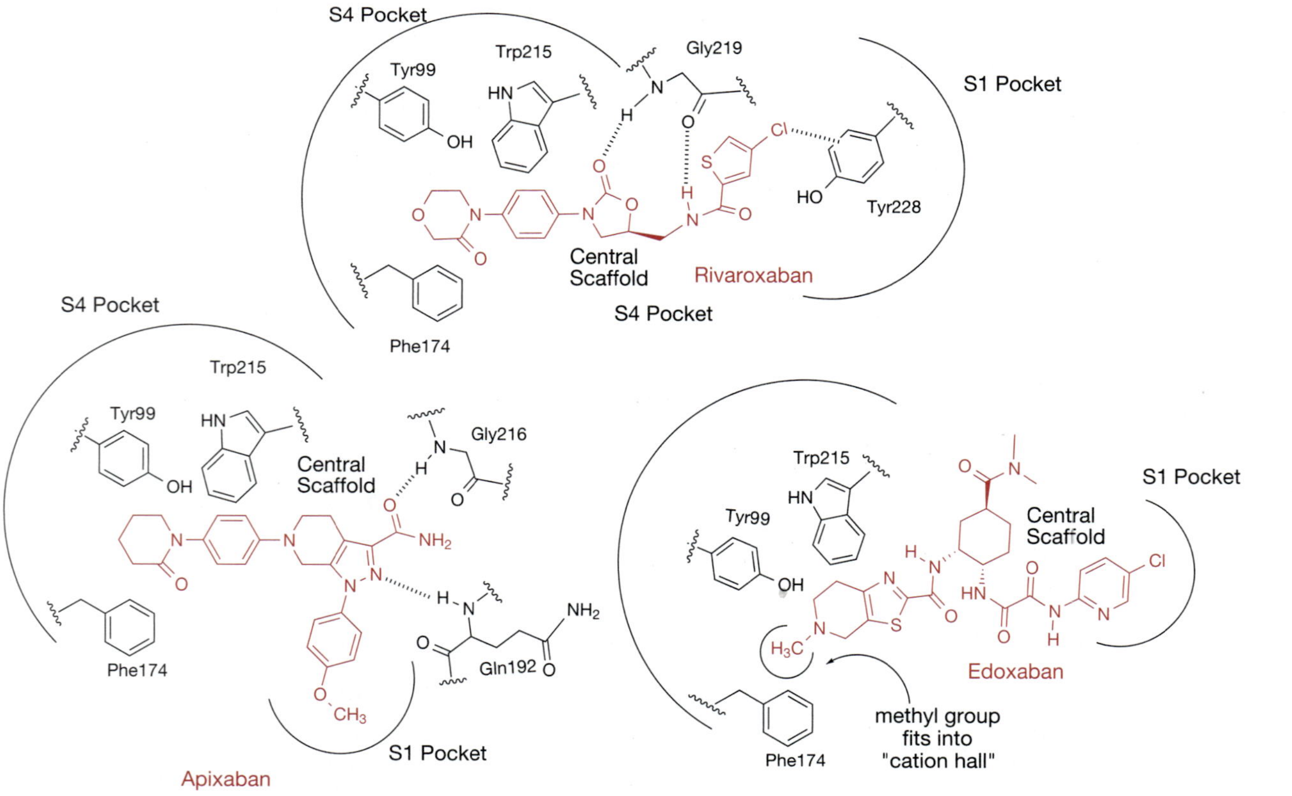

Figure 21.22 Binding of direct factor Xa inhibitors to the factor Xa active site.[166-170] Key amino acids residues/subsites within the factor Xa active site that interact with rivaroxaban, apixaban, and edoxaban are shown in black.

The morpholinone ring of rivaroxaban is situated within the S4 pocket, where it is sandwiched between the side chains of Tyr99 and Phe174.[167] The carbonyl of the morpholinone ring is critical, as the morpholine derivative lacking the carbonyl group is 60 times less potent.[167] The phenyl ring adjacent to morpholinone ring is noncoplanar and extends across the aromatic ring of Trp215.

Apixaban. The central scaffold ring system in apixaban is a unique bicyclic tetrahydropyrazolopyridinone (Fig. 21.22).[169] This bicyclic ring system has minimal interaction with the factor Xa active site, with the pyrazole *N*-2 nitrogen forming a hydrogen bond with the backbone NH of Gln192. The carbonyl oxygen of the carboxamido group at the C-3 position of the pyrazole forms another hydrogen bond with the backbone NH group of Gly216. The central bicyclic ring system orients the *p*-methoxyphenyl group into the S1 pocket. Similar to the morpholinone ring of rivaroxaban, the 6-membered lactam ring of apixaban nestles between Tyr99 and Phe174, while the adjacent phenyl ring is positioned along Trp215. The carbonyl ring of the lactam insures an orthogonal relationship, with the adjacent phenyl ring being key to the optimal fit in the S4 pocket.[169]

Edoxaban. The central scaffold ring system in edoxaban is a cis-1,2-diaminocyclohexane derivative with a dimethylamide group (Fig. 21.22).[170] This positions the 5-chloropyridine-2-yloxalamide group into the S1 pocket and the unique methyltetrahydrothiazolo[5,4-c]pyridine group into the S4 pocket.[166] The tetrahydrothiazolo[5,4-c]pyridine moiety is sandwiched between Tyr99 and Phe174 of the S4 pocket, and the methyl group off the tetrahydropyridine nitrogen fits into what is referred to as the "cation hall" of the S4 pocket.[170] Edoxaban is the only oral direct factor Xa inhibitor that possesses a basic site. It is formulated as the tosylate salt.

METABOLISM

Apixaban Metabolism. Apixaban metabolites represent about 25% of the recovered dose.[171] The main metabolite of apixaban, M1, is the sulfate conjugate of the O-demethylated metabolite, M2 (Fig. 21.23).[171,172] M1 represents about 25% of the area under the curve (AUC) of the parent apixaban, and it is inactive. The remaining minor metabolites, each less than 1%, include O-demethylapixaban (M2), hydroxylapixaban (M7, hydroxylated on the terminal 6-membered lactam ring), and the sulfate conjugate of M7 (M10).

Edoxaban Metabolism. Edoxaban is primarily excreted unchanged. Upon oral administration, approximately 50% of absorbed edoxaban is excreted unchanged in the urine, and 40% is excreted unchanged in the bile.[173-175] The remaining approximately 10% of a dose of edoxaban is metabolized either via hydrolysis, CYP3A4/5, or glucuronidation.[173,174] The major metabolite is the hydrolysis product M4 (Fig. 21.24).[173,174] M4 represents less than 10% of the dose in the plasma. While M4 has anticoagulant activity, it is highly protein bound (80%), and due to its low level, it is not expected to contribute to the pharmacologic effect of edoxaban under normal to moderate renal function.

Rivaroxaban Metabolism. Following oral administration, about 43% of a dose of rivaroxaban is excreted unchanged in the urine (36%) and in feces (7%).[176] P-glycoprotein (P-gp) and breast cancer–resistance protein (BCRP [ABCG2]) are involved with the active renal secretion of rivaroxaban. Over 28% of a dose is excreted in the urine and 17% in the feces as metabolites. The main metabolite excreted both

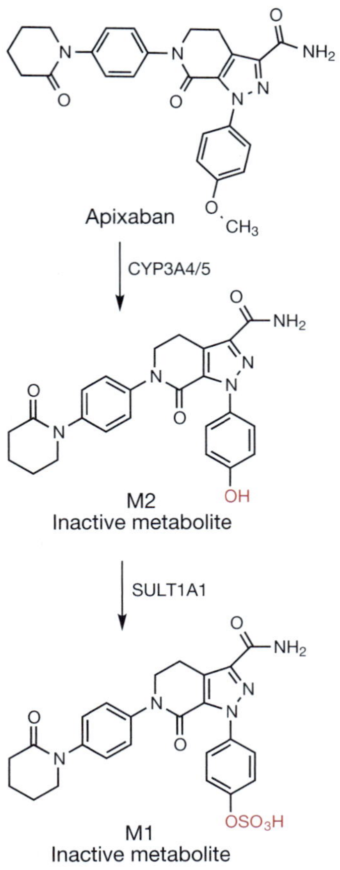

Figure 21.23 Metabolism of apixaban.

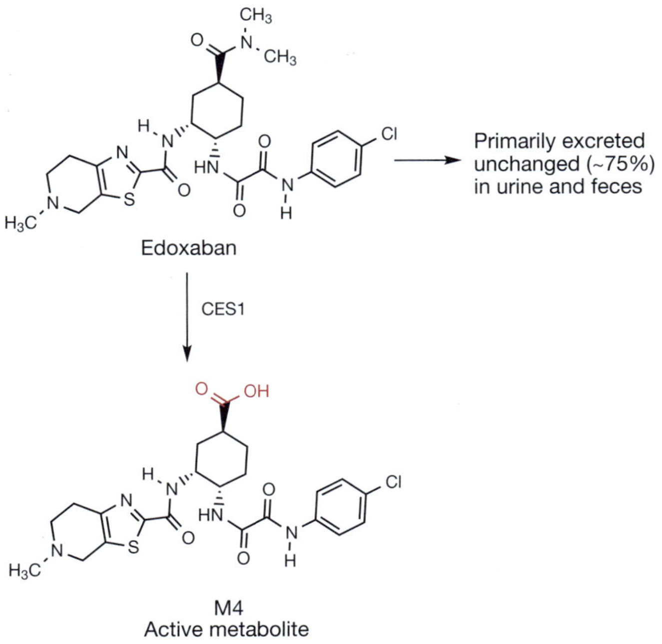

Figure 21.24 Metabolism of edoxaban.

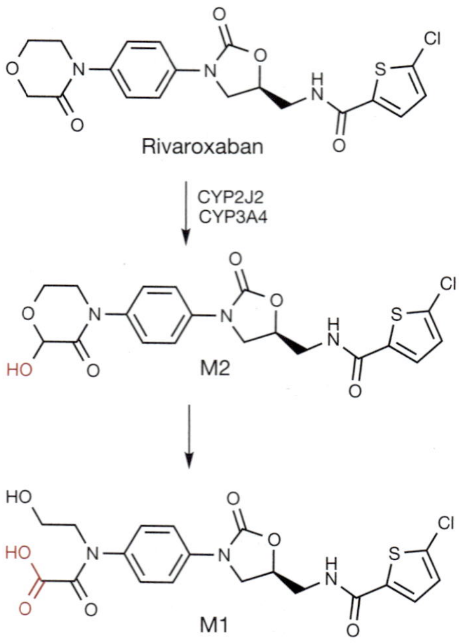

Figure 21.25 Metabolism of rivaroxaban.

in urine (13.1%) and feces (8.9%) is M1 (Fig. 21.25).[177] CYP2J2 and CYP3A4 are the predominant isoforms responsible for M1 formation, with CYP2J2 being the most important.[178]

Pharmacokinetics. The oral bioavailability of apixaban is 51%.[172] Apixaban exists primarily in the plasma unchanged (~70%), and protein binding is 87%. The volume of distribution (V_d) is 21 L, and the terminal elimination half-life is 8 to 13 hours after oral administration. The usual dose of apixaban is 5 mg twice daily for the reduction of stroke and systemic embolism risk in patients with nonvalvular AF.[179] The recommended dose of apixaban is reduced to 2.5 mg twice daily in AF patients, with at least two of the following three characteristics: age of 80 years or older, body weight of 60 kg or less, and serum creatinine greater of 1.5 mg/dL or higher.[179,180] These three characteristics are associated with increased risk of bleeding.[180] In Europe, apixaban is not recommended in patients with creatinine clearance (CrCl) less than 15 mg/mL nor in patients on dialysis.[180] Apixaban is a substrate for CYP3A4/5 and P-gp; therefore, dosage should be decreased with coadministration of strong inhibitors of CYP3A4/5 and P-gp.[172] Apixaban is also a substrate for the BCRP (ABCG2).

The oral bioavailability of edoxaban is 62%.[174] Protein binding of edoxaban is 55%. The V_d is larger than the other two oral factor Xa inhibitors at 107 L, and the elimination half-life is 10 to 14 hours.[174,175] Edoxaban is a substrate for P-gp. For stroke and systemic embolism risk reduction in patients with nonvalvular AF and in the treatment of DVT and PE, the usual dose of edoxaban of 60 mg once daily is recommended to be reduced to 30 mg once daily in patients with CrCl between 15 and 50 mL/min.[181] For the treatment of DVT and PE, the dose should also be reduced in patients who weigh 60 kg or less and in patients taking a strong P-gp inhibitor.[174,175,181] Edoxaban is not recommended in patients with CrCl less than 15 mL/min, due to an increased risk of bleeding. It should also not be used in patients with a CrCl greater than 95 mL/min due to decreased efficacy.[171,181]

Rivaroxaban oral absorption is enhanced when taken with food. The oral bioavailability of rivaroxaban is 80% to 100%, and 92% to 95% is plasma protein bound.[176] Following oral administration, unchanged rivaroxaban is the main compound in the plasma (~90%). The V_d is approximately 50 L, and the elimination half-life of rivaroxaban is 5 to 9 hours.[176] The usual adult recommended dose of rivaroxaban for reduction in risk of stroke in patients in nonvalvular AF is reduced in patients with CrCl of 50 mL/min or less.[182] No dosage adjustment is necessary based on CrCl for reduction of risk of major cardiovascular events in CAD or in reduction of risk of major thrombotic vascular events in PAD. Rivaroxaban is not recommended for use in the treatment or prophylaxis of VTE or PE in patients with CrCl less than 15 mL/min. Pediatric dosing of rivaroxaban is weight-based. Rivaroxaban is a substrate for CYP3A4/5 and P-gp; therefore, coadministration of strong inhibitors of CYP3A4/5 and P-gp should be avoided.[176] Rivaroxaban is also a substrate for the BCRP (ABCG2) transporter.[176]

Like all anticoagulants, the main adverse effect of direct factor Xa inhibitors is bleeding. Table 21.6 is a comparison of pharmacokinetic, physicochemical, and other characteristics of the three direct factor Xa inhibitors.[179,181,182]

Reversal Agent for Rivaroxaban and Apixaban. Andexanet alfa (Andexxa) is an inactivated recombinant coagulation factor Xa product. It is FDA approved for the treatment of rivaroxaban or apixaban toxicity when reversal of anticoagulation is needed due to life-threatening or uncontrolled bleeding. Andexanet alfa is a truncated form of enzymatically inactive human factor Xa.[186] It is catalytically inactive due to a mutation of the serine residue in the protease catalytic triad, which has been substituted with alanine. This renders the protein unable to cleave and activate prothrombin. The modified recombinant protein also lacks the membrane-binding γ-carboxyglutamate domain, which eliminates its ability to bind calcium and assemble into the prothrombinase complex; therefore, it cannot act as a competitive inhibitor of the prothrombinase complex. Andexanet alfa does retain the factor Xa active site, and it can bind to factor Xa inhibitors. Therefore, andexanet alfa acts as a human factor Xa decoy. Factor Xa inhibitors bind to the binding site on andexanet alfa, to a similar affinity as they do to native factor Xa, circumventing their ability to bind to factor Xa. Binding to andexanet alfa reverses the anticoagulant effect of rivaroxaban and apixaban. It is administered IV as a bolus over 15 to 30 minutes followed by an infusion over 2 hours.[187] The anti-factor Xa activity of apixaban and rivaroxaban dramatically decreases at the end of the bolus dose.

Andexanet alfa is formulated as a lyophilized powder for injection in 200 mg vials. The low dose regimen of andexanet alfa requires five vials, and the high dose regimen requires nine vials. Andexxa is sold as a five-vial pack with 200 mg/vial at a wholesale acquisition cost (WAC) of $12,500 for five vials.[188]

Table 21.6 Comparison of Direct Factor Xa Inhibitors[171-182]

Characteristic	Apixaban	Edoxaban	Rivaroxaban
Route of administration	Oral	Oral	Oral
Approved Indications	• Reduction of risk of stroke and systemic embolism in nonvalvular AF • Prophylaxis for DVT and PE following hip or knee replacement surgery • Treatment of DVT and PE • Reduction in the risk of recurrence of DVT and PE	• Reduction of risk of stroke and systemic embolism in nonvalvular AF • Treatment of DVT and PE	• Reduction of risk of stroke and systemic embolism in nonvalvular AF • Treatment of DVT and PE • Reduction in the risk of recurrence of DVT and/or PE • Prophylaxis for DVT and PE following hip or knee replacement surgery • Prophylaxis of VTE in acutely ill medical patients at risk for thromboembolic complications not at high risk of bleeding • Reduction of risk of major CV events in patients with CAD • Reduction of risk of major thrombotic vascular events in patients with PAD • Treatment of VTE and reduction of risk of recurrent VTE in pediatric patients • Thromboprophylaxis in pediatric patients with congenital heart disease after the Fontan procedure
MW (Da)	459.5	548.1	435.9
cLogP[a]	2.2	1.4	2.5
pK_a	Neutral	6.7	Neutral
FXa K_i (nM)	0.08	0.56	0.4
Oral Bioavailability (%)	51	62	80-100
Protein Binding (%)	~87%	55	92-95
V_d (L)	~21	107	~50
Elimination half-life (h)	8-13	10-14	5-9
Major Route(s) of elimination (%)	Urine unchanged ~22 Feces unchanged 34	Urine unchanged 50 Bile unchanged 40	Urine unchanged ~36 Feces unchanged 7
Metabolism (%)	~25	~10	~46

AF, atrial fibrillation; CAD, coronary artery disease; CV, cardiovascular; DVT, deep vein thrombosis; FXa, factor Xa; MW, molecular weight; PAD, peripheral artery disease; PE, pulmonary embolism; V_d, volume of distribution; VTE, venous thromboembolism.

[a]PubChem[183-185]

Direct Thrombin Inhibitors

Whereas heparin inhibits free thrombin, direct thrombin inhibitors can inhibit both free and fibrin-bound thrombin. As their name implies, direct thrombin inhibitors bind directly to thrombin and do not require binding to ATIII to elicit their activity. There are three domains on thrombin: the catalytic site (active site), exosite 1, which binds to substrates such as fibrin, and exosite 2, which is a heparin binding site. Bivalent direct thrombin inhibitors bind to both the thrombin active site and exosite 1. Univalent direct thrombin inhibitors bind only to the thrombin active site. There are three direct thrombin inhibitors currently available; two are intravenous and one is an oral prodrug. There is an increased risk of bleeding with direct thrombin inhibitors.

Bivalirudin

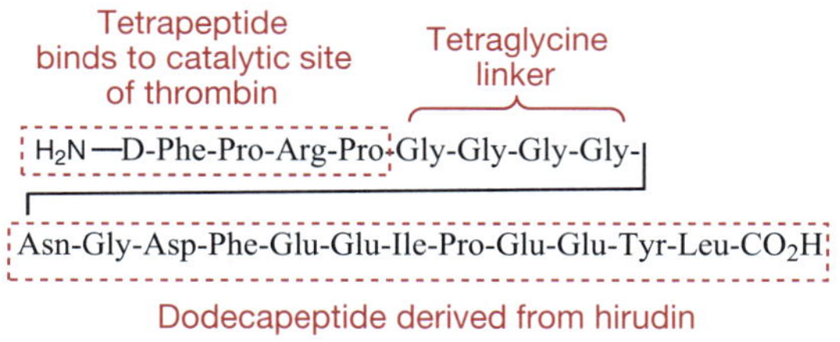

Bivalirudin (Angiomax)

Bivalirudin is a 20-amino acid peptide that acts as a bivalent direct thrombin inhibitor and causes noncompetitive inhibition. Bivalirudin is composed of an N-terminal tetrapeptide that binds to the thrombin catalytic site linked, via

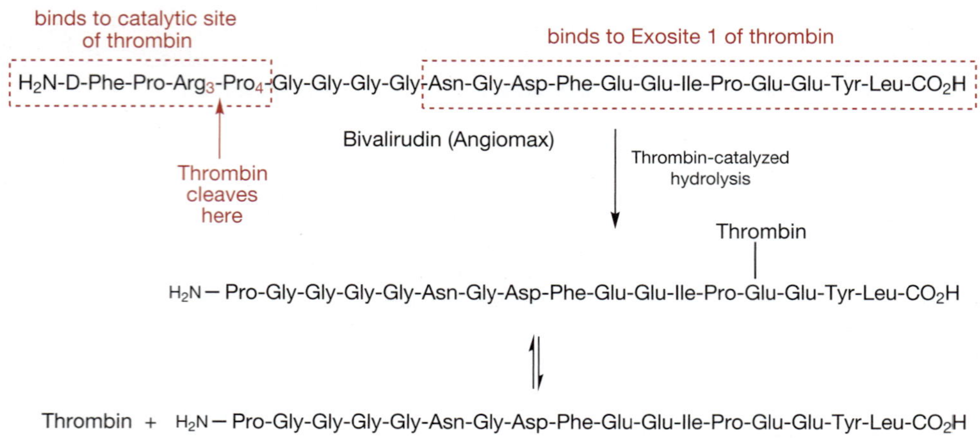

Figure 21.26 Bivalirudin mechanism of action.

four glycine residues, to a C-terminal dodecapeptide derived from hirudin.[189] The direct thrombin inhibitor hirudin is a 65-amino acid protein isolated from the medicinal leech, *Hirudo medicinalis*.[190] After binding to the active site and to exosite 1 of thrombin, bivalirudin is cleaved by thrombin between Arg3 and Pro4 (Fig. 21.26).[189] Upon cleavage, the N-terminus tripeptide dissociates from the thrombin active site, reducing the affinity of the C-terminus dodecapeptide for exosite 1 and converting the remaining peptide to a competitive inhibitor of thrombin. Other substrates, such as fibrinogen, can displace the remnant peptide from exosite 1 regenerating active thrombin.

Bivalirudin is administered intravenously as a bolus followed by continuous infusion for anticoagulation during PCI. It may be used in patients with HIT and HITT. Bivalirudin is monitored with the aPTT. The activated clotting time (ACT) may be used to monitor bivalirudin during the PCI procedure. The half-life of bivalirudin is 25 minutes,[191] which is the shortest plasma half-life of the parenteral anticoagulants. Bivalirudin is mostly hydrolyzed in vivo to inactive metabolites which are renally excreted. Approximately 20% of bivalirudin is excreted unchanged in the urine. Dosing is reduced in patients with renal impairment. There is no reversal agent for bivalirudin.

Argatroban

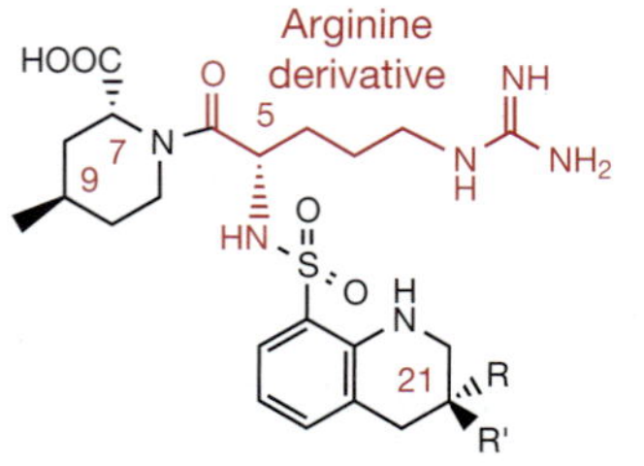

R = CH_3, R' = H: 21*R*-Argatroban
R = H, R' = CH_3: 21*S*-Argatroban

The arginine derivative argatroban is a univalent direct thrombin inhibitor. It is a diastereomeric mixture in a 64:36 ratio of 21*R*- and 21*S*-epimers.[192,193] While both epimers are active thrombin inhibitors, 21*S*-argatroban is twice as potent as 21*R*-argatroban. It is indicated for use in the prevention and treatment of thrombosis in patients with HIT and as an anticoagulant in patients with or at high risk of HIT undergoing PCI.

Argatroban is administered IV as a continuous infusion. It is monitored via the aPTT. The ACT may be used to monitor argatroban during the PCI procedure. The half-life of argatroban is about 46 minutes.[194] Argatroban undergoes hepatic metabolism to M1, the major metabolite (Fig. 21.27).[195] M1, which represents 0% to 20% of the plasma concentration of the parent argatroban, is an active metabolite that retains 20% to 30% of the anticoagulant activity of argatroban.[195,196] CYP3A4/5 is thought to be the enzyme responsible for argatroban hepatic metabolism, although erythromycin does not affect argatroban plasma levels.[194] Approximately 23% and 12% of a dose of argatroban is excreted unchanged in the urine and feces, respectively, within the first 24 hours.[197] Hepatic dysfunction increases plasma concentrations of argatroban and requires dose reduction.[194,196] Argatroban dosing does not require adjustment in patients with renal dysfunction.[194,196]

Argatroban artificially increases the prothrombin time (PT) international normalized ratio (INR) value, which presents a challenge for accurate anticoagulation when the patient is bridged from argatroban to the oral vitamin K antagonist anticoagulant warfarin.[198] There is no reversal agent for argatroban.

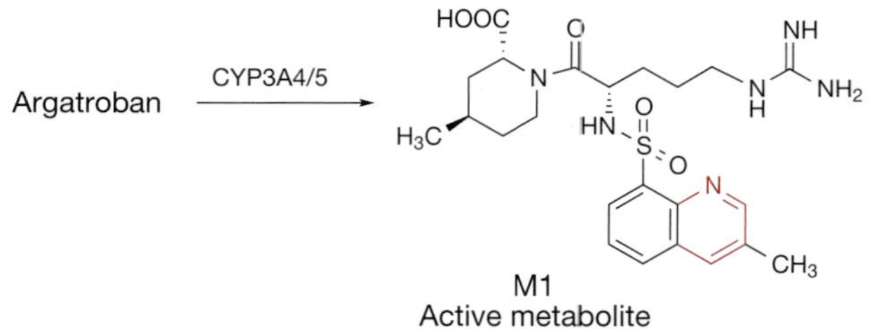

Figure 21.27 Main route of metabolism of argatroban.

Dabigatran Etexilate

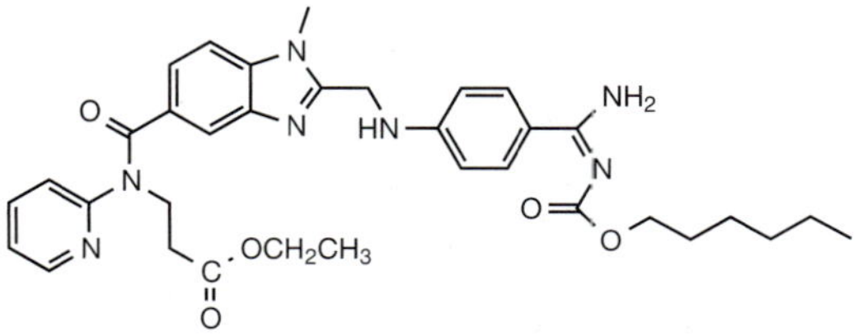

Dabigatran etexilate
(Pradaxa)

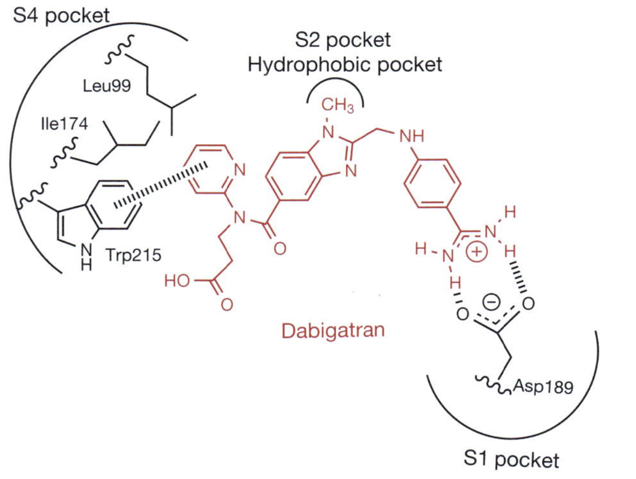

Figure 21.28 Dabigatran, the active form of the prodrug dabigatran etexilate, binding within the thrombin active site. Key amino acid residues within the thrombin active site which interact with dabigatran are shown in black.

Dabigatran etexilate is an oral prodrug of the univalent direct thrombin inhibitor dabigatran. Dabigatran etexilate is categorized as a DOAC, along with the direct factor Xa inhibitors. Dabigatran, the active compound, takes advantage of the S1, S2, and S4 pockets of the thrombin active site (Fig. 21.28).[199] The benzimidazole core ring was found to be an ideal template to direct three key substituents into their correct positions within the S1, S2, and S4 pockets. The active site of thrombin has some similarities to the factor Xa active site. For example, the S1 pocket of thrombin possesses an Asp189 residue. The amidine group of dabigatran forms a bidentate salt bridge with the carboxylate group of Asp189.[199,200] The two atom methylene amino linker between the benzimidazole and the benzamidine ring was the optimal length to position the benzamidine group into the S1 pocket.[199] The remaining binding interactions between dabigatran and the thrombin active site are hydrophobic interactions. The central benzimidazole ring forms hydrophobic interactions with the S2 pocket, while the N-methyl group on the benzimidazole ring nestles perfectly into a small hydrophobic pocket within the S2 pocket.[199,200] In fact, increasing the size of the N-methyl group to ethyl or *n*-propyl reduces activity. The S4 pocket prefers binding to aromatic rings. The carboxamide linker between the benzimidazole and pyridine ring of dabigatran positioned the pyridine ring into the shallow S4 pocket well.[199,200] The pyridine ring is positioned between Leu99 and Ile174 and forms an edge to face π–π interaction with the Trp215 residue in the S4 pocket.[199,200] The propionic acid moiety projects out of the thrombin binding site toward the solvent exposed S3 pocket.[199,200] The carboxylic acid of dabigatran is not interacting with the thrombin active site.[199,200] Studies of thrombin inhibitors showed that the more lipophilic the inhibitor, the greater the decrease in activity, presumably due to increased protein binding.[199] Therefore, the carboxylic acid moiety was added to increase hydrophilicity which decreased protein binding and increased activity; the propionic acid derivative proved optimal.[199]

Dabigatran exists as a zwitterion in the small intestine with the carboxylic acid (pK_a 4.4) and the strongly basic amidine group (pK_a 12.4).[201] It is highly polar with a $\log D_{7.4}$ of −0.6; consequently, it has poor oral absorption and is inactive orally.[202] Therefore, the double prodrug dabigatran etexilate was designed to achieve oral activity. Dabigatran etexilate incorporates an ethyl ester to mask the carboxylic acid, and the amidino group is masked as an *n*-hexylcarbamate increasing the lipophilicity ($\log D_{7.4}$ of 3.7).[199,203]

Metabolism. Upon oral administration, the principal route of metabolism of dabigatran etexilate is sequential hydrolysis to the active metabolite dabigatran (Fig. 21.29).[203] This hydrolysis is rapid and complete and involves two intermediates, BIBR951 and BIBR1087, the result of carbamate hydrolysis and ester hydrolysis, respectively, via serine esterases. The carbamate of dabigatran etexilate is hydrolyzed via intestinal hCE2 to the intermediate BIBR951, followed by ester hydrolysis via hepatic hCE1 to the active metabolite dabigatran.[204] The alternate route of activation of dabigatran etexilate involves hydrolysis of the ethyl ester via hepatic hCE1 to the intermediate BIBR1087, followed by carbamate hydrolysis via hepatic hCE2 to liberate dabigatran.[204]

Approximately 20% of dabigatran is conjugated via glucuronosyltranferases (UGT), primarily UGT2B15, to the active metabolite dabigatran 1-*O*-acylglucuronide (M648) (Fig. 21.29).[202] M648 is unstable and isomerizes to form the 2-*O*-acylglucuronide, the 3-*O*-acylglucuronide, and the 4-*O*-acylglucuronide of dabigatran (Fig. 21.30).[202,205] Dabigatran 1-*O*-acylglucuronide also condenses with urea to form M690.[203] All dabigatran acylglucuronide metabolites are active with antithrombin potency similar to the parent dabigatran. This is a rare example where the glucuronide metabolite has activity. The reason is that the carboxylate moiety of dabigatran does not interact with the binding site of thrombin, but rather is directed outside the thrombin binding site. Therefore, the acylglucuronides do not interfere with thrombin binding.[202]

Pharmacokinetics. The oral bioavailability of dabigatran etexilate is approximately 7%.[203] The plasma protein binding of dabigatran is approximately 35%. Upon oral administration of dabigatran etexilate, the plasma concentration of dabigatran occurs after approximately 1.5 hours. The half-life of dabigatran is 12 to 17 hours.[206] Approximately 80% of dabigatran is excreted unchanged in the urine after IV administration.[203] Less than 4% is excreted as acylglucuronides and derivatives after IV administration.[203] The usual adult recommended dose of dabigatran etexilate for reduction in risk of stroke in patients in nonvalvular AF is 150 mg twice daily and is dependent on renal function.[207,208] The dose is reduced to 75 mg twice daily in patients with CrCl from 15 to 30 mL/min. It is not recommended in patients with CrCl less than 15 mL/min or on dialysis. For the treatment of DVT and PE, prophylaxis of VTE after hip replacement surgery, or to reduce the risk of recurrence of DVT and PE, dosage is not recommended in patients with CrCl of 30 mL/min or less or on dialysis. Dabigatran etexilate is a P-gp substrate. Concomitant administration of P-gp inhibitors increases exposure of dabigatran, requiring a dose reduction or avoiding use depending on renal function.[208]

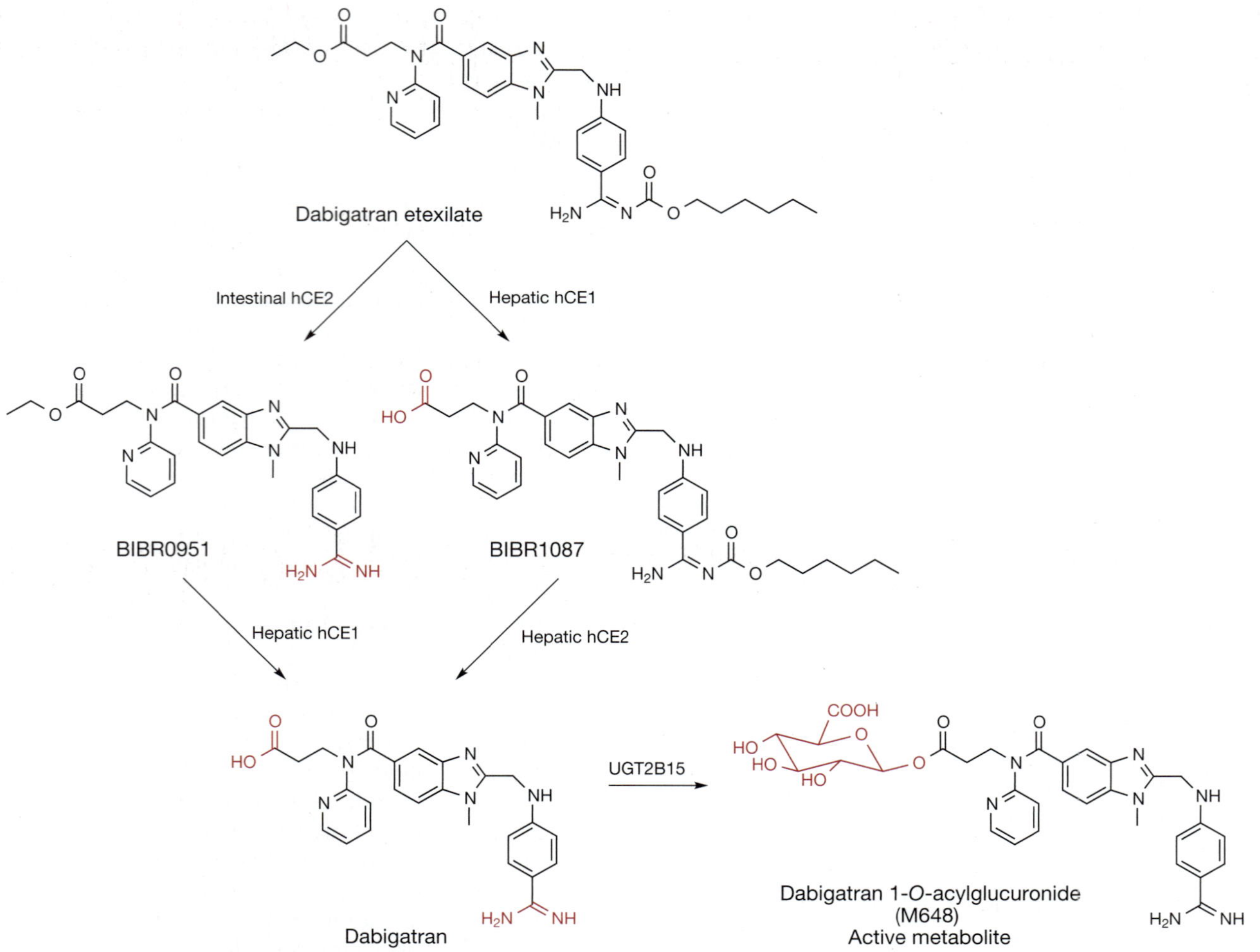

Figure 21.29 Metabolism of dabigatran etexilate. hCE1, human carboxylesterase 1; hCE2, human carboxylesterase 2.

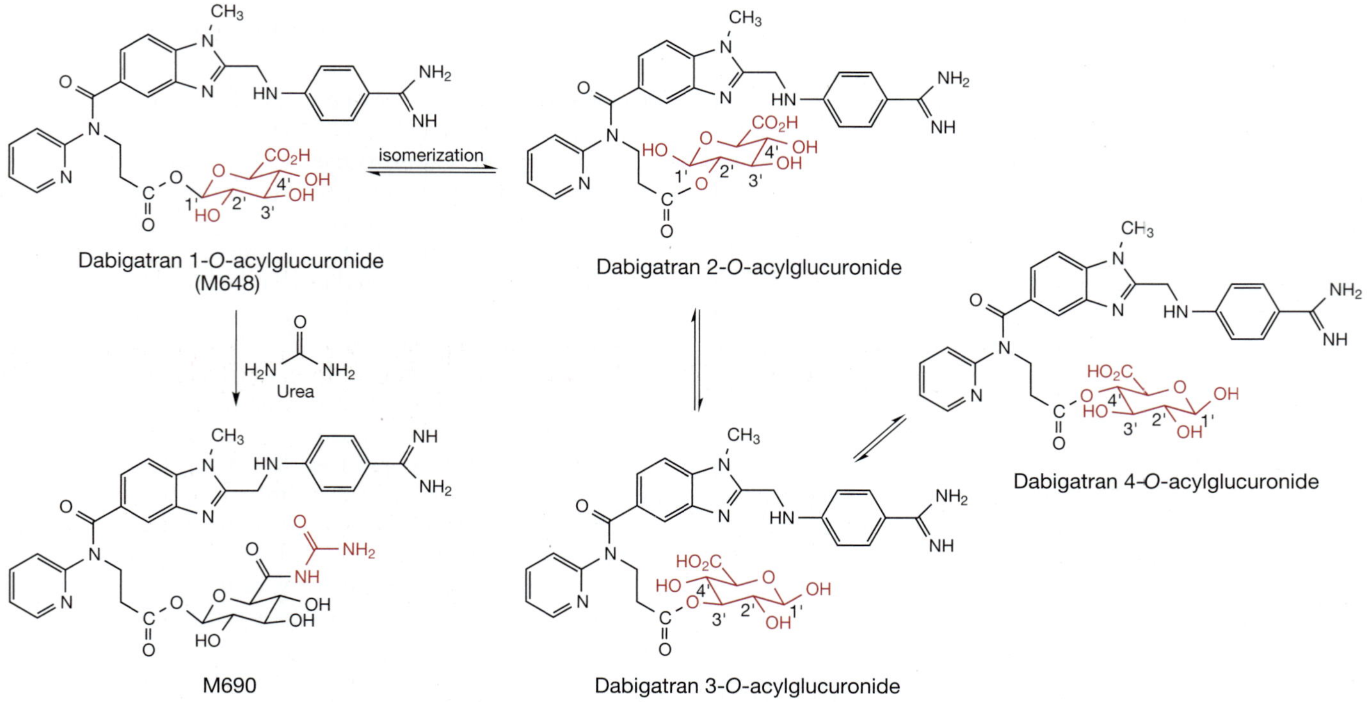

Figure 21.30 Acylglucuronide metabolites of dabigatran.

Table 21.7 Comparison of Direct Thrombin Inhibitors[191,194,204]

Characteristics	Bivalirudin	Argatroban	Dabigatran Etexilate
Tradename	Angiomax	Generic only	Pradaxa
Mode of binding to thrombin	Bivalent	Univalent	Univalent
Route of administration	IV	IV	Oral Prodrug
Thrombin affinity (K_i)	1.9-2.3 nM	5 nM	4.5 nM
Plasma $t_{1/2}$	25 min	46 min	12 h
Main route of clearance	Kidney	Liver	Kidney

IV, intravenous.

Table 21.7 is a comparison of characteristics of the direct thrombin inhibitors.[189,199]

Reversal Agent for Dabigatran. Idarucizumab (Praxbind) is a humanized monoclonal antibody fragment (Fab) that binds to dabigatran and the active acylglucuronides of dabigatran and reverses their anticoagulant effects.[209] The dabigatran binding site on idarucizumab has similarities to the thrombin binding site. The benzamidine group of dabigatran forms a bidentate salt bridge to an aspartate residue of idarucizumab (H:Asp35). The benzimidazole ring of dabigatran participates in a π-stacking interaction with a tyrosine residue (L:Tyr27D) and the pyridine ring forms a T-shaped π-stacking interaction with a tryptophan residue (H:Trp52) of idarucizumab, respectively. The N-methyl group of dabigatran, which forms a key hydrophobic interaction with the S2 pocket of thrombin, does not bind to idarucizumab. The interactions of dabigatran with idarucizumab are reinforced with additional hydrogen bonds and hydrophobic interactions, leading to an astonishingly high affinity of dabigatran for idarucizumab of 2.1 pM.[209] This is approximately 350 times stronger than dabigatran's affinity for thrombin.

The 5-g dose of idarucizumab is administered IV as two 50 mL bolus infusions of 2.5 g each. After administration of one bolus, an analysis of samples from 51 patients who had serious bleeding and 39 patients who required urgent surgery or intervention showed the concentration of unbound dabigatran was less than 20 ng/mL in 89/90 patients.[210] This level of dabigatran produces little or no anticoagulant effect. Praxbind is formulated as a solution for injection in two single-dose 2.5-g/50 mL vials at a WAC of $4,717 for 2 vials.[211]

A summary of the mechanisms of action of drugs that inhibit factor Xa and/or factor IIa is shown in Figure 21.31.

Fast-Track Factor XIa Inhibitors

Factor XIa is an attractive target for anticoagulation because people with congenital factor XIa deficiency have a lower incidence of VTE and cardiovascular events, such as stroke, transient ischemic attacks, and MI, but they do not exhibit spontaneous bleeding.[26,212] Factor XIa plays a limited role in hemostasis, the arrest of bleeding, but it has a more significant role in thrombosis, inappropriate clot formation.[26] Factor XI is activated by thrombin in hemostasis. While factor XI is activated by thrombin in thrombosis, it is also activated by polyphosphate released from activated platelets, NETs released from leukocytes, and extracellular deoxyribonucleic acid (DNA) and ribonucleic acid (RNA) released from NETs. Furthermore, patients with high levels of factor XI are at increased risk for venous thrombosis.[213] There is intense research into drug therapies to inhibit factor XIa activity with the goal to treat or prevent thrombosis with a low risk of bleeding.

Drugs to inhibit factor XIa activity include the dual inhibitor human monoclonal antibody, abelacimab (MAA868). Abelacimab binds to the catalytic domain of both the inactive zymogen factor XI, preventing activation by factor XIIa or thrombin, and to factor XIa.[214] Abelacimab is under clinical investigation as an IV infusion and a once-monthly SC injection.[215,216] Two small-molecule oral factor XIa inhibitors are currently under clinical investigation: milvexian (BMS-986177/JNJ-70033093)[217] and asundexian (BAY 243334).[218]

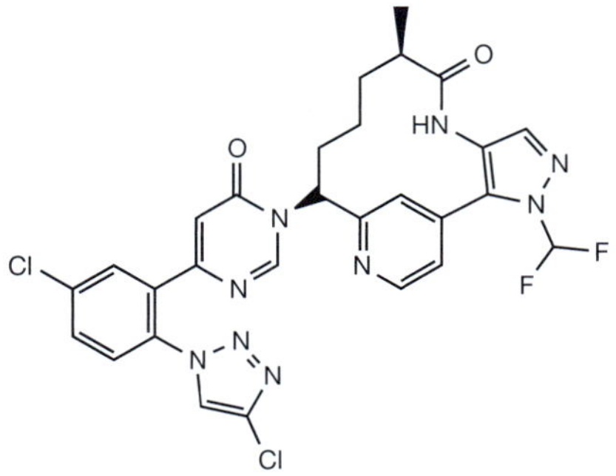

Milvexian
(BMS-986177/JNK-70033093)

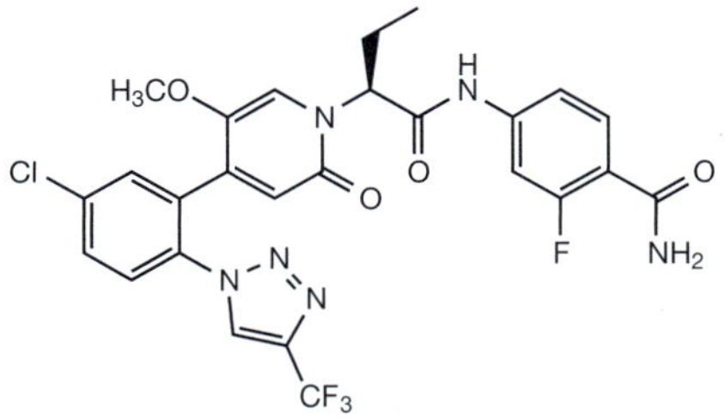

Asundexian
(BAY 2433334)

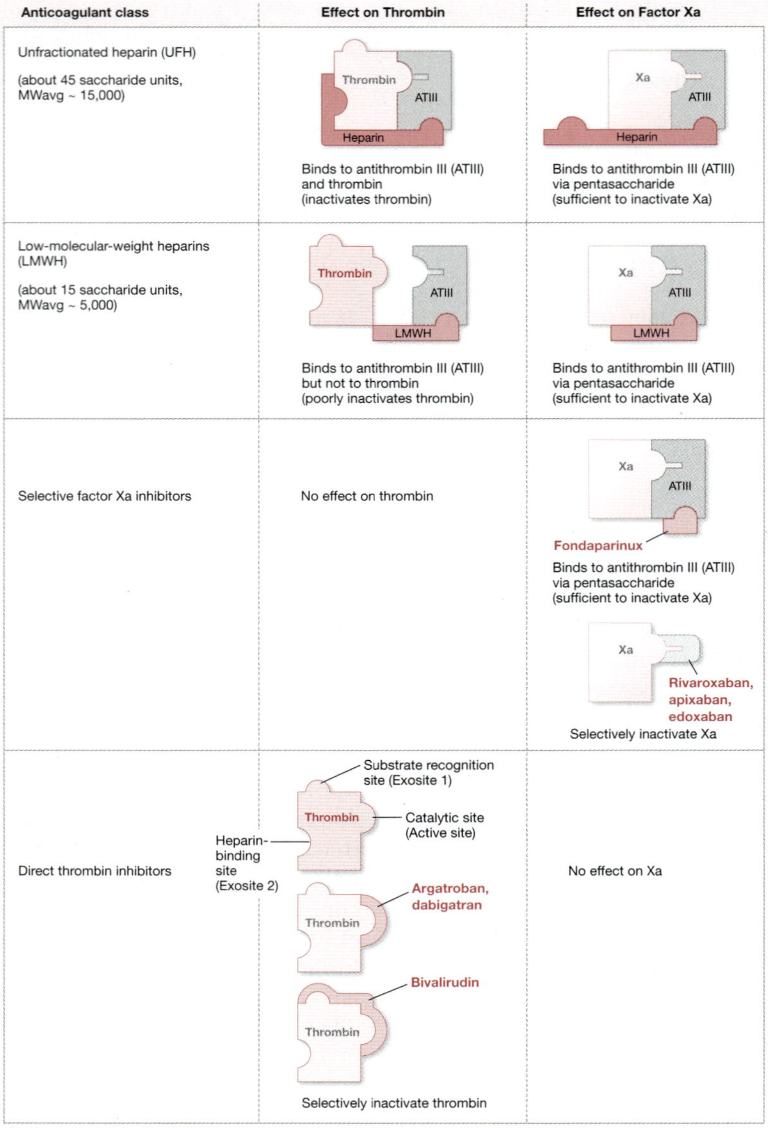

Figure 21.31 Differential effects of unfractionated heparin, low-molecular-weight heparins, selective factor Xa inhibitors, and direct thrombin inhibitors on coagulation factor inactivation. **Effect on thrombin:** To catalyze the inactivation of thrombin, heparin must bind both to antithrombin III via a high-affinity pentasaccharide sequence and to thrombin via an additional 13-saccharide unit. Most of the fragments in low-molecular-weight heparin (LMWH) do not contain a sufficient number of saccharide units to bind thrombin and, therefore, are poor catalysts for thrombin inactivation. Selective factor Xa inhibitors do not inactivate thrombin, while direct thrombin inhibitors only inactivate thrombin. Argatroban and dabigatran bind only to the active (catalytic) site of thrombin, while bivalirudin binds to both the active site and the substrate recognition site (exosite 1) of thrombin. Effect on factor Xa: Indirect inactivation of factor Xa requires only the binding of antithrombin III to the high-affinity pentasaccharide sequence. Since unfractionated heparin, LMWHs, and fondaparinux all contain this pentasaccharide, these drugs are all able to catalyze the inactivation of factor Xa. Rivaroxaban, apixaban, and edoxaban completely inhibit factor Xa by binding to the active site of the enzyme; these drugs bind factor Xa that is complexed with factor Va and Ca^{2+} on phospholipid surfaces. Direct thrombin inhibitors have no effect on factor Xa. (Modified from Armstrong EJ, Golan DE. Pharmacology of hemostasis and thrombosis. In: Golan DE, Armstrong EJ, Armstrong AW, eds. *Principles of Pharmacology: The Pathophysiologic Basis of Drug Therapy.* 4th ed. Wolters-Kluwer; 2017:421, with permission.)

Both milvexian and asundexian take advantage of the S1′ and S2′ pockets factor XIa (Fig. 21.32).[217,218] Both compounds have similar central core rings, a pyrimidinone in milvexian and a 5-methoxypyridinone in asundexian. The pyrimidinone carbonyl oxygen in milvexian forms hydrogen bonds with the backbone nitrogens of Ser195 and Gly193, in the oxyanion hole of factor XIa. The pyrimidinone N1 also forms a hydrogen bond to a water molecule bridging to a hydrogen bond to the backbone nitrogen of Gly216. Similarly, the carbonyl oxygen of the pyridinone ring of asundexian also forms hydrogen bonds with the backbones of Ser195 and Gly193. The 5-methoxy group of the pyridinone ring forms a direct hydrogen bond to the Gly216 backbone, which is a key interaction for potency in asundexian.

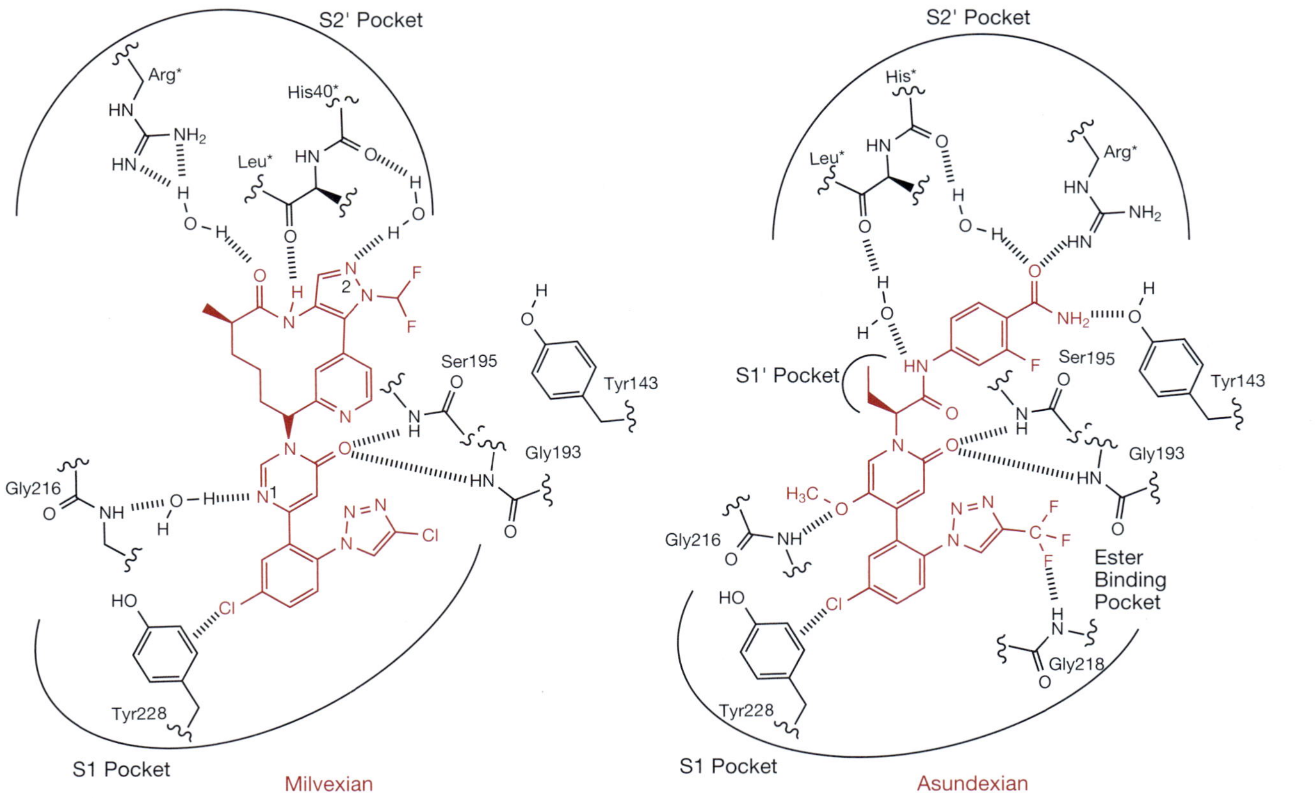

Figure 21.32 Small-molecule oral factor XIa inhibitors milvexian and asundexian binding within the factor XIa active site.[2,18,218] Key amino acid residues within the factor XIa active site which interact with milvexian and asundexian are shown in black. *The Bristol Myers Squibb and Bayer groups use different numbering systems for the amino acid residues in the factor XIa S2' pocket; therefore, the numbers are not included in the figure.

Both milvexian and asundexian possess chlorophenyl rings oriented into the S1 pocket, which interact with Tyr228.[217,218] An additional hydrogen bond between a fluoro group of the trifluoromethyl triazole ring of asundexian occurs with the backbone nitrogen of Gly218 in an area referred to as the ester binding pocket. The (S)-ethyl group of asundexian was the optimal size to fit into the S1' pocket and to minimize opportunity for metabolism.

Both compounds have structural features to ensure key hydrogen bond interactions with the guanidino group of an Arg residue and the backbone of a Leu and His residue in the S2' pocket.[217,218] Milvexian forms a hydrogen bond between the carbonyl oxygen of the macrocycle and a water molecule bridging to two hydrogen bonds with the Arg guanidino group. The macrocyclic lactam nitrogen of milvexian forms a hydrogen bond with the backbone carbonyl oxygen of a Leu residue. The pyrazole N2 nitrogen forms a hydrogen bond to a water molecule, which also forms a hydrogen bond to the carbonyl oxygen of the backbone carbonyl oxygen of a His residue. The nitrogen of the amide linker in asundexian forms a hydrogen bond to a water molecule bridging to a hydrogen bond to the backbone carbonyl oxygen of a Leu residue in the S2' pocket. The carbonyl oxygen of the aryl carboxamide of asundexian forms another hydrogen bond to a water molecule bridging to a hydrogen bond to the backbone carbonyl of a His residue. The carboxamide oxygen also forms a hydrogen bond to the guanidino group of an Arg residue. The nitrogen of the carboxamide in asundexian also forms a hydrogen bond to the phenolic group of Try143.

All three, abelacimab, milvexian, and asundexian, have been granted fast-track designation by the FDA.

Vitamin K Antagonist

Background: Vitamin K Cycle

Synthesis of factors II, VII, IX, and X, along with proteins C and S, require posttranslational γ-carboxylation of glutamate (Glu) residues to form γ-carboxyglutamate (Gla) residues near the N-terminus of the protein structure (Fig. 21.33). Gla residues are necessary for these factors to bind Ca^{2+} to produce the conformation change required to bind to phospholipid surfaces.[219] These are requirements for their ultimate activation. The enzyme required for Glu γ-carboxylation is γ-glutamyl carboxylase (GGCX), which requires the hydroquinone form of vitamin K (vitamin KH_2) as the cofactor. Vitamin KH_2 is a 1,4-naphthoquinone, in the hydroquinone form, with a methyl group at position 2 and a C_{20} phytyl side chain at the 3-position. In the process of the γ-carboxylation of Glu residues in vitamin K–dependent coagulation factors, the vitamin KH_2 cofactor is converted to vitamin K 2,3-epoxide. Vitamin KH_2 is regenerated in a two-step process via the enzyme vitamin

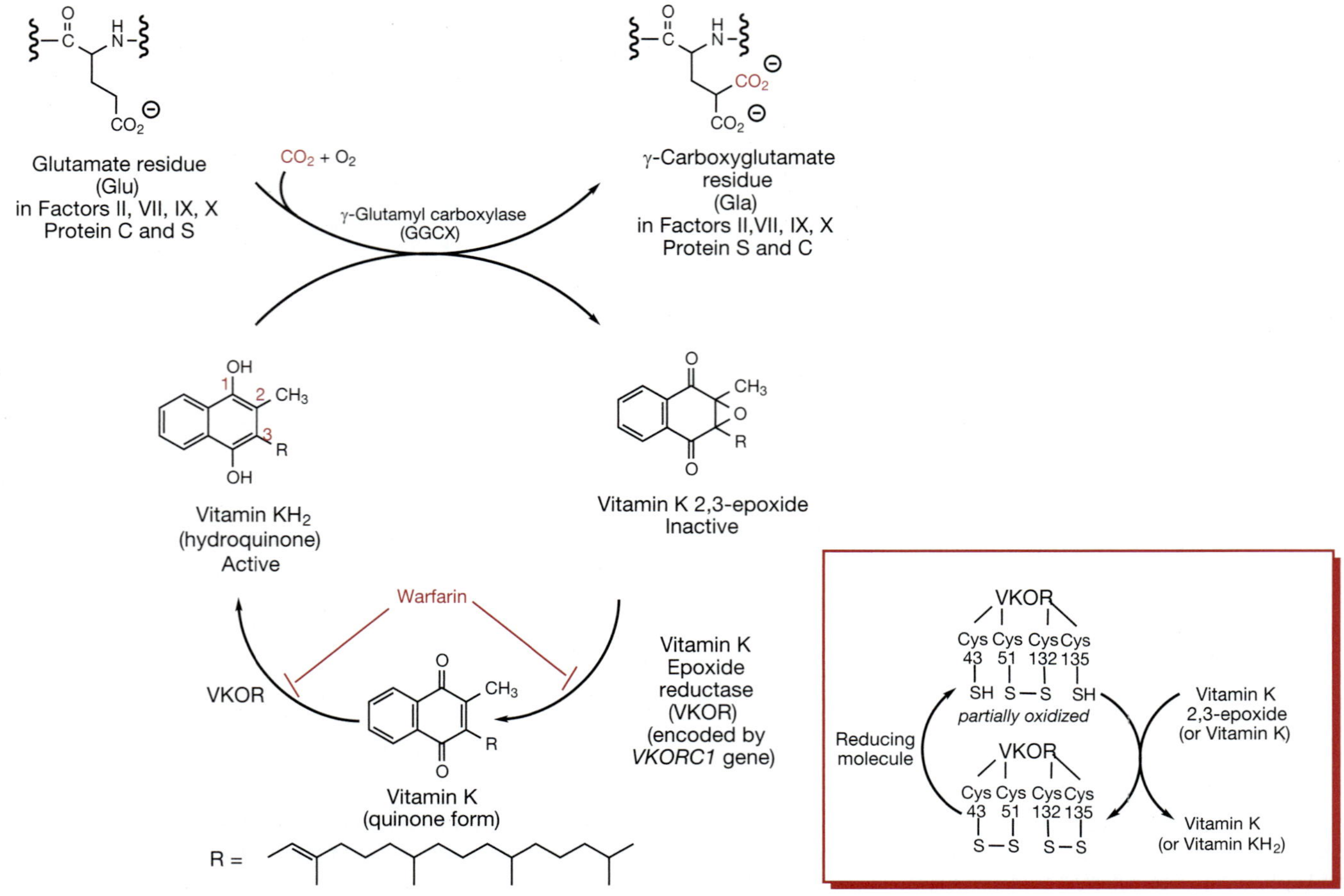

Figure 21.33 Vitamin K cycle.

K epoxide reductase (VKOR).[220-222] VKOR is an endoplasmic membrane oxidoreductase that first reduces vitamin K 2,3-epoxide to the quinone form of vitamin K, followed by further reduction of vitamin K back to vitamin KH_2. Two pairs of cysteine residues within VKOR are critical for the reduction of vitamin K 2,3-epoxide back to vitamin KH_2.[220] VKOR has four transmembrane helices (TMs), forming a catalytic site where one key pair of cysteine residues, Cys132 and Cys135, is located.[222] A β-hairpin loop, extending from TM1 in the endoplasmic reticulum lumen, possesses the other key pair of cysteine residues, Cys43 and Cys51, at the base of each side of the loop. Following is a cap helix that covers the active site. In the process of reducing vitamin K 2,3-epoxide to vitamin K, or vitamin K to vitamin KH_2, two cysteine residues are oxidized. As shown in Figure 21.33, at the beginning of each of the reduction reactions, the two pairs of cysteine residues in the VKOR active site are in a partially oxidized state where Cys43 is a reduced thiol, Cys51 and Cys132 form a disulfide bridge, and Cys135 is a reduced thiol. During the reduction of vitamin K 2,3-epoxide or vitamin K, the cysteine residues are fully oxidized in which both pairs of cysteines form disulfide bonds. To return VKOR to the partially oxidized major form to conduct the reduction reactions, a reducing molecule, yet to be identified, is involved to reduce the Cys43-Cys51 and Cys132-Cys135 disulfide bonds.[222] VKOR is encoded by the *VKORC1* gene. *VKORC1* is genetically polymorphic.

Warfarin

Warfarin is a coumarin derivative (Fig. 21.34). It is an oral vitamin K antagonist (VKA) and the only VKA available in the United States for use as an anticoagulant. The 4-hydroxycoumarin ring of warfarin is acidic because it is the enol form of a 1,3-dicarbonyl compound. It is marketed as the sodium salt. While warfarin is used worldwide, other 4-hydroxycoumarin VKA drugs are available in Europe, including acenocoumarol and phenprocoumon (Fig. 21.34). Flunindione, a 1,3-indanedione VKA, is available in France (Fig. 21.34). The 4-hydroxycoumarin and 1,3-indandione rings of the VKAs are similar to the 1,4-naphthoquinone ring of vitamin K.

Mechanism of Action. Warfarin is a competitive reversible inhibitor of VKOR. Warfarin binds in a central pocket at the active site within VKOR that is predominantly hydrophobic (Fig. 21.35).[222] Key polar interactions between warfarin and the VKOR active site are hydrogen bonds between the 4-hydroxycoumarin ring and Asn80 on TM2 and Tyr139 on TM4 of VKOR.[222,223] Vitamin K forms similar hydrogen bonds between Asn80 and Tyr139 and the 1,4-naphthoquinone ring.[222] The remaining interactions are hydrophobic. The aromatic ring of warfarin forms an important π-stacking interaction with Phe55.[222,224] The coumarin ring fits nicely between Val54 at the top of the VKOR active site and Leu120 at the bottom.[222] The coumarin ring is further

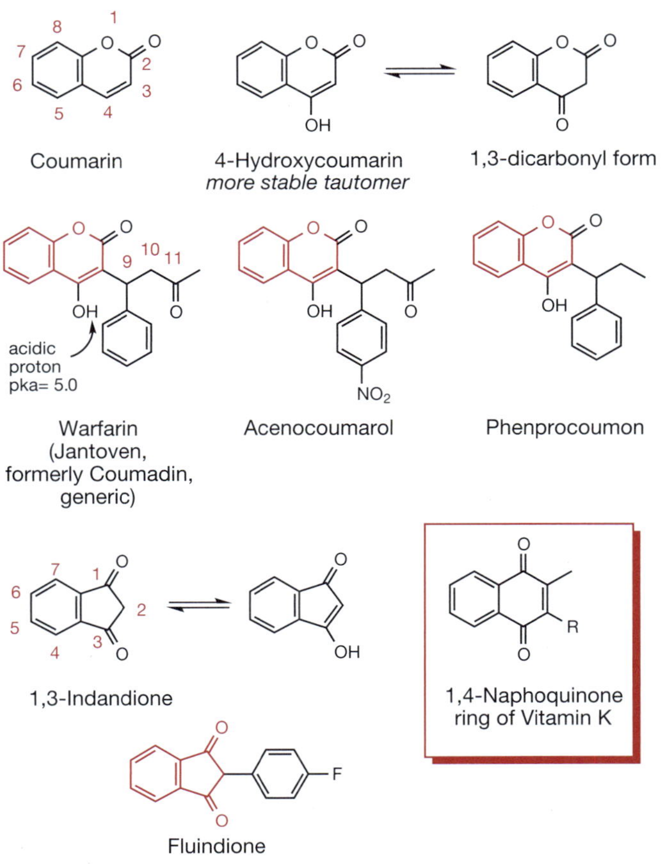

Figure 21.34 Structures of vitamin K antagonists (VKAs).

surrounded by the hydrophobic residues Trp59, Phe63, Leu124, and Leu128 within the central pocket.[222] A similar arrangement within the central pocket occurs around the 1,4-naphthoquinone ring of vitamin K when bound to VKOR.[221] The long phytyl side chain at the 3-position of vitamin K fits in a hydrophobic tunnel formed between TM2 and TM3 within VKOR. Hydrophobic residues, including Phe83, Phe87, and Tyr68, line the tunnel.[222] Warfarin binds to the partially oxidized and fully oxidized forms of VKOR. Warfarin binding to VKOR results in conformational changes, leading to the closed conformation of VKOR, which does not allow the substrates vitamin K 2,3-epoxide or vitamin K to enter the active site. Therefore, γ-carboxylation of Glu residues of vitamin K–dependent coagulation factors does not occur, and anticoagulation ensues. Like all anticoagulants, warfarin is associated with an increased risk of bleeding.

METABOLISM. More than 80% of the *S*-isomer of warfarin is metabolized via CYP2C9 to the major metabolite, *S*-7-hydroxywarfarin and, to a lesser extent, *S*-6-hydroxywarfarin (Fig. 21.36).[225,226] Metabolism by CYP2C19 and CYP3A to various hydroxylated metabolites are minor pathways. Oxidative metabolism also predominates for the *R*-isomer of warfarin, with CYP1A2 and CYP3A4 representing the major routes of metabolism (Fig. 21.36).[225,226] Via CYP1A2, *R*-warfarin is metabolized to its major metabolite *R*-6-hydroxywarfarin and, to a lesser extent, *R*-8-hydroxywarfarin. Oxidation of *R*-warfarin to *R*-10-hydroxywarfarin, via CYP3A4, results in a chiral center, and both enantiomers

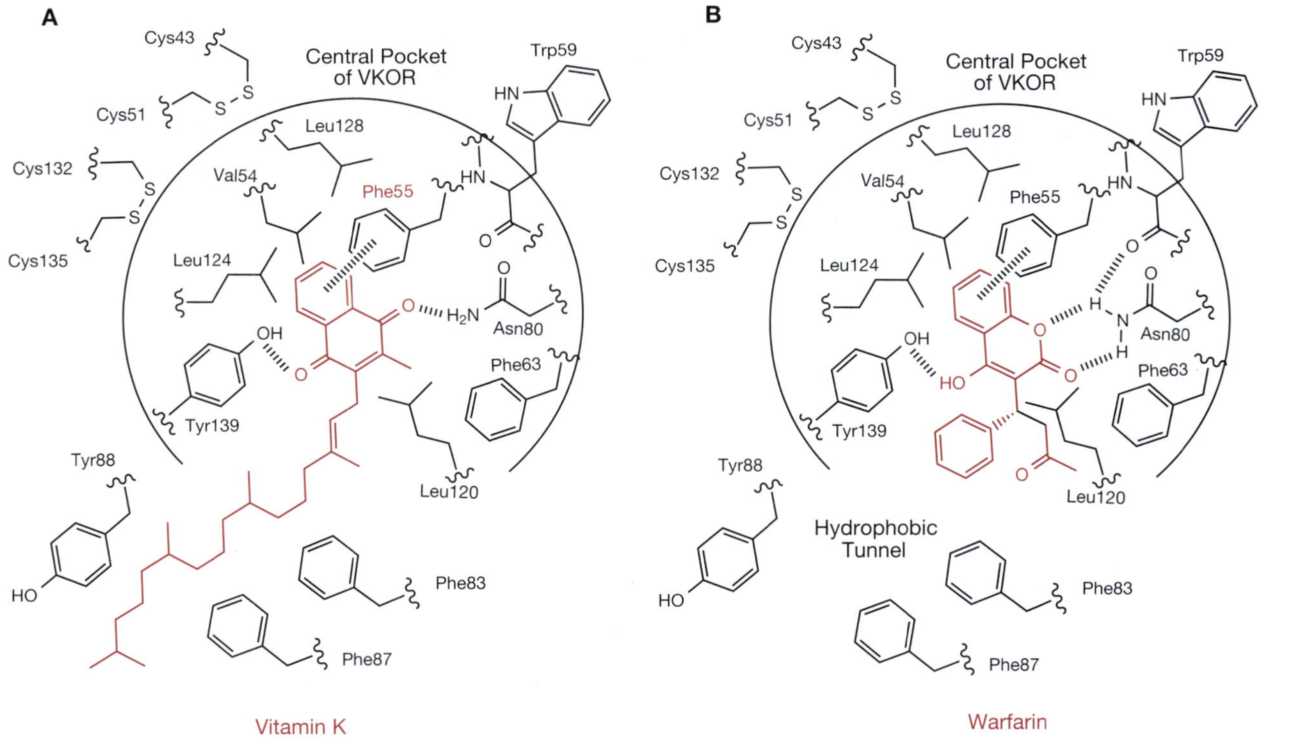

Figure 21.35 Important vitamin K epoxide reductase (VKOR) binding interactions with **(A)** vitamin K and **(B)** warfarin. Key amino acid residues within the VKOR active site that interact with vitamin K and warfarin are shown in black.

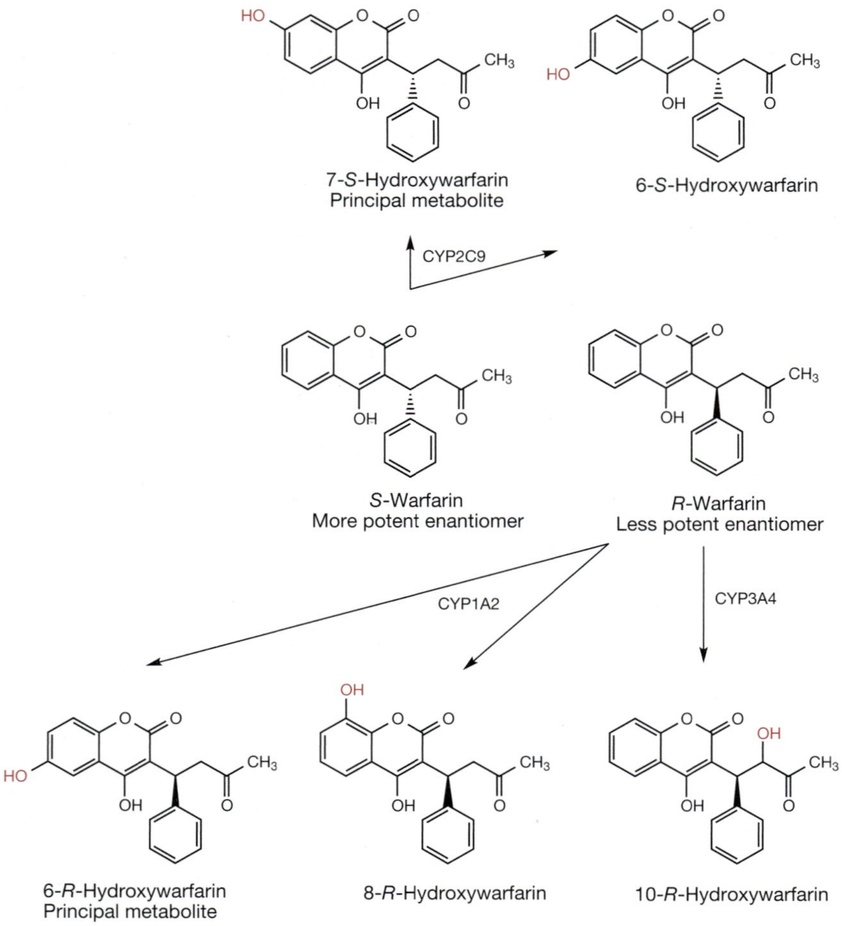

Figure 21.36 Metabolism of warfarin.

are formed. All metabolites are inactive. Hydroxylation of the coumarin ring introduces an unfavorable polar moiety into the hydrophobic binding site with VKOR.[222]

Pharmacokinetics. Warfarin is sold as the racemic mixture. The *S*-isomer is approximately 3 times more potent than the *R*-isomer.[227] The oral absorption of warfarin is rapid, and there is near absolute oral bioavailability. Warfarin is highly protein bound and has a half-life of 36 to 42 hours.[227] The half-lives of the vitamin K–dependent coagulation factors vary widely and are shown in Table 21.8.[227,228] Anticoagulation begins within 24 hours after oral administration of warfarin. Due to the long half-lives of several of the vitamin K–dependent coagulation factors, particularly factor II, the maximum anticoagulant effects are not observed for

Table 21.8 Half-Lives of Vitamin K–Dependent Coagulation Factors

Factor	Half-Life (h)
II	60-72
VII	6
IX	24
X	36

3 to 5 days after warfarin is initiated when all four factors are affected.[227] Warfarin has a narrow therapeutic index and is monitored by the PT measured as the INR. The recommended target INR is 2.0 to 3.0.[229]

Pharmacogenetics and Warfarin Dosing. CYP2C9, which is responsible for more than 80% of the metabolism of the more potent *S*-isomer of warfarin, is genetically polymorphic. *CYP2C9*2* and *CYP2C9*3* are alleles associated with decreased metabolic efficiency of CYP2C9 enzymes. Patients who are carriers of *CYP2C9*2* and *3 may require a dose reduction with warfarin.[230]

A common variant of *VKORC1*, the gene that encodes VKOR, the target enzyme of warfarin action, is -1639G>A (rs9923231). Patients with one or two -1639G>A alleles produce less VKOR than those with the G allele and may require a dose reduction with warfarin.[230]

Drug Interactions That Affect Warfarin Therapy. Warfarin has a narrow therapeutic index, and there are a significant number of drug-drug interactions to consider when patients are on warfarin therapy. Many of the drug interactions reported with warfarin are case studies or based on low-quality evidence, although a recent meta-analysis provides some clarification.[231] Drug interactions that affect warfarin therapy are broadly categorized among several factors: drugs that inhibit or induce the metabolism of warfarin, chiefly CYP2C9, potentially causing an increase or decrease in the INR, respectively; drugs that displace warfarin from plasma protein binding increasing the plasma concentration of free warfarin; antibiotics that inhibit the normal microflora, thereby decreasing vitamin K production and potentiating warfarin activity; and coadministration with antiplatelet drugs, which increases the risk of bleeding with warfarin.[232] Table 21.9 is a selection of drug-drug interactions (DDIs) associated with increasing the risk of bleeding with warfarin therapy for consideration.[231,232] When warfarin is coadministered with PPIs, the risk of bleeding is significantly decreased.[231] Diet may also affect warfarin therapy. Green leafy vegetables, including spinach, kale, and broccoli, are rich in vitamin K. Increasing or decreasing intake of green leafy vegetables may alter a patient's response to a previously stable warfarin dose.

Table 21.9 Examples of Drug Interactions Associated With an Increased Risk of Bleeding With Warfarin[231,232]

Antibiotics, including cephalosporins, penicillins sulfonamides, quinolones
Azole antifungals
Nonsteroidal anti-inflammatory drugs (NSAIDs), including celecoxib
Opioid analgesics
Acetaminophen
Selective serotonin-reuptake inhibitors (SSRIs)
Mirtazapine
Antiplatelet drugs (eg, aspirin, clopidogrel, prasugrel, ticagrelor)

Antidote to Vitamin K–Antagonist Toxicity

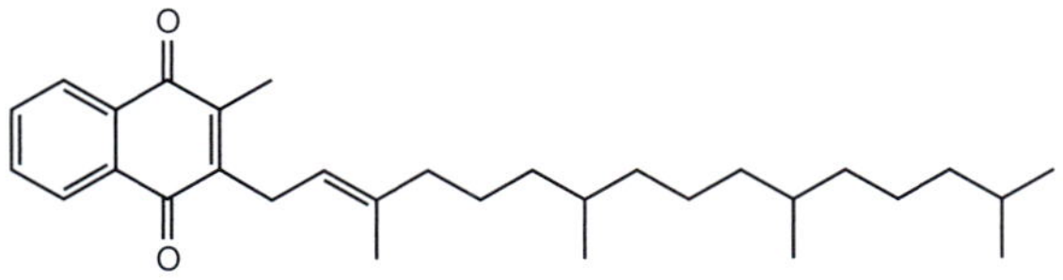

Vitamin K_1
(phytonadione)

For INRs > 10 and no evidence of bleeding in patients taking warfarin, and other VKAs, oral vitamin K1 (phytonadione) is recommended.[229] For patients with VKA-associated major bleeding, 4 factor prothrombin complex combination (4PCC) (Kcentra) is recommended.[233] 4PCC includes human non-activated vitamin K–dependent coagulation factors II, VII, IX, and X, along with the anticoagulants protein C and protein S. Human ATIII and heparin are included in 4PCC to preserve the coagulation factors in their inactive precursor form.[233] 4PCC is administered IV with a slow infusion rate of not more than 8.4 mL/min.[233] The recommended dose is based on factor IX units according to body weight and INR, with a maximum dose of 5,000 units.[233] The WAC of Kcentra is $2.98/unit in 500 and 1,000 unit vials.[234] A dose of 5 to 10 mg of vitamin K_1, as a slow IV infusion, is coadministered with 4PCC in the treatment of bleeding with VKAs.[229] Injectable phytonadione is available as 10 mg/1 mL or 1 mg/0.5 mL in multiple packs for a WAC as low as $42.77 for a 10 mg dose.[235] The vitamin K–dependent coagulation factors within 4PCC are activated in vivo, and the INR returns to or approaches baseline within 30 minutes.[233] While VKOR catalyzes both steps of reduced vitamin K regeneration, it has been suggested that there is an additional vitamin K reductase that catalyzes vitamin K to vitamin KH_2, the second step of reduced vitamin K recycling, in the presence of warfarin.[236] This second vitamin K reductase, yet to be identified, is microsomal, warfarin resistant, and may play a role in vitamin K_1 supplementation for warfarin reversal therapy.[237] However, vitamin K_1 and warfarin both bind to the partially oxidized state of VKOR, and vitamin K_1 is capable of competitively removing warfarin from the VKOR binding site to resume VKOR activity during warfarin toxicity.[237]

BRODIFACOUM POISONINGS

Superwarfarins, including brodifacoum, are used as rodenticides. The superwarfarins are derivatives of warfarin with exceptionally large lipophilic groups off the 3-position of the 4-hydroxycoumarin ring.[238]

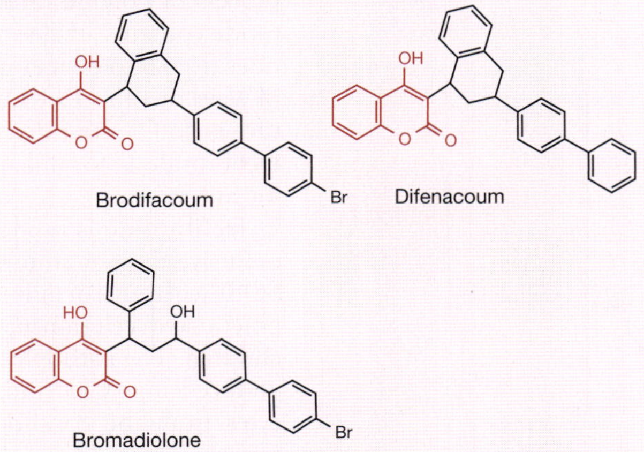

Brodifacoum
Difenacoum
Bromadiolone

(continued)

BRODIFACOUM POISONINGS (*continued*)

The mechanism of action of superwarfarins is inhibition of VKOR. The large lipophilic group imparts increased potency, nearly 100 times the potency of warfarin, and prolonged half-life.[238,239] The interaction of brodifacoum with the binding site of VKOR is shown below.[222] Key amino acid residues within the VKOR active site that interact with brodifacoum are shown in black.

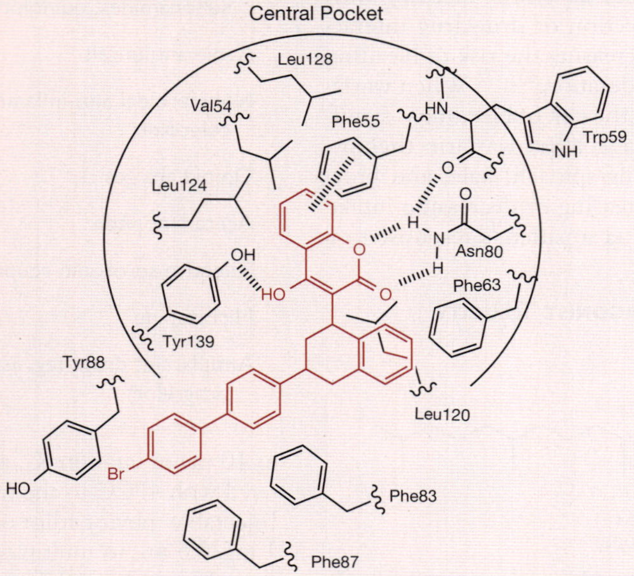

Similar to vitamin K, the long lipophilic group of brodifacoum takes advantage of the hydrophobic tunnel within VKOR, in addition to binding to the central pocket. Compared to warfarin, the enhanced affinity of brodifacoum, and the other superwarfarins, to VKOR leads to its enhanced potency.[221]

The long half-life of superwarfarins is likely due to the enhanced lipophilicity of the long hydrophobic chain, leading to tissue accumulation.[239] The logP value of brodifacoum is 8.5 in comparison to the logP value of 2.3 for warfarin.[239] Furthermore, brodifacoum is minimally metabolized, not renally excreted, and undergoes enterohepatic recycling.[240] The half-life of brodifacoum ranges from 16 to 62 days.[241]

Human poisonings with brodifacoum have occurred. For example, in 2018, in Chicago, Illinois and surrounding counties, more than 150 people presented to hospitals with bleeding due to the use of synthetic cannabinoid products containing superwarfarins. All patient samples tested were positive for brodifacoum.[242,243] Other long-acting VKAs found in patient blood samples included difenacoum and bromadiolone.[243] Along with brodifacoum, warfarin was even found in one sample reported.[243] After initial treatment, the long half-life of brodifacoum requires follow-up therapy with oral vitamin K_1 therapy for several weeks or more to treat brodifacoum toxicity.[240,241]

ANTITHROMBOTIC/PROFIBRINOLYTIC OLIGONUCLEOTIDE

Defibrotide

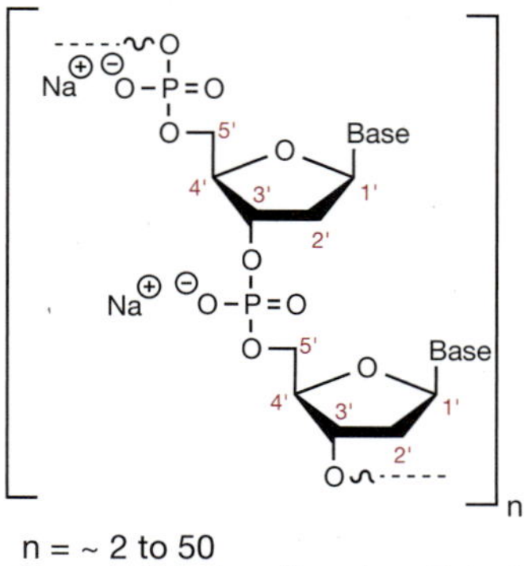

n = ~ 2 to 50
Base = Adenine, Guanine, Cytosine, Thymine

Defibrotide (Defitelio)

Defibrotide is classified as an antisense oligonucleotide (ASO). It is a mixture of deoxyribonucleic acid (DNA) fragments of varying sizes. Derived from a depolymerization process of porcine intestinal mucosal DNA, 90% of defibrotide contains single-stranded phosphodiester oligonucleotides from 9 to 80-mer with an average length of 50-mer and MWavg of 14 to 19 KDa.[244] The remaining 10% of the mixture is double-stranded phosphodiester oligonucleotides.[245] Defibrotide is formulated as the sodium salt in a solution for injection.

Defibrotide is used for the treatment of hepatic veno-occlusive disease/sinusoidal obstruction syndrome (VOD/SOS), with renal or pulmonary dysfunction following hematopoietic stem-cell transplantation (HSCT), both in adults and children. The pathophysiology of VOD/SOS involves toxin-induced injury to sinusoidal endothelial cells and hepatocytes from the conditioning regimens for HSCT.[245] This triggers a cascade of actions, including endothelial cell activation, an inflammatory response, and progressive endothelial cell damage. The result is vasoconstriction, sinusoidal fibrosis, and creation of a prothrombotic-antifibrinolytic environment, which stimulates platelet activation and the formation of fibrin aggregates, potentially causing sinusoid occlusion. Common symptoms of VOD/SOS are hyperbilirubinemia, hepatomegaly, ascites, and weight gain.

Mechanism of Action

The mechanisms of action of defibrotide are myriad, diverse, and not entirely clear. Overall, defibrotide has endothelial protective properties on activated endothelial cells; it reestablishes the thrombotic-fibrinolytic balance and enables endothelial repair.[244,245] It causes vasodilation by increasing NO and PGI_2 and reducing TXA_2. Defibrotide has antithrombotic and profibrinolytic activity due in part by increasing tissue plasminogen activator, TFPI, thrombomodulin, PGI_2 and PGE_2, while reducing plasminogen activator inhibitor-1, platelet activating factor, thrombin, and TXA_2. It also has anti-inflammatory and antiadhesive activities, among other activities.

Pharmacokinetics and Metabolism

Defibrotide is administered intravenously every 6 hours.[246] It is 93% protein bound.[246] The half-life is less than 2 hours.[246] Approximately 5% to 15% of a dose is excreted as unchanged defibrotide in the urine, with the majority excreted within 4 hours of administration. Like all ASO-based drugs, the primary route of metabolism of defibrotide is degradation via endonucleases and exonucleases ultimately to 2′-deoxyribose and the purine and pyrimidine bases.[246] Defibrotide is not a substrate for CYP enzymes.

Adverse Effects

Defibrotide is contraindicated in patients taking anticoagulants or fibrinolytics. In addition to bleeding, the most common adverse effects are hypotension and diarrhea.

Fibrinolytic Drugs

Fibrinolytic, also called thrombolytic, drugs are used to dissolve occlusive clots. The currently marketed fibrinolytic drugs, alteplase, reteplase, and tenecteplase, are all indicated in the treatment of STEMI. Alteplase is FDA approved for additional indications (including AIS, PE), and to restore central venous access patency. In patients with STEMI, current guidelines recommend fibrinolytic therapy, barring no contraindications, when PCI will be delayed by more than 120 minutes.[65] Alteplase is recommended in selected patients with AIS within 3 hours of ischemic stroke symptom onset.[52] The goal of fibrinolytic therapy is dissolution of the offending clot and returning blood flow through the formerly occluded vessel.

Endogenous tPA, secreted by vascular endothelial cells, is composed of 527 amino acids in five domains. Beginning from the N-terminus, the five domains are a fibronectin finger, the epidermal growth factor (EGF) domain, kringle 1 and kringle 2, and a serine protease P domain, which is the site that cleaves plasminogen (Fig. 21.37).[247] The fibronectin finger domain is responsible for the initial binding affinity to fibrin. Kringle 2 also has a binding site to fibrin. Endogenous tPA is N-glycosylated at three sites, Asn117, Asn184,

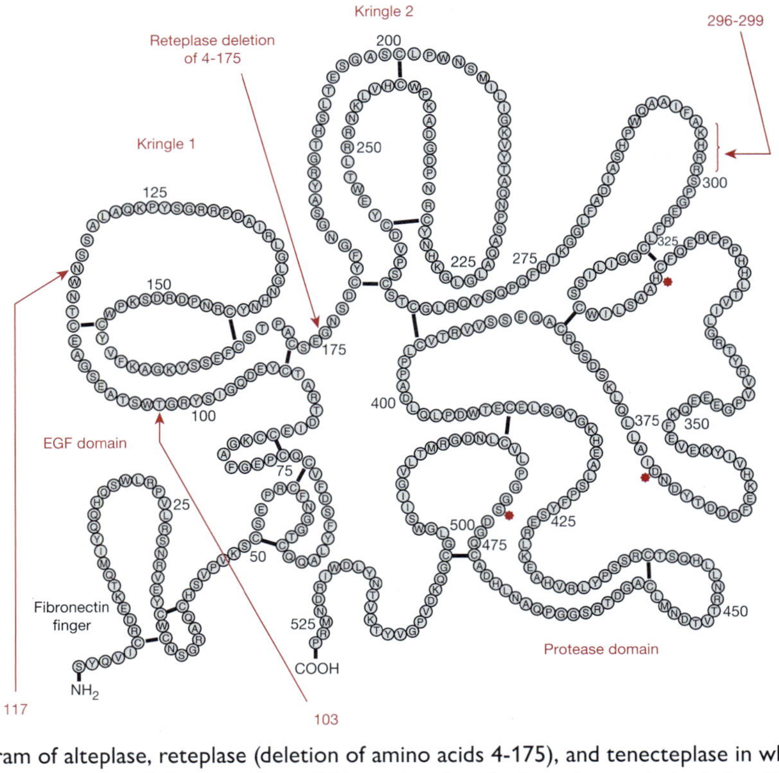

Figure 21.37 Schematic diagram of alteplase, reteplase (deletion of amino acids 4-175), and tenecteplase in which threonine (T) at position 103 is replaced with asparagine, asparagine (N) at position 117 is replaced with glutamine, and the lysine (K), histidine (H), arginine (R), arginine sequence at positions 296-299 is replaced with four alanines. The catalytic triad within the protease domain, His322, Asp371, and Ser478, are each indicated by an asterisk (*). (Adapted with permission from Nordt TK, Bode C. Thrombolysis: newer thrombolytic agents and their role in clinical medicine. *Heart.* 2003;89:1358-1362. With permission from BMJ Publishing Group Ltd.)

and Asn448. As the name implies, tPA binds to the fibrin of a clot and catalyzes the hydrolysis of the Arg561-Val562 bond in fibrin-bound plasminogen to liberate plasmin (see Fig. 21.2). The catalytic activity of fibrin-bound tPA is more than 100 times greater than free tPA.[248] Plasmin digests fibrin into soluble fibrin degradation products. Plasminogen activator inhibitor-1 (PAI-1) irreversibly inhibits tPA. The reactive center loop of PAI-1 binds to the catalytic site of tPA, mimicking the labile bond in plasminogen.[249] The active site Ser478 of tPA attacks the P1-P1′ bond of PAI-1, forming a covalent bond, ultimately resulting in acylation of the tPA serine with P1 of PAI-1.[250] The cationic loop of residues from 296 to 302 and Arg304 of tPA are necessary for PAI-1 recognition.[250]

Alteplase is recombinant tissue plasminogen activator (rtPA) (Fig. 21.37). Reteplase and tenecteplase are variants of rtPA. The fibrinolytic agents all retain the serine protease activity of tPA, cleaving an amide bond between Arg561 and Val562 in fibrin-bound plasminogen converting it to plasmin. The main adverse effect with the fibrinolytic drugs is bleeding, particularly intracerebral hemorrhage.

Alteplase

Alteplase is recombinant tPA from the complementary DNA of endogenous tPA derived from human melanoma cell lines expressed in Chinese hamster ovary (CHO) cells.[251] Alteplase has a short initial plasma half-life of about 5 minutes.[248] Consequently, alteplase is administered as an IV bolus followed by continuous infusion. The short plasma half-life of alteplase is due to rapid clearance by the liver. Alteplase uptake by the liver is receptor-mediated endocytosis via interactions between hepatic glycoprotein receptors and glycosylated and polypeptide domains in alteplase.[251] The fibronectin finger, EGF, and kringle 1 domains play a role in hepatic clearance, as deletion of these domains decreases hepatic clearance.[251] Lysosomal degradation of alteplase within the liver leads to water-soluble metabolites excreted in the urine.[251]

Reteplase

Reteplase is a 355–amino acid single-chain deletion mutant of alteplase expressed in *Escherichia coli*. Reteplase includes the amino acid sequence 1 to 3 and 176 to 527 of alteplase, which includes kringle 2 and the P domain of alteplase only (Fig. 21.37).[247,252] Lacking the fibronectin finger domain, reteplase has reduced binding and selectively to fibrin compared to alteplase.[252] Prokaryotic cells are unable to glycosylate proteins; therefore, reteplase is nonglycosylated. Elimination of the fibronectin finger, EGF, and kringle 1 domains, as well as lack of glycosylation, reduces hepatic elimination, increasing the plasma half-life to 14 to 18 minutes for reteplase.[247,248,252] It is primarily cleared by kidneys. Due to the longer half-life, reteplase is administered as a double IV bolus 30 minutes apart.

Tenecteplase

Tenecteplase is a 527–amino acid variant of alteplase, containing three point mutations, expressed from CHO cells (see Fig. 21.37).[247,253] Thr103 in the kringle 1 domain of alteplase is replaced with Asn in tenecteplase, which provides a new glycosylation site and decreases the rate of clearance.[253] Asn117 in the kringle 1 domain is replaced with a Gln residue, which eliminates a glycosylation site and also reduces the rate of clearance. The third mutation involves replacing the Lys, His, Arg, Arg residues from positions 296 to 299 in the P domain with four Ala residues. This reduces PAI-1 inhibition by removing a key PAI-1 recognition site in tenecteplase. Additionally, substituting the four Ala residues increases fibrin specificity. Collectively, these substitutions increase the half-life of tenecteplase to 20 to 24 minutes, compared to the approximately 5 minute half-life of alteplase. This enables tenecteplase to be dosed as a single bolus. Sometimes tenecteplase is called TNK, as it is a TNK-mutant of alteplase, which refers to the sites of amino acid substitutions, Thr (T), Asn (N), and the four amino acid sequence beginning with Lys (K). Tenecteplase is cleared by the liver.

A comparison of the fibrinolytic drugs available is shown in Table 21.10.[247-257]

Thrombopoietin-Receptor Agonists

Thrombopoietin receptor agonists (TPO-RAs) are used in the treatment of immune thrombocytopenia (ITP) and other forms of thrombocytopenia. ITP is an acquired autoimmune disease characterized by a low platelet count of less than 100,000 cells/mm3 (normal 150,000-400,000).[258] Patients may be asymptomatic or have bleeding complications. While fatal intracranial hemorrhage is rare, other bleeding complications that may occur with ITP include petechiae, purpura, nosebleeds, bleeding from gums, and blood in stool and urine. Fatigue and impaired quality of life are reported in patients with ITP.[258] The pathophysiology of ITP involves IgG autoantibodies, which bind to platelets and megakaryocytes. Platelets bound with autoantibodies are recognize by phagocytes via interaction with Fc gamma receptors (FcγR) and are destroyed by the spleen and liver.[258,259] When bound with autoantibodies, megakaryocytes, which normally produce platelets, are either prevented from maturation or they are destroyed. Consequently, the low platelet count of ITP is due to either impaired production of platelets from megakaryocytes or increased platelet destruction.

Thrombopoietin (TPO) stimulates platelet production via thrombopoietin receptors (TPO-R), also called myeloproliferative leukemia virus receptors (Mpl), located on hematopoietic stem cells, platelets, and megakaryocytes.[259] There are currently four TPO-RAs available, romiplostim, avatrombopag, eltrombopag, and lusutrombopag (Fig. 21.38).[260] Romiplostim binds to the TPO-R in the extracellular domain, the same domain where TPO binds. Avatrombopag, eltrombopag, and lusutrombopag, are oral small-molecule TPO-RAs. All three bind to the transmembrane domain of the TPO-R and participate in a key interaction with His499.[260] Upon TPO-RA binding to the TPO-R, platelet production is induced via Janus kinase 2/signal transducer and activator of transcription 5 (JAK2/STAT5) pathways, among others.[261]

Table 21.10 Comparison of Thrombolytic Drugs[247-257]

Characteristic	Alteplase	Reteplase	Tenecteplase
Tradename	Activase Cathflo Activase	Retavase	TNKase
Indication for use	• AIS • STEMI • PE • Restoration of function to central venous access devices	STEMI	STEMI
Molecular description	rtPA	Single-chain deletion mutant containing amine acid sequence 1-3 and 176-527 of alteplase Nonglycosylated	Three point mutations of alteplase: • Position 103 Asn replaces Thr • Position 117 Gln replaces Asn • Position 296-299 (Lys, His, Arg, Arg) replaced with four Ala residues
Expression source	CHO cells	*Escherichia coli*	CHO cells
Number of amino acids	527	355	527
Plasma $t_{1/2}$ (min)	~5	13-16	20-24
Administration	AIS, STEMI: IV bolus, followed by IV infusion PE: IV infusion	Double IV bolus 30 min apart	Single IV bolus
Route of clearance	Hepatic	Renal/hepatic	Hepatic

AIS, acute ischemic stroke; CHO, Chinese hamster ovary; PE, pulmonary embolism; rtPA, recombinant tissue plasminogen activator; STEMI, ST-elevation myocardial infarction.

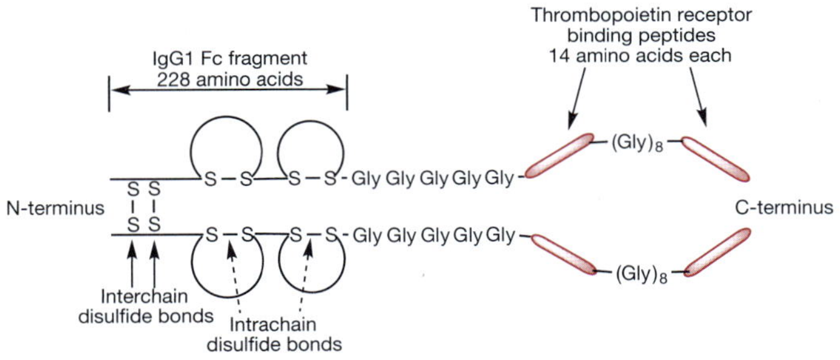

Romiplostim (Nplate)

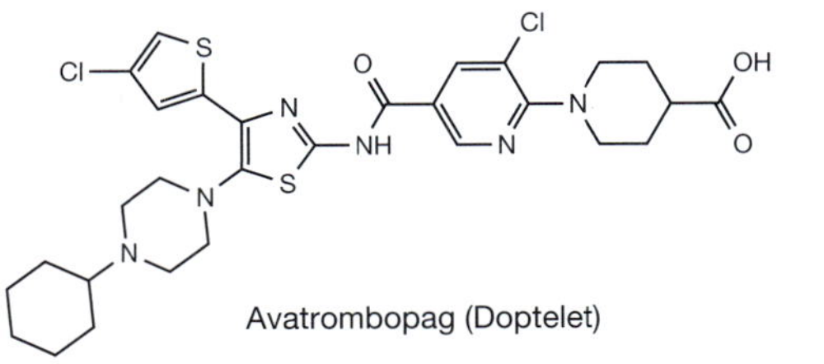

Avatrombopag (Doptelet)

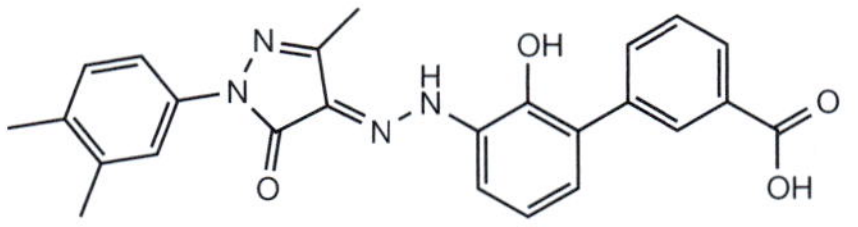

Eltrombopag (Promacta)

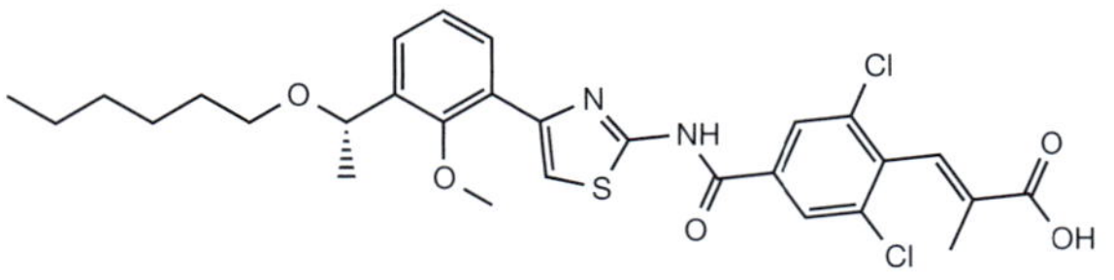

Lusutrombopag (Mulpleta)

Figure 21.38 Thrombopoietin receptor agonists (TPO-RAs).

Romiplostim

Romiplostim is an Fc-peptide fusion protein, or "peptibody," in which a peptide portion that binds and activates the TPO-R is covalently linked to an Fc fragment.[262-267] The peptide portion was chosen based on screening libraries of peptides lacking sequence homology to human thrombopoietin, but had binding affinity to the TPO-R and was capable of activating it.[263] A 14-amino acid peptide was identified, and when two of these peptides are linked by an eight glycine linker, their binding affinity approaches that of recombinant TPO.[262,263] The increased potency of two TPO binding peptides in tandem is thought to be the result of inducing dimerization of the bound TPO receptors necessary for activation.[263] The N-terminus of romiplostim includes the Fc fragment portion composed of two sets of IgG1 heavy chain and kappa light chain constant regions disulfide bonded.[264] The TPO receptor binding peptides separated by eight Gly residues are covalently linked through a five glycine residue linker to the C-terminus of the heavy chain of the Fc region at residue 228.[264] Overall, romiplostim has four peptide sequences that bind to the TPO-R binding site. The function of the Fc fragment is to increase the plasma half-life of romiplostim. Romiplostim is expressed in *Escherichia coli*.

Upon SC administration, the plasma half-life of romiplostim is 1 to 34 days (median 3.5 days).[267] Romiplostim is primarily cleared (~90%) via TPO-R mechanisms and reticuloendothelial clearance.[260,263]

Avatrombopag

Metabolism

The main route of metabolism of avatrombopag is hydroxylation of the 4-position of the cyclohexane ring via CYP2C9 and 3A4 (Fig. 21.39).[260,268] Approximately 43.8% of a dose of avatrombopag is excreted in the feces as 4-hydroxyavatrombopag.[260] The dose of avatrombopag is recommended to be reduced or increased when coadministered with moderate to strong dual inhibitors or inducers of CYP2C9 and CYP3A4, respectively.[268] Avatrombopag has a half-life of approximately 19 hours.[260]

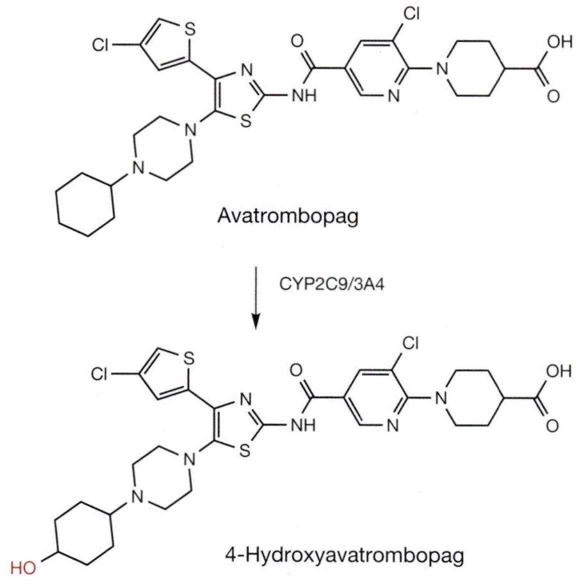

Figure 21.39 Metabolism of avatrombopag.

Eltrombopag

Metabolism

Eltrombopag is extensively metabolized (Fig. 21.40).[269] The main route of metabolism initially involves hydrolysis of the hydrazine bond of the central hydrazone moiety, via gut microbes.[269,270] The two hydrolysis products are quickly absorbed and undergo further conjugation reactions, principally glucuronidation via UGT1A1 and UGT1A3 to glucuronides M3 and M4.[269-271] The M3 metabolite is the *N*-acetylated glucuronide. N-acetylation occurs either before or after glucuronidation. Collectively, M3 and M4 comprise approximately 31% of a dose and are excreted in the urine.[269]

Eltrombopag also undergoes benzylic hydroxylation (M1) via CYP1A2 and CYP2C8.[269,271] M1 forms three glutathione-derived metabolites, likely through an imine methide intermediate.[269] M5 is the glutathione conjugate, M6 is a cysteine derivative, and M7 is a glutamylcysteine derivative. Collectively, M5, M6, and M7 comprise approximately 21% of a dose and are excreted in the feces.[269]

Eltrombopag chelates polyvalent cations, including iron, calcium, aluminum, magnesium, selenium, and zinc, within the central portion of the molecule.[260,261] Chelation decreases oral absorption. Therefore, eltrombopag should be taken 2 hours before or 4 hours after food, such as dairy products, multivitamin supplements, and antacids containing polyvalent cations.[260,271] The half-life of eltrombopag is 21 to 32 hours in healthy patients, and 26 to 35 hours inpatients with ITP.[271] Eltrombopag is a substrate for OATP1B1 and BCRP, and the dose should be lowered with coadministration of other drugs that are substrates for OATP1B1 and BCRP.[271]

Lusutrombopag

Metabolism

The main route of metabolism of lusutrombopag occurs in the liver primarily by CYP4A11 and, to a minor extent, by CYP3A4, via ω-hydroxylation to 6-hydroxylusutrombopag and to M5 via O-dealkylation (Fig. 21.41).[272] The 6-hydroxy metabolite is further metabolized via β-hydroxylation to M4, M6, and M7. M6 is either the O-propanol derivative or the O-acetic acid derivative.[272] M4 and M7 represent 1.53% and 16.9% of the dose in feces. M5 and M6 collectively represent 17.9% of the dose in feces. The effect of cyclosporine, a CYP3A4 inhibitor, on lusutrombopag metabolism was low, suggesting that CYP3A4 does not significantly contribute to its metabolism.[272] Urinary excretion is not an important route of elimination for lusutrombopag nor its metabolites. The half-life of lusutrombopag is 27 hours.[260,273]

Table 21.11 includes a comparison of the TPO-RAs, along with fostamatinib.[260-277,280]

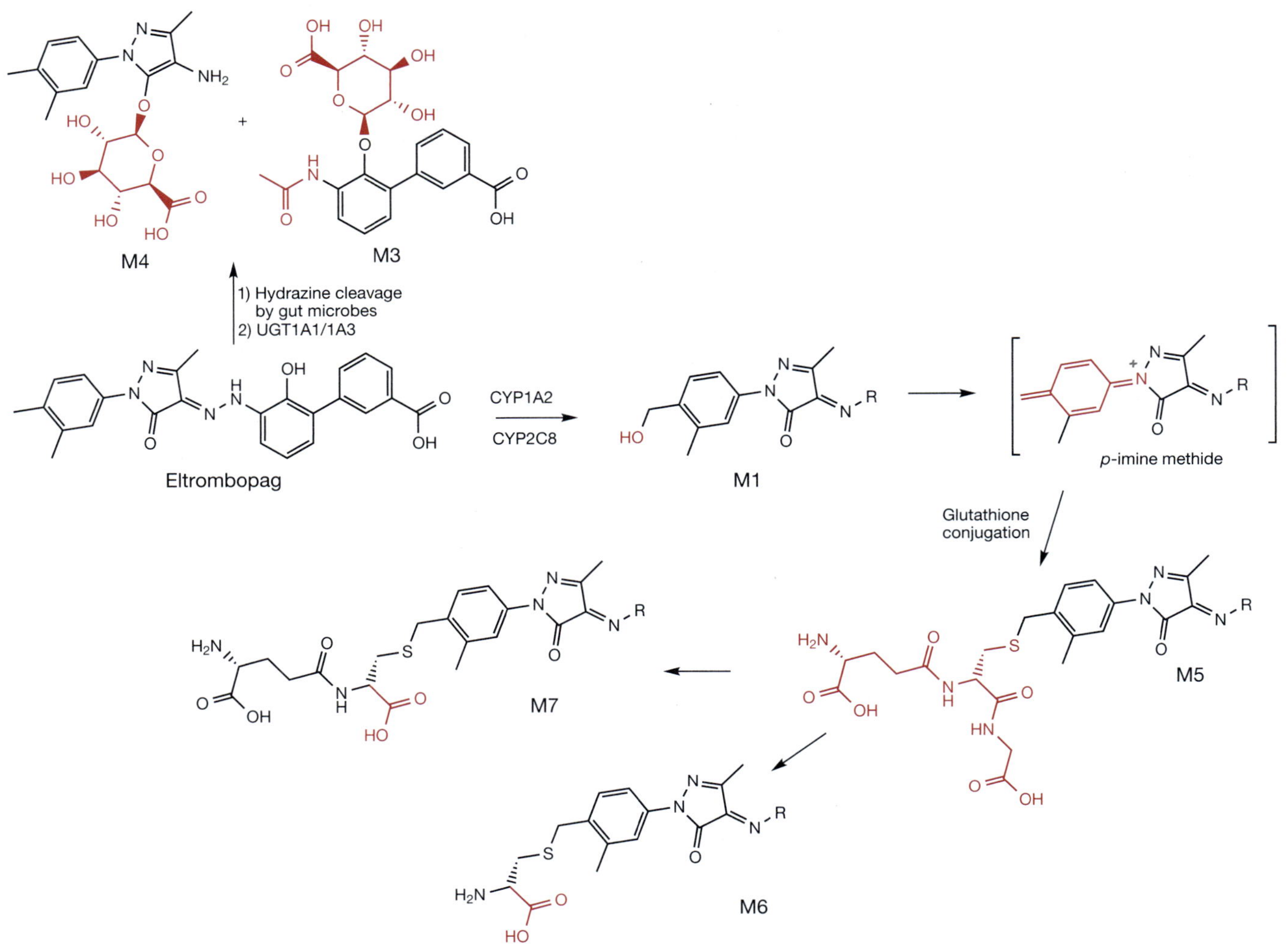

Figure 21.40 Metabolism of eltrombopag.

SPLEEN TYROSINE-KINASE INHIBITOR

Spleen tyrosine kinase (Syk), a cytoplasmic non-receptor tyrosine kinase, is found primarily in hematopoietic cells.[275,276] Syk plays a key role in the signaling of activated FcγRs and B-cell receptors (BCRs).[276] Immune complexes of IgG autoantibodies bound to self-antigens on platelets, as occurs in ITP, activating FcγRs. Activated FcγRs, via Syk signaling, increase phagocytosis of antibody-coated platelets by macrophages in the spleen and/or liver.[258] BCR activation, triggering Syk signaling, stimulates antiplatelet and megakaryocyte autoantibodies by B cells. Inhibition of Syk reduces antibody-mediated destruction of platelets, allowing an increase in platelet count and decreasing the risk of bleeding.

Fostamatinib

Fostamatinib is an oral methylene phosphate prodrug of the Syk inhibitor tamatinib (R406) (Fig. 21.42).[277-279] Tamatinib has low aqueous solubility, necessitating conversion to a water-soluble prodrug to enable adequate dissolution when administered orally.[277] Upon oral administration, the phosphate group of the prodrug fostamatinib is rapidly hydrolyzed via intestinal alkaline phosphatase to the carbinolamine, which spontaneously breaks down to liberate formaldehyde and the active Syk inhibitor, tamatinib (Fig. 21.42).[275,277] Fostamatinib is indicated for the treatment of ITP.[280]

Mechanism of Action

Tamatinib is a competitive inhibitor of ATP at the ATP-binding site on Syk (Fig. 21.43). As a tyrosine kinase, Syk has an N- and a C-terminal lobe, connected by a hinge region. ATP binds at the hinge region. The hinge region of Syk is composed of amino acids 448 to 455.[279] The amino-pyrimidine group of tamatinib forms two hydrogen bonds with the backbone of Ala451 in the hinge region.[279,281] Furthermore, the pyrimidine ring forms a unique hydrogen bond between the unsubstituted aromatic CH group and the backbone carbonyl oxygen of Glu449.[279,281] The trimethoxyphenyl group forms hydrophobic interactions with Gly454 and Pro455 in the hinge region and Leu377 in the Gly-rich loop.[278,279,281] The pyrido-oxazinone ring also participates in hydrophobic interactions with the Gly-rich loop, including with Val385.[278,281]

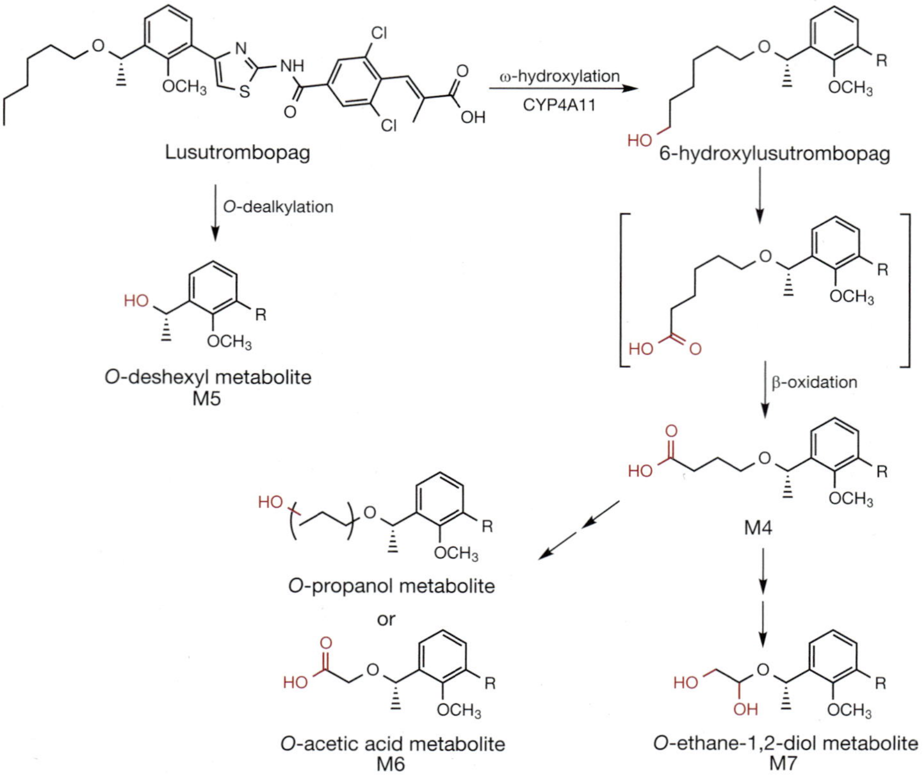

Figure 21.41 Metabolism of lusutrombopag.

Metabolism

Once in the systemic circulation, tamatinib undergoes hepatic metabolism (Fig. 21.44).[277] Via UGT1A9, tamatinib is glucuronidated to the N-glucuronide metabolite M647.[277] M647 is the major urinary metabolite and represents approximately 19% of the administered dose of fostamatinib.[277] Tamatinib is O-dealkylated via CYP3A4 to the *para*-phenolic compound M529. M529 is further metabolized via O-demethylation of the remaining two methoxy groups, followed by *para*-dehydroxylation by anaerobic gut bacteria to form M413, the 3,5-benzene diol derivative of R406. M413 is the major fecal metabolite of fostamatinib. Approximately 80% of a dose of fostamatinib is excreted in the feces as tamatinib and M413.[275,277]

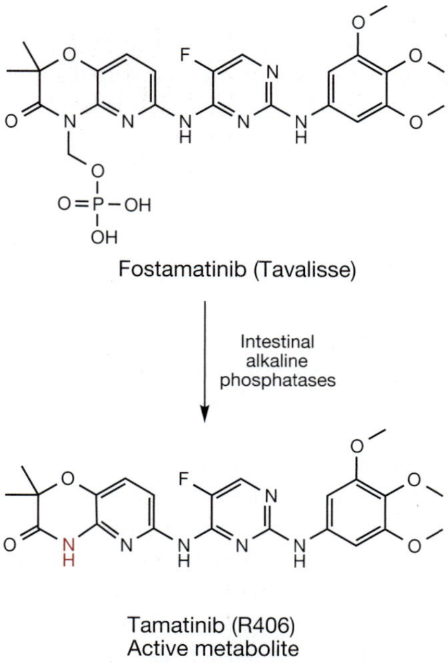

Figure 21.42 Structure of the prodrug fostamatinib and its in vivo activation to the active metabolite tamatinib (R406).

Pharmacokinetics

The absolute bioavailability of tamatinib after a single oral dose of fostamatinib is 55%.[275] The half-life of tamatinib is 12.9 to 20.9 hours.[275] Fostamatinib inhibits P-gp, while

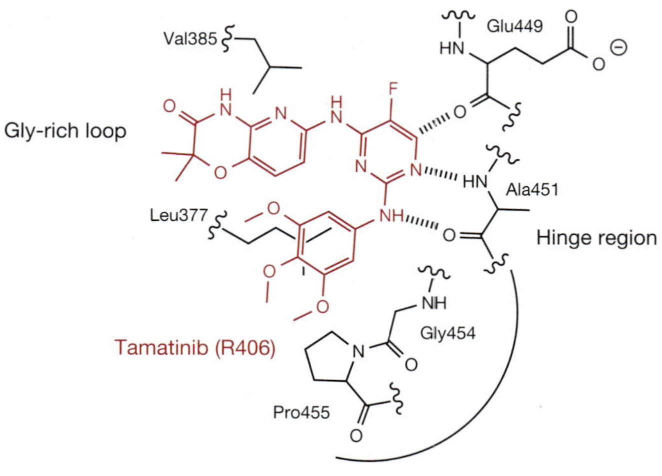

Figure 21.43 Binding interactions of the active metabolite tamatinib, a Syk inhibitor, with the ATP-binding site of Syk. Key amino acid residues within the ATP-binding site of Syk which interact with tamatinib are shown in black. ATP, adenosine triphosphate; Syk, spleen tyrosine kinase.

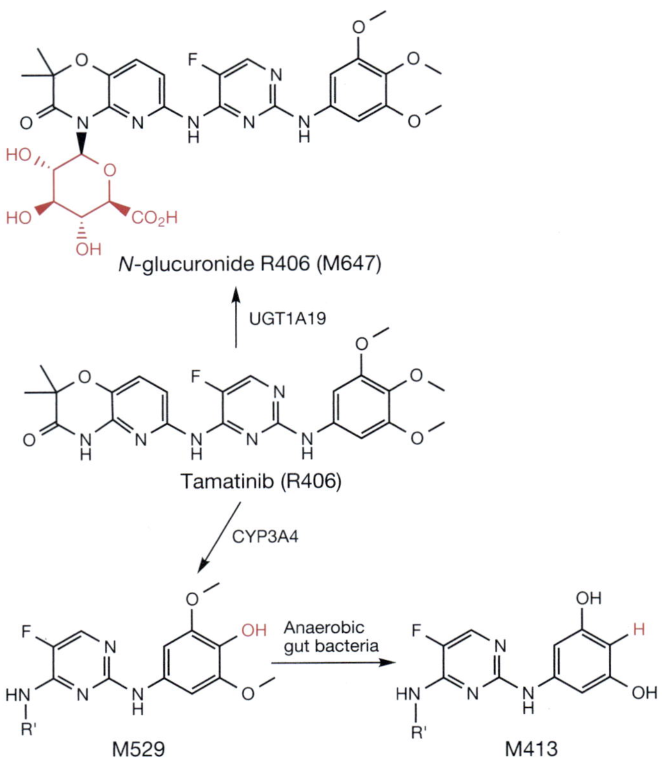

Figure 21.44 Metabolism of tamatinib.

tamatinib is a P-gp substrate. Both fostamatinib and tamatinib inhibit BCRP. This is of particular concern when coadministered with statins, resulting in increased plasma levels of the statin, which increases the risk of statin-induced myopathy.[274] Coadministration of strong inhibitors of CYP3A4 with fostamatinib may increase adverse effects associated with tamatinib.[280] Coadministration of strong inducers of CYP3A4 with fostamatinib is not recommended.[280]

Adverse Effects

The main adverse effects of fostamatinib include hypertension, hepatoxicity, and diarrhea.[280] An increase in blood pressure is due to the off-target inhibitory effects of tamatinib on vascular endothelial growth factor (VEGFR)-1 and VEGFR-2.[275] Monitoring blood pressure and liver function tests with fostamatinib therapy is warranted.[280] Fostamatinib has been shown to cause fetal abnormalities in animal studies and should not be used during pregnancy.[275,280]

Table 21.11 is a comparison of TPO-RAs and fostamatinib in the treatment of thrombocytopenia.[260-277,280]

Fibrinolysis Inhibitors

Plasminogen is a 791–amino acid trypsin-like serine protease glycoprotein that exists in two glycoforms. It consists of seven domains: an N-terminal plasminogen-apple-nematode (PAN) domain, five kringle domains (K1-K5), and a serine protease domain at the C-terminus.[282,283] The K1, K2, K4, and K5 domains contain lysine-binding sites (LBSs) enabling plasminogen to bind to fibrin and other substrates that contain N-terminal lysine residues.[282,284] In intravascular fibrinolysis, single-chain tPA initially binds to fibrin via its fibronectin finger domain. Fibrin-bound tPA activates fibrin-bound plasminogen by cleaving it to the fibrinolytic agent plasmin (see Fig. 21.2). In the process of plasminogen activation, fibrin is degraded, liberating C-terminal Lys residues. Additional binding to fibrin then occurs between the Lys residues on fibrin and a LBS on kringle 2 of tPA.[282] The formation of a ternary complex of fibrin-bound tPA and plasminogen increases the rate of plasminogen activation.[282]

Table 21.11 Comparison of TPO-RAs and Syk Inhibitor in the Treatment of Thrombocytopenia[260-277,280]

Characteristic	Romiplostim	Avatrombopag	Eltrombopag	Lusutrombopag	Fostamatinib
Tradename	Nplate	Doptelet	Promacta	Mulpleta	Tavalisse
Molecular description	Peptibody	Small molecule	Small molecule	Small molecule	Small molecule
Prodrug	No	No	No	No	Yes
MW (Da)	59,000	650	442.5	591.5	580.5 Tamatinib (active form): 407
Mechanism of action	TPO-RA	TPO-RA	TPO-RA	TPO-RA	Syk inhibitor
Binding site target	Extracellular domain	Transmembrane domain	Transmembrane domain	Transmembrane domain	ATP-binding site
Route of administration	SC	Oral	Oral	Oral	Oral

(continued)

Table 21.11 Comparison of TPO-RAs and Syk Inhibitor in the Treatment of Thrombocytopenia[260-277,280] (*continued*)

Characteristic	Romiplostim	Avatrombopag	Eltrombopag	Lusutrombopag	Fostamatinib
Approved Indications	• ITP in adults and children 1 y or older with insufficient response to previous treatment • Hematopoietic syndrome of acute radiation syndrome in adults and children	• Thrombocytopenia in adults with CLD scheduled to undergo a procedure • Chronic ITP with insufficient response to previous treatment in adults	• ITP in adults and children ≥1 y • Hepatitis-C associated thrombocytopenia • Severe aplastic anemia in adults and children ≥2 y	Thrombocytopenia in adults with CLD scheduled to undergo a procedure	Chronic ITP in adults with insufficient response to previous treatment
Dosing frequency	Weekly	Once weekly up to daily	Daily	Daily	Twice daily
Dietary restrictions	No	No	Polyvalent cations	No	No
Plasma $t_{1/2}$	1-35 d (median: 3.5 d)	~19 h	21-32 h	27 h	Tamatinib: 12.9-20.9 h
Metabolism	TPO-Rs and reticuloendothelial clearance	CYP2C9/3A4	Gut microbes; UGT1A1/1A3	CYP4A11	CYP3A4; UGT1A9

CLD, chronic liver disease; ITP, immune thrombocytopenia; SC, subcutaneous; Syk, spleen tyrosine kinase; TPO-R; thrombopoietin receptor; TPO-RA, thrombopoietin-receptor agonist.

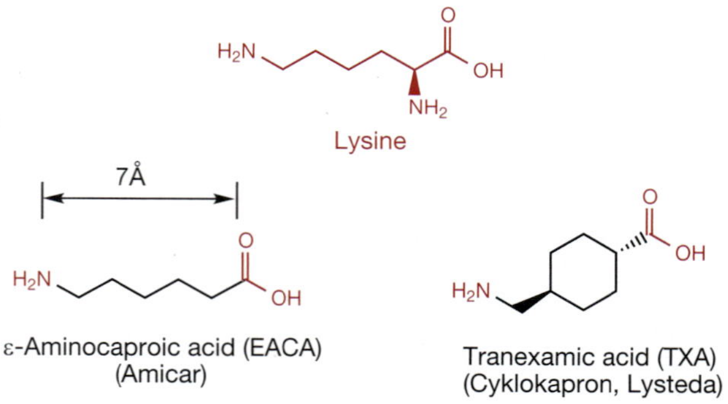

The two fibrinolysis inhibitors available are the lysine analogs ε-aminocaproic acid (EACA) and tranexamic acid (TXA). Both EACA and TXA block plasminogen activation by binding to the LBS on the K1, K2, K4, and K5 domains, mainly on K1, of plasminogen.[282,284] Key features of EACA and TXA include an amine and carboxylic acid separated by an appropriate length. In EACA, the amine and carboxylic acid are approximately 7 Å apart.[282] Increasing or decreasing the length between the amine and carboxylic acid dramatically decreases antifibrinolytic activity. For example, EACA has 10-fold greater antifibrinolytic activity than lysine.[282] The *trans*-relationship of TXA is critical to its activity as the *cis*-stereoisomer is inactive.[282,283] TXA is conformationally restricted, which leads to enhanced potency. TXA is approximately 10-fold more potent than EACA.[283] Figure 21.45 shows key interactions between EACA and TXA and the LBS of K1 of plasminogen.[282] The amino groups of EACA and TXA form salt bridges with Asp137 and Asp139 of K1 of plasminogen. The carboxylate groups of EACA and TXA form electrostatic interactions with Arg117, Try146, Arg153. The hydrophobic central region of each drug—that is, the five methylene central chain of EACA and the core cyclohexyl ring of TXA—forms van der Waals interactions with Phe118, Trp144, Tyr146, and Tyr154.

EACA is indicated as a general fibrinolytic inhibitor.[285] Oral TXA is indicated in the treatment of heavy menstrual bleeding.[286] IV TXA is indicated for treatment of bleeding associated with hemophilia.[287] Both agents are used to stop bleeding or prevent bleeding in a variety of scenarios. For example, IV TXA is used to prevent excess bleeding and the need for blood transfusions after coronary artery surgery.[288] IV TXA is also recommended to reduce postpartum hemorrhage and to treat traumatic bleeding.[289]

Pharmacokinetics

Both EACA and TXA may be administered orally or intravenously. The terminal half-life of EACA is approximately 2 hours.[285] The apparent elimination half-life of TXA is approximately 2 hours, and the mean terminal half-life is approximately 11 hours.[286,287] Renal excretion is the primary route of elimination for EACA and TXA. Nearly all TXA is

Structure Challenge

1. For each of the following drugs, indicate whether it is an antiplatelet drug or anticoagulant and its mechanism of action.

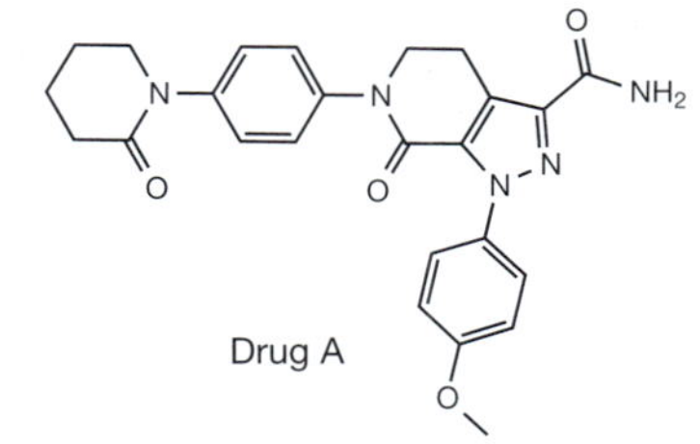

Drug A

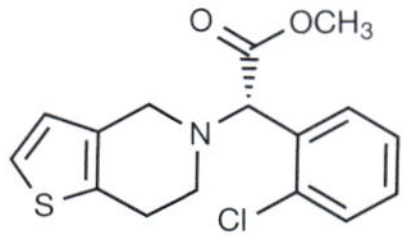

Drug B

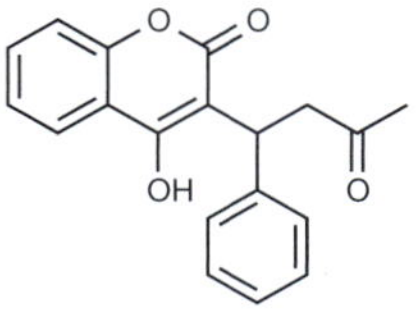

Drug C

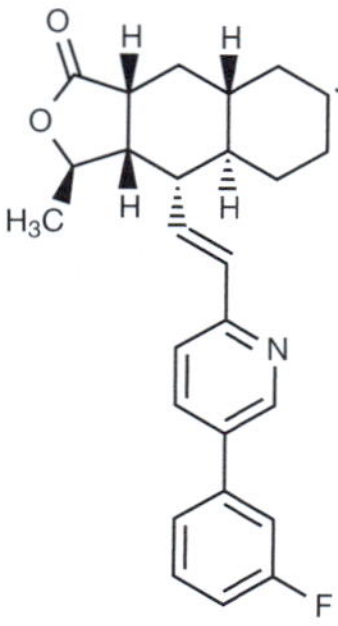

Drug D

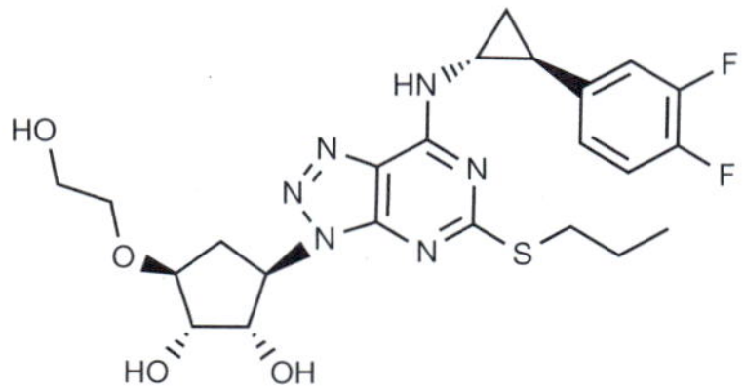

Drug E

2. Which of the following drugs is a prodrug? Select all that apply.

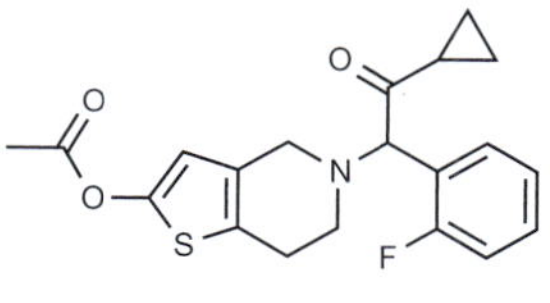

Drug A

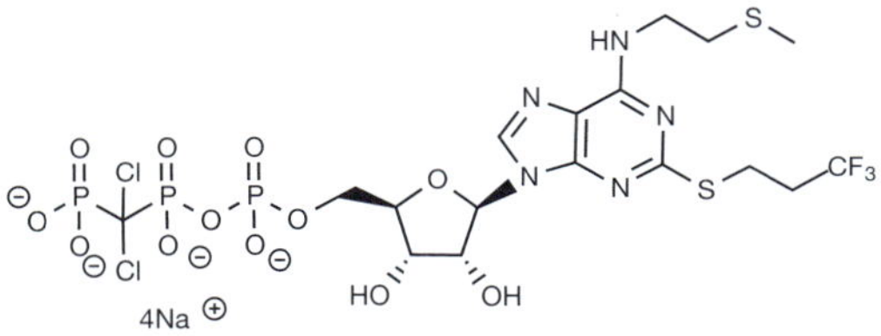

Drug B

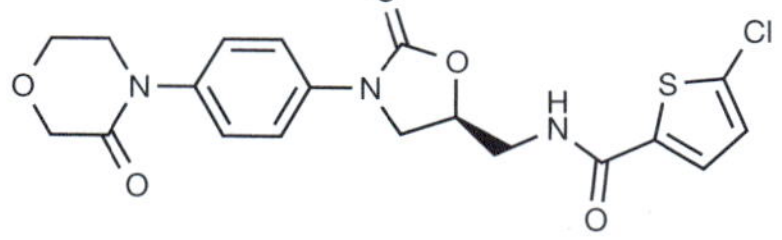

Drug C

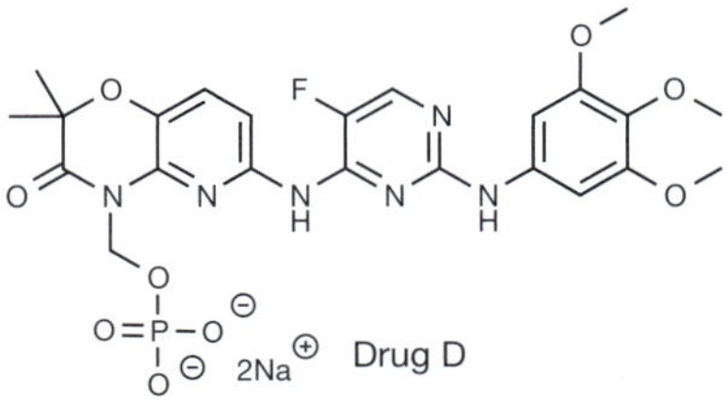

Drug D

3. Idarucizumab binds to which of the following? Select all that apply.

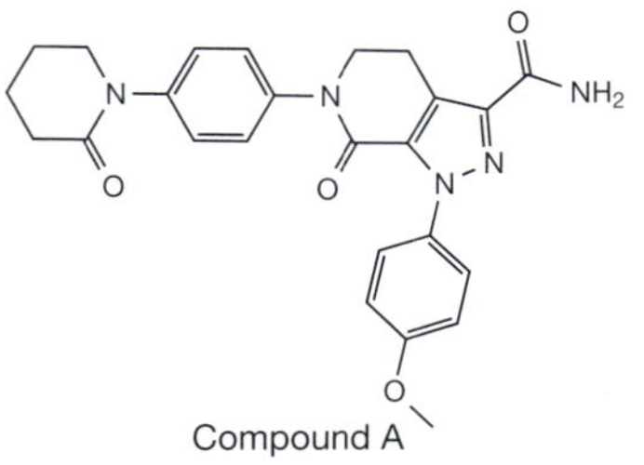

Compound A

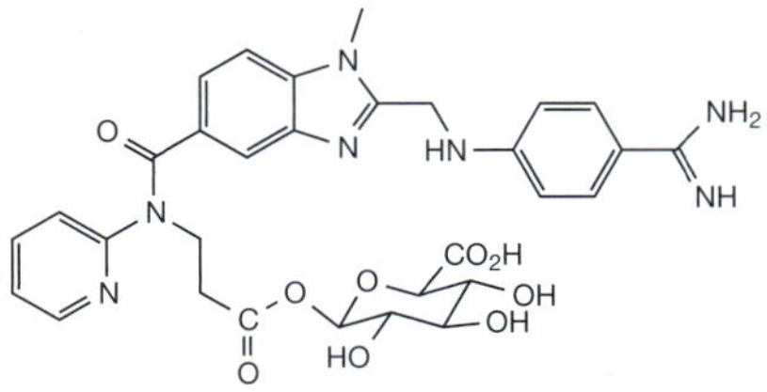

Compound B

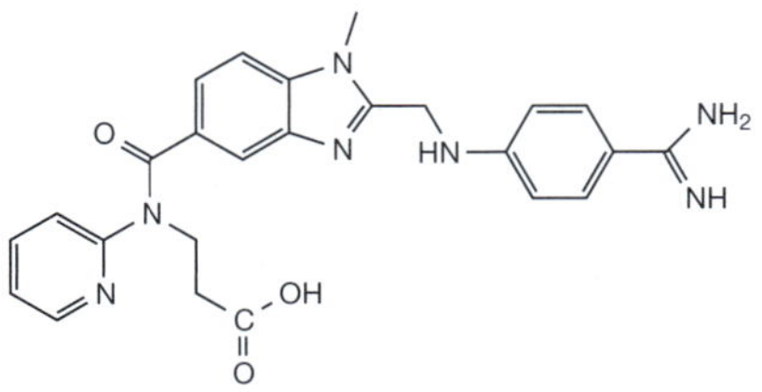

Compound C

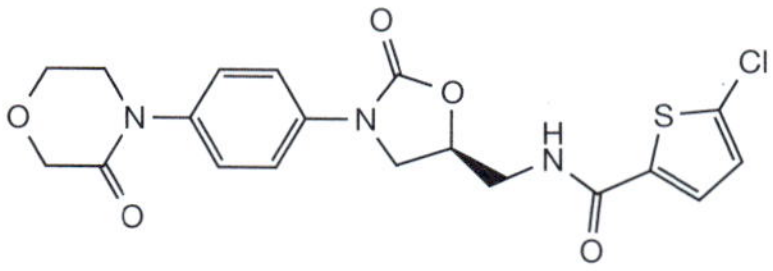

Compound D

Structure Challenge answers found immediately after References.

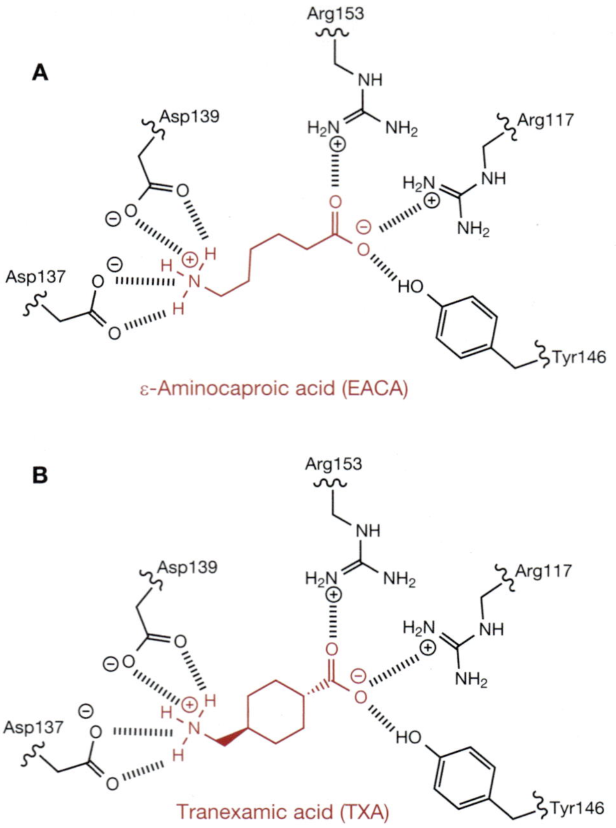

Figure 21.45 Important binding interactions within the lysine-binding site (LBS) of Kringle 1 (K1) of plasminogen with (**A**) ε-aminocaproic acid (EACA) and (**B**) tranexamic acid (TXA).[282] Key amino acid residues within the LBS of K1 in plasminogen that interact with EACA and TXA are shown in black. Not shown are Phe118, Trp144, Tyr146, and Tyr154 of K1 in plasminogen, which participate in van der Waals interactions between the five methylene groups of EACA and the cyclohexyl core of TXA.

excreted unchanged in the urine,[286,287] while 65% of EACA is excreted unchanged in the urine and 11% of the dose is excreted as adipic acid.[285]

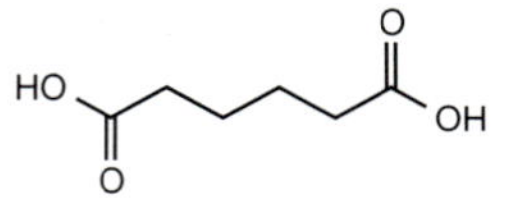

Adipic acid

Adverse Effects

TXA is associated with an increased incidence of seizures.[288]

REFERENCES

1. Golledge J. Update on the pathophysiology and medical treatment of peripheral artery disease. *Nat Rev Cardiol.* 2022;19:456-474.
2. Khurshid S, Trinquart L, Weng LC, et al. Atrial fibrillation risk and discrimination of cardioembolic from noncardioembolic stroke. *Stroke.* 2020;51:1396-1403.
3. Khan F, Tritschler T, Kahn SR, et al. Venous thromboembolism. *Lancet.* 2021;398:64-77.
4. Wolberg AS, Rosendaal FR, Weitz JI, et al. Venous thromboembolism. *Nat Rev Dis Primers.* 2015;1:15006.
5. Cohen AT, Katholing A, Rietbrock S, et al. Epidemiology of first and recurrent venous thromboembolism in patients with active cancer. A population-based cohort study. *Thromb Haemost.* 2017;117:57-65.
6. Middeldorp S, Coppens M, van Haaps TF, et al. Incidence of venous thromboembolism in hospitalized patients with COVID-19. *J Thromb Haemost.* 2020;18(8):1995-2002.
7. Poor HD. Pulmonary thrombosis and thromboembolism in COVID-19. *Chest.* 2021;160:1471-1480.
8. Jimenez D, Garcia-Sanchez A, Rali P, et al. Incidence of VTE and bleeding among hospitalized patients with coronavirus disease 2019: a systematic review and meta-analysis. *Chest.* 2021;159:1182-1196.
9. Fanaroff AC, Lopes RD. COVID-19 thrombotic complications and therapeutic strategies. *Annu Rev Med.* 2023. 74:15-30.
10. Kalaitzopoulos R, Panagopoulos A, Samant S, et al. Management of venous thromboembolism in pregnancy. *Thromb Res.* 2022;211:106-113.
11. Vos T, Lim SS, Abbafati C, et al. Global burden of 369 diseases and injuries in 204 countries and territories, 1990-2019: a systematic analysis for the Global Burden of Disease Study 2019. *Lancet.* 2020;396:1204-1222.
12. World Health Organization. WHO methods and data sources for global burden of disease estimates 2000-2019. Published December 2020. Accessed September 2, 2023. https://cdn.who.int/media/docs/default-source/gho-documents/global-health-estimates/ghe2019_daly-methods.pdf?sfvrsn=31b25009_7
13. Roth GA, Mensah GA, Johnson CO, et al. Global burden of cardiovascular diseases and risk factors, 1990-2019: update from the GBD 2019 study. *J Am Coll Cardiol.* 2020;76:2982-3021.
14. Tsao CW, Aday AW, Armarzooq ZI, et al. Heart disease and stroke statistics-2023 update: a report from the American Heart Association. *Circulation.* 2023;147:e93-e621.
15. Dieleman JL, Cao J, Chapin A, et al. US health care spending by payer and health condition, 1996-2016. *JAMA.* 2020;323:863-884.
16. Christensen EW, Pelzl CE, Hemingway J, et al. Drivers of ischemic stroke hospital cost trends among older adults in the United States. *J Am Coll Radiol.* 2023;20:411-421.
17. Grosse SD, Nelson RE, Nyarko KA, et al. The economic burden of incident venous thromboembolism in the United States: a review of estimated attributable healthcare costs. *Thromb Res.* 2016;137:3-10.
18. Kohn CG, Alberts MJ, Peacock WF. Cost and inpatient burden of peripheral artery disease: Findings from the National Inpatient Sample. *Atherosclerosis.* 2019;286:142-146.
19. Sang Y, Roest M, de Laat B, et al. Interplay between platelets and coagulation. *Blood Revi.* 2021;46:100733.
20. Stojanovski BM, Pelc LA, Zuo X, et al. Zymogen and activated protein C have similar structural architecture. *J Biol Chem.* 2020;295:15236-15244.
21. Gemma L, Rehill AM, Preston RJS. The protein C pathways. *Curr Opin Hematol.* 2022;29:251-258.
22. Gierula M, Salles-Crawley II, Santamaria S, et al. The roles of factor Va and protein S in formation of the activated protein C/protein S/factor Va inactivation complex. *J Thromb Haemost.* 2019;17(12):2056-2068.
23. Gierula M, Ahnström J. Anticoagulant protein S—new insights on interactions and functions. *J Thromb Haemost.* 2020;18:2801-2811.
24. Mast AE, Ruf W. Regulation of coagulation by tissue factor pathway inhibitor: implications for hemophilia therapy. *J Thromb Haemost.* 2022;20:1290-1300.
25. Rezaie AR, Giri H. Anticoagulant and signaling functions of antithrombin. *J Thromb Haemost.* 2020;18:3142-3153.
26. Hsu C, Hutt E, Bloomfield DM, et al. Factor IX inhibition to uncouple thrombosis from hemostasis. *J Am Coll Cardiol.* 2021;78:625-631.

27. Grover SP, Mackman N. Intrinsic pathway of coagulation and thrombosis: insights from animal models. *Arterioscler Thromb Vasc Biol.* 2019;39:331-338.
28. Lin L, Zhao L, Gao N, et al. From multi-target anticoagulants to DOACs, and intrinsic factor inhibitors. *Blood Rev.* 2020;39:100615.
29. Campello E, Henderson MW, Noubouossie DF, et al. Contact system activation and cancer: new insights in the pathophysiology of cancer-associated thrombosis. *Thromb Haemost.* 2018;118:251-265.
30. Raghunathan V, Zilberman-Rudenko J, Olson SR, et al. The contact pathway and sepsis. *Res Pract Thromb Haemost.* 2019;3:331-339.
31. Navarrete S, Solar C, Tapia R, et al. Pathophysiology of deep vein thrombosis. *Clin Exp Med.* 2023;23:645-654.
32. Khan AA, Lip GYH. The prothrombotic state in atrial fibrillation: pathophysiological and management implications. *Cardiovasc Res.* 2019;115:31-45.
33. Fogelstrand P, Borén J. Retention of atherogenic lipoproteins in the artery wall and its role in atherogenesis. *Nutr Metab Cardiovasc Dis.* 2012;22:1-7.
34. Libby P. Inflammation and cardiovascular disease mechanisms. *Am J Clin Nutr.* 2006;83(2):456S-460S.
35. Bentzon JF, Otsuka F, Virmani R, et al. Mechanisms of plaque formation and rupture. *Circ Res.* 2014;114:1852-1866.
36. Head T, Daunet S, Goldschmidt-Clermont PJ. The aging risk and atherosclerosis: a fresh look at arterial homeostasis. *Front Genet.* 2017;8:216.
37. Sakakura K, Nakano M, Otsuka F, et al. Pathophysiology of atherosclerosis plaque progression. *Heart Lung Circ.* 2013;22:399-411.
38. Tabas I, Lichtman AH. Monocyte-macrophages and T cells in atherosclerosis. *Immunity.* 2017;47:621-634.
39. Kamtchum-Tatuene J, Saba L, Heldner MR, et al. Interleukin-6 predicts carotid plaque severity, vulnerability, and progression. *Circ Res.* 2022;131:e22-e33.
40. Ridker PM, MacFayden JG, Thuren T, et al. Residual inflammatory risk associated with interleukin-18 and interleukin-6 after successful interleukin-1β inhibition with canakinumab: further rational for the development of targeted anti-cytokine therapies for the treatment of atherothrombosis. *Eur Heart J.* 2020;41:2153-2163.
41. Gaba P, Gersh BJ, Muller J, et al. Evolving concepts of the vulnerable atherosclerotic plaque and the vulnerable patient: implications for patient care and future research. *Nat Rev Cardiol.* 2023;20:181-196.
42. Libby P, Tabas I, Fredman G, Fisher EA. Inflammation and its resolution as determinants of acute coronary syndromes. *Circ Res.* 2014;114:1867-1879.
43. Libby P, Pasterkamp G, Crea F, et al. Reassessing the mechanisms of acute coronary syndromes: the "vulnerable plaque" and superficial erosion. *Circ Res.* 2019;124:150-160.
44. Fahed AC, Jang IK. Plaque erosion and acute coronary syndromes: phenotype, molecular characteristics and future directions. *Nat Rev Cardiol.* 2021;18:724-734.
45. Narula N, Olin JW, Narula N. Pathological disparities between peripheral artery disease and coronary artery disease. *Arterioscler Thromb Vasc Biol.* 2020;40:1982-1989.
46. Narula N, Dannenberg AJ, Olin JW, et al. Pathology of peripheral artery disease in patients with critical limb ischemia. *J Am Coll Cardiol.* 2018;72:2152-2163.
47. Campbell BCV, De Silva DA, Macleod MR, et al. Ischaemic stroke. *Nat Rev Dis Primers.* 2019;5:70.
48. Chernysh IN, Nagaswami C, Kosolapova S, et al. The distinctive structure and composition of arterial and venous thrombi and pulmonary emboli. *Sci Rep.* 2020;10:5112.
49. Staessens S, Denorme F, Francois O, et al. Structural analysis of ischemic stroke thrombi: histological indications for therapy resistance. *Haematologica.* 2020;105:498-507.
50. Amsterdam EA, Wenger NK, Brindis RG, et al. 2014 AHA/ACC guideline for the management of patients with non-ST-elevation acute coronary syndromes: a report of the American College of Cardiology/American Heart Association Task Force on practice guidelines. *J Am Coll Cardiol.* 2014;64:e139-e228.
51. Jones WS, Mulder H, Wruck LM, et al. Comparative effectiveness of aspirin dosing in cardiovascular disease. *N Engl J Med.* 2021;384:1981-1990.
52. Powers WJ, Rabinstein AA, Ackerson T, et al. Guidelines for the early management of patients with acute ischemic stroke: 2019 update to the 2018 guidelines for the early management of acute ischemic stroke: a guideline for healthcare professionals from the American Heart Association/American Stroke Association. *Stroke.* 2019;50:e344-e418.
53. Patrono C. Aspirin and human platelets: from clinical trials to acetylation of cyclooxygenase and back. *Trends Pharmacol Sci.* 1989;10:453-458.
54. Blobaum AL, Marnett LJ. Structural and functional basis of cyclooxygenase inhibition. *J Med Chem.* 2007;50:1425-1441.
55. Hochgesang GP, Rowlinson SW, Marnett LJ. Tyrosine-385 is critical for acetylation of cyclooxygenase-2 by aspirin. *J Am Chem Soc.* 2000;122:6514-6515.
56. Smith WL, DeWitt DL, Kraemer SA, et al. Structure-function relationships in sheep, mouse, and human prostaglandin endoperoxide G/H synthases. *Adv Prostaglandin Thromboxane Leukot Res.* 1990;20:14-21.
57. Patrono C, Garcia Rodriguez LA, Landolfi R, et al. Low-dose aspiring for the prevention of atherothrombosis. *N Engl J Med.* 2005;353:2373-2383.
58. Pedersen AK, FitzGerald GA. Dose-related kinetics of aspirin. *N Engl J Med.* 1984;311:1206-1211.
59. Grosser T, Fries S, Lawson JA, et al. Drug resistance and pseudoresistance: an unintended consequence of enteric coating aspirin. *Circulation.* 2013;127:377-385.
60. Haastrup PF, Gronlykke T, Jarbol DE. Enteric coating can lead to reduced antiplatelet effect of low-dose acetylsalicylic acid. *Basic Clin Pharmacol Toxicol.* 2015;116:212-215.
61. Raber I, McCarthy CP, Vaduganathan M, et al. The rise and fall of aspirin in the primary prevention of cardiovascular disease. *Lancet.* 2019;393:2155-2167.
62. US Preventive Services Task Force. Aspirin use to prevent cardiovascular disease: US Preventive Services Task Force Recommendation Statement. *JAMA.* 2020;327:1577-1584.
63. Li X, Fries S, Li R, et al. Differential impairment of aspirin-dependent platelet cyclooxygenase acetylation by nonsteroidal antiinflammatory drugs. *Proc Natl Acad Sci U S A.* 2014;111:16830-16835.
64. Catella-Lawson F, Reilly MP, Kapoor SC, et al. Cyclooxygenase inhibitors and the antiplatelet effects of aspirin. *N Engl J Med.* 2001;345:1809-1817.
65. Lawton JS, Tamis-Holland JE, Bangalore S, et al. 2021 ACC/AHA/SCAI guideline for coronary artery revascularization: executive summary: a report of the American College of Cardiology/American Heart Association Joint Committee on clinical practice guidelines. *Circulation.* 2022;145:e4-e17.
66. Levine GN, Bates ER, Bittl JA, et al. 2016 ACC/AHA guideline focused update on duration of dual antiplatelet therapy in patients with coronary artery disease: a report of the American College of Cardiology/American Heart Association Task Force on clinical practice guidelines. *J Am Coll Cardiol.* 2016;68:1082-1115.
67. Tang M, Mukundan M, Yang J, et al. Antiplatelet agents aspirin and clopidogrel are hydrolyzed by distinct carboxylesterases, and clopidogrel is transesterificated in the presence of ethyl alcohol. *J Pharmacol Exp Ther.* 2006;319:1467-1476.
68. Kazui M, Nishiya Y, Ishizuka T, et al. Identification of the human cytochrome P450 enzymes involved in the two oxidative steps in the bioactivation of clopidogrel to its pharmacologically active metabolite. *Drug Metab Dispos.* 2010;38:92-99.

69. Savi P, Zachayus JL, Delesque-Touchard N, et al. The active metabolite of clopidogrel disrupts P2Y12 receptor oligomers and partitions them out of lipid rafts. *Proc Natl Acad Sci U S A.* 2006;103:11069-11074.
70. Algaier I, Jakubowski JA, Asai F, et al. Interaction of the active metabolite of prasugrel, R-138727, with cysteine 97 and cysteine 175 of the human P2Y12 receptor. *J Thromb Haemost.* 2008;6:1908-1914.
71. Farid NA, Kurihara A, Wrighton SA. Metabolism and disposition of the thienopyridine antiplatelet drugs ticlopidine, clopidogrel, and prasugrel in humans. *J Clin Pharmacol.* 2010;50:126-142.
72. Mega JL, Close SL, Wiviott SD, et al. Cytochrome P-450 polymorphisms and response to clopidogrel. *N Engl J Med.* 2009;360:354-362.
73. Brown SA, Pereira N. Pharmacogenomic impact of CYP2C19 variation on clopidogrel therapy in precision cardiovascular medicine. *J Pers Med.* 2018;8:8.
74. Pare G, Mehta SR, Yusuf S, et al. Effects of CYP2C19 genotype on outcomes of clopidogrel treatment. *N Engl J Med.* 2010;363:1704-1714.
75. Doll JA, Neely ML, Roe MT, et al. Impact of CYP2C19 metabolizer status on patients with ACS treated with prasugrel versus clopidogrel. *J Am Coll Cardiol.* 2016;67:936-947.
76. Lee CR, Luzum JA, Sangkuhl K, et al. Clinical Pharmacogenetics Implementation Consortium guidelines for CYP2C19 genotype and clopidogrel therapy: 2022 update. *Clin Pharmacol Ther.* 2022;112:959-967.
77. Plavix. Package insert. Sanofi-Aventis; Revised September 2022. Accessed September 20, 2023. https://products.sanofi.us/plavix/plavix.pdf
78. Kuno T, Fujisaki T, Shoji S, et al. Comparison of unguided de-escalation versus guided selection of dual antiplatelet therapy after acute coronary syndrome: a systematic review and network meta-analysis. *Circ Cardiovasc Interv.* 2022;15(8):e011990.
79. Angiolillo DJ, Gibson CM, Cheng S, et al. Differential effects of omeprazole and pantoprazole on the pharmacodynamics and pharmacokinetics of clopidogrel in healthy subjects: randomized, placebo-controlled, crossover comparison studies. *Clin Pharmacol Ther.* 2011;89:65-74.
80. Frelinger AL, Lee RD, Mulford DJ, et al. A randomized, 2-period, crossover design study to assess the effects of dexlansoprazole, lansoprazole, esomeprazole, and omeprazole on the steady-state pharmacokinetics and pharmacodynamics of clopidogrel in healthy volunteers. *J Am Coll Cardiol.* 2012;59:1304-1311.
81. Melloni C, Washam JB, Jones WS, et al. Conflicting results between randomized trials and observational studies on the impact of proton pump inhibitors on cardiovascular events when coadministered with dual antiplatelet therapy: systematic review. *Circ Cardiovasc Qual Outcomes.* 2015;8:47-55.
82. O'Donague ML, Braunwald E, Antman EM, et al. Pharmacodynamic effect and clinical efficacy of clopidogrel and prasugrel with or without a proton-pump inhibitor: an analysis of two randomised trials. *Lancet.* 2009;374:989-997.
83. Gargiulo G, Costa F, Ariotti S, et al. Impact of proton pump inhibitors on clinical outcomes in patients treated with a 6- or 24-month dual-antiplatelet therapy duration: insights from the PROlonging Dual-antiplatelet treatment after Grading stent-induced Intimal hyperplasia studY trial. *Am Heart J.* 2016;174:95-102.
84. Hobl E, Stimpfl T, Ebner J. Morphine decreases clopidogrel concentrations and effects: a randomized, double-blind, placebo-controlled trial. *J Am Coll Cardiol.* 2014;63:630-635.
85. Hobl E, Reiter B, Schoergenhofer C, et al. Morphine interaction with prasugrel: a double blind, cross-over trial in healthy volunteers. *Clin Res Cardiol.* 2016;105:340-355.
86. Jakubowski JA, Winters KJ, Naganuma H, et al. Prasugrel: a novel thienopyridine antiplatelet agent. A review of preclinical and clinical studies and the mechanistic basis for its distinct antiplatelet profile. *Cardiovasc Drug Rev.* 2007;25:357-374.
87. Wiviott SD, Braunwald E, McCabe CH, et al. Prasugrel versus clopidogrel in patients with acute coronary syndromes. *N Engl J Med.* 2007;357:2001-2015.
88. Effient. Package insert. Cosette Pharmaceuticals; Revised February 2022. Accessed September 21, 2023. https://dailymed.nlm.nih.gov/dailymed/fda/fdaDrugXsl.cfm?setid=69ea2d58-5353-4222-b61f-cab976fa7e5e&type=display
89. Johnston SC, Amarenco P, Denison H, et al. Ticagrelor and aspirin or aspirin alone in acute ischemic stroke or TIA. *N Engl J Med.* 2020;383:207-217.
90. Bhatt DL, Stone GW, Mahaffey KW, et al. Effect of platelet inhibition with cangrelor during PCI on ischemic events. *N Engl J Med.* 2013;368:1303-1313.
91. Arora S, Shemisa K, Vaduganathan M, et al. Premature ticagrelor discontinuation in secondary prevention of atherosclerotic CVD. *J Am Coll Cardiol.* 2019;73:2454-2464.
92. Ingall AH, Dixon J, Bailey A, et al. Antagonists of the platelet P2T receptor: a novel approach to antithrombotic therapy. *J Med Chem.* 1999;42:213-220.
93. Walsh JA, Price MJ. Cangrelor for treatment of arterial thrombosis. *Expert Opin Pharmacother.* 2014;15:565-572.
94. Dovlatova NL, Jakubowski JA, Sugidachi A, et al. The reversible P2Y antagonist cangrelor influences the ability of the active metabolites of clopidogrel and prasugrel to produce irreversible inhibition of platelet function. *J Thromb Haemost.* 2008;6:1153-1159.
95. Springthorpe B, Bailey A, Barton P, et al. From ATP to AZD6140: the discovery of an orally active reversible P2Y12 receptor antagonist for the prevention of thrombosis. *Bioorg Med Chem Lett.* 2007;17:6013-6018.
96. Remko M, Remkova A, Broer R. A comparative study of molecular structure, pKa, lipophilicity, solubility, absorption and polar surface area of some antiplatelet drugs. *Int J Mol Sci.* 2016;17:388.
97. Storey RF, Husted S, Harrington RA, et al. Inhibition of platelet aggregation by AZD6140, a reversible oral P2Y12 receptor antagonist, compared with clopidogrel in patients with acute coronary syndromes. *J Am Coll Cardiol.* 2007;50:1852-1856.
98. Wallentin L, Becker RC, Budaj, et al. Ticagrelor versus clopidogrel in patients with acute coronary syndromes. *N Engl J Med.* 2009;361:1045-1057.
99. Mahaffey KW, Woidyla DM, Carroll K, et al. Ticagrelor compared with clopidogrel by geographic region in the Platelet Inhibition and Patient Outcomes (PLATO) trial. *Circulation.* 2011;124:544-554.
100. Brilinta. Package insert. AstraZeneca Pharmaceuticals; Revised November 2024. Accessed February 11, 2025. https://den8dhaj6zs0e.cloudfront.net/50fd68b9-106b-4550-b5d0-12b045f8b184/565ceafd-fbe3-4573-9c39-19280af566ec/565ceafd-fbe3-4573-9c39-19280af566ec_viewable_rendition__v.pdf
101. Zhou D, Andersson TB, Grimm SW. In vitro evaluation of potential drug-drug interactions with ticagrelor: cytochrome P450 reaction phenotyping, inhibition, induction, and differential kinetics. *Drug Metab Dispos.* 2011;39:703-710.
102. Kubica J, Adamski P, Ostrowska M, et al. Morphine delays and attenuates ticagrelor exposure and action in patients with myocardial infarction: the randomized, double-blind, placebo-controlled IMPRESSION trial. *Eur Heart J.* 2016;37:245-252.
103. Franchi F, Rollini F, Park Y, et al. Effects of methylnaltrexone on ticagrelor-induced antiplatelet effects in coronary artery disease patients treated with morphine. *J Am Coll Cardiol Interv.* 2019;12(16):1538-1549.
104. Holm M, Tornvall P, Henareh L, et al. The MOVEMENT trial. *J Am Heart Assoc.* 2019;8:e010152.
105. Zenklusen I, Hsin C-H, Schilling U, et al. Transition from syringe to autoinjector based on bridging pharmacokinetics and pharmacodynamics of the P2Y12 receptor antagonist selatogrel in healthy subjects. *Clin Pharmacokinet.* 2022;61:687-695.
106. Caroff E, Meyer E, Treiber A, et al. Optimization of 2-phenylpyrimidine-4-carboxamides towards potent, orally bioavailable

and selective P2Y12 antagonists for inhibition of platelet aggregation. *Bioorg Med Chem Lett.* 2014;24:4323-4331.
107. Caroff E, Hubler F, Meyer E, et al. 4-((R)-2-{[6-((S)-3-Methoxypyrrolidin-1-yl)-2-phenylpyrimidine-4-carbonyl]amino}-3-phosphonopropionyl)piperazine-1-carboxylic acid butyl ester (ACT-246475) and its prodrug (ACT-281959), a novel P2Y12 receptor antagonist with a wider therapeutic window in the rat than clopidogrel. *J Med Chem.* 2015;58:9133-9153.
108. Ufer M, Huynh C, Jaap van Lier J, et al. Absorption, distribution, metabolism and excretion of the P2Y12 receptor antagonist selatogrel after subcutaneous administration in healthy subjects. *Xenobiotica.* 2020;50:427-434.
109. Milluzzo RP, Franchina GA, Capodanno D, et al. Selatogrel, a novel P2Y12 inhibitor: a review of the pharmacology and clinical development. *Expert Opin Investig Drugs.* 2020;29:537-546.
110. Armstrong EJ, Golan DE. Pharmacology of hemostasis and thrombosis. In: Golan DE, Armstrong EJ, Armstrong AW, eds. *Principles of Pharmacology: The Pathophysiologic Basis of Drug Therapy.* 4th ed. Wolters-Kluwer Health; 2017:403-432.
111. Morrow DA, Braunwald E, Bonaca MP, et al. Vorapaxar in the secondary prevention of atherothrombotic events. *N Engl J Med.* 2012;366:1404-1413.
112. Qamar A, Morrow DA, Creager MA, et al. Effect of vorapaxar on cardiovascular and limb outcomes in patients with peripheral artery disease with and without conroary artery disease: analysis from the TRA 2°P-TIMI 50 trial. *Vasc Med.* 2020;25:124-132.
113. Chackalamannil S, Xia Y, Greenlee WJ, et al. Discovery of potent orally active thrombin receptor (protease activated receptor 1) antagonists as novel antithrombotic agents. *J Med Chem.* 2005;48:5884-5887.
114. Chackalamannil S, Wang Y, Greenlee WJ, et al. Discovery of a novel, orally active himbacine-based thrombin receptor antagonist (SCH530348) with potent antiplatelet activity. *J Med Chem.* 2008;51:3061-3064.
115. Kosoglou T, Revderman L, Tiessen RG, et al. Pharmacodynamics and pharmacokinetics of the novel PAR-1 antagonist vorapaxar (formerly SCH 530348) in healthy subjects. *Eur J Clin Pharmacol.* 2012;68:249-258.
116. Ghosal A, Lu X, Penner N, et al. Identification of human liver cytochrome P450 enzymes involved in the metabolism of SCH530348 (vorapaxar), a potent oral thrombin protease-activated receptor 1 antagonist. *Drug Metab Dispos.* 2011;39:30-38.
117. Zontivity. Package insert. WraSer Pharmaceuticals; Revised October 2022. Accessed September 21, 2023. https://dailymed.nlm.nih.gov/dailymed/fda/fdaDrugXsl.cfm?setid=f2abe3ed-ed3d-4215-a489-b18341ce85bc&type=display
118. Bledzka K, Smyth SS, Plow EF. Integrin αIIbβ3: from discovery to efficacious therapeutic target. *Circ Res.* 2013;112:1189-1200.
119. Scarborough RM, Gretler DD. Platelet glycoprotein IIb-IIIa antagonists as prototypical integrin blockers: novel parenteral and potential oral antithrombotic agents. *J Med Chem.* 2000;43:3453-3473.
120. Xiao T, Takagi J, Coller BS, et al. Structural basis for allostery in integrins and binding to fibrinogen-mimetic therapeutics. *Nature.* 2004;432:59-67.
121. Scarborough RM, Naughton MA, Teng W, et al. Design of potent and specific integrin antagonists. Peptide antagonists with high specificity for glycoprotein IIb-IIIa. *J Biol Chem.* 1993;268:1066-1073.
122. Hartman GD, Egbertson MS, Halczenk W, et al. Non-peptide fibrinogen receptor antagonists. 1. Discovery and design of exosite inhibitors. *J Med Chem.* 1992;35:4640-4642.
123. Zhu J, Choi WS, McCoy JG, et al. Structure-guided design of a high-affinity platelet integrin αIIbβ3 receptor antagonist that disrupts Mg2+ binding to the MIDAS. *Sci Transl Med.* 2012;4:125ra32.
124. King S, Short M, Harmon C. Glycoprotein IIb/IIIa inhibitors: the resurgence of tirofiban. *Vascul Pharmacol.* 2016;78:10-16.
125. Alton KB, Kosoglou T, Baker S, et al. Disposition of 14C-eptifibatide after intravenous administration to healthy men. *Clin Ther.* 1998;20:307-323.
126. Vickers S, Tehoharides AD, Arison B, et al. In vitro and in vivo studies on the metabolism of tirofiban. *Drug Metab Dispos.* 1999;27:1360-1366.
127. Kleiman NS. Pharmacokinetics and pharmacodynamics of glycoprotein IIb-IIIa inhibitors. *Am Heart J.* 1999;138:263-275.
128. Aster RH. Immune thrombocytopenia caused by glycoprotein IIb/IIIa inhibitors. *Chest.* 2005;127:53S-59S.
129. Platelet Glycoprotein IIb/IIIa in Unstable Angina: Receptor Suppression Using Integrilin Therapy (PURSUIT) Trial Investigators. Inhibition of platelet glycoprotein IIb/IIIa with eptifibatide in patients with acute coronary syndromes. *N Engl J Med.* 1998;339:436-443.
130. Merlini PA, Rossi M, Menozzi A, et al. Thrombocytopenia caused by abciximab or tirofiban and its association with clinical outcome in patients undergoing coronary stenting. *Circulation.* 2004;109:2203-2206.
131. Bougie DW, Wilker PR, Wuitschick ED, et al. Acute thrombocytopenia after treatment with tirofiban or eptifibatide is associated with antibodies specific for ligand-occupied GPIIb/IIIa. *Blood.* 2002;100:2071-2076.
132. Warkentin TE. Drug-induced immune-mediated thrombocytopenia—from purpura to thrombosis. *N Engl J Med.* 2007;356:891-893.
133. Chew DR, Bhatt DL, Topol EJ. Oral glycoprotein IIb/IIIa inhibitors: why don't they work? *Am J Cardiovasc Drugs.* 2001;1:421-428.
134. Bassler N, Loeffler C, Mangin P, et al. A mechanistic model for paradoxical platelet activation by ligand-mimetic alphaIIb beta3 (GPIIb/IIIa) antagonists. *Arterioscler Thromb Vasc Biol.* 2007;27:e9-e15.
135. Jiang J, McCoy JG, Shen M, et al. A novel class of ion displacement ligands as antagonists of the αIIbβ3 receptor that limit conformational reorganization of the receptor. *Bioorg Med Chem Lett.* 2014;24:1148-1153.
136. Rikken AOF, Selvarajah A, Hermanides RS, et al. Prehospital treatment with zalunfiban (RUC-4) in patients with ST- elevation myocardial infarction undergoing primary percutaneous coronary intervention: rationale and design of the CELEBRATE trial. *Am Heart J.* 2023;258:119-128.
137. Liu Y, Shakur Y, Yoshitake M, et al. Cilostazol (Pletal®): dual inhibitor of cyclic nucleotide phosphodiesterase type 3 and adenosine uptake. *Cardiovasc Drug Rev.* 2001;19:369-386.
138. Cilostazol. Package insert. Teva Pharmaceuticals; Revised July 2022. Accessed September 22, 2023. https://dailymed.nlm.nih.gov/dailymed/drugInfo.cfm?setid=a6292311-9cb2-49ff-b8bf-12e2dbd196cd
139. Akiyama H, Kudo S, Shimizu T. The metabolism of a new antithrombotic and vasodilating agent, cilostazol, in rat, dog and man. *Arzneimittelforschung.* 1985;35:1133-1140.
140. Hiratsuka M, Hinai Y, Sasaki, T, et al. Characterization of human cytochrome P450 enzymes involved in the metabolism of cilostazol. *Drug Metab Dispos.* 2007;35:1730-1732.
141. Packer M, Carver JR, Rodeheffer RJ, et al. Effect of oral milrinone on mortality in severe chronic heart failure. *N Engl J Med.* 1991;325:1468-1475.
142. Suri A, Forbes WP, Bramer SL. Effects of CYP3A inhibition on the metabolism of cilostazol. *Clin Pharmacokinet.* 1999;37 (suppl 2):61-68.
143. Suri A, Bramer SL. Effect of omeprazole on the metabolism of cilostazol. *Clin Pharmacokinet.* 1999;37(suppl 2):53-59.
144. Muscatelli SR, Charters MA, Hallstrom BR. Time for an update? A look at current guidelines for venous thromboembolism and knee arthroplasty and hip fracture. *Arthroplast Today.* 2021;10:105-107.
145. Barlow BT, Hannon MT, Waldron JE. Preoperative management of antithrombotics in arthroplasty. *J Am Acad Orthop Surg.* 2019;27:878-886.
146. Key NS, Khorana AA, Kuderer NM, et al. Venous thromboembolism prophylaxis and treatment in patients with cancer: ASCO guideline update. *J Clin Oncol.* 2023;41:3063-3071.

147. Cuker A, Tseng EK, Nieuwlaat R, et al. American Society of Hematology 2021 guidelines on the use of anticoagulation for thromboprophylaxis in patients with COVID-19. *Blood Adv.* 2021;5:872-888.
148. Saad A, Safarzadeh M, Shepherd M. Anticoagulation regimens in pregnancy. *Obstet Gynecol Clin North Am.* 2023;50:241-249.
149. Ortel TL, Neumann I, Ageno W, et al. American Society of Hematology 2020 guidelines for management of venous thromboembolism: treatment of deep vein thrombosis and pulmonary embolism. *Blood Adv.* 2020;4:4693-4738.
150. Lip GYH, Banner A, Boriani G, et al. Antithrombotic therapy for atrial fibrillation: CHEST guidelines and expert panel report. *Chest.* 2018;154:1121-1201.
151. Otto CM, Nishimura RA, Bonow RO, et al. 2020 ACC/AHA guideline for the management of patients with valvular heart disease: a report of the American College of Cardiology/American Heart Association Joint Committee on clinical practice guidelines. *J Am Coll Cardiol.* 2021;77:e25-e197.
152. Linhardt RJ. 2003 Claude S. Hudson Award address in carbohydrate chemistry. Heparin: structure and activity. *J Med Chem.* 2003;46:2551-2564.
153. Baytas SN, Linhardt RJ. Advances in the preparation and synthesis of heparin and related products. *Drug Discov Today.* 2020;25:2095-2109.
154. Hirsh J, Raschke R. Heparin and low-molecular-weight heparin: the seventh ACCP conference on antithrombotic and thrombolytic therapy. *Chest.* 2004;126(3 suppl):188S-203S.
155. Balogh G, Komáromi I, Bereczky Z. The mechanism of high affinity pentasaccharide binding to antithrombin, insights from Gaussian accelerated molecular dynamics simulations. *J Biomol Struct Dyn.* 2020;38:4718-4732.
156. Qiu M, Huang S, Luo C, et al. Pharmacological and clinical application of heparin progress: an essential drug for modern medicine. *Biomed Pharmacother.* 2021;139:111561.
157. Paiardi G, Richter S, Oreste P, et al. The binding of heparin to spike glycoprotein inhibits SARS-CoV-2 infection by three mechanisms. *J Biol Chem.* 2022;298:101507.
158. Hirsh J. Heparin. *N Engl J Med.* 1991;324:1565-1574.
159. Garcia DA, Baglin TP, Weitz JI, et al. Parenteral anticoagulants: antithrombotic therapy and prevention of thrombosis, 9th ed: American College of Chest Physicians evidence-based clinical practice guidelines. *Chest.* 2012;141:e24S-e43S.
160. Salter BS, Weiner MM, Trinh MA, et al. Heparin-induced thrombocytopenia: a comprehensive clinical review. *J Am Coll Cardiol.* 2016;67:2519-2532.
161. Gucinski AC, Boyne MT, Keire DA. Modern analytics for naturally derived complex drug substances: NMR and MS tests for protamine sulfate from chum salmon. *Anal Bioanal Chem.* 2015;407:749-759.
162. Levy JH, Ghadimi K, Kizhakkedathu JN. What's fishy about protamine? Clinical use, adverse reactions, and potential alternatives. *J Thromb Haemost.* 2023;21:1714-1723.
163. Weitz JI. Low-molecular weight heparins. *N Engl J Med.* 1997;337:688-699.
164. Bauer KA, Hawkins DW, Peters PC, et al. Fondaparinux, a synthetic pentasaccharide: the first in a new class of antithrombotic agents—the selective factor Xa inhibitors. *Cardiovasc Drug Rev.* 2002;20:37-52.
165. Schechter I, Berger A. On the active site of proteases. III. Mapping the active site of papain; specific peptide inhibitors of papain. *Biochem Biophys Res Commun.* 1968;32:898-902.
166. Pinto DJP, Smallheer JM, Cheney DL, et al. Factor Xa Inhibitors: next-generation antithrombotic agents. *J Med Chem.* 2010;53:6243-6274.
167. Roehrig S, Straub A, Pohlmann J, et al. Discovery of the novel discovery of the novel antithrombotic agent 5-chloro-N-({(5S)-2-oxo-3- [4-(3-oxomorpholin-4-yl)phenyl]-1,3-oxazolidin-5-yl}methyl) thiophene- 2-carboxamide (BAY 59-7939): an oral, direct factor Xa inhibitor. *J Med Chem.* 2005;48:5900-5908.
168. Perzborn E, Roerig S, Straub A, et al. The discovery and development of rivaroxaban, an oral, direct factor Xa inhibitor. *Nat Rev Drug Discov.* 2011;10:61-75.
169. Pinto DJP, Orwat MJ, Koch S, et al. Discovery of 1-(4-methoxyphenyl)-7-oxo-6-(4-(2-oxopiperidin-1-yl)phenyl)-4,5,6,7-tetrahydro1H-pyrazolo[3,4-c]pyridine-3-carboxamide (apixaban, BMS-562247), a highly potent, selective, efficacious, and orally bioavailable inhibitor of blood coagulation factor Xa. *J Med Chem.* 2007; 50:5339-5356.
170. Nagata T, Yoshino T, Haginoya N, et al. Discovery of N-[(1R,2S,5S)-2-{[(5-chloroindol-2-yl)carbonyl]amino}-5-(dimethylcarbamoyl)cyclohexyl]-5-methyl-4,5,6,7-tetrahydrothiazolo[5,4-c]pyridine-2-carboxamide hydrochloride: a novel, potent and orally active direct inhibitor of factor Xa. *Bioorg Med Chem.* 2009;17:1193-1206.
171. Raghavan N, Frost CE, Yu Z, et al. Apixaban metabolism and pharmacokinetics after oral administration to humans. *Drug Metab Dispos.* 2009;37:74-81.
172. Wong PC, Pinto DJP, Zhang D. Preclinical discovery of apixaban, a direct and orally bioavailable factor Xa inhibitor. *J Thromb Thrombolysis.* 2011;31:478-492.
173. Bathala MS, Masumoto H, Oguma T, et al. Pharmacokinetics, biotransformation, and mass balance of edoxaban, a selective, direct factor Xa inhibitor, in humans. *Drug Metab Dispos.* 2012;40:2250-2255.
174. Parasrampuria DA, Truitt KE. Pharmacokinetics and pharmacodynamics of edoxaban, a non-vitamin K antagonist oral anticoagulant that inhibits clotting factor Xa. *Clin Pharmacokinet.* 2016;55:641-655.
175. Padrini R. Clinical pharmacokinetics and pharmacodynamics of direct oral anticoagulants in patients with renal failure. *Eur J Drug Metab Pharmacokinet.* 2019;44:1-12.
176. Mueck W, Stampfuss J, Kubitza D, et al. Clinical pharmacokinetic and pharmacodynamic profile of rivaroxaban. *Clin Pharmacokinet.* 2014;53:1-16.
177. Weinz C, Schwarz T, Kubitza D, et al. Metabolism and excretion of rivaroxaban, an oral, direct factor Xa inhibitor, in rats, dogs, and humans. *Drug Metab Dispos.* 2009;37:1056-1064.
178. Zhao T, Chen Y, Wang D, et al. Identifying the dominant contribution of human cytochrome P450 2J2 to the metabolism of rivaroxaban, an oral anticoagulant. *Cardiovasc Drugs Ther.* 2022;36:121-129.
179. Eliquis. Package insert. Bristol-Myers Squibb; Revised September 2021. Accessed October 8, 2023. https://packageinserts.bms.com/pi/pi_eliquis.pdf
180. Byon W, Garonzik S, Boyd RA, et al. Apixaban: a clinical pharmacokinetic and pharmacodynamic review. *Clin Pharmacokinet.* 2019;58:1265-1279.
181. Savaysa. Package insert. Daiichi-Sanyo; Revised September 2022. Accessed October 8, 2023. https://dailymed.nlm.nih.gov/dailymed/fda/fdaDrugXsl.cfm?setid=e77d3400-56ad-11e3-949a-0800200c9a66&type=display
182. Xarelto. Package insert. Janssen Pharmaceuticals; Revised February 2023. Accessed October 10, 2023. https://www.janssenlabels.com/package-insert/product-monograph/prescribing-information/XARELTO-pi.pdf
183. National Center for Biotechnology Information. PubChem compound summary for CID 10182969, Apixaban. Accessed October 7, 2023. https://pubchem.ncbi.nlm.nih.gov/compound/Apixaban
184. National Center for Biotechnology Information. PubChem compound summary for CID 10280735, Edoxaban. Accessed October 7, 2023. https://pubchem.ncbi.nlm.nih.gov/compound/Edoxaban
185. National Center for Biotechnology Information. PubChem compound summary for CID 9875401, Rivaroxaban. Accessed October 7, 2023. https://pubchem.ncbi.nlm.nih.gov/compound/Rivaroxaban

186. Lu G, DeGuzman FR, Hollenbach SJ, et al. A specific antidote for reversal of anticoagulation by direct and indirect inhibitors of coagulation factor Xa. *Nat Med.* 2013;19:446-451.
187. Connolly SJ, Crowther M, Eikelboom JW, et al. Full study report of andexanet alfa for bleeding associated with factor Xa inhibitors. *N Engl J Med.* 2019;380:1326-1335.
188. Andexxa. In: *RED BOOK® Online. Merative™ Micromedex®.* Accessed October 10, 2023. http://www.micromedexsolutions.com
189. Warkentin TE. Bivalent direct thrombin inhibitors: hirudin and bivalirudin. *Best Pract Res Clin Haematol.* 2004;17:105-125.
190. Rydel TJ, Ravichandran KG, Tulinsky A, et al. The structure of a complex of recombinant hirudin and human α-thrombin. *Science.* 1990;249:277-280.
191. Robson R, White H, Aylward P, et al. Bivalirudin, pharmacokinetics and pharmacodynamics: effect of renal function, dose, and gender. *Clin Pharmacol Ther.* 2002;71:433-439.
192. Rawson TE, VanGorp KA, Yang J, et al. Separation of 21-(R)- and 21-(S)-argatroban: solubility and activity of the individual diastereoisomers. *J Pharm Sci.* 1993;82:672-673.
193. Colombo D, Ferraboschi P, Grisenti P, et al. Complete ^{1}H and ^{13}C assignments of (21R) and 21S) diastereomers of argatroban. *Magn Reson Chem.* 2008;46:99-102.
194. Swan SK, Hursting MJ. The pharmacokinetics and pharmacodynamics of argatroban: effects of age, gender, and hepatic or renal dysfunction. *Pharmacotherapy.* 2000;20:318-329.
195. Ahmad S, Ahsan A, George M, et al. Simultaneous monitoring of argatroban and its major metabolite using an HPLC method: potential clinical applications. *Clin Appl Thromb Hemost.* 1999;5:252-258.
196. Argatroban. Package insert. Accord Healthcare; Revised November 2022. Accessed October 11, 2023. https://dailymed.nlm.nih.gov/dailymed/drugInfo.cfm?setid=46cdf9e6-839c-49c8-9ee1-c30cfdd9368d
197. Hursting MJ, Alford KL, Becker JCP, et al. Novastan® (brand of argatroban): a small molecule, direct thrombin inhibitor. *Semin Thromb Hemost.* 1997;23:503-516.
198. Koster A, Fischer KG, Harder S, et al. The direct thrombin inhibitor argatroban: a review of its use in patients with and without HIT. *Biologics.* 2007;1:105-112.
199. Hauel N, Nar H, Priepke H, et al. Structure-based design of novel potent nonpeptide thrombin inhibitors. *J Med Chem.* 2002;45:1757-1766.
200. van Ryn J, Goss A, Hauel N, et al. The discovery of dabigatran etexilate. *Front Pharmacol.* 2013;4:1-8.
201. Bloom RA. Environmental assessment: dabigatran etexilate capsules. FDA Center for Drug Evaluation and Research; Published July 16, 2010:1-24; NDA 22-512. Accessed October 12, 2023. https://www.accessdata.fda.gov/drugsatfda_docs/nda/2010/022512Orig1s000EA.pdf
202. Blech S, Ebner T, Ludwig-Schwellinger, et al. The metabolism and disposition of the oral direct thrombin inhibitor, dabigatran, in humans. *Drug Metab Dispos.* 2008;36:386-399.
203. Laizure SC, Parker RB, Herring VL, et al. Identification of carboxylesterase-dependent dabigatran etexilate hydrolysis. *Drug Metab Dispos.* 2013;42:201-206.
204. Ebner T, Wagner K, Wienan W. Dabigatran acylglucuronide, the major human metabolite of dabigatran: in vitro formation, stability, and pharmacological activity. *Drug Metab Dispos.* 2010;38:1567-1575.
205. Shipova M, Armstrong VW, Oellerich M, et al. Acyl glucuronide drug metabolites: toxicological and analytical implications. *Ther Drug Monit.* 2003;25:1-16.
206. Stangier J. Clinical pharmacokinetics and pharmacodynamics of the oral direct thrombin inhibitor dabigatran etexilate. *Clin Pharmacokinet.* 2008;47:285-295.
207. Stangier J, Rathgen K, Stähle H, et al. Influence of renal impairment on the pharmacokinetics and pharmacodynamics of oral dabigatran etexilate. *Clin Pharmacokinet.* 2010;49:259-268.
208. Pradaxa. Package Insert. Boehringer Ingelheim; Revised June 8, 2021. Accessed October 12, 2023. https://content.boehringer-ingelheim.com/DAM/c669f898-0c4e-45a2-ba55-af1e011fdf63/pradaxa%20capsules-us-pi.pdf
209. Schiele F, van Ryn J, Canada K, et al. A specific antidote for dabigatran: functional and structural characterization. *Blood.* 2013;121:3554-3562.
210. Pollack Jr CV, Reilly PA, Eikelboom J, et al. Idarucizumab for dabigatran reversal. *N Engl J Med.* 2015;373:511-520.
211. Praxbind. In: *RED BOOK® Online. Merative™ Micromedex®.* Accessed October 10, 2023. http://www.micromedexsolutions.com
212. Preis M, Hirsch J, Kotler A, et al. Factor XI deficiency is associated with lower risk for cardiovascular and venous thromboembolism events. *Blood.* 2017;129:1210-1215.
213. Meijers JCM, Tekelenburg WLH, Bouma BN, et al. High levels of coagulation factor XI as a risk factor for venous thrombosis. *N Engl J Med.* 2000;342:696-701.
214. Koch AW, Schiering N, Meikko S, et al. MAA868, a novel FXI antibody with a unique binding mode, shows durable effects on markers of anticoagulation in humans. *Blood.* 2019;133:1507-1516.
215. Verhamme P, Yi BA, Segers A, et al. Abelacimab for prevention of venous thromboembolism. *N Engl J Med.* 2021;385:609-617.
216. Yi BA, Freedholm D, Widener N, et al. Pharmacokinetics and pharmacodynamics of abelacimab (MAA868), a novel dual inhibitor of factor XI and factor XIa. *J Thromb Haemost.* 2022;20:307-315.
217. Dilger AK, Pabbisetty KB, Corte JR, et al. Discovery of milvexian, a high-affinity, orally bioavailable inhibitor of factor XIa in clinical studies for antithrombotic therapy. *J Med Chem.* 2022;65:1770-1785.
218. Roehrig S, Ackerstaff J, Jiménez Núñez, et al. Design and preclinical characterization program toward asundexian (BAY 2433334), an oral factor XIa inhibitor for the prevention and treatment of thromboembolic disorders. *J Med Chem.* 2023;66:12202-12224.
219. Ayombil F, Camire RM. Insights into vitamin K-dependent carboxylation: home field advantage. *Haematologica.* 2020; 105:1996-1998.
220. Jin DY, Tie JK, Stafford DW. The conversion of vitamin K epoxide to vitamine K quinone and vitamin K hydroquinone uses the same active site cysteines. *Biochemistry.* 2007;46:7279-7283.
221. Shen G, Cui W, Zhang H, et al. Warfarin traps human vitamin K epoxide reductase in an intermediate state during electron transfer. *Nat Struct Mol Biol.* 2017;24:69-76.
222. Liu S, Li S, Shen G, et al. Structural basis of antagonizing the vitamin K catalytic cycle for anticoagulation. *Science.* 2021;371:eabc5667.
223. Wu S, Chen X, Jin DY, et al. Warfarin and vitamin K epoxide reductase: a molecular accounting for observed inhibition. *Blood.* 2018;132:647-657.
224. Czogalla KJ, Biswas A, Hönig K, et al. Warfarin and vitamin K compete for binding to Phe55 in human VKOR. *Nat Struct Mol Biol.* 2017;24:77-85.
225. Kaminsky LS, Zhang ZY. Human P450 metabolism of warfarin. *Pharmacol Ther.* 1997;73:67-74.
226. Pouncey DL, Hartman JH, Moore PC, et al. Novel isomeric metabolite profiles correlate with warfarin metabolism phenotype during maintenance dosing in a pilot study of 29 patients. *Blood Coagul Fibrinolysis.* 2018;29:602-612.
227. Ageno W, Gallus AS, Wittkowsky A, et al. Oral anticoagulant therapy. *Chest.* 2012;141:e44S-e88S.
228. Weitz JI. Blood coagulation and anticoagulant, fibrinolytic, and antiplatelet drugs. In: Brunton LL, Knollmann BC, eds. *Goodman & Gilman's: The Pharmacological Basis of Therapeutics.* 14th ed. McGraw Hill; 2023. Accessed October 14, 2023. https://accessmedicine.mhmedical.com/content.aspx?sectionid=266700467&bookid=3191#269722571
229. Holbrook A, Schulman S, Witt DM, et al. Evidence-based management of anticoagulant therapy: Antithrombotic Therapy and

Prevention of Thrombosis, 9th ed: American College of Chest Physicians evidence-based clinical practice guidelines. *Chest.* 2012;141:e152S-e184S.
230. Johnson JA, Caudle KE, Gong L, et al. Clinical Pharmacogenetics Implementation Consortium (CPIC) guideline for pharmacogenetics-guided warfarin dosing: 2017 update. *Clin Pharmacol Ther.* 2017;102:397-404.
231. Wang M, Zeraatkar D, Obeda M, et al. Drug-drug interactions with warfarin: a systematic review and meta-analysis. *Br J Clin Pharmacol.* 2021;87:4051-4100.
232. Mar PL, Gopinathannair R, Gengler BE, et al. Drug interactions affecting oral anticoagulant use. *Circ Arrhythm Electrophysiol.* 2022;15:e007956.
233. Reardon DP, Connors JM. Prothrombin complex concentrate (4PCC): a review of its use in reversal of vitamin K antagonists. *Curr Emerg Hosp Med Rep.* 2015;3:50-54.
234. Kcentra. In: *RED BOOK® Online. Merative™ Micromedex®.* Accessed October 17, 2023. http://www.micromedexsolutions.com
235. Phytonadione. In: *RED BOOK® Online. Merative™ Micromedex®.* Accessed October 17, 2023. http://www.micromedexsolutions.com
236. Rishavy MA, Hallgren KW, Wilson L, et al. Warfarin alters vitamin K metabolism; a surprising mechanism of VKORC1 uncoupling necessitates an additional reductase. *Blood.* 2018;131:2826-2835.
237. Liu S, Shen G, Li W. Structural and cellular basis of vitamin K antagonism. *J Thromb Haemost.* 2022;20:1971-1983.
238. Nosal DG, Feinstein DL, Chem L, et al. Separation and quantification of superwarfarin rodenticide diastereomers–bromadiolone, difenacoum, flocoumafen, brodifacoum, and difethiolone-in human plasma. *J AOAC Int.* 2020;103:770-778.
239. Feinstein DL, Akpa BS, Ayee MA, et al. The emerging threat of superwarfarins: history, detection, mechanisms, and countermeasures. *Ann N Y Acad Sci.* 2016;1374:111-122.
240. Nosal DG, van Breemen RB, Haffner JW, et al. Brodifacoum pharmacokinetics in acute human poisoning: implications for estimating duration of vitamin K therapy. *Toxicol Commun.* 2021;5:69-72.
241. Yip L, Stanton NV, Middleberg RA. Vitamin K1 treatment duration in patients with brodifacoum poisoning. *N Engl J Med.* 2020;382:1764-1765.
242. Moritz E, Austin C, Wahl M, et al. Notes from the field: outbreak of severe illness linked to the vitamin K antagonist brodifacoum and use of synthetic cannabinoids-Illinois, March-April 2018. *MMWR Morb Mortal Wkly Rep.* 2018;67:607-608.
243. Kelkar AH, Smith NA, Martial A, et al. An outbreak of synthetic cannibinoid-associated coagulopathy in Illinois. *N Engl J Med.* 2018;379:1216-1223.
244. Pescador R, Capuzzi L, Mantovani M, et al. Defibrotide: properties and clinical use of an old/new drug. *Vascul Pharmacol.* 2013;59:1-10.
245. Richardson PG, Carreras E, Iacobelli M, et al. The use of defibrotide in blood and marrow transplantation. *Blood Adv.* 2018;2:1495-1509.
246. Baker DE, Demaris K, et al. Defibrotide. *Hosp Pharm.* 2016;51:847-854.
247. Hordt TK, Bode C. Thrombolysis: newer thrombolytic agents and their role in clinical medicine. *Heart.* 2003;89:1358-1362.
248. Chester KW, Corrigan M, Schoeffler JM, et al. Making a case for the right '-ase' in acute ischemic stroke: alteplase, tenecteplase, and reteplase. *Expert Opin Drug Saf.* 2019;18:87-96.
249. Sillen M, Declerck PJ. A narrative review on plasminogen activator inhibitor-1 and its (patho)physiological role: to target or not to target? *Int J Mol Sci.* 2021;22:2721.
250. Mican J, Toul M, Bednar, D, et al. Structural biology and protein engineering of thrombolytics. *Comput Struct Biotechnol J.* 2019;17:917-938.
251. Acheampong P, Ford GA. Pharmacokinetics of alteplase in the treatment of ischaemic stroke. *Expert Opin Drug Metab Toxicol.* 2012;8:271-281.
252. Smalling RW. Pharmacological and clinical impact of the unique molecular structure of a new plasminogen activator. *Eur Heart J.* 1997;18:F11-F16.
253. Tanswell P, Modi N, Combs D, et al. Pharmacokinetics and pharmacodynamics of tenecteplase in fibrinolytic therapy of acute myocardial infarction. *Clin Pharmacokinet.* 2002;41:1229-1245.
254. Activase. Package insert. Genentech; Revised September 2022. Accessed October 25, 2023. https://www.gene.com/download/pdf/activase_prescribing.pdf
255. Cathflo Activase. Package insert. Genentech; Revised February 2019. Accessed October 25, 2023. https://www.gene.com/download/pdf/cathflo_prescribing.pdf
256. Retavase. Package insert. Chiesi USA, Inc; Revised April 2022. Accessed October 25, 2023. https://resources.chiesiusa.com/Retavase/RETAVASE_PI.pdf
257. TNKase. Package insert. Genentech; Revised March 2023. Accessed October 25, 2023. https://www.gene.com/download/pdf/tnkase_prescribing.pdf
258. Cooper NC, Ghanima W. Immune thrombocytopenia. *N Engl J Med.* 2019;381:945-955.
259. Zuffrey A, Kapur R, Semple JW. Pathogenesis and therapeutic mechanisms in immune thrombocytopenia (ITP). *J Clin Med.* 2017;6:16.
260. Kuter DJ. The structure, function, and clinical use of the thrombopoietin receptor agonist avatrombopag. *Blood Rev.* 2022;100909.
261. Bussel J, Kulasekararaj A, Cooper N, et al. Mechanisms and therapeutic prospects of thrombopoietin receptor agonists. *Semin Hematol.* 2019;56:262-278.
262. Shimamoto G, Gegg C, Boone T, et al. Peptibodies: a flexible alternative format to antibodies. *MAbs.* 2012;4:586-591.
263. Yang BB, Doshi S, Arkam K, et al. Development of romiplostim for treatment of primary immune thrombocytopenia from a pharmacokinetic and pharmacodynamic perspective. *Clin Pharmacokinet.* 2016;55:1045-1058.
264. Bussel JB, Kuter DJ, George JN, et al. AMG 531, a thrombopoiesis-stimulating protein, for chronic ITP. *N Engl J Med.* 2006;355:1672-1681.
265. Imbach P, Crowther M. Thrombopoietin-receptor agonists for primary immune thrombocytopenia. *N Engl J Med.* 2011;365:734-741.
266. Kuter DJ. Biology and chemistry of thrombopoietic agents. *Semin Hematol.* 2010;47:243-248.
267. Bussel JB, Soff G, Balduzzi A, et al. A review of romiplostin mechanism of action and clinical applicability. *Drug Des Devel Ther.* 2021;15:2243-2268.
268. Doptelet. Package insert. AkaRx; Revised July 2021. Accessed October 26, 2023. https://doptelet.com/themes/pdf/prescribing-information.pdf
269. Deng Y, Madatian A, Wire MB, et al. Metabolism and disposition of eltrombopag, an oral, nonpeptide thrombopoietin receptor agonist, in health human subjects. *Drug Metab Dispos.* 2011;39:1734-1746.
270. Deng Y, Rogers M, Sychterz C, et al. Investigations of hydrazine cleavage of eltrombopag in humans. *Drug Metab Dispos.* 2011;39:1747-1754.
271. Promacta. Package insert. Novartis; Revised March 2023. Accessed October 26, 2023. https://www.novartis.com/us-en/sites/novartis_us/files/promacta.pdf
272. Kawachi T, Ninomiya M, Katsube T, et al. Human mass balance, metabolism, and cytochrome P450 phenotyping of lusutrombopag. *Xenobiotica.* 2021;51:287-296.
273. Mulpleta. Package insert. Shionogi; Revised October 2020. Accessed October 26, 2023. https://www.shionogi.com/content/dam/shionogi/si/products/pdf/mulpleta.pdf

274. Nplate. Package insert. Amgen; Revised February 2022. Accessed October 26, 2023. https://www.pi.amgen.com/-/media/Project/Amgen/Repository/pi-amgen-com/Nplate/nplate_pi_hcp_english.pdf
275. Matsukane R, Suetsugu K, Hirota T, et al. Clinical pharmacokinetics and pharmacodynamics of fostamatinib and its active moiety R406. *Clin Pharmacokinet*. 2022;61:955-972.
276. Cooper N, Ghanima W, Hill Q, et al. Recent advances in understanding spleen tyrosine kinase (SYK) in human biology and disease, with a focus on fostamatinib. *Platelets*. 2023;34:2131751.
277. Sweeney DJ, Li W, Clough J, et al. Metabolism of fostamatinib, the oral methylene phosphate prodrug of the spleen tyrosine kinase inhibitor R409 in humans: contribution of hepatic and gut bacterial processes to the overall biotransformation. *Drug Metab Dispos*. 2010;38:1166-1176.
278. Braselmann S, Taylor V, Zhao H, et al. R406, an orally available spleen tyrosine kinase inhibitor blocks Fc receptor signaling and reduces immune complex-mediated inflammation. *J Pharmacol Exp Ther*. 2006;319:998-1008.
279. Villaseñor AG, Kondru R, Ho H, et al. Structural insights for design of potent spleen tyrosine kinase inhibitors from crystallographic analysis of three inhibitor complexes. *Chem Biol Drug Des*. 2008;73:466-470.
280. Tavalisse. Package insert. Rigel; Revised November 2020. Accessed October 26, 2023. https://www.tavalissehcp.com/downloads/pdf/TAVALISSE-Full-Prescribing-Information.pdf
281. Xie Z, Yang X, Duan Y, et al. Small-molecule kinase inhibitors for the treatment of nononcologic diseases. *J Med Chem*. 2021;64:1283-1345.
282. Steinmetzer T, Pilgram O, Wenzel BM, et al. Fibrinolysis inhibitors: potential drugs for the treatment and prevention of bleeding. *J Med Chem*. 2020;63:1445-1472.
283. Al-Horani RA, Desia UR. Recent advances on plasmin inhibitors for the treatment of fibrinolysis-related disorders. *Med Res Rev*. 2014;34:1168-1216.
284. Wu G, Quek AJ, Caradoc-Davies TT, et al. Structural studies of plasmin inhibition. *Biochem Soc Trans*. 2019;47:541-557.
285. Amicar. Package insert. Akorn; Revised March 2022. Accessed October 27, 2023. https://dailymed.nlm.nih.gov/dailymed/fda/fdaDrugXsl.cfm?setid=2238c70f-b0b5-4755-896b-45b28777b217&type=display
286. Lysteda. Package insert. Ferring; Revised December 2020. Accessed October 27, 2023. https://lysteda.com/wp-content/uploads/2021/03/LYSTEDA-PI-12-2020.pdf
287. Cyclokapron. Package insert. Pfizer; Revised March 2021. Accessed October 27, 2023. https://labeling.pfizer.com/ShowLabeling.aspx?format=PDF&id=556
288. Myles PS, Smith JA, Forbes A, et al. Tranexamic acid in patients undergoing coronary-artery surgery. *N Engl J Med*. 2017;376:136-148.
289. Roberts I, Brenner A, Shakur-Still H. Tranexamic acid for bleeding: much more than a treatment for postpartum hemorrhage. *Am J Obstet Gynecol MFM*. 2023;5:100722.

Structure Challenge Answers

1. A. Anticoagulant, Direct factor Xa inhibitor; B. Antiplatelet drug, Irreversible $P2Y_{12}$ receptor antagonist; C. Anticoagulant, Vitamin K antagonist; D. Antiplatelet drug, PAR-1 antagonist; E. Antiplatelet drug, Reversible $P2Y_{12}$ receptor antagonist
2. A and D
3. B and C

CHAPTER
22

Drugs Used to Treat Diabetic Disorders

S. William Zito and Raghunandan Yendapally

Drugs covered in this chapter:

INSULINS
- Aspart
- Degludec
- Detemir
- Glargine
- Glulisine
- Human insulin
  - NPH
  - Regular insulin
- Lispro

SULFONYLUREAS
- First-generation sulfonylureas
- Acetohexamide
- Chlorpropamide
- Tolazamide
- Tolbutamide

SECOND-GENERATION SULFONYLUREAS
- Glimepiride
- Glipizide
- Glyburide (also known as glibenclamide)

MEGLITINIDES
- Nateglinide
- Repaglinide

BIGUANIDES
- Metformin

THIAZOLIDINEDIONES
- Pioglitazone
- Rosiglitazone
- Troglitazone

A-GLUCOSIDASE INHIBITORS
- Acarbose
- Miglitol
- Voglibose

GLP-1 AGONISTS
- Albiglutide
- Dulaglutide
- Exenatide
- Liraglutide
- Lixisenatide
- Semaglutide
- Tirzepatide

DIPEPTIDYL PEPTIDASE IV INHIBITORS
- Alogliptin
- Linagliptin
- Saxagliptin
- Sitagliptin
- Vildagliptin

AMYLIN AGONISTS
- Pramlintide

SODIUM-GLUCOSE COTRANSPORTER-2 INHIBITORS
- Canagliflozin
- Dapagliflozin
- Empagliflozin
- Ertugliflozin

DOPAMINE AGONIST
- Bromocriptine

BILE ACID SEQUESTRANT
- Colesevelam

Abbreviations

ADA American Diabetes Association
ADP adenosine diphosphate
AGE advanced glycation end product
Aib α-aminoisobutyric acid
AMP adenosine monophosphate
AMPK AMP-activated protein kinase
APP acylaminoacyl carboxypeptidase
ATP adenosine triphosphate
cAMP-PKA cyclic AMP-protein kinase A
CHD coronary heart disease
DAG diacylglycerol
DCCT Diabetes Control and Complications Trial
DHAP dihydroxyacetone phosphate
DKA diabetic ketoacidosis
DNA deoxyribonucleic acid
DPP-IV dipeptidyl peptidase-IV
EDIC Epidemiology of Diabetes Interventions and Complications
FAP fibroblast protein-a

Abbreviations—continued

FDA US Food and Drug Administration
FFA free fatty acid
FPG fasting plasma glucose
FXR farnesoid X receptor (or BAS receptor)
GAPDH glyceraldehyde-3-phosphate dehydrogenase
GFAT glutamine:fructose-6-phosphate amidotransferase
GFR glomerular filtration rate
GI gastrointestinal
GIP glucose-dependent insulinotropic polypeptide
GLN glutamine
GLP-1 glucagon-like peptide-1
GLUT facilitative glucose transporter
GSH glutathione
HbA_{1c} hemoglobin A_{1c}
HDL high-density lipoprotein
HHS hyperosmolar hyperglycemic state
HLA human leukocyte antigen
IDDM insulin-dependent diabetes mellitus
IDE insulin degrading enzyme
IFG impaired fasting glucose
IGT impaired glucose tolerance
IP_3 inositol triphosphate
IRS insulin receptor substrate
IU international unit of enzyme activity
LDL low density lipoprotein
MATE multidrug and toxic compound extrusion transporters
MODY maturity-onset diabetes of youth
NIDDM non-insulin-dependent diabetes mellitus
NADPH nicotinamide adenine dinucleotide phosphate
NPH neutral protamine Hagedorn
OCT organic cation transporter
OGTT oral glucose tolerance test
PARP poly(ADP-ribose) polymerase
PCP prolyl carboxypeptidase
PG plasma glucose
PI3K phosphatidylinositol-3-kinase
PKB phosphokinase B
PKC phosphokinase C
PPAR peroxisome proliferator-activated receptor
QPP quiescent cell proline dipeptidase
ROS reactive oxygen species
RXR retinoidXreceptor
SGLT sodium-glucose cotransporter
SDH sorbitol dehydrogenase
SNAC sodium *N*-(8-[2-hydoxybenzoyl amino] caprylate)
SQ subcutaneous
SUR sulfonylurea receptor
TMD transmembrane domain
TNF-α tumor necrosis factor-α
TZD thiazolidinedione
UGT uridine glucuronyltransferase
VLDL very low density lipoprotein

CLINICAL SIGNIFICANCE

Over the years, many pharmacologic agents have been developed to help manage patients with diabetes, targeting the many different pathophysiologic defects in diabetes. Understanding the structure-activity relationships and physicochemical and biopharmaceutical properties of these various agents has led to the development of more effective and safer medications. These include insulin analogues, sulfonylureas, meglitinides, biguanides, thiazolidinediones, α-glucosidase inhibitors, glucagon-like peptide-1 (GLP-1) agonists, dipeptidyl peptidase IV inhibitors, and sodium-glucose cotransporter-2 inhibitors. Despite this plethora of medications, there remains a need for medications with improved efficacies and pharmacokinetic profiles. A clear understanding of the medicinal chemistry of these agents will help in achieving this goal.

Emily Ambizas, PharmD, MPH

Diabetes Mellitus: Historical Perspectives

Diabetes mellitus is a metabolic disorder characterized by hyperglycemia, where the patient experiences polyuria (frequent urination), polydipsia (extreme thirst), and polyphagia (constant hunger). Physicians have been documenting the signs and symptoms of diabetes for thousands of years. The first description of the symptoms of diabetes is attributed to Hesy-Ra, an Egyptian physician in 1552 BC, in the Ebers Papyrus. Chinese, Greek, and Arab physicians have also described a disease that is characterized by frequent urination and caused emaciation. Aretaeus of Cappadocia in the second century AD provided the first accurate description and coined the term diabetes, which means "siphon" or "run through" in Greek. Galen, also in the second century, described the disease as "diarrhea urinosa" and "dipsakos" (disease of thirst). The term "mellitus" (Latin for honey or sweet) was added to the disease name in the 17th century by Thomas Willis to describe the sweet taste of the urine and to distinguish it from a similar polyuric disease, diabetes insipidus, where the urine was tasteless (insipid). Glucose was identified in the urine of patients with diabetes in 1776 by Matthew Dobson, and glycogen, a polysaccharide in the liver, was identified in 1875 by Claude Bernard.

The role of the pancreas in diabetes was discovered by the experiments of Oskar Minkowski who, in 1889, noted that when the pancreas was removed from a dog, the animal developed all the signs and symptoms of diabetes.[1-4] Small clusters of ductless cells on the pancreas were identified in 1869 by Paul Langerhans, and in 1902 the work of Eugene Opie clearly linked these ductless cells, which by then were called the islets of Langerhans, to diabetes. Although a hypothetical secretion of the islet cells was postulated and called insulin (from insula, or island), it took the work of Frederick Banting, Charles Best, and John Macloud to isolate insulin and use it as a diabetes medication. In 1923, Banting and

Macloud shared the Nobel Prize in medicine, and Banting subsequently shared his prize with Best.[5] Insulin was identified as a protein by Frederick Sanger and Hans Tuppy, who defined its amino acid sequence in 1951.[6,7] The total synthesis of active insulin was accomplished by Katsoyannis et al.[8] In 1942, Janbon et al discovered that sulfonamide 3-(*p*-aminobenzenesulfonamide)-5-isopropylthiadiazole) induced hypoglycemia. This discovery led to the development of small, nonprotein molecules. From this lead compound, carbutamide (1-butyl-3-sulfonylurea) was developed as the first sulfonyl urea used to treat diabetes; however, it was subsequently withdrawn from the market due to its adverse effects on bone marrow.[9]

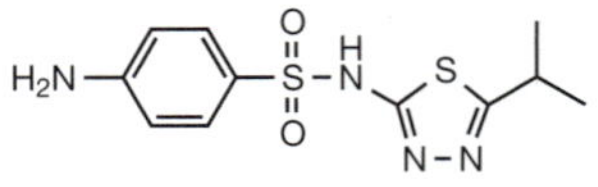
IPTD

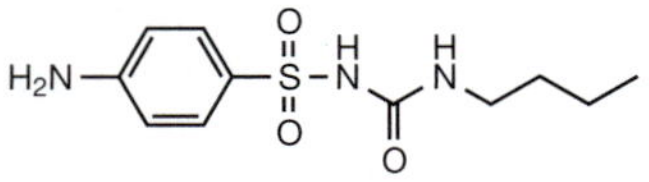
Carbutamide

Types of Diabetes

There are four major types of diabetes: type 1 diabetes, type 2 diabetes, gestational diabetes, and specific types of diabetes, including maturity-onset diabetes of youth (MODY), diabetes secondary to other disease states, and drug- or chemically-induced diabetes.[10,11] Type 1 diabetes was formerly called insulin-dependent diabetes mellitus (IDDM) or juvenile-onset diabetes. It occurs in 5% to 10% of patients[12] and is largely recognized as an autoimmune disease, whereby the β-cells are destroyed by the body's own antibodies. Since the pancreas can no longer produce insulin, patients with type 1 diabetes have an absolute requirement for exogenous insulin.[11]

Type 2 diabetes was formally called non-insulin-dependent diabetes mellitus (NIDDM) or adult-onset diabetes. It accounts for 90% to 95% of adult cases of diabetes. Type 2 diabetes slowly progresses from a state where the patient develops insulin resistance to a state in which the pancreas loses its ability to produce enough insulin to compensate for the insulin resistance of peripheral tissues. In insulin resistance, tissues do not utilize insulin properly. Insulin resistance is associated with a number of physiologic risk factors (hyperinsulinemia, hypertension, dyslipidemia, hypercoagulation, proinflammatory state, and abdominal obesity) and is most commonly referred to as "metabolic syndrome." Nondiabetic patients with metabolic syndrome (Table 22.1) are at high risk for the development of type 2 diabetes, which then gives that patient a 2- to 4-fold greater risk of developing coronary heart disease (CHD) and stroke.[12-15] In addition, outcomes of type 2 diabetes are strongly associated with race, ethnicity, and social determinants of health.[14,16,17]

Gestational diabetes is diagnosed during pregnancy. It occurs more often in women with obesity who have a family history of diabetes and/or are a member of a high-risk ethnic group (African American, Hispanic/Latina, Asian/Pacific Islander, and Native American). Gestational diabetes requires treatment to control hyperglycemia and avoid complications to the infant. Most women return to normal blood glucose levels postpartum; however, there is increased risk of developing diabetes within the next 10 years.[18]

Table 22.1 American Heart Association Definition of Metabolic Syndrome[13]

Central obesity	Waist circumference race and gender specific US men: >40 in US women: >35 in Plus any *two* of the following:
Triglycerides	≥150 mg/dL or if under treatment for this dyslipidemia
HDL cholesterol	Males: <40 mg/dL Females: <50 mg/dL or if under treatment for this dyslipidemia
Blood pressure	≥130/85 mm Hg or if under treatment for hypertension
Fasting plasma glucose	≥100 mg/dL or previously diagnosed type 2 diabetes

HDL, high-density lipoprotein.

MODY is characterized by faulty secretion of insulin, is rare (<5% of type 2), and is associated with a number of genetic defects of β-cell function. These defects are inherited and occur at six loci identified on chromosomes 20q, 7p, 12q, 13q, 17q, and 2q.[11] This form of diabetes is the result of impaired secretion of insulin, and there is no evidence that insulin action on tissue targets is decreased.

Diagnosis of Diabetes

The American Diabetes Association (ADA) has established four criteria for the diagnosis of diabetes.

1. A fasting plasma glucose (FPG) ≥126 mg/dL. Fasting is defined as no caloric intake for at least 8 hours prior to the assessment.
2. A 2 hour plasma glucose (PG) ≥200 mg/dL during an oral glucose tolerance test (OGTT).
3. In patients with overt symptoms of hyperglycemia (polyphagia, polyuria, polydipsia, weight loss), a random PG of ≥200 mg/dL.
4. A hemoglobin A_{1c} (HbA_{1c}) of ≥6.5%.

In addition, the ADA has recognized a prediabetic state for patients who are at risk of developing diabetes. The criteria include an FPG 100 to 125 mg/dL, referred to as impaired fasting glucose (IFG), a 2-hour OGTT of 140 to 199 mg/dL, referred to as impaired glucose tolerance (IGT), and/or an A_{1C} of 5.7% to 6.4%. The A_{1C} is perhaps the most accurate indicator of glucose because it reflects PG levels over the previous 2 to 3 months and is now accepted as the ideal standard for assessing glycemic control.[18-20]

Epidemiology

Diabetes is a global health problem. More than 400 million people worldwide have diabetes. It is predicted that by the year 2040, more than 640 million people will have diabetes.[21]

In 2015, diabetes was the seventh leading cause of death in the United States. The most recent data from the ADA reports that 30.3 million children and adults have diabetes, of which 1.25 million are diagnosed with type 1 diabetes. The number of Americans aged 65 years and older with diabetes is approximately 12 million. The ADA also predicts that 1.5 million new cases of diabetes (both type 1 and type 2) will be diagnosed each year. In 2015, 84.1 million Americans aged 18 years and older had prediabetes. Relatively few patients with diabetes (~0.24%) are younger than age 20, with the majority having type 1 diabetes.

There are race and ethnic differences in the prevalence of diabetes in adults. Figure 22.1 shows that Native American and Indigenous Alaskan populations have the highest prevalence (15.1%) followed closely by non-Hispanic Black populations (12.0%). Hispanic populations, which include Cuban, Mexican American, Central and South American, and Puerto Rican, are similar in prevalence to non-Hispanic Blacks (12.1%). The prevalence of diabetes in Asian American populations is 9.5%, while non-Hispanic White populations have a prevalence of 7.4%.

The risk of death for people with diabetes is twice that for people without the disease.[18] However, diabetes is not likely to be reported as an official cause of death, since death is more likely to be attributed to one of the many complications associated with diabetes, such as heart disease, hypertension, kidney disease, and nervous system disease.

Biochemistry of Diabetes

Regulation of Glucose Homeostasis

Glucose is the primary source of cellular energy, and PG concentration is, therefore, tightly controlled between 65 and 104 mg/dL. Glucose homeostasis is maintained by a number of hormones, the most important being insulin and glucagon. Insulin is secreted by pancreatic β-cells when blood glucose concentration rises. It reduces glucose levels either by inhibiting hepatic glucose production (glycogenolysis and gluconeogenesis) or by increasing glucose uptake into the liver, muscle, and fat tissue. Glucagon is secreted by pancreatic α-cells in response to low concentrations of glucose. It acts principally on the liver and antagonizes the effects of insulin by increasing glycogenolysis and gluconeogenesis. In addition to glucagon, hydrocortisone and catecholamines also raise PG levels.

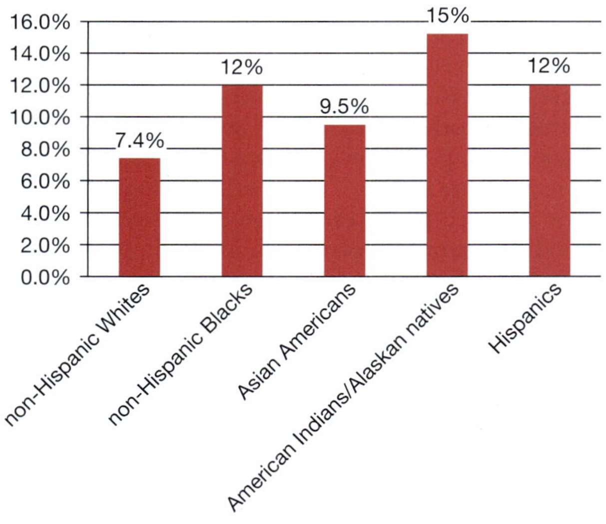

Figure 22.1 Prevalence of diabetes in US adults by race/ethnicity—2019.

Other hormones also function in maintaining normal PG levels. These include amylin, GLP-1, and glucose-dependent insulinotropic polypeptide (GIP). Amylin is actually co-secreted with insulin from β-cells and functions in slowing gastric emptying, which enhances glucose absorption following a meal. GLP-1 and GIP are incretins or gut-derived factors, which have a multitude of effects, primarily promoting the synthesis and secretion of insulin from β cells.[22]

It is surprising that such an essential nutrient as glucose is not freely absorbed from the intestines or by cells that require it for energy. Instead, glucose must be transported across membranes by glucose transporters. The glucose transporters are a family of membrane-bound glycoproteins divided into two main types: sodium-glucose cotransporters (SGLTs) and facilitative glucose transporters (GLUTs). The SGLT1-type is expressed in the absorptive epithelial cells of the intestines and transports glucose against its concentration gradient. SGLT1 is composed of 664 amino acids arranged into 14-transmembranes helices, and both the N- and C-terminals face the extracellular fluid. The SGLT2-type is expressed in the brush border membrane of the kidney and is the major transporter involved in the reabsorption of glucose from the glomerular filtrate. There are as many as six SGLTs found in a variety of tissues, including the liver, brain, lung, and heart.[23]

In contrast to the SGLTs, the GLUT family of transporters is sodium independent and composed of 12 membrane-spanning α-helices connected through extracellular hydrophilic loops. Their N- and C-terminals are located on the cytoplasmic side of the cell membrane. Helices 7, 8, and 11 are believed to form an aqueous pore providing a channel for substrate passage. Mammalian cells have 12 GLUT transporters (GLUTs 1-12). GLUTs 1, 3, and 4 have *d*-glucose specificity, while GLUTs 2 and 5 have specificity for fructose. The GLUT4 transporter is by far the most abundant type, is expressed in adipose tissue and muscle (heart, smooth, and skeletal), and is responsible for insulin-stimulated transport of glucose.[24] Figure 22.2 depicts the GLUT transporter, showing the 12 trans helices and the aqueous pocket, as well as the glycosylation site.

When insulin binds to its receptor on sensitive cells, it sets off a complicated cascade of events involving both phosphatidylinositol-3-kinase (PI3K) and protein kinase Akt or protein kinase B (Akt or PKB) pathways that results in the release of GLUT4 from storage vesicles and its translocation to the cell membrane (Fig. 22.3). The insulin receptor is a transmembrane glycoprotein composed of two α-subunits and two β-subunits linked by disulfide bonds.[25] The α-subunits contain the insulin binding site and are located extracellularly. The β-subunits contain a tyrosine kinase enzyme that is activated by insulin binding–induced autophosphorylation.

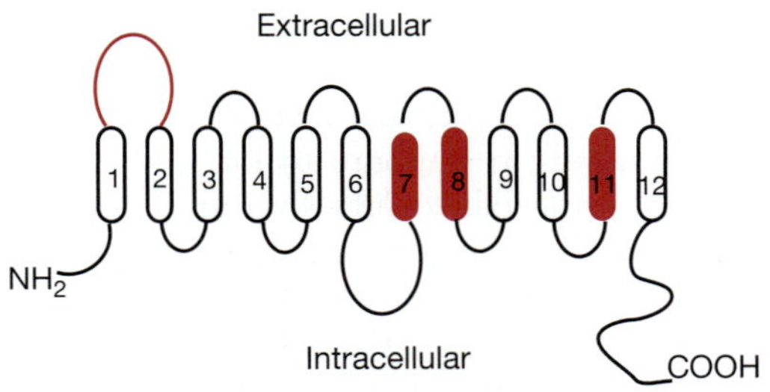

Figure 22.2 Schematic of the GLUT receptor showing the membrane-spanning α-helices (1-12). Helices 7, 8, and 11 (red) are believed to form the hydrophilic channel. The extracellular loop between helices 1 and 2 is the location of glycosylation.

When insulin binds to the receptor's two α-subunits, it enables a conformational change that allows for adenosine triphosphate (ATP) binding to the β-subunit's intracellular domain. ATP binding initiates receptor autophosphorylation, which, in turn, enables the receptor's tyrosine kinase to phosphorylate insulin receptor substrates (IRS). The IRS family of proteins consists of four closely related members (IRS-1 to -4) and a related homolog, Gab-1. These IRS proteins act as intracellular messengers that begin the cascade of events that result in the translocation of GLUT4 to the cell surface, as well as other processes necessary for cell survival.[26]

Pathogenesis of Diabetes

Type 1 Diabetes

It is well established that type 1 diabetes results from immunologic destruction of the insulin-producing β cells of the pancreas. However, it is now understood that type 1 diabetes involves an interplay between genetic susceptibility and certain external triggers such as viruses (mumps, Cosackie B4, enteroviruses), environmental toxins (nitrosamines), or foods (cow's milk proteins, cereals, gluten). Genetic susceptibility to type 1 diabetes is linked to two genes found on chromosome 6. These genes code for the production of human leukocyte antigens (HLAs) DR3 and DR4. Most, but not all, patients with type 1 diabetes express both of these antigens. Interestingly, patients who carry the antigen-producing *HLA-DQA1*0102* or *HLA-DQB1*0602* genes are actually resistant to type 1 diabetes. HLA complex polymorphic alleles are responsible for 40% to 50% of the genetic risk of type 1 diabetes development. The insulin gene (*Ins-VNTR, IDDM 2*) polymorphisms on chromosome 11 and the cytotoxic T lymphocyte–associated antigen-4 gene (*CTLA-4*) on chromosome 2 are responsible for 15% of the genetic predisposition. Type 1 diabetes is characterized by a long preclinical period marked by the presence of immune markers such as circulating antibodies, islet cell antibodies, and insulin autoantibodies. It is not known when the interplay between genetic susceptibility and environmental factors combine to develop the full-blown disease with the resulting absolute insulin deficiency.[27,28]

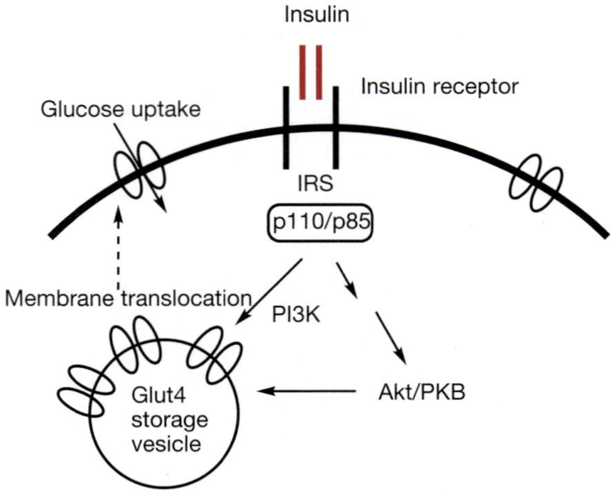

Figure 22.3 Overview of the insulin signaling pathway leading to translocation of the GLUT4 transporter from storage vesicles. Akt, protein kinase Akt; IRS, insulin receptor substrates; p110, catalytic subunit of PI3K; p85, regulatory subunit of PI3K; PI3K, phosphatidylinositol-3-kinase; PKB, protein kinase B.

Type 2 Diabetes

The pathogenesis of type 2 diabetes is complex but typically begins with insulin resistance at target organs such as the liver, muscle, and adipose tissue. In order to compensate, there is initially an increase in insulin production. This hyperinsulinemic state is only temporary, and over time, insulin secretion diminishes due to progressive β-cell deterioration. The combined effect of insulin resistance and β-cell dysfunction results in a diminished capacity to limit hepatic glucose production and the ability to take up and utilize glucose in muscle and adipose tissue.

Insulin resistance is a complex pathologic state that typifies the metabolic syndrome and is likely caused by a number of defects along the insulin signaling cascade. Other factors include increased concentrations of free-fatty acids (FFAs), tumor necrosis factor-α (TNF-α), and the hormone resistin.[29] The increase in plasma FFAs produces insulin resistance by inhibiting glucose uptake and glycolysis in skeletal muscle. It also increases hepatic gluconeogenesis. Both TNF-α and resistin are produced by adipose tissue in greater amounts in patients with obesity and diabetes. TNF-α impairs insulin action while resistin is known to antagonize the effects of insulin.

Increased hepatic glucose production in type 2 diabetes is attributed to both hepatic insulin resistance and increased glucagon levels. β-cells can compensate for insulin resistance by secreting more insulin. The hyperinsulinemic state is only temporary, since β-cells cannot produce the insulin levels required to maintain normal PG levels. Impaired insulin secretion and increased glucagon contribute to continued hepatic glucose output, resulting in elevated fasting blood glucose levels. When insulin resistance can no longer be overcome, transition to type 2 diabetes occurs.[30]

Hyperglycemia can be caused by a number of other mechanisms. Some patients have abnormal hormone levels, including elevated glucagon, somatostatin, growth hormone, hydrocortisone, and epinephrine. Of special importance for the treatment of diabetes is the effect of certain drugs on PG levels. Table 22.2 lists some common drugs that alter PG levels.[31]

Table 22.2 Drugs That Alter Plasma Glucose Levels

Drugs That Increase Plasma Glucose	Drugs That Decrease Plasma Glucose
Acetazolamide	Alcohol (ethanol)
Birth control pills	Anabolic steroids
Atypical antipsychotics: clozapine, olanzapine, risperidone	ACE inhibitors
β-Adrenergic blockers	Chloramphenicol
Caffeine	Fibrates
Calcium channel blockers	Gatifloxacin
Clonidine	MAO inhibitors
Diuretics: thiazides> loop > K^+-sparing	Saquinavir
Glucocorticoids	Warfarin
Niacin	
Phenytoin	
Rifampin	
Thyroid hormones	

ACE, angiotensin-converting enzyme; MAO, monoamine oxidase.

Diabetes Complications

The hyperglycemia so characteristic of diabetes is the result of defects in insulin secretion and/or insulin action, but is also accompanied by impaired fat, carbohydrate, and protein metabolism that progressively leads to chronic microvascular, macrovascular, and neuropathic complications.[32]

Patients with all types of diabetes constantly battle to control their chronic hyperglycemia. If high levels of PG are uncontrolled or poorly controlled, it will result in the development of both acute and chronic pathologies. The short-term effects are usually those symptoms generally associated with type 1 diabetes, such as polydipsia, polyuria, polyphagia, blurred vision, urinary tract infections, weight loss, and fatigue. Although these acute effects are relatively minor, they can lead to two rather serious complications: diabetic ketoacidosis (DKA) and a hyperosmolar hyperglycemic state (HHS).

DKA can be life-threatening. Insulin blocks the action of lipases that hydrolyze stored fats to FFAs. In the patient with diminished or no insulin, the increased serum levels of free fatty acids are oxidized to acetone, acetoacetic acid, and β-hydroxybutyric acid, presumably to make up for lack of glucose for oxidative energy (glycolysis). These keto acids can be metabolized, but in prolonged periods of insulin deficiency, the body cannot keep up with their production and ketoacidosis occurs. Decreased insulin levels also allow unchecked glucagon activity to increase PG by gluconeogenesis and glycogenolysis. The lowering of plasma pH by keto acids, along with hyperglycemia, leads to symptoms of ketoacidosis—vomiting, dehydration, hyperventilation, confusion, and possibly coma and death.

When PG levels exceed 600 mg/dL, increased amounts of glucose are excreted in the urine, leading to development of HHS characterized by dehydration, hyperosmolarity, and electrolyte imbalance. HHS symptoms include tachycardia, dry skin, and orthostatic hypotension which, if not treated, can lead to death in as many as 30% of those afflicted.[22]

The long-term effects of diabetes are serious and often not detected until they become overt. Both microvascular and macrovascular effects occur. The microvascular pathologies involve the retina, renal glomerulus, and peripheral nerves, and as a consequence, diabetes is a leading cause of blindness, end-stage renal disease, and painful neuropathies. The macrovascular effects involve arteries that supply the heart, brain, and lower extremities. Therefore, patients with diabetes have a much higher risk of cardiovascular disease, including atherosclerosis, myocardial infarct, stoke, and limb amputation.[33,34]

The essential question is: how does diabetes result in so many diverse microvascular and macrovascular pathologies? The answer centers around four main molecular mechanisms, all related to the diabetic hyperglycemic state, and all seemingly associated with the overproduction of superoxide radical anion by the mitochondrial electron transport chain. The four biochemical mechanisms are increased polyol pathway flux; increased advanced glycation end-product (AGE) formation; activation of protein kinase C (PKC) isoforms; and increased hexosamine pathway flux.[35,36]

The polyol pathway (Fig. 22.4) involves the reduction of aldehydes generated by reactive oxygen species (ROS) to inactive alcohols and glucose to sorbitol by the enzyme aldose reductase. Aldose reductase is a cytosolic oxidoreductase that utilizes nicotinamide adenine dinucleotide phosphate (NADPH). The sorbitol produced is oxidized by sorbitol dehydrogenase to fructose using NAD^+ as cofactor. When glucose levels are high, the activation of the polyol pathway can deplete reduced glutathione (GSH), leading to cellular oxidative stress. The effect of the polyol pathway flux is implicated in the formation of cataracts, as well as development of peripheral neuropathies.[37]

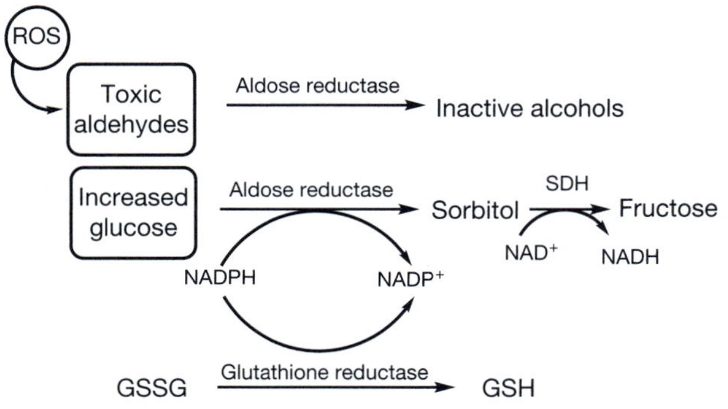

Figure 22.4 Polyol pathway showing the role of aldose reductase in reducing toxic aldehydes and glucose to sorbitol. GSH, reduced glutathione; ROS, reactive oxygen species; SDH, sorbitol dehydrogenase.

Increased levels of AGEs have been found in both retinal blood vessels and renal glomeruli. They arise from intracellular hyperglycemia by the autoxidation of glucose to glyoxal and the subsequent formation of 3-deoxyglucosone and the dephosphorylation of glyceraldehyde-3 phosphate and dihydroxyacetone phosphate to methylglyoxal (Fig. 22.5). These products are often referred to as dicarbonyls, and they react with amino groups of Lys and Arg and the thiol group of Cys to form AGEs. AGEs damage vascular cells and also alter several cellular functions, including gene expression in endothelial cells and macrophages.[38]

Activation of the family of PKC enzymes is brought about by the secondary messenger diacylglycerol (DAG). In hyperglycemic cells, DAG is increased by de novo synthesis involving reduction of dihydroxyacetone phosphate to glycerol-3-phosphate followed by stepwise acylation. PKCs may also be activated indirectly through ligation of AGE receptors and increased activity of the polyol pathway.[36] When increased in cells, PKC is involved in a significant number of biochemical pathways, leading to blood flow abnormalities, vascular permeability and angiogenesis, capillary and vascular occlusion, proinflammatory gene expression, and ROS elevation (Table 22.3). Elevated levels of PKCs, primarily the α- and β-isoforms, have been found in the retina and renal glomeruli of diabetic animals, as well as in cultured vascular cells.[39]

When intracellular glucose levels are in excess, it gets shunted into the hexosamine pathway. In this pathway, fructose-6-phosphate is converted to glucosamine-6-phosphate and then to UDP-*N*-acetylglucosamine by the rate-limiting enzyme glutamine:fructose-6-phosphate amidotransferase (GFAT). UDP-*N*-acetylglucosamine is added to intracellular protein Ser and Thr residues by O-linked *N*-acetylglucosamine transferase (OGT). Since both phosphorylation and OGT acylation compete for the same substrates, the two processes may compete for sites. The increased donation of *N*-acetylglucosamine to Ser and Thr residues on transcription factors leads to alterations in both gene expression and protein function, which, together, contribute to the pathologies of diabetic complications.

Each of the four different pathogenic mechanisms responsible for diabetic micro- or macrovascular complications is activated by a single hyperglycemic event—overproduction of superoxide by the mitochondrial electron transport chain.[36] It is now believed that the overproduction of superoxide activates the four pathogenic pathways (Fig. 22.6). Excess superoxide inhibits the glycolytic enzyme glyceraldehyde-3-phosphate dehydrogenase (GAPDH) through its effect on poly(ADP-ribose) polymerase (PARP). This inhibition causes intermediate metabolites of glycolysis to accumulate. Thus, the inhibition of the conversion of glyceraldehyde-3-phosphate to 1,3-diphosphoglycerate results in increased amounts of dihydroxyacetone phosphate (DHAP), which, in turn, increase the formation of DAG, the intracellular activator of PKC. The increase in DAG also results in the formation of methylglyoxal, the main precursor to AGEs. Earlier in the glycolytic chain, increased levels of fructose-6-phosphate are shunted into the hexosamine pathway, producing UDP-*N*-acetylglucosamine, which, in turn, forms O-linked glycoproteins that affect transcription. Finally, increased amounts of glucose are diverted through the polyol pathway that consumes NADPH and depletes GSH. It was originally thought that superoxide itself directly inhibited GAPDH; however, further investigations revealed that GAPDH is actually inhibited by PARP. PARP is a DNA repair enzyme found in the nucleus. PARP is activated in response to DNA single strand breaks caused by superoxide radicals. Once activated, PARP splits NAD^+ into nicotinic acid and ADP-ribose. PARP then makes polymers of ADP-ribose, which accumulate on GAPDH, inhibiting its activity.[35,40]

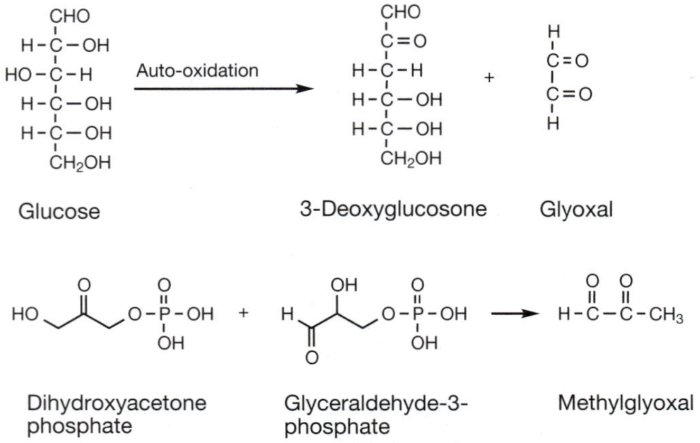

Figure 22.5 Formation of advanced glycation end products (AGEs) precursors, glyoxal, 3-deoxyglucosone, and methylglyoxal.

Table 22.3 Pathologic Consequences of Protein Kinase C Activation

Factor Effected	Pathology
↓ eNOS (endothelial nitric oxide synthase)	Blood flow abnormalities
↑ ET-1 (endothelin-1)	Blood flow abnormalities
↑ VEGF (vascular endothelial growth factor)	Vascular permeability and angiogenesis
↑ Collagen	Capillary occlusion
↑ Fibronectin	Capillary occlusion
↑ PAI-1 (plasminogen activator inhibitor-1)	↓ Fibrinolysis and vascular occlusion
↑ NF-κB (nuclear factor κ-light-chain–enhancer of activated B cells)	Proinflammatory gene expression
↑ NAD(P)H oxidases	Increased ROS and multiple effects

ROS, reactive oxygen species.

Therapeutic Approaches to the Treatment of Diabetes

Diabetes is a complex chronic disease with no cure. Therefore, therapy is directed at controlling hyperglycemia, as well as toward the reduction of the symptoms and morbidities

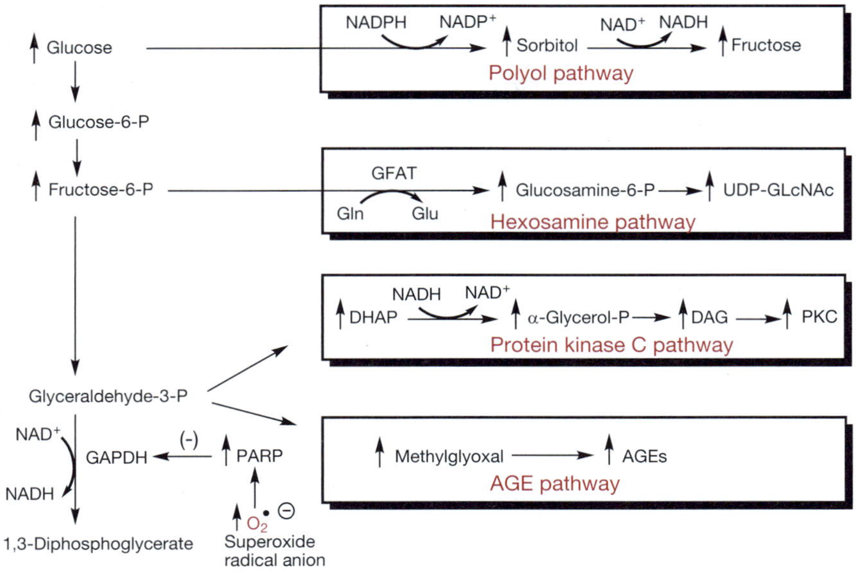

Figure 22.6 Role of hyperglycemia-induced mitochondrial excess superoxide in activation of the four pathways involved in diabetic microvascular and macrovascular damage. AGEs, advanced glycation end products; DAG, diacylglycerol; DHAP, dihydroxyacetone phosphate; GAPDH, glyceraldehyde-3-P dehydrogenase; GFAT, glut-amine:fructose-6-P amidotransferase; GLcNAc, *N*-acetylglucosamine; GLN, glutamine; PARP, poly(ADP-ribose)polymerase; PKC, protein kinase C.

associated with microvascular and macrovascular complications. Early diagnosis and aggressive maintenance of euglycemia will go a long way to moderate the microvascular pathologies.[41,42] However, reduction of the risk for macrovascular pathologies requires management of cardiovascular risk factors, such as smoking cessation, treatment for dyslipidemia, control of hypertension, and antiplatelet therapy. The ADA[43] recommends that appropriate medical care includes setting goals for glycemia, as well as for therapeutic lifestyle changes (diet and exercise) along with control of blood pressure, plasma lipids, and the use of appropriate medications.[44]

Glycemic control assessment involves two primary techniques, patient self-monitoring, and measurement of HbA_{1c}. A_{1C} is perhaps the most accurate indicator of glucose load because it reflects PG levels over the previous 2 to 3 months and is accepted as the gold standard for assessing glycemic control. A_{1C} is formed by the glycosylation of hemoglobin's amino terminal Val residue. This endogenous substance has a half-life equivalent to that of an erythrocyte. The UK Prospective Diabetes Study and the Diabetes Control and Complications Trial/Epidemiology of Diabetes Interventions and Complications (DCCT/EDIC) Study have established that if a patient's A_{1C} is maintained below 7%, the development and progression of neuropathy, nephropathy, retinopathy, and cardiovascular disease in type 1 or 2 patients can be significantly decreased.[32,45]

Pharmacologic treatment for type 1 diabetes requires intensive insulin therapy. The large number of short- and long-acting insulin analogues allows for the use of multiple doses of basal as well as prandial insulin. Therefore, the patient can match their dose of prandial insulin to carbohydrate intake, premeal PG, and anticipated physical activity level. The most common side effect of insulin use is the risk of severe hypoglycemia; however, the development of both quick-acting and long-acting insulin analogues has moderated this adverse effect while maintaining equal A_{1C} lowering.[27]

Medical treatment of type 2 diabetes requires management of hyperglycemia, as measured by the patient's A_{1C} (target <7%). Along with lifestyle interventions, the array of different classes of hypoglycemic drugs offers the provider many different treatment options. Obesity and sedentary lifestyle are the major risk factors for diabetes; therefore, weight loss, dietary changes, and increased physical activity levels should be the initial approach to treating type 2 diabetes. As a matter of fact, patients who have morbid obesity and have undergone weight loss surgery and who have maintained at least a 40-lb weight loss over 5 years effectively show no evidence of disease.[46] When diet and exercise are insufficient to maintain the patient's A_{1C} below 7%, it then becomes necessary to initiate blood glucose–lowering medications. In addition to insulin, there are several classes of oral hypoglycemic agents available. They include the insulin secretagogues (sulfonylureas, meglitinides), biguanides (metformin), insulin sensitizers (thiazolidinedione [TZD], glitazones), α-glucosidase inhibitors, GLP-1 analogues, dipeptidyl peptidase-IV (DPP-IV) inhibitors, amylin agonist, and SGLT2 inhibitors.

It is currently recommended to begin medication therapy with metformin along with lifestyle interventions (Fig. 22.7). If this therapy fails to maintain or sustain glycemic target, another medication should be added, usually one of the other oral hypoglycemic agents. Insulin (intermediate- or long-acting) is indicated for patients who have trouble decreasing their A_{1C} level below 8.5%.

If lifestyle, metformin, and one of the other oral hypoglycemic agents do not result in achievement of target glycemia, the next step is based on individualized glycemic targets based on patients being categorized as either having obesity, at hypoglycemia risk, patient access/cost factors or having severe hypoglycemia, or the patient might present with more than one category. If insulin is initiated, this usually consists of injections of a short- or rapid-acting insulin analogue

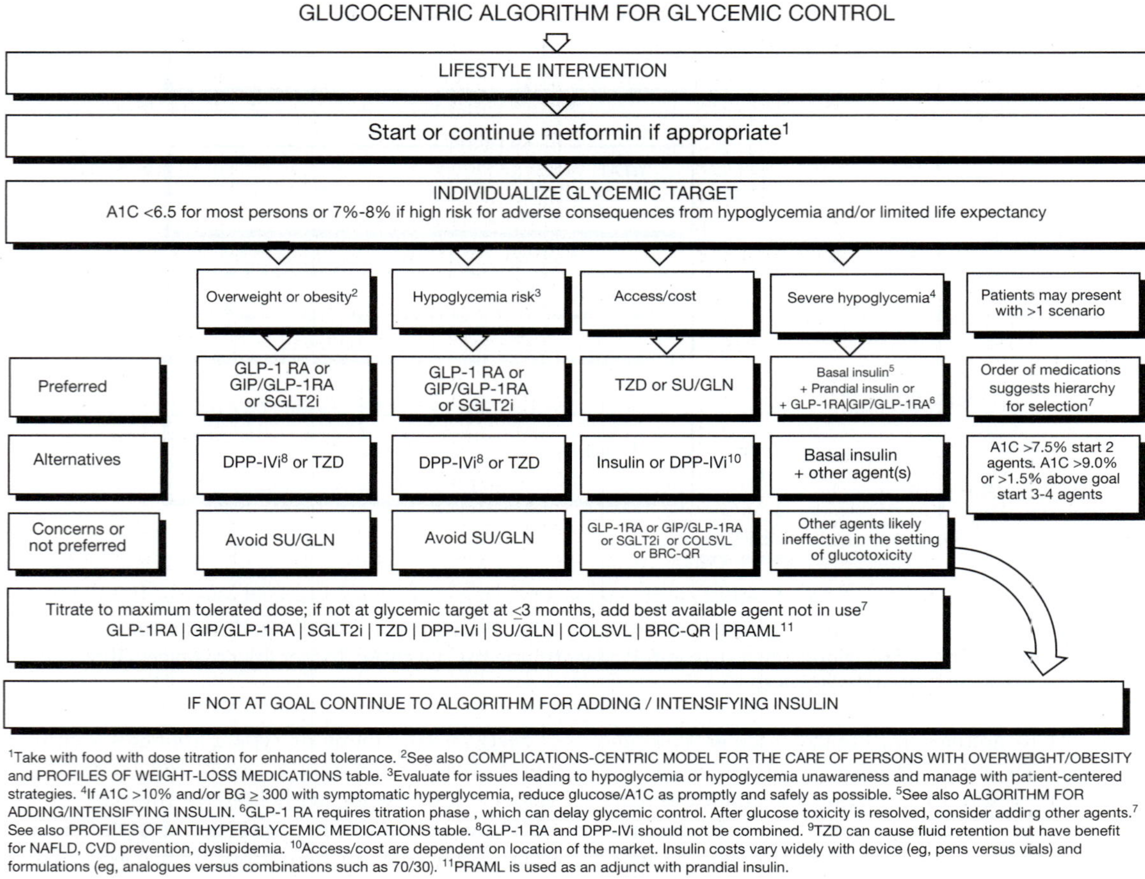

Figure 22.7 Algorithm for glycemic control based on the individualized glycemic target. BRC-QR, bromocriptine-QR; COLSVL, colesevelam; DPP-IVi, dipeptidyl peptidase 4 inhibitor; GIP, glucose-dependent insulinotropic polypeptide; GLN, glitinides; GLP-1 RA, glucose-like peptide 1-receptor agonist; NAFLD, non-alcoholic fatty acid liver disease; PRAML, pramlintide; SGLT2i, sodium-glucose cotransporter-2 inhibitor; SU, sulfonylurea; TZD, thiazolidinedione. (Adapted with permission from Samson SL, Vellanki P, Blonde L. American Association of Clinical Endocrinology consensus statement: comprehensive type 2 diabetes management algorithm—2023 update. *Endocr Pract.* 2023;29(5):305-340.)

given before meals. The preferred oral hypoglycemic agents for patients with obesity are GLP-1 or GIP/GLP-1 agonists or SGLT2 inhibitors. Patients at hypoglycemia risk would use the same preferred agents; however, if access or cost is a factor, TZD or sulfonyl ureas and glitinide could be used. In cases of severe hypoglycemia, basal + prandial insulin or GLP-1 or GIP/GIP-1 agonists are recommended. Alternative medications are DPP-IV inhibitors, TZD, using insulin with other agents. The goal is to reduce blood glucose levels while minimizing adverse effects, especially hypoglycemia. The use of amylin agonists and α-glucosidase inhibitors is generally reserved for those patients who cannot tolerate the first-line drugs because they do not have equivalent glucose-lowering ability, they are relatively expensive, and there are limited clinical data demonstrating effectiveness.[47,48]

Therapeutic Classes of Drugs Used to Treat Diabetes

Insulin

Insulin was isolated by Banting, Best, Collip, and Macleod, from canine pancreas in 1921, and just 5 years later, John Jacob Abel in 1926 was able to crystallize it. As noted previously, Banting and Macleod received the 1923 Nobel Prize for their work, and Banting announced that he would share his prize with Best; Macleod did the same with Collip. In 1958, Sanger received the Nobel Prize for the determination of the amino acid sequence of insulin, and Dorothy Hodgkin received the Nobel Prize in 1964 for determining its three-dimensional structure. The development of an immunoassay for insulin by Solomon Berson and Rosalyn Yallow in 1960 earned Yallow the Nobel Prize in 1977 after Berson's death. Clearly, the awarding of so many Nobel Prizes points to the importance of insulin-related research throughout the 20th century.[49,50]

The insulin molecule is composed of two polypeptide chains (A and B) linked together by two disulfide bonds. There is an additional intramolecular disulfide bond in chain A. The A chain contains 21 amino acid residues, and the B chain has 30 amino acids, giving a molecular weight of 5,734 Da. Insulin is biosynthesized in the β cells of the pancreas from preproinsulin, a 110 amino acid chain with a molecular weight of 12,000 Da. Preproinsulin is cleaved in the endoplasmic reticulum, losing a 24-amino acid unit from the N-terminus. The product is called proinsulin (MW 9,000), which folds to form the disulfide bonds and undergoes further proteolytic modification in the Golgi apparatus, losing four basic amino acids (Arg B31, Arg B32, Lys A64, Arg A65) and releasing a 31-amino acid connector C-chain by the action of prohormone convertases PC 1 and 2 to yield insulin (Fig. 22.8). Insulin is then stored in secretory granules, awaiting release on demand.[51,52]

The biologically active form of insulin is the monomer; however, in solution, insulin can exist as a dimer and hexamer. The hexamer is formed by coordination with two zinc ions and is believed to be the storage form in the granules of the β cells. When released from the granules, the hexamer is diluted in the plasma to nanomolar concentrations and dissociates into monomers. Secretion of insulin is primarily regulated by glucose, but many other nutrients and hormones also play a role. Amino acids, fatty acids, and ketone bodies promote the secretion of insulin. On the other hand, stimulation of α_2-adrenergic receptors on the β-cells inhibits secretion of insulin, while β_2-adrenergic receptor stimulation and vagal nerve stimulation enhance the release of insulin. It follows that any physiologic condition that activates the sympathetic nervous system causes a decrease in the secretion of insulin via stimulation of the α_2-adrenergic receptors and an increased secretion of insulin by the β_2-adrenergic receptors. Such conditions include exercise, hypothermia, surgery, hypoxia, and of course, hypoglycemia. In addition, α_2-adrenergic receptor antagonists will be expected to increase basal insulin levels, while β_2-adrenergic receptor blockers will decrease them.[51]

Insulin secretion results from the metabolism of glucose in the pancreatic β cells. Glucose enters the β cell facilitated by GLUT2 transport, is phosphorylated to glucose-6-phosphate by a specific isoform of glucokinase, and enters glycolysis, ultimately generating ATP. The increase in ATP changes the ratio of ATP to adenosine diphosphate (ADP) and prevents an ATP-sensitive K^+ channel from functioning, which in turn leads to depolarization of the β cells. This prompts activation of a voltage-gated calcium channel, and calcium flows into the β cells. The elevated intracellular calcium concentration causes activation of phospholipases A_2 and C and increased levels of inositol triphosphate (IP_3), an intracellular second messenger. IP_3 facilitates additional release of calcium into the cytosol, and concentrations of calcium are now sufficiently high to promote insulin secretion from the pancreatic β cells. The ATP-sensitive K^+ channel is an octameric heterocomplex consisting of four pore-forming inwardly rectifying K^+ channel subunits (Kir6.2) and four regulatory sulfonylurea receptor subunits (SUR1). ATP binding to Kir6.2 closes the channel. Binding of sulfonylureas and the meglitinides to SUR1 also closes the channel, whereas binding of ADP to SUR1 opens the channel.[53] Therefore, sulfonylurea binding to SUR1 causes the same effect as an increase in the ATP/ADP ratio—closing the channel that leads to the depolarization of the β-cell membrane and the ultimate secretion of insulin (Fig. 22.9).[54,55]

Fifty percent of the insulin secreted from the pancreas is degraded in the liver and never reaches the general circulation. Hepatic degradation of insulin is the result of the action of an insulin degrading enzyme (IDE). IDE is a neutral Zn^{2+} metalloendopeptidase (also known as insulin protease, insulinase, insulysin, insulin-glucagon protease, neutral thiol protease, amyloid-degrading protease, and peroximal protease). As can be inferred from the many names, IDE's action is not limited to the degradation of insulin alone. Therefore, there are still many unanswered questions about the functions of IDE, including evidence that it may have a role in the release of insulin from the pancreas. Insulin is internalized into the hepatocyte by receptor-mediated endocytosis and stored along with its receptor in small vesicles termed "endosomes." Stored insulin is processed through multiple pathways, resulting in degradation or release from the cell intact. Circulatory insulin is filtered by the renal glomeruli and can then be reabsorbed and degraded by the tubules. Insulin is also degraded at the cell surface of insulin-sensitive tissues.[51]

The primary target cells for insulin are the liver, muscle, and adipocytes. Insulin interacts with amino acid residues of the α-subunit of its receptor via key amino acid residues on both the A and B chains. Table 22.4 shows that the N-terminus and C-terminus of the A and B chains are

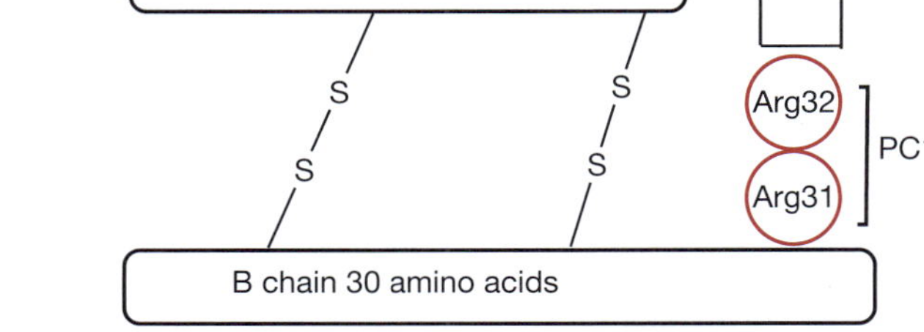

Figure 22.8 Structure of proinsulin. Prohormone convertases (PC1 and 2) cleave dipeptides (red) to form insulin.

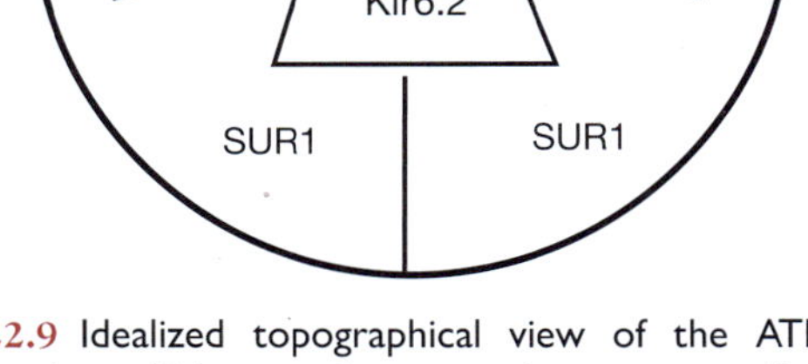

Figure 22.9 Idealized topographical view of the ATP-sensitive potassium channel showing four pore-forming inwardly rectifying potassium subunits (Kir6.2) surrounded by four regulatory sulfonylurea receptor subunits (SUR1).

Table 22.4 Interactions of Insulin Amino Acid Residues With the Insulin Receptor

Chain	N-Terminus	C-Terminus
A	Gly A1, Glu A4, Gln A5	Tyr A19, Asn A21
B	Val B12	Tyr B16, Gly B23, Phe B24, Phe B25, Tyr B26

involved in receptor binding.[51] In addition, it has been determined that insulin also binds to the receptor via an amino acid patch on chain A consisting of Leu A22, Ile A23, Tyr A26, and Phe A27.[56] Insulin binding to its receptor activates a series of intracellular events that lead to translocation of the GLUT4 transporter to the cell surface. The details of this process have previously been described (see Fig. 22.3).

Sources and Stability of Insulin. Historically, patients only had the option of administering either bovine-based or porcine-based insulins. They were viable alternatives to human insulin because the amino acid sequence homology between these species was superb. However, with the availability of biosynthetic and semisynthetic human insulin and its analogues, these sources have fallen into disuse. Human insulin is the least antigenic of the available insulins and tends to be more soluble than nonhuman insulin. Human insulin and insulin analogues are formed by recombinant DNA techniques carried out by inserting the human or a modified human gene for proinsulin into *Escherichia coli, Saccharomyces cerevisiae,* and *Pichia pastoris* (a yeast). Interestingly, transgenic plants (tobacco, lettuce) as well as embryonic stem cells have been suggested as systems to produce insulin. Upon fermentation, these genetically altered organisms produce proinsulin, which is harvested and enzymatically altered to produce insulin. Human insulin can also be produced semisynthetically by enzymatic transpeptidation of pork insulin, which alters position 30 of the B chain with the substitution of Thr for Ala.[22,57]

Only the insulin monomer is able to interact with insulin receptors, and native insulin exists as a monomer only at low, physiologic concentrations (<0.1 μM). However, recent studies indicate the other heteromers of insulin might also be involved.[58] Insulin dimerizes at the higher concentrations (0.6 mM) found in pharmaceutical preparations. At neutral pH and in the presence of zinc ions, hexamers will form. These zinc-associated hexamers are also the storage forms of insulin in β cells. At concentrations greater than 0.2 mM, hexamers form even in the absence of zinc ions. The monomeric form of insulin is the only readily absorbable form, so when insulin is administered subcutaneously (SC) at concentrations wherein dimers and hexamers exist, it is absorbed significantly more slowly.[51]

The importance of zinc ions for stabilizing insulin preparations has been known since the first reported crystallization of insulin in their presence in 1934. Presently, all pharmaceutical preparations are either solutions of zinc insulin or suspensions of insoluble forms of zinc insulin. A longer-acting and more stable form of insulin is protamine zinc insulin, which is prepared by precipitating insulin in the presence of zinc ions and protamine, a basic protein. This precipitate is known to contain two zinc ions per insulin hexamer. A somewhat shorter-acting and more useful preparation is neutral protamine Hagedorn (NPH) insulin, which includes *m*-cresol as a preservative. Six *m*-cresol molecules occupy cavities in the hexamer involving the B1-B8 helix formed by the presence of the *m*-cresol. Later, it was reported that when small additional amounts of zinc ions were added to hexameric two-zinc insulin in neutral acetate buffer, insulin could be made to crystallize in several forms with varying rates of dissolution in water. Thus, the slowly soluble lente insulin is a two-zinc insulin, and the crystalline, more slowly soluble ultralente insulin is a four-zinc form. However, due to declining use, lente insulin and ultralente insulin have been removed from the market.

Fibrils (partially unfolded insulin) are viscous or insoluble insulin precipitates. Shielding of hydrophobic domains is the principal driving force for the aggregation. Further studies revealed that when the exposed hydrophobic domain (A2, A3, B11, and B15) interacts with the normally buried aliphatic residues (A13, B6, B14, and B18) in the hexameric structure, fibrils form. Insulin fibrils do not resuspend on shaking; thus, they are pharmaceutically inactive. Insulin fibril formation is particularly important with the advent of infusion pumps to deliver insulin. In these devices, insulin is exposed to elevated temperatures, the presence of hydrophobic surfaces, and shear forces—all factors that increase insulin's tendency to aggregate. These problems can be overcome if the insulin is prepared with a phosphate buffer or other additives. Another physical stability problem associated with insulin is adsorption to tubing and other surfaces. This normally occurs if the insulin concentration is less than 5 international units (IU)/mL (0.03 mM), and it can be prevented by adding albumin to the dosage form if a dilute insulin solution must be used.[51]

There also are chemical instability issues associated with insulin. For many years, the only rapid-acting form of insulin was a solution of zinc insulin held at pH 2 to 3. If this insulin is stored at 4 °C, deamidation of the Asn at A21 occurs at a rate of 1% to 2% per month. The C-terminal Asn, under acidic conditions, undergoes cyclization to the anhydride, which, in turn, can react with water, leading to deamidation. The anhydride can also react with the N-terminal Phe of another chain to yield a cross-linked molecule. If stored at 25 °C, the inactive deamidated derivative constitutes 90% of the total protein after 6 months (Fig. 22.10).

If insulin is stored at neutral pH, a different reaction may occur. Deamidation occurs on the Asn at B3, and the products, the aspartate- and isoaspartate-containing insulins, are equiactive with native insulin (Fig. 22.10). More problematic transformations are possible, including chain cleavage between Thr A8 and Ser A9 and covalent cross-linking, either with a second insulin chain or with protamine, if present. These processes are relatively slow compared to the deamidations, but they have the potential of leading to products that may cause allergic reactions.[51]

Types of Insulin. The insulin analogues available for the treatment of diabetes are classified according to their rate of onset and duration of action. Structure-activity relationship

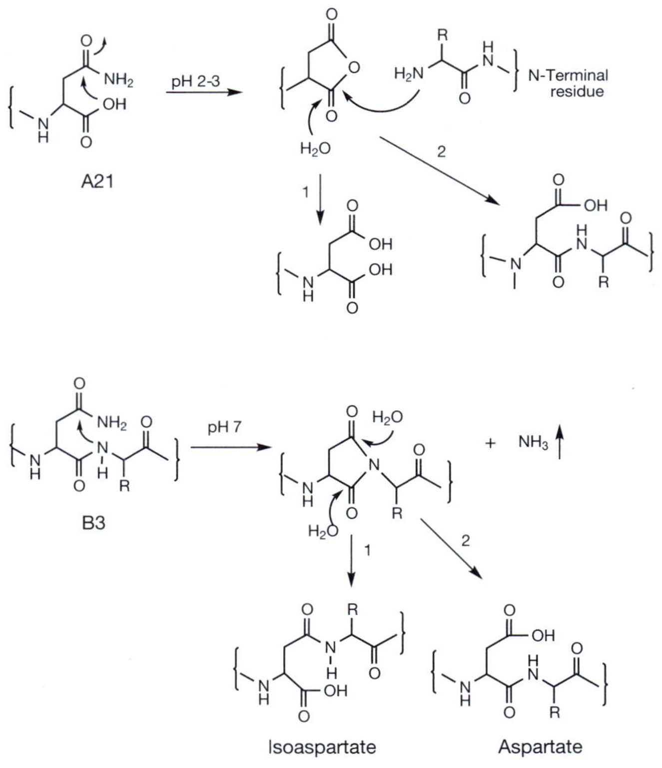

Figure 22.10 Chemical degradation of insulin.

studies revealed that variations in or addition/removal of amino acid residues from the C-terminus of the B chain could influence the rate of dimer formation while not drastically changing the biological activity. Inhibiting dimer formation can allow for rapid-acting insulin. Thus, the various insulin analogues that have been developed have substitutions in, or additions to, the C-terminus of the B chain starting at residue B28. The resulting analogues have either a faster onset or a longer duration of action relative to native insulin. These analogues are all produced by recombinant DNA (deoxyribonucleic acid) technology using a modified DNA template. The available insulin preparations are summarized in Table 22.5.

Rapid-acting insulin analogues include insulin lispro, aspart, and glulisine. All have changes made to the amino acid residues in the C-terminus of the B chain (Table 22.6). In insulin lispro, the B29 Lys is switched with B28 Pro, whereas in insulin aspart, the B28 Pro is changed to an Asp. Glulisine's B3 Val is changed to a Lys, and its B29 Lys is changed to a Glu. These modifications, as previously stated, result in insulin analogues that do not form dimers in solution and dissociate immediately into monomers, producing a very quick onset of action. Pharmacodynamically, lispro, aspart, and glulisine bind as well to insulin receptors as human insulin and have a low mitogenic potency. Mitogenic activity is the ability of insulin to induce cell division and is believed to be associated with insulin's binding to insulin-like growth factor receptors (IGFs I and II).[59] Lispro, aspart, and glulisine have an onset of action within 15 minutes, a peak

Table 22.5 Classification, Appearance, and Pharmacokinetic Properties of Insulin Preparations

Type	Appearance	Onset (h)	Peak (h)	Duration (h)
Rapid-acting				
Lispro	Clear	<0.25	0.5-1.5	3-4
Aspart	Clear	<0.25	0.5-1.5	3-4
Glulisine	Clear	<0.25	0.5-1.5	3-4
Short-acting				
Human insulin	Clear	0.5-1	2-3	4-6
Intermediate-acting				
NPH	Cloudy	2-4	4-12	18-26
Long-acting				
Glargine	Clear	1-4	5-24	20-24
Detemir	Cloudy	1-4	5-24	20-24
Ultralong-acting				
Degludec	Clear	0.5-1.5	NA	>48

NPH, neutral protamine Hagedorn.

activity at 30 to 90 minutes, and a duration of 3 to 4 hours (Table 22.5).

Regular human insulin is the prototype of short-acting insulin. It has an onset of action within 30 to 60 minutes, reaches its peak effect 2 to 3 hours after injection, and has a duration ranging 4 to 6 hours. Its slow onset inconveniently requires it to be administered 30 to 60 minutes before meals, but this property is retained with intravenous (IV) administration, making regular insulin a good choice for IV treatment of diabetes.

Intermediate-acting insulin is prepared by adding stoichiometric amounts of protamine to regular insulin to form a poorly soluble insulin-protamine complex. The complex is known as NPH insulin. NPH insulin has an onset of action of 2 to 4 hours, peak effect at 4 to 12 hours, and duration of 18 to 26 hours after injection. However, most patients get little effect after 13 to 15 hours.[60]

The first long-acting insulin analogue to be introduced to the market was insulin glargine. This analogue results from the replacement of A21 Asn by Gly and the addition of two Arg amino acids to the C-terminus of the B chain (Table 22.6). The resulting analogue has an isoelectric point close to 7, which results in its precipitation on SC injection. Slow dissolution from the site of injection results in an onset of 1 to 4 hours, a peak between 5 and 24 hours, and a duration of 20 to 24 hours that represents a fairly constant release of insulin glargine over 24 hours. It has been demonstrated to be comparable or slightly better than NPH insulin at maintaining or reducing A_{1C} levels without nocturnal hypoglycemia.[61]

Insulin detemir is another long-acting analogue. This analogue results from N-acylation of the B29 Lys with the 14-carbon myristic acid (Table 22.6). The fatty acid side chain binds to plasma albumin to produce a depot, resulting in a longer duration of action. It has approximately the same duration of action as insulin glargine when administered in equivalent doses.

Insulin degludec is an ultra-long-acting insulin that can be administered daily or 3 times a week and is comparable to glargine and detemir in onset and duration of action. Insulin degludec results from the removal of B30 Glu, N-acylation of B29 Lys with *l*-γ-Glu that is acylated with hexadecanedioic acid. The long duration of action of insulin degludec is believed to be due to the combination of (1) the formation of soluble multihexamer assemblies upon SC administration, which slowly release monomers and (2) hexadecandioic acid side chain binding to plasma albumin to produce a depot.[62] An important difference between glargine and determir is that glargine is a clear solution, whereas the others are cloudy. This may be a problem for patients who rely on the physical appearance of their insulin to distinguish NPH from regular, lispro, aspart, glulisine, glargine, or degludec, which are all clear (see Table 22.5).

Different types of insulin may be premixed and are usually prescribed for patients needing a simple insulin treatment plan. For example, insulin glargine is combined with the GLP-1 agonist lixisenatide in Soliqua (Table 22.7). The benefit of using premixed insulin is that rapid-acting and long-acting insulin can be administered at the same time, and can be given twice a day, usually at breakfast and supper. The drawback of using such a regimen is that, to be effective, the amount of carbohydrate to be eaten at each meal is preset. This works best for patients who can follow strict adherence to a consistent schedule of meals and activity and who are able to follow a prescribed diet.[63,64]

Sulfonylureas

The discovery of sulfonylureas as antidiabetic agents resulted from research conducted in 1942 that noted the hypoglycemic effect of sulfonamides used to treat typhoid fever.[65] Subsequent investigations revealed that modifying the sulfonamide antibacterial agents with a urea moiety resulted in sulfonylureas with significant hypoglycemic effects. This led to the discovery of the first generation oral hypoglycemic drugs. These agents include tolbutamide, chlorpropamide, tolazamide, and acetohexamide (Fig. 22.11).

The mechanism of action of all the sulfonylureas is to stimulate the release of insulin from the β cells of the pancreas. These cells metabolize glucose in the mitochondria to produce ATP, which increases the intracellular ratio of ATP/ADP, resulting in the closure of the ATP-sensitive K^+ channel on the plasma membrane. Closure of this channel

Table 22.6 Insulin Analogues

Generic Name	Brand Name	Change in A Chain	Change in B Chain
Lispro	Humalog	None	B28 Pro → Lys B29 Lys → Pro
Aspart	NovoLog	None	B28 Pro → Asp
Glulisine	Apidra	None	B3 Val → Lys B29 Lys → Glu
Glargine	Lantus	A21 Asn → Gly	Add: B31 Arg and B32 Arg
Detemir	Levemir	None	Remove: B30 Thr Add: C14 fatty acid to B29 Lys
Degludec	Tresiba	None	Remove: B30 Thr Acylate B29 Lys with hexadecanedioic acid via a γ-*l*-glutamic acid linker.

Table 22.7 Combination Antidiabetic Medications

Oral Hypoglycemics	Brand Name	Insulin Combinations	Brand Name
Ertugliflozin/sitagliptin	Steglujan	Insulin glargine/lixisenatide	Soliqua
Dapagliflozin/saxagliptin	Qtern	Insulin degludec/liraglutide	Xultophy
Empagliflozin/linagliptin	Glyxambi	Insulin aspart/insulin degludec	Ryzodeg
Empagliflozin/metformin	Synjardy	70% Insulin aspart protamine + 30% insulin aspart	NovoLog 70/30
Canagliflozin/metformin	Invokamet	75% Insulin lispro protamine + 50% insulin lispro	Humalog 75/25
Pioglitazone/glimepiride	Duetact	50% Insulin lispro protamine + 50% insulin lispro	Humalog 50/50
Linagliptin/metformin	Janumet	70% NPH + 30% regular insulin	Humulin 70/30
Linagliptin/metformin XR	Jentadueto		
Sitagliptin/simvastatin	Juvisync		
Saxagliptin/metformin XR	Kombiglyze XR		
Repaglinide/metformin	PrandiMet		
Pioglitazone/metformin	ACTOplus Met		
Rosiglitazone/metformin	Avandamet		

NPH, neutral protamine Hagedorn.

triggers the opening of voltage-sensitive Ca^{2+} channels leading to a rapid influx of Ca^{2+}. Increased intracellular Ca^{2+} causes an alteration in the cytoskeleton and stimulates the translocation of insulin-containing granules to the plasma membrane, allowing the exocytotic release of insulin.[66]

The ATP-sensitive K^+ channel is an octameric heterocomplex consisting of two units of the binding site for both sulfonylureas and ATP, designated as the sulfonylurea receptor type 1 (SUR1) and an inwardly rectifying K^+ channel (Kir6.2) (see Fig. 22.9). The SUR1 subunits consist of three transmembrane domains (TMD 0, 1, and 2), an intracellular loop (L0), and two nucleotide binding domains (NBD1 and 2). The NDB1 is adjacent to the TMD1, and the NBD2 is adjacent to the TMD2 (Fig. 22.12).[67]

The ATP-sensitive K^+ channels are not only found in the plasma membrane of β cells of the pancreas but also in the vasculature (SUR2B) and the cardiac myocytes (SUR2A). The binding of sulfonylureas to vascular and cardiac SURs, like the binding to the β-cell receptors, has a number of physiologic consequences. In cardiac myocytes, sulfonylurea binding to SUR2B prevents the opening of these channels, which, in turn, prevents the reduction of Ca^{2+} influx that results in myocardial cell death. In vascular cells, blocking SUR2B by sulfonylureas increases smooth muscle tone, resulting in decreased blood flow. Both these effects are detrimental to the heart during an ischemic attack.[68] Furthermore, inhibition of SUR2A in the heart prevents ischemic preconditioning. Ischemic preconditioning reduces the size of an infarct and protects against repeated ischemic episodes.[69]

The first generation sulfonylureas structurally differ in the chemical nature of the small lipophilic substituent on the *p*-position of the phenyl ring (R_1 of the pharmacophore; see Fig. 22.11) and the lipophilic alkyl or cycloalkyl substituent on the non–sulfonyl-attached urea nitrogen (R_2 of the pharmacophore). However, these structural modifications did not significantly increase their binding efficiency to the ATP-sensitive K^+ channel; thus, they all require relatively high doses to achieve effectiveness, which increases their potential for adverse events. In addition, the plasma half-life of these first-generation sulfonylureas is fairly long (5-36 hours), which also increases their potential for adverse effects.

The second-generation sulfonylureas developed out of research efforts intended to design hypoglycemic agents with increased potency, a faster rapid onset, shorter plasma half-lives, and longer durations of action. Thus, glyburide (also known as glibenclamide), glipizide, and glimepiride are 50 to 100 times more active than first-generation molecules, with plasma half-lives of 1 to 4 hours and durations of action up to 24 hours. This enhancement of activity is the result of strong binding affinity to the ATP-sensitive K^+ channel associated with the larger *p*-(β-arylcarboxyamidoethyl) group, which replaces the small lipophilic *p*-substituents found in the first-generation agents (see Fig. 22.11). Sulfonylurea binding to the SUR1 subunit is coordinated by the inner helices of the TMD1 and TMD2 domains. Figure 22.13 visualizes the current understanding of the binding of glyburide. The important residues on TDM2 are Asp1245, Thr1242, Arg1246, Asn1245, and Tyr1242; those on TMD1 are Tyr377 and Asp437.[67]

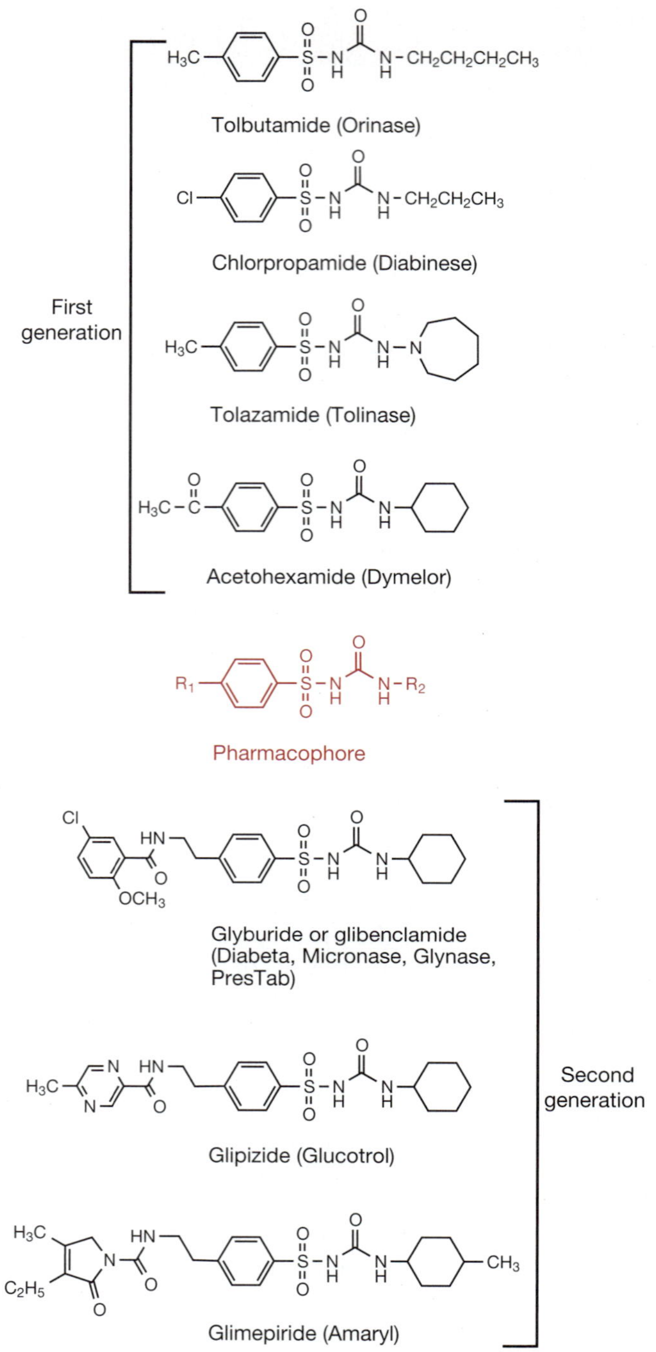

Figure 22.11 First- and second-generation sulfonylurea oral hypoglycemics.

SULFONYLUREA PHARMACOKINETICS AND METABOLISM. Sulfonylureas are highly protein bound, primarily to albumin, which leads to a large volume of distribution (~0.2 L/kg) (Table 22.8). Food can delay the absorption of these drugs, but does not typically affect bioavailability. Metabolism takes place in the liver, and the metabolites are renally excreted.

Glipizide and glyburide are extensively metabolized by oxidation, hydrolysis, and acetylation (Fig. 22.14) into less active or inactive metabolites. Glipizide metabolites are excreted primarily in the urine, whereas glyburide's metabolites are excreted equally in the urine and bile.

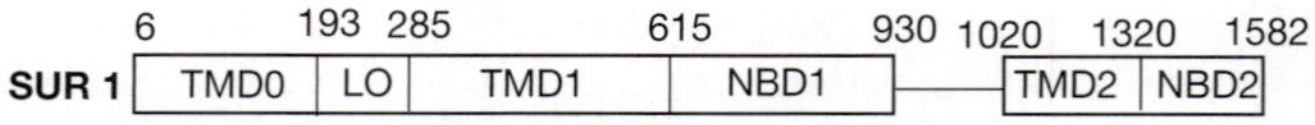

Figure 22.12 Schematic diagram of the sulfonylurea receptor subunits (SUR1) polypeptide. Numbers indicate residue numbers at the beginning and end of the domain.

Glimepiride is metabolized in the liver, primarily by CYP2C9, to the active metabolite M-1 (Fig. 22.15). It is then further metabolized by cytosolic dehydrogenases to the inactive metabolite M-2. Glimepiride is a substrate for OATP1B1 transporter. Therefore, genetic polymorphism of OATP1B1 and CYP2C9 may affect glimepiride's disposition and metabolism.[70]

Meglitinides

Meglitinide is the prototype structure that defines this class of insulin secretagogues. It is the benzoic acid derivative of the nonsulfonylurea moiety of glyburide—that is, the *p*-(β-arylcarboxyamidoethyl group (Fig. 22.16). These agents exert their effects by inducing closure of the ATP-sensitive K^+ channel found on the plasma membrane of the pancreatic β cells.[71,72]

REPAGLINIDE. Repaglinide is an analogue of meglitinide containing additional substituents (*m*-ethoxy, isobutyl, and piperidine ring) added to the basic benzoic acid structure. The aromatic chloro and methoxy groups of meglitinide have been eliminated, and the amide moiety has been transposed. Repaglinide stimulates insulin secretion by binding to three different receptors on the β-cells; one is the SUR1 and the other two receptors have yet to be completely characterized.[71] Repaglinide is not tissue specific and binds well to SUR1, SUR2A, and SUR2B found on cardiac and smooth muscle cells, therefore conferring extra-pancreatic effects in much the same way as sulfonylureas.[73]

Repaglinide has an absolute bioavailability of about 56%.[74] It has a rapid onset of action, and peak plasma concentrations are achieved within 1 hour of administration. Repaglinide has a short duration of action compared to

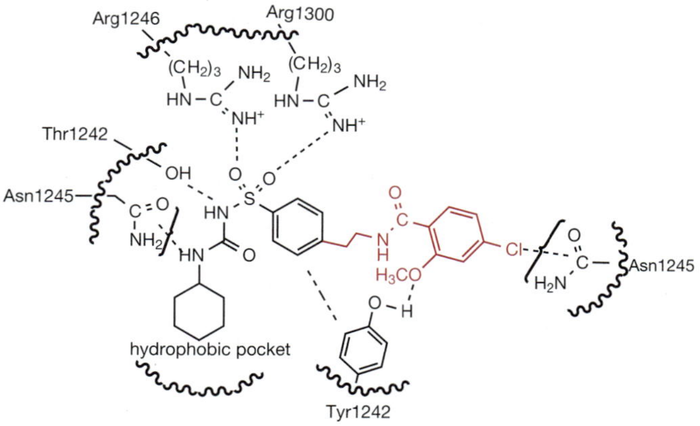

Figure 22.13 Representation of the binding residues for glyburide in the sulfonylurea receptor subunits (SUR1) subdomain. The enhancement of its activity is attributed to the strong binding affinity of the *p*-(arylcarboxyamidoethyl) group (in red) to Asn1245 and Tyr1242.

Table 22.8 Pharmacokinetic Properties of the First-Line Sulfonylureas

Sulfonylurea	Equivalent Dose (mg)	Serum Protein Binding (%)	Half-Life (h)	Duration (h)	Renal Excretion (%)
Glyburide	5	99	1.5-3.0	Up to 24	50
Glipizide	5	92-97	4	Up to 24	68
Glimepiride	2	99	2-3	Up to 24	40

other hypoglycemic drugs. The elimination half-life of repaglinide is about 1 hour. Repaglinide is not associated with the prolonged hyperinsulinemia seen with the sulfonylureas and has fewer side effects, including weight gain and potentially dangerous hypoglycemia. Perhaps, due to these reasons, repaglinide is better tolerated in older patients, than some sulfonylureas.[74] Repaglinide is at least 5-fold more potent than glyburide on intravenous administration and nearly 10-fold more active on oral administration. Repaglinide is oxidatively metabolized by 2C8/3A4 enzymes and directly conjugation with glucuronic acid. The major metabolites are a β-hydroxylated piperidine ring, oxidative opening of the piperine ring, the ortho amination of the unsubstituted phenyl ring, and hydroxylation of the isopropyl moiety.

NATEGLINIDE. Nateglinide is a phenylalanine analogue of meglitinide where the benzoic acid carboxylate group is transposed to the α-carbon of the *N*-ethyl side chain, creating the amino acid functionality. Nateglinide binds selectively to the SUR1 on β cells and has a much lower affinity for cardiac and skeletal muscles.[75] It is a chiral molecule synthesized as the *S*(+)-isomer with traces of the *R*(−)-isomer as an impurity. The *S*(+)-isomer is 100-fold more potent than the *R*(−)-isomer. Nateglinide is a rapidly absorbed insulin secretagogue that has a mechanism of action similar to that of repaglinide, with effects appearing within 20 minutes following oral dosing. Bioavailability is 73%, and it is 98% protein bound, primarily to albumin. Nateglinide is tissue selective, with low affinity for cardiac and skeletal muscles.[76] It is metabolized in the liver, with 16% being excreted unchanged in the urine. The major metabolites are hydroxyl derivatives (CYP2C9, 70%; CYP3A4, 30%) that are further conjugated to glucuronides (Fig. 22.17). The drug has an elimination half-life of 1.5 hours.

Molecular modeling studies have shown a similar conformation between the sulfonylurea hypoglycemics, glyburide and glimepiride, and the meglitinides, which might be important in the interaction of these drugs with the SUR1 on the β-cells. Specifically, these agents display a common U-shape formed by the hydrophobic interaction between the cyclic structures located at the ends of these molecules and a peptide bond at the bottom of the U. Moreover, the inactive analogues of the meglitinides, including the inactive enantiomer of repaglinide, are unable to adopt this U-shape and thus cannot bind effectively to the SUR1.[77]

Biguanides

The use of biguanides can be traced back to medieval times. The plant *Galega officinalis* was not only traditionally used for promoting perspiration during plague epidemics and as a galactogogue in milk-producing farm animals (eg, cows), but it was also prescribed for the relief of frequent urination associated with diabetes. *G. officinalis* has several common

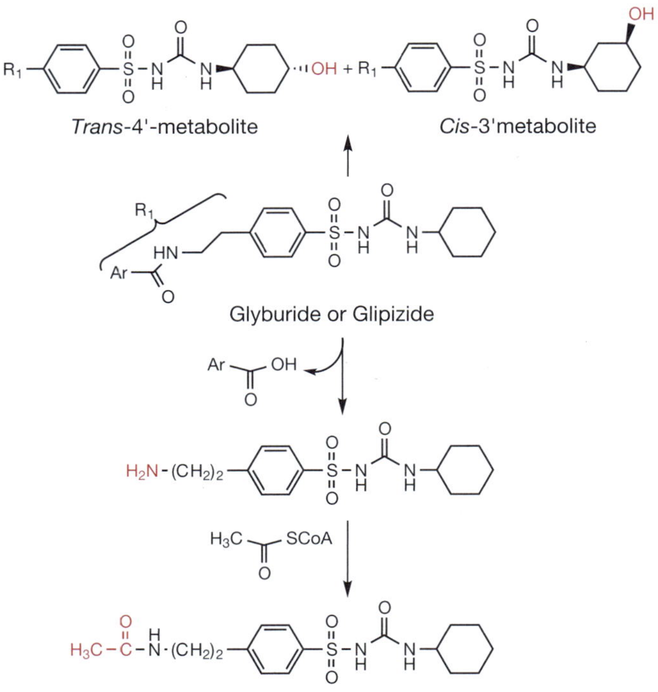

Figure 22.14 Metabolism of glyburide and glipizide.

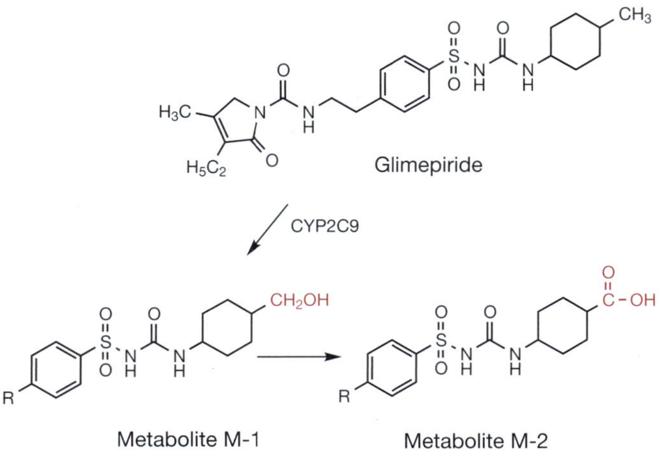

Figure 22.15 Metabolism of glimepiride.

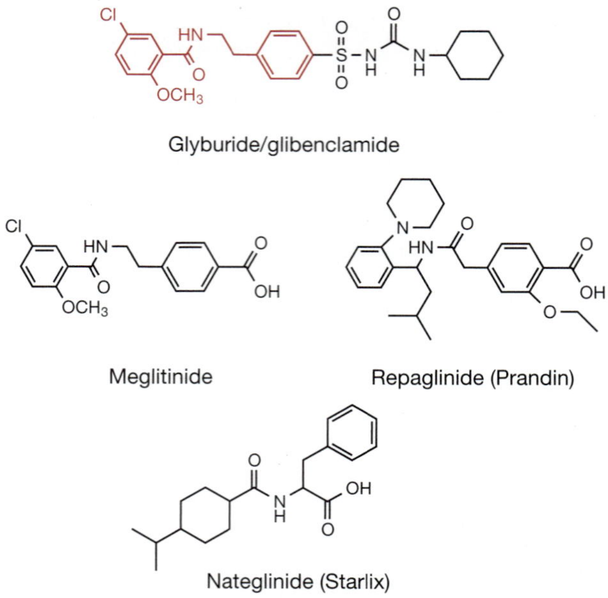

Figure 22.16 Meglitinide hypoglycemic agents.

names, including goat's rue, French lilac, and Italian fitch. This plant contains active compounds, such as galegine (isoamylene guanidine), which were shown to have blood glucose–lowering effects.[78] The hypoglycemic properties of the plant ultimately led to the synthesis of the biguanide compounds. The biguanides are chemically represented by the linkage of two guanidine groups with different side chains. Despite the toxicity associated with guanidine, the biguanides were shown to exert beneficial effects and quickly became available therapeutic agents for diabetes in the 1950s.

Oral hypoglycemic agents from the biguanide chemical class primarily act by reducing hepatic glucose production and by enhancing insulin sensitivity. The mechanism of action of the biguanides is primarily to reduce hepatic glucose output by decreasing gluconeogenesis and stimulating glycolysis. In addition, they affect anabolic pathways such as lipid and cholesterol biosynthesis. These metabolic actions are related to the inhibition of the mitochondrial respiratory chain complex I, as well as the activation of the AMP-activated protein kinase (AMPK) pathway. The biguanides target the mitochondria, where they reduce complex I of the electron transport chain. This results in a reduction in oxidative phosphorylation and, ultimately, a reduction in the synthesis of ATP, which causes AMP levels to rise. Increasing AMP activates AMPK and inhibits cyclic AMP-protein kinase A (cAMP-PKA) and fructose-1,6-bisphosphatase, all resulting in the inhibition of gluconeogenesis.[79] In addition, the activation of AMPK-dependent phosphorylation blocks the breakdown of fatty acids.

Insulin secretion is not directly affected by the biguanides, so they do not cause hypoglycemia. Importantly, biguanides do not induce weight gain, which is very beneficial for patients who are insulin resistant and having obesity.[80] They are also considered to have antihypertriglyceridemic effects and to possess vasoprotective properties, important actions in treating cardiovascular complications.[81]

Approved in 1995, metformin is currently the only available biguanide in the United States and is considered to be the first-line treatment for type 2 diabetes. It is widely used as monotherapy or in combination with other oral antidiabetic agents.[42]

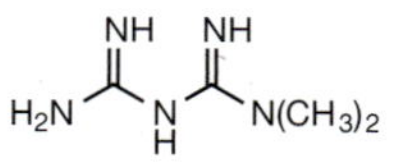

Metformin

Metformin is quickly absorbed from the small intestine. Bioavailability ranges from 50% to 60%, and the drug is not protein bound. Peak plasma concentrations occur at approximately 2 hours. The drug is widely distributed in the body and accumulates in the wall of the small intestine. This depot of drug serves to maintain plasma concentrations, but may also contribute to drug-induced gastrointestinal (GI) distress, lactic acidosis, and diarrhea, the latter of which can be minimized by food intake.[82]

Metformin is excreted in the urine via tubular excretion as an unmetabolized drug, and it has a half-life of approximately 2 to 5 hours; therefore, renal impairment as well as hepatic disease are contraindications for the drug. Since metformin is not metabolized in the liver, drug-drug interactions through the inhibition of metformin transporters (organic cation transporter [OCTs] and multidrug and toxic compound extrusion transporters [MATEs]) are clinically relevant. Genetic polymorphisms in these transporter genes are also likely to have a direct impact on metformin pharmacokinetics and variability in drug responses. Recent

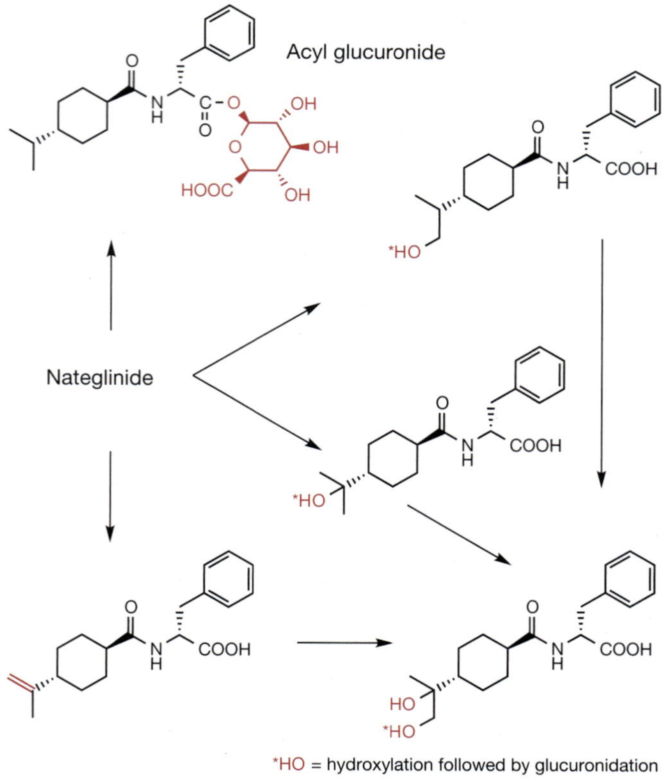

Figure 22.17 Urinary metabolites of nateglinide.

drug-drug interaction studies suggest that proton-pump inhibitors inhibit metformin uptake in vitro by inhibiting OCT proteins OCT1, OCT2, and OCT3. Cimetidine, an H_2 receptor blocker, is a potent inhibitor of MATE1 and an inhibitor of OCT2. Coadministration of metformin and cimetidine will lead to reduced renal tubular secretion and increased systemic exposure to metformin. As a result, it may increase the risk of lactic acidosis associated with metformin. Therefore, it is recommended that metformin's dose be reduced when coadministered with cimetadine.[83] Oral antidiabetic drugs repaglinide and rosiglitazone also inhibited OCT1-mediated metformin transport in vitro. A recent study suggests the potential for a transporter-mediated drug-drug interaction between metformin and specific tyrosine kinase inhibitors (eg, imatinib, nilotinib, gefitinib, and erlotinib; see Chapter 37), which may have clinical implications in the disposition, efficacy, and toxicity of metformin.[84]

Metformin is not recommended for patients with type 2 diabetes who are inclined toward metabolic ketoacidosis induced by certain conditions, including hepatic disease, heart failure, respiratory disease, hypoxemia, severe infection, alcohol abuse, or renal disease.[85]

Peroxisome Proliferator–Activated Receptor Agonists (Insulin Sensitizers)

Activators of peroxisome proliferator–activated receptors (PPARs) in the treatment of insulin resistance and type 2 diabetes mellitus are a much sought after target, since PPARs are central regulators of lipid and carbohydrate metabolism and inflammatory pathways and help maintain homeostasis. They belong to the nuclear hormone receptor superfamily of ligand-activated transcription factors and are closely related to steroid, retinoid, and thyroid hormone receptors (Chapter 7). This receptor family is composed of three members: PPARα, δ, and γ. PPARδ is ubiquitously present in tissues of adult mammals, whereas the α subtype is abundantly present in tissues catalyzing lipid oxidation, which includes the liver, kidney, and heart. PPARγ is primarily expressed in adipose tissue, where it helps control lipid differentiation.[86]

The TZDs are classic examples of PPARγ agonists and are commonly referred to as the "glitazones." These agents were developed when clofibric acid analogues (Chapter 18) were being screened for antihyperglycemic and lipid-lowering activity. Although initially the mechanism of action of the TZDs was unclear, it was soon discovered that they enhanced adipocyte differentiation by activation of the nuclear hormone receptor superfamily, PPAR. Upon binding to PPAR, an endogenous or exogenous ligand induces a conformational change in the receptor, thus stabilizing the interaction with the retinoid X receptor, which, in turn, results in the stimulation of transcription by target genes. The endogenous ligand(s) for PPARγ have not been identified; however, studies suggest that certain arachidonic acid metabolites and long chain unsaturated fatty acids, such as linoleic acid, may be the intrinsic agonists (Fig. 22.18).[86]

PPARγ agonists, such as the glitazones, act by increasing the sensitivity of cells to insulin. The glitazones also decrease both systemic fatty acid production and fatty acid uptake, which contributes to increased sensitization of

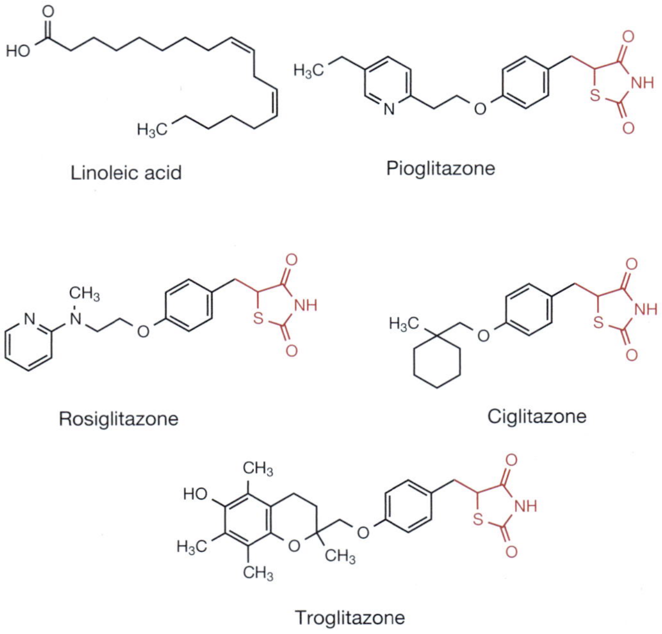

Figure 22.18 Linoleic acid and thiazolidinedione (outlined in red) PPARγ agonists (glitazones).

cells to insulin. Patients with type 2 diabetes are known to have high triglyceride and low HDL levels. The glitazones increase the lipolysis of triglycerides in very low density lipoproteins (VLDLs) and, as a result, increase high density lipoprotein (HDL) levels. They also increase low density lipoprotein (LDL) levels, which could be a major drawback to the use of these drugs.[87,88]

PPARγ activation improves glucose uptake by skeletal muscle and, at the same time, reduces glucose production by slowing gluconeogenesis. Hence, these drugs improve metabolism of glucose not only in patients with diabetes but also in individuals with obesity who have IGT.[86] As mentioned earlier, the first PPARγ agonists to be introduced were the glitazones. The pharmacophore responsible for activity is the thiazolidinedione moiety outlined in red in Figure 22.18. A phenyl ring attached to the thiazolidinone ring via a methylene group is essential for activity and, in many instances, a saturated linker is found to be more potent than the unsaturated counterpart.

The first-generation TZDs include pioglitazone, rosiglitazone, and ciglitazone (Fig. 22.18). The rationale used for the development of these agents was the fact that the structure of troglitazone (the first drug in this class to be marketed) includes the structure of α-tocopherol, an antioxidant that retards the oxidation of LDLs.[89] However, due to severe hepatoxicity and cardiovascular effects, troglitazone has been withdrawn clinically.[87,90] Rosiglitazone is associated with an increased risk of cardiovascular events.[91] Therefore, rosiglitazone is withdrawn from several countries. Pioglitazone is well absorbed orally, with 83% bioavailability.[92] The peak plasma concentration of rosiglitazone is about 1.5 hours. Pioglitazone is metabolized extensively in the liver by CYP2C8 and CYP3A4. These metabolic products result from oxidation at either carbon adjacent to the pyridine ring and are found as various conjugates in the urine and bile (Fig. 22.19).

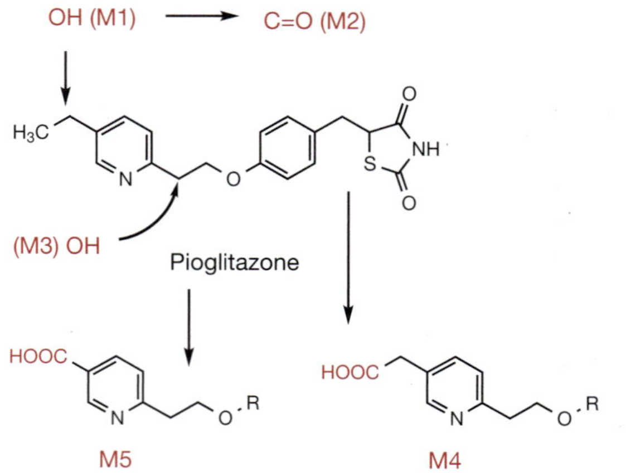

Figure 22.19 Metabolism of pioglitazone.

Metabolites M-1, M-2, and M-3 appear to contribute to the biological activity of pioglitazone.[93]

Recently, dual PPARα/γ agonists have become much sought after targets, and many research groups are actively involved in synthesizing these bioactive compounds as novel antidiabetic agents. The combined activation of PPARα and PPARγ is believed to induce complementary and synergistic action on lipid metabolism, insulin sensitivity, and inflammation control, possibly circumventing or reducing the side effects of PPARγ. To date, there are no PPARα/γ agonists approved for use in the United States. However, saroglitazar is an approved drug in India for the treatment of type 2 diabetes and triglyceridemia in patients whose dyslipidemia is not controlled by statin therapy.[94]

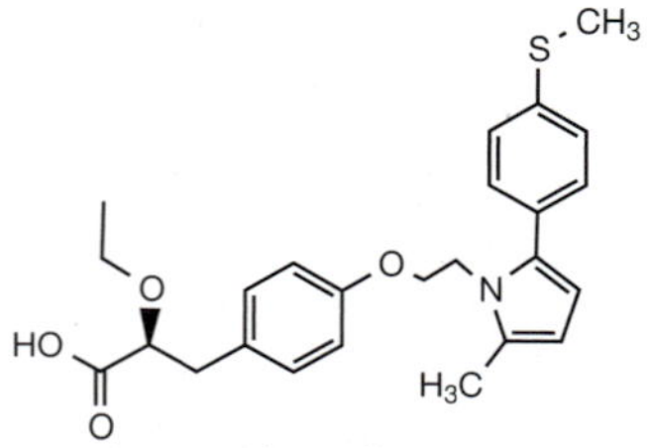

Saroglitazar

α-Glucosidase Inhibitors

α-Amylase and α-glucosidase are key enzymes responsible for the metabolism of carbohydrates. The salivary and pancreatic α-amylases are responsible for the breakdown of complex polysaccharides into oligo- and disaccharides, preparing them for intestinal absorption. α-Glucosidase, which consists of maltase, sucrase, isomaltase, and glucoamylase, is a membrane-bound enzyme present in the brush border of the small intestine and is in relatively high concentrations in the proximal part of the jejunum. This enzyme catalyzes the conversion of the disaccharides sucrose and maltose into glucose. The resulting monosaccharides are then absorbed by the enterocytes of the jejunum and enter systemic circulation, as well as various biochemical pathways for the production of energy.[95] Thus, inhibiting α-glucosidase will delay carbohydrate absorption in the gut by moving undigested disaccharides into the distal sections of the small intestine and colon. The result is the prevention of glucose production, thereby reducing postprandial hyperglycemia. All known α-glucosidase inhibitors act locally and are excreted unchanged in the feces, obviating metabolic drug interactions.[96]

ACARBOSE. The α-glucosidase inhibitors were first introduced in 1996 with the drug acarbose (Fig. 22.20).[97] It is an oligosaccharide obtained from *Actinomyces utahensis* and is the drug of choice in this category. It is a competitive inhibitor of the α-glucosidase enzyme, with a high affinity for sucrase and a lesser affinity for glucoamylase and pancreatic α-amylase in humans.[98] When used in monotherapy, there is no risk of hypoglycemia and weight gain, as seen with the first- and second-generation sulfonylureas. However, GI irritation, bloating, and flatulence caused by fermentation of undigested sugars in the large bowel by intestinal microflora are some drawbacks common to all α-glucosidase inhibitors.[95] These side effects can be minimized to a certain extent by gradual dose titration and the right combination therapy with other orally active hypoglycemic drugs.

VOGLIBOSE AND MIGLITOL. Voglibose and miglitol are other α-glucosidase inhibitors in clinical use for the management of diabetes. α-Glucosidase inhibitors reduce postprandial hyperglycemia to a lesser extent as compared to other oral antidiabetic agents, and clinical trials with acarbose have shown that the reduction in A_{1C} levels is 0.5% to 1% when compared to placebo.[97] These agents are therefore seldom used as monotherapy and frequently find use in combination therapy, especially with sulfonylureas.[98] Apart from diabetes, their use can be extended to the treatment of glycosphingolipid lysosomal storage disease and HIV infections and in the management of certain tumors.[99,100]

Glucagon-Like Peptide 1 Agonists and Dipeptidyl Peptidase IV Inhibitors

Glucagon-like peptide 1 (GLP-1) is a 30–amino acid peptide produced by the posttranslation processing of the

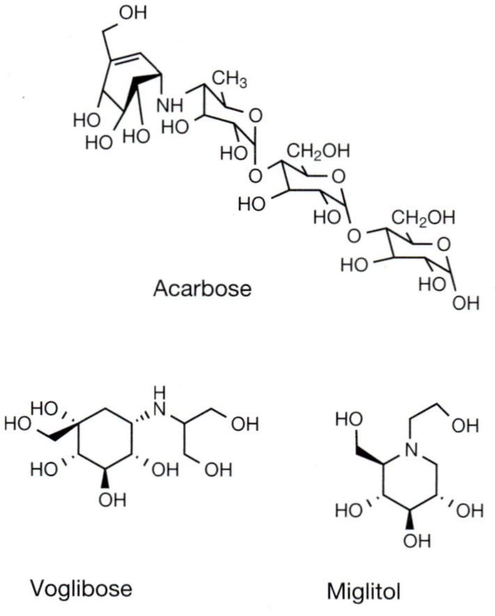

Figure 22.20 Clinically useful α-glucosidase inhibitors.

proglucagon gene and secreted by L-cells of the gut in response to a meal. It exerts control over glucose levels by promoting insulin secretion in a glucose-dependent manner.[101] The role of GLP-1 was first proposed based on the observation that the amount of insulin secreted following an oral glucose dose exceeded that of an equivalent glucose dose administered IV in individuals with and without diabetes.[102] This observation was termed the incretin effect and is the result of two gut hormones: GLP-1 and GIP.[103] GLP-1 secretion from L-cells is similar to that of glucose-induced insulin secretion from pancreatic β cells. Metabolism of glucose in the intestinal L-cells leads to closure of ATP-linked K^+ channels resulting in depolarization of the membrane and entry of Ca^{2+} that leads to the secretion of GLP-1.[104] With an in vivo half-life of 1 to 2 minutes, GLP-1 is rapidly metabolized by an aminopeptidase enzyme, DPP-IV, yielding an inactive peptide that is two amino acids shorter.[105,106] DDP-IV specifically cleaves the peptide bond between alanine and glutamate at positions 8 and 9. It follows that GLP-1 agonists or DDP-IV inhibitors would be effective agents to control blood glucose levels in patients with diabetes.

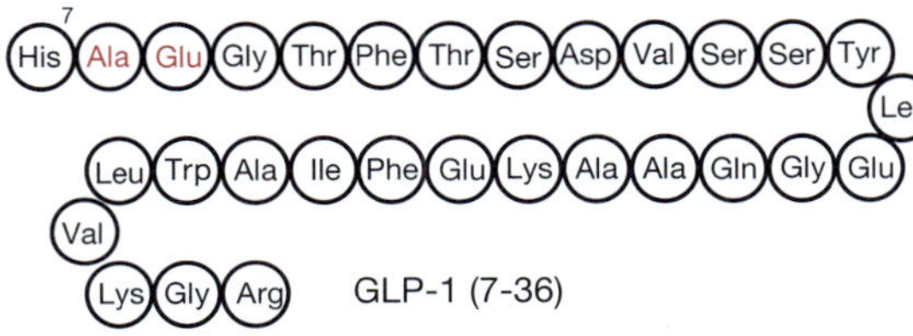

GLP-1 (7-36)

GIP is an incretin secreted by intestinal K cells and cosecreted with GLP-1 after a meal. It appears to work along with GLP-1 in an additive fashion to potentiate insulin secretion from pancreatic β cells. There is a specific GIP receptor found in many tissues, including pancreatic α cells, adipose tissue, bone, and heart. During hyperglycemia, GIP has no effect on glucagon while strongly potentiating insulin secretion. However, GIP increases glucagon levels during fasting and hypoglycemic conditions, while having little or no effect on insulin secretion.[107]

GLP-1 ANALOGUES. GLP-1 is deactivated by DPP-IV, which removes a dipeptide from the N-terminus. One of the principal reasons why GLP-1 is so susceptible to DPP-IV is because it contains an Ala in the penultimate N-terminal position 8. Substitution at this position gives analogues with increased stability. Indeed, substitution of the Ala8 with Thr ($t_{1/2}$ = 197 minutes), Gly ($t_{1/2}$ = 159 minutes), Ser ($t_{1/2}$ = 174 minutes), or α-aminoisobutyric acid (AiB) each gave analogues that are more stable in vitro than GLP-1 ($t_{1/2}$ = 28 minutes) under the same conditions.[108] In fact, the AiB analogue exhibited no degradation even after 6 hours. While such analogues are found to be more stable to DPP-IV in vitro, the in vivo half-life is increased only from 1 to 2 to 3 to 4 minutes, and this is attributed to rapid elimination by the kidneys. Interestingly, these analogues still retained binding affinity to the GLP-1 receptor, with the AiB analogue almost twice as potent as GLP-1.

More useful in vivo analogues, therefore, required both DPP-IV resistance and decreased renal elimination. This was achieved with the introduction into the market in April 2005 of the GLP-1 analogue exenatide as parenteral therapy. Exenatide is a 39-amino acid peptide analogue of GLP-1 (7-36) isolated from the saliva of the Gila monster (*Heloderma suspectum*). It is a GLP-1 receptor–agonist resistant to the action of DPP-IV. It has a Gly8 instead of Ala8 in the penultimate N-terminal position, is 53% homologous to human GLP-1, and has an in vivo half-life of approximately 3 hours.

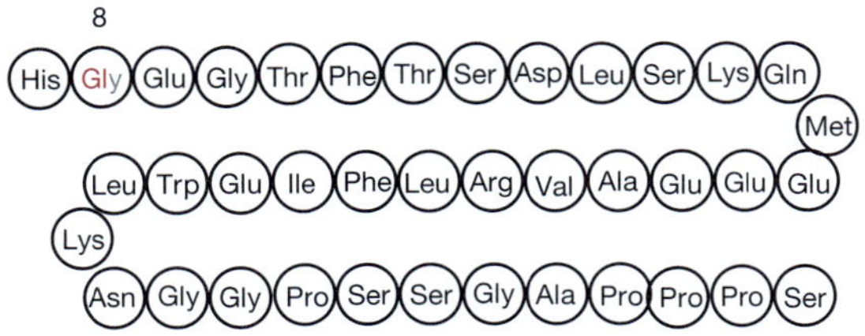

Exenatide
(Byetta)

Exenatide has been shown to reduce A_{1C} levels in sulfonylurea-treated patients with type 2 diabetes and is associated with weight loss.[109] This weight loss is probably due to a decrease in appetite. In *db/db* mice, it increased β-cell mass and delayed the onset of diabetes, indicating that it may even have a prophylactic use.[110]

CURRENTLY MARKETED GLP-1 ANALOGUES.

Liraglutide. Liraglutide, which represents amino acid residues 7 to 37 of GLP-1, was developed from a series of acylated GLP-1 (7-37) derivatives. Several positions of GLP-1 were substituted with different acyl moieties, ranging in length from 12 to 18 carbons. The C_{16} derivative α-*l*-glutamoyl-(*N*-α-hexadecanoyl)-Lys26 Arg34-GLP-1 (liraglutide) was found to have the best combination of albumin binding to retard renal elimination and DPP-IV degradation resistance (due to the replacement of Lys34 with Arg34).[111,112] This analogue of GLP-1 (7-37) has multiple actions in addition to reduction of hyperglycemia, including suppression of inappropriate glucagon secretion, slowing of gastric emptying, and enhancement of β-cell function and mass.[113] Liraglutide was approved by the US Food and Drug Administration (FDA) for marketing under the name Victoza, in 2010. However, because of a possible link to the production of thyroid C-cell tumors, the product label has a black box warning with the recommendation that it be used only in patients for whom the potential benefits outweigh the potential risk.[114]

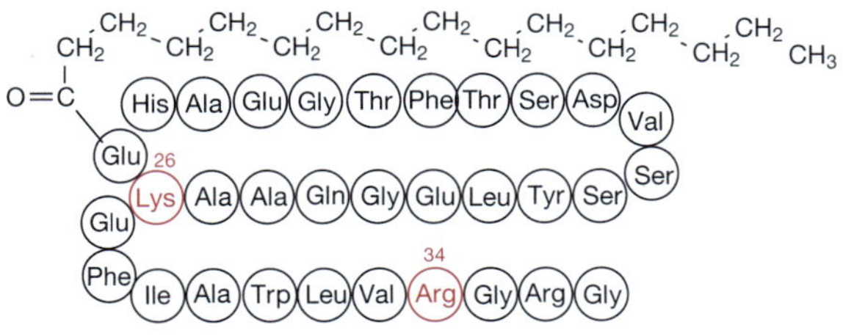

Liraglutide
(Victoza)

Dulaglutide. Dulaglutide is a fusion protein that is prepared by fusing two identical GLP-1 (7-37) analogues (Gly8,

Glu22, Gly36) to a modified IgG4 Fc fragment. The linker is a small peptide joined to the dimer via disulfide bonds.[115] The IgG4 moiety acts to decrease both renal clearance and antigen-antibody formation. It has ~90% amino acid homogeneity to human GLP-1 (7-39).[116]

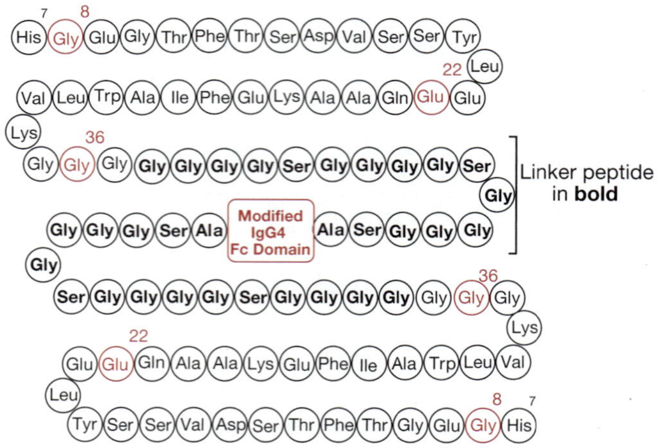

Dulaglutide (Trulicity)

Dulaglutide is administered SQ and is slowly absorbed. It attains peak plasma concentration in about 48 hours and steady state at 2 to 4 weeks. It is administered on a weekly basis and has a half-life of ~5 days. As monotherapy, it has a slightly greater reduction in A_{1C} as compared to metformin, with about the same degree of body weight loss and GI distress. Dulaglutide is metabolized by proteases and not significantly eliminated renally. However, it is not recommended for use by patients with severe kidney dysfunction (glomerular filtration rate [GFR] <30 mL/min).[115]

Albiglutide. Albiglutide is composed of a tandem dimer of an analogue of human GLP-1 (7-37)-Gly8. This construct inhibits DPP-IV metabolism and is covalently bonded to recombinant human albumin. The albumin serves as a carrier protein and substantially reduces renal clearance.[115]

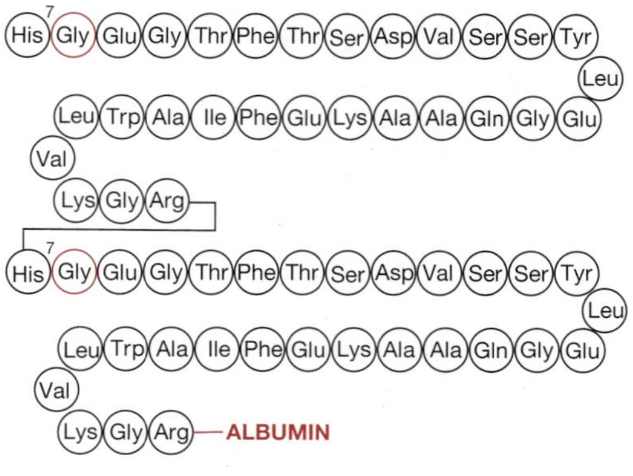

Albiglutide (Tanzeum)

Albiglutide has 97% amino acid homology with human GLP-1. It has a half-life of 6 to 8 days, allowing for weekly SC administration. In monotherapy versus placebo, it lowered A_{1C} by 1.4% without a significant change in body weight. Albiglutide is metabolized by endogenous proteases, and its use is cautioned in patients with compromised renal function (<50 mL/min). Albiglutide has been compared to sitagliptin (discussed later), pioglitazone, liraglutide, and basal insulin in trials. In those trials, albiglutide displayed a modest decrease in A_{1C} or was noninferior to comparators.[117]

Lixisenatide. Lixisenatide was approved in the United States in July 2016. Structurally it is a modified version of exenatide, with one amino acid deleted (Pro38) and a string of six Lys residues added to the Ser at the carboxylic acid terminus. This modification extends the half-life to about 2 to 5 hours and allows for once to twice daily SC administration.

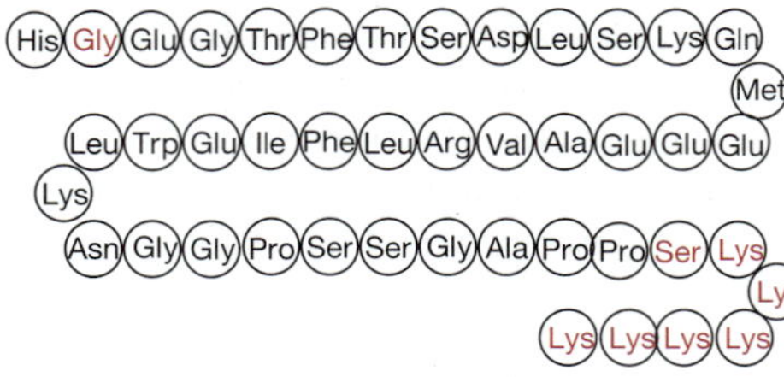

Lixisenatide (Adlyxin)

Lixisenatide has only about 50% amino acid homology to human GLP-1 (7-37). In monotherapy, lixisenatide showed modest A_{1C} decreases (−1.0% to −0.7%), and body weight loss was also minimal (range −0.4 to −0.2 kg).[115] In January 2023, Sanofi discontinued US marketing of lixisenatide for business reasons.

Semaglutide. Semaglutide is a long-acting human GLP-1 analogue ([Aib8, Arg34]-hGLP-1). The amino terminal sequence substitutes Ala8 with the non-human amino, 1-aminoisobutyric acid (Aib8), which allows for resistance to DPP-IV degradation. In addition, Lys26 is derivatized with a C18 fatty diacid using an ADO-linker (8-amino-3,6-dioxooctanoic acid) bridged via a glutamic acid moiety. Semaglutide has a 94% amino acid homology to hGLP-1.[118]

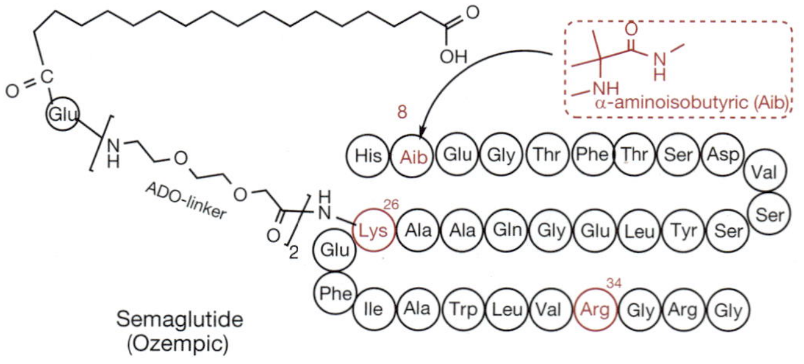

Semaglutide (Ozempic)

As was seen with liraglutide, the fatty acid side chain enhances affinity for albumin; however, in this case, the affinity is 3-fold greater. Therefore, semaglutide exhibits an extremely long half-life of ~165 hours enabling once weekly SC dosing. A once-weekly oral tablet has been developed by co-formulating the peptide with sodium *N*-(8-[2-hydroxybenzoyl amino] caprylate) (SNAC), which acts as a transcellular carrier across GI enterocytes by increasing solubility through higher local pH and decreasing proteolysis. Semaglutide is slowly metabolized by proteolytic cleavage of the peptide backbone and β-oxidation of the fatty acid side chain. Only ~3% is excreted unchanged in the urine.[118]

There are two semaglutide products on the market: Ozempic and Wegovy. Ozempic is approved by the FDA for the treatment of type 2 diabetes, whereas Wegovy was approved in 2021 by the FDA as a treatment for obesity. Since both products contain semaglutide, the only difference between them is in the dosages. Ozempic is approved for treatment of type 2 diabetes with doses between 0.68 and 2.68 mg/mL to bring A_{1C} under control. However, for weight loss Wegovy dosing is 0.25 mg/0.5 mL to 2.4 mg/0.75 mL. Both come in injector pens for subcutaneous (SQ) administration, but Wegovy pens are used once and then disposed whereas Ozempic pens are reusable.

Tirzepatide. Tirzepatide is a 39–amino acid peptide that has dual receptor affinity for both GLP-1 and GIP.[119-121] Tirzepatide is a linear polypeptide based primarily on the native GIP, which is conjugated to a C20 fatty diacid moiety (eicosanedioic acid) via a linker connected to Lys20.[122] Structure activity studies of the interaction of tirzepatide with both the GIP receptor and the GLP-1 receptor show that tirzepatide adopts an α-helical conformation with the N-terminal Tyr1 reaching deep into the transmembrane core of both receptors. The fatty acid moiety is thought to enhance GLP-1 activity. Tirzepatide has two non-coded amino acids (Aib) at positions 2 and 13, which inhibits DDP-4 degradation. The Aib at position 13 specifically contributes to GIP receptor activity. The linkers used in tirzepatide, gamma glutamate and bis-aminodiethoxyacetyl (γGlu-2x Ado), promote peptide flexibility and help optimize receptor biding. These structural features contribute to a long half-life for tirzepatide (116.7 hours) and high albumin affinity.

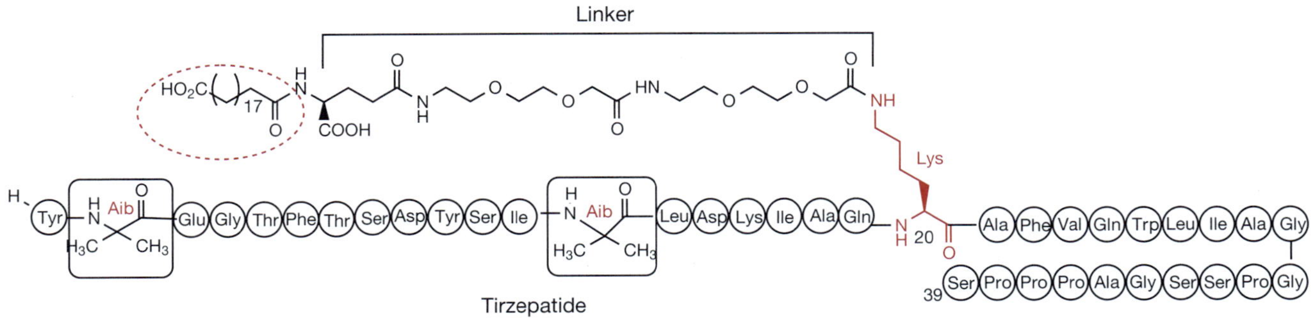

Tirzepatide

The bifunctional action of tirzepatide as an agonist at both the GLP-1 and GIP receptors conveys action as an anti-obesity agent, a hypoglycemic agent, energy balance, and lipid storage. However, the interaction is stronger for GIP versus GLP-1. Tirzepatide was originally approved in 2022 for the treatment of type 2 diabetes. However, it showed an excellent dose-dependent effect on weight reduction and, therefore, was granted Fast Track designation by the FDA for treatment of patients who have obesity and are overweight with metabolic comorbidities.[123]

DPP-IV Inhibitors. The major problem with GLP-1 analogues is their need for SC administration, which may limit patient compliance. Also, GLP-1 analogues, as with any peptide drug, have the potential to be immunogenic. This therefore stimulated the search for small molecule inhibitors of DPP-IV. DPP-IV inhibitors are administered orally, once daily either before or after meals.[124]

DPP-IV is a serine protease that exists in both a membrane-bound and a plasma-soluble form. It is a proline-specific aminopeptidase responsible for the degradation of a number of biologically important peptides other than GLP-1 and GIP. DPP-IV belongs to a family of dipeptidyl peptidase enzymes that include DPP's VI-X, fibroblast protein-a (FAP), acylaminoacyl peptidase (APP), prolyl carboxypeptidase (PCP), and quiescent cell proline dipeptidase (QPP).[125] Since the clinical importance of these other prolyl peptidases has not been established, it is important that inhibitors have specificity for DPP-IV.

There are currently five DPP-IV inhibitors commercially available: sitagliptin, vildagliptin, saxagliptin, linagliptin, and alogliptin. The development of many structural variants has led to the understanding that there is an absolute requirement for a basic amino function in the position equivalent to the penultimate amino acid (Ala) in GLP-1. Most active inhibitors are peptide derivatives of α-aminoacylpyrrolidines or α-aminoacylthiazolidines, which also take advantage of the enzyme's high preference for Pro binding. The most active inhibitors also have an electrophilic group in the 2-position of the pyrrolidine or thiazolidine ring. The most common group is cyano and is present in vildagliptin, saxagliptin, and alogliptin (Fig. 22.21).

Sitagliptin has a piperazine ring fused to a pyrazole in place of the pyrrolidine ring, making it a triazole ring, but it still contains the α-amino acyl moiety and the amide bond. Linagliptin contains a xanthine ring as the central pharmacophore. Alogliptin contains the 2,4-pyrimidine pharmacophore with the essential amino group on the piperidine ring.

All DPP-IV inhibitors bind inside a hydrophobic pocket of DDP-IV made up of Arg125, Glu205, Glu206, Tyr547, Tyr662, Tyr666, Ser630, and Phe357. Their binding residues, however, differ depending on their pharmacophore and the specific moieties attached. Saxagliptin, vildagliptin, and alogliptin contain the cyano group that most likely forms a reversible covalent amidate with the enzyme Ser630, resulting in the deactivation of DPP-IV.[126,127] Figure 22.22 depicts a proposed mechanism for the amidate formation.

All inhibitors bind through ionic interaction with Glu205 and Glu206. The xanthine pharmacophore of linagliptin has a $C_{8\ am}$inopiperidine and an N_7 butynyl substituent for binding to the DPP-IV catalytic site. The aminopiperidine's

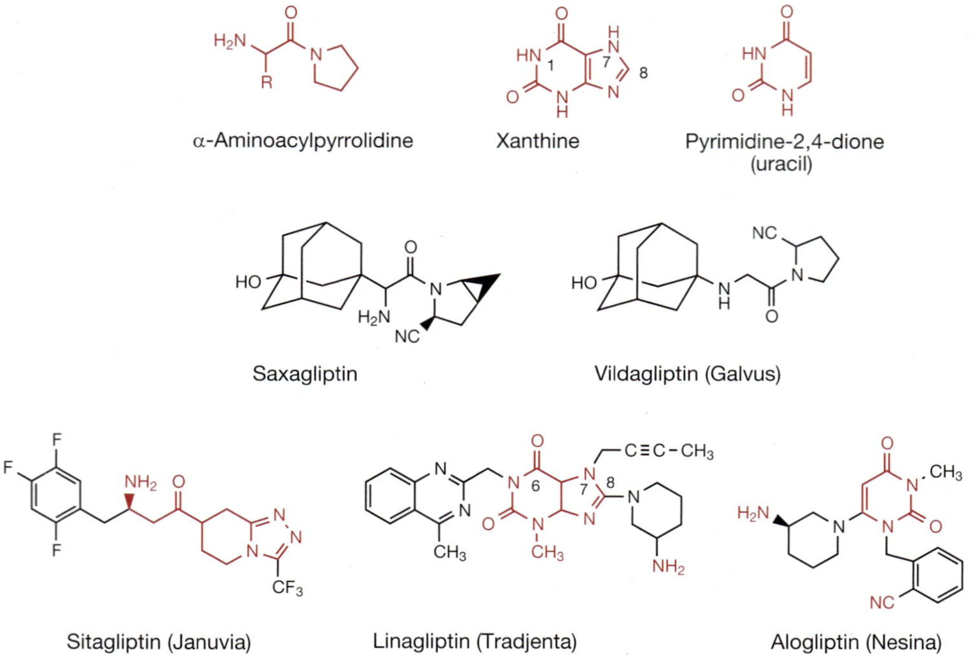

Figure 22.21 α-Aminoacylpyrrolidine, xanthine and uracil pharmacophores, and currently available DPP-IV inhibitors.

primary amino group occupies the recognition site for the amino terminus of GLP-1, and hydrogen bonds with the aforementioned Glu residues. The xanthine is held in place by π stacking with Tyr547. The N_7 butynyl group interacts hydrophobically with Tyr662, Ser630, and Tyr666, and the quinazoline ring interacts by π-stacking with the aromatic ring of Trp629.[126]

Sitagliptin. Sitagliptin was approved by the FDA in 2006 for the treatment of type 2 diabetes, either as monotherapy or in combination with metformin, TDZs, or sulfonylureas. Sitagliptin has good oral bioavailability (87%) with no effect from food. It is protein bound only to about 37%, and 80% is excreted unchanged in the urine. It is important to have high specificity for DPP-IV, as inhibition of DPP-VIII and DPP-IX has been shown to cause severe toxicity in animal studies, including alopecia, thrombocytopenia, splenomegaly, and death. The selectivity of sitagliptin for DPP-IV compared to DPP-VIII and IX is >2,600-fold. Sitagliptin has no effect on glucose levels in healthy patients; however, it reduces A_{1C} about 0.6% to 0.9% in type 2 diabetes. Sitagliptin has a number of side effects, including upper respiratory tract infection, nasopharyngitis, and headache. Patients experience nausea if the drug is taken with metformin, leg swelling when taken with TDZs, and hypoglycemia when administered with a sulfonylurea. There have also been reports of anaphylaxis, angioedema, and rashes, although a causal link has not been established.[128]

Vildagliptin. Vildagliptin was approved in 2008 by the European Medicines Agency for use in the European Union (EU), but the manufacturer has withdrawn its intent to submit it for FDA approval since the FDA demanded additional clinical data, assuring that the skin lesions and kidney impairment observed in animal studies were not seen in humans. Due to these adverse events, vildagliptin is not a first-line treatment for diabetes. In phase III clinical trials, vildagliptin showed good oral bioavailability (85%) and low protein binding (9.3%) and was 21% excreted unchanged in the urine. It has a high specificity for DPP-IV compared to DPP-VIII and IX that ranges from 32- to 250-fold. In clinical trials, no patients discontinued medication because of adverse effects, which is similar to sitagliptin (upper respiratory tract infections, diarrhea, nausea, and hypoglycemia).[128]

Saxagliptin. The FDA approved saxagliptin in 2009. It is 10 times more potent as an inhibitor of DPP-IV than either vildagliptin or sitagliptin. It shows a higher specificity for DPP-IV compared to DPP-VIII and IX (400- and 75-fold, respectively). Trials using doses of 2.5 to 10 mg have shown reductions of A_{1C} of 0.5% to 0.8% with no significant

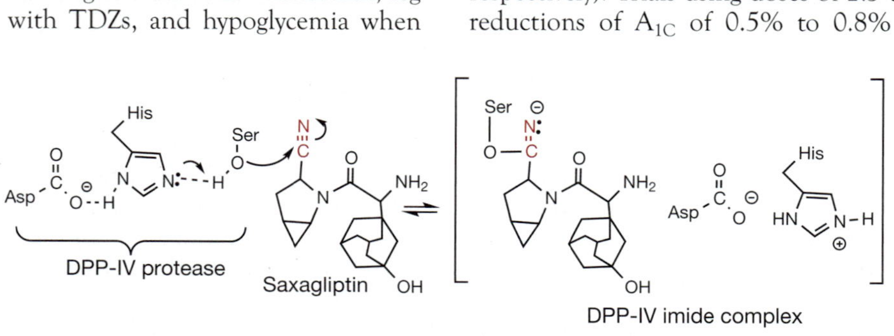

Figure 22.22 Proposed mechanism of reversible inhibition of dipeptidyl peptidase-IV (DPP-IV) by saxagliptin.

weight gain. Saxagliptin was well tolerated, with side effects equivalent to placebo and a very low incidence of hypoglycemia.[128] Saxagliptin is metabolized by CYP3A4 to 5-hydroxy saxagliptin that is half as potent as the parent drug. Therefore, patients should be monitored and/or doses need to be adjusted when CYP3A4 inhibitors (eg, ketoconazole, diltiazem) or inducers (eg, rifampicin) are coadministered.[124]

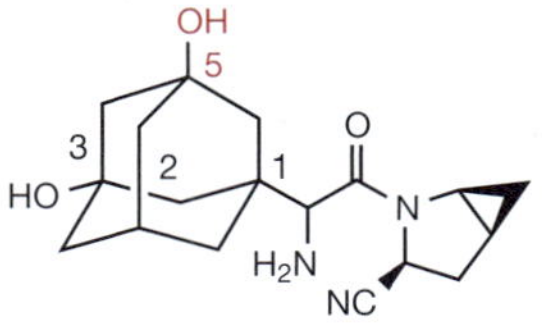

5-Hydroxysaxagliptin

Linagliptin. Linagliptin was approved by the FDA in 2011 as an oral treatment for type 2 diabetes, either as stand-alone medication or in combination with other therapies. Linagliptin should not be prescribed for patients with DKA. Its most common adverse effects are upper respiratory tract infections, stuffy nose, sore throat, muscle pain, and headache. Linagliptin has a high selectivity for DPP-IV over other isoforms of DPP, especially DPP-VIII and DPP-IX. Linagliptin inhibits DDP-IV activity by more than 80% over 24 hours. Linagliptin binds extensively to plasma proteins and is not significantly metabolized. Approximately 85% of the drug excreted unchanged via the feces.[129]

Alogliptin. Alogliptin contains the 2,4-pyrimidinedione pharmacophore with the essential basic amino group on the piperidine ring and the cyano group on the benzyl substituent. The piperidine amino interacts with the Glu205 and Glu206, whereas the pyrimidinedione interacts by π-stacking with Tyr547. The cyano moiety most likely binds to Ser630 in a manner similar to saxagliptin (Fig. 22.22). In addition, the cyanobenzyl group reportedly π-stacks with Tyr662.[126]

Alogliptin was approved by the FDA in 2013 as a standalone medication or in combination with metformin or pioglitazone. When used in combination with metformin, there can be an induction of lactic acidosis. When combined with pioglitazone, there is a warning that it may exacerbate congestive heart failure. A single oral dose is well absorbed with a T_{max} of 1 to 2 hours and a bioavailability of 63%. In clinical trials, it was well tolerated with no dose-limiting toxicity. Alogliptin is eliminated via the kidney, with 60% to 71% of the drug excreted unchanged. Metabolism is a minor elimination pathway, with two minor metabolites M-I and M-II (Fig. 22.23).[130]

The most common adverse reactions (>4%) of patients treated with alogliptin were nasopharyngitis (4.4%), headache (4.2%), and upper respiratory tract infection (4.2%). When in combination with metformin the most common adverse reactions (≥4%) were upper respiratory tract infection (8%), nasopharyngitis (6.8%), diarrhea (5.5%), hypertension (5.5%), headache (5.3%), back pain (4.3%), and urinary tract infection (4.2%). In combination with pioglitazone the most common adverse effects (>4) were nasopharyngitis (4.9%), back pain (4.2%), and upper respiratory tract infection (4.1%).[131]

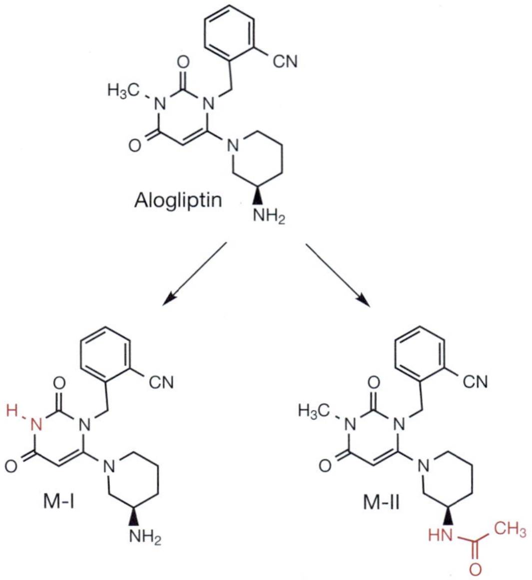

Figure 22.23 Structures of alogliptin and its metabolites M-I (N-demethylated) and M-II (N-acetylated).

Table 22.9 summarizes the pharmacokinetic parameters of the DPP-IV inhibitors, as well as the key metabolic indications. Bioavailability ranges from 30% to 90%, with only linagliptin having significant protein binding.

Amylin Agonists

Amylin is a hormone that consists of a single chain of 37 amino acids. It is released from pancreatic β cells, is co-secreted with insulin, and is primarily involved in controlling postprandial glucose levels. Amylin, like insulin, shows similar fasting and postprandial patterns in healthy individuals by a variety of mechanisms, including, delayed gastric emptying and suppression of glucagon secretion (not normalized by insulin alone), which leads to a suppression of endogenous glucose output from the liver.[132] Amylin also regulates food intake by modulating the appetite center of the brain. The observation that amylin was deficient in both type 1 and type 2 diabetes stimulated research and development of amylin analogues that would be able to control postprandial glucose levels by (1) modulation of gastric emptying, (2) prevention of postprandial rise in glucagon, and (3) inhibition of caloric intake and potential weight gain. Amylin itself is unsuitable as a drug because it aggregates and is insoluble in solution, which encouraged the development of chemical analogues.[133]

PRAMLINTIDE. Pramlintide is a chemical analogue of amylin designed for enhanced water solubility and reduced aggregation liability by replacement of Ala25, Ser28, and Ser29 of the amylin peptide chain with Pro residues.[134] The SQ administration of 15 mg of the drug shows an optimum peak effect within 20 minutes, thus permitting the drug to be used before meals. Pramlintide has a duration of action of 150 minutes, no significant accumulation liability with repetitive administration, and a renal clearance rate of 1 to 2 L/min. The drug is primarily metabolized in the kidneys, with an elimination half-life of 30 to 50 minutes, and should be used with caution in patients with compromised renal function. Pramlintide is

Table 22.9 Selected Pharmacokinetic Parameters of Dipeptidyl Peptidase-IV (DPP-IV) Inhibitors

Inhibitor	Bioavailability	Protein Binding	Metabolism
Sitagliptin (Januvia)	87%	38%	No significant metabolism. 79% excreted unchanged in urine; remainder in feces
Linagliptin (Tradjenta)	30%	70%-80%	No significant metabolism. 90% excreted unchanged; 80% in feces; remainder in urine
Saxagliptin (Onglyza)	67%	<10%	50% of absorbed dose metabolized by CYP3A4 yielding an active metabolite
Vildagliptin (Galvus)	90%	<10%	No significant metabolism. Elimination half-life of ~90 min
Alogliptin (Nesina)	63%	NS	Minimal metabolism (10%-20%) to inactive metabolites; 63% excreted unchanged in urine

used together with insulin for those who are unable to achieve their target postprandial blood sugars on insulin alone.[135,136] Pramlintide delays gastric emptying, suppresses glucagon release, and has a central nervous system anorectic effect via unknown mechanisms. The nucleus accumbens and dorsal vagal complex of the brain have been shown to contain the amylin receptor, which may be involved in the central effects of this hormone. Because of the wide differences between the pH of pramlintide and insulin products (4.0 vs 7.8, respectively), concurrent mixing within the same syringe is not recommended. To avoid severe hypoglycemia with initial drug titration, only short or rapid insulin dosage forms should be used together with pramlintide. In this case, the dose of insulin should be reduced by 50%.[137]

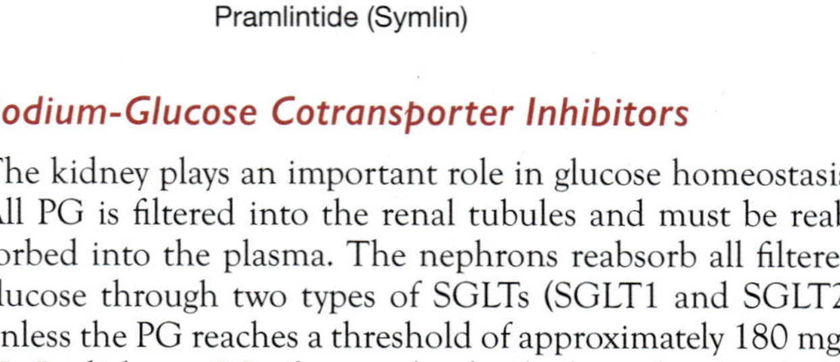

Pramlintide (Symlin)

Sodium-Glucose Cotransporter Inhibitors

The kidney plays an important role in glucose homeostasis. All PG is filtered into the renal tubules and must be reabsorbed into the plasma. The nephrons reabsorb all filtered glucose through two types of SGLTs (SGLT1 and SGLT2) unless the PG reaches a threshold of approximately 180 mg/dL. In diabetes, PG often reaches levels above that threshold, and the urine will then contain glucose. This is called glycosuria, and it is a classic sign of diabetes. In fact, increased excretion of glucose upregulates SGLTs, enhancing, in a negative way, the plasma levels of glucose by as much as 20%.[138]

There are several SGLT transporters; however, the major types are SGLT1 and SGLT2. SGLT2 is expressed in the epithelial cells of the brush border of S1 and S2 segments of the renal tubule. SGLT1 is expressed primarily in the small intestines. SGLT2 reabsorbs 80% to 90% of filtered glucose, whereas the remainder is reabsorbed by SGLT1 in the small intestines. It follows that inhibiting SGLT2 reabsorption of glucose can provide a reduction of hyperglycemia in diabetes. SGLT2 is a transmembrane protein consisting of 672 amino acids arranged in 14 transmembrane (TM) α-helices. TMs 4 to 7 and 10 to 13 form a hydrophilic cavity that is involved in glucose (and other substrate) binding and transport. Glucose and the natural inhibitor phlorizin (Fig. 22.24) bind to Thr156 and Lys157 in TM 4.[139,140]

The development of SGLT2 inhibitors was based on the discovery that phlorizin, an O-glycoside derivative isolated from the bark of the apple tree, increased the amount of glucose in the urine.[141] It was not a good drug candidate since it was quickly hydrolyzed by β-glucosidases in the GI tract. However, it served as a basis for the development of stable glycosides for the inhibition of SGLT2. Phlorizin's aglycone moiety is a 2,4,6-trihydroxyphenyl with a phenyl propanone moiety at position one and the glycoside as a substituent on the 6-hydroxy group. The challenge was to develop structures that were not easily hydrolyzed by β-glucosidases in the gut. This was accomplished by changing the O-glycoside linkage to a C-glycoside linkage, providing the gliflozin pharmacophore. The aglycone portion of this pharmacophore consists of an aryl moiety linked to a benzyl group (see Fig. 22.24). To date, there are four SGLT2 inhibitors approved for the treatment of type 2 diabetes: canagliflozin, dapagliflozin, empagliflozin, and ertugliflozin (see Fig. 22.24). Collectively, they are called the "gliflozins."[142]

CANAGLIFLOZIN. Canagliflozin was approved by the FDA in 2013. It has a 65% bioavailability with a T_{max} of 1 to 2 hours. It is highly bound to plasma proteins (99%). The $t_{1/2}$ is between 10.6 and 13 hours depending on the dose. Its elimination via the feces consists of 41.5% unchanged, 7% as a hydroxylated metabolite, and 3.2% as O-glucuronides (Fig. 22.25). Canagliflozin is also eliminated in the urine (30.5%) as O-glucuronide with <1% as unchanged drug.

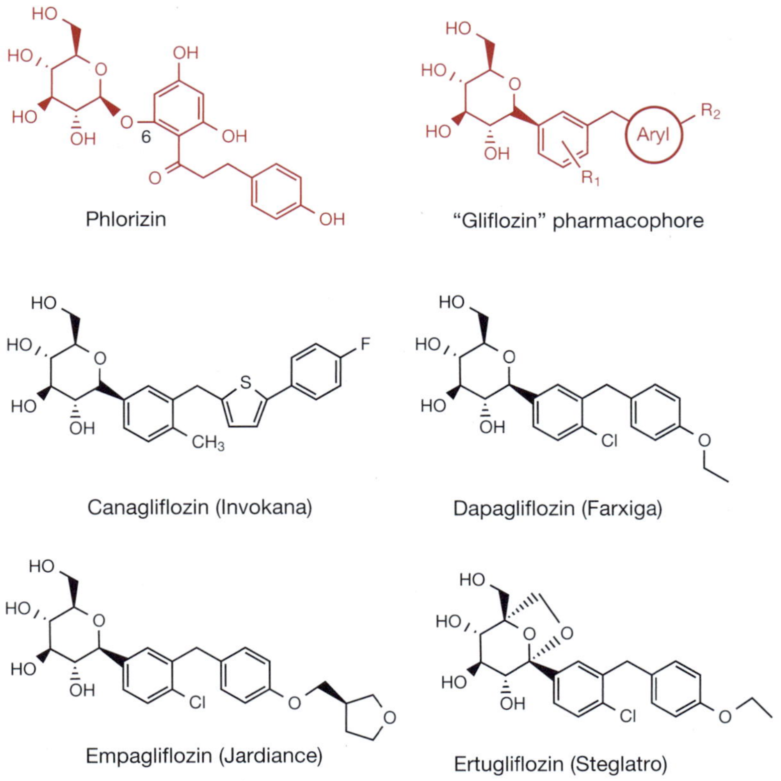

Figure 22.24 Structures of phlorizin, gliflozin pharmacophore, and currently marketed SGLT2 inhibitors.

It is metabolized by both UGT1A9 (uridine glucuronyltransferase) and UGT2B4. In addition, it is metabolized to a minor degree by CYP3A4.[143] It is available in tablet and extended release tablets for monotherapy, as well as in fixed combination with metformin hydrochloride.[144]

DAPAGLIFLOZIN. Dapagliflozin was approved by the FDA in 2014. It binds well to plasma proteins (91%) and has an 80% bioavailability with a T_{max} of 1 to 2 hours. Its mean plasma half-life is 12.9 hours with a 118 L volume of distribution. Dapagliflozin is extensively metabolized, with 73.7% recovered in excreta (72.0% in urine and 1.65% in feces). Metabolic routes included glucuronidation (UGT1A9), dealkylation, and oxidation at various positions to produce desmethyldapagliflozin glucuronides. The major metabolite is 3-O-glucuronide (60.7%), which is eliminated via the kidney. The 2-O-glucuronide was the only other urinary metabolite (Fig. 22.25). As with canagliflozin, dapagliflozin is available in fixed combination tablets with metformin hydrochloride. In 2017, the FDA approved a fixed combination of dapagliflozin with saxaglitin.[144,145]

EMPAGLIFLOZIN. Also in 2014, the FDA approved empagliflozin for the treatment of type 2 diabetes as either monotherapy or in combination with other oral hypoglycemic drugs. It has good selectivity for the SGLT2 receptor (>2,500-fold compared to SGLT1). Empagliflozin is 86% protein bound with 60% oral bioavailability. Its mean plasma half-life is 13.1 hours, with renal excretion as three major glucuronides (2-O-, 3-O-, and 6-O-glucuronide). Glucuronidation occurs via a number of UGTs, including UGT2B7, UGT1A3, UGT1A8, and UGT1A9 (Fig. 22.25). Administered radioactive empagliflozin was recovered in the feces (41% unchanged) and the urine (54%) with about half the radioactivity in the urine as unmetabolized drug.[146] Empagliflozin is also approved for use in fixed combination with metformin and linagliptin.[144]

ERTUGLIFLOZIN. The newest gliflozin to enter the market is ertugliflozin. The FDA approved it in late 2017 for use as monotherapy and as a fixed dose combination with both metformin and sitagliptin. Ertugliflozin is a new structural class of SGLT2 inhibitors incorporating a unique dioxabicyclo[3.2.1]octane ring system (see Fig. 22.24). It is highly selective for the SGLT2 receptor (>2,000-fold compared to SGLT1) and comparable to empagliflozin in its SGLT2 inhibiting action. It demonstrates good concentration-dependent glycosuria after oral administration. Plasma levels peak 1 hour after the administration of a single oral dose with an elimination half-life of 17 hours, making once daily dosing possible. It is 94% bound to plasma protein and, like the other gliflozins, is metabolized by glucuronidation of the hydroxyl groups on the sugar moiety. The two predominant glucuronides are 4-O-glucuronide and 3-O-glucuronide, generated by UGT1A9 (Fig. 22.25). The oxidative pathway through CYP isoforms plays a minor role, yielding monohydroxylated metabolites and a desethyl ertugliflozin.[142]

ROLE OF SGLT2 INHIBITORS IN THE TREATMENT OF TYPE 2 DIABETES. Clinical data have shown that SGLT2 inhibitors are effective as monotherapy. Metformin is the drug of choice for treating patients with diabetes who cannot reduce their A_{1C} under 7 with diet, weight loss, and exercise (Fig. 22.7).

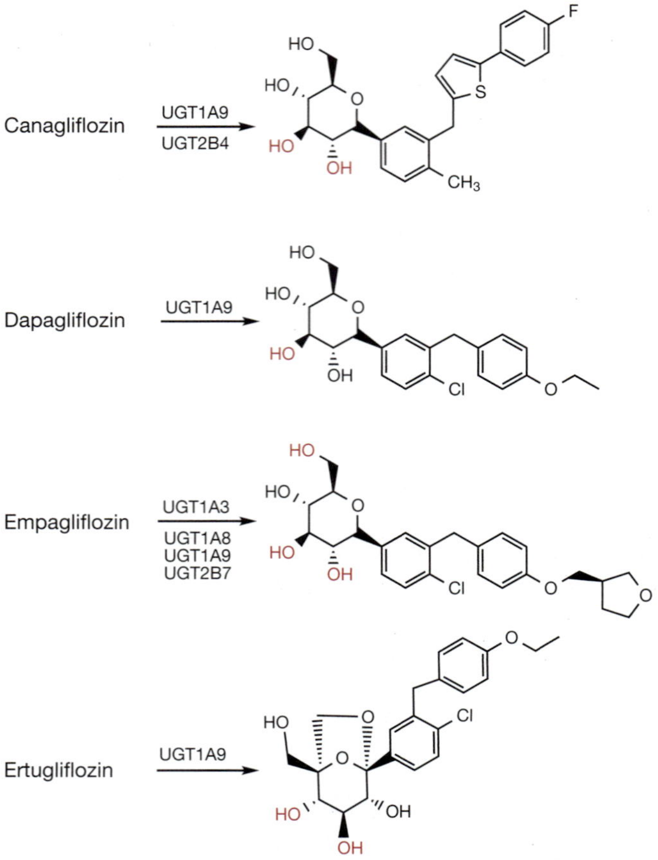

Figure 22.25 Metabolism of canagliflozin, dapagliflozin, empagliflozin, and ertugliflozin by uridine glucuronyltransferases (UGTs). Hydroxyl groups in red denote sites for glucuronidation.

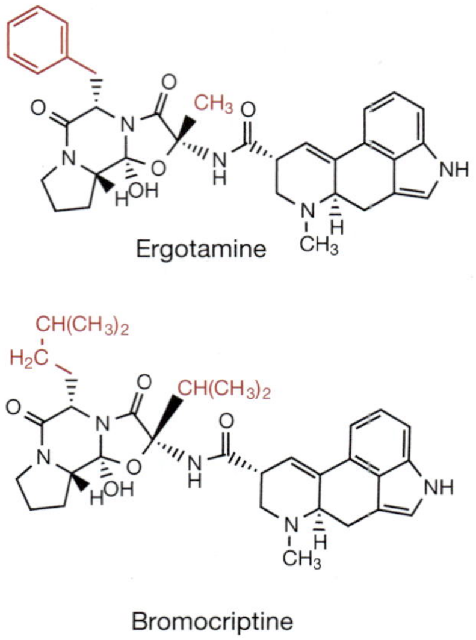

Figure 22.26 Comparison of the structure of bromocriptine to the ergot alkaloid ergotamine. Differences highlighted in red.

This relegates the monotherapy role of the SGLT2 inhibitors for patients who cannot tolerate metformin. SGLT2 inhibitors are also effective as an add-on to any of the other oral hypoglycemics and insulin. When administered once daily, they are well tolerated and do not have any relevant drug-drug interactions. They have a unique mechanism of action since they are insulin independent, which not only promotes reduction in PG but also contributes to weight loss, an improvement in blood pressure, and a low risk of hypoglycemia. This makes them a good choice as an add-on medication for treating patients with type 2 diabetes who have obesity and/or are hypertensive. Since the SGLT2 drugs are relatively new to the clinical arena, the data on long-term safety are lacking. Therefore, as their use increases, post-market surveillance will increase our knowledge in this area.[147] In May 2015, the FDA issued a warning about the risk of diabetic ketoacidosis associated with SGLT2 inhibitors. Although the exact mechanism for this side effect is not completely understood, the plausible mechanisms include reduced insulin levels, increased glucagon secretion, and reduced clearance of ketone bodies.[148]

Miscellaneous Drugs for the Treatment of Type 2 Diabetes

Bromocriptine. Bromocriptine is a dopamine D_2 receptor agonist. It is a structural analogue of ergotamine (Fig. 22.26), and it is primarily used to treat Parkinson disease (Chapter 10). It has a unique mechanism for the treatment of type 2 diabetes since it does not have a specific receptor that mediates its action on glucose and lipid metabolism. Bromocriptine's mechanism of action is believed to augment low hypothalamic dopamine levels and inhibit excessive sympathetic tone within the central nervous system. This reduction results in a decrease in postprandial PG levels due to enhanced suppression of hepatic glucose production (glycogenolysis).

Bromocriptine is administered as the mesylate salt. It is rapidly absorbed within 30 minutes, and its maximum plasma concentration is reached in 60 minutes. Food delays absorption, and there is extensive first-pass metabolism, with only 5% to 10% of the oral dose being bioavailable. It is highly protein bound with an elimination half-life of about 6 hours. It is metabolized in the liver to 20 to 30 metabolites, and 98% of the oral dose is excreted via the biliary route. Adverse effects are common, and dose related. Weakness, depression, and hypotension are frequently observed, along with nausea, vomiting, and diarrhea. Bromocriptine has major drug-drug interactions with 68 drugs, and most importantly, its effect is additive when used in conjunction with antihypertensive agents.[149]

Bile Acid Sequestrants. Colesevelam was found to improve PG control in data from clinical trials for lipid lowering in patients with type 2 diabetes with hypercholesterolemia. The exact mechanism on how colesevelam regulates PG levels is not clearly understood. It is postulated that colesevelam has effects on the farnesoid X receptor (FXR), which may ultimately reduce endogenous glucose production. The FXR is a nuclear receptor found in the liver and intestines. The bile acids are natural ligands for FXR. When activated, FXR translocates to the cell's nucleus, forms a dimer retinoid X receptor (RXR), and binds to hormone response elements on the DNA. This causes either increases or decreases in gene expression (Chapter 7). Colesevelam may also affect the secretion of incretin hormones GLP-1 and GIP, as levels were found to increase in patients administered 1.5 g/day.

Structure Challenge

Use your knowledge of drug pharmacophores presented in this chapter to match the correct drug with its descriptor.

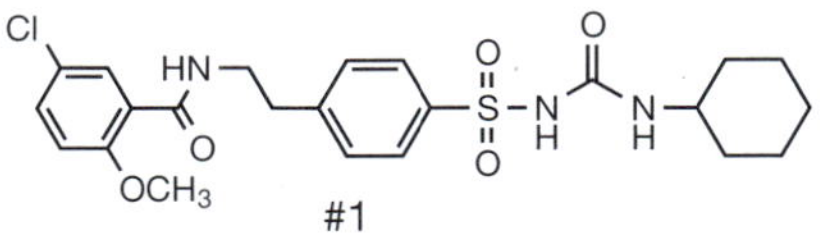
#1

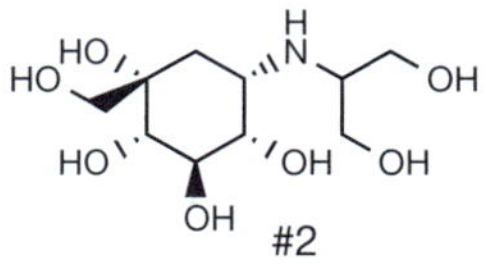
#2

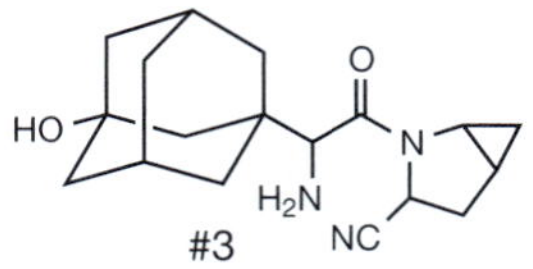
#3

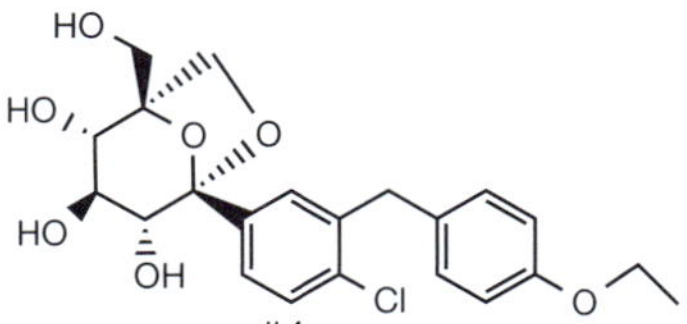
#4

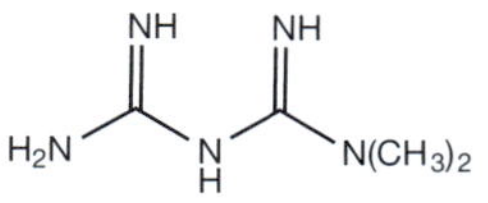
#5

A. Highly basic molecule that has the potential to cause a rare, but life-threatening lactic acidosis
B. Molecule that has structural similarity to glucose and inhibits glucose reabsorption in the kidneys
C. Drug that inhibits the enzyme that hydrolyzes glucagon-like peptide 1
D. Drug that may increase the risk of cardiovascular events
E. Drug that delays carbohydrate absorption from the gut

Structure Challenge answers found immediately after References.

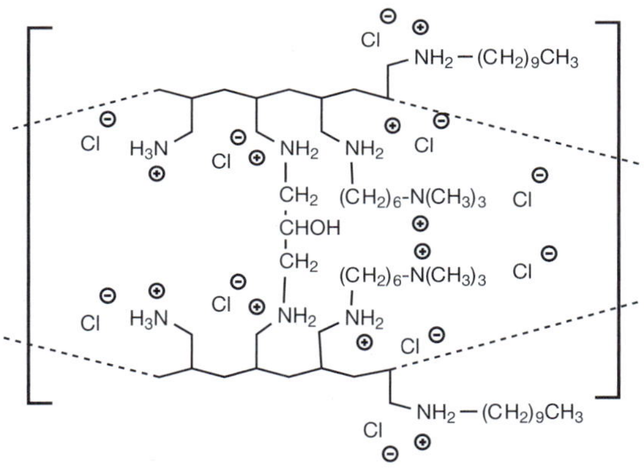
Colesevelam

In patients with type 2 diabetes, colesevelam consistently reduced A_{1C} by ~0.4% when coadministered to patients taking metformin, sulfonylureas, or insulin.[150]

REFERENCES

1. Loriaux DL. Diabetes and the Ebers Papyrus: 1552 B.C. *Endocrinologist.* 2006;16:55-56.
2. Karamanou M, Protogerou A, Tsoucalas G, et al. Milestones in the history of diabetes mellitus: the main contributors. *World J Diabetes.* 2016;7:1-7.
3. Carpenter S, Rigaud M, Barile M, et al. *Possibly* Having *to* Do *with* Diabetes Mellitus. Bard College; 2006:22.
4. Farmer L. Notes on the history of diabetes mellitus. *Bull N Y Acad Med.* 1952;28:408-416.
5. Karamitsos DT. The story of insulin discovery. *Diabetes Res Clin Pract.* 2011;93:S2-S8.
6. Sanger F, Tuppy H. The amino-acid sequence in the phenylalanyl chain of insulin. 1. The identification of lower peptides from partial hydrolysates. *Biochem J.* 1951;49:463-481.
7. Sanger F, Tuppy H. The amino-acid sequence in the phenylalanyl chain of insulin. 2. The investigation of peptides from enzymic hydrolysates. *Biochem J.* 1951;49:481-490.
8. Katsoyannis PG, Tometsko A, Fukuda K. Insulin peptides. IX. The synthesis of the A-chain of insulin and its combination with natural B-chain to generate insulin activity. *J Am Chem Soc.* 1963;85:2863-2865.
9. Sola D, Rossi L, Schianca GP, et al. Sulfonylureas and their use in clinical practice. *Arch Med Sci.* 2015;11:840-848.
10. International Diabetes Federation. *IDF Diabetes Atlas.* 10th ed. International Diabetes Federation; 2021. Accessed July 30, 2023. https://www.diabetesatlas.org
11. Trujillo J, Haines S. Chapter 91 Diabetes mellitus. In: DiPiro JT, Yee GC, Posey LM, Haines ST, Nolin TD, Ellingrod V, eds. *Pharmacotherapy: A Pathophysiologic Approach.* Eleventh edition. McGraw-Hill Education; 2019.
12. Menke A, Orchard TJ, Imperatore G, et al. The prevalence of type 1 diabetes in the United States. *Epidemiology.* 2013;24:773-774.
13. American Heart Association. What is metabolic syndrome? Accessed September 29, 2023. https://cpr.heart.org/-/media/Files/Health-Topics/Answers-by-Heart/What-Is-Metabolic-Syndrome.pdf?rev=95ba140bf7894698a5a90820f38be327
14. Huang PL. A comprehensive definition for metabolic syndrome. *Dis Model Mech.* 2009;2:231-237.
15. Swarup S, Ahmed I, Grigorova Y, et al. Metabolic Syndrome. In: StatPearls [Internet]. Treasure Island (FL): StatPearls Publishing; 2025. Updated March 7, 2024. Available from: https://www.ncbi.nlm.nih.gov/books/NBK459248/
16. Morigny M, Houssier M, Mouisel E, et al. Adipocyte lipolysis and insulin resistance. *Biochimie.* 2016;125:259-266.
17. Walker R, William JS, Egede LE. Influence of race, ethnicity and social determinants of health on diabetes outcomes. *Am J Med Sci.* 2016;351:366-373.
18. Centers for Disease Control and Prevention. National Diabetes Statistics Report. 2020. Accessed July 30, 2023. https://www.cdc.gov/diabetes/pdfs/data/statistics/national-diabetes-statistics-report.pdf

19. WHO. Diabetes. Accessed July 31, 2023. https://www.who.int/health-topics/diabetes#tab=tab_3
20. American Diabetes Association. Classification and diagnosis of diabetes. *Diabetes Care.* 2017;40:S11-S24.
21. Marin-Penalver JJ, Martin-Timon I, Sevillano-Collantes C. Update on the treatment of type 2 diabetes mellitus. *World J Diabetes.* 2016;7:354-395.
22. Helms R, Quan DJ, Herfindal ET, et al. *Textbook of Therapeutics. Drug and Disease Management.* 8th ed. Lippincott Williams & Wilkins; 2006.
23. Yamazaki Y, Harada S, Tokuyama S. Sodium–glucose transporter as a novel therapeutic target in disease. *Eur J Pharmacol.* 2018;822:25-31.
24. Mueckler M, Thorens B. The SLC2 (GLUT) family of membrane transporters. *Mol Aspects Med.* 2013;34:121-138.
25. Kido Y, Nakae J, Accili D. Clinical review 125: the insulin receptor and its cellular targets. *J Clin Endocrinol Metab.* 2001;86:972-979.
26. Haeusler RA, McGraw TE, Accili D. Biochemical and cellular properties of insulin receptor signalling. *Nat Rev Mol Cell Biol.* 2018;19:31-44.
27. Atkinson MA, Eisenbart GS. Type 1 diabetes: new perspectives on disease pathogenesis and treatment. *Lancet.* 2001;358:221-229.
28. Paschou SA, Papadopoulou-Marketou N, Chrousos GP, et al. On type 1 diabetes mellitus pathogenesis. *Endocr Connect.* 2017;7:R38-R46.
29. Moneva MH, Dagogo-Jack S. Multiple drug targets in the management of type 2 diabetes. *Curr Drug Targets.* 2002;3:203-221.
30. Triplitt C, Wright A, Chiquette E. Incretin mimetics and dipeptidyl peptidase-IV inhibitors: potential new therapies for type 2 diabetes mellitus. *Pharmacotherapy.* 2012;26:360-374.
31. Diabetes In Control. 390-Drugs That Can Affect Blood Sugars [Internet]. Available from: https://www.diabetesincontrol.com/wp-content/uploads/2018/03/390-Drugs-That-Can-Affect-Blood-Sugars-F-FF.pdf
32. Nathan DM; DCCT/EDIC Research Group. The diabetes control and complications trial/epidemiology of diabetes interventions and complications study at 30 years: overview. *Diabetes Care.* 2014;37:9-16.
33. American Diabetes Association. Cardiovascular disease and risk management. *Diabetes Care.* 2017;40:S75-S87.
34. American Diabetes Association. Microvascular complications. *Diabetes Care.* 2017;40:S88-S98.
35. Brownlee M. The pathological implications of protein glycation. *Clin Invest Med.* 1995;18:275-281.
36. Brownlee M. Biochemistry and molecular cell biology of diabetic complications. *Nature.* 2001;414:813-820.
37. Lee AY, Chung SS. Contributions of polyol pathway to oxidative stress in diabetic cataract. *FASEB J.* 1999;13:23-30.
38. Degenhardt TP, Thorpe SR, Baynes JW. Chemical modification of proteins by methylglyoxal. *Cell Mol Biol (Noisy-le-grand).* 1998;44:1139-1145.
39. Xia P, Inoguchi T, Kern TS, et al. Characterization of the mechanism for the chronic activation of diacylglycerol-protein kinase C pathway in diabetes and hypergalactosemia. *Diabetes.* 1994;43:1122-1129.
40. Brownlee M. The pathobiology of diabetic complications: a unifying mechanism. *Diabetes.* 2005;54:1615-1625.
41. Bergenstal RM, Bailey CJ, Kendall DM. Type 2 diabetes: assessing the relative risks and benefits of glucose-lowering medications. *Am J Med.* 2010;123:374.e9-374.e18.
42. Qaseem A, Barry MJ, Humphrey LL, et al. Oral pharmacologic treatment of type 2 diabetes mellitus: a clinical practice guideline update from the American College of Physicians. *Ann Intern Med.* 2017;166: 279-290.
43. American Diabetes Association. 6. Glycemic targets: standards of medical care in diabetes—2018. *Diabetes Care.* 2018;41:S55-S64.
44. American Diabetes Association. 4. Lifestyle management: standards of medical care in diabetes—2018. *Diabetes Care.* 2018;41:S38-S50.
45. Fox CS, Golden SH, Anderson C, et al. Update on prevention of cardiovascular disease in adults with type 2 diabetes mellitus in light of recent evidence: a scientific statement from the American Heart Association and the American Diabetes Association. *Diabetes Care.* 2015;38:1777-1803.
46. Pontiroli AE, Folli F, Paganelli M, et al. Laparoscopic gastric banding prevents type 2 diabetes and arterial hypertension and induces their remission in morbid obesity: a 4-year case-controlled study. *Diabetes Care.* 2005;28:2703-2709.
47. American Diabetes Association. Pharmacologic approaches to glycemic treatment. *Diabetes Care.* 2017;40:S64-S74.
48. Samson SL, Vellanki P, Blonde L et al. American Association of Clinical Endocrinology consensus statement: comprehensive type 2 diabetes management algorithm—2023 update. *Endocr Pract.* 2023;29(5):305-340.
49. Kahn CR, Roth J. Berson, Yalow, and the JCI: the agony and the ecstasy. *J Clin Invest.* 2004;114:1051-1054.
50. Bliss M. The Discovery of Insulin. University of Chicago Press; 1984:304.
51. Weiss M, Steiner DF, Philipson LH. Insulin biosynthesis, secretion, structure, and structure-activity relationships. In: De Groot LJ, Chrousos G, Dungan K, et al, eds. *Endotext.* MDText.com, Inc.; 2000. Accessed May 15, 2023. http://www.ncbi.nlm.nih.gov/books/NBK279029/
52. Fu Z, Gilbert ER, Liu D. Regulation of insulin synthesis and secretion and pancreatic beta-cell dysfunction in diabetes. *Curr Diabetes Rev.* 2013;9(1):25-53.
53. Aguilar-Bryan L, Clement JP, Gonzalez G, et al. Toward understanding the assembly and structure of KATP channels. *Physiol Rev.* 1998;78:227-245.
54. Shyng S-L. K_{ATP} channel function: more than meets the eye. *Function (Oxf).* 2022;3(1):zqab070.
55. Ishihara H, Maechler P, Gjinovci A, et al. Islet beta-cell secretion determines glucagon release from neighbouring alpha-cells. *Nat Cell Biol.* 2003;5(4):330-335.
56. Menting J, Whittaker J, Margetts M, et al. How insulin engages its primary binding site on the insulin receptor. *Nature*;493:241-245.
57. Alyas J, Rafiq A, Amir H, et al. Human insulin: history, recent advances, and expression systems for mass production. *Biomed Res Ther.* 2021; 8(9);4540-4561.
58. Lawrence MC. Understanding insulin and its receptor from their three-dimensional structures. *Mol Metab.* 2021;52:101255.
59. Ish-Shalom D, Christoffersen CT, Vorwerk P, et al. Mitogenic properties of insulin and insulin analogues mediated by the insulin receptor. *Diabetologia.* 1997;40:S25-S31.
60. Peyrot M, Bailey TS, Childs BP, et al. Strategies for implementing effective mealtime insulin therapy in type 2 diabetes. *Curr Med Res Opin.* 2018;34(6):1153-1162.
61. Hirsch IB. Insulin analogues. *N Engl J Med.* 2005;352:174-183. Accessed April 6, 2018. http://www.nejm.org/doi/pdf/10.1056/NEJMra040832
62. Jonassen I, Havelund S, Hoeg-Jensen T, et al. Design of the novel protraction mechanism of insulin degludec, an ultra-long-acting basal insulin. *Pharm Res.* 2012;29:2104-2114.
63. Zinman B, Fulcher G, Rao PV, et al. Insulin degludec, an ultra-long-acting basal insulin, once a day or three times a week versus insulin glargine once a day in patients with type 2 diabetes: a 16-week, randomised, open-label, phase 2 trial. *Lancet.* 2011;377:924-931.
64. Bloomgarden ZT. Premixed insulins: a practical guide to their use in type 2 diabetes. *Diabetes Educ.* 2010;36(1):7-14.
65. Loubatières-Mariani M-M. The discovery of hypoglycemic sulfonamides. *J Soc Biol.* 2007;201:121-125.
66. Meglasson MD, Matschinsky FM. Pancreatic islet glucose metabolism and regulation of insulin secretion. *Diabetes Metab Rev.* 1986;2:163-214.

67. Martin GM, Kandasamy B, DiMaio F, et al. Anti-diabetic drug binding site in K channels revealed by Cryo-EM. *eLife.* 2017;6:e31054. doi:10.7554/eLife.31054
68. Thisted H, Johnsen SP, Rungby J. Sulfonylureas and the risk of myocardial infarction. *Metab Clin Exp. 2006*;55:S16-S19.
69. Downey JM. An explanation for the reported observation that ATP dependent potassium channel openers mimic preconditioning. *Cardiovasc Res.* 1993;27:1565.
70. Yang F, Xiong X, Liu Y, et al. CYP2C9 and OATP1B1 genetic polymorphisms affect the metabolism and transport of glimepiride and gliclazide. *Sci Rep. 2018*;8:10994.
71. Malaisse WJ. Stimulation of insulin release by non-sulfonylurea hypoglycemic agents: the meglitinide family. *Horm Metab Res.* 1995;27:263-266.
72. Malaisse WJ. Pharmacology of the meglitinide analogs: new treatment options for type 2 diabetes mellitus. *Treat Endocrinol.* 2003;2:401-414.
73. Proks P, Reimann F, Green N, et al. Sulfonylurea stimulation of insulin secretion. *Diabetes.* 2002;51:S368-S376.
74. Culy CR, Jarvis B. Repaglinide: a review of its therapeutic use in type 2 diabetes mellitus. *Drugs.* 2001;61:1625-1660.
75. Chachin M, Yamada M, Fujita A, et al. Nateglinide, a D-phenylalanine derivative lacking either a sulfonylurea or benzamido moiety, specifically inhibits pancreatic beta-cell-type K(ATP) channels. *J Pharmacol Exp Ther.* 2003;304:1025-1032.
76. Weaver ML, Orwig BA, Rodriguez LC, et al. Pharmacokinetics and metabolism of nateglinide in humans. *Drug Metab Dispos.* 2001;29:415-421.
77. Lins L, Brasseur R, Malaisse WJ. Conformational analysis of non-sulfonylurea hypoglycemic agents of the meglitinide family. *Biochem Pharmacol.* 1995;50:1879-1884.
78. Witters LA. The blooming of the French lilac. *J Clin Invest.* 2001;108:1105-1107.
79. Adak T, Samadi A, Unal AU, et al. A reappraisal on metformin. *Regul Toxicol Pharmacol.* 2018;92:324-332.
80. Augusti KT, Sunil NP, Abraham A, et al. A comparative study on the effects of diet and exercise, metformin and metformin+pioglitazone treatment on NIDDM patients. *Indian J Clin Biochem.* 2007;22:65-69.
81. Bailey CJ. Biguanides and NIDDM. *Diabetes Care.* 1992;15:755-772.
82. Bolen S, Feldman L, Vassy J, et al. Systematic review: comparative effectiveness and safety of oral medications for type 2 diabetes mellitus. *Ann Intern Med.* 2007;147:386-399.
83. Pakkir Maideen NM, Jumale A, Balasubramaniam R. Drug interactions of metformin involving drug transporter proteins. *Adv Pharm Bull.* 2017;7:501-505.
84. Gong L, Goswami S, Giacomini KM, et al. Metformin pathways: pharmacokinetics and pharmacodynamics. *Pharmacogenet Genomics.* 2012;22:820-827.
85. Weisberg LS. Lactic acidosis in a patient with type 2 diabetes mellitus. *Clin J Am Soc Nephrol.* 2015;10:1476-1483.
86. Monsalve FA, Pyarasani RD, Delgado-Lopez F, et al. Peroxisome proliferator-activated receptor targets for the treatment of metabolic diseases. *Mediators Inflamm.* 2013;2013:549627.
87. Schwartz S, Raskin P, Fonseca V, et al. Effect of troglitazone in insulin-treated patients with type II diabetes mellitus. Troglitazone and exogenous insulin study group. *N Engl J Med.* 1998;338:861-866.
88. Suter SL, Nolan JJ, Wallace P, et al. Metabolic effects of new oral hypoglycemic agent CS-045 in NIDDM subjects. *Diabetes Care.* 1992;15:193-203.
89. Parker JC. Troglitazone: the discovery and development of a novel therapy for the treatment of type 2 diabetes mellitus. *Adv Drug Deliv Rev.* 2002;54:1173-1197.
90. Yokoi T. Troglitazone. *Handb Exp Pharmacol.* 2010;196:419-435.
91. Wallach JD, Wang K, Zhang AD, et al. Updating insights into rosiglitazone and cardiovascular risk through shared data: individual patient and summary level meta-analyses. *BMJ.* 2020;368:l7078.
92. Hanefeld M. Pharmacokinetics and clinical efficacy of pioglitazone. *Int J Clin Pract Suppl.* 2001;121:19-25.
93. Jaakkola T, Laitila J, Neuvonen PJ, et al. Pioglitazone is metabolised by CYP2C8 and CYP3A4 in vitro: potential for interactions with CYP2C8 inhibitors. *Basic Clin Pharmacol Toxicol.* 2006;99:44-51.
94. Agrawal R. The first approved agent in the Glitazar's class: saroglitazar. *Curr Drug Targets.* 2014;15:151-155.
95. Cheng AY, Josse RG. Intestinal absorption inhibitors for type 2 diabetes mellitus: prevention and treatment. *Drug Discov Today Ther Strateg.* 2004;1:201-206.
96. Bell DSH. Type 2 diabetes mellitus: what is the optimal treatment regimen? *Am J Med.* 2004;116:23S-29S.
97. Inzucchi SE. Oral antihyperglycemic therapy for type 2 diabetes: scientific review. *JAMA.* 2002;287:360-372.
98. Emilien G, Maloteaux JM, Ponchon M. Pharmacological management of diabetes: recent progress and future perspective in daily drug treatment. *Pharmacol Ther.* 1999;81:37-51.
99. Borges de Melo E, Gomes AS, Carvalho I. α- and β-glucosidase inhibitors: chemical structure and biological activity. *Tetrahedron.* 2006;62:10277-10302.
100. Platt FM, Butters TD. Substrate deprivation: a new therapeutic approach for the glycosphingolipid lysosomal storage diseases. *Expert Rev Mol Med.* 2000;2:1-17.
101. Holst JJ, Orskov C, Nielsen OV, et al. Truncated glucagon-like peptide I, an insulin-releasing hormone from the distal gut. *FEBS Lett.* 1987;211:169-174.
102. Perley MJ, Kipnis DM. Plasma insulin responses to oral and intravenous glucose: studies in normal and diabetic subjects. *J Clin Invest.* 1967;46:1954-1962.
103. Dupre J, Ross SA, Watson D, et al. Stimulation of insulin secretion by gastric inhibitory polypeptide in man. *J Clin Endocrinol Metab.* 1973;37:826-828.
104. Reimann F, Gribble FM. Glucose-sensing in glucagon-like peptide-1-secreting cells. *Diabetes.* 2002;51:2757-2763.
105. Deacon CF, Johnsen AH, Holst JJ. Degradation of glucagon-like peptide-1 by human plasma in vitro yields an N-terminally truncated peptide that is a major endogenous metabolite in vivo. *J Clin Endocrinol Metab.* 1995;80:952-957.
106. Mentlein R, Gallwitz B, Schmidt WE. Dipeptidyl-peptidase IV hydrolyses gastric inhibitory polypeptide, glucagon-like peptide-1(7-36) amide, peptide histidine methionine and is responsible for their degradation in human serum. *Eur J Biochem.* 1993;214:829-835.
107. Christensen M, Vedtofte L, Holst JJ, et al. Glucose-dependent insulinotropic polypeptide: a bifunctional glucose-dependent regulator of glucagon and insulin secretion in humans. *Diabetes.* 2011; 60:3103
108. Deacon CF, Knudsen LB, Madsen K, et al. Dipeptidyl peptidase IV resistant analogues of glucagon-like peptide-1 which have extended metabolic stability and improved biological activity. *Diabetologia.* 1998;41:271-278.
109. Buse JB, Henry RR, Han J, et al. Effects of exenatide (exendin-4) on glycemic control over 30 weeks in sulfonylurea-treated patients with type 2 diabetes. *Diabetes Care.* 2004;27:2628-2635.
110. Wang Q, Brubaker PL. Glucagon-like peptide-1 treatment delays the onset of diabetes in 8 week-old db/db mice. *Diabetologia.* 2002;45:1263-1273.
111. Elbrønd B, Jakobsen G, Larsen S, et al. Pharmacokinetics, pharmacodynamics, safety, and tolerability of a single-dose of NN2211, a long-acting glucagon-like peptide 1 derivative, in healthy male subjects. *Diabetes Care.* 2002;25:1398-1404.
112. Knudsen LB. Glucagon-like peptide-1: the basis of a new class of treatment for type 2 diabetes. *J Med Chem.* 2004;47:4128-4134.
113. Sturis J, Gotfredsen CF, Rømer J, et al. GLP-1 derivative liraglutide in rats with beta-cell deficiencies: influence of metabolic state on beta-cell mass dynamics. *Br J Pharmacol.* 2003;140:123-132.
114. Novo Nordisk Canada Inc. Product monograph including patient medication information: Victoza. Accessed April 6, 2018. http://www.novonordisk.ca/content/dam/Canada/AFFILIATE/www-novonordisk-ca/OurProducts/PDF/victoza-product-monograph.pdf

115. Lovshin JA. Glucagon-like peptide-1 receptor agonists: a class update for treating type 2 diabetes. *Can J Diabetes.* 2017;41:524-535.
116. Glaesner W, Vick AM, Millican R, et al. Engineering and characterization of the long-acting glucagon-like peptide-1 analogue LY2189265, an Fc fusion protein. *Diabetes Metab Res Rev.* 2010;26:287-296.
117. Pratley RE, Nauck MA, Barnett AH, et al. Once-weekly albiglutide versus once-daily liraglutide in patients with type 2 diabetes inadequately controlled on oral drugs (HARMONY 7): a randomised, open-label, multicentre, non-inferiority phase 3 study. *Lancet Diabetes Endocrinol.* 2014;2:289-297.
118. Jensen L, Helleberg H, Roffel A, et al. Absorption, metabolism and excretion of the GLP-1 analogue semaglutide in humans and nonclinical species. *Eur J Pharm Sci.* 2017;104:31-41.
119. Wang L. Designing a dual GLP-1R/GIPR agonist from tirzepatide: comparing residues between tirzepatide, GLP-1, and GIP. *Drug Des Devel Ther.* 2022;16:1547-1559.
120. Coskun T, Sloop KW, Loghin C, et al. LY3298176, a novel dual GIP and GLP-1 receptor agonist for the treatment of type 2 diabetes mellitus: from discovery to clinical proof of concept. *Mol Metab.* 2018;18:3-14.
121. Sun B, Willard FS, Feng D, et al. Structural determinants of dual incretin receptor agonism by tirzepatide. *Proc Natl Acad Sci U S A.* 2022;119(13):e2116506119.
122. Østergaard S, Paulsson JF, Kofoed J, et al. The effect of fatty diacid acylation of human PYY3-36 on Y2 receptor potency and half-life in minipigs. *Sci Rep. 2021*;11(1):21179.
123. Lilly. Lilly receives U.S. FDA Fast Track designation for tirzepatide for the treatment of adults with obesity, or overweight with weight-related comorbidities. Accessed September 29, 2023. https://investor.lilly.com/news-releases/news-release-details/lilly-receives-us-fda-fast-track-designation-tirzepatide
124. Kasina SVS, Baradhi KM. *Dipeptidyl Peptidase IV (DPP IV) Inhibitors.* StatPearls; 2023.
125. Rosenblum JS, Kozarich JW. Prolyl peptidases: a serine protease subfamily with high potential for drug discovery. *Curr Opin Chem Biol.* 2003;7:496-504.
126. Arulmozhiraja S, Matsuo N, Ishitsubo E, et al. Comparative binding analysis of dipeptidyl peptidase IV (DPP-4) with antidiabetic drugs—an Ab initio fragment molecular orbital study. *PLoS One.* 2016;11:e0166275.
127. Metzler WJ, Yanchunas J, Weigelt C, et al. Involvement of DPP-IV catalytic residues in enzyme–saxagliptin complex formation. *Protein Sci.* 2008;17:240-250.
128. Tahrani AA, Piya MK, Kennedy A, et al. Glycaemic control in type 2 diabetes: targets and new therapies. *Pharmacol Ther.* 2010;125:328-361.
129. Blech S, Ludwig-Schwellinger E, Gräfe-Mody EU, et al. The metabolism and disposition of the oral dipeptidyl peptidase-4 inhibitor, linagliptin, in humans. *Drug Metab Dispos.* 2010;38:667-678.
130. Christopher R, Covington P, Davenport, et al. Pharmacokinetics, pharmacodynamics, and tolerability of single increasing doses of the dipeptidyl peptidase-4 inhibitor alogliptin in healthy male subjects. *Clin Ther.* 2008;30:513-527.
131. Takeda. FDA Advisory Committee reviews Takeda's alogliptin EXAMINE cardiovascular safety outcomes trial. Accessed April 7, 2018. https://www.takeda.com/newsroom/newsreleases/2015/fda-advisory-committee-reviews-takedas-alogliptin-examine-cardiovascular-safety-outcomes-trial/
132. Ryan GJ, Jobe LJ, Martin R. Pramlintide in the treatment of type 1 and type 2 diabetes mellitus. *Clin Ther.* 2005;27:1500-1512.
133. Kruger DF, Gloster MA. Pramlintide for the treatment of insulin-requiring diabetes mellitus: rationale and review of clinical data. *Drugs.* 2004;64:1419-1432.
134. Heptulla RA, Rodriguez LM, Bomgaars L, et al. The role of amylin and glucagon in the dampening of glycemic excursions in children with type 1 diabetes. *Diabetes.* 2005;54:1100-1107.
135. Owen SK. Amylin replacement therapy in patients with insulin-requiring type 2 diabetes. *Diabetes Educ.* 2006;32:105S-110S.
136. Pullman J, Darsow T, Frias JP. Pramlintide in the management of insulin-using patients with type 2 and type 1 diabetes. *Vasc Health Risk Manag.* 2006;2:203-212.
137. Singh-Franco D, Robles G, Gazze D. Pramlintide acetate injection for the treatment of type 1 and type 2 diabetes mellitus. *Clin Ther.* 2007;29:535-562.
138. DeFronzo RA, Davidson JA, Del Prato S. The role of the kidneys in glucose homeostasis: a new path towards normalizing glycaemia. *Diabetes Obes Metab.* 2012;14:5-14.
139. Turk E, Wright EM. Membrane topology motifs in the SGLT cotransporter family. *J Membr Biol.* 1997;159:1-20.
140. Reja M, Kinne RK. Identification of phlorizin binding domains in sodium-glucose cotransporter family: SGLT1 as a unique model system. *Biochimie.* 2015;115:187-193.
141. Ehrenkranz JR, Lewis NG, Kahn CR, et al. Phlorizin: a review. *Diabetes Metab Res Rev.* 2005;21:31-38.
142. Cinti F, Moffa S, Impronta F, et al. Spotlight on ertugliflozin and its potential in the treatment of type 2 diabetes: evidence to date. *Drug Des Devel Ther.* 2017;11:2905-2919.
143. Kalra S. Sodium glucose co-transporter-2 (SGLT2) inhibitors: a review of their basic and clinical pharmacology. *Diabetes Ther.* 2014;5:355-366.
144. U.S. Food & Drug Administration. Orange Book: approved drug products with therapeutic equivalence evaluations. Accessed April 10, 2018. https://www.accessdata.fda.gov/scripts/cder/ob/search_product.cfm
145. Kasichayanula S, Liu X, LaCreta F, et al. Clinical pharmacokinetics and pharmacodynamics of dapagliflozin, a selective inhibitor of sodium-glucose co-transporter type 2. *Clin Pharmacokinet.* 2014;53:17-27.
146. Mondick J, Riggs M, Kaspers S, et al. Population pharmacokinetic-pharmacodynamic analysis to characterize the effect of empagliflozin on renal glucose threshold in patients with type 1 diabetes mellitus. *J Clin Pharmacol.* 2018;58:640-649.
147. Solini A. Role of SGLT2 inhibitors in the treatment of type 2 diabetes mellitus. *Acta Diabetol.* 2016;53:863-870.
148. Zurek AM, Yendapally R, Urteaga EM. A review of the efficacy and safety of sodium-glucose cotransporter 2 inhibitors: a focus on diabetic ketoacidosis. *Diabetes Spectr.* 2017;30:137-142.
149. DeFronzo RA. Bromocriptine: a sympatholytic, D2-dopamine agonist for the treatment of type 2 diabetes. *Diabetes Care.* 2011;34:789-794.
150. Handelsman Y. Role of bile acid sequestrants in the treatment of type 2 diabetes. *Diabetes Care.* 2011;34:S244-S250.

Structure Challenge Answers

A-5; B-4; C-3; D-1; E-2.

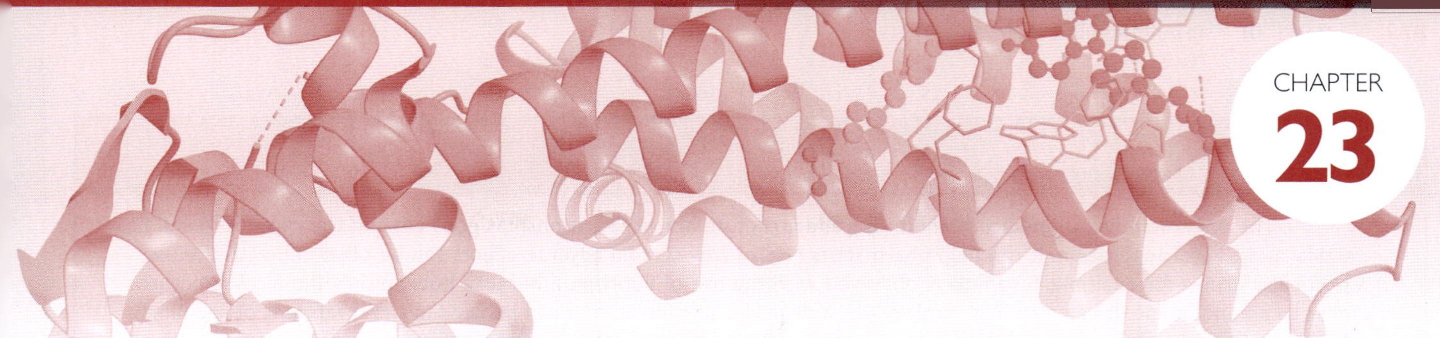

CHAPTER 23

Drugs Used to Treat Obesity

Stacy D. Brown and Thomas L. Lemke

Drugs covered in this chapter:

DRUGS

- Amphetamine
- Benzphetamine
- Diethylpropion
- Icosapent ethyl
- Liraglutide
- Lisdexamfetamine
- Metreleptin
- Naltrexone/bupropion
- Orforglipron
- Orlistat
- Phendimetrazine
- Phenmetrazine
- Phentermine
- Retatrutide
- Semaglutide
- Setmelanotide
- Tirzepatide
- Topiramate
- Triheptanoin

NONNUTRITIVE SWEETENERS AND OTHER FOOD SUBSTITUTES

- Acesulfame-K
- Advantame
- Allulose
- Aspartame
- Brazzein
- Mogrosides
- Neotame
- Rebaudioside A
- Saccharin
- Sucralose
- Thaumatin
- Xylitol

Abbreviations

ACTH adrenocorticotropic hormone
ADO 8-amino-3,6-dioxaoctanoic acid
Aib 1-aminoisobutyric acid
α-MSH α-melanocyte-stimulating hormone
AOM anti-obesity medication
ATP adenosine triphosphate
BMI body mass index
cAMP cyclic adenosine monophosphate
CGL congenital generalized lipodystrophy
CNS central nervous system
CYP450 cytochrome P450
DNA deoxyribo nucleic acid
DP dopamine
DPP-IV dipeptidyl peptidase-IV
DTEase D-tagatose-3-epimerase
EPA eicosapentaenoic acid
FcRn neonatal Fc receptor
FDA U.S. Food and Drug Administration
GABA γ-aminobutyric acid
γGlu γ-glutamate
GI gastrointestinal
GIP gastric inhibitory polypeptide
GIPR gastric inhibitory polypeptide receptor
GLP-1 glucagon-like peptide-1
GLP-1R glucagon-like peptide-1 receptor
GPCR G protein–coupled receptor
GRAS Generally Recognized As Safe
HbA_{1c} Hemoglobin A1C
HSA human serum albumin
IPE icosapent ethyl
LC-FAOD long chain fatty acid oxidation disorders
LEPR leptin receptor
MC4R melanocortin receptor 4
MC4 melanocortin-4
α-MSH α-melanocyte stimulating hormone
NNSs nonnutritive sweeteners
PCSK1 proprotein convertase subtilisin/kexin type 1
PKU phenylketonuria
POMC proopiomelanocortin
RDI recommended daily intake
REDUCE-IT Reduction of Cardiovascular Events With Icosapent Ethyl (IPE)-Intervention
SAR structure-activity relationship
SC subcutaneous
SNAC *N*-[8-(2-hydroxybenzoyl) amino] caprylate
T2D type 2 diabetes
WC waist circumference
WHO World Health Organization
WHR waist-to-hip ratio

CLINICAL SIGNIFICANCE

The understanding of medicinal chemistry and structure-activity relationships goes beyond the classroom and has a practical and clinical application. It can help pharmacists realize why certain adverse effects can be observed with the use of a particular drug—for example, insomnia is observed with the use of bupropion because bupropion's chemical structure is similar to amphetamine. It can also help explain why a drug like spironolactone can be used in the treatment of seemingly unrelated conditions such as acne and polycystic ovarian syndrome because of spironolactone's antagonism to testosterone effects or in treatment of heart failure due to its antagonism to aldosterone.

Rick Hess, PharmD, CDE, BC-ADM, BCACP

Therapeutic Context

Obesity is a chronic disease, with a global rise in prevalence over the last 30 to 40 years, thus garnering it epidemic status.[1] Risk factors for obesity are complex, and include sedentary lifestyle, high sugar/refined carbohydrate diet, as well as genetic, metabolic, and environmental contributors.[2] The United States boasts the highest prevalence of obese population, representing 23% to 38% of adults, varying by state, but that frequency has increased in every country on the globe in the last few decades.[3] Obesity has historically been associated with high income countries, but the prevalence of global free trade, urbanization, economic growth, and the popularity of a westernized diet has translated into the spread of the obesity epidemic to the global stage.[1] Furthermore, adoption of a sedentary lifestyle among more wealthy individuals in low- to middle-income countries has contributed to the development of at least 2% obesity frequency in every country in the world.[4] This increase in obesity in the global community is reflected in Figure 23.1.[1]

The World Health Organization (WHO) defines obesity by body mass index (BMI): individuals with a BMI of more than 25 kg/m^2 are considered overweight and those with more than 30 mg/m^2 are considered obese.[1] However, the WHO recognizes that alternative indicators for obesity may be superior to BMI, as the relationship between BMI and fat may be related to additional factors such as age, sex, and race.[5,6] For example, waist-to-hip ratio (WHR) may be a more accurate reflection of fat distribution, as waist measurement can show variability in subcutaneous and visceral fat, while the hip measurement reflects variation in bone structure and gluteal muscle and fat.[6] This metric and waist circumference (WC) have been shown to better predict risk for type 2 diabetes (T2D).[7,8] Some studies show the superiority of WC over WHR, as the latter can be artificially low if hip circumference is high.[9] While different metrics that define the obese population may be more appropriate depending on the ethnic group,[10] a high BMI has epidemiologic links to cardiovascular disease, diabetes,[11] musculoskeletal diseases,[12,13] dementia,[14] Alzheimer disease,[15] certain cancers,[16] and mortality.[17] Although BMI has long been criticized for its inability to distinguish weight associated with muscle versus fat, it remains the most common metric to define obesity.[18]

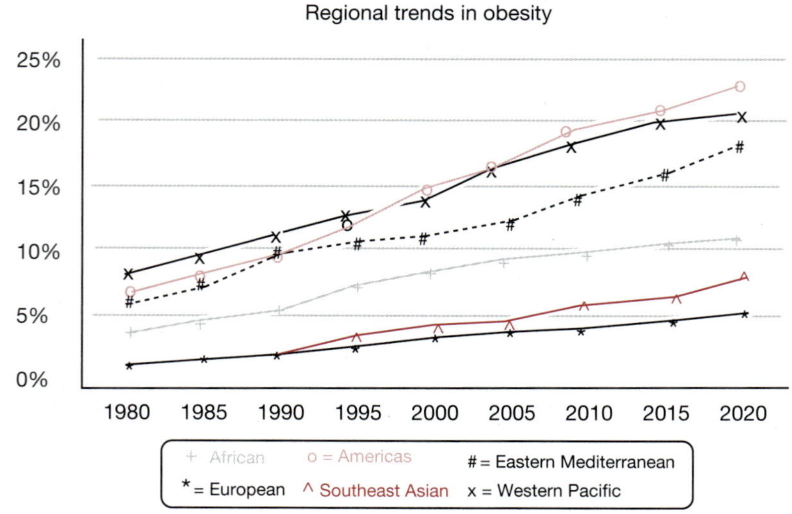

Figure 23.1 Age-standardized prevalence of obesity in adults >20 years old by geographical region and year (ca. 1980-2019). (Data from the Global Burden of Disease Study [Institute for Health Metrics and Evaluation, Seattle, WA].) (From Boutari C, Mantzoros CS. A 2022 update on the epidemiology of obesity and a call to action: as its twin COVID-19 pandemic appears to be receding, the obesity and dysmetabolism pandemic continues to rage on. *Metabolism*. 2022;133:155217.)

Weight reduction can lower risks and complications of other diseases in a dose-related manner,[18] but medicine has faced a significant challenge in managing obesity, even as the underlying hormonal regulation and risk factors have become more thoroughly understood over recent decades.[19] Drivers of obesity treatment are often more cosmetic in nature rather than health driven, to the extent that patients will pursue extreme measures to achieve the desired effect.[20] Despite the significant health gains that might be achieved by a 5% to 10% reduction in weight, this is not often ascetically sufficient to meet patient goals.[21,22] Additionally, patients with obesity face stigma from society and from their health care providers, which may stifle their weight management success.[23]

Obesity poses a significant economic burden, both for individual patients and for the global economy, in terms of health care costs. Several studies have demonstrated a profound economic burden for health care systems when diseases related to obesity and their indirect costs are considered.[24-26] This effect is amplified when the impact is calculated for children and adolescents, for whom obesity will present short- and long-term physical and mental health threats.[27] For example, the lifetime medical cost for fifth graders with obesity in the United States was calculated to be $25 billion higher than that for healthy-weight counterparts.[28] For adult patients, this translates into an annual health care cost of more than $2,500, with the effect felt in every category of care (medication cost, inpatient, outpatient).[29]

Pharmacology Overview

Management of obesity as a disease requires a multifactorial approach, which may include lifestyle changes, behavioral therapy, pharmacotherapy, and, sometimes, surgical intervention.[30,31] Treatment guidelines for anti-obesity medications (AOMs) include BMI cutoffs of at least 30 kg/m^2 or at least 27 kg/m^2 in the presence of comorbidities.[3] Despite the disease prevalence, few drugs are approved by U.S. Food and Drug Administration (FDA) for treatment of obesity. Only eight drugs were approved in the last decade, one of which, lorcaserin, has already been withdrawn due to cancer risk.[30] In general, AOMs work by controlling feeding behavior, increasing energy utilization, or affecting nutrient absorption.

Less than 5% of obesity cases are considered monogenic, associated with a disorder in a single gene.[32] The discovery of leptin in 1994 opened therapeutic doors for individuals whose obesity was associated with leptin deficiency or leptin receptor malfunction.[33] As such, two therapeutic agents used in the treatment of monogenic obesity target the leptin pathway. Setmelanotide is a melanocortin-4 (MC4) receptor agonist, which can work toward reducing hunger and increasing energy expenditure.[34,35] Setmelanotide was approved by the FDA in 2020 for use in patients older than 6 years whose obesity is linked to proopiomelanocortin (POMC), proprotein convertase subtilisin/kexin type 1 (PCSK1), or leptin receptor (LEPR) deficiency. Metreleptin is a leptin analog used in patients with a leptin deficiency due to congenital or acquired lipodystrophy.[3] Both of these products are administered as subcutaneous (SC) injection; thus, injection site reactions were commonly reported adverse events.[36] Of note, these therapies are found ineffective in majority of patients with obesity.[3]

Most FDA-approved AOMs help increase satiety and decrease hunger by affecting targets in the brain and the periphery and are intended for the treatment of nonsyndromic obesity.[37-45] These targets are summarized in Figure 23.2.[3]

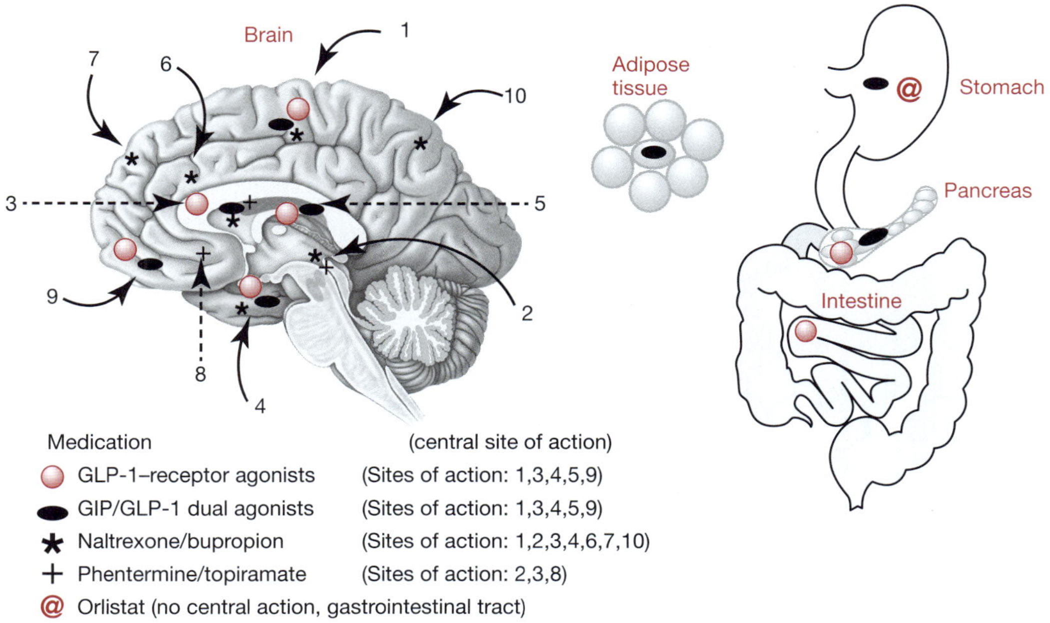

Figure 23.2 Site of action of FDA-approved anti-obesity medications: (1) parietal cortex, (2) hippocampus, (3) hypothalamus, (4) insula, (5) putamen, (6) dorsal anterior cingulate, (7) superior frontal cortex, (8) nucleus accumbens, (9) orbitofrontal cortex, (10) superior parietal cortex. (Modified with permission from Chakhtoura M, Haber R, Ghezzawi M, Rhayem C, Tcheroyan R, Mantzoros CS. Pharmacotherapy of obesity: an update on the available medications and drugs under investigation. *eClinicalMedicine*. 2023;58:101882.)

Historically, sympathomimetics have been used for weight loss due to their tendency to increase satiety and energy expenditure through dopamine release; however, abuse potential and cardiovascular effects have led to the removal of most of these drugs from the market. Phentermine remains, and its lower potency relative to amphetamine give it a lower abuse potential.[46,47] It is used in combination with topiramate, which acts on multiple central nervous system (CNS) targets, including γ-aminobutyric acid (GABA) and glutamate as an agonist and carbonic anhydrase as an inhibitor.[41] Another centrally acting AOM is the combination of naltrexone and bupropion, which work synergistically to decrease food intake by acting on neurotransmitter reuptake and reward pathways.[37,48] The newest AOMs act on glucagon-like peptide-1 receptor (GLP-1) in the CNS and the periphery. This results in decreased appetite and increased insulin sensitivity; thus, these drugs were initially developed for the treatment of T2D.[49] Finally, the only FDA-approved AOM to act solely in the periphery is orlistat, which decreases absorption of dietary fats by inhibiting lipases in the pancreas and gastrointestinal (GI) tract.[50]

A nonpharmacotherapeutic approach for decreasing caloric intake lies in the use of fat and carbohydrate substitutes in the diet. This applies to several molecules detected as "sweet" by human taste receptors, but that, for a variety of reasons, are not metabolized and absorbed.[51] These nonnutritive sweeteners, as well as the fat substitute, olestra, can be consumed without significant contribution to caloric intake.

U.S. Food and Drug Administration–Approved Drugs for the Treatment of Obesity

Setmelanotide

Melanocortin receptors are G protein–coupled receptors (GPCRs) with five subtypes. They mediate feeding and sexual function by interacting with endogenous ligands adrenocorticotropic hormone (ACTH) and melanocortins.[52,53] The melanocortin receptor 4 (MC4R) is of particular interest in the field of obesity, where variants in the gene that codes for MC4R are associated with 1% to 5% of the morbidly obese population.[54] Furthermore, this 332–amino acid peptide has been shown in multiple studies to regulate appetite control within the hypothalamus,[55] ultimately affecting food intake, weight, and insulin sensitivity.[56-58] Dysregulation in the MC4R accounts for 6% to 8% of total obesity cases.[59,60] Agonists of melanocortin receptors are encoded by a single gene, resulting in the generation of proopiomelanocortin, which is converted to α-melanocyte stimulating hormone (α-MSH), ACTH, and other tissue-specific ligands. α-MSH is the endogenous MC4R agonist tetrapeptide with a binding profile that has been well defined to date[61]; thus, drug development in this area has focused on therapeutic peptides or peptidomimetics.[62] Three key acidic residues have been identified in the transmembrane domains of MC4R: Glu100, Asp122, and Asp126, which have been hypothesized to interact with arginine on the side chain of α-MSH.[63]

Four mutations in MC4R have been defined in patients with obesity of monogenic origin. These include Ser127Leu, Ser58Cys, Ile102Thr, and Gly252Ser, all of which impact α binding to MC4R.[64-70] The drug setmelanotide is capable of activating mutated receptors with a 20-fold higher potency than that of α-MSH. This structure, alongside α-MSH, is shown in Figure 23.3.

MECHANISM OF ACTION. Setmelanotide is capable of activating mutated receptors because it can access an allosteric site on transmembrane unit 3 (TM3) that is inaccessible to α-MSH. These interactions have been specifically characterized as polar (Arg^1 on drug to Leu106/Asp111 and His^4 on drug to Asn123) and hydrophobic (Phe^5 on drug to Tyr268/Tyr276). Additionally, setmelanotide interacts with the aforementioned key acidic residues, mimicking α-MSH response.[61]

PHARMACOKINETICS. The peptide nature of setmelanotide necessitates parenteral administration; thus it is given by SC injection. The drug reaches steady state within 2 days, with a 1- to 3-mg daily dose. It has a plasma half-life of 11 hours, is 79.1% bound to plasma proteins, and has a volume of distribution of 48.7 L. The drug's urinary clearance is 4.86 L/h, with a 39% excreted unchanged. Additional metabolism to

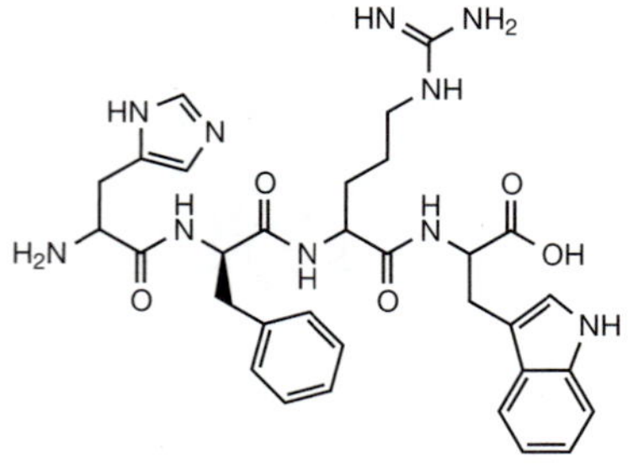

α-MSH tetrapeptide pharmacophore

(NH_2 – His^6 - Phe^7 - Arg^8 - Typ^9 - Ac)

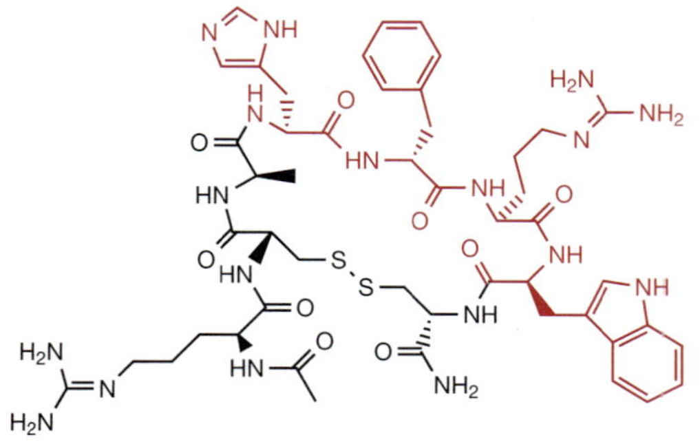

Setmelanotide (Imcivree)

(Ac-Arg-Cys^1-DAla-His-DPhe-Arg-Cys^1NH_2)
S————————S

Figure 23.3 Structures and sequences of setmelanotide and α-MSH. (Modified with permission from Falls BA, Zhang Y. Insights into the allosteric mechanism of setmelanotide (RM-493) as a potent and first-in-class melanocortin-4 receptor (MC4R) agonist to treat rare genetic disorders of obesity through an in silico approach. *ACS Chem Neurosci.* 2019;10:1055-1065. Copyright 2019 American Chemical Society.)

smaller peptides is expected, and no incidence of drug-drug interactions related to protein binding or CYP450s has been reported.[61]

Metreleptin

Leptin is a 167-amino acid, 16-kDa protein produced in adipose tissue that serves as a signaling molecule for energy reserves.[34,71] The LEPR is a class I cytokine receptor with a single transmembrane spanning unit and found in the hypothalamus, pancreas, liver, skeletal muscle, and adipose tissue.[34] Functionally, leptin serves to decrease appetite, decrease insulin secretion, decrease lipogenesis, and increase lipolysis, which serves to modulate weight in non-overweight and non-obese individuals.[72] Mutations in ObR were the first single-gene mutations associated with morbid obesity,[73] thus leptin-related therapies showed potential in individuals expressing these mutations.

Metreleptin is a recombinant human leptin (r-metHuLeptin) analogue produced in *Escherichia coli*.[74] The major sequence difference between leptin and metreleptin is the placement of a methionine residue at the N-terminus, which serves to stabilize the molecule during production.[73,74] Metreleptin is approved for use in congenital generalized lipodystrophy (CGL) and works by reducing feeding behavior and decreasing insulin resistance.[75] Metreleptin does not work in conventional obesity, as circulating leptin is already high in these patients due to high body fat. Additionally, leptin tolerance tends to manifest in obese patients with a normal-functioning ObR.[76] A small number of patients using metreleptin experience an immunogenic response, hypothesized to be associated with the effect that the stabilizing methionine has on the protein's tertiary structure.[77,78]

Metreleptin is administered subcutaneously using weight-based guidelines. It reaches C_{max} in 4 to 4.3 hours and has a half-life of 3.8 to 4.7 hours. Although extensive data on the drug's clearance is not available, the majority of the drug is cleared by the kidney. Because it is a cytokine, it may alter the formation of CYP450 enzymes, which could be clinically relevant to low therapeutic index drugs.[77,78]

Liraglutide/Semaglutide/Tirzepatide (Fig. 23.4)

Glucagon-like peptide-1 (GLP-1) is a 30-amino-acid incretin hormone linked to approximately 70% of insulin secretion in humans. Since its discovery in the early 1990s, its potential in the treatment of T2D has been enthusiastically explored. Administration of exogenous GLP-1 to provoke insulin response is limited by the rapid metabolism of this peptide, contributing to an IV half-life of only 1.5 minutes.[79]

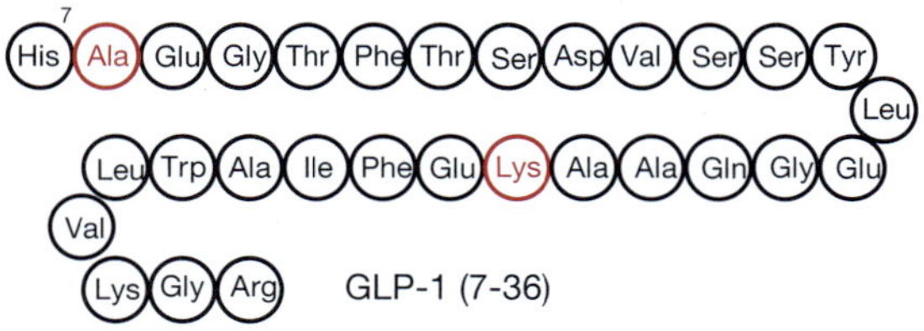

STRUCTURE-ACTIVITY RELATIONSHIP. Early structure-activity relationship (SAR) studies of GLP-1 determined that amino acids in positions 7, 8, 9, 10, 11, 13, 15, 28, and 29 were essential for activity. Additionally, the alanine residue at position 2 was identified as a primary site of attack by dipeptidyl peptidase-IV (DPP-IV).[80] Several investigations into derivation of GLP-1 with fatty acids revealed that removal of the aforementioned amino acids resulted in activity loss of the peptide. Eventually, the lysine residue at position 26 was identified as a point of fatty acid addition, and the Lys34 in native GLP-1 could be substituted for an arginine to restrict fatty acid addition to that position.[81]

The exploration of adding fatty acids to GLP-1 receptor-targeted drugs lies in the interest in human serum albumin (HSA)

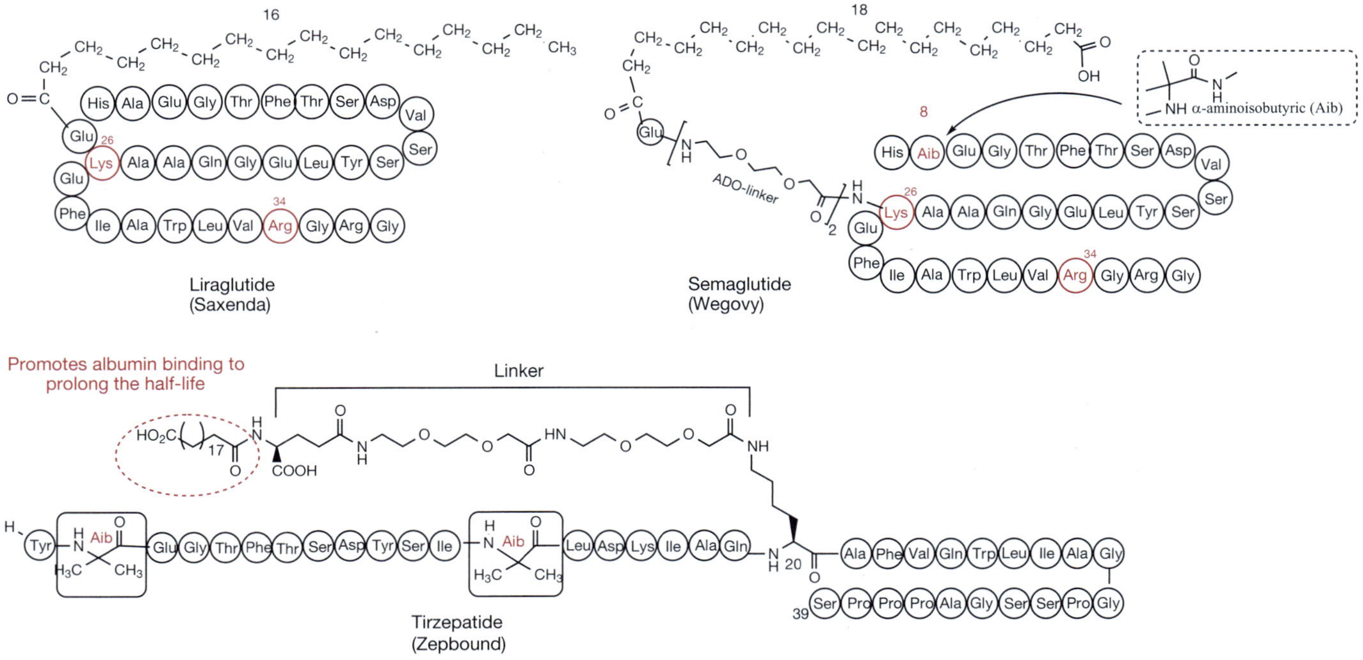

Figure 23.4 Structures of liraglutide, semaglutide, and tirzepatide.

as a potential drug depot for peptides vulnerable to enzymatic degradation. Albumin is a stable and abundant plasma protein with a long half-life, mainly due to its pH-dependent binding to the neonatal Fc receptor (FcRn), which limits its exocytosis.[82] Investigators considered HSA promising for drug binding because of its known behavior to bind steroids and fatty acids, thus facilitating transport of these insoluble solutes through the plasma. For example, C10, C12, C14, C16, and C18 fatty acids have been characterized as binding to seven distinct sites on HSA.[81] The application of binding a peptide to a fatty acid to increase plasma half-life had already played out with insulin detemir, which showed that some of the increase in half-life was due to HSA binding.[83] Albumin has significant capacity, as demonstrated by its high concentration (~0.6 mM) relative to the eventual GLP-1 receptor agonists (20-40 nM).[84]

Liraglutide (see Fig. 23.4). Liraglutide was developed with the goal of retaining as much GLP-1 sequence as possible to sustain receptor potency and decrease risk of immunogenicity. As such, the Lys34 → Arg substitution was made to promote monoacylation as the only amino acid substitution compared to native GLP-1. Fatty acid addition (C16) was optimized at Lys26, with the use of a γ-glutamate (γGlu) linker between the peptide and fatty acid. This modification also served to protect the drug from DPP-IV–facilitated degradation, likely due to steric hindrance and the tendency to engage in reversible binding to HSA. The reversible albumin binding also contributes to the prolonged half-life (11-15 hours) versus native GLP-1, as it promotes self-assembly of liraglutide into a heptapeptide. Selection of liraglutide following extensive SAR studies with different fatty acid lengths, using both mono- and di-acids, concluded that a 16C mono-acid was optimum. Furthermore, the fatty acid length correlates with the pharmacokinetic profile. Finally, the presence of the γGlu linker also played a role in receptor affinity, as omission of this structure resulted in a dramatic decrease in potency.[85] Metabolism of liraglutide mirrors that of other natural amino acids and fatty acids.[81]

Semaglutide (see Fig. 23.4). The goals for the development of semaglutide involved preservation of low immunogenic risk while facilitating once-weekly dosing. As such, the similarity of peptide to GLP-1 was largely preserved. This development was a balancing act between decreasing metabolism and renal clearance of the drug but not promoting excessive HSA binding, which would risk loss of receptor potency. The ultimate development strategy consisted of two parts. Firstly, a key substitution in the peptide sequence involved the replacement of Ala8 with a nonhuman amino acid, 1-aminoisobutyric acid (Aib). This helps restrict DPP-IV cleavage while maintaining sufficient similarity to native GLP-1.[86] Secondly, investigators sought to identify a combination of fatty acid and linker that would help maintain drug-HSA binding but not restrict receptor potency. The water-soluble chemical linker, 8-amino-3,6-dioxaoctanoic acid (ADO), was eventually chosen due to its ability to promote glucagon-like peptide-1 receptor (GLP-1R) affinity in the presence of albumin. The ADO linker, combined with a C18 di-acid, gave the highest combination of GLP-1R potency and half-life, through albumin affinity.[87] The maintenance of semaglutide in its active confirmation is thought to be facilitated through a water-mediated electrostatic interaction between Glu27 and Arg34, as shown in Figure 23.5.

Even though semaglutide contains a nonhuman amino acid and a synthetic linker between fatty acids and drug, metabolic studies indicate that it is fully metabolized like other peptides and fatty acids.[88] Despite the challenges of oral peptide delivery, oral delivery of semaglutide has been explored with the assistance of the permeation enhancer abbreviated as SNAC (*N*-[8-(2-hydroxybenzoyl) amino] caprylate). Pharmacokinetic data indicate very low oral bioavailability, but weight loss and lowering of blood glucose equivalent to subcutaneous semaglutide could still be achieved with the addition of SNAC to the formulation.[89] Data suggests that dissolution and absorption of oral semaglutide occur in the stomach, which helps avoid exposure of the drug to peptidases in the small intestines. Also, SNAC lends to a locally neutral microenvironmental pH, which helps solubilize semaglutide and protect it from peptidase activity in the stomach.[90]

Tirzepatide (see Fig. 23.4). Tirzepatide is a dual agonist of GLP-1 and gastric inhibitory polypeptide (GIP). Its central activity in the hypothalamus is associated with a decrease in food intake, and its peripheral activity contributes to delayed gastric emptying, thus increased satiety.[91] This drug was originally approved in 2022 for the treatment of T2D, but the dose-dependent effect on glycemic control also applied to weight reduction, thus it was granted Fast Track designation by the FDA for treatment of patients with obesity and overweight with metabolic comorbidities.[92]

Structurally, tirzepatide is a 39–amino-acid bifunctional peptide, with shared characteristics of GIP, GLP-1, and semaglutide. However, it does offer advantages over semaglutide related to its different peptide sequence, which contributes to GIP receptor activity, as well as its fatty acid conjugation

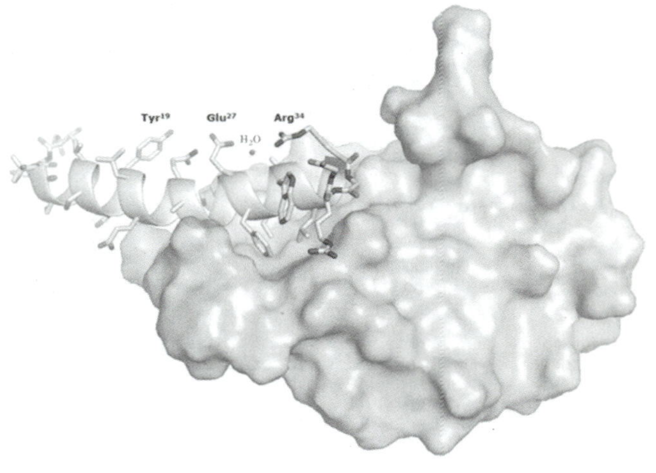

Figure 23.5 Stabilization of semaglutide in active confirmation through a water-mediated electrostatic interaction between Glu27 and Arg34. (Reprinted with permission from Lau J, Bloch P, Schäffer L, et al. Discovery of the once-weekly glucagon-like peptide-1 (GLP-1) analogue semaglutide. *J Med Chem.* 2015;58(18):7370-7380. doi:10.1021/acs.jmedchem.5b00726. Copyright 2015 American Chemical Society.)

and elongation of the C-terminus to include a sequence from exenatide.[93] The structure of tirzepatide is based primarily on native GIP, with a C20 fatty acid moiety (eicosanedioic acid) attached via hydrophobic linkers onto a lysine residue at position 20.[94] The fatty acid moiety is thought to boost GLP-1 activity; however, molecular dynamics investigations show intermittent hydrogen bonding between the fatty acid and gastric inhibitory polypeptide receptor (GIPR), more so than GLP-1R.[94,95] Additionally, there is enough difference between tirzepatide and GLP-1 as to induce less receptor desensitization compared to other GLP-1 receptor agonists.[95] Tirzepatide does contain non-coded amino acids (Aib) at positions 2 and 13. The utilization of Aib at position 2, like semaglutide, circumvents DPP-4 degradation. The Aib at position 13 specifically contributes to GIP activity.[96] The linkers used in tirzepatide, γ-glutamate, and bis-aminoethoxyacetyl (γGlu-2× Ado) promote peptide flexibility and help optimize receptor binding.[93] These structural features contribute to a long half-life for tirzepatide (116.7 hours) and high albumin affinity.[96]

Orforglipron

Orforglipron (LY3502970) is an oral non-peptide GLP-1 receptor agonist. More specifically, it is a partial agonist that has a greater effect on G protein activation and cAMP (cyclic adenosine monophosphate) signaling versus the β-arrestin pathway. This biased signaling, which is also seen with tirzepatide, is hypothesized to lower the possibility of receptor desensitization versus a full agonist.[97] High resolution microscopy studies indicate that orforglipron binds to the upper helical bundle of the GLP-1 receptor, facilitating high receptor occupancy despite its activity as a partial agonist.[98] The half-life of orforglipron (29-49 hours) facilitates once daily dosing. Of note, unlike oral semaglutide, orforglipron does not require absorption enhancers or complex food and drink regimens to drive bioavailability. Clinical trial data supports orforglipron's ability to deliver dose-dependent weight reduction in the ballpark of 7% to 12% after 36 weeks.[97]

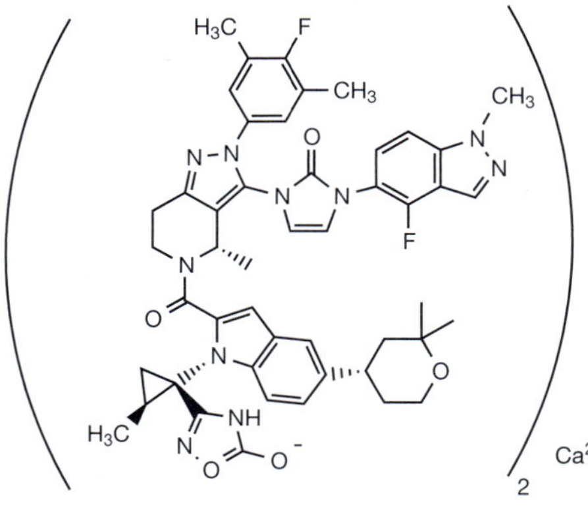

Orforglipron (LY3502970)

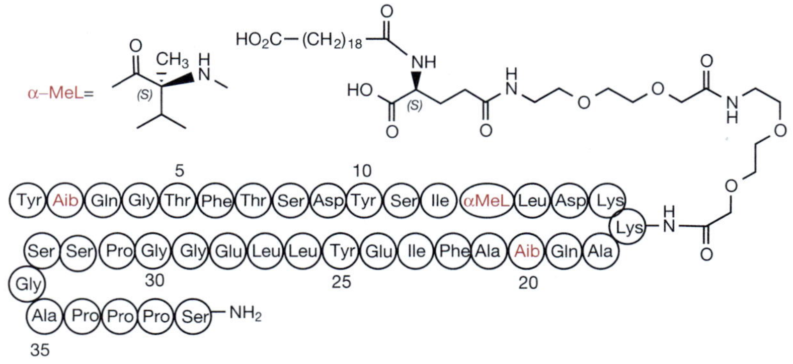

Retatrutide (LY347943)

Retatrutide

Retatrutide (LY3437943) is a "triagonist" drug showing potential for groundbreaking weight reduction in clinical trials. The agonistic targets for this drug encompass GIP, GLP-1, and the glucagon receptor. The success of liraglutide and semaglutide in this space established the applicability of GLP-1 as a target, and tirzepatide validated the efficacy of the addition of GIP receptor agonist to the pharmacologic profile. The inclusion of the glucagon receptor as an additional target for retatrutide was explored because of human data supporting that glucagon receptor agonism could increase energy expenditure.[99] Retatrutide is a fatty acid–acylated 39–amino acid synthetic peptide intended to be administered weekly. Its sequence was engineered from the GIP peptide backbone and has a higher affinity for GIPR and a lower affinity for GLP-1R and glucagon receptors, compared to the native hormones. The peptide contains two different non-coded amino acids found at positions 2, 13, and 20. The use of Aib at position 2 helps protect the peptide from DPP-4 degradation, while the inclusion of this amino acid at position 20 is hypothesized to optimize GIP activity. Position 13 contains an α-methyl-L-leucine (αMeL13), which optimizes both glucagon and GIP activity. A 20C fatty acid is conjugated to lysine at position 17 to facilitate a prolonged half-life and albumin affinity.[100] Retatrutide is in phase II development.

Naltrexone/Bupropion (Contrave)

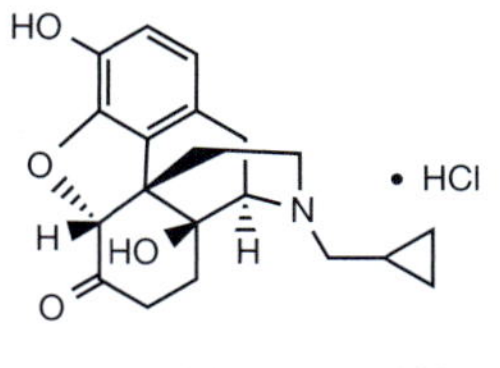

Naltrexone HCl

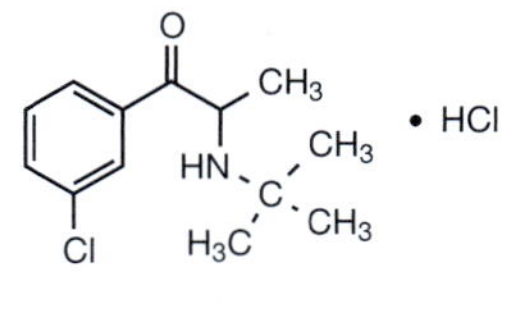

Bupropion HCl

The combination of naltrexone and bupropion is hypothesized to help treat obesity through reducing feeding behaviors, likely through limiting reward pathways in the brain. Naltrexone is a synthetic derivative of oxymorphone, with binding affinity to κ, δ, and μ receptors in the brain as an antagonist.[101] Naltrexone has the highest binding affinity to the μ receptors.[102] Several studies have verified that the presence of the cyclopropylmethyl extension off the nitrogen helps confer antagonist properties to naltrexone.[103] Naltrexone has been used for many years in the treatment of alcohol dependence, due to its limiting effects on endogenous opioid activity. Release of endorphins can occur in anticipation of a reward, or during the rewarding experience, which, in the treatment of obesity, refers to food consumption. As an opioid receptor antagonist, naltrexone would block the response of endogenous opioids, thus limiting the rewarding effects.[104]

Bupropion HCl is an enantiomeric drug with one chiral center, yet there is no therapeutic benefit while administering as a pure enantiomer.[105] Bupropion is structurally related to many amphetamines as an aminopropiophenone that works by inhibiting norepinephrine and dopamine reuptake.[104] Structural features on bupropion specifically linked for dopamine transporter affinity are the secondary amine and halogenation at the meta-position.[106] The limitation on neurotransmitter reuptake is hypothesized to limit food reward. Although data does not support the use of either drug alone for the treatment of obesity, in this drug combination, especially with lifestyle modifications, patients are able to achieve clinically significant weight reduction, defined as more than 5%.[48]

While the mechanism of action for the combination of these drugs is not known, it is thought that the naltrexone-bupropion modulates the homeostatic hypothalamic melanocortin system with the non-homeostatic mesolimbic dopamine (DA) reward system. This action may come about through increased firing frequency of the proopiomelanocortin (POMC) neurons in the hypothalamus by bupropion-releasing α-MSH, which binds to melanocortin-4 receptors (MC4Rs) located in the hypothalamus to decrease food intake and increase energy expenditure. POMC at the same time releases β-endorphin, which inhibits further release of α-MSH by its action on the μ-opioid receptor. The role of naltrexone is to block the μ-opioid receptor, thus inhibiting the negative feedback process.[107]

Topiramate/Phentermine (Qsymia)

Immediate release phentermine and extended release topiramate were the first combination product approved by the FDA for obesity treatment.[108] Phentermine is classified as an "appetite suppressant" due to its pharmacologic effect on neurotransmitters that impact feeding behavior. Phentermine's activity is specifically sympathomimetic in nature, in that it mimics the activity of norepinephrine.[109] Although it has some impact on dopamine transport, its activity at the serotonin transporter is negligible.[110] The structural similarity between phentermine and other amphetamines contributes to its potential for dependence and abuse. Phentermine has a 20-hour half-life, is largely excreted unchanged (≥70%), and metabolized by CYP34A, and has low plasma protein binding (17.5%).[111]

Topiramate has several characterized mechanisms, yet the one that most impacts weight control remains unclear. Topiramate is known to have activity at GABA-A receptors, modulate voltage-gated ion channels, and act as an antagonist at a subtype of glutamate receptors.[108] As an inhibitor of isozymes of carbonic anhydrase, some evidence suggests that this may impact a patient's taste experience.[112] Human studies indicate that reduced caloric intake is the primary factor in topiramate-facilitated weight loss; however, animal studies suggest that increased energy expenditure is also a factor.[113] Structurally, topiramate contains a fructose monosaccharide core with a unique O-alkyl sulfamate group. Modifications of the sulfamate or replacement with carbamate showed a loss of antiepileptic activity, but similar SAR explorations have not been applied to its function in treating obesity.[114] Like phentermine, topiramate is highly excreted unchanged (70%) but has more moderate plasma protein binding (15%-41%) and a longer half-life (65 hours).[108] Topiramate is readily absorbed following oral administration. Common adverse effects include paresthesia, dizziness, visual disturbances, insomnia, constipation, and dry mouth. Topiramate is contraindicated during pregnancy due to the reports of orofacial clefts in the fetus.

Orlistat (Alli, Xenical)

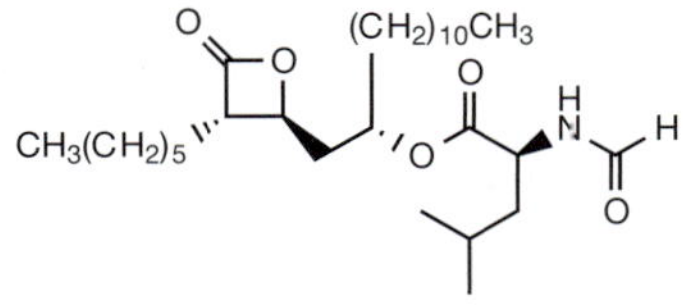

Orlistat

Orlistat, tetrahydrolipstatin, is a semisynthetic derivative of the natural product lipstatin produced by *Streptomyces toxytricini*. The compound acts as an irreversible inhibitor of pancreatic lipase and several other lipases and, as such, prevents the normal metabolic breakdown of fats, leading to reduced absorption of fatty acids from the GI tract.[115,116] Fecal fat loss increases by as much as 30% after treatment with orlistat, thus indicating that reduced activity of intestinal lipases increases the loss of undigested fats. Studies with porcine pancreatic lipase show that acylation of serine 152 is responsible for this inhibition of lipase activity, suggesting a similar mechanism for orlistat in the human intestine.[116] Orlistat itself is not absorbed to any appreciable extent and is excreted from the body via the GI tract. In addition, drug interaction studies indicate that orlistat may interfere with the absorption of a wide spectrum of drugs, such as cyclosporine and some diabetes medications, levothyroxine, and warfarin, and with the fat-soluble vitamins, with the exception of vitamin E.[117]

The most common adverse events were associated with the lack of absorption of fats and consisted of oily stools, spotting bowel movements, stomach pain, and flatulence. A meta-analysis of 16 trials found that 80% of patients treated with orlistat reported at least one GI adverse event.[118] Additionally, it was noted that while on orlistat, obese patients showed a decrease in low-density lipoprotein and total cholesterol levels and that Hemoglobin A_{1C} (HbA_{1c}) levels decreased in patients with T2D.

Orlistat is available as a nonprescription product (Alli, 60 mg taken with each fat-containing meal up to three doses/d) and as a prescription product (Xenical, 120 mg taken with each fat-containing meal up to three doses/d).

Orlistat is used as an adjunct to diet and exercise and can be used for long-term therapy.

Central Nervous System Stimulants Used for Weight Management

The sympathomimetic anorexiants shown in Figure 23.6 are structurally and pharmacologically related to amphetamine and its analogues. The sympathomimetic anorexiants are related to each other through the phenylpropyl amine pharmacophore. Anorexiants are primarily intended to suppress the appetite, but most of the drugs in this class appear not to have a primary effect on appetite. Their appetite-suppressant actions appear to be secondary to CNS stimulation, and as CNS stimulants, they have a potential for abuse or addiction. As a result of the abuse potential, amphetamine itself and many of its analogues have very limited records of safety and efficacy in the treatment of obesity.[119]

Amphetamine (methylphenethylamine) has been tagged for its potential to aid in weight loss since the 1930s.[120] Amphetamine competitively inhibits dopamine and norepinephrine reuptake but induces the release of these neurotransmitters from nerve storage granules. Specifically, the link to increased dopamine signaling is linked to the abuse potential for amphetamine and its related compounds.[119] Amphetamine contains one chiral center, with its *d*-enantiomer shown as the most potent form.[121] Other drugs in this class share this pharmacology. Modifications in structure contribute to affinity differences for norepinephrine versus dopamine reuptake as well as for abuse potential. For example, phentermine, the α-methylated version of amphetamine, has lower overall CNS stimulation versus amphetamine. Substituted amphetamines such as benzphetamine, diethylpropion, phendimetrazine, and phentermine will also have a higher impact on serotonin reuptake compared to amphetamine.[122]

All of the sympathomimetic anorexiants are available as water-soluble salts (ie, hydrochlorides, tartrates, dimesylate).

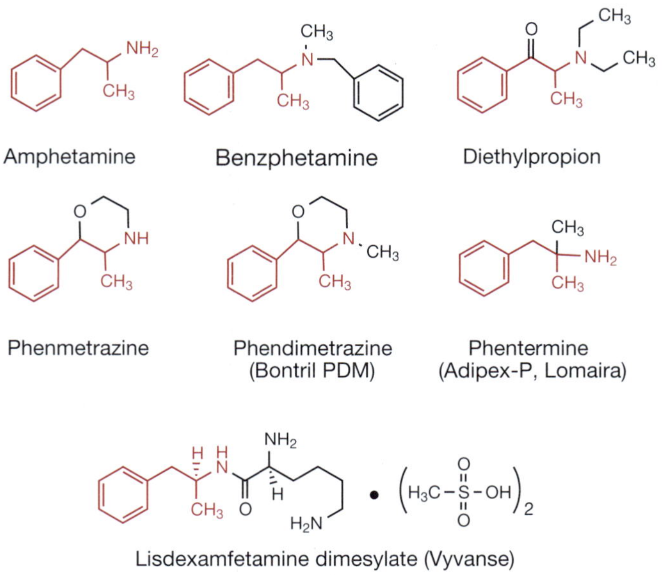

Figure 23.6 Central nervous system stimulants historically used for weight loss.

These compounds are readily absorbed and often extensively metabolized. The sympathomimetics commonly undergo N-dealkylation, where the metabolic products typically retain biological activity.[123,124] Benzphetamine is primarily N-demethylated to *N*-benzylamphetamine and to the minor metabolites, methamphetamine, amphetamine, and their hydroxylated metabolites.[125] The appetite-suppressant effect of diethylpropion is due to its metabolic N-monodeethylation to ethcathinone. Phenmetrazine, a previously approved and withdrawn anorexiant, has been replaced with phendimetrazine, which in turn functions as a prodrug, metabolically giving rise to low levels of phenmetrazine (~30%). Because of the slow conversion to phenmetrazine, the abuse potential of this drug is reported to be less when compared to other amphetamine drugs. Additionally, 30% of the administered drug is excreted unchanged. As with phendimetrazine, lisdexamfetamine is a prodrug, which is metabolized to the active appetite-suppressant drug dextroamphetamine to the extent of ~40%.

Other Drugs Related to Weight Management or Comorbid Conditions

Icosapent Ethyl (Vascepa)

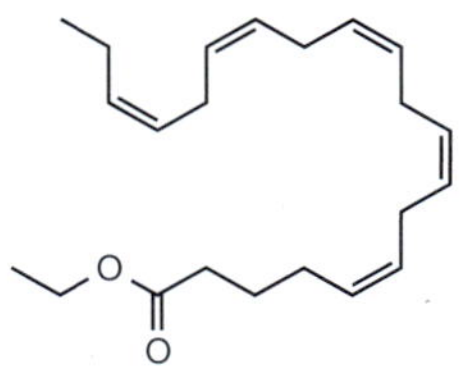

Icosapent ethyl

The potential of omega-3 fatty acids for reduction of serum triglycerides has been studied for many years. Omega-3 fatty acids have been shown to increase fatty acid oxidation and facilitate generation of *N*-acyl taurines.[126,127] As part of the Reduction of Cardiovascular Events With Icosapent Ethyl (IPE)-Intervention trial, the purified ethyl ester of eicosapentaenoic acid (C20:5; EPA) showed promise for reducing triglyceride and protecting against major cardiovascular events in statin-treated patients.[126] This eicosapentaenoic acid ethyl ester, also known as icosapent ethyl (IPE), is used in some patients to reduce overall cardiovascular risk. Once ingested, the ethyl ester form is not readily detectable in the plasma, and is anticipated to be extensively hydrolyzed.[128] Following oral administration of IPE, the peak concentration of EPA in the plasma was detected at 5 to 6 hours, with detection in red blood cells occurring at 8 to 24 hours following dosing. The use of the ethyl ester form contributed to a long plasma half-life of EPA at 70 to 89 hours.[129]

Triheptanoin (Dojolvi)

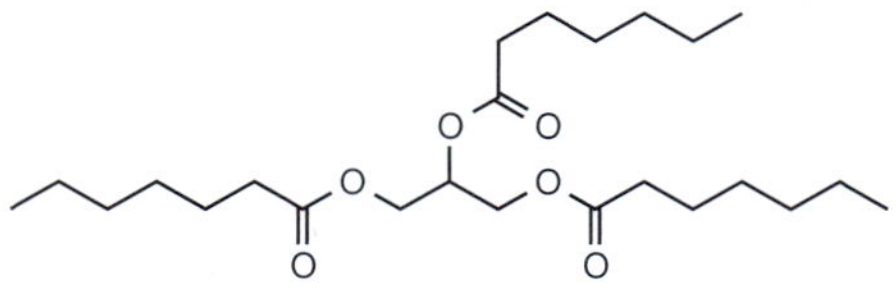

Triheptanoin

Although not specifically used to manage obesity, the drug triheptanoin is used to provide citric acid cycle intermediates for patients with long chain fatty acid oxidation disorders (LC-FAOD). This synthetic triglyceride has three fatty acid chains on a glycerol backbone, which are hydrolyzed by pancreatic lipases to release heptanoate. Heptanoate can be metabolized to acetyl-CoA, propionyl CoA, or four to five-carbon ketone bodies.[130]

Nonnutritive Sweeteners as Food Substitutes

Overview

As indicated, obesity, as a disease, requires a multifactorial approach, which may include lifestyle changes, behavioral therapy, pharmacotherapy, and, sometimes, surgical intervention. From a simplistic viewpoint, overweight and obesity result from the consumption of calories above those needed to fuel the body over an extended period of time (positive energy balance). Thus, behavioral modification in the form of increased physical activity and decreased caloric intake are often coupled with pharmacotherapy in the treatment of obesity. Since carbohydrates (starches, fibers, and sugars) make up 40% to 70% of the human daily caloric intake, a reduction of dietary sugars would arguably be beneficial in the treatment of obesity. Sugars common in our diet include monosaccharides (eg, glucose, fructose, and galactose) and disaccharides (eg, sucrose, lactose, and maltose), both of which are referred to as "free sugars" (Fig. 23.7). It is estimated that the average American adult consumes 64 lb of sucrose per year, while children may consume as much as 140 lb/y. Approximately one-third of sugar is ingested from the table sugar bowl, and two-thirds is found in commercially processed food, mostly as high-fructose corn syrup. Simply deleting or replacing energy-providing nutrients is not going to prevent the excessive caloric intake.[131] However, nonnutritive sugars can be used as alternatives to some of these high caloric sugars. The consumption of sugar has both a physiologic and a psychological basis. The perception of sweetness is detected by GPCRs located in the taste buds on the tongue (T1R2-T1R3 heterodimeric sweet taste receptors), leading to a natural craving of sweet substances. Excessive intake of sucrose or high-fructose corn syrup is directly related to the development of tooth caries and the development of overweight and obesity, and, while obesity is associated with T2D, cardiovascular disease, nonalcoholic liver disease, and cancer,[132] sugars are not directly associated with these latter diseases. Thus, a good approach to health issues is to avoid excessive consumption of carbohydrates, sugars in particular, and replacement is a more palatable strategy than is restraint. Because of the mounting concern regarding overweight and obesity and the need to reduce calorie intake while meeting the desire for sweet substances, nonnutritive sweeteners (NNS) have gained universal acceptance. The replacement of sugars with NNS is not without its critics. It has been suggested that the consumption of sugar-sweetened beverages with NNS could lead to a decreased feeling of satiety, resulting in an increase in intake of calories and an increase in body weight. But a review by Fernstrom argues that "the role of NNSs in weight control is therefore no more or less than meets the eye: used judiciously in the diet, they provide one tool that can help control caloric intake."[133] Supportive documentation has been reported by McGlynn et al[134] that substitution of sugar-sweetened beverages with NNSs appears to be associated with a reduction of body weight, BMI, and percentage of body fat and is an improvement over the replacement of sugar-sweetened beverages with water.

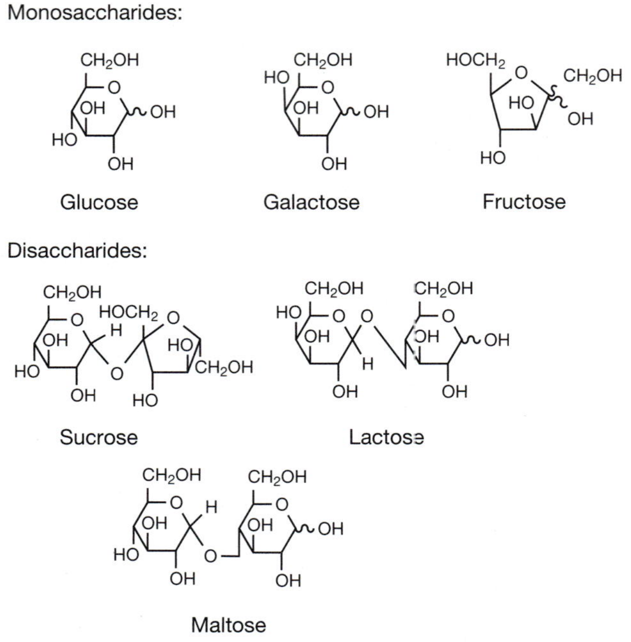

Figure 23.7 Structures of the "free sugars."

Mechanism of Action of Free Sugars and Nonnutritive Sweeteners

As indicated, the sweet-tasting perception is initiated in the oral cavity through the interaction of sweet substances with the T1R2-T1R3 heterodimeric sweet taste sensory GPCRs.[133,135,136] These receptors respond to both "free sugars" (monosaccharide and disaccharides) and many of the NNSs (eg, the synthetic NNSs acesulfame-K, sucralose, aspartame, neotame, and saccharin; the natural NNS proteins monellin, thaumatin, and brazzein; and the natural NNS glycosides steviol and mogroside). It can be concluded that the NNSs produce their effect at the same receptors that are stimulated by the natural sugars. It should be noted that the T1R3-T1R3 receptors can be found in other parts of the human body, namely intestinal cells and pancreatic β cells, but the concentration of NNSs resulting from administering beverages or foods containing the NNSs is unable to stimulate the latter tissue to the same extent that free sugars can.

Nonnutritive Sweeteners

Saccharin (Sweet'N Low) (Fig. 23.8)

The history of saccharin began with its synthesis in 1878, and, over the past 145 plus years, this food additive has been part of the human food scene. Saccharin's history has included a period when it was banned from the market as an

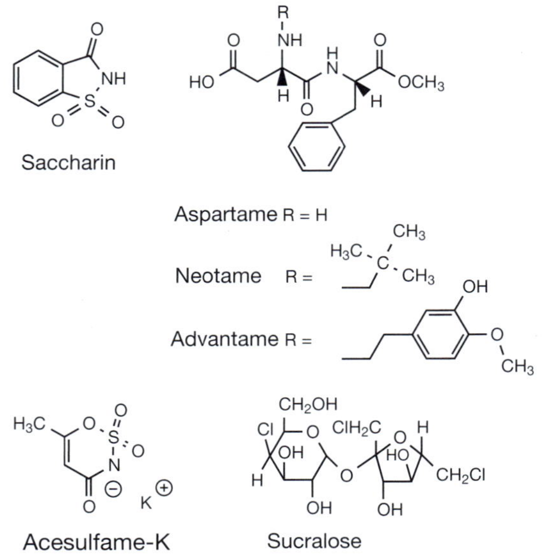

Figure 23.8 Synthetic nonnutritive sweeteners.

adulterant only to be returned as a sugar substitute. It has had limited use directed toward diabetes, carried a warning as a possible carcinogen, and is now openly available for consumer use and a common ingredient in a host of food products. Saccharin's colorful history has been presented in a book titled *Empty Pleasures: The Story of Artificial Sweeteners from Saccharin to Splenda*.[137]

The properties of saccharin include a sweetness 300-fold that of sucrose with zero calories (Table 23.1). Saccharin does have a bitter aftertaste, a fact that makes saccharin less than the ideal NNS, and instability to prolonged heating, thus limiting its use to non-baked products. The bitter aftertaste has been masked by the addition of other sweeteners. The biggest health-related problem associated with saccharin was a scare resulting from the development of bladder cancer in male rats reported in 1977 in a work titled the "Canadian Rat Study." This study resulted in the banning of saccharin by the FDA, but the passage of the Saccharin Study and Labeling Act in 1977 by the U.S. Congress allowed saccharin to remain on the market with the required

Table 23.1 Comparison of Nutritive and Nonnutritive Sweeteners

Nutritive Sweetener		Sweetness	Calories/100 g	Source
Sucrose		100%	All mono- and disaccharides ~370	Natural
Glucose		60%-70%		Natural
Fructose		110%-180%		Natural
Maltose		33%-50%		Natural
Galactose		15%-40%		Natural
Xylitol		100%	~192	Natural
Erythritol		60%-80%	~0	Natural
Allulose (D-Psicose), GRAS list		70%	~0.4	Natural
Nonnutritive Sweetener:		Sweetness × sucrose		
Generic name	Trade name			
Saccharin	Sweet'N Low	300×	0	Synthetic
Aspartame	Equal, NutraSweet, Sugar Twin	200-300×	~0.05	Synthetic
Neotame	Newtame	7,000×	0	Synthetic
Advantame	—	37,000×	0	Synthetic
Sucralose	Splenda	600×	0	Synthetic
Acesulfame-K	Sunett	200×	0	Synthetic
Steviol glycosides	Truvia, Stevia	200-300×	0	Natural
Mogrosides	Monk fruit	300×	0	Natural
Nonnutritive Sweetener, Generally Recognized As Safe (GRAS) list		Sweetness <2% sucrose		
Brazzein, 54 amino acids		37,500×	NA	Natural-protein
Thaumatin II, 207 amino acids		>2,000×	NA	Natural-protein

label that saccharin-containing products were potentially carcinogenic. Saccharin-containing products retained this label until December 2000 when the warning label was removed following presentation of evidence that male rats are unique in that a combination of high bladder pH, high calcium phosphate concentrations, and a specific protein that favors bladder microcrystal formation occurs in the presence of saccharin. These conditions do not exist in humans, and therefore, a threat of saccharin-induced tumors is not possible.[138]

Aspartame, Neotame, and Advantame (Fig. 23.8)

Aspartame, neotame, and advantame are derivatives of the dipeptide of two natural amino acids, L-phenylalanine and L-aspartic acid. In 1965, a chemist working at G.D. Searle & Company discovered that aspartame had an outstanding sweet taste. Coming at a time when saccharin and cyclamate (banned from the U.S. market) were facing intense scrutiny as synthetic NNSs, aspartame was seen as a potentially significant breakthrough in the NNS market. The properties of aspartame included a sweetness 200-fold that of sucrose with no bitter aftertaste. A single serving of aspartame, equivalent to an equally sweet 180-calorie serving of sucrose, contains only 0.1 calories (Table 23.1). Although still not stable upon prolonged heating, aspartame's major attraction was the fact that it was composed of two naturally occurring amino acids. At a time when the consumer was concerned about synthetic, unnatural chemicals, aspartame offered a marketing windfall. Aspartame was first approved for marketing in 1974, but concerns about tumors, brain damage, and testing procedures delayed its introduction to the market until July 1981. By 1985, aspartame was consumed to the extent of 800 million pounds per year, and 2 years later, it was estimated that aspartame appeared in more than 1,200 products.

Aspartame, being a dipeptide, is prone to hydrolytic metabolism, either in the intestine or mucus membrane of the intestinal lining, to produce phenylalanine, aspartic acid, and methanol (Fig. 23.9). This metabolism in turn raised the question of safety of the products formed. Methanol, or wood alcohol, is a potential toxin when absorbed into the bloodstream, where it can be converted into formaldehyde and then to formic acid, which could potentially lead to systemic metabolic acidosis and blindness.[139] It was found that the quantity of formic acid detected in the urine following large doses of aspartame generated less formic acid from the aspartame than that found after consuming some fruit juices.

The second concern for aspartame is the effect of phenylalanine on individuals with phenylketonuria (PKU). PKU is a genetic condition in which children are born with a deficiency of phenylalanine hydroxylase, an enzyme that converts phenylalanine into tyrosine. A lack of this enzyme leads to higher than normal levels of phenylalanine in the blood, which leads to formation of catabolic products such as phenylpyruvate and phenyllactate. These products can result in a reduced level of tyrosine and possibly the neurotransmitters formed from tyrosine (norepinephrine and

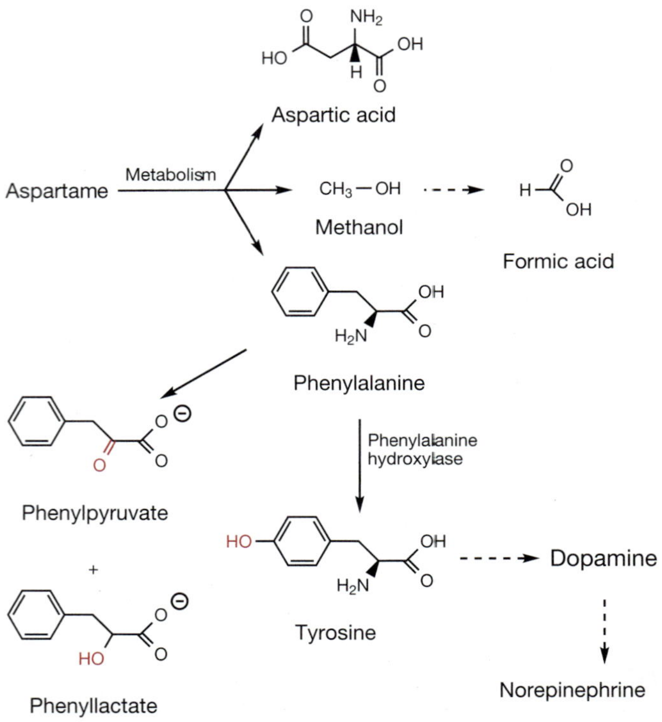

Figure 23.9 **Metabolism of aspartame and its metabolites.**

dopamine). If not diagnosed within a few days of birth, PKU can lead to CNS damage and intellectual disability. The exact cause of the intellectual disability is not known, but it is assumed that one or all of the abnormal conditions cited may have a role in PKU. Although phenylalanine is still essential in patients with PKU, a diet with low phenylalanine levels is important in the prevention of the serious outcomes of excessive phenylalanine. As a result, the consumption of aspartame by women during pregnancy and administering aspartame-containing foods to a child diagnosed with PKU have raised concerns. Studies demonstrated that abusive doses of aspartame (200 mg/kg in an adult or 100 mg/kg in a child) or successive doses of aspartame (three 10 mg/kg doses in a child) did not lead to phenylalanine levels equal to or above those approved for adults or children with PKU.[139] These studies suggested that aspartame-containing foods and beverages are unlikely to have adverse effects on patients with PKU, although there is no reason for infants with or without PKU to be using NNSs. Aspartame-containing foods contain a warning indicating its presence and its potential for harm in patients with PKU.

In 2002, an analog of aspartame, neotame was approved for marketing in the United States (see Fig. 23.8). This compound differs from aspartame by having a dimethylbutyl substituent on the nitrogen of aspartic acid. The result of this substitution is that sweetness is 30-fold greater than aspartame and 7,000- to 13,000-fold greater than sucrose. Metabolism of neotame results in formation of methanol, but significantly less phenylalanine and *N*-dimethylbutylaspartic acid. The nitrogen substitution also decreases the hydrolysis of the dipeptide, and only 20% to 30% of the neotame is absorbed, presumably as the individual amino acids.[140] Since the sweetness of neotame is so much higher than aspartame, a much lower dose would be required to meet the desired sweetness of a neotame-containing food. As a result, it is estimated that the amount of methanol absorbed after an appropriate dose of neotame is approximately 1.3 mg/L, whereas the methanol content from some juices is calculated to be approximately 140 mg/L. The amount of phenylalanine produced from neotame is estimated to be 2.6 mg/d in an adult and 1.5 mg/d in a child, whereas the restricted diet content of phenylalanine for a child with PKU is set at 0.4 to 0.6 g/d, and the average adult consumes 2.5 to 10 g/d of phenylalanine. The amount of phenylalanine obtained from a dose of neotame would have a negligible effect on a patient with PKU. Presently, there do not appear to be any food products where neotame is declared as an ingredient. This may be due, however, to the fact that the amount of neotame used does not meet the FDA's threshold for declaration on food labeling.

In 2014, a third dipeptide derivative, advantame was approved by the FDA as a nonnutritive sweetener. Advantame is considered an ultrahigh-intensity noncaloric sweetener (~20,000 times sucrose), which, because of its sweetness, is not likely to create a problem for PKU patients since the quantity of the drug absorbed and metabolized to phenylalanine would be insignificant (see Fig. 23.8). Advantame is safe and effective when used in coffee, iced tea, other beverages, chewing gum, and yogurt. The drug is rapidly absorbed (~4%-23%) as the demethylated derivative and excreted in the feces.[141]

Acesulfame-K (see Fig. 23.8)

Discovered in 1967, acesulfame-K is an NNS that is approximately 200 times sweeter than sucrose and is heat stable. Therefore, it can be used in cooking and baking (see Table 23.1). The compound is not metabolized and is structurally similar to saccharin. Acesulfame-K is commonly used in combination with other sweeteners due to its bitter aftertaste, a property it has in common with saccharin (both chemicals affect the same bitter receptor).[142] The chemical was approved for use in the United States in 1988 in dry food, and, by 2003, it was approved as a general purpose sweetener, allowing for its added use in carbonated and noncarbonated beverages.

Sucralose (see Fig. 23.8)

Sucralose is a synthetic derivative of sucrose in which three hydroxyl groups have been replaced with chlorine atoms. As a result, the compound is not metabolized by the body but retains the sweet taste of sucrose, and in fact, the sweetness is increased by approximately 600-fold. The chloride substitution, in addition to preventing the metabolism of sucralose, increases stability of the chemical to heat. Sucralose can be used in baking and cooking.[140] In 1999, sucralose was approved as a general purpose sweetener in the United States. Its general purpose use is indicative of its safety, as judged by the FDA. Recently, questions have been raised about environmental accumulation[143] of sucralose and the potential of toxic effects as well as genotoxic effects of both

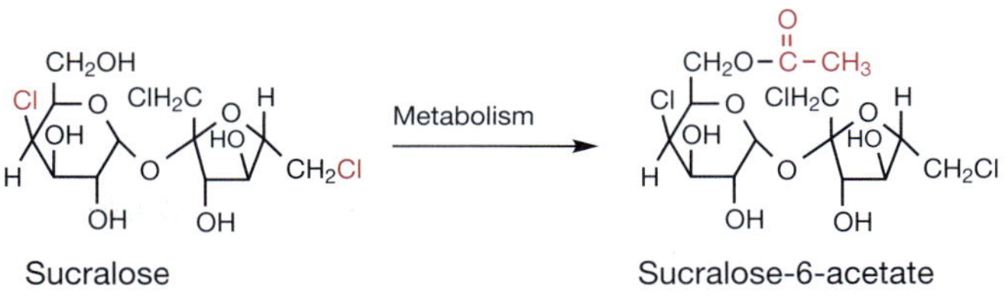

Figure 23.10 Metabolism of sucralose.

sucralose and its metabolite sucralose-6-acetate (an impurity present in sucralose products) (Fig. 23.10), leading to induction of breaks in deoxyribo nucleic acid (DNA), integrity of intestinal barrier function, intestinal epithelium inflammation, oxidative stress, and cancer.[144] Sucralose-6-acetate may also block CYP1A2 and CYP2C19, leading to potential drug-drug interactions. It should be noted that sucralose is the only NNS with a molecular structure containing carbon-chlorine components.

Rebaudioside A (Fig. 23.11)

For many centuries, the leaves of the stevia plant (*Stevia rebaudiana* Bertoni) have been used for their sweet taste,[140,145] but it is not until the last decade has commercial interest in this plant resulted in a marketed product. Two major glycosides possess much of the sweet taste: stevioside and rebaudioside A, which have been developed and introduced to the market as nonnutritive sweeteners. Rebaudioside A, known by the trade name Rebiana or Reb-A, is a diterpene glycoside that possesses a sweetness approximately 200-fold greater than sucrose (see Table 23.1) and has zero calories. As a glycoside, it is prone to acid-catalyzed hydrolysis. At low pH values, stevioside can undergo hydrolysis by intestinal bacterial flora, leading to the formation of steviol, the aglycone component of the rebiosides. Human metabolic studies on stevioside have shown that only trace amounts of stevioside can be detected in the blood, and no steviol is detected. Because steviol has been shown to exhibit positive genetic toxicology as well as the ability to induce chromosome breakage in bacteria, stevioside, stevia extracts, and, to some extent, rebaudioside A have been studied in depth for their safety.[140,145] These studies have concluded that stevioside and rebaudioside A are not genotoxic or carcinogenic in vitro or in vivo and that the only cell-damaging effects of steviol occurred in in vitro studies at excessive concentrations.

In 2008, the FDA approved inclusion of rebaudioside A in the Generally Recognized as Safe (GRAS) list as well as its use in foods and beverages as an NNS. Prior to these approvals, rebaudioside A was available in the United States as a dietary supplement. In the single-component product Truvia, erythritol (a four-carbon polyhydroxy sugar alcohol) is added as a sweetener to mask the aftertaste of licorice, which appears to be associated with rebaudioside A. Erythritol (Fig. 23.11) itself has a caloric content of 0.2 kcal/g. Rebaudioside M is presently under review for inclusion in the GRAS list. The chemical is derived from *Stevia rebaudiana* Bertoni and prepared by fermentation using a yeast from the Saccharomycetaceae family. A significant property of rebaudioside M is that it is pH stable at pH 3 to 8 and heat stable for 1 hour at a temperature of 100 °F.

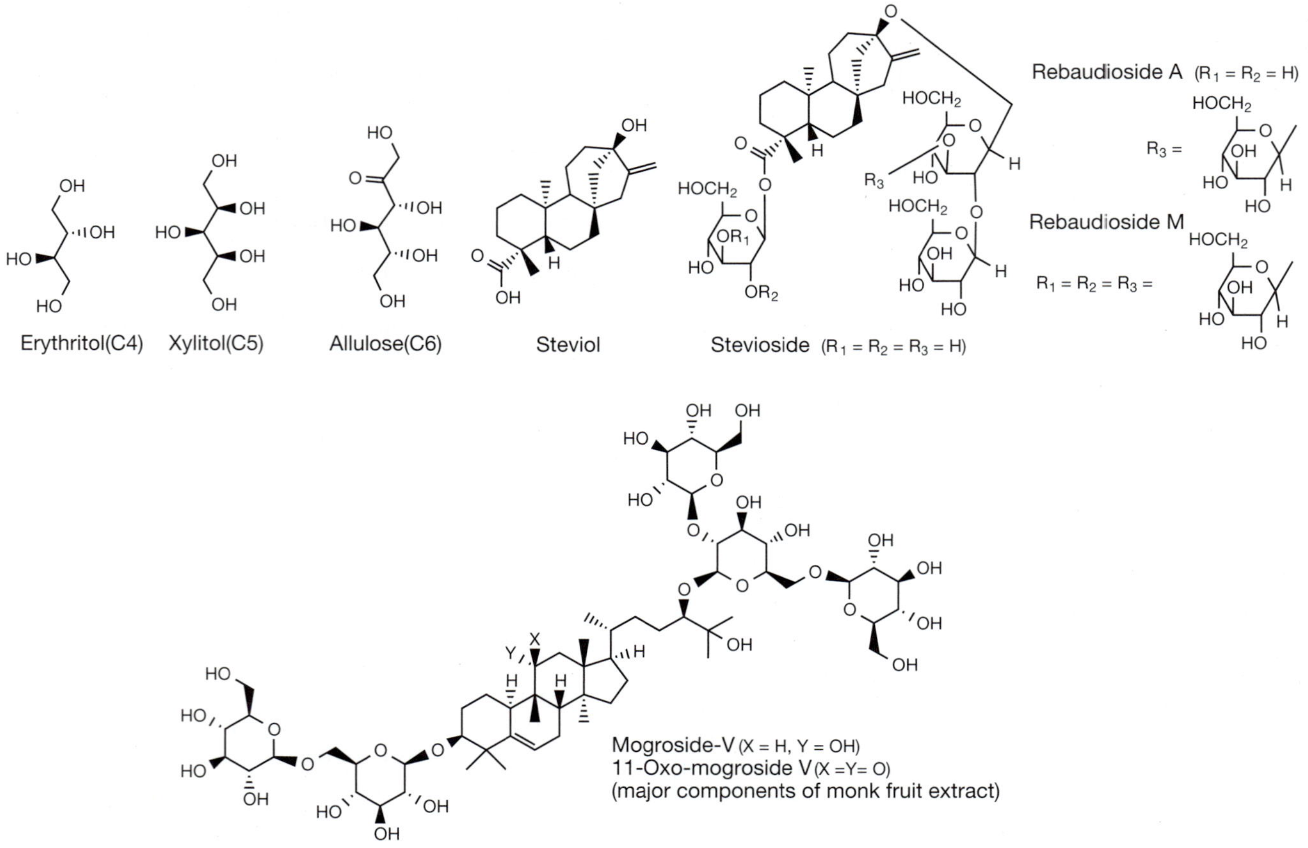

Figure 23.11 Naturally occurring nonnutritive sweeteners.

Xylitol (see Fig. 23.11)

Xylitol is a polyol (a five-carbon polyhydroxy sugar alcohol) with structural similarity to glucose and erythritol. It has been used since the 1960s as a sugar substitute with a sweetness comparable to sucrose but with 40% fewer calories (see Table 23.1). Xylitol is commonly found in chewing gums because it does not promote the development of dental caries or plaque formation and yet satisfies the need for sweetness. This property is due to the fact that the polyols are not metabolized to organic acids in the oral cavity. Xylitol can be added to the gum, and the gum can still be labeled as sugar "free."[140] Xylitol can have a laxative effect due to its poor absorption and water osmotic effect. Xylitol can be consumed by persons with diabetes, and it will not affect blood sugar levels. Xylitol is found naturally in fruits such as raspberries and plums and can be prepared by hydrogenation of xylose, which is found in corncobs and wood pulp.

Allulose (D-Psicose, see Fig. 23.11)

D-Allulose, also known as D-psicose, is the C3 epimer of D-fructose. This sugar can be formed by processing foods containing sucrose or fructose, or can be generated using a variety of strategies, including use of the D-tagatose-3-epimerase (DTEase) family of enzymes.[146] This sugar has been approved by the FDA for general use in foods and is part of the GRAS list (No. 893) of approved food ingredients.

Allulose is a polyol similar to glucose, galactose, fructose, xylitol, and erythritol, but with significantly lower caloric value yet maintaining a relatively high sweetness value (see Table 23.1). There is reason to believe that allulose substitution for the caloric sugars may contribute to anti-obesity and anti-diabetic effects. Studies support its capacity to attenuate postprandial blood glucose, among other potential benefits.[147]

Mogrosides (see Fig. 23.11)

The plant *Siraitia grosvenorii*, found commonly in China and Thailand, is an herbaceous perennial that produces a fruit known as luo han guo or the monk fruit (the fruit was used by Buddhist monks). The fruit is approximately 300 times sweeter than sugar and has been used for generations in cooling drinks and Chinese medicine (see Table 23.1). The fruit is also known as a longevity fruit and comes from Chinese provinces, which are known for their inhabitants living beyond 100 years. The fruit extract has been approved by the FDA for inclusion on the GRAS list, with no known toxicities associated with its use. The major components of the monk fruit are the mogrosides, which are triterpene glycosides. Mogroside V and 11-oxo-mogroside V are the major mogrosides possessing the sweet taste found in the monk fruit. Both of these ingredients have been reported to exhibit antioxidant properties and act as scavengers of reactive oxygen species (ROS).[148,149] In vitro studies suggest that 11-oxo-mogroside V is a more potent scavenger of ROS than mogroside V. Monk fruit has been used to treat a variety of inflammatory conditions, including acute and chronic bronchitis, gastritis, sore throats, and minor stomach and intestinal problems. While generic monk fruit products are available, the initially marketed trade name product Nectresse has been discontinued.

Brazzein and Thaumatin (see Table 23.1)

Brazzein and thaumatin II are recent additions to the GRAS list of FDA-approved substances, allowing for their addition to foods as food additives. Both proteins are considered high-intensity NNSs. Brazzein is isolated from the seed pulp of *Pentadiplandra brazzeana* fruit.[150] The 54-amino acid protein is heat stable (80 °C for 4 hours or 98 °C for 2 hours) and possesses a very intense sweet taste, with little or no aftertaste. Both brassein and thaumatin II are reported to produce their sweetness by binding to the same T1R2-T1R3 heterodimeric sweet taste receptors as reported for the other caloric and noncaloric sweeteners.

Thaumatin II is present in the jelly matrix covering the fruits of *Thaumatococcus daniellii* (Benth) plant. A mixture of sweet proteins is present in this fruit, with thaumatin I and II appearing to be the sweetest. Thaumatin II is a peptide containing 207 amino acids. Like brassein, thaumatin II exhibits thermal stability up to 100 °C. This stability appears to be associated with disulfide bridges in their structures. Thaumatin II is mostly applied as an additive in chewing gum, dairy, pet foods, and animal feeds.

Fat Substitute

Overview

Fats are neutral molecule composed of three fatty acids attached to the alcohol glycerol, thus referred to as triglycerides, and represent a storage and transport form for fatty acids. Fat must be absorbed, transported via the bloodstream either to the cells in tissue where the energy is needed, or to storage sites in adipose cells for future energy needs, and finally moved into a cell's mitochondria for metabolism, with the release of energy in the form of adenosine triphosphate (ATP) units. This process is complicated by the fact that fats themselves cannot be transported across cell membranes due to their low hydrophilicity. Rather, a sequence of hydrolysis and ester formation occurs at various stages in the absorption-transport-storage-utilization process.

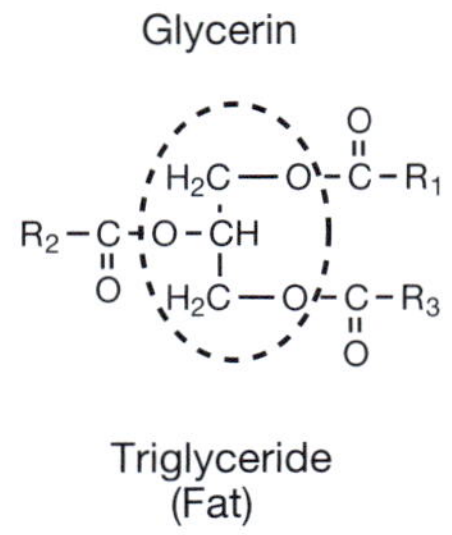

Table 23.2 Fat Substitute/Replacement Products

Carbohydrate-Based	Protein-Based	Fat-Based
Cellulose	Microparticulate protein	Triglycerides-Caprenin
Dextrins	Whey protein	Sucrose-polyesters-Olestra[a]
Grain-based		
Pectin		

[a]Approved by the FDA in 1996, marketed in 1998, and discontinued in 2015/2016 due to poor sales and unacceptable adverse effects.

Fatty acids themselves play multiple biologic roles, including components of the cell wall, usually in the form of phospholipids, glycolipids, and fatty acid acetylated proteins; a high-energy source of calories; and hormone and intracellular messengers. Unfortunately, fats and fatty acids also possess detrimental effects on the human health, and high-fat diets (especially those rich in saturated fat) are thought to increase the risk of heart disease, weight gain, and some forms of cancer.

It is estimated that 35% to 40% of the caloric intake in the United States comes in the form of fat, with greater than 90% of the fat being in the form of triglycerides (free fatty acids, cholesterol, and phospholipids represent the remaining amount of fat in the diet). This amounts to approximately 100 to 150 g/d of triglycerides. The recommended daily intake (RDI) for fat is 65 g/d consisting of 20 g/d of saturated fats and 300 mg of cholesterol. This is based on a 2,000-calorie diet for an adult. It is generally agreed that a high-fat diet (>30% of energy from fat) can induce obesity, but this is not supported by human studies, and the relationship between fat consumption and obesity is not presently clear.[151] It is generally thought that the use of fat substitutes would be beneficial in treating/reducing obesity.

Fat Substitute/Replacement Foods

Fat substitute/replacement substances are defined as foods that have a texture, taste, fewer calories, no health risks, and physical properties of fat. The fat substitutes fit into three chemical classes: carbohydrate-based, protein-based, or fat-based products (Table 23.2). Presently, there are no popular substitute/replacement foods for fats.

Structure Challenge

The following drug is beneficial in the treatment of obesity. Identify the structural components for statements 1 to 4 that were incorporated into the molecule to improve the activity of the drug.

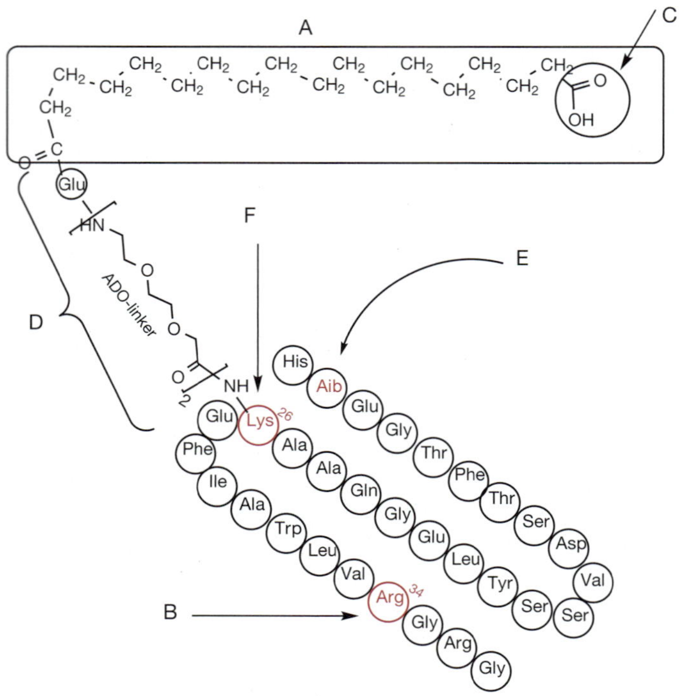

1. Region to increase drug $t_{0.5}$ by promoting albumin affinity: ______
2. Component that improves affinity to GLP-1R in the presence of albumin: _____
3. Site added to the molecule to resist rapid metabolism by DPP-IV: _____
4. Feature retained from liraglutide that assures monoacetylation: ______

Structure Challenge answers found immedictely after References.

REFERENCES

1. Boutari C, Mantzoros CS. A 2022 update on the epidemiology of obesity and a call to action: as its twin COVID-19 pandemic appears to be receding, the obesity and dysmetabolism pandemic continues to rage on. *Metabolism*. 2022;133:155217.
2. Upadhyay J, Farr O, Perakakis N, Ghaly W, Mantzoros C. Obesity as a disease. *Med Clin North Am*. 2018;102(1):13-33.
3. Chakhtoura M, Haber R, Ghezzawi M, Rhayem C, Tcheroyan R, Mantzoros CS. Pharmacotherapy of obesity: an update on the available medications and drugs under investigation. *EClinicalMedicine*. 2023;58:101882.
4. Ameye H, Swinnen J. Obesity, income and gender: the changing global relationship. *Glob Food Sec*. 2019;23:267-281.
5. Ahmad N, Adam SIM, Nawi AM, Hassan MR, Ghazi HF. Abdominal obesity indicators: waist circumference or waist-to-hip ratio in Malaysian adults population. *Int J Prev Med*. 2016;7:82.
6. Seidell JC, Pérusse L, Després JP, Bouchard C. Waist and hip circumferences have independent and opposite effects on cardiovascular disease risk factors: the Quebec Family Study. *Am J Clin Nutr*. 2001;74(3):315-321.
7. Cheng CH, Ho CC, Yang CF, Huang YC, Lai CH, Liaw YP. Waist-to-hip ratio is a better anthropometric index than body mass index for predicting the risk of type 2 diabetes in Taiwanese population. *Nutr Res*. 2010;30(9):585-593.
8. Mamtani MR, Kulkarni HR. Predictive performance of anthropometric indexes of central obesity for the risk of type 2 diabetes. *Arch Med Res*. 2005;36(5):581-589.
9. Kurpad SS, Tandon H, Srinivasan K. Waist circumference correlates better with body mass index than waist-to-hip ratio in Asian Indians. *Natl Med J India*. 2003;16(4):189-192.
10. Lear SA, James PT, Ko GT, Kumanyika S. Appropriateness of waist circumference and waist-to-hip ratio cutoffs for different ethnic groups. *Eur J Clin Nutr*. 2010;64(1):42-61.
11. Singh GM, Danaei G, Farzadfar F, et al. The age-specific quantitative effects of metabolic risk factors on cardiovascular diseases and diabetes: a pooled analysis. *PLoS One*. 2013;8(7):e65174.
12. Jiang L, Rong J, Wang Y, et al. The relationship between body mass index and hip osteoarthritis: a systematic review and meta-analysis. *Joint Bone Spine*. 2011;78(2):150-155.
13. Jiang L, Tian W, Wang Y, et al. Body mass index and susceptibility to knee osteoarthritis: a systematic review and meta-analysis. *Joint Bone Spine*. 2012;79(3):291-297.
14. Anstey KJ, Cherbuin N, Budge M, Young J. Body mass index in midlife and late-life as a risk factor for dementia: a meta-analysis of prospective studies. *Obes Rev*. 2011;12(5):e426-e437.
15. Alford S, Patel D, Perakakis N, Mantzoros CS. Obesity as a risk factor for Alzheimer's disease: weighing the evidence. *Obes Rev*. 2018;19(2):269-280.

16. Lauby-Secretan B, Scoccianti C, Loomis D, Grosse Y, Bianchini F, Straif K. Body fatness and cancer—viewpoint of the IARC Working Group. *N Engl J Med.* 2016;375(8):794-798.
17. Dai H, Alsalhe TA, Chalghaf N, Riccò M, Bragazzi NL, Wu J. The global burden of disease attributable to high body mass index in 195 countries and territories, 1990–2017: an analysis of the Global Burden of Disease study. *PLoS Med.* 2020;17(7):e1003198.
18. Bray GA, Heisel WE, Afshin A, et al. The science of obesity management: an Endocrine Society scientific statement. *Endocr Rev.* 2018;39(2):79-132.
19. Schwartz MW, Seeley RJ, Zeltser LM, et al. Obesity pathogenesis: an Endocrine Society scientific statement. *Endocr Rev.* 2017;38(4):267-296.
20. Kaly P, Orellana S, Torrella T, Takagishi C, Saff-Koche L, Murr MM. Unrealistic weight loss expectations in candidates for bariatric surgery. *Surg Obes Relat Dis.* 2008;4(1):6-10.
21. Foster GD, Wadden TA, Vogt RA, Brewer G. What is a reasonable weight loss? Patients' expectations and evaluations of obesity treatment outcomes. *J Consult Clin Psychol.* 1997;65(1):79-85.
22. Linné Y, Hemmingsson E, Adolfsson B, Ramsten J, Rössner S. Patient expectations of obesity treatment—the experience from a day-care unit. *Int J Obes Relat Metab Disord.* 2002;26(5):739-741.
23. Puhl RM, Latner JD. Stigma, obesity, and the health of the nation's children. *Psychol Bull.* 2007;133(4):557-580.
24. Anis AH, Zhang W, Bansback N, Guh DP, Amarsi Z, Birmingham CL. Obesity and overweight in Canada: an updated cost-of-illness study. *Obes Rev.* 2010;11(1):31-40.
25. Malkin JD, Baid D, Alsukait RF, et al. The economic burden of overweight and obesity in Saudi Arabia. *PLoS One.* 2022;17(3):e0264993.
26. Veiga P. Out-of-pocket health care expenditures due to excess of body weight in Portugal. *Econ Hum Biol.* 2008;6(1):127-142.
27. Ling J, Chen S, Zahry NR, Kao TSA. Economic burden of childhood overweight and obesity: a systematic review and meta-analysis. *Obes Rev.* 2023;24(2):e13535.
28. Finkelstein EA, Graham WCK, Malhotra R. Lifetime direct medical costs of childhood obesity. *Pediatrics.* 2014;133(5):854-862.
29. Cawley J, Biener A, Meyerhoefer C, et al. Direct medical costs of obesity in the United States and the most populous states. *J Manag Care Spec Pharm.* 2021;27(3):354-366.
30. Apovian CM, Aronne LJ, Bessesen DH, et al. Pharmacological management of obesity: an endocrine society clinical practice guideline. *J Clin Endocrinol Metab.* 2015;100(2):342-362.
31. Garvey WT, Mechanick JI, Brett EM, et al. American Association of Clinical Endocrinologists and American College of Endocrinology comprehensive clinical practice guidelines for medical care of patients with obesity. *Endocr Pract.* 2016;22:1-203.
32. Foucan L, Larifla L, Durand E, et al. High prevalence of rare monogenic forms of obesity in obese Guadeloupean Afro-Caribbean children. *J Clin Endocrinol Metab.* 2018;103(2):539-545.
33. Zhang Y, Proenca R, Maffei M, Barone M, Leopold L, Friedman JM. Positional cloning of the mouse obese gene and its human homologue. *Nature.* 1994;372(6505):425-432.
34. Blüher S, Mantzoros CS. Leptin in humans: lessons from translational research. *Am J Clin Nutr.* 2009;89(3):991S-997S.
35. Pierroz DD, Ziotopoulou M, Ungsunan L, Moschos S, Flier JS, Mantzoros CS. Effects of acute and chronic administration of the melanocortin agonist MTII in mice with diet-induced obesity. *Diabetes.* 2002;51(5):1337-1345.
36. Clément K, van den Akker E, Argente J, et al. Efficacy and safety of setmelanotide, an MC4R agonist, in individuals with severe obesity due to LEPR or POMC deficiency: single-arm, open-label, multicentre, phase 3 trials. *Lancet Diabetes Endocrinol.* 2020;8(12):960-970.
37. Billes SK, Sinnayah P, Cowley MA. Naltrexone/bupropion for obesity: an investigational combination pharmacotherapy for weight loss. *Pharmacol Res.* 2014;84:1-11.
38. Farr OM, Tsoukas MA, Triantafyllou G, et al. Short-term administration of the GLP-1 analog liraglutide decreases circulating leptin and increases GIP levels and these changes are associated with alterations in CNS responses to food cues: a randomized, placebo-controlled, crossover study. *Metabolism.* 2016;65(7):945-953.
39. Farr OM, Upadhyay J, Rutagengwa C, et al. Longer-term liraglutide administration at the highest dose approved for obesity increases reward-related orbitofrontal cortex activation in response to food cues: implications for plateauing weight loss in response to anti-obesity therapies. *Diabetes Obes Metab.* 2019;21(11):2459-2464.
40. Gabery S, Salinas CG, Paulsen SJ, et al. Semaglutide lowers body weight in rodents via distributed neural pathways. *JCI Insight.* 2020;5(6):e133429.
41. Husum H, Van Kammen D, Termeer E, Bolwig G, Mathé A. Topiramate normalizes hippocampal NPY-LI in flinders sensitive line "depressed" rats and upregulates NPY, galanin, and CRH-LI in the hypothalamus: implications for mood-stabilizing and weight loss-inducing effects. *Neuropsychopharmacology.* 2003;28(7):1292-1299.
42. Johnson BA. Progress in the development of topiramate for treating alcohol dependence: from a hypothesis to a proof-of-concept study. *Alcohol Clin Exp Res.* 2004;28(8):1137-1144.
43. Rabiner EA, Beaver J, Makwana A, et al. Pharmacological differentiation of opioid receptor antagonists by molecular and functional imaging of target occupancy and food reward-related brain activation in humans. *Mol Psychiatry.* 2011;16(8):826-835.
44. Wang GJ, Tomasi D, Volkow ND, et al. Effect of combined naltrexone and bupropion therapy on the brain's reactivity to food cues. *Int J Obes (Lond).* 2014;38(5):682-688.
45. Wang GJ, Zhao J, Tomasi D, et al. Effect of combined naltrexone and bupropion therapy on the brain's functional connectivity. *Int J Obes (Lond).* 2018;42(11):1890-1899.
46. Baumann MH, Ayestas MA, Dersch CM, Brockington A, Rice KC, Rothman RB. Effects of phentermine and fenfluramine on extracellular dopamine and serotonin in rat nucleus accumbens: therapeutic implications. *Synapse.* 2000;36(2):102-113.
47. Nelson DL, Gehlert DR. Central nervous system biogenic amine targets for control of appetite and energy expenditure. *Endocrine.* 2006;29(1):49-60.
48. Tek C. Naltrexone HCl/bupropion HCl for chronic weight management in obese adults: patient selection and perspectives. *Patient Prefer Adherence.* 2016;10:751-759.
49. Jepsen MM, Christensen MB. Emerging glucagon-like peptide 1 receptor agonists for the treatment of obesity. *Expert Opin Emerg Drugs.* 2021;26(3):231-243.
50. Yanovski SZ, Yanovski JA. Long-term drug treatment for obesity: a systematic and clinical review. *JAMA.* 2014;311(1):74-86.
51. Brown RJ, Rother KI. Clinical review: non-nutritive sweeteners and their role in the gastrointestinal tract. *J Clin Endocrinol Metab.* 2012;97(8):2597.
52. Cone RD, Lu D, Koppula S, et al. The melanocortin receptors: agonists, antagonists, and the hormonal control of pigmentation. *Recent Prog Horm Res.* 1996;51:287-317; discussion 318.
53. Hadley ME, Hruby VJ, Jiang J, et al. Melanocortin receptors: identification and characterization by melanotropic peptide agonists and antagonists. *Pigment Cell Res.* 1996;9(5):213-234.
54. Farooqi IS, Keogh JM, Yeo GSH, Lank EJ, Cheetham T, O'Rahilly S. Clinical spectrum of obesity and mutations in the melanocortin 4 receptor gene. *N Engl J Med.* 2003;348(12):1085-1095.
55. Garfield AS, Li C, Madara JC, et al. A neural basis for melanocortin-4 receptor-regulated appetite. *Nat Neurosci.* 2015;18(6):863-871.
56. Fan W, Boston BA, Kesterson RA, Hruby VJ, Cone RD. Role of melanocortinergic neurons in feeding and the agouti obesity syndrome. *Nature.* 1997;385(6612):165-168.
57. Fan W, Dinulescu DM, Butler AA, Zhou J, Marks DL, Cone RD. The central melanocortin system can directly regulate serum insulin levels. *Endocrinology.* 2000;141(9):3072-3079.

58. Murphy B, Nunes CN, Ronan JJ, et al. Melanocortin mediated inhibition of feeding behavior in rats. *Neuropeptides*. 1998;32(6):491-497.
59. Govaerts C, Srinivasan S, Shapiro A, et al. Obesity-associated mutations in the melanocortin 4 receptor provide novel insights into its function. *Peptides*. 2005;26(10):1909-1919.
60. Santini F, Maffei M, Pelosini C, et al. Melanocortin-4 receptor mutations in obesity. *Advan Clin Chem*. 2009;48:95-109
61. Falls BA, Zhang Y. Insights into the allosteric mechanism of setmelanotide (RM-493) as a potent and first-in-class melanocortin-4 receptor (MC4R) agonist to treat rare genetic disorders of obesity through an in silico approach. *ACS Chem Neurosci*. 2019;10(3):1055-1065.
62. Nargund RP, Strack AM, Fong TM. Melanocortin-4 receptor (MC4R) agonists for the treatment of obesity. *J Med Chem*. 2006; 49(14):4035-4043.
63. Yang YK, Fong TM, Dickinson CJ, et al. Molecular determinants of ligand binding to the human melanocortin-4 receptor. *Biochemistry*. 2000;39(48):14900-14911.
64. Chapman KL, Kinsella GK, Cox A, Donnelly D, Findlay JBC. Interactions of the melanocortin-4 receptor with the peptide agonist NDP-MSH. *J Mol Biol*. 2010;401(3):433-450.
65. Holder JR, Bauzo RM, Xiang Z, Haskell-Luevano C. Structure—activity relationships of the melanocortin tetrapeptide Ac-His-DPhe-Arg-Trp-NH2 at the mouse melanocortin receptors. 1. Modifications at the His position. *J Med Chem*. 2002;45(13): 2801-2810.
66. Hruby VJ, Cai M, Cain J, Nyberg J, Trivedi D. Design of novel melanocortin receptor ligands: multiple receptors, complex pharmacology, the challenge. *Eur J Pharmacol*. 2011;660(1):88-93.
67. Pogozheva ID, Chai BX, Lomize AL, et al. Interactions of human melanocortin 4 receptor with nonpeptide and peptide agonists. *Biochemistry*. 2005;44(34):11329-11341.
68. Roubert P, Dubern B, Plas P, et al. Novel pharmacological MC4R agonists can efficiently activate mutated MC4R from obese patient with impaired endogenous agonist response. *J Endocrinol*. 2010; 207(2):177-183.
69. Sawyer TK, Sanfilippo PJ, Hruby VJ, et al. 4-Norleucine, 7-D-phenylalanine-alpha-melanocyte-stimulating hormone: a highly potent alpha-melanotropin with ultralong biological activity. *Proc Natl Acad Sci U S A*. 1980;77(10):5754-5758.
70. Tan K, Pogozheva ID, Yeo GSH, et al. Functional characterization and structural modeling of obesity associated mutations in the melanocortin 4 receptor. *Endocrinology*. 2009;150(1):114-125.
71. Frederich RC, Hamann A, Anderson S, Löllmann B, Lowell BB, Flier JS. Leptin levels reflect body lipid content in mice: evidence for diet-induced resistance to leptin action. *Nat Med*. 1995;1(12): 1311-1314.
72. Moon HS, Dalamaga M, Kim SY, et al. Leptin's role in lipodystrophic and nonlipodystrophic insulin-resistant and diabetic individuals. *Endocr Rev*. 2013;34(3):377-412.
73. Münzberg H, Morrison CD. Structure, production and signaling of leptin. *Metabolism*. 2015;64(1):13-23.
74. Meehan CA, Cochran E, Kassai A, Brown RJ, Gorden P. Metreleptin for injection to treat the complications of leptin deficiency in patients with congenital or acquired generalized lipodystrophy. *Expert Rev Clin Pharmacol*. 2016;9(1):59-68.
75. Gorden P, Lupsa BC, Chong AY, Lungu AO. Is there a human model for the "metabolic syndrome" with a defined aetiology? *Diabetologia*. 2010;53(7):1534-1536.
76. Heymsfield SB, Greenberg AS, Fujioka K, et al. Recombinant leptin for weight loss in obese and lean adults: a randomized, controlled, dose-escalation trial. *JAMA*. 1999;282(16):1568-1575.
77. Perakakis N, Farr OM, Mantzoros CS. Leptin in leanness and obesity: JACC state-of-the-art review. *J Am Coll Cardiol*. 2021;77(6):745-760.
78. Polyzos SA, Mantzoros CS. Metreleptin for the treatment of lipodystrophy: leading the way among novel therapeutics for this unmet clinical need. *Curr Med Res Opin*. 2022;38(6):885-888.
79. Nauck MA, Heimesaat MM, Orskov C, Holst JJ, Ebert R, Creutzfeldt W. Preserved incretin activity of glucagon-like peptide 1 [7-36 amide] but not of synthetic human gastric inhibitory polypeptide in patients with type-2 diabetes mellitus. *J Clin Invest*. 1993;91(1):301-307.
80. Adelhorst K, Hedegaard BB, Knudsen LB, Kirk O. Structure-activity studies of glucagon-like peptide-1. *J Biol Chem*. 1994;269(9):6275-6278.
81. Knudsen LB, Lau J. The discovery and development of liraglutide and semaglutide. *Front Endocrinol*. 2019;10:155. Accessed June 5, 2023.
82. Andersen JT, Dalhus B, Cameron J, et al. Structure-based mutagenesis reveals the albumin-binding site of the neonatal Fc receptor. *Nat Commun*. 2012;3(1):610.
83. Kurtzhals P, Havelund S, Jonassen I, Markussen J. Effect of fatty acids and selected drugs on the albumin binding of a long-acting, acylated insulin analogue. *J Pharm Sci*. 1997;86(12):1365-1368.
84. Jensen L, Kupcova V, Arold G, Pettersson J, Hjerpsted JB. Pharmacokinetics and tolerability of semaglutide in people with hepatic impairment. *Diabetes Obes Metab*. 2018;20(4):998-1005.
85. Madsen K, Knudsen LB, Agersoe H, et al. Structure—activity and protraction relationship of long-acting glucagon-like peptide-1 derivatives: importance of fatty acid length, polarity, and bulkiness. *J Med Chem*. 2007;50(24):6126-6132.
86. Deacon CF, Nauck MA, Toft-Nielsen M, Pridal L, Willms B, Holst JJ. Both subcutaneously and intravenously administered glucagon-like peptide I are rapidly degraded from the NH2-terminus in type II diabetic patients and in healthy subjects. *Diabetes*. 1995;44(9):1126-1131.
87. Lau J, Bloch P, Schäffer L, et al. Discovery of the once-weekly glucagon-like peptide-1 (GLP-1) analogue semaglutide. *J Med Chem*. 2015;58(18):7370-7380.
88. Jensen L, Helleberg H, Roffel A, et al. Absorption, metabolism and excretion of the GLP-1 analogue semaglutide in humans and nonclinical species. *Eur J Pharm Sci*. 2017;104:31-41.
89. Courrèges JP, Vilsbøll T, Zdravkovic M, et al. Beneficial effects of once-daily liraglutide, a human glucagon-like peptide-1 analogue, on cardiovascular risk biomarkers in patients with type 2 diabetes. *Diabet Med*. 2008;25(9):1129-1131.
90. Buckley ST, Bμkdal TA, Vegge A, et al. Transcellular stomach absorption of a derivatized glucagon-like peptide-1 receptor agonist. *Sci Transl Med*. 2018;10(467):eaar7047.
91. Fukuda M. The role of GIP receptor in the CNS for the pathogenesis of obesity. *Diabetes*. 2021;70(9):1929-1937.
92. Yu Y, Hu G, Yin S, Yang X, Zhou M, Jian W. Optimal dose of tirzepatide for type 2 diabetes mellitus: a meta-analysis and trial sequential analysis. *Front Cardiovasc Med*. 2022;9:990182.
93. Wang L. Designing a dual GLP-1R/GIPR agonist from tirzepatide: comparing residues between tirzepatide, GLP-1, and GIP. *Drug Des Devel Ther*. 2022;16:1547-1559.
94. Coskun T, Sloop KW, Loghin C, et al. LY3298176, a novel dual GIP and GLP-1 receptor agonist for the treatment of type 2 diabetes mellitus: from discovery to clinical proof of concept. *Mol Metab*. 2018;18:3-14.
95. Sun B, Willard FS, Feng D, et al. Structural determinants of dual incretin receptor agonism by tirzepatide. *Proc Natl Acad Sci*. 2022;119(13):e2116506119.
96. Østergaard S, Paulsson JF, Kofoed J, et al. The effect of fatty diacid acylation of human $PYY_{3\text{-}36}$ on Y_2 receptor potency and half-life in minipigs. *Sci Rep*. 2021;11(1):21179.
97. Wharton S, Blevins T, Connery L, et al. Daily oral GLP-1 receptor agonist orforglipron for adults with obesity. *N Engl J Med*. 2023;389(10): 877-888.
98. Kawai T, Sun B, Yoshino H, et al. Structural basis for GLP-1 receptor activation by LY3502970, an orally active nonpeptide agonist. *Proc Natl Acad Sci U S A*. 2020;117(47):29959-29967.
99. Rosenstock J, Frias J, Jastreboff AM, et al. Retatrutide, a GIP, GLP-1 and glucagon receptor agonist, for people with type 2 diabetes: a randomised, double-blind, placebo and active-controlled, parallel-group, phase 2 trial conducted in the USA. *Lancet*. 2023;402(10401):529-544.

100. Coskun T, Urva S, Roell WC, et al. LY3437943, a novel triple glucagon, GIP, and GLP-1 receptor agonist for glycemic control and weight loss: from discovery to clinical proof of concept. *Cell Metab*. 2022;34(9):1234-1247.e9.
101. Blumberg H, Dayton HB. Naloxone, naltrexone, and related noroxymorphones. *Adv Biochem Psychopharmacol*. 1973;8(0):33-43.
102. Froehlich J, O'Malley S, Hyytiä P, Davidson D, Farren C. Preclinical and clinical studies on naltrexone: what have they taught each other? *Alcohol Clin Exp Res*. 2003;27(3):533-539.
103. Selfridge BR, Wang X, Zhang Y, et al. Structure-activity relationships of (+)-naltrexone-inspired Toll-like receptor 4 (TLR4) antagonists. *J Med Chem*. 2015;58(12):5038-5052.
104. Levine AS, Billington CJ. Opioids as agents of reward-related feeding: a consideration of the evidence. *Physiol Behav*. 2004;82(1):57-61.
105. Musso DL, Mehta NB, Soroko FE, Ferris RM, Hollingsworth EB, Kenney BT. Synthesis and evaluation of the antidepressant activity of the enantiomers of bupropion. *Chirality*. 1993;5(7):495-500.
106. Sutton C, Williams EQ, Homsi H, et al. Structure-activity relationships of dopamine transporter pharmacological chaperones. *Front Cell Neurosci*. 2022;16:832536. Accessed June 7, 2023. https://www.frontiersin.org/articles/10.3389/fncel.2022.832536
107. Narayanaswami V, Dwoskin LP. Obesity: current and potential pharmacotherapeutics and targets. *Pharmacol Ther*. 2017;170:116-147.
108. Singh J, Kumar R. Phentermine-topiramate: first combination drug for obesity. *Int J Appl Basic Med Res*. 2015;5(2):157-158.
109. Bray GA. Drug insight: appetite suppressants. *Nat Clin Pract Gastroenterol Hepatol*. 2005;2(2):89-95.
110. Skopp G, Jantos R. Phentermine—a "weighty" or a dangerous substance? *Arch Kriminol*. 2013;231(3-4):116-129.
111. Alexander M, Rothman RB, Baumann MH, Endres CJ, Brasić JR, Wong DF. Noradrenergic and dopaminergic effects of (+)-amphetamine-like stimulants in the baboon *Papio anubis*. *Synapse*. 2005;56(2):94-99.
112. Dodgson SJ, Shank RP, Maryanoff BE. Topiramate as an inhibitor of carbonic anhydrase isoenzymes. *Epilepsia*. 2000;41(S1):35-39.
113. Allison DB, Gadde KM, Garvey WT, et al. Controlled-release phentermine/topiramate in severely obese adults: a randomized controlled trial (EQUIP). *Obesity (Silver Spring)*. 2012;20(2):330-342.
114. Maryanoff BE, Costanzo MJ, Nortey SO, et al. Structure−activity studies on anticonvulsant sugar sulfamates related to topiramate. Enhanced potency with cyclic sulfate derivatives. *J Med Chem*. 1998;41(8):1315-1343.
115. Hadváry P, Lengsfeld H, Wolfer H. Inhibition of pancreatic lipase in vitro by the covalent inhibitor tetrahydrolipstatin. *Biochem J*. 1988;256(2):357-361.
116. Hadváry P, Sidler W, Meister W, Vetter W, Wolfer H. The lipase inhibitor tetrahydrolipstatin binds covalently to the putative active site serine of pancreatic lipase. *J Biol Chem*. 1991;266(4):2021-2027.
117. Heck AM, Yanovski JA, Calis KA. Orlistat, a new lipase inhibitor for the management of obesity. *Pharmacotherapy*. 2000; 20(3):270-279.
118. Padwal R, Li SK, Lau DCW. Long-term pharmacotherapy for obesity and overweight. *Cochrane Database Syst Rev*. 2004;2003(3): CD004094.
119. Fleckenstein AE, Volz TJ, Riddle EL, Gibb JW, Hanson GR. New insights into the mechanism of action of amphetamines. *Annu Rev Pharmacol Toxicol*. 2007;47:681-698.
120. Nathanson MH. The central action of betaaminopropylbenzene (Benzedrine): clinical observations. *J Am Med Assoc*. 1937;108(7):528-531.
121. Heal DJ, Smith SL, Gosden J, Nutt DJ. Amphetamine, past and present—a pharmacological and clinical perspective. *J Psychopharmacol*. 2013;27(6):479-496.
122. Coulter AA, Rebello CJ, Greenway FL. Centrally acting drugs for obesity: past, present, and future. *Drugs*. 2018;78(11):1113-1132.
123. Inoue T, Yasuda T, Suzuki S, Kishi T, Niwaguchi T. The metabolism of 1-phenyl-2-(*N*-methyl-*N*-furfurylamino)propane (furfenorex) in the rat in vivo and in vitro. *Xenobiotica*. 1986;16(2): 109-121.
124. Rothman RB, Baumann MH. Therapeutic potential of monoamine transporter substrates. *Curr Top Med Chem*. 2006;6(17): 1845-1859.
125. Banks ML, Snyder RW, Fennell TR, Negus SS. Role of *d*-amphetamine and *d*-methamphetamine as active metabolites of benzphetamine: evidence from drug discrimination and pharmacokinetic studies in male rhesus monkeys. *Pharmacol Biochem Behav*. 2017;156:30-38.
126. Bhatt DL, Steg PG, Miller M, et al. Cardiovascular risk reduction with icosapent ethyl for hypertriglyceridemia. *N Engl J Med*. 2019;380(1):11-22.
127. Oscarsson J, Hurt-Camejo E. Omega-3 fatty acids eicosapentaenoic acid and docosahexaenoic acid and their mechanisms of action on apolipoprotein B-containing lipoproteins in humans: a review. *Lipids Health Dis*. 2017;16(1):149.
128. Ackman RG. The absorption of fish oils and concentrates. *Lipids*. 1992;27(11):858-862.
129. Braeckman RA, Stirtan WG, Soni PN. Pharmacokinetics of eicosapentaenoic acid in plasma and red blood cells after multiple oral dosing with icosapent ethyl in healthy subjects. *Clin Pharmacol Drug Dev*. 2014;3(2):101-108.
130. Shirley M. Triheptanoin: first approval. *Drugs*. 2020;80(15): 1595-1600.
131. Prinz P. The role of dietary sugars in health: molecular composition or just calories? *Eur J Clin Nutr*. 2019;73(9):1216-1223.
132. Sylvetsky AC, Rother KI. Nonnutritive sweeteners in weight management and chronic disease: a review. *Obesity (Silver Spring)*. 2018;26(4):635-640.
133. Fernstrom JD. Non-nutritive sweeteners and obesity. *Annu Rev Food Sci Technol*. 2015;6:119-136.
134. McGlynn ND, Khan TA, Wang L, et al. Association of low- and no-calorie sweetened beverages as a replacement for sugar-sweetened beverages with body weight and cardiometabolic risk: a systematic review and meta-analysis. *JAMA Netw Open*. 2022;5(3):e222092.
135. Li X, Staszewski L, Xu H, Durick K, Zoller M, Adler E. Human receptors for sweet and umami taste. *Proc Natl Acad Sci U S A*. 2002;99(7):4692-4696.
136. Nelson G, Chandrashekar J, Hoon MA, et al. An amino-acid taste receptor. *Nature*. 2002;416(6877):199-202.
137. De La Pena C. *Empty Pleasures: The Story of Artificial Sweeteners from Saccharin to Splenda*. The University of North Carolina Press; 2010:296.
138. Whysner J, Williams GM. Saccharin mechanistic data and risk assessment: urine composition, enhanced cell proliferation, and tumor promotion. *Pharmacol Ther*. 1996;71(1-2):225-252.
139. Stegink LD. The aspartame story: a model for the clinical testing of a food additive. *Am J Clin Nutr*. 1987;46(1 Suppl):204-215.
140. Kroger M, Meister K, Kava R. Low-calorie sweeteners and other sugar substitutes: a review of the safety issues. *Compr Rev Food Sci Food Saf*. 2006;5(2):35-47.
141. Otabe A, Fujieda T, Masuyama T, Ubukata K, Lee C. Advantame—an overview of the toxicity data. *Food Chem Toxicol*. 2011;49(Suppl 1):S2-S7.
142. Kuhn C, Bufe B, Winnig M, et al. Bitter taste receptors for saccharin and acesulfame K. *J Neurosci*. 2004;24(45):10260-10265.
143. Heredia-García G, Gómez-Oliván LM, Orozco-Hernández JM, et al. Alterations to DNA, apoptosis and oxidative damage induced by sucralose in blood cells of *Cyprinus carpio*. *Sci Total Environ*. 2019;692:411-421.
144. Schiffman SS, Scholl EH, Furey TS, Nagle HT. Toxicological and pharmacokinetic properties of sucralose-6-acetate and its parent sucralose: in vitro screening assays. *J Toxicol Environ Health B Crit Rev*. 2023;26:307-341.
145. Brusick DJ. A critical review of the genetic toxicity of steviol and steviol glycosides. *Food Chem Toxicol*. 2008;46(Suppl 7):S83-S91.

146. Wang Y, Ravikumar Y, Zhang G, et al. Biocatalytic synthesis of D-allulose using novel D-tagatose 3-epimerase from *Christensenella minuta*. *Front Chem*. 2020;8:622325.
147. Franchi F, Yaranov DM, Rollini F, et al. Effects of D-allulose on glucose tolerance and insulin response to a standard oral sucrose load: results of a prospective, randomized, crossover study. *BMJ Open Diabetes Res Care*. 2021;9(1):e001939.
148. Shi H, Hiramatsu M, Komatsu M, Kayama T. Antioxidant property of Fructus Momordicae extract. *Biochem Mol Biol Int*. 1996;40(6):1111-1121.
149. Chen WJ, Wang J, Qi XY, Xie BJ. The antioxidant activities of natural sweeteners, mogrosides, from fruits of *Siraitia grosvenorii*. *Int J Food Sci Nutr*. 2007;58(7):548-556.
150. Farag MA, Rezk MM, Hamdi Elashal M, El-Araby M, Khalifa SAM, El-Seedi HR. An updated multifaceted overview of sweet proteins and dipeptides as sugar substitutes; the chemistry, health benefits, gut interactions, and safety. *Food Res Int*. 2022;162(Pt A): 111853.
151. Hariri N, Thibault L. High-fat diet-induced obesity in animal models. *Nutr Res Rev*. 2010;23(2):270-299.

Structure Challenge Answers

1. A; 2. D; 3. E, 4. B

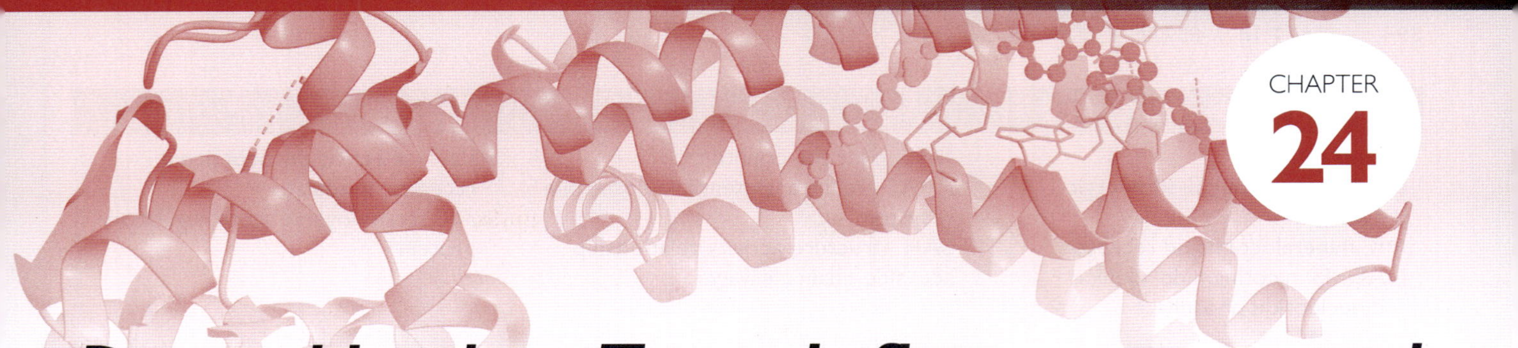

CHAPTER 24

Drugs Used to Treat Inflammatory and Corticosteroid Deficiency Disorders

Michael L. Mohler, Ramesh Narayanan, and James T. Dalton

Drugs covered in this chapter:

GLUCOCORTICOSTEROIDS

- Betamethasone
- Cortisone
- Deflazacort
- Dexamethasone
- Fludrocortisone
- Hydrocortisone
- Methylprednisolone
- Prednisolone
- Prednisone
- Triamcinolone
- Vamorolone

GLUCOCORTICOSTEROIDS USED TOPICALLY OR FOR INHALATION

- Alclometasone dipropionate
- Amcinonide
- Beclomethasone dipropionate
- Budesonide
- Ciclesonide
- Clobetasol propionate
- Clocortolone pivalate
- Desonide
- Desoximetasone
- Diflorasone diacetate
- Flunisolide
- Fluocinolone acetonide
- Fluocinonide
- Fluorometholone
- Flurandrenolide
- Fluticasone propionate
- Halcinonide
- Halobetasol propionate
- Loteprednol etabonate
- Mometasone furoate
- Prednicarbate
- Triamcinolone acetonide

MINERALOCORTICOSTEROIDS

- 11-Desoxycorticosterone
- Aldosterone

ADRENOCORTICOID ANTAGONISTS

- Aminoglutethimide
- Eplerenone
- Finerenone
- Metyrapone
- Mifepristone
- Osilodrostat
- Spironolactone
- Trilostane
- Ulipristal

Abbreviations

ACTH adrenocorticotropic hormone
AKR1C3 aldoketoreductase type 1C3
AUC area under the (plasma concentration over time) curve
BDP beclomethasone dipropionate
17-BMP beclomethasone 17α-monopropionate
21-BMP beclomethasone 21-monopropionate
cAMP cyclic adenosine monophosphate
CoA coactivator
CFC chlorofluorocarbon
COPD chronic obstructive pulmonary disease
CoR corepressor
CRF corticotropin-releasing factor
CYP11B2 11β-hydroxylase
CYP17 17α-hydroxylase
CYP21 21-hydroxylase
DED dry eye disease
des-CIC desisobutyrylciclesonide
21-desDFZ 21-desacetyldeflazacort
DHEA dehydroepiandrosterone
DHT 5α-dihydrotestosterone
DMD Duchenne muscular dystrophy
DME diabetic macular edema
DNA deoxyribonucleic acid
DPI dry powder inhaler
EDS exhalation delivery system
FDA US Food and Drug Administration
GI gastrointestinal
GR glucocorticoid receptor
HFA hydrofluoroalkane
HPA hypothalamic-pituitary-adrenal
HRE hormone response element
3β-HSD 5-ene-3β-hydroxysteroid dehydrogenase
11β-HSD1 type 1 11β-hydroxysteroid dehydrogenase
11β-HSD2 type 2 11β-hydroxysteroid dehydrogenase
17β-HSD3 17β-hydroxysteroid dehydrogenase type 3
17β-HSD5 17β-hydroxysteroid dehydrogenase type 5
HSP heat-shock protein
IL interleukin
IM intramuscular

Abbreviations—continued

IV intravenous
LABA long-acting β-adrenergic agonist
MR mineralocorticoid receptor
NADPH nicotinamide adenine dinucleotide phosphate
OTC over the counter
RAAS renin–angiotensin–aldosterone system
SAR structure-activity relationship
scc side-chain cleavage
SGRM selective glucocorticoid receptor modulator
StAR steroidogenic acute regulatory protein

CLINICAL SIGNIFICANCE

Steroids are widely used in patients for a variety of conditions, and understanding the chemical structure helps direct practitioners' choice of agent. The activity of these medications in the body is largely dependent on the type of receptor activated (glucocorticoid or mineralocorticoid), and the structure of these medications distinguishes the extent of receptor activation. Hydrocortisone is a glucocorticoid, but the absence of mineralocorticoid-abolishing functional groups permits interaction with both glucocorticoid and mineralocorticoid receptors (MRs). This allows adrenal insufficiency in a patient who may not be endogenously making steroids to be managed on one medication instead of treating it with both a glucocorticoid and mineralocorticoid separately.

Emily L. Knezevich, PharmD, BCPS, CDCES, FCCP

INTRODUCTION

The adrenal glands are flattened, cap-like structures located above the kidneys. The inner core (medulla) of the gland secretes catecholamines, whereas the shell (cortex) of the gland synthesizes steroid hormones known as the adrenocorticoids. The adrenocorticoid steroids include the glucocorticoids, which regulate carbohydrate, lipid, and protein metabolism, and the mineralocorticoids, which influence salt balance and water retention. A third class of steroids produced by the adrenal glands is the adrenal androgens, which have a weak androgenic activity in men and women and can serve as precursors to the sex hormones, estrogens, and androgens.

The adrenocorticoids and sex hormones have much in common. All are steroids; consequently, the rules that define their structures, chemistry, and nomenclature are the same. The rings of these biochemically dynamic and physiologically active compounds have a similar stereochemical relationship. Changes in the geometry of the ring junctures usually result in inactive compounds regardless of the biologic category of the steroid. Similar chemical groups are used to render some of these agents water soluble, or active when taken orally, or to modify their absorption.

In addition, the adrenocorticoids and the sex hormones, which include the estrogens, progestins, and androgens (Chapter 25), are mainly biosynthesized from cholesterol, which in turn is synthesized from acetyl–coenzyme A. Cholesterol and steroid hormone catabolism takes place primarily in the liver. Although the products found in the urine and feces depend on the hormone undergoing catabolism, many of the metabolic reactions are similar for these compounds. For example, reduction of double bonds at positions 4 and 5 or 5 and 6, epimerization of 3α-hydroxyl groups, reduction of 3-keto groups to the 3α-hydroxyl function, and oxidative removal of side chains are transformations common to these agents.

The adrenocorticoids have many clinical uses. Glucocorticoids and mineralocorticoids may be used for the treatment of endocrine disorders such as adrenal insufficiency (hypoadrenalism), which results from failure of the adrenal glands to synthesize adequate amounts of the hormones. Major pharmacologic uses of glucocorticoids include the treatment of rheumatoid diseases, acute exacerbations of diseases of the gastrointestinal (GI), nervous, or respiratory systems, symptomatic relief from asthma and allergic conditions, topical application for various dermatologic and ophthalmic diseases, and various hematologic disorders and cancers. Toxicities arise when corticosteroids are used for longer than brief periods, and toxic effects can include glucocorticoid-induced adrenocortical insufficiency, glucocorticoid-induced osteoporosis and diabetes, and generalized protein depletion. Knowledge of the numerous steroid products, structure-activity relationships (SARs), and available dosage forms is necessary in order to maximize the benefits of these drugs for patients and minimize troublesome toxicities.

Despite the similarities in chemical structures and stereochemistry, each class of steroids demonstrates unique and distinctively pleotropic biologic activities. Minor structural modifications to the steroid nucleus, such as changes in or insertion of functional groups at different positions, cause marked changes in physiologic activity. The first part of this chapter focuses on the similarities among the steroids and reviews steroid nomenclature, stereochemistry, and general mechanism of action. The second portion of the chapter focuses on the adrenocorticoids and discusses the biosynthesis, metabolism, medicinal chemistry, pharmacology, and pharmacokinetics of endogenous steroid hormones and synthetic agonists and antagonists, whether steroidal or nonsteroidal agents.

Steroid Nomenclature and Structure

Steroids consist of four fused rings (A, B, C, and D; Fig. 24.1). Chemically, these hydrocarbons are cyclopentanoperhydrophenanthrenes; they contain a five-membered cyclopentane (D) ring plus the three rings of phenanthrene. A perhydrophenanthrene (rings A, B, and C) is the completely saturated derivative of phenanthrene. The polycyclic hydrocarbon known as cholestane will be used to illustrate the numbering system for a steroid (Fig. 24.1). The term "cholestane" refers to a steroid with 27 carbons that includes a side chain of eight carbons at position 17. Numbering begins in ring A at C1 and proceeds around rings A and B to C10, then into ring C beginning with C11, and snakes around rings C and D to C17. The angular methyl groups are numbered 18 (attached to C13) and 19 (attached to C10). Steroid chemists often refer to the series of carbon–carbon bonds from C1-C19 as the steroid backbone or template (Fig. 24.1). The 17-side chain begins with C20, and the numbering finishes in sequential order.

Using the rigid planar representation for drawing the steroid structure (Fig. 24.2A), the basic steroid structure becomes a plane with two surfaces: The top or β surface is pointing out toward the reader, and the bottom or α surface is pointing away from the reader. Hydrogens or functional groups on the β side of the molecule are denoted by solid lines; those on the α side are designated by dotted lines. The 5α notation is used to denote the configuration of the hydrogen atom at C5, which is opposite from the C19 angular methyl group, making the A/B ring juncture *trans* (Fig. 24.2B). The C19 angular methyl group is assigned the

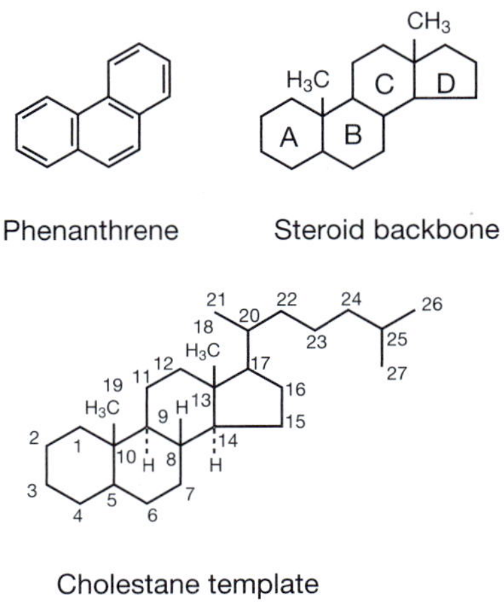

Figure 24.1 Basic steroid structure and numbering system.

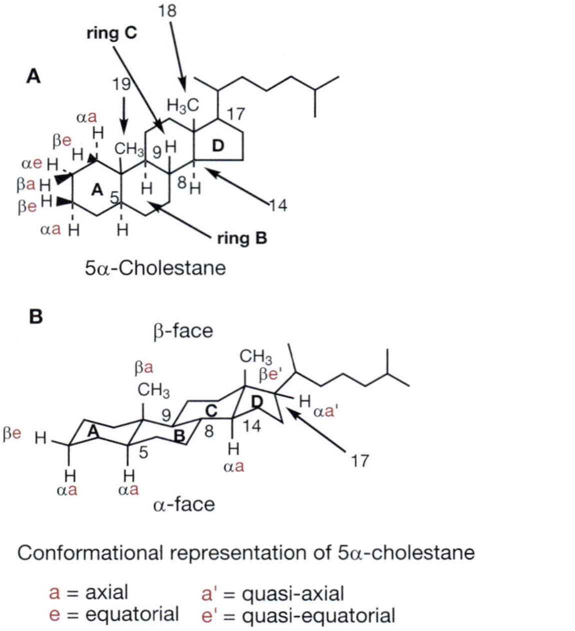

Figure 24.2 Planar (A) and conformational (B) structures of 5α-cholestane.

β side of the molecule. Similarly, the configuration of the 8β and 9α hydrogens (not shown), and the 14α hydrogen and C18 angular methyl group, denote *trans* fusion for rings B/C and C/D. The side chains at position 17 are always β unless indicated by dotted lines or in the nomenclature of the steroid (eg, 17β or 17α).

Cholestane is derived from cholesterol and can be 5α as in sex steroids or 5β as in cholic acids, with the α and β designations referring to the configuration of the hydrogen atom at C5. Just as cyclohexane can be drawn in a chair conformation, the three-dimensional representation for 5α-cholestane is shown by the following conformational formula (Fig. 24.2B). Although cyclohexane may undergo a flip in conformation, steroids are rigid structures with their cyclohexane rings locked into chair conformations. This is because they generally have at least one *trans* fused ring system, and these rings must be diequatorial to each other. In other words, the phenanthrene rings A-C are rigidly held in chair conformations.

Knowing that the angular methyl groups at positions 18 and 19 are β and have an axial orientation (ie, perpendicular to the plane of the rings), the conformational orientation of the remaining bonds of a steroid can be easily assigned. For example, in 5α-cholestane, the C19 methyl group attached at position 10 is always β-axial (βa; on the β-face of the steroid and oriented at a 90° angle to the plane of the steroid); the two bonds at position 3 must be β-equatorial (βe; on the β-face of the steroid and oriented at a slight angle to the plane of the steroid) and α-axial (αa), as indicated. The orientation of the remaining bonds on a steroid may be determined if one recalls that groups on a cyclohexane ring that are positioned on adjacent carbon atoms (vicinal, $-C_1H-C_2H-$) of the ring (ie, 1,2 to each other) are *trans* if their relationship is 1,2-diaxial or 1,2-diequatorial and are *cis*, if their relationship is 1,2-equatorial-axial.

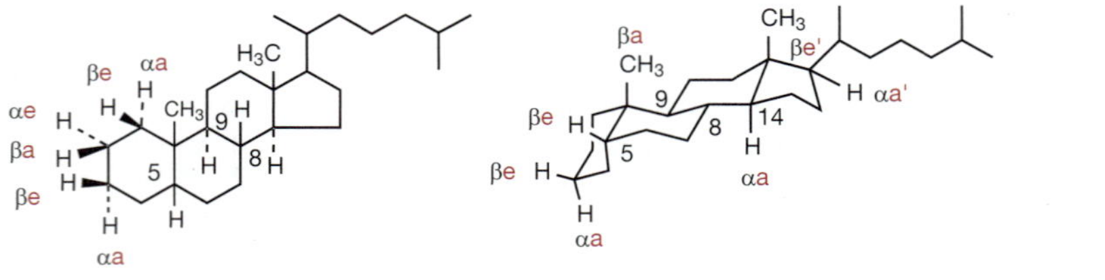

Figure 24.3 Planar and conformational structures of 5β-cholestane.

The *cis* or *trans* relationship of the four rings may be expressed in terms of the steroid backbone. The compound 5α-cholestane (Fig. 24.2) is said to have a *trans-antitrans-antitrans* backbone. In this structure, all the fused rings have *trans* (diequatorial) stereochemistry; in other words, the A/B fused ring, the B/C fused ring, and the C/D fused ring are *trans*. The term *anti* is used in backbone notation to define the orientation of rings that are connected to each other and have a *trans*-type relationship. For example, the bond equatorial to ring B, at position 9, which forms part of ring C, is *anti* to the bond equatorial to ring B, at position 10, which forms part of ring A. 5β-Cholestane (Fig. 24.3) has a *cis-antitrans-antitrans* backbone in which the A/B rings are fused *cis*. The term *syn* is used in a similar fashion as *anti* to define a *cis*-type relationship. No natural steroids exist with a *syn*-type geometry, although such compounds can be chemically synthesized. Thus, the conventional drawing of the steroid nucleus is the natural configuration and does not show the hydrogens at 8β, 9α, or 14α positions. If the carbon at position 5 is saturated, the hydrogen is always drawn as either 5α or 5β. Also, the conventional drawing of a steroid molecule has the C18 and C19 methyl groups shown only as solid lines (no CH_3 drawn).

The stereochemistry of the rings markedly affects the biologic activity of a given class of steroids. Nearly all biologically active steroids have the cholestane-type backbone. For example, the active sex steroids are always the *trans*-configuration across the A-B ring system as seen in 5α-cholestane discussed below, while 5β-cholestanes, as seen in bile acids, are always inactive as sex steroids. In most of the important steroids discussed in this chapter, a double bond is present between positions 4 and 5, or 5 and 6; consequently, there is no *cis* or *trans* relationship between rings A and B. The symbol Δ is often used to designate a carbon–carbon double bond (C=C) in a steroid. If the C=C is between positions 4 and 5, the compound is referred to as a Δ^4-steroid. If the C=C bond is between positions 5 and 6, the compound is referred to as a Δ^5-steroid. If the C=C is between positions 5 and 10, the compound is designated a $\Delta^{5(10)}$-steroid.

Cholesterol (cholest-5-en-3β-ol) is a Δ^5-steroid or, more specifically, a Δ^5-sterol because it is an unsaturated alcohol (Fig. 24.4). Biologically active compounds include members of the 5α-pregnane, 5α-androstane, and 5α-estrane steroid classes (Fig. 24.4). Pregnanes are steroids with 21 carbon atoms. Androstanes contain 19 carbon atoms, and estranes contain 18 carbon atoms, with the C19 angular methyl group at C10 replaced by hydrogen. Numbering is the same as in 5α-cholestane.

The adrenocorticoids (adrenal cortex hormones) are pregnanes and are exemplified by the most potent endogenous glucocorticoid, cortisol (referred to as hydrocortisone in medications), which is an 11β,17α,21-trihydroxypregn-4-ene-3,20-dione (Fig. 24.4). The most potent mineralocorticoid is aldosterone, which is a highly analogous pregnane that lacks the 17α-hydroxy and possesses an aldehyde functionality at C18 (Fig. 24.4). Progesterone (pregn-4-ene-3,20-dione), a female sex hormone synthesized by the corpus luteum, is also a pregnane analogue. The male sex hormones (androgens) are based on the structure of 5α-androstane. Testosterone, an important and naturally occurring androgen, is named 17β-hydroxyandrost-4-en-3-one.

Dehydroepiandrosterone (DHEA) is the major adrenal androgen and is named 3β-hydroxyandrost-5-en-17-one (Fig. 24.4). The estrogens, exemplified by the major endogenous estrogen, 17β-estradiol, are female sex hormones synthesized by the Graafian follicle of the ovaries. These are estrane analogues containing an aromatic A ring. Although the A ring does not contain isolated C=C groups, these analogues are named as if the bonds were in the positions shown in 17β-estradiol. Hence, 17β-estradiol, a typical member of this class of drugs, is named estra-1,3,5(10)-triene-3,17β-diol. Other examples of steroid nomenclature are found throughout this chapter.

Aliphatic side chains at position 17 are always assumed to be β when cholestane or pregnane nomenclature is employed. Hence, the notation 17β need not be used when naming these compounds. If a pregnane has a 17α chain, however, this should be indicated in the nomenclature. Finally, the final "e" in the name for the parent steroid hydrocarbon is always dropped when it precedes a vowel, regardless of whether a number appears between the two parts of the word (eg, note the nomenclature for cholesterol and testosterone vs that for cortisol). For a more extensive discussion of steroid nomenclature, consult the literature.[1]

Mechanism of Steroid Hormone Action

In addition to their structural similarities, adrenocorticoids, estrogens, progestins, and androgens share a common mode of action. They are present in the body only in extremely low

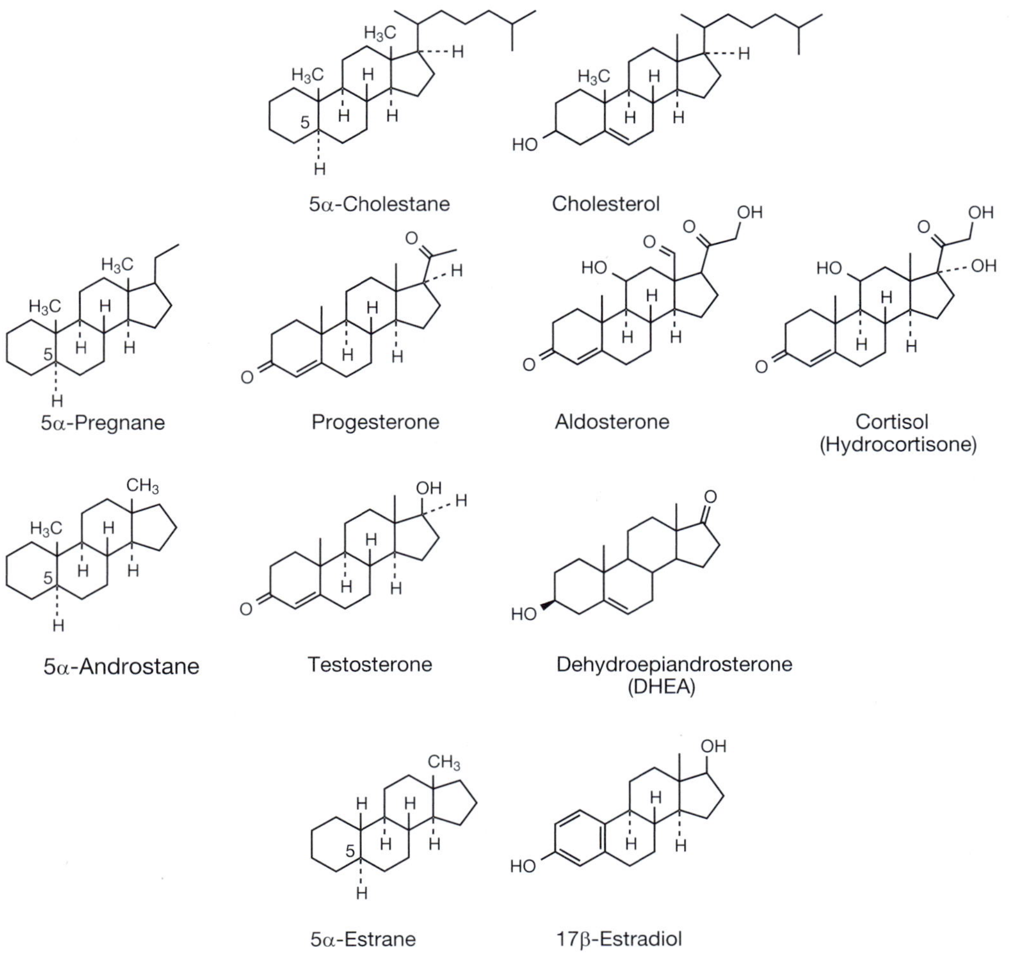

Figure 24.4 Steroid classes and corresponding natural hormones.

concentrations (eg, 0.1-1.0 nmol/L), where they exert potent physiologic effects on sensitive tissues by binding with high affinity to intracellular receptors. Extensive research directed at elucidation of the general mechanism of steroid hormone action has revealed their molecular mechanism of action in great detail, and many reviews have appeared.[2-7] For details on steroid hormone action, the reader is referred to Chapter 7 (Nuclear Receptors).

Briefly, corticosteroids, similar to other steroidal hormones, enter cells by passive diffusion and bind to the ligand-binding domain of glucocorticoid receptors (GRs) and/or mineralocorticoid receptors (MRs), which are present in target cells (Fig. 24.5). GRs and MRs in the absence of ligand are maintained in an inactive conformation by the heat-shock proteins (HSPs) HSP70 and HSP90 and/or corepressors (CoRs; proteins that operate to reduce the rate of gene transcription). Upon ligand binding, the GR and MR undergo conformational changes, which cause HSPs and/or CoRs to dissociate. The steroid-bound receptor then enters the nucleus to bind to deoxyribonucleic acid (DNA) in the regulatory regions of target genes. Several of these DNA elements, also called hormone response elements (HREs), share significant sequence homology that facilitates the binding of various receptors to the same DNA elements. For example, the gene metallothionein 2A (*MT2A*) can be induced by various hormone receptors' binding to a promiscuous response element in the regulatory region of the gene.[8,9] The DNA-bound receptor recruits several coactivators (CoAs; proteins that associate with the receptor to modulate transcription) and other general transcription factors (not shown) to propagate the transcription and translation of target genes, a process known as transactivation (transcriptional activation due to direct binding of the steroid receptor to DNA). The varying degrees of CoR dissociation and CoA association that occur after ligand binding are thought to contribute to differences in the observed pharmacologic activity and tissue selectivity of agonists and antagonists for nuclear receptors, and to be at least partially responsible for the SARs observed between different ligands. The proteins regulated by steroid receptors include enzymes, receptors, and secreted factors that subsequently result in the steroid hormonal response regulating cell function, growth, and differentiation, and playing central roles in normal physiologic processes as well as in many important diseases.

Steroid-receptor complexes have also demonstrated negative regulation of gene expression by interacting at negative response elements, or by transrepression via direct or indirect protein–protein interactions with other known transcriptional proteins such as AP-1 and NFκB.[10,11] In fact, many of the important anti-inflammatory and

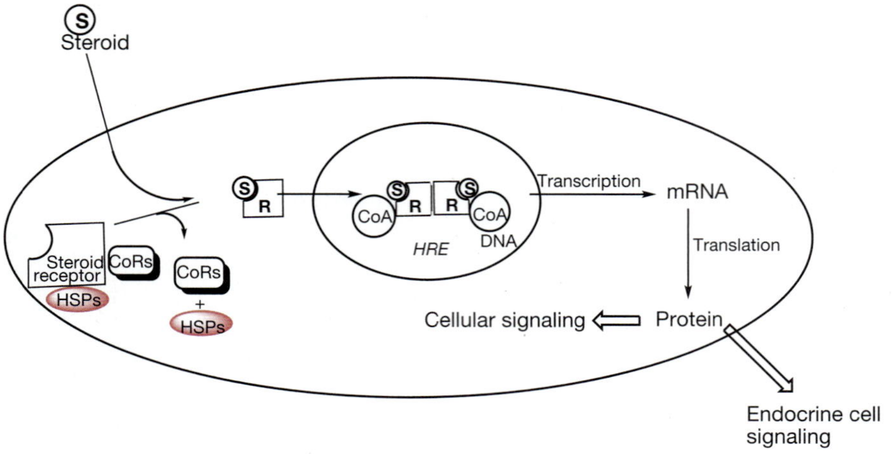

Figure 24.5 General steroid mechanism of action.

immunosuppressive effects of corticosteroids are mediated through transrepression pathways, while some side effects (eg, gluconeogenesis and bone loss) are mediated via transactivation, as described earlier. The transrepression mechanism can also be critical for crosstalk between signaling pathways within the cell and may have an important role in feedback systems. Additional evidence suggests that steroid receptors can activate transcription in the absence of hormone (ligand-independent activation), an effect that appears to depend on the phosphorylation of the receptor via crosstalk with membrane-bound adrenergic and/or growth factor receptors.[12] The interactions necessary for formation of the steroid-receptor complexes and subsequent activation or repression of gene transcription are complicated, involve multistage processes, and leave many unanswered questions. Lastly, non-genomic mechanisms involving cytosolic and/or membrane-bound steroid receptors have been identified to explain rapid onset actions of steroid hormones.[10]

History and Disease States

The importance of the adrenal glands was recognized long ago. Addison disease, Cushing disease, and Conn syndrome are pathologic conditions related to the adrenal cortex and the hormones produced by the gland. Addison disease was named after Thomas Addison, who, in 1855, described a syndrome in which the physiologic significance of the adrenal cortex was emphasized.[13] This disease results from decreased secretion of steroid hormones by the adrenal cortex and is characterized by extreme weakness, anorexia, anemia, nausea and vomiting, low blood pressure, hyperpigmentation of the skin, and mental depression. Addison disease is a rare affliction that affects roughly one in 100,000 people and is seen equally in both sexes and in all age groups.

Conditions of this type, usually referred to as hypoadrenalism, can result from several causes, including atrophy, destruction of the cortex by tuberculosis, or decreased secretion of adrenocorticotropin (adrenocorticotropic hormone [ACTH]) because of diseases of the anterior pituitary (adenohypophysis). Treatment of Addison disease involves hormone replacement therapy.

Cushing disease, or hyperadrenalism, on the other hand, can result from adrenal cortex tumors or increased production of ACTH caused by pituitary carcinoma. Cushing syndrome is also rare, occurring in only two to five individuals for every 1 million people each year. Approximately 10% of newly diagnosed cases are observed in children and teenagers. Cushingoid refers to a constellation of symptoms associated with glucocorticoid excess, including facial puffiness (moon facies), weight gain with truncal obesity but thin arms and legs, thin skin, and muscle weakness. While endogenous Cushing syndrome is rare, iatrogenic or exogenous Cushing syndrome arising from long-term and/or high-dose glucocorticoid therapy is common, emphasizing the need for judicious glucocorticoid selection and dosing.

Conn syndrome is caused by an inability of the adrenal cortex to carry out 17α-hydroxylation during the biosynthesis of the hormones from cholesterol. Consequently, the disease is characterized by a high secretory level of aldosterone, which lacks a 17α-hydroxyl functional group. Hypernatremia, polyuria, alkalosis, and hypertension, which are treatable via MR antagonism (eg, using finerenone, see later), are also observed.[14]

The importance of the adrenocorticoids is most dramatically observed in adrenalectomized animals. Glucocorticoid deficiency symptoms include an increase of urea in the blood, muscle weakness (asthenia), decreased liver glycogen, decreased insulin resistance, and lowered resistance to trauma (eg, cold and mechanical or chemical shock). Mineralocorticoid deficiency symptoms are also present, including electrolyte disturbances, as potassium ions are retained and excretion of Na^+, Cl^-, and water is increased. Adrenalectomy in small animals causes death in a few days.

After Addison's observations in 1855, physiologists, pharmacologists, and chemists from many countries contributed to our understanding of adrenocorticoid structure and function. It was not until 1927, however, that J.M. Rogoff and G.N. Stewart found that extracts of adrenal glands, administered by intravenous (IV) injection, kept adrenalectomized dogs alive.

Since that discovery, similar experiments have been repeated many times. Originally, the biologic activity of the extract was thought to result from a single compound. Later, 47 compounds were isolated from such extracts, and some

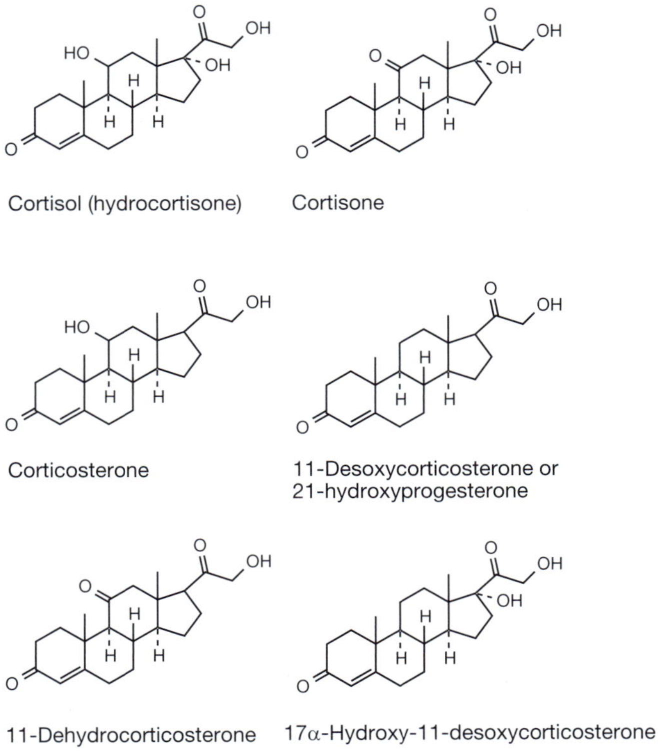

Cortisol (hydrocortisone) — Cortisone — Corticosterone — 11-Desoxycorticosterone or 21-hydroxyprogesterone — 11-Dehydrocorticosterone — 17α-Hydroxy-11-desoxycorticosterone

Figure 24.6 Biologically active corticoids.

were highly active. Among the biologically active corticoids isolated (Fig. 24.6), cortisol (hydrocortisone), cortisone, corticosterone, aldosterone (not shown), 11-desoxycorticosterone (21-hydroxyprogesterone), 11-dehydrocorticosterone (11-keto, 17α-desoxy-cortisol), and 17α-hydroxy-11-desoxycorticosterone were found to be most potent.[15] The biosynthesis of these steroids is described next.

Biosynthesis

Pregnenolone Formation and Conversion to Androgens and Estrogens

In the adrenal glands, cholesterol is converted by enzymatic side-chain cleavage (scc) to pregnenolone, which serves as the biosynthetic precursor of the adrenocorticoids (Fig. 24.7). This biotransformation is performed by a mitochondrial cytochrome P450 enzyme complex. This enzyme complex found in the mitochondrial membrane consists of three proteins: CYP11A1 (also known as $P450_{SCC}$), adrenodoxin, and adrenodoxin reductase[16]. Defects in CYP11A1 lead to a lack of glucocorticoids, feminization, and hypertension. Three oxidation steps are involved in the conversion, and three moles of nicotinamide adenine dinucleotide phosphate (NADPH) and molecular oxygen are consumed for each mole of cholesterol converted to pregnenolone. The first oxidation results in the formation of cholest-5-ene-3β,22*R*-diol (step a), followed by the second oxidation yielding cholest-5-ene-3β,20*R*,22*R*-triol (step b). The third oxidation step catalyzes the cleavage of the C20-C22 bond to produce pregnenolone (step c).

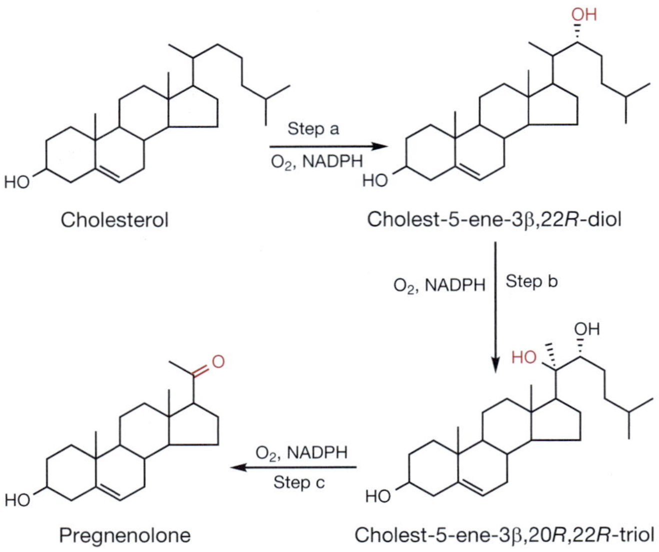

Figure 24.7 Biosynthesis of pregnenolone from cholesterol.

Pregnenolone serves as the common precursor in the formation of the adrenocorticoids and the sex steroid hormones. This C21 steroid is converted via enzymatic oxidations and isomerization of the double bond to a number of physiologically active C21 steroids, including the female sex hormone progesterone and the adrenocorticoids cortisol, corticosterone, and aldosterone (Fig. 24.8), as will be discussed next.

Androgen and estrogen biosynthesis requires oxidative cleavage of the pregnenolone two carbon side chain and subsequent enzymatic oxidations and an isomerization leading to C19 steroids, including the androgens testosterone and 5α-dihydrotestosterone (DHT) (see sex hormone pathway of Fig. 24.8). Specifically, 17α-hydroxylation of pregnenolone by 17α-hydroxylase produces 17α-hydroxypregnenolone (step b). Oxidative cleavage of the two carbon side chain of 17α-hydroxypregnenolone by 17,20-lyase (step j) produces the adrenal androgen dehydroepiandrosterone (DHEA), which serves as the biosynthetic precursors to androgens and estrogens and is present at high serum concentrations as DHEA sulfate in men and women. 3β-HSD (5-ene-3β-hydroxysteroid dehydrogenase) oxidizes and isomerizes DHEA into androstenedione (step c), which can be reduced to testosterone (step g) by testicular17β-HSD3 (17β-hydroxysteroid dehydrogenase type 3). This reaction is catalyzed extratesticularly in men and in women by aldoketoreductase type 1C3 (AKR1C3; also known as 17β-HSD5). Testosterone can be further activated in certain androgenic target tissues, such as skin and prostate, by 5α-reductase, which produces DHT, the most potent endogenous androgen.

The final group of steroids, the C18 female sex hormones, are derived from oxidative aromatization of the A ring of androgens to produce estrogens such as estrone and 17β-estradiol (step h of Fig. 24.8). This oxidative aromatization is performed by aromatase using either androstenedione or testosterone as substrates to produce estrone or 17β-estradiol. The latter is the most potent endogenous estrogen and can be deactivated by metabolism to the former by estradiol dehydrogenase (step i of Fig. 24.8). For further discussion of

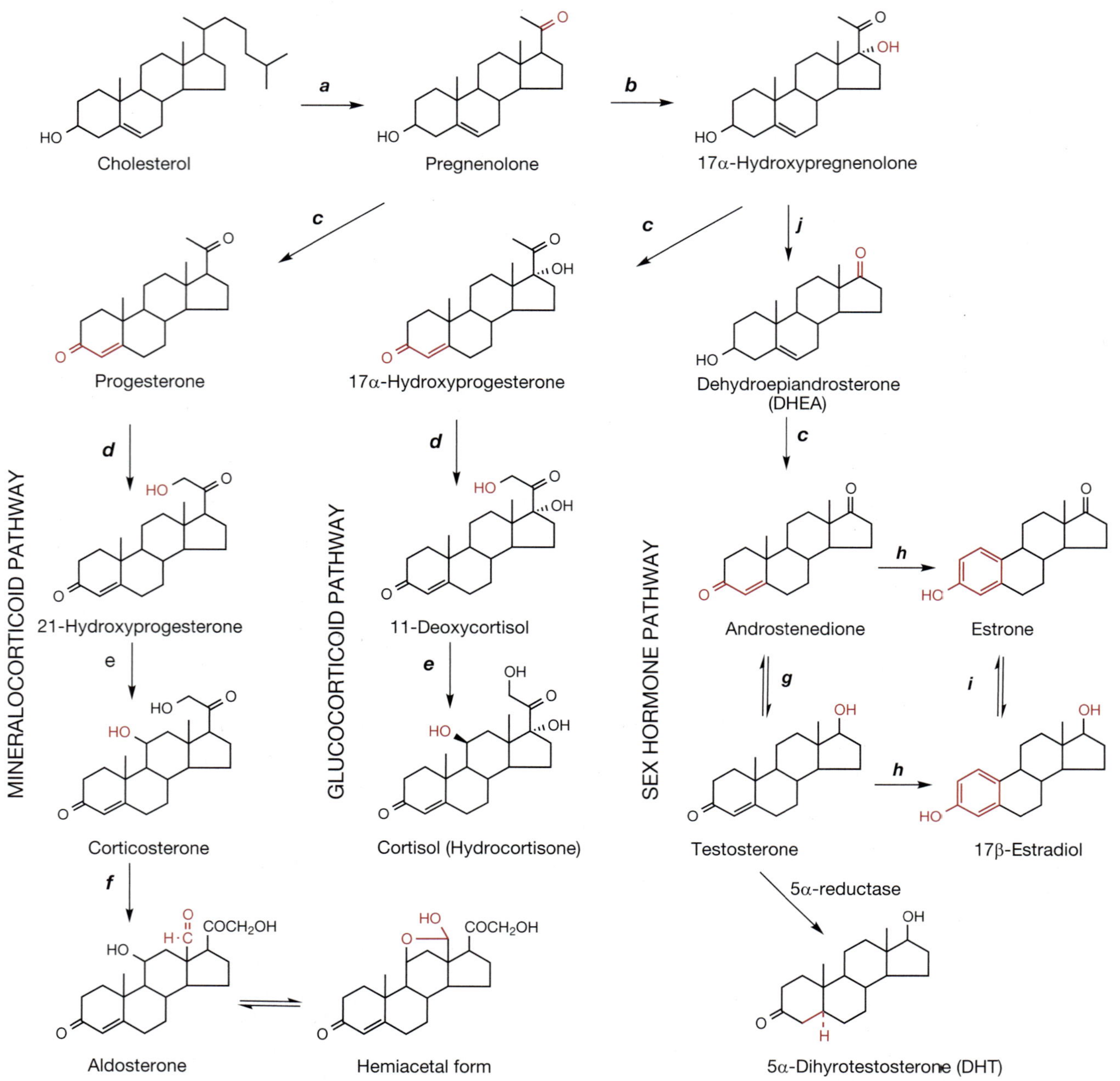

Figure 24.8 Biosynthesis of the adrenocorticoids and sex hormones from cholesterol.

androgens, estrogens, and progestins (eg, progesterone receptor ligands), see Chapter 25.

Pregnenolone to Glucocorticoids and Mineralocorticoids

The biosynthesis of the glucocorticoids and mineralocorticoids is regulated by independent mechanisms. The glucocorticoids, such as cortisol, are biosynthesized and released under the influence of peptide hormones secreted by the hypothalamus and anterior pituitary (adenohypophysis) to activate the adrenal cortex. This relay of activating biochemical events is known as the hypothalamic-pituitary-adrenal (HPA) axis. Removal of the pituitary results in atrophy of the adrenal cortex and a marked decrease in the rate of glucocorticoid formation and secretion. On the other hand, the secretion of the mineralocorticoids, corticosterone, and aldosterone is under the influence of the octapeptide, angiotensin II. Angiotensin II is the active metabolite resulting from the renin (synthesized in the kidney)-catalyzed proteolytic hydrolysis of plasma angiotensinogen (synthesized in the liver) to angiotensin I (no known function) and subsequent proteolysis to angiotensin II. Mineralocorticoid regulation is almost independent of the HPA axis. Hypophysectomized animals have only slightly decreased or unchanged aldosterone levels. Consequently, the electrolyte balance remains nearly normal.

The peptide hormone in the anterior pituitary that influences glucocorticoid biosynthesis is ACTH, whereas the peptide hormone in the hypothalamus is corticotropin-releasing factor (CRF). The production of both ACTH and CRF is regulated by the central nervous system and by a negative corticoid feedback mechanism. CRF is released by the hypothalamus and is transported to the anterior pituitary, where it stimulates the release of ACTH into the bloodstream. ACTH is then transported to the adrenal glands, where it stimulates the biosynthesis and secretion of the glucocorticoids. The circulating levels of glucocorticoids act on the hypothalamus and anterior pituitary to regulate the release of both CRF and ACTH. As the levels of glucocorticoids rise, smaller amounts of CRF and ACTH are secreted, and a negative feedback is observed (HPA suppression). Stimuli, such as pain, noise, and emotional reactions, increase the secretion of CRF, ACTH, and consequently, the glucocorticoids. Once the stimulus is alleviated or removed, the negative feedback mechanism inhibits further production and helps return the body to a normal hormonal balance.[17,18]

ACTH acts at the adrenal gland by binding to a receptor protein on the surface of the adrenal cortex cell to stimulate the biosynthesis and secretion of glucocorticoids. The only steroid stored in the adrenal gland is cholesterol, found in the form of cholesterol esters sequestered in lipid droplets. ACTH stimulates the conversion of cholesterol esters to glucocorticoids by initiating a series of biochemical events through its surface receptor. The ACTH receptor protein is coupled to a G protein that has adenylate cyclase as its second messenger. Binding of ACTH to its receptor leads to activation of adenylate cyclase via the G protein. The result is an increase in intracellular cyclic adenosine monophosphate (cAMP) levels (see Chapter 6). One of the processes influenced by elevated cAMP levels is the activation of cholesterol esterase, which cleaves cholesterol esters and liberates free cholesterol. Another process is the rapid induction of steroidogenic acute regulatory protein (StAR), which transfers cholesterol into the mitochondrial membrane.

Free cholesterol is then converted within mitochondria to pregnenolone via the side-chain cleavage reaction described earlier (Fig. 24.7 and step a of Fig. 24.8). In overview, pregnenolone is converted to adrenocorticoids by a series of enzymatic oxidations and an isomerization of the double bond (see mineralocorticoid and glucocorticoid pathways of Fig. 24.8). The next several enzymatic steps in the biosynthesis of glucocorticoids (middle pathway of Fig. 24.8) occur in the endoplasmic reticulum of the adrenal cortex cell. Hydroxylation of pregnenolone at position 17 by the enzyme 17α-hydroxylase (CYP17) produces 17α-hydroxypregnenolone (step b). The 17α-hydroxyl group is important for adrenocorticoid hormone action, promoting glucocorticoid and diminishing mineralocorticoid activities. In one step, 17α-hydroxypregnenolone is oxidized to a 3-keto intermediate and isomerized to 17α-hydroxyprogesterone by the action of a single enzyme, 5-ene-3β-hydroxysteroid dehydrogenase (3β-HSD) (step c). Another hydroxylation occurs by the action of 21-hydroxylase (CYP21) to give rise to 11-deoxycortisol, which contains the physiologically important ketol ($-COCH_2OH$) side chain at the 17β position (step d). A lack of CYP21 prevents cortisol biosynthesis, diverting excess 17α-hydroxypregnenolone and 17α-hydroxyprogesterone into overproduction of C19 androgens. The final step in the biosynthesis of cortisol is catalyzed by the enzyme 11β-hydroxylase, a mitochondrial cytochrome P450 enzyme complex (CYP11B2). This last enzymatic step (step e) results in the formation of cortisol (hydrocortisone), the most potent endogenous glucocorticoid secreted by the adrenal cortex. Approximately 15 to 20 mg of cortisol are biosynthesized daily. Several reviews provide more detailed discussions about the enzymology and regulation of adrenal steroidogenesis.[16,18-21]

The pathway for the formation of the potent mineralocorticoid molecule aldosterone is similar to that for cortisol and uses several of the same enzymes (mineralocorticoid pathway of Fig. 24.8). The preferred pathway involves the conversion of pregnenolone to progesterone by 3β-HSD (step c). Hydroxylation at position 21 of progesterone by 21-hydroxylase results in 21-hydroxyprogesterone (also known as 11-desoxycorticosterone) (step d). Again, these first conversions occur in the endoplasmic reticulum of the cell, whereas the next enzymatic steps occur in the mitochondria. 11β-Hydroxylase (CYP11B2) catalyzes the conversion of 21-hydroxyprogesterone to corticosterone (step e), which exhibits mineralocorticoid activity. The final two oxidations involve hydroxylations at the C18 methyl group and are catalyzed by 18-hydroxylase (step f). Initially, these reactions produce 18-hydroxycorticosterone (not shown) and then aldosterone, the most powerful endogenous mineralocorticoid secreted by the adrenal cortex. The aldehyde at C18 of aldosterone exists in equilibrium with its hemiacetal form.

Metabolism

Cortisol (hormonally active) and cortisone (the relatively inactive metabolite of cortisol) are biochemically interconvertible by the enzyme 11β-hydroxysteroid dehydrogenase (Fig. 24.9). Two isozymes of 11β-hydroxysteroid dehydrogenase are present: type 1 11β-hydroxysteroid dehydrogenase (11β-HSD1), referred to as the "liver" isozyme, and type 2 11β-hydroxysteroid dehydrogenase (11β-HSD2), referred to as the "kidney" isozyme.[22-24] The 11β-HSD1 isozyme is a bidirectional enzyme, which readily interconverts cortisol and cortisone, and is found in many tissues in the body. This isozyme has an important role in the regulation of hepatic gluconeogenesis in the liver and in fat production in adipose tissues. By contrast, the 11β-HSD2 isozyme is unidirectional, catalyzing the 11β-dehydrogenation of cortisol to cortisone. 11β-HSD2 is present in the placenta and in kidney, specifically the distal convoluted tubules and cortical collecting ducts in the kidney. The 11β-HSD2 isozyme has an important role in the rapid metabolism of cortisol, thus preventing cortisol from binding to the MRs present in the same kidney tissues. A deficiency of 11β-HSD2 is associated with the inherited genetic disease apparent mineralocorticoid excess syndrome, which is characterized by hypertension, excessive salt retention, and hypokalemia caused by the elevated cortisol levels in the kidney.

Cortisol is metabolized by the liver following administration by any route, with a half-life of approximately 1.0 to 1.5 hours.[25] Cortisol is mainly excreted in the urine as inactive O-glucuronide conjugates at the 3 and 21 positions and minor O-sulfate conjugates of urocortisol, 5β-dihydrocortisol, and urocortisone (not shown) (Fig. 24.9). The tetrahydro

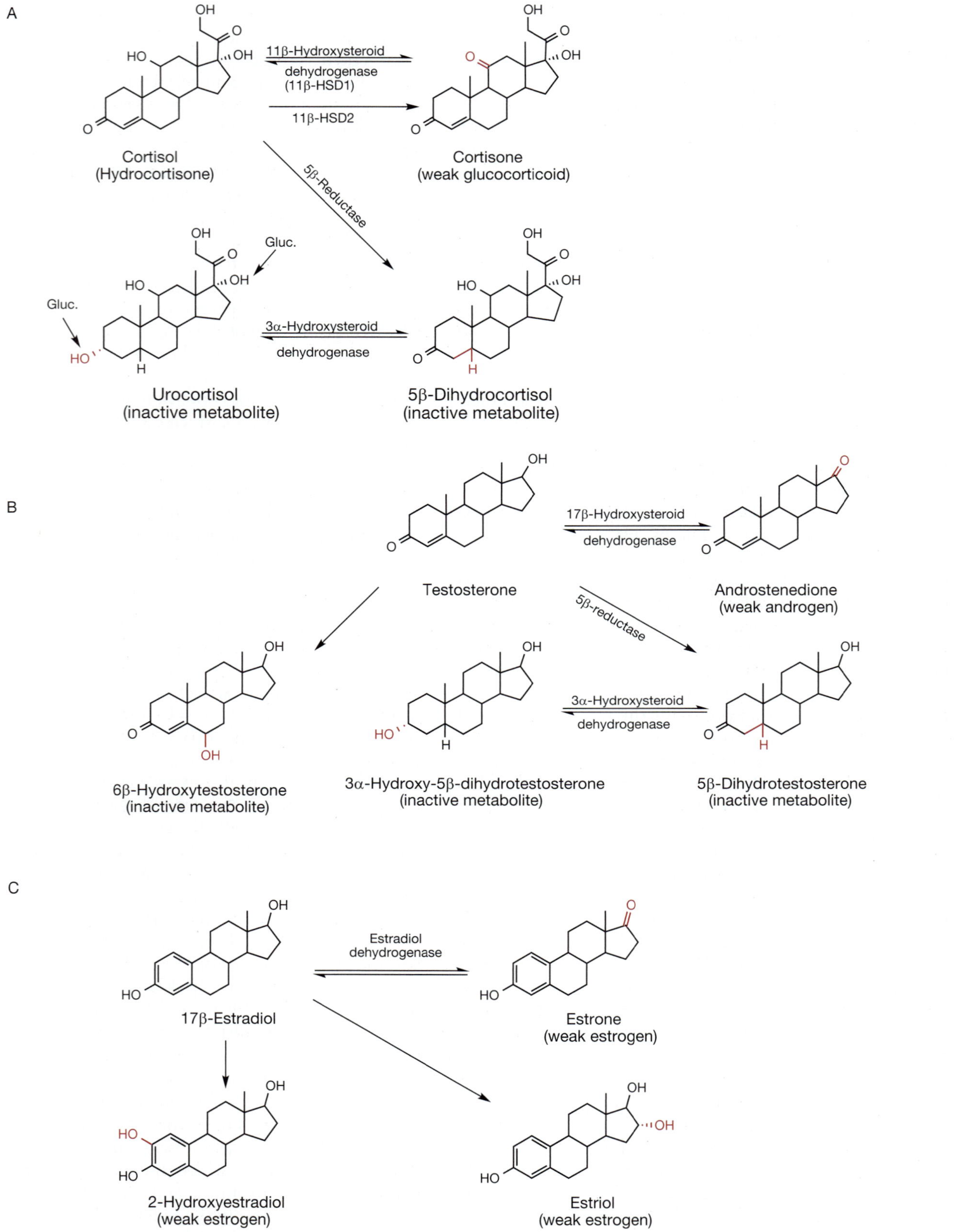

Figure 24.9 Major routes of inactivating metabolism for hydrocortisone (A), testosterone (B), and 17β-estradiol (C). Arrows from Gluc indicate the site of glucuronidation.

metabolite urocortisol is the major metabolite formed and has the 5β-pregnane geometry and 3α-hydroxyl function. The 5β configuration is the same ring geometry for bile acids (eg, obeticholic acid, an agonist of farnesoid X receptor), a class of steroids devoid of adrenocorticoid or sex hormone activities. Several 5β metabolites of this type have been isolated.[26,27]

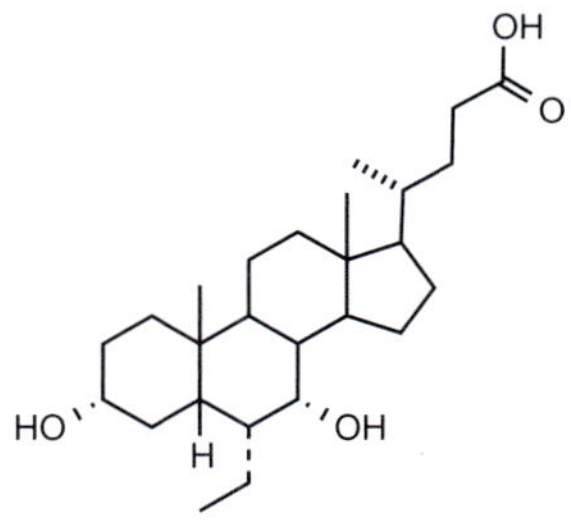

Obeticholic Acid

All of the biologically active adrenocorticoids contain a ketone at the 3-position and a double bond in the 4,5-position. The formation of inactive 5β-metabolites from cortisol is characterized by reduction of the 4,5-double bond to a 5β geometry for rings A and B (a *cis* configuration) by 5β-reductase, which can be further reduced at the 3-ketone by 3α-hydroxysteroid dehydrogenase (3α-hydroxyl configuration) or 3β-hydroxysteroid dehydrogenase (3β-hydroxyl configuration). These reactions represent the major inactivating pathways of metabolism for the glucocorticoids and their endogenous counterparts. Urocortisol and urocortisone are named after cortisol and cortisone, respectively. Oxidation of the 11β-hydroxyl group of many glucocorticoids, including cortisol, prednisolone, and methylprednisolone (but not dexamethasone and other 9α-fluorinated glucocorticoids) by 11β-HSD modulates the activities of these drugs in many tissues and limits their mineralocorticoid activity in the kidneys. Other routes of metabolism include: (1) 6β-hydroxylation (CYP3A4) and reduction of the 20-ketone (eg, prednisolone) to form 20-hydroxyl analogues, (2) oxidation of the 17-ketol side chain to 17β-carboxylic acids, and (3) loss of the 17-ketol side chain, resulting in 11β-hydroxy-17-keto-C19 steroids with the geometry of either 5α-androstane or 5β-androstane (not shown).[18-21] In addition, some ring A aromatic adrenocorticoid metabolites that resemble the estrogens have been isolated (not shown).[28] Biliary and fecal excretion contribute little to the elimination of the adrenocorticoids. The rate of formation of 6β-hydroxycortisol is a biomarker for determining the level of HPA suppression and adrenal insufficiency.

Similarly, testosterone can be metabolically inactivated by 17β-HSDs to androstenedione, a weak androgen, or reduced by 5β-reductases or 3α-hydroxysteroid dehydrogenases to inactive 5β-androstanes and/or 3α-hydroxy metabolites (Fig. 24.9B). It is important to note that 5β-dihydrotestosterone is inactive, while DHT is the most potent endogenous androgen. 6β-hydroxylation of testosterone by CYP3A4 in the liver is responsible for 75% to 80% of cytochrome P450–mediated testosterone metabolism (Fig. 24.9B) Testosterone and its metabolites can also be substrates for direct conjugation via glucuronosyl transferase or sulfotransferase enzymes. Furthermore, androgens can be inactivated by aromatization of testosterone by aromatase to 17β-estradiol or estrone.

Inactivation of the most potent estrogen, 17β-estradiol, occurs primarily via conversion to less potent estrogens, estrone (ie, 17β-dehydrogenation by estradiol dehydrogenase) or estriol (16α-hydroxylation; Fig. 24.9C). Estriol is the major 17β-estradiol metabolite excreted in the urine. 17β-Estradiol and estrone are also metabolized by CYP enzymes in the liver to the catechol, 2-hydroxyestradiol. 17β-Estradiol and its metabolites are rapidly glucuronidated and/or sulfated and eliminated in the urine.

Physiologic Effects of Adrenocorticoids

Glucocorticoids

Corticosteroids influence all tissues of the body and produce numerous and varying effects in cells.[17] These steroids regulate carbohydrate, lipid, and protein biosynthesis and metabolism (glucocorticoid effects), and they influence water and electrolyte balance (mineralocorticoid effects). Hydrocortisone is the most potent glucocorticoid secreted by the adrenal gland, and aldosterone is the most potent endogenous mineralocorticoid. Both naturally occurring glucocorticoids and related, semisynthetic analogues can be evaluated in terms of their ability to sustain life, to stimulate an increase in blood glucose concentrations and a deposition of liver glycogen, to decrease circulating eosinophils,[29] and to cause thymus involution in adrenalectomized animals.[30,31] In addition, corticosteroids can affect immune system functions, inflammatory responses, and cell growth.

The primary physiologic function of glucocorticoids is to maintain blood glucose levels and, thus, ensure glucose-dependent processes critical to life, particularly brain functions. Hydrocortisone and related steroids accomplish this by stimulating the formation of glucose, by diminishing glucose use by peripheral tissues, and by promoting glycogen synthesis in the liver to increase carbohydrate stores for later release of glucose. For glucose formation, glucocorticoids mobilize amino acids and promote amino acid metabolism and gluconeogenesis. These steroids, acting via the GR, induce the production of a variety of enzymes important for glucose formation. The synthesis of tyrosine aminotransferase increases within 30 minutes of glucocorticoid exposure.[32-34] This enzyme promotes the transfer of amino groups from tyrosine to α-ketoglutarate to form glutamate and hydroxyphenylpyruvate. Another amino acid–metabolizing enzyme induced rapidly by glucocorticoids is tryptophan oxidase.[35] This enzyme oxidizes tryptophan to formylkynurenine, which is subsequently converted to alanine. Alanine transaminase is also induced by glucocorticoids.[36] Alanine and, to a lesser extent, glutamate are important for gluconeogenesis in the liver.[37]

Several other enzymes important in gluconeogenesis and glycogen formation are elevated for several hours following glucocorticoid administration; these include glycogen synthase, pyruvate kinase, phosphoenolpyruvate carboxykinase, and glucose-6-phosphate kinase.[17,38,39] The delayed increases in these enzymes suggest that their biosyntheses are not regulated directly by glucocorticoids. In peripheral tissues, glucocorticoid-induced inhibition of phosphofructokinase is observed.[40] This enzyme catalyzes the formation of D-fructose-1,6-diphosphate from D-fructose-6-phosphate during glycolysis. Inhibition of this enzyme decreases glucose utilization by peripheral tissues and results in maintenance of blood glucose levels. Reviews of the multiple effects of glucocorticoids on carbohydrate metabolism have been published.[17,40]

Additional effects of glucocorticoids in the body are preventing or minimizing inflammatory reactions and suppressing immune responses. These steroids interfere with both early events in inflammation (eg, release of mediators, edema, and cellular infiltration) and later stages (eg, capillary infiltration and collagen formation). Only a few of the mechanisms involved in glucocorticoid suppression of inflammation are known. Hydrocortisone will induce the production of lipocortin and related proteins by increasing gene expression through the GR.[41,42] Lipocortin inhibits the activity of phospholipase A_2, which liberates arachidonic acid and leads to the biosynthesis of eicosanoids (eg, prostaglandins and leukotrienes).[43] Lipocortin also mediates the decreased production and release of platelet-activating factor,[44] and glucocorticoids can suppress the expression of interleukin (IL)-1, tumor necrosis factor, inducible nitric oxide synthase,[45-47] and other proinflammatory mediators. These eicosanoids and peptide factors are important as mediators in the inflammatory response. Some of these factors also have important roles in cellular infiltration and capillary permeability in the inflamed region. Suppression of the immune responses is mediated by inhibition of the synthesis and release of important mediators as well. In macrophages, glucocorticoids inhibit IL-1 synthesis and, thus, interfere with proliferation of B lymphocytes, which are important for antibody production.[38] Additionally, IL-1 is important for activation of resting T lymphocytes, which are important for cell-mediated immunity. The activated T cells produce IL-2, the biosynthesis of which is also reduced by glucocorticoids.[48]

Mineralocorticoids

The primary physiologic function of mineralocorticoids is to maintain electrolyte balance in the body by enhancing Na^+ reabsorption and increasing K^+ and H^+ secretion in the kidney. The mechanism of action of aldosterone involves binding of the steroid to the MR and initiation of gene transcription, mRNA biosynthesis, and cognate protein production.[39] A myriad of ligand-specific, tissue-specific, and gene-specific interactions of the MR with CoA and CoR proteins, as well as protein kinase signaling and other nongenomic mechanisms, work in concert to regulate electrolyte homeostasis and water balance.[48,49] Similar effects on cation transport are observed in a variety of secretory tissues, including the salivary glands, sweat glands, and mucosal tissues of the GI tract and the bladder. Aldosterone is the most potent endogenous mineralocorticoid. Deoxycorticosterone is approximately 20-fold less potent than aldosterone. Hydrocortisone exhibits weak mineralocorticoid activity in vivo because of rapid metabolism to cortisone by 11β-hydroxysteroid dehydrogenase.

Summary of Structure-Activity Relationships

The ring conformation and the absolute configuration of hydrocortisone and prednisolone illustrate the all-*trans* (B/C and C/D) backbone that is necessary for activity (Fig. 24.10).

Structural Biology of Adrenocorticoids

As previously pointed out, the adrenocorticoids are classified as either glucocorticoids (which activate the GR, affect intermediary metabolism and are associated with inhibition of the inflammatory process), or mineralocorticoids (which activate the MR and affect electrolyte balance). In fact, most naturally occurring and semisynthetic analogues exhibit both of these actions. The conserved structural features of glucocorticoids (and mineralocorticoids) such as those present in the endogenous ligand hydrocortisone include Δ^4-3-keto, 11β-OH, 17α-OH, and 17β-ketol (20-ketone and 21-OH). Crystal structures of several glucocorticoids reveal a conserved array of polar interactions between the glucocorticoids and GR for each of these conserved features. Furthermore, they help rationalize the importance of groups that have been added to the semisynthetic glucocorticoids to increase GR potency or selectivity over MR. All approved GR agents thus far are steroidal (ie, derivatives of the endogenous agents); however, many nonsteroidal agents have been designed and optimized using these structure-based design techniques. Nonsteroidal agents are highly receptor selective and are generally not metabolized to cross-reactive agents. A nonsteroidal MR antagonist, finerenone, was recently approved, as will be discussed.

As shown using the mometasone furoate:GR co-crystal (4e2j.pdb), the conserved polar interactions include: the binding of the Δ^4-3-ketone to the side chains of Gln570 and Arg611, the 11β-OH to the terminal amide of Asn564, 17α-OH group (present as furoate ester in mometasone furoate) to the side chains of Thr739 (not shown for simplicity) and Gln642, the 20-ketone of the 17β-ketol to the Asn564, and 21-OH (replaced by 21-Cl in mometasone furoate) of the ketol to Thr739 and Gln642 (Fig. 24.11, top panel).

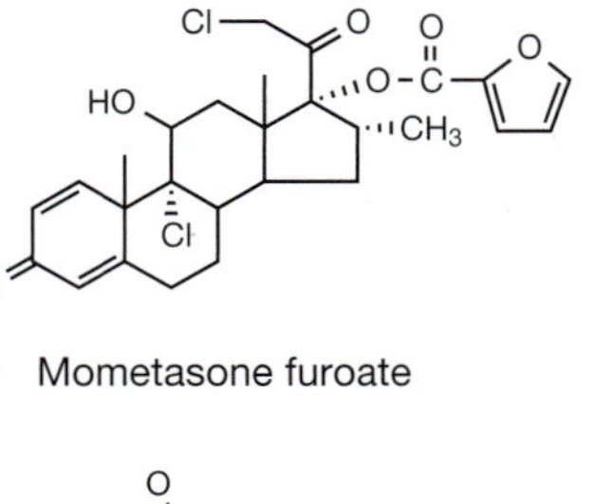

Mometasone furoate

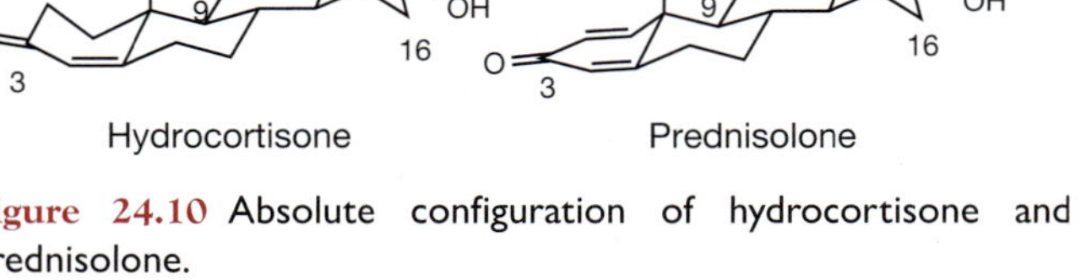

Hydrocortisone Prednisolone

Figure 24.10 Absolute configuration of hydrocortisone and prednisolone.

Furthermore, the crystal structures provide context for understanding the observed SAR of semisynthetic glucocorticoids. For example, it can be seen that the 9α-F/Cl groups inductively activate the hydrogen bond donation of the 11α-OH (all GR agonists). GR tolerates steric bulk on the α-face of the steroid nucleus, particularly at positions 16 and 17. The GR accommodates small groups such as the 16α-methyl of dexamethasone (a 16α-methyl glucocorticoid) and its synthetic derivatives (as discussed in the "Topical Glucocorticoids" section), as well as larger groups such as 16α-,17α-ethers of the triamcinolone (a 16α-OH glucocorticoid) and its synthetic derivatives (eg, the 16α-,17α-acetonides; discussed in the "Topical Glucocorticoids" section) and 17α-esters like the 17α-propionate of betamethasone (a 16β-methyl glucocorticoid).

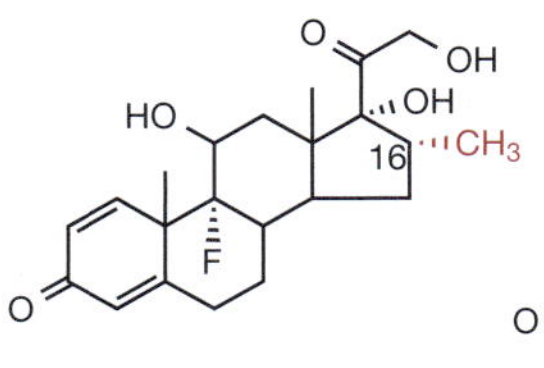

Dexamethasone
(16α-methyl)

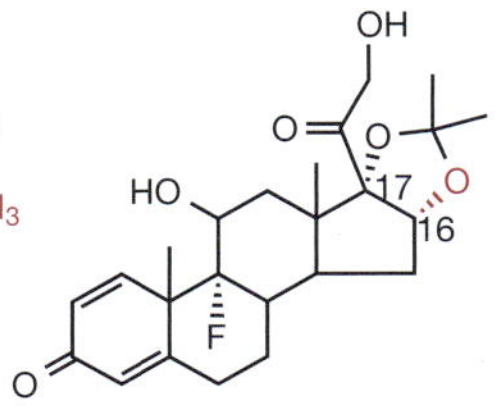

Triamcinolone acetonide
(16α-hydroxy)

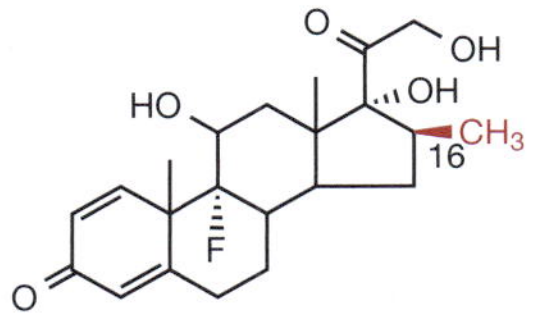

Betamethasone
(16β-methyl)

The ether/ester oxygen atoms form polar interactions with the NH_2 of Gln642 of the GR side chain (Fig. 24.11 [top panel]), and the bulky aromatic or aliphatic substituents form hydrophobic interactions with a large hydrophobic pocket of GR lined by Phe, Ile, Cys, and Met side chains. Examples of bulky α substituents accommodated by GR include the 17α-furoate of mometasone, the 16α,17α-cypionate of amcinonide, or the 16α,17α-acetal of cyclohexanecarboxaldehyde of ciclesonide (discussed in the "Topical Glucocorticoids" section).

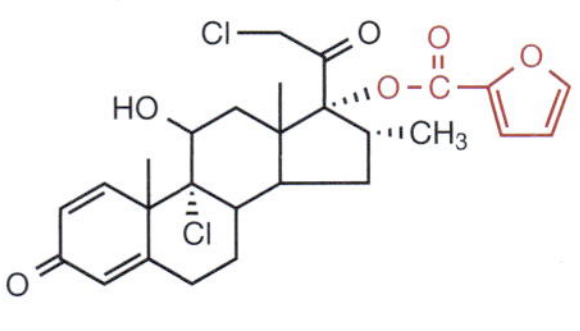

Mometasone furoate

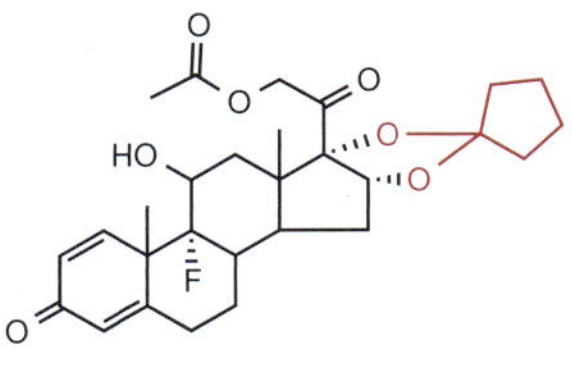

Amcinonide

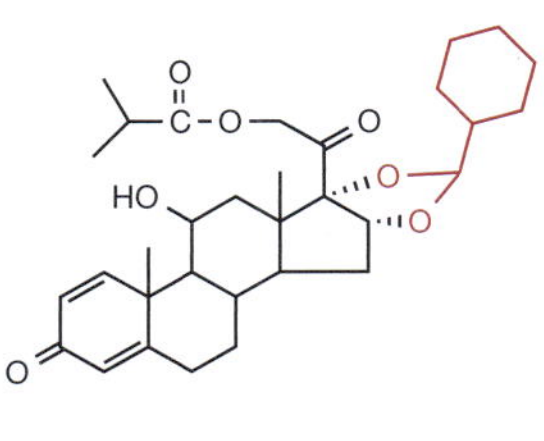

Ciclesonide

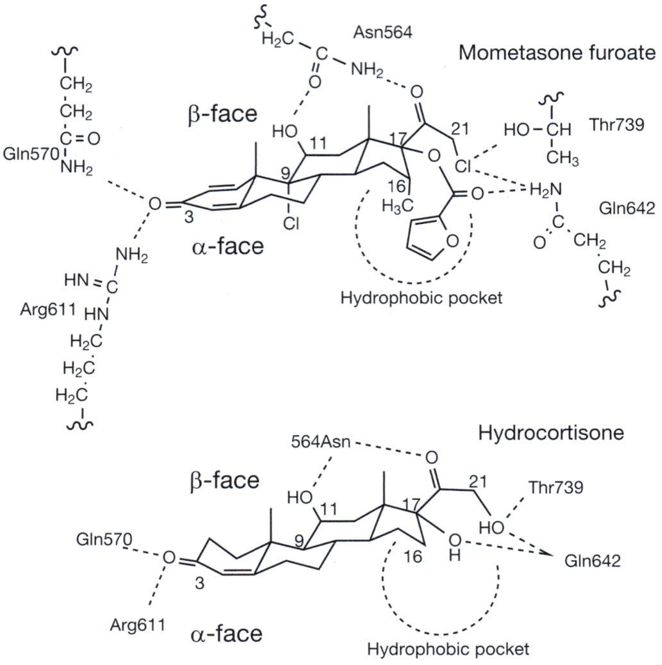

Figure 24.11 Interactions of mometasone furoate and hydrocortisone with glucocorticoid receptor (GR).

Derivation of the 21-OH to halogens (eg, mometasone furoate) or esters (eg, dexamethasone acetate) maintains the interactions with Thr739 or Gln642 of GR. Moreover, 16α- (eg, mometasone furoate [shown]) and 16β-methyl (eg, betamethasone) groups are well accommodated by the GR and enhance its activity.

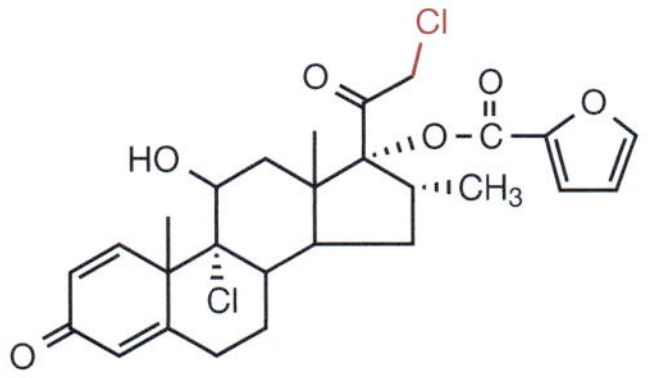

Mometasone furoate

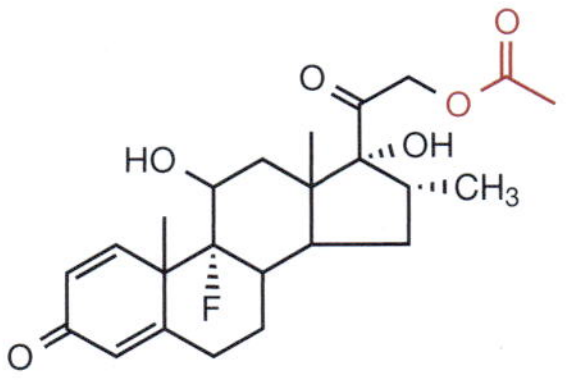

Dexamethasone acetate

The GRs and MRs are members of the nuclear hormone receptor family that also includes other steroid receptors such as androgen receptor, progesterone receptor, and estrogen receptor. The key polar interactions at position 3 (binds to Gln and Arg) and 17α (binds to Thr) are similar across the steroid receptor family. Unsurprisingly, many of the GR interactions described are conserved between GR and MR, as shown by the crystal structure of dexamethasone bound to MR (4uda.pdb). For example, the Δ^4-3-ketone to Gln/Arg side chains interactions (ie, Gln776 and Arg817 in MR) are maintained in MR, as are the 11β-OH to Asn770, 20-ketone to Asn770, and 21-OH to Thr945 (Fig. 24.12). Correspondingly, the 9α-F and 9α-Cl groups, which serve to inductively enhance the 11β-OH hydrogen bond to MR or GR, confer no MR selectivity (eg, fludrocortisone vs hydrocortisone as discussed in the "Systemic Corticosteroids" section). Similarly, the Δ^1 may enhance the Δ^4-3-ketone to Gln/Arg interaction with MR and GR and provides some GR selectivity (eg, prednisolone vs hydrocortisone as discussed in the

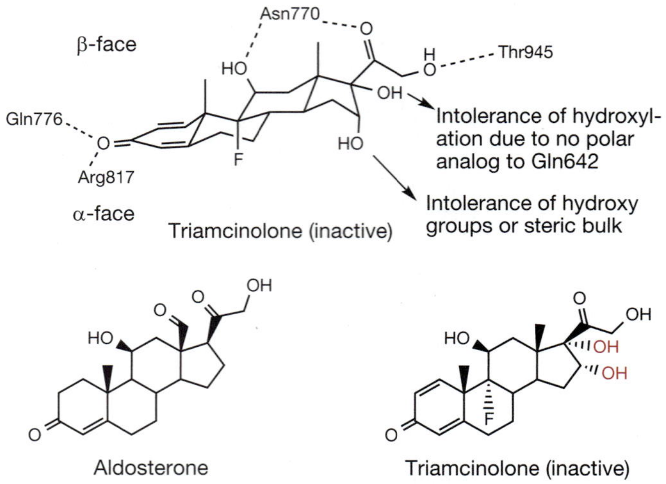

Figure 24.12 Limited interactions of triamcinolone with the mineralocorticoid receptor (MR). Red functional groups are not tolerated by MRs, explaining lack of mineralocorticoid activity in triamcinolone and other glucocorticoids with similar substitution patterns.

"Systemic Corticosteroids" section). Similarly, 21-fluorination increases the activity at both GR and MR with little to no selectivity.

In contrast, the 16α-methylation of dexamethasone (and 16β-methylation of betamethasone) is poorly accommodated by MR, suggesting the inability of MR to form the hydrophobic pocket of GR. Lack of this α-face pocket and, importantly, the absence in MR of an analogue to Gln642 explains the GR selectivity conferred by 16α-hydroxylation (eg, triamcinolone; Fig. 24.12), 17α-hydroxylation (eg, hydrocortisone vs corticosterone), or 16α-,17α-acetals or ketals (eg, triamcinolone acetonide, as shown earlier). Moreover, 6α-methylation (eg, methylprednisolone, as discussed in the "Systemic Corticosteroids" section) is not accommodated in MRs, providing another basis for selectivity; however, halogenation is accommodated. The ability to predict interactions with GR and/or their contributions to GR activity is not the same across all substitution contexts. A more detailed SAR discussion is found in the next section.

Structure-Activity Relationships of Adrenocorticoids

17β-KETOL. The 17β-ketol (–$COCH_2OH$) side chain and the Δ^4-3-ketone functions are found in clinically used adrenocorticoids, and these groups contribute to the potency of these drugs (Figs. 24.11 and 24.12). Modifications of these groups result in derivatives that retain biologic activity. For example, replacement of the 21-OH group with fluorine increases glucocorticoid and sodium-retaining activities, whereas substitution with chlorine or bromine diminishes activity. Some compounds that do not contain the Δ^4-3-ketone system have appreciable activity. It has been suggested that this group makes only a minor contribution to the specificity of action by these drugs or to the steroid-receptor association constant.[50]

INTOLERANCE OF β-SUBSTITUENT BULK. Based on structure-activity studies, the C and D rings, involving positions 11, 12, 13, 16, 17, 18, 20, and 21, are more important for receptor binding than the A and B rings. As a rule, insertion of bulky substituents on the β-side of the molecule abolishes glycogenic activity, whereas insertion on the α-side does not. As discussed earlier, it has been demonstrated that association of these steroids with receptors involves β-surfaces of rings C and D and the 17β-ketol side chain.[50] It is possible, however, that association with the unsubstituted α-surface of rings A, C, and D, as well as with the ketol side chain, is essential for sodium-retaining activity. Many functional groups, such as 17α-OH, 17α-CH_3, 16α-CH_3, 16β-CH_3, 16α-CH_3O, and 16α-OH substituents, abolish or reverse this MR activity in 11-desoxycorticosterone and 11-oxygenated steroids. Discussions of exceptions of these generalities are found in the literature.[50]

Although some steroids cause sodium retention, many have glucocorticoid and either sodium-retaining (MR agonist) or sodium-excreting action. Difficulties in correlating the structures of adrenocorticoids with biologic action are compounded by differences in assay methods, species variation, and mode of drug administration. For example, whereas liver glycogen and anti-inflammatory assays in the rat correlate well, some drugs show high anti-inflammatory action in the rat but little or no antirheumatic activity in humans. The 9α-F analogue fludrocortisone acetate is more active than the 9α-Cl analogue in terms of sodium retention in the dog; the reverse is true in the rat. Although 16α-methylation and 16β-methylation enhance glucocorticoid activity, anti-inflammatory action is increased disproportionately to glycogenic action in both series.

In humans, eosinopenic and hyperglycemic potencies are essentially the same. There is a close correlation in efficacy ratios derived from these tests and antirheumatic potency (Table 24.1). Because the eosinopenic-hyperglycemic activity and antirheumatic potency show excellent agreement, it has been suggested that these assays afford advantages in the preliminary estimation of anti-inflammatory potency.

Structure-activity studies of glucocorticoids have been carried out mainly in animals and are not necessarily applicable to clinical efficacy in man. Relative activity and dose correlations for some of the clinically useful drugs are discussed in the "Systemic Corticosteroids" section.

DOUBLE BONDS. Several other compounds have been studied in animals and used to derive SARs. For example, insertion of a double bond between positions 1 and 2 in hydrocortisone increases glucocorticoid activity. The Δ^1-corticoids have a much longer half-life in the blood than hydrocortisone. Ring A is much more slowly metabolized, but it is oxidatively metabolized at other positions, especially the 6β position and the 17β-ketol, as discussed in the section titled "Prednisone, Prednisolone, and Its Derivatives (Δ^1)." If, however, a double bond is inserted between positions 9 and 11 (noted as $\Delta^{9(11)}$, no oxygen function at 11), a decrease in glucocorticoid activity is generally observed. Vamorolone is a notable $\Delta^{9(11)}$ glucocorticoid that is an exception to this rule in that it retains potent anti-inflammatory activity, but also possesses a unique dissociated corticosteroid activity profile, as discussed in the section entitled "Systemic Corticosteroids." Except for cortisone, which results in an analogue with decreased glucocorticoid activity, a double bond

Table 24.1 Biologic Potencies of Modified Adrenocorticoids in Rats and Humans

	Potency Relative to Hydrocortisone (Cortisol)				
	Rat			Human	
Adrenocorticoid	Thymus Involution	Liver Glycogen Deposition	Eosinopenic Potency	Hyperglycemic Potency	Antirheumatic Potency
Corticosterone	–	0.8	0.06	0.06	<0.1
Prednisone	–	3	–	4	4
Prednisolone	2	3.9	4	4	4
Methylprednisolone	10	11	5	5	5
Triamcinolone	4	47	5	5	5
Paramethasone (6α-Fluoro-16α-methylprednisolone)	–	150	12	12	11
Dexamethasone	56	265	28	28	29
Fludrocortisone acetate	6	9	8	8	10
Fluprednisolone (6α-Fluoro-prednisolone)	6	81	9	9	10
Triamcinolone acetonide	33	242	3	3	3
Flurandrenolone	4	–	1	–	2
Fluorometholone	25	115	10	10	–
Fluocinolone	19	112	5	6	9

Data from Ringer I. Steroidal activity in experimental animals and man. In: Dorfman RI, ed. *Methods of Hormone Research*. Vol 3, Part A. Academic Press; 1964.

inserted between position 6 and 7 generally produces no change in activity.[17]

α-Methylation. Insertion of an α-CH_3 group at positions 2 (in 11β-OH analogues), 6, or 16 increases glucocorticoid activity in animals. Again, insertion of a 2α-CH_3 group into the glucocorticoid almost completely prevents inactivating reduction of the Δ^4-3-ketone system (ie, C=O → C-β-OH) in vivo and in vitro due to steric hindrance.[51-53] Substitutions at positions 4α, 7α, 9α, 11α, and 21 decrease activity.

α-Hydroxylation. Although some analogues, such as vamorolone (discussed later), 16α,17α-isopropylidinedioxy-6α-methylpregna-1,4-diene-3,20-dione, and its 1,2-dihydro derivative, are 11-desoxysteroids and biologically active, the hydrogen bond donating 11β-OH group of hydrocortisone has been demonstrated to be almost an essential drug–receptor interaction.[50] Cortisone, which contains an 11-keto function, is reduced in vivo to hydrocortisone. Insertion of α-OH groups into most other positions (eg, 1, 6, 7, 9, 14, and 16) or reduction of the 20-ketone, however, decreases glucocorticoid activity, in part because of increased hydrophilicity.

The 9α-F group nearly prevents metabolic oxidation of the 11β-OH group to a ketone. Redox metabolism of Δ^4-3-ketone steroids is mainly restricted to the Δ^4-3-ketone, 6 and 16 positions, and 17β-ketol side chains, whereas for 9α-F Δ^4-3-ketone steroids, it is only the 6 and 16 positions and 17β-ketol side chains that are metabolized. Furthermore, the 9α-F group increases glucocorticoid affinity by an inductive effect, which increases the acidic dissociation constant of the 11β-OH group and, thereby, increases the ability of the drug to hydrogen bond to Asn564 of GRs.

α-Fluorination. A 6α-F group also increases glucocorticoid activity, but it has less effect than the 9α-F function on sodium retention. Insertion of 2α-, 11α- (no OH group at 11), or 21-F groups decreases glucocorticoid activity. Of particular interest is a 12α-F group. When this function is inserted into corticosterone, which has no 17α-OH group, it potentiates activity to the same extent as a 9α-F group. However, although a 9α-F group potentiates activity in 16α,17α-dihydroxy steroids, a 12α-F group is inactivating. It has been proposed that intramolecular hydrogen bonding between the 12α-F and 17α-OH groups renders the analogue inactive (Fig. 24.13). Conversion to the 16α,17α-isopropylidinedioxy (acetonide) derivative, which cannot hydrogen bond, restores biologic activity,[54] possibly by providing hydrogen bonding acceptors for the NH_2 of Gln642.

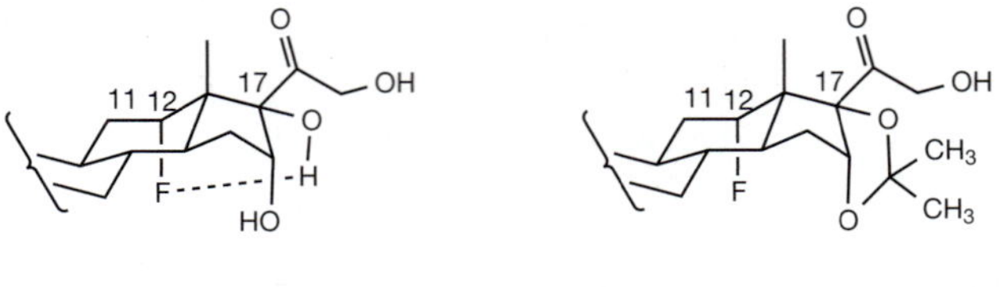

16α-,17α-Dihydroxy (inactive) 16α-,17α-Isopropylidenedioxy (16α-,17α-acetonide) (active)

Figure 24.13 Role of intramolecular hydrogen bonding in glucocorticoid activity.

MINERALOCORTICOID-RECEPTOR ACTIVATION. The mineralocorticoid activity of adrenocorticoids is another action of major significance. Many toxic side effects, making it necessary to withdraw steroid therapy in rheumatoid patients, are a result of this action. Some highly active, naturally occurring mineralocorticoids have no OH function in positions 11 and 17 (eg, aldosterone in Fig. 24.12). In fact, OH groups in any position reduce the sodium-retaining activity of the adrenocorticoids.

9α-F, 9α-Cl, and 9α-Br substitution usually causes increased retention of urinary sodium with an order of activity of F> Cl> Br, but species differences do exist. For these reasons, such compounds are not used internally in the treatment of diseases such as rheumatoid arthritis. Insertion of a 16α-OH group into the molecule affects the sodium retention activity so markedly that it not only negates the effect of the 9α-F, but also causes sodium excretion; see, for example, triamcinolone (Fig. 24.12), as discussed in the "Systemic Corticosteroids" section.

A double bond between positions 1 and 2 (Δ^1-corticoids) also reduces the sodium retention activity of the parent drug. However, this functional group contributes to the parent drug approximately one-fifth the sodium-excreting tendency of a 16α-OH group.[55]

The 12α-F, 2α-CH_3, and 9α-Cl substitutions contribute equally to sodium retention. A 21-OH group, found in all these drugs, contributes to this action to the same degree. Because 21-OH groups also contribute to glucocorticoid activity, it is easy to understand why it is difficult to develop compounds with only one major action.

A 2α-CH_3 group is approximately 3-fold, and a 21-F substituent 2-fold, as effective as unsaturation between positions 1 and 2 in reducing sodium retention. Other substituents reported to inhibit sodium retention include 16α-CH_3, 16β-CH_3, 16α-CH_3O, and 6α-Cl functions. A 17α-OH group, which is present in naturally occurring and semisynthetic analogues, reduces sodium retention to about the same extent as unsaturation between positions 1 and 2. Many of these effects can be rationalized in terms of GR versus MR structural biology (Figs. 24.11 and 24.12), as discussed.

17α-ESTERS OR ETHERS VERSUS 21-ESTERIFICATION/HALOGENATION. Conversion of the 17α-hydroxy to either a 17α-ester or an ether, as with 16α,17α-isopropylidinedioxy (acetonide), greatly enhances the anti-inflammatory potency and GR affinity. However, esterifying the 21-hydroxy group reduces activity and receptor affinity. On the other hand, 21-halogens or 21-halomethylene groups greatly increase topical anti-inflammatory activity with no change or a decrease in mineralocorticoid activity. Perhaps a hydrogen bonding group at position 21 of the naturally occurring 17β-ketol enhances or retains MR affinity, possibly through interaction with Thr945.

PHARMACOLOGIC EFFECTS AND CLINICAL APPLICATIONS

In addition to their natural hormonal actions, the adrenocorticoids have many clinical uses. Glucocorticoids and mineralocorticoids can be used for the treatment of adrenal insufficiency (hypoadrenalism), which results from failure of the adrenal glands to synthesize adequate amounts of the hormones. Adrenocorticoids are also used to maintain patients who have had partial or complete removal of their adrenal glands or adenohypophysis (adrenalectomy and hypophysectomy, respectively).

Two major uses of glucocorticoids are in the treatment of rheumatoid diseases and allergic manifestations. Their use in the treatment of severe asthma is well documented, as is the utility of glucocorticoids in sepsis and acute respiratory distress syndrome.[56,57] They are effective in the treatment of rheumatoid arthritis, acute rheumatic fever, bursitis, spontaneous hypoglycemia in children, gout, rheumatoid carditis, sprue, allergy (including contact dermatitis), and other conditions. The treatment of chronic rheumatic diseases and allergic conditions with glucocorticoids is symptomatic and continuous. Symptoms return after withdrawal of the drug. Because the glucocorticoids can cross the placenta and distribute into milk, their use in pregnant women and new mothers warrants careful consideration of the glucocorticoid selected, route of administration, dose and duration of therapy, and potential effects on the child.

In addition, these drugs are moderately effective in the treatment of ulcerative colitis, dermatomyositis, periarteritis nodosa, idiopathic pulmonary fibrosis, idiopathic thrombocytopenic purpura, regional ileitis, acquired hemolytic anemia, nephrosis, cirrhotic ascites, neurodermatitis, and temporal arteritis. The newer analogues with medium to high potency rankings as discussed in the "Topical Glucocorticoids" section are effective topically in the treatment of psoriasis. Glucocorticoids can be combined with antibiotics to treat pneumonia, peritonitis, typhoid fever, and meningococcemia.

When dosages with equivalent antirheumatic potency are given to patients not previously treated with steroids, the Δ^1-corticoids prednisone and prednisolone promote the same pattern of initial improvement as hydrocortisone. Statistically significant improvements during the first few months of therapy have been similar with prednisone, prednisolone, and hydrocortisone. The results of longer-term therapy have been significantly better with the modified (Δ^1) compounds.

Satisfactory rheumatic control, lost after prolonged hydrocortisone therapy, may be regained in an appreciable number of patients by changing to prednisone, prednisolone, or other synthetic glucocorticoids. Of patients whose conditions deteriorate below adequate levels during hydrocortisone administration, nearly half reach their previous level of improvement using Δ^1-corticoids in doses slightly larger in terms of antirheumatic strength. With further prolongation of steroid therapy, improvement again wanes in some patients, but in other patients, such management is successful for longer than 2 years. In some instances, the improvement is attributed to increased effectiveness of the drug because of correction of salt and water retention; in other instances, there is no adequate explanation.

When these drugs are administered in doses that have similar antirheumatic strengths, the general incidence of adverse reactions with prednisone and prednisolone is about the same as that with hydrocortisone. The compounds differ, however, in their tendencies to induce specific side effects. The incidence and degree of salt and water retention and blood pressure elevation are less with the Δ^1-corticoids. Conversely, these analogues are more likely to promote digestive complaints, peptic ulcer, vasomotor symptoms, and cutaneous ecchymosis.

Although these analogues have unwanted side effects, most clinical investigators prefer the Δ^1-corticoids to hydrocortisone for rheumatoid patients who require steroid therapy. The reasons are that these drugs have a lower tendency to cause salt and water retention and potassium loss, and that they restore improvement in a significant percentage of patients whose therapeutic control has been lost during hydrocortisone therapy.

Most importantly, glucocorticoids should not be withdrawn abruptly in cases of acute infections or severe stress, such as surgery or trauma. Myasthenia gravis, peptic ulcer, diabetes, hyperthyroidism, hypertension, psychological disturbances, pregnancy (first trimester), and infections may be aggravated by glucocorticoid administration. Hormone therapy is contraindicated in these conditions and should be used only with the utmost precaution.

Semisynthetic analogues exhibiting high mineralocorticoid activity are not employed in the treatment of rheumatic disorders because of toxic side effects resulting from a disturbance of electrolyte and water balance. Some newer synthetic steroids (Table 24.1) are relatively free of sodium-retaining activity. They can show other toxic manifestations, however, and eventually may need to be withdrawn.

Glucocorticoids are sometimes used in the treatment of scleroderma, discoid lupus, acute nephritis, osteoarthritis, acute hepatitis, hepatic coma, Hodgkin disease, multiple myeloma, lymphoid tumors, acute leukemia, and chronic lymphatic leukemia, and to alleviate the side effects of chemotherapy and radiation therapy in non-hematologic malignancies. Glucocorticoids may be more or less effective in these diseases, depending on the clinical condition.

Some modified compounds have been recommended for use when other analogues are no longer effective or when it is desirable to promote increased appetite and weight gain (eg, wasting diseases). In contrast, triamcinolone can be used advantageously when salt and water retention (leading to hypertension or cardiac compensation) or excessive appetite and weight gain are problematic in corticosteroid therapy management.

Percutaneous absorption is one factor that must not be overlooked when applying potent anti-inflammatory agents with high mineralocorticoid activity to the skin. Sodium retention and edema occur in patients with dermatitis who apply as much as 75 mg of fludrocortisone acetate (ie, 30 mL of a 0.25% lotion) to the skin in 24 hours. The relative rate of percutaneous absorption, administered as a cream in rats, was triamcinolone acetate ≥ hydrocortisone> dexamethasone, but dexamethasone was deposited in the skin longer than the other two drugs. Hydrocortisone disappeared most rapidly.[58]

Topical Applications

Topical dermatologic products with a low potency ranking have a modest anti-inflammatory effect and are safest for chronic application, as discussed further in the "Topical Glucocorticoids" section. These products are also the safest products for use on the face, with occlusion, and in infants and young children. Those products with a medium potency ranking are used in moderate inflammatory dermatoses, such as chronic hand eczema and atopic eczema, and may be used for a limited duration on the face and intertriginous areas (areas where skin comes into contact with itself, such as the armpits, the groin, and beneath the breasts, which are more prone to infections and rashes because they are warm and often sweaty). High potency preparations are used in more severe inflammatory dermatoses, such as severe eczema and psoriasis. They can be used for a limited duration and for longer periods in areas with thickened skin because of chronic conditions. High potency preparations may also be used on the face and intertriginous areas, but only for a short treatment duration.

Very high–potency products are used primarily as an alternative to systemic corticosteroid therapy when local areas are involved. Examples of conditions for which very high–potency products frequently are used include thick, chronic lesions caused by psoriasis, lichen simplex chronicus, and discoid lupus erythematosus. They may be used for only a short duration of therapy and on small surface areas. Occlusive dressings should not be used with these products. It has been suggested that patients using a lotion or ointment containing these drugs be instructed to apply them sparingly and to spread them lightly over the affected areas. The extent and frequency of applications should be carefully considered. A lotion vehicle is more effective when treating a dermatitis, but a greater degree of percutaneous absorption occurs than when ointments are used.

Intranasal and Inhaled Applications

Pulmonary and nasal bioavailabilities are important determinants for the potential of an inhaled or nasally applied corticosteroid to cause systemic effects because the lung and nasal tissue provide an enormous surface area from which drug absorption can occur into the systemic circulation. The main areas of concern with regard to systemic effects include HPA axis suppression, change in bone mineral density and growth retardation in children, cataracts, and glaucoma. Systemic side effects depend on the dose, administration frequency, and the half-life of the drug, as well as time of day when administered and route of administration. Higher plasma corticosteroid concentrations and a longer half-life will produce greater systemic side effects.[59] The amount of an inhaled or nasal corticosteroid reaching the systemic circulation is the sum of the drug concentration available following absorption from the lungs/nasal mucosa and from the GI tract. The fraction deposited in the mouth will be swallowed, and the systemic availability will be determined by its absorption from the GI tract and the degree of first-pass metabolism.

Delivery devices can produce clinically significant differences in activity by altering the dose deposited in the lung (10%-25%) and, for orally absorbed drugs, the amount deposited in the oropharynx and swallowed (75%-90%). Clinical studies have shown the following relative potency differences: ciclesonide > mometasone furoate > fluticasone propionate> budesonide = beclomethasone dipropionate (BDP) > triamcinolone acetonide = flunisolide (see "Inhaled and Intranasal Glucocorticoids" section for structures and further discussion of these agents). Potency differences can be overcome by giving larger doses of the less potent drug, which increases risks from systemic effects. Adrenal suppression may be associated with high doses of inhaled corticosteroids (>1.5 mg/day, or >0.75 mg/day for fluticasone propionate), although there is a considerable degree of interindividual susceptibility.

All currently used inhaled corticosteroids are rapidly cleared from the body but show varying levels of oral bioavailability, with fluticasone propionate having the lowest (as will be discussed). Following inhalation, there is also considerable variability in the rate of absorption from the lung; pulmonary residence times are greatest for fluticasone propionate and triamcinolone acetonide and shortest for budesonide and flunisolide. Adrenal suppression has been observed when intranasal fluticasone propionate was administered in doses of 200 to 4,000 μg daily for up to 12 months.

Adverse Effects

Although short-term administration of corticosteroids is unlikely to produce harmful effects, these drugs, when used for longer than brief periods, can produce a variety of devastating effects, including glucocorticoid-induced adrenocortical insufficiency, glucocorticoid-induced osteoporosis, and generalized protein depletion.[17] The duration of anti-inflammatory activity of glucocorticoids approximately equals the duration of HPA axis suppression. The durations of HPA axis suppression after a single oral dose of glucocorticoids in one study are shown in Table 24.2. When given for prolonged periods, glucocorticoids suppress the HPA axis, thereby decreasing secretion of endogenous corticosteroids and causing adrenal cortex atrophy. Glucocorticoids inhibit ACTH production by the adenohypophysis, and in turn, this reduces endogenous glucocorticoid production. With time, atrophy of the adrenal glands takes place. The degree and duration of adrenocortical insufficiency produced by the synthetic glucocorticoids is highly variable among patients and depends on the dose, frequency and time of administration, and duration of glucocorticoid therapy. This effect can be minimized by use of alternate-day therapy.

Table 24.2 Effect of an Oral Single Dose on the Duration of HPA Axis Suppression

Adrenocorticoid	Duration of Suppression (d)
Hydrocortisone (250 mg)	1.25-1.5
Cortisone (250 mg)	1.25-1.5
Methylprednisolone (40 mg)	1.25-1.5
Prednisone (50 mg)	1.25-1.5
Prednisolone (50 mg)	1.25-1.5
Triamcinolone (40 mg)	2.25
Dexamethasone (5 mg)	2.75
Betamethasone (6 mg)	3.25

Patients who develop drug-induced adrenocortical insufficiency may require higher corticosteroid dosage when they are subjected to stress (eg, infection, surgery, or trauma). In addition, acute adrenal insufficiency (even death) can occur if the drugs are withdrawn abruptly or if patients are transferred from systemic glucocorticoid therapy to oral inhalation therapy. Therefore, the drugs should be withdrawn very gradually following long-term therapy with pharmacologic doses. Adrenal suppression can persist up to 12 months in patients who receive large doses for prolonged periods. Until recovery occurs, patients may show signs and symptoms of adrenal insufficiency when they are subjected to stress, and replacement therapy may be required. Because mineralocorticoid secretion can be impaired, sodium chloride or a mineralocorticoid should also be administered.

Although side effects and toxicities vary with the drug and, sometimes, with the patient, facial mooning, flushing, sweating, acne, thinning of the scalp hair, abdominal distention, and weight gain are observed with most glucocorticoids. Protein depletion (with osteoporosis and spontaneous fractures), myopathy (with weakness of muscles of the thighs, pelvis, and lower back), and aseptic necrosis of the hip and humerus are other side effects. These drugs can cause psychological disturbances, headache, vertigo, and peptic ulcer, and they can suppress growth in children.

Patients with well-controlled diabetes must be closely monitored and their insulin dosage increased if glycosuria or hyperglycemia ensues either during or following glucocorticoid administration. Patients should also be watched for signs of adrenocorticoid insufficiency after discontinuation of glucocorticoid therapy. Individuals with a history of tuberculosis should receive prophylactic doses of antituberculosis drugs.

Osteoporosis is one of the most serious adverse effects of long-term glucocorticoid therapy. Moderate- to high-dose glucocorticoid therapy is associated with loss of bone and an increased risk of fracture that is most rapid during the initial 6 months of therapy. These adverse effects of glucocorticoids appear to be both dose- and duration-dependent, with oral prednisone doses of 7.5 mg or more daily for 6 months or longer often resulting in clinically important bone loss and increased fracture risk. Bone loss has even been associated with oral inhalation of glucocorticoids and is of great concern in children. Most patients receiving long-term glucocorticoid therapy will develop some degree of bone loss, and more than 25% will develop osteoporotic fractures. Vertebral fractures have been reported in 11% of patients with asthma who are receiving systemic glucocorticoids for at least 1 year, and glucocorticoid-treated patients with rheumatoid arthritis are at increased risk of fractures of the hip, rib, spine, leg, ankle, and foot. Muscle wasting or weakness and atrophy of the protein matrix of the bone resulting in osteoporosis are manifestations of protein catabolism, which can occur during prolonged therapy with glucocorticoids. These adverse effects can be especially serious in debilitated patients, in geriatric populations, and in postmenopausal women who are especially prone to osteoporosis.

To minimize the risk of glucocorticoid-induced bone loss (osteoporosis) and in those with low mineral bone density, the smallest possible effective dose and duration should be used. Topical and inhaled preparations should be used whenever possible. The immunosuppressive effects of glucocorticoids increase the susceptibility to, and mask the symptoms of, infections and can result in activation of latent infection or exacerbation of intercurrent infections. The most common adverse effect of oral inhalation therapy with glucocorticoids is fungal infections of the mouth, pharynx, and occasionally, the larynx. The mineralocorticoid effects are less frequent with synthetic glucocorticoids (except fludrocortisone) than with hydrocortisone but may occur, especially when synthetic glucocorticoids are given in high doses for prolonged periods.

Development of Adrenocorticoid Drugs

Systemic Corticosteroids

The route of administration depends on the disease being treated and the physicochemical, pharmacologic, and pharmacokinetic properties of the drug (Table 24.3). The clinically available adrenocorticoids may be administered by IV or IM injection, oral tablets or solutions, topical formulations, intra-articular or other local parenteral administration, and oral or nasal inhalation (Table 24.4). Several, but not all, of the corticosteroids are used clinically by the oral route, including budesonide, cortisone, deflazacort, dexamethasone, hydrocortisone, methylprednisolone, prednisolone, prednisone, and vamorolone (Fig. 24.14). These corticosteroids are often described as short-acting, intermediate-acting, or long-acting according to their biologic half-life and duration of action (Table 24.3). They are well-absorbed, undergo little first-pass metabolism in the liver, and demonstrate oral bioavailabilities of 70% to 80%, except for triamcinolone (Table 24.5). The larger volume of distribution for methylprednisolone compared to prednisolone is thought to result from a combination of increased lipophilicity, plasma and tissue protein binding, and better tissue penetration. Glucocorticoids vary in the extent to which they are bound to the plasma proteins albumin and corticosteroid-binding globulin (transcortin), but most are highly (>90%) bound (Table 24.5).

Hydrocortisone is extensively bound to plasma proteins, primarily to transcortin, with only 5% to 10% of plasma hydrocortisone unbound. Prednisolone and methylprednisolone (but not the 9α-fluoro analogues betamethasone, dexamethasone, or triamcinolone) have a high affinity for transcortin and, thus, compete with hydrocortisone for this binding protein. The 9α-halo analogues bind primarily to albumin. As with other drugs, only the unbound fraction of the synthetic corticosteroids is biologically active. Glucocorticoids cross the placenta and can be distributed into milk.

The degree of systemic side effects is dose-dependent, related to the half-life of the drug, frequency of administration, time of day when administered, and route of administration. In other words, the higher the plasma corticosteroid concentration and longer the half-life, the greater will be the systemic side effects.[59]

Regardless of the route of administration, all synthetic adrenocorticoids are excreted from the body in a manner similar to the endogenous adrenocorticoids (ie, they are metabolized in the liver and excreted into the urine primarily as glucuronide conjugates but also as sulfate conjugates).[60] In fact, hepatic oxidative metabolism rapidly converts many of the systemic and topical corticosteroids to inactive metabolites and, thus, serves to protect patients from the HPA axis–suppressive effects of these drugs on endogenous steroid production. The corticosteroids are metabolized in many tissues, including the liver, muscles, and red blood cells[18,20,61]; however, the liver metabolizes them most rapidly. The fact that many of the endogenous corticosteroids are rapidly metabolized by the liver precludes their administration by the oral route. Metabolic products can be isolated from the urine and bile and can be formed in tissue preparations in vitro.[62]

Specific Drugs (see Fig. 24.14)

11-Desoxycorticosterone was the first naturally occurring corticoid to be synthesized. Before its isolation from the adrenal cortex, it was prepared by M. Steiger and T. Reichstein.[63] As a result of his synthesis of 11-desoxycorticosterone and other early work with corticoids, Reichstein later shared the Nobel Prize with E.C. Kendall, another chemist who was instrumental in carrying out early steroid syntheses, and with P.S. Hench, a rheumatologist who, in 1929, discovered that cortisone is effective in the treatment of rheumatoid arthritis. Kendall's basic research ultimately led to the synthesis of cortisone from naturally occurring bile acids.[63]

Cortisone, Hydrocortisone, and Their Ester Derivatives. After the synthesis of 11-desoxycorticosterone in 1937, all the corticoids were soon thereafter synthesized and their structures confirmed. The first synthesis of cortisone from methyl 3α-hydroxy-11-ketobisnorcholanate was reported by L.H. Sarett[64] in 1946. Earlier work of Kendall and coworkers involving its preparation from the methyl ester of desoxycholic acid was used in his research.[65] Later, several chemists, including Sarett,[66] Kendall, and M. Tishler, found ways to improve the yields and to decrease the labor involved in the multistep conversion of bile acids to cortisone acetate. In 1949, Merck sold limited quantities of this glucocorticoid to physicians at $200 per gram for treating rheumatoid arthritis. Subsequent improvements in the methods of synthesis reduced the price to $10 per gram by 1951. In 1955, Upjohn used an efficient process involving the synthesis of cortisone acetate from progesterone, with the latter steroid being prepared from diosgenin (a steroid sapogenin isolated

Table 24.3 Pharmacological and Pharmacokinetic Properties for Some Adrenocorticoids

Adrenocorticoid	Oral Glucocorticoid Dose[a] (mg)	Potency Relative to Hydrocortisone		Protein Binding (%)[b]	Half-Life (h)		Duration of Action (d)
		Glucocorticoid Activity[c]	Mineralocorticoid Activity[d]		Plasma	Biologic (tissue)	
Glucocorticoids							
Short-acting:							
Hydrocortisone	20	1	2+	>90	1.5-2.0	8-12	1.0-1.5
Cortisone	25	0.8	2+	>90	0.5	8-12	1.0-1.5
Intermediate-acting:							
Prednisone	5	3.5	1+	>90	3.4-3.8	18-36	1.0-1.5
Prednisolone	5	4	1+	>90	2.1-3.5	18-36	1.0-1.5
Methylprednisolone	5	5	0[e]	>90	>3.5	18-36	1.0-1.5
Triamcinolone	5	5	0[e]	40[f]	2-5	18-36	1.0-1.5
Deflazacort	6	3	0[e]				
Long-acting:							
Dexamethasone	0.75	20-30	0[e]	>90	3.0-4.5	36-54	2.8-3
Betamethasone	0.6	20-30	0[e]	>90	3-5	36-54	2.8-3
Mineralocorticoids							
Fludrocortisone	Not employed	10	10	<90	3.5	18-36	1-2
Aldosterone	Not employed	0.2	800				
11-Desoxycorticosterone	Not employed	0	40				
Corticosterone	IM	0.5	5				

[a]Based on the oral dose of an anti-inflammatory agent in rheumatoid arthritis.

[b]Hydrocortisone binds to transcortin (corticosteroid-binding globulin [CBG]) and to albumin. Prednisone also binds to CBG, but betamethasone, dexamethasone and triamcinolone do not.

[c]Anti-inflammatory, immunosuppressant, and metabolic effects.

[d]Sodium and water retention and potassium depletion effects.

[e]Although these glucocorticoids are considered not to have significant mineralocorticoid activity, hypokalemia and/or sodium and fluid retention may occur depending on the dosage, duration of use, and patient predisposition.

[f]Plasma protein binding for 21-desDFZ.

Table 24.4 Adrenocorticoids: Trade Names and Routes of Administration

Adrenocorticoid	Trade Name	PO	IV	IM or Local Injection	Inhaled or Intranasal	Topical
Alclometasone dipropionate						•
Amcinonide						•
Beclomethasone dipropionate (BDP)	QNASL, Qvar				•	
BDP monohydrate	Beconase AQ				•	
Betamethasone	Celestone	•				
Betamethasone dipropionate	Diprolene, Diprolene AF, Maxivate					•
Betamethasone sodium phosphate	Celestone Soluspan			•		
Betamethasone valerate	BetaVal, Luxiq, Valisone					•
Budesonide	Airsupra, Breztri Aerosphere, Pulmicort TurbuHaler, Pulmicort Respules, Pulmicort Flexhaler, Rhinocort Allergy (OTC)[a]				•	
Budesonide	Entocort EC, Tarpeyo, Uceris[b]	•				•[b]
Ciclesonide	Alvesco, Omnaris, Zetonna				•	
Clobetasol propionate	Clobex, Cormax, Embuline, Olux					•
Clocortolone pivalate	Cloderm					•
Cortisone acetate		•		•		
Deflazacort	Emflaza	•				
Desonide	Desonate, Desowen, Verdeso					•
Desoximetasone	Topicort					•
Dexamethasone	Dexycu Kit[c], Maxidex[c], Ozurdex[c]	•				•[c]
Dexamethasone acetate	Dalalone, Dexasone			•		
Dexamethasone sodium phosphate			•	•		•[c]

(*continued*)

Table 24.4 Adrenocorticoids: Trade Names and Routes of Administration (*continued*)

Adrenocorticoid	Trade Name	PO	IV	IM or Local Injection	Inhaled or Intranasal	Topical
Diflorasone diacetate	ApexiCon E					•
Finerenone	Kerendia	•				
Fludrocortisone acetate		•				
Flunisolide	Aerospan HFA				•	
Fluocinolone acetonide	Capex, Derma-Smoothe, Dermotic, Iluvien[c], Retisert[c], Synlar, Tri-Luma					•
Fluocinonide	Lidex, Vanos					•
Fluorometholone	FML					•[a]
Fluorometholone acetate	Flarex					•[a]
Flurandrenolide	Cordran					•
Fluticasone furoate	Arnuity Ellipta, Veramyst				•	
Fluticasone propionate	ArmonAir Digihaler, Cutivate, Flovent Diskus, Flovent HFA, Flonase Allergy Relief (OTC), Xhance				•	•
Halcinonide	Halog					•
Halobetasol propionate	Duobrii, Ultravate					•
Hydrocortisone	Ala-Cort, Anusol HC, Colocort, Cortef, Texacort	•				•[b]
Hydrocortisone acetate	Cortiform, Micort HC, Pramosone, Proctofoam HC					•[c]
Hydrocortisone buteprate	Pandel					•
Hydrocortisone butyrate	Locoid					•
Hydrocortisone sodium phosphate			•	•		
Hydrocortisone sodium succinate	Solu-Cortef		•	•		
Hydrocortisone valerate						•

Loteprednol etabonate	Alrex, Eysuvis, Inveltys, Lotemax					•
Methylprednisolone	Medrol, Medrol Dose Pack	•				
Methylprednisolone acetate	Depo-Medrol			•		•
Methylprednisolone sodium succinate	Solu-Medrol		•	•		
Mometasone furoate	Elocon					•
Mometasone furoate	Nasonex, Asmanex HFA, Asmanex Twisthaler, Sinuva[d]				•	•
Prednicarbate	Dermatop					•
Prednisolone	Delta-Cortef, Prelone	•				
Prednisolone acetate	Omnipred, Predcor, Predalone	•	•			
Prednisolone acetate	Pred-Mild, Pred-Forte					•[c]
Prednisolone sodium phosphate	Pediapred, Orapred ODT	•	•			•[c]
Prednisone	Rayos	•				
Triamcinolone acetonide		•				
Triamcinolone acetonide	Kenalog, Triderm, Trianex, Delta-Tritex					•
Triamcinolone acetonide	Allernaze, Nasacort Allergy (OTC), Nasacort AQ				•	
Triamcinolone acetonide	Kenalog, Zilretta[e], Triesence[c]		•			
Triamcinolone diacetate			•			
Triamcinolone hexacetonide	Aristospan		•			
Vamorolone	Agamree	•				

IM, intramuscular; IV, intravenous; OTC, over the counter; PO, oral.
[a]Nasal spray is OTC. Aerosol has been discontinued.
[b]Rectal foam for ulcerative colitis.
[c]Ophthalmic formulation (drops, insert, injection, or ointment)
[d]Sinus insert.
[e]Intra-articular injectable extended-release suspension.

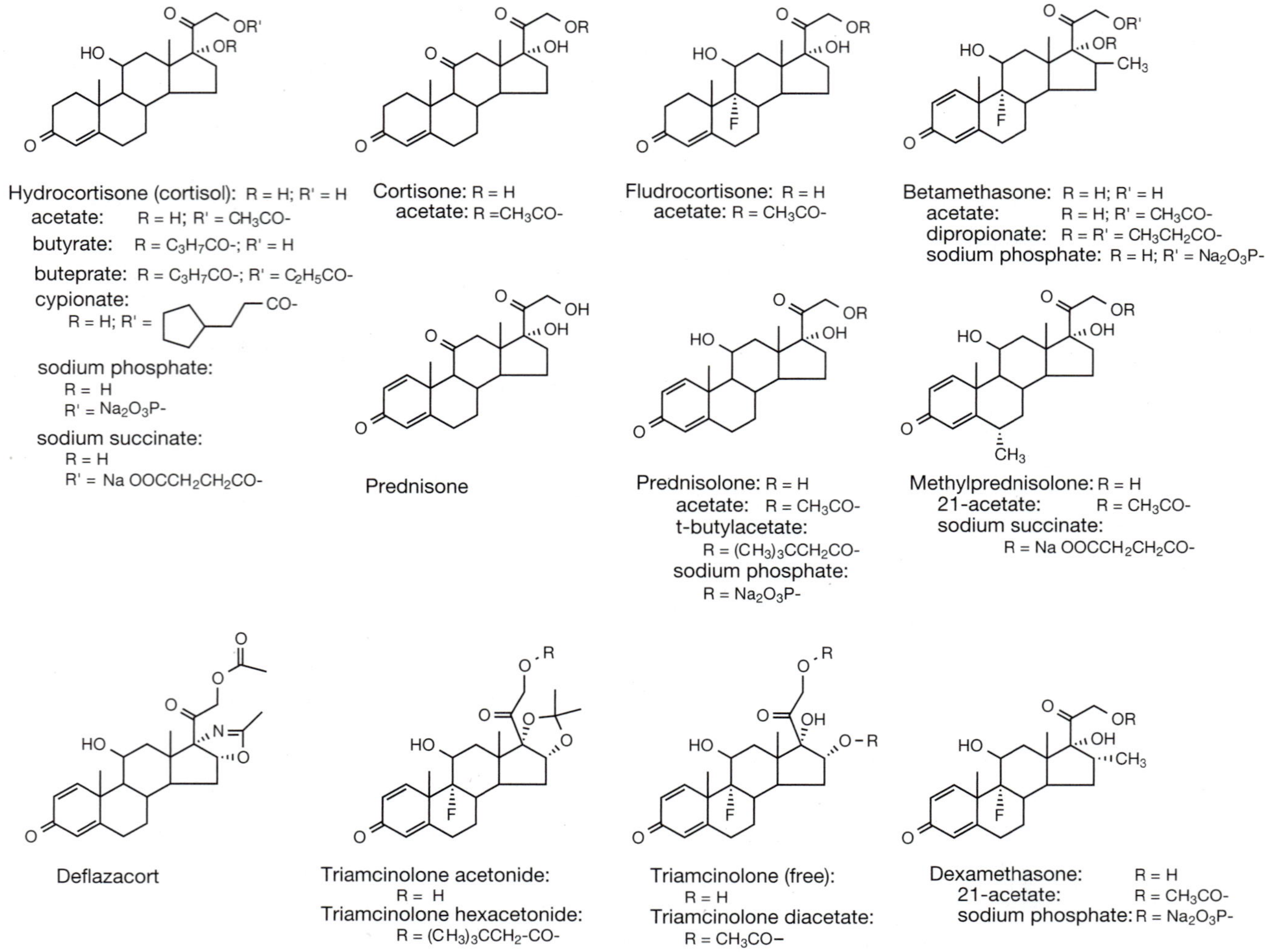

Figure 24.14 Systemic corticosteroids.

from the tubers of the *Dioscorea* wild yam). This further reduced the price to \$3.50 per gram.

Cortisone is administered orally or by intramuscular (IM) injection as its 21-acetate (cortisone acetate). Cortisone acetate or hydrocortisone (acetate) are usually the corticosteroids of choice for replacement therapy in patients with adrenocortical insufficiency because these drugs have both glucocorticoid and mineralocorticoid properties. Following oral administration, cortisone acetate and hydrocortisone acetate are completely and rapidly deacetylated by first-pass esterase metabolism[67]. Much of the oral cortisone, however, is inactivated by oxidative metabolism (Fig. 24.9) before it can be converted to hydrocortisone in the liver.

The pharmacokinetics of hydrocortisone acetate are indistinguishable from those of orally administered hydrocortisone. Oral hydrocortisone is completely absorbed, with a bioavailability of greater than 95% and a half-life of 1 to 2 hours.[25] The metabolism of hydrocortisone (Fig. 24.9) has been previously described. Cortisone acetate is slowly absorbed from IM injection sites over a period of 24 to 48 hours and is reserved for patients who are unable to take the drug orally. The acetate ester derivative demonstrates increased stability and has a longer duration of action when administered by IM injection. Thus, smaller doses can be used. Similarly, hydrocortisone may be dispensed as its 21-acetate (hydrocortisone acetate), which is superior to cortisone acetate when injected intra-articularly. Systemic absorption of hydrocortisone acetate from intra-articular injection sites is usually complete within 24 to 48 hours. When administered intrarectally, hydrocortisone is poorly absorbed.[68,69]

Other ester derivatives that are available include the lipophilic hydrocortisone cypionate [21-(3-cyclopentylpropionate) ester], hydrocortisone butyrate (17α-butyrate ester), hydrocortisone buteprate (17α-butyrate, 21-propionate esters) and hydrocortisone valerate (17α-valerate ester [not shown]), along with water soluble hydrocortisone sodium succinate (21-sodium succinate ester) and hydrocortisone sodium phosphate (the 21-sodium phosphate ester; Fig. 24.14).

- The water-insoluble hydrocortisone cypionate is used orally in doses expressed in terms of hydrocortisone for slower absorption from the GI tract.
- The water-insoluble butyrate, buteprate, and valerate esters are used topically.
- The extremely water-soluble 21-sodium succinate and 21-sodium phosphate esters are used for IV or IM injection in the management of emergency conditions

that can be treated with anti-inflammatory steroids (eg, adrenal crisis during surgery, shock). The phosphate ester is completely and rapidly metabolized by phosphatases, with a half-life of less than 5 minutes.[68] Peak hydrocortisone levels are reached in approximately 10 minutes. The sodium succinate ester is slowly and incompletely hydrolyzed, and peak hydrocortisone levels are attained in 30 to 45 minutes.[68]

After the introduction of cortisone (1948) and, later, hydrocortisone (1951) for the treatment of rheumatoid arthritis, many investigators began to search for superior agents having fewer side effects. When these drugs are used in doses necessary to suppress symptoms of rheumatoid arthritis, they also affect other metabolic processes. Side effects, such as excessive sodium retention and potassium excretion, negative nitrogen balance, increased gastric acidity, edema, and psychosis, are exaggerated manifestations of the normal metabolic functions of the hormones.

It was hoped that a compound with high glucocorticoid and low mineralocorticoid activity could be synthesized. Because it was recognized early from SAR that a carbonyl group at C3, a double bond between carbons 4 and 5, an oxygen (C=O or β-OH) at carbon 11, and a β-ketol side chain at position 17 are necessary for superior glucocorticoid activity, investigators began to synthesize analogues containing these functions. Additional groups were inserted into other positions of the basic steroid structure, with the expectation that these new substituents might modify the glucocorticoid and mineralocorticoid activities of the parent drugs.

Fludrocortisone (9α-Fluoro). A 9α-bromo analogue was prepared that had one-third the glucocorticoid activity of cortisone acetate.[51] Other halogens were introduced into the 9α-position, and it was soon observed that glucocorticoid activity is inversely proportional to the size of the halogen at carbon 9 due to diminishing electron withdrawing effects and increased steric hindrance with the larger halogens. The 9α-fluoro analogue (fludrocortisone; Fig. 24.14) is approximately 11-fold more potent at GRs and even more potent at MRs than cortisone acetate (Table 24.3) due to inductive effects of the fluorine, which enhances the ability of the 11β-OH to hydrogen bond with GR (Asn564) and MRs (Asn770), and inhibition of metabolic oxidation to the less active 11-keto. Fludrocortisone is orally administered as its 21-acetate derivative. When tested clinically in patients with rheumatoid arthritis, it was found to be effective at approximately 1/10 the dose of cortisone acetate. Although glucocorticoid activity is increased 11-fold by insertion of the 9α-fluoro substituent, mineralocorticoid activity is increased 300- to 800-fold. Because of its intense sodium-retaining activity that leads to edema, fludrocortisone is contraindicated in all conditions except those that require a high degree of mineralocorticoid activity.

Fludrocortisone acetate is used orally for mineralocorticoid replacement therapy in patients with adrenocortical insufficiency, such as Addison disease. This drug, introduced in 1954, helped provide the impetus for the synthesis and biologic evaluation of newer halogenated analogues.

Prednisone, Prednisolone, and Their Derivatives (Δ¹). One year after the introduction of fludrocortisone, the Δ^1-corticoids were brought forth into clinical medicine. Investigators at Schering observed that the 1-dehydro derivatives of cortisone and hydrocortisone—namely, prednisone and prednisolone—are more potent antirheumatic and antiallergenic agents than the parent compounds and produced fewer undesirable side effects at lower doses. These compounds are known as Δ^1-corticoids because they contain an additional double bond between positions 1 and 2 (Fig. 24.14).

The Δ^1-corticoids were the first chemical innovation that led to the creation of modified compounds that could be prescribed for rheumatoid arthritis. Both prednisone and prednisolone were found to have adrenocortical activity as measured by eosinopenic response, liver glycogen decomposition, and thymus involution in adrenalectomized mice. In these tests, prednisone and prednisolone were found to be 3- to 4-fold more potent than cortisone and hydrocortisone. Antiphlogistic (anti-inflammatory) strengths in human subjects were similarly augmented, but their electrolyte activities were not proportionately increased (Table 24.3).

The increased potency reflects the effect of the change in geometry of ring A caused by the introduction of C1=C2 on GR affinity and altered pharmacokinetics (primarily metabolism). Although the remaining portions of the steroid are essentially unchanged (except for the less easily visualized molecular perturbations), the conformation of ring A changes from a chair, as in 5α-pregnan-3-one (structure A in Fig. 24.15), to a half-chair (pregn-4-en-3-one; B in Fig. 24.15) and to a flattened boat (pregna-1,4-dien-3-one; C in Fig. 24.15) on introduction of unsaturation.

The order of GR affinity is dexamethasone (10×)> triamcinolone (5×)> methylprednisolone (4×)> prednisolone (2×)> hydrocortisone (1×).[70] The GR binding affinity rank order can be rationalized from SAR observations.

- Addition of the Δ^1 to hydrocortisone to yield prednisolone doubles binding affinity due to A-ring geometry changes discussed earlier, which are likely to improve interaction with Gln570 and Arg611 of GR.
- Addition of 6α-methyl to prednisolone to yield methylprednisolone (Δ^1, 6α-CH_3) again doubles binding affinity (4× hydrocortisone) and provides GR selectivity. Additional benefits of Δ^1 and 6α-methyl groups include prevention of metabolism at the 3-keto and C6 positions.
- Addition of 9α-fluoro to hydrocortisone to yield fludrocortisone also enhances GR and MR affinity through inductive effects on the 11β-OH to enhance interactions with Asn564 (GR) and Asn770 (MR).

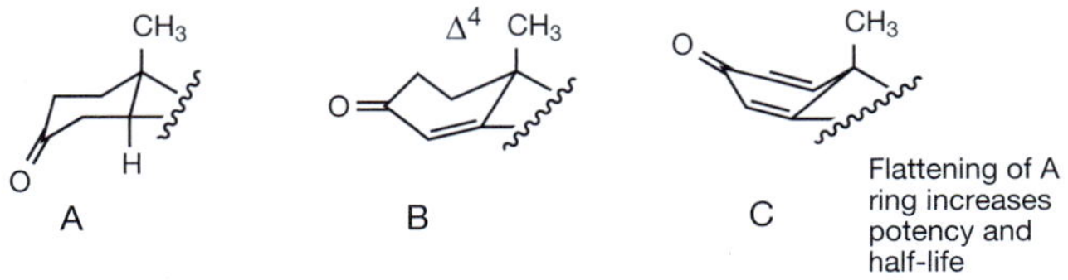

Figure 24.15 Ring A conformations for 5α-pregnan-3-one (A), pregn-4-en-3-one (B), and pregna-1,4-dien-3-one (C). All endogenous and some synthetic glucocorticoids are Δ^4 variants of 5α-pregnane, however, many higher potency glucocorticoids are also Δ^1 variants as depicted in (C).

Inactivating metabolism of 11β-OH to the ketone is also blocked.

- Addition of 16α-substitution provides GR selectivity due to the inability of MR to accommodate bulk or polar groups.
- Addition of 9α-fluoro and 16α-OH to prednisolone (Δ^1) to yield triamcinolone more than doubles the GR affinity (5× hydrocortisone vs 2× for prednisolone) due to an enhanced 11β-OH–Asn564 interaction and introduction of the 16α-OH–Gln642 interaction at the GR. The equivalent of Gln642 is unavailable in MR, explaining the greatly enhanced GR selectivity of triamcinolone relative to prednisolone.
- Changing the 16α-OH of triamcinolone (Δ^1, 9α-F, 16α-OH) to the 16α-methyl of dexamethasone (Δ^1, 9α-F, 16α-methyl) again doubles GR binding affinity (10× hydrocortisone vs 5× for triamcinolone) due to favorable hydrophobic contacts of the 16α-methyl group within a hydrophobic pocket of GR that is not available in MRs.
- The latter two molecules demonstrate that high GR affinity and high GR selectivity are possible through rational substitution of hydrocortisone.

Rank Order of GR Affinity:
Dexamethasone (10×) > triamcinolone (5×) > methylprednisolone (4×) > prednisolone (2×) > hydrocortisone (1×)

Endogenous Hormone

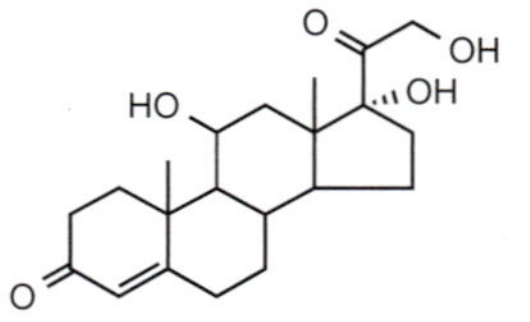

Hydrocortisone (cortisol)

9α-Fluoro

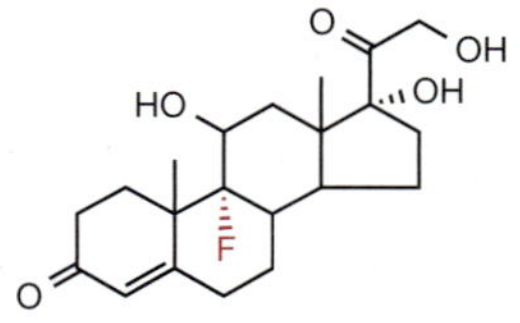

Fludrocortisone

Δ^1 Corticoid

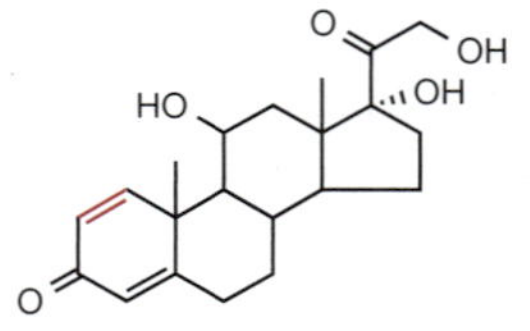

Prednisolone

Δ^1, 6α-methyl

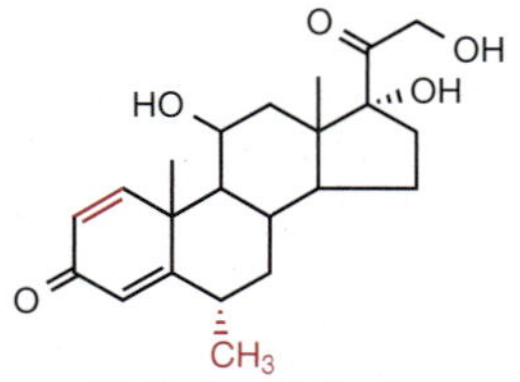

Methylprednisolone

Δ^1, 9α-Fluoro, 16α-hydroxy

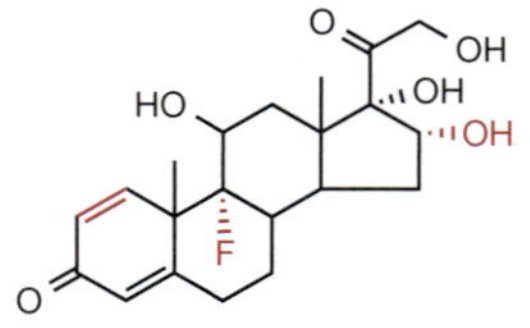

Triamcinolone

Δ^1, 9α-Fluoro, 16α-methyl

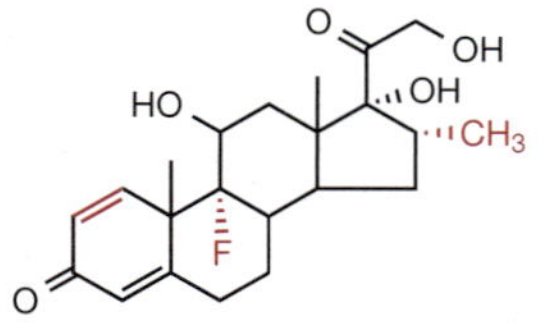

Dexamethasone

When orally administered, prednisone and prednisolone are almost completely absorbed, with a bioavailability of greater than 80% (Table 24.5).[71,72] As with the relationship between cortisone and hydrocortisone, prednisone and prednisolone are also interconvertible by 11β-hydroxysteroid dehydrogenase type 1 (11β-HSD1) in the liver. For practical purposes, prednisone and prednisolone are equally potent and can be used interchangeably. Due to the higher GR affinity afforded by the flattened A-ring and metabolic stabilization of the 3-keto, when prednisone or prednisolone is used in the treatment of rheumatoid arthritis, smaller doses are required than with hydrocortisone. The usual dose is 5 mg 2 to 4 times a day.

Prednisolone is metabolized into a number of more hydrophilic and less active metabolites (Fig. 24.16), except there is greatly decreased reduction of ring A compared with hydrocortisone due to stabilizing extended conjugation. The major metabolites (6β- and 20α/β-hydroxy) are primarily excreted as glucuronide conjugates in the urine.

Prednisolone acetate is available in suspension and ointment forms for external use (Fig. 24.14). As with hydrocortisone, several other 21-esters of prednisolone are available. Prednisolone tebutate (*t*-butylacetate [3,3-dimethylbutyrate]) has been discontinued but was used in suspension form and by injection for the same reasons that the 21-ester derivatives of hydrocortisone are currently employed. Prednisolone tebutate had a long duration of action because of low water solubility and a slow rate of hydrolysis.

Prednisolone sodium phosphate is the water-soluble sodium salt of the 21-phosphate ester. It has a half-life of less than 5 minutes because of rapid hydrolysis by phosphatases.[71-73] Peak plasma levels for prednisolone are attained in approximately 10 minutes following its administration by injection (usual dose of 20 mg intravenously or intramuscularly). Topically, one or two drops of a 0.5% solution may be used 4 to 6 times daily for its anti-inflammatory action in the eye.

As stated in the "Pharmacologic Effects and Clinical Applications" section, Δ^1-corticoids and hydrocortisone in equivalent antirheumatic doses promote the same pattern of initial improvement; however, the results of longer-term therapy are more favorable with the Δ^1 and further modified synthetic corticoids. Studies indicate that the Δ^1-corticoids can be used continuously in patients with rheumatoid arthritis without undue GI distress. Although the Δ^1-corticoids are considered not to have significant mineralocorticoid activity, hypokalemia and sodium and fluid retention can occur depending on the dosage and duration of use.

METHYLPREDNISOLONE (6α-METHYL). Between 1953 and 1962, many derivatives of the Δ^1-corticoids and the halogen-containing analogues (especially 9α-fluorinated compounds) were synthesized, and some became useful clinical agents. Studies with methylcorticoids revealed 2α-methyl derivatives to be inactive, whereas the 2α-methyl-9α-fluoro analogues had potent mineralocorticoid activity.

Methylprednisolone (6α-methyl derivative of prednisolone) was synthesized in 1956 and introduced into clinical medicine (Fig. 24.14). Methylprednisolone is extensively metabolized, with approximately 10% recovered unchanged in the urine.[74] The metabolic pathways include reduction of the C20 ketone, oxidation of 17β-ketol group to C21-COOH and C20-COOH, and 6β-hydroxylation (CYP3A4). Methylprednisolone potentiates glucocorticoid activity with negligible salt retention in short-term therapy (Table 24.3).[75]

In human subjects, the metabolic side effects did not differ appreciably from those of prednisolone. Its activities with respect to nitrogen excretion, ACTH suppression, and reduction of circulating eosinophils were similar to those

Table 24.5 Pharmacokinetics of Commonly Used Oral Adrenocorticoids

Adrenocorticoid	Bioavailability (%)	Half-Life (hours)	Protein Binding (%)	Volume Distribution (L/kg)	LogP (Experimental)	Clearance (mL/min/70 g)
Dexamethasone	78	3.0	90-95	0.2	1.83	260
Hydrocortisone	96	1.7	90	0.5	1.61	400
Methylprednisolone	90	2.3	90-95	1.5	1.76	430
Prednisone	80	3.6	~90	1.0	1.46	250
Prednisolone	82	2.8	90-95	0.7-1.5	1.62	60
Triamcinolone	23	2.96	~90	1.3	1.16	61

of prednisolone. The sodium retention and potassium loss were slightly less than with prednisolone.[76]

Oral methylprednisolone (Medrol) is commonly used for its anti-inflammatory effects in chronic diseases such as arthritis, systemic lupus erythematosus, psoriasis, certain neoplasms, or conditions that affect the eyes, blood cells, intestines or lung to relieve swelling, pain, and allergic-type reactions. It is also available as a dose pack (Medrol Dose Pak) for the treatment of acute asthmatic or allergic exacerbations. The dose pack is designed to provide the high HPA axis suppressing dose needed to resolve the exacerbation and improve patient adherence with the tapering of this dose, which is necessary to avoid adrenal insufficiency crisis when discontinued.

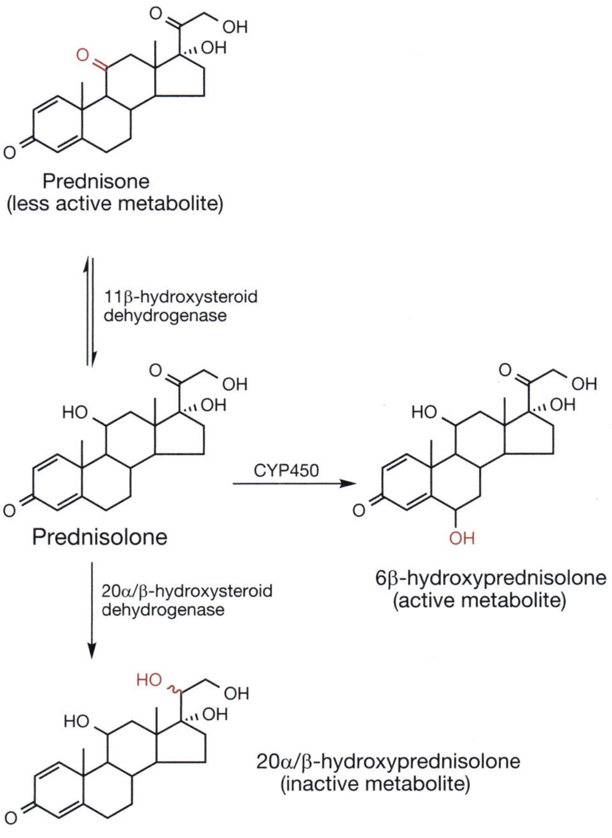

Figure 24.16 Major routes of metabolism for prednisolone.

Methylprednisolone administered parenterally as the 21-acetate ester (Depo-Medrol) is rapidly cleaved to methylprednisolone (Fig. 24.14). IM administration of 80 to 120 mg of methylprednisolone acetate to asthmatic patients provides systemic relief within 6 to 48 hours, which persists for several days to 2 weeks. Intra-articular, soft tissue, or intralesional injection may provide acute local relief of symptoms of rheumatoid arthritis, acute gouty arthritis, or bursitis.

Methylprednisolone is administered intravenously as the water-soluble sodium salt of the 21-succinate ester. The succinate ester is slowly and incompletely hydrolyzed. Peak plasma levels for methylprednisolone are attained in approximately 30 to 60 minutes following IV administration, and approximately 15% of the IV dose is recovered unchanged in the urine.[72,73] CYP3A4 inhibitors, such as the antifungals ketoconazole and itraconazole, can potentiate the effects of methylprednisolone, while CYP3A4 inducers may require methylprednisolone dose increases.

DEFLAZACORT (16α,17α-OXAZOLINE RING). Although prednisone and prednisolone demonstrate increased glucocorticoid potency, there was a need to improve the therapeutic index of these early Δ^1-corticoids. Addition of the 5-membered 16α,17α-oxazoline ring of deflazacort (Fig. 24.14), reminiscent of the acetonide found in triamcinolone, produces an improved side effect profile, with deflazacort demonstrating bone-sparing and carbohydrate-sparing properties as compared to prednisone.[77-79] This is particularly important in long-term administration and/or in pediatric patients. Deflazacort was demonstrated to be effective against various rheumatoid diseases with similar potency as prednisolone and, on the merit of its lessened side effect profile, it was tested in various pediatric populations in the 1990s. It was first approved for use in Europe in 1985 but was not available in the United States until 2017, when it was approved for the treatment of Duchenne muscular dystrophy (DMD) in boys ages 5 years and older. DMD is a rare X-linked muscle wasting disease affecting exclusively young boys.

Deflazacort is rapidly and completely absorbed upon oral administration with a T_{max} of 1 to 2 hours. The 21-acetate of deflazacort is rapidly cleaved by plasma esterases to the active metabolite, 21-desacetyldeflazacort (21-desDFZ).[80] 21-DesDFZ is metabolized in the liver by CYP3A4 to inactive metabolites. The package insert recommends dose reductions of a third if coadministered with moderate or strong CYP3A4 inhibitors and avoiding coadministration with moderate to strong CYP3A4 inducers. Urinary excretion, the primary route of elimination, is almost complete by 24 hours. Studies in children (aged 5-11 years) and adolescents (aged 11-16 years) demonstrated a higher C_{max} and systemic exposures in adolescents. Post-hoc analysis of the phase III study in DMD demonstrated that deflazacort met its primary endpoint of increasing mean muscle strength at 12 weeks, an effect that was durable out to 52 weeks. Furthermore, deflazacort (but not prednisone) increased pulmonary function metrics. Side effects were similar to other corticosteroids and included facial puffiness, weight gain, increased appetite, upper respiratory tract infections, and central obesity. Deflazacort is available as an oral suspension (22.75 mg/mL) or oral tablet (6 mg, 18 mg, 30 mg, and 36 mg).

Triamcinolone (9α-Fluoro, 16α-Hydroxy). The original interest in 16α-hydroxycorticosteroids stemmed from their isolation from the urine of a boy with an adrenal tumor. The desire of chemists to synthesize these corticoids, and the hope that such analogues might have potent biologic activity, furthered their development.[81-83] Insertion of a 16α-hydroxy group into 9α-fluoroprednisolone resulted in triamcinolone, which has glucocorticoid activity equivalent to prednisolone but with decreased mineralocorticoid activity (Table 24.3). In fact, 16α-hydroxy analogues of natural corticoids retain glucocorticoid activity and have a considerably reduced mineralocorticoid activity. Thus, a natural extension of corticoid research involved examination of compounds containing a 9α-fluoro group, a double bond between positions 1 and 2, and a 16α-hydroxy group. Triamcinolone, introduced in 1958, combines the structural features of a Δ^1-corticoid and a 9α-fluoro corticoid plus a 16α-hydroxy group (see Fig. 24.14). As mentioned previously, the 9α-fluoro group increases the anti-inflammatory potency through enhancement of hydrogen bonding between the 11β-OH and Asn564 and inhibition of oxidative metabolism at this site, but also markedly increases the mineralocorticoid potency. This is undesirable if the drug is to be used internally—for example, for the treatment of rheumatoid arthritis. However, by inserting a 16α-hydroxy group into the molecule, one decreases the mineralocorticoid activity due to the lack of a polar H bond accepting residue and/or steric hindrance in MR. These glucocorticoids actually can cause sodium excretion rather than sodium retention.

The lower-than-expected oral anti-inflammatory potency for triamcinolone (Table 24.3; only equipotent to prednisolone despite higher GR affinity) has been attributed to its low oral bioavailability (Table 24.5), in part because of increased hydrophilicity from the 16α-hydroxy group and first-pass metabolism, primarily to its 6β-hydroxy metabolite. Triamcinolone acetonide (16α,17α-acetal with acetone; Fig. 24.14) is active intact and can be taken orally, injected, or topically applied via inhalation or creams/lotions, as discussed later. The 16α,17α-acetonide forms favorable hydrophobic interactions with the hydrophobic pocket of GR, increasing affinity and improving GR selectivity. Triamcinolone diacetate (17α,21-diacetate) and its hexacetonide [16α,17α-acetonide-21-(3,3-dimethylbutyrate)] prodrug esters are administered intramuscularly or intra-articularly for a prolonged release of triamcinolone. Depending on route of administration, triamcinolone diacetate has a duration of action ranging from 1 to 8 weeks, and triamcinolone hexacetonide has a duration of action of 3 to 4 weeks.[84, 85]

On a weight-for-weight basis, the antirheumatic potency of triamcinolone is slightly greater than that of prednisolone (~20%) and approximately the same as that of methylprednisolone (Table 24.3). Initial improvement following administration of triamcinolone is similar to that noted with other compounds. Reports in the literature, however, indicate that the percentage of patients maintained satisfactorily for long periods has been distinctly smaller compared to prednisolone.

Although triamcinolone has an apparently decreased tendency to cause salt and water retention and edema and can even induce sodium and water diuresis, it causes other unwanted side effects, including anorexia, weight loss, muscle weakness, leg cramps, nausea, dizziness, and general malaise.[86] IM triamcinolone is reportedly effective and safe in the treatment of dermatoses. In combination with folic acid antagonists (eg, methotrexate), it is effective in the treatment of psoriasis.[87,88]

Dexamethasone (9α-Fluoro, 16α-Methyl). Research with 16-methyl substituted corticoids was initiated in part because investigators hoped to stabilize the 17β-ketol side chain to metabolism in vivo and improve bioavailability. These studies led to the clinical development of dexamethasone, which combines the structural features of a Δ^1-corticoid and a 9α-fluoro corticoid plus a 16α-methyl group (Fig. 24.14). A 16α-methyl group decreases the reactivity of the 20-keto group to carbonyl reagents and increases the stability of the drug in human plasma in vitro.[89,90] Unlike 16α-hydroxylation, a methyl group increases the anti-inflammatory activity by increasing lipophilicity and, consequently, receptor affinity through bonding to lipophilic residues within a GR hydrophobic pocket. Like the 16α-hydroxyl group, the methyl group markedly reduces the salt-retaining properties of the corticosteroids (Table 24.3).[91-93] The activity of dexamethasone, as measured by glycogen deposition, is 20-fold greater than that of hydrocortisone. It has 5-fold higher anti-inflammatory activity than prednisolone. Clinical data indicate that this compound has 7 times the antirheumatic potency of prednisolone and is roughly 30-fold more potent than hydrocortisone. Its pharmacokinetic parameters are presented in Table 24.5. Routes of metabolism for dexamethasone are similar to those for prednisolone, with the primary 6β-hydroxy metabolite being recovered in urine.[94]

Dexamethasone sodium phosphate is the water-soluble sodium salt of the 21-phosphate ester, with an IV half-life of less than 10 minutes because of rapid hydrolysis by plasma phosphatases.[94] Peak plasma levels for dexamethasone usually are attained in approximately 10 to 20 minutes following an IV administered dose. A similar reaction occurs when the phosphate ester is applied topically. Dexamethasone 21-acetate is a prodrug available as a suspension for IM injection. Dexamethasone is also administered by several other routes (Table 24.4), and is available in tablets, elixir, and ocular formulations.

In practical management of rheumatoid arthritis, 0.75 mg of oral dexamethasone promotes a therapeutic response equivalent to that from 4 mg of triamcinolone or methylprednisolone, 5 mg of prednisolone, and 20 mg of hydrocortisone. Clinical investigations with small groups of patients indicate that this compound could control patients who did not respond well to prednisolone. Over long periods, the improved status of some patients deteriorated.

In summarizing the biologic properties of this drug, it seems clear that, with doses of corresponding antirheumatic strength, this steroid has approximately the same tendency as prednisolone to produce facial mooning, acne, and nervous excitation. Peripheral edema is uncommon (7%) and mild. The more common and most objectionable side effects are excessive appetite and weight gain, abdominal bloating, and distention. The frequency and severity of these symptoms vary with the dose (1 mg maximum for women, and 1.5 mg maximum for men). The longer biologic half-life for dexamethasone significantly increases the potential for glucocorticoid-induced adrenal insufficiency (see "Adverse Effects" section).

The striking increase in potency does not confer a general therapeutic index on dexamethasone that is higher than that of prednisolone. Again, this drug probably is best employed as a special-purpose corticoid. It can be useful when other steroids are no longer effective or when increased appetite and weight gain are desirable. Its efficacy may be increased when it is used in combination with the H_1 antagonist cyproheptadine as an antiallergenic, antipyretic, and anti-inflammatory agent.[92]

BETAMETHASONE (9α-FLUORO, 16β-METHYL). Betamethasone, which differs from dexamethasone only in configuration of the 16-methyl group (Fig. 24.14), was made available for the treatment of rheumatic diseases and dermatologic disorders shortly after the introduction of dexamethasone.[95-98] This analogue, which contains a 16β-methyl group, is as effective as dexamethasone or, perhaps, even slightly more active. Although this drug has been reported to be less toxic than other steroids, some clinical investigators suggest that it is best used for short-term therapy. Toxic side effects, such as increased appetite, weight gain, and facial mooning, occur with prolonged use. A 0.5 mg tablet of betamethasone is equivalent to a 5.0 mg tablet of prednisolone, which is on par with dexamethasone (Table 24.3). Dipropionate and sodium phosphate ester prodrugs are available for topical administration and injection, respectively, the latter in combination with betamethasone acetate.

Selective Glucocorticoid Receptor Modulators

The long-term use of classical glucocorticoids is associated with severe adverse effects (see "Adverse Effects" section), including osteoporosis, hyperglycemia, muscle atrophy or muscle wasting, hypertension, and impaired wound healing. Improved glucocorticoids that demonstrate potent anti-inflammatory activity without these serious side effects would provide a significant therapeutic advance and are the focus of research efforts by the pharmaceutical industry. The molecular mechanism of the GR makes it a particularly suitable target for this effort. The majority of unwanted side effects of the glucocorticoids arise from the interaction of the GR with DNA (ie, GR-mediated transactivation of transcription, referred to as transactivation) to increase protein catabolism, fat storage, glucose production, or bone catabolism, where the anti-inflammatory effects are mediated via protein–protein interactions between the GR and proinflammatory transcription factors (ie, AP-1 and NFκB) that result in repression of the inflammatory response (ie, repression). A variety of GR modulators with the ability to repress inflammation, but with lesser ability to elicit transactivation (dissociated glucocorticoids), have been reported.[99-104]

Early investigations indicate that a variety of different nonsteroidal pharmacophores (eg, pentanamines, pyrazoles, and trans-decalins) bind with high affinity and selectivity to the GR. Importantly, some of these analogues demonstrate preferential ability to repress proinflammatory genes and a lesser ability to induce GR-mediated transcription. The mechanism(s) by which the selective glucocorticoid receptor modulators (SGRMs) promote selective repression of inflammation without the transactivation activity has not been resolved beyond doubt.[101,105] Moreover, the ability to dissociate the activities of glucocorticoids in the clinic has proven difficult and no nonsteroidal SGRMs have been approved for clinical use. Recently however, an initial steroidal dissociated glucocorticoid (see later) was approved for a rare disease, DMD. A better understanding of these and other mechanisms underlying GR agonism may eventually allow the expansion of glucocorticoid therapy into many disease states needing chronic anti-inflammatory therapy without diabetogenic, bone- and muscle-wasting, lipodystrophic, immune suppressive, and other deleterious effects of activating the GR.

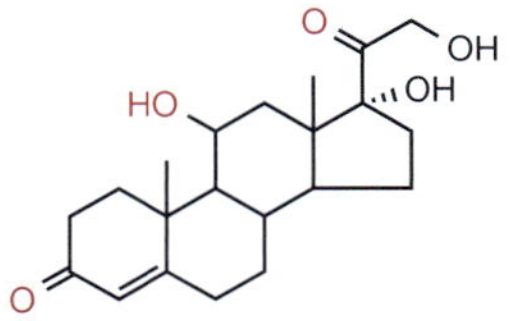

Hydrocortisone (cortisol)

Selected nonsteroidal glucocorticoids

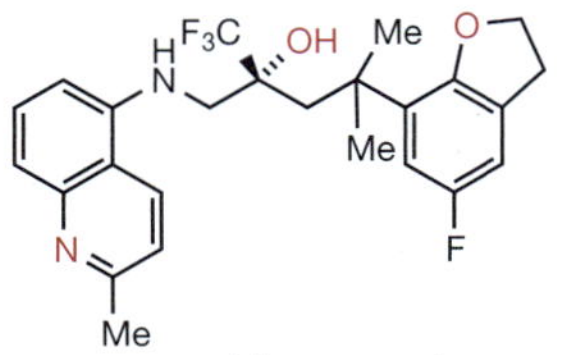

Mapracorat

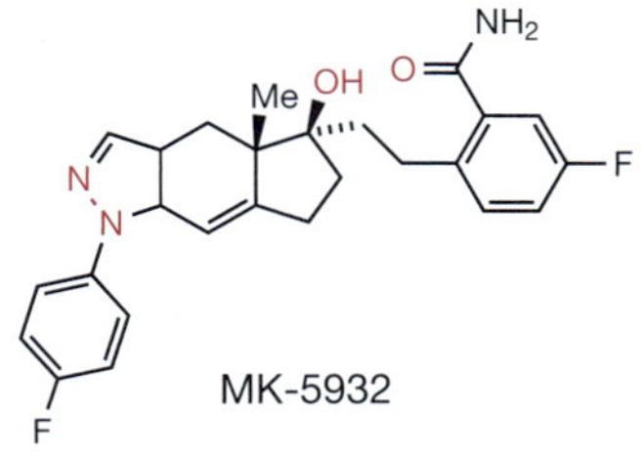

MK-5932

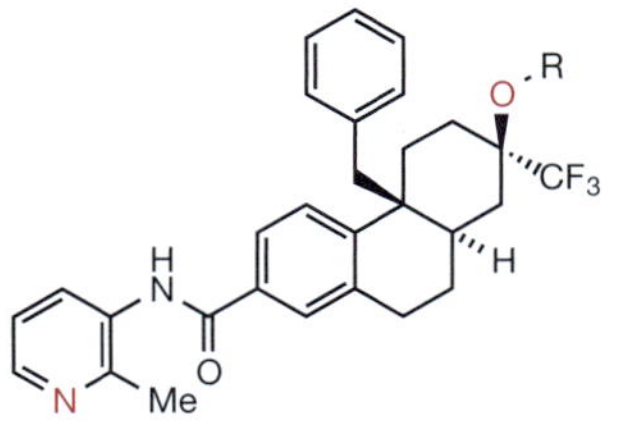

PF-802, R=H
Fosdagrocorat, R = phosphate

Vamorolone ($\Delta^{9(11)}$). Vamorolone (Agamree) was made available in 2023 for the treatment of DMD in boys older than 2 years. Although it is the first dissociated GR agonist to gain US Food and Drug Administration (FDA) approval, its steroidal structure differs from dexamethasone only in the presence of the $\Delta^{9(11)}$ double bond, which precludes the 9α-fluoro and 11β-OH substitutions of dexamethasone. Though this minor structural change did not greatly change the pharmacokinetics and metabolism of vamorolone, which are similar to that of prednisone, it produced a unique dissociated GR agonist and MR antagonist corticosteroid activity profile. Both the GR dissociation and MR antagonism are unlike the DMD standard of care glucocorticoids deflazacort or prednisone.[106] Whereas the absence of the interaction with Asn[770] of MR is consistent with MR antagonism; it is surprising that vamorolone, in the absence of the interaction with Asn[564] of GR, not only retains GR agonist activity, but possesses the ability to separate the different mechanisms of action of GR (ie, dissociated glucocorticoid). Vamorolone is a potent anti-inflammatory agent like traditional corticosteroids, which is the result of repression of proinflammatory genes such as AP-1, NF-κB, etc. However, the advantage of a dissociated glucocorticoid is that it possesses less transactivation of genes related to energy metabolism that typically cause growth retardation and other poorly tolerated side effects in young children.

An early clinical trial (NCT02415439) in healthy volunteers was consistent with the dissociated status of vamorolone. Biomarker assessments indicated reduced occurrence of metabolic disturbance, bone fragility, and immune suppression relative to traditional corticosteroid drugs.[107] Furthermore, the MR antagonism provided the potential to treat DMD-associated cardiomyopathy through modulation of blood pressure. In a phase 2a dose-escalation study in DMD patients, vamorolone efficacy was demonstrated as dose-related improvement in muscle function, with serum marker levels suggestive of bone formation (increased osteocalcin), and less adrenal suppression and insulin resistance compared to typical corticosteroid therapy.[108,109] In a phase 2b study, vamorolone did not change the time-to-stand velocity (the primary endpoint of the study that assessed physical function) from baseline to 30 months in DMD boys aged 4 to 7 years but was associated with maintenance of muscle strength and function up to 30 months, similar to standard of care glucocorticoid therapy. Importantly, vamorolone did not repress growth (ie, had improved height velocity) in this young population compared with standard of care glucocorticoids.[110] In overview, vamorolone is a dissociated anti-inflammatory glucocorticoid and MR antagonist, that exhibited comparable efficacy as prednisone and deflazacort for DMD boys with an improved side effect profile that distinguishes it from these traditional glucocorticoids.[107]

As mentioned, many preclinical dissociated nonsteroidal glucocorticoids have been reported as an attempt to ameliorate the notorious adverse effect profile that limits the scope of traditional steroidal glucocorticoid therapy. Vamorolone offers hope that the scope of glucocorticoid therapy, whether steroidal or nonsteroidal, may yet be expanded through the dissociation of GR agonist therapeutic effects from untoward effects of the GR.

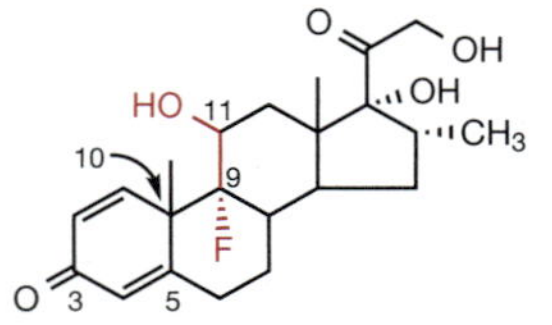

Dexamethasone

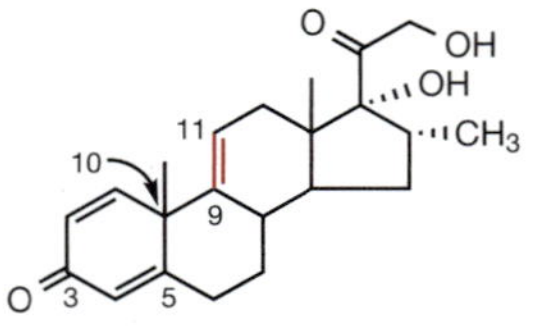

Vamorolone

Topical Glucocorticoids (Figs. 24.17 and 24.18)

Topically applied glucocorticoids are also capable of being systemically absorbed, although to a much smaller extent than orally administered agents. The extent of absorption of topical adrenocorticoids is determined by several factors, including the type of cream or ointment, the condition of the skin to which it is being applied, and the use of occlusive dressings. Previous studies with halobetasol propionate (Fig. 24.17, section [c]) showed that approximately 6% of the drug was systemically absorbed after topical application. Although this is a small fraction of the dose, the very high potency of halobetasol propionate contributed to its ability to cause mild adrenal suppression in some patients. The relative potency of the topical glucocorticoids is commonly determined using topical vasoconstriction assays and is dependent on the intrinsic activity of the drug, its concentration in the formulation, and the vehicle in which it is applied (Table 24.6).

Increased lipophilicity improves penetration through the stratum corneum and can be accomplished by introducing 6α, 7α, and/or 9α halogens, removing the 17α- hydroxy group (eg, desoximetasone; Fig. 24.17, section [b]), masking 16α-, 17α- or 21-hydroxy groups using cyclic ketals (eg, acetonide) or esters (eg, propionate), or replacing the 21-hydroxy group with a halogen, as will be discussed.[111] Once absorbed through the skin, topical corticosteroids are handled through metabolic pathways similar to the systemically administered corticosteroids. They are metabolized, primarily in the liver and are then excreted into the urine or in the bile[112]. The fact that circulating levels of the topical glucocorticoids are often extremely low, in some cases below the level of detection, does not reduce the risk for potential adverse effects from systemic exposure to topical corticosteroids. The structures for the glucocorticoids applied topically are shown in Fig. 24.17 and their relative potencies shown in Table 24.6.

Structurally, the topical glucocorticoids can be segregated based on their 16-position substitution into derivatives of: (a) triamcinolone (16α-hydroxyl), (b) dexamethasone (16α-methyl), (c) betamethasone (16β-methyl), or (d) prednisolone (unsubstituted at the 16-position) (Fig. 24.17). These early template molecules have been modified at the 6, 7, 9, 16, 17, and 21 positions to generate many topical agents with a spectrum of topical potency rankings, allowing tailored glucocorticoid therapy via judicious selection of agents.

Topical dermatologic products with a low potency ranking have a modest anti-inflammatory effect and are safest for chronic application. Those products with a medium potency ranking are used in moderate inflammatory dermatoses treatable with a limited duration of therapy. High

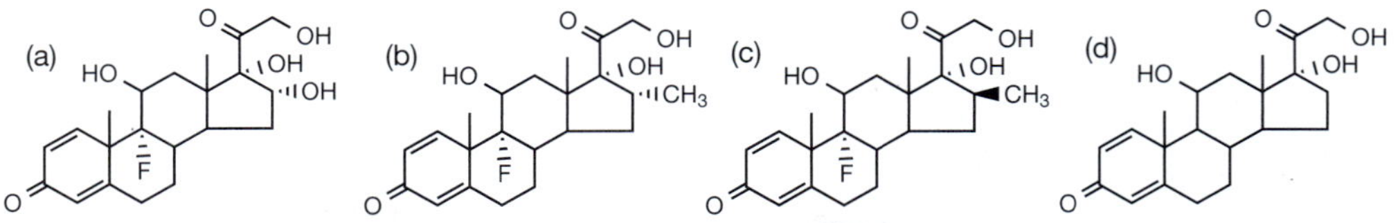

(a) Triamcinolone (b) Dexamethasone (c) Betamethasone (d) Prednisolone

(a)

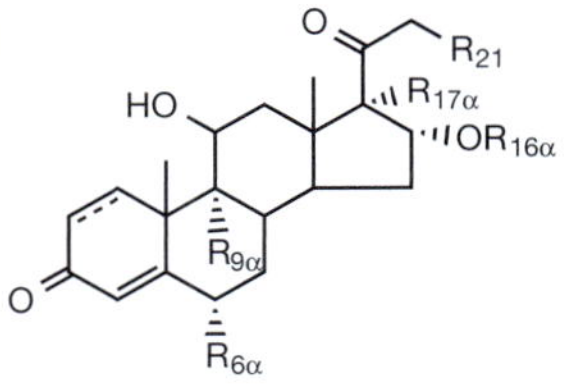

16α-hydroxy derivatives

	Δ^1	$R_{6\alpha}$	$R_{9\alpha}$	$R_{16\alpha}$	$R_{17\alpha}$	R_{21}
Triamcinolone	db	H	F	H	OH	OH
Triamcinolone acetonide	db	H	F	-16,17-acetonide		OH
Flurandrenolide	reduced	F	H	-16,17-acetonide		OH
Fluocinolone acetonide	db	F	F	-16,17-acetonide		OH
Fluocinonide	db	F	F	-16,17-acetonide		$-CO_2CH_3$
Desonide	db	H	H	-16,17-acetonide		OH
Amcinonide	db	H	F	-16,17-cyclo-pentylidenedioxy		$-CO_2CH_3$
Halcinonide	reduced	H	F	-16,17-acetonide		Cl

db = double bond

(b)

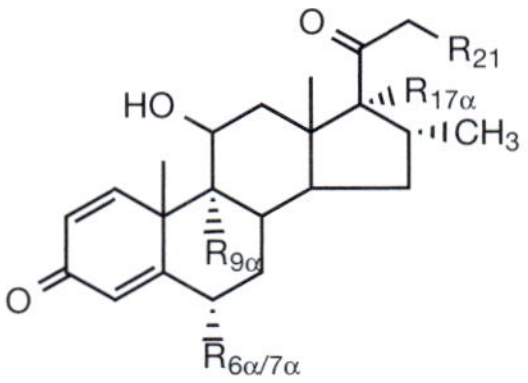

16α-methyl derivatives

	$R_{6/7}$	$R_{9\alpha}$	$R_{16\alpha}$	$R_{17\alpha}$	R_{21}
Dexamethasone	H	F	CH_3	OH	OH
Dexamethasone acetate	H	F	CH_3	OH	$-CO_2CH_3$
Flumethasone	6α-F	F	CH_3	OH	OH
Aclometasone	7α-Cl	H	CH_3	OH	OH
Diflucortolone pivalate	6α-F	F	CH_3	H	pivalate
Clocortolone pivalate	6α-F	Cl	CH_3	H	pivalate
Desoximetasone	H	F	CH_3	H	OH

(c)

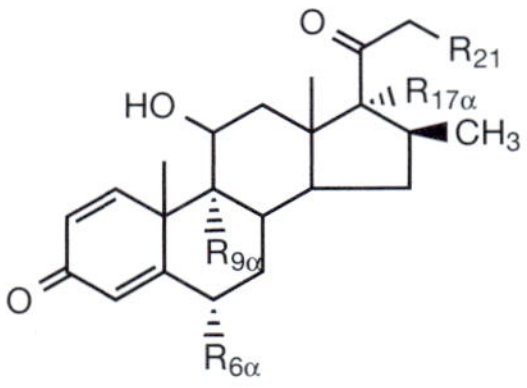

16β-methyl derivatives

	$R_{6\alpha}$	$R_{9\alpha}$	$R_{16\beta}$	$R_{17\alpha}$	R_{21}
Betamethasone	H	F	CH_3	OH	OH
Betamethasone dipropionate	H	F	CH_3	propionate	propionate
Diflorasone diacetate	F	F	CH_3	$-CO_2CH_3$	$-CO_2CH_3$
Beclomethasone	H	Cl	CH_3	OH	OH
Beclomethasone dipropionate (BDP)	H	Cl	CH_3	propionate	propionate
Clobetasol propionate	H	F	CH_3	propionate	Cl
Halobetasol propionate	F	F	CH_3	propionate	Cl

(d)

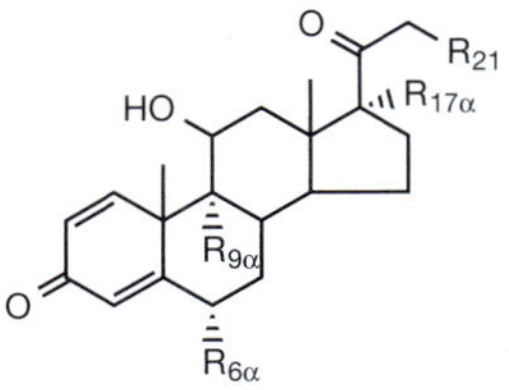

16 unsubstituted derivatives

	$R_{6\alpha}$	$R_{9\alpha}$	$R_{16\beta}$	$R_{17\alpha}$	R_{21}
Prednisolone	H	H	H	OH	OH
Prednisolone acetate	H	H	H	OH	$-CO_2CH_3$
Loteprednol etabonate	H	H	H	-OC(O)OEt	Cl
Fluorometholone acetate	CH_3	F	H	$-CO_2CH_3$	H
Prednicarbate	H	H	H	-OC(O)OEt	propionate

Figure 24.17 Topical corticosteroids.

potency preparations are used in more severe inflammatory dermatoses, but only for a short duration of treatment. Very high-potency products are used primarily as an alternative to systemic corticosteroid therapy when local areas are involved, and for only a short duration of therapy and on small surface areas.

Several inhaled and intranasal corticosteroids shown in Figure 24.18 are also available for topical administration and will be discussed in greater detail in the "Inhaled and Intranasal Glucocorticoids" section. An example is triamcinolone which is usually dispensed for topical use as its more potent and lipophilic 16α,17α-acetonide (Fig. 24.18).

Table 24.6 Potency Ranking for Topical Corticosteroids

Potency Ranking	Topical Corticosteroids
I. Very high potency	Augmented[a] betamethasone dipropionate (lotion, ointment, and gel) Clobetasol propionate Diflorasone diacetate Halobetasol propionate
II. High potency	Amcinonide Augmented[a] betamethasone dipropionate (cream) Betamethasone dipropionate Betamethasone valerate Desoximetasone Diflorasone diacetate Fluocinolone acetonide Fluocinonide Halcinonide Triamcinolone acetonide
III. Medium potency	Betamethasone dipropionate Betamethasone valerate Clocortolone pivalate Fluocinolone acetonide Flurandrenolide Fluticasone propionate Hydrocortisone butyrate Hydrocortisone valerate Loteprednol etabonate Mometasone furoate Triamcinolone acetonide
IV. Low potency	Alclometasone dipropionate Desonide Dexamethasone Dexamethasone sodium phosphate Fluocinolone acetonide Hydrocortisone Hydrocortisone acetate Prednicarbate

The relative potency is based on the drug concentration, type of vehicle used, and the vasoconstrictor assay as a measure of topical anti-inflammatory activity.

[a]Augmented indicates the formulation is designed to penetrate the skin faster, making it more potent than (regular) betamethasone dipropionate.

The acetonide is not cleaved and enhances GR affinity. It is effective in the treatment of psoriasis and other corticoid-sensitive dermatologic conditions. Topically, triamcinolone acetonide is a more potent derivative of triamcinolone and is approximately 8-fold more active than prednisolone. The side effects of the drug, however, have occurred with sufficient frequency to discourage its routine use for rheumatoid patients requiring steroid therapy. The drug can be employed advantageously as a special-purpose steroid for instances in which salt and water retention is a problem

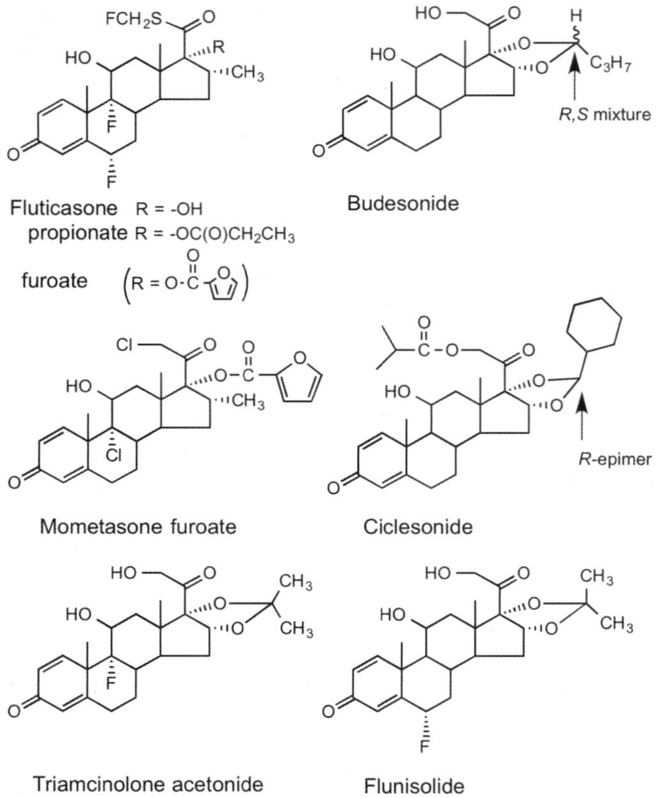

Figure 24.18 Inhaled and intranasal corticosteroids.

(eg, from use of other corticoids, hypertension, or cardiac compensation) or when excessive appetite and weight gain are problems in management.

Triamcinolone acetonide suspension for intravitreal injection (Triesence) was approved for ocular inflammatory conditions unresponsive to topical corticosteroids, and recently intravitreal inserts of triamcinolone acetonide have been investigated in the treatment of diabetic macular edema (DME). An extended-release bioresorbable dexamethasone delivery system (Ozurdex in Tables 24.4 and 24.6) and an extended-release nonbiosorbable fluocinolone acetonide insert (Iluvien in Tables 24.4 and 24.6; see Fig. 24.17 for structure) have both achieved regulatory approval for the treatment of DME. All intravitreal corticosteroids are associated with risks of cataract progression, elevation of intraocular pressure, and endophthalmitis.[113]

Newer synthetic glucocorticoids have incorporated chlorine atoms onto the steroid molecule in place of fluorine substituents. Beclomethasone, a 9α-chloro analogue of betamethasone (Fig. 24.17), is a potent glucocorticoid with approximately half the potency of its fluoro analogue due to less powerful electron withdrawing properties and greater steric bulk. Beclomethasone is used topically as its dipropionate (BDP) derivative in inhalation aerosol therapy for asthma and rhinitis (see "Inhaled and Intranasal Glucocorticoids" section) but not for treatment of steroid-responsive dermatoses[114]. The topical anti-inflammatory potency for BDP is approximately 5,000-fold greater than hydrocortisone, 500-fold greater than betamethasone or dexamethasone, and approximately 5-fold greater than fluocinolone acetonide or triamcinolone acetonide, as measured by vasoconstrictor assay. Alclometasone, the 7α-chloro-9α-unsubstituted derivative of dexamethasone (Fig. 24.17), is a low potency topical glucocorticoid that contains a 7α-chloro group in the B-ring and is available as the 17α-,21-dipropionate.[115] The low potency may partially result from weaker inductive effects of the 7α-chloro group on the 3-keto-Δ4 functional group and absence of 9α-fluoro group inductive effect on 11β-hydroxy. Clocortolone pivalate is a dihalogenated analogue related to dexamethasone and classified as a medium-potency topical agent. The potency is enhanced relative to dexamethasone (Table 24.6) and is likely due to the addition of the 6α-fluoro and increased lipophilicity due to the lack of the 17α-OH. Desoximetasone is another 17α-dehydroxylated dexamethasone derivative that is a high potency topical glucocorticoid.

Additional mono- and difluorinated analogues for topical application include fluorometholone (a 6α-methyl-9α-fluoro-21-dehydroxy derivative of prednisolone for ophthalmic use; fluorometholone (17α-) acetate also used ophthalmically), flurandrenolide (a Δ^1 reduced, 6α-fluoro-9-unsubstituted-16α,17α-acetonide agent related to triamcinolone), fluocinolone acetonide (a 6α,9α-difluoro-16α,17α-acetonide related to triamcinolone), and fluocinonide (a 21-acetate ester of fluocinolone acetonide; Fig. 24.17). These compounds are classified as high- to medium-potency anti-inflammatory agents depending on the concentration and vehicle used (Table 24.6). The acetonide (ketal) derivatives at the 16α,17α-position enhance GR affinity and lipophilicity to provide potent topical anti-inflammatory agents (Table 24.6).

Loteprednol etabonate (Eysuvis among others; Table 24.4) is a 17α-ethyl carbonate, 21-chloro derivative of prednisolone for ophthalmic use. Recently approved for dry eye disease (DED) as Eysuvis, loteprednol etabonate is the only FDA-approved ocular corticosteroid for the treatment of DED. Improved bioavailability at the target site allows therapeutic suppression of the autoimmune responses that drive acute DED flares. Although long-term ophthalmic use of corticosteroids has a risk of increasing intraocular pressure or forming or worsening cataracts, there is increasing use of loteprednol etabonate 0.25% for DED before and/or after cataract or refractive surgery or as induction therapy prior to starting chronic immunomodulatory medication for DED.[116]

Psoriasis is one of the few inflammatory dermatoses that has not responded to routine topical steroid therapy, but these more potent steroids appear to work if a special occlusive dressing is used. In this technique, a thin layer of cream or ointment containing flurandrenolide is applied to the individual patch of psoriasis. The area is then covered with an occlusive pliable plastic film, which traps heat at the site of corticoid application and helps drive the drug into the skin.

Clinical investigations show 0.05% flurandrenolide to be more effective than 1% hydrocortisone acetate and to have approximately the same activity as 0.1% triamcinolone acetonide. Some investigators believe that its greater activity results from an increased biologic half-life secondary to slower metabolism due to the 6α-fluoro group.

Clobetasol propionate, halcinonide, halobetasol propionate, and mometasone furoate are examples of 21-chlorocorticoids in which the 21-chloro group replaces the 21-hydroxyl group (see Figs. 24.17 and 24.18).[117-120] Clobetasol propionate, the 21-chloro analogue of betamethasone 17α-propionate, is approximately eightfold more active as topical anti-inflammatory agent than betamethasone 17α-valerate, the standard of comparison for topical vasoconstrictor/anti-inflammatory activity. Mometasone furoate, a 9α,21-dichloro derivative (see the "Inhaled and Intranasal Glucocorticoids" section) related to dexamethasone, is also approximately 8-fold more active than dexamethasone as a topical anti-inflammatory agent. Thus, substitution of a chlorine (or a fluorine) atom for the 21-hydroxyl group on the glucocorticoids greatly enhances topical anti-inflammatory activity.[118] Clobetasol propionate and halobetasol propionate are classified as very high–potency topical corticosteroid preparations (Table 24.6). HPA axis suppression has occurred following topical application of 2 g of the 0.05% clobetasol propionate ointment or cream (1 mg of clobetasol propionate total) daily. Because of its high potency and potential for causing adverse systemic effects during topical therapy, the usual dosage for very high–potency topical steroids should not be exceeded.

Fluticasone propionate is a dexamethasone derivative that is similar to the 21-chlorocorticoids, except that it has a 17β-fluoromethylcarbothioate group instead of the 17β-ketol group (see "Inhaled and Intranasal Glucocorticoids" section; Fig. 24.18). Although mometasone furoate and fluticasone propionate are very lipophilic and have the highest binding affinity for the GR when compared to triamcinolone acetonide and dexamethasone, their topical potency is listed as medium, in part because of their insolubility and poor dissolution into inflamed tissue.

Several nonfluorinated analogues of triamcinolone acetonide with the potency-enhancing cyclic ketal moieties are marketed, suggesting that halogens are not always necessary for topical activity. These nonfluorinated cyclic ketals include desonide (Fig. 24.17) and the cyclic acetal ciclesonide (see Fig. 24.18). Further, the potency of desonide (low potency) is greatly enhanced in its 9α-fluoro derivative, amcinonide (high potency), by the more lipophilic cyclopentanone (ie, cypionate) ketal and 21-acetate groups of amcinonide. A recent addition to the nonhalogenated prednisolone derivatives is prednicarbate, a 17α,21-diester (17α-ethylcarbonate-21-propionate) derivative of prednisolone (see Fig. 24.17), which is used for the local treatment of corticoid-sensitive skin diseases.[121] Any prednicarbate that is absorbed systemically is readily metabolized by hydrolysis of the 21-ester to its primary and pharmacologically active metabolite, prednisolone-17α ethylcarbonate. This metabolite has a half-life of approximately 1 to 2 hours and is further metabolized by the liver to prednisolone. In vitro binding studies with the GR suggest that the ethyl carbonate metabolite has a receptor binding affinity comparable to that of dexamethasone.[121] The low systemic bioavailability for prednicarbate after dermal application has been attributed to its metabolism to less active prednisolone, which can be a factor for the low systemic side effects of prednicarbate.

Inhaled and Intranasal Glucocorticoids

The potent topical anti-inflammatory effect of glucocorticoids has made them the first-line therapy in controlling airway inflammation. With the exception of vamorolone, approved in 2023 for DMD, it is generally accepted that the anti-inflammatory effects of approved (steroidal) glucocorticoids have not yet been separated from their adverse effects at the receptor level. Therefore, pulmonary and nasal pharmacokinetics become important determinants for the potential of an inhaled or nasally applied corticosteroid to cause systemic effects, because the lung and nasal tissue provide an enormous surface area from which drug absorption can occur into the systemic circulation.[122,123] The main areas of concern with regard to drug-induced systemic effects include HPA axis suppression, change in bone mineral density and growth retardation in children, and cataracts and glaucoma (increased intraocular pressure) in older adults. The degree of systemic side effects increases proportionally to the area under the plasma concentration over time curve (AUC) of the corticosteroid. The AUC increases with longer half-life of the drug, higher dose and frequency of administration, and depends on the route of administration and tissue penetration.[59] Thus, the focus of current research is to develop inhaled/intranasal corticosteroids combined with improved delivery devices that provide the following desirable pharmacokinetic qualities: fast systemic clearance for the portion of the drug that enters the GI tract (ie, high degree of first-pass intestinal/hepatic metabolism), short plasma half-life, lack of active metabolites, high affinity for the GR, and formulated to deliver the drug to the site of action and keep it there. These qualities determine the proportion of the drug that reaches the target cells, as well as the fraction of the dose that reaches the systemic circulation to produce side effects.

Modification of pharmacokinetics through structural alterations has provided several new steroids with a better GR affinity and therapeutic index and lower bioavailability than the older drugs (Fig. 24.18). The new inhaled/intranasal glucocorticoids, all steroids, like mometasone furoate, budesonide, and fluticasone propionate, are more lipophilic than those used in oral and systemic therapy, and have greater affinity for the GR than does dexamethasone as a consequence of their greater lipophilicity.[70] Several of the topical corticosteroids, such as mometasone furoate, beclomethasone dipropionate (BDP), triamcinolone acetonide, and flunisolide, were reintroduced as inhalation and intranasal dosage forms for treatment of respiratory diseases (eg, asthma or rhinitis). Inhaled budesonide and flunisolide are readily absorbed from the airway mucosa into the blood and are rapidly biotransformed in the liver into inactive metabolites. Mometasone furoate and fluticasone propionate are very potent anti-inflammatory steroids with an oral bioavailability of less than 1%. Obviously, the risk of systemic side effects for these newer corticosteroids is greatly reduced when compared with the older glucocorticoids (eg, dexamethasone).

BDP was discovered to be a prodrug cleaved by lung esterases, and this discovery led to the reexamination of other 17α-monoesters as the active form of the corticosteroid esters. The absorption of budesonide, fluticasone propionate, and BDP into the airway tissue was 25- to 130-fold greater than that for dexamethasone and hydrocortisone.[59] The GR affinity and the pharmacokinetic properties for the inhaled and intranasal corticosteroids are listed in Table 24.7.

Recently, multiple inhalation device technologies have been approved as nasal (eg, Optinose Exhalation Delivery System [EDS]) and lung (eg, RespiClick for β-adrenergic bronchodilator) formulations to improve drug delivery to the intended site of action, thereby providing the minimum effective dose to limit systemic (eg, catabolism of muscle/bone) and local (eg, oral or respiratory infections) side effects.[124,125] It is generally recognized that, when administered by oral inhalation, 10% to 30% of a dose of the corticosteroid is deposited in the respiratory tract depending on type of inhaler (ie, metered dose inhaler or dry powder inhaler [DPI]) and spacer used.[126,127] The remainder of the dose is deposited primarily in the mouth and throat to be swallowed into the GI tract, where the drug can be absorbed and metabolized or eliminated unchanged in the feces. Thus, systemic bioavailability of the inhaled/intranasal steroids is determined by the fraction of the dose absorbed from the lungs/nasal mucosa and the GI tract into systemic circulation and the degree of first-pass metabolism.

Although these corticosteroids are very lipid soluble, they display variable degrees of absorption from respiratory and GI tissues, in part because of dissolution problems. When systemically absorbed, they are capable of suppressing the HPA axis and adrenal function with high and chronic dosing regimens.[126,128] Although as much as 40% of the dose for the high potency adrenocorticoids flunisolide, mometasone furoate, fluticasone propionate, or ciclesonide is absorbed into airway and nasal tissues during oral inhalation, the remainder of the drug is swallowed to undergo extensive first-pass metabolism in the liver to essentially inactive metabolites, with no apparent suppression effects on adrenal function with long-term therapy.

Lipophilicity can positively or negatively alter the pharmacokinetic and pharmacodynamic actions of the inhaled/intranasal steroids.[129] The lipophilic substituents attached to the corticosteroid nucleus can improve receptor affinity (Table 24.7), or they can affect pharmacokinetic properties, such as absorption, protein and tissue binding, distribution, and excretion. The inhaled/intranasal corticosteroids are inhaled as microcrystals and need sufficient water solubility to be dissolved in the nasal or lung epithelial tissue for local anti-inflammatory activity to occur. Lipophilicity, however, can delay their rate of dissolution into these tissues, which can be advantageous by prolonging their retention, affecting their onset and duration of action, or a disadvantage by facilitating their transport away from these tissues via mucociliary clearance before full dissolution can occur. The systemic steroids prednisolone and hydrocortisone are less effective as inhaled/intranasal steroids because of their higher water solubility and lower lipophilicity. For inhaled/intranasal steroids, there is a sharp drop in water solubility when the lipophilicity is high [$\log P \geq 4$ ($P = 10{,}000$)], which is the case for BDP, ciclesonide, fluticasone propionate, and mometasone furoate. High lipophilicity correlates well with low oral bioavailability and high protein binding (Table 24.7).

The first topical preparation for rhinitis was dexamethasone sodium phosphate (Decadron Turbinaire), which was propelled by the chlorofluorocarbon Freon. The use of dexamethasone sodium phosphate inhalation aerosol is

Table 24.7 Pharmacokinetics of Inhaled and Intranasal Corticosteroids

Parameters	Beclomethasone Dipropionate (BDP)	Budesonide	Ciclesonide	Flunisolide[a]	Triamcinolone Acetonide	Fluticasone Propionate	Mometasone Furoate
GR binding affinity relative to dexamethasone[b]	0.4 13.5[c] (17-BMP)	9.4 11.2 (22R) 4.2 (22S)	12 (R-epimer) 1200[d] (R-epimer des-CIC)	1.8	3.6	18	25-27
cLogP[e]	4.3 3.2 (17-BMP)	2.9	5.3 3.9 (des-CIC)	2.4	2.2	3.8	4.1
Relative lipophilicity[f]	79,432 25,120 (17-BMP)	3,980	–	2,512	2,515	31,622	50,120
Pulmonary bioavailability	~20%[g]	~39%	~60% (des-CIC)	40%	25%[h]	~30% (aerosol)	<1% (aerosol)
Nasal bioavailability	~20%[g]	<20%	–	50%	25%[h]	13%-16% (powder)	Not detectable (powder)
Oral bioavailability (systemic)	15%-20%	~10%, oral	<1% parent and des-CIC	6%-10%	23%	<2%	<1%
Protein binding	87% (transcortin and albumin)	85%-90% (albumin)	99% <1% (des-CIC)	Moderate (transcortin and albumin)	68%[h] (albumin)	91% (albumin)	90%
Half-life	30 min IV 10 min inhaled 6.5 h IV (17-BMP) 2-7 h inhaled (17-BMP)	2-3 h IV	1 h 6-7 h inhalation (des-CIC)	1-2 h IV	1-2 h IV 1-7 h nasal 3.1 h solution	~7.8 h IV ~14 h inhaled	4-6 h IV Aerosol (not detectable) Inhaled (not detectable)
Metabolism	Lung and liver esterase, liver (CYP3A4) first pass	Liver (CYP3A) first pass	Liver (CYP3A) Lung esterase	Liver first pass	Liver first pass	Liver (CYP3A4) first pass	Liver
Onset of action	3-7 d	2-3 d	2-4 wk (Des-CIC)	3-7 d	4-7 d	2-3 d	7 h
Excretion	Feces, urine 12%-15%	~60% urine ~30% feces	<20% urine ~60% feces	~50% renal ~40% feces	~40% urine ~60% feces	80%-90% feces <5% urine	50%-90% feces 6%-10% urine

17-BMP, beclomethasone 17a-monopropionate; IV, intravenous.

[a]Nasarel and Nasalide (marketed flunisolide preparations) are not bioequivalent. Total absorption of Nasarel was 25% less, and the peak plasma concentration was 30% lower, than that of Nasalide. The clinical significance of this is likely to be small, however, because clinical efficacy is dependent on local effects on the nasal mucosa.

[b]Binding affinity to human glucocorticoid receptors in vitro relative to dexamethasone. Data from Kelly HW. Establishing a therapeutic index for the inhaled corticosteroids. Part 1: pharmacokinetic pharmacodynamic comparison of the inhaled corticosteroids. *J Allergy Clin Immunol*. 1998;102:S36-S51.

[c]Beclomethasone diproprionate is converted in the liver to the more active beclomethasone 17a-monopropionate (17-BMP).

[d]Ciclesonide is hydrolyzed into des-ciclesonide (des-CIC). Relative binding affinity data from Stoeck M, Riedel R, Hochhaus G, et al. In vitro and in vivo anti-inflammatory activity of the new glucocorticoid ciclesonide. *J Pharmacol Exp Ther*. 2004;309(1):249-258.

[e]Clog *P* values were calculated using ChemDraw Version 15.

[f]Measured from reverse-phase high-performance liquid chromatographic technique. Log *k′* data from Brattsand R. What factors determine anti-inflammatory activity and selectivity of inhaled steroids? *Eur Respir Rev*. 1997;7:356-361 were converted to antilogs. *k′* values: water = 1, hydrocortisone = 794, prednisolone = 316, dexamethasone = 400.

[g]Estimated for inhaled BDP aerosol.

[h]Data from oral inhalation administration.

Data from McEvoy GK, ed. *AHFS 2001 Drug Information*. American Society of Health-System Pharmacists; 2001.

not recommended because of the potential for extensive systemic absorption and the long metabolic half-life for dexamethasone after absorption, resulting in an increased risk of adverse effects with usual inhalation doses. Following the oral inhalation of dexamethasone sodium phosphate, a cumulative dose of 1,200 µg/day will result in the systemic absorption of 400 to 600 µg of dexamethasone, which is sufficient to cause HPA axis suppression. Dexamethasone sodium phosphate nasal aerosol delivers 100 µg per metered spray. The total daily adult nasal dose is 1,200 µg.

Triamcinolone acetonide was frequently used by inhalation for the treatment of lung diseases (eg, asthma) until 2010, but is no longer available as an inhalation aerosol. It was discontinued due to the chlorofluorocarbon (CFC) propellant ban, but is still available as an aqueous nasal spray. Glucocorticoids are still commonly administrated as microcrystalline suspensions for pulmonary (inhalation aerosols or dry powders for inhalation) or nasal (aqueous solutions) delivery. Discontinuation of ozone-depleting CFC propellant inhalation products was complete by 2013. They were replaced by a variety of hydrofluoroalkane (HFA) propellant inhalation aerosols, aqueous nasal sprays, DPIs, or other novel delivery devices.

The discontinuation of CFC-based products accelerated the transfer of asthma patients from older inhaled agents such as triamcinolone, flunisolide, and beclomethasone (which are now largely nasal products for rhinitis or nasal polyps) to newer corticosteroids that are better optimized for inhalation therapy such as fluticasone, budesonide, ciclesonide, and mometasone. If monotherapy is ineffective for maintenance treatment, inhaled corticosteroids are commonly used as fixed combination products with long-acting β-adrenergic agonists (LABAs) (see Chapter 31) such as fluticasone propionate/salmeterol, budesonide/formoterol, or mometasone furoate/formoterol combinations.

Recently, Airsupra was the first approved asthma rescue inhaler to contain an inhaled corticosteroid. It is an inhaler that supplies 90 µg albuteral and 80 µg budesonide per inhalation. A single dose is two inhalations or 180 µg of albuterol and 160 µg of budesonide. It is approved for patients with asthma 18 years old and older for the as-needed treatment or prevention of bronchoconstriction and to reduce the risk of exacerbations. Importantly, inclusion of the inhaled corticosteroid was a departure from traditional asthma pharmacotherapeutics in which rescue inhalers (short-acting β-adrenergic agonists such as albuterol whose onset is within a minute or so) were always separated from maintenance inhalers (inhaled corticosteroids optionally including a LABA whose onset was at least hours to days, which is ineffective to provide rescue) to avoid any expectation of immediate effects from a maintenance therapy. Traditionally, maintenance therapy is to be scheduled to avoid the need for rescue inhaler use and its associated cardiovascular side effects of the β-adrenergic agents. However, Airsupra demonstrated increased time to first severe asthma attack requiring at least 3 days of systemic corticosteroids or hospitalization stay of least 24 hours due to asthma as compared to traditional rescue inhaler use (180 µg of albuterol alone), which suggests that providing anti-inflammatory therapy with each minor exacerbation can delay onset of severe asthma attacks.

Specific Drugs (see Fig. 24.18)

Beclomethasone 17α,21-dipropionate. Beclomethasone dipropionate (BDP) is used primarily as an inhalation aerosol therapy (eg, the breath activated Qvar RediHaler) for asthma and rhinitis.[114] A breakthrough in the discovery of new inhalation corticosteroids with reduced risks from systemic absorption was that the 17α-monopropionate ester of beclomethasone (17-BMP) was more active than BDP and beclomethasone 21-monopropionate (21-BMP) esters.[130] Thus, BDP is a prodrug that is rapidly metabolized by esterases in the lung and other tissues to its more active metabolite, 17-BMP, which has 30-fold greater affinity for the GR than BDP due to the introduction of the 21-OH that may bind to Thr739 and Gln642 of GR. Furthermore, 17-BMP has approximately 14-fold greater GR affinity than dexamethasone (Table 24.7),[70] possibly due to polar interactions of 17α-propionate ester oxygens with Gln642 and hydrophobic interactions between the 17α-propionate side chain and 16β-methyl group with distinct regions of GR. 17-BMP is the first monoester to form because the 17-propionate is more sterically hindered than the readily accessible 21-ester.

Whether orally administered or swallowed from inhalation, BDP undergoes rapid first-pass metabolism of the unhindered 21-ester via enzymatic hydrolysis in the liver or GI tract, primarily to 17-BMP but more slowly to 21-BMP and to beclomethasone and other unidentified metabolites and polar conjugates.[131,132] The terminal half-life for 17-BMP is 6.5 hours. The portion of the inhaled dose of BDP that enters the lung is rapidly metabolized to 17-BMP in the respiratory tract before reaching systemic circulation, where it can be further metabolized by the liver. Following oral administration, BDP and its metabolites are excreted mainly in feces via biliary elimination, and 12% to 15% of a 4-mg dose of BDP is excreted in the urine as free and conjugated metabolites. The usual therapeutic dose (<1,200 µg/day) for BDP oral inhalation does not produce systemic glucocorticoid effects, probably because the drug is rapidly metabolized to less active metabolites. At doses greater than 1,200 µg/day, HPA axis suppression has been observed.

The BDP monohydrate nasal suspension is available as an aqueous microcrystalline suspension of BDP, which delivers 42 µg per metered spray. The BDP nasal aerosol or inhalation aerosol consists of a microcrystalline suspension of BDP in HFA-134a (1,1,1,2-tetrafluoroethane) propellant, both of which deliver 40 or 80 µg per metered spray. The total daily adult dose for BDP is 600 µg from the nasal spray or nasal inhaler and 336 to 1,000 µg for the aerosol inhaler. Doses exceeding 2,000 µg/day need to be monitored for HPA axis suppression.

Flunisolide. Flunisolide (6α-fluoro) has higher GR binding affinity, comparable to its fluorination position isomer, triamcinolone acetonide (9α-fluoro), but enhanced pulmonary and nasal bioavailabilities. When administered intranasally or by inhalation, flunisolide (see Fig. 24.18) is rapidly absorbed from nasal or lung tissue (Table 24.7).[133] This corticosteroid is efficiently metabolized by the liver to inactive metabolites with no apparent effects on adrenal function with long-term therapy. Flunisolide that is swallowed undergoes extensive first-pass metabolism in the liver, while that which is absorbed directly from the nasopharyngeal mucosa or lung bypasses this initial metabolism.[134] It is not known if the drug undergoes metabolism in the GI tract. Flunisolide is rapidly hydroxylated by CYP3A4 at the 6β position, followed by elimination of the 6α-fluoro group to its more polar 6β-hydroxy metabolite, which attains plasma concentrations that usually are greater than those for flunisolide.[133, 134]

Following IV administration of flunisolide, the 6β-hydroxy metabolite has 1/100 the potency of flunisolide and a plasma half-life of 3.9 to 4.6 hours. Flunisolide and its 6β-hydroxy metabolite are conjugated in the liver to inactive glucuronides and sulfates. After intranasal administrations of 100 μg, the plasma levels for flunisolide were undetectable within 4 hours. The duration of its systemic effects is short because of its short half-life.

Flunisolide nasal solution (0.025%) is available in an aqueous solubilized form, which delivers 25 μg per spray. The recommended starting dose for adults is two sprays in each nostril twice daily (200 μg per day), with a maximum total daily dose of 400 μg for adults. Flunisolide inhalation aerosol for pulmonary delivery is a microcrystalline suspension in a HFA propellant that delivers 80 μg per metered spray from the built in spacer. The total daily adult inhalation dose for flunisolide is 1,000 μg. Doses exceeding 2,000 μg/day need to be monitored for HPA axis suppression.

Budesonide. Budesonide, another triamcinolone derivative, is a highly potent, nonhalogenated glucocorticoid intended for the local treatment of lung disease and rhinitis. It was designed to have a high ratio between local and systemic effects. Budesonide is composed of a 1:1 mixture of epimers of the 16α,17α-butylacetal, which creates a chiral center (see Fig. 24.18).[135] The 22*R*-epimer binds to the GR with higher affinity than does the 22*S*-epimer (Table 24.7).[70] The butyl acetal chain provided the highest potency for the homologous acetal chains. Its rate of topical uptake into epithelial tissue is more than 100-fold faster than that of hydrocortisone and dexamethasone. Approximately 85% of the orally inhaled dose of budesonide undergoes extensive first-pass hepatic metabolism by CYP3A4 to its primary metabolites, 6β-hydroxybudesonide and 16α-hydroxyprednisolone, which have approximately 1/100 the potency of budesonide.[136,137] This is an important inactivation step in limiting the systemic effect of budesonide on adrenal suppression. Budesonide was metabolized 3- to 6-fold more rapidly than triamcinolone acetonide.

The pharmacokinetics of budesonide after inhalation, oral, and IV administration displayed a mean plasma half-life of 2.8 hours and a systemic bioavailability of approximately 10% after oral administration (Table 24.7).[137] Pulmonary bioavailability is less than 40% after inhalation (70%-75% after correction for the amounts of budesonide deposited in the inhalation device and oral cavity). No oxidative metabolism was observed in the lung. When given by inhalation, 32% of the dose is excreted in the urine as metabolites, 15% is excreted in the feces, and 41% remains in the mouthpiece of the inhaler. Following intranasal administration, very little of intranasal budesonide is absorbed from the nasal mucosa. Much of the intranasal dose (~60%) was swallowed, however, and remained in the GI tract to be excreted unchanged in the feces, whereas that fraction of the intranasal dose that was absorbed was extensively metabolized.

Inhaled budesonide, despite its lower lipophilicity, exhibits greater retention within the airways than other inhaled corticosteroids.[136,137] This unusual behavior for inhaled budesonide has been attributed to the subsequent formation of intracellular fatty acid esters of the 21-hydroxy group of budesonide in the airway and lung tissue.[138,139] Following inhalation, approximately 70% to 80% of budesonide was reversibly esterified by free fatty acids in the airway tissue. These inactive esters behave like an intracellular depot drug by slowly regenerating free budesonide through hydrolysis. Thus, this reversible esterification prolongs the local anti-inflammatory action of budesonide in the airways and may contribute to the high efficacy and safety of budesonide in the treatment of mild asthma when inhaled once daily.

The systemic availability of budesonide in children was estimated to be 6.1% of the nominal dose, and the terminal half-life was 2.3 hours.[140,141] Approximately 6% of the nominal dose reached the systemic circulation of young children after inhalation of nebulized budesonide. This is approximately half the systemic availability found in healthy adults using the same nebulizer.

Budesonide powder for pulmonary inhalation uses micronized dry powder of budesonide only in a turboinhaler (DPI) inhalation-driven device that delivers 200 μg per actuation. Another DPI device, the Flexhaler, delivers 1 mg of micronized formulation containing 90 or 180 μg of micronized budesonide per actuation. The total daily adult dose for budesonide from the DPI is 200 to 800 μg. Full benefit is attained in approximately 1 to 2 weeks. Budesonide ampoules contain 0.25 mg/2 mL, 0.5 mg/2mL, and 1 mg/2mL to be delivered as a sterile solution via a jet nebulizer. Budesonide nasal aerosol, which is now available over the counter (OTC), is supplied as a micronized suspension of budesonide in an aqueous medium, which delivers 32 μg per metered spray. Budesonide inhalation aerosol delivers 80 or 160 μg of budesonide in a fixed combination dose with the LABA formoterol (4.5 μg) using an HFA propellant micronized formulation. Breztri Aerosphere delivers a fixed dose combination of 160 μg budesonide, 4.8 μg formoterol, and 9 μg glycopyrrolate (an anticholinergic agent) as an inhalation aerosol for maintenance therapy of chronic obstructive pulmonary disease (COPD) via two inhalations twice a day.

Ciclesonide. A third-generation nonhalogenated triamcinolone analogue approved in 2006 is ciclesonide (Fig 24.18). Ciclesonide is the 21-isobutyrate ester and the 16α,17α-acetal of the cyclohexanecarboxaldehyde analogue of triamcinolone. It is delivered as the *R*-epimer, which binds to the GR with high affinity (Table 24.7). The 21-isobutyrate ester and 16α,17α-acetal of cyclohexanecarboxaldehyde greatly enhance its lipid solubility. Ciclesonide is a prodrug that is converted locally in airways by carboxylesterases to produce the active metabolite, desisobutyrylciclesonide (des-CIC). With its free C21-OH available to bind (eg, to Thr739), des-CIC has a 100-fold greater relative GR binding affinity than ciclesonide itself (relative GR binding affinities are 1,200 and 12, respectively; dexamethasone is 100). If any ciclesonide or des-CIC enters the circulation, it is highly protein bound (99%) and undergoes extensive first-pass hepatic metabolism by CYP3A4 to 6β-hydroxy metabolites, resulting in very low systemic exposure. Clinical studies demonstrate that ciclesonide is effective as inhalation aerosol therapy for asthma and rhinitis.

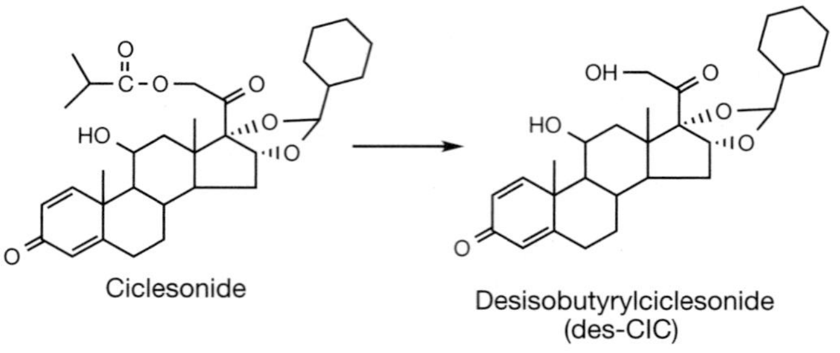

Ciclesonide is supplied as an aqueous inhalation solution pump that dispenses 50 μg per 70 μL spray for seasonal allergies or delivered in solution form via a HFA metered-dose inhaler with a once-daily dosing schedule, which facilitates asthmatic patient compliance. The total daily dose is 200 μg for seasonal allergies and 80 to 160 μg for asthma. In 2012, a new dry nasal aerosol spray was approved that delivers 37 μg of ciclesonide with one spray per nostril daily.

Following inhalation administration, ciclesonide and des-CIC are not detected in the plasma. Ciclesonide has a half-life of less than 1 hour, and des-CIC has a half-life of 6 to 7 hours and an oral bioavailability of less than 1% due to extensive plasma protein binding (Table 24.7). Ciclesonide produces potent anti-inflammatory effects with an onset of action of approximately 2 to 4 weeks. It is extensively metabolized, with less than 20% of the administered dose recovered in the urine as des-CIC. The majority of the oral inhalation for ciclesonide is deposited in the airway passages and swallowed without absorption in the GI tract until eliminated in the feces (~60% of the administered dose is recovered in the feces). These results indicate that inhaled ciclesonide has negligible systemic bioavailability and is extensively metabolized, with reduced risk for causing systemic adrenal suppression effects.

Mometasone Furoate. The development of mometasone furoate resulted from the reexamination of the effect of 17α-ester functionalities on topical anti-inflammatory potency relative to the potent 17α-benzoate ester of betamethasone. The structure-activity relationship study involved substitution of the 17α-benzoate ester with heteroaromatic furoic, thienoic, and pyrrolic esters.[119,142] Of the numerous 17α-heteroaryl esters studied, the 2-furoate ester displayed the greatest increase in potency. Therefore, combining the 17α-(2-furoate) ester with the potency-enhancing effect of the 21-chloro group resulted in mometasone furoate (Fig. 24.18), which is 5- to 10-fold more potent and has a more rapid onset of action than the betamethasone benzoate ester.

Mometasone furoate was originally marketed as a topically applied corticosteroid but because of its low systemic bioavailability, it was found to be more useful in the treatment of allergic disorders and lung diseases.[143] It has the greatest binding affinity for the GR (Table 24.7), followed by fluticasone propionate, budesonide, triamcinolone acetonide, and dexamethasone.[70] Mometasone furoate has strong local anti-inflammatory activity equivalent to that of fluticasone propionate. It has a quick onset of action relative to the other inhaled/intranasal steroids with the least systemic availability and, consequently, the fewest systemic side effects.

Mometasone furoate was detected in the plasma for up to 8 hours after administration of an inhaled aerosolized suspension, with an IV half-life of 4 to 6 hours (Table 24.7) and an oral bioavailability of less than 1% as compared to an intravenous dose. It is extensively metabolized with less than 10% of the administered dose recovered in the urine unchanged.[144] Among the polar metabolites (~80%) and their conjugates (42%) that were recovered were 6β-hydroxymometasone furoate and its 21-hydroxy metabolite. In contrast, following intranasal administration, its plasma concentrations were below the limit of quantification, and the systemic bioavailability by this route was estimated to be less than 1%. The majority of the intranasal dose for mometasone furoate is deposited in the nasal mucosa and swallowed without absorption in the GI tract until eliminated in the feces (~50%-90% of the intranasal dose is recovered in the feces). These results indicate that, like ciclesonide, inhaled mometasone furoate has negligible systemic bioavailability and is extensively metabolized, with reduced risk for causing systemic adrenal suppression effects.

Mometasone furoate nasal suspension is supplied as an aqueous suspension with an atomizing pump that dispenses 50 μg per metered spray. The total daily dose for mometasone furoate is 200 μg. An inhalation powder (Twisthaler) or HFA-based inhalation aerosol delivers 100 or 200 μg of mometasone furoate with a daily dose of 100 μg for children ages 4 to 11 years up to 400 μg for adults. The inhalation aerosol comes as the same doses of mometasone in fixed combinations with LABA formoterol (5 μg).

Fluticasone Propionate:

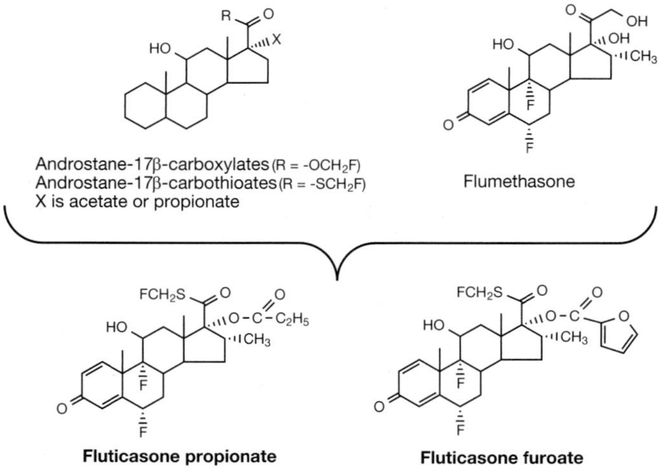

The discovery of fluticasone flowed from the investigation of the androstane 17α-hydroxyl-17β-carboxylates and 17α-hydroxyl-17β-carbothioates, which were designed to be metabolically susceptible to hydrolysis at the 17β position and to have a low systemic bioavailability to minimize systemic glucocorticoid-induced adrenal suppression. The androstane 17α-hydroxyl-17β-carboxylates lacked the 17-ketol group (-$COCH_2OH$) found in most of the systemic corticosteroids. When these 17β-carboxylates were esterified to their 17α/β-diesters, however, they proved to be extremely potent anti-inflammatory corticosteroids, whereas the parent carboxylic acids were inactive.[145] Thus, enzymatic hydrolysis of the 17-carboxylate ester function by intestinal or liver esterases would lead to formation of inactive metabolites. The greatest anti-inflammatory activity was observed with 17α-acetoxy and 17α-propionoxy groups and simple alkyl carboxylate esters, although the fluoromethyl esters showed the highest activity.

Superseding the androstane 17β-carboxylates were the corresponding 17β-carbothioates (thioesters) derived from flumethasone (ie, Δ^1-6α,9α-difluoro-16α-methyl; see Fig. 24.17). The 17β-fluoromethylcarbothioate, when combined with the 17α-propionoxy group, yielded fluticasone propionate (Fig. 24.18).[146] The androstane 17β-carbothioates proved not only to be very potent anti-inflammatory agents but also to exhibit weak HPA suppression in the rat. Both the androstane 17β-carboxylates and the androstane 17β-carbothioates are very lipophilic and exhibit minimal oral bioavailability and very low systemic activity after inhalation because of intestinal and hepatic enzymatic hydrolysis to inactive metabolites, which have 1/2,000 the activity of the parent molecule.[147]

Fluticasone propionate, a trifluorinated glucocorticoid based on the androstane 17β-carbothioate nucleus (see Fig. 24.18), was designed to be metabolically susceptible to hydrolysis and to have a low systemic bioavailability to minimize the systemic effects on plasma hydrocortisone levels. Its susceptibility to metabolic hydrolysis is doubly enhanced by the combination of a thioester and the high electronegativity of the fluorine group. Fluticasone propionate is approximately as lipophilic as BDP, 8-fold more lipophilic than budesonide, and 4-fold more lipophilic than triamcinolone acetonide (Table 24.7). It also displays high in vitro selectivity for the GR and a relative receptor affinity 1.5-fold that of 17-BMP and ciclesonide, about equal to mometasone furoate, 2-fold that of budesonide, 18-fold that of dexamethasone, 10-fold that of flunisolide, and 5-fold that of triamcinolone acetonide.[70] Its relatively tight binding reflects cumulative favorable effects of its substituents such as the inductive effect of the 9α-fluoro group on 11β-OH, the favorable hydrophobic pocket binding effects of the 16α-methyl and 17α-propionate groups, and the ability of the 17β-$FCH_2S(O)C$- group to maintain the hydrogen bonding interactions of the 17β-ketol with GR. The rate of association for fluticasone propionate with the receptor is faster, and the rate of dissociation is slower, than the other corticosteroids. The half-life of the fluticasone propionate active steroid-receptor complex is greater than 10 hours, compared with approximately 5 hours for budesonide, 7.5 hours for 17-BMP, and 4 hours for triamcinolone acetonide.[70]

After topical application to the nasal mucosa or after inhalation, fluticasone propionate produces potent anti-inflammatory effects, with an onset of action of approximately 2 to 3 days. The topical anti-inflammatory potency for fluticasone propionate is approximately equal to that for mometasone furoate, 13-fold greater than that for triamcinolone acetonide, 9-fold greater than that for fluocinolone acetonide, 3-fold greater than that for betamethasone 17α-valerate, and 2-fold greater than that for BDP.[147] Because of its low systemic bioavailability when administered intranasally or by inhalation and nondetectability in plasma, most pharmacokinetic data for fluticasone propionate are based on IV or oral administration (Table 24.7). Its rate of topical uptake into epithelial tissue is more than 100-fold faster than that for hydrocortisone and dexamethasone but is similar to BDP and budesonide.

As a consequence of its high lipophilicity (Table 24.7), fluticasone propionate is very insoluble and, therefore, is poorly absorbed from the respiratory (10%-13%) and GI tracts following nasal inhalation of the drug.[148-150] The majority of the intranasal dose for fluticasone propionate is deposited in the nasal mucosa and swallowed into the GI tract until eliminated in the feces (~80%-90% of the intranasal dose is recovered metabolized and unchanged in the feces). After IV administration, fluticasone propionate displayed a systemic bioavailability of less than 2% and underwent extensive hydrolysis and CYP3A4 first-pass metabolism in the liver, with an elimination half-life of approximately 3 hours. Its primary hydrolysis product is the 17β-carboxylate metabolite, which has 1/2,000 the affinity for the GR and can be recovered from the urine along with other unidentified hydroxy metabolites and their conjugates.

Following oral administration of 1 to 40 mg, fluticasone propionate is poorly absorbed from the GI tract because of hydrolysis and its insolubility, with an oral bioavailability of less than 1%. Pulmonary bioavailability ranges between 16% and 30% depending on the inhalation device used, with an elimination half-life of approximately 14 hours, increasing its potential for drug accumulation with repeated dosing.[150] The long elimination half-life for fluticasone propionate results, in part, from its very high lipophilicity and very poor water solubility and, consequently, slow dissolution into lung tissue. Some suppression of overnight hydrocortisone levels was reported with inhaled fluticasone propionate at higher doses (indicative of HPA axis suppression).[151]

Fluticasone propionate inhalation aerosol is available as a microcrystalline suspension of micronized fluticasone propionate in HFA propellant (Flovent HFA). Each actuation delivers 44, 110, or 220 µg of fluticasone propionate from the mouthpiece. The recommended starting dose of fluticasone propionate aerosol is 88 to 220 µg twice daily with the highest recommended dose of 440 µg. Fluticasone propionate combined with the LABA salmeterol is also available as an HFA-based inhalation aerosol providing 45, 115, and 230 µg each combined with 21 µg of salmeterol.

Fluticasone propionate DPIs deliver the corticosteroid alone (eg, Flovent Diskus or ArmonAir RespiClick) or in fixed combinations with salmeterol (Advair Diskus or AirDuo RespiClick). DPIs come as Diskus plastic inhalers containing a foil blister strip. Each blister on the strip contains a white powder mix that delivers 50, 100, or 250 µg (Flovent Diskus) per inhalation of micronized fluticasone propionate or 100, 250, or 500 µg fluticasone propionate and 72.5 µg salmeterol xinafoate salt (equivalent to 50 µg of salmeterol base) (Advair Diskus). The Diskus dose is 100 to 1,000 µg twice daily for patients aged 12 years and older. After the

Diskus is activated, the powder is dispersed into the airstream created by the patient inhaling through the mouthpiece. The maximum recommended combination dose is 500/50 μg twice daily. The RespiClick DPI formulations deliver the same active ingredients but involve resetting the dry powder dose via opening the mouthpiece cover until a click is heard. RespiClick allowed lowered daily doses of 110 to 464 μg.

Recently introduced is a new digital delivery system called a Digihaler. ArmonAir Digihaler (55, 113, or 232 μg of fluticasone propionate) and AirDuo Digihaler (113 and 14 μg of fluticasone propionate and salmeterol fixed dose combination) are also breath-activated DPIs for maintenance therapy of asthma, but the Digihaler has built-in sensors to help capture inhaler usage data on an app. This data can be shared with health care professionals, whereas the other formulations do not have digital capability to share such data.

Fluticasone furoate, the 2-furoic acid ester of the 17α-hydroxyl group, is available as DPI, alone (Arnuity Ellipta) or combined with the LABA vilanterol (Breo Ellipta). Fluticasone furoate nasal spray is also available (Veramyst). The furoate ester, like the propionate ester, is stable to metabolism, and neither is metabolized to fluticasone.[152] X-ray crystal structures demonstrate that the intact furoate side chain occupies a discrete pocket much more completely than the propionate side chain,[153] conferring fluticasone furoate with higher GR affinity and higher nasal and lung tissue affinity compared to fluticasone propionate.[154,155] The higher tissue affinity translates to enhanced lung residency and once-daily efficacy in asthma.[156] The superior properties of fluticasone furoate allow lowered daily dose for the nasal spray of 110 versus 200 μg for the comparable aqueous fluticasone propionate nasal spray (Flonase). Care should be used to avoid abbreviating either fluticasone furoate or fluticasone propionate as fluticasone (see Fig. 24.18).

Fluticasone propionate available as an anti-allergic nasal spray further contains the histamine antagonist azelastine (Dymista). In addition to the aqueous formulation, a dry nasal fluticasone propionate (Xhance) is actuated by a pump spray into one nostril while simultaneously blowing into the mouthpiece. Recommended adult dosage is one-two sprays per nostril twice daily (total daily dose of 372-744 μg).

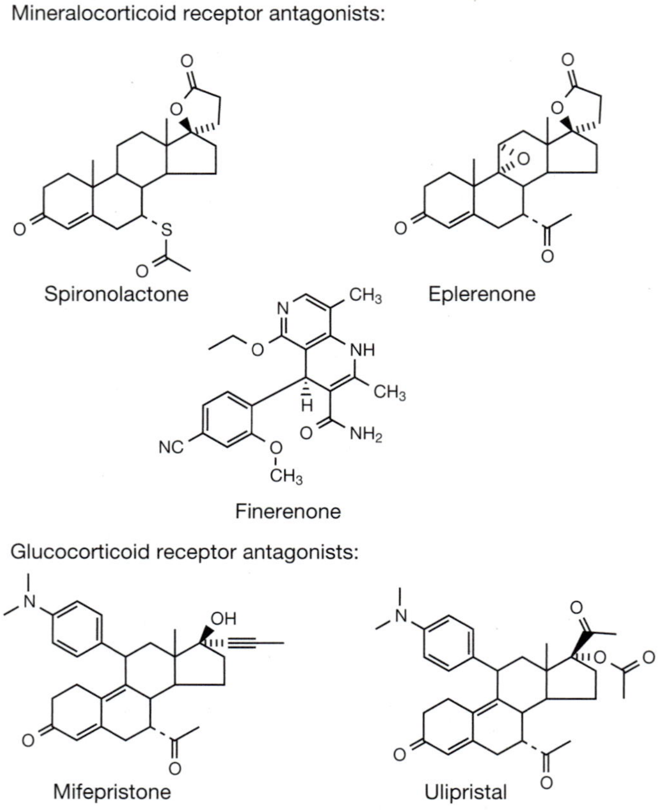

Figure 24.19 Adrenocorticoid receptor antagonists.

ADRENOCORTICOID ANTAGONISTS

Antagonists of adrenocorticoids include agents that compete for binding to steroid receptors (antiglucocorticoids or antimineralocorticoids) and inhibitors of adrenosteroid biosynthesis. The action of adrenal steroids can be blocked by antagonists that compete with the endogenous steroids for binding sites on their respective cytosolic receptor proteins (ie, GR and MR). The antagonist–receptor complexes are unable to stimulate the production of new mRNA and cognate proteins in the target tissues and, thus, are unable to elicit the biologic responses of the hormone agonist. Steroidal MR antagonists, spironolactone and eplerenone (Fig. 24.19) have been known for some time now. Recently, the first nonsteroidal MR antagonist, finerenone (Kerendia), was approved. These agents bind to the MR in the kidney and result in the diuretic response of increased Na^+ excretion and K^+ retention (potassium-sparing diuretics) that are useful in hypertension and heart failure. For the steroidal antagonists, spironolactone and eplerenone, the 3-keto-4-ene A ring is essential for antagonistic activity, and the opening of the lactone ring dramatically reduces activity. The 7α-substituent increases both intrinsic activity and oral activity.[157,158] Progesterone (not shown) has also been shown to possess antimineralocorticoid activity at very high concentrations (10^{-4} molar). Spironolactone was an early very potent MR antagonist approved for hypertension in 1960 but is also a potent androgen receptor (AR) antagonist with only about a 3-fold selectively for MR versus AR. As discussed in Chapter 25, spironolactone is used off-label in some women for acne due to its AR antagonist effects. Its AR antagonist side effects include loss of libido, hair loss, erectile dysfunction, and gynecomastia, which are in addition to MR antagonism untoward effects such as hyperkalemia, depletion of other electrolytes, and muscle cramps.

Eplerenone (Inspra) is a relatively weak MR antagonist but does not suffer from AR antagonism (~20-fold selective). It is approved for resistant hypertension and congestive heart failure after an acute myocardial infarction. Eplerenone binds to the MR and blocks the binding of aldosterone, a component of the renin–angiotensin–aldosterone system (RAAS). Though renin and aldosterone levels increase with eplerenone use, consistent with inhibition of the negative regulatory feedback of aldosterone on renin secretion, the resulting increased plasma renin activity and aldosterone circulating levels do not overcome the effects of eplerenone. Eplerenone selectively binds to human MR relative to human glucocorticoid, progesterone, and androgen receptors. Eplerenone improves survival of stable post-myocardial infarction patients with left ventricular systolic dysfunction defined as left ventricular ejection fraction 40% or lower.

Eplerenone is cleared predominantly by cytochrome P450 (CYP) 3A4 metabolism, with an elimination half-life of 3 to 6 hours. Inhibitors of CYP3A (eg, ketoconazole, saquinavir) increase blood levels of eplerenone. Mean peak plasma concentrations of eplerenone are reached approximately 1.5 to 2 hours following oral administration with an absolute bioavailability of eplerenone of 69% following administration of a 100 mg oral tablet. AUC is dose proportional in the approved dose range of 25 to 100 mg and less than proportional at doses above 100 mg. The plasma protein binding of eplerenone is about 50% (primarily binds α1-acid glycoproteins), with an apparent volume of distribution of more than 42 L. Although it is extensively metabolized, no active metabolites of eplerenone have been identified in human plasma. Following a single oral dose of radiolabeled drug, approximately 32% of the dose was excreted in the feces and approximately 67% was excreted in the urine. Concomitant administration of moderate CYP3A4 inhibitors (erythromycin, saquinavir, verapamil, and fluconazole) requires monitoring of potassium and serum creatinine levels within 3 to 7 days of initiating the CYP3A4 inhibitor. Contraindications include serum potassium higher than 5.5 mEq/L at initiation, creatinine clearance 30 mL/min or lower, or concomitant administration of strong CYP3A inhibitors (eg, ketoconazole, itraconazole, clarithromycin, ritonavir, etc).[159]

Finerenone (Kerendia) is a dihydropyridine (nonsteroidal) MR antagonist with comparable (very high) potency to spironolactone but, unlike spironolactone, it has no cross-reactivity with androgen, progesterone, or GRs. Another advantage compared to the steroidal MR antagonists is that finerenone is distributed equally to renal and cardiac tissue, whereas the steroids are concentrated in the kidneys.[160] Like steroidal agents, finerenone blocks MR-mediated sodium reabsorption and MR overactivation that is believed to contribute to organ fibrosis and inflammation; however, the equal distribution allows blockade of overactivation in both epithelial (eg, kidney) and nonepithelial (eg, heart and blood vessels) tissues. Hence, finerenone is believed to be cardiorenal protective. In 2021, it was approved to reduce the risk of kidney function decline, kidney failure, cardiovascular death, nonfatal heart attack, and hospitalization for heart failure in adults with chronic kidney disease associated with type 2 diabetes mellitus.[161] By binding to the MR receptor, it reduces inflammation, fibrosis, and albuminuria in patients with diabetes and lowered the risk of first onset of kidney failure.[162] Similar to eplerenone, finerenone reduces mortality and morbidity in patients with chronic severe congestive heart failure.[163] Finerenone has similar MR potency as spironolactone but lower incidence of hyperkalemia and other adverse effects compared with both spironolactone and eplerenone.[164]

Finerenone exposure increased proportionally over a dose range of 1.25 to 80 mg (0.06-4 times the maximum approved recommended dosage). The estimated steady-state geometric mean C_{max} and AUC were 160 μg/L and 686 μg*h/L following 2 days of administration of finerenone 20 mg. Finerenone is rapidly (t_{max} of 0.5-1.25 hours) and completely absorbed after oral administration but undergoes metabolism resulting in an absolute bioavailability of 44%. Like eplerenone, there was no clinically significant effect on finerenone AUC following administration with high fat, high calorie food. The terminal half-life of finerenone is about 2 to 3 hours, with volume of distribution and plasma protein binding of 52.6 L and 92% (primarily to serum albumin). Finerenone is primarily metabolized by CYP3A4 (90%) and, to a lesser extent, by CYP2C8 (10%) to inactive metabolites. About 80% of the administered dose is excreted in the urine (<1% as unchanged) and approximately 20% in feces (<0.2% as unchanged). Like eplerenone, finerenone is contraindicated with concomitant strong CYP3A4 inhibitors and renal insufficiency, and risk of hyperkalemia increases with decreased kidney function and higher baseline potassium levels, requiring serum potassium monitoring and dose adjustments as needed. Adverse reactions reported in about 1% of patients on finerenone and more frequently than placebo, including hyperkalemia (14% vs 7% for placebo), hypotension (4.6% vs 3.9% for placebo), and hyponatremia (1.3% vs 0.7% for placebo), which are improved compared to spironolactone and eplerenone.[161]

Theoretically, GR antagonism could have applications in a variety of disease states or conditions involving hypercortisolemia or hyperglycemia; however, long-term GR antagonist therapy could have side effects such as inability to resolve inflammation and/or promotion of autoimmunity. In the absence of an agent that is able to selectively inhibit certain GR biological effects without affecting others, the only approved indication so far is Cushing disease. As discussed, Cushing disease is a rare disease in which the adrenal glands make too much of the endogenous glucocorticoid, cortisol. Steroidal GR antagonists have been described that are derivatives of 19-nortestosterone,[165] such as mifepristone and ulipristal acetate (see Fig. 24.19). Mifepristone was originally developed and approved as an antiprogestin to terminate pregnancy, but also exhibits very effective antagonism of glucocorticoids. Subsequently, it was approved to control hyperglycemia secondary to hypercortisolism in adult patients with endogenous Cushing syndrome who have type 2 diabetes mellitus or glucose intolerance.[166] Ulipristal acetate is a weak antiglucocorticoid that was also approved as a safer abortifacient (potent anti-progestational agent). The abortifacient use of these agents is discussed in more detail in Chapter 25. Nonsteroidal glucocorticoid antagonists have been explored and reviewed previously, but none has been approved for use.[167]

An alternative approach to treating Cushing disease or cushingoid symptoms is to inhibit the adrenocorticoid biosynthetic pathway (see Figs. 24.7 and 24.8). Inhibitors of

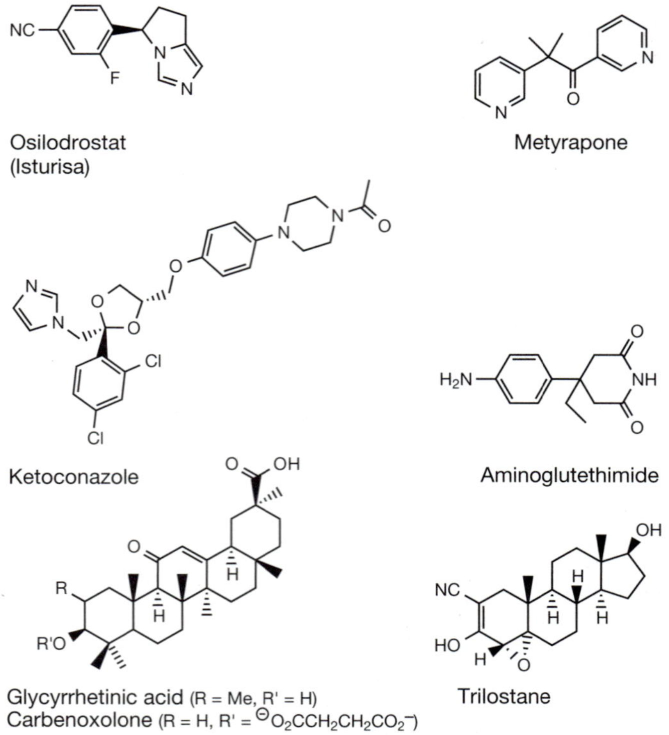

Figure 24.20 Inhibitors of adrenocorticoid biosynthesis or metabolism.

several different enzymes have been described, with the majority of nonsteroidal agents inhibiting one or more of the biosynthetic cytochrome P450 enzyme complexes (Fig. 24.20). Osilodrostat (Isturisa) inhibits cortisol biosynthesis in the adrenal gland via inhibition of 11β-hydroxylase (CYP11B2; step e in Fig 24.8), the enzyme responsible for the final step of cortisol biosynthesis. In vitro, osilodrostat dose-dependently inhibited human CYP11B2 with an IC_{50} value of 2.5 nM. Osilodrostat was approved in 2020 for the treatment of adult patients with Cushing disease for whom pituitary surgery is not an option or has not been curative. Osilodrostat is the first FDA-approved drug to directly address cortisol overproduction. Tested in a Cushing disease population ($N = 137$; there was no healthy population control group), patients were titrated to effect (2 mg up to 30 mg by mouth daily), treated for a specified period of time, and then responders ($N = 71$) were randomized to continued treatment or placebo (discontinuation period). The primary endpoint was the difference between osilodrostat and placebo in the percentage of responders following an 8 week discontinuation period. The study showed that 86% of subjects maintained response when continued on osilodrostat versus 29% for placebo treated subjects.

Osilodrostat is rapidly absorbed (T_{max} of approximately 1 hour) with slightly increasing exposures (increasing AUC and C_{max}) above dose-proportionality within the therapeutic dose range of 1 mg to 30 mg. Though slight reductions in AUC and C_{max} were seen with a high-fat meal, these changes are not considered to be clinically significant, and osilodrostat can be taken with or without food. It has a large volume of distribution (100 L) despite low protein binding (36.4%). The elimination half-life of osilodrostat is approximately 4 hours and the majority is eliminated in the urine (mean: 90.6% of administered dose) as unknown metabolites with only 5.2% as unchanged osilodrostat. Multiple CYP enzymes (ie, CYP3A4, CYP2B6, and CYP2D6) and UDP-glucuronosyltransferases contribute to osilodrostat metabolism, and no single enzyme contributes greater than 25% to the total clearance. The metabolites are not expected to contribute to the pharmacologic effect of osilodrostat.[168]

Like osilodrostat, metyrapone also reduces hydrocortisone (cortisol) biosynthesis primarily by inhibiting 11β-hydroxylase,[169,170] but it also inhibits, to a lesser degree, 18-hydroxylase (step f in Fig. 24.8) and scc (step c in Fig. 24.7). This agent is used to test pituitary-adrenal function and the ability of the pituitary to secrete ACTH.[170] Aminoglutethimide inhibits scc (step c in Fig. 24.7)[170] and has been used as a medical adrenalectomy technique. Several azole antifungal drugs inhibit adrenocorticoid biosynthesis. Ketoconazole is one example of a potent inhibitor of fungal sterol biosynthesis at low concentrations conferring antifungal properties; however, at higher doses, ketoconazole inhibits CYP3A4 in adrenosteroid biosynthesis.[171] Trilostane is a steroidal inhibitor of 3β-hydroxysteroid dehydrogenase ([3β-HSD] step c in Fig. 24.8)[172] and has been used in the treatment of Cushing syndrome.

Adrenocorticoid activity can also be modulated by inhibition of enzymes that catalyze the metabolic interconversions of glucocorticoids. For example, inhibitors of the two 11β-hydroxysteroid dehydrogenase ([11β-HSD1] liver, reversible, and 11β-HSD2, kidney, irreversible) isozymes (Fig. 24.9, part A) exist. Inhibition of the irreversible 11β-HSD2, which converts cortisol to the relatively inactive cortisone, will increase adrenocorticoid activity in target tissues. For example, excessive ingestion of licorice, an extract of the roots of *Glycyrrhiza glabra*, produces undesirable mineralocorticoid-like intoxication (hypertension, excessive salt retention, and hypokalemia). The active components of licorice, glycyrrhetinic acid (Fig. 24.20), and carbenoxolone inhibit both 11β-HSD isozymes,[173] with the undesirable side effects resulting from inhibition of 11β-HSD2 in the kidney. Subtype selective and nonsteroidal inhibitors of the reversible enzyme 11β-HSD1[174,175] are in clinical trials.[176] Such enzyme inhibitors may be useful in the treatment of diseases affected detrimentally by glucocorticoid excess such as metabolic syndrome, cardiovascular disease, or diabetes.[177] In the absence of dissociated GR antagonists, 11β-HSD1 inhibition may represent a mild form of GR antagonism.

ACKNOWLEDGMENT

The authors wish to acknowledge the work of Duane D. Miller, Ph.D. and Dr. Robert W. Brueggemeier, Ph.D. who authored content used within this chapter in a previous edition of this text.

Structure Challenge

The structures of nine drugs discussed in this chapter are provided. Use your knowledge of drug chemistry to identify the agent that would be most appropriate for use in each patient care situation described below.

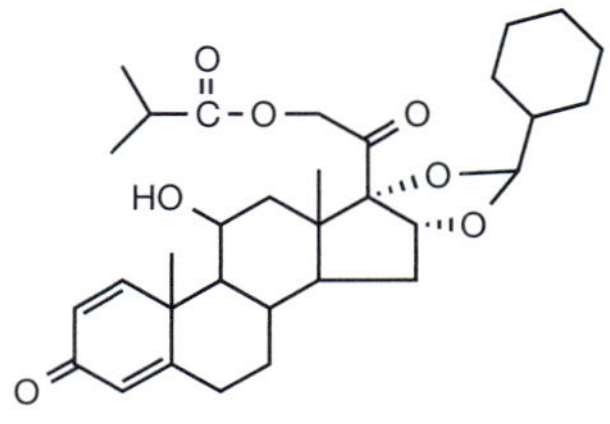

1.

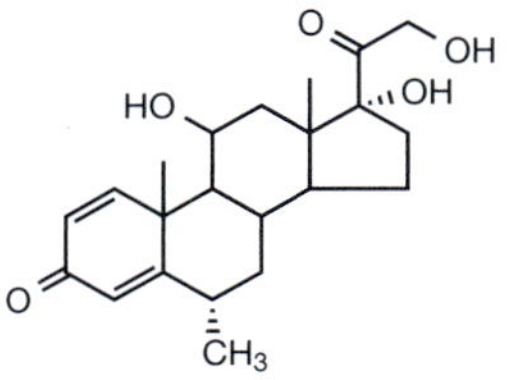

2.

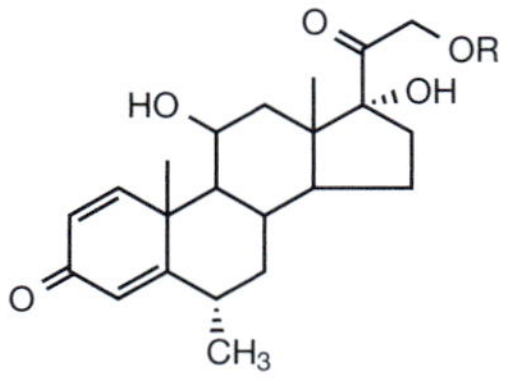

3. R = Na $OOCCH_2CH_2COO$- (sodium succinate)

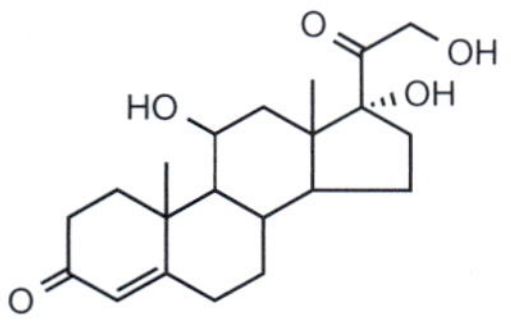

4.

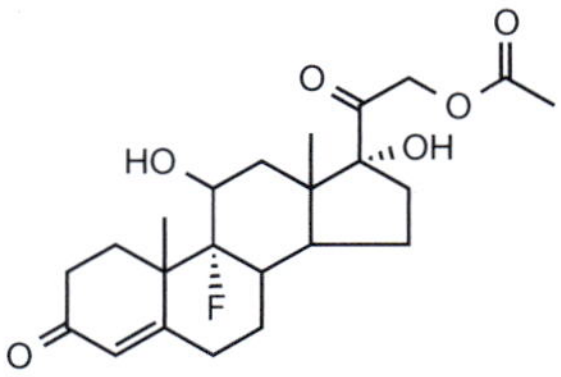

5.

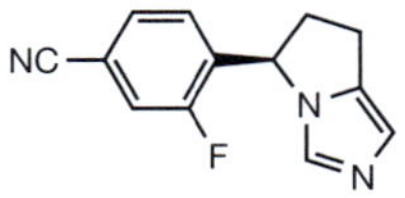

6.

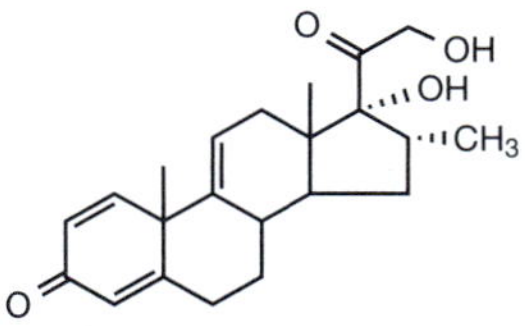

7.

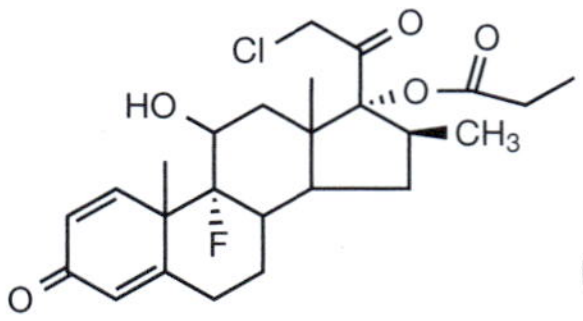

8.

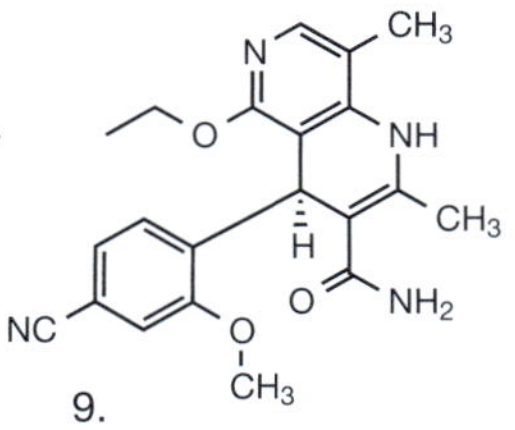

9.

A. An adult patient with Cushing disease for whom pituitary surgery has not been curative ___
B. A newborn diagnosed with classical adrenal hyperplasia characterized by high sodium loss (salt wasting) due to insufficient aldosterone production ___
C. A chronic kidney disease patient with type 2 diabetes who is interested in reducing the risk of further kidney and/or cardiovascular functional decline ___
D. Counseling the parents of a 4 yo patient with Duchenne muscular dystrophy concerned about the growth stunting impact of his current medication and seeking alternative oral therapy ___
E. A military drill sergeant with a job-required “buzz cut” and scalp psoriasis who requires a potent topical glucocorticoid in a shampoo formulation to keep plaques under control ___
F. A 45 yo patient newly diagnosed with adrenal insufficiency secondary to an ablated adrenocortical cancer who requires an injectable glucocorticoid for use in emergencies ___
G. A pharmacist counseling a south Florida vacationer with mild, but itchy, allergic dermatitis from a new sunscreen product on a short-term OTC topical anti-inflammatory agent ___
H. A teenager newly diagnosed with asthma with an active lifestyle seeking oral inhalation therapy with a long-acting steroid he can administer once daily ___
I. An college student with asthma well-maintained on inhalation therapy who needs short-term oral supplementation to participate in a service trip to a community known for high air pollution ___

Structure Challenge answers found immediately after References.

REFERENCES

1. IUPAC-IUB Joint Commission on Biochemical Nomenclature (JCBN). The nomenclature of steroids. Recommendations 1989. *Eur J Biochem*. 1989;186:429-458.
2. Beato M. Gene regulation by steroid hormones. *Cell*. 1989;56:335-344.
3. Carson-Jurica MA, Schrader WT, O'Malley BW. Steroid receptor family: structure and functions. *Endocr Rev*. 1990;11:201-220.
4. Evans RM. The steroid and thyroid hormone receptor superfamily. *Science*. 1988;240:889-895.
5. Ringold G. Steroid hormone action. In: Proceedings of the UCLA Symposium. Januray 17-23, 1987. Liss; 1988.
6. Gustafsson JA, Carlstedt-Duke J, Poellinger L, et al. Biochemistry, molecular biology, and physiology of the glucocorticoid receptor. *Endocr Rev*. 1987;8:185-234.
7. O'Malley B. The steroid receptor superfamily: more excitement predicted for the future. *Mol Endocrinol*. 1990;4:363-369.
8. Narayanan R, Adigun AA, Edwards DP, et al. Cyclin-dependent kinase activity is required for progesterone receptor function: novel role for cyclin A/Cdk2 as a progesterone receptor coactivator. *Mol Cell Biol*. 2005;25:264-277.
9. Sato S, Shirakawa H, Tomita S, et al. The aryl hydrocarbon receptor and glucocorticoid receptor interact to activate human metallothionein 2A. *Toxicol Appl Pharmacol*. 2013;273:90-99.
10. Stahn C, Lowenberg M, Hommes DW, et al. Molecular mechanisms of glucocorticoid action and selective glucocorticoid receptor agonists. *Mol Cell Endocrinol*. 2007;275:71-78.
11. van der Laan S and Meijer OC. Pharmacology of glucocorticoids: beyond receptors. *Eur J Pharmacol*. 2008;585:483-491.

12. Eickelberg O, Roth M, Lorx R, et al. Ligand-independent activation of the glucocorticoid receptor by beta2-adrenergic receptor agonists in primary human lung fibroblasts and vascular smooth muscle cells. *J Biol Chem.* 1999;274:1005-1010.
13. Addison T. *On the Constitutional and Local Effects of Disease of the Suprarenal Capsules.* Classics of Medicine Library; 1980.
14. Murison PJ. Hyperfunctioning adrenocortical diseases. *Med Clin North Am.* 1967;51:883-901.
15. Skoppee CW. *Chemistry of the Steroids.* Butterworths; 1964.
16. Simpson ER. Cholesterol side-chain cleavage, cytochrome P450, and the control of steroidogenesis. *Mol Cell Endocrinol.* 1979; 13:213-227.
17. Schimmer BP, Parker KL. *Adrenocorticotropic Hormones.* McGraw-Hill; 2001.
18. Simpson ER, Waterman MR. Regulation of the synthesis of steroidogenic enzymes in adrenal cortical cells by ACTH. *Annu Rev Physiol.* 1988;50:427-440.
19. Kremers P. Progesterone and pregnenolone 17 alpha-hydroxylase: substrate specificity and selective inhibition by 17 alpha-hydroxylated products. *J Steroid Biochem.* 1976;7:571-575.
20. Miller WL. Molecular biology of steroid hormone synthesis. *Endocr Rev.* 1988;9:295-318.
21. Miller WL, Auchus RJ. The molecular biology, biochemistry, and physiology of human steroidogenesis and its disorders. *Endocr Rev.* 2011;32:81-151.
22. Penning TM. Molecular endocrinology of hydroxysteroid dehydrogenases. *Endocr Rev.* 1997;18:281-305.
23. Tomlinson JW, Walker EA, Bujalska IJ, et al. 11beta-hydroxysteroid dehydrogenase type 1: a tissue-specific regulator of glucocorticoid response. *Endocr Rev.* 2004;25:831-866.
24. White PC, Mune T, Agarwal AK. 11 beta-hydroxysteroid dehydrogenase and the syndrome of apparent mineralocorticoid excess. *Endocr Rev.* 1997;18:135-156.
25. Derendorf H, Mollmann H, Barth J, et al. Pharmacokinetics and oral bioavailability of hydrocortisone. *J Clin Pharmacol.* 1991;31:473-476.
26. Fukushima DK, Leeds NS, Bradlow HL, et al. The characterization of four new metabolites of adrenocortical hormones. *J Biol Chem.* 1955;212:449-460.
27. Romanoff LP, Morris CW, Welch P, et al. The metabolism of cortisol-4-C14 in young and elderly men. I. Secretion rate of cortisol and daily excretion of tetrahydrocortisol, allotetrahydrocortisol, tetrahydrocortisone and cortolone (20alpha and 20beta). *J Clin Endocrinol Metab.* 1961;21:1413-1425.
28. Chang E, Dao TL. Adrenal estrogens. II. Further characterizations of isolated urinary 11beta-hydroxyestradiol. *Biochim Biophys Acta.* 1962;57:609-612.
29. Speirs RS, Meyer RK. A method of assaying adrenal cortical hormones based on a decrease in the circulating eosinophil cells of adrenalectomized mice. *Endocrinology.* 1951;48:316-326.
30. Dorfman RI, Dorfman AS. The relative thymolytic activities of corticoids using the ovariectomized-adrenalectomized mouse. *Endocrinology.* 1961;69:283-291.
31. Ringler I, Brownfield R. The thymolytic activities of 16alpha, 17alpha ketals of triamcinolone. *Endocrinology.* 1960;66:900-902.
32. Kupfer D. Alteration in the magnitude of induction of tyrosine transaminase by glycocorticoids. The effects of phenobarbital, o,p'DDD and beta-diethylaminoethyl diphenylpropylacetate (SKF 525A). *Arch Biochem Biophys.* 1968;127:200-206.
33. Lee KL, Kenney FT. Induction of alanine transaminase by adrenal steroids in cultured hepatoma cells. *Biochem Biophys Res Commun.* 1970;40:469-475.
34. Sereni F, Kenney FT, Kretchmer N. Factors influencing the development of tyrosine-alpha-ketoglutarate transaminase activity in rat liver. *J Biol Chem.* 1959;234:609-612.
35. Feigelson P, Beato M, Colman P, et al. Studies on the hepatic glucocorticoid receptor and on the hormonal modulation of specific mRNA levels during enzyme induction. *Recent Prog Horm Res.* 1975;31:213-242.
36. Kenney F, Lee KL, Reel JR, et al. Regulation of tyrosine alpha-ketoglutarate transaminase in rat liver. IX. Studies of the mechanisms of hormonal inductions in cultured hepatoma cells. *J Biol Chem.* 1970;245:5806-5812.
37. Felig P, Pozefsky T, Marliss E, et al. Alanine: key role in gluconeogenesis. *Science.* 1970;167:1003-1004.
38. Landau BR. Adrenal steroids and carbohydrate metabolism. *Vitam Horm.* 1965;23:2-59.
39. McMahon M, Gerich J, Rizza R. Effects of glucocorticoids on carbohydrate metabolism. *Diabetes Metab Rev.* 1988;4:17-30.
40. Goulding NJ, Godolphin JL, Sharland PR, et al. Anti-inflammatory lipocortin 1 production by peripheral blood leucocytes in response to hydrocortisone. *Lancet.* 1990;335:1416-1418.
41. Peers SH, Smillie F, Elderfield AJ, et al. Glucocorticoid- and non-glucocorticoid induction of lipocortins (annexins) 1 and 2 in rat peritoneal leucocytes in vivo. *Br J Pharmacol.* 1993;108:66-72.
42. Solito E, Parente L. Modulation of phospholipase A2 activity in human fibroblasts. *Br J Pharmacol.* 1989;96:656-660.
43. Parente L, Flower RJ. Hydrocortisone and 'macrocortin' inhibit the zymosan-induced release of lyso-PAF from rat peritoneal leucocytes. *Life Sci.* 1985;36:1225-1231.
44. Beutler B, Cerami A. Cachectin: more than a tumor necrosis factor. *N Engl J Med.* 1987;316:379-385.
45. Goodwin JS, Atluru D, Sierakowski S, et al. Mechanism of action of glucocorticosteroids. Inhibition of T cell proliferation and interleukin 2 production by hydrocortisone is reversed by leukotriene B4. *J Clin Invest.* 1986;77:1244-1250.
46. Lew W, Oppenheim JJ, Matsushima K. Analysis of the suppression of IL-1 alpha and IL-1 beta production in human peripheral blood mononuclear adherent cells by a glucocorticoid hormone. *J Immunol.* 1988;140:1895-1902.
47. Radomski MW, Palmer RM, Moncada S. Glucocorticoids inhibit the expression of an inducible, but not the constitutive, nitric oxide synthase in vascular endothelial cells. *Proc Natl Acad Sci U S A.* 1990;87:10043-10047.
48. Fuller PJ, Yang J, Young MJ. 30 years of the mineralocorticoid receptor: coregulators as mediators of mineralocorticoid receptor signalling diversity. *J Endocrinol.* 2017;234:T23-T34.
49. Harvey BJ, Thomas W. Aldosterone-induced protein kinase signalling and the control of electrolyte balance. *Steroids.* 2018;133:67-74.
50. Bush IE, Mahesh VB. Metabolism of 11-oxygenated steroids. 2. 2-Methyl steroids. *Biochem J.* 1959;71:718-742.
51. Dulin WE, Bowman BJ, Stafford RO. Effects of 2-methylation on glucocorticoid activity of various C-21 steroids. *Proc Soc Exp Biol Med.* 1957;94:303-305.
52. Glenn EM, Stafford RO, Lyster SC, et al. Relation between biological activity of hydrocortisone analogues and their rates of inactivation by rat liver enzyme systems. *Endocrinology.* 1957;61:128-142.
53. Bush IE. Chemical and biological factors in the activity of adrenocortical steroids. *Pharmacol Rev.* 1962;14:317-445.
54. Fried J, Borman A. Synthetic derivatives of cortical hormones. *Vitam Horm.* 1958;16:303-374.
55. Funder JW, Feldman D, Highland E, et al. Molecular modifications of anti-aldosterone compounds: effects on affinity of spirolactones for renal aldosterone receptors. *Biochem Pharmacol.* 1974;23:1493-1501.
56. Meduri GU, Headley AS, Golden E, et al. Effect of prolonged methylprednisolone therapy in unresolving acute respiratory distress syndrome: a randomized controlled trial. *JAMA.* 1998;280: 159-165.
57. Meduri GU, Kanangat S. Glucocorticoid treatment of sepsis and acute respiratory distress syndrome: time for a critical reappraisal. *Crit Care Med.* 1998;26:630-633.
58. Suzuki M. [Percutaneous absorption and systemic distribution of corticosteroids]. *Nihon Hifuka Gakkai Zasshi.* 1982;92:757-776.
59. Derendorf H, Hochhaus G, Meibohm B, et al. Pharmacokinetics and pharmacodynamics of inhaled corticosteroids. *J Allergy Clin Immunol.* 1998;101:S440-S446.

60. Gray CH, Green MA, Holness NJ, et al. Urinary metabolic products of prednisone and prednisolone. *J Endocrinol.* 1956;14:146-154.
61. Burton SD, Byers SO, Friedman M, et al. Hydrocortisone metabolism in the perfused isolated rat liver. *J Clin Endocrinol Metab.* 1957;17:111-115.
62. Glick JH Jr. The isolation of two corticosteroids from cattle bile. *Endocrinology.* 1957;60:368-375.
63. Fieser LF, Fieser M. *Steroids.* Reinhold Publishing Corporation; 1959.
64. Sarett LH. Partial synthesis of pregnene-4-triol-17(beta), 20(beta), 21-dione-3,11 and pregnene-4-diol-17(beta), 21-trione-3,11,20 monoacetate. *J Biol Chem.* 1946;162:601-631.
65. McKenzie BF, Mattox VR, Engel LL, et al. Steroids derived from bile acids: VI. an improved synthesis of methyl 3,8-epoxy-Δ11-cholenate from desoxycholic acid. *J Biol Chem.* 1948;173:271-281.
66. Sarett LH. Preparation of Pregnane-17α,21-diol-3,11,20-trione Acetate. *J Am Chem Soc.* 1949;71:2443-2444.
67. Heazelwood VJ, Galligan JP, Cannell GR, et al. Plasma cortisol delivery from oral cortisol and cortisone acetate: relative bioavailability. *Br J Clin Pharmacol.* 1984;17:55-59.
68. Lima JJ, Jusko WJ. Bioavailability of hydrocortisone retention enemas in relation to absorption kinetics. *Clin Pharmacol Ther.* 1980;28:262-269.
69. Mollmann H, Barth J, Mollmann C, et al. Pharmacokinetics and rectal bioavailability of hydrocortisone acetate. *J Pharm Sci.* 1991;80:835-836.
70. Smith CL, Kreutner W. In vitro glucocorticoid receptor binding and transcriptional activation by topically active glucocorticoids. *Arzneimittelforschung.* 1998;48:956-960.
71. Barth J, Damoiseaux M, Mollmann H, et al. Pharmacokinetics and pharmacodynamics of prednisolone after intravenous and oral administration. *Int J Clin Pharmacol Ther Toxicol.* 1992;30:317-324.
72. Rohatagi S, Barth J, Mollmann H, et al. Pharmacokinetics of methylprednisolone and prednisolone after single and multiple oral administration. *J Clin Pharmacol.* 1997;37:916-925.
73. Mollmann H, Rohdewald P, Barth J, et al. Pharmacokinetics and dose linearity testing of methylprednisolone phosphate. *Biopharm Drug Dispos.* 1989;10:453-464.
74. Vree TB, Verwey-van Wissen CP, Lagerwerf AJ, et al. Isolation and identification of the C6-hydroxy and C20-hydroxy metabolites and glucuronide conjugate of methylprednisolone by preparative high-performance liquid chromatography from urine of patients receiving high-dose pulse therapy. *J Chromatogr B Biomed Sci Appl.* 1999;726:157-168.
75. Spero GB, Thompson JL, Lincoln FH, et al. Adrenal hormones and related compounds. V. Fluorinated 6-methyl steroids. *J Am Chem Soc.* 1957;79:1515-1516.
76. Boland EW. Clinical comparison of the newer anti-inflammatory corticosteroids. *Ann Rheum Dis.* 1962;21:176-187.
77. Ganapati A, Ravindran R, David T, et al. Head to head comparison of adverse effects and efficacy between high dose deflazacort and high dose prednisolone in systemic lupus erythematosus: a prospective cohort study. *Lupus.* 2018;27(6):890-898.
78. Gonzalez-Perez O, Luquin S, Garcia-Estrada J, et al. Deflazacort: a glucocorticoid with few metabolic adverse effects but important immunosuppressive activity. *Adv Ther.* 2007;24:1052-1060.
79. Hahn BH, Pletscher LS, Muniain M. Immunosuppressive effects of deflazacort—a new glucocorticoid with bone-sparing and carbohydrate-sparing properties: comparison with prednisone. *J Rheumatol.* 1981;8:783-790.
80. Assandri A, Buniva G, Martinelli E, et al. Pharmacokinetics and metabolism of deflazacort in the rat, dog, monkey and man. *Adv Exp Med Biol.* 1984;171:9-23.
81. Hirschmann H, Hirschmann FB, Farrel GL. Partial synthesis of 16α,21-diacetoxyprogesterone. *J Am Chem Soc.* 1953;75:4862-4863.
82. Allen WS and Bernstein S. Steroidal cyclic ketals. XII.1 The preparation of Δ16-steroids. *J Am Chem Soc.* 1955;77:1028-1032.
83. Allen WS, Bernstein S. Steroidal cyclic ketals. XX.1 16-hydroxylated steroids. III.2 The preparation of 16α-hydroxyhydrocortisone and related compounds. *J Am Chem Soc.* 1956;78:1909-1913.
84. Hochhaus G, Portner M, Barth J, et al. Oral bioavailability of triamcinolone tablets and a triamcinolone diacetate suspension. *Pharm Res.* 1990;7:558-560.
85. Portner M, Mollmann H, Barth J, et al. [Pharmacokinetics of triamcinolone following oral administration]. *Arzneimittelforschung.* 1988;38:1838-1840.
86. Boland EW. The treatment of rheumatoid arthritis with adrenocorticosteroids and their synthetic analogues: an appraisal of certain developments of the past decade. *Ann N Y Acad Sci.* 1959;82:887-901.
87. Dobes WL. The use of folic acid antagonists and steroids in treatment of psoriasis. *South Med J.* 1963; 56: 187-192.
88. Weiner AL. Intramuscular triamcinolone diacetate therapy of dermatoses: preliminary report. *Antibiot Chemother (Northfield).* 1962;12:360-366.
89. Arth GE, Johnston DBR, Fried J, et al. 16-methylated steroids I. 16α-methylated analogs of cortisone, a new group of anti-inflammatory steroids. *J Am Chem Soc.* 1958;80:3160-3161.
90. Oliveto EP, Rausser R, Weber L, et al. 16-alkylated corticoids. II. 9α-fluoro-16α-methylprednisolone 21-acetate1. *J Am Chem Soc.* 1958;80:4431-4431.
91. Silber RH. The biology of anti-inflammatory steroids. *Ann N Y Acad Sci.* 1959;82:821-828.
92. Sperber PA. Cyproheptadine-dexamethasone combination in the treatment of pruritus. *Curr Ther Res Clin Exp.* 1962;4:70-74.
93. Tolksdorf S. Laboratory evaluation of anti-inflammatory steroids. *Ann N Y Acad Sci.* 1959;82:829-835.
94. Rohdewald P, Mollmann H, Barth J, et al. Pharmacokinetics of dexamethasone and its phosphate ester. *Biopharm Drug Dispos.* 1987;8:205-212.
95. Cohen A, Coldman J. Use of a new corticosteroid in rheumatoid arthritis. *Pa Med J.* 1962;65:347-350.
96. Cohen AI. Treatment of allergy with oral betamethasone in 141 patients. *Antibiot Chemother (Northfield).* 1962;12:91-96.
97. Glyn JH, Fox DB. Preliminary clinical assessment of betamethasone. *Br Med J.* 1961;1:876-877.
98. Nierman MM. Management of steroid-responsive dermatologic disorders with betamethasone. *Clin Med (Northfield).* 1962; 691311-1320.
99. Buijsman RC, Hermkens PH, van Rijn RD, et al. Non-steroidal steroid receptor modulators. *Curr Med Chem.* 2005;12:1017-1075.
100. Cole TJ, Mollard R. Selective glucocorticoid receptor ligands. *Med Chem.* 2007;3:494-506.
101. De Bosscher K. Selective glucocorticoid receptor modulators. *J Steroid Biochem Mol Biol.* 2010;120:96-104.
102. Einstein M, Greenlee M, Rouen G, et al. Selective glucocorticoid receptor nonsteroidal ligands completely antagonize the dexamethasone mediated induction of enzymes involved in gluconeogenesis and glutamine metabolism. *J Steroid Biochem Mol Biol.* 2004;92:345-356.
103. Miner JN, Hong MH, Negro-Vilar A. New and improved glucocorticoid receptor ligands. *Expert Opin Investig Drugs.* 2005;14:1527-1545.
104. Mohler ML, He Y, Wu Z, et al. Dissociated non-steroidal glucocorticoids: tuning out untoward effects. *Expert Opin Ther Pat.* 2007;17:37-58.
105. Sundahl N, Bridelance J, Libert C, et al. Selective glucocorticoid receptor modulation: new directions with non-steroidal scaffolds. *Pharmacol Ther.* 2015;152:28-41.
106. Heier CR, Yu Q, Fiorillo AA, et al. Vamorolone targets dual nuclear receptors to treat inflammation and dystrophic cardiomyopathy. *Life Sci Alliance.* 2019;2:e201800186.
107. Hofman EP, Riddle V, Siegler MA, et al. Phase 1 trial of vamorolone, a first-in-class steroid, shows improvements in side effects via biomarkers bridged to clinical outcomes. *Steroids.* 2018;134:43-52.

108. Conklin LS, Damsker JM, Hoffman EP, et al. Phase IIa trial in Duchenne muscular dystrophy shows vamorolone is a first-in-class dissociative steroidal anti-inflammatory drug. *Pharmacol Res.* 2018;136:140-150.
109. Hoffman EP, Schwartz BD, Mengle-Gaw LJ, et al. Vamorolone trial in Duchenne muscular dystrophy shows dose-related improvement of muscle function. *Neurology.* 2019;93:e1312-e1323.
110. Mah JK, Clemens PR, Guglieri M, et al. Efficacy and safety of vamorolone in Duchenne muscular dystrophy: a 30-month nonrandomized controlled open-label extension trial. *JAMA Network Open.* 2022;5:e2144178.
111. Yohn JJ, Weston WL. Topical glucocorticosteroids. *Curr Probl Dermatol.* 1990;2:31-63.
112. Andersson P, Lihne M, Thalen A, et al. Effect of structural alterations on the biotransformation rate of glucocorticosteroids in rat and human liver. *Xenobiotica.* 1987;17:35-44.
113. Schwartz SG, Scott IU, Stewart MW, et al. Update on corticosteroids for diabetic macular edema. *Clin Ophthalmol.* 2016;10:1723-1730.
114. Brogden RN, Heel RC, Speight TM, et al. Beclomethasone dipropionate. A reappraisal of its pharmacodynamic properties and therapeutic efficacy after a decade of use in asthma and rhinitis. *Drugs.*1984;28:99-126.
115. Green MJ, Berkenkopf J, Fernandez X, et al. Synthesis and structure-activity relationships in a novel series of topically active corticosteroids. *J Steroid Biochem.* 1979;11:61-66.
116. Venkateswaran N, Bian Y, Gupta PK. Practical guidance for the use of loteprednol etabonate ophthalmic suspension 0.25% in the management of dry eye disease. *Clin Ophthalmol.* 2022;16:349-355.
117. Asche H, Botta L, Rettig H, et al. Influence of formulation factors on the availability of drugs from topical preparations. *Pharm Acta Helv.* 1985;60:232-237.
118. Bodor N, Harget AJ, Phillips EW. Structure-activity relationships in the antiinflammatory steroids: a pattern-recognition approach. *J Med Chem.* 1983;26:318-328.
119. Popper TL, Gentles MJ, Kung TT, et al. Structure-activity relationships of a series of novel topical corticosteroids. *J Steroid Biochem.* 1987;27:837-843.
120. Shapiro EL, Gentles MJ, Tiberi RL, et al. 17-Heteroaroyl esters of corticosteroids. 2. 11 beta-hydroxy series. *J Med Chem.* 1987;30:1581-1588.
121. Barth J, Lehr KH, Derendorf H, et al. Studies on the pharmacokinetics and metabolism of prednicarbate after cutaneous and oral administration. *Skin Pharmacol.* 1993;6:179-186.
122. Derendorf H. Pharmacokinetic and pharmacodynamic properties of inhaled corticosteroids in relation to efficacy and safety. *Respir Med.* 1997;91 (suppl A):22-28.
123. Kelly HW. Comparison of inhaled corticosteroids. *Ann Pharmacother.* 1998;32:220-232.
124. Vlckova I, Navratil P, Kana R, et al. Effective treatment of mild-to-moderate nasal polyposis with fluticasone delivered by a novel device. *Rhinology.* 2009;47:419-426.
125. Welch MJ. Pharmacokinetics, pharmacodynamics, and clinical efficacy of albuterol RespiClick() dry-powder inhaler in the treatment of asthma. *Expert Opin Drug Metab Toxicol.* 2016;12:1109-1119.
126. Shaw RJ. Inhaled corticosteroids for adult asthma: impact of formulation and delivery device on relative pharmacokinetics, efficacy and safety. *Respir Med.* 1999;93:149-160.
127. Wales D, Makker H, Kane J, et al. Systemic bioavailability and potency of high-dose inhaled corticosteroids: a comparison of four inhaler devices and three drugs in healthy adult volunteers. *Chest.* 1999;115:1278-1284.
128. Lipworth BJ. Systemic adverse effects of inhaled corticosteroid therapy: a systematic review and meta-analysis. *Arch Intern Med.* 1999;159:941-955.
129. Greiff L, Andersson M, Svensson C, et al. Effects of orally inhaled budesonide in seasonal allergic rhinitis. *Eur Respir J.* 1998;11:1268-1273.
130. Seale JP and Harrison LI. Effect of changing the fine particle mass of inhaled beclomethasone dipropionate on intrapulmonary deposition and pharmacokinetics. *Respir Med.* 1998;92(suppl A):9-15.
131. Harrison LI, Soria I, Cline AC, et al. Pharmacokinetic differences between chlorofluorocarbon and chlorofluorocarbon-free metered dose inhalers of beclomethasone dipropionate in adult asthmatics. *J Pharm Pharmacol.* 1999;51:1235-1240.
132. Lipworth BJ, Jackson CM. Pharmacokinetics of chlorofluorocarbon and hydrofluoroalkane metered-dose inhaler formulations of beclomethasone dipropionate. *Br J Clin Pharmacol.* 1999;48:866-868.
133. Mollmann H, Derendorf H, Barth J, et al. Pharmacokinetic/pharmacodynamic evaluation of systemic effects of flunisolide after inhalation. *J Clin Pharmacol.* 1997;37:893-903.
134. Dickens GR, Wermeling DP, Matheny CJ, et al. Pharmacokinetics of flunisolide administered via metered dose inhaler with and without a spacer device and following oral administration. *Ann Allergy Asthma Immunol.* 2000;84:528-532.
135. Thalen BA, Axelsson BI, Andersson PH, et al. 6 alpha-fluoro- and 6 alpha,9 alpha-difluoro-11 beta,21-dihydroxy-16 alpha,17 alpha-propylmethylenedioxypregn-4-ene-3,20-dione: synthesis and evaluation of activity and kinetics of their C-22 epimers. *Steroids.* 1998;63:37-43.
136. Ryrfeldt A, Andersson P, Edsbacker S, et al. Pharmacokinetics and metabolism of budesonide, a selective glucocorticoid. *Eur J Respir Dis Suppl.* 1982;122:86-95.
137. Szefler SJ. Pharmacodynamics and pharmacokinetics of budesonide: a new nebulized corticosteroid. *J Allergy Clin Immunol.* 1999;104:175-183.
138. Miller-Larsson A, Jansson P, Runstrom A, et al. Prolonged airway activity and improved selectivity of budesonide possibly due to esterification. *Am J Respir Crit Care Med.* 2000;162:1455-1461.
139. Miller-Larsson A, Mattsson H, Hjertberg E, et al. Reversible fatty acid conjugation of budesonide. Novel mechanism for prolonged retention of topically applied steroid in airway tissue. *Drug Metab Dispos.* 1998;26:623-630.
140. Agertoft L, Andersen A, Weibull E, et al. Systemic availability and pharmacokinetics of nebulised budesonide in preschool children. *Arch Dis Child.* 1999;80:241-247.
141. Pedersen S, Steffensen G, Ekman I, et al. Pharmacokinetics of budesonide in children with asthma. *Eur J Clin Pharmacol.* 1987;31:579-582.
142. Shapiro EL, Gentles MJ, Tiberi RL, et al. Synthesis and structure-activity studies of corticosteroid 17-heterocyclic aromatic esters. 1. 9 alpha, 11 beta-dichloro series. *J Med Chem.* 1987;30:1068-1073.
143. Onrust SV, Lamb HM. Mometasone furoate. A review of its intranasal use in allergic rhinitis. *Drugs.* 1998;56:725-745.
144. Affrime MB, Cuss F, Padhi D, et al. Bioavailability and metabolism of mometasone furoate following administration by metered-dose and dry-powder inhalers in healthy human volunteers. *J Clin Pharmacol.* 2000;40:1227-1236.
145. Phillipps GH, Bailey EJ, Bain BM, et al. Synthesis and structure-activity relationships in a series of antiinflammatory corticosteroid analogues, halomethyl androstane-17 beta-carbothioates and -17 beta-carboselenoates. *J Med Chem.* 1994;37:3717-3729.
146. Harding SM. The human pharmacology of fluticasone propionate. *Respir Med.* 1990;84(suppl A):25-29.
147. Johnson M. Development of fluticasone propionate and comparison with other inhaled corticosteroids. *J Allergy Clin Immunol.* 1998;101:S434-S439.
148. Mackie AE, Ventresca GP, Fuller RW, et al. Pharmacokinetics of intravenous fluticasone propionate in healthy subjects. *Br J Clin Pharmacol.* 1996;41:539-542.

149. Mollmann H, Wagner M, Meibohm B, et al. Pharmacokinetic and pharmacodynamic evaluation of fluticasone propionate after inhaled administration. *Eur J Clin Pharmacol.* 1998;53: 459-467.
150. Thorsson L, Dahlstrom K, Edsbacker S, et al. Pharmacokinetics and systemic effects of inhaled fluticasone propionate in healthy subjects. *Br J Clin Pharmacol.* 1997;43:155-161.
151. Rohatagi S, Bye A, Falcoz C, et al. Dynamic modeling of cortisol reduction after inhaled administration of fluticasone propionate. *J Clin Pharmacol.* 1996;36:938-941.
152. Biggadike K. Fluticasone furoate/fluticasone propionate—different drugs with different properties. *Clin Respir J.* 2011;5: 183-184.
153. Biggadike K, Bledsoe RK, Hassell AM, et al. X-ray crystal structure of the novel enhanced-affinity glucocorticoid agonist fluticasone furoate in the glucocorticoid receptor-ligand binding domain. *J Med Chem.* 2008;51:3349-3352.
154. Salter M, Biggadike K, Matthews JL, et al. Pharmacological properties of the enhanced-affinity glucocorticoid fluticasone furoate in vitro and in an in vivo model of respiratory inflammatory disease. *Am J Physiol Lung Cell Mol Physiol.* 2007;293:L660-L667.
155. Valotis A, Hogger P. Human receptor kinetics and lung tissue retention of the enhanced-affinity glucocorticoid fluticasone furoate. *Respir Res.* 2007;8:54.
156. Allen A, Bareille PJ, Rousell VM. Fluticasone furoate, a novel inhaled corticosteroid, demonstrates prolonged lung absorption kinetics in man compared with inhaled fluticasone propionate. *Clin Pharmacokinet.* 2013;52:37-42.
157. Duval D, Durant S, Homo-Delarche F. Effect of antiglucocorticoids on dexamethasone-induced inhibition of uridine incorporation and cell lysis in isolated mouse thymocytes. *J Steroid Biochem.* 1984;20:283-287.
158. Peterfalvi M, Torelli V, Fournex R, et al. Importance of the lactonic ring in the activity of steroidal antialdosterones. *Biochem Pharmacol.* 1980;29:353-357.
159. INSPRA® (eplerenone). Prescribing information. Pfizer Inc.; Revised May 2016.
160. Dymala K. How finerenone compares to other mineralocorticoid receptor antagonists. Pharmacy Times. 2022. Accessed December 7, 2023. https://www.pharmacytimes.com/view/how-finerenone-compares-to-other-mineralocorticoid-receptor-antagonists
161. Kerendia (finerenone). Prescribing information. Bayer HealthCare Pharmaceuticals, Inc.; 2021.
162. Grune J, Beyhoff N, Smeir E, et al. Selective mineralocorticoid receptor cofactor modulation as molecular basis for finerenone's antifibrotic activity. *Hypertension.* 2018;71:599-608.
163. Pitt B, Kober L, Ponikowski P, et al. Safety and tolerability of the novel nonsteroidal mineralocorticoid receptor antagonist BAY 94-8862 in patients with chronic heart failure and mild or moderate chronic kidney disease: a randomized, double-blind trial. *Eur Heart J.* 2013;34:2453-2463.
164. Flores PG, Rodriguez Salazar JD, Nahar BL, Jim B. Finerenone: a novel third-generation mineralocorticoid receptor antagonist. *Cardiol Rev.* 10.109.7/CRD.0000000000000573 (July 11, 2023).
165. Agarwal MK, Hainque B, Moustaid N, et al. Glucocorticoid antagonists. *FEBS Lett.* 1987;217:221-226.
166. Fleseriu M, Biller BM, Findling JW, et al. Mifepristone, a glucocorticoid receptor antagonist, produces clinical and metabolic benefits in patients with Cushing's syndrome. *J Clin Endocrinol Metab.* 2012;97:2039-2049.
167. Mohler ML, He Y, Wu Z, Hong SS, Miller DM. Non-steroidal glucocorticoid receptor antagonists: the race to replace RU-486 for anti-glucocorticoid therapy. *Expert Opin Ther Pat.* 2007;17:59-81.
168. Isturisa (osilodrostat). Prescribing information. Recordati Rare Diseases Inc.; Revised November 2023.
169. Napoli JL, Counsell RE. New inhibitors of steroid 11beta-hydroxylase. Structure–activity relationship studies of metyrapone-like compounds. *J Med Chem.* 1977;20:762-766.
170. Shaw MA, Nicholls PJ, Smith HJ. Aminoglutethimide and ketoconazole: historical perspectives and future prospects. *J Steroid Biochem.* 1988;31:137-146.
171. Sonino N. The use of ketoconazole as an inhibitor of steroid production. *N Engl J Med.* 1987;317:812-818.
172. Potts GO, Creange JE, Hardomg HR, et al. Trilostane, an orally active inhibitor of steroid biosynthesis. *Steroids.* 1978;32:257-267.
173. Monder C, Stewart PM, Lakshmi V, et al. Licorice inhibits corticosteroid 11 beta-dehydrogenase of rat kidney and liver: in vivo and in vitro studies. *Endocrinology.* 1989;125:1046-1053.
174. Buhler H, Perschel FH, Fitzner R, et al. Endogenous inhibitors of 11 beta-OHSD: existence and possible significance. *Steroids.* 1994;59:131-135.
175. Diederich S, Grossmann C, Hanke B, et al. In the search for specific inhibitors of human 11beta-hydroxysteroid-dehydrogenases (11beta-HSDs): chenodeoxycholic acid selectively inhibits 11beta-HSD-I. *Eur J Endocrinol.* 2000;142:200-207.
176. Scott JS, Goldberg FW, Turnbull AV. Medicinal chemistry of inhibitors of 11beta-hydroxysteroid dehydrogenase type 1 (11beta-HSD1). *J Med Chem.* 2014;57:4466-4486.
177. Pereira CD, Azevedo I, Monteiro R, et al. 11beta-hydroxysteroid dehydrogenase type 1: relevance of its modulation in the pathophysiology of obesity, the metabolic syndrome and type 2 diabetes mellitus. *Diabetes Obes Metab.* 2012;14:869-881.

Structure Challenge Answers

A-6, B-5, C-9, D-7, E-8, F-3, G-4, H-1, I-2

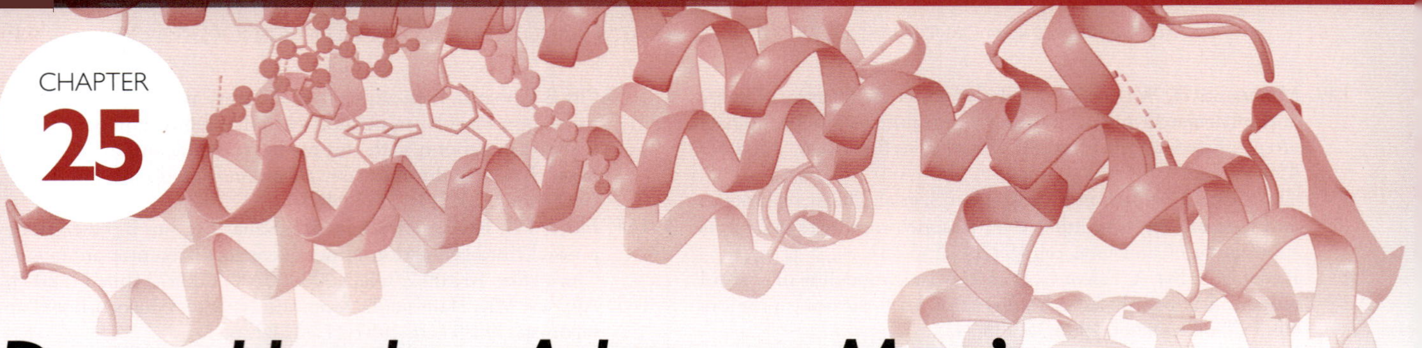

CHAPTER 25

Drugs Used to Advance Men's and Women's Health

Ramesh Narayan, Michael L. Mohler, and James T. Dalton

Drugs covered in this chapter:

Estrogens
- Conjugated estrogens
- Diethylstilbestrol
- Estetrol
- 17β-Estradiol
- Estradiol cypionate
- Estradiol valerate
- Ethinyl estradiol
- Mestranol
- *Nonsteroidal estrogen*
- *Steroidal estrogens*

Progestins
- Desogestrel
- Dienogest
- Drospirenone
- Ethynodiol diacetate
- Etonogestrel
- *First generation*
- *Fourth generation*
- Lynestrenol
- Medroxyprogesterone
- Medroxyprogesterone acetate
- Megestrol acetate
- Norelgestromin
- Norethindrone
- Norethindrone acetate
- Norethynodrel
- Norgestimate
- Norgestrel/levonorgestrel
- Progesterone
- *Second generation*
- Segesterone
- Synthetic progestins
- *Third generation*

Nonpeptidic gonadotropin-releasing hormone receptor antagonist
- Elagolix

Miscellaneous premenopausal drugs
- Bremelanotide
- Brexanolone

Emergency contraceptives and abortifacients
- Carboprost
- Dinoprostone
- Mifepristone
- Misoprostol
- Ulipristal acetate

Infertility drugs
- Clomiphene citrate

Androgens
- Fluoxymesterone
- Methyltestosterone
- Testosterone (oral, transdermal, buccal)
- Testosterone esters

Treatment of menopause

Estrogens
- Conjugated estrogens
- Esterified estrogens
- 17β-Estradiol
- Estropipate

Progestins
- Medroxyprogesterone acetate
- Micronized progesterone

Selective estrogen receptor modulators
- Bazedoxifene
- Ospemifene

Miscellaneous drugs
- Fezolinetant
- Prasterone

Treatment of erectile dysfunction

Phosphodiesterase type 5 inhibitors
- Avanafil
- Sildenafil
- Tadalafil
- Vardenafil

Miscellaneous drug
- Prostaglandin E_1

Treatment of benign prostatic hyperplasia

α_1-Adrenergic antagonists
- Alfuzosin
- Doxazosin
- Silodosin
- Tamsulosin
- Terazosin

5α-Reductase inhibitors
- Dutasteride
- Finasteride

Treatment of acne
- Clascoterone

Treatment of breast cancer

Selective estrogen receptor modulators
- Tamoxifen
- Toremifene

Antiestrogens
- Elacestrant
- Fulvestrant

Aromatase inhibitors
- Anastrozole
- Exemestane
- Letrozole

Treatment of prostate cancer

Gonadotropin-releasing hormone agonists
- Goserelin
- Leuprolide
- Triptorelin

Drugs covered in this chapter:—continued

GONADOTROPIN-RELEASING HORMONE ANTAGONISTS
- Degarelix
- Relugolix

CYP17A1 INHIBITOR
- Abiraterone

ANTIANDROGENS
- Apalutamide
- Bicalutamide
- Darolutamide
- Enzalutamide
- Flutamide
- Nilutamide

Abbreviations

AC-T anthracycline and cyclophosphamide then taxane
ACTH adrenocorticotropic hormone
ADME absorption, distribution, metabolism, and excretion
ADT androgen deprivation therapy
AF-1 activation function-1
AF-2 activation function-2
AI aromatase inhibitor
AIDS acquired immunodeficiency syndrome
AKR1C3 aldoketoreductase type 1C3
AR androgen receptor
5AR 5α-reductase
$5AR_1$ 5α-reductase type 1
$5AR_2$ 5α-reductase type 2
$5AR_3$ 5α-reductase type 3
5ARI 5α-reductase inhibitor
AR-SV androgen receptor splice variant
ATAC Arimidex, Tamoxifen, Alone or in Combination
AUA-SI/I-PSS American Urological Association Symptom Index/ International Prostate Symptom Score
AUC area under the curve
3β-HSD 5-ene-3β-hydroxysteroid dehydrogenase/3-oxosteroid-4,5-isomerase
5β-DHT 5β-dihydrotestosterone
17β-HSD 17β-hydroxysteroid dehydrogenase
17β-HSD3 17β-hydroxysteroid dehydrogenase type 3
17β-HSD5 17β-hydroxysteroid dehydrogenase type 5
BIG Breast International Group
BMD bone mineral density
BPH benign prostatic hyperplasia
BRCA breast cancer susceptibility gene
cAMP cyclic adenosine monophosphate
CAT computed axial tomography
CDK4/6 cyclin-dependent kinase 4/6
CEE conjugated equine estrogens
cGMP cyclic guanosine monophosphate
C_{max} peak serum concentration
COC combined oral contraceptive
CRPC castration-resistant prostate cancer
CSPC castration-sensitive prostate cancer
CYP11A1 cytochrome P-450 side-chain cleavage enzyme
CYP11B2 11β-hydroxylase
CYP17A1 17α-hydroxylase/ 17,20-lyase
CYP19A1 aromatase
CYP21 21-hydroxylase
DCIS ductal carcinoma in situ
DES diethylstilbestrol
DHEA dehydroepiandrosterone
DHT 5α-dihydrotestosterone
DVT deep vein thrombosis
E1 estrone
E2 17β-estradiol
E3 estriol
ED erectile dysfunction
EE ethinyl estradiol
EGFR epidermal growth factor receptor
ER estrogen receptor
ERα estrogen receptor alpha
ERβ estrogen receptor beta
ERE estrogen-response element
FDA U.S. Food and Drug Administration
FSH follicle-stimulating hormone
GABA γ-aminobutyric acid
$GABA_A$ γ-aminobutyric acid receptor subtype A
GI gastrointestinal
GnRH gonadotropin-releasing hormone
GnRH-R gonadotropin-releasing hormone receptor
H12 helix 12
HBA hydrogen bond acceptor
HBD hydrogen bond donor
hCG human chorionic gonadotropin
HER2 human epidermal growth factor receptor type II
HPA hypothalamus-pituitary-adrenal
HPG hypothalamus-pituitary-gonadal
HRE hormone-response element
HRT hormone replacement therapy
HSDD hypoactive sexual desire disorder
IDFS invasive disease-free survival
IM intramuscular
IUD intrauterine device
LBD ligand-binding domain
LH luteinizing hormone
LHRH luteinizing hormone–releasing hormone
LNCaP lymph node carcinoma of the prostate
LUTS lower urinary tract symptoms
MBC metastatic breast cancer
MCR melanocortin receptor
mCRPC metastatic castration-resistant prostate cancer
MFS metastasis-free survival
mHRR mutations of genes that control homologous recombination repair
MPA medroxyprogesterone acetate
MSH melanocyte-stimulating hormone
mTOR mechanistic target of rapamycin
$NADP^+$ nicotinamide adenine dinucleotide phosphate
NADPH nicotinamide adenine dinucleotide phosphate
NAMS North American Menopause Society
NCI National Cancer Institute
NDM TAM *N*-desmethyl tamoxifen
NDM TOR *N*-desmethyl toremifene
NK3 neurokinin-3
nmCRPC nonmetastatic castration-resistant prostate cancer
NO nitric oxide
OC oral contraceptive
4-OH TAM 4-hydroxytamoxifen

Abbreviations—continued

4-OH-NDM TAM 4-hydroxy-N-desmethyl tamoxifen
4-OH-NDM TOR 4-hydroxy-N-desmethyl toremifene
OTC over the counter
P-gp P-glycoprotein
PAP prostatic acid phosphatase
PARP poly(ADP-ribose) polymerase
PD-L1 programmed death-ligand 1
PDE5 phosphodiesterase type 5
PDE5Is phosphodiesterase type 5 inhibitors
PMDD postmenopausal dysphoric disorder
POP progestin-only pill
PPD postpartum depression
PR progesterone receptor
PRE progesterone-response element
PSA prostate-specific antigen
REMS risk evaluation and mitigation strategy
rPFS radiographic progression-free survival
SAR structure-activity relationship
SARM selective androgen receptor modulator
SCC side-chain cleavage
SERD selective estrogen receptor degrader
SERM selective estrogen receptor modulator
SGRM selective glucocorticoid receptor modulator
SHBG sex hormone–binding globulin
TC Taxotere and cyclophosphamide
TNBC triple-negative breast cancer
TOR toremifene
TRT testosterone replacement therapy
UGT UDP-glucuronyltransferase
VCaP vertebral cancer of the prostate
VTE venous thromboembolism
WHI Women's Health Initiative

CLINICAL SIGNIFICANCE

A wide variety of synthetic formulations of estrogens exist in practice, making it confusing for health care providers to select optimal agents for the treatment of various conditions. Understanding the metabolism of estrogens may improve the ability to differentiate a medication's physiologic effects as well as risks associated with treatment. One example of this is the recommended use of transdermal or intravaginal 17β-estradiol as a supplement in postmenopausal women instead of oral treatment, which undergoes hepatic first-pass metabolism, including inactivating (but reversible) oxidation to the 17-keto steroid estrone, irreversible inactivating oxidation at C16 to estriol, and oxidation/methylation to a hypertensive 4-methoxy metabolite. Topical delivery of estradiol results in higher blood levels of active drug and a reduction in the formation of clotting factors, which have been associated with many of the cardiovascular risks tied to the 4-methoxy metabolite of estrogen supplementation.

Emily L. Knezevich, PharmD, BCPS, CDCES, FCCP

INTRODUCTION

This chapter focuses on the physiology, pharmacology, metabolism, and structure-activity relationships (SARs) of therapeutic and emerging classes of drugs that are indicated for use based on sex. Differences in circulating hormones and the anatomy and physiology of reproductive systems differentiate between males and females and provide the basis for numerous endocrine-based therapies that are exclusive for men or women. Although numerous endocrine diseases are common in both men and women, many of which are associated with adrenocorticoids (see Chapter 24), there are also diseases and medical needs that demonstrate sexual dimorphism and require treatment that is exclusive to men or women (Fig. 25.1). Male and female fertility, sexual function, secondary sex characteristics (eg, hair growth and muscle mass), and most endocrine cancers (at least in their early stages) rely on the sex hormones. Female hormonal contraceptives are used widely and represent some of the earliest endocrine therapies employed (second to fourth decades of life), while treatments for benign prostatic hyperplasia (BPH) and erectile dysfunction (ED) in men extend well into the latter decades of the lifespan. The majority of these disorders and their treatments are associated with the male (ie, androgens) or female (ie, estrogens and progestins) sex hormones, their pharmacologic targets (ie, the androgen receptor [AR], estrogen receptors [ERs], and progesterone receptor [PR], respectively), and the tissues that rely on the androgens and estrogens.

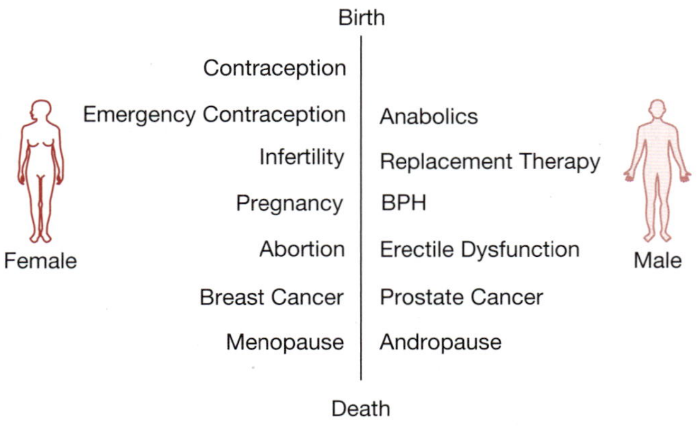

Figure 25.1 Disorders associated with men's and women's health. BPH, benign prostatic hyperplasia.

Sex Hormones

The sex steroid hormones are steroid molecules that are necessary for reproduction in females and males and that affect the development of secondary sex characteristics in both sexes. The sex steroids comprise three classes: estrogens, progestins, and androgens (Fig. 25.2; carbon numbering system is indicated; see Chapter 24 for more detailed discussion of steroid nomenclature and structure). The two principal classes of female sex steroid hormones are estrogens and progestins, and the principal male sex hormone class is androgens. Chemically, the naturally occurring estrogens are C18 steroids, and they have in common an aromatic A ring with a 3-phenolic group that distinguishes them from the other sex steroid hormones. The most potent endogenous estrogen is 17β-estradiol (Fig. 25.2). The naturally occurring progestins are C21 steroids, and they have in common an unsaturated 3-keto-4-ene structure in the A ring and a ketone at the C20 position. The most potent endogenous progestin is progesterone (Fig. 25.2). The naturally occurring androgens are C19 steroids, and they have in common oxygen atoms (as either hydroxyl or ketone groups) at both the C3 and C17 positions. Testosterone is a potent androgen that is found in the blood at higher concentrations than other androgens, whereas 5α-dihydrotestosterone (DHT) (Fig. 25.2; note *trans* A/B ring fusion) is a more potent metabolite of testosterone that is formed in certain androgen target tissues, including the prostate and scalp.

All three classes of endogenous steroids are present in both males and females. The production and circulating plasma levels of estrogens and progestins are higher in females, and the production and circulating plasma levels of androgens are higher in males. Although estrogens are regarded as female hormones, their circulating levels are only a fraction of serum androgen levels. While serum 17β-estradiol in premenopausal women is in the picogram/milliliter range, serum androgen levels are in the nanogram/milliliter range. This discrepancy between the level and activity reflects that the estrogens rely more on local synthesis from androgens by aromatization. In endocrine tissues, cholesterol is the steroid that is stored and converted to estrogens, progestins, or androgens when the tissue is stimulated by a gonadotropic hormone.

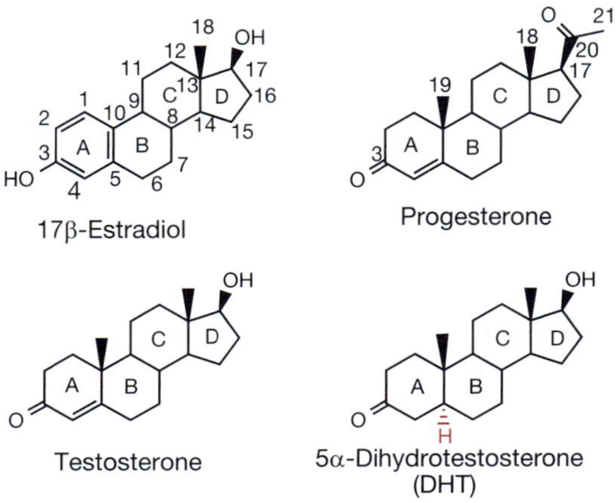

Figure 25.2 Steroidal sex hormones.

Sexual Hormone Biosynthesis and Metabolism

Biosynthesis

The major pathways for the biosynthesis of the sex steroid hormones are summarized in Figure 25.3, and the synthesis of adrenocorticoids is discussed later (see also Chapter 24 and Fig. 24.8). Briefly, cholesterol is stored in endocrine tissues and is converted to androgens, estrogens, or progestins when the tissue is stimulated by a gonadotropic hormone. Androgens (male sex hormones) primarily are synthesized from cholesterol in the testes, whereas estrogens are biosynthesized chiefly in the ovary in premenopausal and mature women and in adipose tissue in men and postmenopausal women.[1] Androgens are intermediates in the biosynthesis of estrogens. In the liver, lower potency androgens are formed from C21 steroids. During pregnancy, the placenta is the main source of estrogen biosynthesis and pathways for production change.[2,3] Small amounts of these hormones are also synthesized by the adrenal cortex, the hypothalamus, and the anterior pituitary in both sexes.

Luteinizing hormone (LH), a gonadotropic hormone produced and secreted by the anterior pituitary gland, binds to its receptor on the surface of the Leydig cells of the testis, or theca cells in the ovary, to initiate testosterone, and progesterone and estrogen biosynthesis, respectively. As in other endocrine cells, the binding of gonadotropin (ie, LH) activates the G_s signal transduction pathway, increasing intracellular cyclic adenosine monophosphate (cAMP) levels via activation of adenylyl cyclase. One of the processes influenced by elevated cAMP levels is the activation of cholesterol esterase, which cleaves cholesterol esters and liberates free cholesterol. The free cholesterol is then converted in mitochondria to pregnenolone via the cholesterol side-chain cleavage (SCC) reaction catalyzed by a mitochondrial cytochrome P450 enzyme complex found in the mitochondrial membrane. The complex consists of three proteins: CYP11A1 (also known as $P450_{SCC}$), adrenodoxin, and adrenodoxin reductase (step a of Fig. 25.3; see also Chapter 24 and Fig. 24.7). Pregnenolone is converted by 17α-hydroxylase to 17α-hydroxypregnenolone (step b) in the endoplasmic reticulum and then to dehydroepiandrosterone (DHEA; a C19 steroid) via 17,20-lyase (step j), which involves cleavage of the C17 to C20 carbon-carbon bond and loss of the 17β-acetyl side chain.[4] Steps b and j are catalyzed by the same bifunctional enzyme CYP17A1. Progesterone can be formed from pregnenolone via the action of another bifunctional enzyme 5-ene-3β-hydroxysteroid dehydrogenase/3-oxosteroid-4,5-isomerase (3β-HSD), which catalyzes the 5-ene-3β-hydroxysteroid dehydrogenase and 3-oxosteroid-4,5-isomerase reactions (step c). This same enzyme is responsible for the conversion of DHEA to the 17-ketosteroidal androgen, androstenedione (step c).

Testosterone is formed in the testes by the reduction of the 17-ketone of androstenedione by 17β-hydroxysteroid dehydrogenases (17β-HSD), but the reaction is reversible (step g in Fig. 25.3); that is, testosterone and androstenedione are metabolically interconvertible. 17β-Hydroxysteroid dehydrogenase type 3 (17β-HSD3) is largely responsible for

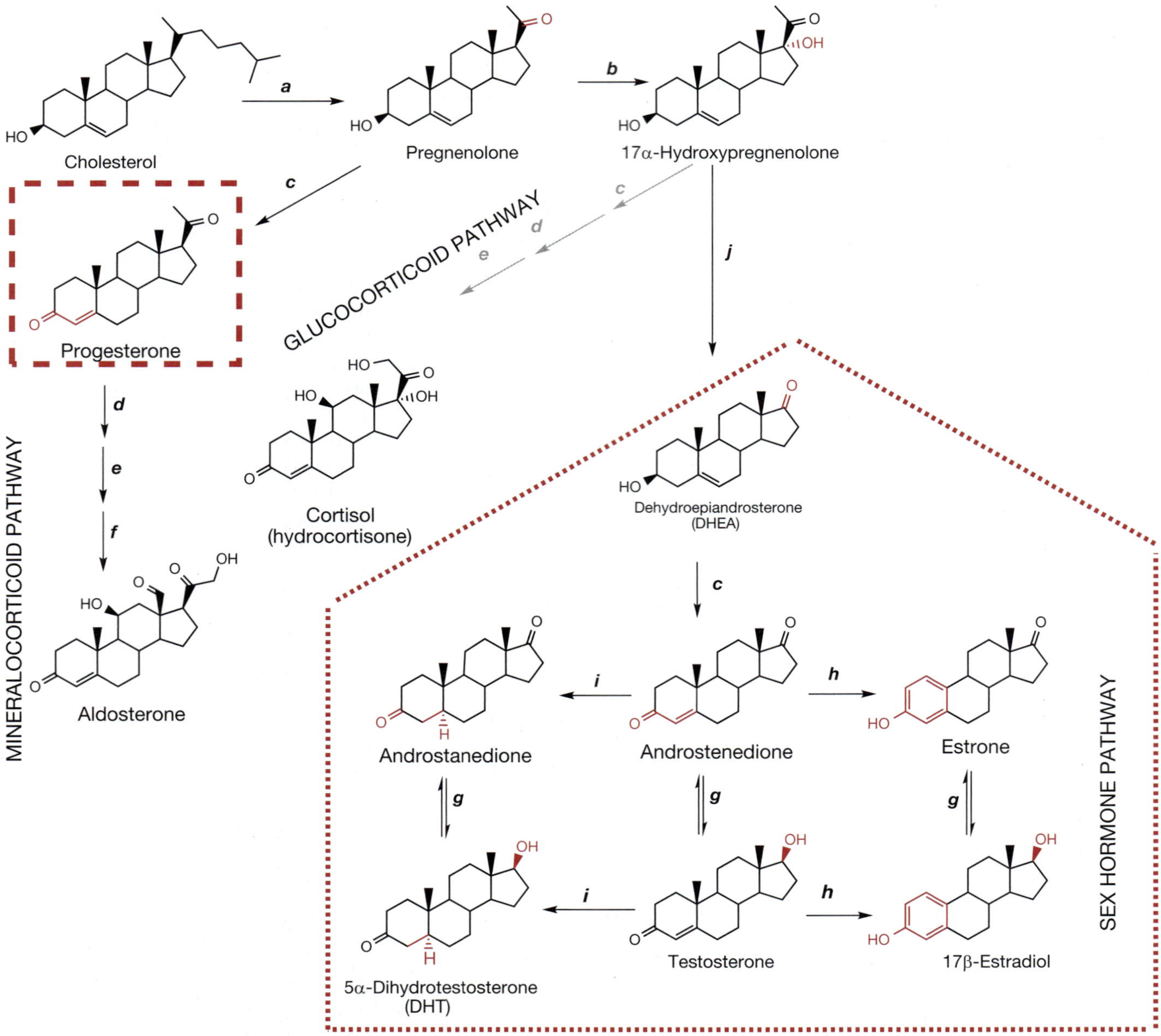

Figure 25.3 Biosynthesis of the adrenocorticoids and sex hormones from cholesterol. The enzymes involved in these biosynthetic pathways are (a) a mitochondrial cytochrome P450 enzyme complex consisting of three proteins: CYP11A1 (also known as P450SCC), adrenodoxin, and adrenodoxin reductase; (b) 17α-hydroxylase (CYP17A1); (c) 5-ene-3β-hydroxysteroid dehydrogenase/3-oxosteroid-4,5-isomerase (3β-HSD); (d) 21-hydroxylase (CYP21); (e) 11β-hydroxylase (CYP11B2); (f) 18-hydroxyase; (g) 17β-hydroxysteroid dehydrogenases (17β-HSDs); (h) aromatase (CYP19A1); (i) 5α-reductase (5AR); and (j) 17,20-lyase (CYP17A1).

the conversion of androstenedione to testosterone in the testes, while type 5 (also known as aldoketoreductase 1C3) is thought to predominate in peripheral (eg, adipose tissue and prostate) conversion of androstenedione to testosterone. Loss of the C19 angular methyl group and aromatization of the A ring of testosterone or androstenedione is catalyzed by the microsomal cytochrome P450 enzyme complex, called aromatase, and results in the C18 steroids—namely, 17β-estradiol or estrone, respectively (step h). 17β-Estradiol and estrone are also metabolically interconvertible and catalyzed by 17β-HSD (step g) but involve different isozymes of 17β-HSD than those responsible for the conversion of androstenedione to testosterone and androstenedione to DHT.

The most potent endogenous androgen is the 5α-reduced steroid, DHT, which is biosynthesized by two 5α-reductase (5AR) isoforms, types 1 and 2 (step i). Type 1 5AR ($5AR_1$) is expressed predominantly in sebaceous glands of the skin, scalp, and liver and is responsible for approximately one-third of the circulating DHT (Fig. 25.3). Type 2 5AR ($5AR_2$) is found primarily in the prostate, seminal vesicles, epididymides, genital skin (scrotum), hair follicles, and liver, and it is responsible for two-thirds of the circulating DHT. Approximately 6% to 8% of testosterone is converted to DHT. Conversion to DHT amplifies the action of testosterone by 3 to 5 times because of the greater binding affinity of DHT as compared to testosterone for the AR.[5]

Progesterone is biosynthesized and secreted by the corpus luteum of the ovary during the luteal phase of the reproductive cycle. LH binds to the LH receptor on the surface of the ovarian cells to initiate progesterone biosynthesis. As in other endocrine cells such as adrenal cortical cells, the binding of LH results in an increase in intracellular cAMP levels via activation of a G_s protein and adenylyl cyclase. One of the processes influenced by elevated cAMP levels is the activation of cholesterol esterase, which cleaves cholesterol esters and liberates free cholesterol. The free cholesterol is then converted in mitochondria to pregnenolone via the cholesterol SCC reaction (step a of Fig. 25.3), and progesterone is formed from pregnenolone by the action of 3β-HSD, as discussed previously for 17β-estradiol (and adrenocorticoids) (step c).

Metabolism

The metabolic transformations of androgens, estrogens, and progesterone are similar in many ways (Fig. 25.4). In most cases, metabolic transformations occur predominantly on the A or D ring through phase I hydroxylations followed by phase II conjugation reactions (sulfonation or glucuronidation being most common). The stereochemistry of the A/B ring junction upon reduction plays a key three-dimensional (3D) conformational role in how these hormones can bind to their respective receptors (Fig. 25.4). By adding a 17α-ethinyl group onto 17β-estradiol, oxidation via first-pass metabolism is prevented, allowing for an orally active compound to be used in oral contraceptives. Understanding inactivating metabolic transformations is pivotal to understanding why medicinal chemists have added substituents at key positions to prevent their occurrence.

Androgen Metabolism. Testosterone can be metabolized in either its target tissues or the liver[6-8] as shown in Figure 25.3. In androgen target tissues, testosterone can be converted to physiologically active metabolites. In the prostate gland, skin, and liver,[9] testosterone is reduced to DHT by 5AR (types 1 and 2).[10] On the other hand, a small amount of testosterone (0.3%) also can be converted to 17β-estradiol by aromatase through cleavage of the C19 methyl group and aromatization of ring A, which mainly occurs in adipose tissue in men. This process also occurs in premenopausal ovaries. In men, approximately 80% of the circulating estrogen arises from aromatization of testosterone in the adipose tissue,[11] with the other 20% being secreted by the Leydig cells in the testes.[12] Both 5α-reduction and aromatization are irreversible processes.

In addition to these pathways to active metabolites, testosterone can also be inactivated in the liver through (1) 6β-oxidation to an inactive hydroxyl metabolite or (2) 5β-reduction to an inactive cholic acid metabolite (5β-DHT), then possibly 3α-reduction (see also panel B of Fig. 24.9 in Chapter 24 on Adrenocorticoids). Hydroxylated testosterone metabolites are glucuronidated and renally eliminated. Further, testosterone can be metabolized to androstenedione through oxidation of the 17β-OH group, which can be further converted to another inactive cholic acid metabolite, etiocholanolone, through 5β- and 3-keto reduction (Fig. 25.4). The 5β-reduction of testosterone to its *cis* A/B ring juncture conformation (eg, 5β-DHT and etiocholanolone) explains its complete loss of activity because the *cis* A/B ring no longer has an affinity for the AR. Most of the other metabolites mentioned earlier undergo extensive glucuronidation as well (eg, of the 3α- and/or 17β-OH groups) either in the target tissues or in the liver[13] and are excreted in the urine.

After the administration of radiolabeled testosterone, approximately 90% of the radioactivity is found in the urine, and 6% is recovered in the feces through biliary excretion and enterohepatic recycling.[14] Major urinary metabolites include androsterone and its 5β-diastereoisomer etiocholanolone, both of which are inactive metabolites, demonstrating double bond reduction and 3α-hydroxylation as the major metabolic pathway. They are excreted mainly as glucuronide conjugates or, to a lesser extent, as sulfate conjugates.[13] Following oral administration of testosterone, extensive first-pass hepatic metabolism (90% of oral dose) severely limits oral bioavailability and produces a plasma half-life of less than 30 minutes. However, testosterone is commonly delivered in many parenteral dosage forms, and there are ongoing efforts to develop oral dosage forms of testosterone that better circumvent first-pass hepatic metabolism. The primary class of enzymes that glucuronidate androgens to inactive water-soluble metabolites is the UDP-glucuronyltransferase (UGT) subfamily 2B or UGT2B.[15]

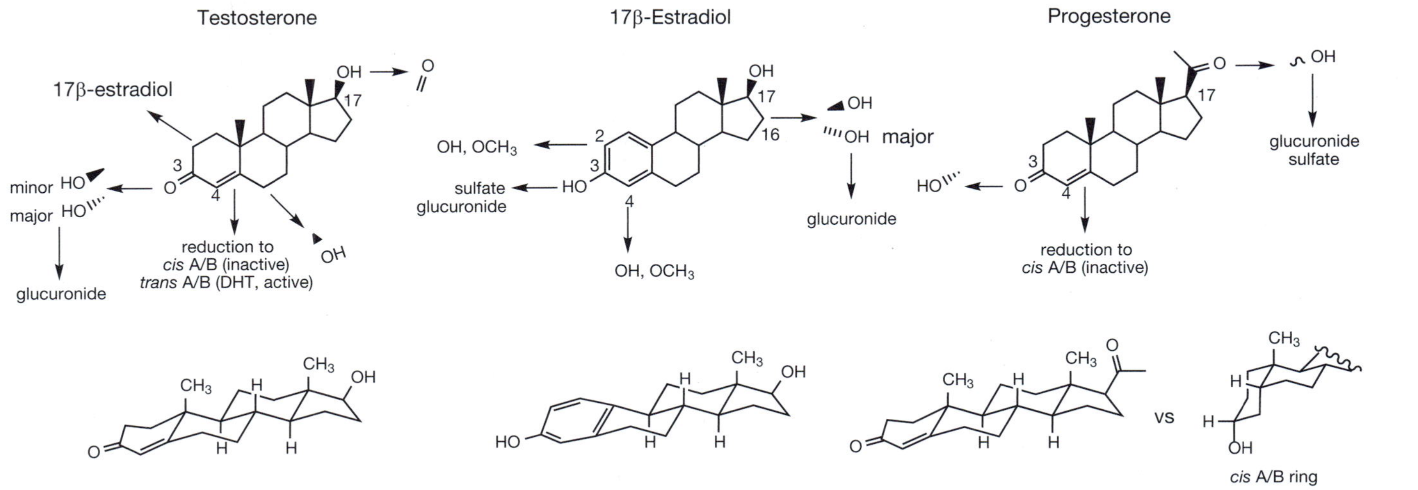

Figure 25.4 General metabolic pathways for androgens, estrogens, and progestins.

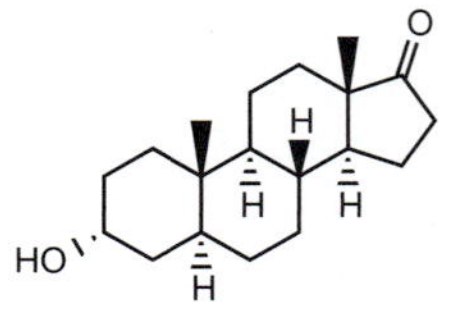

Androsterone

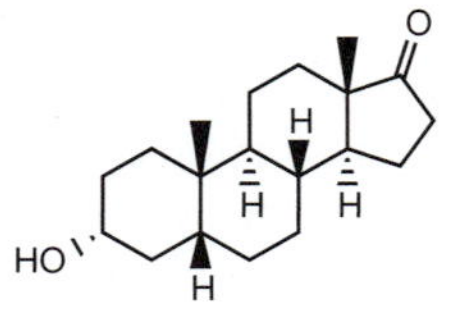

5β-Androsterone (etiocholanolone)

Estrogen Metabolism. The endogenous estrogens, estrone (E1) and 17β-estradiol (E2), are biochemically interconvertible via the actions of opposing 17β-HSD isozymes, one of which is alternatively referred to as estradiol dehydrogenase, that yield the same metabolic products (Fig. 25.5).[16-18] These hormones are metabolized mainly in the liver and largely excreted as water-soluble glucuronide and sulfate conjugates. Other tissues such as the kidneys and intestines are also involved.

Many metabolites have been isolated from urine, but to date, no one has been able to account for all the radioactivity of an administered dose of ^{14}C-labeled 17β-estradiol. The major metabolites are shown in Figure 25.4. Both 17β-estradiol and estrone are converted by CYP3A4 to yield estriol (estra-1,3,5[10]-triene-3,16α,17β-triol; E3). Estriol (Fig. 25.5) is found in the urine as the glucuronide conjugate. Estrogens are also oxidized by CYP3A4 at positions *ortho* to the 3-phenolic group to provide catechol estrogens, 2-hydroxyestrogens and 4-hydroxyestrogens. These metabolites are unstable in vivo, rapidly converted to 2-methoxyestrogen and 4-methoxyestrogen metabolites, and further to glucuronide, sulfate, and glutathione conjugates (Fig. 25.4). These compounds are also found in comparatively large amounts in the urine.[16-18] The catechol estrogens will bind to ERs and produce weak-to-moderate estrogenic effects. These catechol steroids have also been shown to be produced in certain central nervous system (CNS) tissues such as those in the pituitary and hypothalamus, suggesting possible neuroendocrine functions. The formation, metabolism, and biologic effects of catechol estrogens have been reviewed.[19]

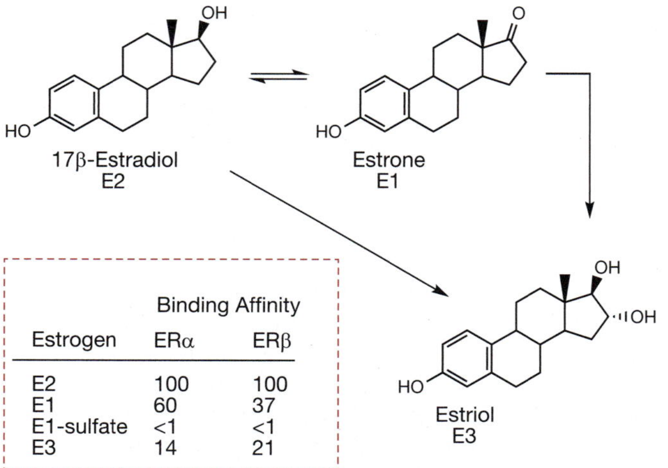

Estrogen	Binding Affinity ERα	ERβ
E2	100	100
E1	60	37
E1-sulfate	<1	<1
E3	14	21

Figure 25.5 Estrogens and their relative binding affinity to ERα and ERβ. Erα, estrogen receptor alpha; Erβ, estrogen receptor beta.

Progesterone Metabolism. Progesterone, the female sex hormone synthesized by the corpus luteum, is metabolized in part by routes similar to those for the adrenocorticoids. Progesterone is mainly excreted as conjugates of 5β-pregnane-3α,20-diol. Reduction of the 20-ketone to an alcohol, reduction of the 4,5-double bond resulting in 5β (ie, *cis*) ring fusion geometry, and reduction of the 3-ketone to the 3α-configuration characterize the production of 5β-pregnane-3α,20-diol from progesterone (Fig. 25.4). Minor pathways of metabolism in the liver can occur, with the side chain at position 17 removed and pathways similar to those for the metabolism of androgens observed.

Understanding Hormone Pharmacotherapy Based on the Hypothalamus-Pituitary-Gonadal Axis

The male and female reproductive cycle is regulated by the endocrine system and CNS via the hypothalamus-pituitary-gonadal (HPG) axis (Fig. 25.6). Gonadotropin-releasing hormone (GnRH), also known as luteinizing hormone–releasing hormone (LHRH), is a decapeptide that is synthesized in the hypothalamus, secreted, and acts on the GnRH receptor (GnRH-R) on the anterior pituitary gland. The anterior pituitary gland releases follicle-stimulating hormone (FSH) and LH, glycoproteins of approximately 29,000 molecular weight that are each made of an identical α-subunit (92 amino acids) with differences in the β-subunits that will bind, respectively, to their receptors (FSH or LH) on the testes/ovary (gonads). In the male, the role of FSH is to stimulate spermatogenesis in Sertoli cells of testes in addition to testes development, while the role of LH is to stimulate testosterone production from cholesterol in the Leydig cells. In the female, FSH stimulates the growth of follicles, while LH induces luteinization of the ruptured follicle leading to corpus luteum formation. In granulosa cells of the ovary, FSH can regulate expression of aromatase, which converts androgens into estrogens, while LH acts on the theca cells to stimulate the synthesis of androstenedione. The production and release of androgens and estrogens from the ovaries/testes allow these hormones to have tissue-specific effects by binding to their respective hormone receptors and resulting in the transcription and translation of proteins that can result in altered cell function. These hormones also exhibit negative feedback regulation, which allows for their precise control of hormone levels.

Knowledge of this axis and the role of hormonal negative feedback can be used to understand how various therapeutic agents work. Disorders of the HPG axis can arise due to increases or decreases in the concentrations of the sex steroids, known as hypergonadism or hypogonadism, respectively. Changes in concentrations of sex steroids or their effects can lead to infertility, precocious puberty, or delayed puberty. A woman's reproductive cycle can be modulated to prevent pregnancy by using estrogen and progestin agonists as oral or parenteral contraceptive agents. GnRH agonists can help treat central precocious puberty when given in a pulsatile manner, mimicking the normal decapeptide. GnRH or GnRH agonists given in a continuous manner can lead to high concentrations and

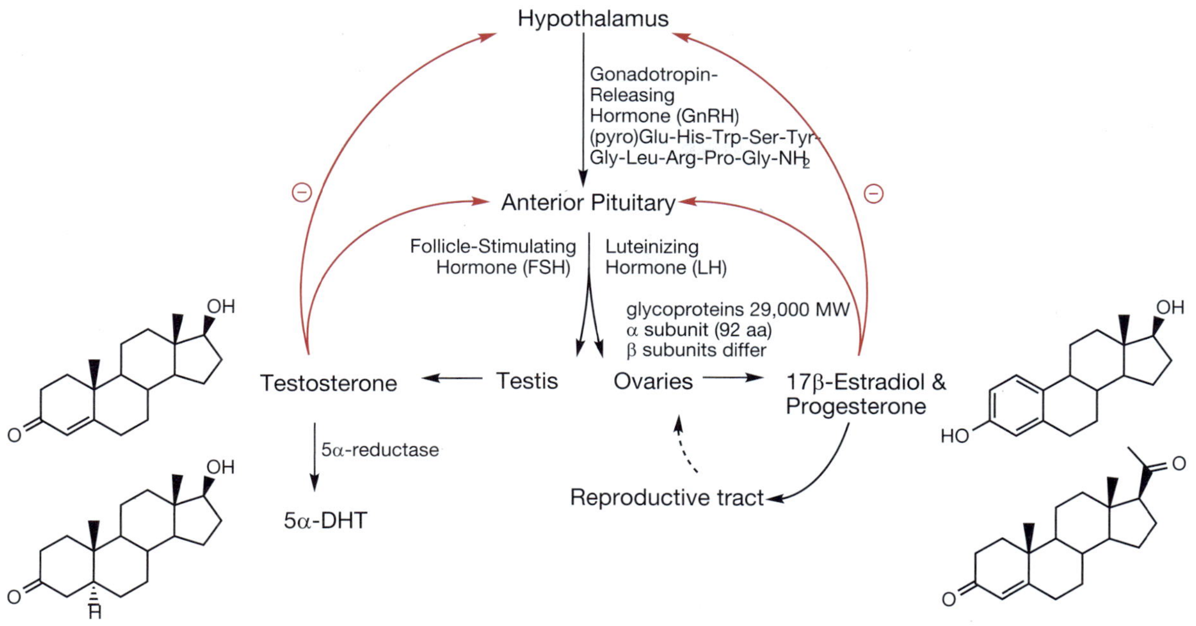

Figure 25.6 Negative feedback role on the hypothalamus-pituitary-testes/ovary axis and reproductive tract interrelationships.

downregulation of the GnRH-R, which decreases androgen and estrogen levels and thus can be used in the treatment of hormone-dependent prostate and breast cancers. GnRH antagonists given continuously also inhibit the HPG axis, block androgen synthesis for the treatment of prostate cancer, and block estrogen synthesis for the treatment of painful endometriosis. Exogenous supply of FSH and LH can allow an endocrinologist to control hormone production and ovarian function, resulting in hyperstimulation for egg retrieval for in vitro fertilization to address infertility problems. Tracking of the LH surge can be used by women in over-the-counter (OTC) ovulation kits to estimate the timing of ovulation to increase the chances of achieving pregnancy. Progesterone is known as the hormone of pregnancy, and progesterone antagonists can be used to terminate pregnancy. Higher concentrations of progestin antagonists can be used in emergency contraception when taken within 72 hours of unprotected intercourse to prevent pregnancy. During menopause, estrogen and progesterone levels fall, giving rise to menopausal side effects that can be alleviated by exogenous administration of agonists of these hormones. Inhibition of the conversion of testosterone to the more potent androgen DHT reduces the size of the prostate to decrease symptoms of BPH in the aging male. ER or AR antagonists can be useful in the treatment of hormone-dependent breast and prostate cancers, respectively.

This chapter primarily discusses hormonal pharmacotherapy approaches used to modulate a woman's fertility (contraceptive agents, infertility, emergency contraception), to improve quality of life in men and women's health (male hypogonadism, andropause, menopause, ED, BPH), and to treat hormone-dependent cancers (breast, prostate).

Drugs Used in Modulating Women's Fertility

Estrogens: Physiology, Actions, and Structure-Activity Relationships

Discovery of Estrogens

Allen and Doisy[20] showed in 1923 that an extract of ovaries can produce estrus. Soon thereafter, it was found that a good source of estrogen is in the urine of pregnant women. Estrone [3-hydroxyestra-1,3,5(10)-trien-17-one; E1] was the first crystalline estrogen to be isolated from a natural source. Two other C18 estrogen steroids, 17β-estradiol (E2) and estriol (E3), were later isolated and characterized to round out what are considered to be the three classic estrogens (Fig. 25.5).[21,22]

Estrogen Physiology

Female Sex Hormones and the Reproductive Cycle. The ovarian cycle, the preparation of endocrine tissues and release of oocytes, the menstrual cycle, and the preparation and maintenance of the uterine lining, occur concurrently and govern the female reproductive process.[23,24] During the follicular phase of the ovarian cycle, GnRH secreted by the hypothalamus stimulates the release of LH and FSH from the anterior pituitary, which, in turn, act on the ovaries to regulate the expression of sex hormones (mainly 17β-estradiol) and two protein complexes (activin and inhibin) that govern the reproductive cycle. As the name implies, FSH promotes the initial development of the immature Graafian follicle in the ovary. FSH cannot induce ovulation but must work in conjunction with LH. The combined effect is to promote follicle growth and increase secretion of 17β-estradiol.

Growing follicles begin to produce high levels of 17β-estradiol, which acts in concert with activin and inhibin in a negative feedback system to inhibit the production of FSH and stimulate the output of LH. The level of LH rises to a sharp peak at the midpoint, signaling the end of the follicular phase and causing rupture of the follicle and release of its mature oocyte (ovulation). In contrast, FSH reaches its highest level during menses, falls to a low level during and after ovulation, and then increases again toward the onset of menses.

Once ovulation has taken place, LH induces luteinization of the ruptured follicle, which leads to corpus luteum formation. After luteinization has been initiated, there is an increase in progesterone levels from the developing corpus luteum, which, in turn, suppresses the production of LH. Once the corpus luteum is complete, it begins to degenerate toward menses, and the levels of progesterone and 17β-estradiol decline. LH levels remain low during menses. The major events are summarized in Figure 25.7.

The endometrium, the mucous membrane lining of the uterus, transitions through different phases that depend on the steroid hormones secreted by the ovary. During the follicular phase, which lasts approximately 12 to 14 days, the endometrium undergoes proliferation owing to estrogenic stimulation. The luteal phase follows ovulation, lasts about 14 to 16 days, and ends at menses. During the luteal phase, the endometrium shows secretory activity needed for implantation of a fertilized ovum (if present), and cell proliferation declines.

In the absence of pregnancy, the levels of 17β-estradiol and progesterone decline; this leads to sloughing of the endometrium. This, together with the flow of interstitial blood through the vagina, is called menses and lasts for 4 to 6 days. Because the 17β-estradiol and progesterone levels are now low, the hypothalamus releases more GnRH, and the cycle begins again. The reproductive cycle in the female extends from the onset of menses to the next period of menses, with a regular interval varying from 20 to 35 days; the average length is 28 days.

If pregnancy occurs, the menstrual cycle is interrupted because of the release of a fourth gonadotropin. In human pregnancy, the gonadotropin produced by the placenta is referred to as human chorionic gonadotropin (hCG). hCG maintains and prolongs the life of the corpus luteum. The hCG level

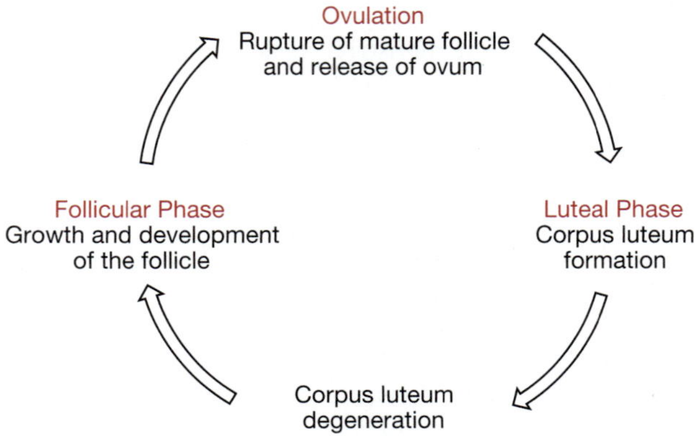

Figure 25.7 Ovarian cycle.

in the urine rises to the point where it can be detected after 14 days and reaches a maximum around week 7 of pregnancy. After this peak, the hCG concentration falls to a constant level, which is maintained throughout pregnancy.

The corpus luteum, because of hCG stimulation, provides an adequate level of steroidal hormones to maintain pregnancy during the first 9 weeks. After this period, the placenta can secrete the required level of estrogen and progestational hormones to maintain pregnancy. The levels of estrogen and progesterone increase during pregnancy and finally reach their maximal concentrations a few days before parturition (birth). Because the level of hCG in the urine rises rapidly after conception, it serves as the basis for many pregnancy tests.

Sexual maturation, or the period in which cyclic menstrual bleeding begins to occur, is reached between ages 10 and 17; the average age is 13. The period of irregular menstrual cycles (perimenopause) before the cessation of menses (menopause) usually occurs between ages 45 and 55.

Menopause. Menopause is defined as the cessation of the menstrual cycle due to the loss of ovarian function, which results in negligible levels of 17β-estradiol and progesterone. The average age of menopause is 51 years, and 90% of women are menopausal by age 55 years. By 2020, the U.S. population entering perimenopause (ages 45-54) and menopause (ages 55-64) was projected to be 20.6 and 22.1 million, respectively.[25] Perimenopause typically begins 3 to 5 years before menopause but can last up to 10 years. It is due to the sporadic failure of ovarian follicles (follicular atresia) and a decrease in estrogen levels, and without a corpus luteum, the progesterone levels also decrease. FSH levels are high during this time, and total androgens decrease. Unopposed estrogen and lack of progesterone cause endometrial buildup, resulting in heavier flow in early perimenopause. The length of the cycle is irregular, shorter or longer, and eventually with skipped periods.

Menopausal symptoms are due to negligible levels of 17β-estradiol as the ovaries are no longer functional. The predominant estrogen produced in this stage is estrone. It is produced in largest amounts in adipose tissue but also from muscle and the adrenal gland. In these tissues, androstenedione is converted to the weaker estrogen estrone by the action of aromatase. Due to the decline of estrogens, menopausal symptoms can be treated by exogenous administration of estrogen alone (for women without a uterus) or in combination with a progestin (for women with an intact uterus) to help improve quality of life, but recommendations depend on age in relationship to the onset of menopause. If the replacement dose of exogenous estrogen is too high, side effects such as nausea/vomiting, breast tenderness, weight gain, and vaginal bleeding will develop. Progesterone is known as the hormone of pregnancy in premenopausal women, but it and synthetic progestins can have negative effects (eg, fluid retention, breast tenderness) in menopause. However, unopposed estrogen usage in women with an intact uterus has been shown to cause endometrial hyperplasia and increase the risk of endometrial cancer. Thus, progestins protect the uterus and are included in hormone replacement therapy (HRT) when women have an intact uterus.

Mechanisms of Estrogen Action

Molecular Interactions. Steroidal estrogens were first isolated in the 1920s, but the presence of their cognate receptor was not reported until 1962.[26,27] The earliest searches for a biochemical mechanism of action of 17β-estradiol focused on the female reproductive tissues, since estrogens localize and produce dramatic and selective responses in these tissues. Using labeled 17β-estradiol, Jensen and Jacobson[27] showed that uptake of 17β-estradiol is rapid and that 17β-estradiol is retained to a high degree in the uterus and vagina.

The biochemical mechanism of estrogen action is the regulation of gene expression and subsequent induction of protein biosynthesis via specific, high-affinity ERs, as described in Chapter 7 (Nuclear Receptors).[28] ER subtype α (ERα) was successfully cloned in 1986 and was considered to be the sole ER until 1996 when a homologous but novel ER, ERβ, was cloned from a rat prostate.[29] This receptor demonstrated subnanomolar affinity for 17β-estradiol and offered a plausible explanation for the residual ER activity detected in existing ERα knockout mouse models.[30-32] Disparate tissue expression, combined with further development of ER knockout models, elucidated overlapping but distinct biologic roles for these sister receptors.[33-35] Receptor-binding sites for 17β-estradiol are located in the cytoplasm and nucleus of target cells[36-39] and exhibit both high affinity (K_D = 10^{-11}–10^{-10} M) and low capacity. Binding to the ERs is specific. The uptake of [2,4,6,7-^{3}H]-17β-estradiol by the receptors can be inhibited by pretreatment with unlabeled 17β-estradiol or diethylstilbestrol (DES; a nonsteroidal ER agonist). Pretreatment with testosterone, cortisol, or progesterone does not inhibit binding of radiolabeled 17β-estradiol. The binding is stereospecific because 17α-estradiol, which differs from 17β-estradiol in the configuration of the hydroxyl group at carbon 17, does not prevent the binding of 17β-estradiol to the ERs.[40]

The two ERs differ in size, with ERα having 595 amino acids and ERβ having 485 amino acids. 17β-Estradiol and other endogenous estrogens have similar affinities for both ERα and ERβ (Fig. 25.5, Table 25.1), whereas nonsteroidal estrogenic compounds and antiestrogens have differing affinities between ERα and ERβ.[41] Subtype selectivity is possible to attain via antiperiplanar substitution of the linking element between the hydroxyl groups.

As discussed in Chapter 7 for steroid hormone receptors, when 17β-estradiol binds to the ER, a conformational change of the 17β-estradiol receptor complex occurs and results in interactions of this complex with particular hormone-response element (HRE) regions of the cellular DNA, referred to as estrogen-response elements (EREs). Binding of the complex to ERE results in the initiation of transcription of the DNA sequence (activation of estrogen-dependent genes) to produce messenger RNA (mRNA). Finally, the elevated levels of mRNA lead to an increase in protein synthesis in the endoplasmic reticulum. Steroidal hormone receptors also repress certain genes, revealing a complex and tissue-dependent program of transcriptional control that is sensitive to regulation by cross talk with other signaling pathways. For example, levels of PRs increase in uterine tissue in response to ER-ERE binding, thus preparing the tissue for the actions of progesterone on the uterus during the later half of the reproductive cycle.[42,43]

Table 25.1 Relative Binding Affinities of Endogenous and Exogenous Estrogens

Estrogen	ERα-Binding Affinity	ERβ-Binding Affinity
17β-Estradiol (E2)	100	100
Estrone (E1)	60	37
Estrone sulfate	<1	<1
Estriol (E3)	14	21
4-Hydroxy-estradiol	13	7
2-Hydroxy-estradiol	7	11
Coumestrol	94	185
Genistein	5	36
Tamoxifen	7	6
4-Hydroxytamoxifen	178	339
Clomiphene	25	12
Diethylstilbestrol	468	295

ER, estrogen receptor.

Based on Kuiper GG, Carlsson B, Grandien K, et al. Comparison of the ligand binding specificity and transcript tissue distribution of estrogen receptors alpha and beta. *Endocrinology*. 1997;138:863-870.

In addition to the conventional ER actions mentioned earlier, a third ER was identified in 2005. This ER, a G protein coupled receptor, is localized in the cell membrane and is called GPR30.[44] GPR30 promotes rapid actions of estrogens and has been identified to be responsible for various rapid physiologic and pharmacologic actions of estrogens that are mediated through activation of signaling pathways. In addition to GPR30, ER is also activated by various post-translational mechanisms induced by growth factors and kinases. This rapid activation of GPR30 by ligands or ligand-independent activation of ER by post-translational mechanisms and growth factors is called nongenomic activation. This nongenomic or ligand-independent action of ER has been found to be common in the nuclear receptor family.

Although ERα and ERβ are synthesized by two different genes, the PR isoforms, PR-B and PR-A, are synthesized by the same gene as a result of alternate splicing. PR-A lacks the first 164 amino acids of PR-B, with the rest of the receptor being completely identical. Despite the sequence homology, PR-A and PR-B have distinct functions, with PR-A under several conditions functioning as a dominant suppressor of PR-B.

Physiologic Effects. Estrogens act on many tissues, such as those of the reproductive tract, breast, bone, and CNS. ERα is expressed at high levels in several normal tissues classically associated with estrogenic activity, including the uterus, ovary (theca cells), bone, and breast. ERα is also expressed at high levels in the prostate (stroma) and brain. ERβ is found at its highest levels in the normal colon, prostate (epithelium), ovary (granulosa cells), bone marrow, and brain, with smaller amounts reported in the uterus, bladder, lung, and testis.[45,46] ERα appears to mediate the ability of 17β-estradiol to provide negative (endocrine) feedback in the HPG axis in the brain and to slow bone resorption and maintain bone mineral density (BMD).

The primary physiologic action of estrogens is to stimulate the development of secondary sex characteristics, including growth of hair, softening of skin, growth of breasts, widening of the hips, and distribution of fat in the thighs, hips, and buttocks. Estrogens also stimulate the growth and development of the female reproductive tract, including the uterus, oviduct, cervix, and vagina. The proliferative changes that occur in the endometrium and myometrium upon administration of exogenous estrogens resemble those that take place naturally. Bleeding often follows withdrawal of the estrogens. The growth and development of tissues in the reproductive tract of animals, in terms of actual tissue weight gained, are not seen for as long as 16 hours after administration of the estrogen, although some biochemical processes in the cell are affected immediately. The growth response produced in the uterus by estrogens is temporary, and the maintenance of such growth requires the hormone to be available almost continuously. The initial growth induced by the estrogen is, therefore, of limited duration, and atrophy of the uterus occurs if the hormone is withdrawn.

Another physiologic effect of estrogens, observed within 1 hour of administration, is edema in the uterus. During this period, vasodilation of the uterine pre- and postcapillary arterioles occurs, and there is an increase in permeability to plasma proteins. These effects appear to occur predominantly in the endometrium and not to any great extent in the myometrium.[47] Correspondingly, endometriosis can result from prolonged exposure to estrogens or hormone imbalances among the sex hormones.

Another target of estrogens is breast tissue. Estrogens stimulate the proliferation of breast cells and promote the growth of hormone-dependent mammary carcinoma. Because breast cancer is the most common cancer among women, considerable research has been focused on understanding breast cancer and the factors that influence its development. 17β-Estradiol will stimulate gene expression and the production of several proteins in breast cancer cells via the ER mechanism. These proteins include both intracellular proteins important for breast cell function and growth and secreted proteins that can influence tumor growth and metastasis. Intracellular proteins include enzymes needed for DNA synthesis, such as DNA polymerase, thymidine kinase, thymidylate synthetase, and dihydrofolate reductase.[48,49] PRs are induced in breast cells by estrogens,[50] and the content of both ERs and PRs is utilized clinically as markers for hormone responsiveness of the breast cancer in determining hormonal therapy.[51]

Pharmacology, Side Effects, and Clinical Applications

Estrogens are used in a wide variety of menstrual disturbances, such as amenorrhea, dysmenorrhea, and oligomenorrhea. They are also effective in failure of ovarian development, acne, and senile vaginitis. For example, a nonsteroidal estrogen is now used in dyspareunia (painful sexual intercourse), as is discussed later. After childbirth, estrogens have been used to suppress lactation. One of the most widespread uses of estrogens is in birth control. HRT and selective estrogen receptor modulators (SERMs) have been used in osteoporosis because it is thought that an estrogen deficiency in postmenopause can lead to this serious disorder of the bone. One of the primary therapeutic uses is in the treatment of menopausal symptoms, such as hot flashes, chilly sensations, dizziness, fatigue, irritability, and sweating. For many women, menopause does not cause much discomfort; in some, however, both physical and mental discomfort may occur and can usually be prevented through estrogen therapy. Because of feminizing effects, estrogen therapy in males is limited.

Nausea appears to be the main side effect of estrogen therapy; other adverse effects include vomiting, anorexia, and diarrhea. If small doses are used to initiate therapy, and the dose is gradually increased, most of the side effects can be avoided. Excessive doses of estrogens inhibit the development of bones in young patients by accelerating epiphyseal closure.

When estrogens are given in large doses over long periods of time, they can inhibit ovulation because of their feedback action; inhibition of the release of FSH from the anterior pituitary results in inhibition of ovulation. Administration of these drugs may promote sodium chloride retention; the result is retention of water and subsequent edema. This effect, however, is less pronounced than with glucocorticoids. More detailed information on the pharmacology and toxicology of estrogens can be found in published reviews.[52-55]

Clomiphene for Infertility. Clomiphene citrate (first approved in 1967) is an effective first-line treatment used to induce ovulation in anovulatory women. Clomiphene is a nonsteroidal antiestrogenic triphenylethylene derivative like tamoxifen (discussed later). It is administered as a mixture of stereoisomers in approximately a 3:2 ratio of the *trans*-clomiphene (enclomiphene) and *cis*-clomiphene (zuclomiphene) enantiomers, each with unique pharmacology. The more potent *trans*-isomer is responsible for the ovulation-inducing actions.

In the early follicular phase, plasma estrogen serves as a negative feedback inhibitor to the hypothalamus and anterior pituitary. Clomiphene (oral, 50 mg) is taken by women for 5 days starting on the second to fifth day after the onset of menses. Most (52%) women ovulate in response to 50 mg treatment of clomiphene; however, a titration may be necessary to determine the lowest effective dose for an individual woman, as doses can range daily from 50 to 250 mg.[56] Higher doses may be necessary in women with greater body mass indexes (BMIs). By binding to and antagonizing the ER, clomiphene prevents 17β-estradiol from exerting its negative feedback in the hypothalamus. Compensatory mechanisms by the hypothalamus result in increased pulsatile secretions of GnRH secretions and increases of LH and FSH secretion from the pituitary, which, in turn, increase ovarian follicular activity.[56] The LH surge occurs 5 to 12 days after the last dose of clomiphene.

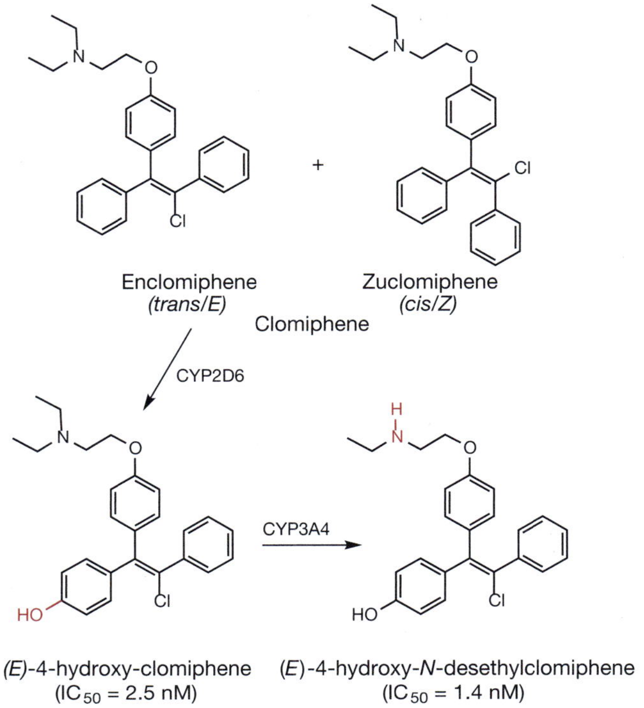

Major metabolites are the *trans* (*E*) metabolites shown above
100× more potent at ER

Clomiphene has been shown to exhibit both estrogen agonist and antagonist properties.[57] In humans, it is usually considered to be an antiestrogen (competitive ER antagonist), and in rats and other species, it is considered to be a mixed agonist/antagonist.[57] The estrogenic properties of clomiphene are generally seen only when endogenous estrogen levels are extremely low. By using a cell-based transcription assay, clomiphene has been shown to act as an agonist or antagonist via ERα depending on 17β-estradiol concentration. Serum concentrations of clomiphene in women taking a therapeutic dose are reported to be 10^{-9} to 10^{-7} M. Clomiphene acted as a complete antagonist (at 10^{-8} M) of ERα in the presence of lower concentrations of 17β-estradiol (10^{-12} M), but not at higher concentrations (10^{-10} M).[58] Clomiphene exhibits a more pronounced antagonist effect at ERβ, as it eliminated the estrogenic activity of 17β-estradiol even at the higher concentrations of 10^{-10} M.

Clomiphene is readily absorbed, reaches peak concentrations in ~6 hours, is metabolized predominately by liver via CYP2D6 and CYP3A4,[59] undergoes enterohepatic recycling, and is eliminated in feces (42%) and urine (8%). It has a half-life of approximately 5 days. Enclomiphene is metabolically activated to (*E*)-4-hydroxylated metabolites produced via CYP2D6 followed by CYP3A4 to afford (*E*)-4-hydroxy-clomiphene and (*E*)-4-hydroxy-*N*-desethylclomiphene (*trans* metabolites). The *trans* metabolites are the major active metabolites of clomiphene and are at least 100 times more potent at the ER than their parent compound. The median inhibitory concentration (IC_{50}) values for inhibition of 17β-estradiol for ER were reported as 2.5 nM for (*E*)-4-hydroxy-clomiphene and 1.4 nM for (*E*)-4-hydroxy-*N*-desethylclomiphene.[60] These results demonstrate that clomiphene is a prodrug with similar metabolic pathways as tamoxifen and toremifene (TOR) (discussed later).

The most common side effects of treatment with clomiphene are ovarian enlargement (14%), hot flashes (10%), bloating (≤6%), and visual disturbances (2%, reversible upon discontinuation).[61,62] Relatively common with clomiphene usage is the 8% increased risk of multiple gestation for anovulatory women due to the development of multiple follicles. Although rare, women should be cautioned about ovarian hyperstimulation syndrome that may begin within 24 hours of treatment but may be most severe 7 to 10 days after therapy.

A woman who does not conceive after three to four successful clomiphene-induced ovulation cycles should be further evaluated for other infertility causes, especially if older than age 35. Clomiphene can be given in combination with metformin, glucocorticoids, and exogenous gonadotropins when clomiphene-only treatment proves unsuccessful for ovulation.

Structure-Activity Relationships

Analyses of the biologic activities of both steroidal and nonsteroidal estrogens, in vitro investigations with subcellular fractions containing ERs, and x-ray crystallography studies on the ligand-binding domain (LBD) of the ERs have resulted in an extensive knowledge of the SARs for estrogens.[54,63-65] These studies demonstrated the high affinity and specificity of the most potent endogenous estrogen, 17β-estradiol. There are two polar interactions between 17β-estradiol and ERs, which are essential for all estrogens to bind ERα or ERβ: (1) The phenoxy substituent at C3 (or other hydrogen bond donor if nonsteroidal) of the steroid nucleus (or other hydrophobic, often rigid and/or planar linking element) interacts with ER amino acids Glu353, Arg394, and a conserved/structural water molecule, and (2) the 17β-hydroxyl (or other hydrogen bond acceptor) interacts with His524 (see Fig. 25.8). Importantly, the distance between the two polar groups of the estrogen ligand must be approximately the same as 17β-estradiol and connected by an often rigid and/or planar hydrophobic connecting group, as illustrated with *trans*-DES.

For optimal estrogenic activity, the distance between the oxygen atoms of the two hydroxyl groups is in the range of 10.3 to 12.1 Å. The region of the ER that binds the cyclopentano D ring is flexible and can conform to ligands with different distances (eg, 10.3 Å for 17β-estradiol and 12.1 Å for DES). Many other potent steroidal and nonsteroidal estrogens conform to the described requirements, but there seem to be few restrictions on the types of linking groups that can be employed. Further, these requirements apply to both ER subtypes as the illustrated amino acids are the same. However, ERβ selectivity can be attained by antiperiplanar substitution of the linking element that would extend toward amino acids that vary between ERα and ERβ.[41] Although many preclinical ERβ agonists exist, none have been U.S. Food and Drug Administration (FDA) approved.

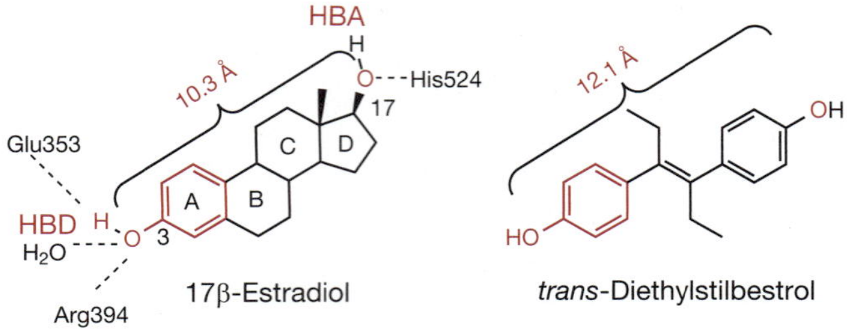

Pharmacophore
1. Phenol bioisostere
2. Flat, hydrophobic spacer
3. HBA

	Binding Affinity	
Estrogen	ERα	ERβ
E2	100	100
DES	468	295

Figure 25.8 Estrogen pharmacophore with important binding interactions to the estrogen receptor (ER) are shown. The C3-phenol of 17β-estradiol interacts with the shown amino acids and structural water molecule and acts as both a hydrogen bond donor (HBD) and a hydrogen bond acceptor (HBA), and the 17β-OH acts as an HBA from the amino acid shown. The amino acid numbering shown reflects binding to ERα. Relative binding affinity to ERα and ERβ are given. DES, diethylstilbestrol; ERα, estrogen receptor alpha; ERβ, estrogen receptor beta.

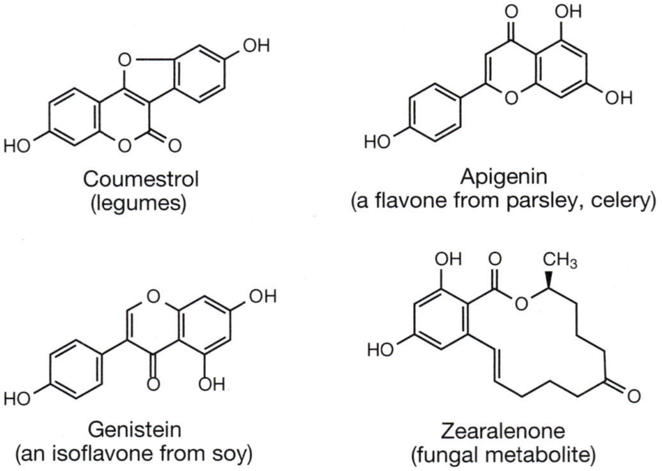

	Binding Affinity	
Estrogen	ERα	ERβ
E2	100	100
Coumestrol	94	185
Genistein	5	36

Figure 25.9 Xenoestrogens and their relative binding affinity to ERα and ERβ. ERα, estrogen receptor alpha; ERβ, estrogen receptor beta.

Substituents on the estrogen steroidal nucleus significantly modify estrogenic activity. On the aromatic A ring, any functionality at the C1 position greatly reduces activity, and only small groups can be accommodated at the 2 and 4 positions. Insertion of hydroxyl groups at positions 6, 7, and 11 reduces activity. Removal of the oxygen function from position 3 or 17 or epimerization of the 17-hydroxyl group of estradiol to the α-configuration results in a less active estrogenic substance.[66] Introduction of unsaturation into the adjacent cyclohexane B ring similarly reduces potency. Substituents at the 11β-position can be well tolerated; for example, 11β-methoxy or 11β-ethyl has significantly greater affinity for ER compared to 17β-estradiol. Modifications at the 17α and 16 positions can lead to enhanced activity. Ethinyl or vinyl groups provide the greatest activity, while highly polar groups are poorly tolerated. At the 16 position, moderate size and polarity are tolerated.

Many compounds of natural origin have estrogenic activity including nonsteroidal xenobiotics consumed as food by humans and livestock (Fig. 25.9).[67] Naturally occurring estrogens are found in a number of plants, such as legumes (coumestrol), parsley/celery (apigenin), soy (genistein), or corn/oats (zearalenone).[68] Since these are natural products, they are sold over the counter in products, such as Estroven that contains soy isoflavones. Generally, phytoestrogens are weak nonselective estrogens believed to provide some relief for postmenopausal women, but there is controversy about their safety and efficacy relative to HRTs using purified and potent estrogens. Although not well studied, it is advisable for those with a history of breast cancer to avoid large amounts of phytoestrogens in foods and supplements.

Steroidal Estrogens

Endogenous Estrogens and Their Analogs

17β-Estradiol is the most potent endogenous estrogen, exhibiting high affinity for the ER and high potency when administered parenterally. The naturally occurring estrogens are only weakly active when administered orally, as they are thought to be rapidly absorbed from the intestine but can be degraded by microorganisms in the gastrointestinal (GI) tract.[69] The endogenous estrogens are promptly metabolized by the liver to a great extent, resulting in the observed low therapeutic effectiveness when administered orally. Comparative ER potencies for endogenous estrogens (17β-estradiol, estrone, and estriol) are shown in Figure 25.5. The observed in vivo biologic activity varies with the mode of administration of the estrogens. The order of activity of the three naturally occurring steroids when administered subcutaneously (SC) is 17β-estradiol > estrone > estriol. The order changes to estriol >17β-estradiol > estrone when the drugs are administered orally.[70] Also, metabolic conjugation (phase II metabolism) may produce estrogens that retain some of their activity; it has been reported that estrone sulfate (used as the piperazine salt estropipate; Fig. 25.10) is actually more active than the original hormone when administered orally to rats. The modified drug also retains some activity in humans but is considered a prodrug that will undergo cleavage to estrone.[71,72]

Owing to limited oral bioavailability, 17β-estradiol is administered via once- or twice-weekly transdermal patches (eg, Minivelle, Vivelle-Dot, Menostar, and Climara), gels (eg, Divigel, Estrogel, Elestrin), creams (eg, Estrace), vaginal inserts (eg, Imvexxy, Estring), and a spray (eg, Evamist) for the prevention of postmenopausal osteoporosis, treatment

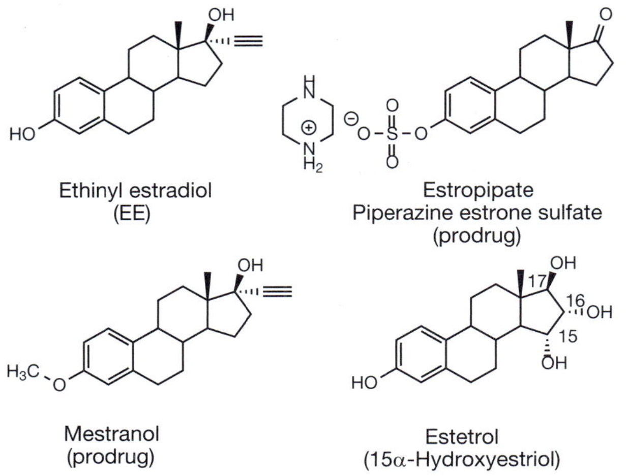

Figure 25.10 Orally active steroidal estrogens.

of moderate-to-severe vasomotor symptoms associated with menopause (eg, hot flashes), and treatment of moderate-to-severe symptoms of vulvar and vaginal atrophy associated with menopause. Transdermal patches are preferably placed on the lower abdomen or buttocks but should not be applied to the breast. Systemic levels of 17β-estradiol concentrations vary by product and the route of administration and remain generally low (ranging from ~10 to 100 pg/mL) because of the rapid hepatic metabolism of the hormone once it enters the circulatory system.[73,74]

Chemical modifications have led to better orally effective estrogens. One successful method of overcoming the rapid inactivation of 17β-estradiol by the liver has been to stabilize the alcoholic function at C17β with an appropriate substituent. Ethinyl estradiol (EE) [17α-ethynyl-1,3,5(10)-estratriene-3,17β-diol] (Fig. 25.10) is an estrogenic substance that is very potent when taken orally.[75] EE was synthesized in 1939, is a highly effective oral estrogen due to improved hepatic and intestinal pharmacokinetics, and is the predominantly used estrogen in oral contraceptives. Mestranol, a 3-methoxy ether and orally active prodrug of EE, is also found in some oral contraceptives.[76] EE or mestranol combined with synthetic progestins produces a synergistic suppression of the hypothalamus and pituitary production of FSH and LH, preventing follicular development, ovulation, and implantation.

EE and mestranol are rapidly and nearly completely absorbed in the stomach. Peak serum concentration (C_{max}) values of EE and mestranol are achieved in 1 and 4 hours, respectively. In both cases, EE accumulates in the endometrium and ovary compared to plasma. EE is also found in fat and bound to plasma proteins that produce a large volume of distribution. EE is largely converted to various glucuronide and sulfate conjugates of its ethynylated (2-methoxy, unchanged, 16β-hydroxy, 2-hydroxy, and 6α-hydroxy) and de-ethynylated (estrone [E1], 17β-estradiol [E2], estriol [E3], and 2-methoxy) metabolites.[77] Thirty-nine percent of radioactivity of EE appears in urine and 53% in feces over a 7- to 10-day period.[77] The high fecal radioactivity is largely due to the biliary excretion of sulfate and glucuronide metabolites. Enterohepatic recycling occurs as the biliary metabolites are excreted into the intestines, hydrolyzed by microorganisms back to EE, and then reabsorbed and returned to the

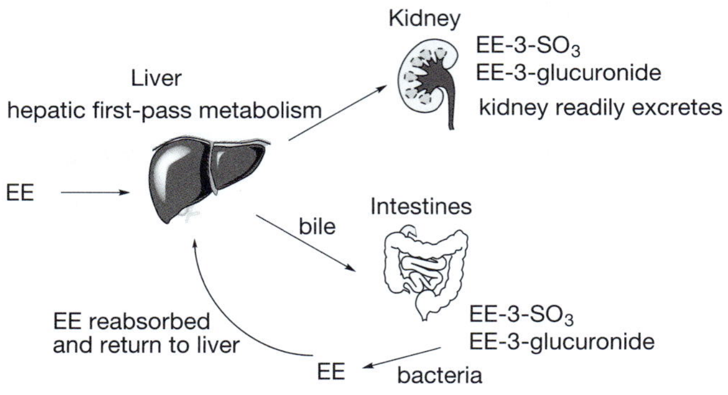

Figure 25.11 Enterohepatic recycling of estrogens using ethinyl estradiol (EE) as an exemplary estrogen.

liver (Fig. 25.11). The oral activity of EE results because it is much less susceptible than 17β-estradiol to hepatic first-pass metabolism and microbial degradation.

Estetrol is a naturally occurring estrogen, identified as 15α-hydroxyestriol, synthesized in both male and female fetal liver tissue during human pregnancy. The hormone is present in maternal urine within 9 weeks of pregnancy, entering the circulation through the placenta. The levels of conjugated and unconjugated estetrol are reported to be much higher in fetal plasma and amniotic fluid than in the mother's plasma. Early studies with estetrol indicated weak estrogenic activity suggesting minimal pharmacologic value. Recently, estetrol combined with the synthetic progestin drospirenone (Nextstellis, discussed later) has been approved as an oral contraceptive. Estetrol is chemically quite stable in vitro, and it exhibits high water solubility in comparison with 17β-estradiol; its octanol/water partition coefficient of 1.5 makes it approximately 100 times less lipophilic than 17β-estradiol. Estetrol has high selectivity for the ER with minimal binding to nearly all other tested human receptors.

Estetrol undergoes minimal metabolism, resulting in a long half-life in vivo. The drug has not been shown to be converted to other estrogenic agents, but rather the major routes of metabolism consist of phase II glucuronidation and sulfation via UGT2B7 (16-glucuronide). Estetrol is primarily excreted unchanged via the urine (69%) and feces (~22%). The reported half-life for estetrol is 27 hours.[78]

Ester derivatives (ie, 17β-valerate and 17β-cypionate) of the naturally occurring and synthetic estrogens have been used to prolong estrogenic action (Fig. 25.12). In contrast to the 17α-ethinyl derivatives that are administered orally, the 17β-ester derivatives of estrogens are given intramuscularly (IM) in an oil vehicle that may produce durable estrogenic effects for up to 4 weeks as the ester is slowly hydrolyzed in vivo at the site of injection to release the free hormone. The 17β-valerate (Delestrogen) and 17β-cyclopentylpropionate (cypionate, Depo-Estradiol) esters of 17β-estradiol are the most commonly used products. The 17β-valerate is also used in combination with the progestin dienogest as an oral contraceptive (Natazia).

A 3-acetate ester of E2 (Fig. 25.12) is available for therapeutic use as a cured silicone elastomer vaginal ring (eg, Femring) that is inserted into the vagina for the treatment of moderate-to-severe vasomotor symptoms or vulvar and vaginal atrophy due to menopause. The exact position of

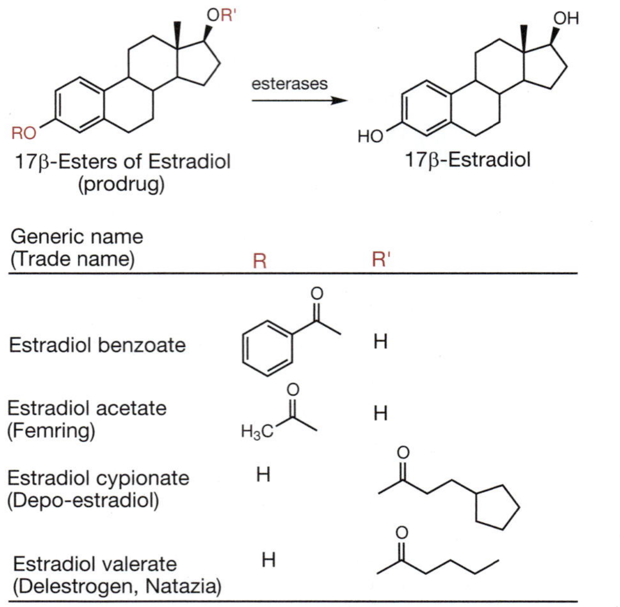

Figure 25.12 Esterified synthetic estrogens used for long-term estrogen therapy.

the ring is not critical to its function. The elastomeric ring surrounds a central core designed to release 0.10 mg of 17β-estradiol per day for 3 months until removal. A 3-benzoate ester of 17β-estradiol is no longer used therapeutically.

Equine Estrogens

Conjugated, water-soluble forms of naturally occurring estrogens obtained from the urine of pregnant mares, such as Premarin (oral or cream) and Menest (oral), are utilized therapeutically, mainly to treat postmenopausal symptoms. Horses produce two unique estrogenic compounds, equilin [3-hydroxyestra-1,3,5(10),7-tetraene-17-one] and equilenin [estra-1,3,5(10),6,8-pentaen-3-ol-17-one], and secrete them in the urine as sodium sulfate conjugates (Fig. 25.13). Estrone and other estrogen metabolites are secreted into the urine as well. Premarin contains six estrogen metabolites as active ingredients, including ~50% to 65% sodium estrone sulfate,

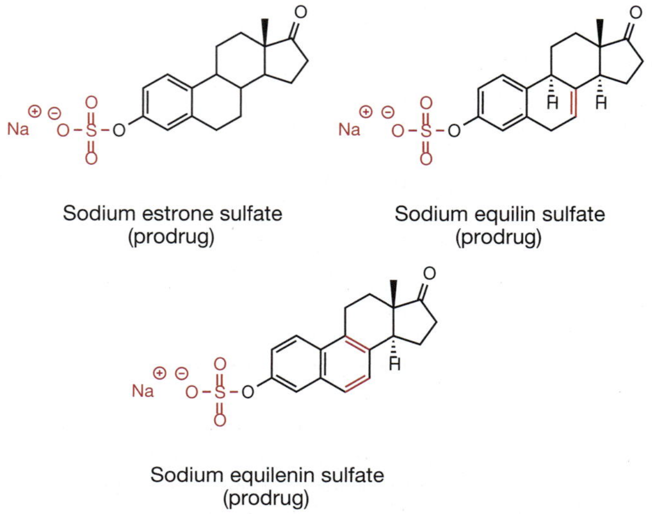

Figure 25.13 Conjugated estrogens.

~20% to 35% sodium equilin sulfate, and four other conjugated estrogens in lesser amounts. Menest is composed of not less than 90% of two conjugated estrogens derived synthetically, sodium estrone sulfate (75%-85%) and sodium equilin sulfate (6%-15%), in addition to 17α-estradiol.[79] Another sulfate conjugate that is orally effective is estropipate (ie, piperazine salt of estrone sulfate; Fig. 25.10). This derivative has the same actions and uses as the conjugated naturally occurring estrogens. In an in vivo assay comparing the induction of estrogen-dependent genes following oral administration to postmenopausal women, EE is about 100 times more potent than conjugated estrogen preparations, 500 times more potent than 17β-estradiol and estrone sulfate, and 650 times more potent than 17β-estradiol valerate when administered orally.[80]

NONSTEROIDAL ESTROGEN: DIETHYLSTILBESTROL

The scarcity of natural estrogen hormones led chemists to prepare synthetic materials that could be used as substitutes. *trans*-DES (see Fig. 25.8) was first prepared in 1939 and was approved by the FDA in 1941 to treat menopausal symptoms. *trans*-DES has 10 times the estrogenic potency of the *cis*-isomer because it resembles more closely the natural estrogen, 17β-estradiol.[81] Although many stilbene derivatives have been prepared since, the *trans*-isomer of DES remains one of the most active nonsteroidal estrogens known.[82,83]

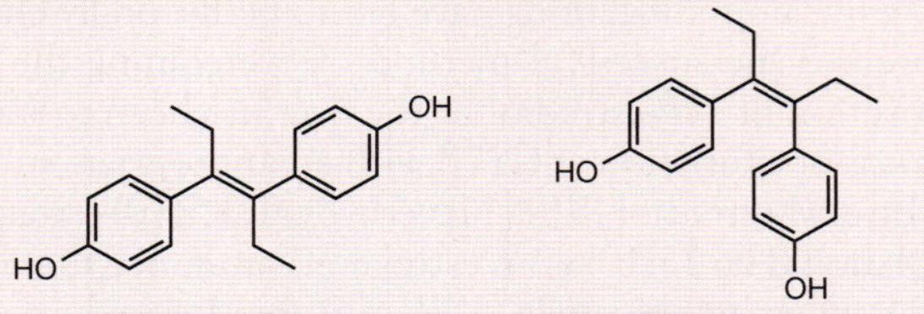

trans-Diethylstilbestrol *cis*-Diethylstilbestrol

The therapeutic use of DES expanded greatly through the 1960s, being prescribed to prevent miscarriage, premature labor, and related complications of pregnancy. In 1971, a landmark study linking clear cell adenocarcinoma, a type of cancer of the cervix and vagina, in women exposed to DES prior to birth led FDA to urge doctors to stop prescribing the drug to pregnant women. Surprisingly, the FDA did not ban or discontinue DES at that time. Although its use dropped precipitously, an estimated 5 to 10 million pregnant women and children born of these pregnancies had already been exposed to DES and similar drugs between 1941 and 1971.[84,85] The consequences of this prenatal exposure were widespread as the daughters of women who used DES during pregnancy, commonly called DES daughters, have ~40 times the risk of developing clear cell adenocarcinoma, and ~1 in every 1,000 actually developed the disease. DES daughters also appeared to have a higher incidence of breast cancer, fertility problems, and early menopause.[86,87] There appeared to be few if any effects on the sons of women who used DES during pregnancy. DES, along with the thalidomide tragedy in Europe, remains a somber reminder of the importance and need for harmonized global regulations regarding studies required to characterize the safety and efficacy of new drugs.

Progestins

Discovery of Progestins

Once ovulation has taken place, the tissue remaining from the ruptured follicle forms the corpus luteum, which has the important function of preparing for and maintaining pregnancy if it occurs. Fraenkel[88] first observed in 1903 that removal of the corpus luteum shortly after conception results in termination of the pregnancy. In 1914, Pearl and Surface[89] showed that the corpus luteum can prevent ovulation in animals. In 1929, Corner and Allen[90] developed a method of assay for progestational activity. By 1934, the progestational hormone progesterone (Fig. 25.14) had been isolated by several research groups, and by 1937, it had been shown that pure progesterone alone can maintain pregnancy in animals.[70,91]

The most abundant pregnane steroid found in the urine during pregnancy is 5β-pregnane-3α,20-diol (Fig. 25.14), present as its glucuronide conjugate, which is also the main excretory product of exogenous progesterone. Note the *cis* A/B ring junction makes this metabolite devoid of progestational activity.[92] This conjugated substance can serve as an index of the corpus luteum and placental activity, and a premature drop in its level in the urine may be a warning of possible miscarriage.

Synthetic Progestins

The five structural classes of synthetic progestins are shown in Figure 25.15 and include derivatives of (1) progesterone (pregnane), (2) 17α-hydroxyprogesterone (pregnane), (3) testosterone (androstane), (4) 19-nortestosterone (estrane), and (5) gonane and miscellaneous agents.

Pregnanes (Classes 1 and 2). Progesterone (class 1), an important hormone for maintaining pregnancy and normal menstrual bleeding, is used to treat disorders in these areas. Owing to its ability to prevent ovulation during pregnancy and thicken the cervical mucus (thus acting as a sperm barrier), it is considered a natural contraceptive.[93] Early efforts focused on identifying a good source of progesterone. Synthetic procedures were devised for the production of progesterone from naturally occurring steroids, including diosgenin, ergosterol, and bile acids. The natural hormone, however, has many drawbacks, including a relatively low activity when

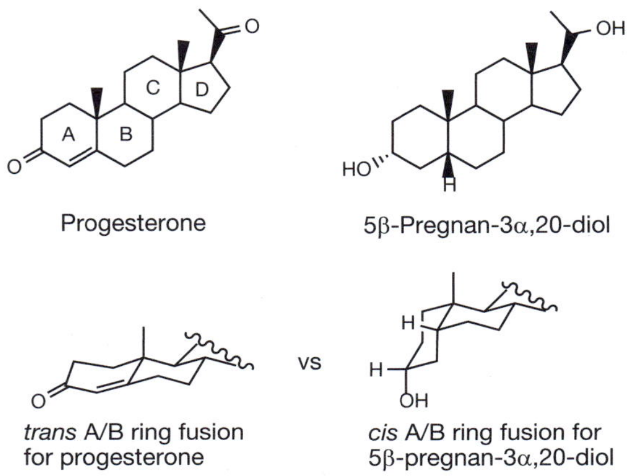

Figure 25.14 The conformation of progesterone and its predominant metabolite.

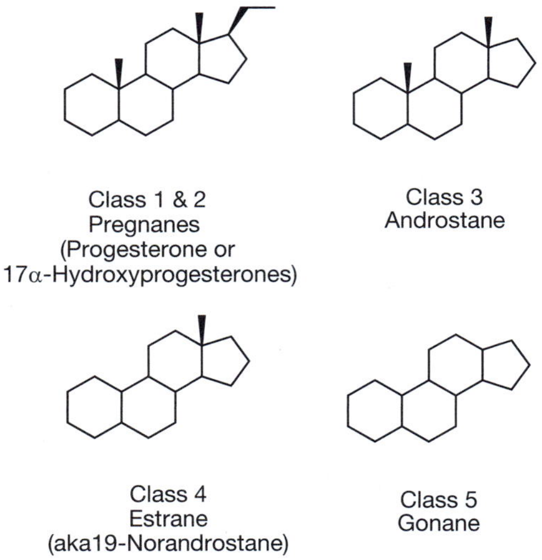

Figure 25.15 Steroidal ring systems present in the five structural classes of synthetic progestins.

orally administered due to poor absorption and almost complete first-pass metabolism in the liver. Progesterone is available today as capsules (Prometrium), vaginal gels (Crinone), vaginal suppositories (Endometrin), creams for transdermal delivery (9EC-RX Progesterone), and an IM injection in oil (various suppliers) for the treatment of secondary amenorrhea and the prevention of endometrial hyperplasia in postmenopausal women who are also taking conjugated estrogens. Adding progesterone to conjugated estrogen therapy has been shown to reduce the risk of endometrial cancer in women using unopposed estrogens.[94] Progesterone is predominantly administered parenterally for therapeutic effects, and even the injection must be repeatedly administered over relatively short periods for best results.

A variety of orally active, 17α-acyl derivatives of progesterone that maintain the 3-keto-4-ene and the 20-keto pharmacophoric elements were developed (Fig. 25.16). Although many of the early structural modifications of progesterone led to weakly active or inactive progestational agents, it was eventually shown that derivatives of 17α-hydroxyprogesterone (class 2) such as 17α-acetoxyprogesterone had some activity when administered orally, even though the parent compound, 17α-hydroxyprogesterone, was inactive.[95] A second derivative of 17α-hydroxyprogesterone, the 17α-caproate ester (Fig. 25.16), was available for therapeutic use via IM or SC injection (Makena) to reduce the risk of preterm birth in women[96] who had a history of spontaneous preterm birth, but FDA withdrew approval in 2023 for lack of efficacy. The 17α-acyl analogs are not prodrugs of progesterone but, rather, slow the metabolism of the 20-one to increase their duration of action compared to progesterone.

Further structural modifications of 17α-acetoxyprogesterone enhanced its oral contraceptive action. In most instances, these modifications are carried out at the C_6 position. Substituents in this position hinder metabolism of the unsaturated A ring and increase lipid solubility, resulting in an enhanced biologic effect.[97] Among the first of these interesting analogs of 17α-acetoxyprogesterone to be used in progestational therapy was medroxyprogesterone acetate

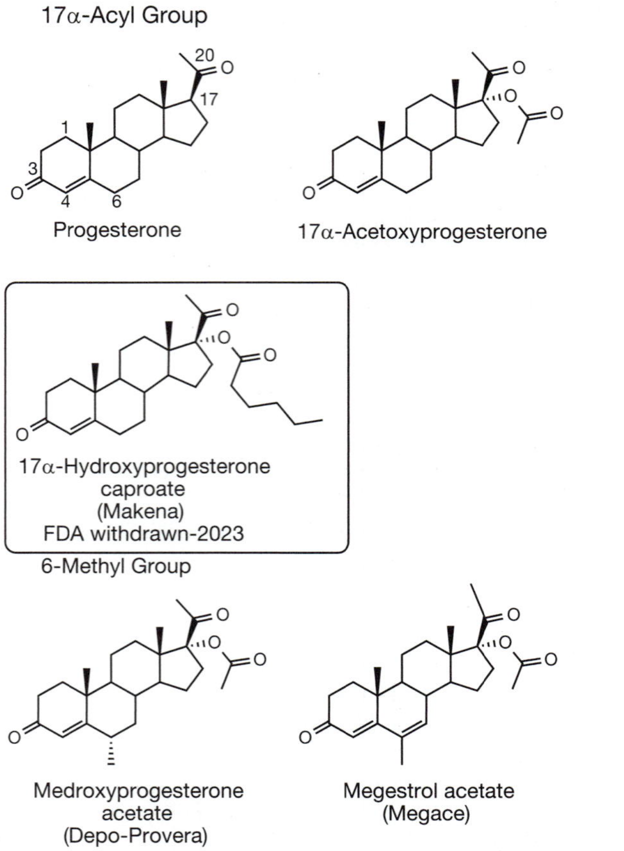

Figure 25.16 Progestins based upon the pregnane nucleus (class 2), which are 17α-acyl derivatives. FDA, Food and Drug Administration.

(MPA; 6α-methyl-17β-hydroxy-4-pregnene-3,20-dione 17-acetate) (Fig. 25.16), the active pharmaceutical ingredient in Depo-Provera (SC or IM injection) and Provera (oral tablets).[98] MPA binds the PR with a similar affinity to progesterone.[99]

Progestational activity is further enhanced in 6-substituted 17α-acetoxyprogesterones when a double bond is introduced between positions 6 and 7. Megestrol acetate (6-methyl-17α-hydroxy-4,6-pregnadiene-3,20-dione 17-acetate; Megace) is a typical example of a clinically useful progestin.

Androstanes (Class 3). The first synthetic progestin to be used to any extent was synthesized from male sex hormones (androstanes). Ethisterone (17α-ethynyl-17β-hydroxyandrost-4-en-3-one; prepared in 1937), which is 17α-ethinyl testosterone, proved to be an effective oral progestin and weak androgen and became useful in the treatment of menstrual dysfunction (Fig. 25.17).[100,101] Recall that the unsaturated 17α-ethinyl group also enhanced the activity of the female sex steroid 17β-estradiol. 17α-Methyltestosterone also demonstrates some weak progestin activity. Similar to what was seen for the estrogens, 17α-substituents block metabolism to the 17-one, thereby allowing oral activity. Several molecular modifications of ethisterone led to enhanced progestational activity. For example, introduction of a methyl group in the 6α-position, as in dimethisterone, provided an active analog (Fig. 25.17).[22] Ethisterone, therefore, paved the way for the synthesis of other progestins that did not have a typical progesterone-type C17β side chain.

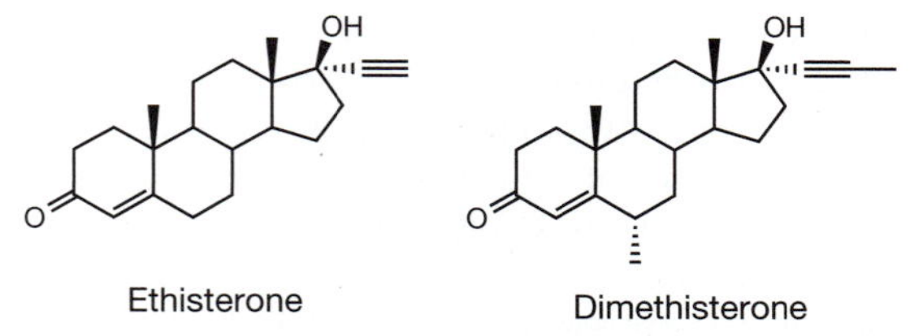

Figure 25.17 Progestins based upon the androstane nucleus (class 3), which are 17α-substituted testosterone derivatives.

19-Norandrostanes or Estranes (Class 4). A second breakthrough was made in 1944 when Ehrenstein[102] discovered that the C19 methyl group on steroids is not necessary for progestational activity. In fact, his work showed that loss of the C19 methyl (from a compound he thought was progesterone) produced 19-nor-14β,17α-pregn-4-ene-3,20-dione, an estrane with activity equal to or greater than that of parenterally administered progesterone.

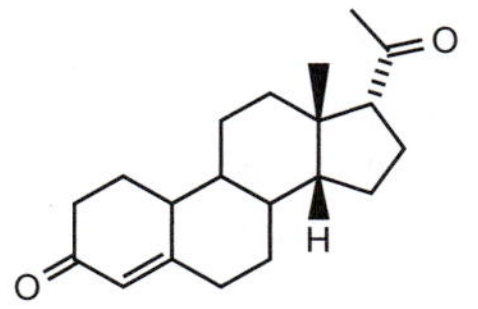

19-Nor-14β,17α-preg-4-ene-3,20-dione

This work led to intensive attempts to prepare orally active progestins that were devoid of estrogenic and androgenic activities. In 1953, 19-norprogesterone was synthesized[103] and differed from the natural hormone only in replacement of the C19 angular methyl group by hydrogen (not shown). This analog was 8 times as active as progesterone when administered parenterally to rabbits and was the most potent progestin known. The addition of the 17α-ethinyl group to the 19-norsteroids (ie, estranes) resulted in two potent and orally active progestins, namely, norethindrone (17α-ethynyl-17β-hydroxyestr-4-en-3-one) and norethynodrel [17α-ethynyl-17β-hydroxyestr-5(10)-en-3-one] (Fig. 25.18).[24] The progestational activity of norethynodrel is about one-tenth that of norethindrone, and both compounds appear to have weak estrogenic activity. These two substances were among the first 19-norsteroids (19-nor is synonymous with missing 19-methyl) to be used clinically for progestin-related hormonal disorders. Importantly, they also afforded a method, when used with estrogens such as mestranol, for control of conception and ultimately led to the development and widespread introduction of oral contraceptives. The first oral contraceptive, Enovid, was a combination of mestranol and norethynodrel and was introduced in 1960.

The usefulness of norethynodrel and norethindrone for therapy of irregular menses and as oral contraceptive agents provided the impetus to continue research in the area of 19-norsteroids. Another 19-norsteroid reported to be effective and exhibit few side effects is ethynodiol diacetate (17α-ethynylestr-4-ene-3,17β-diol-3,17-diacetate) (Fig. 25.18). This drug has been used as an oral progestin.[104]

Since the discovery of the first generation of 19-nortestosterone derivatives (estranes), referred to as class 4 herein, multiple new generations of norsteroids have been

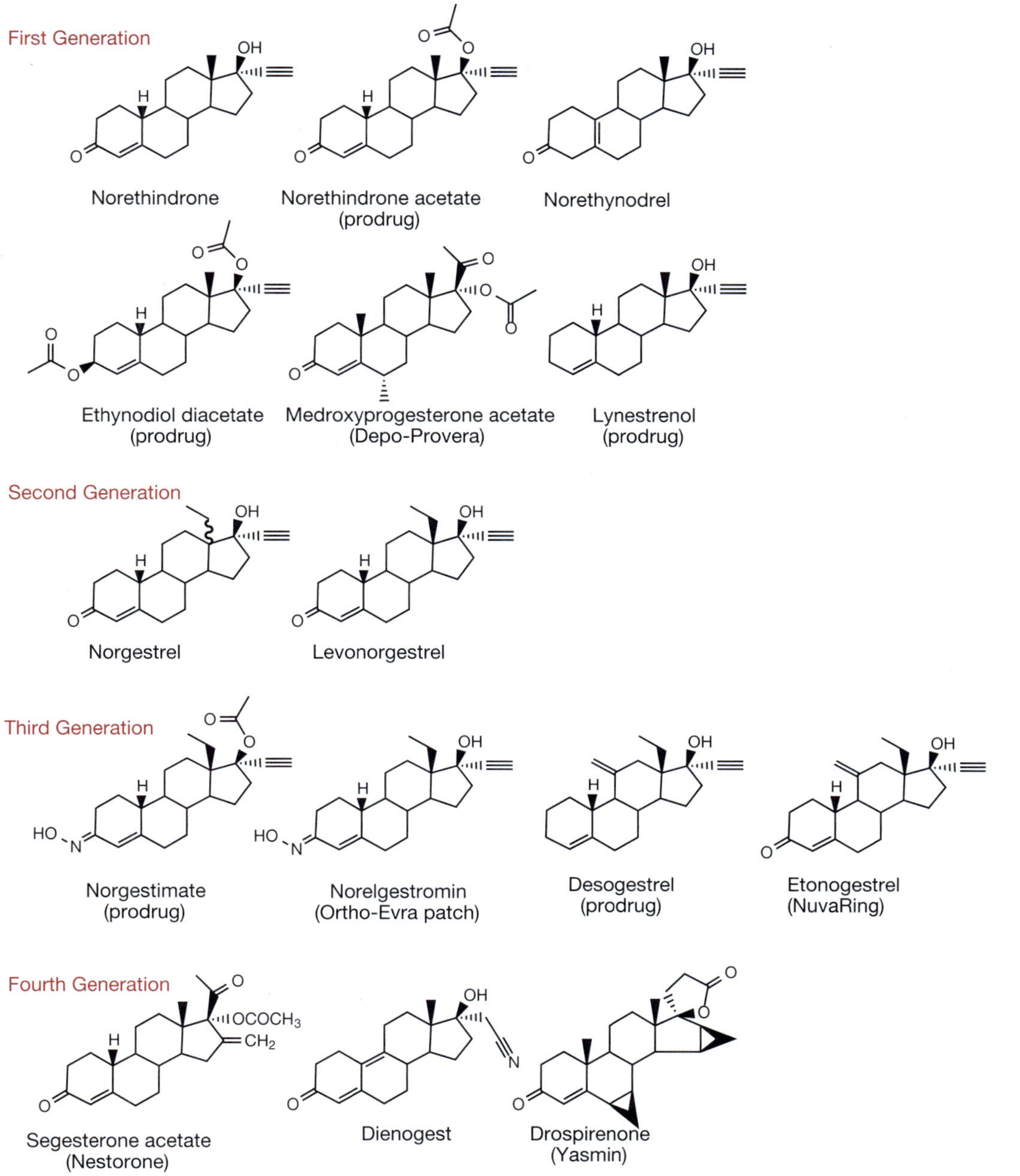

Figure 25.18 Progestins based upon the androstane (class 3) or estrane (class 4) nucleus ordered by generation.

discovered. For example, replacement of the 18-methyl group of norethindrone with an ethyl group resulted in a second generation of progestins, represented by norgestrel (a racemic mixture of the dextronorgestrel and levonorgestrel; rac-13-ethyl-17α-ethynyl-19-nortestosterone). The dextro-stereoisomer of norgestrel is inactive, while levonorgestrel is biologically active and one of the most widely used progestins in oral contraceptives. Third-generation progestins are analogs of levonorgestrel, including the active progestins norelgestromin (metabolized to levonorgestrel) and etonogestrel and their respective prodrugs norgestimate and desogestrel. Fourth-generation progestins include segesterone, dienogest, and drospirenone. Segesterone and drospirenone have therapeutic use in combination with an estrogen as contraceptives.

Structure-Activity Relationships

Currently available progestins are restricted to molecules with a steroid nucleus. Klimstra has pointed out that it is difficult to compare progestins on the basis of studies reported in the literature because there are many ways to evaluate activity.[101] Two of the most common methods of measuring uterine glandular development are Clauberg and McGinty tests. Other biologic evaluations of the progestins include their effect on uterine carbonic anhydrase, inhibition of gonadotropin hormones, delay of parturition, and their ability to maintain pregnancy in a spayed female animal. Substances should be evaluated in the same laboratory as the resulting data are more consistent and thus more informative.

Androstane Derivatives. Ethisterone (Fig. 25.17), the first androgenic compound found to be effective, has about one-third the activity of progesterone in women when taken SC but is 15 times as active when taken orally. Because this analog is closely related to testosterone, it has androgenic activity. Removal of the methyl group at position 19 leads to norethindrone (Fig. 25.18), which has 5 to 10 times more progestational activity. The activity of norethindrone may be increased further by substituting a chlorine atom at position 21 (not shown) or by adding a methyl group at carbon 18 (norgestrel; see Fig. 25.18). Ethynodiol diacetate is an extremely potent oral progestin; it is more active orally than parenterally and is effective as an oral contraceptive when combined with an estrogen.

Further unsaturation of the B or C ring of 19-androstane derivatives enhances progestational activity, as does the introduction of halogen or methyl substituents in the 6α or 7α-position. Acetylation of the 17β-OH of norethindrone to produce norethindrone acetate (see Fig. 25.18) results in a longer duration of action due to the need for hydrolysis of the active alcohol. Removal of the keto function of norethindrone at C_3 gives lynestrenol (17-ethynylestr-4-en-17β-ol; never marketed in the United States), which retains potent progestational activity and is free of androgenic effects. This hormone is used in combination with an estrogen as a contraceptive agent.

Pregnane Derivatives. Some of the potent orally administered progestins are pregnane derivatives. Like androstane-derived progestins, the activity of 17α-hydroxyprogesterones (see Fig. 25.16) is enhanced by unsaturation at positions 6 and 7 and substitution of a methyl group or a halogen at C_6. Activity may be further increased by introducing a CH_3 group at C_{11}. These substitutions likely prevent metabolic reduction of the C_3 and C_{20} carbonyl groups as well as metabolic oxidation at C_6. Substitution of a fluoro group at C_{21} (not shown) prevents hydroxylation at this point (which would generate a glucocorticoid; see Chapter 24) and enhances oral effectiveness.

The adrenocortical hormone 21-hydroxyprogesterone (see Chapter 24, Fig. 24.8) and the precursor of progesterone, pregnenolone (see Fig. 25.3), have no progestational activity.[103] However, because the progestins share the same steroid backbone as adrenocorticoids, androgens, and estrogens, cross-reactivity with other members of the nuclear hormone receptor family is common.[105]

Progestin Antagonists

The use of an antiprogestin (ie, competitive PR antagonist) as an abortifacient agent for interfering with the early phases of pregnancy has been approved in the United States since 2000. The first antiprogestin, mifepristone,[106] contains an 11β-(4-dimethylaminophenyl) side chain believed to destabilize the PR agonist conformation. However, mifepristone also demonstrates potent antiglucocorticoid activity.[106] Additional antiprogestin analogs, such as ulipristal (see "Emergency Contraception and Abortifacients" section), exhibit lowered antiglucocorticoid activity[107] and have been developed and approved as emergency contraceptives.

LEGAL ISSUES IN PREGNANCY TERMINATION AND DETERRENCE

In 2022, the U.S. Supreme Court overturned *Roe v Wade*, reversing what had been considered a "constitutional right" to an abortion in the United States. State legislatures subsequently began passing laws that either affirmed or restricted women's reproductive health decision-making authority within the State, leading to a time of impassioned debate. The Supreme Court decision did not render unconstitutional the use of pharmacotherapeutic estrogen-progestin combination or progestin-only contraceptives (preventing sperm fertilizing an ovum), high-dose progestin emergency contraception (preventing ovulation), or abortifacients (progestin antagonists with or without prostaglandins; preventing implantation and inducing expulsion of the implanted embryo). Their decision, and those of the States, is likely to increase the importance of these agents as more women may rely on pharmacologic means to prevent or terminate pregnancies. This includes the first nonprescription daily progestin-only oral contraceptive, Opill, approved in 2023, and an OTC nonhormonal vaginal gel contraceptive, Phexxi, approved in 2020. The latter is a combination of lactic acid, citric acid, and potassium bitartrate that works by maintaining an acidic vaginal pH, which negatively impact sperm motility.

Emergency Contraception and Abortifacients (Progestin Antagonists and/or Prostaglandins)

Abortifacient Emergency Contraception. The first approved abortifacient to end an early pregnancy was Mifeprex, the combination of mifepristone (2000), a progestin antagonist, given with a prostaglandin, misoprostol. In 2016, the use of Mifeprex was revised by the FDA to be approved to end a pregnancy through 70 days of gestation using 200 mg of mifepristone on day 1 of therapy, then 24 to 48 hours later 800 μg of misoprostol taken buccally, with health care provider follow-up 7 to 14 days later (Fig. 25.19). To ensure safe use, this form of postconception and implantation contraception can only be prescribed and dispensed by, or under the supervision, of a health care provider participating in a risk evaluation and mitigation strategy (REMS) program. Mifepristone acts as an antiprogestin by preventing or reversing implantation. During pregnancy, the compound sensitizes the myometrium of the uterus to the contraction-inducing activity of prostaglandins. Many women (44.1%) in the U.S. trials expelled the products of conception within 4 hours after taking misoprostol and 62.8% experienced expulsion within 24 hours after the misoprostol administration.[108,109] Mifeprex has a black box warning for very rare but serious and sometimes fatal infections and bleeding. The 2016 approval was intended to address the safety concerns for the mother.

Two prostaglandins, PGE_2 (dinoprostone) and carboprost, an analog of $PGF_{2\alpha}$, have been used as abortifacients (Fig. 25.19). The $PGF_{2\alpha}$ analog is injected into the amniotic sac, whereas PGE_2 is given by vaginal suppository to induce abortion.

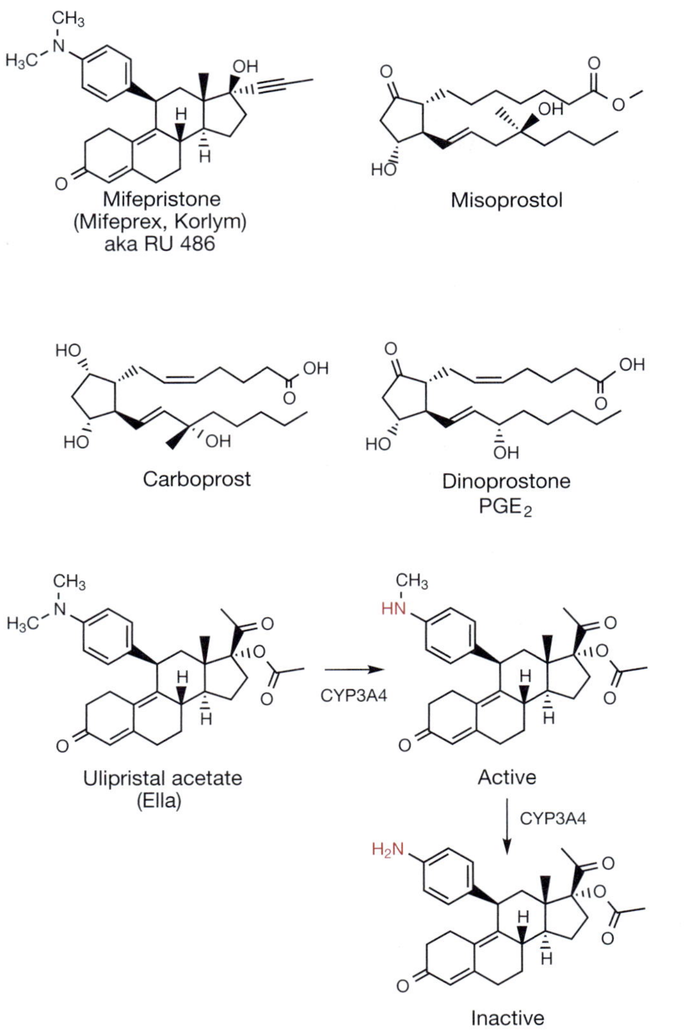

Figure 25.19 Emergency contraceptives and abortifacients.

In 2010, ulipristal acetate (Ella, Fig. 25.19) was approved as an emergency contraceptive that can cut the chances of becoming pregnant by about two-thirds (from 5.6% expected to 1.9% observed with a 30 mg dose of ulipristal acetate) for at least 120 hours after a contraceptive failure or unprotected sex. Ulipristal acetate is not intended for routine use as a contraceptive and is not indicated for termination of an existing pregnancy. It works as an antiprogestin by delaying ovulation or preventing implantation of a fertilized ovum. A rapid return to fertility is likely following treatment with ulipristal acetate, which may interfere pharmacologically with the progestin component of oral contraceptives, requiring barrier methods of contraception for subsequent acts of intercourse that occur in that same menstrual cycle. Oral contraceptive agents with progestins may impair the ability of ulipristal acetate to delay ovulation, and women should start or resume oral contraceptives no sooner than 5 days after taking ulipristal acetate. Ulipristal acetate is metabolized to mono *N*-desmethylulipristal acetate, an active metabolite, and inactive *N,N*-didesmethylulipristal acetate by CYP3A4. Correspondingly, CYP3A4 inducers (600 mg rifampin) significantly decreased the ulipristal area under the plasma concentration-time curve (area under the curve [AUC]) by 93%. Ulipristal is also extremely sensitive to CYP3A4 inhibitors with 400 mg ketoconazole daily for 7 days increasing ulipristal acetate AUC by 5.9-fold.

Nonabortifacient Emergency Contraception. A high-dose progestin "morning-after pill" containing only levonorgestrel was approved in 1982 based on its ability to reduce pregnancy rates from the expected 8% with no contraceptive use to approximately 1%[110] if taken less than 72 hours after intercourse, and better efficacy if taken sooner. Clinical studies showed that 84% of expected pregnancies were prevented with a single 1.5 mg dose of levonorgestrel, as compared to only 79% when levonorgestrel was administered as two doses of 0.75 mg administered 12 hours apart. All of the available formulations (Plan B One Step, My Way, Aftera, and others) now provide 1.5 mg of levonorgestrel as an emergency contraceptive indicated for the prevention of pregnancy following unprotected intercourse or contraceptive failure. These should be taken orally as one 1.5 mg tablet as soon as possible within 72 hours after unprotected intercourse. If vomiting occurs within 2 hours of taking, patients are advised to consider redosing. In 2009, it became available OTC to women older than age 17 and, after legal challenge, in 2013 became available OTC to all women of reproductive potential. In 2022, the FDA approved amendments to the package insert to indicate Plan B works by inhibiting or delaying ovulation and the midcycle hormonal changes, not as an abortifacient (progestin antagonist). This medication, and presumably the multiple approved generics thereof, is ineffective if the woman is already pregnant. Approximately 31% of women experience heavier menstrual bleeding after ingesting the 1.5 mg dose.

Mechanism of Progestin Action

MOLECULAR INTERACTIONS. The uterus is the primary site of progesterone action in females. Once the endometrium proliferates and becomes dense under the influence of estrogens, the levels of progesterone rise. This hormone inhibits the proliferation of the endometrium and initiates the secretory phase of the reproductive cycle. During this stage, the endometrium becomes edematous and glycogen increases in the epithelium of the endometrium.

In an attempt to understand the cellular transformations induced by progesterone that involve gene expression, O'Malley, Schrader, and colleagues studied the effects of progesterone on the chick oviduct, a particularly useful biologic system for the examination of the mechanism of action of progesterone.[111] These studies on PRs extend into mammalian systems as well.[112] The PR consists of two hormone-binding proteins, receptors A and B.[113,114] Biologically active PRs are present in the nucleus of target cells, whereas inactive receptors have been found in the cytosol as a complex with heat shock protein (HSP) 70 and HSP 90,[115] similar to inactive glucocorticoid complexes (see Chapter 24). The nuclear PR heterodimer binds progesterone with high affinity, resulting in a conformational change in the complex and PR dimerization. The steroid receptor complex interacts with HRE regions of the cellular DNA, referred to as progesterone-response elements (PREs), and initiates (activates genes) or abrogates (represses genes) transcription of the DNA sequence to stimulate or inhibit synthesis of the cognate mRNA. This complex and tissue-dependent program of transcriptional control is also sensitive to regulation by cross talk with other signaling pathways. Administration of progesterone to estrogen-stimulated chicks resulted in the synthesis of the specific oviduct protein, avidin. In mammals, uteroglobin (a small secretory protein of the uterus) and the enzyme estradiol dehydrogenase have been identified as proteins induced by progesterone.

Physiologic Effects. Progesterone has many biologic functions. The primary site of the physiologic action of progesterone is the uterus. The hormone acts on both the endometrium (inner mucous lining) and myometrium (muscle mass) of the uterus. It acts on the endometrium, which has been primed by estrogens, to induce the secretory phase, during which the endometrial glands grow and secrete large amounts of carbohydrates that will possibly be used by the fertilized ovum as a source of energy. The primary function of progesterone with respect to the myometrium is to stop the spontaneous rhythmic contractions of the uterus. The effects of progesterone on the uterus are to prepare the endometrium for reception, implantation, and maintenance of the fertilized ovum and to suppress the myometrial contractions so that the embryo is not dislodged from the uterus.

The corpus luteum is the primary source of progesterone for the first third of pregnancy. Subsequently, the developing placenta is the major source of progesterone and estrogens. Both hormones are secreted continually in large amounts until parturition. The high levels of progesterone produced by the corpus luteum and placenta during pregnancy act upon the hypothalamus through the negative feedback system to prevent the formation of new ova. In addition, this steroid hormone is important for the maintenance of pregnancy. Thus, progesterone is often referred to as the "hormone of pregnancy."

Extragenital effects of progesterone, except when secreted in large amounts, are slight. Progesterone is natriuretic, probably because of antagonism of aldosterone. Subsequently, increased sodium excretion stimulates the secretion of aldosterone, which affects sodium retention. Progesterone is also catabolic because it increases the total nitrogen excretion brought about by catabolism of amino acids.[116]

The main feedback effects of progesterone in the CNS are thought to occur in the hypothalamus; causing inhibition of pituitary secretion.[23] PRs have been identified in the hypothalamus and are involved in this feedback inhibition. Prior administration of estrogens or progestins does not appear to inhibit ovulation induced by exogenous gonadotropins. Progesterone appears to have a biphasic feedback effect on ovulation. During the first few hours after administration of this hormone, ovulation is produced and then these effects are inhibited. It appears that the effects of progesterone are reversed as time passes.

Additional actions of progesterone and progesterone metabolites in the CNS have been identified. The identification of various C21 and C19 steroids and enzymatic processes for their production in brain tissues led investigators to suggest that these steroids have a possible function in the CNS.[117] Two 5α-reduced metabolites of progesterone, pregnanolone (3α-hydroxy-5α-pregnan-20-one) and its hydroxy derivative (3α,21-dihydroxy-5α-pregnan-20-one), have been shown to bind to the γ-aminobutyric acid (GABA) receptor subtype A ($GABA_A$) complex at 10^{-8} M concentrations and potentiate GABA responses.[118,119] Another C21 metabolite found in CNS tissues is pregnenolone sulfate, which demonstrates an inhibitory activity on the $GABA_A$ receptor complex.[120] The physiologic relevance of these progestin metabolites in CNS function remains to be determined.

Development of the alveolar sacs in the mammary gland during pregnancy is stimulated by progesterone and estrogens, but lactation does not occur until after the levels of these hormones fall at parturition. Progesterone also increases the basal temperature and decreases the motility of the fallopian tubes. It has been suggested that the temperature-raising effect of progesterone may be due to increased body heat resulting from reduced sweating. This effect is not unique to progesterone; other steroids in the pregnane and androstane series can also produce it.[121] In large doses, progesterone can produce weak analgesia and general anesthesia.

Pharmacology, Side Effects, and Clinical Applications. The mechanism controlling ovarian secretion of progesterone involves the release of LH from the anterior pituitary during ovulation. The LH induces progesterone secretion from the corpus luteum during the second half of the menstrual cycle. As stated earlier, the high levels of progesterone produced by the corpus luteum and placenta during pregnancy act upon the hypothalamus through the negative feedback system to prevent the formation of new ova (see Figs. 25.6 and 25.7). This information led to studies involving progesterone and its analogs as contraceptives.[52,122] If conception does not occur, the corpus luteum regresses and progesterone production decreases. This finally leads to sloughing of part of the endometrium during menstruation.

Progesterone, and more recently its synthetic analogs, has been used to treat dysmenorrhea, endometriosis, functional uterine bleeding, and amenorrhea. Progesterone (eg, Endometrin [progesterone] Vaginal Insert) and its derivatives have been used as assisted reproduction therapy to support early pregnancy, although not always successfully.[123] This seems to be a reasonable use because progesterone is considered a pregnancy-supporting hormone. Because abortion is not always due to a hormonal deficiency, however, progestin treatment has not been as successful as predicted, as evidenced by the aforementioned withdrawal of approval by the FDA of the synthetic progestin, Makena (see Fig. 25.16).

Historically, early pregnancy could be diagnosed by giving the combination of an estrogen and a progestin for several days and then withdrawing it. If bleeding occurs in a few days, the patient is not pregnant. Progesterone has also been used in the treatment of carcinoma of the endometrium. The major use of progestins is in combination with estrogens as a contraceptive.

Among the side effects seen with progestins are nausea and vomiting, drowsiness, spotting, and irregular bleeding; these may occur when these drugs are taken for a short time. With prolonged therapy, a greater incidence of side effects may be seen, including edema and weight gain, breast discomfort, breakthrough bleeding, decreased libido, and masculinization of the female fetus.

Miscellaneous Premenopausal Drugs: Bremelanotide and Brexanolone

Two nonhormonal drugs were approved in 2019 to treat distinct disorders in premenopausal women: bremelanotide (Vyleesi) and brexanolone (Zulresso). Bremelanotide is a seven-membered cyclic peptide and melanocortin receptor (MCR) agonist that is indicated for the treatment of premenopausal women with acquired, generalized hypoactive sexual desire disorder (HSDD). Bremelanotide is not indicated for HSDD in postmenopausal women, or in men, and is not indicated to enhance sexual performance. The MCRs are a series of receptors: MCR1, MCR4, MCR3, MCR5, and MCR2 in order of potency. MCR2 is the receptor for adrenocorticotropic hormone (ACTH; see Chapter 24). Only MCR3 and MCR4 are expressed in the brain. The melanocortins are a group of peptide hormones, which include ACTH and melanocyte-stimulating hormones (α-, β-, and γ-MSH), among others. Bremelanotide acts as an agonist at the MCR3 and MCR4 receptors. Why agonism of the MCR3 and MCR4 receptors in the brain leads to improvement in hypoactive sexual desire is not known. These two receptors are found throughout the CNS and are primarily related to food intake and energy homeostasis. However, one theory is that bremelanotide stimulates dopamine in the medial preoptic area, which is known to be involved in sexual behavior of a number of animals.

Available as 1.75 mg/0.3 mL single-dose solution in a prefilled autoinjector, bremelanotide is administered 1.75 mg SC as needed at least 45 minutes before sexual activity. It should not be administered more than once in 24 hours or more than eight doses/month. The drug should be discontinued after 8 weeks if symptoms do not improve. After a 1.75 mg SC dose, bremelanotide is 100% bioavailable with a T_{max} of 1 hour. The C_{max} is 72.8 ng/mL, and the AUC is 276 ng h/mL. Its mean volume of distribution is 25.0 ± 5.8 L. Following a single SC dose, the mean terminal half-life of bremelanotide is 2.7 hours (range, 1.9-4.0 hours) and the mean (± standard deviation) clearance (CL/F) is 6.5 ±1.0 L/h. Since it is a peptide, it is metabolized by multiple hydrolyses of its amide bonds. Bremelanotide is eliminated via both the kidneys and feces (64.8% and 22.8%, respectively).[124]

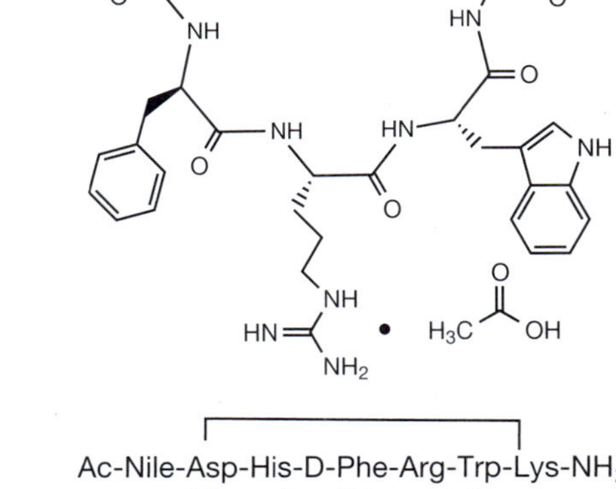

Ac-Nile-Asp-His-D-Phe-Arg-Trp-Lys-NH2
Bremelanotide acetate

Ac-Ser-Tyr-Ser-Met-Glu-His-Phe-Arg-Trp-Gly-Lys-Pro-Val
α-Melanocortin

Brexanolone (Zulresso) is the first FDA-approved drug, specifically for the treatment of postpartum depression (PPD) in adult females. Brexanolone is a synthetic neuroactive steroid with the same chemical structure as the endogenous neuroactive steroid allopregnanolone. Endogenous allopregnanolone levels decrease after childbirth and can be replaced by administration of the structurally identical brexanolone. Allopregnanolone exhibits activity as a barbiturate-like, positive allosteric modulator of both synaptic and extrasynaptic $GABA_A$ receptors. Brexanolone, therefore, can enhance the activity of the receptor to cause calcium channels to open more often and for longer periods of time. These subunit sites are distinct from those associated with benzodiazepines. In addition to the decrease in allopregnanolone, $GABA_A$ receptor levels and expression are decreased and downregulated throughout pregnancy. It is believed that decreases of allopregnanolone and $GABA_A$ may be related to PPD. Therefore, brexanolone can facilitate a return of $GABA_A$ receptor levels to the norm of postpartum.

Brexanolone has low oral bioavailability (<5%) and is, therefore, administered as a continuous intravenous (IV) infusion over a total period of 60 hours (2.5 days). The prescribed maximum dose is 90 μg/kg/h with the following dosing regimen: 30 μg/kg/h for 4 hours, 60 μg/kg/h for 20 hours, 90 μg/kg/h for 28 hours, 60 μg/kg/h for 4 hours, and 30 μg/kg/h for 4 hours. Brexanolone is approved by the FDA contingent on an REMS program and is, therefore, limited to administration at certified health care facilities. Its volume of distribution is approximately 3 L/kg and is highly protein bound (99%). Brexanolone is metabolized by non-cytochrome (CYP) enzymes that result in keto reduction (aldoketoreductases at the C20 keto), glucuronidation (UGT), and sulfonation (sulfotransferase). All metabolites are inactive. Metabolites are eliminated in the feces (47%) and urine (42%), with <1% eliminated as unchanged drug. The terminal half-life is ~9 hours, and plasma clearance is ~1 L/h/kg. Clinical trials have demonstrated that brexanolone is generally well tolerated. Its most common adverse effects include dizziness, sedation/somnolence, xerostomia, loss of consciousness, and hot flushes.[125,126]

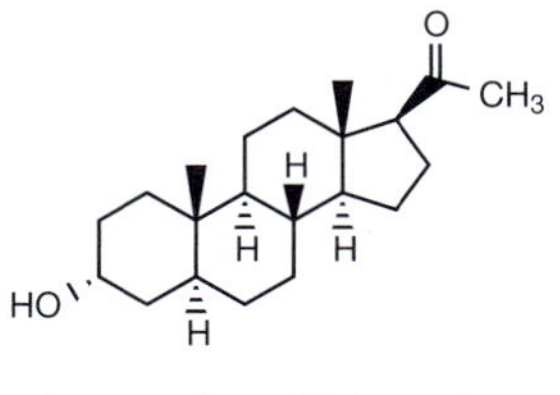

Brexanolone (Zulresso)

Nonpeptidic Gonadotropin-Releasing Hormone Receptor Antagonist: Elagolix

GnRH or LHRH is a decapeptide central regulator of the reproductive system via the HPG axis. As discussed later, increased levels of GnRH stimulate the release of FSH and LH, and estrogens and progesterone. These hormones stimulate the growth of estrogen- (or progesterone-) dependent tissues, such as the uterus and breast. However, agonist and antagonist peptide drugs binding GnRH-Rs have long been available to treat breast and prostate cancers but are not orally bioavailable due to solubility problems and instability to acid pH. Further, GnRH agonists are associated with a clinically relevant "flare" reaction (due to initial hypersecretion of HPG hormones) lasting 1 to 2 weeks in which sex steroidogenesis is initially stimulated, exacerbating any estrogen-dependent diseases or conditions. However, GnRH antagonists immediately suppress the HPG axis without the untoward effects of the flare reaction. Bone loss on long-term use of a GnRH agonist is another side effect not seen with a GnRH antagonist.

Elagolix was the first orally active, nonpeptide GnRH antagonist approved (relugolix now also approved; see "Treatment of Prostate Cancer" section) and directly suppresses the HPG axis via inhibition of GnRH-Rs in the hypothalamus. This allows suppression of estrogen- and progesterone-dependent tissues. It is a highly potent (K_D = 54 pM) antagonist of the human GnRH-R and suppresses LH in castrated macaques after oral administration.[127] The safety profile and oral dosing have allowed the expansion of GnRH antagonist therapy to include nonmalignant conditions (such as endometriosis or uterine fibroids) by maintaining estrogen at low, but not necessarily menopausal, levels. For example, Orilissa is an FDA-approved (2018) elagolix (150 mg daily or 200 mg twice daily [bid]) oral tablet for pain associated with endometriosis in premenopausal women, the first and only pill specifically approved for endometriosis pain relief. Endometriosis is an extrauterine growth of endometrial glands that affects about 8% of premenopausal women. This inflammatory condition has a tremendous impact on patients' lives due to pelvic pain, such as nonmenstrual pelvic pain and dyspareunia. Previously, drugs approved for endometriosis included peptide GnRH agonists, two progestins (depot MPA and norethindrone acetate), and the androstane analog danazol.

Similarly, Oriahnn is an elagolix (300 mg) combination product with 17β-estradiol (1 mg) and norethindrone acetate (0.5 mg) approved for another unique indication, treating heavy menstrual bleeding caused by leiomyomas (uterine fibroids) in premenopausal women. The combination product has a morning combination capsule and an evening capsule of 300 mg of elagolix. Uterine fibroids are extremely common benign tumors in premenopausal women, with a prevalence of 70% and 80% in Caucasian and African American women, respectively, by age 50. Previously, the only approved agent was leuprolide acetate, a peptide GnRH agonist.

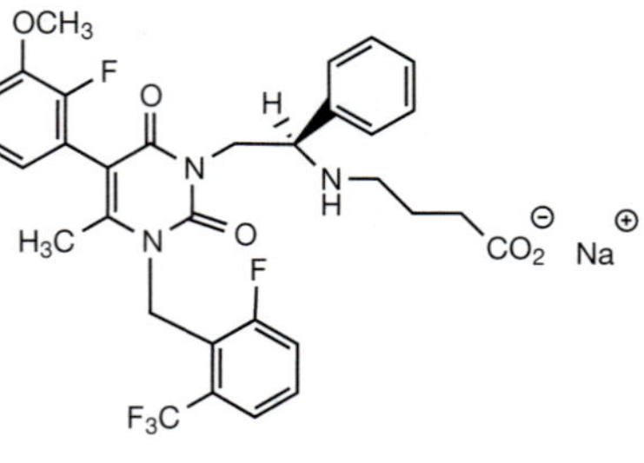

Elagolix sodium

At steady state, elagolix has a T_{max} of 1 hour, a C_{max} (ng/mL) of 574, and an AUC_{24h} of 1,292 ng h/mL. It is 80% bound to serum proteins and a large volume of distribution (>20 L/kg). The elimination half-life is about 6 hours, and it has an apparent clearance rate of 120 L/h. Elagolix is metabolized not only by CYP3A4 but also by other CYP enzymes and UGT. Elagolix is primarily eliminated via biliary excretion in the feces of the unchanged drug (26%) and the O-demethyl metabolite (38%), with the remainder eliminated as multiple metabolites. The most common adverse effects of elagolix include nausea, headache, hot flashes, and night sweats, with minor effects on mood disorder and bone loss, which are recommended to be monitored. Warnings for both the single agent and combination product include bone loss, suicidal ideation and mood disorders, and hepatic impairment. The combination also has a warning of increased risk of thrombotic and thromboembolic disorders due to the estrogen component.[128]

Female Hormonal Contraceptives

Pincus and his colleagues initiated the use of steroidal hormones in oral contraception (OC) in the early 1950s.[129] Early findings in animals were extended to human subjects in Haiti and Puerto Rico, and such investigations showed that a combination of estrogen and progestin prevents conception.[130] Oral contraceptives were approved in the 1960s that contained nonselective progestins and much higher (mg) doses of estrogen than are used today (μg); thus, the side effects of OCs have been reduced over time. Although early forms of OCs explored estrogen only and estrogen then progestin used sequentially, all current OCs are combination (estrogen plus progestin) OC (COC) or progestin-only contraceptives (discussed later as progestin-only pill [POP]) formulations. A plethora of oral contraceptives (Table 25.2) combining progestin and estrogen are now available for therapeutic use worldwide. Their pharmacokinetic properties are summarized in Table 25.3.

Combination Oral Contraceptives

COC regimens are fixed daily doses of an estrogen and a progestin coadministered in a single tablet for 20 or 21 days followed by hormone-free pills (possibly containing iron or folic acid [eg, levomefolate] supplements) for typically 7 or 8 days to complete a 28-day regimen. The 28-day cyclic regimens are continued for as long as contraception is desired. The hormone-free period allows for a 5-day menstrual period. The predominant estrogen in COCs is EE with mestranol and estradiol valerate also available. Typical doses of EE are 30 or 35 μg, but some products contain low (≤20 μg) or high (~50 μg) EE doses based on patient needs to either limit estrogenic side effects or ensure adequate contraceptive efficacy. The progestin component of COCs is the major differentiating factor among COC products. The steroid hormone receptor selectivity, pharmacology (eg, agonist vs antagonist), and relative potencies vary greatly across the progestins employed in COCs. Some progestins (eg, norgestrel, levonorgestrel, MPA) possess androgen side effects, such as acne, oily skin/scalp, weight gain, increased libido, and hirsutism. In some cases, known off-target effects such as antiandrogen (norethindrone, norgestimate) or

Table 25.2 Combination Oral Contraceptives: Estimated Relative Progestin/Estrogen/Androgen Activity

Type of Oral Contraceptive	Trade Name	Estrogen		Progestin		Estrogen Activity	Progestin Activity	Androgen Activity
		Estrogen	Dose (μg)	Progestin	Dose (mg)			
Monophasic (one hormone dose over a cycle)	Apri, Desogen, Emoquette, Enskyce, Ortho-Cept, Reclipsen, Solia	EE	30	Desogestrel	0.15	Intermediate	High	Low
	Beyaz,[a] Gianvi, Loryna, Nikki, Vestura, Yaz	EE	20	Drospirenone	3	Intermediate	High	None
	Ocella, Safyral,[a] Syeda, Yasmin, Zarah	EE	30	Drospirenone	3	Intermediate	High	None
	Kelnor, Zovia	EE	35	Ethynodiol diacetate	1	Low	High	Low
	Zovia	EE	50	Ethynodiol diacetate	1	Intermediate	High	Low
	Aubra, Aviane, Delyla, FaLessa,[a] Falmina, Lessina, Lutera, Orsythia, Sronyx	EE	20	Levonorgestrel		Low	Low	Low
	Altavera, Chateal, Kurvelo, Levora, Marlissa, Portia	EE	30 (28 d)	Levonorgestrel	0.15	Intermediate	Intermediate	Intermediate
	Introvale, Jolessa, Quasense	EE	30 (91 d)	Levonorgestrel	0.15	Low	Intermediate/high	Intermediate/high
	Amethyst, Lybrel	EE	20	Levonorgestrel	0.09	Low	Intermediate/high	Intermediate/high
	Balziva, Briellyn, Femcon FE, Gildagia, Ovcon, Philith, Vyfemla, Wymzya FE, Zenchent, Zenchent FE	EE	35	Norethindrone	0.4	Intermediate	Low	Low
	Brevicon, Modicon, Necon, Nortrel, Wera	EE	35	Norethindrone	0.5	Low	Low	Low
	Generess FE, Layolis FE	EE	25	Norethindrone	0.8	Intermediate	Low	Low
	Alyacen, Cyclafem, Dasetta, Necon, Norinyl, Nortrel, Ortho-Novum, Pirmella	EE	35	Norethindrone	1	Intermediate	Intermediate	Intermediate
	Necon, Norinyl	Mestranol	50	Norethindrone	1	Intermediate	Intermediate	Intermediate
	Gildess, Gildess FE, Junel, Junel FE, Larin, Larin FE, Loestrin, Loestrin FE, Lomedia FE, Microgestin, Microgestin FE, Minastrin FE, Tarina FE	EE	20	Norethindrone acetate	1	Low	Intermediate/high	Intermediate/high

(*continued*)

Table 25.2 Combination Oral Contraceptives: Estimated Relative Progestin/Estrogen/Androgen Activity (*continued*)

Type of Oral Contraceptive	Trade Name	Estrogen: Estrogen	Estrogen: Dose (μg)	Progestin: Progestin	Progestin: Dose (mg)	Estrogen Activity	Progestin Activity	Androgen Activity
	Gildess, Gildess FE, Junel, Junel FE, Larin, Larin FE, Loestrin, Loestrin FE, Microgestin, Microgestin FE	EE	30	Norethindrone acetate	1.5	Low	Intermediate/high	Intermediate/high
	Estarylla, Mono-Linyah, MonoNessa, Ortho-Cyclen, Previfem, Sprintec	EE	35	Norgestimate	0.25	Intermediate	Low	Low
	Cryselle, Elinest, Low-Ogestrel	EE	30	Norgestrel	0.3	Intermediate	Intermediate	Intermediate
	Ogestrel	EE	50	Norgestrel	0.5	High	High	High
Biphasic (two hormone doses over a cycle)	Azurette, Kariva, Kimidess, Pimtrea, Mircette, Viorele	EE	20/10	Desogestrel	0.15	Intermediate		Low
	Amethia Lo, Camrese Lo, LoSeasonique	EE	20/10	Levonorgestrel	0.1	Low	Intermediate/high	Intermediate/high
	Amethia, Ashlyna, Camrese, Daysee, Seasonique	EE	30/10	Levonorgestrel	0.15	Low	Intermediate/high	Intermediate/high
	Necon	EE	35/35	Norethindrone	0.5/1	Intermediate	Intermediate	Low
	Lo Loestrin FE, Lo Minastrin FE	EE	10/10	Norethindrone	1	Low	Intermediate/high	Intermediate/high
Triphasic (three hormone doses over a cycle)	Ortho Tri-Cyclen Lo	EE	25	Norgestimate	0.18/0.215/0.25	Intermediate	Low	Low
	Enpresse, Levonest, Myzilra, Trivora	EE	30/40/30	Levonorgestrel	0.05/0.075/0.125	Intermediate	Low	Low
	Ortho Tri-Cyclen, Tri-Estarylla, Tri-Previfem, TriNessa, Tri-Linyah, Tri-Sprintec	EE	35	Norgestimate	0.18/0.215/0.25	Intermediate	Low	Low
	Aranelle, Leena, Tri-Norinyl	EE	35	Norethindrone	0.5/1/0.5	Low	Low	Low
	Alyacen, Cyclafem, Dasetta, Necon, Nortel, Ortho-Novum, Pirmella	EE	35	Norethindrone	0.5/0.75/1	Intermediate	Intermediate	Low
	Estrostep FE, Tilia FE, Tri-Legest FE	EE	20/30/35	Norethindrone acetate	1	Low	Intermediate/high	Intermediate/high
	Caziant, Cesia, Cyclessa, Velivet	EE	25	Desogestrel	0.1/0.125/0.15	Intermediate	Intermediate	Low
Quadriphasic (four hormone doses over a cycle)	Natazia	Estradiol valerate	3/2/2/1	Dienogest	0/2/3/0	Intermediate	High	Low
	Quartette	EE	20/25/30/10	Levonorgestrel	0.15/0.15/0.15/0	Low	Intermediate/high	Intermediate/high

EE, ethinyl estradiol; FE, contains iron.

[a]Also contains levomefolate.

Based on Facts and Comparisons. *Oral Contraceptives Monograph*. http://fco.factsandcomparisons.com/lco/action/doc/retrieve/docid/fc_dfc/5546102

Table 25.3 Pharmacokinetic Properties for Some Estrogenic and Progestational Agents

Drug	Protein[a] Binding	Oral Bioavailability	Biotransformation	Elimination Half-Life (h)	Time to Peak Conc. (h)	Peak Serum Conc. (ng/mL)	Elimination (%)	
							Renal[b]	Fecal
17β-Estradiol	50%-80%	Poor	Hepatic[c]	20 min		0.1-0.2	90	
Ethinyl estradiol (EE)	98%	40%	Hepatic	26 (6-20)	1-2	33		
Progesterone Oral 200 mg micronized IM 45 mg IM 90 mg Vaginal gel 45 mg	>90%	<10%	Hepatic	<5 min 10 wk 19.6 34.8	2-4 28 9.2 6.8	24.3 39.1 53.8 14.9	50-60 10	
Medroxyprogesterone acetate: Oral 10 mg IM 150 mg/mL every 3 mo	>90%	High	Hepatic IM no hepatic	30 50 d	2-4 3 wk	19-35 1-7	15-22	45-80
Megestrol acetate Oral 160 mg Oral 600 mg	>90		Hepatic	38 (13-104)	2-3 2-3	200 753	66	20
Norgestrel	>90%	60%	Hepatic	20	24		45	32
Levonorgestrel 3/12/60 mo implants 216 mg loading dose[d]	>90	60	No hepatic	16 (8-30)	24	1,6 first week, then 0.26-0.4	45	32
Desogestrel (Desogen) (as 3-keto-desogestrel)	>90	76	Hepatic to active 3-ketodesogestrel	12-58	1-2	2-6	43	50
Norethindrone	>80	65	Hepatic	8 (5-14)	0.5-4.0	5-10	50	20-40
Norethindrone acetate	>80	65	Hepatic	8 (5-14)	0.5-4.0	5-10	50	20-40
Norgestimate as (desacetylnorgestimate)	>50-60 >90	60	Hepatic to desacetyl-norgestimate	37	1-2	0.5-0.7	47	37

Data from USP Drug Information 2000', which is in keeping with Pharmacokinetic Properties data tables in other chapters of the 9th edition.

IM, intramuscular.

[a]Sex hormone–binding globulin (SHBG) synthesis is stimulated by estrogens and inhibited by androgens: Levels are twice as high in women as in men. Progesterone binds strongly to cortisol-binding globulin (CBG; 17.7%) and SHBG (0.6%) and weakly to albumin (79.3%). Absorption is the rate-limiting step for the elimination half-life. Levonorgestrel: free, 1.1% to 1.7%; SHBG, 92% to 62%; and albumin, 37.56%; but suppresses SHBG by 33%. Norethindrone: free, 3.5%; SHBG, 35.5%; and albumin, 61%. Medroxyprogesterone does not bind SHBG. 3-Keto-desgestrel, 64%; albumin, 32%. Norgestimate >90% protein bound; not SHBG.

[b]Renal metabolites are primarily conjugates.

[c]Hepatic indicates hepatic first-pass metabolism.

[d]A mean dose of 35 μg levonorgestrel is released daily.

antimineralocorticoid (drospirenone) activities can be therapeutic in patients with acne or postmenopausal dysphoric disorder (PMDD), respectively. In other cases, COC intolerance can be addressed by changing the progestin component (Table 25.4).

The progestin dose is also variable but in the low to submilligram (mg) range. Estrogen and progestin dose is another differentiating factor between COCs with low- and high-dose estrogen products mentioned earlier. Further, the dose of estrogen or progestin can be static or vary multiple times during the 28-day regimen. The original COCs employed static doses of estrogen and progestin (ie, estrogen to progestin dose and ratio was fixed throughout each cycle), which are now termed *monophasic regimens*. Efforts to more closely replicate the normal menstrual cycle and/or limit the side effects of COCs have led to the development of biphasic, triphasic, or quadraphasic formulations where the estrogen and/or progestin doses change 2 to 4 times during the 28-day regimen. Consistent with reproductive physiology, often the progestin dose is lower in the initial follicular phase but increases during the luteal phases, whereas the EE dose optionally stays the same or decreases as the menstrual period is approached (Table 25.2).

The length of the active hormone pill period is another COC differentiating factor. Extended cycle products that provide 24 days of hormone therapy (eg, Yaz) with only a 4-day hormone-free period and continuous cycle (ie, no hormone-free period) (eg, Lybrel) formulations reduce or eliminate menstrual bleeding and may be beneficial when patients present with a history of dysmenorrhea or menstrual (ie, estrogen withdrawal) migraine headaches.[131] Nextstellis is the only approved 24-day active, 4-day placebo product with estetrol (14.2 mg; 15α-hydroxyestriol; Fig. 25.10), a weak ER agonist naturally occurring in the body during pregnancy and manufactured from a plant source, in combination with drospirenone (3 mg).

Moreover, Yaz 24/4 is FDA approved for PMDD, purportedly due to the strong antimineralocorticoid effects of the progestin drospirenone.[131] An enormous assortment of COC products is engendered by the combination of variables reviewed earlier, affording the practitioner the opportunity to rationally select an initial COC for a patient or optimize the COC to patient preferences and/or needs. Although extremely popular, in some cases, a COC is not the optimal hormonal contraception for a particular patient, and other options are described later.

Progestin-Only Pills

POPs employ a small daily dose of the progestin with prescription products using 0.35 mg of norethindrone (0.35 mg) daily (eg, Micro-Nor or Nor-QD and bioequivalents thereof). Recently, the FDA approved Opill (0.075 μg norgestrel) tablets as the first daily oral contraceptive available for nonprescription use to prevent pregnancy. POPs are continuous hormone OCs (ie, there is no hormone-free period during the 28-day regimen and no break between regimens). POPs suppress ovum release and promote thickening of the cervical mucus, which makes it difficult for sperm to reach the ovum. Further, no estrogen is given at any time that reduces some of the risks associated with the use of estrogens. POPs may be recommended for breastfeeding patients or patients intolerant of or contraindicated to estrogens. Unlike COCs, the time of day of dosing POPs must be consistent, as efficacy is compromised in POPs if the dose is delayed by more than 2 to 3 hours from normal. In such cases, barrier contraception

Table 25.4 Achieving Proper Hormonal Balance in Oral Contraceptive Agents

Estrogen		Progestin		Androgen[a]
Excess	**Deficiency**	**Excess**	**Deficiency**	**Excess**
• Nausea • Bloating • Cervical mucorrhea • Polyposis • Melasma • Hypertension • Migraine headache • Increase in breast size • Breast fullness or tenderness • Edema • Urinary tract infection • Uterine enlargement • Uterine fibroid growth	• Early or midcycle breakthrough bleeding • Increased spotting • Hypomenorrhea • Nervousness • Vaginitis atrophic • Vasomotor symptoms	• Increased appetite • Depression • Fatigue • Hypertension • Hypoglycemia symptoms • Hypomenorrhea • Libido decrease • Vaginal yeast infections • Breast regression	• Late breakthrough bleeding • Amenorrhea • Dysmenorrhea • Hypermenorrhea	• Acne • Cholestatic jaundice • Edema • Hirsutism • Libido increase • Oily skin and scalp • Rash and pruritus

From Facts and Comparisons. *Oral Contraceptives Monograph.* http://fco.factsandcomparisons.com/lco/action/doc/retrieve/docid/fc_dfc/5546102
[a]Result of androgenic activity of progestins.

(eg, condom) is recommended for 48 hours. Another major disadvantage of POPs is that irregular bleeding is common, especially during the first 18 months of therapy.

As noted, the major POP advantage is the absence of estrogen excess side effects reported with the combination methods, including serious thromboembolic episodes such as cerebrovascular accidents or other estrogenic side effects such as enlarged, tender, and/or cystic breasts, hypermenorrhea, spider veins, irritability, edema, bloating, and nausea. Other serious conditions predisposed by estrogens are increased risk of myocardial infarction, hepatic adenomas, hypertension, severe congenital hyperlipidemia, gallbladder disease, breast cancer, and altered carbohydrate metabolism. In addition to a current pregnancy, a history of any of the aforementioned conditions or heavy smoker more than 35 years old is also considered contraindication to COC use, possibly suggesting POP or progestin-only parenteral methods to avoid these estrogenic effects.

Parenteral Hormonal Contraceptives

A variety of parenteral contraceptives are now available to deliver hormones via transdermal patch, vaginal ring, IM or SC depot injection, SC implant, or progesterone-impregnated intrauterine device (IUD). Although similar or identical estrogens and progestins are employed, parenteral administration alters drug exposure. For example, the systemic AUC of EE from COC (30 μg) is 21.9 versus 35.8 and 10.6 ng h/mL for patch (20 μg) and ring (15 μg), respectively. This indicates that relatively high systemic EE levels are achieved from the patch (possibly due to avoidance of first-pass effects) while low systemic EE levels are achieved from ring, qualifying the latter as a low estrogen-dose contraceptive method when compared to COC.[132] A few specific parenteral products are discussed next.

Patch. Daily transdermal delivery of 20 μg EE and 150 μg of norelgestromin (metabolized to levonorgestrel in liver) is achieved by Xulane patches, which are applied weekly for 3 weeks and then no patch for 1 week. Patches typically adhere well to trunk and arm (they should not be applied to the breast) despite water/soap exposure. If the patch falls off, patients should replace it within 24 hours. Efficacy is 99% but lower in women weighing more than 90 kg. As mentioned, higher levels of EE suggest the possibility of increased risk of thromboembolism.

Vaginal Ring. Transvaginal delivery of 15 μg/d of EE and continuous release of etonogestrel (0.12 mg/ring) are achieved by NuvaRing, a clear and colorless flexible polymer ring. One ring remains in position for 3 weeks and then no ring for 1 week; if the ring falls out, it can be replaced within 3 hours. The ring formulation provides comparable efficacy to other methods despite the low levels of hormones in the product, which is probably attributable to rapid absorption and no first-pass effect. NuvaRing produces continuous and relatively low steady-state drug levels, suggesting that this product may be side-effect sparing.

A second option, Annovera, is a flexible silicon ring containing 17.4 mg EE and 103.0 mg segesterone that can be used continuously for 1 year (thirteen 28-day cycles). The ring must remain in place continuously for 21 days and then be removed by the patient for 7 days to complete one cycle. This system is unique in that it can be removed and replaced (ie, reusable) for 1 year, which may make this a good option for women in low-resource settings where access to health care may be problematic.

Intramuscular and Subcutaneous Injections. Depot injections are intermediate-term contraceptive products that use MPA (150 mg IM as Depo-Provera or 104 mg SC as Depo-SubQ Provera) every 3 months (every 11-13 weeks). Advantages include lack of estrogen-related adverse effects, amenorrhea, and prevention of endometrial cancer. Disadvantages include weight gain, irregular bleeding, and risk of prolonged infertility and/or side effects due to the 3-month duration. They also require a health care provider visit every 3 months.

Subcutaneous Implants. Long-term (up to 3 years) contraception is achieved by Nexplanon, which involves implantation of a single ethylene vinylacetate rod (4 cm × 2 mm; which is removable) that delivers 67 μg daily of etonogestrel. Advantages include comparable efficacy in patients who are obese (unlike COCs and patches) and ensure patient adherence. Further, ease of implantation and removal is much improved compared to Norplant (discontinued; Norplant was relatively large and more difficult to implant/remove). Disadvantages include the possibility of progestin excess side effects including weight gain, depression, fatigue, decreased libido, and breast size, as well as bleeding irregularities.

Intrauterine Devices. Several brand names of levonorgestrel-impregnated IUDs (Mirena, Liletta, Skyla) release 13.5 to 20 μg of levonorgestrel daily, which is not systemically absorbed. Nonetheless, local progestin thickens cervical mucus and inhibits sperm motility. The IUD may remain in place for up to 3 to 7 years, depending on which product is used, with no delay in fertility upon discontinuation. Limitations include that it must be implanted by a health care professional and is recommended after having at least one child.

HOW TO TAILOR CONTRACEPTIVE REGIMEN TO PATIENT NEEDS

Approximately 10 million women use hormonal contraceptives, with the duration of therapy varying from one or two cycles to up to 30 years. Hormonal contraception is highly effective when consistently and correctly used, leading to only 5% of unintended pregnancies, whereas 95% of unintended pregnancies result from lack of or inconsistent contraceptive use. Unintended pregnancies in the first year with perfect use of COC are only 0.3% versus 8% for typical use, which takes into account human error. Nonhormonal contraception methods such as withdrawal, rhythm, and symptothermal vary in typical use failure rates from 29% (spermicide) to 15% (condom), demonstrating the superiority of hormonal methods.

Hormonal contraceptives have a variety of immediate side effects (Table 25.4) and drug-drug interactions (DDIs) and should be avoided in certain patient populations. Choice of hormonal contraceptive should consider any symptoms of estrogen, progestin, or androgen excess or deficiency. For example, acne is an androgen excess symptom and, if present, could be treated by an antiandrogenic progestin containing COC, such as Estrostep (norethindrone acetate), Ortho Tri-Cyclen (norgestimate), or Yaz (drospirenone). Estrogen excess or deficiency symptoms can be corrected by employing low or high EE formulations, respectively.

Selection of hormonal contraception should also be made in view of age, life/family goals, potential for DDIs, and risk factors revealed by family history or social history. For example, age in excess of 35 years, family or personal history of cardiovascular problems and coagulopathies, and/or personal history of smoking may predispose patients to estrogenic thromboembolic events, elevating the need to consider progestin-only hormonal contraception methods. OCs are known to interact with multiple anticonvulsants and some antibiotics that are CYP3A4 inducers, which, possibly due to induction of first-pass metabolism, lower EE (or progestin) to subtherapeutic levels. Although high-dose estrogen COC may be an option, a parenteral hormonal contraceptive may be optimal. Broad-spectrum antibiotics such as tetracyclines, metronidazole, and quinolones may cause worrisome breakthrough bleeding with COCs as a consequence of perturbed microbial EE metabolism that returns EE to bloodstream via enterohepatic recycling; backup contraception may be warranted.

Potential recommendations based on patient-specific criteria include:

- Weight (>90 kg): Start with 35 μg EE or more; avoid patch; consider implant.
- Very young age: Start with 20 μg EE.
- Predisposed to therapeutic nonadherence: Consider parenteral therapy.
- Not planning a near-term pregnancy within 1 to 3 years: Consider long-acting parenteral therapy.
- Breakthrough/dysfunctional bleeding, history of ovarian cyst or endometriosis, and/or DDI risk: Consider a high-dose EE.

Drugs Used in Hormone Replacement Therapy for Menopause

Menopause Symptoms and Treatment Approaches

After menopause, the ovaries atrophy and 17β-estradiol and progesterone are no longer produced. Physiologic changes occur, including vasomotor symptoms (hot flashes, night sweats, flushing, palpitations, and anxiety), psychological changes (depression, mood swings, memory or concentration changes, fatigue, and irritability), vaginal atrophy and decreased vaginal elasticity, decreased libido, dyspareunia (painful intercourse), urinary tract changes (atrophy of bladder epithelium, stress urinary incontinence, shortening of urethra), risk of cardiovascular disease, bone loss and osteoporosis, and loss of skin elasticity. These menopausal symptoms can greatly affect a women's quality of life.

Menopausal symptoms can be alleviated by pharmacologic therapies, such as HRT. Nonpharmacologic therapies including lifestyle changes, diet, exercise, and stress reduction can also help to a lesser extent. Due to negative, insufficient, or inconclusive data, the North American Menopause Society (NAMS) does not currently recommend cooling techniques, avoidance of triggers, exercise, yoga, relaxation, or OTC supplements and herbal therapies.[133] NAMS recommends cognitive-behavioral therapy using the FDA-approved selective serotonin reuptake inhibitor paroxetine (Brisdelle, 7.5 mg) as an effective nonhormonal prescription therapy to alleviate vasomotor symptoms.[133] At this time, the use of soy isoflavones, weight loss, and mindfulness-based stress reduction may be beneficial but should be recommended with caution.[133]

The presence of an intact uterus is a major factor governing the choice to use estrogens either alone or in combination with a progestin as HRT. Therapy with an estrogen alone in women with an intact uterus has been shown to cause endometrial hyperplasia and increase the risk of endometrial cancer. Thus, the addition of progestin protects the uterus and is included in HRT in these women. Conversely, progestins can have negative effects on menopausal women. The decision of whether to use HRT by patients should be done in consultation with their physician and/or pharmacist to take patient-relevant risk factors into account.

Since the findings of the Women's Health Initiative (WHI) were released in 2002, U.S. women have decreased their usage of HRT.[134] The objective of the WHI trial was to determine if long-term use of HRT in postmenopausal women (average age 64 years) reduces risks of heart disease, breast cancer, colon cancer, and fractures. The results of this trial have been since used inappropriately to make therapeutic decisions for women having symptoms during peri- or menopausal years.[134] Based on WHI findings, the use of HRT is supported in menopausal women, ages 50 to 59 years, who are experiencing symptoms and have a low risk of breast cancer or cardiovascular disease. Women who initiate HRT within 10 years of menopause to help alleviate bothersome menopausal symptoms are not at increased risk of cardiovascular disease.

Using the WHI data, a benefit and risk assessment of two hormone therapy formulations was carried out (conjugated equine estrogens [CEE] alone and CEE + MPA) in women ages 50 to 59 years (Table 25.5).[134] The risks and benefits were expressed as the difference in the number of events (number in the hormone therapy group minus the number in the placebo group) per 1,000 women over 5 years. For women on CEE alone, a risk existed for deep vein thrombosis (DVT), which had 2.5 more events per 1,000 women than placebo. Benefits were seen in the CEE-alone trial, as negative values show decreased number of events per 1,000 women compared to placebo. Whether on CEE alone or in combination with MPA, benefits for this group of women were seen with diabetes, death from any cause, all fractures, and cancers including colorectal. Additional benefits of

Table 25.5 Benefits and Risks of Two Formulations (CEE + MPA; CEE Alone) in the WHI for Women (Ages 50-59 years)

	Trial[a]	
Disease	**CEE + MPA**	**CEE – Alone**
Deep vein thrombosis	5.0	2.5
Coronary heart disease	2.5	−5.5
Stroke	2.5	−0.5
Breast cancer	3.0	−2.5
Colorectal cancer	−0.5	−1.5
All cancers	−0.5	−4.0
All fractures	−12.0	−8.0
Death from any cause	−5.0	−5.5
Diabetes	−5.5	−13.0

CEE, conjugated equine estrogens; MPA, medroxyprogesterone acetate.
[a]Difference given is the number of events per 1,000 women over 5 years. That is, the number in the hormone therapy group minus the number in the placebo group. A positive number illustrates a risk, and a negative number illustrates a benefit.
Based on Manson JE, Kaunitz AM. Menopause management–getting clinical care back on track. *N Engl J Med.* 2016;374:803-806.

CEE alone included protection from breast cancer, stroke, and coronary heart disease. Increased risks were seen in the CEE with or without MPA group for DVT, but only in the CEE with MPA group were risks seen for coronary heart disease, stroke, and breast cancer. These risks were no more than five events per 1,000 women above the placebo group.

Patients and physicians need to work together to determine options for managing menopausal symptoms. A free mobile app has been developed by the NAMS called MenoPro to aid patients and physicians with treatment options.[135] Starting HRT more than 10 years after menopause can increase the risk of cardiovascular disease and other side effects. It is not recommended to initiate systemic HRT more than 10 years after menopause due to risks of coronary heart disease, stroke, venous thromboembolism (VTE), and dementia.[136] A low-dose vaginal estrogen (nonsystemic) is safe to use more than 10 years after menopause.[136]

Estrogens Used Alone in Hormone Replacement Therapy

The estrogens used in oral HRT include 17β-estradiol and mixtures of sulfate esters of estrone and its derivatives (collectively known as conjugated estrogens or esterified estrogens) (Table 25.6). The structures of the conjugated estrogens used in estrogen replacement therapy are shown in Figure 25.13 and represent mixtures of water-soluble phase II metabolites (sulfate esters) of naturally occurring estrogens obtained from the urine of pregnant mares or prepared synthetically. These metabolites are prodrugs that are unable to bind to the ER. However, when orally administered, the sulfates are hydrolyzed in the intestines to the phenols, which can weakly bind to the ER.

In 1941, Ayerst, McKenna, and Harrison introduced Premarin, the name coined from *pre*gnant *mar*e ur*in*e with subsequent FDA approval in 1942. Premarin was a top-selling prescription drug, and it has been estimated that more than 30 billion doses have been dispensed, with yearly sales reaching over $1 billion. Premarin revenues in the United States have been decreasing due to decreases in prescription volume.[137] The other oral estrogens that are approved for estrogen replacement therapy are synthetically derived and include 17β-estradiol, piperazine salt of estrone sulfate, or mixtures of sodium sulfate esters of weak estrogens (estrone, equilin, or derivatives).

Doses for oral administration of estrogen are typically 60% to 80% lower than those used for OCs, as the smallest dose needed to relieve symptoms is the goal. Treatment typically will start with a low dose of estrogen (Table 25.7) and increase depending on the needs of the patient to maximize symptom relief while minimizing side effects. Estrogen

Table 25.6 Estrogens Used Alone in Hormone Replacement Therapy

Product	Generic	Trade Name	Components
Estrogen (oral)	Estrogens (conjugated/equine, systemic)	Premarin	Sodium estrone sulfate (~50%-65%) Sodium equilin sulfate (~20%-35%) Sodium 17α-dihydroequilin sulfate Sodium 17α-estradiol sulfate Sodium 17β-dihydroequilin sulfate
	Estrogens (esterified)	Menest	Sodium estrone sulfate (75%-85%) Sodium equilin sulfate (6%-15%) Other estrogen components (~10%)
	Estropipate	Ogen	Piperazine estrone sulfate
	Estradiol (Systemic)	Estrace	17β-Estradiol, micronized

Femtrace, Enjuvia, Estratab, and Cenestin were all discontinued.
From Facts and Comparisons. *Conjugated estrogens (systemic) monograph; esterified estrogens oral monograph; estropipate (piperazine estrone sulfate) oral monograph.* Accessed April 17, 2018. http://fco.factsandcomparisons.com/lco/action/doc/retrieve/docid/fc_dfc/5546102

Table 25.7 Daily Dose Treatment Options of Estrogen for Postmenopausal Use

	Treatment		
Estrogen	Standard Dose (mg)	Low Dose (mg)	Ultra-Low Dose (mg)
17β-Estradiol, micronized	1	0.5	0.25
Conjugated equine estrogens (CEE)	0.625	0.45	0.3
17β-Estradiol, transdermal	0.1	0.05	0.014
Ethinyl estradiol (EE)		0.005	

products are available in many formulations, including oral, transdermal (patch, gel, emulsion, spray), and vaginal (insert, tablet, ring, cream) (Table 25.8). The estrogens present in these various formulations include 17β-estradiol, micronized 17β-estradiol, 17β-estradiol acetate, estropipate (piperazine estrone sulfate), CEE, and esterified estrogens. The approximate equivalent estrogen doses for postmenopausal use are given in Table 25.9.[138] Due to first-pass metabolism, orally administered estrogens are transformed into estrone and estriol metabolites. 17β-Estradiol acetate and CEE are prodrugs and will be active upon hydrolysis of the acetate or sulfate esters of the A ring phenol.

Estrogen and Progestin Combinations Used in Hormone Replacement Therapy

Estrogens are given in combination with progestins for women with an intact uterus, and available products are listed in Table 25.8. The lowest dose progestin should be administered that prevents endometrial hyperplasia. If the dose is too low, breakthrough bleeding will result. The progestins used in HRT include micronized progesterone, MPA, norethindrone acetate (first generation), levonorgestrel (second generation), norgestimate (third generation), and drospirenone (fourth generation) (Table 25.8). Adverse effects of progestins in HRT include premenopausal symptoms of irritability and depression, headaches, bloating, weight gain, and irregular bleeding. Newer progestins are better tolerated than MPA, which has shown more adverse reactions (increased DVT and cardiovascular risk and worsening lipid profile).

The progestins used in combination with estrogens in HRT are shown in Figures 25.16 and 25.18. Progesterone has low oral bioavailability due to poor absorption and almost complete first-pass metabolism in the liver. It is also light sensitive. Micronized progesterone demonstrates increased oral absorption. MPA is a 6α-methyl-17α-acetoxy derivative of progesterone given in combination with CEE (Prempro, Premphase). Both of these structural changes prevent metabolism: 17α-acetoxy slows metabolic reduction of 20-ketone to the alcohol, and 6α-methyl slows metabolism of the 3-keto-4-ene system.

Norethindrone acetate is a first-generation 19-nortestosterone derivative based upon the estrane nucleus and is given in combination with either 17β-estradiol (Activella,

Table 25.8 Hormone Replacement Therapy Products[139]

Category	Trade Name	Components	Dosage Form	Frequency of Dosing
Estrogen (oral)	Estrace	17β-Estradiol (micronized)	Tablet	Once daily
	Menest	Esterified estrogens	Tablet	Once daily
	Ogen	Estropipate	Tablet	Once daily
	Premarin	CEE	Tablet	Once daily
Estrogen (transdermal)	Alora	17β-Estradiol	Patch (matrix)	Twice weekly
	Climara	17β-Estradiol	Patch (matrix)	Once weekly
	Divigel, Elestrin	17β-Estradiol	Gel (topical)	Once daily
	Estraderm	17β-Estradiol	Patch (reservoir)	Twice weekly
	EstroGel	17β-Estradiol	Gel (topical)	1 pump once daily
	Evamist	17β-Estradiol	Spray (topical)	Initially 1 spray daily; may increase to 2-3 sprays if needed
	Menostar	17β-Estradiol	Patch (matrix)	Once daily for osteoporosis
	Vivelle, Vivelle-Dot	17β-Estradiol	Patch (matrix)	Twice weekly

Table 25.8 Hormone Replacement Therapy Products (*continued*)

Category	Trade Name	Components	Dosage Form	Frequency of Dosing
Estrogen (vaginal)	Imvexxy	17β-Estradiol	Vaginal inserts for manual placement	Once daily for 2 wk, then twice weekly
	Vagifem	17β-Estradiol	Vaginal tablets placed by applicator	Once daily for 2 wk, then twice weekly
	Estring	17β-Estradiol	Ring	Once every 90 d
	Femring	Estradiol acetate	Ring	Once every 3 mo (systemic)
	Premarin	CEE	Cream	Daily
Progestin (oral)	Aygestin	Norethindrone acetate	Tablet	Once daily
	Prometrium	Progesterone (micronized)	Capsule	Once daily
	Provera	MPA	Tablet	Once daily
Estrogen + progestin (oral)	Activella	17β-Estradiol/norethindrone acetate	Tablet	Once daily
	Angeliq	17β-Estradiol/drospirenone	Tablet	Once daily
	Femhrt	EE/norethindrone acetate	Tablet	Once daily, continuously
	Prefest	17β-Estradiol/norgestimate	Tablet	Once daily, sequentially
	Premphase	CEE/MPA	Tablet	Once daily, sequentially, cyclic
Estrogen + SERM (oral)	Duavee	CEE/bazedoxifene	Tablet	Once daily
Estrogen + progestin (transdermal)	Climara Pro	17β-Estradiol/levonorgestrel	Patch (matrix)	Once weekly
	CombiPatch	17β-Estradiol/norethindrone acetate	Patch (matrix)	Twice weekly

EE, ethinyl estradiol; CEE, conjugated equine estrogens; MPA, medroxyprogesterone acetate; SERM, selective estrogen receptor modulator.

Based on Facts and Comparisons. *Conjugated estrogens (systemic) monograph; esterified estrogens oral monograph; estropipate (piperazine estrone sulfate) oral monograph*. Accessed April 17, 2018 http://fco.factsandcomparisons.com/lco/action/doc/retrieve/docid/fc_dfc/5546102; and also based on Straight Healthcare. *Female hormone medications*. Accessed April, 2018. http://www.straighthealthcare.com/female-hormone-medications.html

CombiPatch) or EE (Femhrt). It is a prodrug and rapidly deacetylated to norethindrone after oral administration. The presence of the 17α-alkynyl group blocks metabolism to 17-ketone, increases progestational activity, and decreases androgenic activity. The absence of the 19β-methyl group increases progestational activity. 19-Nortestosterone derivatives have their primary activity as progestins but do possess some androgenic activity.

Levonorgestrel is a second-generation 19-nortestosterone derivative that possesses an 18β-ethyl instead of methyl group. It is given in combination with 17β-estradiol as a transdermal patch (Climara Pro). The 18β-ethyl group decreases androgenic activity while increasing progestational activity; however, second-generation progestins have the most androgenic activity as compared to other generations. In efforts to decrease androgenic activity, an isosteric replacement of an oxime for the 3-keto group of levonorgestrel resulted in the third-generation progestin known as norgestimate. Norgestimate is a prodrug that undergoes cleavage of 17β-ester to the active 17β-hydroxyl group in the intestine and liver. The oxime is active and able to bind to the PR for progestational activity, but it is also metabolized into the 3-keto group in the liver. Norgestimate is given in combination with 17β-estradiol (Prefest). Drospirenone is a fourth-generation progestin and is given orally in combination with 17β-estradiol (Angeliq) and does not possess androgenic activity.

Nonoral routes of administration of estrogens as single hormone replacement agents (transdermal and vaginal)

Table 25.9 Approximate Equivalent Doses of Estrogen for Postmenopausal Use

Route	Estrogen	Dose
Oral	17β-Estradiol	1.0 mg
	Conjugated equine estrogens (CEE)	0.625 mg
	Esterified estrogens	0.625 mg
	Estropipate	0.625 mg
	Ethinyl estradiol (EE)	0.005-0.015 mg
Transdermal	17β-Estradiol patch	0.05 mg
	17β-Estradiol gel	1.5 mg/2 metered doses

Based on Menopause Practice: A Clinician's Guide. 5th ed. North American Menopause Society; 2014.

offer the advantage of bypassing first-pass metabolism and are also recommended for women at increased risk for VTE.[139,140] Femring is a vaginal ring made of a central core of the prodrug 17β-estradiol acetate, which delivers a high enough dose for relief of systemic symptoms even though vaginal delivery. Vaginal atrophy can be treated with vaginal delivery of estrogens, which can relieve local or systemic side effects depending on the dose.

Selective Estrogen Receptor Modulators Used in Hormone Replacement Therapy

SERMs are nonsteroidal molecules that possess a unique pharmacology in which they behave as an ER agonist in some tissues and as an ER antagonist in other tissues. The first SERMs discovered were the ER antagonists tamoxifen and TOR that are used exclusively for the treatment of breast cancer (discussed later). However, the search for the optimal SERM continued into the early 21st century and resulted in the discovery and development of two SERMs, bazedoxifene and ospemifene, which are used in HRT.

Bazedoxifene, a third-generation SERM, is combined with CEE in an oral product (Duavee). It was approved in 2013 for the treatment of menopausal vasomotor symptoms in addition to the prevention of postmenopausal osteoporosis in women with a uterus (Fig. 25.20).[141] It is the first nonprogestin drug for use in menopausal women with an intact uterus, as usually they need to take a progestin with the estrogen. Bazedoxifene is a mixed ER agonist/antagonist that acts as an ER agonist in bone and cardiovascular system and relieves menopausal symptoms but acts as an antagonist in the breast and uterus, thus reducing the risk of endometrial hyperplasia that can occur with CEE.[141,142] The use of bazedoxifene in combination with CEE for up to 2 years has not indicated an increased risk of breast cancer.[143]

Bazedoxifene is a 2-phenylindole analog of the benzothiophene raloxifene (see "Selective Estrogen Receptor Modulators" section and Figures therein) and can be envisioned to bind similarly to ERα due to the isosteric placement of the three phenyl rings compared to *trans*-stilbenes (Fig. 25.20). Bazedoxifene undergoes extensive glucuronidation on the indole alcohol to form 5-bazedoxifene glucuronide with little to no CYP-mediated metabolism detected in plasma.[144] The concentration of the glucuronide is 10-fold higher than the unchanged drug in plasma. Because it undergoes glucuronidation by the UGT enzyme in the intestinal tract and liver, metabolism of bazedoxifene may be increased by UGT inducers (rifampin, phenobarbital, carbamazepine, phenytoin). Relief of hot flashes (both severity and frequency) was seen after 4 weeks of therapy.[145]

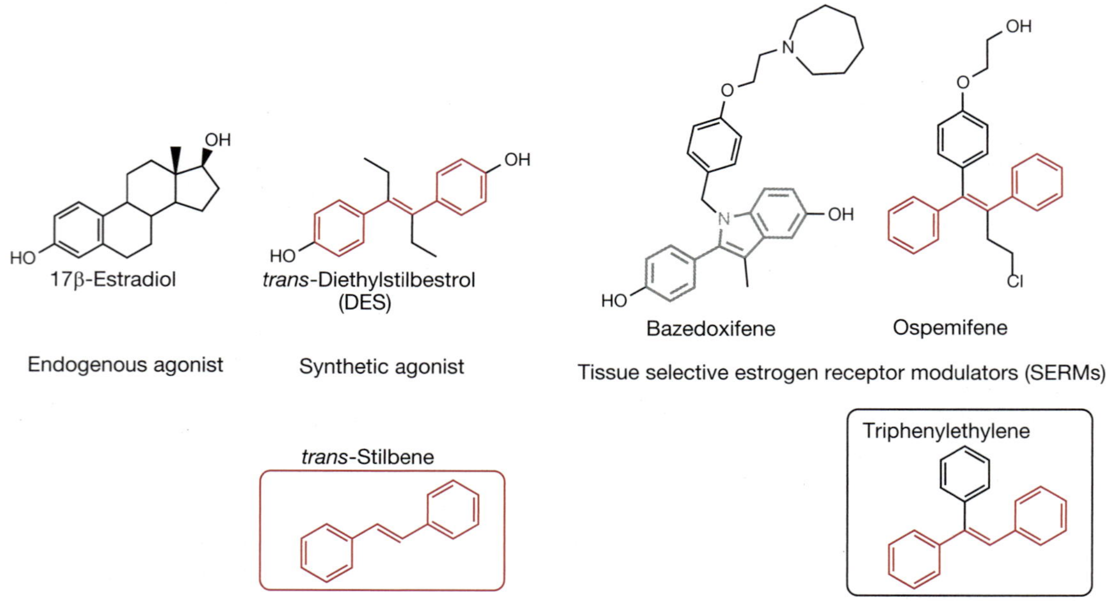

Figure 25.20 17β-Estradiol, nonsteroidal agonist DES, and two SERMs used in hormone replacement therapy. The *trans*-stilbene element of DES and triphenylethylenes like ospemifene are highlighted in red. Bazedoxifene replaces the *trans*-stilbene with a 2-phenylindole (shown in gray) moiety to bioisosterically place the hydroxyl groups of 17β-estradiol.

Bazedoxifene has poor bioavailability (~6%), has elimination half-life of 33 hours for the unchanged drug, is excreted primarily in feces (~85%), has time to peak concentration of ~2.5 hours, and is a P-glycoprotein (P-gp) substrate.[142,144] It is extensively protein bound (98%-99%) in vitro, but not to sex hormone–binding globulin (SHBG). Bazedoxifene is expected to undergo enterohepatic recycling from the gut back to systemic circulation; therefore, a decrease in its systemic exposure can be postulated if given in combination with drugs that interfere with the recycling process.[144]

In postmenopausal women, estrogen deficiency causes not only physical changes in the vagina but also thinning of vaginal secretions and vaginal tissue, reduced blood flow, and decreased elasticity and, therefore, can result in impaired sexual function due to difficult or painful sexual intercourse (dyspareunia). The symptoms of vulvar and vaginal atrophy can affect quality of life, and treatment options can include estrogen replacement therapy, HRT, vaginal moisturizers and lubricants, or SERMs. Ospemifene (Osphena, approved 2013) is a SERM recommended for postmenopausal women suffering from moderate-to-severe dyspareunia with vaginal atrophy or vaginal dryness; however, the use should be avoided if a history or suspicion of breast cancer exists.[146] Ospemifene is a triphenylethylene and a metabolite of TOR (see discussion later in this chapter). By binding to the ER, it is an agonist in vaginal epithelial tissue and stimulates endometrial tissue to relieve symptoms of dyspareunia. As it has estrogenic agonist effects in the endometrium, there is an increased risk of endometrial hyperplasia and endometrial cancer in women with a uterus who use unopposed estrogens. This risk can be decreased when a progestin is added to estrogen therapy. Ospemifene has estrogen antagonist activity in breast and uterus.

Ospemifene undergoes hepatic metabolism by CYP3A4 (major), CYP2C9 (major), and CYP2C19 (minor) to form 4-hydroxyospemifene and is excreted predominantly in feces (75%) and, to a lesser extent, in the urine (7%; <0.2% as unchanged drug). It has increased bioavailability when taken with food by 2- to 3-fold, and its peak concentration in serum occurs at ~2 hours. Ospemifene binds extensively to plasma proteins (>99%) and has a half-life of ~26 hours. Fluconazole increases serum concentrations of ospemifene. After 12 weeks of therapy, a significant decrease in vaginal dryness and dyspareunia is seen.[147]

Miscellaneous Drugs for Menopause-Related Symptoms: Prasterone and Fezolinetant

Prasterone (DHEA, Intrarosa) was approved in 2016 for the treatment of severe pain during sexual intercourse in women (dyspareunia) due to vulvar and vaginal atrophy associated with menopause. It is administered as an intravaginal insert (6.5 mg) once daily at bedtime. While the mechanism of action of prasterone is unknown, it is known that it is metabolized to testosterone and 17β-estradiol. Serum concentrations of DHEA, testosterone, and 17β-estradiol were observed to increase following vaginal administration of the drug, demonstrating 100%, 10%, and 50% higher AUC values after 7 days of daily prasterone. The role of each of these metabolites is yet to be determined in the relief of dyspareunia. Postmenopausal women with a history of breast cancer should be cautioned when using prasterone, as 17β-estradiol is a metabolite.

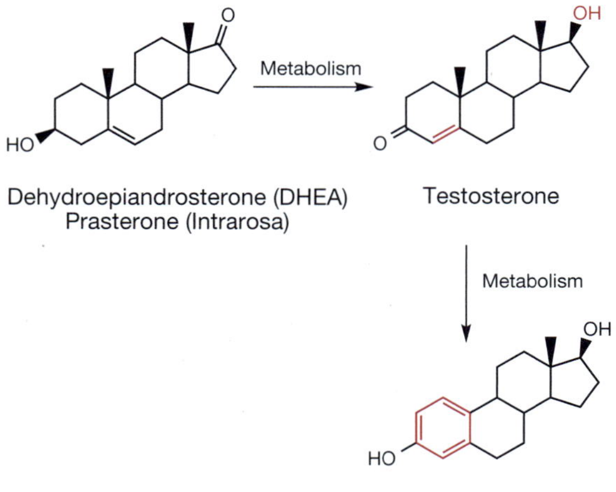

Dehydroepiandrosterone (DHEA)
Prasterone (Intrarosa)
Testosterone
17β-Estradiol

Fezolinetant (Veozah) was recently approved as a nonhormonal therapy for severe vasomotor symptoms in postmenopausal women. Fezolinetant is a neurokinin-3 (NK3) receptor antagonist that binds to NK3 receptor and inhibits neurokinin B binding on kisspeptin/neurokinin B/dynorphin neurons.[148,149] Adverse side effects include abdominal pain, diarrhea, insomnia, back pain, and elevated liver values. It is primarily excreted by kidneys.

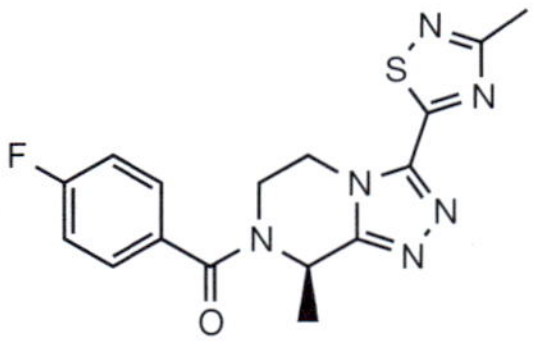

Fezolinetant
(Veozah)

Drugs Used in the Treatment of Androgen Insufficiencies

Androgens

Discovery of Androgens

One of the earliest and most unusual experiments with testicular extracts was carried out in 1889 by the French physiologist Charles Brown-Séquard. He administered such an extract to himself and reported that he felt an increased vigor and capacity for work.[150] In 1911, Pézard showed that extracts of testicular tissue increase comb growth in capons.[151] Early attempts to isolate pure male hormones from the testes failed because only small amounts are present in this tissue.

The earliest report of an isolated androgen was presented by Butenandt[152] in 1931. He isolated 15 mg of crystalline androsterone (see "Androgen Metabolism" section for structure) from 15,000 L of human male urine. A second crystalline compound, DHEA (see discussion on prasterone for structure), which has weak androgenic activity, was isolated by Butenandt and Dannenberg[153] in 1934. During the following year, testosterone was isolated from bull testes by David et al[154] This hormone was shown to be 6 to 10 times more active than androsterone.

Shortly after testosterone was isolated, Butenandt and Hanisch[155] reported its synthesis. In that same year, extracts of urine from males were shown to cause nitrogen retention (a measure of protein anabolism) as well as the expected androgenic effects.[156] Many steroids with androgenic activity have subsequently been synthesized. Steroid hormones may have many potent effects on various tissues, and slight chemical alterations of androgenic steroids may increase some of these effects without altering others.

Testosterone was the first androgen to be used clinically for its anabolic activity. Because of its androgenic action, testosterone is limited in its use in humans, especially females, as an anabolic steroid. Many steroids were synthesized in an attempt to separate the androgenic and the anabolic actions. Because testosterone had to be given parenterally, it was also desirable to find orally active agents.

Although many anabolic steroids have been synthesized and FDA approved, only testosterone, 17α-methyltestosterone, and several testosterone esters remain available in the United States for prescription use. Despite a rich exploration of the SARs of steroidal agents for the AR, most synthetic androgens have been supplanted by other classes of agents and/or withdrawn from the market by their manufacturers. Anabolic agents are also subject to abuse by athletes due to their performance-enhancing properties, contributing further to their out-of-favor status among the medical community. In the United States, most of the androgens and anabolic steroid products are subject to control by the U.S. Federal Controlled Substances Act as amended by the Anabolic Steroid Control Act of 1990 as Schedule III drugs.

Androgen Physiology

The overall physiologic effects of endogenous androgens are contributed by testosterone and its active metabolites, DHT and 17β-estradiol. Testosterone and DHT execute their actions predominantly through the AR, which belongs to the nuclear receptor superfamily and functions as a ligand-dependent transcription factor. Circulating testosterone is essential for the differentiation and growth of male accessory reproductive organs (eg, prostate and seminal vesicles), control of male sexual behavior, and the development and maintenance of male secondary characteristics that involve muscle, bone, larynx, and hair. Healthy young adult men produce approximately 3 to 10 mg of testosterone per day, with circulating serum levels ranging from approximately 500 to 1,000 ng/dL in eugonadal (normal) men. Circulating testosterone and 17β-estradiol participate in the feedback regulation of androgen production by the HPG axis, as shown in Figure 25.21. Testosterone, LH, and GnRH (also known as LHRH) constitute the elements of a negative feedback control mechanism, whereby testosterone controls its own release. Low circulating testosterone levels increase the

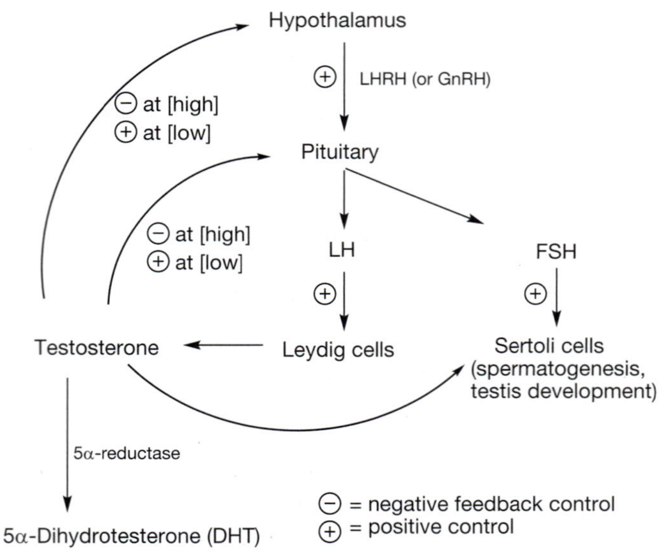

Figure 25.21 Hypothalamic-pituitary-testicular axis. FSH, follicle-stimulating hormone; LH, luteinizing hormone.

hypothalamic secretion of GnRH, which leads to increased production of LH and, consequently, increased testosterone production by the Leydig cells. More than 95% of circulating testosterone is synthesized and secreted by the Leydig cells in the testes. GnRH is released from the hypothalamus in short, intermittent pulses every 2 hours and at greater magnitude in the morning, which, in turn, stimulates the pulsatile secretion of LH and FSH from the pituitary. Thus, testosterone secretion likewise is pulsatile and diurnal, with the highest concentration occurring at approximately 8:00 AM and the lowest at approximately 8:00 PM.

In the testis, FSH directly interacts with FSH receptors expressed in Sertoli cells and stimulates spermatogenesis, whereas LH indirectly stimulates spermatogenesis through testosterone synthesized by Leydig cells. Testosterone and its aromatized metabolite (17β-estradiol) negatively regulate circulating levels of testosterone by their actions in the hypothalamus and pituitary. Activin and inhibin produced by Sertoli cells stimulate or inhibit, respectively, the secretion of FSH from the pituitary.[157] High concentrations of intratesticular testosterone are essential for the initiation and maintenance of spermatogenesis, as evidenced by the infertility of hypogonadal men. Results from both animal models and humans, however, support the idea that both FSH and testosterone are required to achieve quantitative and qualitative spermatogenesis.

In older men, especially those older than age 60 years, testosterone levels often remain relatively constant, without the morning pulses observed in young adult men. Average serum testosterone concentrations in older men peak in the morning, with daily ranges of approximately 300 to 550 ng/dL by age 70 years. The diurnal cycling is blunted as men age.[158] In women, testosterone levels range from 15 to 100 ng/dL. Starting at approximately age 40 years, testosterone levels drop by approximately 10% every decade in men. In the normal functioning of the male hormonal system, 97% to 98% of plasma testosterone is bound to SHBG, essentially making it unavailable to the body's tissues due to the high binding affinity of testosterone for SHBG. The remaining 2% to 3% is known as "bioavailable" or free testosterone. Serum concentrations of SHBG increase with age in men, resulting in a corresponding decrease in free testosterone as men age. Free testosterone levels in serum are positively correlated with muscle strength and BMD in older adults but negatively correlated with fat mass.[159]

Androgens also are needed for the development of secondary sex characteristics. The male voice deepens because of thickening of the laryngeal mucosa and lengthening of the vocal cords. In both men and women, they play a role first in stimulating the growth of hair on the face, arms, legs, and pubic areas and later in the recession of the male hairline. The fructose content of human semen and both the size and secretory capacity of the sebaceous glands also depend on the levels of testosterone.

Testosterone causes nitrogen retention by increasing the rate of protein synthesis and muscle mass while decreasing the rate of protein catabolism. The positive nitrogen balance, therefore, results from both decreased catabolism and increased anabolism of proteins that are used in male sex accessory apparatus and muscle. The actions of androgen in the reproductive tissues, including prostate, seminal vesicle, testis, and accessory structures, are known as the androgenic effects, whereas the nitrogen-retaining effects of androgen in muscle and bone are known as the anabolic effects. Although the precise mechanism of androgen action on muscle remains unknown, the common hypothesis is that testosterone directly promotes muscle protein synthesis, as evidenced by the lack of effects of dutasteride, a 5AR inhibitor (5ARI), on muscle mass in healthy men when coadministered with testosterone.[160] Evidence supports the idea that testosterone supplementation increases muscle protein synthesis in men.[161] Also, androgen-induced increases in muscle mass appear to arise from muscle fiber hypertrophy rather than hyperplasia (ie, cellular enlargement rather than cellular proliferation).[162]

The thickness and linear growth of bones are stimulated and later limited by testosterone because of closure of the epiphyses. Androgens affect BMD by changing overall osteoblast (bone-forming cell) activity and osteoclast (bone-resorbing cell) activity, resulting from changes in the total number of each cell type and individual cell functional capacity.[163,164] Androgens seem to have the ability to decelerate the bone remodeling cycle and tilt the focal balance of that cycle toward bone formation. The loss of androgens is thought to increase the rate of bone remodeling by removing the restraining effects on osteoblastogenesis and osteoclastogenesis.

Mechanisms of Androgen Action

Testosterone, DHT, and other androgens execute their actions predominantly through the AR. The AR is mainly expressed in androgen target tissues, such as the prostate, skeletal muscle, liver, and CNS, with the highest expression level being observed in the prostate, adrenal gland, and epididymis.[165] Testosterone is thought to be largely responsible for initiation of AR action in muscle, bone, brain, and bone marrow, whereas DHT plays a major role in genitalia, prostate, skin, and hair follicles due to the higher expression of 5AR enzymes. The mechanism of action of the AR is similar to that of the other nuclear receptors and has been described in detail in Chapter 7.

Besides the genomic pathway, the nongenomic pathway of AR has also been reported in oocytes,[166] skeletal muscle cells,[167] osteoblasts,[168,169] and prostate cancer cells.[170,171] As compared to the genomic pathway, the nongenomic actions of steroid receptors are characterized by the rapidity of the action, which varies from seconds to an hour or so, and by interaction with plasma membrane–associated signaling pathways.[172] Nevertheless, the structural basis for nongenomic action is direct interactions between AR and cytosolic proteins from different signaling pathways, which could be closely related to the ligand-induced conformational change of the LBD or, indirectly, the N-terminal domain. Functionally, the nongenomic action of androgens involves either rapid activation of kinase signaling cascades or modulation of intracellular calcium levels, which could be related to stimulation of gap junction communication, neuronal plasticity, and aortic relaxation.[173] Separation of the genomic and nongenomic functions of steroid receptors using specific ligands was also proposed as a strategy to achieve tissue selectivity.[172,174]

In the past decade, splice variants of AR (AR-SVs) have gained attention due to their oncogenic role in advanced prostate cancer.[175] Patients who have been treated with antiandrogens or inhibitors of the AR axis express AR-SVs, and the expression correlates with an aggressive phenotype and shorter progression-free and overall survival. Considering that the AR-SVs lack LBD, the AR-SVs cannot be inhibited by LBD-binding AR antagonists, making the cancers expressing AR-SVs hard to treat. The response of patients expressing AR-SVs to chemotherapy has also been inconsistent.[176,177]

Male Hypogonadism

Male hypogonadism (testosterone deficiency) is the inability of the testes to produce sufficient testosterone to maintain sexual function, muscle strength, BMD, and fertility (spermatogenesis). Primary hypogonadism refers to a disorder of the testes, wherein LH and/or FSH are elevated and the testes fail to produce sufficient testosterone. LH and FSH levels are generally normal or low in men classified as having secondary hypogonadism, indicating that the problem resides in the brain (ie, hypothalamic-pituitary failure to stimulate testicles to produce testosterone). Klinefelter syndrome (a chromosomal abnormality resulting in testicular dysfunction), cryptorchidism (failure of the testes to descend), and/or physical damage (eg, torsion) are disorders associated with very low or absent serum testosterone levels.

Aging-related androgen insufficiency is a physiologic condition characterized by the inability of the testes to produce sufficient testosterone as men age, resulting in deficits in sexual function, muscle strength, BMD, and fertility (spermatogenesis). One in five men older than 50 years will exhibit symptoms of this condition. In men, there is a gradual decline of approximately 1% per year in the production of testosterone beginning around age 40 years. For most men, testosterone levels naturally decline with advancing age but still remain within the physiologic range throughout their lifetimes, causing no significant problems. Approximately 20% of men older than age 60 years and 30% to 40% of men older than 80 years have plasma testosterone levels indicative of hypogonadism (<280-300 ng/dL). Symptoms of aging-related androgen insufficiency may include lethargy or decreased energy, decreased libido or interest in sex, ED, muscle weakness and aches, inability to sleep, hot flashes, night sweats, depression, infertility, thinning of bones or bone loss, and cardiovascular disease. Studies show that a decline in testosterone actually can put men at risk for other health problems, such as heart disease, metabolic syndrome, and weak bones. Psychological stress, alcohol abuse, injuries or surgery, medications, obesity and infections, tobacco, and drugs, such as decongestants, antihypertensives, tranquilizers, statins, or antiseizure agents, can contribute to the onset of these conditions. There is no way of predicting who will experience the symptoms of androgen insufficiency that are of sufficient severity to seek medical help; neither is it predictable at what age the symptoms of aging-related androgen insufficiency will occur in a particular individual. Each individual's symptoms may also be different. Because all this happens at a time of life when many men begin to question their values, accomplishments, and direction in life, it is often difficult to realize that the changes occurring are related to more than just external conditions. Now that men are living longer, there is heightened interest in aging-related androgen insufficiency, its risks for other health problems, and its treatment.

Testosterone and structurally related steroidal androgens have been used for decades to treat male hypogonadism, Klinefelter syndrome, anemia secondary to chronic renal failure, aplastic anemia, protein wasting diseases associated with cancer, burns, traumas, acquired immunodeficiency syndrome (AIDS), short stature, breast cancer (as an antiestrogen), and hereditary angioedema. However, many of the synthetic anabolic steroid agents have been discontinued such that their use for wasting conditions, anemia, and cancer is no longer possible. This is partially due to not only serious hepatotoxicity and poor public image of anabolic steroids as drugs of abuse but also the recent development of more effective therapies (eg, erythropoietin, aromatase inhibitors [AIs], and taxanes) leading to decreased demand for synthetic anabolic steroids.

An area where a variety of formulations of testosterone and testosterone esters still find increasing use is testosterone replacement in hypogonadal men. Although severe hypogonadism is uncommon, aging-related androgen insufficiency is much more frequent. Low endogenous testosterone concentrations are associated with sarcopenia and frailty arising from decreased fat-free mass, lessened muscle strength, and reduced BMD (osteoporosis). Low testosterone concentrations are also associated with decreased sexual libido and ED. More than 30 million men older than 40 years in the United States are estimated to have ED. Although androgens are not essential for erection,[178] transdermal and IM testosterone replacement therapy (TRT) is often employed in hypogonadal men with ED.[179] Furthermore, selective phosphodiesterase type 5 inhibitors (PDE5Is) that increase penile blood flow are considered to be the treatment of choice for men with ED. HRT with testosterone in aging men also improves body composition, bone and cartilage metabolism, and memory and cognition, and it even decreases cardiovascular risk.[180]

Testosterone Replacement Therapy

The acceptance of TRT has been hampered by the lack of orally active preparations with good efficacy and, particularly, a safe profile.[181] Progress has been limited over the past three decades in developing synthetic molecules that could separate the desirable physiologic functions normally regulated by endogenous androgens from the undesirable or dose-limiting side effects. The abuse of synthetic anabolic steroids by athletes and body builders has contributed to the general perception of certain undesirable side effects, such as aggressive behavior, liver toxicity, acne, or impotency.

Current formulations for TRT largely include IM or SC injectable formulations of testosterone esters, transdermal delivery formulations (scrotal or nonscrotal patches, gels, topical solution, and pellet implants), buccal or nasal mucosal delivery formulations, and, recently, several lipid matrix-assisted oral formulations of testosterone undecanoate. Marketed injectable forms of testosterone esters (eg, testosterone enanthate, cypionate, and undecanoate) can produce undesirable fluctuations in testosterone blood levels, with supraphysiologic concentrations early and subphysiologic levels toward the end of the period before the next injection. These fluctuations provide an unsatisfactory benefits profile and, in some cases, undesired side effects. Skin patches provide a better blood-level profile of testosterone, but skin irritation and daily application limit the usefulness and acceptability of this form of therapy. Topical gels are widely used for TRT but must be cautiously used in homes with children due to the risk of virilization. Oral preparations such as fluoxymesterone and 17α-methyltestosterone (structures are discussed later) are only sparingly used because of concerns about liver toxicity linked to the 17α-alkyl group and because of somewhat lower efficacy.[181] Thus, these oral androgens are generally considered to be obsolete and do not represent a viable form of therapy.

Benefits and Risks of Testosterone Replacement Therapy

Multiple large-scale and long-term clinical trials of TRT have been conducted in aging men to evaluate the risk-benefit ratio, but no agreement exists (Table 25.10) (for review, see Hijazi and Cunningham[182] and Rhoden and Morgentaler[181]). The potential benefits of TRT include an increase in BMD and improvement in muscle mass and strength, cognitive function, mood, and sexual function. The potential risks of TRT, however, including those in the cardiovascular system, blood (eg, hematocrit and hemoglobin levels), and prostate, are routinely experienced. Because the long-term effects of TRT in otherwise healthy men remain unclear, guidelines published by the Endocrine Society recommend a general policy that TRT not be offered to older men with low serum testosterone levels and that TRT only be used in men with clinically significant symptoms of androgen deficiency and serum total testosterone concentrations approaching 200 ng/dL.[183]

Table 25.10 Testosterone Replacement Therapy

Benefits	Risks
Improved sexual performance and desire	Stimulated growth of preexisting prostate cancer
More energy and improved quality of life	Greater chance for benign prostatic hyperplasia
More energy and sense of well-being	Increased hemoglobin levels to above the physiologic range
Increased bone mineral density	Problems with voiding; symptoms include poor urine flow and hesitancy before urinating
Improved muscle mass and strength	
Improved (lower) low-density lipoprotein profile	Increased potential for liver damage from oral preparations Sleep apnea (stopping of breathing during sleep)
Decreased irritability and depression	Breast tenderness and swelling (gynecomastia)
Improved cognitive function	Testicular shrinkage (testicular atrophy)
Increased hemoglobin levels to the physiologic range	Infertility (decreased spermatogenesis) Skin reaction from patches or gel
Thickened body hair and skin	Pain, soreness, or bruising from injection Increased fluid retention Increased skin problems (acne, oily skin) Increased body hair

Clearly, TRT is beneficial for hypogonadal men with androgen insufficiency to restore sexual function and muscle strength, to prevent bone loss, and to protect against heart disease (atherosclerosis).[181] Increasing testosterone levels with TRT, however, may pose problems by stimulating the growth of the prostate. Long-term TRT could cause prostate gland enlargement, which might exacerbate BPH or fuel the growth of prostate cancer that is already present and could cause breast enlargement in men (gynecomastia). This is especially worrisome because of the high prevalence of BPH in older men and the possibility that many men may have prostate cancer that is undiagnosed. In fact, men with a palpable prostate nodule, a prostate-specific antigen (PSA) level greater than 4 ng/mL, or severe lower urinary tract symptoms (LUTSs) associated with BPH are usually advised to avoid TRT.

In older men, testosterone effects on muscle mass and strength have not been consistent or impressive, possibly because of the low dosages used in clinical trials. The high correlation between the dose (and serum concentration) and the anabolic actions of androgen in muscle suggests that androgen administration of higher doses in older men may significantly increase muscle mass and strength, but high doses might increase the adverse effects and the aromatization of testosterone to estrogen.[184]

Types of Testosterone Replacement Therapy

Several types of TRT exist. Choosing a specific therapy depends on the patient's preference of a particular delivery system, the side effects, and the cost. Types include injection, transdermal, buccal mucosal, and oral (Table 25.11).

INJECTION. Orally administered testosterone is ineffective in the treatment of male androgen insufficiency syndromes due to extensive presystemic first-pass metabolism. IM injections bypass the problems of first-pass metabolism. IM injections are depot formulations of testosterone esters that undergo differing rates of in vivo ester hydrolysis to release free testosterone over an extended period of time. Typically, the depot esters are administered IM into a large muscle once every 2 to 4 weeks depending on the depot ester used (Table 25.11). They are safe, effective, and the least expensive androgen preparations available. Besides being painful, the major disadvantage with the IM route for the depot esters is that testosterone serum concentrations exhibit a saw-toothed pattern, with supraphysiologic levels within 2 to 4 days following the IM injection and subphysiologic levels before the next injection. This can lead to fluctuation in mood and libido and increased risk of polycythemia. A more satisfactory physiologic replacement therapy without the fluctuations in free testosterone serum levels would be to administer a lower IM dose (ie, 100 mg) on a weekly or biweekly schedule. IM injection of testosterone or its esters causes local irritation. The rate of absorption for IM products may be erratic.

Esters of testosterone prepared for IM administration include the 17β-propionate, 17β-enanthate, and the cypionate (17β-cyclopentylpropionate) (Fig. 25.22). Testosterone enanthate (not currently available) and cypionate demonstrate comparable pharmacokinetics. Testosterone enanthate is formed by esterification of the 17β-hydroxy group of testosterone with heptanoic acid, while testosterone cypionate is formed with cyclopentane propionic acid. Sterile solutions of these esters are available in a suitable vegetable oil, such as cottonseed oil. Unlike oral testosterone, with a half-life of 10 to 100 minutes, IM testosterone administration avoids first-pass metabolism and exhibits a longer duration due to

Table 25.11 Testosterone Products and Properties

Product	Trade Name	Onset of Peak Response	Duration of Action	Time to Peak Conc.	Time to Steady-State Conc.	Dose (mg)	Frequency of Dosing	Oral Bioavailability (%)	Elimination Half-life
Methyltestosterone	Android Testred Virilon Oreton Methyl	—	24 h	2 h	—	10-50	Daily	70	3 h
Testosterone undecanoate	Jatenzo (po) Tlando (po)	6 h	12 h	2-6 h	—	150-250	Twice daily	~3	3 h
Testosterone cypionate	Depo-Testosterone	6-24 h (IM)	2-4 wk	24 h	—	50-400	2-4 wk	—	8 d
Testosterone enanthate	Andro-LA Andryl Delatestryl Delatest Everone Testamon Xyosted (SC)	6-24 h (IM)	2-4 wk (IM)	24 h (IM); 12 h (SC)	—	50-400 (IM); 50-100 (SC)	2-4 wk (IM); Weekly (SC)	—	8 d (IM)
Testosterone pellets	Testopel	1-2 mo	3-6 mo	1 mo	1-2 wk	150-450	3-6 mo	—	—
Testosterone solution	Axiron	14 d	24 h	2-4 h	14 d	60	24	—	—
Transdermal patches	Androderm	3-6 mo	24 h	2-4 h	2-3 d	2-5	24 h	—	10-100 min
Transdermal gels	AndroGel Fortesta Testim Vogelxo	3-6 mo	5 d	4 (2-6) h	2-3 d	50-100	24 h	—	10-100 min
Testosterone nasal gel	Natesto	<1 mo	4-6 h	40 min	2-3 d	11	Thrice daily	—	10-100 min
Buccal mucosal	Striant	—	24 h	5 (0.5-12) h	2-3 d	30	Every 12 h	—	6 h

IM, intramuscular; PO, orally; SC, subcutaneous.

From Thompson Healthcare, Inc. Micromedex healthcare series. http://www.Thompsonhc.com

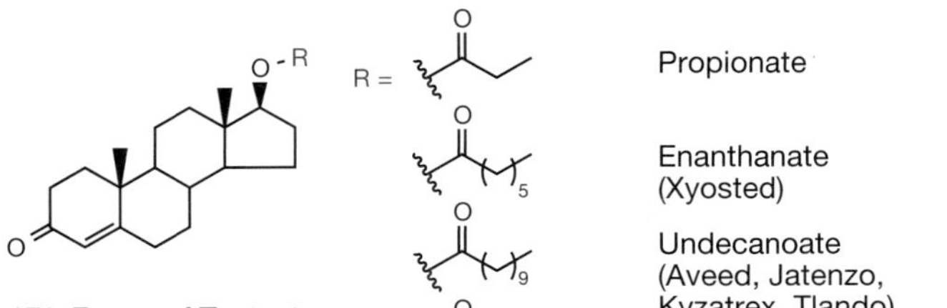

17β-Esters of Testosterone (prodrug)

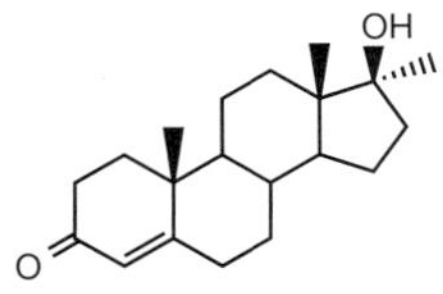

17α-Methyltestosterone

Figure 25.22 Androgenic derivatives of testosterone.

the slow hydrolysis and release of testosterone from the depot injection site. Generally, the concentration of SHBG in plasma determines the distribution of testosterone between free and bound forms. The bulky cypionate and enanthate esters of testosterone have durations of action of up to 2 to 4 weeks, whereas the shorter propionate ester (not currently available) has a shorter duration of action of 1 to 2 weeks. Doses may be adjusted by aiming for midphysiologic (400-600 ng/dL) testosterone values after 1 week or at the low end (300-400 ng/dL) just before the next injection is due.

An SC option of testosterone enanthate (Xyosted) was approved in 2017 as a 50, 75, or 100 mg per 0.5 mL autoinjection given once weekly. Advantages compared to IM formulations include less painful injections and fewer fluctuations in testosterone levels compared with IM; however, it is more expensive and reportedly can increase blood pressure.

IMPLANT. SC implantation of testosterone pellets (Testopel) is much less flexible for dose adjustment as compared to transdermal, oral, or IM injection. Fat-soluble pellets containing 75 mg of testosterone can be implanted SC on the anterior abdominal wall or buttocks to deliver testosterone over a 3- to 4-month period. Recommended doses range from 150 to 450 mg implanted SC every 3 to 6 months. The longer duration of action of the pellets is accompanied by a larger dose requirement as compared to weekly or biweekly IM injections. Approximately one-third of the material from the pellet is absorbed in the first month, one-fourth in the second month, and one-sixth in the third month. Adequate effects from the pellets can occasionally continue for as long as 6 months.

TRANSDERMAL. Transdermal TRT systems are, perhaps, the most commonly used systems for delivering testosterone to bypass the rapid first-pass metabolism associated with oral testosterone. Clinical studies have shown that these formulations are effective forms of testosterone replacement, with peak response within 3 to 6 months. The use of the transdermal formulation should be discontinued if the desired response is not reached within this time period. Skin irritation is more common with the transdermal formulations, with more than 50% experiencing some form of skin irritation at some point during the treatment. Pretreatment with corticosteroid creams (not with the ointment) has been shown to reduce the severity and incidence of skin irritation without significantly affecting testosterone absorption from the formulation. With the transdermal formulations, testosterone levels are maintained within physiologic values, and a beneficial effect on general mood and sexual functioning is generally observed. A serum concentration in the midphysiologic range (400-600 ng/dL) is the goal.

Matrix-Type Transdermal Systems. This type of patch (scrotal patch; Testoderm) must be applied to dry, clean (shaven) scrotal skin, which is 5 to 30 times more permeable to testosterone than other skin sites, every 24 hours to produce an adequate testosterone plasma concentration. The matrix system is described as a "drug-in-adhesive film," in which the drug is located on the adhesive layer of the film; thus, it is thinner and less bulky than the reservoir system. The advantage of the matrix system is that it produces supraphysiologic levels of DHT because of the high 5AR enzyme activity of the scrotal tissue. The patches have an occlusive backing that prevents sex partners from coming in contact with the active drug. A matrix transdermal system will not produce adequate serum testosterone concentrations if applied to nonscrotal skin. Serum testosterone concentrations are reached in approximately 2 to 4 hours. Although testosterone is absorbed throughout a 24-hour period, concentrations do not simulate the circadian rhythm of endogenous testosterone in normal (eugonadal) males. Within 24 hours after application of the matrix system, serum testosterone concentration gradually falls to 60% to 80% of the peak concentration, and when the system is removed, testosterone serum concentration declines to baseline within 2 hours. Inadequate scrotal size and adherence problems are limitations. Skin irritation does occur in those with sensitive scrotal skin.

Reservoir-Type Transdermal Systems. Reservoir-type patches (nonscrotal patch; Androderm, Testoderm TTS) are not applied to scrotal skin but, rather, to the abdomen, back, thighs, or upper arms every 24 hours (see Table 25.11 for dosage strengths). This type of patch is membrane controlled for the drug to diffuse continuously over 24 hours from the reservoir into the skin. Thus, this type of patch is thicker than the matrix (scrotal) patch. The patches have an occlusive backing that prevents sex partners from coming in contact with the active drug. The site of the application is rotated at 7-day intervals between applications to lessen skin reactions at the same application site. The advantage of the reservoir transdermal system is that it achieves normal testosterone circadian rhythm as seen in younger men, peaking in the morning and decreasing throughout the rest of the day. The reservoir-type patch, when applied to nonscrotal skin, produced physiologic DHT and 17β-estradiol serum concentrations. Steady-state serum concentrations of testosterone, which are approximately 10 times baseline values, are reached in about 6 hours (range, 4-10 hours depending on patch application location), which then fall to 60% to 80% of the peak serum concentration within 24 hours after application of the transdermal system. Thus, physiologic serum testosterone concentrations are maintained over 24 hours with this type of patch. Drug accumulation does not occur with repeated applications. When the system is removed, testosterone serum concentrations decline to baseline within 2 hours. A usual dose for the reservoir-type transdermal results in the systemic absorption of 2 to 10 mg daily in hypogonadal men.

Topical Solution. Topical testosterone solutions are also approved for TRT. For example, Axiron (Accurx Pharma; approved in 2010 but subsequently discontinued) delivered 30 mg per pump actuation applied to each axilla (60-mg total dose) once daily at the same time in the morning. This topical application allowed for dose decreases (30 mg or one actuation) or increases (90 or 120 mg via three or four actuations) based on serum testosterone concentration. On the skin, the ethanol and isopropyl alcohol evaporate, leaving testosterone and octisalate (a photostabilizer used in many sunscreens). The skin acts as a reservoir from which testosterone is released into the systemic circulation over time. In general, steady-state serum concentrations are achieved by approximately 14 days of daily dosing. Topical solutions present the risk of transfer of testosterone to household contacts (131% increased testosterone AUC with intentional skin-to-skin contact), which may be mitigated by the use of axillary application and wearing of a T-shirt after application (13% increased testosterone AUC with intentional contact through a T-shirt). Though Axiron has been discontinued, multiple generic topical solutions of testosterone are still available.[185]

Gels. Testosterone gel (AndroGel, Testim, Fortesta, and generics) is a 1% testosterone hydroalcoholic gel that provides continuous transdermal delivery of testosterone for 24 hours once the gel is rubbed into the skin on the lower abdomen, upper arm, or shoulder. It should not be applied to scrotal tissue (Table 25.11). Because there is a continuous release of testosterone over 24 hours, the normal circadian rhythm is not observed. As the gel dries, approximately 10% of the testosterone is absorbed through the skin. Gel application of TRT appears to cause fewer skin reactions than those that occur with the patches. Men should avoid showering or bathing for several hours after an application to ensure adequate absorption. A potential side effect of the gel is the possibility of transferring the medication to a partner; Skin-to-skin contact should be avoided either until the gel is completely dry or by covering the area after an application. Skin-to-skin contact with children is of particular concern and is included as a black box warning for these products. Following the application of 5 g of gel, which will deliver 50 mg of testosterone, the mean peak testosterone concentrations are reached in approximately 2 hours, which are about 2 to 3 times the baseline values. For optimum results, the gel is best applied in the evening to allow maximum concentration to occur early in the morning hours. Doses of the gel may be adjusted by aiming for mid-physiologic (400-600 ng/dL) testosterone values after 1 week. When the gel treatment is discontinued, plasma testosterone levels remain in the physiologic range for 24 to 48 hours, then return to their pretreatment levels within 5 days following the last application. An increase in serum testosterone can be observed within 30 minutes of application. Serum concentrations approximate the steady-state level by the end of the first 24 hours and are at steady state by the second or third day of dosing.

NASAL GEL. Natesto is a metered-dose nasal gel that supplies 5.5 mg of testosterone per 0.122 g intranasal actuation. The drug is given by two actuations, one per nostril, 3 times a day to provide physiologic amounts of testosterone to the systemic circulation. Reportedly, some patients found thrice-daily nasal gels more convenient than once-daily transdermal gels. Testosterone levels should be monitored by 1 month after initiation. If the testosterone levels are consistently below 300 ng/dL or above 1,050 ng/dL, then Natesto should be discontinued, and alternative TRT considered. Natesto is not recommended for patients younger than 18 or older than 65 years, or in patients with chronic nasal conditions or altered nasal anatomy (nasal/sinus surgery or mucosal inflammatory disorders). The maximum concentration for Natesto is achieved rapidly at approximately 1 hour after administration and returns to predose levels by 4 to 6 hours (half-life from 10 to 100 minutes). The unique, pulsatile pharmacokinetic profile is believed to have limited impact on the HPG axis, with substantial trough time preserving LH, FSH, and endogenous testosterone production.[186] In clinical studies, 90% of hypogonadal patients ($N = 73$) had a C_{avg} within the normal range (300-1,050 ng/dL) on day 90 of Natesto administration as described earlier. However, some adverse effects seen may be related to the nasal site of application, such as runny nose, nosebleeds, nose pain, sore throat, cough, and sinus infection.

BUCCAL MUCOSAL. Striant is a gel-like drug product that adheres to the gumline, which softens to deliver physiologic amounts of testosterone to the systemic circulation, thereby producing circulating testosterone concentrations in hypogonadal males that approximate physiologic levels seen in healthy young men (400-700 ng/dL). One buccal system (30 mg) is applied to the gum region bid, morning and evening, approximately 12 hours apart. Because there is a continuous release of testosterone over 24 hours, the normal circadian rhythm is not observed. Peak serum testosterone concentrations are reached within 10 to 12 hours and are stable within a few days of initiating the buccal preparation. The buccal preparation is difficult for patients to get used to, because the side effects may include gum irritation or pain, bitter taste, and headache. A study found that this form of TRT delivers a steadier dose of testosterone throughout the day without significant adverse effects, comparable to the gel.

ORAL. Orally administered testosterone is ineffective in the treatment of male androgen deficiency syndromes because of extensive presystemic first-pass metabolism, primarily to inactive 17-ketosteroids, etiocholanolone and androsterone, and androstenediol (not shown) metabolites in the GI mucosa during absorption and in the liver (Fig. 25.23). Oral administration is generally thought to result in supraphysiologic elevations and undesirable variability in serum testosterone and DHT concentrations. The serum half-life of testosterone is less than 30 minutes. Generally, the amount of SHBG determines the distribution of testosterone between free and bound forms. Approximately 90% of a dose

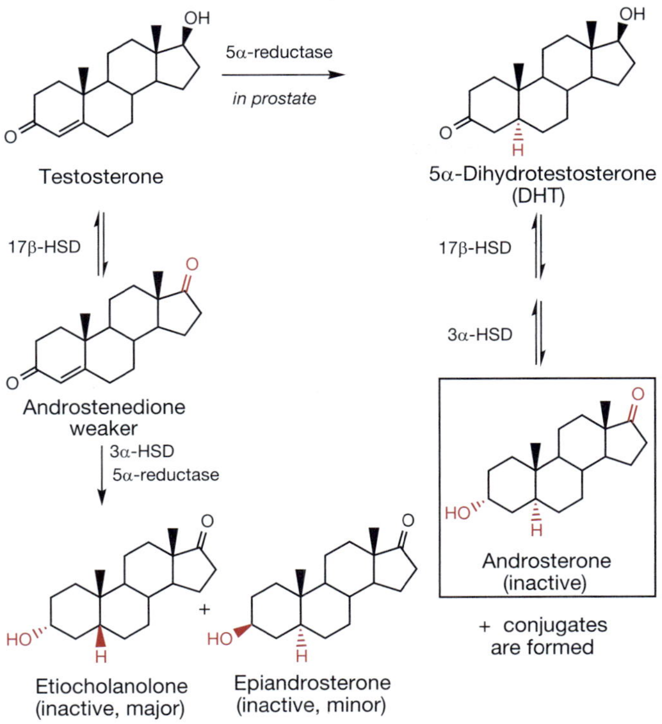

Figure 25.23 Testosterone metabolism. HSD, hydroxysteroid dehydrogenase.

of testosterone is metabolized, and its metabolites are excreted in the urine primarily as glucuronide conjugates, with approximately 6% of a dose being excreted in the feces as unmetabolized testosterone. Comparative dosage ranges for testosterone and its currently available synthetic preparations are shown in Table 25.11. Taking testosterone orally (Android, Testred), in the form of methyltestosterone, is not recommended for long-term replacement. Oral testosterone may cause an unfavorable cholesterol profile and increase the risk of blood clots and heart and liver problems.

The androgenic activity of lipophilic long-chain ester testosterone 17β-undecanoate (Andriol, Jatenzo, Kyzatrex, Tlando) (Fig. 25.22) has been attributed to the formation of testosterone via systemic ester hydrolysis of lymphatically transported testosterone undecanoate.[187] Its oral bioavailability was approximately 3%. Lymphatically transported testosterone undecanoate accounted for between 90% and 100% of the systemically available ester, and 83% to 85% of the systemically available testosterone resulted from systemic hydrolysis of lymphatically transported testosterone undecanoate. These data demonstrate that intestinal lymphatic transport of testosterone undecanoate produces increased systemic exposure of testosterone by avoiding the extensive first-pass hepatic metabolism responsible for the inactivation of testosterone after oral administration.

New oral formulations of testosterone undecanoate have recently been approved, presenting an opportunity for oral TRT. Lymphatic uptake is enhanced by the use of novel lipid matrices within the dosage form to enhance oral bioavailability. These novel formulations enjoy the convenience of bid oral dosing, allowing easy reversibility and no risk of transmission of testosterone to household contacts. However, these formulations are expensive, have food-dependent absorption, GI side effects (nausea and diarrhea), and a consistent but mild hypertensive effect (~5-10 mm Hg). Considerably lower liver toxicity is a major advantage compared to previous oral formulations of testosterone and its 17α-alkylated synthetic derivatives (discussed next).[188]

Synthetic Derivatives of Testosterone

Some of the early studies with androgens included structural modifications of the naturally occurring hormones to avoid first-pass metabolism. Blocking the metabolism of the 17β-hydroxy group with substituents in the 17α-position resulted in androgens with an increased bioavailability and duration of action when given orally. Although many synthetic steroidal androgens have been synthesized, tested, and approved, as discussed in the "Structure-Activity Relationships of Steroidal Androgens" section, currently only methyltestosterone (Fig. 25.22) and various 17β-esters remain available from legal sources in the United States. The long-term use of 17α-alkylated oral androgens has been associated with hepatotoxic effects, including cholestasis, transient hepatitis, and liver cancer.

The synthesis of 17α-methyltestosterone made available a compound that was orally active[189] in daily doses between 10 and 50 mg (Android, Testred), which achieves serum concentrations similar to a 400-mg oral dose of testosterone. Unfortunately, 17α-methyltestosterone is the only synthetic steroid not currently withdrawn from the market. The presence of a 17α-alkyl group reduces susceptibility to hepatic oxidative metabolism, thereby increasing oral bioavailability (~70%). Following oral administration, methyltestosterone is well absorbed from the GI tract, with a half-life of approximately 3 hours. This drug has the androgenic and anabolic activities of testosterone. Although orally active, it is more effective when administered sublingually. The alkylated oral androgens are seldom used due to their potential hepatotoxicity.

Adverse Effects

TRT can have undesirable side effects depending on the type of delivery system used. The adverse effects from oral testosterone include stomach upset, headache, acne, increased hair growth on the face or body, jaundice (liver toxicity), anxiety, change in sex drive, sleeplessness, increased urination, depression, enlargement of breasts, and increased frequency and duration of erections.[181,183,184] Breast enlargement can develop because the exogenous testosterone may lead to increased conversion to 17β-estradiol via aromatase. Other adverse effects include water retention, liver toxicity, cardiovascular disease, sleep apnea, and prostate enlargement. These risks are relatively uncommon when the dosage is closely monitored to maintain physiologic serum testosterone concentrations. TRT is contraindicated in men with carcinoma of the breast or with known or suspected BPH or carcinoma of the prostate. Therefore, pretreatment screening for any prostate dysfunction is mandatory before starting TRT.

Structure-Activity Relationships of Steroidal Androgens (Mostly Discontinued)

Most of the synthetic steroidal androgens in this section were discontinued from use; however, the AR remains a viable target for clinical therapy, and its SAR is discussed here as it may find novel clinical applications in the future. Complete dissociation of anabolic and androgenic effects has not been reported with a steroidal nucleus, and many of the actions of anabolic steroids are similar to those of endogenous androgens. Until the discovery of nonsteroidal androgens (discussed later for SARMs and antiandrogens), it was believed that a substance must contain a steroid skeleton to have androgenic activity.[190] Oxygen functional groups normally occurring at positions 3 and 17 of the steroid ring system are not essential, because the basic nucleus, 5α-androstane, has androgenic activity. This appears to be the minimal structural requirement for hormonal activity of steroids. For derivatives of etiocholane, in which the hydrogen is in the 5β-position, thereby affording a *cis* A/B ring juncture, no active androgens and anabolic agents are known.[190] Generally, ring expansion (to form homo derivatives by inserting a methylene group into one of the rings in the steroid nucleus) or ring contraction (by removing a methylene group) significantly reduces or destroys the androgenic and anabolic activities.

Introduction of a 3-ketone function or a 3α-OH group enhances androgenic activity. A hydroxyl group in the 17α-position of androstane contributes no androgenic or anabolic activity. Importantly, no known substituent can approach the effectiveness of a 17β-OH group. Evidence indicates that the longer acting esters (still used clinically as discussed) of the 17β-OH compounds are hydrolyzed in vivo to the free alcohol, which is the active species. The 17β-oxygen atom is important for attachment to the receptor site, while 17α-alkyl groups are important for preventing metabolic changes at this position.[189] Such 17α-substituents render the compounds orally active.

Increasing the length of the alkyl side chain beyond ethyl at the 17α-position, however, resulted in decreased activity, and the incorporation of other substituents, such as the 17α-ethinyl group, produced compounds with useful progestational activity (progestins), such as ethisterone (Fig. 25.17). Attaching an isoxazole ring to ethisterone produced danazol (Danatrol, Danocrine; still available), which exhibited potent antigonadotropic properties (blocks the action of LH and/or FSH), weak androgen and anabolic properties, and no estrogen or progestin activity.

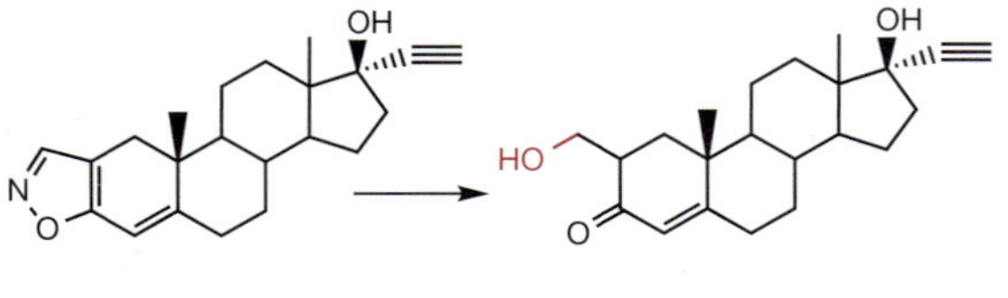

Danazol

2-Hydroxymethylethisterone
(Danazol metabolite)

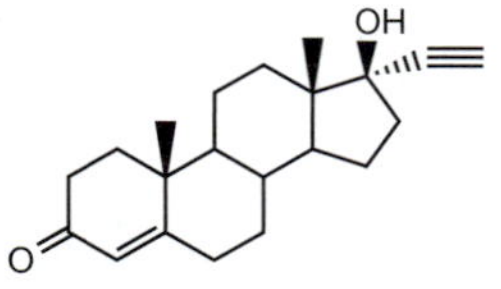

Ethisterone

As a gonadotropin inhibitor, danazol suppresses the surge of LH and FSH from the pituitary, thus suppressing ovarian steroidogenesis. For this reason, it is used in the treatment of endometriosis. Previous treatment of endometriosis had been surgical or medical, with progestins or a combination of estrogen and progestin; and recently the nonsteroidal and nonpeptidic GnRH inhibitor elagolix has been approved (discussed earlier). Danazol is metabolized by CYP3A4 to its inactive metabolite, 2-hydroxymethylethisterone.

Several modifications of 17α-methyltestosterone lead to potent, orally active anabolic agents. Two hydroxylated analogs include oxymesterone and oxymetholone (Fig. 25.24; both discontinued). These drugs have at least 3 times the anabolic and half the androgenic activity of testosterone.[189]

Halogen substitution produces compounds with decreased activity, except when inserted into position 4 or 9. By substituting a 9α-fluoro group onto an analog of 17α-methyltestosterone, fluoxymesterone (discontinued; Fig. 25.24) has 20 times the anabolic and 10 times the androgenic activity of 17α-methyltestosterone (Fig. 25.22).[189] Fluoxymesterone is also associated with sodium and water

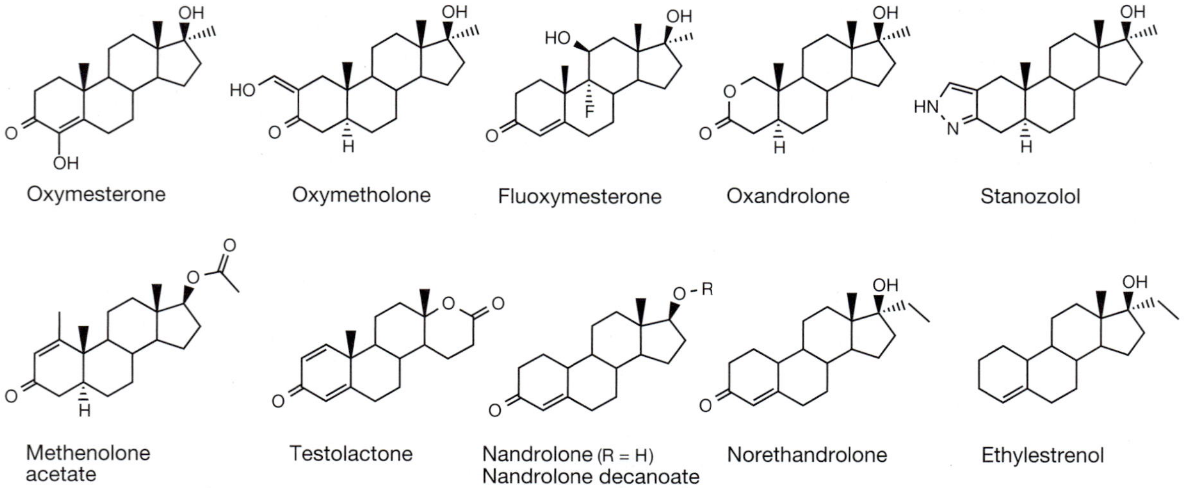

Figure 25.24 Anabolic steroids that have been discontinued from use.

retention likely due to the 11β-hydroxyl group common in adrenocorticoids (Chapter 24), which could lead to edema. Replacement of a carbon atom in position 2 by oxygen has produced the only clinically successful heterocyclic steroid, oxandrolone (discontinued), among a number of oxasteroids (not shown) and azasteroids (stanozolol; discontinued) (Fig. 25.24). Some of the 2-oxasteroids are potent anabolic agents. Oxandrolone contains a lactone in the A ring (oxygen bioisostere of ring A) and, therefore, is susceptible to in vivo hydrolysis. It has 3 times the anabolic activity of 17α-methyltestosterone but exhibits slight androgenic activity.[191] A pyrazole heterocyclic compound used for its anabolic effects was stanozolol.[191]

Introduction of a sp^2-hybridized carbon atom into the A ring of 5α-androstane–based agents, such as in methenolone acetate and testolactone (both discontinued; Fig. 25.24), renders the ring more planar, and in turn, this may be responsible for greater anabolic activity. Further, alkylation at the 1, 2, 7, and 18 positions of the androstane molecule generally increases anabolic activity.[189] Methenolone acetate is an example of such a Δ^1-1-methyl 5α-androstane with potent anabolic activity that does not have an alkyl substituent at the 17α-position.

Testolactone (discontinued), an 18-oxasteroid, is a 19-oxoandrostenedione analog, with ring D being a six-membered lactone ring (no 17α-alkylation). Although testolactone possesses some anabolic activity with weak androgenic effects, it was used primarily in the treatment of breast cancer as a noncompetitive irreversible inhibitor of aromatase.[192]

The 19-norandrogens (removal of the 19-CH_3 from C_{10} of the 5α-androstane nucleus), such as nandrolone and its decanoate and phenpropionate 17β-esters (all discontinued; Fig. 25.24), were of interest because these agents seem to produce a more favorable ratio of anabolic to androgenic activity, leading to favorable tissue-building properties (eg, myoanabolic). In animal assays, 19-nortestosterone (nandrolone) has about the same anabolic activity as the propionate ester of testosterone, but its androgenic activity is much lower. Because nandrolone showed some separation of anabolic and androgenic activities, related analogs were synthesized and biologically investigated. Two of the more potent members of the series are norethandrolone and ethylestrenol (both discontinued; Fig. 25.24). Norethandrolone has a better ratio of anabolic to androgenic activity than either 19-nortestosterone (nandrolone) or 17α-methyl-19-nortestosterone (not shown).[193] Both androgenic and progestational side effects have been observed with this agent. Ethylestrenol is more potent than norethandrolone.

Nandrolone phenpropionate and nandrolone decanoate are esters of 19-nortestosterone, as shown in Figure 25.24. When administered IM, slow in vivo hydrolysis of the ester occurs, releasing free 19-nortestosterone over a prolonged period. Nandrolone decanoate is the longer acting ester intended for deep IM injection, preferably into the gluteal muscle, and was used in the treatment of anemia associated with renal insufficiency. Nandrolone phenpropionate has a shorter duration of action than decanoate and was used in the treatment of metastatic breast cancer (MBC) in women.

Vida[189] has extensively reviewed the replacement of various hydrogens on the androgen steroid skeleton by other functional groups. It appears that certain substitutions at positions 1, 2, 7, 17, and 18 may result in compounds with favorable activities that could be of clinical importance.

Abuse of Steroidal Anabolic Agents to Enhance Athletic Performance

Performance-enhancing substances are now a point of major interest for athletes, government, and news media. These substances are having a major impact on sports and the public in general. A great deal of interest has recently been shown in illicit "designer" anabolic steroids for their high muscle-building effects, as shown in Figure 25.25. Tetrahydrogestrinone (THG) and desoxymethyltestosterone brought a great deal of interest to the performance-enhancing area, because their use was very difficult to detect.[194,195] THG is thought to have been derived from gestrinone, a substance that has been used for the treatment of a variety of gynecologic disorders. THG is also related to trenbolone, which has been used by bodybuilders and ranchers to build up cattle before marketing. Before THG, both gestrinone and trenbolone had been on the banned anabolic steroid list of the International Olympic Committee. THG was very difficult to trace, however, because it was unstable under the normal conditions of testing for anabolic steroids. Once a suitable assay was developed, it was possible to go back and test samples of athletes around the world, and several were found to have taken THG. The Designer Anabolic Steroid Control Act of 2014 had these agents and other designer steroids added to the list of previously defined anabolic steroids. More recently, dehydrochloromethyltestosterone (DHCMT) has garnered attention in antidoping, due to its detected use among athletes and the presence of a long-term metabolite facilitating its detection months after ingestion.[196]

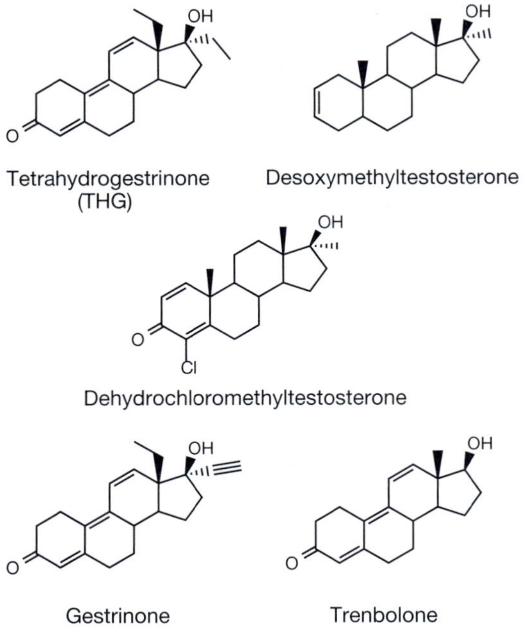

Figure 25.25 Illegal anabolic agents.

Nonsteroidal Androgens

Selective Androgen Receptor Modulators

The successful marketing and clinical application of SERMs raised the possibility of developing selective ligands for other members of the nuclear receptor superfamily. The concept of selective androgen receptor modulator (SARM)[197,198] emerged more recently; namely, a compound that is an antagonist or weak agonist in the prostate but agonist in the bone and muscle and is orally available with low hepatotoxicity. For an ideal SARM, the antagonist or weak agonist activity in the prostate will reduce concern for the potential to stimulate nascent or undetected prostate cancer or exacerbate existing BPH, whereas the strong agonist activity in the muscle and bone can be used to treat muscle-wasting conditions, hypogonadism, and/or aging-related frailty. Agonist activity in the breast provides an approach to the treatment of AR-positive breast cancer. SARMs have reached clinical development but are still looking for a therapeutic indication.

SARM pharmacophores include *N*-arylpropanamide,[198] bicyclic hydantoin,[199] tricyclic quinolines,[200] and tetrahydroquinoline[201] analogs, as shown in Figure 25.26. These nonsteroidal AR ligands are not substrates for aromatase or 5AR but exhibit affinity as full AR agonists in anabolic organs (eg, muscle and bone) and as partial AR agonists in androgenic tissues (eg, prostate and seminal vesicles).

STRUCTURE-ACTIVITY RELATIONSHIPS FOR THE *N*-ARYLPROPANAMIDES. The majority of published preclinical research has focused on a series of *N*-arylpropanamide analogs as AR agonists or partial agonists, using the key structural elements of bicalutamide, an androgen antagonist.[198,202]

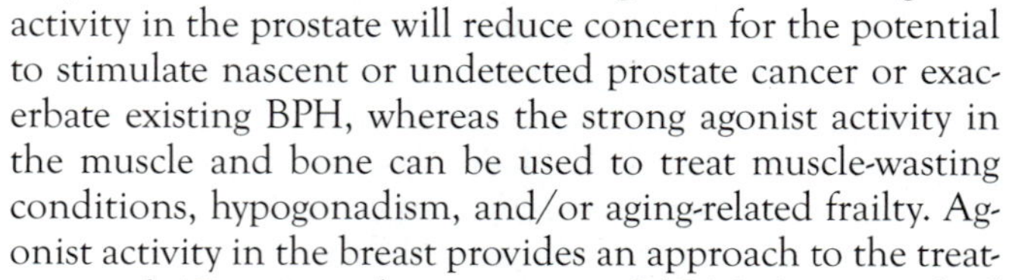

SARM Comparison

A series of chiral ether analogs of bicalutamide, which bear electron-withdrawing groups (see variable X of the *N*-arylpropanamides structure) in the A ring and a fluoro or acetylamino substituent at the *para* position in ring B (variable R) demonstrated high in vitro AR-binding affinity and reduced in vivo androgenicity but retained full anabolic activity in castrated male rats.[203,204] The sulfide analogs (replacement of ether oxygen with sulfur) exhibited greater AR-binding affinity, except that hepatic oxidation of the sulfur to sulfoxides (not shown) or sulfones (like bicalutamide) led to rapid in vivo inactivation and reduced efficacy.

For ether analogs, replacing the aromatic ring A with an aryl heterocycle failed to retain AR-binding affinity; however, a heterocyclic B ring was tolerated. Small size electron-withdrawing moieties at R, such as fluoro, chloro, nitro, or cyano groups, are optimum. Because aromatic nitro groups are associated with hepatotoxicity, they were replaced with a nonreducible electron-withdrawing cyano group. The dicyano (X and R) gave the most potent and efficacious *N*-arylpropanamide SARM with favorable

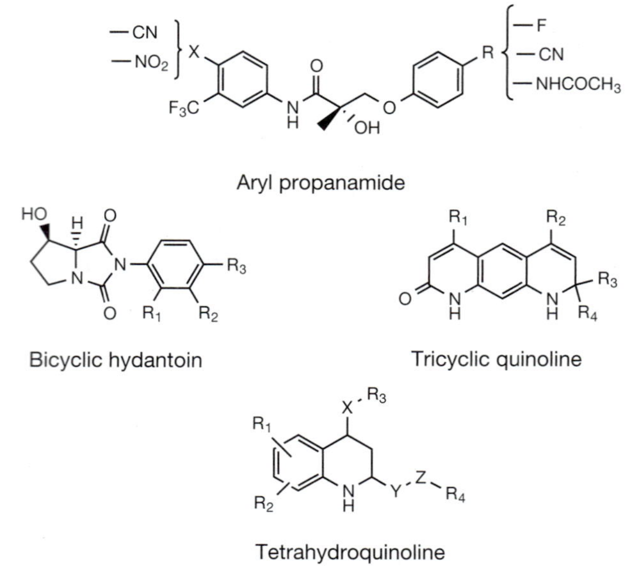

Figure 25.26 Selective androgen receptor modulators (SARMs).

pharmacokinetic properties. As evidenced from SAR studies, minor differences in ligand structure can lead to either agonist or antagonist activity. Full or partial agonist binding to AR is influenced by stereoisomeric conformation as well as by steric and electronic effects of the substituents. Molecular modeling of *N*-arylpropanamide AR ligands was used in conjunction with pharmacology, pharmacodynamics, pharmacokinetics, and metabolism to examine and optimize structural properties.

Results from in vitro and in vivo animal studies suggest that the therapeutic promise of SARMs as treatment for muscle wasting, osteoporosis, hormonal male contraception, BPH, and/or breast cancer—without unwanted side effects associated with testosterone—may be realized.[205] The AR specificity and lack of side effects intrinsic to the steroidal backbone such as steroid receptor cross-reactivity, metabolic activation by 5AR and/or aromatase, and hepatotoxicity clearly distinguish these drugs from their steroidal predecessors and open the door for expanded clinical use of androgens.

DRUGS USED FOR THE TREATMENT OF ERECTILE DYSFUNCTION

The National Institutes of Health Consensus Development Panel on Impotence defined ED as the inability to achieve or maintain an erection sufficient for satisfactory sexual performance that may substantially influence quality of life. It is estimated that 10 to 30 million U.S. men and more than 100 million men worldwide experience some form of ED.[206] This condition is strongly associated with age, and according to the community-based Massachusetts Male Aging Study, the prevalence of ED in men between ages 40 and 70 years is 52%.[207] The general classification of ED includes psychogenic ED (eg, depression, psychological stress, relationship problems, and performance anxiety), organic ED (eg, diabetes, hypertension, spinal cord injuries, and some medications), and mixed psychogenic and organic ED.

Treatment options for men with ED have changed significantly over the past three decades and have progressed from psychosexual therapy and penile prostheses (1970s) through revascularization, vacuum constriction devices, and intracavernosal injection therapy (1980s) to transurethral and oral drug delivery (1990s). In 2023, FDA approved the first ever OTC ED gel, Eroxon, which in clinical trials was found effective in 65% of men who used this gel. Applying the gel to the tip of the penis achieved an erection within 10 minutes and maintained it long enough to have sex. Eroxon stimulates nitric oxide release and vasodilation nonpharmacologically due to cooling effects of solvents in the gel. Eroxon's place in ED therapy is still unknown. Similar to Eroxon, common first-line prescription ED drugs like tadalafil (Cialis) and sildenafil (Viagra) are oral agents that elevate nitric oxide and vasodilation in the corpus cavernosum by PDE5 inhibition and take around 30 minutes to work. If the PDE5Is (or Eroxon) are not effective, then the cause may be low libido, and men should have their testosterone serum levels checked (in some instances, TRT may help to resolve ED). Other alternative drugs currently available for the treatment of ED include prostaglandin E_1, which is given by injection at the base of the penis or by suppository into the tip of the penis as well as the α1-adrenergic blocker and the nonselective PDE inhibitor papaverine. Apomorphine is a dopamine agonist that can be used for treating ED but, in humans, has the undesirable emetic side effect. Some selective dopamine D4 agents are now being investigated for treatment of ED. Vacuum devices and penile implants are also available.

Phosphodiesterase Inhibitors

The currently available first- and second-generation oral PDE5Is, sildenafil, tadalafil, vardenafil, and avanafil, have emerged as the first-line prescription treatment for ED because of patient convenience, safety, and clinical efficacy and have markedly improved the quality of life in men with ED of various etiologies. The introduction of the first PDE5I, sildenafil citrate (Viagra), in 1998 revolutionized the treatment of men with ED of a broad-spectrum of etiologies and acknowledged the need for pharmacologic agents in the treatment of ED.[208] With the recognition of the prevalence of ED by the public and the effectiveness of agents like sildenafil, there was an increased effort in the search for new agents with fewer side effects that led to the development of the second-generation PDE5Is, vardenafil (2003), tadalafil (2003), and avanafil (2012), which have since been introduced into the world market at differing potencies and pharmacokinetics (Fig. 25.27).

Sildenafil (Viagra)

In 1998, sildenafil was the first selective PDE inhibitor to be approved and found to be effective in treating ED.[208] Sildenafil is 16-fold more selective for PDE5 as compared to PDE6, which is found in the photoreceptors of the human retina. In vitro metabolism studies for sildenafil have shown that the primary metabolite, *N*-desmethylsildenafil, and the minor metabolite, oxidative opening of the piperazine ring, are mediated by CYP3A4, CYP2C9, CYP2C19, and CYP2D6 (Fig. 25.27). The estimated relative contributions to clearance were 79% for CYP3A4, 20% for CYP2C9, and less than 2% for CYP2C19 and CYP2D6. These results demonstrate that CYP3A4 is the primary cytochrome mediating *N*-demethylation and that drugs inhibiting CYP3A4 likely impair sildenafil biotransformation and clearance. The pharmacokinetics of radiolabeled sildenafil were consistent with rapid absorption, first-pass metabolism, and primarily fecal elimination of *N*-demethylated metabolites. The absorption of sildenafil following oral administration was rapid (<0.5 hours), whereas the oral bioavailability was approximately 38% as a result of first-pass metabolism. Starting doses of 50 mg of sildenafil should be taken approximately 1 hour before sexual activity; however, it may be

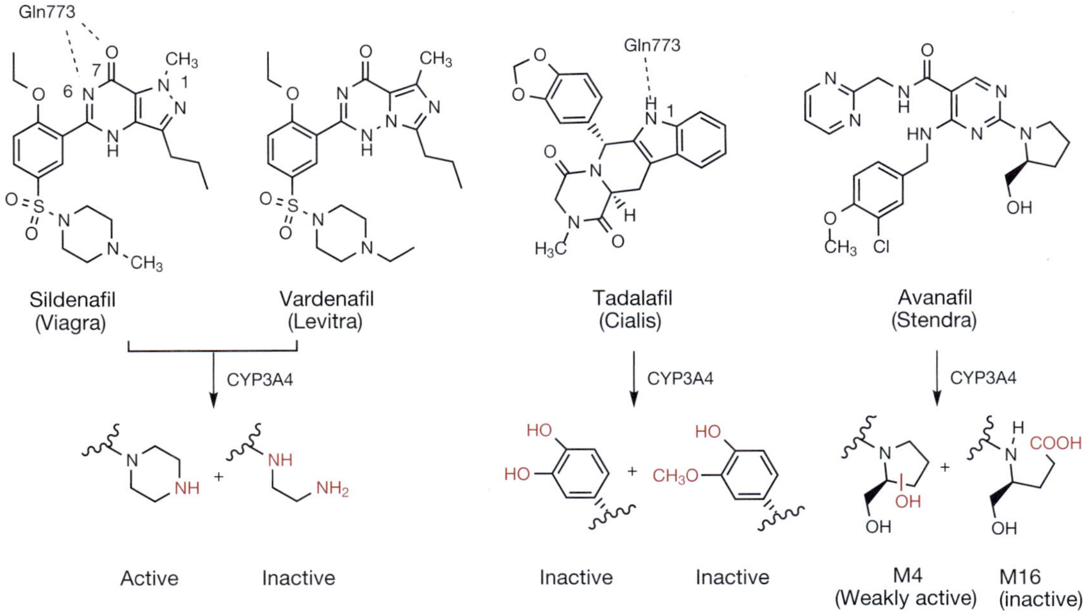

Figure 25.27 Phosphodiesterase 5 inhibitors and primary metabolites.

taken anywhere from 30 minutes to 4 hours before sexual activity. Dosage may be decreased (25 mg) or increased (100 mg) based upon efficacy and tolerability with maximum once per day frequency. If taken after a high-fat meal, sildenafil may take longer to start working.

Vardenafil (Levitra)

Vardenafil was the second agent to be marketed and had the advantage that its onset time was not reduced by taking the medication on a full stomach (Table 25.12).[209,210] It is ~20 times more potent as an inhibitor of PDE5 (mean IC_{50} = 0.084 nM) than sildenafil and 48 times more potent than tadalafil, with a greater selectivity (>14,000 times) for human PDE5 than for human PDE2, PDE3, and PDE4 and moderate selectivity (>1,000 times) for PDE1 (Table 25.13).[211-213] Starting doses of 10 mg of vardenafil should be taken approximately 1 hour before sexual activity. Dosage may be decreased (5 mg) or increased (20 mg) based upon efficacy and tolerability. It may be taken with or without food, but its effects are reduced following a fatty meal. Vardenafil is also available as a 10-mg disintegrating oral tablet (Staxyn), which is more rapidly absorbed than oral tablets (Levitra) and provides higher systemic exposure than Levitra. Maximum dosage is 10 mg/d (Staxyn) or 20 mg/d (Levitra).

Tadalafil (Cialis)

Tadalafil was the third agent to be released and can be taken on a full stomach without slowing the onset (Table 25.12).[209] It has a much longer duration of action, lasting up to 48 hours, compared with sildenafil and vardenafil, which last for approximately 4 hours. The longer half-life of tadalafil results in a lengthened period of responsiveness as compared to sildenafil and vardenafil. This longer therapeutic window requires fewer time constraints for the effectiveness of tadalafil and has been interpreted as being advantageous through providing the option for more spontaneous sexual activity. Because of its long half-life, however, tadalafil has been detected in plasma even 5 days after oral administration. This suggests the possibility of accumulation if taken

Table 25.12 Some Properties and Pharmacokinetics of the PDE5Is

Drugs	Sildenafil	Vardenafil	Tadalafil	Avanafil
Trade Name	**Viagra**	**Levitra**	**Cialis**	**Stendra**
cLog P^a	1.8	2.18	2.36	2.78
Oral bioavailability (%)	38-40	15 (8-25)	~36	
Onset of action (h)	<0.5	<1	0.5-1	0.25
Duration of action (h)	<4	<1	<36	
Protein binding (%)	96	94	94	99
Time to peak concentration (h)	0.5-2	0.5-3	0.5-6	0.5-0.75 (fasting) 1.12-1.25 (high-fat meal)
Volume of distribution (L/kg)	105	208	63	
Peak plasma concentration (nmol/L)	1-2	0.03	0.84	
Elimination half-life (h)	3-5	4-5	18	5
Metabolism	3A4 (major)	3A4 (major)	3A4 (primary)	3A4 (major)
	2C9 (minor)	2C9 (minor)		2C9 (minor)
Active metabolites	*N*-Desmethyl	*N*-Desethyl	None	M4
Excretion (%)				
Fecal Renal	~80 ~13	>90 <10	~60 ~35	~62 ~21
PDE5 IC_{50} (nM)[200]	1.6	0.084	4	5.2

IC_{50}, median inhibitory concentration; met, metabolite; PDE, phosphodiesterase.
[a]www.drugbank.ca. Accessed July 15, 2025.

Table 25.13 Selectivity of PDE5Is for PDE1-11 Isozymes

	PDE vs PDE5 Selectivity (Fold Difference)			
PDE	Sildenafil	Vardenafil	Tadalafil	Avanafil
1	375	1,012	10,500	10,192
2	39,375	273,810	>25,000	9,808
3	16,250	26,190	>25,000	>19,231
4	3,125	14,296	14,750	1,096
5	1	1	1	1
6	16	21	550	121
7	13,750	17,857	>25,000	5,192
8	>62,500	1,000,000	>25,000	2,308
9	2,250	16,667	>25,000	>19,231
10	3,375	17,857	8,750	1,192
11	4,875	5,952	25	>19,231

PDE5I, phosphodiesterase type 5 inhibitor.

Based on Kotera J, Mochida H, Inoue H, et al. Avanafil, a potent and highly selective phosphodiesterase-5 inhibitor for erectile dysfunction. *J Urol.* 2012;188:668-674.

regularly and in short intervals, which may result in an increased risk of side effects with the excessive use of this PDE5I. The 3,4-methylenedioxy substitution on the phenyl ring was significant for increasing its potency as a PDE5I. Optimization of the chain on the piperazinedione ring resulted in no significant change in IC_{50}. Tadalafil is a highly potent PDE5I (IC_{50} = 4 nM), with high selectivity for PDE5 versus PDE1 through PDE4.[213,214] The PDE6/PDE5 selectivity ratio is 550 (Table 25.13).

Avanafil (Stendra)

Avanafil is a pyrimidine derivative and is the latest PDE5I to be approved. It exhibits higher potency for PDE5 than other PDEs and high PDE5 selectivity (>100-fold for PDE6; >1,000-fold for PDE4, PDE8, and PDE10; >5,000-fold for PDE2 and PDE7; >10,000-fold for PDE1, PDE3, PDE9, and PDE11) (Table 25.13).[214] It is a competitive inhibitor of cGMP binding to PDE5 (K_I of 4.3 nM).[214] Avanafil was found to show potent PDE5 inhibitory activity (IC_{50} = 5 nM) with the (*S*)-enantiomer of the 2-hydroxymethyl group on the pyrrolidine ring being 7-fold more potent than its (*R*)-enantiomer (IC_{50} = 36 nM).[215] Avanafil showed higher selectivity against PDE6 than sildenafil and vardenafil (121-fold vs 15- to 21-fold) but less than tadalafil (550-fold). The onset of action appears to be shorter (15 minutes),[216] which can add to its convenience and offers a major advantage during sexual activity. Avanafil is extensively metabolized in the liver predominantly by CYP3A4 and to a minor extent by CYP2C isoforms to produce an active metabolite called M4 (PDE5 inhibitory activity 10% of avanafil) and is responsible for about 4% of pharmacologic activity. The M16 metabolite is inactive and represents about 29% of the parent.[217] Its terminal half-life is 5 hours with the majority excreted in the feces. Dosage adjustments are not necessary based upon hepatic or renal function, age, or gender.[218]

Structure-Activity Relationships

PDE5Is are nonhydrolyzable competitive inhibitors of cGMP. The modified purine ring of sildenafil and vardenafil is thought to mimic the guanine ring systems of cGMP, with the other substituents acting as the ribose and phosphate of cGMP when binding to the PDE. The chemical similarities and distinct differences between PDE5Is regarding their selectivity for inhibition of PDE5 in preference to the 10 other PDE isoforms give rise to pharmacokinetic differences that affect the efficacy profile of these compounds. The obvious difference for the four drugs is the heterocyclic ring systems used to mimic the purine ring of cGMP. Although the heterocyclic ring systems and the N-substituent (ethyl vs methyl) attached to the piperazine side chain (Fig. 25.27) are the only two structural differences between sildenafil and vardenafil, these differences do not explain why vardenafil has a more than 20 times greater potency than sildenafil for inhibiting PDE5. An SAR analysis for the difference in potency between sildenafil and vardenafil revealed that the methyl/ethyl group on the piperazine moiety plays very little role in the potency difference for inhibiting PDE5, whereas the differences in the heterocyclic ring systems play a critical role in higher potency for vardenafil.[211,212]

A comparison of the in vitro inhibition values (IC_{50}) reveals that each drug inhibits PDE5 in the nanomolar range with vardenafil exhibiting higher potency (vardenafil > tadalafil > sildenafil > avanafil) (Table 25.13).[211,214] Selectivity of each drug for PDEs has been determined.[214] The low PDE5/PDE6 selectivity ratio suggests that at therapeutic doses, sildenafil is only approximately 16-fold more selective for PDE5 as for PDE6, which is an enzyme found in the photoreceptors of the human retina. PDE5 and PDE6 are more similar in terms of amino acid sequences and pharmacologic properties as compared to other PDEs. This lower PDE5/PDE6 selectivity ratio toward PDE6 for sildenafil indicates it is more likely to inhibit PDE6, which is presumed to be the cause of transient color vision abnormalities observed with high doses or plasma levels of sildenafil. A 3D homology model of PDE5 with tadalafil suggests reasons why sildenafil causes visual disorders because of its poor selectivity but tadalafil does not. It suggests that sildenafil binds to PDE6 and PDE5 in a similar pattern and thus may account for its similar inhibitor potencies toward PDE5 and PDE6. The high selectivity of tadalafil for PDE5 versus PDE6 may result from two key amino acid residues in the catalytic sites that vary (Val782 and Leu804 in PDE5 and their corresponding Val738 and Met760 in PDE6).[219] Tadalafil binds PDE6 in a different pattern from sildenafil. Sildenafil forms two hydrogen bonds from the N^6 and O^7 of the pyrazolo-pyrimidine ring to Gln773 in PDE6, while only the N_1 of the indole ring of tadalafil can have a single hydrogen bond to Gln773, giving rise to its lower affinity for PDE6 (Fig. 25.27).[219]

Mechanism of Action

The physiologic mechanism to achieve penile erection is mediated via a nitric oxide (NO)/cyclic guanosine monophosphate (cGMP) pathway (Fig. 25.28). Sexual stimulation is required for a response to treatment with PDE5Is. During sexual stimulation, parasympathetic neurons and vascular endothelial cells release NO, which activates soluble guanylyl cyclase, thereby increasing the level of cGMP in the corpus cavernosum and relaxation (vasodilation) of vascular smooth muscle. PDE5 is a cGMP-specific hydrolyzing enzyme and is present at high concentrations in the smooth muscle of the penile corpus cavernosum.[220,221] One of the more effective methods for elevating cGMP levels in this tissue is to use PDE5Is. Other PDE isoenzymes also found in the human cavernous smooth muscle include PDE3 (cGMP-inhibited PDE) and PDE4 (cAMP-specific PDE). Thus, inhibitors of PDE, especially PDE5, have been shown to be an effective means for treating ED by enhancing and maintaining erections during sexual stimulation through sustaining sufficient cellular levels of cGMP in both the corpus cavernosum and the blood vessels supplying it. The increased vasodilation of the corporeal sinusoids allows more blood flow into the penis, thereby enhancing an erection.

Pharmacokinetics

PDE5Is have only limited oral bioavailability because of extensive presystemic metabolism in the intestine and hepatic first-pass metabolism via the CYP3A isoform family (Table 25.12).[209] They are rapidly absorbed after oral administration and reach peak plasma concentrations within 15 to 60 minutes. Avanafil has the fastest onset of action, which allows the patient to take the drug 15 minutes prior to sexual activity and offers a major advantage. Rapid absorption and lipophilicity are considered to be a prerequisite for their rapid onset of efficacy and sexual satisfaction. Sildenafil, vardenafil, and tadalafil are rapidly absorbed, but with a significant difference in their mean bioavailability of approximately 15% for vardenafil and ~40% for sildenafil and tadalafil. The administration of a high-fat meal had no significant effect on the rate and extent of absorption of tadalafil but did decrease the rate of absorption for the other three, which is consistent with their calculated lipophilicity (Table 25.12). It remains unclear whether food has any effect on their absorption and therapeutic efficacy. They are all highly protein bound (≥94%), with free plasma concentration fractions of only 4% to 6%. The elimination half-life and duration of action for PDE5Is are similar (~5 hours), with exception of tadalafil, which has a long duration of action (<36 hours) and half-life of 18 hours, suggesting that it is predominately metabolized by hepatic CYP3A4 to catechol metabolites, with minimal presystemic metabolism.

The major route of elimination for the PDE5Is is hepatic metabolism, with renal excretion of unmetabolized drug accounting for 1% or less of the elimination pathways (Fig. 25.27).[209] CYP3A4 is the major drug-metabolizing enzyme for the four PDE5Is. CYP2C9, CYP2C19, and CYP2D6, however, also contribute to the metabolism of sildenafil, and CYP2C9 contributes to the metabolism of vardenafil. Both sildenafil and vardenafil have active metabolites that reach plasma concentrations high enough to contribute to the overall efficacy and safety profile of their parent-drug molecules.

The larger differences in their volumes of distribution, together with the substantial differences in their systemic clearance, result in distinct differences in their elimination half-lives: 3 to 5 hours for sildenafil, vardenafil, and avanafil, compared with approximately 18 hours for tadalafil.

Hepatic CYP3A and CYP2C activity has been described as being age dependent, with reduced activity being exhibited in older patients compared to young individuals. This decrease in metabolic activity is reflected by a corresponding increase in plasma concentrations of PDE5Is, warranting dose reductions for sildenafil and vardenafil in older patients. Similarly, ethnicity-dependent differences in the pharmacokinetics of PDE5Is may be expected based on known ethnic differences in CYP3A4/5 activity. Gender differences in pharmacokinetics have not been described for any of the PDE5Is. Severe renal impairment resulted in an increase in plasma concentrations for sildenafil, vardenafil, and tadalafil, and this warrants dose reductions for sildenafil and tadalafil in the affected patient population. Avanafil has not been studied in patients with severe renal disease or on renal dialysis. However, clinical studies of avanafil showed that only minimal changes in avanafil exposure occurred in patients with mild-to-moderate renal impairment.

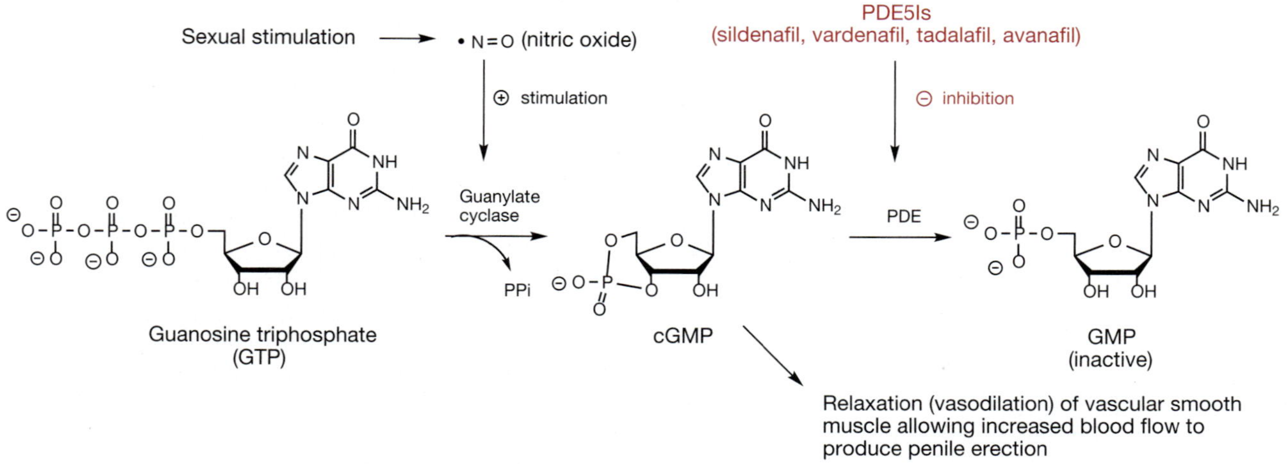

Figure 25.28 Mechanism of action of phosphodiesterase 5 inhibitors (PDE5Is). cGMP, cyclic guanosine monophosphate.

Drug-Drug Interactions

PDE5Is have not been identified as CYP inhibitors, including CYP3A or CYP2C. Because metabolism via CYP3A is the major elimination pathway for PDE5Is, all inducers and inhibitors of CYP3A activity have the potential to interfere with the elimination of these drugs. This DDI potential has only been verified clinically for inducers of CYP3A activity, specifically for the effect of rifampicin on tadalafil.[209] The strong inhibitors of CYP3A4 (ritonavir, indinavir, saquinavir, erythromycin, and ketoconazole) increased the plasma levels of sildenafil, vardenafil, tadalafil, and avanafil. Grapefruit juice, a selective inhibitor of CYP3A intestinal metabolism, also increased the plasma concentrations of sildenafil and vardenafil, but not of tadalafil. Grapefruit juice is likely to increase avanafil exposure; however, specific interactions have not been determined. Ritonavir, a strong CYP3A4 and CYP2C9 inhibitor, resulted in increases in vardenafil's AUC (49-fold), C_{max} (13-fold), and half-life (26 hours) and avanafil's AUC (2- and 13-fold) and half-life (9 hours). This is most likely a consequence of the simultaneous inhibition of both CYP3A4 and CYP2C9, the major metabolism pathways for both. The effect of ritonavir on sildenafil was much less pronounced than vardenafil (11 times), because other compensatory CYP-mediated metabolism pathways were still available. Ritonavir increased the plasma levels for tadalafil (CYP3A4) by approximately 3 times.

Adverse Effects

PDE5Is are generally safe, effective, and well tolerated in patients. The most commonly reported side effects include headaches, flushing, dizziness, visual disturbance (sildenafil), and nasal congestion. There are no significant differences in the efficacy of sildenafil, vardenafil, and avanafil when the recommended maximal doses are used.[222] It is suggested that some of these side effects result from the inhibition of other PDEs, including the isoform PDE6.[209,223] The search is on for even more selective ED agents to see if additional side effects can be eliminated. If one is taking α-adrenergic blockers for high blood pressure, one should consult a physician before using the agents together.[209] Other vasodilators associated with regulating the intracellular levels of cGMP, such as nitroglycerin, should not be used in combination with the PDE5Is.

Prostaglandin E_1

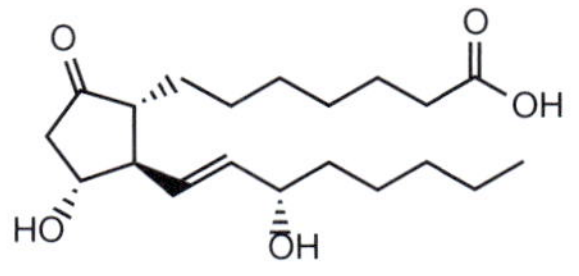

Alprostadil
PGE_1

PGE_1 (alprostadil) is approved for the intracavernosal (Caverject, Edex) or intraurethral suppository (Muse) treatment of ED. A three-drug combination of PGE_1, papaverine, and phentolamine sometimes is used as an intracavernosal injection to achieve a synergistic action. ED that is medication induced or caused by endocrine problems, such as hypogonadism or hyper- or hypothyroidism, should be evaluated and appropriately treated before PGE_1 treatment is considered. PGE_1 is produced endogenously to relax vascular smooth muscle and cause vasodilation by activating the adenylyl cyclase/cAMP pathway. Recent studies show that cAMP is important in the PGE_1 relaxation of penile erectile tissue and vasodilation of penile resistance arteries.[224] Moreover, agents that stimulate the release of cAMP also cross-activate the NO/cGMP cascade.

When administered by intracavernosal injection or as an intraurethral suppository, PGE_1 acts locally to relax the smooth muscle of the corpora cavernosa and the cavernosal arteries. Swelling, elongation, and rigidity of the penis result when arterial blood rapidly flows into the corpus cavernosum to expand the lacunar spaces. The entrapped blood reduces the venous blood outflow as sinusoids compress against the tunica albuginea. Adding papaverine and phentolamine to the PGE_1 regimen synergistically increases arterial blood flow via separate mechanisms. Papaverine relaxes the sinusoid and the smooth muscle of the helicine arteries, whereas phentolamine relaxes arterial smooth muscle and blocks both the α-adrenergic receptors that inhibit an erection. PGE_1 is rapidly metabolized within the urethra, prostate, and corpus cavernosum to 7α-hydroxy-5,11-diketotetranorprosta-1,16-dioic acid and 5α,7α-dihydroxy-11-ketotetranor-prostane-1,16-dioic acid (not shown).[225] The major route of excretion of PGE_1 metabolites is via the kidney. Its elimination half-life is 5 to 10 minutes. If any alprostadil is systemically absorbed, it is metabolized by a single pass through the lungs. The onset of action is within 10 minutes, and the time to peak effect is less than 20 minutes. The duration of action is 1 to 3 hours for the intracavernosal injection and 30 to 60 minutes for the intraurethral suppository.

MALE OSTEOPOROSIS

Osteoporosis is a common condition in men that usually develops after age 70 years and affects approximately 2 million U.S. men.[226] Osteoporosis occurs less frequently in men because of greater skeletal bone mass during growth (ie, greater bone size). Approximately 20% to 25% of all hip fractures occur in men, however, and the age-adjusted prevalence of vertebral deformities appears to be similar in men and women. Currently, bisphosphonates (alendronate and risedronate) are the therapy of choice for increasing BMD to decrease the risk of fracture in the treatment of male osteoporosis, and a short course of parathyroid hormone (1-34; teriparatide) may be indicated for men with very low BMD or for those in whom bisphosphonate therapy is unsuccessful. Denosumab (Prolia) is also indicated in men with osteoporosis at high risk for fracture, defined as a history of osteoporotic fracture, or multiple risk factors for fracture; or patients who have failed or are intolerant to other available osteoporosis therapy. Medical castration (eg, GnRH agonists and antagonists discussed in this chapter) and antiandrogen therapy for the treatment of prostate cancer, hypogonadism, and diabetes are some of the risk factors for osteoporosis and fracture. Vitamin D and calcium have been shown to help improve BMD. TRT is controversial, except in men who clearly have hypogonadism and low levels of testosterone; in those men, treatment with testosterone appears to increase bone density.

Drugs Used for Benign Prostatic Hyperplasia

Prostate problems are common in older men, particularly those ages 50 years and above. An individual may have prostate problems for a number of reasons, including an infection of the prostate (prostatitis), a noncancerous enlargement of the prostate (BPH), or prostate cancer, the second most common cancer in men. BPH is the most common disease of the prostate, occurring in 50% to 60% of men in their 60s and up to 80% to 90% of men over age 70 years.[227] Prostate problems are often discovered by men themselves. The signs of prostate problems include a frequent urge to urinate, blood in the urine, painful or burning urination, difficulty urinating, or inability to urinate.

BPH is the noncancerous asymmetric proliferation of the prostate gland that can restrict the urethra as it passes through the prostate. Thus, the major problem associated with BPH is LUTSs. The symptoms of BPH stem from obstruction of the urethra by an enlarged prostate and the gradual loss of bladder function, which results in incomplete emptying of the bladder. The two categories of symptoms of BPH include obstructive and irritative. Obstructive symptoms result from factors that reduce bladder emptying (eg, hesitancy, straining, weak urine stream, dribbling, and urinary retention). Irritative symptoms typically occur late in the disease course and result from long-term obstruction of bladder (eg, urinary frequency, urgency, incontinence, dysuria, hematuria, and nocturia). The quality of life can be significantly compromised when BPH symptoms wake up the patient every 1 to 2 hours at night to void (nocturia). The enlarging prostate increases the adrenergic tone of the prostate in patients with BPH, which results in further tightening of the urethra. The consequence of this obstruction can include urinary retention (and can in some cases lead to emergency catheterization), stagnant urine retention leading to urinary infections, and even hydronephrosis.

Short questionnaires exist (American Urological Association Symptom Index/International Prostate Symptom Score [AUA-SI/I-PSS]) that allow practitioners to assess the severity of symptoms regarding urine storage, voiding, and quality of life and make treatment recommendations.[228,229] Management of BPH depends on the severity of symptoms and can range from active surveillance, pharmacotherapy (α_1-adrenergic antagonists, 5ARIs, or combination), and surgical/laser reduction of prostate. When partial obstruction is present, urinary retention can also be brought on by alcohol, cold temperatures, a long period of immobility, or the ingestion of OTC cold or allergy medicines that contain a sympathomimetic decongestant or anticholinergic drug. It is important to ask patients if BPH symptoms worsen when on OTC cold or allergy medications, as they may experience acute, severe urinary retention that requires catheterization. First-generation antihistamines can cause urinary retention due to their anticholinergic effects, while the decongestant pseudoephedrine, an α_1 agonist, promotes further tightening on the urethra.

Although the cause of BPH is not well understood, it occurs mainly in older men and it does not develop in men whose testes were removed before puberty. Before and during adulthood, DHT plays a critical role in determining prostate size, and multiple lines of evidence suggest the importance of DHT in the development of BPH.[230,231] Men who do not produce DHT do not develop BPH.[232] For instance, BPH does not develop in males with certain $5AR_2$ mutations or in males with very low levels of androgen because of prepubertal castration or hypopituitarism-related hypogonadism. Moreover, clinical treatment of BPH either by chemical or surgical castration or by inhibition of $5AR_2$ (eg, finasteride or dutasteride) induces apoptosis of epithelial cells, which, in turn, significantly decreases the volume of the prostate.[231]

The role of age-dependent changes in the intraprostatic hormonal environment in the development of BPH was evaluated.[233] Despite the aging-related decrease in testosterone and intraprostatic DHT production, an increased 17β-estradiol/DHT ratio was observed in the aging human prostate, which can be relevant to the development of BPH. As men age, the concentration of free testosterone in the blood decreases due to increases in SHBG, while the concentrations of 17β-estradiol increase due to aromatization in adipose tissue. Animal studies have suggested that BPH may result from the increased concentration of 17β-estradiol or DHT within the gland, which promotes cell growth.[234] Furthermore, 17β-estradiol is capable of inducing precancerous lesions and prostate cancer in aging dogs.[235] Therefore, TRT in older men raises concern regarding acceleration of BPH and/or prostate cancer due to the possible aromatization of the exogenous testosterone.

Surgical procedures are often used to reduce a large prostate mass, but there are early pharmacologic treatments for BPH, including α_1-adrenergic antagonists and 5ARIs.

α_1-Adrenergic Antagonists

Often the first-line treatment for LUTS and BPH, the α_1-adrenergic antagonists treat the increased adrenergic tone of the sympathetic nervous system by relaxing the muscles at the neck of the bladder and in the prostate, thereby reducing the pressure on the urethra and increasing the flow of urine.[236] They do not cure BPH but, rather, help to alleviate some of the symptoms. For moderate symptoms of BPH, α_1-adrenergic antagonists are often used due to their faster onset of symptom relief as compared with 5ARIs. They can also be used in combination with 5ARIs when prostate volume is large (>40 g), as α_1-adrenergic antagonists do not decrease prostate volume. Approximately 60% of men find that symptoms improve significantly within the first 2 to 3 weeks of treatment with an α_1-antagonist. Alfuzosin, tamsulosin, and silodosin are used exclusively as first-line α_1-adrenergic antagonists for the treatment of BPH, while doxazosin and terazosin have also been used to treat high blood pressure. Prazosin, another α_1-antagonist, is not indicated for the treatment of BPH. Tamsulosin, alfuzosin, and silodosin are uroselective α_1-adrenergic antagonists developed specifically to treat BPH. When BPH and ED are present, α_1-adrenergic antagonists are used in combination with a phosphodiesterase inhibitor.

Classes of α_1-Adrenergic Antagonists

QUINAZOLINES. Alfuzosin (2003), terazosin (1987), and doxazosin (1990) are nonselective α_1-adrenergic antagonists, each bearing a 4-amino-6,7-dimethoxyquinazoline ring system (Fig. 25.29). They differ at the two-position of the quinazoline ring, having either a piperazine ring (terazosin and doxazosin) or open-chain amine analog (alfuzosin). The first selective quinazoline α_1-blocker discovered in the late 1960s was prazosin (not shown), a commonly used antihypertensive agent that is not recommended for BPH due to multiple doses per day and significant cardiovascular adverse effects. Prazosin is a derivative of terazosin and differs only with respect to a furan ring in place of the hydrofuran of terazosin. Other structural differences exist between the approved quinazolines including the different acyl groups attached to the nitrogen of either the piperazine ring or the open-chain analog. The differences in these groups afford dramatic differences in some of the pharmacokinetic properties of these agents (Table 25.14). Perhaps most significant are the long half-lives (10-22 hours) and durations of action (18-48 hours) for these drugs that permit once-a-day dosing and generally lead to increased patient compliance.

Alfuzosin, lacking the piperazine ring, is a first-line uroselective drug for the treatment of BPH, but with no utility in treating hypertension because it has fewer cardiovascular effects than terazosin and doxazosin. It is hepatically metabolized by 7-*O*-demethylation and *N*-dealkylation, primarily by CYP3A4, to inactive metabolites. In patients with moderate or severe hepatic insufficiency, a reduction in clearance resulted in a 3 to 4 times increase in its plasma concentration, which may require a reduction in dose.

Doxazosin is extensively metabolized by 7-*O*-demethylation, hydroxylation of the benzodioxan ring, and oxidation of the piperazine ring to active metabolites in the liver catalyzed by CYP3A4. In patients with renal insufficiency, the elimination half-life was not significantly different from healthy volunteers.

Terazosin is similarly metabolized via 7-*O*-demethylation and *N*-dealkylation to four metabolites: 6-*O*-demethyl terazosin and 7-*O*-demethyl terazosin, the piperazine derivative of terazosin, and the diamine metabolite of the piperazine compound. Terazosin and doxazosin require dose titration to minimize orthostatic hypertension and dizziness.

CATECHOLAMINE-SULFONAMIDE. Tamsulosin exhibits uroselectivity for the α_{1A}-adrenergic receptor and is a first-line drug for the treatment of BPH, with no utility for treating hypertension due to lower affinity for vascular α_{1B}-adrenergic receptor. Food decreases oral absorption of tamsulosin; thus, it should be taken on an empty stomach. Tamsulosin is *O*-deethylated by CYP3A4 to phenolic metabolites that are conjugated with glucuronic acid or sulfate before renal excretion, and by *O*-demethylation and 3′-hydroxylation to catechol metabolites that are also glucuronidated or sulfonated. Tamsulosin should be avoided in patients with severe sulfa allergies due to the presence of the aryl sulfonamide.

INDOLE CARBOXAMIDE. Silodosin is the most uroselective of the α_1-adrenoceptor antagonists, demonstrating 160- and 50-fold higher affinity for binding to α_{1A}-adrenoceptors as compared to α_{1B}- and α_{1D}-adrenoceptors.[237] Silodosin undergoes extensive metabolism through glucuronidation, alcohol and aldehyde dehydrogenase, and CYP3A4. The glucuronide conjugate (formed via direct glucuronidation of the alcohol) of silodosin is active, has a longer half-life (24 hours) than the parent drug, and achieves a plasma exposure (AUC) 4 times higher than that of silodosin.

Mechanism of Action

α_1-Adrenoceptors are widely distributed in the human body and play important physiologic roles (see Chapter 6). There are three α_1-adrenoceptor subtypes (α_{1A}, α_{1B}, and α_{1D}). Two of these receptors (α_{1A} and α_{1D}) have been shown to mediate smooth muscle contraction. α_{1A}-Adrenoceptors are expressed in prostate and urethral tissue, while α_{1D}-adrenoceptors are expressed mainly in the detrusor muscle of the bladder and the sacral region of the spinal cord. In BPH, α_1-antagonists block adrenergic receptor activation causing relaxation of the prostate smooth muscle and provide relief

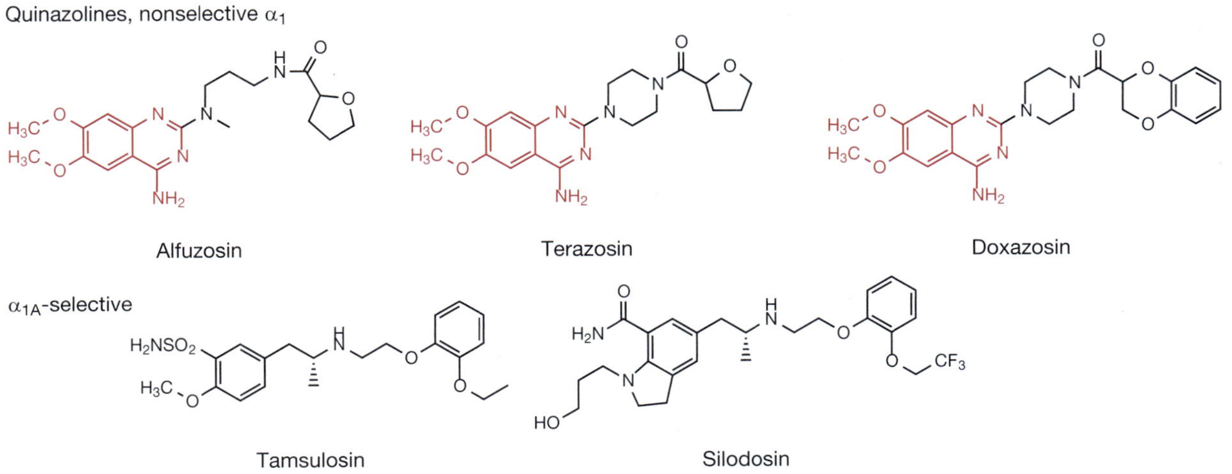

Figure 25.29 α1-Adrenergic antagonists for the treatment of benign prostatic hyperplasia.

Table 25.14 Some Properties and Pharmacokinetics of the α-Adrenergic Antagonists

Drug	Alfuzosin	Terazosin	Doxazosin	Tamsulosin	Silodosin
Trade Name	**Uroxatral**	**Hytrin**	**Cardura**	**Flomax**	**Rapaflo**
cLog *P*[a]	1.19	1.12	2.53	3.05	2.96
Oral bioavailability (%)	49 fed	90	65 (54-59 XL)	>90 fasted	32
Onset of action (wk)[b]	<2	2	1-2	1	<1
Duration of action (h)	>48	>18	>24	>24	24
Protein binding (%)	82-90	90-94	98	94-99	97
Time to peak concentration (h)	8	1	2-3 (8-9 XL)	4-5 fasting/6-7 fed	3
Volume of distribution (L/kg)	3.2	25-30	1.0-3.4	16	49.5
Elimination half-life (h)	10	12	22 (15-19 XL)	9-15	13
		14 older adult		14-15 older adult	
Cytochrome isoforms	3A4 (inactive metabolites)	—	3A4 (active metabolites)	3A4, 2D6	3A4
Excretion (%)[c] Feces	69/–	60/20 feces	63/5	21/–	55/–
Urine	24/11	40/10	9/4.8	76/<10	34/–
Ki (nM) for α_{1A}	2.4	2.5	2.7	0.5	1.0

XL, extended-release tablet formulation.
[a]www.drugbank.ca. Accessed July 15, 2025.
[b]Time for improvement in urine flow observed.
[c]% given as metabolites/unchanged.

from the symptoms of LUTS. The vast majority of α-adrenoceptors expressed in the prostate are of the α_{1A} (70%) and α_{1D} subtypes (27%). The α_{1B}-adrenoceptor is known to be important in the regulation of blood pressure.[238] The predominant expression of the α_{1A}-adrenoceptor subtype in the prostatic stromal region and urethral smooth muscle cells led to the design of drugs with uroselectivity for this receptor subtype. Thus, alfuzosin (an aminoquinazoline), tamsulosin (an *N*-substituted, catecholamine-related sulfonamide), and silodosin (a substituted indole carboxamide) were designed for the treatment of BPH (Fig. 25.29).[231] Doxazosin and terazosin, along with prazosin, were originally used as antihypertensives but also were found to be effective for the treatment of BPH based on their common mechanism of action. Comparisons of the affinities (K_i, nM) of the α_{1A}-adrenoceptor antagonists (Table 25.14) did not show substantial differences for the quinazoline α_{1A}-antagonists (alfuzosin, doxazosin, and terazosin), but some uroselectivity for tamsulosin and silodosin was observed.[236,237,239] In vivo studies showed that those α_{1A}-adrenoceptor antagonists without in vitro adrenoceptor subtype selectivity, such as alfuzosin and doxazosin, showed uroselectivity (terazosin was not uroselective), whereas tamsulosin, which exhibited in vitro selectivity for the α_{1A}-adrenoceptor, did not show the expected in vivo uroselectivity.[240] Silodosin, the most recent addition to this class of drugs, showed both in vitro and in vivo uroselectivity. However, these differences between in vitro and in vivo studies suggest that these drugs modify urethral pressures in a manner that is not directly correlated with their selectivity for the cloned α_{1A}-adrenoceptor subtypes. It is apparent that the existing α_{1A}-adrenoceptor antagonists have different in vivo pharmacologic profiles that are not yet predictable from their receptor based on the current state of knowledge regarding the α_{1A}-adrenoceptor classification.[240]

Tamsulosin, alfuzosin, and silodosin are first-line drugs for the treatment of BPH and have no utility in treating hypertension because they have fewer cardiovascular effects than terazosin and doxazosin. Some of the basic physicochemical and pharmacokinetic properties of the α_1-antagonists are summarized in Table 25.14. Improvements in urine flow occur 4 to 8 hours after the first dose and in BPH symptoms within 1 week.

Adverse Reactions

In patients with BPH, the most common adverse effects for α_1-adrenergic antagonists are related to abnormal ejaculation and orthostatic hypotension, with vasodilation, dizziness, headache, and tachycardia also occurring in some patients during the first 2 weeks of treatment.[241] Therefore, a dose titration is usually required, especially in patients taking doxazosin or terazosin, or older than 60 years. These cardiovascular side effects are attributed to a nonselective blockade of α_1-adrenoceptors present in vascular smooth muscle in addition to the required blockade of α_1-adrenoceptors in prostate. No first-dose effect and fewer vasodilatory adverse events have been reported with silodosin and the sustained-release formulations of other drugs, which occur more frequently with the immediate-release formulation. At higher doses, orthostatic hypotension occurs more frequently. The first-dose phenomenon of orthostatic hypotension and syncope has been reported occasionally in older adult patients and in those concurrently receiving calcium antagonists, diuretics, and β-blockers. Concomitant use of the α_1-adrenoceptor antagonists with PDE5Is (used commonly for ED in older men) is associated with a higher risk for dizziness and symptomatic hypotension.

5α-Reductase Inhibitors

The 5ARIs work by suppressing the production of intraprostatic DHT, thereby reducing the size of the prostate.[233] When the prostate volume is large, finasteride and dutasteride are the most commonly used drugs, either alone or in combination with α_1-adrenergic antagonists. Unlike α_1-antagonists, 5ARIs are able to reverse BPH to some extent and so may delay the need for surgery. Several months (6-12) of treatment may be needed before the benefit is noticed by the patient; thus, the patient needs to be encouraged to stay on the medication.

The discovery of the 5ARI finasteride by Merck is an interesting drug discovery story that received inspiration from male pseudohermaphrodites who have an error in the gene that encodes for $5AR_2$.[242,243] This genetic disease was of inspiration to scientists at Merck because the male pseudohermaphrodites had $5AR_2$ deficiency, decreased DHT levels, small prostates throughout life and did not develop BPH, male-pattern baldness (androgenic alopecia), or acne. Except for the associated urogenital defects that were present at birth, no other clinical abnormalities related to 5AR deficiency were observed in these individuals. Thus, scientists hypothesized that DHT was the causative agent. If they could recreate the decreased levels of DHT in men, they hoped they might be able to prevent BPH, acne, and hair loss. In 1992, finasteride was approved for symptomatic treatment of BPH (Proscar, 5 mg) and in 1997, it received approval for androgenic alopecia (Propecia, 1 mg). Dutasteride (Avodart, 0.5 mg) was approved in 2010. 5ARIs may be used to prevent progression of LUTS secondary to BPH only when prostatic enlargement is present and, as previously noted, can take 6 to 12 months for clinical benefit to be felt by patient. Because the clinical efficacy of 5ARIs can be modest at best, 5ARIs can be given in combination with the α_{1A}-adrenergic antagonist for additive effects. Dutasteride is available in combination with tamsulosin (Jalyn). 5ARIs may cause decreases in serum PSA concentration in the presence of prostate cancer. 5ARIs are not approved for prostate cancer prevention, but clinical trials have shown they can reduce low-grade prostate cancer by nearly 20%. FDA approval for prostate cancer prevention was rejected as it was also shown there was an increase in high-grade prostate cancer with 5ARIs.[244]

Mechanism of Action of 5α-Reductase Inhibitors

The development of BPH requires a combination of intraprostatic DHT and the aging process. Although not elevated in BPH, levels of DHT in the prostate remain at physiologic levels with aging despite a decrease in serum testosterone. Inhibitors of DHT biosynthesis can result in a decrease in both circulating and target tissue (prostate and skin) DHT concentrations, thus blocking its androgenic action in these tissues. The critical enzyme targeted for DHT biosynthesis inhibition is 5AR, which converts testosterone into the more active metabolite DHT (Fig. 25.30). Three different isozymes of 5AR have been reported: $5AR_1$, $5AR_2$, and $5AR_3$, and their basic biology and role in human diseases are reviewed.[245] $5AR_1$ is predominantly expressed in the skin, liver, brain, and prostate, while $5AR_2$ is present in prostate, seminal vesicles, skin, liver, and hair follicles. The mechanism for testosterone reduction to DHT is shown in Figure 25.30 and

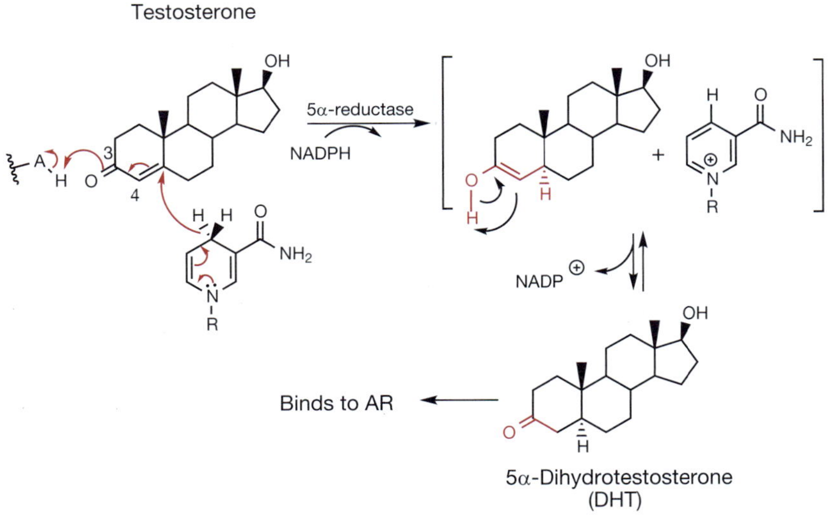

Figure 25.30 Conversion of testosterone into DHT by 5α-reductase.

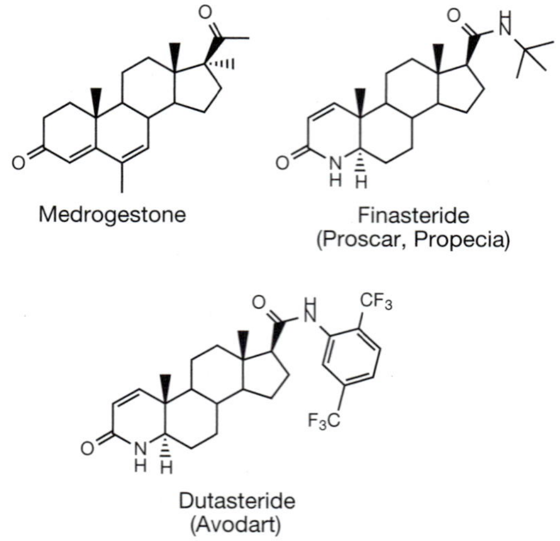

Figure 25.31 5α-Reductase inhibitors.

involves a hydride transfer from the cofactor NADPH to the 5α-position of testosterone, leading to an enol intermediate that can undergo enzyme-mediated tautomerization to form the products of DHT and oxidized form of nicotinamide adenine dinucleotide phosphate ($NADP^+$).

The first agent to demonstrate 5AR inhibition was a progestin analog, medrogestone (Fig. 25.31).[246] Two azasteroid-17-amide derivatives of medrogestone have been developed as potent competitive inhibitors of 5AR and approved for the treatment of BPH: finasteride, a selective inhibitor of $5AR_2$,[247,248] and dutasteride, a more potent but nonselective inhibitor of $5AR_1$ and $5AR_2$ (Fig. 25.31).[249] Inhibition of $5AR_2$ suppresses the metabolism of testosterone to DHT, resulting in significant decreases in serum and intraprostatic DHT concentrations.[248-250]

Finasteride and dutasteride are competitive inhibitors of 5AR that also have the ability to work as mechanism-based inhibitors to inactivate 5AR through an apparent irreversible modification of the enzyme.[251,252] They exhibit differing selectivity for 5AR. The inhibition constants (IC_{50}), in Table 25.15, suggest that finasteride is 30 times more selective for $5AR_2$, whereas dutasteride appears to be approximately 2 times more potent as an inhibitor of $5AR_2$ as compared to $5AR_1$. Finasteride binds to 5AR where testosterone normally binds and accepts a hydride transfer from NADPH to the 1α-position of the A ring of finasteride, forming an enol intermediate (Fig. 25.32). Due to the presence of the 4-aza group, the enol does not tautomerize to the keto group, but rather is postulated to form an enolate that can attack the electrophilic $NADP^+$ still present to form an enzyme-bound, dihydrofinasteride-NADP adduct that slowly releases dihydrofinasteride with a half-life of 1 month.[251] Finasteride and dutasteride are 4-aza steroids with a 1-ene and *trans* A-B ring junction and are thought to mimic the pathway of testosterone reduction to DHT. It was found that lipophilic groups at the 17β-position improve biologic activity.[253] The

Table 25.15 Some Properties and Pharmacokinetics of the 5α-Reductases

Drugs	Finasteride	Dutasteride
Tradename	Proscar	Avodart
cLog P^a	3.53	5.45
Oral bioavailability (%)	65 (26-170)	60 (40-94)
Onset of action (h)	<24	—
Duration of action (h)	—	>5 wk
Protein binding (%)	90	99
Time to peak concentration (h)	—	2-3
Volume of distribution (L/kg)	76 (44-96)	300-500
Elimination half-life (h)	5-6 (ages 18-60 y)	5 wk
	>8 (ages ≥70 y)	
Cytochrome isoforms	3A4	3A4
Active metabolites	None	6′-OH
Excretion (%) feces/urine	57/40 as metabolites	40/5 as metabolites
IC_{50} (nM)	313 (type 1)	3.9 (type 1)
	11 (type 2)	1.8 (type 2)

[a]www.drugbank.ca. Accessed July 15, 2025.

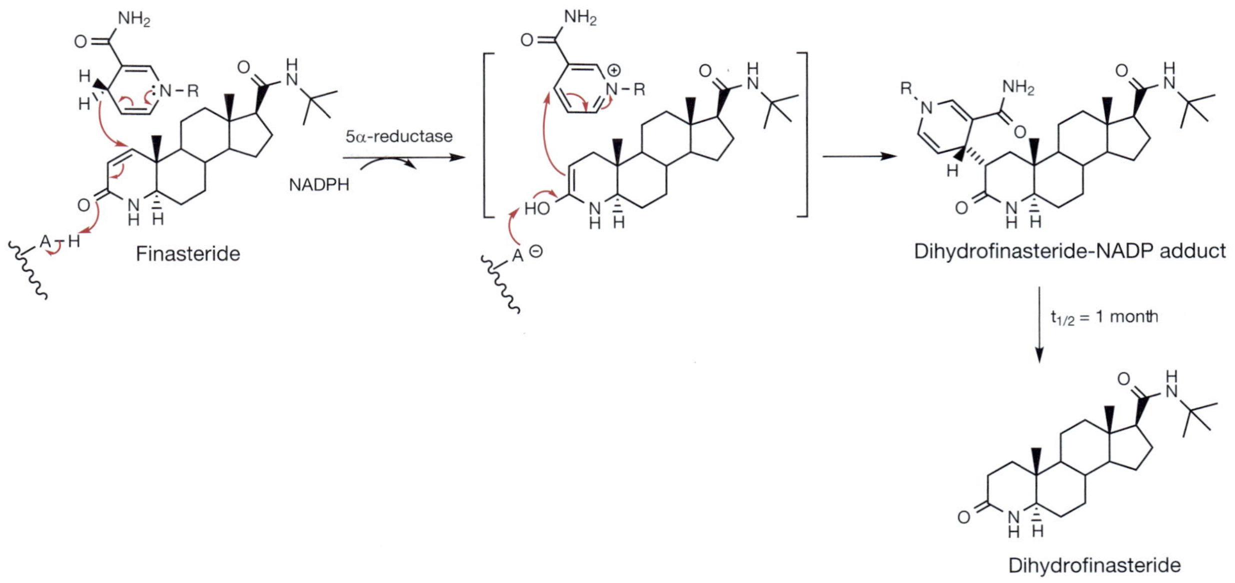

Figure 25.32 Mechanism-based inactivation of 5α-reductase by finasteride.

mechanism-based inhibition explains the exceptional potency and specificity of finasteride and dutasteride in the treatment of BPH. This concept of mechanism-based inhibition may have application to the development of other inhibitors of pyridine nucleotide–linked enzymes.

The 5ARIs are most effective in patients with large prostates (>40 g) and can decrease the production of DHT by 50% to 70%. A disadvantage of 5ARIs is their slow onset of action, as it can take 6 to 12 months to exert their maximum clinical effect. Common adverse effects of these agents include decreased libido, impotence, and ejaculation disorders, which can be bothersome in sexually active patients. 5ARIs can be useful to increase urinary flow rate, decrease prostate volume, prevent acute urinary retention, and avoid surgery in patients with BPH. However, if combined with α_1-antagonists, patients get better resolution of their symptoms. BPH can also be treated with 5ARIs together with PDE5Is. For example, 5 mg finasteride combined with 5 mg tadalafil in a fixed-dose combination (Entadfi), approved in 2021 for the signs and symptoms of BPH for up to 26 weeks of therapy, may also benefit patients with coexisting ED. Entadfi is the only BPH drug that does not have a risk of sexual side effects.

Finasteride (Proscar)

The selective inhibition of the $5AR_2$ isozyme by finasteride produces a rapid reduction in serum DHT concentration, reaching 65% suppression within 24 hours of administering a 1 mg oral tablet.[254] At steady state, finasteride suppresses DHT levels by approximately 70% in serum and by as much as 85% to 90% in the prostate. The remaining DHT in the prostate likely is the result of $5AR_1$. The mean circulating levels of testosterone and 17β-estradiol remained within their physiologic concentration range. Long-term therapy with finasteride can reduce clinically significant end points of BPH, such as acute urinary retention or need for surgery. Finasteride is most effective in men with large prostates (>40 g). Finasteride has no affinity for the AR and no androgenic, antiandrogenic, estrogenic, antiestrogenic, or progestational effects.

PHARMACOKINETICS. The mean oral bioavailability of finasteride is 65%, as shown in Table 25.15, and is not affected by food.[254] Approximately 90% of circulating finasteride is bound to plasma proteins.[255] Finasteride has been found to cross the blood-brain barrier (BBB), but levels in semen were undetectable (<0.2 ng/mL). Finasteride is extensively metabolized in the liver, primarily via CYP3A4, to two major metabolites: monohydroxylation of the *t*-butyl side chain, which is further metabolized via an aldehyde intermediate to the second metabolite, a monocarboxylic acid (Fig. 25.33). The metabolites show approximately 20% of the 5AR inhibition of finasteride.[255] The mean terminal half-life is approximately 5 to 6 hours in men ages 18 to 60 years and 8 hours in men older than age 70 years. Following an oral dose of finasteride, approximately 40% of the dose was excreted in the urine as metabolites and approximately 57% in the feces. Even though the elimination rate of finasteride is decreased in the older patients, no dosage adjustment is necessary. No dosage adjustment is necessary in patients with renal insufficiency. A decrease in the urinary excretion of metabolites was observed in patients with renal impairment, but this was compensated for by an increase in fecal excretion of metabolites. Caution should be used during administration to patients with liver function abnormalities because finasteride is metabolized extensively in the liver. Finasteride can be absorbed through the skin. As such, tablets, especially broken ones, should not be handled by women who are pregnant or could become pregnant due to a risk of fetal exposure.

Dutasteride (Avodart)

Similar to finasteride, dutasteride is a competitive and mechanism-based inhibitor not only of $5AR_2$ but also of $5AR_1$ isoenzyme, with which stable enzyme-NADP adduct complexes are formed, inhibiting the conversion of testosterone to DHT.[252] The suppression of both $5AR_1$ and $5AR_2$

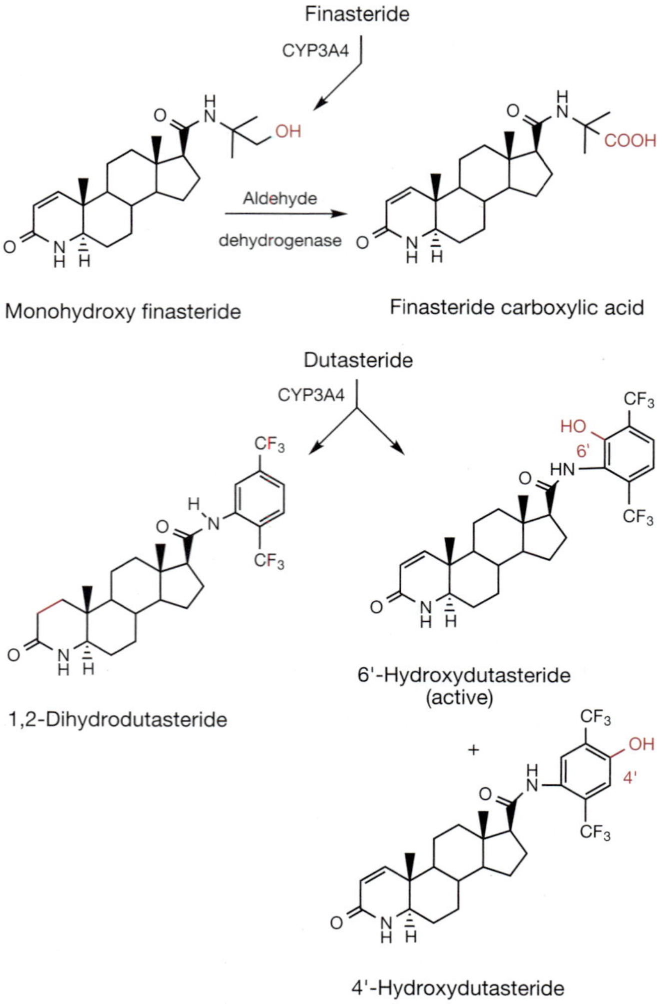

Figure 25.33 Metabolites of finasteride and dutasteride.

isoforms results in greater and more consistent reduction of plasma DHT than that observed for finasteride.[256-258] The more effective dual inhibition of $5AR_1$ and $5AR_2$ isoforms lowers circulating DHT to a greater extent than with finasteride and shows advantages in treating BPH and other disease states (eg, prostate cancer) that are DHT dependent.

The maximum effect of 0.5-mg daily doses of dutasteride on the suppression of DHT is dose dependent and is observed within 1 to 2 weeks. After 2 weeks of 0.5-mg daily dosing, median serum DHT concentrations were reduced by 90%, and after 1 year, the median decrease in serum DHT was 94%.[257,258] The median increase in serum testosterone was 19% but remained within the physiologic range. The drug also reduced serum PSA by approximately 50% at 6 months and total prostate volume by 25% at 2 years. Dutasteride produced improvements in quality of life and peak urinary flow rate and reduction of acute urinary retention without the need for surgery. The main side effects are ED,[259] decreased libido, gynecomastia, and ejaculation disorders. Long-term use (>4 years), however, did not reveal increased onset of sexual side effects. A combination product (Jalyn) containing dutasteride (0.5 mg) and tamsulosin (0.4 mg) was approved by the FDA (2010) based on clinical studies showing that the combination was more effective than either monotherapy as assessed by prostate symptom score and maximal urine flow rates. The decreased adrenergic tone associated with tamsulosin and long-term reduction in prostate size (obstruction) associated with dutasteride provide rapid and sustained symptomatic relief for men with BPH.

Pharmacokinetics. Following oral administration, peak plasma concentrations of dutasteride occur in approximately 2 to 3 hours, with a bioavailability of approximately 60% (Table 25.15), and no meaningful reduction in absorption occurs with food.[254,256,260] Dutasteride is highly bound to plasma proteins by 99%. The concentrations of dutasteride in semen averaged approximately 3 ng/mL, with no significant effects on DHT plasma levels of sex partners. Dutasteride is extensively metabolized in humans by CYP3A4 to three major metabolites: 4′-hydroxydutasteride and 1,2-dihydrodutasteride, which are less potent than parent drug, and 6′-hydroxydutasteride, which is comparable to the parent drug as an inhibitor of both $5AR_1$ and $5AR_2$ (Fig. 25.33). Dutasteride is excreted mainly (40%) in feces as dutasteride-related metabolites. The terminal elimination half-life of dutasteride is approximately 5 weeks. Because of its long half-life, systemic concentrations remain detectable for up to 4 to 6 months after discontinuation of treatment. No dose adjustment is necessary in older adult patients, even though its half-life increased with age from approximately 170 hours in men aged 20 to 49 years to 300 hours in men older than age 70 years.[254,261] No adjustment in dosage is necessary for patients with renal impairment. Like finasteride, dutasteride can be absorbed through the skin. As such, dutasteride capsules should not be handled by women who are pregnant or who could become pregnant.

Drug-Drug Interactions

Because finasteride and dutasteride are metabolized primarily by CYP3A4, the CYP3A4 inhibitors, such as ritonavir, ketoconazole, verapamil, diltiazem, cimetidine, and ciprofloxacin, may increase these drugs' blood levels and, possibly, cause DDIs. Clinical drug interaction studies have shown no pharmacokinetic or pharmacodynamic interactions between dutasteride and tamsulosin or terazosin, warfarin, digoxin, and cholestyramine.

Phytotherapy

A number of plant extracts are popularly used to alleviate BPH, although formal evidence that they are effective is often scanty.[261,262] Current guidelines from the AUA do not recommend dietary supplements or combination phytotherapeutic agents for the management of LUTS secondary to BPH.[229] However, extracts of the saw palmetto berry (*Serenoa repens*) are widely used for the treatment of BPH, often as an alternative to pharmaceutical agents. It has been thought that a 160-mg bid dose of saw palmetto extract was approximately as effective as 5ARIs over time. However, increasing doses of a saw palmetto fruit extract did not reduce LUTS more than placebo in clinical trials.[262] Other Western herbs that have been investigated for the treatment of BPH include pumpkin seeds (*Cucurbita pepo*), nettle root (*Urtica *dioica* or *Urtica urens*), bee pollen (particularly that from the rye plant), African potato (tubers of *Hypoxis rooperi*), and the African tree *Pygeum africanum*, also known as *Prunus africanum*. A detailed discussion of phytotherapy can be found in Chapter 40 of the seventh edition of this book.

Treating Skin Conditions With Inhibitors of the Androgen Receptor Axis

Acne vulgaris is an example of an androgen-dependent condition affecting ~80% of adolescents and young adults of both sexes ages 11 to 30 years, when hormone levels surge.[263] The effects of androgens are exaggerated in the skin due to the high expression of 5AR. Sebocytes, the cells within the sebaceous glands of the face, are exquisitely sensitive to DHT and produce the oily secretion known as sebum. The excessive production of oils, which must be expelled from the hair follicle, can result in plugged and infected hair follicles producing multiple comedos (pimples), collectively referred to as acne,[264] an inflammatory condition of the skin.[265] Due to the importance of androgens (and estrogens) in the pubertal development from adolescence to adults, the use of systemic antiandrogens (eg, AR inhibitors not approved for acne such as flutamide and finasteride) is precluded in the affected population. Other classes of agents approved for acne exist, such as combined oral contraceptives (females only) or spironolactone (an aldosterone receptor antagonist; see Chapter 24), but also suffer from systemic effects that limit their scope of use. Androgen-dependent growth and developmental processes are robust in youth, without pathology in most tissues, and are necessary to thrive. However, acne and seborrhea (excessively oily skin) are associated in the short term with social insecurities and long-term sequelae in the form of facial scars, which would be preventable and treatable with an antiandrogen if its effects could be localized to the sebaceous gland or skin, such as through a topical therapy that does not penetrate the skin.[266]

Similarly, topical therapies could be used to prevent or treat androgenic alopecia (baldness) by blocking hyperandrogenicity in the hair follicle. Androgenic alopecia affects ~50% of Caucasian males by midlife and up to 90% by 80 years old. Minoxidil (a topical vasodilator) and finasteride (a systemic 5ARI) are FDA approved for alopecia but require 4 to 12 months of treatment to produce a therapeutic effect, and only arrest hair loss in most with mild-to-moderate hair regrowth in 30% to 60%. The slow and limited efficacy of approved therapies that produce unwanted sexual side effects due to systemic exposure leaves androgenic alopecia and other hyperandrogenic dermatologic diseases in need of local inhibition of the AR axis.

Recently, clascoterone (Winlevi), a steroidal antiandrogen with anti-inflammatory activity, was approved as 1% topical cream (applied to affected area bid) for the treatment of acne vulgaris in patients aged 12 years and above. Clascoterone is cortexolone 17α-propionate, which is an 11-deoxy derivative of endogenous glucocorticoid hormone hydrocortisone or cortisol (see Chapter 24), which helps to rationalize the anti-inflammatory activity. Clascoterone blocks the sebum-producing and inflammatory cytokine production effects of DHT in the sebaceous gland. Clascoterone was able to reduce the number and severity of inflammatory and noninflammatory lesions in patients with acne vulgaris without significant hypothalamus-pituitary-adrenal (HPA) axis suppression in most patients (only seen 5% and 9% of patients at 30 minutes and 14 days postapplication), illustrating its limited systemic exposure. Following 2 weeks of topical administration of the cream (on average 6 g applied bid) to adult patients with acne vulgaris, clascoterone can be detected with a C_{max} in the plasma of 4.5 ng/mL. The 17α-propionate side chain of clascoterone is metabolically cleaved by unknown esterases to produce cortexolone (11-deoxycortisol) as its primary metabolite, whose plasma concentration is very low, generally below the limit of quantitation (0.5 ng/mL).[267] Clascoterone is also being tested for alopecia but is not yet available for that indication.

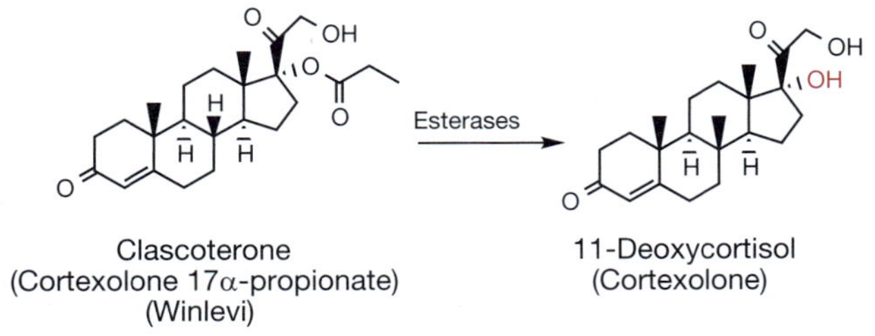

Treatment of Prostatitis

Prostatitis is a broad term used to identify inflammation of the prostate gland associated with LUTSs in men.[268] Prostatitis rarely occurs in males younger than 30 years; however, it is a common problem in older males, being described as acute bacterial prostatitis, chronic bacterial prostatitis, or nonbacterial prostatitis. Because antimicrobial drug penetration is generally poor into the prostate gland, with poor efficacy of the antimicrobial agents and long duration of treatment, a 30% to 40% failure rate occurs with common treatment modalities. Three major factors determine the diffusion and concentration of antimicrobial agents in prostatic fluid and tissue: the lipid solubility of the antimicrobial agent, its dissociation constant (pK_a), and the percentage of plasma protein binding. The physiologic pH of human prostatic fluid is 6.5 to 6.7, but it increases in chronic prostatitis, ranging from 7.0 to 8.3.[269] A greater concentration of antimicrobial agents in the prostatic fluid occurs in the presence of a pH gradient across the membrane separating plasma from prostatic fluid. Of the available antimicrobial agents, β-lactam drugs have a low pK_a and poor lipid solubility and thus penetrate poorly into prostatic fluid, except for some cephalosporins. Good to excellent penetration into prostatic fluid and tissue has been demonstrated with many antimicrobial agents, including tobramycin, tetracyclines, macrolides, fluoroquinolones, sulfonamides, and nitrofurantoin. The diagnosis and therapy of prostatitis remains a challenge. Because prostatitis usually requires prolonged therapy, patients must understand the importance of compliance, and physicians should screen for drug interactions that may decrease compliance and efficacy.

Acute bacterial prostatitis is the least common of the prostate infections and is usually accompanied by a urinary tract infection with positive cultures. The symptoms include sudden onset of fever, chills, and low back pain, as well as complaints of urinary obstruction (eg, dysuria, nocturia, urgency, frequency, and burning) and urinary irritation (eg, hesitancy, straining, dribbling, weak stream, and incomplete emptying). The most commonly prescribed antimicrobials for acute bacterial prostatitis are trimethoprim/sulfamethoxazole, doxycycline, fluoroquinolones, ciprofloxacin, ofloxacin, and norfloxacin (see Chapter 32). The concentrations of these antimicrobial agents in the prostatic fluid are 2 to 3 times that in plasma, thus achieving adequate concentrations in prostatic tissues to eradicate the most common causative pathogens. The recommended duration of treatment for acute bacterial prostatitis is 4 to 6 weeks. A short-course therapy is not recommended because of the risk of relapse or progression to chronic bacterial prostatitis.

Chronic bacterial prostatitis occurs when acute bacterial prostatitis has been inadequately treated because of pathogen resistance, relapse, or short-course therapy or because of blocked drainage of secretions from the prostate. Most men with chronic prostatitis will have had a previous bout of acute prostatitis. The most common clinical feature of chronic prostatitis is recurrent urinary tract infections and the symptoms and complaints of acute bacterial prostatitis. Fluoroquinolones, trimethoprim-sulfamethoxazole, doxycycline, and nitrofurantoin are used in the management of chronic prostatitis. Chronic prostatitis warrants at least 10 to 12 weeks of therapy. Poor clinical outcomes, however, have been observed because of poor diffusion of antimicrobials into the prostate.

Nonbacterial prostatitis is the most common type of prostatitis. It occurs more frequently than bacterial prostatitis, with the same signs and symptoms as bacterial prostatitis, except that prostatic fluid cultures are negative for the presence of bacteria. Inflammation is evident on prostate gland examination. Treatment includes minocycline, doxycycline, or erythromycin. Treatment duration is approximately 2 to 4 weeks.

Drugs Used for the Treatment of Hormone-Dependent Cancers (Breast, Prostate)

As men and women age, hyperproliferation of sexual organs such as the breast and prostate tends to occur under the influence of endogenous estrogens and androgens, commonly leading to malignancies originating in these tissues. Breast and prostate cancers are both extremely common cancers, having an increased incidence with age and being predominantly dependent on hormones for their growth. Hormone-dependent cancers tend to be slower growing cancers than other solid malignancies, particularly in early-stage disease, where the disease may be considered as treatable and curable. Staging is based on the size and extent of spread of disease, with early stage considered as stage 1 (small; confined to the organ of origin), stage 2 (bigger; confined to the organ of origin and/or nearby lymph nodes may be involved), and stage 3 (any size; considered locally advanced because of spread to regions close to the organ of origin). Stage 3 has not spread to distant organs but is at higher risk for progression to stage 4, which is distantly metastatic or advanced disease. Advanced disease (stage 4) indicates that the disease is no longer early stage and is most commonly used to describe cancers that cannot be cured even with optimal treatment and response.

Whereas surgical hormone ablation and chemotherapy were once the main treatment options, better understanding of the underlying biology of these cancers has allowed modern treatments to be more personalized, especially for breast cancer. Suppression of the ER or AR axis, respectively, has remained the cornerstone of therapy and produced many targeted hormonal therapies to improve the overall survival and quality of life of patients with breast or prostate cancer. Further, earlier interventions to prevent or delay disease recurrence and progression and rational sequencing of newer agents have become more common, contributing to improved prognosis for these hormone-dependent cancers. Nonetheless, many of the commonly used agents are less than optimal, possessing low potency, intrinsic agonism, dosing-limiting side effects, and/or poor absorption, distribution, metabolism, and excretion (ADME) properties. Development of resistance to these directed hormonal therapies is common. Consequently, the treatment of hormone-refractory breast and prostate cancers is still a significant unmet medical need, leaving room for improvement of existing therapeutic classes or circumvention of their resistance, as well as extension of the anticancer armamentarium to novel therapeutic classes that are less susceptible to the development of resistance.

Hormone-Dependent Breast Cancer

Personalized Medicine in Breast Cancer

In the United States, the lifetime risk of developing breast cancer is one in eight, with the greatest incidence in women older than age 60 years.[270] It is the second leading cause of death from cancer in women (lung cancer is number one). Breast cancer is a diverse collection of diseases that are connected by the formation of tumors in breast tissue. Upon presentation with a breast tumor, in addition to typical staging of the cancer in terms of T (tumor size/aggressiveness/location), N (spread to regional lymph nodes), and M (presence of distant metastasis), the prognosis and treatment regimen are largely determined by the types of drug targets that are present in the tumor as determined by its molecular phenotype. The diversity of molecular targets in breast cancer allows for personalized pharmacotherapy. The majority of breast cancers (~80%) express high levels of the hormone receptors ERα and PR, congruent with their origins as hyperproliferative milk duct linings. These breast cancers that depend on the ERα to grow are referred to herein as ER-positive breast cancer (also commonly referred to as hormone receptor–positive breast cancer) and can be treated with antiestrogen treatments. Typically, ER-positive breast cancer is a better prognosis disease, particularly when the PR is also highly expressed and HER2 (human epidermal growth factor receptor [EGFR] type II) is absent. Hormone-dependent breast cancer (ie, ER-positive breast cancer that is responsive to a variety of hormone therapies) is the main focus of this chapter.

Other Breast Cancers

Approximately 25% to 30% of breast cancers[271] are HER2 positive, meaning that they overexpress proteins of the EGFR family. These are more aggressive forms of breast cancer with a poorer prognosis because EGFR activates signaling pathways that promote tumor progression and resistance to treatment.[272] In addition to antiestrogens if ER positive, the mainstay of directed therapies for HER2-positive tumors is the use of monoclonal antibodies such as trastuzumab (1998), pertuzumab (2013), ado-trastuzumab emtansine (2013), or fam-trastuzumab deruxtecan-nxki (2022; uniquely approved for HER2 low breast cancer) that flag the tumor cell for destruction by the body's immune system (ie, antibody-dependent cellular cytotoxicity). Further, the latter two employ trastuzumab-directed delivery of chemotherapy to tumor cells (Chapters 37 and 38). It is also possible to inhibit the kinase function of EGFR using small molecule kinase inhibitors. For example, lapatinib (2007) was approved in breast cancer, and more recently, neratinib (2017) (Chapter 37) was approved in early-stage breast cancer after a woman has completed 1 year of trastuzumab. In 2020, tucatinib combined with trastuzumab and capecitabine was approved in advanced unresectable or metastatic HER2-positive breast cancer. Unfortunately, resistance can develop to targeted antiestrogen and/or HER2 therapies, and the number of effective pharmacotherapeutic tools starts to diminish, leaving salvage therapies and chemotherapies as the only remaining options.

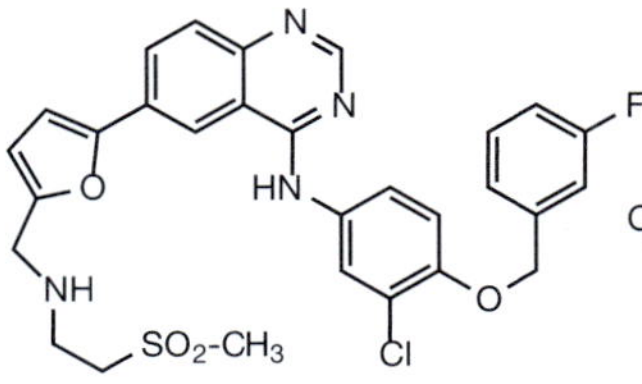

Lapatinib

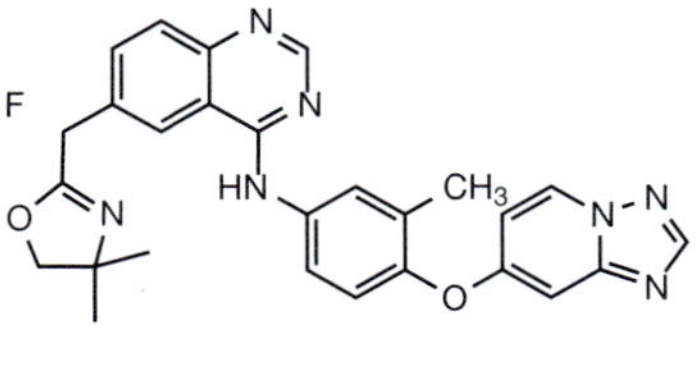

Tucatinib

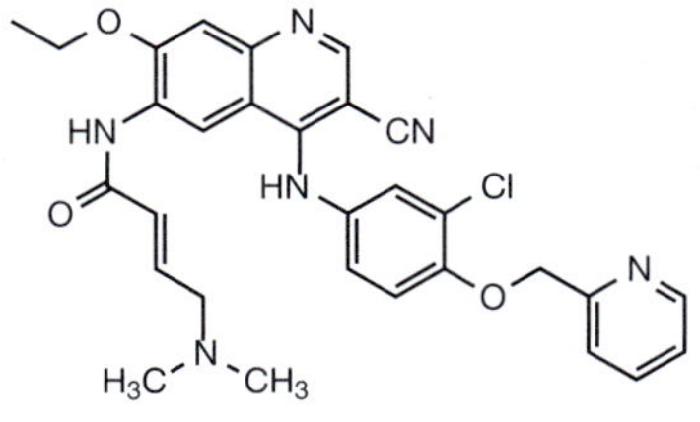

Neratinib

Unfortunately, approximately 15% to 20% of breast cancers upon presentation are triple-negative breast cancers (TNBCs) that do not express any of ERα, PR, or HER2, indicating the lack of responsiveness to traditional targeted drug therapy options. TNBC is also characterized by more aggressive tumors and poorer prognosis, and TNBC treatment traditionally has been almost entirely dependent on chemotherapy. Recently, the FDA has approved a couple of novel directed therapy or personalized medicine approaches that are nonhormonal in nature for TNBC. In 2021, a programmed death-ligand 1 (PD-L1)-directed therapy, pembrolizumab (Keytruda), was approved in combination with chemotherapy for neoadjuvant treatment of high-risk, early-stage TNBC whose tumors express PD-L1. The PD-L1-targeted therapy is then continued as a single agent as adjuvant treatment after surgery. The other recently approved directed therapy is an antibody-drug conjugate, sacituzumab govitecan-hziy (Trodelvy), that delivers chemotherapy to Trop-2 (a transmembrane glycoprotein encoded by the *Tacstd2* gene) positive cells as third-line therapy for unresectable locally advanced or metastatic TNBC (see Chapters 37 and 38). Other attempts for directed therapies include AR-directed therapies,[273] as TNBC is commonly AR positive. However, there are at least six subtypes of TNBC, and responses to these or other targeted therapies are not likely to be univocal[274] across all subtypes. There is also hope that genotyping may be helpful in some patients with TNBC.

Genotyping

Genotyping has long been used to screen women who may be genetically predisposed to developing breast cancer. It is another diagnostic or prognostic tool that can be used to determine the availability of therapies. For example, certain women are predisposed to develop breast cancer based on the presence of germline (ie, inherited) mutations in the breast cancer susceptibility genes (*BRCA*) type 1 (*BRCA1*) or *BRCA2*.[275] A couple of SERMs (discussed in detail below), tamoxifen in 1999 and raloxifene in 2007, were approved for the primary prevention of breast cancer in patient populations who are at high risk based on family history and/or genotype considerations.[276,277] However, hysterectomy or prophylactic mastectomy was often considered in these patients as a more definite preventive. Olaparib (Lynparza) and talazoparib (Talzenna), inhibitors of the enzyme poly(ADP-ribose) polymerase (PARP) (Chapter 37), are approved for patients with advanced ER-positive and HER2-negative breast cancer with certain inherited *BRCA* mutations who have received previous therapy.[278] Olaparib is also indicated in high-risk early breast cancers with inherited *BRCA* mutant that are HER2 negative. Further, there is hope that PARP inhibitors may be helpful in TNBC with inherited *BRCA1* mutations, which accounts for ~80% of TNBC.

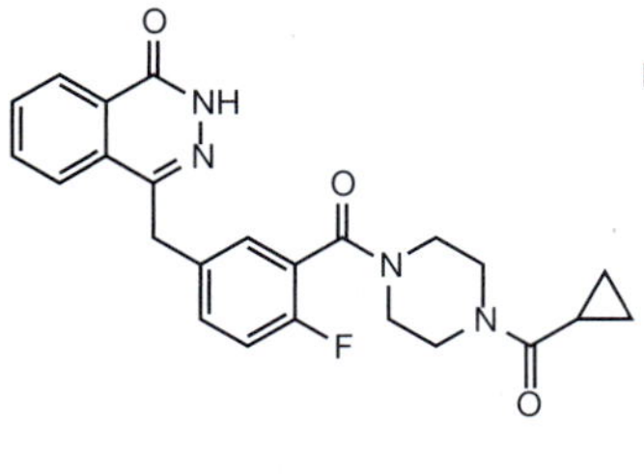

Olaparib

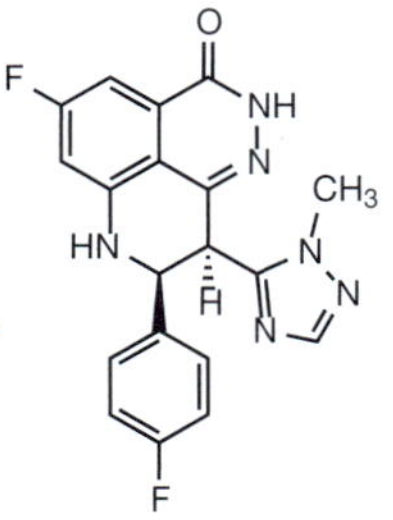

Talazoparib

Endocrine Therapy for Estrogen Receptor–Positive Breast Cancer

The endogenous female hormone 17β-estradiol is the natural ligand for ERα and ERβ. ERα's primary role is support of the gender dimorphic female characteristics including primary sexual features, such as growth of the mammary glands. Unfortunately, ERα-dependent hyperproliferation of breast tissue (and uterus) is common, affecting ~80% of the one in eight women who develop breast cancer in their lifetime. Suppression of ER signaling is the central feature in the treatment of ER-positive breast cancer and can be accomplished by (1) direct tissue-selective inhibition of the ER by SERMs (tamoxifen, TOR, or raloxifene); (2) suppression of endogenous estrogen synthesis, centrally in pre- or perimenopausal women by the GnRH agonist (goserelin), which suppresses ovarian production, or peripheral suppression in postmenopausal women by AIs (exemestane, anastrozole, letrozole); or (3) pure antiestrogen activity, including ER degradation by selective estrogen receptor degraders (SERDs) fulvestrant or elacestrant.

While the prognosis of most patients with early-stage ER-positive breast cancer is relatively good compared to nonhormonal cancers, adjuvant hormone therapy failures do occur, resulting in recurrence, including distant metastases (ie, advanced breast cancer). Metastatic or advanced breast cancer, whether hormone naïve or progressive despite endocrine therapy, is often still ER positive and still dependent on the ER axis for growth. The treatment of early or advanced breast cancer is rapidly evolving from the use of an endocrine monotherapy such as SERM or AI or SERD as first-line agents (initial therapy), to combinations of an endocrine therapy with kinase inhibitors, especially the cyclin-dependent kinase 4/6 (CDK4/6) inhibitors (palbociclib [2015], ribociclib [2017], or abemaciclib [2017]). Second-line therapies (therapies used following progression on first-line therapies) now include the mechanistic target of rapamycin (mTOR) inhibitor (everolimus [2012]) or the phosphoinositide 3-kinase (PI3KCA) inhibitor (alpelisib [2019]). These combination therapies that delay progression of advanced breast cancer compared to endocrine therapy alone have all but supplanted the use of endocrine therapy alone in late breast cancer. As mentioned later, CDK4/6 inhibitors combined with endocrine therapies are starting to be approved in certain early breast cancer settings.

Treatment of Early Hormone Receptor–Positive Breast Cancer. For the sake of clarity, early hormone receptor–positive breast cancer is uncomplicated locally invasive breast cancer or noninvasive breast cancer (ie, not metastatic). The initial treatment of hormone receptor–positive breast cancer, in the absence of HER2, depends largely on the staging of the tumor. In the absence of distant metastasis, surgical excision such as lumpectomy, which is now favored over radical mastectomy, followed by radiation therapy are common primary treatments. In view of further prognostic criteria such as patient age, tumor lymph node status, tumor size (>1 cm), and aggressiveness (eg, mitotic index, Ki67 staining levels, and the results of gene expression profile[s]), a decision is made with regard to whether adjuvant (treating in the absence of observable active disease) chemotherapy would be beneficial to lower the probability of recurrence. Noninvasive breast cancer (ie, ductal carcinoma in situ [DCIS]) and the lowest risk invasive carcinoma presenting as a nonaggressive small tumor with no spread to lymph nodes may not warrant adjuvant chemotherapy. For low- to moderate-risk invasive breast cancers, chemotherapy is typically four cycles of the dose-intensive taxane docetaxel (Taxotere) and cyclophosphamide (regimen known as TC), whereas good evidence suggests that higher risk breast cancers should receive six cycles of sequential anthracycline and cyclophosphamide followed by a taxane (AC-T)[279] despite the cardiac toxicity of anthracyclines (Chapter 36). Unfortunately, chemotherapy only offers a modest benefit in terms of overall survival.

A complex array of risk factors, including various biomarkers such as gene expression profiling by OncotypeDx[280] or PAM50[281] aid in risk assessment and inform decisions regarding whether adjuvant chemotherapy is warranted. There is now strong evidence that genes beyond *BRCA1/2* confer markedly increased risk of breast and/or ovarian cancers, such as *CDH1*, *PALB2*, *PTEN*, and *TP53*.[282] Gene expression profiling to predict recurrence likelihood is recommended in patients with large tumors that are node negative and all node-positive patients.[283] Neoadjuvant (ie, before initial treatment with surgery/radiation) chemotherapy is considered in patients with TNBC and HER2-positive patients, but rarely in ER-positive patients.

RISK FACTORS OR PROGNOSIS INDICATORS IN EARLY-STAGE HORMONE RECEPTOR–POSITIVE BREAST CANCER

There is still great uncertainty as to which patient with early-stage breast cancer is likely to progress. As such, there is poor insight as to which patient would benefit from adjuvant chemotherapy. However, the following is a nonexhaustive listing of potential risk factors[284]:

Potentially Favorable Prognosis: Increased Chance of Less Aggressive and/or Treatment-Responsive Tumor

- ER or PR positive, particularly when both are highly expressed
- ER or PR positive, especially in tumors that are HER2 negative
- HER2 positive, especially in tumors that are ER/PR negative
- Radiologic initial presentation (eg, on mammogram) is favorable.

Potentially Unfavorable Prognosis: Increased Risk of Aggressive and/or Treatment-Resistant Tumor

- Triple negative (not hormone receptor positive)
- ER and/or PR negative
- HER2 positive, especially in tumors that are also ER/PR positive
- Young age at diagnosis and/or family history of breast cancer
- Clinical initial presentation (eg, the cancer progressed until symptomatic issues such as pain or necrosis caused the patient to seek medical care)
- High nuclear grade, indicating abnormal cell nuclei in tumor versus normal breast tissue
- Positive or close margins, which are postsurgical evidence of residual tumor
- Tumor burden to include large size (>1 cm) tumor and/or multiple tumors
- *BRCA* mutation positive, which indicates difficult tumor biology (now targeted) and is often associated with young diagnostic age
- Sentinel node positive, indicative of dedifferentiated and potentially metastatic disease
- Obesity, which can elevate aromatase levels and limits healthy activity post-treatment

Adjuvant hormonal therapy or endocrine therapy, however, is associated with huge benefits for the vast majority of ER-positive (but not ER-negative) patients in terms of preventing recurrence (eg, in the ipsilateral or contralateral breast or distance metastasis) and improving overall survival. Adjuvant hormonal therapy should only be considered optional in DCIS or small and node-negative invasive carcinoma. All other ER-positive patients will be advised to receive adjuvant hormonal therapy. Historically, the main classes of endocrine therapies in the adjuvant setting are monotherapy with SERMs or AIs. However, FDA recently approved a CDK4/6 inhibitor (abemaciclib; discussion in the "Advanced or Metastatic Breast Cancer: Endocrine and Targeted Therapies" section) for adjuvant therapy of early breast cancer (2021) in combination with tamoxifen or an AI in those with high risk for recurrence (node positive and a Ki67 score ≥20%). A similar approval with another CDK4/6 inhibitor, ribociclib, may soon occur. Again, many criteria can factor into the selection of which agent(s) to choose, but a few overriding factors include menopausal status, risk factors for progression, and tolerance of side effects.

Tamoxifen is preferred for adjuvant therapy of DCIS. Tamoxifen, a SERM, is typically prescribed for pre- and perimenopausal patients as adjuvant therapy of locally invasive carcinoma. Further, premenopausal patients will also receive ovarian suppression with a GnRH agonist, goserelin (Zoladex), being approved for this indication. Perimenopausal patients should be ovarian suppressed and then treated long term with adjuvant AI or SERM. Tamoxifen is typically regarded as having less severe side effects but also inferior ability to prevent recurrence compared to an AI. AIs have become favored as adjuvant monotherapy in postmenopausal locally invasive carcinoma, which is the majority of hormone-dependent breast cancers.[285] Usually, patients are treated in the adjuvant setting with a 5- to 10-year course of SERM (predominantly tamoxifen) or AI (most commonly letrozole or anastrozole), sometimes crossing over at some point; however, the introduction of approved combinations of endocrine therapy with various protein kinase inhibitors may change the therapeutic landscape.

Selective Estrogen Receptor Modulators. Since the discovery of the first nonsteroidal estrogen, DES, in 1938 many estrogenic scaffolds have been discovered and explored (Fig. 25.34). The structure of DES belies the simplicity of the pharmacophore for producing ligands of the ER(s). The basic precept is to position two phenol groups approximately the same distance apart, as in 17β-estradiol. There seem to be few restraints on the nature of the element linking the phenols, allowing tremendous chemodiversity[41,46]; however, most linking elements are rigidified to orient the phenolic groups in a similar manner as the steroidal backbone. In the course of SAR explorations in the 1960s, it was discovered that addition of steric bulk with a pendant basic amine group to the linking element produced compounds with tissue-selective antagonism in vivo. For example, addition of the *N,N*-dimethyl(aminoethyl)phenoxy side chain to DES produced tamoxifen, which was the first SERM to be FDA approved. Further, addition of a chlorine atom to the ethyl group of tamoxifen produced another FDA-approved SERM, TOR. Historically, these are referred to as antiestrogens due to their use as antagonists of breast tissue growth and utility in treating breast cancer; however, they retain some intrinsic agonist activity as seen in their action in the bone and uterus. The basic pharmacophoric elements of an

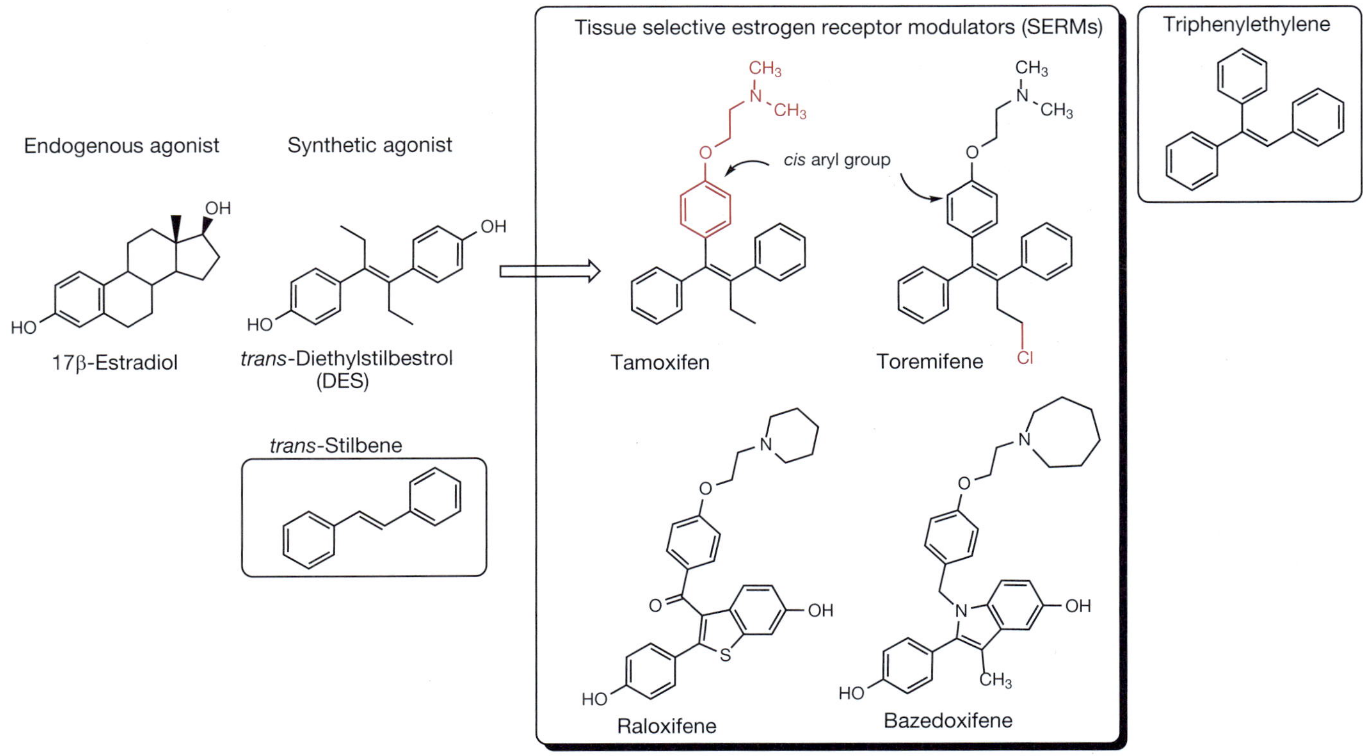

Figure 25.34 17β-Estradiol, nonsteroidal agonist DES, and various SERMs.

SERM or antiestrogen are (1) three aromatic groups rigidly held in place by a nonsteroidal linking element; (2) the *trans*-aryl groups must bear either a phenol group or bioisostere, or be metabolized to an active phenolic metabolite; and (3) the *cis*-aryl group must be composed of a phenoxy group linked by a linear alkyl chain (usually ethyl) to a basic tertiary amine. These pharmacophoric features are apparent in the structures of FDA-approved SERMs: tamoxifen, TOR, raloxifene, and bazedoxifene (see also Chapter 27) (Fig. 25.34).

SERMs, as a class, possess a unique pharmacology in which they behave as an ER agonist in some favorable estrogenic tissues (eg, bone and cardiovascular system) and as an ER antagonist in sexual tissues (eg, the breast and variably and incompletely in the uterus). Triphenylethylene SERMs exhibit a moderately strong and persistent binding to the ER, producing antiestrogen receptor complexes described later as ERα antagonist conformations. These complexes are believed to translocate into the nucleus of target cells, but normal estrogen transcriptional processes are altered. Hence, antiestrogens interfere with estrogen-dependent tumor growth by competing with estrogens for the receptor site and thereby altering the normal estrogenic processing of genetic information within the nucleus. The result is downregulation of transcription of estrogen-dependent genes, leading to decreased expression of estrogen-dependent proteins, resulting in inhibition of estrogen-dependent tumor growth.

Although the full mechanism of action is not completely understood, the molecular basis for tissue selectivity is apparent from crystallographic studies of the LBD. For example, the DES-ERα LBD co-crystal structure (3ERD.pdb)[64] demonstrated that DES binds analogous to 17β-estradiol (ie, the ligand is well accommodated by the ERα, which completely encloses it within a ligand-binding pocket) (Fig. 25.35). Importantly, steroidal agonists and synthetic agonists such as DES promote the formation of, and stabilize, the agonist conformation of ERα in which the C-terminal helix 12 (H12) folds in toward the helical barrel structure of the LBD and encloses the ligand. In the agonist conformation, the activation function-2 (AF-2) located on the exterior of ERα is able to bind to coactivators, recruit the preinitiation complex to ERE sites, and activate transcription of estrogen-driven genes. In contrast, for the antagonist conformations, as seen

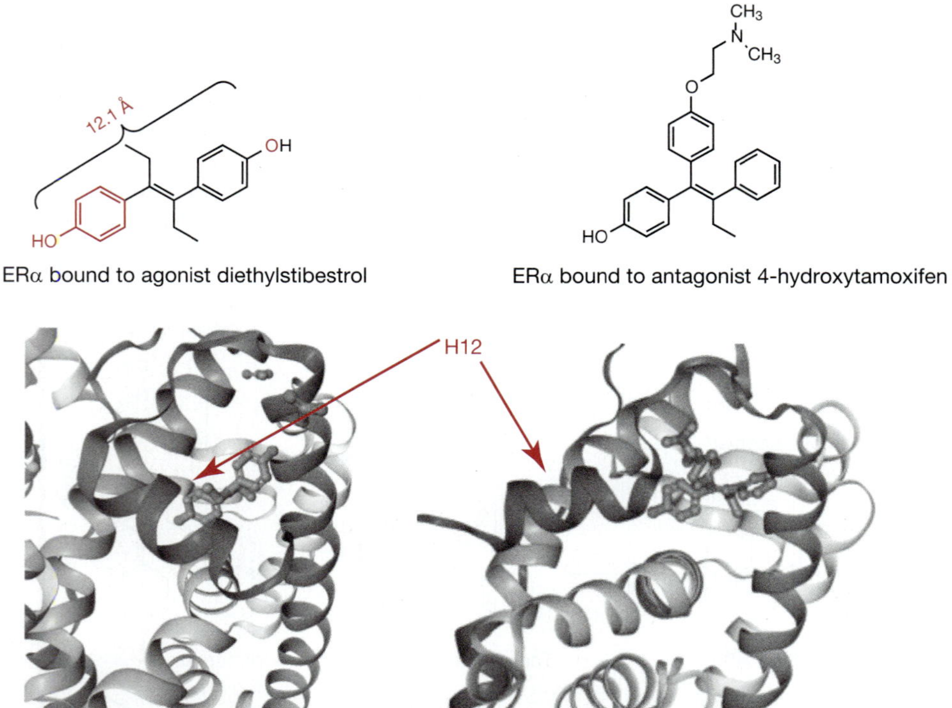

Figure 25.35 Agonist and antagonist conformations of estrogen receptor alpha (Erα). The left panel demonstrates the agonist conformation of the ERα ligand-binding domain (LBD) when bound to diethylstilbestrol, whereas the right panel demonstrates the antagonist conformation when bound to 4-hydroxytamoxifen. A key difference is the orientation of helix 12 (H12; indicated by red arrows). H12 is a short segment of helix located at the C-terminus of the LBD. In the agonist conformation, H12 folds toward the ligand and completely encloses the ligand within the barrel-shaped binding pocket. Externally, the activation function-2 of the agonist conformation forms a coactivator interaction site such that ERα recruits coactivators and activates ERα-dependent transcription. In the antagonist conformation, the basic amino side chain together with the *cis*-aryl group is not accommodated by the receptor. Instead, the ligand protrudes toward the exterior of the receptor. H12 is pushed into an alternate orientation, which recruits corepressors in breast and uterine tissues, but still acts as an agonist in other tissues such as bone.

with 4-hydroxytamoxifen (4-OH-TAM; active metabolite of tamoxifen) (3ERT.pdb),[65] the entire ligand is not accommodated within the interior of the receptor (Fig. 25.35). Instead, the basic amine side chain protrudes to the exterior of the ERα helical barrel. The SERM pushes H12 away from the coactivator-binding site, preventing coactivator binding and AF-2 function in some tissues, resulting instead in recruitment of corepressors in these tissues (breast and uterus). The antiestrogenic and some of the estrogen-like actions of SERMs can be explained by the different conformations of their ERα complexes, which attract coactivators and/or corepressors (cumulatively cofactors) that are different depending on the cellular context. In this model, the receptor and cofactors would be differentially expressed across SERM target tissues, leading to pleiotropic outcomes.[286] Alternatively, ERα could be modulated by different concentrations of ERβ at different sites. It has been suggested that ERβ could enhance estrogen-like gene activation through a protein-protein interaction at AP-1 (*fos* and *jun*) sites.[287]

At present, it is not entirely clear how SERM action is modulated at each target tissue. Indeed, more than one mechanism may occur. This pleiotropic pharmacology can be characterized as the dissociation in vivo of the favorable effects of ERα on bone, heart, and brain, from unfavorable growth stimulatory effects of ERα on breast and uterus, which is characteristic of SERMs. Similar tissue-selective dissociation of other nuclear hormone receptor effects has been seen with the AR (SARMs)[205] and glucocorticoid receptor (GR) (SGRMs [selective glucocorticoid receptor modulators]).[288,289] However, there are no approved SARM products yet. Tissue-selectivity and anticancer effects have also been sought using agonists of ERβ, which has a distinct tissue distribution and often opposes the growth stimulatory effects of ERα.[41]

Tamoxifen (Nolvadex). Tamoxifen is an example of a compound that was designed for one indication and, upon failure, was steered toward another indication where it has become the first targeted and the most prescribed anticancer therapy in history. In the early 1960s, tamoxifen was initially discovered as part of a fertility-control program as a successful postcoital contraceptive in rats and was considered as a possible "morning-after pill." However, the reproductive pharmacology of tamoxifen is species specific, and in women, it induced ovulation (central antagonist action) rather than reducing fertility (central agonist action). Also in the 1960s, the hormone dependency of breast cancer was further substantiated by the presence of ERα (ERβ was not discovered until 1996) in breast cancers, prompting Dr Arthur L. Wadpole to encourage the clinical investigation of tamoxifen in patients with breast cancer. In 1977, tamoxifen was FDA approved for the treatment of MBC and has since been approved for adjuvant hormone therapy of ER-positive breast cancer and chemoprevention in women at high risk for breast cancer.[290] Further, tamoxifen replaced endocrine ablative surgery in both pre- and postmenopausal patients with advanced breast cancer. For decades, tamoxifen was the endocrine treatment of choice for all stages of breast cancer. Over time, AIs have gained favor as a first-line treatment in many settings due to increased efficacy and cost-effectiveness,[291] but tamoxifen remains the treatment of choice for premenopausal patients and those with DCIS, and a viable first-line option in almost any ER-positive early breast cancer.

Unfortunately, tamoxifen retains some intrinsic agonist activity, and therapy commonly results in tamoxifen resistance and the need to switch to other endocrine therapies, as discussed earlier. The emergence of tamoxifen resistance seems to be most problematic in patients who are obese where, even if gonadal estrogen synthesis is ablated by GnRH agonists, fat cells produce estrogens via aromatase that is highly expressed in adipose tissue. Further, low-adherence patients have shorter time to recurrence, so it is very important to counsel patients to continue taking it on a daily basis throughout their course of therapy.

Tamoxifen citrate therapy was associated with serious and life-threatening events, including uterine malignancies, stroke, pulmonary embolism, and DVT,[292] with thromboembolic event risk higher when used in combination with cytotoxic agents. Careful risk-benefit evaluation is advised in patients predisposed to thrombotic events. Further, vasomotor and gynecologic problems, including sexual dysfunction, are common with tamoxifen and can be rationalized as symptoms of chemically induced menopause. Fatty liver[293] and occasionally severe liver diseases, myalgias, and eye disorders (eg, cataracts and retinopathy) have been reported. Fatigue and asthenia have been reported very commonly. Excessive vaginal bleeding or severe pelvic discomfort should be followed up to assess for endometrial cancer versus postmenopausal symptoms.

Tamoxifen is a prodrug that is thought to require metabolic activation by CYP2D6 to produce the 4-OH TAM metabolite (Fig. 25.36). Underscoring the overarching importance of the phenolic OH to activity, tamoxifen and 4-OH TAM are also metabolized by CYP3A4 to the essentially inactive *N*-desmethyl tamoxifen (NDM TAM; similar activity as tamoxifen) metabolite and the active 4-hydroxy-*N*-desmethyl tamoxifen (4-OH-NDM TAM; known as endoxifen in the literature) metabolite, respectively. These active metabolites bind to the ER with up to 30-fold greater affinity than tamoxifen, and this increased potency for ER binding translates into enhanced antiestrogen activity.[294,295] Since plasma levels of 4-OH-NDM TAM in patients with functional CYP2D6 frequently exceed the levels of 4-OH TAM, it seems likely that 4-OH-NDM TAM is at least as important as 4-OH TAM to the overall activity of this drug.[295] Consequently, efficacy is lowered by low or null CYP2D6 activity found in patients harboring certain CYP2D6 alleles, for example, CYP2D6*10/*10.[296] Guidelines suggest consideration of patient genotyping before adjuvant tamoxifen in early breast cancer, and if a poor metabolizer genotype is found, then initiating AI (with ovarian suppression if pre- or perimenopausal) instead of tamoxifen.[297] Further, coadministration with CYP2D6 inhibitors (eg, fluoxetine, duloxetine, bupropion, and especially paroxetine) can lead to persistent reduction in the plasma concentrations of the active phenolic metabolites. Concurrent chronic use of CYP2D6 inhibitors should be avoided if possible. Although there is still controversy regarding this DDI,[298] pragmatism dictates avoidance of 2D6 inhibitors in general. If antidepressants are

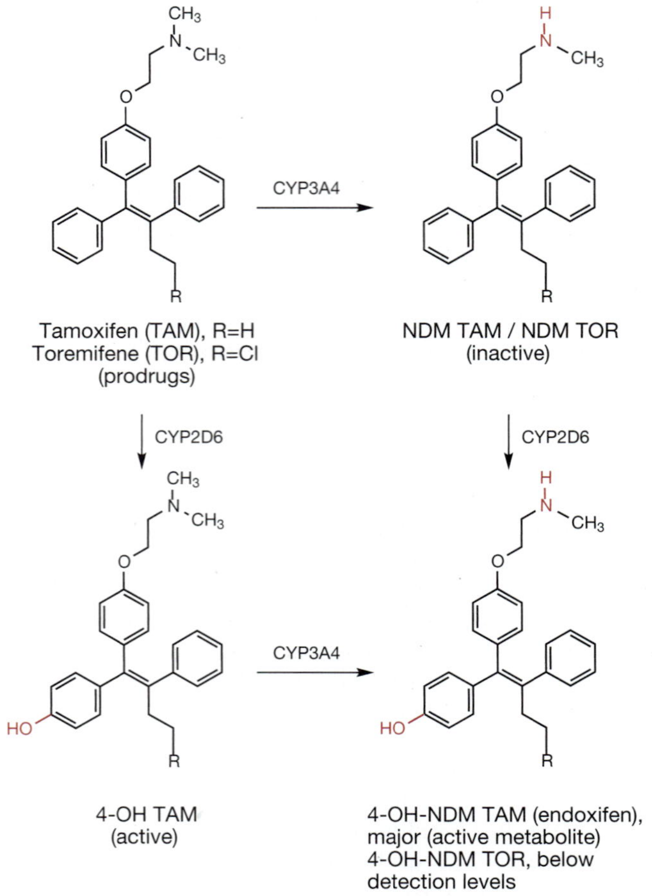

Figure 25.36 Metabolism of tamoxifen (TAM) and toremifene (TOR); NDM, *N*-desmethyl.

warranted, those with the lowest inhibitory impact on 2D6 (eg, sertraline, citalopram, escitalopram, venlafaxine) should be prescribed.[299]

Tamoxifen citrate is dosed daily as 20- to 40-mg tablets, employing the lowest effective dose. In early disease, a 5-year regimen is recommended, and it should not be taken at the same time as AIs. Tamoxifen is rapidly and well absorbed (~100%) from the GI tract with C_{max} of 3 to 7 hours and has a large volume of distribution (20 L/kg) owing to plasma protein binding. High concentrations are found in the uterus and breast tissue. As described earlier, tamoxifen is metabolized by CYP2D6 and CYP3A4 to active metabolites. Systemic concentrations vary considerably between patients, possibly due in part to genetic polymorphisms, and these variations can affect efficacy and metabolite levels. Tamoxifen undergoes extensive enterohepatic recycling and is eliminated mostly in the feces (26%-65%) due to bile excretion. The terminal elimination half-life of tamoxifen is 5 to 7 days with an extremely wide range of 3 to 21 days.[300,301]

Toremifene (Fareston). TOR, approved in 1997, is another triphenylethylene SERM that differs from tamoxifen by the addition of a chlorine atom to the ethyl side chain (Fig. 25.36). The goal of TOR development was to improve the safety profile while retaining the efficacy of tamoxifen, although studies to date suggest similar safety profiles. TOR is indicated for the treatment of MBC in postmenopausal women with ER-positive or unknown tumors. Despite a number of clinical trials and over 500,000 patient-years of use, many oncologists have limited familiarity with TOR. Some in vitro evidence suggests that, unlike tamoxifen, TOR is not a prodrug that requires CYP2D6 activation and that the use of TOR in patients with genetically low or null CYP2D6 activity should be investigated.[302,303] The chlorine atom of TOR was postulated to sterically clash with the CYP2D6 catalytic pocket when the TOR substrate is oriented for 4-hydroxylation. Further, no 4-hydroxy-*N*-desmethyl toremifene (4-OH-NDM TOR) metabolite was detected in the clinical samples evaluated.[302] The endometrial cancer side effect of tamoxifen, which is not as prevalent with TOR, could be due to the more active 4-hydroxylated tamoxifen metabolites. The pharmacokinetics of TOR, with the exceptions in the metabolism noted earlier (ie, not a substrate for CYP2D6) and later, are comparable to tamoxifen.

TOR is rapidly and well absorbed orally, has a large apparent volume of distribution (580 L) due to extensive albumin binding, is extensively metabolized by CYP3A4 to *N*-desmethyl toremifene (NDM TOR) (Fig. 25.37), autoinduces its own CYP3A4-mediated metabolism (a property also exhibited by tamoxifen), and has a terminal elimination half-life of 5 days. In addition to potential resistance to CYP2D6-catalyzed aromatic hydroxylation, another metabolic divergence from tamoxifen is that TOR is deaminated to form deaminohydroxy-TOR, known as ospemifene (Osphena), which is an FDA-approved SERM for dyspareunia (Fig. 25.37).[304]

Notably, a black box warning for QT prolongation exists for TOR, but not for tamoxifen, although the two drugs likely have the same effect. Coadministration of drugs known to prolong the QT interval and strong CYP3A4 inhibitors

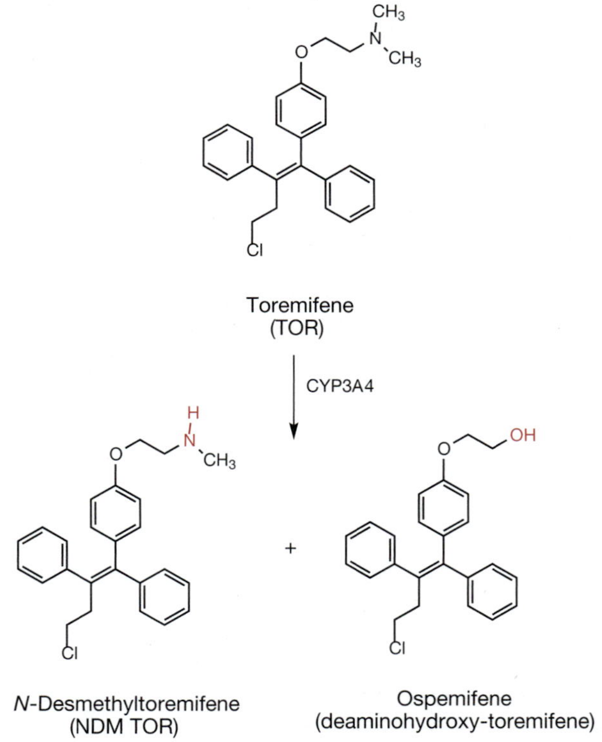

Figure 25.37 Metabolism of toremifene (TOR). NDM, *N*-desmethyl.

should be avoided. Efficacy of TOR for the indicated disease state (advanced breast cancer) seems comparable to tamoxifen, and the safety profile is at least not worse, suggesting that TOR may serve as a reasonable alternative to tamoxifen when antiestrogens are applicable.[305] Studies in the adjuvant setting (which is off-label for TOR) also indicated comparable efficacy.[305]

The search for the optimal SERM continued into the early 21st century with not only two notable successes but also a few failures.[306] Raloxifene hydrochloride (Evista) is a benzothiophene SERM (see Fig. 25.34) that was originally indicated for the prevention and treatment of osteoporosis in postmenopausal women. In 2007, raloxifene was FDA approved as a chemopreventive agent to reduce the risk of developing invasive breast cancer in postmenopausal women with osteoporosis and postmenopausal women at high risk for invasive breast cancer (Chapter 27). Similarly, bazedoxifene, an indole SERM (see Fig. 25.20), was approved in 2007 for the prevention and treatment of postmenopausal osteoporosis when administered with conjugated estrogens. Ospemifene was approved in 2013 for postmenopausal women experiencing dyspareunia. These latter SERMs were considered safer with regard to uterine adverse effects, allowing their use in nononcologic indications (eg, as antiresorptives in the bone or for climacteric symptoms).

Aromatase Inhibitors. The structures of endogenous estrogens differ most notably from androgens and other endogenous steroids in the A ring of the steroidal nucleus. The unique requirement of estrogens to have an aromatic A ring allows the inhibition of estrogen biosynthesis without affecting androgen, progesterone, or adrenocorticoid biosynthesis. All mammalian estrogens (except equine estrogens) are aromatized as their last step in biosynthesis by the action of the enzyme aromatase, which converts androstenedione and testosterone to estrone and 17β-estradiol, respectively (Fig. 25.38). In view of the requirement for A-ring aromatization and the incomplete blockade of estrogen action by tamoxifen, an alternative approach was hypothesized, which indirectly blocked the ER axis by decreasing estrogen production, whether gonadal (ovarian) or peripheral (adipose).[307]

Aromatization is energetically expensive, and unlike androgen or adrenocorticoid biosynthesis, there is no redundant or salvage metabolic pathways to achieve aromatization of estrogens. Consequently, levels of endogenous estrogens can be very successfully lowered by potent AIs, which

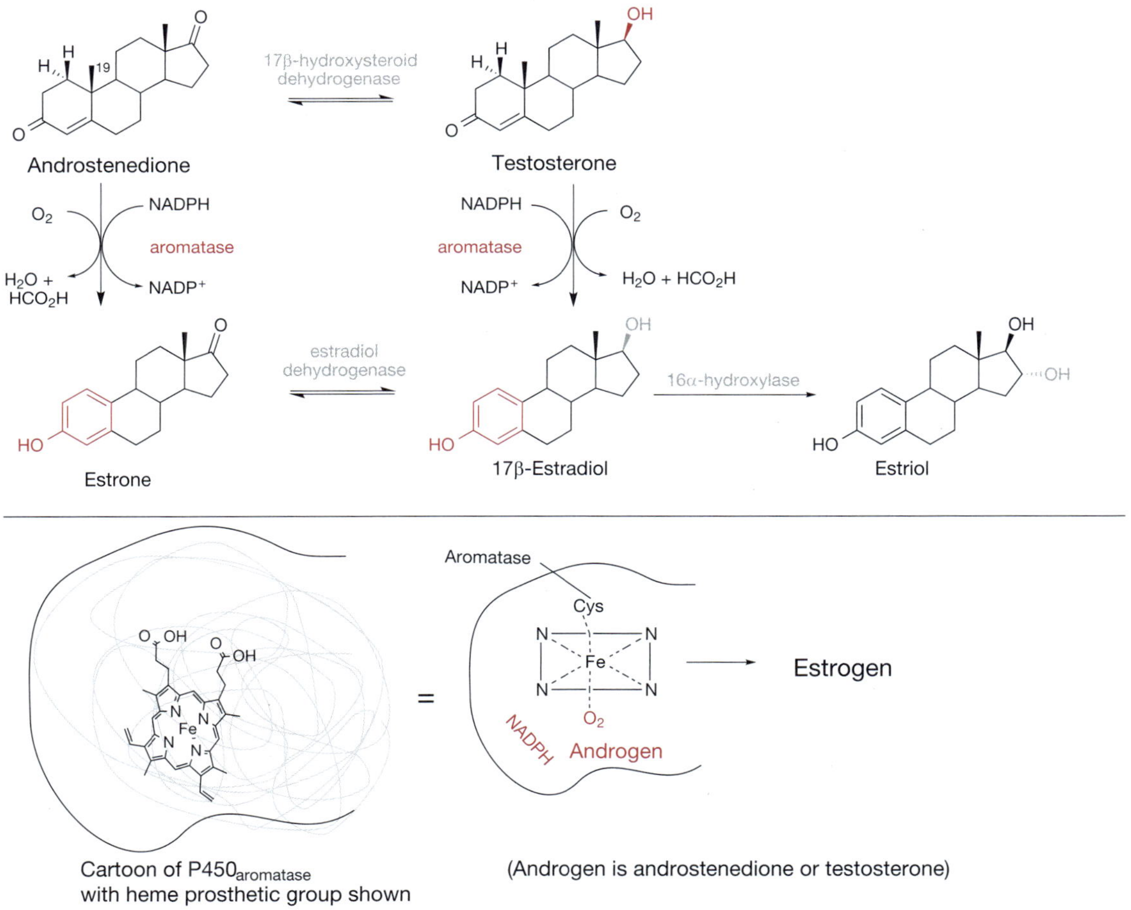

Figure 25.38 Aromatization of androgens to estrogens by aromatase. Top panel: Androstenedione and testosterone are converted by aromatase to the estrogens estrone and 17β-estradiol via an energetically unfavorable reductive dealkylation process, as is shown in red. Biotransformations by other enzymes are shown in gray. Bottom panel: The binding pocket of aromatase contains a heme prosthetic group, which is directly involved in the catalytic conversion of androgens to estrogens. Aromatase inhibitors bind strongly to the iron (Fe) atom of the heme group, prevent androgen binding, and inhibit enzyme turnover.

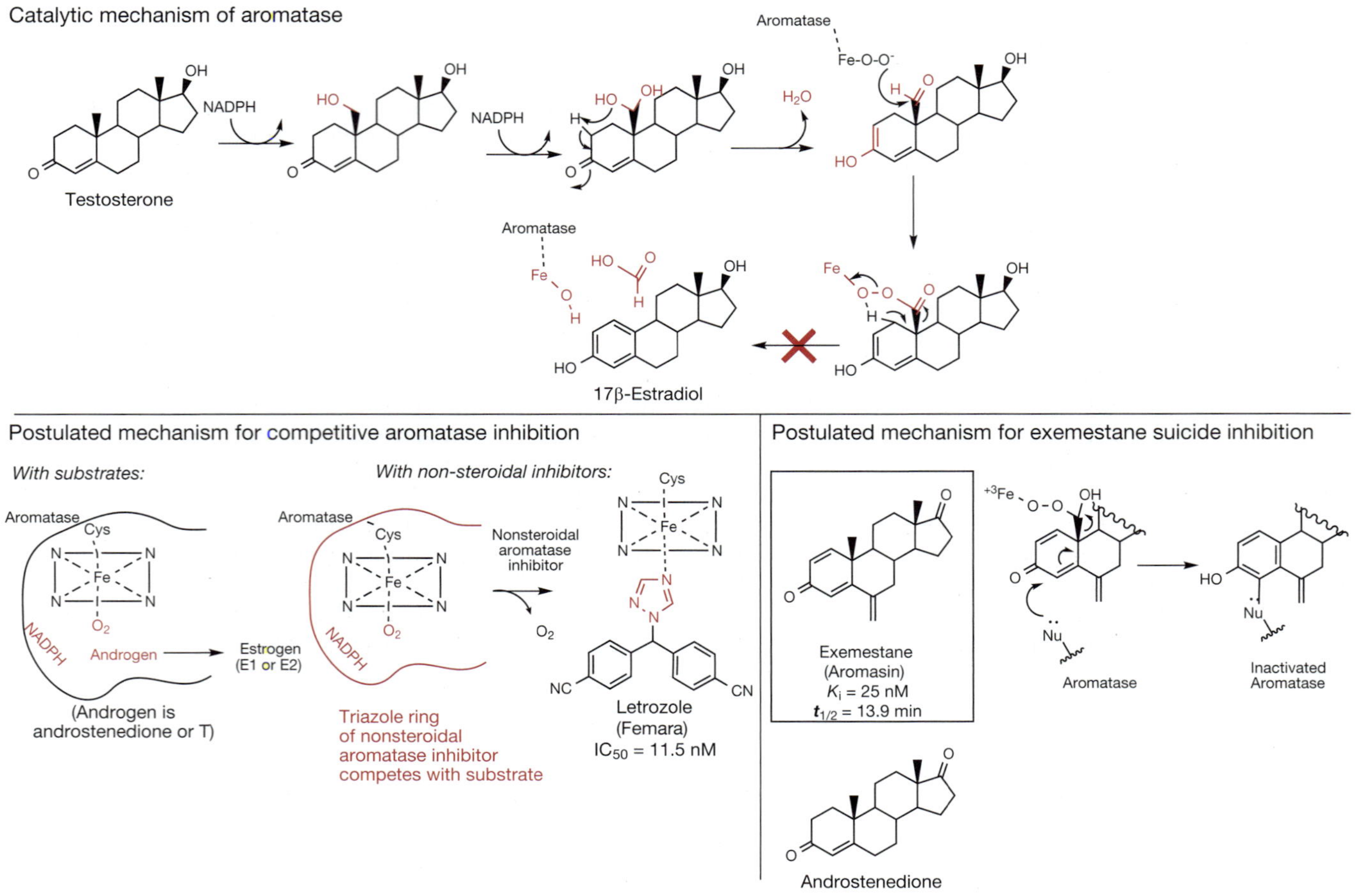

Figure 25.39 Catalytic mechanism of aromatase and postulated mechanisms for its reversible and irreversible inhibition. Top panel: The catalytic mechanism involves two successive NADPH-dependent hydroxylations of the C19 methyl group followed by the 2β-hydrogen elimination as H_2O, which allows the enolization of the 3-keto group. Aromatization is completed by the attack of the activated oxygen atom of the ferric oxide cofactor on the C19 aldehyde, positioning the other oxygen atom to accept the 1β-hydrogen from the steroid and simultaneously eliminating the C19 group as formate. Bottom left panel: Reversible agents bind tightly and competitively with androgen substrate to the iron atom of the heme. Bottom right panel: Exemestane resembles androstenedione allowing the enzyme to form the gem-diol intermediate; however, the 3-keto-$\Delta^{1,4}$ A ring is aromatized as it captures a nucleophile from the enzyme, thus irreversibly inactivating the enzyme.

indirectly suppress the ER axis in estrogen-dependent breast cancers. Aromatase utilizes three moles of NADPH and O_2 for each mole of estrogen formed, suggesting that aromatization involves three successive hydroxylations (Fig. 25.39, top panel).[308] The first two occur at the 19-methyl group of androgens to produce a C19 *gem* diol, a hydrated form of the C19 aldehyde. This is followed by the simultaneous elimination of the 19-methyl group as formate (HCO_2H) and aromatization of the A ring. Reversible AIs are triazoles that bind tightly with the Fe atom of the heme group to act as competitive inhibitors of aromatase (Fig. 25.39, bottom panel). Two reversible competitive nonsteroidal AIs are available, letrozole and anastrozole, and these are the most commonly used as breast cancer endocrine therapy. An irreversible "suicide" inhibitor of aromatase, exemestane, is also approved (Fig. 25.40).

Originally approved for MBC, AIs are now a standard treatment for all postmenopausal patients and are effective as monotherapy in the adjuvant and first-line metastatic settings. It is important not to use AIs in premenopausal patients because the reduction in estrogen levels will induce the expression of ovarian aromatase. The recent favor of AIs over tamoxifen in the postmenopausal setting derives from the adverse partial estrogenic effects of tamoxifen, resulting in incomplete blockage of estrogen action and the development of tamoxifen resistance.[307] It is recommended that postmenopausal women who have completed a 5-year regimen of tamoxifen for the treatment of early-stage, ER-positive breast cancer consider extending their treatment with an AI. It has not yet been definitively established what the optimum duration of treatment should be or whether

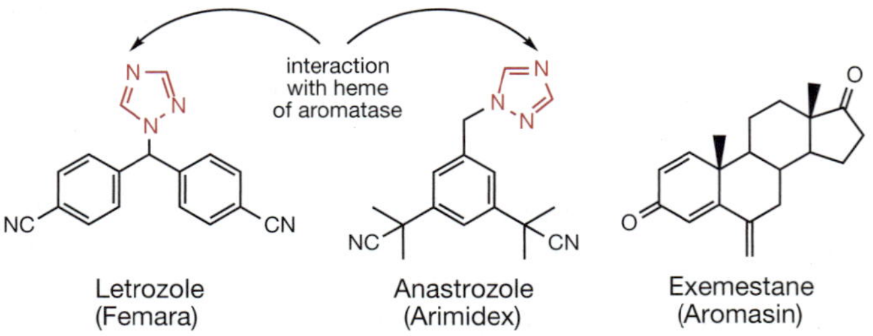

Figure 25.40 Nonsteroidal and steroidal aromatase inhibitors.

an AI should supplant or be sequenced after tamoxifen therapy. AIs are associated with a lower risk of endometrial cancer and thromboembolic events but with higher rates of fractures and myalgia as compared to tamoxifen. Unfortunately, resistance to AIs also occurs as a result of pathogenic cross talk with kinase receptor cell growth pathways,[307] ushering in the recent advent of CDK4/6 inhibitor therapies, which were initially indicated for advanced breast cancer (discussed later). Endocrine and CDK4/6 inhibitor combination therapies are now the recommended first line in advanced disease, supplanting AI monotherapy.

Letrozole (Femara). Letrozole was originally approved in 1997 as monotherapy for the treatment of advanced breast cancer in postmenopausal women with disease progression following antiestrogen therapy (Fig. 25.40); however, guidelines for first-line therapy in advanced disease now recommend combinations of CDK4/6 inhibitors with an AI or SERD (fulvestrant). Letrozole monotherapy is still prevalent and favored in the adjuvant setting where there is an annual 2% to 4% chance that the cancer might return or recur. For example, extended adjuvant letrozole monotherapy, both after 5 years of recurrence-free tamoxifen and as initial adjuvant therapy in early breast cancer, can cut recurrence rates in half. The latter approval was based on a clinical trial (Breast International Group [BIG] 1-98) comparing 5 years of tamoxifen monotherapy to 5 years of letrozole monotherapy. Compared to tamoxifen, letrozole had a lower risk for contralateral breast cancer recurrence, greater time to distant metastasis, and trended toward an overall survival benefit.[309,310] Similar trials also demonstrated that indirect inhibition of the ER axis by the lowering of endogenous estrogen levels with letrozole was significantly more efficacious than tamoxifen in the neoadjuvant (before any treatment), adjuvant (after treatment but in the absence of evidence of disease), extended adjuvant (switching from tamoxifen to letrozole in the absence of disease), and advanced (metastatic or refractory disease) settings[311] and that such uses were cost effective.[312]

Letrozole is a nonsteroidal reversible (type I) inhibitor of aromatase that binds via its 1,2,4-triazole ring to the enzyme's heme group (Fig. 25.39, bottom left panel). Letrozole suppresses the plasma concentration of estrone, estrone sulfate, and 17β-estradiol by 75% to 95% in a dose-dependent manner, with maximal suppression achieved in 2 to 3 days. This is achieved without accumulation of adrenal androgen substrates and without effects on adrenal steroidogenesis. Letrozole inhibits aromatase expressed in the gonads, brain, adipose tissue, and the tumor itself. Letrozole also reduces uterine weight and regresses estrogen-dependent tumors as effectively as ovariectomy.

Letrozole is administered orally (2.5 mg daily) and is completely and rapidly absorbed from the GI tract, and absorption is not affected by food. However, when taken with palbociclib, it should be administered with a fatty meal to increase the CDK4/6 inhibitor absorption. Steady state is reached in 2 to 6 weeks. Steady-state plasma concentrations are 1.5 to 2 times higher than predicted from concentrations following single dosing, suggesting a slight nonlinearity of daily dosing of 2.5 mg; however, accumulation does not continue. It is slowly metabolized (CYP3A4 and CYP2A6) to an inactive carbinol metabolite that is subsequently glucuronidated and eliminated renally. Ninety percent of radioactive letrozole is recovered in the urine. Letrozole strongly inhibits CYP2A6 and moderately inhibits CYP2C19. The only notable DDI is that coadministration with tamoxifen resulted in 38% reduction in plasma letrozole,[313] probably due to CYP3A4 induction by tamoxifen; however, clinical efficacy studies do not support the concurrent use of these agents.

Moderate hepatic impairment increased letrozole AUC values by 37% in normal subjects; thus, patients with breast cancer with severe impairment are expected to be exposed to higher serum levels of letrozole. Letrozole increases the risk of osteoporosis and commonly causes hot flashes and night sweats. An increased incidence of hypercholesterolemia also has been documented. Overall, the side-effect profile of letrozole compared to tamoxifen is more striking for their similarities than their differences, with most adverse events reported at comparable levels. Common adverse events for both (letrozole vs tamoxifen) included hot flashes (33.7% vs 38.0%), night sweats (14.1% vs 16.4%), and weight gain (10.7% vs 12.9%). Arthralgia (21.1% vs 13.4%) and bone fractures (5.6% vs 4.0%) were reported more frequently following treatment with letrozole. Bone loss appears manageable through bisphosphonate therapy[314] and, more recently, denosumab (Xgeva).

Anastrozole (Arimidex). Anastrozole is FDA approved for a similar set of indications in postmenopausal women as letrozole, including initial adjuvant therapy in early breast cancer,[315] first line in advanced breast cancer or MBC, and second line in advanced disease with disease progression following tamoxifen therapy. As noted earlier, monotherapies in late disease are largely supplanted by CDK4/6 inhibitor combinations.

The registration trial for the initial adjuvant therapy indication, Arimidex, Tamoxifen, Alone or in Combination (ATAC), tested anastrozole (1 mg) and tamoxifen (20 mg) monotherapy for 5 years, along with the combination of the two; however, the combination arm was discontinued for lack of efficacy superior to tamoxifen alone. The two monotherapy arms demonstrated statistically significant disease-free survival for anastrozole at 68 and 120 months of treatment. Decreased long-term recurrence with anastrozole treatment was demonstrated in the hormone receptor–positive population (84% of trial patients) analyzed at 120 months, meaning 5 years after discontinuation of treatment. Anastrozole patients presented with 735 recurrence events versus 924 for tamoxifen. This established the superiority of anastrozole compared to tamoxifen in the adjuvant setting, which is similar to letrozole. In the advanced breast cancer registration trials, anastrozole seemed to produce similar objective tumor response rates and time to tumor progression statistics as tamoxifen. Direct head-to-head clinical trials comparing letrozole to anastrozole have not been published.[316]

Letrozole is the only AI to demonstrate consistent superiority to tamoxifen in the neoadjuvant and first-line advanced breast cancer settings.[311,317] In direct comparisons with anastrozole, letrozole is significantly more potent in aromatase inhibition in vitro and suppresses estrogen to a greater degree than anastrozole in the serum and breast tumor.[318] Further, it is more efficacious as second-line endocrine therapy in advanced breast cancer or MBC as measured by clinical response.[319] However, a recent trial concluded that letrozole was not significantly superior in efficacy or safety compared with anastrozole in postmenopausal patients with hormone receptor–positive, node-positive early breast cancer.[320]

Anastrozole, a benzyltriazole (see Fig. 25.40), is another potent and highly selective, nonsteroidal reversible (type I) AI in which coordination of the triazole ring with the heme iron atom allows potent inhibition of aromatase (see Fig. 25.39, bottom left panel).[321,322] Similar to letrozole, anastrozole inhibits aromatase expressed in all tissues and oral 1 mg daily dosing reduced 17β-estradiol by ~70% within 24 hours and by ~80% by 14 days. Anastrozole is rapidly (C_{max} 2 hours) and well absorbed orally. Food reduces the rate, but not overall extent, of anastrozole absorption. Linear pharmacokinetics were observed from 1 to 20 mg. Metabolism to inactive metabolites occurs by N-dealkylation to produce triazole as the major circulating metabolite, but hydroxylation and glucuronidation were also observed. Hepatic metabolism accounts for 85% of anastrozole elimination, and the terminal elimination half-life is approximately 50 hours.[321] Side effects are similar to letrozole and include adverse changes in hip and lumbar spine BMD and increased fractures (10% vs 7%), and elevated cholesterol (9% vs 3.5%) relative to tamoxifen. Unlike letrozole, the anastrozole package insert reported higher incidence of ischemic cardiovascular events than tamoxifen (17% vs 10%), including angina pectoris (2.3% vs 1.6%), and advises that risks and benefits be considered before initiating anastrozole in preexisting ischemic heart disease. However, more recent meta-analysis disputes this conclusion.[316] Based on clinical and pharmacokinetic results from the ATAC trial, tamoxifen should not be administered with either anastrozole or letrozole.

Exemestane (Aromasin). Exemestane is a steroid-based, irreversible (type II) AI (see Fig. 25.40). It is approved as monotherapy for adjuvant therapy after 2 to 3 years of tamoxifen to complete 5 consecutive years of adjuvant therapy in hormone receptor–positive early breast cancer. In this role, at 34.5 months after initiation, exemestane reduced initial disease recurrence events to 9.06% compared to 12.94% for tamoxifen alone. However, overall survival was comparable at 119 months. Unlike letrozole and anastrozole, exemestane is not approved as first-line adjuvant therapy. Unlike other AIs, exemestane is indicated in advanced breast cancer in combination with the mTOR inhibitor everolimus (Chapter 37). Along with other AIs, it is indicated as monotherapy in advanced breast cancer following tamoxifen failure, although this indication may be becoming obsolete, given the recommended use of CDK4/6 inhibitors combined with endocrine therapy in early and first-line advanced settings.

Exemestane resembles androstenedione in structure, acting as a false substrate and thereby binding irreversibly to aromatase as a suicide inhibitor (Fig. 25.39, bottom right panel). Because this agent has high binding affinity and specificity for aromatase, it is able to suppress the activity of this enzyme by 97.7% (anastrozole, 92%-96%; letrozole, 98%).[323] Exemestane is administered orally (25 mg daily) after a meal. Only 42% of radiolabeled exemestane was absorbed from the GI tract with a terminal half-life of about 24 hours. Absorption of exemestane was improved when taken following a high-fat meal, with increases in AUC and C_{max} of 59% and 39%, respectively. Approximately 90% of a dose is bound to plasma proteins, including albumin and α_1-acid glycoprotein. Exemestane undergoes extensive metabolism by CYP3A4, and to a minor extent by aldoketoreductases. Dosage adjustments may be necessary if given concomitantly with a CYP3A4 inducer.[323] For example, 600 mg rifampicin for 14 days decreased C_{max} and AUC by 41% and 54%, respectively, in healthy postmenopausal volunteers; however, the CYP3A4 inhibitor ketoconazole had no effect. The initial steps in metabolism are oxidation of the methylene group at position 6 and reduction of the 17-keto, which are inactive or reduced potency metabolites. Radioactive exemestane is excreted equally in the urine and feces (42% each). Adverse reactions reported in patients with early breast cancer (exemestane vs tamoxifen) include hot flashes (21.2% vs 19.9%), arthralgia (14.6% vs 8.6%), and fatigue (16.1% vs 14.7%), which is similar to other AIs. BMD is also lowered by exemestane, and patients should be evaluated for calcium or vitamin D deficiencies.

Bone Health in Hormone-Dependent Cancers. Patients with breast cancer in general have a high prevalence of vitamin D deficiency, resulting in bone loss that can be exacerbated by the use of chemotherapy, AIs, and/or pure antiestrogens. In contrast, tamoxifen and other SERMs increase BMD compared to placebo. Bone health is extremely important in breast cancer, not just to prevent fractures but also to prevent metastasis to the bone. The most common site of metastasis is the bones of the hip and vertebral column where the metastases form lytic lesions and cause compression fractures of vertebrae. Patients with breast cancer should be encouraged to take calcium and vitamin D supplements and should consider the use of antiresorptive agents such as denosumab, which is largely supplanting the use of bisphosphonates in breast and prostate cancers.

Case Study 1

CASE

HP is a 45-year-old female patient with obesity whose menopausal status is unknown and who presents with a large 2.5-cm tumor with a high mitotic index in the left breast near the chest wall close to her heart, making radiation therapy difficult. Molecular phenotyping demonstrates 99% ER staining, 75% PR staining, and HER2-negative status. Genotyping does not reveal known pathogenic mutations in the *BRCA1/2* genes. OncoTypeDx suggests a high recurrence score. The sentinel lymph nodes are reported as negative and no further efforts are put into detecting metastatic lesions, but the patient complains of

Case Study 1 (continued)

hip pain. Radical double mastectomy with reconstruction is elected as surgery leaving no breast tissue to irradiate. Following a four-cycle adjuvant TC chemotherapy regimen of docetaxel (Taxotere) and cyclophosphamide, HP is initiated on tamoxifen 20 mg daily.

A. Rationalize whether HP should have been considered for the six-cycle adjuvant chemotherapy regimen of TC followed by anthracyclines.
B. Rationalize possible reasons why HP should or should not receive tamoxifen as adjuvant endocrine therapy? What further information would be needed to decide? What other therapies should be considered for HP, and why?
C. By 18 months after initiating tamoxifen therapy, HP reports severe hip pain and musculoskeletal pain in the torso that does not seem to heal. An ultrasound at the gynecologist did not reveal any metastases in the viscera but a strikingly low platelet count.

What is likely to be happening to HP?

Case Solution found immediately after References.

Advanced or Metastatic Breast Cancer: Endocrine and Targeted Therapies. Unfortunately, even though uncomplicated early breast cancer can be thought of as very treatable and curable, Kaplan-Meier curves of ER-positive breast cancers undergoing adjuvant therapy have a steep survival drop-off for the initial 2 years following surgery and/or initial adjuvant chemotherapy. After this initial higher mortality phase, there is about a 2% to 4% recurrence rate per year despite adjuvant therapies. Despite extensive prognostic testing, there is still little insight as to why some patients relapse almost immediately whereas others do well for decades. Overall, approximately 30% of patients with early breast cancer eventually progress to advanced breast cancer or MBC. Further, a certain percentage of ER-positive breast cancers present as advanced or distantly metastatic cancers, which is associated with poorer prognosis. Breast cancer usually spreads to the bones (most common), liver, lungs, or brain (worst effect on quality of life and prognosis). At this point, it is considered stage 4 breast cancer. Goals of treatment of stage 4 breast cancer or MBC therapy include extending overall survival, maintaining quality of life, and delaying the use of chemotherapy.

Treatment of MBC is less personalized than early breast cancer where multiple therapeutic targets (ER/PR/HER2) are defined as well as newer genotype-guided therapy. The previous notwithstanding, the 21st century has seen an ongoing renaissance in the treatment of advanced breast cancer. Originally, tamoxifen and TOR were used in advanced breast cancer, as well as salvage therapies such as the progestogens megestrol acetate or medroxyprogesterone or androgens such as fluoxymesterone or oxandrolone. However, responses were short-lived, and clinicians resorted to chemotherapy. In the early 21st century, AIs were commonly given as first-line therapy or following recurrence on tamoxifen. Likewise, fulvestrant was approved in 2002 for advanced breast cancer following disease progression on antiestrogen therapy.

CDK4/6 inhibitors:

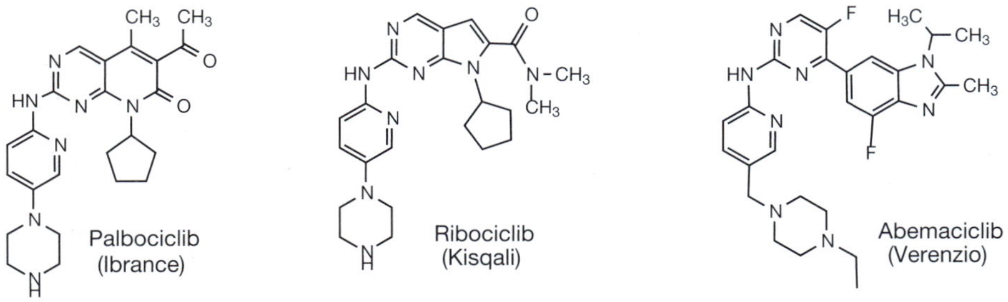

mTOR inhibitor

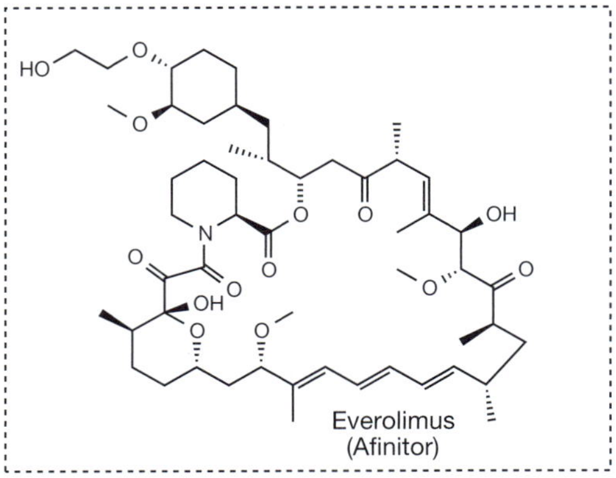

PIK3CA inhibitor

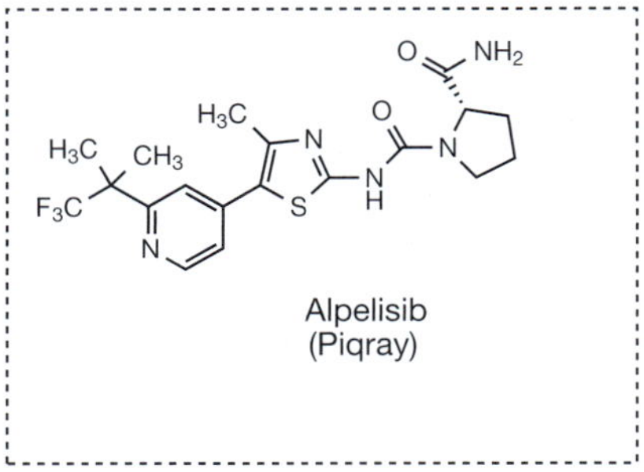

Since 2012, four kinase inhibitors (everolimus, an mTOR inhibitor) and palbociclib, ribociclib and abemaciclib (CDK4/6 inhibitors) have been approved for advanced hormone receptor–positive breast cancer and HER2-negative breast cancer, mostly as specific combinations with the endocrine therapies discussed earlier or fulvestrant, but also as monotherapy. The kinase inhibitor therapies have improved upon the efficacy of AIs and fulvestrant (discussed later) in early and advanced breast cancers. These combination therapies take advantage of the improved understanding of the interactions between hormone signaling pathways and other important tumor growth factors. Kinase inhibitors modulate hormone signaling and interfere with resistance mechanisms that are yet to be fully understood.

Initially approved for endocrine failures in postmenopausal MBC, CDK4/6 inhibitor combinations with endocrine therapies have gained favor and are now the recommended first-line therapy in MBC, with ever expanding indications to now include combination therapies for early or adjuvant breast cancer (abemaciclib) and treatment of pre- and perimenopausal women and men (all three CDK4/6 inhibitors), and monotherapy (abemaciclib). The indications for each CDK4/6 inhibitor for advanced breast cancer as of 2023 are summarized next.

Palbociclib in combination with letrozole or fulvestrant is indicated in advanced disease as initial (first-line) therapy for endocrine treatment failures in postmenopausal women or men or, more recently, regardless of menopausal status. Though rare, male breast cancer is seen with an incidence of 1 in 833 men. The label expansion broadening its use regardless of menopausal status now includes pre- and perimenopausal women, which, according to Pfizer, represent about 17% of the patients with ER-positive HER2-negative breast cancer. Treatment of pre- and perimenopausal women should be in combination with an approved GnRH agonist.

A second CDK4/6 inhibitor, ribociclib, is indicated as first-line endocrine-based therapy in advanced breast cancer or MBC in combination with an AI for premenopausal women or in combination with fulvestrant for postmenopausal women. Like palbociclib, label expansions include pre- and perimenopausal women and men. Like abemaciclib, the possibility of approval for early breast cancer is being considered based on a phase III clinical trial, NATALEE (NCT03701334), which included 5,100 men and women with stage 2a, 2b, or stage 3 (early disease), as opposed to stage 4 (advanced) breast cancer. Results suggest improved invasive disease-free survival (IDFS) that was generally consistent across stratification factors and other subgroups.[324,325]

A third CDK4/6 inhibitor, abemaciclib, is uniquely approved for adjuvant therapy of early breast cancer in combination with tamoxifen or an AI, but this is limited thus far to cancers at high risk for recurrence (node positive and a Ki67 score ≥20%). Ribociclib was studied in a broader group, suggesting it might be approved as adjuvant therapy without such limitations. Further abemaciclib approvals in the advanced or metastatic setting include use in combination with an AI as first-line endocrine therapy for postmenopausal women and men, or in combination with fulvestrant for endocrine therapy failures. Abemaciclib is also uniquely approved as monotherapy in those who previously received endocrine therapy and chemotherapy.

In addition to differences in approved indications, CDK4/6 inhibitors also differ in the primary side effects observed, which can be substantial with palbociclib and ribociclib commonly having dose-limiting suppressions of white blood cell counts (eg, neutropenia) and abemaciclib commonly having dose-limiting and clinically severe diarrhea. CDK4/6 inhibitors consistently improve objective response rates and progression-free survival.[326] However, they suffer from a lack of biomarkers to aid in patient selection or therapeutic monitoring.[327]

An example of personalized medicine in the treatment of advanced breast cancer, alpelisib (Piqray; 2019), is a PI3KCA inhibitor that is approved in combination with fulvestrant for postmenopausal women and men with ER-positive HER2-negative, *PIK3CA*-mutated advanced breast cancer following progression on, or after, an endocrine-based treatment. Approximately 40% of patients with ER-positive HER2-negative advanced breast cancer possess certain activating mutations in the gene *PIK3CA*[328] detectable by an approved companion diagnostic, an indicator of poor prognosis including resistance to endocrine therapy.[329] These are the patients who are candidates for alpelisib in combination with fulvestrant. This personalized medicine combination therapy attempts to ameliorate dysregulated tumor growth in certain patients with advanced breast cancer but comes with some severe side effects. For example, rashes (52%) including severe rashes and skin-sloughing syndromes called severe cutaneous adverse reactions are common. Severe cutaneous adverse reactions include Stevens-Johnson syndrome, erythema multiforme, and toxic epidermal necrolysis. Also, clinically significant laboratory abnormalities including increased blood glucose levels were common (79%), often requiring diet restrictions and coadministration of metformin. For more information on these classes of kinase inhibitors, see Chapter 37.

Despite recent changes in treatment guidelines and recommendations, some patients with MBC may be better suited to receive endocrine therapy only as the first line in the advanced setting in order to avoid the added toxicities of the kinase therapies described earlier. These patients include those with comorbidities (patients with diabetes may be contraindicated with alpelisib) or who are clinically fragile and older adults.[330]

Pure Antiestrogens or Selective Estrogen Receptor Degraders. Despite the fact that 30% to 40% of patients with advanced breast cancer respond to tamoxifen therapy, this response only lasts for 12 to 18 months. Tamoxifen resistance is caused, in part, by its intrinsic ER agonist activity. In addition, tamoxifen only inhibits the AF-2 activation pathway but does not affect transcription promoted by activation function-1 (AF-1). Pure antiestrogens do not possess any intrinsic estrogenic activity in any target tissue or cellular context and, therefore, offer an additional avenue of treatment when resistance to tamoxifen occurs. In addition, because they are devoid of estrogenic action, these agents cannot be classified as SERMs. In addition to potent inhibition of ER, this class of endocrine therapy is believed to degrade the ER at the protein level, blocking endocrine activation by removal of the primary target of estrogen-dependent tumor growth. Correspondingly, this class has been termed *selective ER degraders* (SERDs).

Fulvestrant (Faslodex)

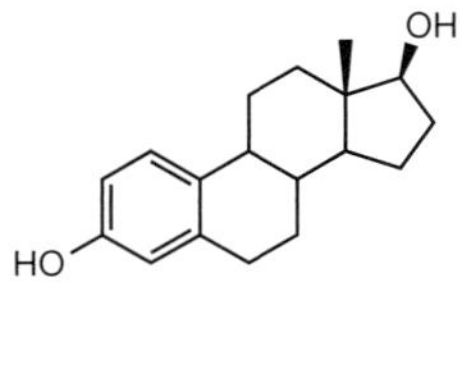

17β-Estradiol

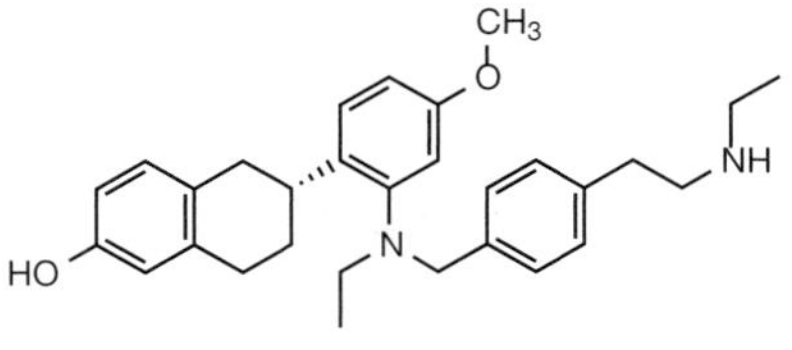

Elacestrant (Orserdu)

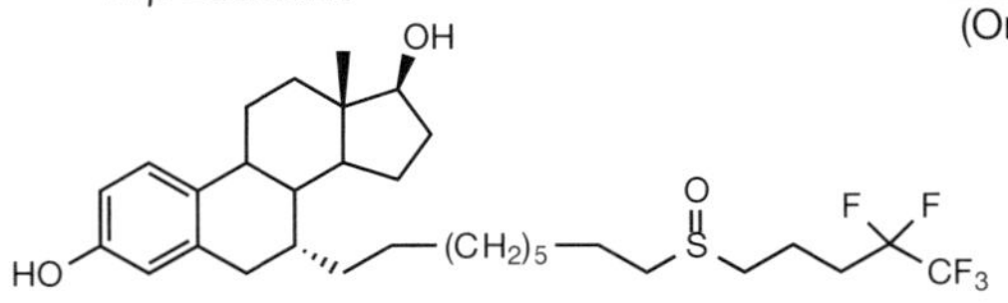

Fulvestrant

Fulvestrant is a pure antiestrogen devoid of ER agonist activity and has high ER-binding affinity comparable to 17β-estradiol. It has multiple effects on ER signaling such as blocking dimerization and nuclear localization of the ER, and reducing cellular levels of ER (ie, acts as a SERD),[331] although the significance of this latter mechanism has been disputed.[332] Despite SERD activity, fulvestrant resistance develops due to compensatory activation of ERα-independent growth factor signaling and stimulation of downstream kinases, which are at least partially addressed by CDK4/6 inhibition and/or alpelisib (*PIK3CA* inhibitor). Fulvestrant is not orally active because of poor aqueous solubility, but instead requires painful monthly injections with large-bore needles needed to administer the drug product that uses thick oils to dissolve fulvestrant. Nonetheless, its approved indications for MBC continue to expand.

Fulvestrant is effective in preventing the growth of tamoxifen-resistant breast cancers in both the laboratory[333] and clinical trials.[334] Recently, CDK4/6 inhibitors palbociclib and abemaciclib combined with endocrine therapy, including fulvestrant, have been recommended as first- or second-line treatment for MBC. As such, patients who progressed to advanced disease on adjuvant AI may receive fulvestrant combined with CDK4/6 inhibitor as their first line in the advanced or MBC setting. Fulvestrant was originally approved for postmenopausal women as monotherapy following SERM therapy for the treatment of ER-positive MBC that has continued to progress or treatment of hormone-naïve advanced breast cancer.[335] As mentioned, fulvestrant combined with the *PIK3CA* inhibitor alpelisib is also approved for certain patients with *PIK3CA*-mutated MBC following disease progression after endocrine failure. Pre- and perimenopausal women treated with these combinations should be treated with GnRH agonists as well. In 2023, fulvestrant combined with the AKT inhibitor capivasertib (Truqap) was approved for advanced hormone receptor–positive breast cancer that has certain specific biomarker alterations (PIK3CA, AKT1, or PTEN) that collectively occur in up to 50% of these patients.[336] Although first-line CDK4/6 inhibitors and ER-targeting therapies are frequently used in this setting, resistance is common, underscoring the need for additional endocrine therapy–based options.

Fulvestrant is a 17β-estradiol analog with a long hydrophobic side chain in the 7α-position. Fulvestrant has poor oral bioavailability owing to very poor solubility, despite metabolic protection on the end of the hydrophobic side chain. As a result, it is administered as a painful 500 mg IM injection once a month. Fulvestrant is 99% plasma protein bound with lipoproteins and SHBG contributing. Metabolism of fulvestrant follows biotransformation pathways similar to endogenous steroids producing both active and less active metabolites. Metabolites include aromatic hydroxylation followed by glucuronic acid and sulfate conjugation at the 2, 3, and 17 positions, and oxidation of the side-chain sulfoxide.[337] Side effects appear to be minimal and include several arthralgias, GI symptoms, headache, and hot flashes. There is no clinical evidence of uterine stimulation or laboratory evidence of stimulation of endometrial carcinoma models.[338] Fulvestrant should not be administered to women who are pregnant, who are taking anticoagulants, or who have thrombocytopenia.

Elacestrant (Orserdu). Since fulvestrant was the only SERD approved by FDA and it has to be administered IM, there was a need for an orally active ER degrader. Several groups have advanced molecules in this space to the clinic. In 2023, FDA approved elacestrant for the treatment of ER-positive HER2-negative estrogen receptor 1 gene (*ESR1*)-mutated advanced or MBC with disease progression following at least one line of endocrine therapy. Elacestrant is recommended for *ESR1*-mutated patients (~48% of these patients) as second-line therapy in the metastatic setting, for example, following progression of the patient with MBC on combined endocrine (AI or fulvestrant) and CDK4/6 inhibitor therapy. EMERALD, a phase III randomized, open-label trial, enrolled 478 postmenopausal women and men with ER-positive HER2-negative MBC who have progressed on prior hormonal therapy or CDK4/6 inhibitor. Of the 478 patients, 228 had mutations of *ESR1*, the gene expressing ERα, which is the hormone receptor that drives ER-positive breast cancer growth. The elacestrant-treated patients had a hazard ratio of 0.55 and progression-free survival of 3.8 months compared to 1.9 months in the fulvestrant or AI group. Elacestrant degraded ER and inhibited ER activity in vitro and in vivo and inhibited the growth of ER-positive breast cancer xenografts.[339] Breast cancer that metastasizes to the brain is associated with greatly diminished quality of life and poor prognosis. Unlike other approved agents, elacestrant crosses the BBB and inhibits ER activity, suggesting that it may retard metastasis to the brain or treat preexisting brain metastases.

Unlike fulvestrant, elacestrant possesses a nonsteroidal chemical structure and oral bioavailability; like fulvestrant, it functions as an ER pure antagonist. Its ER-binding mode is similar to SERMs in that there are the two groups mimicking the hydroxyls of the endogenous ligand, 17β-estradiol, that are rigidly oriented by a nonsteroidal core structure. Elacestrant employs a chiral tetrahydronaphthalen-2-ol substituted by 4-methoxyphenyl as the core structure for this purpose. The phenyl portion of this core is connected to a side chain containing two basic nitrogens, which provide the much-needed aqueous solubility to allow oral bioavailability and daily oral dosing via 86- or 345-mg film-coated tablets, which should not be split or crushed. Like fulvestrant, elacestrant is an ER antagonist that binds to ERα and inhibits 17β-estradiol–mediated cell proliferation in

ER-positive HER2-negative breast cancers at concentrations inducing proteasomal pathway–mediated degradation of ERα protein. Elacestrant demonstrated in vitro and in vivo antitumor activity, including in ER-positive HER2-negative breast cancer models that were resistant to fulvestrant and CDK4/6 inhibitors and those harboring *ESR1* mutations.

Elacestrant is recommended at an oral dosage of 345 mg once daily with food and achieves steady state within 6 days with a mean C_{max} of 119 ng/mL and $AUC_{0\text{-}24h}$ of 2,440 ng h/mL. Elacestrant exhibits only 10% oral bioavailability but rapid absorption with T_{max} of 1 to 4 hour and nonlinear C_{max} and AUC over a dose range from 43 to 862 mg once daily. Importantly, a food effect is seen when administered with a high-fat meal (800-1,000 calories, 50% fat), with C_{max} and AUC increased by 42% and 22%, respectively, compared to fasted administration, hence the requirement to take with food. Elacestrant is highly plasma protein bound (>99%) producing an estimated apparent volume of distribution of 5,800 L. Elacestrant has an elimination half-life of 30 to 50 hours. About one-third of a dose is eliminated unchanged in the feces (34% unchanged), while metabolism occurs primarily by CYP3A4 and, to a lesser extent, by CYP2A6 and CYP2C9, to metabolites eliminated in the feces (82% of total radioactivity in feces) or urine (7.5% of radioactivity; <1% unchanged). The most commonly reported adverse effects seen in the registration trial were musculoskeletal pain (41%), followed by GI problems such as nausea (35%) and vomiting (19%), and fatigue (26%). The 86-mg tablet allows for dose reduction if adverse effects are not tolerable. No significant DDIs were detected in phase I trials.

Treatment of Prostate Cancer

Prostate cancer is the most common noncutaneous cancer and remains the second leading cause of cancer death and the most commonly diagnosed cancer in U.S. men, with ~288,300 estimated new cases and ~34,700 estimated deaths in 2023.[340] The growth and maintenance of the prostate is dependent on the endogenous androgens testosterone and DHT. As men age, the growth of the prostate can become pathogenic due to either BPH or prostate cancer, which is typically an adenocarcinoma. Prostate cancer incidence on biopsy is approximately the same as a man's age (ie, a 50-year-old has ~50% chance of latent prostate cancer and a 90-year-old has 90% chance of latent prostate cancer). However, men castrated before puberty (eunuchs) or men with inherited deficiency of $5AR_2$, in which testosterone cannot be converted into DHT, do not develop prostate cancer. Correspondingly, prostate cancer pharmacotherapies primarily block the AR axis. Because prostate cancer typically grows slowly and causes no symptoms, serum PSA test is most often used to screen for prostate cancer. The limited potential benefits and significant potential for harm (due to false positives) of screening for prostate cancer via digital rectal examination or serum PSA prompted changes to prostate cancer clinical guidelines and suggest that physicians should not use PSA to screen for prostate cancer in average-risk men under age 50, men over age 69, or men with a life expectancy of less than 10 to 15 years.

Treatment of prostate cancer is guided by three initial analyses: (1) staging of the tumor(s) by Gleason score; (2) staging of the cancer following typical tumor/node/metastasis analysis, and (3) PSA biomarker levels and their changes over time. After initial workup, about 40% of prostate cancers present with low-grade, low-volume tumor and slow PSA doubling time. These patients are considered to have a good prognosis. For these low-risk patients, therapeutic intervention is trending toward active surveillance because of a popular belief that this population is overtreated, with in excess of 1,410 patients treated to prevent one death.[341] Moreover, bothersome side effects caused by surgical and radiation therapies used in early prostate cancer include urinary incontinence and impotence. Another 20% of prostate cancers present with high-grade, high-volume tumor and fast PSA doubling times. The prognosis for these patients is relatively poor, and pharmacotherapy is clearly indicated in these high-risk patients. Another 40% have a mixture of favorable and unfavorable prognostic indicators, making the decision whether to treat these patients less clear and discussion of risks and benefits with the patient necessary.

Importantly, consistent with PSA screening having fallen out of favor,[342] more patients are presenting with advanced disease. Advanced-stage disease, including metastatic castration-sensitive prostate cancer (mCSPC), has been increasing by about 5% per year in recent years.[340] The expected rise in morbidity and mortality may be offset to

Case Study 2

Four months later, HP presents to the oncologist in extreme and debilitating pain and using a walking aid. Computed axial tomography (CAT) scans show large lytic lesions in the painful hip and lytic lesions in multiple vertebrae, most prominently at T7 and T12, where the spinal canal has been encroached due to multiple pathologic fractures collapsing the spinal column. Radiation therapy of the vertebra is successful at shrinking the tumor, and HP's functional status improves. Despite reported adherence with adjuvant tamoxifen, bone biopsy reveals MBC, which is still ER and PR positive and HER2 negative. Serum estrogen levels are reported as well above menopausal levels. Further, testing reveals a mutation in the *PIK3CA* gene.

A. In addition to therapies for advanced breast cancer, what other issues does HP have that require immediate therapy, and what should be the agents chosen?
B. What classes of targeted therapies are available to HP for the advanced breast cancer? What is your targeted treatment, and what is your rationale?
C. Should chemotherapy be considered?

Case Solution found immediately after References.

some extent by the recent advances in the pharmacotherapy, including the use of combination hormonal therapies earlier in the natural history of the disease. While metastatic prostate cancer remains a lethal disease, improvements in overall survival through combination therapies have resulted in a renaissance in the entire landscape for clinicians caring for men with advanced metastatic prostate cancer. At present, there is limited data-driven evidence regarding optimal agent combination or sequence, but, where possible, 2023 AUA guidelines are mentioned in this text.[340]

Traditional treatments for localized (early) prostate cancer include active surveillance, surgery (radical prostatectomy), and external beam radiation, whereas advanced prostate cancer (locally advanced or metastasized disease) treatments also include systemic pharmacologic approaches. Chemical or surgical castration has been the cornerstone for advanced prostate cancer since the discovery of the role of androgens in prostate cancer by Huggins and Hodges in 1941.[343] Initial pharmacotherapy for advanced prostate cancer has traditionally been androgen deprivation therapy (ADT) such as GnRH superagonists or, more recently, antagonists, but the trend is for secondary hormonal suppression to be introduced early in the natural history of the disease. Advanced disease is initially controlled by suppression of gonadal androgens, but eventually, relapse occurs despite castration levels of testosterone, a condition referred to as castration-resistant prostate cancer (CRPC). Secondary hormonal therapies (discussed under "Castration-Resistant Prostate Cancer" section) concurrent with ADT were shown to extend survival in nonmetastatic castration-resistant prostate cancer (nmCRPC; see "Apalutamide" section) and metastatic CRPC (mCRPC; see "Abiraterone" and "Enzalutamide" sections), and even castration-sensitive prostate cancer (CSPC; see "Abiraterone" and "Darolutamide" sections). Secondary hormonal therapies can directly and competitively bind and antagonize the AR; for example, enzalutamide, apalutamide, or darolutamide can be used to suppress the AR axis in CSPC or when the AR axis is reactivated in CRPC. Alternatively, suppression of androgen biosynthesis by lyase inhibitors abiraterone or ketoconazole can also suppress the reactivated AR axis.

With increased therapeutic options in CRPC, the pharmacotherapy in advanced CSPC is changing to include these agents. Preliminarily, it is suggested that younger and healthier patients who have a greater chance of dying from prostate cancer rather than other causes should be considered as candidates for ADT plus docetaxel and/or ADT plus secondary hormonal therapies, whereas older and unhealthy patients with lower life expectancies may still be candidates for ADT only. For example, the addition of chemotherapy with docetaxel (six cycles) upon initiation of standard of care has been shown to increase overall survival and reportedly should become standard of care in M1 (metastatic) disease.[344] Recent data with secondary hormonal therapies in the pre-CRPC setting will be discussed later. How these agents will be integrated with other agents for advanced prostate cancer therapy is still yet to be seen.

Unfortunately, prostate cancer progresses while taking ADT in virtually all patients who have metastatic disease and in many patients with nonmetastatic disease.[344] CRPC is prostate cancer that progresses despite testosterone levels less than 50 ng/dL, the level considered as castration by FDA. Disease progression can be observed as increasing PSA while taking ADT (biochemical recurrence)[345] or progressive disease on imaging. Biochemical recurrence is defined as a PSA doubling time of less than 12 months, and recommended treatment is observation or offering a clinical trial. In the absence of observed advanced disease, there is no consensus on when to start systemic therapy. Traditionally, ADT was considered as the treatment of choice in biochemical recurrence in patients at high risk for progression. However, recent data support the use of combined ADT (leuprolide) plus secondary hormonal therapy (enzalutamide) or enzalutamide monotherapy.[346]

CRPC can be symptomatic or asymptomatic and metastatic (mCRPC) or nonmetastatic (nmCRPC), affecting the recommended pharmacotherapies. In general, CRPC is treated with ADT plus secondary hormonal therapies. However, resistance to secondary hormonal therapies is also inevitable with cross-resistance being prevalent. Once CRPC no longer responds to secondary hormonal therapy, then chemotherapy with docetaxel should be considered, followed by cabazitaxel if unresponsive. Moreover, immunotherapy (sipuleucel-T) improves survival in asymptomatic CRPC, and radium-223 improves overall survival in men with mCRPC that has spread to the bones. Many of the recently approved agents as monotherapy for CRPC improve overall survival but only by about 4 months in the CRPC setting; whereas metastasis-free survival (MFS) benefits are much longer in the premetastatic setting, as discussed. This indicates that comprehensive studies on proper sequencing or rational combinations of these therapies are needed to maximize pharmacotherapeutic benefits. The modest survival benefits also emphasize the need for the discovery and exploration of novel pharmacotherapies for CRPC with less susceptibility to the development of resistance.

Treatment of Advanced or Metastatic Castration-Sensitive Prostate Cancer

Gonadotropin-Releasing Hormone Therapy. Huggins and Hodges won the 1966 Nobel Prize for describing the relationship between testosterone and prostate cancer, having shown in 1941 that marked reductions in serum testosterone by castration or estrogen treatment caused metastatic prostate cancer to regress.[343] ADT has remained an important component in the treatment of prostate cancer since then. Testicular surgery (bilateral orchiectomy) to prevent testosterone production was once the most common treatment for advanced prostate cancer and is still used by some today but is associated with physical and psychological discomforts. Although this surgery is not a cure, it delays the advance of the disease. Chemical castration to achieve ADT is now the cornerstone of therapy with the goal of reducing serum testosterone to below 50 ng/dL, although some suggest that this threshold should be even lower (eg, <20 ng/dL). In the 1940s, ADT pharmacotherapy was commonly achieved with DES an estrogen that suppressed testicular testosterone synthesis via a feedback mechanism involving ERs in the brain. DES is now seldom used due to the introduction of GnRH therapies in the 1980s.[347]

Modern ADT involves the use of analogs of GnRH that possess greater potency than the natural GnRH hormone. These superagonists bind to GnRH-Rs in the pituitary and cause an initial increase in LH and FSH, and, subsequently, increased testosterone[348] synthesis in testes. The initial androgen surge occurs within the first 3 to 7 days and can be associated with a clinical flare (eg, increases in prostate volume, bone pain, and spinal cord compression).[349] While combined androgen blockade through concomitant antiandrogen (eg, flutamide) to block flare symptoms was once common practice, it is now disfavored. Continuous overstimulation of GnRH-Rs desensitizes the gonadotroph cells and downregulates GnRH-R expression, resulting in decreased LH synthesis and nearly abrogating testicular steroidogenesis. More succinctly, gonadal androgen synthesis is suppressed via feedback inhibition of the HPG axis (see Fig. 25.6). Castration levels of testosterone (ie, <50 ng/dL) are attained within 2 to 4 weeks after initiation and maintained long term.

The GnRH agonists (see Fig. 25.41), commonly referred to as GnRH superagonists or LHRH agonists, are administered in a continuous, nonpulsatile manner, which is in contrast to the pulsatile release of the endogenous hormone GnRH. Further, they bind with higher affinity to GnRH-Rs in the pituitary than does the endogenous hormone, cumulatively causing a durable effect in the majority of patients upon constant or intermittent dosing.[350] A wide variety of GnRH agonists have been approved, not just for ADT in prostate cancer but also for use in other indications such as ovarian suppression in breast cancer (nonpulsatile) or dosed in a pulsatile manner for central precocious puberty, as will be reviewed separately. Unfortunately, up to 12% of patients fail to achieve castration levels of testosterone and up to 37% fail to achieve levels <20 ng/dL. Also, breakthrough testosterone levels that increase into the range of 20 to 50 ng/dL were reported in 32% of patients receiving a GnRH agonist[351] and shortened time to progression to CRPC.[352]

Gonadotropin-Releasing Hormone Agonists. GnRH agonists approved for use in prostate cancer include leuprolide (Lupron), goserelin (Zoladex), and triptorelin (Trelstar). For prostate cancer, these are given via high-dose and constant (nonpulsatile) release formulations. GnRH agonists are peptidic agents that mimic the natural peptide hormone GnRH and consist of an approximately 9- or 10-amino acid segment of GnRH modified to stabilize the N- and C-terminus. Further, modifications at the 6 and 10 positions of the decapeptide block enzyme cleavage sites and increase agonist activity (Fig. 25.41). For example, the first site can be blocked by replacing glycine 6 (Gly6) with a hydrophobic D-amino acid such as D-leucine in leuprolide, D-serine modified with a *t*-Bu group in goserelin, or D-tryptophan in triptorelin. Another enzyme cleavage site can be blocked by eliminating Gly10, as is seen in both leuprolide and goserelin. Changes in GnRH structure at other amino acid positions decrease activity. A variety of depot formulations for SC or IM administration of leuprolide, goserelin, or triptorelin are available, with durations of action ranging from 1 to 6 months.

Leuprolide (Lupron). Leuprolide acetate (Lupron) is the synthetic nonapeptide 5-oxo-L-prolyl-His-Trp-Ser-Tyr-D-leucyl-Leu-Arg-*N*-ethyl-L-prolinamide acetate salt (where 5-oxo-L-prolyl is the same as PyroGlu in Fig. 25.41; PyroGlu is pyroglutamic acid, a chemical degradation product of N-terminal glutamine). Leuprolide acetate is inactive orally but can be administered SC or, more commonly, as a monthly IM depot injection that allows constant slow

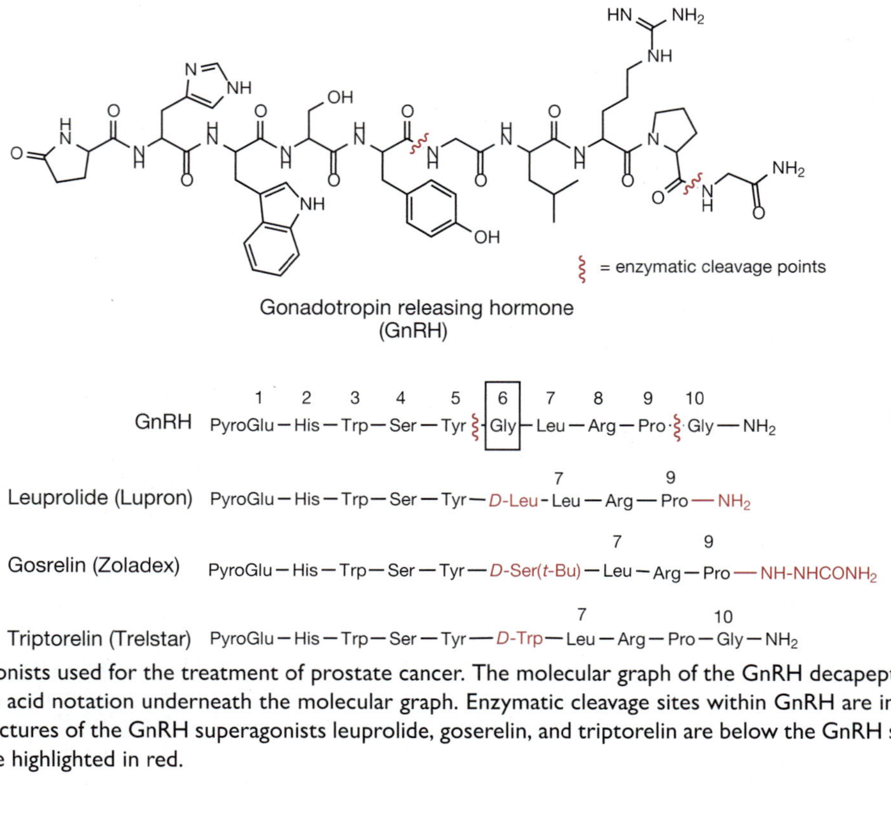

Figure 25.41 GnRH agonists used for the treatment of prostate cancer. The molecular graph of the GnRH decapeptide is shown at the top of the figure with amino acid notation underneath the molecular graph. Enzymatic cleavage sites within GnRH are indicated therein. Amino acid notation of the structures of the GnRH superagonists leuprolide, goserelin, and triptorelin are below the GnRH structure. Modifications at positions 6 and 10 are highlighted in red.

release. The 3.75 mg depot formulation is rapidly absorbed, producing a C_{max} of 4.6 to 10.2 ng/mL at 4 hours. Two days after dosing, plasma concentrations were maintained at about 0.3 ng/mL for about 4 to 5 weeks. Once released into the plasma, the steady-state volume of distribution was about 27 L, with a terminal elimination half-life of about 3 hours. Metabolism involves enzymatic cleavage to smaller inactive peptides, with only 5% of the intact peptide eliminated in the urine.

Goserelin (Zoladex). Goserelin acetate (Zoladex) is also a synthetic nonapeptide: 5-oxo-L-prolyl-His-Trp-Ser-Tyr-D-Ser(t-Bu)-Leu-Arg-Pro-Azgly-NH_2 acetate (where 5-oxo-L-prolyl is the same as PyroGlu in Fig. 25.41, and where Azgly is azaglycine). It is available as an SC injectable implant administered every 28 days (3.6 mg [breast cancer or prostate cancer]) or 12 weeks (10.8 mg [prostate cancer]). The implant is a biodegradable polymer (D,L-lactic and glycolic acids copolymer) that provides rapid initial absorption and constant release over the indicated time periods. For example, for the 3.6 mg depot, mean serum concentrations gradually rise to reach a peak of about 3 ng/mL around 15 days after administration and then decline to approximately 0.5 ng/mL by the end of the treatment period. For the 10.8 mg depot, mean serum concentrations increase to a peak of about 8 ng/mL within the first 24 hours and then decline rapidly up to day 4. Thereafter, mean concentrations remain relatively stable in the range of about 0.3 to 1 ng/mL up to the end of the treatment period. After release into the plasma, goserelin has a large volume of distribution (44 L) and is eliminated similarly to leuprolide as inactive peptides in the urine with only 20% as unchanged peptide.

Triptorelin (Trelstar). Triptorelin pamoate (Trelstar), a synthetic decapeptide 5-oxo-L-prolyl-His-Trp-Ser-Tyr-D-tryptophyl-Leu-Arg-L-prolylglycine amide (where 5-oxo-L-prolyl is the same as PyroGlu in Fig. 25.41) is available as a single IM depot injection in either buttock delivering 3.75, 11.25, or 22.5 mg every 4, 12, or 24 weeks. It is 100-fold more active than native GnRH in vitro. Like leuprolide depot, SC triptorelin serum concentrations peak rapidly within 1 to 3 hours after injection with any of the mentioned doses with a volume of distribution of 30 to 33 L. Elimination is via a three-compartment model; however, metabolic pathways are unknown as no metabolites of triptorelin have been identified, presumably due to complete degradation. It is eliminated by both liver and kidneys with 42% excreted in the urine as an intact peptide, which increased to 62.3% in patients with liver disease.

Gonadotropin-Releasing Hormone Antagonist

Relugolix (Orgovyx). *Relugolix* (Orgovyx), approved in 2020, is the first oral form of ADT approved for advanced prostate cancer in decades. Unlike all previous GnRH mimetics used for ADT, relugolix is a nonpeptide small molecule GnRH-R antagonist (similar to elagolix approved for uterine fibroids discussed earlier). Relugolix, provided as 120 mg film-coated tablets for oral administration, rapidly reduced LH, FSH, and testosterone concentrations after the recommended loading dose of 360 mg and a 120 mg daily dose. Out of 622 patients, 56% had testosterone concentrations at castrate levels (<50 ng/dL) by the first sampling timepoint at day 4, and 97% maintained castrate levels of testosterone through 48 weeks. Consistent with the GnRH antagonist mechanism of action, the onset to castration is sooner than GnRH agonists, and notably without the untoward and potentially dangerous clinical flare. In the HERO trial, relugolix achieved 91% castration rates by day 8 versus leuprolide castration rates of only 82% by day 29. Relugolix also achieved lower testosterone serum levels than leuprolide, with 95% versus 57% achieving testosterone levels of less than 20 ng/dL (subcastration levels) by day 29. Side effects with relugolix are similar to other forms of ADT, such as hot flashes, flushing of the skin, increased weight, decreased sex drive, and difficulties with erectile function, with the important exception that relugolix was more than 50% less likely than leuprolide to cause serious cardiac events, such as stroke and myocardial infarction. Also, upon discontinuation of daily oral relugolix for 90 days, testosterone recovered to eugonadal levels to a greater extent than leuprolide administered by long-term release injection. Unlike all other forms of ADT (the agonists already discussed and the antagonist peptide degarelix discussed later), there is no painful injection nor requirement for administration in a health care environment. Unlike the long-term release injections, adverse effects, if intolerable, can be reversed rapidly upon discontinuation with this daily oral tablet. In summary, relugolix has the advantages of daily oral administration at home, mechanistic advantages of a GnRH antagonist such as no flare, faster castration onset, and greater extent of testosterone serum levels suppression to less than 20 ng/mL while mitigating the cardiac liability surrounding ADT. Conversely, compliance with daily dosing is critical to the success of relugolix therapy. Accordingly, relugolix is a novel agent that has the potential to become a new standard of care for men with advanced prostate cancer in need of ADT.[127]

After single oral doses of relugolix in the range of 60 to 360 mg, linear pharmacokinetics were observed with regard to C_{max} and AUC; whereas multiple doses in the range of 20 to 180 mg demonstrated disproportionate increases in C_{max}, but not in AUC. The accumulation of relugolix upon once-daily administration is approximately 2-fold. The mean absolute bioavailability is about 12% with no food effect observed and a median T_{max} of 2.25 hours. Plasma protein binding of relugolix is 68% to 71%, primarily to albumin and, to a lesser extent, to α1-acid glycoprotein. The mean effective half-life of relugolix is 25 hours and mean total clearance of 29.4 L/h with a renal clearance of 8 L/h. Relugolix is extensively metabolized after oral administration to metabolites predominantly excreted in the feces (~81% of total; 4.2% as unchanged) with a minor excretion route to the urine (4.1% total; 2.2% as unchanged). Relugolix is metabolized primarily by CYP3A and, to a lesser extent, by CYP2C8 in vitro and is a substrate for P-gp. Coadministration with erythromycin (P-gp and moderate CYP3A inhibitor) increased the AUC and C_{max} of relugolix by 6.2-fold, whereas rifampin (P-gp and strong CYP3A inducer) decreased the AUC and C_{max} of relugolix by 55% and 23%, respectively. This suggests the possibility of DDIs with either inhibitors or inducers of P-gp or CYP3A.

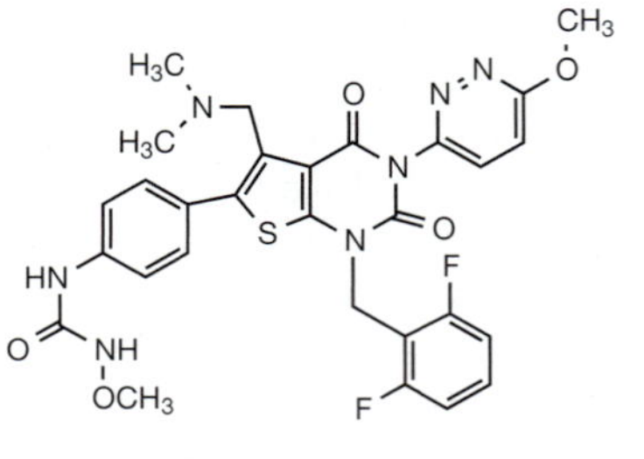

Relugolix
(Orgovyx)

Degarelix (Firmagon). Degarelix acetate (Firmagon), approved in 2012, is another GnRH antagonist for use in the treatment of advanced prostate cancer. It effectively replaced abarelix, a predecessor, which was voluntarily withdrawn from the market in 2005 due to unfavorable efficacy compared to GnRH agonists. Like relugolix, degarelix competes reversibly with the endogenous GnRH for GnRH-R binding on the pituitary gonadotroph cells and directly suppresses LH and consequently testosterone production, producing chemical castration. Unlike relugolix, it is a peptide that requires high-volume injections that frequently cause pain or injection site reactions.

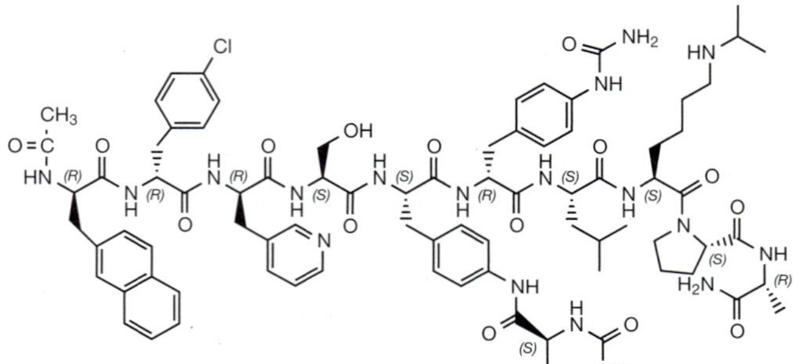

Degarelix
(Firmagon)

Like relugolix, degarelix as an antagonist does not produce an initial surge in pituitary LH or testicular androgen production as is observed with the GnRH agonists, so no clinical flare is manifested. As such, approximately 96% (vs 0% for leuprolide 7.5 mg) of men achieve castration levels of serum testosterone within 3 days and 99% within 14 days (vs 18% for leuprolide) after receiving their first (loading) dose of 240 mg of degarelix (administered as two SC injections of 120 mg). Lower maintenance doses of degarelix (80 mg) are administered every 28 days thereafter to maintain castration. Medical castration rates from days 28 to 364 were comparable to leuprolide 7.5-mg depot in advanced prostate cancer, with each achieving more than 95% efficacy. SC administration forms a depot from which degarelix is released to the circulation. After the 240 mg SC dose (with 40 mg/mL concentration product; or 6 mL injection volume), the C_{max} occurred within 2 days. Pharmacokinetic behavior is strongly influenced by its concentration in the injection solution; however, only the 40-mg/mL concentration is approved.

Degarelix is widely distributed throughout the total body water, and in vitro plasma protein binding is estimated to be more than 90% (distribution volume >1,000 L). Degarelix is subject to peptide hydrolysis during passage through the hepatobiliary system and is mainly excreted as peptide fragments in the feces. Terminal elimination half-life of the SC depot injection is 53 days due to very slow release from the depot. Approximately 20% to 30% was renally excreted, whereas 70% to 80% was excreted via hepatobiliary excretion. The most common adverse effect was injection site reactions (28% pain and 17% erythema vs <1% for leuprolide). Most other adverse effects were similar to leuprolide.

ADT with GnRH agonists or antagonists significantly reduces serum testosterone levels, thereby depriving prostate cancer cells of their primary signal for growth (testosterone and DHT) and alleviating or easing the symptoms associated with advanced prostate cancer. However, GnRH agonists and antagonists are not cures for prostate cancer. They are considered palliative care. Periodic monitoring of PSA and serum testosterone levels is recommended. Failure of one mode of ADT cannot be compensated for by changing to another. Instead, once castration resistance develops, a secondary hormonal suppression and/or chemotherapy can be added, if not already in use, to again suppress the AR axis or suppress tumor growth.

The testosterone deficiency associated with ADT produces a variety of untoward and adverse effects, which increase the morbidity of and affect the quality of life of ADT patients. Increased risk morbidities are due to bone and cardiometabolic complications, such as osteoporosis and fractures, cardiovascular disease (with the possible exception of relugolix) including strokes and acute myocardial infarctions, weight gain, insulin resistance, hyperlipidemia, and diabetes. Adverse quality of life issues include, among others, genital atrophy, ED, decreased mood and mentation, hot flashes and gynecomastia.[353-355] After induction of castration, some low-risk patients can be considered for intermittent ADT to limit iatrogenic morbidity and cost with comparable overall survival rates; however, this practice may lose favor in view of the availability of relugolix with its ease of administration and mitigated cardiac risk.[356] Intermittent ADT candidates include those with a robust PSA response and/or if the prostate cancer is asymptomatic.

Treatment of Castration-Resistant Prostate Cancer

Nearly one-third of patients with prostate cancer develop metastatic disease, and about 80% to 90% of those metastatic patients will have good initial responses to treatments such as surgery, radiation or other local therapy, and systemic pharmacotherapies such as ADT or combinations of ADT with secondary hormonal suppression or docetaxel. However, most patients with advanced prostate cancer will go on to develop progressive disease,[357] where they present with increasing PSA or progression observed on imaging despite ongoing ADT, possibly combined with chemotherapy or secondary hormonal therapies. Once castration resistance is verified through testosterone-level testing, then pharmacotherapy depends on whether the disease is asymptomatic or symptomatic and nonmetastatic (nmCRPC) or metastatic (mCRPC) in view of the pharmacotherapeutic history.

Recently, the CRPC therapeutic landscape has been rapidly expanding. For example, until 2010, the only pharmacotherapy for CRPC was docetaxel; however, six new agents have been approved in the past decade to include (in order): sipuleucel-T, cabazitaxel, abiraterone, enzalutamide, Ra-223, apalutamide, and darolutamide. Most of these were approved in a CRPC setting following progression on docetaxel, but some have subsequently gained approvals and/or quality of life benefits for earlier stage disease, as discussed next for each agent. Although there are a variety of agents, improvements in CRPC survival are typically by only ~4 months, suggesting the need for exploration of optimal sequencing and/or earlier intervention in order to improve outcomes or delay progression for patients with advanced and castration-resistant prostate cancer using existing agents. Novel therapies that are less susceptible to the development of resistance are also needed.

Immunotherapy. Sipuleucel-T (Provenge), originally termed a *therapeutic cancer vaccine* but now referred to as an immunotherapy similar to programmed death-ligand agents, was approved for the treatment of asymptomatic or minimally symptomatic mCRPC in 2010. Sipuleucel-T was the first immunotherapy and utilizes an autologous cellular immunotherapy approach. Peripheral blood mononuclear cells, a type of white blood cell that includes antigen-presenting cells, are removed from the patient's blood through leukapheresis at a treatment center. These cells are then activated ex vivo (outside the body) at a separate laboratory with a recombinant fusion protein (PA2024) so that the cells recognize and target prostate cancer cells. Next, the modified cells are reinfused into the patient. The modified cells, together with the immune system of the patient, find and destroy prostate cancer cells. Although the precise mechanism of action is unknown, sipuleucel-T is designed to induce an immune response targeted against prostatic acid phosphatase (PAP), an antigen expressed in most prostate cancers. Since PAP is only found on prostatic cells, this leads to a localized treatment.[358] However, there is no PSA response or other biomarker to monitor therapy. The treatment course comprises infusions at weeks 0, 2, and 4 that each deliver a minimum of 50 million autologous $CD54^+$ cells activated with PAP-granulocyte-macrophage colony-stimulating factor. Infusions are associated with a high prevalence (~70%) of acute infusion reactions that can be managed via premedication with oral acetaminophen and an antihistamine, such as diphenhydramine, approximately 30 minutes prior to administration.

Clinical trials with sipuleucel-T demonstrated a 4-month improvement in survival as compared to placebo[359] in asymptomatic mCRPC. It has been suggested that patients whose cancer is less advanced generally have a more "active" immune system and may benefit the most from this treatment. However, thus far, the expense, narrow indication, and the inconvenience of the workflow (leukapheresis at a specialty clinic, ex vivo cell activation, and reinfusion) have hampered exploration of other indications with little clinical data to suggest indication expansion.[360] Nonetheless, information on its optimal use in combination and/or sequenced with other approved agents is awaited.[358]

Secondary Hormonal Therapies and Chemotherapy. Last century, disease that progressed despite ongoing ADT was termed *androgen-independent prostate cancer*, suggesting that AR was no longer operant in the growth mechanisms of the prostate cancer. In 2004, a discovery in recurrent prostate cancer revealed that AR was expressed at levels that were comparable to androgen-stimulated benign prostate.[361] Further, endogenous testosterone levels were also at normal levels in the recurrent prostate cancer tissue, with ongoing AR axis activation observable as high expression of AR target genes such as PSA in the recurrent cancer. The conclusion was that the AR axis was reactivated despite castration levels of serum testosterone.[361] Importantly, the recurrent prostate cancer, retermed as CRPC, should be sensitive to suppression of the AR axis if more potent agents could be discovered. Many novel AR signaling inhibitor therapies for CRPC were designed and trialed.[362] This stimulated a renaissance in the exploration of secondary hormonal therapies that resulted in the discovery and approval of several new agents such as abiraterone (Zytiga), enzalutamide (Xtandi), apalutamide (Erleada), and darolutamide (Nubeqa).

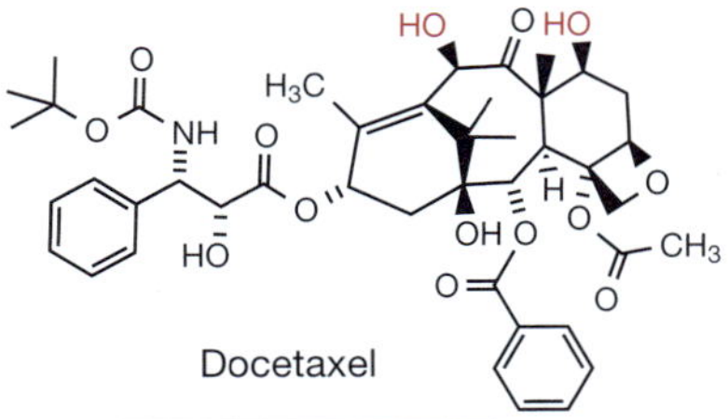
Docetaxel

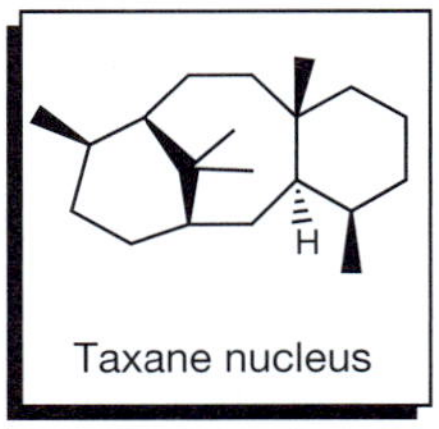
Taxane nucleus

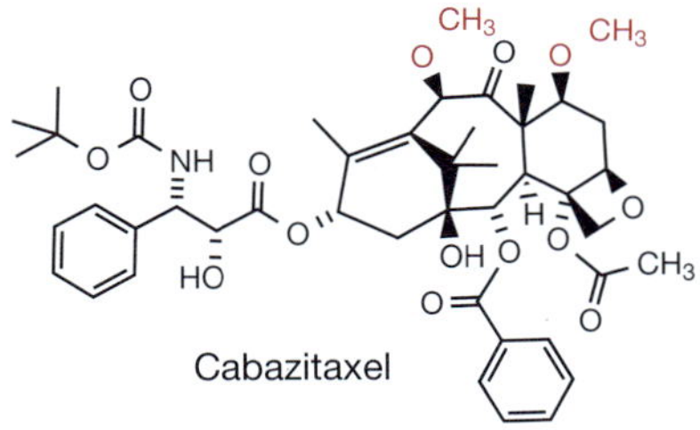
Cabazitaxel

Contemporaneously, advances were being made in chemotherapy for "androgen-independent" prostate cancer. The only FDA-approved chemotherapy for advanced prostate cancer was mitoxantrone (Novantrone), which was approved because it improved pain in approximately one-third of symptomatic patients. However, there was no evidence for a survival advantage. In 2004, docetaxel (Taxotere; Chapter 36) in combination with prednisone became the first chemotherapeutic agent to show increased survival to 18.9 months, or approximately 2 months longer as compared to treatment with mitoxantrone and prednisone.[363] Infusions of 75 mg/m^2 of docetaxel over 1 hour once every 3 weeks in combination with 5 mg of prednisone bid for 10 cycles became the standard of care once metastatic patients were demonstrated hormone refractory (ie, ADT and older generation antiandrogens were ineffective). Today, these patients would be classified as mCRPC. In 2011, a cabazitaxel (Jevtana; Chapter 36) dose of 25 mg/m^2

every 3 weeks in combination with 5 mg oral prednisone bid was approved as second line after docetaxel exposure or failure in mCRPC.[364] In this population, median survival was 15.1 months for cabazitaxel versus 12.7 months for mitoxantrone, demonstrating a second survival benefit after docetaxel. In 2017, a lowered dose of 20 mg/m^2 every 3 weeks with prednisone was approved.[365] However, the lowered dose may not be appropriate if used in combination with the strong CYP3A4 inducer enzalutamide due to the possibility of subtherapeutic exposure to cabazitaxel, a CYP3A4 substrate.[366]

Once a patient has become resistant to AR axis inhibition and taxane-based chemotherapy, there are limited systemic therapeutics available to treat their disease. One approach to help these patients, lutetium Lu-177 vipivotide tetraxetan (Pluvicto), approved in 2023, is indicated for the treatment of prostate-specific membrane antigen (PSMA)-positive[367] mCRPC, that is, PSMA-positive mCRPC that has become resistant to AR axis inhibition and taxane-based chemotherapy. Pluvicto, a type of personalized medicine, uses a complementary diagnostic imaging agent, Locametz, after radiolabeling with gallium-68 for the identification of PSMA-positive lesions. PSMA is highly expressed in more than 80% of patients with prostate cancer, providing a biomarker for determining who is a candidate for treatment. It is the first FDA-approved targeted radioligand therapy for eligible patients with mCRPC that combines a targeting compound (ligand) with a therapeutic radioisotope (a radioactive particle) to specifically bind to and image the prostate cancer and produce local radiation therapy. The phase III VISION trial demonstrated that patients with PSMA-positive mCRPC previously treated with AR pathway inhibition and taxane-based chemotherapy who received Pluvicto plus standard of care had improved radiographic progression-free survival (rPFS; the time from randomization to the first objective evidence of radiographic progression) and overall survival compared to standard of care alone.[368] Moreover, ~30% of patients receiving Pluvicto plus standard of care demonstrated an overall radiographic response compared to 2% for standard of care alone.

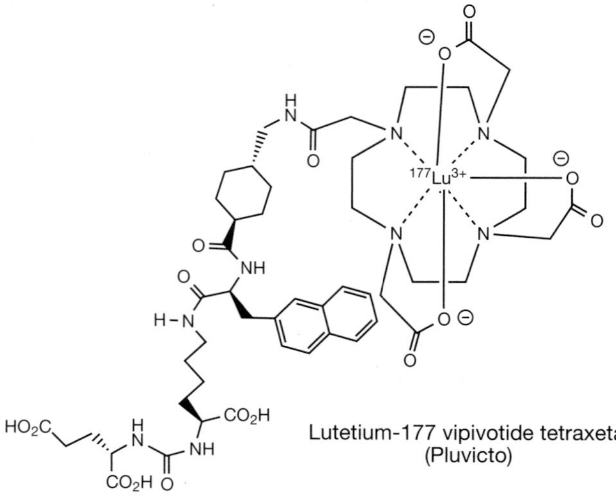

Lutetium-177 vipivotide tetraxetan (Pluvicto)

Inhibitors of Androgen Biosynthesis. Although the antiandrogens bicalutamide (Casodex), nilutamide (Nilandron), and flutamide (Eulexin) were approved in the late 1990s for advanced prostate cancer, these agents were weak AR antagonists that had a limited ability to suppress the AR axis. Consequently, there was still a large unmet need to provide highly potent AR signaling inhibitors to serve as secondary hormonal suppression in CRPC where androgens were demonstrated to be elevated intratumorally despite the castrate environment (<50 ng/dL testosterone in plasma)[361] produced by ADT, regardless of whether ADT consisted of GnRH agonist or antagonist or orchiectomy. Subsequently, the source of these extragonadal androgens was discovered to be intratumoral, and adrenal biosynthetic pathways (among other minor sources) contributed sufficient endogenous androgens to reactivate the AR axis and sustain prostate tumor growth as CRPC despite ongoing ADT. This left open the possibility of suppressing the AR axis by blocking endogenous biosynthesis. Unlike estrogen biosynthesis, androgen biosynthesis can occur via redundant biosynthetic pathways (see Figs. 25.3 and 25.42; note that enzymes ***b*** and ***j*** are the same protein, CYP17A1). Further, mutant ARs in CRPC cells are promiscuously activated by weak adrenal androgens and glucocorticoids, not just testosterone and DHT. Consequently, simply blocking the last step in the testosterone/DHT synthetic pathway, as was possible for estrogens (see "Aromatase Inhibitors" section), was not available as an effective treatment modality. Instead, androgen biosynthesis must be blocked at an early and common step to these redundant pathways, as discussed later for the lyase (CYP17A1) inhibitor abiraterone.

Inhibitors of a variety of other enzymes within the redundant biosynthesis pathways have been evaluated to reduce androgen biosynthesis, but none have advanced to the drug development stage. For example, inhibitors of 17β-HSD (enzyme ***g*** in Fig. 25.3) type 3 (gonadal 17β-HSD3)[369] or type 5 (peripheral 17β-HSD5 [17β-hydroxysteroid dehydrogenase type 5]; also known as AKR1C3 [aldoketoreductase type 1C3])[370] exist, but there is no clinical evidence to support their use. Further, inhibitors of 5AR (enzyme ***i*** in Figure 25.3) were approved for BPH, but when examined for chemoprevention of prostate cancer, were officially advised against by FDA due to more aggressive phenotype cancers in those where chemoprevention failed.

CYP17A1 Inhibitors. 17α-Hydroxylase/17,20-lyase (CYP17A1 or CYP17; sometimes just called lyase) is a bifunctional enzyme, which converts pregnenolone into 17α-hydroxypregnenolone (hydroxylase) and subsequently cleaves the 17β side chain (lyase) of this C21 steroid to produce the C19 sex steroid precursor DHEA. These steps are marked with red Xs in Figure 25.42. Inhibition of CYP17A1 blocks the synthesis in both the glucocorticoid and sex hormone pathways due to the common intermediate, 17α-hydroxypregnenolone, and increases the synthesis in the mineralocorticoid pathway, the only alternative for the resulting elevated levels of pregnenolone. The result is inhibition of androgen biosynthesis in the adrenals, prostatic tumor tissues, and testes, leading to decreased levels of weak intermediate androgens, testosterone, and DHT (and 17β-estradiol), but also decreased hydrocortisone levels requiring supplementation with glucocorticoids. Further, the mineralocorticoid excess produces side effects, including hypertension, potassium secretion, and fluid retention, which must be monitored.

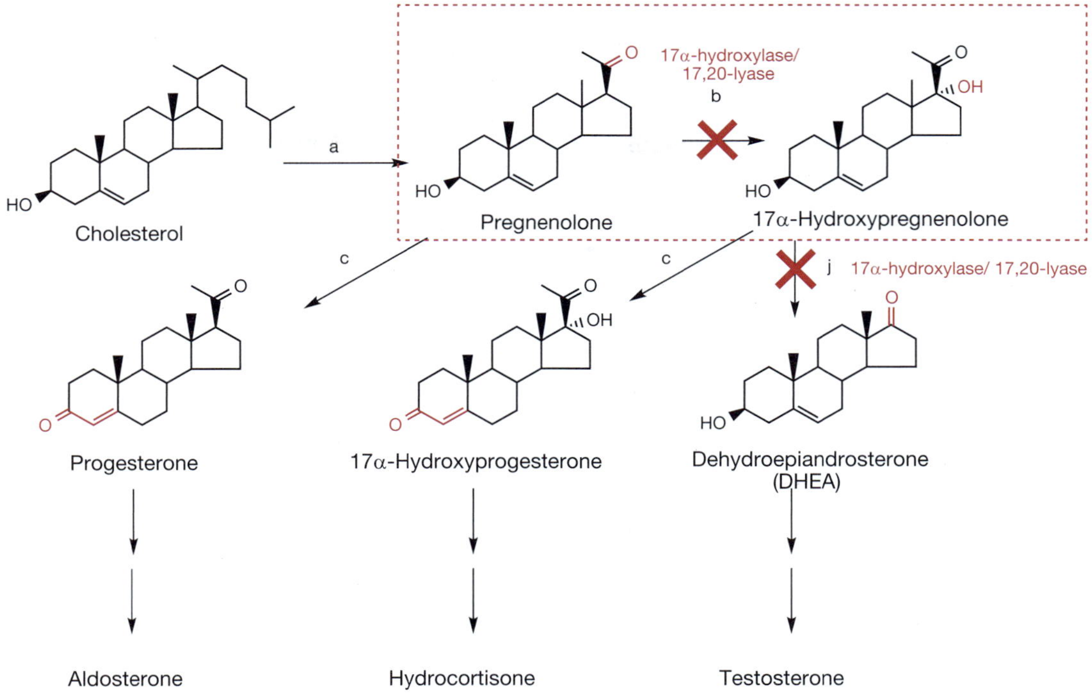

Figure 25.42 Inhibition of androgen synthesis by CYP17A1 inhibitors. Lyase inhibitors block conversion of cholesterol to the precursor of glucocorticoids and androgens through their actions to prevent the formation of 17α-hydroxypregnenolone (step b above) and DHEA (step j above). (a) A mitochondrial cytochrome P450 enzyme complex consisting of three proteins: CYP11A1 (also known as P450SCC), adrenodoxin, and adrenodoxin reductase; (b) 17α-hydroxylase (CYP17A1); (c) 5-ene-3β-hydroxysteroid dehydrogenase/3-oxosteroid-4,5-isomerase (3β-HSD); and (j) 17,20-lyase (CYP17A1).

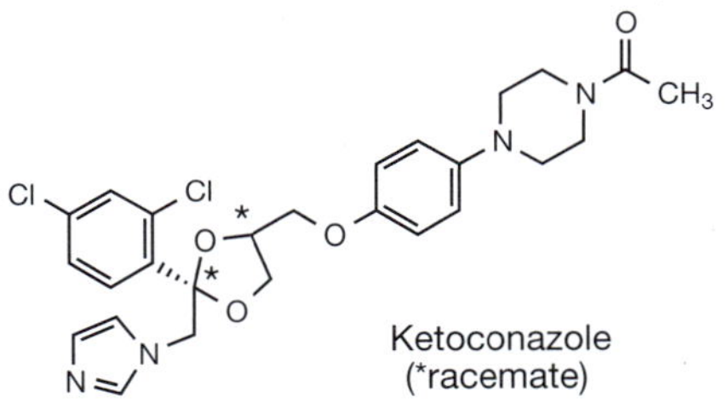

An early CYP17A1 inhibitor (17α-hydroxylase IC_{50} = 76 nM) that was used in patients with metastatic prostate cancer[371] was the antifungal agent ketoconazole. Ketoconazole's role in prostate cancer was supplanted by the approval of abiraterone acetate (Zytiga) plus prednisone in 2011 for patients with mCRPC previously treated with docetaxel. Whereas ADT abrogates only gonadal testosterone production, abiraterone (the active metabolite of the abiraterone acetate prodrug, Fig. 25.43) potently inhibits both the hydroxylase and lyase enzymatic actions of CYP17A1, blocking adrenal and tumoral androgen production. Consequently, abiraterone acetate, added to ongoing ADT, was able to effectively suppress the reactivated AR axis in CRPC. Abiraterone acetate (1,000 mg; four 250 mg tablets daily) plus prednisone (5 mg bid) resulted in increased overall survival for docetaxel-pretreated patients, with a median survival benefit of about 4 months (14.8 vs 10.9 months for placebo). In 2012, the indication was expanded to mCRPC in general (ie, not requiring previous chemotherapy), based on median rPFS (16.5 vs 8.3 months with prednisone alone) and a trend toward improved overall survival.[372]

In 2018, the FDA expanded the indication for abiraterone acetate (1,000 mg) in combination with prednisone (5 mg bid) plus ongoing ADT to include metastatic high-risk CSPC earlier in the natural history of prostate cancer. Approval was based on benefits on overall survival (median overall survival not estimable vs 34.7 months for placebo)

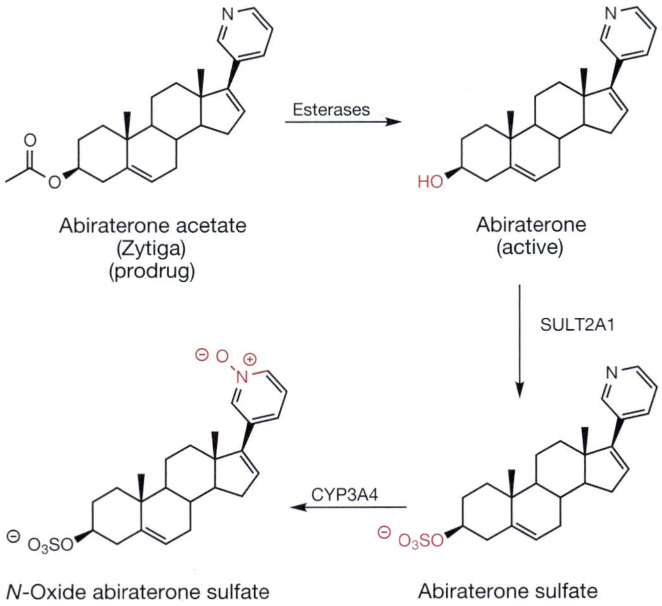

Figure 25.43 Structure of the CYP17A1 inhibitor abiraterone, its activation, and metabolism.

and time to initiation of chemotherapy (median time not reached vs 38.9 months for placebo).[373]

Abiraterone acetate (Fig. 25.43) is a steroidal prodrug, which is rapidly and completely cleaved by unspecified esterases into the active 3β-hydroxy metabolite abiraterone. An oral dose of 1,000 mg daily of abiraterone acetate without food is recommended (combined with 5 mg prednisone bid). Following oral administration of the inactive prodrug, maximum plasma concentrations of abiraterone were reached in 2 hours. Due to poor solubility, there is a dramatic and inconsistent food effect on absorption, with 5- to 7-fold increases with a low-fat (7% fat, 300 calories) meal versus 10- to 17-fold increases with a high-fat (57%, 825 calories) meal. Due to unreliable efficacy and intolerable untoward effects from such wide variations, food is to be avoided for at least 1 hour before and 2 hours after dosing. Abiraterone is highly bound (>99%) to the plasma protein albumin and α-1 acid glycoprotein, producing an apparent volume of distribution of 19,669 L. The two main circulating metabolites of abiraterone are abiraterone sulfate and *N*-oxide abiraterone sulfate, which are products of SULT2A1 and CYP3A4, respectively. The terminal elimination half-life of abiraterone is 12 hours, with 88% of the radioactive dose recovered in feces. The major compounds present in feces are unchanged abiraterone acetate and abiraterone (55% vs 22%).

The side effect and DDI profiles for abiraterone are substantial. In subjects with mild or moderate hepatic impairment, abiraterone systemic exposures were significantly increased and terminal elimination half-life prolonged to 18 hours. For patients with baseline moderate hepatic impairment, dose reduction to 250 mg is recommended. Further, all patients must be monitored for development of hepatotoxicity. Abiraterone is an inhibitor of CYP2D6, and coadministration with narrow therapeutic index CYP2D6 substrates should be avoided. Due to the expected mineralocorticoid excess, prescribers are warned to control hypertension and correct hypokalemia before treatment and monitor for symptoms of mineralocorticoid excess, such as fluid retention or increased blood pressure. Risk-benefit analysis should be performed in cardiovascular disease, and safety in patients with class III or IV heart failure has not been established. Due to the expected adrenocortical insufficiency, daily abiraterone acetate must be taken together with oral prednisone 5 mg bid. Further, the prednisone dose may need to be increased before, during, and after stressful events.

In 2018, a new microparticle formulation of abiraterone acetate, Yonsa, was approved for patients with mCRPC in combination with methylprednisolone (4 mg bid) and concurrent ADT. Compared to Zytiga, Yonsa had improved abiraterone acetate dissolution rates and oral bioavailability while decreasing the effects of food on efficacy. For example, 500 mg (four tablets at 125 mg each) of Yonsa had similar absorption as 1,000 mg (four tablets at 250 mg each) Zytiga and therapeutic bioequivalence based on PSA and testosterone suppressions. Other than dosing and food effects (taken with or without food), the drug profiles for Yonsa and Zytiga are essentially identical.

In 2023, FDA approved abiraterone acetate in fixed-dose combination tablet with niraparib (Akeega), a PARP inhibitor, for patients with mCRPC with deleterious or suspected deleterious *BRCA*-positive mCRPC, as detected by an FDA-approved test. Like other abiraterone therapies, patients must also take prednisone separately with Akeega therapy. The MAGNITUDE study prospectively identified a subpopulation of mCRPC with the aforementioned mutations and demonstrated significant improvement in rPFS in this subpopulation when given the Akeega tablet plus prednisone compared with abiraterone acetate and prednisone alone. This approval, and the approval of enzalutamide plus talazoparib discussed later, is example of personalized medicine therapy now available for certain high-risk late-stage prostate cancer populations.[374]

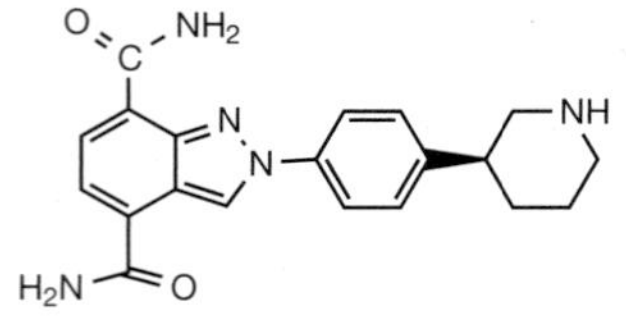

Niraparib
(combined with abiraterone acetate plus prednisone for *BRCA-positive mCRPC)*

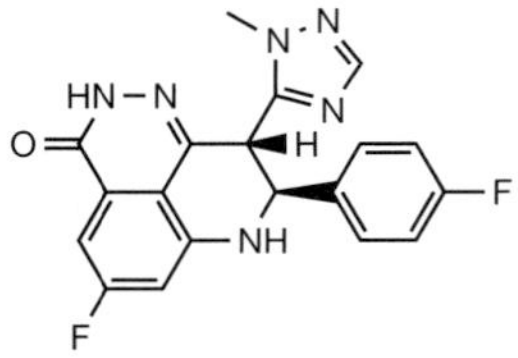

Talazoparib
(combined with enzalutamide for mutated homologous recombination repair-positive mCRPC)

Antiandrogens (Competitive Androgen Receptor Antagonists). Secondary hormonal therapy to suppress the reactivated AR axis in patients with CRPC can also be achieved by antiandrogens that compete with endogenous androgens for binding, thereby antagonizing the AR. Early nonsteroidal antiandrogens such as bicalutamide, flutamide, and nilutamide were approved for advanced prostate cancer as combined androgen blockade with ADT (Fig. 25.44). However, as mentioned, these first-generation antiandrogens suffered from low-potency activities and intrinsic agonism, particularly of mutant ARs present in many CRPCs. Although termed pure antagonists, these first-generation agents were later demonstrated to have less favorable antiandrogen activity profiles than more recently approved antiandrogens, as discussed later, and have been largely supplanted. For example, advances in the understanding of AR biology in CRPC allowed the development of the second-generation antiandrogens, including enzalutamide and apalutamide, that are more potent in vitro (AR binding and antagonism) and in vivo (inhibition of lymph node carcinoma of the prostate (LNCaP)/AR or other CRPC xenograft growth), and possessed novel antiandrogenic properties such as inhibition of AR nuclear translocation (Fig. 25.44). Importantly, enzalutamide extended overall survival in the mCRPC setting and apalutamide extended the MFS in nmCRPC. Both were demonstrated as preclinically and clinically superior compared to bicalutamide, the most efficacious of the first-generation antiandrogens.

Clinical Use of Second-Generation Antiandrogens

Enzalutamide (Xtandi) and Apalutamide (Erleada). Abiraterone acetate (combined with ADT and prednisone) was approved in 2011 for mCRPC following docetaxel, but it only extended survival by ~4 months. Enzalutamide in combination with ADT was approved for the same indication in 2012 and was expanded to include chemotherapy-naïve mCRPC in 2014. Enzalutamide (plus ADT) demonstrated the ability to improve the overall survival of docetaxel-pretreated (18.4 vs 13.6 months for placebo) or chemotherapy-naïve (35.3 vs 31.3 months for placebo) patients. Further, this combination demonstrated superiority over bicalutamide in rPFS in chemotherapy-naïve patients (19.5 vs 13.4 months for bicalutamide). Although the overall survival benefits of enzalutamide and abiraterone (and other newer agents used in prostate cancer) may seem to be short, the benefit to quality of life should not be overlooked. The indication for enzalutamide (Xtandi) combined with ADT was expanded to the nmCRPC setting based on extended MFS to 36.6 versus 14.7 months with ADT alone and trended toward overall survival benefit.[375] The indication was further expanded to mCSPC based on results from ARCHES, a randomized phase III study that evaluated 1,150 men with mCSPC and met its primary end point of rPFS. As mentioned earlier, an example of personalized medicine recently approved in 2023 involves the combination of enzalutamide and talazoparib (Talzenna), another PARP inhibitor, for mCRPC with certain specified mutations of genes that control homologous recombination repair (mHRR). These mHRR genes are associated with aggressive disease and poor prognosis, and the combination improves outcomes for this population.[374]

In 2018, apalutamide was approved for nmCRPC (also called M0 CRPC) by also demonstrating improved MFS in patients with CRPC who were confirmed nonmetastatic and had a PSA doubling time of less than 10 months. Concomitant ADT and apalutamide in this population provided dramatically improved MFS of 40.51 months compared to 16.2 months for placebo plus ADT. However, no overall survival benefit has yet been reported.[376] In 2019, the indication was expanded to include mCSPC based on improvements in overall survival and rPFS.

As can be seen, the use of these agents earlier in the natural history of prostate cancer delays the onset of metastasis by almost 2 years, improving the prognosis of men with nmCRPC. The approval of abiraterone acetate in high-risk CSPC provides further hope that secondary hormonal therapy can dramatically delay progression of disease if used earlier.

Darolutamide (Nubeqa). The second-generation AR antagonists were extremely successful in extending the progression-free and overall survival (if metastatic) or MFS (if not metastatic) of patients affected by mCSPC, or metastatic or nonmetastatic CRPC. However, both enzalutamide and apalutamide have seizurogenic effects due to their ability to cross the BBB and subsequently inhibit the $GABA_A$ in the brain. Darolutamide is a potent AR antagonist that is comparable to other second-generation AR antagonists in preclinical models. However, it does not cross the BBB and is likely to have minimal to no seizurogenic effect. Darolutamide was approved for nmCRPC in combination with ADT based on significant improvement in MFS in the ARAMIS trial, with a median of 40.4 months versus 18.4 months for placebo plus ADT.[377] In 2022, darolutamide was approved in combination with ADT and docetaxel for mCSPC based on the ARASENS trial, which showed a significant overall survival benefit with darolutamide plus ADT and docetaxel compared to ADT and docetaxel.[378]

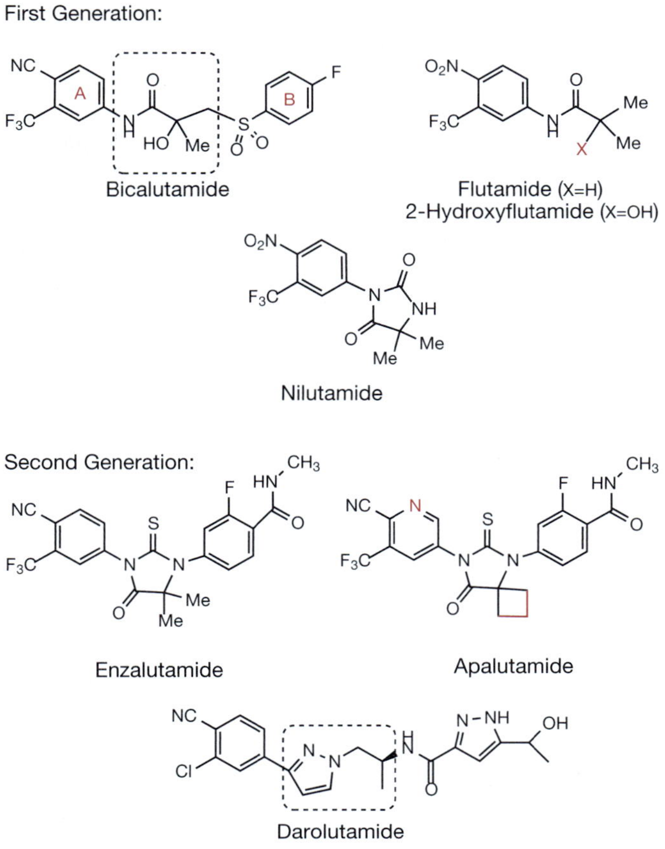

Figure 25.44 First- and second-generation nonsteroidal antiandrogens. The linear propanamide of bicalutamide and its bioisostere in darolutamide are enclosed by the boxes.

Structural Elements of a Nonsteroidal Antiandrogen. Nonsteroidal AR ligands generally contain an electron-deficient aniline A ring that is most often *m*-CF_3 or Cl and *p*-CN or NO_2 substituted. Bicalutamide and flutamide contain a linear propanamide segment attached to the aniline *N*-atom of the A ring. In the hydantoin (nilutamide) or thiohydantoins (enzalutamide and apalutamide), the propanamide segment has been cyclicized into a five-membered ring. In some cases, the propanamide or its analog is a linking segment, which also attaches to a substituted aromatic B ring, as seen in bicalutamide, enzalutamide, and apalutamide (Fig. 25.44). Darolutamide can be thought of as a diaryl propanamide like bicalutamide in which the amide is replaced with a pyrazole ring (Fig. 25.44). Perhaps, the amide NH of darolutamide behaves like OH of bicalutamide or hydroxyflutamide.

All antiandrogens bind to the same binding site on the LBD of AR with a similar predicted binding mode. Although the antagonist conformation of wild-type AR (wtAR) has never been crystallized, the agonist conformation of AR LBD-escape mutants bound to first-generation antiandrogens can be used to rationalize the binding contacts of the conserved structural elements of antiandrogens. Similar to ER in breast cancer, AR-escape mutants emerge in prostate cancer upon antiandrogen use and confer antiandrogen resistance. Antiandrogen binding to escape mutant AR reactivates the AR axis. For example, the use of bicalutamide results in Trp741 mutating to Leu741 (Trp741Leu or W741L), and flutamide use results in the Thr877Ala (T877A) mutation. The conserved A ring of antiandrogens has polar interactions with Gln711 and Arg752 via the *para* cyano or nitro substituents of the A ring. Similarly, the NH and carbinol OH of bicalutamide and hydroxyflutamide (active metabolite of flutamide) bind to Leu704 and Asn705 of AR as seen in the bicalutamide:W741L (1z95.pdb)[379] and hydroxyflutamide:T877A (2ax6.pdb)[379] LBD co-crystal structures, respectively. This latter aspect of the binding mode is not available to enzalutamide and apalutamide, and docking attempts into the cited escape mutants fail (personal experience), suggesting the second-generation antiandrogens cannot be accommodated by the known AR agonist conformations of the first-generation antiandrogens. The divergent antiandrogenicity profile of the thiohydantoins may be explained, in part, by the induction of different AR conformations. Unfortunately, as discussed next, cross-resistant escape mutants for the secondary hormonal therapies (enzalutamide, apalutamide, and abiraterone) are also known and cause clinical failures, such as the Phe876Leu_Thr877Ala double mutant (F876L_T877A).

Pharmacodynamics and Pharmacokinetics of Enzalutamide and Apalutamide. Enzalutamide and apalutamide are thiohydantoin antiandrogens discovered in the same laboratory, differing only slightly in structure and possessing largely parallel pharmacokinetics and pharmacodynamics. These agents were discovered while screening for antiandrogens that displayed full and pure antagonism, unlike bicalutamide, in AR overexpressing models of CRPC. Enzalutamide and apalutamide bind tightly and competitively with ^{18}F-16βF-DHT to AR, with 21.4 and 16.0 nM affinities compared to 11.5 nM for ^{18}F-16βF-DHT and 160 nM for bicalutamide (7- to 10-fold weaker) in a whole-cell–binding assay. The thiohydantoins are pure antagonists of wtAR that produced no agonism of AR-dependent genes such as PSA, even in wtAR overexpressing models of CRPC[380] (eg, LNCaP/AR cells). However, the weaker binding antagonist bicalutamide acted as an agonist in prostate cancer cells overexpressing wtAR and could not effectively antagonize R1881, a steroidal agonist commonly used in preclinical research. Bicalutamide acted similarly in vertebral cancer of the prostate (VCaP) prostate cancer cells (another cell line that overexpresses full-length AR and also expresses an AR-V7–truncated mutant[381]), stimulating cellular proliferation and only partially antagonizing R1881-induced cellular proliferation. The thiohydantoins (including RD-162 [not shown])[382] had no intrinsic stimulatory properties and were also full antagonists in VCaP cells. Further, thiohydantoins inhibit the nuclear translocation of AR, producing nuclear-to-cytoplasmic ratios of 3.0 (enzalutamide) and 2.5 (apalutamide) versus 29 and 14 for R1881 and bicalutamide, and 0.7 for vehicle, helping to rationalize the relatively high intrinsic agonism of bicalutamide in cells that overexpress the AR as compared to thiohydantoins. Importantly, both enzalutamide and apalutamide are able to regress (shrink) CRPC xenografts in vivo, whereas bicalutamide activity was limited to growth inhibition (only 1/10 tumors treated with bicalutamide regressed >50% vs 8/10 for apalutamide) despite 3-fold lower plasma levels.

Apalutamide appears to be more potent than enzalutamide in vivo. It was more potent preclinically in regressing LNCaP/AR xenografts, requiring a 30-mg/kg dose to achieve tumor volume reduction of more than 50% in 13 of 20 tumors as compared to a dose of 100 mg/kg of enzalutamide to achieve similar efficacy (>50% reduction of 12/20 tumors). Apalutamide also demonstrated slightly better MFS in nmCRPC humans (as discussed earlier). Increased seizure activity was observed clinically for both drugs owing to their shared inhibition of $GABA_A$ receptors in the brain. The incidence of seizures was 2.2% for enzalutamide in patients with predisposing risk factors, such as the use of seizure threshold lowering agents, history of head/brain injury, or cerebrovascular accident or transient ischemic attack, in early clinical trials. The incidence of seizures was lower (0.5% and 0.2% for enzalutamide and apalutamide, respectively) in later clinical trials that excluded predisposed patients. Patients experiencing new-onset seizures on either of these drugs must permanently discontinue their use.

Following daily oral administration with or without food, enzalutamide (160 mg as four 40 mg tablets) and apalutamide (240 mg as four 60 mg tablets) are rapidly (C_{max} of 1 and 2 hours, respectively) and completely absorbed. Steady state is achieved in 4 weeks with minimal daily fluctuations (1.25 and 1.63 peak-to-trough ratios) and significant accumulation ratios relative to single dosing (8.3- and 5-fold). Both are highly plasma protein bound.

Enzalutamide and apalutamide are metabolized by CYP2C8 and CYP3A4 to NDM active metabolites, with 30% and 40% of total steady-state AUC being unchanged drug and 49% and 37%, respectively, being active metabolite. The metabolites are equipotent and have one-third the activity of their parent, contributing significantly to overall activity. Apalutamide is reported to autoinduce its metabolism via CYP3A4. The terminal elimination half-lives are long at 5.8 and 3 days, as shown in Table 25.16. Excretion of radioactivity following single-dose oral administration of enzalutamide or apalutamide is slow, with 85% and 65% recovered by 77 and 70 days, respectively, largely in the urine at 71% and 65% versus 14% and 24% in feces, mostly as inactive metabolites. Single doses of gemfibrozil, a CYP2C8 inhibitor, increased thiohydantoin levels by 220% (AUC of enzalutamide plus metabolite) and 68% (AUC of apalutamide). Both thiohydantoins significantly reduced levels of CYP3A4 (midazolam), CYP2C9 (S-warfarin), and CYP2C19 (omeprazole) substrates, suggesting the avoidance of coadministration of narrow therapeutic index substrates of these enzymes. Shared untoward effects compared to placebo include falls and fractures, hot flash, and hypertension, with apalutamide generally having increased prevalence commensurate with increased AR potency.

Pharmacodynamics and Pharmacokinetics of Darolutamide. *Like* the other antiandrogens, darolutamide is an AR antagonist that competitively inhibits endogenous androgen binding, AR nuclear translocation, and AR-mediated transcription. Unlike the thiohydantoins enzalutamide and apalutamide, darolutamide does not cross the BBB nor does it activate the HPG axis to increase serum testosterone.[383] In addition, darolutamide functions as a PR antagonist in vitro. Darolutamide was designed to overcome enzalutamide resistance via pan-antagonism of escape mutations in vitro, and in vivo inhibits xenograft growth and suppresses intratumoral PSA levels in enzalutamide-resistant M49F LNCaP cells, which harbor the F876L_T877A double mutant.[384]

Table 25.16 Some Properties and Pharmacokinetics of the First- and Second-Generation Antiandrogens

Drugs	Bicalutamide	Flutamide	Nilutamide	Enzalutamide	Apalutamide	Darolutamide
Trade Name	**Casodex**	**Eulexin**	**Nilandron**	**Xtandi**	**Erleada**	**Nubeqa**
cLog *P*[a]	2.7	3.27	1.74	3.75	3.05	3.0
Oral bioavailability (%)	80-90	—	100	100	100	30
Onset of action (wk)[b]	8-12	2-4	1-2	—	—	—
Duration of action	8 d	3 mo to 2.5 y	1-3 mo	—	—	—
Protein binding (%)	96	94-96	80-84	97-98	96	92
Time to peak concentration (h)	31	2-3	1-4	0.5-3	2	4
Elimination half-life	~6 d	8 h (10 h for active metabolite)	40-60 h	5.8 d (7.8-8.6 for active metabolite)	~3 d	20 h
Cytochrome isoforms	3A4	1A2	Flavin mono-oxygenase, CYP2C	2C8	2C8, 3A4	3A4
Active metabolites	None	2-Hydroxy	Yes	*N*-Desmethyl	*N*-Desmethyl	Keto-darolutamide
Excretion: Feces (%) Urine (%)	43 34 (glucuronide)	<10 28	<10% 62	14% 71	24 65	32 63

[a]www.drugbank.ca. Accessed July 15, 2025.

[b]Time for significant improvement in prostate-specific antigen (PSA) or other biomarkers.

Darolutamide is composed of two pharmacologically active compounds ([*S*,*R*]-darolutamide and [*S*,*S*]-darolutamide), which convert into the metabolically active metabolite keto-darolutamide (Fig. 25.45).

Even though darolutamide displayed advantages compared to the thiohydantoins such as increased in vitro potency, lack of CNS penetration, and preclinical ability to overcome bicalutamide and thiohydantoin resistance, it is important to note that current data do not clearly demonstrate better clinical outcomes with darolutamide compared to enzalutamide or apalutamide.[383] This is despite darolutamide having three major active components (including the active keto metabolite), their very distinct chemical structures compared to the thiohydantoins, and the absence of known escape mutations. It has been postulated that a major cause of secondary hormonal therapy cross-resistance, including darolutamide resistance, is the upregulation of the constitutively active AR-V7 truncation mutant or similarly truncated AR mutants that lack the LBD,[385] as discussed next.

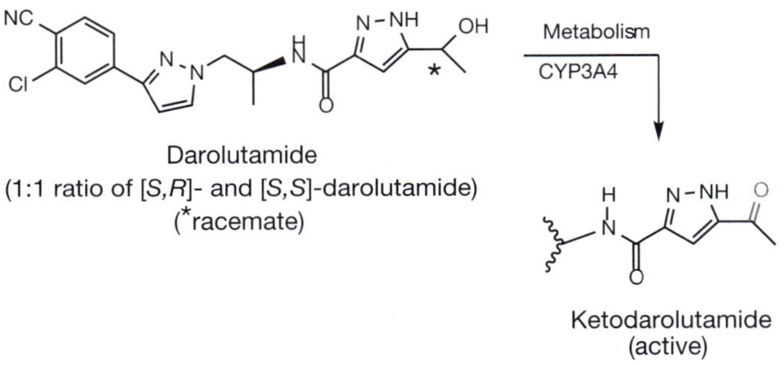

Figure 25.45 Metabolism of the components of darolutamide to the active metabolite keto-darolutamide.

Darolutamide is available as 300-mg tablets administered as two tablets bid for a 1,200-mg total daily dose. It is taken with food in order to increase the AUC and C_{max} values observed with a high-fat meal. Patients should also concurrently receive ADT. Administration of the 1,200-mg daily dose yields a C_{max} of 4.79 mg/L reached in 4 hours and an AUC_{12h} of 52.82 µg h/mL from 0 to 12 hours, with steady state reached in 2 to 5 days. Darolutamide taken with food is 30% bioavailable (Table 25.16), which is increased 2- to 5-fold compared to without food. Darolutamide is 92% protein bound, primarily to serum albumin, and exhibits an apparent volume of distribution of 119 L after IV administration. The effective half-life of darolutamide is approximately 20 hours in patients, and its clearance following IV administration is 116 mL/min. As mentioned, the darolutamide racemate is composed of two active diastereomers that are metabolized primarily by CYP3A4 to a single active metabolite, keto-darolutamide; whereas other metabolites result from glucuronidation by UGT1A9 and UGT1A1 to *O*- and *N*-glucuronides.[386] The total exposure of keto-darolutamide in plasma is 1.7-fold higher compared to darolutamide. Both parent and metabolite are 63.4% excreted via the urine (~7% unchanged) and 32.4% in the feces (~30% unchanged), as shown in Table 25.16. Qualitatively, the adverse effect profile of darolutamide is similar to enzalutamide and apalutamide, but several adverse effects are less prevalent than the thiohydantoins, such as less fatigue (12.1% for darolutamide vs 33% and 30.4% for enzalutamide and apalutamide), hypertension (6.6% vs 12.0% and 24.8%), falls (4.2% vs 11.0% and 15.6%), and mental impairment (0.9% vs 5.0% and 5.1%). Another advantage of darolutamide over enzalutamide and apalutamide might be the lessened risk of DDIs with darolutamide due to the lack of inhibition of the most common CYP enzymes.

Resistance to Secondary Hormonal Therapies. Given the cross-resistance among secondary hormonal therapies such as abiraterone acetate and antiandrogens, there remains an unmet clinical need in CRPC who have progressed following secondary hormonal therapy. Already resistance mechanisms to thiohydantoin therapy have evolved, including cross-resistance to apalutamide and enzalutamide, and possibly abiraterone acetate, as conferred by F876L point mutant or F876L_T877A double mutant.[387] At the time of writing, no escape point mutations for darolutamide have been prominently reported. Similar to escape mutants of the first-generation antiandrogens (eg, T877A for flutamide and W741L or W741C for bicalutamide, among other LBD mutations), these mutants operate as agonist switch mutations in which the antiandrogen acts as an agonist when binding to their escape mutant at high concentration. Consequently, antiandrogen-withdrawal syndrome is observed clinically and is defined as tumor regression or symptomatic relief on cessation of antiandrogen therapy. Cross-resistance between the different modes of secondary hormonal therapy has been observed, and no FDA approvals exist to guide their sequential use. Although darolutamide was tested preclinically to overcome enzalutamide resistance, there is not yet any clinical evidence suggesting that darolutamide will maintain activity if sequenced after enzalutamide or apalutamide. Various sequential and combinatorial approaches are being explored clinically.[388,389]

A major cause of secondary hormonal cross-resistance is the upregulation of the constitutively active AR truncation mutants, which lack the LBD. Without the LBD, all currently approved antiandrogens cannot bind to and inhibit these AR-escape mutants,[385] nor would decreased levels of endogenous androgens due to abiraterone treatment be successful. AR-V7 is the most prominently studied of the constitutively active AR truncation mutants and is believed to play an important role in treatment failures in late-stage prostate and breast cancers.[390] Correspondingly, next-generation inhibitors of the AR axis will require targeting of binding sites outside the LBD as has been previously reviewed.[391,392]

First-Generation Antiandrogens

Bicalutamide (Casodex). Bicalutamide is a biaryl propanamide (Fig. 25.44) given at a dosage of 50 mg once daily in combination with ADT (GnRH analog or surgical castration) for the treatment of advanced prostate cancer in the United States. Bicalutamide is a racemate, and its antiandrogenic activity resides almost exclusively in the (*R*)-enantiomer, which has an approximately 4-fold higher affinity for the prostate AR than hydroxyflutamide (discussed next). The (*S*)-enantiomer has no antiandrogenic activity. (*R*)-Bicalutamide is slowly absorbed, but absorption is unaffected by food.[393] It has a terminal elimination half-life of 1 week and accumulates approximately 10-fold in plasma during daily administration (Table 25.16). (*S*)-Bicalutamide is much more rapidly absorbed and cleared from plasma. At steady state, the plasma levels of (*R*)-bicalutamide are 100 times higher than those of (*S*)-bicalutamide. Although mild-to-moderate hepatic impairment does not affect its pharmacokinetics, evidence suggests slower elimination of (*R*)-bicalutamide in subjects with severe hepatic impairment.[393] Bicalutamide metabolites are excreted almost equally in urine and feces, with little or no unchanged drug excreted in urine. Unmetabolized drug predominates in the plasma. (*R*)-Bicalutamide is cleared almost exclusively by CYP3A4-mediated metabolism, but glucuronidation is the predominant metabolic route for (*S*)-bicalutamide.

Flutamide (Eulexin). Flutamide is a propanamide lacking the B ring of bicalutamide (Fig. 25.44). After oral administration (the usual dose is 250 mg every 8 hours), flutamide is completely absorbed from the GI tract and undergoes extensive first-pass metabolism by CYP1A2 to its major metabolite, 2-hydroxyflutamide (see Fig. 25.44), and its hydrolysis product, 3-trifluoromethyl-4-nitroaniline (not shown).[394] 2-Hydroxyflutamide is a more powerful antiandrogen in vivo, with higher affinity for the receptor than flutamide.[395] 2-Hydroxyflutamide has a terminal elimination half-life of approximately 10 hours (see Table 25.16). These studies show the principal role of CYP1A2 in the metabolism of flutamide to 2-hydroxyflutamide, with minor contribution from CYP3A4. 2-Hydroxyflutamide inhibits the metabolism of flutamide and both 2- and 4-hydroxylation of 17β-estradiol. Flutamide is a pure antagonist, whereas 2-hydroxyflutamide is a more potent AR antagonist but also can activate AR-escape mutants at higher concentrations, as discussed earlier.[395] These findings raise the possibility that increased conversion of flutamide to 2-hydroxyflutamide or accumulation of 2-hydroxyflutamide in cells may contribute to the anomalous responses to flutamide that were observed in some advanced prostate cancers. Rare reports of liver failure have been associated with flutamide, mandating regular monitoring of liver function tests in men taking flutamide therapy.

Nilutamide (Nilandron). Nilutamide (Fig. 25.44) is a hydantoin analog of flutamide that is completely absorbed after oral administration, with a mean terminal elimination half-life of approximately 50 hours (see Table 25.16).[396] Daily oral doses of nilutamide range from 150 to 300 mg/d. One of the methyl groups attached to the hydantoin ring is stereoselectively hydroxylated to a chiral metabolite, which subsequently is oxidized to its carboxylic acid metabolite. Less than 2% of nilutamide is excreted unchanged in the urine. In vitro, the nitro group of nilutamide was reduced to the amine and hydroxylamine moieties by nitric oxide (NO) synthases, a flavin monooxygenase system.[397] This reduction proceeds via the formation of a nitro anion free radical or via its reduction to its hydroxylamino derivative, which could explain some of the poorly investigated toxic effects of this drug,[398] which overshadow the therapeutic effects.

Testicular Cancer

Testicular cancer develops in the testicles and, according to the National Cancer Institute (NCI), accounts only for approximately 1% of all cancers in men. The American Cancer Society estimates about 9,760 new cases of testicular cancer diagnosed and about 500 deaths from testicular cancer in 2024 with an increasing incidence for several decades.[399] Compared with prostate cancer, testicular cancer is relatively rare. It is most common among males aged 15 to 40 years and is approximately 4-fold more common in White men than in Black men.

Nearly all testicular tumors originate from germ cells, the specialized sperm-forming cells within the testicles. These tumors fall into one of two types, seminomas or nonseminomas.[400] Seminomas account for approximately 40% of all testicular cancer and are made up of immature germ cells. Seminomas are slow growing and tend to stay localized in the testicle for long periods. Nonseminomas arise from more mature, specialized germ cells and tend to be more aggressive than seminomas. According to the American Cancer Society, 60% to 70% of patients with nonseminomas have cancer that has spread to the lymph nodes. α-Fetoprotein is a tumor-associated marker in blood for testicular cancer. Its measurement can help to show how well the chemotherapeutic drugs are working.

Because seminomas are slow growing, they tend to stay localized and are usually diagnosed at stage 1 (confined to testicles) or stage 2 (spread to lymph nodes). Treatment might be a combination of testicle removal, radiation, or chemotherapy. Most nonseminomas are not diagnosed at stage 1. Advanced (stage 3, metastasized to other tissues) testicular seminomas, as well as stage 2 and stage 3 nonseminomas, are usually treated with multidrug chemotherapy. The majority of cases are stage 1 when first identified; stage 3 cases are relatively rare.

Chemotherapy is the standard treatment, with or without radiation, when the cancer has spread to other parts of the body. The drugs approved to treat testicular cancer include ifosfamide, etoposide, vinblastine, bleomycin, and cisplatin (Chapter 36). Cisplatin is usually given in combination with bleomycin and etoposide or other chemotherapy drugs following surgery or radiation therapy. Testicular cancer has one of the highest cure rates of all cancers, essentially 100% at stage 1. Approximately 90% of men with advanced testicular cancer can be cured, according to the NCI. Because testicular cancer is curable when detected early, the NCI recommends regular monthly testicular self-examination after a hot shower, when the scrotum is looser, feeling for lumps or enlargement.

Acknowledgments

The authors wish to acknowledge the work of Jennifer L. Whetstone, PhD; Duane D. Miller, PhD; and Robert W. Brueggemeier, PhD, who authored content used within this chapter in a previous edition of this text.

Structure Challenge

The structures of 15 drugs discussed in this chapter are provided. Use your knowledge of medicinal chemistry to identify the indicated hormone or select the appropriate drug as described in the following.

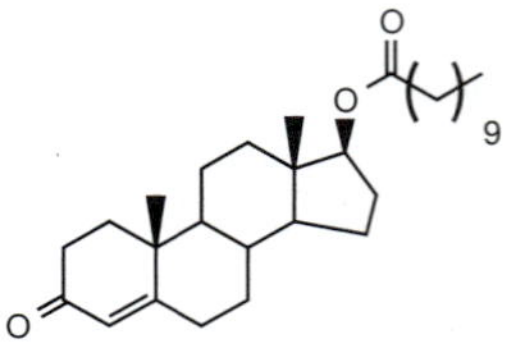

1

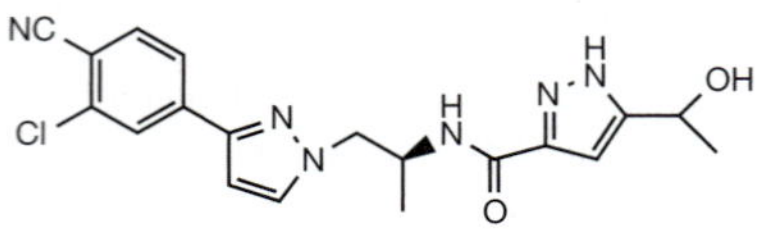

2

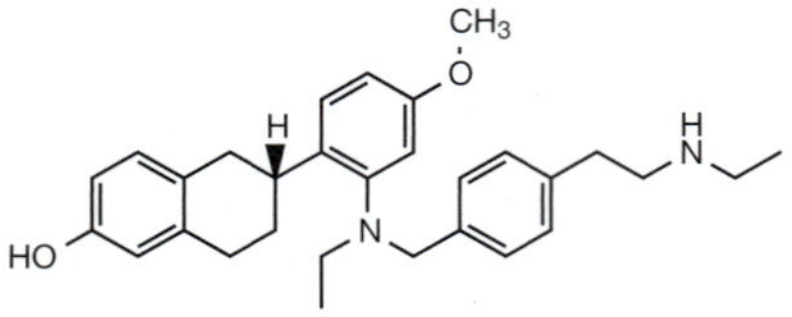

3

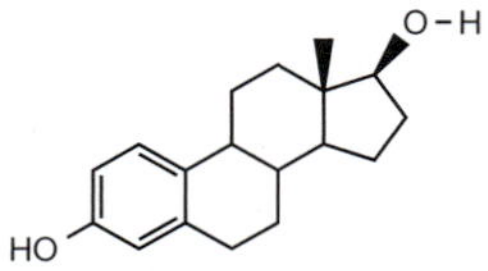

4

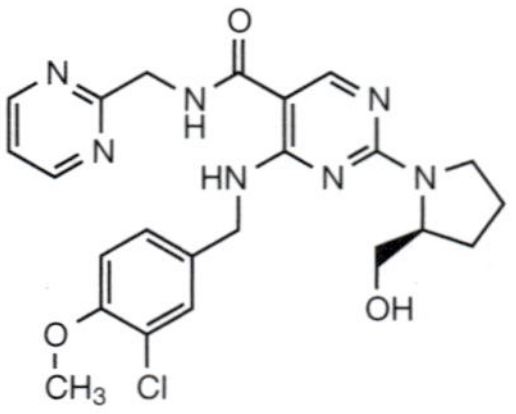

5

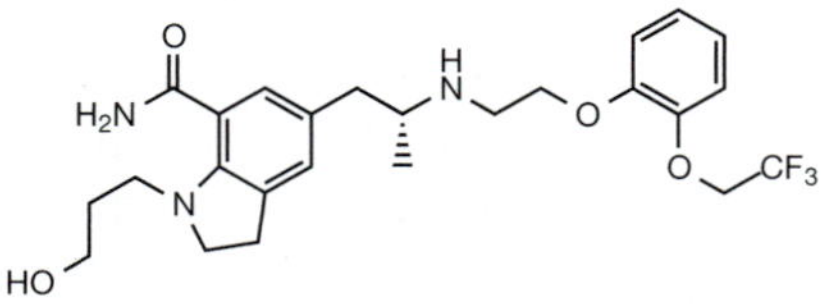

6

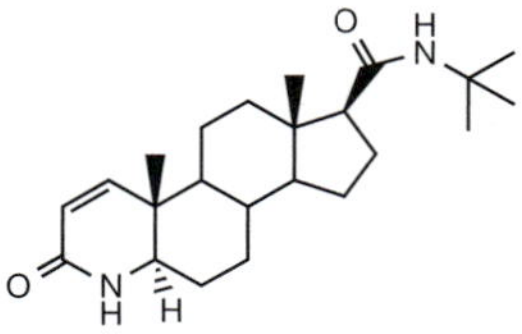

7

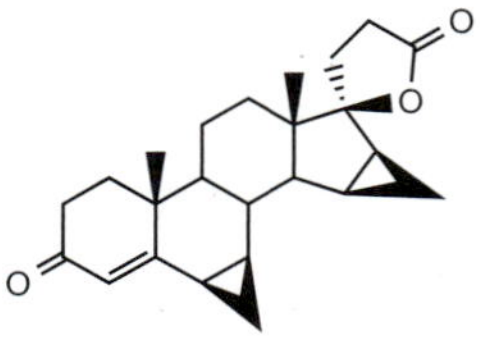

8

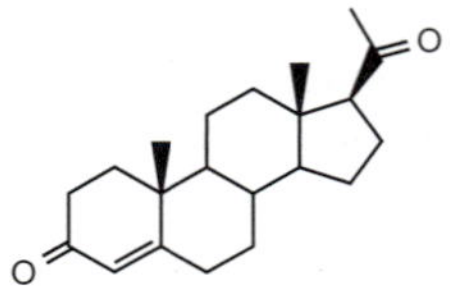

9

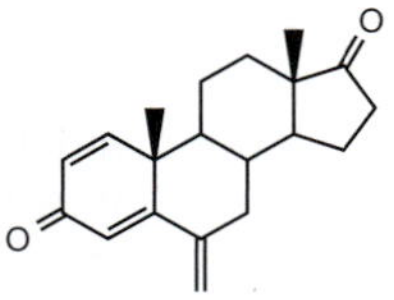

10

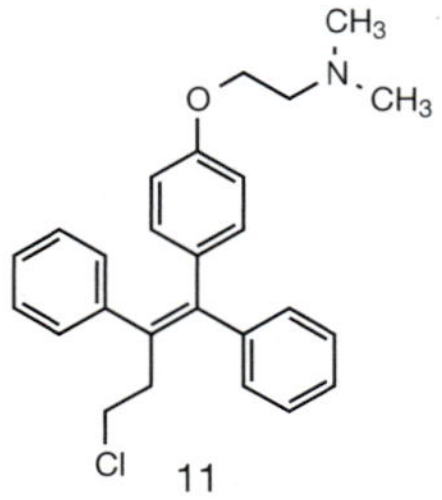

11

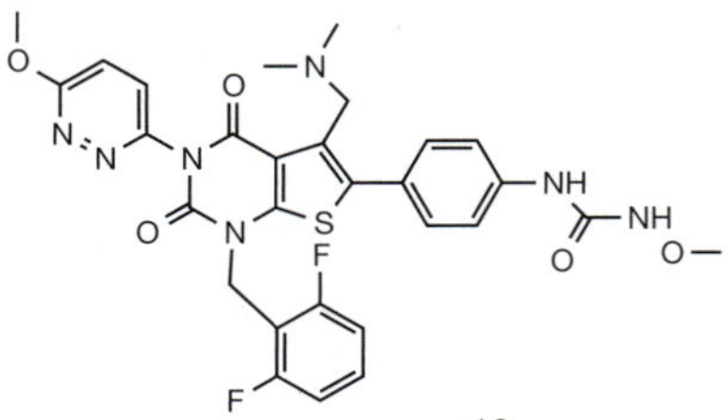

12

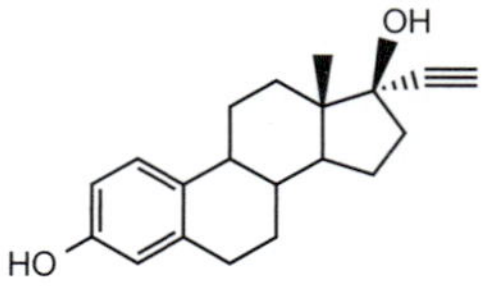

13

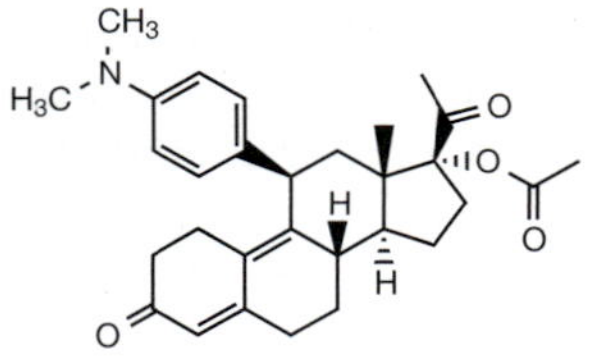

14

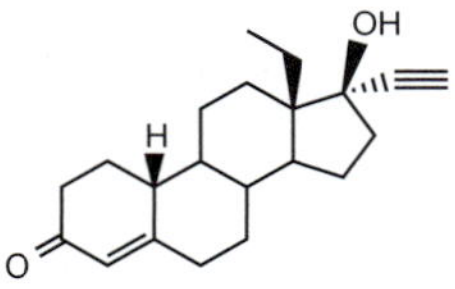

15

A. Novel progestin of value in PMDD due to its antimineralocorticoid action. __
B. Endogenous steroid most critical to the maintenance of pregnancy. ___
C. SERM that might possibly be of particular value in a patient with ER-positive breast cancer who is a poor 2D6 metabolizer. ___
D. 19-Nor contraceptive progestin with structural features designed to lower estrogenic and androgenic adverse effects. ___
E. Most uroselective α-adrenergic antagonist used for BPH. ___
F. Endogenous estrogen given by nonoral routes due to inactivating first-pass metabolism. __
G. Ester of testosterone recently approved for oral TRT. __

Structure Challenge (continued)

H. Phosphodiesterase inhibitor used in ED. __
I. Nonsteroidal AR antagonist used in prostate cancer. __
J. Commonly used and orally active estrogen that, unlike 17β-estradiol, is metabolized primarily by phase 2 conjugation. __
K. Steroidal AI used in the treatment of breast cancer. __
L. α-Reductase inhibitor used for androgenic alopecia. __
M. Steroid receptor antagonist that induces a short-term impairment of fertility if taken within 120 hours of unprotected sex or failure of a contraceptive system, which also temporarily counteracts the protection provided by oral contraceptives. __
N. First oral GnRH antagonist to be used as ADT for prostate cancer. __
O. Oral nonsteroidal SERD used in breast cancer. __

Structure Challenge answers found immediately after References.

REFERENCES

1. Simpson ER, Merrill JC, Hollub AJ, et al. Regulation of estrogen biosynthesis by human adipose cells. *Endocr Rev.* 1989;10:136.
2. Fishman J, Brown JB, Hellman L, et al. Estrogen metabolism in normal and pregnant women. *J Biol Chem.* 1962;237:1489-1494.
3. Gurpide E, Angers M, Vande Wiele RL, et al. Determination of secretory rates of estrogens in pregnant and nonpregnant women from the specific activities of urinary metabolites. *J Clin Endocrinol Metab.* 1962;22:935-945.
4. Nakajin S, Hall PF. Microsomal cytochrome P-450 from neonatal pig testis. Purification and properties of A C21 steroid side-chain cleavage system (17 alpha-hydroxylase-C17,20 lyase). *J Biol Chem.* 1981;256:3871.
5. Liao S, Liang T, Fang S, et al. Steroid structure and androgenic activity: specificities involved in the receptor binding and nuclear retention of various androgens. *J Biol Chem.* 1973;248:6154-6162.
6. Brueggemeier RW. Male sex hormones, analogues, and antagonists. In: Burger A, Abraham DJ, eds. *Burger's Medicinal Chemistry and Drug Discovery.* 6th ed. Wiley; 2003.
7. Dorfman RI, Ungar F. *Metabolism of Steroid Hormones.* Academic Press; 1965.
8. Thigpen AE, Silver RI, Guileyardo JM, et al. Tissue distribution and ontogeny of steroid 5 alpha-reductase isozyme expression. *J Clin Invest.* 1993;92:903-910.
9. Russell DW, Berman DM, Bryant JT, et al. The molecular genetics of steroid 5 alpha-reductases. *Recent Prog Horm Res.* 1994;49:275-284.
10. Johansen KL. Testosterone metabolism and replacement therapy in patients with end-stage renal disease. *Semin Dial.* 2004;17:202-208.
11. Vermeulen A, Kaufman JM, Goemaere S, et al. Estradiol in elderly men. *Aging Male.* 2002;5:98-102.
12. Fotherby K, James F, Atkinson L, et al. Studies in the aromatization of a synthetic progestin. *J Endocrinol.* 1972;52:v-vi.
13. Dorfman RI, Hamilton JB. Urinary excretion of androgenic substances after intramuscular and oral administration of testosterone propionate to humans. *J Clin Invest.* 1939;18:67-71.
14. Taylor W, Scratcherd T. Steroid metabolism in the rabbit. Biliary and urinary excretion of metabolites of [4-14-C]testosterone. *Biochem J.* 1967;104:250-253.
15. Barbier O, Belanger A. The cynomolgus monkey (Macaca fascicularis) is the best animal model for the study of steroid glucuronidation. *J Steroid Biochem Mol Biol.* 2003;85:235-245.
16. Brown JB. The determination and significance of the natural estrogens. *Adv Clin Chem.* 1960;3:157-233.
17. Diczfalusy E, Lauritzen C. *Oestrogene Beim Menschen.* Springer; 1961.
18. Breuer H. Metabolism of the natural estrogens. *Vitam Horm.* 1962;20:285.
19. Merriam GR, Lipsett MB, John E; Fogarty International Center for Advanced Study in the Health Sciences. *Catechol Estrogens.* Raven Press; 1983.
20. Allen E, Doisy EA. Landmark article Sept 8, 1923. An ovarian hormone. Preliminary report on its localization, extraction and partial purification, and action in test animals. By Edgar Allen and Edward A. Doisy. *JAMA.* 1983;250:2681-2683.
21. Williams C, Stancel GM. Estrogens and progestins. In: Goodman LS, Gilman A, Hardman JG, Gilman AG, Limbird LE, eds. *Goodman & Gilman's the Pharmacological Basis of Therapeutics.* 9th ed. McGraw-Hill, Health Professions Division; 1996:1411-1440.
22. Ruentiz PC. Female sex hormones and analogs. In: Burger A, Wolff ME, eds. *Burger's Medicinal Chemistry and Drug Discovery.* Vol 4. 5th ed. Wiley; 1995:553-558.
23. Harris GW, Naftolin F. The hypothalamus and control of ovulation. *Br Med Bull.* 1970;26:3-9.
24. Jaffe RB, et al. Chapter 1. In: Lednicer D, ed. *Contraception: The Chemical Control of Fertility.* M. Dekker; 1969:xiv, 269 p.
25. U.S. Census Bureau. Population Division. 2017 National Population Projections Tables: Main Series (Table 2: Projected 5-Year Age Groups and Sex Composition: Main Projections Series for the United States, 2017-2060). Accessed April 10, 2018. https://census.gov/data/tables/2017/demo/popproj/2017-summary-tables.html
26. MacGregor JI, Jordan VC. Basic guide to the mechanisms of antiestrogen action. *Pharmacol Rev.* 1998;50:151-196.
27. Jensen EV, Jacobson HI. Basic guides to the mechanism of estrogen action. *Recent Prog Horm Res.* 1962;18:387-414.
28. Greene GL, Gilna P, Waterfield M, et al. Sequence and expression of human estrogen receptor complementary DNA. *Science.* 1986;231:1150-1154.

29. Green S, Walter P, Kumar V, et al. Human oestrogen receptor cDNA: sequence, expression and homology to v-erb-A. *Nature.* 1986;320:134-139.
30. Couse JF, Curtis SW, Washburn TF, et al. Analysis of transcription and estrogen insensitivity in the female mouse after targeted disruption of the estrogen receptor gene. *Mol Endocrinol.* 1995;9:1441-1454.
31. Kuiper GG, Enmark E, Pelto-Huikko M, et al. Cloning of a novel receptor expressed in rat prostate and ovary. *Proc Natl Acad Sci U S A.* 1996;93:5925-5930.
32. Lubahn DB, Moyer JS, Golding TS, et al. Alteration of reproductive function but not prenatal sexual development after insertional disruption of the mouse estrogen receptor gene. *Proc Natl Acad Sci U S A.* 1993;90:11162-11166.
33. Couse JF, Korach KS. Estrogen receptor null mice: what have we learned and where will they lead us? *Endocr Rev.* 1999;20:358-417.
34. Curtis Hewitt S, Couse JF, Korach KS. Estrogen receptor transcription and transactivation: estrogen receptor knockout mice: what their phenotypes reveal about mechanisms of estrogen action. *Breast Cancer Res.* 2000;2:345-352.
35. Deroo BJ, Korach KS. Estrogen receptors and human disease. *J Clin Invest.* 2006;116:561-570.
36. Gorski J, Welshons WV, Sakai D, et al. Evolution of a model of estrogen action. *Recent Prog Horm Res.* 1986;42:297.
37. Chan L, O'Malley BW. Mechanism of action of the sex steroid hormones (third of three parts). *N Engl J Med.* 1976;294:1430.
38. Chan L, O'Malley BW. Mechanism of action of the sex steroid hormones (second of three parts). *N Engl J Med.* 1976;294:1372.
39. Chan L, O'Malley BW. Mechanism of action of the sex steroid hormones (first of three parts). *N Engl J Med.* 1976;294:1322.
40. Noteboom WD, Gorski J. Stereospecific binding of estrogens in the rat uterus. *Arch Biochem Biophys.* 1965;111:559.
41. Mohler ML, Narayanan R, Coss CC, et al. Estrogen receptor beta selective nonsteroidal estrogens: seeking clinical indications. *Expert Opin Ther Pat.* 2010;20:507-534.
42. Ing NH, Tornesi MB. Estradiol up-regulates estrogen receptor and progesterone receptor gene expression in specific ovine uterine cells. *Biol Reprod.* 1997;56:1205-1215.
43. Rasmussen KR, Whelly SM, Barker KL. Estradiol regulation of the synthesis of uterine proteins with clusters of proline- and glycine-rich peptide sequences. *Biochim Biophys Acta.* 1988;970:177-186.
44. Revankar CM, Cimino DF, Sklar LA, et al. A transmembrane intracellular estrogen receptor mediates rapid cell signaling. *Science.* 2005;307:1625-1630.
45. Shughrue PJ, Lane MV, Scrimo PJ, et al. Comparative distribution of estrogen receptor-alpha (ER-alpha) and beta (ER-beta) mRNA in the rat pituitary, gonad, and reproductive tract. *Steroids.* 1998;63:498-504.
46. Veeneman GH. Non-steroidal subtype selective estrogens. *Curr Med Chem.* 2005;12:1077-1136.
47. Hechter O, Halkerston IDK. *The Hormones.* Vol 5. Academic Press; 1964.
48. Aitken SC, Lippman ME. Hormonal regulation of de novo pyrimidine synthesis and utilization in human breast cancer cells in tissue culture. *Cancer Res.* 1983;43:4681-4690.
49. Aitken SC, Lippman ME. Effect of estrogens and antiestrogens on growth-regulatory enzymes in human breast cancer cells in tissue culture. *Cancer Res.* 1985;45:1611-1620.
50. Horwitz KB, McGuire WL. Estrogen control of progesterone receptor in human breast cancer: correlation with nuclear processing of estrogen receptor. *J Biol Chem.* 1978;253:2223.
51. Lippman ME. In: Williams RH, Wilson JD, eds. *Williams Textbook of Endocrinology.* 9th ed. Saunders; 1998:1675-1692.
52. Murad F, Kuret JA. Estrogens and progestins. In: Goodman LS, Gilman A, eds. *Goodman and Gilman's the Pharmacological Basis of Therapeutics.* Pergamon Press; 1990:1384-1412.
53. Deghenghi R, Givner ML. Chapter 29. In: Wolff ME, ed. *Burger's Medicinal Chemistry.* Vol 2. 6th ed. Wiley; 1979.
54. Bentley PJ. *Endocrine Pharmacology: Physiological Basis and Therapeutic Applications.* Cambridge University Press; 1980.
55. Gruber CJ, Tschugguel W, Schneeberger C, et al. Production and actions of estrogens. *N Engl J Med.* 2002;346:340-352.
56. Practice Committee of the American Society for Reproductive Medicine. Use of clomiphene citrate in infertile women: a committee opinion. *Fertil Steril.* 2013;100:341-348.
57. Clark JH, Guthrie SC. Agonistic and antagonistic effects of clomiphene citrate and its isomers. *Biol Reprod.* 1981;25:667-672.
58. Kurosawa T, Hiroi H, Momoeda M, et al. Clomiphene citrate elicits estrogen agonistic/antagonistic effects differentially via estrogen receptors alpha and beta. *Endocr J.* 2010;57:517-521.
59. Kim MJ, Byeon JY, Kim YH, et al. Effect of the CYP2D6*10 allele on the pharmacokinetics of clomiphene and its active metabolites. *Arch Pharm Res.* 2018;41:347-353.
60. Murdter TE, Kerb R, Turpeinen M, et al. Genetic polymorphism of cytochrome P450 2D6 determines oestrogen receptor activity of the major infertility drug clomiphene via its active metabolites. *Hum Mol Genet.* 2012;21:1145-1154.
61. Choi SH, Shapiro H, Robinson GE, et al. Psychological side-effects of clomiphene citrate and human menopausal gonadotrophin. *J Psychosom Obstet Gynaecol.* 2005;26:93-100.
62. Clomid (Clomiphene) [prescribing information]. Sanofi-Aventis US LLC; 2017.
63. Anstead GM, Carlson KE, Katzenellenbogen JA. The estradiol pharmacophore: ligand structure-estrogen receptor binding affinity relationships and a model for the receptor binding site. *Steroids.* 1997;62:268-303.
64. Brzozowski AM, Pike AC, Dauter Z, et al. Molecular basis of agonism and antagonism in the oestrogen receptor. *Nature.* 1997;389:753-758.
65. Shiau AK, Barstad D, Loria PM, et al. The structural basis of estrogen receptor/coactivator recognition and the antagonism of this interaction by tamoxifen. *Cell.* 1998;95:927-937.
66. Baran JS. A synthesis of 11-beta-hydroxyestrone and related 16- and 17-hydroxyestratrienes. *J Med Chem.* 1967;10:1188-1190.
67. Murkies AL, Wilcox G, Davis SR. Clinical review 92: phytoestrogens. *J Clin Endocrinol Metab.* 1998;83:297-303.
68. Heftmann E. *Steroid Biochemistry.* Academic Press; 1970.
69. Baker JM, Al-Nakkash L, Herbst-Kralovetz MM. Estrogen-gut microbiome axis: physiological and clinical implications. *Maturitas.* 2017;103:45-53.
70. Fieser LF, Feiser M. *Steroids.* Reinhold Publishing Corporation; 1959.
71. Kupperman HS, Blatt MH, Wiesbader H, et al. Comparative clinical evaluation of estrogenic preparations by the menopausal and amenorrheal indices. *J Clin Endocrinol Metab.* 1953;13:688-703.
72. Grant GA, Beall D. Studies on estrogen conjugates. *Recent Prog Horm Res.* 1950;5:307.7.
73. Chetkowski RJ, Meldrum DR, Steingold KA, et al. Biologic effects of transdermal estradiol. *N Engl J Med.* 1986;314:1615.
74. Judd H. Efficacy of transdermal estradiol. *Am J Obstet Gynecol.* 1987;156:1326.
75. Inhoffen HH, Hohlweg W. New per os-effective female hipofisis gland hormone derivatives: 17-aethinyl-oesteridol and pregnen-in-on-3-ol-17. *Naturwissenschaften.* 1938;26:96-96.
76. Colton FB, Nysted LN, Riegel B, et al. 17-Alkyl-19-Nortestosterones. *J Am Chem Soc.* 1957;79:1123-1127.
77. Helton ED, Goldzieher JW. The pharmacokinetics of ethynyl estrogens: a review. *Contraception.* 1977;15:255-284.
78. Coelingh-Bennink HJ, Holinka CF, Diczfalusy E. Estetrol review: profile and potential clinical applications. *Climacteric.* 2008;11 (suppl 1):47-58.
79. Menest (Estrogens, Esterified) [prescribing information]. Monarch Pharmaceuticals; 2011.
80. Helgason S, Damber MG, von Schoultz B, et al. Estrogenic potency of oral replacement therapy estimated by the induction of pregnancy zone protein. *Acta Obstet Gynecol Scand.* 1982;61:75-79.
81. Solmssen UV. Synthetic estrogens and the relation between their structure and their activity. *Chem Rev.* 1945;37:481-598.
82. Rubin M, Wishinsky H. Functional variants of diethylstilbestrol. *J Am Chem Soc.* 1944;66:1948-1950.

83. Dodds EC, Golberg L, Lawson W, et al. Estrogenic activity of alkylated stiloestrols. *Nature*. 1938;142:34.
84. Exposure in utero to diethylstilbestrol and related synthetic hormones. Association with vaginal and cervical cancers and other abnormalities. *JAMA*. 1976;236:1107-1109.
85. Giusti RM, Iwamoto K, Hatch EE. Diethylstilbestrol revisited: a review of the long-term health effects. *Ann Intern Med*. 1995;122:778-788.
86. Hoover RN, Hyer M, Pfeiffer RM, et al. Adverse health outcomes in women exposed in utero to diethylstilbestrol. *N Engl J Med*. 2011;365:1304-1314.
87. Palmer JR, Wise LA, Hatch EE, et al. Prenatal diethylstilbestrol exposure and risk of breast cancer. *Cancer Epidemiol Biomarkers Prev*. 2006;15:1509-1514.
88. Fraenkel S. Die Function des Corpus luteum. *Arch f Gynaek*. 1903;68:438-545.8.
89. Pearl R, Surface FM. Effect of corpus luteum substance upon ovulation in the fowl. *J Biol Chem*. 1914;19:263.
90. Corner GW, Allen WM. Physiology of the corpus luteum II. Production of a special uterine reaction (progestational proliferation) by extracts of the corpus luteum. *Am J Physiol*. 1929;88:326-339.
91. Makepeace AW, Weinstein GL, Friedman MH. The effect of progestin and progesterone on ovulation in the rabbit. *Am J Physiol*. 1937;119:512-516.
92. Heftmann E, Mosettig E. *Biochemistry of Steroids*. Reinhold Publishing Corporation; 1960.
93. Djerassi C. Steroid oral contraceptives. *Science*. 1966;151:1055.
94. Greenblatt RB, Gambrell RD Jr, Stoddard LD. The protective role of progesterone in the prevention of endometrial cancer. *Pathol Res Pract*. 1982;174:297-318.
95. Davis ME, Wied GL. 17-Alpha-hydroxyprogesterone-caproate: a new substance with prolonged progestational activity: a comparison with chemically pure progesterone. *J Clin Endocrinol Metab*. 1955;15:923-930.
96. Siegel I. Conception control by long-acting progestogens: preliminary report. *Obstet Gynecol*. 1963;21:666-668.
97. Klopper A. Developments in steroidal hormonal contraception. *Br Med Bull*. 1970;26:39-44.
98. Babcock JC, Gutsell ES, Herr ME, et al. 6-Alpha-methyl-17-alpha-hydroxyprogesterone 17-acylates—a new class of potent progestins. *J Am Chem Soc*. 1958;80:2904-2905.
99. Dong Y, Roberge JY, Wang Z, et al. Characterization of a new class of selective nonsteroidal progesterone receptor agonists. *Steroids*. 2004;69:201-217.
100. Ruzicka L, Hofmann K. Se hormones XXIV. On the disposition of acetylene in the 17-constant keto group of trans-androsterone and delta(5)-trans-dehydro-androsterone. *Helv Chim Acta*. 1937;20:1280-1282.
101. Klimstra PD. Progestational agents. *Am J Pharm Educ*. 1970;34:630.
102. Ehrenstein M. Investigations on steroids VIII lower homologs of hormones of the pregnane series 10-nor-11-desoxycorticosterone acetate and 10-norprogesterone. *J Org Chem*. 1944;9:435-456.
103. Djerassi C, Miramontes L, Rosenkranz G. Steroids. XLVIII.1 19-Norprogesterone, a potent progestational hormone. *J Am Chem Soc*. 1953;75:4440-4442.
104. Pincus G, Garcia CR, Paniagua M, Shepard J. Ethynodiol diacetate as a new, highly potent oral inhibitor of ovulation. *Science*. 1962;138:439-440.
105. Africander DJ, Storbeck KH, Hapgood JP. A comparative study of the androgenic properties of progesterone and the progestins, medroxyprogesterone acetate (MPA) and norethisterone acetate (NET-A). *J Steroid Biochem Mol Biol*. 2014;143:404-415.
106. Agarwal MK, Hainque B, Moustaid N, et al. Glucocorticoid antagonists. *FEBS Lett*. 1987;217:221.
107. Melis GB, Piras B, Marotto MF, et al. Pharmacokinetic evaluation of ulipristal acetate for uterine leiomyoma treatment. *Expert Opin Drug Metab Toxicol*. 2012;8:901-908.
108. Mifeprex (Mifepristone) [prescribing information]. Danco Laboratories; 2016.
109. Cytotec (Misoprostol) [prescribing information]. Pfizer; 2017.
110. Plan B (Levonorgestrel) [prescribing information]. Teva Pharmaceuticals USA Inc; 2017.
111. O'Malley BW, McGuire WL, Kohler PO, et al. Studies on the mechanism of steroid hormone regulation of synthesis of specific proteins. *Recent Prog Horm Res*. 1969;25:105.
112. Carson-Jurica MA, Schrader WT, O'Malley BW. Steroid receptor family: structure and functions. *Endocr Rev*. 1990;11:201.
113. Gronemeyer H, Turcotte B, Quirin-Stricker C, et al. The chicken progesterone receptor: sequence, expression and functional analysis. *EMBO J*. 1987;6:3985.
114. Misrahi M, Atger M, d'Auriol L, et al. Complete amino acid sequence of the human progesterone receptor deduced from cloned cDNA. *Biochem Biophys Res Commun*. 1987;143:740.
115. Carson-Jurica MA, Lee AT, Dobson AW, et al. Interaction of the chicken progesterone receptor with heat shock protein (HSP) 90. *J Steroid Biochem*. 1989;34:1.
116. Fotherby K. The biochemistry of progesterone. *Vitam Horm*. 1964;22:153-204.
117. Baulieu EE. *Steroid Hormone Regulation of the Brain: Proceedings of an International Symposium Held at the Wenner-Gren Center, Stockholm 27-28 October*. Pergamon Press; 1981.
118. Majewska MD, Harrison NL, Schwartz RD, et al. Steroid hormone metabolites are barbiturate-like modulators of the GABA receptor. *Science*. 1986;232:1004.
119. Morrow AL, Suzdak PD, Paul SM. Steroid hormone metabolites potentiate GABA receptor-mediated chloride ion flux with nanomolar potency. *Eur J Pharmacol*. 1987;142:483.
120. Baulieu EE, Robel P. Neurosteroids: a new brain function? *J Steroid Biochem Mol Biol*. 1990;37:395.
121. Rothchild I. The physiologic basis for the temperature raising effect of progesterone. In: Salhanick HA, Kipnis DM, Vande Wiele RL, eds. *Metabolic Effects of Gonadal Hormones and Contraceptive Steroids*. Plenum Press; 1969:668.
122. Drill VA. *Oral Contraceptives*. McGraw-Hill; 1966.
123. Lewis JJ, Crossland J. *Lewis's Pharmacology*. 4th ed. Williams and Wilkins; 1970.
124. Vyleesi (bremelanotide) [prescribing information]. AMAG Pharmaceuticals, Inc.; 2019.
125. Dacarett-Galeano DJ, Diao, X. Brexanolone: a novel therapeutic in the treatment of postpartum depression. *Am J Psychiatry Resid J*. 2019;15:2-4.
126. Meltzer-Brody S, Colquhoun H, Riesenberg R, et al. Brexanolone injection in post-partum depression: two multicentre, double-blind, randomized, placebo-controlled, phase 3 trials. *Lancet*. 2018;392:1058-1070.
127. Struthers RS, Nicholls AJ, Grundy J, et al. Suppression of gonadotropins and estradiol in premenopausal women by oral administration of the nonpeptide gonadotropin-releasing hormone antagonist elagolix. *J Clin Endocrinol Metab*. 2009;94:545-551.
128. Shebley M, Polepally AR, Nader A, et al. Clinical pharmacology of elagolix: an oral gonadotropin-releasing hormone receptor antagonist for endometriosis. *Clinical Pharmacokinetics*. 2020;59:297-309.
129. Pincus G. Control of conception by hormonal steroids. *Science*. 1966;153:493.
130. Pincus G, Garcia CR, Rock J, et al. Effectiveness of an oral contraceptive; effects of a progestin-estrogen combination upon fertility, menstrual phenomena, and health. *Science*. 1959;130:81-83.
131. Schindler AE. Non-contraceptive benefits of oral hormonal contraceptives. *Int J Endocrinol Metab*. 2013;11:41-47.
132. van den Heuvel MW, van Bragt AJ, Alnabawy AK, et al. Comparison of ethinylestradiol pharmacokinetics in three hormonal contraceptive formulations: the vaginal ring, the transdermal patch and an oral contraceptive. *Contraception*. 2005;72:168-174.
133. Nonhormonal management of menopause-associated vasomotor symptoms 2015 position statement of The North American Menopause Society. *Menopause*. 2015;22:1155-1172; quiz 1173-1154.

134. Manson JE, Kaunitz AM. Menopause management–getting clinical care back on track. *N Engl J Med.* 2016;374:803-806.
135. Manson JE, Ames JM, Shapiro M, et al. Algorithm and mobile app for menopausal symptom management and hormonal/non-hormonal therapy decision making: a clinical decision-support tool from The North American Menopause Society. *Menopause.* 2015;22:247-253.
136. The Nams Hormone Therapy Position Statement Advisory Panel. The 2017 hormone therapy position statement of The North American Menopause Society. *Menopause.* 2017;24:728-753.
137. Pfizer Inc. 2017 Pfizer Financial Report to Shareholders. Accessed April 11, 2018. https://investors.pfizer.com/financials/annual-reports/default.aspx
138. *Menopause Practice, a Clinician's Guide.* 5th ed. North American Menopause Society; 2014.
139. Tremollieres F, Brincat M, Erel CT, et al. EMAS position statement: managing menopausal women with a personal or family history of VTE. *Maturitas.* 2011;69:195-198.
140. Stuenkel CA, Davis SR, Gompel A, et al. Treatment of symptoms of the menopause: an Endocrine Society Clinical Practice Guideline. *J Clin Endocrinol Metab.* 2015;100:3975-4011.
141. Pickar JH, Yeh IT, Bachmann G, et al. Endometrial effects of a tissue selective estrogen complex containing bazedoxifene/conjugated estrogens as a menopausal therapy. *Fertil Steril.* 2009;92:1018-1024.
142. Duavee (Conjugated Estrogens and Bazedoxifene Acetate) [prescribing information]. Pfizer Inc; 2017.
143. Pickar JH, Komm BS. Selective estrogen receptor modulators and the combination therapy conjugated estrogens/bazedoxifene: a review of effects on the breast. *Post Reprod Health.* 2015;21:112-121.
144. Shen L, Ahmad S, Park S, et al. In vitro metabolism, permeability, and efflux of bazedoxifene in humans. *Drug Metab Dispos.* 2010;38:1471-1479.
145. Pinkerton JV, Utian WH, Constantine GD, et al. Relief of vasomotor symptoms with the tissue-selective estrogen complex containing bazedoxifene/conjugated estrogens: a randomized, controlled trial. *Menopause.* 2009;16:1116-1124.
146. Stuenkel CA, Santen RJ. An introduction to the Endocrine Society Clinical Practice Guideline on treatment of symptoms of the menopause. *Post Reprod Health.* 2016;22:6-8.
147. Bachmann GA, Komi JO, Ospemifene Study G. Ospemifene effectively treats vulvovaginal atrophy in postmenopausal women: results from a pivotal phase 3 study. *Menopause.* 2010;17:480-486.
148. Neal-Perry G, Cano A, Lederman S, et al. Safety of fezolinetant for vasomotor symptoms associated with menopause: a randomized controlled trial. *Obstet Gynecol.* 2023;141:737-747.
149. Johnson KA, Martin N, Nappi RE, et al. Efficacy and safety of fezolinetant in moderate to severe vasomotor symptoms associated with menopause: a phase 3 RCT. *J Clin Endocrinol Metab.* 2023;108:1981-1997.
150. Brown-Sequard CE. Des effects produits chez Phomme par des injections sous cutanées d'un liquide retire des testicules frais de cobaye et de chien. *CR Seanc Soc Biol.* 1889;1:420-430.
151. Pezard A. Sur la determination des caractéres sexuels secondaire chez les gallinacés. *C R H Acad Sci.* 1911;153:1027-1043.
152. Butenandt A. Chemical investigation of the sex hormones. *Angew Chem.* 1931;44:905-908.
153. Butenandt AH, Dannenberg H. Androsterone, a crystalline male sex hormone. III. Isolation of a new physiologically inert sterol derivative from male urine, its relationship to dehydroandrosterone and androsterone. *Z Physiol Chem.* 1934;229:192-208.
154. David K, Dingemanse E, Freud J, et al. Crystalline male hormone from testes (testosterone), more active than androsterone prepared from urine or cholesterol. *Z Physiol Chem.* 1935:281-282.
155. Butenandt A, Hanisch G. Testosterone. Transformation of dehydroandrosterone into androstenediol and testosterone; a way to the preparation of testosterone from cholesterol. *Chem Ber.* 1935;68B:1859-1862.
156. Kochakian CD, Murlin JR. Effect of male hormone on the protein and energy metabolism of castrate dogs. *J Nutr Biochem.* 1935;10:437-459.
157. Vale W, Wiater E, Gray P, et al. Activins and inhibins and their signaling. *Ann NY Acad Sci.* 2004;1038:142-147.
158. Bremner WJ, Vitiello MV, Prinz PN. Loss of circadian rhythmicity in blood testosterone levels with aging in normal men. *J Clin Endocrinol Metab.* 1983;56:1278-1281.
159. van den Beld AW, de Jong FH, Grobbee DE, et al. Measures of bioavailable serum testosterone and estradiol and their relationships with muscle strength, bone density, and body composition in elderly men. *J Clin Endocrinol Metab.* 2000;85:3276-3282.
160. Bhasin S, Travison TG, Storer TW, et al. Effect of testosterone supplementation with and without a dual 5α-reductase inhibitor on fat-free mass in men with suppressed testosterone production: a randomized controlled trial. *JAMA.* 2012;307(9):931-939.
161. Ferrando AA, Sheffield-Moore M, Yeckel CW, et al. Testosterone administration to older men improves muscle function: molecular and physiological mechanisms. *Am J Physiol Endocrinol Metab.* 2002;282:E601-E607.
162. Bhasin S. Testosterone supplementation for aging-associated sarcopenia. *J Gerontol A Biol Sci Med Sci.* 2003;58:1002-1008.
163. Manolagas SC, Kousteni S, Jilka RL. Sex steroids and bone. *Recent Prog Horm Res.* 2002;57:385-409.
164. Wiren KM. Androgens and bone growth: it's location, location, location. *Curr Opin Pharmacol.* 2005;5:626-632.
165. Gao W, Bohl CE, Dalton JT. Chemistry and structural biology of androgen receptor. *Chem Rev.* 2005;105:3352-3370.
166. Lutz LB, Jamnongjit M, Yang WH, et al. Selective modulation of genomic and nongenomic androgen responses by androgen receptor ligands. *Mol Endocrinol.* 2003;17:1106-1116.
167. Estrada M, Espinosa A, Muller M, et al. Testosterone stimulates intracellular calcium release and mitogen-activated protein kinases via a G protein-coupled receptor in skeletal muscle cells. *Endocrinology.* 2003;144:3586-3597.
168. Kousteni S, Bellido T, Plotkin LI, et al. Nongenotropic, sex-nonspecific signaling through the estrogen or androgen receptors: dissociation from transcriptional activity. *Cell.* 2001;104:719-730.
169. Zagar Y, Chaumaz G, Lieberherr M. Signaling cross-talk from G beta(4) subunit to Elk-1 in the rapid action of androgens. *J Biol Chem.* 2004;279:2403-2413.
170. Kampa M, Papakonstanti EA, Hatzoglou A, et al. The human prostate cancer cell line LNCaP bears functional membrane testosterone receptors that increase PSA secretion and modify actin cytoskeleton. *FASEB J.* 2002;16:1429-1431.
171. Unni E, Sun S, Nan B, et al. Changes in androgen receptor nongenotropic signaling correlate with transition of LNCaP cells to androgen independence. *Cancer Res.* 2004;64:7156-7168.
172. Norman AW, Mizwicki MT, Norman DP. Steroid-hormone rapid actions, membrane receptors and a conformational ensemble model. *Nat Rev Drug Discov.* 2004;3:27-41.
173. Simoncini T, Genazzani AR. Non-genomic actions of sex steroid hormones. *Eur J Endocrinol.* 2003;148:281-292.
174. Kousteni S, Chen JR, Bellido T, et al. Reversal of bone loss in mice by nongenotropic signaling of sex steroids. *Science.* 2002;298:843-846.
175. Maughan BL, Antonarakis ES. Clinical relevance of androgen receptor splice variants in castration-resistant prostate cancer. *Curr Treat Options Oncol.* 2015;16:57.
176. Antonarakis ES, Lu C, Luber B, et al. Androgen receptor splice variant 7 and efficacy of taxane chemotherapy in patients with metastatic castration-resistant prostate cancer. *JAMA Oncol.* 2015;1:582-591.
177. Zhang G, Liu X, Li J, et al. Androgen receptor splice variants circumvent AR blockade by microtubule-targeting agents. *Oncotarget.* 2015;6:23358-23371.
178. Bancroft J, Wu FC. Changes in erectile responsiveness during androgen replacement therapy. *Arch Sex Behav.* 1983;12:59-66.

179. Arver S, Dobs AS, Meikle AW, et al. Improvement of sexual function in testosterone deficient men treated for 1 year with a permeation enhanced testosterone transdermal system. *J Urol.* 1996;155:1604-1608.
180. Oettel M. Testosterone metabolism, dose-response relationships and receptor polymorphisms: selected pharmacological/toxicological considerations on benefits versus risks of testosterone therapy in men. *Aging Male.* 2003;6:230-256.
181. Rhoden EL, Morgentaler A. Risks of testosterone-replacement therapy and recommendations for monitoring. *N Engl J Med.* 2004;350:482-492.
182. Hijazi RA, Cunningham GR. Andropause: is androgen replacement therapy indicated for the aging male? *Annu Rev Med.* 2005;56:117-137.
183. Bhasin S, Cunningham GR, Hayes FJ, et al. Testosterone therapy in men with androgen deficiency syndromes: an Endocrine Society clinical practice guideline. *J Clin Endocrinol Metab.* 2010;95:2536-2559.
184. Basaria S, Coviello AD, Travison TG, et al. Adverse events associated with testosterone administration. *N Engl J Med.* 2010;363:109-122.
185. Axiron (topical testosterone) [prescribing information]. Eli Lilly and Company; 2017.
186. Gronski MA, Grober ED, Gottesman IS, et al. Efficacy of nasal testosterone gel (Natesto®) stratified by baseline endogenous testosterone levels. *J Endocrin Soc.* 2019;3:1652-1662.
187. Shackleford DM, Faassen WA, Houwing N, et al. Contribution of lymphatically transported testosterone undecanoate to the systemic exposure of testosterone after oral administration of two Andriol formulations in conscious lymph duct-cannulated dogs. *J Pharmacol Exp Ther.* 2003;306:925-933.
188. Bhat SZ, Dobs AS. Testosterone replacement therapy: a narrative review with a focus on new oral formulations. *touchREV Endocrinol.* 2022;18:133-140.
189. Vida JA. *Androgens and Anabolic Agents: Chemistry and Pharmacology.* Academic Press; 1969.
190. Segaloff A, Gabbard RB. 5 Alpha-androstane–an androgenic hydrocarbon. *Endocrinology.* 1960;67:887-889.
191. Arnold A, Potts GO, Beyler AL. The ratio of anabolic to androgenic activity of 7:17-dimethyltestosterone, oxymesterone, mestanolone and fluoxymesterone. *J Endocrinol.* 1963;28:87-92.
192. Cocconi G. First generation aromatase inhibitors–aminoglutethimide and testolactone. *Breast Cancer Res Treat.* 1994;30:57-80.
193. Kicman AT. Pharmacology of anabolic steroids. *Br J Pharmacol.* 2008;154:502-521.
194. Catlin DH, Sekera MH, Ahrens BD, et al. Tetrahydrogestrinone: discovery, synthesis, and detection in urine. *Rapid Commun Mass Spectrom.* 2004;18:1245-1049.
195. Jasuja R, Catlin DH, Miller A, et al. Tetrahydrogestrinone is an androgenic steroid that stimulates androgen receptor-mediated, myogenic differentiation in C3H10T1/2 multipotent mesenchymal cells and promotes muscle accretion in orchidectomized male rats. *Endocrinology.* 2005;146:4472-4478.
196. Sobolevsky T, Rodchenkov G. Detection and mass spectrometric characterization of novel long-term dehydrochloromethyltestosterone metabolites in human urine. *J Steroid Biochem Mol Biol.* 2012;128(3-5):121-127.
197. Negro-Vilar A. Selective androgen receptor modulators (SARMs): a novel approach to androgen therapy for the new millennium. *J Clin Endocr Metab.* 1999;84:3459-3462.
198. Dalton JT, Mukherjee A, Zhu ZX, et al. Discovery of nonsteroidal androgens. *Biochem Biophys Res Commun.* 1998;244:1-4.
199. Balog A, Salvati ME, Shan WF, et al. The synthesis and evaluation of [2.2.1]-bicycloazahydantoins as androgen receptor antagonists. *Bioorg Med Chem Lett.* 2004;14:6107-6111.
200. Higuchi RI, Edwards JP, Caferro TR, et al. 4-Alkyl- and 3,4-dialkyl-1,2,3,4-tetrahydro-8-pyridono[5,6-g]quinolines: potent, nonsteroidal androgen receptor agonists. *Bioorg Med Chem Lett.* 1999;9:1335-1340.
201. Zhi L, Tegley CM, Marschke KB, et al. Switching androgen receptor antagonists to agonists by modifying C-ring substituents on piperidino[3,2-g]quinolinone. *Bioorg Med Chem Lett.* 1999;9:1009-1012.
202. Tucker H, Crook JW, Chesterson GJ. Nonsteroidal antiandrogens. Synthesis and structure-activity relationships of 3-substituted derivatives of 2-hydroxypropionanilides. *J Med Chem.* 1988;31:954-959.
203. Yin D, He Y, Perera MA, et al. Key structural features of nonsteroidal ligands for binding and activation of the androgen receptor. *Mol Pharmacol.* 2003;63:211-223.
204. He Y, Yin D, Perera M, et al. Novel nonsteroidal ligands with high binding affinity and potent functional activity for the androgen receptor. *Eur J Med Chem.* 2002;37:619-634.
205. Mohler ML, Bohl CE, Jones A, et al. Nonsteroidal selective androgen receptor modulators (SARMs): dissociating the anabolic and androgenic activities of the androgen receptor for therapeutic benefit. *J Med Chem.* 2009;52:3597-3617.
206. Albersen M, Orabi H, Lue TF. Evaluation and treatment of erectile dysfunction in the aging male: a mini review. *Gerontology.* 2012;58(1):3-14.
207. Feldman HA, Goldstein I, Hatzichristou DG, et al. Impotence and its medical and psychosocial correlates: results of the Massachusetts male aging study. *J Urol.* 1994;151:54-61.
208. Boolell M, Allen MJ, Ballard SA, et al. Sildenafil: an orally active type 5 cyclic GMP-specific phosphodiesterase inhibitor for the treatment of penile erectile dysfunction. *Int J Impot Res.* 1996;8:47-52.
209. Gupta M, Kovar A, Meibohm B. The clinical pharmacokinetics of phosphodiesterase-5 inhibitors for erectile dysfunction. *J Clin Pharmacol.* 2005;45:987-1003.
210. Porst H, Rosen R, Padma-Nathan H, et al. The efficacy and tolerability of vardenafil, a new, oral, selective phosphodiesterase type 5 inhibitor, in patients with erectile dysfunction: the first at-home clinical trial. *Int J Impot Res.* 2001;13:192-199.
211. Saenz de Tejada I, Angulo J, Cuevas P, et al. The phosphodiesterase inhibitory selectivity and the in vitro and in vivo potency of the new PDE5 inhibitor vardenafil. *Int J Impot Res.* 2001;13:282-290.
212. Corbin JD, Beasley A, Blount MA, et al. Vardenafil: structural basis for higher potency over sildenafil in inhibiting cGMP-specific phosphodiesterase-5 (PDE5). *Neurochem Int.* 2004;45:859-863.
213. Kotera J, Mochida H, Inoue H, et al. Avanafil, a potent and highly selective phosphodiesterase-5 inhibitor for erectile dysfunction. *J Urol.* 2012;188:668-674.
214. Kuan J, Brock G. Selective phosphodiesterase type 5 inhibition using tadalafil for the treatment of erectile dysfunction. *Expert Opin Inv Drug.* 2002;11:1605-1613.
215. Sakamoto T, Koga Y, Hikota M, et al. The discovery of avanafil for the treatment of erectile dysfunction: a novel pyrimidine-5-carboxamide derivative as a potent and highly selective phosphodiesterase 5 inhibitor. *Bioorg Med Chem Lett.* 2014;24:5460-5465.
216. Goldstein I, McCullough AR, Jones LA, et al. A randomized, double-blind, placebo-controlled evaluation of the safety and efficacy of avanafil in subjects with erectile dysfunction. *J Sex Med.* 2012;9:1122-1133.
217. Stendra (Avanafil) [package insert]. Mist Pharmaceuticals, LLC; 2017.
218. Kyle JA, Brown DA, Hill JK. Avanafil for erectile dysfunction. *Ann Pharmacother.* 2013;47:1312-1320.
219. Huang YY, Li Z, Cai YH, et al. The molecular basis for the selectivity of tadalafil toward phosphodiesterase 5 and 6: a modeling study. *J Chem Inf Model.* 2013;53:3044-3053.
220. Setter SM, Iltz JL, Fincham JE, et al. Phosphodiesterase 5 inhibitors for erectile dysfunction. *Ann Pharmacother.* 2005;39:1286-1295.
221. Pissarnitski D. Phosphodiesterase 5 (PDE 5) inhibitors for the treatment of male erectile disorder: attaining selectivity versus PDE6. *Med Res Rev.* 2006;26:369-395.

222. Corona G, Rastrelli G, Burri A, et al. The safety and efficacy of Avanafil, a new 2(nd) generation PDE5i: comprehensive review and meta-analysis. *Expert Opin Drug Saf.* 2016;15:237-247.
223. Kloner RA. Cardiovascular effects of the 3 phosphodiesterase-5 inhibitors approved for the treatment of erectile dysfunction. *Circulation.* 2004;110:3149-3155.
224. Beckman TJ, Abu-Lebdeh HS, Mynderse LA. Evaluation and medical management of erectile dysfunction. *Mayo Clin Proc.* 2006;81:385-390.
225. Mcdonaldgibson WJ, McDonald R, Greaves MW. Prostaglandin-E1 metabolism by human plasma. *Prostaglandins.* 1972;2:251.
226. Kamel HK. Male osteoporosis—new trends in diagnosis and therapy. *Drug Aging.* 2005;22:741-748.
227. Bushman W. Etiology, epidemiology, and natural history of benign prostatic hyperplasia. *Urol Clin North Am.* 2009;36:403-415,
228. Barry MJ, Fowler FJ Jr, O'Leary MP, et al. The American Urological Association symptom index for benign prostatic hyperplasia. *J Urol.* 2017;197:S189-S197.
229. American Urological Association. Management of lower urinary tract symptoms attributed to benign prostatic hyperplasia: AUA guidelines. Accessed March 17, 2025. http://www.auanet.org/guidelines-and-quality/guidelines/benign-prostatic'hyperplasia-(bph)-guideline
230. Tan SY, Antonipillai I, Murphy BE. Inhibition of testosterone metabolism in the human prostate. *J Clin Endocrinol Metab.* 1974;39:936-941.
231. Andriole G, Bruchovsky N, Chung LWK, et al. Dihydrotestosterone and the prostate: the scientific rationale for 5 alpha-reductase inhibitors in the treatment of benign prostatic hyperplasia. *J Urol.* 2004;172:1399-14232.
232. Lee M, Sharifi R. Benign prostatic hyperplasia: diagnosis and treatment guideline. *Ann Pharmacother.* 1997;31:481-486.
233. Tarter TH, Vaughan ED. Inhibitors of 5 alpha-reductase in the treatment of benign prostatic hyperplasia. *Curr Pharm Design.* 2006;12:775-783.
234. Shibata Y, Ito K, Suzuki K, et al. Changes in the endocrine environment of the human prostate transition zone with aging: simultaneous quantitative analysis of prostatic sex steroids and comparison with human prostatic histological composition. *Prostate.* 2000;42:45-55.
235. Liang T, Cascieri MA, Cheung AH, et al. Species differences in prostatic steroid 5 alpha-reductases of rat, dog, and human. *Endocrinology.* 1985;117:571.
236. Martin DJ. Preclinical pharmacology of alpha(1)-adrenoceptor antagonists. *Eur Urol.* 1999;36:35-41.
237. Tatemichi S, Tomiyama Y, Maruyama I, et al. Uroselectivity in male dogs of silodosin (KMD-3213), a novel drug for the obstructive component of benign prostatic hyperplasia. *Neurourol Urodyn.* 2006;25:792-799; discussion 800-791.
238. Cavalli A, Lattion AL, Hummler E, et al. Decreased blood pressure response in mice deficient of the alpha(1b)-adrenergic receptor. *Proc Natl Acad Sci U S A.* 1997;94:11589-11594.
239. Amadesi S, Varani K, Spisani L, et al. Comparison of prazosin, terazosin and tamsulosin: functional and binding studies in isolated prostatic and vascular human tissues. *Prostate.* 2001;47:231-238.
240. Foglar R, Shibata K, Horie K, et al. Use of recombinant alpha(1)-adrenoceptors to characterize subtype selectivity of drugs for the treatment of prostatic hypertrophy. *Eur J Pharmacol.* 1995;288:201-207.
241. Michel MC. The forefront for novel therapeutic agents based on the pathophysiology of lower urinary tract dysfunction: alpha-blockers in the treatment of male voiding dysfunction—how do they work and why do they differ in tolerability? *J Pharmacol Sci.* 2010;112:151-157.
242. Cordes EH. *Hallelujah Moments: Tales of Drug Discovery.* Oxford University Press; 2014.
243. Stoner E. The clinical development of a 5 alpha-reductase inhibitor, finasteride. *J Steroid Biochem Mol Biol.* 1990;37:375-378.
244. Liss MA, Thompson IM. Prostate cancer prevention with 5-alpha reductase inhibitors: concepts and controversies. *Curr Opin Urol.* 2018;28:42-45.
245. Azzouni F, Godoy A, Li Y, et al. The 5 alpha-reductase isozyme family: a review of basic biology and their role in human diseases. *Adv Urol.* 2012;2012:530121.
246. Peterson CM. Progestogens, progesterone antagonists, progesterone, androgens—synthesis, classification, and uses. *Clin Obstet Gynecol.* 1995;38:813-820.
247. Rasmusson GH, Reynolds GF, Steinberg NG, et al. Azasteroids: structure-activity relationships for inhibition of 5 alpha-reductase and of androgen receptor binding. *J Med Chem.* 1986;29:2298.
248. McConnell JD, Wilson JD, George FW, et al. Finasteride, an inhibitor of 5 alpha-reductase, suppresses prostatic dihydrotestosterone in men with benign prostatic hyperplasia. *J Clin Endocrinol Metab.* 1992;74:505.
249. Djavan B, Milani S, Fong YK. Dutasteride: a novel dual inhibitor of 5 alpha-reductase for benign prostatic hyperplasia. *Expert Opin Pharmacol.* 2005;6:311-317.
250. Vermeulen A, Giagulli VA, De Schepper P, et al. Hormonal effects of an orally active 4-azasteroid inhibitor of 5 alpha-reductase in humans. *Prostate.* 1989;14:45.
251. Bull HG, GarciaCalvo M, Andersson S, et al. Mechanism-based inhibition of human steroid 5 alpha-reductase by finasteride: enzyme-catalyzed formation of NADP-dihydrofinasteride, a potent bisubstrate analog inhibitor. *J Am Chem Soc.* 1996;118:2359-2365.
252. Stuart JD, Lee FW, Noel DS, et al. Pharmacokinetic parameters and mechanisms of inhibition of rat type 1 and 2 steroid 5 alpha-reductases: determinants for different in vivo activities of GI198745 and finasteride in the rat. *Biochem Pharmacol.* 2001;62:933-942.
253. Bakshi RK, Rasmusson GH, Patel GF, et al. 4-Aza-3-oxo-5 alpha-androst-1-ene-17 beta-N-aryl-carboxamides as dual inhibitors of human type 1 and type 2 steroid 5 alpha-reductases. Dramatic effect of N-aryl substituents on type 1 and type 2 5 alpha-reductase inhibitory potency. *J Med Chem.* 1995;38:3189-3192.
254. Steiner JF. Clinical pharmacokinetics and pharmacodynamics of finasteride. *Clin Pharmacokinet.* 1996;30:16-27.
255. Proscar (Finasteride) [package insert]. Merck Sharp & Dohme; 2013.
256. Frye SV. Discovery and clinical development of dutasteride, a potent dual 5 alpha-reductase inhibitor. *Curr Top Med Chem.* 2006;6:405-421.
257. Dolder CR. Dutasteride: a dual 5-alpha reductase inhibitor for the treatment of symptomatic benign prostatic hyperplasia. *Ann Pharmacother.* 2006;40:658-665.
258. Roehrborn CG, Boyle P, Nickel JC, et al. Efficacy and safety of a dual inhibitor of 5-alpha-reductase types 1 and 2 (dutasteride) in men with benign prostatic hyperplasia. *Urology.* 2002;60:434-441.
259. Corona G, Tirabassi G, Santi D, et al. Sexual dysfunction in subjects treated with inhibitors of 5alpha-reductase for benign prostatic hyperplasia: a comprehensive review and meta-analysis. *Andrology.* 2017;5:671-678.
260. Avodart (Dutasteride) [package insert]. GlaxoSmithKline; 2014.
261. Buck AC. Is there a scientific basis for the therapeutic effects of *Serenoa repens* in benign prostatic hyperplasia? Mechanisms of action. *J Urol.* 2004;172:1792-1799.
262. Barry MJ, Meleth S, Lee JY, et al. Effect of increasing doses of saw palmetto extract on lower urinary tract symptoms: a randomized trial. *JAMA.* 2011;306:1344-1351.
263. Husein-ElAhmed, H. Management of acne vulgaris with hormonal therapies in adult female patients. *Dermatol Ther.* 2015;28(3):166-172.
264. Beylot C, Auffret N, Poli F, et al. Propionibacterium acnes: an update on its role in the pathogenesis of acne. *J Eur Acad Dermatol Venereol.* 2014;28:271-278.
265. Gollnick HP, Dreno B. Pathophysiology and management of acne. *J Eur Acad Dermatol Venereol.* 2015;29(suppl 4):1-2.

266. Valente Duarte De Sousa IC. New and emerging drugs for the treatment of acne vulgaris in adolescents. *Expert Opin Pharmacother.* 2019;20(8):1009-1024.
267. Mazzetti A, Moro L, Gerloni M, et al. Pharmacokinetic profile, safety, and tolerability of clascoterone (cortexolone 17-alpha propionate, CB-03-01) topical cream, 1% in subjects with acne vulgaris: An open-label phase 2a study. *J Drugs Dermatol.* 2019;18(6):563.
268. Stevermer JJ, Easley SK. Treatment of prostatitis. *Am Fam Physician.* 2000;61:3015-3022, 3025-3016.
269. Charalabopoulos K, Karachalios G, Baltogiannis D, et al. Penetration of antimicrobial agents into the prostate. *Chemotherapy.* 2003;49:269-279.
270. Swanson GM. Breast-cancer risk-estimation—a translational statistic for communication to the public. *J Natl Cancer Inst.* 1993;85:848-849.
271. Slamon DJ, Godolphin W, Jones LA, et al. Studies of the HER-2/neu proto-oncogene in human breast and ovarian cancer. *Science.* 1989;244:707-712.
272. Segovia-Mendoza M, Gonzalez-Gonzalez ME, Barrera D, et al. Efficacy and mechanism of action of the tyrosine kinase inhibitors gefitinib, lapatinib and neratinib in the treatment of HER2-positive breast cancer: preclinical and clinical evidence. *Am J Cancer Res.* 2015;5:2531-2561.
273. Anestis A, Karamouzis MV, Dalagiorgou G, et al. Is androgen receptor targeting an emerging treatment strategy for triple negative breast cancer? *Cancer Treat Rev.* 2015;41:547-553.
274. Abramson VG, Lehmann BD, Ballinger TJ, et al. Subtyping of triple-negative breast cancer: implications for therapy. *Cancer.* 2015;121:8-16.
275. Welcsh PL, King MC. BRCA1 and BRCA2 and the genetics of breast and ovarian cancer. *Hum Mol Genet.* 2001;10:705-713.
276. Grann VR, Jacobson JS, Whang W, et al. Prevention with tamoxifen or other hormones versus prophylactic surgery in BRCA1/2-positive women: a decision analysis. *Cancer J Sci Am.* 2000;6:13-20.
277. King MC, Wieand S, Hale K, et al. Tamoxifen and breast cancer incidence among women with inherited mutations in BRCA1 and BRCA2: National Surgical Adjuvant Breast and Bowel Project (NSABP-P1) Breast Cancer Prevention Trial. *JAMA.* 2001;286:2251-2256.
278. First PARP inhibitor Ok'd for breast cancer. *Cancer Discov.* 2018;8:256-257.
279. Swain SM, Jeong JH, Geyer CE Jr, et al. Longer therapy, iatrogenic amenorrhea, and survival in early breast cancer. *N Engl J Med.* 2010;362:2053-2065.
280. Albain KS, Barlow WE, Shak S, et al. Prognostic and predictive value of the 21-gene recurrence score assay in postmenopausal women with node-positive, oestrogen-receptor-positive breast cancer on chemotherapy: a retrospective analysis of a randomised trial. *Lancet Oncol.* 2010;11:55-65.
281. Ohnstad HO, Borgen E, Falk RS, et al. Prognostic value of PAM50 and risk of recurrence score in patients with early-stage breast cancer with long-term follow-up. *Breast Cancer Res.* 2017;19:120.
282. Daly MB, Pilars R. NCCN guidelines insights: genetic/familial high-risk assessment: breast, ovarian, and pancreatic, version 1.2020. *JNCCN.* 2020;18:380-391.
283. Pomponio M, Keele K, Hilt E, et al. Impact of 21-gene expression assay on clinical outcomes in node-negative $\leq$ T1b breast cancer. *Ann Surg Oncol.* 2020;27(5):1671-1678.
284. Rudloff U, Jacks LM, Goldberg JI, et al. Nomogram for predicting the risk of local recurrence after breast-conserving surgery for ductal carcinoma in situ. *J Clin Oncol.* 2010;28:3762-3769.
285. Breast International Group 1-98 Collaborative Group; Thurlimann B, Keshaviah A, et al. A comparison of letrozole and tamoxifen in postmenopausal women with early breast cancer. *N Engl J Med.* 2005;353:2747-2757.
286. Wijayaratne AL, Nagel SC, Paige LA, et al. Comparative analyses of mechanistic differences among antiestrogens. *Endocrinology.* 1999;140:5828-5840.
287. Paech K, Webb P, Kuiper GG, et al. Differential ligand activation of estrogen receptors ERalpha and ERbeta at AP1 sites. *Science.* 1997;277:1508-1510.
288. Schacke H, Berger M, Rehwinkel H, et al. Selective glucocorticoid receptor agonists (SEGRAs): novel ligands with an improved therapeutic index. *Mol Cell Endocrinol.* 2007;275:109-117.
289. Mohler ML, He Y, Wu Z, et al. Dissociated non-steroidal glucocorticoids: tuning out untoward effects. *Expert Opin Ther Pat.* 2007;17:37-58.
290. Fisher B, Costantino JP, Wickerham DL, et al. Tamoxifen for prevention of breast cancer: report of the National Surgical Adjuvant Breast and Bowel Project P-1 Study. *J Natl Cancer Inst.* 1998;90:1371-1388.
291. Okubo I, Kondo M, Toi M, et al. Cost-effectiveness of letrozole versus tamoxifen as first-line hormonal therapy in treating postmenopausal women with advanced breast cancer in Japan. *Gan To Kagaku Ryoho.* 2005;32:351-363.
292. Day R, Ganz PA, Costantino JP, et al. Health-related quality of life and tamoxifen in breast cancer prevention: a report from the National Surgical Adjuvant Breast and Bowel Project P-1 Study. *J Clin Oncol.* 1999;17:2659-2669.
293. Wickramage I, Tennekoon KH, Ariyaratne MA, et al. CYP2D6 polymorphisms may predict occurrence of adverse effects to tamoxifen: a preliminary retrospective study. *Breast Cancer (Dove Med Press).* 2017;9:111-120.
294. Borgna JL, Rochefort H. Hydroxylated metabolites of tamoxifen are formed in vivo and bound to estrogen receptor in target tissues. *J Biol Chem.* 1981;256:859-868.
295. Johnson MD, Zuo H, Lee KH, et al. Pharmacological characterization of 4-hydroxy-*N*-desmethyl tamoxifen, a novel active metabolite of tamoxifen. *Breast Cancer Res Treat.* 2004;85:151-159.
296. Sirachainan E, Jaruhathai S, Trachu N, et al. CYP2D6 polymorphisms influence the efficacy of adjuvant tamoxifen in Thai breast cancer patients. *Pharmacogenomics Pers Med.* 2012;5:149-153.
297. Goetz MP, Sangkuhl K, Guchelaar HJ, et al. Clinical pharmacogenetics implementation consortium (CPIC) guideline for CYP2D6 and tamoxifen therapy. *Clin Pharmacol Ther.* 2018;103(5):770-777.
298. Donneyong MM, Bykov K, Bosco-Levy P, et al. Risk of mortality with concomitant use of tamoxifen and selective serotonin reuptake inhibitors: multi-database cohort study. *BMJ.* 2016;354:i5014.
299. Juurlink D. Revisiting the drug interaction between tamoxifen and SSRI antidepressants. *BMJ.* 2016;354:i5309.
300. Tamoxifen Citrate [package insert]. Watson Laboratories; 2011.
301. Reid JM, Goetz MP, Buhrow SA, et al. Pharmacokinetics of endoxifen and tamoxifen in female mice: implications for comparative in vivo activity studies. *Cancer Chemother Pharmacol.* 2014;74:1271-1278.
302. Kim J, Coss CC, Barrett CM, et al. Role and pharmacologic significance of cytochrome P-450 2D6 in oxidative metabolism of toremifene and tamoxifen. *Int J Cancer.* 2013;132:1475-1485.
303. Vogel CL, Johnston MA, Capers C, et al. Toremifene for breast cancer: a review of 20 years of data. *Clin Breast Cancer.* 2014;14:1-9.
304. Palacios S, Cancelo MJ. Clinical update on the use of ospemifene in the treatment of severe symptomatic vulvar and vaginal atrophy. *Int J Womens Health.* 2016;8:617-626.
305. Mao C, Yang ZY, He BF, et al. Toremifene versus tamoxifen for advanced breast cancer. *Cochrane Database Syst Rev.* 2012;2012:CD008926.
306. Vogelvang TE, van der Mooren MJ, Mijatovic V, et al. Emerging selective estrogen receptor modulators: special focus on effects on coronary heart disease in postmenopausal women. *Drugs.* 2006;66:191-221.
307. Chumsri S, Howes T, Bao T, et al. Aromatase, aromatase inhibitors, and breast cancer. *J Steroid Biochem Mol Biol.* 2011;125:13-22.
308. Fishman J, Raju MS. Mechanism of estrogen biosynthesis. Stereochemistry of C-1 hydrogen elimination in the aromatization of 2 beta-hydroxy-19-oxoandrostenedione. *J Biol Chem.* 1981;256:4472-4477.

309. Femara (Letrozole) [prescribing information]. Novartis; 2017.
310. Cohen MH, Johnson JR, Justice R, et al. Approval summary: letrozole (Femara® tablets) for adjuvant and extended adjuvant postmenopausal breast cancer treatment: conversion of accelerated to full approval. *Oncologist.* 2011;16:1762-1770.
311. Simpson D, Curran MP, Perry CM. Letrozole: a review of its use in postmenopausal women with breast cancer. *Drugs.* 2004;64:1213-1230.
312. Dunn C, Keam SJ. Letrozole: a pharmacoeconomic review of its use in postmenopausal women with breast cancer. *Pharmacoeconomics.* 2006;24:495-517.
313. Morello KC, Wurz GT, DeGregorio MW. Pharmacokinetics of selective estrogen receptor modulators. *Clin Pharmacokinet.* 2003;42:361-372.
314. Monnier A. Adjuvant trials: aromatase inhibitors in early breast cancer–are they alike? *Cancer Treat Rev.* 2006;32:532-540.
315. Howell A, Cuzick J, Baum M, et al. Results of the ATAC (Arimidex, Tamoxifen, Alone or in Combination) trial after completion of 5 years' adjuvant treatment for breast cancer. *Lancet.* 2005;365:60-62.
316. Zhao X, Liu L, Li K, et al. Comparative study on individual aromatase inhibitors on cardiovascular safety profile: a network meta-analysis. *Onco Targets Ther.* 2015;8:2721-2730.
317. Berry J. Are all aromatase inhibitors the same? A review of controlled clinical trials in breast cancer. *Clin Ther.* 2005;27:1671-1684.
318. Dixon JM, Renshaw L, Langridge C, et al. Anastrozole and letrozole: an investigation and comparison of quality of life and tolerability. *Breast Cancer Res Treat.* 2011;125:741-749.
319. Rose C, Vtoraya O, Pluzanska A, et al. An open randomised trial of second-line endocrine therapy in advanced breast cancer: comparison of the aromatase inhibitors letrozole and anastrozole. *Eur J Cancer.* 2003;39:2318-2327.
320. Smith I, Yardley D, Burris H, et al. Comparative efficacy and safety of adjuvant letrozole versus anastrozole in postmenopausal patients with hormone receptor-positive, node-positive early breast cancer: final results of the randomized phase III Femara versus Anastrozole Clinical Evaluation (FACE) trial. *J Clin Oncol.* 2017;35:1041-1048.
321. Higa GM, al Khouri N. Anastrozole: a selective aromatase inhibitor for the treatment of breast cancer. *Am J Health Syst Pharm.* 1998;55:445-452.
322. Higa GM. Altering the estrogenic milieu of breast cancer with a focus on the new aromatase inhibitors. *Pharmacotherapy.* 2000;20:280-291.
323. Higa GM. Exemestane: treatment of breast cancer with selective inactivation of aromatase. *Am J Health Syst Pharm.* 2002;59:2194-2201; quiz 2202-2194.
324. Slamon DJ, Fasching PA, Hurvitz S. Rationale and trial design of NATALEE: a phase III trial of adjuvant ribociclib + endocrine therapy versus endocrine therapy alone in patients with HR+/HER2- early breast cancer. *Ther Adv Med Oncol.* 2023;15:17588359231178125.
325. Slamon DJ, Stroyakovskiy D, Yardley DA, et al. Ribociclib and endocrine therapy as adjuvant treatment in patients with HR+/HER2- early breast cancer: primary results from the phase III NATALEE trial. *J Clin Oncol.* 2023;41(suppl 17):LBA500.
326. Hu X, Huang W, Fan M. Emerging therapies for breast cancer. *J Hematol Oncol.* 2017;10:98.
327. Reinert T, Barrios CH. Optimal management of hormone receptor positive metastatic breast cancer in 2016. *Ther Adv Med Oncol.* 2015;7:304-320.
328. Cancer Genome Atlas Network. Comprehensive molecular portraits of human breast tumours. *Nature.* 2012;490:61-70.
329. André F, Ciruelos E, Rubovszky G, et al. Alpelisib for *PIK3CA*-mutated, hormone receptor–positive advanced breast cancer. *NEJM.* 2019;380:1929-1940.
330. Blancas I, Olier C, Conde V, et al. Real-world data of fulvestrant as first-line treatment of postmenopausal women with estrogen receptor-positive metastatic breast cancer. *Sci Rep.* 2021;11(1):4274.
331. Howell A. Pure oestrogen antagonists for the treatment of advanced breast cancer. *Endocr Relat Cancer.* 2006;13:689-706.
332. Wardell SE, Marks JR, McDonnell DP. The turnover of estrogen receptor alpha by the selective estrogen receptor degrader (SERD) fulvestrant is a saturable process that is not required for antagonist efficacy. *Biochem Pharmacol.* 2011;82:122-130.
333. Brunner N, Frandsen TL, Holst-Hansen C, et al. MCF7/LCC2: a 4-hydroxytamoxifen resistant human breast cancer variant that retains sensitivity to the steroidal antiestrogen ICI 182,780. *Cancer Res.* 1993;53:3229-3232.
334. Howell A, DeFriend DJ, Robertson JF, et al. Pharmacokinetics, pharmacological and anti-tumour effects of the specific anti-oestrogen ICI 182780 in women with advanced breast cancer. *Br J Cancer.* 1996;74:300-308.
335. Bross PF, Cohen MH, Williams GA, et al. FDA drug approval summaries: fulvestrant. *Oncologist.* 2002;7:477-480.
336. Howell SJ, Casbard A, Carucci M, Ingarfield K, et al. Fulvestrant plus capivasertib versus placebo after relapse or progression on an aromatase inhibitor in metastatic, oestrogen receptor-positive, HER2-negative breast cancer (FAKTION): over all survial, updated progression free survival, and expanded biomarker analysis from a randomized, phase 2 trial. *Lancet Oncol.* 2022;23(7) 851-864.
337. Faslodex (Fulvestrant) [prescribing information]. AstraZeneca; 2017.
338. O'Regan RM, Cisneros A, England GM, et al. Effects of the antiestrogens tamoxifen, toremifene, and ICI 182,780 on endometrial cancer growth. *J Natl Cancer Inst.* 1998;90:1552-1558.
339. Wardell SE, Nelson ER, Chao CA, et al. Evaluation of the pharmacological activities of RAD1901, a selective estrogen receptor degrader. *Endocr Relat Cancer.* 2015;22:713-724.
340. Lowrance W, Dreicer R, Jarrard DF, et al. Updates to advanced prostate Cancer: AUA/SUO guideline (2023). *J Urol.* 2023;209;1082-1090.
341. Schroder FH, Hugosson J, Roobol MJ, et al. Screening and prostate-cancer mortality in a randomized European study. *N Engl J Med.* 2009;360:1320-1328.
342. Qaseem A, Barry MJ, Denberg TD, et al; Clinical Guidelines Committee of the American College of Physicians. Screening for prostate cancer: a guidance statement from the Clinical Guidelines Committee of the American College of Physicians. *Ann Intern Med.* 2013;158(10):761.
343. Huggins C, Hodges CV. Studies on prostatic cancer—I. The effect of castration, of estrogen and of androgen injection on serum phosphatases in metastatic carcinoma of the prostate. *Cancer Res.* 1941;1:293-297.
344. Vale CL, Burdett S, Rydzewska LHM, et al. Addition of docetaxel or bisphosphonates to standard of care in men with localised or metastatic, hormone-sensitive prostate cancer: a systematic review and meta-analyses of aggregate data. *Lancet Oncol.* 2016;17:243-256.
345. Roberts WB, Han M. Clinical significance and treatment of biochemical recurrence after definitive therapy for localized prostate cancer. *Surg Oncol.* 2009;18:268-274.
346. Freedland SJ, de Almeida Luz M, De Giorgi U. Improved outcomes with enzalutamide in biochemically recurrent prostate cancer. *N Engl J Med.* 2023;389:1453-1465.
347. Wattenberg CA. Carcinoma of the prostate gland, and benefits of diethylstilbestrol or orchiectomy. *Mo Med.* 1945;42:482-485.
348. Tolkach Y, Joniau S, Van Poppel H. Luteinizing hormone-releasing hormone (LHRH) receptor agonists vs antagonists: a matter of the receptors? *BJU Int.* 2013;111:1021-1030.
349. Schroder F, Crawford ED, Axcrona K, Payne H, Keane TE. Androgen deprivation therapy: past, present and future. *BJU Int.* 2012;109(suppl 6):1-12.
350. Oesterling JE. LHRH agonists—a nonsurgical treatment for benign prostatic hyperplasia. *J Androl.* 1991;12:381-388.
351. Morote J, Planas J, Salvador C, et al. Individual variations of serum testosterone in patients with prostate cancer receiving androgen deprivation therapy. *BJU Int.* 2009;103:332-335; discussion 335.

352. Morote J, Orsola A, Planas J, et al. Redefining clinically significant castration levels in patients with prostate cancer receiving continuous androgen deprivation therapy. *J Urol.* 2007;178:1290-1295.
353. Lepor H, Shore ND. LHRH agonists for the treatment of prostate cancer: 2012. *Rev Urol.* 2012;14:1-12.
354. Allan CA, Collins VR, Frydenberg M, et al. Androgen deprivation therapy complications. *Endocr Relat Cancer.* 2014;21:T119-T129.
355. Trost LW, Serefoglu E, Gokce A, et al. Androgen deprivation therapy impact on quality of life and cardiovascular health, monitoring therapeutic replacement. *J Sex Med.* 2013;10(suppl 1):84-101.
356. Schulman C, Cornel E, Matveev V, et al. Intermittent versus continuous androgen deprivation therapy in patients with relapsing or locally advanced prostate cancer: a phase 3b randomised study (ICELAND). *Eur Urol.* 2016;69:720-727.
357. Zhang TY, Agarwal N, Sonpavde G, et al. Management of castrate resistant prostate cancer-recent advances and optimal sequence of treatments. *Curr Urol Rep.* 2013;14:174-183.
358. Mulders PF, De Santis M, Powles T, et al. Targeted treatment of metastatic castration-resistant prostate cancer with sipuleucel-T immunotherapy. *Cancer Immunol Immunother.* 2015;64: 655-663.
359. Kantoff PW, Higano CS, Shore ND, et al. Sipuleucel-T immunotherapy for castration-resistant prostate cancer. *N Engl J Med.* 2010;363:411-422.
360. Hu R, George DJ, Zhang T. What is the role of sipuleucel-T in the treatment of patients with advanced prostate cancer? An update on the evidence. *Ther Adv Urol.* 2016;8:272-278.
361. Mohler JL, Gregory CW, Ford OH 3rd, et al. The androgen axis in recurrent prostate cancer. *Clin Cancer Res.* 2004;10:440-448.
362. Mohler ML, Coss CC, Duke CB III, et al. Androgen receptor antagonists: a patent review (2008-2011). *Expert Opin Ther Pat.* 2012;22:541-565.
363. Tannock IF, de Wit R, Berry WR, et al. Docetaxel plus prednisone or mitoxantrone plus prednisone for advanced prostate cancer. *New Engl J Med.* 2004;351:1502-1512.
364. de Bono JS, Oudard S, Ozguroglu M, et al. Prednisone plus cabazitaxel or mitoxantrone for metastatic castration-resistant prostate cancer progressing after docetaxel treatment: a randomised open-label trial. *Lancet.* 2010;376:1147-1154.
365. Jevtana (Cabazitaxel) [prescribing information]. Sanofi-Aventis; 2018.
366. Belderbos BPS, Bins S, van Leeuwen RWF, et al. Influence of enzalutamide on cabazitaxel pharmacokinetics: a drug-drug interaction study in metastatic castration-resistant prostate cancer (mCRPC) patients. *Clin Cancer Res.* 2018;24:541-546.
367. Hupe MC, Philippi C, Roth D, et al. Expression of prostate-specific membrane antigen (PSMA) on biopsies is an independent risk stratifier of prostate cancer patients at time of initial diagnosis. *Front Oncol.* 2018;8:623.
368. Fizazi K, Herrmann K, Krause BJ, et al. Health-related quality of life and pain outcomes with [177Lu]Lu-PSMA-617 plus standard of care versus standard of care in patients with metastatic castration-resistant prostate cancer (VISION): a multicentre, open-label, randomised, phase 3 trial. *Lancet Oncol.* 2023;24:597-610.
369. Ning X, Yang Y, Deng H, et al. Development of 17beta-hydroxysteroid dehydrogenase type 3 as a target in hormone-dependent prostate cancer therapy. *Steroids.* 2017;121:10-16.
370. Penning TM, Tamae D. Current advances in intratumoral androgen metabolism in castration-resistant prostate cancer. *Curr Opin Endocrinol Diabetes Obes.* 2016;23:264-270.
371. Barrie SE, Potter GA, Goddard PM, et al. Pharmacology of novel steroidal inhibitors of cytochrome P450(17-alpha) (17-alpha-hydroxylase C17-20 lyase). *J Steroid Biochem.* 1994;50:267-273.
372. Ryan CJ, Smith MR, de Bono JS, et al. Abiraterone in metastatic prostate cancer without previous chemotherapy. *N Engl J Med.* 2013;368:138-148.
373. Fizazi K, Tran N, Fein L, et al. Abiraterone plus prednisone in metastatic, castration-sensitive prostate cancer. *N Engl J Med.* 2017;377:352-360.
374. Slootbeek PHJ, Overbeek JK, Ligtenberg MJL, et al. PARPing up the right tree; an overview of PARP inhibitors for metastatic castration-resistant prostate cancer. *Cancer Lett.* 2023;577:216367.
375. Hussain M, Fizazi K, Saad F, et al. PROSPER: a phase 3, randomized, double-blind, placebo (PBO)-controlled study of enzalutamide (ENZA) in men with nonmetastatic castration-resistant prostate cancer (M0 CRPC). *J Clin Oncol.* 2018;36:3.
376. Smith MR, Saad F, Chowdhury S, et al. Apalutamide treatment and metastasis-free survival in prostate cancer. *N Engl J Med.* 2018;378(15):1408-1418.
377. Fizazi K, Shore N, Tammela TL, et al. Darolutamide in nonmetastatic, castration-resistant prostate Cancer. *N Engl J Med.* 2019;380(13):1235-1246.
378. Smith MR, Hussain M, Saad F, et al. Darolutamide and survival in metastatic, hormone-sensitive prostate cancer. *N Engl J Med.* 2022;386:1132-1142.
379. Bohl CE, Gao W, Miller DD, et al. Structural basis for antagonism and resistance of bicalutamide in prostate cancer. *Proc Natl Acad Sci U S A.* 2005;102(17):6201-6206.
380. Clegg NJ, Wongvipat J, Joseph JD, et al. ARN-509: a novel antiandrogen for prostate cancer treatment. *Cancer Res.* 2012;72: 1494-1503.
381. Krause WC, Shafi AA, Nakka M, et al. Androgen receptor and its splice variant, AR-V7, differentially regulate FOXA1 sensitive genes in LNCaP prostate cancer cells. *Int J Biochem Cell Biol.* 2014;54:49-59.
382. Makkonen H, Kauhanen M, Jaaskelainen T, et al. Androgen receptor amplification is reflected in the transcriptional responses of vertebral-cancer of the prostate cells. *Mol Cell Endocrinol.* 2011;331:57-65.
383. Bastos AD, Antonarakis ES. Darolutamide for castration-resistant prostate cancer. *Onco Targets Ther.* 2019;12:8769-8777.
384. Borgmann H, Lallous N, Ozistanbullu D, et al. Moving towards precision urologic oncology: targeting enzalutamide-resistant prostate cancer and mutated forms of the androgen receptor using the novel inhibitor darolutamide (ODM-201). *Eur Urol.* 2018;73:4-8.
385. Chen H, Dong K, Ding J, et al. CRISPR genome-wide screening identifies PAK1 as a critical driver of ARSI cross-resistance in prostate cancer progression. *Cancer Lett.* 2024;587:216725.
386. Taavitsainen P, Prien O, Kähkönen M, et al. Metabolism and mass balance of the novel nonsteroidal androgen receptor inhibitor darolutamide in humans. *Drug Metab Dispos.* 2021;49(6):420-433.
387. Joseph JD, Lu N, Qian J, et al. A clinically relevant androgen receptor mutation confers resistance to second-generation antiandrogens enzalutamide and ARN-509. *Cancer Discov.* 2013;3:1020-1029.
388. Rathkopf DE, Antonarakis ES, Shore ND, et al. Safety and antitumor activity of apalutamide (ARN-509) in metastatic castration-resistant prostate cancer with and without prior abiraterone acetate and prednisone. *Clin Cancer Res.* 2017;23:3544-3551.
389. Galletti G, Leach BI, Lam L, Tagawa ST. Mechanisms of resistance to systemic therapy in metastatic castration-resistant prostate cancer. *Cancer Treat Rev.* 2017;57:16-27.
390. Tien AH, Sadar MD. Treatments targeting the androgen receptor and its splice variants in breast cancer. *Int J Mol Sci.* 2024;25(3):1817.
391. Mohler ML, Sikdar A, Ponnusamy S, et al. An overview of next-generation androgen receptor-targeted therapeutics in development for the treatment of prostate cancer. *Int J Mol Sci.* 2021;22(4):2124.
392. Mohler ML, Dalton JT. Modulation of the androgen receptor axis. In: *Burger's Medicinal Chemistry and Drug Discovery.* 8th ed. John Wiley & Sons, Inc; 2021.
393. Cockshott ID. Bicalutamide: clinical pharmacokinetics and metabolism. *Clin Pharmacokinet.* 2004;43:855-878.
394. Shet MS, McPhaul M, Fisher CW, et al. Metabolism of the antiandrogenic drug (Flutamide) by human CYP1A2. *Drug Metab Dispos.* 1997;25:1298-1303.

395. Marugo M, Bernasconi D, Miglietta L, et al. Effects of dihydrotestosterone and hydroxyflutamide on androgen receptors in cultured human breast cancer cells (EVSA-T). *J Steroid Biochem Mol Biol*. 1992;42:547-554.
396. Creaven PJ, Pendyala L, Tremblay D. Pharmacokinetics and metabolism of nilutamide. *Urology*. 1991;37:13-19.
397. Ask K, Decologne N, Ginies C, et al. Metabolism of nilutamide in rat lung. *Biochem Pharmacol*. 2006;71:377-385.
398. Ask K, Dijols S, Giroud C, et al. Reduction of nilutamide by NO synthases: implications for the adverse effects of this nitroaromatic antiandrogen drug. *Chem Res Toxicol*. 2003;16:1547-1554.
399. American Cancer Society. Key statistics for testicular cancer. Accessed April 4, 2024. https://www.cancer.org/cancer/types/testicular-cancer/about/key-statistics.html#
400. McGlynn KA, Devesa SS, Sigurdson AJ, et al. Trends in the incidence of testicular germ cell tumors in the United States. *Cancer*. 2003;97:63-70.

Case Solution 1

A. HP has several risk factors for early recurrence and poor prognosis, including large tumor size (2.5 cm), unfavorable oncotype score, obesity (high aromatase production), and high mitotic index. HP should probably be presented with the option of the six cycles of chemotherapy consisting of AC-T, anthracycline, and cyclophosphamide then taxane with clear explanation of the risks and benefits.

B. Tamoxifen is a valid selection for HP, but AIs tend to have better prevention of recurrence in postmenopausal patients. From the initial workup, the menopausal status of the patient is not certain, so endogenous 17β-estradiol levels should be followed from diagnosis through surgery and adjuvant chemo. Ovarian suppression should be considered if estrogen levels are not menopausal. Following ovarian suppression, tamoxifen is generally considered standard of care for premenopausal patients, but AIs are favored in postmenopausal.

C. The most common site of metastasis is the bone and commonly the hip (and spine), which was painful on initial presentation, but not evaluated. (Although not the best diagnostic test, ultrasound suggests no visceral metastasis.) Breast cancer tumors grow in the bone marrow and particularly in weak bone, and the low platelet count suggests the possibility of metastasis to the bone. HP should be referred to her oncologist immediately.

Case Solution 2

A. 1. Bone-protective agents are needed to prevent further pathologic fractures. In addition to calcium and vitamin D supplements, bisphosphonates have been used historically. However, denosumab has largely supplanted bisphosphonate use in breast and prostate cancer.
   2. Encourage HP to do physical therapy to strengthen bones.
   3. Stabilizing the spinal column to prevent further disability, for example, kyphoplasty might be considered.

B. Tamoxifen resistance is common, and many AIs have been approved for endocrine failures. Letrozole and/or anastrozole are approved as monotherapies in tamoxifen-resistant patients. However, outcomes are improved, and guidelines now recommend the addition of a CDK4/6 inhibitor to the AI. For example, palbociclib and abemaciclib are approved for endocrine therapy failures in combination with an AI. Letrozole may have the most clinical data to support its use, but anastrozole could also be considered. Fulvestrant is also indicated for endocrine failures as monotherapy or combined with palbociclib or abemaciclib, which also improves outcomes over monotherapy. Though a *PIK3CA* gene mutation is detected, the alpelisib combined with fulvestrant combination is not approved for first-line therapy and should be reserved until progression on one of the endocrine therapies outlined earlier. Importantly, the observation of estrogen levels above those expected for postmenopausal patients suggests that HP is either pre- or perimenopausal and should be on a GnRH agonist such as goserelin and further supports the use of an AI to help further suppress estrogen synthesis.

C. No. The cancer is still ER positive. So endocrine therapies should be considered first.

Structure Challenge Answers

A-8, B-9, C-11, D-15, E-6, F-4, G-1, H-5, I-2, J-13, K-10, L-7, M-14, N-12, O-3.

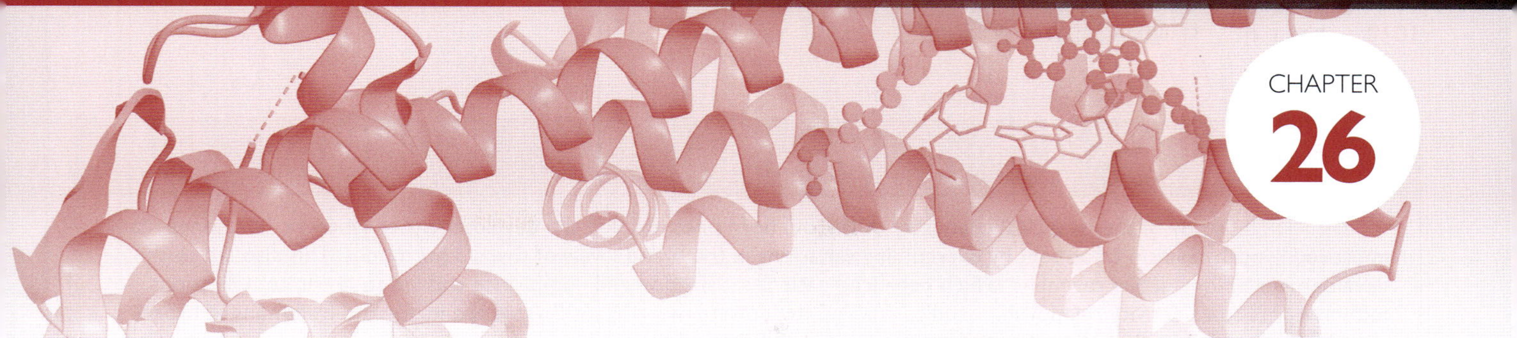

CHAPTER 26

Drugs Used to Treat Thyroid Disorders

Rami A. Al-Horani

Drugs covered in this chapter:

DRUGS FOR TREATMENT OF HYPOTHYROIDISM
- Levothyroxine sodium
- Liothyronine sodium
- Liotrix
- Natural thyroid hormone preparations

DRUGS FOR TREATMENT OF HYPERTHYROIDISM
- 1-Methyl-2-mercapto-imidazole (methimazole)
- Carbimazole
- Iodine and radioactive iodine
- Ionic inhibitors
- Propylthiouracil

DRUGS FOR THYROID CARCINOMA
- Cabozantinib
- Dabrafenib
- Entrectinib
- Larotrectinib
- Lenvatinib
- Pralsetinib
- Radioactive iodine
- Selpercatinib
- Selumetinib
- Sorafenib
- Trametinib
- Vandetanib
- Vemurafenib

Abbreviations

ADHD attention-deficit/hyperactivity disorder
AMP adenosine monophosphate
BCRP breast cancer resistance protein
ClO_4^- perchlorate
CTLA-4 cytotoxic T-lymphocyte antigen 4
DIT 3,5-diiodo-L-tyrosine
EGF epidermal growth factor
EGFR epidermal growth factor receptor
ERK extracellular signal-related kinase
FMO flavin-containing monooygenase
GPCR G protein-coupled receptor
GRTH generalized resistance to thyroid hormone
HSA human serum albumin
I^- iodide
IGF-1 insulin-like growth factor-1
LAO L-amino acid oxidase
MAO monoamine oxidase
MAP mitogen activated protein
MCT8 monocarboxylate transporter 8
MEK mitogen-activated extracellular signal-regulated kinase
MIT 3-monoiodo-L-tyrosine
MMI 1-methyl-2-mercapto-imidazole (methimazole)
NADPH nicotinamide adenine dinucleotide phosphate
NIS sodium/iodide symporter
ODC ornithine decarboxylase
OTC over the counter
PD-1 programmed cell death 1
PTU propylthiouracil
RET rearranged during transfection
rT_3 reverse T_3 (3,3′,5′-triiodo-L-thyronine)
RTHs resistance to thyroid hormones
RXRs retinoic acid X receptors
SCN^- thiocyanate
SULT sulfotransferase
T_2 3,3′-diiodo-L-thyronine
T_3 3,5,3′-triiodo-L-thyronine, triiodothyronine
T_4 3,5,3′,5′-tetraiodo-L-thyronine, thyroxine
TBG thyroxine-binding globulin
TBPA thyroxine-binding prealbumin
TcO_4^- pertechnetate
TGF-β transforming growth factor-β
THRs thyroid hormone receptors
TPO thyropyroxidase
TREs thyroid-response elements
TRH thyroid-releasing hormone
TSH thyroid-stimulating hormone
TTR transthyretin
UGT uridine 5′-diphosphateglucuronyltransferase
VEGFR vascular endothelial growth factor receptor

CLINICAL SIGNIFICANCE

The study of the medicinal chemistry of thyroid hormones enabled the development of synthetic hormones that improved hypothyroidism treatment by overcoming variations in the blood levels of thyroid hormones. This also led to the development of long-acting regimens, which enhanced patient satisfaction and compliance and led to fewer complications. Extensive structure-activity relationship studies enabled the development of antithyroid agents for the treatment of hyperthyroidism and tyrosine kinase inhibitors for the treatment of thyroid cancer. Understanding the medicinal chemistry aspects of thyroid-targeting drugs is critical to address the need to adjust doses in certain patient population, to avoid potential drug-drug interactions, and to manage potential chemistry-driven side effects.

Ahlam Ayyad, PharmD

Introduction

The thyroid (Greek *thyreos*, shield, and *eidos*, form) gland is located in the front of the trachea between the cricoid cartilage and the suprasternal notch. It is composed of two lobes linked by an isthmus. The thyroid gland is a highly vascular tissue, with a normal size of 12 to 20 g. Four parathyroid glands are located posterior to each pole of the thyroid gland. Although the word "thyroid" was first introduced by Wharton,[1] the first clue about its function was described by Baumann[2] as the only mammalian organ that can incorporate iodine into organic substances. The thyroid gland produces two related hormones: thyroxine (T_4) and triiodothyronine (T_3). Thyroid hormones are virtually important for every organ system. By binding to thyroid hormone receptors (THRs), T_4 and T_3 play a critical role in cell differentiation and organogenesis during development and help maintain thermogenic and metabolic homeostasis in adults.

Anatomically, the thyroid gland possesses numerous spherical follicles, forming the thyroid follicular cells that surround secreted colloid, a proteinaceous fluid containing large amounts of thyroglobulin, which is the protein precursor of the thyroid hormones. The follicular cells are polarized: the apical surface faces the follicular lumen, and the basolateral surface faces the bloodstream. Demand for thyroid hormones is regulated by thyroid-stimulating hormone (TSH), which has its receptor on the basolateral surface of the follicular cells. The binding event results in thyroglobulin being reabsorbed from the follicular lumen into the cytoplasm where it undergoes proteolysis, yielding thyroid hormones for secretion into the bloodstream. It is worth mentioning here that the thyroid's *para*follicular cells produce calcitonin, which is not an important endogenous hormone but can serve as a therapeutic agent in hypercalcemia and osteoporosis.

Reservoirs of thyroid hormones in the thyroid gland and blood support consistent hormone availability. The hypothalamic-pituitary-thyroid axis is very sensitive to small changes in circulating thyroid hormone concentrations, and peripheral free thyroid hormone levels are maintained within a narrow range via alterations in thyroid hormone secretion. In this axis, hypothalamic thyroid-releasing hormone (TRH) stimulates the thyrotrope cells of the anterior pituitary gland to produce TSH, which subsequently stimulates thyroid hormone synthesis and secretion. Evidently, TSH is the set point in this axis. Reduced levels of thyroid hormones increase basal TSH production and enhance TRH-mediated stimulation of TSH. High thyroid hormone levels rapidly and directly suppress TSH gene expression and inhibit TRH stimulation of TSH secretion, indicating that thyroid hormones are the dominant regulator of TSH production. Thyroid hormones act via a negative feedback loop predominantly through the thyroid hormone receptor β_2 to inhibit the production of TRH and TSH.

Patients typically seek medical care for evaluation of symptoms due to either abnormal thyroid hormone levels or nodular or diffuse thyroid gland enlargement. Contemporary understandings of the physiology of thyroid glands as well as the pathophysiology of thyroid disorders have led to several medical interventions that have helped alleviate patients' symptoms and improve the quality of their lives. This chapter presents the biochemical and physiologic aspects of thyroid hormones as well as the chemical and pharmacologic aspects of the therapeutic agents used to treat various thyroid disorders.

Biosynthesis, Transport, Metabolism, and Excretion of Thyroid Hormones

Thyroid Hormones

Thyroid hormones are iodinated amino acids derived from L-tyrosine. They are synthesized in the thyroid gland's follicular cells and stored as iodinated amino acids of thyroglobulin. The first identified major thyroid hormone was named as L-thyroxine, the structure of which was established to be 3,5,3′,5′-tetraiodo-L-thyronine (T_4; Fig. 26.1). Initially, it was thought that all the hormonal activity of thyroid tissue can be accounted for by its T_4 content. Nonetheless, subsequent studies revealed that crude thyroid preparations demonstrated greater calorigenic activity than what can be accounted for by their T_4 contents. Therefore, the presence of another thyroid hormone was debated, and was finally detected, isolated, and synthesized by Gross and Pitt-Rivers in 1952.[3] The second principal hormone

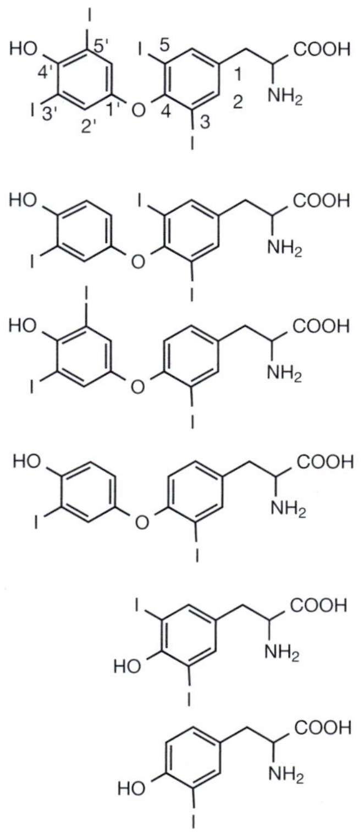

Thyroxine (T_4)
3,5,3',5'-Tetraiodo-L-thyronine

Thyroxine (T_3)
3,5,3'-Triiodo-L-thyronine

Thyroxine T_3 (rT_3)
3,3',5-Triiodo-L-thyronine

(T_2)
3,3'-Diiodo-L-thyronine

(DIT)
3,5-Diiodo-L-tyrosine

(MIT)
3-Monoiodo-L-tyrosine

Figure 26.1 Chemical structures of iodinated molecules of the thyroid gland.

is 3,5,3′-triiodo-L-thyronine (T_3; Fig. 26.1). T_3 is derived mainly from T_4 by the action of deiodinase enzymes outside the thyroid. This implied that the body could use a dose of T_4 to produce its own T_3 as demonstrated in athyreotic humans. This led to the practice of effective replacement in hypothyroidism with T_4 only. The thyroid gland also contains relatively significant quantities of 3,5-diiodo-L-tyrosine (DIT) and 3-monoiodo-L-tyrosine (MIT; Fig. 26.1). Furthermore, there are small amounts of 3,3′-diiodo-L-thyronine (T_2) and 3,3′,5′-triiodo-L-thyronine (reverse T_3 [rT_3]), yet none of them appears to possess significant hormonal activity. Structurally, coupling of the outer ring of one 3,5-diiodo-L-tyrosine (DIT) molecule to the phenolic oxygen of a second DIT molecule would result in T_4 formation, whereas coupling of the outer ring of one MIT molecule to the phenolic oxygen of a DIT molecule would result in T_3 formation. The two couplings are typically accompanied by a loss of alanine moiety.

Biosynthesis of Thyroid Hormones

Thyroglobulin and iodine are two important molecular species for the biosynthesis of thyroid hormones. On the one hand, thyroglobulin serves as the matrix for the synthesis of T_4 and T_3 as well as the storage form of the hormones and iodide. Thyroglobulin is a large glycoprotein of 660 kDa, accounting for approximately one-third of the gland's weight. It carries an average of six tyrosine residues as MIT, five residues as DIT, 0.3 residues as T_3, and one residue as T_4. Accordingly, it is estimated that a 20-g thyroid gland stores roughly 7.8 mg of T_4 and 2 mg of T_3 and that the normal human thyroid gland stores sufficient T_4 to maintain an euthyroid status for 2 months without new biosynthesis. On the other hand, iodine is an essential component of thyroid hormones. Iodine consists 65% of T_4 weight and 58% of T_3 weight. The iodine substituents play a major role in the conformational preferences for T_4 and T_3 given their steric bulkiness. The thyroid hormones are the only iodine-containing molecules with established physiologic significance in vertebrates. Iodine ingested in the diet is absorbed through the small intestine cells and reaches the systemic circulation in the form of iodide ion (I^-). The iodide ion is then actively transported to the thyroid gland, where it is concentrated, oxidized, and then incorporated into thyroglobulin to form MIT and DIT and later T_4 and T_3. Thyroglobulin is stored in the follicular lumen and must reenter the cell, where the process of proteolysis liberates thyroid hormones into the bloodstream, where specific binding proteins shuttle them to the target tissues.

The biosynthesis of T_4 and T_3 is largely regulated by TSH (also known as thyrotropin), which promotes the synthesis of thyroglobulin, hydrogen peroxide, and Thyropyroxidase (TPO). The biosynthesis of thyroid hormones is dependent on the exogenous supply of iodine. The thyroid gland is unique in that it is the only body tissue capable of storing iodine in large quantities (~25% of the body's supply) and incorporates it into hormones. The biosynthesis of thyroid hormones involves the following sequence of events: (1) active uptake of iodide by follicular cells, (2) oxidation of iodide and formation of iodotyrosines, (3) formation of iodothyronines from iodotyrosines, (4) proteolysis of thyroglobulin and release of T_4 and T_3 into the blood stream, and (5) conversion of T_4 to T_3. These steps are depicted in Figure 26.2 and summarized in the following sections.[4]

Active Uptake of Iodide by Follicular Cells

The first step in the biosynthesis of thyroid glands is the uptake of the iodide from the bloodstream by the thyroid gland. Normally, the iodide concentration in the blood is very low (0.2-0.4 μg/dL; ~15-30 nM). This steady state concentration in the blood is the result of an equilibrium state between iodide input and iodide output. The iodide input is provided by dietary iodide, leaked iodide from the thyroid gland, and the reclaimed hormonal iodide from peripheral tissues. The iodide output is given by the thyroid gland uptake, renal elimination, and limited biliary excretion. Iodide metabolism is simplified in Figure 26.3.

The mechanism by which the iodide enters the thyroid gland is active transportation. Iodide is actively transported through the basolateral membrane via a sodium/iodide symporter (NIS) from the extracellular space into the thyroid follicular cell against an electrochemical gradient, driven by the coupled transport of sodium. As a result, the ratio of $[\text{iodide}]_{\text{thyroid}}/[\text{iodide}]_{\text{plasma}}$ is usually between 20 and 50 and can exceed 100 when the gland is stimulated. Structurally related anions such as perchlorate (ClO_4^-), thiocyanate (SCN^-), and pertechnetate (TcO_4^-) are competitive inhibitors of iodine transport. In addition, bromine, fluorine,

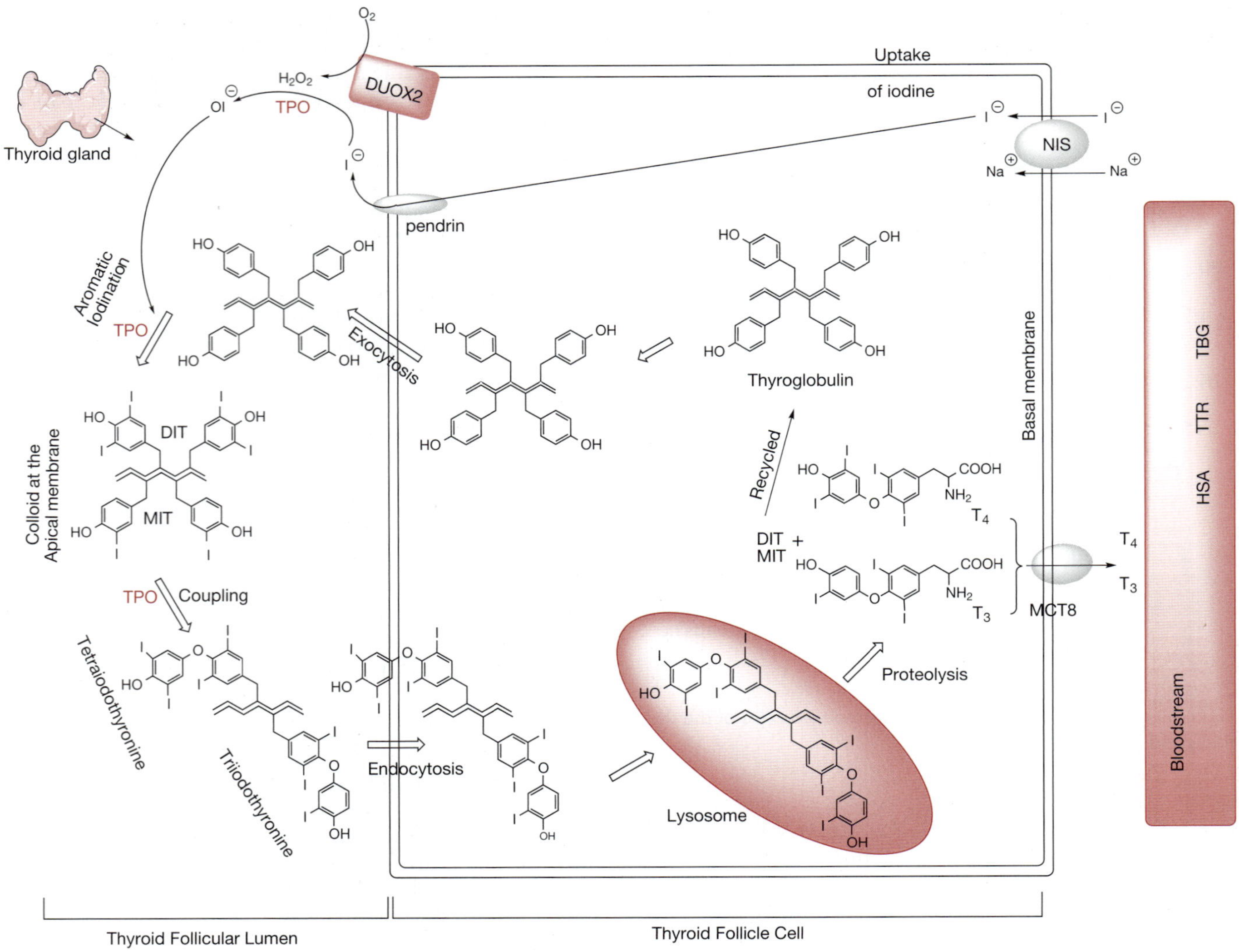

Figure 26.2 Summary of the major pathways for the biosynthesis and secretion of the thyroid hormones. When thyrotropin (TSH) binds to its receptor at the basal membrane of the follicle cell, the biosynthesis of thyroglobulin is stimulated, as that of TPO and the production of hydrogen peroxide. Noniodinated thyroglobulin is synthesized by the rough endoplasmic reticulum and secreted through the apical membrane into the follicular lumen. Iodide enters the cell via NIS and is then transported to the lumen by pendrin-assisted exocytosis. In the lumen, iodide is oxidized by hydrogen peroxide (H_2O_2)/TPO to form OI^-, followed by TPO-catalyzed aromatic iodination of thyroglobulin's tyrosine residues resulting in the formation of diiodotyrosyl (DIT) and monotyrosyl (MIT) residues. Hydrogen peroxide is produced at the apical membrane by the action of DUOX2. Two adjacent DIT residues are subsequently coupled to form tetraiodothyronine residues (thyroglobulin attached T_4), whereas DIT and MIT are coupled to make triiodothyronine residues (thyroglobulin attached T_3). Although shown as sequential reactions, aromatic iodination and coupling reaction occur simultaneously. Low plasma levels for T_4 cause the iodinated thyroglobulin to be re-absorbed via endocytosis process into the follicle cell, where complete proteolysis occurs by lysosomal enzymes to mainly T_4 and T_3, and to lesser extent DIT, MIT, and noniodinated residues. T_4 can be de-iodinated to T_3 inside the cell. Both T_4 and T_3 are secreted by the cell into the blood and shuttled to peripheral tissues by TBG, TTR, and/or HSA. Although MIT and DIT are released, they do not leave the gland, but they are selectively de-iodinated and recycled to form new thyroglobulin. (Modified from the 8th edition of this textbook as well as reference[112].)

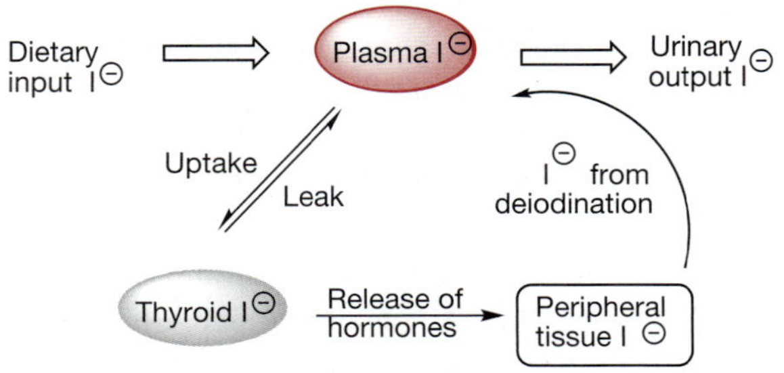

Figure 26.3 Simplified scheme of iodide metabolism.

and under certain circumstances, lithium, block iodide transport into the thyroid gland.[5,6] Importantly, NIS is most highly expressed in the thyroid gland, with low levels present in the lactating breast, placenta, and salivary glands. This iodide transport process is highly regulated, allowing adaptation to changes in dietary intake. Decreased iodine levels increase the amount of NIS and stimulate uptake, whereas elevated iodine levels suppress NIS expression and uptake. The selective expression of NIS in thyroid gland permits isotopic scanning, treatment of hyperthyroidism, and ablation of thyroid cancer with radioisotopes of iodine, without significantly affecting other organs.

Oxidation of Iodide and Formation of Iodotyrosines

After the inorganic iodide enters the thyroid follicular cell, it is escorted through the cell to the apical membrane, where it is transported into the follicular lumen by pendrin (an anion exchange protein) and potentially other proteins. Iodide must next be oxidized to a higher oxidation state in order to serve as an iodinating agent. Located on the luminal side of the apical membrane, TPO, a membrane-bound heme enzyme, catalyzes the oxidation of the iodide utilizing hydrogen peroxide as oxidizing agent, and the resulting iodinating form is thought to be hypoiodite (OI^-).[7] TPO also catalyzes the iodination of tyrosine residues to form MIT and DIT residues in thyroglobulin, in a process referred to as organification of iodine. TPO activity is influenced by TSH.

Importantly, the oxidizing agent, hydrogen peroxide, is considered to be the limiting agent in the oxidation of iodide and the aromatic iodination of tyrosine residues, together known as oxidative iodination. The first study that identified the role of hydrogen peroxide was published in 1975 and described decreased hydrogen peroxide generation in human thyroid nodules with defective iodide organification. The source of luminal hydrogen peroxide was later characterized as a thyrocyte apical membrane enzyme that utilizes NADPH as electron donor. Subsequent studies identified the thyrocyte hydrogen peroxide-generating enzymes as members of the NADPH oxidase family. The proper identities of the enzymes were finally established in 2000 by protein purification and sequencing as well as by thyroid cDNA library screening. The enzymes were initially thought to be thyroid-specific, and thus, were named thyroid oxidases. However, the proteins were later identified in other tissues and their names were modified to dual oxidase 1 and 2 (DUOX1/2) to reflect their dual oxidase and peroxidase activities. The major source of hydrogen peroxide in the thyroid follicle is DUOX2.[8] The generation of hydrogen peroxide is controlled by iodide. Limited iodide concentration permits efficient hormone synthesis, whereas abundant iodide concentration limits hormone synthesis. Hydrogen peroxide deficiency has been proposed as a contributing factor to goiter and decreased aromatic iodination in euthyroid patients, as suggested by the restoration of normal organification of the thyroid homogenates from these patients following the in vitro addition of a hydrogen peroxide-generating system.

Coupling of Iodotyrosine Residues

The iodotyrosines (MIT and DIT) in thyroglobulin are then coupled via an ether linkage in a reaction that is also catalyzed by TPO at the apical membrane. Either T_4 or T_3 can be produced by this reaction, depending on the number of iodine atoms present in the iodotyrosines. Coupling the two rings of DIT residues results in the formation of T_4, whereas coupling MIT with DIT results in the formation of T_3. As shown in Figure 26.2, a tyrosyl residue donates its iodinated phenyl moiety as a DIT radical to become the outer ring of the iodothyronine amino acid at an acceptor site, leaving dehydroalanine at the donor site. The location of the iodotyrosyl residues within thyroglobulin creates an optimal spatial alignment for the coupling reactions. Considering the two steps, aromatic iodination and tyrosine residue coupling are both oxidative in nature and take place simultaneously.

Proteolysis of Thyroglobulin and Release of Iodothyronines

When there is a demand for thyroid hormones, their release is initiated by endocytosis of the thyroglobulin colloid from the follicular lumen at the apical surface of the follicular cell, with the participation of a thyroglobulin receptor megalin. This engulfed thyroglobulin appears as intracellular colloid droplets and fuses with digestive lysosomes containing proteases. TSH enhances the degradation of thyroglobulin by increasing the activity of lysosomal thiol endopeptidases, which yield hormone-containing intermediates that are further processed by exopeptidases. Eventually, thyroglobulin proteolysis yields MIT, DIT, T_3, and T_4. Although MIT and DIT are released, they do not leave the gland, but they are selectively de-iodinated and recycled to form new thyroglobulin. The iodide is again converted into the oxidized form to drive subsequent iodination. A defect in the recyclization of MIT and DIT may lead to hypothyroidism and goiter. T_3 and T_4 are secreted by the gland to the systemic circulation.

Conversion of T_4 to T_3

T_4 is the major hormone that is released by the thyroid gland. It is released at a rate that is 8 to 10 times faster than the rate of T_3 release. Nevertheless, T_4 is considered as a prohormone, and, because it has a longer half-life than that of T_3, much higher levels of T_4 than that of T_3 are in circulation. In most extrathyroidal tissues, the conversion of T_4 to T_3 is essential for the physiologic action of thyroid hormones. In these tissues, about 33% of the secreted T_4 undergoes 5′-deiodination to form T_3, and another 40% undergoes deiodination of the inner ring to produce the inactive molecule rT_3.[9] About 80% of T_3 is derived from the circulating T_4. The 5′-deiodination of T_4 is a reductive process catalyzed by a group of 5′-deiodinases found in various tissues.

Three types of 5′-deiodinases are known and distinguished from each other, based on location, substrate specificity, and susceptibility to inhibitors. Type I 5′-deiodinase is found in the liver and kidney and catalyzes inner and outer ring deiodination, including T_4 to T_3. Type II 5′-deiodinase is present in brain and pituitary and catalyzes mainly outer ring deiodination, including T_4 to T_3. Type III 5′-deiodinase is found in the brain, skin, and placenta and is the principal source of rT_3.[10]

Although T_3 is secreted by the thyroid gland, metabolism of T_4 by 5′-deiodination of the outer ring in the peripheral tissues contributes to about 80% of circulating T_3, whereas the 5′-deiodination of the inner ring produces the metabolically inactive rT_3. Under normal physiologic conditions, about 40% of T_4 is metabolized to T_3 and rT_3, and about 20% is metabolized via other pathways, such as hepatic glucuronidation, resulting in a metabolite excreted in the bile.

Table 26.1 Comparative Aspects of Thyroid Hormones

Parameter	T_4	T_3
Daily production	80-100 μg	30-40 μg
$[Total]_{plasma}$	5-12 μg/dL	80-175 ng/dL
$[Free]_{plasma}$	0.8-2.0 ng/dL	2-4 pg/mL
Free fraction in plasma (%)	0.02	0.3
Intracellular fraction (%)	15	65
V_d (L)	10	40
Plasma $T_{1/2}$	7 d	20 h
Turnover (%/day)	10	56

T_3 has a much higher affinity for the nuclear thyroid hormone receptor (THR) compared with T_4, and it is about five times more active than T_4. Comparative quantitative aspects of thyroid hormone metabolism are provided in Table 26.1.

Transport of Thyroid Hormones in Blood

About 95% of iodine exists in the circulation as organic iodine and the rest exists as iodide. Most (90%-95%) organic iodine is T_4, and the rest is T_3. Given their high hydrophobicity, the thyroid hormones are transported in the blood in strong, noncovalent association with several carrier proteins. In fact, 99% of thyroid hormones in blood are bound to plasma proteins, but they can rapidly be liberated to enter peripheral cells. These proteins include thyroxine-binding globulin (TBG), transthyretin (TTR), human serum albumin (HSA), and lipoproteins. It appears that thyroid hormone binding to these proteins serves multiple purposes. Binding of thyroid hormones to plasma proteins protects the hormones from metabolism and excretion, resulting in their long half-lives in the circulation. It can also protect against sudden changes in thyroid hormone production and degradation as well as against iodine deficiency. Lastly, binding proteins may also serve as extrathyroidal storage sites for thyroid hormones, which is necessary to maintain appropriate distribution among tissues. Essential to the regulation of thyroid function is the free hormone concept because only the unbound hormone has metabolic activity. Given the high binding affinity of thyroid hormones to plasma proteins, variations in the affinities of the hormone-protein interactions or in the concentrations of these proteins have major effects on the total serum hormone levels. Certain drugs and different pathophysiologic conditions can change the binding of thyroid hormones to plasma proteins and the amounts of these proteins. Pharmacists should be able to identify potential drug-drug or drug-disease interactions involving thyroid hormones to provide quality pharmaceutical care.

Thyroxine-Binding Globulin

TBG is the major carrier of thyroid hormones. The protein is encoded by a single gene on the X chromosome, and is produced and cleared by the liver. It is a glycoprotein with a mass of ~63 kDa and a single iodothyronine-binding site. It has a very high affinity for T_4 (K_d is ~10^{-10} M and stoichiometry of 1:1) compared to T_3. Steroid hormones have a remarkable effect on TBG. Estrogen prolongs the biologic half-life of TBG, and thus, it results in increased plasma concentrations of thyroid hormones. Testosterone has the opposite effect.[11] In children and adolescents, this has an implication in diseases with a severe sex hormone overproduction related to age as well as pregnancy and the use of contraceptive in young girls.

Transthyretin

TTR is also known as thyroxine-binding prealbumin, a retinol-binding protein. TTR binds only ~15% to 20% of the circulating thyroid hormones despite the fact its serum concentration is 20-fold higher than that of TBG. TTR binds only T_4, and not T_3, with a K_d value of ~10^{-7} M. Apparently, TTR is responsible for the immediate delivery of T_4. It is also the major thyroid hormone-binding protein in cerebrospinal fluid (CSF). The protein is synthesized in the liver and choroid plexus, and subsequently, is released into blood and CSF, respectively. Each protein molecule has two binding sites for thyroid hormones. Only 0.5% of the circulating TTR is occupied by T_4 with a rapid turnover half-life of 2 days. Importantly, changes in TTR concentration have a relatively minor effect on the serum concentration of serum iodothyronines.

Human Serum Albumin

Human Serum Albumin (HSA) is a 66.5-kD protein synthesized by liver. HSA binds a wide variety of endogenous and exogenous molecules, including hormones and drugs, particularly those with hydrophobic domains. Therefore, the binding of thyroid hormones to HSA is largely nonspecific. Of the several iodothyronine-binding sites on HSA, only one appears to have a relatively high affinity for T_4 and T_3. Yet, these are 10,000-fold inferior to that of TBG. Given the low affinity of thyroid hormones to HAS, its contribution to thyroid hormone transport is relatively minor. Even the most subtle fluctuations in serum concentration of HSA have no significant effects on thyroid hormone levels.[12]

Lipoproteins

Lipoproteins transport a minor fraction of the circulating T_4 and, to some extent, T_3.[13] The affinity for T_4 to lipoproteins appears to be similar to its affinity to TTR. The binding site for thyroid hormones is on apolipoprotein A1 and is different from that of cellular protein receptors.

Metabolism and Excretion

Although thyroid hormones are mainly metabolized by deiodination, other metabolic transformations may happen concurrently. As usual, the primary goal of metabolism is to increase the hydrophilicity of resulting metabolites to promote their excretion renally or through the biliary system. T_4 is eliminated slowly from the body, with a half-life of 6 to 8 days. In hyperthyroidism, the half-life is shortened to 3 to 4 days, whereas in hypothyroidism, it may be 9 to 10 days. In conditions associated with increased binding to TBG, such as pregnancy, clearance is retarded. The opposite effect is observed when binding to

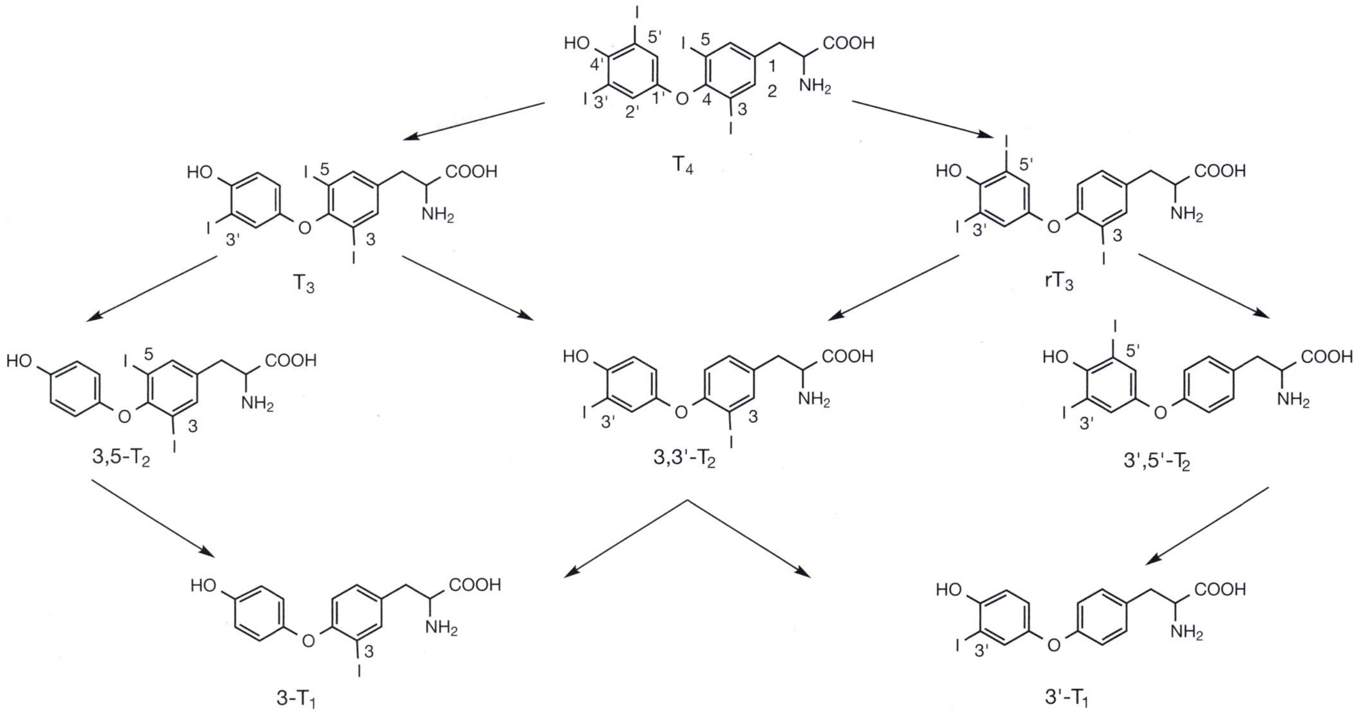

Figure 26.4 Metabolic pathways of deiodination of the iodothyronines by deiodinases. (Modified from reference.[112])

protein is inhibited by certain drugs. T_3, which is less avidly bound to protein, has a half-life of about 18 to 24 hours.

Considering deiodination transformations (Fig. 26.4), the outer ring of the prohormone T_4 can be de-iodinated by 5′-deiodinase, resulting in the formation of T_3, which is biologically active. The inner ring of T_4 can be de-iodinated, resulting in the formation of rT_3, which has no known activity. T_3 and rT_3 can be further de-iodinated at 5-position or 5′-position, respectively, to result in the formation of 3,3′-diiodothyronine. Other metabolic transformations include conjugation of the phenolic group of the outer ring of T_3 and T_4 with glucuronic acid or sulfonate group. These conjugation reactions take place primarily in the liver and, to a lesser extent, in the kidney. On the one hand, the iodothyronine glucuronides are rapidly excreted in bile, but after hydrolysis in the intestine by bacterial β-glucuronidases, part of the released iodothyronine is reabsorbed via the enterohepatic circulation. A portion of the conjugated iodothyronine reaches the colon unchanged, where it is hydrolyzed and eliminated in feces as free molecules. On the other hand, the sulfonates of T_4 and T_3 are normal components of human serum. Although T_3 sulfonate does not bind to nuclear receptors, and therefore, it lacks intrinsic biologic activity, sulfonation of iodothyronines is an important metabolic step in determining their disposal. For example, the majority of normal T_3 disposal occurs via T_3 sulfonate formation. Sulfonation has been also thought of as a mechanism to facilitate the deiodination of iodothyronines. It has been suggested that the function of sulfonation is to deactivate the thyroid hormones so that iodine can be reused for thyroid hormone synthesis. This intriguing idea is supported by the demonstration that the sulfonation of T_4 and T_3, as well as other metabolites, strongly promotes hepatic deiodination.[14]

Ether linkage cleavage is also a mechanism for thyroid hormone degradation, presumably a minor pathway, and one potential product is diiodotyrosine. It is catalyzed by peroxidases and can become an important pathway during infections. Oxidative deamination or decarboxylation of the alanine side chains of T_4 and T_3 are also possible metabolic transformations. Deamination results in the formation of acetic acid derivatives, while decarboxylation results in the formation of the corresponding amine derivatives. The quantity, activity, and contribution to the overall hormonal activity in humans of those derivatives represent an active area of research.[15] The reactions by which thyroid hormones are metabolized are summarized in Figure 26.5.

Physiologic Actions of Thyroid Hormones

Thyroid Hormone and Cellular Membrane

Thyroid hormones enter cells by passive diffusion as well as via specific transporters, which include monocarboxylate 8 transporter (MCT8), MCT10, and organic anion-transporting polypeptide 1C1. After passing through the cellular membrane, thyroid hormones act primarily by binding to nuclear receptors to affect gene expression. They also have nongenomic actions by directly acting on blood vessels and heart via integrin receptors or by stimulating mitochondrial enzymatic responses.

Nuclear Thyroid Hormone Receptors

Thyroid hormone action is mediated largely by the binding of T_3 to THRs, which are members of the nuclear receptor

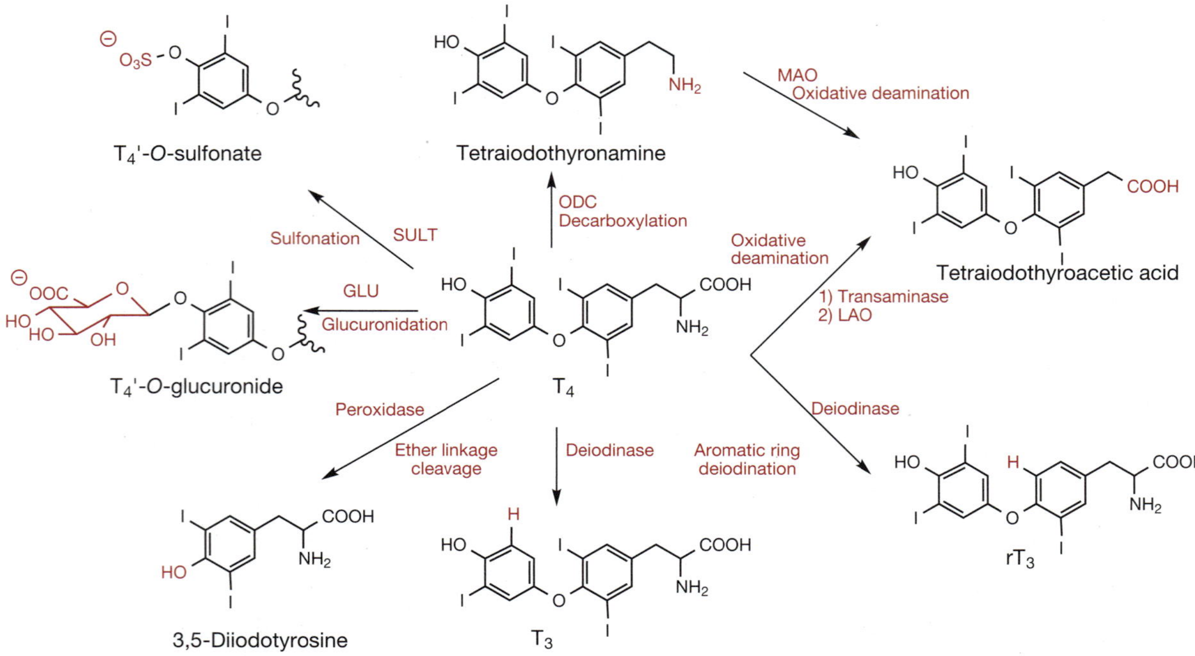

Figure 26.5 Metabolic pathways of T_4. LAO, L-amino acid oxidase; MAO, monoamine oxidase; ODC, ornithine decarboxylase; SULT, sulfotransferase; UGT, uridine 5′-diphosphateglucuronyltransferase. T_3 undergoes similar metabolic pathways.

superfamily of transcription factors. Thyroid hormones bind with high affinity to nuclear THRs α and β. Both THRα and THRβ are expressed in most tissues. THRα is particularly abundant in brain, muscle, heart, kidneys, and gonads, whereas THRβ expression is relatively high in the pituitary and liver. The THRs have the classic nuclear receptor structure of an N-terminal domain, a centrally located zinc finger DNA-binding domain, and a ligand-binding domain that occupies the C-terminal of the protein. They bind to specific DNA sequences known as thyroid-response elements (TREs), in target genes. The receptors bind as homodimers or as heterodimers with retinoic acid X receptors (RXRs). The activated receptor can either stimulate gene transcription or inhibit transcription, depending on the nature of the regulatory elements in the target gene. T_3 is bound with 10 to 15 times greater affinity than T_4, which explains its increased potency. Although T_4 is more abundant than T_3, THRs are occupied mainly by T_3, indicating T_4 to T_3 conversion by peripheral tissues. After binding to THRs, T_3 induces conformational changes in the receptors that modify its interactions with accessory transcription factors. In the absence of T_3 binding, the aporeceptors "unbound THRs" bind to co-repressor proteins that inhibit gene transcription. T_3 promotes the dissociation of the co-repressors and allows the recruitment of co-activators that increase transcription.

Physiologic Effects

Most cells and organs are responsive to the action of thyroid hormones. In general, when the thyroid hormones bind to their nuclear receptors, they activate the genes for increasing metabolic rate and thermogenesis. Increasing metabolic rate involves increased oxygen and energy consumption. Furthermore, their effects depend on protein synthesis as well as potentiation of the secretion and action of growth hormone.

Thyroid hormones are critical for the development and functioning of skeletal, nervous, and reproductive tissues. Thyroid hormones play a critical role in brain development.[16] Thyroid hormones also help with brain maturation by promoting axonal growth and the formation of the myelin sheath.[17] Thyroid deprivation in early life results in irreversible mental retardation and dwarfism. Thyroid hormones are also necessary for both obligatory thermogenesis and adaptive thermogenesis.[18] Thyroid hormones increase the basal metabolic rate. They enhance Na^+/K^+-ATPase expression in different tissues, resulting in elevated oxygen consumption, respiration rate, and body temperature. Depending on the metabolic status, they can promote lipid synthesis or lipolysis. Thyroid hormones stimulate the metabolism of carbohydrates and the anabolism of proteins. Thyroid hormones can also induce catabolism of proteins at high doses. Thyroid hormones do not necessarily change the blood glucose level, yet they can cause increased glucose reabsorption, gluconeogenesis, glycogen synthesis, and glucose oxidation.[19]

In the heart, thyroid hormones have a permissive effect on catecholamines. They increase β-receptors' expression, which subsequently increase heart rate, stroke volume, cardiac output, and contractility.[20] In skeletal muscles, thyroid hormones promote the development of type II muscle fibers, which are fast-twitch muscle fibers capable of fast and powerful contractions. Thyroid hormones also stimulate the respiratory centers, leading to increased oxygenation because of high perfusion.

As far as the skeleton, thyroid hormones act synergistically with growth hormone to stimulate bone growth in children. They induce chondrocytes, osteoblasts, and osteoclasts. Childhood hypothyroidism leads to decreased linear growth, delayed bone age, and epiphyseal dysgenesis.[21] Childhood thyrotoxicosis can cause decreased final height. Adulthood thyrotoxicosis accelerates bone turnover and can increase the risk of osteoporosis. Thyroid hormones also stimulate the expression of hepatic low-density lipoprotein (LDL) receptors and reduce apolipoprotein B levels through non-LDL receptor pathways, which is the reason that hypercholesterolemia is a characteristic of hypothyroidism.

Regulation of Thyroid Hormone Biosynthesis

The amount of circulating thyroid hormones in biologic fluids and in tissues remains constant owing to the relatively long biologic half-life of the thyroid hormones, the regulation by the hypothalamus-pituitary system, and the availability of iodide. Although T_4 represents the main secreted thyroid hormone with a biologic half-life of 1 week and binding potential to plasma proteins of 99.9%, research suggests that T_3 is more potent than T_4. In fact, T_4 is generally considered as a prohormone. Therefore, factors that affect the conversion of T_4 to T_3 in peripheral tissue by deiodinases are highly relevant.

The thyroid gland is under a direct control of the pituitary gland hormone TSH (also known as thyrotropin), a 31-kD glycoprotein composed of α and β subunits; the α subunit is common to the other glycoprotein hormones (luteinizing hormone, follicle-stimulating hormone, human chorionic gonadotropin), whereas the TSH β subunit is unique to TSH. TSH is secreted in a pulsatile manner and in a circadian pattern that is opposite to the cortisol circadian pattern, implying that cortisol reduces TSH secretion. TSH increases the synthesis and secretion of thyroid hormones. Binding of TSH to its G protein-coupled receptor (GPCR) on the plasma membrane of thyroid cells stimulates the G_s-adenylyl cyclase-cyclic AMP pathway. Higher concentrations of TSH activate the G_q-PLC pathway. GPCRs are presented in more detail in Chapter 6.

TSH secretion is largely dictated by the hypothalamic peptide TRH. TRH is a tripeptide (L-pyroglutamyl-L-histidyl-L-proline amide) biosynthesized by the hypothalamus and secreted into the hypophyseal-portal circulation, and, eventually, it interacts with TRH receptors on thyrotropes of the anterior pituitary. TRH binding to its GPCR receptor stimulates the G_q–PLC–IP_3–Ca^{2+} pathway, activates protein kinase C, and ultimately stimulates the synthesis and release of TSH. TSH secretion is also dictated by the concentration of free thyroid hormones in the circulation. On the one hand, elevated thyroid hormone inhibits the transcription of genes encoding for TRH and TSH. This suppresses the secretion of TSH, and subsequently, the release of thyroid hormones in a classical feedback inhibition. On the other hand, reduced thyroid hormone secretion by the thyroid gland causes an increased secretion of TSH. Figure 26.6 illustrates some aspects of the feedback inhibition regulation mechanism as well as the chemical structure of TRH.

The amount of iodide available for hormone synthesis is also an important regulator of the gland function. In the

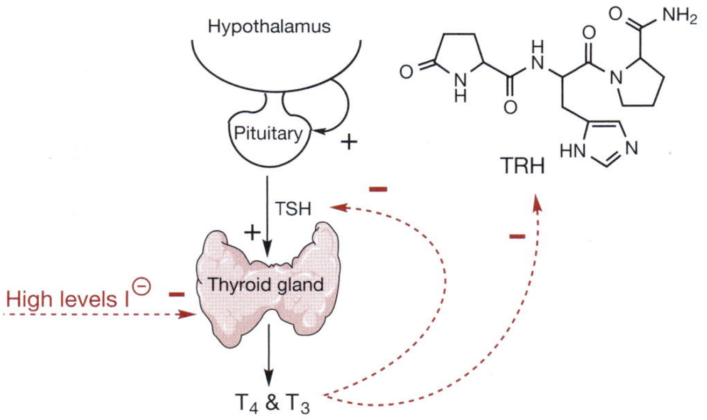

Figure 26.6 Hypothalamic-pituitary-thyroid axis from which thyroid hormones are released is promoted by TRH from the hypothalamus and then TSH from the pituitary. The figure also illustrates the feedback inhibition regulation mechanism by thyroid hormones as well as the chemical structure of TRH.

case of iodide deficiency, thyroid hormones biosynthesis is decreased, which triggers TSH secretion via a feedback mechanism. The rise in TSH concentration stimulates the biosynthesis of thyroid hormones by increasing the iodide pump efficiency and the biosynthesis of thyroglobulin as well as TPO. When iodide deficiency is severe, a persistent rise in TSH is observed, which results in thyroid gland overgrowth. In the case of excessive circulating iodide, the absolute amount of iodide in thyroid gland remains tentatively constant. Furthermore, there is an increase in the amount of the iodide leaked from the gland and a decrease in the iodide taken up by the gland. In addition, there may be a decrease in the formation of iodinated thyroglobulin residues and in the release of hormones from the gland. The decrease in the formation of iodinated thyroglobulin residues that takes place with excessive amounts of iodide is known as Wolff-Chaikoff block.[22] This phenomenon is caused by the interaction between iodide and NADPH, which decreases follicular NADPH and hydrogen peroxide needed for TPO activation.[23] When iodide is given pharmacologically in milligram quantities, the decrease in thyroid hormone release lasts only a few weeks.

The activity of deiodinases reflects the thyroid status. In hypothyroidism, there is a decrease in hepatic 5′-deiodinase I but an increase in 5′-deiodinase II activity.[23] After hepatic disease,[24] renal damage,[25] chronic illnesses,[26] or starvation,[27] there is a decrease in T_3 and rT_3, suggesting a reduced activity of 5′-deiodinase I. The mechanism of deiodinase control appears to be complex and may involve adrenergic aspects, given the inhibitory effects of propranolol (β-blocker) and prazosin (α_1-blocker) on 5′-deiodinase I[28] and 5′-deiodinase II,[29] respectively. Furthermore, the rapid change in the deiodinase activity observed after asphyxia suggests c-AMP-mediated regulation.[30]

Several other factors may also influence the secretion of thyroid hormones. For example, a cold environment triggers TSH secretion, which subsequently enhances thyroid hormones release. This is in line with the established role of the thyroid gland in sparking body heat production. Moreover, several growth factors also influence thyroid hormone synthesis. These include insulin-like growth factor 1 (IGF-1), transforming growth factor β (TGF-β), epidermal growth factor, endothelins, and various cytokines. These factors are important in selected disease states. For example, increased levels of growth hormone and IGF-1 are associated with goiter and predisposition to multinodular goiter. Certain cytokines and interleukins are produced in autoimmune thyroid disease and induce thyroid growth, while others promote apoptosis.

Thyroid Diseases and Therapeutic Interventions

Thyroid diseases are associated with either inadequate production (hypothyroidism) or overproduction (hyperthyroidism) of thyroid hormones. Generally, thyroid dysfunction is one of the most common endocrine diseases encountered in clinical practice. For example, about 12% of the US population is likely to be affected by a thyroid disorder in their lifetime.[31] Women are up to 10 times more likely to experience thyroid disorders than men, and thyroid disorders can have a significant impact on a woman's health, contributing to complications pertaining to menstruation, fertility, and pregnancy. As far as the cost of disease burden, direct health care costs in the United States for women older than age 18 years being treated for thyroid disease in the year of 2008 were estimated at $4.3 billion. Although abnormally low or high levels of thyroid hormones can be tolerated for a long time, there are obvious symptoms and signs of overt thyroid dysfunction. While nonpharmacologic interventions such as diet and dietary supplements may assist in the management of symptoms of certain thyroid diseases,[32,33] therapeutic interventions are often needed and involve the use of certain medications or procedures.

Thyroid Diseases: Hypothyroidism

Hypothyroidism is the most common disorder of thyroid function. Severe cases of hypothyroidism are known as myxedema. Hypothyroidism resulting from iodine deficiency remains a common problem worldwide. However, chronic autoimmune thyroiditis, also known as Hashimoto thyroiditis, accounts for most cases of hypothyroidism in areas of iodine sufficiency. Hashimoto thyroiditis is characterized by circulating antibodies targeting thyroid peroxidase and, sometimes, thyroglobulin. These conditions are examples of thyroid gland failure, also known as "primary hypothyroidism." Autoimmune hypothyroidism can be associated with goiter (goitrous thyroiditis) or minimal residual thyroid tissue (atrophic thyroiditis). The mean annual incidence rate of autoimmune hypothyroidism is up to 4 per 1,000 women and 1 per 1,000 men. It is more common in certain populations, such as Japanese, which can be attributed to genetic factors and chronic exposure to a high iodine diet. In the Third National Health and Nutrition Examination Survey III, levels of serum TSH and total T_4 were measured in a representative sample of adolescents and adults who neither were taking thyroid medication nor reported histories of thyroid disease. About 3.9% had subclinical hypothyroidism (serum TSH >4.5 mIU/L, and T_4 normal), and 0.2% had clinically significant hypothyroidism (TSH >4.5 mIU/L, and T4 <4.5 mcg/dL).[34] Central hypothyroidism may also occur. It occurs much less often and results from reduced stimulation of the thyroid gland by TSH attributed to pituitary failure, known as "secondary hypothyroidism," or hypothalamic failure, known as "tertiary hypothyroidism." Congenital hypothyroidism occurs at birth in about 1 in 2,000 to 4,000 newborns, and it is a significantly preventable cause of intellectual disability.[35,36]

Other causes of acquired hypothyroidism include thyroid ablation, thyroid surgery, ^{131}I treatment for hyperthyroidism, exposure to external beam radiation therapy for head and neck cancers, and medications such as amiodarone, lithium, and tyrosine kinase inhibitors.[37] Antithyroid medications such as propylthiouracil and methimazole may produce hypothyroidism. Pregnant women can develop hypothyroidism, hyperthyroidism, thyroid nodule, goiter, and thyroid cancer. Overt hypothyroidism and hyperthyroidism during pregnancy are responsible for adverse obstetric and neonatal complications. Postpartum thyroiditis can develop during the first 6 to 12 months after delivery in women who were euthyroid during pregnancy.[38]

Frequently occurring symptoms of hypothyroidism include fatigue, lethargy, mental slowness, depression, cold intolerance, dry skin, muscle aches and stiffness, constipation, mild weight gain, fluid retention, irregular menses, and infertility. Common signs include goiter in case of primary hypothyroidism, bradycardia, hypertension, nonpitting edema, delayed relaxation phase of the deep tendon reflexes, dry and cool skin, and facial puffiness. Elevated levels of bad cholesterol (LDL) are also a problem. Deficiency of thyroid hormone in newborns causes feeding problems, constipation, sleepiness, and failure to thrive. If not treated promptly, impairment of mental development becomes irreversible, known as congenital hypothyroidism (formerly known as cretinism). Childhood hypothyroidism weakens linear growth and bone maturation. Because the signs and symptoms of hypothyroidism are nonspecific, diagnosis requires the finding of reduced or low-normal serum free T_4 and/or an elevated serum level of TSH.[31,39]

Treatment of Hypothyroidism

Goals of therapeutic interventions in hypothyroidism are to alleviate symptoms, restore thyroid hormone levels, minimize the long-term damage to organs, prevent serious complications such as myxedema coma and heart disease, prevent neurologic deficits in newborns and children, and improve overall quality of life. Although there are no specific nonpharmacologic treatments for the management of hypothyroidism, the control of foods with goitrogenic properties may help in the management of certain conditions. Particularly, there is growing evidence supporting the use of selenium in a variety of hypothyroid conditions.[32] Inadequate dietary iodine intake represents a major global cause of subclinical and overt symptomatic hypothyroidism, and thus, dietary intake should be considered.[40] The World Health Organization recommends a daily dietary iodine intake of 150 μg for adults, 200 μg for pregnant and lactating women, and 50 to 120 μg for children.[41]

Thyroid Replacement Therapy

Therapeutically, hypothyroidism is typically treated with thyroid hormone replacement. Thyroid hormone drugs are natural or synthetic preparations. These preparations contain the sodium salt of T_4 known as levothyroxine (Levoxyl and Synthroid), the sodium salt of T_3 known as liothyronine (Cytomel), or the natural combination of T_4 and T_3 (Armour Thyroid). Natural hormonal preparations include desiccated thyroid and thyroglobulin. Desiccated thyroid is derived from domesticated animals used by humans for food, which can be either bovine (cow) or porcine (pig) thyroid; thyroglobulin is derived from the pig's thyroid glands. The United States Pharmacopeia (USP) has standardized the total iodine content of natural preparations. Thyroid USP contains no less than 0.17% and no more than 0.23% iodine, and thyroglobulin contains no less than 0.7% organically bound iodine. Iodine content is an indirect indicator of the true hormonal biologic activity. A large number of organic and inorganic molecules affect thyroid hormone formation by interfering with the iodide uptake into follicular cells, inhibiting TPO, preventing thyroid hormone binding to plasma proteins, or affecting deiodinases. Therefore, treating hypothyroidism must include limiting or modifying the dose regimen of these other molecules that are concurrently used for therapeutic, diagnostic, or experimental purposes. Overall, hormone replacement remains to be the established therapy in the treatment of various forms of hypothyroidism, from goiter and cretinism to the complete absence of thyroid function in myxedema.

Natural Thyroid Hormone Preparations (Armour Thyroid, NP Thyroid)

Natural preparations include desiccated thyroid and thyroglobulin. Desiccated thyroid is derived from domesticated animals used by humans for food; thyroglobulin is derived from porcine thyroid glands. Upon oral administration, MIT, DIT, T_3, T_4 are released by the proteolytic activity of digestive enzymes. Potency is dependent on iodine content and is somewhat variable among different preparations. The shelf life of desiccated thyroid is not exactly known, but its potency is better preserved if the preparation is kept under anhydrous conditions.

Desiccated thyroid preparations (Thyroid USP) are essentially acetone powders of bovine or porcine thyroid glands compressed into oral tablets. A diluent is usually present because the preparations (especially of porcine origin) commonly exceed the iodine content of 0.17% to 0.23% required by the USP. Because the iodine in these preparations is in the form of iodinated tyrosine or thyronine residues, the preparation efficacy is attributed to the hormones that are released by the action of intestinal proteases. Desiccated preparations are reported to have a ratio of T_4 and T_3 similar to the ratio in humans (about 4:1). Desiccated preparations are less expensive than synthetic ones, but have been shown to produce variable blood levels of T_4 and T_3 because of variabilities between and within animal sources of thyroid gland. Although many aspects are similar for partially purified thyroglobulin, the total and relative amounts of T_3 and T_4 are different. Importantly, the use of desiccated thyroid is hardly justified over synthetic preparations, given the disadvantages of protein antigenicity, product instability, variable hormone concentrations, and difficulty in laboratory monitoring. High amounts of T_3 can be found in some thyroid extracts and may produce significant elevations in T_3 levels and toxicity. Nonetheless, a large-scale assessment of patient satisfaction with hormone replacement found that patients were more satisfied with desiccated thyroid than with T_4 or T_4/T_3 combination. Approximate equivalence of desiccated thyroid 60 mg (one grain) to 80 to 100 μg of T_4, and approximately 37.5 μg of T_3 has been reported.

As a point of regulation, the U.S. Food and Drug Administration (FDA) recently designated the natural thyroid hormone preparations as biologics, requiring a Biologics License Application (BLA) by 2029.

Synthetic Thyroid Hormones

Synthetic, crystalline thyroid hormones are more uniformly absorbed than natural preparations and contain more accurately measured amounts of active ingredients. T_4, T_3, and T_4/T_3 mixture are commonly used. Importantly, the shelf life of synthetic hormones is ~2 years, particularly if they are stored in dark bottles to minimize spontaneous deiodination. Table 26.2 describes some properties and pharmacokinetics of T_4 (Levothyroxine) and T_3 (Liothyronine).

Levothyroxine Sodium (Levoxyl and Synthroid)

The chemistry and mechanism of action are identical to those of endogenous T_4 and have been presented. The drug can be used orally or parenterally. Levothyroxine sodium is approved as replacement or supplemental therapy in congenital or acquired hypothyroidism of any etiology. Specific indications include primary (thyroidal), secondary (pituitary), and tertiary (hypothalamic) hypothyroidism. Levothyroxine monotherapy is recommended as the preferred thyroid preparation for the treatment of hypothyroidism. It is also approved for use as an adjunct to surgery and radioiodine therapy in the management of thyrotropin-dependent well-differentiated thyroid cancer. Injectable forms are also available to treat myxedema coma. Levothyroxine is the preferred treatment of maternal hypothyroidism. There are 11 different tablet strengths, ranging from 25 to 300 μg, which allows individual dosing.[42,43]

Potentially life-threatening cardiovascular effects may occur with levothyroxine.[44] Several dose-related mechanisms are proposed, including abnormal myocardial response to catecholamines and increased number and sensitivity of adrenergic receptors in the cardiovascular system.[45,46] Precautions should be taken when the medication is given to older adult patients as well as patients with thyroid hypersensitivity, diabetes, or osteoporosis. The drug is contraindicated in patients with uncorrected adrenal insufficiency. A boxed warning exists against the use of all forms of thyroid gland hormones as treatment for obesity or for weight loss.

Following oral administration, onset of action is 3 to 5 days, and peak therapeutic effect may require 4 to 6 weeks. Following intravenous administration, peak therapeutic effect takes place within 6 to 8 hours. Oral

Table 26.2 Some Properties and Pharmacokinetics for Levothyroxine and Liothyronine[a]

Parameter	Levothyroxine	Liothyronine
Trade name	Levoxyl Synthroid	Cytomel Triostat
pKa (phenolic)[b]	4.7	6.9
CLogP[b]	3.5	2.6
Oral bioavailability	Capsules, tablets 40%-80%; Solution 98% Fasting increases absorption, soybean and infant formula decrease absorption, dietary fiber decreases bioavailability	Tablet 95%
Time to peak concentration	2-4 h	1-2 h
Peak response	Several weeks in hypothyroidism	2-3 d
Volume of distribution	8.7-9.7 L	41-45 L
Protein binding	>99%	Not firmly bound
Metabolism	Mainly hepatic: ~80%, deiodination to T_3, conjugation, and undergoes enterohepatic recirculation	Hepatic, and primarily to de-iodinated and conjugated metabolites
Elimination half-life	6-8 d 3-4 d (hyperthyroidism) 9-10 d (hypothyroidism)	Adult 25 h, pediatric 7 h 16-49 h in euthyroid patients 1.4 d in hypothyroid patients 0.6 d in hyperthyroid patients
Total body clearance	0.84-1.37 L/d	20-36 L/d
Excretion	Primarily renal (50%), it decreases with age Feces (20%-50%), ~20% unchanged fecal excretion	Primarily renal (76%-83%)

[a]Merative Micromedex 2023.
[b]ChemDraw Professional 22.0.0.

absorption is erratic (40%-80%). Reported bioavailability in fasting state is 79% to 81%. Absorption may decrease by age, specific foods, and drugs. Given the amino acid nature of levothyroxine, concomitant administration of positively charged drugs such as bile acid sequestrants (colesevelam, cholestyramine, and colestipol) or negatively charged drugs such as polystyrene sulfonate and sucralfate should be avoided, and an appropriate time gap should be allowed. Furthermore, polyvalent-containing preparations may chelate with the amino acid moiety of levothyroxine, resulting in compromised oral absorption. Therefore, therapy modification is advised with concurrent use of calcium-containing, iron-containing, or magnesium-containing preparations. Taking levothyroxine with enteral nutrition may cause reduced bioavailability and may lower serum thyroxine levels. Soybean flour, grapefruit juice, espresso coffee, cottonseed meal, walnuts, and dietary fiber may interfere with absorption of levothyroxine from the gastrointestinal (GI) tract. Levothyroxine should be taken in the morning on an empty stomach at least 30 minutes before food or at night 3 to 4 hours after the last meal.[42,47]

More than 99% is bound to plasma proteins, including thyroxine-binding globulin, thyroxine-binding prealbumin, and albumin. Time to peak in serum is 2 to 4 hours. Because of its binding to plasma carrier proteins, crystalline levothyroxine sodium salt has a slower onset of action than crystalline T_3 or a desiccated thyroid preparation. Its administration leads to a greater increase in serum T_4 but a lesser increase in serum T_3 compared to USP thyroid.[48] Levothyroxine is metabolized as described by deiodination (to T_3) and conjugation (glucuronidation and sulfonation). The drug undergoes enterohepatic recirculation. Elimination half-life is dependent on patient status, and it is 6 to 8 days, 9 to 10 days, and 3 to 4 days in euthyroid, hypothyroid, and hyperthyroid patients, respectively. The major route of elimination is the urine, which decreases with age. About 20% is eliminated unchanged in feces.

Liothyronine Sodium (Cytomel and Triostat)

The chemistry and mechanism of action are identical to those of endogenous T_3 and have been presented. The drug can be used orally or parenterally. Liothyronine sodium is approved as replacement therapy in primary, secondary, and tertiary, congenital, or acquired hypothyroidism. It is also used as a diagnostic agent in suppression tests to differentiate suspected mild hyperthyroidism or thyroid gland autonomy. Intravenous liothyronine sodium is also available to treat myxedema coma. It can be used off-label for antidepressant augmentation.[49]

Following oral administration, onset of action is within a few hours, and peak response is achieved within 2 to 3 days. The drug is well absorbed (95% in 4 hours). Its elimination half-life is 16 to 49 hours, and is eliminated primarily in the urine. Accordingly, liothyronine is more frequently used for thyroid hormone replacement when a rapid onset of action is desired, such as in myxedema coma, or if rapid termination of action is desired, such as when preparing a patient with thyroid cancer for ^{131}I therapy. It is also potentially used in patients with heart diseases. Liothyronine is less desirable than levothyroxine for chronic therapy due to the higher cost, more frequent dosing, and transient elevations of serum T_3 concentrations.[50]

Liotrix (Thyrolar)

A synthetic mixture of T_4 and T_3, around 4:1 by weight, is also available. The combination is used to treat hypothyroidism and to diagnose thyroid disorders. It is also used in the treatment or prevention of various types of euthyroid goiters, including thyroid nodules, subacute or chronic lymphocytic thyroiditis, multinodular goiter, and in the management of thyroid cancer. It has also been used in combination with antithyroid agents for the treatment of thyrotoxicosis to prevent goitrogenesis and hypothyroidism.

Conformational Properties of Thyroid Hormones and Their Analogs

The importance of the diphenyl ether conformation for the biologic activity of thyroid hormones was first proposed by Zenker and Jorgensen.[51,52] Using computational work, they showed that a perpendicular orientation of the aromatic rings of 3,5-diiodothyronines would be favored to minimize steric clashes between the bulky 3,5-iodines and the 2′,6′-hydrogens. In the perpendicular orientation, the 3′- and 5′-positions of the outer ring are not conformationally equivalent, and the 3′-iodine of T_3 could be oriented either distally (away from) or proximally (close to) the alanine side chain of the inner ring (Fig. 26.7). This is true because of the free rotation around the ether bridge. Accordingly, to identify whether the distal or proximal 3′-iodine is favored, analogs of 3′,5′-dimethyl-3,5-diiodothyronine were synthesized with an alkyl group at 3′-position, alkyl or iodine group at 5′-position, and a methyl group at 2′-position to block the rotation around the ether bridge. The analogs were then evaluated in the antigoiter assay. Analogs with a locked distal 3′-substitutent were 2′,3′dimethyl-3,5-DL-diiodothyronine (derivative I) and O-(4′-hydroxy-1′-naphthyl)-3,5-DL-diiodotyrosine (derivative II). Analogs with locked proximal 5′-substituent were 2′,5′dimethyl-3,5-DL-diiodothyronine (derivative III) and 2′-methyl-3,5,5′-DL-iodothyronine (derivative IV). All structures are given in Figure 26.7. The antigoiter activities

Table 26.3 Effectiveness of Distal and Proximal Thyroid Hormone Derivatives in Antigoiter Assay

Derivative[a]	Dose (mg/kg/d)	%T_4 Activity
I	0.025	50
II	0.013	>100
III	2.3	<1
IV	0.5	2

[a]See text and Figure 26.7 for the specific description and structures of derivatives I-IV.

of these derivatives are presented in Table 26.3 and suggest that the distal 3′-substitution is favorable for thyromimetic activity.[53,54]

In addition to being perpendicular to the inner ring, the outer ring can assume a *cisoid* or *transoid* orientation relative to the alanine side chain (see Fig. 26.7). Although the bioactive conformation of the alanine side chain in thyroid hormone analogs is yet to be determined, the conformations appear to be energetically similar, given their natural existence in thyroid active structures as determined by x-ray crystallography.[55] The synthesis of conformationally locked cyclic or unsaturated analogs may allow the evaluation of the bioactivity of the *cisoid* and *transoid* conformers.

Transthyretin Receptor Model and Thyroid Analogs Design

An important model that has been utilized to assist in designing thyromimetics is the TTR receptor or thyroxine-binding prealbumin (TBPA) model. TTR is a serum and CSF protein carrier of thyroid hormones as well as vitamin A (retinol). TTR is secreted by the liver into the blood as well as by the choroid plexus into the CSF. It was originally named prealbumin, given its behavior on electrophoresis gels, but later the name was changed when it was discovered to transport thyroxine and retinol.

Importantly, TTR has been found to bind as much as 27% of plasma T_3.[56] The amino acid sequence of the TTR-T_3 binding site is known, and the protein has therefore served as a tentative model of the T_3 receptor. This model portrays T_3 placed in an envelope near the axis of symmetry of the TTR dimer. Hydrophobic residues, such as Leu and Ala, form pockets to accommodate the 3,5,3′- and 5′-positions of T_3, whereas the hydrophilic groups of Ser and Thr residues, hydrogen bonded to water, are between the 3′- substituent and the phenolic group at position-4′. For example, this model has been used to devise the design of 3′-acetyl-3,5-diiodothyronine as a new thyroid receptor-binding agent (Fig. 26.8). Despite the fact that the formation of a receptor-phenol hydrogen bond is precluded by the presence of a strong intramolecular hydrogen bond between the 3′-acetyl- and 4′-hydroxyl group, which resulted in reduced affinity to

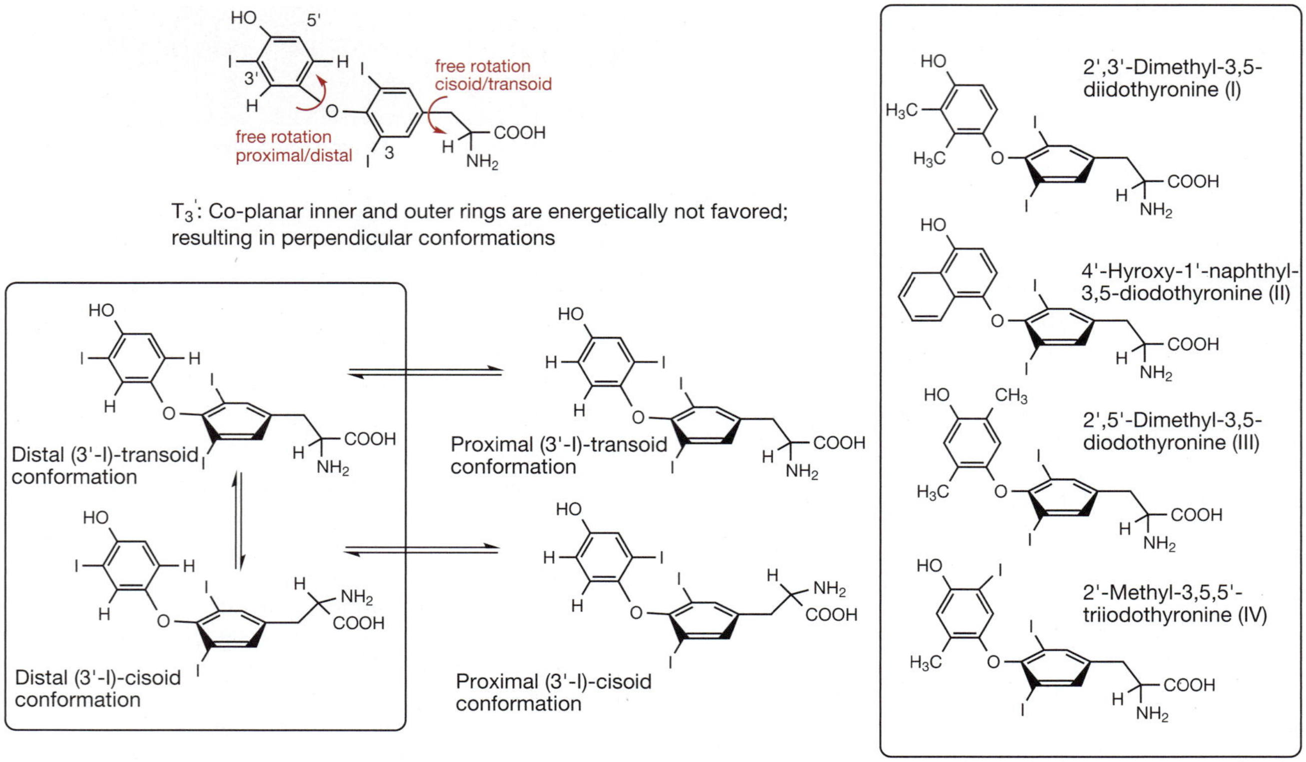

Figure 26.7 Co-planar orientation of the two rings in thyroid hormones (in this case T_3) is not energetically favored. Free rotations around the designated bonds result in the formation of distal and proximal orientations, considering the 3′-position as well as *cisoid* and *transoid* conformations of the alanine side chain. The distal conformations of T_3 are favored as indicated by the results of antigoiter assay for T_3 derivatives (I-IV). See Table 26.3 for results. Note that amino acid groups are presented in a neutral form for simplicity, although they may exist in ionized forms under physiologic conditions.

the T_3-receptor in isolated rat hepatic nuclei, the agent demonstrated that thyromimetic activity (assessed by its ability to induce rat hepatic glycerol-3-phosphate dehydrogenase and increased oxygen uptake by liver slices) was roughly equal to that of T_3.[57,58]

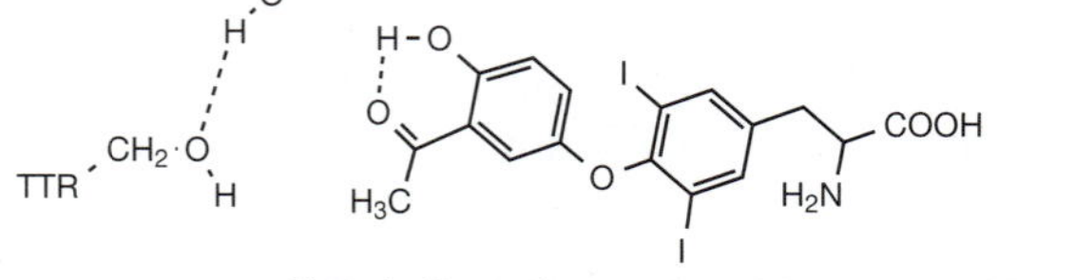

3'-Deiodinated, acetylated derivative of T_3

Figure 26.8 Depiction of a potential hydrogen bond interaction between the phenolic group at position-4′ of T_3 based on a TTR receptor model. Using the same model, it was demonstrated that 3′-deiodinated, acetylated derivative of T_3 may lose such interaction to intramolecular hydrogen bonding between the same phenolic group and the adjacent carbonyl oxygen of the acetyl group, which suggested a weaker affinity for the new derivative. Although that was the case, the new derivative demonstrated thyromimetic activity that was roughly equal to that of T_3 in a rat model.

Structure-Activity Relationships of Thyroid Hormone Analogs

The chemical synthesis and biologic evaluation of a large number of T_3 and T_4 analogs enabled medicinal chemists to understand how chemical structural features dictate thyroid hormonal activity. Such evolving understanding is essential to ultimately develop more clinically relevant molecules, in the near future. In general, single ring derivatives such as DIT and its aliphatic and alicyclic ether derivatives showed no T_4-like activity in the rat antigoiter test, the method most often used to determine thyromimetic activity in vivo.[59,60] Only analogs with the appropriately substituted phenyl-X-phenyl scaffold have demonstrated significant thyroid hormonal activity. The key findings are summarized in Table 26.4 and are described in following sections, considering modifications in five structural domains: (1) aliphatic side chain, (2) 3-and 5-substituents of the inner ring, (3) the bridging atom, (4) 3′- and 5′-substituents of the outer ring, and (5) 4′-substituent (phenolic) of the outer ring.

Modifications of the Aliphatic Side Chain

The naturally occurring thyroid hormones are biosynthesized from L-tyrosine, and thus, they possess the L-alanine side chain. The L-isomers of T_4 and T_3 (molecules 1 and 3 in Table 26.4) are more active than the corresponding D-isomers (molecules 2 and 4). In the case of T_4, the L-isomer is about 6-fold more potent than the corresponding D-isomer. However, the L-isomer of T_3 is about 13.5-fold more potent than the corresponding D-isomer. Interestingly, L-T_3 is 5.5-fold more potent than L-T_4,

Table 26.4 Structure-Activity Relationship of Thyromimetics

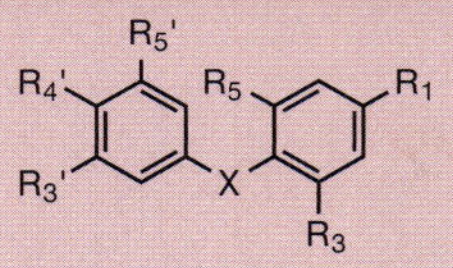

Analog	R_1	R_3	R_5	X	$R_{3'}$	$R_{5'}$	$R_{4'}$	Antigoiter Activity[a]
1 (L-T_4)	L-Ala	I	I	O	I	I	OH	100
2 (D-T_4)	D-Ala	I	I	O	I	I	OH	17
3 (L-T_3)	L-Ala	I	I	O	I	H	OH	550
4 (D-T_3)	D-Ala	I	I	O	I	H	OH	41
5	COOH	I	I	O	I	I	OH	0.1
6	COOH	I	I	O	I	H	OH	0.4
7	CH_2COOH	I	I	O	I	I	OH	50
8	CH_2COOH	I	I	O	I	H	OH	36
9	$(CH_2)_2COOH$	I	I	O	I	I	OH	15
10	$(CH_2)_2COOH$	I	I	O	I	H	OH	20
11	$(CH_2)_3COOH$	I	I	O	I	I	OH	4
12	$(CH_2)_3COOH$	I	I	O	I	H	OH	5
13	$(CH_2)_2NH_2$	I	I	O	I	I	OH	0.6
14	$(CH_2)_2NH_2$	I	I	O	I	H	OH	6
15	L-Ala	H	H	O	I	I	OH	<0.01
16	L-Ala	H	H	O	I	H	OH	<0.01
17	DL-Ala	Br	Br	O	I	H	OH	93
18	L-Ala	Br	Br	O	iPr	H	OH	166
19	L-Ala	Me	Me	O	Me	H	OH	3
20	L-Ala	Me	Me	O	iPr	H	OH	20
21	DL-Ala	iPr	iPr	O	I	H	OH	0
22	DL-Ala	sBu	sBu	O	I	H	OH	0
23	DL-Ala	I	I	-	I	I	OH	0
24	DL-Ala	I	I	S	I	H	OH	132
25	DL-Ala	I	I	CH_2	I	H	OH	300
26	L-Ala	I	I	O	H	H	OH	5
27	L-Ala	I	I	O	OH	H	OH	1.5
28	L-Ala	I	I	O	NO_2	H	OH	<1
29	DL-Ala	I	I	O	F	H	OH	6
30	L-Ala	I	I	O	Cl	H	OH	27
31	DL-Ala	I	I	O	Br	H	OH	132
32	L-Ala	I	I	O	Me	H	OH	80
33	L-Ala	I	I	O	Et	H	OH	517

(continued)

Table 26.4 Structure-Activity Relationship of Thyromimetics (*continued*)

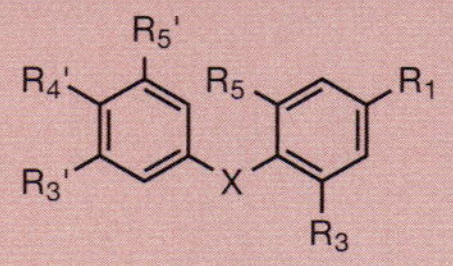

Analog	R_1	R_3	R_5	X	$R_{3'}$	$R_{5'}$	$R_{4'}$	Antigoiter Activity[a]
34	L-Ala	I	I	O	iPr	H	OH	786
35	L-Ala	I	I	O	nPr	H	OH	200
36	DL-Ala	I	I	O	Phe	H	OH	11
37	DL-Ala	I	I	O	F	F	OH	2.3
38	L-Ala	I	I	O	Cl	Cl	OH	21
39	L-Ala	I	I	O	I	H	NH_2	<1.5
40	DL-Ala	I	I	O	I	H	H	>150
41	DL-Ala	I	I	O	Me	H	CH_3	0
42	L-Ala	I	I	O	I	H	OCH_3	225

[a]See Ekins[56] and Ahmad et al.[57] In vivo activity in rats relative to L-T_4 = 100% or DL-T_4 = 100% for goiter prevention.

whereas D-T_3 is 2.5-fold more potent than D-T_4. Moreover, although the carboxylate and amino groups are important for activity, it appears that the carboxylate group is more important than the amino group. For example, the T_4 analog lacking the amino group (analog 9) is about 7-fold less potent than L-T_4 (hormone 1) but is equipotent to D-T_4 (analog 2). In contrast, T_4 analog lacking the carboxylate group (analog 13) is about 167-fold less potent than Ll-T_4 and about 28-fold less potent than D-T_4. A similar trend is seen with T_3 analogs. The T_3 analog lacking the amino group (analog 10) is about 27.5-fold less potent than L-T_3 (hormone 3) but is only 2-fold less potent than D-T_3 (analog 4). In contrast, the T_3 analog lacking the carboxylate group (analog 14) is about 92-fold less potent than L-T_3 and about 7-fold less potent than D-T_3. Interestingly, the distance between the carboxylate group and the inner ring is also important, and a one-atom linker to make an acetic acid side chain appears to be the optimal distance in the two series of T_4 analogs and T_3 analogs (analogs 7 and 8). Analogs with no linker (carboxylate group directly connected to the ring—ie, benzoic acid derivatives, analogs 5 and 6) possess very poor antigoiter activity. Analogs with longer linkers (ie, two-atom propanoic acid derivatives, analogs 9 and 10) and three-atom butanoic acid derivatives (analogs 11 and 12) possess relatively weak antigoiter activity. Lastly, analogs of T_3 in which the alanine side chain is transposed with 3-iodine substituent or occupies the 2-position were inactive in the rat antigoiter test,[61] suggesting the critical spatial *para* relationship between the alanine side chain and the outer ring—that is, alanine side chain is at 1-position and the outer ring is at 4-position.

Modification of the Inner Ring

The inner ring is also labeled the α-ring, and it is substituted with two iodine substituents at the 3- and 5-positions in both T_4 and T_3. As shown in Table 26.4, the removal of these iodine substituents led to analogs 3′,5′-T_2 (analog 15) or 3′-T_1 (analog 16) that lack T_4-like activity. The loss of activity was attributed to the loss of the perpendicular orientation of the diphenyl ether conformation. Interestingly, replacement of the iodine substituents on the inner ring with two bromine substituents maintained the antigioter activity. For example, the racemic, 3,5-dibromo analog of T_3 (analog 17) possesses substantial activity. Analogs with other halogen substituents (such as chlorine or iodine) have not been reported. However, the replacement of iodine substituents with alkyl groups such as isopropyl (analog 21) or sec-butyl (analog 22) resulted in inactive analogs. The substantial difference in the activity between DL-T_3 analogs is very interesting, given that iodine and bromine substituents as well as isopropyl and sec-butyl substituents are large and lipophilic ones and placed at the appropriate positions to attain the required perpendicular orientation of the two rings. This may suggest that iodine (or bromine) substituents at the 3- and 5-positions are not only essential because of their lipophilic and steric contributions, but it is also because of their electronic contribution. Iodine and bromine are electron-withdrawing groups in contrast to the alkyl groups, which are electron-releasing groups. This may indicate that having an electronically deficient inner ring is preferable for antigoiter activity.

Modifications of the Bridging Atom

Several analogs were synthesized in which the ether oxygen bridge has been removed or replaced by another atom. The analogs were evaluated in the rat antigoiter test. The biphenyl analog of T_4 (analog 23), which was formed by the removal of the oxygen bridge, was completely inactive. The inactivity is attributed to the drastic change in the shape of the analog, which assumes a coplanar (flat) orientation rather than the perpendicular orientation found in the natural thyroid hormones. Furthermore, in a bivalent classical bioisosterism exercise, replacement of the ether oxygen with thioether (analog 24), or with a methylene group (analog 25) resulted in analogs with greatly enhanced antigoiter activity. These results have challenged the Niemann quinoid theory, which postulates that the ability of the molecule to form a quinoid structure in the phenolic ring is essential for thyromimetic activity and have emphasized the important of the three-dimensional structure of the hormones and analogs and their ability to fit the receptor. Lastly, it appears that attempts to replace the ether oxygen with an amino group or carbonyl group in T_4 and T_3 analogs have been unsuccessful.[62,63]

Modifications of the Outer Ring

The outer ring, also called the β-ring, of the thyronine scaffold is essential for hormonal activity. Variations in 3′- and/or 5′- substituents have dramatic effects on biologic activity and the affinity for the nuclear receptor. The unsubstituted L-T_2 (analog 26) possesses 20-fold less activity than L-T_4 and 110-fold less activity than T_3. Substitution at 3′-position by hydroxyl (analog 27) or nitro (analog 28) groups almost abolishes the activity owing to a lowered lipophilicity and intramolecular hydrogen bonding with the 4′-hydroxyl.[64] In contrast, substitution by halogen or alkyl groups results in an increase in thyromimetic activity in a proportional relation to bulkiness and lipophilicity of the substituent (F $<$Cl $<$Br $<$ I and CH_3 $<CH_2CH_3$ $<CH[CH_3]_2$). 3′-Isopropylthyronine (analog 34) is the most potent analog known with about 1.4-fold activity of L-T_3. However, 3′-n-propylthyronine (analog 35) is only about 0.25-fold as active as 3′-isopropylthyronine, suggesting size restriction at 3′-position. This is further supported by the fact that 3′-phenylthyronine (analog 36) possesses very weak activity. In relation to the monosubstituted 3′-fluorothyronine (analog 29) and 3′-chlorothyronine (analog 30), the disubstituted 3′,5′-difluorothyronine (analog 37) and 3′,5′-dichlorothyronine (analog 38) have reduced thyromimetic activity. The decrease in activity has been attributed to the increase in 4′-hydroxyl ionization, which increases binding to TBG, the primary carrier of thyroid hormones in human plasma.[65] In general, a substituent at the 5′-position significantly reduces antigoiter activity in a direct proportion to its size.

An interesting SAR can be deduced by comparing the activity of analogs 32 and 34 with those of analogs 19 and 20. Replacing the 3,5-di-iodo substituents of analog 32 with the 3,5-di-methyl substituents of analog 19 resulted in about 27-fold decrease in the activity. Likewise, replacing the 3,5-di-iodo substituents of analog 34 (which is the most potent analog in this series) with the 3,5-di-methyl substituents of analog 20 resulted in about a 39-fold decrease in the activity. This highlights the importance of the two iodine substituents of the inner ring over those of the outer ring. In fact, 3′-isopropyl-3,6-dimethyl-thyronine (analog 20) appears to have the ability to cross the placental membrane and exerts thyromimetic effects in the fetus after administration to the mother. This can become useful in treating fetal thyroid hormone deficiencies or in enhancing lung development, immediately before premature birth, by stimulating the lung to synthesize special phospholipid surfactants, which ensure sufficient functioning of the infant's lungs at birth.[66]

Modifications of the Phenolic Group of the Outer Ring

The weakly ionized phenolic group at the 4′-position appears to be essential for thyromimetic activity. Replacement of the hydroxyl group with an amino group (analog 39) almost abolishes the activity. Likewise, replacing the hydroxyl group with a lipophilic nonionizable group such as methyl (analog 41) also renders the resulting analog inactive. Interestingly, the 4′-unsubstituted analog (analog 40) exhibits substantial activity, suggesting a potential 4′-hydroxylation as an activating metabolic transformation. Lastly, the 4′-methoxy analog (analog 42) also shows substantial activity, suggesting a potential oxidative O-demethylation at position-4′ as another activating metabolic transformation. Overall, if this position is substituted with a hydroxyl group or any other group that can be transformed to a hydroxyl group, the analog continues to have substantial activity.

Another important contribution of this group is to pharmacokinetics. The pKa of the 4′-phenolic group is 4.7 for T_4 resulting in a significant ionization at physiologic pH, which leads to a stronger affinity to plasma proteins and a longer plasma half-life. In contrast, the pKa of the 4′-phenolic group is 6.9 for T_3, resulting in less ionization at physiologic pH, which leads to a weaker affinity to plasma proteins and a shorter plasma half-life.

Thyroid Diseases: Hyperthyroidism

Hyperthyroidism refers to overproduction of thyroid hormones by the thyroid gland. In the National Health and Nutrition Examination Survey III, 0.7% of participants had subclinical hyperthyroidism, and 0.5% had clinically significant hyperthyroidism (TSH $<$0.1 mIU/L, and T_4 $>$13.2 μg/dL).[34] The prevalence of suppressed TSH values peaks in people ages 20 to 39 years, declines in those 40 to 79 years, and increases again in those who are 80 years and older. Abnormal TSH levels were more common among women.

Hyperthyroidism can be attributed to Graves disease, an autoimmune disorder in which thyroid-stimulating antibody directed against the thyrotropin receptor elicits the same biologic response as TSH. Graves disease is also associated with other autoimmune diseases. Sudden increases in iodine intake may precipitate Graves disease, and there is a 3-fold increase in Graves disease occurrence in the postpartum period. Drug-induced Graves disease may occur after highly active antiretroviral therapy or alemtuzumab treatment and following treatment with nivolumab and pembrolizumab, immune-checkpoint inhibitors. Importantly, exposure of tissues to excessive levels of T_4, T_3, or both results in thyrotoxicosis.[67] The major causes of thyrotoxicosis are hyperthyroidism caused by Graves disease, toxic multinodular goiter, and toxic adenomas.

Signs and symptoms of hyperthyroidism can include palpitations; feeling shaky and/or nervous; weight loss despite increased appetite; diarrhea and/or more frequent bowel movements; thin, warm, moist skin; intolerance to heat and excessive sweating; insomnia; enlarged thyroid gland; hair loss and change in hair texture; menstrual changes; and muscle weakness. A characteristic exophthalmos associated with Graves disease is demonstrated as an infiltrative ophthalmopathy and is considered an autoimmune-mediated inflammation of the periorbital connective tissue and extraocular muscles.[68]

Treatment of Hyperthyroidism

Goals of therapeutic interventions in hyperthyroidism are to eliminate excess thyroid hormone levels, to normalize free T_4 and TSH concentrations in tissues, to minimize symptoms and long-term consequences, and to improve the overall quality of the patient's life. Toward these goals, several molecules can directly or indirectly interfere with the synthesis, release, or action of thyroid hormones. Medications that are used in the treatment of hyperthyroidism include antithyroid drugs, which directly interfere with the synthesis of thyroid hormones, high concentrations of iodine which decrease the release of thyroid hormones and may decrease their synthesis, and radioactive iodine, which damages the thyroid gland with ionizing radiation. Ionic inhibitors, which block the iodide transport mechanism, as well as adjunct therapeutics are also used.

Antithyroid Drugs

History. In 1928, it was observed that rabbits fed a diet composed largely of cabbage often developed goiters, which was attributed to the presence of precursors of the thiocyanate ion in cabbage leaves. Later, phenylthiourea and sulfaguanidine, a sulfonamide antimicrobial agent, were shown to produce *goiter*. Investigation of thiourea derivatives suggested that rats became hypothyroid despite hyperplastic changes in their thyroid glands. Furthermore, no new hormone was detected, and the goitrogen had no visible effect on the thyroid gland following the administration of thyroid hormones or hypophysectomy. This indicated that the goiter was a compensatory response resulting from the induced state of hypothyroidism, and that the principal action of the compounds was to inhibit the biosynthesis of thyroid hormone.

Thioamides. The thioamides (–N–C=S), also known as thionamides and thiocarbamides, are major drugs for the treatment of thyrotoxicosis and hyperthyroidism. The thiocarbamide group is essential for antithyroid activity. The most clinically useful thioamides are thioureylenes, which are five- (thioimidazole) or six-membered (thiouracil) heterocyclic derivatives of thiourea and include 1-methyl-2-mercaptoimidazole (methimazole, MMI), carbimazole, and propylthiouracil (PTU) (Fig. 26.9). Methimazole and propylthiouracil are more widely used in the United States. Carbimazole appears to be used more in the United Kingdom. Carbimazole is considered a prodrug, which is, after absorption, converted to the active form, methimazole. Activation takes place via ester hydrolysis followed by decarboxylation. Methimazole is about 10 times more potent than propylthiouracil, and is the drug of choice in adults and children. However, the additional ability of PTU to inhibit the peripheral enzyme 5′-deiodinase has made it the drug of choice in emergency treatment of thyroid storm.[69] Doses of PTU in excess of 300 mg are effective and almost completely block the peripheral production of T_3.[70]

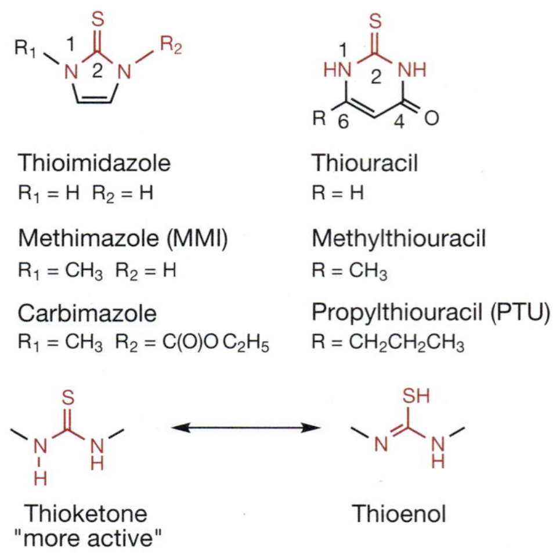

Figure 26.9 Chemical structures of thioureylene-based antithyroid agents, including MMI, carbimazole, and PTU. Thioketone tautomer is a more active antithyroid form.

The thioamides act by several mechanisms. The major action is to prevent hormone synthesis by inhibiting TPO-catalyzed reactions and by blocking iodine organification. Furthermore, they block coupling of the iodotyrosines. They do not block uptake of iodide by the gland, and they do not affect the thyroid hormone release. Inhibition of TPO was described to be irreversible when the drug-to-iodide ratio is high, and reversible when the drug:iodide is low. Moreover, PTU but not methimazole also inhibits the peripheral deiodination of T_4 and T_3. Since the biosynthesis is affected, the onsets of their actions are slow, requiring 3 to 4 weeks before T_4 stores are significantly depleted. Importantly, the uptake of these drugs into the thyroid gland is stimulated by TSH and inhibited by iodide.

Structurally, these drugs may exist as thioketone or thioenol tautomers, the former of which appears to be the more effective form. A number of studies has reported on the SARs of the thiouracils and other related compounds as inhibitors of the outer ring deiodinase.[71] These studies indicated that a C-2 thioketone/thioenol group and an unsubstituted N−1 position are essential for the activity. The enolic hydroxyl group at C-4 in PTU and the presence of large lipophilic alkyl groups at C-5 and C-6 positions enhance the inhibitory activity. For example, methylthiouracil ($R=CH_3$) was found to have less than one-tenth the antithyroid activity of PTU ($R=(CH_2)_2CH_3$). Methimazole possesses more potent TPO inhibitory activity than PTU, and it is longer acting. Nevertheless, it does not have the ability to inhibit peripheral deiodinases, presumably because of the methyl substituent at the N−1 position.

Methimazole is the drug of choice for hyperthyroidism. It is effective when given as a single daily dose and is less toxic than PTU. Methimazole has a relatively long plasma and intrathyroidal half-life and long duration of action. Due to a Black Box warning about severe hepatitis, PTU should be reserved for use during the first trimester of pregnancy, in thyroid storm, and in those experiencing adverse reactions to methimazole, other than agranulocytosis or hepatitis. The usual starting dose for methimazole is 15 to 40 mg/d. The usual starting dose of PTU is 100 mg every 8 hours.

Pharmacokinetics. Absorption of methimazole after oral administration is rapid and extensive with an absolute bioavailability of about 95% and a T_{max} ranging from 0.25 to 4.0 hours. C_{max} is slightly higher in hyperthyroid patients. The apparent volume of distribution of methimazole is about 20 L. Following oral administration, methimazole is highly concentrated in the thyroid gland. Intrathyroidal methimazole levels are about two to 5 times higher than peak plasma levels and continue to be high for 20 hours after ingestion. Methimazole exhibits negligible protein binding, existing primarily as a free drug in the serum.[72]

Methimazole is extensively metabolized by the liver, mainly by CYP450 and flavin-containing monooygenase (FMO) enzyme systems. Several metabolites have been identified. The 3-methyl-2-thiohydantoin metabolite was reported to demonstrate antithyroid activity in animals, and thus, may partially explain the prolonged duration of action despite methimazole's relatively short half-life. Several metabolites have been investigated for methimazole-induced hepatotoxicity. Both glyoxal and N-methylthiourea have established cytotoxicity and are known metabolic products of methimazole's dihydrodiol intermediate. Sulfenic and sulfinic acid derivatives of methimazole are thought to be the ultimate toxicants responsible for hepatotoxicity, though their origin is unclear. Figure 26.10 depicts the metabolism of methimazole.[73,74] Urinary excretion of unmetabolized methimazole has been reported to be 7% to 12%. Elimination via feces appears to be limited. Enterohepatic circulation also appears to play a role in the elimination of methimazole and its metabolites, as significant amounts of these substances are found in the bile post-administration. The elimination half-life is about 5.5 hours, while its primary active metabolite has a half-life approximately three times longer than its parent drug. Renal impairment does not appear to alter the half-life of methimazole, but patients with hepatic impairment showed an increase in half-life proportional to the impairment severity.

PTU is rapidly absorbed, reaching peak serum levels after 1 hour. Its bioavailability of 50% to 80% may be due to partial absorption or a significant hepatic first-pass effect. PTU has a short elimination half-life of 1.5 hours. It exhibits significant plasma protein binding of 80%. Its volume of distribution approximates total body water with accumulation in the thyroid gland. Most of the ingested dose of PTU is excreted by the kidney as the inactive glucuronide within 24 hours.

The two drugs cross the placental barrier leading to fetal hypothyroidism, so caution must be employed when using these drugs in pregnancy. The two drugs are classified as FDA pregnancy category D. PTU is preferable during the first trimester of pregnancy because it is more strongly protein-bound, and thus, crosses the placenta less readily. Furthermore, although rarely, methimazole has been associated with congenital malformations. The two drugs are secreted in low concentrations in breast milk but are considered safe for the nursing infant.

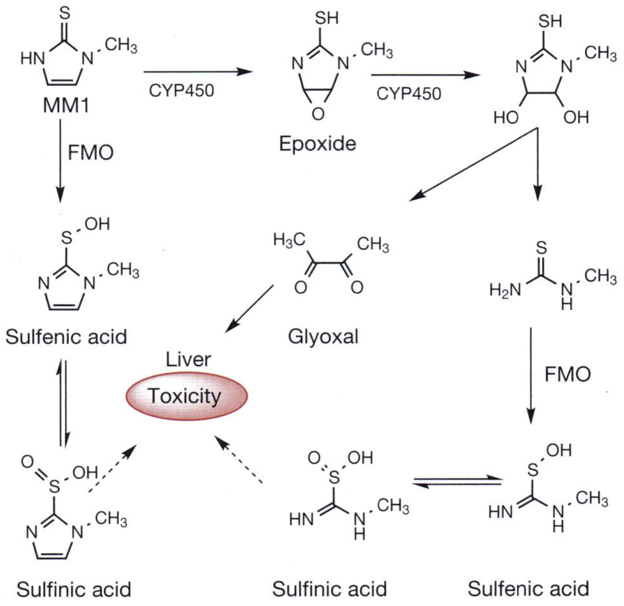

Figure 26.10 Proposed 1-methyl-2-mercaptoimidazole (MMI) metabolites. Reactive intermediates formed during MMI metabolism may bind to macromolecular targets and cause toxicity or might be detoxified by nucleophilic molecules such as glutathione.

Adverse Reactions. Adverse reactions occur in 3% to 12% of treated patients. Most reactions occur early, especially nausea and GI distress. An altered sense of taste or smell may occur with methimazole. The most common adverse effect is a maculopapular pruritic rash (4%-6%), at times accompanied by fever. Rare adverse effects include an urticarial rash, exfoliative dermatitis, a lupus-like reaction, vasculitis, hypoprothrombinemia, lymphadenopathy, polyserositis, and acute arthralgia. An increased risk of severe hepatitis, sometimes resulting in death, has been reported with PTU (Black Box warning). Cholestatic jaundice is more common with methimazole than PTU. Asymptomatic elevations in transaminase levels can also occur. The most life-threatening complication is agranulocytosis (granulocyte count <500 cells/mm^3). It occurs in 0.1% to 0.5% of patients taking thioamides, but the risk may be increased in older patients and usually within the first 90 days in those receiving high dose of methimazole. The reaction is usually rapidly reversible when the drug is discontinued.

Iodine and Radioactive Iodine. Iodide is the oldest treatment for thyroid gland disorders. Elevated concentrations of iodide can affect several functions of the thyroid gland. Iodide limits its own transport and inhibits the synthesis of iodotyrosines and iodothyronines (Wolff-Chaikoff effect).[75]

An important clinical effect of high iodide plasma concentration is the inhibition of thyroid hormones release. This action is effective and rapid in severe thyrotoxicosis. The effect is exerted directly on the thyroid gland and can be demonstrated in euthyroidism as well as hyperthyroidism. Vascularity of the thyroid gland is also reduced, the gland becomes much firmer, the cells become smaller, and colloid reaccumulates in the follicles as iodine concentration increases. It has been suggested that excess iodide might change the conformation of thyroglobulin, making it less susceptible to proteolysis. The maximal effect occurs after 10 to 15 days of continuous therapy.

The iodide preparations are also used in the preparation for thyroidectomy and, in combination with an antithyroid drug, in the treatment of thyrotoxic crisis. In thyroid surgery, the preparations are administered for about 2 weeks to ensure decreased vascularity and firming of the gland. Strong iodine solution (Lugol solution) consists of 5% iodine and 10% potassium iodide, yielding a dose of about 8 mg of iodine/drop. Potassium iodide saturated solution is also available, containing 50 mg/drop. The most frequent side effects are hypersensitivity reactions (skin rashes, fever, rhinitis, and conjunctivitis), salivary gland swelling, "iodism" (metallic taste, burning mouth and throat, sore teeth and gums, symptoms of a head cold, and sometimes stomach upset and diarrhea), and gynecomastia.

Another use of iodide preparations is to protect the thyroid gland from the consequences of exposure to radioactive iodine following a military exposure or nuclear accident. Because the uptake of radioactive iodine is inversely proportional to the serum concentration of stable iodine, the daily administration of 30 to 100 mg of iodine will significantly decrease the thyroid uptake of radioisotopes. Typical doses include 16 to 36 mg (two to six drops) of Lugol solution or 50 to 100 mg (one to two drops) of potassium iodide saturated solution three times a day. Potassium iodide products (Thyroshield) are available over the counter (OTC) to use in the event of a radiation emergency and block the uptake of radioiodine into the thyroid gland. The adult dose is 2 mL (130 mg) every 24 hours.

Although others exist, ^{123}I and ^{131}I isotopes are used for the diagnosis and treatment of thyroid diseases. The former is a short-lived γ-emitter with a half-life of 13 hours and is used in diagnostic studies. The latter has a half-life of 8 days and emits both γ-rays and β particles. ^{131}I is used therapeutically to destroy an overactive or enlarged thyroid (hyperthyroidism)[76] and in thyroid cancer for thyroid ablation and treatment of metastatic disease. The chemical behavior of the radioactive iodine isotopes is similar to that of the stable isotope, ^{127}I. ^{131}I is rapidly and selectively trapped by the thyroid gland. There, it is incorporated into the iodinated amino acids and is deposited in the colloid of the follicles. Thus, the destructive β particles originate within the follicle and act almost exclusively on the parenchymal cells of the thyroid, with little or no damage to surrounding tissue. With properly selected doses of ^{131}I, it is possible to destroy the thyroid gland completely without detectable injury to adjacent tissues.

Advantages of radioiodine include the ease of administration, effectiveness, low expense, and absence of pain. The main adverse effect of the use of radioactive iodine is the high incidence of delayed hypothyroidism. Although cancer death rate is not increased after radioiodine therapy, some studies suggest a potential increase in specific types of cancer (stomach, kidney, and breast). Radioactive iodine treatment can induce radiation thyroiditis. In most patients, there can be worsening of symptoms of hyperthyroidism. Rare cardiac manifestations (atrial fibrillation or ischemic heart disease) and thyroid storm can happen. Radioactive iodine should not be administered to pregnant women or nursing mothers because it passes through the placenta and destroys the fetal thyroid gland, and it is excreted in breast milk.

Radioiodine whole-body scan and serum thyroglobulin measurement are commonly used as follow-up testing in patients with thyroid cancer. Both follow-up tests require a hypothyroid state. For thyroid cells to take up labeled iodine, thyrotropin must be available, and for the pituitary to supply it, the body must be free of thyroid hormones. This means that patients must completely stop taking medication for several weeks before the scan day. This results in severe hypothyroidism. To make the follow-up tests easier, thyrogen (thyrotropin α for injection), a recombinant human thyrotropin that stimulates the thyroid gland-like endogenous TSH to produce thyroid hormone, is used. The effect of TSH activation of thyroid cells is to increase uptake of radioiodine to allow scan detection or radioiodine killing of thyroid cells. TSH activation also leads to the release of thyroglobulin by thyroid cells. Thyroglobulin functions as a tumor marker that is detected in blood specimens. Thyrogen has been shown to significantly enhance the sensitivity of thyroglobulin testing in patients maintained on thyroid hormone therapy. It allows patients with thyroid cancer to avoid the debilitating effects of hypothyroidism when undergoing radioiodine imaging scans during diagnostic testing or as adjunctive treatment for radioiodine ablation.

Other compounds containing organic iodide have also been used therapeutically for hyperthyroidism. These include various radiologic contrast media that share a triiodo-aminobenzene and mono-aminobenzene ring with a propionic acid chain. The effect of these preparations is a result of inhibiting thyroid hormone release as well as competitive inhibition of 5′-deiodinase. These agents are no longer available in the United States.

IONIC INHIBITORS. Anions such as perchlorate (ClO_4^-), pertechnetate (TcO_4^-), thiocyanate (SCN−), and fluoroborate (BF_4-) can block the iodide uptake by the thyroid gland via competitive inhibition of the iodide transport mechanism. All are monovalent hydrated anions of a size similar to that of iodide. Given that these effects are competitive, they can be overcome by large doses of iodides, and hence, their effectiveness can be unpredictable. Thiocyanate qualitatively differs from others. It is not concentrated by the thyroid gland but, in large amounts, may block the organification of iodine.

Perchlorate is 10 times as active as thiocyanate. Perchlorate salts occur both naturally and through manufacturing. They have been used as a medicine for more than 50 years to treat thyroid gland disorders. Potassium perchlorate has clinically been used to block the thyroidal reuptake of iodide in patients with iodide-induced hyperthyroidism such as amiodarone-induced hyperthyroidism. Perchlorate can also be used to displace inorganic iodide from the thyroid gland in a diagnostic test of iodide organification. Perchlorate, in doses of 750 mg daily, has been used in the treatment of Graves disease. In Europe, perchlorate has been used for surgical preparation and for the long-term treatment of thyrotoxicosis. In the United States, the use of perchlorate was drastically curtailed after aplastic anemia, and severe renal damage was reported following its use. In fact, the US Environmental Protection Agency has issued substantial guidance and analysis concerning the impact of perchlorate use on the environment and in drinking water.[77] Another ion that may have an effect on thyroid gland is lithium. Lithium decreases secretion of T_4 and T_3, which can cause overt hypothyroidism in some patients who use lithium for the treatment of mania.

Radioactive pertechnetate ($^{99m}TcO_4^-$) anion is an important radiopharmaceutical agent for the study and imaging of the thyroid gland, including its morphology, function, and vascularity. Its advantages include the short half-life of 6 hours and the low radiation exposure of the patients. $^{99m}TcO_4^-$ has comparable charge/radius ratio to iodide, and thus, it is similarly incorporated into the thyroid gland. Yet, it is not incorporated into thyroglobulin. Sodium pertechnetate cannot pass through the blood-brain barrier. It is eliminated renally after injection, and patients are recommended to drink plenty of water to expedite the elimination of the radionuclide, after scanning is over. In contrast to iodide, these anions do not undergo intrathyroidal metabolism after they are trapped.

ADJUNCT THERAPY. Because many of the manifestations of hyperthyroidism are mediated by β-adrenergic receptors, β-blockers without intrinsic sympathomimetic activity such as metoprolol, propranolol, and atenolol are effective therapeutic adjuncts in the management of thyrotoxicosis since many of these symptoms mimic those associated with sympathetic stimulation. Propranolol has been the β-blocker most widely studied and used in the therapy of thyrotoxicosis. β-blockers cause clinical improvement of hyperthyroid symptoms but do not typically alter thyroid hormone levels. Propranolol at doses greater than 160 mg/d may also reduce T_3 levels ~20% by inhibiting the peripheral conversion of T_4 to T_3. Antiadrenergic agents such as centrally acting sympatholytics (clonidine) and calcium-channel antagonists (diltiazem) may have some role in the symptomatic treatment of hyperthyroidism. Therapeutic plasmapheresis is an effective alternative treatment option to prepare for ablative treatment in patients that have side effects or who do not respond to antithyroid drugs.[78]

Traditionally, corticosteroids, radiation therapy, and surgical correction have been the mainstays of therapy for Graves ophthalmopathy. Rituximab, tocilizumab, and teprotumumab-trbw (Tepezza) have been assessed in randomized clinical trials.[79] In 2020, FDA approved teprotumumab, a monoclonal anti-insulin-like growth factor I receptor antibody, for the treatment of thyroid eye disease.[80]

Resistance to Thyroid Hormones

As mentioned, thyroid hormone action is mediated by the nuclear TRs TRα and TRβ, which are encoded by the *THRA* and *THRB* genes, respectively. The first form of resistance to thyroid hormones (RTHs) is generalized resistance to thyroid hormone (GRTH), which is caused by mutations in *THRB* (resistance to TRβ), resulting in elevated serum levels of the thyroid hormones and a TSH level that is inappropriately normal or slightly elevated. The second form is caused by *THRA* mutations (resistance to TRα), leading to a low serum TSH and slightly low free T_4 level.[81-83]

In GRTH, most affected individuals are clinically euthyroid. Some patients are present with goiter, stunted growth, delayed maturation, attention-deficit/hyperactivity disorder (ADHD), and tachycardia. The disorder is familial in 75% of cases, and inheritance is autosomal dominant. In most patients with GRTH, the increased levels of T_3 and T_4 appear to compensate for the receptor defect, and treatment is unnecessary. In some children, administration of thyroid hormones may be necessary to correct defects in growth or mental development. Occasionally, individuals with GRTH have symptoms of mild hyperthyroidism. If the hyperthyroid state is causing significant symptoms, therapy with β-blockers, antithyroid drugs, or radioactive iodine can be considered.

Individuals with resistance to TRα have delayed growth, failed tooth eruption, constipation, low intellectual function, and decreased heart rate. These clinical features are consistent with an abnormal TRα protein, which is expressed predominantly in the skeleton, heart, and likely the intestine. Changes in thyroid function tests include a low-normal free T_4, high-normal or elevated T_3, and normal TSH. Thyroxine treatment appears to alleviate some of the clinical manifestations of patients with RTH caused by TRα mutations.

Thyroid Diseases: Cancer

Thyroid carcinoma is the most common malignancy of the endocrine system. The majority of thyroid cancers are differentiated tumors from the thyroid follicular cells and are classified as papillary or follicular carcinomas. Most of these carcinomas are adequately treated by surgery, radioiodine, and levothyroxine to suppress TSH. However, a small fraction progresses, in which case, systemic therapy with kinase inhibitors may be appropriate. Anaplastic thyroid carcinomas are undifferentiated tumors of the thyroid follicular cells. They are highly aggressive with an average life expectancy of only 6 months from the time of diagnosis. Few thyroid cancers originate from the parafollicular cells that produce calcitonin. These are known as medullary thyroid carcinoma. Because they derive from parafollicular cells, they are not responsive to radioiodine or TSH suppression. The first-line therapy for this type is surgery.

The incidence of thyroid cancer has increased from 4.9 to more than 15 cases per 100,000 individuals in the United States over the past 30 years. Nonetheless, disease-specific mortality has only minimally increased. Current trends in thyroid cancer care focus on avoiding overdiagnosis, limiting surgery, radioiodine, surveillance for low-risk tumors, and identifying patients at higher recurrence risk for more aggressive treatment and monitoring. Thyroid cancer is twice as common in women as in men, yet male gender is associated with a more serious prognosis. Prognosis is worse in older persons (>65 years).

Treatment of Thyroid Cancer

Radioactive Iodine

Most well-differentiated thyroid carcinomas accumulate very limited amounts of iodine. Stimulation of iodine uptake with TSH is required to effectively treat metastases.[84,85] Endogenous TSH stimulation is promoted by withdrawal of thyroid hormone replacement therapy. To achieve adequate stimulation of endogenous TSH (>30 mIU/L), levothyroxine (half-life of 7 days) therapy should be held for about 4 weeks. Liothyronine, which has a much shorter half-life, can be used in the first half of levothyroxine withdrawal to mitigate the symptoms of hypothyroidism. An ablative dose of ^{131}I (30-150 mCi) is administered, and a repeat total-body scan is obtained several days to 1 week later. Recombinant thyrotropin α (recombinant human TSH) can be used instead of thyroid hormone withdrawal to prepare patients for radioiodine ablation of thyroid remnant tissue or to test the capacity of thyroid tissue to take up radioactive iodine and to secrete thyroglobulin.

Thyroid Cancer Chemotherapeutics: Tyrosine Kinase Inhibitors

Tyrosine kinase inhibitors are used when surgery, ^{131}I, TSH suppression, and external beam radiotherapy are inadequate. Tyrosine kinases are important enzymes for the modulation of growth factor signaling. Dysregulated tyrosine kinases play an important role in many neoplastic diseases, including thyroid cancer. Inhibiting tyrosine kinases restricts their effect on cell division and cell longevity. Generally, tyrosine kinase inhibitors target the ATP-bind site of the catalytic domain of several oncogenic tyrosine kinases. For a complete discussion about tyrosine kinase inhibitors, see Chapter 37.

Importantly, the choice of systemic therapies is guided by somatic mutation testing of the primary tumor or a metastasis. Patients with tumors that contain *NTRK* or *RET* driver mutations (fusion genes with different partners) can be treated with specific small-molecule inhibitors such as larotrectinib (Vitrakvi) or entrectinib (Rozlytrek) for *NTRK* fusions[86] or selpercatinib (Retevmo) or pralsetinib (Gavreto) for *RET* fusions.[87] Nevertheless, these mutations are relatively rare in thyroid cancer. In the absence of *NTRK* or *RET* driver mutations, lenvatinib (Lenvima) or sorafenib (Nexavar), multikinase inhibitors, can be used. These drugs are relatively promiscuous; however, vascular endothelial growth factor receptors (VEGFR) are important targets. Multikinase inhibitors are antiangiogenics and can prolong progression-free survival.

The most common driver mutation in papillary thyroid cancer is *BRAF V600E*. Vemurafenib (Zelboraf) and dabrafenib (Tafinlar) specifically inhibit this kinase and have efficacy in *BRAF*-mutated papillary thyroid cancer.[88] Several papillary and follicular cancer driver mutations including *NTRK*, *RET*, and *BRAF V600E* fusions and RAS mutations activate the mitogen activated protein (MAP) kinase pathway. Treatment with dabrafenib or vemurafenib and/or a MEK inhibitor such as trametinib (Mekinist) or selumetinib (Koselugo), for several weeks, appears to have the potential to restore radioiodine uptake and facilitate radioiodine therapy in some of these tumors.[89,90]

The combination of dabrafenib and trametinib is FDA approved for anaplastic carcinomas that harbor *BRAF V600E*.[91] As mentioned, surgery is the first-line treatment for medullary thyroid carcinomas. Yet, *RET*-driven medullary thyroid carcinomas that progress despite surgery can be treated with a selective RET kinase inhibitor such as selpercatinib or pralsetinib. The multikinase inhibitors vandetanib (Caprelsa) and cabozantinib (Cometriq) also have efficacy and can be prescribed without considering *RET* gene mutational status.[92] The chemical structures and classification of kinase inhibitors used in thyroid carcinoma are provided in Figure 26.11.

Larotrectinib.[93,94] Larotrectinib is a disubstituted pyrazolo [1,5-a]pyrimidin-3-yl derivative. It is an orally available kinase inhibitor, which, upon administration, binds to tropomyosin receptor kinase, thereby preventing neurotrophin-tropomyosin receptor kinase interaction and tropomyosin-receptor kinase activation. This results in both the induction of cellular apoptosis and the inhibition of cell growth in tumors that overexpress tropomyosin receptor kinase. The drug is a substrate and inhibitor of CYP3A4 and is a substrate of p-glycoprotein and breast cancer resistance protein (BCRP). Its major metabolite is O-glucuronide.

Entrectinib.[95] Entrectinib is a disubstituted indazole derivative. It is an orally bioavailable inhibitor of the tyrosine kinases tropomyosin receptor kinases A, B and C, *C-ros oncogene 1*, and anaplastic lymphoma kinase. Upon administration, entrectinib binds to and inhibits these kinases, which results in a disruption of the associated signaling pathways. This leads to an induction of apoptosis and an inhibition of tumor cell proliferation in tumor cells that express these kinases. The drug is metabolized hepatically by CYP3A4. The major metabolite is the N-demethylated form of the piperazine domain. This metabolite is active and is a substrate of p-glycoprotein and BCRP.

Selpercatinib and Pralsetinib. Selpercatinib[96] is an orally bioavailable selective inhibitor of wild-type, mutant, and fusion products involving the proto-oncogene receptor tyrosine kinase rearranged during transfection (RET). Selpercatinib selectively binds to and targets wild-type RET as well as various RET mutants and RET-containing fusion products. This results in an inhibition of cell growth of tumor cells that exhibit increased RET activity. In addition, selpercatinib binds to and inhibits vascular endothelial growth factor (VEGF) receptors 1 to 3 and fibroblast growth factor receptors 1 to 3. The drug is substrate of CYP3A4, p-glycoprotein, and BCRP.

Likewise, pralsetinib[97] is an orally bioavailable selective inhibitor of mutant forms of and fusion products involving the proto-oncogene receptor tyrosine kinase RET. The drug has a complex hepatic metabolism. Metabolism is primarily by CYP3A4 and, to a lesser extent, by CYP2D6 and

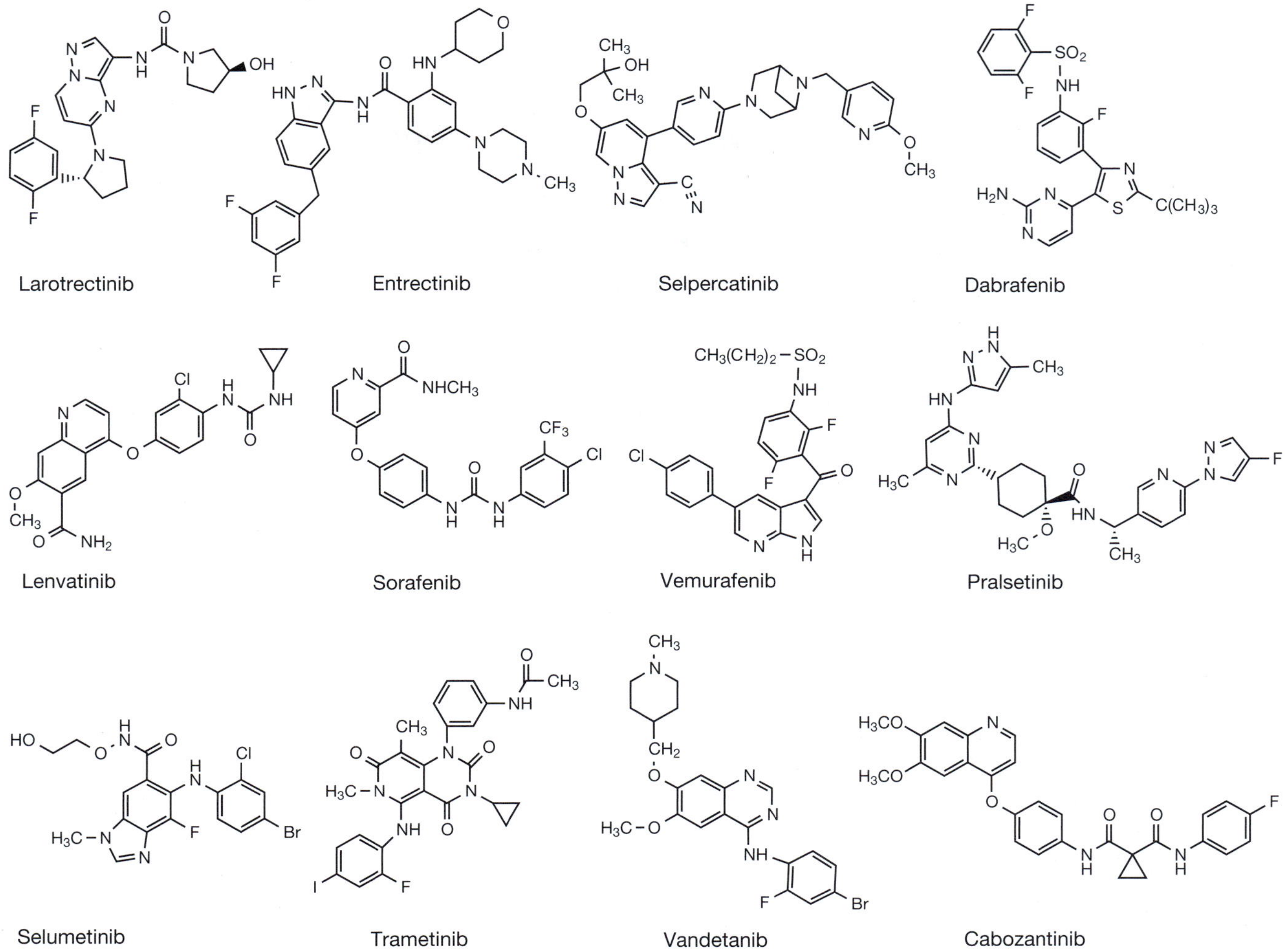

Figure 26.11 Kinase inhibitors used in the treatment of thyroid cancers.

CYP1A2. Oxidative metabolites and glucuronide conjugates have been identified, yet their activity remains unknown.

LENVATINIB.[98] Lenvatinib is a member of the class of quinolines that is the carboxamide of 4-(3-chloro-4-[(cyclopropylcarbamoyl)amino]phenoxy)-7-methoxyquinoline-6-carboxylic acid. A multikinase inhibitor and orphan drug used (as its mesylate salt) for the treatment of various types of thyroid cancer that do not respond to radioiodine. The drug is an orally bioavailable receptor tyrosine kinase inhibitor of VEGF receptors 1 to 3 and other receptor tyrosine kinases, including fibroblast growth factor receptor, platelet-derived growth factor receptor α, KIT, and RET. Lenvatinib is metabolized by the liver enzyme CYP3A4 to desmethyllenvatinib (M2). M2 and lenvatinib itself are oxidized at the quinoline ring by aldehyde oxidase to substances called M2′ and M3′, the main metabolites in the feces. Another metabolite, also mediated by a CYP enzyme, is the *N*-oxide M3. Non-enzymatic metabolization also occurs.

SORAFENIB.[99] Sorafenib targets vascular endothelial growth factors, platelet-derived growth factor receptors, and RAF kinases. It is a phenyl urea derivative in which one of the nitrogens is substituted by a 4-chloro-3-trifluorophenyl group while the other is substituted by a phenyl group, which is further substituted at the para-position by (2-[methylcarbamoyl]pyridin-4-yl)oxy group. It is available for oral use as the tosylate salt. Sorafenib is an oral multi-kinase inhibitor that is used in the therapy of advanced renal cell, liver, and thyroid cancer. It is extensively metabolized by CYP3A4 (*N*-oxide, active) followed by *O*-glucuronidation.

VEMURAFENIB.[100] Vemurafenib is *1H*-pyrrolo[2,3-b]pyridine derivative, which is substituted at position-5 by a *para*-chlorophenyl group and at position-3 by a 3-amino-2,6-difluorobenzoyl group, the amino group of which has undergone formal condensation with propane-1-sulfonic acid to give the corresponding sulfonamide. Vemurafenib is a potent and highly selective oral kinase inhibitor of some mutated forms of BRAF serine-threonine kinase, including BRAF V600E. It is metabolized by CYP3A4, and the metabolites make up 5% of the components in plasma. The parent compound makes up for the remaining 95%.

DABRAFENIB.[101] Dabrafenib is a difluorinated orally bioavailable inhibitor of BRAF protein, which plays a role in regulating the MAP kinase/ERKs (extracellular signal-related kinases) signaling pathway, which may be constitutively activated due to *BRAF* gene mutations. It is orally available as the mesylate salt. The metabolism of dabrafenib is primarily mediated by CYP2C8 and CYP3A4 to form hydroxy-dabrafenib (active) of the *t*-butyl group. Hydroxy-dabrafenib is further oxidized via CYP3A4 to form carboxy-dabrafenib and subsequently excreted in bile and urine. Carboxy-dabrafenib is decarboxylated to form desmethyl-dabrafenib (active); desmethyl-dabrafenib may be reabsorbed from the gut. Desmethyl-dabrafenib is further metabolized by CYP3A4 to oxidative metabolites.

TRAMETINIB.[102] Trametinib is an orally used pyridopyrimidine derivative that is developed as dimethyl sulfoxide solvate. Trametinib is a reversible, allosteric inhibitor of mitogen-activated extracellular signal-regulated kinase 1 (MEK1) and MEK2 activation and of MEK1 and MEK2 activity. Trametinib inhibits *BRAF* V600E mutation-positive melanoma cell growth in vitro and in vivo, and, when used in combination with dabrafenib, there is greater and prolonged inhibition compared with either drug alone. Trametinib is metabolized predominantly via deacetylation alone or with monooxygenation or in combination with glucuronidation biotransformation pathways in vitro. Deacetylation is likely mediated by hydrolytic enzymes, such as carboxyl-esterases or amidases.

SELUMETINIB.[90] Selumetinib is an orally active, small-molecule benzimidazole derivative. It is an ATP-independent inhibitor of MEK1/2. MEK1/2 proteins are upstream regulators of the extracellular signal-related kinase (ERK) pathway. Both MEK and ERK are critical components of the RAS-regulated RAF-MEK-ERK pathway, which is often activated in different types of cancers. The drug is hepatically metabolized, primarily by CYP3A4. *N*-Desmethyl selumetinib is the major metabolite. It is 3 to 5 times more potent than the parent drug.

VANDETANIB AND CABOZANTINIB. Vandetanib is an orally bioavailable 4-anilinoquinazoline derivative. Vandetanib is a potent inhibitor of the VEGF receptor, epidermal growth factor (EGF) receptor, and RET (*re*arranged during *t*ransfection) tyrosine kinases.[103] Unchanged vandentanib and metabolites vandetanib *N*-oxide and *N*-desmethyl vandetanib were detected in plasma, urine, and feces. *N*-Desmethyl-vandetanib is primarily produced by CYP3A4, and vandetanib-*N*-oxide is primarily produced by flavin-containing monooxygenase enzymes FMO1 and FMO3.

Cabozantinib[104] is an oral nonspecific tyrosine kinase inhibitor. Structurally, it has quinoline, diamide, and fluorobenzene moieties, and sold as the malate salt. It inhibits tyrosine kinase activity of RET, MET, VEGFR 1-3, KIT, TRKB, FLT-3, AXL, ROS1, TYRO3, MER, and TIE-2. Cabozantinib is metabolized mostly by CYP3A4 and, to a minor extent, by CYP2C9. Both enzymes produce an *N*-oxide metabolite with unknown activity.

Drugs Affecting Thyroid Function: Implications for Drug-Drug and Drug-Food Interactions

The presence of environmental goitrogens was earlier suggested by the resistance of endemic goiters to iodine prophylaxis and iodide treatment in Italy and Colombia. Previously, outbreaks of hypothyroidism have pointed toward calcium as a source of waterborne goitrogenicity, and it is presently believed that calcium is a weak goitrogen that can cause latent hypothyroidism to come to the surface. Along these lines, lithium salts have been used as safe adjuncts in the initial treatment of thyrotoxicosis.[105] Lithium is concentrated by the thyroid gland,[106] with a thyroid-to-serum ratio of more than 2:1, suggesting active transport. Lithium inhibits adenylate cyclase, which forms cAMP. Inhibition of the formation of cAMP eventually inhibits processes involved in thyroid hormone release. Inhibition of thyroid hormone secretion by lithium has proved to be a useful adjunct in the treatment of hyperthyroidism.[107]

In the view of the role of cysteine residues in the conformation of thyroglobulin, the action of TPO, and the deiodination of T_4, the effect of sulfur-containing molecules on thyroid hormone formation is hardly surprising. Several naturally occurring sulfur compounds are derived from glucosinolates (also known as thioglucosides), which are present in food such as cabbage, turnips, mustard seed, salad greens, and radishes (many of them from *Brassica* or *Cruciferae*) as well as in the milk of cows grazing in areas containing *Brassica* weeds. Chemically, glucosinolates can primarily give rise to isothiocyanate, which has a similar size to iodide and competes with it for uptake by thyroid gland. Its goitrogenic effect can be reversed by iodide intake. Goitrin (5-*R*-vinyloxazolidine-2-thione) is a potent naturally occurring thyroid peroxidase inhibitor that reduces the production of thyroid hormones and thought to be the cause of a mild goiter endemic to Finland.[108] In rats, goitrin appears to actively be taken up by the thyroid gland and appears to inhibit the coupling of thyroglobulin diiodotyrosyl residues.[109] However, many researchers believe that the goitrogenic effect of goitrin-containing plants is attributed to the additive effects of all goitrogenic components present.

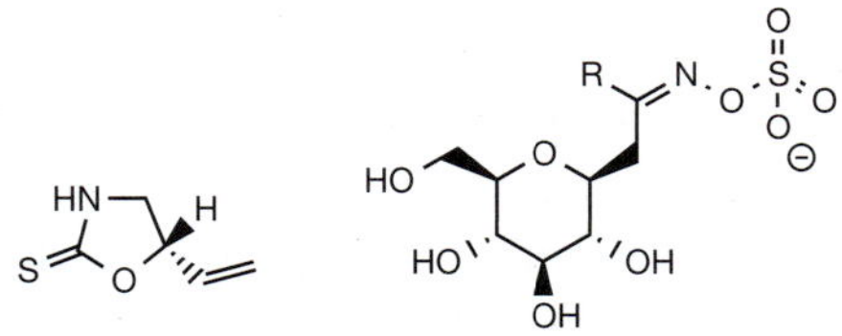

Goitrin

Glucosinolate "general structure"

In addition to environmental goitrogens, there is a growing list of medications that adversely affect thyroid function or interpretation of the results of standard thyroid laboratory testing. These medications are commonly used preparations, ranging from OTC supplements to advanced medical therapy, and include antiarrhythmic agents, antineoplastic agents, and glucocorticoids.[110] Several mechanisms are responsible as listed in Table 26.5. For example, mitotane (Lysodren) causes hypothyroidism in most patients treated for adrenocortical carcinoma. Patients present with subnormal free T_4 levels and a blunted thyrotroph response to TRH, findings that are consistent with central hypothyroidism. Immune checkpoint inhibitors, including those that inhibit cytotoxic T-lymphocyte antigen 4 (CTLA-4)

Table 26.5 Drug Effects on the Thyroid Gland and Its Hormones

Effect	Example
Interference with endogenous thyroid function	Disruption of hypothalamic-pituitary control Increased or decreased thyroid hormone production or release Enhanced thyroid autoimmunity or destructive thyroiditis Changes in thyroid hormone-binding proteins Displacement of thyroid hormone from binding proteins Inhibition of thyroid hormone activation Increased thyroid hormone metabolism or elimination
Interference with thyroid hormone therapy	Decreased tablet dissolution or thyroid hormone absorption Decreased free thyroid hormone levels Increased thyroid hormone metabolism or elimination
Interference with thyroid laboratory testing in euthyroid persons	Incorrect increase or decrease of thyroid hormone levels Incorrect low serum thyrotropin levels Incorrect increased thyrotropin-receptor antibody levels

and programmed cell death 1 (PD-1) receptor, have a variety of adverse endocrine effects. Hypophysitis occurs more frequently with CTLA-4 inhibitors such as ipilimumab (Yervoy), whereas primary thyroid dysfunction is seen more often with PD-1 inhibitors. The synthetic retinoid bexarotene (Targretin), an antineoplastic agent used for the treatment of cutaneous T cell lymphoma, induces rapid and profound thyrotropin suppression, leading to overt central hypothyroidism in 40% to 70% of treated patients, with recovery of normal function within weeks after drug discontinuation. These effects occur through the direct action of bexarotene on pituitary thyrotrophs and by enhancing thyroid hormone metabolism through nondeiodinase pathways such as sulfation. Interestingly, several categories of drugs exert suppressive effects on thyrotropin release without significantly affecting circulating T_4 levels, including glucocorticoids, dopamine agonists, somatostatin analogues, and metformin. Although suppression in patients receiving these agents is insignificant, a low thyrotropin level with a normal free T_4 level may be confused with subclinical hyperthyroidism.

As mentioned, excess intrathyroidal iodine inhibits thyroid hormone synthesis, resulting in the Wolff-Chaikoff effect. Common drug sources of excess iodine include (i) iodinated contrast agents used for computed tomography and cholecystography; (ii) medications with a high iodine content such as amiodarone (Nexterone, antiarrhythmic agent) and topical povidone-iodine; and (iii) OTC preparations and supplements, including expectorants, vaginal douches, and kelp (Fig. 26.12). In particular, amiodarone is 37.3% iodine by weight. It undergoes partial deiodination, releasing approximately 7 mg of iodide per 200-mg tablet, which is about 45 times the recommended daily intake of 150 $\mu\gamma$ for men and nonpregnant women. In addition to inducing hypothyroidism in susceptible patients, iodine from amiodarone causes hyperthyroidism in some patients, a disorder known as type 1 amiodarone-induced thyrotoxicosis.

Newer drugs that promote immune system targeting of cancer cells also increase the risk of autoimmune disorders. Primary thyroid dysfunction is reported in about 5% to 10% of patients treated with CTLA-4 inhibitors, 10% to 20% of those treated with PD-1 inhibitors, and more than 20% of patients treated with combination therapy. The use of nonspecific immunostimulatory cytokines such as interleukin-2 and interferon-α in patients with metastatic renal-cell carcinoma, melanoma, or hepatitis C results in thyroid dysfunction in 15% to 50% of patients, with varying degrees of hypothyroidism preceded by thyrotoxicosis. For example, alemtuzumab (Campath) is a humanized monoclonal antibody against the cell-surface antigen CD52. Treatment with alemtuzumab leads to a substantial depletion of circulating B cells and T cells and a high rate of thyroid autoimmunity in patients with multiple sclerosis. Furthermore, targeted cancer therapy involving tyrosine kinase or multikinase inhibitors has been associated with an increased risk of thyroiditis.

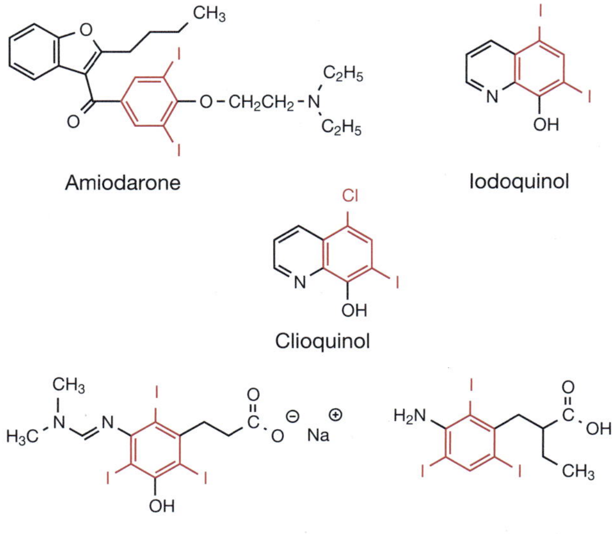

Figure 26.12 Chemical structures of iodine-containing therapeutics and contrast agents that impact thyroid gland hormone physiology.

Several drugs lead to an increase in thyroxine-binding globulin, including oral estrogen and selective estrogen-receptor modulators, mitotane, methadone, and fluorouracil. In contrast, reduction in this protein occurs with the use of glucocorticoids, androgens, and niacin. Either way, these drugs can substantially affect the free amount of thyroxine. Drug-induced displacement of thyroid hormone from binding proteins occurs with the antiepileptic agents of phenytoin and carbamazepine, salsalate and some other nonsteroidal anti-inflammatory drugs, high-dose furosemide, and heparin preparations. The clinical importance of these interactions is usually negligible. In the case of antiepileptic agents and heparin, the effects primarily involve alterations in laboratory testing of thyroid function.

Conversion of T_4 to T_3 is inhibited by several drugs, including amiodarone, dexamethasone, propranolol at high doses, the cholecystographic agents ipodate and iopanoic acid (see Fig. 26.12), and the antithyroid drug propylthiouracil. Amiodarone inhibits T_3 generation both within the pituitary and in the periphery. Dexamethasone inhibition of T_4-to-T_3 conversion is exploited therapeutically in the treatment of patients with severe thyrotoxicosis.

Bile acid sequestrants such as cholestyramine, colestipol, and colesevelam reduce thyroid hormone levels, presumably by interfering with the recycling of thyroid hormone in the enterohepatic circulation. Treatment with drugs that induce glucuronidation enzymes, including phenobarbital, carbamazepine, phenytoin, and rifampin, sometimes necessitates an increase in the dose of levothyroxine. Tyrosine kinase inhibitors also appear to augment thyroid hormone metabolism. A study of sorafenib in levothyroxine-dependent patients with thyroid cancer showed that 26 weeks after the start of treatment, there was evidence of accelerated levothyroxine inactivation through augmented type 3 deiodinase activity. Remarkably, glucagon-like peptide 1 receptor agonists, which are used to manage type 2 diabetes mellitus and obesity, have been shown to cause increased risk of all thyroid cancer and medullary thyroid cancer.[111]

Thyroid hormone tablets taken orally require an acid environment for dissolution before being transported to the small bowel for absorption. About 60% to 80% of levothyroxine is absorbed within 2 to 4 hours after an oral dose in the fasting state. Daily use of proton-pump inhibitors such as omeprazole (Prilosec) is associated with an increased levothyroxine requirement. This need is met by either increasing the levothyroxine dose or switching to a liquid preparation. Along these lines, there are many drugs that interfere with GI absorption of thyroid hormone including ferrous sulfate, calcium carbonate, aluminum hydroxide, sucralfate, bile acid sequestrants, and raloxifene. Taking thyroid hormone 4 hours before ingesting any of these medications or moving the levothyroxine dose to bedtime is recommended. An empty stomach is advised, since even soy formula, milk, or coffee can impair absorption.

Several drugs are associated with abnormal results of laboratory tests of the thyroid in euthyroid persons. These drugs are presented in Table 26.6. Lastly, both hyperthyroidism and hypothyroidism can affect the pharmacokinetics and efficacy of concurrent drugs as well as the frequency of adverse effects. A striking example includes warfarin (Coumadin, oral anticoagulant), with a counterintuitive lower dose requirement during hyperthyroidism as a result of accelerated turnover of vitamin K-dependent clotting factors. Another example is statins, which are associated with an increased risk of myopathy in the presence of hypothyroidism. Hyperthyroidism accelerates the metabolism of many drugs, including propranolol, cardiac glycosides, and glucocorticoids, and conversely, hypothyroidism delays clearance of these drugs.

Overall, drugs interact with the thyroid gland or its hormones via diverse mechanisms. Drugs may also alter the results of thyroid laboratory tests in a manner that artifactually mimics Graves disease, central hypothyroidism, and central hyperthyroidism. Awareness of these potential interactions allows pharmacists to monitor patients for them, intervene when appropriate, and avoid unnecessary testing and treatment.

Table 26.6 Drugs and Micronutrients That Cause Incorrect Thyroid Test Results in Euthyroid Individuals

	Test Results			
Drug	**Thyrotropin**	**T_3**	**Free T_4**	**Mimicked Conditions**
Amiodarone	High end normal	Low end normal	High	Thyroid hormone resistance Thyrotropin-secreting pituitary adenoma
Biotin	Low	High	High	Primary hyperthyroidism
Carbamazepine Oxcarbazepine Phenytoin	Normal	Low end normal	Low	Central hypothyroidism
Heparin(s)	Normal	High	High	Thyroid hormone resistance Thyrotropin-secreting pituitary adenoma
Salsalate	Normal	Low end normal	Low end normal	Central hypothyroidism

Clinical Case

Rami A. Al-Horani, PhD

CASE PRESENTATION

AB, 35-year-old women with no history of thyroid problems presented to the clinic with symptoms of fatigue, weight gain, hair loss, constipation, and anxiety. She also reported partially impaired memory at times. She is otherwise healthy with no history of medication except for the occasional use of antacids to manage hyperacidity. AB also reported the use of multivitamin/multimineral supplement. Her mother has a history of thyroid fluctuations, and her father has thyroid carcinoma. AB recently delivered a baby and returned to work a few weeks afterward. Initially, she attributed her fatigue to her long sleepless nights attending to her newborn. Nevertheless, her duplicated lab results indicated that she has substantially elevated TSH (100 mIU/L, normal range is 0.04-5 mIU/L) and a low free T_4 (<0.5 ng/dL, normal range is 0.9-1.8 ng/dL) in addition to a positive TPO antibody test. Her physician diagnosed her with severe hypothyroidism attributed to recent pregnancy. She was advised to start levothyroxine replacement therapy. The endocrinologist prescribed Synthroid at a daily dose of 125 μg. The dose is to be adjusted later as her condition improves. The endocrinologist also advised the patient to take the medicine at bedtime.

OUTCOME

After 1 month, the patient's TSH decreased to 15 mIU/L. After 2 months, the patient's TSH was normal with a value of 0.08 mIU/L and an elevated free T_4 of 1.3 ng/dL. The patient was considered responsive and became euthyroid, and after 3 months she started to feel less fatigue and lost considerable weight. The endocrinologist discussed a long-term plan with the patient, which comprises adjusted diet and decreased dose of Synthroid that is adequate to sustain her euthyroid status.

What are the other thyroid hormone replacement therapy preparations available? Why did the endocrinologist prescribe Synthroid for this patient? Why did the endocrinologist advise the patient to take Synthroid at bedtime?

ACKNOWLEDGMENTS

The author wishes to acknowledge Ali R. Banijamali, PhD, who authored content used within this chapter in a previous edition of this text.

Clinical Case

Rami A. Al-Horani, PhD

MEDICINAL CHEMISTRY-DRIVEN DECISION MAKING

Given the lab test results of AB, oral thyroid hormone replacement therapy is essential to treat her chronic hypothyroidism. There are several approved thyroid hormone replacement brands available, including natural and synthetic ones.

Natural desiccated preparations (Armour Thyroid, NP Thyroid) are reported to have a ratio of T_4 and T_3 similar to the ratio in humans (about 4:1). Desiccated preparations have been shown to produce variable blood levels of T_4 and T_3 because of variabilities between and within animal sources of thyroid gland. Although many aspects are similar for partially purified thyroglobulin, the total and relative amounts of T_3 and T_4 are different. Natural preparations are also associated with the disadvantages of protein antigenicity, product instability, and difficulty in laboratory monitoring. Furthermore, high amounts of T_3 can be found in some thyroid extracts and may produce significant elevations in T_3 levels and toxicity. Thus, natural preparations are not an optimal choice for this patient.

Synthetic thyroid preparations, on the other hand, have more predictable pharmacodynamic and pharmacokinetic properties. In particular, liotrix (Thyrolar) contains a mixture of T_3 and T_4, liothyronine sodium (Cytomel) contains the sodium salt of T_3, levothyroxine sodium (Levoxyl and Synthroid) contains the sodium salt of T_4. Considering the synthetic mixture of liotrix, our body converts T_4 to the more active hormone T_3, yet this conversion can be variable, resulting in substantial potential of variability in pharmacodynamics. Therefore, the synthetic mixture of thyroid hormones is not an optimal choice to treat chronic hypothyroidism in this patient.

(continued)

Clinical Case (continued)

When deciding between liothyronine sodium (which contains the sodium salt of T_3) and levothyroxine sodium (which contains the sodium salt of T_4), we should consider the pharmacokinetic aspects of the two synthetic preparations and the impact of the additional iodine substituent in T_4, rather their hormonal activity itself. Given the additional lipophilic substituent, T_4 (cLogP = 3.5) is more lipophilic than T_3 (cLogP = 2.6). This appears to cause T_4 to extensively bind to plasma proteins (>99%), whereas T_3 does not bind as much. As a result, the synthetic T_4 preparation has a slower clearance rate (0.84-1.37 L/d) than that of the synthetic T_3 preparation (20-36 L/d) as well as a longer elimination half-life (6-8 days; it becomes longer in hypothyroidism) than that of the synthetic T_3 preparation (7-25 hours). Therefore, synthetic T_4 preparations such as Synthroid, in this condition, are more suitable to orally treat chronic hypothyroidism because they promote better patient adherence and compliance, in addition to the lack of pharmacokinetic and pharmacodynamic variability.

The patient was advised to take her medication at bedtime to avoid potential interactions with the magnesium and/or calcium components of antacids as well as potential interactions with the iron component of the multimineral supplement. The multivalent cations in this preparation can form insoluble complexes with the amino acid moiety of T_4, which may result in poor absorption and lack of therapeutic effect.

REFERENCES

1. Harington CR. Biochemical basis of thyroid function. *Lancet.* 1935;225:1261-1266.
2. Baumann E. Uber das normale Vorkommen von Jod in Tierkorper. *Zeitschr f Physiol Chem.* 1896;21:319.
3. Gross J, Pitt-Rivers R. The identification of 3:5:3′-L-triiodothyronine in human plasma. *Lancet.* 1952;1(6705):439-441.
4. Koenig RJ, Brent GA. Thyroid and antithyroid drugs. In: Brunton LL, Knollmann BC, eds. *Goodman & Gilman's: The Pharmacological Basis of Therapeutics.* 14th ed. McGraw Hill; 2023:941-958.
5. Kogai T, Brent GA. The sodium iodide symporter (NIS): regulation and approaches to targeting for cancer therapeutics. *Pharmacol Ther.* 2012;135:355-370.
6. Portulano C, Paroder-Belenitsky M, Carrasco N. The Na^+/I^- symporter (NIS): mechanism and medical impact. *Endocr Rev.* 2014;35(1):106-149.
7. Taurog A. Hormone synthesis: thyroid iodine metabolism. In: Braverman L, Utiger R, eds. *Werner & Ingbar's The Thyroid: A Fundamental and Clinical Text.* 8th ed. Lippincott Williams & Wilkins; 2000:61-85.
8. Szanto I, Pusztaszeri M, Mavromati M. H_2O_2 metabolism in normal thyroid cells and in thyroid tumorigenesis: focus on NADPH oxidases. *Antioxidants (Basel).* 2019;8(5):126.
9. Chopra IJ, Solomon DH, Chopra U, et al. Pathways of metabolism of thyroid hormones. *Recent Prog Horm Res.* 1978;34:521-567.
10. Visser TJ, Docter R, Krenning EP, Hennemann G. Regulation of thyroid hormone bioactivity. *J Endocrinol Invest.* 1986;9(suppl 4): 17-26.
11. Krassas GE, Rivkees SA, Kiess W, eds. *Diseases of the thyroid in childhood and adolescence.* In: *Pediatric and Adolescent Medicine.* Vol 10. Karger; 2007:80-103.
12. Hollander CS, Bernstein G, Oppenheimer JH. Abnormalities of thyroxine binding in analbuminemia. *J Clin Endocrinol Metab.* 1968;28:1064-1066.
13. Benvenga S, Robbins J. Lipoprotein-thyroid hormone interactions. *Trends Endocrinol Metab.* 1993;4(6):194-198.
14. Strott CA. Sulfonation and molecular action. *Endocr Rev.* 2002;23(5):703-732.
15. Wu SY, Green WL, Huang WS, Hays MT, Chopra IJ. Alternate pathways of thyroid hormone metabolism. *Thyroid.* 2005;15(8): 943-958.
16. Abduljabbar MA, Afifi AM. Congenital hypothyroidism. *J Pediatr Endocrinol Metab.* 2012;25:13-29.
17. Mughal BB, Fini JB, Demeneix BA. Thyroid-disrupting chemicals and brain development: an update. *Endocr Connect.* 2018;7(4): R160-R186.
18. Mullur R, Liu YY, Brent GA. Thyroid hormone regulation of metabolism. *Physiol Rev.* 2014;94:355-382.
19. Müller MJ, Seitz HJ. Thyroid hormone action on intermediary metabolism. Part I: respiration, thermogenesis and carbohydrate metabolism. *Klin Wochenschr.* 1984;62(1):11-18.
20. Grais IM, Sowers JR. Thyroid and the heart. *Am J Med.* 2014;127: 691-698.
21. Wojcicka A, Bassett JH, Williams GR. Mechanisms of action of thyroid hormones in the skeleton. *Biochim Biophys Acta.* 2013;1830(7): 3979-3986.
22. Wolff J, Chaikoff IL. Plasma inorganic iodide as a homeostatic regulator of thyroid function. *J Biol Chem.* 1948;174(2):555-564.
23. Virion A, Michot JL, Deme D, Pommier J. NADPH oxidation catalyzed by the peroxidase/H_2O_2 system. Iodide-mediated oxidation of NADPH to iodinated NADP. *Eur J Biochem.* 1985;148(2): 239-243.
24. McConnon J, Row VV, Volpé R. The influence of liver damage in man on the distribution and disposal rates of thyroxine and triiodothyronine. *J Clin Endocrinol Metab.* 1972;34(1):144-151.
25. Lim VS, Fang VS, Katz AI, Refetoff S. Thyroid dysfunction in chronic renal failure. A study of the pituitary-thyroid axis and peripheral turnover kinetics of thyroxine and triiodothyronine. *J Clin Invest.* 1977;60(3):522-534.
26. Carter JN, Eastmen CJ, Corcoran JM, Lazarus L. Inhibition of conversion of thyroxine to triiodothyronine in patients with severe chronic illness. *Clin Endocrinol (Oxf).* 1976;5(6):587-594.
27. Spaulding SW, Chopra IJ, Sherwin RS, Lyall SS. Effect of caloric restriction and dietary composition of serum T_3 and reverse T_3 in man. *J Clin Endocrinol Metab.* 1976;42(1):197-200.
28. Heyma P, Larkins RG, Campbell DG. Inhibition by propranolol of 3,5,3′-triiodothyronine formation from thyroxine in isolated rat renal tubules: an effect independent of beta-adrenergic blockade. *Endocrinology.* 1980;106(5):1437-1441.
29. Silva JE, Larsen PR. Adrenergic activation of triiodothyronine production in brown adipose tissue. *Nature.* 1983;305(5936):712-713.
30. Zenker N, Chacon MA, Tildon JT. Mode of death effect on rat liver iodothyronine 5′ deiodinase activity: role of adenosine 3′,5′ monophosphate. *Life Sci.* 1984;35(22):2213-2217.
31. Sawka AM, Carty SE, Haugen BR, et al. American Thyroid Association Guidelines and Statements: past, present, and future. *Thyroid.* 2018;28(6):692-706.
32. Ventura M, Melo M, Carrilho F. Selenium and thyroid disease: from pathophysiology to treatment. *Int J Endocrinol.* 2017;2017: 1297658.
33. Liontiris MI, Mazokopakis EE. A concise review of Hashimoto thyroiditis (HT) and the importance of iodine, selenium, vitamin D and gluten on the autoimmunity and dietary management of HT patients. Points that need more investigation. *Hell J Nucl Med.* 2017;20(1):51-56.
34. Hollowell JG, Staehling NW, Flanders WD, et al. Serum TSH, T(4), and thyroid antibodies in the United States population

(1988 to 1994): National Health and Nutrition Examination Survey (NHANES III). *J Clin Endocrinol Metab.* 2002;87(2):489-499.
35. Zimmermann MB. Iodine deficiency. *Endocr Rev.* 2009;30:376-408.
36. Esfandiari NH, McPhee SJ. Thyroid disease. In: Hammer GD, McPhee SJ, eds. *Pathophysiology of Disease: An Introduction to Clinical Medicine.* 8th ed. McGraw Hill; 2019. Accessed February 26, 2025. Available from: Access Medicine.
37. Torino F, Corsello SM, Longo R, et al. Hypothyroidism related to tyrosine kinase inhibitors: an emerging toxic effect of targeted therapy. *Nat Rev Clin Oncol.* 2009;6(4):219-228.
38. Moleti M, Mauro MD, Alibrandi A, et al. Postpartum thyroiditis in women with euthyroid and hypothyroid Hashimoto's thyroiditis antedating pregnancy. *J Clin Endocrinol Metab.* 2020; 105(7):dgaa197.
39. Jameson J, Mandel SJ, Weetman AP. Hypothyroidism. In: Loscalzo J, Fauci A, Kasper D, et al, eds. *Harrison's Principles of Internal Medicine.* 21th ed. McGraw Hill; 2022. Accessed February 26, 2025. Available from: Access Pharmacy.
40. Hatch-McChesney A, Lieberman HR. Iodine and iodine deficiency: A comprehensive review of a re-emerging issue. *Nutrients.* 2022;14(17):3474.
41. World Health Organization. Recommended iodine levels in salt and guidelines for monitoring their adequacy and effectiveness. Nutrition Unit. 1996. Accessed July, 2023. https://apps.who.int/iris/handle/10665/63322
42. Jonklaas J, Bianco AC, Bauer AJ, et al; American Thyroid Association Task Force on Thyroid Hormone Replacement. Guidelines for the treatment of hypothyroidism: prepared by the American thyroid association task force on thyroid hormone replacement. *Thyroid.* 2014;24(12):1670-1751.
43. Fleseriu M, Hashim IA, Karavitaki N, et al. Hormonal replacement in hypopituitarism in adults: an Endocrine Society Clinical Practice Guideline. *J Clin Endocrinol Metab.* 2016;101(11): 3888-3921.
44. Klein I, Danzi S. Thyroid disease and the heart. *Circulation.* 2007;116(15):1725-1735.
45. Akashi YJ, Nef HM, Möllmann H, et al. Stress cardiomyopathy. *Annu Rev Med.* 2010;61:271-286.
46. Zeitjian V, Moazez C, Saririan M, et al. Manifestation of non-ST elevation myocardial infarction due to hyperthyroidism in an anomalous right coronary artery. *Int J Gen Med.* 2017; 10:409-413.
47. Garber KR, Cobin RH, Gharib H, et al; American Association of Clinical Endocrinologists and American Thyroid Association taskforce on hypothyroidism in adults. Clinical practice guidelines for hypothyroidism in adults: cosponsored by the American Association of Clinical Endocrinologists and the American Thyroid Association. *Endocr Pract.* 2012;18(6):988-1028.
48. Jackson IM, Cobb WE. Why does anyone still use desiccated thyroid USP? *Am J Med.* 1978;64(2):284-288.
49. Aronson R, Offman HJ, Joffe RT, Naylor CD. Triiodothyronine augmentation in the treatment of refractory depression. A meta-analysis. *Arch Gen Psychiatry.* 1996;53(9):842-848.
50. Dong BJ. Thyroid & antithyroid drugs. In: Katzung BG, ed. *Basic & Clinical Pharmacology.* 16th ed. McGraw Hill; 2024. Accessed February 26, 2025. Available from: Access Pharmacy.
51. Malm J, Grover GJ. Thyroid hormones and thyromimetics. In: Abraham DJ, Rotella DP, eds. *Burger's Medicinal Chemistry.* 7th ed. Vol 4. Wiley; 2010:189-222.
52. Zenker N, Jorgensen EC. Thyroxine analogs. I. Synthesis of 3,5-diiodo-4-(2′-alkylphenoxy)-DL-phenylalanines. *J Am Chem Soc.* 1959;81(17):4643-4647.
53. Jorgensen EC, Zenker N, Greenberg C. Thyroxine analogues. III. Antigoitrogenic and calorigenic activity of some alkyl substituted analogues of thyroxine. *J Biol Chem.* 1960;235:1732-1737.
54. Jorgensen EC, Lehman PA, Greenberg C, Zenker N. Thyroxine analogues. VII. Antigoitrogenic, calorigenic, and hypocholesteremic activities of some aliphatic, alicyclic, and aromatic ethers of 3, 5-diiodoty-rosine in the rat. *J Biol Chem.* 1962;237:3832-3838.
55. Cody V. Thyroid hormones: crystal structure, molecular conformation, binding, and structure-function relationships. *Recent Prog Horm Res.* 1978;34:437-475.
56. Ekins R. Methods for the measurement of free thyroid hormones. In: Ekins R, Faglia G, Pennisi F, et al, eds. *International Symposium on Free Thyroid Hormones.* Excerpta Medica; 1979:7-29.
57. Ahmad P, Fyfe CA, Mellors A. Parachors in drug design. *Biochem Pharmacol.* 1975;24(10):1103-1110.
58. Benson MG, Ellis D, Emmett JC, et al. 3′-Acetyl-3,5-diiodo-L-thyronine: a novel highly active thyromimetic with low receptor affinity. *Biochem Pharmacol.* 1984;33(20):3143-3149.
59. Jorgensen EC, Lehman PA. Thyroxine analogs. V. Synthesis of some 1- and 2-naphthyl ethers of 3,5-diiodo-DL-tyrosine. *J Org Chem.* 1961;26(3):897-900.
60. Mussett MV, Pitt-Rivers R. The physiologic activity of thyroxine and triiodothyronine analogs. *Metabolism.* 1957;6(1):18-25.
61. Jorgensen EC, Reid JA. Thyroxine analogues. XI. Structural isomers of 3,5,3′-triiodo-DL-thyronine. *J Med Chem.* 1964;7:701-705.
62. Tripp SL, Block FB, Barile G. Synthesis of methylene-and carbonyl-bridged analogs of iodothyronines and iodothyroacetic acids. *J Med Chem.* 1973;16(1):60-64.
63. Mukherjee R, Block P. Thyroxine analogues: synthesis and nuclear magnetic resonance spectral studies of diphenylamines. *J Chem Soc C.* 1971;9(2):1596-1600.
64. Leeson PD, Ellis D, Emmett JC, et al. Thyroid hormone analogues. Synthesis of 3′-substituted 3,5-diiodo-L-thyronines and quantitative structure-activity studies of in vitro and in vivo thyromimetic activities in rat liver and heart. *J Med Chem.* 1988;31(1):37-54.
65. Jorgensen EC. Thyroid hormones and analogs II. Structure-activity relationships. In: Li CH, ed. *Hormonal Proteins and Peptides.* Vol 6. Academic Press; 1978:107-204.
66. Gluckman PD, Ballard PL, Kaplan SL, Liggins GC, Grumbach MM. Prolactin in umbilical cord blood and the respiratory distress syndrome. *J Pediatr.* 1978;93(6):1011-1014.
67. Ross DS, Burch HB, Cooper DS, et al. 2016 American Thyroid Association Guidelines for diagnosis and management of hyperthyroidism and other causes of thyrotoxicosis. *Thyroid.* 2016;26: 1343-1421.
68. Dosiou C, Kossler AL. Thyroid eye disease: navigating the new treatment landscape. *J Endocr Soc.* 2021;5:1-13.
69. Morreale de Escobar G, Escobar del Rey F. Extrathyroid effects of some antithyroid drugs and their metabolic consequences. *Recent Prog Horm Res.* 1967;23:87-137.
70. Cooper DS, Saxe VC, Meskell M, Maloof F, Ridgway EC. Acute effects of propylthiouracil (PTU) on thyroidal iodide organification and peripheral iodothyronine deiodination: correlation with serum PTU levels measured by radioimmunoassay. *J Clin Endocrinol Metab.* 1982;54(1):101-107.
71. Visser TJ, van Overmeeren E, Fekkes D, Docter R, Hennemann G. Inhibition of iodothyronine 5'-deiodinase by thioureylenes; structure-activity relationship. *FEBS Lett.* 1979;103(2):314-318.
72. Jansson R, Lindström B, Dahlberg PA. Pharmacokinetic properties and bioavailability of methimazole. *Clin Pharmacokinet.* 1985;10(5):443-450.
73. Heidari R, Niknahad H, Jamshidzadeh A, Eghbal MA, Abdoli N. An overview on the proposed mechanisms of antithyroid drugs-induced liver injury. *Adv Pharm Bull.* 2015;5(1):1-11.
74. Mizutani T, Yoshida K, Murakami M, et al. Evidence for the involvement of N-methylthiourea, a ring cleavage metabolite, in the hepatotoxicity of methimazole in glutathione-depleted mice: structure-toxicity and metabolic studies. *Chem Res Toxicol.* 2000;13(3):170-176.
75. Pramyothin P, Leung AM, Pearce EN, Malabanan AO, Braverman LE. Clinical problem-solving. A hidden solution. *N Engl J Med.* 2011;365(22):2123-2127.
76. Alexander EK, Larsen PR. High dose of (131)I therapy for the treatment of hyperthyroidism caused by Graves' disease. *J Clin Endocrinol Metab.* 2002, 87:1073-1077.

77. Agency for Toxic Substances and Disease Registry, U.S. Department of Health and Human Services. *Toxicological Profile for Perchlorates*. U.S. Department of Health and Human Services. 2005.
78. Simsir IY, Ozdemir M, Duman S, et al. Therapeutic plasmapheresis in thyrotoxic patients. *Endocrine*. 2018;62(1):144-148.
79. Kamboj A, Lee MS, McClelland CM. Medical management of thyroid eye disease. *Int Ophthalmol Clin*. 2023;63(2):81-89.
80. Douglas RS, Kahaly GJ, Patel A, et al. Teprotumumab for the treatment of active thyroid eye disease. *N Engl J Med*. 2020;382(4):341-352.
81. Persani L, Campi I. Syndromes of resistance to thyroid hormone action. *Exp Suppl*. 2019;111:55-84.
82. Pappa T, Refetoff S. Human genetics of thyroid hormone receptor beta: resistance to thyroid hormone beta (RTHβ). *Methods Mol Biol*. 2018;1801:225-240.
83. Briet C, Bouhours-Nouet N, Illouz F, Prunier-Mirebeau D, Rodien P. TRα mutations in human. *Methods Mol Biol*. 2018;1801:241-245.
84. Haugen BR, Alexander EK, Bible KC, et al. 2015 American Thyroid Association management guidelines for adult patients with thyroid nodules and differentiated thyroid cancer: The American Thyroid Association Guidelines Task Force on Thyroid Nodules and Differentiated Thyroid Cancer. *Thyroid*. 2016;26:1-133.
85. Haugen BR, Sherman SI. Evolving approaches to patients with advanced differentiated thyroid cancer. *Endocr Rev*. 2013;34:439-455.
86. Dunn DB. Larotrectinib and entrectinib: TRK inhibitors for the treatment of pediatric and adult patients with NTRK gene fusion. *J Adv Pract Oncol*. 2020;11(4):418-423.
87. Zhao L, Mei Q, Yu Y, et al. Research progress on RET fusion in non-small-cell lung cancer. *Front Oncol*. 2022;12:894214.
88. Crispo F, Notarangelo T, Pietrafesa M, et al. BRAF inhibitors in thyroid cancer: clinical impact, mechanisms of resistance and future perspectives. *Cancers (Basel)*. 2019;11(9):1388.
89. Rissmann R, Hessel MH, Cohen AF. Vemurafenib/dabrafenib and trametinib. *Br J Clin Pharmacol*. 2015;80(4):765-767.
90. Markham A, Keam SJ. Selumetinib: first approval. *Drugs*. 2020;80(9):931-937.
91. The U.S. Food and Drug Administration. FDA approves dabrafenib plus trametinib for anaplastic thyroid cancer with BRAF V600E mutation. Accessed June 29, 2023. https://www.fda.gov/drugs/resources-information-approved-drugs/fda-approves-dabrafenib-plus-trametinib-anaplastic-thyroid-cancer-braf-v600e-mutation
92. Subbiah V, Cote GJ. Advances in targeting RET-dependent cancers. *Cancer Discov*. 2020;10(4):498-505.
93. Loxo Oncology, Inc. Vitrakvi (larotrectinib) capsules for oral use and oral solution [product information]. Revised November 2018. U.S. Department of Health and Human Services, Food and Drug Administration. Accessed on June 29, 2023. www.accessdata.fda.gov/drugsatfda_docs/label/2018/210861s000lbl.pdf
94. U.S. Department of Health and Human Services, Food and Drug Administration. FDA approves an oncology drug that targets a key genetic driver of cancer, rather than a specific type of tumor [FDA News Release]. U.S. Department of Health and Human Services, Food and Drug Administration. Published November 26, 2018. Accessed on June 29, 2023. www.fda.gov/NewsEvents/Newsroom/PressAnnouncements/ucm626710.htm
95. Al-Salama ZT, Keam SJ. Entrectinib: first global approval. *Drugs*. 2019;79(13):1477-1483.
96. Markham A. Selpercatinib: first approval [published correction appears in drugs. 2021 Jan;81(1):181]. *Drugs*. 2020;80(11):1119-1124.
97. Markham A. Pralsetinib: first approval. *Drugs*. 2020;80(17):1865-1870.
98. Scott LJ. Lenvatinib: first global approval. *Drugs*. 2015;75(5):553-560.
99. White PT, Cohen MS. The discovery and development of sorafenib for the treatment of thyroid cancer. *Expert Opin Drug Discov*. 2015;10(4):427-439.
100. Bollag G, Tsai J, Zhang J, et al. Vemurafenib: the first drug approved for BRAF-mutant cancer. *Nat Rev Drug Discov*. 2012;11(11):873-886.
101. Ballantyne AD, Garnock-Jones KP. Dabrafenib: first global approval. *Drugs*. 2013;73(12):1367-1376.
102. Wright CJ, McCormack PL. Trametinib: first global approval. *Drugs*. 2013;73(11):1245-1254.
103. Commander H, Whiteside G, Perry C. Vandetanib: first global approval. *Drugs*. 2011;71(10):1355-1365.
104. Duke ES, Barone AK, Chatterjee S, et al. FDA approval summary: cabozantinib for differentiated thyroid cancer. *Clin Cancer Res*. 2022;28(19):4173-4177.
105. Turner JG, Brownlie BE, Sadler WA, Jensen CH. An evaluation of lithium as an adjunct to carbimazole treatment in acute thyrotoxicosis. *Acta Endocrinol (Copenh)*. 1976;83(1):86-92.
106. Berens SC, Wolff J, Murphy DL. Lithium concentration by the thyroid. *Endocrinology*. 1970;87(5):1085-1087.
107. Temple R, Berman M, Robbins J, Wolff J. The use of lithium in the treatment of thyrotoxicosis. *J Clin Invest*. 1972;51(10):2746-2756.
108. Langer P, Michajlovskij N. Effect of naturally occurring goitrogens on thyroid peroxidase and influence of some compounds on iodide formation during the estimation. *Endocrinol Exp*. 1972;6(2):97-103.
109. Elfving S. Studies on the naturally occurring goitrogen 5-vinyl-2-thiooxazolidone. Metabolism and antithyroid effect in the rat. *Ann Clin Res*. 1980;Suppl 28:1-47.
110. Burch HB. Drug effects on the thyroid. *N Engl J Med*. 2019;381(8):749-761.
111. Bezin J, Gouverneur A, Pénichon M, et al. GLP-1 receptor agonists and the risk of thyroid cancer. *Diabetes Care*. 2023;46(2):384-390.
112. Mondal S, Raja K, Schweizer U, Mugesh G. Chemistry and biology in the biosynthesis and action of thyroid hormones. *Angew Chem Int Ed Engl*. 2016;55(27):7606-7630.

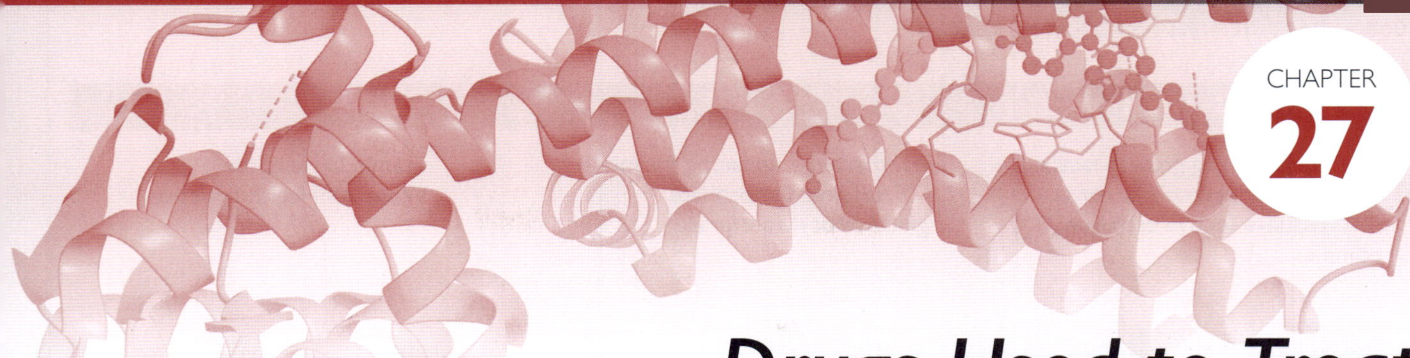

CHAPTER 27

Drugs Used to Treat Calcium-Dependent Disorders

Robin M. Zavod

Drugs covered in this chapter:

Selective estrogen receptor modulators
- Bazedoxifene acetate
- Raloxifene hydrochloride
- Tamoxifen

Bisphosphonates
- Alendronate sodium
- Disodium
- Ibandronate sodium
- Pamidronate
- Risedronate sodium
- Zoledronic acid

Calcitonin

PTH analogues
- Abaloparatide
- Teriparatide

Monoclonal antibody
- Denosumab
- Romosozumab

Calcium mimetics
- Cinacalcet hydrochloride
- Etelcalcetide

Inorganic salts
- Calcium salts

Abbreviations

AF-2 activation factor-2
ATP adenosine triphosphate
BMD bone mineral density
BMU basic multicellular unit
BRONJ bisphosphonate-related osteonecrosis of the jaw
cAMP cyclic adenosine monophosphate
CaSR calcium-sensing receptor
CAT catalase
CT calcitonin
CYP450 cytochrome P-450
DAG diacylglycerol
DIOP drug-induced osteoporosis
DKK-1 dickkopf-1
DNA deoxyribonucleic acid
ER estrogen receptor
ERE estrogen responding element
ERT estrogen replacement therapy
FDA US Food and Drug Administration
FGF23 fibroblast growth factor 23
FPPS farnesyl pyrophosphate synthetase
GnRH gonadotropin releasing hormone
GPCR G protein–coupled receptor
GSK-3β glycogen synthase kinase-3β
HDL2-C high-density lipoprotein 2 cholesterol
IGF-1 insulin-like growth factor 1
IL-6 interleukin-6
IM intramuscular
IP_3 inositol triphosphate
IU international units
IV intravenous
LDL-C low-density lipoprotein cholesterol
LRP5/6 low-density lipoprotein coreceptor–related proteins 5/6
MBF modeling-based formation
mEq milliequivalent
M-CSF macrophage colony-stimulating factor
NFκB nuclear factor κ-light-chain-enhancer of activated B cells
$1,25(OH)_2D_3$ 1,25-dihydroxycholecalciferol
$25(OH)D_3$ 25-hydroxycholecalciferol
OPG osteoprotegerin
PKA phosphokinase A
PLC phospholipase C
PPARγ(2) peroxisome proliferator-activated receptor γ2
PPi pyrophosphate
PTH parathyroid hormone
PTHR1 parathyroid hormone receptor type 1
PTHrP parathyroid hormone–related protein
RANKL receptor activator of nuclear factor-κB ligand
RBF remodeling-based formation
REMS risk evaluation and mitigation strategy
RRE raloxifene-responding element
SAR structure-activity relationship
SC subcutaneous
SERM selective estrogen receptor modulator
SHBG sex hormone–binding globulin
SOD superoxide dismutase

Abbreviations—continued

TGFβ transforming growth factor β
TNF-α tumor necrosis factor α
TSEC tissue-selective estrogen complex
TSH thyroid-stimulating hormone
UGT uridine diphosphate glucuronosyltransferase
VDR vitamin D receptor
WHI Women's Health Initiative

CLINICAL SIGNIFICANCE

Taking a "drug holiday" is not typically included in a treatment plan for patients diagnosed with chronic diseases. The need to maintain consistent therapeutic drug levels, short drug half-life, and rebound effects are several of the many factors that prevent clinicians from being able to offer a scheduled, temporary, purposeful break from a medication to their patients. A drug holiday is actually feasible for those taking bisphosphonates to treat osteoporosis. Why is this possible? Drug structure evaluation, as championed by medicinal chemists, provides a simple explanation. The bisphosphonates have a high affinity for the bone, as they mimic natural pyrophosphate (PPi) in their ability to chelate calcium and get incorporated into the bone matrix. Since the bone is virtually unsaturable, prolonged bisphosphonate treatment results in significant drug accumulation. This allows for continual drug release for months or perhaps even years after treatment is stopped with continued antifracture benefit.

Jill S. Borchert, PharmD

INTRODUCTION

Three primary hormones—calcitonin (CT), parathyroid hormone (PTH), and vitamin D—control the homeostatic regulation of calcium and its principle counterion, inorganic phosphate. Homeostatic control of these ions is essential not only for the moderation of longitudinal bone growth and bone remodeling but also for blood coagulation, neuromuscular excitability, plasma membrane structure and function, muscle contraction, glycogen and adenosine triphosphate (ATP) metabolism, neurotransmitter/hormone secretion, and enzyme catalysis.[1] In an average 70-kg adult, approximately 1 kg of calcium is found, approximately 45% is bound to plasma proteins, 15% is bound to anions, and approximately 40% is in the free or ionized form.[2] The primary calcium salt in the hydroxyapatite crystalline lattice of teeth and bones is $Ca_{10}(PO_4)_6(OH)_2$. Similarly, approximately 500 to 600 g of phosphate are present, 85% of which is in the bone. The normal plasma concentration of calcium is approximately 4.5 to 5.7 mEq/L, 50% of which is protein bound. The remainder of the calcium is either complexed to corresponding counterions (46%) or exists in its ionized form (4%). Only the ionized form of calcium is tightly hormonally regulated.[1] Because serum calcium concentrations fluctuate, so do the plasma levels of the hormones associated with calcium homeostasis. Serum phosphorous levels vary with age, diet, and hormonal status. The most common form of phosphate in the blood (pH 7.4) is HPO_4^{2-}.

The bone is composed of two distinct tissue structures: cortical (compact) bone and trabecular (cancellous) bone.[3] Eighty percent of the skeleton is composed of the cortical bone (eg, long bones such as the humerus, radius, and ulna), which is a relatively dense tissue (80%-90% calcified) that provides structure and support.[3,4] Bone marrow cavities, flat bones, and the ends of long bones are all composed of the trabecular bone, which is considerably more porous (5%-20% calcified). To maintain healthy, well-mineralized bone, a continuous process of bone resorption (loss of ionic calcium from bone) and bone formation occurs along the bone surface in the trabecular bone, and tunnels through the bone in cortical bone.[3] There are similar amounts of bone lost from both types of the bone for the first 10 years after menopause. Thereafter, more cortical bone is lost.[3] In terms of calcium turnover in the bone, approximately 500 mg is removed and replaced daily.

Both inorganic and organic components are present in the bone. The highly crystalline inorganic component is hydroxyapatite, and the collagen matrix comprises the major portion (90%) of the organic component. The collagen matrix serves as the foundation for hydroxyapatite mineralization. Osteocalcin and osteonectin are minor organic constituents that promote binding of hydroxyapatite and calcium to the collagen matrix and regulate the rate of bone mineralization, respectively.[5]

In general, peak bone mass occurs between ages 30 and 40 years and is dependent on genetic factors as well as proper intake of calcium, maintenance of quality nutrition, and participation in weight-bearing exercise.[6] Thereafter, peak bone mass progressively declines at the rate of 0.3% to 0.5% of the cortical bone per year.[3] After menopause, bone loss is accelerated (2% per year in the spine)[6] for a period of 5 to 10 years due to estrogen loss. This can result in up to a 30% decrease in bone mineral density (BMD).

Hormonal Regulation of Serum Calcium Levels

Complex interrelationships among the three hormones (parathyroid, CT, and vitamin D) control calcium homeostasis (serum concentrations of ionic calcium) and their target organs (bone, kidney, and intestine). Figure 27.1 tracks the intake, utilization, and excretion of 1,000 mg calcium and the relative contributions of each of these three hormones. It is important to note that calcium homeostasis is achieved only if active vitamin D as well as sufficient levels of both PTH and CT are present. In addition to these three hormones, fibroblast growth factor 23 (FGF23) and the calcium-sensing receptor (CaSR) also contribute to calcium homeostasis.[2] FGF23 is a hormone that inhibits reabsorption of phosphate and kidney-based vitamin D activation.[7]

Calcitonin

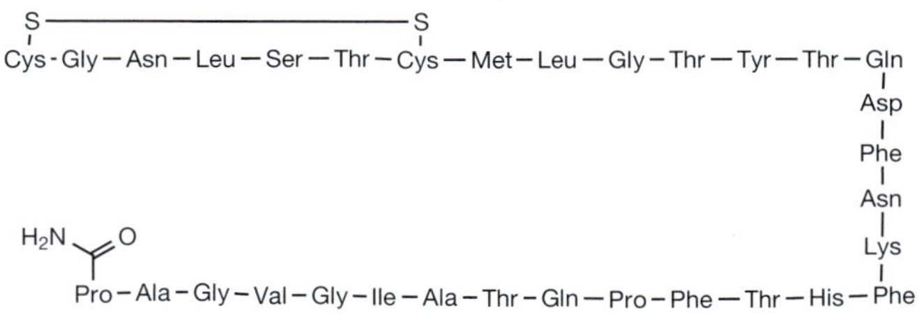

Human calcitonin

Human CT is a 32-amino acid peptide (molecular weight, 3,527 Da) biosynthesized in the parafollicular "C" cells within the thyroid gland. This hormone contains a critical disulfide bridge between residues 1 and 7, with the entire amino acid sequence required for biologic activity. The carboxy-terminal residue is a proline amide. "Procalcitonin," a precursor peptide, has been identified and proposed to facilitate intracellular transport and secretion. CT is secreted in response to elevated serum calcium concentrations (>9 mg/100 mL) and serves to oppose the hormonal effects of PTH. In response to a hypercalcemic state, increased CT secretion drives serum calcium concentrations down via stimulation of urinary excretion of both calcium and phosphate, prevention of calcium resorption from the bone via inhibition of osteoclast activity, and inhibition of intestinal absorption of calcium. When serum calcium concentrations are low (hypocalcemia), the release of CT is slowed.

Parathyroid Hormone

PTH is biosynthesized as a 115-amino acid preprohormone in the rough endoplasmic reticulum of the parathyroid gland and is cleaved to the prohormone (90 amino acids) in the cisternal space of the reticulum (Fig. 27.2). The active hormone is finally produced (84 amino acids; molecular weight, 9,500 Da) in the Golgi complex and is stored in secretory granules in the parathyroid gland. This gland is exquisitely sensitive to serum calcium concentrations and is able to monitor these levels via CaSR. These cell surface receptors react to micromolar changes in the concentration of ionized calcium in the serum.[8] Binding of calcium to these receptors facilitates activation of phospholipase C (PLC) and, ultimately, inhibition of PTH secretion. The relatively short-acting PTH is secreted from the parathyroid gland chief cells in response to a hypocalcemic state and serves to oppose the hormonal effects of CT.[1] Unlike CT, the biologic activity of PTH resides solely in residues 1 to 34 in the amino terminus.

PTH decreases renal excretion of calcium, indirectly stimulates intestinal absorption of calcium, and, in combination with active vitamin D, promotes bone resorption. PTH stimulates bone resorption by several mechanisms:

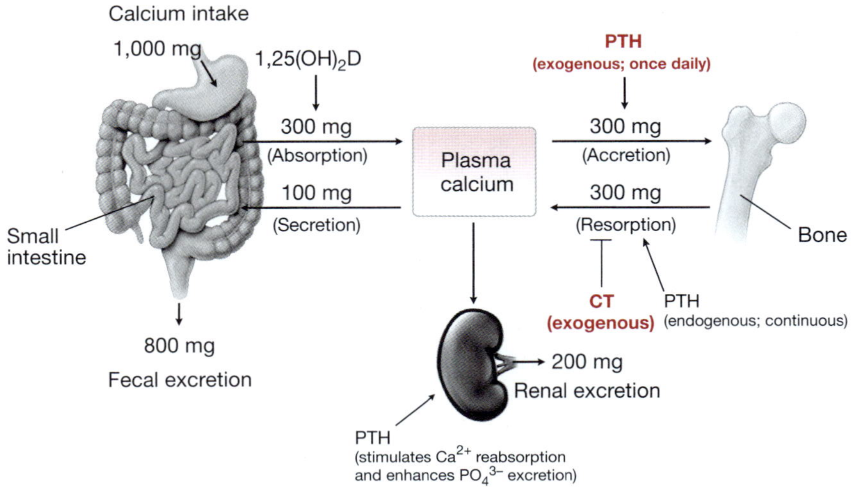

Figure 27.1 Calcium homeostasis; the fate of 1,000 mg of calcium. In a state of whole-body calcium balance, the fluxes of calcium include net uptake of 200 mg/d from the gastrointestinal (GI) tract and excretion of 200 mg/d by the kidneys. Calcitriol [$1,25(OH)_2D$] enhances absorption of Ca^{2+} from the GI tract. Continuous secretion of parathyroid hormone (PTH) increases bone formation and (even more) bone resorption and stimulates renal tubular reabsorption of calcium; both effects raise plasma Ca^{2+}. Exogenous calcitonin (CT) inhibits bone resorption. (Adapted with permission from Slovik DM, Armstrong EJ. Pharmacology of bone mineral homeostasis. In: Golan DE, Armstrong EJ, Armstrong AW, eds. *Principles of Pharmacology: The Pathophysiologic Basis of Drug Therapy*. 4th ed. Wolters Kluwer Health; 2017.)

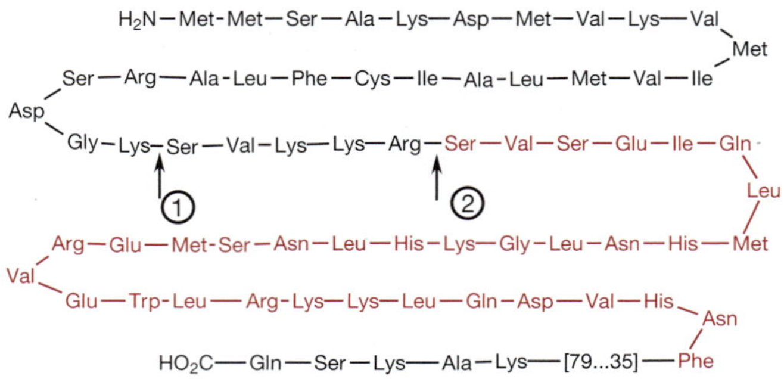

Figure 27.2 Preproparathyroid hormone is the 115–amino acid protein indicated earlier. Cleavage at site 1 gives rise to proparathyroid hormone (89 amino acids), while cleavage at site 2 gives parathyroid hormone (PTH, 84 amino acids). The protein shown in *red* is teriparatide (34 amino acids).

(1) transformation of osteoprogenitor cells into osteoclasts is stimulated in the presence of PTH, (2) PTH promotes the deep osteocytes to mobilize calcium from perilacunar bone, and (3) surface osteocytes are stimulated by PTH to increase the flow of calcium out of the bone. In addition, the secretion of PTH stimulates the biosynthesis, activation, and release of the third hormone associated with calcium homeostasis, vitamin D. When serum calcium concentrations are high, the release of PTH is inhibited.

Vitamin D

Derived from cholesterol, vitamin D is biosynthesized from its prohormone cholecalciferol (D_3), the product of solar ultraviolet irradiation of 7-dehydrocholesterol in the skin.[9] In 1966, it was first recognized that vitamin D must undergo activation via two oxidative metabolic steps (Fig. 27.3). The first oxidation to 25-hydroxycholecalciferol [25(OH)D_3: calcidiol; Rayaldee] occurs in the endoplasmic reticulum of the liver and is catalyzed by vitamin D 25-hydroxylase. This activation step is not regulated by plasma calcium concentrations. The major circulating form (10-80 μg/mL) is 25(OH) D_3, which is also the primary storage form of vitamin D. In response to a hypocalcemic state and the secretion of PTH, a second oxidation step is activated in the mitochondria of the kidney, catalyzed by vitamin D 1α-hydroxylase.[9] The product of this reaction, 1,25-dihydroxycholecalciferol [1,25$(OH)_2D_3$: 1,25-calcitriol; Rocaltrol] is the active form of vitamin D. Its concentration in the blood is 1/500 that of its mono-hydroxylated precursor. The biosynthesis of vitamin D is tightly regulated based on the serum concentrations of calcium, phosphate, PTH, and active vitamin D.[9]

Sterol-specific cytoplasmic receptor proteins (vitamin D receptor) mediate the biologic action of vitamin D.[9] The active hormone is transported from the cytoplasm to the nucleus via the vitamin D receptor, and because of the interaction of the hormone with target genes, a variety of proteins are produced that stimulate the transport of calcium in each of the target tissues. Active vitamin D works in concert with PTH to enhance active intestinal absorption of calcium, to stimulate bone resorption, and to prohibit renal excretion of calcium.[9] If serum calcium or 1,25-calcitriol concentrations

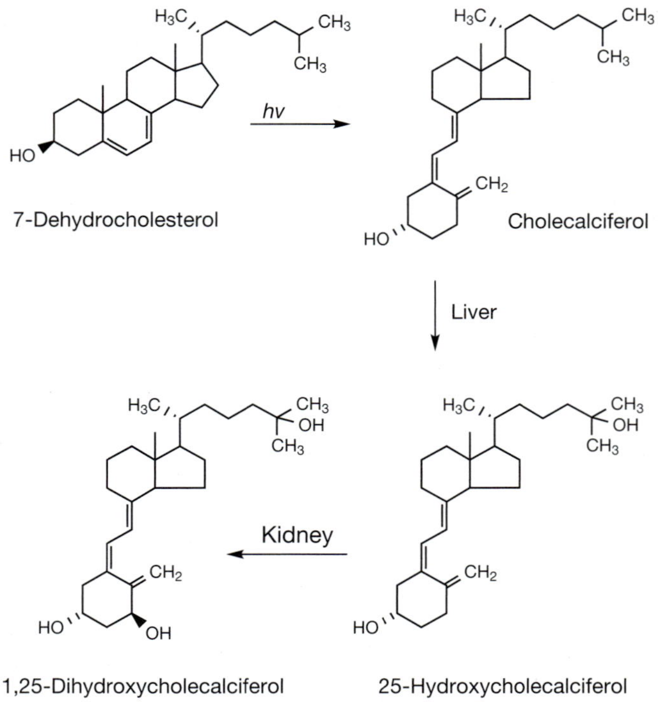

Figure 27.3 Bioactivation of vitamin D.

are elevated, then vitamin D 24-hydroxylase (in renal mitochondria) is activated to oxidize 25(OH)D_3 to inactive 24,25-dihydroxy-cholecalciferol and to further oxidize active vitamin D to the inactive 1,24,25-trihydroxylated derivative. Both the 1,24,25-trihydroxylated and the 24,25-dihydroxylated products have been found to suppress PTH secretion as well. Several factors have been identified in the regulation of the biosynthesis of vitamin D, including low phosphate concentrations (stimulatory) as well as pregnancy and lactation (stimulatory). In addition, FGF23 (produced by osteoblasts and osteocytes) suppresses vitamin D activation in the kidney.[7]

Normal Physiology

During growth periods in childhood and early adulthood, bone formation characteristically exceeds bone loss. In young adulthood, bone formation and bone resorption are nearly equal. After the age of 40 years, however, bone resorption is slightly greater than bone formation, and this results in a gradual decline in skeletal mass. Osteoblasts, osteoclasts, and osteocytes are the three types of cells that make up the bone remodeling unit or bone metabolizing unit and, therefore, are largely responsible for the bone remodeling process.[10]

Traditionally, the bone remodeling process has been thought of as two opposing iterative activities: bone resorption and bone formation. Bone resorption is launched when osteocytes and those cells that line the bone surface release cytokines and growth factors (Fig. 27.4). These endogenous substances signal osteoblasts to release receptor activator of nuclear factor-κB (NFkB) ligand RANK-ligand [RANKL].[10,11] This ligand interacts with and activates its receptor (RANK)

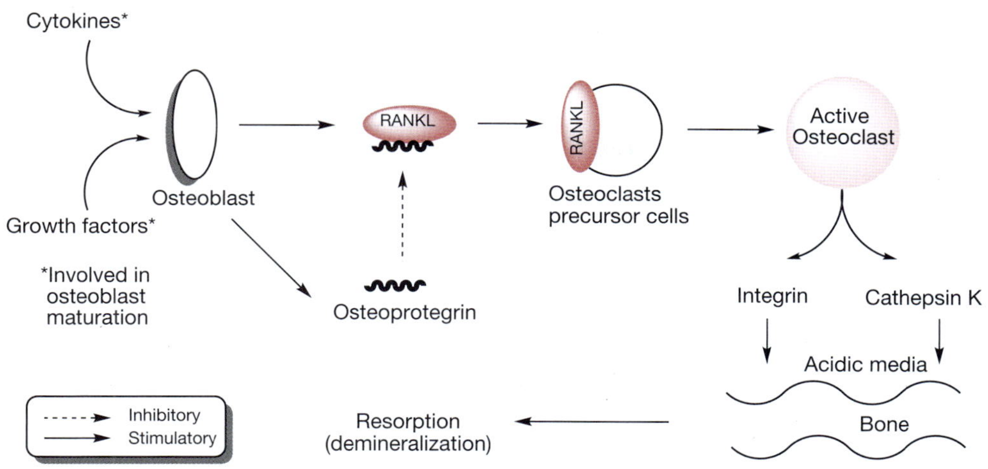

Figure 27.4 Bone resorption involving receptor activator of nuclear factor-κB ligand (RANKL).

found on (1) the surface of osteoclast precursor cells, which stimulates osteoclast differentiation, and (2) the surface of mature osteoclasts, which promotes activation.[10] Receptor activation regulates differentiation of the major skeletal cell types—osteoclasts, osteoblasts, osteocytes, and chondrocytes.

Osteoblasts, which are of mesenchymal origin and are formed in the bone marrow, stimulate bone formation.[6] In the maturation process, osteoblasts undergo multiple cell divisions and, in so doing, express the gene products that are needed to form the bone matrix or osteoid as well as those products responsible for mineralization of that tissue.[10,11] Biosynthesis of the bone matrix protein occurs in the rough endoplasmic reticulum.[4] Multiple endogenous substances are involved in osteoblast maturation, including many cytokines (interleukins [ILs] and granulocyte-macrophage colony-stimulating factor [M-CSF]) as well as hormones and growth factors.

Not only are osteoblasts involved in bone formation, but they also have a role in limiting bone resorption. Produced by osteoblasts, osteoprotegerin (OPG), a RANK receptor homolog, binds to RANKL, and thereby prevents its interaction with its RANK receptors on the osteoclast.[10,11] As a result, osteoclast differentiation and bone resorption are inhibited.[11]

Recently, bone modeling, remodeling, and regulation of bone resorption and bone formation have been portrayed as components of a functional basic multicellular unit (BMU) and not as separate processes. The BMU contains all bone cells interacting with their progenitors, T cells, and bone matrix components.[10] The BMU is composed of three zones: the osteoclasts are found in the "cutting cone," followed by the reversal zone (reversal cells and osteoblasts), and then a closing zone, where osteocytes are located. Focal coupling is the transfer of information within these units to link bone reabsorption with the laying down of the new bone.[10]

A number of signaling pathways are involved in focal coupling, including mechanical signals that are detected by the osteocyte–bone lining cells that modulate cell apoptosis and survival as well as the anabolic Wnt pathway.[10] The Wnt signaling pathway has two branches: the canonical Wnt-β-catenin pathway (important in bone remodeling) and the noncanonical pathway. In the canonical pathway, Wnt binds to low-density lipoprotein coreceptor–related proteins 5/6 (LRP5/6) as well as a specific Frizzled coreceptor. This interaction facilitates phosphorylation of LRP5/6. Axin then binds to this phosphorylated receptor complex. The axin complex inhibits glycogen synthase kinase-3β (GSK-3β), the enzyme that degrades β-catenin. Accumulation of β-catenin increases bone mass. When sclerostin binds to LRP5/6, Wnt is unable to bind, and the LRP5/6-Frizzled coreceptor complex does not form and is not phosphorylated. Axin no longer inhibits GSK-3β and β-catenin undergoes phosphorylation. The phosphorylated β-catenin is now eligible for degradation and is no longer available to increase bone mass.[12-14]

Disease States Associated With Abnormal Calcium Homeostasis

Osteoporosis

Osteoporosis is a skeletal disease characterized by loss of bone mass as well as microarchitectural deterioration of bone tissue. This disease is associated with increased bone fragility and susceptibility to fracture. It is a condition characterized not by inadequate bone formation but, rather, by a deficiency in the production of well-mineralized bone mass. Whereas no medical cause typically is evident in primary osteoporosis,[15] secondary osteoporosis classically stems from medical illness or medication use. There are two types of primary adult osteoporosis: postmenopausal and age-related (Table 27.1).[5,12,15] In postmenopausal primary osteoporosis, there is an accelerated rate of bone loss via enhanced resorption at the onset of menopause. In this form of the disease, the loss of trabecular bone is 3-fold greater than the loss of cortical bone. This disproportionate loss of bone mass is the primary cause of the vertebral crush fractures and the wrist and ankle fractures experienced in postmenopause. In age-related primary osteoporosis, the degree of bone loss is similar in both trabecular and cortical bone and is caused by decreased bone formation by the osteoblasts.[5]

Drug- or disease-induced osteoporosis, otherwise known as secondary osteoporosis (Table 27.2), accounts for up to

Table 27.1 Classification of Osteoporosis

Etiology	Primary (Postmenopausal) Increased Osteoclast Activity and Bone Resorption	Primary (Age-Related) Decreased Osteoblast Activity and Bone Formation; Decreased Gastrointestinal Calcium Absorption	Secondary Drug Therapies; Disease States
Typical age at diagnosis (y)	50-75	>70	Any age
Gender ratio (women:men)	6:1	2:1	1:1
Typical fracture site	Vertebrae, distal radius	Femur, neck, hip	Vertebrae, hip, extremities
Bone morphology	Decreased trabecular bone	Decreased trabecular and normal cortical bone	Decreases cortical bone
Rate of bone loss (per year)	2%-3%	0.3%-0.5%	Variable

From Hansen LB, Vondracek SF. Prevention and treatment of non-postmenopausal osteoporosis. *Am J Health Syst Pharm*. 2004;61:2637-2656.

30% of the cases of vertebral fractures reported annually. It can be caused by a variety of factors, including long-term suppression of osteoblast function, inhibition of calcium absorption from the gut, altered vitamin D metabolism, or excessive loss of calcium in the urine.[12] Disease states or pharmacologic therapies that result in estrogen deficiency, hyperparathyroidism, hyperthyroidism, or hypogonadism have been correlated with the development of osteoporosis.[12] Drug-induced osteoporosis (DIOP) is associated with the use of glucocorticoids, thyroid hormone replacement, lithium, antiepileptic agents, selective serotonin reuptake inhibitors, proton pump inhibitors, thiazolidinediones, aromatase inhibitors, gonadotropin-releasing hormone agonists, and immunosuppressive therapy.[5,12,16-19] See Table 27.3 for a list of the drug-specific mechanisms.[16]

After estrogen deficiency related to menopause, long-term therapy with glucocorticoids represents the most prevalent cause of drug-induced osteoporosis. As much as 3% to 27% of total bone loss can occur within the first 6 to 12 months of glucocorticoid therapy.[19] From a mechanistic perspective, glucocorticoids cause an initial increase in bone resorption as a result of their ability to increase RANKL and M-CSF. This results in an increase in osteoclastogenesis and a decrease in osteoclast apoptosis. With the ability of the glucocorticoids to have an impact on numerous biochemical pathways, including an increase in

Table 27.2 Representative Causes of Secondary Osteoporosis

Gastrointestinal disorders	Anorexia nervosa, chronic liver disease, pancreatic disease, primary biliary cirrhosis, malabsorption syndromes (eg, celiac disease, Crohn disease, gastric bypass, bariatric surgery, short bowel disease)
Nutritional excesses or deficiencies	Calcium deficiency, vitamin D inadequacy, protein deficiency, excess vitamin A, parenteral nutrition, high salt intake
Endocrine-based disorders	Acromegaly, diabetes (types 1 and 2), disease-related elevated hormone levels (Cushing syndrome, hyperthyroidism, hyperparathyroidism), disease-related suppressed hormone levels (androgen insensitivity, athletic amenorrhea, premature menopause)
Genetic disorders	Cystic fibrosis, glycogen storage diseases, osteogenesis imperfecta, hemochromatosis, Gaucher disease, porphyria
Other disorders	Chronic obstructive pulmonary disease, hemophilia, myeloma, AIDS/HIV, end-stage renal disease, sarcoidosis, depression, multiple sclerosis, congestive heart failure
Drugs	Corticosteroids, aromatase inhibitors, thiazolidinediones, anticonvulsants, barbiturates, heparin, chemotherapeutic agents, lithium, proton pump inhibitors, selective serotonin reuptake inhibitors

AIDS, acquired immunodeficiency syndrome; HIV, human immunodeficiency virus.

From Cosman F, de Beur SJ, LeBoff MS, et al. Clinician's guide to prevention and treatment of osteoporosis. *Osteoporos Int*. 2014;25:2359-2381; Aibar-Almazán A, Voltes-Martínez A, Castellote-Caballero Y, Afanador-Restrepo DF, Carcelén-Fraile MDC, López-Ruiz E. Current status of the diagnosis and management of osteoporosis. *Int J Mol Sci*. 2022;23:9465; Ilias I, Milionis C, Zoumakis E. An overview of glucocorticoid-induced osteoporosis. In: Feingold KR, Anawalt B, Blackman MR, et al, eds. *Endotext* [Internet]. MDText.com, Inc; 2000. Updated March 19, 2022. https://www.ncbi.nlm.nih.gov/books/NBK278968/

Table 27.3 Mechanisms Related to Drug-Induced Osteoporosis

Osteoporosis-Causing Mechanism	Drug Class	Mediators and Pathways Involved
Decrease intestinal Ca^{2+} absorption	Proton pump inhibitors Iron supplements Thyroid hormone	TSH
Decrease intestinal Ca^{2+} absorption; increase osteoclast proliferation; increase vitamin D metabolism	Antiepileptic drugs	RANKL, DKK-1
Stimulate osteoclasts; suppress osteoblasts	Heparin	OPG
Promote osteoclast differentiation and bone resorption; decrease osteoblastogenesis; decrease bone formation	Thiazolidinediones	PPAR-γ, IGF-1
Reduce ovarian production of estrogen	GnRH agonists Aromatase inhibitors Selective serotonin reuptake inhibitors Medroxyprogesterone acetate Chemotherapy	OPG, RANKL, M-CSF, TGFβ, IL-1, TNF
Stimulate osteoclast differentiation, proliferation, and activation; inhibit differentiation of osteoblasts; stimulate osteoblast and osteocyte apoptosis	Glucocorticoids	RANKL, M-CSF, OPG, DKK-1, TGFβ, IGF-1, SOD, CAT, Caspase 3

CAT, catalase; DKK-1, dickkopf-1; IGF-1, insulin-like growth factor 1; IL-1, interleukin-1; M-CSF, macrophage colony-stimulating factor; GnRH, gonadotropin releasing hormone; OPG, osteoprotegerin; PPAR-γ, peroxisome proliferator-activated receptor γ; RANKL, receptor activator of nuclear factor-κB ligand; SOD, superoxide dismutase; TGFβ, transforming growth factor β; TNF, tumor necrosis factor; TSH, thyroid-stimulating hormone.

Adapted from Wang LT, Chen LR, Chen KH. Hormone-related and drug-induced osteoporosis: a cellular and molecular overview. *Int J Mol Sci.* 2023;24(6):5814.

peroxisome proliferator-activated receptor γ2 [PPARγ(2)] signaling and a decrease in Wnt signaling protein, there is a decrease in osteoblast formation and function, an increase in osteoblast apoptosis result, and a decrease in bone formation.[19]

Additional risk factors associated with osteoporosis are presented in Table 27.4.

The International Osteoporosis Foundation estimates that there will be a 68% increase in the number of fractures by 2040. In individuals aged 55 and older worldwide, 37 million fractures occur on an annual basis, which translates to 70 fractures/min. This foundation estimates that one in three women and one in five men older than age 50 years will experience a fracture.[20] As compared to non-Hispanic White adults, non-Hispanic Black adults generally have higher BMD, a lower fracture rate, and a lower frequency of osteoporosis. Within Hispanic adults, the evidence is unclear. Albeit with limited data available, Asian populations typically have lower BMD, a higher frequency of osteoporosis, and lower fracture rates compared to non-Hispanic White adults.[21] The prevalence of this condition and poor adherence reports (70% of patients diagnosed as being at risk for osteoporosis and receiving drug therapy do not continue therapy after 1 year) continue to position osteoporosis and low bone mass as significant health concerns in the United States.[21]

Table 27.4 Lifestyle and Genetic Risk Factors for Osteoporosis

Lifestyle Factors	Genetic Factors
Smoking	Female
Sedentary lifestyle/immobilization	Family history
Milk intolerance	Small frame
Excessive caffeine	Early menopause
Excessive alcohol	
Nulliparity	
Excessive thinness/weight loss	

Reprinted from Springer: From Cosman F, de Beur SJ, LeBoff MS, et al. Clinician's guide to prevention and treatment of osteoporosis. *Osteoporos Int.* 2014;25:2359-2381.

Osteopetrosis

Osteopetrosis, also known as "marble bone disease," describes a group of heritable disorders that are centered on a defect in osteoclast-mediated bone resorption. There are two autosomal recessive forms and two autosomal dominant forms (types I and II) of osteopetrosis.[22] It is generally characterized by abnormally dense, brittle bone and increased skeletal mass. Unlike osteoporosis, this disorder results from defective osteoclast development or function (eg, defective pumps, chloride channels, and carbonic anhydrase II proteins), which influences both the shape and structure (density) of the bone.[22] In very extreme cases, the medullary cavity, which houses bone marrow, fills with new bone, and production of hematopoietic cells, is hampered.

Like osteoporosis, this disease can be detected radiographically and appears as though there is a "bone within a bone."

Hypocalcemia

Hypocalcemia can be caused by PTH deficiency, high PTH levels, due to vitamin D deficiency, chronic kidney disease and pseudohypoparathyroidism, various pharmacologic agents (eg, bisphosphonates, denosumab, cinacalcet, cisplatin, foscarnet), and miscellaneous disorders (eg, acidosis/alkalosis, severe sepsis, hypomagnesemia, acute pancreatitis).[2] CT release is inhibited under conditions of hypocalcemia. This results in an elevation of PTH biosynthesis and release and indirectly causes an increase in the production of vitamin D. As a result, serum calcium concentrations increase. In the absence of CT, osteoclast activity is unregulated; therefore, bone resorption is accelerated. Acute hypocalcemia is best treated with IV calcium gluconate or IV calcium chloride, whereas chronic hypocalcemia is best remedied with oral calcium and vitamin D supplements.

Hypercalcemia

Hypercalcemia is primarily caused by excess PTH and secondarily due to malignancy.[23] A state of hypercalcemia (Table 27.5) promotes CT biosynthesis and release. As a result, PTH biosynthesis and its secretion are inhibited, as is the production of active vitamin D. As a result, serum calcium concentrations decrease. In the presence of CT, osteoclast activity is inhibited, so bone resorption is slowed. In acute cases of hypercalcemia, CT may be administered, though the effect is limited to a few days.[23] Hypercalcemia is most often treated with saline infusion to promote diuresis, reducing gastrointestinal (GI) absorption and decreasing bone resorption.[23]

Hypoparathyroidism

Hypoparathyroidism is caused by decreased serum PTH concentrations. It is characterized by hypocalcemia, hyperphosphatemia, reduced levels of circulating vitamin D, and low serum calcium concentrations. This condition is typically a complication of a thyroidectomy or head/neck surgery.[24] Administration of intravenous (IV) or oral calcium and active vitamin D serves to acutely correct plasma calcium levels.[24]

Pseudohypoparathyroidism

In this disease state, levels of PTH are normal or even elevated; however, serum calcium concentrations are low. End-organ insensitivity to PTH has been proposed to be the cause of the hypocalcemic state. Treatment of this condition with calcium and vitamin D has proven to be successful.

Hyperparathyroidism

Increased levels of PTH lead to moderate to severe increases in serum calcium concentrations as a result of a significant loss of calcium from the bone.[2] Deposits of calcium salts in soft tissue, as well as formation of renal calculi, can also result from this hormonal imbalance. Surgery is the treatment of choice for primary hyperparathyroidism. Treatment of this condition with bisphosphonates and cinacalcet is appropriate for certain patients.[25] The vitamin D analogues paricalcitol (Zemplar) and doxercalciferol (Hectorol) are used for both prevention and treatment of hyperparathyroidism secondary to chronic renal failure. They have been shown to reduce PTH levels by an average of 30% after 6 weeks of treatment. Whereas paricalcitol is a fully active form of vitamin D, doxercalciferol requires activation by the liver.

Treatment of secondary hyperparathyroidism with vitamin D therapy is problematic, however, because it often leads to hypercalcemia, hyperphosphatemia, or both because of increased intestinal absorption of both calcium and phosphorous. In patients with chronic renal failure, CaSR agonists (eg, cinacalcet) can limit progression of hyperparathyroidism and growth of the parathyroid gland.[26]

Rickets and Osteomalacia

Rickets (in children) and osteomalacia (in adults) are bone diseases characterized by poor bone mineralization. The most common cause of rickets is due to a nutritional deficiency in vitamin D. It is characterized by a defect in the mineralization and widening of the epiphyseal plates.[27] There are other causes of rickets, including disease caused

Table 27.5 Calcium Homeostasis–Related Disorders

Type of Disorder	Treatment	Examples
Disorders leading to hypercalcemia	Fluids, low-calcium diet, sulfate, glucocorticoids, calcitonin, EDTA	Hyperparathyroidism Hypervitaminosis D Sarcoidosis Neoplasia Hyperthyroidism Immobilization Paget disease of the bone
Disorders of bone remodeling	Bisphosphonates, calcitonin, estrogen, calcium, fluoride, PTH + vitamin D	Osteoporosis

EDTA, ethylenediaminetetraacetic acid; PTH, parathyroid hormone.

by genetic defects, drug-induced rickets, and rickets secondary to liver disease.[27]

There are three types of rickets: calcipenic, phosphopenic, and rickets due to inhibited mineralization. Calcipenic rickets is due to a nutritional deficiency of calcium, which may be coupled with a vitamin D deficiency. Phosphopenic rickets is caused by chronic low serum-phosphate levels, either from impaired intestinal absorption or from increased renal loss.[27] Rickets that is due to inhibited mineralization typically stems from hereditary hypophosphatasia, first-generation bisphosphonates, and aluminum and fluoride toxicity.[27]

Vitamin D dependent–related rickets is caused by several types of factors, including defects in the biosynthesis of vitamin D (1,25-dihydroxy vitamin D; types IA and IB), a defect in the vitamin D receptor ([VDR] type IIA), or a defect in the interactions between vitamin D and its receptor.[27] Type IA rickets is characterized by a defect in converting 25-hydroxyvitamin D to 1,25-dihydroxyvitamin D, whereas type IB rickets is associated with a 25-hydroxylase deficiency.

Congenital hypophosphatemic rickets is characterized by a defect in bone mineralization caused by hypophosphatemia (secondary to renal phosphate loss). There are two subclasses of this type of rickets, FGF23-dependent hypophosphatemic rickets, and FGF23-independent hypophosphatemic rickets.[27]

The increased use of milk substitutes (eg, soy), extended breast feeding without vitamin D supplementation, inadequate consumption of vitamin D fortified foods, and significantly less exposure to sunlight has led to a rise in rickets in the Americas, Europe, and the Middle East. Rickets due to calcium deficiency is still considered to be a worldwide health problem, especially in Africa and Asia.[27] Vitamin D supplementation (to improve intestinal absorption of calcium and mineralization of the bone) as well as oral calcium supplementation are required to treat these diseases. For vitamin D deficiency–based rickets, a single dose treatment (stoss therapy) is composed of an oral or subcutaneous injection of 100,000 to 600,000 international units (IU) of vitamin D for infants older than 1 month.[27] It is recommended that this is followed by weekly doses of 50,000 IU of vitamin D_2 or D_3, with daily maintenance doses of 400 to 600 IU. This type of rickets can also be treated with multiple smaller age-dependent doses (1,000-5,000 IU) followed by daily maintenance doses of 400 IU.[27]

In addition to the classical environmental or nutritional cause of these diseases, both osteomalacia and rickets can have a pharmacologic origin as a result of chronic treatment with anticonvulsants (phenobarbital and phenytoin) or glucocorticoids. These drugs induce the cytochrome P450 isozymes responsible for catalyzing the inactivation of vitamin D via 25-hydroxylation.

Paget Disease of the Bone

Paget disease of the bone (Table 27.6) is characterized by excessive bone resorption, followed by replacement of the normally mineralized bone with soft, poorly mineralized tissue.[28] It has been determined that the osteoclasts have an abnormal structure, are hyperactive, and are present at elevated levels. The axial skeleton is typically targeted (spine, pelvis, and skull).[28] Patients afflicted with this painful condition often suffer from multiple compression fractures. Osteoclasts producing interleukin-6 (IL-6) and genetic predisposition are two of the causes of this disease.[28] Administration of CT as well as oral calcium and phosphate supplements had been the treatment of choice until the bisphosphonates pamidronate disodium (IV) and risedronate sodium (oral tablet) were approved by the US Food and Drug Administration (FDA). Daily administration of risedronate sodium (see later discussion of bisphosphonates) results in a decreased rate of bone turnover and a decrease in the levels of serum alkaline phosphatase, a biochemical marker of bone turnover.[10] A significant advantage to treatment with the bisphosphonates is long-term suppression of the disease. Calcium supplementation, which often is necessary in these patients, must be dosed separately from risedronate sodium because calcium- and aluminum- or magnesium-containing antacids interfere with absorption of the bisphosphonates.

Table 27.6 Percent of Elemental Calcium Content in Various Salts

Salt	Calcium (%)	Elemental Calcium (mg/tablet)
Calcium carbonate	40	
Tums (500 mg chewable)		200 mg
Os-Cal 500 (1,250 mg tablet)		500 mg
Viactive (1,250 mg chewable)		500 mg
Tribasic calcium phosphate	39 27 23	
Posture (1,565.2 mg tablets)		600 mg
Calcium citrate	21	
Citrical (950 mg tablets)		200 mg
Citrical Liquitab (2,376 mg effervescent tablets)		500 mg
Calcium lactate	13	
Generics (325 mg tablets)		42 mg
Generics (650 mg tablets)		84 mg
Calcium gluconate	9.3	
Generics (500 mg tablets)		46.5 mg
Generics (650 mg tablets)		60.4 mg
Calcium glubionate	6.5	
Neo-Calglucon (1.8 g/5 mL syrup)		115 mg/5 mL

Camacho PM, Petak SM, Binkley N, et al. American Association of Clinical Endocrinologists/American College of Endocrinology clinical practice guidelines for the diagnosis and treatment of postmenopausal osteoporosis—2020 update. *Endocr Pract.* 2020;26(suppl 1):1-46.

Drug Therapies Used to Treat Osteoporosis

Agents used in the treatment and prevention of osteoporosis are categorized as antiresorptive agents or bone-forming agents depending on their primary mechanism of action.[12] For most of the effective therapies, bone mass is observed to increase for the first few years of treatment. Eventually, however, all the pits or lacunae will be filled in with new bone, and no additional increase in bone mass will occur. Antiresorptive agents have been shown to increase bone mass by as much as 8% to 9% at the lumbar spine and 3% to 6% in the femoral neck. Once a diagnosis of osteoporosis and the likely cause has been established, it is important to consider both patient fracture history and general medical history when selecting the appropriate treatment for a given patient.[5,12]

Antiresorptive Agents

Estrogen Analogues—Estrogen Replacement Therapy

Mechanism of Action. The precise mechanism by which estrogen prevents bone resorption has not been elucidated; however, it continues to be associated with inhibition of osteoclast activity, promotion of osteoblast activity, regulation of the RANK/RANKL/OPG system, apoptosis of osteoclasts, and regulation of cytokines and other growth factors. Estrogen improves calcium absorption, promotes CT biosynthesis, and increases vitamin D receptors on osteoclasts. Although the primary mechanism of action remains unclear and its use may be considered controversial at best, ERT (ie, 17β-estradiol, estrone sodium sulfate, or 17-ethinyl estradiol) has value in the treatment and prevention of osteoporosis.[5]

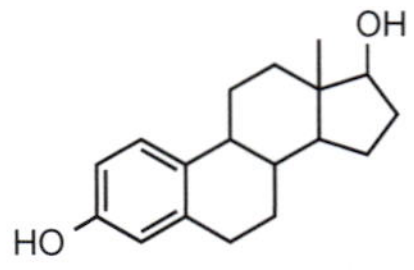

17β-estradiol

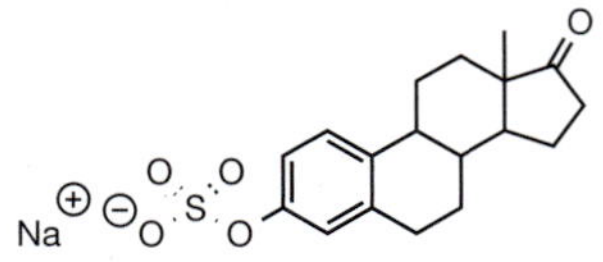

Estrone sodium sulfate

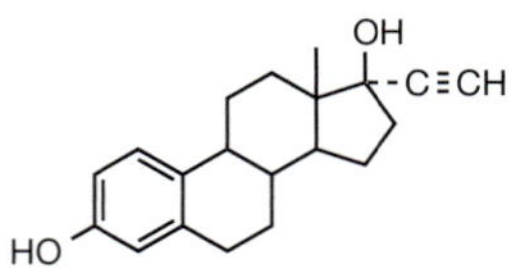

17-Ethinyl estradiol

In light of the findings of the Women's Health Initiative (WHI) study,[29] the FDA recommends the use of short-term, low-dose hormone replacement therapy (estrogen and progestin) in the prevention of osteoporosis only in select cases. Studies conducted since the release of WHI report have contested these conclusions, as patients taking low-dose oral and transdermal formulations are less likely to experience breast cancer, endometrial hyperplasia, coronary artery disease, and venous thromboembolism.[30] The pharmacokinetics of the estrogens are covered in detail in Chapter 25.

Therapeutic Effects. The WHI study reported that a 5-year course of treatment with hormone replacement therapy led to a 34% decrease of risk of clinical vertebral fracture and hip fractures and a 23% decrease in other types of osteoporetic fractures.[29] The minimum dose required and that which is considered to be standard therapy is 0.625 mg/d of conjugated estrogens (Premarin); however, a 0.3-mg/d dose of esterified estrogen (eg, Menest) has been shown to be adequate for the prevention of osteoporosis.[5] Estrogen replacement therapy (ERT) is also available as transdermal patches (eg, 17β-estradiol: Climara, Dotti, Lyllana, Menostar, Minivelle, Vivelle-Dot).

Selective Estrogen Receptor Modulators

Tamoxifen Citrate and Raloxifene Hydrochloride (Evista). Tamoxifen citrate, classified chemically as a triarylethylene, is a selective estrogen receptor modulator (SERM). As an antiestrogenic agent in breast tissue, it is indicated for the treatment of breast cancer in both men and women, as adjuvant therapy in the treatment of axillary node–negative or -positive breast cancer following partial or full mastectomy as well as for breast cancer risk reduction in high-risk patients. Raloxifene hydrochloride (Evista), a benzothiophene derivative, is a semirigid analogue of tamoxifen (Fig. 27.5) that is indicated for reduction of invasive breast cancer in menopausal women who are at high risk.

Raloxifene hydrochloride, the first SERM approved for the prevention of osteoporosis in postmenopausal women, acts as an estrogen agonist on receptors in osteoblasts and osteoclasts but as an antagonist at breast and uterine estrogen receptors. This selective action means that this agent does not increase the risk of endometrial or breast cancer, as is the case with long-term tamoxifen therapy. Because this agent does not have a stimulatory effect at its receptors on most tissues, it does not prevent the hot flashes and other symptoms of menopause as estrogen does.[5,29] Raloxifene also has a positive influence on cardiovascular risk markers via decreasing low-density lipoprotein cholesterol (LDL-C),

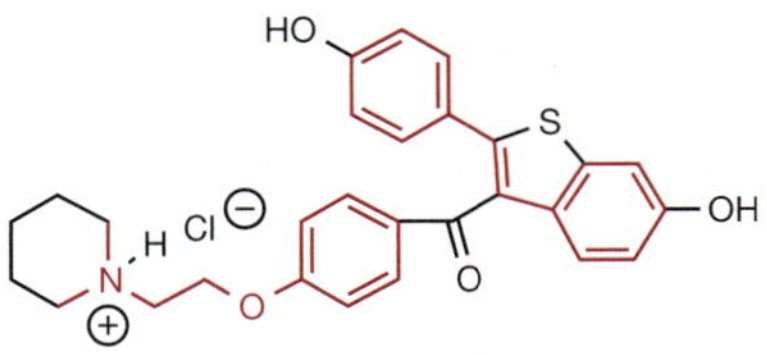

Raloxifene hydrochloride (Evista)

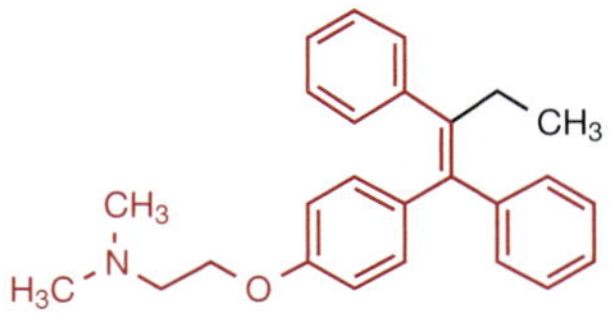

Tamoxifen (Nolvadex)

Figure 27.5 Structures of raloxifene and tamoxifen highlighting the structural similarity between the two drugs.

fibrinogen, lipoprotein A, and increasing high-density lipoprotein 2 cholesterol (HDL2-C).[31] There are boxed warnings associated with raloxifene due to an increased risk of death due to stroke for postmenopausal women or for those with an increased risk of major coronary events. There are additional warnings for an increased risk of deep vein thrombosis and pulmonary embolism.[32]

Therapeutic Action. Raloxifene hydrochloride decreases the risk of vertebral fracture by 41% and nonvertebral fractures by 39% over 3 years.[31] It has additional direct actions on the bone, including decreasing the resorptive activity of osteoclasts by up to 50%, IL-6 production, and production of tumor necrosis factor α (TNF-α) by 30%.[33] Raloxifene hydrochloride should not be administered in combination with cholestyramine (decreased absorption), warfarin (prothrombin times and international normalized ratios must be monitored more closely), and those drugs that are highly protein bound, such as clofibrate, diazepam, ibuprofen, indomethacin, and naproxen.[32]

Structure-Activity Relationship. From a structural perspective, the only pure antiestrogens are 7α-substituted estrogens.[32] In the triarylethylene class of agents (eg, tamoxifen), the phenol or g ring system is critical for interaction with the portion of the estrogen receptor (ER) protein referred to as the activation factor-2 (AF-2) region because it mimics the essential C3 phenol group found in estrogen.[32] This interaction initiates a change in protein conformation to the form of the receptor able to interact with a specific deoxyribonucleic acid (DNA) sequence known as the estrogen responding element (ERE). As a result, activation of a specific group of genes occurs, and protein biosynthesis ensues. The orientation of the three aryl rings in a propeller type of arrangement also is important for tight receptor binding and biologic activity.[32] In raloxifene hydrochloride, the substituted benzothiophene ring mimics the estrogen A ring; however because of the presence of a semirigid, amine-containing side chain, raloxifene is unable to interact with AF-2.[32] As a result, interaction with ERE is prevented, and antiestrogenic action is observed in reproductive tissues. The raloxifene hydrochloride–ER complex, in concert with specific adapter proteins, is also able to interact with and activate a raloxifene-responding element (RRE). Activation of this DNA sequence facilitates activation of another group of genes responsible for the production of proteins that allows for agonist action in nonreproductive tissues.[32]

Pharmacokinetics. Raloxifene hydrochloride is rapidly absorbed following oral administration, with an estimated 60% absorption, but it has a very low bioavailability (2%), associated with extensive phase II metabolism. The metabolites are excreted via the bile, with potential enterohepatic recycling that could account for the interaction with cholestyramine. Supportive of the enterohepatic recycling is the half-life of 28 hours. It is extensively protein bound (95%). Metabolism of raloxifene hydrochloride occurs to a great extent in the intestine and consists of glucuronide conjugation catalyzed by uridine diphosphate glucuronosyltransferase (UGT).[33] The UGT1A family is responsible for intestinal human metabolism, as shown in Figure 27.6. Efflux by intestinal cells of the resulting glucuronide occurs via P-glycoprotein and multidrug resistance–related protein. The combination of rapid metabolism and efflux can account for the low bioavailability.

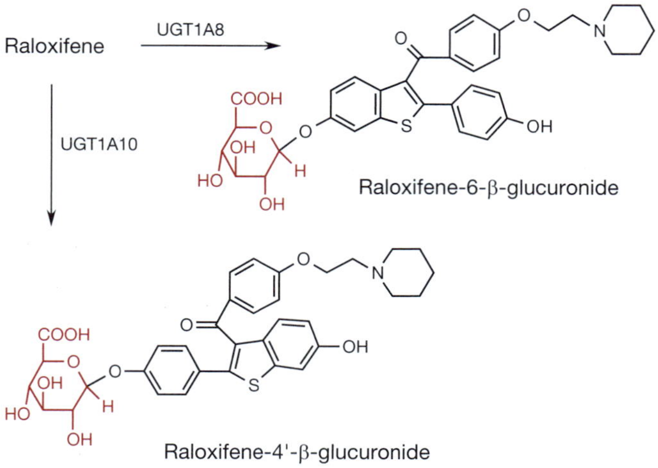

Figure 27.6 Metabolism of raloxifene. UGT, uridine diphosphate glucuronosyltransferase.

Bazedoxifene Acetate. Bazedoxifene acetate is an indole-based third-generation SERM used in combination with conjugate estrogens (Duavee) for the prevention of postmenopausal osteoporosis and for the treatment of moderate to severe vasomotor symptoms associated with menopause. It is recommended for patients who cannot or refuse to take bisphosphonates due to issues related to either tolerability or safety[34] who have an intact uterus. For those patients who anticipate the need for long-term therapy, bazedoxifene may be an appropriate alternative to avoid the effects of long-term bisphosphonate therapy. It can also be used in the prevention of glucocorticoid-induced osteoporosis.[34]

Therapeutic Action. This combination of agents is referred to as a tissue-selective estrogen complex (TSEC). It acts as an estrogen agonist at the bone and as an estrogen antagonist at the uterus and breast.[35] Bazedoxifene acetate displaces 17β-estradiol from ERs and has excellent binding affinity for the receptor itself (both ERα and ERβ). It is less ERα selective than raloxifene and exhibits 10-fold less affinity for ERα than 17β-estradiol. Unlike raloxifene hydrochloride, this agent does not cause hot flashes at the doses required to have a beneficial effect on the bone.

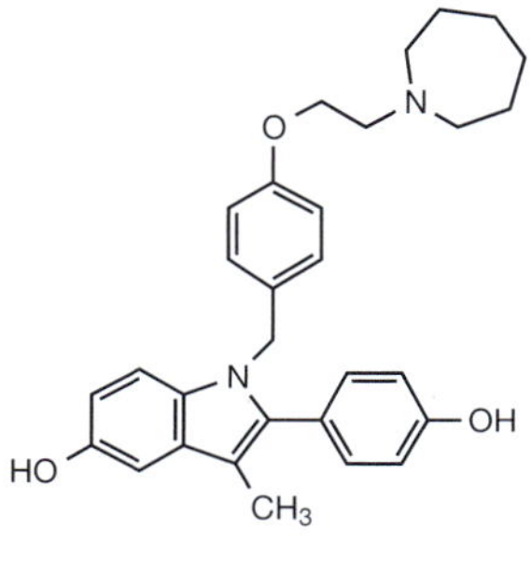

Bazedoxifene

Pharmacokinetics. The absolute bioavailability of this agent is approximately 6% and is it is extensively bound to

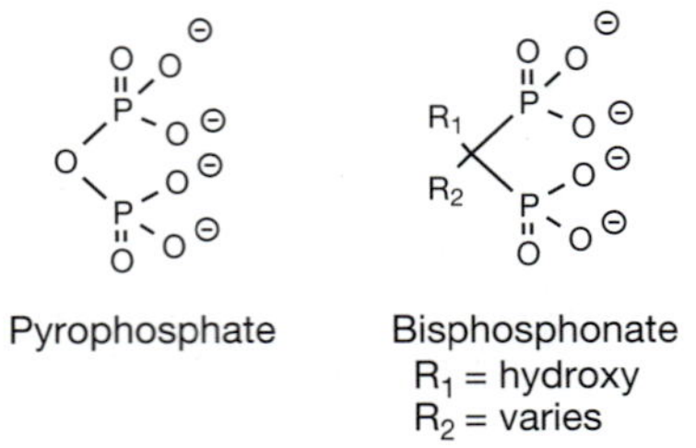

Figure 27.7 Bisphosphonate structure-activity relationships.

plasma proteins (98%-99%), but not sex hormone–binding globulin (SHBG). In combination with conjugated estrogens, this agent is administered orally (once daily) with or without meals. Calcium and vitamin D supplements are important adjunct therapy. Given that estrogens are at least partially metabolized by CYP3A4, this combination agent should not be given concurrently with inducers or inhibitors of this isoform. Glucuronidated metabolites of bazedoxifene have been isolated; therefore, agents that induce UGT (eg, rifampin, carbamazepine) should also be avoided.[35] This combination agent is eliminated via urinary and biliary routes and is not recommended in patients with renal or hepatic impairment or in pregnant women. The primary adverse effects include muscle spasms, dizziness, nausea, diarrhea, and dyspepsia as well as neck and throat pain. Given the inclusion of an estrogen component, it is prudent to monitor for any signs or symptoms of cardiovascular effects.[35]

Bisphosphonates

MECHANISM OF ACTION. The bisphosphonates are synthetic in origin and are designed to mimic PPi, in which the oxygen in P-O-P is replaced with a carbon atom to create a nonhydrolyzable backbone (Fig. 27.7).[36] Because PPi is a normal constituent of the bone, these analogues selectively target the hydroxyapatite portion of the bone. Mechanistically, the bisphosphonates can be split into two categories. The nonnitrogen bisphosphonates (eg, clondronate; Fig. 27.8) most closely mimic PPi and get incorporated into nonhydrolyzable ATP analogues via amino acyl tRNA synthetases. The resulting nonhydrolyzable nucleotides accumulate within osteoclasts and negatively impacts the energy metabolism of the cell. This initiates osteoclast apoptosis, and there is a corresponding decrease in bone breakdown. The nitrogen-containing bisphosphonates (eg, alendronate, pamidronate, ibandronate; Fig. 27.8) operate by a distinctly different mechanism and are much more potent antiresorptive agents. This is largely accomplished via inhibition of the mevalonate pathway (specifically farnesyl pyrophosphate synthetase [FPPS]), and interferes with protein prenylation within osteoclasts, as well as via inhibition of ATP-dependent enzymes (impairing cellular energetics). FPPS contributes to the biosynthesis of Ras, Rho, and Rac, proteins that are essential for osteoclast cell processes.[37] By these mechanisms, the bisphosphonates can limit bone turnover and allow the osteoblasts to form well-mineralized bone without opposition.[36]

STRUCTURE-ACTIVITY RELATIONSHIPS. From a structural perspective, the nitrogen-containing bisphosphonates have been proposed to have specific molecular interactions with their biologic target for drug action, FPPS, and structure-activity relationships (SARs) have been elucidated. The central carbon of the geminal phosphonate has been substituted with a variety of functional groups to yield a large family of compounds with differing physicochemical and biologic properties.[37] The SAR studies (see Fig. 27.7) have concluded that a hydroxyl substituent (R_1) maximizes the affinity of the agent for the hydroxyapatite as well as

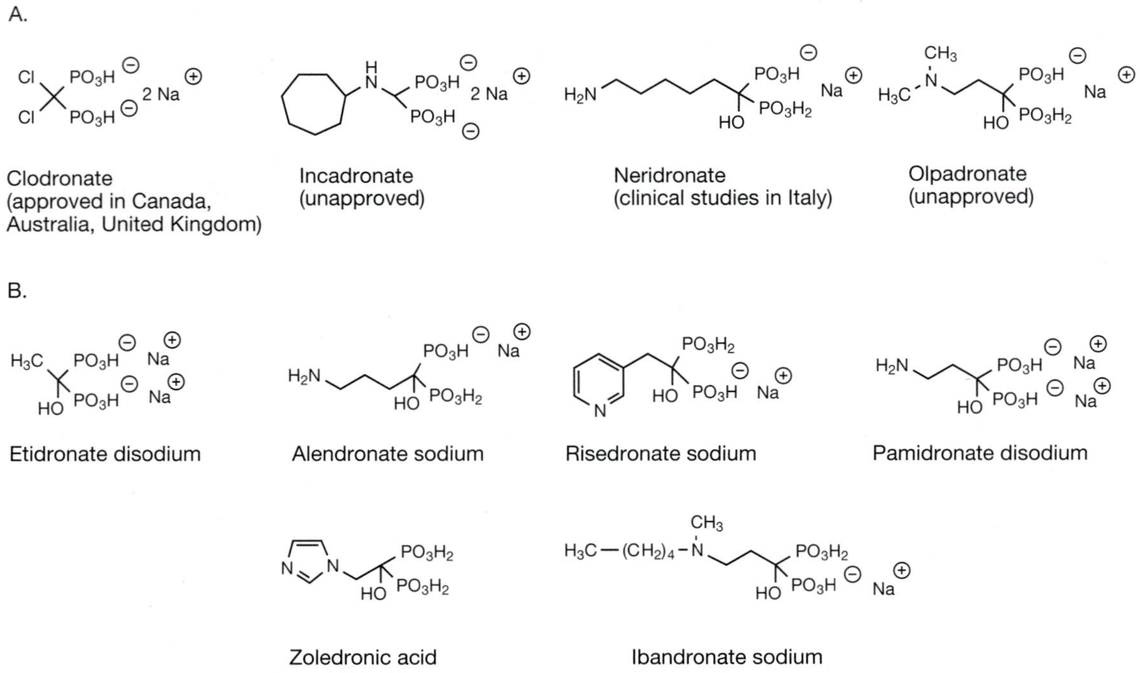

Figure 27.8 Bisphosphonates: unapproved (A) and approved and used clinically (B).

improves the antiresorptive character of the agent. The bisphosphonate itself, as well as the hydroxyl group at R_1, should be included as critical SAR features due to their ability to act as a bone "hook." Because structural variation of R_2 has a significant effect on potency, it can be surmised that R_2 interacts at an "active site" and participates in a specific molecular interaction within a carbocation binding site within the biologic target.

The character of the R_2 substituent varies widely and clearly has a significant influence on the potency of this class of compounds (see Fig. 27.8). The R_2 amino–substituted bisphosphonates (pamidronate disodium, alendronate sodium, and neridronate) are more potent than etidronate disodium and clodronate disodium (not available in the United States). The R_2 3-carbon amino linear chain for alendronate sodium is more potent than the R_2 2-carbon derivative pamidronate disodium and the R_2 6-carbon analogue neridronate.[37] Alkylation of the amine functional group improves potency as is demonstrated by compounds with N-substituted amino alkyls at R_2 (eg, olpadronate, ibandronate sodium) and those that contain rings at R_2 (eg, risedronate sodium, incadronate, zoledronic acid). A specific hydrophobic interaction in the active site of FPPS has been proposed for the R_2 substituent.[37] The third-generation analogues contain a basic heterocyclic side chain at R_2 tethered to the central carbon by a variety of linkages (potency: NH > CH_2 > S > O).[37]

PHARMACOKINETICS. To date, four generations of bisphosphonates have been developed for the treatment of osteoporosis (see Fig. 27.8). Absorption of these agents from the gut is quite poor (1%-5%) because of their polar nature, and as a therapeutic class, they have limited cellular penetration.[38] A significant portion of the actual absorbed dose is taken up specifically by the bone within 4 to 6 hours, and the rest is exclusively excreted by the kidney. Uptake of these agents in the bone is concentrated in areas of the bone that are actively undergoing remodeling.[38] Between the selective uptake and the rapid rate of clearance, the bisphosphonates enjoy a short circulating half-life and very limited drug exposure to nontarget tissues.[37] Because the bisphosphonates are released only from the bone when the bone is resorbed, they have a tissue half-life of 1 to 10 years; however, these agents remain pharmacologically active only while they are exposed on bone resorption surfaces.[38]

SPECIFIC DRUGS

Alendronate Sodium (Fosamax). The second-generation agent alendronate sodium was the first bisphosphonate agent approved by the FDA for the prevention and treatment of osteoporosis and Paget disease of the bone and is 1,000-fold more potent than etidronate disodium (see Fig. 27.8).[39] Alendronate sodium is also indicated for the treatment of glucocorticoid-induced osteoporosis and male osteoporosis. This derivative, when dosed continuously (5-10 mg/d for osteoporosis and 40 mg/d for Paget disease of the bone) and given with oral calcium supplements (500 mg/d), produced well-mineralized bone and significantly improved BMD (7% in the spine and 4% in the hip) within 18 months.[6] In addition, the vertebral fracture rate was shown to decrease by 47%. A side effect associated with alendronate sodium, chemical esophagitis, has been attributed to inadequate intake of water and lying down after taking the medication. Specific patient instructions were developed to limit the incidence of upper gastrointestinal problems and include (1) taking the medication with 6 to 8 ounces of water on arising in the morning; (2) remaining in an upright position for at least 30 minutes after taking the medication; and (3) delaying drinking other liquids/eating for at least 30 minutes, if not 1 to 2 hours, to allow maximal absorption of the agent.[39] The bioavailability of alendronate decreases by 60% in the presence of food. To maximize absorption, calcium supplements and any aluminum- or magnesium-containing antacids should be dosed separately from agents in this class. These agents are not recommended in patients with renal impairment (serum creatinine, <2.5 mg/dL) or has a history of esophageal disease, gastritis, or peptic ulcer.[5] This agent can be orally administered daily or weekly. In an attempt to address the inconvenience associated with tablet administration, a once-weekly, 70-mg buffered effervescent formulation of alendronate is available (Binosto). A long-term controlled release formulation using a variety of types of hydrogel loaded with alendronate is under investigation.[40]

Risedronate Sodium (Actonel). The third-generation agent risedronate sodium has been approved for both the prevention and treatment of osteoporosis (both postmenopausal and in men), Paget disease of the bone, and glucocorticoid-induced osteoporosis (see Fig. 27.8).[41] Risedronate sodium is 1,000- to 5,000-fold more potent than etidronate disodium. At the end of an 18-month study, 53% of patients who took risedronate sodium for 2 months remained in remission, as compared to 14% of patients who took etidronate disodium, an earlier-generation bisphosphonate (no longer available in the United States), for 6 months. Oral administration of this agent suffers from the same problems as that of other bisphosphonate agents. Risedronate sodium should not be given to patients with creatinine clearance of less than 30 mL/min. A once-weekly, delayed-release formulation (Atelvia) is available and is taken immediately after breakfast with 4 oz of water, while remaining in an upright position for 30 minutes post-administration. Other oral formulations of risedronate sodium include tablets to be consumed daily (5 mg), weekly (35 mg), and monthly (75 mg on each of 2 consecutive days, or 150 mg once).[41]

Ibandronate Sodium (Boniva). Ibandronate sodium is approved for the treatment and prevention of osteoporosis in postmenopausal women and has a mechanism of action that is identical to the other bisphosphonate agents (see Fig. 27.8). Administered daily (2.5 mg) with the same administration restrictions as the other bisphosphonates, ibandronate sodium has been clinically shown to reduce the risk of vertebral fractures by 62%.[42] If administered on an intermittent basis (20 mg), it reduces the risk of vertebral fractures by 50%. Ibandronate sodium (2.5 mg daily), along with 500 mg of supplemental calcium, has been clinically shown to increase BMD in the hip (1.8%), femoral neck (2.0%), and lumbar spine (3.1%). A 150-mg formulation has been approved by the FDA for once-monthly administration as well as a 3-mg IV formulation for quarterly administration.

The oral bioavailability of this agent is extremely poor (0.6%) and is adversely affected by the presence of food, beverages other than water, and other medications, including calcium or vitamin D supplements and antacids.[42] Because of the increased calcium content in mineral water, patients should not take this medication with this type of water. Drugs that inhibit gastric acid secretion (eg, H_2 antagonists, proton pump inhibitors) actually promote ibandronate sodium absorption. Like the other agents in this therapeutic class, ibandronate sodium is not metabolized, and that which is not bound to bone (40%-50% of the absorbed dose) is eliminated renally unchanged. It does not inhibit the cytochrome P-450 (CYP450) isozymes. This agent does not require dosage adjustment for patients with hepatic impairment or mild to moderate renal impairment (creatinine clearance, >30 mL/min). Ibandronate sodium should not be prescribed for patients with severe renal impairment (creatinine clearance, <30 mL/min).[42]

Zoledronic Acid (Reclast). Zoledronic acid is approved for the treatment of glucocorticoid-induced osteoporosis and prevention and treatment of postmenopausal osteoporosis, male osteoporosis, and Paget disease of the bone (see Fig. 27.8). For the treatment of osteoporosis, zoledronic acid is formulated as a 5-mg, once-yearly IV infusion. The frequency of IV infusion decreases to 5 mg every 2 years for the prevention of osteoporosis. In order to prevent hypocalcemia, concomitant calcium (1,500 mg) and vitamin D (800-1,000 IU) intake and/or supplementation is recommended in patients being treated for osteoporosis. On the day of treatment, patients should drink at least two glasses of water and eat normally. Dose adjustments for renally impaired patients may be necessary.

Osteonecrosis of the jaw, a unique adverse effect for zoledronic acid, has been reported in patients receiving IV bisphosphonate therapy.[43] The majority of the patients who developed bisphosphonate-related osteonecrosis of the jaw (BRONJ) were undergoing chemotherapy (typically for multiple myeloma, breast, prostate, or lung cancers), taking corticosteroids, and had undergone a dental procedure (eg, tooth extraction). The FDA recommends that patients receive a thorough dental examination before initiation of IV bisphosphonate therapy and that they avoid invasive dental work during treatment. Patients taking bisphosphonates are recommended to stop the bisphosphonate 2 months before undergoing an invasive dental procedure and to restart once jaw healing is complete.[43]

There have also been reports of an increase in risk of atypical femur fracture in patients undergoing long-term bisphosphonate therapy.[44] In addition, an increase in the risk of developing esophageal cancer has surfaced in patients with approximately 5 years of oral bisphosphonate use. Because of these adverse effects, it is recommended that clinicians weigh the benefits against the potential risks.

ADDITIONAL BISPHOSPHONATE DOSAGE FORMS

A unique formulation of alendronate sodium, FOSAMAX PLUS D, includes 70 mg of alendronate sodium and 2,800 or 5,600 IU of vitamin D_3 (ie, a 7-day supply of both the bisphosphonate and vitamin D). This formulation should not be used in patients with severe kidney disease or low serum calcium levels and should not be the only therapy used to correct a vitamin D deficiency.

Risedronate sodium with calcium carbonate (Actonel with Calcium) represents an additional type of packaging for this class of agents. It addresses the Surgeon General's Report on Bone Health and Osteoporosis, which states that treatments for osteoporosis need to be made simpler and more structured. Sold in units that contain a 1-month supply, each week of therapy includes a total of seven tablets, including one 35-mg tablet of risedronate and six 500-mg tablets of calcium carbonate.

Calcitonin (Miacalcin)

Calcitonin (see earlier discussion) has been approved for the treatment of postmenopausal osteoporosis (after a minimum of 5 years postmenopausal), hypercalcemia of malignancy, and Paget disease of the bone (when intolerance to bisphosphonates occurs).[45] The CT isolated from salmon is the preferred source, because it has greater receptor affinity and a longer half-life than the human hormone.[45]

STRUCTURE-ACTIVITY RELATIONSHIPS. CT is commercially available as synthetic "calcitonin-salmon," which contains the same linear sequence of 32 amino acids as occurs in natural salmon CT. Calcitonin-salmon differs structurally from human CT at 16 of 32 amino acids (see Fig. 27.9 for primary structural differences between human and salmon calcitonin). A disulfide bond (Cys1-Cys7) is required for biological activity.

PHARMACOKINETICS. The pharmacologic activity of the CTs is the same, but calcitonin-salmon is approximately 50-fold more potent on a weight basis than human calcitonin

Salmon CT (S—S disulfide bond between Cys1 and Cys7):

Cys-Ser—Asn—Leu—Ser—Thr—Cys-Val—Leu—Gly—Lys—Leu—Ser—Gln—Glu—Leu—His—Lys—Leu—Gln—
(1, 5, 10, 15, 20)

Thr-Tyr—Pro—Arg—Thr—Asn—Thr—Gly—Ser—Gly—Thr—Pro-NH_2
(25, 30)

Human CT (S—S disulfide bond between Cys1 and Cys7):

Cys-Gly—Asn—Leu—Ser—Thr—Cys-Met—Leu—Gly—Thr—Tyr—Thr—Gln—Asp-Phe—Asn—Lys—Phe—His—
(1, 5, 10, 15, 20)

Thr-Phe—Pro—Gln—Thr—Ala—Ile—Gly—Val—Gly—Ala—Pro-NH_2
(25, 30)

Figure 27.9 Primary structures of salmon and human calcitonin (CT). Similarities are highlighted in *red*.

with a longer duration of action. The duration of action for calcitonin-salmon is 8 to 24 hours following intramuscular (IM) or subcutaneous (SC) administration and 0.5 to 12.0 hours following IV administration. The parenteral dose required for the treatment of osteoporosis is 100 IU/day.[45] Calcitonin-salmon is readily metabolized in the kidney, with an elimination half-life calculated at 43 minutes. As a result, the intranasal dose required is 200 IU/day.

Therapeutic Application. CT therapy requires the concomitant oral administration of elemental calcium (500 mg/day, see Table 27.6). Clinical studies have shown that the combination of intranasal calcitonin-salmon (200 IU/day), oral calcium supplementation (>1,000 mg/day of elemental calcium), and vitamin D (400 IU/d) has decreased the rate of new fractures by more than 75% and has improved vertebral BMD by as much as 3% annually.[45] Calcitonin prevents the abnormal bone turnover characteristic of Paget disease of the bone and has antiresorptive activity. Side effects are significantly more pronounced when calcitonin-salmon is administered by injection and can include nausea, vomiting, anorexia, and flushing.[45] Because calcitonin-salmon is protein in nature, the possibility of a systemic allergic reaction (eg, bronchospasm, tongue swelling, and anaphylactic shock) should be considered, and appropriate measures for treatment of hypersensitivity reaction should be readily available. Although calcitonin-salmon does not cross the placenta, it may pass into breast milk. Calcitonin-salmon is a possible alternative to ERT; however, only limited evidence suggests that it has efficacy in women who already have fractures. Resistance to calcitonin-salmon can result from the development of neutralizing antibodies.[45]

In addition to its antiresorptive action via suppression of osteoclast activity, calcitonin-salmon exhibits a potent analgesic effect and has provided considerable relief to those patients suffering from the pain associated with Paget disease of the bone and osteoporosis. The mechanism of this analgesic effect is still unknown, though evidence exists that calcitonin decreases the number of serotonin transporters, increases expression of serotonin receptors and decreases sodium channel transcription.[45] The potency of this analgesic effect has been demonstrated to be 30- to 50-fold that of morphine in selected patients. Calcitonin is preferred over estrogen and bisphosphonates when treatment of both osteoporosis and related bone pain is warranted.

PTH Analogues

Bone-Forming Agents

Teriparatide (Forteo)

Teriparatide is approved for the treatment of postmenopausal osteoporosis in patients who have a high risk of fracture, for the treatment of glucocorticoid-induced osteoporosis, and to increase bone mass in men with primary or hypogonadal osteoporosis who have a high risk of fracture.[46] Teriparatide is recombinant human PTH 1-34 (see Fig. 27.2), the biologically active portion of the endogenously produced preprohormone. Unlike the bisphosphonates, which are classified as bone restorative agents, teriparatide is the first approved bone-forming agent.

Mechanism of Action. Teriparatide is an agonist at the parathyroid hormone type 1 receptor (PTHR1), a G protein–coupled receptor (GPCR). Receptor activation leads to a prolonged response to the cyclic adenosine monophosphate (cAMP) second messenger. This receptor is also activated by parathyroid hormone–related peptide (PTHrP).[46] Bone formation is possible because of the ability of this agent to increase the number of osteoblasts. Although teriparatide enhances the function of both osteoclasts and osteoblasts, the exposure incidence dictates its effect on the skeleton. If administered once daily or intermittently, teriparatide preferentially enhances osteoblastic function (via an upregulation of the expression of pro-osteoblastic growth factors insulin-like growth factor 1 [IGF-1], fibroblast growth factor 2, and downregulation of the Wnt antagonist sclerostin),[46] and bone formation occurs. Continuous exposure to endogenous PTH may result in poor skeletal composition because of enhanced osteoclast-mediated bone resorption (via increasing the expression of pro-osteoclastic cytokines, including RANKL, and M-CSF.)[46] After 18 months of treatment, lumbar BMD increased up to 12% in postmenopausal women. After 10 months of treatment, 53% of men had an increase of 5% or greater in spine BMD. The risk for developing new vertebral fractures was reduced by 65% after 18 months of treatment, and the number of nonvertebral fragility fractures was reduced by 53%.[46] There is limited evidence that teriparatide can regrow jawbone that has been damaged by osteonecrosis and periodontitis.

Pharmacokinetics. Administered as a once daily 20-μg SC injection in the anterior thigh or abdominal wall, teriparatide is a clear, colorless liquid. Concurrent calcium (1,000 mg) and vitamin D (400 IU) supplementation is recommended. Teriparatide is rapidly absorbed, demonstrates 95% bioavailability, and is quickly eliminated via both hepatic and extrahepatic routes.[46] The half-life is 1 hour when administered SC. Metabolic studies have not been performed on teriparatide; however, the entire PTH preprohormone has been shown to undergo enzyme-mediated transformations in the liver. Dizziness, nausea, and leg cramps are the most commonly reported adverse side effects.[46]

Temporary increases in serum calcium levels occur following administration of teriparatide. As a result, this agent is contraindicated in patients who are predisposed to hypercalcemia. Teriparatide should not be prescribed to patients with Paget disease of the bone, children, young adults, women who are pregnant or nursing, and patients who have received skeletal radiation therapy.[5] While there is an increased basal risk for osteocarcoma,[46] there is no longer a boxed warning associated with teriparatide.

Abaloparatide (Tymlos)

H-Ala-Val-Ser-Glu-His-Gln-Leu-Leu-His-Asp-Lys-Ser-Ile-Gln-Asp-Leu-Arg-Arg-Arg-Glu-Leu-

-Glu-Lys-Aib-Lys-Leu-His-Thr-Ala-NH_2

Abaloparatide

Abaloparatide was approved in April 2017 for the treatment of osteoporosis in postmenopausal women at high risk for fracture. It has been shown to reduce the risk of vertebral and nonvertebral fractures regardless of age, timeframe post menopause, prior fracture history, and BMD at the start of treatment. After 18 months of treatment, there was a 43% reduction in nonvertebral fracture risk compared to the 28% decrease observed with teriparatide.[47] Vertebral fracture risk was decreased by 86% and 80%, respectively. The previously issued boxed warning for an increased risk of osteosarcoma has been removed; however, caution is still advised. As with teriparatide, therapy is not recommended to exceed a total of 2 years in a patient's lifetime.[47]

Structure-Activity Relationship. Abaloparatide is a 34–amino acid synthetic analogue of PTHrP (1-34). It retains 76% sequence homology with human PTHrP (1-34) and 41% homology with PTH (1-34).

Mechanism of Action. PTHR1 interacts with two endogenous ligands, PTH and PTHrP, and can adopt two conformations, R° and RG.[48] As a PTHR1 agonist, abaloparatide has greater selectivity for the RG PTHR1 conformation. Whereas activation of the RG conformation of PTH1R leads to receptor signaling that is short-lived, activation of the R° conformation yields a more long-lived response. As an agonist, this agent stimulates the Gs-mediated cAMP pathway that activates PLC and phosphokinase A (PKA), which in turn activates osteoblast activity.[47] Given that intermittent PTH receptor activation generally is associated with a bone-forming response, it is no surprise that abaloparatide promotes bone formation with less bone resorption and hypercalcemia than found with PTH (1-34).[49]

Pharmacokinetics. Abaloparatide is administered as a once daily 80-μg subcutaneous injection. Supplementation with calcium and vitamin D is recommended should dietary intake be compromised. It has a mean half-life of 1 hour, which allows nearly complete clearance prior to the next injection (hence being considered intermittent vs continuous dosing).[47] It is 36% bioavailable and is largely renally eliminated as peptide fragments. Dosage adjustment is not required in patients with severe renal impairment. It has not been shown to inhibit or induce CYP450 enzymes and is 70% bound by plasma proteins.[47] Adverse effects include hypercalciuria, dizziness, nausea, upper respiratory tract infection, and headache.[47] Patients are also at risk for developing hypercalcemia and, therefore, should not be administered to those diagnosed with primary hyperparathyroidism or other hypercalcemic conditions. Antidrug antibodies were present in 49% of patients taking abaloparatide.

Monoclonal Antibody–Based Therapies

RANKL Inhibitor

Denosumab (Prolia, Xgeva). Denosumab is approved for the treatment of osteoporosis in postmenopausal women and men at high risk for fracture as well as those who have giant cell tumor of the bone, hypercalcemia of malignancy, glucocorticoid-induced osteoporosis, or bone loss due to androgen deprivation or use of aromatase inhibitors. Studies show that denosumab is more effective in improving BMD (4%-7%) than weekly administration of alendronate (5%).[49] Denosumab is reported to reduce the risk of vertebral fraction (68%), hip fracture (40%), and nonvertebral facture (20%).[49]

Mechanism of Action. Denosumab is a fully human IgG2 monoclonal antibody to RANKL, where it functions as a RANKL inhibitor (see Fig. 27.4). The RANKL receptor is expressed on the surface of osteoclasts and osteoclast precursors. When bound to its receptor, RANKL promotes the formation and activation of osteoclasts. To balance the effects of RANKL, osteoblasts produce OPG, which binds to RANKL and prevents it from binding to and activating its receptor, modulating the production and activation of osteoclasts.[49] When an individual develops osteoporosis, this balance is disrupted, and RANKL overwhelms OPG activity, causing significant bone loss. Denosumab was designed to mimic the biochemical effects of OPG.

Pharmacokinetics. Denosumab is administered once every 6 months as a subcutaneous injection for the treatment of osteoporosis.[49] It has a bioavailability of 62%.[49] The mean elimination half-life is 28 days, and clearance and volume of distribution are proportional to body weight. Renal impairment has no effect on its pharmacokinetics. This agent has been associated with adverse events, including hypocalcemia and osteonecrosis of the jaw.[49]

Sclerostin Inhibitors

Romosozumab (Evenity). Romosozumab is indicated for the treatment of osteoporosis in postmenopausal women at a high risk of fracture, multiple risk factors for fracture, failure of first line anti-osteoporosis therapy, and intolerance to anti-osteoporetic therapy.[13] The FRActure study in postmenopausal women with ostEoporosis (FRAME) study showed that after 1 year of monthly romosozumab administration followed by 1 year of denosumab therapy, there was a 75% relative reduction in the risk of new vertebral fracture compared with placebo.[50] In the FRAME EXTENSION study showed that after 1 year of monthly romosozumab administration followed by 2 years of denosumab therapy, there was relative risk reduction observed in new vertebral fractures (66%), clinical fractures (27%), and nonvertebral fracture (21%).[51] Another sclerostin antibody, blosozumab (Eli Lilly), is under investigation.

Mechanism of Action. Romosozumab is an IgG2 antibody to sclerostin, a Wnt antagonist. It has both antiresorptive and osteoanabolic activity.[12] It has an effect on both components associated with bone formation: (1) remodeling-based formation (RBF) and (2) modeling-based formation (MBF). The initial effect is activation of bone lining cells on both cancellous and cortical bone. This causes bone formation on the non-resorbed surface of the bone (MBF). MBF then decreases, and a corresponding increase in the antiresorptive effect (RBF) occurs, ultimately resulting in a slow increase in BMD.[13,14]

Pharmacokinetics. Romosozumab is administered as a once-monthly 210-mg SC injection for 1 year. Discontinuation of the drug is recommended after 1 year. Nonlinear pharmacokinetics is evident. An increase in body weight decreases romosozumab exposure. Adequate intake of both calcium and vitamin D is recommended. The risk of hypocalcemia is highest in patients with severe renal impairment and in those on dialysis. Common adverse effects include headache, nasopharyngitis, arthralgia, and injection site pain and erythema.[13] There is a boxed warning due to the potential risk of adverse cardiac events (eg, myocardial infarction, stroke, cardiovascular death).[13] Romosozumab is contraindicated in pregnant and lactating women, and those at high risk for cardiovascular disease or cerebrovascular disease.[13]

Inorganic Salts

Calcium Salts. Appropriate intake of calcium during childhood, adolescence, and early adulthood increases peak BMD and may reduce the overall risk of developing osteoporosis. For those who are at low risk of developing osteoporosis and have adequate BMD, consumption of the recommended amounts of calcium (1,300 mg/d of elemental calcium for teenagers, 1,000 mg/d for premenopausal women and men, and 1,200 mg/d for postmenopausal women) typically is sufficient to prevent bone loss.[52] This often can be accomplished by eating a well-balanced diet. For patients with established osteoporosis or areas of poorly mineralized bone, calcium supplementation alone is not sufficient to reverse the bone loss or to significantly improve mineralization of the bone.[53]

The actual amount of elemental calcium that is present in the available calcium salts varies considerably; however, no one particular salt has been identified as an exceptional source of elemental calcium (Table 27.6).[39] Absorption of calcium from the gastrointestinal tract (25%-40%) improves under acidic conditions; therefore, those medications that change the acidic environment of the stomach (eg, H_2 antagonists, proton pump inhibitors) have an adverse effect on calcium absorption. Total daily doses of elemental calcium that exceed 500 mg should be spaced out over the day to improve absorption.[5] The more water soluble and, therefore, more easily absorbed salts (eg, citrate, lactate, gluconate) are less dependent on the acidic environment for appropriate absorption[5] and would be appropriate alternatives for patients who produce low levels of acid. Calcium carbonate is a poorly soluble form of calcium, but it is inexpensive and only requires the patient to take a few tablets per day with acidic food or beverages like citrus juice.

Drug Therapies Used to Treat Hyperparathyroidism

Increased levels of PTH lead to moderately to severely elevated serum calcium concentrations and alterations in phosphorous metabolism.[25] To modulate the levels of PTH released from the parathyroid gland chief cells, regulation of CaSR sensitivity is required. An agonist at this receptor, a calcimimetic, serves to activate the receptor, whereas an antagonist at this receptor is classified as a calcilytic. There are two types of calcimimetic agents: agonists that activate the CaSR directly (type I) (eg, calcium, other divalent cations), and those that are positive allosteric modulators (type II).[54] The type II calcimimetics sensitize the CaSR to calcium. When calcium binds and activates the extracellular portion of the CaSR, the resulting cascade of intracellular signaling suppresses the secretion of PTH, causing a decrease in serum calcium levels.

Cinacalcet Hydrochloride (Sensipar)

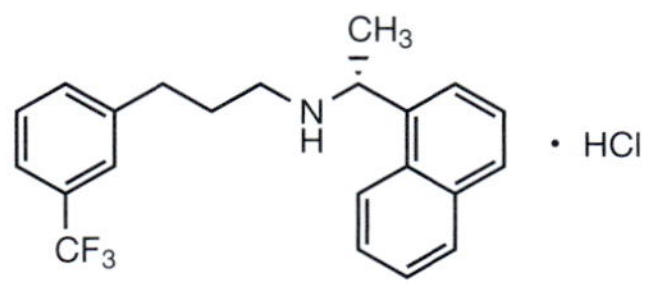

Cinacalcet hydrochloride (Sensipar)

Mechanism of Action

Cinacalcet hydrochloride is a second-generation calcimimetic approved for the treatment of secondary hyperparathyroidism in patients with end-stage kidney disease and for calciphylaxis in patients with advanced kidney disease or on dialysis. Cinacalcet binds to the transmembrane region of CaSR located on the chief cells of the parathyroid gland. After receptor activation, inhibition of cAMP accumulation occurs and stimulation of the phosphoinositide-PLC results. Production of the inositol triphosphate (IP_3) and diacylglycerol (DAG) second messengers leads to influx of calcium intracellularly, and ultimately the secretion of PTH is inhibited.[26] In the presence of cinacalcet, not only is a decrease in PTH levels observed, but a decrease in serum calcium and phosphorous levels is also observed. This represents a significant therapeutic advantage over vitamin D–based treatments for secondary hyperparathyroidism.[55] It can be used alone, with vitamin D and/or with a phosphate binder.[55]

Pharmacokinetics

Administered orally once daily with food, cinacalcet has an initial half-life of 6 hours and a terminal half-life of 30 to 40 hours. It is 93% to 97% bound to plasma proteins, and absorption is enhanced when taken with a high-fat meal. Cinacalcet is metabolized primarily by CYP3A4, less so by CYP2D6 and CYP1A2.[54] It is a strong inhibitor of CYP2D6. Caution is advised for coadministration with an inhibitor of either CYP3A4 or with drugs that are primarily metabolized by CYP2D6. While no dosage adjustment is required for renal impairment, patients with moderate to severe hepatic impairment should be monitored.[55] Common adverse effects include nausea and vomiting.

Etelcalcetide (Parsabiv)

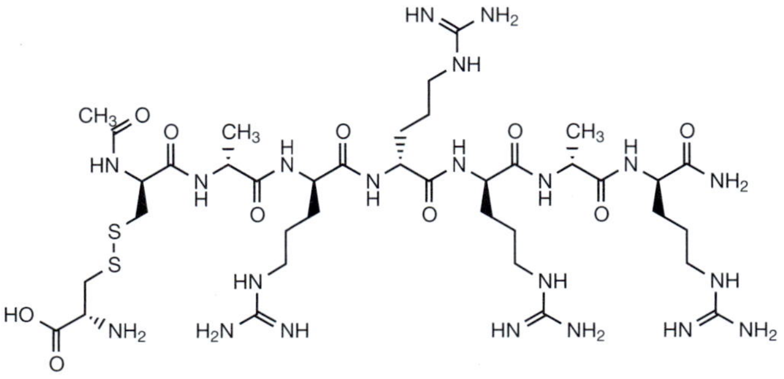

Etelcalcetide

Mechanism of Action

Etelcalcetide is a second-generation type II calcimimetic approved for the treatment of secondary hyperparathyroidism in patients with chronic kidney disease who receive dialysis. This agent is a long-acting 8–amino acid peptide CaSR agonist that is associated with allosteric receptor activation on the parathyroid gland chief cells. Activation occurs once a disulfide bridge forms between the amino terminal D-cysteine present in etelcalcetide and Cys482 of the CaSR.[56] Unlike cinacalcet, there is slight direct CaSR activation by etelcalcetide under low-calcium conditions. This indicates that etelcalcetide can act as both a direct agonist (minor mechanism) and as an allosteric modulator of CaSR (major mechanism). PTH levels decreased 50% more than what was observed when cinacalcet was administered.[57]

Pharmacokinetics

IV injection of etelcalcetide is administered 3 times weekly via the venous line of the hemodialysis blood circuit at the conclusion of hemodialysis.[58] In the plasma, a covalent albumin peptide conjugate forms between the D-cysteine in the drug molecule and Cys34 found within serum albumin. Etelcalcetide is not metabolized by CYP450 enzymes.[58] Renal elimination is significant, and the terminal elimination half-life is 18.4 hours.[58] The primary adverse effect was an asymptomatic reduction in plasma calcium levels, muscle spasms, diarrhea, nausea, and symptomatic hypocalcemia.[58]

Drug Therapies Used to Treat Hypercalcemia of Malignancy

Zoledronic Acid

Mechanism of Action

Zoledronic acid, a bisphosphonate, is approved for the treatment of hypercalcemia of malignancy, a metabolic complication that can be life-threatening (see Fig. 27.8). The primary indication is for adjunct use in patients with multiple myeloma and those with bone metastases from solid tumors.[59] Hypercalcemia of malignancy can occur in up to 50% of patients diagnosed with multiple myeloma, leukemia, and non-Hodgkin lymphoma.[23] This condition arises when chemical moieties produced by the tumor cause overstimulation of osteoclasts. When there is an increase in bone degradation, there is a concomitant release of calcium into the plasma. When serum concentrations of calcium rapidly elevate, the kidneys are unable to handle the overload, and hypercalcemia results. This can lead to dehydration, nausea, vomiting, fatigue, and confusion. Zoledronic acid effectively decreases plasma calcium concentrations via inhibition of bone resorption (inhibition of osteoclastic activity and induction of osteoclast apoptosis).[59] It also prevents the increase in osteoclastic activity caused by tumor-based stimulatory factors.

Cancer treatment–induced bone loss is a major adverse effect associated with endocrine-based cancer therapies. These therapies may depress ovarian function (eg, goserelin acetate), decrease ER activation (eg, ER antagonist), and/or inhibit estrogen biosynthesis (eg, aromatase inhibition) all of which will lead to significant bone loss. Zoledronic acid has demonstrated efficacy in reducing or delaying these complications.

Pharmacokinetics

Zoledronic acid is a white, crystalline powder that is available in vials for reconstitution for IV infusion over at least 15 minutes. It does not undergo metabolic transformation and does not inhibit CYP450 enzymes.[59] Clearance of this agent is dependent on the patient's creatinine clearance, not on dose. Serum creatinine levels should be evaluated prior to every treatment. Zoledronic acid is contraindicated in patients with severe renal impairment.

Zoledronic acid should not be mixed with infusion solutions that contain calcium (eg, lactated Ringer solution) and should be administered via IV infusion in its own line. Because of the possibility of a serious deterioration in renal function, the manufacturer requires strict adherence to the infusion duration of no less than 15 minutes.[59]

Pamidronate Disodium

Pamidronate disodium, a second-generation bisphosphonate, is 100-fold more potent than etidronate disodium for the treatment of moderate or severe hypercalcemia of malignancy (see Fig. 27.8).[5] It has also been approved for the treatment of moderate to severe Paget disease of the bone and for osteolytic bone metastases of breast cancer and osteolytic lesions of multiple myeloma.[60] When used to treat bone metastases, pamidronate disodium decreases osteoclast recruitment, decreases osteoclast activity, and increases osteoclast apoptosis.[60] Mechanistically, it is identical to the other nitrogen-containing bisphosphonates (eg, alendronate). Administered by IV infusion, a single dose is typically sufficient for the treatment of hypercalcemia and Paget disease of the bone. In the treatment of osteolytic lesions of multiple myeloma, monthly administration is indicated.[60]

Pharmacokinetics

Pamidronate disodium is cleared renally and, therefore, is contraindicated in patients with impaired renal function. As with other bisphosphonates, there is a risk of osteonecrosis of the jaw, and patients are advised against invasive dental procedures.[60]

Drug Therapy Used in the Treatment of Hypoparathyroidism

Parathyroid Hormone [rhPTH 1-84] (Natpara)

Mechanism of Action

Natpara has an orphan drug designation to treat (along with calcium and vitamin D) the hypocalcemia associated with hypoparathyroidism (see Fig. 27.2). Structurally identical to endogenous PTH, the recombinant human PTH is administered once daily as an SC injection. Although Natpara shares a common mechanism of action with teriparatide, it has been suggested that the C-terminal region may possess valuable biologic activity mediated by a novel receptor that specifically interacts with this portion of the peptide hormone.

Representative examples of the common side effects include tingling or burning sensation (paresthesia), hypocalcemia, headache, and nausea.[61] Due to the increase in the reported incidence of osteosarcoma in male and female rats, Natpara is available only through a restricted program (NATPARA REMS–Risk Evaluation and Mitigation Strategy).

Pharmacokinetics

Administered subcutaneously, Natpara has an absolute bioavailability of 53%. Degradation by hepatic cathepsins yields fragments that are renally eliminated. Dosage adjustment is not required in patients with mild to moderate liver or kidney impairment.

Natpara will negate the effects of alendronate and, therefore, they should not be used in combination.[61] The effectiveness of digoxin is reduced if administered in patients diagnosed with hypocalcemia. Patients should be monitored for calcium levels and digoxin toxicity when taking Natpara.

Structure Challenge

Vitamin D activation is a two-step process (below) regardless of whether vitamin D_2 (from plants) is consumed or D_3 (from animals and skin biosynthesis) is consumed or produced.

1. If a patient is diagnosed with severe renal disease, which of the two activation steps will likely be impacted?
2. Impaired vitamin D activation will have what kind of impact on bone mineralization?
3. Vitamin D deactivation is catalyzed by which enzyme?

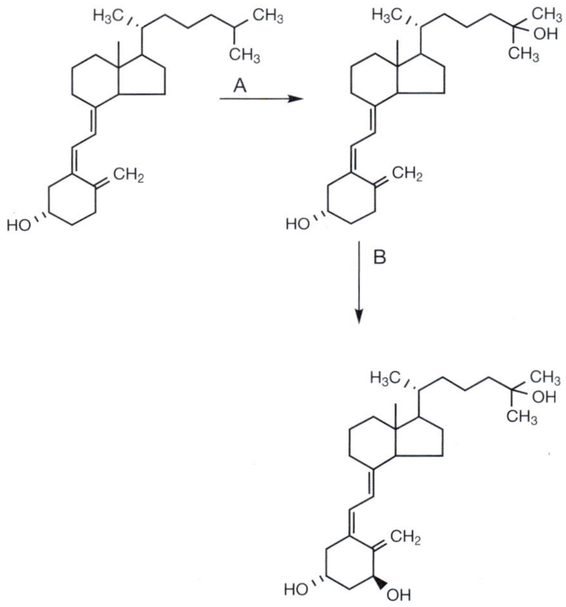

4. The following two vitamin D analogues are commercially available. Determine which, if any, activation steps must still occur for the analogue to be completely active.

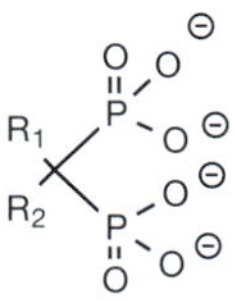

Many of the bisphosphonates in Figure 27.8 are used in the treatment of osteoporosis. Consider those structures as you answer the following questions.

5. Which functional group maximizes the affinity of the drug for the hydroxyapatite and improves the antiresorptive activity?
6. Which functional groups act as the bone "hook"?
7. The functional group at R_2 varies considerably and influences the potency of the drug. Provide a pair of examples of functional group variations at R_2 and the effect on potency.
8. What are the two mechanisms by which these agents are effective in the treatment of osteoporosis?
9. Analyze each of the approved drug structures and determine which drugs work by each of the two mechanisms identified in Question #8.
10. Analyze each of the unapproved drug structures and determine which drugs work by each of the two mechanisms identified in Question #8.

Structure Challenge answers found immediately after References.

REFERENCES

1. Copp DH. Calcitonin: discovery, development, and clinical application. *Clin Invest Med.* 1994;17:268-277.
2. Goyal A, Anastasopoulou C, Ngu M, et al. Hypocalcemia. In: *StatPearls* [Internet]. StatPearls Publishing; 2024. Updated October 15, 2023. https://www.ncbi.nlm.nih.gov/books/NBK430912/
3. Ott SM. Cortical or trabecular bone: what's the difference? *Am J Nephrol.* 2018;47(6):373-375.
4. Christenson RH. Biochemical markers of bone metabolism: an overview. *Clin Biochem.* 1997;30:573-593.
5. Cosman F, de Beur SJ, LeBoff MS, et al. Clinician's guide to prevention and treatment of osteoporosis. *Osteoporos Int.* 2014;25:2359-2381.
6. Khosla S, Riggs BL. Pathophysiology of age-related bone loss and osteoporosis. *Endocrinol Metab Clin North Am.* 2005;34:1015-1030.
7. Erben RG. Physiological actions of fibroblast growth factor-23. *Front Endocrinol.* 2018;9:267. https://www.frontiersin.org/journals/endocrinology/articles/10.3389/fendo.2018.00267
8. Brown EM, Gamba G, Riccardi D, et al. Cloning and characterization of an extracellular Ca^{2+}-sensing receptor from bovine parathyroid. *Nature.* 1993;366:575-580.
9. Nair R, Maseeh A. Vitamin D: the "sunshine" vitamin. *J Pharmacol Pharmacother.* 2012;3:118-119.
10. Bolamperti S, Villa I, Rubinacci A. Bone remodeling: an operational process ensuring survival and bone mechanical competence. *Bone Res.* 2022;10:48. https://www.nature.com/articles/s41413-022-00219-8
11. Rosen CJ. The epidemiology and pathogenesis of osteoporosis. In: Feingold KR, Anawalt B, Blackman MR, et al, eds. *Endotext* [Internet]. MDText.com, Inc; 2000. Updated June 21, 2020. https://www.ncbi.nlm.nih.gov/books/NBK279134/
12. Aibar-Almazán A, Voltes-Martínez A, Castellote-Caballero Y, Afanador-Restrepo DF, Carcelén-Fraile MDC, López-Ruiz E. Current status of the diagnosis and management of osteoporosis. *Int J Mol Sci.* 2022;23:9465.
13. Aditya S, Rattan A. Sclerostin inhibition: a novel target for the treatment of postmenopausal osteoporosis. *J Midlife Health.* 2021;12:267-275.
14. MacNabb C, Patton D, Hayes JS. Sclerostin antibody therapy for the treatment of osteoporosis: clinical prospects and challenges. *J Osteoporos.* 2016;2016:6217286.
15. Hansen LB, Vondracek SF. Prevention and treatment of non-postmenopausal osteoporosis. *Am J Health Syst Pharm.* 2004;61:2637-2656.
16. Wang LT, Chen LR, Chen KH. Hormone-related and drug-induced osteoporosis: a cellular and molecular overview. *Int J Mol Sci.* 2023;24(6):5814.
17. Gray SL, LaCroix AZ, Larson J, et al. Proton pump inhibitor use, hip fracture and change in bone mineral density in postmenopausal women. *Arch Intern Med.* 2010;170:765-771.
18. Riche DM, King ST. Bone loss and fracture risk associated with thiazolidinedione therapy. *Pharmacotherapy.* 2010;30:716-727.
19. Ilias I, Milionis C, Zoumakis E. An overview of glucocorticoid-induced osteoporosis. In: Feingold KR, Anawalt B, Blackman MR, et al, eds. *Endotext* [Internet]. MDText.com, Inc; 2000. Updated March 19, 2022. https://www.ncbi.nlm.nih.gov/books/NBK278968/
20. International Osteoporosis Foundation. Epidemiology of osteoporosis and fragility fractures. https://www.osteoporosis.foundation/facts-statistics/epidemiology-of-osteoporosis-and-fragility-fractures
21. Noel SE, Santos MP, Wright NC. Racial and ethnic disparities in bone health and outcomes in the United States. *J Bone Miner Res.* 2021;36(10):1881-1905.
22. Sobacchi C, Schulz A, Coxon FP, Villa A, Helfrich MH. Osteopetrosis: genetics, treatment and new insights into osteoclast function. *Nat Rev Endocrinol.* 2013;9(9):522-536.
23. Walker MD, Shane E. Hypercalcemia: a review. *JAMA.* 2022;328(16):1624-1636.
24. Pasieka JL, Wentworth K, Yeo CT, et al. Etiology and pathophysiology of hypoparathyroidism: a narrative review. *J Bone Miner Res.* 2022;37(12):2586-2601.
25. Dandurand K, Ali DS, Khan AA. Primary hyperparathyroidism: a narrative review of diagnosis and medical management. *J Clin Med.* 2021;10(8):1604. doi:10.3390/jcm10081604
26. Cinacalcet. Prescribing information. Amgen; Revised August 2011. Accessed July 9, 2024. https://www.accessdata.fda.gov/drugsatfda_docs/label/2011/021688s017lbl.pdf
27. Biasucci G, Donini V, Cannalire G. Rickets types and treatment with vitamin D and analogues. *Nutrients.* 2024;16(3):416.
28. Banaganapalli B, Fallatah I, Alsubhi F. et al. Paget's disease: a review of the epidemiology, etiology, genetics, and treatment. *Front Genet.* 2023;14:1131182.
29. Rossouw JE, Anderson GL, Prentice RL, et al. Risks and benefits of estrogen plus progestin in healthy postmenopausal women. Principal results from the Women's Health Initiative randomized controlled trial. *JAMA.* 2002;288:321-333.
30. Levin VA, Jiang S, Kagan R. Estrogen therapy for osteoporosis in the modern era. *Osteoporos Int.* 2018;29:1049-1055.
31. Harris ST, Watts NB, Genant HK, et al. Effect of risedronate treatment on vertebral and nonvertebral fractures with postmenopausal osteoporosis. Vertebral Efficacy with Risedronate Therapy (VERT) study group. *JAMA.* 1999;282(14):1344-1352.
32. Evista. Prescribing information. Eli Lilly; Revised September 2007. Accessed July 1, 2024 https://www.accessdata.fda.gov/drugsatfda_docs/label/2007/022042lbl.pdf
33. Rey JR, Cervino EV, Rentero ML, et al. Raloxifene: mechanism of action, effects on bone tissue, and applicability in clinical traumatology practice. *Open Orthop J.* 2009;3:14-21.
34. Cho SK, Kim H, Lee J, et al. Effectiveness of bazedoxifene in preventing glucocorticoid-induced bone loss in rheumatoid arthritis patients. *Arthritis Res Ther.* 2021;23(1):176.
35. Goldberg T, Fidler B. Conjugated estrogens/bazedoxifene (Duavee): a novel agent for the treatment of moderate-to-severe vasomotor symptoms associated with menopause and the prevention of postmenopausal osteoporosis. *P T.* 2015;40:178-182.
36. Rogers MJ, Crockett JC, Coxon FP, et al. Biochemical and molecular mechanisms of action of bisphosphonates. *Bone.* 2011;49:34-41.
37. Ebetino FH, Hogan AM, Sun S, et al. The relationship between the chemistry and biological activity of the bisphosphonates. *Bone.* 2011;49(1):20-33.
38. Cremers S, Papapoulas S. Pharmacology of bisphosphonates. *Bone.* 2011;49:42-49.
39. Camacho PM, Petak SM, Binkley N, et al. American Association of Clinical Endocrinologists/American College of Endocrinology clinical practice guidelines for the diagnosis and treatment of postmenopausal osteoporosis—2020 update. *Endocr Pract.* 2020;26(suppl 1):1-46.
40. Nafee N, Zewail M, Boraie N. Alendronate-loaded, biodegradable smart hydrogel. A promising injectable depot formulation for osteoporosis. *J Drug Target.* 2018;26:565-575.
41. Eastell R, Walsh JS, Watts NB, et al. Bisphosphonates for postmenopausal osteoporosis. *Bone.* 2011;49:82-88.
42. Ibandronate Sodium. Prescribing information. Apotex; Revised January 2017. Accessed July 9, 2024. https://www.apotex.com/products/us/downloads/pre/iban_psin_3mg3ml_ins_3ml_usa.pdf
43. Khan AA, Morrison A, Hanley DA, et al; International Task Force on Osteonecrosis of the Jaw. Diagnosis and management of osteonecrosis of the jaw: a systematic review and international consensus. *J Bone Miner Res.* 2015;30(1):3-23.
44. U.S. Food and Drug Administration. Drug safety communication safety update for osteoporosis drugs, bisphosphonates, and atypical fractures. Updated February 6, 2017. Accessed May 9, 2024. https://www.fda.gov/Drugs/DrugSafety/ucm229009.htm
45. Srinivasan A, Wong FK, Karponis DK. Calcitonin: a useful old friend. *J Musculoskelet Neuronal Interact.* 2020;20(4):600-609.

46. Teriparatide. Prescribing information. Alvogen; Revised November 2023. Accessed July 9, 2024. https://dailymed.nlm.nih.gov/dailymed/drugInfo.cfm?setid=1b007339-dd0d-f019-5e0a-9b1b0f75011c
47. Tymlos. Prescribing information. Radius; Revised April 2017. Accessed May 9, 2024. https://www.accessdata.fda.gov/drugsatfda_docs/label/2017/208743lbl.pdf
48. Hattersley G, Dean T, Corbon BA, et al. Binding selectivity of abaloparatide for PTH-type-1-receptor conformations and effects on downstream signaling. *Endocrinology*. 2016;157:141-149.
49. Prolia. Prescribing information. Amgen; Revised March 2024. Accessed July 9, 2024. https://www.pi.amgen.com/-/media/Project/Amgen/Repository/pi-amgen-com/Prolia/prolia_pi.pdf
50. Cosman F, Crittenden DB, Adachi J, et al. Romosozumab treatment in postmenopausal women with osteoporosis. *N Engl J Med*. 2016;37(16):1532-1543.
51. Lewiecki EM, Dinavahi RV, Lasaretti-Castro M, et al. One year of romosozumab followed by two years of denosumab maintains fracture risk reductions: results of the FRAME extension study. *J Bone Miner Res*. 2019;34:419-428.
52. Institute of Medicine (US) Committee to Review Dietary Reference Intakes for Vitamin D and Calcium; Ross CA, Taylor CL, Yaktine AL, eds. *Dietary Reference Intakes for Calcium and Vitamin D*. National Academies Press (US); 2011. Accessed May 9, 2024. https://www.ncbi.nlm.nih.gov/books/NBK56050/#summary.s5
53. Black DM, Rosen CJ. Postmenopausal osteoporosis. *N Engl J Med*. 2016;374:254-262.
54. Pereira L, Meng C, Marques D, et al. Old and new calcimimetics for treatment of secondary hyperparathyroidism: impact on biochemical and relevant clinical outcomes. *Clin Kidney J*. 2018;11:80-88.
55. Sensipar. Prescribing information. Amgen; Revised December 2019. Accessed May 9, 2024. https://www.pi.amgen.com/-/media/Project/Amgen/Repository/pi-amgen-com/sensipar/sensipar_pi_hcp_english.pdf
56. Alexander ST, Hunter T, Walter S, et al. Critical cysteine residues in both the calcium-sensing receptor and the allosteric activator AMG 416 underlie the mechanism of action. *Mol Pharmacol*. 2015;88:853-865.
57. Hamano N, Komaba H, Fukagawa M. Etelcalcetide for the treatment of secondary hyperparathyroidism. *Expert Opin Pharmacother*. 2017;18:529-534.
58. Parsabiv. Prescribing information. Amgen; Revised February 2017. Accessed May 9, 2024. https://www.accessdata.fda.gov/drugsatfda_docs/label/2017/208325Orig1s000Lbledt.pdf
59. Zoledronic Acid Injection. Prescribing information. Sagent Pharmaceuticals; Revised March 2016. Accessed July 1, 2024. https://www.accessdata.fda.gov/drugsatfda_docs/label/2016/203231s011lbl.pdf
60. Pamidronate Disodium. Prescribing information. Bedford Laboratories; 2009. Accessed May 9, 2024. https://www.accessdata.fda.gov/drugsatfda_docs/label/2009/021113s008lbl.pdf
61. Natpara. Prescribing information. Takeda Pharmaceuticals USA, Inc; Revised February 2023. Accessed May 10, 2024. https://www.shirecontent.com/PI/PDFs/Natpara_USA_ENG.pdf

Structure Challenge Answers

Vitamin D activation is a two-step process (see later) regardless of whether vitamin D_2 (from plants) is consumed or D_3 (from animals and skin biosynthesis) is consumed or produced.

1. Step B
2. Active vitamin D is required for calcium absorption. If less vitamin D is activated, then there will be less calcium absorbed, and bone mineralization will be poor.
3. Vitamin D deactivation is catalyzed by vitamin D 24-hydroxylase.
4. Paracalcitol does not require any additional activation. Doxercalciferol requires 25 hydroxylation catalyzed by vitamin D 25-hydroxylase in the liver.

Many of the bisphosphonates in Figure 27.8 are used in the treatment of osteoporosis. Consider those structures as you answer the following questions.

5. A hydroxyl group at R_1 maximizes the affinity of the drug for the hydroxyapatite and improves the antiresorptive activity.
6. The bisphosphonate and the R_1 hydroxyl group act as the bone "hook."
7. Amino-substituted (R_2) bisphosphonates are more potent than etidronate, which has an R_2 methyl substituent. A three-carbon-chain amino-substituted (R_2) bisphosphonate is more potent than the two-carbon-chain amino-substituted (R_2) bisphosphonate.
8. Mechanism #1: Mimics pyrophosphate (PPi) and gets incorporated into nonhydrolyzable adenosine triphosphate (ATP) analogues. These nucleotides accumulate within osteoclasts and decrease their activity.

Mechanism #2: Inhibit farnesyl pyrophosphate synthetase (FPPS) and interfere with protein prenylation within osteoclasts. They also inhibit ATP-dependent enzymes.

Mimics pyrophosphate Incorporated into nonhydrolyzable ATP	FPPS Inhibitors
Etidronate	Alendronate
	Ibandronate
	Pamidronate
	Risedronate
	Zoledronic acid
Mimics pyrophosphate Incorporated into nonhydrolyzable ATP	FPPS Inhibitors
Clodronate	Incadronate
	Neridronate
	Olpadronate

CHAPTER 28

Drugs Used to Treat Gastrointestinal and Genitourinary Disorders

Sabesan Yoganathan

Drugs covered in this chapter:

H_2-RECEPTOR ANTAGONISTS
- Cimetidine
- Famotidine
- Nizatidine

PROTON PUMP INHIBITORS
- Dexlansoprazole
- Esomeprazole
- Lansoprazole
- Omeprazole
- Pantoprazole sodium
- Rabeprazole sodium
- Tenatoprazole

OTHER ANTIULCER AGENTS
- Bismuth subsalicylate
- Dexpanthenol
- Metoclopramide
- Misoprostol
- Prostaglandin E_1
- Sucralfate
- Vonoprazan

ANTIEMETICS AND IRRITABLE BOWEL SYNDROME DRUGS
- Alosetron
- Amisulpride
- Dolasetron
- Granisetron
- Linaclotide
- Ondansetron
- Palonosetron
- Plecanatide
- Prochlorperazine
- Promethazine
- Renzapride
- Tegaserod
- Tropisetron

SMALL-MOLECULE THERAPY FOR INFLAMMATORY GASTROINTESTINAL DISEASES
- Etrasimod
- Ozanimod
- Tofacitinib
- Upadacitinib

MONOCLONAL ANTIBODY FOR INFLAMMATORY GI DISEASES
- Adalimumab
- Certolizumab
- Golimumab
- Infliximab
- Vedolizumab

MUSCARINIC AGONISTS
- Bethanechol
- Cevimeline
- Pilocarpine

MUSCARINIC ANTAGONISTS
- Atropine
- Darifenacin
- Fesoterodine
- Mirabegron
- Oxybutynin
- Scopolamine
- Solifenacin
- Tolterodine
- Trospium chloride
- Vibegron

Abbreviations

AC adenylyl cyclase
AcCoA acetyl-coenzyme A
Ach acetylcholine
AChE acetylcholinesterase
ATPase adenosine triphosphatase
AUC area under the (plasma concentration) curve
cAMP cyclic adenosine monophosphate
CD Crohn's disease
ChT choline transporter

Abbreviations—continued

ChAT choline acetyltransferase
CNS central nervous system
CoA coenzyme A
CTZ chemoreceptor trigger zone
CYP450 cytochrome P450
CYP2C19 cytochrome P450 family 2 subfamily C member 19
DDIs drug-drug interactions
DEO dealkylated desethyl metabolite
EC enterochromaffin cells
ECL enterochromaffin-like cells
EM extensive metabolizer
FDA US Food and Drug Administration
GERD gastroesophageal reflux disease
GI gastrointestinal
GPCR G protein–coupled receptor
GSH glutathione
GU genitourinary
5-HT 5-hydroxytryptamine (serotonin)
IBD inflammatory bowel disease
IBS irritable bowel syndrome
IM intermediate metabolizer
JAK Janus kinase
MAb monoclonal antibody
mAChR muscarinic acetylcholine receptor
MAO monoamine oxidase
MS multiple sclerosis
nAChR nicotinic acetylcholine receptor
NDMA *N*-nitrosodimethylamine
NSAID nonsteroidal anti-inflammatory drug
OAB overactive bladder
OTC over the counter
PG prostaglandin
P-gp P-glycoprotein
PLC phospholipase C
PLP pyridoxal phosphate
PM poor metabolizer
PPI proton pump inhibitor
S1P sphingosine-1-phosphate
SARs structure-activity relationships
SNAP synaptosomal-associated protein
STATs signal transducers and activators of transcription
TNF-α tumor necrosis factor alpha
TYK2 tyrosine kinase 2
UC ulcerative colitis
UM ultrafast metabolizer
VAMP vesicle-associated membrane protein
VAT vesicular acetylcholine transporter

CLINICAL SIGNIFICANCE

Pharmacists frequently encounter patients with gastrointestinal issues across different practice settings. Understanding the structural relationships between these compounds is crucial for pharmacists to make informed decisions about drug therapy. As chemical structure determines drug action and drug metabolism, a clear understanding of the chemical basis of a specific drug class is a fundamental aspect of pharmacy profession. For instance, a patient not responding to omeprazole may be a rapid CYP2C19 (cytochrome P450 family 2 subfamily C member 19) metabolizer and could benefit from esomeprazole, which is metabolized by CYP2C19 at a slower rate. This understanding has led to the development of drugs with improved efficacy and receptor selectivity while reducing side effects, empowering pharmacists to choose the most suitable treatment for their patients.

Emily M. Ambizas, PharmD

INTRODUCTION

Gastrointestinal Disorders

Gastrointestinal (GI) disorders are broadly characterized by illnesses associated with upper GI tract (esophagus, stomach, and duodenum) and lower GI tract (small and large intestine) and/or diseases associated with the liver, gallbladder, and pancreas. In general, GI disorders are (1) structural, (2) malabsorptive, (3) inflammatory, and/or (4) neoplastic in nature. The most common GI diseases include acid reflux, peptic ulcer, inflammation-associated diseases, constipation, infection, diarrhea, celiac disease, and cancer. These diseases substantially diminish the quality of life and are a huge economic burden in terms of health care costs. GI diseases affect close to 70 million people in the United States annually, and more than 200,000 deaths are related to GI diseases. Moreover, the direct and indirect cost of managing GI diseases in the United States has been estimated to be $142 billion per year.[1,2] This chapter focuses on drugs that are clinically used for the treatment of acid reflux, peptic ulcer, irritable bowel syndrome (IBS), inflammatory bowel disease (IBD), and nausea and vomiting. Many other drug classes covered elsewhere in this text are also used for the treatment of other GI disorders, including infections and cancer.

Gastroesophageal reflux disease (GERD) is one of the most common GI disorders and affects a significant number of people in the United States and worldwide.[3,4] GERD is typically associated with the esophageal mucosa being continuously exposed to gastric secretions. This often occurs when the lower esophageal sphincter relaxes, and the duration of esophageal acid exposure is considerably prolonged. Typically, when gastric secretions enter the esophagus, innate clearing mechanisms limit the duration of exposure by rapidly pushing the refluxed content into the stomach. Additionally, bicarbonate-rich secretions by esophageal glands help neutralize the residual acid trapped within the mucosa. Since GERD is associated with gastric acid reflux and associated symptoms, most treatment options are directed toward reducing the acidic nature of the refluxate. An effective therapeutic option should heal esophageal damage while providing symptomatic relief. Current therapy for acid reflux–related GI diseases focuses on inhibiting biological pathways that directly or indirectly play a role in stomach acid secretion. Two such pathways involve inhibition of the histamine H_2 receptor and inhibition of the proton pump (H^+/K^+-adenosine triphosphatase [ATPase]) in the stomach. Selective muscarinic receptor antagonists and prokinetic agents can also be used for the treatment of GERD.[5,6]

Other common GI disorders include IBS and IBD. Ulcerative colitis (UC) and Crohn's disease (CD) are two examples of IBD, which are chronic diseases of the GI tract caused by inflammation in the gut mucosal tissue.[7] The pathogenesis of IBD is linked to multiple inflammatory cell types, including neutrophils, macrophages, and lymphocytes. In most cases, modulation of inflammation in the GI tract is a viable approach that provides symptomatic treatment of IBDs.[8] Additionally, serotonergic agents and anti-inflammatory monoclonal antibodies have also been considered as useful therapeutic options for the treatment of IBDs.

Genitourinary Disorders

The genitourinary (GU) system consists of the genital or reproductive organs and urinary system. Some of the primary functions of the GU system include (1) excretion of cellular waste products, (2) regulation of blood volume via conservation or excretion of fluids, (3) regulation of electrolytes, (4) balancing pH via regulation of H^+ and HCO_3^- ions reabsorbed or excreted, (5) arterial blood pressure control via regulation of sodium excretion and renin secretion, and (6) erythropoietin secretion. Taken together, the GU system plays an important role in maintaining homeostasis. Several pathologic conditions are associated with the GU tract, ranging from infections, inflammation, dysuria, nocturia, and kidney-related diseases. The focus of this chapter is on managing urination frequency from an overactive bladder with the use of antimuscarinic agents. Other chapters within this text provide more detailed discussions on therapeutic agents used as diuretics (Chapter 19) and for the treatment of GU tract infections (Chapter 32) and inflammation (Chapter 24).

Overactive bladder (OAB) is characterized as symptoms of urgency to urinate, with or without urge urinary incontinence. This happens because the detrusor muscle is overactive and inconsistently contracts. The smooth muscle in bladder is controlled by the parasympathetic nervous system and, more specifically, by the action of acetylcholine (ACh) on the muscarinic acetylcholine receptor (mAChR). There are several subtypes of the mAChR (see Chapter 6), and the M_2 and M_3 subtypes are mainly present in the urinary bladder. Although the M_2 subtype is the predominant mAChR in the bladder, the M_3 subtype appears to play a more important role in directly mediating detrusor contraction.[9] Inhibition of these receptors in the urinary bladder results in decreased bladder contraction, providing relief from OAB. Several antimuscarinic agents have been developed from the structure-activity relationships (SARs) of atropine, a natural alkaloid and antimuscarinic agent. The detailed structure, function, and SARs of this class of medicinal agents are discussed later in this chapter.

Histamine and Histamine Receptors

Histamine plays an important role in mediating biochemical responses through different signaling pathways. Its action on endothelial cells and vascular smooth muscle cells results in the symptoms of allergic reactions, and it also acts on parietal cells to stimulate gastric acid secretion.[10,11] Inhibition of the histamine-based signaling pathway in specific tissues has been proven to be an effective approach to treat allergic reactions or GI disorders.

Histamine is a basic compound with an imidazole ring and a primary amine motif. The imidazole has a pK_a value of 5.80, and the aliphatic amine has a pK_a value of 9.40. Due to its basic nature, histamine protonates to form cations at physiological pH, including a monocation (major) and a dication (minor). Both species are considered biologically active. When the imidazole ring of histamine is protonated, it tautomerizes, forming a mixture of the N^{τ}-H tautomer and N^{π}-H tautomer with a ratio of 4:1, respectively. Chemical modifications of the imidazole ring change the rate of formation of one or the other tautomer.[12,13] More specifically, the electronic nature of the substituent at the 4-position (eg, CH_3 vs Cl) changes the proportion existing as the N^{τ}-H tautomer. The electron-withdrawing chlorine substitution provides 12% of the N^{τ}-H tautomer versus 70% for the electron donating 4-methylhistamine. Additionally, this change in composition decreases agonist potency, indicating that tautomeric composition is important in the agonist-receptor interaction.[13]

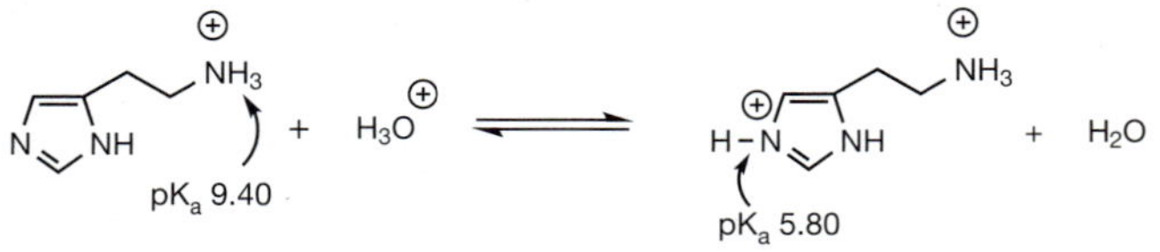

pKa of histamine

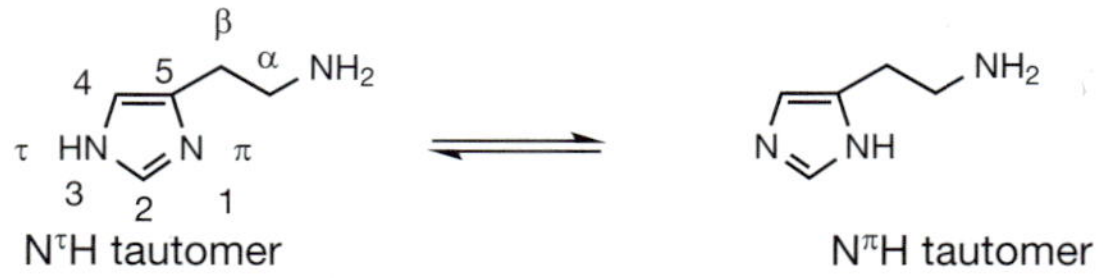

Tautomers of histamine

Histamine exists as both *trans* and *gauche* conformations in solution (Fig. 28.1),[13] and studies have shown that the conformational isomerism impacts selectivity toward the different histamine receptors (H_1, H_2, H_3, and H_4).[13] Although histamine has no chiral centers, the selectivity toward the receptor binding arises from its ability to form the *trans/gauche* conformational isomers. Based on experimental

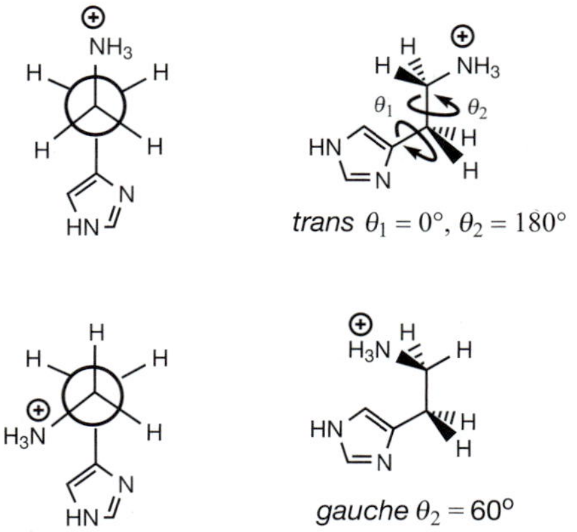

Figure 28.1 Conformers of histamine.

studies done using conformationally restricted analogues of histamine, it is evident that *trans* conformer selectively binds to H_1 and H_2 receptors, while the *gauche* conformer binds to the H_3 receptor. Synthesis and evaluation of histamine analogues have yielded some important information about the SAR of histamine. Introduction of alkyl groups typically produces compounds with reduced activity toward H_1 and H_2 receptors. Introduction of a methyl group at the 2- or 4-position produces selective compounds toward the H_1 receptor and H_2 receptor, respectively. However, imidazole N-substitution produces inactive compounds. Additionally, modification of the aliphatic amine through substitution decreases histamine's activity ($R\text{-}NH_2 > R\text{-}NHMe > R\text{-}NMe_2 > R\text{-}N^+Me_3$) at both H_1 and H_2 receptors.[13,14]

Histamine is synthesized in various tissues, including mast cells, parietal cells of the gastric mucosa, and neurons in the central nervous system (CNS) and periphery. The biosynthesis of histamine occurs in the Golgi apparatus of these cells via an enzymatic decarboxylation of histidine. A decarboxylase enzyme utilizes pyridoxal phosphate (PLP) as a cofactor to convert L-histidine into histamine (Fig. 28.2). The reaction mechanism for this process involves condensation of histidine with PLP, which forms an imine intermediate. Subsequently, loss of the carboxylate group in the form of carbon dioxide generates the histamine-PLP adduct. Finally, histamine is released from PLP via hydrolysis of the intermediate. This type of PLP-dependent decarboxylation of amino acids is a common catalytic transformation known to generate amino acid–derived endogenous small molecules. Based on the mechanism of histamine biosynthesis, α-fluoromethylhistidine was identified as an inhibitor of histidine decarboxylase.[15] Although this small molecule was a useful tool to inhibit histamine biosynthesis, such an approach has not yielded any successful drug leads for the treatment of histamine-induced disorders, including peptic ulcer or motion sickness.

Once histamine is released from mast cells or parietal cells, its physiological effect is mediated by binding to the various histamine receptors. The histamine receptors belong to the G protein–coupled receptor (GPCR) family, which are a diverse family of transmembrane proteins (see Chapter 6).[16] Histamine plays a central role in immune responses and regulates physiological function in the gut as well as in the CNS. Due to its important role in various physiological functions that relates to several diseases, histamine receptors have been targeted for the treatment of many disorders. In fact, scientist Daniel Bovet was awarded the 1957 Nobel Prize for Physiology or Medicine for his work on substances that inhibit the action of histamine, called "antihistamines." Histamine's role in allergy and inflammation is extensively discussed in Chapter 29. Drugs for the treatment of allergy and inflammatory disorders target the H_1 receptor, whereas drugs that target the H_2 receptor inhibit acid secretion in the stomach. As noted previously, this chapter focuses on the H_2 receptor and its role in GI disorders.[17]

In addition to H_2 receptors, the proton pump found in the canaliculus of parietal cells of the gastric mucosa is also commonly targeted for the treatment of GI disorders. Activation of H_2 histamine, M_3, and gastrin receptors initiates a stimulatory signaling pathway for acid secretion. The H_2 receptor acts through the cyclic adenosine monophosphate (cAMP)–dependent pathway, while M_3 and gastrin receptors act via the Ca^{2+} dependent pathway to activate the proton pump. Once activated and facilitated by a trio of anionic residues (Asp824, Glu820, and Glu795), the proton pump exchanges cytoplasmic H^+ and extracytoplasmic K^+ ions across the gastric membrane to maintain an acidic pH in the stomach (Fig. 28.3).[17-19] The proton pump is Cys-rich, containing a total of 28 of these nucleophilic residues, and at least two will be critical to the action of the inhibitors used in the treatment of gastric ulcers (discussed later).

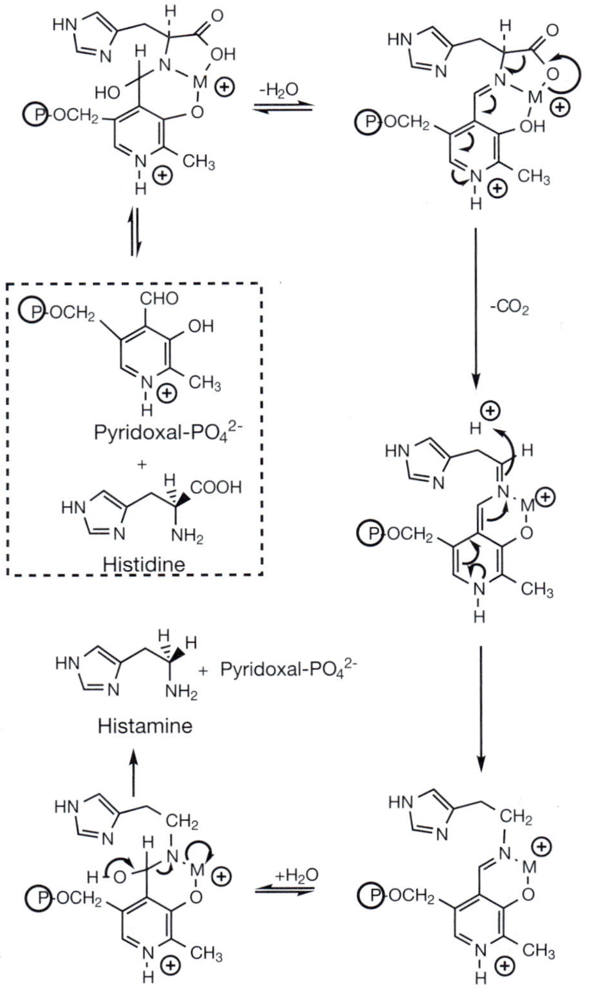

Figure 28.2 Biosynthesis of histamine.

Drugs Used for the Treatment of Gastrointestinal Disorders, Including Ulcer and Gastroesophageal Reflux Disease

As noted earlier, gastric acid secretion occurs at the level of parietal cells in the gastric mucosa. Remarkably, these cells can secrete up to 3 L of gastric juice daily, where the hydrochloric acid can drop the pH to approximately 1. The parietal cells contain receptors for ACh, histamine, and gastrin, which are signal molecules that stimulate acid production. ACh binds to the muscarinic receptor (M_3 subtype), and histamine binds to the H_2 receptor on parietal cells to stimulate acid secretion.

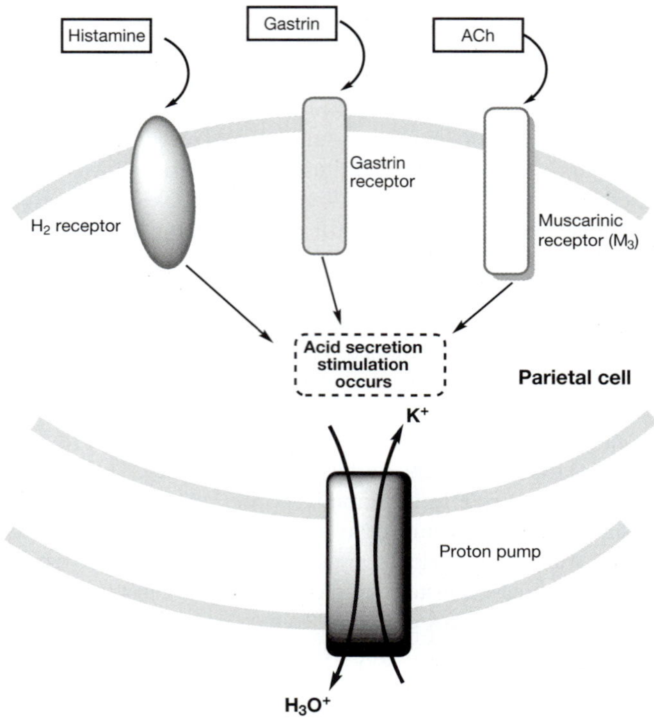

Figure 28.3 Physiologic mechanism of gastric acid secretion in parietal cells.

It is proposed that gastrin also mediates acid secretion indirectly via the release of histamine from enterochromaffin-like (ECL) cells. Although the receptor stimulation and gastric acid secretion steps are highly regulated, in many cases *Helicobacter pylori* infection has been associated with hypersecretion of gastric acid.[20] Such an event is likely to contribute to gastric mucosal deterioration and can lead to gastric ulceration.

Antacids

Patients suffering from mild dyspepsia and/or gastric acid–induced disorders typically find relief with the use of nonprescription antacids. These have been used for centuries, at least until the advent of H_2 antihistamines and proton pump inhibitors (PPIs). However, common antacids continue to be used by patients as readily available remedies for intermittent heartburn. Antacids are weak inorganic bases that neutralize stomach acid to generate water and a metal-containing chloride salt. Some of the common antacids are pharmaceutical formulations containing sodium bicarbonate, calcium carbonate, magnesium hydroxide, and aluminum hydroxide (Table 28.1). Both sodium bicarbonate and calcium carbonate may cause belching or metabolic alkalosis due to the production of carbon dioxide (CO_2). Additionally, excessive intake of calcium carbonate with calcium-rich dairy products can lead to hypercalcemia and potential renal insufficiency. Magnesium- and aluminum-based antacids may impact bowel function. Since both magnesium and aluminum are absorbed and excreted by the kidneys, intake of these antacids must be limited in patients with renal insufficiency.

Table 28.1 Composition of Selected Antacids

Product	Composition (mg)[a]
Tablets	
Rolaids—regular strength	$CaCO_3$—550 $Mg(OH)_2$—110
Rolaids—advanced	$CaCO_3$—1,000 $Mg(OH)_2$—200 Simethicone—40
Tums—regular strength	$CaCO_3$—500
Tums—extra strength	$CaCO_3$—750
Maalox	$CaCO_3$—600
Gelusil	$Mg(OH)_2$—200 $Al(OH)_3$—200 Simethicone—25
Liquids	
Milk of magnesia	$Mg(OH)_2$—400
Mylanta—maximum strength	$Mg(OH)_2$—400 $Al(OH)_3$—400 Simethicone—40
Maalox—therapeutic concentrate	$Mg(OH)_2$—300 $Al(OH)_3$—600

[a]mg per tablet or 5 mL liquid.

H_2 Antihistamines

The role of H_2 receptors in GI disorders directly relates to their role in the stimulation and secretion of stomach acid. Histamine binds to H_2 receptors on parietal cells, which results in activation of adenylyl cyclase. Activation of this enzyme increases intracellular cAMP, which in turn activates kinases that stimulate the proton pump. Cimetidine, famotidine, and nizatidine are the three H_2 antihistamines currently available for clinical use (Fig. 28.4).[21] These agents are available over the counter (OTC) and used for the treatment of gastric ulcers, GERD, and upper GI bleeding. H_2 antihistamines are considered inverse agonists that block the basal level activity of H_2 receptors by promoting a shift from an active to an inactive conformation.[22]

Structural Features and Mechanism of Action of H_2 Antihistamines

The H_2 antihistamines were designed based on extensive medicinal chemistry research on the partial agonists that are structurally similar to histamine. Cimetidine was the first drug developed for clinical use in the treatment of heartburn and peptic ulcers.[23] Cimetidine has an imidazole ring that mimics the structural feature of histamine. Introduction of a C_4 methyl group afforded selectivity toward the H_2 receptor by stabilizing the N^{τ}-H tautomer required for receptor recognition.

All three clinically used H_2 antihistamines have a thioether-containing four-atom side chain, a heterocyclic structure with a basic functional group, and a guanidine

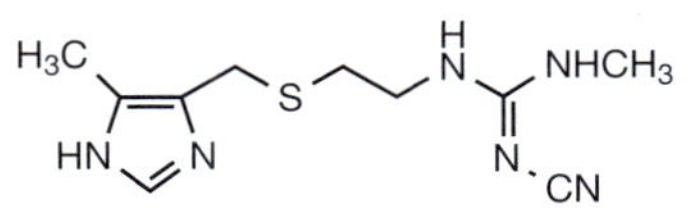

Cimetidine (Tagamet)

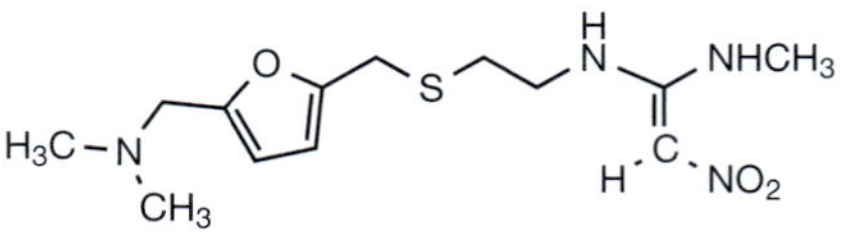

Ranitidine (Zantac)
[removed from the market by US FDA]

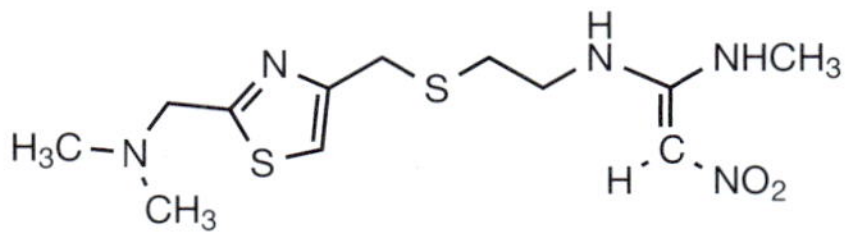

Nizatidine (Axid)

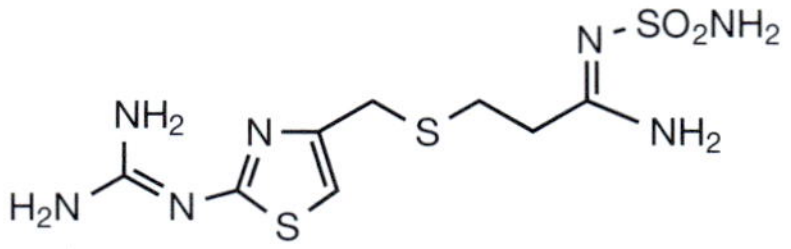

Famotidine (Pepcid)

Figure 28.4 H_2-receptor antihistamines.

group with different substituents. The sulfur atom in the side chain increases potency compared to carbon or oxygen analogues. The guanidine moiety is substituted with an electron-withdrawing group (ie, cyano, nitro, sulfonamido) that significantly decreases the basicity of the guanidine; thus, the guanidine group is not protonated under physiologic conditions. Initial structure-based research that led to the discovery of cimetidine showed that protonation of the guanidine group abolishes H_2 antagonist activity. Based on the binding model of ranitidine with the H_2 receptor, it has been shown that the basic amino group attached to (or, in the case of cimetidine, a component of) the heterocycle interacts with Asp98 via an ionic interaction, and the guanidine NH forms a hydrogen bond with Asp186 within the binding pocket.[24] Through these interactions, these drugs prevent histamine binding, and thus, inhibit the action of H_2 receptors. Cimetidine has an imidazole ring; however, other heterocyclic motifs (ie, furan, thiazole) are utilized to generate famotidine, and nizatidine. These newer structures have a basic amine or guanidine motif attached to these heterocycles because a basic group is necessary for binding.

Metabolism and Drug Interactions of H_2 Antihistamines

Cimetidine and famotidine undergo first-pass metabolism, and their oral bioavailability is 40% to 60% in patients with GI issues (Fig. 28.5). On the other hand, nizatidine has a high oral bioavailability (90%). The half-lives of these three H_2 antihistamines are between 1 and 4 hours, and they are generally excreted unaltered in urine. The primary metabolic pathways can involve oxidation of the sulfur atom, the nitrogen atom of the amine functional group, and C-H oxidation (Fig. 28.5). Cimetidine undergoes both thioether oxidation to the sulfoxide and oxidation at the C_4 methyl group to yield a hydroxylated metabolite. Nizatidine undergoes negligible metabolic transformations. Famotidine is primarily metabolized via an S-oxidation (Fig. 28.5). Except for nizatidine, metabolites of H_2 antihistamines do not contribute to the therapeutic properties of the parent drug.[25]

Drug interactions of H_2 antihistamines are certainly a concern, especially with cimetidine.[26] Cimetidine's imidazole ring inhibits CYP450-dependent oxidation of drugs, causing an increased duration of action of several agents. Based on this observation, other members of this class of drugs were specifically developed with different heterocyclic motifs to prevent their ability to inhibit CYP450. Cimetidine is also a known inhibitor of renal tubular secretion of some drugs (ie, procainamide), where other members of the class show little or no effect.

Specific Drugs

Famotidine is the most commonly utilized OTC H_2 antihistamine for the relief of GI distress, and is described in more detail next, along with the historically relevant agent cimetidine. The third H_2 antagonist, nizatidine is a "patchwork" of structural features found in other antagonists. Although ranitidine was available as an effective H_2 antagonist, the US Food and Drug Administration (FDA) requested it to be removed from clinical use in 2020. The medication contained *N*-Nitrosodimethylamine (NDMA) as a contaminant, and the amount of

Metabolites of cimetidine:

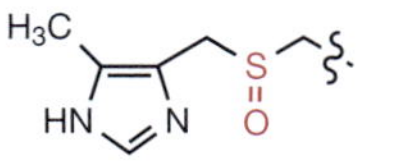

Cimetidine sulfoxide

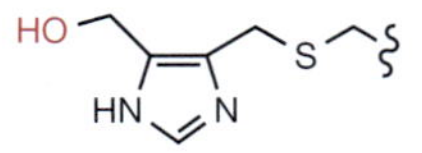

4-Hydroxymethyl cimetidine

Metabolites of nizatidine:

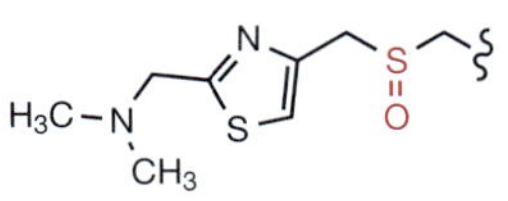

Nizatidine sulfoxide

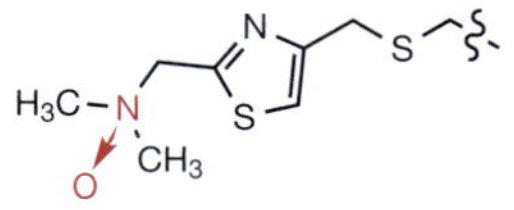

Nizatidine *N*-oxide

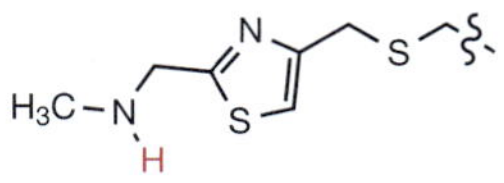

Monodesmethyl nizatidine

Metabolite of famotidine:

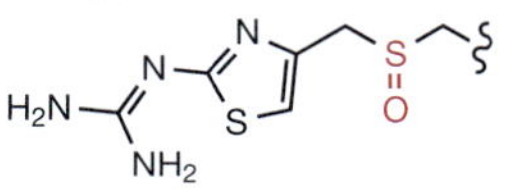

Famotidine sulfoxide

Figure 28.5 Major metabolites of H_2 antihistamines.

NDMA in ranitidine was shown to increase over time. Due to the concern that ranitidine use may result in unacceptable levels of NDMA, it was withdrawn from the market.

Cimetidine. As mentioned, cimetidine was the first H_2 antagonist developed and is an OTC drug available for the treatment of acid reflux and related GI disorders. It is available in tablet form (200, 300, 400, 600, or 800 mg). An injection formulation (cimetidine hydrochloride injection, 300 mg/2 mL) is also available by prescription for administration by providers in a clinic setting. The 4-methylimidazole ring mimics the imidazole motif found in histamine, and, due to conformational preference driven by the stabilization of the N^{τ}-H tautomer, it is more selective toward the H_2 receptor. Additionally, the nonionizable cyanoguanidine motif is key to high H_2-receptor affinity and antagonistic activity, and it is held at the proper distance from the anchoring cationic nitrogen of the imidazole ring by the methylthioethyl connecting chain. The electron-withdrawing sulfur atom in this chain also helps stabilize the N^{τ}-H tautomer required for receptor recognition. Cimetidine has an oral bioavailability of 60% to 70%, and about 20% is bound to plasma protein. The estimated elimination half-life is about 2 hours, and about 40% to 80% of drug is excreted in the urine in unaltered form.[27]

Cimetidine undergoes hepatic metabolic transformation, providing the sulfoxide and 4-hydroxymethyl metabolites shown in Figure 28.5. One of the major clinical limitations is the reversible inhibition of CYP enzymes, which occurs through competition for heme iron (Fe^{2+}) binding between cimetidine's imidazole ring and the identical ring of a His residue on the CYP protein.[28] This leads to many drug-drug interactions (some of them serious), particularly in older adults who commonly take many CYP vulnerable drugs. It inhibits the hepatic metabolism of warfarin, phenytoin, propranolol, lidocaine, and diazepam, to name a few, leading to increased plasma level of these drugs and the risk of serious or potentially fatal toxicity.[29,30]

Following administration, cimetidine is widely distributed in various tissues; thus, it exhibits some adverse effects, including dizziness, headache, drowsiness, and nausea. The later generation H_2 antagonists, to some extent, address some of these adverse effects, primarily by the replacement of the CYP-inhibiting imidazole ring with aromatic isosteres less capable (but not incapable) of competing with the CYP His residue for heme Fe^{2+}.

Famotidine. Famotidine is another H_2 antagonist that is used for the treatment of GERD, duodenal ulcers, and stomach ulcers. It is available as a tablet as well as in the form of injection. In the United States, 10 and 20 mg tablets are available OTC. A prescription is required for higher doses and the injectable formulation. Famotidine has a 2-guanidothiazole ring in place of the imidazole ring found in cimetidine, and this basic guanidine provides the cation needed for anchoring to the H_2 receptor Asp98. The second guanidine moiety attached to the ethylthiomethyl connecting chain is modified via the addition of an electron-withdrawing sulfonamide group, which lowers the basicity of this guanidine moiety and improves potency by ensuring a lack of positive charge at physiologic pH. Famotidine is about 7.5 times more potent than famotidine and about 20 times more potent than cimetidine.[31]

Famotidine is not completely absorbed, providing a bioavailability of about 40% to 45% when orally administered. About 15% to 20% of the drug is bound to plasma protein. Famotidine has an elimination half-life of 4.5 hours, and a large portion (65%-70%) is eliminated via renal excretion. Famotidine is metabolized by CYP enzymes, and the only metabolite identified is the famotidine sulfoxide (Fig. 28.5). Unlike cimetidine, this drug does not exhibit significant inhibitory effect on CYP enzyme activity, indicating minimal drug-drug interactions (DDIs).

Nizatidine. Nizatidine is the third H_2 antagonist and designed from the SAR of famotidine and ranitidine. The design is based on the incorporation of the thiazole ring of famotidine, the basic dimethylaminomethyl and neutral diaminonitroethene moiety of ranitidine, and the methylthioethyl connecting chain found in all marketed H_2 antagonists. These structural modifications contribute positively to overcome different drug-drug interactions and adverse effects observed with other members. Unlike the binding of famotidine, nizatidine's receptor binding is characterized as competitive binding. Yet, the mechanism of action is similar to all three drugs, in which gastric acid suppression and reduction of pepsin secretion are achieved in an indirect fashion. While famotidine and cimetidine exhibit low to moderate oral bioavailability, nizatidine is completely absorbed following oral administration. Nizatidine undergoes minor modification via S-oxidation, N-oxidation, and N-dealkylation (Fig. 28.5). The N-monodesmethyl metabolite of nizatidine exhibits about 61% of the H_2 antihistaminic activity of the parent drug.[25] Nizatidine has a half-life of 1 to 2 hours, and the drug and its metabolites are excreted through renal filtration.

Proton Pump Inhibitors

A second class of drugs that are commonly and more frequently used in the treatment of peptic ulcer disease is the PPIs.[32] This class of drugs covalently inhibits the gastric H^+/K^+-ATPase that is responsible for secretion of stomach acid in parietal cells of the gastric mucosa.[33,34] The gastric proton pump is very similar to Na^+/K^+-ATPase,[19] and also similar in structure and function to the H^+/K^+-ATPase found in osteoclasts, which play an important role in bone resorption. PPIs enable healing of peptic ulcer, erosive esophagitis, GERD, GERD-related laryngitis, Barrett esophagus, and Zollinger-Ellison syndrome, as well as the infection caused by *H. pylori*, with the latter in combination with antibiotics.[33,34]

Since the H^+/K^+-ATPase–mediated process is the final step in gastric acid secretion, inhibiting this enzyme is considered the most effective approach to acid suppression. PPI discovery began with the early investigation of timoprazole. This compound is a pyridylmethylsulfinylbenzimidazole, which is the conserved pharmacophore for subsequently developed PPIs. Based on its acid-dependent activity, it was identified as an acid-activated prodrug. Omeprazole was later synthesized and, in 1989, became the first drug of this class available for clinical use.[35] Other clinically available PPIs include lansoprazole, dexlansoprazole, esomeprazole, pantoprazole sodium, and rabeprazole sodium (Fig. 28.6). Dexlansoprazole and esomeprazole are enantiomerically pure forms of lansoprazole and omeprazole, respectively. Omeprazole and lansoprazole are both also marketed as racemic mixtures.

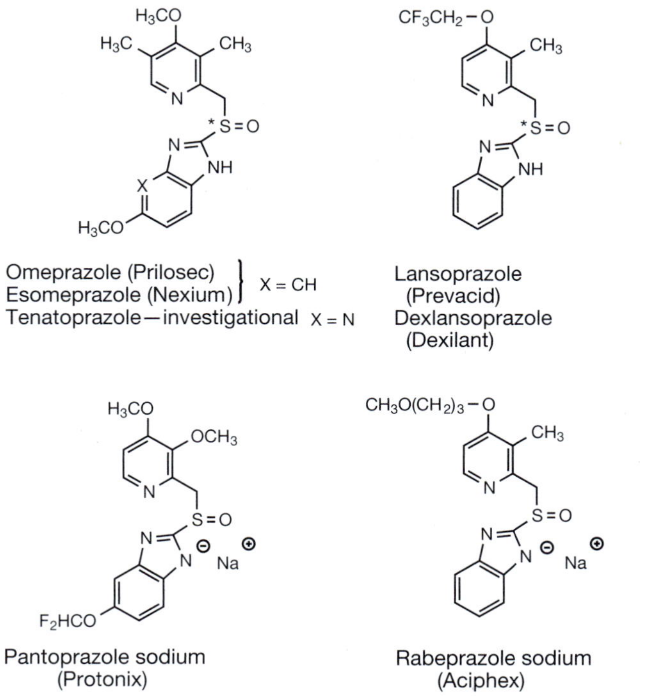

Figure 28.6 Proton pump inhibitors.

Structural Features and Mechanism of Action of Proton Pump Inhibitors

The 2-pyridylmethylsulfinylbenzimidazole motif is conserved in all members of the PPI family, as it is necessary for bioactivity through acid-catalyzed decomposition to the reactive sulfenic acid and sulfenamide structures. Typically, the structural modifications are done on the pyridine ring or at the benzo component of the benzimidazole to generate drugs with differing levels of acid stability, which impacts duration of proton pump inhibiting action. The investigational drug, tenatoprazole is slightly different in that it has an imidazopyridine isostere, instead of the traditional benzimidazole scaffold.

PPIs are weak bases with a pyridine pK_a between 3.8 and 4.9, which enables them to selectively accumulate through ion trapping in the stimulated parietal cell (pH ~1.0). This acidic environment-selective accumulation of PPIs is an important property that contributes to their selectivity and activity. As mentioned, PPIs are prodrugs, and acid-catalyzed activation generates the active form of the drug. The active form has electrophilic sulfenic acid and sulfenamide sulfur atoms capable of reacting with the thiol group of a Cys residue of the ATPase, forming a covalent adduct.[36] Covalent inhibition of the proton pump results in inactivation of the catalytic function of this enzyme.[19]

The chemical mechanism of activation of omeprazole and subsequent covalent interaction is described in Figure 28.7.[33] All PPIs follow a similar mechanism of action. The N_3 atom in the imidazole ring is an exceptionally weak base, with a pK_a <0.8, and is first protonated under the very low pH of the parietal cell through proton transfer from pyridine N_1 atom. Nucleophilic attack by the unionized pyridine nitrogen at the benzimidazole C_2 atom (made electron deficient by the cationic N_3 atom) generates a highly electrophilic and unstable electrophilic spiro intermediate, which rearranges to generate the sulfenic acid intermediate that preferentially forms the inactivating disulfide bond with the proton pump Cys (Fig. 28.7). The following step involves loss of water and the formation of a reactive sulfenamide intermediate, which can also covalently modify the Cys thiol of the proton pump.[36]

Within the proton pump, several different Cys residues are potential sites for covalent modification. The different substituents on the pyridine or benzimidazole ring of PPIs determine which Cys residue the drug preferentially reacts with, which subsequently determines the permanency of the covalent attachment, as discussed later. Electron-donating groups on the C_5 position of the benzimidazole ring enhance reactivity by increasing the extent of benzimidazole N_3 protonation and the strength of the δ^+ charge on the carbon at the C_2 position of the benzimidazole moiety. Electron-donating groups at the C_4 position of the pyridine ring increase the nucleophilicity of the pyridine nitrogen, enhancing the rate at which the N_1

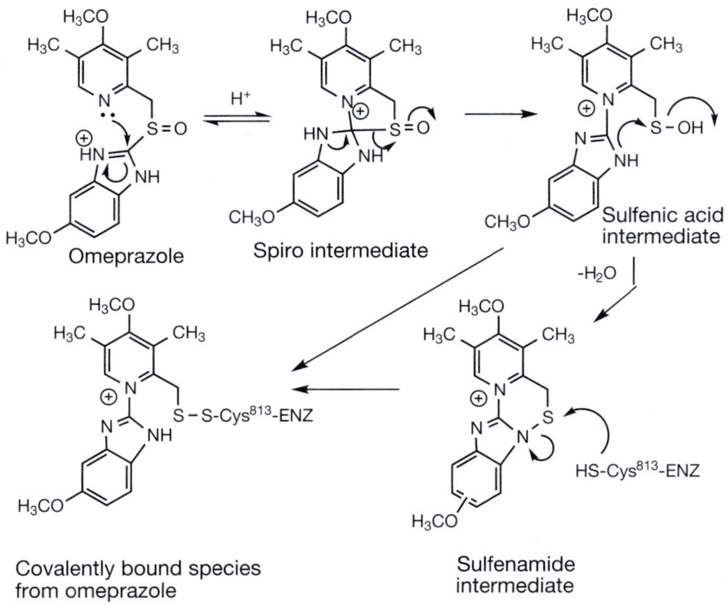

Figure 28.7 Acid-catalyzed activation of omeprazole to reactive sulfenic acid and sulfenamide.

atom attacks the electrophilic benzimidazole C_2 atom. Conversely, electron-withdrawing groups at either site have been shown to decrease reactivity.[37]

All PPIs can react with the readily accessible Cys813 of the ATPase. It has been observed that activated molecules of omeprazole can bind to either Cys813 or Cys892 of the proton pump.[37,38] Similarly, lansoprazole is known to covalently modify Cys813 or Cys321. Pantoprazole, the most sluggish-reacting of the PPIs, can react with either Cys813 or the more deeply recessed and less-accessible Cys822. Although PPIs are covalently bound to the proton pump, the interaction with accessible Cys residues can be reversed by reduced glutathione (GSH). The disulfide bond formed between the drug and receptor can be cleaved by this endogenous reducing agent, regenerating the essential Cys thiol of the pump and prompting the excretion of the drug fragment as a glutathione conjugate. Due to low concentration of GSH in the body, regeneration of proton pumps inhibited through Cys813 is incomplete. Pantoprazole binding is found to be less susceptible to GSH-mediated removal. These observations suggest that modification of Cys813 is more easily reversed, providing a fast phase of recovery, while modification of Cys822 is difficult to reverse, as GSH may not easily reach this site.[37]

Since the activation and rearrangement of PPIs take place at a strongly acidic pH, all of the oral formulations of PPIs have been developed to be acid-stable. This allows for better dissolution and absorption of PPIs (typically enteric-coated formulations) from the intestines. Both lansoprazole (enteric-coated) and omeprazole (either enteric-coated or formulated with $NaHCO_3$) are available in granular form. This allows for the drug to be absorbed readily with minimal drug destruction in the stomach. Rearrangement selectively occurs in the acidic environment of the canaliculus within parietal cells after the drug is absorbed from the intestine and delivered to that target site. Typically, the half-life of PPIs is relatively short (~1 hour); however, the duration of action is long (~20-48 hours) because of their ability to irreversibly inhibit the proton pump.

The benzimidazole N_1 atom is typically nonionizable at physiological pH and considered neutral in nature. However, as noted in Figure 28.6, the benzimidazole N_1 atom within PPIs is slightly acidic due to the electron-withdrawing property of the attached sulfinyl moiety. Due to this change in acidity, PPIs can be made into salt forms when the benzimidazole N_1 atom ionizes (loses proton) through treatment with strong base and becomes paired with the resultant metal cation (eg, Na^+ or Mg^{2+}). Due to this property, some of the PPIs are marketed in the salt form, which provides improved aqueous solubility.

Metabolism and Drug Interactions

CYP enzymes in the liver extensively metabolize all PPIs, with CYP2C19 and CYP3A4 isoforms catalyzing most of the oxidations. The investigational drug tenatoprazole is an exception, in that it is less readily metabolized, yielding a longer plasma half-life of 7 to 9 hours. Excretion of PPI metabolites is predominantly renal. The CYP2C19 metabolizer phenotype determines the extent of metabolic transformation of PPIs. The three common phenotypes include extensive metabolizers (EM, "normal," *1 allele), ultrafast metabolizers (UMs, *17 allele), and poor metabolizers (PMs, *2 and *3 alleles).[39] About 3% of Whites and 15% to 20% of Asians are considered PMs.[37,39] Omeprazole is found to exhibit significant inhibition of CYP2C19, and it may increases the plasma concentration of other drugs that are substrates for this isoform (ie, diazepam) when administered at the same time. Lansoprazole is also found to inhibit CYP2C19 at therapeutically relevant concentration and exhibits DDIs.

Omeprazole undergoes five possible metabolic transformations: (1) CYP2C19-catalyzed hydroxylation of the 5′-methyl group on the pyridine ring, (2) CYP3A4-catalyzed hydroxylation of the 3′-methyl group on the pyridine ring (3) CYP3A4-catalyzed sulfone formation, (4) CYP2C19-catalyzed 5-O-demethylation, and (5) a nonenzymatic reduction of sulfoxide (Fig. 28.8). Among these pathways,

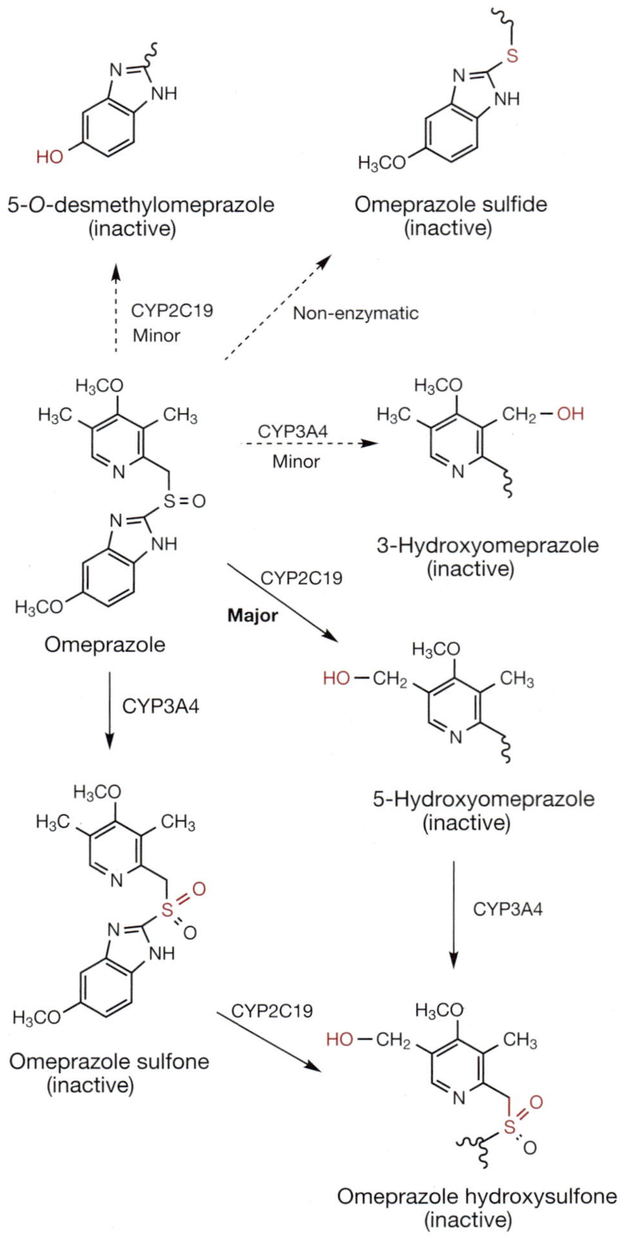

Figure 28.8 Omeprazole metabolism. (Adapted from Roche VF. The chemically elegant proton pump inhibitors. *Am J Pharm Educ.* 2006;70[5]:101, with permission.)

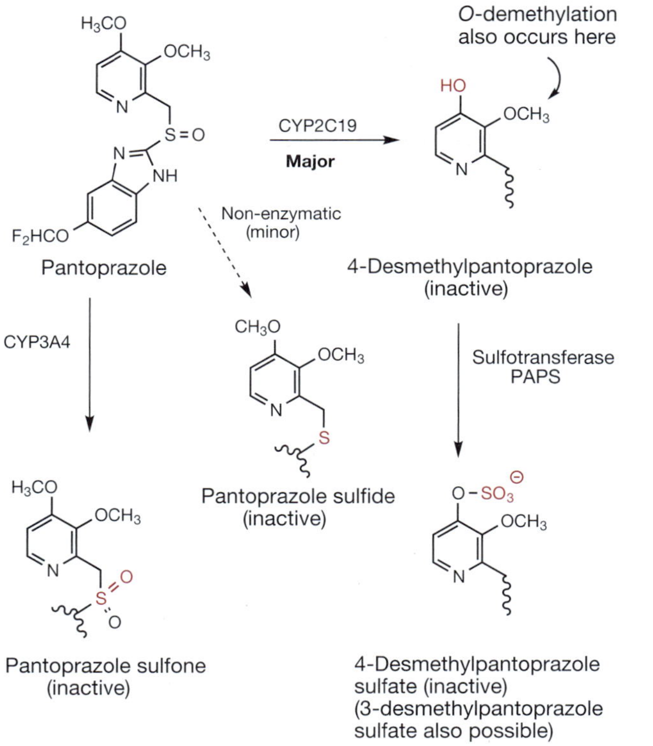

Figure 28.9 Pantoprazole metabolism. (Adapted from Roche VF. The chemically elegant proton pump inhibitors. *Am J Pharm Educ.* 2006;70[5]: 101, with permission.)

5′-hydroxylation and sulfone formation are identified as the two major metabolic pathways. Pantoprazole is metabolized into the O-desmethyl metabolite, pantoprazole sulfone, and pantoprazole thioether (a minor metabolite). The 4-desmethylpantoprazole is further modified via phase 2 metabolic transformation into 4-desmethylpantoprazole sulfate (Fig. 28.9). Lansoprazole also undergoes sulfone and thioether formation similar to pantoprazole. Additionally, a major pathway involves 5-hydroxylation of the benzimidazole motif (Fig. 28.10). Finally, rabeprazole is metabolized to generate sulfone, thioether, and demethylated derivatives. The desmethylrabeprazole thioether further undergoes oxidation to yield the carboxylic acid derivative as well (Fig. 28.11).[33,40,41]

The thioether metabolite of rabeprazole has been shown to undergo oxidation by microsomal enzymes (CYP2C19 and CYP3A4) under experimental conditions to generate the parent drug with the regenerated sulfoxide moiety. Rabeprazole is found to exhibit significantly fewer drug interactions as compared to other PPIs; however, its thioether metabolite, which is formed via a nonenzymatic pathway, does inhibit CYP2C19, CYP2C9, CYP2D6, and CYP3A4.[42,43] Although the pyridyl-5-methyl group readily oxidized by CYP2C19 is not present in rabeprazole, lansoprazole, and pantoprazole, other sites in each of these drugs are modified by the same enzyme.

Similar to clinically available PPIs, investigational tenatoprazole also undergoes hepatic metabolism. The *S*-isomer of tenatoprazole is predominantly metabolized by CYP3A4 and the *R*-isomer is metabolized by CYP2C19.[44]

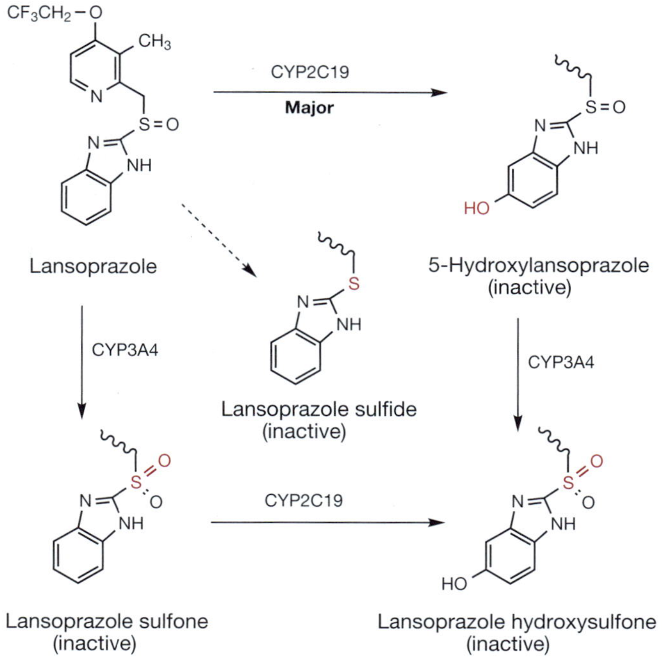

Figure 28.10 Lansoprazole metabolism. (Adapted from Roche VF. The chemically elegant proton pump inhibitors. *Am J Pharm Educ.* 2006;70[5]:101, with permission.)

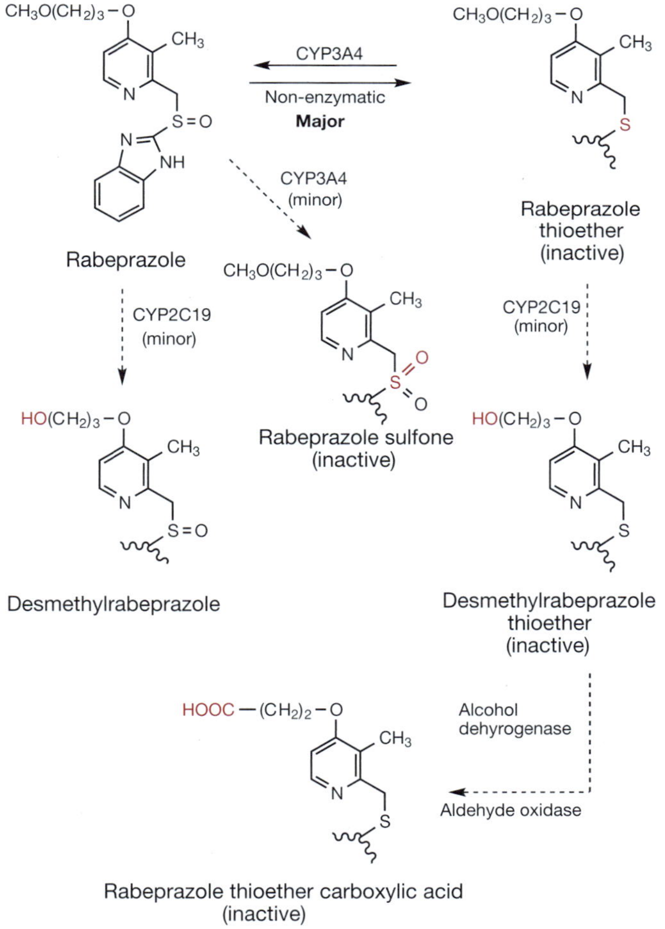

Figure 28.11 Rabeprazole metabolism. (Adapted from Roche VF. The chemically elegant proton pump inhibitors. *Am J Pharm Educ.* 2006;70[5]:101, with permission.)

The structure of all PPIs contains a sulfoxide (also called sulfinyl) group where the sulfur atom is chiral. The stereochemistry of this functional group plays an important role in the pharmacological activity and metabolic profile. The *R*-enantiomer of omeprazole is metabolized more rapidly by CYP2C19 than the *S*-enantiomer. Thus, the single enantiomer, esomeprazole, provides improved bioavailability in those individuals who are EM or UM CYP2C19 metabolizers. Systemic drug exposure, or area under the plasma concentration curve (AUC), is greater for esomeprazole compared to racemic omeprazole in EM and UM patients. Therefore, duration of drug exposure is extended and the gastric pH achieved from therapy is more than 4. All of this correlates with improved healing rates.

Lansoprazole is metabolized by CYP2C19 and CYP3A4 in the liver. The CYP2C19 genotype has been shown to influence the metabolism of *S*-lansoprazole to a greater extent than the *R*-enantiomer. Since the potency of both enantiomers is equal, the use of *R*-lansoprazole would be more desirable, as it has less interpatient variability. Pantoprazole is metabolized by CYP2C19, and via a subsequent sulfonation pathway. It is less susceptible to CYP3A4-catalyzed metabolism. The enantiomers of pantoprazole are also differentially affected by the CYP2C19 genotype.[44] Rabeprazole, on the other hand, is less sensitive to CYP-catalyzed metabolism.

Omeprazole and esomeprazole are both substrates and strong inhibitors of the CYP2C19 isoform, and they compete with drugs that depend on this isoform for metabolic activation or clearance while limiting the availability of the isoform. For example, clopidogrel is an antiplatelet prodrug that is activated by CYP2C19 and is commonly prescribed to patients who have suffered a stroke or have a high risk of ischemia.[45] These patients may also be prescribed a PPI due to higher risk of GI ulceration from clopidogrel therapy. In this case, omeprazole and esomeprazole should be avoided because inhibition of CYP2C19 will inhibit clopidogrel activation and put patients at a risk for a potentially fatal cardiovascular event.[46] Lansoprazole has been a suitable option for patients when a PPI and clopidogrel need to be co-administered but pantoprazole, the weakest CYP2C19 inhibitor of the PPIs, is now considered the preferred agent.[32] In addition, due to the possibility of PPIs interfering with bone remodeling, prolonged usage of PPIs (>1 year) is likely to increase the risk of bone fracture. Additionally, recent studies have indicated that PPI use is linked to chronic kidney disease. Since the use of PPIs is frequently extended beyond recommended durations, the risk of renal toxicity may be higher than normally anticipated.[47,48] The exact mechanism of damage is unclear at this stage.

The reason for the discovery and development of enantiomers of omeprazole and lansoprazole relates to their different metabolic profile and efficacy. The interest in developing single enantiomers as drugs has been at the forefront of medicinal chemistry and drug discovery. The single bioactive enantiomer of a drug, if it exists, provides more specificity and generally less toxicity than a racemic mixture. The development of improved chemical methods to synthesize pure enantiomers and the ability to investigate each enantiomer against a specific disease model have facilitated the development of enantiomerically pure drugs. During such investigations, "isomeric ballast" is used as an informal term to describe the enantiomer that is less active or inactive (also called the distomer). On the other hand, the eutomer is the pharmacologically active, or most active, enantiomer.

In the case of PPIs, both enantiomers are biologically active because the activated form has no chiral center (the chiral sulfoxide is converted into achiral structures upon activation). The difference is related to their metabolic conversion by CYP2C19 and CYP3A4. In the case of omeprazole (racemic mixture), the AUC of the *S*-enantiomer exhibits an activity difference of 3-fold between EM and PM patients, where the *R*-enantiomer shows about a 7.5-fold difference. This indicates that omeprazole (*R*-isomer) exhibits more significant variability between patients and potentially improved therapeutic outcomes in PMs.[49,50] Dexlansoprazole is the *R*-enantiomer of lansoprazole, and it has a higher plasma concentration than the *S*-enantiomer due to less rapid inactivating metabolism. *S*-Pantoprazole has been shown to be more potent than the *R*-enantiomer, and its pharmacokinetic profile is less dependent on CYP2C19 genotype. Therefore, although pantoprazole is marketed as a racemic mixture, the *S*-enantiomer is considered to have pharmacokinetic and pharmacodynamic advantages for clinical use. In the case of racemic rabeprazole, the *R*-enantiomer is more potent than the *S*-enantiomer, providing a superior pharmacokinetic profile.

Another major GI issue where PPIs can have therapeutic value relates to infection by *H. pylori*, which is likened to peptic ulcer in a majority of patients.[51] *H. pylori* infects the gastric mucosa and produces ammonia and CO_2 in order to withstand the acidic pH. The process involves hydrolysis of urea by the bacterial enzyme urease. Once a diagnosis has been made to show that *H. pylori* infection is the cause, eradication regimens involve a combination of PPI and antibiotics. Typically, PPIs with amoxicillin and clarithromycin or metronidazole are recommended. More details on bacterial infections and available antibiotics to treat them are discussed in Chapter 32.

Specific Drugs (Fig. 28.6)

The chemistry, reactivity, and metabolism of the clinically available PPIs have been discussed earlier, but three of the more commonly used and/or kinetically unique drugs are summarized in greater depth in the following sections.

OMEPRAZOLE. The pyridine substituents of omeprazole (and esomeprazole) promote the nucleophilicity of the N_1 atom through electron release via π (methoxy) and σ (methyl) bonds. Protonation of the benzimidazole N_3 atom (with subsequent enhancement of the electrophilic character of the adjacent C_2 atom) is augmented by the electron-releasing property of the C_5-methoxy group, resulting in a readily activated drug that inactivates the proton pump predominantly through covalent interaction with Cys813. Recovery through reduced GSH and *de novo* protein synthesis yields a duration of approximately 20 hours, although it can range up to 72 hours.

Absorption of the enteric-coated oral dosage form is rapid, and bioavailability ranges from 30% to 40%. Activity often begins within 1 hour. Omeprazole is 96% protein bound, and a magnesium salt formulation is available.[32,52] The combination product with sodium bicarbonate (Zegerid) does not require that omeprazole be enteric coated because the bicarbonate increases gastric pH from the normal (close to 1) to 4.2 to 5.2. At this elevated pH, the benzimidazole N_3 atom will not protonate and the nucleophilic attack by the pyridine N_1 atom cannot occur. Thus, the drug is safe from premature activation in the stomach. In addition, without an enteric coating, once the drug reaches the intestine, absorption can proceed immediately.

Pantoprazole Sodium. Pantoprazole sodium is marketed as a racemic mixture of *R*- and *S*-enantiomers. It is a prescription drug and available for oral administration (20, 40 mg) and intravenous (IV) administration. Pantoprazole has two electron-releasing methoxy groups conjugated with the pyridine ring. While the σ electron-withdrawing effect of the C_3 methoxy group can impact the pyridine N_1 atom, the nitrogen atom is still reasonably and sufficiently nucleophilic for the drug to be activated at the acidic canalicular pH. However, the strongly electron-withdrawing difluoromethyl substitution at the benzimidazole C_5 atom is instrumental in lowering the pK_a of the benzimidazole N_3 atom, which decreases the extent of protonation and detracts from the δ^+ character of the benzimidazole C_2 atom. This significantly slows nucleophilic attack by the pyridine N_1 nucleophile, which is a requirement for drug activation. Pantoprazole is the most sluggishly activated PPI of those currently marketed, and this is directly related to its long duration. Despite a short half-life of approximately 1 to 2 hours,[32] pantoprazole in its active form has time to reach and bind to a deeply recessed and less-accessible Cys822 within the proton pump. Since the inactivated pump cannot be rescued by reduced GSH, the therapeutic effect lasts for a longer period of time (47 hours) than other PPIs (~20 hours).[37]

Since PPIs are sensitive to stomach acid, pantoprazole sodium is available as an enteric-coated tablet, where the drug release begins only after the tablet leaves the stomach. Bioavailability of pantoprazole is about 77%, and it takes about 2 to 3 hours to reach maximum plasma level. A significant percentage (98%) of this drug is bound to plasma proteins. Pantoprazole undergoes hepatic metabolic clearance by the action of CYP2C19 and CYP3A4 (Fig. 28.9). Studies have shown that there are no significant drug interactions observed with pantoprazole in combination with other common drugs metabolized by CYP2C19, 3A4, 2D6, or 1A2.

Dexlansoprazole. Dexlansoprazole is the newest PPI introduced for the treatment of gastric acid–related GI diseases. It is the *R*-enantiomer of lansoprazole, marketed as a dual delayed release pharmaceutical formulation. The variation in CYP2C19 genotype influences the metabolism of *S*-lansoprazole to a greater extent than the *R*-enantiomer. Thus, dexlansoprazole is more desirable, as it has less interpatient variability. It is available as a 30- or 60-mg capsules for use. The recommended regimen for nonerosive GERD in adult is 30 mg twice daily for 4 weeks. A 60 mg twice-daily regimen is recommended for healing of erosive esophagitis for about 8 weeks.

As noted, dexlansoprazole is formulated with a dual delayed release formulation using two different copolymer-coated granules. These are pH-sensitive granules, and about 25% of the drug is released within 2 hours and the other 75% is released at 4 to 5 hours from the distal intestine.[53] While the resulting duration does not quite mimic that of twice-daily dosing and distress from nocturnal acid rebound can still occur, dexlansoprazole is more likely to provide "round the clock" coverage as compared to a simple enteric-coated formulations like racemic lansoprazole or omeprazole. By 6.5 hours postadministration, the canaliculus "residence time" of isomerically pure dexlansoprazole is approximately twice that of the racemic mixture. Like other PPIs, since dexlansoprazole lowers the pH of stomach contents, absorption of drugs that depend on low gastric pH can be negatively affected, including ampicillin esters, digoxin, and ketoconazole.

Potassium-Competitive Acid Blocker

As discussed in previous section, stomach acid secretion is regulated by the action of gastric H^+/K^+-ATPase. Although PPIs have revolutionized the field in treating gastric acid–related illnesses, several limitations still exist. Some of the limitations relates to relative slow onset of action, inability to suppress night-time acid secretion, and unpredictable pharmacokinetics due to genetic polymorphisms of CYP enzymes. To address some or all the clinical limitations, scientists are constantly looking for an alternative strategy to develop a more efficacious drug class. A viable strategy is to develop a potassium-competitive acid blocker. The mechanism of proton secretion by gastric H^+/K^+-ATPase involves an equal amount of potassium ion transported into the cytoplasm of the parietal cells. Studies have shown that competitive inhibition of the availability of extracellular potassium ion is beneficial in blocking acid secretion. Vonoprazan was approved by the FDA in 2022 for treating *H. pylori* infection, in combination with antibiotics.[54] It is a reversible, potassium-competitive acid blocker that blocks the availability of potassium ions for the proton pump. The drug is available in tablet form for oral administration, and in co-packaged form with either amoxicillin or clarithromycin for the treatment of *H. pylori* infection. Vonoprazan is a pyrrole derivative and has a basic methylamino group connected to the pyrrole motif. Based on the chemical structure, vonoprazan is stable to acidic pH and readily absorbed, reaching C_{max} by about 2 hours.[54] The advantage of vonoprazan over classical PPIs relates to of its ability to inhibit active and resting proton pumps. Vonoprazan is considered more potent and longer acting than traditional PPIs, providing superior therapeutic effect. Therefore, it is under investigation for an alternative therapy for the treatment of reflux or erosive esophagitis. The drug is largely metabolized by CYP3A4 isoform and, to some extent, is sensitive to metabolism by CYP2B6, CYP2C19, CYP2D6, and SULT2A1 (Fig. 28.12).[55,56] The metabolites are identified as pharmacologically inactive. Due to observed CYP interaction, vonoprazan is known to inhibit various CYP isoforms, including CYP3A4/5 and CYP2C19. Moreover, similar to some of the PPIs, vonoprazan is known to interact with CYP2C19, which may lead to interindividual variability.[55,56]

Prokinetic Agents

Gastrointestinal hypomotility is linked to various GI disorders, including GERD, gastroparesis IBS, and colonic pseudoobstruction. One approach to managing

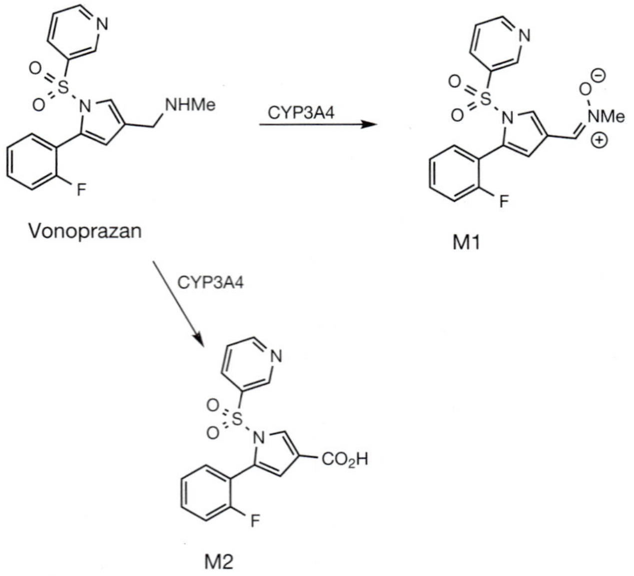

Figure 28.12 Structures of vonoprazan and its metabolites.

these pathological events is administration of prokinetic agents.[57,58] This class of drugs stimulates and facilitates GI motility. Increased gastric emptying takes place via drug-induced peristalsis, which improves the symptoms of the earlier-mentioned GI disorders. Traditionally, prokinetic agents are classified into three categories: (1) agents that target cholinergic or serotonin (5-HT_4) receptors, (2) agents that target dopamine or opioid receptors, and (3) agents with agonistic activity on GI hormone receptors (motilin receptor agonists or somatostatin agonists). This section only focuses on selected prokinetic agents, namely metoclopramide, dexpanthenol, and tegaserod (Fig. 28.13).

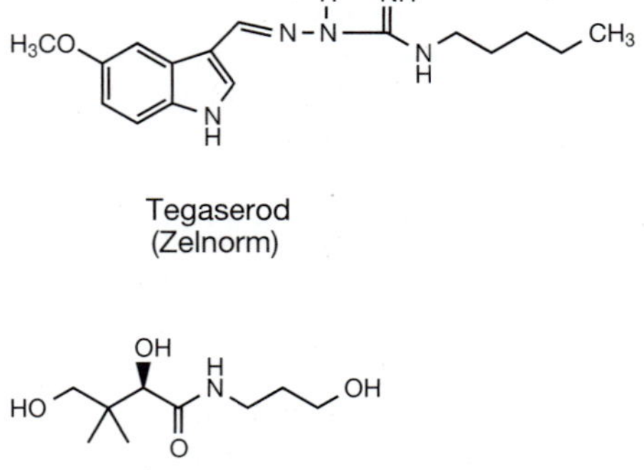

Figure 28.13 Examples of prokinetic agents.

The reader is directed toward specific sections within this chapter for more details on how cholinergic and serotonin (5-HT) receptors are targeted for the treatment of various GI disorders.

Metoclopramide

Metoclopramide is a procainamide derivative that does not exhibit antiarrhythmic or topical anesthetic activity, and that was initially developed as an antiemetic agent. Later, its ability to stimulate upper GI tract motility was realized, and it was used as a drug for improving gastric emptying. Metoclopramide is either orally administered or injected to alleviate GERD, diabetic gastropharesis, and chemotherapy-induced nausea and vomiting. Metoclopramide exhibits an agonistic effect at 5-HT_4 receptors and an antagonistic effect at dopamine D_2 and 5-HT_3 receptors. Inhibition of dopamine secretion by metoclopramide increases the release of ACh in the myenteric plexus in the GI tract and increases GI motility.[57] However, some of the adverse effects caused by this agent are also related to D_2 antagonistic effects, particularly in the CNS, where patients may develop irreversible tardive dyskinesia. To prevent potential complications, metoclopramide treatment is often restricted to less than 3 months and discontinued at the first observation of involuntary muscle movement. Metoclopramide should not be given to patients who take monoamine oxidase (MAO) inhibitors, tricyclic antidepressants, or phenothiazines due to the risk for serious DDIs.

CYP and phase 2 conjugating enzymes metabolize metoclopramide to a significant extent. Some of the commonly observed metabolites include the N-deethylated derivative (CYP2D6), N-oxidation (CYP2D6), and glucuronide and sulfate conjugates of the aryl amine (Fig. 28.14).[59]

Dexpanthenol and Tegaserod

Dexpanthenol is used for paralytic ileus and intestinal atonia. The administration is IM for these conditions. Dexpanthenol is the alcohol analogue of endogenous pantothenic acid, a precursor of coenzyme A (CoA). The biosynthesis of ACh requires CoA, and as previously emphasized, ACh plays an important role in controlling GI muscle movement.

Tegaserod is also a selective 5-HT_4 partial agonist and has been shown to be an effective prokinetic agent. It is clinically used for the treatment of IBS.[60] A more detailed discussion on IBS is given in a later section of this chapter.

Other Prokinetic Agents

Several other prokinetic agents structurally similar to metoclopramide are available outside the United States and/or are in clinical trials. Some of these include prucalopride, mosapride, and itopride. These are used for either chronic constipation or gastritis.[61-63] Prucalopride and mosapride are 5-HT_4 receptor agonists while itopride is an acetylcholinesterase (AChE) inhibitor and D_2 receptor antagonist. Centrally active dopamine antagonists provide an antiemetic property, while peripherally these antagonists stimulate GI tract motility.[64,65]

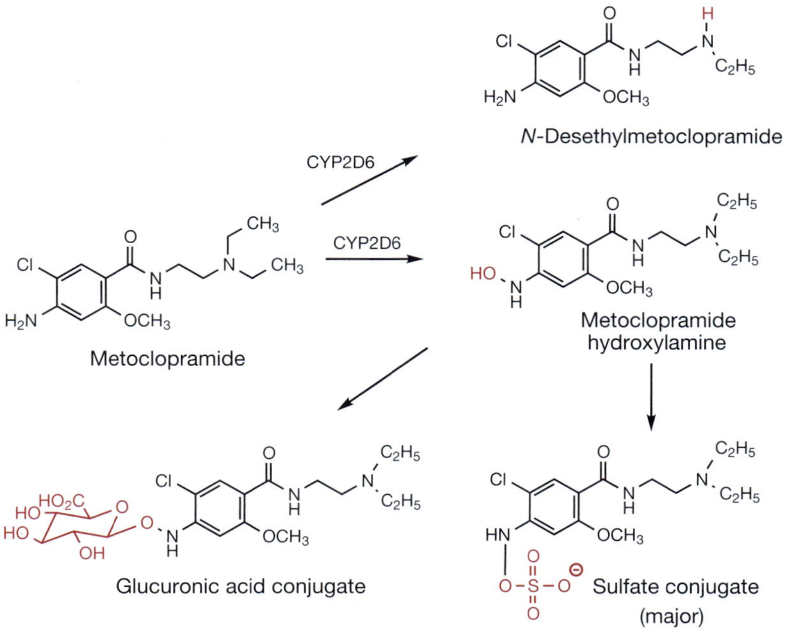

Figure 28.14 Metabolism of metoclopramide.

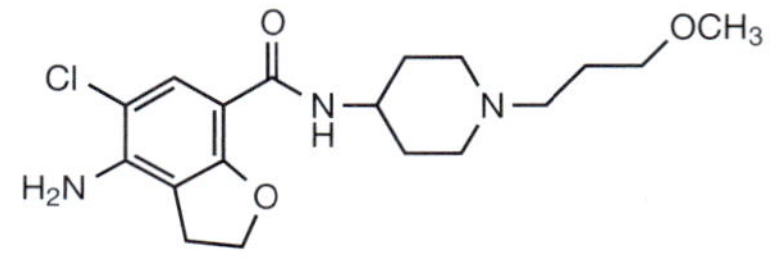

Prucalopride

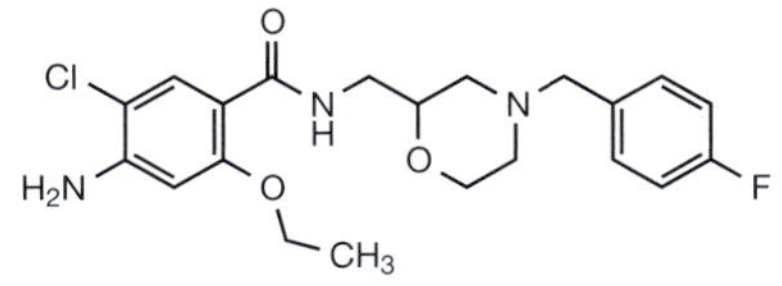

Mosapride

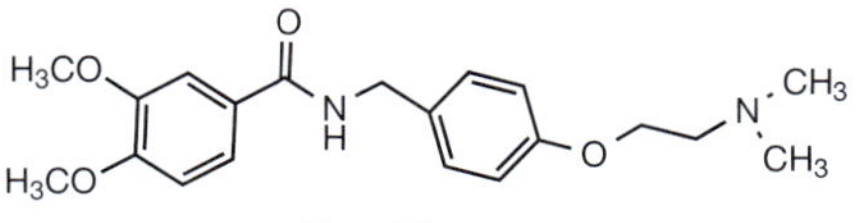

Itopride

Prostaglandins

Prostaglandins (PGs) exhibit antisecretory effects by inhibiting adenylyl cyclase activity in parietal cells. This in turn results in inhibition of gastric acid secretion. Additionally, PGs stimulate secretion of mucus and bicarbonate to prevent acid-related erosion in the GI tract.[66] Endogenous PG E_1 and a more stable synthetic derivative, misoprostol, exhibit cytoprotective effects. The active form of this class of molecules has a terminal carboxylic acid, so misoprostol, a methyl ester, is a prodrug with the advantage of oral bioavailability. The ester is hydrolyzed to the corresponding bioactive carboxylic acid in the bloodstream. Other structural differences are at the C_{15} and C_{16} carbon atoms. PG E_1 has a secondary hydroxyl group at the C_{15} position, while misoprostol has a tertiary hydroxyl group at the C_{16} position. The C_{16} hydroxyl group is stable to oxidation compared to the allylic secondary alcohol at C_{15} position of PG E_1. Combined with the need for hydrolytic activation, this prolongs duration of action.

Misoprostol reduces the basal levels of gastric acid secretion, resulting in GI mucosal protection.[67] In terms of GI disorders, misoprostol has been recommended for the treatment of duodenal ulcers that are unresponsive to traditional H_2 antagonists. Due to its ability to induce smooth muscle contraction, misoprostol's adverse effects relate to diarrhea and abdominal pain. It is contraindicated in pregnant women due to its ability to stimulate uterine contraction. In the United States, misoprostol can be administered in combination with nonsteroidal anti-inflammatory drugs (NSAIDs) because it reduces the risk of gastric ulceration associated with extended use of NSAIDs.[66]

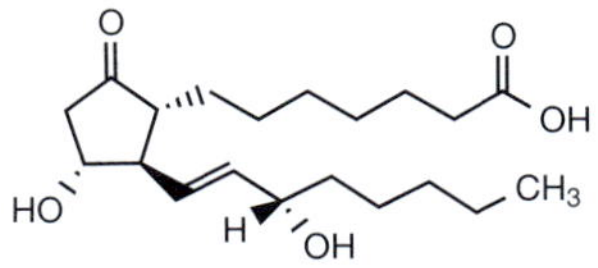

Prostaglandin E_1

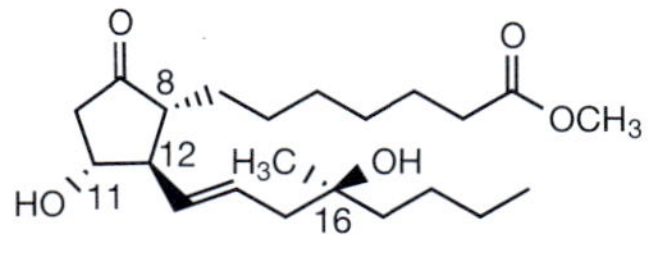

Misoprostol

Gastrointestinal Mucosal Protectants

Sucralfate

Sucralfate is a poly-sulfuric acid ester of sucrose complexed with aluminum hydroxide and is used in gastric ulcer disease.[68,69] These poorly dissociated complexes are insoluble in the stomach. The physical complex sits in the crater of the ulcerated area and serves as a physical and chemical barrier to protect the ulcer from erosion by enzymes and bile salts in the stomach. The chemical barrier is the result of the basic metal hydroxide neutralization of gastric acid. It is also observed that sucralfate stimulates PG synthesis and bicarbonate release, which may be beneficial in peptic ulcers. Systemic absorption of sucralfate is negligible, but it reduces the absorption of other drugs, such as H_2 antihistamines, quinolone antibiotics, phenytoin, and warfarin.[70] As aluminum is part of this complex, there is a risk of aluminum accumulation from absorbed material in patients with renal impairment.

Bismuth Subsalicylate

Bismuth-based preparations, such as bismuth subsalicylate, exhibit a similar protective effect as sucralfate and by a similar mechanism. A combination therapy involving an H_2 antihistamine, antibiotic (metronidazole, tetracycline), and potassium bismuth subsalicylate is used as a second-line option for *H. pylori* eradication and treatment of associated ulcers.

ANTIEMETIC AGENTS

Serotonergics

Serotonin is one of the prominent neurotransmitters that has generated remarkable interest in drug development.[71] Although its physiologic importance was underappreciated in the early days, later it became an important focus of scientific and clinical investigation. Serotonin has been associated with many disorders, including anxiety, depression, drug abuse, cardiovascular disorders, sexual behavior, appetite control, gastric motility, nausea, and irritable bowel disorders.[72] This section discusses the role of serotonin and its receptors in nausea and IBD.

Serotonin (5-hydroxytryptamine [5-HT]) was discovered independently in the United States and in Italy. In addition to various homeostatic physiologic actions, 5-HT is also associated with certain mental/behavioral disorders. This was realized due to 5-HT being structurally similar to a hallucinogenic agent, (+)-lysergic acid diethylamide (LSD). This drug was shown to be a potent 5-HT receptor agonist at certain receptor subtypes and an antagonist at others. With the development of sophisticated biochemical methods, substantial research has been undertaken to understand the structure and function of 5-HT receptors and the physiologic roles of 5-HT.[73,74]

To date, seven distinct families or subtypes of 5-HT receptors have been discovered, which are designated as 5-HT_1 to 5-HT_7. Within each subtype, several subpopulations of receptors are also known.[75] All 5-HT receptors are GPCRs except for 5-HT_4, which belongs to the Cys-loop–containing ligand-gated ion channels (see Chapter 6).[19,76] This chapter specifically focuses on drugs developed to target 5-HT_3 and 5-HT_4 receptors closely associated with GI disorders.[77-80]

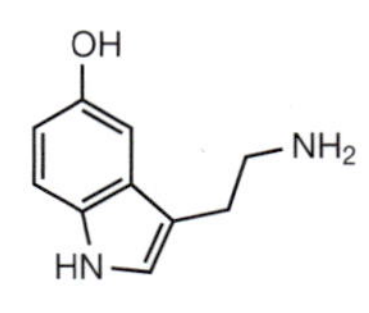

Serotonin

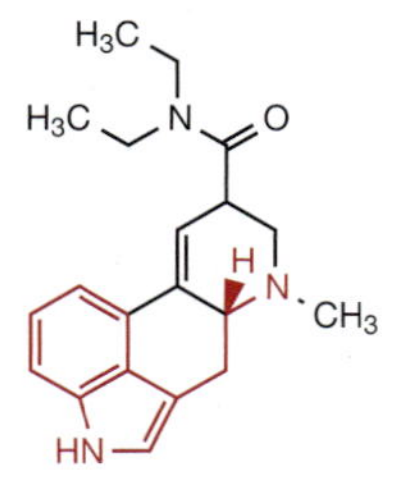

(+)-Lysergic acid diethylamide

The biosynthesis of 5-HT begins with the hydroxylation of dietary tryptophan by tryptophan hydroxylase, which generates 5-hydroxytryptophan (5-HTP). Subsequently, a nonselective amino acid decarboxylase called 5-HTP decarboxylase converts 5-HTP into 5-HT. The major metabolic pathway involves oxidative deamination by MAO to the corresponding aldehyde, which further undergoes oxidation to the carboxylic acid or reduction to the primary alcohol (Fig. 28.15). In addition, acylation of 5-HT by *N*-acetyltransferase occurs to yield *N*-acetylserotonin. It is interesting to note that O-methylation of acetylated 5-HT generates melatonin, the endogenous hormone associated with circadian rhythms and sleep. From a drug discovery standpoint, it is important to realize that each step in 5-HT biosynthesis and metabolism, along with the understanding of the nature of important receptor interactions, is a potential target for drug development.

5-HT_3 Antagonists

A large proportion of 5-HT is found in the GI tract, where it regulates physiologic functions and changes.[81] 5-HT is

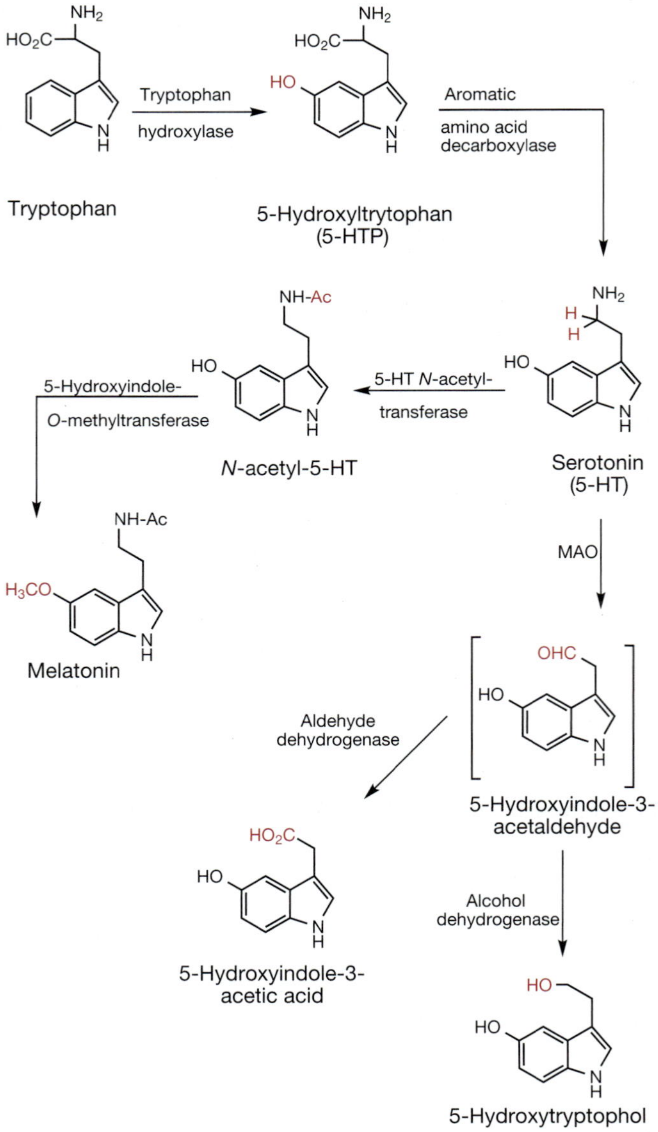

Figure 28.15 Biosynthesis and catabolism of serotonin (5-HT).

found in the mucosal enterochromaffin cells (EC), which release 5-HT to activate 5-HT_3 and 5-HT_4 receptors. Stimulation of 5-HT_3 receptors inhibits gastric secretions and stimulates ion migrating motor complexes in the gut.[77] This enhances the intestinal secretions to facilitate bowel movements. Activation of intestinal 5-HT_3 receptors also stimulates antral contractions and vagal afferent nerves which induce nausea. It is understood that chemotherapy agents induce nausea, at least in part, through the release of large amount of 5-HT in the EC, which stimulates vagal afferent nerves and initiates the vomiting reflex. Several 5-HT_3 receptor antagonists have been developed as antiemetics to inhibit this process (Fig. 28.16).

Structural Features and Mechanism of Action

Ondansetron, palonosetron, granisetron, alosetron, dolasetron, and tropisetron are the clinically available 5-HT_3 receptor antagonists (Fig. 28.16). The first-generation agents can be categorized into three major structural classes: (1) carbazole derivatives, (2) indazole derivatives, and (3) indole derivatives. Palonosetron is a second-generation agent that is highly selective toward the 5-HT_3 receptor.

The first selective 5-HT_3 antagonist (bemesetron) was developed based on the structure of cocaine, which was previously shown to weakly inhibit the 5-HT_3 receptor and exhibit an antiemetic property.[79] The tropane core from cocaine is an important structural feature and retained in many of the early 5-HT_3 antagonists, including tropisetron. This nitrogen-containing heterocycle was slightly modified to introduce similar-looking bicyclic cores to generate newer members of this class of agents, including granisetron, dolasetron, and palonosetron. Both ondansetron and alosetron have an imidazole or similar amine-containing heterocyclic structure.

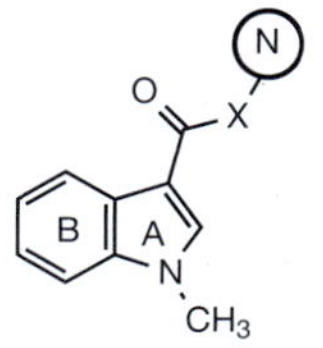

Figure 28.17 General pharmacophore model for 5-HT_3 antagonists.

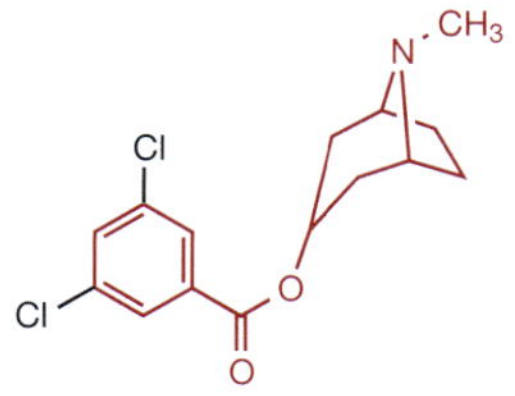

Bemesetron
(cocaine core is highlighted in red)

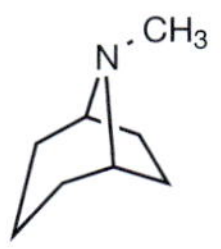

Tropane core

Based on the SAR of 5-HT_3 antagonists, a number of structural features have been identified as important motifs for receptor binding.[79,82,83] A proposed pharmacophore model is provided in Figure 28.17. It has been speculated that ring A may not be required for binding but, rather, acts as a spacer between ring B and the carbonyl oxygen atom. Ring B may be more important for binding and associated hydrophobic binding regions have been proposed. An aromatic centroid (A)-to-oxygen distance of 3.3 to 3.5 Å is thought to be optimal. Distances calculated from the terminal amine to the oxygen atom, and from the terminal amine to centroid A, are 5.1 to 5.2 Å and 6.7 to 7.2 Å, respectively.

As mentioned previously, the cocaine scaffold was an inspiration for the design of early 5-HT_3 antagonists. The tropane or amine-containing bicyclic motifs are linked to the aromatic component via an ester or amide bond. The aromatic

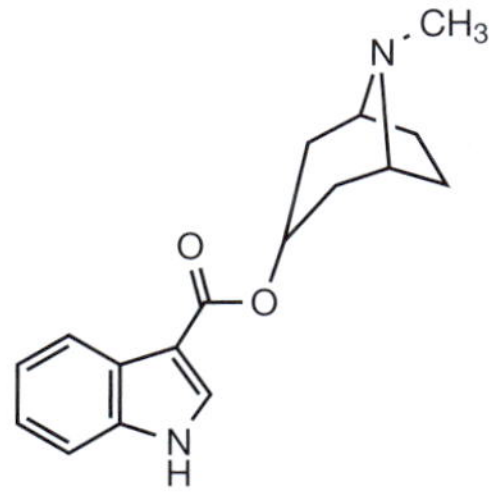

Tropisetron
(Novaban)

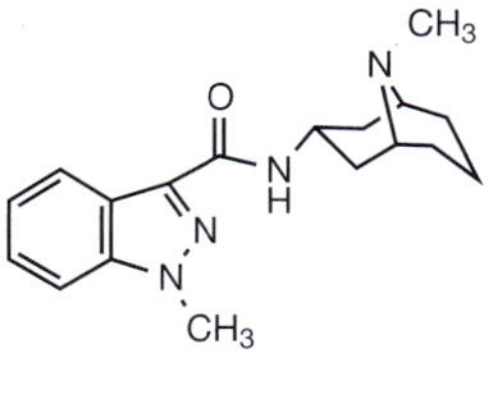

Granisetron
(Kytril)

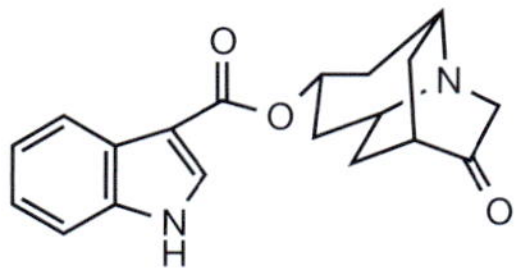

Dolasetron
(Anzemet)

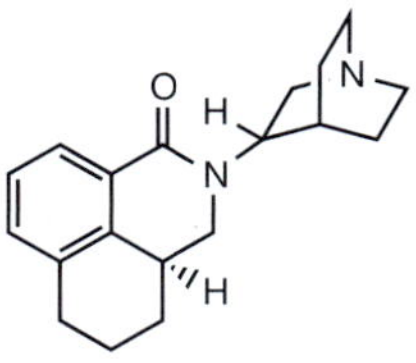

Palonosetron
(Aloxi)

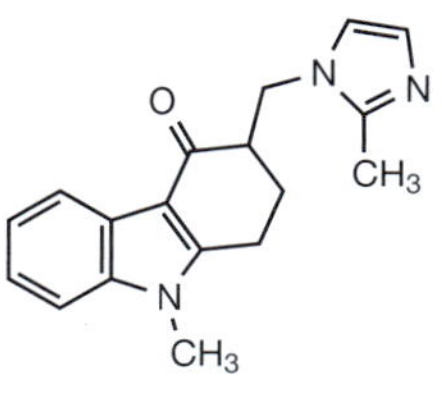

Ondansetron
(Zofran)

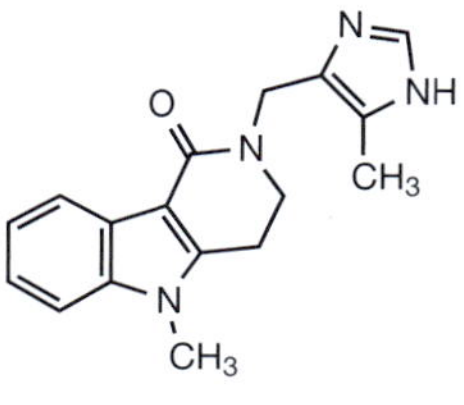

Alosetron
(Lotronex)

Figure 28.16 5-HT_3 receptor antagonists.

component has a fused benzene ring and nitrogen heterocycle as part of the indole, indazole, or carbazole core. The distance between the aromatic ring segment and the terminal basic amine is optimal at 6.7 Å. The nitrogen heterocycle of the aromatic ring moiety is important to provide the needed electron density for the observed cation-π interaction with Arg55 of the 5-HT_3 receptor. Based on proposed pharmacophoric models, the aromatic ring segment is also involved in hydrophobic interactions. Additionally, the carbonyl oxygen of the amide bond forms a water-mediated hydrogen bond, and the amine-containing ring (in protonated form) forms a cation-π interaction with Trp183 and Tyr193 (Fig. 28.18).[84]

Palonosetron (Fig. 28.16), a more recent 5-HT_3 antagonist, also contains a similar pharmacophore, yet it has a longer half-life (40 hours) and greater receptor binding affinity compared to first-generation agents. The stronger binding affinity can be attributed to the following drug-receptor interactions: (1) a hydrogen bond between Tyr153 and the carbonyl oxygen of the amide group of palonosetron, which is consistent with the role of this residue interacting with 5-HT, and (2) a cation-π interaction of the quinuclidine nitrogen (in its protonated form) with Tyr153 and Trp183. The precision of the angle and distance of these functional groups within palonosetron is proposed to be crucial for its high binding affinity.[85]

Currently available 5-HT_3 receptor antagonists are important in the treatment of chemotherapy- and radiation-induced nausea and vomiting. These are unavoidable and often dose-limiting adverse effects for patients undergoing such treatments. Many of the 5-HT_3 antagonists exhibit comparable efficacy and safety, yet their pharmacologic and pharmacokinetic properties are different.[86-89] The half-lives of these drugs vary widely. The selection of a specific agent relates, in part, to the emetogenic potential and properties of the chemotherapeutic regimen, the patient's ability to tolerate adverse effects, and patient history. The metabolic profile of the drug also plays a role in selecting the most suitable drug for a specific population of patients.

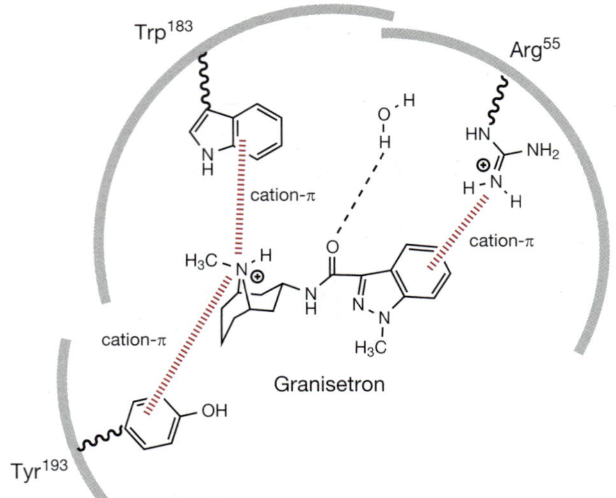

Figure 28.18 Proposed binding interactions of granisetron with the 5-HT_3 receptor.

Ondansetron is a competitive, reversible antagonist of 5-HT_3 receptor, whereas granisetron, tropisetron, and palonosetron produce an insurmountable antagonism.[89] Ondansetron has an alkylimidazole moiety as the nitrogen-containing heterocycle, and a ketone moiety between the aromatic segment and the nitrogen-containing heterocycle (Fig. 28.16). The other members of this class have a tertiary alkyl amine–containing heterocycle (a stronger base) and an amide or ester moiety (a better hydrogen bond acceptor). Based on these structural features, it is highly likely that granisetron, tropisetron, and palonosetron can make stronger cation-π and hydrogen bond interactions, which are key interactions for tighter receptor binding.

Ondansetron also has some affinity for the 5-HT_1 (B and C subtypes), α-adrenergic, and opioid receptors, while dolasetron is considered a very selective 5-HT_3 receptor antagonist. Dolasetron readily undergoes a reduction by carbonyl reductase to generate hydrodolasetron, which is an active metabolite with a half-life of 4 to 8 hours. The bioavailability of orally administered dolasetron is high and makes it a therapeutically useful option for those who can tolerate oral medications. Although IV administration was available in earlier times, the FDA suspended this mode of administration in 2010 due to the risk of hemodynamically unstable tachyarrhythmia. The mechanism of this adverse effect is related to slowing or delaying of cardiac depolarization by sodium or potassium channel blockade.[90]

Selected pharmacokinetic properties of common 5-HT_3 antagonists are summarized in Table 28.2.

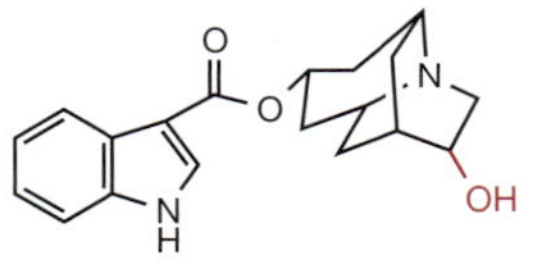

Hydrodolasetron

Metabolism

Although all 5-HT_3 receptor antagonists exhibit a similar mechanism of action, their structural differences alter their binding affinities and pharmacokinetic profiles. Dolasetron undergoes reduction of the carbonyl group by carbonyl reductase and aryl hydroxylation and N-oxidation catalyzed by CYP2D6 and CYP3A4. As indicated previously, hydrodolasetron is an active metabolite that exhibits about 20 to 60 times greater 5-HT_3 receptor affinity than dolasetron.[91,92] Granisetron is primarily metabolized by CYP3A4 to the N-demethylated metabolite and by CYP1A1 to the 7-hydroxy derivative.[93] Chemical inhibitors of CYP3A4, such as ketoconazole, affect the metabolism of granisetron. Palonosetron typically undergoes an N-oxidation and 6S-hydroxylation. Well-known genetic variations in CYP2D6 are known to produce patients who are intermediate metabolizers (IMs), PMs, or UMs related to this isoform, and this affects the metabolic profile of 5-HT_3 antagonists, leading to inconsistent therapeutic response and risk of adverse effects. In addition to the phase 1 metabolic transformations, most of the 5-HT_3 receptor antagonists also undergo phase 2 transformations, including glucuronidation and

Table 28.2 Pharmacokinetic Properties of 5-HT_3 Antagonists

Parameters	Ondansetron (Zofran)	Dolasetron (Anzemet)	Granisetron (Kytril)	Alosetron (Lotronex)	Palonosetron (Aloxi)	Tropisetron (Navoban)
cLog P (calc)[a]	2.35	2.33	1.88	1.21	2.55	3.14
Bioavailability (%)	56-70[d]	Hydrodolasetron: 60-80	60[d]	50-60[b,c]	NA (administered IV)	60 (60-100)
Protein binding (%)	70-76	Hydrodolasetron: 70-80	65	82	62	71
Volume of distribution (L/kg)	PO: 2.2-2.5	Hydrodolasetron: PO: 5.8-10	PO: 3.9	PO: 70 (65-95)	IV: 6.8-12.5	IV: 500
		PO: 6-7				
Elimination half-life (h)	PO: 3-6	PO: <10 min	IV: 4-5	PO: 1.5-2.0	PO: 30-40	EM: PO: 6-8
	Older adults: PO: 11	Hydrodolasetron: PO: 4-9	PO: ~6			PM: PO: 30
Metabolism	Hydroxylation	Reduction of carbonyl	N-Demethylation	6-Hydroxylation	N-oxidation	Hydrolysis
	Glucuronidation	Hydroxylation	Hepatic	N-Demethylation	6S-Hydroxylation	Glucuronidation
	Hepatic	N-Demethylation			Hepatic: 50%	
Metabolizing enzyme	CYP3A4	Carbonyl reductase	CYP3A4	CYP2C9: 30%	CYP2D6	CYP2D6
	CYP2D6	CYP2D6		CYP3A4: 20	CYP3A4	
		CYP3A4 (*N*-oxide)		CYP1A2: 10%	CYP1A2	
Time to peak plasma concentration (h)	PO: 1-2	Hydrodolasetron IV: <0.5	PO: 2-3	PO: 0.5-2	IV: injected over 30 sec	EM: PO: 3
		Hydrodolasetron PO: <1				PM: PO: 4
Excretion (%)	Urine metabolites (40-60)	Urine metabolites (45)	Urine metabolites (48)	Urine metabolites (70)	Urine metabolites (80)	Urine metabolites (~70)
	Feces metabolites (25)	Feces metabolites (30)	Feces metabolites (38)	Feces metabolites (25)		Feces metabolites (~15)
	Unchanged (<10)	Unchanged hydrodolasetron (60)	Unchanged (<10)	Unchanged (<10)	Unchanged (40)	Unchanged (<10)
Duration (h)	-	-	8-24	1-10	>24	-

EM, extensive metabolizer; IM, intramuscular; IV, intravenous; PM, poor metabolizer; PO, oral.
[a]www.drugbank.ca. Accessed July 16, 2025.
[b]First-pass metabolism.
[c]Food delays absorption and peak plasma concentrations.
[d]Food increases extent of absorption.

sulfate conjugation. The phase 2 metabolites are excreted in the urine, in addition to 10% to 60% of the unmodified parent drug.

Specific Drugs

The 5-HT_3 antagonists described in the following sections are the two most prescribed antiemetics in this class.

ONDANSETRON. Ondansetron is a carbazole-based 5-HT_3 antagonist indicated for the prevention of chemotherapy-induced nausea/vomiting in adults and in children 4 years and older. It is available for oral and IV administration. Based on a proposed receptor binding model, the carbazole interacts with the 5-HT_3 receptor via hydrophobic and cation-π interactions. The weakly basic methylimidazole moiety, in a protonated state, can form a cation-π interaction with conserved active site Tyr and Trp residues.[84] Ondansetron is a reversible antagonist and exhibits relatively weaker binding compared to other members, perhaps due to reduced basicity of the imidazole nitrogen.

Ondansetron is primarily metabolized by CYP3A4 and follows a secondary metabolic pathway catalyzed by CYP1A2, CYP2D6, and CYP2E1. Significant drug-drug interactions based on this metabolic profile are known. Major metabolic reactions include aryl hydroxylation at positions 6, 7, or 8, and demethylation of the carbazole nitrogen.[94] There has not been any reported major adverse effect linked to ondansetron besides headache.

PALONOSETRON. Palonosetron is the most recent 5-HT_3 antagonist approved for therapeutic use. Despite having an aryl ring, an amide bond, and a nitrogen heterocycle like all members of this therapeutic class, it is structurally slightly different than other classic 5-HT_3 antagonists. It has a tricyclic aryl amide linked to a quinuclidine ring via the amide nitrogen. Based on the binding models with the receptor, the stronger cation-π interaction introduced by the highly basic quinuclidine (in its protonated form) and the conformation achieved by the rigid tricyclic core within this molecule may help explain its strong binding affinity. Palonosetron is available as capsules (0.5 mg) and as IV injection (0.25 mg/5 mL). It is currently used for the prevention of cancer chemotherapy-induced nausea and vomiting in adult and geriatric patients. It has the longest half-life of about 40 hours among clinically used 5-HT_3 antagonists. Palonosetron is well distributed in tissues and exhibits moderate plasma protein binding.[95] Its metabolism is primarily hepatic, and CYP2C9, CYP3A4, and CYP1A2 are the common isoforms responsible for its biotransformation.[96] DDIs based on CYP3A4 vulnerability are less common than with ondansetron, and it can be a viable alternative when serious or otherwise significant interactions rule out ondansetron use.

Other Antiemetic Agents

Although several 5-HT_3 antagonists are available as antiemetic agents for the treatment of nausea and vomiting, promethazine and prochlorperazine are three other agents with non-5-HT_3 mechanisms that are commonly used as well. Some of these agents are very useful for the prevention and treatment of postoperative nausea and vomiting in patients who has gone through surgery under general anesthesia. Postoperative vomiting often leads to dehydration, electrolyte imbalance, and other complications among patients. These difficulties negatively impact patients' smooth recovery from a surgery. Muscarinic and dopamine receptors are two other druggable targets to prevent/treat nausea and vomiting.

Promethazine

Promethazine is a phenothiazine derivative and falls in the category of a tricyclic H_1-antihistamine (see Chapter 29). Phenothiazine antihistamines have a short, branched carbon chain between the nonbasic phenothiazine nitrogen and the basic aliphatic amine. The branched side chain is an important structural difference between promethazine and antipsychotic phenothiazines, which have a straight chain connection between nitrogen atoms. In addition to being used to reverse the symptoms of allergic reaction (a common H_1 antihistamine indication), promethazine is widely used for the treatment of nausea and vomiting associated with anesthesia, and for the treatment of motion sickness. The sedative properties of H_1 antihistamines have been instrumental in treating nausea caused by analgesic drugs and/or chemotherapeutics.

For patients at high risk of postoperative nausea and vomiting, combination therapy including granisetron and promethazine has been shown to be more effective than promethazine alone. Promethazine is also an antagonist at muscarinic (M1) and dopamine (D2) receptors, and these actions contribute to its antiemetic action. However, these nonspecific actions cause several adverse effects, including dystonic reactions and neuroleptic malignant syndrome. A high percentage of absorbed promethazine undergoes first-pass hepatic N-glucuronidation and sulfoxidation, leading to relatively low absolute bioavailability. Additionally, promethazine undergoes CYP2D6-catalyzed aryl-oxidation and dealkylation, where the methyl group or the entire aminoalkyl chain is lost from the tricyclic structure (Fig. 28.19).[97]

Prochlorperazine

Prochlorperazine is a D_2-antagonist and belongs to the phenothiazine class of compounds. It also exhibits mild H_1 antihistaminic activity, although that activity is kept low by the aromatic Cl atom. Inhibition of D_2-receptors in the chemoreceptor trigger zone (CTZ) is the primary mechanism leading to the observed antiemetic property of this agent.

Structurally, prochlorperazine has a chlorinated tricyclic phenothiazine core, and the aliphatic amino group is a three-carbon chain attached to an *N*-methylpiperazine motif. Prochlorperazine is closely related to the first antipsychotic agent, chlorpromazine, which has a dimethyl amine motif at the alkyl side chain. It is known to exhibit lower sedative and anticholinergic effects than other D_2-antagonists, activities attributed to the phenothiazine component of the structure. Similar to promethazine, prochlorperazine also undergoes significant first-pass metabolism, including aryl-oxidation, sulfoxidation, and N-dealkylation (Fig. 28.20).[98]

Amisulpride

Amisulpride is a selective D_2- and D_3-receptor antagonist. It is available as an IV formulation and approved in the United

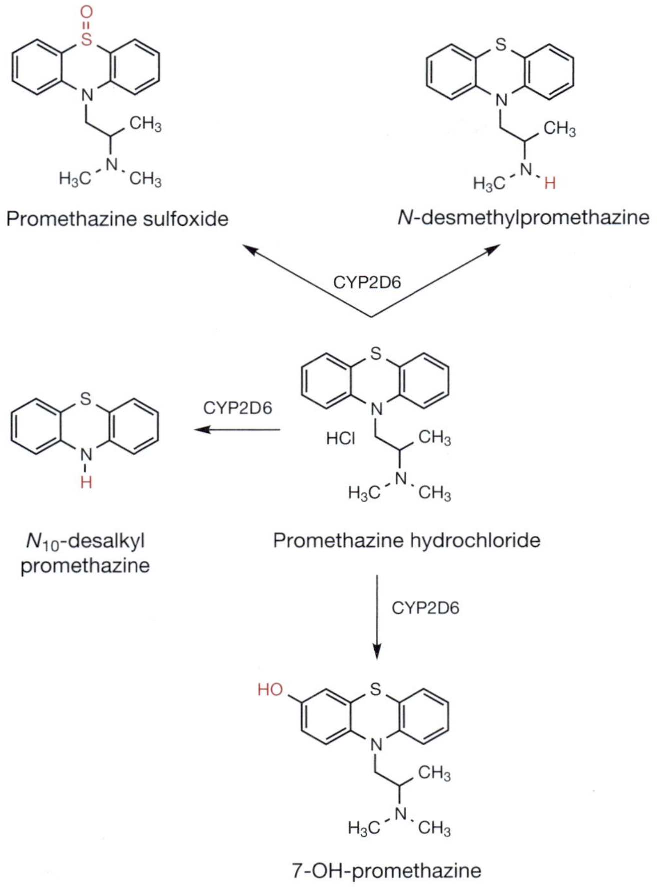

Figure 28.19 Metabolism of promethazine.

States for the prevention and treatment of postoperative nausea and vomiting in adults.[99,100] Amisulpride is a structural analogue of the benzamide antiemetic drugs, namely metoclopramide. It is also a *para*-amino analogue of sulpiride, which is a first-generation antipsychotic agent (Chapter 11).

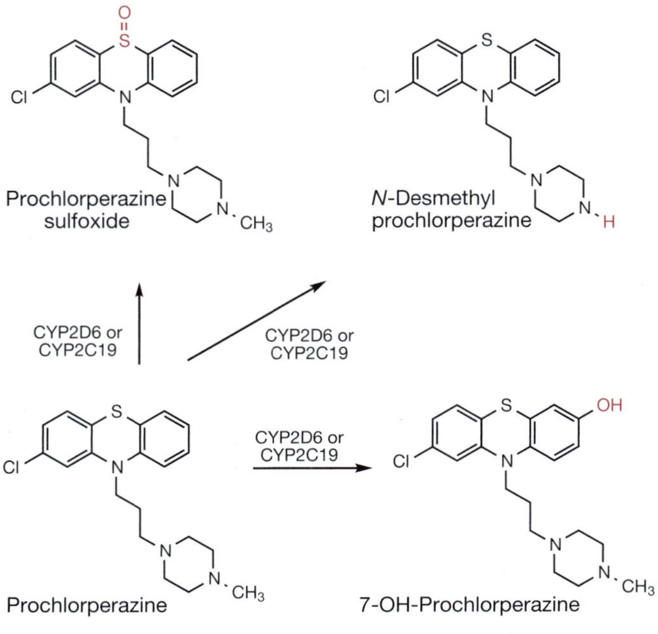

Figure 28.20 Metabolism of prochlorperazine.

Amisulpride has a sulfonyl-anisamide structure and a basic *N*-ethyl pyrrolidine motif. Although the pyrrolidine group has a stereogenic carbon, the drug is available as a racemic mixture. The drug inhibits the dopamine-2 receptors in the CTZ, and dopamine-3 receptors in the area postrema, to provide the therapeutic effect. Inhibition of presynaptic dopamine receptors is achieved at low doses, while postsynaptic dopamine receptor inhibition is achieved at high doses. Amisulpride is administered alone or in combination with other clinically available antiemetic agents. A 5-mg dosage is available for the prevention of postoperative nausea and vomiting, and a 10-mg dosage is available for the treatment to be administered after a surgical procedure. Amisulpride has a mean elimination half-life of 4 to 5 hours, and primarily excreted via the kidneys (~58%). Metabolic evaluation in vitro indicates that amisulpride does not inhibit or induce many of the common CYP enzymes. However, it has been identified as a substrate for P-glycoprotein (P-gp) and BCRP.[99,100]

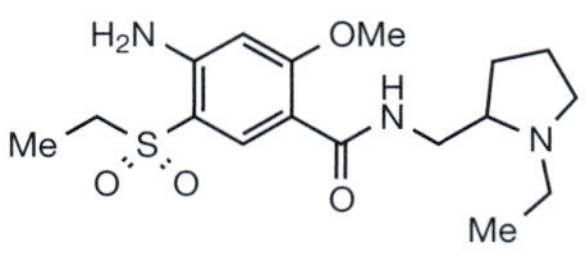

Amisulpride

Irritable Bowel Syndrome and Treatment Options

IBS is often a debilitating GI disorder that affects a significant proportion of the population in the United States and worldwide.[101] The difficulty in managing IBS with limited therapeutic interventions affects the quality of life of millions of people.[102] It has been estimated that about 1.4 million people in the United States are affected by IBS, and the economic impact associated with diagnosis and care is substantial.[103]

IBS is described as a disorder of the brain-GI tract connection, where GI motility is affected, and the sensitivity of the gut is heightened. The symptoms include cramping, abdominal pain, bloating, and diarrhea or constipation.[58,102,104] Based on the symptoms, IBS can be designated as diarrhea predominant (IBS-D), constipation predominant (IBS-C), or a third category, where patients experience diarrhea alternating with constipation (IBS-A).[105] The management of IBS has been guided by a better understanding of the pathology of the disorder, collaborative physician-patient relationships, and judicious use of treatment options based on symptoms. In general, only those patients suffering from severe symptoms are treated with medications.

Serotonin Receptor-Antagonists and Agonists

Until recently, available treatment options for IBS were limited by poor efficacy or adverse effects. Typically, laxatives, antispasmodics and smooth muscle relaxants, and tricyclic antidepressants are used, but with limited patient satisfaction.

However, important drug targets that have emerged for the treatment of IBS are $5HT_3$ and $5\text{-}HT_4$ receptors.

Alosetron

$5\text{-}HT_3$ receptor stimulation causes increased motility, secretion, and excitation in the gut. Thus, $5\text{-}HT_3$ antagonists can reduce colonic transit and improve fluid absorption. Alosetron (Fig. 28.15), a $5\text{-}HT_3$ antagonist, is one of the agents used for IBS treatment. Since $5\text{-}HT_3$ antagonists can inhibit the action of $5\text{-}HT_3$ receptors on extrinsic afferent neurons, they can decrease the visceral pain associated with IBS as well.[58,103,105-107]

Tegaserod

On the other hand, $5\text{-}HT_4$ receptors mediate the initiation of peristalsis through a coupled process with $5\text{-}HT_{1p}$ receptors. Tegaserod (Fig. 28.13), a prokinetic agent discussed earlier, is a partial agonist of presynaptic $5\text{-}HT_4$ receptors, which entered clinical use for the treatment of IBS in 2002.[108] It is an aminoguanidine indole derivative of 5-HT. Tegaserod accelerates small bowel and colonic transit in patients with IBS. It is absorbed readily, and peak plasma concentrations are reached in approximately 1 hour. It is significantly bound to plasma proteins (98%), more specifically to α1-acid glycoprotein. In terms of metabolism, tegaserod undergoes acid-catalyzed hydrolysis in the stomach to cleave the indole component from the aminoguanidine chain and form an aldehyde. Hepatic oxidation further converts the aldehyde metabolite into the inactive 4-methoxyindole-3-carboxylic acid. Tegaserod is also modified by phase 2 metabolism to yield the three isomeric N-glucuronides.[109,110]

Although tegaserod is an efficacious drug for the treatment of IBS, it was removed from the US market due to increased risk of myocardial infractions or stroke. In the past, it was only available through a restricted distribution program for life-threatening circumstances. However, as of 2019, tegaserod has been reintroduced for the treatment of IBS-C in women younger than 65 years who have no history of cardiovascular ischemic diseases and those who have no more than one risk factor for cardiovascular diseases.

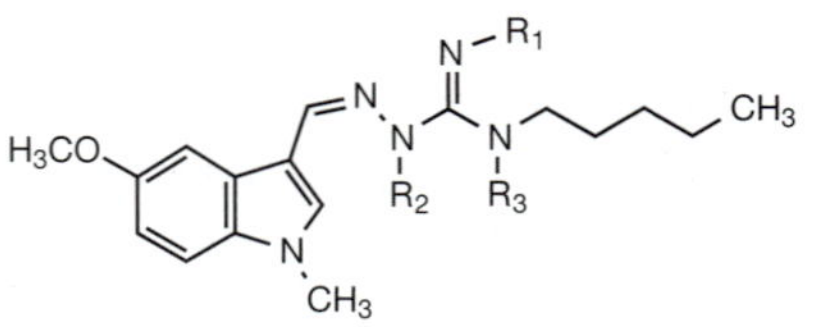

Tegaserod glucuronide—M1 (R_1 = glucuronide, $R_2 = R_3$ = H)

Tegaserod glucuronide—M2 ($R_1 = R_3$ = H, R_2 = glucuronide)

Tegaserod glucuronide—M3 ($R_1 = R_2$ = H, R_3 = glucuronide)

Glucuronide =

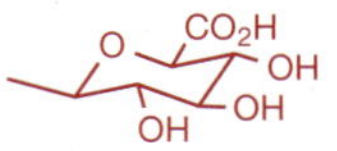

Renzapride

Renzapride is another example of a $5\text{-}HT_4$ agonist that is useful as a gastroprokinetic and an antiemetic agent. It is currently an investigational drug and has the potential to be useful for the treatment for IBS. It stimulates GI tract motility and has been shown to be potentially effective for IBS-C and IBS-A. Renzapride is a benzamide derivative and structurally similar to metoclopramide. The structure retains the biologically important tertiary amine in the form of a bulky bicyclic amine. Renzapride is predominantly metabolized by CYP enzymes to the N-oxide, which exhibits reduced binding affinity to $5\text{-}HT_4$ receptors.[111]

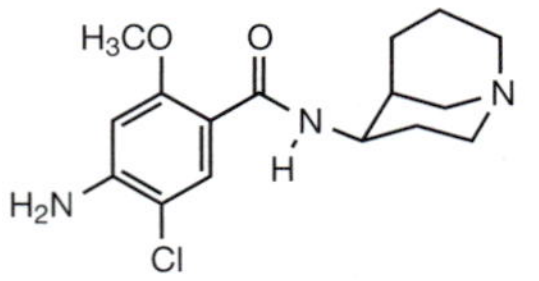

Renzapride

Guanylyl Cyclase-C Agonists

Agonists of guanylyl cyclase-C have been useful therapeutic options for IBS-C and chronic idiopathic constipation. Plecanatide and linaclotide are two peptide-derived agonists of this enzyme approved for therapeutic use.[112] Guanylyl cyclase-C is expressed mainly in the GI neurons, and the binding of endogenous guanylin and uroguanylin regulates water and electrolyte transport in the gut. Guanylin is a 15–amino acid peptide with defined secondary structure. It is secreted in the colon, and binding to its receptor induces chloride secretion and decreases intestinal fluid absorption, which causes diarrhea. This process is similar to the binding of enterotoxins in the gut, which leads to diarrhea.[113] Uroguanylin is a 16–amino acid oligopeptide that is secreted in the duodenum and proximal small intestine. This peptide ligand functions in a similar fashion to guanylin.[114] Based on the structure and biological role of these endogenous ligands, both plecanatide and linaclotide have been developed into therapeutic agents.[115]

Plecanatide is a structural analogue of uroguanylin that is 16 amino acids long. The structural change involves modification of the third residue of uroguanylin into glutamic acid. All Cys residues within the structure are preserved, as they all are involved in the formation of disulfide bonds to generate the secondary structure. Linaclotide is a peptide mimic of endogenous guanylin and uroguanylin that is a 14-amino acid synthetic peptide.

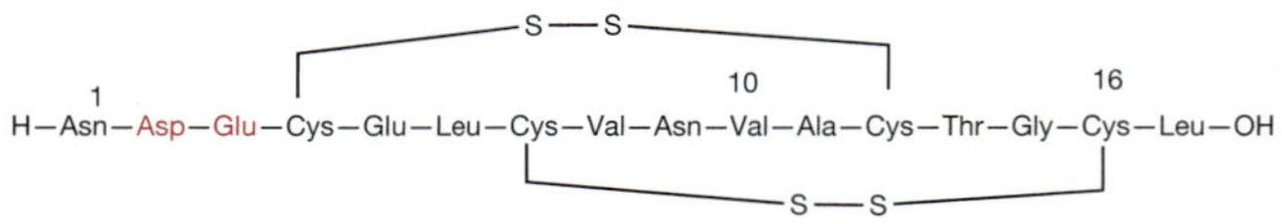

Plecanatide
(Trulance)

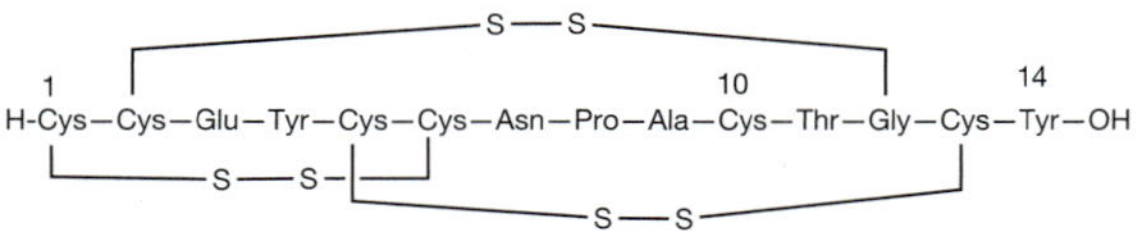

Linaclotide
(Linzess)

Systemic absorption of these agents after oral administration is minimal; however, since these agents act on receptors present on the apical side of the endothelium of GI tract, there is no need for them to be systemically absorbed. The acidic residues (Asp2 and Glu3) of plecanatide are important for binding to the receptor, and optimal binding is observed at pH 5. One of the limitations of peptide agents is metabolic instability in the GI tract and, as one can expect, plecanatide and linaclotide are degraded by intestinal proteases. Linaclotide is an effective drug; however, it has a boxed warning against use in children younger than 6 years, and it is not recommended for patients who are 6 to 18 years old due to a high risk of dehydration.

Sphingosine-1-Phosphate Receptor Modulators for Irritable Bowel Disease Treatment

Sphingosine-1-phosphate (S1P) is a lysophospholipid signaling molecule and binds to five different cell-surface GPCRs (S1P1 to S1P5).[116] Some of these receptors, including S1P1, are widely distributed in various tissues. Since S1P receptor activation plays a key role in lymphocyte egress, S1P1 modulators have attracted interest as useful anti-inflammatory medicines.[116,117] Fingolimod is the first S1P receptor modulator developed for the treatment of relapsing-remitting multiple sclerosis (MS). For more details on fingolimod, a sphingosine analogue, readers are referred to Chapter 10 of this textbook. Due to its autoimmune modulation effect, fingolimod is under investigation as a potential therapeutic agent for treating UC. Ozanimod and etrasimod are two synthetic S1P receptor modulators that are available for the treatment of UC.[117] These drugs bind to the S1P receptor with high affinity and block the extent of lymphocyte egress, which leads to a reduction of lymphocyte count in the peripheral blood. A general structural design of S1P receptor modulators contains a polar head group that mimics the phosphate motif and a hydrophobic tail group. Ozanimod is available in capsule form and exhibits an approximate T_{max} of 6 to 8 hours. The mean plasma half-life is 21 hours, and the drug is largely excreted as various inactive metabolites. Ozanimod is extensively metabolized by ADH/ALDH, MOA-B, and CYP enzymes to a series of active and inactive metabolites. A CYP3A4 catalyzed removal of hydroxy-ethyl motif and subsequent deamination leads to an active metabolite.[117]

Etrasimod is the second S1P receptor modulator approved by the FDA for the treatment of moderate to severely active UC. It competitively binds to S1P1, S1P4, and S1P5, while exhibiting considerably low affinity toward S1P2 and S1P3.[117] Etrasimod has notable structural similarity to another S1P receptor targeting autoimmune modulator, siponimod, which is used for the management of MS (Chapter 10). Etrasimod has a polar, ionizable carboxylic acid head group connected to a cyclopenta[b]indole heterocycle. The aryl-ring units provide an extended hydrophobic scaffold for this drug. Etrasimod exhibits high plasma protein binding, where approximately 98% is plasma protein bound. Additionally, it has a long plasma elimination half-life of 30 hours. Drug metabolism is primarily due to CYP2C8, CYP2C9, and CYP3A4, while a minor contribution is related to CYP2C19 isoform. The carboxylic acid is a site for UGT-catalyzed conjugation during phase II metabolism.[117]

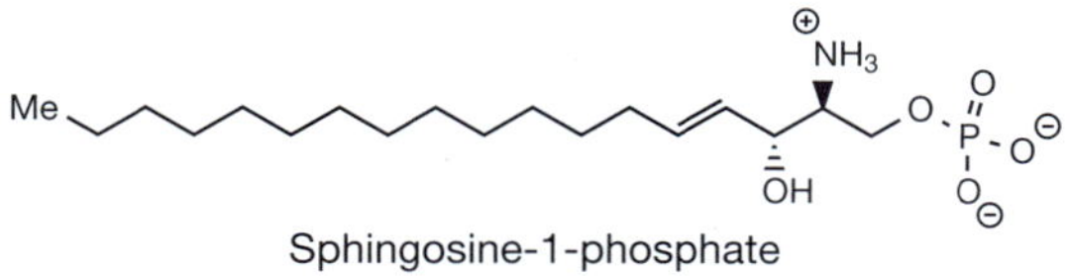

Sphingosine-1-phosphate

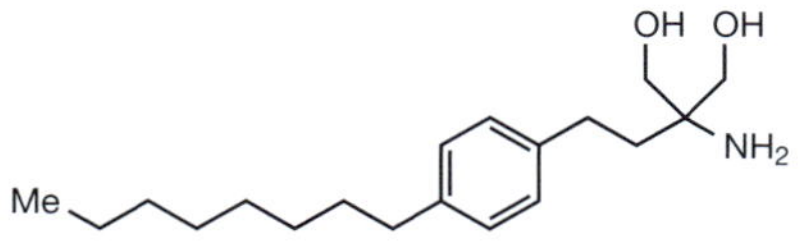

Fingolimod
(under investigation)

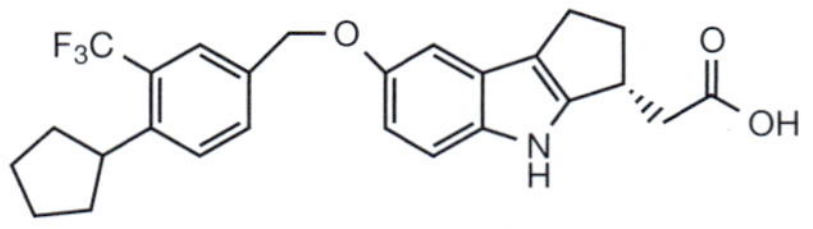

Etrasimod (Velsipity)

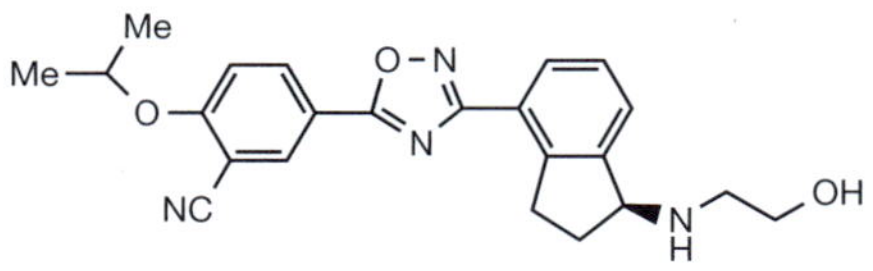

Ozanimod
(Zeposia)

Janus Kinase Inhibitors

IBDs are characterized by chronic inflammation of the GI tract, which is related to an immunological imbalance of the intestinal mucosa.[7,8,118] The cells of the adaptive immune system are observed to respond against self-antigens that lead to inflammatory conditions. It is also associated with an imbalance in the gut microflora. CD and UC are the most common types of IBD and are very prevalent in the world population.[119-121] The pathophysiological mechanism of IBD is not well understood; however, substantial efforts have been dedicated to discovering drugs to target inflammatory pathways.

Investigation of various druggable targets for the treatment of autoimmune disorders led to the discovery of the Janus kinase (JAK) family as a viable target to develop new drugs. The JAK family of enzymes (JAK1, JAK2, JAK3, and tyrosine kinase 2 [TYK2]) are important intracellular enzymes linked to proinflammatory signaling mediated by various cytokines.[122] JAK inhibitors are under development for treating various autoimmune diseases, including rheumatoid arthritis, psoriasis, myelofibrosis, and IBD.[123,124] More specifically, activation of signal transducers and activators of transcription (STATs) in T cells is linked to the pathogenesis of CD. Tofacitinib is a pan-JAK inhibitor approved for the treatment of rheumatoid arthritis and psoriatic arthritis. Fedratinib has been clinically available since 2019 for the treatment of myelofibrosis and thrombocythemia. Upadacitinib, a JAK1-selective inhibitor is FDA-approved and has been available for the treatment of rheumatoid arthritis since 2019.[123] Although JAK inhibitors are classically approved for rheumatoid arthritis, their clinical use for the treatment of IBD is being appreciated in the field.[123,124] Tofacitinib, a broad JAK inhibitor with inhibitory activity toward JAK1, JAK3, and tyrosine kinases outside JAK family, was approved for the treatment of UC in adults. It is currently being investigated as a treatment option for moderate to severe cases of CD. Tofacitinib has a half-life of 3 hours and undergoes extensive hepatic metabolism (70% of drug). The drug is mainly metabolized by CYP3A5 and, to some extent, by CYP2C19. Common metabolic pathways identified include oxidation of the pyrrolopyrimidine and piperidine rings, N-demethylation, and glucuronic acid conjugation.[125,126] Upadacitinib is the second reversible and selective JAK1 inhibitor approved for the treatment of both UC and CD. It exhibits 74% more selectivity toward JAK1 over JAK2. It has a longer half-life than tofacitinib (8 to 14 hours). Drug elimination heavily depends on hepatic metabolism (80% of drug) and metabolized by CYP3A4 and CYP2D6.[126] With the success of these two JAK inhibitors, one can anticipate the discovery and development of newer drugs for the treatment of IBD in the future.

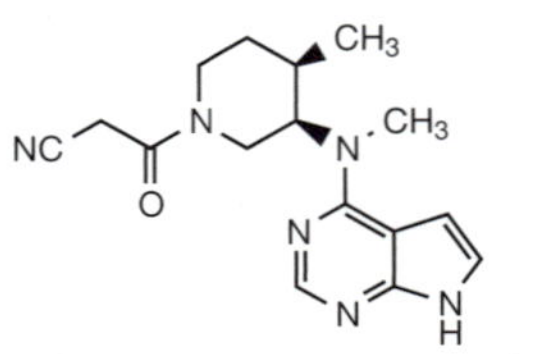

Tofacitinib (Xeljanz)

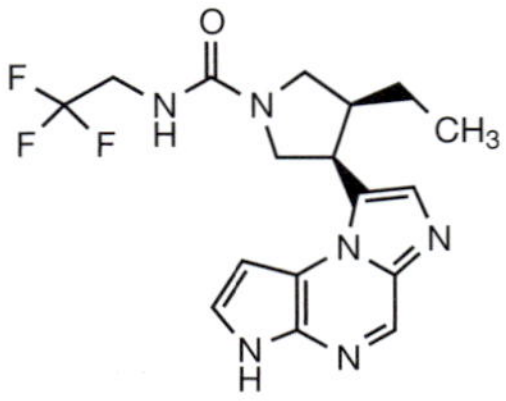

Upadacitinib (Rinvoq)

Monoclonal Antibodies

Given the role of tumor necrosis factor alpha (TNF-α) as a proinflammatory cytokine and its ability to promote production of other proinflammatory cytokines, chemokines, and adhesion molecules (eg, α4β7-integrin), this pathway is a highly investigated target for IBD drug development. To date, various monoclonal antibodies (MAbs) have been developed against the offending proinflammatory molecules named earlier as treatment options. Given the pleiotropic effect of TNF-α, therapeutic agents targeting TNF-α are being developed for the treatment of IBD.

An antibody is a large Y-shaped protein that is used by immune system to neutralize pathogens (see Chapters 5 and 38). A MAb is a monovalent antibody, and it binds to an epitope on an antigen. MAbs are one of the fastest growing classes of therapeutics agents, and about 30 are currently in clinical use (see Chapter 38). In recent years, several MAbs have been developed for the treatment of IBS by targeting some of the key proinflammatory molecules as well as integrins, a specific type of cell surface adhesion protein.[127-129-130]

Adalimumab, certolizumab, infliximab, and golimumab are the four clinically available anti-TNF-α MAbs that are prescribed to achieve clinical remission from moderate to severe CD, and in adults to induce and sustain remission from UC (Table 28.3). All carry a boxed warning relative to the risk of developing serious or life-threatening infection and/or malignancies.[125] Vedolizumab is an MAb that targets the adhesion protein integrin a4b7, rather than TNF-α. Due to its unique mechanism of action, it has been shown to exhibit gut-selective anti-inflammatory activity. Vedolizumab is approved for the treatment of moderate to severe UC or CD, and as an alternative option for patients who do not respond to MAb treatments that target TNF-α.[131] Although it carries no boxed warning, there is a risk of infection, leukoencephalopathy, and hepatotoxicity associated with its use.

MAbs target inflammatory pathways to treat diseases linked to autoimmune response. In this regard, they are also useful therapies for other inflammatory diseases, including rheumatoid arthritis, psoriatic arthritis, and ankylosing spondylitis. As noted, one of the concerning adverse effects is the risk of serious infections, including tuberculosis. Since anti-inflammatory MAbs compromise immune function, a patient's ability to fight infections becomes difficult.

Although MAbs have been developed to target various diseases, developing novel, safe, and efficacious drugs of this type is very challenging. Some of the challenges include (1) the use of inefficient biological models for generating human antibodies, (2) a lack of efficacy for targeted diseases, and (3) the cost-effectiveness associated with MAb-based treatment. Current efforts are focused on addressing one or more of these limitations. It seems that, with new technologies and expanding knowledge, future MAb treatment options can be more efficacious and much more personalized to address the need of individual patients.[132]

Table 28.3 Monoclonal Antibodies for the Management of Ulcerative Colitis and Crohn's Disease

Name	Antibody Type	Mechanism of Action	Indication
Adalimumab (Humira)	Recombinant	Anti-tumor necrosis factor alpha (anti-TNF-α)	Crohn's disease and ulcerative colitis
Certolizumab (Cimzia)	Humanized (pegylated)	Anti-TNF-α	Crohn's disease
Infliximab (Remicade)	Chimeric	Anti-TNF-α	Crohn's disease and ulcerative colitis
Golimumab (Simponi)	Human	Anti-TNF-α	Ulcerative colitis
Vedolizumab (Entyvio)	Humanized	Anti-α4β7 integrin	Crohn's disease and ulcerative colitis

Agents That Impact Gastrointestinal and Genitourinary Smooth Muscle and Glands

Cholinergic Nervous System

ACh is released by cholinergic neurons in the autonomic nervous system and somatic nervous system and by some neurons in the CNS.[133,134] Cholinergic receptors are classified as either muscarinic (mAChR) or nicotinic (nAChR) based on their affinity for the naturally occurring alkaloids muscarine and nicotine, respectively (Fig. 28.21).[135] The mAChR is the receptor of relevance for cholinergic drugs targeting the GI and GU systems.

Parasympathetic nerve activities stimulate GI and urinary tract muscle contraction and relaxation of vascular smooth muscle and lower heart contractility. Direct-acting cholinergic agonists bind directly to receptors, whereas inhibitors of AChE indirectly stimulate cholinergic receptors by increasing the concentration of the ACh neurotransmitter in the synapse. AChE is responsible for hydrolyzing ACh into choline and acetate, that latter of which can supplement pools needed to generate cofactors like acetyl coenzyme A. Cholinergic antagonists have affinity for cholinergic receptors; however, they cannot stimulate them. ACh-mediated activation of cholinergic receptors in parasympathetic nervous system is a therapeutically important process, and the pathway has been extensively investigated for drug discovery.[136]

Acetylcholine Biosynthesis Metabolism and Stereochemistry

ACh biosynthesis, storage, release, and metabolism are illustrated in Figure 28.22.[136] The biosynthesis of this important neurotransmitter begins in the cholinergic neuron, where the transfer of an acetyl group from acetyl-CoA to choline is catalyzed by choline acetyltransferase. When ACh is hydrolyzed by AChE in the synaptic space, the generated choline is transported into the neurons to be used for ACh biosynthesis. Most newly synthesized ACh is kept in cytosolic storage vesicles in presynaptic nerve endings. The release of ACh into the synapse is triggered by an action potential that opens voltage-gated calcium channels, allowing influx of calcium ion and exocytotic release of ACh. Once released, ACh in the synapse binds with cholinergic receptors and produces a response.

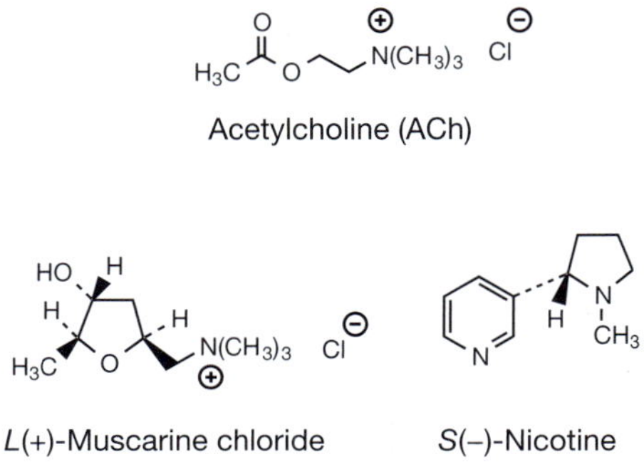

Figure 28.21 Structures of naturally occurring cholinergic agonists.

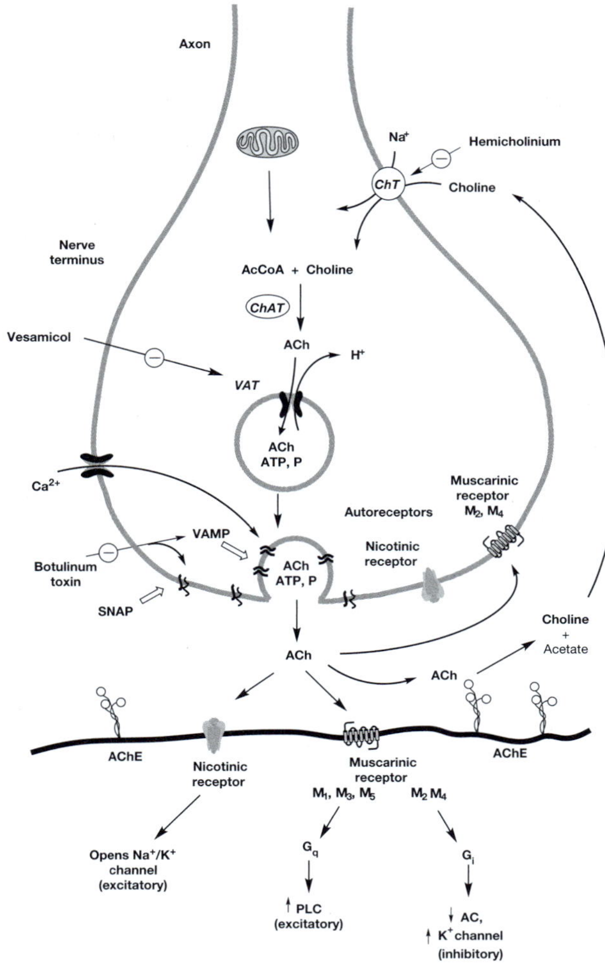

Figure 28.22 Cholinergic neuron site of biosynthesis, storage, release, and receptor activation. AC, adenylyl cyclase; AcCoA, acetyl-coenzyme A; ChT, choline transporter; ChAT, choline acetyltransferase; PLC, phospholipase C; SNAP, synaptosomal-associated protein; VAMP, vesicle-associated membrane protein; VAT, vesicular acetylcholine transporter.

Although ACh is an achiral molecule, the stereochemical impact resides in conformational isomerism. Four of the most commonly studied conformations of ACh are shown in Figure 28.23. Based on the activity of ACh analogues, it is likely that the less-favored anticlinal conformation binds to the mAChR.[137]

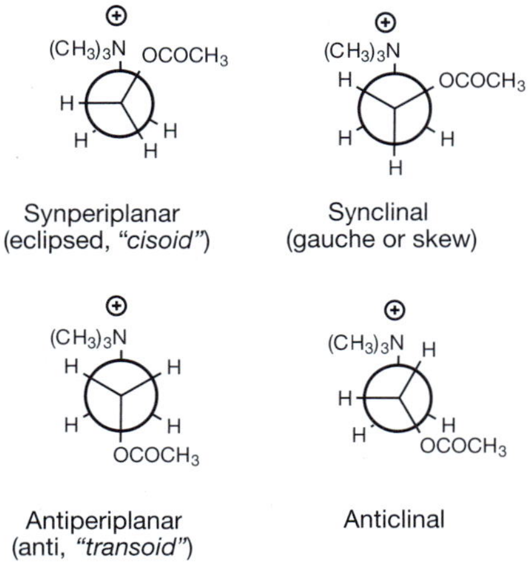

Figure 28.23 Conformational isomers of acetylcholine.

Muscarinic Cholinergic Receptors

As noted, multiple mAChR subtypes exist and are designated as M_1 through M_5.[135,138] All are GPCRs (Chapter 6).[16] Activation of M_3 receptors found in smooth muscle stimulates contraction, and activation in glands stimulates secretion. Understanding their effect on smooth muscle of the bladder has led to the development of M_3 receptor antagonists as therapeutic agents for OAB (discussed later). Although M_3 receptors are also found in the CNS, their concentration is much lower than other receptor subtypes in that tissue. When these receptor subtypes are activated in smooth muscle and secretary glands, it leads to inhibition of potassium and calcium channels.

Structure-Activity Relationship of Acetylcholine and Its Analogues

The synthetic design for many cholinergic agonists and antagonists comes from the SAR of ACh analogues. The structure of ACh can be divided into three segments to explain the SAR: (1) the acyloxy group or acetyl group, (2) the ethylene group that connects the acyloxy and quaternary ammonium motif, and (3) the quaternary ammonium group.[139] Briefly, a cationic amine is important for muscarinic agonist activity.[139] Replacement of a single methyl group of ACh with a longer alkyl group (ie, ethyl, propyl) lowers the muscarinic activity, as does sequential replacement of each methyl group with hydrogen to generate tertiary, secondary, or primary amine analogues.[140] The "Rule of Five" by Ing[139] states that there should be no more than five atoms between the cationic nitrogen and the terminal hydrogen atom (eg, on the acetyl group of ACh) for optimal mAChR binding and stimulation. Methyl substituents on the ethylene chain are permitted, and methacholine (the β-methyl analogue of ACh) exhibits muscarinic activity that is equal to ACh and has improved selectivity toward the mAChR over the nAChR. The *S*-isomer of chiral methacholine is 20 times more active at the mAChR than the *R*-enantiomer and is also much more slowly hydrolyzed by AChE due to both steric hindrance and a less electrophilic carbonyl carbon. Modification of the terminal acyloxy group (eg, extending the length to propionyl or butanoyl) provides less-effective agonists, as expected based on Ing's Rule of Five.[139] However, conversion of the acetate ester to a carbamate retains high mAChR affinity, as discussed next.

As noted, ACh is rapidly degraded by AChE and ubiquitous plasma esterases via the hydrolysis of the acetyl group. To improve the stability of ACh in the synapse, analogues have been developed by replacing the ester functionality with a hydrolytically more stable isostere. Carbamates are esters derived from carbamic acid (and therefore are hybrids of an ester and an amide) and are much more stable to hydrolysis compared to simple esters. Using this bioisosteric replacement strategy, carbachol and bethanechol have been developed, which are the carbamate derivatives of ACh and methacholine, respectively. The conversion of a terminal acetate to a carbamate is tolerated at the mAChR, and so these are both potent direct-acting cholinergic agonists with improved stability to AChE and other esterases. Once they do hydrolyze, they reversibly inactivate AChE by carbamylating the catalytic Ser residue responsible for its hydrolyzing action, allowing ACh to enjoy a longer duration in cholinergic synapses.

The SARs for mAChR agonists are developed based on the binding interactions of ACh with its receptor. The oxygen atoms of the acetate ester moiety form a hydrogen bond with an active site Asn residue, while the quaternary ammonium nitrogen forms an ionic interaction with active site Asp residue. The methyl groups occupy the hydrophobic pockets within the receptor. Considering the importance of these interactions, the SARs of mAChR agonists can be summarized as follows: (1) they contain a quaternary ammonium functional group with a permanent positive charge,[139,140] (2) improved binding and agonist potency is achieved when the onium nitrogen is substituted with small alkyl groups, with methyl group being optimal,[135] (3) an ester-like oxygen atom that can be a hydrogen bond acceptor at the mAChR is required, and (4) the quaternary ammonium nitrogen and the oxygen atom should be connected by a two-carbon bridge (Fig. 28.24).[141]

Muscarinic Receptor Agonists

Since mAChRs play a crucial role in regulating GI and urinary tract functions, agonists can be used to reestablish smooth muscle tone of the GI and urinary tract following

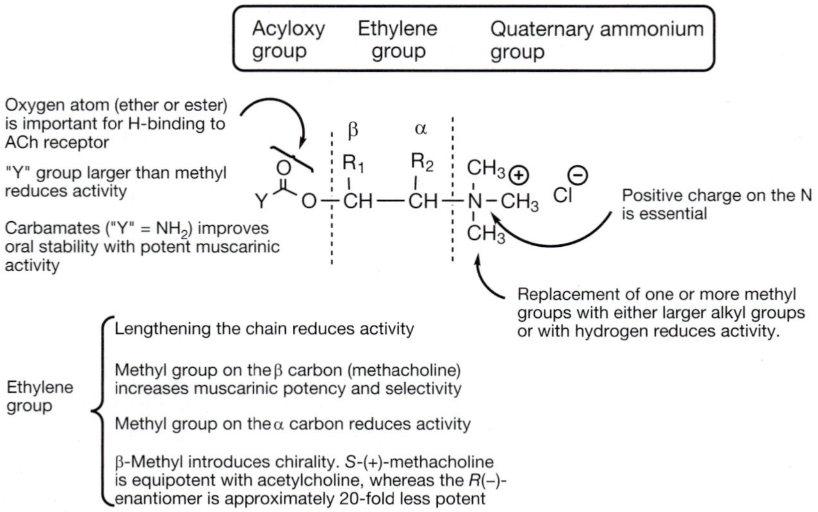

Figure 28.24 Structure-activity relationship summary for muscarinic agonists.

surgical procedures. These agents can relieve abdominal distention and urinary retention and stimulate glandular secretions. To be therapeutically useful in treating GI and GU disorders, they must have a sufficiently long duration of action, and the close structural analogues of ACh, methacholine, and carbachol do not qualify. However, bethanechol can be used in the treatment of postsurgical and postpartum urinary retention, and two mAChR analogues that are structurally distinct from ACh have some therapeutic utility in treating dry mouth (a GI disorder) (Fig. 28.25).

Specific Drugs

Bethanechol Chloride. Bethanechol chloride is the carbamate analogue of methacholine and a selective agonist at the mAChR. Its localized action (ammonium head), direct action selectivity (β-methyl), and prolonged duration (carbamate and β-methyl) make it useful for the treatment of postsurgical and postpartum urinary retention and abdominal distension. Similar to carbachol, the carbamate functional group makes this drug hydrolytically stable and, when it does hydrolyze, it reversibly inhibits AChE through Ser carbamylation. It is an orally administered drug and, due to concern about more system-wide cholinergic effects, it is not given by IV or IM injection. Some of the more serious adverse effects associated with this drug relate to cardiovascular events and bronchoconstriction. Because it is administered orally and retained locally, adverse events are uncommon.

Pilocarpine. Pilocarpine is a natural alkaloid isolated from *Pilocarpus jaborandi* that exhibits potent muscarinic agonistic activity. It was discovered in 1876, and the *N*-methylimidazole-containing lactone structure was determined in 1901. The naturally occurring compound is 3*S*,4*R*-(+)-pilocarpine, and the specific stereochemistry is important for bioactivity. Pilocarpine exhibits affinity for the M_3 receptor subtype.

Pilocarpine is available as tablets, ophthalmic solution, and gel. It is a useful drug for the treatment of dry mouth caused by radiation therapy based on the activity of cholinergic agents as sialagogues (salivation inducers). Due to its lactone motif, the α-stereocenter (C_3 position) is sensitive to epimerization when stored in solution. The epimerized product is called isopilocarpine. The lactone functionality is also susceptible to hydrolysis, yielding pilocarpic acid as the inactive product. Epimerization is expected to be a problem only if the drug is improperly stored. One approach to enhancing in vitro stability is conversion of the lactone into a carbamate, which increases the lactone moiety's hydrolytic stability and minimizes the extent of epimerization.

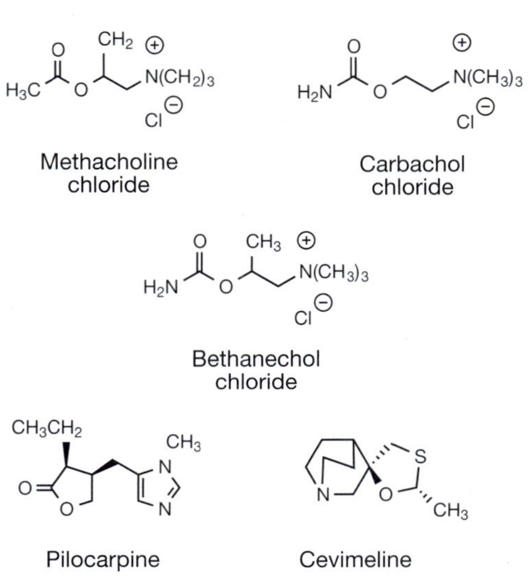

Figure 28.25 Muscarinic agonists.

Cevimeline. Cevimeline is a nonclassic agonist of the mAChR. It is derived from a cyclic amine called quinuclidine. Cevimeline exhibits affinity for M_1 receptors in the CNS and M_3 receptors in epithelial tissue of lacrimal and salivary glands. It is administered orally for the treatment of dry mouth and acts in the same manner as pilocarpine. Some of the important contraindications to the use of these mAChR agonists include asthma, GU or GI tract obstructions, and peptic acid–related illnesses. The metabolic profile of cevimeline includes CYP2D6-, CYP3A3-, and CYP3A4-catalyzed oxidations. The thioether is oxidized to the sulfoxide, and the amine is converted to the *N*-oxide. It is also metabolized by phase 2 glucuronidation.

Muscarinic Receptor Antagonists

Muscarinic antagonists competitively and reversibly bind to mAChR and prevent the binding of ACh. It is proposed that binding of muscarinic antagonists induces a conformational change in the receptor that is different from the conformation induced by agonists and uncouples the receptor from its G protein. By blocking ACh access to the mAChR, antimuscarinic agents decrease the contraction of smooth muscle of the GI and urinary tracts and reduce gastric, mucociliary, and salivary secretions. Due to their relaxant effect, they are useful therapeutic agents for the treatment of smooth muscle spasm and OAB. Since they also reduce gastric secretions, they were at one time useful therapeutic agents for the management of peptic ulcers. However, these drugs lost their place in clinical practice due to the introduction of more effective H_2 antagonists and PPIs (as previously discussed).

A recent study has illuminated the mode of binding of antimuscarinics with the M_2 receptor. It is proposed that binding of sterically bulky molecules (ie, muscarinic antagonists) blocks the activation-related contraction of the binding pocket, which locks the M_2 receptor in an inactive conformation (Fig. 28.26).[142] This leads to the observed antagonistic activity.

Antimuscarinic agents exhibit several predictable adverse effects based on their inhibition of ACh-induced actions, including blurred vision, photophobia, dry mouth, and difficulty in urination. Antimuscarinics that act centrally are sedative, which can be viewed as either an adverse effect or, when needed to avoid motion sickness, a therapeutic benefit (eg, scopolamine, discussed next). Taken together, the effect of antimuscarinic agents has been very useful in treating various

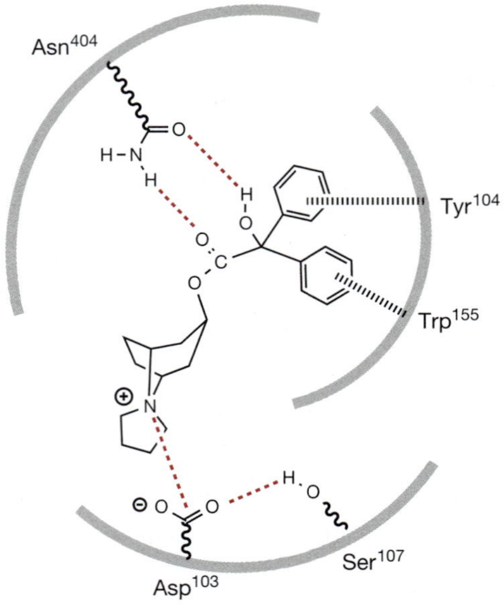

Figure 28.26 Proposed binding interactions of a model anticholinergic drug (3-quinuclidinyl benzilate) with the M_2 receptor.

GI and GU disorders,[136] and selected agents are available as both prescription-based and OTC drugs.

Alkaloids from Solanaceae Family—Atropine and Scopolamine

Atropine and scopolamine are two natural products from the plant family *Solanaceae* and the earliest known anticholinergic agents. They are competitive mAChR antagonists and prevent the action of ACh and other direct- and indirect-acting muscarinic agonists. While they are not used in the treatment of GI or GU disorders, they served as the template for the design of new antimuscarinics that are structurally similar, and their chemistry is briefly summarized later.

Atropine is a tropine ester of tropic acid (Fig. 28.27). The tertiary amine functionality within this molecule makes it a basic drug, and it is clinically available as the sulfate salt. The naturally occurring (−)-hyoscyamine undergoes racemization during isolation and yields the racemic mixture of (+) and (−)-isomers known as atropine. The tropic acid component has the stereogenic center that undergoes racemization. The bicyclic tropane-scaffold is the other preserved component of these natural products. Atropine has been used as a preoperative agent to reduce secretions prior to a surgery. Following administration of atropine sulfate, approximately half is excreted in the urine in its parent form, while the remainder is excreted as the *N*-demethylated noratropine metabolite, the *N*-oxide, and hydrolysis products.

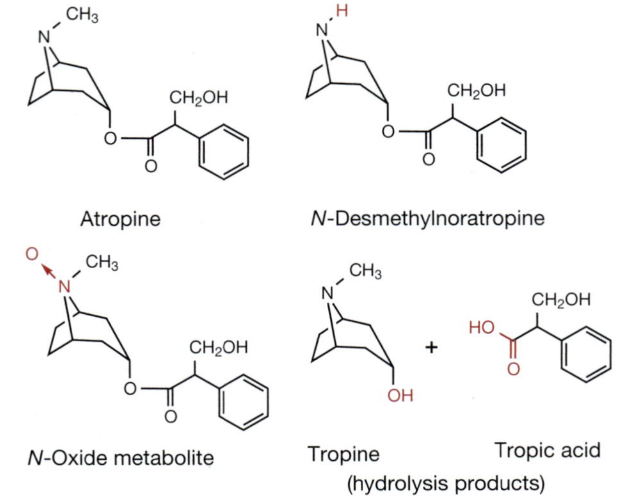

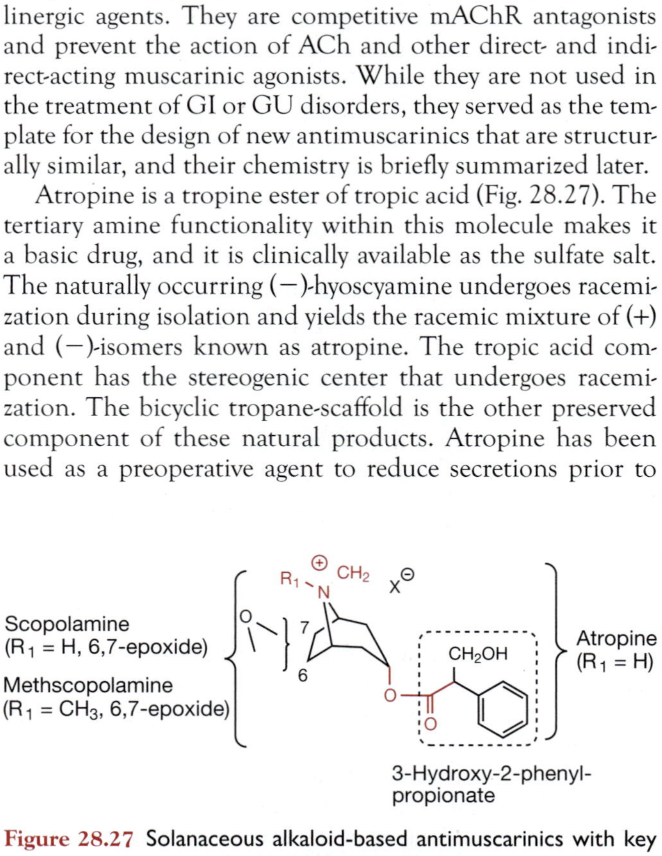

Figure 28.27 Solanaceous alkaloid-based antimuscarinics with key structural features of acetylcholine (Ach) highlighted in red.

The other natural alkaloid, scopolamine ((−)-hyoscine) is structurally very similar to atropine. It is also a tropane ester of tropic acid, but the tropane core in scopolamine has a 6,7-epoxide functionality (Fig. 28.27). Scopolamine is available as the hydrobromide salt for clinical use. The interesting pharmacologic difference between atropine and scopolamine is that atropine is a CNS stimulant and scopolamine is a CNS depressant. Scopolamine is clinically used for the treatment of iritis, uveitis, and Parkinsonism. Scopolamine is extensively metabolized by hepatic enzymes via phase 1 reactions that are similar to atropine metabolism and through glucuronide conjugation of the hydroxyl group.[143]

Structural Features and Structure-Activity Relationships

The SAR of atropine has provided the structural information needed for designing synthetic antimuscarinic agents. As discussed, the ester- and the nitrogen-containing functional groups of the endogenous mAChR ligand ACh are important for binding. Similarly, the ester and tertiary amine group found in atropine and scopolamine are important structural features. Antimuscarinics bind to the mAChR in a similar fashion to ACh, where the ester group forms a hydrogen bond with a conserved active site Asn residue, and the quaternary ammonium nitrogen forms an ionic interaction with conserved active site Asp residue. Both of these interactions are shown in Figure 28.26. Additionally, several aromatic residues within the active site, such as Phe, Trp, and Tyr, provide additional hydrophobic regions for stronger binding affinity of antimuscarinics.[142] Although the ester and amine groups within atropine are separated by more than two carbons (unlike in ACh), the conformation assumed by the tropane ring places these two functional groups close to each other, with a distance similar to that found in ACh. The key structural difference between ACh and atropine is the size of the acyl portion.

Based on the proposal that sterically larger molecules tend to block mAChR and behave as antagonists, several analogues of atropine have been designed and synthesized as potential antimuscarinic agents. Based on the structural modifications and bioactivity profile, it was evident that most potent mAChR antagonists contain two lipophilic ring substitutions on the acyl group (α to the carbonyl group of the ester). Antimuscarinic SAR that describes the impact of substituents on the antimuscarinic pharmacophore is briefly summarized next.[136,144]

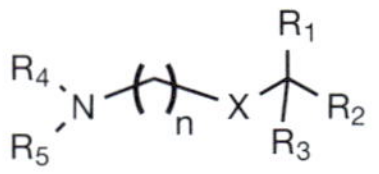

Antimuscarinic pharmacophore

- R_1 and R_2 should be carbocyclic or heterocyclic rings and bind to the mAChR through hydrophobic and/or π stacking interactions with active site Tyr, Phe, and Trp residues that lie outside the ACh binding pocket (see Fig. 28.26).[144] Optimal potency is observed when one ring is aromatic and the other is saturated. Typically, five- or six-membered ring substituents are optimal. Analogues containing larger ring structures, such as naphthalene, tend to be inactive, perhaps due to increased steric bulk.
- The R_3 substituent is variable, with a hydrogen atom, a hydroxy group, a hydroxymethyl group, or a carboxamide group all acceptable. H-bonding hydroxy or hydroxymethyl substituents are optimal and can be a substituent on the R_1 or R_2 ring system. These groups interact with a conserved Asn residue within the mAChR active site through two hydrogen bonding interactions.
- The connecting functional group "X" in most analogues is an ester, mimicking ACh. However, ether and carbon X moieties also produce active compounds. The nature of the connecting group allows antimuscarinic agents to be chemically classified as aminoalkyl esters, aminoalkyl ethers, or aminoalcohols. The nitrogen is typically a quaternary ammonium species (most potent) or a tertiary amine. The tertiary amine will be extensively protonated at physiological pH to generate the cationic species needed for ionic interaction with the conserved active site Asp residue.
- R_4 and R_5 are typically small alkyl groups such methyl, ethyl, propyl, or isopropyl. Some compounds contain a cyclic motif to yield the quaternary nitrogen.
- Due to molecular flexibility, the distance between the nitrogen atom of the tertiary or quaternary amine and the ring-substituted carbon seems to be less critical for activity. Normally, the linking chain is two (optimal) to four carbons.

Synthetic Muscarinic Antagonists

As discussed earlier, the atropine scaffold has been used as the structural model for developing the SAR for the synthetic antimuscarinic agents. Because the outer regions of the mAChR are largely hydrophobic in nature, they bind more strongly than ACh and in a competitive manner. The most common synthetic antimuscarinic agents used to treat OAB are given in Figure 28.28. There are representatives from the aminoalkyl ester class (solifenacin, oxybutynin, trospium chloride) and modified aminoalcohols (X = carbon) where the OH has been replaced by an aromatic ether substituent (tolterodine, fesoterodine) or an amide (darifenacin). These agents all follow the classic SAR, where a tertiary amine or quaternary ammonium motif and a bulky hydrophobic structure are present.[145,146]

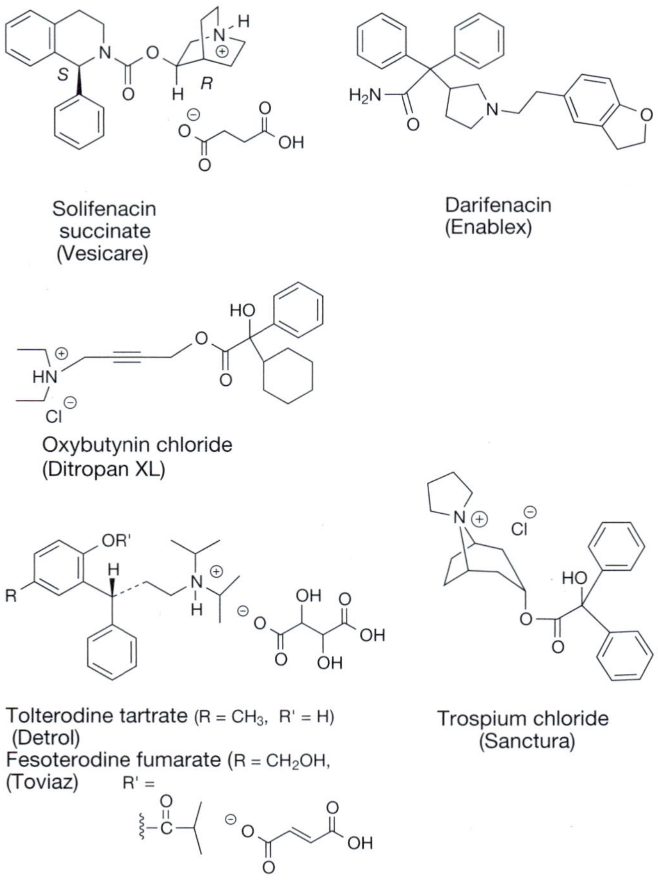

Figure 28.28 Antimuscarinics used in overactive bladder.

Therapeutic Use in Overactive Bladder

OAB is associated with urinary frequency or nocturia. It is a common health disorder that affects the quality of life for many and can be successfully treated with antimuscarinics.[147] As discussed earlier, antimuscarinics decrease smooth muscle contraction in the bladder by acting on M_2 or M_3 subtypes.[148,149] The common mAChR antagonists used for the treatment of OAB are oxybutynin, trospium chloride, tolterodine, fesoterodine, darifenacin, and solifenacin (Fig. 28.28).[150] These agents are also able to control GI motility and secretions by inhibiting the effects of parasympathetic activity in the gut. Antimuscarinics reduce gastric and salivary gland secretions by acting on the M_1 subtype; however, they produce pronounced adverse effects due to their nonselective binding to other muscarinic receptor subtypes.

While they were once widely used to manage peptic ulcer disease, their utility in that disease state has significantly declined.

Chemically, trospium chloride contains a quaternary ammonium motif that is permanently cationic, so it is generally not well absorbed from the GI tract. The remainder of the antimuscarinics used in OAB possess a basic tertiary amine motif and, therefore, exist in both cationic and unionized base forms in the gut. They are better absorbed relative to the quaternary ammonium salt. Moreover, the change provides better systemic distribution regardless of the route of administration. The tertiary amine–containing drugs also cross the blood-brain barrier very well, leading to central adverse effects.

Although these are all effective antimuscarinic agents, their nonspecific binding to mAChR subtypes causes several predictable adverse effects, including xerostomia (dry mouth), blurred vision, constipation, and dyspepsia. Binding of antimuscarinics to receptors in CNS causes drowsiness, dizziness, and confusion. Oxybutynin is the oldest mAChR antagonist clinically used for the treatment of OAB. Improved formulations and delivery methods (ie, transdermal delivery, extended-release formulations) have been developed to minimize generally observed unwanted actions. Solifenacin and darifenacin show selectivity toward M_3 receptors, giving a desirable ratio of efficacy to adverse effects.[151]

The pharmacological properties and receptor-subtype selectivity of the synthetic antimuscarinics used in OAB are given in Table 28.4.

Table 28.4 Antimuscarinic Agents Used in Overactive Bladder

Name	Calculated[a] Log P	Half-Life (h)	Metabolism	Comments
Trospium chloride (Sanctura)	-	20	Hydrolysis; conjugation	High affinity for M_1 and M_3 receptors; lesser affinity for M_2
Oxybutynin (oral: Ditropan and Ditropan XL; transdermal: Oxytrol)	4.44 (Log P)	2-5	CYP3A4; hydrolysis; N-dealkylation	Nonselective muscarinic antagonist
Solifenacin (Vesicare)	3.96 (Log P)	55	4-(*R*)-Hydroxy (active); *N*-glucuronide; *N*-oxide; 4*R*-hydroxy-*N*-oxide	Selective M_3 antagonist
Tolterodine (Detrol)	5.12 (Log P)	2-4 (extensive metabolizers); 9.6 (poor metabolizers)	Primary pathway: CYP2D6 (primary); 7% of Whites and 2% of African Americans lack CYP2D6; CYP3A4 is the primary pathway in the latter. Metabolites: 5-hydroxymethyl (active), 5-carboxylic acid, *N*-dealkylated-5-carboxylic acid	Nonselective muscarinic antagonist
Fesoterodine fumarate (Toviaz)	5.70 (Log P)	7	Hydrolysis to 5-hydroxymethyl tolterodine, followed by CYP2D6 and CYP3A4 to give carboxy, carboxy-N-desisopropy, N-desisopropyl metabolites	Prodrug of 5-hydroxymethyl tolterodine, a nonselective muscarinic agonist
Darifenacin (Enablex)	4.54 (Log P)	-	CYP2D6 (primary; see "tolterodine" in this table); hydroxylation of the dihydrobenzofuran; ring opening (dihydrobenzofuran); N-dealkylation	Selective M_3 antagonist

[a]www.drugbank.ca. Accessed July 16, 2025. (values for quaternary compounds are not listed).

Metabolism

The synthetic anticholinergic agents discussed here are all extensively metabolized by hepatic enzymes and, if they contain an ester linkage, undergo both enzymatic (plasma esterase) and nonenzymatic (acidic or basic pH) hydrolysis. One of the most common hepatic oxidation reactions of antimuscarinic agents is N-oxidation. Since many of these compounds possess a tertiary amine group, CYP enzyme–catalyzed oxidation leads to an inactive N-oxide metabolite. Another common reaction is oxidative N-dealkylation. A summary of common metabolic reactions for selected anticholinergic agents is given in Table 28.4 and Figure 28.29. To illustrate the metabolic reactions in this class of agents, some common metabolic transformations are summarized here. Several of the phase 1 metabolites undergo conjugation via phase 2 metabolic transformations.[146]

- Trospium is predominantly metabolized via hydrolysis.
- Darifenacin is oxidized by CYP2D6 and CYP3A4 to generate a phenolic hydroxyl group and a ring-opened carboxylic acid metabolite (Fig. 28.29). An *N*-dealkylated metabolite is generated via the action of CYP3A4.[152]
- Tolterodine (active) and fesoterodine (a tolterodine prodrug) undergo CYP2D6-mediated oxidation and esterase-mediated hydrolysis, respectively, to a common active benzylic alcohol metabolite that is further oxidized by CYP3A4 and 2D6 to an inactive carboxylic acid. The *N*-dealkylated metabolite of tolterodine and fesoterodine is inactive.
- Solifenacin is converted into the inactive *N*-oxide by the action of CYP3A4. A benzylic oxidation of solifenacin yields the corresponding hydroxy metabolite, which is active. The hydroxy metabolite subsequently forms an inactive glucuronide conjugate and is excreted.
- Oxybutynin is metabolized by CYP3A4 to the corresponding dealkylated metabolite, which retains biological activity. The carboxylic acid metabolite generated via hydrolysis is pharmacologically inactive.

Specific Drugs

OXYBUTYNIN. Oxybutynin is one of the oldest mAChR antagonists used in OAB. It relaxes bladder urothelium, calms overactive detrusor smooth muscle contractions, and interferes with cholinergic neurotransmission in bladder afferent pathways, resulting in a decrease in urinary urgency and frequency.[138] While the M_2 mAChR subtype is most prevalent in human bladder, M_3 is viewed as the critical receptor mediating the therapeutic utility of antimuscarinics in OAB.[150]

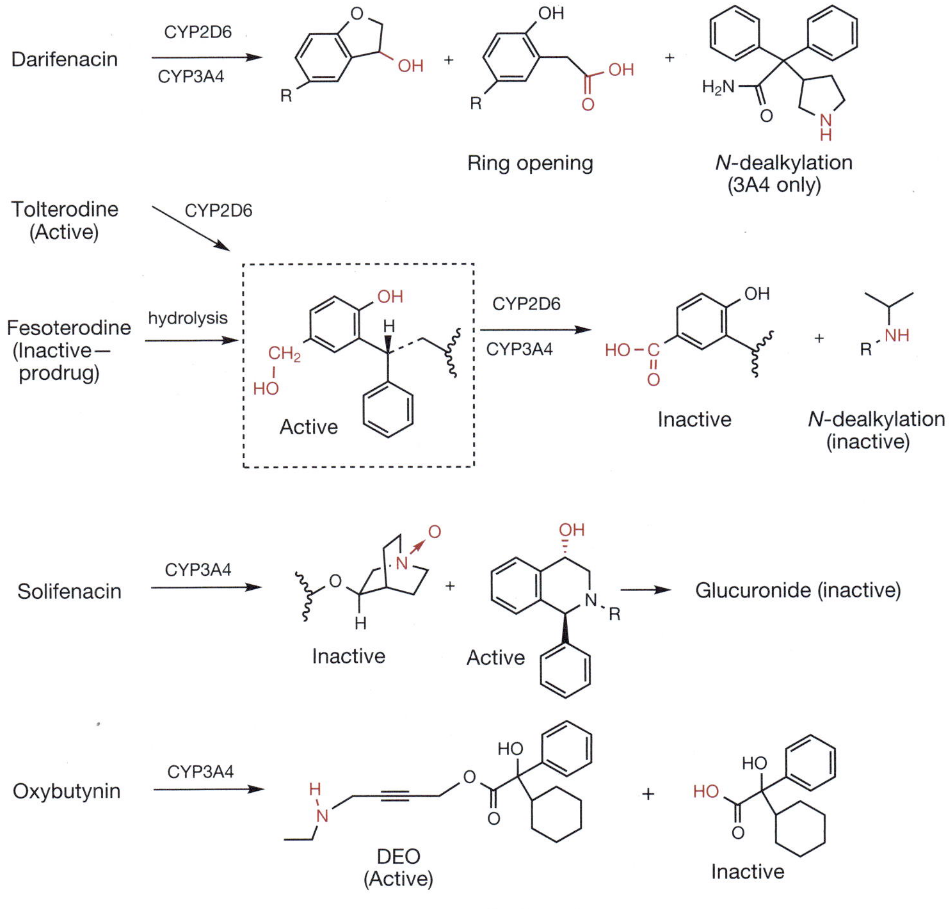

Figure 28.29 Metabolism of selected antimuscarinics.

The dealkylated desethyl metabolite (DEO, Fig. 28.29) noted earlier is generated in both gut and liver and binds with high affinity to salivary mAChRs (M_1 and M_3 subtypes[153,154]), resulting in a high incidence of dry mouth which can limit patient acceptability.[150,153] While the parent drug has low affinity for the M_2 subtype,[155] the DEO metabolite is deemed responsible for the potential induction of cardiac arrhythmias (an M_2 effect[145]) that negatively impacts adherence.[155] In fact, it has been estimated that between 43% and 83% of women patients stop antimuscarinic therapy (including oxybutynin, which carries the highest risk of adverse effects) within a month of initiation.[156]

Oxybutynin is marketed as the racemic mixture, but its antimuscarinic action is isolated to the *R*-isomer.[154] It is over 99% protein bound. In addition to tablet and syrup formulations, extended-release tablets and transdermal gel and patch dosage forms that limit DEO formation (and, therefore, adverse effects) are clinically available.[150,156] With regard to therapeutic efficacy, oxybutynin immediate- and extended-release formulations are comparable and statistically equivalent to tolterodine and darifenacin (see later).[150,154] Combination therapy that includes oxybutynin (eg, in combination with solifenacin or tolterodine) has been shown to provide symptom relief superior to the partner product alone.[156] The transdermal gel and patch formulations have demonstrated efficacy compared to placebo, and patients may experience mild-moderate application site pruritus from their use.[150]

OAB incidence rises as patients age,[150] and caution must be used when treating older adults, particularly frail older adults, as antimuscarinic agents can negatively impact gait stability and cognition.[153,156] Oxybutynin in particular has been associated with serious decreases in attention and cognitive function due to central M_1 receptor antagonism, and the benefits of its use in vulnerable patients should clearly outweigh the risks. Safer choices include the quaternary trospium chloride (which does not penetrate the blood-brain barrier) and the M_3-selective antagonist darifenacin, which also has a low level of CNS accumulation due to active efflux from the brain via P-gp (Fig. 28.28).[156]

Oxybutynin, and all antimuscarinic OAB agents, should be used with extreme caution or be avoided altogether in patients with urinary obstructions, compromised GI motility, or uncontrolled narrow angle glaucoma. This agent can exacerbate gastroesophageal reflux, which can be a use-limiting adverse effect in patients already suffering from GERD.

DARIFENACIN. Darifenacin is an M_3 selective antimuscarinic that acts quickly to improve OAB symptoms, often within the first week of therapy. It is available in extended-release tablets and costs more per dose than any of the other orally available OAB options.[154] Dry mouth and constipation are its most commonly observed adverse effects, but they are normally not severe enough to prompt discontinuation.[150,154] As alluded to, cognition impairment with darifenacin use is not significantly different from placebo,[150,156] and its safety and tolerability in patients older than age 65 years have been documented.[157]

Darifenacin is metabolized by both CYP3A4 and 2D6 (Fig. 28.29). Manufacturer dosing guidelines recommend a downward adjustment when darifenacin is co-administered with strong CYP3A4 inhibitors, but the caution does not apply to co-administered CYP2D6 inhibitors.[154] It is highly protein bound, and the inactive metabolites are excreted in both the urine and feces.

TOLTERODINE/FESOTERODINE. Tolterodine and fesoterodine are structurally related nonselective aminoalkyl antimuscarinics (Fig. 28.28). While the former contains a phenolic OH essential to pharmacological action, the latter is an inactive isobutyrate ester of that phenol and must hydrolyze to provide therapeutic utility. The hydrolyzing enzymes are nonspecific esterases. As shown in Figure 28.29, tolterodine undergoes CYP2D6-mediated benzylic hydroxylation to provide the identical active metabolite, 5-hydroxymethyltolterodine (5-HMT), and the elimination half-life in 2D6 PMs rise from 2 to 10 hours (immediate-release tablet) and from 7 to 18 hours (extended-release capsule). As shown in Figure 28.29, the active 5-HMT metabolite is inactivated by both CYP3A4 and 2D6. Excretion of both drugs and their metabolites is predominantly renal, and the presence of 5-HMT in the urinary bladder has been proposed to potentially play a role in their therapeutic action.[155]

Tolterodine binds to mAChRs in the bladder and submaxillary gland with approximately equal affinity, although the binding to bladder receptors is more prolonged. The 5-HMT metabolite preferentially binds to the M_3 receptor in bladder.[150] As noted earlier, tolterodine has OAB efficacy comparable to oxybutynin with a much lower risk of adverse effects, although the incidence of dry mouth is significantly higher than placebo.[150] Once-daily administration of the extended-release capsule formulation is claimed to be slightly more effective in attenuating urinary urge incontinence than twice-daily administration of the immediate-release tablets and may result in less dry mouth.[154] Tolterodine (but not fesoterodine) can prolong the QT interval at therapeutic doses and must be used with care in patients vulnerable to arrhythmia.[154] While tolterodine is over 96% protein bound, 5-HMT is only modestly sequestered by albumin (36%-54%).[155]

Pharmacokinetics of Fesoterodine is less complex than that of tolterodine, given its lack of dependence on the highly polymorphic CYP2D6 for the generation of the active 5-HMT metabolite. Hydrolysis to this active metabolite is rapid and complete, and the elimination half-life of the extended-release tablet (the only formulation marketed) is 7 hours. A head-to-head comparison of the OAB therapeutic efficacy of 8 mg fesoterodine versus 4 mg extended-release tolterodine showed fesoterodine to be superior in decreasing urinary urge incontinence episodes, increasing the ability of the bladder to hold urine and providing patients with a perceived enhanced physical and emotional quality of life.[158] Neither fesoterodine nor 5-HMT concentrates in the CNS due to limited blood-brain barrier penetration and active efflux from central sites by P-gp.[150] In contrast, tolterodine is not a P-gp substrate and the risk of cognitive impairment would conceivably be higher.[157] However, the safety of tolterodine in the elderly is generally viewed as comparable with younger patient populations.[159]

SOLIFENACIN. Solifenacin enjoys a high M_3 receptor selectivity and, thus, is less problematic for patients with OAB as far as M_1- and M_2-mediated adverse reactions are concerned.[150] Its primary mechanism of action is inhibition of detrusor smooth muscle contraction, and it is marketed as the pure 1*S*, 3*R*-isomer (see Fig. 28.28). Efficacy studies have given it the edge over tolterodine in terms of urinary urgency, frequency, and urinary urge incontinence episodes. The OAB efficacy is viewed as comparable to fesoterodine.[150] In addition to decreasing daytime urinary frequency and urge incontinence, solifenacin provides therapeutic benefit to patients experiencing nocturia.[154]

Solifenacin has a decreased incidence of dry mouth when compared to tolterodine. The drug is not a P-gp substrate, but no worsening of cognition impairment in mildly impaired elders has been observed, likely due to its high M_3 selectivity.[150,156] However, the AUC can increase between 20% and 25% in older adults,[160] which may put them at risk for other adverse effects. Like tolterodine, prolongation of the QT interval is possible.[154] Patient adherence to the prescribed regimen of solifenacin has been found to be higher than for other antimuscarinic agents.[155]

Solifenacin is available as immediate-release tablets and has a prolonged elimination half-life of 45-68 hours. Like most OAB antimuscarinics, solifenacin is strongly protein bound (>98%).[160] CYP3A4 is the principal isoform involved in its metabolism and, like darifenacin, the manufacturer recommends decreasing the dose if strong CYP3A4 inhibitors must be co-administered.[154] The most abundant metabolite, 4*R*-hydroxysolifenacin (see Fig. 28.29) is comparatively active with the parent structure but is unlikely to contribute to therapeutic efficacy due to its low concentration.[161] The *N*-oxides of the 4*R*-hydroxymetabolite (generated by CYP3A4) and the parent drug (generated by multiple CYP isoforms) are inactive.

TROSPIUM CHLORIDE. While not used clinically to the extent of the other drugs described in this section, trospium chloride bears mentioning because it is the only quaternary amine antimuscarinic available for OAB. It has the highest affinity for all mAChR subtypes and is a powerful inhibitor of bladder and detrusor smooth muscle contractions.[150] Immediate-release tablets and extended-release capsules are marketed, and dry mouth and constipation are the major adverse effects. The extended-release dosage form has an elimination half-life of 35 hours (~15 hours longer than the immediate-release formulation) and maintains efficacy over 24 hours.[150,162] Trospium is effective in patients experiencing nocturia.

As a quaternary amine, trospium chloride's ability to penetrate membranes is poor. Oral absorption is less than 10%,[162] and it does not cross the blood-brain barrier. While ester hydrolysis can occur, the majority of a dose is excreted unchanged in the feces.

β-Adrenergic Agonists

Mirabegron

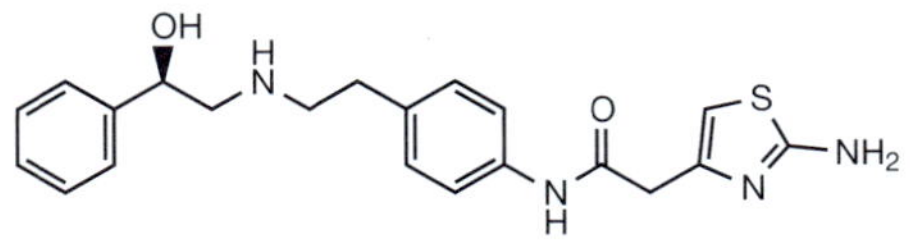

Mirabegron
(Myrbetriq)

Mirabegron is an orally active agent for the treatment of OAB. It is a potent β_3-adrenoreceptor agonist that activates receptors in bladder tissue and causes dose-dependent detrusor relaxation. Once administered, it is rapidly absorbed and well distributed. A large percentage (71%) is bound to plasma proteins. The fat content of the food affects the bioavailability of mirabegron. Several metabolic pathways have been identified through which mirabegron is metabolized, including dealkylation, oxidation, hydrolysis, and glucuronidation. The various oxidative biotransformations are linked to the activity of CYP3A4, CYP2D6, and alcohol dehydrogenase. Due to its dependence on CYP2D6, polymorphism of CYP2D6 causes pharmacokinetic differences among PM, EM, and UM phenotypes.[163,164]

Vibegron

Vibegron is another orally active β_3-adrenoreceptor agonist available for the treatment of OAB. It exhibits notable structural similarity to mirabegron. Vibegron is designed to contain a pyrrolidine ring to mimic the secondary amine, and a fused heterocyclic structure, in place of the thiazole group in mirabegron. Vibegron is a selective agonist of the human β_3-adrenoreceptor, and it shows much lower binding toward β_1- and β_2-receptors. Following oral administration of a 75-mg tablet, maximum absorption is observed within 1 to 3 hours. There was no significant change in pharmacokinetics observed when vibegron is taken in various types of food. Vibegron has an effective half-life is approximately 31 hours. Based on the chemical structure, oxidation is a common transformation linked to drug metabolism. Vibegron is metabolized by CYP3A4. It is not identified as an inhibitor or inducer of major CYP enzymes. Additionally, very low risk of drug-drug interaction is observed based on CYP enzyme activity. In vitro studies showed that vibegron is a substrate for P-gp, but not an inhibitor of P-gp activity.[165,166]

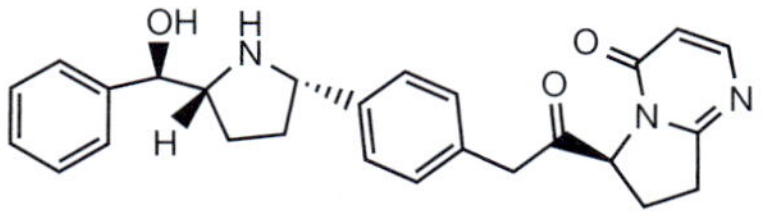

Vibegron (Gemtesa)

Structure Challenge

Based on your knowledge about the pharmacophore and drug action of the following therapeutic agents/structures, answer the following questions.

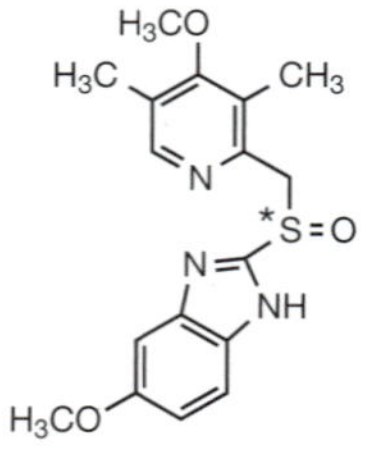

1

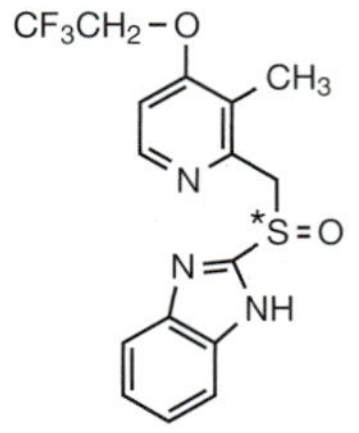

2

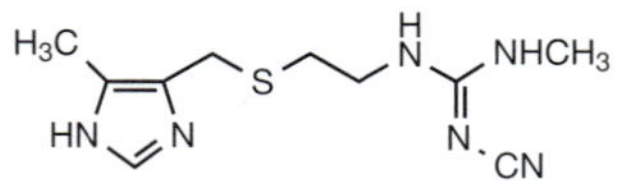

3

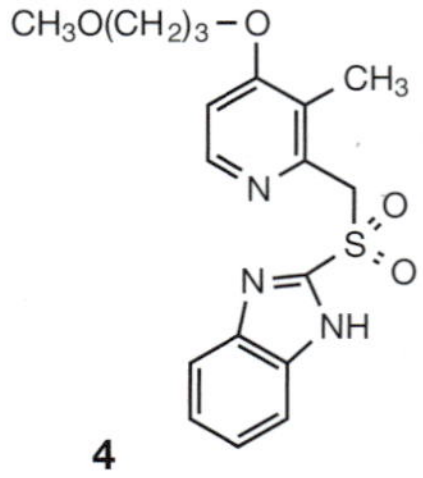

4

A. Which drug is designed based on structural features of histamine and considered an H_2-antihistamine?
B. Based on your knowledge about the mechanism of drug action of the given structures, which molecules inhibit the gastric H^+/K^+-ATPase?
C. Select all structures that can act as a covalent inhibitor of the gastric proton pump.
D. Describe the mechanism of acid-catalyzed activation of Drug 1.
E. Considering SAR and mechanism of action, would you expect structure 4 to be an effective inhibitor of gastric proton pump?
F. Describe the metabolic pathway that generates structure 4.

Structure Challenge answers found immediately after References.

REFERENCES

1. Everhart JE, Ruhl CE. Burden of digestive diseases in the United States part I: overall and upper gastrointestinal diseases. *Gastroenterology*. 2009;136:376-386.
2. Everhart JE, Ruhl CE. Burden of digestive diseases in the United States part II: lower gastrointestinal diseases. *Gastroenterology*. 2009;136:741-754.
3. Katz PO, Gerson LB, Vela MF. Guidelines for the diagnosis and management of gastroesophageal reflux disease. *Am J Gastroenterol*. 2013;108:308-328.
4. Sobieraj DM, Coleman SM, Coleman CI. US prevalence of upper gastrointestinal symptoms: a systematic literature review. *Am J Manag Care*. 2011;17:e449-e458.
5. Vakil N. New pharmacological agents for the treatment of gastroesophageal reflux disease. *Rev Gastroenterol Disord*. 2008;8:117-122.
6. Sharkey KA, MacNaughton WK. Pharmacotherapy for gastric acidity, peptic ulcer, and gastroesophageal reflux disease. In: Brunton LL, Hilal-Dandan R, Knollmann BC, eds. *Goodman & Gilman's the Pharmacological Basis of Therapeutics*. 13th ed. McGraw-Hill Medical; 2018:909-920.
7. Kaser A, Zeissig S, Blumberg RS. Inflammatory bowel disease. *Annu Rev Immunol*. 2010;28:573-621.
8. D'Haens GR, Sartor RB, Silverberg MS, et al. Future directions in inflammatory bowel disease management. *J Crohns Colitis*. 2014;8:726-734.
9. Chapple CR, Yamanishi T, Chess-Williams R. Muscarinic receptor subtypes and management of the overactive bladder. *Urology*. 2002;60:82-88; discussion 88-89.
10. Parsons ME, Ganellin CR. Histamine and its receptors. *Br J Pharmacol*. 2006;147(suppl 1):S127-S135.
11. Pino-Angeles A, Reyes-Palomares A, Melgarejo E, et al. Histamine: an undercover agent in multiple rare diseases? *J Cell Mol Med*. 2012;16:1947-1960.
12. Zhang M-Q, Leurs R, Timmerman H. Histamine H1-receptor antagonists. In: Wolff ME, ed. *Burger's Medicinal Chemistry and Drug Discovery*. 5th ed. John Wiley & Sons; 1997:495-559.
13. Cooper DG, Young RC, Durant GJ, et al. Histamine receptors. In: Emmett JC, ed. *Comprehensive Medicinal Chemistry: The Rational Design, Mechanistic Study and Therapeutic Application of Chemical Compounds*. Vol 3. Pergamon Press; 1990:343-421.
14. Watanabe T, Yamatodani A, Maeyama K, et al. Pharmacology of a-fluoromethylhistidine, a specific inhibitor of histidine decarboxylase. *Trends Pharmacol Sci*. 1990;11:363-367.
15. Moya-Garcia AA, Pino-Angeles A, Gil-Redondo R, et al. Structural features of mammalian histidine decarboxylase reveal the basis for specific inhibition. *Br J Pharmacol*. 2009;157:4-13.
16. Katritch V, Cherezov V, Stevens RC. Structure-function of the G protein-coupled receptor superfamily. *Annu Rev Pharmacol Toxicol*. 2013;53:531-556.
17. Nelson WL. Antihistamines and related antiallergic and antiulcer agents. In: Lemke TL, Williams DA, Roche VF, Zito SW, eds. *Foye's Principles of Medicinal Chemistry*. 7th ed. Lippincott Williams & Wilkins; 2012:1045-1072.
18. Hoogerwerf WA, Pasricha PJ. Pharmacotherapy of gastric acidity, peptic ulcers, and gastroesophageal reflux disease. In: Hardman JG, Limbird LE, Mollinoff PB, et al., eds. *Goodman and Gilman's the Pharmacological Basis of Therapeutics*. 11th ed. McGraw-Hill; 2005:968.
19. Shin JM, Munson K, Vagin O, et al. The gastric HK-ATPase: structure, function, and inhibition. *Pflugers Arch*. 2009;457:609-622.
20. Pace F, Porro GB. Gastroesophageal reflux and Helicobacter pylori: a review. *World J Gastroenterol*. 2000;6:311-314.
21. Jones AW. Perspectives in drug development and clinical pharmacology: the discovery of histamine H1 and H2 antagonists. *Clin Pharmacol Drug Dev*. 2016;5:5-12.
22. Roberts S, McDonald IM. Inhibitors of gastric acid secretion. In: Abraham DJ, ed. *Burger's Medicinal Chemistry and Drug Discovery*. 6th ed. Wiley-Interscience; 2003:85-127.
23. Ganellin CR. Discovery of cimetidine. In: Roberts SM, Price AH, eds. *Medicinal Chemistry: The Role of Organic Chemistry in Drug Research*. Academic Press; 1985:93-118.
24. Gantz I, DelValle J, Wang LD, et al. Molecular basis for the interaction of histamine with the histamine H2 receptor. *J Biol Chem*. 1992;267:20840-20843.

25. Price AH, Brogden RN. Nizatidine—a preliminary review of its pharmacodynamic and pharmacokinetic properties, and its therapeutic use in peptic-ulcer disease. *Drugs*. 1988;36:521-539.
26. Penston J, Wormsley KG. Adverse reactions and interactions with H2-receptor antagonists. *Med Toxicol*. 1986;1:192-216.
27. Lin JH. Pharmacokinetic and pharmacodynamic properties of histamine H2-receptor antagonists. Relationship between intrinsic potency and effective plasma concentrations. *Clin Pharmacokinet*. 1991;20:218-236.
28. Stadel R, Yang J, Nalwalk JW, et al. High-affinity binding of [3H] cimetidine to a heme-containing protein in rat brain. *Drug Metab Dispos*. 2008;36:614-621.
29. Sedman AJ. Cimetidine-drug interactions. *Am J Med*. 1984;76: 109-114.
30. Breen KJ, Bury R, Desmond PV, et al. Effects of cimetidine and ranitidine on hepatic drug metabolism. *Clin Pharmacol Ther*. 1982;31:297-300.
31. Berardi RR, Tankanow RM, Nostrant TT. Comparison of famotidine with cimetidine and ranitidine. *Clin Pharm*. 1988;7:271-284.
32. Strand DS, Kim D, Peura DA. 25 years of proton pump inhibitors: a comprehensive review. *Gut Liver*. 2017;11:27-37.
33. Roche VF. The chemically elegant proton pump inhibitors. *Am J Pharm Educ*. 2006;70:101.
34. Robinson M. Proton pump inhibitors: update on their role in acid-related gastrointestinal diseases. *Int J Clin Pract*. 2005;59:709-715.
35. Lindberg P, Brandstrom A, Wallmark B, et al. Omeprazole: the first proton pump inhibitor. *Med Res Rev*. 1990;10:1-54.
36. Jana K, Bandyopadhyay T, Ganguly B. Revealing the mechanistic pathway of acid activation of proton pump inhibitors to inhibit the gastric proton pump: a DFT study. *J Phys Chem B*. 2016;120:13031-13038.
37. Shin JM, Sachs G. Pharmacology of proton pump inhibitors. *Curr Gastroenterol Rep*. 2008;10:528-534.
38. Shin JM, Cho YM, Sachs G. Chemistry of covalent inhibition of the gastric (H^+, K^+)-ATPase by proton pump inhibitors. *J Am Chem Soc*. 2004;126:7800-7811.
39. Scott SA, Sangkuhl K, Shuldiner AR, et al. PharmGKB summary: very important pharmacogene information for cytochrome P450, family 2, subfamily C, polypeptide 19. *Pharmacogenet Genomics*. 2012;22:159-165.
40. Andersson T. Pharmacokinetics, metabolism and interactions of acid pump inhibitors—focus on omeprazole, lansoprazole and pantoprazole. *Clin Pharmacokinet*. 1996;31:9-28.
41. Andersson T. Single-isomer drugs—true therapeutic advances. *Clin Pharmacokinet*. 2004;43:279-285.
42. Ishizaki T, Horai Y. Review article: cytochrome P450 and the metabolism of proton pump inhibitors–emphasis on rabeprazole. *Aliment Pharmacol Ther*. 1999;13(suppl 3):27-36.
43. Shin JM, Kim N. Pharmacokinetics and pharmacodynamics of the proton pump inhibitors. *J Neurogastroenterol Motil*. 2013;19:25-35.
44. Zhou Q, Yan XF, Pan WS, et al. Is the required therapeutic effect always achieved by racemic switch of proton-pump inhibitors? *World J Gastroenterol*. 2008;14:2617-2619.
45. Huang B, Huang Y, Li Y, et al. Adverse cardiovascular effects of concomitant use of proton pump inhibitors and clopidogrel in patients with coronary artery disease: a systematic review and meta-analysis. *Arch Med Res*. 2012;43:212-224.
46. Drepper MD, Spahr L, Frossard JL. Clopidogrel and proton pump inhibitors–where do we stand in 2012? *World J Gastroenterol*. 2012;18:2161-2171.
47. Hung SC, Liao KF, Hung HC, et al. Using proton pump inhibitors correlates with an increased risk of chronic kidney disease: a nationwide database-derived case-controlled study. *Fam Pract*. 2018;35:166-171.
48. Lazarus B, Chen Y, Wilson FP, et al. Proton pump inhibitor use and the risk of chronic kidney disease. *JAMA Intern Med*. 2016;176:238-246.
49. Lind T, Rydberg L, Kyleback A, et al. Esomeprazole provides improved acid control vs. omeprazole in patients with symptoms of gastro-oesophageal reflux disease. *Aliment Pharmacol Ther*. 2000;14:861-867.
50. Andersson T, Weidolf L. Stereoselective disposition of proton pump inhibitors. *Clin Drug Investig*. 2008;28:263-279.
51. Souza RC, Lima JH. Helicobacter pylori and gastroesophageal reflux disease: a review of this intriguing relationship. *Dis Esophagus*. 2009;22:256-263.
52. Omeprazole. *Drug Facts and Comparisons. Facts & Comparisons eAnswers [database online]*. Wolters Kluwer Health, Inc; 2005. *Accessed November 07, 2018*.
53. Metz DC, Vakily M, Dixit T, et al. Review article: dual delayed release formulation of dexlansoprazole MR, a novel approach to overcome the limitations of conventional single release proton pump inhibitor therapy. *Aliment Pharmacol Ther*. 2009;29:928-937.
54. Gunaratne AW, Hamblin H, Clancy A, et al. Combination of antibiotics and vonoprazan for the treatment of *Helicobacter pylori* infections-exploratory study. *Helicobacter*. 2021;26:e12830.
55. Echizen H. The first-in-class potassium-competitive acid blocker, vonoprazan fumarate: pharmacokinetic and pharmacodynamic considerations. *Clin Pharmacokinet*. 2016;55:409-418.
56. Graham DY, Dore MP. Update on the use of vonoprazan: a competitive acid blocker. *Gastroenterology*. 2018;154:462-466.
57. Acosta A, Camilleri M. Prokinetics in gastroparesis. *Gastroenterol Clin North Am*. 2015;44:97-111.
58. Gershon MD. Review article: serotonin receptors and transporters—roles in normal and abnormal gastrointestinal motility. *Aliment Pharmacol Ther*. 2004;20(suppl 7):3-14.
59. Livezey MR, Briggs ED, Bolles AK, et al. Metoclopramide is metabolized by CYP2D6 and is a reversible inhibitor, but not inactivator, of CYP2D6. *Xenobiotica*. 2014;44:309-319.
60. Patel S, Berrada D, Lembo A. Review of tegaserod in the treatment of irritable bowel syndrome. *Expert Opin Pharmacother*. 2004;5:2369-2379.
61. Curran MP, Robinson DM. Mosapride in gastrointestinal disorders. *Drugs*. 2008;68:981-991.
62. Frampton JE. Prucalopride. *Drugs*. 2009;69:2463-2476.
63. Holtmann G, Talley NJ, Liebregts T, et al. A placebo-controlled trial of itopride in functional dyspepsia. *N Engl J Med*. 2006;354:832-840.
64. Quigley EM. Prokinetics in the management of functional gastrointestinal disorders. *J Neurogastroenterol Motil*. 2015;21:330-336.
65. Quigley EMM. Prokinetics in the management of functional gastrointestinal disorders. *Curr Gastroenterol Rep*. 2017;19:53.
66. Wallace JL. Prostaglandins, NSAIDs, and gastric mucosal protection: why doesn't the stomach digest itself? *Physiol Rev*. 2008;88:1547-1565.
67. Collins PW. Misoprostol: discovery, development, and clinical applications. *Med Res Rev*. 1990;10:149-172.
68. Nagashima R, Yoshida N. Sucralfate, a basic aluminum salt of sucrose sulfate. I. Behaviors in gastroduodenal pH. *Arzneimittelforschung*. 1979;29:1668-1676.
69. Nagashima R, Yoshida N, Terao N. Sucralfate, a basic aluminum salt of sucrose sulfate. II. Inhibition of peptic hydrolysis as it results from sucrose sulfate interaction with protein substrate, serum albumins. *Arzneimittelforschung*. 1980;30:73-76.
70. Marks IN. Sucralfate: worldwide experience in recurrence therapy. *J Clin Gastroenterol*. 1987;9(suppl 1):18-22.
71. Frazer A, Hensler JG. Serotonin. In: Siegel GJ, Agranoff BW, Albers RW, et al, eds. *Basic Neurochemistry*. Raven Press; 1993:283-308.
72. Langlois M, Fischmeister R. 5-HT4 receptor ligands: applications and new prospects. *J Med Chem*. 2003;46:319-344.
73. Glennon RA, Dukat M. Serotonin receptors and drugs affecting serotonergic neurotransmission. In: Lemke TL, Williams DA, Roche VF, et al, eds. *Foye's Principles of Medicinal Chemistry*. 6th ed. Lippincott Williams & Wilkins; 2008:415-443.
74. Nichols DE, Nichols CD. Serotonin receptors. *Chem Rev*. 2008;108: 1614-1641.
75. Hoyer D, Clarke DE, Fozard JR, et al. International union of pharmacology classification of receptors for 5-hydroxytryptamine (serotonin). *Pharmacol Rev*. 1994;46:157-203.
76. Lameh J, Cone RI, Maeda S, et al. Structure and function of G-protein coupled receptors. *Pharm Res*. 1990;7:1213-1221.
77. Barnes NM, Hales TG, Lummis SCR, et al. The 5-HT3 receptor—the relationship between structure and function. *Neuropharmacology*. 2009;56:273-284.

78. Bockaert J, Claeysen S, Compan V, et al. 5-HT4 receptors. *Curr Drug Targets CNS Neurol Disord*. 2004;3:39-51.
79. Gaster LM, King FD. Serotonin 5-HT3 and 5-HT4 receptor antagonists. *Med Res Rev*. 1997;17:163-214.
80. Glennon RA, Dukat M. Serotonin receptors and drugs affecting adrenergic neurotransmission. In: Lemke TL, Williams DA, Roche VF, Zito SW, eds. *Foye's Principles of Medicinal Chemistry*. 7th ed. Lippincott Williams & Wilkins; 2012:365-396.
81. Gershon MD. 5-Hydroxytryptamine (serotonin) in the gastrointestinal tract. *Curr Opin Endocrinol Diabetes Obes*. 2013;20:14-21.
82. Gozlan H. 5-HT3 receptors. In: Olivier B, van Wijngaarden I, Soudin W, eds. *Serotonin Receptors and Their Ligands*. Elsevier; 1997:221-258.
83. Heidempergher F, Pillan A, Pinciroli V, et al. Phenylimidazolidin-2-one derivatives as selective 5-HT3 receptor antagonists and refinement of the pharmacophore model for 5-HT3 receptor binding. *J Med Chem*. 1997;40:3369-3380.
84. Kesters D, Thompson AJ, Brams M, et al. Structural basis of ligand recognition in 5-HT3 receptors. *EMBO Rep*. 2013;14:49-56.
85. Price KL, Lillestol RK, Ulens C, et al. Palonosetron-5-HT3 receptor interactions as shown by a binding protein cocrystal structure. *ACS Chem Neurosci*. 2016;7:1641-1646.
86. Aapro M, Blower P. 5-Hydroxytryptamine type-3 receptor antagonists for chemotherapy-induced and radiotherapy-induced nausea and emesis—can we safely reduce the dose of administered agents? *Cancer*. 2005;104:1-13.
87. de Wit R, Aapro M, Blower PR. Is there a pharmacological basis for differences in 5-HT3-receptor antagonist efficacy in refractory patients? *Cancer Chemother Pharmacol*. 2005;56:231-238.
88. Jordan K, Kasper C, Schmoll HJ. Chemotherapy-induced nausea and vomiting: current and new standards in the antiemetic prophylaxis and treatment. *Eur J Cancer*. 2005;41:199-205.
89. Aapro M. Optimising antiemetic therapy: what are the problems and how can they be overcome? *Curr Med Res Opin*. 2005;21:885-897.
90. Roberts SM, Bezinover DS, Janicki PK. Reappraisal of the role of dolasetron in prevention and treatment of nausea and vomiting associated with surgery or chemotherapy. *Cancer Manag Res*. 2012;4:67-73.
91. Obach RS. Pharmacologically active drug metabolites: impact on drug discovery and pharmacotherapy. *Pharmacol Rev*. 2013;65:578-640.
92. Reith MK, Sproles GD, Cheng LK. Human metabolism of dolasetron mesylate, a 5-HT3 receptor antagonist. *Drug Metab Dispos*. 1995;23:806-812.
93. Nakamura H, Ariyoshi N, Okada K, et al. CYP1A1 is a major enzyme responsible for the metabolism of granisetron in human liver microsomes. *Curr Drug Metab*. 2005;6:469-480.
94. Pritchard JF. Ondansetron metabolism and pharmacokinetics. *Semin Oncol*. 1992;19:9-15.
95. Navari RM. Palonosetron for the treatment of chemotherapy-induced nausea and vomiting. *Expert Opin Pharmacother*. 2014;15:2599-2608.
96. Stoltz R, Parisi S, Shah A, et al. Pharmacokinetics, metabolism and excretion of intravenous [l4C]-palonosetron in healthy human volunteers. *Biopharm Drug Dispos*. 2004;25:329-337.
97. Huang M, Gao JY, Zhai ZG, et al. An HPLC-ESI-MS method for simultaneous determination of fourteen metabolites of promethazine and caffeine and its application to pharmacokinetic study of the combination therapy against motion sickness. *J Pharm Biomed Anal*. 2012;62:119-128.
98. Finn A, Collins J, Voyksner R, et al. Bioavailability and metabolism of prochlorperazine administered via the buccal and oral delivery route. *J Clin Pharmacol*. 2005;45:1383-1390.
99. Kang C, Shirley M. Amisulpride: a review in post-operative nausea and vomiting. *Drugs* 2021;81:367-375.
100. Smyla N, Koch T, Eberhard LHJ, et al. An overview of intravenous amisulpride as a new therapeutic option for the prophylaxis and treatment of postoperative nausea and vomiting. *Expert Opin Pharmacother*. 2020;21: 517-522.
101. Khan S, Chang L. Diagnosis and management of IBS. *Nat Rev Gastroenterol Hepatol*. 2010;7:565-581.
102. Camilleri M. Pharmacology of the new treatments for lower gastrointestinal motility disorders and irritable bowel syndrome. *Clin Pharmacol Ther*. 2012;91:44-59.
103. Fayyaz M, Lackner JM. Serotonin receptor modulators in the treatment of irritable bowel syndrome. *Ther Clin Risk Manag*. 2008;4:41-48.
104. Dinning PG, Smith TK, Scott SM. Pathophysiology of colonic causes of chronic constipation. *Neurogastroenterol Motil*. 2009;21(suppl 2):20-30.
105. Camilleri M. Current and future pharmacological treatments for diarrhea-predominant irritable bowel syndrome. *Expert Opin Pharmacother*. 2013;14:1151-1160.
106. Gershon MD, Tack J. The serotonin signaling system: from basic understanding to drug development for functional GI disorders. *Gastroenterology*. 2007;132:397-414.
107. Hornby PJ. Drug discovery approaches to irritable bowel syndrome. *Expert Opin Drug Discov*. 2015;10:809-824.
108. Layer P, Keller J, Loeffler H, et al. Tegaserod in the treatment of irritable bowel syndrome (IBS) with constipation as the prime symptom. *Ther Clin Risk Manag*. 2007;3:107-118.
109. Vickers AE, Zollinger M, Dannecker R, et al. In vitro metabolism of tegaserod in human liver and intestine: assessment of drug interactions. *Drug Metab Dispos*. 2001;29:1269-1276.
110. Chiu SH, Huskey SW. Species differences in N-glucuronidation. *Drug Metab Dispos*. 1998;26:838-847.
111. Meyers NL, Hickling RI. Pharmacology and metabolism of renzapride: a novel therapeutic agent for the potential treatment of irritable bowel syndrome. *Drugs R D*. 2008;9: 37-63.
112. Love BL, Johnson A, Smith LS. Linaclotide: a novel agent for chronic constipation and irritable bowel syndrome. *Am J Health Syst Pharm*. 2014;71:1081-1091.
113. Currie MG, Fok KF, Kato J, et al. Guanylin: an endogenous activator of intestinal guanylate cyclase. *Proc Natl Acad Sci U S A*. 1992;89:947-951.
114. Hamra FK, Forte LR, Eber SL, et al. Uroguanylin: structure and activity of a second endogenous peptide that stimulates intestinal guanylate cyclase. *Proc Natl Acad Sci U S A*. 1993;90:10464-10468.
115. Corsetti M, Tack J. Linaclotide: a new drug for the treatment of chronic constipation and irritable bowel syndrome with constipation. *United European Gastroenterol J*. 2013;1:7-20.
116. McGinley MP, Cohen JA. Sphingosine-1-phosphate receptor modulators in multiple sclerosis and other conditions. *Lancet*. 2021;398:118-1194.
117. Choden T, Cohen NV, Rubin DT. Sphingosine-1-phosphate receptor modulators: the next wave of oral therapeutics in inflammatory bowel disease. *Gastroenterol Hepatol*. 2022;18:265-271.
118. de Mattos BR, Garcia MP, Nogueira JB, et al. Inflammatory bowel disease: an overview of immune mechanisms and biological treatments. *Mediators Inflamm*. 2015;2015:1-11.
119. Ordas I, Eckmann L, Talamini M, et al. Ulcerative colitis. *Lancet*. 2012;380:1606-1619.
120. Sandborn WJ, Feagan BG, Lichtenstein GR. Medical management of mild to moderate Crohn's disease: evidence-based treatment algorithms for induction and maintenance of remission. *Aliment Pharmacol Ther*. 2007;26:987-1003.
121. Sartor RB. Mechanisms of disease: pathogenesis of Crohn's disease and ulcerative colitis. *Nat Clin Pract Gastroenterol Hepatol*. 2006;3:390-407.
122. Danese S, Argollo M, Le Berre C, et al. JAK selectivity for inflammatory bowel disease treatment: does it clinically matter? *Gut*. 2019;68:1893-1899.
123. Flamant M, Rigaill J, Paul S, et al. Advances in the development of Janus kinase inhibitors in inflammatory bowel disease: future prospects. *Drugs*. 2017;77:1057-1068.
124. Rogler, G. Efficacy of JAK inhibitors in Crohn's Disease. *J Crohns Colitis*. 2020;14:S746-S754.
125. Dowty ME, Lin J, Ryder TF, et al. The pharmacokinetics, metabolism, and clearance mechanisms of Tofacitinib, a Janus kinase inhibitor, in human. *Drug Metab Dispos*. 2014;42:759-773.
126. Lefevre PLC, Casteele NV. Clinical pharmacology of Janus kinse inhibitors in inflammatory bowel disease. *J Crohns Colitis*. 2020;14:S725-S736.
127. Jovani M, Danese S. Vedolizumab for the treatment of IBD: a selective therapeutic approach targeting pathogenic a4b7 cells. *Curr Drug Targets*. 2013;14:1433-1443.

128. Khanna R, Preiss JC, MacDonald JK, et al. Anti-IL-12/23p40 antibodies for induction of remission in Crohn's disease. *Cochrane Database Syst Rev*. 2015:CD007572.
129. Shah B, Mayer L. Current status of monoclonal antibody therapy for the treatment of inflammatory bowel disease. *Expert Rev Clin Immunol*. 2010;6:607-620.
130. Sofia MA, Rubin DT. The impact of therapeutic antibodies on the management of digestive diseases: history, current practice, and future directions. *Dig Dis Sci*. 2017;62:833-842.
131. Soler D, Chapman T, Yang LL, et al. The binding specificity and selective antagonism of vedolizumab, an anti-alpha4beta7 integrin therapeutic antibody in development for inflammatory bowel diseases. *J Pharmacol Exp Ther*. 2009;330:864-875.
132. Liu JK. The history of monoclonal antibody development—progress, remaining challenges and future innovations. *Ann Med Surg (Lond)*. 2014;3:113-116.
133. Katzung BG. Introduction to autonomic pharmacology. In: Katzung BG, ed. *Basic and Clinical Pharmacology*. 11th ed. McGraw-Hill; 2009:77-94.
134. Changeux JP, Devillers-Thiery A, Chemouilli P. Acetylcholine receptor: an allosteric protein. *Science*. 1984;225:1335-1345.
135. Lukas RJ, Bencherif M. Heterogeneity and regulation of nicotinic acetylcholine receptors. *Int Rev Neurobiol*. 1992;34:25-131.
136. Fifer EK. Drugs affecting cholinergic neurotransmission. In: Lemke TL, Williams DA, Roche VF, Zito SW, eds. *Foye's Principles of Medicinal Chemistry*. 7th ed. Lippincott Williams & Wilkins; 2012:309-339.
137. Armstrong PD, Cannon JG, Long JP. Conformationally rigid analogues of acetylcholine. *Nature*. 1968;220:65-66.
138. Caulfield MP, Birdsall NJ. International Union of Pharmacology. XVII. Classification of muscarinic acetylcholine receptors. *Pharmacol Rev*. 1998;50:279-290.
139. Ing HR. The structure-action relationships to the choline group. *Science*. 1949;109:264-266.
140. Ing HR, Kordik P, Williams DP. Studies on the structure-action relationships of the choline group. *Br J Pharmacol Chemother*. 1952;7:103-116.
141. Holton P, Ing HR. The specificity of the trimethylammonium group in acetylcholine. *Br J Pharmacol Chemother*. 1949;4:190-196.
142. Haga K, Kruse AC, Asada H, et al. Structure of the human M2 muscarinic acetylcholine receptor bound to an antagonist. *Nature*. 2012;482:547-551.
143. Renner UD, Oertel R, Kirch W. Pharmacokinetics and pharmacodynamics in clinical use of scopolamine. *Ther Drug Monit*. 2005;27:655-665.
144. Ariens EJ. Receptor theory and structure activity relationships. *Adv Drug Res*. 1966;3:235-285.
145. Tzefos M, Dolder C, Olin JL. Fesoterodine for the treatment of overactive bladder. *Ann Pharmacother*. 2009;43:1992-2000.
146. Malhotra B, Gandelman K, Sachse R, et al. The design and development of fesoterodine as a prodrug of 5-hydroxymethyl tolterodine (5-HMT), the active metabolite of tolterodine. *Curr Med Chem*. 2009;16:4481-4489.
147. Jayarajan J, Radomski SB. Pharmacotherapy of overactive bladder in adults: a review of efficacy, tolerability, and quality of life. *Res Rep Urol*. 2013;6:1-16.
148. Chapple C, Khullar V, Gabriel Z, et al. The effects of antimuscarinic treatments in overactive bladder: a systematic review and meta-analysis. *Eur Urol*. 2005;48:5-26.
149. Chapple CR, Khullar V, Gabriel Z, et al. The effects of antimuscarinic treatments in overactive bladder: an update of a systematic review and meta-analysis. *Eur Urol*. 2008;54:543-562.
150. Yamada S, Ito Y, Nishijima S, et al. Basic and clinical aspects of antimuscarinic agents used to treat overactive bladder. *Pharmacol Ther*. 2018;189:130-148.
151. Chapple CR, Rechberger T, Al-Shukri S, et al. Randomized, double-blind placebo- and tolterodine-controlled trial of the once-daily antimuscarinic agent solifenacin in patients with symptomatic overactive bladder. *BJU Int*. 2004;93:303-310.
152. Skerjanec A. The clinical pharmacokinetics of darifenacin. *Clin Pharmacokinet*. 2006;45:325-350.
153. Fonseca AM, Meinberg MF, Monteiro MV, et al. The effectiveness of anticholinergic therapy for overactive bladders: systematic review and meta-analysis. *Rev Bras Ginecol Obstet*. 2016;38:564-575. doi:10.1055/s-0036-1594289
154. Hesch K. Agents for treatment of overactive bladder: a therapeutic class review. *Proc (Bayl Univ Med Cent)*. 2007;20:307-314.
155. Mansfield KJ. Role of fesoterodine in the treatment of overactive bladder. *Open Access J Urol*. 2009;2:1-9.
156. Marcelissen T, Rashid T, Lopes TA, et al. Oral pharmacologic management of overactive bladder syndrome: where do we stand? *Eur Urol Focus*. 2019;5:1112-1119. doi:10.1016/j.euf.2018.03.011
157. McFerren SC, Gomelsky A. Treatment of overactive bladder in the elderly female: the case for trospium, oxybutynin, fesoterodine and darifenacin. *Drugs Aging*. 2015;32:809-819.
158. Herschorn S, Swift S, Guan Z, et al. Comparison of fesoterodine and tolterodine extended release for the treatment of overactive bladder: a head-to-head placebo-controlled trial. *BJU Int*. 2010;105:58-66.
159. Tolterodine. *Drug Facts and Comparisons. Facts & Comparisons eAnswers [database online]*. Wolters Kluwer Health, Inc; 2005. Accessed November 07, 2018.
160. Solifenacin. *Drug Facts and Comparisons. Facts & Comparisons eAnswers* [database online]. Wolters Kluwer Health, Inc; 2005. Accessed November 07, 2018.
161. Doroshyenko O, Fuhr U. Clinical pharmacokinetics and pharmacodynamics of solifenacin. *Clin Pharmacokinet*. 2009;48:281-302.
162. Trospium chloride. *Drug Facts and Comparisons. Facts & Comparisons eAnswers* [database online]. Wolters Kluwer Health, Inc; 2005. Accessed November 07, 2018.
163. Sacco E, Bientinesi R. Mirabegron: a review of recent data and its prospects in the management of overactive bladder. *Ther Adv Urol*. 2012;4:315-324.
164. Sacco E, Bientinesi R, Tienforti D, et al. Discovery history and clinical development of mirabegron for the treatment of overactive bladder and urinary incontinence. *Expert Opin Drug Discov*. 2014;9:433-448.
165. Edmondson SD, Zhu C, Kar NF et al. Discovery of vibegron: a potent and selective beta-3 adrenergic receptor agonist for the treatment of overactive bladder. *J Med Chem*. 2016;59:609-623.
166. Rechberger T, Wróbel A. Evaluating vibegron for the treatment of overactive bladder. *Expert Opin Pharmacother*. 2021;22:9-17.

Structure Challenge Answers

A. 3
B. 1 and 2
C. 1 and 2
D. The sulfoxide motif is converted into sulfenic acid via an acid-catalyzed initial step. Subsequently, sulfenic acid converts into a reactive sulfenamide intermediate and covalently reacts with Cys thiol of the gastric proton pump.
E. Structure 4 is a metabolilte after CYP enzyme catalyzed oxidation and considered pharmacologically inactive.
F. Structure 4 is generated via a CYP3A4 catalyzed oxidation. Sulfoxide group is converted into sulfone.

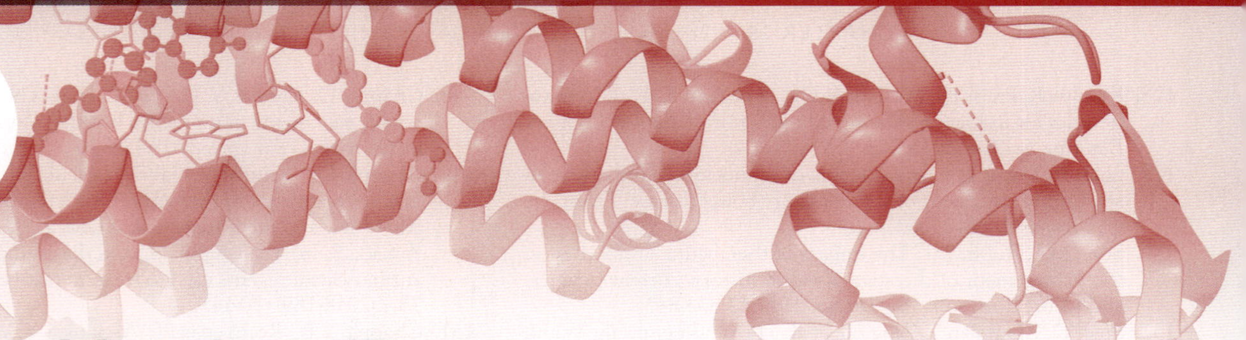

CHAPTER

29

Drugs Used to Treat Allergic Disorders

Rami A. Al-Horani

Drugs covered in this chapter:

H1-ANTIHISTAMINES

- Acrivastine
- Alcaftadine
- Antazoline (topical)
- Azelastine
- Bepotastine
- Brompheniramine (dexbrompheniramine)
- Buclizine
- Carbinoxamine
- Cetirizine (levocetirizine)
- Chlorcyclizine
- Chlorpheniramine (dexchlorpheniramine)
- Clemastine
- Cyclizine
- Cyproheptadine
- Desloratadine
- Dimethindene (oral and topical)
- Diphenhydramine (dimenhydrinate)
- Doxylamine
- Emedastine
- Epinastine
- Fexofenadine
- Hydroxyzine
- Ketotifen
- Levocabastine
- Loratadine
- Meclizine
- Olopatadine
- Pheniramine
- Promethazine
- Trimeprazine
- Tripelennamine
- Triprolidine

MAST-CELL STABILIZERS

- Cromolyn
- Lodoxamide
- Nedocromil

Abbreviations

ALDH aldehyde dehydrogenase
AO aldehyde oxidase
ATP adenosine triphosphate
BBB blood-brain barrier
CNS central nervous system
DAG 1,2-diacylglycerol
DAO diamine oxidase
ECL enterochromaffin-like
FcεRI high-affinity Fc immunoglobulin E receptor
GI gastrointestinal
GPCRs G protein–coupled receptors
HDC histidine decarboxylase
HMT histamine *N*-methyltransferase
IgE immunoglobulin E
IP_3 inositol-1,4,5-trisphosphate
MAO-B monoamine oxidase B
MRGPR Mas-related G protein–coupled receptor
MRGPRX2 a mast cell–specific member of MRGPR superfamily
PIP_2 phosphatidylinositol-4,5-bisphosphate
PLP pyridoxal phosphate
PNS peripheral nervous system
PRT phosphoribosyl transferase
SAM *S*-adenosylmethionine
SAR structure-activity relationship
TM transmembrane
XO xanthine oxidase

CLINICAL SIGNIFICANCE

H_1-antihistamines are classified into first and second generations. Knowledge of their chemical structures and physicochemical properties enables pharmacists to identify best therapeutic options, in clinical settings, to meet patients' treatment needs. Minor structural changes can increase or decrease antihistaminic, anticholinergic, and sedative properties, as well as many other pharmacokinetic and pharmacodynamic aspects of these medications, which enables therapy optimization. For instance, enhanced anticholinergic activity may be preferred in the case of rhinorrhea; however, little-to-no anticholinergic activity may be ideal for older adults.

Ahlam Ayyad, PharmD

INTRODUCTION

Allergic disorders or hypersensitivity reactions are generally exaggerated immune reactions to foreign antigens. Using Gell and Coombs classification,[1] hypersensitivity reactions are divided into four types (I-IV). This chapter focuses on drugs used for the treatment of disorders resulting from type I hypersensitivity reactions, also known as immediate hypersensitivity. Type I reactions lie behind all atopic disorders such as allergic asthma, atopic dermatitis, rhinitis, and conjunctivitis as well as many allergic disorders such as anaphylaxis, urticaria, some cases of angioedema, latex allergy, and some food allergies. The terms atopy and allergy are frequently used interchangeably; nevertheless, they are different. Atopy is an exaggerated immunoglobulin E (IgE)–mediated immune response; however, allergy is any exaggerated immune response to a foreign antigen regardless of mechanism. Therefore, all atopic disorders are considered allergic, but not all allergic disorders are atopic.[2]

Type I hypersensitivity reactions develop within 1 hour following exposure to antigen. These reactions are IgE-mediated reactions in which antigen binds to IgE on tissue mast cells and blood basophils (Fig. 29.1), triggering the

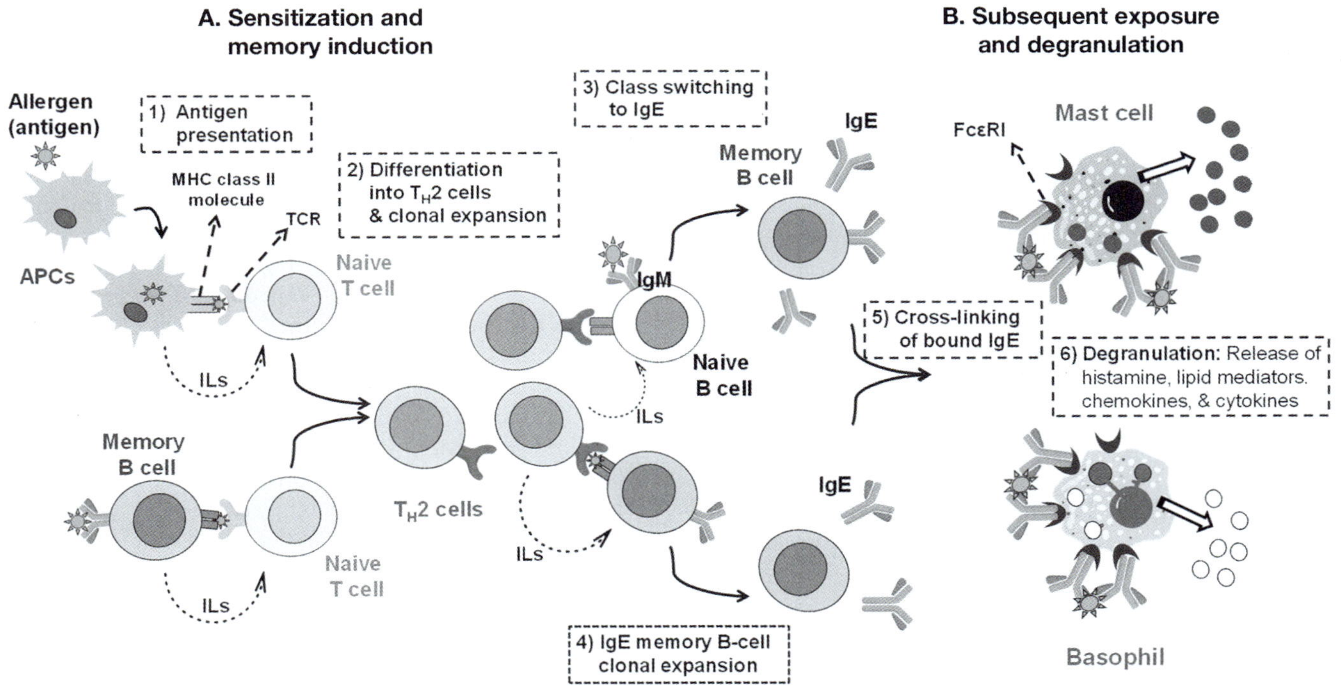

Figure 29.1 Mechanism of type I allergic reactions. A. Sensitization to allergen (antigen) and development of specific B-cell and T-cell memory. Following endocytosis, antigen-presenting cells (APCs) facilitate antigen presentation. Differentiation of naive T cells and clonal expansion of allergen-specific T helper 2 (T_H2) cells lead to the production of certain interleukins (ILs), which induce immunoglobulin class switching from IgM (naive B cells) to IgE (memory B cells) and clonal expansion of IgE-bound memory B-cell populations. IgE at the surface of allergen-specific IgE-bound B cells further facilitates antigen presentation. "Sensitization" occurs upon binding of the specific IgE antibodies to FcεRI receptors (high-affinity receptor for IgE) on mast cells or basophils. B. Subsequent exposure to the allergen leads to crosslinking of mast-cell and basophil cell-surface FcεRI-bound IgE, which results in cellular degranulation and the release of histamine, lipid mediators (prostaglandin D, leukotrienes, and platelet-activating factor), chemokines, and other cytokines, and to the immediate symptoms of allergic disorders. FcεRI, high-affinity Fc immunoglobulin E receptor; IgE, immunoglobulin E; IgM, immunoglobulin M; ILs, interleukins; MHC, major histocompatibility complex; TCR, T-cell receptor; T_H2, T helper 2 cells.

release of pre-synthesized mediators (including histamine, chemotactic factors and proteases) as well as the synthesis of new ones (including leukotrienes, prostaglandins, cytokines, and platelet-activating factor). These mediators cause vasodilation, capillary hyperpermeability, smooth muscle spasm, mucus hypersecretion, and tissue infiltration with various inflammatory cells such as eosinophils and type 2 helper T cells. Importantly, complex environmental, genetic, and site-specific factors contribute to the development of IgE-mediated allergies. Along these lines, allergens that induce type I IgE-mediated immune responses are almost always low-molecular-weight proteins, and many are attached to airborne particles. Examples of allergens are dust mites, animal dander, pollens, molds, household chemicals, latex, insect saliva and venom, as well as certain foods and drugs.

Pathophysiology of Allergic Disorders of Type 1 Hypersensitivity Reactions

Upon allergen binding to IgE of mast cells and basophils, histamine is released from intracellular granules. Given that mast cells are most concentrated in the skin, lungs, and gastrointestinal (GI) mucosa, symptoms of allergy are clearly presented by these organs. Among the many released chemicals, histamine is the primary mediator of clinical allergy and atopy. Histamine causes (1) local vasodilation-mediated erythema; (2) capillary hyperpermeability and edema; (3) vasodilated arterioles mediated by neuronal reflex mechanisms, causing redness; (4) excessively stimulated sensory nerves, causing itching; (5) smooth muscle contraction in the airways (bronchospasm) and in the GI muscles (abdominal cramps); and (6) increased salivary, nasal, and bronchial gland secretions. Furthermore, since histamine is a potent arteriolar dilator, it can cause serious hypotension. Cerebral vasodilation may cause vascular headaches. Histamine-mediated capillary hyperpermeability also permits the loss of plasma and plasma proteins from the vascular space, which can worsen circulatory shock. This loss triggers a compensatory catecholamine release from adrenal gland, which may further worsen symptoms. As a result, type I hypersensitivity allergic disorders can be associated with upper respiratory tract symptoms of sneezing, rhinorrhea, and nasal congestion; lower respiratory tract symptoms of wheezing and dyspnea; and excessive itching of the eyes, nose, and skin. Signs may include conjunctival hyperemia and edema, sinus pain, urticaria, dermatitis, skin lichenification, and angioedema.

Allergic Rhinitis and Conjunctivitis

When John Bostock first described "hay fever," also known as allergic rhinitis or seasonal rhinitis, in 1819, it was a rarely seen condition.[3] Today, the incidence of allergies has reached epidemic proportions in industrialized nations. In the United States and other industrialized countries, allergic rhinitis is very common, affecting 10% to 30% of children and adults.[4] The cost associated with treating allergic rhinitis is substantial and increases with disease severity and comorbidity. Recently, the annual cost of treating allergic rhinitis in the United States was estimated to be more than $4.6 billion.[5] In addition to these costs, there are indirect costs associated with both absenteeism and compromised productivity at work and school as well as medical costs associated with comorbidities. Allergic rhinitis can also have adverse effects on social life and academic performance, especially when treated with an antihistamine that produces sedation. Reports indicate that allergic rhinitis annually accounts for about 2.5% of all clinician visits, on average 6 million lost workdays, 2 million lost schooldays, and 28 million restricted workdays.

Addressing this condition early can have significant clinical benefits toward improving the patient's quality of life while decreasing comorbid disorders such as asthma, rhinosinusitis, allergic conjunctivitis, and sleep apnea. Allergic rhinitis may occur seasonally or throughout the year (ie, perennial rhinitis). Patients can have a combination of seasonal and perennial rhinitis. Generally, allergic rhinitis patients have itching (eye, nose, throat), sneezing, rhinorrhea, and nasal and sinus obstruction, which may cause frontal headaches. Sinusitis is a frequent complication. Coughing and wheezing may also occur.

Allergic conjunctivitis, or ocular allergy, is estimated to annually affect at least 20% of the population, and the incidence is increasing.[6] It is predominantly a disease of young adults. Symptoms appear to decrease with age, although severe symptoms can continue in some older patients. Allergic conjunctivitis typically accompanies other allergic diseases, particularly allergic rhinitis.[7] Asthma and atopic dermatitis are other common comorbidities.

Depending on the severity, allergic disorders can be treated by one or a combination of the following medication: (1) oral or topical antihistamines (H_1-receptor blockers or, more accurately, inverse agonists), (2) mast-cell degranulation inhibitors (histamine release inhibitors), (3) local/nasal glucocorticoids, and (4) leukotriene receptor antagonists. Treatment with antihistamines and/or nasal glucocorticoids appears to show good clinical outcomes. This chapter will focus on the use of antihistamines and mast-cell degranulation inhibitors.

Glucocorticoid nasal sprays can be first-generation (beclomethasone, flunisolide, triamcinolone, and budesonide) or second-generation (fluticasone propionate or furoate, mometasone furoate, and ciclesonide) preparations. Second-generation agents are preferred because they are equally efficacious and potentially carry a lower risk of systemic effects owing to their limited bioavailability. These agents are discussed in Chapter 24. Leukotriene receptor antagonists, such as montelukast, are used in the management of asthma. Montelukast also has efficacy in allergic rhinitis but should be used only when other treatments are not effective or not tolerated due to the risk of mental health adverse effects. Leukotriene receptor antagonists are discussed in Chapter 31. Other medications that can be used are vasoconstrictors/nasal decongestants (Chapter 30), bronchodilators such as ipratropium bromide (Chapter 31), and a short course of systemic glucocorticoids.

Immune desensitization can also be used to induce tolerance by exposing the patient to allergen in gradually increasing injectable or oral doses, or in sublingually administered high doses. Desensitization is indicated when allergen exposure cannot be avoided and/or drug treatment is insufficient. Lastly, parenteral biologics such as omalizumab (Xolair) and dupilumab (Dupixent) can be used. Omalizumab, an anti-IgE monoclonal antibody that is approved for asthma and chronic urticaria, was shown to reduce daily nasal symptoms and improve quality of life in patients with uncontrolled allergic rhinitis.[8] Dupilumab, an anti-interleukin-4 receptor α monoclonal antibody that is approved for asthma and chronic rhinosinusitis with nasal polyposis, also improves symptoms of allergic rhinitis.[9]

Key Player: Histamine

Given its structural similarity to the natural amino acid histidine and the natural alkaloid pilocarpine, histamine [2-(imidazole-4-yl)ethylamine] (Fig. 29.2) was first synthesized in 1907 by Windaus and Vogt.[10] Three years later, histamine was discovered to be produced by ergot[11] and as a product of bacterial decarboxylation of histidine.[12] That same year, the pharmacological actions of histamine were reported by Sir Henry Dale and his colleagues at the Wellcome Laboratories.[13] They noted that histamine produced smooth muscle contractions, decreased blood pressure and, in some species, produced effects similar to those of anaphylactic shock. However, it was not until 1927, when Best and his colleagues isolated histamine (named after the Greek word for tissue, *histos*) from samples of liver and lungs, that this amine was found to be a natural constituent of the body.[14] Dale and Laidlaw made the crucial observation that histamine injection into mammals caused a shocklike reaction and proposed its role in mediating symptoms of anaphylaxis.[15]

Histamine is biosynthesized in many tissues, including: (1) mast cells, basophils, and lymphocytes to promote allergic and inflammatory responses; (2) gastric enterochromaffin-like (ECL) cells to stimulate gastric acid secretion; and (3) CNS histaminergic neurons to function as a neurotransmitter. In many tissues, histamine acts as an autacoid (local hormone), a molecule that is secreted locally to modulate the activity of nearby cells.

In humans, histamine actions in different tissues are mediated through four distinct receptors, designated as H_1-H_4. They belong to the superfamily of G protein–coupled receptors (GPCRs) (Table 29.1). These receptors are hepta-helical transmembrane (TM) molecules that transduce extracellular signals to intracellular second messenger systems via G proteins (Chapter 6). Molecules acting at each of the four histamine receptors are identified in Figure 29.2. The H_1-receptors appear to be closely related to muscarinic receptors, which may explain the anticholinergic effects of some of the first-generation H_1-antihistamines described later, whereas the H_2-receptors resemble 5-HT_1 receptors. H_3- and H_4-receptors are not closely related to the either of these receptors. The H_3-receptors are found in the neurons of peripheral and central nervous systems (PNS and CNS, respectively), bronchioles, and GI tract. Binding of histamine to H_3-receptors in the CNS decreases the release of histamine, acetylcholine, dopamine, and serotonin. H_3-receptors partly prevent excessive

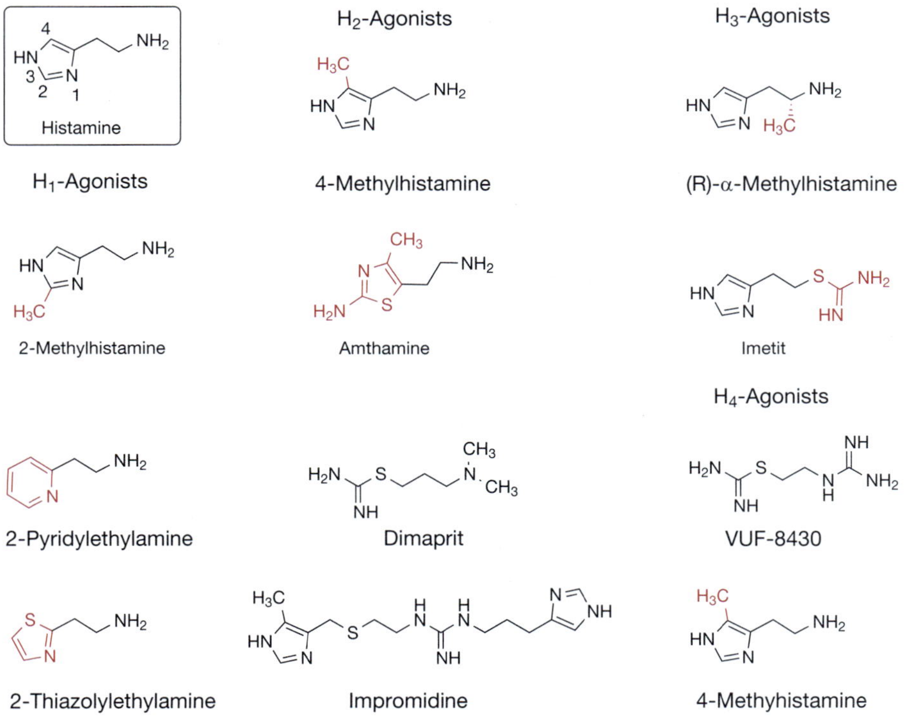

Figure 29.2 Structure of histamine and examples of H_1, H_2, H_3, and H_4 agonists. Figure 29.2 4-Methylhistamine, originally identified as specific H_2-agonist, has a much higher affinity for H_4-receptor. Dimaprit is also partial H_4-agonist. Impromidine is not only among the most potent H_2-agonists but also is an antagonist at H_1- and H_3-receptors and a partial agonist at H_4-receptors. (R)-α-Methylhistamine and imetit are high-affinity agonists of H_3-receptors and lower-affinity agonists at H_4-receptors.

Table 29.1 Characteristics of Histamine Receptors: Structures, Functions, and Effects

Characteristic	H_1	H_2	H_3	H_4
Amino acids	487	359	329-445 (isoforms)	390
Signaling	$G_{q/11}$; activates phospholipase C, ↑ IP_3 and DAG	G_s; stimulates adenylate cyclase, ↑ cAMP	$G_{i/o}$; inhibits adenylate cyclase, ↓ cAMP	$G_{i/o}$; ↓ cAMP, ↑ intracellular Ca^{2+}
Tissue distribution	a. Vascular smooth muscle b. Endothelial cells c. Lung d. Peripheral nerves	Gastric parietal cells, cardiac muscle, mast cells, CNS	CNS: pre and postsynaptic	Cells of hematopoietic origin
Effect[a]	a. Dilation (arterioles and venules) Vasoconstriction b. Contraction and separation of endothelial cells c. Bronchoconstriction d. Afferent sensitization	↑ HCl secretion, slight increase in heart rate and contractility	Neurotransmitter	Chemotaxis/ Inflammation
Clinical response[a]	a. Erythema b. Edema c. Asthma-like symptoms d. Itching, pain	Heartburn, peptic ulcer disease	Cognitive processes, circadian rhythms, wakefulness	
Representative agonist	2-CH_3-histamine	Amthamine	(*R*)-α–CH_3-histamine	4-CH_3-histamine
Representative antagonist	Diphenhydramine	Cimetidine	Pitolisant	JNJ7777120

cAMP, cyclic adenosine monophosphate; CNS, central nervous system; DAG, 1,2-diacylglycerol; IP_3, inositol-1,4,5-trisphosphate.
[a]Lettered items refer back to the similarly tagged items in the Tissue Distribution cell.

bronchoconstriction and are important in controlling neurogenic inflammation. H_4-receptors are located in leukocytes, bone marrow, lung, colon, spleen, liver, and hippocampus, and have a role in the differentiation of myeloblasts and promyelocytes and in eosinophil chemotaxis. Therapeutically, histamine receptors are being targeted by antihistamines to treat allergic disorders (H_1-antihistamines), GI acidity disorders (H_2-antihistamines), and narcolepsy (H_3-antihistamines). No H_4-antihistamines have been approved thus far for clinical use, although trials for their use as antiallergic, anti-inflammatory, and anti-hyperalgesic medications are ongoing. Interestingly, H_1-antihistamines were considered for years as traditional receptor antagonists. With the recognition that all histamine receptors have some constitutive activity, it is now established that the first- and second-generation "H_1-antagonists" are functioning as inverse agonists.

Histamine Chemistry and Structure-Activity Relationships

Structurally, histamine possesses a basic imidazole ring (pK_a = 5.80) connected to a primary aliphatic amino group (pK_a = 9.40) by an ethylene bridge. At the physiological pH of 7.4, histamine exists in three forms: unionized (1%), mono-cation (96%), and di-cation (3%). At lower pH values, a much larger proportion of the di-cation will exist. While the mono- and di-cation forms are often considered the biologically active species, it is the unprotonated free base form that is believed to penetrate biological membranes.[16] Considering the ionizable hydrogen of the imidazole ring, histamine generally exists as two tautomers, Nτ-H and Nπ-H, which are numbered according to Black and Ganellin[17] (Fig. 29.3).

In aqueous solution, the mono-cation exists as a mixture of the two tautomers (Fig. 29.4). The N^{τ}-H/N^{π}-H tautomer ratio of the mono-cation is 4.2, and thus, about 80% exits as

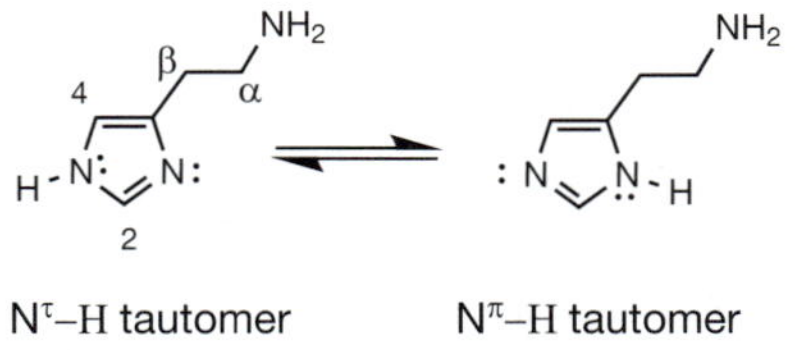

Figure 29.3 Conformers of histamine.

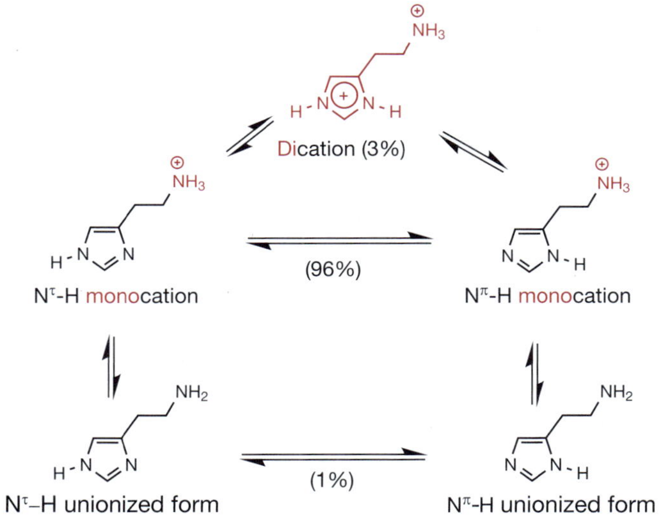

Figure 29.4 Ionization states and tautomerizaton of histamine.

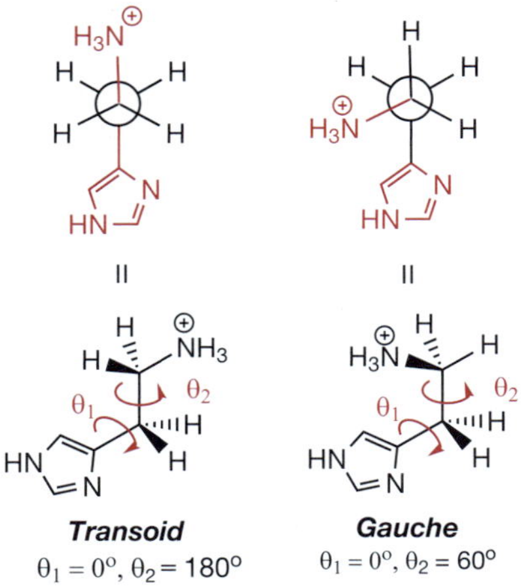

Figure 29.5 *Transoid* and *gauche* conformers of histamine.

N^{τ}-H and 20% as N^{π}-H.[16] Studies using the Hammett equation suggest that the tautomeric preference is influenced by the electron-withdrawing nature of the amine-containing side chain. The N^{τ}-H tautomer is also preferred for the free base in aqueous solution. Interestingly, while the monocationic hydrobromide salt crystallizes as the N^{τ}-H tautomer, the free base crystallizes as the N^{π}-H tautomer. However, the crystalline forms are conformationally "frozen" and cannot be related to their tautomeric stability under equilibrating conditions. These findings for the mono-cation and the unionized free base forms are supported by molecular orbital calculations on isolated molecules. The tautomeric ratios differ with different 4-substituted histamine analogues. As the N^{τ}-H/N^{π}-H tautomer ratio decreases on going from 4-methylhistamine (70%) to 4-chlorohistamine (12%), a similar decrease is observed for agonist potency. One interpretation of this is that the N^{τ}-H tautomer might be important for agonist interaction with histamine receptors. Structure-activity analysis suggests that the active form of histamine at both the H_1 and H_2-receptors is the N^{τ}-H tautomer of the mono-cation.[18,19]

Furthermore, both *anti-* (or *transoid*) and *gauche* conformations of histamine can exist in solution (Fig. 29.5). It has been suggested that the *trans* conformation is preferred at H_1- and H_2-receptors since both α- and β-methylhistamine, which exist predominately in the gauche conformation due to steric hindrance, exhibit greatly reduced agonist activity at both H_1- and H_2-receptors. Interestingly, α-methylhistamine and other conformationally restricted histamine analogues that predominately exist in the *gauche* conformation have been shown to be active H_3-agonists.[17-20]

Methylation of histamine at different positions results in different effects. For example, 2-methylhistamine and 4-methylhistamine are selective H_1- and H_2-agonists, respectively. However, methyl substitution at the N^{τ}- or N^{π}-positions of the imidazole ring produces nearly inactive molecules. Methylation of the aliphatic amine also results in successively decreased activity (ie, the corresponding primary amine is the most active and the quaternary ammonium is the least active at H_1- and H_2-receptors). Overall, structure-activity relationship (SAR) studies of histamine indicate that, for binding to the two receptors H_1 and H_2, a protonated primary amine is essential to interact with the corresponding acidic amino acids (Asp107 in H_1 and Asp98 in H_2), which will be predominantly anionic at physiological pH. As noted earlier, the N^{τ} -H tautomer appears to be the preferred ligand for the two receptors. Once recognized, a charge relay system involving a series of proton transfers between histamine and its receptor results in tautomerization to N^{π} -H form and receptor activation (Fig. 29.6).[17-21]

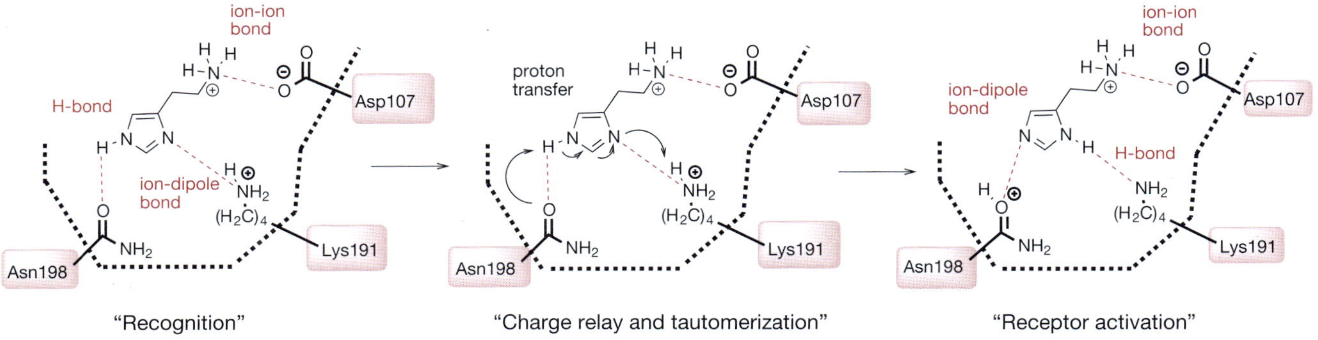

Figure 29.6 Histamine binding and activation of the H_1-receptor.

Histamine Physiology

Histamine Biosynthesis and Metabolism

In mammalian cells, histamine is biosynthesized in the Golgi apparatus of mast cells and basophils by a single step decarboxylation of the natural amino acid L-histidine. The biotransformation is catalyzed by pyridoxal phosphate (PLP)–dependent L-histidine decarboxylase (HDC).[22] The mechanism of this biotransformation is illustrated in Figure 29.7 and is similar to that seen for other α-amino acids, involving the HDC-PLP aldehyde-imine (aldimine), a Schiff base formed between Lys305 on HDC and its coenzyme PLP.[23] The amino group of the substrate L-histidine displaces Lys305 of HDC to produce a new aldimine of L-histidine-PLP, which undergoes decarboxylation, releasing carbon dioxide and the aldimine of histamine-PLP. Next, another displacement biotransformation involving Lys305 of HDC takes place to release histamine, the product, and regenerate the original aldimine HDC-PLP. The mechanism-based inhibitor, α-fluoromethylhistidine, can decrease the rate of histamine biosynthesis, and thus, deplete cells of histamine.[24] In theory, inhibition of histamine biosynthesis might be of use in the treatment of allergic inflammatory disorders, peptic ulcers, or motion sickness, yet the lack of selectivity of this approach limits its clinical utility.

Upon release, histamine is rapidly metabolized via both Phase 1 and Phase 2 metabolic reactions (Fig. 29.8). One pathway involves N^{τ}-methylation of the imidazole ring, which is catalyzed by histamine *N*-methyltransferase (HMT). The methyl group is donated by the coenzyme *S*-adenosylmethionine (SAM) so as to give the corresponding inactive 3-methylhistamine, which subsequently undergoes oxidative deamination by either diamine oxidase (DAO) or monoamine oxidase B (MAO-B) to produce the corresponding aldehyde. The produced aldehyde is subsequently oxidized by aldehyde dehydrogenase (ALDH), aldehyde oxidase (AO), or xanthine oxidase (XO) to afford the corresponding 3-methylimidazole acetic acid. Likewise, histamine can first undergo oxidative deamination and aldehyde oxidation to afford imidazole acetic acid then conjugation to afford the corresponding ribonucleoside. All metabolites are renally eliminated.

Histamine Storage and Release

Histamine is stored in many tissues throughout the body, but most is found in the secretory granules of circulating basophils and tissue-bound mast cells. Given the basic nature of histamine, it is complexed in its mono-cationic conjugate form with chondroitin sulfate, a negatively charged glycosaminoglycan, in basophils, and with heparin, another negatively charged glycosaminoglycan, in mast cells.[25] Non–mast cell sites of histamine formation include the epidermis, ECL cells of the gastric mucosa, neurons within CNS, and cells in regenerating or rapidly growing tissues. The turnover rate of histamine in secretory granules is slow (in the range of days to weeks). However, the turnover is rapid at the non-mast cell sites because histamine is released continuously rather than stored. Non–mast cell sites of histamine production contribute significantly to the daily excretion of histamine metabolites in the urine. Because HDC is an inducible enzyme, histamine biosynthesis in non–mast cells is subject to regulation.

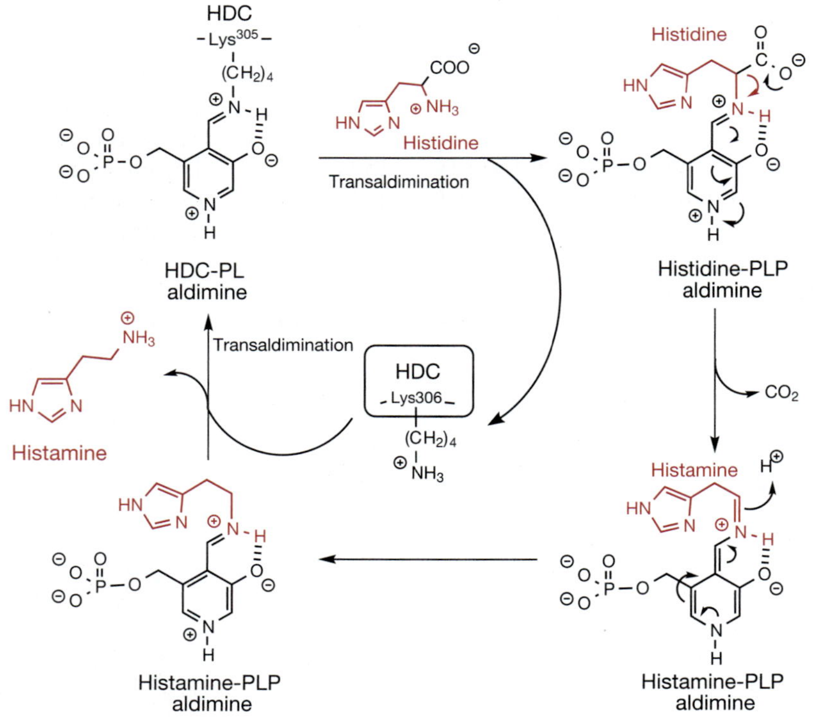

Figure 29.7 Histidine decarboxylase–catalyzed biosynthesis of histamine from amino acid L-histidine. HDC, histidine decarboxylase; PL, pyridoxal; PLP, pyridoxal phosphate.

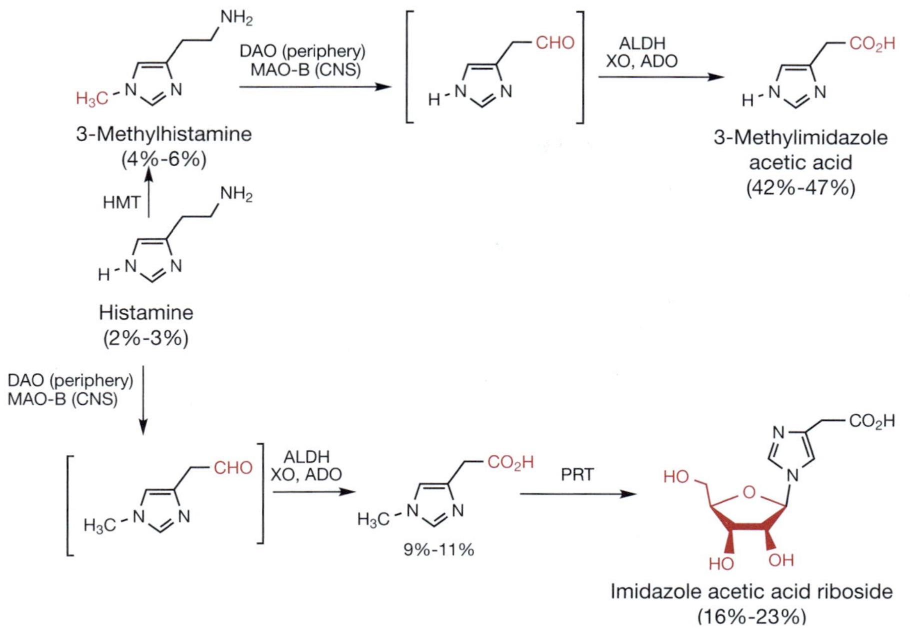

Figure 29.8 Histamine metabolism. Metabolites are renally eliminated. ALDH, aldehyde dehydrogenase; AO, aldehyde oxidase; DAO, diamine oxidase; HMT, histamine *N*-methyltransferase; MAO-B, monoamine oxidase B; PRT, phosphoribosyl transferase; XO, xanthine oxidase.

The tissue-bound form of histamine is not biologically active. Histamine can be released from secretory granules by several mechanisms. The immunologic mechanism, triggered by allergic reactions, anaphylaxis, cellular trauma, and cold, is responsible for the most important pathophysiological mechanism of mast cell and basophil histamine release. When the appropriate antigen binds to IgE antibodies attached to the surface membranes of these cells, cellular degranulation takes place explosively. This mechanism of release requires energy and calcium and leads to the simultaneous release of histamine, adenosine triphosphate (ATP), and other mediators in the granules.[26] As a mediator of immune and inflammatory reactions, histamine plays an important role in allergic responses (IgE-mediated type I hypersensitivity reactions). These reactions are also referred to as immediate hypersensitivity reactions because they occur within an hour of initial exposure to antigen. As shown in Figure 29.1, in this type of reaction, the allergen (antigen) must penetrate an epithelial surface of skin or nasal mucosa, or it could be delivered systemically, as with penicillin allergy. With the aid of T_H2 cells, the antigen comes in contact with B lymphocytes and stimulates production of IgE antibodies, which are specific for a particular antigen. "Sensitization" occurs upon binding of the specific IgE antibodies to high-affinity Fc immunoglobulin E receptor (FcεRI) receptors on mast cells or basophils. Once sensitized with IgE antibodies, immune cells are able to recognize and quickly respond to the next exposure to the antigen. Upon subsequent exposure, antigen binds and cross-links the IgE/FcεRI receptor complexes leading to degranulation and release of histamine and other inflammatory mediators. Released histamine activates H_1-receptors on vascular smooth muscle and endothelial cells, leading to the early stage of the inflammatory response (ie, increased local blood flow and vascular hyperpermeability). Other immune cells are required for prolonged inflammation. Histamine-induced local vasodilation provides other immune cells with greater access to the injured area, and vasodilation aids movement of the immune cells into the tissue.[27]

Histamine Release Induced by Drugs, Peptides, Venoms, and Other Agents

An immune response is not always required for mast-cell degranulation. Disruption of mast cells by chemicals or trauma can lead to degranulation. Mechanical injury and many chemical compounds can promote the release of histamine from mast cells without prior sensitization. This is most likely to occur following intravenous (IV) injections of organic basic molecules in their water-soluble salt forms, such as the nicotinic blocker tubocurarine and opioid analgesics like morphine. Succinylcholine, some antibiotics, radiocontrast media, and certain carbohydrate plasma expanders may also provoke this response. Although the released histamine facilitates access of macrophages and other immune cells to the damaged area to initiate the repair process, this phenomenon is of clinical concern and may account for unexpected anaphylactoid reactions.

Furthermore, basic polypeptides often are effective histamine releasers, and their potency generally increases with the number of basic groups that can become cationic at physiological pH. For instance, bradykinin is a poor histamine releaser, whereas kallidin (Lysbradykinin) and substance P, with more positively charged amino acids, are more active. Some venoms, such as that of the wasp, contain potent histaminereleasing peptides.[28] Basic polypeptides released upon tissue injury constitute pathophysiological stimuli for secretion of histamine from mast cells and basophils.

Within seconds of the IV injection of a histamine liberator, human subjects experience a burning, itching sensation in the palms of the hand and in the face, scalp, and ears. This effect is soon followed by a feeling of intense warmth. The skin reddens and the color rapidly spreads over the trunk. Blood pressure falls, the heart rate accelerates, and the subject usually complains of headache. Shortly after, crops of hives usually appear on the skin and blood pressure recovers. Nausea, hypersecretion of gastric acid, colic-like pain, and moderate bronchospasm also frequently occur. The effect becomes less intense with successive administrations of the secretagogue, as mast cell stores of histamine are depleted. Histamine liberators do not deplete histamine from non–mast cell sites.

Importantly, the mechanism by which basic secretagogues release histamine potentially involves a direct interaction with MRGPRX2, a mast cell–specific member of the Masrelated G protein–coupled receptor (MRGPR) superfamily. Two proteins in the X family, MRGPRX1 and MRGPRX2, interact with a variety of positively charged compounds, transducing signals that result in itch and pain. Activation of MRGPRX2 on mast cells appears to provide a route for histamine release that is independent of the traditional IgE pathway and potentially accounts for some adverse drug reactions. Thus, MRGPRX2 inhibitors can be a potential treatment of pseudo-allergic and inflammatory diseases.[29,30]

Histamine Receptors

As mentioned, all histamine receptors, H_1-H_4, are GPCRs and are widely distributed throughout the body (Table 29.1). This chapter will focus on the H_1-receptor. It is found on bronchial and vascular smooth muscle, chondrocytes, endothelial cells, eosinophils, monocytes, macrophages, hepatocytes, dendritic cells, B and T lymphocytes, and nerve cells. Stimulation of the H_1-receptor results in vasodilation, edema, bronchoconstriction, itching, and pain. It also affects maturation of cells of the immune system, altering their activation, chemotactic, and effector functions.[31,32] The human H_1-receptor gene encodes for a 487-amino acid GPCR of seven TM domains, N-terminal glycosylation sites, phosphorylation sites for protein kinase A and C, and a large intracellular loop rich in Ser and Thr residues.[33,34] There is about 40% homology between the human H_1-receptor and muscarinic M_1- and M_2-receptors. Site-directed mutagenesis studies suggested that Asp107 in TM3 domain coordinates with the protonated aliphatic amine of histamine, whereas the Nτ-nitrogen and the Nπ-nitrogen of histamine interact with Asn198 and Lys191 of TM5 domain, respectively.[34,35]

H_1-receptor signal transduction involves $G_{q/11}$-coupled activation of phospholipase C and its subsequent hydrolysis of phosphatidylinositol-4,5-bisphosphate (PIP_2) to form the second messengers inositol-1,4,5-trisphosphate (IP_3) and 1,2-diacylglycerol (DAG). The former molecule is an intracellular messenger that opens ligand-gated calcium channels on the endoplasmic reticulum, leading to intracellular calcium release, while the latter messenger activates protein kinase C (see Table 29.1).

H_1-ANTIHISTAMINES

Discovery

After the discovery of histamine, researchers at the Pasteur Institute attempted to synthesize antagonists to better understand its physiological role. In 1933, the first compound reported as an antihistamine by Ungar, Parrot, and Bovet was the adrenolytic benzodioxan, piperoxan (933F) (Fig. 29.9),[36] which blocked the effect of histamine on the guinea pig ileum. This was followed shortly by the report of structurally related aryl ethers such as the thymol ether 929F, which protected the guinea pig from the lethal effects of histamine-induced anaphylaxis.[37] The latter compound proved to be too toxic for clinical development, but replacement of the ether oxygen by an amino group led to the discovery of aniline ethylene diamine derivatives. For his work on antihistamines and curare, Bovet was awarded the 1957 Nobel Prize for Physiology or Medicine. The work on anilino compounds was followed up in France in collaboration with Rhone-Poulenc and, independently during the war years (1939-1945), by researchers in the United States. The first antihistamine to be used in humans in 1942 was Antergan (phenbenzamine, RP 2339), but this was subsequently replaced by Neoantergan (mepyramine, pyrilamine, RP 2786) (see Fig. 29.9), which is still used topically to counteract the unpleasant effects of histamine release in the skin.

Many other antihistamines followed. For example, diphenhydramine was synthesized in 1943, and shortly after, in 1947, orphenadrine was introduced. The hydrochloride salt of orphenadrine is used in the treatment of Parkinson disease, and the citrate salt is used as a muscle relaxant. In the same years, Searle and Company modified diphenhydramine to reduce drowsiness. Dimenhydrinate, the 8-chlorotheophylline salt of diphenhydramine, serendipitously cured a patient of long-standing motion sickness. This benefit was proven in a clinical trial in 1949, in which

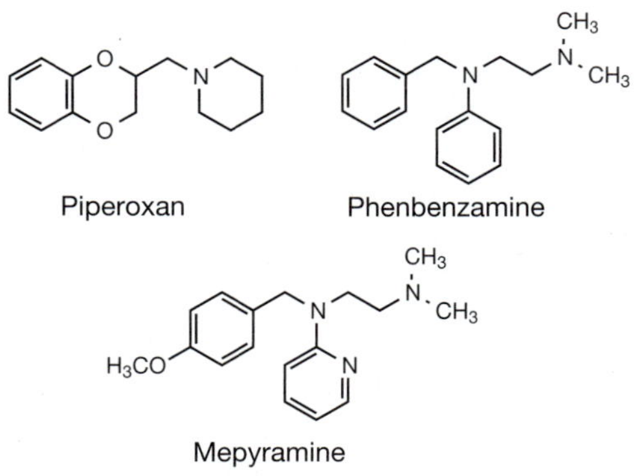

Figure 29.9 Chemical structures of early antihistamines.

25% of the troops crossing the Atlantic from New York who received a placebo experienced seasickness compared with only 4% of those receiving dimenhydrinate. Cyclizine was developed in the 1960s. It proved to be long acting and was used during the first manned flight to the moon by the National Aeronautics and Space Administration to control space sickness. It is no longer approved for use in the United States, although its derivative, hydroxyzine, remains in use.[38,39]

In the 1970s, terfenadine was synthesized as a tranquilizer, but it lacked CNS penetration. Yet, its peripheral antihistaminic effects proved useful. In 1989, more than 773 adverse reactions to terfenadine were reported, ranging from prolonged QT intervals to convulsions in cases of supratherapeutic ingestions. In 1992, the US Food and Drug Administration (FDA) issued a warning for the risk of torsades de pointes with terfenadine (a cardiotoxic CYP3A4 substrate) when administered with CYP3A4 inhibitors. Fexofenadine, its active and non-toxic metabolite, was marketed instead.[38]

Although the aforementioned antihistamines have been shown to be useful for the treatment of allergic and inflammatory disorders, they do not antagonize the effects of histamine on the stomach (increased gastric acid secretion) or the heart (positive chronotropic and inotropic effects). These observations led to assumption that there was more than one histamine receptor and ultimately led to the discovery of H_2-receptors and the development of selective H_2-antagonists. Subsequently, H_3-receptors have been reported, which function as presynaptic autoreceptors and heteroreceptors. As autoreceptors in the CNS, they presynaptically control the biosynthesis and release of histamine, whereas, as heteroreceptors, they control release of other neurotransmitters. H_3-receptors affect cognitive processes, circadian rhythms, and wakefulness. Lastly, H_4-receptors have been primarily found on eosinophils and mast cells where they are involved in inflammatory responses.

Inverse Agonists Versus Pure Antagonists

Historically, H_1-antihistamines have been considered as pure H_1-receptor antagonists that are lacking intrinsic efficacy in the absence of an agonist. Initially, this designation was supported by the parallel shift (along the *x*-axis) in concentration–response relationships in tracheal smooth muscle. Nevertheless, advances in histamine pharmacology have demonstrated that not all of these antihistamines are antagonists. Rather, many of them are inverse agonists. In the absence of histamine or another ligand, H_1-receptors exist in equilibrium between two conformational states, active and inactive. With no ligand bound, the receptor exhibits constitutive activity.[39] When histamine binds to the receptor as an agonist, the receptor equilibrium shifts toward the active state. However, when an antihistamine binds, the receptor equilibrium shifts toward the inactive state, and activity is reduced. The term "inverse agonists" is used because these structures preferentially bind to the inactive conformation of the H_1-receptor and reduce its constitutive activity, even in the absence of histamine. This is in contrast to classical antagonists, which bind to both the active and inactive receptor conformations, inhibiting the ability of histamine to reach the H_1-receptor active site.

First Generation Versus Second Generation

Generally speaking, H_1-antihistamines can be either first or second generation. First-generation antihistamines can be divided into several chemical subclasses (see "First-Generation H1-Antihistamines (Generally Sedative)" section). They have variable efficacy in the treatment of allergic disorders, and also exhibit many side effects through interaction with adrenergic, cholinergic, dopaminergic, and serotonergic receptors. Although adverse CNS effects vary according to the class, they almost always include drowsiness, decreased cognitive function, sedation, and somnolence. CNS depression is so pronounced with some agents that they are marketed as over the-counter (OTC) sleep aids, rather than as treatment for allergic disorders. Furthermore, peripheral anticholinergic effects include blurred vision, dry mouth and eyes, urinary retention, and constipation. Other undesirable effects include muscle spasm, anxiety, confusion, irritability, tremor, appetite stimulation, and tachycardia. Weight gain (attributed to H_1- and serotonergic blocking properties) and orthostatic hypotension (attributed to α-blocking effect) can also be problematic in some patients. Because of the potential for significant anticholinergic and CNS depressant effects, the first-generation antihistamines are considered potentially inappropriate for use in children and older adults.

The numerous adverse effects associated with first-generation H_1-antihistamines, ranging from annoying to serious, often limit their clinical use. Current thoughts on the sedative properties of the first-generation antihistamines are that they are attributed to their H_1-antihistamine and anticholinergic effects in CNS. Structural modifications of the early first-generation antihistamines resulted in a "second generation" of antihistamines that have limited access to CNS because they are more polar amphoteric molecules and/or are substrates for the permeability glycoprotein (P-glycoprotein) transporter system, which causes their efflux from the CNS. The structural modifications also enhanced the selectivity of molecules in the second generation to H_1-receptors over other receptors such as cholinergic (muscarinic), adrenergic, or even serotonergic receptors, which further improved their safety profiles. Development of the second-generation antihistamines has been a breakthrough in the treatment of allergic rhinitis and similar conditions. These agents exhibit separation of the peripheral H_1-antihistamine activity from the CNS depressant and anticholinergic side effects and have improved the quality of life of patients with allergies.

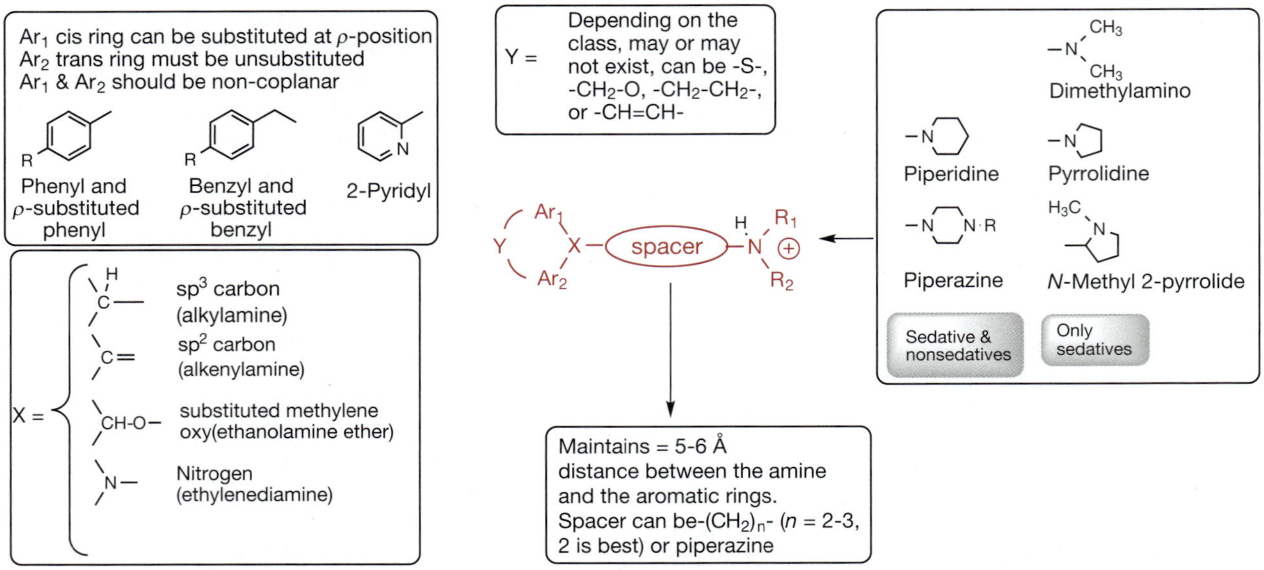

Figure 29.10 General structure of first-generation antihistamines.

First-Generation H_1-Antihistamines (Generally Sedative)

Structure-Activity Relationship Studies

Because H_1-antihistamines, referred to simply as antihistamines, do not bind with all of the same H_1-receptor residues as histamine, their structures are distinctly different. A general structure for antihistamines is given in Figure 29.10. A representation of their binding to the H_1-receptor is given in Figure 29.11. The only binding residue all antihistamines have in common with histamine is Asp107. Two hydrophobic receptor areas are important to antihistamine binding. One contains Phe432 and the other includes Trp158.[21]

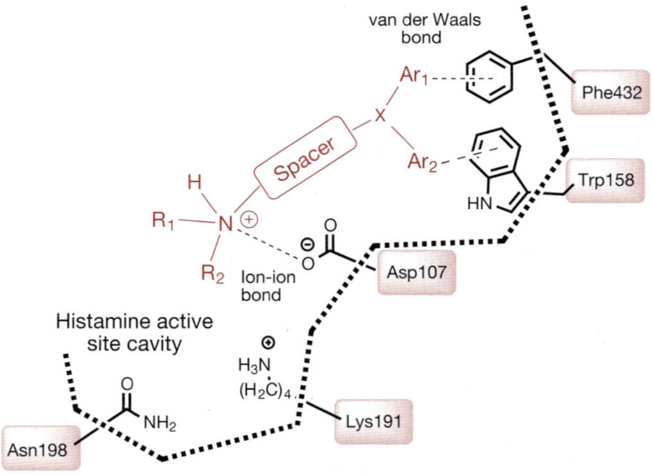

Figure 29.11 Representation of antihistamine binding to the H_1-receptor.

The first-generation antihistamines can be divided into five chemical subclasses: (1) ethylenediamines, (2) ethanolamine ethers (aminoalkyl ethers), (3) piperazines (cyclizines), (4) alkylamines (propylamines or pheniramines), and (5) tricyclic antihistamine (phenothiazines and other tricyclics). SAR studies indicated that the terminal nitrogen must be basic and is most often a tertiary dimethyl-substituted amine. Antihistaminic activity is best when the substitution is with small alkyl groups to minimize steric hindrance to ion-ion anchoring at the H_1-receptor Asp107. Methyl substitution is better than ethyl, but sterically constrained five- to six-membered nonaromatic heterocycles (pyrrolidine, piperidine, and piperazine) have been used. The pK_a of these groups usually ranges from 8.5 to 10.3; thus, they will be significantly cationic at physiological pH and able to form an electrostatic bond with anionic Asp107.

The spacer unit is generally unsubstituted and is two to three atoms in length. Branching enhances activity only in phenothiazine antihistamines. The spacer maintains a 5- to 6-Å distance between the cationic center and the aromatic rings. The moiety to which the two terminal aryl groups are attached is labeled as X, and it will have either carbon or nitrogen as the atom of attachment. This moiety determines the subclass of antihistamines. For example, alkylamines involve saturated or unsaturated carbon, ethanolamine ethers involve substituted methyleneoxy, and ethylenediamines involve saturated nitrogen. If the aryl groups are different, the saturated carbon X becomes chiral, and in most cases, the *S*-isomer is the active form.

Diaryl substitution is required for high H_1-receptor affinity and may be seen in both first- and second-generation antihistamines. The two aryl groups in Ar_1-X-Ar_2 moiety must be non-coplanar or able to become non-coplanar in order to exhibit substantial receptor affinity.[40] The ring that orients *trans* to the cationic amine binds to a sterically restricted receptor area that includes Phe432. This aromatic moiety (phenyl or 2-pyridyl) must be unsubstituted. A 2-pyridyl group in place of a phenyl often increases antihistaminic activity while reducing anticholinergic and sedative properties. The ring that orients *cis* to the cationic amine binds via van der Waals forces to a receptor area that includes Trp158. Substituted aryl or arylmethyl (benzyl) moieties are acceptable. The bulkier ring (substituted) assumes the required *cis* orientation via free rotation in sp^3 alkylamines, ethanolamine ethers, and ethylenediamines. However, this ring must be synthetically placed in *cis* orientation in rigid sp^2 alkylamines. Importantly, substituents on the aryl rings should not be hydrophilic. Lipophilic substituents enhance activity by increasing distribution. Duration increases if the substituent also blocks inactivating metabolism. When substituted in the *p*-position of the aryl moiety that orients in a *cis* fashion, an increase in antihistaminic activity, as well as a decrease in anticholinergic activity, is generally observed, while *o*-substitution decreases H_1-receptor affinity and favors anticholinergic activity. Benzyl-like groups are commonly seen in the ethylenediamine class but are only allowed for the *cis*-orienting ring. The two aromatic rings may or may not be linked via a bridge, Y. This connection is seen in the tricyclic antihistamines, for example, phenothiazines (Y = -S-), dibenzoheptanes (Y = $-CH_2-CH_2-$), or dibenzoheptenes (Y = -CH=CH-). While there are several antihistamines in clinical use today, several antihistamines were discontinued or became less frequently used. The structures of latter group are presented to highlight interesting structural features.

DISCONTINUED OR LESS COMMONLY USED ANTIHISTAMINES OF STRUCTURAL INTEREST[a]

DISCONTINUED OR "LESS COMMONLY" USED DRUGS OF STRUCTURAL INTEREST

Ethylenediamine H_1-antihistamines

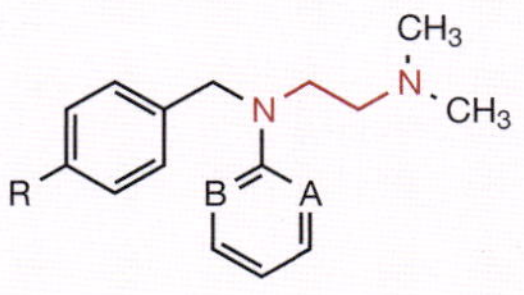

Phenbenzamine
(R = H, A = B = CH)

Tripelennamine
(R = H, A = N, B = CH)

Thonzylamine
(R = OCH_3, A = B = N)

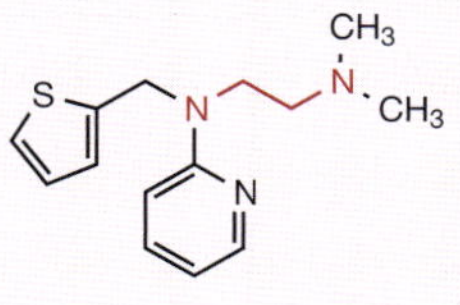

Methapyrilene

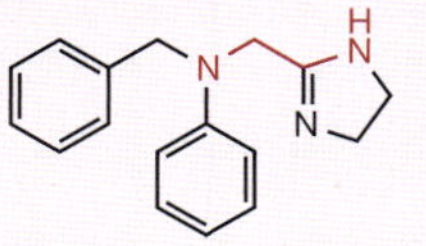

Antazoline

Unsaturated alkylamine H_1-antihistamines

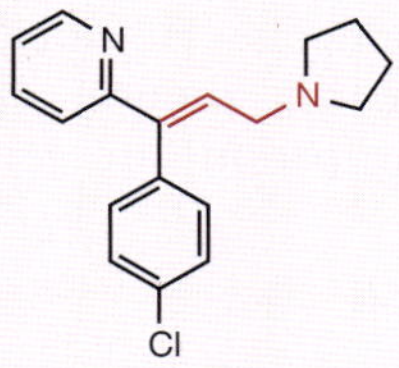

E-Triprolidine

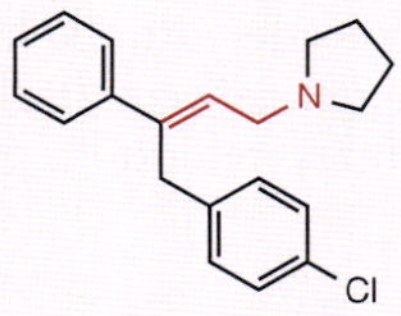

E-Pyrrobutamine

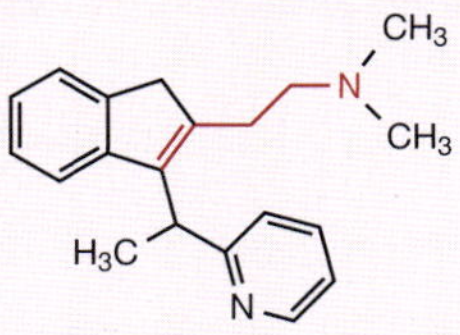

Dimethindene

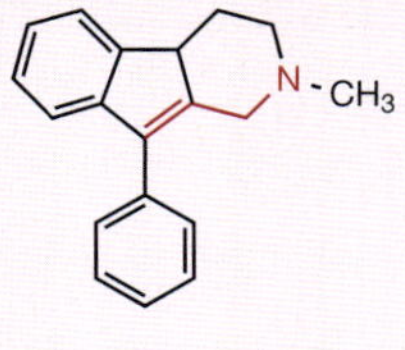

Phenindamine

Piperazine H_1-antihistamines

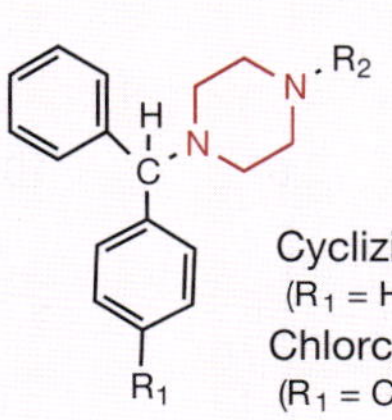

Cyclizine
(R_1 = H, R_2 = CH_3)
Chlorcyclizine
(R_1 = Cl, R_2 = CH_3)

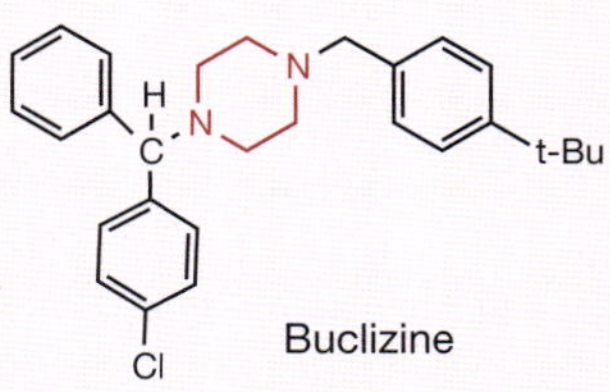

Buclizine

Tricyclic phenothiazine H_1-antihistamines

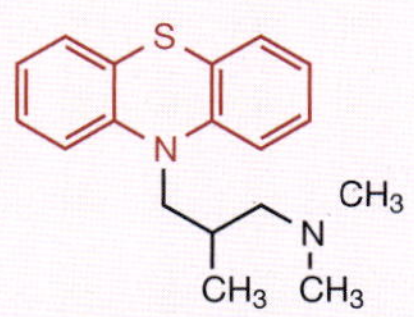

Methdilazine

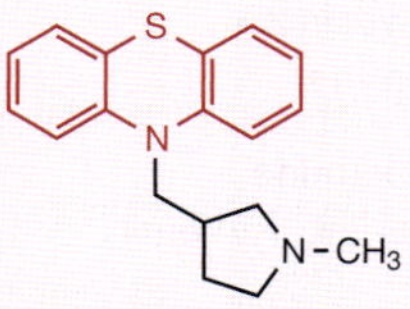

Trimeprazine

[a]Few may still available in combination.

Ethylenediamines

The ethylenediamine antihistamines were the earliest to find clinical use. With the exception of antazoline, which contains an amidine as part of an imidazoline ring, compounds in this series possess two nitrogen atoms separated by a two-carbon spacer. Examples of bioisosteric aromatic ring replacements (eg, pyridine, pyrimidine, furan, thiazole) can be seen in this class, although no such antihistamines are currently marketed in the United States. As a class, ethylenediamines exhibit low antihistaminic and anticholinergic effects and moderate sedative effects. Although tripelennamine (see Discontinued or Less Commonly Used Antihistamines of Structural Interest) is still available, the ethylenediamines find little clinical use today. There are limited data on the pharmacokinetics and metabolism of the ethylenediamines, and the first-generation antihistamines in general. As a representative example, tripelennamine undergoes *N*-demethylation, aryl hydroxylation, *N*-oxide formation, and glucuronic acid conjugation.[41,42]

Ethanolamine Ethers (Aminoalkyl Ethers)

Diphenhydramine, a benzhydryl (diphenylmethyl) ether, is considered the prototype of this class and continues to be widely used. Several *p*-substituted phenyl ring analogues of diphenhydramine have been developed (CH_3, OCH_3, Cl, Br), as have 2-pyridyl aromatic ring bioisosteres (Table 29.2).

The antihistaminic effect of the ethanolamine ethers is generally considered to be low to moderate. However, their anticholinergic effects (tachycardia, dry mouth, blurred vision, urinary retention, and constipation) are generally considered to be high. Interestingly, their central anticholinergic effects have enabled the use of some members of this class (and potentially other classes) in the management of Parkinson disease because they partially restore the balance between dopamine and acetylcholine in certain brain areas. Furthermore, some of ethanolamine ethers are used as over-the-counter sleep aids because they produce a moderate to high degree of sedation (attributed to central antihistamine and anticholinergic effects), have relatively short half-lives, and enjoy a wide safety margin. Their sedative properties require that they be used with caution in the elderly, when taking other sedative agents or consuming alcohol, and when engaging in activities that require alertness (eg, operating dangerous machinery). They can also reach the chemoreceptor trigger zone, producing good antiemetic effects. Diphenhydramine is formulated with 8-chlorotheophylline to form the organic salt dimenhydrinate, which is used over the counter to prevent and/or treat motion sickness and postoperative nausea and vomiting. The stimulant 8-chlorothiophylline is used to overcome the sedative properties of diphenhydramine.

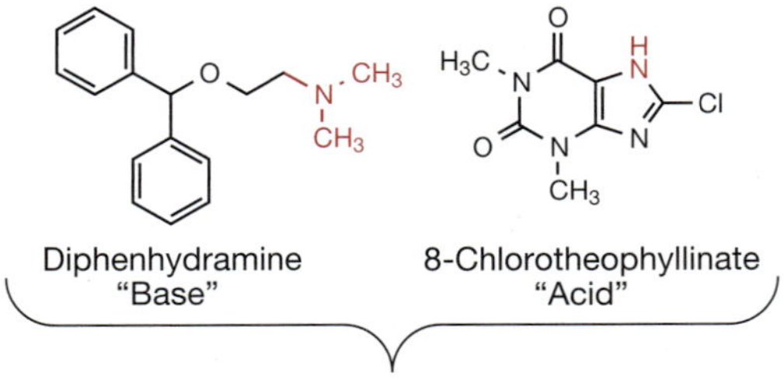

Dimenhydrinate

Table 29.2 Ethanolamine Ether Antihistamines

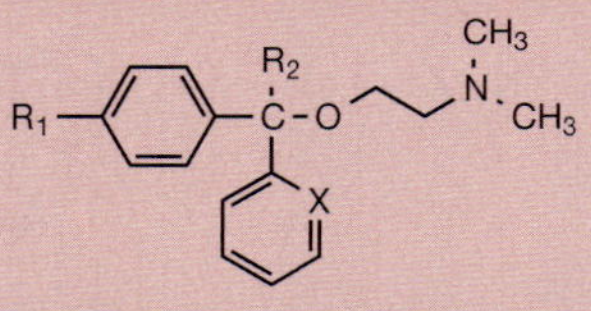

Drug	Salt	R_1	R_2	X	pK_a[a]	cLogP[a]	$T_{0.5}$[b] (h)
Diphenhydramine (Benadryl) Dimenhydrinate (Dramamine)	HCl, citrate, tannate, 8-Chlorotheophyllinate	H	H	CH	9.44	3.45	4-8
Carbinoxamine (Karbinal ER; RyVent)	Maleate	Cl	H	N	9.35 5.23	2.67	10-20
Doxylamine	Succinate	H	CH_3	N	9.39 5.23	2.35	7-13
Clemastine	Fumarate	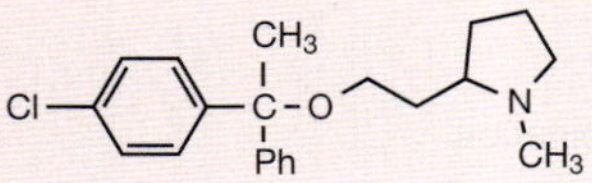			9.65	5.45	21

[a]pK_a and cLogP (calculated LogP) from ChemDraw 22.0.0.

[b]From Baselt RC. *Disposition of Toxic Drugs and Chemicals in Man.* 11th ed. Biomedical Publications; 2017 (monographs and references therein) or Micromedex.

Substituting the α-carbon (benzyl carbon) with a methyl group, as in doxylamine (Table 29.2), increases the hypnotic effect to a level comparable with secobarbital. Selectivity for the H_1-receptor over the muscarinic receptor is affected by the substitution of the *cis*-aromatic ring (with respect to the amine). With *ortho*-alkyl substituted analogues, rotation of the two aromatic rings is restricted, and decreased antihistaminic and increased anticholinergic activity is observed, particularly as the size of the alkyl group increases. In contrast, *para*-substitution results in decreased anticholinergic activity along with an increase in antihistaminic activity. Both *ortho-* and *para*-substitutions introduce chirality into the molecule, and enantiomeric differences in activity and receptor affinity are observed.

SPECIFIC DRUGS (TABLE 29.2)

Diphenhydramine. Diphenhydramine is a tertiary amine-containing drug with a pK_a of 9.44. Therefore, it is predominately ionized at physiological pH and exhibits high water solubility (1 g/mL). Its HCl salt is available in several dosage forms that can be used orally, parenterally, and topically. It is approved for symptomatic relief of allergic symptoms caused by histamine release, including allergic rhinitis and allergic dermatosis. It can also be used as an adjunct to epinephrine in the treatment of anaphylaxis. Given its sedative effect, it is used to treat occasional insomnia. It is used for the prevention or treatment of motion sickness and for the management of drug-induced extrapyramidal symptoms (eg, dystonia) and Parkinsonian syndrome, alone or in combination with centrally acting anticholinergic agents. It can also be used as an antitussive and for the treatment of common cold.

Diphenhydramine undergoes extensive oxidative N-dealkylation to the secondary and primary amines, followed by deamination and oxidation to form diphenylmethoxyacetic acid (Fig. 29.12). The primary amine metabolite undergoes phase 2 conjugation to form the N-glucuronide, while the carboxylic acid metabolite is likely excreted as a glycine or glutamine conjugate.[42] Only about 1% of an oral dose of diphenhydramine is excreted unchanged, with about 64% excreted as metabolites in the urine.[43] Its elimination half-life is 4 to 8 hours in young adults, but it is significantly extended to 13.5 hours in the elderly. The onset of action after an oral dose of diphenhydramine is 15 to 60 minutes, with a duration of action of 4 to 6 hours for allergic reactions. Its bioavailability is about 65%. Protein binding varies from 76% to 85%. The volume of distribution varies from 292 to 480 L/70 kg.[44]

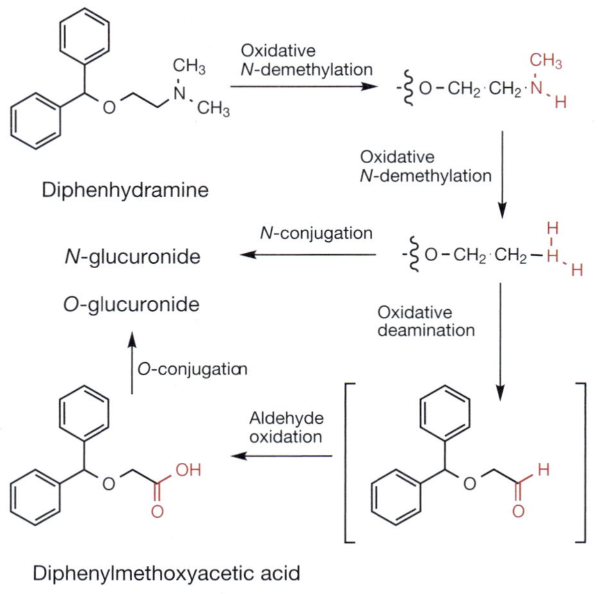

Figure 29.12 Diphenhydramine metabolism.

Diphenhydramine is associated with the known adverse effects of all first-generation antihistamines, including dry mouth, blurred vision, and sedation. These effects may be exaggerated in the elderly due to their slower rate of elimination in this often hepatically and renally compromised population. Concurrent use with CNS depressants may increase the risk of CNS and respiratory depression. Thus, patients should avoid use while driving, while operating dangerous machinery, or whenever it is essential to remain alert. Use along with other anticholinergic agents may increase the risk for paralytic ileus. Interestingly, diphenhydramine has been shown to inhibit the metabolism of CYP2D6 substrates. One such interaction is its inhibition of β-blocker metabolism, such as metoprolol metabolism in extensive 2D6 metabolizers. In this population, the negative chronotropic and inotropic effects are prolonged, resulting in excessive drops in heart rate and blood pressure.[45]

Carbinoxamine. Carbinoxamine is a potent antihistaminic agent that is marketed as the racemate of the maleate salt. The (S)-enantiomer is the more potent isomer. Carbinoxamine is more lipophilic than diphenhydramine by the virtue of its *p*-chlorine substituent, which blocks potential aromatic oxidation metabolism at this site, resulting in increased potency and longer duration of action. Since *p*-substitution results in decreased anticholinergic activity along with an increased antihistaminic activity, carbinoxamine is less sedative than diphenhydramine and it is almost exclusively used for allergic rhinitis. Its side effects and drug interactions are similar to other ethanolamine antihistamines. Carbinoxamine appears to undergo extensive metabolic transformation since no parent drug is found in the urine.

Doxylamine. Like carbinoxamine, doxylamine also has two basic nitrogen atoms with pK_a values similar to those of carbinoxamine (see Table 29.2). It is marketed as the succinate salt of the more basic aliphatic amine and is primarily used as a sleep-inducing agent, as the α-methyl group enhances antimuscarinic action and sedative potential. It is also indicated for allergic rhinitis and for symptom control in the common cold, and in combination with pyridoxine for pregnancy-associated nausea and vomiting. It is also combined with acetaminophen, codeine, and/or dextromethorphan for pain and cold and flu symptoms. It is comparable to diphenhydramine in potency as an antihistamine, and its hypnotic potential is comparable to secobarbital and pentobarbital.

Doxylamine is well absorbed orally, and its absorption is unaffected by food. Its LogP is 2.34, and, despite the addition of the α-methyl, it is less lipophilic than diphenhydramine due to the bioisosteric replacement of phenyl ring of diphenhydramine with the more polar 2-pyridyl ring. Its onset and duration for treatment of insomnia are 30 minutes and 3 to 6 hours, respectively, with a mean elimination half-life of 13.11 hours.[46] The half-life is increased in geriatric and pediatric patients. There are few studies examining the metabolism of doxylamine in man, but it is known to be excreted in the urine as unchanged doxylamine, the desmethyl and didesmethylated metabolites, and the *N*-acetyl conjugates.[47]

Clemastine. Clemastine fumarate has some unique features compared to other clinically available ethanolamine ethers. While it has a *p*-chlorophenyl ring similar to carbinoxamine, and a quaternary, methyl substituted benzhydryl carbon similar to doxylamine, it is also a homolog with one extra carbon between the ether oxygen and the tertiary amine. The additional carbon atom in the spacer is accepted because the molecule is flexible enough to "bend" to ensure the appropriate 5- to 6-Å distance between anchoring cationic amine and the receptor-binding aromatic moieties. In addition, the 2-position of the pyrrolidine ring is chiral. Because clemastine possesses two chiral centers, it exists as four stereoisomers (two enantiomeric pairs and four diastereomeric pairs) (Table 29.3). The (*R*,*R*)-enantiomer is in clinical use and is the most potent of the four possible isomers. The chiral center at the benzhydryl carbon appears to influence receptor selectivity to a greater extent than the asymmetric pyrrolidine carbon.[48]

Table 29.3 Stereoisomers of Clemastine

Stereoisomers	ED_{50} (mg/kg)[a]	pA_2[b]
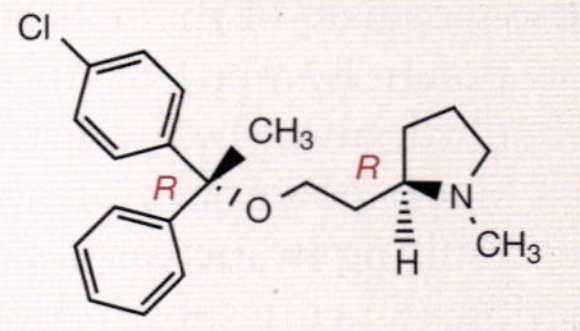	0.04	9.45
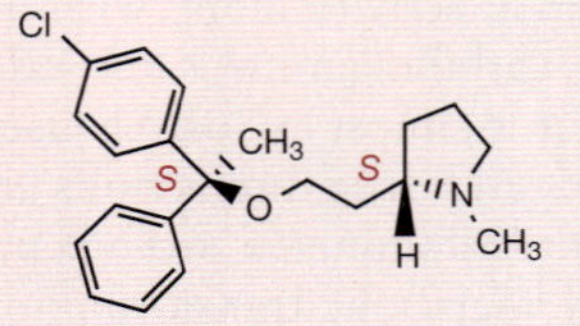	5.0	7.99
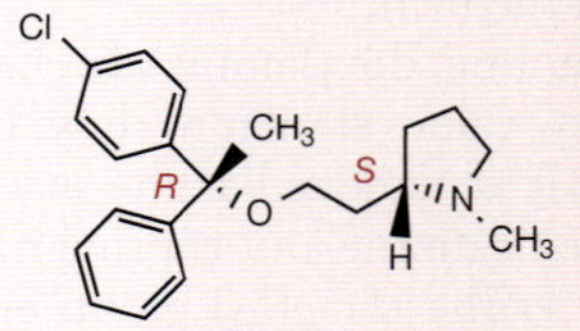	0.28	9.44
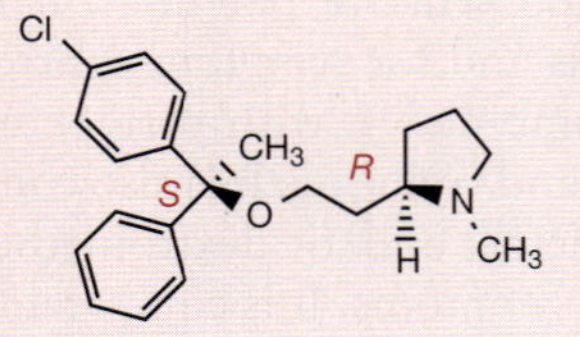	11.0	8.57

Note: The (*R*,*R*) and (*S*,*S*) isomers, as well as the (*R*,*S*) and (*S*,*R*) isomers, are enantiomers (mirror images). However, the (*R*,*R*) and the (*R*,*S*) or the (*S*,*R*) isomers are diastereomers (non-mirror imagines). Likewise, the (*S*,*S*) isomer is diastereomeric with the (*S*,*R*) and (*R*,*S*) isomers.

[a] ED_{50} for a lethal dose of histamine in guinea pigs.

[b] The negative log of the molar concentration of an antagonist that requires doubling the concentration of an agonist in order to elicit the original submaximal response obtained in the absence of the antagonist.

Clemastine is approved for the treatment of allergic rhinitis, urticaria, and angioedema as well as the common cold, hay fever, and upper respiratory allergies. Clemastine is well absorbed following oral administration and has an onset of 2 hours. It is primarily excreted renally with an elimination half-life of 21 hours. Its duration of action with multiple dosing is 10 to 12 hours. Clemastine undergoes extensive metabolism. The major urinary metabolite (M3) is the product of oxidative O-dealkylation (Fig. 29.13). A number of oxidative metabolites and dehydration products are also formed.[49] Its side effects and drug interactions are similar to others in this class and primarily involve its anticholinergic effects and sedation. Thus, like the others, it should be used with caution in the elderly, when operating machinery, or taking other anticholinergic drugs or CNS depressants.

Alkylamines (Propylamines)

The X atom in the general structure of antihistamines (see Fig. 29.10) can be a carbon atom. This atom can be either sp3 to afford propylamine derivatives (Table 29.4) or sp2 to give an olefinic propene derivatives (see Discontinued or Less Commonly Used Antihistamines of Structural Interest), with the *E*-isomer being more potent than the *Z*-isomer. The more active *E*-isomer places the bulkier of the two aromatic rings *cis* to the protonated amine, allowing the unsubstituted *trans* ring to reach the sterically restricted binding site on the H_1-receptor. In the case of phenindamine, both

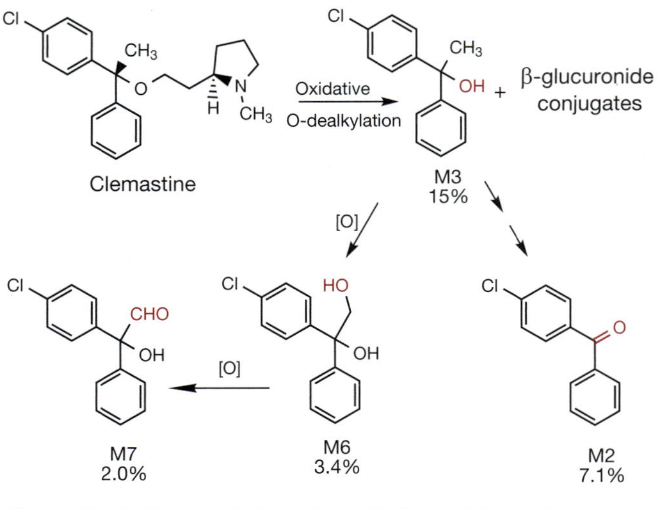

Figure 29.13 Reported phase 1 metabolites of clemastine.

Table 29.4 Alkylamine Antihistamines

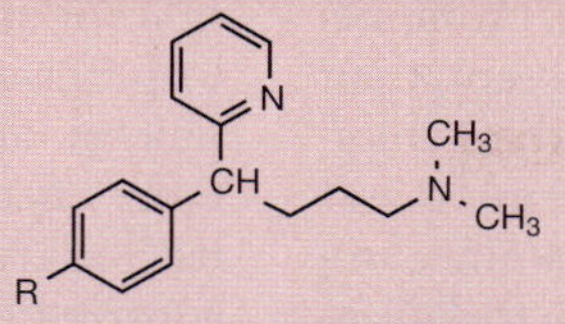

Drug	Salt	R	pK_a[a]	cLogP[a]	$T_{0.5}$[b] (h)
Pheniramine	Maleate	H	10.02	2.96	16-19
Chlorpheniramine (Aller-Chlor, Chlor-Trimeton)	Maleate	Cl	10.01	3.68	20
Brompheniramine	Maleate Tannate	Br	10.01	3.83	25

[a]pK_a and cLogP (calculated LogP) from ChemDraw 22.0.0.
[b]From Baselt RC. *Disposition of Toxic Drugs and Chemicals in Man.* 11th ed. Biomedical Publications; 2017 (monographs and references therein) or Micromedex.

aromatic rings are unsubstituted and would be accepted at either site. The saturated propylamines are often referred to as pheniramines. Three of these, pheniramine (*p*-H), chlorpheniramine (*p*-Cl), and brompheniramine (*p*-Br), are currently in clinical use. The halogen-substituted analogues exhibit much greater potency, likely due to an increase in lipophilicity and, potentially, inhibition of aromatic oxidative metabolism. They have good antihistaminic properties and a long duration of action, and thus, have been widely used for the OTC treatment of allergic rhinitis, often in combination with decongestants, expectorants, antitussives, and analgesics.

The *p*-halo–substituted pheniramines generally produce less sedation than the ethylenediamines and ethanolamine ethers. In addition, they exhibit relatively fewer anticholinergic effects in comparison to the ethanolamine ethers. Those in clinical use have a 2-substituted pyridine ring, making them chiral. Racemic chlorpheniramine and brompheniramine were the most widely used antihistamines until the nonsedating second-generation antihistamines were introduced.

Structural and Stereochemical Effects. In tissue-based assays, the *E*-isomers of the olefinic derivatives exhibit a much greater potency than the corresponding *Z*-isomers. For example, the *E*-isomers of pyrrobutamine and triprolidine are 165- and 1,000-fold more potent, respectively, than their *Z*-isomers. As noted earlier, studies with molecules with varying degrees of conformational restriction (eg, dimethindene and phenindamine) suggested that the receptor requires a 5- to 6-Å distance between the binding site for the cationic tertiary aliphatic amine and one of the aromatic rings,[50,51] and that the binding sites for the two aromatic moieties differ in their degree of steric restriction.

Potency differences between the enantiomers of the pheniramine derivatives have also been observed. In radioligand displacement and tissue-based assays, the (+)-*S*-enantiomer of chlorpheniramine (Ar = Cl-Ph, 2-pyridyl) exhibits 200- to 1,000-fold greater affinity for H_1-receptors than its (−)-*R*-enantiomer. The (+)-*S*-enantiomer also shows greater selectivity for H_1-receptors relative to muscarinic and adrenergic receptors, and it is also more potent. Both chlorpheniramine and brompheniramine, and their dextro-isomers, have been used as the maleate or tannate salts in OTC and prescription products. They are sometimes formulated with decongestants, expectorants, antitussives, and analgesics.

Specific Drugs (Table 29.4)

Chlorpheniramine. Chlorpheniramine is used for the treatment of allergic rhinitis and symptoms associated with the common cold in adults and children older than age 6 years. Off-label uses include atopic dermatitis, urticaria, psoriasis, and mastocytosis. It exhibits low sedative effects, some anticholinergic effects, and moderate-to-high antihistaminic effects. While its average half-life is about 20 hours, it can vary from 12 to 43 hours depending on the individual and urine pH. The lipophilicity and inhibition of oxidative metabolism contributed by the *p*-chloro group contribute to the longer half-life. Chlorpheniramine undergoes oxidative N-dealkylation to form the mono- and di-demethylated amines, as well as other oxidized products. On chronic administration of 4 mg, urinary metabolites have been reported to include unchanged drug (13%), mono-demethylated (13%), and di-demethylated (6%) amines over a 24-hour period.[52] Deamination has not been reported for chlorpheniramine.

Chlorpheniramine maleate is primarily marketed as a racemic mixture, often in combination with a decongestant. Although not as widely used, the (+)-enantiomer, dexchlorpheniramine maleate, is also available. The dose of the (+)-isomer is half that of the racemic mixture since the (−) isomer in the racemic mixture is significantly less active. It is available as oral, single, and extended-release tablets and as an oral solution.

Brompheniramine. Brompheniramine is indicated for the treatment of allergic rhinitis, as an adjunct to epinephrine for anaphylaxis, urticaria, urticarial transfusion reaction, and vasomotor rhinitis. Because a bromo substituent imparts greater lipophilicity than a chloro substituent, brompheniramine is more lipophilic, and therefore more potent, than chlorpheniramine. It also has a longer half-life than chlorpheniramine; 20 and 25 hours for chlorpheniramine and brompheniramine, respectively. Like chlorpheniramine, brompheniramine undergoes mono- and di-*N*-demethylation. Unlike chlorpheniramine, it also undergoes deamination followed by oxidation to the diarylpropionic acid. It is eliminated as a phase 2 glycine conjugate.

Pheniramine. Pheniramine is not available in the United States as a single-ingredient product. It is marketed for ophthalmic use in combination with naphazoline for the treatment of ocular inflammatory conditions. A nasal spray containing phenylephrine is also available. It is found in several oral extended-release tablet or capsule formulations and oral liquids for the treatment of nasal and sinus congestion. Other ingredients in these oral products may include phenylephrine, phenylpropanolamine, guaifenesin, sodium salicylate, dextromethorphan, codeine, or hydrocodone. Like its halogen-substituted analogues, pheniramine undergoes oxidative N-dealkylation to the mono- and di-dealkylated amines.[53,54]

Piperazines

Examination of the structure of the piperazine class of first-generation H_1-antihistamines (Table 29.5) reveals substantial similarities with the ethylenediamines and bioisosteric similarities with the ethanolamine ethers. The two nitrogen atoms found in the ethylenediamines are incorporated into a piperazine ring in this class, thus providing a two-carbon separation between the nitrogen atoms as seen in straight chain ethylendiamines. The diaryl-substituted methylene or benzhydryl group is attached to one nitrogen atom of the piperazine ring. The other nitrogen, a basic aliphatic amine, is attached to an alkyl or arylalkyl group.

Members of this class include hydroxyzine, meclizine, buclizine, cyclizine, and chlorcyclizine (see Discontinued or Less Commonly Used Antihistamines of Structural Interest for the last three members). The piperazines are moderately potent as antihistamines, and they exhibit significant anticholinergic side effects. Because of their ability to penetrate the CNS, they also cause sedation and psychomotor and cognitive dysfunction. They are among the more effective antihistamine-based antiemetics and can be used to treat motion sickness. Their anticholinergic actions contribute to this therapeutic action. While teratogenicity has been observed in rodents, this has not been confirmed in humans. Nevertheless, these agents should be used with caution in pregnant women and children.

Specific drugs (Table 29.5)

Hydroxyzine. Hydroxyzine is marketed as the hydrochloride (intramuscular and oral) and pamoate (oral) salt forms. The former hydrophilic salt may afford fast action, whereas the latter lipophilic salt may afford extended action. While it is rarely used as an antihistamine because of its sedative properties, it is used pre- and postoperationally for nausea, anxiety, pruritus, and allergic rhinitis. It is also used as a sedative agent for stress-related agitation. Phase 1 metabolites of hydroxyzine are illustrated in Figure 29.14. The terminal hydroxymethyl group of hydroxyzine undergoes sequential oxidation by cytosolic alcohol dehydrogenase and ALDH to provide the active carboxylic-acid metabolite, cetirizine (see Second-Generation H_1-Antihistamines (Generally Nonsedative); approved by the FDA in 1995). Oxidative O-dealkylation and N-dealkylation of the ether side chain gives the ethanolamine and norhydroxyzine analogues, respectively. N-dealkylation at the benzhydryl carbon affords *p*-chlorobenzophenone. Reduction of the latter gives the corresponding secondary alcohol. *p*-Hydroxylation (aromatic oxidation) of the phenyl ring of *p*-chlorobenzophenone also occurs to yield the corresponding phenol. Similar metabolic patterns occur for others in this class.

Meclizine. Meclizine is an analogue of hydroxyzine in which the hydroxy ether side chain has been replaced with a 3-methylbenzyl group. The 3-methylbenzyl significantly increases lipophilicity relative to hydroxyzine. It is marketed

Table 29.5 Piperazine Antihistamines

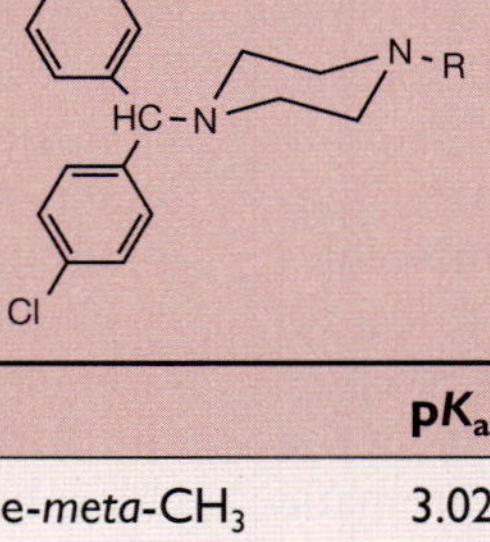

Drug	Salt	R	pK_a[a]	cLogP[a]	$T_{0.5}$[b] (h)
Meclizine (Antivert)	HCl, di-HCl	$-CH_2$-Phe-*meta*-CH_3	3.02 (R-substituted), 8.36	6.73	5-6
Hydroxyzine (Vistaril)	HCl, pamoate	$-CH_2CH_2OCH_2CH_2OH$	3.00 (R-substituted), 8.25	5.61	13-27

[a]pK_a and cLogP (calculated LogP) from ChemDraw 22.0.0.
[b]From Baselt RC. *Disposition of Toxic Drugs and Chemicals in Man.* 11th ed. Biomedical Publications; 2017 (monographs and references therein) or Micromedex.

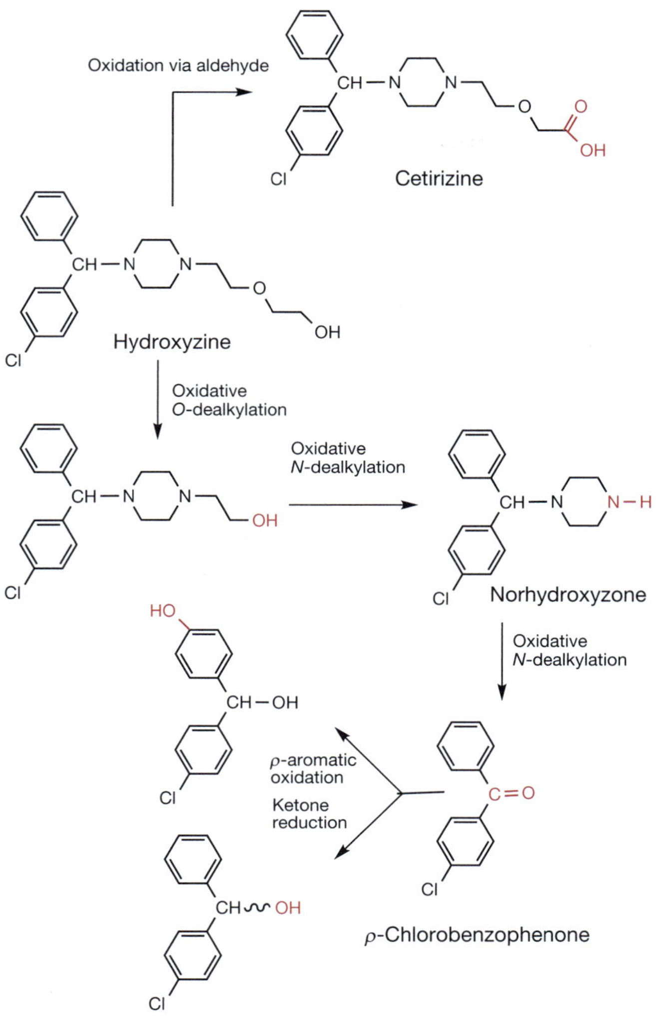

Figure 29.14 Reported phase 1 metabolites of hydroxyzine.

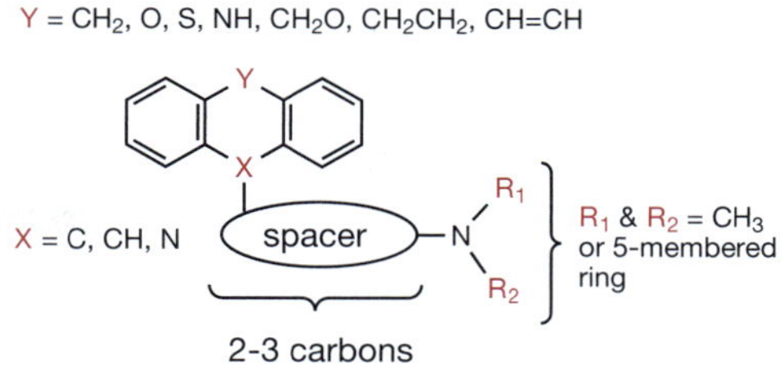

Figure 29.15 General structure of tricyclic antihistamines.

as both hydrochloride and dihydrochloride salts. It is metabolized via N-dealkylation similar to hydroxyzine to afford normeclizine, which has the same structure as norhydroxyzine and has only minimal pharmacological activity. Meclizine is almost exclusively used for motion sickness and vertigo. The chloro substituent blocks inactivating aromatic oxidation, and thus, it increases distribution and potency and provides a longer duration of action.

Tricyclic Antihistamines

Connecting the two aromatic rings found in the earlier-mentioned classes of first-generation antihistamines affords active tricyclic H_1-antihistamines. The two rings may be connected via a heteroatom such as sulfur or oxygen, or with a one- or two-carbon chain (Fig. 29.15 and Table 29.6). Molecules with a phenothiazine ring system (Y = S, X = N) were the earliest tricyclic antihistamines. The aromatic rings in antihistaminic phenothiazines (such as promethazine) are unsubstituted and have a branched two- or three-carbon aliphatic amine side chain attached to the nonbasic diarylamine. Antipsychotic phenothiazines differ in that they have an electron-withdrawing substituent on one of the aromatic rings and possess a three-carbon, unbranched aliphatic amine side chain. Tricyclic antihistamines are typically used to treat nausea and vomiting associated with

Table 29.6 Tricyclic First-Generation Antihistamines

Drug	Salt	pK_a[a]	cLogP[a]	$T_{0.5}$[b] (h)
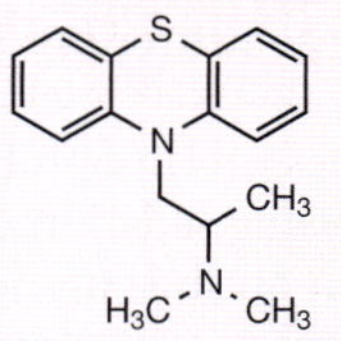 Promethazine (Phenergan)	HCl	9.29	4.60	10-20
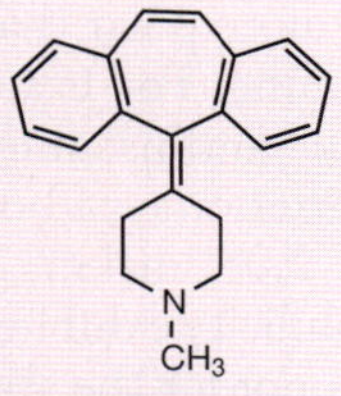 Cyproheptadine	HCl	9.61	5.30	20-70

[a] pK_a and cLogP (calculated LogP) from ChemDraw 22.0.0.
[b] From Baselt RC. *Disposition of Toxic Drugs and Chemicals in Man.* 11th ed. Biomedical Publications; 2017 (monographs and references therein) or Micromedex.

anesthesia and motion sickness, and for their antipruritic effect in the treatment of urticaria.

There are important conformational and stereochemical effects that should be considered when evaluating the antihistaminic activity of phenothiazines. Connecting the two aromatic rings results in steric restrictions. These rings are not flat or co-planar; however, they are slightly puckered. These possible conformations may rapidly interconvert, but in some cases, the interconversion is slow, resulting in conformational enantiomers (ie, atropoisomers).[55,56] These have been studied with cyproheptadine, doxepin, and hydroxylated metabolites of loratadine (discussed next).[57] The pharmacological potency is significantly different (9- to 60-fold) for the conformational enantiomers of 3-methoxycyproheptadine as antihistaminic, antiserotonergic, and anticholinergic agents. The (−)-isomer retains the antihistaminic, antiserotonergic, and appetite-stimulant effects, while the (+)-isomer shows greater anticholinergic potency.

Replacement of the sulfur atom of the phenothiazine ring system with a two-carbon unsaturated or saturated bridge produced related compounds cyproheptadine and azatadine (not available in the United States), respectively. Replacement with $-CH_2$-O-affords doxepin, a tricyclic antidepressant with antihistamine activity.

SPECIFIC DRUGS (TABLE 29.6)

Promethazine. Promethazine is a good antiemetic with high antihistaminic and anticholinergic effects. While it can be used for its antihistaminic effects to treat allergic rhinitis, it is used more often as a sedative, an antiemetic in the prevention of motion sickness, and pre- and postoperatively to prevent and treat nausea and vomiting associated with surgical procedures. It is sometimes used to potentiate the pain-relieving effects of analgesics. It is marketed in oral tablets, syrups, and solutions, and is also available by injection or as rectal suppositories. Promethazine metabolism has not been extensively studied in man, but the metabolites norpromethazine (N-demethylation) and the sulfoxide have been reported.

While promethazine is approved for use with caution in children older than 2 years, the lowest dose possible should always be used. In 2006, the FDA issued a warning for pediatric promethazine use, as fatal respiratory depression was reported in patients under 2 years. Patients of any age with compromised respiratory function should not use promethazine. The drug also increases the seizure risk in patients with seizure disorders.[21] It is also associated with severe tissue injury, including gangrene, at the site of injection. Although α-receptor blocking effects can be demonstrated by many antihistamines, it is more commonly exhibited by those in the phenothiazine group, such as promethazine. This action may cause orthostatic hypotension in susceptible individuals. Lastly, owing to their ability to block sodium channels in excitable membranes in the same fashion as procaine and lidocaine, promethazine is actually more potent than procaine as a local anesthetic. Promethazine (and diphenhydramine) are occasionally used to produce local anesthesia in patients allergic to conventional local anesthetic drugs.

Cyproheptadine. Cyproheptadine is piperidine-containing antihistamine and can be considered an analogue of phenothiazine in which the sulfur is replaced with an unsaturated ethylene bridge. Similarities may also be seen with the olefinic alkylamines, where the two aromatic rings are connected through an unsaturated ethylene bridge. In addition to its antihistaminic activity, cyproheptadine exhibits moderate anticholinergic and low sedative effects. FDA-approved uses include allergic conjunctivitis and rhinitis, dermatologic urticaria, hypersensitivity to blood or plasma, urticaria due to cold, and vasomotor rhinitis. It also acts as a serotonin antagonist, which explains its ability to stimulate appetite. While appetite stimulation and weight gain are not approved uses, it is used "off-label" to promote weight gain in conditions where this is needed, such as cancer and cystic fibrosis. Off-label indications also include nightmare attenuation in patients with posttraumatic stress disorder and prevention of migraine headaches in children and teens.

Cyproheptadine is a long-acting antihistamine with an elimination half-life of 16 hours owing to its lipophilicity (large volume of distribution) and its potentially extensive binding to plasma proteins. It is eliminated as unchanged drug (1%) or quaternary ammonium glucuronide (10%), and the remainder as metabolites resulting from N-demethylation, aromatic hydroxylation, heterocyclic ring oxidation, and conjugation. No metabolism at the ethylene bridge was reported.[58]

Second-Generation H_1-Antihistamines (Generally Nonsedative)

Selectivity and Lack of Significant Central Nervous System Effect

The introduction of second-generation, nonsedating H_1-antihistamines in the 1980s improved the quality of life of patients suffering from allergic conditions. These antihistamines have greater selectivity for peripheral H_1-receptors and are relatively free from adverse CNS effects, as well as from anticholinergic, antiserotonergic, and antiadrenergic effects.[59] Their lack of sedative properties is likely due to a greatly reduced ability to penetrate the blood-brain barrier (BBB). This is attributed to their affinity for the drug efflux P-glycoprotein transporter or the organic anion transporter[60] and/or because of their poor partitioning characteristics resulting from being amphoteric and existing as zwitterions at physiological pH.[59]

While the first-generation antihistamines are lipophilic amines that readily penetrate the BBB, causing sedation as a side effect, most of the second-generation antihistamines possess both the basic amine required for activity as well as a carboxylic acid group. As a result, these agents exist as zwitterions at physiological pH and are more polar than those agents containing only the basic amine. For example, the cLogP value of the first-generation antihistamine hydroxyzine is 4.00 while cetirizine, its zwitterionic carboxylic-acid metabolite, has a cLogP value of 2.08, making it much less lipophilic. The decrease in lipophilicity exhibited by cetirizine would be even greater if it was not for the ability of the carboxylate anion to fold around and form an intramolecular ionic bond with the protonated amine. Thus,

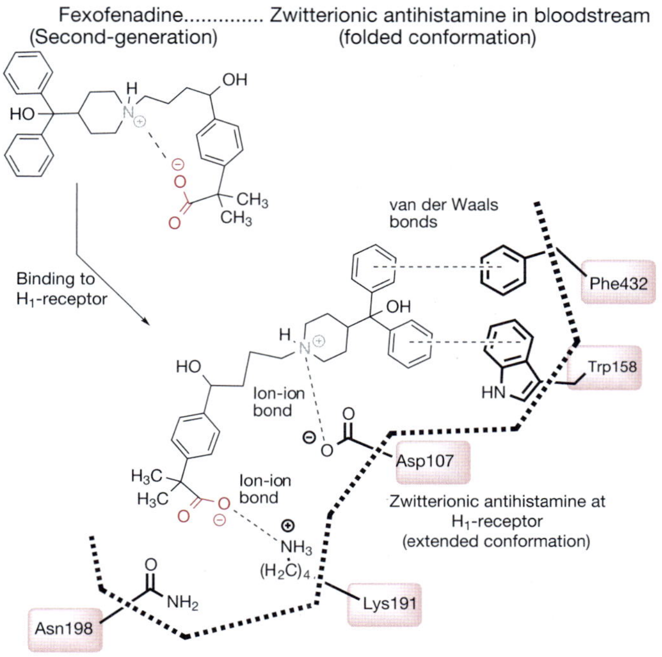

Figure 29.16 Zwitterionic antihistamine binding at the H_1-receptor. (From Lemke TL, Zito SW, Roche VF, Williams DA, eds. Antihistamines and related antiallergic and antiulcer agents. In: *Essentials of Foye's Principles of Medicinal Chemistry*. Wolters Kluwer; 2017:408-432.)

these zwitterionic molecules exhibit lower CNS penetration and an improved side-effect profile. The CNS activity of the second-generation agents varies from 0% (fexofenadine) to 30% (cetirizine).

The carboxylic acid group also contributes to enhanced H_1-receptor affinity, as it can form an ionic bond with Lys191 of the receptor.[61] This contributes to the slow receptor dissociation kinetics seen with these agents. As presented in Figure 29.16, the folded conformation predominates in the bloodstream, and this minimizes affinity for CNS transporting proteins. Affinity for central P-glycoprotein efflux protein is high, so molecules that passively enter the brain are readily pumped out. At the peripheral H_1-receptors, the extended conformation allows two ionic interactions with charged receptor residues to form. The ionic binding, especially with Lys191, is strong and augments antihistamine potency.[21]

Interestingly, there is a large variation in the structures of the second-generation antihistamines. For some, structural similarities with first-generation agents are readily apparent, while for others they are not obvious. Importantly, the large *N*-substituents found on these agents when compared to the first-generation antihistamines may contribute to their lack of affinity for cholinergic, α-adrenergic, and serotonergic receptors.

Historically, extensive clinical use of astemizole and terfenadine revealed that simultaneous use with drugs that are inhibitors of or co-substrates for CYP3A4 is associated with cardiac QT prolongation, precipitating a life-threatening ventricular arrhythmia known as torsades de points.[62] This adverse effect is associated with blockade of the hERG gene product, a subunit of an inward-rectifying cardiac potassium channel (I_{Kr}).[63,64] The arrhythmias are observed at high concentrations of astemizole and terfenadine, such as when they are concurrently used with inhibitors of CYP3A4 (including grapefruit juice, ketoconazole or macrolide antibiotics like erythromycin) or with competing CYP3A4 substrates. This is not a class effect and is only associated with astemizole and terfenadine. Both are no longer marketed in the United States.

Withdrawn from the US market because of cardiotoxicity

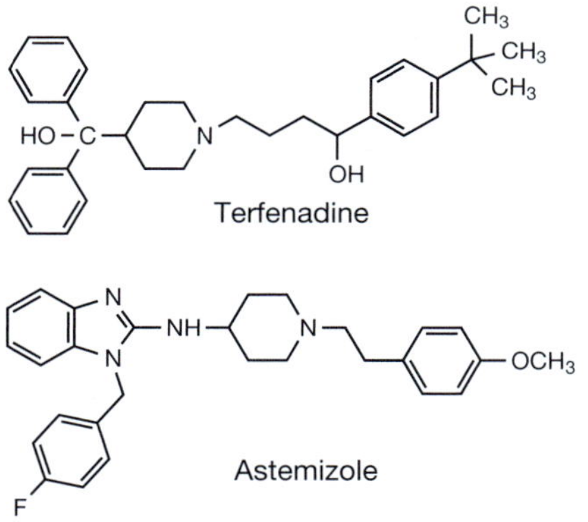

Specific Drugs Used Systemically (Fig. 29.17 and Table 29.7)

Fexofenadine. The story of the marketing of fexofenadine is both a tale of serendipity and a reinforcement of pharmacists' professional responsibility. Fexofenadine was

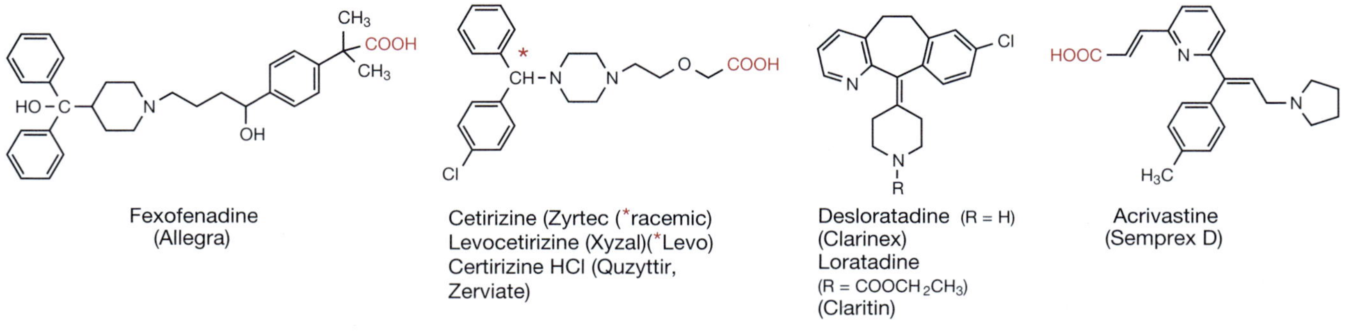

Figure 29.17 Second-generation antihistamines used for their systemic action. They may be marketed in salt form and/or in combination with decongestants.

Table 29.7 Second-Generation Antihistamines Used for Peripheral Systemic Actions

Drug	pK_a[a]	cLogP[a]	Oral Bioavailability (%)[b]	Onset of Action[b] (h)	$T_{0.5}$ (h)[b]	Plasma Protein Binding (%)[b]	Metabolism[b]	Excretion[b]	Duration of Action (h)[b]
Fexofenadine (Allegra)	9.57, 4.34	1.96	~33	1-3	14-18	60-70	<10%	80% feces 11% urine (unchanged)	12-24
Cetirizine (Zyrtec)	2.98, 8.25, 3.08	2.08	70	<1	8.3	93	Limited, hepatic	10% feces (unchanged) 70% urine (50% unchanged)	24
Levocetirizine (Xyzal)	2.98, 8.25, 3.08	2.08	85	<1	7-8 (adult) 5.7 (children)	91-95	<14%	13% feces 85% urine (80% unchanged)	Up to 32
Acrivastine	9.09, 3.94	1.46	Significant	<1	1.5-1.9	50	Minimal, hepatic	13% feces 84% urine (67% unchanged)	12
Loratadine (Claritin)	5.0	5.05	Significant	1-3	8.4-18.2	97-99	CYP3A4 and CYP2D6 (active metabolite)	40% feces 40% urine (metabolites)	24-48
Desloratadine (Clarinex)	9.22	3.83	Significant	<1	19-40 (adult) 16-19 (children)	82-97	CYP2C8 (active metabolite)	46.5% feces 40.6% urine (metabolites)	Up to 24

[a] pK_a and cLogP (calculated LogP) from ChemDraw 22.0.0.
[b] From Baselt RC. *Disposition of Toxic Drugs and Chemicals in Man*. 11th ed. Biomedical Publications; 2017 (monographs and references therein) or Micromedex.

discovered as an active metabolite of terfenadine (Seldane), which was the first nonsedative antihistamine to be marketed in the United States and, as such, a blockbuster. It was known to be highly cardiotoxic, but in most individuals it was readily converted via CYP3A4 and cytosolic enzymes to non-cardiotoxic metabolites. These metabolites not only retained the nonsedative properties of terfenadine, but the carboxylic acid metabolite also exhibited antihistaminic action up to 4 times that of the parent drug. However, given the fatal risk of torsades des pointes and cardiac arrest when given to vulnerable patients (such as those with hepatic disease) and/or when co-administered drugs or foods that inhibit CYP3A4, a Black Box warning was issued. In 1996, a study conducted by Georgetown University researchers revealed that approximately one-third of practitioners in selected Washington DC area pharmacies dispensed terfenadine along with erythromycin without comment or warning when presented with simultaneous prescriptions. The study received much attention in the professional literature and lay press, and within 3 years, terfenadine was withdrawn from the US market. The event served as a good reminder of the pharmacists' critical role in protecting the public health. Interestingly, the manufactures of terfenadine took clinical and economic advantage of their understanding of terfenadine metabolism to bring the non-cardiotoxic carboxylic-acid metabolite to the market as fexofenadine (Allegra, the Italian word for "happy"). Allegra has enjoyed significant success and has been joined by other second-generation antihistamines that owe their nonsedating properties to their zwitterionic chemical nature, which prevents their accumulation in the CNS.

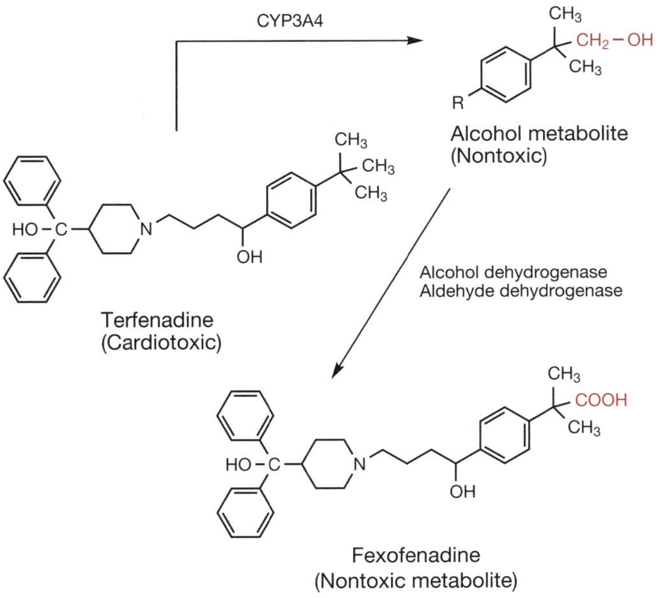

Metabolism of terfenadine and discovery of fexofenadine

Fexofenadine is a piperidine-containing, long-acting (>12 hours), selective H_1-antihistamine that shows little affinity for the cholinergic, adrenergic, or serotonergic receptors. The bulky *N*-phenylbutanol group is believed to be, at least in part, responsible for the high H_1-receptor selectivity. The enantiomers of terfenadine have been shown to have approximately equal activity,[65] but there are little data on the activity of the enantiomers of fexofenadine. However, the drug efflux transporter P-glycoprotein and organic anion transporter proteins may show some stereoselectivity because higher plasma concentrations are seen for the *R*-enantiomer. The *N*-phenylbutanol group is linked to affinity for the P-glycoprotein efflux pump and, thus, reduced CNS accumulation. Fexofenadine is primarily eliminated unchanged, with 80% appearing in the feces and 11% in the urine.

Cetirizine and Levocetirizine. Cetirizine is the carboxylic acid metabolite formed upon oxidation of the primary alcohol of the first-generation antihistamine hydroxyzine.[66] It is a piperazine-containing and amphoteric antihistamine. It has a long duration of action and no cardiotoxicity. Although many consider cetirizine to have decreased sedative effects, they are not absent. The claimed decrease in sedation is potentially the result of its amphoteric nature. The *R*-enantiomer is now marketed as levocetirizine, and its affinity for the H_1-receptor is more than 30-fold greater than that of the *S*-enantiomer and its receptor dissociation rate is more than 20-fold slower.[67] Therefore, most antihistaminic properties observed with cetirizine are likely due to the *R*-enantiomer. Levocetirizine is largely excreted unchanged (77%) in the urine, with eight minor products of oxidation and glucuronide conjugation.[68]

Acrivastine. Acrivastine is a second-generation, acrylic acid-substituted analogue of the first-generation antihistamine triprolidine. Its CNS penetration is limited, and it is less sedating than triprolidine. It is used in combination with the decongestant pseudoephedrine in seasonal rhinitis. Urinary excretion products include unchanged drug, the product of reduction of the double bond in the acrylic acid side chain, and some unidentified products. The reduction product is pharmacologically active but probably contributes little to overall activity because it is a minor product compared to the parent. Acrivastine requires more frequent dosing (about 4 times a day) because it has the shortest duration of action among all systemically used second-generation antihistamines. This perhaps is attributed to its high hydrophilicity given the acrylic side chain and significant extent of conjugated unsaturation.

Loratadine and Desloratadine. Loratadine and its active metabolite desloratadine are also piperidine-containing antihistamines. Loratadine, in particular, is unique because it does not have a basic amine. Rather, it has a carbamate group although, as described next, that moiety will be lost to first-pass metabolism to provide the expected basic amine before the drug reaches the general circulation. The two drugs are peripherally selective, nonsedating antihistamines used for treatment of idiopathic urticarial and chronic and seasonal allergic rhinitis. They have structural similarities with first-generation tricyclic antihistamines and tricyclic antidepressants.

Desloratadine is the descarboethoxy metabolite of loratadine, and it has a longer half-life (17-27 hours) than the parent drug (3-20 hours). Thus, with the continuous use, its plasma concentration exceeds that of loratadine. The potency of desloratadine is greater than that of loratadine as both an inhibitor of histamine release and as a H_1-antihistamine. Because of its longer half-life, greater potency, and essentially complete generation from loratadine on first-pass metabolism, desloratadine likely contributes significantly to the overall activity of loratadine. When compared to first-generation antihistamines, desloratadine has a 100-fold slower receptor dissociation rate.[69]

The metabolic removal of the carbamate group of loratadine to afford the des-carboethoxy analogue desloratadine is not via direct hydrolysis. Rather, it involves oxidation by CYP2D6 and CYP3A4 at the methylene group of the carbamate (Fig. 29.18).[70] This unstable hydroxylated intermediate readily undergoes O-deethylation and decarboxylation to give the corresponding active secondary amine, desloratadine. CYP2C8-catalyzed aromatic hydroxylation of desloratadine provides another active metabolite. Inactivation through glucuronic acid conjugation of the phenol completes the major loratadine/desloratadine metabolic pathway. Other hydroxylated aliphatic and aromatic metabolites, and their glucuronide conjugates, have been identified.

As noted, orally administered loratadine is extensively converted to desloratadine on first pass through the liver. Thus, little, if any, loratadine parent drug reaches the general circulation or H_1-receptors. Concurrent use of loratadine or desloratadine with CYP3A4 inhibitors or competitive substrates does not lead to significant drug-drug interactions (DDIs), and they both lack effects on hERG potassium ion channels in the heart. Desloratadine does not penetrate the CNS in significant concentration and has a long half-life, 17 to 27 hours in humans, with about 41% of an administered dose being excreted in the urine and 47% in the feces over a 10-day period.[71,72]

Topical H_1-Antihistamines (Ophthalmic and Nasal)

Therapeutic Applications. Ocular allergic reactions are common in seasonal allergy patients given the high density of mast cells in the conjunctiva as well as the significant

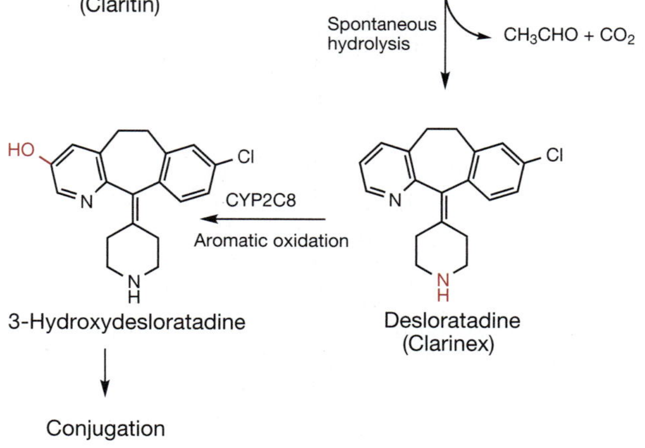

Figure 29.18 Metabolism of loratadine.

concentration of histamine in the tear film. Several H_1-antihistamines have been formulated for topical application in the eye to relieve itching, congestion of the conjunctiva, and erythema (Fig. 29.19 and Table 29.8).[73] When delivered topically, sedation is minimized. The first topical ocular antihistamines were antazoline and pheniramine, first-generation agents in the ethylenediamine and alkylamine class, respectively. They are used in combination with sympathomimetic vasoconstrictors. Only about 1% to 5% of the antihistamine penetrates the cornea when topically applied. Most of the drug is systemically absorbed via the conjunctiva and nasal mucosa as well as from being swallowed upon tear duct and nasal drainage.

The more recently developed second generation ocular antihistamines exhibit slow receptor dissociation kinetics and have a long duration of action. The relationship between the partitioning characteristics of an antihistamine and its receptor affinity suggests that a particular range of lipophilicity is best for topical ocular antihistamines with minimum ocular irritation.[74] The most effective antihistamines are those with a log D near 1.0 ± 0.5 at physiological pH. Their water-soluble salts are associated with a low incidence of ocular irritation. The only contraindication to their use is hypersensitivity to the drug or a formulation component.

Specific Drugs (See Fig. 29.19 and Table 29.8)

Ketotifen. Ketotifen[73] is a tricyclic, piperidine-containing antihistamine with significant structural similarities to cyproheptadine. It has a bioisosteric thiophene ring in place of the benzene ring, and the bridge between the two aromatic rings is saturated and oxidized to a ketone at the benzylic position. It is a potent, selective dual-acting H_1-antihistamine that, in addition to blocking the H_1-receptor, also stabilizes mast cells and prevents degranulation of eosinophils.

Ketotifen is used in the United States as OTC ophthalmic drops for the treatment and prevention of itching associated with allergic conjunctivitis, and it is used systemically in other countries for seasonal allergic rhinitis, hay fever, and asthma. When it is used topically, action starts within minutes. Systemically used ketotifen undergoes metabolic N-dealkylation to give norketotifen as well as N-oxidation to produce an *N*-oxide metabolite. Reduction of the exocyclic double bond produces dihydroketotifen. Glucuronic acid conjugation at the tertiary amine gives the quaternary *N*-glucuronide.

Olopatadine. Olopatadine is a tricyclic, amphoteric dibenzoxepin antihistamine. It is formulated for topical use in the eye to treat allergic conjunctivitis and as a nasal spray for nasal symptoms of allergic rhinitis. It is a dual-acting antihistamine since it also exhibits mast cell–stabilizing properties—that is, it inhibits release of other inflammatory mediators from mast cells. Olopatadine is highly specific for H_1-receptors over H_2, H_3, α-adrenergic, dopaminergic, serotonergic, and muscarinic receptors. It has a rapid onset (<30 minutes) and long duration of action, which is indicative of high receptor affinity and slow dissociation kinetics. The elimination half-life of olopatadine following intranasal administration is 8 to 12 hours and following ophthalmic administration is 3 hours. The carboxylic acid-containing

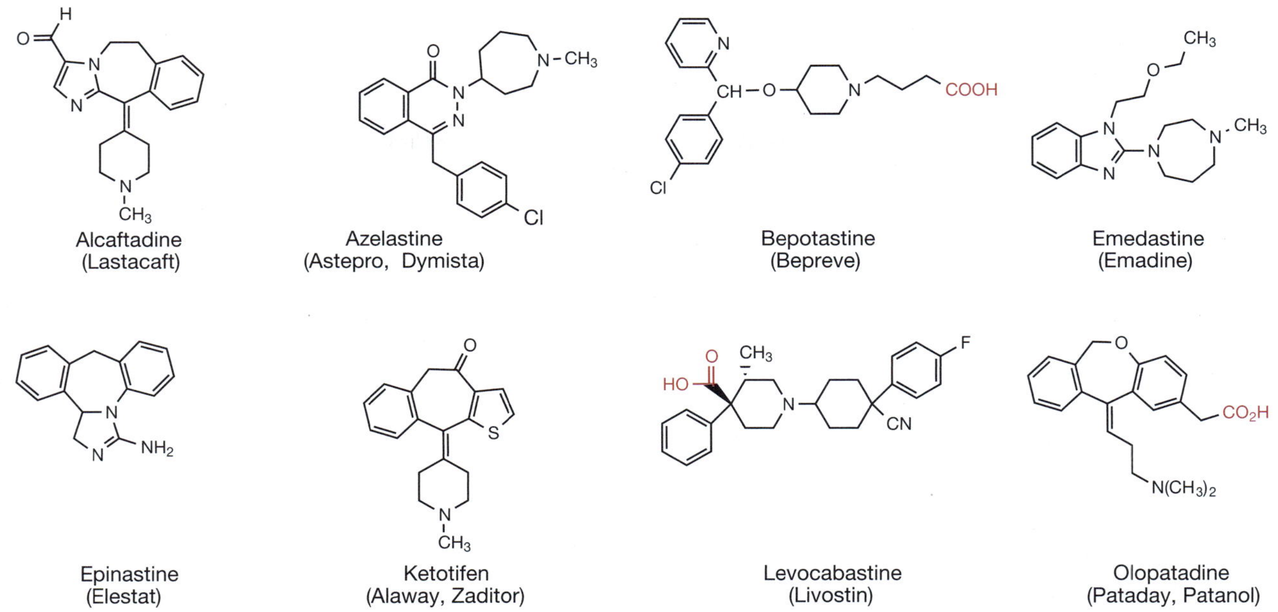

Figure 29.19 Second-generation antihistamines used for their local action.

aromatic substituent potentially contributes to its lack of muscarinic effects. At physiological pH, olopatadine exists as a zwitterion, which contributes to the drug's limited access to CNS. The carboxylate group of the *Z*-isomer, which fixes the terminal amine on the same molecular side of the structure, could form an ionic bond with protonated amine side chain. When binding to the receptor, the carboxylic acid extends out of the binding pocket and interacts with Lys191 and Tyr108.[61]

Table 29.8 Second-Generation Antihistamines Used Topically

Drug	pK_a[a]	cLogP[a]	$T_{0.5}$ (h)[b]
Ketotifen fumarate (Alaway)	9.05	3.59	7-27
Olopatadine HCl (Pataday)	9.85, 4.20	1.09	9-10
Alcaftadine (Lastacaft)	9.08	2.45	2
Epinastine HCl	11.98	2.15	12
Emedastine Difumarate (Emadine)	8.87	2.30	3-8
Azelastine HCl (Astepro)	9.31	4.01	22
Bepotastine besilate (Bepreve)	9.52, 3.47	0.28	3-7
Levocabastine HCl (Livostin)	9.35, 2.75	1.86	35-40

[a]pK_a and cLogP (calculated LogP) from ChemDraw 22.0.0.
[b]From Baselt RC. *Disposition of Toxic Drugs and Chemicals in Man.* 11th ed. Biomedical Publications; 2017 (monographs and references therein) or Micromedex.

Olopatadine is only metabolized to a minor extent. In a 48-hour, single-dose study using labeled olopatadine in healthy adults, urine collection afforded parent drug (63%-72%), *N*-desmethylolopatadine (1%), and olopatadine-*N*-oxide (3%).[75] Approximately 17% of a radiolabeled oral dose of olopatadine is excreted in the feces.

Alcaftadine. Alcaftadine is a tricyclic, piperidine-containing antihistamine. It is an aldehyde-substituted imidazobenzazpine H_1-blocker related to other tricyclic H_1-antihistamines. It is indicated for treatment of allergic conjunctivitis, and also inhibits both histamine release from mast cells and eosinophil activation. The aldehyde group on the imidazole ring is metabolically oxidized to the active carboxylic-acid metabolite and is excreted in the urine.

Epinastine. Epinastine is a tetracyclic antihistamine containing a dibenzazepine tricyclic system fused with a dihydroimidazole-amine moiety. Embedded within the structure is a basic guanidine moiety that is more basic than the typical aliphatic amine (pK_a ~12 vs pK_a ~9, respectively), assuring a persistent cationic charge for anchoring to the H_1 receptor. It is indicated for treatment of allergic conjunctivitis. Activity starts within 5 minutes, and its elimination half-life is 12 hours. Epinastine is selective for the H_1-receptor but also has some affinity for histamine H_2-receptors, adrenergic α-receptors, and 5-HT_2 receptors. In humans, it is eliminated largely unchanged in the urine (25%) and feces (70%).

Emedastine. Emedastine is a disubstituted benzimidazole H_1-antihistamine. Like other topical antihistamines, it has also been shown to stabilize mast cells. It is formulated for ophthalmic administration for treatment of allergic conjunctivitis. Emedastine is metabolized to two inactive phenols (5- and 6-hydroxyemedastine) via aromatic oxidation, emedastine-*N*-oxide, and conjugates of the phenols. It has an elimination half-life of 2 to 6.6 hours, with approximately 44% of an oral dose recovered in the urine. Only 3.6% is excreted as the parent drug over 24 hours.[76]

Azelastine. Azelastine is a disubstituted phthalazine-1(2*H*)-one dual-acting antihistamine. It is used as a nasal spray and as eye drops in the United States for seasonal and perennial allergic rhinitis, allergic conjunctivitis, and vasomotor rhinitis. In Europe, it is available for systemic treatment of seasonal allergies and asthma. Azelastine undergoes oxidative N-dealkylation to give the active metabolite, *N*-desmethylazelastine, which has a half-life twice that of the parent (parent half-life of 22-25 hours vs metabolite half-life of 42-54 hours).

Bepotastine. Bepotastine is an amphoteric *N*-substituted piperidine H_1-antihistamine structurally related to the aminoalkyl ethers. Similarities to cetirizine and fexofenadine are also readily apparent. It is formulated as an ophthalmic solution for treatment of allergic conjunctivitis. In addition to its antihistaminic properties, it also inhibits the release of histamine from mast cells. In a 24-hour study following a single oral dose in Japanese men, the parent drug was eliminated (76%-88%) in the urine along with an unidentified metabolite (1%).[77]

Levocabastine. Levocabastine is a highly substituted amphoteric, piperidine-containing H_1-antihistamine. An *N*-cyclohexylpiperidine derivative with unique cyano and *p*-fluorophenyl substituents, it is structurally dissimilar from other antihistamines. It appears to lack significant antiserotonergic, antidopaminergic, or anticholinergic activity, while α-adrenergic antagonism has been observed only at very high doses in animals. The antihistaminic potency of levocabastine is greater than that of other H_1-antihistamines. Its ophthalmic solution has been effective in alleviating histamine-induced conjunctivitis. Hepatic metabolism is minimal, and the drug is mainly eliminated in urine (75%-80%; 65%-70% is excreted unchanged and 10% as the glucuronide metabolite). Its onset of action is 15 minutes, and its elimination half-life is 33 to 40 hours.[78]

HISTAMINE RELEASE INHIBITORS (MAST-CELL STABILIZERS)

Background and Mechanism of Action

Khellin, a chromone found in the fruit of *Ammi visnaga* (also known as toothpick weed), possesses bronchodilatory activity and has been used as a spasmolytic in the Mediterranean region.[79] Subsequently, cromolyn sodium was developed while studying a large number of bis-chromones. Other agents in this class include nedocromil and lodoxamide (see Table 29.9).

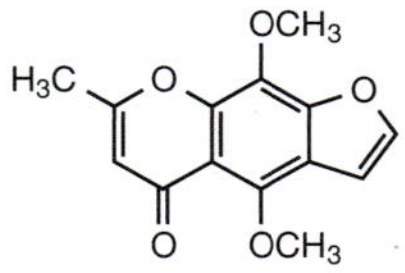

Khellin
(a lead natural product from *Ammi visnaga*)

Table 29.9 Mast-Cell Stabilizers

Drug	pK_a[a]	cLogP[a]	$T_{0.5}$ (h)[b]	Major Excretion[b]
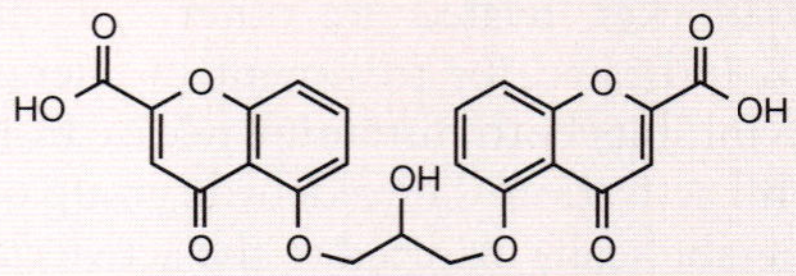 Cromolyn (NasalCrom) (sodium salt)	2.58, 13.24, 2.58	1.48	1.5	30%-50% (urine) >70% (feces) [unchanged]
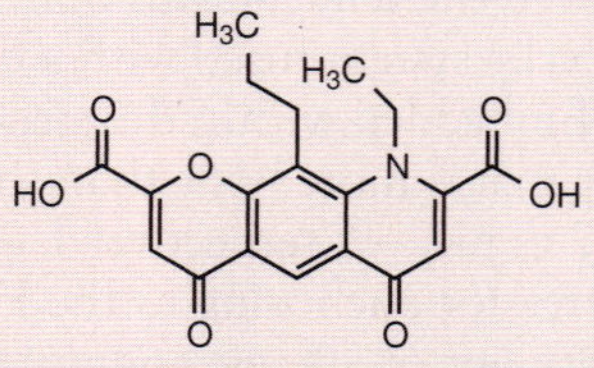 Nedocromil (Alocril) (sodium salt)	2.43, 3.08	1.50	~3.3	70% (urine) 30% (feces) [unchanged]
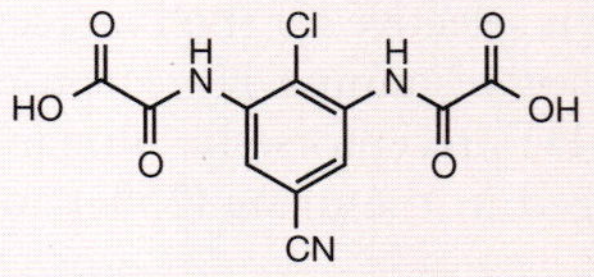 Lodoxamide (Alomide) (tromethamine salt)	0.97, 0.97	−2.24	8.5	urine

[a]pK_a and cLogP (calculated LogP) from ChemDraw 22.0.0.
[b]From Baselt RC. Disposition of Toxic Drugs and Chemicals in Man. 11th ed. Biomedical Publications; 2017 (monographs and references therein) or Micromedex.

These agents are classified as mast-cell stabilizers because they prevent the release of histamine and other mediators from mast cells and other inflammatory cells associated with allergy and asthma. While they prevent bronchospasm, they do not reverse antigen-induced bronchoconstriction. They exhibit no intrinsic bronchodilatory, antihistaminic, anticholinergic, glucocorticoid, vasoconstrictor, or other systemic activity. Mast-cell stabilizers also inhibit activation and release of allergy mediators from eosinophils, macrophages, neutrophils, monocytes, and platelets.[80]

Mechanistically, the majority of the mast-cell stabilizers stimulate protein kinase C–catalyzed phosphorylation of serine residues of moesin, a protein involved in the bridging of actin cytoskeleton and cell membranes. Upon phosphorylation, a conformational change in moesin promotes its association with actin and other proteins of the secretory granules, leading to immobilization of the granules and inhibition of their exocytosis. Another proposed mechanism involves inhibition of antigen-induced calcium ion influx into mast cells. This stabilizes the cells and prevents release of histamine, leukotrienes, and other inflammatory mediators that are involved in allergic reactions.[81] There is evidence to suggest that lodoxamide may also act by inhibiting eosinophil infiltration, possibly decreasing the number of T_H2 cells.

Specific Drugs (see Table 29.9)

CROMOLYN. Cromolyn is a synthetic bis-chromone carboxylic-acid derivative that is marketed as the sodium salt. The two chromone moieties are linked together via a glycerol bridge. The drug is available in several dosage forms. Cromolyn nasal solution is approved for the treatment of allergic rhinitis. Cromolyn nebulized solution is indicated for preventing and managing asthma and exercise-induced bronchospasm. Ophthalmic cromolyn is indicated for the treatment of vernal keratitis, conjunctivitis, and keratoconjunctivitis. Oral cromolyn is indicated for the symptomatic management of mastocytosis, a rare disorder that involves abnormal elevation of mast cell density in the skin, bone marrow, and/or internal organs. To be effective, cromolyn must be administered at least 30 minutes prior to antigen exposure. Overuse can lead to development of tolerance.

The medication's bioavailability is variable: inhalation (8%), nasal (7%), oral (1%), and ophthalmic (up to 0.03%). The drug is not metabolized, has an elimination half-life of 80 to 90 minutes, and is eliminated unchanged in urine and feces.

NEDOCROMIL. Nedocromil is a pyranoquinolone dicarboxylic acid derivative related to cromolyn in both structure and mechanism. Its sodium salt is formulated as an ophthalmic solution for the prevention of seasonal and perennial allergic conjunctivitis. Systemic absorption from the eye is minimal. The drug is not metabolized, has an elimination half-life of 1.5 to 3.3 hours, and is eliminated unchanged in urine and feces.

LODOXAMIDE. Lodoxamide is a bis-(2-oxoacetic acid) derivative with some structural similarities to both cromolyn and nedocromil. It is marketed as the tromethamine (1,1,1-tris(hydroxymethyl)aminomethane salt. It is used as an ophthalmic solution for the treatment of vernal conjunctivitis and vernal keratitis. The drug has an elimination half-life of 8.5 hours and is primarily eliminated unchanged in the urine.

ACKNOWLEDGMENT

The author wishes to acknowledge the work of E. Kim Fifer, PhD, who authored content used within this chapter in a previous edition of this text.

Structure Challenge

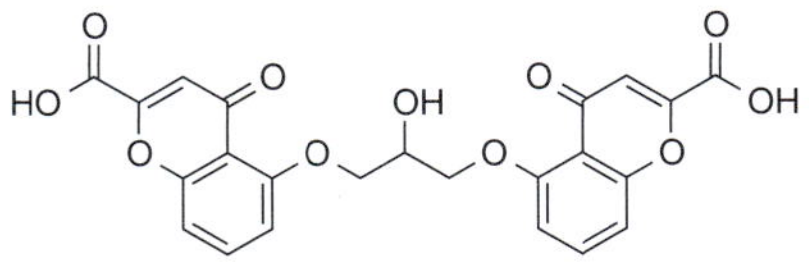

I

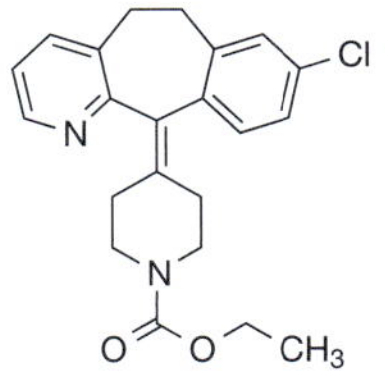

II

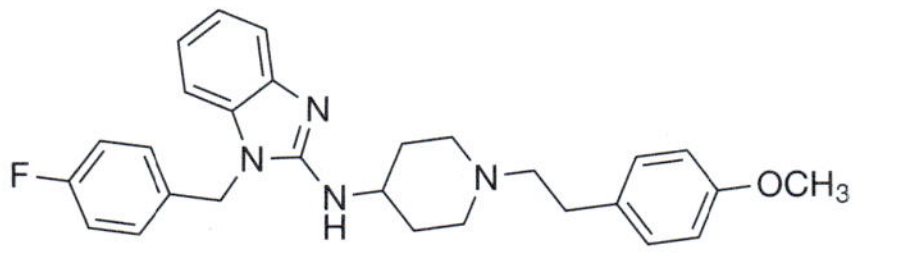

III

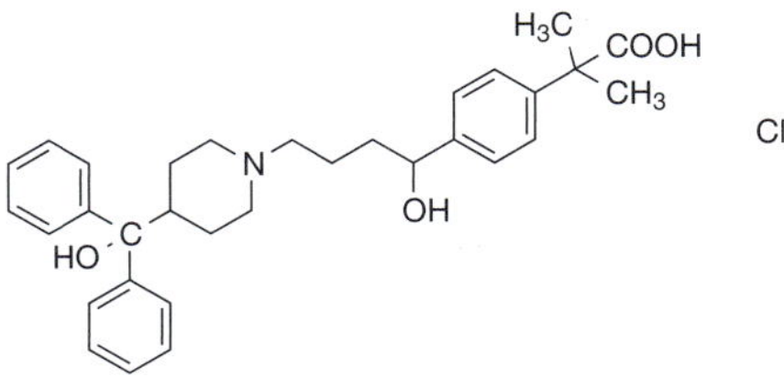

IV

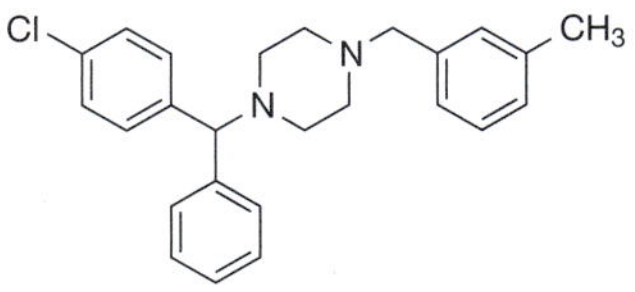

V

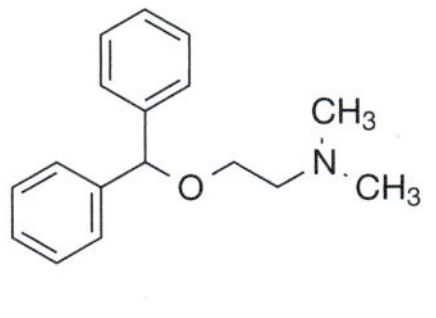

VI

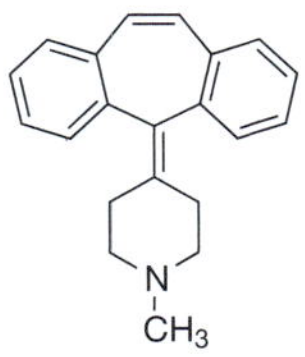

VII

The structures of seven antiallergic drugs are provided later. Use your understanding of SARs to identify the appropriate agent(s) for each of the following situations.

(continued)

Structure Challenge (continued)

1. Which antiallergic would be best for a patient who is worried about motion sickness while cruising the Caribbean for her honeymoon?
2. Which antiallergic should be avoided by a patient who suffers from benign prostate hyperplasia?
3. Which antiallergic would be best for a patient who is working as a long-distance truck driver for goods transportation across states?
4. Which antiallergic is metabolized to an active metabolite with a longer elimination half-life than the parent? Describe its metabolism.
5. Which antiallergic is sometime used to stimulate appetite resulting in weight gain?
6. Which antiallergic(s) is(are) classified as nonsedative amphoteric antihistamine(s)?
7. Which antiallergic is best to use as OTC sleep aid? If the same drug is to be used for motion sickness what can be done to mitigate its sedative properties?
8. Which antiallergic(s) is(are) eliminated mostly unchanged in the urine? Which is(are) metabolized by oxidative N-demethylation?
9. Which antiallergic(s) is(are) to be avoided when the patient is being treated for respiratory tract infection using erythromycin?
10. Which antiallergic would be best to be proactively considered in a patient with a history of seasonal allergies and exercise-induced asthma planning a hiking vacation during spring break?
11. Which antiallergic is prepared as an alkaline salt (ie, sodium salt)? How will this drug likely be applied?

Structure Challenge answers found immediately after References.

REFERENCES

1. Weiss ME, Adkinson NF. Immediate hypersensitivity reactions to penicillin and related antibiotics. *Clin Allergy*. 1988;18:515-540.
2. Larché M, Akdis CA, Valenta R. Immunological mechanisms of allergen-specific immunotherapy. *Nat Rev Immunol.* 2006;6(10): 761-771.
3. Ramachandran M, Aronson JK. John Bostock's first description of hayfever. *J R Soc Med.* 2011;104:237-240.
4. Wheatley LM, Togias A. Clinical practice. Allergic rhinitis. *N Engl J Med.* 2015;372(5):456-463.
5. Roland LT, Wise SK, Wang H, Zhang P, Mehta C, Levy JM. The cost of rhinitis in the United States: a national insurance claims analysis. *Int Forum Allergy Rhinol.* 2021;11(5):946-948.
6. Rosario N, Bielory L. Epidemiology of allergic conjunctivitis. *Curr Opin Allergy Clin Immunol.* 2011;11(5):471-476.
7. Bousquet J, Khaltaev N, Cruz AA, et al. Allergic rhinitis and its impact on asthma (ARIA) 2008 update (in collaboration with the World Health Organization, GA(2)LEN and AllerGen). *Allergy.* 2008;63 suppl 86:8-160.
8. Yu C, Wang K, Cui X, et al. Clinical efficacy and safety of omalizumab in the treatment of allergic rhinitis: a systematic review and meta-analysis of randomized clinical trials. *Am J Rhinol Allergy.* 2020;34(2):196-208.
9. Weinstein SF, Katial R, Jayawardena S, et al. Efficacy and safety of dupilumab in perennial allergic rhinitis and comorbid asthma. *J Allergy Clin Immunol.* 2018;142(1):171-177.
10. Windaus A, Vogt W. Synthesis of iminazolylethylethylamine. *Chem Ber.* 1907;40:3691-3698.
11. Barger G, Dale HH. 4β-Aminoethylglycoxaline (β-iminazolylethylamine) and the other active principles of ergot. *J Chem Soc Trans.* 1910;97:2592-2595.
12. Ackermann D. About the bacterial degradation of histidine. *Hoppe-Seyler's J Physiol Chem.* 1911;65:504-510.
13. Dale HH, Laidlaw PP. The physiological action of β-imidazolylethylamine. *J Physiol.* 1910;41:318-344.
14. Best CH, Dale HH, Dudley HW, et al. The nature of the vaso-dilator constituents of certain tissue extracts. *J Physiol.* 1927; 62(4):397-417.
15. Emanuel MB. Histamine and the antiallergic antihistamines: a history of their discoveries. *Clin Exp Allergy.* 1999;29(suppl 3):1-11.
16. Ganellen CR. The tautomer ratio of histamine. *J Pharm Pharmacol.* 1973;25:787-792.
17. Black JW, Ganellin CR. Naming of substituted histamines. *Experientia.* 1974;30:111-113.
18. Ganellin CR. Imidazole tautomerism of histamine derivatives. In: Bergmann ED, Pullman B, eds. *Molecular and Quantum Pharmacology.* D. Reidel Publishing Company; 1974:43-44.
19. Ganellin CR. Chemistry and structure-activity relationships of drugs acting at histamine receptors. In: Ganellin CR, Parsons ME, eds. *Pharmacology of Histamine Receptors.* John Wright & Sons; 1982:10-102.
20. Cooper DG, Young RC, Durant GJ, et al. Histamine receptors. In: Emmett JC, ed. *Comprehensive Medicinal Chemistry: The Rational Design, Mechanistic Study, and Therapeutic Application of Chemical Compounds.* Vol 3. Membranes and Receptors. Pergamon Press; 1990:343-421.
21. Antihistamines and related antiallergic and antiulcer agents. In: Lemke TL, Zito SW, Roche VF, Williams DA, eds. *Essentials of Foye's Principles of Medicinal Chemistry.* Wolters Kluwer; 2017:408-432.
22. Moya-Garcia AA, Pino-Angeles A, Gil-Redondo R, et al. Structural features of mammalian histidine decarboxylase reveal the basis for specific inhibition. *Br J Pharmacol.* 2009;157:4-13.
23. Wu F, Yu J, Gehring H. Inhibitory and structural studies of novel coenzyme-substrate analogs of human histidine decarboxylase. *FASEB J.* 2008;22:890-897.
24. Watanabe T, Yamatodani A, Maeyama K, et al. Pharmacology of α-fluoromethylhistidine, a specific inhibitor of histidine decarboxylase. *Trends Pharmacol Sci.* 1990;11:363-367.
25. Mulloy B, Lever R, Page CP. Mast cell glycosaminoglycans. *Glycoconj J.* 2017;34(3):351-361.

26. Katzung BG. Histamine, serotonin & the ergot alkaloids. In: Katzung BG, Todd WV, eds. *Basic & Clinical Pharmacology*. 12th ed. McGraw Hill; 2012:273-293.
27. Chambers C, Kvedar JC, Armstrong AW. Histamine pharmacology. In: Golan DE, Tashjian AH, Armstrong EJ, et al, eds. *Principles of Pharmacology: The Pathophysiologic Basis of Drug Therapy*. 3rd ed. Wolters Kluwer; 2018:765-775.
28. Johnson AR, Erdos EG. Release of histamine from mast cells by vasoactive peptides. *Proc Soc Exp Biol Med*. 1973;142:1252-1256.
29. McNeil BD. Minireview: Mas-related G protein-coupled receptor X2 activation by therapeutic drugs. *Neurosci Lett*. 2021;751:135746.
30. McNeil BD. MRGPRX2 and adverse drug reactions. *Front Immunol*. 2021;12:676354.
31. Jutel M, Akdis M, Akdis CA. Histamine, histamine receptors and their role in immune pathology. *Clin Exp Allergy*. 2009;39: 1786-1800.
32. Simons FE, Akdis CA. Histamine and H1-antihistamines. In: Adkinson NF, Bochner BS, Busse WW, eds. *Middleton's Allergy: Principles and Practice*. 7th ed. Mosby; 2009:1517-1547.
33. Bakker RA, Timmerman H, Leurs R. Histamine receptors: specific ligands, receptor biochemistry, and signal transduction. In: Simons FE, ed. *Histamine and H1-Antihistamines in Allergic Disease*. 2nd ed. Marcel Dekker; 2002:27-64.
34. Bruysters M, Pertz HH, Teunissen A, et al. Mutational analysis of the histamine H1-receptor binding pocket of histaprodifens. *Eur J Pharmacol*. 2004;487(1-3):55-63.
35. Luers R, Smit MJ, Tensen CP, et al. Site-directed mutagenesis of the histamine H1-receptor reveals a selective interaction of asparagine 207 with subclasses of H1-receptor agonists. *Biochem Biophys Res Commun*. 1994;201:295-301.
36. Forneau E, Bovet D. Recherches sur l'action sympathicolytique d'un nouveau derive du dioxane. *Arch Int Pharmacodyn*. 1933; 46:178-191.
37. Bovet D, Staub A-M. Action protectrice des éthers phénoliques an cours de l'intoxication histaminique. *C R Soc Biol (Paris)*. 1937;124: 547-549.
38. Sneader W. Drugs originating from the screening of organic chemicals. In: Sneader W, ed. *Drug Discovery: A History*. John Wiley & Sons; 2005:403-431.
39. Simons FE. Advances in H_1-antihistamines. *N Engl J Med*. 2004;351: 2203-2217.
40. Ahlquist RP. A study of the adrenotropic receptors. *Am J Physiol*. 1948;153:586-600.
41. Lijinsky W, Rueber MD, Blackwell BN. Liver tumors induced in rats by oral administration of the antihistaminic methapyrilene hydrochloride. *Science*. 1980;209:817-819.
42. Baselt RC. *Disposition of Toxic Drugs and Chemicals in Man*. 11th ed. Biomedical Publications; 2017 (monographs and references therein).
43. Glazko AJ, Dill WA, Young RM, et al. Metabolic disposition of diphenhydramine. *Clin Pharmacol Ther*. 1974;16:1066-1076.
44. Spector R, Choudhury AK, Chiang CK, et al. Diphenhydramine in orientals and caucasians. *Clin Pharmacol Ther*. 1980;28:229-234.
45. Hamelin BA, Bouayad A, Méthot J, et al. Significant interaction between the nonprescription antihistamine diphenhydramine and the CYP2D6 substrate metoprolol in healthy men with high or low CYP2D6 activity. *Clin Pharmacol Ther*. 2000;67:466-477.
46. Videla S, Lahjou M, Guibord P, et al. Food effects on the pharmacokinetics of doxylamine hydrogen succinate 25 mg film-coated tablets: a single-dose, randomized, two-period crossover study in healthy volunteers. *Drugs R D*. 2012;12:217-225.
47. Ganes DA, Midha KK. Identification in in vivo acetylation pathway for N-dealkylated metabolites of doxylamine in humans. *Xenobiotica*. 1987;17:993-999.
48. Ebnöther A, Weber HP. Synthesis and absolute konfiguration von clemastine und seiner isomeren [Synthesis and absolute configuration of clemastine and its isomers]. *Helv Chim Acta*. 1976; 59:2462-2468.
49. Choi MH, Jung BH, Chung BC. Identification of urinary metabolites of clemastine after oral administration to man. *J Pharm Pharmacol*. 1999;51:53-59.
50. Towart R, Sautel M, Moret E, et al. Investigation of the antihistaminic action of dimethindene maleate (Fenistil) and its optical isomers. In: Timmerman H, van der Goot H, eds. *Agents Actions Supplements*. Vol 33. New Perspectives in Histamine Research. Birkhäuser; 1991:403-408.
51. Hanna PE, Ahmed AE. Conformationally restricted analogs of histamine H1 receptor antagonists: trans- and cis-1,5-diphenyl-3-dimethylaminopyrrolidine. *J Med Chem*. 1973;16:963-968.
52. Kabasakalian P, Taggart M, Townley E. Urinary excretion of chlorpheniramine and its N-demethylated metabolites in man. *J Pharm Sci*. 1968;57:856-858.
53. Witte PU, Irmisch R, Hajdu P. Pharmacokinetics of pheniramine (Avil®) and metabolites in healthy subjects after oral and intravenous administration. *Int J Clin Pharmacol Ther Toxicol*. 1985;23:59-62.
54. Kabasakalian P, Taggart M, Townley E. Urinary excretion of pheniramine and its N-demethylated metabolites in man—comparison with chlorpheniramine and brompheniramine data. *J Pharm Sci*. 1968;57:621-623.
55. Piwinski JJ, Wong JK, Chan TM, et al. Hydroxylated metabolites of loratadine: an example of conformational diastereomers due to atropisomerism. *J Org Chem*. 1990;55:3341-3350.
56. Otsuki I, Ishiko J, Sakai M, et al. Pharmacological activities of doxepin hydrochloride in relation to its geometrical isomers. *Oyo Yakuri*. 1972;6:973-984.
57. Remy DC, Rittle KE, Hunt CA, et al. (+)- and (−)-3-Methoxycyproheptadine. A comparative evaluation of the antiserotonin, antihistaminic, anticholinergic, and orexigenic properties with cyproheptadine. *J Med Chem*. 1977;20:1681-1684.
58. Porter CC, Arison BH, Gruber VF, et al. Human metabolism of cyproheptadine. *Drug Metab Dispos*. 1975;3(3):189-197.
59. Simons FE, Simons KJ. Histamine and H1-antihistamines: celebrating a century of progress. *J Allergy Clin Immunol*. 2011; 128:1139-1150.
60. Chen C, Hanson E, Watson JW, et al. P-glycoprotein limits the brain penetration of nonsedating but not sedating H1-antagonists. *Drug Metabol Dispos*. 2003;31:312-318.
61. Shimamura T, Shiroishi M, Weyland S, et al. Structure of the human histamine H1 receptor complex with doxepin. *Nature*. 2011;475(7354):65-70.
62. Soldovieri MV, Miceli F, Taglialatela M. Cardiotoxic effects of antihistamines: from basics to clinics (...and back). *Chem Res Toxicol*. 2008;21:997-1004.
63. Aronov AM. Predictive in silico modeling for hERG channel blockers. *Drug Discov Today*. 2005;10:149-155.
64. Pearlstein R, Vaz R, Rampe D. Understanding the structure-activity relationship of the human ether-a-go-go-related gene cardiac K^+ channel. A model for bad behavior. *J Med Chem*. 2003;46:2017-2022.
65. Zhang MQ, Caldirola P, Timmerman H. Chiral manipulation of drug selectivity: studies on a series of terfenadine-derived dual antagonists of H1-receptors and calcium channels. *Agents Actions*. 1994;41:C140-C142.
66. Curran MP, Scott LJ, Perry CM. Cetirizine: a review of its use in allergic disorders. *Drugs*. 2004;64:523-561.
67. Gillard M, Van Der Perren C, Moguilevsky N, et al. Binding characteristics of cetirizine and levocetirizine to human H1 histamine receptors: contribution of Lys191 and Thr194. *Mol Pharmacol*. 2002;61:391-399.
68. Benedetti MS, Plisnier M, Kaise J, et al. Absorption, distribution, metabolism and excretion of [14C]levocetirizine, the R enantiomer of cetirizine, in healthy volunteers. *Eur J Clin Pharmacol*. 2001;57:571-582.
69. DuBuske LM. Pharmacology of desloratadine: special characteristics. *Clin Drug Investig*. 2002;22(suppl 2):1-11.

70. Yumibe N, Huie K, Chen KJ, et al. Identification of human liver cytochrome P450 enzymes that metabolize the nonsedating antihistamine loratadine. Formation of descarboethoxyloratadine by CYP3A4 and CYP2D6. *Biochem Pharmacol.* 1996;51:165-172.
71. Ramanathan R, Reyderman L, Kulmatycki K, et al. Disposition of loratadine in healthy volunteers. *Xenobiotica.* 2007;37: 753-769.
72. Ramanathan R, Reyderman L, Su AD, et al. Disposition of desloratadine in healthy volunteers. *Xenobiotica.* 2007;37:770-787.
73. Bielory L, Lien KW, Bigelsen S. Efficacy and tolerability of newer antihistamines in the treatment of allergic conjunctivitis. *Drugs.* 2005;65:215-228.
74. Sharif NA, Hellberg MR, Yanni JM. Antihistamines, topical ocular. In: Wolff ME, ed. *Burger's Medicinal Chemistry and Drug Discovery.* 5th ed. John Wiley & Sons, Inc; 1997:255-279.
75. Roland PS, Marple BF, Wall GM. Olopatadine nasal spray for the treatment of allergic rhinitis. *Expert Rev Clin Immunol.* 2010;6(2): 197-204.
76. Brunner M, Kletter K, Assandi A. Pharmacokinetic and mass balance study of unlabeled and 14C-labeled emedastine difumarate in healthy volunteers. *Xenobiotica.* 2002;32:761-770.
77. Yokota H, Mizuuchi H, Maki T, et al. Phase I study of TAU-284—single oral dose administration in healthy male volunteers. *J Clin Ther Med.* 1997;4:1137-1153.
78. Dechant KL, Goa KL: Levocabastine. A review of its pharmacological properties and therapeutic potential as a topical antihistamine in allergic rhinitis and conjunctivitis. *Drugs.* 1991;41:202-224.
79. Edwards AM, Holgate ST. The chromones: cromolyn sodium and neodocromil sodium. In: Adkinson NF, Bochner BS, Busse WW, et al, eds. *Middleton's Allergy: Principles and Practice.* 7th ed. Mosby; 2009:1591-1601.
80. Zhang T, Finn DF, Barlow JW, et al. Mast cell stabilisers. *Eur J Pharmacol.* 2016;778:158-168.
81. Cook EB, Stahl JL, Barney NP, et al. Mechanisms of antihistamines and mast cell stabilizers in ocular allergic inflammation. *Med Chem Rev.* 2004;1:333-347.

Structure Challenge Answers

1. **Antiallergic V.** The piperazines are moderately potent as antihistamines, and they exhibit significant anticholinergic side effects. Because of their ability to penetrate the central nervous system (CNS), they also cause sedation and psychomotor and cognitive dysfunction. They are among the more effective antihistamine-based antiemetics and can be used to treat motion sickness.
2. **Antiallergic VI.** Antihistamines with strong anticholinergic activity are generally contraindicated in benign prostate hyperplasia because of concerns for developing acute urinary retention. VI is ethanolamine with no *para*-substituent or 2-pyridyl group; thus, it possesses strong anticholinergic effect.
3. **Antiallergics II or IV.** They are the least sedative (or nonsedative). The former is loratadine with significant affinity for P-glycoprotein, and the latter is fexofenadine with an amphoteric structure that impedes its ability to penetrate BBB.
4. **Antiallergic II.** It is metabolized by oxidative O-dealkylation followed by spontaneous decarboxylation. The complete metabolic pathway is given in Figure 29.18.
5. **Antiallergic VII.** It is a centrally acting, tricyclic antihistamine with neither para-substituent nor 2-pyridyl group, which demonstrates significant serotonin antagonist activity, explaining its ability to stimulate appetite.
6. **Antiallergic IV.** It possesses a carboxylic acid group and a basic amine group; thus, its ability to generate a zwitterion at physiological pH impedes its ability to penetrate the BBB.
7. **Antiallergic VI.** It can penetrate BBB and has both significant antihistamine and anticholinergic effects, both of which contribute to its sedative properties and its use as OTC sleep aid. To be used for motion sickness, it is combined with the CNS stimulant 8-chlorotheophylline. See the monograph on diphenhydramine.
8. **Antiallergics I** and **IV** are highly polar (water-soluble) because the former is di-acidic, and the latter is amphoteric. Thus, they are mostly eliminated in urine without significant metabolism. Antihistamines VI and VII are hepatically metabolized by oxidative N-demethylation.
9. **Antiallergic III.** Erythromycin is a CYP3A4 inhibitor that increases the concentration of antihistamine III, which possesses significant affinity for the hERG channel, leading to life-threatening QT prolongation (cardiac arrhythmia: torsades de pointes).
10. **Antiallergic I** is a mast-cell stabilizer that can be used as a nebulized and/or nasal solution to proactively prevent the release of histamine, preventing an episode of seasonal allergies.
11. **Antiallergic I** has an acidic carboxylic acid moiety that can readily react with metal hydroxides (eg, NaOH) to generate a water-soluble basic salt. It is generally used locally via inhalation as a mast-cell stabilizer.

SECTION 6

Drugs Impacting Ocular, Nasal, and Pulmonary Systems

CHAPTER 30

Drugs Used to Treat Ocular and Nasal Disorders

Srikanth Kolluru

Drugs covered in this chapter:

ACETYLCHOLINESTERASE INHIBITORS (ANTICHOLINESTERASES)
- Echothiophate iodide

α_1-ADRENERGIC AGONISTS
- Naphazoline
- Oxymetazoline
- Phenylephrine
- Tetrahydrozoline
- Xylometazoline

α_2-ADRENERGIC AGONISTS
- Apraclonidine
- Brimonidine

β-ADRENERGIC RECEPTOR BLOCKERS
- Betaxolol
- Carteolol
- Levobunolol
- Timolol

CARBONIC ANHYDRASE INHIBITORS
- Acetazolamide
- Brinzolamide
- Dorzolamide
- Methazolamide

MIXED-ACTING SYMPATHOMIMETICS

PHENYLPROPANOLAMINES
- (−)-Ephedrine
- (+)-Pseudoephedrine

MUSCARINIC AGONISTS
- Acetylcholine
- Carbachol chloride
- Pilocarpine

PROSTAGLANDIN AGONISTS
- Bimatoprost
- Latanoprost
- Latanoprostene bunod
- Omidenepag isopropyl
- Tafluprost
- Travoprost

RHO KINASE INHIBITORS
- Netarsudil

TOPICAL OPHTHALMIC NONSTEROIDAL ANTI-INFLAMMATORY DRUGS
- Bromfenac
- Flurbiprofen
- Ketorolac tromethamine
- Nepafenac

TOPICAL OPHTHALMIC STEROIDS
- Dexamethasone
- Difluprednate
- Fluorometholone
- Fluorometholone acetate
- Loteprednol etabonate
- Prednisolone acetate
- Prednisolone sodium phosphate

TOPICAL OPHTHALMIC ANTIHISTAMINES
- Alcaftadine
- Azelastine
- Bepotastine
- Cetirizine
- Epinastine
- Ketotifen
- Olopatadine
- Pheniramine

OPHTHALMIC DRUGS TO TREAT DRY EYE
- Cyclosporine
- Lifitegrast
- Loteprednol etabonate
- Lotilaner
- Perfluorohexyloctane
- Varenicline

Abbreviations

AChE acetylcholinesterase
AChEI acetylcholinesterase inhibitor
BBB blood-brain barrier
CA carbonic anhydrase
CAI carbonic anhydrase inhibitor
cAMP cyclic adenosine monophosphate
CNS central nervous system
COMT catechol-*O*-methyltransferase
COPD chronic obstructive pulmonary disease
COX cyclooxygenase
CYP2C19 cytochrome P450 family 2 subfamily C member 19
DAG 1,2-diacylglycerol
DED dry eye disease
DFB 6α,9-difluoroprednisolone 17-butyrate
EPI epinephrine
FDA US Food and Drug Administration
GABA-Cls γ-aminobutyric acid–gated chloride channels
GDP guanosine diphosphate
GPCR G protein–coupled receptor
GR glucocorticoid receptor
GTP guanosine triphosphate
Gi G-inhibitory
G_s G-stimulatory
ICAM-1 intercellular adhesion molecule-1
IgE immunoglobulin E
IOP intraocular pressure
IP_3 inositol 1,4,5-triphosphate
JNK c-Jun N-terminal kinase
LFA-1 lymphocyte function-associated antigen 1
L-DOPA L-dihydroxyphenylalanine
mAChR muscarinic acetylcholinergic receptor
MAO monoamine oxidase
MAOI monoamine oxidase inhibitor
MLCK myosin light chain kinase
nAChR nicotinic acetylcholinergic receptor
NE norepinephrine
NET norepinephrine-reuptake transporter
NLF nasolacrimal reflex
NSAID nonsteroidal anti-inflammatory drug
OMD omidenepag
OTC over the counter
ROCK rho kinase
SAR structure-activity relationship
TMD transmembrane domain
TMD-7 transmembrane domain 7
TPP trigeminal parasympathetic pathway

CLINICAL SIGNIFICANCE

The principles of medicinal chemistry are directly relevant to the development of nasal and ocular products. Drugs must be carefully designed with a balance of water and lipid solubility to ensure efficient absorption through the nasal mucosa or ocular tissues. Additionally, these formulations must be isotonic and have an appropriate pH to prevent patient discomfort or irritation. To maintain stability, many of these products also include preservatives. The application of medicinal chemistry is crucial in creating products with these essential characteristics.

Marsha McFalls, PharmD, MSEd, RPh

INTRODUCTION

Congestion is an abnormal accumulation of fluids in tissues, leading to swollen membranes, dilated blood vessels, and blockade of passages. Vasodilation widens gaps between cells lining blood vessels, allowing fluids to escape to the surrounding tissue causing itching, sneezing, runny nose, and watery eyes. If congestion is untreated, it may facilitate infections via the movement of mucus from the nose to throat (causing throat infection) and accumulation of fluids in the sinus cavities (causing sinus infections). Congestion can be responsible for anywhere from mild discomfort to a life-threatening situation. Nasal congestion may also lead to headaches, sleep apnea, snoring, and interfere with hearing and speech. Risk factors for nasal congestion include allergic rhinitis, influenza, gastroesophageal reflux disorder,[1] sinus infection, deviated septum, drug addiction, enlarged adenoids, hormonal changes, nasal polyps, nonallergic rhinitis, occupational asthma, respiratory syncytial virus, stress, thyroid disorders, seasonal allergies, and common cold.[2] Allergic rhinitis is the most common cause for nasal congestion and affects about 60 million people each year in the United States.[3,4] In 2021, 25.7% of adults and 18.9% of children were diagnosed with seasonal allergies in the United States.[5] Nasal congestion may also occur due to structural abnormalities of the nose and nasal septum, enlargement of adenoids, and nasal tumors.

Ocular congestion is associated with burning, pain, itchy, swollen, and watery eyes. Common causes for ocular congestion include allergic conjunctivitis, infection, glaucoma, migraine, sinus infection, and influenza. Seasonal allergic rhinoconjunctivitis affects about 16% of the US population annually.[6] Nasal or ocular decongestants help relieve discomfort caused by congestion, but the root cause may need treatment with other medications. The pathophysiology of nasal congestion involves inflammation, vasodilation, increased venous engorgement, increased nasal secretions, and edema. It may also alter sensory perception and the physical structure of the nasal passage.[7]

Therapeutic Classes of Drugs Used to Treat Nasal and Ocular Congestion

Treating the two common causes, vasodilation and inflammation, is critical to help relieve nasal and ocular congestion. Smooth muscle tone of vasculature is maintained through a balance between the sympathetic and the parasympathetic nervous systems with opposing functions. Sympathetic activation causes vasoconstriction, and parasympathetic activation inhibits vasoconstriction. Vasodilation is due to the shift of balance to the parasympathetic nervous system over the sympathetic nervous system. Congestion can be treated by constricting the dilated vasculature, which brings cells together and reduces fluid leakage. Thus, drugs that are agonists at adrenergic receptors or antagonists at cholinergic receptors can be used in the treatment of congestion disorders. Due to several systemic adverse effects and availability of safer alternatives, cholinergic antagonists are no longer used for treating congestion disorders.

A second symptom of congestion disorders is inflammation, due to the release of inflammatory substances such as inflammatory prostaglandins, interleukins, histamine, leukotrienes, and various other hormones. Antihistamines play a big role and are used widely in treating nasal congestion. Antihistamines are discussed in detail in Chapter 29. Drugs discussed in this chapter target adrenergic receptors, cholinergic receptors, or pathways responsible for the synthesis or release of inflammatory autacoids.

α_1-Adrenergic Agonists

Understanding the role of adrenergic receptors, their distribution in tissues, and the binding of endogenous substrates such as norepinephrine (NE) and epinephrine (EPI) is essential to address the value of using α_1-adrenergic receptor agonists to relieve nasal and ocular congestion.

Vascular smooth muscles of the nasal pathway and the eye are rich in α_1-adrenergic receptors. Activation of α_1-receptors causes smooth muscle contraction and vasoconstriction that is needed for treating congestion. Detailed information about various adrenergic receptors in the body is discussed in Chapter 19, while tissue distribution and physiologic functions of α_1-receptor activation are listed in Table 30.1. Except in the vasculature of skeletal muscles, α_1-receptors are widely distributed in arterioles and veins throughout the body.

As indicated, vasodilation widens the gap between endothelial cells lining blood vessels, allowing fluids to escape to the surrounding tissue, causing congestion. Therefore, agonists at α_1-adrenergic receptors can constrict blood vessels, thereby reducing the amount of fluid release. However, adrenergic receptors are widely distributed in various tissues and organs as well as on the neurons of both the peripheral and central nervous system (CNS). Because of their wider distribution, patients taking certain oral or other systemic adrenergic agonists may experience systemic adverse effects such as hypertension. Caution must be exercised while administering oral adrenergic agonists to treat congestion disorders in patients with hypertension. Since the target site is vascular smooth muscles in the nose and eye, the topical administration is the most preferred route of drug delivery for both nasal and ocular decongestants.

Table 30.1 Tissue Distribution and Physiologic Effects of the Activation of Adrenergic α_1-Receptors

Organ	Physiologic Effects of α_1-Receptors
Eye	
Iris radial muscle contraction	Dilation—mydriasis
Upper eyelid tarsal smooth muscle	Contraction—lifts eyelid
Arterioles	
	Contraction-decreases ocular redness, decreases nasal congestion, increases blood pressure
Veins	
	Contraction-decreases ocular redness, decreases nasal congestion, increases blood pressure
Stomach and intestine	
Sphincters	Contraction—closes sphincters
Glandular secretions	
Lacrimal glands	Increases
Salivary glands	Increases
Bronchial	Decreases
Pancreatic gland	Decreases
Mucosal	Decreases
Sweat	Increases
Bladder sphincter	Contraction—closes
Sex organs—male (seminal track)	Ejaculation
Uterus	Contraction—premature labor

Endogenous Substrates Norepinephrine and Epinephrine

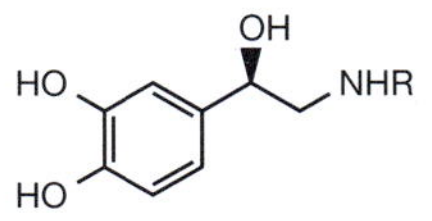

Norepinephrine, R = H
Epinephrine, R = CH_3

NE and EPI are members of a class of pharmacologically active substances known as catecholamines. The catecholamine structure is composed of an ethanolamine bound to a 3′,4′ dihydroxy phenyl group. Most adrenergic drugs are catecholamine derivatives.

Biosynthesis and Metabolism Norepinephrine. Biosynthesis of NE takes place within the adrenergic neurons, whereas biosynthesis of EPI occurs within the chromaffin cells of the adrenal medulla. The general biosynthetic pathway[8] is illustrated in Figure 30.1. Starting with L-tyrosine, the enzyme tyrosine hydroxylase catalyzes the hydroxylation at the *meta* position of tyrosine to form a catechol, L-dihydroxyphenylalanine (L-DOPA). This is the rate-limiting step in NE biosynthesis. The activity of tyrosine hydroxylase is inhibited by the negative feedback mechanism upon excessive synthesis of NE.[9]

Decarboxylation of L-DOPA by L-DOPA decarboxylase, also known as aromatic L-amino acid decarboxylase, leads to the synthesis of dopamine. Dopamine is further hydroxylated on the β-carbon by dopamine β-hydroxylase, giving rise to NE. NE is converted to EPI by N-methylation catalyzed by phenylethanolamine *N*-methyltransferase. Two major enzymes, monoamine oxidase (MAO) and catechol-O-methyltransferase (COMT), metabolize NE. MAO converts a primary amine into an aldehyde through oxidative deamination. COMT metabolizes via selective transfer of a methyl group on to the *meta*-hydroxyl function of the catechol moiety. Drugs that are resistant to both MAO and COMT metabolism are expected to have a longer duration of action. Since both metabolizing enzymes are abundantly present in the body, drugs inhibiting any one of the two enzymes may not improve their duration of action. General metabolic pathways for NE are given in Figure 30.2. Refer to Chapters 19, 20, or 31 for a detailed discussion.

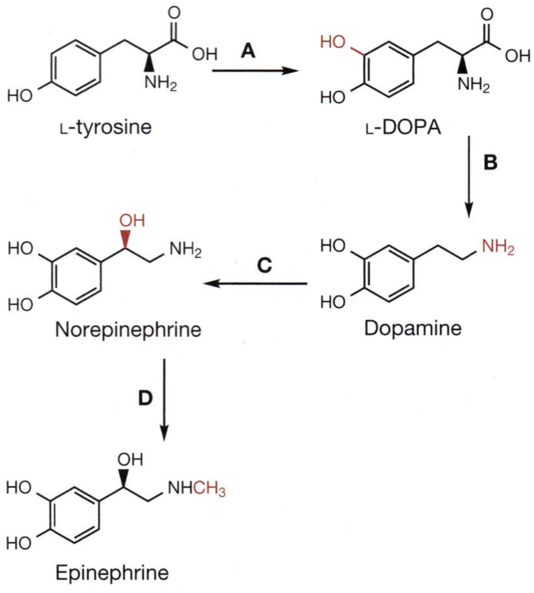

A = Tyrosine hydroxylase; B = Aromatic L-amino acid decarboxylase; C = Dopamine β-hydroxylase; D = Phenylethanolamine *N*-methyl transferase.

Figure 30.1 Biosynthesis of norepinephrine and epinephrine. L-DOPA, L-dihydroxyphenylalanine.

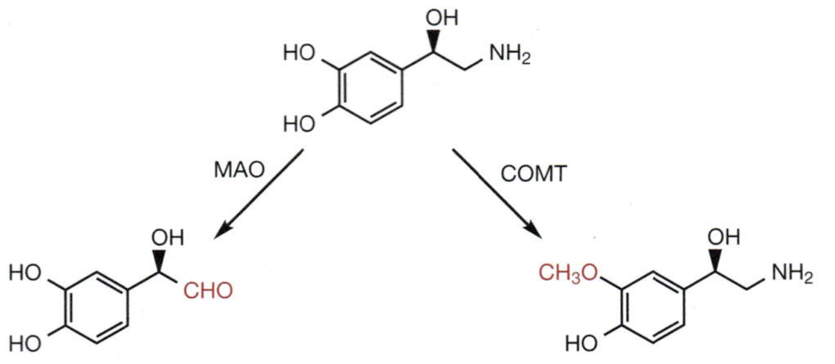

Figure 30.2 General metabolism of norepinephrine. COMT, catechol-*O*-methyltransferase; MAO, monoamine oxidase.

Adrenergic Receptors

Adrenergic receptors are classified into α- and β- adrenoreceptors. α-Receptors are further classified into the α_1 and α_2 subtypes, and β-adrenoceptors are classified into β_1, β_2, and β_3 subtypes. Currently, three types of α_1-adrenoceptors (α_{1A}, α_{1B}, and α_{1D}) and three subtypes of α_2 receptors (α_{2A}, α_{2B}, and α_{2C}) have been identified.[10] α_1-Receptors are predominantly postsynaptic, G_q-coupled receptors and are found in the vascular smooth muscles and the CNS. α_1–Receptor stimulation activates phospholipase C, which increases cellular levels of inositol 1,4,5- triphosphate (IP3) and 1,2-diacylglycerol (DAG). Released IP_3 induces the opening of the voltage-gated calcium channels allowing the influx of calcium. This leads to the activation of myosin light chain kinase (MLCK), which in turn phosphorylates myosin filaments of smooth muscles, causing muscle contraction. DAG also contributes to smooth muscle contraction by activating cytosolic protein kinase C. Consequently, agonists at α_1-adrenergic receptors cause vasoconstriction, thereby having utility in treating shock, nasal congestion, and ocular redness (also called conjunctival hyperemia). Nasal and ocular decongestants are most commonly administered topically to avoid systemic adverse effects such as hypertension. Furthermore, stimulation of α_1-adrenergic receptors in the upper eyelid, via topical application of agonists, causes contraction of the upper eyelid tarsal smooth muscle and opening of the eye. α_2-Receptors are presynaptic and G-inhibitory (G_i) coupled. α_2-Receptor stimulation inhibits adenylyl cyclase, which decreases intracellular cyclic adenosine monophosphate (cAMP). This action inhibits the release of NE from presynaptic terminals, leading to reduced blood pressure as well as reduced intraocular pressure (IOP). α_2-Adrenergic agonists, therefore, have therapeutic utility in treating hypertension and glaucoma, among other indications. Stimulation of α_2-receptors found in the ciliary epithelium of the eye reduces aqueous humor production, thereby reducing IOP. Additionally, stimulation of α_2-receptors on small vessels in the eye, via application in an ophthalmic solution, causes vasoconstriction and is used to treat ocular redness.

β_1- and β_2-receptors are predominantly postsynaptic and G-stimulatory (G_s) coupled. Stimulation activates adenylyl cyclase, which increases intracellular cAMP. β_1-receptors are primarily present in the myocardium of the heart. Stimulation results in increased chronotropic (heart rate) and inotropic (force of contraction) effects. β_2-receptors are found in the lungs, uterus, vascular smooth muscle, and skeletal

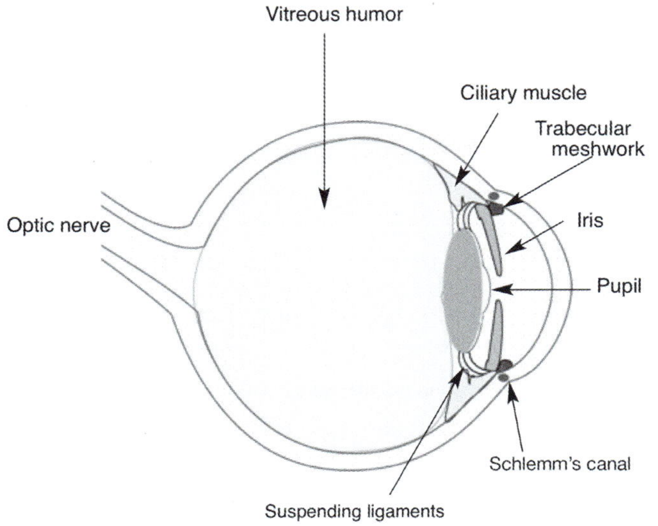

Figure 30.3 Diagram of the eyeball and key components of the eye.

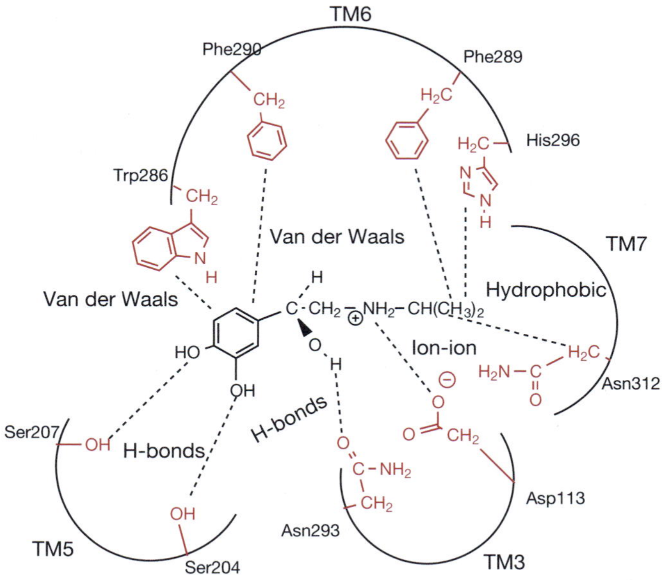

Figure 30.4 Isoproterenol–human β_2-adrenergic receptor binding interactions.

muscle. β_2-receptors are also present in the ciliary muscle and ciliary epithelium of the eye. Activation leads to ciliary muscle relaxation, dilation of the pupil (mydriasis), and increased aqueous humor production, thereby increasing IOP (Fig. 30.3). Thus, β-blockers have found utility in the treatment of ocular hypertension. Nonselective β-blockers such as timolol, carteolol, levobunolol, and selective β_1-blocker betaxolol are currently used in the treatment of glaucoma. Only adrenergic agonists that target α-receptors are used for treating nasal and ocular congestion.

Adrenergic Receptor Ligand Interactions

All adrenergic receptors are G protein–coupled receptors (GPCRs). In all of the adrenoceptors, the agonist/antagonist recognition site is located within the membrane-bound portion of the receptor. This binding site is within a pocket formed by the membrane-spanning regions of the peptide. The adrenergic receptor site was identified based on the mutational studies and the crystal structure of the β_2 adrenoceptor with isoproterenol. These studies identified the key amino acid residues and their interactions with the ligand functional groups at the adrenergic receptor site. Figure 30.4 illustrates binding sites for isoproterenol bound to the human β_2-receptor. Isoproterenol shows interactions with amino acid residues from transmembrane domains (TMDs) 3, 5, 6, and 7.

Asp113 in TMD3 of the β_2-receptor exhibits ionic or a salt bridge binding with the positively charged amine functional group of adrenergic agonists. This is a common interaction among all adrenergic receptors. Serine amino acid residues at 204 and 207 positions of TMD5 show hydrogen bonds with the catechol hydroxyl groups.[11,12] Ser204 interacts with the *meta*-hydroxyl group of the ligand, whereas Ser207 interacts specifically with the *para*-hydroxyl group of the catechol. Phe290 and Trp286 residues of TMD6 show van der Waals interactions with the catechol ring. Phe289, His296 of TMD6, and Asn312 of TMD7 show hydrophobic interactions with the isopropyl group of isoproterenol. In the case of α-receptors, TMD7 does not have any involvement in the agonist interactions due to a smaller hydrophobic pocket in the region of the isopropyl group. This is a significant difference between α- and β-receptors. Therefore, drugs having smaller substituents on the nitrogen such as hydrogen or methyl groups bind to both α- and β-receptors, whereas nitrogen substituents larger than the methyl group shifts their selectivity to β-receptors.

When the *N*-alkyl group is isopropyl or larger, the agonist completely loses α-activity, leaving behind only β-activity. Other critical binding sites within the α-receptors are similar to those seen in β-receptors.

General Mechanism of Action of Adrenergic Agonists

There are three categories of adrenergic agonists based on their mechanism of action: direct-acting, indirect-acting, and mixed-acting adrenergic agonists. As the name itself indicates, direct-acting agonists bind directly to the adrenergic receptors and elicit intrinsic activity similar to NE. They can be selective to adrenergic receptor subtypes. Indirect-acting adrenergic agonists act by inhibiting metabolism of NE, inhibiting reuptake of NE from the synapse or increasing the release of NE from synaptic vesicles. All these mechanisms increase the amount of NE at the synaptic cleft and its time spent at the receptor site. Therefore, indirect-acting agonists are nonselective to receptor subtypes, as NE activates all adrenergic receptors. Mixed-acting adrenergic agonists act by the combination of both direct and indirect mechanisms.

Specific Adrenergic Receptor Agonists Used in the Treatment of Congestion Disorders

Epinephrine

EPI is an endogenous adrenergic agonist synthesized in the adrenal medulla. It binds and activates all adrenergic receptors, eliciting responses similar to NE. It has a poor oral bioavailability due to extensive metabolism by MAO and COMT enzymes. Despite its limitations, EPI occasionally finds use as a nasal decongestant owing to its agonistic activity at α-adrenergic receptors. Activation of α_1-adrenergic receptors in the dilated blood vessels of the mucous membranes causes vasoconstriction and reduces nasal congestion. EPI has a limited clinical utility for treating congestion disorders due to rebound congestion. Its onset of action is about 5 minutes, with a duration of action less than 1 hour. Since it has a catechol functional group, it rapidly undergoes oxidation to produce a potentially toxic *o*-quinone metabolite in aqueous conditions or when exposed to light or oxygen. Therefore, it is formulated in combination with antioxidants and must be stored away from light. It must be used with caution in patients with cardiovascular disease or diabetes, as it may cause hypertension upon systemic absorption.

Phenylephrine

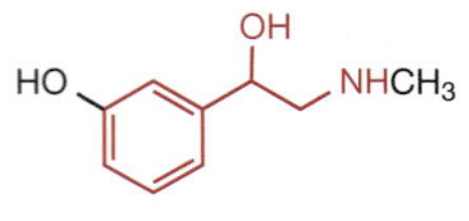

Phenylephrine

Phenylephrine has a phenylethanolamine pharmacophore. The presence of the 3′-phenolic hydroxyl moiety improves α_1-receptor selectivity while decreasing β-receptor binding. As a result, phenylephrine has minimal cardiac stimulatory properties. Phenylephrine is found in over-the-counter (OTC) decongestant cold medications. It is not a substrate for COMT unlike EPI and, hence, the duration of action is longer than EPI. Its oral bioavailability is less than 10% because of its hydrophilic properties and intestinal metabolism by MAO and 3′-O-glucuronidation/sulfate conjugation. Phenylephrine as an oral formulation is used to treat nasal and sinus congestion as well as to relieve symptoms such as sneezing, lacrimation, and itchy eyes. The US Food and Drug Administration (FDA) advisory committee has recently concluded that this drug may work no better than placebo. The FDA is expected to remove phenylephrine from orally administered OTC nasal decongestants following a period of public comment. Phenylephrine preparations are applied topically to the eye to constrict the dilated blood vessels of bloodshot eyes. During surgery, a higher dose phenylephrine formulation is used to dilate pupil.

Oral decongestants can cause systemic adverse effects such as tachycardia, hypertension, and CNS adverse effects (eg, tremors, anxiety, and insomnia). Hence, in patients with hypertension, phenylephrine use in combination with oral decongestants must not exceed 5 days. Phenylephrine is also used to treat itching and congestion caused by allergic conjunctivitis.

2-Arylimidazoline α_1-Agonists

The imidazoline derivatives shown in Figure 30.5 are selective α_1-agonists with vasoconstrictor/vasopressor activity.[13] Arylimidazoline analogues are structurally very different from traditional adrenergic agonists and NE/EPI. The α-adrenoceptors can accommodate a very diverse assortment of ligand structures.

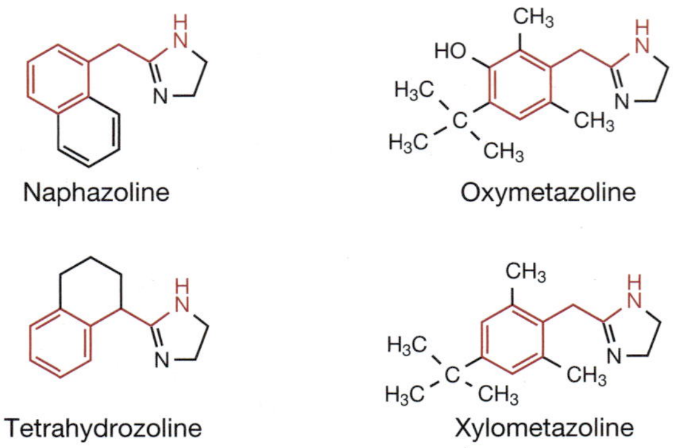

Figure 30.5 Imidazoline α_1-adrenergic agonists.

Structure-Activity Relationships. The imidazolines contain a one-carbon bridge between the C-2 of the imidazoline ring (pK_a range, 10-11) and a phenyl substituent. The phenylethylamine pharmacophore exists within the heterocyclic arylimidazoline structures, as indicated in Figure 30.5.

Lipophilic substitution (eg, methyl) on the phenyl ring *ortho* to the methylene bridge appears to be required for agonist activity at α_1- and α_2-receptors.[14] Presumably, the bulky lipophilic groups attached to the phenyl ring at the *para* positions provide selectivity for the α_1-receptor by diminishing affinity for α_2-receptors. The arylimidazolines do not have a chiral center unlike most adrenergic agonists. Quaternization of the imidazoline nitrogen or replacement of nitrogen with another heteroatom (eg, oxygen) significantly reduces activity.

Imidazoline derivatives bind differently at the adrenergic α_1-receptor active site compared to the phenylethanolamines. The arylimidazolines bind more like antagonists through van der Waals interactions with Phe308 and Phe312 in the transmembrane domain 7 (TMD-7) (Fig. 30.6A). This could be the reason for their partial agonistic properties. Mutations at either Phe308 or Phe312 significantly reduces imidazoline's agonist affinity compared to phenylethanolamines or EPI at the adrenergic α_1-receptors.[15] The lipophilic functional groups on the aryl ring of imidazolines show essential van der Waals interactions with Phe308 and Phe312 in the TM-7. These groups are also responsible for their selectivity for α_1-receptors. The orientation of arylimidazolines at the α_1-receptor is in sharp contrast to epinephrine binding, where the phenyl ring is oriented toward TM-5 (Fig. 30.6B). The nitrogen atom on the imidazole ring undergoes protonation under physiologic pH and shows the required ionic bonding with Asp106 on TM3. A general overview of structure-activity relationship (SAR) studies for arylimidazolines is given in Figure 30.7.

Pharmacokinetics. Arylimidazoline adrenergic agonists are highly ionic in nature. They are widely used in topical preparations as nasal decongestants and eye drops for conditions associated with the common cold, influenza, sinusitis, allergic and nonallergic rhinitis, and upper respiratory tract infections (Table 30.2). Due to potent vasoconstrictor activity, they are not used systemically.

Upon topical administration, oxymetazoline is minimally absorbed into the systemic circulation. The absorbed

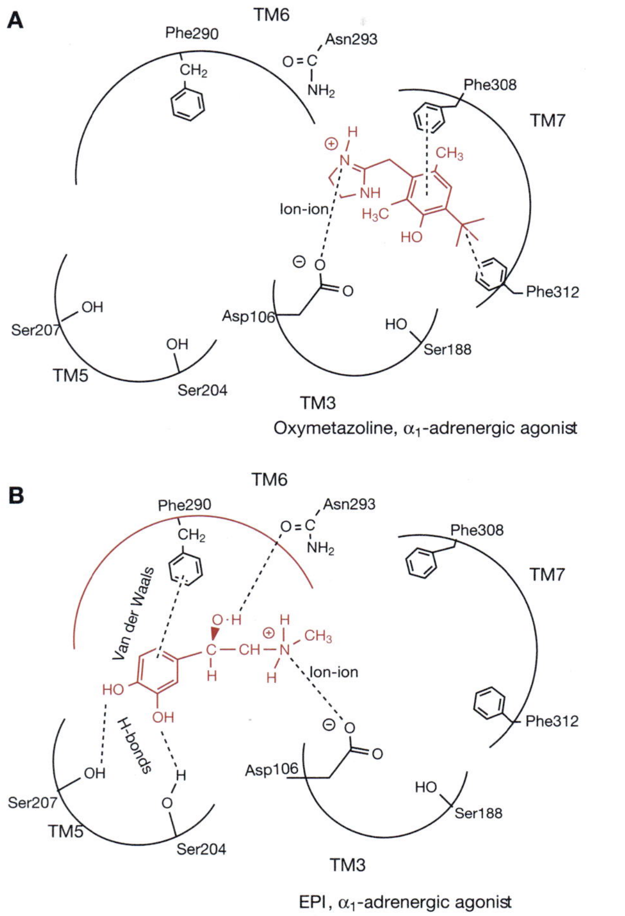

Figure 30.6 Representation of oxymetazoline and epinephrine (EPI) binding to the α_1-adrenergic receptor pocket. A. Oxymetazoline, α_2-arylimidazoline α_1-adrenergic agonist binding to the receptor pocket, as compared to (B), EPI binding to the same receptor pocket.

drug is metabolized by CYP2C19 (cytochrome P450 family 2 subfamily C member 19), resulting in hydroxylation of the *t*-butyl group to produce a monohydroxy derivative. The resultant phenolic hydroxyl group is conjugated via uridine diphosphate glucuronosyltransferase (UGT)-mediated glucuronidation. An imidazole metabolite produced through CYP2C19-catalyzed oxidative dehydrogenation of the imidazoline ring has been reported, as shown in Figure 30.8. Furthermore, oxymetazoline has the potential to undergo bioactivation, resulting in the formation of a reactive toxic intermediate. However, this intermediate is subsequently converted into glutathione conjugates in the liver, via glutathione S-transferase and glutathione (GSH).[16,17]

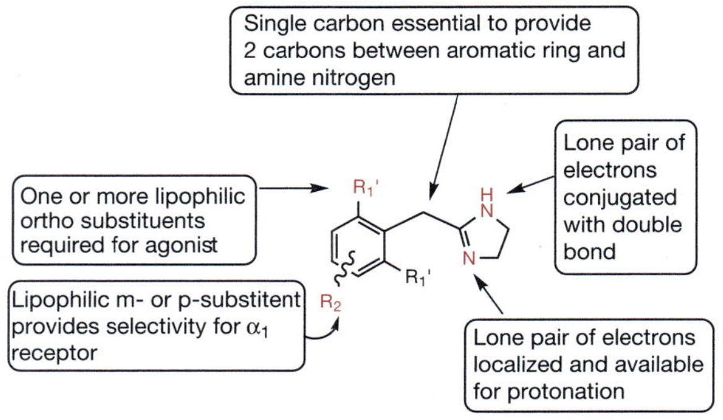

Figure 30.7 Structure-activity relationship (SAR) of arylimidazoline agonists.

Clinical Application

The duration of action of topical α_1-adrenergic agonists used in nasal and ocular decongestants differ significantly. Phenylephrine has a short duration of action of less than 4 hours; naphazoline and tetrahydrozoline have intermediate duration of action of approximately 4 to 6 hours; and oxymetazoline and xylometazoline have a longer duration of action of nearly 12 hours. Prolonged use of these medications will lead to rebound congestion, which may be severe.[13] Their use should be restricted to less than 5 days, and patient counseling on rebound congestion upon prolonged usage should occur. Caution must be exercised while using in an elderly population or patients with cardiovascular disease, glaucoma, and diabetes.[18] It should be noted that these products are often found in combination with an antihistamine (ie, pheniramine).

α_2-Agonists for Ocular Redness

The α_2-adrenergic agonist brimonidine is available as an OTC 0.025% ophthalmic solution/drops (Lumify) indicated for the treatment of ocular redness.

Mixed-Acting Sympathomimetics

Mixed-acting sympathomimetics are common ingredients in many cold medications with oral decongestant formulations. These are commonly given in combination with antihistamines. The systemic sympathomimetic products generally have a slower onset but longer duration of action compared to topical decongestants and do not cause irritation to the nasal membranes or rebound congestion after completion of the therapy as is seen with topical decongestants.

PHENYLPROPANOLAMINES

Mechanism of Action. The mixed-acting sympathomimetics with the phenylpropanolamine pharmacophore lack substituents on the phenyl ring (Fig. 30.9). This makes them both direct- and indirect-acting agonists. Their direct action stems from binding to both α- and β-adrenoceptors, while their indirect action results from displacing NE from the synaptic vesicles or reuptake inhibition, thereby increasing NE concentration at the adrenergic receptors. Because NE stimulates both α- and β-adrenoceptors, indirect activity cannot be selective. These drugs are more frequently used as oral decongestants. The stereochemistry of the various substituents can also play a role in determining the extent of direct/indirect activity. For example, ephedrine and pseudoephedrine have the same substitution pattern (Fig. 30.9), but substitution at both chiral carbons produces four stereoisomers.

Racemic (±)-ephedrine is a mixture of the *erythro* enantiomers 1*R*,2*S* and 1*S*,2*R*, whereas the *threo* pair of enantiomers, 1*R*,2*R* and 1*S*,2*S*, are found in racemic pseudoephedrine (ψ-ephedrine). (−)-Ephedrine is the naturally occurring

Table 30.2 Imidazoline α_1- and α_2-Adrenergic Agonists in Over-the-Counter Vasoconstrictors

Generic Name	Nasal Decongestant: Trade Names	Dosage Form	Duration of Action (h)	Eye Drops: Trade Names	Dosage Form
α_1-Adrenergic agonists					
Xylometazoline	Otrivine	Spray	12	NA	NA
Oxymetazoline	Afrin, Dristan, Mucinex Sinus-Max, Vicks Sinex, Zicam	Spray	12	Upneeq[a]	Drops/solution
Tetrahydrozoline	NA	NA	4-6	Visine A.C., Rohto Digi-Eye	Drops/solution
Naphazoline	NA	NA	4-6	Clear Eyes, Rohto Cool, Rohto Cool Max, Rohto Cool Relief, Rohto Max Strength, Rohto Optic Glow	Drops/solution
α_2-Adrenergic agonists					
Brimonidine	NA	NA	8	Lumify	Drops/solution

NA, not available.
[a]Upneeq is a prescription ophthalmic drop/solution for the treatment of low-lying eyelids.

stereoisomer and has the 1*R*,2*S* absolute configuration with a mixed activity on both α- and β-receptors and some indirect activity. Its 1*S*,2*R*-(+)-enantiomer exhibits primarily indirect activity. 1*S*,2*S*-(+)-Pseudoephedrine has virtually no direct receptor activity, but acts via indirect activity.

Specific Drugs

(−)-Ephedrine. Ephedrine (see Fig. 30.9) is a natural product isolated from several species of ephedra plants, used for centuries in Chinese folk medicine. Its occurrence in ephedra represents approximately 80% to 90% of the alkaloid content. Other alkaloids also found include (+)-pseudoephedrine (10%-15%) and *N*-methylephedrine (2%-5%). Ephedrine's sympathomimetic activity was not recognized until 1917, and the pure drug was used clinically even before epinephrine and NE were isolated and characterized. Ephedrine does not have any phenolic substituents, making it a mixed-acting adrenergic agonist. It has good oral bioavailability stemming from the lack of a catechol function and, therefore, is not a substrate for COMT. Additionally, ephedrine is not metabolized by MAO due to the presence of an α-methyl group, which sterically hinders metabolism by MAO. Lacking hydrogen-bonding phenolic substituents, ephedrine is more lipophilic and crosses

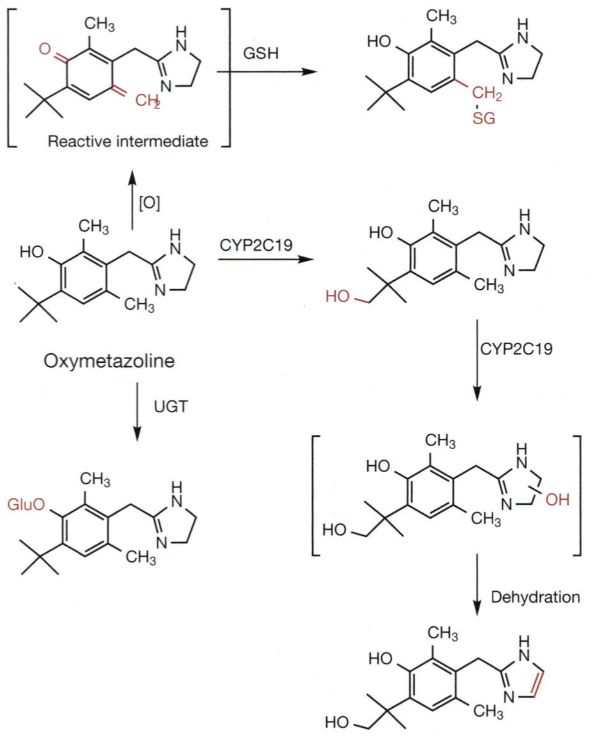

Figure 30.8 Metabolism of oxymetazoline. GSH, glutathione; UGT, uridine diphosphate glucuronosyltransferase.

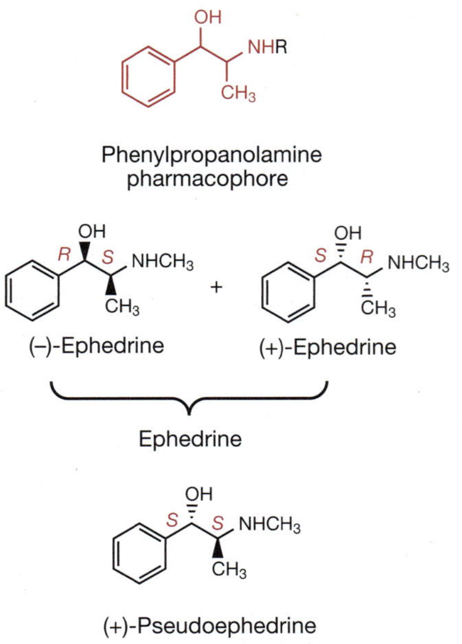

Figure 30.9 Ephedrine and pseudoephedrine.

the blood-brain barrier (BBB) far better than the catechol-containing agonists, thus causing CNS adverse effects. Because of its ability to penetrate the BBB, ephedrine has also been used as a CNS stimulant. Ephedrine is widely used for many of the same indications as EPI, including use as a bronchodilator, vasopressor, cardiac stimulant, and nasal decongestant.

(+)-Pseudoephedrine. Pseudoephedrine (see Fig. 30.9), as previously discussed, is the *threo* (S,S) diastereomer of ephedrine, with virtually no direct activity and fewer CNS adverse effects than ephedrine. (+)-Pseudoephedrine is widely used as a nasal decongestant. The most common adverse effects of pseudoephedrine include restlessness, nausea, vomiting, weakness, and headache. Currently its sale is restricted because it can be used in the illicit manufacture of the widely abused drug methamphetamine. Pseudoephedrine is sold from behind the counter to control its availability. Pseudoephedrine is available in both sustained as well as controlled release formulations. Due to the vasoconstriction effects of pseudoephedrine, it is used with caution in patients with hypertension. It might antagonize the actions of antihypertensive drugs such methyldopa, carvedilol, and labetalol. It is contraindicated in combination with monoamine oxidase inhibitors (MAOIs), as it can lead to life-threatening hypertension.

Intranasal Corticosteroids

Sneezing, nasal congestion, and rhinorrhea are the common symptoms of allergic rhinitis and occur in response to the release of histamine, prostaglandins, and leukotrienes following exposure to external allergens. The nasal steroids have proven effective in reducing inflammation arising from the exposure to allergens as well as relieve the symptoms of congestion and mucus production.

Mechanism of Action. Steroids work through a multitude of mechanisms, including inhibition of immunoglobulin E (IgE)–dependent release of histamine and inhibition of the synthesis and release of cytokines and chemokines from T-lymphocytes, epithelial cells, eosinophils, and mast cells.[19] The exact mechanism of action of the intranasal corticosteroids remains unclear.

Structure-Activity Relationship Studies. The steroid basic structure has the cyclopentanoperhydrophenanthrene nucleus with specific functional groups essential for both glucocorticoid and mineralocorticoid activity. These include the unsaturation and a ketone in ring A, free β-hydroxyl groups at C-11 in ring C, and a ketol and hydroxyl groups at the C-17 side chain. By esterifying at the C-21 hydroxyl, a prodrug can be produced (Figure 30.10).

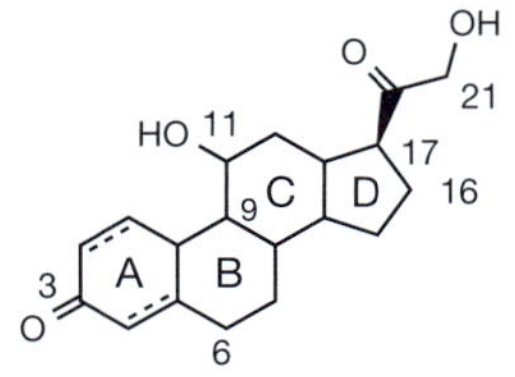

Basic nucleus required for gluco- and mineralocorticoid activity

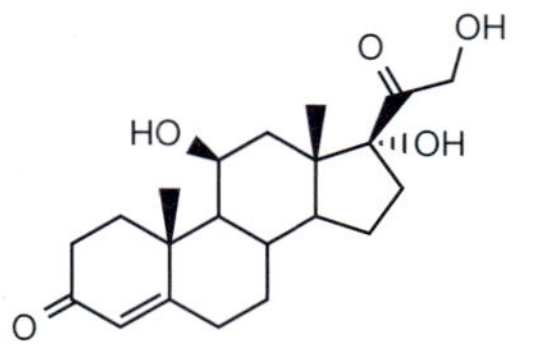

Hydrocortisone

Additionally, this position is commonly used to adjust the lipophilicity of the drug, thereby the duration of action. Substituents at other locations also affect lipophilicity and activity such as a methyl substitution at C-6 position and substitution at C-16. Both of these substitutions abolish mineralocorticoid activity, leaving behind only glucocorticoid activity. Lipophilic halogen substitutions at C-9 increases both glucocorticoid and mineralocorticoid activity, whereas halogen substitution at C-6 increases only glucocorticoid activity without altering mineralocorticoid activity.[20] Hydrocortisone represents the prototype corticosteroid.

The commonly used nasal corticosteroids include beclomethasone dipropionate and beclomethasone dipropionate monohydrate, budesonide, ciclesonide, fluticasone furoate, fluticasone propionate, mometasone furoate monohydrate, and triamcinolone acetonide (Fig. 30.10).

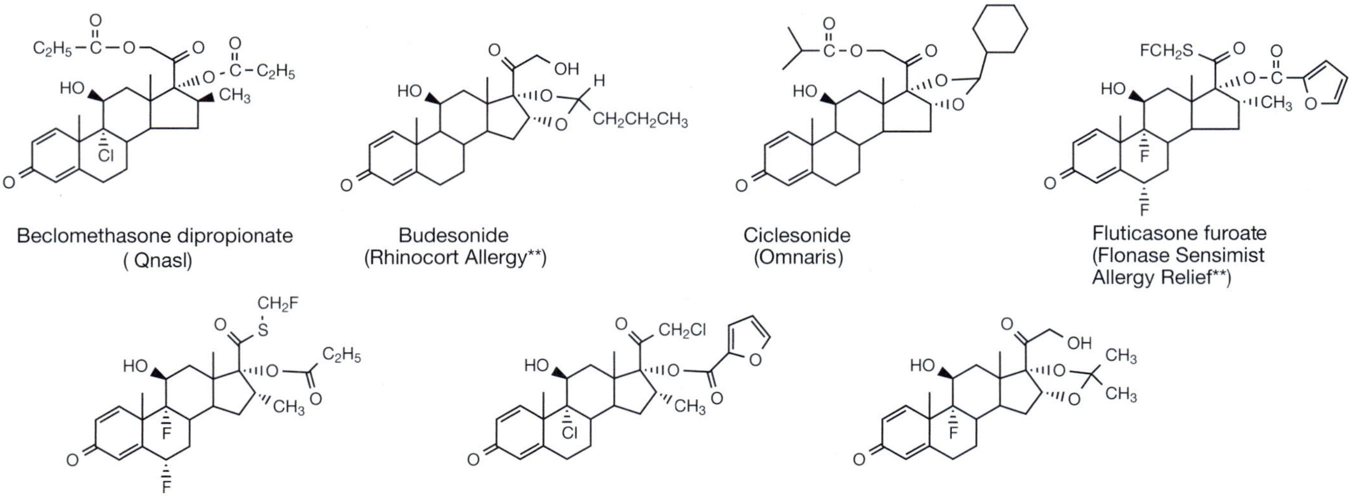

Beclomethasone dipropionate (Qnasl)

Budesonide (Rhinocort Allergy**)

Ciclesonide (Omnaris)

Fluticasone furoate (Flonase Sensimist Allergy Relief**)

Fluticasone propionate (Flonase Allergy Relief**)

Mometasone furoate (Nasonex 24HR Allergy**)

Triamcinolone acetonide (Nasacort Allergy 24 Hour**)

**Indicates products that are available over-the-counter

Figure 30.10 Intranasal corticosteroids.

Pharmacokinetics. Intranasal corticosteroids are generally available as nasal sprays, as their action is on the tissue of the nasal passage. While the benefit of the intranasal corticosteroids for treatment of allergic rhinitis is local, varying amounts of the administered drug is swallowed and absorbed from the intestinal tract. As a result, plasma levels of the administered drug can be measured, and systemic drug metabolism does occur to some extent. Additionally, several corticosteroids are prodrugs (ie, beclomethasone dipropionate and ciclesonide). The C-21 ester group must be metabolized to a free alcohol, which is the active form, and as a result, awareness of the active form of the drug as well as the metabolism of the corticosteroids is important (Fig. 30.11).[21-23] An exception to this is that both fluticasone and mometasone are active as such, even without a free -OH group at C-21 position.

As indicated in Figure 30.10, the intranasal corticosteroids are available as prescription products as well as OTC products. Its local adverse effects include nasal irritation, burning, stinging, sore throat, and (in rare cases) bleeding. The benefits of nasal steroids are seen only after 2 to 3 weeks. Detailed steroidal drugs mechanism, SAR, and metabolism are discussed in Chapters 24 and 31.

Drugs Used for Treating Glaucoma

Glaucoma is the leading cause for irreversible vision loss due to damage to the optic nerve head. There are two types of glaucoma, open-angle glaucoma and angle-closure glaucoma. Open-angle glaucoma is most commonly seen in the United States. The pathophysiology of glaucoma is not clearly understood, but the optic neuropathy is associated with the increase in the IOP. Therefore, the drugs that help reduce IOP can prevent or delay optic nerve damage, leading to blindness. It is estimated about 70 million people worldwide are affected by glaucoma, with nearly 10% being classified as bilaterally blind.[24] An estimated 6 million people worldwide may go blind by 2020, if untreated. In a majority of cases, glaucoma is asymptomatic until which time the diagnosis and treatment become quite difficult. Major risk factors include high IOP, advanced age, hypertension, diabetes, and thin central cornea.[25]

Under normal conditions, aqueous humor from the eye flows out through the trabecular network. In open-angle glaucoma, the trabecular network is blocked internally, whereas in angle-closure glaucoma, it is blocked by the iris (see Fig. 30.3). When the trabecular network is blocked, IOP increases, leading to damage to the optic nerve head, interfering with the transmission of optical images to the brain. Increased pressure in the eye is manifested via eye pain, headache, and blurred vision. Genetic anomalies may also lead to glaucoma. There are approximately 15 genes identified that contribute to the development of glaucoma. The major treatment goal for glaucoma is to reduce the IOP, which has been shown to delay or prevent the disease onset and progression. Prostaglandin analogues are used as first-line agents to treat glaucoma. Muscarinic agonists, β-blockers, α_2-adrenergic agonists, and carbonic anhydrase inhibitors (CAIs) are also used.[26] In most cases, the ophthalmic drugs are administered topically. Absorption and duration of action for topical ophthalmic formulations can be adjusted by varying the formulation or vehicle used. Topical medications work either by increasing the outflow of aqueous humor (prostaglandin analogues, adrenergic and cholinergic agonists) or by reducing aqueous humor production (α_2–adrenergic agonists, β-blockers, and CAI). The various classes of drugs used are discussed later.

α_2-Adrenergic Agonists—Their Role in Treatment of Glaucoma

Agonist action at α_2-receptors in the eye reduces IOP by decreasing the aqueous humor production and increasing its outflow thus reducing the IOP. The α_2-receptors are presynaptic receptors present on the outer membrane of the nerve termini within the eye. The α_2-receptor serves as a sensor and modulator of the quantity of neurotransmitter present in the synapse. Thus, during periods of rapid nerve firing and neurotransmitter release, the α_2-receptor is stimulated and causes an inhibition of further release of neurotransmitter. This is a well-characterized mechanism for modulation of neurotransmission. But not all α_2-receptors are presynaptic, and the physiologic significance of postsynaptic α_2-receptors is less well understood.[27] The α_2-receptor can use more than one effector system depending on the location of the receptor. The best-understood effector system of the α_2-receptor appears to be similar to that of the β-receptors, except that linkage via a G protein (G_i) leads to inhibition of adenylyl cyclase instead of activation.

α_2-Adrenoceptors are comprised of three subtypes α_{2A}, α_{2B}, and α_{2C}, and agonists at these sites find clinical utility in a number of indications including the treatment of glaucoma, when applied topically to the eye. Brimonidine is also formulated as an ophthalmic solution for the treatment of ocular redness. Clonidine, was introduced as an antihypertensive drug, an effect attributed to its action on central α_{2A}-adrenoceptors.[28] The imidazolines, which include clonidine, are effective in the treatment of glaucoma through their α_2-adrenergic agonist activity are shown in Figure 30.12.

Imidazoline α_2-Receptor Agonists. Structural modification of the previously reported nasal decongestant arylimidazolines in which the aryl and imidazoline are connected by a CH_2 group (X = CH_2; Fig. 30.12) is replaced with an -NH- group gave rise to the arylaminoimidazolines class (X = NH; Fig. 30.12). Unlike the nasal decongestant arylimidazolines which possess α_1-agonist activity (Fig. 30.5) the newly discovered drugs exhibit α_2-receptors agonist activity.

Clonidine is the prototype α_2-agonist. By replacing the CH_2 with a NH gives rise to a guanidine functional group. Clonidine in the uncharged form exists as a pair of tautomers with the physiochemical properties of pK_a of 8.3 and a log $D_{pH\ 7.4}$ = 1.03.

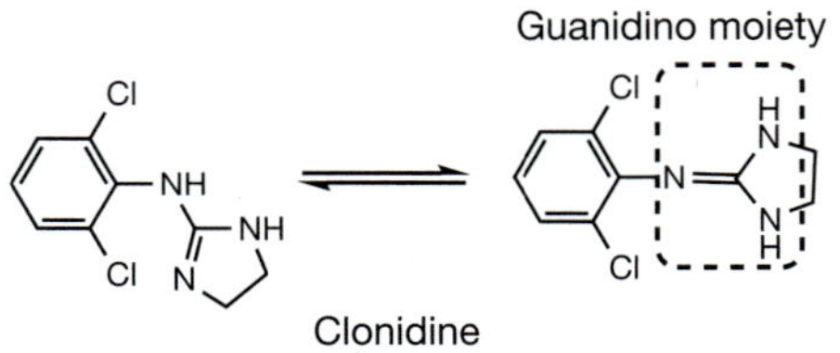

Clonidine

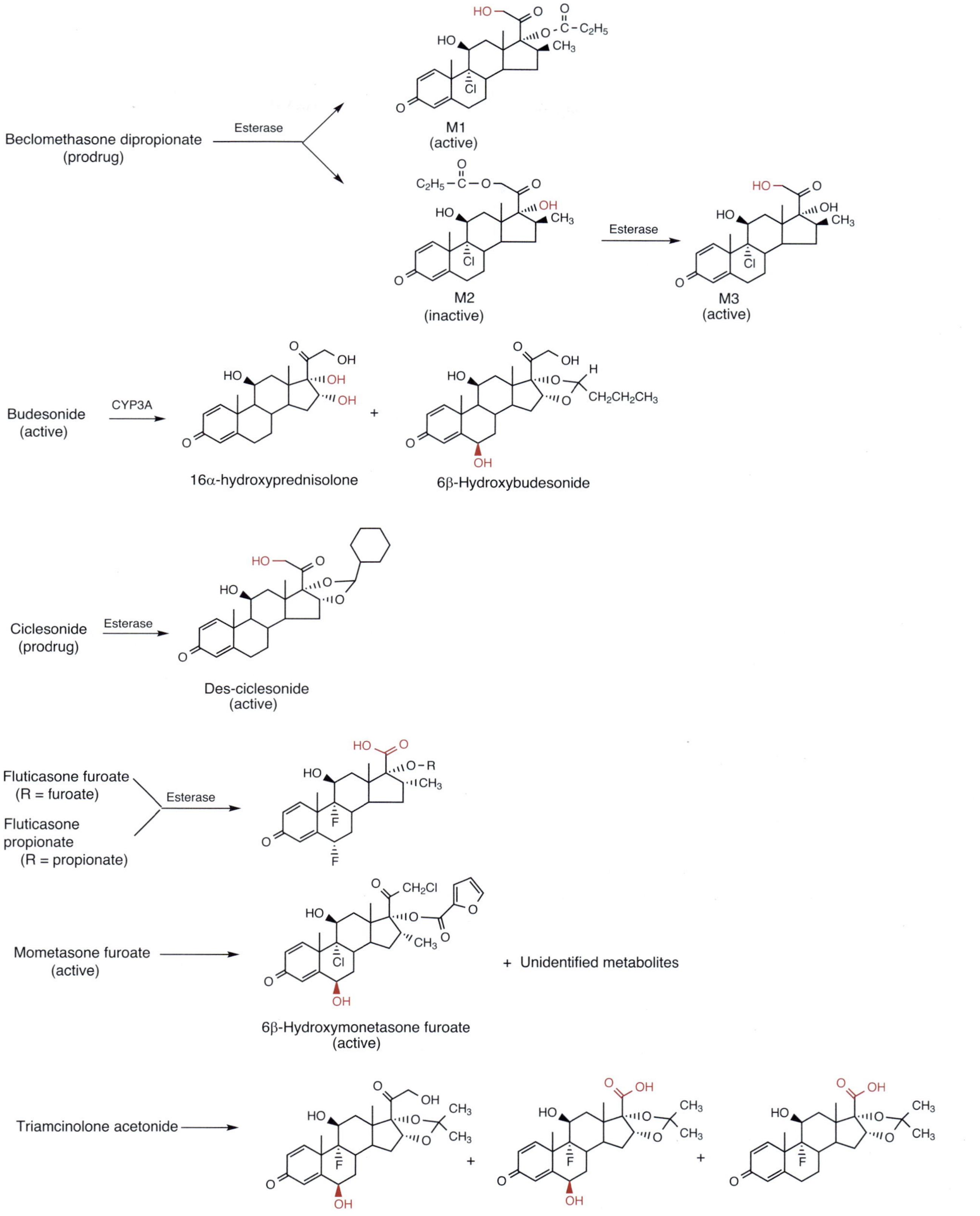

Figure 30.11 Metabolism of intranasal corticosteroids.

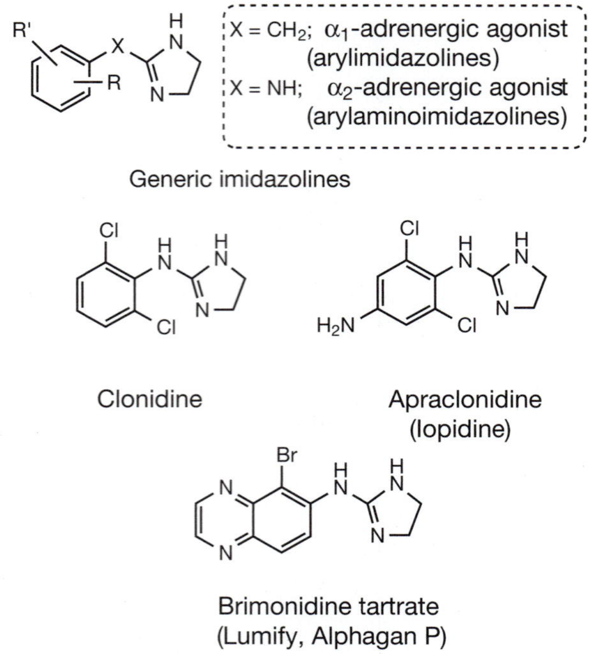

Figure 30.12 Imidazoline α_2-adrenergic agonists.

The pK_a value indicates an approximately 80% ionization at physiologic pH, and the log D is the result of the lipophilic *ortho*-dichloro substituents on the phenyl ring.

While developed as a potential nasal decongestant, clonidine was found to possess hypotensive activity along with potential therapeutic benefit of reducing high IOP in glaucoma. Because of the high lipophilicity, the drug has the ability to cross the BBB, causing significant CNS effects which has limited its utility for treating glaucoma. This led to the development of its close analogues apraclonidine and brimonidine (see Fig. 30.12).

Apraclonidine and Brimonidine. Apraclonidine (pK_a = 9.22; log $D_{pH\ 7.4}$ = 0.01) is highly ionized at physiologic pH and is significantly more polar, and as a result, it does not cross the BBB as readily making a good candidate for treating glaucoma with fewer CNS adverse effects. Brimonidine (pK_a = 7.4; log $D_{pH\ 7.4}$ = 0.49) is lipophilic enough to cross BBB causing fatigue and/or drowsiness in some patients.

Both drugs, through stimulation of α_2-receptors in the eye, reduces production of aqueous humor and enhances its outflow, thus reducing IOP. They also have a neuroprotective effect apparently through α_{2A}-receptors located in the retina.[29,30] Apraclonidine's primary mechanism of action is due to a reduction of aqueous humor formation, whereas brimonidine lowers IOP by reducing aqueous humor production and increasing uveoscleral outflow. Brimonidine is approximately 1,000-fold more selective for α_2-receptors than are clonidine or apraclonidine. It exhibits minimal cardio stimulatory effects. Although both are applied topically to the eye, measurable quantities of these drugs are detectable in plasma, so caution must be employed when cardiovascular agents are coadministered. Plasma brimonidine levels peaked within 1 to 4 hours and declined with a systemic half-life of approximately 3 hours. Apraclonidine and brimonidine, have a duration of action of 4 and 8 hours, respectively, requiring twice or thrice daily dosing. That is why they are considered second-line agents for treating glaucoma after the introduction of prostaglandin analogues. Both drugs are contraindicated in patients receiving MAOI therapy. Tricyclic antidepressants have been shown to reduce the therapeutic effects of apraclonidine. Major adverse effects of apraclonidine include discomfort, hyperemia, and pruritus in the eye. Major adverse effects of brimonidine include allergic conjunctivitis, conjunctival hyperemia, and eye pruritus.

β-Adrenergic Receptor Blockers

Mechanism of Action. As previously discussed, IOP can be reduced by decreasing the production of aqueous humor from the ciliary body or increasing the outflow from the anterior chamber through the trabecular network. β-Adrenergic receptor blockers decrease the aqueous humor production by blocking β-adrenergic receptors on the ciliary body. β-Adrenergic receptors are of three subtypes, β_1, β_2, and β_3. Apart from the eye, these receptors are distributed in other organs such as β_1-receptors in cardiac smooth muscle, β_2-receptors in bronchioles, and β_3- receptors in adipose tissue and in the bladder. β-blockers that are currently used in the treatment of glaucoma include betaxolol, carteolol, levobunolol, and timolol. All of these are nonselective β-blockers except for betaxolol, which is a selective β_1-blocker.

Structure-Activity Relationships. All β-blockers used in the treatment of glaucoma have an aryloxypropanolamine pharmacophore. These agents are more potent β-blockers than the corresponding arylethanolamines. In addition to the use of β-blockers for the treatment of glaucoma these drugs have found widespread use in treating hypertension (see Chapter 19).

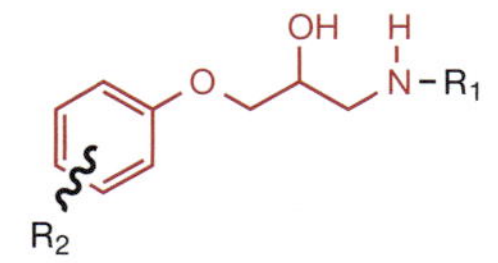

Aryloxypropanolamine pharmacophore

For maximum effectiveness in receptor binding, the hydroxy group in aryloxypropanolamines must occupy the same region in space as it does for the phenylethanolamine agonists in the *R* absolute configuration. Because of the insertion of an oxygen atom in the side chain of the aryloxypropanolamines, the Cahn-Ingold-Prelog priority of the substituents around the asymmetric carbon changes, and the isomer with the required special arrangement now has the *S* absolute configuration. A general overview of the SAR is given in Figure 30.13. Understanding SAR is crucial for elucidating the pharmacologic properties and optimizing the efficacy of these agents in receptor binding.

Substitution at the 4 position of the aryl group results in selectivity as β_1-blockers (Fig. 30.14).

Pharmacokinetics. In general, the ophthalmic aryloxypropanolamine β-blockers have a rapid onset (1-2 hours) and duration of action (verses other β-blockers) ranging

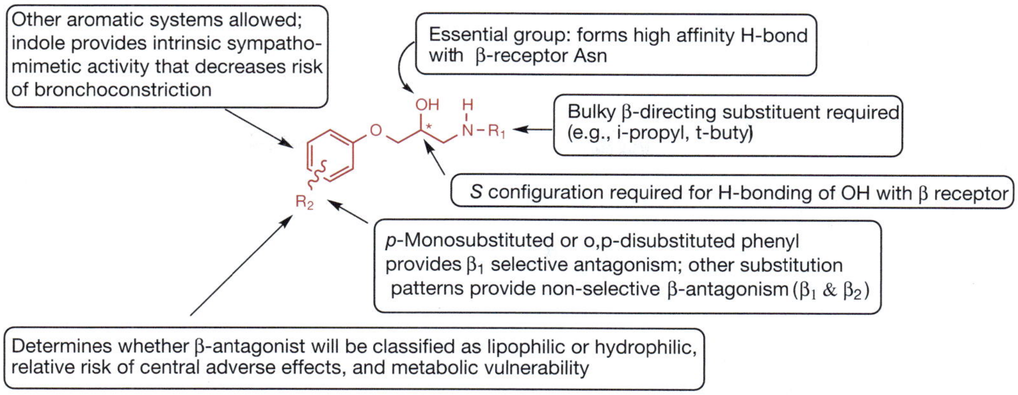

Figure 30.13 Aryloxypropanolamine β-adrenergic antagonist structure-activity relationship (SAR).

from 12 to 24 hours and are normally administered 1 or 2 times daily.[31] While some systemic absorption is possible, this is usually minimal and as a result little is reported concerning metabolism or excretion.

Adverse Effects. Dose-dependent follicular conjunctivitis is a common adverse effect.[26] Systemic absorption of β-blockers used in treating glaucoma may present adverse effects associated with their binding elsewhere in the body such as bradycardia (β_1), bronchospasms (β_2) as well as other adverse effects including depression, fatigue and ocular dryness. Some of these adverse effects can be lowered or avoided by closing the eyelid for at least 1 minute after administering the topical formulation that prevents systemic absorption through the nasolacrimal duct. Betaxolol, being a selective β_1-blocker, presents fewer respiratory adverse effects.[32] In general, β-blockers are contraindicated in patients with bronchial asthma, chronic obstructive pulmonary disease (COPD), sinus bradycardia, or cardiac failure. Coadministration of oral β-blockers may lead to additive effects. β-blockers were previously considered first-line therapy for glaucoma until the advent of prostaglandin analogue therapy.

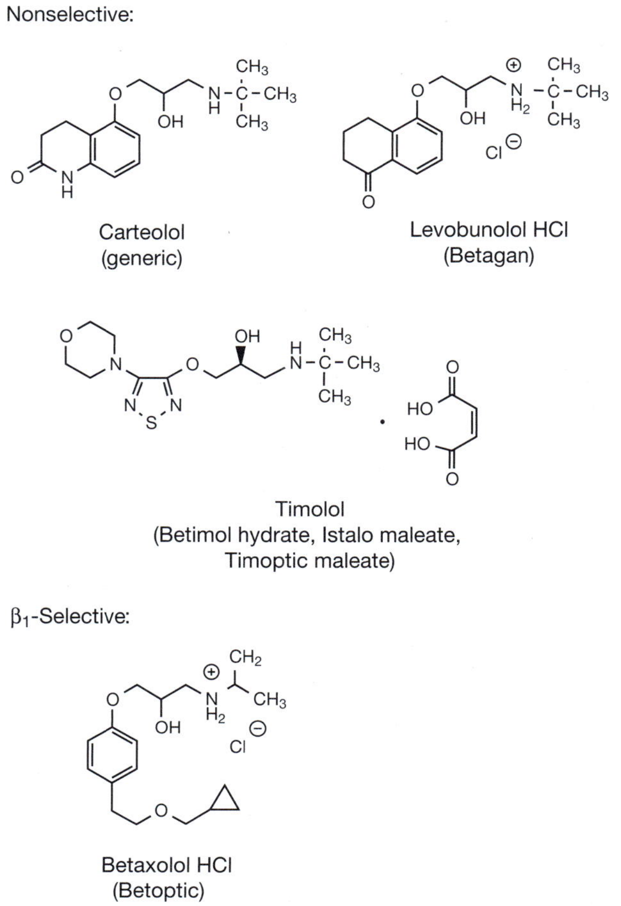

Figure 30.14 β-Blockers used in the treatment of glaucoma.

Prostaglandin Analogues

Prostaglandin (PG) analogues are the first-line therapy for glaucoma. Bimatoprost, latanoprost, latanoprostene bunod, omidenepag isopropyl, tafluprost, and travoprost (Fig. 30.15) are currently indicated for treating glaucoma or ocular hypertension.

Mechanism of Action. As indicated, an increase in the ocular pressure is one of the major causes of optic nerve damage in patients with primary open-angle glaucoma. This is due to the increase in the production and/or decrease in the outflow of aqueous humor in the eye. In the normal eye, outflow of aqueous humor occurs mostly through the trabecular meshwork while the uveoscleral pathway (also referred to as the unconventional outflow pathway) is a minor pathway. The prostaglandin derivatives increase the aqueous humor outflow from the anterior chamber of the eye thereby reducing IOP, but the exact mechanism is presently unknown. The action of these drugs include agonistic binding at the prostaglandin F (PGF) receptor, an action similar to that of the natural ($PGF^{2\alpha}$), but there is mounting evidence that these drugs may act through a mimicking action on the uveoscleral pathway. The relative affinity of prostaglandins for PGF receptor are $PGF^{2\alpha} > PGD_2 > PGE_2 > PGI_2 = TXA_2$. The PGF receptor is a GPCR and is a G_q type. On activation, this receptor couples to G protein Rho via G_q-independent mechanisms resulting in the activation of phospholipase C, which causes muscle contraction.[33] PGF receptors are found in the ciliary muscle and trabecular meshwork cells of the eye and, on activation, lead to

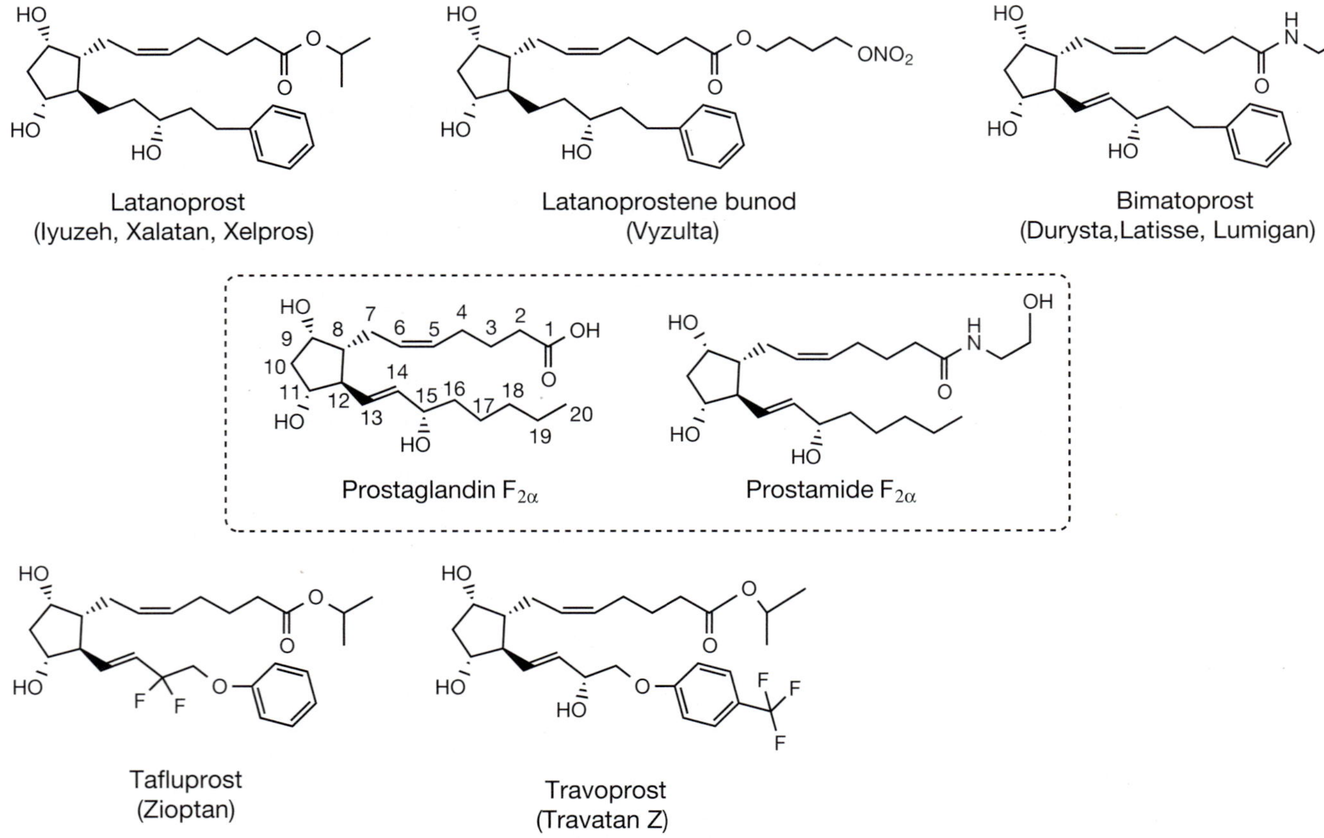

Figure 30.15 Prostaglandin analogues.

a widening and drainage of the channels (uveoscleral pathway), increasing the outflow of aqueous humor from the anterior chamber through the Schlemm canal. Prostaglandin analogues reduce IOP by 25% to 30%.

Specific Drugs

Latanoprost. Latanoprost is a $PGF^{2\alpha}$ analogue, which is formulated as a sterile, isotonic, buffered aqueous solution. Latanoprost is a prodrug, which is rapidly metabolized in the cornea by esterase to produce the active metabolite latanoprost acid (Fig. 30.16). Latanoprost acid is thought to produce an outflow of aqueous humor through the uveoscleral pathway via binding to prostaglandin $F_{2\alpha}$ receptors. This is considered a non-conventional mechanism for lowering IOP. Further metabolism of latanoprost acid occurs in the liver via successive β-oxidations the first of which results in removal of two carbons (dinor) and then two additional carbons (tetranor) to give an acid, which can exist as a lactone (these same metabolic reactions occur with all four of the prostaglandin derivatives [Fig. 30.15]). The only metabolites found in the urine are oxidative products.[34] The plasma half-life of latanoprost is approximately 17 minutes. Reduction of IOP starts within 3 to 4 hours and peaks after 8 to 12 hours. The drug is indicated to treat elevated IOP in patients with open-angle glaucoma or ocular hypertension.

A second prodrug source of latanoprost acid is the drug latanoprostene bunod (Fig. 30.16). Like latanoprost, latanoprostene bunod rapidly undergoes esterase metabolism following application to the eye producing latanoprost acid which increases outflow of aqueous humor. Additionally, butanediol mononitrate is formed (Fig. 30.16). The butanediol mononitrate is further metabolized to produce nitric oxide (NO) a compound which is reported to lower IOP via a conventional outflow of aqueous humor through the trabecular meshwork/Schlemm canal. Latanoprostene bunod, therefore, is considered a dual-acting glaucoma treatment drug which produces improved lowering of IOP. The drug (0.024% concentration) is administered as a single drop once daily for 28 days. Common adverse effects include eye irritation, conjunctival hyperemia, eye pain, and installation site pain.[35]

Bimatoprost. Bimatoprost is also a prostaglandin $F_{2\alpha}$ analogue (see Fig. 30.15), indicated for treating ocular hypertension. Unlike latanoprost, tafluprost, and travoprost the amide nature of this drug results in a significantly more stable product, which is active in its own right.[36,37] It has been suggested that bimatoprost may be active by virtue of its ability to interfere with the biosynthesis of prostamide $F_{2\alpha}$ at a yet to be defined PGF receptor. An agonist at this receptor might be expected to increase the aqueous humor outflow via the uveoscleral pathway without effecting production of aqueous humor. In addition to its stability the amide helps improve the lipophilicity, which facilitate absorption through the corneal membrane. There is no indication that bimatoprost is hydrolyzed in the eye nor is the activity due to bimatoprost acid formation unlike the action of latanoprost acid or travoprost acid.[38] Bimatoprost is well absorbed through the cornea reaching peak plasma concentration within 10 minutes. It is highly bound to plasma protein (88%) and is eliminated within 90 minutes

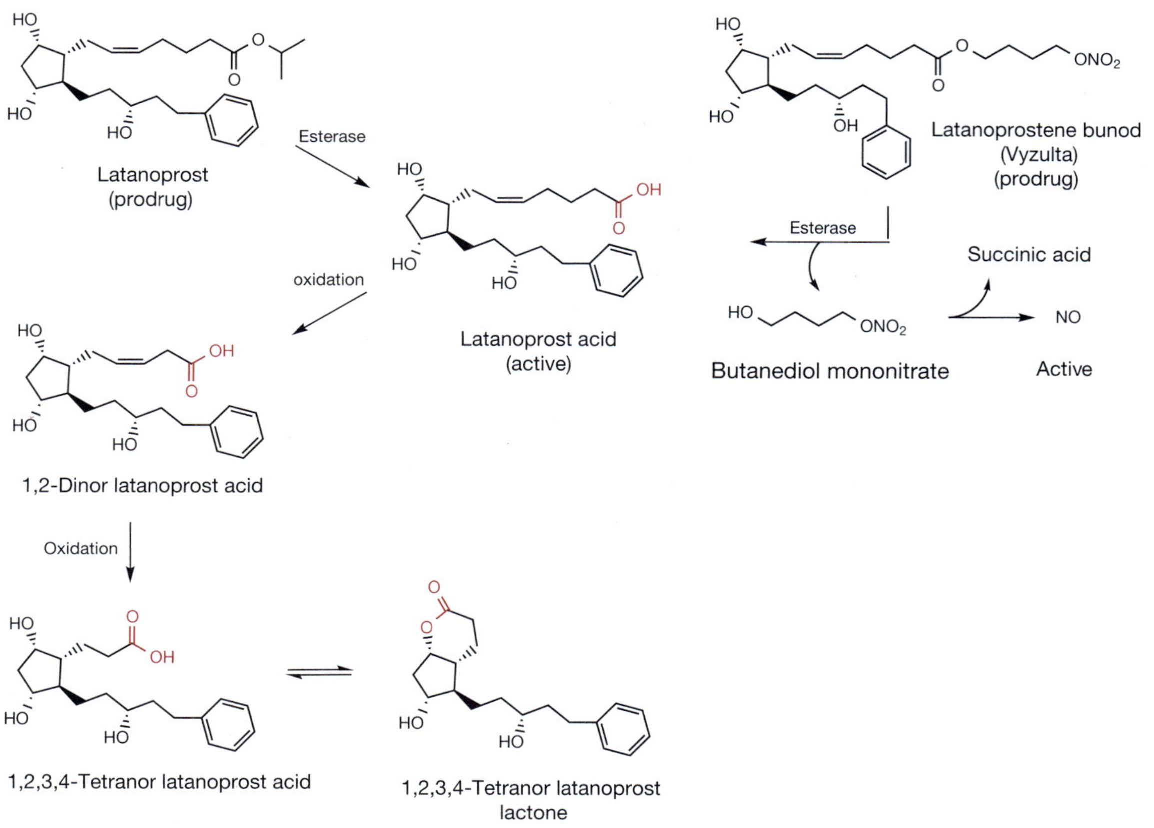

Figure 30.16 Metabolism of latanoprost.

of administration. Bimatoprost is metabolized by oxidation, *N*-deethylation, and glucuronidation. It is a substrate of CYP3A4. Bimatoprost is available as 0.01% and 0.03% solutions.

Common adverse effects associated with bimatoprost include eye irritation, hyperpigmentation of the iris, periorbital tissue and eyelashes, eyelash growth, and conjunctival hyperemia. One of the significant side effects of bimatoprost is increasing length and thickness of eyelashes. In 2008, it was approved by the FDA for cosmetic use of lengthening and darkening of eyelashes under the brand name Latisse.

Travoprost. Travoprost is an isopropyl ester prodrug, which is converted to an active acid metabolite by esterases in the eye. It follows similar a metabolism and elimination profile as latanoprost (see Fig. 30.16). Travoprost metabolism includes β-oxidation to give 1,2-dinor travoprost acid and 1,2,3,4-tetranor travoprost acid. Further, oxidation of the 15-OH group as well as reduction of the 13,14 double bond have also been reported.[39]

Tafluprost. The design of tafluprost was based upon the replacement of both the 15-hydroxy and hydrogen with two fluorides with the intent of decreasing the potential for 15-hydroxydehydrogenase catalyzed oxidation. In addition, this replacement results in increased lipophilicity to improve corneal absorption. As with latanoprost and travopost, tafluprost is a prodrug which is rapidly hydrolyzed to the active tafluprost acid. As indicated in Figure 30.16, β-oxidation leads to the 1,2-dinor and then 1,2,3,4-tetranor tafluprost.[40,41]

Tafluprost is the only preservative-free prostaglandin analogue; thus, it is packaged in unit dose, to be discarded after single use. It is a lipophilic ester, which readily crosses the cornea (~75% absorption in rats). Its onset of action is 2 to 4 hours with maximal effect reaching after 12 hours. The drug is administered once daily. No CYP enzymes are involved in its metabolism.

Clinical Application. Once-daily dosing and fewer systemic adverse effects make prostaglandin analogues first-line agents. Maximum therapeutic effect is reached in 2 weeks. PGF receptors are also highly expressed in dermal papillae, which increases the eyelash growth, one of the major adverse effects reported for prostaglandin analogues.[42] However, this side effect is temporary and will be relieved after discontinuation of the therapy. Other common adverse effects include pigmentation on the iris and eyelashes, redness, stinging, hyperemia, ocular inflammation, and ocular pruritus. These medications should be avoided in patients with active intraocular inflammation. Due to instability, prostaglandin analogues should be stored away from light below room temperature.[43] Patients should be advised to discard any unused medication after 4 to 6 weeks.

Omidenepag Isopropyl (Omlonti). Omidenepag isopropyl has recently been approved for the treatment of IOP in patents with open-angle glaucoma. Unlike the prostaglandin analogues, this non-prostaglandin is a selective E-prostanoid subtype 2 (EP2) agonist. Omidenepag isopropyl is a prodrug which after application to the corneal tissue, the drug undergoes metabolism via esterase into the active drug

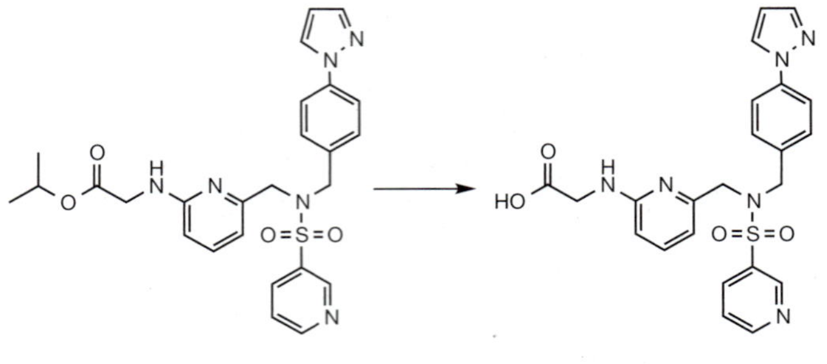

Omidenepag isopropyl
(Omlonti)
(prodrug)

Omidenepag (OMD
(active)

Figure 30.17 Metabolic activation of omidenepag.

omidenepag (OMD) (Fig. 30.17). OMD is a selective binder to EP2 receptors acting as an agonist with little or no effect on other prostanoid receptors.[44] Binding to EP2 receptor leads to aqueous humor outflow via trabecular and uveoscleal outflow pathways. The drug is administered as a topical once-daily 0.002% solution with minimal yet different adverse effects from those exhibited by the prostaglandin agonists.

Rho Kinase Inhibitors

Rho kinases (ROCKs) are serine/threonine kinases that act as effectors for Rho proteins. There are two types of Rho kinases, ROCK1 and ROCK2. ROCK1 is an important downstream effector for Rho-GTP protein. Rho proteins (RhoA, RhoB, RhoC) are small G proteins bound to guanosine diphosphate (GDP) in their inactive state. Upon external stimuli, GDP is converted into guanosine triphosphate (GTP). Rho proteins are active when bound to GTP. The active Rho-GTP protein binds to Rho kinase at the Rho binding pocket. Rho kinase phosphorylates a number of downstream proteins including myosin light chain. All these actions result in a contractile state of the cells increasing their stiffness and smooth muscle contraction. Due to the increase in contractile nature of cells in the trabecular meshwork, changes in the extracellular matrix composition and/or a decrease in the conductance of the inner wall endothelial cells of Schlemm canal in the eye leads to clogging and buildup of IOP. Rho kinase inhibitors can help relax these muscles by reducing cell contraction, stiffness and decreasing the concentration of fibrosis related proteins, thereby increasing aqueous humor outflow through the trabecular meshwork.[45]

Aqueous humor outflow occurs in two ways, conventional trabecular outflow and unconventional uveoscleral pathway. Ninety percent of the aqueous humor outflow occurs through the trabecular meshwork. Traditional glaucoma drugs work by increasing the aqueous humor outflow through the unconventional uveoscleral pathway without having much effect on the clogged trabecular meshwork. In contrast, a Rho kinase inhibitor works to unclog the trabecular meshwork, increasing aqueous humor outflow. Due to this unique mechanism of action, a Rho kinase inhibitor can be used in combination with other classes of glaucoma drugs. It has also been suggested that ROCK inhibitors could have a dual mechanism of action.[46]

A second mechanism reported involves inhibition of norepinephrine-reuptake transporter (NET) in ciliary body synapses causing vasoconstriction of arteries that supply blood to ciliary body, which in turn reduces aqueous humor production.

Rho kinase inhibitors have found a number of clinical uses including the treatment of glaucoma and cerebral vasospasm among several others. These are the newest class of drugs used for treating high IOP associated with glaucoma or ocular hypertension. Netarsudil is the first Rho kinase inhibitor to enter the US market. Several other Rho kinase inhibitors are currently under development.

NETARSUDIL

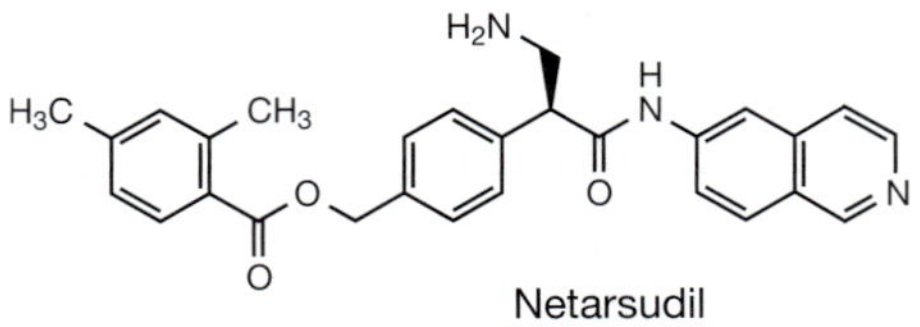

Netarsudil
(Rhopressa)

Mechanism of Action. Netarsudil is approved for treating elevated IOP in open-angle glaucoma and ocular hypertension.[47] Similar to the use of prostaglandin esters to improve corneal drug absorption, it is administered as a prodrug, which undergoes hydrolysis by esterases present in the eye to produce the active metabolite M1 (Fig. 30.18). Netarsudil-M1 is an active inhibitor of ROCK 1 and ROCK 2. In vitro studies have shown that netarsudil-M1 is approximately 5-fold more active than netarsudil. It does not appear that M1 possess NET inhibition activity in humans but studies are continuing.[48]

Conjunctival hyperemia is a common adverse effect seen. Less common adverse effects include corneal verticillata, instillation site pain, and conjunctival hemorrhage. Netarsudil is administered once daily.

The FDA has recently approved the fixed combination of netarsudil and latanoprost (Rocklatan) for the treatment of open-angle glaucoma or ocular hypertension as a once-daily product. Both netarsudil and latanoprost have previously been approved as single agents.

Carbonic Anhydrase Inhibitors

Carbonic anhydrase (CA) is an important enzyme in the body, which regulates secretions and fluid transport. Of the several different families of CAs (ie, α-CA, β-CA) that have been identified, α-CA is found in humans. CAs have minimal sequence similarity among themselves

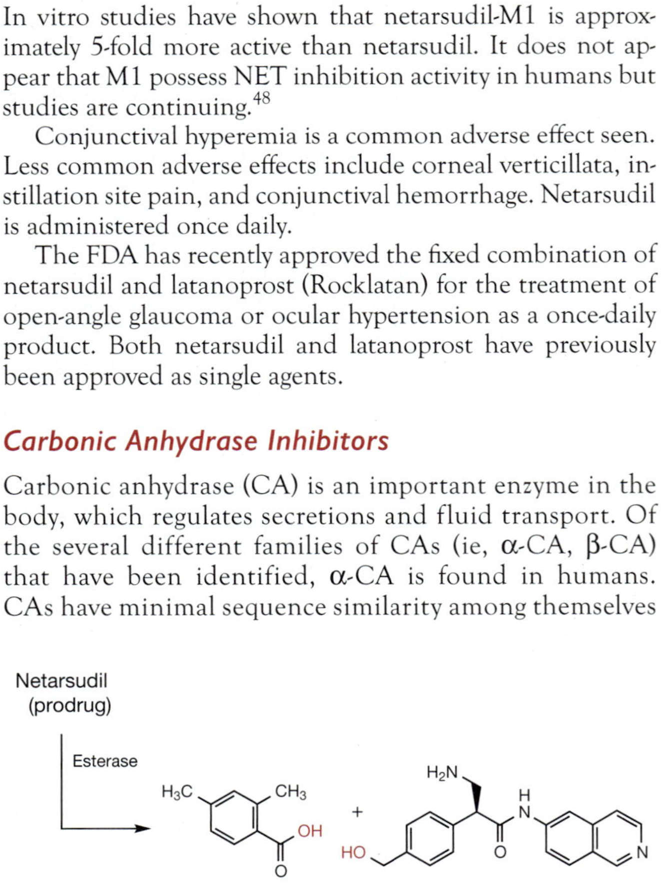

Netarsudil-M1
(Active)

Figure 30.18 Metabolism of netarsudil.

with 10 different isoforms of α-CA having been identified. They are present throughout the body and with various functions based on tissue location. Carbonic anhydrase II (CA II) which belongs to the α-CA family, is highly expressed in the ciliary body of the eye, where its role is to regulate aqueous humor production through pH changes. CA rapidly interconverts carbon dioxide and water into dissociated carbonic acid, bicarbonate and a hydrogen ion, and thus regulates fluid pH. Due to its wide array of functions in the body, systemic use of CA inhibitors (CAIs) is expected to cause numerous biologic effects

$$CO_2 + H_2O \underset{\text{anhydrase}}{\overset{\text{Carbonic}}{\rightleftharpoons}} HCO_3^{\ominus} + H^{\oplus}$$

In the treatment of glaucoma, the development of topical CAIs holds appeal, aiming to mitigate the potential for systemic effects. Unfortunately, topical application of CAIs is less effective compared to oral formulations. Of the drugs available, the first-generation inhibitors, acetazolamide and methazolamide, are used as systemic drugs, while the second-generation drugs, dorzolamide and brinzolamide, are available in topical dosage forms (Fig. 30.19).

Mechanism of Action. As indicated, CA converts water and carbon dioxide to carbonic acid. CA is a zinc-metalloenzyme, which has zinc (Zn) in its catalytic site. The Zn prosthetic ion is coordinated to three histidine residues as well as a water molecule (Fig. 30.20).[49]

Glutamine (Gln92) and threonine (Thr199) are key catalytic amino acids within CA's catalytic site, facilitating the binding of carbon dioxide and facilitating the generation of carbonic acid. The resulting dissociated carbonic acid brings about a change in pH and the movement of sodium ions that eventually promotes fluid secretion.[49] CAIs interfere with interactions of a water molecule with zinc ion as well as prevent carbon dioxide from entering the active site through their interactions with the threonine amino acid. Binding interactions of the CAI dorzolamide in the CA active site is shown in Figure 30.20B. All CAIs used in the treatment of glaucoma are sulfonamide derivatives. As seen in Figure 30.20, the sulfonamide functional group exhibits

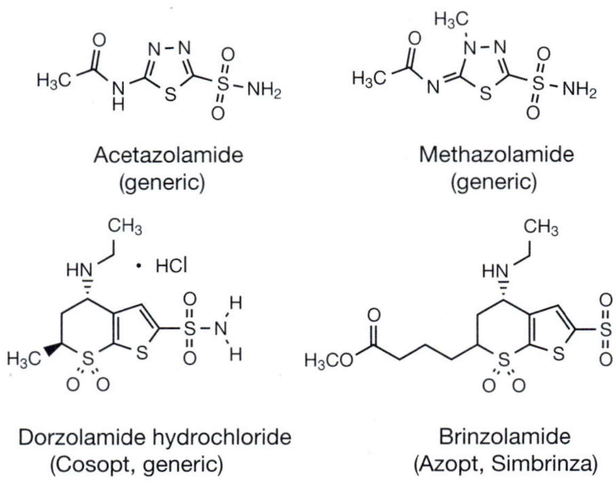

Figure 30.19 Carbonic anhydrase inhibitors.

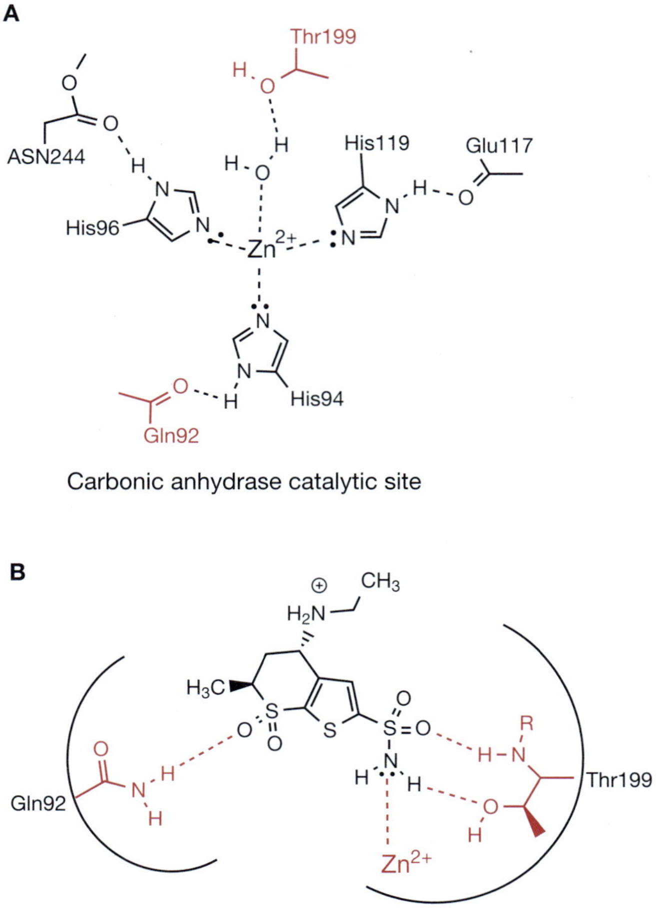

Figure 30.20 A. Carbonic anhydrase catalytic site. B. The binding interactions of dorzolamide at the carbonic anhydrase catalytic site.

key hydrogen-bonding interaction with Thr199 amino acid as well as chelation to the zinc metal. The alicyclic sulfone oxygen also shows hydrogen-bonding interaction with the Gln92.[49]

Specific Drugs

Acetazolamide and Methazolamide. Acetazolamide and methazolamide are potent first-generation CAIs, which are administered orally. They effectively inhibit most of the CA isoforms (see Fig. 30.19). These medications decrease the aqueous humor production reducing IOP by 25% to 30%. Because of their poor solubility, they are unable to pass through the cornea to reach the ciliary body, which limits their use. Most of the acetazolamide is excreted unchanged while methazolamide undergoes N-dealkylation to produce an active metabolite. Both drugs are indicated for the treatment of refractory glaucoma that does not respond to β-adrenergic antagonists or prostaglandin analogues. In general, due to systemic adverse effects, they have been replaced with topical agents.

Dorzolamide and Brinzolamide. Dorzolamide and brinzolamide are second-generation CAIs, developed as topical formulations (see Fig. 30.19). They selectively inhibit CA II. Their pharmacokinetic profiles suggest a more favorable ability to cross the cornea and reach the ciliary body, the location of CA enzymes. Both of these drugs have a good hydrophilic/lipophilic balance. Upon topical application, more than 50% of the drug is absorbed with significant amounts reaching systemic circulation where the drug is absorbed by red blood cells. It should be noted that 90% of body's CA is stored in red blood cells. Both drugs are extremely effective in inhibiting CA in ciliary bodies (~100% inhibition). Dorzolamide and brinzolamide undergoes N-deethylation catalyzed by CYP2B1/2, CYP2E2, and CYP3A to produce the corresponding desethyl active metabolites (Fig. 30.21). These drugs and their metabolites are eliminated through the kidneys.[50]

The second-generation CAIs are devoid of most systemic adverse effects unlike first-generation drugs. Common adverse effects include stinging, burning of the eye, blurred vision, pruritus, and bitter taste. Brinzolamide produces less stinging/burning adverse effects but more blurred vision in comparison to dorzolamide. Additional adverse effects associated with dorzolamide include contact allergy, nephrolithiasis, anorexia, depression, dementia, and irreversible corneal decompensation in patients with established corneal problems.

Muscarinic Agonists

Several muscarinic agonists continue to be used in the treatment of ocular conditions. They are also called "miotics" as they induce miosis.

Mechanism of Action. Interaction of cholinergic agonists with muscarinic acetylcholinergic receptors (mAChRs) leads to well-defined pharmacologic responses depending on the tissue or organ in which the receptor is located. These responses include contractions of smooth muscle, vasodilation, increased secretion from exocrine glands, miosis, and decreased heart rate and force of contraction. Muscarinic receptors are G protein–coupled receptors (GPCRs) of five types M_1 through M_5, of which M_3 muscarinic receptors are highly populated in the ciliary body and iris sphincter of the eye.[51] Signal transduction at the stimulatory M_3 mAChR occurs via coupling with a $G_{q/11}$ protein that is involved with mobilization of intracellular calcium. Agonist binding to this receptor results in activation of phospholipase C, with subsequent production of the second messengers, DAG and inositol 1,4,5-triphosphate (IP_3). Stimulation of IP_3 ion channel receptors leads to release of intracellular calcium from the endoplasmic reticulum. The DAG produced, along with calcium, activates protein kinase C, which phosphorylates proteins to afford ciliary muscle contraction in the eye causing miosis. This opens up the trabecular meshwork allowing the aqueous humor to flow out, thus lowering IOP. Topical muscarinic agonists are used for reducing the IOP in treating glaucoma and ocular hypertension. They also find utility in inducing miosis during surgery.

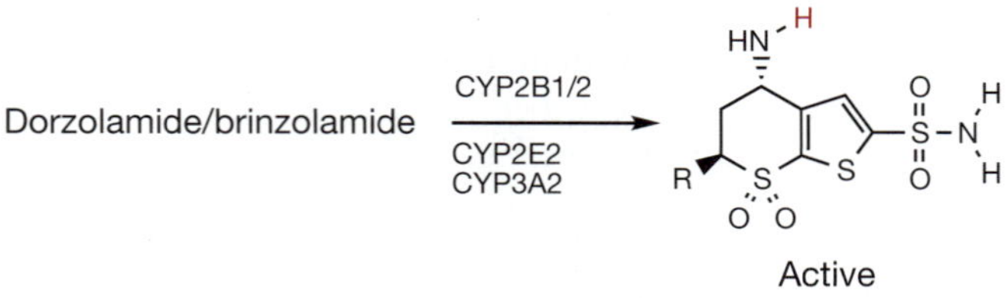

Figure 30.21 Metabolism of dorzolamide and brinzolamide.

Acetylcholine. Acetylcholine is the prototypical muscarinic and nicotinic agonist because it is the physiologic chemical neurotransmitter for the cholinergic nervous system. However, it is a poor therapeutic agent due to its lack of specificity for both nicotinic acetylcholinergic receptors (nAChRs) and mAChRs. In addition, the chemical properties associated with the ester and the quaternary ammonium functional group create potential problems. Although very stable in the solid crystalline form, ACh undergoes rapid hydrolysis in aqueous solution. This hydrolysis is accelerated in the presence of catalytic amounts of either acid or base. For this reason, acetylcholine cannot be administered orally due to rapid hydrolysis in the gastrointestinal tract. Even when administered parenterally, its pharmacologic action is fleeting as a result of hydrolysis by butyrylcholinesterase (also known as pseudocholinesterase or plasma cholinesterase) in serum. The quaternary ammonium functional group of acetylcholine imparts excellent water solubility, but quaternary ammonium salts are poorly absorbed across lipid membranes due to their high hydrophilic and ionic character. Thus, even if acetylcholine were stable enough to be administered orally, it would be poorly absorbed. When used during ocular surgery to produce complete miosis, acetylcholine is available as a powder to be reconstituted as an intraocular solution for injection. It must be directly instilled into the anterior chamber. It cannot be administered topically because it is not lipophilic enough to penetrate the cornea, and it must be reconstituted immediately before instillation into the eye due to its hydrolytic liability. It is therefore not used in the treatment of glaucoma.

Structure-Activity Relationship. The classic SAR for muscarinic agonist activity is summarized in Figure 30.22. Key SAR points are listed as follows:

- The molecule must possess a nitrogen atom capable of bearing a positive charge, preferably a quaternary ammonium salt.
- For maximum potency, the size of the alkyl groups substituted on the nitrogen should not exceed the size of a methyl group.
- The molecule should have an oxygen atom, preferably an ester-like oxygen, capable of participating in a hydrogen bond.
- There should be a two-carbon unit between the oxygen atom and the nitrogen atom.

Specific Drugs

Carbachol Chloride (Miostat)

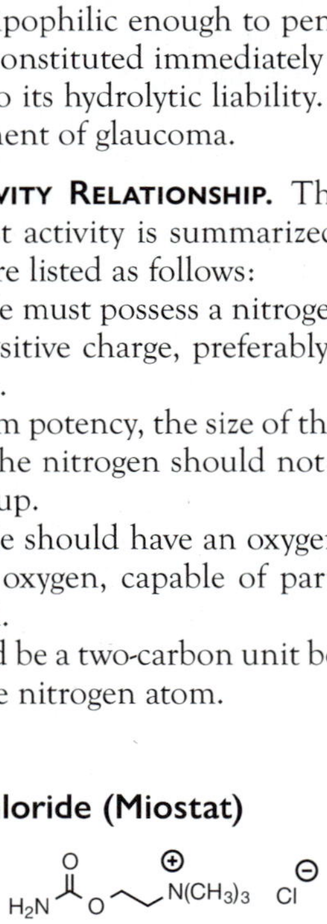

Carbachol
(Miostat)

Carbachol, the carbamate analogue of acetylcholine, exhibits affinity for both mAChRs and nAChRs. Because it is a carbamate, carbachol is more resistant toward acid-, base-, or enzyme acetylcholinesterase (AChE)–catalyzed hydrolysis than acetylcholine. It is also reported to exhibit weak anticholinesterase activity. Both of these actions work to prolong the duration of action of carbachol. Carbachol is

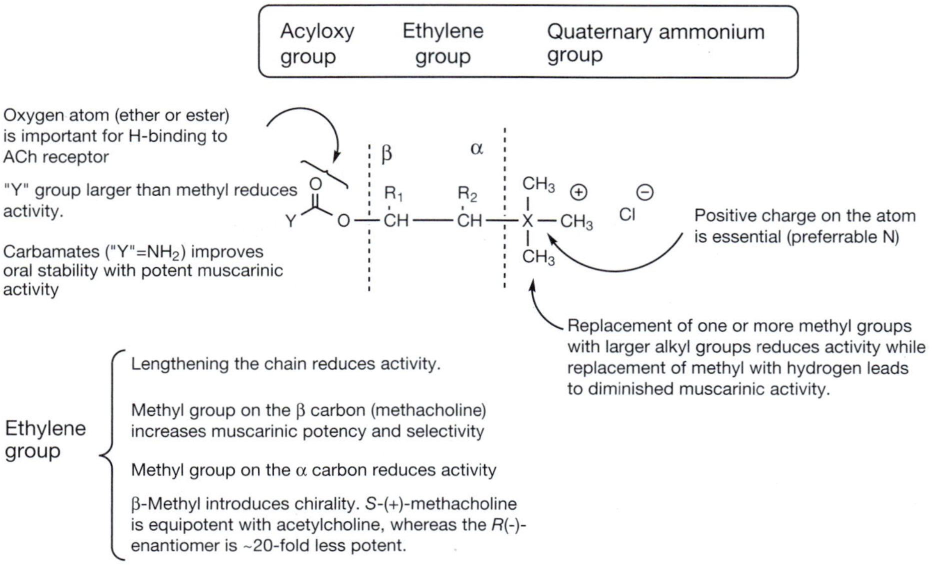

Figure 30.22 Summary of muscarinic agonists' structure-activity relationship (SAR).

available as an intraocular solution. Carbachol is used for the induction of miosis in ocular surgery and to reduce IOP during the first 24 hours after cataract surgery.

Pilocarpine Hydrochloride (Vuity)

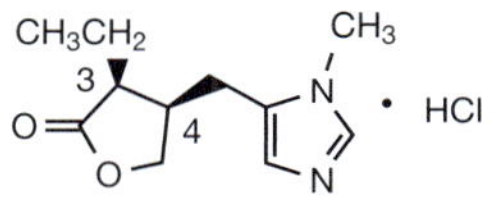

3*S*,4*R*-pilocarpine hydrochloride
(Isopto Carpine)

Pilocarpine hydrochloride, the salt of an alkaloid obtained from *Pilocarpus jaborandi*, is a selective M_3 mAChR agonist that does not adhere to the traditional SAR of muscarinic agonists. It possesses two chiral centers at C-3 and C-4. Thus, four optical isomers (two enantiomeric pairs) are possible, and of these, the naturally occurring alkaloid is 3*S*,4*R*-(+)-pilocarpine, with a pK_a of 6.8 and a log $D_{7.4}$ of 1.03.

Pilocarpine is marketed as tablets (for treatment of dry mouth and dry eye disease [DED]) and an ophthalmic solution. It penetrates the eye well and is the miotic of choice for open-angle glaucoma and to terminate acute angle-closure attacks. Because pilocarpine is a lactone, its solutions are subject to (1) hydrolysis to afford the pharmacologically inactive pilocarpic acid and (2) base-catalyzed epimerization at C-3 in the lactone to give isopilocarpine, an inactive stereoisomer of pilocarpine (Fig. 30.23).

Epimerization is not believed to be a serious problem if the drug is properly stored. Its solutions can be stored at room temperature. Pilocarpine is metabolized by esterases as well as CYP2A6. It is also an inhibitor of CYP2A6. Given the low amounts of pilocarpine, systemic absorption upon topical administration is minimal and is not expected to show significant drug-drug interactions. Pilocarpine is approved for treating elevated ocular pressure in patients with ocular hypertension or open-angle glaucoma, the management of acute angle-closure glaucoma, the prevention of postoperative elevated IOP associated with laser surgery, and induction of miosis.[52]

Acetylcholinesterase Inhibitors

Acetylcholine esterase inhibitors inhibit the metabolism of acetylcholine by AChE. Thus, inhibition of hydrolysis by AChE increases the concentration of acetylcholine in the synapse and results in potentiation and/or prolonged activation of both muscarinic and nicotinic effects.

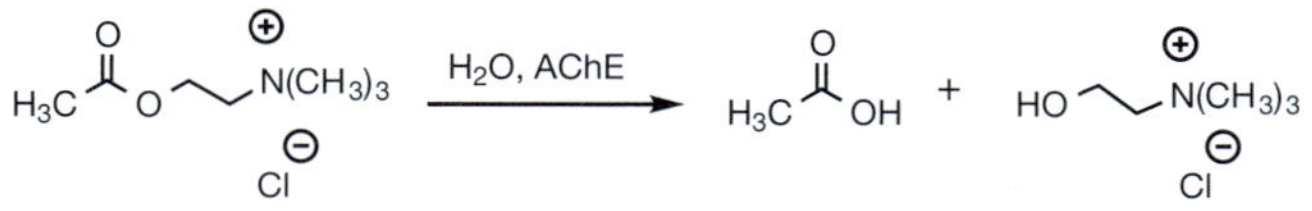

Acetylcholine Acetic acid Choline

Acetylcholinesterase inhibitors (AChEIs), sometimes referred to as anticholinesterases, are classified as indirect cholinomimetics because their principal mechanism of action does not involve binding to cholinergic receptors but indirectly increasing the synaptic concentration of acetylcholine. AChEIs are used in open-angle glaucoma to decrease IOP by stimulating contraction of the ciliary muscle and sphincter of the iris. This facilitates outflow of aqueous humor via the canal of Schlemm.

Mechanism of Acetylcholinesterase-Catalyzed Hydrolysis of Acetylcholine

The active site of AChE consists of the ester binding site (at which hydrolysis of the ester occurs) and an "anionic

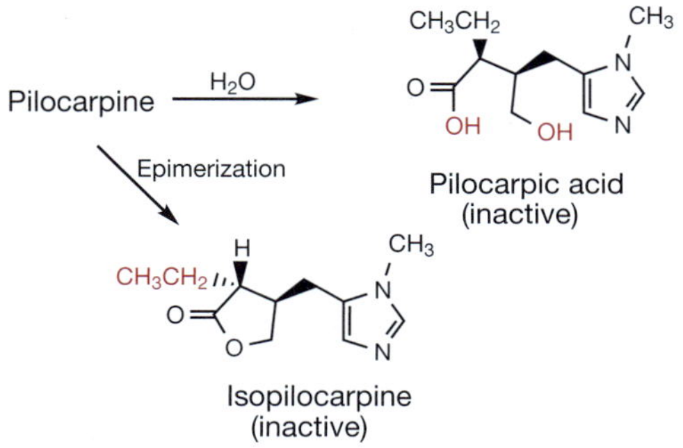

Figure 30.23 Chemical instabilities of pilocarpine.

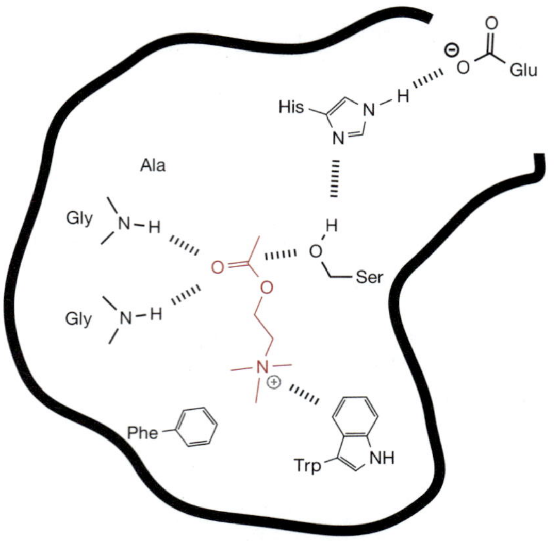

Figure 30.24 Binding of acetylcholine to catalytic site of acetylcholinesterase; role of serine and histidine residues is illustrated.

binding site" (where the cationic nitrogen of acetylcholine binds) (Fig. 30.24).

Instead of a regular ionic bond, the quaternary nitrogen of acetylcholine binds to the π-electrons of a tryptophan residue forming a cation–π bonding interaction.[53] Like other serine hydrolases, the functional catalytic unit of AChE is composed of a catalytic triad of glutamate, histidine, and serine at the ester binding site.[54,55] During hydrolysis the serine amino acid is acetylated. The acylated enzyme then undergoes rapid hydrolysis to regenerate the active form of AChE and a molecule of acetic acid.

Hydrolysis of the acylated enzyme (deacylation) is important in the development of AChEIs. If the enzyme becomes acylated by a functional group (ie, carbamyl or phosphate) that is more stable toward hydrolysis than a carboxylate ester, the enzyme remains inactive for a longer period of time. Application of this chemical principle regarding rates of hydrolysis led to discovery and design of two classes of AChEIs, the reversible inhibitors and the irreversible inhibitors.

Reversible Inhibitors of Acetylcholinesterase

PHYSOSTIGMINE

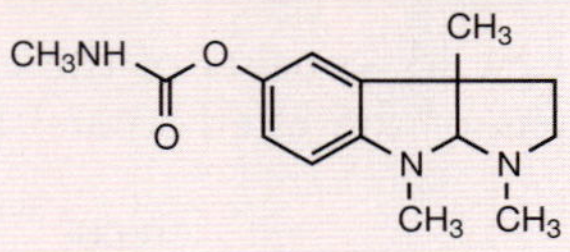

Physostigmine

For many years, physostigmine was a marketed drug available for the treatment of glaucoma. Physostigmine has exceptionally high affinity ($K_i \sim 10^{-9}$ M) for the catalytic site of AChE where it acted as a reversible AChEI. The carbamylated AChE was regenerated very slowly. Because physostigmine is lipophilic, it was able to diffuse across lipophilic membranes including the blood-brain barrier. Physostigmine is no longer marketed in the United States as an ophthalmic formulation.

Irreversible Inhibitors of Acetylcholinesterase

Mechanism of Action. The chemical logic involved in the development of AChEIs was to synthesize compounds that would be substrates for AChE and result in an acylated enzyme more stable to hydrolysis than a carboxylate ester. Phosphate esters are very stable to hydrolysis even more so than many amides. Application of this chemical property to the design of AChEIs led to derivatives of phosphoric, pyrophosphoric, and phosphonic acids that are effective inhibitors of AChE. These act as inhibitors by the same mechanism as the previously available carbamate inhibitor physostigmine, except that they form phosphate esters with the enzyme. The rate of hydrolysis of the phosphorylated enzyme is very slow with its rate being measured in hours (eg, the half-lives for diethyl phosphates are ~8 hours). Because of their exceptionally longer duration of action, these compounds, are referred to as irreversible inhibitors of AChE. Knowledge of the chemical mechanisms associated with irreversible inhibition of AChE has led to the development of a series of phosphoester insecticides (ie, malathion, parathion, chlorpyrifos, etc) as well as the development of deadly phosphorus-derived chemical warfare "nerve agents," one of which is sarin.

Echothiophate Iodide (Phospholine Iodide)

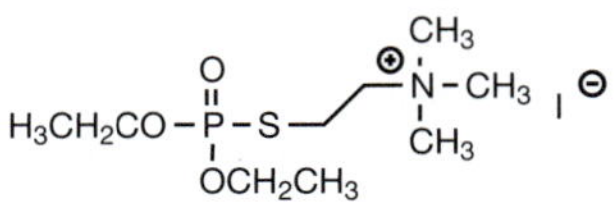

Echothiophate iodide
(Phospholine iodide)

Echothiophate iodide has found therapeutic application for the treatment of glaucoma and strabismus. Echothiophate is applied topically as a solution and is the only irreversible AChEI for the treatment of glaucoma. The decrease in IOP observed which can last up to 4 weeks. Phosphoester AChEIs exhibit cataractogenic properties; thus, their use should be reserved for patients who are refractory to other forms of treatment (ie, short-acting miotics, β-blockers, epinephrine, and, possibly, CAIs). Because of its toxicity, echothiophate is not used for its systemic action. Adverse effects include stinging, burning, lacrimation, eyelid muscle twitching, reddening, and blurred vision.

Topical Ophthalmic Nonsteroidal Anti-Inflammatory Drugs

There has been considerable interest in the safety and effectiveness of topical ophthalmic nonsteroidal anti-inflammatory drugs (NSAIDs) for treatment of inflammation of the anterior segment of the eye (the cornea, iris, ciliary body, and lens) as a result of corneal damage from diclofenac ophthalmic solution.[56] Since 1999, several replacement ophthalmic NSAID products have been introduced including flurbiprofen ophthalmic solution, ketorolac tromethamine ophthalmic solution, bromfenac ophthalmic solution, and nepafenac ophthalmic suspension for postoperative pain and inflammation after cataract extraction or from corneal refractive surgery (Fig. 30.25). Pharmacokinetic

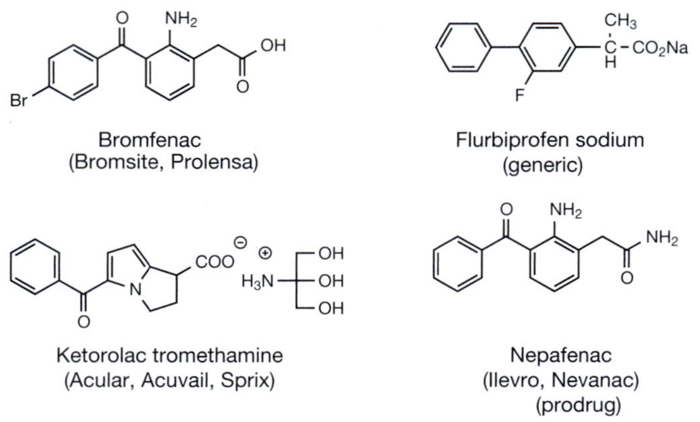

Figure 30.25 Topical nonsteroid anti-inflammatory drugs (NSAIDs).

and physicochemical properties for diclofenac, flurbiprofen, and ketorolac are reported in Chapter 17 (Table 17.3). Systemic toxicity from topical NSAIDs is rare due to minimal absorption, but there are some reports of asthma exacerbations with the use of ophthalmic NSAIDs.[54] Thus, their use should be avoided in patients allergic to NSAIDs. Most common ocular toxicities include burning, irritation, and conjunctival hyperemia. Prolonged use may result in corneal thinning, ulcerations, and corneal perforations in susceptible individuals.[57]

Mechanism of Action. NSAIDs are competitive and reversible inhibitors of two closely related cyclooxygenase (COX) enzymes, COX-1 and COX-2. These are the rate-limiting enzymes in the synthesis of the inflammatory prostaglandins PGE_2 and $PGF_{2\alpha}$ and the vasoactive prostanoids thromboxane A2 (TXA2) and prostacyclin (PGI_2) (Fig. 30.26).

COX-1 is constitutively expressed, meaning it is continually present, while COX-2 is inducible and actively expressed during inflammatory episodes. COX-2 is the ideal target for NSAIDs, as it is the enzyme expressed and active in pathological states; however, most anti-inflammatory NSAIDs in clinical use are nonselective in their action. The optimal structural features for all nonselective NSAIDs that promote high affinity binding at the COX active site include (1) an acidic functional group with pK_a between 3 and 6 (ie, anionic at pH 7.4) and (2) one or two aromatic rings that can achieve a noncoplanar orientation with respect to one another. Functional groups that add lipophilicity to the compounds (thus enhancing distribution through membranes) or which block degradative metabolism will increase potency and duration of action.

Specific Drugs

Nepafenac. Nepafenac (Fig. 30.25) is unique among ophthalmic NSAIDs. It is an amide prodrug that requires intraocular hydrolysis to the more active amfenac, a potent nonselective COX inhibitor (Fig. 30.27). An important factor in the design of NSAIDs as topical ophthalmic drugs is the degree of penetration through the corneal epithelium. Corneal absorption of an NSAID into the anterior segment depends on its lipid solubility and degree of ionization (pH range of normal tears 6.5-7.6). Due to the inherent water solubility and the degree of ionization of phenylalkanoic acid NSAIDs (pK~4), it would be predicted that these agents would have limited ability to penetrate corneal epithelium. However, nepafenac as an unionized amide prodrug would be expected to readily penetrate the corneal epithelium and enter into all ocular tissues including aqueous humor, iris, ciliary body, and retina.[58] In a rabbit model, corneal permeability of nepafenac was approximately 19- and 28-fold greater than bromfenac and ketorolac, respectively.[59] Another important factor for nepafenac is that the drug has no inherent COX inhibition activity before absorption.

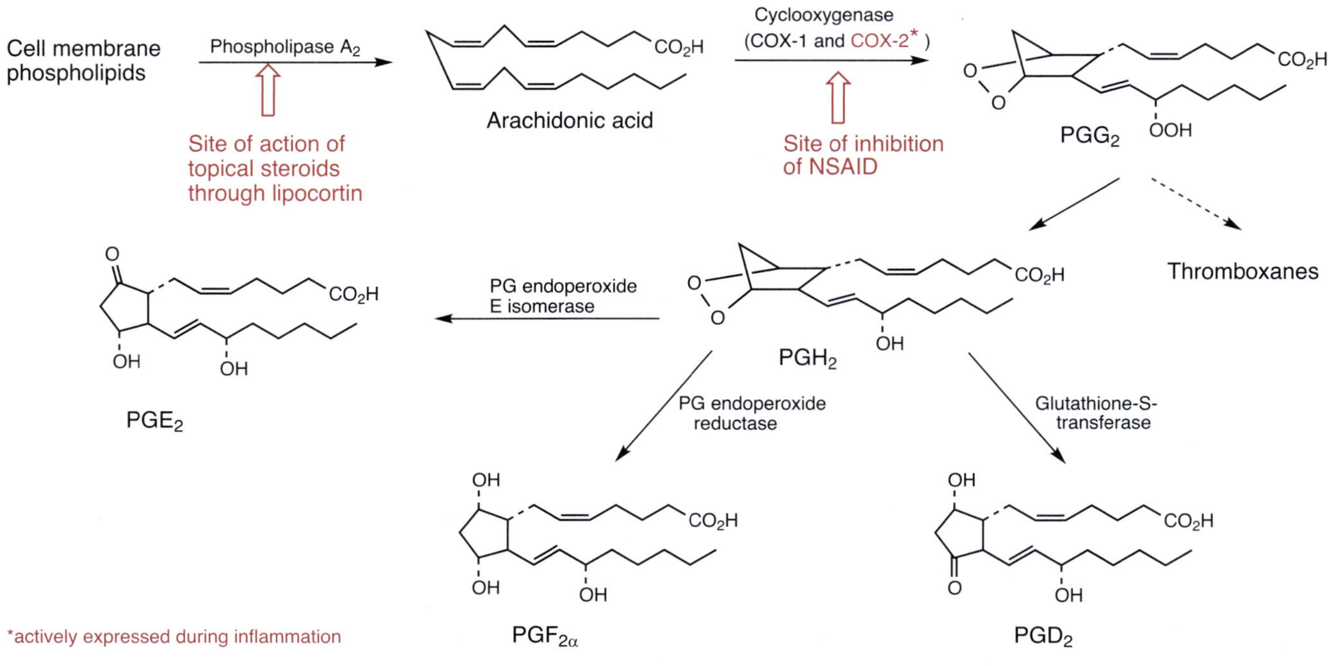

Figure 30.26 Biosynthesis of prostaglandins from arachidonic acid. NSAID, nonsteroidal anti-inflammatory drug; PG, prostaglandin.

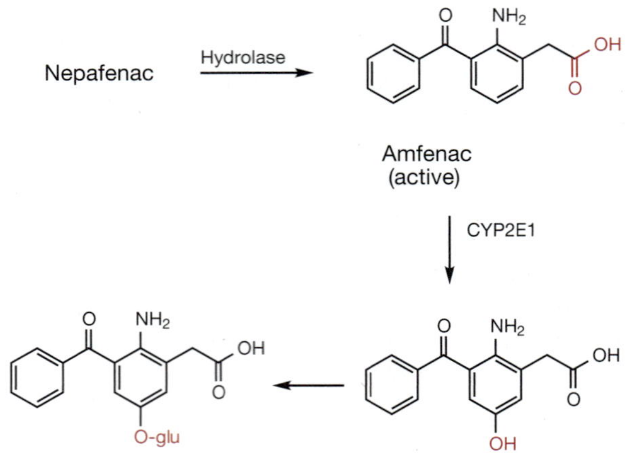

Figure 30.27 Metabolic activation and metabolism of nepafenac.

Mechanism of Action. Nepafenac exhibits weak COX inhibition. However, its active metabolite, amfenac inhibits both COX-1 and COX-2 prostaglandin synthesis for up to 6 hours, with greater selectivity for COX-2 than does ketorolac. The COX-2/COX-1 ratio was approximately 9-fold that of ketorolac, which suggests greater COX-2 anti-inflammatory activity for nepafenac than with ketorolac ophthalmic suspensions.[58] Nepafenac exhibited a longer duration of action than ketorolac.

Pharmacokinetics. Nepafenac is rapidly absorbed when administered topically as a 0.1% ophthalmic suspension. Amfenac has high affinity (~95%) for serum albumin proteins. Following topical application, the onset of napafenac is approximately 15 minutes and the duration of action is greater than 8 hours. Small quantifiable plasma concentrations of nepafenac and amfenac have been observed in subjects in 2 to 3 hours after topical application. In rabbits, nepafenac conversion to active metabolite is seen mostly in the retina, the iris and ciliary body and minimal conversion in the cornea.[59] Bioactivation of nepafenac in aqueous humor appears to be negligible; however, it is possible that nepafenac could undergo water hydrolysis once reaching the aqueous humor.[60] Amfenac undergoes CYP2E1-catalyzed oxidation followed by conjugation to its glucuronide (Fig. 30.27). The major route of elimination is via the urine.

Bromfenac. Bromfenac is a nonselective COX inhibitor approved for the treatment of postoperative inflammation and reduction of ocular pain in patients who had undergone cataract surgery (see Fig. 30.25).[61] It is available as 0.07% ophthalmic solution with once-daily dosing starting 1 day before and continuing until 14 days after the surgery. It has minimal systemic absorption. Most common adverse effects include anterior chamber inflammation, foreign body sensation, eye pain, photophobia, and blurred vision.

Therapeutic Use. The ophthalmic dosage forms of these drugs are used to treat postoperative pain and inflammation associated with cataract surgery. Additionally, they might have value to reduce swelling and stinging sensations following cataract surgery or corneal refractory surgery.

Topical ophthalmic nepafenac is also approved for use as a preoperative agent. The dosage is one drop 2 to 4 times a day for 2 weeks following the surgery. The topical application is preferred over systemic dosing due to the higher ocular drug concentration that can be gained as well as a reduction in adverse effects. In general, there are minimal adverse effects and few if any drug-drug interactions.

These two ophthalmic NSAIDs or a topical steroid anti-inflammatory (difluprednate ophthalmic) are commonly prescribed with a fluoroquinolone ophthalmic antimicrobial solution (besifloxacin, moxifloxacin, or gatifloxacin) following cataract surgery.

Topical Ophthalmic Steroids

Topical ophthalmic steroids are commonly used for the management of inflammation due to external injury, allergies, ocular surgeries, and infections. Topical steroidal drugs that are currently used for treating ocular inflammation are dexamethasone, difluprednate, fluorometholone, fluorometholone acetate, loteprednol etabonate, prednisolone acetate, and prednisolone sodium phosphate (Fig. 30.28).

MECHANISM OF ACTION. During ocular injury or infection, the body releases prostaglandins causing inflammation, vasodilation, miosis, and increased aqueous humor production. The mechanism of action of the topical ophthalmic steroids is not totally understood. They are believed to act by inhibiting phospholipase A_2, an enzyme that catalyzes the first

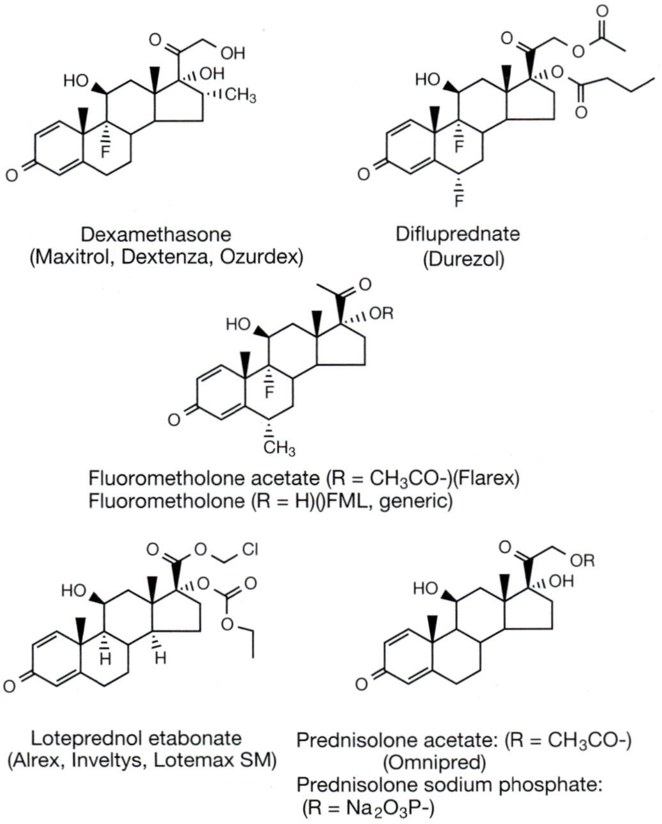

Figure 30.28 Topical ophthalmic steroids.

step in the biosynthesis of prostaglandins (see Fig. 30.26). Furthermore, it is suggested that glucocorticoids induce the production of lipocortin and related proteins by increasing gene expression through activation of the glucocorticoid receptor (GR). The inhibition of phospholipase A_2 blocks the release of arachidonic acid leading to reduction in the inflammatory prostaglandins and thromboxanes. Through the action of lipocortin, other inflammatory responses can be reduced such as cellular infiltration and capillary permeability, which adds to the inflammatory condition. For more details concerning the steroidal mechanism of action, the reader is referred to Chapter 24.

PHARMACOKINETICS. The most unique of the topical ophthalmic steroids is loteprednol etabonate, which was developed with the goal of being an effective agent for treatment of various ocular inflammatory conditions (ie, giant papillary conjunctivitis, seasonal allergic conjunctivitis, uveitis, inflammation, DED, and pain following cataract surgery) with minimal adverse effects. Common to topical ophthalmic steroids is the development of cataracts and IOP elevation upon long-term use. Loteprednol etabonate is a lipophilic drug that penetrates the cornea and exhibits strong affinity for the GR. However, the drug is rapidly metabolized to an inactive metabolite without the adverse effects reported for other ophthalmic steroids as shown in Figure 30.29.[62]

Dexamethasone is available as a 0.1% ophthalmic suspension (Maxidex), in a 0.4-mg ophthalmic insert (Dextenza), for insertion into the lower lacrimal punctum, and in a 0.7-mg intravitreal implant (Ozurdex).

Difluprednate is a lipophilic prodrug indicated for the treatment of inflammation and pain associated with ocular surgery. The drug is rapidly deacetylated to the active drug 6α,9-difluoroprednisolone 17-butyrate (DFB). Fluorometholone is available as such or as its 17α- acetate ester, fluorometholone acetate. Fluorometholone acetate is more lipophilic which helps facilitate corneal transport.

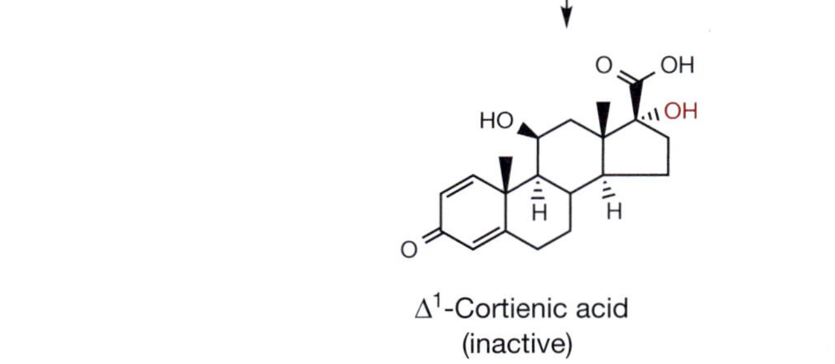

Figure 30.29 Metabolism of loteprednol etabonate.

THERAPEUTIC APPLICATION. The topical ophthalmic steroids are used for the management of inflammation due to external injury, allergies, ocular surgeries, and infections. The therapy is usually started immediately after the refractive surgery and tapered off over a few days to weeks and sometimes months. They may have better anti-inflammatory effects when combined with NSAIDs than as a monotherapy in treating cystoid macular edema. The biggest concern results from prolonged usage, which may result in glaucoma with damage to the optic nerve. Prolong usage may also suppress the immune response increasing the possibility of a secondary ocular infection. These drugs are contraindicated in viral infections of cornea and conjunctiva, varicella and mycobacterial as well as fungal infections of eye.

Topical Antihistamines

The topical antihistamines are formulated with the intent of being used directly in the eye for treatment of allergic conjunctivitis. They play an important role in providing quick symptomatic relief. The ophthalmic antihistamines most commonly used are shown in Figure 30.30.

MECHANISM OF ACTION. Topical antihistamines used in the treatment of allergic conjunctivitis are all potent H_1 inverse agonists. They also have a certain degree of inhibition of H_2 and H_4 receptors. The eyelids and conjunctiva are rich in mast cells, which upon exposure to allergens produce IgE leading to mast cell degranulation releasing inflammatory mediators including histamine. The activation of histamine receptors present in the conjunctival epithelium and goblet cells of the upper eyelid leads to redness, tearing, eyelid swelling, and associated symptoms (often referred to as early phase symptoms). Antihistamines, such as pheniramine, bepotastine, and cetirizine, act by antagonizing histamine action at H_1 receptors thereby alleviating early phase symptoms of allergic conjunctivitis. These early phase symptoms can also be inhibited by preventing IgE-mediated mast cell degranulation. Several dual-acting drugs are available such as azelastine, epinastine, alcaftadine, ketotifen, and olopatadine, which act by both blocking H_1 receptors as well as stabilizing mast cells from degranulation. This dual-acting therapy has improved patient compliance and management of allergic conjunctivitis.[63] One of the newer drugs, alcaftadine also works as an inverse agonist at H_4 receptors resulting in inhibition of the recruitment of immune cells and release of inflammatory chemokines and cytokines.[64] Burning is a very commonly seen adverse effect with dual-acting drugs.[60] Topical antihistamine pheniramine is available in combination with adrenergic α_1 agonist naphazoline. Most common side effects seen with ophthalmic antihistamines include burning, stinging, and headache.

PHARMACOKINETICS. Less than 10% of the topically administered antihistamines crosses corneal membrane and enters into the aqueous humor and ocular structures. A large amount of drug escapes into the systemic circulation via conjunctiva and scleral routes. Higher corneal absorption is observed for drugs having higher lipophilicity.

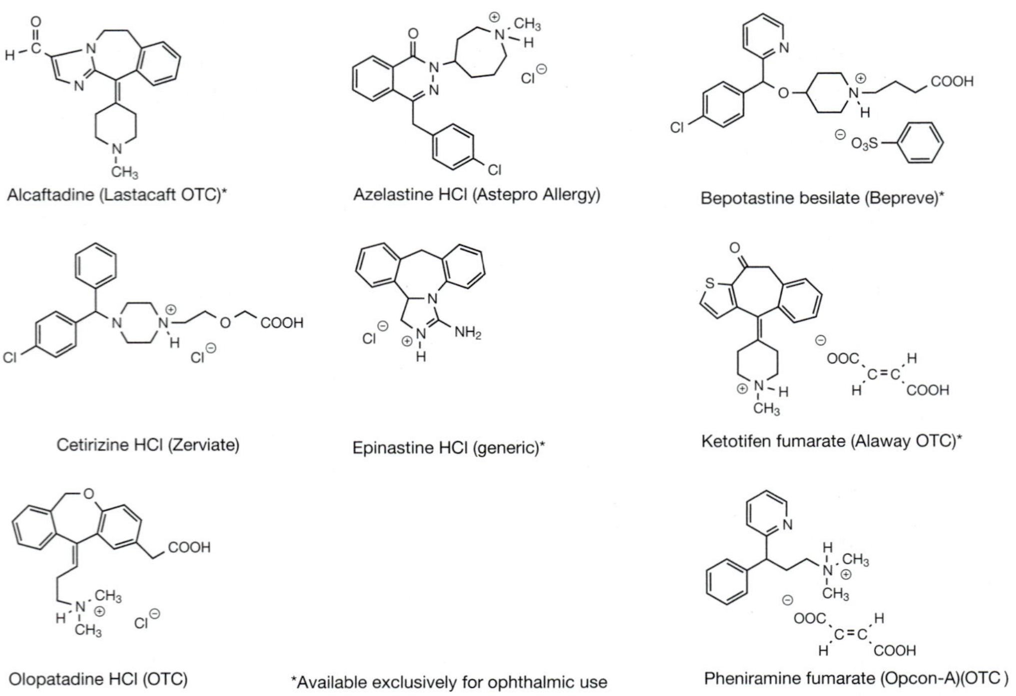

Figure 30.30 Topical antihistamines.

However, systemic side effects are very rarely observed with ophthalmic antihistamines due to the low doses. Minor systemic side effects observed include dry mouth, nausea, headache, and dizziness. Onset of action for ophthalmic antihistamines is much faster compared to oral antihistamines, ranging from 3 to 15 minutes with a duration of action ranging from 8 to 12 hours. Due to their high lipophilic nature, H_1 antihistamines dissociate very slowly from the receptor site providing longer duration of action. Metabolites of various topical antihistamines are shown in Figure 30.31.

Therapeutic Application. Topical antihistamines are commonly used to treat mild to moderate symptoms associated with seasonal and perennial allergic conjunctivitis. They are used alone or in combination with mast cell stabilizers or α_1-adrenergic agonists (vasoconstrictors). Topical antihistamines are contraindicated in patients with closed-angle glaucoma, as they may increase IOP through pupillary dilation. Prophylactic treatment of ocular antihistamines also proved beneficial. Dosing parameters are shown in Table 30.3.

Dry Eye Disease

Dry eyes are reported as a condition in which tears are not able to adequately lubricate the eyes. The tears may be produced in insufficient amounts or be of poor-quality leading to an uncomfortable feeling of dryness, stinging or burning sensation in the eyes of the patient. It is estimated that DED may affect more than 16 million Americans. The patient experiencing DED may report sensitivity to light, redness in the eyes, a feeling of something in the eye or eyes, blurred vision, or eye fatigue.

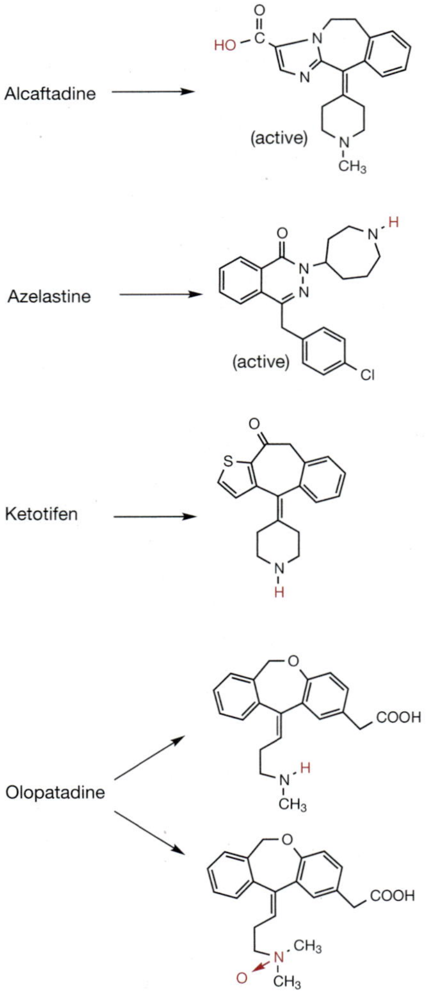

Figure 30.31 Metabolism of topical antihistamines.

Table 30.3 Dosing Parameters for Topical Antihistamines

Topical Antihistamine	Ophthalmic Solution Strengths	Ophthalmic Dosing (Drops Each Eye)	Nasal Solution Strengths	Nasal Dosing (Each Nostril)
Alcaftadine	0.25%	1/daily	NA	NA
Azelastine	0.05%	1/twice daily	137 μg/spray 15%	1-2 sprays twice daily
Bepotastine	1.5%	1/twice daily	NA	NA
Cetirizine	0.24%	1/twice daily	NA	NA
Epinastine	0.05%	1/twice daily	NA	NA
Pheniramine	0.135%	1-2/4 times daily		
Ketotifen	0.025%	1/twice daily	NA	NA
Olopatadine	0.1%, 0.2%	1/daily (0.2%) 1/twice daily (0.1%)	0.6%	2 sprays twice daily

NA, not available.

DED is a multifactorial disease and the underlying cause is not always apparent; although, inflammation of the ocular surface seems to be a major contributor to DED. The tear film loses its homeostasis resulting in tear film instability and hyperosmolarity, ocular surface inflammation and damage, and neurosensory abnormalities. Contributing to DED is the fact that decreased tear production is associated with aging, underlying disease states such as eye allergy, Sjögren syndrome, systemic lupus erythematosus, thyroid disorders, infections, use of certain types of medications (eg, antihistamines, decongestants, antidepressants, and even preservatives such as benzalkonium chloride), and atmospheric conditions (dry air, wind, smoke).

The film itself is composed of lipids, water, and mucin. The lipid component is a product of the meibomian glands located in the eyelids.[65,66] The benefit of the lipid component is that it reduces tear evaporation. The aqueous layer arises from the lacrimal glands found in the orbits and conjunctiva. Mucins are glycoproteins produced by conjunctival goblets cells. The mucins help the spread of the tear film and regulate the surface tension of the tear film.

The complexity of the tear film and the variety of potential causes leading to DED has led to an assortment of medications that are labeled as DED medications with these drugs working through various mechanisms of action.

Ophthalmic Drugs for Dry Eyes

Cyclosporine (Cequa, Restasis, Verkazia). Tear hyperosmolarity appears to be a major contributor to some forms of DED. The hyperosmolarity produces damage to the surface of the epithelium, which increases the release of a complex series of immunologic events including proinflammatory cytokines and chemokines which ultimately leads to cellular damage.[67] Within T cells, calcium binds to cytosolic protein calmodulin forming calcineurin (calcium–calmodulin-activated serine/threonine-specific protein phosphatase complex). The calcineurin complex undergoes dephosphorylation and the dephosphorylated product enters the nucleus of the T cells increasing gene coding and transcription of interleukin 2 (IL-2) and inflammatory cytokines.[68]

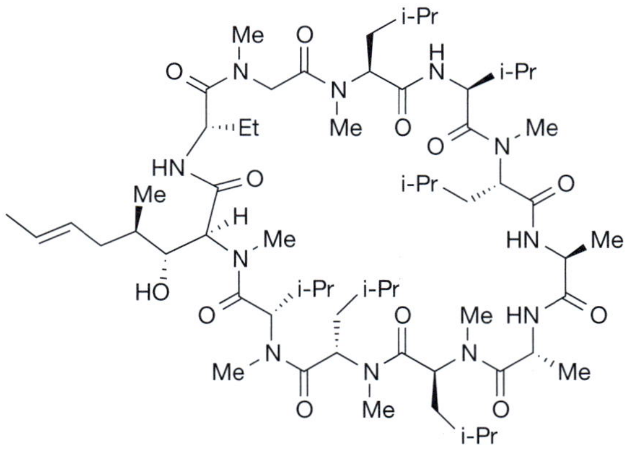

Cyclosporine, also referred to as cyclosporine A or ciclosporin, is a naturally occurring cyclic polypeptide first isolated in 1971 from the fungus *Tolypocladium inflatum.* The drug is a neutral lipophilic agent with very poor water solubility. Cyclosporine is a calcineurin inhibitor that exerts immunomodulatory action by blocking T cell infiltration, activation and subsequent release of inflammatory cytokines and chemokines (such as IL-1β, TNFα, intercellular adhesion molecule-1 [ICAM-1], and vascular cell adhesion molecule-1). Cyclosporine also inhibits p38 and c-Jun N-terminal kinase (JNK) activation, which leads to reduced IL-2 production. Reduced IL-2 levels further block the function of effector T cells.

A second action of cyclosporine is thought to involve a reduction of epithelial mitochondrial permeability and reduces conjunctival epithelial cell death.[69] Cyclosporine increases tear production in patients with DED who are refractory to conservative treatments such as ocular lubricants.

Cyclosporine, because of its lipophilicity, exhibits poor absorption that is improved when formulated as a solution or emulsion. Cyclosporine emulsion (Restasis) consists of cyclosporine 0.05%, glycerin (2.2%), castor oil (1.25%), polysorbate 80 (1%), carbomer copolymer type A (0.05%), purified water (to 100%) with sodium hydroxide for pH adjustment; Cyclosporine emulsion (Verkazia) is composed of cetalkonium chloride, glycerol, medium-chain triglycerides, poloxamer 188, sodium hydroxide to adjust pH, tyloxapol (nonionic polymer) and water for injection. Two solution formulations are available: the first solution (Cequa) consists of cyclosporine 0.9%, polyoxyl hydrogenated castor oil, octoxynol-40, polyvinylpyrrolidone, sodium phosphate dibasic anhydrous, water for injection, with either sodium hydroxide or hydrochloric acid to adjust pH; while a second solution (Vevye) is 0.1% cyclosporine dissolved in perfluorobutylpentane and anhydrous ethanol.

The adverse effects of cyclosporine include instillation site pain, conjunctival hyperemia, blepharitis, and eye irritation. These side effects are said to be the reason that cyclosporine is often discontinued by the patient.

Lifitegrast (Xiidra)

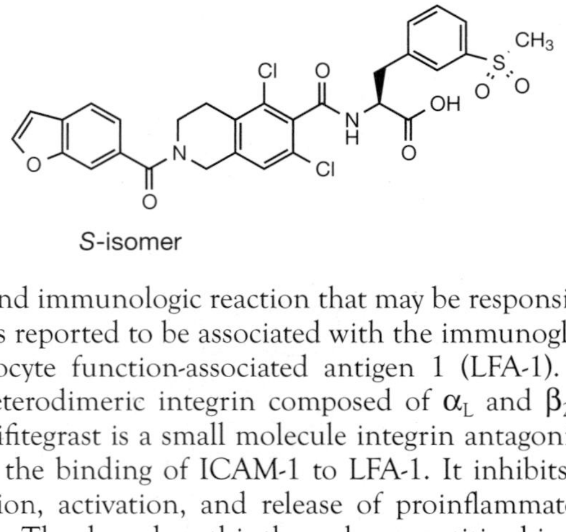

S-isomer

A second immunologic reaction that may be responsible for DED is reported to be associated with the immunoglobulin lymphocyte function-associated antigen 1 (LFA-1). LFA-1 is a heterodimeric integrin composed of α_L and β_2 subunits. Lifitegrast is a small molecule integrin antagonist that blocks the binding of ICAM-1 to LFA-1. It inhibits T cell migration, activation, and release of proinflammatory cytokines. The drug does this through competitive binding to the LFA-1 α_L subunit.[70] The actual mechanism of action in DED is presently not fully known.

Lifitegrast is dissolved in a phosphate-buffered saline as a 5% solution and administered as one drop twice daily. At this concentration the product is nearly equal to human tears. The product comes in a single-use foil pouch. The pouch should be protected from light, can be stored at room temperature, and should not be opened until ready to use. Adverse side effects of lifitegrast include instillation site irritation and decreased visual acuity. Contact lenses should be removed prior to use.

Loteprednol etabonate (Alrex, Eysuvis, Inveltys, Lotemax)

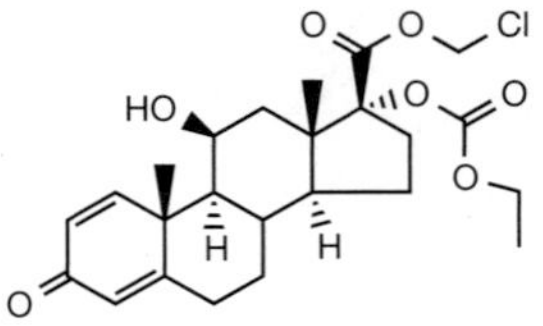

Loteprednol etabonate, as previously indicated was developed as a topical ophthalmic steroid, is now also used for the treatment of DED along with seasonal allergic conjunctivitis. It is available in a non-settling gel formulation (0.5%), which does not require shaking and thus gives a uniform dose.[71,72]

The uniqueness of this drug is shown in Figure 30.28 and is discussed in the topical ophthalmic steroids section. See the earlier discussion for additional information.

Lotilaner (Xdemvy)

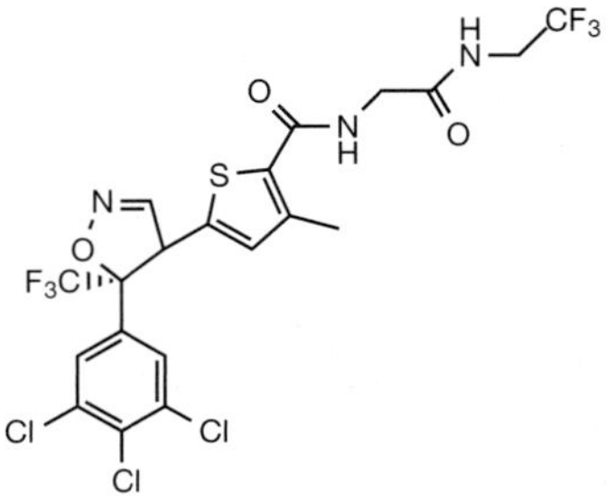

Occasionally, the itchiness of the eye which may be thought to be DED actually presents itself as inflammation of the eyelids and is referred to as blepharitis. It has been reported that 60% to 70% of the cases of dry eyes are associated with blepharitis. The disease is commonly the result from clogging of the oil glands near the base of the eyelids. On the other hand, blepharitis may result from an infection of the eyelid either by *Staphylococcus aureus* or *Demodex folliculorum*. The latter condition is the result of an ectoparasite referred to as a mite, which causes Demodex blepharitis. In Demodex blepharitis, a gelatinous debris surrounding the base of the eyelash is present and is referred to as lash-cuffing collarettes. The collarettes consist of lipids, keratin, Demodex eggs, and dead Demodex mites. The mite is extremely small (~0.3 mm), making it difficult to identify and thus the disease is difficult to diagnosis.[73] Epidemiologic studies suggest that a high percentage of patients with blepharitis (>60%) have Demodex blepharitis. The presence of *Demodex folliculorum* mite infestation is associated with upregulation of proinflammatory cytokines and chronic inflammation.

Recently, lotilaner has been FDA approved for the treatment of Demodex blepharitis.[74] Lotilaner is considered an ectoparasiticide, which is effective via inhibition of γ-aminobutyric acid–gated chloride channels (GABA-Cls) as well as inhibition of glutamate-gated chloride channels.[75] Lotilaner (available as the S-enantiomer, which is 100 times more active than the R-enantiomer) is reported to act as a noncompetitive antagonist of the GABA-Cls, preventing the transfer of chloride ions across cell membranes. The binding of the drug to GABA-Cls leads to mite paralysis and death. Lotilaner is selective in its action without inhibition of mammalian GABA-Cls.

Following ophthalmic application, the drug is found to be highly bound to plasma proteins (>99%) with an effective half-life of 11 days.[74] Lotilaner is available in a 0.25% solution which is administered as one drop in each eye twice daily for 6 weeks. The extended use is because the Demodex life cycle is approximately 3 weeks. Lotilaner and is well tolerated with a minimum of reported adverse effects (instillation site stinging and burning).

Perfluorohexyloctane (Miebo)

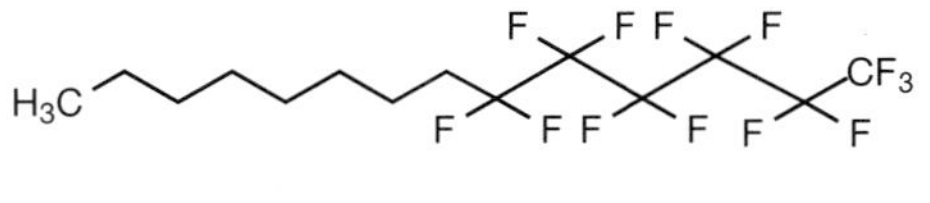

As indicated, DED is a condition that can occur following a loss of homeostasis of the tear film. Depending on the underlying cause of DED, artificial tear products represent the simplest treatment; although, there is very little evidence that such products are truly effective. A protective response to DED involves ophthalmic trigeminal sensory nerve activation that increases blinking and tearing. There is evidence that transient receptor potential melastatin subtype 8 (TRPM8) of the corneal cold-thermoreceptors may also play a role in regulation of tearing and blinking with innervation occurring in the CNS.

The recently introduced prescription drug perfluorohexyloctane may produce relief through a combination of mechanisms for the treatment of DED. Perfluorohexyloctane is a polyfluorinated hydrocarbon that is chemically inert and possesses the properties of being colorless, hydrophobic, and with a density greater than water. As a non-aqueous liquid, microbial growth would not be expected and therefore adding a preservative is not important in its formulation. When applied topically, the drug is reported to reduce eye dryness by forming a uniform film layer over the tear layer thus reducing evaporation.[76] In addition, the tear film thickness is reported to increase. It has also been reported that perfluorohexyloctane produces corneal surface temperature changes facilitating heat exchange between corneal tissue and the environment to reduce corneal temperature (~1 °C). This in turn may activate TRPM8 cold-thermosensitive channels of cold thermoreceptor nerves and increase tearing and blinking rates. These effects would be expected to relieve the symptoms of DED.

Perfluorohexyloctane is instilled one drop 4 times a day with a minimal adverse reaction of blurred vision (<4%).

Varenicline Tartrate (Tyrvaya)

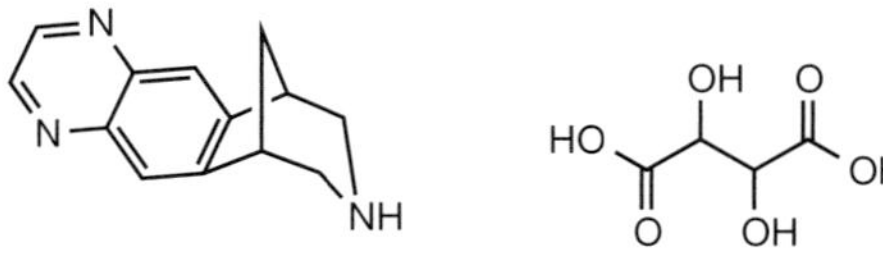

A novel approach to the treatment of DED is to increase tear film production via neuroactivation of the nasolacrimal reflex (NLF). This reflex, also known as the trigeminal parasympathetic pathway (TPP), is reported to be responsible for as much as one-third of tear film production. Intranasal neurostimulation of the NLR/TPP is noninvasive and represents the mechanism of action of the newly introduced nasal spray formulation of the drug varenicline. The exact mechanism of action of varenicline remains unknown although it has been suggested that its action is associated with the ability to bind to nicotinic acetylcholine receptors (nAChR) on trigeminal sensory nerve endings located within the anterior nasal cavity.[77] Varenicline exhibits high affinity for various human neuronal nAChR subtypes including α4β2, where it acts as partial agonist. A second study reported that reduction of conjunctival goblet cell area and perimeter results in degranulation and release of mucins into tear film which in turn promotes water retention to provide a protective barrier.[78] This action is associated with nerve stimulation of goblet cells through TPP.

The pharmacokinetics of varenicline consists of a rapid onset of action (detection in the plasma within 5 minutes) after a single intranasal dose into each nostril of varenicline solution (0.03 mg/spray). The drug is administered twice daily reaching peak concentration within 2 hours with a half-life of approximately 19 ~19 ± 10 10 hours. Varenicline is excreted in the urine primary unchanged (92%). The most common adverse effect is sneezing.

Structure Challenge

Several agents used to treat ocular or nasal disorders, or to facilitate ocular surgery, are drawn as follows. Evaluate their structures and identify which drug (or drugs) is being described in each of the following list.

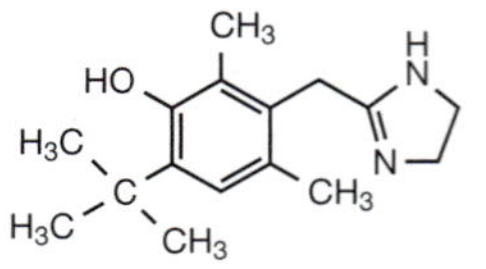

A

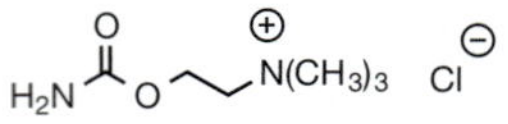

B

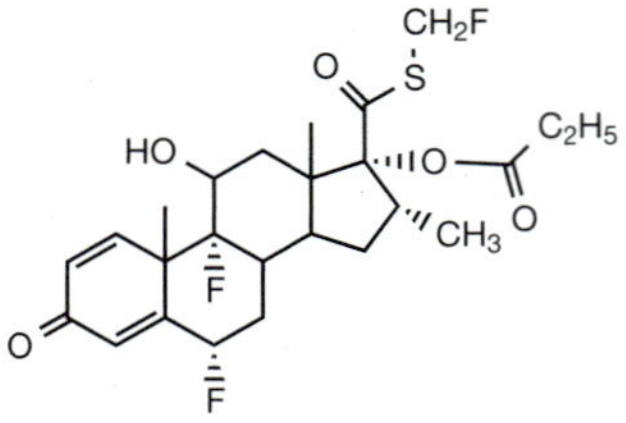

C

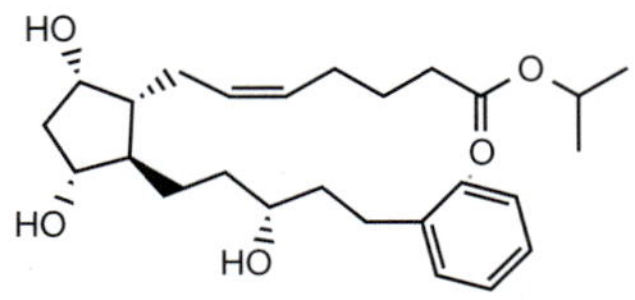

D

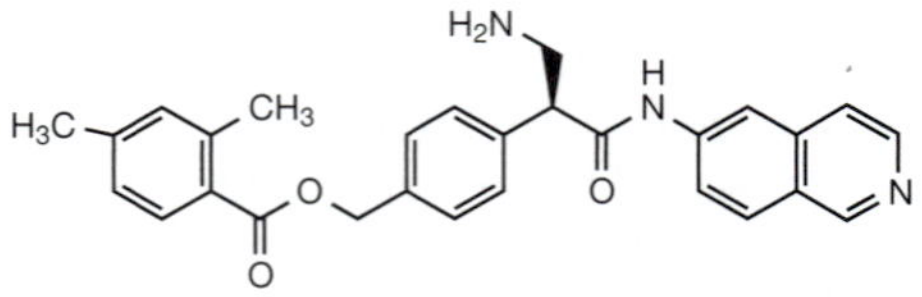

E

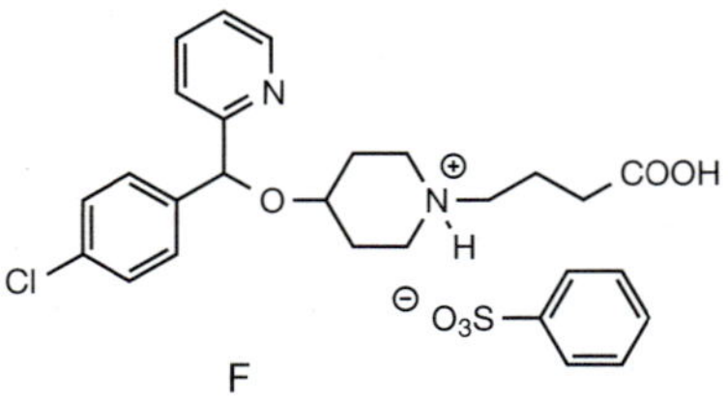

F

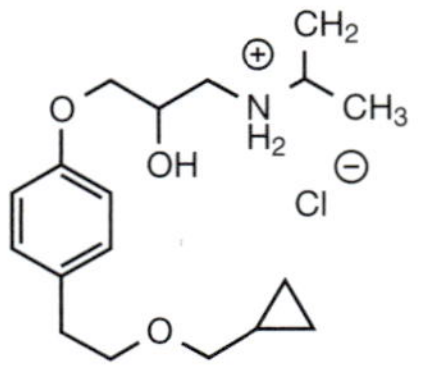

G

1. Lowers intraocular pressure in patients with glaucoma by facilitating aqueous humor outflow via a prostaglandin receptor-mediated mechanism.
2. Has the potential to induce a mechanism-based decrease in heart rate and systemic blood pressure when administered to patients with glaucoma.
3. Miotic agent used topically in ocular surgery that would be water soluble regardless of the pH of the aqueous vehicle.
4. Glaucoma agent that targets kinase enzymes in the trabecular meshwork to facilitate aqueous humor outflow.
5. Topical antihistamine used to decrease ocular itch in patients with allergic conjunctivitis.
6. Therapeutic agent effective in decreasing the red appearance of irritated eyes, lifting the eyelids in patients with low-lying lids, and relieving mild nasal congestion via the same mechanism.
7. Most effective topical agent to treat chronic allergic rhinitis.
8. Most likely to decompose after prolonged exposure to light or high pH.
9. Potentially vulnerable to metabolic hydrolysis (Select all correct answers).
10. Of these in question 9, which must be metabolically hydrolyzed in order to be active? (Select all correct answers.)

Structure Challenge answers found immediately after References.

REFERENCES

1. Pacheco-Galvan A, Hart SP, Morice AH. Relationship between gastro-oesophageal reflux and airway diseases: the airway reflux paradigm. *Arch Bronconeumol.* 2011;47:195-203.
2. Mayo Clinic Staff. Nasal congestion: causes. *Mayo Clinic.* March 2, 2023. Accessed February 24, 2025. https://www.mayoclinic.org/symptoms/nasal-congestion/basics/causes/sym-20050644
3. Bush RK. Etiopathogenesis and management of perennial allergic rhinitis: a state-of-the-art review. *Treat Respir Med.* 2004;3:45-57.
4. Meltzer EO, Blaiss MS, Derebery MJ, et al. Burden of allergic rhinitis: results from the pediatric allergies in America survey. *J Allergy Clin Immunol.* 2009;124:S43-S70.
5. Center for Disease Control and Prevention/National Center for Health Statistics. Allergies. Updated February 1, 2023. Accessed August 29, 2024. https://www.cdc.gov/nchs/fastats/allergies.htm
6. Meltzer EO, Farrar JR, Sennett C. Findings from an online survey assessing the burden and management of seasonal allergic rhinoconjunctivitis in US patients. *J Allergy Clin Immunol Pract.* 2017;5:779-789.e6.
7. Naclerio RM, Bachert C, Baraniuk JN. Pathophysiology of nasal congestion. *Int J Gen Med.* 2010;3:47-57.
8. Von Euler US. Synthesis, uptake, and storage of catecholamines in adrenergic nerves: the effect of drugs. In: Blaschko H, Marshall E, eds. *Catecholamines.* Springer; 1972:186-230.
9. Kaufman S, Nelson TJ. Studies on the regulation of tyrosine hydroxylase activity by phosphorylation and dephosphorylation. In: Dahlstrom A, Belmaker RH, Sandler M, eds. *Progress in Catecholamine Research. Part A: Basic Aspects and Peripheral Mechanisms.* Alan R Liss; 1988:57-60.
10. Harrison JK, Pearson WR, Lynch KR. Molecular characterization of alpha 1- and alpha 2-adrenoceptors. *Trends Pharmacol Sci.* 1991;12:62-67.
11. Strader CD, Candelore MR, Hill WS, et al. Identification of two serine residues involved in agonist activation of the beta-adrenergic receptor. *J Biol Chem.* 1989;264:13572-13578.
12. Strader CD, Sigal IS, Register RB, et al. Identification of residues required for ligand binding to the beta-adrenergic receptor. *Proc Natl Acad Sci U S A.* 1987;84:4384-4388.
13. Melvin TA, Patel AA. Pharmacotherapy for allergic rhinitis. *Otolaryngol Clin North Am.* 2011;44:727-739.

14. Nichols AJ, Ruffolo RRJ. Structure–activity relationships for α-adrenoceptor agonists and antagonists. In: Ruffolo RRJ, ed. *Alpha-Adrenoceptors: Molecular Biology, Biochemistry, and Pharmacology*. Karger; 1991:75-114.
15. Waugh DJ, Gaivin RJ, Zuscik MJ, et al. Phe-308 and Phe-312 in transmembrane domain 7 are major sites of alpha 1-adrenergic receptor antagonist binding. Imidazoline agonists bind like antagonists. *J Biol Chem*. 2001;276:25366-25371.
16. Mahajan MK, Uttamsingh V, Daniels JS, et al. In vitro metabolism of oxymetazoline: evidence for bioactivation to a reactive metabolite. *Drug Metab Dispos*. 2011;39:693-702.
17. Mahajan MK, Uttamsingh V, Gan LS, et al. Identification and characterization of oxymetazoline glucuronidation in human liver microsomes: evidence for the involvement of UGT1A9. *J Pharm Sci*. 2011;100:784-793.
18. Kushnir NM. The role of decongestants, cromolyn, guaifenesin, saline washes, capsaicin, leukotriene antagonists, and other treatments on rhinitis. *Immunol Allergy Clin North Am*. 2011;31:601-617.
19. Nelson HS. Mechanisms of intranasal steroids in the management of upper respiratory allergic diseases. *J Allergy Clin Immunol*. 1999;104:S138-S143.
20. Bush IE. Chemical and biological factors in the activity of adrenocortical steroids. *Pharmacol Rev*. 1962;14:317-445.
21. Teng XW, Cutler DJ, Davies NM. Mometasone furoate degradation and metabolism in human biological fluids and tissues. *Biopharm Drug Dispos*. 2003;24:321-333.
22. Sahasranaman S, Issar M, Hochhaus G. Metabolism of mometasone furoate and biological activity of the metabolites. *Drug Metab Dispos*. 2006;34:225-233.
23. Roberts JK, Moore CD, Ward RM, et al. Metabolism of beclomethasone dipropionate by cytochrome P450 3A enzymes. *J Pharmacol Exp Ther*. 2013;345:308-316.
24. Weinreb RN, Aung T, Medeiros FA. The pathophysiology and treatment of glaucoma: a review. *JAMA*. 2014;311:1901-1911.
25. Quigley HA, Broman AT. The number of people with glaucoma worldwide in 2010 and 2020. *Br J Ophthalmol*. 2006;90:262-267.
26. Weinreb RN, Leung CK, Crowston JG, et al. Primary open-angle glaucoma. *Nat Rev Dis Primers*. 2016;2:16067.
27. Timmermans PB, van Zwieten PA. Alpha 2 adrenoceptors: classification, localization, mechanisms, and targets for drugs. *J Med Chem*. 1982;25:1389-1401.
28. Kanagy NL. Alpha(2)-adrenergic receptor signalling in hypertension. *Clin Sci (Lond)*. 2005;109:431-437.
29. Wheeler LA, Woldemussie E. Alpha-2 adrenergic receptor agonists are neuroprotective in experimental models of glaucoma. *Eur J Ophthalmol*. 2001;11(suppl 2):S30-S35.
30. Wheeler LA, Gil DW, WoldeMussie E. Role of alpha-2 adrenergic receptors in neuroprotection and glaucoma. *Surv Ophthalmol*. 2001;45(suppl 3):S290-S294; discussion S295-S296.
31. Frishman WH, Fuksbrumer MS, Tannenbaum M. Topical ophthalmic beta-adrenergic blockade for the treatment of glaucoma and ocular hypertension. *J Clin Pharmacol*. 1994;34:795-803.
32. Gupta D, Chen PP. Glaucoma. *Am Fam Physician*. 2016;93:668-674.
33. Ricciotti E, FitzGerald GA. Prostaglandins and inflammation. *Arterioscler Thromb Vasc Biol*. 2011;31:986-1000.
34. Sjoquist B, Stjernschantz J. Ocular and systemic pharmacokinetics of latanoprost in humans. *Surv Ophthalmol*. 2002;47(suppl 1):S6-S12.
35. Weinreb RN, Realini T, Varma R. Latanoprostene bunod, a dual-acting nitric oxide donating prostaglandin analog for lowering of intraocular pressure. *US Ophthalmic Rev*. 2016;9(2):80-87.
36. Woodward DF, Krauss AH, Chen J, et al. The pharmacology of bimatoprost (Lumigan). *Surv Ophthalmol*. 2001;45(suppl 4):S337-S345.
37. Brubaker RF. Mechanism of action of bimatoprost (Lumigan). *Surv Ophthalmol*. 2001;45(suppl 4):S347-S351.
38. Shafiee A, Bowman LM, Hou E, et al. Ocular pharmacokinetics of bimatoprost formulated in DuraSite compared to bimatoprost 0.03% ophthalmic solution in pigmented rabbit eyes. *Clin Ophthalmol*. 2013;7:1549-1556.
39. Travatan Z. Package insert. Novartis; Revised 2023. Accessed August 30, 2024. https://dailymed.nlm.nih.gov/dailymed/drugInfo.cfm?setid=028455e0-ae77-4213-8819-3b58ef7d6a14
40. Liu Y, Mao W. Tafluprost once daily for treatment of elevated intraocular pressure in patients with open-angle glaucoma. *Clin Ophthalmol*. 2013;7:7-14.
41. Fukano Y, Kawazu K. Disposition and metabolism of a novel prostanoid antiglaucoma medication, tafluprost, following ocular administration to rats. *Drug Metab Dispos*. 2009;37:1622-1634.
42. Woodward DF, Jones RL, Narumiya S. International Union of Basic and Clinical Pharmacology. LXXXIII: classification of prostanoid receptors, updating 15 years of progress. *Pharmacol Rev*. 2011;63:471-538.
43. Johnson TV, Gupta PK, Vudathala DK, et al. Thermal stability of bimatoprost, latanoprost, and travoprost under simulated daily use. *J Ocul Pharmacol Ther*. 2011;27:51-59.
44. Tanna AP, Johnson M. Rho kinase inhibitors as a novel treatment for glaucoma and ocular hypertension. *Ophthalmology*. 2018;125(11):1741-1756.
45. Matsu M, Matsuoka Y, Ma Tanito M. Efficacy and patient tolerability of omidenepag isopropyl in the treatment of glaucoma and ocular hypertension. *Clin Ophthalmol*. 2022;16:1269-1279.
46. Ren R, Li G, Le TD, et al. Netarsudil increases outflow facility in human eyes through multiple mechanisms. *Invest Ophthalmol Vis Sci*. 2016;57:6197-6209.
47. Sturdivant JM, Royalty SM, Lin CW, et al. Discovery of the ROCK inhibitor netarsudil for the treatment of open-angle glaucoma. *Bioorg Med Chem Lett*. 2016;26:2475-2480.
48. Wang RF, Williamson JE, Kopczynski C, et al. Effect of 0.04% AR-13324, a ROCK, and norepinephrine transporter inhibitor, on aqueous humor dynamics in normotensive monkey eyes. *J Glaucoma*. 2015;24:51-54.
49. Smith GM, Alexander RS, Christianson DW, et al. Positions of His-64 and a bound water in human carbonic anhydrase II upon binding three structurally related inhibitors. *Protein Sci*. 1994;3:118-125.
50. Martens-Lobenhoffer J, Banditt P. Clinical pharmacokinetics of dorzolamide. *Clin Pharmacokinet*. 2002;41:197-205.
51. Gil DW, Krauss HA, Bogardus AM, et al. Muscarinic receptor subtypes in human iris-ciliary body measured by immunoprecipitation. *Invest Ophthalmol Vis Sci*. 1997;38:1434-1442.
52. Vuity. Package insert. AbbVie; Revised March 28, 2023. Accessed August 23, 2024. https://dailymed.nlm.nih.gov/dailymed/drugInfo.cfm?setid=8d806897-8a2a-4518-8c68-0ec3b778de50
53. Ordentlich A, Barak D, Kronman C, et al. Dissection of the human acetylcholinesterase active center determinants of substrate specificity. Identification of residues constituting the anionic site, the hydrophobic site, and the acyl pocket. *J Biol Chem*. 1993;268:17083-17095.
54. Shafferman A, Kronman C, Flashner Y, et al. Mutagenesis of human acetylcholinesterase. Identification of residues involved in catalytic activity and in polypeptide folding. *J Biol Chem*. 1992;267:17640-17648.
55. Zhang Y, Kua J, McCammon JA. Role of the catalytic triad and oxyanion hole in acetylcholinesterase catalysis: an ab initio QM/MM study. *J Am Chem Soc*. 2002;124:10572-10577.
56. Gaynes BI, Onyekwuluje A. Topical ophthalmic NSAIDs: a discussion with focus on nepafenac ophthalmic suspension. *Clin Ophthalmol*. 2008;2:355-368.
57. Aragona P, Tripodi G, Spinella R, et al. The effects of the topical administration of non-steroidal anti-inflammatory drugs on corneal epithelium and corneal sensitivity in normal subjects. *Eye (Lond)*. 2000;14(pt 2):206-210.
58. Gamache DA, Graff G, Brady MT, et al. Nepafenac, a unique nonsteroidal prodrug with potential utility in the treatment of trauma-induced ocular inflammation: I. Assessment of anti-inflammatory efficacy. *Inflammation*. 2000;24:357-370.

59. Ke TL, Graff G, Spellman JM, et al. Nepafenac, a unique nonsteroidal prodrug with potential utility in the treatment of trauma-induced ocular inflammation: II. In vitro bioactivation and permeation of external ocular barriers. *Inflammation.* 2000;24:371-384.
60. Walters T, Raizman M, Ernest P, et al. In vivo pharmacokinetics and in vitro pharmacodynamics of nepafenac, amfenac, ketorolac, and bromfenac. *J Cataract Refract Surg.* 2007;33:1539-1545.
61. Prolensa. Package insert. Bausch & Lomb; Revised 2023. Accessed August 30, 2024. https://pi.bausch.com/globalassets/pdf/PackageInserts/Pharma/prolensa-insert.pdf
62. Comstock TL, Paterno MR, Bateman KM, et al. Safety and tolerability of loteprednol etabonate 0.5% and tobramycin 0.3% ophthalmic suspension in pediatric subjects. *Paediatr Drugs.* 2012;14:119-130.
63. del Cuvillo A, Sastre J, Montoro J, et al. Allergic conjunctivitis and H1 antihistamines. *J Investig Allergol Clin Immunol.* 2009;19(suppl 1):11-18.
64. Gong H, Blaiss MS. Topical corticosteroids and antihistamines-mast cell stabilizers for the treatment of allergic conjunctivitis. *US Ophthalmic Rev.* 2013;6:78-85.
65. Farrand KF, Fridman M, Stillman IO, et al. Prevalence of diagnosed dry eye disease in the United States among adults aged 18 years and older. *Am J Ophthalmol.* 2017;182(10):90-98.
66. Golden MI, Meyer JJ, Patel MC. Dry eye syndrome. In: *StatPearls* [Internet]. StatPearls Publishing; 2024. https://www.ncbi.nlm.nih.gov/books/NBK430685/
67. Periman LM, Mah FS, Karpecki PM. A review of the mechanism of action of cyclosporine A: the role of cyclosporine a in dry eye disease and recent formulation developments. *Clin Ophthalmol.* 2020;14:4187-4200.
68. Wang P, Heitman J. The cyclophilins. *Genome Biol.* 2005;6(7):226.
69. Ames P, Galor A. Cyclosporine ophthalmic emulsions for the treatment of dry eye: a review of the clinical evidence. *Clin Investig (Lond).* 2015;5(3):267-285.
70. Haber SL, Benson V, et al. Lifitegrast: a novel drug for patients with dry eye disease. *Ther Adv Ophthalmol.* 2019;11:1-8.
71. Amon M, Busin M. Loteprednol etabonate ophthalmic suspension 0.5%: efficacy and safety for postoperative anti-inflammatory use. *Int Ophthalmol.* 2012;32(5):507-517.
72. Beckman K, Katz J, Majmudar P, et al. Loteprednol etabonate for the treatment of dry eye disease. *J Ocul Pharmacol Ther.* 2020;36(7):497-511.
73. Rhee MK, Yeu E, Barnett M, et al. *Demodex* blepharitis: a comprehensive review of the disease, current management, and emerging therapies. *Eye Contact Lens.* 2023;49(8):311-318.
74. Syed YY. Lotilaner ophthalmic solution 0.25%: first approval. *Drugs.* 2023;83(16):1537-1541.
75. Rufener L, Danelli V, Bertrand, et al. The novel isoxazoline ectoparasiticide lotilaner (Credelio): a non-competitive antagonist specific to invertebrates γ-aminobutyric acid-gated chloride channels (GABACls). *Parasit Vectors.* 2017;10:530.
76. Delicado-Miralles M, Velasco E, Diaz-Tahocos, et al. Deciphering the action of perfluorohexyloctane eye drops to reduce ocular discomfort and pain. *Front Med (Lausanne).* 2021;8:709712.
77. Frampton JE. Varenicline solution nasal spray: a review in dry eye disease. *Drugs.* 2022;82:1481-1488.
78. Dieckmann GM, Cox SM, Lopez MJ, et al. A single administration of OC-01 (varenicline solution) nasal spray induces short-term alterations in conjunctival goblet cells in patients with dry eye disease. *Ophthalmol Ther.* 2022;11(4):1551-1561.

Structure Challenge Answers

1. D: Lowers intraocular pressure in glaucoma patients by facilitating aqueous humor outflow via a prostaglandin receptor-mediated mechanism.
2. G: Has the potential to induce a mechanism-based decrease in heart rate and systemic blood pressure when administered to patients with glaucoma.
3. B: Miotic agent used topically in ocular surgery that would be water soluble regardless of the pH of the aqueous vehicle.
4. E: Glaucoma agent that targets kinase enzymes in the trabecular meshwork to facilitate aqueous humor outflow.
5. F: Topical antihistamine used to decrease ocular itch in patients with allergic conjunctivitis.
6. A: Therapeutic agent effective in decreasing the red appearance of irritated eyes, lifting the eyelids in patients with low-lying lids, and relieving mild nasal congestion via the same mechanism.
7. C: Most effective topical agent to treat chronic allergic rhinitis.
8. A: Most likely to decompose after prolonged exposure to light or high pH.
9. B, C, D, E: Potentially vulnerable to metabolic hydrolysis.
10. D, E: Must be metabolically hydrolyzed in order to be active.

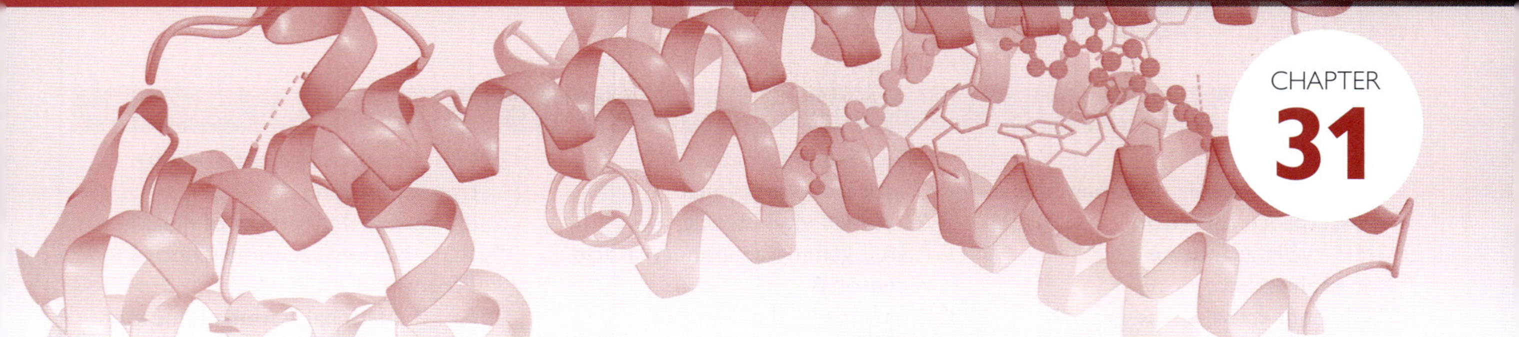

CHAPTER 31

Drugs Used to Treat Pulmonary Disorders

Carolyn Friel

Drugs covered in this chapter:

DRUGS USED FOR TREATING ASTHMA AND COPD

ADRENOCORTICOIDS
- Beclomethasone dipropionate
- Budesonide
- Ciclesonide
- Dexamethasone
- Flunisolide
- Fluticasone propionate/furoate
- Hydrocortisone
- Methylprednisolone
- Mometasone furoate
- Prednisolone
- Triamcinolone acetonide

β_2-ADRENERGIC AGONISTS
- Albuterol sulfate
- Arformoterol tartrate
- Epinephrine (adrenalin)
- Formoterol fumarate
- Metaproterenol sulfate
- Olodaterol
- Salmeterol xinafoate
- Terbutaline sulfate
- Vilanterol trifenatate

ANTIMUSCARINICS
- Aclidinium bromide
- Glycopyrrolate bromide
- Ipratropium hydrobromide
- Revefenacin
- Tiotropium bromide
- Umeclidinium bromide

LEUKOTRIENE MODIFIERS
- Montelukast
- Zafirlukast
- Zileuton

MAST CELL DEGRANULATION INHIBITORS
- Cromolyn sodium (sodium cromoglycate)
- Nedocromil sodium

METHYLXANTHINES
- Caffeine
- Theophylline

MONOCLONAL ANTIBODIES
- Benralizumab
- Dupilumab
- Mepolizumab
- Omalizumab
- Reslizumab
- Tezepelumab-ekko

PHOSPHODIESTERASE INHIBITORS
- Roflumilast

SMOKING-CESSATION MEDICATIONS
- Bupropion
- Nicotine
- Varenicline

DRUGS USED TO TREAT CYSTIC FIBROSIS

CFTR CORRECTORS
- Elexacaftor
- Lumacaftor
- Tezacaftor

CFTR POTENTIATORS
- Ivacaftor

DRUGS USED TO TREAT IDIOPATHIC PULMONARY FIBROSIS
- Nintedanib
- Pirfenidone

DRUGS USED TO TREAT PULMONARY ARTERIAL HYPERTENSION

PROSTACYCLIN RECEPTOR AGONISTS
- Epoprostenol
- Iloprost
- Selexipag
- Treprostinil

ENDOTHELIN RECEPTOR ANTAGONISTS
- Ambrisentan
- Bosentan
- Macitentan

PDE-5 INHIBITORS
- Sildenafil
- Tadalafil

SOLUBLE GUANYL-CYCLASE STIMULATORS
- Riociguat

Abbreviations

AAT α-1 antitrypsin
ABC ATP binding cassette
ACh acetylcholine
ACOS asthma-COPD overlap syndrome
AECs alveolar epithelial cells
AMP adenosine monophosphate
ATP adenosine triphosphate
AUC area under the curve
AV atrioventricular
BBB blood brain barrier
BLTRs leukotriene B4 receptors
BPH benign prostatic hyperplasia
cAMP cyclic adenosine monophosphate

Abbreviations—continued

CF cystic fibrosis
CFTR cystic fibrosis transmembrane conductance regulator
cGMP cyclic guanosine monophosphate
CTGF connective-tissue growth factor
CDC Centers for Disease Control and Prevention
C_{max} maximum plasma concentrations
C_{avg} average concentrations
COMT catechol *O*-methyl transferase
COPD chronic obstructive pulmonary disease
CAT chronic obstructive pulmonary disease assessment test
CRF corticotrophin-releasing factor
cryo-EM cryo-electron microscopy
cysLT cysteinyl leukotriene
cysLT1 cysteinyl leukotriene receptor 1
CysLTRs cysteinyl leukotriene receptors
CYP cytochrome
des-CIC ciclesonide
DDIs drug-drug interactions
DNA doxyribonucleic acid
DNRI dopamine/NE-reuptake inhibitor
DPI dry powder inhaler
EOS eosinophil count
ET-1 endothelin 1
ETI elexacaftor, tezacaftor, and ivacaftor
ETR endothelin receptor
ETR_A endothelin receptor A
ETR_B endothelin receptor B
EPI epinephrine
ERAs endothelin receptor antagonists
FcεRI high-affinity Fc immunoglobulin E receptor
FDA US Food and Drug Administration
FEV_1 forced expiratory volume in 1 second
FLAP 5-lipoxygenase–activating protein
FF fluticasone furoate
FP fluticasone propionate
FVC forced vital capacity
$GABA_A$ gamma-aminobutyric acid receptor A
GD guanosine diphosphate
GERD gastroesophageal reflux disorder
GI gastrointestinal
GINA Global Initiative for Asthma
GOLD Global Initiative for Chronic Lung Disease
GPCRs G protein–coupled receptors
GR glucocorticoid receptor
Gs stimulatory G protein
GTP guanosine triphosphate
HDAC2 histone deacetylase type 2
HETE hydroperoxyeicosatetraenoic acid
HPA hypothalamus–pituitary–adrenal
HRE hormone-response element
ICS inhaled corticosteroid
IFN interferon
IL interleukin
IP prostacyclin receptor
Ig immunoglobulin
IgE immunoglobulin E
IL interleukin
IPF idiopathic pulmonary fibrosis
IV intravenous
ISO isoproterenol
L-DOPA L-dihydroxyphenylalanine
LABA long-acting β_2-adrenergic agonist
LAMA long-acting muscarinic antagonist
LBD ligand binding domain
LTs leukotrienes
MAbs monoclonal antibodies
MAO monoamine oxidase
MDI metered dose inhaler
mMRC modified Medical Research Council dyspnea questionnaire
NBD nucleotide-binding domain
NSAIDs nonsteroidal anti-inflammatory drugs
NE norepinephrine
NETosis neutrophil extracellular trap formation
NIH National Institutes of Health
NACP National Asthma Control Program
NAEPP National Asthma Education and Prevention Program
NBD nucleotide-binding domain
NK natural killer
NO nitric oxide
NRT nicotine replacement therapy
OCTN1 organic cation/carnitine transporter 1
OCTN2 organic cation/carnitine transporter 2
OTC over the counter
PAH pulmonary arterial hypertension
PDE phosphodiesterase
PDE4 phosphodiesterase-4
PDE5 Phosphodiesterase-5
PDE5i phosphodiesterase-5 inhibitors
PDGF platelet-derived growth factor
PE pulmonary embolism
PEF peak expiratory flow
REMS Risk Evaluation and Mitigation Strategy
SABA short-acting β_2-adrenergic agonist
SAMA short-acting muscarinic antagonist
SC subcutaneous
sGC soluble guanylate cyclase
SRS-A slow-reacting substance of anaphylaxis
T-bet T-box transcription factor
TGF-β1 transforming growth factor beta-1
Th helper T cells
TM transmembrane
TMDs transmembrane domains
TSLP thymic stromal lymphopoietin
UGT1A glucuronyl transferase
VEGF vascular endothelial growth factor

CLINICAL SIGNIFICANCE

The science of medicinal chemistry continues to pave the way for advancements in drug therapy for respiratory diseases. Newer compounds for asthma and chronic obstructive pulmonary disease (COPD) interact with receptors to allow for quicker relief from shortness of breath and longer protection against exacerbations than drugs from just a decade prior. Monoclonal antibodies, engineered to precisely attack targets of airway inflammation, have dramatically improved the lives of patients suffering from severe asthma. For cystic fibrosis (CF), medicinal chemistry has facilitated the development of therapeutic molecules that help unclog malfunctioning chloride channels, resulting in better lung function, reduced disease flares, and longer lives for these patients. Medicinal chemistry has had a similarly powerful impact for other respiratory illnesses discussed in this chapter, including tobacco use disorder, idiopathic pulmonary fibrosis (IPF), and pulmonary hypertension. Gains and breakthroughs in medicinal chemistry have radically transformed how clinicians prescribe and monitor drugs for respiratory disease, and treatment guidelines are constantly being updated to keep up with the flood of new agents entering the market. Advancements in medicinal chemistry continue to lessen respiratory disease burden for patients worldwide.

Dinesh Yogaratnam, PharmD

Introduction

The respiratory system is composed of the mouth, nose, lungs, trachea, bronchi, bronchioles, alveoli, and diaphragm, all of which collectively play a role in exchanging oxygen and carbon dioxide. Oxygen is necessary for every cell in the body. Any factor influencing lung function directly affects one's quality of life. Smoking, infections, and exposure to air pollution are recognized as primary contributors to respiratory disorders.

Diseases of the respiratory system fall into three major categories: (1) obstructive, (2) restrictive, and (3) pulmonary vascular diseases. Obstructive disorders include asthma and COPD. Restrictive pathophysiology diseases include IPF, asbestosis, and neuromuscular diseases. Pulmonary embolism (PE) and pulmonary arterial hypertension (PAH) are examples of pulmonary vascular disorders.[1] Pulmonary function can also be affected by bacterial or viral infections as well as malignancy.

This chapter focuses on asthma, COPD, CF, and PAH. Drugs that are used to treat lung cancer are covered in Chapters 36 and 37; drugs used to treat pulmonary infections are covered in Chapter 32 (antibacterial agents), Chapter 33 (antiviral agents), Chapter 34 (antifungal agents), and Chapter 35 (parasitic agents).

Medicinal Chemistry of Inhaled Agents

As many of the drugs in this chapter are administered via inhalation, a discussion of this method of administration is warranted. Inhalation therapy offers several advantages when treating pulmonary disorders. First, the drug is delivered directly to the site where it is needed. This results in a quicker onset of action, reduced systemic exposure, and a lower overall dose administered to the patient. For example, albuterol 100 to 200 μg by inhalation is equivalent to an oral dose of 2 to 4 mg.[2] The lower dose leads to diminished off-target binding, fewer drug-drug interactions (DDIs), and potentially fewer side effects. Avoiding first-pass metabolism is beneficial but it is important to note that the lung is continually exposed to toxic substances and has an extensive enzyme processing system for both phase I and phase II metabolism. The cytochrome (CYP) isoforms in the lung (including CYP1A1 (increased in smokers), CYP1B1, CYP2B6, CYP2E1, CYP2J2, CYP2A6, and CYP3A5) have been identified thus far. The lungs also express aldehyde oxidase, epoxide hydrolase, esterases, UGT1A (glucuronyl transferase), and glutathione *S*-transferase.[2,3] Thus drug metabolism within the lung contributes to clearance. Drugs may also be removed by mucociliary clearance.

There are three main devices used for delivering drugs via inhalation, metered dose inhalers (MDIs), dry-powder inhalers (DPIs), and nebulizer therapy. MDIs utilize a propellant gas to deliver the drug either as a fine suspension or a solution in a carrier solvent. Drugs used in solutions need to have excellent solubility and stability in the solvent. Typical solvents used are water and ethanol. Suspensions need to have uniform, small particle sizes (<5 μm) to reduce the amount that gets deposited on the oropharynx and swallowed. Drugs in suspensions are in crystalline form and not dissolved; therefore, patients must be properly counseled to shake the canister to ensure the correct dose is actuated from the device. The propellant gas is either norflurane (HFA134a) or apaflurane (HFA227ea). Both of these are greenhouse gases that contribute to global warming, and manufacturers are searching for alternatives with lower environmental impacts.[4]

A DPI is a breath-activated device that does not use any propellant. The drug is prepared as a crystalline solid typically combined with a carrier with good flow properties. Most current DPIs are formulated with lactose as the carrier. Anaphylactic reactions in patients with severe milk protein allergies have been reported. Patients with milk protein allergies generally avoid lactose-containing powders that may potentially be contaminated with milk protein. Another issue with lactose is that it is not chemically inert. It can react with primary and, to a lesser extent, secondary amines, via a Maillard reaction; thus, it must be avoided in drugs with these functional groups. Mannitol appears to be the most promising replacement carrier for lactose, as it has an established low toxicity profile and low hygroscopicity.[2] The medications for DPI devices are often dispensed as capsules to insert in the inhaler. Patients should always be trained in the use of their device and told not to swallow the capsule.

The last mechanism used for delivering drugs to the lungs is nebulizer therapy. A nebulizer uses compressed air to deliver the aqueous drug solution in a mist for inhalation. The mist is delivered via a mask or oral mouthpiece. The drug must be soluble and stable in the aqueous solution. Solutions are available with preservatives such as benzalkonium chloride or may be packaged as individual preservative-free unit doses. Although patients would prefer to mix multiple nebulizer medications for simultaneous nebulizer therapy, very little research has been conducted on compatibility. Changes in pH and osmolarity may affect the physicochemical compatibility of mixtures. Particle size and lung deposition may also change when multiple drugs are mixed in a nebulizer. This is an area that needs continuous research as new products are developed.[5] Nebulizers have the disadvantage that they are larger and usually require an electrical outlet, although portable battery-operated types are available. They are good choices for older adults, those with mobility impairments, and children because they do not require coordinating inhalation with pressing an actuation button on an MDI or a DPI.

ASTHMA

Epidemiology

Asthma has been known since antiquity. The word asthma is a Greek noun derived from the verb *aazein*, meaning to exhale with an open mouth. Symptoms of the medical condition were described by Hippocrates in the *Corpus Hippocraticum*. The best clinical description of asthma from antiquity was offered by the physician Aretaeus of Cappadocia, who practiced in the first century AD. He described asthma and noted its association with a "thick and viscid phlegm caused by coldness and humidity of the pneuma" as well as its association with exercise.[6] The earliest literary reference to asthma can be found in Homer's *Iliad*, where it was used to denote breathlessness or panting.[7]

In 2021, the US Centers for Disease Control and Prevention (CDC) reported that 7.7% of the United States population has received a diagnosis of asthma. Asthma prevalence for children under 18 is 6.5%, while the prevalence in adults over age 18 years is 8.0%. The prevalence in males is less than 18 years is 7.3% and males over 18 years is 6.2%, while the prevalence in females less than 18 years is 5.6% and females over 18 years is 9.7%. Among all ages, the prevalence is 5.7% in Hispanic persons, 7.7% in White persons, and 11.0% in Black persons. Asthma prevalence also differed by poverty level. Asthma was more prevalent among persons with family incomes lower than 100% of the US Census Bureau's poverty level threshold (10.4%) than among persons with family incomes at or above 450% of the poverty level threshold (6.8%).[8]

Although all-age asthma prevalence has risen from 7.4% in 2001 to 7.7% in 2021, the prevalence of asthma attacks, emergency department visits, and the rate of hospitalizations decreased during this period. For children with asthma, the percentage who had at least one asthma attack per year decreased from 61.7% in 2001 to 38.7% in 2021. For adults with asthma, the percentage who had at least one asthma attack per year declined from 53.8% in 2001 to 39.6% in 2021. Similarly, the rate of asthma-related emergency department visits declined from 62.6 per 10,000 population in 2001 to 29.8 per 10,000 in 2020. The rate of asthma deaths has also declined from 15.0 per million population in 2001 to 10.6 deaths per million population in 2021, which equated to 3,517 deaths in 2021.[9] The substantial burden of asthma led the CDC to create the National Asthma Control Program (NACP) in 1999. The NACP leads a coordinated public health response to control asthma through national and state surveillance systems, funding public health programs, training health professionals, and educating individuals with asthma.[10] The overall decline in morbidity and mortality is a testimony to the success of programs such as this and better recognition and treatment of asthma.

Asthma imposes a considerable financial impact on patients, families, employers, and the US health care system, due to direct costs (such as medical expenses) and indirect costs (such as productivity losses). A cross-sectional analysis conducted on data from the Medical Expenditure Panel Survey (2010-2017) examined the medical costs of patients aged 11 years and above with asthma. The findings revealed that, on average, individuals with asthma incurred annual direct medical costs of $4,333 more per person compared to those without asthma. On average, persons with asthma missed 1.27 more workdays and 0.87 more school days, compared to a person without asthma. When asthma was classified as mild, moderate, or severe, the number of missed days per year was 0.76, 2.31, and 7.19 respectively, clearly showing that the severity of asthma affects absenteeism. Annual direct medical costs were also associated with asthma severity with $3,305 in mild, $7,250 in moderate, and $9,175 in severe asthma. These outcomes show that controlling the severity of asthma can reduce the economic and social burden of asthma.[11]

Asthma is a worldwide problem affecting over a quarter of a billion people. In 1993, the World Health Organization and the US National Heart, Lung, and Blood Institute joined forces to create the Global Initiative for Asthma (GINA), to enhance global awareness, prevention, and management of asthma. Asthma is estimated to be responsible for 1,000 deaths per day worldwide.[12]

Etiology, Signs, and Symptoms

Asthma is characterized by a fluctuating history of respiratory symptoms, including wheezing, shortness of breath, chest tightness, and cough, which change in both frequency and severity. Asthma is a complicated disease that presents with different signs and symptoms, but it is usually characterized by chronic airway inflammation and intermittent expiratory airflow restriction.[13]

Asthma phenotypes, which represent identifiable clusters of demographic, clinical, and pathophysiologic characteristics, are studied to provide information on progression and guide specific treatment responses.[14] Typical asthma phenotypes include (1) Allergic asthma, triggered by allergens like pollen, dust mites, mold, or animal dander. Patients with atopic diseases such as hay fever or eczema have a higher risk of developing asthma.[15] This is the most common form of asthma. (2) Nonallergic asthma is not related to allergen exposure but is often triggered by irritants or infections. Occupational asthma is a type of nonallergic asthma that is exacerbated by exposure to an irritant or sensitizer in the work environment. Industries with high occupational asthma include car manufacturing, construction, painting, printing, textile manufacturing, and pharmaceutical manufacturing.[16] Some of the known irritants include polyurethane foam, paint, ink, varnishes, rubber, glues, and over 40 different drugs.[16,17] (3) Exercise-induced asthma is when symptoms occur during or after physical activity. (4) Obesity-related asthma, which is related to weight and metabolic factors. (5) Drug-exacerbated asthma, which can be induced by specific drugs such as aspirin, nonsteroidal anti-inflammatory drugs (NSAIDs), or β-blockers. (6) Age-stratified asthma categorizes patients based on when they were initially diagnosed with asthma, distinguishing between early-onset asthma, which is usually diagnosed in childhood, and late-onset asthma, which is when asthma is diagnosed after age 35. (7) Severity-stratified asthma is usually determined retrospectively based on symptoms, exacerbations, and the treatment required to control symptoms.[18] Currently only age and severity of symptoms are used in treatment guidelines. Most asthma phenotypes were found to have weak correlations with specific pathological processes or treatment responses.[13]

The etiology of asthma is believed to be a combination of environmental and genetic factors. Although asthma has a genetic component, the multifactorial nature of the disease makes it difficult to predict who will develop asthma. The recurrence risk of asthma in children with one affected parent is around 25%, whereas the risk if both parents are affected is around 50%. Twin studies have shown that if one identical twin develops asthma, the concordance for asthma in the other twin is not 100%, but around 75%, suggesting that environmental and other risk factors contribute to the risk.[19] All forms of asthma are characterized by an exaggerated hypersensitivity response to an offending agent. These agents can be allergens, pollution, tobacco smoke, or environmental triggers such as exercise.

Pathogenesis of Asthma

Asthma is a complex disease characterized by airway inflammation, hyperresponsiveness, and airflow obstruction. Its exact causes are complex and not fully understood but involve the interplay of genetic factors, environmental factors, and immune dysregulation. Asthma is induced by the stimulation of different inflammatory cells. T lymphocytes, B lymphocytes, mast cells, eosinophils, neutrophils, macrophages, and dendritic cells have all been found to play a role in asthma. When naïve T cells are exposed to an allergen (an antigen), they differentiate into effector T cells also known as helper T cells (Th). Five major T helper cell subsets have been identified. In asthma, there is often an imbalance of the activity of the different subsets. These effector T cells influence innate immune cells, macrophages, eosinophils, mast cells, and B cells. These innate immune cells produce inflammatory cytokines and chemokines that exacerbate the immune response leading to airway muscle contraction, mucus secretion, airway hyperresponsiveness, and obstruction. An imbalance between Th1 and Th2 cells results in characteristic allergic asthmatic inflammation. Th1 cells, when triggered by interleukin (IL) 12 and interferon (IFN)-γ, become activated through the T-box transcription factor (T-bet) and the STAT4 signal pathway. This activation leads to the promotion of type 1 immunity by generating cytokines such as IL-2, IFN-γ, and lymphotoxin-α. Th1 cells play a dual role in asthma by suppressing Th2 cell activation to limit eosinophilic inflammation while promoting neutrophilic inflammation. On the other hand, Th2 cells, stimulated by IL-4 through the GATA3 and STAT6 signal, secrete cytokines like IL-4, IL-5, and IL-13. The IL-13 cytokine triggers B cells to produce immunoglobulin E (IgE), leading to mucus secretion, airway hyperresponsiveness, and allergic responses, exacerbating asthma (Fig. 31.1). Additionally, mast cell degranulation after exposure to an allergen or cold air releases histamine. Histamine can bind to the H1 receptor in smooth muscle and lead to airway obstruction via smooth muscle constriction, bronchial hypersecretion, and airway mucosal edema. Both mast cell numbers and histamine concentrations were reported to be higher in the bronchoalveolar lavage fluid of patients with asthma compared to patients without asthma.[20] The breakdown of arachidonic acid in the lipoxygenase pathway produces leukotrienes (Fig. 31.2). These leukotrienes C_4, D_4, and E_4 produce bronchoconstriction, mucus secretions, and airway edema. Chronic inflammation of the lungs can lead to remodeling, resulting in hyperplasia and hypertrophy of the airway smooth muscle cells, including mucus-secreting goblet cells.[21] Effective management of asthma requires a comprehensive approach that includes identification and avoidance of triggers, pharmacological therapy with bronchodilators and anti-inflammatory agents, and patient education.

Diagnosis of Asthma

Over- and underdiagnosis of asthma occurs due to the lack of confirmed blood biomarkers and objective lung function tests that exclude other causes. There is no single test that can diagnose asthma. The clinical evaluation includes a history of respiratory symptoms such as cough, wheezing, and shortness of breath. This history should include the time of day of symptoms, as asthma is often worse at night and in the early morning. Triggering events such as allergen exposure or exercise-induced symptoms should be noted.[13] The diagnosis of asthma is supported by spirometry testing, which measures both the capacity of the lungs and the speed at which air can be forced out of the lungs. An increase in the forced expiratory volume in 1 second (FEV_1) recorded by spirometry 15 minutes after administration of

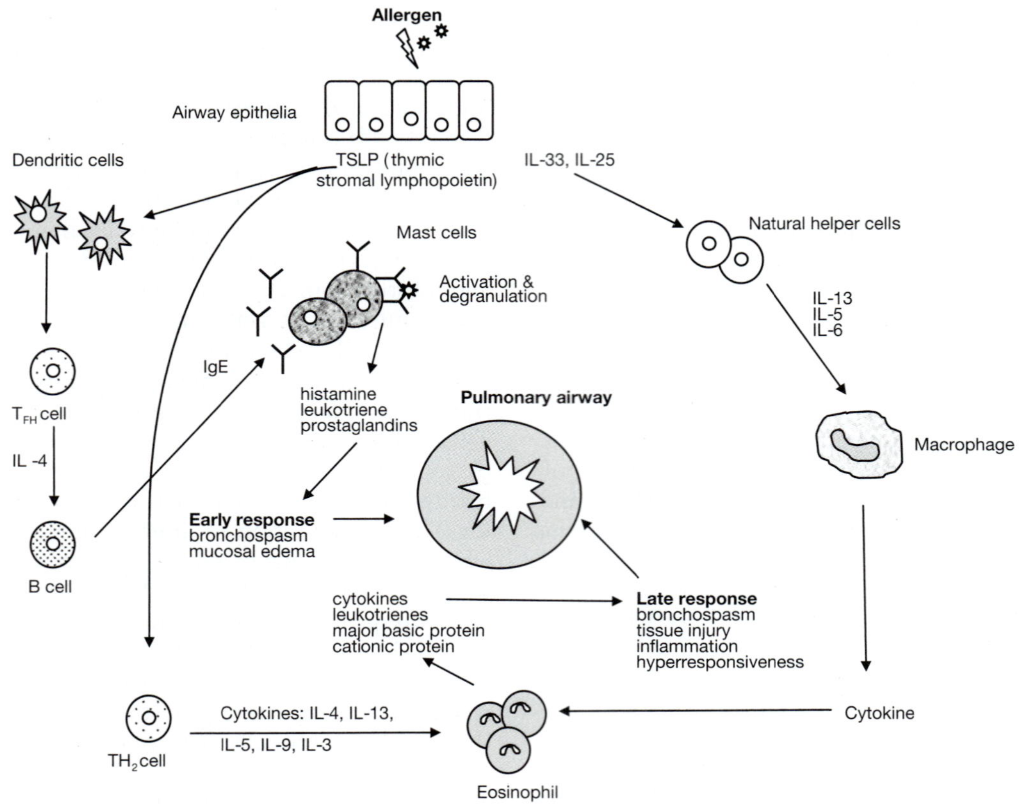

Figure 31.1 Asthma pathogenesis. IgE, immunoglobulin E; IL, interleukin; TSLP, thymic stromal lymphopoietin.

a bronchodilator supports the diagnosis of asthma. As per the GINA 2023 guidelines, in adults, an increase of over 200 mL and 12% from the pre-bronchodilator (baseline) FEV_1 is indicative of asthma. In children, an increase of more than 12% from the predicted FEV_1 value supports an asthma diagnosis.[13]

Asthma is a variable condition, so bronchodilator reversibility may not be evident during initial lung function testing. If it is not detected in the initial spirometry test, it should be retested at later visits when the patient is experiencing symptoms and has not taken bronchodilator medications. If spirometry testing is unavailable, another option is to have the patient track their peak expiratory flow (PEF) every morning and evening for 2 weeks. Diurnal PEF variability is calculated by subtracting the lowest reading from the highest reading for each day, dividing the result by the mean of the highest and lowest readings for the day, and then averaging these results over 1 week. Excessive diurnal PEF variability is defined as a mean variability of more than 10% in adults or more than 13% in children.

In individuals suspected of having asthma with normal expiratory airflow and no significant reversibility, a bronchoprovocation test with methacholine or mannitol can be used to reveal airway hyperresponsiveness, which supports an asthma diagnosis. Bronchodilators should be withheld before the challenge test.

Ideally, variable expiratory airflow limitation should be demonstrated before starting asthma inhaler treatment. Confirming the diagnosis becomes more challenging once inhaler treatment has begun. However, asthma diagnosis can also be confirmed if there is a clinically significant improvement in FEV_1 (by >12% and >200 mL) or in PEF by more than 20% after 4 weeks of inhaled corticosteroid (ICS) treatment.[13]

Therapeutic Approaches to the Treatment and Management of Asthma

Both the National Asthma Education and Prevention Program (NAEPP) and GINA publish strategies for the management and treatment of asthma. The NAEPP publishes updates to their guidelines after extensive vetting by expert panels, which require about 6 years between updates. The GINA updates are updated every year and thus can incorporate new evidence quicker. The NAEPP published a partly updated clinicians' guideline in 2020 and GINA in 2023.[13,22] The 2023 GINA guidelines recommend a personalized approach by the clinician for individualized care. This includes assessment of inhaler technique and adherence, patient goals, modifiable risk factors, and comorbidities. Adjustments to the patient's management are based on these assessments. These include education, treatment of modifiable risk factors, and both pharmacological and nonpharmacological strategies. This is a continuous management cycle for personalized asthma care and includes reviewing the patient's side effects, individual goals, and satisfaction with treatment outcomes. The treatment of

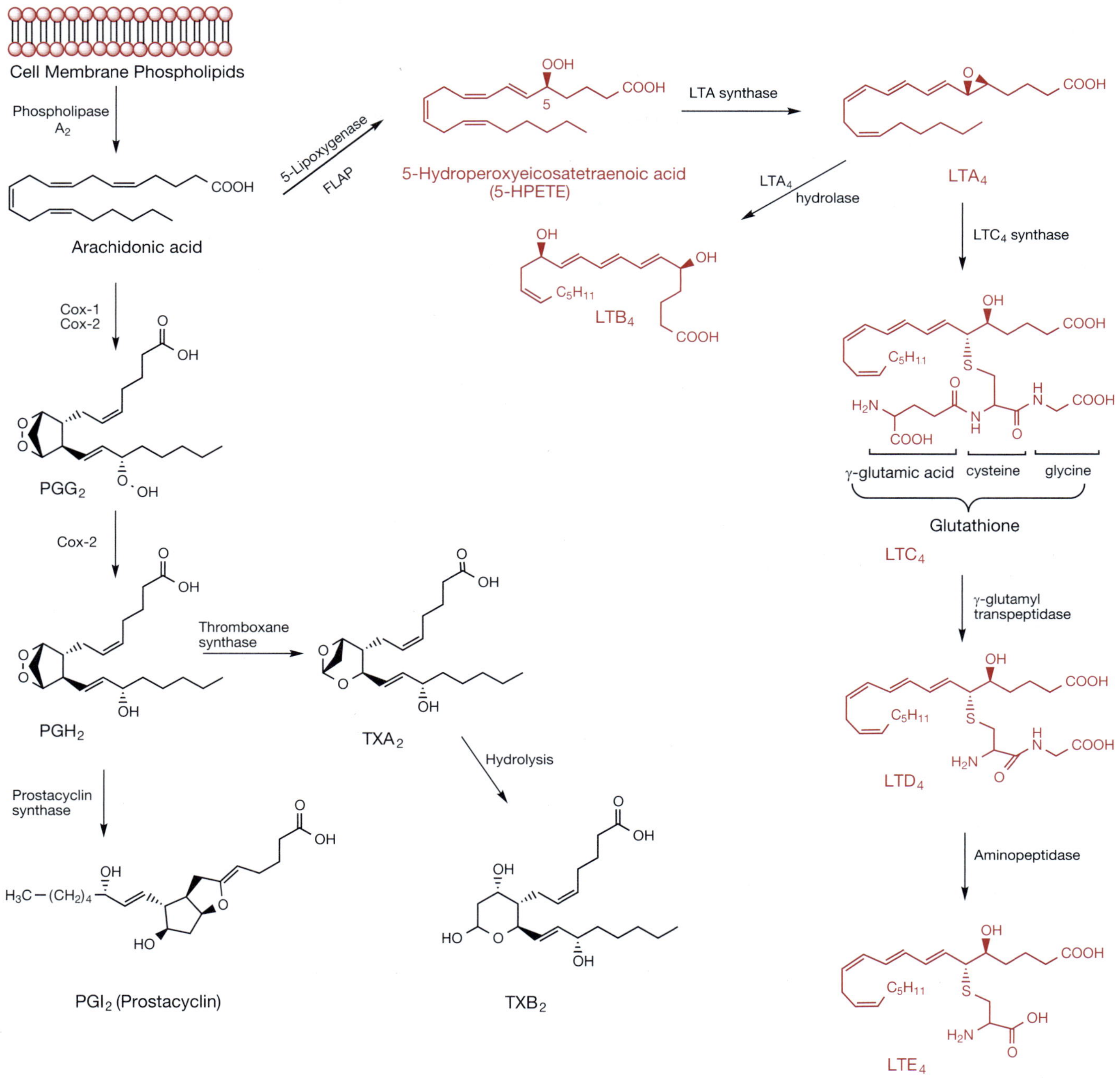

Figure 31.2 Arachidonic acid cascade in relation to pulmonary disorders. FLAP, 5-lipoxygenase activating protein; LT, leukotriene; PG, prostaglandin, TX, thromboxane.

asthma differs slightly between the NAEPP and the GINA guidelines, and clinicians can consult both for guidance. Both guidelines place the patient into steps based on the severity of symptoms with recommended therapy at each step. Alternative therapies are also listed to aid individualized therapy. GINA management strategies are age-based, with guidelines for adults and adolescents, children between ages 5 and 11, and children ages 0 to 4 (www.ginasthma.org).[13] Treatment of adults and adolescents in Steps 1 and 2 begins with as-needed ICS-formoterol. This differs from the NAEPP guidelines, which begin Step 1 in adults with as-needed short-acting β_2-adrenergic agonist (SABA) and add daily or as-needed ICS in Step 2. This change to the GINA guidelines was based on a study that showed that using low-dose ICS-formoterol prn reduces the risk of severe exacerbations and emergency room visits by 65% compared with SABA-only treatment.[23] Both guidelines move through the stepwise approach by adding therapy that targets the inflammation and the bronchoconstriction of asthma. Inhaled corticosteroids were referred to as controller medications in the past but both treatment guidelines now include prn (as needed) use of ICS as an anti-inflammatory reliever taken when symptoms occur and before exercise or allergen exposure. For breakthrough symptoms, additional relievers in both guidelines include SABAs. Over-use of SABA increases the risk of asthma exacerbations. Both treatment guidelines include corticosteroids, SABAs, long-acting β_2-adrenergic agonists (LABAs), and long-acting muscarinic antagonists (LAMAs). Clinicians should refer to these guidelines for details on the steps and up-to-date protocols.

Therapeutic Classes of Drugs Used to Treat Asthma and Chronic Obstructive Pulmonary Disease

Adrenergic Receptors

Adrenergic receptors have been studied extensively and divided into two major groups designated as α and β. The adrenergic receptors are pharmacologically classified as α or β based on their interaction with norepinephrine (NE), epinephrine (EPI), and the adrenergic agonist prototype, isoproterenol.[24] NE and EPI are nonselective and interact with all adrenergic receptors, while isoproterenol selectively interacts with both the β_1- and β_2-receptors.

The α_1-, α_2-, and β-adrenergic receptors have been further divided into three receptor subtypes based on their organ distribution and physiologic activities. Therefore, there are now a total of nine adrenergic receptor subtypes, but the most important in relation to the treatment of asthma and COPD are the β_1 and β_2 subtypes that are found primarily in the heart and the lung, respectively.[25] As may be deduced from Table 31.1, adrenergic agonists that are selective for the β_2 subtype will cause bronchial dilation and be expected to relieve the bronchospasm of an asthmatic attack. Nonselective β-agonists, however, will have stimulatory cardiac effects and, therefore, would have limited use in cardiac patients with asthma.

Table 31.1 Physiologic Response in Relationship to β-Receptor Subtype and Organ Site

Receptor Subtype	Organ Location	Agonist Response
β_1	Heart	Increased rate and force
		Increased conduction velocity
β_2	Bronchiole smooth muscle	Dilation
	Intestine	Decreased motility
	Liver	Increased gluconeogenesis
		Increased glycogenolysis
	Uterus	Contraction
	Lungs	Bronchial dilation
β_3	Bladder	Relaxation detrusor muscle

The endogenous substrates for the adrenergic receptors are EPI and NE. EPI was isolated from sheep adrenal glands and given the name "adrenalin" by Jokichi Takamine in 1900.[26] EPI is the classic "fight or flight" hormone synthesized in the chromaffin cells of the adrenal medulla in response to stress (Fig. 31.3).

Activation of α_1-receptors on smooth muscle cells in blood vessels leads to vasoconstriction and an increase in blood pressure, heart rate, and myocardial contractility. α_1-Agonists are used as vasopressors (Chapter 19). EPI's action at α_2-receptors can lead to a reduction in sympathetic outflow by inhibiting the release of NE from presynaptic nerve terminals. The β_1-receptors are primarily found in the heart. EPI stimulates the β_1-receptors in the sinoatrial node of the heart, leading to an increased rate of depolarization and an elevated heart rate. The β_1-agonists also increase the contractility of the myocardium. This positive inotropic effect strengthens the force with which the heart contracts, leading to an increased stroke volume. The conductivity of the electrical impulses through the atrioventricular (AV) node of the heart is also increased, facilitating coordination of the atrial and ventricular contractions (positive dromotropic effect). The net result of β_1-agonists on the heart is an increase in cardiac output, the volume of blood pumped by the heart per unit of time. EPI also acts on β_2-receptors found in the smooth muscle tissue, including those in the lungs, blood vessels, and skeletal muscle. EPI causes vasodilation in the blood vessels supplying skeletal muscle when it activates β_2 receptors. This increased blood flow enhances oxygen delivery to muscles and supports increased physical activity. In the liver, EPI, through β_2 receptor activation, stimulates glycogenolysis (breakdown of glycogen into glucose) and gluconeogenesis (formation of glucose from non-carbohydrate sources). This contributes to an increased availability of glucose in the bloodstream to provide energy for the body during times of increased demand. Activation of β_2 receptors can also lead to relaxation of the smooth muscle in the uterus. The activation of β_2 receptors in the smooth muscle of the bronchioles leads to relaxation of the smooth muscle, resulting in bronchodilation. The most effective bronchodilators are β_2 agonists. The β_3 receptor is the least studied β adrenergic receptor but is a promising target for conditions such as overactive bladder.[27] A summary of β-receptor organ location and action is provided in Table 31.1.

The β-adrenergic agonists may also cause transient but significant hypokalemia in some patients.[28] The β_2-adrenergic agonists increase the flow of potassium into the cell via the Na^+/K^+-ATPase pump. This can be utilized advantageously for the emergency treatment of hyperkalemia as both (intravenous) IV and inhalation β_2-agonists (in conjunction with insulin and glucose) are effective at reducing serum concentrations of potassium.[29,30]

Chemistry and Biochemistry of Norepinephrine and Epinephrine

Chemically, NE is classified as a catecholamine. A catechol is a 1,2-dihydroxybenzene, and NE is a β-hydroxyethylamino-3,4-dihydroxybenzene. In chemistry, the term "nor" means without a methyl group; thus "nor"epinephrine is simply

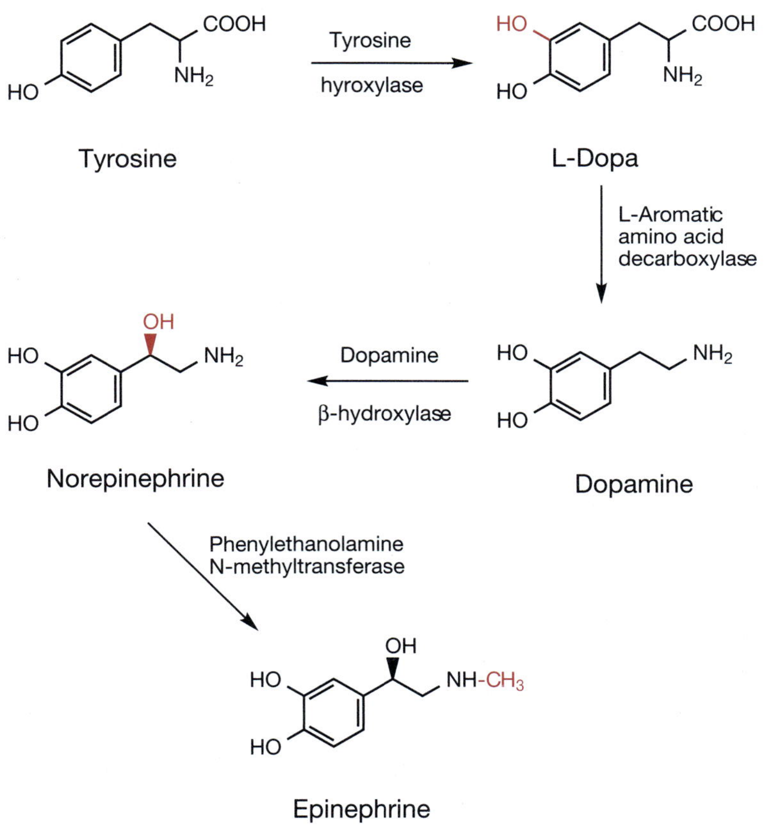

Figure 31.3 Biosynthesis of norepinephrine and epinephrine from tyrosine. L-DOPA, L-dihydroxyphenylalanine.

epinephrine without the methyl group. Physiologically, they behave as bases, being more than 99% protonated at pH 7.4 (amine $pK_a = 9.6$) and function as an ionized acid. The weakly acidic phenols have pK_a values of approximately 9 and remain predominantly unionized at physiologic pH.

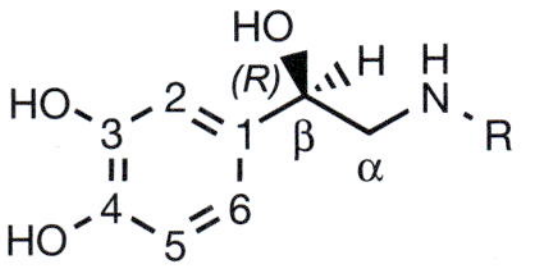

Norepinephrine R=H
Epinephrine R=CH_3

NE is biosynthesized in the neurons of both the central nervous system (CNS) and the autonomic nervous system, whereas EPI is formed in and secreted from the chromaffin cells of the adrenal medulla. Both NE and EPI are derived from L-tyrosine by a series of enzyme-catalyzed reactions (Fig. 31.3 depicts the overall pathway). Tyrosine hydroxylase hydroxylates the *m*-position of L-tyrosine, producing L-dihydroxyphenylalanine (L-DOPA), and is the rate-limiting step. The L-DOPA is then decarboxylated by L-aromatic amino acid decarboxylase to form dopamine, which is converted to NE by the action of dopamine β-hydroxylase. Dopamine β-hydroxylase is found in storage vesicles of the nerve ending, and the NE formed is stored there until it is released into the synaptic cleft upon nerve depolarization. In the chromaffin cells, the formed NE is converted to EPI by N-methylation catalyzed by phenylethanolamine *N*-methyltransferase.

Termination of Neurotransmission

Stimulated adrenergic neurons release NE into the synaptic cleft, which then binds reversibly with receptors to produce a characteristic adrenergic response. Termination of the adrenergic response occurs primarily by reuptake (uptake-1) into the presynaptic neuron; however, diffusion away from the receptors and extracellular metabolism also occur to a limited extent. The NE that is taken back up into the pr-esynaptic neuron is either used again as a neurotransmitter or is metabolized by mitochondrial monoamine oxidase (MAO). The extraneuronal NE that diffuses away from the neurons is either metabolized by catechol *O*-methyl transferase (COMT) in situ or reaches the circulatory system and is metabolized by COMT and MAO in various tissues, most importantly the liver, gastrointestinal (GI) tract, and the lungs. Figure 31.4 depicts the possible metabolic pathways for both NE and EPI. It is important to note that agonists that are resistant to MAO and/or COMT have greater oral bioavailability and a longer duration of action.

Adrenergic Receptor Structure and Agonist Interactions

The adrenergic receptors are members of the guanine nucleotide-binding regulatory protein–coupled receptor family more commonly referred to as G protein–coupled receptors (GPCRs; see Chapter 6). They affect biologic activity by releasing second messenger molecules inside the cell after agonist binding. This process of signal transduction is

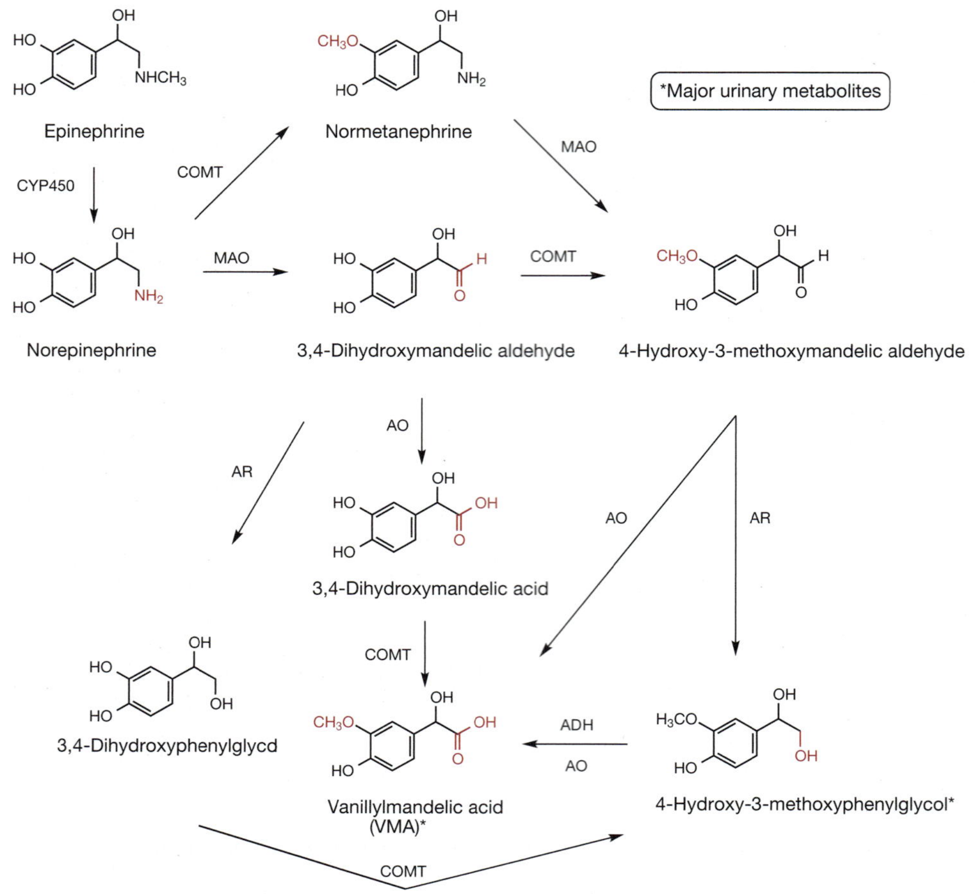

Figure 31.4 Metabolic pathways for norepinephrine and epinephrine. ADH, alcohol dehydrogenase; AO, aldehyde oxidase; AR, aldehyde reductase; COMT, catachol-*O*-methyltransferase; CYP, cytochrome; MAO, monoamine oxidase.

common to neurotransmitter receptors found in the muscarinic, serotonergic, dopaminergic, and adrenergic systems. All GPCRs are structurally similar, being composed of seven transmembrane (TM1-TM7) helix bundles. The helices are connected by short stretches of hydrophilic residues, which form multiple loops in the intracellular and extracellular domains. The G proteins (α,β,γ) are embedded in the inner membrane and interact with the TM domains through interactions with the Gα protein (Fig. 31.5).[31]

When a β-adrenergic agonist binds to the receptor on the cell membrane, it induces a conformational change in the receptor protein, allowing it to interact with a G protein, typically Gs (stimulatory G protein), exchanging guanosine diphosphate (GDP) for guanosine triphosphate (GTP) within the G protein. Once activated, the Gs protein dissociates into its α and βγ subunits. The α subunit then activates adenylate cyclase, which catalyzes the conversion of ATP to cyclic AMP (cAMP). This increase in cAMP levels subsequently activates protein kinase A, which phosphorylates numerous proteins, leading to downstream cellular responses (Fig. 31.6). The intracellular phosphodiesterases (PDEs) hydrolyze cAMP to form AMP and terminate its action.

A great deal of research has been done to identify the binding residues of the adrenergic receptors. Molecular modeling

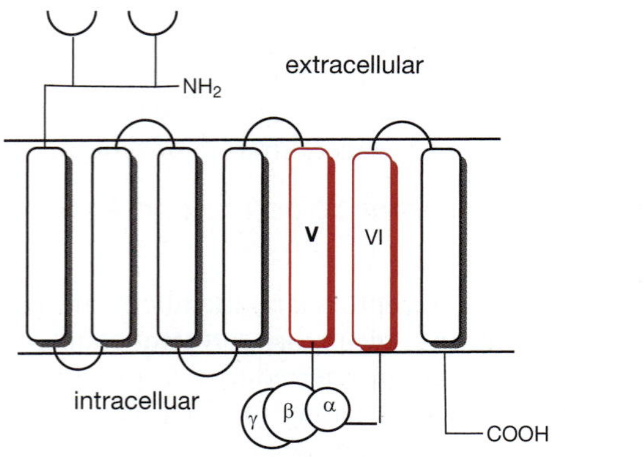

Figure 31.5 Representation of the G protein–coupled receptor.

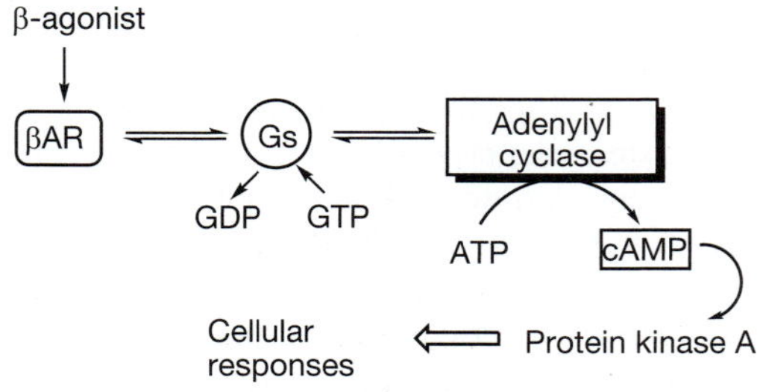

Figure 31.6 β-Adrenergic receptor (β-AR) G-protein coupling to adenylyl cyclase. ATP, adenosine triphosphate; cAMP, cyclic adenosine monophosphate; GDP, guanosine diphosphate; Gs, G proteins; GTP, guanosine triphosphate.

methods have been used to construct three-dimensional models for agonist complexes with the β_2-adrenergic receptor. The picture that has emerged is that NE binds ionically via its protonated amine to Asp113 in helix 3 and hydrogen bonds to both hydroxyls of the catechol ring with Ser204 and Ser207 in helix 5. That binding limits configurational and rotational freedoms, which allows reinforcing van der Waals interactions between the aromatic ring with residues Phe290 in helix 6 and Val114 in helix 3. The N-alkyl substituents are believed to fit into a pocket formed between aliphatic residues in helix 6 and helix 7. Stereochemistry also plays an important role in receptor binding. The β-carbon in NE/EPI is chiral and can be either R or S in configuration. Endogenous NE/EPI exists in the R configuration so that the β-hydroxy is oriented toward the receptor Asn293 (Fig. 31.7).[32] This bond is deemed essential at β-receptors, and every direct-acting β agonist (including the β_2-selective agonists used in asthma) will have a β–OH group.

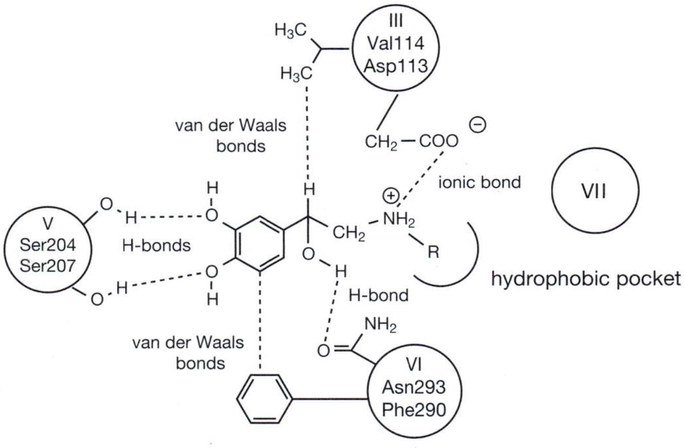

Figure 31.7 Ligand binding to key residues in the adrenergic receptor.

Adrenergic Agonist Structure-Activity Relationships

The fundamental pharmacophore for all adrenergic agonists is a substituted β-phenylethylamine (as in EPI and NE). The nature and number of substituents on the pharmacophore influence whether an analogue will be direct acting, indirect acting, or have a mixture of direct and indirect action. In addition, the nature and number of substituents also influences the specificity for the β-receptor subtypes. Direct-acting adrenergic agonists bind the β-adrenergic receptors similar to NE/EPI, producing a sympathetic response. Indirect-acting agonists cause their effect by several mechanisms. They can stimulate the release of NE from the presynaptic terminal, inhibit the reuptake of released NE, or inhibit the metabolic degradation of NE by neuronal MAO (ie, MAO inhibitors). Mixed-acting agonists work as their name implies (ie, they have both direct and indirect abilities).

Relationship of Structure to α- or β-Receptor Selectivity

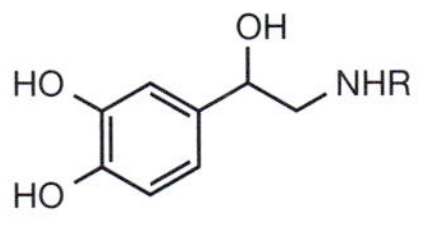

Norepinephrine (NE) R = H

Epinephrine (EPI) R = CH_3

Isoproterenol (ISO) 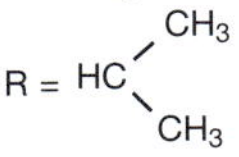

The R substituent on the amino group determines α- or β-receptor selectivity. As was noted earlier, when the R substituent is changed from hydrogen (NE) to methyl (EPI) to isopropyl (isoproterenol [ISO]), the receptor affinity transitions from nonselective (NE/EPI) to β-selective (ISO). Increasing bulkiness greater than a methyl on the amino nitrogen imparts selectivity for the β receptor. When the substituent is a *t*-butyl, there is a complete loss of α-receptor affinity and selectivity for the β_2 receptor. Selectivity is contingent on the administered dose, and at high doses, selectivity can be lost.

There are no marketed β_2 agonists with substituents on the α carbon. Substituents on the α-carbon inhibit MAO, but they show nonselective adrenergic agonist activity at both the α and β adrenergic receptors. The β carbon is chiral, and the *R* and *S* enantiomers bind to different residues on the receptor. The binding of the OH to the Asn293 residue in TM6 of the β_2-receptor favors the R conformation; thus, newer drugs coming onto the market have this stereochemistry (Fig. 31.8).[33]

For an adrenergic agonist to demonstrate significant β_2-receptor selectivity, there needs to be, in addition to the bulky *N*-substituent, an appropriately substituted phenyl ring. The currently marketed adrenergic agonists contain either a resorcinol ring, a salicyl alcohol moiety, a *m*-formamide group, or a quinoline-based 6-hydroxybenzoxazine-3-one or 8-hydroxybenzquinolin-2-one group (Fig. 31.9). In addition, these ring configurations are resistant to COMT metabolism and will increase the duration of action.

Specific Adrenergic Drugs Used to Treat Asthma and Chronic Obstructive Pulmonary Disease

Adrenergic agonists used to treat both asthma and COPD are classified by their duration of action. As noted, all of these drugs were developed using EPI as the starting point. The SABAs and the LABAs can be seen in Figure 31.8. Highlighted in red is the core structure shared with EPI.

Epinephrine (Adrenalin)

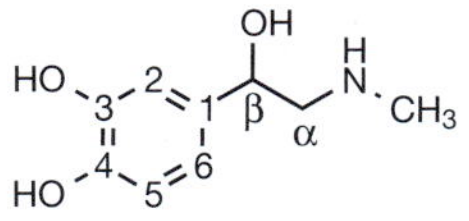

Epinephrine

The combination of the catechol nucleus, the β-hydroxy group, and the N-methyl gives EPI direct action and high affinity for all adrenergic receptors. EPI is biosynthesized as R EPI although synthetic EPI is marketed as the racemic mixture. EPI and all other catechols are susceptible to oxidation, especially in the presence of base and/or light,

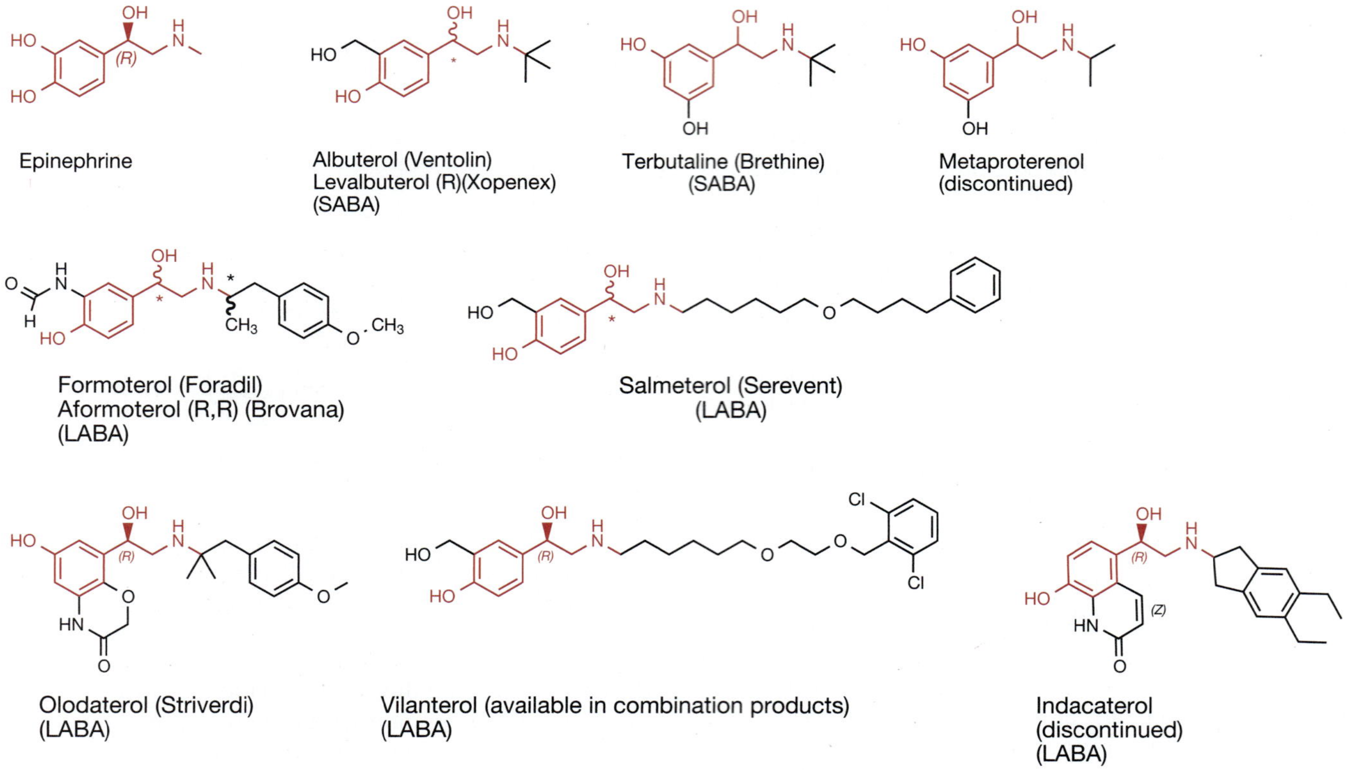

Figure 31.8 Short-acting β_2-agonists (SABAs) and long-acting β_2-agonists (LABAs) in relationship to epinephrine.

quickly decomposing to inactive quinones. Therefore, all catechol-containing drugs are stabilized with antioxidants and dispensed in air-tight amber containers.

EPI is ultimately metabolized by COMT and MAO to 3-methoxy-4-hydroxymandelic acid (vanillylmandelic acid), which is excreted as the sulfate or glucuronide conjugate in the urine (see Fig. 31.4). Only a very small amount is excreted unchanged.

EPI is available over the counter (OTC) as a MDI (Primatene Mist). As a nonselective α- and β-receptor agonist, it is intentionally absent from current asthma guidelines due to cardiac stimulation. Despite strong statements to the US Food and Drug Administration (FDA) from the medical

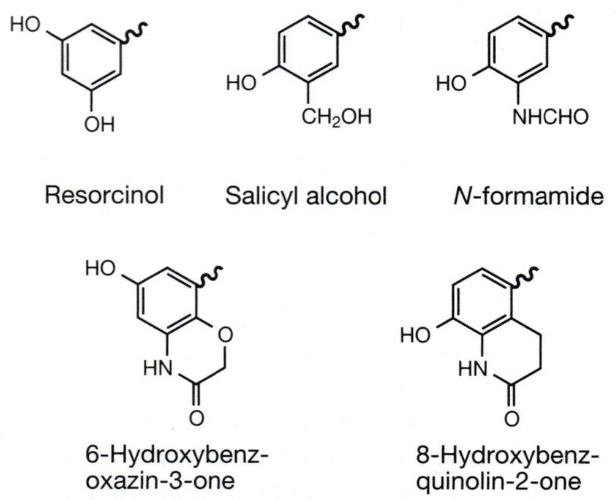

Figure 31.9 Ring configurations that contribute to β_2-receptor selectivity.

community against its continued availability, it remains available OTC.[34]

Intramuscular (IM) or IV EPI is indicated for acute asthma associated with anaphylaxis and angioedema. It is not recommended for any other asthma exacerbation.[12] It is typically administered intramuscularly in the emergency department because of ease of administration and quick onset. Due to metabolism, the duration of action is only 20 to 30 minutes. So patients must be monitored while receiving EPI therapy. Patients who administer IM EPI outside of a medical setting must seek medical care after administration.

Intravenous EPI administration is indicated only for (1) adult patients with hypotension associated with septic shock, (2) induction and maintenance of mydriasis during intraocular surgery, and (3) the treatment of allergic reactions including anaphylaxis. Adverse effects include headache, palpitations, tachycardia, sweating, nausea and vomiting, respiratory difficulty, dizziness, tremor, apprehension, and anxiety. Arrhythmias, including fatal ventricular fibrillation and rapid rises in blood pressure leading to cerebral hemorrhage, have occurred. There is little evidence to support using EPI in the treatment of asthma.

Metaproterenol Sulfate

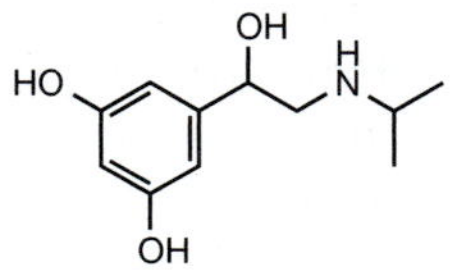

Metaproterenol

Metaproterenol is a direct-acting resorcinol analogue of isoproterenol. With both hydroxyl groups in the "meta" position, "meta" proterenol is no longer a catechol and is not metabolized by COMT. The N-isopropyl substitution limits MAO metabolism and enhances the selectivity for β-receptors.[24] Absorption studies in humans following oral administration indicate that less than 10% of the drug is absorbed intact. It is the least potent and selective of the β_2-selective agonists, and although still an FDA-approved drug, it has been discontinued by all manufacturers due to the availability of more effective and selective β_2-agonists.

Terbutaline Sulfate

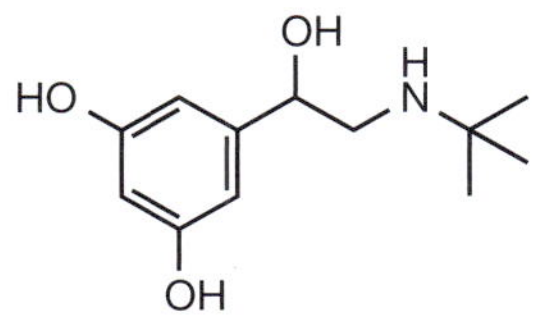

Terbutaline

Terbutaline is the N-*t*-butyl analogue of metaproterenol and, as such, would be expected to have better β_2-selectivity and potency. When compared to metaproterenol, terbutaline has a 3-fold greater potency at the β_2-receptor. It is resistant to COMT but vulnerable to intestinal and hepatic sulfonation. It is slowly metabolized by MAO and thus has good oral bioavailability, with a similar onset and duration of action to metaproterenol. Terbutaline is available as tablets, parenteral solutions, and solutions for nebulized inhalation. Adverse effects are similar to other direct-acting β_2-selective agonists but with a greater incidence of palpitations. An IV bolus followed by a continuous infusion of terbutaline is used as a second-line therapy in acute asthma attacks in pediatric patients.[12] It may be used as the first line during albuterol shortages.[13]

Albuterol

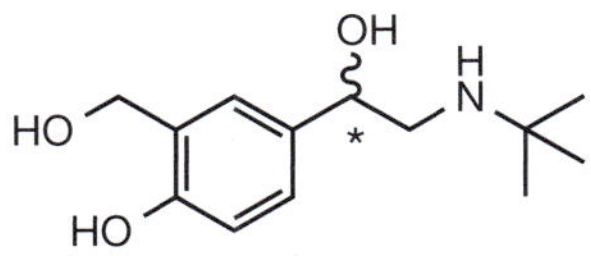

Albuterol (Ventolin)
Levalbuterol (*R*)(Xopenex)

Albuterol (also known as salbutamol) has the *N*-*t*-butyl and a salicyl alcohol phenyl ring, which gives it optimal β_2-selectivity. It is only a partial agonist at the β_2-receptor as it does not form as many hydrogen bonds with the receptor as the full agonist isoproterenol.[35] The non-catechol isostere inhibits COMT metabolism, and the N substitution inhibits metabolism by MAO. Neither the 3-*O*-methylated phenol metabolite nor the aldehyde metabolite is formed.[36] Albuterol is available as a tablet, MDI, and a solution for nebulization. Orally administered albuterol has a bioavailability of about 44%.[37] First-pass hepatic biotransformation leads to the major metabolite, the inactive 4′-*O*-sulfate, which is eliminated in the urine (Fig. 31.10).[36] Several

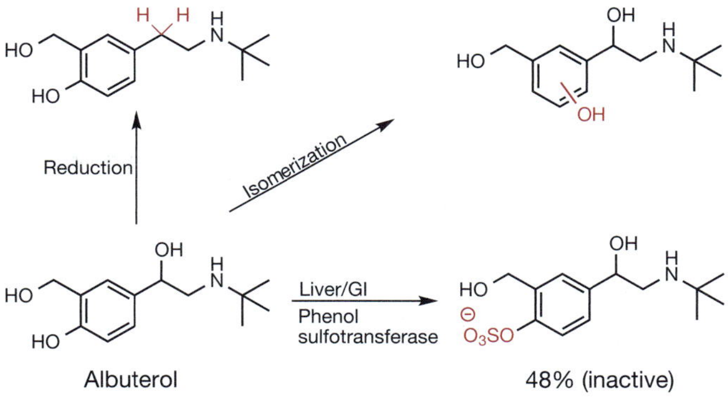

Figure 31.10 Metabolism of albuterol. GI, gastrointestinal.

minor albuterol metabolites have also been identified using human respiratory and liver cell culture studies.[37] Albuterol and its metabolites are eliminated by renal excretion. Its onset by inhalation is within 5 minutes, and it has a duration of action between 4 and 8 hours. It currently is the SABA drug of choice for relief of the acute bronchospasm of an asthmatic attack.

Levalbuterol is the *R*-(−)-enantiomer of albuterol and is available as a solution to be administered via nebulizer and as an MDI (Xopenex HFA). The *R* enantiomer is the active form of the drug; thus, the dose administered from the MDI form of racemic albuterol (90 μg) is twice the dose delivered by the *R* enantiomer (45 μg).[38-40] Studies with the *R*/*S* enantiomers of albuterol have shown that the *S*-enantiomer can be proinflammatory, exacerbating airway reactivity to a variety of spasmogens and, thereby, enhancing bronchiolar smooth muscle contraction. This opposes the bronchodilation effects of the *R*-enantiomer levalbuterol. The metabolism of levalbuterol has been shown to produce 11 metabolites, including the 4-*O*-sulfate (Fig. 31.10).[36] Metabolic isomerization is seen in other drug classes (NSAIDs and tetracyclines) and may diminish the benefit of single isomer therapy. It has not been determined if this occurs with levalbuterol. Clinically, levalbuterol has not shown a statistical benefit over racemic albuterol in either asthma treatment or cardiac side effects.[41,42] As discussed, β_2-adrenergic agonists may also be used with insulin and glucose to move potassium into cells. By redistributing potassium, they can be used to treat hyperkalemia.

Salmeterol Xinafoate

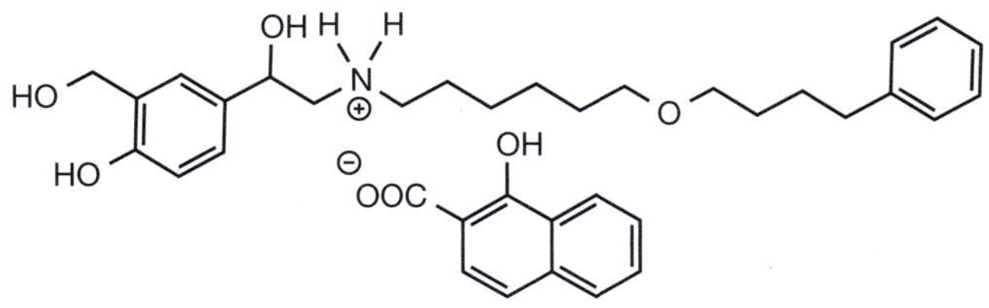

Salmeterol xinafoate (Serevent Diskus)

Salmeterol is at least 50 times more selective for β_2-receptors than albuterol and, like albuterol, it is a partial agonist at the β_2-receptor. It has an N-phenylbutoxyhexyl substituent, a β-hydroxy group, and a salicyl alcohol phenyl ring for optimal β_2-receptor selectivity and potency. It is resistant to both MAO and COMT and has an increased lipophilicity compared to albuterol (LogP 4.2 vs 0.9 respectively). All inhaled drugs are initially deposited on the mucosal lining fluid. They need to dissolve in this aqueous environment before diffusing through different tissue components deeper into the bronchial wall. The high lipophilicity of salmeterol delays the onset of action but is proposed to increase the deposition of the drug in the smooth muscle cells of the bronchi.[43] The x-ray crystal structure of salmeterol bound to the β_2 receptor shows that the long aryloxyalkyl tail binds to an extracellular vestibule of the β_2 adrenergic receptor, the exosite. Sequence differences between the exosite of β_1AR and β_2AR explain the high receptor-subtype selectivity of salmeterol. Both the increased lipophilicity and additional binding site not accessible to EPI nor albuterol provide the structural basis for the pharmacological specificity and long duration of action of salmeterol.[44,45]

Inhaled salmeterol has limited systemic absorption with minimal plasma concentrations peaking at 20 minutes and no accumulation with repeated doses. The metabolism of salmeterol is mainly through CYP3A4 benzylic hydroxylation. Despite low plasma levels of the inhaled dose, concurrent ingestion of a CYP3A4 inhibitor such as ketoconazole can cause a significant increase in the plasma level of salmeterol.[45]

Salmeterol is utilized as a DPI that contains lactose. As previously discussed, patients with milk protein allergy should avoid lactose-containing powders that may be contaminated with milk protein. Salmeterol is approved for the maintenance treatment of bronchospasm associated with COPD. The onset of action after a single dose averages 40 minutes, and the duration of bronchodilation was seen for 12 hours.[44,45] LABA monotherapy, without ICS, increases the risk of asthma-related hospitalizations and asthma-related deaths.[45] Salmeterol is therefore only used in combination therapy for the treatment of asthma. The available combination inhalers are listed in Table 31.2.

Formoterol Fumarate

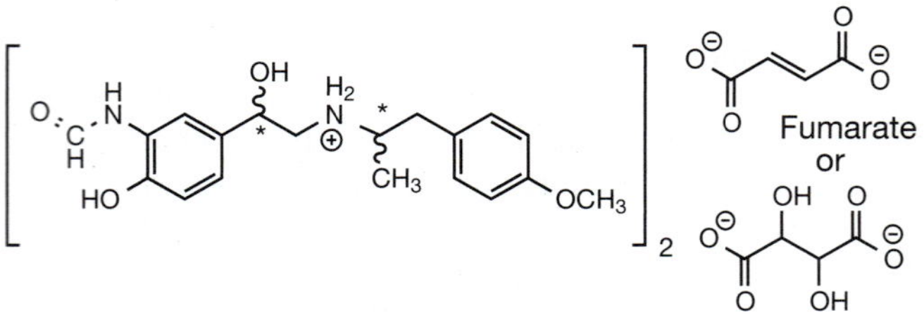

Formoterol fumarate (Perforomist)
Arformoterol (*R,R*) tartrate (Brovana)

Formoterol has an *N*-isopropyl-*p*-methoxyphenyl group, a β hydroxyl, and a unique *m*-formamide as the catechol bioisostere, all of which provide selectivity for β_2-receptors. It is resistant to MAO and COMT, placing it in the LABA class. The main metabolite formed is the glucuronide of the phenol on the drug. Sulfation also occurs on the phenol of the parent drug and after the formamide group is hydrolyzed. O-demethylation of the methoxy group also occurs followed by glucuronidation.[46] Phase 1 oxidation involves four cytochrome P450 isoenzymes (CYP2D6, CYP2C19, CYP2C9, and CYP2A6).[47]

Formoterol has a more rapid onset as compared to salmeterol (5 minutes vs ~40 minutes) while maintaining the same 12-hour duration of action. The quicker onset is believed to be a result of formoterol's greater water solubility (calculated LogP = 1.91 vs 4.2 for salmeterol), allowing it to move through the aqueous mucosal lining fluid and bind to the receptor sites quickly.[43] The moderate lipophilicity still allows it to stay localized in the lungs.[43] Its long duration of action is due to the formation of a highly stable formoterol–β_2-receptor complex. This complex is entirely within the orthosteric binding pocket and does not extend to the exosite inhabited by salmeterol.[48] It is a full agonist and as a LABA it is not indicated to be used alone for the treatment of asthma. Combination products are seen in Table 31.2. Formoterol is available as a lactose containing

Table 31.2 Combination Inhalers for Asthma/Chronic Obstructive Pulmonary Disease Treatment

β_2 Agonist	Antimuscarinic	Corticosteroid	Brand Name	FDA Approval
Albuterol sulfate	Ipratropium		Combivent Respimat	COPD
Vilanterol	Umeclidinium		Anoro Ellipta	COPD
Olodaterol	Tiotropium		Stiolto Respimat	COPD
Formoterol	Glycopyrrolate		Bevespi aerosphere	COPD
Formoterol	Aclidinium		Duaklir Pressair	COPD
Salmeterol		Fluticasone Propionate	Advair	Asthma/COPD
Formoterol		Budesonide	Symbicort	Asthma/COPD
Vilanterol		Fluticasone Furoate	Breo Ellipta	Asthma/COPD
Albuterol		Budesonide	Airsupra	Asthma
Formoterol fumarate		Mometasone furoate	Dulera	Asthma
Vilanterol	Umeclidinium	Fluticasone furoate	Trelegy Ellipta	Asthma/COPD
Formoterol	Glycopyrrolate	Budesonide	Breztri	COPD

DPI and a nebulizer solution and is indicated for the maintenance treatment of bronchoconstriction in patients with COPD, including chronic bronchitis and emphysema.

Formoterol has two asymmetric centers and, therefore, can exist in four possible enantiomers. The *R,R*-enantiomer is active and reported to be 1,000 times more active than the S,*S*-enantiomer and twice as potent as racemic formoterol. The *R,R*-enantiomer is available as a nebulizer inhalation solution under the name arformoterol (Brovana), undergoes the same metabolism, and is only indicated for the treatment of COPD.[49]

Olodaterol

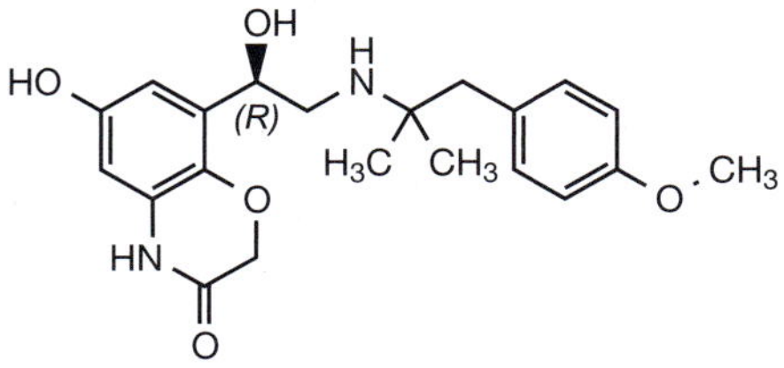

Olodaterol (Striverdi)

Olodaterol has a β_2-directing *N*-isobutyl joined to a *p*-methoxyphenyl ring (aralkyl substituent), an enantiomerically pure R conformation of the β-OH, and a unique 6-hydroxybenzoxazine-3-one ring that provides selectivity for the β_2-receptors. The *m*-orientation of the phenolic OH group relative to the ethanolamine moiety of the pharmacophore is believed to contribute to the observed selectivity. It is resistant to both COMT and MAO making it a long-acting agonist. It is metabolized to an *O*-demethylated product by CYP2C9 and 2C8. Both olodaterol and its O-demethylated metabolite form glucuronides. Concurrent administration of potent CYP2C8 and 2C9 inhibitors such as ketoconazole increases plasma concentrations of olodaterol by 70%, but no dosage adjustments are recommended.

Olodaterol's long duration of action is enhanced by its fast and high-affinity association with the β_2-receptor. Olodaterol forms a stable complex when bound to the β_2AR with a dissociation half-life greater than 17 hours. This provides a rationale for the 24-hour duration of action and once-daily dosing. It is administered via an MDI and is approved for the treatment of COPD as well as in combination products shown in Table 31.2. Like all LABAs, without an inhaled corticosteroid (ICS), it is contraindicated in patients with asthma. The most common adverse reactions include nasopharyngitis, upper respiratory tract infection, bronchitis, cough, rash, diarrhea, and arthralgia.

Vilanterol

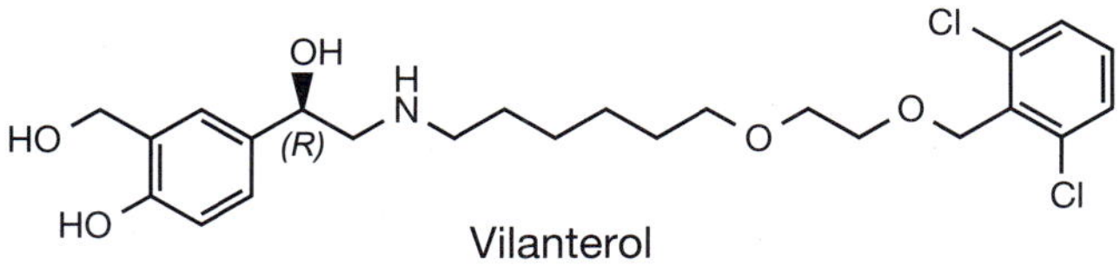

Vilanterol

Vilanterol is an LABA that is structurally similar to salmeterol, having the salicyl alcohol ring system and a β-hydroxy group in the active, R configuration. The *N*-phenylbutoxy moiety of salmeterol is changed to a dichlorobenzyloxyethyl group. This combination confers a greater intrinsic activity and better direct-acting β_2-receptor selectivity than albuterol or salmeterol.[50] Its long duration of action (24 hours) suggests that vilanterol has strong binding to the β_2-receptor. Docking experiments demonstrated strong H-bonding in transmembrane helix 5 between Ser207 and its phenolic hydroxy group, as well as between Asn293 and the benzylic hydroxy, interactions common to all β_2 agonists. Asp113 in transmembrane 5 also shows the anticipated ionic interaction with the cationic amine. In addition, the central ether oxygen H-bonds to Asn318 of transmembrane 7, and the benzylic ether can H-bond with the Ser in transmembrane 3 and an Asn of transmembrane 7, enhancing vilanterol's receptor affinity. In addition to the long duration of action, vilanterol has a rapid onset of action.[50] It undergoes extensive first-pass metabolism to compounds with minimal β_2 agonist activity, suggesting reduced systemic side-effects of absorbed drug. The major metabolic pathway is via CYP3A4-mediated O-demethylation to a primary alcohol and 2,6-dichlorobenzoic acid. The alcohol metabolite retains only a very small β_2-receptor agonist activity.[51] Vilanterol serum drug concentration is increased by 70% when administered concurrently with potent CYP3A4 inhibitors. Vilanterol is available only in combination products with corticosteroids and muscarinic antagonists listed in Table 31.2. When combined with fluticasone, caution should be exercised when used with strong CYP3A4 inhibitors since both drugs are substrates for CYP3A4. Combination products are approved for the treatment of asthma or COPD as indicated.

Antimuscarinics

Acetylcholine (ACh) serves as the endogenous neurotransmitter for the parasympathetic nervous system, which is present in both the autonomic and central nervous systems. Within these systems, parasympathetic nerve fibers can be categorized based on their response to muscarine or nicotine stimulation. Nicotine, derived from *Nicotiana tabacum*, stimulates preganglionic fibers in both the parasympathetic and sympathetic systems, as well as somatic motor fibers in the skeletal system. Muscarine, obtained from the poisonous mushroom *Amanita muscaria*, stimulates postganglionic parasympathetic fibers with receptors located on autonomic effector cells. The CNS contains fibers with both nicotinic and muscarinic receptors.

This section focuses primarily on drugs that inhibit muscarinic fibers (antimuscarinics). Blocking these fibers leads to cardiovascular, mydriatic, antispasmodic, antisecretory, and bronchodilatory effects, making them of interest in treating respiratory disorders.

Biochemistry and Metabolism of Acetylcholine

ACh is the primary parasympathetic neurotransmitter that induces bronchoconstriction in the airways. ACh is produced through the transfer of an acetyl group from acetyl coenzyme A to choline, a reaction catalyzed by choline acetyltransferase within presynaptic cholinergic

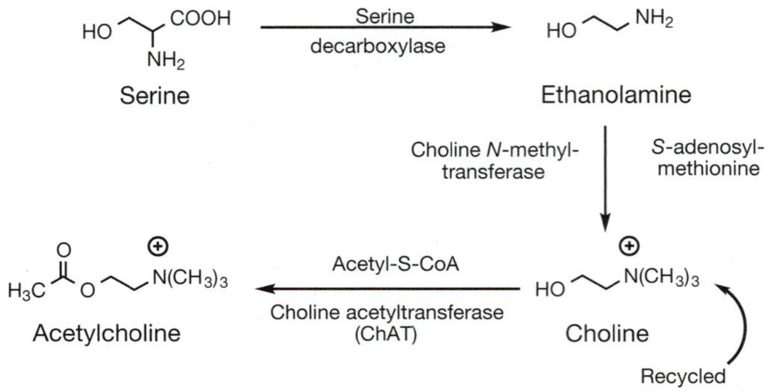

Figure 31.11 Biosynthesis of acetylcholine.

neurons. The majority of the choline needed for ACh synthesis is obtained through uptake from the synaptic space. This choline is recycled upon hydrolysis of ACh by acetylcholinesterase, an enzymatic protein bound to the neuronal membrane. Once synthesized, ACh is stored in vesicles and released upon stimulation. ACh and its synthesizing enzyme are found throughout the airways (Fig. 31.11).

The duration of action of ACh is very short because it is rapidly hydrolyzed by the acetylcholinesterase present on postsynaptic terminals in the synaptic space. ACh binds in the pocket of the enzyme and is hydrolyzed by the catalytic triad in the esteratic site. It is hydrolyzed into acetic acid and choline. The positive charge on the nitrogen helps bring the ACh molecule deep into the active-site gorge within acetylcholinesterase. A combination of cation-π interactions and cation-anion interactions helps guide ACh to the catalytic triad and place the ester in position to be attacked by the Ser hydroxyl (Fig. 31.12).[52]

Once bound, the hydrolysis involves two hydrolytic steps. The first step is the hydrolysis of ACh by nucleophilic attack at the carbonyl carbon by the Ser hydroxy group, which liberates choline and leaves the enzyme acetylated. A triad formed between Glu, His, and the Ser at the catalytic site activates the Ser for the nucleophilic attack. The second step is the hydrolysis of the acetylated enzyme by water to regenerate the free enzyme. The water is activated by hydrogen bonding to the His residue, which increases the nucleophilic character of the oxygen of water. The activated water

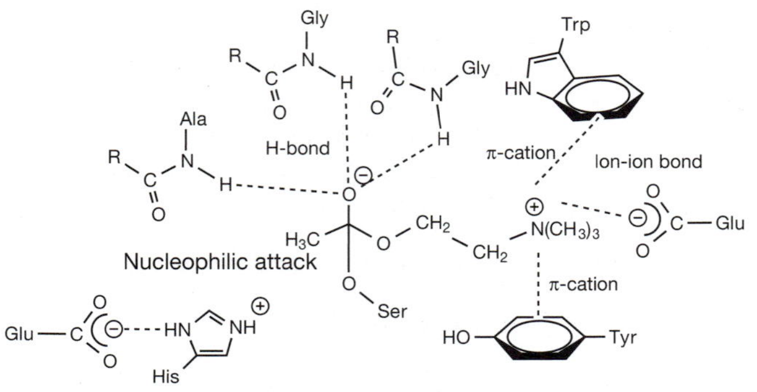

Figure 31.12 Binding of acetylcholine in the catalytic site of acetylcholinesterase.

attacks the electrophilic carbonyl carbon of the acetyl group to generate acetic acid and regenerate the free hydroxy group of Ser (Fig. 31.13).[53]

Methacholine Challenge Test

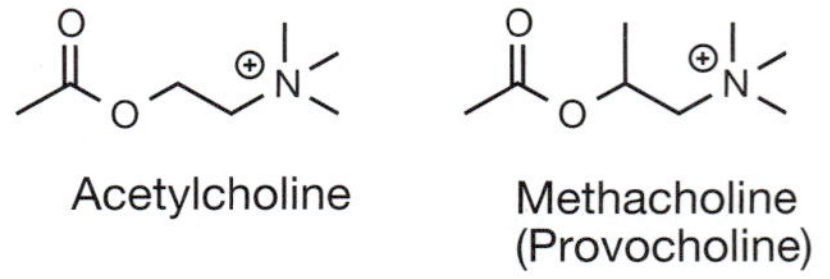

Methacholine is used in the bronchial challenge test to detect bronchial airway hyperreactivity. Patients with asthma are more sensitive to methacholine-induced bronchoconstriction than healthy subjects, which is the pharmacological basis of the test. Prior to the test, patients should not use SABAs (for 6 hours), LABAs (for 36 hours), short-acting muscarinic antagonist (SAMAs) (for 12 hours), or LAMAs (for ≥168 hours) or oral theophylline or caffeinated beverages (12-48 hours). Methacholine is a synthetic choline ester that binds as an agonist at all muscarinic receptors. The methyl group on the β carbon provides selectivity for muscarinic receptors compared to nicotinic receptors. It is a potent bronchoconstrictor and must be used in a pulmonary function clinic by trained health care practitioners. Patients will perform a spirometry test baseline and then will receive increasing doses of methacholine followed by FEV_1 measurements. A challenge test is considered positive if methacholine causes a 20% or greater decrease in FEV_1 compared to the mean baseline. Methacholine is provided as a powder that must be diluted before use in a nebulizer. Once reconstituted, the solution is stable for up to 2 weeks under refrigeration. Health care providers must take precautions not to inhale the powder while reconstituting, or allow it to be released into the room air.[54]

Muscarinic Receptor Structure and Agonist/Antagonist Interactions

The muscarinic receptors are members of the superfamily of G protein–coupled receptors (see Chapter 6). They consist of seven transmembrane helices and are linked to their G protein through interaction with the second and third intracellular loops. There are five receptor subtypes, designated M_{1-5}, and the odd-numbered receptors (M_1, M_3, and M_5) are coupled to the G_q/G_{11} class. This class of receptors activates intracellular phospholipase C to hydrolyze phosphatidylinositol 4,5-diphosphate (PIP_2) to diacylglycerol (DAG) and inositol triphosphate (IP3) as membrane-bound and intracellular second messengers, respectively. The even-numbered receptors (M_2 and M_4) are coupled to the G_i/G_o class, which mediates the inhibition of adenylyl cyclase (Fig. 31.14).

The muscarinic receptors in the bronchial tree are mainly M_1, M_2, and M_3 subtypes. The M_3 subtype predominates in the airway smooth muscles of the bronchial tree. Activation of the M_3 subtype in airway smooth muscle causes bronchoconstriction, airway remodeling, mucus secretion, and inflammation. The M_2 receptor subtype is prejunctional and

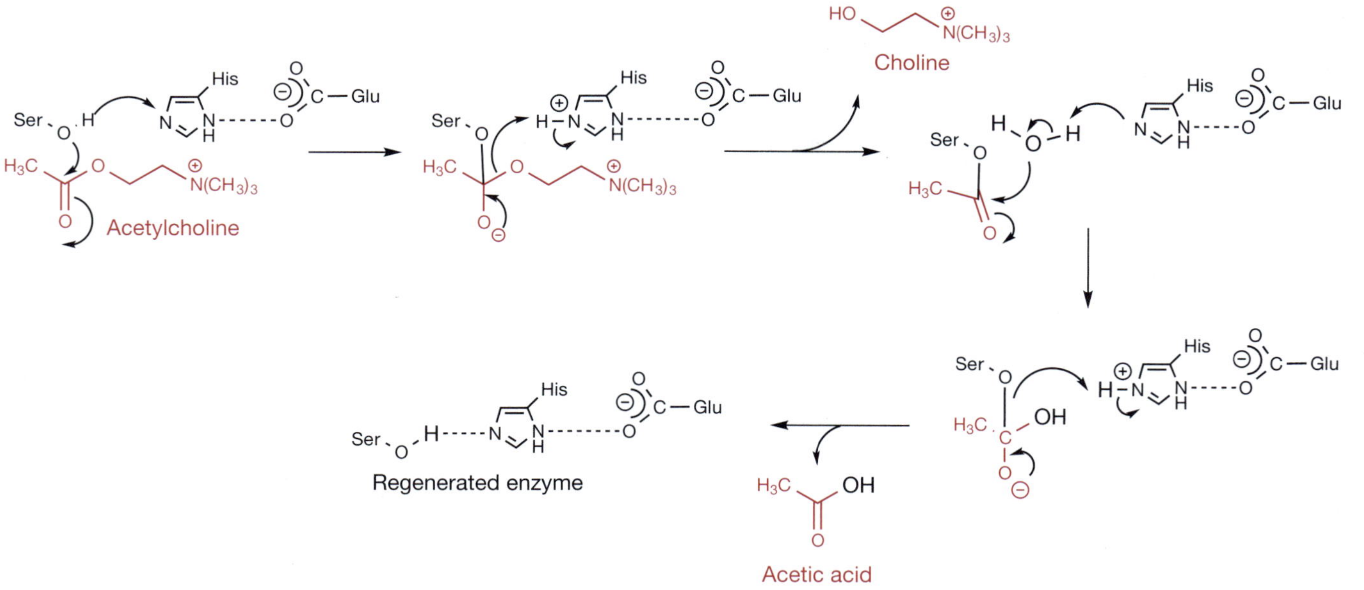

Figure 31.13 Hydrolysis of acetylcholine by acetylcholinesterase triad glutamate, histidine and serine, to form choline and acetic acid.

acts as an autoreceptor responsible for ACh release. The M_2 subtype is the predominant muscarinic receptor in the heart and, thus, stimulating this receptor leads to the adverse effects of tachycardia and prolonged QT interval.[55] Activation of the postganglionic presynaptic M_2 autoreceptors in the lung actually protects against vagally induced bronchoconstriction through feedback mechanisms. Thus, the ideal drug would behave as an antagonist at the M_3 receptors but have limited effect on the M_2 receptors. The crystal structures of the M_2 and the M_3 receptors show a critical difference in the orthosteric binding pocket that can be utilized to design compounds with optimized M_3 binding. There is only one residue in the binding pocket that is not identical, M_2 has a Phe, while M_3 has a Leu.[56] SAMAs such as ipratropium block the M_3 receptor, but they unfortunately block the M_2 inhibitory neuronal receptor, which can cause vagally induced bronchoconstriction. Long-acting antimuscarinics (LAMAs) overcome this effect by prolonged binding at the M_3 receptor with faster dissociation from the M_2 receptors, thus prolonging the duration of bronchodilator effect.[57] LAMAs, specifically tiotropium and aclidinium, have shown a beneficial effect on mucus hypersecretion and improving the rate of mucociliary clearance and the severity of cough.[58] Table 31.3 lists the physiologic action of the M_3 receptors.

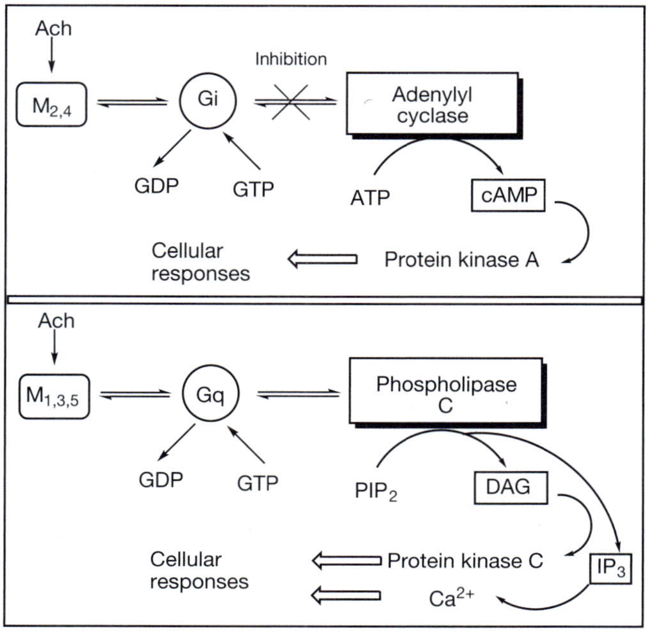

Figure 31.14 Comparison of the role of G protein in odd- and even-numbered muscarinic receptors. ATP, adenosine triphosphate; cAMP, cyclic adenosine monophosphate; DAG, diacylglycerol; GDP, guanosine diphosphate; GTP, guanosine triphosphate; IP_3, inositol triphosphate; PIP_2, phosphatidylinositol biphosphate.

Affinity labeling and mutagenic studies have established that ACh binds to its receptor in a narrow region of the circular arrangement of the seven transmembrane helices approximately 10 to 15Å away from the membrane surface. The quaternary cationic nitrogen of ACh binds to the anionic carboxylate of an Asp located in helix 3. As depicted in Figure 31.15, the ionic interaction is stabilized by hydrogen bonding with a Tyr in helix 5 and a Thr in helix 5. It is postulated that muscarinic antagonists bind to the Asp and contain hydrophobic substituents that bind within a hydrophobic pocket in the receptor, which does not allow the change in conformation needed to transfer the agonist signal to the coupled G protein[59] (see "Structure-Activity Relationships of Antimuscarinic Agents" section).

Structure-Activity Relationships of Antimuscarinic Agents

The structural pharmacophore for the SAMAs and the LAMAs (Fig. 31.16) is based on the alkaloid atropine.

Table 31.3 Physiologic Action Associated with the M_3 Muscarinic Receptors

M_3-Receptor Expression	M_3-Agonist Effect
Iris circular muscle	Contracts (miosis)
Ciliary muscle	Contracts
Sinoatrial node	Decelerates
Atrial muscle	Decelerates contraction
Bronchiole smooth muscle	Bronchoconstriction
Endothelium	Release NO vasodilation
Smooth muscle	Contracts
Epithelial cells	Increase secretions
Salivary glands	Increase secretions
Mac, Lym, Neu, Eos	Cytokine production

Eos, eosinophil; Lym, lymphocyte; Mac, macrophage; Neu, neutrophil.

With only one exception (umeclidinium), all currently used antimuscarinics are amino alcohol esters. On the carbon α to the ester, R_1 is substituted with an OH or a CH_2OH. The docking studies of antimuscarinics show that both the hydroxyl group and the ester form hydrogen bonds with Asn on helix 6.[56] Substituents R_2 and R_3 are either both aromatic rings (usually phenyl or thiophene) or one aromatic ring and one alicyclic ring. Selectivity for the M_3 receptor over the M_2 receptor can be modified by optimizing these two rings. As discussed,

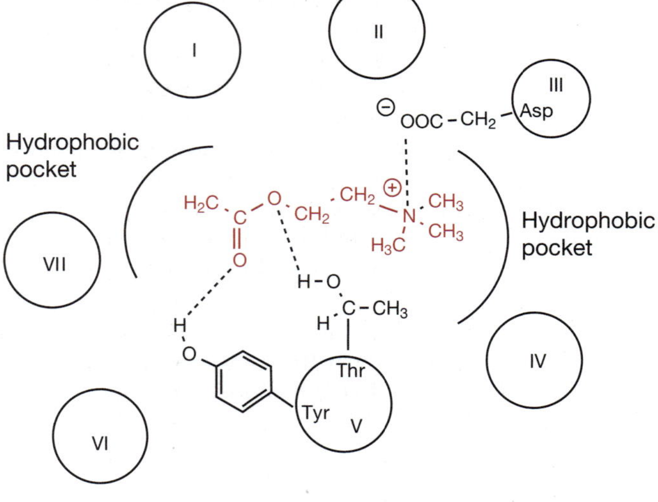

Figure 31.15 Acetylcholine binding to residues in the muscarinic receptor.

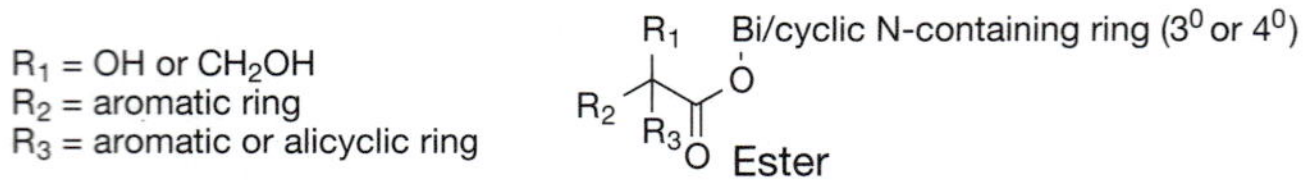

Figure 31.16 Pharmacophore for antimuscarinic agents.

exploiting the single Leu-Phe difference in extracellular loop 2 can afford M_3 selective antagonists. The ester is connected to various nitrogen-containing rings based on atropine. Nitrogen can be substituted with alkyl groups (tertiary and quaternary amines are the most active). When the nitrogen is made quaternary, the molecule loses its oral bioavailability but leads to compounds that can be administered effectively by inhalation with minimal absorption.

The classic chemical prototype for antimuscarinic drugs is atropine, an alkaloid from the deadly nightshade family *Atropa belladonna*. Antimuscarinics have been used since antiquity to treat asthma. The ancient Egyptian *Ebers Papyrus*, compiled in approximately 1550 BC, included a remedy of using henbane on hot stones to create smoke for inhalation.[60] Henbane contains hyoscyamine, atropine, tropane, and scopolamine.[61] Throughout the Middle Ages, the deadly nightshade shrub was used as a medical source of atropine.[62] The design of muscarinic antagonists using atropine as its pharmacophore is evident in Figure 31.17. Atropine contains the amino alcohol ester with a -CH_2OH at R_1, a phenyl ring at R_2, and a hydrogen at R_3. The bicyclic ring system is a tropane, a seven-membered carbon ring system connected at carbon 1 and 5 with a nitrogen substituted with a methyl. When the methyl is removed, it is known as a nortropane; when carbon 3 is substituted with a hydroxyl group, it is known as a tropine ring. Atropine is a tropine ring that has been esterified at position 3.[63]

Atropine is not approved for use in asthma or COPD, but it is used as an antimuscarinic agent. It is marketed as the racemic mixture and used to reduce saliva and fluid in the respiratory tract during surgery, as a parasympatholytic to increase blood pressure (Chapter 19, and as an antidote to nerve gas/insecticide poisoning Chapter 28).

Although atropine does not have a quaternary nitrogen, the conjugate acid of the tertiary amine has a calculated pK_a of 10.3.[64] Therefore, it is protonated at physiologic pH and can bind to the anionic Asp residue in the muscarinic receptor. Atropine is nonselective and competitively blocks the binding of ACh to M_1, M_2, M_3, M_4, and M_5 receptor subtypes.

Scopolamine (see Fig. 31.17) is atropine with an added epoxide formed by the addition of an oxygen between carbons 6 and 7 on the tropine ring. It is effective for motion sickness[65] and postoperative nausea and vomiting. It has good transdermal bioavailability and is available in a patch formulation. It is presumed to work by antagonizing the M_1 receptors in either the vestibular system or the medulla oblongata, the vomiting center of the brain.[66]

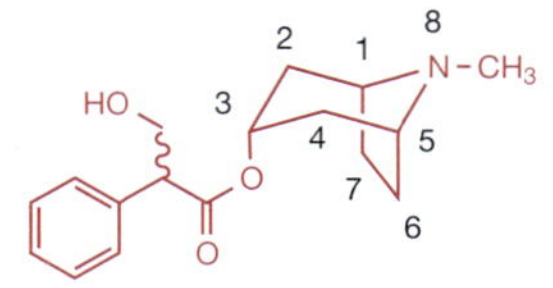

Atropine
(nonselective muscarinic antagonist)

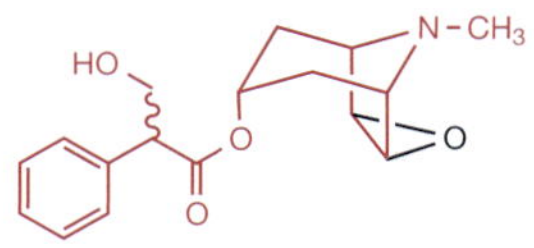

Scopolamine
(used for motion sickness)

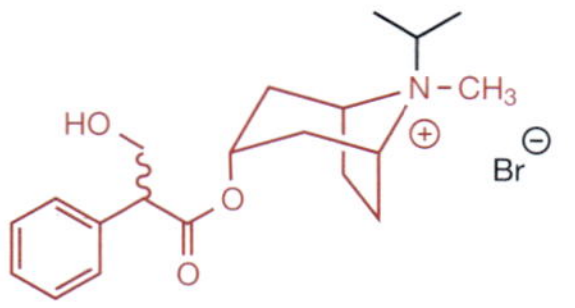

Ipratropium bromide
(Atrovent) SAMA

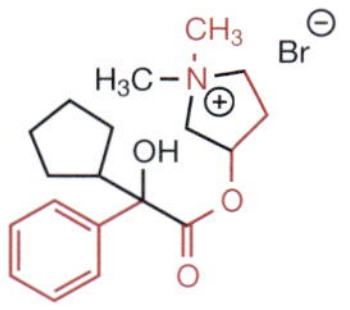

Glycopyyrolate bromide
(Combination inhalers/LAMA)

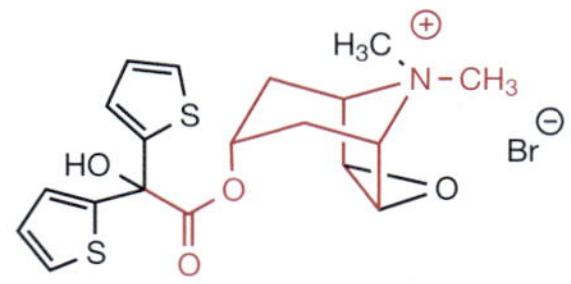

Tiotropium bromide
(Spiriva) LAMA

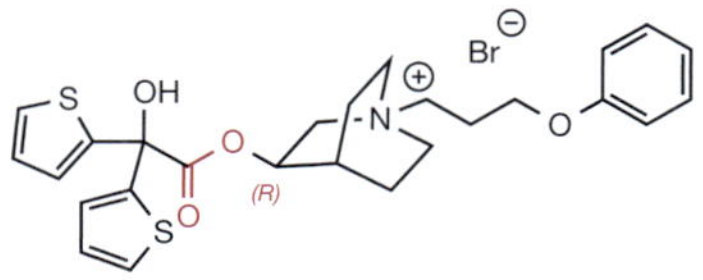

Aclidinium bromide
(Tudorza Pressair) LAMA

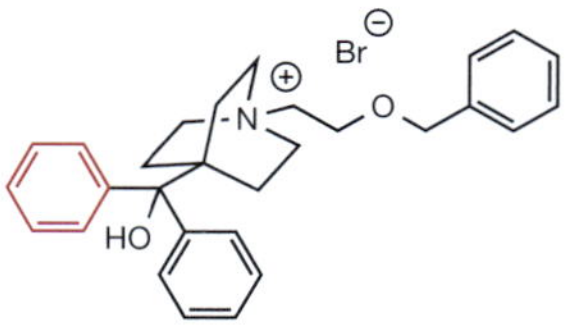

Umeclidinium bromide
(Incruse Ellipta) LAMA

Figure 31.17 Muscarinic antagonists and their relationship to atropine. LAMA, long-acting muscarinic antagonist; SAMA, short-acting muscarinic antagonist.

Specific Antimuscarinic Drugs Used to Treat Asthma and Chronic Obstructive Pulmonary Disease

Ipratropium Hydrobromide

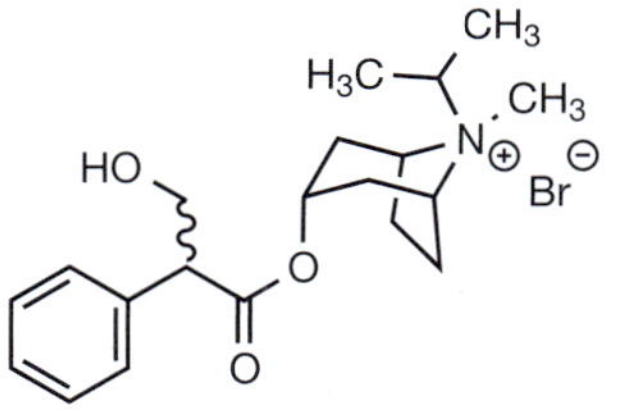

Ipratropium bromide
(Atrovent)

Ipratropium was developed from atropine by the addition of an isopropyl (thus the Ipr in the name), to the nitrogen to form a quaternary nitrogen. The cationic nature makes it highly hydrophilic and poorly absorbed from the lungs after inhalation via solution or aerosol; therefore, the bronchodilation effect can be considered to be a local, site-specific effect. The drug can pass through the airway epithelia via uptake by organic cation/carnitine transporters OCTN1 and OCTN2.[67] Inhaled ipratropium has a 15-minute onset of action and a short duration of action (<4 hours); therefore, it is typically dosed 4 times a day. The short duration of action is due to its very quick dissociation from the M_3 receptor.[2] It is available as an MDI and as a solution for nebulizer treatment for COPD. Ipratropium is also available as a nasal spray for the relief of rhinorrhea associated with the common cold and perennial rhinitis. It is currently the only SAMA used. Much of an inhaled dose is swallowed and excreted without significant absorption. It does not penetrate the blood brain barrier (BBB). The little ipratropium that reaches the circulation is minimally protein-bound and is partially metabolized by esterase to inactive products. Most adverse effects from ipratropium are common to antimuscarinics and include blurred vision, dry mouth, tachycardia, urinary retention, and headache. Patients should be careful to protect their eyes if using nebulizer treatments because it can increase intraocular pressure as well as precipitate acute angle closure glaucoma.[68]

Tiotropium Bromide

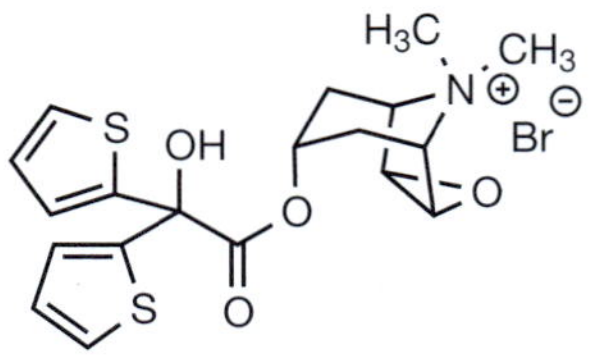

Tiotropium bromide
(Spiriva)

Tiotropium has an R_1 alcohol and both the R_2 and R_3 substituents of the pharmacophore (Fig. 31.16) substituted with thiophene. It is the N-methyl derivative of the scopolamine ring system, which includes the 6,7 epoxide. Although a quaternary nitrogen, approximately 33% of the inhaled dose reaches systemic circulation. The oral bioavailability of any inadvertently swallowed dose is only 2%. As a LAMA, tiotropium is approved for once-daily maintenance treatment for both COPD and asthma, although at different dosages. It is available as a DPI, a solution-based MDI inhaler, and in combination inhalers (see Table 31.2). Inhaled tiotropium has a 30-minute onset but a much longer duration than ipratropium (24 hours vs <4 hours, respectively). The long duration of action can be inferred by its long residence time on the M_3 receptor with a dissociation half-life of 35 hours.[2] Approximately 74% of an experimental IV dose of tiotropium was excreted unchanged in the urine. The remaining fraction of tiotropium was metabolized through ester hydrolysis, oxidation by CYP3A4 and CYP2D6 followed by glutathione conjugation to a variety of metabolites.[69] Tiotropium has an adverse reaction profile similar to that of ipratropium, with dry mouth being the most common adverse effect; however, blurred vision, tachycardia, urinary difficulty, headache precipitation, and exacerbation of narrow-angle glaucoma have been reported.[69]

Aclidinium Bromide

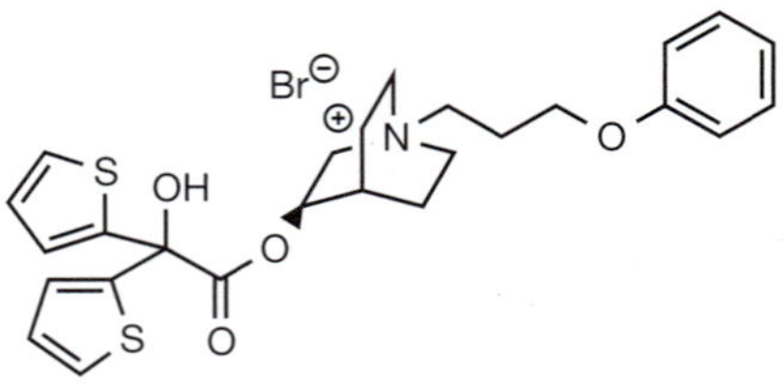

Aclidinium bromide
(Tudorza Pressair)

Aclidinium bromide is structurally related to tiotropium in that the R_1, R_2, and R_3 groups are identical. The tropine ring has been replaced by a quinuclidine ring system. This ring system is also known as a 1-azabicyclo[2,2,2]-octane ring system. The nitrogen is a bridgehead for the three cyclohexane rings that adopt boat conformations. Aclidinium has equal affinity for the M_2 versus the M_3 receptor but much higher residence on the M_3 receptor. This kinetic selectivity for the M_3 versus the M_2 muscarinic receptors is desirable, as it reduces M_2 cardiac inhibition, which leads to tachycardia.[70] Aclidinium is a long-acting bronchodilator with a quick onset of action and is classified as a LAMA. The bioavailability of a single inhaled dose is approximately 5%.[71] It undergoes rapid hydrolysis of its ester in plasma to form inactive acid and alcohol components, with a half-life of 2.4 minutes. In comparison, more than 70% of tiotropium remains intact in plasma after 1 hour. The short half-life, combined with the lack of antimuscarinic activity of its hydrolysis products, suggests that aclidinium may have reduced antimuscarinic side effects. In addition to hydrolysis, aclidinium also undergoes CYP metabolism, yielding a monooxygenated phenyl ring and the loss of one of the thienyl rings, mediated by 3A4 and 2D6 CYP isoforms. Due to the low plasma levels, aclidinium is not expected to have any DDIs with drugs metabolized by CYPs. In a clinical trial with patients with mild to severe COPD, aclidinium demonstrated significant elevation of FEV_1 from baseline, producing sustained bronchodilation over 24 hours. Aclidinium is manufactured as a DPI that contains lactose so the same warnings for patients with hypersensitivity reactions to milk proteins previously discussed apply. Post-marketing studies have reported typical anticholinergic side effects such as blurred vision, urinary retention, tachycardia, and nausea. Immediate hypersensitivity reactions have also been reported.[72]

Umeclidinium Bromide

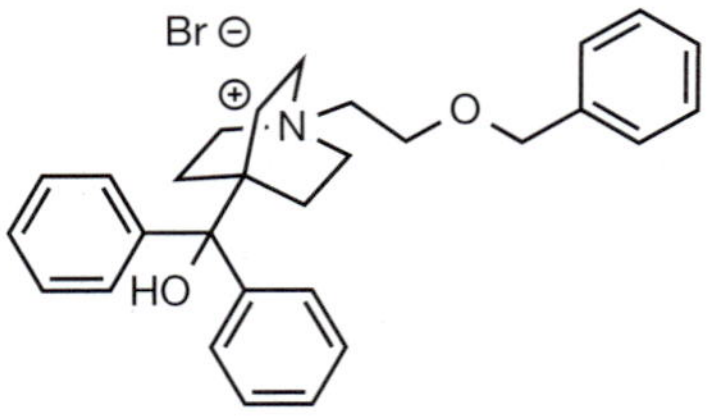

Umeclidinium bromide
(Incruse Ellipta)

Umeclidinium is a LAMA approved for the long-term maintenance treatment of airflow obstruction in patients with COPD. The R_1 group is an alcohol; the R_2 and R_3 groups are phenyl rings. It uses the same octane bicyclic ring system as aclidinium but the attachment of the R_1, R_2, R_3 α carbon is directly to the bridgehead carbons of the bicyclic ring system. The ether on the nitrogen has also shifted in umeclidinium versus aclidinium. Umeclidinium is a competitive, reversible antagonist with affinity for all muscarinic receptors. Like all LAMAs, it shows a longer residence time on the M_3 receptor compared to the M_2 receptor (half-life values 82 and 9 minutes respectively) and clinical trials showed no significant tachyphylaxis.[73]

Upon inhalation, umeclidinium stays localized in the lung, and plasma levels are insignificant. Following experimental IV administration, the drug is highly bound to plasma proteins (89%). Umeclidinium is a substrate for P-glycoprotein as well as CYP2D6, with O-dealkylated, hydroxylated, and glucuronidated metabolites being formed. Following oral administration, elimination occurs primarily in the feces (98%), suggesting poor bioavailability.[73] Umeclidinium may worsen acute narrow-angle glaucoma as well as urinary retention, especially in patients with prostate hyperplasia or bladder-neck obstruction. Umeclidinium is used alone as a lactose containing DPI or in combination products (see Table 31.2).

Glycopyrrolate Bromide

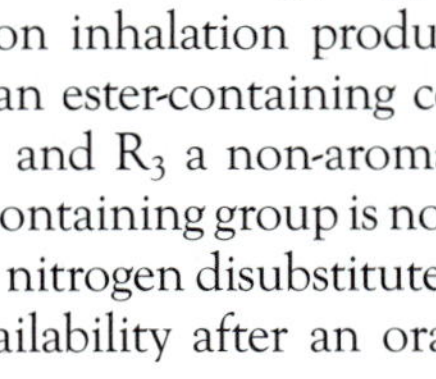

Glycopyrrolate bromide

Glycopyrrolate (also known as glycopyrronium) is a LAMA used in combination inhalation products for the treatment of COPD. This is an ester-containing compound with an R_1 alcohol, R_2 phenyl, and R_3 a non-aromatic cyclohexane. The quaternary amino containing group is not a bicyclic but a pyrrolidine ring with the nitrogen disubstituted with methyl groups. As such the bioavailability after an oral dose is low (~3%).

Despite this, it is available as both a tablet and liquid formulation to decrease secretions during surgery or to decrease salivary secretions. It has also been approved for use as a topical cloth for the treatment of primary axillary hyperhidrosis (excessive underarm sweating). A nebulizer form is FDA-approved but is no longer marketed due to low usage; inhaled forms are currently available only in combination products (see Table 31.2). Glycopyrrolate competitively and reversibly inhibits the action of ACh at all muscarinic receptors, with greater affinity for the M_1 and M_3 subtypes. The 3*S*, 2*R* enantiomer was found to be the most potent but it is marketed with no stereochemistry at either chiral center defined.[74] It undergoes minimal ester hydrolysis in the liver and is excreted in both the urine and bile. Only a slight increase in total systemic exposure is seen in patients with moderate renal impairment. Glycopyrrolate, as with all anticholinergics, should be used with caution in patients with glaucoma, benign prostatic hyperplasia (BPH), diabetes, and myasthenia gravis.

Revefenacin

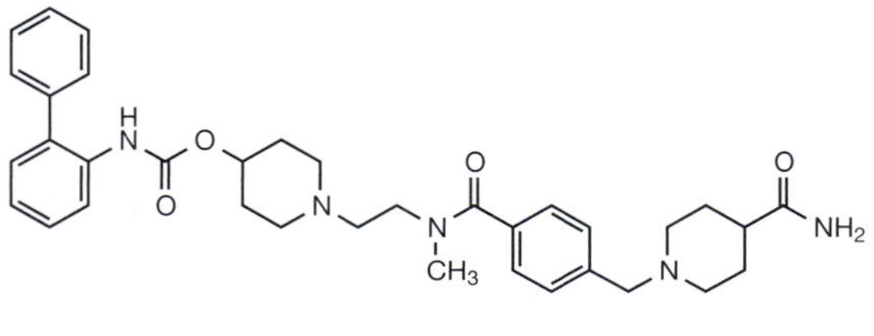

Revefenacin
(Yupelri)

Revefenacin is a LAMA that is available as a nebulizer solution indicated for the once-daily treatment of COPD. Revefenacin has a novel structure that deviates from those seen in Figure 31.17. It uses a biphenyl carbamate to replace the R_1, R_2, R_3 and ester groups seen in the pharmacophore. It also does not have a bicyclic ring with a quaternary nitrogen but contains two tertiary cyclic amines, with predicted pK_as of approximately 8.6. It is presumed that the larger structure accesses parts of the M_3 receptor that other drugs do not, but there is currently no published model of revefenacin in its binding pocket. The inhalation solution is packaged as individual unit doses at a pH of 5.0. The acidic pH favors the protonated form of the drug that remains soluble in the solution. Revefenacin has kinetic selectivity for the M_3 receptor over the M_2 receptor, displaying a longer dissociation half-life at M_3 receptors (82 minutes) than M_2 receptors (6.9 minutes).[75] It has a rapid onset and demonstrated sustained bronchodilation for more than 24 hours. Oral bioavailability is very low (3%); thus, systemic side effects of inadvertently swallowed revefenacin are minimal.[76] The two main metabolites are the hydrolysis product of the terminal formamide to the carboxylic acid (M2 ~14%) and the *N*-dealkylated and reduced parent compound at the carbon β to the central amide (M10) (Fig. 31.18).[76] The hydrolysis product had a 10-fold lower binding affinity for the M_3 receptor compared to revefenacin, this and its low receptor occupancy suggests minimal activity.[76] No dosage adjustment is required in patients with renal impairment. Adverse effects were reported to be minimal and are similar to

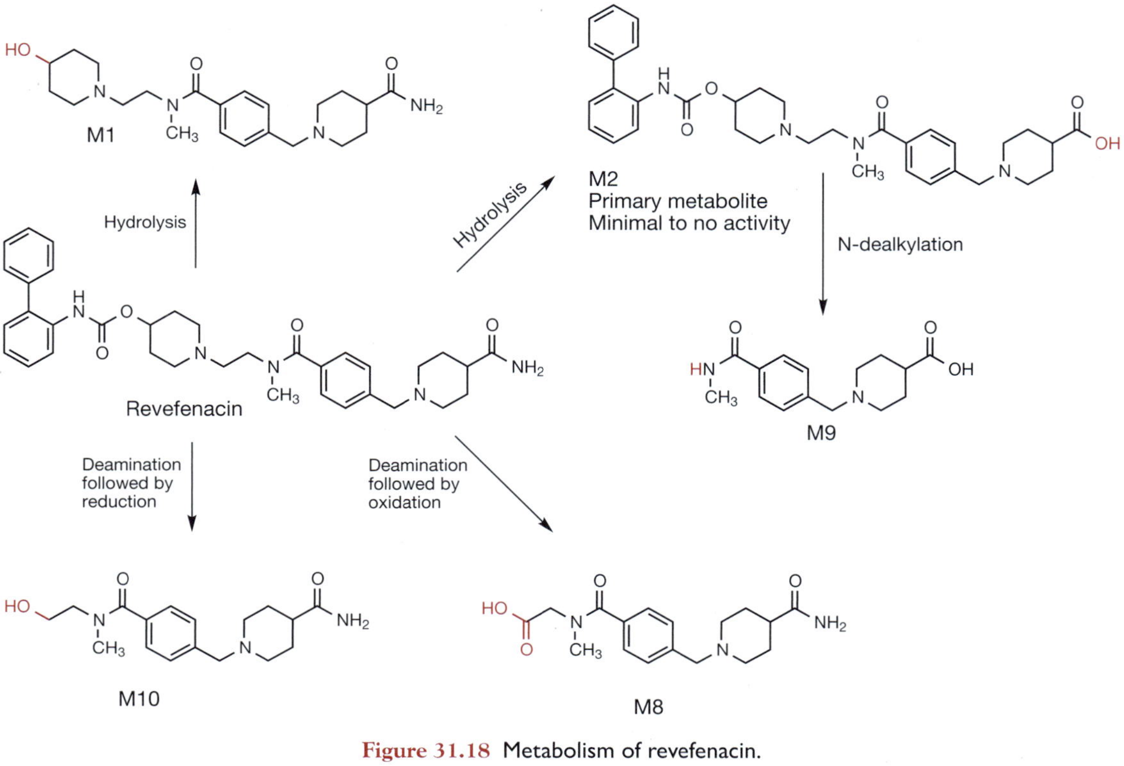

Figure 31.18 Metabolism of revefenacin.

other anticholinergic agents such as nasopharyngitis, cough, upper respiratory tract infections, headache, back pain, and dry mouth.

Methylxanthines

The methylxanthines naturally occur in coffee (*Coffea arabica*), cacao/chocolate (*Theobroma cacao*), and tea (*Camellia sinensis*).[77] The major methylxanthines are caffeine, theophylline, and theobromine, and they differ in the position and number of methyl groups on their xanthine ring system (Fig. 31.19). The amount of methylxanthines in coffee, tea, and chocolate varies widely based on the preparation and source. An 8-ounce cup of coffee contains about 100 mg of caffeine, an 8-ounce cup of tea about 30 to 50 mg, 12 ounces of caffeinated sodas contain about 30 to 40 mg, and an energy drink may contain from 40 to 250 mg per 8 ounces. A 1-oz bar of dark chocolate contains about 130 mg of theobromine, while a 1-oz bar of milk chocolate contains about 44 mg.[78]

Caffeine has been used in neonatal intensive care units to treat apnea of prematurity for over 50 years. Caffeine is a stimulant of the respiratory and central nervous systems, thus increasing respiratory rate and minute volume. It is FDA-approved to use either orally or intravenously since the oral bioavailability approaches 100%. It is metabolized at R_2 by N-demethylation by CYP1A2 (major metabolite 70%) followed by N-acetylation by N-acetyltransferase.[79] Due to the immaturity of the hepatic enzymes and renal function in neonates, the half-life of caffeine is prolonged. In adults, the half-life of caffeine is 3 to 6 hours, whereas in neonates its half-life is approximately 100 hours.[80]

Theophylline is available but not recommended for use in asthma. Its importance has declined greatly since it has a narrow therapeutic window, which requires close patient monitoring and periodic blood level determination to avoid serious side effects. Multiple studies are currently investigating low-dose theophylline in combination with other treatment modalities.

Theophylline Mechanism of Action and Metabolism

Despite being used for over 100 years, the precise mechanism by which theophylline induces bronchodilation remains unclear. There are two commonly proposed mechanisms of action of theophylline. The first is as a nonselective phosphodiesterase (PDE) inhibitor. There are more than 11 families of PDEs, and studies in animals suggest that theophylline inhibits PDE3 and, to a lesser extent, PDE4. Theophylline inhibits the hydrolysis of cAMP and cyclic guanosine monophosphate (cGMP), thus maintaining the downstream activity of PKA, inhibiting TNF-α and inhibiting leukotriene synthesis. In vitro studies have demonstrated theophylline's inhibition of PDEs, and x-ray crystallographic studies have identified the specific binding residues that interact with methylxanthines. The second mechanism is as a nonselective adenosine receptor antagonist, inhibiting bronchoconstriction. Other possible effects of methylxanthines include the modulation of Gamma-aminobutyric acid A ($GABA_A$) receptors and the activation of histone deacetylase isoenzyme type II (HDAC2).[81] The activation of HDAC2 results in switching off an activated inflammatory gene. This may be why a benefit was seen when theophylline was used as an add-on therapy in patients with COPD already on ICS therapy.[82]

The nonselective action of theophylline is also responsible for its side effect profile. The low potency requires high plasma levels for therapeutic efficacy and the need for therapeutic blood level monitoring. The PDE inhibition leads to side effects such as nausea, vomiting, and headaches, and the adenosine antagonism leads to cardiac stimulation and seizures. Because theophylline has only weak efficacy in asthma, it is no longer recommended for use. It also has limited use in COPD. The GOLD Report for COPD states that it has a minor bronchodilator effect compared with placebo in stable COPD, and the addition of theophylline to salmeterol therapy produces a greater improvement in FEV_1 than salmeterol alone; it was ineffective in other combinations.[57]

Chemically, theophylline is 1,3-dimethylxanthine and contains both an acidic and a basic nitrogen (N7 and N9, respectively; see Fig. 31.19). Physiologically, it behaves as an acid ($pK_a = 8.6$), and its poor aqueous solubility can be enhanced by salt formation with organic bases. Theophylline is metabolized by a combination of C-8 oxidation by xanthine oxidase and N-demethylation by CYP1A2 and CYP3A4 to yield methyluric acid metabolites (Fig. 31.20). The major urinary metabolite is 1,3-dimethyl uric acid, which is produced by multiple pathways, including xanthine oxidase, CYP1A2, and CYP2E1.[83]

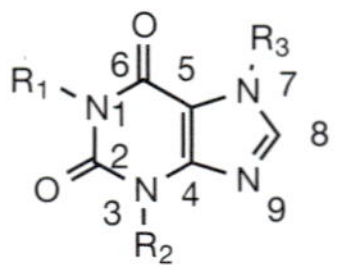

	R_1	R_2	R_3
Caffeine	CH_3	CH_3	CH_3
Theophylline	CH_3	CH_3	H
Theobromine	H	CH_3	CH_3

Figure 31.19 Structural differences between the methylxanthines.

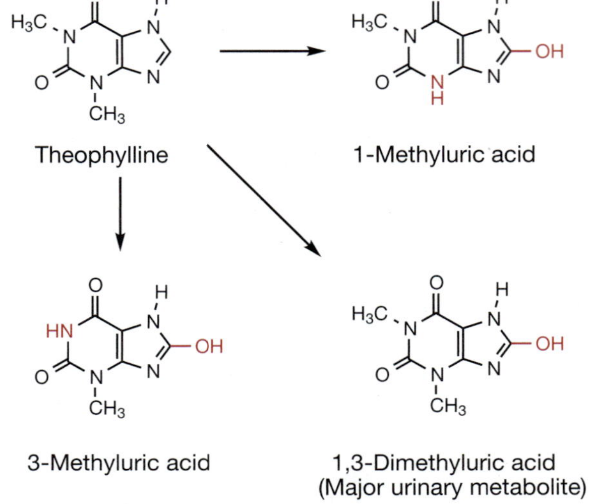

Figure 31.20 Metabolism of theophylline.

Methylxanthine Drugs Used to Treat Asthma

Theophylline

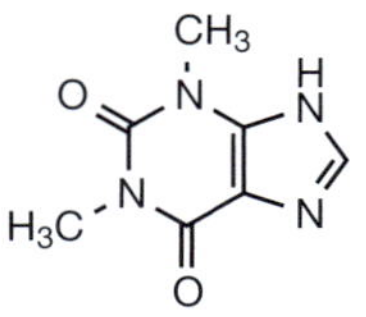

Theophylline
Molecular weight: 180.17

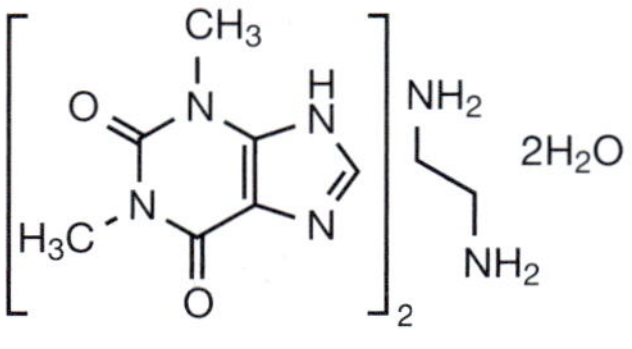

Aminophylline
Molecular weight 456.46

Theophylline has a modest bronchodilator effect compared with placebo in stable COPD. No benefit was found when theophylline was used alone or in combination with corticosteroids on the number of exacerbations of COPD.[57] The primary indication for theophylline is as an add-on controller medication for the treatment of bronchospasm of severe COPD. In addition to bronchodilation effects, theophylline dilates pulmonary blood vessels, acts centrally to stimulate respiration, acts as a diuretic, increases gastric acid secretion, and inhibits uterine contractions. Dosing requires the determination of plasma levels, with 10 to 20 μg/mL associated with the lowest incidence of side effects. Theophylline overdose can result in a quick onset of ventricular arrhythmias, convulsions, or even death without any warning. Many drugs increase the plasma concentration of theophylline, including quinolone and macrolide antibiotics, nonselective β-blockers, ephedrine, calcium channel blockers, cimetidine, and oral contraceptives. Many manufacturers have discontinued producing theophylline, and it is only available in tablet form. Aminophylline is theophylline in a 2:1 ratio with ethylenediamine dihydrate. It is currently only available as a solution for IV injection. Care must be taken to correctly calculate the equivalent dose when switching a patient from theophylline to aminophylline or vice versa.

Adrenocorticoids Used to Treat Asthma and Chronic Obstructive Pulmonary Disease

The major classes of steroids include the corticosteroids (the glucocorticoids and mineralocorticoids) and the sex steroids (the progestins, the androgens, and the estrogens).

The corticosteroids are formed in the adrenal cortex; thus, they are also referred to as adrenocorticoids and they are subdivided into glucocorticoids and mineralocorticoids. The glucocorticoids are so named because they affect glucose homeostasis, but they also have significant anti-inflammatory activity. The mineralocorticoids affect sodium and water retention. The reproductive organs in both the male and female produce steroid hormones, which are responsible for the differentiation of the sex characteristics. This chapter will cover the glucocorticoids used in the treatment of asthma and COPD.

Steroid Nomenclature

The basic structure of a steroid is a tetracyclic (Rings A, B, C, and D) cyclopentanoperhydrophenanthrene, referred to as the steroid nucleus, as depicted in Figure 31.21. The addition of methyl groups at C10 and C13 and of an ethyl group at C17 to the steroid nucleus gives a 21-carbon base structure called pregnane. All glucocorticoids are substituted pregnanes (see Chapter 24). Rings A, B, and C are in the chair conformation in pregnane, and all ring junctions are *trans*. The glucocorticoids all have a double bond at C4 and have a rigid backbone with β (above) and α (below) faces. When dexamethasone is drawn in three dimensions (Fig. 31.21), the position of the substituents in either the α or β face is clear, as is the all-*trans* ring B, C, D backbone. When a double bond is between consecutive carbon numbers (eg, C-4 and C-5), only the first carbon number is noted using the δ designation (Δ^4). If a double bond is between nonconsecutive carbon numbers (eg, C-9 and C-11) both numbers would be indicated for clarity ($\Delta^{9(11)}$). The substituents and their location on either the α or β face are important for binding. The active form of glucocorticoids has hydroxy groups at C11, C17, and C21 as well as 3- and 20-keto groups. For example, hydrocortisone is Δ^4-11β,17α,21-trihydroxy-3,20-pregnenedione (see Fig. 31.21).

Steroid Biosynthesis and Secretion

Adrenocorticoids are biosynthesized from cholesterol. Cholesterol levels are intricately regulated by a balance between dietary intake and endogenous biosynthesis. The adrenocorticoid biosynthesis pathway is shown in Figure 31.22. Of note is the central branching role played by pregnenolone, leading to both classes of the adrenocorticoids.

Once formed, the adrenocorticoids are secreted into the circulatory system, and circulating levels are maintained via a feedback mechanism (Fig. 31.23). When circulating levels are low, the hypothalamus secretes corticotrophin-releasing factor (CRF). In turn, CRF stimulates the anterior pituitary to secrete adrenocorticotrophic hormone, which stimulates

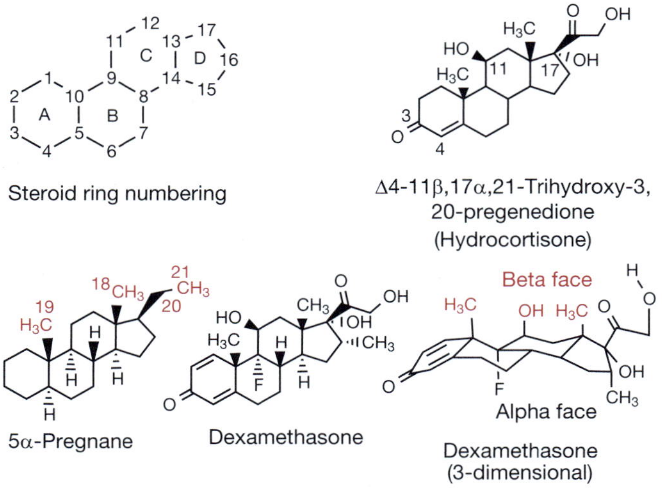

Figure 31.21 Basic skeletons for steroid structures, numbering and nomenclature.

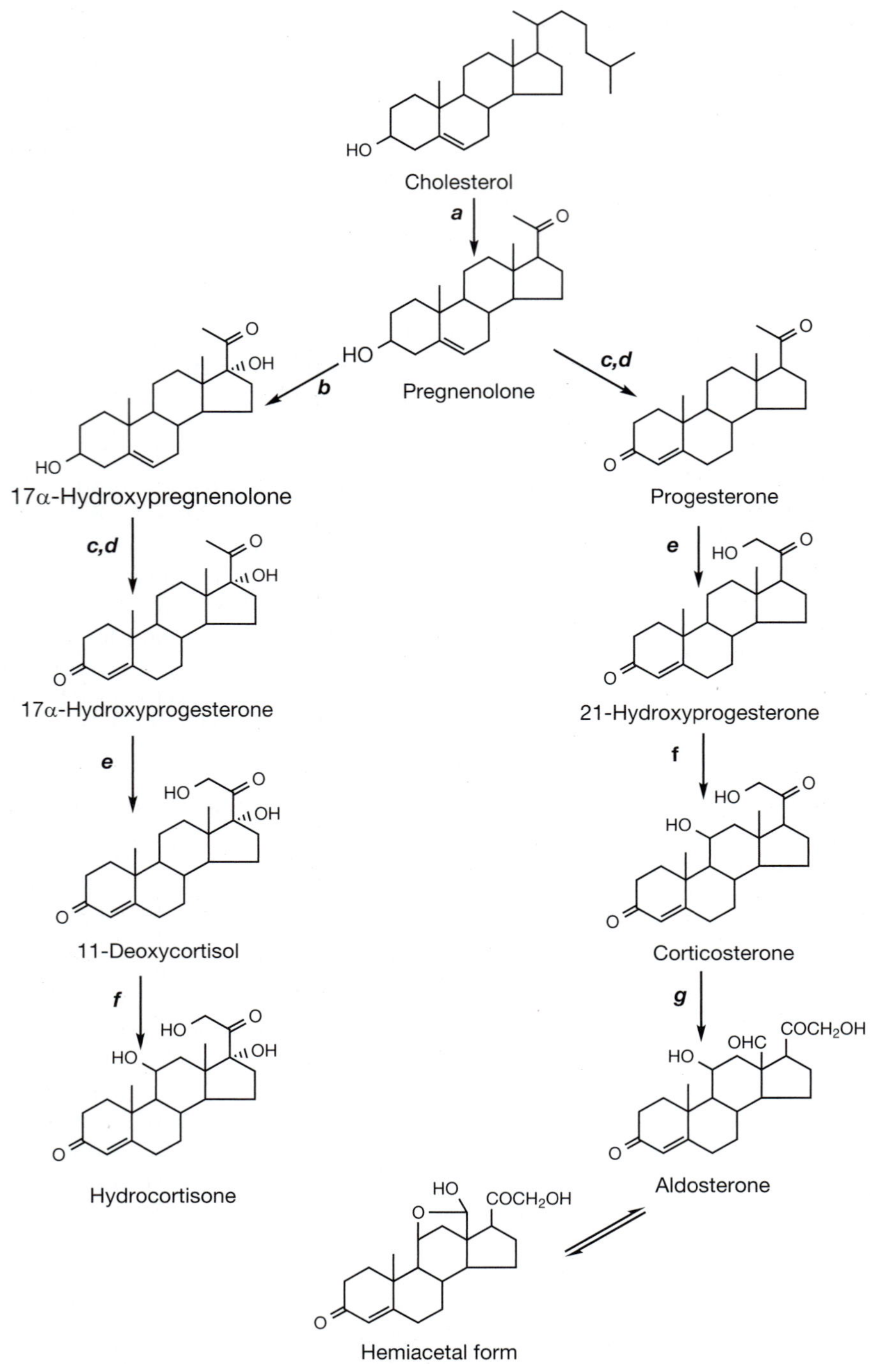

Figure 31.22 Biosynthesis of the adrenocorticoids from cholesterol. The enzymes involved are (a) side chain cleavage enzyme, (b) 17α-hydroxylase, (c) 5-ene-3β-hydroxy-steroid dehydrogenase, (d) 3-oxosteroid-4,5-isomerase, (e) 21-hydroxylase, (f) 11β-hydroxylase, and (g) 18-hydroxylate.

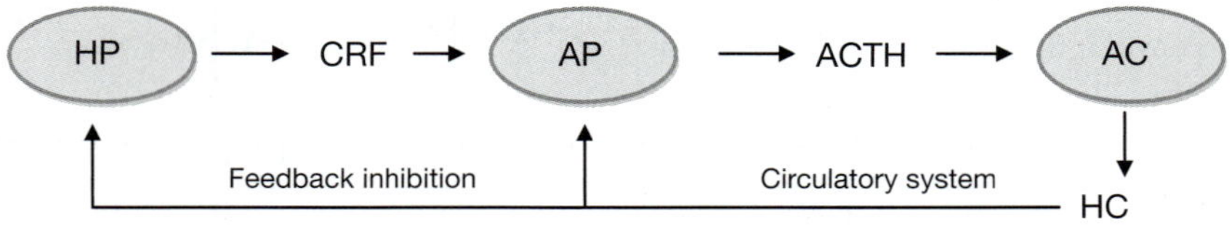

Figure 31.23 Mechanism of adrenocorticoid secretion and control. AC, adrenal cortex; ACTH, adrenocorticotrophic hormone; AP, anterior pituitary; CRF, corticotrophin-releasing factor; HC, hydrocortisone; HP, hypothalamus.

the adrenal cortex to synthesize and secrete the adrenocorticoids (mainly hydrocortisone and aldosterone). When circulating levels of the adrenocorticoids are sufficiently high, they induce a feedback inhibition of CRF secretion from the hypothalamus and adrenocorticotrophic hormone release from the anterior pituitary gland. It should be noted that chronic use of steroids inhibits the adrenal cortex from producing glucocorticoids. This is known as hypothalamus–pituitary–adrenal (HPA) axis suppression. If steroid therapy is stopped abruptly, the lack of endogenous glucocorticoids can be life-threatening. A slow and gradual taper off of exogenous steroid therapy is warranted to allow the HPA axis to recover.

Glucocorticoid Mechanism of Action

The glucocorticoids are nuclear receptor hormones affecting gene transcription. Figure 31.24 summarizes the steps involved in turning on gene transcription. Circulating glucocorticoids enter the target cell by simple diffusion because they are relatively lipophilic (eg, LogP hydrocortisone = 1.61). The glucocorticoid receptor resides in the cytoplasm bound to its chaperone protein complex. The glucocorticoid receptor has three distinct regions: the amino terminus for trans-activating functions (eg, nuclear translocation, phosphorylation, and other protein interactions), a central region for binding to DNA (deoxyribonucleic acid), and the carboxy terminus ligand-binding domain (LBD), where the glucocorticoids bind. When the glucocorticoid binds to its receptor, the heat shock protein is released, resulting in a conformational change in the steroid-receptor complex. The glucocorticoid-receptor complex then translocates into the nucleus of the cell, through nuclear pores. The DNA binding region of the glucocorticoid receptor contains eight Cys amino acid residues that coordinate two zinc ions that form peptide loops called zinc fingers. The zinc finger domains bind to specific sequences of DNA called hormone-response elements (HREs), which are located in the promoter areas of hormone-responsive genes. The HRE motif of DNA stabilizes the dimerization of the glucocorticoid-receptor complex, placing each subunit in adjacent binding grooves. The dimers recruit cofactors, leading to gene transcription.[84] The genes activated by glucocorticoids include anti-inflammatory proteins such as Annexin A-1 (= lipocortin I), secretory leukocyte protease inhibitor, and mitogen-activated protein kinase phosphatase.[85] Annexin A-1 inhibits the enzyme phospholipase A_2, which catalyzes the breakdown of membranes to release arachidonic acid, the first step in the arachidonic acid cascade that results in the production of inflammatory prostaglandins and leukotrienes (see Fig. 31.2). Therefore, inhibition of phospholipase A_2 ultimately results in the reduction of the inflammatory prostaglandins and leukotrienes.[86] The binding of glucocorticoids may also have a transpression activity and block the production of proteins.

Another consequence of glucocorticoids involves inhibition of genes that regulate the expression of inflammatory cytokines, including IL1 through IL-6, IL-8, IL-10, IL-13, GM-CSF, TNFα, and IFN-γ.[86] IL-1 stimulates the proliferation of T and B lymphocytes that are responsible for the production of the cytokines and antibodies, which in turn are important in the inflammatory and immune responses to antigens. The glucocorticoids, by their ability to inhibit IL-1, cause a decrease in T and B lymphocytes, leading to immunosuppression; therefore, they must be used with caution in patients with infection. Glucocorticoids can also work through nongenomic mechanisms and directly inhibit the release of histamines and other autocoids from mast cells.[87]

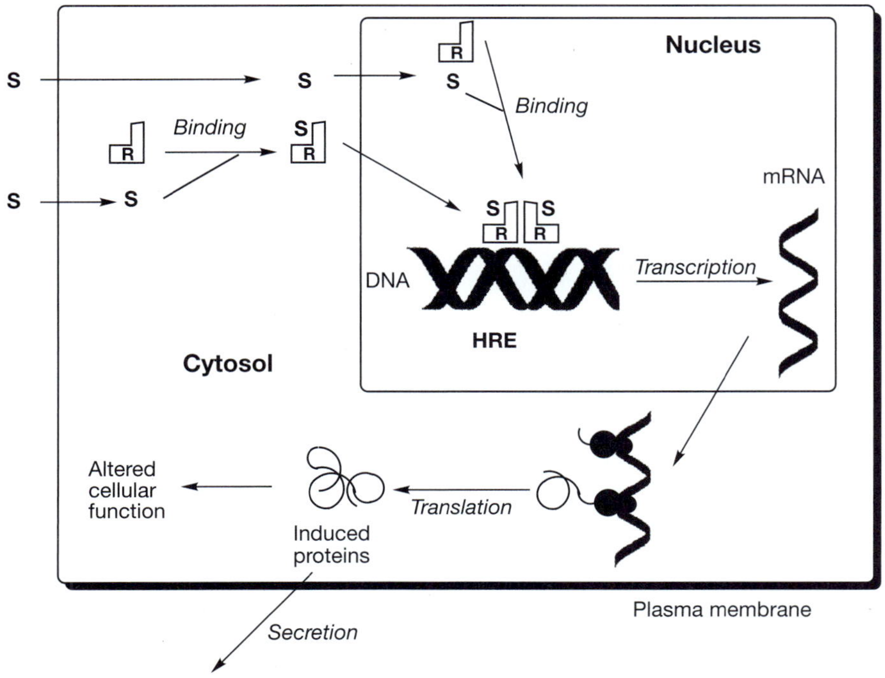

Figure 31.24 Mechanism of steroid hormone action. HRE, hormone response element; R, receptor; S, steroid.

Despite their anti-inflammatory capabilities, glucocorticoid therapy has limitations. They increase blood glucose levels, body weight, and redistribute body fat. They also have adverse effects such as osteoporosis, atherosclerosis, hypertension, and increased risks for infections. Additionally, they have known effects on the CNS such as mood swings, euphoria, and depression. Some patients also exhibit resistance to therapy, referred to as glucocorticoid resistance. This can be inherited through mutations in the *NR3C1* gene or acquired due to chronic glucocorticoid treatment. Glucocorticoid resistance has been observed in 4% to 10% of asthma patients, and most patients with COPD having sepsis.[88]

Receptor Structure and Glucocorticoid Binding

The glucocorticoid receptor is a member of the nuclear receptor superfamily and has three components as discussed: an N-terminus, a central DNA binding domain, and a C-terminal LBD. The LBD of all the steroid receptors consists of 11 α-helices and 4 β-strands. X-ray crystallographic structural analysis, however, has revealed a unique binding pocket in the glucocorticoid receptor, which makes it distinct from the estrogen receptor, androgen receptor, and mineralocorticoid receptor. When a glucocorticoid binds to its receptor, it is completely enclosed within a pocket formed by α helices 3, 4, 5, 6, 7, and 10 and β-strands 1 and 2.

The strong binding affinity for the glucocorticoids is a result of the hydrophobic and hydrophilic interactions with amino acid residues in the ligand binding domain (LBD). Nearly every atom of the glucocorticoid contacts one or more amino acid residues. The most significant contacts are the hydrogen bonding between the hydrophilic groups on the glucocorticoid structure (Fig. 31.25). The carbonyl group on ring A acts as a H-acceptor to both Arg611 and the amide of Gln570. The hydroxyls at C-11 and C-21 are H-donors to the side chain carbonyl oxygen of Asn564. The C-17 hydroxy group hydrogen bonds with Gln642, and the C-20 carbonyl oxygen bonds with Thr739. Glucocorticoid binding to the LBD releases the heat shock protein and stabilizes the receptor in an active form capable of dimerization subsequent to HRE site binding.[89]

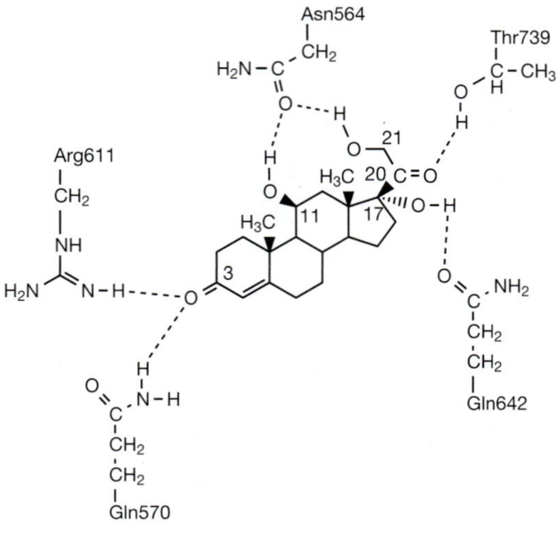

Figure 31.25 Important glucocorticoid receptor–ligand-binding residues.

Glucocorticoid Structure-Activity Relationships

There are essential structural features that are necessary for glucocorticoid activity. The natural glucocorticoids also interact with the mineralocorticoid receptor and, therefore, will have salt-retaining properties. A large number of synthetic analogues have been prepared to decrease the mineralocorticoid effects in favor of increasing the relative glucocorticoid (anti-inflammatory) action of the steroids. In addition, many derivatives are prepared to enhance pharmacokinetic parameters, most notably the synthesis of lipophilic and hydrophilic esters.

Functional groups that are essential for both mineralocorticoid and glucocorticoid activity include the pregnane skeleton with an all-*trans* backbone, the A-ring enone system (Δ^4-3-one), and the 17β-ketol side chain (C-20-keto-C-21-hydroxy). The C-21 hydroxy group must be free for both mineralocorticoid and glucocorticoid activity. Exceptions to this rule are the C-21-chloro and C-20-fluoromethylthio ester ($-SCH_2F$) derivatives that retain anti-inflammatory activity when applied topically or by inhalation. Systemic glucocorticoids that are used for their anti-inflammatory effects and that have both glucocorticoid and mineralocorticoid activities are hydrocortisone, cortisone, prednisone, and prednisolone.

Figure 31.26 specifies the different modifications that have been made to the fundamental structure of pregnanes in order to enhance their anti-inflammatory effects (glucocorticoid activity) while minimizing or eliminating their tendency to cause salt retention (mineralocorticoid activity) when administered in therapeutic doses.

Anti-inflammatory activity is greatly increased by flattening ring A by adding a double bond at C-1 (Δ^1). Anti-inflammatory activity is also increased by adding a hydroxy group at C-11β. A 17α-hydroxy increases both activities, as does 9α-fluoro or 9α-chloro. Mineralocorticoid activity is substantially eliminated by 16α- or 16β-methyl groups, a 16α-hydroxy group, or a 16α,17α-acetonide. A C-6α-methyl group only slightly enhances the anti-inflammatory activity, whereas a C-6α-fluoro doubles the anti-inflammatory effect. By combining a variety of these substituents, multiple synthetic compounds have been marketed with enhanced glucocorticoid activity and reduced mineralocorticoid activity.

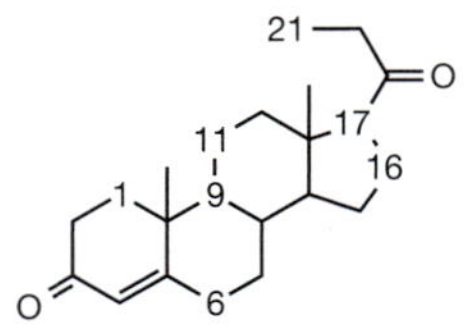

Increases glucocorticoid and mineralcorticoid activity	Increases glucocorticoid activity	Decreases mineralocorticoid activity
17α-OH	Δ^1 (1 ene)	6α-CH_3
9α-F	6α-F>>6α-CH_3	16α or 16β-CH_3
9α-Cl	11β-OH	16α,17α-acetonide
21-OH	16α or 16β-CH_3	16α-OH

Figure 31.26 Glucocorticoid structure-activity relationships.

Table 31.4 Inhaled Corticosteroid Binding Affinity

Drug	Receptor Binding Affinity Relative to Dexamethasone
Dexamethasone	100
Beclomethasone dipropionate	53 1,345 active metabolite)
Budesonide	935
Ciclesonide (des-CIC) MDI	12 (1,200)
Flunisolide MDI	190
Fluticasone propionate DPI	1,775
Fluticasone furoate DPI	2,989
Mometasone furoate	2,100
Triamcinolone acetonide MDI	233

DPI, dry powder inhaler; MDI, metered dose inhaler.
Adapted with permission from Matera MG, Rinaldi B, Calzetta L, Rogliani P, Cazzola M. Pharmacokinetics and pharmacodynamics of inhaled corticosteroids for asthma treatment. *Pulm Pharmacol Ther.* 2019;58:101828.

When used at high doses and for extended periods, mineralocorticoid side effects can occur. Table 31.4 lists the binding affinity of a number of glucocorticoids compared to dexamethasone.[90] Binding affinity of dexamethasone is given the standard affinity of 100 for comparison, and this is used as a proxy for potency. Most glucocorticoids in the table have a higher affinity to the receptor compared to dexamethasone. Fluticasone furoate (FF) has the highest affinity while the parent drug ciclesonide had the lowest affinity. The metabolite of ciclesonide, desisobutyryl-ciclesonide, shows a 100-fold greater binding activity than ciclesonide.[90]

The addition of a double bond between carbon 9 and 11 yields novel steroids with interesting receptor affinity, a number of these are in development.[89] Vamorolone has this 9,11 double bond and has anti-mineralocorticoid activity and acts as a partial agonist of the glucocorticoid receptor with transrepression activities but limited transactivation activities.[91] It is only approved for Duchenne muscular dystrophy, and a full discussion is beyond the scope of this chapter.

Glucocorticoid Metabolism

If one or more of the essential functional groups on the glucocorticoid skeleton are modified by metabolism, glucocorticoid activity will be lost. There are three major metabolic reactions that will eliminate glucocorticoid activity. They are ring A reductions, C-17 oxidation, and C-11 keto-enol isomerization. Reduction of the ring A 3-keto to a 3α-hydroxy by 3α-hydroxysteroid dehydrogenase and the reduction of the 4,5-double bond by 5β-reductase to produce the A/B *cis*-fused ring give rise to inactive metabolites (Fig. 31.27). Oxidation of the C-17 side chain to produce a 17-keto steroid requires both the C-17 hydroxy group and a free C-21 hydroxy group. Esterification of one or both will inhibit this metabolism and prolong the duration of action. The rapid in vivo equilibrium that exists between cortisone (11-keto) and hydrocortisone (11β-hydroxy) is catalyzed by 11β-hydroxysteroid dehydrogenase and produces the keto form that is inactive but also regenerates the hydroxy form that is highly glucocorticoid enhancing and found on all glucocorticoids. Figure 31.27 summarizes the metabolism of hydrocortisone.

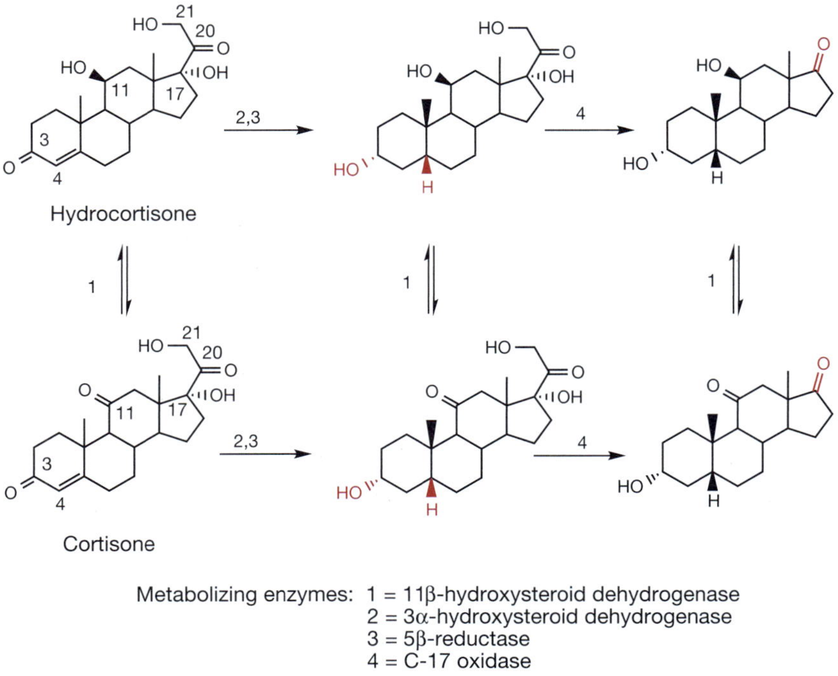

Figure 31.27 Metabolic pathways for hydrocortisone.

Synthetic Steroid Esters

The glucocorticoids are lipophilic despite having at least three hydroxy groups. The hydroxy groups can be esterified with an appropriate acid that will either enhance or decrease lipophilicity. The C-21 hydroxy group is the most accessible and, therefore, is the easiest to esterify. The C-17 hydroxy group is easily esterified, but because it is slightly hindered by the C-17 side chain, it will react more slowly. The C-11 hydroxy group is highly hindered by the C-10 and C-13 methyl groups and will not react with acids to form esters. In addition, esterification affects both receptor affinity and glucocorticoid metabolism. Because the C-21 hydroxy must be free to hydrogen bond to the Arg564 in the glucocorticoid receptor, C-21 esters are prodrugs requiring hydrolysis to become active. Also, the C-17 hydroxy group needs to be free to be metabolically oxidized; therefore, esterification of the C-17 hydroxy group inhibits oxidation to the C-17 keto group and prolongs the duration of action. Duration also is prolonged because the lipophilic glucocorticoid esters do not concentrate in the urine (ie, they undergo tubular reabsorption after glomerular filtration).

The lipophilicity of a glucocorticoid can be enhanced by esterification with lipophilic acids. The increased LogP may slow dissolution and pulmonary absorption and enhance residence time in the lungs, leading to less frequent dosing. The fact that C-21 lipophilic esters are prodrugs means that they have longer durations of action. They also have a slower onset because the lipophilic esters generally are bulky and retard hydrolytic enzymes.

These lipophilic prodrugs can be administered orally to treat a variety of conditions, by inhalation to treat asthma and COPD, and topically to treat dermatitis. When administered orally, their longer duration of action means that they can be given less frequently, which often results in better patient adherence. When administered topically, C-21 lipophilic ester prodrugs are activated by hydrolysis by skin esterases.[92] Figure 31.28 shows the structures of the most common C-21 lipophilic esters found on commercially available glucocorticoids.

Diesters and ketals provide a further enhancement of log P and an increased duration of action because they are slowly metabolized (Fig. 31.29). Diesters are formed at C-21 and at either the C-17α or, if present, the C-16α hydroxyl groups, although 16α is a more sterically constrained position compared to 17α. Diesters and hexacetonides are prodrugs due to the esterification of the C-21-OH. Esters at C-17α or C-16α are active and intact.

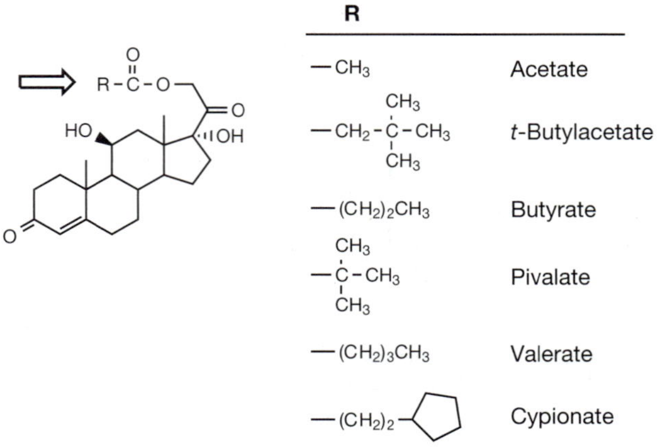

Figure 31.28 Common lipophilic esters of glucocorticoids.

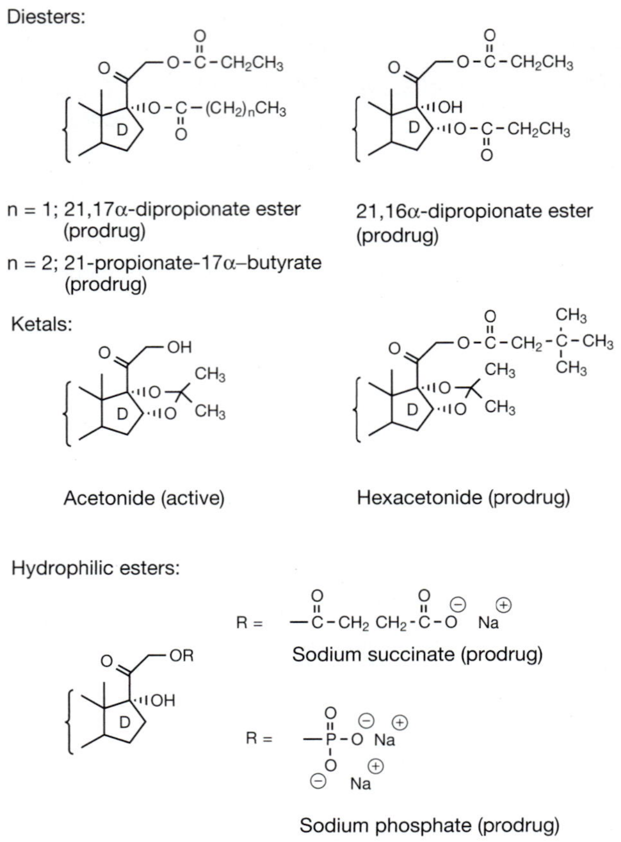

Figure 31.29 Examples of glucocorticoid lipophilic diesters and ketals and hydrophilic esters.

A ketal is a cyclic derivative formed between hydroxy groups on adjacent carbons and a carbonyl carbon of a ketone. The most common ketal found in glucocorticoids is called an acetonide and is the condensation product formed between the C-16α and C-17α hydroxy groups and the carbonyl carbon of acetone (CH_3COCH_3) (Fig. 31.29). Ketals with a free C-21 hydroxy group are active. If the acetonide is found along with a C-21-t-butylacetate ester, it is named a hexacetonide; the "hex" refers to the total number of carbons found in the butylacetate group. The hexacetonides are prodrugs and must hydrolyze at C-21 to become active.

Esterification also can be used to increase the hydrophilicity of the glucocorticoids, making them water-soluble prodrugs. The synthetic approach here is to use either a dicarboxylic acid or phosphoric acid to condense with the C-21 hydroxy group (Fig. 31.29). This places an ionizable group (a carboxylate or phosphate) on the prodrug, yielding water-soluble esters. These derivatives are used to prepare aqueous injectable products that can be administered intramuscularly or IV.

Hydrophilic glucocorticoid prodrugs have a rapid onset because they are readily hydrolyzed by plasma esterases. In contrast to the lipophilic prodrugs, their water solubility allows them to be easily excreted through the kidney, resulting in a shorter duration of action. Hydrophilic prodrugs have more systemic side effects because of the wide distribution that comes from their high solubility in the blood. Along with their ability to be injected IV, this property makes them useful in asthmatic emergencies (ie, status asthmaticus) when the patient is unable to take oral medication.

Glucocorticoid Drugs Used to Treat Asthma

Systemic Glucocorticoids[93]

Hydrocortisone

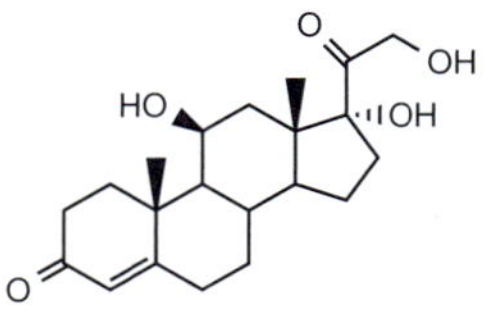

Hydrocortisone
Δ^4-11β,17α,21-Trihydroxy-3,20-pregnenedione
(Cortisol)

Hydrocortisone is endogenous, and it has both glucocorticoid and mineralocorticoid activity. Functional groups that are essential for both mineralocorticoid and glucocorticoid activity include the pregnane skeleton with an all-*trans* backbone, the A-ring Δ^4-3-one system, and the 17β-ketol side chain. The glucocorticoid activity is enhanced by the C-11β and C-17α hydroxy groups. Hydrocortisone can be used to treat severe asthmatic attacks, and oral administration is as effective as IV. IV administration may be necessary if patient is unable to swallow, is vomiting, or is intubated. Due to its mineralocorticoid activity, it is not recommended for patients with hypertension.

Prednisolone

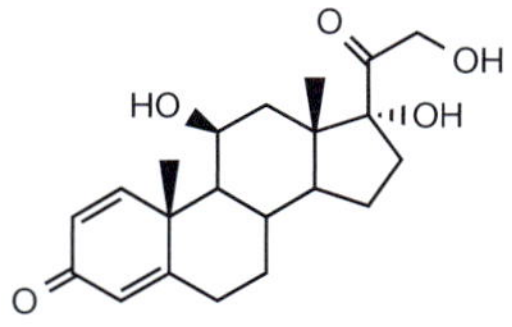

Prednisolone
$\Delta^{1,4}$-11β,17α,21-trihydroxy-pregnadiene-3,20-dione

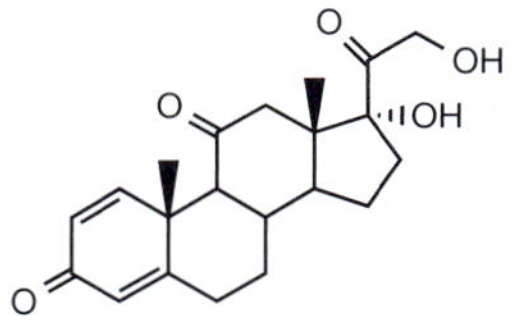

Prednisone
$\Delta^{1,4}$-17α,21-dihydroxy-pregnadiene-3,11,20-trione

Prednisolone is hydrocortisone with an additional Δ^1 double bond. This forms an A-ring that is conjugated from C-1 to C-5, and the trigonal coplanar sp^2 hybridized carbons flatten the ring to increase glucocorticoid action at the expense of mineralocorticoid activity. Prednisolone has 4-fold the glucocorticoid activity of hydrocortisone while having approximately half its mineralocorticoid activity. In addition, prednisolone has an increased duration of action compared to hydrocortisone because the extra double bond in ring A retards metabolic reduction.

Prednisolone can be used to treat severe asthmatic attacks and is available in tablet form or liquid form for children. The C-21 sodium phosphate ester is available for parenteral use. A nonester prodrug of prednisolone is prednisone. It is the 11-keto analogue of prednisolone and must be converted in vivo to the active 11β-hydroxy metabolite, which is necessary to serve as an H-donor in a hydrogen bond to Asn564 in the glucocorticoid receptor. Prednisone should not be used in patients with hepatic dysfunction, because their ability to reduce the 11-keto group with 11β-hydroxysteroid dehydrogenase to the active metabolite may be impaired.

When orally administered, prednisone and prednisolone are almost completely absorbed, with a bioavailability greater than 80%. Prednisolone is metabolized into several hydrophilic and less active metabolites. The major metabolites (6β- and 16β-hydroxy analogues) are primarily excreted as glucuronide conjugates in the urine.

Methylprednisolone

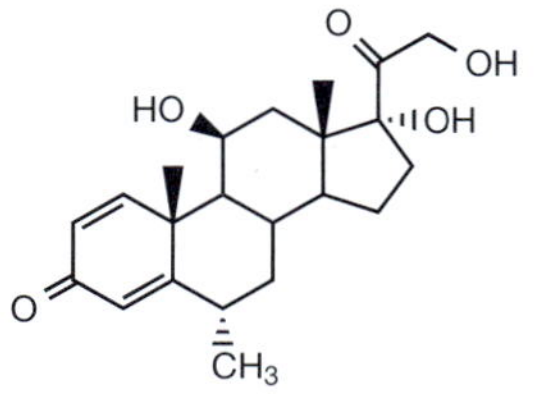

Methylprednisolone
$\Delta^{1,4}$-6α-methyl-11β,17α,21-trihydroxy-pregnadiene-3,20-dione
(Medrol)

Adding a 6α-methyl group to prednisolone increases the glucocorticoid activity and effectively abolishes mineralocorticoid action. It has 5-fold the glucocorticoid activity of hydrocortisone (25% more than prednisolone) and none of its mineralocorticoid properties. The administration of methylprednisolone IV is included in the GINA guidelines for the initial management of asthma exacerbations in children aged 5 years and younger.[13] Methylprednisolone is administered intravenously as its water-soluble sodium salt of the 21-succinate ester. The succinate ester is slowly and incompletely hydrolyzed, and peak plasma levels are attained in approximately 30 to 60 minutes.

Methylprednisolone is extensively metabolized in the liver primarily via CYP3A4. The metabolic pathways include oxidation of the C-11-OH to the ketone, reduction of the C-20 ketone, 6β-hydroxylation, and 6,7 dehydrogenation.[94] Coadministration with CYP3A4 inhibitors can potentiate the effects of methylprednisolone, and CYP3A4 inducers can increase hepatic clearance, which may necessitate dose adjustments.

Dexamethasone

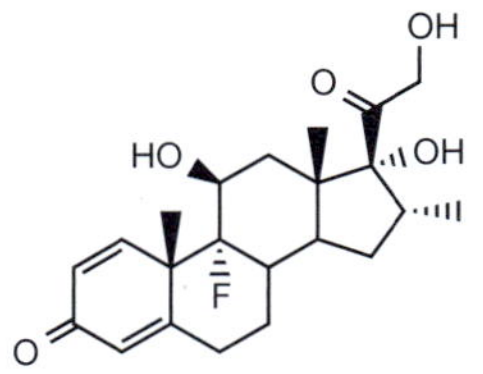

Dexamethasone
$\Delta^{1,4}$-9-α–fluoro-11β,17α,21-trihydroxy-16α-methylpregnadiene-3,20-dione

Dexamethasone is a potent glucocorticoid having approximately 30 times the glucocorticoid potency of hydrocortisone with minimal mineralocorticoid activity. The 9α-F group increases potency at the glucocorticoid receptor and, as an electron withdrawing group, decreases the metabolism by

11β-hydroxysteroid dehydrogenase. This gives dexamethasone a long duration of action (36-72 hours). The 16α-methyl group decreases the binding to the mineralocorticoid receptor, thus decreasing mineralocorticoid-related side effects such as sodium and fluid retention. It also increased binding at the glucocorticoid receptor. The stereochemistry of the 16-methyl is not important as both the α and β methyl are tolerated. Betamethasone has the same structure as dexamethasone, but the 16 methyl is in the β face. It is available only as a topical cream. Dexamethasone is available as a tablet, solution, and IV/IM formulations. Dexamethasone, hydrocortisone, prednisolone, and prednisone are all used as systemic oral corticosteroids in the emergency management of asthma.[95] Dexamethasone undergoes typical glucocorticoid metabolism by CYP3A4 to the 6α-OH and 6β-OH metabolites, oxidation at the 11β-OH, and reduction of the C-20 carbonyl.[96]

Side Effects. Systemic administration of glucocorticoids can result in a large number of adverse effects on prolonged use. As previously stated, there is the serious risk of HPA axis suppression, requiring the slow tapering of the dose. In addition, glucocorticoids can affect the following systems:

- cardiovascular (thromboembolism, hypertension, and arrhythmias)
- immune system (immunosuppression, worsening of existing tuberculosis, fungal, bacterial, viral, or parasitic infection)
- infections (more serious or even a fatal course of chickenpox or measles can occur in susceptible patients)
- CNS (seizures, depression, and steroid psychosis)
- dermatologic (acne, thin fragile skin, hair thinning, and impaired wound healing)
- endocrine (decreased glucose tolerance, menstrual irregularities, and suppression of growth in children)
- GI (pancreatitis, increased appetite, nausea, and peptic ulcer)
- musculoskeletal (muscle weakness, steroid myopathy, and osteoporosis)
- ophthalmic (cataracts, increased intraocular pressure, and glaucoma)
- electrolyte disturbances (sodium and fluid retention, and hypokalemic alkalosis)
- other (weight gain, abnormal fat deposits, moon face)

Glucocorticoids for Inhalation[93]

Beclomethasone Dipropionate

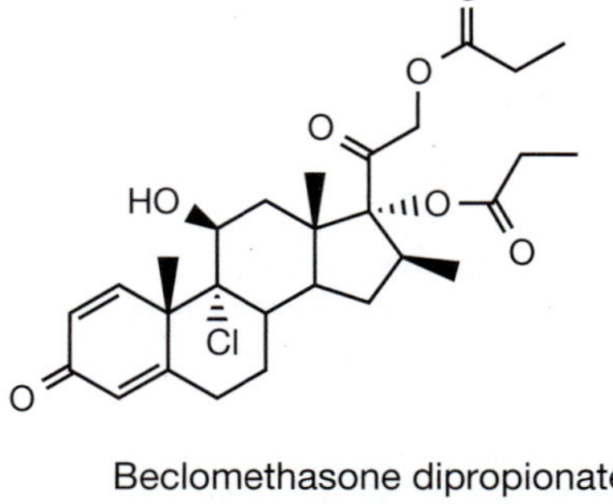

Beclomethasone dipropionate
9α-Chloro-16β-methyl-11β-hydroxypregna-1,4-diene-3,20-dione 17α,21-dipropionate
(QVAR)

Beclomethasone dipropionate is a lipophilic diester prodrug that, when inhaled, shows a systemic bioavailability of approximately 20%. While the 9α-chloro substituent normally increases both glucocorticoid and mineralocorticoid activity, the 16β-methyl group essentially abolishes mineralocorticoid action, resulting in potent anti-inflammatory activity with little or no salt-retaining effects. The main adverse effects are headache, sinusitis, and sinus pain. Beclomethasone dipropionate is hydrolyzed in the lungs and liver by esterases to form three metabolites. The C21 ester is hydrolyzed to form the active 17α-monopropionate derivative. The 17α ester is metabolized to form the 17α hydroxyl C21-monopropionate. Less commonly, both esters are metabolized by esterases. Beclomethasone 17α-monopropionate has 30-fold greater affinity for the GR than when both esters are metabolized. When only the 17α ester is metabolized, the compound is essentially inactive.[97] CYP3A4 and CYP3A5 present in both the liver and lung metabolize beclomethasone via β-hydroxylation at C-6 and dehydrogenation at C-6,7. Beclomethasone dipropionate and its metabolites are mainly excreted in the feces, with less than 10% of the drug and metabolites excreted in the urine.

Budesonide

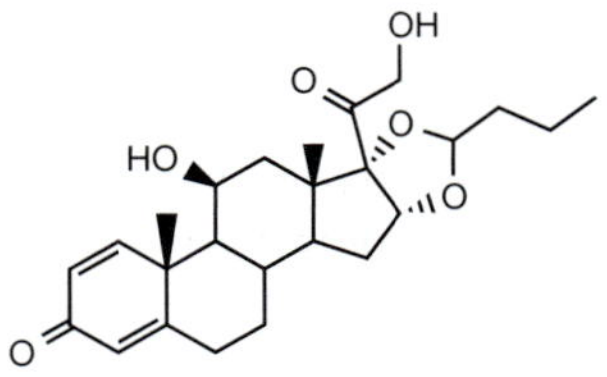

Budesonide
16α,17α-[(*R,S*-butylidenebis(oxy)]-11β,21-dihydroxypregna-1,4-diene-3,20-dione
(Pulmacort turbuhaler, Respules)

Budesonide is an acetal formed between the 16α,17α-dihydroxy groups and butanal. It is a nonhalogenated glucocorticoid with decreased mineralocorticoid activity due to the presence of the 16α-17α ketal. In receptor affinity studies, the acetal C-22 *R*-epimer was twice as active as the *S* but it is marketed as the racemic mixture. Because the C-21 hydroxy is free, budesonide is not a prodrug and is active as administered.

Systemically absorbed budesonide is highly protein-bound and metabolized by CYP3A4 to 6β-hydroxybudesonide in the liver. Carbon 22 of the ketal is hydroxylated to form an intermediary that is further metabolized to 16α-hydroxyprednisolone. Both metabolites have less than 1% of the glucocorticoid activity of the parent compound.[98] It is known that the polar 16α-OH decreases glucocorticoid affinity (the complimentary receptor residues are lipophilic), and activity can be retained only if augmented by other glucocorticoid-enhancing groups (eg, 9α-F as found in triamcinolone, discussed later). Inhaled budesonide is excreted mainly as metabolites via both feces and urine. Approximately 60% of an IV radiolabeled dose was recovered in the urine. Twenty minutes after an inhalation, up to 70% to 80% is reversibly esterified by free fatty acids in the airway tissue. These inactive long chain esters behave like an intracellular depot drug by slowly regenerating free budesonide. Thus, esterification prolongs the local anti-inflammatory action of budesonide in the airways allowing for once-daily dosing despite the relatively short plasma half-life of 4.5 hours.[99] Budesonide is available as a powder delivered as an aerosol or as a suspension for nebulizer inhalation or in combination products (see Table 31.2).

Ciclesonide

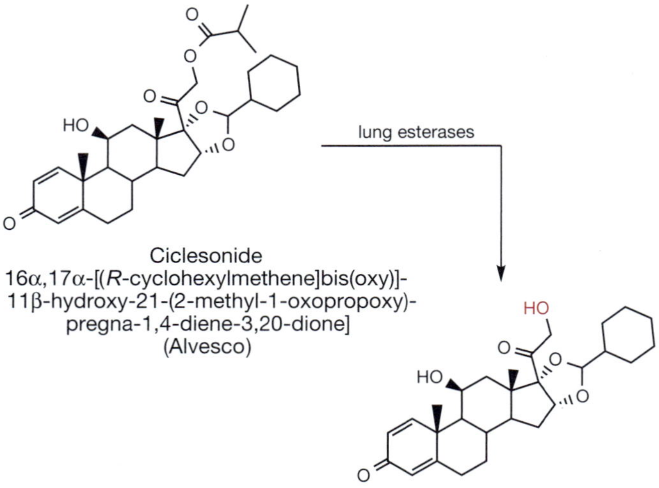

Ciclesonide
16α,17α-[(*R*-cyclohexylmethene]bis(oxy)]-11β-hydroxy-21-(2-methyl-1-oxopropoxy)-pregna-1,4-diene-3,20-dione]
(Alvesco)

Desisobutyrylciclesonide
(active metabolite)

Ciclesonide is a glucocorticoid with an acetal formed at positions C16α and C17α with cyclohexylcarboxaldehyde. A 16α–oxygen atom, including the one found in glucocorticoid acetals, decreases mineralocorticoid activity. In addition, ciclesonide has a Δ^1 that retards ring A reduction, promoting a longer duration of action, and increasing glucocorticoid action at the expense of mineralocorticoid activity through conformational influences, as previously described. Ciclesonide is a prodrug that is converted to the active C-21-OH (>100×) desisobutyrylciclesonide (des-CIC) via esterases in the lung. It is reported to have a relative potency equivalent to beclomethasone dipropionate (Table 31.4). In vitro and in vivo studies show that the des-CIC metabolite forms reversible conjugates with fatty acids (des-CIC-oleate and des-CIC-palmitate) that act as reservoirs for the active metabolite in the lungs. This may support the once-daily dosing regimen of ciclesonide.[100] Lung deposition on inhalation is 52%, and the oral bioavailability is less than 1%, presumably due to low GI absorption and high first-pass metabolism. Desisobutyrylciclesonide is metabolized in the liver to polar metabolites mainly hydroxylated des-CIC.[101] Ciclesonide is available as an HFA MDI (Alvesco) and a nasal spray (Omnaris) for the treatment of hay fever.

Flunisolide

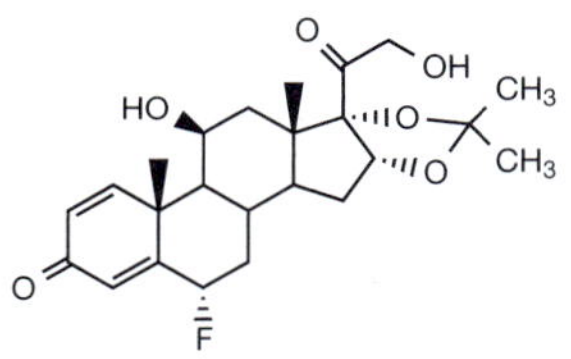

Flunisolide
6α-Fluoro-11β,21-dihydroxy-16α,17α-(acetonide)-pregna-1,4-diene-3,20-dione

Inhaled forms of flunisolide are approved, but only available in a nasal form in the United States. Flunisolide is an active acetone ketal (acetonide) with a 6α-fluoro group and a free C-21 hydroxyl group. As with other acetonides, the 16α-oxygen decreases mineralocorticoid activity and the 6α-fluoro group increases glucocorticoid activity. Flunisolide is metabolized by CYP3A4 to the Δ^6-flunisolide, 21-carboxyflunisolide, and the defluorinated 6β-OH flunisolide.[98] This, along with the rapid elimination of both flunisolide and its hydroxy metabolite as glucuronides, greatly limits systemic exposure. Flunisolide is available as a nasal spray for allergic rhinitis.

Fluticasone Propionate and Fluticasone Furoate

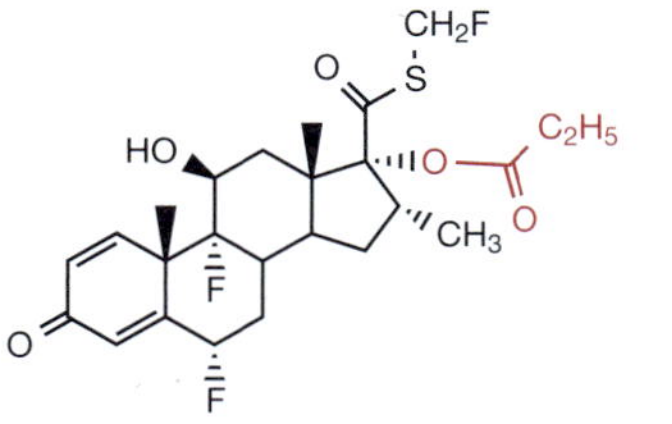

Fluticasone propionate
17β-carbothiolate-20-*S*-(fluoromethyl) 6α,9-difluoro-17α-proprionate-11β–hydroxy-16α-methyl-1,4-diene

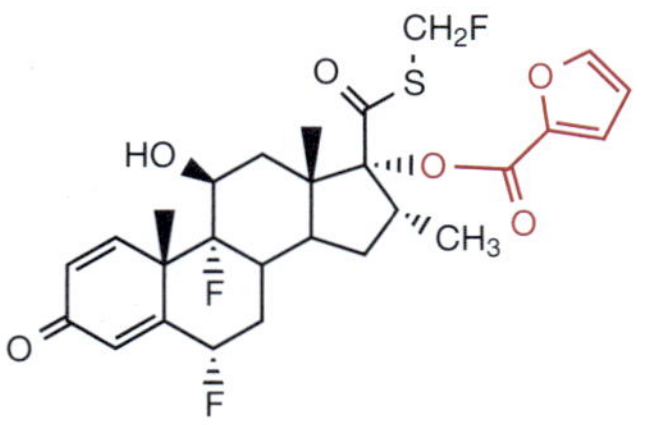

Fluticasone furoate
17β-carbothiolate-20-*S*-(fluoromethyl)-6α,9-difluoro-17α–[(2-furanyl-carbonyl)-oxy]-11β–hydroxy-16α-methyl-1,4-diene

Fluticasone propionate (FP) and fluticasone furoate (FF) are two distinct drugs. The unusual naming convention that gives the 17α ester substituent its own name leads to confusion. The fluticasone 17α esters are stable and are not metabolized; thus, they are unique drugs that bind at the GR with their ester intact.[102] Neither FP nor FF are prodrugs.

The 9α-fluoro group of fluticasone increases both glucocorticoid and mineralocorticoid activities. The 6α-fluoro group enhances only the glucocorticoid binding.

The 17β position of both FP and FF is substituted with a unique fluoromethyl thioester. This group also binds specifically to the GR. The x-ray crystal docking studies have shown that the fluoromethylthio fluorine of FP and FF makes favorable electrostatic interaction with the Asn564 in this pocket. The thioester is stable in lung tissue but is rapidly metabolized in the liver to the inactive carboxylic acid. This results in an oral bioavailability of less than 1%. This is a good example of an ante-drug strategy.[2] Evidence suggests that the thioester is not cleaved by esterases but by CYP3A4.[98] The main metabolite is the inactive 17β-carboxylic acid, which is eliminated through both the feces and the urine.

As stated earlier, in addition to the 17β pocket, there is a 17α hydrophobic pocket on the GR. The 17α pocket that binds the FP and FF esters shows a clear binding preference for the FF ester. Thus FF has 60% greater binding affinity than FP for the 17α binding pocket.[103] The enhanced potency is reflected in Table 31.4. FF has a longer duration of action in experimental models. The efficacy of FF 100 μg/d was comparable to that of medium and high dose FP (500-1,000 μg/d).[104] Fluticasone furoate and propionate show a similar time to effect onset, reaching their efficacy plateau at approximately 2 weeks.

Fluticasone propionate (FP) is available in aerosol and powder inhalation formulations. FF is available in combination forms (see Table 31.2). Confusingly, the adult form of OTC Flonase uses FP (Flonase) while the pediatric form of the OTC Flonase (Fluticasone Sensimist) uses FF.

Mometasone Furoate

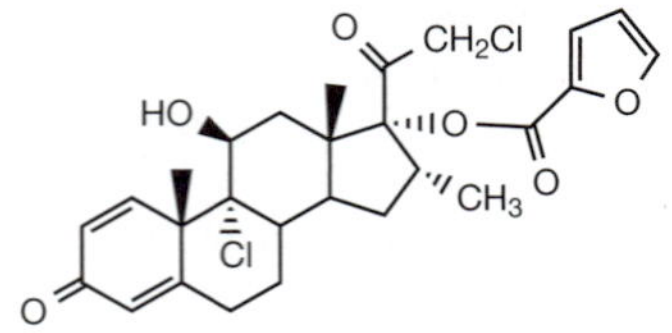

Mometasone furoate
9α,21-dichloro-17α-[(2-furanylcarbonyl)oxy]-11β-hydroxy-16α-methylpregna-1,4-diene-3,20-dione
(Asmanex Twisthaler)

Mometasone furoate contains a C-9α-Cl, a C-21 chloro substituent, and a furoic acid ester at C-17α results in high glucocorticoid receptor affinity. As with beclomethasone, while the 9α-chloro group is known to increase both glucocorticoid and mineralocorticoid activity, the 16α-methyl eliminates mineralocorticoid action in the same way beclomethasone's 16β-methyl does. It is extensively metabolized undergoing 17α ester hydrolysis, 6β-hydroxylation, and C21 hydroxylation with the loss of the chloro substituent.[105] Inhaled mometasone furoate is mainly excreted in the feces (~74%) as metabolites and only minimally excreted in the urine (~8%). It has a relatively long half-life in the lung and is administered once daily, usually in the evening. It is currently only available in inhaled form in combination with LABAs (see Table 31.2).[106]

Triamcinolone Acetonide

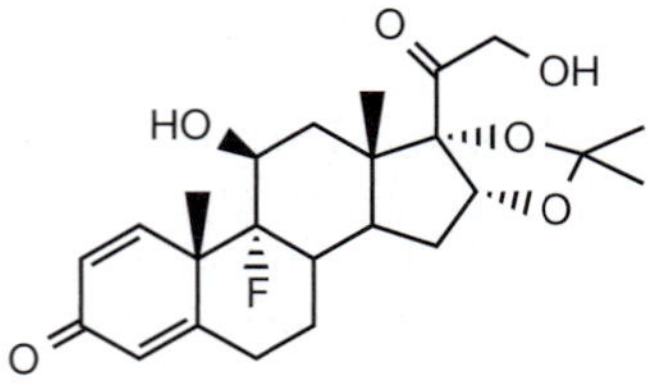

Triamcinolone acetonide
9α-Fluoro-11β,21-dihydroxypregna-1,4-diene-3,20-dione-16α,17α-acetonide (Nasacort)

Triamcinolone acetonide has the 16α,17α acetonide, which abolishes most mineralocorticoid activity. The 9α-fluoro group, known to increase both the glucocorticoid and the mineralocorticoid activities, essentially promotes only glucocorticoid action in drugs with mineralo-abolishing functional groups. Triamcinolone acetonide has low GR affinity compared to other inhaled glucocorticoids. It is still an FDA-approved medication but no longer manufactured as an MDI. It is currently available only as a nasal spray. It is metabolized in the liver to a number of metabolites, including 6β-hydroxytriamcinolone acetonide and the C-21 carboxy-6β-hydroxytriamcinolone acetonide, both of which are readily excreted via the kidneys. The C-21 nortriamcinolone has also been identified as a metabolite.[98] The acetonide is highly resistant to hydrolytic cleavage and remains intact during metabolic transformation. Triamcinolone acetonide is excreted mainly as metabolites in the urine (40%) and feces (60%), with less than 1% being excreted unchanged.[107]

Mast Cell–Degranulation Inhibitors

The discovery that a Middle Eastern herb, *Ammi visnaga* (Khella, Bishop's weed), had mild bronchodilation effects led to the isolation of the benzopyrone (a chromone), khellin. Khellin had only weak bronchodilator effects, so synthetic analogues were prepared in an attempt to enhance the bronchodilation. Dr Roger Altounyans, who was experimenting on himself with these analogues, discovered that if inhaled before an asthmatic attack, it could attenuate the symptoms.[108] The active compound was identified as a bischromone and named cromolyn sodium (Fig. 31.30).

This class of compounds is known as mast cell stabilizers or mast cell degranulation inhibitors. They prevent the release of histamine, leukotrienes, prostaglandins, and other inflammatory autocoids by interaction with the sensitized mast cell before antigenic challenge. They do not inhibit the binding of IgE to the mast cell or the antigen to IgE. The exact mechanism of action is still not completely understood; however, it is clear that inhibition of the role of calcium in the degranulation process is involved. Several membrane and cellular proteins that bind cromolyn sodium are known to regulate intracellular calcium levels, including basophilic membrane protein, nucleoside diphosphate kinase, S100 proteins, calgranulins B and C, and annexins I through V.[109,110] They are FDA-approved for asthma, allergic rhinitis, allergic eye conditions as well as systemic mast cell disease (mastocytosis). They are not immediate acting so they cannot treat acute asthma attacks.

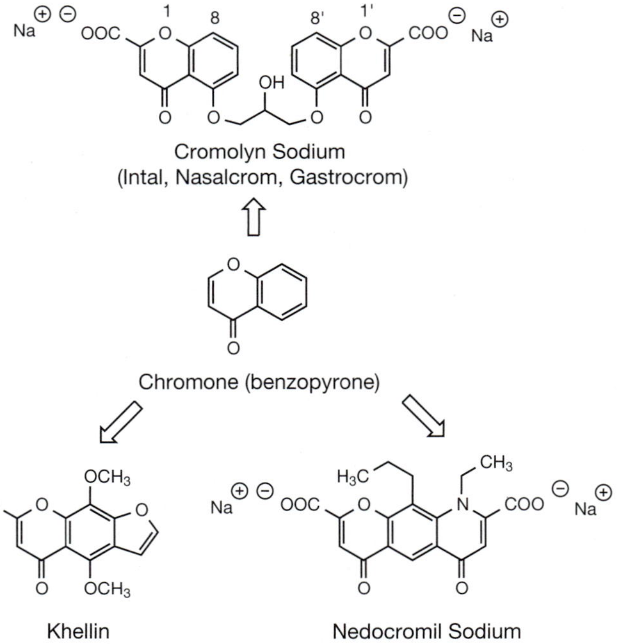

Figure 31.30 Structures of several chromone mast cell stabilizers.

Mast Cell Stabilizers Used to Treat Asthma

Cromolyn Sodium

Cromolyn sodium is a bischromone that contains the fundamental benzopyrone moiety of khellin (see Fig. 31.30). The two chromone rings are necessary for activity and must be coplanar, with a linking chain of no longer than six carbons. If one changes the linking chain to positions 8 and 8′, coplanarity cannot be maintained, and the compound loses all activity. Cromolyn sodium is poorly absorbed from the lungs (~8%), insignificantly from the eye (~0.07%), and approximately 1% from the GI tract. It takes 2 to 6 weeks for onset of action. The majority of the drug is eliminated in the feces unabsorbed (98%).[111] Cromolyn appears to have a role in neutrophilic asthma and may relieve cough in resistant asthma.[112] For the treatment of asthma, cromolyn sodium is available as a solution for both intranasal and inhalation administration. There is also an oral concentrate that is primarily used to treat mastocytosis.

Nedocromil Sodium

Nedocromil sodium was developed by replacing the furan ring of khellin with a substituted pyridinone ring (see Fig. 31.30). In vitro, nedocromil sodium inhibits the release of inflammatory response mediators from a variety of cells, including neutrophils, mast cells, macrophages, and platelets. The MDI form of nedocromil sodium is no longer available in the United States because it used a chlorofluorocarbon (CFC) as a propellant. An ophthalmic solution is available to treat allergy symptoms.

Leukotriene Modifiers

It has been known since 1939 that slow-reacting substance of anaphylaxis (SRS-A) produced a slowly developing, long-lasting contraction of isolated guinea pig jejunum and that this same substance was associated with the pathophysiology of asthma.[113] Subsequently, it was determined that SRS-A was a mixture of three Cys-leukotrienes (LTs): LTC_4, LTD_4, and LTE_4. These leukotrienes were so named because they had three conjugated double bonds ("trienes") and a cysteine in their structure. They are formed from membrane-derived arachidonic acid, as seen in Figure 31.2. Determination of the chemical structure of these biologically active compounds led to the development of inhibitors of their biosynthesis, as well as receptor antagonists that are useful in the treatment of asthma.[114]

Biosynthesis of Leukotrienes

The leukotrienes occur in a variety of inflammatory cells that are abundant in asthma, including eosinophils, mast cells, and macrophages. They are derived from arachidonic acid via a branch of the common pathway to the prostacyclins and thromboxanes. Figure 31.2 depicts the biosynthetic pathway. Arachidonic acid is produced by the action of phospholipase A_2 on cell membranes. Unlike the prostacyclins and thromboxanes, excess arachidonic acid does not activate the leukotriene pathway. The first step in the conversion of arachidonic acid to leukotrienes is controlled by 5-lipoxygenase–activating protein (FLAP), which helps localize arachidonic acid to the active site of 5-lipoxygenase, which converts it to 5-HPETE. This unstable peroxide intermediate is quickly converted by the elimination of water to form LTA_4. The unstable epoxide is quickly metabolized by (1) LTA_4 hydrolase to LTB_4 and (2) LTC_4 synthase to the glutathione adduct, LTC_4. LTC4 can also stimulate the synthesis of prostacyclin.[115] Cleavage of γ-glutamic acid by γ-glutamyl transpeptidase converts LTC_4 to LTD_4, which in turn is converted to LTE_4 by the removal of Gly under the action of dipeptidase. LTE_4 is the most stable of the leukotrienes thus is the most abundant found in biologic fluids. LTD_4 is the most potent bronchoconstrictor with the fastest onset of action. While LTB_4 has no bronchoconstrictive activity, it is a potent neutrophil chemotactic agent.[114]

Leukotriene Receptors

LTs act as endogenous agonists for two distinct GPCR families; the LTB_4 receptors (BLTRs), BLT_1R and BLT_2R, and cysteinyl LT receptors (CysLTRs), $CysLT_1R$ and $CysLT_2R$.[116] The BLTRs share very little sequence similarity to the CysLTRs and $CysLT_1R$ and $CysLT_2R$ only share 38% primary amino acid sequence identity. As GPCRs, they consist of seven transmembrane-spanning helices that activate intracellular signaling pathways in response to their endogenous ligands (LTC_4, LTD_4, and LTE_4). There is a slight difference in ligand-binding affinities between the two cysteine receptors. The $cysLT_1$ receptors have an affinity profile of LTC4 > LTD4 > LTE4, whereas the $cysLT_2$ receptors show an affinity profile of $LTC_4 = LTD_4 > LTE_4$. Both receptor types are found in the lungs and the spleen. The $cysLT_1$ receptor is also found in the placenta and small intestines, whereas the $cysLT_2$ receptor is also in the heart, lymph nodes, and brain. The incomplete overlap of tissue distribution, along with distinct ligand-binding properties, suggests $cysLT_1$ and $cysLT_2$ receptors might serve different functions in vivo.[116] Because the $cysLT_1$ receptors are inhibited by selective antagonists, they have importance in the treatment of leukotriene-related bronchoconstriction in asthma.

There are two leukotriene receptors for LTB_4, designated as BLT_1 and BLT_2. They are also GPCRs and are expressed in mast cells. There is growing evidence supporting the involvement of BLT_1 and BLT_2 receptor activation in the pathophysiology of asthma. BLT_1 receptors are also expressed in bronchial fibroblasts, neutrophils, and macrophages. BLT_1 receptors are upregulated in steroid-resistant inflammatory cells potentially involved in causing inflammation.[90] Developing therapies to antagonize LTB_4/BLT_1 action could provide a promising treatment for steroid-resistant asthma. There are currently no inhibitors of BLT_1 nor $cysLT_2R$.[117]

Leukotriene-Modifier Drugs

Two approaches to the development of leukotriene modifiers have been taken. The first approach was to block their biosynthesis by designing compounds that inhibit one or more of the enzymes involved in their biochemical pathway. The second approach was to identify antagonists with selective affinity for the $cysLT_1$ receptor.

Leukotriene-Biosynthesis Inhibitors

Despite over 3,000 articles in PubMed on 5-lipoxygenase inhibitors, only one drug, Zileuton has made it to the market. An alternate developing target is the 5-lipoxygenase-activating protein (FLAP), which also targets the first step in leukotriene synthesis (see Fig. 31.2). There are currently several compounds in phase II clinical trials, but none on the market.[118]

ZILEUTON

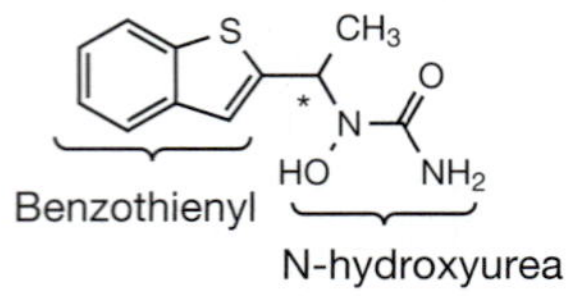

Zileuton

Zileuton is the only lipoxygenase inhibitor to be marketed. It inhibits the initial step in the formation of all leukotrienes, including LTA_4, LTB_4, LTC_4, LTD_4, and LTE_4 (Fig. 31.2). Zileuton chelates the active site iron in the 5-lipoxygenase enzyme to inhibit its activity.[119] It is the benzothienylethyl derivative of *N*-hydroxyurea and is marketed as the racemic mixture, as both isomers are pharmacologically active. The *N*-hydroxyurea group is essential for inhibitory activity, with the benzothienyl group contributing to its overall lipophilicity. Zileuton is rapidly absorbed after oral administration and is 93% protein-bound. Metabolism occurs in the liver, with the inactive *O*-glucuronide of the N-hydroxyl being the major metabolite. GI microflora produce the N-dehydroxylated metabolite, which inactivates some of the drug prior to absorption. Glucuronidation is stereoselective, with the *S*-isomer (major metabolite) being metabolized and eliminated about 4 times more quickly.[90] Greater than 90% of an oral dose is bioavailable, and 95% is excreted as metabolites in the urine. The short 2.5-hour half-life of the immediate-release formulation led to the development of an oral, controlled-release formulation with twice daily dosing.

Zileuton is a weak inhibitor of CYP1A2 and increases the plasma levels of propranolol, theophylline, and R-warfarin, and dosing of these drugs should be monitored in patients taking one or more in combination with zileuton. The most serious side effect of zileuton is the elevation of liver enzymes; if symptoms of liver dysfunction (eg, nausea, fatigue, pruritus, jaundice, or flu-like symptoms) occur, the drug should be discontinued.[120] Zileuton is used as an alternative to LABAs, and in addition to ICSs, for the treatment of moderate persistent asthma.

Leukotriene Receptor Antagonists

The search for leukotriene receptor antagonists began without the aid of ligand-receptor binding data and took three distinct approaches: (1) design of leukotriene structural analogues, (2) exploration of quinoline analogues, and (3) random screening from compound libraries.[121] Based on this background, synthetic efforts resulted in the development of montelukast and zafirlukast as $cysLT_1$ receptor antagonists. The x-ray crystal structure of the $cysLT_1$ receptor bound to two structurally different antagonists has since been published.[122] Figure 31.31 shows how zafirlukast binds the $cysLT_1$ receptor. The ligand-binding pocket is deep inside the TM domain, Y104 and Y249 make extensive polar interactions with the sulfonamide, the toluene group points toward TM6 and TM7 making hydrophobic interactions. The endogenous agonist LTD4 was also modeled in this structure and binds to the same site, also forming a hydrogen bond with Y249. The bonds of zafirlukast to $cysLT_1$ are weak, and the availability of this structure should lead to the rational design of better leukotriene antagonists. Leukotriene receptor antagonists are included in both the GINA guidelines and NAEPP guidelines for therapy in asthma.

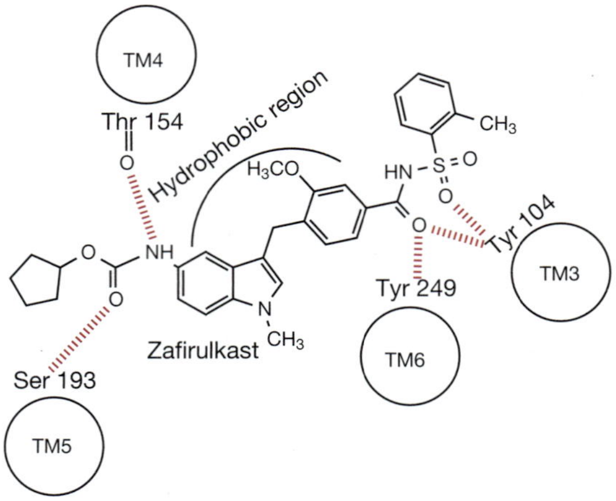

Figure 31.31 Cysteinyl leukotriene receptor (cysLT1) bound to zafirlukast.

MONTELUKAST SODIUM

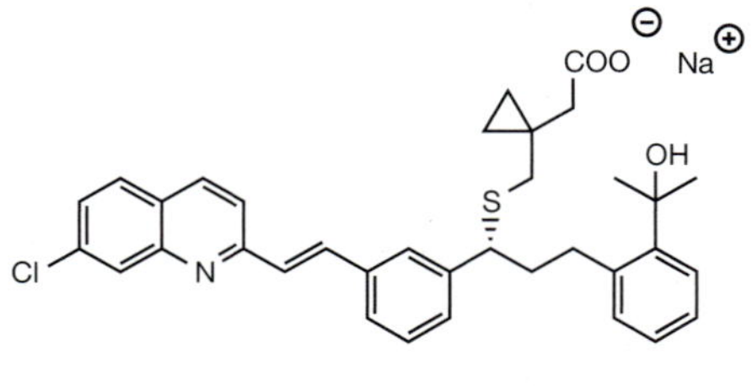

Montelukast (Singulair)

Montelukast sodium is a high-affinity, selective antagonist of the $cysLT_1$ receptor that was developed from quinoline derivatives that were weak antagonists. Several changes can be made to the structure without the loss of activity. These include changing the double bond between the two aromatic rings to an ether linkage, reducing the quinoline ring, changing the chlorine to fluorine, and/or exchanging the sulfur for an amide group.[121] It is rapidly absorbed orally, with a bioavailability of 64%. Montelukast is 99% bound to plasma proteins and is metabolized extensively in the liver. Figure 31.32 shows the primary metabolic pathway for montelukast in humans.[123] CYP3A4 oxidizes the sulfur and the C21 benzylic carbon, whereas CYP2C9 is selectively responsible for methyl hydroxylation. More than 86% of an oral dose is eliminated as metabolites through the bile. Montelukast did not demonstrate any significant adverse effects greater than placebo in clinical trials; however, because

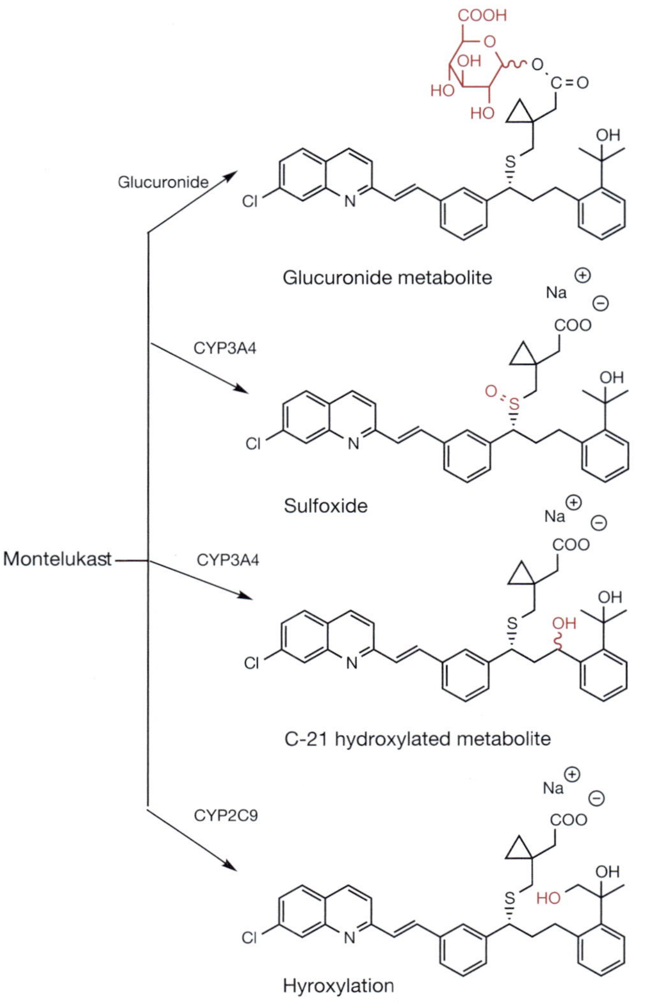

Figure 31.32 Metabolism of montelukast.

CYP450 enzymes metabolize it, its plasma levels should be monitored when coadministered with CYP450-inducing drugs, such as phenobarbital, rifampin, and phenytoin. Montelukast is also an inhibitor of CYP2C8. Montelukast is available in tablet or chewable tablet forms as well as granules for administration mixed with food. According to the GINA guidelines, LTRAs are less effective than ICS. Health care professionals should counsel patients about the risks of neuropsychiatric events and serious mental health effects associated with montelukast.[124]

ZAFIRLUKAST

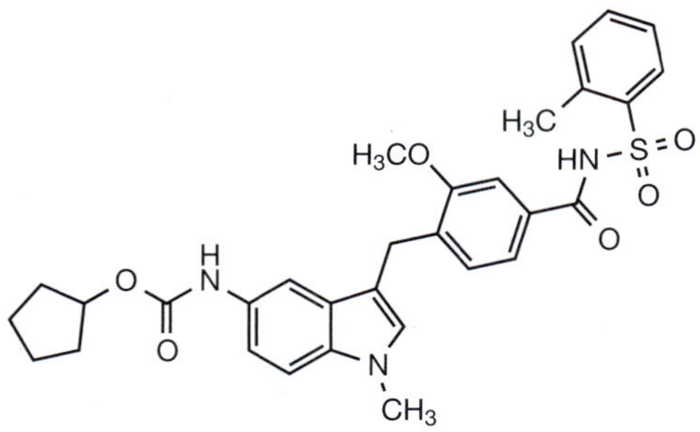

Zafirlukast

Zafirlukast, like montelukast, is a selective antagonist for the cysLT$_1$ receptor and antagonizes the bronchoconstrictive effects of all leukotrienes (LTC$_4$, LTD$_4$, and LTE$_4$). As discussed, it has been co-crystalized in the cysLT$_1$ receptor (see Fig. 31.31). It is well absorbed orally; however, food will decrease its absorption by as much as 40%. Zafirlukast is metabolized in the liver by CYP2C9 and CYP3A4 to hydroxylated metabolites and undergoes carbamate hydrolysis followed by N-acetylation.[125] Additionally, zafirlukast is known to produce an idiosyncratic hepatotoxicity in susceptible patients. This may be due to the formation of an electrophilic α, β-unsaturated iminium intermediate evidenced by the formation of a glutathione adduct on the methylene carbon bridging the indole ring to the methoxyphenyl moiety of the molecule.[126] This reactive intermediate may also form adducts with the CYP3A4 and CYP2C9 enzymes inhibiting their function. Thus, zafirlukast inhibits its own metabolism. Figure 31.33 summarizes the metabolism of zafirlukast. More than 90% of its metabolites are excreted in the feces, with the remainder found in the urine. It should be used with caution in patients taking other drugs metabolized by these enzymes.

Monoclonal Antibodies

The pathophysiology of allergic asthma, as already discussed, ultimately results in the production of allergen-specific IgE by activated B lymphocytes. The IgE binds to high-affinity FcεRI receptors on mast cells. The site where IgE binds to the receptor is located on the Fc fragment area of the C-ε-3

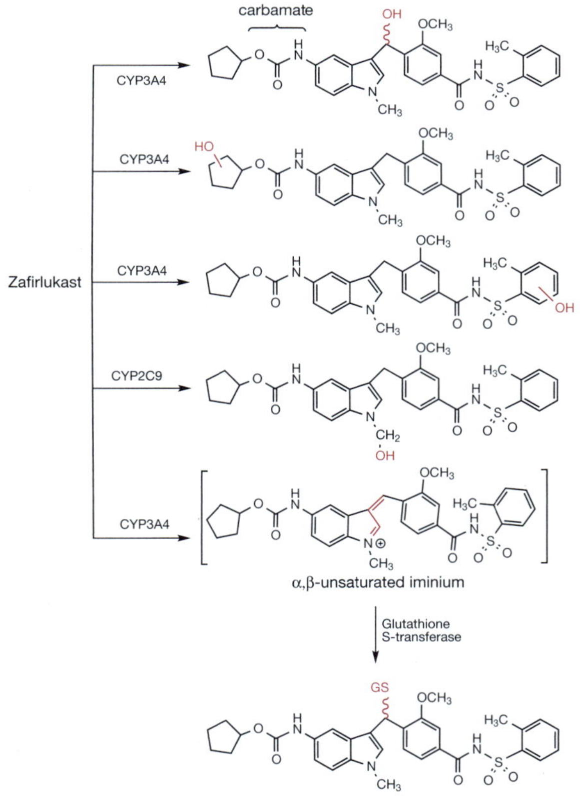

Figure 31.33 Metabolism of zafirlukast.

region, hence the acronym FcεRI (Fig. 31.34A). Subsequent allergen exposure causes cross-linking of bound IgE molecules, which triggers degranulation of these cells and results in the release of asthma mediators. Monoclonal anti-IgE antibody development is designed to moderate the role of IgE in activating mast cells, thereby decreasing the severity of allergic asthmatic attacks, and may also have beneficial effects in treating seasonal allergic rhinitis. Since monoclonal antibodies (MAbs) work to suppress the immune response, they may influence the immune response against some infections, such as helminth infections, by inhibiting immune signaling. It is advised that infections are treated and resolved before initiating MAb therapy.

The success of IgE antibodies that moderate the role of mast cells has stimulated the development of antibodies to cytokines involved in the asthmatic inflammatory processes. There are now MAbs to IL-4 and IL-5, cytokines responsible for the growth and differentiation, recruitment, activation, and release of eosinophils. The naming of MAbs provides clues to their target, source, and potential immunogenicity. MAb nomenclature is evolving and is based on a specific structure developed by the International Nonproprietary Names (INN) Working Group under the direction of the World Health Organization. The old naming structure used for the drugs in this chapter consists of a Prefix, Substem A, Substem B, and a Suffix. The Prefix does not follow any specific criteria and only serves to distinguish MAbs from one another. The Suffix used was MAb, noting the drug is a monoclonal antibody. The Substem A denotes the target of the antibody, and Substem B specifies the source (organism) from which the antibody is derived, providing insight into possible immunogenicity. For example, OMALIZUMAB has a Prefix OMA with Substem A as –LI, meaning its target is the immune system. Substem B is –ZU, meaning it is humanized; therefore, it will have diminished immunogenicity compared to murine-derived antibodies.[127] The large number of INN requests for dugs with the suffix -mabs led to the adoption of very long, similar sounding names that have the potential to lead to medication errors. The term -mab has thus been discontinued for any drug approved after 2021 and four new suffixes have been developed.[127] As all the MAbs discussed below are large protein structures, their chemical structures are omitted. For example, the chemical formula of dupilumab is $C_{6512}H_{10066}N_{1730}O_{2052}S_{46}$.

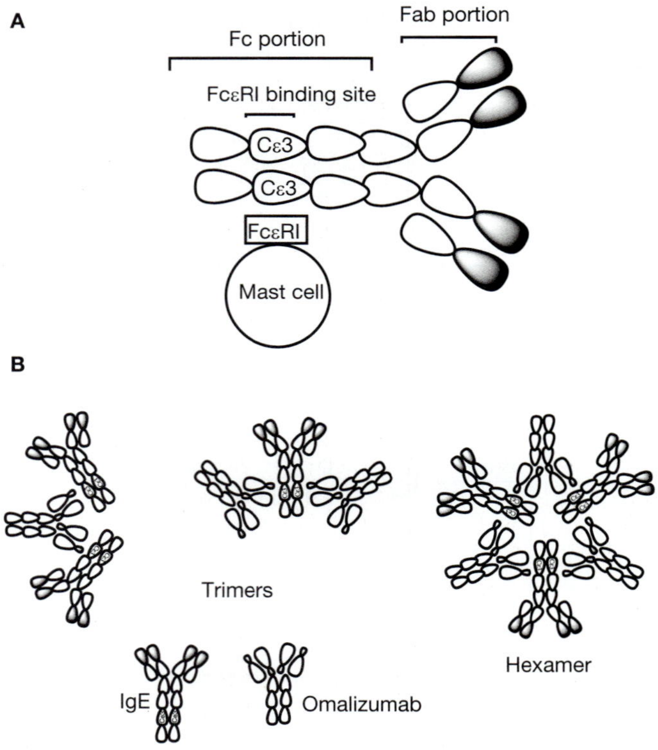

Figure 31.34 A. Graphic representation of immunoglobulin E (IgE) binding to the high-affinity Fc immunoglobulin E receptor (FcεRI) on a mast cell. B. Graphic representation of immune complexes formed between omalizumab. Hexamers predominate when components are in a 1:1 ratio, and the trimers predominate when one of the components is in excess.

Omalizumab

Omalizumab was the first monoclonal antibody used for the add-on treatment of allergic asthma.[128] It is a humanized antibody containing only 5% murine residues; thus, it has a low risk of eliciting immune reactions. Omalizumab selectively binds to the two Cε3 domains of human IgE forming trimeric or hexameric IgE/anti-IgE immune complexes (Fig. 31.34B). These immune complexes were found to be soluble and can be removed by the mononuclear phagocytic system.

In vitro, omalizumab has been shown to complex with free IgE, forming trimers consisting of a 2:1 and 1:2 complexes of IgE:omalizumab. In addition, larger complexes are also formed consisting of a 3:3 ratio of each (Fig. 31.34B). Omalizumab inhibits the binding of IgE to the FcεRI on the surface of dendritic cells, basophils, and mast cells. Thus, omalizumab effectively neutralizes free IgE. Clinical improvement in patients was seen if the mean serum-free IgE decrease was at least 35%. The decrease of available IgE also causes the downregulation of FcεRI receptors on the mast cell surface, resulting in a decrease of IgE bound to the mast cell.

The main clinical role for omalizumab is in the treatment of allergic asthma. It is approved for the treatment of adults and pediatric patients aged 6 years and older whose symptoms are not controlled with inhaled glucocorticoids and who have a positive skin test for airborne allergens. The bioavailability after subcutaneous administration is 62%, with slow absorption resulting in peak serum levels from a single dose in 7 to 8 days. Steady-state plasma concentration is reached in 14 to 29 days with multiple dosing regimens.

The elimination of omalizumab is not clearly understood; however, studies have determined that intact IgE is excreted via the bile and that omalizumab-IgE complexes are cleared faster than uncomplexed omalizumab and more slowly than free IgE. This means that, over time, total IgE concentrations (free and complexed) increase because the complex is cleared more slowly. The metabolism of omalizumab is not known, and the clearance of the complex is similar to the hepatic elimination of another immunoglobulin, IgG. The reticuloendothelial system degrades IgG, and it is believed that the same process occurs for the omalizumab-IgE complex. In patients with asthma, the serum elimination half-life averaged 26 days.[129] Omalizumab is available in two forms. For in-office use, a lyophilized powder that needs to be reconstituted is available. For home use, a prefilled syringe is available. All monoclonal antibodies need to be stored in the refrigerator.

Benralizumab

Benralizumab (Fasenra) is an IL-5 receptor antagonist. The IL-5 receptor is highly expressed in eosinophils, basophils, and mast cells and contains monomeric α and dimeric β subunits. High-affinity binding of IL-5 to IL-5Rα initiates the interaction between α and βc receptor subunits, inducing dimerization. This process initiates tyrosine phosphorylation-dependent activation, subsequently triggering the activation of signal transducers and activators of transcription, which transcriptionally activate genes involved in eosinophil proliferation and survival. Benralizumab binds to the α subunit of the IL-5R, expressed on the surface of eosinophils and basophils. This inhibits dimerization and signal transduction, resulting in inhibition of IL-5 receptor expressed cells. Natural killer (NK) cells can cause apoptosis of these targeted eosinophils and basophils through antibody-dependent cell-mediated cytotoxicity. IL-5 is the major cytokine responsible for the maturation and survival of eosinophils, and high levels of eosinophils are implicated in severe treatment-resistant asthma. Thus, benralizumab's reduction of eosinophil viability and proliferation can alleviate asthma symptoms.[130]

As the name indicates, benralizumab targets the immune system (substem A –li) and is humanized (substem B –zu). It is indicated as an add-on medication for the treatment of severe asthma in adults and children aged 12 years and up with an eosinophilic phenotype. It is administered subcutaneously in a 30-mg dose every 4 weeks for the first three doses and then once every 8 weeks. It has approximately 58% bioavailability with an elimination half-life of 15 days (nonrenal). It undergoes proteolytic degradation throughout the body. Adverse reactions include immunological development of antibodies, headache, pharyngitis, and fever. It is available as a 30 mg/mL solution in prefilled syringes.[131]

Mepolizumab

Mepolizumab (Nucala) is an IL-5 antagonist monoclonal antibody (IgG1k) indicated as add-on therapy for adult and pediatric patients aged 6 years and older with severe asthma and with an eosinophilic phenotype. It acts by binding to IL-5 and inhibits its binding to the IL-5 receptor complex expressed on the eosinophil cell surface. This results in a reduction in eosinophil production and survival. However, the exact mechanism of action is not clearly established. It also has the same nomenclature, with the –li and –zu substems indicating its immune system targeting and humanized structure.

Mepolizumab is administered subcutaneously in a dose of 100 mg every 4 weeks. It is 80% bioavailable with a 3.6 L volume of distribution. Like benralizumab, it is metabolized by proteases and not renally excreted. It has a terminal half-life of 16 to 22 days. The most significant adverse reactions are headache and injection site irritation. Other adverse effects include fatigue, pruritus, eczema, and infections (influenza and urinary tract infections). For subcutaneous (SC) administration, the lyophilized powder is diluted to 100 mg/mL concentration using sterile water for injection.[132]

Reslizumab

Reslizumab (Cinqair) is an IL-5 antagonist MAb, similar to benralizumab and mepolizumab, indicated for add-on maintenance therapy for patients with severe asthma. It has the same nomenclature, with the –li and –zu substems indicating its immune system targeting and humanized structure. It is administered by IV infusion at a 3-mg/kg dose every 4 weeks. Approximately 0.3% of patients experienced anaphylaxis; thus it must be administered in a health care setting. Similar to other Mabs, it is metabolized by proteases. It has a 5 L volume of distribution and a terminal half-life of approximately 24 days. Reslizumab has fewer adverse effects compared to both benralizumab and mepolizumab, with the major toxicities being antigenicity, myalgia, and oropharyngeal pain.[133]

Dupilumab

Dupilumab (Dupixent) is a human monoclonal IgG4 antibody that targets IL-4 and IL-13 signaling by binding specifically to the IL-4Rα subunit shared by the IL-4 and IL-13 receptor complexes. It inhibits IL-4 signaling via the type I receptor and both IL-4 and IL-13 signaling through the type II receptor. This action blocks inflammatory responses induced by IL-4 and IL-13, crucial in asthma pathogenesis, involving various cell types expressing IL-4Rα (such as mast cells, eosinophils, macrophages, lymphocytes, epithelial cells, and goblet cells). This antagonism inhibits the signaling of inflammatory mediators, including chemokines, nitric oxide, and IgE.

Dupilumab is a fully human ("u"-mab) monoclonal IgG4 antibody produced by recombinant DNA technology targeting the immune system ("l"umab). Dupilumab is indicated as an add-on maintenance treatment for patients aged 6 years and older with moderate-to-severe asthma characterized by an eosinophilic phenotype or with oral corticosteroid-dependent asthma. However, the drug is not indicated for relief of acute bronchospasm or status asthmaticus. Dosing is weight-based for patients under age 12, and severity based in adults. A one-time SC loading dose is followed by a SC injection every 4 weeks. The estimated volume of distribution is approximately 4.8 L.[134] Elimination is expected to be through proteases although it has not been characterized. The half-life was approximately 15.5 days for patients with asthma.[135]

The most common side effects include upper respiratory infections, injection site reactions, eye and eyelid inflammation, oropharyngeal pain, cold sores in the mouth/lips, and arthralgia.[134] A retrospective multicenter cohort study compared the effectiveness of dupilumab, mepolizumab, and benralizumab in adult patients with difficult-to-control asthma, using electronic health records and claims-based databases. The study concluded that among patients newly initiated on biologic therapy for difficult-to-control asthma, dupilumab showed a lower rate of asthma exacerbations in the year following initiation compared to mepolizumab or benralizumab.[136]

Tezepelumab-ekko

Tezepelumab-ekko (Tezspire) is a thymic stromal lymphopoietin (TSLP) blocker, human monoclonal antibody (IgG2λ). TSLP was originally identified as an IL-2 family cytokine produced by thymic stromal cells but is now known to be secreted by many cells, including epithelial cells, airway smooth muscle cells, keratinocytes, fibroblasts, mast cells, and macrophages. TSLP is an upstream cytokine and blocking its action decreases biomarkers associated with asthma inflammation including eosinophils, IgE, IL-5, and IL-13. Its mechanism is not fully understood but it has shown efficacy in reducing asthma exacerbations and improving lung function in patients with severe asthma. It may have a disease-modifying effect by targeting one of the underlying mechanisms of allergic inflammation.[137] It is approved for adults and children aged 12 years and older for severe asthma. It is administered subcutaneously once every 4 weeks.

Chronic Obstructive Pulmonary Disease

Definition and Epidemiology

COPD is a group of progressive lung diseases, including emphysema and chronic bronchitis. It usually is the result of an abnormal inflammatory response to airborne toxic chemicals. Cigarette smoking is the dominant cause of COPD in adults. Other types of tobacco (eg, pipe, cigar) and marijuana are also risk factors for COPD.[57] Asthma is considered to be a disease entity unto itself and is not included in the definition of COPD. However, asthma is a risk factor for developing COPD. Adults with asthma have a 12-fold higher risk of developing COPD compared to those without asthma.[57] Both COPD and asthma are considered inflammatory diseases; however, the nature of the inflammation is different. Asthma is associated with the release of inflammatory mediators from mast cells and eosinophils, whereas chronic bronchitis is primarily associated with neutrophils and emphysema with alveoli damage. In addition, asthma is more often than not allergenic, whereas chronic bronchitis and emphysema have no allergic component and are usually due to smoking. Although they are different diseases, patients can present with both asthma and COPD, this is sometimes referred to as Asthma-COPD overlap syndrome (ACOS). The GOLD recommendation is for patients with both diseases to follow asthma guidelines.[57]

Patients with COPD display a variety of symptoms, ranging from chronic productive cough to severe dyspnea requiring hospitalization. Other chronic illnesses, including cardiac, endocrine, and renal disease, often occur along with COPD. COPD is estimated to affect over 380 million people worldwide.[138] In the United States, COPD was the sixth leading cause of death in 2021. In 2021, it was estimated that 6.4% of adults in the United States have COPD. The age-adjusted prevalence of COPD varied between states and ranged from a high of 12.3% in West Virginia to a low of 3.0% in Hawaii. Although women have a slightly higher age-adjusted prevalence of COPD versus men, they have a lower death rate (98 vs 116.2 deaths per 100,000).[139] COPD is recognized as a global health problem. In 2017 the National Institutes of Health (NIH) and the World Health Organization developed the Global Initiative for Chronic Lung Disease (GOLD) guidelines, which present yearly updates on evidence-based recommendations for the treatment of COPD.[57]

Pathogenesis

Emphysema and chronic bronchitis are the two main subtypes of COPD. Both emphysema and chronic bronchitis often occur together although symptoms from one disease may be more prevalent. Smoking is the most important risk factor for developing COPD. Emphysema primarily involves damage to the alveoli. Cigarette smoke or occupational irritants can trigger the release of elastase from neutrophils. This protease breaks down elastin, a structural component of lung tissue. Elastin allows the alveoli to remain stretchy, and when it is removed, the alveoli become stiff. Usually, elastase levels are counterbalanced by the protein α-1 antitrypsin (AAT), which inhibits elastase function by forming a 1:1 complex with it.[140] This protein may not be present in sufficient quantities in patients with COPD, and a rare genetic condition called α-1 antitrypsin deficiency predisposes patients to early-onset emphysema. Patients with a genetic deficiency of AAT can be treated with an IV infusion of exogenous AAT through clinical trials.[141] Cigarette smoke or pollutants can also generate reactive oxygen species that expose the alveoli to oxidative damage leading to further inflammation. The anti-oxidant *N*-acetylcysteine is effective in reducing exacerbations and modestly improving health status.[142]

Chronic bronchitis is caused by the repeated irritation of the lining of the larger airways by cigarette smoke or other toxins. This leads to hypertrophy and hyperplasia of goblet cells, resulting in excessive mucus production. Chronic inflammation results in narrowing of the airways. Drugs targeting inflammation, such as corticosteroids or phosphodiesterase-4 (PDE4) inhibitors, can help reduce airway inflammation and mucus production in chronic bronchitis. In chronic bronchitis, the cilia in the airway may be impaired and unable to clear the excessive mucus. Patients often exhibit cyanosis due to inadequate oxygen exchange resulting from narrowed, inflamed, mucus-filled airways, leading to hypoxia. Repeated respiratory infections and exacerbations of COPD are common. Mucolytic agents like carbocysteine may help improve mucus clearance. According to the 2024 GOLD guidelines, COPD should be suspected in patients with chronic cough, dyspnea, a history of recurrent lower respiratory tract infections, and/or a history of exposure to risk factors. To be diagnosed with COPD, it is mandatory that spirometry testing shows the presence of non-fully reversible airflow obstruction (ie, FEV_1/forced vital capacity [FVC] < 0.7 post-bronchodilation).[57]

Pharmacotherapy

Medications used to treat COPD have been included in the previous section on asthma. The reader should review the latest version of the GOLD criteria for therapeutic advice as recommendations change every year (https://goldcopd.org). The GOLD criteria of 2024 pharmacotherapy treatment is based on the goals of reduced symptoms and reduced exacerbations. The patient's preference and ability to use inhalers correctly must also be assessed. Initial pharmacotherapy is based on the patient's GOLD group (A, B, or E). Patients are assigned based on the number and severity of exacerbations they have had per year, their blood eosinophil count (EOS), the modified Medical Research Council dyspnea questionnaire (mMRC) score, and the COPD Assessment Test (CAT) score. Group A patients have had 0 or 1 moderate exacerbation that did not lead to hospitalization, an mMRC between 0 and 1 and a CAT score less than 10. Group B patients have had 0 or 1 moderate exacerbations that did not lead to hospitalization, an mMRC score greater or equal to 2 and a CAT score greater or equal to 10. The only criteria required to be placed in Group E is two or more moderate exacerbations or one or more exacerbation that led to hospitalization.

The initial treatment for Group A patients is a bronchodilator. The choice of initial bronchodilator is based on its effect on breathlessness. Either a short-acting or a long-acting inhaler is acceptable based on affordability, availability, and the patient's perceived response. A long-acting inhaler is preferred over a short-acting inhaler, and either a LAMA or LABA is recommended. Either one is acceptable as the GOLD guidelines acknowledge that there is no high-quality evidence to support initial pharmacological treatment in newly diagnosed patients with COPD. Initial treatment for Group B is a LABA and LAMA or a combination product. Initial treatment for Group E is a LABA and LAMA with an added ICS if blood EOS is greater than or equal to 300 cells per microliter. The use of LABA/ICS combination is not encouraged, as the LABA/LAMA/ICS combination has been shown to be superior. Combination inhalers are listed in Table 31.2. Treatment regimen adjustments are made following the review of symptoms, assessment of inhaler technique, and evaluation of adherence. Rescue short-acting bronchodilators should be prescribed to all patients for immediate relief of symptoms.[57]

Phosphodiesterase Inhibitors

PDEs break down cyclic nucleotides like cAMP and cGMP. By inhibiting PDE, the increased cAMP and cGMP levels lead to physiologic effects depending on the type of PDE inhibited. There are 11 families of PDEs. Other chapters cover PDE3 inhibitors (such as milrinone), which are used in heart failure, and PDE5 inhibitors, such as sildenafil to treat erectile dysfunction. Theophylline and caffeine, nonselective PDE inhibitors, have already been covered. This section of the chapter will focus on PDE4 inhibitors. Inflammatory cells like T and B cells, monocytes, neutrophils, and eosinophils play a significant role in releasing inflammatory cytokines. In asthma, eosinophils are a key inflammatory cell involved in pathogenesis. By inhibiting PDE4, which is highly expressed in eosinophils, PDE4 inhibitors can reduce the release of inflammatory mediators from these cells, leading to the attenuation of asthma symptoms. Similarly, in COPD, neutrophils are prominent inflammatory cells contributing to disease progression. PDE4 inhibitors can inhibit neutrophil activation and the release of inflammatory cytokines, thereby exerting anti-inflammatory effects in the lungs of patients with COPD. There are three PDE4 subtypes (PDE4A, PDE4B, and PDE4D) found in inflammatory cells, with PDE4B being predominant. Therefore, efforts in this area have been directed toward the development and synthesis of selective PDE4 inhibitors. Progress in the development of PDE4 inhibitors has been slow because of a lack of clinical efficacy and dose-limiting side effects such as nausea, diarrhea, and headache. There is some evidence to suggest that the isoform PDE4D is responsible for the GI effects of the PDE4 inhibitors. Research is ongoing to find a more selective compound or an inhaled PDE4 inhibitor that can avoid the toxicity-limiting GI effects of this class.[143] To date, only one PDE4 inhibitor, roflumilast, has made it to the market.

Roflumilast

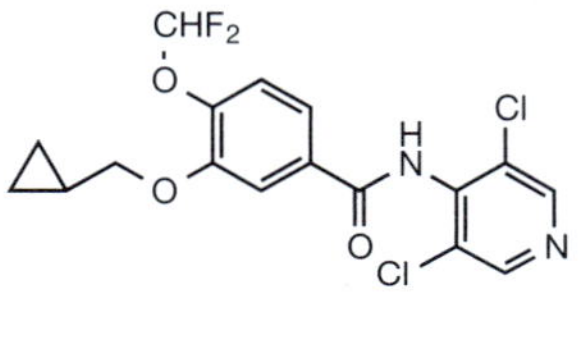

Roflumilast
(Daliresp)

Roflumilast (Daliresp) is indicated for patients with COPD who continue to have exacerbations following treatment with LABA + LAMA + ICS, particularly if they have had one hospitalization for bronchitis in the previous year.[57] Roflumilast has anti-inflammatory efficacy against a number of effector cells, including macrophages, eosinophils, neutrophils, and lymphocytes.[144] The active site of the PDE4 enzyme contains three pockets; a hydrophobic pocket (M) that binds metal (Mg^{2+} and Zn^{2+}) and coordinates water, a hydrophilic pocket (S) filled with water molecules, and a pocket (Q) that contains glutamine to selectively bind the purine of the nucleotide. Roflumilast binds to the active site through interactions with both the Q pocket and the M pocket. The oxygens of the dialkoxyphenyl bond to the NH of the γ-carboxamide group of the Gln in the Q pocket. The difluoromethoxy group and the cyclopropyl group are also accommodated in the Q pocket, resulting in hydrophobic interactions. The nitrogen of the dichloropyridyl group of roflumilast forms one hydrogen bond with a water molecule coordinated to the Mg^2+ within the M pocket.[145]

Roflumilast is administered as a tablet and is well absorbed with a half-life of 10 hours. It is metabolized in the liver by CYP3A4 and CYP1A2 to its major metabolite, the N-oxide derivative, which is about 1/10th as active as a PDE4 inhibitor but has a longer plasma half-life of 20 hours and may contribute to its activity (Fig. 31.35).[144] Roflumilast has been shown to penetrate the BBB, and treatment is associated with an increase in psychiatric adverse reactions, including depression.[146]

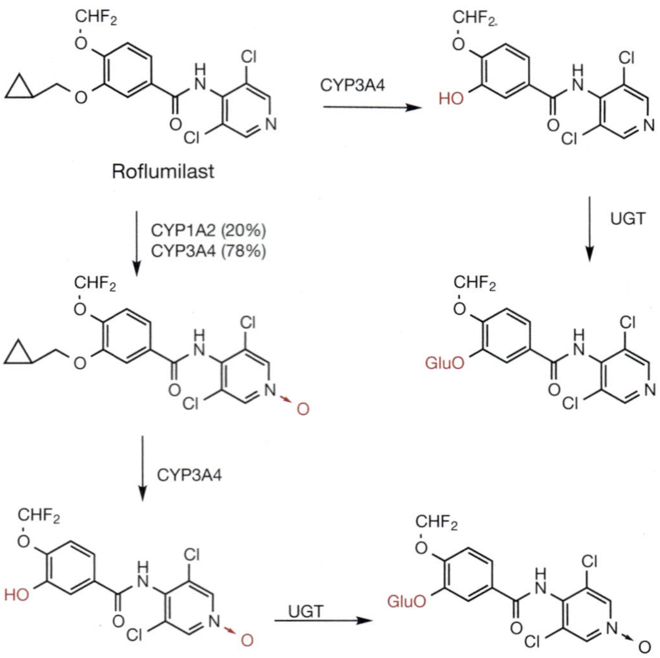

Figure 31.35 Roflumilast metabolism. UGT, uridine diphosphate glucuronosyltransferase.

Smoking Cessation

Cigarette smoking is responsible for approximately one in every five deaths in the United States annually. Among these deaths, approximately 278,544 are males, while 201,773 are females, underscoring the impact of smoking on all genders. Smokers face a significant reduction in life expectancy, with their lifespan cut short by at least 10 years compared to nonsmokers. Quitting smoking before the age of 40 decreases the risk of death from smoking-related diseases by approximately 90%. Most adult cigarette smokers want to quit. In 2018, 55.1% of adult smokers (21.5 million) said that they had attempted to quit in the past year. Unfortunately, only 7.5% of adult smokers successfully quit. Less than a third of adult cigarette smokers use counseling or cessation medications approved by the FDA when trying to quit. Withdrawal from nicotine in addicted people can lead to craving, nervousness, irritability, anxiety, increased appetite, headache, and fatigue. Studies have shown that maintaining smoke-free homes is associated with improved quit attempts, higher rates of smoking cessation, and reduced relapse rates.[147] Patients who utilized counseling and/or FDA-approved smoking cessation medications including nicotine, varenicline, and bupropion reported a higher success rate (up to 60%).[147,148]

Nicotinic Receptor

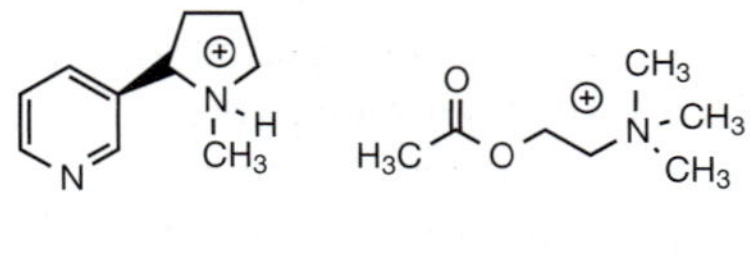

Nicotine Acetylcholine

Nicotine, the primary addictive component in tobacco, exerts its effects by binding to nicotinic acetylcholine receptors (nAChRs) distributed throughout the central and peripheral nervous systems. Nicotinic receptors are cholinergic receptors but are distinct from muscarinic receptors. While muscarinic receptors are G-protein–coupled (Chapter 6), nAChRs are cation-selective ligand-gated ion channels (see Chapter 8). Upon binding of an agonist, such as ACh or nicotine, the nAChR undergoes conformational changes that lead to the selective permeability of cations, including Na^{2+}, K^{+}, and/or Ca^{2+} ions, resulting in an inward flow of these ions. The focus of this section is on neuronal nicotinic receptors, not peripheral receptors, as this is the primary site of action of drugs used in smoking cessation. Nicotine binds nAChRs in the mesolimbic dopamine region of the brain. Activation leads to the release of neurotransmitters such as dopamine, serotonin, and NE, which are involved in the brain's reward pathways. The release of dopamine, in particular, contributes to the pleasurable sensations associated with smoking. Chronic exposure to nicotine can lead to upregulation of the nAChRs, requiring higher doses of nicotine to achieve the same effects. The activation of the nAChRs is a key factor in the addictive nature of smoking and the difficulty of quitting.

Nicotinic receptors are pentameric structures consisting of various combinations of 17 known subunits (10 αs, four βs, γ, δ, and ε subunits), resulting in multiple subtypes and complex pharmacology. Each of the five subunits contains an extracellular domain, a transmembrane domain composed of four transmembrane helices (TM1-TM4) with TM2 helices lining the ion pore, and an intracellular domain. Seventeen genes have been identified that encode for the nAChR subunits and 12 genes encode for those expressed in the brain.[149] Two of the most researched neuronal nAChR subtypes involved in nicotine addiction are the $(\alpha4)_2(\beta2)_2$ α5, and $(\alpha4)_3(\beta2)_2$ receptors. Figure 31.36

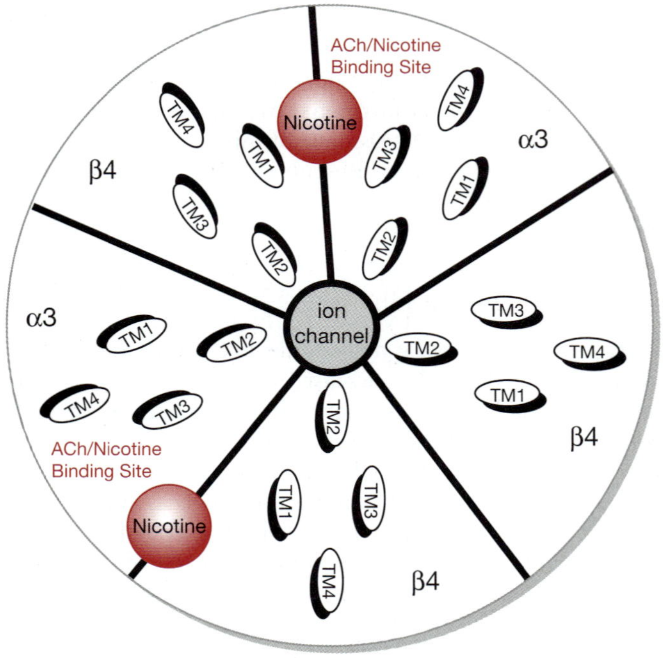

Figure 31.36 α3β4 NEURONAL nicotinic acetylcholine receptor.

shows the putative binding site of nicotine on an $(\alpha3)_2(\beta4)_3$ nicotinic receptor that is also expressed in brain areas that affect reward circuits.[150] Superimposing the nicotinic binding site of the $(\alpha3)_2(\beta4)_3$ over the $(\alpha4)_3(\beta2)_2$ receptor showed a conserved binding site for nicotine and ACh.

Two nicotine molecules bind at the interfaces of the α3 and β4 subunits in a highly conserved region of the extracellular domain. Tyrosine, tryptophan, and leucine amino acids from both the α3 subunit (Y93, W149, Y190, and Y197) and the β4 subunit (W59, L123, and L121) contribute to this pocket. The basic pyrrolidine nitrogen of nicotine forms a hydrogen bond with the backbone carbonyl of W149 as well as a cation-π interaction with the aromatic side chain of this same residue. Multiple ordered water-bridging bonds have also been identified. The precise binding location of nicotine at different receptor subtypes may inform the development of novel drugs to treat nicotine addiction. Additionally, identifying genetic variants associated with cessation success or failure may guide precision medicine therapy.[151]

Nicotine Replacement Therapy

Nicotine. Nicotine replacement therapy (NRT), in combination with behavioral and/or pharmacotherapy, has the best cessation results.[147,152] NRT therapy helps patients quit smoking by allowing them to maintain a nicotine level to prevent withdrawal craving, while they gradually reduce the dose of nicotine over time. This therapy does not expose patients to the additional toxic chemicals found in cigarette smoke. Nicotine replacement products include OTC nicotine patches, gum, lozenges, and prescription nasal spray and inhaler formulations.

Nicotine gum is available in 2-mg and 4-mg doses. Unlike cigarettes, which deliver nicotine within 2 minutes, nicotine's buccal absorption from gum is much slower, taking 15 to 30 minutes. Nicotine is a weak base (with a pK_a of 8.0) and is most effectively absorbed when in its unionized form. To enhance nicotine absorption in the mouth, the gum is formulated with bases such as calcium carbonate, sodium carbonate, and sodium bicarbonate. This will increase the mouth's pH to around 8.5 instead of the normal 6.5 to 7.5.[153,154] Studies have shown that the 4-mg dose of nicotine gum has a higher success rate in aiding smoking cessation. It was found that there was no significant difference in effectiveness between starting the gum 4 weeks before the quit date or starting it on the quit date.[152] Nicotine lozenges, available in the same strengths as the gum, are also formulated with a buffering agent. Compared to the gum, they offer about twice the maximum concentration (C_{max}) and area under the curve (AUC) of nicotine in the bloodstream, with a similar elimination half-life.[155]

The NRT transdermal patches come in multiple strengths, and patients should select a starting patch strength based on the number of cigarettes they smoke per day. After 4 to 6 weeks of smoking abstinence, patients should taper the dose every 2 to 4 weeks as tolerated. Patch sites should be rotated daily to reduce skin irritation. The NRT 21 mg/24 h patch exhibited lower maximum plasma concentrations (C_{max}), and average concentrations (C_{avg}) of nicotine compared to controlled smoking of one cigarette every half hour. Nicotine values for C_{max} and C_{avg} for the NRT patch were approximately half those observed with controlled smoking.[156] Patients should be informed that used nicotine patches still contain a toxic amount of nicotine and must be disposed of properly to prevent accidental poisoning of children and pets.

The nicotine nasal spray provides a fast onset, typically within 3 minutes, and closely mimics the rapid increase in nicotine levels observed with smoking. The recommended dosage is one spray, containing 0.5 mg of nicotine in each nostril (totaling 1 mg), to be used as needed. Users can administer up to four doses per hour up to 40 doses per day. Approximately 53% of the dose is absorbed, aiming to approximate the nicotine intake from smoking a single cigarette. Research indicates that using the nasal spray doubles the likelihood of successfully quitting smoking when compared to using a placebo.[152]

A nicotine inhaler (Nicotrol 10 mg/cartridge) is also available. The inhaler uses the active S-isomer of nicotine, which is the prevalent form in tobacco. Although patients puff on the inhaler, like a cigarette, most of the nicotine gets deposited in the mouth, with only 5% reaching the lungs. Peak arterial concentrations are reached in about 15 minutes and reach about one-eighth the level achieved with cigarette smoking.[157]

Absorbed nicotine is metabolized (Fig. 31.37) primarily by CYP2A6. The major metabolites are cotinine (15%) and the 3′trans-hydroxycotinine derivative (45%). Nicotine and its metabolites are rapidly excreted via the kidney, with a half-life of 2 hours.

Bupropion

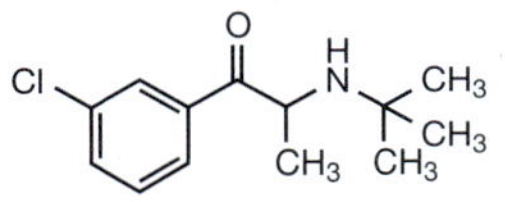

Bupropion

Bupropion was the first non-nicotine based agent approved for smoking cessation. It is also an antidepressant that acts as a weak dopamine/NE-reuptake inhibitor (DNRI) at the presynaptic neuronal membrane. In addition, bupropion also inhibits the nAChR, giving it antinicotinic activity and utility as a medication for smoking cessation.

Bupropion has a half-life of about 21 hours and is extensively metabolized, with less than 1% being excreted in the urine unchanged. The elimination half-life of the active metabolites may exceed that of bupropion. Bupropion is administered as a racemic mixture of *S*- and *R*-bupropion and metabolism is stereospecific. *S*-bupropion has a higher clearance than *R*-bupropion. It is metabolized extensively in the liver by the CYP system and many other enzymes. The primary metabolite is hydroxybupropion, which is half as active as bupropion and cyclizes to an active phenylmorpholinol structure (Fig. 31.38). The 2*S*,3*S* enantiomer of the pheynylmorpholinol metabolite (named radafaxine) was evaluated as an antidepressant but did not reach the market. Racemic threohydrobupropion and erythrohydrobupropion also formed and are both 20% as active as the parent drug. In addition, bupropion and its metabolites

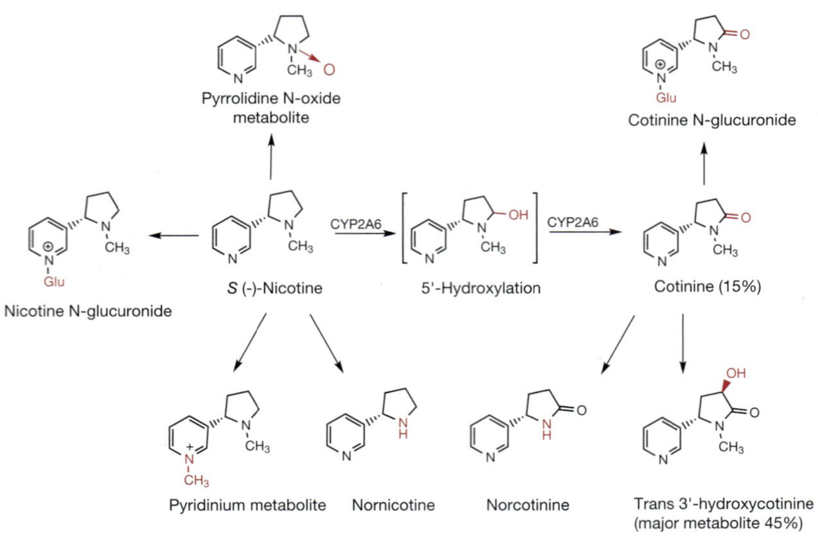

Figure 31.37 Nicotine metabolism.

inhibit CYP2D6 and may reduce the clearance of drugs metabolized by this isoform.[158,159]

Bupropion is available in a 150-mg sustained-release tablet, usually taken twice a day with therapy beginning 1 to 2 weeks before the anticipated quit date. The drug demonstrates a number of adverse reactions and side effects, including headache, confusion, dry mouth, dizziness, decreased libido, hallucinations, unusual thoughts and behaviors, and an increased risk of seizures.

VARENICLINE. Varenicline was developed as a partial agonist of neuronal nicotinic receptors. As a partial agonist, it behaves as an antagonist in the presence of a full agonist like nicotine, but in the absence of nicotine, it will behave as an agonist and mitigate withdrawal symptoms. Varenicline was developed based on the structure of cytisine. Cytisine is a naturally occurring α4β2 nAChR partial agonist, isolated from the seed of the Laburnum tree (*Cytisus laburnum*).[160] Cytisine has been used as a nicotine replacement for over 100 years in Europe and is still an affordable and effective smoking cessation aid available throughout Europe and Canada.[161,162] Varenicline was synthesized using cytisine as the starting point for development. Binding to the nicotinic receptor was known to require an ammonium headgroup at physiological pH and a π-system. Cytisine was first modified with a nitro benzene, which had excellent affinity for the nicotinic receptor. This compound was an effective partial agonist and was expanded to a quinoxaline ring to produce varenicline. This aromatic and flat extension proved to increase the affinity to the nicotinic receptor and maintain partial agonist activity (Fig. 31.39).

Varenicline is FDA-approved as an aid to smoking cessation.[162,163] It is well absorbed (~90%), and oral bioavailability is unaffected by food. Maximum plasma levels occur within 3 to 4 hours, and protein binding is approximately 20%. Varenicline undergoes minimal metabolism and is almost exclusively excreted unchanged in the urine. The elimination half-life is about 24 hours. Adverse events include nausea, insomnia, vivid dreams, drowsiness, constipation, and headaches.[164]

Patients should begin taking varenicline for smoking cessation 1 week before their quit date or begin varenicline and then quit smoking between days 8 and 35 of treatment.

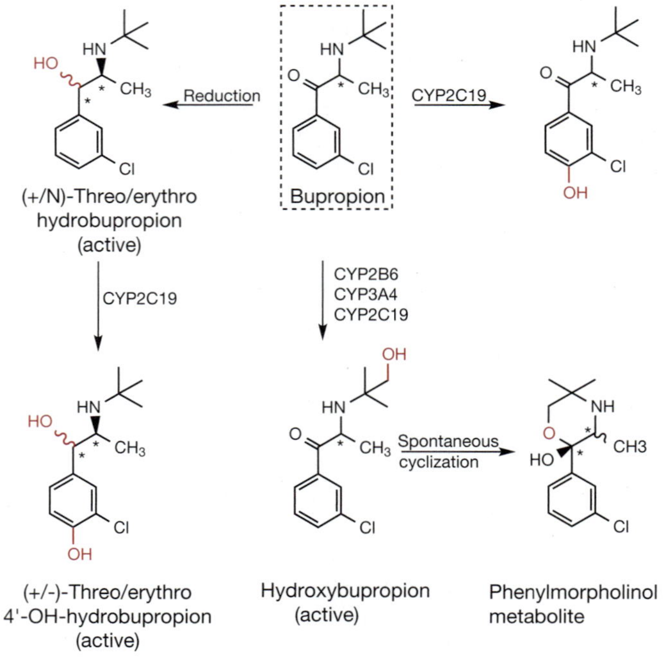

Figure 31.38 Metabolic pathways of bupropion. All metabolites undergo extensive glucuronidation.

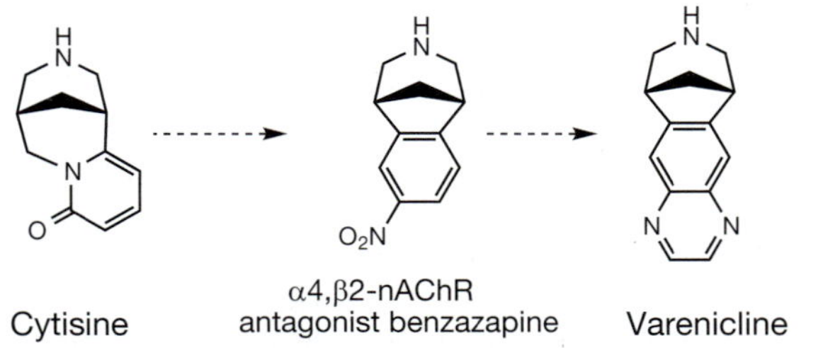

Figure 31.39 Development of varenicline from cytisine. nAChR, nicotinic acetylcholine receptors.

Patients start on day 1 with a 0.5-mg dose and titrate up to 1 mg twice daily, as prescribed. Quitting success rate is greatly enhanced when taken along with NRT.[165,166]

Cystic Fibrosis

CF is an inherited life-threatening genetic disorder that damages the lungs, pancreas, liver, and other organs. CF is an autosomal recessive disorder; thus, patients who develop CF inherit two faulty cystic fibrosis transmembrane conductance regulator (CFTR) genes, one from each parent. It is estimated that there are 40,000 children and adults with CF in the United States, with approximately 1,000 new cases diagnosed every year.[167] CF affects cells that produce mucus, sweat, and digestive juices. People with CF have a sticky mucus buildup in their digestive system and lungs, making breathing difficult and increasing their susceptibility to bacterial infections. Mucus clogging in the airways also leads to inflammation and injury to the lung tissue. CF may be diagnosed through newborn screening or later in life through a combination of clinical evaluation, genetic testing, and the sweat test. The sweat test measures the amount of salt in the sweat after the application of pilocarpine. A high salt level indicates CF.

Drugs that are utilized for treating patients with CF can be classified into two major classes: (1) drugs that are used to treat common sequelae of CF such as inflammation, constipation, glucose intolerance, infection, osteoporosis, and congestion due to thickened mucus, and (2) drugs that modulate the effect of gene mutations. Chronic inflammation and infection in the lungs lead to neutrophil recruitment. Neutrophils release DNA as part of their defense mechanism used to trap and clear bacteria through a process called NETosis (neutrophil extracellular trap formation), which increases mucus viscoelasticity.[168] Congestion is treated with an inhaled recombinant human DNAase enzyme named Dornase Alfa and hypertonic saline, both of which are used as mucus thinners. Dornase Alfa breaks up mucus by cutting DNA strands and has been shown to reduce pulmonary exacerbations. Hypertonic saline thins dehydrated mucus through osmotic forces by increasing sodium levels in the airways and drawing fluid into the mucus, making it easier to clear.[169]

Bacteria, fungi, and viruses can all cause infections in persons with CF. The airways should be sampled for infection at each clinic visit. CF microbiologists should be part of the CF team to identify pathogens and effective antimicrobials. Tobramycin and aztreonam are available as inhaled formulations, to treat patients with CF infected with *Pseudomonas aeruginosa*. Over half of patients with CF have chronic *Pseudomonas* infections.[170] Inhaled colistin is available in Europe for *Pseudomonas* infections and is currently in phase III trials to test effectiveness in people with CF in the United States. *Aspergillus fumigatus* and other fungi are common in children and adults with CF. If triazoles are used as antifungals, doses of CFTR modulators must be adjusted due to CYP-induced DDIs.

Approximately 85% of patients with CF have exocrine pancreatic insufficiency and need pancreatic enzyme replacement therapy. Normally, the pancreas secretes digestive enzymes and bicarbonate, but in CF, this is reduced due to mucus obstructing the pancreatic ducts and fibrosis. Therapy with pancreatic enzymes is used to treat malabsorption and malnutrition.[171] Treatment with CFTR modulators may also improve pancreatic exocrine function. Due to pancreatic damage, people with CF should be screened for diabetes annually and treated appropriately.

The second class of drugs includes those that modulate the effect of mutated genes responsible for the development of CF. The CFTR regulator protein is produced from the CFTR gene, is a member of the ATP binding cassette (ABC) transporter family, and works as an ATP-gated chloride ion channel. Its structure includes an N-terminal motif known as the lasso motif, two transmembrane domains (TMDs) that create a pathway for anion conduction, two cytoplasmic nucleotide-binding domains (NBDs) responsible for ATP binding and hydrolysis, and a regulatory domain that allows channel opening when phosphorylated. Its normal function is to regulate the flow of chloride ions and water in and out of cells (Fig. 31.40). This regulation is crucial to maintain the correct fluid balance in the cells lining the airways and other organs such as the pancreas, liver, and intestines. Over 1,700 mutations have been identified, and the Clinical and Functional Translation of CFTR organization (cftr.org) maintains a curated database of variants and whether the variant or variant combination leads to CF.[172] The faulty gene translates into a defective CFTR protein. These mutations cause reduced chloride and water release, resulting in mucus thickening, the hallmark of CF (Fig. 31.40). Table 31.5 lists some of the currently known CFTR mutations along with the damage they cause, the percent of patients with those mutations, and the drug classes available to treat the specific mutations.[172,173]

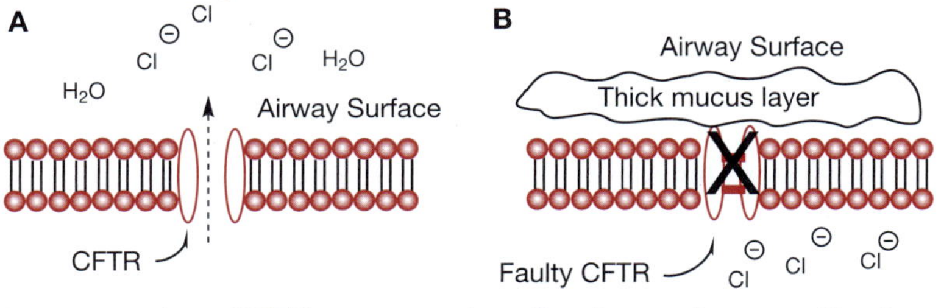

Figure 31.40 A. Normal conductance regulator (CFTR) protein on the cell surface working as a chloride ion channel allowing for salt and water balance in airways. B. Defective CFTR protein resulting from genetic mutations.

Table 31.5 CFTR Mutation Classification, Outcomes, and Potential Therapy

Class	Class I	Class II	Class III	Class IV	Class V
Example mutations	G542X, W1282X, R553X	F508del, N1303K, I507 del, E56K, P67L, E92K, R170G, L206W, V232D, F508G, A561E	G551D, S549N,G178R, S549N, S549R, G551S, G1244E, S1251N, S1255P, G1349D	D1152H, R347P, R117H	3849+10kbC→T, 2789+5G→A, A455E
% of patients with mutation	22%	88%	6%	6%	5%
Result of mutation	Production mutations that include non-sense proteins and shortened protein, no CFTR created	Processing mutation leads to misfolded protein and reduced protein moving to cell surface	Gating mutation, channel gate does not open	Conduction mutation, faulty channel	Some splice mutations, not enough CFTR made
Drug classes used	Read-through compounds	Correctors	Potentiators	Potentiators	Potentiators
Example drugs used	Clinical trials with aminoglycosides/ derivatives	Tezacaftor, Lumacaftor, Elexacaftor	Ivacaftor	Ivacaftor	Ivacaftor

CFTR, cystic fibrosis transmembrane conductance regulator.

CFTR Modulators

CFTR modulators are divided into three classes, based on their function as either CFTR potentiators, correctors, or amplifiers. Amplifiers increase the amount of CFTR messenger RNA and, thus, the amount of protein made. Currently there are no CFTR amplifiers on the market, but there are several drugs in phase II clinical trials.

CFTR Potentiators

Depending on the type of mutation, a patient may have nonfunctioning, faulty functioning or a reduction in CFTR protein levels. CFTR potentiators enhance the residual activity of faulty CFTR channels and enhance normal CFTR channel activity, thereby increasing chloride ion transport.

IVACAFTOR

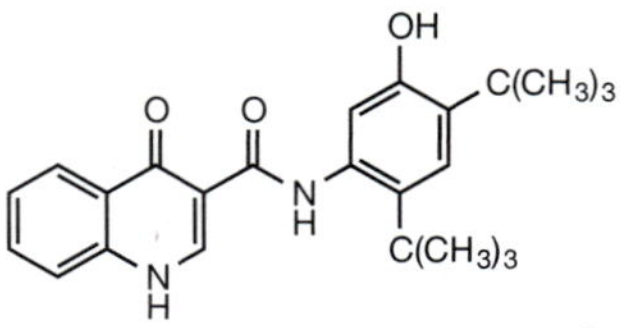

Ivacaftor (Kalydeco)

Ivacaftor was the first CFTR modulator approved for the treatment of CF. Ivacaftor is approved for infants as young as 1 month who have at least one copy of 97 mutations that have been shown to be responsive. Most of these variants are Class III variants (Table 31.5). The list of mutations that respond to specific CFTR modulators is updated regularly. For the most up-to-date information on which mutations are approved for use with specific drugs or combinations, the reader is directed to check the FDA website. The superiority of the triple combination, elexacaftor, tezacaftor, and ivacaftor (ETI) (Ivacaftor is the "I" in ETI brand name Trikafta), has supplanted other modulator combinations in eligible patients.[174] Ivacaftor facilitates chloride transport by potentiating the channel open probability of the CFTR protein. The precise mechanism is not fully understood, but it is theorized that it could involve either decoupling the gating cycle and ATP hydrolysis cycle, or enhancing the ATP-dependent opening rate while reducing the closing rate.[175] A cryo-electron microscopy (cryo-EM) structure of the Δ508 CFTR shows that ivacaftor binds in a cleft formed by TM helices 4, 5, and 8 about halfway through the lipid bilayer. TM helix 8 is the hinge region involved in gating of the channel and ivacaftor stabilizes the open configuration of the pore.[176] Ivacaftor is classified as a potentiator because it does not induce a change in the structure of the protein; it only stabilizes the correct folding, thus potentiating its action. Ivacaftor, tezacaftor, and elexacaftor all bind at different sites on the protein and work synergistically to form a functional CFTR channel.[176] All three drugs bind within the transmembrane domain of the channel protein, and their binding is described below.

Ivacaftor is orally effective, highly bound to plasma proteins (99%), and exhibits an effective half-life of about 15 hours.[174] It is metabolized by CYP3A4/5 to metabolites M1 and M6 (Fig. 31.41).[177] Metabolite M1 is active and retains about 15% of activity, M6 is considered inactive. Because

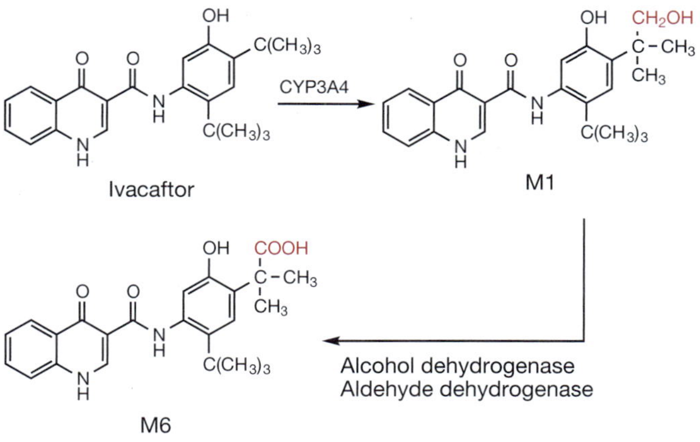

Figure 31.41 Metabolism of ivacaftor.

ivacaftor is primarily used as the combination therapy (ETI), the pharmacokinetic parameters and metabolism must be considered simultaneously. The majority of the dose of all three drugs in ETI is eliminated through the feces as metabolites. For all three compounds, there is little recovered drug found in the urine, indicating that renal excretion is not a major elimination pathway. Metabolism of all components of ETI occurs primarily in the liver via CYP3A4/5, thus drugs that inhibit or induce CYP3A4 may lead to DDIs.[174] Drugs that are commonly coadministered in patients with CF such as anti-infective agents, anti-reflux medication and immunosuppressants are the focus of the clinically relevant DDIs covered. Rifampin, a strong CYP3A4 inducer will increase the metabolism of ETI components and may reduce effectiveness. The AUC of ivacaftor was found to decrease by 89% when used with rifampin, thus coadministration of strong CYP3A4 inducers such as rifampin, rifabutin, phenobarbital, or carbamazepine is not recommended with ivacaftor. Strong CYP3A4 inhibitors, such as itraconazole, will increase ETI levels. Several clinical trials confirm that azole antifungals increase the AUC of all three of the ETI components. Ketoconazole resulted in an 8.5-fold AUC increase of ivacaftor monotherapy. Itraconazole was found to increase the AUC of elexacaftor by 2.8, ivacaftor 15.6-fold, and tezacaftor 4.5-fold. The limitations of the fixed-dose combinations make reduction in the individual drugs complicated and thus require expert guidance for adjustments.[174]

The most common adverse effects include headache, upper respiratory infections, stomach pain, and diarrhea. The drug may also result in increased levels of liver transaminases and increased cataracts in children.

CFTR Correctors

About 90% of patients with CF have at least one copy of the F508del mutation, resulting in the deletion of a Phe at position 508 (ΔF508), which causes the misfolding of the CFTR protein in the cytoplasm and prevents it from moving onto the cell surface. As noted previously, this is the most common mutation responsible for CF. CFTR correctors help defective CFTR fold correctly and translocate to the cell surface.

Lumacaftor

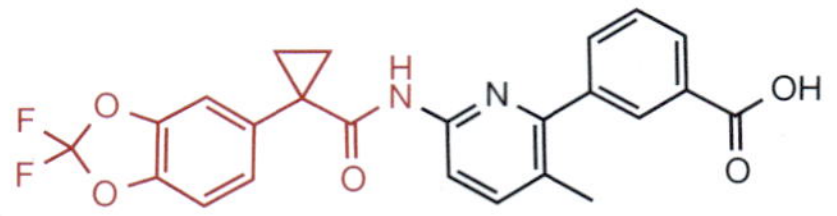

Lumacaftor

Lumacaftor is indicated in combination with ivacaftor (combination brand Orkambi) to treat CF in patients 1 year and older who have two copies of the CFTR F508del mutation in their CFTR gene. Lumacaftor is reported to act by increasing the amount of ΔF508-CFTR protein delivered to the cell surface through suppression of misfolding. This leads to a partial restoration of chloride ion transport. If ΔF508-CFTR protein does not misfold, then proteolytic degrading enzymes will not recognize it. The cryo-EM Δ508 CFTR receptor bound to lumacaftor alone shows that it binds to a hydrophobic pocket and stabilizes TM domain 1, but is insufficient alone to correct the misfolding of Δ508 CFTR. Lumacaftor fills this binding site on TM domain 1 formed by TM helices 1, 2, 3, and 6 and stabilizes the four helixes by linking them together. It prevents degradation and increases the overall probability of a fully folded and functional CFTR. The combination of lumacaftor and elexacaftor (not a clinically available combination) had a greater effect in forming a functional CFTR than either did alone.[170] By positively impacting CFTR protein conformational stability, lumacaftor increases mature protein transport to the cell surface, where the coadministered ivacaftor subsequently potentiates the opening and function of the chloride ion channel.

Lumacaftor undergoes minimal metabolism and is excreted primarily unchanged in the feces. Lumacaftor is a strong inducer of CYP3A. When administered as the combination product with ivacaftor, lumacaftor greatly decreases the serum concentration of ivacaftor. Both lumacaftor and ivacaftor exhibit significantly increased absorption when administered with fatty foods (lumacaftor double and ivacaftor triple). Like ivacaftor, lumacaftor is 99% bound to plasma proteins, and the most common adverse effects involve the GI (nausea, diarrhea, flatulence) and respiratory tract (upper respiratory tract infection, rhinorrhea, influenza). Elevations in blood phosphokinase bilirubin-transaminases are also noted.

Tezacaftor

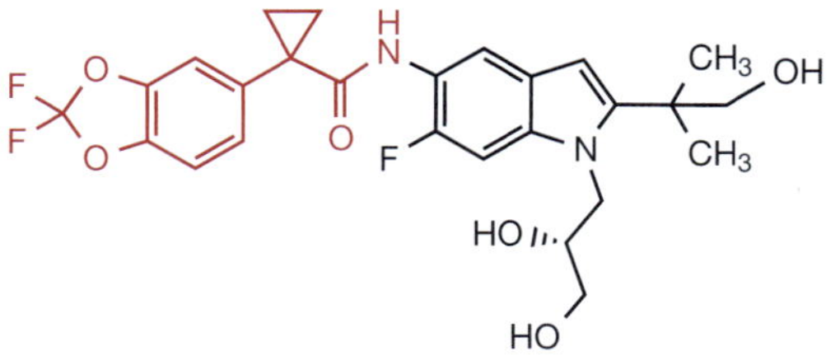

Tezacaftor

Tezacaftor is a CFTR corrector drug for use in combination with ivacaftor in patients aged 6 and over with two copies of the F508del mutation (Combination brand name Symdeko) and in combination with ivacaftor and elexacaftor (tezacaftor is the "T" in ETI brand name Trikafta) in patients aged 2 years or over with one or two copies of the F508del mutation or one F508del and one mutation in a list of 177 specified mutations.[141] Tezacaftor's mechanism of action is similar to that of lumacaftor; it is a corrector that helps the CFTR protein form the correct shape, move to the cell surface, and stay there longer. It binds and stabilizes TM domain 1 in the same manner as lumacaftor, and the structural similarities leading to this are colored red in both molecules. Like the CFTR modifiers discussed thus far, tezacaftor is approximately 99% bound to plasma proteins. It is metabolized extensively by CYP3A4/5 to the three major metabolites M1, M2, and M5 (Fig. 31.42).[177,178] Metabolite M1 is active with a potency similar to that of the parent drug, M2 is less active, and M5 is inactive. Dosage adjustments are needed when coadministered with CYP3A4 inducers or inhibitors. Tezacaftor is also a substrate of the hepatic uptake transporter OATP1B1, and it is possible for inhibitors of this transporter, such as cyclosporine, to reduce the hepatic uptake and clearance of tezacaftor. The majority of the dose (72%) is excreted in the feces unchanged or as the M2 metabolite.

Elexacaftor

Elexacaftor is the "E" component of ETI and is only available in the triple combination drug Trikafta. It is a CFTR corrector. It is used as the racemic mixture although the S enantiomer has been found to be more potent.[176] Trikafta is approved for patients aged 2 years and older who are either homo- or heterozygous for the F508del-CFTR mutation or have at least one copy of 177 specified mutations on the FDA website. This is estimated to represent 90% of patients with CF. Trikafta received FDA fast-track approval as well as priority review in 2019 and has been life-changing for people with CF. Elexacaftor has a dual mechanism of action improving both CFTR folding and ion conductance. As already described, the three drugs in Trikafta bind to three distinct sites on the Δ508CFTR protein and synergistically work to correct the misfolding. Elexacaftor was found to bind to the Δ508CFTR on a shallow, surface binding site. It interacts with TM helix 11 through van der Waals interactions of the lipophilic CF_3 tail end of the molecule and forms a salt bridge between arginine 1102 of TM11 and the acidic sulfonamide nitrogen (pK_{acalc} = 4.9). It also forms electrostatic interactions between the sulfonyl oxygens and the lasso motif amino acids serine 18 and arginine 21.[176]

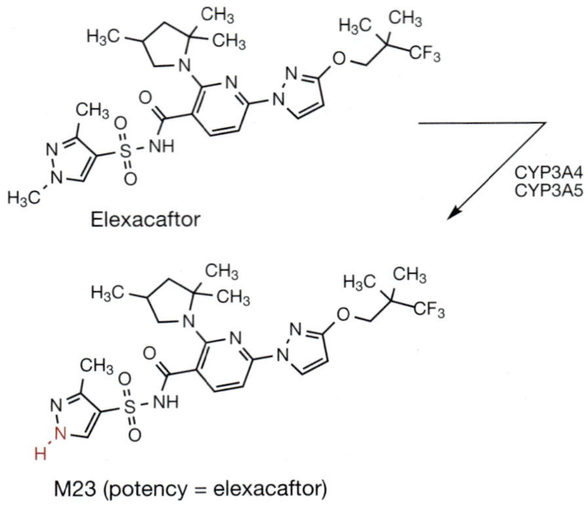

Figure 31.43 Metabolism of elexacaftor.

Structurally it is a lipophilic molecule with a calculated LogP of 5.8. Its primary metabolite in human plasma (about 17% of the dose) is the *N*-demethylated pyrazole, M23, which has similar potency as the parent structure (Fig. 31.43). The oral bioavailability is approximately 80%. The AUC of elexacaftor is increased 1.9 to 2.5-fold following a moderate-fat meal; therefore, it is recommended to give Trikafta with fat-containing food. It is eliminated in the feces (87%) and has an effective half-life of 29 hours.[179]

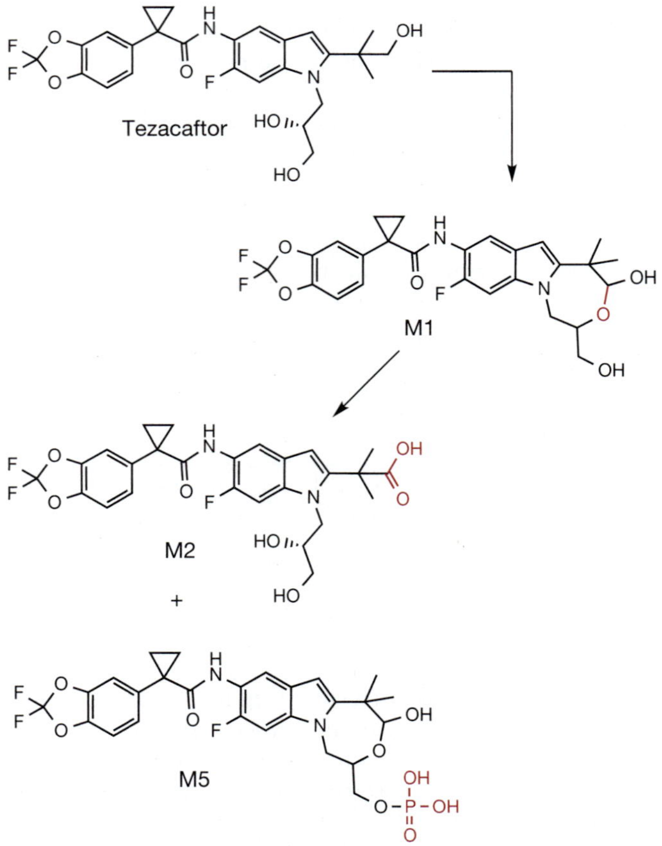

Figure 31.42 Metabolism of tezacaftor.

Idiopathic Pulmonary Fibrosis

Idiopathic pulmonary fibrosis (IPF) is a slow, progressive, irreversible disease that leads to scarring of the interstitial tissue of the lungs. The etiology and pathophysiology are not fully understood. It is believed that repetitive alveolar epithelial cell injury and dysregulated repair lead to scarring around the alveoli, which prevents oxygen absorption, and thus it becomes harder to breathe.

The pathogenesis of IPF is believed to be due to maladapted repair processes of the repeatedly damaged alveolar epithelial cells (AECs). There are two types of AECs: type I and type II. Type I AECs line the majority of the alveolar surface on the basement membrane. The repetitive exposure over time to microinjuries from infections, inhaled toxins, and gastroesophageal reflux aspirations leads to damage of the AECs. Under normal conditions, when type I AECs are damaged, type II AECs undergo hyperproliferation and lead the recovery process. The recovery process involves many chemokines such as TGF-β1, platelet-derived growth factor (PDGF), vascular endothelial growth factor (VEGF), and fibroblast growth factor (FGF). Under normal conditions, the repair mechanisms regenerate type I AECs, but under pathologic conditions, the dysfunctional type II AECs continue the repair process, leading to an inflammatory phase, which recruits IL-1 and TNF-α, leading to tissue remodeling. The dysregulated type II AECs also stimulate the production of TGF-β1. This cytokine is a pro-fibrotic mediator promoting epithelial cell apoptosis, epithelial mesenchymal transition, epithelial cell migration, and the production of other profibrotic mediators such as VEGF and connective-tissue growth factor (CTGF).[180]

Typical IPF symptoms include shortness of breath, dry cough, and clubbing of the tips of the fingers or toes. Smoking is thought to be the most common risk factor, and all patients are encouraged to quit. Approximately 50,000 new cases of IPF are diagnosed per year in the United States. It is more prevalent in men, with most patients diagnosed between ages 50 and 70. Other risk factors include environmental and occupational exposure to noxious chemicals, gastroesophageal reflux disorder (GERD), genetic predisposition, and epigenetic alterations.[181] Survival times following a diagnosis are influenced by the severity of the disease at the time of diagnosis. There is no cure for IPF, but symptoms may be treated to enhance quality of life. Typical therapy consists of oxygen supplementation, pulmonary rehabilitation, and lung transplant, along with treating comorbidities such as GERD. There are currently two FDA-approved drugs to treat IPF: nintedanib and pirfenidone.

Nintedanib (Ofev)

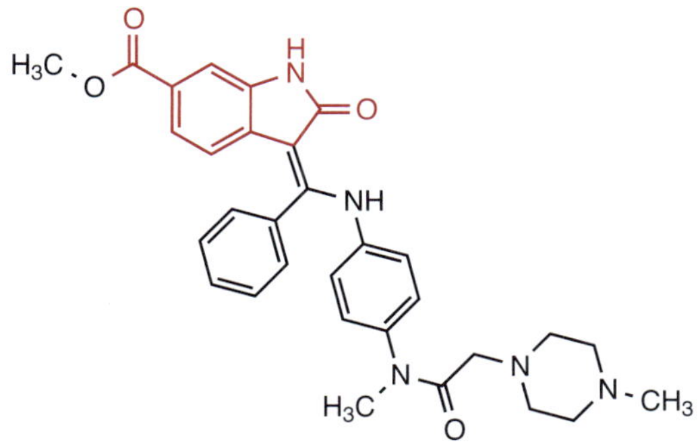

Nintedanib
(Ofev)

Nintedanib is an oral anti-fibrotic agent that has been shown to decrease the rate of fibrosis in the lungs. It is a multiple tyrosine kinase inhibitor that targets VEGF receptors 1, 2, and 3; FGF receptors 1, 2, and 3; and PDGF receptors α and β. The destructive effects of IPF are associated with these growth factors, which require tyrosine kinases for signal transduction. The oxoindoline-carboxylate structure, highlighted in red, mimics the purine of ATP, and competitively binds to the intracellular ATP binding site of the tyrosine receptor kinase. The X-ray crystal structure of the intracellular domain of human FGFR-1 shows that both oxygens (in red) are able to form hydrogen bonds with amino acids in the hinge region of the tyrosine kinase receptor.[182]

Nintedanib is reported to exhibit a low bioavailability (~5%) due to high P-glycoprotein transport. Mean plasma protein binding is 98%, with albumin being the major binding protein. The major metabolites of nintedanib found in the plasma are the carboxylic acid metabolite (32%) generated from the acetate ester hydrolysis, and its glucuronide (30%), both of which are eliminated in the feces. Other metabolites were found in low concentrations in the plasma, such as the CYP3A4 *N*-demethylelated piperazine (4%), which are also eliminated in the feces.[183] Low CYP metabolism indicates that oxidative metabolism via CYPs is minimal; thus, DDIs with CYP metabolized drugs should be negligible. The urinary excretion of nintedanib and metabolites was only 1% of the dose; thus, nonrenal elimination is responsible for the clearance. Administration of nintedanib with the potent P-gp inhibitor ketoconazole increased the AUC of nintedanib by 61%. Therefore, patients should be monitored if a P-gp inhibitor is being coadministered.[183] Common adverse effects following oral administration are GI (diarrhea, nausea, abdominal pain, vomiting) and an increase in liver transaminases. Major cardiovascular events were also reported in a small number of patients.

Pirfenidone

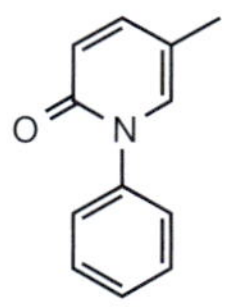

Pirfenidone (Esbriet)

Pirfenidone (Esbriet) is approved for the treatment of IPF. Pirfenidone and nintedanib have similar efficacy, and pirfenidone is often an add-on therapy to patients currently on nintedanib. There are currently no markers to monitor treatment response, and efficacy of treatment response beyond 2 years for either drug is unknown. Pirfenidone is available orally and should be taken with food to enhance absorption and decrease GI side effects. The mechanism of action of pirfenidone is not known. Pirfenidone appears to exhibit its antifibrotic effects by inhibiting fibroblast proliferation and collagen synthesis through decreased expression of TGFβ, although no molecular target or mechanism has been confirmed.[184] Pirfenidone is an example of a drug that was approved because of a therapeutic need even though no molecular target was identified. Studies in mice suggest that pirfenidone is rapidly absorbed, completely metabolized (as shown in Figure 31.44), and readily excreted in the urine following oral administration (terminal half-life in mice

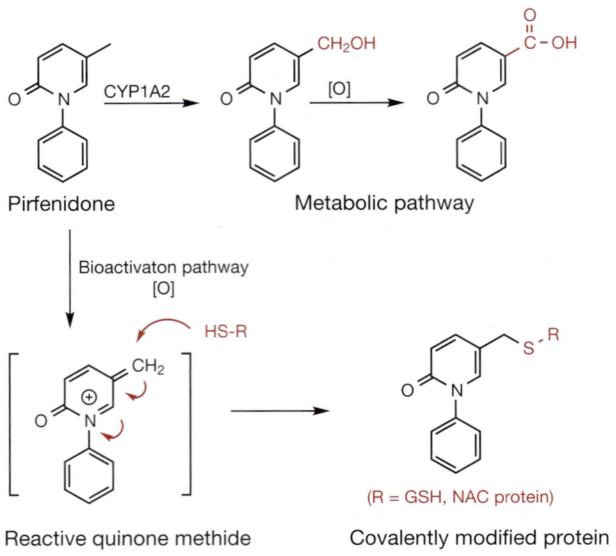

Figure 31.44 Metabolism of pirfenidone.

following IV administration is 8.6 minutes). The drug is rapidly distributed to most tissues and penetrates the blood brain barrier.[185] Approximately 80% of pirfenidone was excreted in the urine as parent drug or metabolite.[186] Metabolism consists of benzylic hydroxylation followed by cytosolic oxidation to the carboxylic acid.

Pirfenidone has similar GI side effects to nintedanib. It also displays a high incidence of photosensitivity reactions (9%). These photosensitivity reactions may be the result of covalent protein modifications of an electrophilic reactive quinone methide intermediary of pirfenidone.[187] It is also not known if the reactive quinone methide is responsible for its mechanism of action since the drug target has not been identified.

Pulmonary Arterial Hypertension

PAH is a progressive and life-threatening condition characterized by elevated blood pressure in the arteries that supply the lungs. The increased pressure in the pulmonary arteries is due to increased vascular resistance. Thickening of the pulmonary artery wall, sustained vasoconstriction, and the overabundance of many inflammatory mediators lead to remodeling of the pulmonary endothelium and vascular smooth muscle. This results in reduced blood flow and a reduced oxygen supply. Patients have an excessive hemodynamic load on the right ventricle leading to reduced cardiac output and signs of systemic congestion such as fatigue, syncope, and edema. Treatment focuses on symptomatic treatment and targeted therapies to reduce afterload of the right ventricle.

PAH is a rare disease, with a prevalence of 15 to 55 cases per million people, affecting females more frequently than males.[188] The disease may be heritable due to a gene mutation, or it may be idiopathic. Median survival time of untreated PAH patients is about 3 years, whereas treated patients survive about 7 years. PAH therapies target one of three pathways that are out of balance in patients with PAH; no treatment is curative. The three pathways with current treatments are: (1) the prostacyclin pathway treated with prostacyclin mimetics/receptor agonists, which stimulate cAMP production; (2) the endothelin pathway treated with endothelin receptor antagonists (ERAs), which mitigate effects of excess endothelin; and (3) the nitric oxide (NO) pathway, treated with phosphodiesterase-5 inhibitors (PDE5i) and soluble guanylate cyclase stimulators (sGCS).

Endothelial cells cover the pulmonary blood vessels and secrete vasoactive molecules, which interact with the underlying vascular smooth muscle to determine the diameter of the pulmonary vessels (Fig. 31.45). Pulmonary vasodilation is mediated by cAMP and cGMP. PGI_2 (prostacyclin) is a vasoactive prostaglandin highly expressed in pulmonary vascular endothelial cells and formed from the metabolism of arachidonic acid (see Fig. 31.2). PGI_2 binding to the prostanoid IP receptor activates the adenylyl cyclase enzyme, which converts AMP to cAMP. Cyclic AMP increases protein kinase activity, leading to several physiologic events, including vasodilation. Reduced levels of prostacyclin synthase (and, therefore, PGI_2) are observed in PAH patients (see Fig. 31.2). The IP receptor offers an excellent drug target for treating PAH.

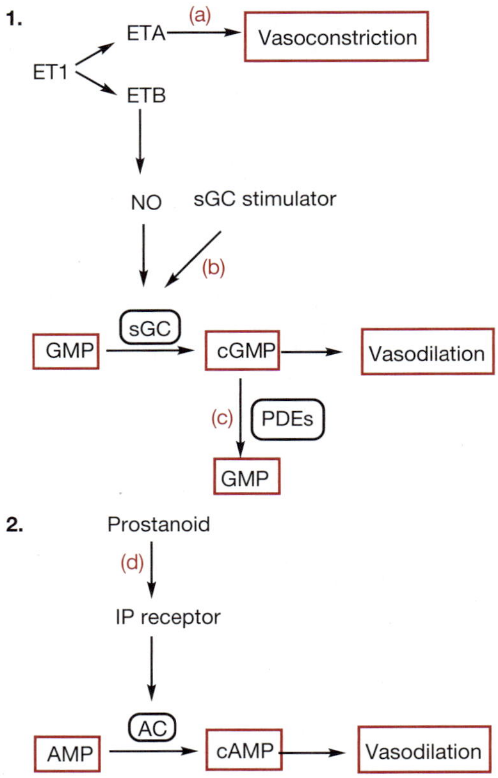

Figure 31.45 Various pathways of vasodilation in pulmonary arteries along with drug targets for the currently available drugs. (1) cGMP-mediated vasodilation pathway; (2) cAMP-mediated vasodilation pathway; (a) endothelic receptor antagonist; (b) sGC stimulator; (c) phosphodiesterase-5 inhibitors; (d) prostacyclin receptor agonists. AC, adenylyl cyclase; AMP, adenosine monophosphate; ET1, endothelin-1; ETA, endothelin receptor A; ETB, endothelin receptor B; cGMP, cyclic guanosine monophosphate; GTP, guanosine triphosphate; IP, prostacyclin receptor; NO, nitric oxide; sGC, soluble guanylyl cyclase; PDE, phosphodiesterase.

Cyclic GMP–mediated vasodilation is initiated by NO. Endothelin-1 (ET-1) is an endogenous vasoconstrictor produced in the pulmonary vascular smooth muscles that facilitates smooth muscle proliferation. ET-1 binds to two subtype receptors, ET_A and ET_B receptors. Binding at ET_A receptors leads to vasoconstriction and smooth muscle proliferation, whereas ET_B binding leads to vasodilation via activating the NO-cGMP pathway catalyzed by the guanylyl cyclase enzyme (see Fig. 31.45). ET_A receptors are overexpressed in vascular smooth muscles of PAH patients, and antagonists at ET_A receptors could help alleviate PAH symptoms. Direct activators of the soluble guanylyl cyclase (sGC) enzyme are also clinically available to treat PAH.

Cyclic GMP and cAMP are metabolized by PDE enzymes to GMP and AMP, respectively. Phosphodiesterase-5 (PDE5) is highly expressed in lungs and, hence, PDE5 inhibitors provide therapeutic benefit in PAH patients.[188] The PDE5i drugs used in PAH include sildenafil and tadalafil, which are covered in more detail in Chapter 25.

Therapeutic Classes of Drugs Used for Treating Pulmonary Arterial Hypertension

Prostacyclin Receptor Agonists

The prostacyclin agonists were the first drugs developed to treat PAH. Prostacyclin is synthesized from arachidonic acid through the cyclooxygenase pathway (see Fig. 31.2). It is a potent vasodilator. PGI_2 is an endogenous prostacyclin that activates IP receptors resulting in vasodilation along with antiproliferative and anticoagulant effects. Prostacyclin synthetase is downregulated in patients with PAH, leading to decreased levels of PGI_2. Hence, agonists at prostacyclin receptors help alleviate symptoms in patients by compensating for the loss of endogenous PGI_2. Prostacyclin receptor agonists are available in oral, inhaled, and parenteral (IV or SC) formulations.

PGI_2 ANALOGUES. Epoprostenol sodium, iloprost, and treprostinil are synthetic PGI_2 (prostacyclin) analogues, while selexipag is a non-prostanoid that binds to the prostacyclin receptor (IP). All are indicated for the treatment of PAH.

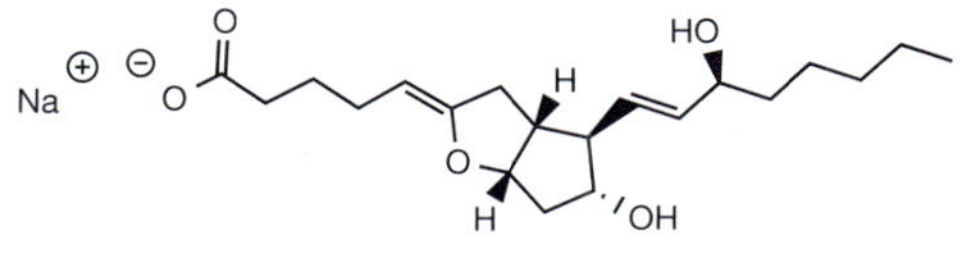

Epoprostenol sodium = PGI_2
(Flolan, Veletri)

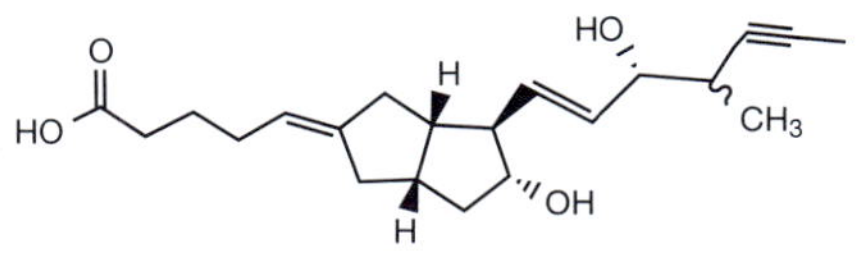

Iloprost
(Ventavis)

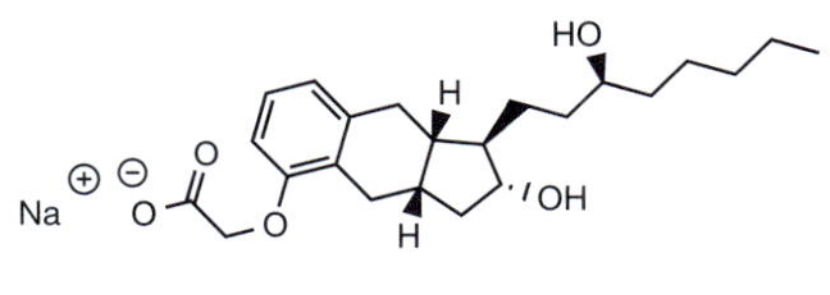

Treprostinil sodium
(Remodulin)

Epoprostenol (Flolan) is the sodium salt form of PGI_2. It is highly unstable, with a half-life of less than 5 minutes. It is administered as an IV solution or through a surgically placed central venous catheter. Due to the short half-life, patients are instructed to have backup pumps and drug available. Epoprostenol undergoes metabolism to inactive 6-keto-$PGF_{1\alpha}$ (Prostaglandin F1α [nonenzymatic]) and 6,15-diketo-13,14-dihydro-$PGF_{1\alpha}$ (Fig. 31.46).

Iloprost (Ventavis) is a synthetic analogue of PGI_2. It is available in Europe as an injectable formulation, and in the United States as an inhaled solution for use with a pulmonary drug delivery device. The improved half-life of 20 to 30 minutes allows for q2 hour dosing. The FDA approved an injectable form of iloprost (Aurlumyn) for the treatment of severe frostbite.

Treprostinil is available as an injectable (Remodulin), inhaled (Tyvaso), and oral tablet (Orenitram) formulation. Treprostinil has a longer half-life of 4 hours and improved stability compared to epoprostenol. Remodulin is a parenteral formulation, with continuous SC infusion being the preferred mode. Tyvaso, the DPI inhalation form, is scheduled every 4 hours. This is less frequently needed compared to iloprost and leads to better patient compliance.[189] The oral formulation uses diolamine as the salt and osmotic tablet technology. The tablet is coated with a semipermeable membrane that absorbs water. The tablet contents are released when the hydrostatic pressure within the tablet forces the drug across the membrane at a controlled, near zero-order rate. The oral bioavailability is approximately 17%. The tablet does not dissolve. So patients should be counseled to expect to see it in the feces. Treprostinil undergoes extensive first-pass metabolism, with only 1% of the drug eliminated unchanged. It undergoes metabolism by CYP2C8 and to a lesser extent by 2C9 (Fig. 31.47).[190]

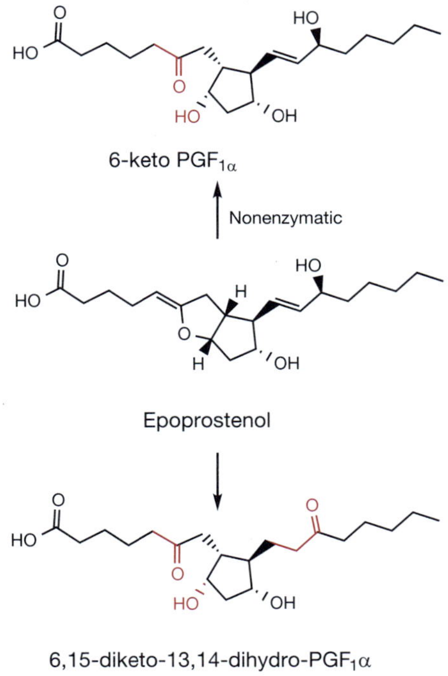

Figure 31.46 Metabolism of epoprostenol. PGF, prostaglandin F.

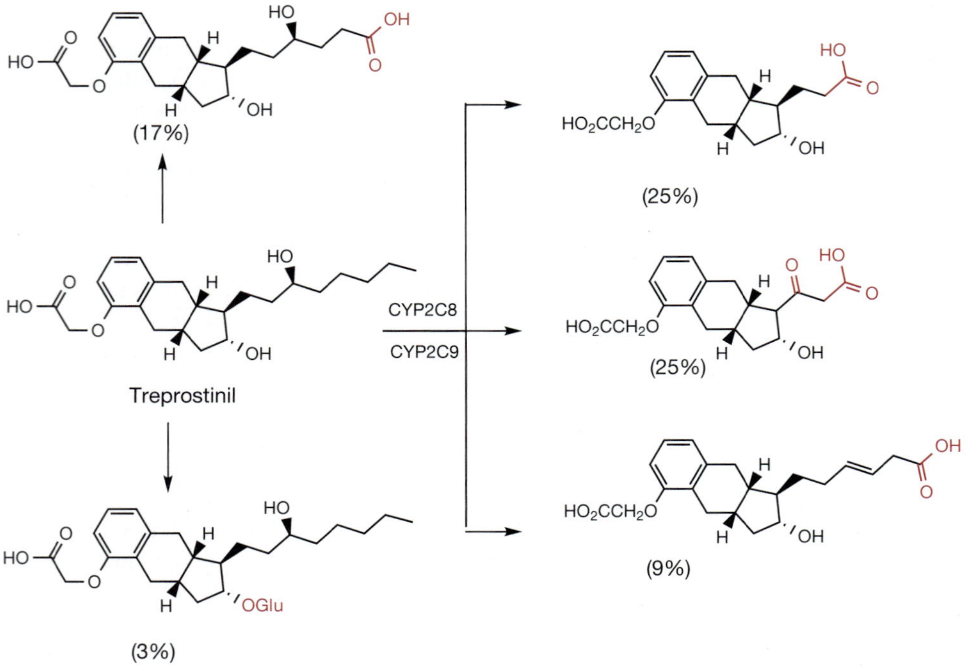

Figure 31.47 Metabolism of treprostinil.

PGI_2 is a powerful inhibitor of platelet aggregation. So, apart from vasodilation, these agonists also possess a strong anticoagulant effect. Hence, caution must be observed in patients with bleeding risk. The most common adverse reactions are dizziness, jaw pain, headache, musculoskeletal pain, and nausea/vomiting, and all drugs are generally associated with vasodilation effects such as flushing and syncope. Therapy should not be abruptly stopped, or patients run the risk of rebound PAH.

SELEXIPAG

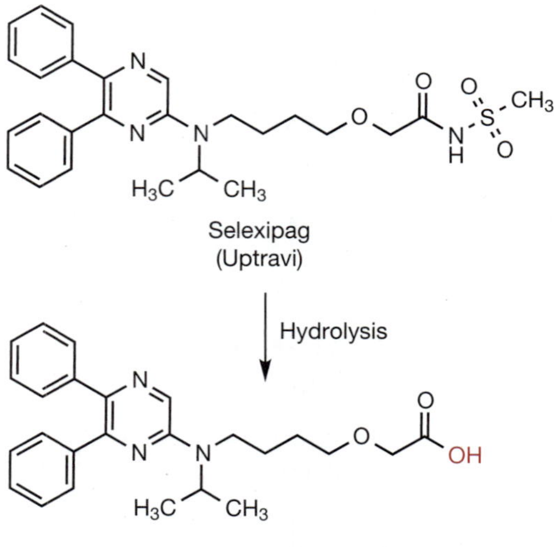

Selexipag (Uptravi) is the first nonprostanoid IP receptor agonist developed. It is approved for the treatment of PAH, and is available in both an oral and intravenous formulation. Selexipag is rapidly absorbed following oral administration and rapidly hydrolyzed by liver carboxylesterase to its active metabolite. The metabolite is approximately 37-fold more potent based on binding to the IP receptor. Both selexipag and its active metabolite undergo hydroxylation by CYP2C8 at the para position of the phenyl ring. CYP2C8 also catalyzes dealkylation reactions.[191] Concomitant use of strong CYP2C8 inhibitors such as gemfibrozil is contraindicated. Maximum plasma concentrations of selexipag and its metabolite are reached within 3 hours, and the terminal half-life for the active metabolite is 6.2 to 13.5 hours. When administered with food, absorption is reduced, as is the blood level of the metabolite, but adverse effects are also significantly reduced. The major route of elimination is the hepatobiliary route, with 93% of a radiolabeled dose recovered in the feces. The common adverse effects reported for selexipag include headache, diarrhea, jaw pain, and nausea.

Endothelin-Receptor Antagonists

The endothelins (ETs) consist of three different isoforms (ET-1, ET-2, and ET-3), with ET-1 being the most clinically significant. ET-1 is a potent vasoactive compound produced by vascular endothelial cells. The lungs are a major source of endothelin, and plasma levels of ET-1 are raised in both lung tissue and plasma in patients with PAH. Endothelin has two G-protein receptors ETR_A and ETR_B (endothelin receptor A and endothelin receptor B, respectively). When ET-1 binds to ETR_A, vasoconstriction results; when it binds to ETR_B, it activates the release of nitric oxide and prostacyclin and inhibits apoptosis. The expression of both ETR_A and ETR_B in patients with PAH is increased while the proportion remains constant (60% ETR_A and 40% ETR_B).[192] The biology of ETR function is highly complex, but dual blockade of both ETR_A and ETR_B resulted in maximal reduction of sensitivity to ET-1 and improved clinical outcomes in patients with PAH.

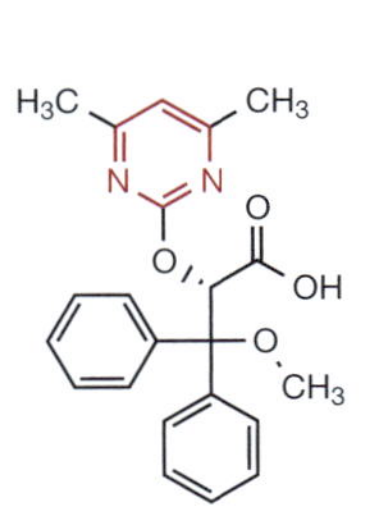

Ambrisentan
(Letairis)

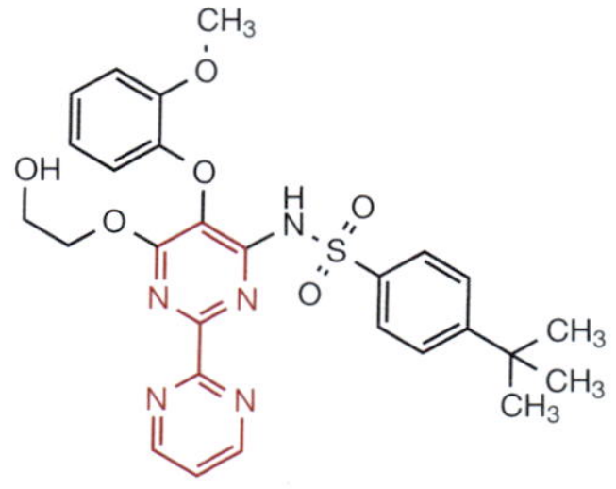

Bosentan
(Tracleer)

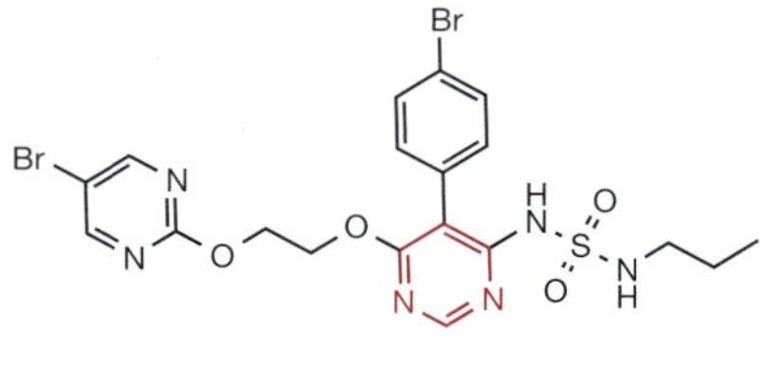

Macitentan
(Opsumit)

Macitentan, Ambrisentan, and Bosentan

All three FDA-approved ERAs, Macitentan (Opsumit), Bosentan (Tracleer) and Ambrisentan (Letairis) block both ETR_A and ETR_B. Bosentan has a slightly higher affinity for ETR_A than ETR_B. Macitentan exhibits a 50-fold selectivity for ETR_A, while ambrisentan has the highest selectivity for the ETR_A receptor (>4,000-fold).[193] The clinical impact of the selectivity is not known.

All three drugs have chemical similarity. They all contain one or more substituted pyrimidines, and they each have a required acidic functional group and multiple hydrophobic (aromatic or acyl) groups. The acidic functional group differs among them: bosentan has a sulfonamide, macitentan contains a sulfamide, and ambrisentan has a carboxylic acid. Bosentan was the first drug approved and was discovered through high throughput screening, not rational drug design.[194] Subsequently the x-ray crystal structure of the drug bound to ETR_B showed that bosentan occupies the same binding site as the terminal 3 amino acids of ET-1. The sulfonamide of bosentan binds to a positively charged pocket of the receptor occupied by two lysines and an arginine. These same amino acids are involved in binding the terminal carboxylic acid of the endogenous ligand ET-1. The hydrophobic functional groups of bosentan were found to mimic the terminal three amino acids (Il-19, Ile20, and Trp21) of ET-1 and bind to the same hydrophobic binding pocket.[195] Bosentan is available as a twice daily oral tablet. Hepatotoxicity is a concern, and patients are required to have their liver function monitored. Bosentan is metabolized by CYP2C9 and CYP3A4 and has a terminal half-life of about 5 hours.

Ambrisentan is approved as a once-daily tablet and may be started with the PDE5 inhibitor tadalafil for improved outcomes. It is highly bound to plasma proteins and metabolized through CYP3A4, CYP2C19, and UGTs. The only clinically relevant DDI found thus far is with cyclosporine. Cyclosporine increases ambrisentan exposure, necessitating an ambrisentan dose reduction. It has an effective half-life of about 9 hours.

Macitentan was specifically developed to have a longer half-life than bosentan and a better hepatic safety profile. Converting the sulfonamide to a sulfamide decreased the acidity ($pK_a = 6.2$) yet increased the drug's target affinity, not through charge-charge interactions (Arg_{326} in ETR_A) but through hydrophobic interactions in a sub-pocket of the receptor. It was also determined that the second pyrimidine ring could be removed without a loss of potency.[194] Macitentan is administered 10 mg daily in tablet form. The drug undergoes primarily CYP3A4 metabolism to an active and several inactive metabolites (Fig. 31.48), and DDIs may be expected if coadministered with CYP3A4 inhibitors or inducers.[196] The elimination half-life of macitentan is approximately 16 hours and the active metabolite approximately 48 hours.

Peripheral edema is one of the consequences of PAH, and this may worsen with ERAs. Increased fluid retention may necessitate a discontinuation of the ERA. The most common adverse effects of ERAs consist of respiratory tract infections and anemia. All three FDA-approved drugs have been shown to cause embryo-fetal toxicity in animals. They are contraindicated in pregnancy and may only be administered to female patients through a restricted Risk Evaluation and Mitigation Strategy (REMS) program.

Phosphodiestase-5 Inhibitors

PDEs metabolize cGMP and cAMP, important mediators for vasodilation. PDE5 is highly expressed in pulmonary vascular smooth muscle cells of patients with PAH. Inhibiting PDE5 extends the duration of cGMP and cAMP and promotes vasodilation. Sildenafil and tadalafil are the two PDE5 inhibitors approved for treating patients with PAH. Tadalafil has a longer half-life, allowing once-daily dosing rather than the 3 times daily dosing for sildenafil. Detailed mechanism and metabolism information for this class of drugs can be found in Chapter 25.

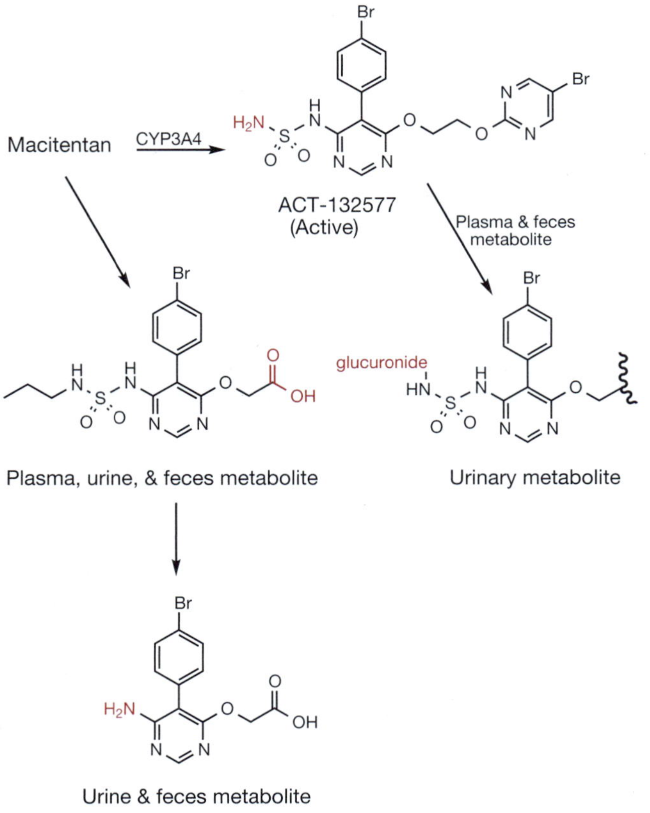

Figure 31.48 Metabolism of macitentan.

Soluble Guanylyl Cyclase Stimulators

RIOCIGUAT (ADEMPAS)

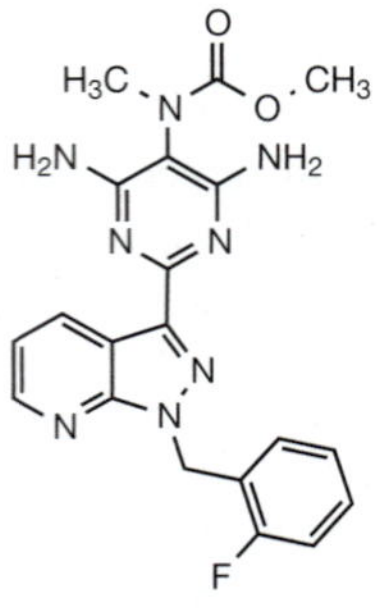

Riociguat
(Adempas)

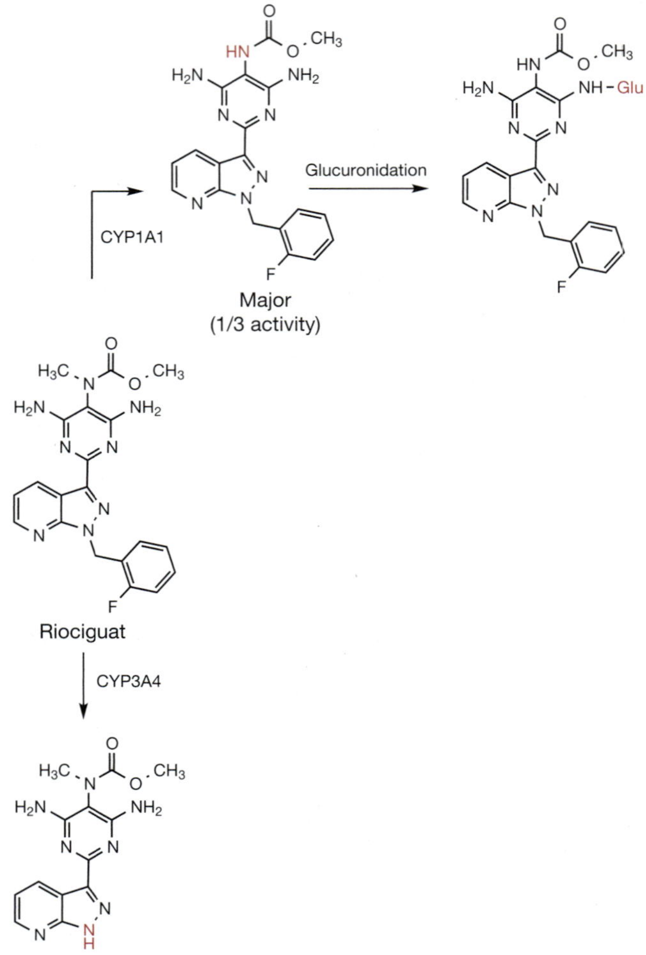

Figure 31.49 Metabolism of riociguat.

The PDE inhibitors sildenafil and tadalafil block the metabolism of cGMP and, thus, increase the nitric oxide-cGMP pathway, while soluble guanylyl cyclase (sGC) stimulators directly enhance cGMP production. Soluble guanylyl cyclase consists of one α and one β subunit, which contains a heme (Fe^{2+}) moiety. When the endogenous substrate for sGC, nitric oxide (NO), binds to the Fe^{2+}, it causes the cleavage of an Fe^{2+}-histidine bond, likely causing the conformational change required to activate the catalytic site, which converts GTP to cGMP, initiating vasodilation.[197] Riociguat is indicated for the treatment of PAH and has two mechanisms of actions. It binds to the sGC in the presence of NO to enhance the activity of sGC increasing the formation of cGMP. It can also bind to sGC without NO to directly stimulate the conformational change required to activate its catalytic site and thereby convert GTP to cGMP. The diaminopyrimidine group of riociguat binds to the sGC through polar interactions with a β1 cysteine. The terminal methylcarbamate of riociguat binds to α1 arginine.[198] These and other interactions keep the sGC in the active state.

Riociguat is available as an oral tablet dosed 3 times a day. It has a bioavailability of 94%, and 95% of the drug is bound to plasma albumin and α1-acidic glycoprotein. It is metabolized by CYP1A1 (major metabolite, a third as active), CYP3A4, CYP2C8, and CYP2J2 (Fig. 31.49).[199] Concomitant use with strong CYP inhibitors such as azole antifungals or HIV protease inhibitors may result in hypotension; thus, a lower dose may be indicated.[200] It is also a substrate of P-glycoprotein/ABCB1. CYP1A1 is induced by cigarette smoke, making riociguat subtherapeutic in chronic smokers. Its elimination half-life is about 12 hours, and it is excreted almost equally via the feces and urine. Common side effects seen are headache, dizziness, dyspepsia, nausea, diarrhea, and anemia. It is contraindicated in pregnancy due to fetal toxicity seen in rat studies and is only available through REMS programs.

Structure Challenge

Objective: Based on your knowledge of pK_a and pH, and the formulation of buccal nicotine discussed in this chapter, answer the following questions.

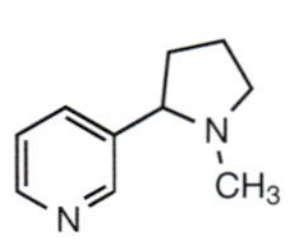

Nicotine

A 45-year-old patient, attempting to quit smoking for the third time, is prescribed buccal nicotine lozenges to manage withdrawal symptoms. The patient finds the taste of the buccal nicotine lozenges unpleasant and decides to consume orange juice while the lozenge is dissolving in his mouth to mask the taste. He comes to the pharmacy counter for a consult.

1. You first review the package insert and it lists two pK_as. The first pK_a listed is 3.4 and the second is 8.1. Assign the pK_as to the correct functional groups. Which pK_a belongs to the pyrrolidine nitrogen?

   A. 3.4
   B. 8.1

Structure Challenge (continued)

2. What will be the outcome of the patient's decision to consume orange juice with the buccal nicotine?

   A. Enhanced absorption of nicotine leading to increased side effects due to protonated pyridine
   B. Enhanced absorption of nicotine leading to increased side effects due to protonated pyrrolidine
   C. Decreased absorption of nicotine reducing the therapeutic effect due to protonated pyridine
   D. Decreased absorption of nicotine reducing the therapeutic effect due to protonated pyrrolidine

3. The patient returns to the pharmacy and mentions that they took your advice to stop using orange juice to mask the taste of the nicotine in the buccal lozenge. They state that the bitter taste bothers them so much that they decided to just swallow the lozenge whole. We will assume the pH of their stomach is approximately 2. What will the charge on nicotine be in the stomach?

   A. +2
   B. +1
   C. 0
   D. −1
   E. −2.

Objective: Based on your knowledge of the SARs required for glucocorticoid activity discussed in this chapter, answer the following question.

4. The metabolism of inhaled Steroid X below forms the following three metabolites. Which metabolite is inactive?

   A. Metabolite A
   B. Metabolite B
   C. Metabolite C

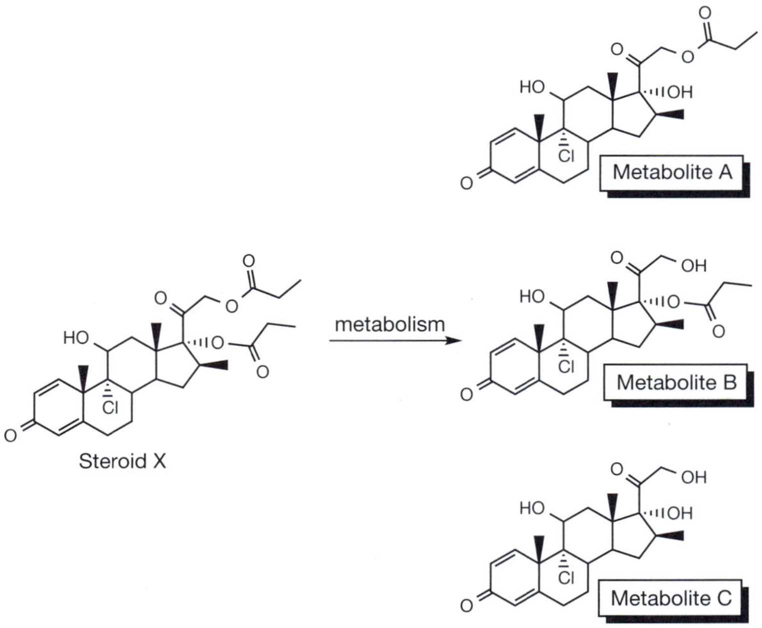

Structure Challenge answers found immediately after References.

ACKNOWLEDGEMENTS

The author wishes to acknowledge the work of S. William Zito PhD and Srikanth Kolluru PhD who authored components of the content used within this chapter in a previous edition of this text.

REFERENCES

1. Levy BD. Approach to the patient with disease of the respiratory system. In: Loscalzo J, Fauci A, Kasper D, Hauser S, Longo D, Jameson JL, eds. *Harrison's Principles of Internal Medicine.* 21st ed. McGraw-Hill Education; 2022. Accessed March 12, 2025. https://accessmedicine-mhmedical-com.ezproxymcp.flo.org/content.aspx?bookid=3095&sectionid=263546227
2. Pasqua E, Hamblin N, Edwards C, Baker-Glenn C, Hurley C. Developing inhaled drugs for respiratory diseases: a medicinal chemistry perspective. *Drug Discov Today.* 2022;27(1):134-150.
3. Castell JV, Teresa Donato M, Gómez-Lechón MJ. Metabolism and bioactivation of toxicants in the lung. The in vitro cellular approach. *Exp Toxicol Pathol.* 2005;57:189-204.
4. Buttini F, Glieca S, Sonvico F, Lewis DA. Metered dose inhalers in the transition to low GWP propellants: what we know and what is missing to make it happen. *Expert Opin Drug Deliv.* 2023;20(8):1131-1143.
5. Chen Y, Du S, Zhang Z, et al. Compatible stability and aerosol characteristics of Atrovent® (ipratropium bromide) mixed with salbutamol sulfate, terbutaline sulfate, budesonide, and acetylcysteine. *Pharmaceutics.* 2020;12(8). doi:10.3390/pharmaceutics12080776
6. Karamanou M, Androutsos G. Aretaeus of Cappadocia and the first clinical description of asthma. *Am J Respir Crit Care Med.* 2011;184(12):1420-1421.
7. Marketos SG, Ballas CN. Bronchial Asthma in the Medical Literature of Greek Antiquity. *J Asthma.* 1982;19(4):263-269.
8. Centers for Disease Control and Prevention. Asthma: most recent national asthma data. Updated May 2023. Accessed September 22, 2023. https://www.cdc.gov/asthma/most_recent_national_asthma_data.htm
9. National Center for Environmental Health. Asthma surveillance in the United Stated, 2001-2021. Accessed September 22, 2023. https://www.cdc.gov/asthma/Asthma-Prevalence-US-2023-508.pdf
10. Centers for Diasease Control and Prevention. CDC's National Asthma Control Program: an investment in America's health. Accessed July 5, 2025. https://stacks.cdc.gov/view/cdc/133926/cdc_133926_DS1.pdf
11. Song HJ, Blake KV, Wilson DL, Winterstein AG, Park H. Medical costs and productivity loss due to mild, moderate, and severe asthma in the United States. *J Asthma Allergy.* 2020;13:545-555.
12. Levy ML, Bacharier LB, Bateman E, et al. Key recommendations for primary care from the 2022 Global Initiative for Asthma (GINA) update. *NPJ Prim Care Respir Med.* 2023;33(1):7.
13. Global Initiative for Asthma. Global strategy for asthma management and prevention. 2023. www.ginasthma.org
14. Haldar P, Pavord ID, Shaw DE, et al. Cluster analysis and clinical asthma phenotypes. *Am J Respir Crit Care Med.* 2008;178(3):218-224.
15. Chabra R, Gupta M. Allergic and environmentally induced asthma. In: *StatPearls* [Internet]. StatPearls Publishing; 2024.
16. Valverde-Monge M, Fernández-Nieto M, López VB, et al. Novel causes of drug-induced occupational asthma. *J Allergy Clin Immunol Pract.* 2019;7(2):740-742.e1.
17. U.S. Department of Labor. Occupational asthma. Occupational Safety and Health Administration (OSHA). https://www.osha.gov/occupational-asthma
18. Reddel HK, Bacharier LB, Bateman ED, et al. Global initiative for asthma strategy 2021: executive summary and rationale for key changes. *J Allergy Clin Immunol Pract.* 2022;10(1):S1-S18.
19. Thomsen SF. Genetics of asthma: an introduction for the clinician. *Eur Clin Respir J.* 2015:2.
20. Shinde V, Wankhede P, Vyawahare N. Asthma: cells involved in the pathophysiology of asthma. *J Assoc Chest Physicians.* 2023;11(1):10-18.
21. Barnes PJ. Pulmonary pharmacology. In: Brunton LL, Knollmann BC, eds. *Goodman & Gilman's: The Pharmacological Basis of Therapeutics.* 14th ed. McGraw-Hill Education; 2023. Accessed March 12, 2025. https://accessmedicine-mhmedical-com.ezproxymcp.flo.org/content.aspx?bookid=3191&sectionid=269308304
22. Cloutier MM, Baptist AP, Blake KV, et al. 2020 Focused updates to the asthma management guidelines: report from the National Asthma Education and Prevention Program Coordinating Committee Expert Panel Working Group. *J Allergy Clin Immunol Pract.* 2020;146(6):1217-1270.
23. Crossingham I, Turner S, Ramakrishnan S, et al. Combination fixed-dose beta agonist and steroid inhaler as required for adults or children with mild asthma. *Cochrane Database Syst Rev.* 2021;5(5):CD013518.
24. Garzon-Siatoya WT, Carrillo-Martin I, Chiarella SE, Gonzalez-Estrada A. State-of-the-art beta-adrenoreceptor agonists for the treatment of asthma. *Expert Opin Pharmacother.* 2022;23(2):243-254.
25. Bylund DB, Eikenberg DC, Hieble JP, et al. International Union of Pharmacology nomenclature of adrenoceptors. *Pharmacol Rev.* 1994;46(2):121.
26. Parascandola J. Abel, Takamine, and the isolation of epinephrine. *J Allergy Clin Immunol.* 2010;125(2):514-517.
27. Schena G, Caplan MJ. Everything you always wanted to know about β(3)-AR * (* but were afraid to ask). *Cells.* 2019;8(4):357.
28. Moratinos J, Reverte M. Effects of catecholamines on plasma potassium: the role of alpha- and beta-adrenoceptors. *Fundam Clin Pharmacol.* 1993;7(3-4):143-153.
29. Mandelberg A, Krupnik Z, Houri S, et al. Salbutamol metered-dose inhaler with spacer for hyperkalemia: how fast? how safe? *Chest.* 1999;115(3):617-622.
30. Montassier E, Legrand M, Rossignol P, Potel G. Hyperkalemia in the emergency department: consider the use of nebulized salbutamol. *Am J Emerg Med.* 2019;37(5):1004.
31. Rasmussen SG, DeVree BT, Zou Y, et al. Crystal structure of the β2 adrenergic receptor-Gs protein complex. *Nature.* 2011;477(7366):549-555.
32. Ring AM, Manglik A, Kruse AC, et al. Adrenaline-activated structure of β2-adrenoceptor stabilized by an engineered nanobody. *Nature.* 2013;502(7472):575-579.
33. Jozwiak K, Toll L, Jimenez L, Woo AY, Xiao RP, Wainer IW. The effect of stereochemistry on the thermodynamic characteristics of the binding of fenoterol stereoisomers to the beta(2)-adrenoceptor. *Biochem Pharmacol.* 2010;79(11):1610-1615.
34. Sadreameli SC, Brigham EP, Patel A. The surprising reintroduction of Primatene Mist in the United States. *Ann Am Thorac Soc.* 2019;16(10):1234-1236.
35. Yang F, Ling S, Zhou Y, et al. Different conformational responses of the β2-adrenergic receptor-Gs complex upon binding of the partial agonist salbutamol or the full agonist isoprenaline. *Natl Sci Rev.* 2020;8(9):nwaa284.
36. Ye F, Liu S, Yang Y, et al. Identification of the major metabolites of (R)-salbutamol in human urine, plasma and feces using ultra high performance liquid chromatography coupled with quadrupole time-of-flight mass spectrometry. *J Sep Sci.* 2019;42(20):3200-3208.
37. Nakpheng T, Songkarak S, Suwandecha T, Sritharadol R, Chunhachaichana C, Srichana T. Evidences for salbutamol metabolism by respiratory and liver cell lines. *Drug Metab Pharmacokinet.* 2017;32(2):127-134.
38. Proair HFA (albuterol sulfate). Package insert. IVAX Pharmaceuticals; Revised February 2019. Accessed December 21, 2023. https://www.accessdata.fda.gov/drugsatfda_docs/label/2019/021457s036lbl.pdf

39. Xopenex (levalbuterol tartrate). Package insert. Sunovion Pharmaceuticals Inc; Revised July 2012. Accessed May 20, 2023. https://www.accessdata.fda.gov/drugsatfda_docs/label/2012/021730s024lbl.pdf
40. Delmotte P, Sanderson MJ. Effects of albuterol isomers on the contraction and Ca2+ signaling of small airways in mouse lung slices. *Am J Respir Cell Mol Biol.* 2008;38(5):524-531.
41. Maly G, Mudge S, Brown P. Do inhaled levalbuterol and racemic albuterol have different cardiac effects? *Evidence-Based Pract.* 2016;19(2):15.
42. Jat KR, Khairwa A. Levalbuterol versus albuterol for acute asthma: a systematic review and meta-analysis. *Pulm Pharmacol Ther.* 2013;26(2):239-248.
43. Lötvall J. Pharmacological similarities and differences between β2-agonists. *Respir Med.* 2001;95:S7-S11.
44. Masureel M, Zou Y, Picard L-P, et al. Structural insights into binding specificity, efficacy and bias of a β2AR partial agonist. *Nat Chem Biol.* 2018;14(11):1059-1066.
45. Salmeterol (Serevent Diskus). Package insert. GlaxoSmithKline; Revised October 2022. Accessed December 21, 2023. https://gskpro.com/content/dam/global/hcpportal/en_US/Prescribing_Information/Serevent_Diskus/pdf/SEREVENT-DISKUS-PI-MG-IFU.PDF
46. Rosenborg J, Larsson P, Tegnér K, Hallström G. Mass balance and metabolism of hformoterol in healthy men after combined i.v. and oral administration–mimicking inhalation. *Drug Metabol Dispos.* 1999;27(10):1104-1116.
47. Cheer SM, Scott LJ. Formoterol. *Am J Respir Med.* 2002;1(4):285-300.
48. Zhang Y, Yang F, Ling S, et al. Single-particle cryo-EM structural studies of the β2AR–Gs complex bound with a full agonist formoterol. *Cell Discov.* 2020;6(1):45.
49. Brovana (arformoterol tartrate). Package insert. Sunovion Pharmaceuticals Inc; Revised 2014. Accessed February 25, 2024. https://www.accessdata.fda.gov/drugsatfda_docs/label/2014/021912s013lbl.pdf
50. Cazzola M, Page CP, Calzetta L, Matera MG. Pharmacology and therapeutics of bronchodilators. *Pharmacol Rev.* 2012;64(3):450-504.
51. Harrell AW, Siederer SK, Bal J, et al. Metabolism and disposition of vilanterol, a long-acting adrenoceptor agonist for inhalation use in humans. *Drug Metab Dispos.* 2013;41(1):89-100.
52. Dvir H, Silman I, Harel M, Rosenberry TL, Sussman JL. Acetylcholinesterase: from 3D structure to function. *Chem Biol Interact.* 2010;187(1-3):10-22.
53. Pinho BR, Ferreres F, Valentão P, Andrade PB. Nature as a source of metabolites with cholinesterase-inhibitory activity: an approach to Alzheimer's disease treatment. *J Pharm Pharmacol.* 2013;65(12):1681-1700.
54. Provocholine (Methacholine chloride). Package insert. Methapharm Inc; Revised November 2019. Accessed February 24, 2024. https://www.accessdata.fda.gov/drugsatfda_docs/label/2019/019193s021lbl.pdf
55. Ora J, Coppola A, Cazzola M, Calzetta L, Rogliani P. Long-acting muscarinic antagonists under investigational to treat chronic obstructive pulmonary disease. *J Exp Pharmacol.* 2020;12:559-574.
56. Liu H, Hofmann J, Fish I, et al. Structure-guided development of selective M3 muscarinic acetylcholine receptor antagonists. *Proc Natl Acad Sci U S A.* 2018;115(47):12046-12050.
57. Global Initiative for Chronic Obstructive Lung Disease. 2024 Gold Report: Global strategy for the diagnosis, management, and prevention of chronic obstructive pulmonary disease. Accessed February 28, 2024. https://goldcopd.org/2024-gold-report/
58. Calzetta L, Ritondo BL, Zappa MC, et al. The impact of long-acting muscarinic antagonists on mucus hypersecretion and cough in chronic obstructive pulmonary disease: a systematic review. *Eur Respir Rev.* 2022;31(164):210196.
59. Wess J, Blin N, Mutschler E, Blüml K. Muscarinic acetylcholine receptors: structural basis of ligand binding and G protein coupling. *Life Sci.* 1995;56(11-12):915-922.
60. Jackson M. "Divine stramonium": the rise and fall of smoking for asthma. *Med Hist.* 2010;54(2):171-194.
61. Alizadeh A, Moshiri M, Alizadeh J, Balali-Mood M. Black henbane and its toxicity–a descriptive review. *Avicenna J Phytomed.* 2014;4(5):297-311.
62. Moulton BC, Fryer AD. Muscarinic receptor antagonists, from folklore to pharmacology; finding drugs that actually work in asthma and COPD. *Br J Pharmacol.* 2011;163(1):44-52.
63. Griffin WJ, Lin GD. Chemotaxonomy and geographical distribution of tropane alkaloids. *Phytochemistry.* 2000;53(6):623-637.
64. Domańska U, Pobudkowska A, Pelczarska A, Gierycz P. pKa and solubility of drugs in water, ethanol, and 1-octanol. *J Phys Chem B.* 2009;113(26):8941-8947.
65. Spinks A, Wasiak J. Scopolamine (hyoscine) for preventing and treating motion sickness. *Cochrane Database Syst Rev.* 2011; 2011(6):CD002851.
66. Riad M, Hithe CC. Scopolamine. In: *StatPearls.* StatPearls Publishing; Updated May 23, 2023. Accessed February 28, 2024. https://www.ncbi.nlm.nih.gov/books/NBK554397/
67. Nakamura T, Nakanishi T, Haruta T, Shirasaka Y, Keogh JP, Tamai I. Transport of ipratropium, an anti-chronic obstructive pulmonary disease drug, is mediated by organic cation/carnitine transporters in human bronchial epithelial cells: implications for carrier-mediated pulmonary absorption. *Mol Pharm.* 2010;7(1):187-195.
68. Kola M, Hacıoğlu D, Erdöl H, Türk A. Bilateral acute angle closure developing due to use of ipratropium bromide and salbutamol. *Int Ophthalmol.* 2018;38(1):385-388.
69. Spiriva (tiotropium bromide). Package insert. Boehringer Ingelheim International GmbH; November 2021. Accessed February 8, 2024. https://www.accessdata.fda.gov/drugsatfda_docs/label/2014/021936s000lbl.pdf
70. Gavaldà A, Ramos I, Carcasona C, et al. The in vitro and in vivo profile of aclidinium bromide in comparison with glycopyrronium bromide. *Pulm Pharmacol Ther.* 2014;28(2):114-121.
71. Ortiz S, Flach S, Caracta C, Gil EG, Jansat JM. Safety and tolerability of aclidinium administered intravenously and absolute bioavailability of inhaled aclidinium in healthy male participants. *J Clin Pharmacol.* 2012;52(6):819-827.
72. Tudorza Pressair (aclidinium bromide). Package insert. Astra Zeneca; Revised March 2019. Accessed February 9, 2024. https://www.accessdata.fda.gov/drugsatfda_docs/label/2019/202450s012lbl.pdf
73. Manickam R, Asija A, Aronow WS. Umeclidinium for treating COPD: an evaluation of pharmacologic properties, safety and clinical use. *Expert Opin Drug Saf.* 2014;13(11):1555-1561.
74. Chabicovsky M, Winkler S, Soeberdt M, Kilic A, Masur C, Abels C. Pharmacology, toxicology and clinical safety of glycopyrrolate. *Toxicol Appl Pharmacol.* 2019;370:154-169.
75. Heo Y-A. Revefenacin: first global approval. *Drugs.* 2019;79(1):85-91.
76. Bourdet DL, Yeola S, Hegde SS, Colson P-J, Barnes CN, Borin MT. Revefenacin absorption, metabolism, and excretion in healthy subjects and pharmacological activity of its major metabolite. *Drug Metab Dispos.* 2020;48(12):1312-1320.
77. U.S. Food and Drug Administration. Consumer updates: spilling the beans: how much caffeine is too much? Updated September 2023. Accessed February 25, 2024. https://www.fda.gov/consumers/consumer-updates/spilling-beans-how-much-caffeine-too-much
78. Shively C, Tarka Jr S. Methylxanthine composition and consumption patterns of cocoa and chocolate products. *Prog Clin Biol Res.* 1984;158:149-178.
79. Arnaud M, Welsch C. Theophylline and caffeine metabolism in man. In: Rietbrock N, Woodcock BG, Staib, AH, eds. *Theophylline and Other Methylxanthines.* Vol 3. Vieweg and Teubner Verlag; 1982:135-148.
80. Abdel-Hady H, Nasef N, Shabaan AE, Nour I. Caffeine therapy in preterm infants. *World J Clin Pediatr.* 2015;4(4):81-93.
81. Kutryb-Zając B, Kawecka A, Nasadiuk K, et al. Drugs targeting adenosine signaling pathways: a current view. *Biomed Pharmacother.* 2023;165:115184.

82. Barnes PJ. Theophylline. *Pharmaceuticals (Basel).* 2010;3(3):725-747.
83. Whirl-Carrillo M, Huddart R, Gong L, et al. An evidence-based framework for evaluating pharmacogenomics knowledge for personalized medicine. *Clin Pharmacol Ther.* 2021;110(3):563-572.
84. Timmermans S, Vandewalle J, Libert C. Dimerization of the glucocorticoid receptor and its importance in (patho)physiology: a primer. *Cells.* 2022;11(4):684. doi:10.3390/cells11040683
85. Ingawale DK, Mandlik SK. New insights into the novel anti-inflammatory mode of action of glucocorticoids. *Immunopharmacol Immunotoxicol.* 2020;42(2):59-73.
86. Perretti M, Dalli J. Resolution pharmacology: focus on pro-resolving annexin a1 and lipid mediators for therapeutic innovation in inflammation. *Annu Rev Pharmacol Toxicol.* 2023;63(1):449-469.
87. Zhou J, Liu DF, Liu C, et al. Glucocorticoids inhibit degranulation of mast cells in allergic asthma via nongenomic mechanism. *Allergy.* 2008;63(9):1177-1185.
88. Timmermans S, Souffriau J, Libert C. A general introduction to glucocorticoid biology. review. *Front Immunol.* 2019;10:1545.
89. Frank F, Ortlund EA, Liu X. Structural insights into glucocorticoid receptor function. *Biochem Soc Trans.* 2021;49(5):2333-2343.
90. Matera MG, Rinaldi B, Calzetta L, Rogliani P, Cazzola M. Pharmacokinetics and pharmacodynamics of inhaled corticosteroids for asthma treatment. *Pulm Pharmacol Ther.* 2019;58:101828.
91. Heier CR, Yu Q, Fiorillo AA, et al. Vamorolone targets dual nuclear receptors to treat inflammation and dystrophic cardiomyopathy. *Life Sci Alliance.* 2019;2(1):e201800186.
92. Bätz FM, Klipper W, Korting HC, et al. Esterase activity in excised and reconstructed human skin—biotransformation of prednicarbate and the model dye fluorescein diacetate. *Eur J Pharm Biopharm.* 2013;84(2):374-385.
93. Hobson A. *The Medicinal Chemistry of Glucocorticoid Receptor Modulators.* SpringerBriefs in Molecular Science. Springer Nature; 2023.
94. Matabosch X, Pozo OJ, Monfort N, et al. Urinary profile of methylprednisolone and its metabolites after oral and topical administrations. *J Steroid Biochem Mol Biol.* 2013;138:214-221.
95. Cai K-J, Su S-Q, Wang Y-G, Zeng Y-M. Dexamethasone versus prednisone or prednisolone for acute pediatric asthma exacerbations in the emergency department: a meta-analysis. *Pediatr Emerg Care.* 2021;37(12):e1139-e1144.
96. Gentile DM, Tomlinson ES, Maggs JL, Park BK, Back DJ. Dexamethasone metabolism by human liver in vitro. Metabolite identification and inhibition of 6-hydroxylation. *J Pharmacol Exp Ther.* 1996;277(1):105-112.
97. Roberts JK, Moore CD, Ward RM, Yost GS, Reilly CA. Metabolism of beclomethasone dipropionate by cytochrome P450 3A enzymes. *J Pharmacol Exp Ther.* 2013;345(2):308-316.
98. Moore CD, Roberts JK, Orton CR, et al. Metabolic pathways of inhaled glucocorticoids by the CYP3A enzymes. *Drug Metabol Dispos.* 2013;41(2):379-389.
99. Van Den Brink KIM, Boorsma M, Staal-van den Brekel AJ, Edsbäcker S, Wouters EF, Thorsson L. Evidence of the in vivo esterification of budesonide in human airways. *Br J Clin Pharmacol.* 2008;66(1):27-35.
100. Nave R, Watz H, Hoffmann H, Boss H, Magnussen H. Deposition and metabolism of inhaled ciclesonide in the human lung. *Eur Respir J.* 2010;36(5):1113-1119.
101. Nave R, Fisher R, Zech K. In vitro metabolism of ciclesonide in human lung and liver precision-cut tissue slices. *Biopharm Drug Dispos.* 2006;27(4):197-207.
102. Biggadike K. Fluticasone furoate/fluticasone propionate—different drugs with different properties. *Clin Respir J.* Jul 2011;5(3):183-184.
103. Biggadike K, Bledsoe RK, Hassell AM, et al. X-ray crystal structure of the novel enhanced-affinity glucocorticoid agonist fluticasone furoate in the glucocorticoid receptor–ligand binding domain. *J Med Chem.* 2008;51(12):3349-3352.
104. Zhong Y, Li L, Chen R, Zheng Q. Quantitative comparison of dose–effect and time–course of fluticasone furoate and fluticasone propionate in adult and adolescent patients with persistent asthma: a systematic review and meta-analysis. *Respirology.* 2022;27(3):194-201.
105. Derendorf H, Daley-Yates P, Pierre L, Efthimiou J. Bioavailability and metabolism of mometasone furoate: pharmacology versus methodology. *J Clin Pharmacol.* 2002;42(4):383-387.
106. Mometasone furoate and formoterol fumarate dihydrate inhalation aerosol (Dulera). Package insert. Merck and Co, Inc; Revised June 2017. Accessed February 25, 2024. https://www.accessdata.fda.gov/drugsatfda_docs/label/2017/022518s021lbl.pdf
107. Heffler E, Madeira LNG, Ferrando M, et al. Inhaled corticosteroids safety and adverse effects in patients with asthma. *J Allergy Clin Immunol Pract.* 2018;6(3):776-781.
108. Minutello K, Gupta V. Cromolyn sodium. In: *Statpearls* [Internet]. StatPearls Publishing; 2023. https://www.ncbi.nlm.nih.gov/books/NBK557473/
109. Oyama Y, Shishibori T, Yamashita K, et al. Two distinct anti-allergic drugs, amlexanox and cromolyn, bind to the same kinds of calcium binding proteins, except calmodulin, in bovine lung extract. *Biochem Biophys Res Commun.* 1997;240(2):341-347.
110. Okada M, Tokumitsu H, Kubota Y, Kobayashi R. Interaction of S100 proteins with the antiallergic drugs, olopatadine, amlexanox, and cromolyn: identification of putative drug binding sites on S100A1 protein. *Biochem Biophys Res Commun.* 2002;292(4):1023-1030.
111. Zhang T, Finn DF, Barlow JW, Walsh JJ. Mast cell stabilisers. *Eur J Pharmacol.* 2016;778:158-168.
112. Mirsadraee M, Sabbagh Sajadieh Z, Ghafari S, Tavakoli A, Sabbagh Sajadieh S. Cromolyn, a new hope for limited treatment of neutrophilic asthma: a phase II randomized clinical trial. *Tanaffos.* 2019;18(3):208-214.
113. Kellaway C, Trethewie E. The liberation of a slow-reacting smooth muscle-stimulating substance in anaphylaxis. *Q J Exp Physiol Cogn Med Sci.* 1940;30(2):121-145.
114. Samuelsson B, Dahlén SE, Lindgren JA, Rouzer CA, Serhan CN. Leukotrienes and lipoxins: structures, biosynthesis, and biological effects. *Science.* 1987;237(4819):1171-1176.
115. Ibe BO, Campbell WB. Synthesis and metabolism of leukotrienes by human endothelial cells: influence on prostacyclin release. *Biochim Biophys Acta.* 1988;960(3):309-321.
116. Luginina A, Gusach A, Lyapina E, et al. Structural diversity of leukotriene G-protein coupled receptors. *J Biol Chem.* 2023;299(10):105247.
117. Dakhama A, Collins ML, Ohnishi H, et al. IL-13-producing BLT1-positive CD8 cells are increased in asthma and are associated with airway obstruction. *Allergy.* 2013;68(5):666-673.
118. Haeggström JZ, Newcomer ME. Structures of leukotriene biosynthetic enzymes and development of new therapeutics. *Annu Rev Pharmacol Toxicol.* 2023;63:407-428.
119. Rossi A, Pergola C, Koeberle A, et al. The 5-lipoxygenase inhibitor, zileuton, suppresses prostaglandin biosynthesis by inhibition of arachidonic acid release in macrophages. *Br J Pharmacol.* 2010;161(3):555-570.
120. Zyflo CR (Zileuton). Package insert. Chiesi USA; Revised December 2018. Accessed February 16, 2024. https://www.accessdata.fda.gov/drugsatfda_docs/label/2018/022052s014lbl.pdf
121. Palomer A, Pascual J, Cabré F, García ML, Mauleón D. Derivation of pharmacophore and CoMFA models for leukotriene D(4) receptor antagonists of the quinolinyl(bridged)aryl series. *J Med Chem.* 2000;43(3):392-400.
122. Luginina A, Gusach A, Marin E, et al. Structure-based mechanism of cysteinyl leukotriene receptor inhibition by antiasthmatic drugs. *Sci Adv.* 2019;5(10):eaax2518.
123. Chiba M, Xu X, Nishime JA, Balani SK, Lin JH. Hepatic microsomal metabolism of montelukast, a potent leukotriene D4 receptor antagonist, in humans. *Drug Metab Dispos.* 1997;25(9):1022-1031.
124. Paljarvi T, Forton J, Luciano S, Herttua K, Fazel S. Analysis of neuropsychiatric diagnoses after montelukast initiation. *JAMA Netw Open.* 2022;5(5):e2213643.

125. Savidge R, Bui K, Birmingham B, Morse J, Spreen R. Metabolism and excretion of zafirlukast in dogs, rats, and mice. *Drug Metab Dispos*. 1998;26(11):1069-1076.
126. Kassahun K, Skordos K, McIntosh I, et al. Zafirlukast metabolism by cytochrome P450 3A4 produces an electrophilic α,β-unsaturated iminium species that results in the selective mechanism-based inactivation of the enzyme. *Chem Res Toxicol*. 2005;18(9):1427-1437.
127. Guimaraes Koch SS, Thorpe R, Kawasaki N, et al. International nonproprietary names for monoclonal antibodies: an evolving nomenclature system. *MAbs*. 2022;14(1):2075078.
128. Pelaia C, Calabrese C, Terracciano R, de Blasio F, Vatrella A, Pelaia G. Omalizumab, the first available antibody for biological treatment of severe asthma: more than a decade of real-life effectiveness. *Ther Adv Respir Dis*. 2018;12:1753466618810192.
129. Xolair (Omalizumab injection). Package insert. Genentech; Revised April 2021. Accessed February 23, 2024. https://www.accessdata.fda.gov/drugsatfda_docs/label/2021/103976s5238lbl.pdf
130. Pelaia C, Vatrella A, Bruni A, Terracciano R, Pelaia G. Benralizumab in the treatment of severe asthma: design, development and potential place in therapy. *Drug Des Devel Ther*. 2018;12:619-628.
131. Fasenra (Benralizumab). Package insert. AstraZeneca AB; Accessed February 23, 2024. https://www.accessdata.fda.gov/drugsatfda_docs/label/2017/761070s000lbl.pdf
132. Nucala (Mepolizumab). Package insert. GlaxoSmithKline LLC; Revised March 2023. Accessed February 23, 2024. https://www.accessdata.fda.gov/drugsatfda_docs/label/2023/125526Orig1s021,761122Orig1s011Corrected_lbl.pdf
133. Cinqair (Reslizumab injection). Package insert. Teva Pharmaceuticals; Revised March 2016. Accessed February 23, 2024. https://www.accessdata.fda.gov/drugsatfda_docs/label/2016/761033lbl.pdf
134. Dupixent (Dupilumab). Package insert. Regeneron Sanofi Genzyme; Revised June 2022. Accessed February 29, 2024. https://www.accessdata.fda.gov/drugsatfda_docs/label/2022/761055s042lbl.pdf
135. Yan L, Wang B, Chia YL, Roskos LK. Population pharmacokinetic modeling of benralizumab in adult and adolescent patients with asthma. *Clin Pharmacokinet*. 2019;58(7):943-958.
136. Kearney CM, Sangani R, Shankar D, et al. Comparative effectiveness of mepolizumab, benralizumab and dupilumab among patients with difficult-to-control asthma: a multicenter retrospective propensity-matched analysis. *Ann Am Thorac Soc*. 2024;21(6):866-874.
137. Hoy SM. Tezepelumab: first approval. *Drugs*. 2022;82(4):461-468.
138. Iheanacho I, Zhang S, King D, Rizzo M, Ismaila AS. Economic burden of chronic obstructive pulmonary disease (COPD): a systematic literature review. *Int J Chron Obstruct Pulmon Dis*. 2020;15:439-460.
139. Liu Y, Carlson SA, Watson KB, Xu F, Greenlund KJ. Trends in the prevalence of chronic obstructive pulmonary disease among adults aged ≥18 years—United States, 2011-2021. *MMWR Morb Mortal Wkly Rep*. 2023;72:1250-1256. doi:10.15585/mmwr.mm7246a1
140. Engelmaier A, Weber A. Sensitive and specific measurement of alpha(1)-antitrypsin activity with an elastase complex formation immunosorbent assay (ECFISA). *J Pharm Biomed Anal*. 2022;209:114476.
141. Brantly ML, Lascano JE, Shahmohammadi A. Intravenous alpha-1 antitrypsin therapy for alpha-1 antitrypsin deficiency: the current state of the evidence. *Chronic Obstr Pulm Dis*. 2018;6(1):100-114.
142. Dekhuijzen PN, van Beurden WJ. The role for N-acetylcysteine in the management of COPD. *Int J Chron Obstruct Pulmon Dis*. 2006;1(2):99-106.
143. Gomes F, Cheng S-L. Pathophysiology, therapeutic targets, and future therapeutic alternatives in COPD: focus on the importance of the cholinergic system. *Biomolecules*. 2023;13(3):476.
144. Lahu G, Nassr N, Hünnemeyer A. Pharmacokinetic evaluation of roflumilast. *Expert Opin Drug Metab Toxicol*. 2011;7(12):1577-1591.
145. Moussa BA, El-Zaher AA, El-Ashrey MK, Fouad MA. Synthesis and molecular docking of new roflumilast analogues as preferential-selective potent PDE-4B inhibitors with improved pharmacokinetic profile. *Eur J Med Chem*. 2018;148:477-486.
146. Jabaris SG, Sumathy H, Kumar RS, Narayanan S, Thanikachalam S, Babu CS. Effects of rolipram and roflumilast, phosphodiesterase-4 inhibitors, on hypertension-induced defects in memory function in rats. *Eur J Pharmacol*. 2015;746:138-147.
147. Mersha AG, Eftekhari P, Kennedy M, Gould GS. Factors associated with quitting among smoking cessation medication-assisted smokers and ex-smokers: a cross-sectional study in Australia. *Prev Med Rep*. 2023;32:102168.
148. Centers for Disease Control and Prevention. Smoking and tobacco use. Data and Statistics; Office on Smoking and Health, National Center for Chronic Disease Prevention and Health Promotion; Updated November 2, 2023. https://www.cdc.gov/tobacco/index.html
149. Bertrand D, Terry AV. The wonderland of neuronal nicotinic acetylcholine receptors. *Biochem Pharmacol*. 2018;151:214-225.
150. Gharpure A, Teng J, Zhuang Y, et al. Agonist selectivity and ion permeation in the $\alpha3\beta4$ ganglionic nicotinic receptor. *Neuron*. 2019;104(3):501-511.e6.
151. Jones SK, Wolf BJ, Froeliger B, Wallace K, Carpenter MJ, Alberg AJ. A systematic review of genetic variation within nicotinic acetylcholine receptor genes and cigarette smoking cessation. *Drug Alcohol Depend*. 2022;239:109596.
152. Pajai DD, Paul P, Reche A. Pharmacotherapy in tobacco cessation: a narrative review. *Cureus*. 2023;15(2):e35086.
153. Russell MA, Feyerabend C, Cole PV. Plasma nicotine levels after cigarette smoking and chewing nicotine gum. *Br Med J*. 1976;1(6017):1043-1046.
154. Nicorelief (nicotine polacrilex gum). Human OTC drug label. Atlantic Biologicals Corp; Revised September 2016. Accessed March 2, 2024. https://dailymed.nlm.nih.gov/dailymed/index.cfm?setid=4d1b1bf9-e0ea-48de-a83c-daddbac3ea21
155. Azzopardi D, Ebajemito J, McEwan M, et al. A randomised study to assess the nicotine pharmacokinetics of an oral nicotine pouch and two nicotine replacement therapy products. *Sci Rep*. 2022;12(1):6949.
156. Gupta SK, Hwang SS, Causey D, Rolf CN, Gorsline J. Comparison of the nicotine pharmacokinetics of Nicoderm (nicotine transdermal system) and half-hourly cigarette smoking. *J Clin Pharmacol*. 1995;35(10):985-999.
157. Nicotrol (nicotine inhalant). Package insert. Pfizer; Revised August 2019. Accessed March 2, 2024. https://www.accessdata.fda.gov/drugsatfda_docs/label/2019/020714s018lbl.pdf
158. Wilkes S. The use of bupropion SR in cigarette smoking cessation. *Int J Chron Obstruct Pulmon Dis*. 2008;3(1):45-53.
159. Nadia OB, Jessica BLL, Zeruesenay D. Stereoselective metabolism of bupropion to active metabolites in cellular fractions of human liver and intestine. *Drug Metab Dispos*. 2023;51(1):54.
160. Dale HH, Laidlaw PP. The physiological action of cytisine, the active alkaloid of laburnum (Cytisus laburnum). *J Pharmacol Exp Ther*. 1912;3(3):22.
161. Jordan CJ, Xi ZX. Discovery and development of varenicline for smoking cessation. *Expert Opin Drug Discov*. 2018;13(7):671-683.
162. Karnieg T, Wang X. Cytisine for smoking cessation. CMAJ. 2018;190(19):E596.
163. Coe JW, Brooks PR, Vetelino MG, et al. Varenicline: an $\alpha4\beta2$ nicotinic receptor partial agonist for smoking cessation. *J Med Chem*. 2005;48(10):3474-3477.
164. Singh D, Saadabadi A. Varenicline. In: *StatPearls* [Internet]. StatPearls Publishing; 2024. Updated December 14, 2022. https://www.ncbi.nlm.nih.gov/books/NBK534846
165. Musa R, Haddad I, Thomas A, Karakattu S, El Abbassi A. Combined nicotine replacement therapy (nicotine patch) and varenicline vs varenicline alone for smoking cessation: a systematic review and meta-analysis. *Chest*. 2021;160(4):A2458.
166. Rábade-Castedo C, de Granda-Orive JI, Riesco-Miranda JA, et al. Clinical practice guideline of Spanish Society of Pneumology and Thoracic Surgery (SEPAR) on pharmacological treatment of tobacco dependence 2023. *Arch Bronconeumol*. 2023;59(10):651-661.

167. Cystic Fibrosis Foundation. About cystic fibrosis guide. 2024. https://www.cff.org/intro-cf/about-cystic-fibrosis
168. Khan MA, Ali ZS, Sweezey N, Grasemann H, Palaniyar N. Progression of cystic fibrosis lung disease from childhood to adulthood: neutrophils, neutrophil extracellular trap (NET) formation, and NET degradation. *Genes*. 2019;10(3):183.
169. Figueira MF, Ribeiro CMP, Button B. Mucus-targeting therapies of defective mucus clearance for cystic fibrosis: a short review. *Curr Opin Pharmacol*. 2022;65:102248.
170. Burgel P-R, Southern KW, Addy C, et al. Standards for the care of people with cystic fibrosis (CF); recognising and addressing CF health issues. *J Cyst Fibros*. 2024;23(2):187-202.
171. Durie P, Baillargeon JD, Bouchard S, Donnellan F, Zepeda-Gomez S, Teshima C. Diagnosis and management of pancreatic exocrine insufficiency (PEI) in primary care: consensus guidance of a Canadian expert panel. *Curr Med Res Opin*. 2018;34(1):25-33.
172. The Clinical and Functional Translation of CFTR. @ Copyright 2011 US CF Foundation, Johns Hopkins University, The Hospital for Sick Children. Updated April 7, 2023. http://cftr2.org
173. Veit G, Avramescu RG, Chiang AN, et al. From CFTR biology toward combinatorial pharmacotherapy: expanded classification of cystic fibrosis mutations. *Mol Biol Cell*. 2016;27(3):424-433.
174. Hong E, Shi A, Beringer P. Drug-drug interactions involving CFTR modulators: a review of the evidence and clinical implications. *Expert Opin Drug Metab Toxicol*. 2023;19(4):203-216.
175. Fohner AE, McDonagh EM, Clancy JP, Whirl Carrillo M, Altman RB, Klein TE. PharmGKB summary: ivacaftor pathway, pharmacokinetics/pharmacodynamics. *Pharmacogenet Genomics*. 2017;27(1):39-42.
176. Fiedorczuk K, Chen J. Molecular structures reveal synergistic rescue of Δ508 CFTR by Trikafta modulators. *Science*. 2022;378(6617):284-290.
177. Donakonda M, Indrakanti S, Pasala PK, Desari M, Kammari S. A rapid RP-HPLC method for the simultaneous estimation of Ivacaftor and Tezacaftor and in silico study of their metabolitic products. *Future J Pharm Sci*. 2021;7(1):1-14.
178. Symdeko (tezacaftor/ivacaftor tablets). Package insert. Vertex Pharmaceuticals Inc; Revised August 2023. Accessed March 8, 2024. https://pi.vrtx.com/files/uspi_tezacaftor_ivacaftor.pdf
179. U.S. Food and Drug Administration. Multi-discipline review, Elexacaftor/Tezacaftor/Ivacaftor. Center for Drug Evaluation and Research. https://www.accessdata.fda.gov/drugsatfda_docs/nda/2019/212273Orig1s000MultidisciplineR.pdf
180. Sgalla G, Iovene B, Calvello M, Ori M, Varone F, Richeldi L. Idiopathic pulmonary fibrosis: pathogenesis and management. *Respir Res*. 2018;19(1):32.
181. Herberts MB, Teague TT, Thao V, Sangaralingham LR, Henk HJ, Hovde KT, Dempsey TM, Limper AH. Idiopathic pulmonary fibrosis in the United States: time to diagnosis and treatment. *BMC Pulm Med*. 2023;23(1):281. doi:10.1186/s12890-023-02565-7.
182. Wollin L, Wex E, Pautsch A, et al. Mode of action of nintedanib in the treatment of idiopathic pulmonary fibrosis. *Eur Respir J*. 2015;45(5):1434-1445.
183. Wind S, Schmid U, Freiwald M, et al. Clinical pharmacokinetics and pharmacodynamics of nintedanib. *Clin Pharmacokinet*. 2019;58(9):1131-1147.
184. Suckling CJ. The allure of targets for novel drugs. *RSC Med Chem*. 2024;15:472-484.
185. Aimo A, Cerbai E, Bartolucci G, et al. Pirfenidone is a cardioprotective drug: mechanisms of action and preclinical evidence. *Pharmacol Res*. 2020;155:104694.
186. Rubino CM, Bhavnani SM, Ambrose PG, Forrest A, Loutit JS. Effect of food and antacids on the pharmacokinetics of pirfenidone in older healthy adults. *Pulm Pharmacol Ther*. 2009;22(4):279-285.
187. Zhou S, Li W, Tian M, et al. Metabolic activation of pirfenidone mediated by cytochrome P450s and sulfotransferases. *J Med Chem*. 2020;63(15):8059-8068.
188. Humbert M, Sitbon O, Guignabert C, et al. Treatment of pulmonary arterial hypertension: recent progress and a look to the future. *Lancet Respir Med*. 2023;11(9):820-835.
189. Burger CD, Wu B, Classi P, Morland K. Inhaled treprostinil vs iloprost: comparison of adherence, persistence, and health care resource utilization in patients with pulmonary arterial hypertension. *J Manag Care Spec Pharm*. 2023;29(1):101-108.
190. U.S. Food Drug Administration. Clinical pharmacology and biopharmaceutics review, Treprostinil. Center for Drug Evaluation and Research; 2011. https://www.accessdata.fda.gov/drugsatfda_docs/nda/2013/203496Orig1s000ClinPharmR.pdf
191. Gnerre C, Segrestaa J, Seeland S, et al. The metabolism and drug–drug interaction potential of the selective prostacyclin receptor agonist selexipag. *Xenobiotica*. 2018;48(7):704-719.
192. Shao D, Park JES, Wort SJ. The role of endothelin-1 in the pathogenesis of pulmonary arterial hypertension. *Pharmacol Res*. 2011;63(6):504-511.
193. Croxtall JD, Keam SJ. Ambrisentan. *Drugs*. 2008;68(15):2195-2204.
194. Boss C, Bolli MH, Gatfield J. From bosentan (Tracleer®) to macitentan (Opsumit®): the medicinal chemistry perspective. *Bioorg Med Chem Lett*. 2016;26(15):3381-3394.
195. Shihoya W, Nishizawa T, Yamashita K, et al. X-ray structures of endothelin ETB receptor bound to clinical antagonist bosentan and its analog. *Nat Struct Mol Biol*. 2017;24(9):758-764.
196. Bruderer S, Hopfgartner G, Seiberling M, et al. Absorption, distribution, metabolism, and excretion of macitentan, a dual endothelin receptor antagonist, in humans. *Xenobiotica*. 2012;42(9):901-910.
197. Follmann M, Ackerstaff J, Redlich G, et al. Discovery of the soluble guanylate cyclase stimulator vericiguat (BAY 1021189) for the treatment of chronic heart failure. *J Med Chem*. 2017;60(12):5146-5161.
198. Liu R, Kang Y, Chen L. Activation mechanism of human soluble guanylate cyclase by stimulators and activators. *Nat Commun*. 2021;12(1):5492.
199. Tiwari SS, Chavan BB, Kushwah BS, et al. In vitroand in vivo investigation of metabolic fate of riociguat by HPLC-Q-TOF/MS/MS and in silico evaluation of the metabolites by ADMET predictor™. *J Pharm Biomed Anal*. 2019;164:326-336.
200. Kenny M, Clarke MM, Pogue KT. Overview of riociguat and its role in the treatment of pulmonary hypertension. *J Pharm Pract*. 2022;35(3):437-444.

Structure Challenge Answers

1. B.
2. D.
3. A.
4. A.

SECTION 7

Drugs Impacting Infectious and Neoplastic Disease Processes

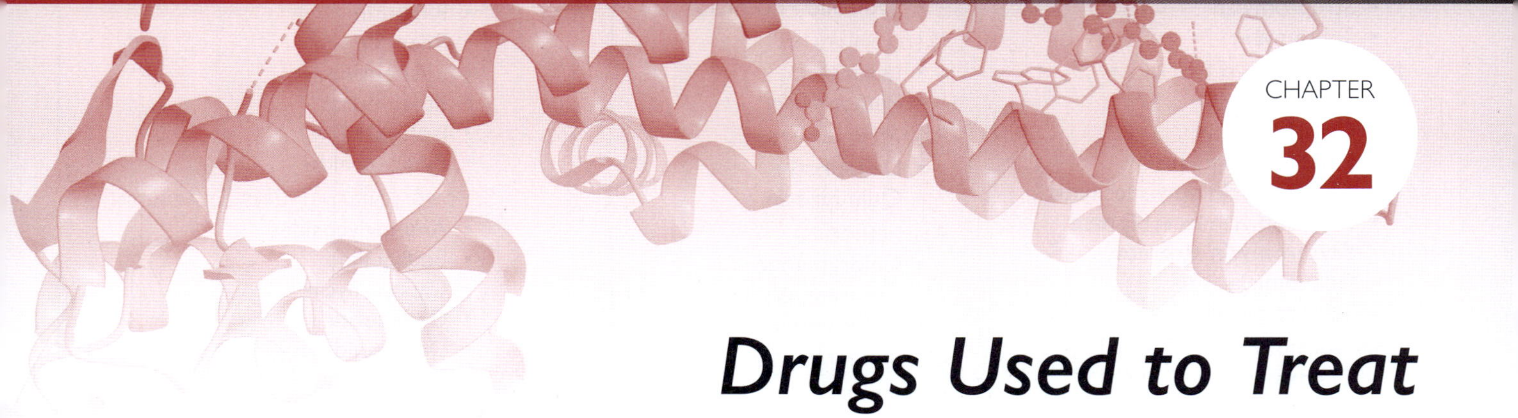

CHAPTER

32

Drugs Used to Treat Bacterial Infections

Jozef Stec and Kirk E. Hevener

Drugs covered in this chapter:

CELL ENVELOPE DISRUPTORS

β-LACTAM ANTIBIOTICS

PENICILLIN CLASS
- Amoxicillin
- Ampicillin
- Dicloxacillin
- Nafcillin
- Oxacillin
- Penicillin G
- Penicillin salts
- Penicillin V
- Piperacillin

β-LACTAMASE INHIBITORS
- Avibactam
- Clavulanate
- Durlobactam
- Relebactam
- Sulbactam
- Tazobactam
- Vaborbactam

CEPHALOSPORINS
- Cefaclor
- Cefadroxil
- Cefazolin
- Cefdinir
- Cefepime
- Cefiderocol
- Cefixime
- Cefotetan
- Cefoxitin
- Cefpodoxime proxetil
- Cefprozil
- Ceftaroline fosamil
- Ceftazidime
- Ceftobiprole
- Ceftolozane
- Ceftriaxone
- Cefuroxime
- Cephalexin

CARBAPENEMS
- Ertapenem
- Imipenem/cilastatin
- Meropenem

MONOBACTAMS
- Aztreonam

GLYCOPEPTIDES, LIPOGLYCOPEPTIDES, AND LIPOPEPTIDES
- Dalbavancin
- Daptomycin
- Oritavancin
- Telavancin
- Vancomycin

POLYMYXINS
- Colistin (Polymyxin E)
- Polymyxin B_1
- Polymyxin B_2

BACITRACIN

DNA DISRUPTORS

SULFONAMIDES AND TRIMETHOPRIM
- Silver sulfadiazine
- Sulfacetamide
- Sulfadiazine (oral)
- Sulfamethoxazole
- Trimethoprim

QUINOLONE CLASS
- Besifloxacin
- Ciprofloxacin
- Delafloxacin
- Gatifloxacin
- Levofloxacin
- Moxifloxacin
- Ofloxacin
- Ozenoxacin

NITROIMIDAZOLES
- Metronidazole
- Nitrofurantoin
- Secnidazole
- Tinidazole

PROTEIN SYNTHESIS DISRUPTORS

AMINOGLYCOSIDES
- Amikacin
- Gentamicin
- Kanamycin A
- Neomycin

Drugs covered in this chapter:—continued

- Paromomycin
- Plazomicin
- Spectinomycin
- Streptomycin
- Tobramycin

Macrolides and ketolides
- Azithromycin
- Clarithromycin
- Erythromycin base
- Erythromycin ethylsuccinate
- Erythromycin lactobionate
- Erythromycin stearate
- Fidaxomicin
- Telithromycin

Lincosamides
- Clindamycin
- Lincomycin

Tetracyclines, aminomethylcyclines, fluorocyclines, and glycylcyclines
- Demeclocycline
- Doxycycline
- Eravacycline
- Minocycline
- Omadacycline
- Sarecycline
- Tetracycline
- Tigecycline

Oxazolidinones
- Linezolid
- Tedizolid
- Tedizolid Phosphate

Pleuromutilins
- Lefamulin
- Retapamulin

Streptogramins
- Dalfopristin
- Quinupristin

Amphenicols
- Chloramphenicol
- Chloramphenicol palmitate
- Chloramphenicol succinate

Other antibacterials

Mupirocin

Urinary antiseptics
- Fosfomycin
- Methenamine

Monoclonal antibodies
- Bezlotoxumab

Fecal bacteriotherapy
- Fecal microbiota, live-jslm (Rebyota)
- Fecal microbiota spores, live-brpk (VOWST)

Antimycobacterial agents

First-line antitubercular agents
- Ansamycins
- Rifabutin
- Rifampin
- Rifapentine
- Ethambutol
- Isoniazid
- Pyrazinamide

Second-line antitubercular agents
- Aminoglycosides
- Bedaquiline
- Capreomycin
- Cycloserine
- Delamanid
- Ethionamide
- Fluoroquinolones
- Linezolid
- *p*-Aminosalicylic acid
- Pretomanid

Non-tubercular antimycobacterials
- Clofazimine
- Dapsone
- Thalidomide

Abbreviations

6-APA 6-aminopenicillanic acid
7-ACA 7-aminocephalosporanic acid
AAC aminoglycoside acetylase
ABC ATP-binding cassette
ABSSSI acute bacterial skin and skin structure infection
ACP acyl carrier protein
ADMET absorption, distribution, metabolism, and excretion-toxicity
AG arabinogalactan
AIDS acquired immunodeficiency syndrome
ALIS amikacin liposome inhalation suspension
ANT aminoglycoside nucleotidyltransferase
APH aminoglycoside phosphorylase
ART antiretroviral therapy
ATP adenosine triphosphate
ATS American Thoracic Society
AUC area under the curve
CABP community-acquired bacterial pneumonia
CDAD *C. difficile*–associated diarrhea
CDC U.S. Centers for Disease Control and Prevention
CDI *C. difficile* infection
CF cystic fibrosis
CLSI Clinical and Laboratory Standards Institute
CNS central nervous system
COMT catechol-*O*-methyltransferase
COPD chronic obstructive pulmonary disease
CPK creatine phosphokinase
CRE carbapenem-resistant Enterobacterales
CSF cerebrospinal fluid
DARQ diarylquinoline
DBO diazabicyclo[3.2.1]octane
DCS D-cycloserine
DDI drug-drug interaction
Ddn deazaflavin F_{420}-dependent nitroreductase
DDRP DNA-directed RNA polymerase
DDS diaminodiphenyl sulfone
DHFR dihydrofolate reductase
DHP-1 dehydropeptidase-I
DHPS dihydropteroate synthase
DOT directly observed therapy
DP diaminopimelic acid
DPA decaprenylphosphoryl-D-arabinose
DPR decaprenylphosphoryl-D-ribose
DprE1 decaprenylphosphoryl-D-ribose oxidase
DprE2 decaprenylphosphoryl-D-2-keto erythropentose reductase
DPX decaprenylphosphoryl-2-keto-β-D-erythro-pentofuranose
DS drug susceptible
ELISA enzyme-linked immunosorbent assay
EMA European Medicines Agency
EMB ethambutol
ENL erythema nodosum leprosum
EON EMB-induced optic neuropathy
ER extended release
ERS European Respiratory Society
ESBL extended-spectrum β-lactamase

Abbreviations—continued

ESCMID European Society of Clinical Microbiology and Infectious Diseases
ETH ethionamide
FAS fatty acid synthase
FDA U.S. Food and Drug Administration
Fgd1 F420-dependent glucose-6-phosphate dehydrogenase
GABA γ-aminobutyric acid
GI gastrointestinal
GTP guanosine triphosphate
HABA L-hydroxyaminobutyryl amide
hERG human Ether-à-go-go-Related Gene
HIV human immunodeficiency virus
HMG-CoA 3-hydroxy-3-methylglutaryl coenzyme A
HTS high-throughput screening
IDSA Infectious Diseases Society of America
IgG1 immunoglobulin G1
Ikr rectifier potassium current
IL interleukin
IM intramuscular
INH isoniazid
IR immediate release
IRB institutional review board
IV intravenous
KPC *Klebsiella pneumoniae* carbapenemases
LAM lipoarabinomannan
L-DAB L-α,γ-diaminobutyric acid
LPS lipopolysaccharides
LTBI latent tuberculosis infection
MABC *M. abscessus* complex
MAC *Mycobacterium avium* complex
MAO monoamine oxidase
MBC minimum bactericidal concentration
MBL metallo-β-lactamase
MDR multidrug resistant
MDR-TB multidrug-resistant tuberculosis
MIC minimum inhibitory concentration
MmpL3 mycobacterial membrane protein Large 3
MOA mechanism of action
mRNA messenger RNA
MRSA methicillin-resistant *S. aureus*
Msm *Mycobacterium smegmatis*
MSSA methicillin-susceptible *S. aureus*
Mtb *Mycobacterium tuberculosis*
MTT methylthiotetrazole
NAD nicotinamide adenine dinucleotide
NADH reduced nicotinamide adenine dinucleotide
NAG *N*-acetylglucosamine
NAM *N*-acetylmuramic acid
NO nitric oxide
NPET nascent peptide exit tunnel
NSAID nonsteroidal anti-inflammatory drug
NTM nontuberculous mycobacteria
PABA *p*-aminobenzoic acid
PAE post-antibiotic effect
PAS *p*-aminosalicylic acid
PBP penicillin-binding protein
PCP *P. jirovecii* pneumonia
PCR polymerase chain reaction
PEP phosphoenolpyruvate
Pgp P-glycoprotein
POA pyrazinoic acid
PRSP penicillin-resistant *S. pneumoniae*
PTC peptidyl transferase center
PZA pyrazinamide
PZase pyrazinamidase
RFB rifabutin
RIA radioimmunoassay
RIF rifampin
RIPE rifampin, isoniazid, pyrazinamide, and ethambutol
RNAP RNA polymerase
RNS reactive nitrogen species
ROS reactive oxygen species
RPT rifapentine
rRNA ribosomal RNA
SAR structure-activity relationship
SDA 4,4′-sulfonyldianiline
SNP single-nucleotide polymorphism
SPIND single patient Investigational New Drug
SSRI selective serotonin reuptake inhibitor
STM streptomycin
TB tuberculosis
TCA tricyclic antidepressant
TDM therapeutic drug monitoring
Th T helper
TMM trehalose monomycolate
TMP-SMX trimethoprim-sulfamethoxazole
TNF-α tumor necrosis factor-α
tRNA transfer RNA
UR upstream region
UTI urinary tract infection
VFS vancomycin flushing syndrome
VISA vancomycin intermediate *S. aureus*
VRE vancomycin-resistant enterococci
VRSA vancomycin-resistant *Staphylococcus aureus*
WHO World Health Organization
XDR-TB extensively drug-resistant tuberculosis

CLINICAL SIGNIFICANCE

The management of bacterial infections poses a consistent challenge for clinicians throughout their careers. Antimicrobial resistance changes daily, with significant variability between geographic locales and treatment centers. Each infection provides a distinct overlap of host, microbiologic, and pathogenesis factors requiring a patient-specific approach. An appreciation and knowledge of drug-specific properties allows for informed decision-making and individualized patient care. Medicinal chemistry knowledge is foundational in understanding many of the pharmacokinetic and pharmacologic principles of antimicrobial agents.

Brandon Hawkins, PharmD

Introduction

Naturally occurring antibiotics are organic molecules produced by soil bacteria and fungi. These microbial metabolites serve not only as weapons when the microbes need to compete with other microorganisms for habitat and food, but they also play a vital role in macronutrient acquisition.[1] Synthetic substances (ie, obtained by means of chemical synthesis) that interfere with the growth of microorganisms are referred to as antimicrobial agents. Those with activity specific to bacteria are referred to as antibacterial agents. Often such antibacterial agents are derived from chemical modification of naturally occurring antibiotics and are therefore referred to as "semisynthetic" antibacterials. In the case of semisynthetic agents, the utility of natural antibiotics is improved through rational chemical manipulation of the original structure, leading to broader antimicrobial spectrum, greater potency, decreased toxicity, more convenient administration, and other pharmacokinetic advantages. Natural antibiotics and synthetic/semisynthetic antimicrobial agents, in small doses, inhibit the growth of or kill other microorganisms without causing serious toxicity to the host. This is referred to as selective toxicity, and it is a key concept in drug action. Antibiotics are among the most frequently prescribed medications today, although microbial resistance due to evolutionary pressure, socioeconomic factors, and inappropriate medication use threatens their continued efficacy.

Bacteria, parasites, viruses, and fungi represent the four major types of microorganisms, and their combined number on earth is over 10 billion times the number of stars in the universe.[2] Despite their large number, only about one in a billion microbial species is a human pathogen, and approximately 1,400 human pathogens have been described thus far.[3] The great majority of the known microorganisms are generally harmless to the host and, in some cases, can provide several benefits, for example, some bacteria support host's immune system and improve intestinal digestion. This type of bacteria is referred to as commensal bacteria. With their estimated total count of 5×10^{30}, bacteria occupy practically every environment, spreading from 7 miles beneath the ocean floor up to 40 miles high in the atmosphere.[4] An average human being carries similar or even higher number of bacterial cells when compared to their own cells, which is ~30 trillion cells.[3] These bacteria can primarily be found in the gastrointestinal (GI) tract, genitourinary system, and on the skin. All our internal fluids, organs, and body structures are sterile under normal circumstances, and the presence of bacteria or other microorganisms in these places is diagnostic evidence of an infection. In immunocompetent individuals, many infections are usually mild because the host immune system prevents the development of illness and thus pharmacologic treatment may not be necessary. However, in the case of immunocompromised individuals and/or when serious infection has been developed, appropriate therapeutic intervention is required. Bacterial infections have plagued humankind for millennia, leading to high morbidity and mortality rates, and they continue to be a global health threat even today. In 2019 alone, there was an estimated 7.7 million deaths worldwide due to bacterial infections, which equals 1 in 8 of all global deaths.[5] Only three bacterial diseases–tuberculosis (TB), pneumonia, and meningitis–are responsible for more than half of those reported deaths.

History

Humankind has been subject to infection by microorganisms since before recorded history. One of the first traces of bacterial infection came from bone fragments of vertebrate bearing the tuberculous changes (Pott disease) that date back to ~8000 BCE and are also found in human remains from the Neolithic era.[6] One presumes that humankind has been searching for suitable therapy for nearly as long, as evidenced by clusters of pollen grains from 28 species of flowers, including 7 medicinal herbs, that were found next to 60,000-year-old bones of Neanderthals at the Shanidar Cave in northern Iraq. Also, seeds of the mildly psychoactive areca nut (*Areca catechu*) dated 7000 to 5500 BCE were found in the Spirit Cave in northwestern Thailand.[7] Although one can find indications in ancient medical writings as well as folkloric use of plant and animal preparations, these factors were inefficiently applied, and thus they often failed. Until the discovery of bacteria by van Leeuwenhoek in 1676 and subsequent understanding of their role in infection about 150 years later, there was little hope for rational therapy.

In 1882, Robert Koch announced the discovery of tubercle bacilli, which was a breakthrough in understanding bacterial infections. A few years later, he formulated postulates that constitute the basis of modern bacteriology, which are still used today to assess whether a microorganism causes a particular disease. Koch's four postulates state that a microorganism causing certain disease:

1. must be found in abundance in hosts suffering from the specific disease but is absent in healthy individuals.
2. must be isolated from a diseased organism and grown in pure culture.
3. must be able to cause disease when introduced into a new healthy host.
4. must be re-isolated from the deliberately infected host and identified as being identical to the original infectious agent.

Following these rules, a chain of evidence connecting cause and effect was forged between certain microorganisms and specific infectious diseases. This work laid the foundation for today's prevention and rational therapy of infectious diseases.

The era of modern anti-infective agents started in 1907 with the synthesis of the organoarsenic compound Salvarsan (arsphenamine) in Paul Ehrlich's laboratory.[8] Salvarsan was introduced in 1910, and it was the first modern antimicrobial chemotherapeutic agent used to treat syphilis and trypanosomiasis. Following the discovery of Salvarsan, the concept of "selective toxicity" was coined and pertains to the identification and validation of drug targets in metabolic pathways (enzymes) that are essential for the invasive organism but absent or nonessential in the human host.[9] This concept has also been referred to as a "magic bullet," a "silver bullet," or "one drug, one target." Ehrlich's pioneering drug discovery efforts paved the way for the "golden era of antibiotics," which was initiated with the discovery of penicillin (1928) by Alexander Fleming and synthetic sulfonamides (prontosil, 1932) by Gerhard Domagk.[10,11] The well-known observation of a clear zone of inhibition (lysis) in a bacterial colony surrounding a colony of contaminating airborne *Penicillium* mold by Alexander Fleming in England in 1928 and the subsequent experiments with purified penicillin in 1940 by Florey and Chain, along with technology for mass production of this antibiotic, forever revolutionized medicine.[12] Since the first successful clinical trial of penicillin in early 1940s, penicillin has been recognized as the most efficient life-saving drug ever discovered. It is estimated to have saved approximately 100 million lives. In rapid succession, deliberate searches of the metabolic products of a wide variety of soil microbes led to the discovery of tyrothricin (1939), streptomycin (STM; 1943), chloramphenicol (1947), chlortetracycline (1948), neomycin (1949), erythromycin (1952), and rifampin (RIF; 1963). These discoveries ushered in the age of the so-called miracle drugs. The discovery of antibiotics is widely considered to be one of the top five discoveries/inventions of the 20th century.

Microbes of soil origin to this day remain one of the most fruitful sources of antibiotics, although the specific means employed for their discovery are more sophisticated today than those employed 80 years ago. Initially, extracts of fermentations were screened simply for their ability to inhibit the growth or kill pathogenic microorganisms in vitro. Those that displayed this property were subsequently evaluated in more complex pharmacologic and toxicologic tests in attempts to discover clinically useful agents. Today, thousands of such extracts from increasingly unusual microbes are tested each year, and the tests now include sophisticated assays for agents operating through specific biochemical mechanisms or possessing particular properties.

Combinatorial chemical synthesis coupled with high-throughput screening (HTS) makes it possible today to screen hundreds of thousands to millions of compounds for antimicrobial activity in a brief period of time. This is coupled with dramatic advances in all the relevant sciences, including engineering, robotics, and automation. The rapid progress in genomics and proteomics is predicted to have a significant impact not only on discovering new and effective antibiotics but also on combating drug resistance and expanding personalized medicine. The genomes of *Haemophilus influenzae* and *Mycoplasma genitalium* were sequenced in 1995, and currently thousands of microbial genomes have been deciphered and are publicly available.[13-15] The whole-genome sequencing technique allows the identification of essential genes whose expression products (predominantly proteins) are indispensable for microbial survival and thus constitute viable targets for antimicrobial drug discovery and development.[16] However, these exciting new possibilities have yet to yield the expected practical results due to the inherent complexity of the modern drug discovery and approval process.[17,18]

Antibacterial Nomenclature

The names given to antimicrobials and antibiotics are highly varied, yet some helpful unifying conventions are followed. For example, the penicillins are derived from fungi and have names ending in the suffix -cillin, as in the drug ampicillin. The cephalosporins are likewise fungal products, although their names mostly begin with the prefix cef- (or sometimes, following the English convention, ceph-). The agents belonging to the carbapenem drug class carry the suffix -penem, whereas the names of β-lactamase inhibitors predominantly end with the suffix -bactam. The synthetic fluoroquinolones typically end in the suffix -floxacin. Although helpful in many respects, this nomenclature does result in many related substances possessing quite similar names. This in turn can make differentiating them difficult. Most of the remaining antibiotics are produced by fermentation of soil microorganisms belonging to various *Streptomyces* spp. By convention, these have names ending in the suffix -mycin, as in STM. Some prominent antibiotics are produced by fermentation of various soil microbes known as *Micromonospora* spp. These antibiotics have names ending in -micin (eg, gentamicin).

Historically, the terms "broad spectrum" and "narrow spectrum" had specific clinical meaning, with broad spectrum referring to an antibacterial agent possessing activity against both gram-positive and gram-negative organisms, and narrow spectrum referring to agents with activity limited to specific bacterial species or genera.[19] However, the rapid and widespread emergence of microbes resistant to single or even multiple agents has made these terms less meaningful. Nonetheless, it is still valuable to remember that some antibacterial families have the potential of inhibiting a wide range of bacterial genera belonging to both gram-positive and gram-negative cultures and so are called broad spectrum (such as the tetracyclines). Others inhibit only a few bacterial genera and are termed narrow spectrum (such as the glycopeptides, typified by vancomycin with activity limited to gram-positive organisms).

Bacterial Pathogen Identification

A wide variety of clinical microbiology techniques have been developed to identify the causative agents of bacterial infection.[20,21] Phenotypic methods include microscopic morphology, macroscopic morphology, and biochemical testing. Genotypic methods identify the bacteria using DNA or RNA sequencing methods, while immunologic methods use antibodies specific to bacterial antigens for bacterial identification. Cell morphology visualized by microscopy can help to distinguish general classes of bacteria such as cocci (spheres), bacilli (rod-like), and spirochetes (twisted, helical). Subclasses may also be distinguishable, including staphylococci (clusters), streptococci (bead-like chains), diplococci (pairs), and streptobacilli (chains). Staining tests can be used to further distinguish bacteria by the composition of their cell envelope and associated structural components.

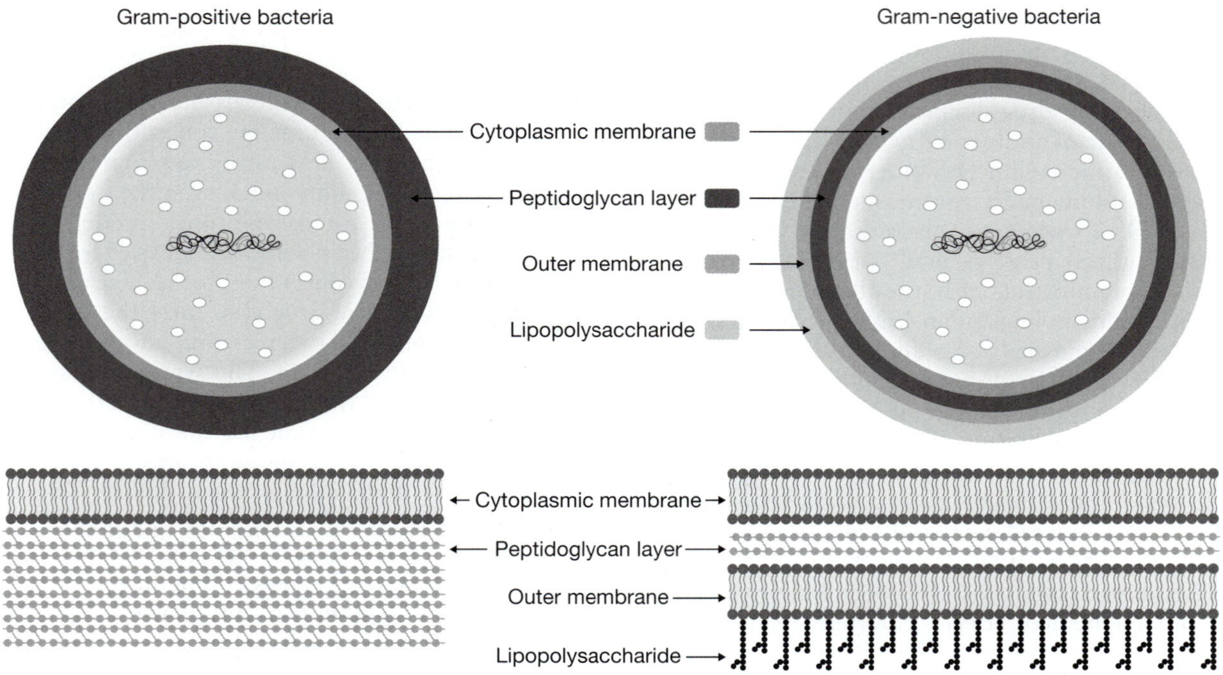

Figure 32.1 Cell envelope characteristics of gram-positive and gram-negative bacteria. (Adopted without change from Allaf MM, Peerhossaini H. Cyanobacteria: model microorganisms and beyond. *Microorganisms*. 2022;10(4):696, under a Creative Commons license.)

The Gram stain was developed by Hans C.J. Gram in 1884 and is commonly used to distinguish between bacteria with a single cell membrane and thick cell wall (gram positive) and bacteria with two cell membranes separated by a thinner cell wall (gram negative) (Fig. 32.1). Other types of staining tests have been developed to identify mycobacteria (acid-fast stain), flagellated bacteria, and spirochetes. Macroscopic morphology methods classify bacteria based on the media required for growth and the visualized characteristics of bacterial colonies growing on culture plates (shape, size, edge characteristics, color, opacity, elevation, surface characteristics, consistency).

Additional microbiology diagnostic tests have been developed to identify bacterial species more specifically by their biochemical characteristics. The catalase test has been used to distinguish gram-positive staphylococci (catalase positive) from gram-positive streptococci (catalase negative). The coagulase test is used to distinguish *Staphylococcus aureus* (coagulase-positive) from coagulase-negative staphylococci such as *Staphylococcus epidermidis*. Other biochemical tests include the β-glucuronidase test for *Escherichia coli*, the oxidase test, the indole test, lactose fermentation, citrate utilization, and bile solubility. Although dependable, many of these tests require bacterial culture, which can be time consuming. To circumvent this downside, various non-culture genotypic and immunologic methods have been developed that are faster, more sensitive, and can be utilized with bacteria that are difficult to culture.

Immunologic tests, or immunoassays, detect bacterial antigens (ie, molecules from the microorganism that can trigger host's immune response) or host antibodies (molecules produced by the host's immune system) that are released in response to the antigens from the invasive pathogen. These tests are rapid, inexpensive, and can often be applied directly to clinical samples; however, they can have poor specificity. Immunologic tests include agglutination tests, precipitation tests, Western blot tests, and fluorescent antibody tests. The radioimmunoassay (RIA) and enzyme-linked immunosorbent

GRAM STAIN

Hans C.J. Gram, a Danish microbiologist, developed the Gram staining method for staining bacteria so that they were more readily visible under the microscope. The term has proven to be particularly useful in describing antibiotics as well, because antibiotics are conveniently classified by their activity against microorganisms depending on their reaction to this method. Gram-positive microorganisms are stained purple by contact with a methyl violet-iodine process. This is largely a consequence of their lack of an outer membrane and the nature of the thick cell wall surrounding them. Gram-negative microorganisms do not retain the methyl violet-iodine stain when washed with alcohol but rather are colored pink when subsequently treated with the red dye safranin. The lipopolysaccharides (LPS) on their outer membrane apparently are responsible for the staining behavior of gram-negative cells. Since the Gram stain is dependent on the outer layers of bacterial cells and this also strongly influences the ability of antimicrobial agents to reach their cellular targets, knowing the Gram staining behavior of infectious bacteria helps one decide which antimicrobial might be effective in therapy. Not all bacteria can be stained by the Gram procedure. These often require special staining processes for visualization. Among the more prominent of these for our purposes are the mycobacteria (the causative agents of TB, for example). These very waxy cells are called acid fast and are stained by a carbol fuchsin mixture.

assay (ELISA) are immunoassays with improved sensitivity. Nucleic acid–based tests for detection and identification of bacteria are extremely sensitive but can be costly and require special instrumentation. Amplified nucleic acid tests typically rely on polymerase chain reaction (PCR) or other types of nucleic acid amplification techniques to identify genetic material specific to bacterial species. Non-amplified nucleic acid tests utilize DNA or RNA probes to identify specific bacteria and can be used directly with clinical samples. These nucleic acid–based tests have the advantage of being used to simultaneously identify the presence of genes related to antibacterial resistance, which in turn allows for more rapid and precise selection of an appropriate therapeutic agent. Lastly, proteomic approaches have been recently developed to identify bacteria and other microorganisms. The method involves the use of tandem mass spectrometry to identify proteins specific to bacterial species and is rapid, highly accurate, and can be employed in a high-throughput manner.

ANTIBACTERIAL SUSCEPTIBILITY TESTING

The modern clinical application of Koch's discoveries to the selection of an appropriate antibiotic involves sampling infectious material from a patient before instituting anti-infective chemotherapy, culturing the microorganism on suitable growth media, and identifying its genus and species. The bacterium in question is then grown in the presence of several antibiotics to identify those that will inhibit its growth and determine the effective drug concentration. The Clinical and Laboratory Standards Institute (CLSI) has standardized methods for performing antibacterial susceptibility testing. The most common susceptibility test is the minimum inhibitory concentration (MIC), which is the lowest concentration of antibacterial drug that will inhibit the visible, in vitro growth of bacteria after incubation for a specific period of time. The choice of antibacterial agent is then made from those agents, with MIC values reflecting drug levels that are achievable in vivo without deleterious (toxic) effects. These values are established by the CLSI and are known as MIC breakpoints. MIC values are typically determined using either broth microdilution assay or the E-test (Fig. 32.2). The broth microdilution assay uses serial dilutions of the test drug in a microplate well with media and the bacteria being tested. Bacterial growth is indicated by culture turbidity, with the MIC determined as the well with the lowest drug concentration and no visible bacterial growth. The proprietary Epsilometer test, or E-test, uses a plastic strip embedded with a gradient drug concentration that can be placed on a solid media culture with the bacteria under investigation.[22] A zone of growth inhibition near the test strip is used to determine the drug's MIC value.

Another convenient experimental test to determine bacterial drug susceptibility is the disk diffusion test, or Kirby-Bauer test.[23] This test involves the use of sterile filter paper disks infused with fixed doses of antibacterials that are placed on culture plates with the bacteria of interest. Clear zones of growth inhibition are measured after a set period, with larger inhibition zones reflecting a more effective antibacterial against the bacterium. Testing variables, including test medium, test organism concentration,

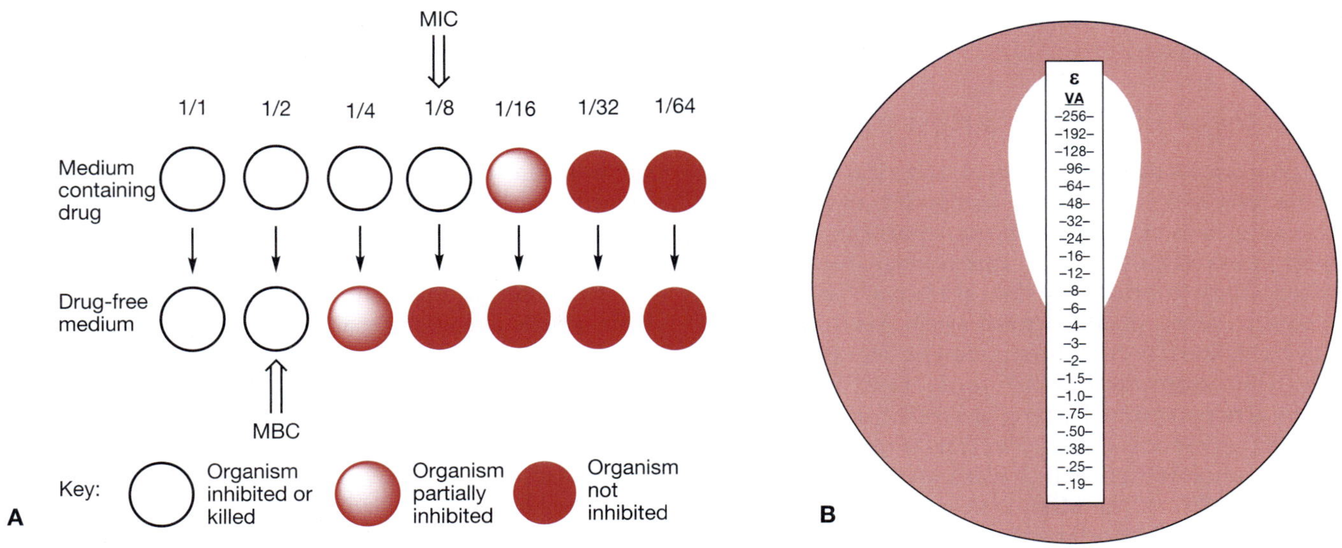

Figure 32.2 Clinical minimum inhibitory concentration (MIC) determination methods. A. Broth microdilution method. In the first row of wells, a serially decreasing amount of antibacterial is added to a suitable growth medium that has been inoculated with a microorganism. Following incubation, microbial growth is detected by turbidity. The last concentration that produces no visible growth is determined to be the MIC (1/8). Next a sample is taken from each well and placed in fresh medium (second row). In tubes where the organisms were killed by the drug there is no resumption of growth. Where the organisms were inhibited but not killed, removal of drug allows for resumption of growth. The last concentration that produces no visible growth under these conditions is determined to be the minimum bactericidal concentration (MBC) (1/2). B. Epsilometer test (E-test). A strip impregnated with decreasing concentrations of an antibacterial is placed onto an agar plate growing a specific microorganism. Drug concentrations are indicated on the test strip. The concentration where bacterial growth resumes is determined to be the MIC.

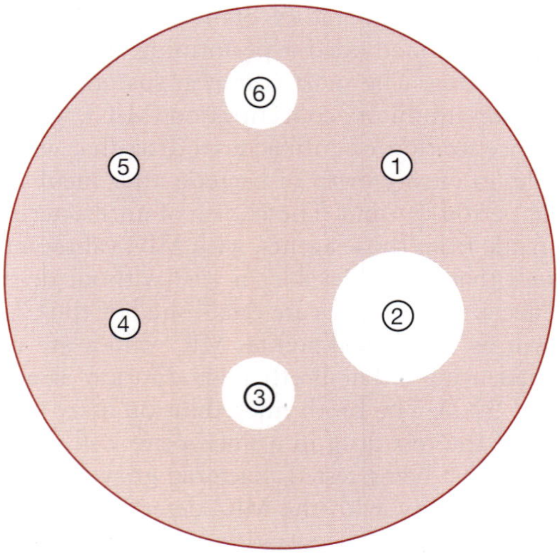

Figure 32.3 Kirby-Bauer disk diffusion. Looking down upon a Petri dish containing solidified nutrient agar to which had been added a suspension of a bacterial species. Next, six filter paper disks containing six different antimicrobials were added followed by overnight incubation. The antimicrobials in disks 1, 4, and 5 were inactive. Of the active agents in disks 2, 3, and 6, antibiotic 2 was much more active, as the microorganism was not able to grow as near this impregnated disk.

antibacterial concentration, are standardized by the CLSI. If performed properly, the growth inhibition zone size is predictive of bacterial sensitivity to the antibacterial agent. This method is illustrated in Figure 32.3. In addition to dilution and diffusion methods, specialized methods can be used to identify specific bacterial resistance mechanisms such as the presence of β-lactamase, which can impact the efficacy of the β-lactam antibiotics.

Bactericidal Versus Bacteriostatic

The pharmacodynamic concepts of bactericidal agents that kill bacteria and bacteriostatic agents that slow or inhibit bacterial growth at specific concentrations can be a useful in vitro method for classifying antibacterial agents but have limited utility in predicting clinical efficacy.[24] It should be noted that nearly all antibacterial agents have the capacity to be bactericidal if the concentration or dose is sufficiently high. The designations "cidal" and "static" refer to the agent's actions against bacteria at specific concentrations. Formally, an agent is classified as cidal if its minimum bactericidal concentration (MBC) is at least 4-fold greater than the agent's MIC.[25] The MBC is defined as the lowest concentration of an antibacterial agent required to kill a bacterium, where the MIC is the lowest concentration of an agent required to inhibit bacterial growth. Generally, antibacterial classes considered to be bactericidal include the aminoglycosides, β-lactams, fluoroquinolones, and certain peptide antibacterials, while bacteriostatic classes include tetracyclines, glycylcyclines, lincosamides (clindamycin), macrolides, oxazolidinones (linezolid), and sulfonamides. It should be noted that agents may be cidal against some bacteria and static against others. In addition to the agent's concentration, other factors such as the agent's pharmacokinetics, the organism's characteristics (gram-positive vs gram-negative), the site of infection, and nutrient and oxygen requirements can influence the cidal versus static designation. It was previously believed that bactericidal agents should be favored for treating infections occurring in patients with immune suppression (ie, immunocompromised); however, an abundance of clinical data does not support this dogma.[24] The most important factors predicting positive therapeutic outcomes with a specific antibacterial agent are the pharmacokinetics of the agent and the achievement of appropriate drug concentrations at the infection site.

Bacterial Resistance and Tolerance

Resistance

Bacterial resistance occurs when a microorganism possesses the ability to bypass or overcome the effect of the applied antibacterial agent.[26] Resistance can either be intrinsic (present before exposure to a drug) or acquired (develop after exposure to a drug).[27] Resistance of bacteria to the effects of antimicrobial agents develops easily in both the laboratory and the clinic and constitutes an ever-increasing public health threat. While the development of acquired resistance due to exposure to antibacterial agents is well established, more recently it has emerged that other, unrelated, drug classes such as antidepressants also help bacteria resist antibiotics.[28] Some common molecular mechanisms of bacterial resistance include the enzymatic inactivation of the antibacterial agent, decreased permeability of the cell envelope to the agent, efflux of the agent from the cell, alteration of the target or binding site, protection of the target, overproduction of the target, bypass of the inhibited pathway, and sequestration of the antibacterial agent (Fig. 32.4).

Many of these molecular resistance mechanisms may be present in a bacterium prior to drug exposure and contribute to intrinsic resistance. Resistance mechanisms may also be acquired by genetic mutations driven by selective pressure from antibacterial exposure such as "point mutations" in genes encoding the drug target protein that result in decreased affinity of the agent for the molecular target. Larger scale genetic alterations that can result in resistance development include DNA inversions, insertions, deletions, and transpositions. Bacteria can also acquire genetic material from other microorganisms in their environment that permit them to acquire resistance, such as resistance plasmids (R factors), naked DNA sequences, bacteriophages, and transposable genetic elements.[29] This latter mechanism is referred to as horizontal gene transfer. Plasmid DNA carrying resistance genes may migrate within the cell from plasmid to plasmid or from plasmid to chromosome by a process known as transposition. Plasmids migrate from cell to cell by conjugation (passage through a sexual pilus), transduction (carriage by a virus vector), or transformation (uptake of exogenous DNA from the environment). The potential for bacteria to rapidly acquire resistance traits provides strong rationale for conservative but aggressive application of appropriate antibacterial chemotherapy.

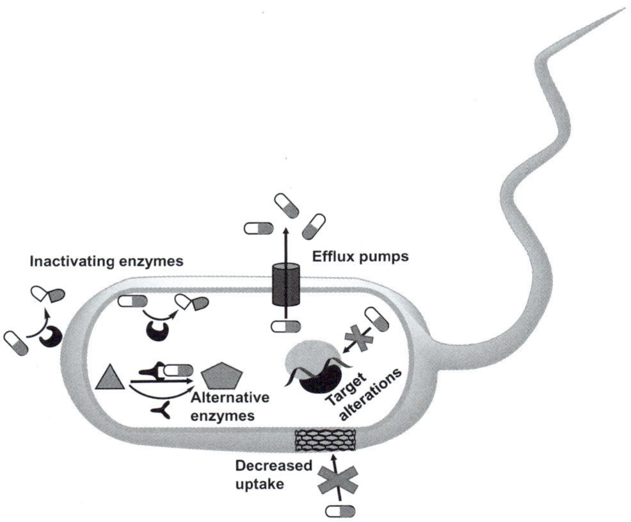

Figure 32.4 General mechanisms of bacterial resistance. (Adapted with permission from Wistrand-Yuen E, Knopp M, Hjort K, et al. Evolution of high-level resistance during low-level antibiotic exposure. *Nat Commun.* 2018;9:1599. doi:10.1038/s41467-018-04059-1 under a Creative Commons Attribution 4.0, http://creativecommons.org/licenses/by/4.0/)

Heteroresistance, Tolerance, and Persistence

Resistance is broadly considered to be the ability of bacteria to replicate, or grow, in the presence of an antibacterial agent. This is typically demonstrated by increased MICs of the antibacterial agent against the resistant organism. When the entire bacterial population can survive at higher antibacterial concentrations, or higher MICs, this is referred to as classical, or homogeneous, resistance. In some cases, a subpopulation of bacteria within a larger population sensitive to an antibacterial possesses a resistance phenotype. This is referred to as "heteroresistance" and can be difficult to detect by standard MIC tests, which will reflect the activity of the agent against the entire population. Heteroresistance can result in treatment failures as the selected antibacterial agent affects only the susceptible population allowing the resistant subpopulation to outgrow.[30] Unlike resistance, "tolerance" is the ability of bacteria to survive exposure to an antibiotic without a corresponding increase in the MIC. Tolerance occurs when the bacteria survive longer during antibacterial exposure reflected by lower bacterial kill rates. Tolerant bacteria can survive a typical antibacterial treatment period, resulting in treatment failure. Lastly, a special type of tolerance is known as "persistence." This occurs when a subpopulation of bacterial cells can survive antibacterial exposure, or have a slower kill rate, versus the larger population. Persistence can be considered "heterotolerance." Molecular mechanisms for tolerance and persistence can include cell dormancy, reduced metabolic rates, and reduced adenosine triphosphate (ATP) levels.

THERAPEUTIC CONSIDERATIONS

Empiric Versus Definitive Therapy

Fundamental to the selection of an appropriate antimicrobial agent for the treatment of an infectious disease is an appreciation that individual species of bacteria are associated with specific infectious diseases and that specific antibacterial agents (or classes of antibacterials) are more likely to be effective against these organisms than others. This understanding forms the basis for what is known as "empiric therapy," or treatment selected based on experience without definitive knowledge of the infecting organism or its resistance characteristics. Empiric treatments are often selected based on the initial characterization of the infecting organism (if available), the presentation (characteristics) of the illness, the most likely infecting organism based on patient history and community trends, and the known spectrum of activity of the antibacterial medication under consideration. For example, community-acquired urinary tract infections (UTIs) in otherwise healthy individuals are typically caused by gram-negative *E. coli*, which are usually susceptible to the combination drug co-trimoxazole, which contains sulfamethoxazole and trimethoprim. Similarly, skin infections often result from gram-positive staphylococci, which are susceptible to certain β-lactam antibiotics. The use of a "broad-spectrum" antibacterial agent for empiric treatment is common as there is an increased likelihood that the infecting organism will be susceptible. It should be noted, however, that the spectrum of activity of the selected agent should only be as broad as required to cover the most likely organism causing the disease to limit the development of resistance. "Definitive therapy" involves the rational selection of an antibacterial agent or agents following the identification of the infecting organism and the characterization of its antibacterial susceptibility. A key factor in the selection of definitive therapy is choosing an antibacterial agent with as narrow a spectrum as possible that ideally covers only the bacteria identified to minimize the development of resistance. This may involve switching the patient from a broader spectrum empiric agent to a narrower spectrum agent that covers the specific infectious organism.

Combination Therapy

It is usually desirable to select the best single antimicrobial agent with as narrow a spectrum of activity as possible to cover the most likely infecting organism. However, in certain cases, it may be necessary to use two or more antibacterial agents to ensure the best empiric coverage. An example of such a situation would be the use of multiple antibacterial agents to treat intra-abdominal infections, which are often polymicrobial, or the use of additional agents to cover atypical bacterial pathogens in community-acquired pneumonia. Another reason for choosing combination therapy is to prevent the development of microbial resistance. An example of this is the use of multiple antimycobacterial agents to treat TB, which is caused by *Mycobacterium tuberculosis* (Mtb). It is known that Mtb grows very slowly, can develop persistence, and can develop mutations rapidly due to high bacterial densities at the infection sites (eg, in the lungs), which altogether leads to high-degree resistance. There are several considerations when selecting antibacterial agents to use in combination therapy. First, the mechanisms of action of the selected antibacterial agents should usually be different: for example, the use of a β-lactam combined with an aminoglycoside or a fluoroquinolone. The β-lactam antibiotics[31] interfere with bacterial cell wall formation and thus facilitate the passage of the other agent that in turn interferes with intracellular processes, such as protein or nucleic acid biosynthesis. A second consideration is whether there is potential antagonism between the two agents under consideration that would result in decreased antibacterial efficacy. Antagonism may be physicochemical, such as the chemical incompatibility of β-lactam antibiotics with aminoglycosides. Aminoglycosides possess basic (amino) functional groups that chemically deactivate β-lactams (discussed later). This typically precludes their mixing together in the same intravenous (IV) bag or administering together, although they still can be used empirically if administered separately. Antagonism can also be mechanistic, where the mode of action of one agent interferes with the mode of action of another. For example, there have been reports of antagonism when bacteriostatic agents are used in combination with bactericidal agents, such as the use of a penicillin with a tetracycline.[31] However, the clinical significance of this interaction has been debated. Another consideration for combination therapy is to select agents with non-overlapping toxicity profiles to avoid increased adverse effects.

When recommending a combination therapy, the potential for a synergistic or additive effect of the combination is sought. Several types of antibacterial combinations result in a synergistic effect. One common mechanism of antibacterial synergy is the use of an antibacterial agent in combination with a drug that will prevent its metabolism or degradation. The best example of this scenario is the use of β-lactamase inhibitors combined with β-lactam antibiotics. β-Lactamase is an enzyme produced by resistant bacteria that can destroy β-lactam antibiotics. Another mechanism of antibacterial synergy is the combination of antibacterials that inhibit different steps in the same metabolic pathway. This is known as "sequential blocking." A good example of this is the use of trimethoprim, an inhibitor of dihydrofolate reductase (DHFR), with sulfamethoxazole, an inhibitor of dihydropteroate synthase (DHPS). The DHPS and DHFR enzymes catalyze key steps in the bacterial folate biosynthesis pathway. Another mechanism of antibacterial synergy is the use of antibacterials that inhibit different targets in different pathways, such as the combined use of β-lactam antibiotics with aminoglycosides discussed earlier. Lastly, the use of efflux pump inhibitors combined with antibacterials known to be pumped out of bacterial cells can also result in a synergistic effect. This latter mechanism has been the focus of recent studies.[32] Other factors influencing the decision to use combination therapy may include the higher cost of the treatment, higher pill burden that usually impacts patient's compliance, increased likelihood of adverse effects, and the potential to drive the emergence of resistance in noninfecting organisms in the environment or microbiome.

Pharmacokinetics and Pharmacodynamics

An understanding of the interplay between pharmacokinetic (how the body acts on a drug) and pharmacodynamic (how a drug acts on the body) characteristics of antibacterial agents is critical in the selection of an appropriate agent for successful antibacterial therapy. Pharmacokinetic considerations that may affect the selection of an appropriate antibacterial agent include whether and to what extent a drug is absorbed upon oral administration, how a drug is distributed in the body, if and to what extent the drug is metabolized by the body, and how fast and through which route the drug is eliminated from the body. Antibacterial agents with poor oral absorption are typically only available in parenteral formulations (subcutaneous, intramuscular [IM], IV, and intrathecal), and generally are not suitable for use in an outpatient setting. However, an antibacterial agent with poor oral absorption still can be used for the treatment of GI infections without showing systemic adverse effects. For example, the polymyxin antibiotic colistin must be administered IV, IM, or topically for systemic or topical infections. However, when it is administered orally, its action is local, is limited to the GI tract, and can be used for bowel decontamination. However, parenteral formulations may be desirable in critical patients in a hospital setting as desirable drug levels can be reached much faster and thus concerns associated with oral absorption are avoided. The distribution of an antibacterial agent in the body is another consideration as some drugs may need to penetrate specific tissues to be effective. Examples include bone tissue in osteomyelitis, central nervous system (CNS) infections, the prostate tissue in prostatitis, and the lung tissue in TB. Penicillins, for example, penetrate the prostate tissue poorly while fluoroquinolones have excellent prostate tissue distribution; hence, the latter would be a better choice for prostate infection. The volume of distribution of a drug is a common measure of how extensively it distributes in the body, with high volumes of distribution indicating a large level of drug distribution. An example of how this property is used clinically is the use of antibacterials with low volumes of distribution, and hence higher blood levels, to treat blood infections or bacteremia. The extent of metabolism and route of elimination of an antibacterial can also influence its selection. Drugs with low metabolism and renal elimination are useful for the treatment of kidney and bladder infections. An example of such is the drug nitrofurantoin, a urinary antiseptic that is poorly metabolized and rapidly eliminated by the kidney. In a different scenario, patients with renal failure should not be administered antibacterial agents that are primarily eliminated in the urine, unless dose adjustments and therapeutic drug monitoring (TDM) are additionally considered. Other factors that may influence selection of an antibacterial therapeutic include the microenvironment of the infected tissue such as oxygen tension and pH. For example, aminoglycosides require an oxygen-dependent system to penetrate bacterial cells and thus are less useful to treat infections in low-oxygen microenvironments, such as abscesses. Other pharmacokinetic factors that may impact antibacterial efficacy include the extent of the agent's serum protein binding and whether the agent displays linear or nonlinear pharmacokinetics.[33]

Similarly, there are many pharmacodynamic properties of antibacterial agents that must be considered when selecting an appropriate medication for the treatment of an infection. Antibacterial agents can kill bacteria following differing pharmacodynamic principles. The killing activity of the β-lactam antibiotics, for example, is dependent on the duration of time the concentration of a drug stays above the drug's MIC level. This is known as "time-dependent killing." Aminoglycosides, however, have killing activity that correlates to how high the drug concentration is relative to the drug's MIC. This is known as "concentration-dependent killing." These pharmacodynamic properties will influence the choice of dosing regimen for the selected antibacterial agent(s). Another pharmacodynamic property that is relevant to drug selection and drug dosing is called the post-antibiotic effect (PAE). This refers to a period of time after the antibacterial agent's concentration has fallen below the MIC, but the growth of the infecting bacteria is still inhibited. This effect is dependent on the class of antibacterial, the duration of exposure to the antibacterial, and the bacterial species being treated. Antibacterial classes with reported PAEs include aminoglycosides, fluoroquinolones, and tetracyclines.[34] This pharmacodynamic property is considered desirable in many cases and will influence how the antibacterial medication is dosed.

Other Factors

Other factors that may influence therapeutic decision-making in antibacterial selection include dosage forms available, drug costs, geography, the bacteria's mode of growth, the patient's medical history and immune status, and the duration of treatment. While some medications are available in both oral and parenteral formulations, it is common for an antibacterial agent to only be available in one or the other dosage form. As mentioned, for critically ill patients, a parenteral formulation is often desirable, but when their condition improves, they are often switched to an oral formulation. If an oral formulation is not available for a given medication, then the patient will receive an alternative antimicrobial that has similar activity and is available for oral administration. For many patients, medication cost is a significant consideration. A newer, and therefore very often higher cost, agent may not be affordable, thus prescribing such medication would certainly impact patient compliance. This is an area of health care where the pharmacist is in an ideal position to help the physician choose an alternative agent with similar efficacy but lower cost. The patient's location can also impact therapeutic decision-making. For example, patients may not have access to health systems or home health care for parenteral doses of antibacterials in rural settings, necessitating the selection of alternative oral formulations. Additionally, patients living in economically challenged parts of the globe are inherently at risk of not having access to proper health care services and thus antimicrobial therapy. Another factor that may influence antibacterial treatment is the presence of bacterial biofilms. Planktonic bacteria are free-living and actively replicating, and thus easier to kill using antibacterial agents. Bacteria can also form biofilms, which are surface-adhered structures consisting of bacteria in a glycoprotein matrix that are often dormant and thus more difficult to kill with the available antibacterial medications. Treatment of bacterial biofilms often requires mechanical intervention along with use of combination therapy including antibacterials that have improved penetration, such as macrolides, tetracyclines, and oxazolidinones.[35] The patient's immune status may also influence the selection of antibacterial agents. This is because immune suppressed patients are more likely to have infections with unusual bacterial etiologies, which will impact the selection of empirical treatment. For example, patients with T-cell deficiency may present with lung infections caused by atypical pathogens such as TB or *Pneumocystis pneumonia*, in addition to the typical pneumococcal pneumonia. The patient's past and current medical history is another key factor while carefully selecting an adequate antimicrobial therapy in order to avoid drug-drug interactions (DDIs) and antagonistic effects between drug classes. Lastly, the duration of treatment may impact the selection of antibacterial agent. Oral agents are significantly more preferable for longer, outpatient treatment regimens, while parenteral agents are preferred for short-term treatment of critically ill patients. Shorter courses of antibacterials are desirable whenever possible to minimize both adverse effects to the patient and the development of bacterial resistance. If a longer course (>7 days) is required, it may be necessary to select an agent with a decreased adverse effect profile and longer duration of action, thus allowing for less frequent administration and affordable price.

MECHANISTIC CLASSES

Cell Envelope–Disrupting Agents

Bacterial Cell Envelope

Bacterial cells are enclosed in a unique cell envelope comprised of one or more lipid membranes and a rigid cell wall composed of peptidoglycan (which protects the cells from lysis due to osmotic pressure) and often additional components such as lipoproteins and LPS. This differs significantly from mammalian cells, which consist of a single lipid membrane that is comprised of lipids distinct from those composing the bacterial cell membranes. This distinct bacterial cell envelope affords several attractive targets for selective chemotherapy of bacterial infection, including enzymes responsible for biosynthesis, restructuring, and maintenance of the bacterial cell wall, as well as the unique components of the bacterial cell membranes. Three of the main functions of the bacterial cell wall are (1) to provide a semipermeable barrier interfacing with the external environment through which only desirable substances may pass; (2) to provide a sufficiently strong barrier that maintains the cell shape, contributes to cell motility, and protects the cellular integrity from changes in the osmotic pressure of its environment;

and (3) to prevent digestion by host enzymes and other environmental stressors. The components of the cell wall are constructed within the cell, with the final assembly taking place outside of the inner membrane. This makes the enzymes involved in late steps of cell wall biosynthesis more vulnerable to inhibition because they are at or near the cell surface. Individual bacterial species usually differ in specific details relating to the components and construction of their cell wall. The general cell wall morphology for gram-positive and gram-negative bacteria is described next.

Gram-Positive Bacteria

The cell wall of gram-positive bacteria is a simpler construct than that of gram-negative organisms. A schematic representation is shown in Figure 32.5. On the outside of the cell wall is a set of characteristic carbohydrates and proteins that together make up the antigenic determinants that differ from species to species and that also allow the bacteria to adhere to target cells. In some bacteria, there may also be a lipid-rich capsule external to the cell wall (not shown in the figure). The cell wall is primarily composed of peptidoglycan, a spongy, gel-forming layer consisting of a series of alternating sugars (*N*-acetylglucosamine, NAG, and *N*-acetylmuramic acid, NAM) connected in a long chain by (1,4)-β linkages (Fig. 32.6). NAM units in different strands are further connected with a peptide linker composed of serval amino acids. This connection occurs via amide bond created between the respective NAM's lactic acid carboxy group and amino group at the N-terminus of the peptide linker. In *S. aureus*, which is representative of gram-positive organisms, the amino acids comprising the peptide linker are L-alanine-D-glutamate-L-lysine-D-alanine. The D-stereochemistry of the glutamate and alanine residues is notable and serves to protect the bacteria from peptidoglycan hydrolysis by peptidases in the host, which cannot recognize amino acids with D-stereochemistry as all amino acids in mammalian organisms have the opposite, L-configuration.

The early steps in the biosynthesis of the peptidoglycan result in formation of a complex polymeric sheet composed

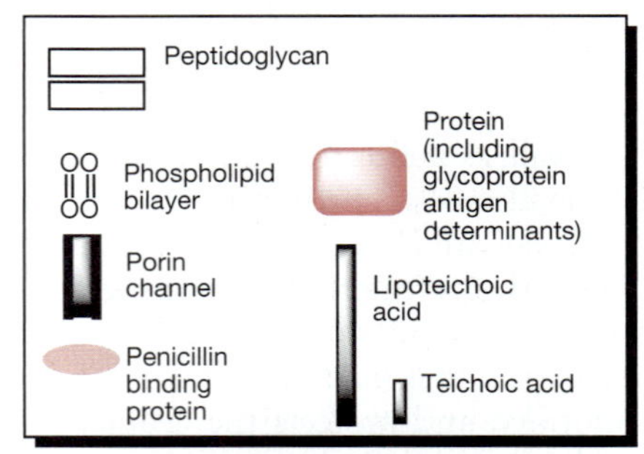

Figure 32.5 Major features of the gram-positive bacterial cell wall.

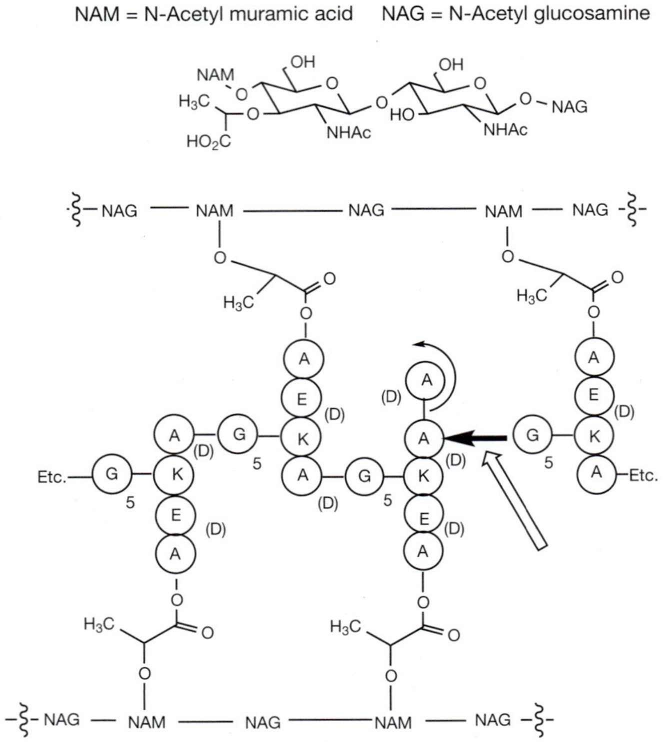

Figure 32.6 Peptidoglycan cross-linking process in bacterial cell wall. The last glycine residue in the pentaglycyl linker replaces terminal D-alanine.

of NAM-NAG strands, which is then cross-linked by peptides to form a thickened, more rigid, and mature layer. As shown in Figure 32.6, in *S. aureus*, the unreacted (ie, non-cross-linked) peptide sequence attached to NAM (via the aforementioned amide bond with lactic acid group) is L-Ala-D-Glu-L-Lys-D-Ala-D-Ala. The cross-linking is achieved by connecting via a pentaglycyl linker of the lysine residue in one tetrapeptide unit appended to the respective NAM-NAG strand with the penultimate D-alanine residue and thus simultaneous expulsion of the ultimate D-alanine residue from the adjacent pentapeptide of a neighboring NAM-NAG strand. This last step is an enzyme-catalyzed transamidation by which the terminal amino moiety on the last glycine unit of the A strand displaces the terminal D-Ala unit on the nearby B strand (Fig. 32.6). The cell wall transamidase, a so-called penicillin-binding protein (PBP), forms a transient covalent bond during the synthesis phase with a serine hydroxyl group in the active site of the enzyme. Completion of the catalytic cycle involves displacement of the enzyme by a glycine residue from the pentaglycyl linker, which regenerates the enzyme. This linkage process gives the wall additional rigidity and strength, which protects the cell against osmotic stress. The completed cell wall also accounts for the characteristic morphologic shape of gram-positive bacteria (spherical cocci and rod-like bacilli, for example). The transamidation reaction in cell wall formation is an extremely sensitive process to the inhibitory action of β-lactam antibiotics. It is also the target of the glycopeptide antibiotics such as vancomycin. The peptidoglycan layer is traversed by complex glycophospholipids called teichoic and teichuronic acids, which play a role in both cell wall integrity and bacterial pathogenesis. Antibacterial compounds can penetrate the gram-positive cell envelope significantly better than the gram-negative cell envelope discussed later.

Beneath the peptidoglycan layer is the bacterial cell membrane composed of a unique lipid bilayer in which several important proteins such as transporters and enzymes are embedded. The inner membrane and its protein components provide the principal barrier to uptake of antibiotics. Among these proteins are the molecular targets for the β-lactams, the PBPs.[36] These are enzymes that are important for cell wall formation and remodeling. There are several different types of PBPs (PBP-1a, PBP-1b, PBP-2, PBP-2a, PBP-3, etc), whose presence and function are dependent on the species of bacteria.[37] β-Lactam antibiotics bind to these proteins and kill bacteria by preventing the biosynthesis of a functional cell wall. The different β-lactam antibiotics display different patterns of binding and inhibition of the various PBPs. Interference with the function of PBPs by β-lactam antibiotics prevents normal cell wall growth and repair, which results in serious problems for bacteria, particularly young cells needing to grow and mature cells needing to repair damage or to divide.

GRAM-NEGATIVE BACTERIA. In the case of gram-negative bacteria, the cell wall is more complex (Fig. 32.7). The cell envelope of these bacteria is composed of both outer and inner lipid membranes separated by a thinner peptidoglycan layer relative to gram-positive bacteria. The periplasmic space between the outer and inner lipid membranes contains a thin layer of peptidoglycan. The inner lipid membrane is phospholipid-rich and embeds several proteins with various functions important to the cell, including the PBPs that are targeted by the β-lactam antibiotics. Other inner membrane proteins are involved in transport, energy, and biosynthesis. Many gram-negative bacteria express proteins that actively pump out antibiotics from the cell, a process known as "efflux," which can counteract the action of therapeutics and lead to resistance development. The outer lipid membrane differs significantly from the inner membrane and contains complex LPS that encode antigenic responses, cause septic shock, provide serotype, and influence morphology. This exterior layer also contains several enzymes and porin channels, which are transmembrane channels composed of several polypeptide subunits through which molecules can diffuse into the cell. Many porin channels allow the transit of distinct types of small molecules, while others contain specific receptors that allow only specific molecules to pass. Porins are critical to the entry of antibacterial drugs into the gram-negative cell. The size, shape, charge, and lipophilic character of antibacterials can affect their ability to pass through porin channels. Because of the more complex architecture of the cell envelope, antibacterial agents have greater difficulty penetrating into the cell of gram-negative bacteria.

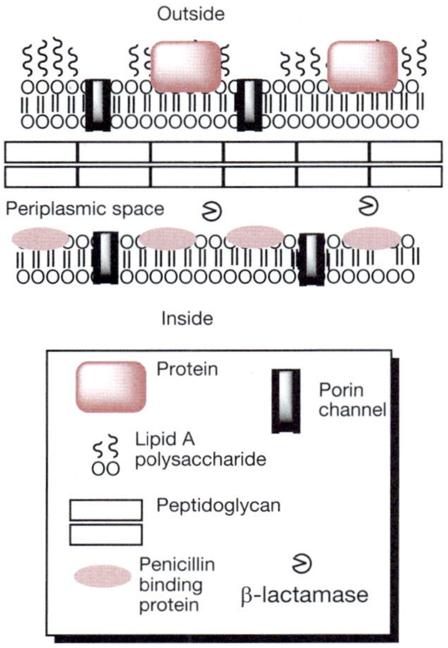

Figure 32.7 General morphologic components of the gram-negative bacterial cell wall.

β-Lactam Antibiotics

The name lactam is given to cyclic amides and is analogous to the name lactone given to cyclic esters. In organic chemistry nomenclature, the carbon atom immediately adjacent to the carboxylic acid functional group is designated as α, and the subsequent carbon atoms are designated as β, γ, and so on. Thus, a β-lactam is a cyclic amide with four atoms in its ring. The contemporary name for this ring system is azetidinone. This structural feature was rare when it was found within the core structure of the penicillins, so the name β-lactam came to be a generic descriptor for the whole class of antibiotics. Ultimately, this ring proved to be the main component of the pharmacophore, so the term possesses not only chemical but also medicinal significance. The penicillin subclass of β-lactam antibiotics is characterized by the presence of a substituted five-membered thiazolidine ring fused to the β-lactam ring. This fusion and the chirality of the β-lactam ring result in the molecule roughly possessing a "V" shape. This drastically interferes with the planarity of the lactam bond and inhibits resonance of the lactam nitrogen with its carbonyl group. Consequently, the β-lactam ring is much more reactive and thus more sensitive to nucleophilic attack when compared with normal planar amides.

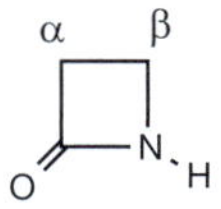

β-lactam
azetidinone

PENICILLINS. The medicinal classifications, chemical structures, generic names, and brand names (when available) are shown in Table 32.1.

History. The general story describing the serendipitous discovery of the penicillins was discussed earlier. The earliest penicillins were produced by fungi from media constituents. The heterobicyclic nucleus of 6-aminopenicillanic acid (6-APA) is constructed in a biosynthetic process catalyzed by enzymes. The side chain attached to the 6-amino group

Table 32.1 Commercially Available Penicillins

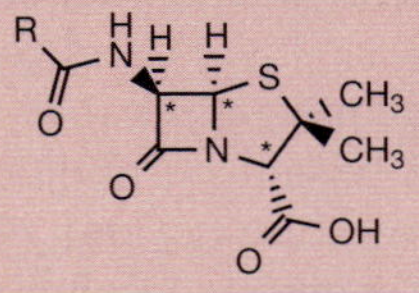

Generic Names	Trade Names	R-group
Fermentation-Derived (Natural) Penicillins		
6-Aminopenicillanic acid		H
Benzylpenicillin (Penicillin G)	Pfizerpen, Bicillin L-A, Bicillin C-R	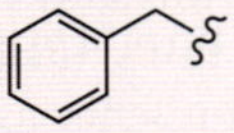
Phenoxymethylpenicillin (Penicillin V)	Penicillin - VK	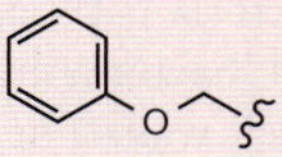
Anti-Staphylococcal (β-Lactam-Resistant) Penicillins		
Nafcillin	Nallpen	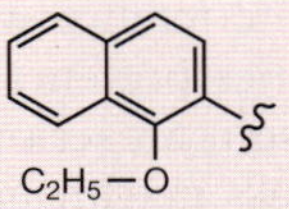
Oxacillin (X = Y = H)	Bactocill	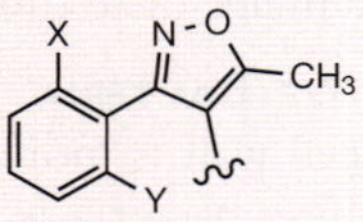
Dicloxacillin (X = Y = Cl)	N/A	
Amino-Penicillins (Broad-Spectrum)		
Ampicillin	Unasyn (with sulbactam)	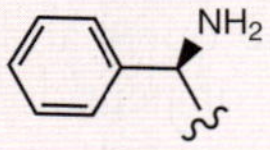
Amoxicillin	Amoxil, Larotid, Augmentin (with clavulanate)	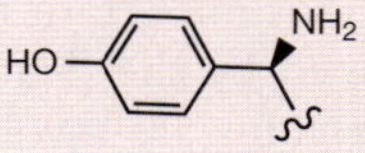
Anti-Pseudomonal (Extended-Spectrum) Penicillins		
Piperacillin	Zosyn (with tazobactam)	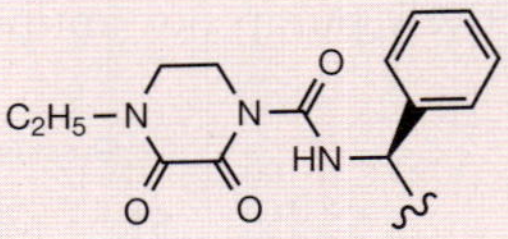

was added essentially intact from media constituents. It was discovered that certain arylacetic acids, when added to the medium, were used to form the side chain amide moiety and that this was very important for stability and breadth of spectrum.[38] It was later discovered that exclusion of such materials from the medium allowed the production of 6-APA without a side chain.[39] Chemists could subsequently further elaborate the advance building block (6-APA) by adding a wider variety of side chains without being limited by the specific requirements of the fungal enzymes. With this breakthrough, the penicillin field expanded to include orally active, broad-spectrum, and enzymatically stable penicillins.

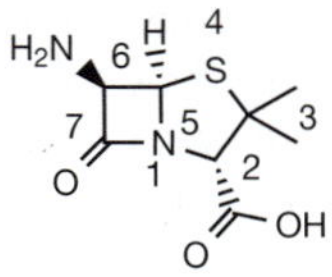

Isolation of Penicillins. The original fermentation-derived penicillins were produced by growth of the fungus *Penicillium chrysogenum* on complex solid media, with the result that they were mixtures differing from one another in the identity of the side chain moiety. When a sufficient supply of phenylacetic acid is present in liquid media, it is preferentially incorporated into the molecule to produce mainly benzylpenicillin (penicillin G). Use of phenoxyacetic acid instead yields phenoxymethylpenicillin (penicillin V). More than two dozen different penicillins have been made by following this methodology, but penicillin G and V are the only two medications that continue to have clinical use to this date. Complete exclusion from the medium of the organic acids serving as the side chain precursors provides rather in modest yield the fundamental penicillin nucleus, 6-APA. By itself, 6-APA has only a weak antibacterial activity, but when substituted on its primary amino group with a suitable carboxylic acid to give amide side chains, the resulting potency and antibacterial spectrum are profoundly enhanced. With this key precursor isolated, limitations caused by enzyme specificities in the biosynthesis could be readily overcome by employing partial chemical synthesis, that is, semisynthesis.

Nomenclature and Classification. The nomenclature of the penicillins can be complex. The Chemical Abstracts Service is definitive and unambiguous but too complex for ordinary use (Fig. 32.8). For example, the chemical name for benzylpenicillin sodium is monosodium (2S,5R,6R)-3, 3-dimethyl-7-oxo-6-(2-phenylacetamido)-4-thia-l-azabicyclo[3.2.0] heptane-2-carboxylate. A simpler system has been widely adopted by scientists and practitioners that involves taking the repeating unit, that is, carbonyl-6-APA, and adding to it the trivial chemical name stemming from the side chain moiety. Therefore, the use of names such as benzylpenicillin and phenoxymethylpenicillin makes practical sense. There are three asymmetric centers in the penicillin core structure as indicated by the asterisks in Table 32.1. This absolute stereochemistry must be preserved to observe useful antibiotic activity.

Chemical Properties. The sodium and potassium salts of penicillins are crystalline, hygroscopic, and water soluble. They can be administered orally or parentally. When they are kept dry, they are stable for an extended period of time. On the contrary, they hydrolyze rapidly when in solution. Their best stability is noted at pH values between 5.5 and 8, especially at pH 6.0 to 7.2. The procaine and benzathine salts of benzylpenicillin (discussed later), on the other hand, are water insoluble as they are weak salts created by a weak organic acid (penicillin) and a weak organic base. When administered by IM injection, these compounds dissolve and enter the bloodstream slowly. Hence, they are useful as depot or repository injections when sustained blood levels are desirable.

The most unstable bond in the penicillin molecule is the highly strained and reactive β-lactam amide bond. This bond cleaves moderately slowly in water unless heated, but it breaks down at a fast pace in alkaline solutions to produce penicilloic acid, which readily decarboxylates to produce penilloic acid, which is further degraded to penilloaldehyde and penicillamine (Fig. 32.9). Penicilloic acid has a negligible tendency to reclose to the corresponding penicillin; therefore, this reaction is essentially irreversible under physiologic conditions. Because the β-lactam ring is an essential portion of the pharmacophore, its hydroxide-mediated hydrolysis completely deactivates the antibiotic. A significant degree of hydrolysis also takes place in the liver. The bacterial enzyme, β-lactamase, also catalyzes this reaction (ie, β-lactam ring opening) and therefore it constitutes the principal mechanism of bacterial resistance in the clinic. Organic alcohols and amines bring about the same cleavage reaction, but in this case the decomposition products are the corresponding esters and amides, which obviously are inactive. If mixed together or coformulated, a chemical interaction of the β-lactam ring with a specific primary amino functional group of aminoglycoside antibiotics is of clinical relevance as it inactivates penicillins and cephalosporins. This concept will be discussed later in the chapter. Of note, the host's proteins can also serve as the nucleophiles in this reaction to produce antigenic conjugates that are responsible for the reported penicillin allergies. Small molecules that are not inherently antigenic but react with proteins to produce antigens in this manner are called haptens. Although rare, the commercially available penicillin salts may be contaminated with small amounts of these antigenic penicilloyl proteins derived from reaction with proteins encountered in their fermentative production or by high-molecular-weight self-condensation–derived polymers resulting from high-concentration penicillins, which then react with themselves. Both classes of impurities are antigenic and may sensitize some patients.

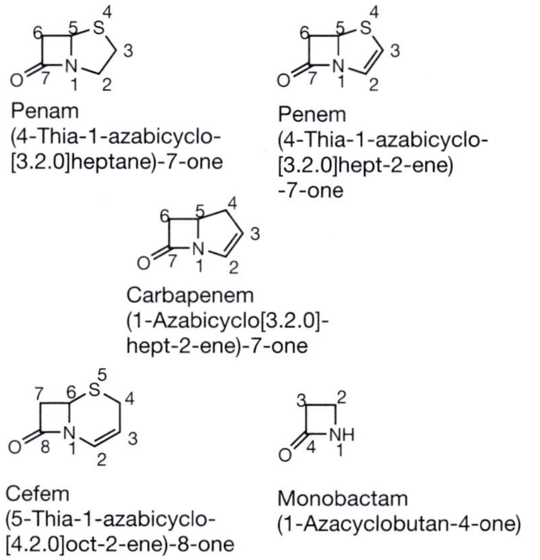

Figure 32.8 Ring and numbering systems of β-lactam scaffolds.

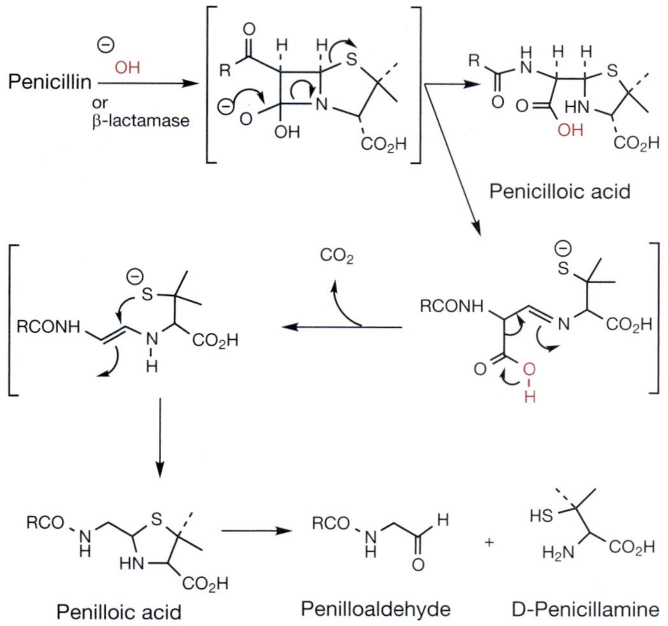

Figure 32.9 Instability of penicillins to nucleophiles.

In acidic solutions, the hydrolysis of penicillins is complex. Hydrolysis of the β-lactam bond can be shown through

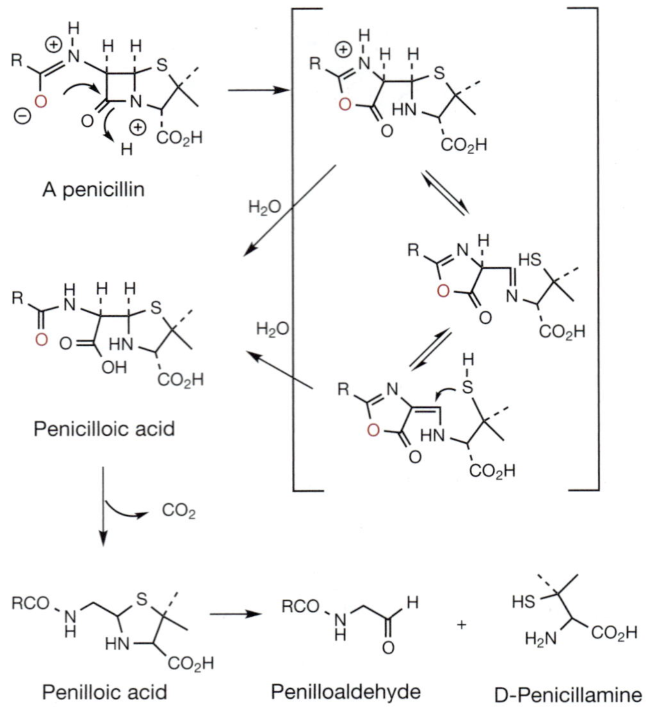

Figure 32.10 Instability of penicillins in acid. Hydrolysis involves the C_6 side chain.

kinetic analysis to involve participation of the side chain amide oxygen. The rate of this reaction differs widely depending on the nature of the R group. The major final by-products of the acid-mediated degradation are penicillamine, penilloic acid, and penilloaldehyde (Fig. 32.10). The intermediate penicillenic acid is highly unstable and undergoes rapid hydrolysis to the corresponding penicilloic acid.

An alternate pathway involves sulfur ejection to a product that in turn fragments to liberate the penicilloic acid. Penicilloic acid readily decarboxylates to penilloic acid. The latter hydrolyzes to produce penilloaldehyde and penicillamine (itself used clinically as a chelating agent). Several related fragmentations to a variety of other products were indicated to take place. None of these products has antibacterial activity. At gastric pH (~2.0) and a temperature of 37 °C, the half-life of benzylpenicillin is measured in minutes.

Mechanism of Action. The molecular mode of action of the β-lactam antibiotics is a selective and irreversible inhibition of the enzymes processing the developing peptidoglycan layer (Fig. 32.11). Just before the cross-linking occurs in peptidoglycan, the peptide pendant from the lactate carboxyl of a muramic acid unit terminates in a D-alanyl-D-alanine unit. The terminal D-alanine residue is exchanged for a glycine unit on an adjacent strand in a reaction catalyzed by a cell wall transamidase. This enzyme is one of the PBPs (carboxypeptidases, endopeptidases, and transpeptidases) that normally reside in the bacterial inner membrane and perform construction, repair, and housekeeping functions, maintaining cell wall integrity, and playing a vital role in cell growth and division. They differ significantly between species and even individual strains, and this fact is used to rationalize different potency and morphologic outcomes following β-lactam attack on the different bacteria. The cell wall transamidase uses a serine hydroxyl group to attack the penultimate D-alanine thus forming a covalent ester bond, while the terminal D-alanine is released by this action and diffuses away. The enzyme-peptidoglycan ester bond is attacked by the free amino end of a pentaglycyl linker of an adjacent strand, regenerating the transpeptidase's active site for further catalytic action and producing a new amide bond, which connects two adjacent strands together.

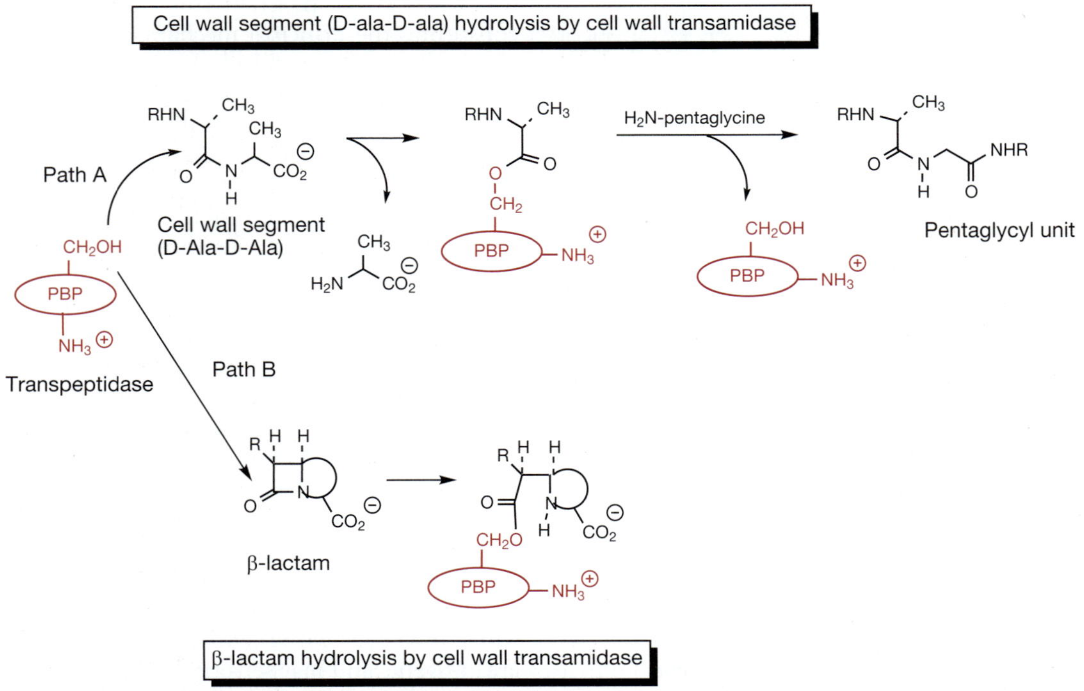

Figure 32.11 Cell wall cross-linking and mechanism of action of β-lactams. Path A represents the normal cross-linking mechanism. Path B illustrates the reaction of β-lactam antibiotics with the penicillin-binding protein (PBP).

The three-dimensional geometry of the active site of the enzyme (PBP) perfectly accommodates the shape and separation of the amino acids of its substrate. Because the substrate has an unnatural D-stereochemistry at the critical residues, this enzyme is not expected to attack host peptides or even other bacterial peptides composed of natural amino acids. The penicillins and the other β-lactam antibiotics have a structure that closely resembles that of the acylated D-alanyl-D-alanine. The enzyme therefore mistakenly accepts the penicillins as though they were its endogenous substrate. The highly strained β-lactam ring is much more reactive than a standard amide moiety, particularly when fused into the appropriate bicyclic system. The intermediate acyl-enzyme complex, however, is structurally different from the ordinary intermediate and thus hydrolysis does not break down the penicillin. In the case of penicillins, a bulky heterocyclic moiety is still covalently bound to PBP and cannot diffuse away as the natural terminal D-alanine unit does. This presents a steric barrier that the nearby pentaglycyl unit cannot overcome and thus prevents the enzyme's active site from being regenerated and the peptidoglycan's peptide units from being cross-linked. The result is an inactivated enzyme and a defective cell wall. The strain energy release obtained via the PBP enzymatic β-lactam bond cleavage is so pronounced that there is virtually no tendency for the reaction to reverse. Water is also an insufficient nucleophile and therefore it cannot hydrolyze the complex to regenerate PBP. Thus, the cell wall transamidase is stoichiometrically inactivated. The gaps produced in peptidoglycan by this covalent interference of penicillins with PBP are not filled in because the enzyme has been permanently inactivated. The resulting cell wall is structurally weak and subject to osmotic stress. Cell lysis can result, and the cell rapidly dies assisted by another class of bacterial enzymes, the autolysins.[40]

Pharmacokinetic and Pharmacodynamic Properties. The pharmacokinetic properties of the penicillins have been well characterized.[41] As discussed in the structure-activity relationship (SAR) section, penicillin V, the aminopenicillins (ampicillin and amoxicillin), and dicloxacillin are acid stable and thus are orally absorbed to an acceptable extent for oral dosage. Absorption of these penicillins is rapid, with peak plasma concentrations achieved in 30 minutes to 2 hours, depending on the agent. After oral absorption, the penicillins are distributed widely in the body except for the eye, prostate tissue, and uninflamed meninges. However, penicillins can distribute into the CNS if the meninges are inflamed. A portion of a penicillin dose is metabolized (10%-50%, depending on the specific agent), with the remaining amount being eliminated in the urine unchanged. Protein binding of the penicillins is highly variable and dependent on the lipophilicity of the specific agent. As an example, it can range from 20% for amoxicillin to 96% for dicloxacillin. With respect to the pharmacodynamic properties of the penicillins, the class in general is classified as bactericidal with time-dependent killing. Most penicillins exhibit a weak to absent PAE. Therapeutically, the time-dependent killing and weak PAE of the penicillins mean that the drugs are more effective with extended or continuous infusions versus intermittent dosing (when dosed parenterally).

Table 32.2 Improved Acid Stability and Absorption of Substituted Penicillins

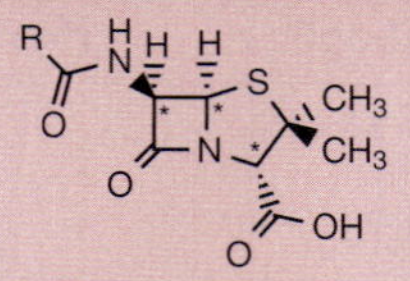

Drug	R	% Absorption Intact Drug
Benzylpenicillin (Pen G)	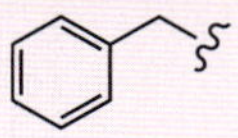	15-30
Phenoxypenicillin (Pen V)	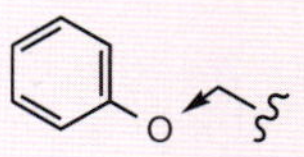	60
Ampicillin	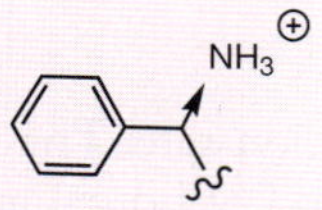	33-54
Amoxicillin	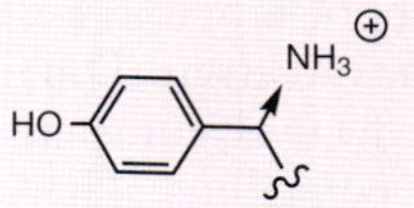	74-80

Structure-Activity Relationship. The chemical substituents attached to the penicillin nucleus can significantly influence the stability of the penicillins as well as their spectrum of activity. It is important to recognize whether the structural changes affect drug stability on the shelf or in the GI tract (in vivo), improve stability toward degradation by β-lactamase enzymes, or expand the spectrum of activity. The substitution of a side chain R group on the primary amine of 6-APA with an electron-withdrawing group acts as an "electron sink" that decreases the electron density on the side chain carbonyl oxygen, which protects these penicillins in part from an acid-promoted degradation. This structural modification has clinical implications because it allows these compounds to survive passage through the stomach without acid degradation and improves the oral absorption of the intact drugs. The degree of absorption under fasting conditions is shown in Table 32.2. Additionally, in vitro degradation reactions of penicillins can be retarded by keeping the pH of solutions between 6.0 and 6.8 and by refrigerating them. Metal ions such as mercury, zinc, and copper catalyze the degradation of penicillins so their contact with penicillin solutions shall be avoided. The lids of containers used today are commonly made from inert materials, in part to minimize such problems.

Increased lipophilicity of the side chain of a penicillin contributes to increased serum protein binding (Table 32.3). While this can measurably reduce the effective concentration of the drug in whole blood, the clinical impact is low. The degree of serum protein binding of the penicillins has relatively little influence on their half-lives. The penicillins are actively excreted into the urine via an active transport system for weak acids, and the rate of release from their protein-bound form is sufficiently rapid that the controlling

Table 32.3 Lipophilicity and Protein Binding of Penicillins

Penicillin	cLogP	Protein Binding (%)
Penicillin G	1.74	60
Penicillin V	1.94	80
Ampicillin	−1.20	20
Amoxicillin	−1.87	20
Nafcillin	3.53	90
Oxacillin	2.05	90
Dicloxacillin	2.98	96
Piperacillin	1.36	48

rate is the kidney secretion rate. The serum half-life of penicillin G is about 0.4 to 0.9 hours, and that of phenoxymethylpenicillin is about 0.5 hours. Both are excreted into the urine by tubular excretion. The drug probenecid, when present, competes effectively for excretion and thus prolongs the half-life of the penicillins. Therefore, to modulate/enhance their half-lives, the combinations of a penicillin with probenecid have been used in the past therapeutically.

The stability of the penicillins toward β-lactamase is influenced by bulkiness in the acyl group attached to the primary amine. β-Lactamase are much less tolerant to the presence of steric hindrance near the side chain amide bond than are the PBPs. The stability of methicillin (discontinued in the United States) toward the action of β-lactamases is an excellent example of the impact of such structural modification. When the aromatic ring is attached directly to the side chain carbonyl and both ortho positions are substituted by methoxy groups, β-lactamase stability results (Fig. 32.12). Movement of one of the methoxy groups to the para position or replacing one of them with a hydrogen yields a derivative that is sensitive to β-lactamases. Introducing a methylene between the aromatic ring and 6-APA likewise produces a β-lactamase-sensitive agent (Fig. 32.12). These findings support the hypothesis that the degree of penicillin resistance to β-lactamase degradation is predominantly based on the degree of steric hindrance at this key position in the structure. Further examples of this effect are seen in the structure of nafcillin, oxacillin, and dicloxacillin, which bear the designation of anti-staphylococcal (β-lactamase-resistant) penicillins due to their activity against methicillin-susceptible *S. aureus* (MSSA), which expresses β-lactamases (Table 32.1).

Resistance. The first literature reports of a penicillinase (now referred to as β-lactamase) were published in 1940.[42] This phenomenon was rare at the time and caused no particular alarm. Resistance to β-lactam antibiotics is now quite common and has become alarming. There are several mechanisms of bacterial resistance to β-lactam antibiotics. The first is the expression of β-lactamase enzymes (usually serine proteases) that catalyze the hydrolysis of the β-lactam bond and inactivate β-lactam antibiotics to penicilloic acids before they can reach and interact with the PBPs (Fig. 32.13). They resemble the cell wall transamidase, which is the usual target of β-lactams. However, hydrolytic regeneration of the active site is much faster with β-lactamases when compared to the cell wall transamidases (PBPs), so that the enzyme can perform many cycles; thus, a comparatively small amount of β-lactamase can destroy a large amount of β-lactams. With gram-positive bacteria, such as staphylococci, the β-lactamases are usually shed continuously into the medium and meet the drug outside the cell wall (Fig. 32.5). They are biosynthesized in significant quantities. With gram-negative bacteria, a more conservative course is followed. In this case, the β-lactamases are secreted into the periplasmic space between the inner and outer membrane, so while still distal to the PBPs, they do not readily escape into the medium and therefore there is no need for their frequent production (Fig. 32.7). Numerous β-lactamases with various antibiotic substrate specificities have been identified. Diverse classification systems are used for β-lactamases, and they have been

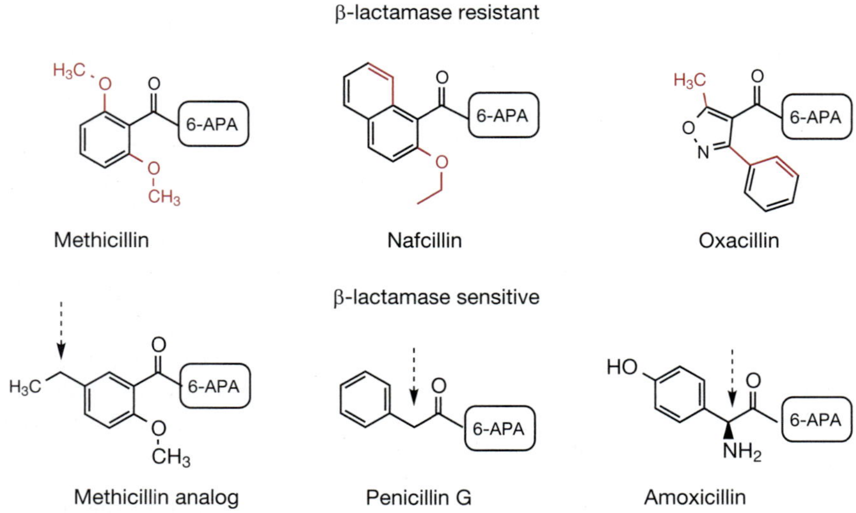

Figure 32.12 β-Lactamase-resistant/sensitive structural features.

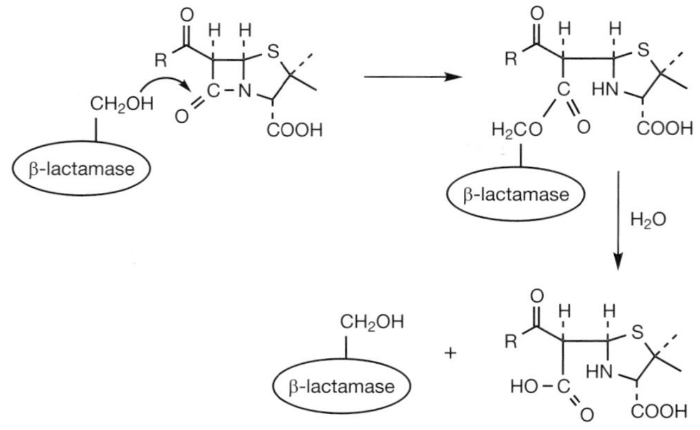

Figure 32.13 β-Lactamase-catalyzed hydrolysis of penicillins.

extensively reviewed.[37] The clinical relevance of β-lactamases is becoming increasingly important as more destructive examples known as extended-spectrum β-lactamases (ESBLs) become more commonly encountered. These β-lactamases are capable of inactivating many previously stable β-lactams. This is an intensive area of research and is frequently updated as new information is discovered.[43] Elaboration of β-lactamases is often R-factor mediated and, in some cases, is even induced by the presence of β-lactam antibiotics.

Another mechanism of resistance found in gram-positive bacteria is thickening of the cell wall. This also affects other cell wall–active antibiotics such as the glycopeptides. Bacteria can also express PBPs that have decreased binding affinity for β-lactam antibiotics. An example of such is the expression of PBP-2a by *S. aureus*, which resulted in methicillin resistance and coined the term "methicillin-resistant *S. aureus*" (MRSA). Gram-negative bacteria have additional unique mechanisms of resistance related to their different cell envelope. In these bacteria, the outer membrane acts as an additional barrier to cell penetration by antibiotics. In gram-negative pathogens, the antibacterial agents often traverse the cell envelope by means of porin channels (discussed earlier). This in turn can substantially affect the design of gram-negative-acting β-lactam drugs as there are restrictions on the shape, size, composition, charge, and rigidity for them to be able to access the porin channels.[44] Gram-negative organisms can alter their cell permeability to decrease drug penetration. This is often achieved by reduction in the expression of the porin channels or by mutations in the porins that affect antibiotic accessibility. The expression of efflux pumps by gram-negative bacteria that can rapidly expel antibiotics from the cell before they can act on their targets is another resistance mechanism. There are now a large variety of efflux pumps with varying levels of activity against the β-lactam antibiotics.[45]

Adverse Effects and Allergenicity. The most common adverse effect reported for the penicillins is hypersensitivity, and this drug class ranks among the highest for reported drug allergy. Even up to 10% of patients report having an allergic reaction to penicillins.[46] The true rate of penicillin allergy is difficult to determine due to confusion between adverse effects of the drugs and true hypersensitivity. Penicillin hypersensitivity commonly presents as rash, fever, and bronchospasm (difficulty breathing). Severe reactions can produce exfoliative dermatitis, Stevens-Johnson syndrome, angioedema, and anaphylaxis, which may result in cardiovascular collapse, shock, and death. A patient's history may be helpful in determining a penicillin allergy and reported past hypersensitivity should be reason for caution in using drugs from this class. Skin tests are available if there is doubt about the potential for hypersensitivity. Cross-sensitivity to other β-lactam classes (cephalosporins, carbapenems) can occur and they should be used with caution in patients with confirmed penicillin hypersensitivity. Alternative antibacterial classes, such as macrolides, lincosamides, and tetracyclines, may be considered if β-lactam hypersensitivity is a strong concern. The penicillin hypersensitivity stems from the formation of covalent haptens between penicillins and their penicilloyl degradation products with proteins in the body. The "major determinant" for this reaction is the penicilloic acid formed when the β-lactam ring is cleaved. Other penicillin degradation products can also act as haptens and are the "minor determinants."

Other adverse effects of the penicillins are rare and relatively mild. This drug class can cause bone marrow suppression and granulocytopenia. Hepatitis has been reported with oxacillin and nafcillin. Impaired platelet aggregation has been reported for penicillin G and piperacillin. Adverse effects from orally administered penicillins can include nausea, vomiting, and diarrhea. Of note, amoxicillin has a lower rate of GI effects. Adverse effects from injectable formulations can include phlebitis (IV formulations) and pain (IM formulations). Intrathecal injections of penicillins can produce encephalopathy and should be avoided. Inadvertent IV administration of the IM depot penicillin formulations (procaine and benzathine salts) can produce severe reactions including hallucinations, seizures, and cardiorespiratory arrest.

Individual Penicillins. The penicillins are classified herein by using the common scheme of spectrum of activity and resistance to β-lactamase inactivation.

Natural (Fermentation-Derived) Penicillins

Benzylpenicillin (Penicillin G). Benzylpenicillin, or penicillin G, is one of two fermentation-derived penicillins currently used in practice. This agent is highly susceptible to inactivation by β-lactamase enzymes and has poor oral bioavailability due to its acid instability. Notwithstanding this, the drug is still frequently used and is available in both IV and IM (discussed later) dosage forms. It is used regularly for the treatment of infections caused by gram-positive streptococci, which remain largely susceptible, though penicillin-resistant strains of *Streptococcus viridans* and *Streptococcus pneumoniae* are emerging. It can also be used against sensitive strains of *Enterococcus faecalis* and *Corynebacterium diphtheriae*. Penicillin G is active against spirochetes, including *Leptospira* spp. (leptospirosis), *Borrelia burgdorferi* (Lyme disease), and *Treponema pallidum* (syphilis). It is active against *Neisseria meningitidis* and certain anaerobic gram-positive organisms. The drug is inactive against most staphylococci due to their production of β-lactamase and is universally inactive against gram-negative bacteria. As with most antibiotics, susceptibility tests should be performed because many formerly susceptible microorganisms have now become resistant.

Phenoxymethylpenicillin (Penicillin V). Penicillin V is the second natural penicillin used clinically. The drug is produced by fermentation where the medium is enriched in phenoxyacetic acid. It can also be prepared by semisynthesis. The phenoxy side chain of penicillin V is electron withdrawing and, as discussed, this increases its acid stability, allowing the drug to be used orally (Table 32.1). Like penicillin G, it is highly susceptible to deactivation by β-lactamases. With a few exceptions, the spectrum of activity of penicillin V is the same as that of penicillin G. The ability to give the drug orally allows for outpatient use and hence this drug is preferred over penicillin G, which requires IV or IM injections, in noncritical infections. Like penicillin G, penicillin V is active against most streptococci, though resistance is emerging in *S. viridans* and *S. pneumoniae.* Unlike penicillin G, penicillin V is not active against *E. faecalis*. It also lacks activity against *Leptospira* spp. and is less active than penicillin G against anaerobic bacteria.

Penicillin Salts. The natural penicillins are often administered as water-soluble sodium or potassium salts (eg, Pen-VK). In some cases, however, it may be desirable to use a slow-release depot (or repository) formulation. This allows parenteral penicillin G to be used in patients with noncritical infections who do not require hospitalization. For these situations, penicillin G is available in two water-insoluble salt formulations using procaine or benzathine (*N,N′*-dibenzylethylenediamine). The formulations are given by IM injection, which results in a slow absorption into the system and sustained drug concentrations over prolonged periods. Though they possess different physicochemical properties (solubility) due to their salt formulations, their spectrum of antibacterial activity is unchanged. Examples of their use include the treatment of *T. pallidum* (syphilis) infection and the prevention of rheumatic fever, a complication that can occur from group A streptococcal infection. It should be noted that serious toxicity can occur if either of the depot formulations is inadvertently given IV.

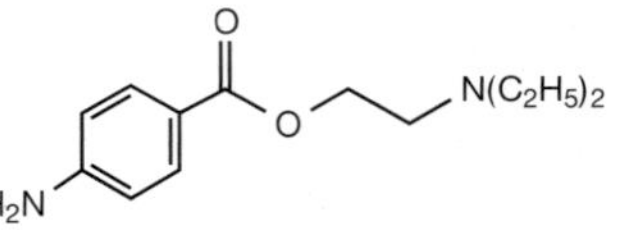

Procaine

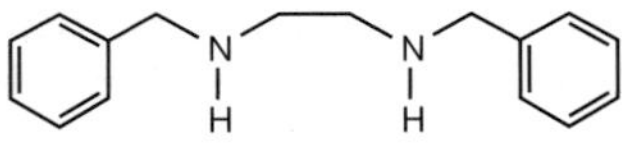
Benzathine

β-Lactamase-Resistant (Anti-Staphylococcal) Penicillins

Methicillin. Discovered in 1960, methicillin was the first β-lactamase-resistant agent to reach the clinic (Fig. 32.12).[47] The bulky ortho methoxy groups on methicillin's side chain imparted resistance to β-lactamases produced by staphylococci (see SAR discussion), and this SAR insight led to the discovery of several other β-lactamase-resistant penicillins. Though the spectrum of activity was limited to specific gram-positive aerobes (staphylococci, streptococci), it represented an effective therapy against these organisms. Methicillin was removed from the US market due to its high adverse effect profile (interstitial nephritis) and the availability of safer agents resistant to β-lactamase. Though no longer used clinically, the term MRSA is still frequently used to describe staphylococci that express PBP-2a, which imparts resistance to the anti-staphylococcal penicillins.

Nafcillin. Nafcillin has a 2-ethoxynaphthyl side chain (Table 32.1). This bulky group serves to inhibit destruction by β-lactamases analogous to methicillin. As discussed earlier, increased steric bulkiness in the side chain leads to a β-lactamase-resistant drug. The nafcillin side chain is not electron withdrawing, so the drug is not acid stable and thus cannot be given orally. The spectrum of activity of nafcillin is narrow and limited to susceptible staphylococci and streptococci.[48] Nafcillin's activity against streptococci is weaker compared to the natural penicillins; therefore it is considered an alternative agent for the treatment of streptococcal infections. An increasing number of staphylococci are now MRSA and resistant to nafcillin and other agents in this subclass.

Oxacillin and Dicloxacillin. The isoxazole ring on the side chain of oxacillin and dicloxacillin is a bioisosteric replacement for the benzene ring of penicillin G (Table 32.1). The side chains of both these agents possess sufficient steric bulk adjacent to the carbonyl group to impart β-lactamase resistance like nafcillin. Because the isoxazole ring has some electron-withdrawing character, these two agents have improved acid stability and can be administered orally. The addition of two chlorine substituents to the 3′-phenyl group in dicloxacillin imparts additional steric bulk and acid stability. Approximately 33% of an administered oxacillin dose is orally absorbed versus 37% of an administered dicloxacillin dose. While oral dosage forms of oxacillin, dicloxacillin, and cloxacillin (a related agent with a single chlorine substituent that is no longer on the US market) have previously been available, currently only dicloxacillin has a marketed oral formulation. The spectrum of activity of these agents is like nafcillin and is limited to susceptible gram-positive staphylococci and streptococci.[49] They have no activity against gram-negative or anaerobic organisms and show weaker activity against streptococci compared to the natural penicillins.

Broad-Spectrum or Amino-Penicillins

Ampicillin. The first member of this group, ampicillin, is a benzylpenicillin analog in which one of the hydrogen atoms of the side chain methylene has been replaced with a primary amino group to produce an R-phenylglycine moiety (see Table 32.1). In addition to significant acid stability enhancing its oral bioavailability, the antimicrobial spectrum is shifted so that many common gram-negative pathogens are sensitive to ampicillin. This is believed to be due to enhanced binding to gram-negative PBPs (PBP-1b and PBP-3) and greater penetration of ampicillin into gram-negative bacteria facilitated by the positively charged primary amine.[50] The acid stability is believed to be caused by the electron-withdrawing character of the protonated primary amine group reducing the side chain carbonyl participation in hydrolysis of the β-lactam bond as well as to the comparative difficulty of bringing another positively charged species (H_3O^+) into the vicinity of the protonated amino group. The oral activity is also enhanced by active uptake by the dipeptide transporters.[51]

Ampicillin unfortunately lacks stability toward β-lactamases and resistance to this drug is common. Coadministration with a β-lactamase inhibitor (discussed later) significantly expands the drug's spectrum of activity. Ampicillin alone has activity against gram-positive species including *E. faecalis*, certain *Streptococcus* spp., *C. diphtheriae*, *Listeria monocytogenes*, and several anaerobes. Ampicillin's gram-negative spectrum is limited to *Proteus mirabilis*, *B. burgdorferi* (Lyme disease), *Kingella* spp., *Leptospira* spp., *N. meningitidis*, and *Pasteurella multocida*. Combination of ampicillin with the β-lactamase inhibitor sulbactam (Unasyn) expands the spectrum of activity to include staphylococci species, *E. coli*, *Klebsiella* spp., *H. influenzae*, *Moraxella catarrhalis*, and *Bacteroides fragilis*.

Amoxicillin. Amoxicillin is a structurally close analog of ampicillin in which the para-phenolic hydroxyl group has been introduced into the side chain phenyl moiety (see Table 32.1). This modification adjusted the isoelectric point of the drug to a more acidic value and is believed to be partially responsible, along with the intestine dipeptide transporter, for the enhanced blood levels obtained with amoxicillin when compared to ampicillin (see Table 32.2). Better oral absorption leads to less disturbance of the normal GI flora and, therefore, less drug-induced diarrhea. The antimicrobial spectrum and clinical uses of amoxicillin are approximately the same as those of ampicillin. The addition of the β-lactamase inhibitor clavulanic acid (discussed later) to amoxicillin gives a combination (Augmentin) in which the clavulanic acid serves to protect amoxicillin to a considerable extent against β-lactamases. This expands the spectrum of activity to include organisms and strains that produce β-lactamases like the expanded spectrum of ampicillin already discussed.

Extended-Spectrum (Anti-Pseudomonal) Penicillins

Piperacillin. Piperacillin is an ampicillin derivative in which the side chain amino group has been converted by chemical processes to a substituted urea derivative (see Table 32.1). This ampicillin analog is referred to as an acyl ureidopenicillin. It preserves the gram-positive activity of ampicillin but has expanded gram-negative activity to include *Pseudomonas aeruginosa*. It is believed that the added side chain moiety mimics a longer segment of the peptidoglycan chain than ampicillin does. This cell wall fragment is usually a tetrapeptide, so there is expected to be room for an extension in this direction. This would possibly give more points of attachment to the PBPs, and these features may be responsible for this drug's enhanced antibacterial properties. Piperacillin has negligible oral absorption and is used parenterally to treat key gram-negative organisms including *E. coli*, *Klebsiella* spp., *Morganella morganii*, *P. aeruginosa*, and *B. fragilis*.[52] While piperacillin is marketed as an individual agent, it is most often used in combination with the β-lactamase inhibitor (Zosyn) to further expand its spectrum of activity to include β-lactamase-expressing species.

Summary. The penicillins ushered in the era of powerful antibiotics and their use transformed the practice of antimicrobial chemotherapy. A significant percentage of the population that is alive today owes their longevity and relative freedom from morbidity to the use of these agents. The pace of discovery has fallen off dramatically, and with the exception of pivmecillinam, no new penicillin has been introduced into the market for many years. Recent β-lactam research has instead focused on advanced-generation cephalosporins and carbapenems, as discussed further.

NEW DRUG APPROVAL—PIVMECILLINAM (PIVYA)

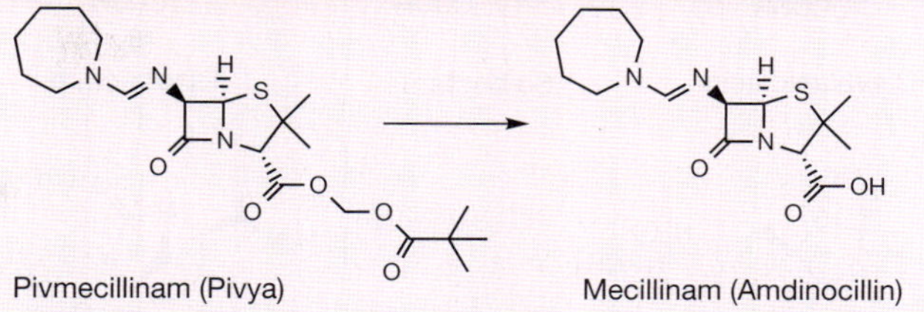

Pivmecillinam (Pivya) Mecillinam (Amdinocillin)

Pivmecillinam, or amdinocillin pivoxil, marketed as Pivya, was approved by the U.S. Food and Drug Administration (FDA) in April 2024 for the treatment of uncomplicated UTIs in women. Pivmecillinam, marketed in Europe for more than 40 years, is an orally active prodrug of the parenteral agent, mecillinam. This drug is considered an extended-spectrum aminopenicillin and possesses activity against ESBL-producing strains of *E. coli* and other organisms causing UTIs. Pivmecillinam is rapidly converted in vivo to mecillinam, which possesses activity against ESBL-producing bacterial by a "collateral sensitivity" mechanism, whereby development of bacterial resistance to one drug leads to sensitivity of the organism to another.[53]

β-Lactamase Inhibitors. The most common mechanism of bacterial resistance to the β-lactam antibiotics is the expression of enzymes that can deactivate these antibiotics by catalytically opening the key β-lactam ring, the so-called β-lactamases. Discovered in the early 1940s and initially named "penicillinases,"[42] the number and type of β-lactamases have significantly expanded to include enzymes capable of inactivating cephalosporins ("cephalosporinases") and carbapenems ("carbapenemases").[54] The number of β-lactamases that have been identified is now several thousand. Mechanistically, there are two general types: serine β-lactamases and metallo-β-lactamases (MBLs). They are further categorized into four classes based on molecular and functional classifications. To overcome this resistance mechanism, a variety of β-lactamase inhibitors have been developed that can be broadly categorized into three chemical classes: β-lactams, diazabicyclo[3.2.1]octane (DBO), and boronic acids (Fig. 32.14).

Clavulanic Acid. Clavulanic acid was identified as an inhibitor of β-lactamases in 1977.[55] It is a natural product that was isolated from a *Streptomyces* spp. Along with the related agents sulbactam and tazobactam (Fig. 32.14), clavulanic acid (or clavulanate, the ionized form) possesses a β-lactam ring system lacking the characteristic side chain of the β-lactam antibiotics. The agent does possess weak antibacterial activity but is notable for its strong, irreversible inhibition of serine β-lactamases. Like the activity of the β-lactam antibiotics against PBPs, clavulanic acid is believed to acylate the active site serine residue of β-lactamases, resulting in mechanism-based, irreversible inhibition (or suicide enzyme inhibition). A proposed mechanism for the irreversible inhibition of β-lactamases by clavulanic

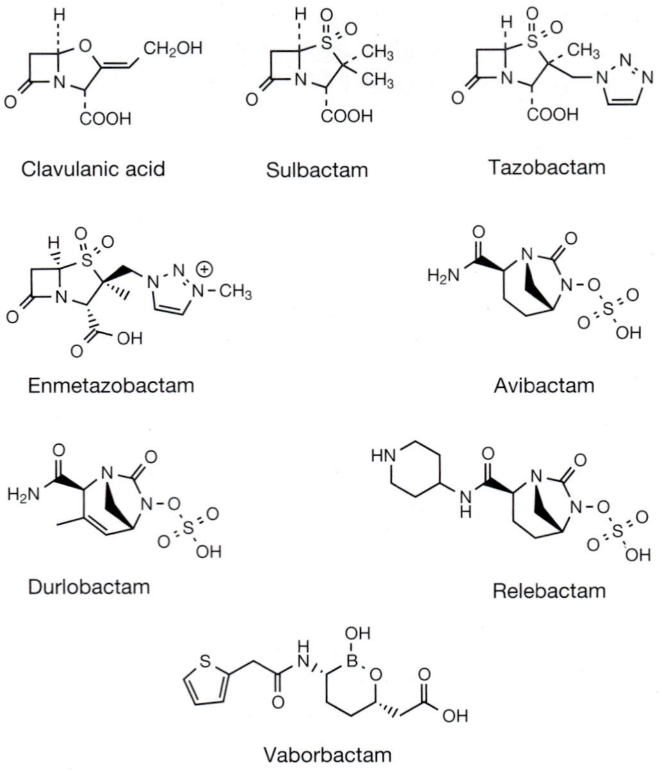

Figure 32.14 β-Lactamase inhibitors.

acid, and the other β-lactam scaffold agents, is shown in Figure 32.15.[56] Clavulanic acid is marketed in combination with amoxicillin (Augmentin) to extend the spectrum of activity of that agent.

Sulbactam. Like clavulanate, sulbactam possesses a β-lactam scaffold and it is also an irreversible inhibitor of serine β-lactamases (Fig. 32.14). It is a 6-desaminopenicillin sulfone produced by partial chemical synthesis from 6-APA. The oxidation of the sulfur atom to a sulfone extends the spectrum of β-lactamase inhibition, but partly decreases the potency. Interestingly, sulbactam alone has modest activity against *Acinetobacter baumannii* and a combination with another β-lactamase inhibitor, durlobactam (discussed later), has recently been approved for the treatment of *Acinetobacter* infections. Sulbactam is also used in combination with ampicillin (Unasyn) to extend the spectrum of activity of ampicillin in a parenteral formulation. There are no oral formulations of sulbactam.

Tazobactam. Like sulbactam, tazobactam is a sulfone derivative of penicillanic acid. It has a triazole ring substituted at the 3-position. Tazobactam has low antibacterial activity alone. Its spectrum of β-lactamase inhibition is similar to that of sulbactam, but it has greater potency that is similar to clavulanic acid. Tazobactam is used in combination with piperacillin (discussed earlier) to extend this agent's spectrum of activity to include β-lactamase-expressing staphylococci, gram-negative enteric bacteria, and many anaerobic bacteria. Tazobactam is also combined with ceftolozane (discussed later) to expand this agent's spectrum of activity to include multidrug-resistant *P. aeruginosa* and other resistant organisms.

Enmetazobactam. Enmetazobactam, formerly AAI101, is the newest β-lactamase inhibition. It was approved by the FDA in February 2024 in combination with cefepime hydrochloride and marketed as Exblifep for the treatment of complicated UTIs. Enmetazobactam is an *N*-methylated zwitterionic analog of tazobactam. The net neutral charge facilitates bacterial cell penetration. When combined with cefepime (discussed later), also a zwitterion, enmetazobactam restores cefepime's activity against ESBL-producing strains of Enterobacteriaceae. Enmetazobactam is reported to possess activity against ESBLs that are resistant to tazobactam, possibly due to stronger binding to the ESBL active site.[57] This drug combination product is considered a "carbapenem-sparing" treatment for infections caused by ESBL-expressing Enterobacteriaceae.

Avibactam. Avibactam represents the first in a new structural class of β-lactamase inhibitors, namely bridged diazabicyclo[3.2.1]octanes (Fig. 32.14).[58] Avibactam does not possess a β-lactam structure and inhibits β-lactamases by a mechanism unique from clavulanate, sulbactam, and tazobactam. The drug is believed to covalently carbamylate the β-lactamase enzyme, a reaction that slowly reverses back to the intact avibactam (Fig. 32.16). Interestingly, the avibactam-β-lactamase complex is stable to hydrolytic cleavage, which would normally deactivate the drug.[59,60] Avibactam has improved activity against β-lactamases compared to the β-lactam scaffold inhibitors including β-lactamases that can inactivate cephalosporins and carbapenems, so-called ESBLs. Avibactam is currently marketed in combination with

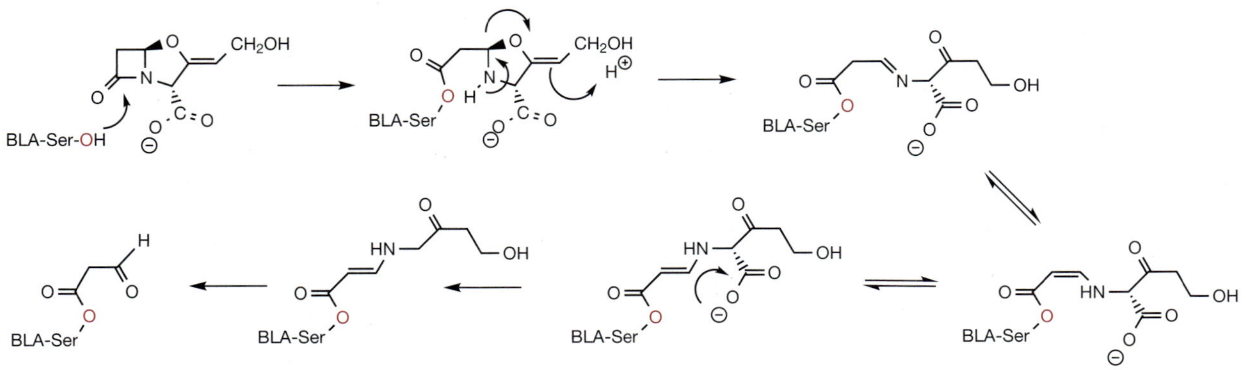

Figure 32.15 Speculative mechanism for irreversible inactivation of β-lactamase by clavulanic acid. BLA, β-lactamase.

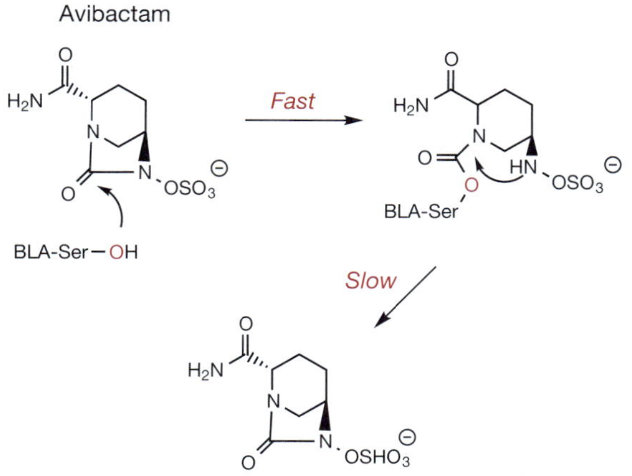

Figure 32.16 Mechanism of avibactam inhibition of β-lactamase. BLA, β-lactamase.

ceftazidime (Avycaz) (discussed later) to extend this agent's spectrum of activity to include bacteria expressing serine β-lactamases in class A, class C, and variable activity against class D. Avibactam is not an inhibitor of class B MBLs. It is also not an inhibitor of transpeptidase enzymes and thus does not possess intrinsic antibacterial activity. The discovery and characterization of DBOs with dual transpeptidase/β-lactamase activity is currently an active area of research.

Relebactam. Relebactam is the second agent in the DBO class of β-lactamase inhibitors. Its mechanism of β-lactamase inhibition is similar to avibactam. The spectrum of β-lactamase inhibition of relebactam is similar to avibactam, extending to class A and class C ESBLs, with variable activity against class D carbapenemases. Like avibactam, relebactam has no activity against class B MBLs. Relebactam is marketed in combination with imipenem (Recarbrio) (discussed later), a carbapenem antibiotic, for the treatment of ESBL-producing gram-negative organisms and *P. aeruginosa* strains resistant to imipenem alone.

Durlobactam. Durlobactam is the third DBO agent to be approved and one of the newest β-lactamase inhibitor to enter the clinical market. It is marketed in combination with sulbactam for the treatment of resistant *Acinetobacter* infections. Sulbactam is a β-lactamase inhibitor possessing a β-lactam scaffold and intrinsic activity against *A. baumannii*. Combination with durlobactam allows for use against *Acinetobacter* spp. that express β-lactamases that can deactivate sulbactam. Mechanistically, durlobactam inhibits β-lactamases similar to avibactam and relebactam. The spectrum of β-lactamase inhibition of durlobactam is expanded relative to avibactam and relebactam to include class D β-lactamases, in addition to class A and class C enzymes. This additional activity is attributed to the 3-methyl-3-ene moiety of durlobactam, which was added to form an additional hydrophobic binding interaction with class D β-lactamases. The drug is inactive against class B MBLs. Interestingly, durlobactam has also been shown to inhibit the PBP-2 transpeptidases of some bacteria, which contributes to the reported in vitro antibacterial activity of this agent against *E. coli* and some other bacterial species.[61]

Vaborbactam. Vaborbactam represents the third marketed chemical class of β-lactamase inhibitor, boronic acids or boronates (Fig. 32.14). This agent possesses a boronic acid heterocyclic structure that can form reversible covalent bonds with serine β-lactamases. The heterocyclic structure is believed to give the compound specificity for bacterial enzymes (ie, β-lactamases) versus human serine hydrolases.[62] Vaborbactam has activity against class A and class C β-lactamases, in particular class A *Klebsiella pneumoniae* carbapenemases (KPCs), but poor activity against class D β-lactamases. It does not inhibit class B MBLs. It is marketed in combination with the carbapenem drug meropenem to extend the agent's spectrum of activity to include KPC-producing gram-negative bacteria such as carbapenem-resistant Enterobacterales (CRE).[63] Vaborbactam does not possess any appreciable intrinsic antibacterial activity.

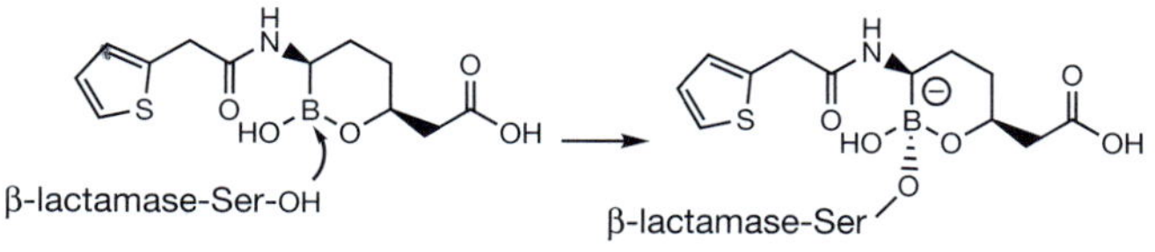

Cephalosporins

History. In contrast to the discovery of the penicillins, in which the first agent had such outstanding biologic antibiotic properties that it entered clinical use with comparatively little modification, the cephalosporins are remarkable for the level of persistence required before their initial discovery yielded clinical applications. Abraham and Newton described the structure of the first cephalosporin, cephalosporin C.35.[64] The compound was interesting because, although it was not very potent, it had activity against some penicillin-resistant cultures due to its stability to β-lactamases. Cephalosporin C is not potent enough to be a useful antibiotic, but removal, through chemical means, of the natural side chain produced 7-aminocephalosporanic acid (7-ACA), which, analogous to 6-APA, could be fitted with unnatural side chains (Fig. 32.17). Because cephalosporin C.35 was stable to many activity-destroying β-lactamases, its core nucleus, 7-ACA, was substituted with a wide variety of synthetic side chains, and several generations of clinically useful analogs have resulted. Later work produced the carbapenems, monobactams, and β-lactamase inhibitors.[65-67]

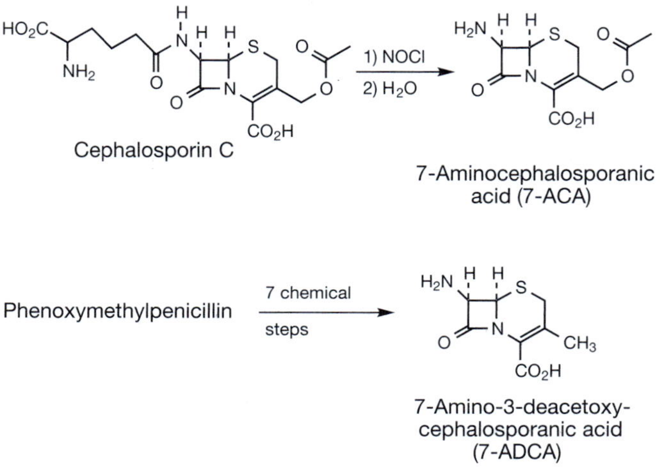

Figure 32.17 Chemical preparation of 7-ACA and 7-ADCA.

Many thousands of these compounds have been prepared by partial or total chemical synthesis, and a significant number of these remain on the market many years after their discovery. They differ from one another in antimicrobial spectrum, β-lactamase stability, absorption from the GI tract, metabolism, stability, and adverse effects as detailed later.

Nomenclature and Classification. Most cephalosporins have generic names beginning with cef- or ceph-. This is convenient for classification but makes discriminating between individual members a true memory test. The cephalosporins are classified by a trivial nomenclature system loosely derived from the chronology of their introduction but more closely related to their antimicrobial spectrum. The first-generation cephalosporins are primarily active in vitro against gram-positive cocci (including β-lactamase-producing *S. aureus* and *S. epidermidis*), group A β-hemolytic streptococci (*Streptococcus pyogenes*), group B streptococci (*Streptococcus agalactiae*), and nonresistant *S. pneumoniae*. They are not effective against MRSA. They are not significantly active against gram-negative bacteria, although some strains of *E. coli*, *K. pneumoniae*, *P. mirabilis*, and *Shigella* spp. may be sensitive.[68] The second-generation cephalosporins generally retain the anti–gram-positive activity of the first-generation agents but have improved anti–gram-negative activity to include *H. influenzae* and *M. catarrhalis*. Some strains of *E. coli*, *Klebsiella*, *Moraxella*, *Proteus*, and *Serratia* may also be sensitive. Cefotetan and cefoxitin also have activity against some anaerobic species, including *B. fragilis*.[69] The third-generation agents have comparable activity to first-generation agents against gram-positive organisms including *S. aureus* (including β-lactamase-producing strains) and streptococci and improved gram-negative activity relative to the first- and second-generation agents to include sensitive strains of *Citrobacter* and *Enterobacter*.[70] They are often useful against nosocomial multidrug-resistant (MDR) hospital-acquired strains. Ceftazidime, often referred to as a third-generation agent, possesses activity against *P. aeruginosa*. This agent is discussed under "Anti-Pseudomonal Cephalosporins" section. Additional anti-pseudomonal cephalosporins include cefepime (often referred to as fourth generation), ceftolozane, and cefiderocol. Lastly, anti-MRSA cephalosporins uniquely possess activity against MRSA infections that express PBP-2a. These "advanced-generation" cephalosporins possess expanded activity to particularly problematic organisms and may be combined with a β-lactamase inhibitor to further expand their activity to include resistant organisms, as discussed later.

Chemical Properties. The cephalosporins have their β-lactam ring fused to a six-membered dihydrothiazine ring, in contrast to the penicillins where the β-lactam ring is fused to a five-membered thiazolidine ring. Because of the larger ring, the β-lactam ring of the cephalosporins is less strained and, in consequence, less reactive toward PBPs. However, much of the reactivity loss is made up by the addition of an olefinic linkage (double bond) at $C_{2,3}$ and a methylene-acetoxy or other leaving group at C_3. When the β-lactam ring is opened by hydrolysis, the leaving group can be ejected, carrying away the developing negative charge. This greatly reduces the energy required for the process and drives the reaction with PBPs. Thus, the facility with which the β-lactam bond of the cephalosporins is broken is modulated both by the nature of the C_7 substituent (analogous to the penicillins) as well as the nature of the C_3 substituent and its ability to serve as a leaving group. Considerable support for this hypothesis comes from the finding that isomerization of the olefinic linkage to $C_{3,4}$ leads to great losses in antibiotic activity. In practice, most cephalosporins are comparatively unstable in aqueous solutions, and the pharmacist is often directed to keep injectable preparations frozen before use. As carboxylic acids, they form water-soluble sodium salts, whereas the protonated acids are comparatively water insoluble.

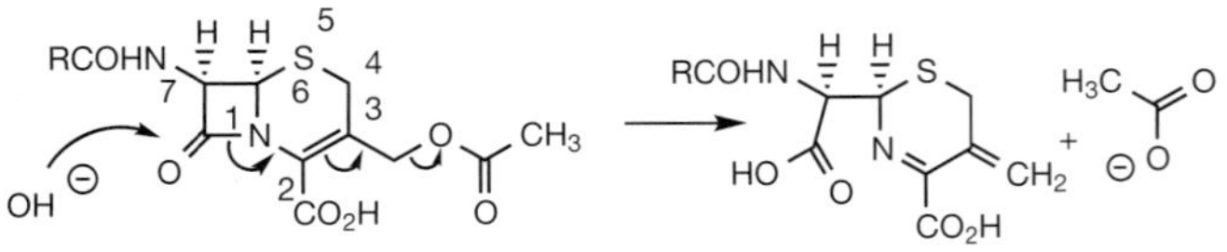

The principal chemical instability of the cephalosporins is associated with β-lactam bond hydrolysis. Ejection of the C_3 substituent following β-lactam bond cleavage is usually drawn for convenience as though this is an unbroken (concerted) process. However, ejection of the side chain may at certain times and with specific cephalosporins involve a discrete intermediate with the β-lactam bond broken, but the C_3 substituent not yet eliminated, while other cephalosporins have nonejectable C_3 substituents. The methylthiotetrazole (MTT) group, found in some cephalosporins (eg, cefotetan), is capable of elimination. When this happens, this moiety is believed to be responsible in part for clotting difficulties and acute alcohol intolerance in certain patients. The role of the C_7 side chain in all of these processes is clearly important, but active participation of the amide moiety in a manner analogous to the penicillins is rarely specifically involved. The same considerations that modulate the chemical stability of cephalosporins are also involved in dictating β-lactamase sensitivity, potency, and allergenicity.

Mechanism of Action. The cephalosporins are believed to act in a manner analogous to that of the penicillins by binding to the PBPs followed by cell lysis (Fig. 32.11).

Pharmacokinetic and Pharmacodynamic Properties. Like the penicillins, the pharmacokinetic properties of the cephalosporins have been well characterized.[71] As discussed later, the 7-position side chain (analogous to the 6-position side chain of the penicillins) influences acid stability and oral absorption. Additionally, the side chain at the 3-position appears to influence oral bioavailability, with cephalosporins containing poor leaving groups at this position (ie, methyl groups, vinyl groups, or simply hydrogens) possessing improved oral bioavailability. Early cephalosporins with an acetyl group at the 3-position were subject to enzymatic hydrolysis in vivo. The resulting molecule, with a hydroxy methyl moiety at the 3-position, possessed poor activity and potential for chemical rearrangement. There are no longer any cephalosporins with this side chain marketed for clinical use. Certain cephalosporins possess lipophilic ester prodrug formulations at the 2-position carboxyl group to improve oral bioavailability. Examples include cefuroxime axetil and cefpodoxime proxetil, discussed further. Generally, the cephalosporins are well distributed in the body, a notable exception being the cerebrospinal fluid (CSF). Their plasma protein binding is highly variable, ranging from 7% to 90%, depending on the agent. The cephalosporins are rapidly eliminated, primarily by renal route, and dosage adjustments are often required in patients with renal dysfunction. The third-generation cephalosporin, ceftriaxone, is notable for its longer half-life and high biliary elimination. The pharmacodynamic properties of the cephalosporins are similar to those of the penicillins. They are bactericidal in vitro, with time-depending killing. They generally exhibit a weak to absent PAE.

Structure-Activity Relationship. As with the penicillins, various molecular changes to the cephalosporin scaffold can improve in vitro stability, antibacterial activity, and stability toward β-lactamases.[72] The addition of an amino and a hydrogen to the α and α′ positions, respectively, results in a basic compound that is protonated under the acidic conditions of the stomach. The ammonium ion improves the stability of the β-lactam of the cephalosporin, similar to that of the amino-penicillins, leading to orally active drugs. The 7β-amino group is essential for antimicrobial activity, whereas replacement of the 7α-hydrogen (X = H) with an alkoxy (X = OR) results in improvement of the antibacterial activity of the cephalosporin, notably anaerobic activity. Agents with this structural motif are known as "cephamycins." A 7α-methoxy derivative can also improve stability toward β-lactamase in specific cephalosporins. Cephalosporins possessing the dihydrothiazine ring (Y = S) display greater antibacterial activity than those possessing a dihydrooxazine ring (Y = O), but the dihydrooxazine agents show increased stability toward β-lactamase. The 6α-hydrogen is essential for biologic activity. Finally, antibacterial activity is generally improved when Z is a 5-membered heterocycle versus a 6-membered heterocycle.

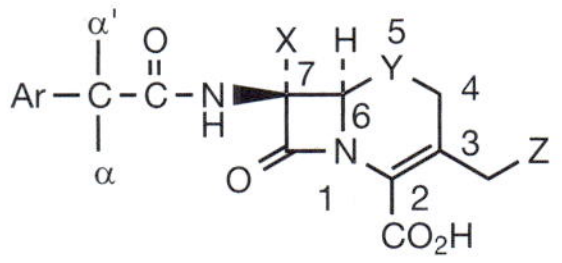

In a study examining the stability of cephalosporins toward β-lactamase, it was noted that the following changes improved β-lactamase resistance: (1) the L-isomer of an α-amino α′-hydrogen derivative of a cephalosporin was 30 to 40 times more stable than the D-isomer; (2) the addition of an alkoxy-oxime to the α- and α′-positions increased stability nearly 100-fold; and (3) the Z-oxime was as much as 20,000-fold more stable than the E-oxime (Fig. 32.18).[72] These changes have been incorporated into a number of marketed and experimental cephalosporins, including the second-generation agent, cefuroxime, and most third- and advanced-generation cephalosporins.

Resistance. Like the penicillins, cephalosporins can be hydrolyzed by β-lactamase enzymes, which constitutes a

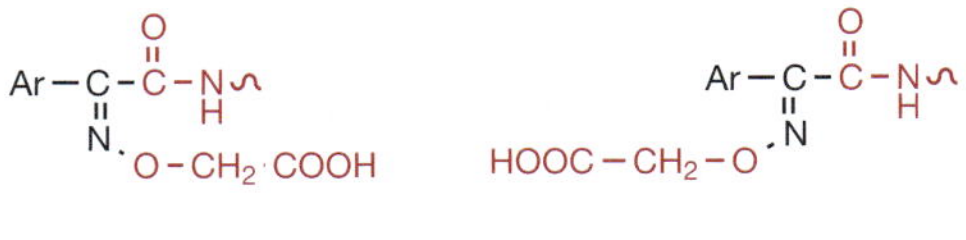

Figure 32.18 Z- and E-oxime configuration.

primary mechanism of bacterial resistance toward this drug class. However, the cephalosporins possess intrinsic resistance to the earlier β-lactamases expressed by staphylococci that rendered penicillins inactive, the so-called "penicillinases." Unfortunately, some bacteria have evolved the ability to express "cephalosporinases" and ESBLs that can render cephalosporins inactive. Some β-lactamases are constitutive (chromosomally encoded) in certain strains of gram-negative bacteria (*Citrobacter*, *Enterobacter*, *Pseudomonas*, and *Serratia*) and their expression is normally repressed. However, expression of these β-lactamases can be induced by exposure to specific β-lactam antibiotics (eg, imipenem, cefotetan, and cefoxitin).

Adverse Effects and Allergenicity. Aside from mild to severe allergic reactions, the most commonly experienced cephalosporin toxicities are mild and temporary nausea, vomiting, and diarrhea associated with disturbance of the normal flora. Rarely, a life-threatening pseudomembranous colitis diarrhea associated with the opportunistic and toxin-producing anaerobic pathogen, *Clostridioides difficile*, can be experienced. Rare blood dyscrasias, which can even include aplastic anemia, can also be seen. Cephalosporins containing a MTT side chain are associated with prolonged bleeding times and a disulfiram-like acute alcohol intolerance. Only the agent cefotetan, possessing this chemical moiety, remains in clinical use in the United States. Allergenicity is less commonly experienced and is less severe with cephalosporins than with penicillins. Cephalosporins are frequently administered to patients who have had a mild or delayed penicillin reaction; however, cross-allergenicity is possible, and this should be done with caution for patients with a history of penicillin allergy. Patients who have had a rapid and severe reaction to penicillins should not be treated with cephalosporins. In situations where there are no alternative agents, sensitivity testing can be performed prior to beginning cephalosporin therapy.

Individual Cephalosporins. The structures of the first- and second-generation cephalosporins are shown in Table 32.4, and the structures of the third-generation and advanced-generation cephalosporins are shown in Table 32.5.

First-Generation Cephalosporins

Cefazolin. Cefazolin has the natural acetyl side chain at the 3-position of cephalosporin C replaced by a thio-linked thiadiazole ring. This group is an activating leaving group but is not subject to the inactivating hydrolysis reaction of acetyl groups described earlier. At the 7-position, it possesses a tetrazoyl-methylene moiety. Like most cephalosporins, cefazolin is primarily eliminated by the kidneys and the dose should be reduced in the presence of renal impairment. It is relatively unstable and should be protected from heat and light. Due to its intrinsic resistance to penicillinases, cefazolin is a preferred agent for the treatment of staphylococcal infection. The drug is also active against most species of *Streptococcus* and non-ESBL-producing strains of *E. coli*, *Klebsiella* spp., *Proteus* spp., and *Kingella* spp.

Cephalexin. Incorporation of the ampicillin-like side chain at the 7-position confers oral activity to cephalexin. The drug does not possess an activating leaving group at the 3-position, thus potency may be somewhat diminished, although this is mitigated by the low potential for metabolic

Table 32.4 Commercially Available First- and Second-Generation Cephalosporins

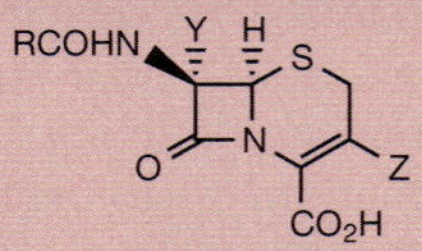

Generic Names	R	Y	Z
First-Generation Agents			
Cefazolin	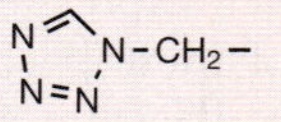	H	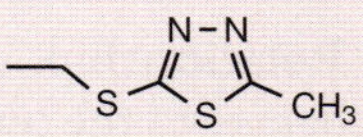
Cephalexin	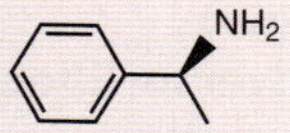	H	—CH_3
Cefadroxil	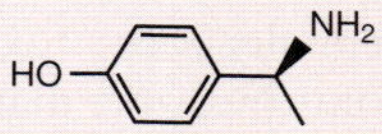	H	—CH_3
Second-Generation Agents			
Cefuroxime	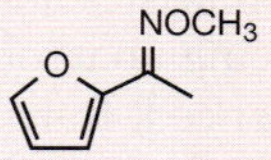	H	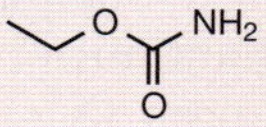
Cefoxitin	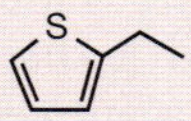	OCH_3	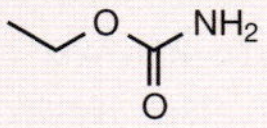
Cefotetan	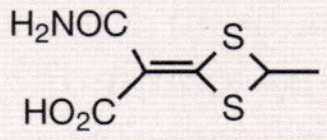	OCH_3	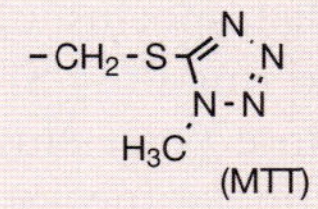
Cefaclor	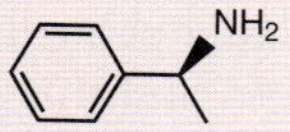	H	Cl
Cefprozil	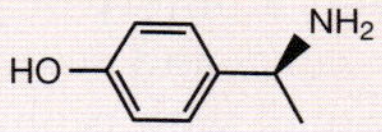	H	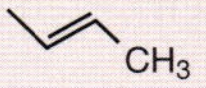

MTT, methylthiotetrazole.

deactivation at this position. It is rapidly and nearly completely (90%) absorbed from the GI tract. Interestingly, while the use of the ampicillin side chain in the cephalosporins improves oral bioavailability, it does not result in a comparable shift in the antimicrobial spectrum. Cephalexin is active against gram-positive staphylococci, with slightly less potency than cefazolin, and most gram-positive streptococci (with the exception of *S. pneumoniae*). Relative to cefazolin, the potency of cephalexin against gram-negative organisms (*E. coli*, *Klebsiella*, *Proteus*, and *Kingella*) is decreased and the drug has limited utility against these organisms.[68]

Cefadroxil. Cefadroxil has an amoxicillin-like side chain at the 7-position and is also orally active. Approximately 90% of the administered dose is absorbed. Cefadroxil has a longer biologic half-life than cephalexin, allowing dosing every 12 hours (vs every 6 hours). This agent has comparable antimicrobial activity to cephalexin, though it has retained activity against *Proteus* spp.

Second-Generation Cephalosporins. These cephalosporins are characterized by improved activity against gram-negative bacteria, particularly *H. influenzae*, relative to the first-generation agents, with similar gram-positive activity. Modifications to the 7-position, α- and β-orientations, are primarily responsible for the improved spectrum (Table 32.4). A subset of second-generation cephalosporins, known as "cephamycins," possess a methoxy at the 7-position in the α-orientation. These agents have activity against the anaerobic organism, *B. fragilis*. The second-generation cephalosporins with oral activity are characterized by ampicillin- or amoxicillin-like side chains at the 7-position and a metabolically stable side chain at the 3-position. The addition of a lipophilic ester at the 2-position carboxyl group as a prodrug moiety also improves oral bioavailability (eg, cefuroxime axetil).

Cefuroxime. Cefuroxime has a Z-oriented methoxyimino moiety as part of its C_7 side chain (Table 32.4). This conveys considerable resistance to the attack by many β-lactamases, although the drug is susceptible to ESBLs. This effect is believed to result from the steric hindrance and thus protective effect provided by this group. The carbamoyl moiety at C_3 is intermediate in metabolic stability between the native acetyl moiety and the thiotetrazoles. A prodrug formulation as an axetil ester ([acetyloxy]ethyl ester), cefuroxime axetil, results in improved oral bioavailability due to enhanced lipophilicity. The terminal ester of the prodrug moiety is cleaved metabolically, and the resulting

Table 32.5 Commercially Available Third- and Advanced-Generation Cephalosporins

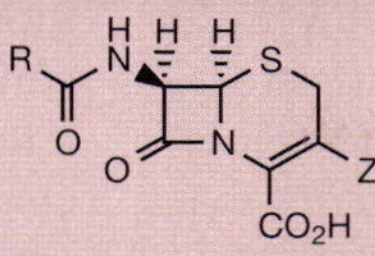

Generic Names	Trade Names	R	Z
Third-Generation Agents			
Ceftriaxone	N/A	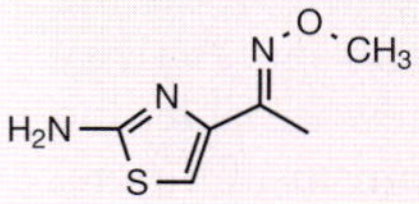	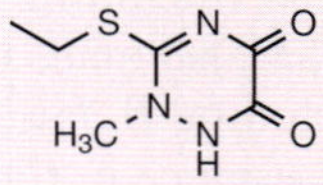
Cefixime	Suprax	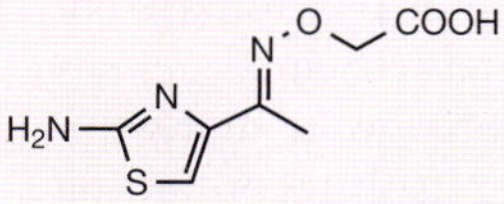	
Cefdinir	N/A	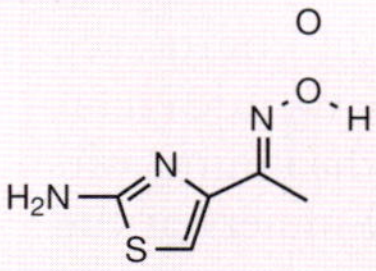	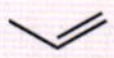
Cefpodoxime	N/A	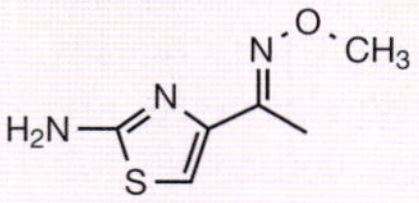	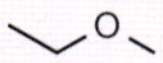
Anti-Pseudomonal Agents			
Ceftazidime	Tazicef, Avycaz (with avibactam)	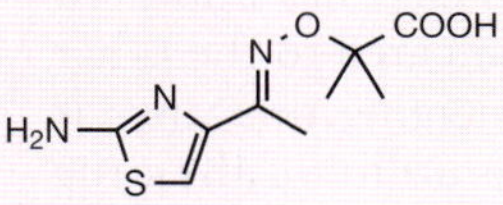	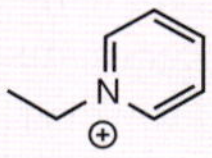
Cefepime	N/A	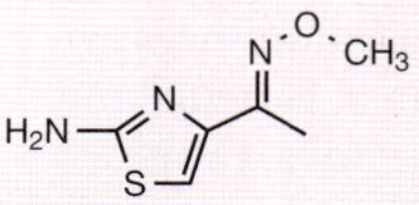	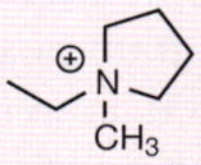
Ceftolozane	Zerbaxa (with tazobactam)	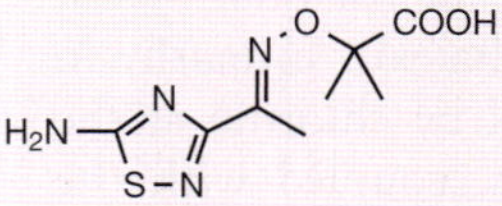	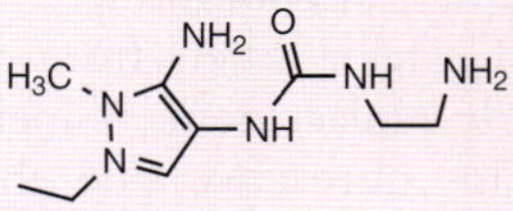
Cefiderocol	Fetroja	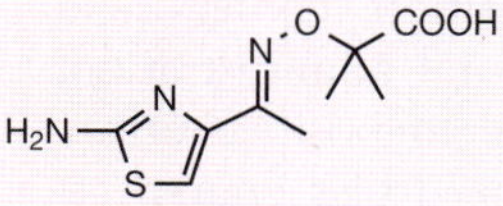	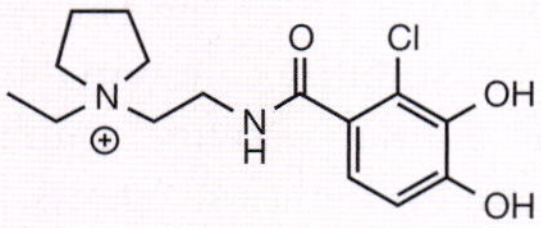
Anti-MRSA Agents			
Ceftaroline fosamil	Teflaro	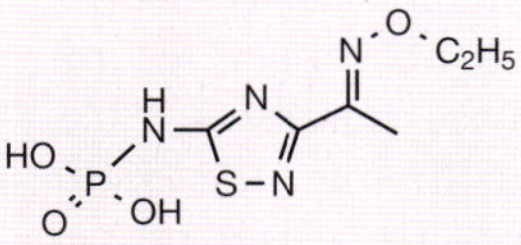	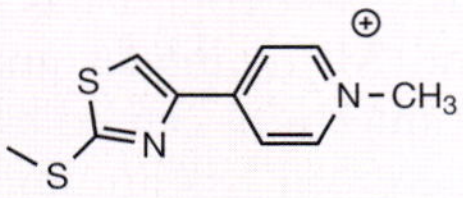
Ceftobiprole medocaril	Zevtera, Mabelio	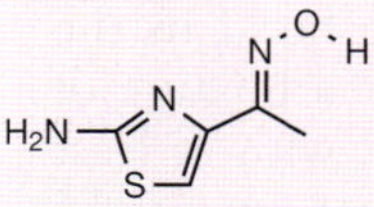	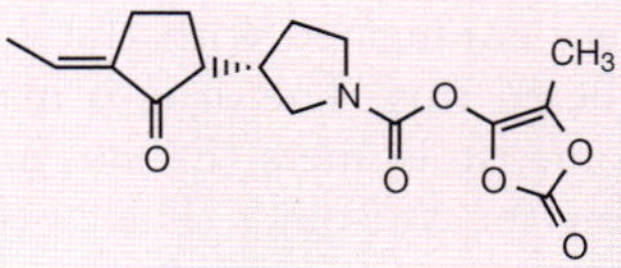

MRSA, methicillin-resistant *Staphylococcus aureus.*

intermediate form loses acetaldehyde spontaneously to produce cefuroxime itself. Like other second-generation agents, cefuroxime has improved activity against *H. influenzae* and has retained activity against nonresistant strains of staphylococci and streptococci. It also has activity against *E. coli*, certain *Klebsiella* spp., and *Proteus* spp. Cefuroxime axetil is additionally indicated as an alternative agent for the treatment of Lyme disease (*B. burgdorferi*).[73]

Cefoxitin. The most novel chemical feature of cefoxitin is the possession of an α-oriented methoxy group in place of the normal H-atom at C_7. This increased steric bulk conveys additional stability against β-lactamases. The inspiration for these functional groups was provided by the discovery of the naturally occurring antibiotic cephamycin C derived from fermentation of *Streptomyces lactamdurans*.[74] Cephamycin C itself has not seen clinical use but provided the structural clue that led to useful agents such as cefoxitin and cefotetan (discussed next). As previously mentioned, agents that contain this 7α-methoxy group are commonly referred to as cephamycins. Cefoxitin is active against gram-positive staphylococci and streptococci, and gram-negative bacteria including *H. influenzae*, *E. coli* (including some ESBL-producing strains), *Klebsiella* spp., *M. morganii*, and *Proteus* spp. Activity against anaerobes, including *B. fragilis*, is now variable due to the emergence of resistance in these organisms. Of note, cefoxitin is able to induce the expression of β-lactamase enzyme in some bacteria, particularly *Enterobacter* spp.

Cefotetan. Cefotetan is another cephamycin representative with an unusual dithietane ring (sulfur-containing four-membered ring) in the 7-position side chain (see Table 32.4). The second carboxyl group in the C_7 side chain allows the formulation of this agent as a disodium salt. The *N*-methylthiotetrazole (NMTT, or MTT) moiety at the 3-position is a reactive leaving group that enhances potency and prevents metabolism but is associated with increased bleeding and a "disulfiram-like" reaction when patients are exposed to alcohol. The bleeding effect is believed to be due to inhibition of vitamin K metabolism, which leads to hypoprothrombinemia.[75] Like cefoxitin, cefotetan has improved activity against anaerobic organisms compared to the other second-generation agents. However, emerging resistance is now limiting the activity and therefore utility of the drug against these organisms. Cefotetan has a similar spectrum of activity to cefoxitin against gram-positive and gram-negative organisms but has improved activity against *Serratia* and *M. catarrhalis*. Like cefoxitin, it is stable to a range of β-lactamases but is also an inducer in some bacteria.

Cefaclor. Cefaclor differs from cephalexin primarily in the bioisosteric replacement of methyl by chlorine at the 3-position. This unreactive side chain, coupled with the ampicillin-like side chain at the 7-position, confers acid and metabolic stability, allowing for oral administration. Cefaclor has similar activity against gram-positive organisms as the first-generation agents. The drug's gram-negative spectrum is less than other second-generation agents and is limited to *Proteus* spp. It has variable activity against *H. influenzae* and *M. catarrhalis* and is no longer recommended to treat infections caused by these organisms.

Cefprozil. Cefprozil has an amoxicillin-like side chain at the 7-position, and at the 3-position, there is a propenyl moiety conjugated with the 2,3-double bond in the six-membered ring. The drug is marketed as a mixture of both geometric isomers (E/*trans* and Z/*cis*), with at least 90% being the *cis* isomer. The *cis* isomer is reported to be significantly more active against gram-negative organisms than the *trans* isomer.[76] Cefprozil has similar activity to cefaclor against gram-positive organisms, with the exception of viridans group streptococci, against which it is inactive. Cefprozil has improved activity over cefaclor against gram-negative organisms, including activity against *H. influenzae*, non-ESBL-producing *E. coli*, *Klebsiella* spp., *Kingella* spp., and *M. catarrhalis*.

Third-Generation Cephalosporins

Ceftriaxone. Ceftriaxone has the same C_7 side chain moiety as cefotaxime and ceftizoxime, but the C_3 side chain consists of a metabolically stable and activating thiotriazinedione in place of the natural acetyl group. The C_3 side chain is sufficiently acidic that at normal pH, it forms an enolic sodium salt, and thus the commercial product is a disodium salt. Ceftriaxone is active against a broad range of gram-negative organisms, including non-ESBL-producing *E. coli*, *Klebsiella* spp., *M. morganii*, *Proteus* spp., *H. influenzae*, *Kingella* spp., *M. catarrhalis*, and *N. meningitidis*. It is useful for many severe infections and notably in the treatment of some *N. meningitidis* CNS infections. This drug has a longer half-life than many cephalosporins, approximately 8 hours, which allows for once to twice daily dosing, depending on the indication. It is also notable because a significant amount of the drug is eliminated by biliary secretion, which can lead to adverse effects that include biliary sludging and gallstones. It is stable to many β-lactamases but is sensitive to some inducible chromosomal β-lactamases.[77]

Cefixime. Cefixime possesses a β-lactamase-stabilizing Z-oximino acidic ether at C_7 and a vinyl group, analogous to the propenyl group of cefprozil, at the C_3 position. This is believed to contribute strongly to the oral activity of the drug. Cefixime has anti–gram-negative activity intermediate between that of the second-generation and third-generation agents described previously. It is poorly active against staphylococci because it does not bind satisfactorily to a specific PBP (PBP-2).[78]

Cefpodoxime Proxetil. Cefpodoxime proxetil is a prodrug. It is cleaved enzymically to isopropanol, carbon dioxide, acetaldehyde, and cefpodoxime in the gut wall.[79] It has improved anti–*S. aureus* activity over cefixime and is used to treat pharyngitis, UTI, upper and lower respiratory tract infections, otitis media, skin and soft tissue infections, and gonorrhea.

Cefdinir. Cefdinir has an unsubstituted Z-oxime in its C_7 side chain, the consequence of which is attributed to its somewhat enhanced anti–gram-positive activity. It has a vinyl moiety attached to C_3 that is associated with its oral activity. Cefdinir, like cefpodoxime, has improved activity over cefixime against non-MRSA. It has activity similar to cefixime and cefpodoxime against gram-negative bacteria.

Anti-Pseudomonal Cephalosporins

Ceftazidime With Avibactam. Ceftazidime possesses a more complex oxime moiety containing two methyl groups and a carboxylic acid. This group conveys even more pronounced β-lactamase stability and improved gram-negative activity to include *P. aeruginosa*. The C_3 side chain has been replaced by a charged pyridinium moiety. The latter considerably enhances water solubility and also highly activates the β-lactam bond toward cleavage. It is not stable under some conditions, such as in the presence of aminoglycosides and vancomycin. It is also unstable in sodium bicarbonate solutions. Resistance is mediated by chromosomally mediated β-lactamases and also by decreased penetration into target bacteria. Ceftazidime has recently been marketed in combination with avibactam, a novel, broad-spectrum β-lactamase inhibitor (see earlier discussion), in a product (Avycaz) to treat complicated UTIs caused by ESBL-producing organisms, such as *E.*

coli and *Klebsiella* spp. It is also used for complicated intra-abdominal infections in combination with metronidazole and hospital/ventilator-associated pneumonia due to susceptible gram-negative bacteria.[80]

Cefepime. Cefepime contains a Z-methoxyimine and an aminothiazolyl group at C_7, broadening its spectrum and increasing its β-lactamase stability. A quaternary *N*-methylpyrrolidine group at C_3 facilitates penetration into gram-negative bacteria. Often referred to as a fourth-generation cephalosporin, cefepime has improved gram-negative activity to include *P. aeruginosa* and *Citrobacter* spp., while retaining the gram-negative spectrum seen with the third-generation agents. Similar to other anti-pseudomonal cephalosporins, the gram-positive spectrum is diminished, though cefepime does possess improved *S. aureus* activity (MSSA) over ceftazidime and other third-generation agents. Cefepime is used IM and IV against UTIs, skin and skin structure infections, pneumonia, and intra-abdominal infections.[81]

Ceftolozane With Tazobactam. Ceftolozane is a ceftazidime analog with a thiadiazole replacing ceftazidime's thiazole ring at the C_7 position. Additionally, a quaternary pyrazole substituted with a 2-aminoethyl-ureido functional group resides at the C_3 position. Similar to ceftazidime, the bulky oxime group at the C_7 position improves stability of this drug to β-lactamases, while the positively charged C_3 moiety and the 7-aminothiadiazole improve activity against gram-negative organisms. Ceftolozane is reported to be active against bacteria resistant to ceftazidime via β-lactamase production, suggesting its greater stability to β-lactamases.[82] Ceftolozane has expanded activity against gram-negative organisms relative to third-generation cephalosporins, including activity against *P. aeruginosa* and *Citrobacter* spp., but has limited gram-positive activity. The gram-negative spectrum is further improved to cover ESBL-producing *E. coli* and *Klebsiella* spp. by the combination of this drug with the β-lactamase inhibitor, tazobactam (discussed earlier), in a product marketed as Zerbaxa in the United States. This drug is approved to treat complicated UTIs, hospital/ventilator-associated pneumonia, and, in combination with metronidazole, for the treatment of complicated intra-abdominal infections.[83]

Cefiderocol. Cefiderocol is a novel "siderophore" cephalosporin with an improved penetration of gram-negative bacteria. Referred to as a "trojan horse strategy," the amide-linked 3-chloro-catechol group at the C_3 position mimics a natural iron-binding siderophore and allows the drug to be actively transported into gram-negative bacteria. The catechol is not rapidly metabolized by catechol-O-methyltransferase (COMT) after administration because the electron-withdrawing chlorine substituent lowers the pK_a of the adjacent catechol hydroxyl group such that the group is deprotonated at physiologic pH. COMT has less affinity for the anionic catechol than the neutral species.[84] The C_7 substituent of cefiderocol mimics that seen in ceftazidime, with the larger oxime group conferring improved β-lactamase resistance while the C_7 amino-thiazole and C_3 pyrrolidinium group improve gram-negative activity. Because of its unique cell penetration mechanism, cefiderocol has activity against gram-negative bacteria with multiple resistance mechanisms, including decreased porin channels, drug efflux, and the production of β-lactamases. This drug has poor gram-positive activity and is inactive against staphylococci and streptococci. However, the drug has excellent gram-negative activity against Enterobacterales, including ESBL, KPC, and MBL-producing organisms, and *P. aeruginosa*.

Anti–Methicillin-Resistant. *Staphylococcus aureus* Cephalosporins

Ceftaroline Fosamil. Ceftaroline fosamil possesses high affinity for resistance-conferring PBP-2a in *S. aureus* and moderate affinity for PBP-2*x* in *S. pneumoniae*, affording the drug antibacterial activity against MRSA and penicillin-resistant *S. pneumoniae* (PRSP).[85] In MRSA, PBP-2a has low affinity for β-lactam antibiotics because it can adopt a "closed" conformation in which the active site is not accessible to β-lactams. The active site is believed to open during catalysis when an allosteric site is activated by binding cell wall components. Ceftaroline has the ability to trigger opening of the active site and subsequent inhibition of PBP-2a by mimicking the cell wall components that bind to the allosteric site.[86] Ceftaroline fosamil is an N-phosphono prodrug formulated for improved aqueous solubility. After parenteral administration, the phosphate group is cleaved, yielding the active ceftaroline. Ceftaroline has excellent activity against gram-positive organisms, including most strains of staphylococci and streptococci and gram-negative activity similar to third-generation cephalosporins (eg, ceftriaxone). It is not active against *P. aeruginosa*, and the drug can be inactivated by ESBLs. Ceftaroline is approved in the United States for the treatment of skin and skin structure infections caused by MRSA as well as community-acquired pneumonia.

Ceftobiprole Medocaril. Ceftobiprole possesses high affinity for PBP-2a of MRSA and PBP-2*x* in PRSP affording the drug excellent activity against gram-positive staphylococci and streptococci. It has similar gram-negative activity to ceftaroline and third-generation cephalosporins. While ceftobiprole has reported activity against ceftazidime-susceptible *P. aeruginosa*, it is not currently approved or recommended for the treatment of *P. aeruginosa* infection.[87-89] The drug is susceptible to hydrolysis by ESBLs. Ceftobiprole is marketed as the medocaril prodrug for improved aqueous solubility. Cleavage of the ester on the C_3 group after parenteral administration yields the active ceftobiprole, which possesses a novel pyrrolidinone-3-ylidenemethyl group at C_3. Ceftobiprole was approved in the United States in April 2024 under a priority review, fast track program for *S. aureus* bloodstream infection, acute bacterial skin and skin structure infection (ABSSSI), and community-acquired bacterial pneumonia (CABP). It is also approved in the EU, Switzerland, and Canada for CABP and hospital-acquired pneumonia.

Summary. With their broader spectrum of antibacterial activity relative to the penicillins and intrinsic resistance to penicillinases, the cephalosporins have come to dominate β-lactam chemotherapy, despite often lacking oral activity. As cephalosporin drug discovery is still highly active, the introduction of additional agents in this class of β-lactams in the future is likely. Infections of the upper and lower respiratory tract, skin and related soft tissue, urinary tract, bones, and joints, as well as septicemias, endocarditis, intra-abdominal, and bile tract infections caused by susceptible organisms are usually responsive to cephalosporins. When gram-positive bacteria are involved, a first-generation agent is preferred, or alternatively an advanced-generation anti-MRSA cephalosporin. When gram-negative bacteria are involved, third-generation or anti-pseudomonal cephalosporins are preferred. Gram-positive enterococci are universally resistant to cephalosporins, and alternative agents are recommended in these cases.

Carbapenems

History. Thienamycin (Fig. 32.19), the first of the carbapenem subclass of β-lactams, was isolated from *Streptomyces cattleya* in 1976.[90] It was shown to possess promising activity against gram-positive and gram-negative bacteria and at the same time resistance to β-lactamase enzymes. Structurally, the carbapenem scaffold differs from the penicillin scaffold by the replacement of the sulfur atom with a methylene group at the 4-position and the addition of 2,3-double bond, hence the carb- and -ene- in their name. Also notable is the stereochemistry inversion at the 6-position of the carbapenem scaffold relative to the penicillin scaffold.

Structure-Activity Relationship. The carbapenems are water soluble, which facilitates gram-negative cell entry via porin channels. As a result of the substitution of the penicillin sulfur atom with the smaller carbon at the 4-position and the incorporation of the 2,3-double bond, the carbapenem ring system is highly strained and very susceptible to reactions cleaving the β-lactam bond, including reactions between two molecules resulting in inactivation (Fig. 32.19). Thienamycin is particularly susceptible to water-mediated decomposition and thus had limited clinical use. At C_6, there is a 2-hydroxyethyl group attached with α-stereochemistry, which is opposite to the stereochemistry found in penicillins and cephalosporins. Thus, the absolute stereochemistry of the carbapenem scaffold is 5R,6S. The C_6 side chain is believed to play a role in resistance of the carbapenems to β-lactamases as the trans-1-hydroxyethyl moiety displaces water required for hydrolysis of the β-lactam ring in the β-lactamase active site.[91] These structural differences result in an overall improved binding and reactivity to PBPs over the penicillins and cephalosporins, and an increased resistance to hydrolysis by β-lactamases, which translates to expanded activity against problematic organisms including *P. aeruginosa* and *A. baumannii*.[92] Notably, however, none of the currently marketed carbapenems have activity against MRSA.

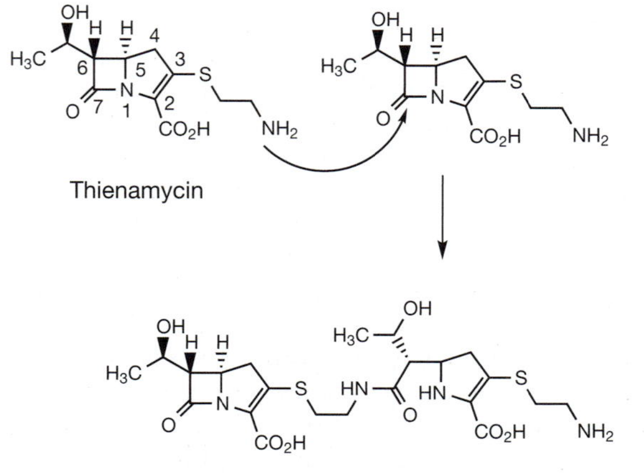

Figure 32.19 Inactivation of thienamycin via intermolecular reaction.

Resistance. Although the carbapenems are intrinsically resistant to many β-lactamases, including AmpC and ESBLs, there has been recent emergence of carbapenemase-type β-lactamases in some bacteria that can confer resistance to this class. A notable example of such is KPC. Additionally, carbapenems are susceptible to MBLs produced by some gram-negative organisms (eg, *Stenotrophomonas maltophilia*). In addition to the production of carbapenemases, resistance in gram-negative organisms can arise from decreased permeability of the outer membrane by decreased expression of porin channels or efflux mechanisms. In gram-positive organisms, resistance to the carbapenems is often mediated by alterations to PBPs from mutations.

Individual Carbapenems

Imipenem. Imipenem (Table 32.6) is a thienamycin analog with a modified 3-position side chain. The modification of the side chain to an amidine versus primary amine results in improved stability of the drug. Imipenem, like thienamycin, penetrates very well through porins and is very stable, even inhibitory, to many β-lactamases. Imipenem is not orally active. Renal dehydropeptidase-l (DHP-1) metabolizes imipenem through hydrolysis of the β-lactam and deactivates the drug. To counteract this undesirable effect, an inhibitor of this enzyme, cilastatin, is coadministered with imipenem to protect it from the degradation.[92] Inhibition of human DHP does not have deleterious consequences to the patient, making this combination highly efficacious.

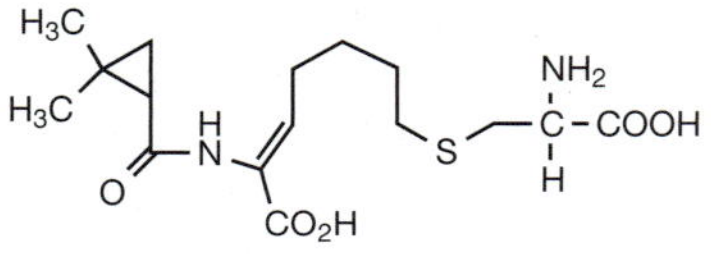

Cilastatin

Table 32.6 Commercially Available Carbapenems

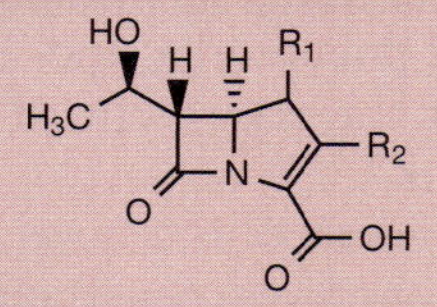

Generic Names	Trade Names	R_1	R_2
Imipenem	Primaxin Recarbrio	H	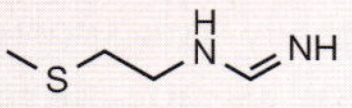
Ertapenem	Invanz	CH_3	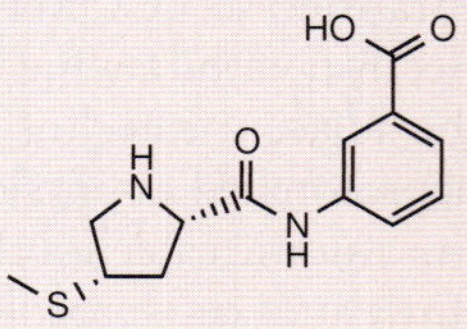
Meropenem	Merrem Vabomere	CH_3	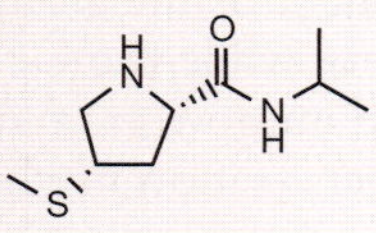

The combination of imipenem and cilastatin (Primaxin) is approximately 25% serum protein bound. The drug penetrates well into most tissues after parenteral administration, except for the CSF, and it is subsequently excreted in the urine. Imipenem/cilastatin is used to treat a wide variety of infections caused by aerobic and anaerobic gram-negative bacilli, including ESBL producers and *P. aeruginosa*, and gram-positive staphylococci and streptococci. The drug is not active against KPC or MBL-producing organisms nor against MRSA. Common adverse effects are irritation at the infusion site, fever, rash, nausea, and vomiting. A greater concern is the ability of imipenem, and other carbapenems, to induce seizures. Risk factors for seizure development include impaired renal function, preexisting CNS disease or infection, and use of large doses.[93]

A recently approved combination product of imipenem/cilastatin with the β-lactamase inhibitor relebactam (discussed earlier) is now marketed in the United States as Recarbrio. The combination with relebactam extends the spectrum of activity to include KPC-producing organisms, *E. coli* and *Klebsiella* spp. This drug is approved for the treatment of hospital/ventilator-associated pneumonia, complicated UTIs, and complicated intra-abdominal infections.

Meropenem. Meropenem (Table 32.6) possesses a complex side chain at C_3 consisting of a thio-linked basic pyrrolidine ring. Similar to other carbapenems, a basic moiety at the C_3 position increases gram-negative activity. The drug also has a chiral methyl group at C_4 in the β-orientation. This methyl group conveys intrinsic resistance to hydrolysis by DHP-1.[94] As a consequence, this drug can be administered as a single agent for the treatment of severe bacterial infections. The spectrum of activity of meropenem is similar to imipenem and includes coverage of *P. aeruginosa*. The common adverse effects are similar to imipenem/cilastatin. While the drug is reported to have a similar risk of seizures to imipenem,[95] no drug-related seizures were reported in several clinical trials.[96] A combination product of meropenem with the β-lactamase inhibitor, vaborbactam (Vabomere), is now approved in the United States. Like Recarbrio, this combination with a β-lactamase inhibitor extends the spectrum of activity to include KPC-producing organisms. Vabomere is approved for use in the treatment of complicated UTIs.[97]

Ertapenem. Ertapenem (Table 32.6) possesses a complex side chain at C_3 that includes a basic pyrrolidine and an amide-linked benzoate moiety. This modification results in a longer half-life versus imipenem and meropenem, allowing the drug to be administered once daily. As with meropenem, a 4β-methyl group confers stability toward DHP-1. The spectrum of activity of ertapenem is more limited when compared with imipenem and meropenem, primarily because it lacks activity against *P. aeruginosa* and *Enterococcus* spp.[98] Ertapenem is also more susceptible to carbapenemases than imipenem and meropenem. The drug is approved for use in the treatment of community-acquired pneumonia, complicated UTIs, pelvic infections, and skin and skin structure infections.

The carbapenem class of antibiotics is under intensive investigation, and several analogs are currently in various phases of preclinical investigation, including tebipenem and sulopenem, both esterified oral prodrug formulations. Tebipenem pivoxil is an oral prodrug carbapenem that is currently available in Japan,[99] and sulopenem etzadroxil is another oral prodrug that is coadministered with probenecid to further improve systemic concentrations after oral administration.

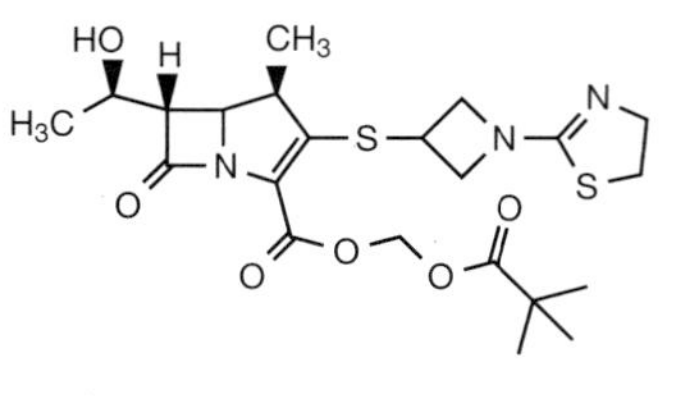

Tebipenem pivoxil

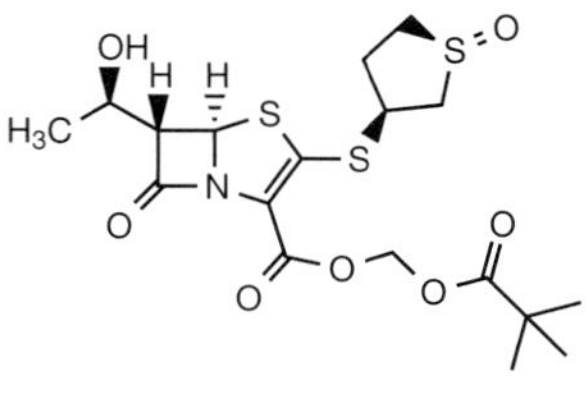

Sulopenem etzadroxil

Monobactams

Aztreonam

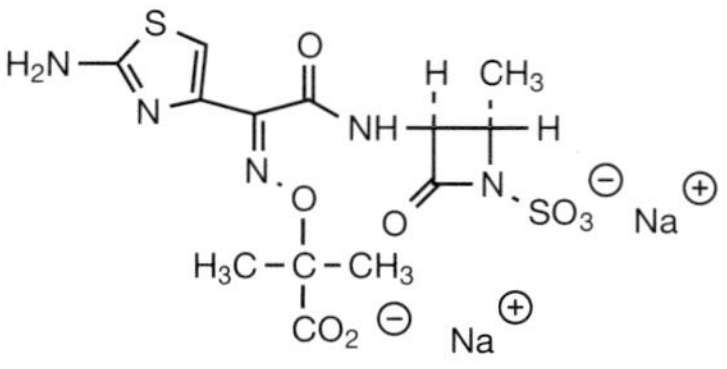

Aztreonam disodium (Azactam)

Fermentation of unusual microorganisms led to the discovery of a class of monocyclic β-lactam antibiotics named monobactams.[66,67] None of the natural molecules proved to be clinically important, but the group served as the inspiration for the synthesis of aztreonam. Marketed as the disodium salt, aztreonam is a synthetic parenteral agent with antibacterial activity almost exclusively restricted to gram-negative organisms. Aztreonam's molecular mode of action is closely similar to that of the penicillins, cephalosporins, and carbapenems, the action being characterized by strong affinity for PBP-3. Additionally, the drug is capable of inactivating some β-lactamases and is resistant to inactivation by MBLs. This latter feature is highly clinically relevant as all marketed β-lactamase inhibitors are inactive against MBLs. Aztreonam has no activity against clinically relevant gram-positive bacteria or anaerobes, but possesses broad gram-negative activity, including some MBL-producing organisms and *P. aeruginosa*. The drug is not active against ESBL- and KPC-producing organisms.

Whereas the principal side chain at C_3 is identical to that of ceftazidime and cefiderocol, the sulfamic acid moiety attached to the β-lactam ring was unprecedented. Remembering the comparatively large size of sulfur atoms, this assembly may sufficiently spatially resemble the corresponding C_2 carboxyl group of the precedent β-lactam antibiotics to confuse the PBPs. The strongly electron-withdrawing character of the sulfamic acid group may also render the β-lactam bond more vulnerable to hydrolysis. In any case, the monobactams demonstrate that a fused ring is not essential for antibiotic activity. The α-oriented methyl group at C_2 and the Z-oxime are associated with the stability of aztreonam toward β-lactamases. The protein binding is moderate (~50%), and the drug is nearly unchanged by metabolism. Aztreonam is given by injection and is primarily excreted in the urine. The primary clinical use of aztreonam is against severe infections caused by gram-negative microorganisms, especially those acquired in the hospital. These are mainly urinary tract, upper respiratory tract, bone, cartilage, abdominal, obstetric, and gynecologic infections, and septicemias. The drug is well tolerated, and adverse effects are infrequent.[100] An important clinical aspect of this drug is that cross-allergenicity with other β-lactam antibiotics is rare, so the drug can be used safely in most patients with reported allergies to other β-lactams. An important exception is patients with confirmed allergies specifically to ceftazidime or cefiderocol, which possess identical side chains to aztreonam.

Glycopeptides, Lipoglycopeptides, and Lipopeptides

A variety of cyclic peptides are utilized for their antibiotic properties. Typically, physiologically relevant peptides are linear; however, several bacterial species produce antibiotic mixtures of cyclic peptides that include uncommon amino acids and common amino acids with the unnatural D absolute stereochemistry. An example of a common unnatural amino acid is L-α,γ-diaminobutyric acid (L-DAB) that is present in polymyxins. Cyclic peptides may also possess an appended fatty acid chain. One of the consequences of this unusual architecture is that these peptide agents are not as easily metabolized. They are usually water soluble and are highly lethal to susceptible bacteria because they attach themselves to the bacterial membranes and interfere with their semi-permeability so that essential metabolites leak out and undesirable substances pass in. Unfortunately, they can also be toxic in humans, so their use is often reserved for serious situations where there are few alternatives or to topical uses. Bacteria are rarely able to develop significant resistance to this group of antibiotics. They are generally unstable, so solutions should be protected from heat, light, and extremes of pH.

Polymyxins

Polymyxin B. Polymyxin B is a combination of several structurally related polymyxins, B_1, B_2, B_3, and B_6, with the major components being B_1 and B_2 (Fig. 32.20). The drug is produced by the fermentation of *Bacillus polymyxa* and is primarily active against gram-negative microorganisms. Polymyxin B possesses affinity for the negatively charged outer membrane of gram-negative bacteria by virtue of the positively charged amino acids in the drug's cyclic peptide group.[101] Binding to the membrane results in membrane disruption and a destabilized outer membrane. The lipophilic "tail" moiety of polymyxin inserts into the bacterial membrane and further disrupts its integrity. The resulting leakage of cell contents produces a bactericidal effect. The drug is primarily used topically, often formulated with bacitracin and/or neomycin due to a high adverse effect profile that includes nephrotoxicity. However, IM and IV formulations as the sulfate salt are available for the treatment of serious, MDR infections caused by gram-negative pathogens.

Colistin (Polymyxin E). Colistin, or polymyxin E, is another cyclic polypeptide with a lipophilic tail (Fig. 32.20), chemically related to polymyxin B. Structurally, the only difference is the substitution of the D-phenylalanine residue in the peptide ring with a D-leucine. The mechanism of action

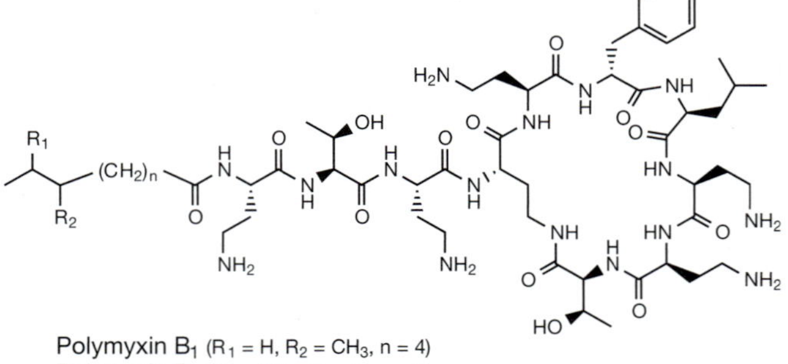
Polymyxin B_1 (R_1 = H, R_2 = CH_3, n = 4)
Polymyxin B_2 (R_1 = CH_3, R_2 = H, n = 3)

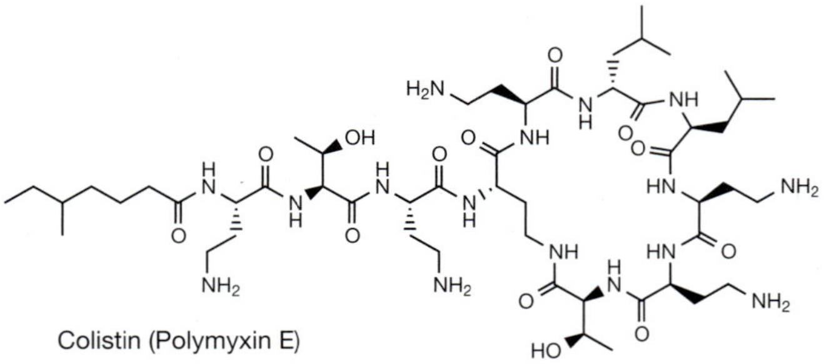
Colistin (Polymyxin E)

Figure 32.20 Polymyxin antibiotics.

(MOA) and antibacterial spectrum of colistin are the same as those of polymyxin B. Colistin can be administered topically or orally (for bowel decontamination) as colistin sulfate, or by inhalation or parenterally as the prodrug colistimethate sodium. The prodrug formulation incorporates a methane sulfonate group to each of the compound's four lysine residues for improved solubility. Similar to polymyxin B, colistin is associated with a high adverse effect rate, including nephrotoxicity, and parenteral use is considered the last resort for MDR gram-negative infections. Colistin is preferred over polymyxin B for the treatment of UTIs and, unlike polymyxin B, can be given by inhalation for pneumonia caused by MDR gram-negative pathogens.

Bacitracin

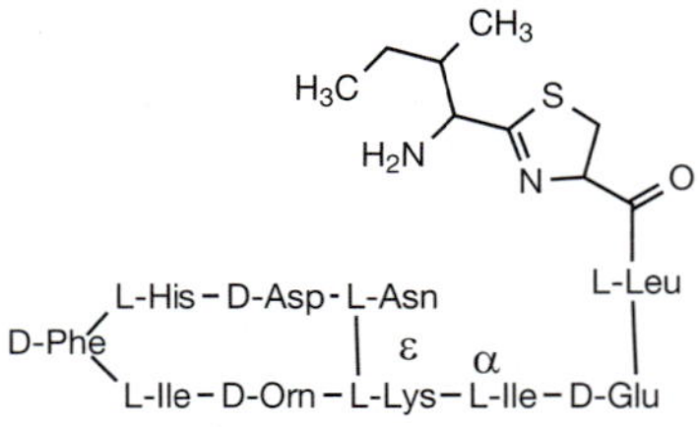
Bacitracin A

Bacitracin is a mixture of similar peptides produced by fermentation of the bacterium *Bacillus licheniformis.* The A component predominates. Unlike the polymyxins described earlier, bacitracin is primarily active against gram-positive organisms, including staphylococci, streptococci, and *Clostridium* spp. Its molecular MOA is believed to be the inhibition of peptidoglycan biosynthesis at a late stage (likely at the dephosphorylation of the phospholipid carrier step) and disruption of plasma membrane function.[102] The drug is used topically in ophthalmic and dermatologic formulations, sometimes in combination with neomycin and/or polymyxin B.

An IM formulation of bacitracin was previously used in infants with pneumonia and empyema caused by resistant staphylococci, but this product has been withdrawn due to significant risk of nephrotoxicity and anaphylaxis.[103]

Vancomycin. Vancomycin is produced by the fermentation of *Amycolatopsis orientalis.* It has been available in the United States for over 60 years, but its popularity has increased significantly with the emergence of MRSA in the early 1980s. Chemically, vancomycin is a glycosylated tricyclic heptapeptide core composed of unusual amino acids, several of which contain aromatic rings cross-linked by aryl ether bonds into a rigid molecular framework (Table 32.7). Vancomycin's spectrum of activity is limited to gram-positive organisms, including enterococci, staphylococci, and streptococci. It is a preferred agent for the treatment of infections caused by *E. faecalis*, MRSA, and viridans streptococci, though vancomycin-resistant enterococci (VRE) have now emerged.

Mechanism of Action. Vancomycin inhibits bacterial cell wall biosynthesis by binding to the D-alanine-D-alanine building block and preventing it from being incorporated into the cell wall by PBP-mediated peptidoglycan cross-linking. There is some evidence that the active species is a homodimer of two vancomycin units. The binding site for its target is a peptide-lined cleft having high affinity for acetyl-D-alanyl-D-alanine and related peptides through five hydrogen bonds (Fig. 32.21).[104] The result of this interaction is downstream inhibition of both transglycosylases (inhibiting the linking between muramic acid and acetyl glucosamine units) and transpeptidase (inhibiting peptide cross-linking) activities in cell wall biosynthesis (Fig. 32.11). Thus, vancomycin functions like a peptide receptor and interrupts bacterial cell wall biosynthesis at the same step as does the β-lactams but by a different mechanism.

Resistance. Vancomycin resistance did not begin to emerge until after this drug had been used for several decades. VRE was first reported in 1986, strains of *S. aureus* with reduced susceptibility were first reported in 1997 (now referred to as "vancomycin intermediate *S. aureus*," or VISA), and fully vancomycin-resistant *S. aureus* (VRSA) was first reported in 2002.[105] The mechanism of resistance in VISA organisms was demonstrated to be a thickened cell wall impeding access of the drug to the site of action. This can be overcome by increasing the vancomycin dosage. The mechanism of resistance in VRE and VRSA has been confirmed to be the alteration of the target D-alanine-D-alanine cell wall precursor to D-alanine-D-lactate. Vancomycin has decreased affinity for D-Ala-D-Lac due to the loss of one hydrogen bond (Fig. 32.21). The reason that it took nearly 30 years for full vancomycin resistance to emerge, when resistance to other antibiotics emerges quite quickly (2-4 years), is because vancomycin uniquely binds to an enzyme substrate to prevent the enzyme's action, instead of binding directly to a target enzyme or receptor, which can readily evolve mutations to prevent drug binding. In fact, the genetic mechanism of vancomycin resistance is quite complex and involves five gene products: two "sensor" genes to detect the presence of vancomycin and turn on three other genes that produce two enzymes to synthesize D-Ala-D-Lac and one enzyme to destroy the pool of D-Ala-D-Ala in the cell.[106]

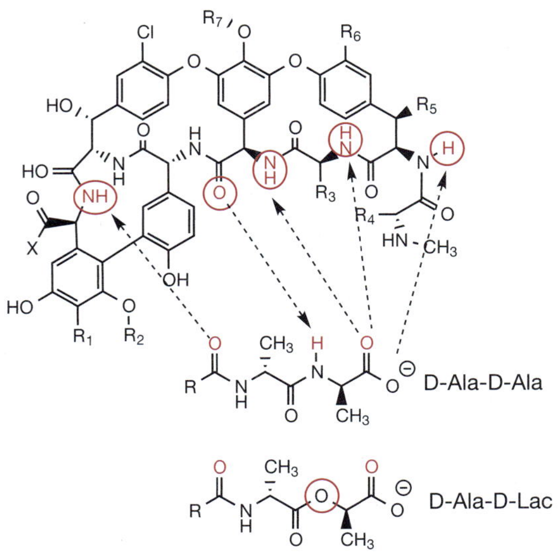

Figure 32.21 Binding of glycopeptide antibiotics to bacterial cell wall D-alanine-D-alanine moiety and resistance-conferring D-alanine-D-lactate.

Therapeutic Applications. Vancomycin has very low oral absorption and cannot be given orally to treat systemic infection. A marketed oral formulation, Vancocin, is used to treat GI infections caused by *C. difficile*. Parental formulations are used to treat infections caused by susceptible gram-positive pathogens, including MRSA and MRSE (*S. epidermidis*) septicemia, endocarditis, skin and soft tissue infections, and infections associated with venous catheters.[107] Vancomycin is also used as an alternative agent for MSSA in the case of penicillin allergy.

Adverse Effects. Parenteral administration of vancomycin is associated with infusion-related adverse events. These are especially prevalent with higher doses and a rapid infusion rate. Rapid infusion rate has been shown to cause anaphylactoid reactions, including hypotension, wheezing, dyspnea, urticaria, and pruritus. A significant erythematic rash, referred to as a "vancomycin infusion reaction," can also occur. These events are much less frequent with a slower infusion rate. In addition to the danger of infusion-related events, higher doses of vancomycin can cause nephrotoxicity and auditory nerve damage. The risk of these effects is increased with elevated, prolonged concentrations, so vancomycin use should be monitored and potentially dose adjusted in patients with impaired renal function. The ototoxicity may be transient or permanent and more commonly occurs in patients on high doses, those who have underlying hearing loss, and those treated concomitantly with other ototoxic agents (ie, aminoglycosides).[107] Vancomycin can also cause vancomycin flushing syndrome (VFS), previously referred to as "red man's syndrome." This is an adverse reaction resulting in pruritus and an erythematous rash on the upper part of the body, including the torso, neck, and face.

Telavancin, Dalbavancin, and Oritavancin. Telavancin, dalbavancin, and oritavancin are semisynthetic derivatives of vancomycin, known as "lipoglycopeptides," that have altered substituents at several positions in the scaffold, including the addition of a lipid tail at the R_8 position (Table 32.7).[108-110]

Table 32.7 Structure of the Glycopeptide and Lipoglycopeptide Antibiotics

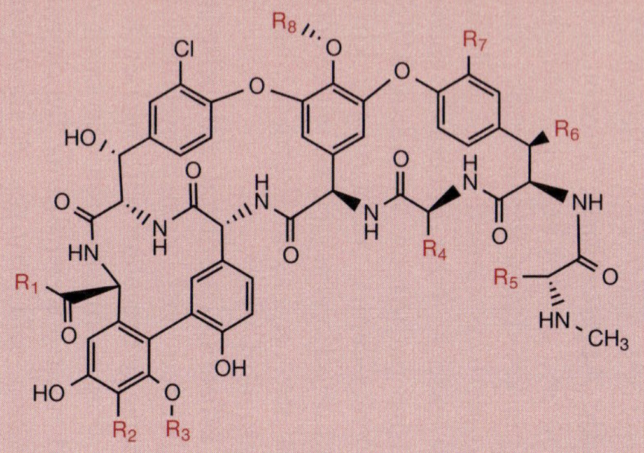

	R_1	R_2	R_3	R_4	R_5	R_6	R_7	R_8
Dalbavancin (Dalvance)	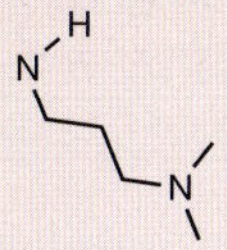	H	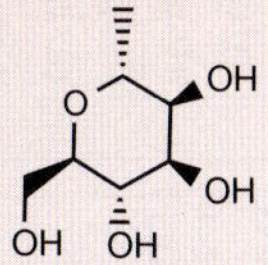	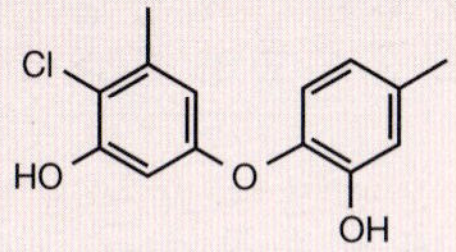		H	H	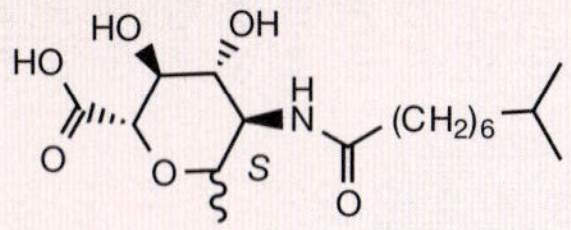
Telavancin (Vibativ)	OH	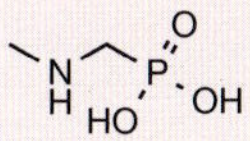	H	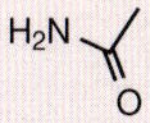	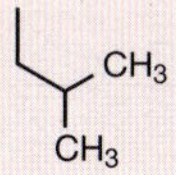	OH	Cl	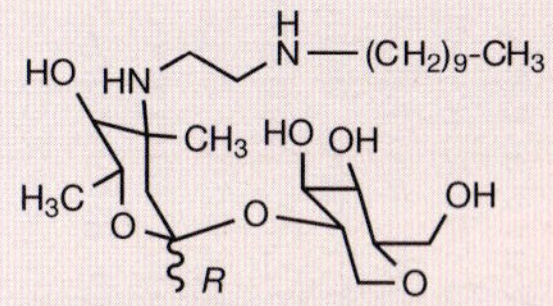
Vancomycin (Vancocin)	OH	H	H	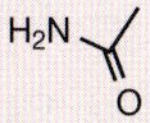	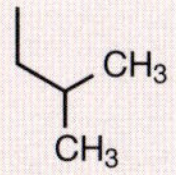	OH	Cl	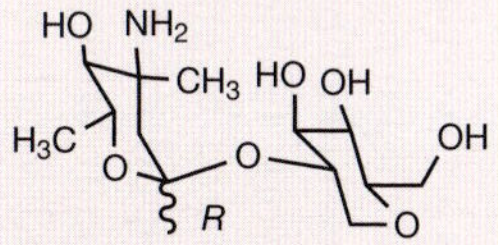
Oritavancin (Orbactiv)	OH	H	H	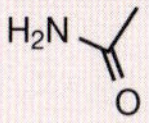	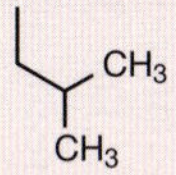	OH	Cl	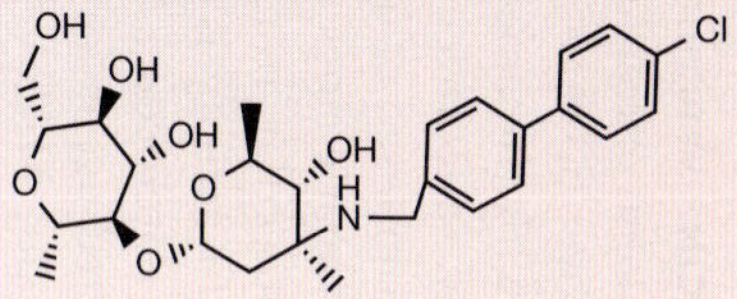

These changes have an effect on the half-life of the derivatives that allows for less frequent dosing of these drugs. Telavancin is dosed once per day versus every 6 to 12 hours for vancomycin dosing. Dalbavancin and oritavancin with their long half-lives of ~14.5 days and ~10 days, respectively, can be given as a single-dose therapy. Although they inhibit cell wall biosynthesis in the same manner as that of vancomycin, it appears that the structural changes also cause disruption of cell membrane integrity (similar to a detergent) as part of their mechanism. Oritavancin also binds to the pentaglycyl bridging structure to further inhibit peptidoglycan cross-linking.[110] These additional mechanisms may account for retention of oritavancin's antibacterial activity against some vancomycin-resistant organisms. For example, oritavancin has activity against VRE organisms, while telavancin has variable activity against these organisms, and vancomycin and dalbavancin have no activity. Similar to vancomycin, these agents possess no activity against gram-negative pathogens.

The lipoglycopeptides are indicated for the treatment of skin and skin structure infections by susceptible gram-positive organisms, including MRSA. Telavancin is also indicated for hospital- or ventilator-acquired bacterial pneumonia when alternative treatments are not suitable. A special note of caution with dalbavancin is that the drug should only be administered in D5W (dextrose) infusions as the drug can precipitate in saline infusions. Like vancomycin, telavancin and dalbavancin require dose adjustment with renal impairment. Oritavancin does not require adjusted doses for mild or moderate renal impairment. Both dalbavancin and telavancin are highly bound to plasma proteins (>90%), while vancomycin is poorly bound (10%-55%). Dalbavancin and oritavancin produce GI effects (nausea, vomiting, diarrhea) and rash, whereas telavancin causes renal toxicity and QT prolongation. These agents can also produce infusion-related toxicities, so slow infusion is recommended to reduce the toxicities.

Daptomycin

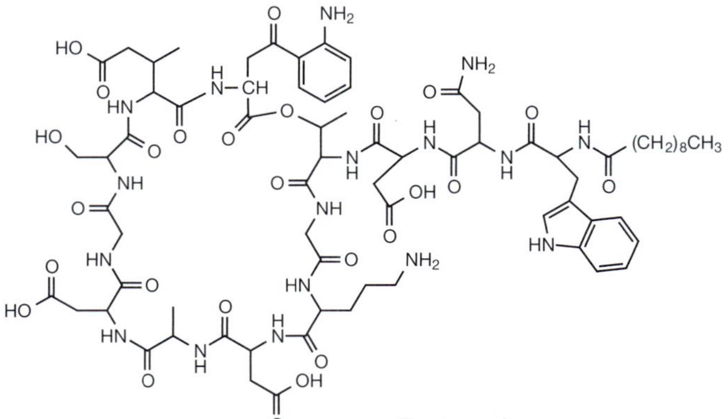

Daptomycin

Daptomycin is a fermentation product of *Streptomyces roseosporus*. It is a lipopeptide antibiotic with a cyclic structure.[111] This agent is primarily active against gram-positive pathogens; a notable exception is the viridans streptococci, against which daptomycin is inactive. It is active against VRE and staphylococci. Daptomycin is not active against any clinically relevant gram-negative organisms. The bactericidal activity of daptomycin stems from its binding to bacterial cell membranes resulting in membrane depolarization that ultimately disrupts protein, DNA, and RNA synthesis. Daptomycin is approved for use in the treatment of complicated skin and skin structure infections, *S. aureus* bacteremia, and *S. aureus* endocarditis. Daptomycin cannot be used for the treatment of bacterial pneumonias as the drug is inactivated by lung surfactant. Resistance to daptomycin has been reported and is attributed to increases in the cell surface cationic charge that repels daptomycin from binding.[112] Patients should be monitored by serum creatine phosphokinase (CPK) testing because some incidence of myopathy has been reported, more frequently at higher doses. Because of this, the administration of statin drugs is recommended to be halted during daptomycin therapy. Daptomycin is administered as an IV injection, has relatively high plasma protein binding (89%-94%), and this agent is eliminated primarily via the kidney, so minor dose adjustment may be necessary in cases of renal insufficiency.[113]

DNA-Disrupting Agents

DNA-disrupting agents produce their antibacterial action by interfering with various essential processes in DNA synthesis, replication, or repair. Antibacterial classes falling within this general category include the sulfonamide antibacterials, trimethoprim, the quinolone/fluoroquinolone antibacterials, and the nitroimidazole antibacterials. It is interesting to note that each of these classes is considered fully "synthetic," meaning they have not been derived or modeled after any natural product. As such, they cannot be properly called "antibiotics" and are referred to as "antibacterials."

Sulfonamides

The antibacterial properties of the sulfonamides were discovered in the mid-1930s after an incorrect hypothesis, but after observing the results carefully and drawing correct conclusions. Prontosil rubrum, a red dye, was one of a series of dyes examined by Gerhard Domagk of Bayer Company in Germany in the belief that it might be taken up selectively by certain pathogenic bacteria and not by human cells, in a manner analogous to a Gram stain, and thus serve as a selective poison to kill these cells.[11] The dye, indeed, proved active in vivo against streptococcal infections in mice. Curiously, it was not active in vitro. Trefouel and others soon showed that the urine of prontosil rubrum–treated animals was bioactive in vitro.[114] Fractionation led to identification of the active substance as p-aminobenzenesulfonic acid amide (sulfanilamide), a colorless cleavage product formed by reductive liver metabolism of the administered dye. This conversion also occurs in the gut where it is mediated by the azoreductase of the gut bacteria. Today, we would call prontosil rubrum a prodrug.

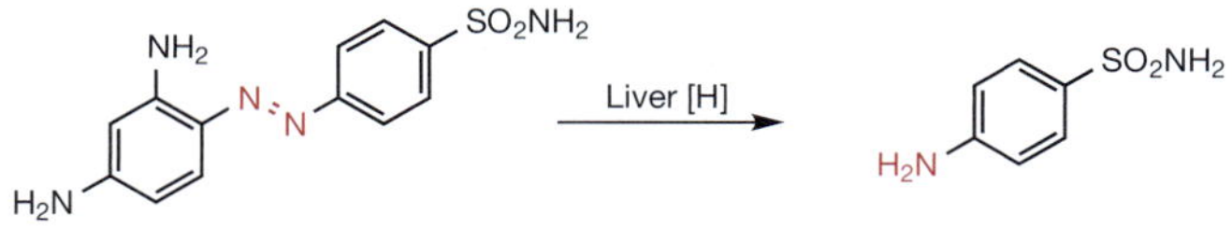

Prontosil rubrum Sulfanilamide

The discovery of sulfanilamide's in vivo antibacterial properties ushered in the modern anti-infective era, and

Domagk was awarded a Nobel Prize for Medicine in 1939. Once a mainstay of antimicrobial chemotherapy, the sulfonamides have decreased significantly in popularity with the introduction of newer and more effective classes of antibacterials. The relative inexpensiveness of the sulfonamides is one of their more attractive features and accounts for much of their persistence on the market. While their use as first-line agents has seen significant decline, it should be noted that sulfonamide or sulfonamide combination products are the preferred agents for infections caused by several pathogens, including *Nocardia* spp., *Klebsiella granulomatis*, *S. maltophilia*, and *Pneumocystis jirovecii* (a fungal pathogen).

Mechanism of Action. The sulfonamides are bacteriostatic when administered to humans in achievable doses. They inhibit the enzyme DHPS, an important enzyme needed for the biosynthesis of folic acid derivatives and, ultimately, the thymidine required for DNA.[115] They act by competing at the active site with *p*-aminobenzoic acid (PABA), a normal structural component of folic acid derivatives. PABA is otherwise incorporated into the developing tetrahydrofolic acid molecule by enzyme-catalyzed condensation with 6-hydroxymethyl-7,8-dihydropterin pyrophosphate to form 7,8-dihydropteroate and pyrophosphate (Fig. 32.22). Thus, sulfonamides may also be classified as antimetabolites. Indeed, the antimicrobial efficacy of sulfonamides can be reversed by adding significant quantities of PABA into the diet (in some multivitamin preparations and as metabolites of certain local anesthetics) or into the culture medium. Most susceptible bacteria are unable to take up preformed folic acid from their environment and convert it to a tetrahydrofolic acid, but, instead, synthesize their own folates de novo. Folates are essential intermediates for the biosynthesis of thymidine without which bacteria cannot multiply. Thus, inhibition of the DHPS is bacteriostatic. Humans are unable to synthesize folates from component parts, lacking the necessary enzymes (including DHPS), and folic acid is supplied to humans in the diet. Sulfonamides consequently have no similarly lethal effect on human cell growth, and the basis for the selective antibacterial activity of sulfonamides is therefore obvious.

In a few strains of bacteria, however, the situation is somewhat more complex. In those cases, sulfonamides are attached to the dihydropteroate diphosphate in place of the normal PABA. The resulting unnatural product, however, is not capable of undergoing the next necessary reaction, condensation with glutamic acid. This false metabolite is also an enzyme inhibitor, and the net result is inability of the bacteria to multiply when the folic acid in their cells is used up, and further nucleic acid biosynthesis becomes impossible. The net result is the same, but the molecular basis of the effect is somewhat different in these strains (Fig. 32.22). Bacteria that can uptake preformed folic acid into their cells are intrinsically resistant to sulfonamides.

Structure-Activity Relationships. The basis of the structural resemblance of sulfonamides to PABA is clear. The functional group that differs between the two molecules is the carboxyl of PABA and the sulfonamide moiety of sulfanilamide. The strongly electron-withdrawing character of the aromatic SO_2 group makes the nitrogen atom to which it is directly attached partially electropositive. This, in turn, increases the acidity of the hydrogen atoms attached to the nitrogen so that this functional group is slightly acidic ($pK_a = 10.4$). The pK_a of the carboxyl group of PABA is approximately 4.9. It was soon found that replacement of one of the NH_2 hydrogens by an electron-withdrawing heteroaromatic ring enhanced the acidity of the remaining hydrogen and dramatically enhanced potency. With suitable groups in place, the pK_a is reduced to the same range as that of PABA itself. Not only did this markedly increase the antibacterial potency of the product, but it also dramatically increased

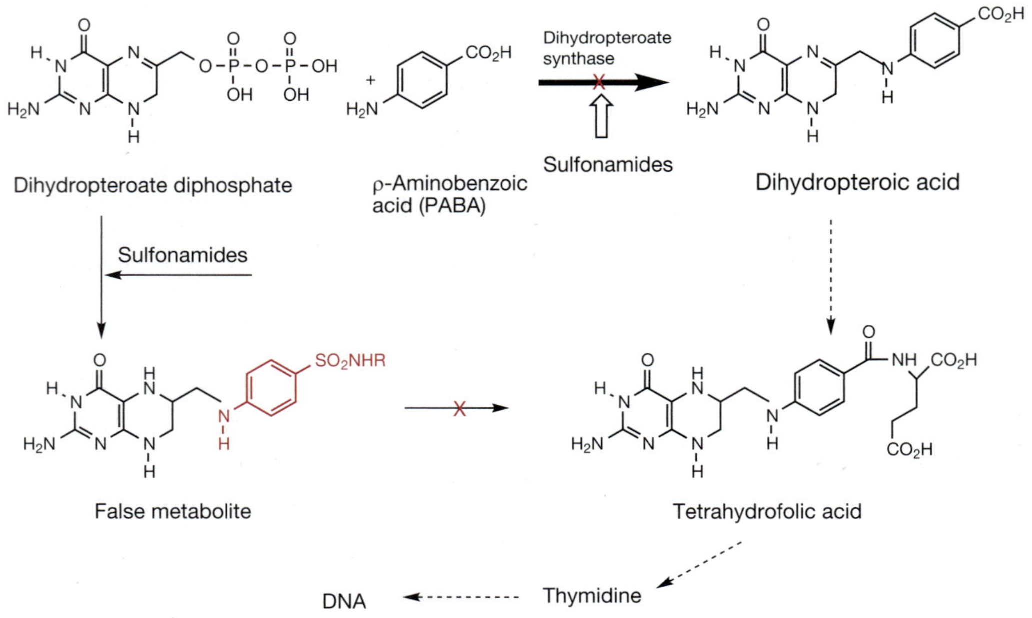

Figure 32.22 Microbial biosynthetic pathway leading to tetrahydrofolic acid synthesis and major site of action (↑) of sulfonamides as well as site of action seen in some bacteria (←), resulting in incorporation of sulfanilamide as a false metabolite.

the water solubility under physiologic conditions. The pK_a of sulfamethoxazole, one of the sulfonamides in present use, is approximately 5.6. The poor water solubility of the earlier sulfonamides led to occasional crystallization in the urine (crystalluria) and resulted in kidney damage because the molecules were unionized at urine pH values. It is still recommended to drink increased quantities of water to avoid crystalluria when taking certain sulfonamides, but this form of toxicity is now comparatively uncommon with the agents used today because they form sodium salts that are at least partly ionized and hence reasonably water soluble at urinary pH values. Sulfonamides are poorly tolerated on injection, however, because these salts are corrosive to tissues. Structural variation among the clinically useful sulfonamides is restricted primarily to installation of various heterocyclic aromatic substituents on the sulfonamide nitrogen.

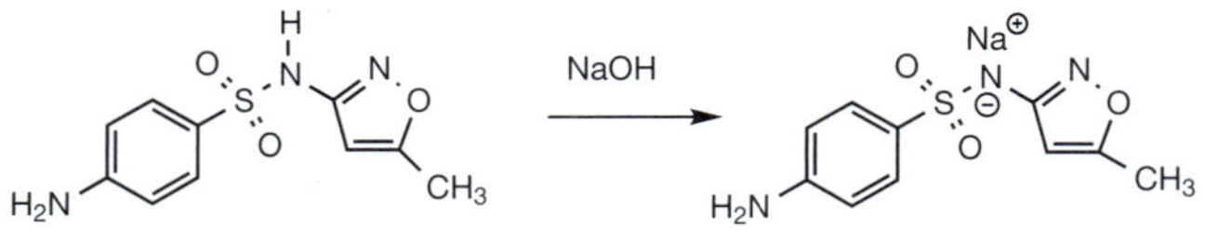

Sulfamethoxazole p*K*a = 5.6   Sodium Sulfamethoxazole

Pharmacokinetics and Resistance. The orally administered sulfonamides are well absorbed from the GI tract, distributed widely in the body, and excreted by the kidney. The drugs vary in their binding to plasma proteins (sulfisoxazole 30%-70%, sulfamethoxazole 70%) and, as such, may displace other protein-bound drugs as well as bilirubin. The latter phenomenon disqualifies them for use in late-term pregnancy because they can cause neonatal jaundice. Sulfonamides are partly deactivated by acetylation at N_4 and hepatic glucuronidation of the aniline nitrogen atom.[116] Plasmid-mediated resistance development is common, particularly among gram-negative microorganisms, and usually takes the form of decreased sensitivity of DHPS or increased production of PABA.[117]

Therapeutic Applications. Of the thousands of sulfonamides that have been evaluated, only a few are still available and are often used in combination with other agents. The prescribed sulfonamides (Table 32.8) include sulfamethoxazole, marketed in combination with trimethoprim (discussed next) as oral and injectable formulations, sulfadiazine marketed as an oral tablet and a topical silver salt formulation, sulfacetamide marketed as topical and ophthalmic sodium salt formulations, and sulfasalazine, a prodrug marketed in oral formulations for anti-inflammatory indications. Sulfamethoxazole (with trimethoprim) has a comparatively broad antimicrobial spectrum covering both gram-positive and gram-negative pathogens but is not considered a first-line agent for many of these infections. Susceptible organisms generally include staphylococci (including MRSA), *L. monocytogenes*, *Nocardia* spp., *Serratia* spp., *Yersinia* spp., *H. influenzae*, *Kingella* spp., *Legionella* spp., and *S. maltophilia*.[118] The remaining sulfonamides are not typically used systemically for bacterial infections. Sulfadiazine is used orally primarily in combination with other agents for the treatment of protozoal infection and topically as the silver salt for the prevention of infection in burn patients. It is effective against a broad range of bacteria and fungi. Sulfacetamide is used topically, often in combination, to treat skin infections (acne, seborrheic dermatitis) and in ophthalmic preparations as an alternative agent for bacterial conjunctivitis. Sulfasalazine is used primarily for its anti-inflammatory properties to treat rheumatoid arthritis, ulcerative colitis, and Crohn disease. It is available in oral formulations.

Table 32.8 Clinically Relevant Sulfonamides

General Sulfonamide Scaffold

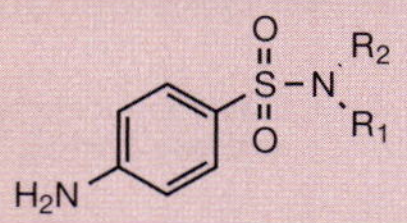

Drug: Generic name	R_1	R_2	pK_a
Sulfisoxazole acetyl[a] (prodrug)	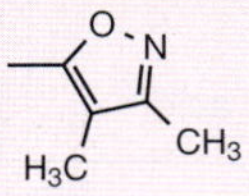	$-C(=O)-CH_3$	5.6 after hydrolysis
Sulfamethoxazole	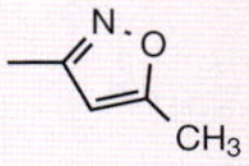	—H	5.0
Sulfadiazine	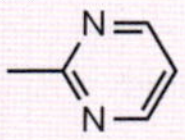	—H	6.52
Silver sulfadiazine	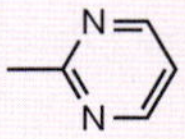	$\ominus$ $\oplus$ Ag	
Sulfacetamide sodium	$-C(=O)-CH_3$	$\ominus$ $\oplus$ Na	5.4 free acid
Sulfasalazine	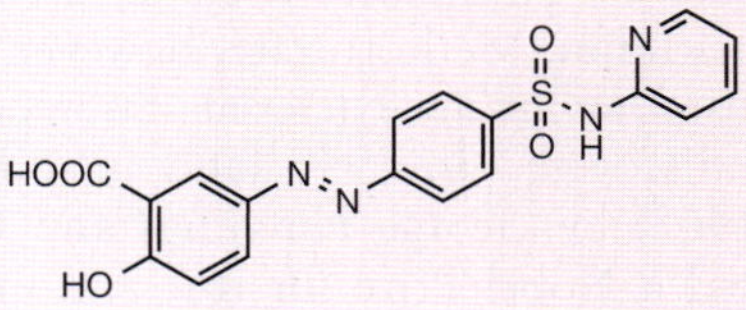		

[a]No longer marketed in the United States (aka sulfafurazole).

Adverse Effects. Allergic reactions are the most common and take the form of rash, photosensitivity, and drug fever. Less common problems are kidney and liver damage, hemolytic anemia, and other blood problems. The most serious adverse effect is the Stevens-Johnson syndrome characterized by sometimes fatal erythema multiforme and ulceration of mucous membranes of the eye, mouth, and urethra.[116] Fortunately, these effects are rare.

Trimethoprim

Mechanism of Action. The target of trimethoprim is DHFR that catalyzes a reduction reaction two steps after DHPS in the bacterial folate biosynthesis pathway. This enzyme converts dihydrofolic acid to tetrahydrofolic acid (Fig. 32.23). Similar to DHPS, this enzyme is involved in an essential step in the bacterial biosynthesis of tetrahydrofolic acid, which serves as an important cofactor essential for supplying one-carbon units in thymidine and DNA biosynthesis. DHFR is also found in mammals, where exogenous (dietary) folic acid is reduced to dihydrofolic acid,

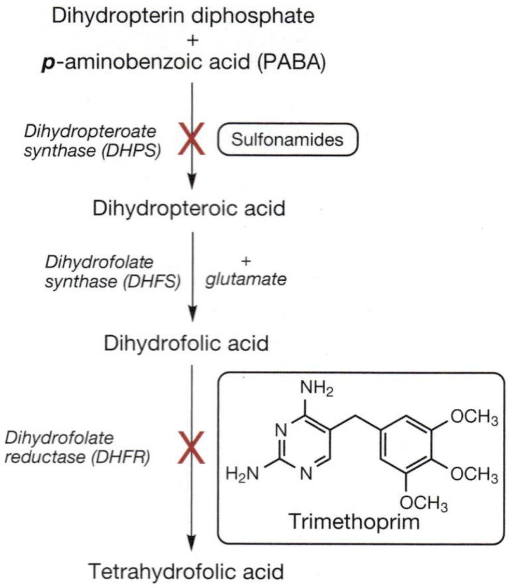

Figure 32.23 Trimethoprim targets the DHFR enzyme, two steps after the DHPS step in the bacterial folate biosynthesis pathway.

the DHFR substrate. Inhibition of this key enzyme had been widely studied in attempts to find anticancer agents by starving rapidly dividing cancer cells of needed DNA precursors. Antifolates such as methotrexate arose from such studies. Methotrexate, however, is much too toxic to be used as an antibacterial. Subsequently, trimethoprim was discovered in 1948 (and introduced for clinical use in 1962) by George Hitchings and Gertrude Elion (who shared a Nobel Prize for this and other contributions to chemotherapy in 1988).[119] This inhibitor prevents tetrahydrofolic acid biosynthesis and results in bacteriostasis. Trimethoprim's selectivity between bacterial and mammalian DHFRs results from the subtle but significant structural differences between the prokaryotic and eukaryotic variants of this enzyme. Whereas the bacterial enzyme and the mammalian enzyme both efficiently catalyze the conversion of dihydrofolic acid to tetrahydrofolic acid, the bacterial enzyme is sensitive to inhibition by trimethoprim by up to 100,000 times lower concentrations than is vertebrate enzyme.[120] This difference explains the useful selective toxicity of trimethoprim.

Therapeutic Application. Trimethoprim can be used as a single agent clinically for the oral treatment of uncomplicated UTIs caused by susceptible bacteria (predominantly community-acquired *E. coli* and other gram-negative rods).[121] However, it is most commonly used in a 1:5 fixed concentration ratio with the sulfonamide sulfamethoxazole (Bactrim, Septra, Septra DS). This combination is not only synergistic in vitro but is less likely to induce bacterial resistance than either agent alone. It is rationalized that microorganisms not completely inhibited by sulfamethoxazole at the DHPS step will be unlikely to pass the decreased amount of substrate through a subsequent blockade of DHFR. This synergistic strategy of inhibiting two different steps in the same essential metabolic pathway is called "sequential blocking" and is very difficult for a native microorganism to overcome. This is because it is very unlikely that a microorganism would be able to successfully mutate both target enzymes during a course of therapy. However, if the organism is already resistant to either drug at the outset of therapy, much of the advantage of the combination may be lost.

The pairing of these two antibacterial agents was based on pharmacokinetic factors. For such a combination to be useful in vivo, the two agents must arrive at the necessary tissue compartment where the infection is at the correct time and in the right ratio. In this context, the optimum ratio of these two agents in vitro is 1:20. Administration of the 1:5 combination of the two drugs orally produces the desired 1:20 ratio in the body once steady state is reached.[116] This combination, sometimes referred to as TMP-SMX or "co-trimoxazole," is used to treat a wide range of susceptible bacteria (discussed earlier), causing uncomplicated UTIs, prostatitis, shigellosis, traveler's diarrhea, community-acquired MRSA, acute exacerbations of chronic bronchitis, and *P. pneumonia*.[116] The most frequent adverse effects of trimethoprim-sulfamethoxazole are rash, nausea, and vomiting. Blood dyscrasias are less common, as is pseudomembranous colitis (caused by non–antibiotic-sensitive opportunistic gut anaerobes, often *C. difficile*).[116] Despite significant efforts, no structurally related analog has emerged to be sufficiently good in order to compete with trimethoprim.

Resistance. Bacterial resistance to trimethoprim is increasingly common. In pneumococcal infections, it can result from a single amino acid mutation (Ile100 to Leu100) in the DHFR enzyme. Overexpression of DHFR by *S. aureus* has also been reported in resistant strains.[117]

Quinolones

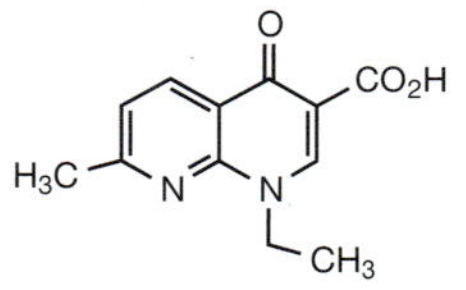

Nalidixic acid

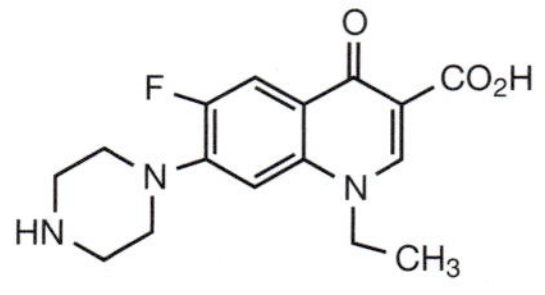

Norfloxacin

The quinolone antimicrobials comprise a group of synthetic substances possessing in common an N_1-alkylated 3-carboxypyrid-4-one ring fused to another aromatic ring, which itself carries other substituents. The first quinolone to be marketed, nalidixic acid, was serendipitously discovered as a by-product of chloroquine synthesis and was used for the treatment of UTIs. It has since been discontinued. Nalidixic acid was classified as a first-generation quinolone based on its spectrum of activity and pharmacokinetic properties. The spectrum of activity was limited to a small number of gram-negative organisms. Thus, the quinolones were of little clinical significance until the discovery that the addition of a fluoro group to the 6-position of the basic nucleus greatly increased the desired biologic activity.[122,123] Agents that contain the 6-fluoro-substitution are referred to as fluoroquinolones and represent an important therapeutic class of antimicrobials. Norfloxacin was approved for use in 1986 and represented the first of the second-generation quinolones; it was considered to be broad spectrum and equivalent in potency

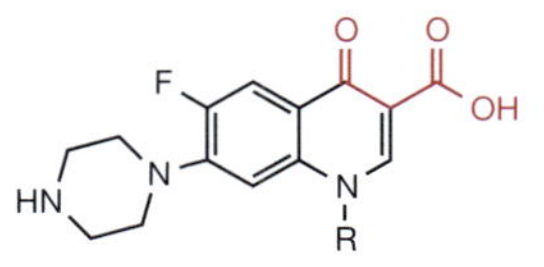

Ciprofloxacin (Cipro)

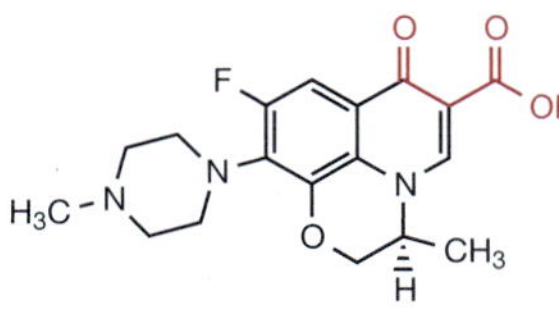

Ofloxacin (Racemic)(generic)
Levofloxacin (1-*S*)(Levaquin)

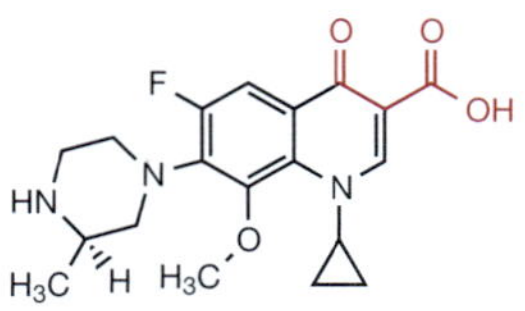

Gatifloxacin (Zymaxid)

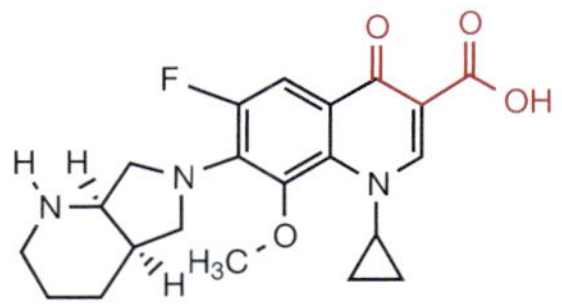

Moxifloxacin (Avelox)

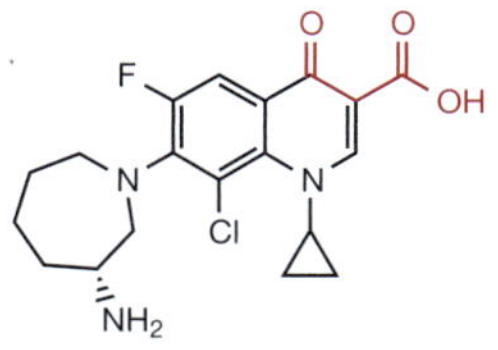

Besifloxacin (Besivance)

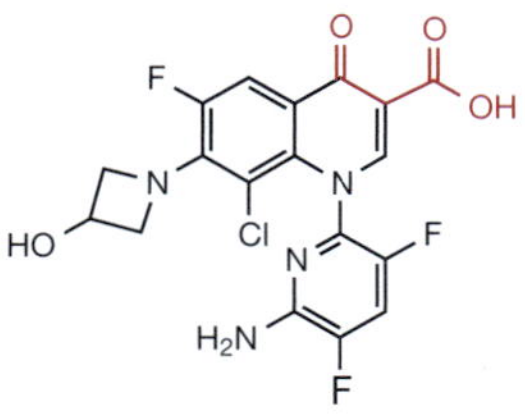

Delafloxacin (Baxdela)

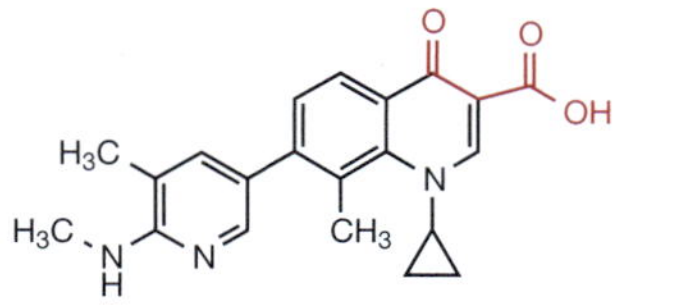

Ozenoxacin (Ozanex, Xepi)

Figure 32.24 US-marketed fluoroquinolones.

to many of the fermentation-derived antibiotics.[122] It has also now been discontinued for use in the United States. Following the introduction of norfloxacin, intense research ensued, and over a thousand analogs have now been made. Fluoroquinolones currently marketed in the United States include the second-generation agents ciprofloxacin and ofloxacin; the third-generation agents levofloxacin and gatifloxacin; the fourth-generation agents moxifloxacin, delafloxacin, and besifloxacin; and the advanced-generation agent ozenoxacin (Fig. 32.24). Of these, gatifloxacin and besifloxacin are only marketed in ophthalmic formulations, while ozenoxacin is only marketed in a topical cream formulation.

Mechanism of Action. The quinolones are rapidly bactericidal, largely as a consequence of dual inhibition of DNA gyrase and topoisomerase IV, key bacterial enzymes that dictate the conformation of DNA.[123,124] Using the energy generated by ATP hydrolysis, DNA is progressively wound about itself in a positive supercoil. In the absence of ATP, the process is reversed, relaxing the molecule. It must also be partially unwound during transcription and replication so that the cell has access to the genetic information it contains. This requires reversible conformational changes so that it can be stored properly, unwound, replicated, repaired, and transcribed on demand. DNA gyrase alters the conformation of DNA by catalyzing transient double-strand cuts, passing the uncut portion of the molecule through the gap, and resealing the molecule back together (Fig. 32.25).[123] In this way, DNA gyrase alters the degree of twisting of DNA by introducing negative DNA supercoils releasing tensional stress in the molecule. DNA topoisomerase IV, on the other hand, decatenates (unties) enchained daughter DNA molecules produced through replication of circular DNA.[123] Inhibition of DNA gyrase and topoisomerase IV makes a cell's DNA inaccessible and leads to cell death, particularly if the cell encounters other toxic effects at the same time. Different quinolones inhibit these essential enzymes to different extents, which explains some of the differences in the spectrum of activity of the fluoroquinolones. Topoisomerase IV

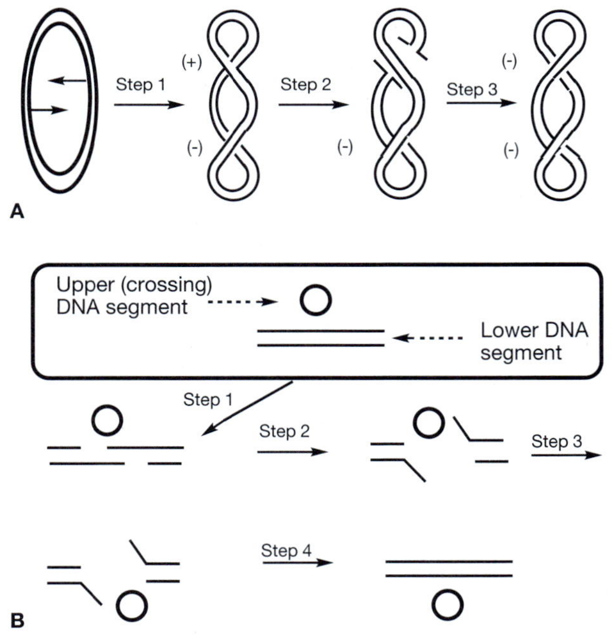

Figure 32.25 Schematic depicting supercoiling of circular DNA catalyzed by DNA gyrase. A. View from the top: Step 1, stabilize positive node. Step 2, break both strands of the back segment. Step 3, pass unbroken segment through the break and reseal on the front side. B. View from the side: Step 1, staggered cuts in each strand. Step 2, gate opens. Step 3, transverse segment passed through the break. Step 4, reseal cut segment.

seems more important to some gram-positive organisms, and DNA gyrase seems more important to some gram-negative organisms. Humans shape their DNA with a topoisomerase II, an analogous enzyme to DNA gyrase that, however, does not bind quinolones at normally achievable doses, so the clinically used fluoroquinolones have significantly decreased toxicity against host cells.

Structure-Activity Relationship. The structural features of the quinolones strongly influence the antimicrobial, pharmacokinetic, and toxicity properties of this class of drugs.[125,126] The essential pharmacophore for activity is the 3-carboxy-4-keto-1,4-dihydropyridine nucleus. The carboxylate and the ketone are present in all quinolones (Fig. 32.24) and are reported to be involved in binding to the DNA/DNA-gyrase enzyme complex. Reduction of the 2,3-double bond or the 4-keto group inactivates the molecule, and substitutions at C_2 are not tolerated as they interfere with enzyme-substrate complexation. Fluoro-substitution at the C_6 position greatly improves antimicrobial activity by increasing the lipophilicity of the molecule, which in turn improves the drug's penetration through the bacterial cell wall. The C_6 fluoro also increases the DNA gyrase/topoisomerase IV inhibitory action. Heterocyclic substitution at C_7 improves the spectrum of activity especially against gram-negative organisms. The piperazinyl (ciprofloxacin) and pyrrolidinyl (moxifloxacin) derivatives represent the most significant antimicrobial improvement. Unfortunately, the piperazinyl group at C_7 also increases binding to CNS γ-aminobutyric acid (GABA) receptors, which accounts for CNS adverse effects. Alkyl substitution on the piperazine nitrogen (ofloxacin and levofloxacin) is reported to decrease binding to GABA. Incorporation of a non-ionizable group at C_7 results in a weakly acidic compound with ionized/non-ionized states dependent on the pH and improved activity under acidic conditions (delafloxacin).[127]

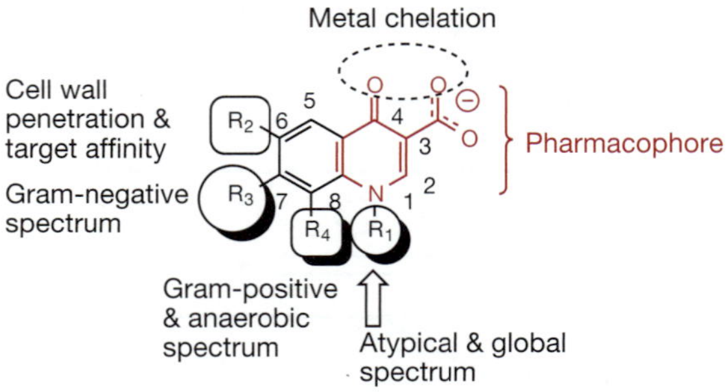

The addition of a fluorine at C_8 further improves drug absorption and half-life, but also increases drug-induced photosensitivity. Substitution of a methoxy group at C_8 reduces the photosensitivity (moxifloxacin and gatifloxacin). Substitution of a chlorine at C_8 is reported to improve activity against gram-positive and anaerobic organisms (besifloxacin and delafloxacin).[128] The cyclopropyl substitution at N_1 appears to broaden activity of the quinolones to include activity against atypical bacteria including *Mycoplasma*, *Chlamydia*, and *Legionella* spp. Substitution of a bulkier, di-fluorinated ring system at N_1 also improves antimicrobial potency, including against organisms that have shown resistance to other fluoroquinolones (delafloxacin).[128] The introduction of a third ring to the nucleus of the quinolones gives rise to ofloxacin. Additionally, ofloxacin has an asymmetric carbon at the $C_{3'}$ position. The S-(-)-isomer (levofloxacin) is twice as active as ofloxacin and 8 to 128 times more potent than the R-(+)-isomer resulting from increased binding to the DNA gyrase. Finally, a chemical incompatibility common to all the quinolones involves the ability of these drugs to chelate polyvalent metal ions (Ca^{2+}, Mg^{2+}, Zn^{2+}, Fe^{2+}, Al^{3+}), resulting in decreased solubility and reduced drug absorption. Chelation occurs between the metal and the 3-carboxylic acid and 4-keto groups. Agents containing polyvalent metals should be administered separately from the quinolones (eg, antacids, iron salts).

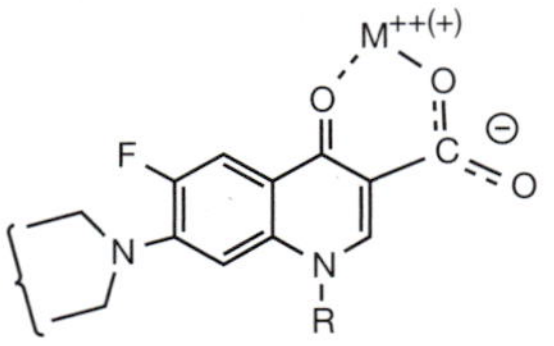

Pharmacokinetics. The fluoroquinolones are well absorbed following oral administration, with excellent bioavailability ranging from 60% to 99% among the agents marketed for systemic use. The maximum plasma concentration is usually reached within a few hours, and the drugs are moderately bound to plasma protein (30%-84%), leading to comparatively long half-lives. Early generation quinolones were rapidly excreted into the urine, which limited their therapeutic application to UTIs, whereas the newer agents are distributed to alveolar macrophages, bronchial mucosa, epithelial lining fluid, and saliva, thus improving their use in various systemic infections.

Therapeutic Applications. The quinolones therapeutically fall into one of four classifications (Table 32.9). The specific drugs within each classification include nalidixic acid and cinoxacin as first-generation agents, both of which have been discontinued in the United States. The second-generation quinolones include norfloxacin and ciprofloxacin. Ciprofloxacin has a broader spectrum of activity and is used for UTIs, bone and joint injections, treatment and exposure prophylaxis for anthrax, shigellosis, and infectious diarrhea caused by susceptible organisms.[129] Ciprofloxacin is also used in combination with metronidazole (discussed later) for treating intra-abdominal infections. The third-generation quinolones include levofloxacin and gatifloxacin, the latter now only marketed in an ophthalmic formulation. They have broad-spectrum activity that includes respiratory and enteric pathogens. Levofloxacin is used in the treatment of bacterial exacerbation of chronic bronchitis and community-acquired pneumonia.[130] Levofloxacin is also used to treat respiratory infections caused by *Legionella*, *Chlamydia*, and *Mycoplasma* as well as other nosocomial pneumonias. Additional indications for levofloxacin include skin and skin structure infections and acute sinusitis caused by *S. pneumoniae*, *H. influenzae*, and *M. catarrhalis*.[130] The fourth-generation quinolones include moxifloxacin, delafloxacin, and besifloxacin, the latter only marketed in an ophthalmic formulation. They have broad spectrum of activity against respiratory and enteric pathogens and

Table 32.9 Therapeutic Classification of Quinolones

Generation	Characteristics
First Generation	• Poor serum and tissue concentration; not valuable for systemic infections • Lack activity against *Pseudomonas aeruginosa*, gram-positive organisms, and anaerobes
Second Generation	• Adequate serum and tissue concentration; good for systemic infections • Active against gram-negative organisms including *P. aeruginosa*[a]; weak activity against *Streptococcus pneumoniae*; no activity against *Streptococcus aureus* or anaerobes
Third Generation	• Extended $t_{1/2}$ permits once-daily dosing • Active against *S. pneumoniae*, MSSA, and atypical bacteria; less active against *P. aeruginosa*; not active against MRSA
Fourth Generation	• Improved activity against anaerobes and aerobic gram-positive and gram-negative organisms • Delafloxacin is active against MRSA and *P. aeruginosa*, moxifloxacin lacks activity against these organisms.
Advanced Generation (ozenoxacin)	• Des-fluoro quinolones with excellent gram-positive activity, including MRSA • Active against some fluoroquinolone-resistant pathogens due to low drug efflux • Reduced potential for joint toxicities

[a]Increasing resistance now limits clinical use of second-generation fluoroquinolones against *P. aeruginosa*.
MRSA, methicillin-resistant *Staphylococcus aureus*; MSSA, methicillin-susceptible *Staphylococcus aureus*.

improved activity against anaerobic pathogens, including *B. fragilis*.[131] Delafloxacin has greater activity against gram-positive organisms, including MRSA, and possesses activity against *P. aeruginosa*. Moxifloxacin and levofloxacin are also recommended as second-line agents for TB as an off-label use.[130,131] The advanced-generation agent, ozenoxacin, is notable for its lack of a C_6 fluoro-substituent. It is available only in topical formulations and possesses excellent activity against gram-positive organisms, including MRSA, but limited gram-negative activity. Ozenoxacin is resistant to drug efflux and thus possesses activity against some fluoroquinolone-resistant pathogens.[132]

Resistance. Resistance to the quinolones is becoming more frequent and is associated with spontaneous mutations in genes (*gyrA* and *gyrB*) that encode for the quinolone target protein, DNA gyrase, and genes (*parC* and *parE*) that encode for topoisomerase IV.[133] A single mutation can lead to low-level resistance, whereas mutations in more than one gene lead to high-level resistance. This mechanism of resistance would be expected to produce differing levels of cross-resistance within the class of quinolones. In addition, there are suggestions that resistance may be associated with an increase in drug efflux or a decrease in outer membrane permeability affecting drug influx.[133] Such a mechanism of resistance would be expected to be more common in gram-negative organisms with a more complex cell wall than in gram-positive organisms with their cell envelope.

Adverse Effects. The quinolone class is associated with significantly more adverse effects than the β-lactam and macrolide classes, including several notable toxicities. For this reason, there has been a general overall decline in the use of quinolone antibacterials over the last decade. The FDA has now issued several safety announcements related to serious quinolone adverse effects including disabling and potentially permanent side effects of the tendons, muscles, joints, nerves, and CNS. A warning was also issued regarding the use of quinolones in patients with aortic aneurysm or risk of aortic aneurysm. Currently, the FDA advises systemic quinolone antibacterials be reserved for the treatment of uncomplicated UTI, acute bacterial sinusitis, or acute exacerbation of chronic bronchitis in patients with no other treatment options and where the benefits outweigh the risks. Systemic quinolones should also not be used in patients with myasthenia gravis. They are associated with a proconvulsant action, especially when coadministered with nonsteroidal anti-inflammatory drugs (NSAIDs). Other CNS problems include hallucinations, insomnia, and visual disturbances. Some patients also experience diarrhea, vomiting, abdominal pain, and anorexia.

The quinolones are associated with erosion of the load-bearing joints of young animals. As a precaution, these drugs are not used casually in children younger than 16 years or in sexually active females of childbearing age. Exceptions to this are the use of ciprofloxacin and levofloxacin for anthrax and ciprofloxacin for pyelonephritis in pediatric patients 1 year and older. They are also potentially damaging in the first trimester of pregnancy because of a risk of severe metabolic acidosis and of hemolytic anemia. Some of the quinolones may potentiate the action of theophylline and should be monitored closely. They also have been linked to QT prolongation and may increase the risk of torsades de pointes when used with other QT-prolonging agents such as some antiarrhythmic agents.[129-131,134,135] The high adverse effect profile of the quinolone antibacterials has led to the removal of many systemic agents from the US market in recent years, including gatifloxacin (hypo- and hyperglycemia), grepafloxacin (cardiac toxicity), temafloxacin (kidney and liver toxicity), trovafloxacin (liver toxicity), enoxacin, gemifloxacin, finafloxacin, lomefloxacin, and sparfloxacin.

Nitroheteroaromatic Compounds

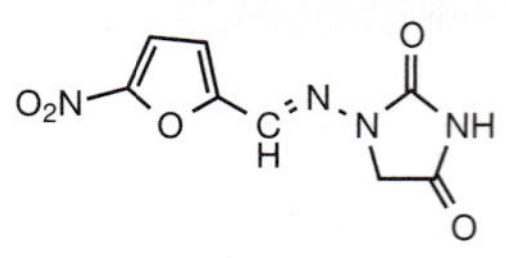

Nitrofurantoin
(Furadantin, Macrodantin)

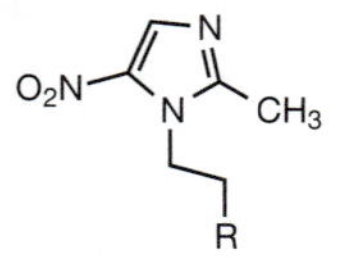

Metronidazole, (Flagyl) R = OH
Tinidazole (Fasigyn) R = $SO_2C_2H_5$

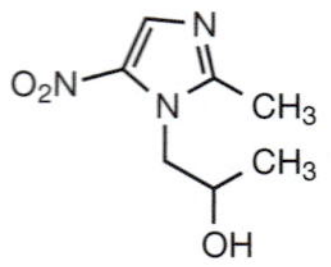

Secnidazole
(Solosec)

NITROFURANTOIN. Nitrofurantoin, a widely used oral antibacterial nitrofuran, has been available since 1953. It is used for prophylaxis or treatment of acute UTIs when kidney function is not impaired, and it inhibits kidney stone growth. Nausea and vomiting are common side effects. This is avoided in part by slowing the rate of absorption of the drug through use of wax-coated macrocrystal formulations (Macrodantin, Macrobid). Nitrofurantoin is activated by enzymatic nitro reduction in bacteria to give reactive nitrogen species (RNS) that effectively damage bacterial DNA.[136] There is a very low level of acquired resistance to this agent in bacteria. Nitrofurantoin is well absorbed following oral administration (~90%) and rapidly eliminated in the urine. It has low tissue penetration and, for this reason, is used only for UTIs and uncomplicated cystitis. It is active against *E. coli* and enterococci, but inactive against *Proteus* spp., *Pseudomonas* spp., and *Enterobacter* spp. Common adverse effects include nausea, vomiting, and diarrhea. Severe side effects that can be experienced when using this drug include acute pulmonary toxicity, peripheral neuropathy, hemolytic anemia, liver toxicity, and fertility impairment.[137]

NITROIMIDAZOLES. Metronidazole is a nitroimidazole antibacterial and antiprotozoal agent that, similar to nitrofurantoin, is reduced in microbes to produce the highly reactive forms of the drug. In anaerobic and microaerophilic organisms, metronidazole's nitro group is reduced to reactive nitro free radical, nitroso, nitroso free radical, and hydroxylamine sequentially, which produce a damaging effect to the microbe's DNA.[138] Because this reductive activation process does not occur in aerobic species, the clinical use of metronidazole is limited to anaerobic (or microaerophilic) organisms, including *C. difficile*, *Bacteroides* spp., *Gardnerella* spp., and protozoal species causing amebiasis, trichomoniasis, and giardiasis. Metronidazole is used to treat bacterial vaginosis, pelvic inflammatory disease, in combination therapies for bowel infections, in combination therapies for *Helicobacter pylori* infection, intestinal and extraintestinal amebiasis, acne rosacea (topically), trichomonas infection, and as alternative treatment for *C. difficile* and giardiasis.[139] Metronidazole use is associated with taste disturbances, "furry tongue," nausea, allergic rashes, and CNS disturbances, including convulsions in some patients, and peripheral neuropathy with prolonged use. Metronidazole is also associated with "disulfiram-like" reactions, which include nausea, vomiting, flushing, tachycardia, and shortness of breath. For this reason, alcohol should be avoided when taking this drug.

Tinidazole, another nitroimidazole, has been introduced primarily as an antibacterial and antiprotozoal agent.[140] Because of the similarities in structure and action, tinidazole is believed to have the same MOA as metronidazole. It is currently approved for the treatment of amebiasis, giardiasis, trichomoniasis, and bacterial vaginosis. An advantage of tinidazole over metronidazole is its longer half-life, which allows for once-daily dosing, versus 3 to 4 times a day for metronidazole. Adverse effects of tinidazole include dysgeusia or metallic taste (due to the presence of sulfone functional group), nausea, anorexia, and vomiting. Like metronidazole, tinidazole can cause disulfiram-like adverse reactions when alcohol is consumed.

Secnidazole was introduced to the US market in 2017 for the treatment of bacterial vaginosis in adult women and trichomoniasis in adults. It is administered orally as granules that are swallowed whole in applesauce, yogurt, or pudding. It is believed to work by the same mechanism as other nitroimidazoles and, while initially reported not to cause a disulfiram-like reaction, there have been postmarketing reports of such. It is now recommended that alcohol be avoided during treatment and for 2 days after completion of therapy.[141]

Protein Synthesis–Disrupting Agents

Basis for Selectivity

Once the bacterial cell wall is traversed, complex cellular machinery deeper within the cell becomes available for targeting by antibacterial agents. Some of the most successful antibacterial classes exert their lethal effects on bacteria by inhibiting ribosome-mediated protein biosynthesis. At first glimpse, this may seem problematic because eukaryotic organisms also construct their essential proteins on ribosomal organelles and the sequence of biochemical steps is closely analogous to that in prokaryotic microorganisms. At a molecular level, however, the apparent anomaly resolves itself because the detailed architecture of prokaryotic ribosomes is rather different, and the prokaryotic translation differs substantially from the eukaryotic process (Table 32.10).

In *E. coli*, for example, the 70S ribosomal particle is composed not only of three RNA molecules, but also of 55 different structural and functional proteins arranged in a nonsymmetrical manner. The small (30S) subunit has a 16S ribosomal RNA (rRNA) molecule and 21 different proteins. The large subunit (50S) has a 23S rRNA, a 5S rRNA, and 34 proteins. The X-ray crystal structure of the components of the bacterial ribosome has been determined.[142,143] This was a landmark achievement given the small size and high complexity of this organelle. The picture is still not complete but allows one to unravel the molecular details not only of how proteins are biosynthesized but also where important antibiotics bind when they interrupt this process. The functioning parts of the ribosome organize and catalyze some portions of the biosynthetic cycle. The transfer RNA

Table 32.10 Comparison of Prokaryotic and Eukaryotic Translation

Feature	Prokaryotes	Eukaryotes
Timing with regard to transcription, pace	Synchronous, faster process	Asynchronous, slower process
Ribosomes, structure and location	30S + 50S = 70S, cytoplasm	40S + 60S = 80S, attached to endoplasmic reticulum
mRNA structure and location	Polycistronic, cytoplasm	Monocistronic, nucleus (subsequently released to cytoplasm)
mRNA, stability	Less stable (half-life of seconds to minutes)	More stable (half-life of minutes to hours)
Initiation factors	Three factors are involved	At least 12 factors are involved
Termination factors	Two release factors	Two release factors
Energy	GTP	GTP

GTP, guanosine triphosphate; mRNA, messenger RNA.

(tRNA) molecules bind roughly at the interface where the 50S and 30S subunits come together. The codon-anticodon interaction with messenger RNA (mRNA) takes place in the 30S subunit, while the incoming amino acid and the growing peptide chain are accommodated in the 50S subunit. It was believed for decades that the antibiotics bind to ribosomal proteins; however, it is now known that they bind to the rRNA instead (Fig. 32.26).

Interference with bacterial protein biosynthesis prevents ordinary physiologic processes such as cellular growth and division, repair, defense, and survival, which results in bacteriostatic or bactericidal effect that is clinically utilized. At therapeutic doses, antibiotics do not bind to or interfere with the function of eukaryotic 80S ribosomal particles. The basis for the selective toxicity of these antibiotics is therefore apparent.

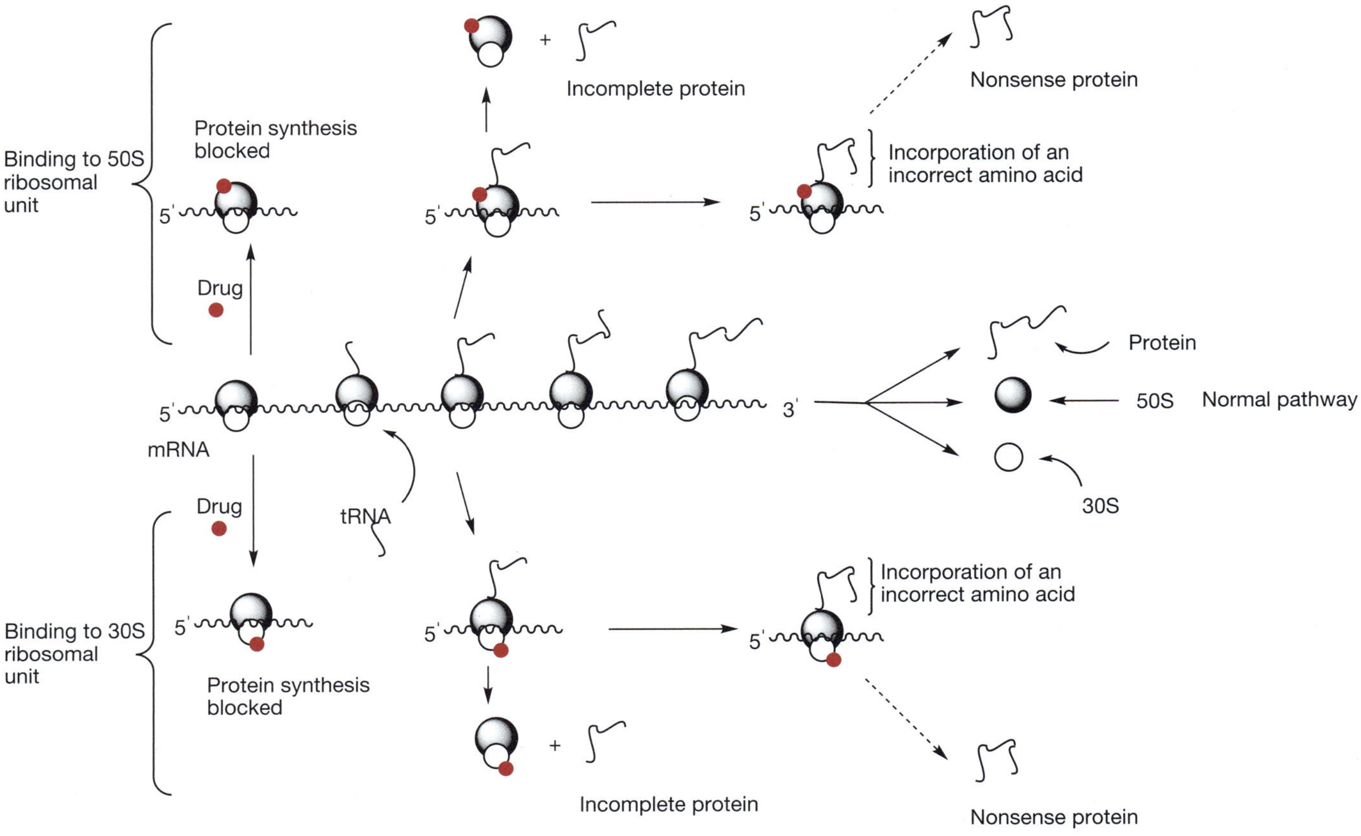

Figure 32.26 General mechanism of action of drugs that block protein synthesis by binding to ribosomal components.

Aminoglycosides/Aminocyclitols

Chemical Properties. The aminoglycoside/aminocyclitol class of antibiotics contains the 1,3-diaminoinositol pharmacophore represented by streptamine, 2-deoxystreptamine, spectinamine, or streptidine [also known as N^1,N^3-bis(aminoiminomethyl)streptamine] (Fig. 32.27). Several of the alcoholic functions of the 1,3-diaminoinositol are substituted through glycosidic bonds with characteristic amino sugars to form pseudo-oligosaccharides. The chemistry, spectrum, potency, toxicity, and pharmacokinetics of these agents are a function of the specific identity of the diaminoinositol unit and the arrangement and identity of the attachments. The various aminoglycoside antibiotics are largely water soluble across the pH scale, are basic, and thus form acid salts; due to the high hydrophilicity, they are not absorbed in significant amounts from the GI tract; and they are excreted in high concentrations in the urine following injection as the active form. When the kidneys are not functioning efficiently, the dose needs to be adjusted accordingly to prevent accumulation of the drug to toxic levels. When given orally, their action is confined to the GI tract. Aminoglycosides are also used topically as solutions or ointments for ophthalmic infections. They can be given IM but are more commonly delivered by IV infusion. In addition, tobramycin is available for inhalation to treat *P. aeruginosa* infections in patients with cystic fibrosis (CF) and has led to improved pediatric treatment outcomes and improved patient compliance.[144,145] In 2018, the FDA also approved liposomal amikacin for inhalation use as part of a combination antibacterial drug regimen in the treatment of *Mycobacterium avium* complex (MAC) pulmonary disease in adults who have limited or no alternative treatment options.[146,147] Inhalation route of administration results in significantly reduced toxicity to the patient. Overall, the aminoglycoside/aminocyclitol antibiotics have intrinsically broad antimicrobial spectra, but their toxicity potential limits their clinical use to infections caused by gram-negative bacteria. Due to their high hydrophilicity, they are widely distributed in extracellular fluids, have low levels of protein binding, and synergize with a variety of other antibacterial classes.

Mechanism of Action. The aminoglycosides are bactericidal and often produce a prolonged PAE due to a combination of toxic effects. At therapeutic doses, they bind with high affinity to the A-site on the 16S rRNA portion of the 30S ribosomal subunit, impairing the proofreading function of the ribosome.[148] A conformational change occurs in the peptidyl A-site of the ribosome upon aminoglycoside binding. This leads to mistranslation of RNA templates and the selection of wrong amino acids and the formation of so-called nonsense proteins that cause damage to the cell membrane and other cellular compartments (Fig. 32.26). More recent data revealed that aminoglycosides bind not only to the small, 30S ribosomal subunit but also to the large, 50S subunit.[149,150] Some aminoglycosides can also interfere with protein synthesis by blocking the elongation step or by directly inhibiting initiation.

The unnatural (ie, prematurely terminated and nonsense) proteins have erratic folding patterns, are dysfunctional, and negatively impact functions of the bacterial membrane. Their presence destroys the semi-permeability of the membrane, and this damage cannot be repaired without de novo programmed protein biosynthesis. Among the substances that can enter the bacterial cell due to the damaged membrane are additional, large quantities of aminoglycoside. At these increased concentrations, protein biosynthesis ceases altogether. These combined effects are devastating to the target bacterial cells. Aminoglycosides are highly polar drugs, and cellular permeability through diffusion is expected to be low. However, they are able to penetrate the cell wall of gram-negative bacteria through interesting process of passive and active transport. First, due to their polycationic nature aminoglycosides bind through electrostatic interactions to negatively charged phospholipids and LPS.[148] This initial binding results in displacement of magnesium ions, which are responsible for cross-bridging and stabilization of the lipid components of the bacterial membrane.[148] Removal of the Mg^{2+} ions leads to disruption of the outer membrane, enhanced permeability, and initiation of aminoglycoside uptake.[148] On the contrary, elevated concentrations of Mg^{2+} stabilize the outer membrane and therefore inhibit the intracellular uptake of aminoglycosides. These ions are, therefore, partially incompatible therapeutically. Subsequent passage through the cytoplasmic membrane is dependent on electron transport and energy generation. While aminoglycoside/aminocyclitol antibiotics are relatively selective at therapeutic doses, their higher concentrations can lead to inhibition of eukaryotic protein biosynthesis.[151,152]

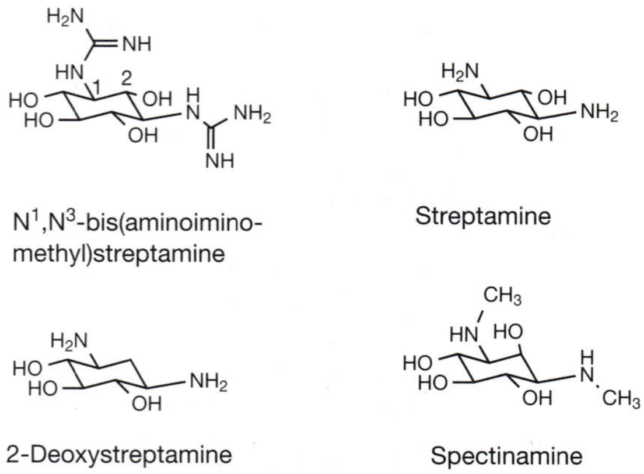

Figure 32.27 1,3-Diaminoinositol moieties present in aminoglycosides.

Bacterial Resistance. Bacterial resistance to aminoglycoside antibiotics in the clinic is most commonly conferred due to enzymatic modification of the drug molecule, target site modification, and efflux.[148] Bacterial elaboration of R-factor-mediated enzymes that *N*-acetylate (aminoglycoside acetyltransferase), *O*-phosphorylate (aminoglycoside phosphotransferase), and *O*-adenylate (aminoglycoside nucleotidyltransferase [ANT]) specific functional groups prevent the aminoglycosides from binding to their ribosomal targets (Fig. 32.28). In some cases, rational chemical deletion of the functional groups that are targeted and modified by these enzymes yields a molecule that still shows an antibiotic action but is no longer a substrate for these enzymes. These semisynthetic agents with intrinsically broader spectrum of activity and

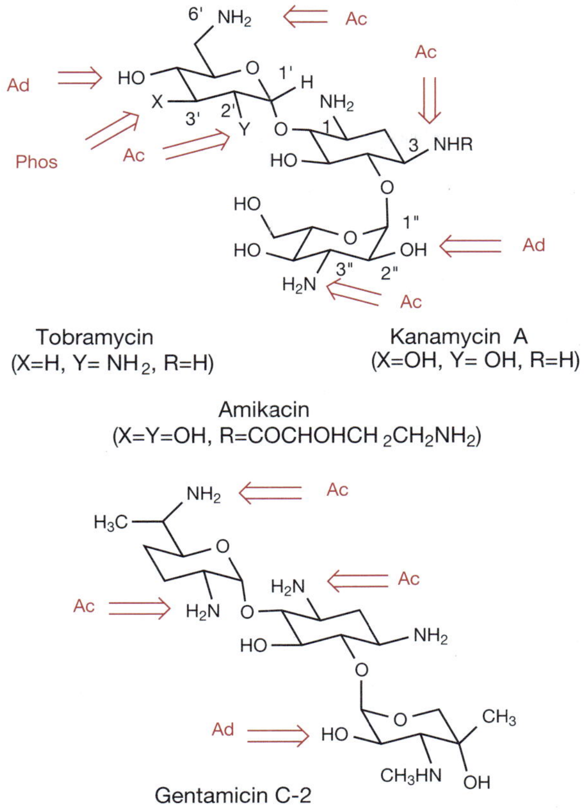

Figure 32.28 Commercially important 2-desylstreptamine-containing aminoglycosides. Some points of inactivating attack by specific R-factor-mediated enzymes are indicated by the following: Ac, acetylation; Ad, adenylation; Phos, phosphorylation. APH(3′)-1, for example, is an acronym for an enzyme that phosphorylates aminoglycosides at the 3′-OH position.

improved absorption, distribution, metabolism, and excretion-toxicity (ADMET) properties constitute an important treatment option. In other cases, bioisosteric replacement of functional groups and/or implementation of novel functional groups retains bioactivity of the medications and at the same time converts them to be poorer substrates for the R-factor-mediated enzymes. It is important to note that resistance developed in this way is not necessarily class-wide; therefore, susceptibility testing with multiple aminoglycosides should be used. Resistance can also stem from point mutations of the ribosomal A-site. These involve single-nucleotide residues at specific positions.[152] The substituent at position 6′ of the aminoglycoside, the number of protonated amino groups, and the linkage between the sugar rings and the central deoxystreptamine moiety are particularly important for the interactions with rRNA.

Adverse Effects. The adverse effects associated with the use of aminoglycosides involve toxicity to functions mediated by the eighth cranial nerve, most commonly exemplified by dose-dependent, irreversible hearing loss, which can be vestibular and/or cochlear.[153] Their use can also lead to renal tubular toxicity (nephrotoxicity), which in turn leads to decrease in glomerular function. However, renal effects associated with the use of aminoglycosides are generally reversible.[153] These toxic effects are related to the drug's blood levels and are apparently mediated by the special affinity of these aminoglycosides to kidney cells and to the sensory cells of the inner ear.[154] The effects may have a delayed onset, thus making them more dangerous because the patient can be injured significantly before symptoms appear, hence the product insert for these medications includes a boxed warning. Less commonly, curare-like neuromuscular blockade can exaggerate the muscle weakness in patients with myasthenia gravis and Parkinson disease.[155] In current practice, all of these toxic phenomena are well known; therefore, creatinine clearance should be determined and the dose adjusted downward accordingly to alleviate the unwanted adverse effects.

Therapeutic Application. Intrinsically, aminoglycosides have broad antibiotic spectra against aerobic gram-positive and gram-negative bacteria, but they are reserved for use in serious infections caused by gram-negative organisms because of their serious toxicities that are often delayed in onset. They are active against gram-negative aerobes such as *Acinetobacter* spp., *Citrobacter* spp., *Enterobacter* spp., *E. coli*, *Klebsiella* spp., *Proteus* spp., *Providencia* spp., *P. aeruginosa*, *Salmonella* spp., *Serratia* spp., and *Shigella* spp.[153] Of note is the application of the newest aminoglycoside, plazomicin, for the treatment of CRE- and ESBL-producing gram-negative bacteria.[156] Indications for this drug class include both empirical and directed treatment. In empirical therapy, aminoglycosides should not be used for more than 2 days, due to toxicity to the patient, whereas for directed treatment, aminoglycoside use for longer than 48 hours is acceptable.[153] Given the fact that aminoglycosides demonstrated effectiveness in MDR gram-negative pathogens, they are indicated for empiric therapy in patients with severe illness such as infective endocarditis, sepsis, complicated intra-abdominal infections, and complicated genitourinary infections.[153] Several of those aminoglycosides such as amikacin, STM, and kanamycin A are also important agents in the treatment of resistant TB, although kanamycin A is no longer marketed in the United States but is available in other countries. Spectinomycin differs from the others in its antimicrobial spectrum; however, it has been discontinued in the United States but is used to treat gonorrhea in other countries. Some of the aminoglycoside antibiotics with clinical application are illustrated in Figure 32.28, along with some of their sites of enzyme-mediated inactivation.

Overall, due to their relatively poor tissue penetration, aminoglycosides are not preferred choices for monotherapy. They are often used in combination therapy for infections caused by gram-negative organisms. If no other options are available, aminoglycosides can be used in synergy combination with β-lactam antibiotics for the treatment of endocarditis. TDM is required to ensure that plasma concentrations are sufficiently high for effective antimicrobial treatment and at the same time minimize the serious adverse effects (especially nephrotoxicity). Dosing is based on ideal body weight for several of these agents. It has been shown that higher doses given less frequently have equal effectiveness as traditional dosing but are associated with a lower risk for adverse reactions in comparison to conventional therapy.[157]

Specific Agents

Amikacin. Amikacin is a semisynthetic analog of the natural product kanamycin A (Fig. 32.28). Interestingly, the L-hydroxyaminobutyryl amide (HABA) moiety attached to N_3 inhibits adenylation and phosphorylation in the distant amino sugar ring (at $C_{2'}$ and $C_{3'}$) even though the HABA substituent is not where the enzymatic reaction takes place. This effect is attributed to decreased binding of this drug to the R-factor-mediated enzymes. With this change, the potency and spectrum are strongly enhanced while bacterial resistance is reduced; therefore, amikacin is used for the treatment of serious infections (eg, bone infection, respiratory tract infection, endocarditis, bloodstream infection, intra-abdominal infection, CNS infection, skin and soft tissue infection) caused by gram-negative organisms, including *Pseudomonas*, *E. coli*, *Proteus*, *Providencia*, *Klebsiella*, *Enterobacter*, *Serratia*, and *Acinetobacter*. Many strains of gram-negative organisms that are resistant to other members from this class have been shown to be sensitive to amikacin in vitro. Amikacin is also a second-line agent used for the treatment of multidrug-resistant tuberculosis (MDR-TB) in combination with other medications. In addition, amikacin is also used to treat other infections caused by MAC and nontuberculous mycobacteria (NTM) (eg, *Mycobacterium abscessus*).

This medication is administered predominantly as an IV or IM injection, but other routes of administration (eg, intraperitoneal, intrathecal, and intraventricular) are also possible. As mentioned previously, the liposomal formulation of amikacin (Arikayce) was FDA-approved in 2018 for oral inhalation in the treatment of MAC pulmonary disease in adult patients. Time to peak is strongly associated with the route of administration and it can be achieved in 0.5 hours for IV injection and 1 hour for IM injection. Average elimination half-life is approximately 2 hours in adults but it can be significantly extended (17-150 hours) in patients with renal failure. The drug is largely (>94%) eliminated in its active form in the urine.

DISCOVERY AND ISOLATION OF KANAMYCIN

Kanamycin was isolated from *Streptomyces kanamyceticus* in 1957 as a mixture of three chemicals: kanamycin A, B, and C, in which kanamycin A is the main component. Kanamycin A was one of the first aminoglycosides used in the clinic for several decades. Moreover, it serves as an advanced intermediate in the semisynthesis of amikacin (Fig. 32.28). Although it was used as an IV or IM injection (as a sulfate salt) for the treatment of infections caused by various pathogens, it mostly gained recognition as a second-line agent for the treatment of resistant strains of Mtb, the causative agent of TB. However, because of its toxicity and the emergence of resistant organisms, kanamycin A is no longer marketed in the United States, but it is still an important antibacterial agent utilized in many countries, especially those located in the developing regions of the world.

Tobramycin. Tobramycin is one component of a mixture produced by fermentation of *Streptomyces tenebrarius* (Fig. 32.28). Lacking the $C_{3'}$ hydroxyl group, it is not a substrate for APH(3′)-I and -II, and thus has an intrinsically broader spectrum than kanamycin. It is a substrate, however, for adenylation at $C_{2'}$ by ANT(2′) and acetylation at C_3 by AAC(3)-I and -II and at $C_{2'}$ by AAC(2′) (Fig. 32.28). It is used parenterally for the treatment of difficult infections, as listed for amikacin. It is also used for the treatment of pneumonia caused by various bacteria in adult and pediatric patients. Tobramycin is also available as ophthalmic drops (Tobrex) to treat superficial eye infections and oral inhalation (Bethkis, Kitabis Pak, Tobi) for the management of CF in adults and pediatric patients (age >6 years) with *P. aeruginosa*. Tobramycin's route of administration and pharmacokinetic properties are similar to those described for amikacin.

Gentamicin. Gentamicin is a mixture of several antibiotic components produced by the fermentation of *Micromonospora purpurea* and other related soil microorganisms (hence its name is spelled with an "i" instead of a "y"). Gentamicins C-l, C-2, and C-1a are most prominent (gentamicin C-2 is shown in Fig. 32.28). Gentamicin was one of the first antibiotics to have significant activity against *P. aeruginosa* infections. This water-loving opportunistic pathogen is frequently encountered in burns, pneumonias, and UTIs, and it is highly virulent. As noted earlier, some of the functional groups that serve as targets for R-factor-mediated enzymes are missing in the structure of gentamicin, so their antibacterial spectrum is enhanced. They are, however, inactivated through $C_{2'}$ adenylation by enzyme ANT(2′) and acetylation at $C_{6'}$ by AAC(6′), at C_1 by AAC(1)-I and -II, and at $C_{2'}$ by AAC(2′). Gentamicin is often combined with other anti-infective agents, and an interesting incompatibility has been uncovered. With certain β-lactam antibiotics, the two drugs react with each other so that *N*-acylation on C_1 of gentamicin by the β-lactam antibiotic takes place, thus inactivating both antibiotics (Fig. 32.29). The two agents should not, therefore, be mixed in the same solution and should ideally be administered into different tissue compartments to prevent this detrimental interaction. This incompatibility is likely to be associated with other aminoglycoside antibiotics as well. Gentamicin is used for sepsis, meningitis, UTIs, respiratory tract infections, peritonitis, bone infections, and skin and soft tissue infections caused by susceptible gram-negative bacteria. Ophthalmic gentamicin is used for the topical treatment of ocular bacterial infections, including conjunctivitis, whereas topical gentamicin is used for the treatment of various primary and secondary skin infections. Gentamicin's route of administration and pharmacokinetic properties are similar to those of amikacin.

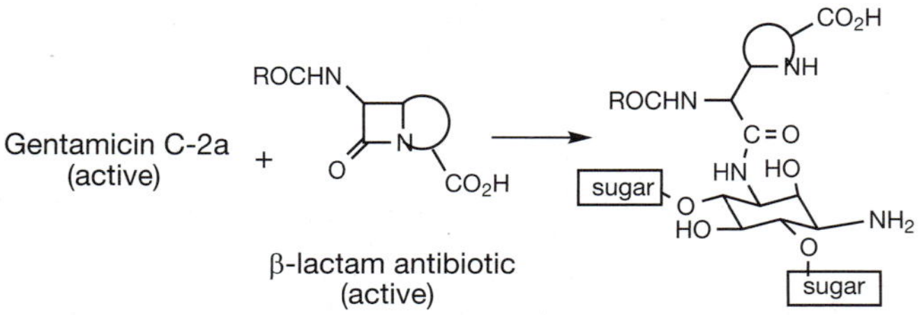

Figure 32.29 Chemical drug-drug incompatibility between gentamicin C-2a and β-lactams.

Streptomycin

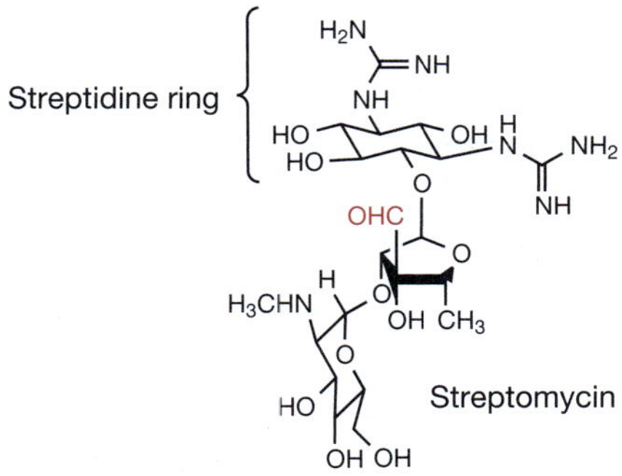

STM is produced by fermentation of *Streptomyces griseus* and several related soil microorganisms. Selman Waksman and his student Albert Schatz by the end of 1943 refined STM as the first clinically useful aminoglycoside antibiotic effective against *M. tuberculosis*. The structure was proposed and later confirmed by Kuehl and coworkers in 1948.[158] STM was also the first antibiotic to be effective and clinically useful in the treatment of TB, a devastating disease with no cure at that time. Waksman received the Nobel Prize in 1952 for his discovery of STM.[155] STM differs from the typical aminoglycosides as it carries a modified pharmacophore in that the diaminoinositol unit is a streptidine moiety. Additionally, STM has an axial hydroxyl group at C_2 and two highly basic guanidino groups at C_1 and C_3 in place of the primary amine moieties of 2-deoxystreptamine. It is possible that the particular pharmacophore of STM accounts in large measure for its unusual antibacterial spectrum. Another molecular feature, the α-hydroxyaldehyde moiety, is a center of instability such that STM cannot be sterilized by autoclaving, so STM sulfate solutions that need sterilization are made by ultrafiltration. Modification of the α-streptose portion of STM that contains the aldehyde group has been extensively studied. Reduction of the aldehyde to the corresponding alcohol results in a compound referred to as dihydrostreptomycin, which has activity comparable to STM but with a greater potential for producing delayed, severe deafness. Oxidation of the aldehyde to a carboxyl group or conversion to Schiff base derivatives (eg, oxime, semicarbazone, or phenylhydrazone) results in inactive analogs. Oxidation of the methyl group in α-streptose to the corresponding hydroxymethyl group gives an active analog that has no advantage over STM. Modification of the aminomethyl group in the glucosamine portion of the molecule by demethylation or by replacement with larger alkyl groups reduces activity, whereas removal or modification of either guanidine in the streptidine nucleus also decreases activity. STM is administered as an IM injection, with time to peak being achieved within 1 to 2 hours. The elimination half-life ranges between 2 and 5 hours and it is prolonged in patients with renal impairment. The majority of the dose (up to 89%) is excreted unchanged in the urine.

STM is rarely used today as a single agent due to the apparent toxicity and resistance developed over the decades to this agent. Combination drug therapy was partially successful in reducing this problem, but over time, resistance has greatly reduced the value of STM as a chemotherapeutic agent for the treatment of TB. Permeability barriers can result in STM not being transported through the cytoplasmic membrane, but the evidence appears to suggest that enzymatic inactivation of STM via *N*-acetylation, *O*-phosphorylation, and *O*-adenylation of specific functional groups represents the major problem. The adenylyltransferase enzymes catalyze adenylation of the C_3 hydroxyl group in the *N*-methylglucosamine moiety to give the O-3-adenylated metabolite, and phosphotransferase phosphorylates the same C_3 hydroxyl to give the O-3-phosphorylate metabolite. The result of these chemical modifications is that the produced metabolites will not bind to bacterial ribosomes and the drug's bioactivity is lost. Additional resistance mechanism includes two changes within the ribosome: first, S12 protein undergoes a change in which the lysine present at amino acids 43 and 88 in ribosomal protein S12 is replaced with arginine or threonine; second, the pseudoknot conformation of 16S rRNA, which results from intramolecular base pairing between GCC bases in regions 524 to 526 of the rRNA to CGG bases in regions 505 to 507, is perturbed.[159] It is thought that S12 protein stabilizes the pseudoknot, which is essential for 16S rRNA function.

ORALLY USED AMINOGLYCOSIDES

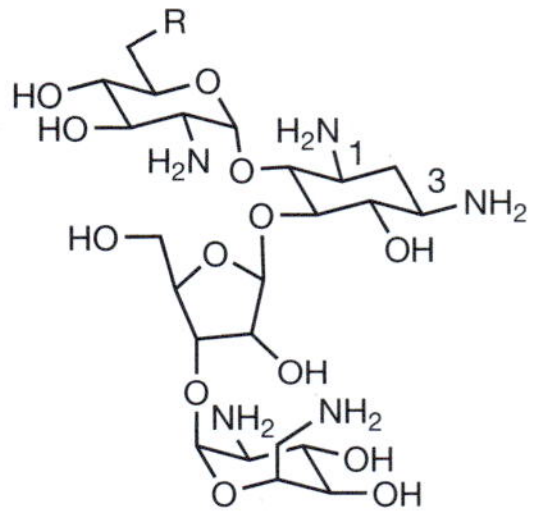

Neomycin B, R = NH_2
Paromomycom, R = OH

Neomycin finds some oral use for the suppression of gut flora in preparation for bowel surgery. Paromomycin (Humatin) is also used orally for the treatment of amoebic dysentery. Amoebas are persistent pathogens causing chronic diarrhea and are acquired most frequently by travelers who consume food supplies contaminated with human waste.

Neomycin. Neomycin is a mixture of three compounds (neomycin A, B, and C) produced by fermentation of *Streptomyces fradiae*, with neomycin B predominating.[160] Although it is not normally considered to have systemic absorption when administered orally, neomycin now has a boxed warning related to systemic toxicities due to absorption in ulcerated or denuded areas of the GI tract.[161] It is also found in nonprescription ointments (in combination with polymyxin B and/or glucocorticoids) for topical use in the treatment of bacterial skin infections. When applied to intact skin, the drug is not absorbed, but if applied to large, denuded areas, systemic absorption occurs with the potential to cause toxic adverse effects, hence the boxed warning.

Paromomycin. Paromomycin (Humatin) is produced by *Streptomyces rimosus* var. *paromomycinus*. It is a hydroxy (R = OH) analog of neomycin B that represents cyclitol, a cycloalkane containing at least three hydroxyl groups each attached to a different ring carbon atom. It is currently the only aminoglycoside on the US market that is not accompanied with boxed warning. Paromomycin also shows antiprotozoal activity.

Newer Aminoglycosides

PLAZOMICIN

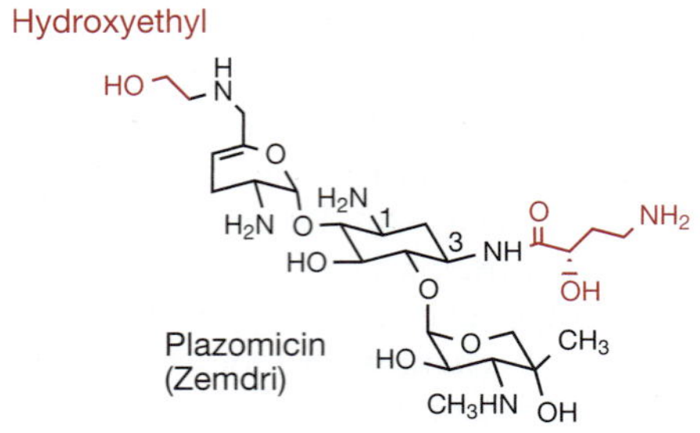

Plazomicin (Zemdri) is considered a next-generation aminoglycoside that is resistant to many aminoglycoside-modifying enzymes. It was approved in 2018 for the treatment of complicated UTIs in adults. It has been demonstrated to be effective in infections associated with *E. coli*, *K. pneumoniae*, *P. mirabilis*, and *Enterobacter cloacae*.[162]

Plazomicin is a semisynthetic derivative of another aminoglycoside sisomicin, which was isolated from *Micromonospora*, and it is structurally and pharmacologically related to gentamicin. Addition of the HABA group and a hydroxyethyl side chain to the sisomicin structure resulted in plazomicin.[163] This antibiotic reaches its peak plasma concentrations right after the IV infusion is completed, and the half-life ranges between 3 and 4 hours. It is exclusively excreted in the urine. The modified structure and improved pharmacokinetic properties make plazomicin a suitable choice for the treatment of CRE- and ESBL-producing gram-negative microorganisms.

Macrolide Antibiotics

The term "macrolide" is derived from the characteristic large lactone (cyclic ester) ring found in these antibiotics. Although a 14-membered macrocyclic skeleton is the most prevalent in the approved and clinically used macrolide antibiotics in the United States, other ring sizes such as the 12- and 16-membered macrocycles found in the first-generation natural products and the 15-membered second-generation semisynthetic derivatives (eg, azithromycin) are well known.[164] Macrolide antibiotics with 16-membered rings are generally popular outside the United States. However, one example, tylosin (Tylan), finds extensive use in veterinary medicine in the United States. The clinically important antibiotics in the macrolide family (Fig. 32.30) have two or more characteristic sugars (usually cladinose and desosamine) attached to the 14-membered ring. One of these sugars usually carries a substituted amino group, so their overall chemical character is weakly basic with a pK_a range between 8 and 9. The free base form of macrolide antibiotics is not very water soluble; however, the use of water- and lipid-soluble salts can alter the solubility. As shown in Figure 32.30, lactobionic acid increases water solubility, whereas stearic acid decreases solubility. The 12- and 14-membered ring macrolides are postulated to be biosynthesized via the route of acetyl-coenzyme A with the addition of malonyl-coenzyme A into the growing chain or the alternative biosynthetic pathway based on direct incorporation of propionic acid units.[165,166] More recently, butyric acid has been identified as a precursor involved in the biosynthesis of 16-membered ring macrolide antibiotics.[167] Upon construction of the macrocyclic ring (Fig. 32.31), the two hydroxyl groups on C_3 and C_5 are glycosylated.

CHEMICAL PROPERTIES. The early macrolides of the erythromycin class are chemically unstable due to rapid acid-catalyzed internal cyclic ketal formation between the C_6 hydroxyl group and C_9 ketone group, leading to inactivity (Fig. 32.32). This reaction is promoted in the acidic

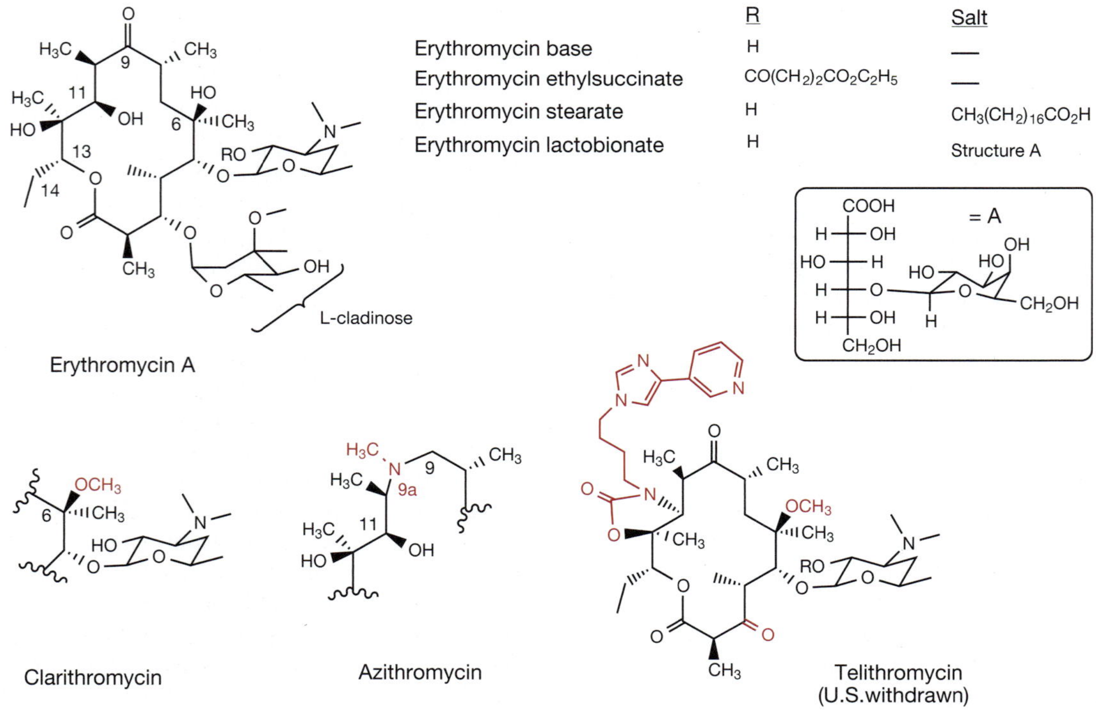

Figure 32.30 Clinically important macrolide antibiotics.

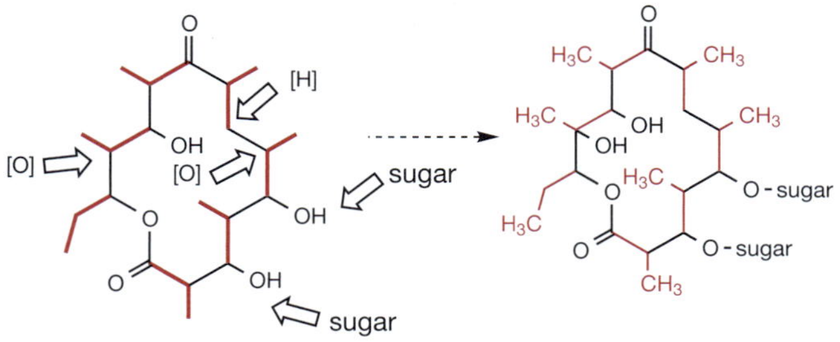

Figure 32.31 Biosynthetic pathway to erythromycins from propionic acid units. (↑ refers to modifications to the basic ring skeleton.)

environment of the GI tract, and thus it has clinical implications. Most acid-susceptible macrolides are administered in enteric-coated tablets to minimize the unwanted decomposition of the drug and thus significantly decrease the negative effects of the decomposition by-products on the GI tract. Newer analogs have been prepared semisynthetically that are chemically resistant to this reaction and have become very popular in the clinic.[168] Many macrolides have an unpleasant taste, which is partially overcome by applying water-insoluble dosage forms that also reduce acid instability and help alleviate the aforementioned GI adverse effects, such as gut cramps.

Mechanism of Action. The macrolides interfere with programmed ribosomal protein biosynthesis via binding to the 23S rRNA and occupying a site within the nascent peptide exit tunnel (NPET) adjacent to the peptidyl transferase center (PTC) in the large 50S ribosomal subunit (Fig. 32.26).[164] More specifically, they interact via hydrogen bonding with a nucleobase of the 23S rRNA, and their binding is additionally stabilized by tight packing of the hydrophobic face of the lactone ring against rRNA nucleotides.[164] This binding results in extremely low dissociation

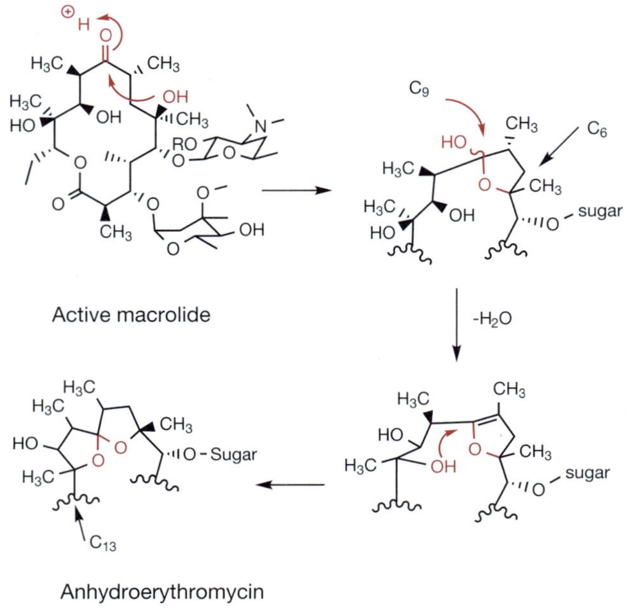

Figure 32.32 Acid-catalyzed intramolecular ketal formation with erythromycin.

rate constants for some macrolides, thus making them almost irreversibly bound to the ribosome.[164] This in turn prevents the growing peptide from becoming longer than a few residues, subsequently resulting in the dissociation of peptidyl tRNA molecules. Although the macrolides are generally considered to produce a bacteriostatic effect, depending on the specific organism and the drug's concentration, they may also be bactericidal. Chloramphenicol and the clinically used lincosamides (clindamycin and lincomycin) bind in the same vicinity, leading to extensive cross-resistance among all these agents.

Resistance. Bacterial resistance primarily occurs in bacteria that possess R-factor enzymes that methylate a specific guanine residue on their rRNA. While this makes the bacteria somewhat less efficient at protein biosynthesis, they are comparatively poor binders of macrolides.[169] The erythromycin-producing soil organism uses the same ribosomal methylation technique to protect itself against the toxic effects of its own metabolite.[169] This leads to the speculation that the origin of some antibiotic resistance genes may lie in the producing organism itself and that this genetic material is acquired by other bacteria via a variety of mechanisms. Other possibilities to inactivate this class of agents include phosphorylation of the 2′-hydroxyl of the sugar by phosphotransferases and hydrolysis of the macrocyclic lactone by esterases. A second mechanism of resistance is associated with the mutation of adenine to guanine that occurs in domain V at A2058. This change results in a 10,000-fold reduction of binding capacity of erythromycin and clarithromycin to the 23S rRNA. Some bacterial strains, however, appear to be resistant to macrolides due to the operation of an active efflux process in which the drug is expelled from the cell at the cost of energy.[169] The efflux proteins belong mainly to Mef and Msr families and counteract the drug's action by working as antiporters and thus exchange the bound macrolide with a proton (Mef) or by offering ribosome protection by binding, displacing, and chasing the bound drug from the ribosome.[164] Intrinsic resistance of gram-negative bacteria is primarily caused by lack of penetration through their cell wall as the ribosomes isolated from these organisms are often inhibited by the macrolide antibiotics.

Adverse Effects and Drug Interactions. DDIs with macrolides are comparatively common and usually involve inhibition of CYP3A4 isoform of the cytochrome P450 oxidase superfamily.[170] Moreover, some of the macrolide antibiotics (erythromycin and clarithromycin) are thought to be metabolized by CYP3A4 in the liver and they also inhibit CYP3A4 by forming inactive complexes with this metabolizing enzyme through their nitrosoalkane metabolites.[171] There is also evidence suggesting that these interactions are intensified by the inhibition of the ATP-dependent efflux pump, P-glycoprotein (Pgp).[170,172] The result of these effects on CYP3A4 and Pgp can have severely negative consequences for the patient as increased drug concentration and thus enhanced potential toxicity over time is observed. Examples are seen with the concurrent use of macrolides and 3-hydroxy-3-methylglutaryl coenzyme A (HMG-CoA) reductase inhibitors (also known as statins). The combination use of erythromycin and simvastatin results in a 6-fold increase in the area under the curve (AUC) of simvastatin. Similar to this, concomitant use of erythromycin and lovastatin results in rhabdomyolysis possibly due to both decreased metabolism and efflux of lovastatin.[171] In general, macrolide antibiotics are known to cause QT prolongation due to binding to and blocking the rapid component of the delayed rectifier potassium current (IKr) encoded by the human Ether-à-go-go-Related Gene encoding the α-subunit of K^+ ion channel (hERG), hence their potential to cause cardiac arrhythmias. Additionally, use of this class of agents is associated with hepatotoxicity and GI disturbance, the latter being greater with clarithromycin and erythromycin.

Therapeutic Application. Overall, the macrolides are orally bioavailable, relatively well tolerated, and are considered to have a broad spectrum of activity against many gram-positive bacteria. Therefore, they are often used for the treatment of various mild-to-moderate bacterial infections, which include pneumonia, sinusitis, pharyngitis, and tonsillitis. Due to their favorable properties, macrolides are also used in uncomplicated skin infections and otitis media in pediatric patients.[173]

Macrolide antibiotics are used for the treatment of upper and lower respiratory tract and soft tissue infections primarily caused by gram-positive microorganisms like *S. pyogenes* and *S. pneumoniae*, Legionnaires' disease, prophylaxis of bacterial endocarditis caused by *S. viridans* (although contraindicated in patients with existing cardiac arrhythmia), otitis media caused by *H. influenzae* (in combination with sulfonamide), mycoplasma pneumonia, and MAC infections in patients with acquired immunodeficiency syndrome (AIDS) (in combination with aminoglycosides, rifamycins, or other agents).[174] The utility of the macrolides against upper respiratory tract infections is enhanced by their affinity for these tissues. Tissue levels in the upper respiratory tract are often several times higher than those seen in the blood. In addition to the abovementioned application, they are used for the treatment of certain sexually transmitted diseases, such as gonococcal and chlamydial infections.[173] Clarithromycin is also used to treat gastric ulcers due to *H. pylori* infection as a component of multidrug cocktails.

Specific Agents

Erythromycin Base, Esters, and Salts

Erythromycin Base (Erythromycin, Eryc, Erygel). The original natural product (Fig. 32.30) was isolated from *Saccharopolyspora erythraea* (formerly *Streptomyces erythraeus*) and is available in various dosage forms and strengths: tablets, capsules, and delayed-release pellets for oral administration; gels, solutions, and swabs for topical applications; and an ophthalmic ointment.[175] It is prescribed for the treatment of various infections caused by gram-positive, gram-negative, and other microorganisms. The most common dose for adult patients is 250 mg every 6 hours taken 1 hour before meals, whereas pediatric uses are based on the child's age, body weight, and severity of the infection.[175] The drug has significant plasma protein binding of 73% to 81%, time to peak of approximately 4 hours, and half-life of 1.5 to 2 hours. It undergoes extensive hepatic CYP3A4-mediated metabolism to give the *N*-demethylation product, which is predominantly excreted in bile.

Erythromycin Ethylsuccinate (EryPed, Ery-Tab, E.E.S.). Erythromycin ethylsuccinate (Fig. 32.30) is a mixed double-ester prodrug in which one carboxyl group of succinic acid esterifies the $C_{2'}$ hydroxyl of erythromycin and the other ethanol (Fig. 32.30). This prodrug is frequently used as an oral, cherry-flavored suspension for pediatric use largely to mask the bitter taste of the drug. Film-coated tablets are predominantly prescribed for older children and adults. Time to peak after oral administration is between 0.5 and 2.5 hours and it might be delayed when the medications are taken with food. Hepatic dysfunction manifested by increased liver enzymes and hepatocellular and/or cholestatic hepatitis (with or without jaundice) was reported in patients receiving oral erythromycin ethylsuccinate.[176,177]

Erythromycin Stearate. Erythromycin stearate (Fig. 32.30) is a lipid-soluble salt form of erythromycin. This decreases the water solubility and aqueous dissolution of erythromycin and helps mask the taste of the drug and enhances its stability in the stomach. It is available as film-coated tablets for oral administration (250 mg every 6 hours; or 500 mg every 12 hours) taken in the fasting state or immediately before meal.[178] Peak concentrations are achieved within 3 hours.

Erythromycin Lactobionate. Erythromycin lactobionate (Fig. 32.30) is a salt with enhanced water solubility that is used as an IV injection for the treatment of various infections. The injections are usually administered every 6 hours, and this route of administration ensures the fastest peak plasma concentrations that are achieved in 1 hour.

Clarithromycin. Clarithromycin differs from erythromycin in that the C_6 hydroxy group has been converted semisynthetically to a methyl ether (Fig. 32.30). The C_6 hydroxy group is involved in the unwanted process initiated by protons at lower pH, leading to internal cyclic ketal formation in erythromycin that results in drug inactivation (Fig. 32.32). This ketal, or one of the products of its subsequent degradation, is also associated with GI discomfort and cramping. Conversion of the C_6 hydroxyl group to a methyl ether significantly decreases the nucleophilicity of the functional group, enhances the lipophilicity of the drug, and prevents internal ketal formation. This chemical change not only gives better blood levels through chemical stabilization, but also results in less gastric upset. An extensive saturable first-pass liver metabolism of clarithromycin leads to formation of its C_{14} hydroxy analog, which has even greater antimicrobial potency, especially against *H. influenzae*.[179] Immediate-release (IR) and extended-release (ER) formulations are available and applied as follows: 500 mg of IR every 12 hours or 1 g of ER once daily. These formulations also impact the time to peak parameter, which is 2 to 3 hours for IR and 5 to 8 hours for ER. The modest bioavailability of ~50% dictates the most common dose to be 500 mg. However, for mild infections, lower and less frequent dosage is applied. In early 2018, the FDA issued a safety communication before prescribing clarithromycin to patients with heart disease as increased risk of heart problems or even death can occur years later following use of this medication.

Azithromycin (Zithromax, Zithromax Tri-Pak/Z-Pak, AzaSite, Klarity-A). Azithromycin, also referred to as an "azalide" due to the presence of nitrogen atom, was formed by the semisynthetic conversion of erythromycin to a ring-expanded analog in which an *N*-methyl group has been inserted between carbons 9 and 10 and the carbonyl moiety is thus absent (Fig. 32.30). Due to the ring expansion achieved through the means of synthetic medicinal chemistry, azithromycin has therefore a 15-membered lactone ring. Since the C_9 ketone group is absent, the new functionality does not form a cyclic internal ketal with the hydroxyl group on C_6. Therefore, azithromycin is not only more stable to acid degradation than erythromycin but also it has a considerably longer half-life (68-72 hours in adults), attributed to greater and longer tissue penetration, allowing once-a-day dosing. This antibiotic is available in several dosage forms including oral tablet and suspension, IV injection, and ophthalmic drops. The oral dosage forms have moderate bioavailability (34%-52%, but it is increased for the suspension when taken with food), moderate plasma protein binding (~50%), and about half of the dose is excreted unchanged in the bile. A popular treatment schedule with azithromycin is to take 500 mg in a single loading dose on the first day followed by either 250 mg once daily on days 2 to 5 or 500 mg once daily for 3 days. This is especially convenient for patients who present challenges with compliance. An oral suspension may be administered with or without food whereas the tablet, if administered with food, produces decreased GI adverse effects. Azithromycin tends to be a broader spectrum agent than either erythromycin or clarithromycin. Azithromycin has a significant PAE against a number of pathogens.[180] Azithromycin is now commonly the first choice for treatment of infections that require a macrolide.

Fidaxomicin (Dificid)

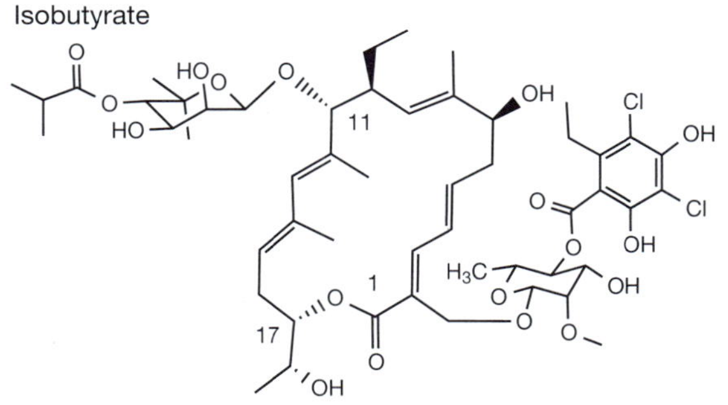

Fidaxomicin (Dificid)

Fidaxomicin is a unique 18-membered macrolide isolated from the fermentation broth of *Dactylosporangium aurantiacum*. It is poorly absorbed upon oral administration, and it is primarily used to treat *C. difficile*–associated diarrhea (CDAD). *C. difficile* releases toxins, which can cause bloating and diarrhea that in turn can be life threatening. The narrow spectrum of activity and high effectiveness of cure rate (88%) of patients suffering from this microorganism lead to minimal disruption of normal intestinal flora whereas the lack of oral absorption leads to minimal systemic adverse effects.[181] The MOA is distinct from other macrolides, in that fidaxomicin exerts its bactericidal activity via noncompetitive inhibition of the DNA-directed RNA polymerase (DDRP), thus interfering with protein synthesis. Hydrolysis of the isobutyl ester on the C_{11} sugar by intestinal enzymes produces a metabolite that still retains significant activity, although lower than that of the parent compound.[182]

DEVELOPMENT OF KETOLIDES

Extensive research efforts in the macrolide antibiotic class have been focused on attempts to reduce their side effects and to broaden their antimicrobial spectra. The ketolides are a group of agents that are characterized by oxidation of the 3-hydroxyl group to a ketone (hence the name of this drug class). These new derivatives turned out to be active against a significant number of erythromycin-resistant microorganisms, including azithromycin-resistant strains due to the enhanced binding at ribosome facilitated by the *N*-aryl-alkyl side chain appended on C_{11}.

Telithromycin (Fig. 32.30) was approved for oral treatment of community-acquired pneumonia, acute bacterial exacerbations of chronic bronchitis, and acute sinusitis in 2004. However, significant controversy about the safety of this agent arose after approval by the FDA, which ultimately led to the removal of two indications, issuing an additional warning information about liver toxicity (which can be fatal) and a boxed warning regarding use in patients with myasthenia gravis. The drug was withdrawn from the US market shortly after the decision by the FDA. The toxicity reported for telithromycin appears to be associated with the pyridine portion of the molecule and the antagonist action of the drug on cholinergic receptors (due to structural similarity of the imidazole-pyridine moiety with nicotine).

Lincosamides

Mechanism of Action and Chemical and Absorption, Distribution, Metabolism, and Excretion-Toxicity Properties. The lincosamides (Fig. 32.33) contain an unusual 8-carbon sugar, a thiomethyl amino-octoside (O-thiolincosamide), that is linked by an amide bond to 1-methyl-4-propylpyrrolidine-2-carboxylic acid (4-n-propyl hygric acid). Due to the tertiary nitrogen atom in the pyrrolidine ring, lincosamides are weakly basic and form clinically useful salts with hydrochloric acid. Although they are chemically distinct from the macrolide antibiotics, lincosamides possess many pharmacologic similarities with them. The lincosamides bind to 50S ribosomal subunit, thus affecting the process of peptide chain initiation. Since they bind at a site that partly overlaps with the macrolide binding site, these two drug classes essentially have the same molecular MOA and thus show cross-resistance (Fig. 32.26). Chemical conversion of the lincomycin's C_7 hydroxyl group into chlorine gives a semisynthetic derivative, clindamycin, that is both more lipophilic and more active.[183] The medications undergo extensive hepatic metabolism resulting primarily in *N*-demethylation and *S*-oxidation. The *N*-desmethyl and sulfoxide metabolites have insignificant antimicrobial activity and are excreted in the bile. The lincosamide medications are generally considered as

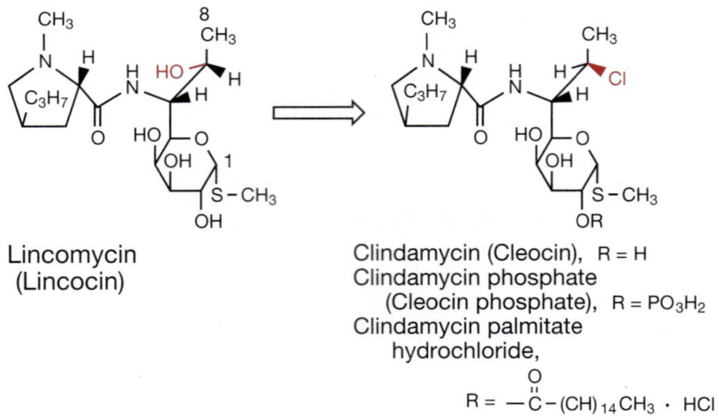

Figure 32.33 Structures of the approved lincosamides.

broad-spectrum bacteriostatic antibiotics that are particularly active against gram-positive bacteria including some anaerobes. The agents from this drug class are accompanied with a boxed warning as CDAD and severe colitis were reported with their use.

Specific Agents

Lincomycin (Lincocin). Lincomycin (Fig. 32.33) is a natural product isolated from fermentations of *Streptomyces lincolnensis.* This agent is indicated for the treatment of serious infections caused by sensitive strains of streptococci, pneumococci, and staphylococci. It is generally reserved for patients with penicillin allergy. It is administered as an IV, IM, or subconjunctival ocular injection and has an elimination half-life of approximately 5 hours. The natural product serves as the starting material for the synthesis of clindamycin. An SN2 nucleophilic substitution reaction inverts the R-stereochemistry of the C_7 hydroxyl to a C_7 chloroderivative with an S-stereochemistry.

Clindamycin (Cleocin, Cleocin Phosphate, Clindacin, Clindagel, Clindesse, Xaciato). Clindamycin (Fig. 32.33) is more active and lipophilic than lincomycin, and thus, it is better absorbed following oral administration. When taken orally as a hydrochloride salt, it is rapidly absorbed from the GI tract to the extent of 90%. Clindamycin palmitate hydrochloride for oral solution is a prodrug of clindamycin that lacks the bitter taste, but it must be hydrolyzed in the GI tract before it is active. It is obtained by converting the C_2 hydroxyl into an ester with palmitic acid, a 16-carbon saturated fatty acid. The orally administered medication is vastly bound (94%) to plasma proteins, achieves peak plasma concentration in approximately 1 hour, and has an elimination half-life in adults of ~3 hours (extended to 3.5-5 hours in older adults). Additional dosage forms and routes of administrations include IV and IM injection of a sterile phosphate solution; foam, gel, lotion, solution, and pledget for topical use; as well as cream, gel, and suppository for vaginal use. Clindamycin is used for the treatment of septicemia, intra-abdominal, lower respiratory, gynecologic, bone and joint, and skin and skin structure infections. It is also used to treat streptococcal pharyngitis, acne vulgaris, bacterial vaginosis, and severe pelvic inflammatory disease.[184] Clindamycin is also very useful in gynecology for patients with endometritis and bacterial vaginosis and in dentistry for prophylactic uses against endocarditis.[184] This medication can be used to treat babesiosis, anthrax, and malaria and also showed effectiveness against MRSA. Clindamycin has excellent activity against *Propionibacterium acnes* when applied topically.[185] The improved bioactivity and tissue penetration of clindamycin are associated with various unwanted adverse effects such as CDAD (requiring a boxed warning), severe colitis, GI problems (nausea, vomiting, cramps, and drug-related diarrhea).[185] Vaginal pain for the formulations used vaginally as well as burning sensation of skin and oily skin for topical applications were reported. Inducible clindamycin resistance (iMLS$_B$ phenotype) D-test to treat S. *aureus* infections must be performed in order to detect inducible clindamycin resistance in staphylococci for the optimum treatment of patients.[186]

The lincosamide pharmacophore is currently a subject of intensive medicinal chemistry and drug discovery research that led recently to the identification of two viable preclinical candidates, iboxamycin and cresomycin, that possess improved activity, spectrum, and efficacy against MDR bacteria.[187,188]

Tetracyclines, Aminomethylcyclines, Fluorocyclines, and Glycylcyclines

The traditional tetracycline drug class comprised several medications that were widely prescribed across the globe. To date, only a few of the original agents still find applications in clinical practice. Of the agents, demeclocycline, doxycycline, minocycline, and tetracycline are still frequently prescribed in the United States. Within the last two decades, many of the originally approved tetracycline antibiotics were replaced with newer derivatives that are more effective against drug-resistant bacterial strains (Table 32.11). These agents were developed through rational modifications of the original tetracycline skeleton to provide modified pharmacophores referred to as aminomethylcyclines, fluorocyclines, and glycylcyclines. In general, this family of antibiotics is characterized by a highly functionalized, partially reduced tetracene ring system (also known as naphthacene that possesses four linearly fused six-membered aromatic rings) from which both the drug's class name and numbering system are derived (Fig. 32.34A).

Chemical Properties. The tetracyclines are amphoteric substances with three pK_a values revealed by titration (2.8-3.4, 7.2-7.8, and 9.1-9.7) and have an isoelectric point at about pH 5. The basic function is the C_4-α-dimethylamino group. The conjugated phenolic enone system extending from C_{10} to C_{12} is associated with the pK_a at about 7.5, whereas the conjugated trione system extending from C_1 to C_3 in ring A is nearly as acidic as acetic acid (pK_a ~3).[189] The amphoteric nature of these medications leads to formation of zwitterion at physiologic pH, which additionally impacts their water solubility. The resonating systems in the tetracycline skeleton can be drawn in a number of essentially equivalent ways with the double bonds in alternate positions. The formulae normally shown are those settled upon by popular convention. The molecular architecture of tetracycline core along with the conjugated system of

Table 32.11 Clinically Important Tetracyclines and Their Derivatives

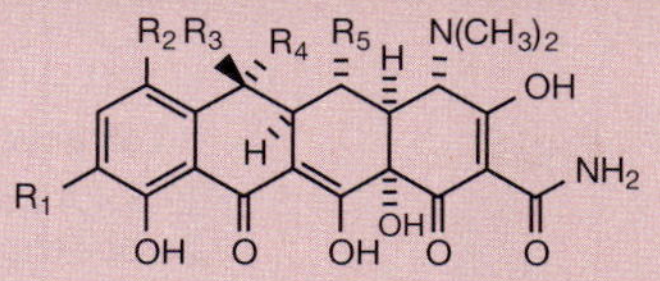

Generic Name	Trade Name	R_1	R_2	R_3	R_4	R_5
Tetracyclines						
Tetracycline	Generic	H	H	OH	CH_3	H
Demeclocycline	Generic	H	Cl	OH	H	H
Doxycycline	Avidoxy, Doryx MPC, Doxy 100 Mondoxyne NL, Oracea, TargaDOX, Vibramycin	H	H	H	CH_3	OH
Minocycline	Arestin, Amzeeq, Minocin, Solodyn, Zilxi	H	$N(CH_3)_2$	H	H	H
Aminomethylcyclines						
Omadacycline	Nuzyra	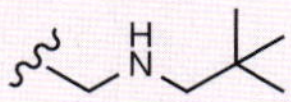	$N(CH_3)_2$	H	H	H
Sarecycline	Seysara	H	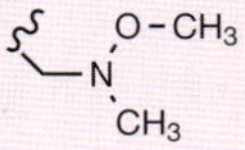	H	H	H
Glycylcycline and Fluorocyclines						
Eravacycline	Xerava	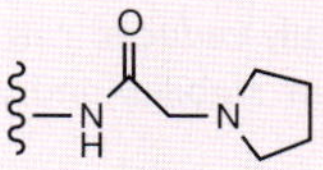	F	H	H	H
Tigecycline	Tygacil	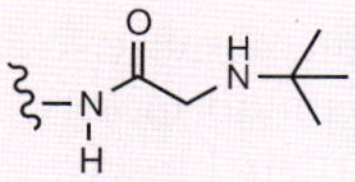	$N(CH_3)_2$	H	H	H

double bonds makes tetracycline a very adaptive molecule, capable of easily modifying itself through tautomerism in response to various chemical environments.[190] In theory, there are 64 possible tautomers, two of which are shown in Figure 32.34B.

Chelation. Chelation is an important chemical process associated with the use of tetracyclines and it has serious clinical implications. The acidic functions of the tetracyclines can form salts through chelation with metal ions. The salts created with polyvalent metal ions, such as Fe^{2+}, Fe^{3+}, Ca^{2+}, Mg^{2+}, and Al^{3+}, are all quite insoluble at neutral pH (Fig. 32.34B). This insolubility is not only inconvenient for the preparation of solutions, but also interferes with achieving therapeutic blood levels upon oral administration. Consequently, the tetracyclines are incompatible with coadministered multivalent ion-rich antacids, and concomitant consumption of daily products rich in calcium ion is also contraindicated.[189] When concomitant oral therapy with tetracyclines and incompatible metal ions needs to be implemented, a time gap in administration of these products must be introduced, usually either should be taken 1 hour before or 2 hours after the tetracyclines. Furthermore, the bones, of which the teeth are the most visible, are calcium-rich structures and during their formation, they readily bind and accumulate tetracyclines in proportion to the amount and duration of therapy. Because the tetracyclines are yellow to dark orange in color, this leads to a progressive and essentially permanent discoloration of teeth that, in advanced cases, makes them even brown. The intensification of discoloration with time is thought to be a photochemical process. This is a cosmetically unattractive adverse effect but it does not seem to be deleterious except in extreme cases where so much antibiotic is taken up that the structure of bone is mechanically weakened. To avoid this scenario, tetracyclines are normally not recommended for children.[189]

Epimerization. The behavior of tetracyclines in solution depends on several factors, including pH and the dielectric constant of the solvent. Tetracyclines could undergo four deprotonations leading to 64 tautomers, which directly

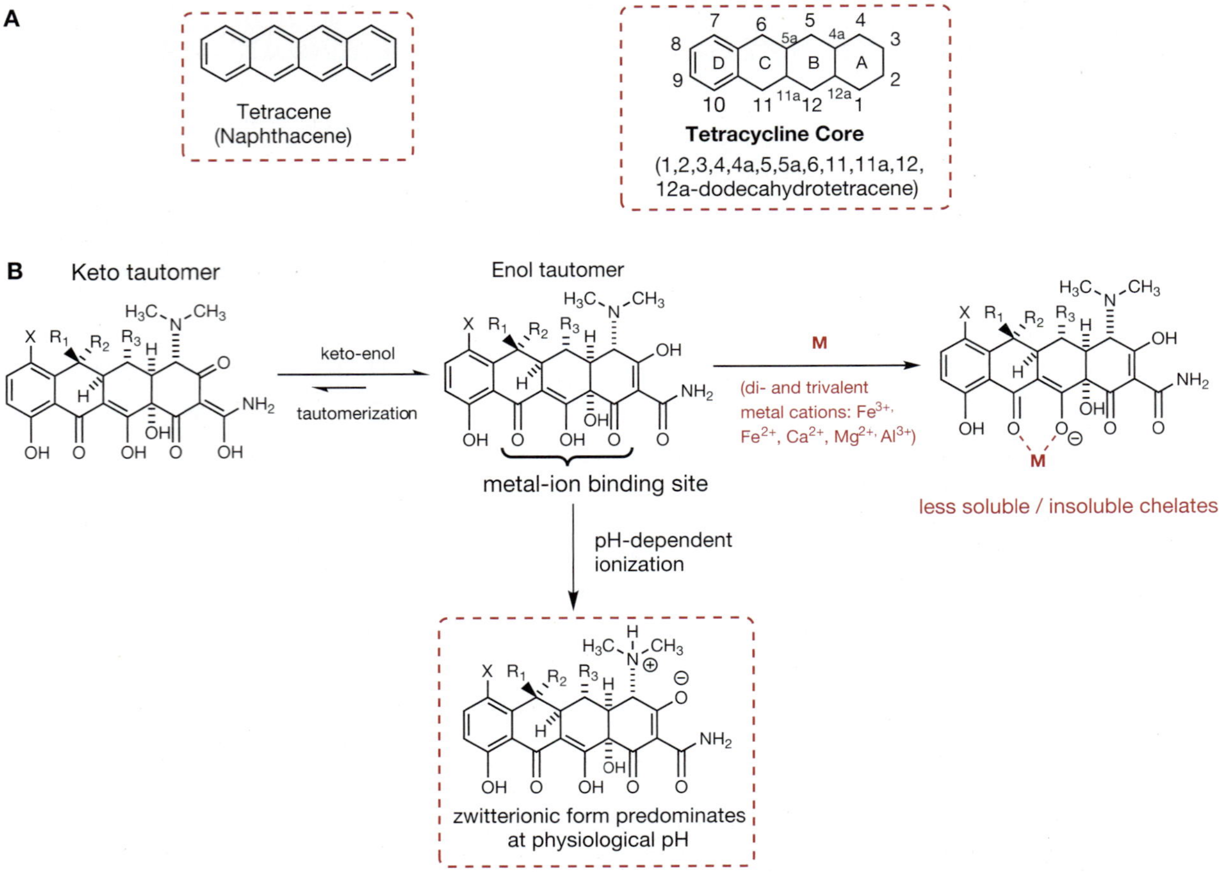

Figure 32.34 A. Structure of tetracene and its partially reduced ring system to obtain tetracycline pharmacophore. B. Structural and physicochemical properties of tetracyclines impacting their stability and water solubility: keto-enol tautomerization, chelation of metal cations, and formation of zwitterion.

impacts their chemical stability and biologic activity.[190] The α-stereo orientation of the C_4 dimethylamino moiety of the tetracycline skeleton is essential for their bioactivity. The presence of the tricarbonyl system of ring A allows enolization involving loss of the C_4 hydrogen (Fig. 32.35). Re-protonation can take place from either the top or bottom surface of the molecule. Re-protonation from the top of the enol regenerates the parent tetracycline. Re-protonation from the bottom, however, produces the inactive 4-epitetracycline. At equilibrium, the mixture consists of nearly equal amounts of the two diastereomers.

Dehydration. Most of the natural tetracyclines have a tertiary and a benzylic hydroxyl group at the C_6 position in the C-ring. This function has the ideal geometry for acid-catalyzed dehydration involving the C_{5a} α-oriented hydrogen (antiperiplanar conformation). The resulting product is a more stable naphthalene derivative (ie, rings D and C are aromatic). Favorable energetic reasons drive the reaction, thus resulting in the aromatization of ring C (Fig. 32.36). $C_{5a,6}$-anhydrotetracycline is much deeper in color than tetracycline and is biologically inactive.

Not only can inactive 4-epitetracyclines dehydrate to produce 4-epianhydrotetracyclines, but also anhydrotetracycline can epimerize to produce the same product. This degradation product is toxic to the kidneys and produces a Fanconi-like syndrome that is manifested by electrolyte imbalance

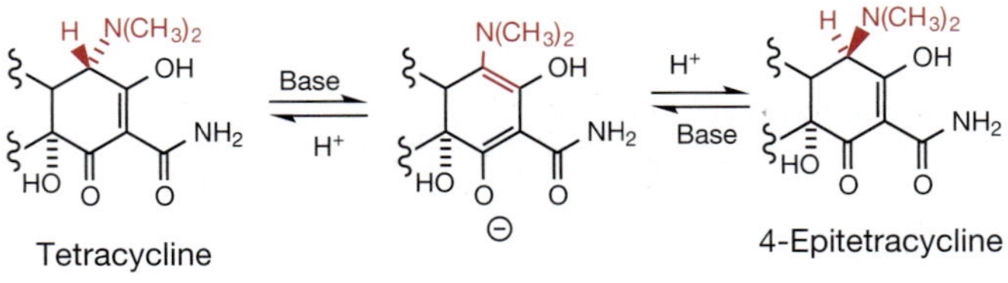

Figure 32.35 Epimerization of tetracyclines.

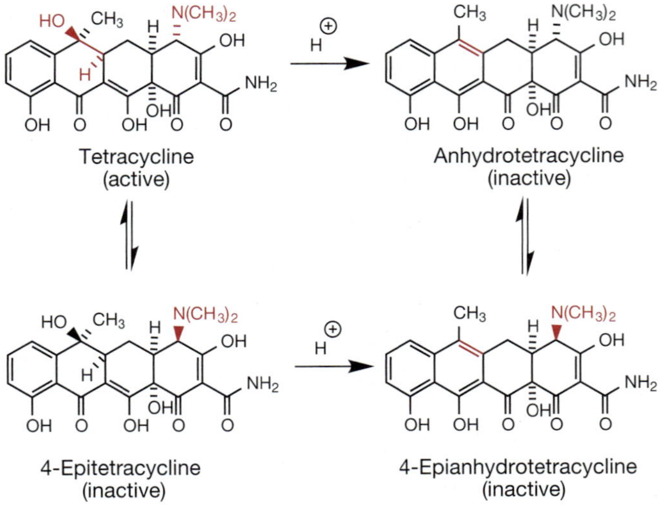

Figure 32.36 Acid-catalyzed instability of tetracyclines.

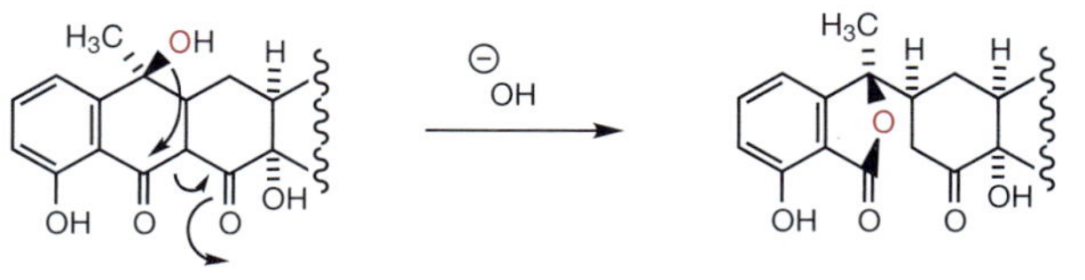

Figure 32.37 Base-catalyzed instability of tetracyclines.

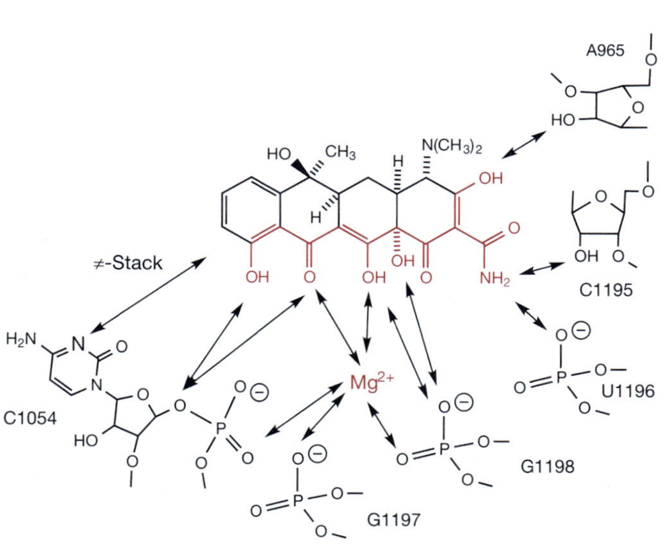

Figure 32.38 Schematic representation of the primary binding site for a tetracycline and the sugar phosphate groups of 16S ribosomal RNA, which also involves a magnesium ion and the critical functional groups on the "southern" and "eastern" face of the tetracycline. (Redrawn and modified from Brodersen DE, Clemons WM Jr, Carter AP, MorganWarren RJ, Wimberly BT, Ramakrishnan V. The structural basis for the action of the antibiotics tetracycline, pactamycin, and hygromycin B on the 30S ribosomal subunit. *Cell*. 2000;103:1143-1154.)

and induces tubular impairment, which in extreme cases has been fatal.[191,192] Tetracyclines that do not have the C_6-hydroxyl group, such as minocycline and doxycycline as well as the newer agents, cannot undergo dehydration and thus are free of this chemical instability and resulting toxicity.

Cleavage in Base. Another undesirable degradation reaction involving the benzylic C_6-hydroxyl group is cleavage of the C-ring in alkaline solutions at or above pH 8.5 (Fig. 32.37). In this environment, the C_6 oxygen is involved in a nucleophilic attack on the C_{11} ketone group. The lactonic product, an isotetracycline, is inactive. The clinical impact of this degradation under normal conditions has not been fully elucidated.

Phototoxicity. Certain tetracyclines, most notably those with a C_7-chlorine, absorb ultraviolet light at a particular wavelength (320-400 nm) spectrum found in sunlight or artificial sunlight. This leads to the destabilization of the compounds and destruction of their structure, resulting in the formation of reactive oxygen species (ROS). The generated oxygen radicals have damaging effects on cell membranes that are often manifested by skin irritation, erythema, and sunburn. This phenomenon is broadly referred to as phototoxicity. Patients should be advised to be cautious about exposure to sunlight for at least the first few doses to avoid potentially severe sunburn. This effect is comparatively rare with most of the tetracyclines that are currently used.[191]

Mechanism of Action. The tetracyclines of clinical importance interfere with protein biosynthesis at the ribosomal level, leading to a bacteriostatic effect. They inhibit bacterial protein synthesis by preventing the association of aminoacyl-tRNA with the bacterial mRNA-ribosome complex.[189] More specifically, the tetracycline antibiotics bind to a binding pocket composed of several nucleobases in the 16S rRNA and protein S7 within the 30S subunit (Fig. 32.26). Such interaction of the antibiotic with the ribosomal component causes wide-ranging structural changes in 16S rRNA.[189] In addition to this, several studies have indicated the complexity of the tetracycline-ribosome interactions and the apparent sites for drug interaction in the ribosome may not necessarily reflect the actual binding site. The points of contact with the rRNA are those associated with the observed antibiosis, with the surprising exception of the dimethylamino functional group (Fig. 32.38). This group is known to be essential for activity but does not appear to bind to the target in the X-ray structures that are available.[193-195] Once the tetracycline binds, it inhibits subsequent binding of aminoacyl-tRNA to the ribosome, resulting in termination of peptide chain growth. Overall, the association of tetracyclines with the ribosome is reversible, which explains the bacteriostatic effect of this drug class. Additionally, the relatively planar layout of the B, C, and D rings along with higher lipophilicity of certain tetracyclines provides opportunity for their trapping in the hydrophobic environment of the cytoplasmic membrane, thus impacting the integrity and disrupting its function.[189] The tetracyclines have been also shown to impact mitochondria by promoting mitonuclear protein imbalance and mitochondrial dysfunction across eukaryotic kingdoms due to the evolutionary relationship between mitochondria and proteobacteria.[196]

Resistance. As in the case of other drug classes, resistance to traditional tetracyclines is well established in a number of pathogenic, opportunistic, and commensal bacteria. The most common way of developing tetracycline resistance is via acquisition of new genes (associated with plasmids or transposons) referred to as tetracycline resistance (*tet*) genes and oxytetracycline resistance (*otr*) genes, which code for energy-dependent efflux of these drugs or for proteins that protect bacterial ribosomes from the action of tetracyclines.[189] The action of unusual ribosomal protection proteins is associated with their binding to and exerting conformational change on the ribosomes by using guanosine triphosphate (GTP). The alteration in ribosomal conformation prevents tetracycline from binding to the ribosome but it does not impact the binding of aminoacyl-tRNA to the acceptor site of the ribosome, thus allowing for protein synthesis. It has been shown that the bacterial protein synthesis proceeds even in the presence of tetracycline at concentrations that would normally inhibit translation.[189] Additionally, the protection proteins can induce dissociation of the tetracycline from the ribosome.[189] Some bacteria acquire resistance by mutations, which alter the permeability of the porins and/or

LPS in the outer membrane, change the regulation of innate efflux systems, alter the 16S rRNA,[189] or enzymatically inactivate the tetracycline antibiotic.[189]

Adverse Effects. In addition to the adverse effects mentioned earlier, the tetracyclines are associated with common GI effects such as nausea, vomiting, and diarrhea. Additionally, some drugs produce specific unwanted effects. Minocycline can cause CNS effects such as dizziness and vertigo, whereas doxycycline can cause esophageal irritation. Rapid administration or prolonged IV use can lead to infusion site reactions and thrombophlebitis; therefore, the oral route of administration is preferred. At higher doses or in special situations (eg, IV use during pregnancy), the tetracyclines can also bind to the mammalian 80S ribosomes and produce a significant antianabolic effect. In cases of significant renal impairment, higher serum levels of tetracyclines can lead to azotemia. Additionally, inducers of cytochrome P450 (CYP450) metabolism (ie, RIF, barbiturates, carbamazepine) increase the metabolism of tetracyclines (especially doxycycline), so the dose of the tetracycline may require adjustment.[191]

Therapeutic Application. Tetracyclines are classified as broad-spectrum bacteriostatic agents that have been widely employed in the clinic, veterinary medicine, and agriculture. The older first- and second-generation agents (doxycycline, minocycline, and tetracycline) have a broad spectrum; however, they are inactive against *Pseudomonas*, *Enterococcus*, and anaerobes. The more recently approved novel third-generation tetracycline derivatives (eravacycline, omadacycline, and tigecycline) have even broader spectrum (including most gram-positive and gram-negative anaerobes) than the first- and second-generation agents. The only exception to this is sarecycline, which is a third-generation, narrow-spectrum tetracycline antibiotic with negligible or low activity against many gram-negative and anaerobic bacteria. Because of the resistance phenomenon and the comparative frequency of troublesome adverse effects, the first- and second-generation drugs nowadays are rarely the first choice of treatment. Overall, the tetracycline-containing medications are used in the management and treatment of a variety of infectious diseases. They can treat rickettsial diseases, ehrlichiosis, anaplasmosis, leptospirosis, amebiasis, actinomycosis, nocardiosis, brucellosis, melioidosis, tularemia, chlamydial infections, pelvic inflammatory disease, syphilis, traveler's diarrhea, early Lyme disease, acne, Legionnaire's disease, and Whipple disease. They cover *Borrelia recurrentis*, *Mycobacterium marinum*, *Mycoplasma pneumoniae*, *S. aureus* (including MRSA), *Vibrio vulnificus*, and in some cases VRE.[197] *Meningococcal* prophylaxis is also achievable. Although rare, their other indications include rosacea, bullous dermatoses, sarcoidosis, Kaposi sarcoma, pyoderma gangrenosum, hidradenitis suppurativa, Sweet syndrome, α_1-antitrypsin deficiency, panniculitis, pityriasis lichenoides chronica, rheumatoid arthritis, scleroderma, cancer, and cardiovascular diseases.[197]

Specific Agents. The structures and brand names of the currently available tetracyclines can be found in Table 32.11.

Tetracycline. Tetracycline is produced by fermentation of *Streptomyces aureofaciens* and *S. rimosus* or by catalytic hydrogenation of chlortetracycline. It is administered orally with a usual dose of 500 mg twice daily. It is recommended to be taken on an empty stomach (eg, 1 hour prior to or 2 hours after meals). As previously discussed, serum concentrations of all tetracyclines may be decreased if taken with dairy products, antacids, and other cation-containing products and thus should be taken at least 1 to 2 hours prior to or 4 hours after these products. Absorption, after oral administration, can reach up to 88%, with time to peak 2 to 4 hours, and elimination half-life ranging between 6 and 11 hours. Up to 60% of the dose is excreted in feces, and up to 30% in the urine. Since the renal excretion of this agent is significantly affected by the state of renal function, dose adjustment is needed for patients with renal failure.

Demeclocycline. Demeclocycline lacks the C_6-methyl of tetracycline and contains C_7-chloro atom, hence the prefix demeclo- in the name of this medication. It is produced by a genetically altered strain of *S. aureofaciens*. Because the C_6 hydroxy group is a secondary alcohol, it is more chemically stable than tetracycline toward the unwanted dehydration. The absorption for a fasting adult is 66% but will be decreased if taken with food and/or cation-containing products. The time required to achieve peak plasma concentrations is approximately 4 hours, elimination half-life 10 to 16 hours, and it is largely excreted unchanged in the urine and feces.

Doxycycline (Avidoxy, Doryx MPC, Doxy 100, Mondoxyne NL, Oracea, TargaDOX, Vibramycin). Doxycycline is produced semisynthetically from tetracyclines and contains a C_5 hydroxy group instead of C_6. Besides minocycline, it is the most widely prescribed agent from the tetracycline family. It is also the most phototoxic compound of the series. Doxycycline is available as capsules and tablets (immediate and delayed release) for oral administration and as an IV injection, which are bioequivalent, but the oral route is preferred. Although labeling of some manufacturers recommends administration on an empty stomach, this agent is generally recommended to be taken with meals to decrease GI upset. Also, the oral dosage forms are recommended to be followed with at least 8 ounces (240 mL) of water and have patients sit up for at least 30 minutes after taking the medication in order to reduce the risk of esophageal irritation and ulceration. Doxycycline is almost completely absorbed from the GI; however, coconsumption with food or milk will reduce the absorption by 20%. The time to achieve peak plasma concentrations is dictated by the type of the tablet, and ranges from 1.5 to 4 hours for IR and 2.8 to 3 hours for delayed-release tablets. This drug's elimination half-life is between 18 and 22 hours, permitting once-a-day dosing for mild infections. It is excreted partly in the feces and partly in the urine.

Minocycline (Arestin, Amzeeq, Minocin, Minolira, Solodyn, Zilxi). Minocycline is an important antibiotic produced by semisynthesis from demeclocycline. It contains the C_7 dimethylamino group and at the same time lacks the C_6 alcohol functionality, which altogether makes this derivative much more lipophilic than its precursors and leads to a quick and nearly quantitative absorption from the GI tract. Elimination half-life of this drug is 16 hours, which can be substantially increased in patients with hepatic and/or renal failure. The elimination half-life is longer after IV injection, and it spans between 15 and 23 hours. The orally administered medicine is taken once or twice daily with or without food, but it shall be taken with plenty of fluids to reduce the risk of esophageal irritation and ulceration. As in the previous cases, the time to achieve peak plasma concentrations for oral minocycline depends on the type of formulation, and can range from 1 to 3 hours for regular tablet, 1 to 4 hours for a capsule, and 3.5 to 4 hours for ER tablet. This medication is widely prescribed for the treatment of diverse infections. It is available as periodontal microspheres, pellet-filled capsules, tablets and ER tablets, IV injection, aerosol, and foam.

Omadacycline (Nuzyra). Omadacycline represents a novel derivative of tetracyclines and is classified as an aminomethylcycline due to the presence of the *N*-substituted aminomethyl group appended on C_9 carbon of the aromatic ring D.[198] Also, carbons C_5 and C_6 of the tetracycline core are unsubstituted. These structural modifications resulted in improvement of various pharmacokinetic properties, broader spectrum, and enhanced activity against drug-resistant bacterial strains due to increased resistance toward the efflux-mediated process moderated by multidrug resistance pumps. Omadacycline is used as an oral tablet and IV injection. A loading dose is required, and the maintenance dosing (once daily) differs between IV (100 mg) and PO (300 mg). The difference in doses is explained by the rather modest bioavailability of 34.5% upon oral administration. Food and drinks other than water will further decrease absorption of this drug; therefore, omadacycline is recommended to be taken on an empty stomach. Time to peak is achieved in approximately 0.5 hours for IV injection and 2.5 hours for oral administration, and elimination half-life oscillates around 16 hours. Most of the drug (up to 84%) is excreted in the feces.

Sarecycline (Seysara). Similar to omadacycline, sarecyclin is an aminomethylcycline possessing an *N*-methoxy-*N*-methyl aminomethyl functional group on the C_7 carbon.[199] Sarecyclin is administered as an oral tablet and achieves its peak plasma concentrations between 1.5 and 2 hours. It may be administered with or without food, but it should be taken with lots of fluids for the same reasons as minocycline. It has a relatively long elimination half-life of 21 to 22 hours and is excreted nearly in equal portions in the feces and urine. Sarecyclin differs from other tetracyclines by its narrow spectrum of activity against gram-positive anaerobic *Cutibacterium acnes* and skin organisms such as staphylococci and streptococci.

Tigecycline (Tygacil). The increased incidence of resistance developed toward first- and second-generation tetracyclines led to renewed research efforts to identify novel agents with improved properties. This effort led to the discovery of a new class of antibiotics referred to as glycylcyclines that are structurally closely related to the tetracyclines but have broader spectrum of activity and lack many of the clinical resistance issues.[200,201] They are characterized by having an additional *N*-alkyl-glycylamido group at the C_9 position of ring D. Tigecycline is the first-in-class agent to be marketed. It is administered IV and has an elimination half-life of 27 hours for a single dose and 42 hours for multiple doses. It is eliminated predominantly unchanged in the feces (major) and urine (minor). Like the other tetracyclines administered IV, tigecycline can cause injection site pain and inflammation. Its other adverse effects are similar to those described for tetracyclines, with GI effects (diarrhea, nausea, vomiting) being most pronounced. Tigecycline is accompanied with a boxed warning due to an increase in mortality rates. Therefore, this medication should be reserved for use in situations when alternative treatments are not suitable.

Eravacycline (Xerava). Eravacycline is classified as a fluorocycline due to the presence of C_7 fluoro-substituent.[202] It also possesses a pyrrolidinoacetamido group. This is similar to tigecycline and contains a C_9 glyclamido substituent with the nitrogen atom embedded in the pyrrolidine ring. Eravacycline has a spectrum of action, therapeutic applications, and adverse effects profile similar to those of tigecycline but is not accompanied with boxed warning. It is also administered IV and excreted predominantly as CYP3A4 metabolism products in the feces (major) and urine (minor). As such, both medications do not require dose adjustment in patients with renal dysfunction as their renal elimination is the minor route. Additionally, the half-life of eravacycline is approximately 20 hours, which is shorter than that of tigecycline.

Oxazolidinones

Oxazolidinone is a five-member heterocyclic ring that gives rise to three possible isomers (stemming from the different arrangements of oxygen atom, NH, and the carbonyl group), with 2-oxazolidinone being investigated the most in medicinal chemistry and drug discovery (Fig. 32.39).[203] Linezolid was the pioneer drug containing an oxazolidinone ring as the pharmacophore that was approved by the FDA in 2000 and subsequently served as a chemical template for the discovery and development of other agents containing this pharmacophore.

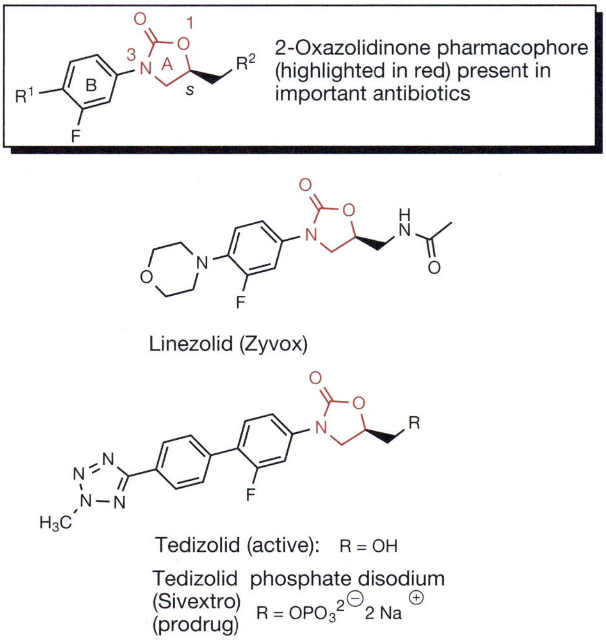

Figure 32.39 2-Oxazolidinone pharmacophore and structures of the therapeutically important oxazolidinone antibiotics.

Mechanism of Action and Structure-Activity Relationship. The oxazolidinone drug class contains fully synthetic antibacterials that are primarily effective against gram-positive bacteria. They are bacteriostatic against enterococci and staphylococci with a short PAE, and also show bactericidal activity against some streptococcal species.[204] The 5-(S)-stereochemistry of the oxazolidinone ring (A) is essential for activity, which is further improved with C_5 acylaminomethyl group and an *N*-(m-fluoro)phenyl moiety (ring B). This pharmacophore has been broadly explored as a chemical scaffold for the development of several antibiotics that seem to be more active and safer than the parent compound, linezolid. To date, a number of oxazolidinones have reached various phases of clinical trials as prospective anti-TB medications for use in combination therapy.[205] Linezolid and tedizolid (including the phosphate prodrug) are the only representatives of this drug class that have been approved for use in the United States.[206] Tedizolid is more potent than linezolid on susceptible strains due to the presence of additional aromatic rings that enhance its interactions with the ribosome.

The MOA of the oxazolidinones is associated with inhibition of protein synthesis; however, this occurs at a stage different from that reported for the other protein synthesis inhibitors. The oxazolidinones inhibit the initiation of protein synthesis by binding to the A-site pocket of the 50S subunit at the PTC and interacting extensively with several nucleotides of the 23S rRNA located in close proximity. This prevents the formation of a functional initiation ternary complex including *N*-formylmethionyl-tRNA (tRNAfMet), mRNA, and the 50S subunit.[204,207] The net result of this interaction is that translation of the mRNA is prevented. The other prominent inhibitors of bacterial ribosomal protein biosynthesis bind to and inhibit after the formation of the functional initiation complex. In those cases, mRNA translation begins, but elongation of the growing peptide chain is blocked.

Resistance. To date, three different oxazolidinone resistance mechanisms have been described.[206] The first mechanism involves the point mutation G2576T single-nucleotide polymorphism (SNP) in the domain V of 23S rRNA genes that ultimately affects the peptidyl transferase domain of 23S rRNA.[208,209] The second mechanism involves the acquisition of the ribosomal methyltransferase gene designated as "*cfr* gene" (chloramphenicol-florfenicol resistance gene). This gene is responsible for encoding a methyltransferase that modifies position A-2503 in bacterial 23S rRNA and thus confers resistance to five classes of antibiotics: phenicols, lincosamides, oxazolidinones, pleuromutilins, and streptogramin A.[210] The third mechanism depends on mutations in *rplD* and *rplC* genes encoding 50S ribosomal proteins L4 and L3, respectively, which are essential and indispensable components for the formation of PTC.[211] In general, resistance to linezolid is more common than to tedizolid as the latter agent is newer. Tedizolid retains activity on strains carrying the cfr mechanism of resistance because it contains the less sterically hindered (when compared to linezolid's acetamido group) hydroxymethyl group, which enables its binding to the methylated ribosomes.[204] In vitro data demonstrated that tedizolid retained activity against cfr isolates, which suggests that this drug might be an effective alternative against some linezolid-resistant pathogens, most notably *S. aureus*.[212] Gram-negative microorganisms are intrinsically resistant to oxazolidinones due to the presence of endogenous efflux pumps that keep those agents from accumulating in the cells.

Adverse Effects and Drug Interactions. The adverse effects consist of bone marrow suppression in the case of prolonged administration (>2-3 weeks), with related thrombocytopenia, anemia, and decreased hemoglobin concentration. However, all of these blood abnormalities are reversible and return to baseline values within 10 to 14 days after the end of the treatment.[206] Oxazolidinones also interact with mitochondrial ribosomes to inhibit protein synthesis, which is most likely the molecular basis for their undesirable myelosuppressive, neurotoxic, and metabolic effects (lactic acidosis).[204] Of high concern is the observed peripheral and optic neuropathy that may occur in the case of prolonged treatment. Improvement or complete recovery of optic neuropathy typically occurs with discontinuation of therapy, but the peripheral neuropathy can be irreversible. GI effects (especially diarrhea) are associated with this drug class. Both agents are weak inhibitors of monoamine oxidase (MAO); therefore, patients should be cautious about eating tyramine-containing foods. To avoid serotonin syndrome, coadministration with selective serotonin reuptake inhibitors (SSRIs), tricyclic antidepressants (TCAs), and buspirone is unadvisable. Additionally, due to their MAO inhibitory activity, oxazolidinones may enhance the hypoglycemic effect of agents with blood glucose–lowering activity.

Therapeutic Application. Linezolid has proven antimicrobial activity against a broad range of susceptible and resistant gram-positive bacteria, including activity against MRSA with intermediate resistance to glycopeptides like vancomycin. It is approved for the treatment of bacterial pneumonia, skin and skin structure infections, and VRE infections, including infections complicated by bacteremia.[213] Linezolid is recommended for empirical therapy against MRSA in hospitalized adult patients with complicated skin and soft tissue infection, for community-associated MRSA skin and soft tissue infection, and MRSA-associated purulent and non-purulent cellulitis. It can also be used as an alternative option for MRSA in hospitalized pediatric patients.[213] Linezolid is also used off-label as a component of combination therapy against MDR-TB.[214] Tedizolid has a spectrum of activity very similar to that of linezolid. However, as previously mentioned, it may have activity against some linezolid-resistant gram-positive cocci. Tedizolid phosphate is a prodrug of tedizolid and has a similar microbial spectrum but is specifically approved for the treatment of acute skin and soft tissue infections.[215]

Specific Agents

Linezolid (Zyvox). Linezolid contains the morpholine heterocyclic ring in the para position of the ring B, hence the prefix line- in the name of this medication (Fig. 32.39).[216] It is administered orally as a tablet and oral suspension as well as an IV injection. It is rapidly and extensively absorbed with nearly 100% bioavailability. This medication is not extensively plasma protein bound (31%), achieves peak plasma concentration within 1 to 2 hours, and has a half-life of approximately 5 hours in adults. It is largely metabolized through morpholine ring oxidation to two inactive metabolites: an aminoethoxy acetic acid metabolite and a hydroxyethyl glycine metabolite. The majority of the dose (>80%) is eliminated in the urine (~30% as the parent drug and ~50% as the metabolites).

Tedizolid Phosphate (Sivextro). Tedizolid's B ring has been sequentially extended in the para position with additional phenyl and tetrazole rings, hence the prefix te- in the name of this agent (Fig. 32.39). It is a newer derivative of linezolid that has enhanced activity, longer elimination half-life (~12 hours), high bioavailability (~91%), high plasma protein binding (up to 90%), and lower incidence of adverse effects (especially serotonin syndrome), which altogether result in tedizolid's administration of 200 mg tablet once daily versus 600 mg tablet every 12 hours for linezolid. Contrary to linezolid, tedizolid is vastly (>80%) excreted in the feces and has slightly longer time to peak (~3 hours).

Tedizolid phosphate[215] is a phosphate prodrug of tedizolid approved for IV infusion over 1 hour, hence it has time to peak of approximately 1 to 1.5 hours.

Pleuromutilins

(+)-Pleuromutilin is a naturally occurring diterpene that is produced by the members of basidiomycetes (Fig. 32.40). Originally, it was isolated from *Pleurotus mutilus* (currently known as *Clitophilus scyphoides*), which is an edible mushroom.[217] Currently, *Clitophilus passeckerianus* is the basidiomycete fungus employed in commercial production of pleuromutilin, which is utilized as an advanced intermediate in the semisynthesis of pleuromutilin analogs that are approved antibiotics for therapeutic use.[218] The antibacterial effect of pleuromutilin against *S. aureus* was discovered in 1951, which initiated exploration of this pharmacophore from the pharmaceutical perspective leading to tiamulin, a first-in-class drug that was approved in 1979 for veterinary use.[219] Subsequently, this scaffold received less attention especially in the competitive landscape of several other classes of antibiotics that were vigorously researched and developed at that time. However, in light of the rapidly growing antibiotic resistance, the pleuromutilin scaffold has drawn new interest and motivation to develop successful derivatives for the treatment of infections in humans. The extensive research efforts resulted in the first medication in this class, retapamulin, that received FDA approval for human applications and marketing in 2007. Over a decade later, in 2019, another pleuromutilin, lefamulin, with enhanced activity and properties was approved by the FDA (Fig. 32.40).

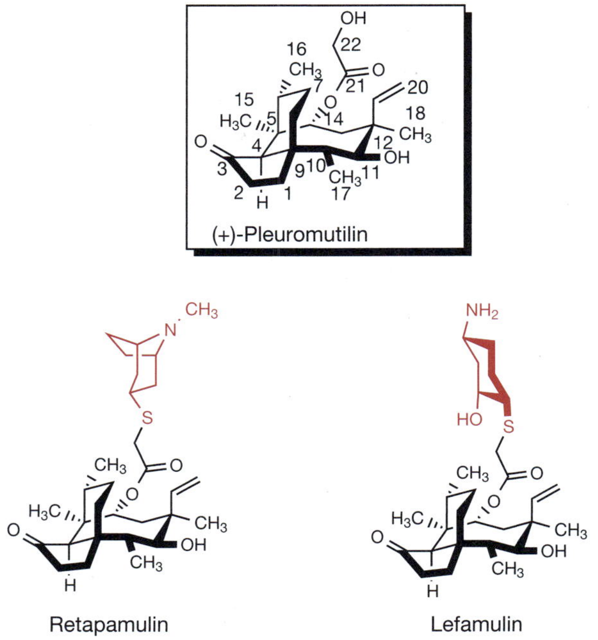

Figure 32.40 Structures of the natural product (+)-pleuromutilin and its semisynthetic derivatives that found therapeutic uses.

Mechanism of Action and Structure-Activity Relationship. Pleuromutilin and its analogs consist of the crucial, tricyclic mutilin core that includes 3-cyclopentenone, cyclohexane, and cyclooctane fused rings. The latter ring is functionalized with several methyl, C_{11} hydroxyl, C_{12} vinyl, and C_{14} α-hydroxyacetate groups. The α-hydroxyester provided the basis for structural modifications introduced at the C_{22} hydroxyl group to yield thousands of pleuromutilin analogs, many of which showed significantly improved activity and became approved agents for use in humans and animals whereas others are in pre- and clinical development. The C_{22} hydroxyl group has been replaced with a thioether that further extends the side chain and contains either primary or tertiary amino group.

Pleuromutilins inhibit bacterial protein synthesis by binding to the central part of domain V of the 23S rRNA in the 50S ribosomal subunit at the PTC. This prevents the correct positioning of the CCA ends (that carry amino acids) of tRNAs for peptide transfer in the A- and P-site, which inhibits peptide bond formation and exerts antibacterial action.[220-222] The interaction at the ribosome involves binding of the C_{14} extension and the tricyclic core to the P- and A-sites of the PTC, respectively.[223] The C_{14} side chain binds to the ribosome via H-bonding created with the C_{21} carbonyl oxygen and the sulfur atom. Some hydrophobic interactions also take place. The tricyclic core binds via H-bond created with the C_{11} hydroxyl and it is additionally anchored via hydrophobic forces.[223] In the case of lefamulin, an additional hydrogen bond is formed between the primary amine located within the C_{14} extension and the molecular target, which leads to a tighter binding pocket that is in turn reflected in significantly higher activity of this drug, including efficacy against drug-resistant pathogens.[223]

Resistance. Pleuromutilins are associated with low rates of resistance development, which is one of the most important characteristics of this drug class. Additionally, they show minimal cross-resistance with other antibiotics that act by interfering with the ribosomal protein synthesis. Nevertheless, the bacterial resistance to pleuromutilins has been identified and described, and it occurs via three distinctive mechanisms. These include mutations in 23S rRNA and *rplC* genes encoding the ribosomal protein L3, and methylation of the nucleotide by Cfr methyltransferase, both of which directly impact binding of these agents. The third mechanism depends on drug efflux by ATP-binding cassette (ABC) transporters.[223]

Therapeutic Application. The pleuromutilin drug class displays high activity against gram-positive and fastidious gram-negative pathogens as well as against mycoplasmas and intracellular organisms, such as *Chlamydia* spp. and *Legionella pneumophila*. Pleuromutilins are not affected by resistance to other major antibiotic classes, such as macrolides, fluoroquinolones, tetracyclines, and β-lactam antibiotics, which makes them a valuable therapeutic option for the treatment of various infections.[224] Additionally, they show synergistic effect in combination with other antimicrobial agents.[225] This drug class produces bacteriostatic effect; however, substantial increase in the drug's concentration might lead to a bactericidal effect.

Specific Agents

Retapamulin. Retapamulin's side chain has been elaborated by appending the 8-methyl-8-azabicyclo[3.2.1] octane skeleton to the sulfur atom (Fig. 32.40). This medication has been approved for use in adults and children age 9 months and older for the treatment of impetigo caused by MSSA and *S. pyogenes*. Impetigo is a highly contagious infection found mostly in children involving the upper layers of the skin and spread through close contact.[226] Retapamulin is applied as a topical ointment, and it is well tolerated. Its use is accompanied with minimal adverse events, which are mostly limited to application-site irritation and eczema. The drug does not appear to have systemic absorption to any great degree when applied topically, although it is a substrate for CYP3A4 and undergoes mono-oxygenation and di-oxygenation to multiple metabolites.[226]

Lefamulin. Lefamulin is the newest representative of this drug class that has the aminocyclohexanol ring embedded within the thioether moiety. Due to the presence of a primary amine, it easily forms salts. This agent has been approved as an acetate salt for oral (tablet) and IV (solution) administration. It is indicated for the treatment of CABP in adults caused by various susceptible microorganisms. Generally, this medication is well tolerated, although diarrhea (after oral) and injection site reaction (after IV) were the major adverse reactions reported. Lefamulin has poor bioavailability (25%) that is additionally decreased by food. Therefore, this agent should be taken at least 1 hour before or 2 hours after a meal and accompanied by drinking 8 ounces of water. Its high protein binding (~95%-97%) and average half-life of ~8 hours allow this drug to be administered once every 12 hours. It achieves peak plasma concentration within 2 hours after taking the drug orally and undergoes hepatic, CYP3A4-mediated metabolism followed by elimination in the feces (77%-88% of the dose).

Streptogramins

Quinupristin and Dalfopristin (Synercid)

Mechanism of Action and Chemical Properties. Quinupristin and dalfopristin are semisynthetic derivatives of the natural products pristinamycin IA and pristinamycin IIA, respectively (Fig. 32.41). They are produced by *Streptomyces pristinaespiralis* as well as other microorganisms, therefore other names are also associated with these compounds. They represent streptogramin-type antibiotic, and like several other members of this family (such as virginiamycin, mikamycin, and vernamycin), these molecules constitute a mixture of two structurally different chemical components. Pristinamycin IA is a branched cyclic hexadepsipeptide (ie, a peptide in which at least one amide group is replaced by the corresponding ester group) of streptogramin B group, whereas pristinamycin IIA has the structure of a polyunsaturated cyclo-peptidic macrolactone belonging to the A group of streptogramins (Fig. 32.41).[227] These natural products are coproduced by *S. pristinaespiralis* in a ratio of 30:70 (w/w), respectively. Since they show synergistic antimicrobial activity, they are often referred to as synergimycins.[227] Quinupristin was obtained from pristinamycin IA in a semisynthetic approach by adding the bicyclic tertiary amine, quinuclidine, via thioether linker. On the other hand, pristinamycin IIA was utilized in the semisynthesis of dalfopristin by introducing the respective side chain composed of *N,N*-diethyl-(phenylsulfonyl)ethan-1-amine.

Each of the natural products binds to the bacterial 50S ribosomal subunit and inhibits the elongation process of the bacterial protein synthesis. As such, their independent action results only in moderate bacteriostatic activity. However, when both agents are given as a combination, they

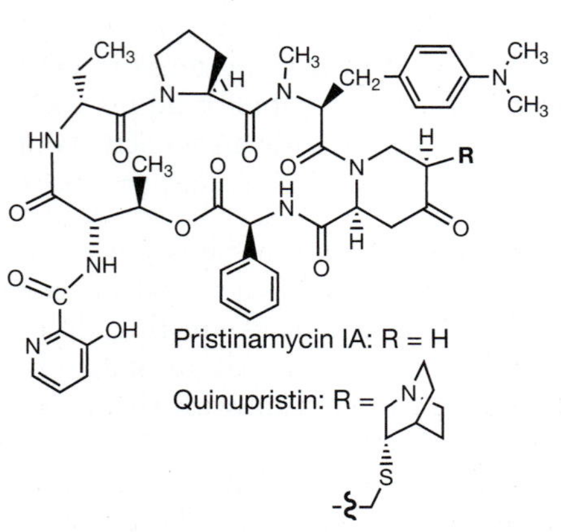

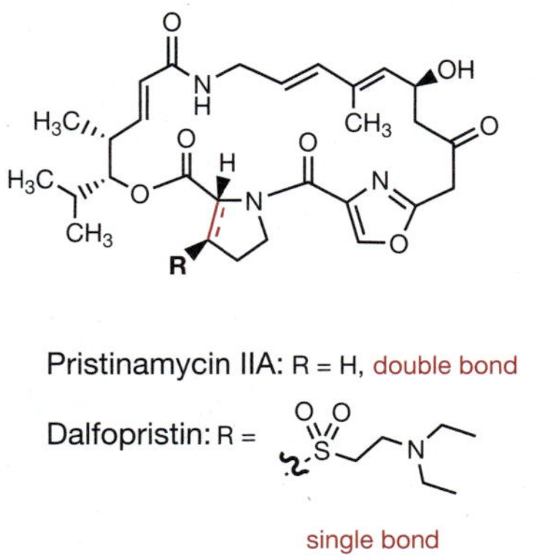

Figure 32.41 Structures of the natural streptogramin-type antibiotics and their semisynthetic derivatives: quinupristin and dalfopristin.

show synergistic action that leads to a potent bactericidal activity, which can be enhanced even up to 100 times than that of the separate components.[227] The marketed combination drug, Synercid, is composed of quinupristin/dalfopristin in a ratio of 30:70 (w/w). This reflects the proportion in which the original natural products are coproduced. Both components work synergistically to induce strong bactericidal effect. Dalfopristin inhibits the early phase of protein synthesis while quinupristin inhibits the late phase of protein synthesis. Because the MOA of Synercid differs from that of other major classes of antibacterial agents, there is practically no cross-resistance between Synercid and these agents. Resistance to both counterparts of Synercid has been identified and reported.[228]

Therapeutic Application and Absorption, Distribution, Metabolism, and Excretion-Toxicity. The combination of the streptogramins quinupristin and dalfopristin has been approved for IV use in the treatment of infections caused by complicated skin and skin structure infections caused by MSSA or *S. pyogenes*. However, the use of this drug is accompanied by poor tolerance, frequent need for administration via central line, and high potential for DDIs. Synercid is a strong inhibitor of the CYP3A4 isozyme, and several drug interactions are to be expected. Therapeutic-level monitoring of cyclosporine should be performed when used concomitantly with Synercid.[228] Although this drug does not appear to prolong the QTc interval, it inhibits the metabolism of several agents that have been shown to have this effect, so their concomitant administration should be avoided. Synercid can also produce several other adverse effects including infusion site reactions (pain and/or reaction to infusion, local inflammation and/or edema) and GI effects (nausea, vomiting, diarrhea).[228] Quinupristin and dalfopristin are converted to several metabolites that are active. For quinupristin, two major metabolites are conjugated (one with glutathione and one with cysteine) and for dalfopristin one non-conjugated metabolite is formed by drug hydrolysis.[228] Biliary excretion is the principal route for fecal elimination, with approximately 80% of the dose being eliminated in this manner. The half-life of those agents is short and lasts less than 1 hour for each of them.

Chloramphenicol

Mechanism of Action and Chemical Properties. Chloramphenicol was originally produced by fermentation of *Streptomyces venezuelae*, but its comparatively simple chemical structure soon resulted in several efficient total chemical syntheses. It represents the phenylpropanoid skeleton with the two chiral carbon atoms giving rise to four diastereomers, only one of which (1R,2R) is significantly active (Fig. 32.42). Chloramphenicol is a neutral substance and only moderately soluble in water. Its two nitrogen atoms, an amide and a nitro group, are non-basic under physiologic conditions. The name of this natural product partly reflects the dichloromethyl group present in its structure, hence the prefix chlor-. Chloramphenicol was the first broad-spectrum oral antibiotic used in the United States (1947) and was once popular, including veterinary applications. Potentially severe blood dyscrasia has greatly decreased its use in North

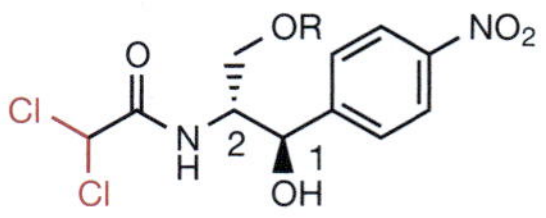

Chloramphenicol: R = H

Chloramphenicol sodium hemisuccinate:

R =
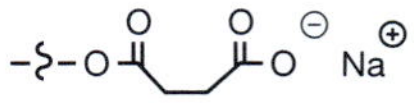

Figure 32.42 Chloramphenicol and its prodrug form, sodium hemisuccinate.

America; however, its low cost and appreciable efficacy still make it a popular choice in many countries in the world where it can often be purchased over the counter without a prescription.

Chloramphenicol is bacteriostatic by virtue of inhibition of protein biosynthesis in both bacterial and, to a lesser extent, the host ribosomes. Chloramphenicol binds to the 50S ribosomal subunit and inhibits the attachment of tRNA to the A-site on the 50S ribosome (Fig. 32.26).[229] Resistance is mediated by several R-factor enzymes that catalyze acetylation of the secondary and, to some extent, the primary hydroxyl groups in the aliphatic side chain.[230] These products no longer bind to the bacterial ribosomes and thus are inactive. Also, bacterial multidrug efflux system exists that expels chloramphenicol from the bacterial cell, as well as an increase in the ribosome biosynthesis machinery to counteract the drug's action has been reported.[231]

Absorption, Distribution, Metabolism, and Excretion-Toxicity. When given orally, chloramphenicol is rapidly and completely absorbed with a bioavailability of 80% but has rather a short half-life (1.5-3.5 hours). It is mainly excreted in the urine in the form of its metabolites, which are C_3 and C_1 glucuronides (up to 90%), and to a lesser extent, its deamidation product and the product of dehalogenation as well as reduction of the nitro group (the latter primarily occurs in the gut and is performed by the normal bacterial flora).[232] These metabolites are all inactive. Chloramphenicol potentiates the activity of some other medications by weakly inhibiting CYP2C9-mediated metabolism in the liver. Such agents include anticoagulant coumarins, sulfonamides, oral hypoglycemics, and phenytoin.[232]

Two prodrug forms of chloramphenicol are available (only the IV injectable form is available in the United States). Since the drug is intensively bitter, a C_3 palmitate prodrug (cleaved in the duodenum to liberate the active component) has been introduced for use as a pediatric oral suspension. Chloramphenicol's poor water solubility has been largely overcome by its conversion to the C_3 hemisuccinate, which easily forms a water-soluble sodium salt (Fig. 32.42). This prodrug is cleaved in the body by tissue (lung, liver, kidney) and plasma esterases to produce active chloramphenicol. Because cleavage in muscles is slow, this prodrug is used IV rather than IM.

Toxicities prevent chloramphenicol from being more widely used. Serious and fatal blood dyscrasias (aplastic anemia, hypoplastic anemia, thrombocytopenia, and granulocytopenia) are associated with the use of this agent, hence the boxed warning.[232] The more serious form is a pancytopenia of the blood, which is believed to be caused by one of the reduction products of the aromatic nitro group that may result in a radical and other toxic reactive species. The so-called "gray" or "gray baby" syndrome, a form of cardiovascular collapse, is encountered when chloramphenicol is given to young infants (especially premature infants) whose liver glucuronidation is underdeveloped, and thus successive drug doses will lead to rapid accumulation of the drug due to impaired metabolism and excretion.

Therapeutic Applications. Chloramphenicol is a broad-spectrum antibiotic with activity against gram-positive, gram-negative, and anaerobic bacteria. Despite its potentially serious limitations, chloramphenicol is an effective drug when prescribed and used with proper caution. Its particular value is in typhoid fever, *Haemophilus* infections (especially epiglottitis and meningitis, when given along with ampicillin), rickettsial infections, and in cases when less toxic agents turned out to be ineffective or contraindicated against susceptible organisms. Safer antibiotics should be used prior to initiating therapy with chloramphenicol. The medication is about 60% serum protein bound and diffuses well into tissues, especially into inflamed CSF, and therefore it is of high value in the treatment of meningitis. It also penetrates well into lymph nodes and mesenteric ganglions, rationalizing its usefulness in typhoid fever.

Other Antibacterials. This group of antibiotics consists of a miscellaneous collection of structural types whose narrow range of applicability and/or toxicities secured them a more specialized place in antimicrobial chemotherapy than all the agents discussed thus far. They are generally reserved for use in special circumstances and/or for particular purposes.

Mupirocin

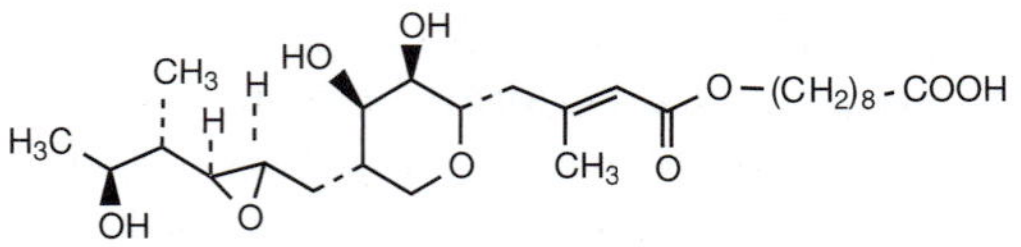

Mupirocin

Mechanism of Action and Chemical Properties. Mupirocin is a member of a group of lipid acids produced by fermentation of *Pseudomonas fluorescens*. Mupirocin is a mixture of several pseudomonic acids, with pseudomonic acid A constituting greater than 90% of the mixture.[233] The other components of the mixture are pseudomonic acids B, C, and D, which share a similar chemical structure and antimicrobial spectrum.[204] In general, pseudomonic acid A is composed of two substantially different moieties, the left-hand side monic acid (which is a C_{17} polyketide) and the right-hand side 9-hydroxy-nonanoic acid (which is a C_9 fatty acid) that are connected via an ester bond. This agent acts by binding reversibly to bacterial isoleucyl tRNA synthetase, an enzyme that catalyzes the formation of isoleucyl tRNA from isoleucine and tRNA. This prevents incorporation of isoleucine into protein chains, thus resulting in the inhibition of bacterial protein synthesis.[204] Due to the unique MOA, there is no cross-resistance between mupirocin and other antimicrobial agents. However, bacterial resistance to this agent has been identified, and it develops through the alterations of the synthase target such that the enzyme still functions but does not bind mupirocin.

Therapeutic Applications and Absorption, Distribution, Metabolism, and Excretion-Toxicity. Mupirocin displays a broad spectrum of activity against many gram-positive bacteria and it also shows in vitro activity against certain gram-negative bacteria. This agent is bacteriostatic at low concentrations, but it becomes bactericidal at concentrations achieved when administered locally.[204] Mupirocin is used only topically as systemic use would result in a rapid and vast hydrolysis of the ester to give an inactive monic acid, which is then excreted in the urine. Mupirocin is available as a topical ointment for the treatment of impetigo due to *S. aureus* and *S. pyogenes* and as a cream for the treatment of secondarily infected traumatic skin lesions caused by these pathogens.[234,235] In general, the adverse reactions are minimal due to topical application of this agent. Stinging of the skin, localized burning and/or pain as well as headache are the adverse reactions that have been associated with the use of this medication.

Urinary Antiseptics

Fosfomycin

Mechanism of Action and Chemical Properties. Fosfomycin is a small-molecule natural product produced by *S. fradiae* and other *Streptomyces* spp. It was discovered in 1969 and soon after was recognized for its antimicrobial effects.[236] Due to its simple chemical structure, the total synthesis of this natural product has been easily achieved. Fosfomycin mimics the structure of phosphoenolpyruvate (PEP), which is a natural substrate required for the biosynthesis of peptidoglycan (Fig. 32.43A). Fosfomycin acts through creating a covalent bond with the sulfhydryl group of cysteine 115 that is located in the active site of the bacterial UDP-*N*-acetylglucosamine-3-enolpyruvyltransferase enzyme also known as MurA (Fig. 32.43B). This enzyme catalyzes an essential biosynthetic step involving the interaction of PEP with UDP-NAG to give an intermediate that is subsequently converted (via MurB enzyme) into UDP-NAM, an essential component of peptidoglycan.[237,238] The net outcome of the action of MurA and MurB enzymes is the resulting ether of lactic acid side chain within NAM that serves as a point of attachment for the pentapeptide stem structure (L-Ala-D-Glu-L-Lys-D-Ala-D-Ala), which in turn is cross-linked with the pentaglycyl bridging segment by the action of PBPs to afford a mature peptidoglycan polymer (Fig. 32.43C). As such, alkylation of MurA by fosfomycin inactivates the enzyme, which directly results in the inhibition of peptidoglycan biosynthesis and a bactericidal effect. Although this agent is very hydrophilic, and it can be ionized depending on the pH, it passes through the bacterial cell wall via two carrier-dependent systems that actively transport fosfomycin. The α-glycerophosphate permease transport system (GlpT) for which α-glycerophosphate is the natural substrate has been shown to uptake fosfomycin. The second system is

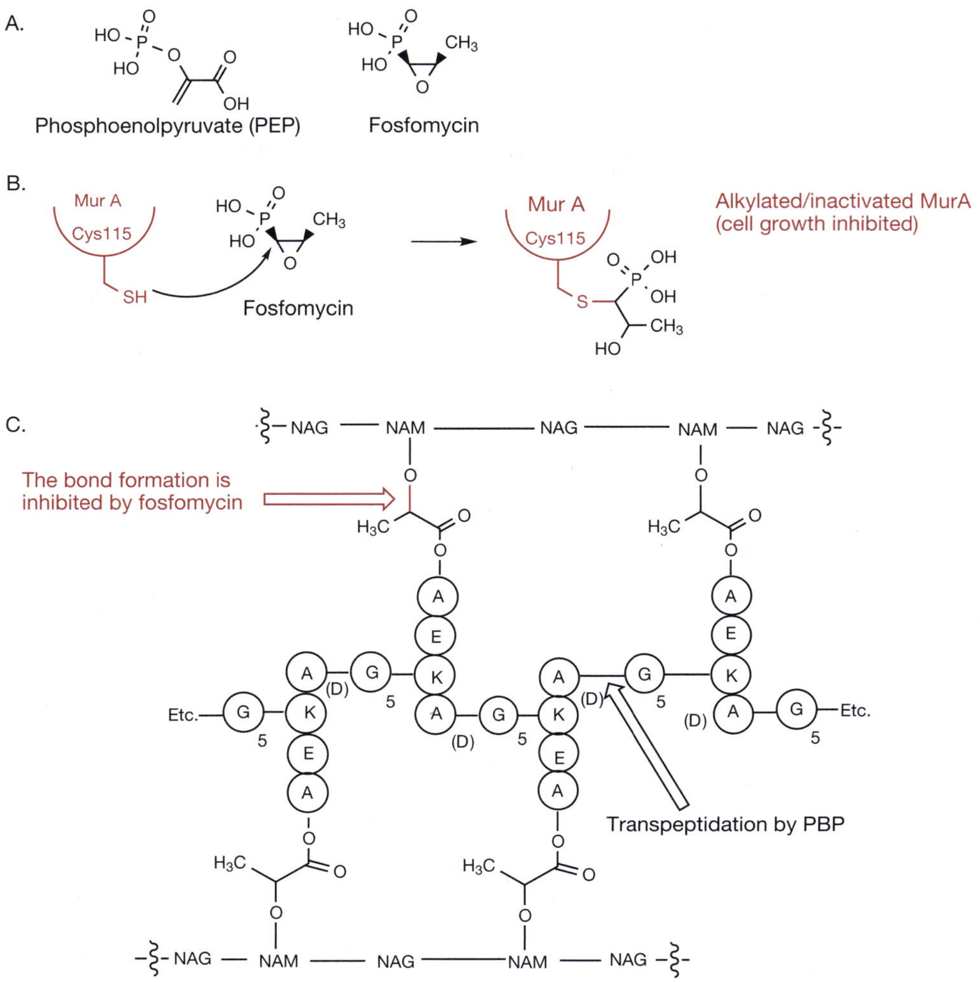

Figure 32.43 A. Structures of phosphoenolpyruvate (PEP) and fosfomycin. B. Covalent inhibition of cysteine 115 in MurA by fosfomycin. C. Overall impact of fosfomycin on peptidoglycan biosynthesis. NAG, *N*-acetylglucosamine; NAM, *N*-acetylmuramic acid; PBP, penicillin-binding protein.

the hexose phosphate uptake system (UhpT), which also transports this drug into the cell of some bacteria.

Resistance. Resistance mechanisms to fosfomycin have been developed by bacteria. Those include mutations in genes encoding the GlpT and UhpT drug uptake systems, mutations in the fosfomycin target gene encoding MurA enzyme, upregulation of gene expression leading to MurA overproduction, as well as production of fosfomycin-modifying enzymes (especially metalloenzymes) that inactivate the drug by converting it to di- and triphosphates, conjugating via nucleophilic addition (in the same manner as MurA reacts with the drug) of glutathione or bacillithiol, and opening the epoxide (oxirane) ring via hydrolysis.[237]

Therapeutic Applications and Absorption, Distribution, Metabolism, and Excretion-Toxicity. Fosfomycin has a broad spectrum of activity, and it shows high efficacy against various gram-positive and gram-negative bacteria, including MDR organisms. It has been approved for oral administration as a suspension (mixed with water). Although fosfomycin is rapidly absorbed, its bioavailability is only 37% when taken by a fasting patient. Food, especially high-fat meals, decreases absorption to 30% and increases time to peak to approximately 4 hours (from 2 hours when taken on an empty stomach). This agent is eliminated predominantly in the urine and has variable elimination half-life ranging from 3 to 8 hours. Fosfomycin is indicated for the treatment of uncomplicated UTIs (acute cystitis) in women due to susceptible strains of *E. coli* and *E. faecalis*.[239] It may also be used off-label to treat chronic bacterial prostatitis. Fosfomycin is accompanied with various adverse effects, such as GI effects (abdominal pain, dyspepsia, nausea, and diarrhea), CDAD, and hypersensitivity reactions (immediate and delayed) that may range from skin rash to rare cases of anaphylaxis and even anaphylactic shock.

Methenamine (Hiprex)

Mechanism of Action and Chemical Properties. Methenamine is a heterocyclic organic compound readily produced at large scale by reacting ammonia with formaldehyde. It has a cage-like structure similar to that of adamantane (Fig. 32.44). Nitrogen atoms are placed on the four vertices, which are linked by six methylene ($-CH_2-$) linkers, hence the alternative names: hexamethylenetetramine, hexamine.

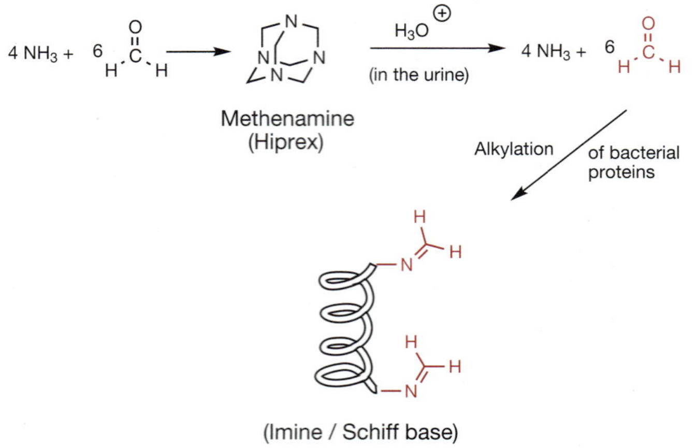

Figure 32.44 Synthesis of methenamine, its breakdown at low pH in the urine, and subsequent alkylation of bacterial proteins.

Methenamine can be viewed as a prodrug that is bioactivated non-enzymatically at lower pH. In the acidic pH of the urine, methenamine breaks down to formaldehyde and ammonia. The resulting formaldehyde has a nonspecific bactericidal action and alkylates proteins and nucleic acids within the bacteria.[240] In an alkaline environment, methenamine is practically inactive. Therefore, to aid in providing an acidic environment and thus promoting the formation of formaldehyde in the urine, methenamine is available in two salt formulations created with organic acids: hippurate (1 g twice daily) and mandelate (1 g 4 times daily).[240]

Therapeutic Applications and Absorption, Distribution, Metabolism, and Excretion-Toxicity. Methenamine is administered orally as a tablet, and it is rapidly absorbed from the GI. If the tablet is not protected by an enteric coating, up to 30% of the dose will be hydrolyzed and inactivated in the stomach. It achieves its peak concentration within 1 to 2 hours and has a half-life of approximately 4 hours. Due to the site of action, it is excreted in the urine. The following adverse reactions have been associated with the use of methenamine: GI (dyspepsia, nausea, abdominal pain, vomiting, diarrhea), dermatologic (skin rash), CNS (headache), genitourinary (bladder pain, blood in the urine), and back pain.

Because almost all bacteria are susceptible to the action of formaldehyde, the resistance to methenamine practically does not develop. As such, this medication is particularly useful in suppressing recurrent or chronic UTIs.[241] However, *Proteus* spp. produce urease, an enzyme that hydrolyzes urea to ammonia and carbon dioxide, thereby alkalinizing the urine and creating an environment where the bacteria can survive.[242] Therefore, methenamine is less effective against *Proteus* spp.

Monoclonal Antibodies

Bezlotoxumab (Zinplava). Bezlotoxumab is a human immunoglobulin G1 (IgG1) monoclonal antibody, which acts by binding to and neutralizing the toxic effects of *C. difficile* toxin B (but not toxin A). It has been approved by the FDA to reduce the recurrence of *C. difficile* infection (CDI) in adults and pediatric patients ages 1 year and older who are currently treated for CDI with antibacterial drug regimen but are at a high risk for CDI recurrence.[243] Bezlotoxumab is not an antibacterial drug and therefore is not indicated solely for the treatment of CDI. As a biologic agent, it is not suitable for oral administration (due to degradation in the GI) and therefore this medication must be given as an IV infusion for over 60 minutes. It has an elimination half-life of ~19 days and undergoes metabolism through protein catabolism. Worsening of heart failure, heart failure, infusion-related reaction, nausea, fever, and headache are the major adverse reactions.

Fecal Bacteriotherapy

More recently, an emphasis was placed on restoration of the intestinal microbiota balance (ie, eubiosis) to support gut homeostasis following antibiotic treatment. In recent years, two products with such properties have been approved for the prevention of recurrence of CDI in individuals 18 years of age and older after they completed antibiotic treatment of recurrent CDI infection. This therapy is approved for prophylaxis of CDI, and it shall not be used for the treatment of CDI.

Fecal Microbiota, Live-jslm (Rebyota). Fecal microbiota, live-jslm is the first microbiome-based live biotherapeutic agent. It was approved by the FDA in 2022. It is administered rectally as a single dose of 150 mL within 24 to 72 hours after completion of *C. difficile* treatment regimen.[244] Rebyota can be considered as fecal transplant therapy that is used to restore intestinal eubiosis in patients. It is generally well tolerated with GI adverse effects such as abdominal pain and distention, diarrhea, flatulence, and nausea being observed.

Fecal Microbiota Spores, Live-brpk (VOWST). This product contains live purified Firmicutes spores that are formulated as a capsule. The capsule should be swallowed whole, without opening, to prevent disintegration. The spores modulate bile acid concentrations and restore short chain fatty acids, which subsequently induces colonization resistance to *C. difficile* and restores intestinal eubiosis.[245] This agent was approved in 2023 by the FDA for oral administration to be taken as four capsules once daily for 3 consecutive days, beginning 2 to 4 days after completion of *C. difficile* treatment.[246] No food or drink should be consumed at least 8 hours prior to the first dose. The subsequent doses should be taken on an empty stomach before the first meal of the day. The major adverse effect is abdominal distention. Others include constipation, diarrhea, flatulence, and nausea.

Antimycobacterial Agents

Introduction

Mycobacteria are a genus of acid-fast bacilli belonging to Mycobacteriaceae, which include the organisms responsible for TB and leprosy as well as several other, less common diseases. Mycobacteria tend to be slow growing and difficult to stain pathogens and, when they are stained with basic dye, can resist decolorization with acid alcohol. The staining characteristics relate to the abnormally high lipid content of the cell wall. In fact, detailed understanding of the morphology and biochemistry of the cell wall (cell envelope) of the mycobacterium reveals the secret to many of the characteristics of this genus of organisms. The cell envelope is unique in both morphologic structure and functional complexity.

ANTIBACTERIAL VACCINES

Vaccines are an effective and proven way of protecting people's lives against harmful diseases, especially infections caused by viruses and bacteria. Uromune (also known as MV140) is a novel, polyvalent bacterial vaccine that has been approved in several countries for the prevention of recurrent UTIs in females, and it is currently in clinical trials/under development in many other countries, including the United States (phase 2).[247] It is a sublingual, mucosal-based bacterial vaccine composed of a suspension of whole-cell heat-inactivated bacteria (300 Formazin Turbidity Units) in glycerol, sodium chloride, artificial pineapple flavoring, and water that upon administration (two sprays under the tongue once daily for 3 months) induces protective immunity in the bladder for up to 9 months.[248] The putative MOA of this vaccine is that it induces antibody production and activates human dendritic cells to generate T helper (Th) cells Th1 and Th17 as well as the cytokine interleukin-10 (IL-10), all of which produce anti-inflammatory T-cell responses in secondary lymphoid organs and locally in the bladder.[248]

It has been suggested that the cell envelope is responsible for mycobacterium pathogenicity (virulence), multiple drug resistance, cell permeability, immunoreactivity, and inhibition of antigen responsiveness, as well as disease persistence and recrudescence. Therefore, it is apparent that significant effort has been put forth to define the chemical structure of the mycobacterial cell envelope. In result, over the past several decades, successful chemotherapeutic agents were developed that act by inhibiting the biosynthesis of cell envelope.

The mycobacterial cell envelope contains, on the interior surface, a cytoplasmic membrane like that found in most bacteria. A conventional peptidoglycan layer affording the organism rigidity appears next. The plasma membrane and the peptidoglycan layer are separated with a periplasmic space in which are present β-lactamases. This layer is composed of alternating *N*-acetyl-D-glucosamines (NAG) linked to *N*-glycolyl-D-muramic acids (Mur, an *N*-glycolyl analog of NAM) through 1-4 linkages that, in turn, is attached to the peptide linker composed of D-alanine (A), D-glutamine (Q), meso-diaminopimelic acid (DP), and L-alanine (A). A novel disaccharide phosphodiester linker made up of *N*-acetyl-D-glucosamine and rhamnose connects the muramic acid to polygalactan and polyarabinose chains, which constitute the arabinogalactan (AG) layer of the cell envelope. The AG layer is covalently linked to the unusually long-chain (C_{60}-C_{90}) mycolic acid residues, which constitute the so-called inner leaflet of the mycobacterial outer membrane. Noncovalently bound to the mycolates are various complex lipids such as the phthiocerol lipids and the glycopeptidolipids, respectively, which form the outer leaflet.[249] Lastly, spanning from the interior, embedded in the plasma membrane, to the exterior is the lipoarabinomannan (LAM) polymer. As indicated, this unit is composed of polyarabinose, polymannan, and various lipids attached through a phosphatidylinositol moiety (Fig. 32.45).[250,251]

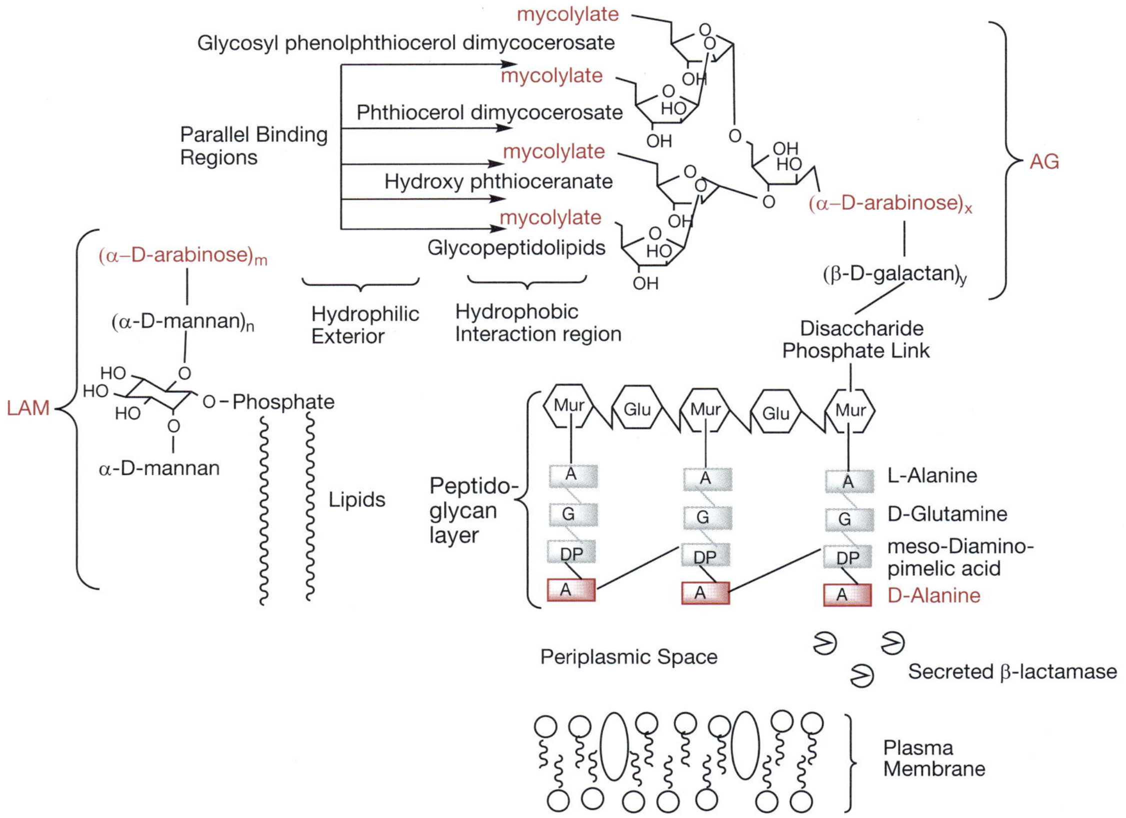

Figure 32.45 Diagrammatic representation of the cell wall/cell envelope of mycobacterium with drug sites of action highlighted in red. AG, arabinogalactan; LAM, lipoarabinomannan.

Specific Diseases

Tuberculosis. TB is a disease that has been known from the earliest recorded history and is a current global epidemic. Egyptian mummies dated 2050 to 500 BC were shown to contain DNA of Mtb, the causative agent of TB.[252] Throughout the centuries, various terms were used for TB, including consumption, wasting disease, scrofula, king's evil, the white death, and the great white plague. Although pulmonary TB is the most common form of the infection, other organs can also be infected. This includes the CNS (TB meningitis), cervical lymph nodes or lymph nodes, skin (systemic lupus erythematosus), bones and joints (Pott disease), kidneys, and the urinary tract. TB that has disseminated to multiple organs is referred to as miliary TB, and it is the most fatal form of the disease. Mtb is an acid-fast, aerobic bacillus with the previously discussed, unusual composition of the cell wall. The cell wall has a high lipid content, resulting in a high degree of hydrophobicity and resistance to alcohol, acids, alkali, and various disinfectants. After staining with a dye, the cell wall of Mtb cannot subsequently be decolorized with an acid wash, thus the characteristic of being an acid-fast bacillus. According to the World Health Organization's (WHO's) Global Tuberculosis Report 2024, approximately 10.8 million people (~5.9 million males, ~3.6 million females, and ~1.3 million children) developed TB worldwide in 2023, and 1.25 million people died from TB in the same year.[253] This ranks TB as the leading cause (replacing COVID-19) of mortality from an infectious disease and one of the top 10 causes of death worldwide. Before 1984, only 10% of the organisms isolated from patients with TB were resistant to any drug. In 1984, 52% of the organisms were resistant to at least one drug, and 32% were resistant to more than one drug. MDR-TB is associated with resistance to the two most potent first-line anti-TB drugs, isoniazid (INH) and RIF. In recent decades, patients are also being diagnosed with extensively drug-resistant tuberculosis (XDR-TB), a condition in which the organism is resistant to either INH or RIF, any fluoroquinolone, and at least one of the second-line injectable drugs. As a result of MDR-TB and XDR-TB, isolates of Mtb should be tested for antimicrobial susceptibility as drug resistance has been encountered in patients who have never been treated with any of the anti-TB drugs.

Nontuberculous Mycobacterial Infections

Leprosy (Hansen Disease). Leprosy (Hansen disease) is recognized as a chronic granulomatous infection caused by *Mycobacterium leprae*. The disease can consist of lepromatous leprosy, tuberculoid leprosy, or a condition with characteristics between these two poles and referred to as borderline leprosy. The disease is more common in tropical countries but is not limited to warm climate regions. Over the last four decades, more than 17 million people received medical treatment to counteract this infectious disease.[254] In 2022 alone there were 174,087 new cases, of which 67,657 (39%) were among females.[254] Children appear to be the most susceptible patient population, but the signs and symptoms do not usually occur until much later in life as the incubation period for M. *leprae* is usually 3 to 5 years and can even be as long as 20 years. In the past several years, the number of cases reported in the United States was consistently below 200. Their diagnosis is often delayed because health care providers are either unaware of the symptoms or misdiagnose the condition as the disease is rare in the United States. The disease is contagious, but the infectiousness is relatively low. Person-to-person contact appears to be how the disease is spread, with entrance into the body occurring through the skin or the mucosa of the upper respiratory tract. Skin and peripheral nerves are the most susceptible regions to the attack. Without the involvement of nerves, Hansen disease would be practically a minor skin disease. The first signs of the disease consist of hypopigmented or hyperpigmented macules. Anesthetic or paresthetic patches can be additionally experienced by the patient. Neural involvement in the extremities leads ultimately to muscle atrophy, resorption of small bones, and spontaneous amputation. When facial nerves are involved, corneal ulceration and blindness can occur. The identification of M. *leprae* in skin or blood samples is not always possible, but the detection of the antibody to the organism is an effective diagnostic test, especially for the lepromatous form of the disease.

Mycobacterium avium-intracellulare and Mycobacterium abscessus. Complexes *Mycobacterium avium* and *Mycobacterium intracellulare* are atypical acid-fast bacilli that are ubiquitous in the environment and considered usually to be nonpathogenic in healthy, immunocompetent individuals. However, in immunocompetent patients with structural lung disease, an isolated pulmonary infection is usually observed.[174] On the contrary, in immunocompromised individuals, these and possibly other unidentified mycobacteria may cause severe, life-threatening infections. In patients with human immunodeficiency virus (HIV) infection, the two principal forms of MAC infection are disseminated disease and focal lymphadenitis.[174] It is also a very common opportunistic infection behind candidal esophagitis and primary *P. jirovecii* pneumonia (PCP) reported in patients with AIDS. Before the availability of effective antiretroviral medications, the incidence of MAC in persons with advanced immunosuppression not receiving MAC prophylaxis was reported to range between 20% and 40%.[174] With the widespread use of effective antiretroviral therapy (ART), the incidence has decreased to less than 2 cases per 1,000 persons. Overall, lungs are the organ most affected by MAC in patients without HIV, but the infection can involve the bone marrow, lymph nodes, liver, and blood in patients with HIV. The $CD4^+$ T-lymphocyte count is used as a predictor for risk of disseminated MAC; a count of less than 50 cells/mm^3 in an HIV-infected person (adult or adolescent) is an indication of a potential infection and a recommendation for chemoprophylaxis. Another concern is the increasing prevalence of M. *abscessus* complex (MABC) infections among patients with structural lung diseases such as chronic obstructive pulmonary disease (COPD) and CF.[255,256] The MAC and MABC organisms grow within macrophages; therefore, the drug must be capable of penetrating the macrophage. Treatment of MAC and MABC, both prophylactically and for diagnosed infections, requires the use of multidrug regimen, and in the case of disseminated MAC, the therapy is for the life of the patient.

General Approaches to Drug Therapy

The mycobacteria have several characteristics in common, but it is important to recognize that the respective species vary widely in their susceptibility to the different drug classes. Some species such as Mtb are very slow growing, with a doubling time of approximately 24 hours, whereas others, such as *Mycobacterium smegmatis* (Msm), double in 2 to 3 hours. The pathogenic mycobacterial species can be divided into organisms that are actively metabolizing and rapidly growing; semidormant bacilli, which exhibit spurts of metabolism; bacilli that can survive at low pH and exhibit low metabolic activity; and dormant cells, the so-called persisters. The latter characteristic is the most problematic and responsible for treatment failures. Most of the currently used anti-TB drugs are those that are effective against actively metabolizing and rapidly growing bacilli. Thus, successful chemotherapy calls for medications with bactericidal action against all stages of the organisms, especially against the dormant, persister cells. The use of combination therapy based on agents with different mechanisms of action for an extended period of time is the widely used approach to successful treatment outcomes.

Drug Therapy for Tuberculosis

The effectiveness of the adopted drug therapy for the treatment of TB has been greatly hampered by the development of MDR-TB and XDR-TB and the lack of new classes of drugs. In fact, no new agents have been developed for drug-susceptible (DS) TB in the last 60 years. The medications that have been approved in the last two decades are second-line agents for the treatment of MDR-TB and XDR-TB, and they are accompanied with serious adverse effects. The only change in the treatment of TB has been the strategy of using directly observed therapy (DOT) short-course, with an emphasis on patient-centered care.[257] Currently, the short-course treatment consists of a four-drug cocktail comprised of RIF (also known as rifampicin), isoniazid, pyrazinamide, and ethambutol (RIPE) for a 2-month "intensive phase" followed by a 4-month or 7-month "continuation phase" with the two most powerful TB chemotherapeutics, INH and rifampicin (for a total of 6-9 months of treatment).[258] Additionally, patient compliance continues to be a serious problem for the lengthy course of therapy, which in turn contributes to the development of bacterial resistance.

First-Line Antitubercular Agents

Isoniazid

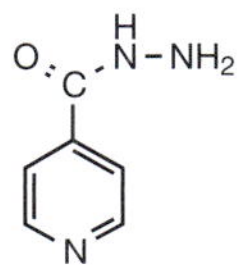

Isoniazid

INH (or H) is a synthetic antibacterial agent that represents an aromatic hydrazide and shows bactericidal action against Mtb. Its inhibitory effects against intracellular and extracellular bacilli were discovered in 1952, and it is generally considered to be the first drug widely adopted for the treatment of Mtb infections. It should be noted that STM and p-aminosalicylic acid (PAS) were discovered earlier; however, their use as anti-TB agents was substantially compromised by the development of bacterial resistance. INH's action is bactericidal against replicating organisms, but it appears to be only bacteriostatic at best against semidormant and dormant populations. After treatment with INH, Mtb loses its acid fastness, which is a direct indication that this agent interferes with the biosynthesis of mycobacterial cell wall.

Structure-Activity Relationship. INH is a simplified name for isonicotinic acid hydrazide, a compound composed of the pyridine heteroaromatic ring and unsubstituted hydrazide functional group. A plethora of derivatives of nicotinaldehyde, isonicotinaldehyde, and substituted isonicotinic acid hydrazides, various INH prodrugs, and even analogs of the isonicotinyl-nicotinamide adenine dinucleotide (NAD) adduct have been prepared and investigated for their antitubercular activity. INH hydrazones were found to possess activity, but these compounds were shown to be unstable in the GI tract, releasing the active INH. Thus, it would appear that their activity resulted from the liberated INH stemming from the acid-promoted hydrolysis of the hydrazone at lower pH in the stomach rather than the actual derivatives of INH.[259,260] Substitution of the hydrazine portion of INH with alkyl or aryl substituents resulted in a mixed series of active and inactive derivatives. Substitution of the N_1 hydrogen with alkyl groups (R^1 = alkyl) destroyed the activity; however, substitution of the N_2 position resulted in active compounds (R^2 and/or R^3 = alkyl; R^1 = H). Although many of the derivatives showed good in vitro activity and safety, none of them was ultimately superior in vivo when compared to INH.

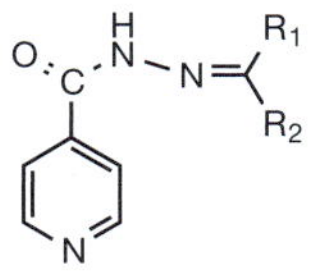

Isoniazid hydrazones

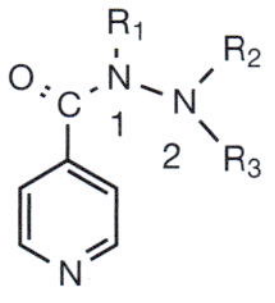

Isoniazid hydrazides

Mechanism of Action. INH is a prodrug that is activated through an oxidation reaction catalyzed by an endogenous enzyme, the catalase-peroxidase katG.[261] This enzyme converts INH to highly reactive, isonicotinoyl radical, which rapidly reacts with NADH to create a covalent adduct. This adduct acts as a slow, tight-binding, competitive inhibitor of the enoyl-acyl carrier protein (enoyl-ACP) reductase (InhA) enzyme, which ultimately inhibits the biosynthesis of mycolic acids. Evidence in support of this mechanism of activation of INH reveals that INH-resistant isolates have decreased catalase activity, and that the loss of catalase activity is associated with the deletion of the catalase gene, *katG*. Furthermore, reintroduction of the gene into resistant organisms results in restored sensitivity of the organism to the drug. Reaction of INH with catalase-peroxidase results in the formation of isonicotinaldehyde, isonicotinic acid, and isonicotinamide, which can be accounted for through formation of the reactive intermediate species isonicotinoyl radical and isonicotinic peroxide (Fig. 32.46).[262]

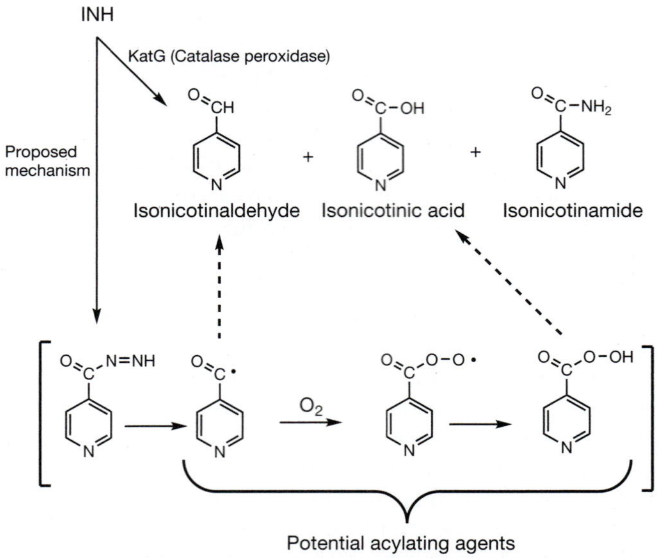

Figure 32.46 Reaction products formed from catalase-peroxidase reaction with isoniazid (INH).

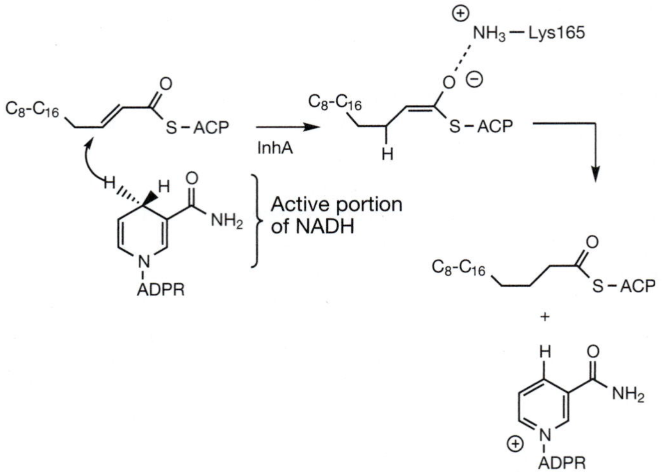

Figure 32.48 Enoylthioester (ACP, acyl carrier protein) reduction catalyzed by an InhA enzyme (enoyl-acyl carrier protein reductase) with NADH (reduced nicotinamide adenine dinucleotide) as the cofactor.

Mycolic acids (Fig. 32.47) are the primary lipid component of the thick, waxy mycobacterial cell wall. They provide an effective barrier that prevents various xenobiotics and hydrophilic molecules from penetration into the cell.[263,264] The enzyme InhA, encoded by the *inhA* gene, is an NADH-dependent, enoyl-ACP reductase involved in double-bond reduction during elongation steps in the biosynthesis of the long-chain mycolic acids (Fig. 32.48). INH specifically inhibits the biosynthesis of fatty acids longer than 26 carbon atoms. It should be noted that the mycolic acids are α-alkylated β-hydroxylated lipids having a "short" α-chain of 20 to 26 carbons and a "long" meromycolyl chain of 40 to 60 carbons. It has been proposed that INH is activated to an electrophilic species that acylates the 4-position of the NADH cofactor (Fig. 32.49). The acylated NADH (isonicotinyl-NAD) acts as a slow, tight-binding, competitive inhibitor of InhA. In result, the essential reduction step of unsaturated fatty acids does not take place, and the biosynthesis of the mycolic acids is therefore inhibited.[265,266]

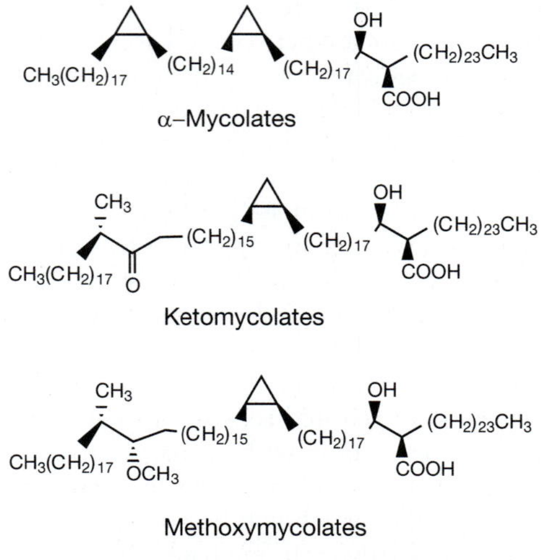

Figure 32.47 Representative structures of mycolic acids.

Resistance. The mechanism of resistance to INH appears to be a complex process, possibly involving mutations in multiple genes including *katG* and *inhA*. It is possible that different mutations result in different degrees of resistance. This seems to be especially true in MDR-TB. A high level of resistance is reported to occur through katG mutation especially at codon 315, which leads to a Ser315 to Thr315 substitution in KatG enzyme, thus preventing INH from activation and conferring a high-level INH resistance.[267] Mutations in regulatory regions of *inhA* cause a rather low-level resistance, which can be overcome with application of high doses of INH.[268] An additional mechanism of resistance comes from mutations in the *Ndh* gene encoding NADH dehydrogenase of the respiratory chain. Defects in this enzyme result in lowering the rate of NADH oxidation and thus increasing the intracellular NADH/NAD^+ ratio. The increased amount of NADH is thought to prevent formation of isonicotinyl-NAD or may even promote displacement of the isonicotinic acyl NADH from InhA enzyme.[269]

Absorption, Distribution, Metabolism, and Excretion-Toxicity. INH is readily absorbed following oral administration and achieves peak plasma concentrations within

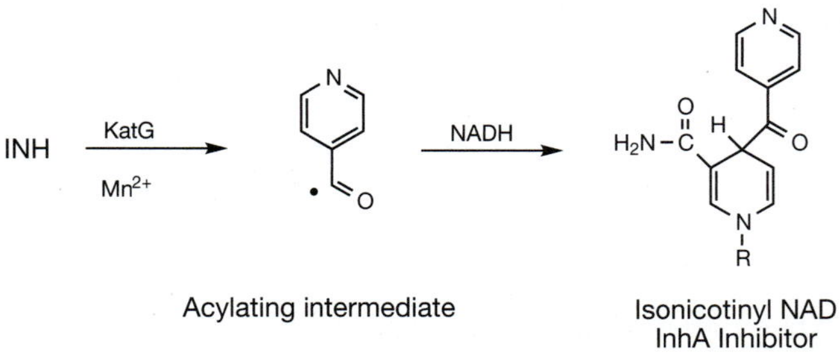

Figure 32.49 Activated INH acylates NADH of NADH-dependent enoyl-acyl protein (InhA). INH, isoniazid; NADH, reduced nicotinamide adenine dinucleotide.

1 to 2 hours. It is available as a tablet and oral solution/syrup. Food and various antacids, especially aluminum-containing antacids, can decrease and/or delay the absorption; therefore, this medication is recommended to be taken on an empty stomach. The drug is well distributed to body tissues, including infected tissues. A long-standing concern about the use of INH during preventive therapy for latent tuberculosis infection (LTBI) has been the high incidence of hepatotoxicity, which can be severe and sometimes fatal. This has led to a boxed warning. A study has concluded that excluding patients older than 35 years and when relevant clinical monitoring is employed, the rate of hepatotoxicity is relatively low.[270] The risk of hepatotoxicity is associated with increasing age (the highest is for persons ages 50-64 years), and, for unknown reasons, it appears to be higher in females, particularly Black and Hispanic females. When oral therapy is not possible or the GI adverse effects are high, INH can also be administered as an IM injection.

INH is extensively metabolized to inactive metabolites (Fig. 32.50).[271,272] The major metabolite is *N*-acetylisoniazid. The enzyme responsible for acetylation, cytosolic *N*-acetyltransferase, is located primarily in the liver and small intestine and it is produced under genetic control in an inherited autosomal fashion. Individuals who possess high concentrations of the enzyme are referred to as fast (or rapid) acetylators, whereas those with low concentrations are slow acetylators. About 50% of Black and White patients are "slow acetylators." East and Southeast Asian patients and native people from Alaska and Canada have higher chances to be fast acetylators.[273] The half-life of this medication in fast acetylators ranges between 0.5 and 1.5 hours, whereas in slow acetylators it is extended to 2 to 5 hours. This phenomenon may result in a need to adjust the dosage for those patients. Other metabolites include isonicotinic acid, which is found in the urine as a glycine conjugate, and hydrazine. In general, even up to 95% of the dose of INH is excreted in the urine. Isonicotinic acid can also result from hydrolysis of *N*-acetylisoniazid, but in this case the second product of hydrolysis is *N*-acetylhydrazine, which is a toxic metabolite. Mono-*N*-acetylhydrazine is acetylated by *N*-acetyltransferase to the inactive *N*-diacetyl product. This reaction occurs more rapidly in rapid acetylators. The formation of *N*-acetylhydrazine is a significant problem as this compound has been associated with hepatotoxicity that can occur during INH therapy. *N*-acetylhydrazine has been postulated to serve as a substrate for microsomal CYP2E1 isoform, resulting in the formation of a reactive intermediate, an acetyl radical that covalently modifies liver proteins by acetylation, thus leading to liver necrosis.[274] It has been suggested that an *N*-hydroxylamine intermediate is formed in the first instance followed by homolytic bond cleavage, which subsequently results in the reactive species, the acetyl radical (Fig. 32.51). The acetyl radical rapidly acylates liver proteins, thus leading to changes in liver function, which is manifested as an increased serum transaminases, hyperbilirubinemia, jaundice, and hepatitis. Since the CYP2E1 isoform is induced by alcohol, daily users of alcohol have significantly increased risk of hepatitis. Moreover, formation of this unwanted acetyl radical is linked to peripheral neuropathy caused by this agent. Other neurologic effects that have been reported for INH include paresthesia, sensory impairment, seizures, optic neuritis, and encephalopathy. To alleviate the undesirable cytotoxic reactions resulting from formation of the acetyl radical, concomitant administration of pyridoxine (vitamin B_6) is often recommended.

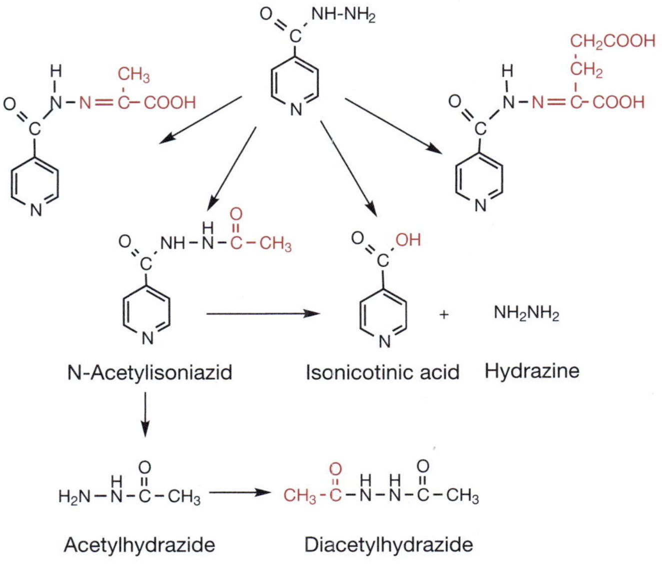

Figure 32.50 Metabolism of isoniazid.

Rifamycin Antibiotics. The rifamycins are members of the ansamycin class of natural products produced by *Streptomyces mediterranei*. The molecules in this chemical class are characterized by the presence of an aliphatic chain forming a bridge or a handle (*ansa* from the Latin) between two nonadjacent positions of an aromatic moiety. While investigating the biologic activity of the naturally occurring rifamycins (B, O, and S), a spontaneous reaction gave the biologically active rifamycin SV, which was later isolated from natural sources. Rifamycin SV was the original rifamycin antibiotic chosen for clinical development. Semisynthetic derivatives are prepared via conversion of the natural rifamycins to 3-formylrifamycin, which is then derivatized with various hydrazines to give products such as RIF (and/or R), rifapentine (RPT), and rifabutin (RFB). These semisynthetic derivatives have significant benefits over previously investigated rifamycins in that they are orally bioavailable, are highly effective against a variety of both gram-positive and gram-negative organisms, and have high clinical efficacy in the treatment of TB. The rifamycin class of antibiotics is active against both growing and slow metabolizing, nongrowing bacilli.

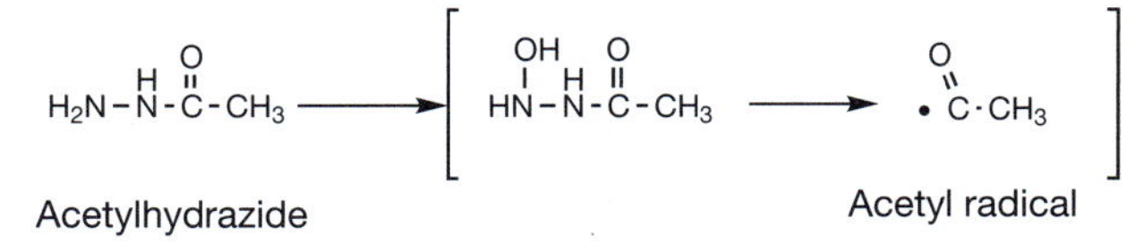

Figure 32.51 Reactive (acetylating) metabolite of isoniazid that causes hepatotoxicity and other adverse effects.

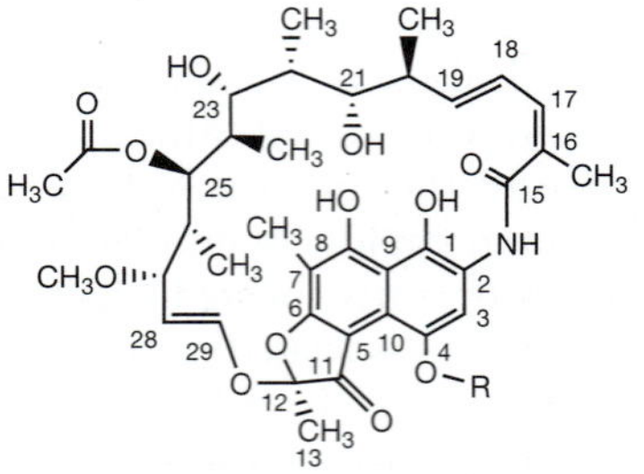

Rifamycin B: R = CH_2COOH
Rifamycin SV: R = H

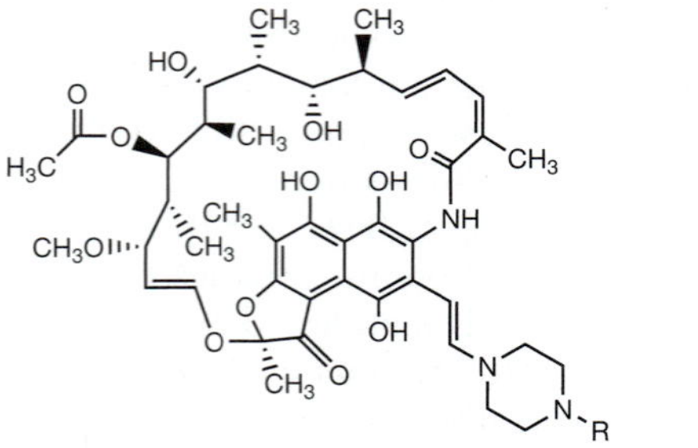

Rifampin (RIF, Rifadin, Rimactane): R = CH_3
Rifapentine (RFT, Priftin): R =
Rifabutin (RFB): R =

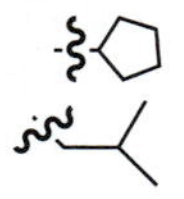

Structure-Activity Relationship. A large number of derivatives of the naturally occurring rifamycins have been prepared and investigated for inhibitory activity of Mtb growth.[275] From these compounds, the following generalizations can be made concerning the SAR: (1) free –OH groups are required at C_1, C_8, C_{21}, and C_{23}; (2) these groups appear to be positioned in a direction that is crucial for interaction with the molecular target, bacterial DDRP (Fig. 32.52); (3) acetylation of C_{21} and/or C_{23} produces inactive compounds; (4) reduction of the double bonds in the ansa ring results in a progressive decrease in activity; and (5) opening of the macro ring gives inactive compounds.[276] The latter two changes greatly affect the conformational structure of the rifamycins, which in turn decreases binding to DDRP. Substitutions at C_3 or C_4 were extensively explored and provided compounds with varying degrees of antibacterial activity. The substitutions at these positions also appear to affect transport across the bacterial cell wall.

Mechanism of Action. The rifamycins inhibit bacterial DDRP by binding to the β-subunit deep within the DNA/RNA channel, thus directly blocking the path of the elongating RNA.[277] This class of medications is highly active against rapidly dividing intracellular and extracellular bacilli. RIF is active against DDRP from both gram-positive and gram-negative bacteria, but because of poor penetration of the cell wall of gram-negative organisms by RIF, the drug has less value in infections caused by such organisms. The naphthalene ring of the rifamycins engages via π-π stacking interactions with an aromatic amino acid ring in the DDRP protein (Fig. 32.52).[278] The DDRP is a metalloenzyme that contains two zinc atoms. It is further postulated that the oxygens at C_1 and C_8 of the rifamycins' aromatic moiety chelate to a zinc atom, which increases the binding to DDRP. Lastly, the oxygens at C_{21} and C_{23} form strong hydrogen bonds to the DDRP. The net result of binding of the rifamycins to DDRP is the inhibition of the RNA synthesis. Specifically, the drug's binding takes place more than 12 Å away from the active site. This blocks transcription at or shortly after (when the transcript becomes 2 to 3 nucleotides in length) the initiation of an RNA chain by the polymerase, but it does not block the elongation of chains already initiated.[277,279] Additional evidence for this MOA comes from the observation that the inhibitory activity of rifamycins is maximal on free enzymes (not bound to DNA); therefore, they inhibit the initiation rather than elongation step of RNA synthesis.[280]

Resistance. Resistance develops when a mutation occurs in the gene responsible for the β-subunit of the RNA polymerase (RNAP; *rpoB* gene), leading to a change in the structure of the β-subunit of RNAP and causing an inability of the antibiotic to readily bind to the RNAP.[281,282] Approximately 90% to 95% of RIF-resistant isolates acquired their resistance through this mechanism.[283] The mutations take place in various regions of the gene and result in various degrees of sensitivity to this antibiotic, several of which were associated with high-level RIF resistance.[283] Additionally, cross-resistance among rifamycins has been a topic of controversy and the current evidence indicates that complete cross-resistance among the three agents RIF, RPT, and RFB does exist.[284] Intrinsic resistance mechanisms involve permeability or efflux/influx pump mechanisms.[284] Other bacteria are intrinsically resistant to RIF due to the composition of their cell wall and lower permeability. Some *Mycoplasma* spp. possess RNAP that is refractory to RIF.[284]

Absorption, Distribution, Metabolism, and Excretion-Toxicity. The rifamycin class of antibiotics are reddish orange, crystalline compounds with zwitterionic properties.

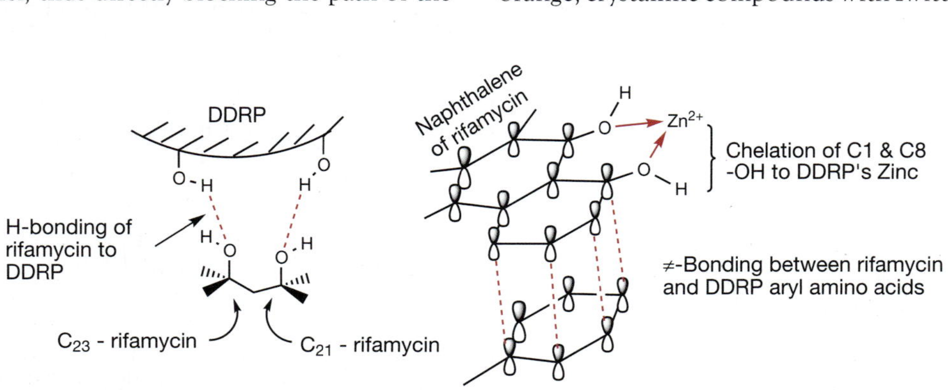

Figure 32.52 Binding of rifamycin to DNA-dependent RNA polymerase (DDRP).

The presence of the phenolic groups results in acidic properties (pK_a ~1.7 in water), whereas the piperazine moiety gives basic properties (pK_a ~7.9 in water). These compounds are prone to acid-promoted hydrolysis of the hydrazone moiety, giving rise to 3-formylrifamycin SV. They might also be prone to air oxidation of the 1,4-phenolic groups in the naphthalene ring to give the *p*-quinone (ie, $C_{1,4}$ quinone) (Fig. 32.53). The rifamycins and their metabolites are excreted in the urine, stools (biliary excretion), saliva, sweat, and tears. Because these agents have dye characteristics, discoloration of all body fluids ranging from reddish orange to reddish brown is directly associated with the use of those agents. This is an important patient counseling point as discoloration of the tears and sweat may cause permanent staining of contact lenses and clothing. Additionally, discoloration of the saliva, urine, and stools might be concerning to patients undergoing therapy with those agents who additionally were not warned about these adverse effects. Other commonly encountered adverse effects include stomach upset or pain, nausea, vomiting, loss of appetite, diarrhea, headache, joint pain, skin rash, or itching.

The three approved agents are generally readily absorbed from the intestine, although food in the GI tract can affect absorption. RIF's absorption can be delayed or even reduced by food in the intestine; therefore, this medication is recommended to be taken on an empty stomach.[272] In terms of RPT, high-fat meals increase its AUC and C_{max} levels. On the contrary, high-fat meals delay the absorption of RFB without impacting the extent of its absorption.[285] These agents do not seem to interfere with the absorption of other antitubercular medications, but there are conflicting reports on whether INH affects the absorption of RIF.[272]

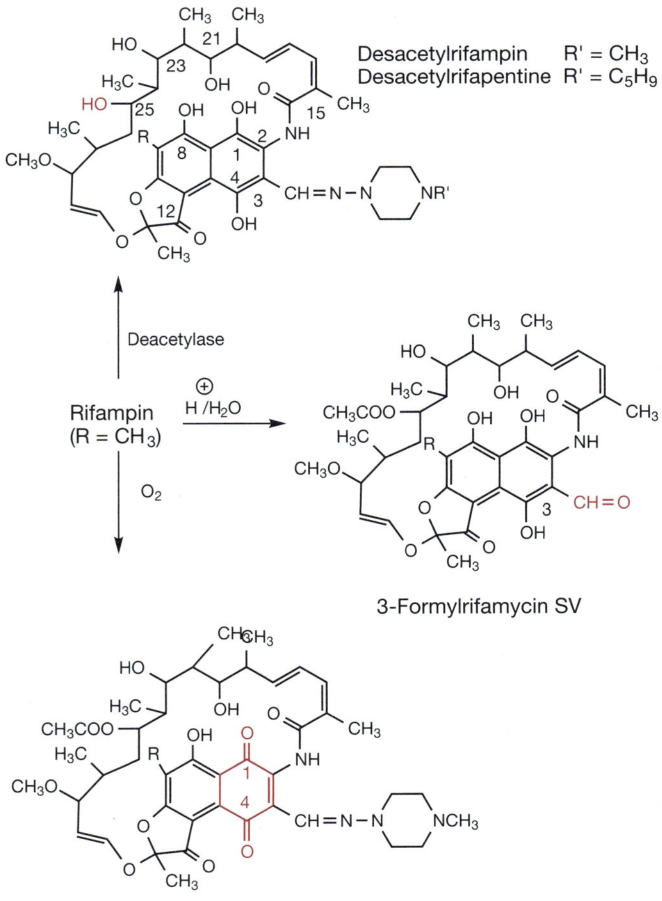

Figure 32.53 Metabolism and in vitro reactions of rifampin.

The major metabolism of RIF, RPT, and RFB occurs via deacetylation, which takes place at the C_{25} acetate (Fig. 32.53). The resulting metabolites, desacetyl-RIF, desacetyl-RPT, and desacetyl-RFB, are still active antibacterial agents. The majority of desacetyl-RIF and desacetyl-RPT metabolites are found in feces, although the glucuronide conjugate of desacetyl-RIF can be found in the urine as well. On the other hand, the desacetyl-RFB metabolite is predominantly excreted in the urine. 3-Formylrifamycin SV has been reported as a second metabolite after administration of those agents. This product is thought to arise in the gut from an acid-catalyzed hydrolysis reaction of the hydrazone linker in the respective agents. The 3-formylrifamycin is reported to possess a broad spectrum of antibacterial activity.[286]

Specific Agents

Rifampin (Rifampin, Rifadin, Rimactane). With the introduction of RIF in Italy in 1968, the duration of combination therapy for the treatment of TB was significantly reduced from 18 to 9 months. RIF is nearly always used in combination with other antitubercular agents for the treatment of active TB infection and LTBI, although one of the approaches to the treatment of LTBI short-course therapy is based on a 4-month treatment with only RIF. It is available as an oral capsule and IV injection. It achieves peak plasma concentrations in approximately 2 hours after oral administration and has a half-life of 2 to 3.5 hours in adults, but its duration of action (due to MOA) is longer and is estimated to last even up to 24 hours. It is bound to plasma proteins to the extent of 80%. In addition to the adverse effects listed for the entire drug class, RIF is associated with hepatotoxicity, CDI and C. *difficile* colitis, hematologic effects (eg, hemolytic anemia, hemorrhage, leukopenia, thrombocytopenia), pneumonitis, and in rare cases hypersensitivity reactions. RIF is known to be a strong inducer of hepatic CYP3A4 and CYP2C19 isoforms and a weak to moderate inducer for several other CYP enzymes. This creates potential for DDIs by decreasing the effectiveness of various agents including oral contraceptives, corticosteroids, warfarin, quinidine, methadone, zidovudine, clarithromycin, and the azole antifungal agents. In addition, RIF increases the expression of Pgps, which in turn increases the efflux of various drugs. Because RIF decreases the effectiveness of protease inhibitors and nonnucleoside reverse transcriptase inhibitors used in the treatment of HIV, the U.S. Centers for Disease Control and Prevention (CDC) has recommended avoidance of RIF in the treatment of patients infected with HIV presently on these HIV therapies.

Rifapentine (Priftin). RPT was approved by the FDA in 1998 for the treatment of active and latent pulmonary TB. The drug's major advantage over RIF is the fact that when used in combination therapy, RPT can be administered twice weekly during the "initial intensive" phase of therapy, followed by once-a-week administration during the "continuation" phase (Table 32.12). In contrast, RIF normally is administered once daily during both the "initial intensive" phase and the "continuation" phase. Because relapse and the emergence of resistant strains of bacteria are often associated with poor patient adherence, reduced dosing and frequency of administration as well as decreased pill burden are expected to increase patient compliance and thus improve treatment outcomes. RPT is readily absorbed following oral administration and is highly bound to plasma proteins (98% vs 80% for RIF). To improve the absorption and exposure, RPT is recommended to be taken with food. On the other hand, crushing the tablet results in 26% lower exposure when compared to taking the whole tablets. Related to the higher plasma binding, RPT has a longer mean elimination half-life (~17 hours for the parent compound and ~24 hours for the desacetyl metabolite) in comparison with the half-life reported for RIF (~2-3.5 hours). However, RPT has a significantly longer time to peak, which can span 3 to 10 hours. Approximately 70% of the drug is excreted in the feces, which is comparable with the elimination of RIF (60%-65% in feces). RPT is generally considered to be more active than RIF. Additionally, it causes milder and fewer adverse effects than RIF and can be used in patients with varying degrees of hepatic dysfunction without the need for dose adjustment.[287] This drug is only a moderate inducer of CYP3A4, and therefore its potential for DDI is lower when compared to RIF.

Rifabutin. RFB was approved for the treatment of both Mtb and MAC infections in 1992. RFB can be used as the first-line treatment for TB in lieu of RIF; however, this is not commonly practiced due to its higher cost. RFB is more commonly used in patients coinfected with both Mtb and

Table 32.12 Group of Medications Used for the Treatment of DS-, MDR-TB, and XDR-TB

Drug Class and Group		Generic (Brand) Name	Dose and Frequency[a]
First-line	Group 1	Isoniazid	300 mg, daily regimen 900 mg, BID or TID regimen
		Rifampin or Rifampicin (Rifampin, Rifadin)	600 mg, daily regimen
		Pyrazinamide	3 g, daily regimen
		Ethambutol[b] (Myambutol)	800 mg-1.6 g, daily regimen 1.2-2.4 g, TID regimen 2-4 g, BID regimen
		Rifapentine (Priftin)	600 mg twice weekly during initial phase and then once weekly during continuation phase
		Rifabutin	300 mg, daily regimen
Second-line	Group 2: Injectable aminoglycosides and polypeptides	Streptomycin	1 g, daily regimen 1.5 g, BID or TID regimen
		Amikacin	15 mg/kg, daily regimen 25 mg/kg, TID regimen
		Capreomycin	15 mg/kg, daily regimen 25 mg/kg, TID regimen
	Group 3: Oral and injectable fluoroquinolones	Moxifloxacin	400 mg, daily regimen
		Levofloxacin	750 mg-1 g, daily regimen
	Group 4: Miscellaneous agents	*p*-Aminosalicylic acid	8-12 g, daily regimen
		Cycloserine	250-750 mg, daily regimen
		Ethionamide (Trecator)	250-500 mg, daily regimen
		Linezolid (Zyvox)	600 mg, daily regimen
		Bedaquiline (Sirturo)	400 mg once daily for 2 wk, followed by 200 mg 3 times weekly
		Pretomanid	200 mg, daily regimen

[a]Doses are provided for adult patients.

[b]Dose should be based on lean body weight.

BID, twice-daily dosing; DS-TB, drug-susceptible tuberculosis; MDR-TB, multidrug-resistant tuberculosis; TID, thrice-daily dosing; XDR-TB, extensively drug-resistant tuberculosis.

HIV, a clinical scenario when RIF causes DDI with the ART.[288] There are less DDIs reported among HIV ART with RFB than with RIF.[288] RFB is taken as a capsule once daily as part of an appropriate combination regimen. It is readily absorbed to the extent of ~53% and it can be taken with food, which reduces the GI adverse effects. The plasma protein binding of RFB is ~85% and this drug achieves peak plasma concentration within 2 to 4 hours, whereas its terminal elimination half-life is 45 hours. Apart from the aforementioned adverse reactions common for the entire drug class, the use of RFB is also accompanied with skin rash, leukopenia, neutropenia, thrombocytopenia, and various GI effects.

PYRAZINAMIDE

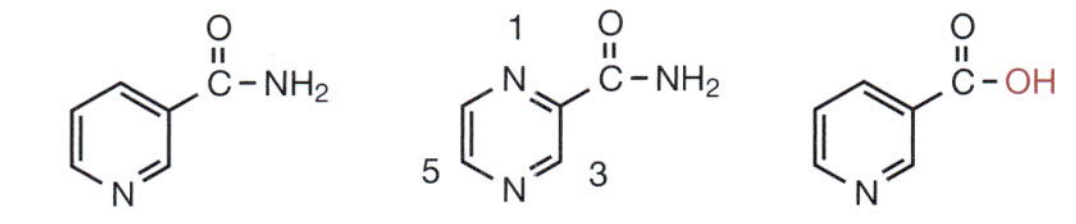

Nicotinamide Pyrazinamide (PZA, Z) Pyrazinoic acid (POA)

Similarly to INH, the bioactivity of pyrazinamide (pyrazine-2-carboxamide, PZA and/or Z) against Mtb was first recognized in 1952.[289] PZA was discovered while investigating analogs of nicotinamide. PZA is a bioisostere of nicotinamide and possesses bacteriostatic or bactericidal action against Mtb depending on the drug's concentration. PZA has become one of the most popular antitubercular medications even though resistance develops relatively quickly to this agent. The clinical utility of this agent stems from the fact that PZA kills non-replicating persisters, which other TB drugs fail to eliminate. Therefore, this agent became an essential component of the combination therapy for the treatment of TB.[289] The activity of PZA is pH dependent with good in vivo activity at pH below 5.5, while at neutral pH this compound is nearly inactive.

Structure-Activity Relationship. PZA contains pyrazine, a heterocyclic aromatic organic compound with 1,4-nitrogen atoms, and an amide group. Due to its structural simplicity and thus easiness for chemical modifications, a wide series of derivatives have been synthesized and screened against Mtb. However, those structural modifications of PZA have proven to be rather ineffective in developing analogs with increased biologic activity. Most substitutions on the pyrazine ring or the use of alternate heterocyclic aromatic rings has resulted in compounds with reduced activity.[290] The replacement of the amide group turned out to be mostly unsuccessful. The only derivatives that showed good promise to compete with the parent drug were the *N*-monosubstituted, α-alkyl branched analogs of PZA bearing a 5-Cl atom on the aromatic ring: tert-butyl 5-chloropyrazinamide and 2′-(2′-methyldecyl) 5-chloropyrazinamide.[291] Overall, the requirements for successful analogs include: (1) provision for hydrophilicity to allow sufficient plasma concentrations such that the drug can be delivered to the site of infection, (2) appropriate lipophilicity to allow penetration into the mycobacterial cell, and (3) susceptibility to hydrolysis such that the prodrug is unaffected by the "extracellular" enzymes but is readily hydrolyzed inside the Mtb's cell at the site of action.

Mechanism of Action. The MOA of PZA remains debatable to this date. The mostly accepted MOA of this agent includes its intracellular conversion to pyrazinoic acid (POA) that is mediated by Mtb's pyrazinamidase (PZase, also known as nicotinamidase).[282] Support for this mechanism comes from the fact that mutation in the PZase gene (*pncA*) results in PZA-resistant strains of Mtb.[282,292] POA has been shown to possess biologic activity at acidic pH (<5.5). This is because upon conversion of PZA in POA (a moderately strong acid with a pK_a of 2.9) by the cytoplasmic PZase, POA gets out of the cell through passive diffusion and a deficient efflux mechanism in Mtb. If the extracellular pH is acidic, the POA gets protonated and thus becomes neutral, which allows the uncharged protonated pyrazinoic acid (POA) to readily permeate through the cell wall back inside the mycobacterial cell. This leads to accumulation of POA over time inside the Mtb cells. This in turn causes cytoplasmic acidification that leads to inhibition of vital enzymes that are associated with fatty acid synthase (FAS) type I fatty acid biosynthesis responsible for the production of mycolic acids.[289] At neutral or alkaline pH, 99.9% of POA is in its charged (ie, ionized) form, which cannot pass through the Mtb's thick cell wall, hence the lack of efficacy observed for this agent at higher pH. In addition to the postulated inhibition of FAS I complex, POA could also de-energize the membrane by collapsing proton motive force and affect membrane transport, thus inhibiting protein and RNA synthesis, trans-translation, and possibly pantothenate/coenzyme A required for persister survival.[289] The more recently published research results indicate, however, that POA acts as an uncoupler of oxidative phosphorylation and therefore disruption of proton motive force is the primary MOA of this agent.[293]

Resistance. Mutations in the *pncA* gene encoding PZase are by far the main mechanism through which Mtb acquires resistance toward PZA. Those mutations impact the protein PZase, which is involved in the conversion of the prodrug PZA to the active form POA. Mutations in the drug target rpsA encoding ribosomal protein S1, which in turn is involved in the process of trans-translation, was recently identified in some PZA-resistant strains. Additionally, overexpression of *rpsA* resulted in decreased efficacy of PZA. Very recently, *panD* mutations were also found in some PZA-resistant Mtb strains. The gene *panD* encodes aspartate decarboxylase, an enzyme that is involved in the synthesis of β-alanine, which in turn serves as a precursor for pantothenate and coenzyme A biosynthesis. The latter processes are crucial for survival and pathogenesis in vivo of Mtb.[289]

Absorption, Distribution, Metabolism, and Excretion-Toxicity. PZA is administered orally as a tablet, and it is readily and well absorbed from the GI tract. It reaches its peak plasma concentration within 2 hours and its half-life in adult patients is 9 to 10 hours. PZA undergoes extensive hepatic metabolism, with the major metabolic route being hydrolysis by hepatic microsomal PZase to give POA, which then is often oxidized by xanthine oxidase to 5-hydroxypyrazinoic acid (Fig. 32.54). PZA is not affected by the presence of food in the GI tract and shows rather minimal DDI with other agents, one of which is enhanced hepatotoxic effect of RIF. PZA is generally well tolerated with hepatotoxicity, GI effects (anorexia, nausea, vomiting), dysuria, dermatitis, and skin rash being reported for the use of this agent.

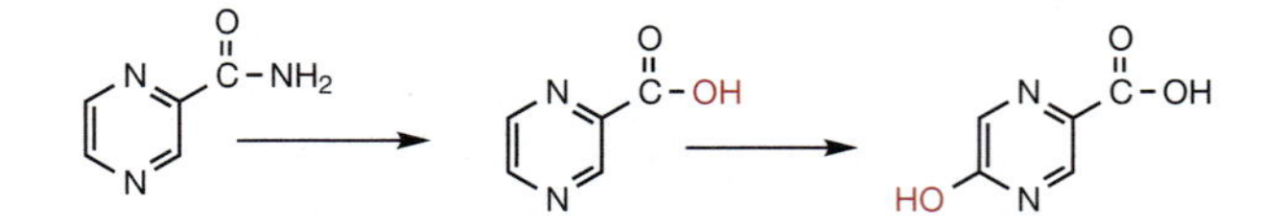

Pyrazinamide Pyrazinoic acid 5-Hydroxypyrazinoic acid

Figure 32.54 Metabolism of pyrazinamide.

Therapeutic Application. PZA has gained acceptance as an essential component of combination therapy for the treatment of TB. The drug is active against semidormant intracellular tubercle bacilli that are not affected by other agents.[257,287] PZA also retains its activity against nonreplicating persister bacilli. The introduction of PZA combinations has further reduced the time of treatment to 6 months from the previous 9-month therapy.

ETHAMBUTOL (MYAMBUTOL)

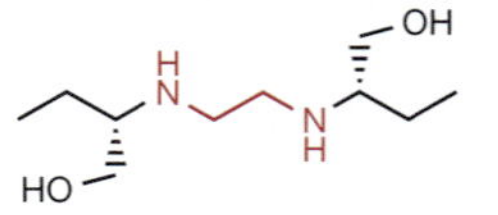

Ethambutol
(Emb, E, Myambutol)

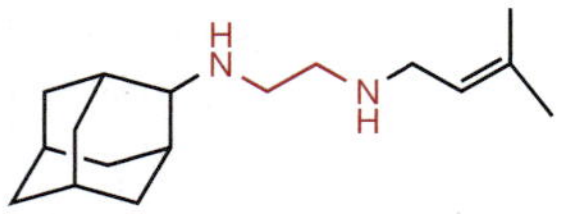

SQ109

Ethambutol (EMB and/or E) is composed of two 1-butanol molecules connected via the ethylenediamine linker. It therefore represents an ethylenediiminobutanol scaffold that contains two constitutionally symmetrical stereogenic carbons, which give rise to four possible stereoisomers. However, only the (+)-(*S,S*)-enantiomer is marketed, which is 200- to 500-fold more active than the opposite (–)-(*R,R*)-enantiomer. The difference in activity between the two enantiomers suggests a stereospecific binding of EMB at its molecular target.

Structure-Activity Relationship. An extensive number of analogs of EMB have been prepared and investigated, but ultimately none has proven to be superior to EMB. Extension of the ethylenediamine chain, replacement of either nitrogen, increasing the size of the nitrogen substituents, and moving the location of the alcohol groups provided derivatives with decreased activity. However, recent efforts focused on modifying the EMB scaffold provided a new series of compounds based on the ethylenediamine linker that showed novel mode of action against Mtb. Among those compounds, SQ109 turned out to be the most prominent inhibitor of the mycobacterial membrane protein Large 3 (MmpL3), which is a transporter of mycolic acids in the form of trehalose monomycolate (TMM) from the cytoplasm into the periplasmic space.[294] MmpL3 is an essential drug target, and its effective inhibition is associated with the bactericidal activity of SQ109, a novel agent that is currently being evaluated in phase 2 clinical trials.[295]

Mechanism of Action. While the MOA of EMB remains to be fully elucidated, recent evidence indicates inhibition of the arabinosyl transferases (embA, embB, and embC) by EMB, which in turn prevents the formation of the cell wall components AG and LAM as well as interference with cell division.[296] In addition to the usual peptidoglycan portion of the cell wall, the mycobacteria have a unique outer envelope consisting of arabinofuranose and galactose (AG), which is covalently attached to the peptidoglycan and an intercalated framework of LAM. The AG portion of the cell wall is highly branched and contains distinct segments of galactan and distinct segments of arabinan. At various locations within the arabinan segments (terminal and penultimate), the mycolic acids are attached to the $C_{5'}$ position of arabinan.[297,298] One action of arabinosyl transferase[297,298] is to catalyze the polymerization of D-arabinofuranose, thus leading to AG formation (Fig. 32.55).[299,300] EMB mimics arabinan, resulting in a buildup of the arabinan precursor β-D-arabinofuranosyl-L-monophosphoryldecaprenol, and as a result the synthesis of both AG and LAM is compromised (Fig. 32.55).[301] This would explain the bacteriostatic nature of EMB and therefore the necessity to use it in combination with other agents in order to observe bactericidal effect. This MOA also accounts for the synergism seen between EMB and intracellularly acting agents, such as RIF. Damage to the cell wall created by EMB improves the cell penetration of the intracellular drugs, resulting in increased biologic activity.

Resistance. The mechanism of resistance to EMB involves a gene overexpression of arabinosyl transferase, which is controlled by the *embCAB* operon (*embC, embA, and embB*).[302] The majority of EMB-resistant isolates carry mutations within *embB*, primarily at codon 306 (*embB306*), as well as certain mutations within the upstream region (UR) of *embA* also confer resistance to EMB.[303] However, the acquisition of resistance mechanisms to EMB seems to be more complex as some other mutations that occurred within the aforementioned *embAB* region yielded EMB-susceptible isolates. On the contrary, there were no mutations identified within this particular region in some isolates that were still resistant to the action of EMB, which implies the involvement of other resistance mechanisms. More recently, hypermethylation and in consequence downregulation of *mbtD* and *celA1* genes was reported to produce in vitro mono-EMB-resistant strains.[304]

Absorption, Distribution, Metabolism, and Excretion–Toxicity. EMB is a water-soluble, bacteriostatic agent that is readily absorbed (~80%) after oral administration (as a tablet). The majority of the administered EMB dose is excreted unchanged (~50% in the urine and ~20% in the feces), whereas a small portion (no more than 20%) of the dose undergoes

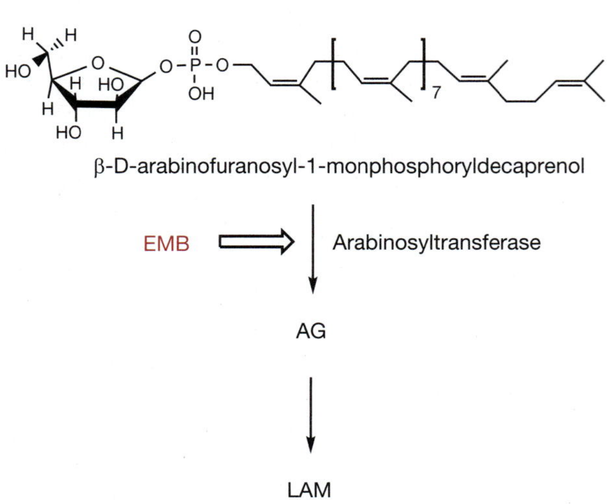

Figure 32.55 Site of action of ethambutol (EMB) in cell wall synthesis. AG, arabinogalactan; LAM, lipoarabinomannan.

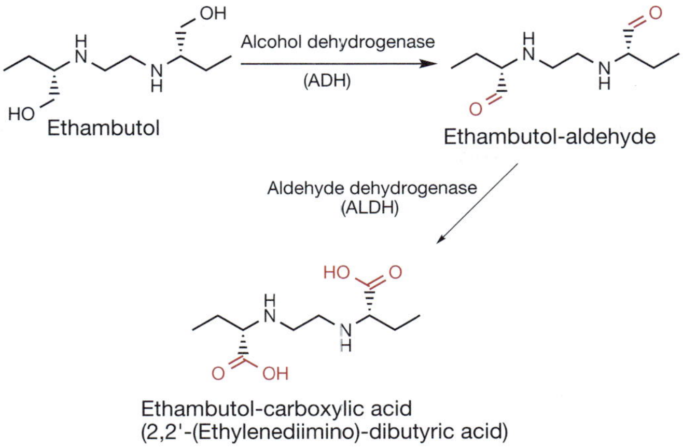

Figure 32.56 Hepatic metabolism of ethambutol.

hepatic metabolism to yield inactive metabolites that are excreted in the urine (Fig. 32.56). EMB achieves peak plasma concentration within 2 to 4 hours and its elimination half-life is approximately 2.5 to 3.5 hours. However, in patients with renal disease, the elimination half-life might be substantially prolonged to 7 to 15 hours. This agent is only moderately bound to plasma proteins (20%-30%). EMB is associated with several adverse effects such as GI (abdominal pain, anorexia, gastric distress, nausea, and vomiting), hematologic (leukopenia, neutropenia, thrombocytopenia), hepatotoxicity, nephritis, and acute kidney injury as well as confusion, disorientation, dizziness, headache, and malaise. EMB is also known to cause optic neuropathy in a dose-dependent manner (not always reversible on discontinuation of the therapy) due to suspected chelation of copper or zinc cations in human mitochondria. The EMB-induced optic neuropathy (EON) includes painless loss of central vision and cecocentral scotomas in the visual field. As a result, this medication was not prescribed in the past for use in children under 5 years. However, the latest guidelines recommend ethambutol for children and adolescents between three months and 16 years of age with non-severe pulmonary TB disease.[305]

Second-Line Antitubercular Agents

Several medications that represent distinct pharmacophores and mechanisms of action are used as second-line agents for the treatment of MDR-TB and XDR-TB, retreatment, or when a patient develops intolerance to the first-line agents. Some of these agents (and their respective drug classes) have already been discussed extensively in the previous sections of this chapter. These are STM and amikacin (aminoglycosides), moxifloxacin and levofloxacin (fluoroquinolones), and linezolid (oxazolidinone). Additional second-line anti-TB medications that are further discussed later include: ethionamide (ETH), PAS, cycloserine, capreomycin, bedaquiline, and pretomanid.

Ethionamide (Trecator)

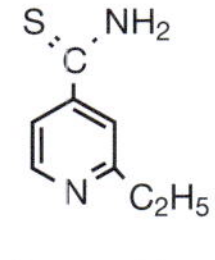

Ethionamide
(ETH, Trecator)

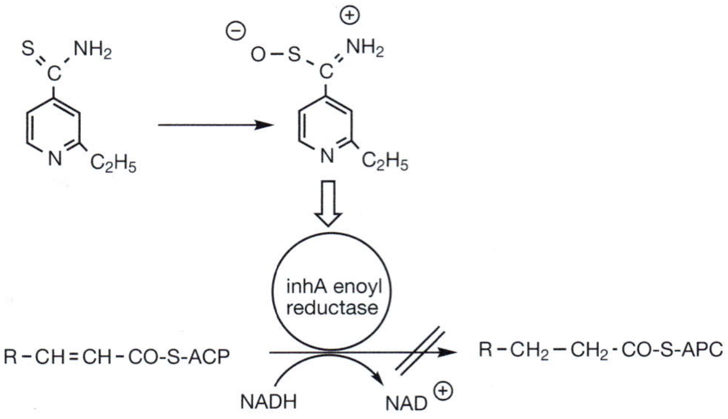

Figure 32.57 Mechanism of action of ethionamide.

The synthesis of analogs of isonicotinamide, which is a regioisomer of nicotinamide, resulted in the discovery of a new agent, ETH, that has been proven to be bactericidal against Mtb and *M. leprae*. The MOA of ETH is thought to be identical to INH, although the pathway of activation is distinct from that of INH.[266,306,307] ETH is a prodrug that is converted via oxidation by ethA, an Mtb's mono-oxygenase enzyme similar to katG, to give the active ETH sulfoxide that is suspected to undergo further conversions to give an acylating agent, which in turn creates adduct with NADH and subsequently inactivates the enoyl-ACP reductase/inhA enzyme (Fig. 32.57). Similar to INH, resistance to ETH arises from mutations in *ethA* and *inhA* genes. Moreover, mutations in the gene encoding the inhA reductase confer cross-resistance between INH and ETH.[308]

ETH may be bacteriostatic or bactericidal in action, depending on the drug's concentration and Mtb's susceptibility. ETH is administered orally as a tablet followed by an essentially complete absorption. However, this agent is not well tolerated in a single large dose (>500 mg). The GI irritation (abdominal pain, diarrhea, metallic taste, nausea, vomiting) can be reduced by administration with meals. It achieves peak plasma concentrations within 1 hour and has a short elimination half-life of approximately 2 hours. Less than 1% of the drug is excreted in the free form, with the remainder of the drug appearing as one of the six metabolites. Among the metabolites are ETH sulfoxide, 2-ethylisonicotinamide, and the *N*-methylated-6-oxodihydropyridines (compounds A, B, and C in Fig. 32.58).[309] In addition to the aforementioned GI disturbances, additional adverse effects can include CNS (depression, dizziness, drowsiness, headache), hepatitis, hypothyroidism, hypersensitivity, blurred vision, and erectile dysfunction. It also has been shown that INH may increase the serum concentration of ETH and vice versa.

p-Aminosalicylic Acid

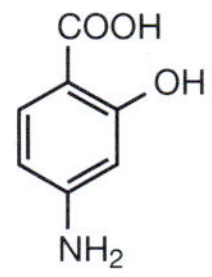

p-Aminosalicylic acid

PAS was synthesized and evaluated by Dr Jorgen Lehmann around the same time that the discovery of STM

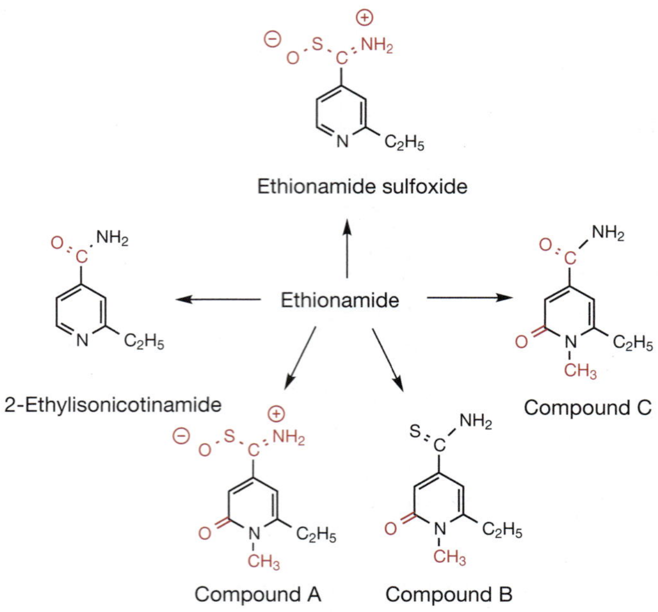

Figure 32.58 Metabolism of ethionamide.

was reported. However, due to the Second World War, Dr Lehmann was unaware of the isolation of STM, and he also did not publish his results regarding the anti-TB efficacy of PAS until 1950. PAS, once a popular component of anti-TB therapy, is nowadays used as a second-line agent. A combination of bacterial resistance along with pronounced adverse effects has greatly reduced the therapeutic value of PAS over the past few decades. Although there were several proposals to explain the MOA of PAS, more recent evidence suggests that this agent acts as an antimetabolite interfering with the incorporation of PABA into folic acid (Fig. 32.59), similar to the sulfonamides previously discussed.[310] The resistance developed by Mtb to PAS occurs due to the overexpression of the *dfrA* gene that encodes DHFR. Recently a putative functional analog of DHFR, which is a bifunctional enzyme riboflavin biosynthesis protein (RibD), has been identified and overexpression of *ribD* gene encoding this enzyme led to PAS-resistant isolates.[310]

PAS is administered orally as a packet containing granules with a delayed-release formulation, hence the time to peak of this agent is approximately 6 hours. The packet should not be used if it appears swollen or the granules have lost their tan color and turned dark brown or purple. PAS is readily absorbed (>90%) and more than 50% of the dose undergoes hepatic metabolism via acetylation and by conjugation with glucuronic acid and glycine at the carboxyl group. The unchanged drug and its metabolites are predominantly (>80%) excreted in the urine. Renal impairment prolongs the elimination half-life, which normally is very short (~0.5-2.5 hours). PAS is moderately bound to plasma proteins to the extent of 60%. As a bacteriostatic agent, PAS is used at a dose of 8 to 12 g/d in combination with other anti-TB agents, which causes considerable GI irritation (abdominal pain, diarrhea, nausea, vomiting). In addition, hypersensitivity reactions can occur in patients, with some of these reactions being life threatening. PAS is contraindicated in patients with known hypersensitivity to aminosalicylic acid. When coadministered with INH, PAS is found to reduce the acetylation of INH, itself being the substrate for acetylation, thus increasing the plasma levels of INH.[311] This action can be of high importance to patients who are so-called rapid (or fast) acetylators.

D-CYCLOSERINE

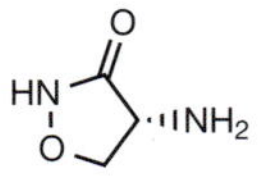

Cycloserine (DCS)

D-Cycloserine (DCS) is a natural product isolated from *Streptomyces orchidaceus* as the D-(+)-enantiomer. DCS is a cyclic, rigid analog of D-alanine that is active against microbes as the single D-enantiomer. DCS exerts its pharmacologic action by inhibiting two key enzymes, D-alanine racemase (Alr) and D-Ala:D-Ala ligase. D-Alanine is a critical component of the peptidoglycan layer in the mycobacterial cell wall. Mycobacteria can use naturally occurring L-alanine and convert this enantiomer into the opposite D-alanine via the action of an enzyme known as D-alanine racemase. The resulting D-alanine is coupled with itself to form a D-alanine-D-alanine dimer by the action of D-Ala:D-Ala ligase. This complex is subsequently incorporated into the peptidoglycan of the mycobacterial cell wall (Fig. 32.60). DCS, as a close structural analog of D-alanine, inhibits the binding of D-alanine to both enzymes and its subsequent incorporation into the peptidoglycan (Fig. 32.60).[312] The inactivation of Alr is thought to proceed via a mechanism-based irreversible route, which leads to forming an adduct with the pyridoxal 5′-phosphate cofactor, thus resulting in bacterial death.[313] Resistance is often associated with an overexpression of D-alanine racemase.

DCS is administered orally as a capsule with or without food. Its good absorption (up to 90%) is accompanied with a wide distribution, including the CSF, bile, ascitic, pleural, and synovial fluids. Its serum peak concentration is achieved within 4 to 8 hours, and its half-life oscillates around 12 hours. Two-thirds of the dose is eliminated unchanged in the urine. Unfortunately, DCS is accompanied with various adverse effects. DCS binds to neuronal *N*-methylaspartate receptors, and in addition to this, it affects the synthesis and metabolism of GABA, leading to a complex CNS adverse effects/neurotoxicity (eg, amnesia, behavioral changes, coma, confusion, seizure, tremor, vertigo). This agent also causes peripheral neuropathy; therefore, concomitant use of pyridoxine is recommended. Heart failure and increased serum transaminases have also been reported when using DCS. Vitamin B_{12} and folic acid supplementation may be needed for the duration of therapy with this medication. As a second-line agent, DCS should only be used when other drugs become less effective and it must be used in combination therapy, not as a single medication for the treatment of TB.

Modification of the structure of DCS afforded various analogs (eg, terizidone), which is used in other countries.[314]

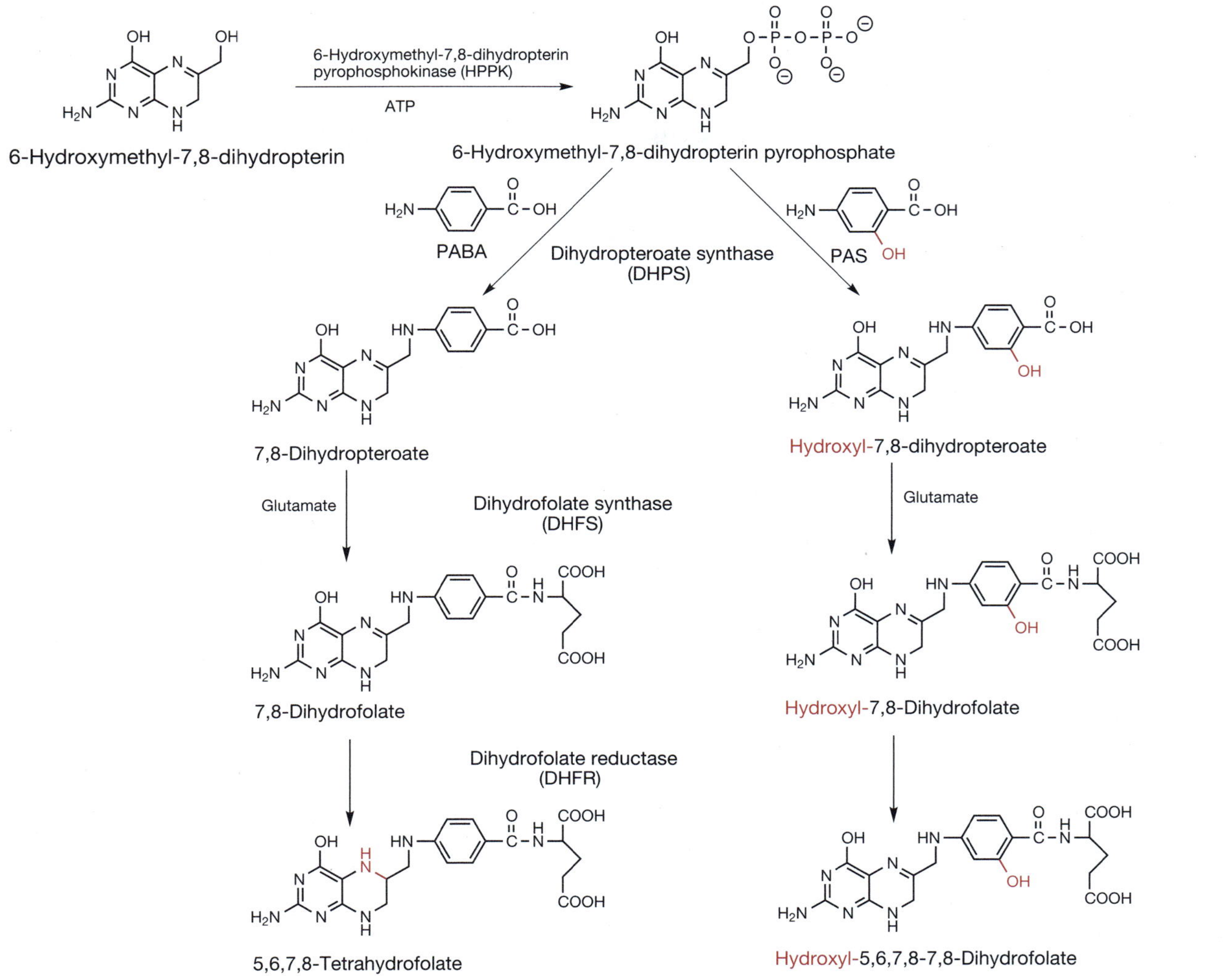

Figure 32.59 Conversion of *p*-aminosalicylic acid (PAS) into antimetabolite, which inhibits bacterial dihydrofolate reductase.

Capreomycin

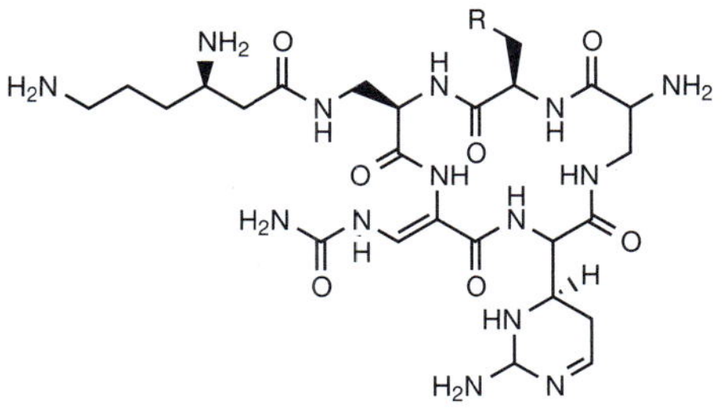

Capreomycin IA: R = OH
Capreomycin IB: R = H

Capreomycin is a mixture of four cyclic polypeptides, of which capreomycin IA and IB make up 90% of the mixture. Capreomycin is produced by *Streptomyces capreolus*, and it is structurally related to another antibiotic from this class, viomycin (discontinued in the United States). The MOA of capreomycin still remains to be fully elucidated; however, more recently additional information became available about capreomycin's mode of action. The ribosomal proteins L12 and L10 bind together to constitute the stalk of the 50S ribosomal subunit, which then recruits the initiation and elongation factors necessary for the translation process. Capreomycin inhibits the L12-L10 interaction and therefore interferes with the bacterial protein synthesis.[315] As a polypeptide, capreomycin must be administered parenterally via IV or IM injection, with the latter route being preferred. It achieves peak plasma concentrations within 1 to 2 hours,

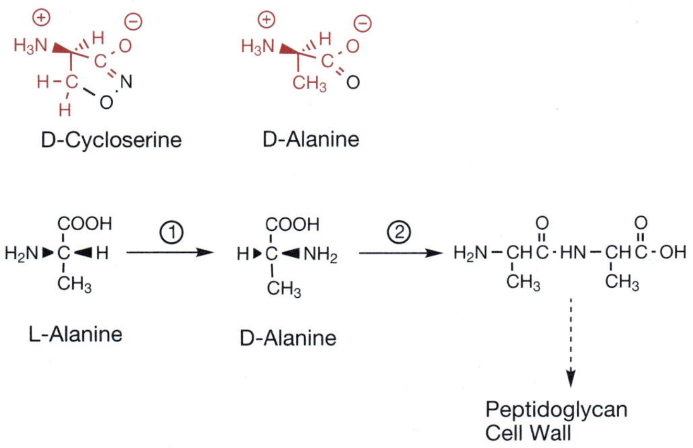

Figure 32.60 Sites of action of D-cycloserine: 1, D-alanine racemase and 2, D-alanine ligase.

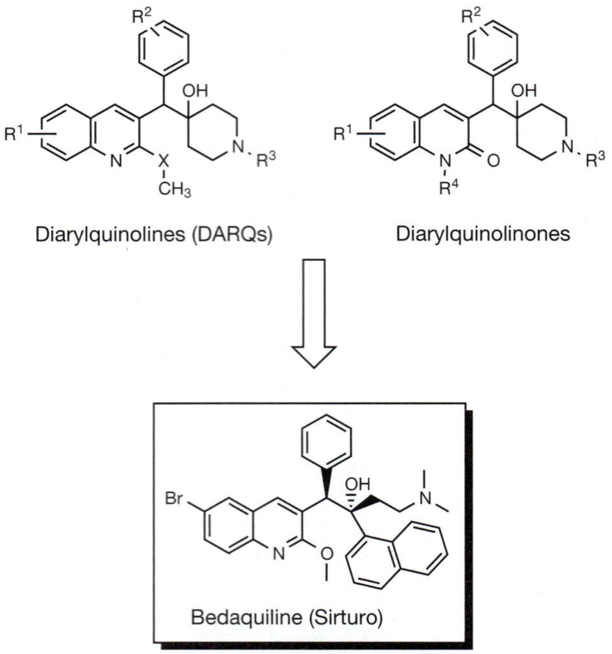

Figure 32.61 Pharmacophores of the diarylquinolines (DARQs) and diarylquinolinones that led to discovery of bedaquiline.

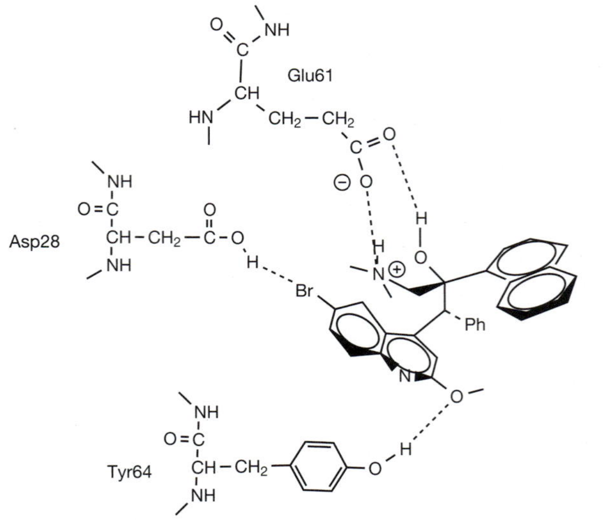

Figure 32.62 Binding of bedaquiline and amino acids in adenosine triphosphate (ATP) synthase C-subunit of *Mycobacterium tuberculosis.*

and about half of the dose is eliminated unchanged in the urine within 12 hours. As a second-line bacteriostatic antitubercular drug, it is reserved for use against drug-resistant infections and in cases of prior treatment failure. The drug should not be given as a single agent; therefore, it is often used in combination with EMB, INH, and/or other medications. Reported toxicity of capreomycin includes renal damage, auditory/hearing loss, and worse clinical outcomes (ie, decreased effectiveness and increased mortality), hence the boxed warning. Additional adverse effects include thrombocytopenia, injection site reaction, and allergic reactions.

Bedaquiline (Sirturo). Bedaquiline is a novel diarylquinoline (DARQ) compound that was approved in 2012 for the treatment of MDR-TB in combination with previously established anti-TB agents.[316-318] Initial HTS of a library with small molecules using Msm as the surrogate of Mtb led to identification of two novel pharmacophores: DARQ and diarylquinolinone (Fig. 32.61). These two scaffolds underwent medicinal chemistry structure optimization to yield bedaquiline, the first-in-class anti-TB drug that was approved by the FDA in the last four decades.[319] The success of bedaquiline has initiated focused research efforts to discover second-generation DARQs possessing improved ADMET properties, some of which are currently investigated at various stages of the clinical trials.[320,321] Bedaquiline is a time-dependent mycobacterial growth inhibitor that acts via binding to the C-ring of the mycobacterial ATP synthase, thus blocking the electrochemical gradient energy source (Fig. 32.62).[319,322-324] This is a unique MOA compared to the other antitubercular drugs used prior to bedaquiline's approval; thus, cross-resistance is low and allows bedaquiline to be used against drug-resistant strains of Mtb in combination with other agents. Additionally, this medication has been shown to have strong bactericidal and sterilizing properties. Bedaquiline also displays activity against NTM strains including *M. abscessus*, *M. avium*, *Mycobacterium fortuitum*, and *Mycobacterium kansasii*; however, this agent is not approved for clinical use in patients diagnosed with these infections.

Bedaquiline is formulated as a fumarate salt for oral administration as a tablet. Maximum plasma concentrations are observed 5 hours after dosing and are more than 99.9% bound to plasma proteins.[319] Food increases the bioavailability of bedaquiline by approximately 2-fold, and thus it is recommended to be taken with meals. This agent is primarily metabolized through CYP3A4 *N*-dealkylation to give the *N*-monodesmethyl metabolite (M2). This metabolite is approximately 4 to 6 times less potent against whole-cell Mtb; however, its impact on clinical efficacy is not significant. Elimination occurs primarily through the feces, with negligible amount (≤0.001%) of the drug being excreted unchanged in the urine. The mean terminal elimination half-life of bedaquiline and its M2 metabolite is approximately 5.5 months, which most likely reflects the slow release of the parent drug and its metabolite from the peripheral tissues. The use of bedaquiline is accompanied with several serious adverse effects. These include GI (nausea, anorexia), cardiovascular (chest pain, prolonged QT interval on electrocardiogram), hepatic (hepatotoxicity, increased serum transaminases), CNS (headache), hemoptysis (ie, cough with blood), arthralgia, and skin rash. The QT prolongation along with an increased risk of death warrant marketing of this drug with a boxed warning.

Nitrodihydroimidazooxazoles. Pretomanid and delamanid are the newest anti-TB medications that represent bicyclic 4-nitroimidazoles, and more specifically nitrodihydroimidazooxazoles (Fig. 32.63). They are derived from 2-ethyl-5-nitro-2,3-dihydro[2-1b]imidazo-oxazole, more commonly known as CGI-17341, which served as a prototype compound for the development of this class of antimycobacterial agents.[325] CGI-17341 in turn is considered to be an advanced analog of the natural product azomycin, which is a 2-nitroimidazole known for its inhibitory action against

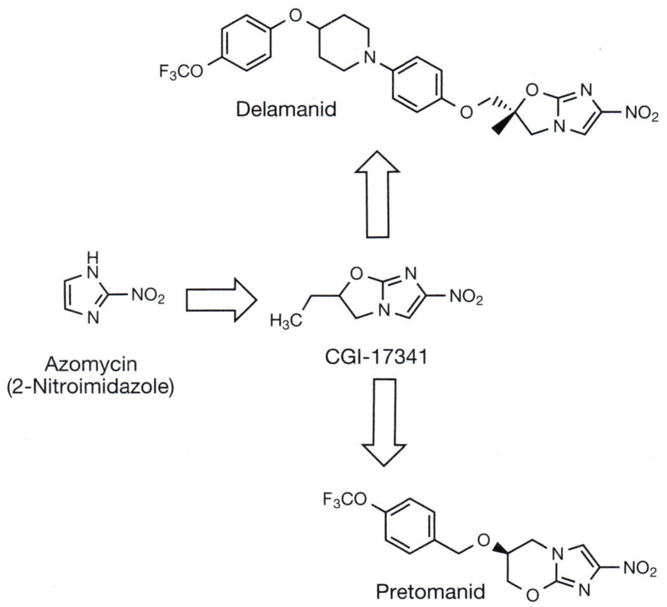

Figure 32.63 Evolution of the nitrodihydroimidazooxazole pharmacophore.

anaerobic bacteria and protozoa. A derivative of CGI-17341 provided pretomanid. This drug was approved by the FDA in 2019, thus making it the newest anti-TB agent on the US market. Another CGI-17341 derivative, delamanid, received conditional approval from the European Medicines Agency (EMA) in 2013 for the treatment of MDR-TB. Clinical studies have shown that delamanid has high potency, low risk for DDIs, and good tolerability.[326] Currently, this medication is in phase 3 clinical trials in the United States.

Both agents are efficacious against actively replicating MDR strains of Mtb as well as non-replicating, hypoxic Mtb strains. However, pretomanid is considered to be a safer medication than delamanid. These medications are prodrugs that require bioactivation via deazaflavin F_{420}-dependent nitroreductase (Ddn) to give RNS such as nitric oxide (NO).[327] Many different metabolites are formed during the prodrug activation step, and some of them are suspected to be unstable and short lived; thus, they are toxic to the mycobacterial cell. During the aerobic growth, these agents have been shown to affect the biosynthesis of the cell wall, with an observed reduction in cell wall components such as mycolate intermediates implying that they might inhibit the formation of methoxy-mycolic and keto-mycolic acids. More recently however, an enzyme required for the synthesis of AG, the decaprenylphosphoryl-D-2-keto erythropentose reductase (DprE2) subunit of decaprenylphosphoribose-2′-epimerase, has been identified as a putative molecular target for this drug class.[327] Moreover, there is evidence that some of the reactive species stemming from the Ddn-mediated activation of delamanid and pretomanid create an adduct with NADH, which then is suspected to serve as the inhibitor of DprE2 enzymatic function.[327] The decaprenylphosphoribose-2′-epimerase is a heteromeric protein composed of decaprenylphosphoryl-D-ribose oxidase (DprE1)-DprE2 complex that catalyzes the two-step epimerization reaction of decaprenylphosphoryl-D-ribose (DPR) into decaprenylphosphoryl-D-arabinose (DPA) involving the ketone intermediate, decaprenylphosphoryl-2-keto-β-D-erythro-pentofuranose (DPX) (Fig. 32.64).[327] The first oxidation step of DPR to DPX is mediated by the DprE1 subunit of the epimerase, whereas the second reduction step of DPX to DPA is performed by the DprE2 subunit of the epimerase. DPA is a key precursor that serves as the donor of arabinose, which is a necessary component for the synthesis of arabinans that in turn contributes to the AG layer in the Mtb's cell wall. The activation mechanism of these prodrugs is dependent on the F_{420} redox cycle. The F420-dependent glucose-6-phosphate dehydrogenase (Fgd1) catalyzes the oxidation of glucose-6-phosphate to 6-phosphogluconolactone, thus generating F_{420}-H_2. This coenzyme is subsequently oxidized by Ddn in the reduction of pretomanid or delamanid to yield the active forms of these drugs and at the same time regenerate F_{420} (Fig. 32.64).[327] The action of pretomanid and delamanid during the non-replicating phase under anaerobic (hypoxic) conditions is based on releasing NO, which subsequently serves as bacterial respiratory poison interfering with electron flow and ATP homeostasis.[327] Resistance to these agents, both laboratory-generated and identified in clinical isolates of Mtb, arises due to mutations in either *Ddn* gene (encoding the nitroreductase) or one of five other genes: *fbiA*, *fbiB*, *fbiC*, *fbiD*, or *fgd1*, all of which are essential in prodrug activation. FbiA, FbiB, FbiC, and FbiD are involved in the synthesis of F_{420} coenzyme, whereas Fgd1 regenerates the reduced form of the F_{420} for further cycles with Ddn.[327,328]

Tablets of pretomanid are administered orally and are recommended to be taken with high-fat meals for better absorption. On average, this medication achieves peak plasma concentrations within 4.5 hours, and its elimination half-life is approximately 16 hours. Pretomanid undergoes multiple reductive and oxidative pathways with CYP3A4 being responsible for ~20% of the metabolism. Therefore, there is potential for DDI of this agent with strong inducers/inhibitors of CYP3A4 isoform. The metabolites are subsequently excreted in the urine (53%) and feces (38%). Pretomanid is bound to plasma proteins to the extent of 86%. There are several serious concerns related to adverse effects of this drug. These include myelosuppression (including anemia, leukopenia, pancytopenia, and thrombocytopenia), peripheral (including severe form) and optic neuropathy, lactic acidosis, QT prolongation, hepatic effects, headache, dermatologic effects (acne vulgaris, skin rash, pruritus), and GI (nausea, vomiting, dyspepsia, decreased appetite, abdominal pain) and musculoskeletal pain. Many of those adverse effects are related to the MOA of this agent and its activation to reactive species.

FLUOROQUINOLONES. The fluoroquinolones (Fig. 32.24) are a broad-spectrum class of antibacterials that have been demonstrated to have bactericidal activity against a wide range of gram-negative and gram-positive pathogens, including *M. tuberculosis*, *M. kansasii*, *Mycobacterium xenopi*, *M. fortuitum*, MAC, and *M. leprae*. Refer to previous discussions in this chapter about their MOA, SAR, and ADMET properties. The structural requirements for activity against mycobacterium and, specifically, for activity against the MAC have been explored.[329,330] It is known that nonfluorinated quinolones are inactive against mycobacteria. In addition, it has been reported

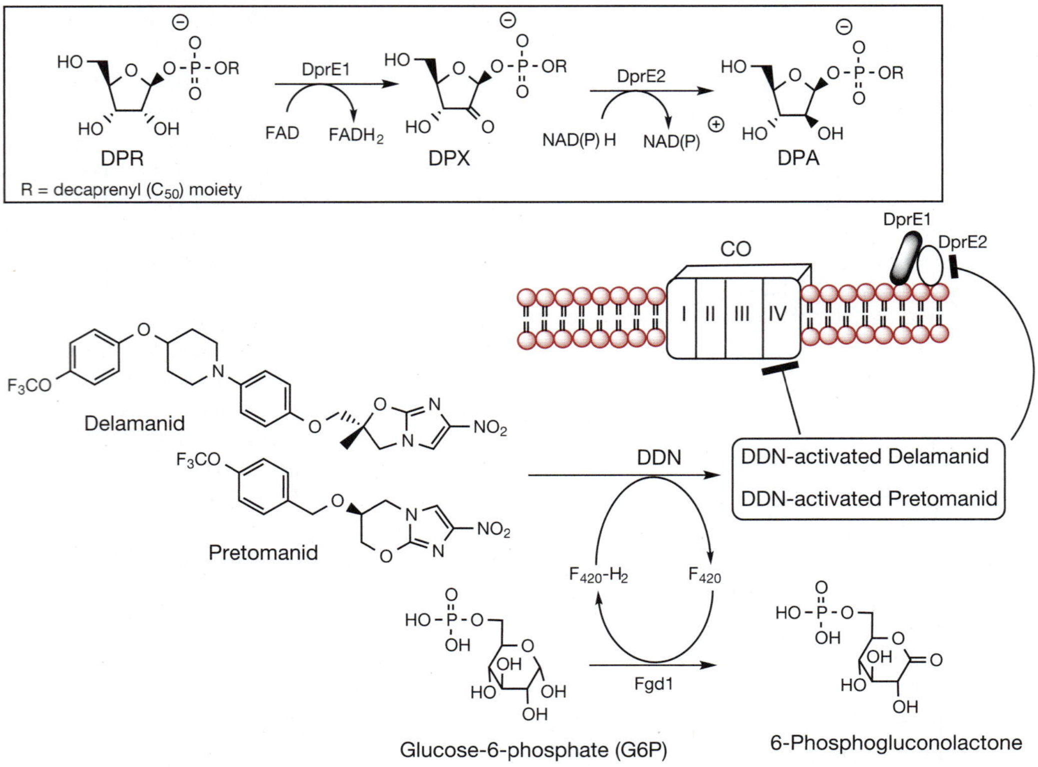

Figure 32.64 Mechanism of action of nitrodihydroimidazooxazoles: pretomanid and delamanid. CO, cytochrome oxidase; DDN, deazaflavin F_{420}-dependent nitroreductase; DPA, decaprenylphosphoryl-D-arabinose; DPR, decaprenylphosphoryl-D-ribose; DprE1, decaprenylphosphoryl-D-ribose oxidase; DprE2, decaprenylphosphoryl-D-2-keto erythropentose reductase; DPX, decaprenylphosphoryl-2-keto-β-D-erythro-pentofuranose; F_{420}/F_{420}-H_2, oxidized/reduced coenzyme; Fgd1, F420-dependent glucose-6-phosphate dehydrogenase. (Adapted from Abrahams KA, Batt SM, Gurcha SS, et al. DprE2 is a molecular target of the anti-tubercular nitroimidazole compounds pretomanid and delamanid. *Nat Commun.* 2023;14:3828. doi:10.1038/s41467-023-39300-z under a Creative Commons Attribution 4.0, http://creativecommons.org/licenses/by/4.0/)

that certain functional groups or substructures within the quinolone skeleton improve activity toward the MAC (biophores), whereas other fragments deactivate the quinolones (biophobes). The important structural features acting as biophores include: (1) a cyclopropyl ring at the N_1 position, (2) fluorine atoms at positions C_6 or C_8, and (3) a C_7 heterocyclic (piperazine or pyrrolidine) substituent. Excessive lipophilicity at N_1 can decrease activity (ie, 2,4-difluorobenzene). Several C_8 methoxy-substituted fluoroquinolones have been reported with superior activity over earlier quinolones.[331,332] Currently, moxifloxacin and levofloxacin are used as components of combination therapy for the treatment of resistant TB.

Therapeutic Considerations for the Treatment of Tuberculosis

Apart from drug-sensitivity and resistance factors, various stages and forms of the infectious organism have been identified that require special consideration when selecting the appropriate anti-TB therapy regimen. The actively growing stage of the organism can find the bacteria either in an extra- or intracellular location. A stage of the organism, which is classified as the very slowly metabolizing bacteria, exists in a relatively acidic environment. Mtb can be in a dormant stage, which is difficult to treat and eradicate. Finally, the organism can exhibit a stage in which it is dormant, followed by spurts of growth. As noted in the discussion of specific agents, one stage or another can be more or less susceptible to a particular drug based on the abovementioned characteristics. It is also recognized that organisms from some geographic regions can show a low incidence of drug resistance, whereas those from other regions have a high incidence of drug resistance.

For patients who developed an active TB infection due to drug-sensitive organisms and exhibit low rates of drug resistance, the American Thoracic Society (ATS) as well as the CDC recommend several treatment regimens. One of the most frequently prescribed is the RIPE TB treatment regimen based on a minimum 26-week treatment period, consisting of an initial 2-month (8-week) so-called "initial intensive phase," followed by a continuation phase of either 4 or 7 months. During the initial phase, the regimens use a combination of the four first-line medications: INH, RIF, PZA, and EMB. Once the Mtb isolate is known to be fully susceptible, PZA and EMB can be discontinued. Several drug options exist for the continuation phase of treatment.[333] In most cases, the continuation phase will last 4 or 7 months (for the total of 6-9 months of the treatment). The drug combination of INH and RIF is predominantly used during this phase. However, if isolated resistance to INH has been documented, INH is discontinued and the treatment continues with the other three agents (RIF, PZA, EMB) for 6 months. Additionally, therapy must be extended if the patient remains culture-positive after 2 months of treatment or has cavitary disease. DOT is the standard approach to patient care for TB treatment in the United States and around the world, as after the initial 2 weeks of daily dosing, the regimen can be adjusted to 3 or even 2 times per week. Patients on the DOT regimen need to take the medications in the presence of an assigned DOT worker, and those who are on the twice-weekly dosing must not miss any of those doses. Patients on self-administered medication therapy shall take the prescribed medications on a daily basis. The same group of medications is recommended for patients with both TB and HIV coinfection. The "cardinal rules" for all TB regimens are as follows: (1) obtain drug susceptibility information as soon as possible, (2) begin therapy with the four first-line drugs, (3) adjust the regimen based on the obtained drug susceptibility tests and DOT/self-administered approach, and (4) addition of more medications (at least two, usually the injectables) will be needed in the case that the initially recommended regimen is failing.[334] Newer regimens are currently being proposed to shorten the duration of the therapy to 4 months. One such regimen is RIPE that has been modified to 16-week therapy for the treatment of non-severe, presumed isoniazid- and rifampin-susceptible TB in children. In this case, all four medications are used for 8 weeks during the intensive phase (ETB still might be excluded based on local guidelines) followed by 8-week continuation phase with INH and RIF.[305] Another regimen includes RPT, moxifloxacin, INH, and PZA for the first 8 weeks and is continued for additional 9 weeks without PZA in the case of isoniazid-susceptible, rifampin-susceptible TB in adults.[305] In all cases when INH is included in the therapy, pyridoxine (vitamin B6, 25 -50 mg/d) should be given to all patients in order to prevent isoniazid-induced neuropathy. LTBI is usually treated with a combination of INH and rifamycin (RPT or RIF) for 3 months or only RIF for 4 months or INH monotherapy for 6 to 9 months.

High-risk patients are adults and children with HIV infection, close contacts of infectious cases, and those with fibrotic lesions on chest radiographs. Adverse effects when using INH over a long treatment period can be a serious problem. INH can cause severe liver damage, and the drug should be removed if serum aminotransferase activity increases to 3- to 5-fold the normal level, or the patient develops symptoms of hepatitis. Peripheral neuropathy can be seen with INH therapy. This condition can be prevented by coadministration of pyridoxine. Persons who are presumed to be infected with INH-resistant organisms should be treated with RIF and other medications and INH should be discontinued. Hepatitis, thrombocytopenia, and nephrotoxicity can be seen with RIF therapy. RIF is thought to potentiate the hepatitis caused by INH. GI upset and staining effects caused by RIF are bothersome but of minor importance. Although drug-sensitive TB has been successfully treated, the extended period of treatment and low patient adherence have in part led to the development of drug-resistant TB, both MDR-TB and XDR-TB. In such situations, a new treatment paradigm has become necessary. For treatment of MDR-TB a five- to six-drug regimen is commonly used (Table 32.12).[335,336] The particular regimen should be based on drug susceptibility testing or previous treatment history. With dual mycobacterium resistance to INH and RIF, a combination of an aminoglycoside from group II drugs, a fluoroquinolone from group III drugs, along with EMB and PZA from group I, and ETH from group IV, can be used at the indicated doses and frequency.[337] If resistance to all group I agents is reported, then various agents from group IV are added to the previously indicated drug list of an aminoglycoside, a fluoroquinolone, and ETH. In the case of MDR-TB and XDR-TB infections, the treatment usually continues for 18 to 20 (or even 24) months and the success rate for survival and full recovery is dependent on many different factors. The most recently updated guidelines[305] allow to implement the shortened, 26-week therapy regimen for the treatment of: a) rifampin-resistant, fluoroquinolone-susceptible TB with BPaLM Regimen: Bedaquiline (400 mg daily for 2 wk, then 200 mg three times/wk for subsequent 24 wk), Pretomanid (200 mg daily), Linezolid (600 mg daily), Moxifloxacin (400 mg daily); b) rifampin-resistant, fluoroquinolone-resistant TB with BPaL Regimen: Bedaquiline (400 mg daily for 2 wk, then 200 mg three times/wk for subsequent 24 wk), Pretomanid (200 mg daily), Linezolid (600 mg daily).[305]

Drug Therapy for Leprosy (Hansen Disease)

DAPSONE

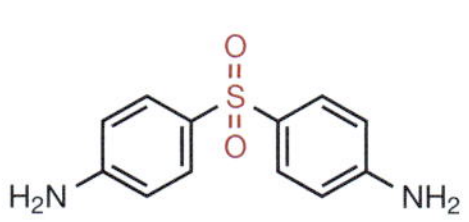

Dapsone

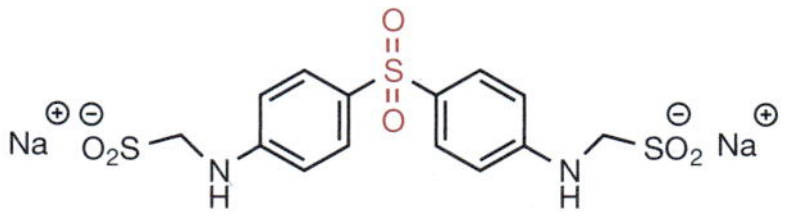

Sulfoxone sodium
(prodrug of dapsone)

The diaryl sulfones represent the major class of agents used to treat leprosy. The initial discovery of the sulfones came about because of studies directed at exploring the SAR of the sulfonamides. A variety of additional chemical modifications have produced several other active agents, but none has proved to be more beneficial than the original lead compound known as dapsone or its chemical names 4,4′-sulfonyldianiline (SDA) and diaminodiphenyl sulfone (DDS). Dapsone, which is a symmetrical sulfone, was first synthesized in 1908 (just 1 year after Salvarsan was discovered) and introduced into the treatment of leprosy around 1945. Several derivatives of dapsone have been prepared to increase the desired bioactivity. Bioisosteric replacement of one of the benzene rings provided a wide series of analogs. Although still active, they were mostly less effective than dapsone. Substitution with various functional groups on the aromatic ring afforded analogs with improved ADMET properties, such as increased water solubility and thus decreased GI irritation; however, those derivatives also had reduced activity. A successful structure modification was based on adding methanesulfinate groups to the anilines, which resulted in sulfoxone sodium, a prodrug of dapsone. This water-soluble form of dapsone is hydrolyzed in vivo to produce dapsone. Sulfoxone sodium was used in individuals who were unable to tolerate dapsone because of GI irritation, but the prodrug is no longer marketed in the United States. Chemical modifications of dapsone continue to be pursued with the intent of finding newer agents useful for the treatment of resistant strains of *M. leprae*.[338] Dapsone is a bacteriostatic agent that is thought to act in a similar manner to the antibacterial sulfonamides, namely, through competitive inhibition of the incorporation of PABA into folic acid. Both dapsone and clofazimine (discussed later) have significant anti-inflammatory actions, which may or may not play a role in the antimicrobial action. The anti-inflammatory action can

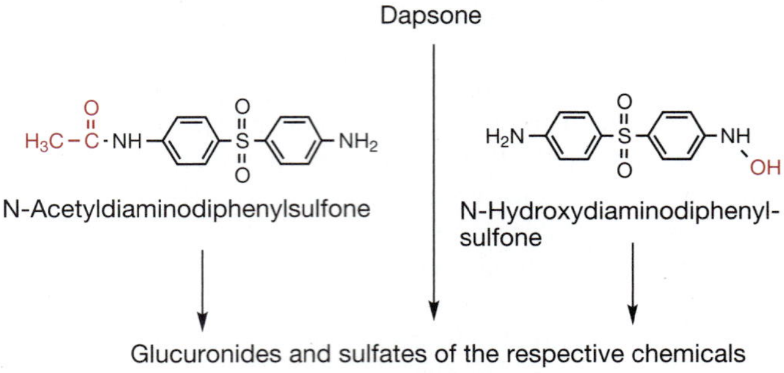

Figure 32.65 Metabolites of dapsone.

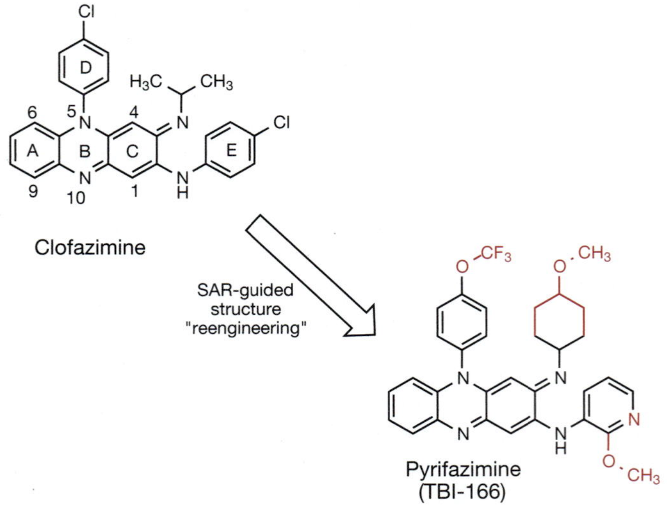

Figure 32.66 Structure of clofazimine and its newer derivative pyrifazimine, which is evaluated in a clinical trial. SAR, structure-activity relationship.

also be a beneficial effect offsetting the complication of erythema nodosum leprosum (ENL) seen in some patients. The anti-inflammatory action can come about by inhibition of myeloperoxidase-catalyzed reactions.[339]

Dapsone is applied topically as a gel of various strength and orally as a tablet. The oral formulation results in a rapid and almost complete absorption, although dapsone has poor water solubility. The time to peak of this agent is in the range between 4 and 8 hours, and its elimination half-life is approximately 28 hours in adults. Although dapsone is bound to plasma protein up to 90%, it is distributed throughout the body. It undergoes hepatic metabolism via acetylation and hydroxylation to form multiple metabolites (Fig. 32.65). The major metabolic product of dapsone results from *N*-acetylation in the liver by *N*-acetyltransferase. Dapsone is also *N*-hydroxylated to the hydroxylamine derivative. These metabolic reactions are catalyzed by CYP3A4 isoforms. Neither of these compounds possesses significant leprostatic activity, although *N*-acetyldiaminodiphenylsulfone can be deacetylated back to dapsone. Up to 85% of the dose is excreted in the urine. Products found in the urine consist of small amounts of dapsone (up to 15%), the metabolites *N*-acetyldiaminodiphenylsulfone and *N*-hydroxydiaminodiphenylsulfone, and glucuronide and sulfates of each of these substances (Fig. 32.65). Consideration should be given when prescribing dapsone as this agent causes blood dyscrasias (including methemoglobinemia, hemolytic anemia, neutropenia, and agranulocytosis), hepatic effects (increased serum transaminases, hepatic failure, hyperbilirubinemia), and hypersensitivity reactions that may be delayed. Additionally, pancreatitis, acute kidney injury, or eosinophilic pneumonitis might occur. Due to the low water solubility, GI effects such as abdominal pain, nausea, and vomiting are common. Dapsone may also cause male infertility.

CLOFAZIMINE. Clofazimine is a phenazine-based compound known as a water-insoluble dye (dark-red crystals) that was synthesized in the 1950s as an anti-TB agent. However, its use became more popular in the treatment of leprosy (Fig. 32.66). The name of this agent is related to the pharmacophore (phenazine) and the functional groups (chlorine and imine) present in this drug. It is classified as a secondary drug and commonly used as a component of a multidrug therapy for the treatment of leprosy. Clofazimine was first used to treat advanced leprosy unresponsive to dapsone or STM in 1966. Since 2004, clofazimine is not commercially available in the United States; however, there are two mechanisms by which physicians can acquire this drug. The first mechanism is through Novartis Pharmaceuticals Corporation, which currently produces clofazimine sold under the trade name Lamprene for patients with NTM infections who are eligible for the Novartis NTM program. In this case, Novartis is the sponsor of a clofazimine expanded access program in the United States for patients ages 18 years and older. The second mechanism is for patients who are not eligible for the Novartis NTM program. In this case, the FDA may authorize access to clofazimine under a single patient Investigational New Drug (SPIND), but all the regulatory criteria must be met. The patient's health care provider works with their local institutional review board (IRB) (eg, the patient's hospital) to complete and submit a SPIND to the FDA for the individual patient who requires clofazimine treatment. Upon approval, the same health care provider will need to contact Novartis in order to obtain clofazimine.[340]

Several studies were directed toward understanding of the SAR of clofazimine.[341-343] Substituents on the imino group at position 3, *p*-chloro substitution on the phenyl rings D and E, and substituents at position 8 have been investigated. The imino group at C_3 appears to be essential, with activity increased when the imino group is substituted with alkyl and cycloalkyl groups. Halogens installed on the para position of the two phenyls enhance lipophilicity and thus activity but are not essential to the overall bioactivity of this compound. The following order of activity has been reported: Br> Cl> CH_3> EtO > H or F. In the analogs studied, the increased activity correlates well with pro-oxidative activities of the molecule (eg, ability to generate superoxide anion) as well as increased lipophilicity. In the past two decades, clofazimine attracted renowned interest as a prospective agent for combination therapy for the treatment of MDR-TB and XDR-TB. Therefore, there are several clinical trials ongoing with this agent. Moreover, the intriguing SAR of this agent provided the basis for so-called "SAR-guided structure reengineering" that resulted in pyrifazimine (TBI-166), which is clofazimine's newer derivative with similar activity but significantly improved ADMET properties (Fig. 32.67). Pyrifazimine is currently in phase 2 clinical trial for the treatment of pulmonary TB.[344]

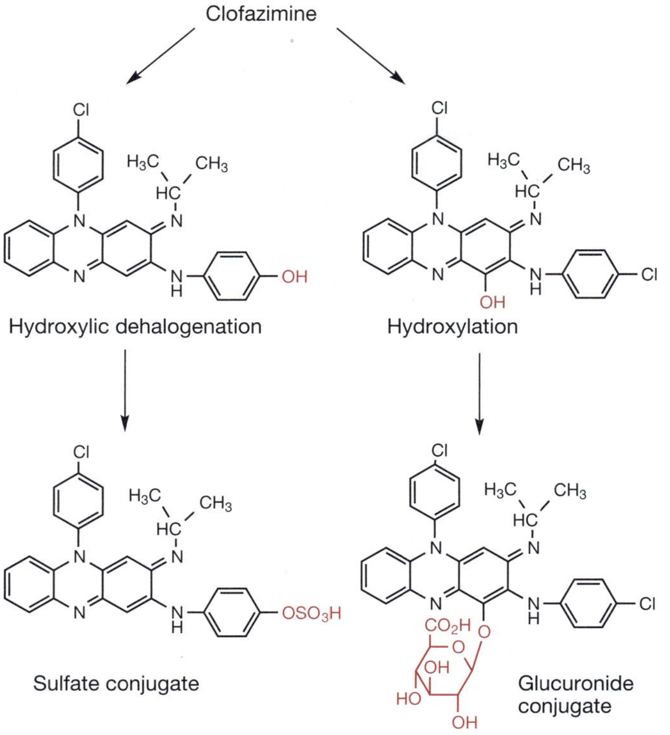

Figure 32.67 Human metabolic products of clofazimine.

The MOA of clofazimine remains unclear; however, many studies have shown that clofazimine may act via at least two different mechanisms of actions: (1) microbial intracellular redox cycling, thus producing ROS such as H_2O_2 and superoxide, and (2) disruption of membrane integrity via interaction with bacterial membrane phospholipids.[345] The molecule possesses direct antimycobacterial and immunosuppressive properties. It has been shown that clofazimine increases prostaglandin synthesis and the generation of antimicrobial reactive oxidants from neutrophils, which can play a role in the observed antileprosy effects. The host cell defense can be stimulated by clofazimine, resulting in the generation of oxidants such as the superoxide anion, which in turn could have a lethal effect on the microorganism.[346,347]

Clofazimine is administered orally as a capsule and has modest absorption ranging between 45% and 62% when taken with food. If administered in a fasting state, the absorption is decreased. Clofazimine is highly lipophilic and therefore deposits primarily in fatty tissues, hence its half-life may last even up to 69 days. Crystalized deposits of this drug have been found in many organs and tissues throughout the body, including lymph nodes, adrenals, subcutaneous fat, liver, spleen, small intestine, muscles, bones, and skin. Since clofazimine is a pigment, its use leads to pigmentation of the skin. In addition, discoloration (pink, red, or brownish black) of the feces, eyelid lining, sputum, sweat, tears, and urine has been seen. Various metabolites of clofazimine have been identified, but these account for less than 1% of the administered dose. The lack of higher concentrations of the metabolites can partially result from the slow elimination of clofazimine from the body, which has an estimated half-life of 8.8 to 69 days. There appears to be some discrepancy as to the structures of the metabolites.[343] The most recent studies suggest the presence of two conjugates, with the possibility of various intermediates (Fig. 32.67). Clofazimine is thought to undergo oxidative dehalogenation on 2-chloroaniline, followed by 4-hydroxylation and sulfate conjugation. Hydroxylation of the C_1 position followed by glucuronic acid conjugation represents another metabolic pathway.[348]

Thalidomide (Thalomid)

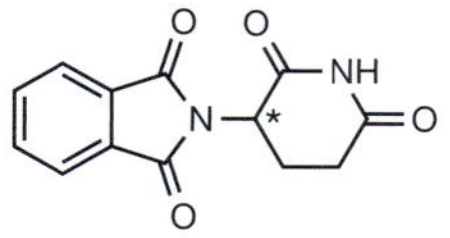

Thalidomide (Thalomid)

The development of painful, tender, inflamed, subcutaneous nodules that can last 1 or 2 weeks but can reappear and last for extended periods of time is seen in a number of diseases. In the case of leprosy, the condition is referred to as ENL, and it appears to be a hypersensitivity reaction. While it can appear in nontreated patients, it is most commonly observed as a complication of the chemotherapy used for the treatment of leprosy. In addition to painful nodules, the patient can experience fever, malaise, wasting, vasculitis, and peripheral neuritis. This condition has been successfully treated with thalidomide. Thalidomide has been approved by the FDA for the treatment of ENL and is considered to be the drug of choice.[349] The mechanism whereby thalidomide produces relief is thought to be associated with the drug's immunomodulatory ability to control inflammatory cytokines. Specifically, thalidomide inhibits the synthesis and release of tumor necrosis factor-α (TNF-α), which is synthesized and released in excess by blood mononuclear cells and appears in the serum during ENL. Concentrations of TNF-α drop when the patient is treated with thalidomide. In addition to the treatment of ENL, thalidomide has been reported to exhibit beneficial effects in the treatment (off-label) of aphthous ulcers in patients who are HIV positive and patients with chronic graft-versus-host disease, Waldenström macroglobulinemia, systemic light chain amyloidosis, and multiple myeloma.

Thalidomide is a very well-known and potent teratogenic agent. It has a boxed warning and a history of an estimated 10,000 deformed infants born to mothers who used the drug during pregnancy to treat morning sickness. It can be used safely in postmenopause, but strict controls are required for females of childbearing age. Evidence suggests that thalidomide is also present in the semen of males; therefore, the use of condoms by male patients is required for up to 28 days following discontinuation of therapy during sexual contact with females of childbearing potential. Thalidomide is administered orally as a capsule (of various strength) followed by good but slow absorption. It takes between 2 and 5 hours to achieve peak plasma concentrations, and its elimination half-life ranges between 5.5 and 7.5 hours. It undergoes minimal metabolism and up to 92% of the dose is excreted in the urine. It is moderately bound to plasma proteins to the extent of 66%. Apart from being teratogenic, thalidomide also has an increased risk of thromboembolic events such as deep venous thrombosis and pulmonary embolism; therefore, its use is accompanied with a boxed warning. This agent can additionally cause peripheral edema, hyperglycemia, asthenia, tremor, pneumonia as well as various GI (constipation, dyspepsia, nausea) and CNS (anxiety, dizziness, fatigue, paresthesia) adverse effects.

Rifampin (Rifampin, Rifadin, Rimactane). RIF is a first-line antitubercular drug that has already been discussed in this chapter. Its actions against *M. leprae* parallel those effects reported for Mtb. Currently, RIF is used off-label in combination with dapsone, and in some situations clofazimine, for the treatment of Hansen disease.

Therapeutic Considerations for Leprosy. Since its introduction in the mid-1940s, dapsone has proved to be the single most effective agent in the treatment of leprosy. This drug was initially used as monotherapy despite the recognition that resistant strains were beginning to emerge; however, since 1977, monotherapy with dapsone is no longer recognized as an acceptable method for the treatment of leprosy. Today, combination chemotherapy is the method of choice. The combination consists of RIF (600 mg daily), dapsone (100 mg daily), and clofazimine (50 mg daily added for patients with multibacillary leprosy, which is defined as more than five skin lesions). Therapy is continued for at least 2 years, or as long as skin smears are positive, and the patient is kept under supervision for 5 years following completion of chemotherapy. A similar regimen (excluding clofazimine) is recommended for treatment of paucibacillary leprosy (defined as five or fewer skin lesions) except that treatment is continued for 1 year and the patient is kept under observation for an additional 2 years.[350,351] It should be noted that the patient is noninfectious within 72 hours of starting the treatment; therefore, after taking only a few doses of the prescribed medications, the patient does not need to be isolated from family and friends. Other combinations that have been reported also included minocycline. Outside the United States, ofloxacin and clarithromycin have been suggested as alternative agents for the combination therapy.[352] An important aspect of therapy for leprosy involves the treatment of peripheral nerve damage. The nerve damage can be treated with steroids, such as prednisolone. For severe cases, however, thalidomide is used.

Drug Therapy for Mycobacterium avium Complex

MAC is a term used to describe multiple NTM species, which cannot be distinguished by the traditional microbiology laboratory testing and genetic testing is required. MAC-caused infections are ubiquitous and have been reported on all inhabited continents. In the United States, the prevalence varies from 1.4 to 6.6 individuals per 100,000 in a population, and females are on average 1.6 times more impacted than males.[353] Drug therapy for the treatment of MAC (and other NTM) is based on the clinical practice guidelines published in 2020 by a panel of experts from the ATS, the European Respiratory Society (ERS), the European Society of Clinical Microbiology and Infectious Diseases (ESCMID), and the Infectious Diseases Society of America (IDSA).[354] These guidelines were based on the prior information published in 2007 by ATS/IDSA, which constituted the main approach to the treatment and prophylaxis of MAC.[355]

In general, in patients with macrolide-susceptible MAC pulmonary disease, a three-drug regimen (including a macrolide and EMB) over a regimen with two drugs (a macrolide and EMB alone) is recommended. Additionally, a three-drug regimen that includes a macrolide over a three-drug regimen without a macrolide is recommended with azithromycin-based rather than clarithromycin-based treatment regimens. Patients with noncavitary nodular/bronchiectatic macrolide-susceptible MAC pulmonary disease should be placed on a 3 times per week macrolide-based regimen as opposed to patients with cavitary or severe/advanced nodular bronchiectatic MAC disease who should receive a daily macrolide-based regimen. For patients with cavitary or advanced/severe bronchiectatic or macrolide-resistant MAC pulmonary disease, parenteral amikacin or STM should be included in the initial treatment regimen. In the case of patients with newly diagnosed MAC, neither inhaled amikacin (parenteral formulation) nor amikacin liposome inhalation suspension (ALIS) should be used as a part of the initial treatment regimen. However, for patients who have failed the treatment after at least 6 months of guideline-based therapy, the addition of ALIS to the treatment regimen is recommended. It is also suggested that the treatment continues for at least 12 months after culture conversion.[356]

The general guidelines pertinent to drug selection and doses are:[355]

a. For most patients with nodular/bronchiectatic MAC disease, a 3-times-weekly regimen of clarithromycin (1,000 mg) or azithromycin (500 mg), RIF (600 mg), and EMB (25 mg/kg) is recommended.
b. For patients with fibrocavitary MAC lung disease or severe nodular/bronchiectatic disease, a daily regimen of clarithromycin (500-1,000 mg) or azithromycin (250 mg), RIF (600 mg) or RFB (150-300 mg), and EMB (15 mg/kg) with consideration of 3-times-weekly amikacin or STM early in therapy is recommended. Patients should be treated until culture negative on therapy for 1 year.
c. Therapy for disseminated MAC disease should include clarithromycin (1,000 mg/d) or azithromycin (250 mg/d) and EMB (15 mg/kg/d) with or without RFB (150-350 mg/d). Therapy can be discontinued with resolution of symptoms and reconstitution of cell-mediated immune function.
d. Prophylaxis of disseminated MAC disease should be given to adults with AIDS with $CD4^+$ T-lymphocyte counts less than 50 cells/μL. Azithromycin 1,200 mg/wk or clarithromycin 1,000 mg/d has proven efficacy. RFB 300 mg/d is also effective but less well tolerated.

All the agents recommended for the treatment of MAC have been already discussed along with their respective drug classes in the previous sections of this chapter.

ACKNOWLEDGMENTS

This chapter is based on Chapter 29 of the 8th edition written by Dr Elmer J. Gentry, Dr E. Jeffrey North, and Dr Robin M. Zavod. The authors gratefully acknowledge these authors' previous work as well as for reusing several figures from that chapter, some of which were created by Dr Victoria F. Roche. Useful discussions with Dr Thomas L. Lemke and Dr Marc Harrold while writing and revising this chapter are acknowledged.

Structure Challenge

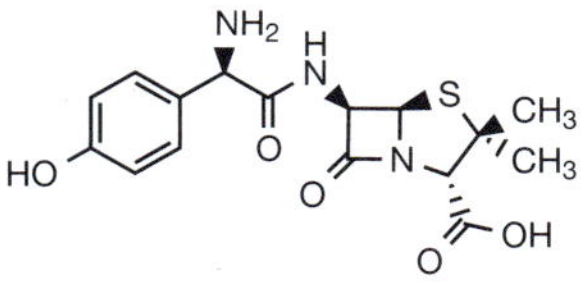

Structure A

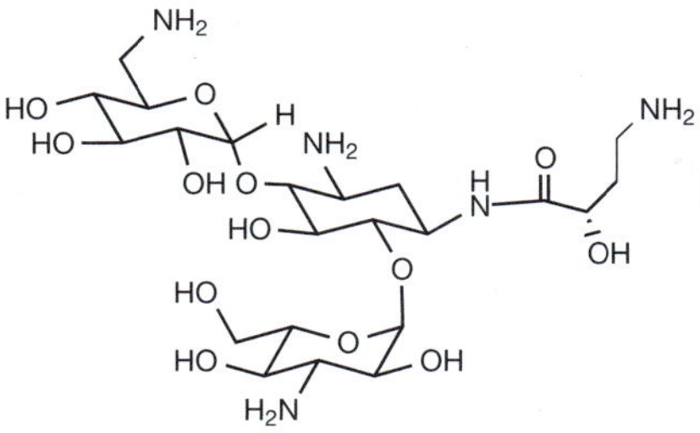

Structure B

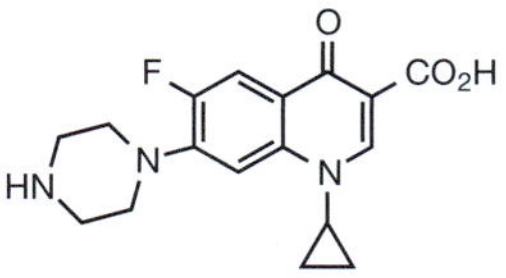

Structure C

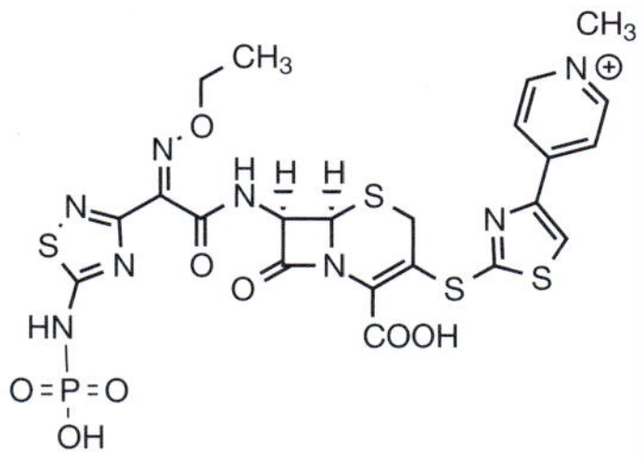

Structure D

Consider the structures A to D, and based on the information presented in this chapter, answer the following questions:

1. Which major class of antibiotics is represented by each of the structures?
2. Which compounds contain a β-lactam pharmacophore?
3. Which of the compounds disrupts the following bacterial processes: (a) cell wall biosynthesis, (b) protein biosynthesis, (c) nucleic acids topology?
4. What are the discrete molecular targets of the compounds A to D?
5. Which of the compounds is a prodrug?
6. Which of the compounds are available as an IV injection? Why?
7. Which of the compounds have the potential to cause: (a) hypersensitivity reactions, (b) nephrotoxicity, (c) tendonitis? Why?
8. Which of the presented agents needs to be combined with clavulanic acid in order to retain activity against bacteria-producing β-lactamase?
9. The intracellular uptake of which medication is inhibited by the elevated concentration of Mg^{2+} ions?
10. Which of the compounds chelates polyvalent metal ions such as Ca^{2+}, Mg^{2+}, Zn^{2+}, Fe^{2+}, Al^{3+}? Why?
11. Why should medication B not be physically mixed and/or coformulated with a β-lactam antibiotic?
12. What are some of the most common mechanisms that microbes have developed to counteract the antibiotic action of the agents A to D?

Structure Challenge answers found immediately after References.

REFERENCES

1. McRose DL, Newman DK. Redox-active antibiotics enhance phosphorus bioavailability. *Science*. 2021;371(6533):1033-1037.
2. Microbiology by numbers. *Nat Rev Microbiol*. 2011;9(9):628.
3. Balloux F, van Dorp L. Q&A: What are pathogens, and what have they done to and for us? *BMC Biol*. 2017;15(1):91.
4. Whitman WB, Coleman DC, Wiebe WJ. Prokaryotes: the unseen majority. *Proc Natl Acad Sci U S A*. 1998;95(12):6578-6583.
5. GBD 2019 Antimicrobial Resistance Collaborators. Global mortality associated with 33 bacterial pathogens in 2019: a systematic analysis for the Global Burden of Disease Study 2019. *Lancet*. 2022;400(10369):2221-2248.
6. Herzog H. History of tuberculosis. *Respiration*. 1998;65(1):5-15.
7. Sneader W. *Drug Discovery: A History*. John Wiley & Sons, Ltd; 2005.
8. Neu HC, Gootz TD. Antimicrobial chemotherapy. In: Baron S, ed. *Medical Microbiology*. 4th ed. University of Texas Medical Branch at Galveston; 1996.
9. Strebhardt K, Ullrich A. Paul Ehrlich's magic bullet concept: 100 years of progress. *Nat Rev Cancer*. 2008;8(6):473-480.
10. Fleming A. On the antibacterial action of cultures of a penicullum, with special reference to their use in the isolation of B. influenza. *Br J Exp Pathol*. 1929;10:226-236.
11. Domagk G. Ein Beitrag zur Chemotherapie der bakteriellen Infektionen. *Dtsch Med Wochenschr*. 1935;61:250-253.
12. Gaynes R. The discovery of penicillin—new insights after more than 75 years of clinical use. *Emerg Infect Dis*. 2017;23(5):849-853.
13. Fleischmann RD, Adams MD, White O, et al. Whole-genome random sequencing and assembly of Haemophilus influenzae Rd. *Science*. 1995;269(5223):496-512.
14. Complete Microbial Genomes. Accessed November 2023. https://www.ncbi.nlm.nih.gov/genome/microbes/
15. Fraser CM, Gocayne JD, White O, et al. The minimal gene complement of Mycoplasma genitalium. *Science*. 1995;270(5235):397-403.
16. Zhang R, Ou HY, Zhang CT. DEG: a database of essential genes. *Nucleic Acids Res*. 2004;32(Database issue):D271-272.
17. Payne DJ, Gwynn MN, Holmes DJ, et al. Drugs for bad bugs: confronting the challenges of antibacterial discovery. Review. *Nat Rev Drug Discov*. 2007;6(1):29-40.
18. Ayon NJ. High-throughput screening of natural product and synthetic molecule libraries for antibacterial drug discovery. *Metabolites*. 2023;13(5).
19. Ory EM, Yow EM. The use and abuse of the broad spectrum antibiotics. *JAMA*. 1963;185:273-279.
20. Varadi L, Luo JL, Hibbs DE, et al. Methods for the detection and identification of pathogenic bacteria: past, present, and future. *Chem Soc Rev*. 2017;46(16):4818-4832.
21. Murray PR. The clinician and the microbiology laboratory. In: Bennett JE, Dolin R, Blaser MJ, eds. *Mandell, Doublas, and Bennett's Principles and Practice of Infectious Disease*. 8th ed. Elsevier, Inc.; 2015:191-223:chap 16.
22. Glupczynski Y, Labbe M, Hansen W, et al. Evaluation of the E test for quantitative antimicrobial susceptibility testing of Helicobacter pylori. *J Clin Microbiol*. 1991;29(9):2072-2075.

23. Bauer AW, Kirby WM, Sherris JC, et al. Antibiotic susceptibility testing by a standardized single disk method. *Am J Clin Pathol.* 1966;45(4):493-496.
24. Wald-Dickler N, Holtom P, Spellberg B. Busting the myth of "static vs cidal": a systemic literature review. *Clin Infect Dis.* 2018;66(9):1470-1474.
25. Barry AL, Craig WA, Nadler H, et al. *M26-A Methods for Determining Bactericidal Activity of Antimicrobial Agents.* 1st ed. Clinical and Laboratory Standards Institute; 1999.
26. Almagro-Moreno S. How bacterial pathogens emerge. *Am Sci.* 2022;110(3):162-169.
27. Reygaert WC. An overview of the antimicrobial resistance mechanisms of bacteria. *AIMS Microbiol.* 2018;4(3):482-501.
28. How DL. How antidepressants help bacteria resist antibiotics. *Nature.* 2023. doi:10.1038/d41586-023-00186-y.
29. Toleman MA, Walsh TR. Combinatorial events of insertion sequences and ICE in Gram-negative bacteria. *FEMS Microbiol Rev.* 2011;35(5):912-935.
30. Band VI, Weiss DS. Heteroresistance: a cause of unexplained antibiotic treatment failure? *PLoS Pathog.* 2019;15(6):e1007726.
31. Ocampo PS, Lazar V, Papp B, et al. Antagonism between bacteriostatic and bactericidal antibiotics is prevalent. *Antimicrob Agents Chemother.* 2014;58(8):4573-4582.
32. Sharma A, Gupta VK, Pathania R. Efflux pump inhibitors for bacterial pathogens: From bench to bedside. *Indian J Med Res.* 2019;149(2):129-145.
33. Bulitta JB, Kinzig M, Jakob V, et al. Nonlinear pharmacokinetics of piperacillin in healthy volunteers—implications for optimal dosage regimens. *Br J Clin Pharmacol.* 2010;70(5):682-693.
34. Spivey JM. The postantibiotic effect. *Clin Pharm.* 1992;11(10): 865-875.
35. Wu H, Moser C, Wang HZ, et al. Strategies for combating bacterial biofilm infections. *Int J Oral Sci.* 2015;7(1):1-7.
36. Wise EM, Jr., Park JT. Penicillin: its basic site of action as an inhibitor of a peptide cross-linking reaction in cell wall mucopeptide synthesis. *Proc Natl Acad Sci U S A.* 1965;54(1):75-81.
37. Kong KF, Schneper L, Mathee K. Beta-lactam antibiotics: from antibiosis to resistance and bacteriology. *APMIS.* 2010;118(1):1-36.
38. Behrens OK, Corse JW, Jones RG, et al, inventors; Eli Lilly & Co., assignee. Process and culture media for producing new penicillins. US patent 2,479,297. United States patent US2479295. August 16, 1949. 1949.
39. Peter DF, Charles NJH, Newbolt RG, inventors. Recovery of solid 6-amino-penicillanic acid. US patent 2,941,995. United States patent US2479295. August 16, 1949. 1960.
40. Tomasz A, Waks S. Mechanism of action of penicillin: triggering of the pneumococcal autolytic enzyme by inhibitors of cell wall synthesis. *Proc Natl Acad Sci U S A.* 1975;72(10):4162-4166.
41. Barza M, Weinstein L. Pharmacokinetics of the penicillins in man. *Clin Pharmacokinet.* 1976;1(4):297-308.
42. Abraham EP, Chain E. An enzyme from bacteria able to destroy penicillin. 1940. *Rev Infect Dis.* 1988;10(4):677-678.
43. Husna A, Rahman MM, Badruzzaman ATM, et al. Extended-spectrum beta-lactamases (esbl): challenges and opportunities. *Biomedicines.* 2023;11(11):2937.
44. Richter MF, Drown BS, Riley AP, et al. Predictive compound accumulation rules yield a broad-spectrum antibiotic. *Nature.* 2017;545(7654):299-304.
45. Van Bambeke F, Balzi E, Tulkens PM. Antibiotic efflux pumps. *Biochem Pharmacol.* 2000;60(4):457-470.
46. Joint Task Force on Practice Parameters; American Academy of Allergy, Asthma and Immunology; American College of Allergy, Asthma and Immunology; Joint Council of Allergy, Asthma and Immunology. Drug allergy: an updated practice parameter. *Ann Allergy Asthma Immunol.* 2010;105(4):259-273.
47. Fairbrother RW, Taylor G. Sodium methicillin in routine therapy. *Lancet.* 1961;1(7175):473-476.
48. Nafcillin. Package insert. Baxter Healthcare Corp; 2007.
49. Dicloxacillin. Package insert. Teva Pharmaceuticals USA Inc; 2022.
50. Brown DG, May-Dracka TL, Gagnon MM, et al. Trends and exceptions of physical properties on antibacterial activity for Gram-positive and Gram-negative pathogens. *J Med Chem.* 2014;57(23):10144-10161.
51. Ganapathy ME, Brandsch M, Prasad PD, et al. Differential recognition of beta-lactam antibiotics by intestinal and renal peptide transporters, PEPT 1 and PEPT 2. *J Biol Chem.* 1995;270(43):25672-25677.
52. Zosyn (piperacillin and tazobactam). Package insert. Pfizer Inc; 2017.
53. Rosenkilde CEH, Munck C, Porse A, et al. Collateral sensitivity constrains resistance evolution of the CTX-M-15 beta-lactamase. *Nat Commun.* 2019;10(1):618.
54. Bush K. Past and present perspectives on beta-lactamases. *Antimicrob Agents Chemother.* 2018;62(10):e01076-18.
55. Reading C, Cole M. Clavulanic acid: a beta-lactamase-inhibiting beta-lactam from Streptomyces clavuligerus. *Antimicrob Agents Chemother.* 1977;11(5):852-857.
56. Padayatti PS, Helfand MS, Totir MA, et al. High resolution crystal structures of the trans-enamine intermediates formed by sulbactam and clavulanic acid and E166A SHV-1 beta-lactamase. *J Biol Chem.* 2005;280(41):34900-34907.
57. Papp-Wallace KM, Bethel CR, Caillon J, et al. Beyond piperacillin-tazobactam: cefepime and aai101 as a potent beta-lactam-beta-lactamase inhibitor combination. *Antimicrob Agents Chemother.* 2019;63(5)
58. Drawz SM, Papp-Wallace KM, Bonomo RA. New beta-lactamase inhibitors: a therapeutic renaissance in an MDR world. *Antimicrob Agents Chemother.* 2014;58(4):1835-1846.
59. Lahiri SD, Johnstone MR, Ross PL, et al. Avibactam and class C beta-lactamases: mechanism of inhibition, conservation of the binding pocket, and implications for resistance. *Antimicrob Agents Chemother.* 2014;58(10):5704-5713.
60. Lahiri SD, Mangani S, Durand-Reville T, et al. Structural insight into potent broad-spectrum inhibition with reversible recyclization mechanism: avibactam in complex with CTX-M-15 and Pseudomonas aeruginosa AmpC beta-lactamases. *Antimicrob Agents Chemother.* 2013;57(6):2496-2505.
61. Durand-Reville TF, Guler S, Comita-Prevoir J, et al. ETX2514 is a broad-spectrum beta-lactamase inhibitor for the treatment of drug-resistant Gram-negative bacteria including Acinetobacter baumannii. *Nat Microbiol.* 2017;2:17104.
62. Hecker SJ, Reddy KR, Totrov M, et al. Discovery of a cyclic boronic acid beta-lactamase inhibitor (rpx7009) with utility vs class a serine carbapenemases. *J Med Chem.* 2015;58(9):3682-3692.
63. Zhanel GG, Lawrence CK, Adam H, et al. Imipenem-relebactam and meropenem-vaborbactam: two novel carbapenem-beta-lactamase inhibitor combinations. *Drugs.* 2018;78(1):65-98.
64. Abraham EP, Newton GG. The structure of cephalosporin C. *Biochem J.* 1961;79(2):377-393.
65. Nagarajan R, Boeck LD, Gorman M, et al. Beta-lactam antibiotics from Streptomyces. *J Am Chem Soc.* 1971;93(9):2308-2310.
66. Imada A, Kitano K, Kintaka K, et al. Sulfazecin and isosulfazecin, novel beta-lactam antibiotics of bacterial origin. *Nature.* 1981;289(5798):590-591.
67. Sykes RB, Cimarusti CM, Bonner DP, et al. Monocyclic beta-lactam antibiotics produced by bacteria. *Nature.* 1981;291(5815):489-491.
68. Keflex (cephalexin). Package insert. Pragma Pharmaceuticals LLC; 2018.
69. Cuchural GJ Jr, Tally FP, Jacobus NV, et al. Comparative activities of newer beta-lactam agents against members of the Bacteroides fragilis group. *Antimicrob Agents Chemother.* 1990;34(3):479-480.
70. Rocephin (ceftriaxone). Package insert. Roche; 2004.
71. Bergan T. Pharmacokinetic properties of the cephalosporins. *Drugs.* 1987;34(suppl 2):89-104.

72. Dunn GL. Ceftizoxime and other third-generation cephalosporins: structure-activity relationships. *J Antimicrob Chemother.* 1982;10(suppl C):1-10.
73. Ceftin (cefuroxime). Package insert. GlaxoSmithKline; Updated 2019. Accessed March 1, 2024. https://www.accessdata.fda.gov/drugsatfda_docs/label/2019/050605s051,050672s037lbl.pdf
74. Wildman GT, Datta R, inventors. Isolation of antibiotic cephamycin C. US patent 4,137,405. United States patent US2479295. August 16, 1949. 1979.
75. Shearer MJ, Bechtold H, Andrassy K, et al. Mechanism of cephalosporin-induced hypoprothrombinemia: relation to cephalosporin side chain, vitamin K metabolism, and vitamin K status. *J Clin Pharmacol.* 1988;28(1):88-95.
76. Wiseman LR, Benfield P. Cefprozil. A review of its antibacterial activity, pharmacokinetic properties, and therapeutic potential. *Drugs.* 1993;45(2):295-317.
77. Neu HC, Meropol NJ, Fu KP. Antibacterial activity of ceftriaxone (Ro 13-9904), a beta-lactamase-stable cephalosporin. *Antimicrob Agents Chemother.* 1981;19(3):414-423.
78. Brogden RN, Campoli-Richards DM. Cefixime. A review of its antibacterial activity. Pharmacokinetic properties and therapeutic potential. *Drugs.* 1989;38(4):524-550.
79. Borin MT. A review of the pharmacokinetics of cefpodoxime proxetil. *Drugs.* 1991;42(suppl 3):13-21.
80. Sharma R, Park TE, Moy S. Ceftazidime-avibactam: a novel cephalosporin/beta-lactamase inhibitor combination for the treatment of resistant gram-negative organisms. *Clin Ther.* 2016;38(3):431-444.
81. Maxipime (cefepime). Package insert. Hospira; 2012.
82. Takeda S, Nakai T, Wakai Y, et al. In vitro and in vivo activities of a new cephalosporin, FR264205, against Pseudomonas aeruginosa. *Antimicrob Agents Chemother.* 2007;51(3):826-830.
83. Zhanel GG, Chung P, Adam H, et al. Ceftolozane/tazobactam: a novel cephalosporin/beta-lactamase inhibitor combination with activity against multidrug-resistant gram-negative bacilli. *Drugs.* 2014;74(1):31-51.
84. Ohi N, Aoki B, Kuroki T, et al. Semisynthetic beta-lactam antibiotics. III. Effect on antibacterial activity and comt-susceptibility of chlorine-introduction into the catechol nucleus of 6-[(R)-2-[3-(3,4-dihydroxybenzoyl)-3-(3-hydroxypropyl)-1-ureido]-2-phenylacetamido]penicillanic acid. *J Antibiot.* 1987;40(1):22-28.
85. Kosowska-Shick K, McGhee PL, Appelbaum PC. Affinity of ceftaroline and other beta-lactams for penicillin-binding proteins from Staphylococcus aureus and Streptococcus pneumoniae. *Antimicrob Agents Chemother.* 2010;54(5):1670-1677.
86. Villegas-Estrada A, Lee M, Hesek D, et al. Co-opting the cell wall in fighting methicillin-resistant Staphylococcus aureus: potent inhibition of PBP 2a by two anti-MRSA beta-lactam antibiotics. *J Am Chem Soc.* 2008;130(29):9212-9213.
87. Dauner DG, Nelson RE, Taketa DC. Ceftobiprole: A novel, broad-spectrum cephalosporin with activity against methicillin-resistant Staphylococcus aureus. *Am J Health Syst Pharm.* 2010; 67(12):983-993.
88. Del Pozo JL, Patel R. Ceftobiprole medocaril: a new generation beta-lactam. *Drugs Today (Barc).* 2008;44(11):801-825.
89. Davies TA, Page MG, Shang W, et al. Binding of ceftobiprole and comparators to the penicillin-binding proteins of Escherichia coli, Pseudomonas aeruginosa, Staphylococcus aureus, and Streptococcus pneumoniae. *Antimicrob Agents Chemother.* 2007;51(7):2621-2624.
90. Kahan JS, Kahan FM, Goegelman R, et al. Thienamycin, a new beta-lactam antibiotic. I. Discovery, taxonomy, isolation and physical properties. *J Antibiot.* 1979;32(1):1-12.
91. El-Gamal MI, Brahim I, Hisham N, et al. Recent updates of carbapenem antibiotics. *Eur J Med Chem.* 2017;131:185-195.
92. Birnbaum J, Kahan FM, Kropp H, et al. Carbapenems, a new class of beta-lactam antibiotics. Discovery and development of imipenem/cilastatin. *Am J Med.* 1985;78(6A):3-21.
93. Primaxin (imipenem and cilastatin). Package insert. Merck & Co. Inc; 2016.
94. Tsuji M, Ishii Y, Ohno A, et al. In vitro and in vivo antibacterial activities of S-4661, a new carbapenem. *Antimicrob Agents Chemother.* 1998;42(1):94-99.
95. Cannon JP, Lee TA, Clark NM, et al. The risk of seizures among the carbapenems: a meta-analysis. *J Antimicrob Chemother.* 2014;69(8):2043-2055.
96. Norrby SR, Gildon KM. Safety profile of meropenem: a review of nearly 5,000 patients treated with meropenem. *Scand J Infect Dis.* 1999;31(1):3-10.
97. Vabomere (meropenem and vaborbactam). Package insert. Melinta Therapeutics, LLC; 2017.
98. Zhanel GG, Wiebe R, Dilay L, et al. Comparative review of the carbapenems. *Drugs.* 2007;67(7):1027-1052.
99. Kobayashi R, Konomi M, Hasegawa K, et al. In vitro activity of tebipenem, a new oral carbapenem antibiotic, against penicillin-nonsusceptible Streptococcus pneumoniae. *Antimicrob Agents Chemother.* 2005;49(3):889-894.
100. Azactam (aztreonam). Package insert. Bristol-Myers Squibb Co; 2022.
101. Khondker A, Dhaliwal AK, Saem S, et al. Membrane charge and lipid packing determine polymyxin-induced membrane damage. *Commun Biol.* 2019;2:67.
102. Stone KJ, Strominger JL. Mechanism of action of bacitracin: complexation with metal ion and C 55 -isoprenyl pyrophosphate. *Proc Natl Acad Sci U S A.* 1971;68(12):3223-3227.
103. Federal Register. Determination that bacitracin for injection, 10,000 Units/Vial and 50,000 Units/Vial, was withdrawn from sale for reasons of safety or effectiveness. U.S. Department of Health and Human Services; 2022:56680-56681.
104. Barna JC, Williams DH. The structure and mode of action of glycopeptide antibiotics of the vancomycin group. *Annu Rev Microbiol.* 1984;38:339-357.
105. Sievert DM, Rudrik JT, Patel JB, et al. Vancomycin-resistant Staphylococcus aureus in the United States, 2002-2006. Case Reports. *Clin Infect Dis.* 2008;46(5):668-674.
106. Selim S. Mechanisms of gram-positive vancomycin resistance (Review). *Biomed Rep.* 2022;16(1):7.
107. Vancocin (Vancomycin). Package insert. ANI Pharmaceuticals, Inc; 2017.
108. Higgins DL, Chang R, Debabov DV, et al. Telavancin, a multifunctional lipoglycopeptide, disrupts both cell wall synthesis and cell membrane integrity in methicillin-resistant Staphylococcus aureus. *Antimicrob Agents Chemother.* 2005;49(3):1127-1134.
109. Dalvance (dalbavancin). Package insert. Allergan USA Inc; 2021.
110. Orbactiv (oritavancin). Package insert. Melinta Therapeutics Inc; 2022.
111. Tally FP, DeBruin MF. Development of daptomycin for gram-positive infections. *J Antimicrob Chemother.* 2000;46(4):523-526.
112. Stefani S, Campanile F, Santagati M, et al. Insights and clinical perspectives of daptomycin resistance in Staphylococcus aureus: A review of the available evidence. *Int J Antimicrob Agents.* 2015;46(3):278-289.
113. Cubicin (daptomycin). Package insert. Merch & Co. Inc; 2022.
114. Trefouel J, Trefouel J, Nitti F, et al. Activite du p-aminophenylsulfamide sur les infections streptococciques experimentales de la souris et du lapin. *C R Soc Biol.* 1935;120:756-758.
115. Anand N. Sulfonamides: structure-activity relationships and mechanism of action. In: Hitchings GH, ed. *Inhibition of Folate Metabolism in Chemotherapy Handbook of Experimental Pharmacology (Continuation of Handbuch der experimentellen Pharmakologie).* Springer; 1983.
116. Bactrim Tablets and Double Strength Tablets. Package insert. AR Scientific; Revised June 13, 2013.
117. Skold O. Sulfonamides and trimethoprim. *Expert Rev Anti Infect Ther.* 2010;8(1):1-6.
118. Masters PA, O'Bryan TA, Zurlo J, et al. Trimethoprim-sulfamethoxazole revisited. *Arch Intern Med.* 2003;163(4):402-410.

119. Hitchings GH, Elion GB. Pyrimidine derivatives as antagonists of pteroylglutamic acid. *J Biol Chem*. 1948;174(2):765.
120. Roberts VA, Dauber-Osguthorpe P, Osguthorpe DJ, et al. A comparison of the binding of the ligand trimethoprim to bacterial and vertebrate dihydrofolate reductases. *Israel J Chem*. 1986;27(2):198-210.
121. Trimethoprim tablets. Package insert. Novitium Pharma LLC; 2022.
122. Andriole VT. The quinolones: past, present, and future. *Clin Infect Dis*. 2005;41(suppl 2):S113-S119.
123. Drlica K, Zhao X. DNA gyrase, topoisomerase IV, and the 4-quinolones. *Microbiol Mol Biol Rev*. 1997;61(3):377-392.
124. Cheng G, Hao H, Dai M, et al. Antibacterial action of quinolones: from target to network. *Eur J Med Chem*. 2013;66:555-562.
125. Domagala JM. Structure-activity and structure-side-effect relationships for the quinolone antibacterials. *J Antimicrob Chemother*. 1994;33(4):685-706.
126. Blondeau JM. Fluoroquinolones: mechanism of action, classification, and development of resistance. *Surv Ophthalmol*. 2004;49 (suppl 2):S73-78.
127. Tulkens PM, Van Bambeke F, Zinner SH. Profile of a novel anionic fluoroquinolone-delafloxacin. *Clin Infect Dis*. 2019;68(suppl 3):S213-S222.
128. Turban A, Guerin F, Dinh A, et al. Updated review on clinically-relevant properties of delafloxacin. *Antibiotics (Basel)*. 2023; 12(8).
129. Cipro (ciprofloxacin). Package insert. Bayer HealthCare Pharmaceuticals LLC; 2023.
130. Levaquin (levofloxacin). Package insert. Janssen Pharmaceuticals Inc; 2023.
131. Avelox (moxifloxacin). Package insert. Bayer HealthCare Pharmaceuticals Inc; 2023.
132. Lopez Y, Tato M, Espinal P, et al. In vitro activity of Ozenoxacin against quinolone-susceptible and quinolone-resistant gram-positive bacteria. *Antimicrob Agents Chemother*. 2013;57(12): 6389-6392.
133. Hooper DC, Jacoby GA. Mechanisms of drug resistance: quinolone resistance. *Ann N Y Acad Sci*. 2015;1354(1):12-31.
134. Kang J, Wang L, Chen XL, et al. Interactions of a series of fluoroquinolone antibacterial drugs with the human cardiac K+ channel HERG. *Mol Pharmacol*. 2001;59(1):122-126.
135. Hussen NHA, Qadir SH, Rahman HS, et al. Long-term toxicity of fluoroquinolones: a comprehensive review. *Drug Chem Toxicol*. 2023:1-12.
136. Tu Y, McCalla DR. Effect of activated nitrofurans on DNA. *Biochim Biophys Acta*. 1975;402(2):142-149.
137. Macrodantin (nitrofurantoin). Package insert. Alvogen, Inc; 2022.
138. Dingsdag SA, Hunter N. Metronidazole: an update on metabolism, structure-cytotoxicity and resistance mechanisms. *J Antimicrob Chemother*. 2018;73(2):265-279.
139. Flagyl (metronidazole). Package insert. Chartwell RX, LLC; 2023.
140. Tindamax (tinidazole). Package insert. Mission Pharmacal Co; 2021.
141. Solosec (secnidazole). Package insert. Lupin Pharmaceuticals, Inc; 2022.
142. Schuwirth BS, Borovinskaya MA, Hau CW, et al. Structures of the bacterial ribosome at 3.5 A resolution. *Science*. 2005;310(5749):827-834.
143. Selmer M, Dunham CM, Murphy FVt, et al. Structure of the 70S ribosome complexed with mRNA and tRNA. *Science*. 2006;313(5795):1935-1942.
144. Ratjen F, Moeller A, McKinney ML, et al. Eradication of early P. aeruginosa infection in children <7 years of age with cystic fibrosis: the early study. *J Cyst Fibros*. 2019;18(1):78-85.
145. Blasi F, Carnovale V, Cimino G, et al. Treatment compliance in cystic fibrosis patients with chronic Pseudomonas aeruginosa infection treated with tobramycin inhalation powder: the FREE study. *Respir Med*. 2018;138:88-94.
146. Shirley M. Amikacin liposome inhalation suspension: a review in mycobacterium avium complex lung disease. *Drugs*. 2019;79(5):555-562.
147. Olivier KN, Griffith DE, Eagle G, et al. randomized trial of liposomal amikacin for inhalation in nontuberculous mycobacterial lung disease. *Am J Respir Crit Care Med*. 2017;195(6):814-823.
148. Krause KM, Serio AW, Kane TR, et al. Aminoglycosides: an overview. *Cold Spring Harb Perspect Med*. 2016;6(6):a027029.
149. Wasserman MR, Pulk A, Zhou Z, et al. Chemically related 4,5-linked aminoglycoside antibiotics drive subunit rotation in opposite directions. *Nat Commun*. 2015;6:7896.
150. Frazier AD, Champney WS. Impairment of ribosomal subunit synthesis in aminoglycoside-treated ribonuclease mutants of Escherichia coli. *Arch Microbiol*. 2012;194(12):1033-1041.
151. Jana S, Deb JK. Molecular understanding of aminoglycoside action and resistance. *Appl Microbiol Biotechnol*. 2006;70(2):140-150.
152. Magnet S, Blanchard JS. Molecular insights into aminoglycoside action and resistance. *Chem Rev*. 2005;105(2):477-498.
153. Block M, Blanchard DL. Aminoglycosides. In: *StatPearls* [Internet]. StatPearls Publishing; 2024.
154. Kahlmeter G, Dahlager JI. Aminoglycoside toxicity—a review of clinical studies published between 1975 and 1982. *J Antimicrob Chemother*. 1984;13(suppl A):9-22.
155. Warner WA, Sanders E. Neuromuscular blockade associated with gentamicin therapy. *JAMA*. 1971;215(7):1153-1154.
156. Hooper DC. Extended-spectrum beta-lactamases. In: Connor RF, ed. *UpToDate*. Wolters Kluwer; 2024.
157. Barclay ML, Begg EJ, Hickling KG. What is the evidence for once-daily aminoglycoside therapy? *Clin Pharmacokinet*. 1994;27(1):32-48.
158. Kuehl FA Jr, Peck RL. Streptomyces antibiotics; structure of streptomycin. *J Am Chem Soc*. 1948;70(7):2325-2330.
159. Finken M, Kirschner P, Meier A, et al. Molecular basis of streptomycin resistance in Mycobacterium tuberculosis: alterations of the ribosomal protein S12 gene and point mutations within a functional 16S ribosomal RNA pseudoknot. *Mol Microbiol*. 1993;9(6):1239-1246.
160. Fan Q, Huang F, Leadlay PF, et al. The neomycin biosynthetic gene cluster of Streptomyces fradiae NCIMB 8233: genetic and biochemical evidence for the roles of two glycosyltransferases and a deacetylase. *Org Biomol Chem*. 2008;6(18):3306-3314.
161. Masur H, Whelton PK, Whelton A. Neomycin toxicity revisited. *Arch Surg*. 1976;111(7):822-825.
162. Walkty A, Adam H, Baxter M, et al. In vitro activity of plazomicin against 5,015 gram-negative and gram-positive clinical isolates obtained from patients in Canadian hospitals as part of the CANWARD study, 2011-2012. *Antimicrob Agents Chemother*. 2014;58(5):2554-2563.
163. Aggen JB, Armstrong ES, Goldblum AA, et al. Synthesis and spectrum of the neoglycoside ACHN-490. *Antimicrob Agents Chemother*. 2010;54(11):4636-4642.
164. Dinos GP. The macrolide antibiotic renaissance. *Br J Pharmacol*. 2017;174(18):2967-2983.
165. Staunton J, Wilkinson B. Biosynthesis of erythromycin and rapamycin. *Chem Rev*. 1997;97(7):2611-2630.
166. Birch AJ, Djerassi C, Dutcher JD, et al. Studies in relation to biosynthesis. Part XXXV. Macrolide antibiotics. Part XII. Methymycin. *J Chem Soc*. 1964:5274-5278.
167. Yan X, Dong Y, Gu Y, et al. Effect of precursors and their regulators on the biosynthesis of antibiotics in actinomycetes. *Molecules*. 2024;29(5):1132.
168. Fiese EF, Steffen SH. Comparison of the acid stability of azithromycin and erythromycin A. *J Antimicrob Chemother*. 1990;25(suppl A):39-47.
169. Roberts MC, Sutcliffe J, Courvalin P, et al. Nomenclature for macrolide and macrolide-lincosamide-streptogramin B resistance determinants. *Antimicrob Agents Chemother*. 1999;43(12): 2823-2830.

170. Westphal JF. Macrolide-induced clinically relevant drug interactions with cytochrome P-450A (CYP) 3A4: an update focused on clarithromycin, azithromycin and dirithromycin. *Br J Clin Pharmacol*. 2000;50(4):285-295.
171. Fohner AE, Sparreboom A, Altman RB, et al. PharmGKB summary: macrolide antibiotic pathway, pharmacokinetics/pharmacodynamics. *Pharmacogenet Genomics*. 2017;27(4):164-167.
172. Eberl S, Renner B, Neubert A, et al. Role of p-glycoprotein inhibition for drug interactions: evidence from in vitro and pharmacoepidemiological studies. *Clin Pharmacokinet*. 2007;46(12):1039-1049.
173. Patel PH, Hashmi MF. Macrolides. In: *StatPearls* [Internet]. StatPearls Publishing; 2024.
174. Currier JS. Mycobacterium avium complex (MAC) infections in persons with HIV. In: Connor RF, ed. *UpToDate*. Wolters Kluwer; 2023.
175. Cunha JP. Eryc—erythromycin delayed-release. WebMD. June 9, 2022. RxList Accessed April 1, 2022. https://www.rxlist.com/eryc-drug.htm
176. Ery-Ped (erythromycin ethyl succinate). Package insert. Arbor Pharmaceuticals, Inc; 2022.
177. E.E.S. (erythromycin ethyl succinate) tablet and oral suspension. Prescribing Information. Arbor Pharmaceuticals, Inc; July 2013.
178. Cunha JP. Erythrocin Stearate. WebMD. December 15, 2022. RxList Accessed April 1, 2022. https://www.rxlist.com/erythrocin-stearate-drug.htm
179. Ferrero JL, Bopp BA, Marsh KC, et al. Metabolism and disposition of clarithromycin in man. *Drug Metab Dispos*. 1990;18(4):441-446.
180. Zithromax (azirthromycin). Package insert. Pfizer Inc; 2023.
181. Golan Y, Epstein L. Safety and efficacy of fidaxomicin in the treatment of Clostridium difficile-associated diarrhea. *Therap Adv Gastroenterol*. 2012;5(6):395-402.
182. Dificid (fidaxomicin). Package insert. Merck & Co. Inc; 2022.
183. Spizek J, Rezanka T. Lincomycin, clindamycin and their applications. *Appl Microbiol Biotechnol*. 2004;64(4):455-464.
184. Murphy PB, Bistas KG, Patel P, et al. Clindamycin. In: *StatPearls* [Internet]. StatPearls Publishing; 2024.
185. Cleocin (clindamycin). Package insert. Pharmacia & Upjohn Co. LLC; 2022.
186. Prabhu K, Rao S, Rao V. Inducible clindamycin resistance in Staphylococcus aureus isolated from clinical samples. *J Lab Physicians*. 2011;3(1):25-27.
187. Mitcheltree MJ, Pisipati A, Syroegin EA, et al. A synthetic antibiotic class overcoming bacterial multidrug resistance. *Nature*. 2021;599(7885):507-512.
188. Wu KJY, Tresco BIC, Ramkissoon A, et al. An antibiotic preorganized for ribosomal binding overcomes antimicrobial resistance. *Science*. 2024;383(6684):721-726.
189. Chopra I, Roberts M. Tetracycline antibiotics: mode of action, applications, molecular biology, and epidemiology of bacterial resistance. *Microbiol Mol Biol Rev*. 2001;65(2):232-260.
190. Duarte HA, Carvalho S, Paniago EB, et al. Importance of tautomers in the chemical behavior of tetracyclinesdagger. *J Pharm Sci*. 1999;88(1):111-120.
191. Tetracycline. Package insert. Breckenridge Pharmaceutical, Inc; 2023.
192. Karatzas A, Paridis D, Kozyrakis D, et al. Fanconi syndrome in the adulthood. The role of early diagnosis and treatment. *J Musculoskelet Neuronal Interact*. 2017;17(4):303-306.
193. Brodersen DE, Clemons WM Jr, Carter AP, et al. The structural basis for the action of the antibiotics tetracycline, pactamycin, and hygromycin B on the 30S ribosomal subunit. *Cell*. 2000;103(7):1143-1154.
194. Pioletti M, Schlunzen F, Harms J, et al. Crystal structures of complexes of the small ribosomal subunit with tetracycline, edeine and IF3. *EMBO J*. 2001;20(8):1829-1839.
195. Anokhina MM, Barta A, Nierhaus KH, et al. Mapping of the second tetracycline binding site on the ribosomal small subunit of E.coli. *Nucleic Acids Res*. 2004;32(8):2594-2597.
196. Moullan N, Mouchiroud L, Wang X, et al. Tetracyclines disturb mitochondrial function across eukaryotic models: a call for caution in biomedical research. *Cell Rep*. 2015;10(10):1681-1691.
197. Shutter MC, Akhondi H. Tetracycline. In: *StatPearls* [Internet]. StatPearls Publishing; 2024.
198. Draper MP, Weir S, Macone A, et al. Mechanism of action of the novel aminomethylcycline antibiotic omadacycline. *Antimicrob Agents Chemother*. 2014;58(3):1279-1283.
199. Rusu A, Buta EL. The development of third-generation tetracycline antibiotics and new perspectives. *Pharmaceutics*. 2021;13(12).
200. Goldstein FW, Kitzis MD, Acar JF. N,N-dimethylglycyl-amido derivative of minocycline and 6-demethyl-6-desoxytetracycline, two new glycylcyclines highly effective against tetracycline-resistant gram-positive cocci. *Antimicrob Agents Chemother*. 1994;38(9):2218-2220.
201. Sum PE, Petersen P. Synthesis and structure-activity relationship of novel glycylcycline derivatives leading to the discovery of GAR-936. *Bioorg Med Chem Lett*. 1999;9(10):1459-1462.
202. Kunz Coyne AJ, Alosaimy S, Lucas K, et al. Eravacycline, the first four years: health outcomes and tolerability data for 19 hospitals in 5 U.S. regions from 2018 to 2022. *Microbiol Spectr*. 2024;12(1):e0235123.
203. Fernandes GFS, Scarim CB, Kim SH, et al. Oxazolidinones as versatile scaffolds in medicinal chemistry. *RSC Med Chem*. 2023;14(5):823-847.
204. van Bambeke F, Mingeot-Leclercq M-P, Glupczynski Y, et al. Mechanisms of action. In: Cohen J, Powderly WG, Opal SM, eds. *Infectious Diseases*. Elsevier; 2017:1162-1180.e1.
205. Bendre AD, Peters PJ, Kumar J. Tuberculosis: past, present and future of the treatment and drug discovery research. *Curr Res Pharmacol Drug Discov*. 2021;2:100037.
206. Foti C, Piperno A, Scala A, et al. Oxazolidinone antibiotics: chemical, biological and analytical aspects. *Molecules*. 2021;26(14):4280.
207. Colca JR, McDonald WG, Waldon DJ, et al. Cross-linking in the living cell locates the site of action of oxazolidinone antibiotics. *J Biol Chem*. 2003;278(24):21972-21979.
208. Sinclair A, Arnold C, Woodford N. Rapid detection and estimation by pyrosequencing of 23S rRNA genes with a single nucleotide polymorphism conferring linezolid resistance in Enterococci. *Antimicrob Agents Chemother*. 2003;47(11):3620-3622.
209. Lincopan N, de Almeida LM, Elmor de Araujo MR, et al. Linezolid resistance in Staphylococcus epidermidis associated with a G2603T mutation in the 23S rRNA gene. *Int J Antimicrob Agents*. 2009;34(3):281-282.
210. Li SM, Zhou YF, Li L, et al. Characterization of the multi-drug resistance gene cfr in methicillin-resistant staphylococcus aureus (MRSA) strains isolated from animals and humans in China. *Front Microbiol*. 2018;9:2925.
211. Klitgaard RN, Ntokou E, Norgaard K, et al. Mutations in the bacterial ribosomal protein l3 and their association with antibiotic resistance. *Antimicrob Agents Chemother*. 2015;59(6):3518-3528.
212. Rodriguez-Avial I, Culebras E, Betriu C, et al. In vitro activity of tedizolid (TR-700) against linezolid-resistant staphylococci. *J Antimicrob Chemother*. 2012;67(1):167-169.
213. Azzouz A, Preuss CV. Linezolid. In: *StatPearls* [Internet]. StatPearls Publishing; 2024.
214. Lee M, Lee J, Carroll MW, et al. Linezolid for treatment of chronic extensively drug-resistant tuberculosis. *N Engl J Med*. 2012;367(16):1508-1518.
215. Sivextro (tedizolid phosphate). Package insert. Merck & Co., Inc; 2022.
216. Zyvox (linezolid). Package insert. Pfizer & Upjohn, Inc; 2023.
217. Mishra S, Singh J, Singh V. Types and applications of potential antibiotics produced by fungi. In: Abd-Elsalam KA, Mohamed HI, eds. *Fungal Secondary Metabolites*. Elsevier; 2024:493-517.
218. de Mattos-Shipley KMJ, Foster GD, Bailey AM. Insights into the classical genetics of Clitopilus passeckerianus—the pleuromutilin producing mushroom. *Front Microbiol*. 2017;8:1056.

219. Eyal Z, Matzov D, Krupkin M, et al. A novel pleuromutilin antibacterial compound, its binding mode and selectivity mechanism. *Sci Rep*. 2016;6(1):39004.
220. Yan K, Madden L, Choudhry AE, et al. Biochemical characterization of the interactions of the novel pleuromutilin derivative retapamulin with bacterial ribosomes. *Antimicrob Agents Chemother*. 2006;50(11):3875-3881.
221. Davidovich C, Bashan A, Auerbach-Nevo T, et al. Induced-fit tightens pleuromutilins binding to ribosomes and remote interactions enable their selectivity. *Proc Natl Acad Sci U S A*. 2007;104(11):4291-4296.
222. Champney WS, Rodgers WK. Retapamulin inhibition of translation and 50S ribosomal subunit formation in Staphylococcus aureus cells. *Antimicrob Agents Chemother*. 2007;51(9):3385-3387.
223. Goethe O, Heuer A, Ma X, et al. Antibacterial properties and clinical potential of pleuromutilins. *Nat Prod Rep*. 2019;36(1):220-247.
224. Paukner S, Riedl R. Pleuromutilins: potent drugs for resistant bugs-mode of action and resistance. *Cold Spring Harb Perspect Med*. 2017;7(1):a027110.
225. Dong CL, Li LX, Cui ZH, et al. synergistic effect of pleuromutilins with other antimicrobial agents against Staphylococcus aureus in vitro and in an experimental galleria mellonella model. *Front Pharmacol*. 2017;8:553.
226. Altabax (retapamulin). Package insert. Amirall, LLC; 2023.
227. Mast Y, Weber T, Golz M, et al. Characterization of the 'pristinamycin supercluster' of Streptomyces pristinaespiralis. *Microb Biotechnol*. 2011;4(2):192-206.
228. Monarch Pharmaceuticals, Inc. Synercid (quinupristin and dalfopristin) [package insert]. U.S. Food and Drug Administration; Revised August 2010. Accessed April 15, 2024. www.accessdata.fda.gov/drugsatfda_docs/label/2012/050747s014,050748s013lbl.pdf
229. Oong GC, Tadi P. Chloramphenicol. In: *StatPearls* [Internet]. StatPearls Publishing; 2024.
230. Shaw WV, Packman LC, Burleigh BD, et al. Primary structure of a chloramphenicol acetyltransferase specified by R plasmids. *Nature*. 1979;282(5741):870-872.
231. Fernandez M, Conde S, de la Torre J, et al. Mechanisms of resistance to chloramphenicol in Pseudomonas putida KT2440. *Antimicrob Agents Chemother*. 2012;56(2):1001-1009.
232. Chloramphenicol. Package insert. Fresenius Kabi USA, LLC; 2016.
233. Parenti MA, Hatfield SM, Leyden JJ. Mupirocin: a topical antibiotic with a unique structure and mechanism of action. *Clin Pharm*. 1987;6(10):761-770.
234. GlaxoSmithKline. Bactroban Ointment (mupirocin) [package insert]. U.S. Food and Drug Administration; Revised March 2017. Accessed April 15, 2024. www.accessdata.fda.gov/drugsatfda_docs/label/2017/050591s034lbl.pdf
235. GlaxoSmithKline. Bactroban Cream (mupirocin) [package insert]. U.S. Food and Drug Administration; Revised March 2017. Accessed April 15, 2024. www.accessdata.fda.gov/drugsatfda_docs/label/2017/050746s021lbl.pdf
236. Falagas ME, Vouloumanou EK, Samonis G, et al. Fosfomycin. *Clin Microbiol Rev*. 2016;29(2):321-347.
237. Silver LL. Fosfomycin: mechanism and resistance. *Cold Spring Harb Perspect Med*. 2017;7(2).
238. de Oliveira MVD, Furtado RM, da Costa KS, et al. Advances in UDP-N-acetylglucosamine enolpyruvyl transferase (MurA) covalent inhibition. *Front Mol Biosci*. 2022;9:889825.
239. Forest Pharmaceuticals, Inc. Monurol (fosfomycin) [package insert]. U.S. Food and Drug Administration; Revised July 2007. Accessed April 15, 2024. www.accessdata.fda.gov/drugsatfda_docs/label/2008/050717s005lbl.pdf
240. Chwa A, Kavanagh K, Linnebur SA, et al. Evaluation of methenamine for urinary tract infection prevention in older adults: a review of the evidence. *Ther Adv Drug Saf*. 2019;10:2042098619876749.
241. Methenamine. In: *LiverTox–Clinical and Research Information on Drug-Induced Liver Injury*. National Institute of Diabetes and Digestive and Kidney Diseases. Updated January 2021. Accessed April 15, 2024. https://www.ncbi.nlm.nih.gov/books/NBK567340/
242. Jamil RT, Foris LA, Snowden J. Proteus mirabilis infections. In: *StatPearls* [Internet]. StatPearls Publishing; 2024.
243. Merck Sharp & Dohme, LLC. Zinplava (bezlotuxumab) [package insert]. U.S. Food and Drug Administration; Revised May 2023. Accessed April 15, 2024. www.accessdata.fda.gov/drugsatfda_docs/label/2023/761046s012lbl.pdf
244. Rebiotix, Inc. Rebyota (fecal microbiota, live - jslm) [package insert]. U.S. Food and Drug Administration; Revised December 2022. Accessed April 15, 2024. www.fda.gov/media/163587/download
245. Soveral LF, Korczaguin GG, Schmidt PS, et al. Immunological mechanisms of fecal microbiota transplantation in recurrent Clostridioides difficile infection. *World J Gastroenterol*. 2022;28(33):4762-4772.
246. Seres Therapeutics, Inc. Vowst (Fecal microbiota spores, live-brpk) [package insert]. U.S. Food and Drug Administration; Revised April 2024. Accessed April 15, 2024. www.fda.gov/media/167579/download?attachment
247. Uromune in Treating Recurrent Urinary Tract Infections in Women, NCT04096820. ClinicalTrials.gov; 2022. Accessed April 15, 2024. clinicaltrials.gov/study/NCT04096820
248. Nickel JC, Doiron RC. An effective sublingual vaccine, MV140, safely reduces risk of recurrent urinary tract infection in women. *Pathogens*. 2023;12(3)359.
249. Ly A, Liu J. Mycobacterial virulence factors: surface-exposed lipids and secreted proteins. *Int J Mol Sci*. 2020;21(11)3985.
250. McNeil MR, Brennan PJ. Structure, function and biogenesis of the cell envelope of mycobacteria in relation to bacterial physiology, pathogenesis and drug resistance; some thoughts and possibilities arising from recent structural information. *Res Microbiol*. 1991;142(4):451-463.
251. Jackson M. The mycobacterial cell envelope-lipids. *Cold Spring Harb Perspect Med*. 2014;4(10).
252. Zink AR, Sola C, Reischl U, et al. Characterization of Mycobacterium tuberculosis complex DNAs from Egyptian mummies by spoligotyping. *J Clin Microbiol*. 2003;41(1):359-367.
253. Global tuberculosis report. 2024. World Health Organization. Accessed March 2024. https://www.who.int/teams/global-tuberculosis-programme/tb-reports/global-tuberculosis-report-2024
254. Yang J, Li X, Sun Y, et al. Global epidemiology of leprosy from 2010 to 2020: a systematic review and meta-analysis of the proportion of sex, type, grade 2 deformity and age. *Pathog Glob Health*. 2022;116(8):467-476.
255. Prevots DR, Shaw PA, Strickland D, et al. Nontuberculous mycobacterial lung disease prevalence at four integrated health care delivery systems. *Am J Respir Crit Care Med*. 2010;182(7):970-976.
256. Park IK, Olivier KN. Nontuberculous mycobacteria in cystic fibrosis and non-cystic fibrosis bronchiectasis. *Semin Respir Crit Care Med*. 2015;36(2):217-224.
257. Zhang Y. The magic bullets and tuberculosis drug targets. *Annu Rev Pharmacol Toxicol*. 2005;45:529-564.
258. Treatment of TB Disease. U.S. Centers for Disease Control. Updated March 22, 2023. Accessed April 15, 2024. https://www.cdc.gov/tb/topic/treatment/tbdisease.htm
259. Bavin EM, James B, Kay E, et al. Further observations on the antibacterial activity to Mycobacterium tuberculosis of a derivative of isoniazid, omicron-hydroxybenzal isonicotinylhydrazone (nupasal-213). *J Pharm Pharmacol*. 1955;7(12):1032-1038.
260. Bavin EM, Drain DJ, Seiler M, et al. Some further studies on tuberculostatic compounds. *J Pharm Pharmacol*. 1952;4(11):844-855.
261. Zhang Y, Heym B, Allen B, et al. The catalase-peroxidase gene and isoniazid resistance of Mycobacterium tuberculosis. *Nature*. 1992;358(6387):591-593.

262. Johnsson K, Schultz PG. Mechanistic studies of the oxidation of isoniazid by the catalase peroxidase from Mycobacterium tuberculosis. *J Am Chem Soc*. 2002;116(16):7425-7426.
263. Dubnau E, Chan J, Raynaud C, et al. Oxygenated mycolic acids are necessary for virulence of Mycobacterium tuberculosis in mice. *Mol Microbiol*. 2000;36(3):630-637.
264. Glickman MS, Cox JS, Jacobs WR Jr. A novel mycolic acid cyclopropane synthetase is required for cording, persistence, and virulence of Mycobacterium tuberculosis. *Mol Cell*. 2000;5(4):717-727.
265. Quemard A, Sacchettini JC, Dessen A, et al. Enzymatic characterization of the target for isoniazid in Mycobacterium tuberculosis. *Biochemistry*. 1995;34(26):8235-8241.
266. Johnsson K, King DS, Schultz PG. Studies on the mechanism of action of isoniazid and ethionamide in the chemotherapy of tuberculosis. *J Am Chem Soc*. 2002;117(17):5009-5010.
267. van Soolingen D, de Haas PE, van Doorn HR, et al. Mutations at amino acid position 315 of the katG gene are associated with high-level resistance to isoniazid, other drug resistance, and successful transmission of Mycobacterium tuberculosis in the Netherlands. *J Infect Dis*. 2000;182(6):1788-1790.
268. Bollela VR, Namburete EI, Feliciano CS, et al. Detection of katG and inhA mutations to guide isoniazid and ethionamide use for drug-resistant tuberculosis. *Int J Tuberc Lung Dis*. 2016;20(8): 1099-1104.
269. Miesel L, Rozwarski DA, Sacchettini JC, et al. Mechanisms for isoniazid action and resistance. *Novartis Found Symp*. 1998;217: 209-220; discussion 220-221.
270. Nolan CM, Goldberg SV, Buskin SE. Hepatotoxicity associated with isoniazid preventive therapy: a 7-year survey from a public health tuberculosis clinic. *JAMA*. 1999;281(11):1014-1018.
271. Weber WW, Hein DW. Clinical pharmacokinetics of isoniazid. *Clin Pharmacokinet*. 1979;4(6):401-422.
272. Holdiness MR. Clinical pharmacokinetics of the antituberculosis drugs. *Clin Pharmacokinet*. 1984;9(6):511-544.
273. Sabbagh A, Darlu P, Crouau-Roy B, et al. Arylamine N-acetyltransferase 2 (NAT2) genetic diversity and traditional subsistence: a worldwide population survey. *PLoS One*. 2011;6(4):e18507.
274. Timbrell JA, Mitchell JR, Snodgrass WR, et al. Isoniazid hepatoxicity: the relationship between covalent binding and metabolism in vivo. *J Pharmacol Exp Ther*. 1980;213(2):364-369.
275. Lancini G, Zanchelli W. Structure-activity relationship in rifamycins. In: Perlman D, ed. *Structure–Activity Relationship Among the Semisynthetic Antibiotics*. Academic Press; 1977.
276. Bacchi A, Pelizzi G, Nebuloni M, et al. Comprehensive study on structure-activity relationships of rifamycins: discussion of molecular and crystal structure and spectroscopic and thermochemical properties of rifamycin O. *J Med Chem*. 1998;41(13):2319-2332.
277. Campbell EA, Korzheva N, Mustaev A, et al. Structural mechanism for rifampicin inhibition of bacterial RNA polymerase. *Cell*. 2001;104(6):901-912.
278. Arora SK. Correlation of structure and activity in ansamycins: structure, conformation, and interactions of antibiotic rifamycin S. *J Med Chem*. 1985;28(8):1099-1102.
279. Parker J. Antibiotic-resistance mutants. In: Maloy S, Hughes K, eds. *Brenner's Encyclopedia of Genetics*. Academic Press; 2013:138-139.
280. Bury-Moné S. Antibacterial therapeutic agents: antibiotics and bacteriophages. In: Caplan M, ed. *Reference Module in Biomedical Sciences*. Elsevier; 2014. doi:10.1016/B978-0-12-801238-3.00244-0
281. Levin ME, Hatfull GF. Mycobacterium smegmatis RNA polymerase: DNA supercoiling, action of rifampicin and mechanism of rifampicin resistance. *Mol Microbiol*. 1993;8(2):277-285.
282. Blanchard JS. Molecular mechanisms of drug resistance in Mycobacterium tuberculosis. *Annu Rev Biochem*. 1996;65:215-239.
283. Li MC, Lu J, Lu Y, et al. rpoB Mutations and effects on rifampin resistance in Mycobacterium tuberculosis. *Infect Drug Resist*. 2021;14:4119-4128.
284. Goldstein BP. Resistance to rifampicin: a review. *J Antibiot*. 2014;67(9):625-630.
285. Narang PK, Lewis RC, Bianchine JR. Rifabutin absorption in humans: relative bioavailability and food effect. *Clin Pharmacol Ther*. 1992;52(4):335-341.
286. Reith K, Keung A, Toren PC, et al. Disposition and metabolism of 14C-rifapentine in healthy volunteers. *Drug Metab Dispos*. 1998;26(8):732-738.
287. Keung AC, Eller MG, Weir SJ. Pharmacokinetics of rifapentine in patients with varying degrees of hepatic dysfunction. *J Clin Pharmacol*. 1998;38(6):517-524.
288. Crabol Y, Catherinot E, Veziris N, et al. Rifabutin: where do we stand in 2016? *J Antimicrob Chemother*. 2016;71(7):1759-1771.
289. Zhang Y, Shi W, Zhang W, et al. Mechanisms of pyrazinamide action and resistance. *Microbiol Spectr*. 2013;2(4):1-12.
290. Kushner S, Dalalian H, Sanjurjo JL, et al. Experimental chemotherapy of tuberculosis. II. The synthesis of pyrazinamides and related compounds1. *J Am Chem Soc*. 2002;74(14):3617-3621.
291. Bergmann KE, Cynamon MH, Welch JT. Quantitative structure-activity relationships for the in vitro antimycobacterial activity of pyrazinoic acid esters. *J Med Chem*. 1996;39(17):3394-3400.
292. Scorpio A, Zhang Y. Mutations in pncA, a gene encoding pyrazinamidase/nicotinamidase, cause resistance to the antituberculous drug pyrazinamide in tubercle bacillus. *Nat Med*. 1996;2(6):662-667.
293. Fontes FL, Rooker SA, Lynn-Barbe JK, et al. Pyrazinoic acid, the active form of the anti-tuberculosis drug pyrazinamide, and aromatic carboxylic acid analogs are protonophores. *Front Mol Biosci*. 2024;11:1350699.
294. Tahlan K, Wilson R, Kastrinsky DB, et al. SQ109 targets MmpL3, a membrane transporter of trehalose monomycolate involved in mycolic acid donation to the cell wall core of Mycobacterium tuberculosis. *Antimicrob Agents Chemother*. 2012;56(4): 1797-1809.
295. Hoelscher M. Evaluation of SQ109, high-dose rifampicin, and moxifloxacin in adults with smear-positive pulmonary TB in a MAMS design, NCT01785186. ClinicalTrials.gov. Updated September 20, 2017. Accessed April 21, 2024. https://clinicaltrials.gov/study/NCT01785186
296. Zhang L, Zhao Y, Gao Y, et al. Structures of cell wall arabinosyltransferases with the anti-tuberculosis drug ethambutol. *Science*. 2020;368(6496):1211-1219.
297. Daffe M, Brennan PJ, McNeil M. Predominant structural features of the cell wall arabinogalactan of Mycobacterium tuberculosis as revealed through characterization of oligoglycosyl alditol fragments by gas chromatography/mass spectrometry and by 1H and 13C NMR analyses. *J Biol Chem*. 1990;265(12):6734-6743.
298. Wolucka BA, McNeil MR, de Hoffmann E, et al. Recognition of the lipid intermediate for arabinogalactan/arabinomannan biosynthesis and its relation to the mode of action of ethambutol on mycobacteria. *J Biol Chem*. 1994;269(37):23328-23335.
299. Mikusova K, Slayden RA, Besra GS, et al. Biogenesis of the mycobacterial cell wall and the site of action of ethambutol. *Antimicrob Agents Chemother*. 1995;39(11):2484-2489.
300. Lee RE, Mikusova K, Brennan PJ, et al. Synthesis of the arabinose donor β-D-arabinofuranosyl-1-monophosphoryldecaprenol, development of a basic arabinosyl-transferase assay, and identification of ethambutol as an arabinosyl transferase inhibitor. *J Am Chem Soc*. 2002;117(48):11829-11832.
301. Khoo KH, Douglas E, Azadi P, et al. Truncated structural variants of lipoarabinomannan in ethambutol drug-resistant strains of Mycobacterium smegmatis. Inhibition of arabinan biosynthesis by ethambutol. *J Biol Chem*. 1996;271(45):28682-28690.
302. Belanger AE, Besra GS, Ford ME, et al. The embAB genes of Mycobacterium avium encode an arabinosyl transferase involved in cell wall arabinan biosynthesis that is the target for the antimycobacterial drug ethambutol. *Proc Natl Acad Sci U S A*. 1996;93(21):11919-11924.

303. Li MC, Chen R, Lin SQ, et al. Detecting ethambutol resistance in Mycobacterium tuberculosis isolates in China: a comparison between phenotypic drug susceptibility testing methods and DNA sequencing of embAB. *Front Microbiol.* 2020;11:781.
304. Wu Z, Tan Q, Zhang C, et al. mbtD and celA1 association with ethambutol resistance in Mycobacterium tuberculosis: A multi-omics analysis. *Front Cell Infect Microbiol.* 2022;12:959911.
305. Saukkonen JJ, Duarte R, Munsiff SS, et al. Updates on the treatment of drug-susceptible and drug-resistant tuberculosis: an official ATS/CDC/ERS/IDSA clinical practice guideline. Am J Respir Crit Care Med. 2025;211(1):15-33.
306. Banerjee A, Dubnau E, Quemard A, et al. inhA, a gene encoding a target for isoniazid and ethionamide in Mycobacterium tuberculosis. *Science.* 1994;263(5144):227-230.
307. Vale N, Gomes P, Santos HA. Metabolism of the antituberculosis drug ethionamide. *Curr Drug Metab.* 2013;14(1):151-158.
308. Vilcheze C, Weisbrod TR, Chen B, et al. Altered NADH/NAD+ ratio mediates coresistance to isoniazid and ethionamide in mycobacteria. *Antimicrob Agents Chemother.* 2005;49(2):708-720.
309. Auclair B, Nix DE, Adam RD, et al. Pharmacokinetics of ethionamide administered under fasting conditions or with orange juice, food, or antacids. *Antimicrob Agents Chemother.* 2001;45(3):810-814.
310. Zheng J, Rubin EJ, Bifani P, et al. para-Aminosalicylic acid is a prodrug targeting dihydrofolate reductase in Mycobacterium tuberculosis. *J Biol Chem.* 2013;288(32):23447-23456.
311. Abulfathi AA, Donald PR, Adams K, et al. The pharmacokinetics of para-aminosalicylic acid and its relationship to efficacy and intolerance. *Br J Clin Pharmacol.* 2020;86(11):2123-2132.
312. Caceres NE, Harris NB, Wellehan JF, et al. Overexpression of the D-alanine racemase gene confers resistance to D-cycloserine in Mycobacterium smegmatis. *J Bacteriol.* 1997;179(16):5046-5055.
313. de Chiara C, Homsak M, Prosser GA, et al. D-Cycloserine destruction by alanine racemase and the limit of irreversible inhibition. *Nat Chem Biol.* 2020;16(6):686-694.
314. van der Walt ML, Shean K, Becker P, et al. Treatment outcomes and adverse drug effects of ethambutol, cycloserine, and terizidone for the treatment of multidrug-resistant tuberculosis in South Africa. *Antimicrob Agents Chemother.* 2020;65(1):e00744-20.
315. Lin Y, Li Y, Zhu N, et al. The antituberculosis antibiotic capreomycin inhibits protein synthesis by disrupting interaction between ribosomal proteins L12 and L10. *Antimicrob Agents Chemother.* 2014;58(4):2038-2044.
316. Wong EB, Cohen KA, Bishai WR. Rising to the challenge: new therapies for tuberculosis. *Trends Microbiol.* 2013;21(9):493-501.
317. Hoffmann H, Kohl TA, Hofmann-Thiel S, et al. Delamanid and bedaquiline resistance in Mycobacterium tuberculosis ancestral Beijing genotype causing extensively drug-resistant tuberculosis in a Tibetan refugee. *Am J Respir Crit Care Med.* 2016;193(3):337-340.
318. Bonnet M, Bastard M, du Cros P, et al. Identification of patients who could benefit from bedaquiline or delamanid: a multisite MDR-TB cohort study. *Int J Tuberc Lung Dis.* 2016;20(2):177-186.
319. Andries K, Verhasselt P, Guillemont J, et al. A diarylquinoline drug active on the ATP synthase of Mycobacterium tuberculosis. *Science.* 2005;307(5707):223-227.
320. Global Alliance for TB Drug Development. Evaluate safety, tolerability, PK of TBAJ-876 in healthy adults, NCT04493671. ClinicalTrials.gov. Updated November 21, 2022. Accessed April 24, 2024. https://clinicaltrials.gov/study/NCT04493671
321. TBAJ-876. TB Alliance. Accessed April 15, 2024. https://www.tballiance.org/portfolio/compound/tbaj-876
322. Koul A, Dendouga N, Vergauwen K, et al. Diarylquinolines target subunit c of mycobacterial ATP synthase. *Nat Chem Biol.* 2007;3(6):323-324.
323. Cole ST, Alzari PM. Microbiology. TB—a new target, a new drug. *Science.* 2005;307(5707):214-215.
324. Segala E, Sougakoff W, Nevejans-Chauffour A, et al. New mutations in the mycobacterial ATP synthase: new insights into the binding of the diarylquinoline TMC207 to the ATP synthase C-ring structure. *Antimicrob Agents Chemother.* 2012;56(5):2326-2334.
325. Ashtekar DR, Costa-Perira R, Nagrajan K, et al. In vitro and in vivo activities of the nitroimidazole CGI 17341 against Mycobacterium tuberculosis. *Antimicrob Agents Chemother.* 1993;37(2):183-186.
326. Xavier AS, Lakshmanan M. Delamanid: a new armor in combating drug-resistant tuberculosis. *J Pharmacol Pharmacother.* 2014;5(3):222-224.
327. Abrahams KA, Batt SM, Gurcha SS, et al. DprE2 is a molecular target of the anti-tubercular nitroimidazole compounds pretomanid and delamanid. *Nat Commun.* 2023;14(1):3828.
328. Rifat D, Li SY, Ioerger T, et al. Mutations in fbiD (Rv2983) as a novel determinant of resistance to pretomanid and delamanid in Mycobacterium tuberculosis. *Antimicrob Agents Chemother.* 2020;65(1).
329. Jacobs MR. Activity of quinolones against mycobacteria. *Drugs.* 1995;49(suppl 2):67-75.
330. Renau TE, Sanchez JP, Gage JW, et al. Structure-activity relationships of the quinolone antibacterials against mycobacteria: effect of structural changes at N-1 and C-7. *J Med Chem.* 1996;39(3):729-735.
331. Miyazaki E, Miyazaki M, Chen JM, et al. Moxifloxacin (BAY12-8039), a new 8-methoxyquinolone, is active in a mouse model of tuberculosis. *Antimicrob Agents Chemother.* 1999;43(1):85-89.
332. Zhao BY, Pine R, Domagala J, et al. Fluoroquinolone action against clinical isolates of Mycobacterium tuberculosis: effects of a C-8 methoxyl group on survival in liquid media and in human macrophages. *Antimicrob Agents Chemother.* 1999;43(3):661-666.
333. Nahid P, Dorman SE, Alipanah N, et al. Official American Thoracic Society/Centers for Disease Control and Prevention/Infectious Diseases Society of America clinical practice guidelines: treatment of drug-susceptible tuberculosis. *Clin Infect Dis.* 2016;63(7):e147-e195.
334. Taylor HG. The tuberculosis epidemic and the pharmacist's role. *Am Pharm.* 1992;NS32(7):41-44.
335. Nuermberger EL, Spigelman MK, Yew WW. Current development and future prospects in chemotherapy of tuberculosis. *Respirology.* 2010;15(5):764-778.
336. Caminero JA, Sotgiu G, Zumla A, et al. Best drug treatment for multidrug-resistant and extensively drug-resistant tuberculosis. *Lancet Infect Dis.* 2010;10(9):621-629.
337. Mase SR, Chorba T. Treatment of drug-resistant tuberculosis. *Clin Chest Med.* 2019;40(4):775-795.
338. Dhople AM. In vitro and in vivo activity of K-130, a dihydrofolate reductase inhibitor, against Mycobacterium leprae. *Arzneimittelforschung.* 1999;49(3):267-271.
339. van Zyl JM, Basson K, Kriegler A, et al. Mechanisms by which clofazimine and dapsone inhibit the myeloperoxidase system. A possible correlation with their anti-inflammatory properties. *Biochem Pharmacol.* 1991;42(3):599-608.
340. Expanded Access to Clofazimine. U.S. Food & Drug Administration. Updated 11/15/2023. Accessed April 28, 2024. https://www.fda.gov/about-fda/center-drug-evaluation-and-research-cder/expanded-access-clofazimine.
341. Arutla S, Arra GS, Prabhakar CM, et al. Pro- and anti-oxidant effects of some antileprotic drugs in vitro and their influence on super oxide dismutase activity. *Arzneimittelforschung.* 1998;48(10):1024-1027.
342. Liu B, Liu K, Lu Y, et al. Systematic evaluation of structure-activity relationships of the riminophenazine class and discovery

of a C2 pyridylamino series for the treatment of multidrug-resistant tuberculosis. *Molecules*. 2012;17(4):4545-4559.
343. O'Sullivan JF, Conalty ML, Morrison NE. Clofazimine analogues active against a clofazimine-resistant organism. *J Med Chem*. 1988;31(3):567-572.
344. Early bactericidal activity safety pulmonary tuberculosis Pyrifazimine (TBI-166), NCT04670120. U.S. National Library of Medicine. Updated September 20, 2021. Accessed April 28, 2024. https://clinicaltrials.gov/study/NCT04670120.
345. Cholo MC, Mothiba MT, Fourie B, et al. Mechanisms of action and therapeutic efficacies of the lipophilic antimycobacterial agents clofazimine and bedaquiline. *J Antimicrob Chemother*. 2017;72(2):338-353.
346. Savage JE, O'Sullivan JF, Zeis BM, et al. Investigation of the structural properties of dihydrophenazines which contribute to their pro-oxidative interactions with human phagocytes. *J Antimicrob Chemother*. 1989;23(5):691-700.
347. Franzblau SG, White KE, O'Sullivan JF. Structure-activity relationships of tetramethylpiperidine-substituted phenazines against Mycobacterium leprae in vitro. *Antimicrob Agents Chemother*. 1989;33(11):2004-2005.
348. Krishna DR, Mamidi RN, Hofmann U, et al. Characterization of clofazimine metabolites in humans by HPLC-electrospray mass spectrometry. *Arzneimittelforschung*. 1997;47(3):303-306.
349. Stirling D, Sherman M, Strauss S. Thalidomide. A surprising recovery. *J Am Pharm Assoc (Wash)*. 1997;NS37(3):306-313.
350. Lockwood DN, Kumar B. Treatment of leprosy. *BMJ*. 2004;328(7454):1447-1448.
351. Finch RG, Greenwood D, Whitley RJ, et al. *Antibiotic and Chemotherapy*. 9th ed. Saunders; 2010.
352. Cruz R, Buhrer-Sekula S, Penna MLF, et al. Leprosy: current situation, clinical and laboratory aspects, treatment history and perspective of the uniform multidrug therapy for all patients. *An Bras Dermatol*. 2017;92(6):761-773.
353. Akram SM, Attia FN. Mycobacterium avium complex. In: *StatPearls* [Internet]. StatPearls Publishing; 2024.
354. Daley CL, Iaccarino JM, Lange C, et al. Treatment of nontuberculous mycobacterial pulmonary disease: an official ATS/ERS/ESCMID/IDSA clinical practice guideline. *Clin Infect Dis*. 2020;71(4):905-913.
355. Griffith DE, Aksamit T, Brown-Elliott BA, et al. An official ATS/IDSA statement: diagnosis, treatment, and prevention of nontuberculous mycobacterial diseases. *Am J Respir Crit Care Med*. 2007;175(4):367-416.
356. Daley CL, Iaccarino JM, Lange C, et al. Treatment of nontuberculous mycobacterial pulmonary disease: an official ATS/ERS/ESCMID/IDSA clinical practice guideline. *Eur Respir J*. 2020;56(1).

Structure Challenge Answers

1. A: penicillins, B: aminoglycosides, C: fluoroquinolones, D: cephalosporins.
2. A and D.
3. a: A and D, b: B, c: C.
4. A and D: PBPs, B: 16S RNA of the 30S subunit, C: DNA gyrase and topoisomerase IV.
5. D.
6. B, C, and D (due to their polarity/ionization and associated water solubility).
7. a: A and D (formation of covalent adducts/haptens with host proteins), b: B (potential for accumulation in the kidneys), c: C (depletion of chondrocytes that constitute cartilage).
8. A.
9. B.
10. C (V-fork-like structure created by the adjacent carboxylic acid and ketone functional groups possessing lone pairs of electrons on oxygen atoms).
11. Due to inactivation of the β-lactam core by the nucleophilic nature of functional groups present in aminoglycosides.
12. Modification of PBPs and/or overexpression of β-lactamases for A and D; acetylation/phosphorylation/adenylation of drug's functional groups and/or point mutations of the ribosomal A-site for B; spontaneous mutations in genes encoding DNA gyrase/topoisomerase IV and/or efflux pumps for C. For more examples, please Figure 32.4 and specific paragraphs on resistance for each of the respective drug classes.

CHAPTER 33

Drugs Used to Treat Viral Infections

Marc W. Harrold and Lauren A. O'Donnell

Drugs covered in this chapter:

Drugs for herpesvirus infections
- Acyclovir
- Docosanol
- Famciclovir
- Penciclovir
- Trifluridine
- Valacyclovir

Drugs for cytomegalovirus infections
- Cidofovir
- Foscarnet
- Ganciclovir
- Letermovir
- Maribavir
- Valganciclovir

Drugs for influenza infections
- Amantadine
- Baloxavir marboxil
- Oseltamivir
- Peramivir
- Rimantadine
- Zanamivir

Drugs for COVID-19 infections
- Molnupiravir
- Nirmatrelvir and ritonavir
- Remdesivir

Drugs for respiratory syncytial virus infections
- Nirsevimab
- Palivizumab
- Ribavirin

Drugs for hepatitis B infections
- Adefovir dipivoxil
- Entecavir
- Pegylated interferon-α-2a/2b
- Telbivudine

Drugs for hepatitis C infections

NS3/4A protease inhibitors
- Glecaprevir
- Grazoprevir
- Paritaprevir
- Voxilaprevir

NS5A protein inhibitors
- Elbasvir
- Ledipasvir
- Ombitasvir
- Pibrentasvir
- Velpatasvir

NS5B polymerase inhibitors
- Dasabuvir
- Sofosbuvir

Drugs for human immunodeficiency virus infections

Nucleoside reverse transcriptase inhibitors
- Abacavir
- Didanosine
- Emtricitabine
- Lamivudine
- Stavudine
- Tenofovir
- Zidovudine

Nonnucleoside reverse transcriptase inhibitors
- Delavirdine
- Doravirine
- Efavirenz
- Etravirine
- Nevirapine
- Rilpivirine

HIV integrase strand transfer inhibitors
- Bictegravir
- Cabotegravir
- Dolutegravir
- Elvitegravir (and cobicistat)
- Raltegravir

HIV protease inhibitors
- Atazanavir
- Darunavir
- Fosamprenavir
- Indinavir
- Lopinavir
- Nelfinavir
- Ritonavir
- Saquinavir
- Tipranavir

Drugs preventing entry
- Enfuvirtide
- Ibalizumab
- Lenacapavir
- Maraviroc

HIV capsid inhibitors
- Fostemsavir

Antidiarrheal
- Crofelemer

Drugs for smallpox
- Tecovirimat

Abbreviations

acyclo-GMP acyclo-guanosine monophosphate
acyclo-GDP acyclo-guanosine diphosphate
AIDS acquired immune deficiency syndrome
ALT alanine aminotransferase
ARDS acute respiratory distress syndrome
ART antiretroviral therapy
ARV antiretroviral
AST aspartate aminotransferase
ATP adenosine triphosphate
BCRP breast cancer–resistance protein
CaCC calcium-activated chloride channels
cAMP cyclic adenosine monophosphate
CCD catalytic core domain
CDC Centers for Disease Control and Prevention
cDNA complementary DNA
CFTR cystic fibrosis transmembrane conductance regulator
CMV cytomegalovirus
CNS central nervous system
CPK creatine phosphokinase
CPSF6 cleavage and polyadenylation specificity factor subunit 6
DAA direct-acting antivirals
DANA 2-deoxy-2,3-dehydro-N-acetylneuraminic acid
dATP deoxyadenosine triphosphate
dCTP deoxycytidine triphosphate
dGTP deoxyguanosine triphosphate
dTMP deoxythymidine monophosphate
dTTP deoxythymidine triphosphate
EBOV Ebola virus
EBV Epstein-Barr virus
EUA Emergency Use Authorization
FDA US Food and Drug Administration
GI gastrointestinal
HA hemagglutinin
HAART highly active antiretroviral therapy
H1N1 hemagglutinin type 1 and neuraminidase type 1
HBV hepatitis B virus
HCC hepatocellular carcinoma
HCV hepatitis C virus
HIV human immunodeficiency virus
HSV-1 herpes simplex virus type 1
HSV-2 herpes simplex virus type 2
IC_{50} half-maximal inhibitory concentration
ICTV International Committee on Taxonomy of Viruses
IgG1k human immunoglobulin G1 kappa
IM intramuscular
INSTI integrase strand transfer inhibitor
IV intravenous
JAK Janus-activated kinase
mAbs monoclonal antibodies
MERS-CoV Middle Eastern respiratory syndrome coronavirus
M^{pro} main protease
mRNAs messenger RNAs
NA neuraminidase
NHC N^4-hydroxycytidine
NMDA N-methyl-D-aspartate
NNRTI nonnucleoside reverse transcriptase inhibitor
NRTI nucleoside reverse transcriptase inhibitor
NS nonstructural
Nup153 nucleoporin 153
OAT organic acid transporter
OATP organic anion-transporting polypeptide
OCT2 organic cation transporter 2
PA polymerase acidic protein
PEG-IFN-α pegylated interferon alpha
PFA phosphonoformic acid
P-gp permeability glycoprotein
PI protease inhibitor
PP_i pyrophosphate
Pre-mRNA pre-messenger RNA
QTc corrected QT interval
RDRP RNA-dependent RNA polymerase
RDV-TP remdesivir triphosphate
RMP ribavirin monophosphate
RSV respiratory syncytial virus
RT reverse transcriptase
RTP ribavirin triphosphate
SAR structure-activity relationship
SARS-CoV-2 severe acute respiratory syndrome coronavirus 2
UGT UDP-glucuronyltransferase
VZV varicella-zoster virus

CLINICAL SIGNIFICANCE

Antiviral agents are a heterogeneous group of antimicrobial agents that exhibit various mechanisms of action, such as inhibiting viral enzymes and surface proteins, as well as serving as nucleoside analogues. The medicinal chemistry of these agents predicts characteristics such as potency and tolerability, which are important when clinically selecting antiviral regimens. Various prodrugs such as valacyclovir and valganciclovir used for treatment of human herpesviruses provide clinically significant differences in oral bioavailability and clinical efficacy. For certain viral infections such as hepatitis and human immunodeficiency virus (HIV), preferred therapeutic agents have a structural design and mechanism of action that provides a higher barrier to resistance than other agents. A detailed understanding of these characteristics can help clinicians select optimal, individualized antiviral treatment regimens.

Anthony J. Guarascio, PharmD, BCPS, BCIDP

Introduction

Essentially every living organism on the planet, including animals, insects, bacteria, and plants, can be infected by viruses. Viruses are among the smallest of microscopic infectious agents. Despite their relatively small size, viruses cause substantial diseases, with over 260 viruses known to infect humans.[1] Some viral diseases, such as polio and smallpox, have been recognized for centuries.[2] New viruses, such as Zika virus and severe acute respiratory syndrome coronavirus 2 (SARS-CoV2), continue to emerge and spread in the human population, often spilling over from animal species. Even with the advances in immunizations and antiviral therapies, viruses continue to present an outstanding challenge to human health.

Although viruses are biological entities, it is debated whether viruses are alive. It can be argued that a virus does not qualify as a true life-form, as it cannot move or replicate on its own power. However, when a virus enters a permissive host cell, the infected cell is forced to make new copies of the invading virus, demonstrating a clear reproductive plan. As such, all viruses are obligate intracellular parasites, meaning that they can only reproduce within a cell. A single viral particle, or virion, is equipped with a genome that encodes for the building blocks of new progeny and, depending on the type of virus, various viral proteins that help complete its life cycle. However, viruses are utterly dependent on the host cell to provide the necessary resources (eg, nucleotides, amino acids, carbohydrates) and machinery (eg, ribosomes for protein translation) to produce new viral particles.

Viruses are simple organisms compared to the size and complexity of a human cell, yet viruses are significant causative agents for human disease. As such, viruses represent a major challenge in drug discovery. Antiviral agents typically differ from most other drugs, as they involve inhibition of unique viral enzymes or processes that are particular to a certain virus, in contrast to modulation of a human receptor or enzyme. In addition, viruses excel at adaptation. Resistance to existing therapies often develops over time. Thus, the discovery of new antiviral agents is a critical ongoing effort in medicinal chemistry.

Virus Structure and Classification

Viruses are remarkably diverse in terms of size, structure, genome organization, and host range, but they do share key features. Since all viruses exist as obligate cellular parasites, they do not need to possess the complex biochemical machinery that is characteristic of higher organisms. However, they do have a defined macromolecular structure that is designed to protect them from the environment and facilitate their entry into cells. The basic subunit of a virus is its genome, which is composed of either DNA or RNA. The genome is shielded from the environment by a protective protein coat called a capsid. The combination of the nucleic acid core and the capsid is termed the nucleocapsid, and in some cases, this comprises the entire virus. In other cases, the nucleocapsid is surrounded by a lipid-containing membrane, or an envelope, that the virus acquires by budding through the host cell membrane.

Viral taxonomy is complex, and viruses are classified according to a number of factors, including morphology of the capsid (icosahedral, helical, or complex), the type of genome (eg, DNA vs RNA, single-stranded vs double-stranded, positive vs negative sense), the presence or absence of an envelope (enveloped vs nonenveloped or naked), and replication strategy. Today, virus taxonomy is defined by the genetic and protein sequences of the virus, which is standardized and updated by the International Committee on Taxonomy of Viruses (ICTV).[3] Viruses are separated into major groups called families, with names that end in the suffix *-viridae*, and then into genera that end in *-virus*. For instance, variola virus, which causes smallpox, is in the family *Poxviridae*, and in the genus *Orthopoxvirus*. Aside from the scientific classification, some viruses are known by more common names that reflect the disease state that they cause (eg, SARS-CoV2) or the geographic locale where they were first identified (ie, West Nile virus, Zika virus), although this naming practice is no longer applied to new viruses due to the stigma associated with naming a pathogen after a place.[4]

Infectious Cycle

The ultimate goal of any virus is to produce new copies of itself. Since viruses lack the machinery to generate new viral particles, the production of new viruses can only occur within a host cell. The infectious cycle is the process by which a virus enters a cell, produces new viral genomes and proteins, and ultimately assembles and releases new viral particles. These newly made viral particles are then free to infect other cells and continue the cycle of infection. Unlike cell division seen with human or bacterial cells, where one cell divides into two daughter cells, one virus can produce hundreds or even thousands of new progeny from a single infectious cycle. Although the infectious cycle of each virus is unique, there are eight general steps that all viruses must complete. These steps are described in Table 33.1 and exemplified using an enveloped virus in Figure 33.1. Importantly, antiviral agents have been designed to interfere with many of these steps, depending on the virus.

Attachment, Entry, and Uncoating

To initiate the infectious cycle, the virus must enter the host cell, but it is too large to simply diffuse across the plasma membrane of the cell. The first step in the infectious cycle occurs when the virus binds to the surface of the target cell. This process is known as attachment (step 1). A virus cannot attach randomly to any cell it may encounter. Rather, attachment is a specific process that is mediated by interactions between an attachment or "spike" protein on the surface of the virus and one or more receptors on the plasma membrane of the host cell. The attachment step is important for determining the tropism, or host range, of the virus. For instance, HIV first attaches to a cellular protein called CD4, which is expressed on $CD4^+$ helper T cells. The specificity

Table 33.1 Steps in the Viral Infectious Cycle

	Step	Characteristics
1	Attachment	Specific binding between proteins on the surface of the viral particle and host cell surface receptors
2	Entry	Viral particle crosses the cell membrane to enter the host cell. For enveloped viruses, entry occurs by fusion of the viral envelope with a host cell membrane. For nonenveloped viruses, entry occurs by penetration (eg, endocytosis)
3	Uncoating and genome release	Viral genome and associated proteins are released into the host cell
4	Transcription of viral RNAs	Depends on the type of viral genome. For positive-sense RNA viruses, the genome is translated directly into viral proteins without further modification. For DNA viruses and other RNA viruses, the genome must be transcribed into positive-sense RNA to be used as viral mRNAs
5	Translation of viral proteins	Viral RNAs are translated into proteins by host cell ribosomes
6	Genome replication	Synthesis of the appropriate viral DNA or RNA
7	Assembly/ maturation	New viral particles are assembled, and the viral genome is packaged within the particle. Many viruses then undergo maturation to further process the viral proteins and become infectious
8	Egress	Release of the new viral particle from the host cell. For enveloped viruses, egress will include budding and release from a cellular membrane. For nonenveloped viruses, egress may include lysis of the host cell or exit via cellular pathways (eg, microvesicles)

of HIV for CD4 leads to infection and destruction of helper T cells in the body, ultimately causing immunosuppression.

Once the virus has physically bound to the cell surface, it must use an entry mechanism to get inside of the cell (step 2). Many factors contribute to entry mechanisms with the presence or absence of a viral envelope playing a key role. For enveloped viruses, the envelope can directly fuse with the plasma membrane of the cell, or the virus may be taken up by receptor-mediated endocytosis, where the envelope ultimately fuses at the endosomal membrane. For nonenveloped viruses, the particle is typically endocytosed into the cell after binding to its cellular receptor. Either during or following entry, an uncoating step releases the nucleocapsid or viral genome into the cell, thereby allowing the genome to be transported to the cellular compartment where transcription and replication will occur (step 3).

Gene Expression and Replication

Once released safely into a host cell, the viral genome serves two purposes: (1) to encode for viral proteins (steps 4 and 5) and (2) to serve as a template for replicating new copies of the genome (step 6). The strategies used to accomplish these steps vary widely among the viruses, and the type of genome (ie, DNA vs RNA) dictates the steps that must be followed. However, for all viruses, the viral genes must be expressed as messenger RNAs (mRNAs) to be translated into viral proteins.[5] Later on, we describe the steps for viral gene expression and

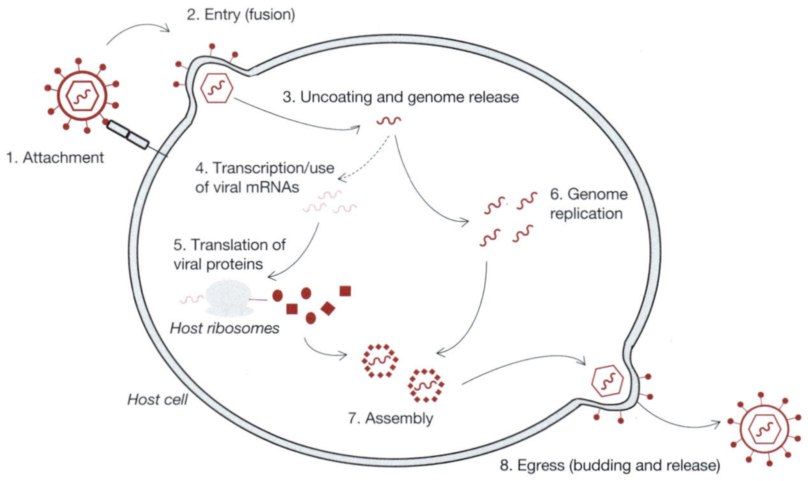

Figure 33.1 Example of the infectious cycle for an enveloped virus.

genome replication based on the type of genome (ie, double-stranded DNA, single-stranded RNA) that the virus carries.

Most DNA viruses (ie, human papillomavirus, herpesviruses) contain double-stranded DNA as their genome, similar to the DNA of host cells.[6] Thus, DNA viruses often use host cell machinery to produce mRNA directly. The transcription of viral genes is tightly timed once the virus has entered the cell. Early viral genes are expressed first and encode for factors needed for genome replication and for commandeering functions of the host cell. Late genes are then expressed, which encode for structural proteins (ie, capsids, surface glycoproteins) that are used to build the complete viral particle. Most double-stranded DNA viruses replicate in the host nucleus and thus use transcriptional enzymes of the host (ie, DNA-dependent RNA polymerase) to synthesize mRNA. This mRNA is then translated to form viral proteins, including enzymes (eg, DNA-dependent DNA polymerase) used to produce copies of the DNA genome. Although single-stranded DNA viruses are abundant in the environment, they are less commonly associated with human disease. However, as modern sequencing approaches are applied to virus identification, new single-stranded DNA viruses have been discovered that may prove to be significant in human disease.[7]

Compared to the DNA viruses, RNA viruses have evolved a wide variety of replication strategies. The single-stranded RNA viruses can be divided into three groups based on their genomes and replication strategies: positive-sense RNA viruses, negative-sense RNA viruses, and retroviruses. In all three groups, the RNA genome must serve two functions: to encode for viral proteins and to be copied into RNA genomes for new virus particles. RNA viruses (ie, Dengue virus, SARS-CoV2) that have genomes capable of directly being used as mRNA are by convention termed as positive-sense RNA viruses. In most cases, the positive-sense RNA genome binds to the host ribosome shortly after entering the cell, where it is translated and used to produce a single polypeptide called the polyprotein. The polyprotein is then cleaved by autocatalysis and proteases to separate the required viral proteins. Following the initial translation of the positive-sense strand, it serves as a template for the synthesis of a negative-sense strand via a viral RNA-dependent RNA polymerase (RDRP). This negative-sense RNA strand can then be transcribed by RDRP to produce additional positive-sense RNA strands that serve as mRNA transcripts and as genomes for new viruses. Because cells do not possess RDRP, this enzyme represents a unique target for antiviral therapy.

Negative-sense RNA viruses (ie, influenza virus, measles virus) carry a single-stranded RNA genome that is in the opposite orientation of mRNA transcripts. As such, it cannot be directly translated at host ribosomes, but must first be converted to a positive-sense form. All negative-sense RNA viruses package RDRP in the viral particle so that the genome can be quickly transcribed to viral mRNA transcripts upon entry into the cell. Unlike the positive-sense RNA viruses, viral mRNA is not translated into polyproteins, and thus viral proteases are not required. Ultimately, the RDRP produces a full-length positive-sense RNA strand that is complimentary to the genome, which is then used as a template to make multiple copies of the negative-sense viral genome. The new viral genomes and proteins can then be assembled to form a new infectious viral particle.

The third group of RNA viruses is known as retroviruses and includes HIV. The HIV particle includes two copies of a positive-sense RNA genome. This RNA genome serves as a template for the formation of double-stranded viral DNA. Host cells do not have an enzyme that can transcribe DNA from an RNA template. Thus, HIV carries reverse transcriptase (RT) to mediate the transcription of viral DNA from the RNA genome. The resulting double-stranded DNA is translocated to the nucleus, where the viral integrase enzyme incorporates the genome-length viral DNA into the host genome. The viral genome can remain latent for long periods, but it can also be expressed to make progeny viral RNAs, a process that is catalyzed by host RNA polymerase II. The transcription of viral RNAs from the integrated genome ultimately leads to the production of the building blocks for new viral particles.

Assembly and Egress

Once the new viral proteins and genomes have been synthesized, viral particles can be built in the assembly step (step 7). The new viral genome is packaged into the protective capsid along with any viral enzymes necessary for replication in the next infectious cycle. Depending on the virus, the newly assembled viral particle may also undergo a maturation step to process and arrange the viral proteins in a final, infectious form. The assembly reaction is often tied to the egress of the virus from the host cell (step 8). Nonenveloped viruses (ie, polyomaviruses, rhinoviruses) complete their maturation by assembling into their corresponding viral particles within the cell nucleus or cytoplasm. In most cases, death of the host cell is required to release the new viral particles.[8] For enveloped viruses (ie, negative-sense RNA viruses), the new viral particles must capture a piece of the host cell membrane when exiting the cell. The viral attachment proteins and glycoproteins contain signal sequences that cause them to be inserted into the host cell membrane. Viral matrix proteins align on the inner surface of the host cell membrane through interactions with the attachment proteins. The nucleocapsid then binds to the matrix proteins on the inner surface of the membrane, with the matrix proteins acting as a bridge between the envelope and the nucleocapsid. The matrix proteins are also the driving force in the budding process, where the new viral particle exits the cell and acquires the lipid envelope. Viral budding can have a variety of effects on the host cell, ranging from destruction of the cell to minimal noncytolytic effects. Step 8 in Figure 33.1 shows the budding of an enveloped virus, with minimal damage to the host cell.

Viral Pathogenesis

Clinical disease develops through a complex series of events that varies between viruses and individual patients, and a complete discussion of viral pathogenesis is beyond the scope of this chapter. However, in general, the symptoms of a viral infection arise from cell death or damage by the virus and/or from the effects of the immune response against the infection (immunopathology). When new viruses are produced, the host cellular metabolism may be completely directed to the production of viral products, resulting in impaired function or even destruction of the cell. Some symptoms of infection, such as malaise and anorexia, are due to the natural immune response. The sequelae of the infection may linger even after the infection is resolved if cell types that do not regenerate effectively (eg, neurons) are damaged. The range of these responses may be either local or systemic, depending on the tropism of the virus, the vulnerability of the host cells, and the extent of the immune response.

Ultimately, the outcomes for the host can include succumbing to the infection, developing a chronic or latent infection, or recovery. In chronic infections, the virus can be continuously detected at low levels, and either mild or no clinical symptoms may present (eg, hepatitis C virus [HCV]). Latent infections are those in which the virus persists for extended periods of time in an inactive form (eg, herpesviruses). Intermittent flare-ups of clinical disease can occur, during which time infectious virus can be detected. Subclinical infections are those that give no overt sign of their presence. Humoral and cell-mediated immunity, interferon and other cytokines, and other host defense factors are common mediators of recovery and begin to develop very soon after infection. Information regarding specific viral infections is provided throughout this chapter.

General Concepts in the Development of Antiviral Drugs

The strategy involved in the design of antiviral drugs is similar to that used in the design of antibacterial, antifungal, and antiparasitic drugs. Specifically, the development of antiviral drugs is focused on identifying inhibitors of enzymes or processes that are vital to viral particles and not present in human cells. In some cases, viral particles contain a target enzyme that is similar to a human enzyme; however, in these situations, there is sufficient difference between the human and viral isoforms to provide selectivity. By focusing on viral-specific enzymes or processes, these drugs avoid interfering with required human enzymatic pathways and avoid specific types of toxicity. Unfortunately, by focusing on viral-specific pathways, it is possible for the virus to develop resistance.[9,10] The continuing identification of new targets for antiviral agents provides new avenues for the discovery of small-molecule therapies. The drugs discussed in this chapter can be generally placed into one of five different categories, as follows:

1. Drugs that disrupt the entry of viral particles into human cells.
2. Drugs that mimic normal purine or pyrimidine nucleosides or nucleotides.
3. Drugs that inhibit viral transcription by mechanisms different than nucleoside and nucleotide mimics.
4. Drugs that interfere with the processing of viral proteins and the assembly of viral particles.
5. Drugs that prevent the release of newly formed viral particles from cell surface membranes.

Structural Analogues of Purines and Pyrimidine

Structural analogues of naturally occurring purines and pyrimidines are primarily used to treat viral infections and specific types of cancer; however, they can also be used to treat fungal and parasitic infections.[11-13] These structural analogues can also be referred to as antimetabolites. Prior to the discussion of the drugs used to treat specific viral infections, it is important to review three key concepts: (1) the differences between nucleosides and nucleotides, (2) the general mechanisms of DNA and RNA polymerases, and (3) the general types of chemical alterations that are made to normal purines and pyrimidines.

Nucleosides are composed of a nitrogenous base and a sugar molecule. Naturally occurring bases are either adenine, guanine, cytosine, uracil, or thymine, and the sugar molecule is either ribose or deoxyribose. Nucleotides are similar to nucleosides but also contain one, two, or three phosphate molecules. Examples of nucleosides and nucleotides are shown in Figure 33.2 with adenosine and cytidine monophosphate. As shown in these two examples, nucleotides are much more water soluble than nucleosides due to the presence of ionizable phosphate functional groups. While both nucleosides and nucleotides contain sufficient water solubility to dissolve in aqueous environments, nucleotides lack the required lipid solubility to adequately traverse the gastrointestinal (GI) membrane. As a result, most purine and pyrimidine analogues are marketed as either their nucleosides or as an esterified nucleotide to allow for a better lipid/water balance and a better oral absorption. A more thorough explanation for the need of a balance between lipid and water solubility can be found in Chapter 2 or other resources.[14]

While nucleosides or esterified nucleotides are preferred over the ionized nucleotides for oral administration, it should be noted that in order for these drugs to be active, they must be converted to their respective nucleotides. Thus, all antiviral drugs that are structural analogues of the natural purines or pyrimidines are prodrugs that must be activated by phosphorylation, hydrolysis, and/or other metabolic pathways prior to exerting their activity. This is because the enzymes that they inhibit require all three structural features (nitrogenous base, sugar, and phosphates) in order to meet their binding requirements.[11-13] As will be discussed in this chapter, some drugs are active at the monophosphate level,

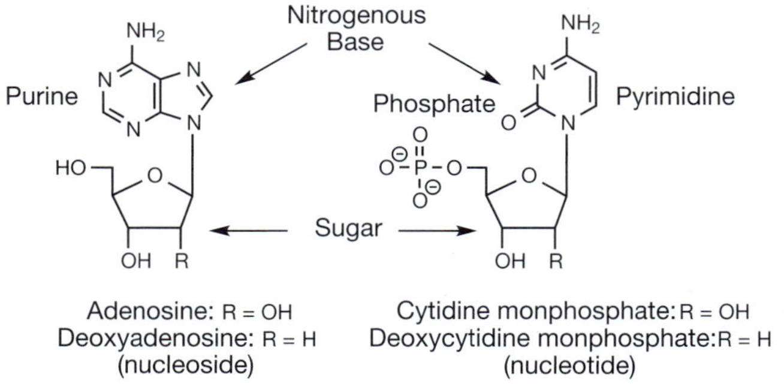

Figure 33.2 Examples of nucleosides and nucleotides.

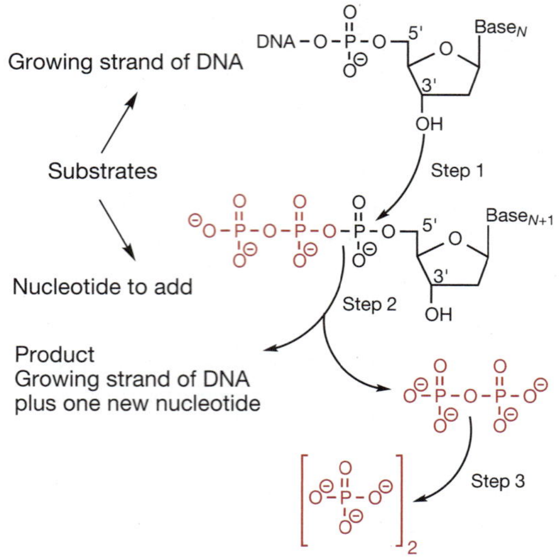

Figure 33.3 General mechanism of DNA and RNA polymerases. The role of pyrophosphate is highlighted in red.

while others are active at the triphosphate level. In order for a purine or pyrimidine analogue to be incorporated into DNA or RNA, it must be converted to its respective triphosphate. DNA and RNA polymerase enzymes add nucleoside triphosphates to growing DNA or RNA strands and contain specific binding regions for the nucleic acid base, the sugar, and the triphosphate. A general overview of this mechanism is shown in Figure 33.3.[15] In this mechanism, the terminal 3′-OH group of growing DNA or RNA strand is involved in a nucleophilic attack on the innermost phosphate group of the nucleotide that is to be added (step 1). This forms a link between the newly added nucleotide and the growing DNA or RNA strand and releases a molecule of pyrophosphate (PP_i) (step 2). The released PP_i is important in this reaction because its subsequent hydrolysis to two inorganic phosphate molecules releases energy that drives the reaction in the forward direction (step 3). In evaluating this mechanism, it should be easy to see that nucleoside triphosphates are required. One of the phosphate groups is required to serve as a bridge between other nucleotides, and the other two are required to form PP_i and participate in an essential hydrolysis. It should also be noted that DNA and RNA are polymers and that it is essential for the sugars to have a 3′-OH and a 5′-OH group to link the nucleotides.

In order to convert a naturally occurring purine or pyrimidine nucleotide into an enzyme inhibitor, alterations are primarily made in either the nitrogenous bases or in the sugars. The general strategy is to alter either the electronics or the steric factors in the nucleotides, such that these analogues are able to bind to their target enzymes and then cause disruption of their normal function. These alterations are usually seen in the purine and pyrimidine bases or the ribose and deoxyribose sugars. Alteration of the phosphate bonds that link the nucleotides is rare but can occur. The individual alterations will be discussed with each drug and/or drug class; however, there are specific strategies that are repeated using a variety of structural modifications.

Herpesviruses

Herpesviruses are a family of enveloped, double-stranded DNA viruses with over 100 species identified.[16] Of these, there are eight herpesviruses that infect humans (Table 33.2). Herpesviruses are responsible for many common diseases, although many infections are subclinical. A key feature of herpesviruses is the ability to induce life-long latent infections after an initial acute phase of infection. The latent state allows for the virus to persist in a host with the potential for

Table 33.2 Herpesviruses of Humans

Number	Common Name and Abbreviation	Disease States
Human herpesvirus 1	Herpes simplex virus type 1 (HSV-1)	Oral and genital herpes, encephalitis, congenital infections
Human herpesvirus 2	Herpes simplex virus type 2 (HSV-2)	Genital herpes (predominately), oral herpes, encephalitis, congenital infections
Human herpesvirus 3	Varicella-zoster virus (VZV)	Chicken pox, shingles, postherpetic neuralgia
Human herpesvirus 4	Epstein-Barr virus (EBV)	Mononucleosis, Burkitt lymphoma, risk factor for multiple sclerosis
Human herpesvirus 5	Cytomegalovirus (CMV)	Esophageal, respiratory, and hepatic infections; retinitis; congenital infections
Human herpesvirus 6A and 6B	HHV-6A and HHV-6B	Exanthema subitum (roseola infantum, sixth disease)
Human herpesvirus 7	HHV-7	Exanthema subitum (roseola infantum, sixth disease)
Human herpesvirus 8	Kaposi sarcoma–associated herpesvirus (KSHV)	Kaposi sarcoma, multicentric Castleman disease, primary effusion lymphoma

reactivation of viral replication and disease when the host experiences stress or impaired immunity. As such, patients who are immunocompromised are at particular risk of complications from herpesvirus infections.

Herpesviruses are large viruses encoding from 80 to 200 proteins, which offers many potential targets for antiviral therapy.[17] At the time of this publication, antiviral agents are available for four of the eight herpesviruses. Here, we introduce the salient features for each of the herpesviruses that can be treated with antiviral drugs, with the remaining human herpesviruses addressed in Table 33.2.[18,19]

Herpes Simplex Viruses

Herpes simplex virus types 1 and 2 (HSV-1 and HSV-2, respectively) are common infections with 70% to 90% seropositivity to HSV-1 and 15% to 20% seropositivity to HSV-2 in adults, although many infections are subclinical.[20] Herpes labialis (cold sores) and genital herpes infections are most often caused by HSV-1 and HSV-2, respectively. However, an increasing number of genital herpes infections are caused by HSV-1. HSV-1 infections typically occur earlier in life and can be passed by close contact with infected skin, such as a parent kissing a child. HSV-2 infections are spread mostly through sexual contact. These viruses initially infect epithelial cells in the skin, causing painful blisters or sores typical of HSV infections. Latency is then established in the ganglia of nerves that innervate the site of the primary infection. The virus can be reactivated by a number of factors, including emotional stress, ultraviolet light, and hormonal changes. Upon reactivation, new viral particles are produced, allowing for release of the virus from the neuron and reinfection of epithelial cells. Viral shedding may or may not be associated with a recurrence of skin lesions, and as such, asymptomatic transmission is feasible. Although there is no cure for HSV-1 or HSV-2, treatment of active infections can reduce the duration of symptoms and reduce recurrence.

HSV-1 and HSV-2 are also important causes of congenital infections. HSV-1 can be transmitted to newborns during delivery or from family members or caregivers who are shedding virus, whereas HSV-2 is usually transmitted during delivery. In neonates, these viruses are often more invasive than in older hosts and are associated with severe infections, including ocular infections, encephalitis, and visceral infections (eg, lungs and liver).[21] Although HSV causes significant illness and mortality in newborns, treatment of neonatal HSV infections is associated with improved survival and prognosis.

Varicella-Zoster Virus

Varicella-zoster virus (VZV) is a highly contagious herpesvirus that was ubiquitous in the pre-vaccine era. Today, effective vaccines are available for children or seronegative adults to prevent primary infection and chicken pox and for adults with prior VZV infection to prevent shingles and postherpetic neuralgia. Transmission of VZV typically occurs through respiratory droplets or direct contact with skin lesions caused by the virus. Primary VZV infection results in chicken pox, which is characterized by a diffuse, blister-like rash and is typically acquired in childhood. Although chicken pox is usually benign, rare but serious complications, including pneumonia and encephalitis, can occur.

As the primary infection resolves, VZV establishes latency in the spinal ganglia, where it remains for the life of the host. In many individuals, the virus remains quiescent, and disease does not recur. However, if VZV exits latency and reactivates, shingles (herpes zoster) results, which is characterized by a painful rash along the skin that is innervated by the infected neuron. Postherpetic neuralgia may follow the rash, where pain persists after the skin has healed due to damage to the neurons. Shingles is most common in older adults because the immune memory to VZV wanes over time. However, immunosuppression (eg, HIV infection, immunosuppressive therapy) or even stress can permit reactivation of VZV. Antiviral therapy can be used to reduce the duration of shingles outbreaks and to treat the more serious complications of chicken pox.

Cytomegalovirus

Cytomegalovirus (CMV) is a common herpesvirus across the globe. In the United States, CMV seroprevalence is estimated to be between 60% and 70%, with higher estimates in many lower-income countries.[22] Transmission can occur across the placenta or during delivery to newborns, via saliva or urine, or by sexual contact. Most CMV infections are robustly controlled by the immune system and are asymptomatic. After the primary infection resolves, CMV establishes latency in hematopoietic progenitor cells in the bone marrow, where the viral genome is maintained as the cells mature into monocytes and dendritic cells.[23] Although latency is life-long, most healthy patients do not experience reactivation during their lifetime.

While CMV infections are mostly subclinical, they can cause severe disease in newborns and patients who are immunocompromised.[24] CMV is the most common congenital infection in the United States, affecting 1 in 200 births.[25] The infection is a leading cause of birth defects and is associated with low birth weight, hearing loss, intellectual and developmental impairments, and retinitis. Hosts who are immunocompromised (eg, patients with HIV, solid organ transplant and hematopoietic cell transplant recipients) are susceptible to disease from reactivation of the virus. CMV infection is disseminated in patients who are immunosuppressed, leading to GI disease, pneumonia, and retinitis.[25] There are a number of antiviral drugs available to treat and/or control CMV infection for both newborns and patients who are immunocompromised.

Antiviral Drugs to Treat Herpes Viral Infections

Acyclovir and Valacyclovir

Acyclovir (Fig. 33.4) is a synthetic analogue of deoxyguanosine in which the deoxyribose sugar is replaced with an acyclic chain. The acyclic chain can overlap with either ribose or deoxyribose, but it lacks the 2′ and 3′ carbon atoms and most importantly, the 3′-OH group. Valacyclovir (Fig. 33.4)

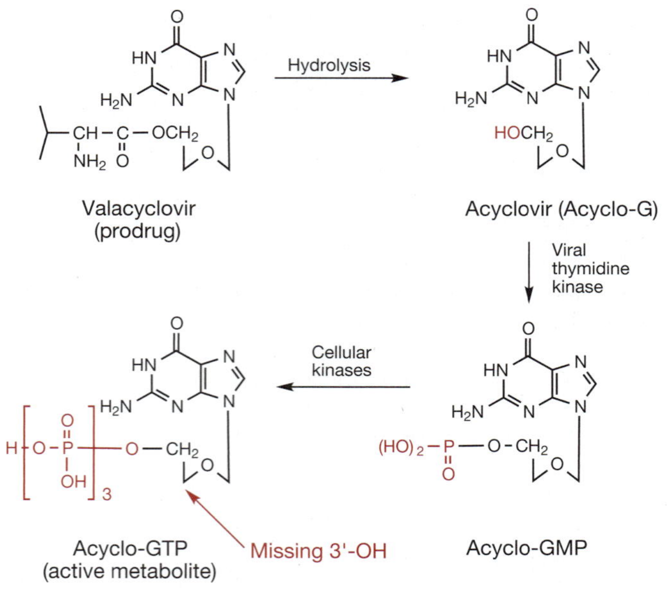

Figure 33.4 Conversion of valacyclovir and acyclovir to their active metabolite.

is a prodrug of acyclovir in which the surrogate 5′-OH group is esterified with a valine amino acid.[26] Both drugs are approved for the treatment of viral infections caused by HSV, CMV, and VZV.[27,28]

Mechanism of Action

Acyclovir and valacyclovir have the same mechanism of action in treating susceptible viral infections since the oral administration of valacyclovir produces acyclovir via the hydrolysis of the valine ester. As shown in Figure 33.4, acyclovir is initially converted to acyclo-guanosine monophosphate (acyclo-GMP) by viral thymidine kinase once it has entered the viral particle.[29-31] This phosphorylation reaction occurs faster within cells infected by HSV and other viruses than in normal human cells because acyclovir is a poor substrate for the normal human cell thymidine kinase. Acyclovir is further converted to acyclo-guanosine diphosphate (acyclo-GDP) and acyclo-guanosine triphosphate (acyclo-GTP) by a normal cellular enzyme called guanosine monophosphate kinase. The viral DNA polymerase is competitively inhibited by acyclo-GTP with a lower half-maximal inhibitory concentration (IC_{50}) than that for cellular DNA polymerase. Once acyclo-GTP is incorporated into the viral DNA strand, further elongation of the DNA chain is immediately terminated due to the lack of a 3′-OH group. As shown in Figure 33.3, DNA and RNA polymerase enzymes require the presence of a 3′-OH group to act as a nucleophile in the subsequent reaction.

The selectivity of acyclovir for HSV-infected cells as compared to uninfected cells is due to both activation by HSV thymidine kinase and a preferential uptake of acyclovir by herpes-infected cells as compared to uninfected cells. These effects result in a higher concentration of acyclo-GTP in the viral particle and a high therapeutic index between HSV-infected cells as compared to normal cells. Acyclovir significantly reduces DNA synthesis in virus-infected cells without significantly disturbing the active replication of uninfected cells.[29-31]

Resistance to acyclovir can occur due to mutations of the viral-encoded thymidine kinase that fail to effectively convert acyclovir to acyclo-GMP. Resistance rarely develops in patients who are immunocompetent, and almost all acyclovir-resistant viral infections are seen in patients who are immunocompromised. Since valacyclovir is a prodrug of acyclovir; patients resistant to acyclovir will also be resistant to valacyclovir.[27,32]

Common Adverse Effects and Drug Interactions

Acyclovir and valacyclovir are generally well tolerated, and adverse effects are dependent on the route of administration. Valacyclovir is administered orally, while acyclovir can be administered orally, intravenously, and topically. The most common adverse effects seen with oral administration are GI effects, headache, and malaise. The intravenous (IV) administration of acyclovir can cause phlebitis, inflammation at the infusion site, and reversible renal impairment. Additional adverse effects seen with the IV administration of acyclovir include myalgia, rash, and central nervous system (CNS) effects. Application-site reactions can occur with topical acyclovir. Drug interactions are uncommon.[27,28]

Receptor Binding and Structure-Activity Relationship

The active metabolite of both acyclovir and valacyclovir is acyclo-GTP (see Fig. 33.4). This antimetabolite mimics the naturally occurring deoxyguanosine triphosphate (dGTP) and is able to bind to the viral DNA polymerase in a similar fashion as dGTP. The presence of the 5′-triphosphate allows acyclo-GTP to be incorporated into the growing viral DNA strand; however, the absence of a 3′-OH group causes chain termination. Thus, in evaluating the structure of acyclo-GMP, there are three key structural features that allow it to bind and inhibit viral DNA polymerase: (a) a guanidine base that is recognized by the polymerase, (b) a 5′-triphosphate that allows it to initially act as a substrate for the polymerase, and (c) a lack of a 3′-OH group that prevents further polymerization.

Physicochemical and Pharmacokinetic Properties

Acyclovir is a weak base due to the presence of the substituted purine ring. The bioavailability of acyclovir is 15% to 30%, and its plasma protein binding ranges from 9% to 33%. Approximately 70% is excreted unchanged in the urine by both glomerular filtration and tubular secretion, and approximately 15% is metabolized through oxidation to an inactive metabolite, 9-carboxymethoxymethylguanine. The half-life of acyclovir is approximately 3 hours in patients with normal renal function. In an individual with renal diseases, the half-life of the drug is prolonged. Therefore, acyclovir dosage adjustment is necessary for patients with renal impairment.

Valacyclovir is an amino acid ester prodrug of acyclovir and is more basic than acyclovir due to the presence of the primary amine. The oral bioavailability of valaciclovir is considerably greater than that of oral acyclovir. As previously mentioned, it is rapidly converted to acyclovir and thus has similar pharmacokinetic parameters.[26,28,33]

Famciclovir and Penciclovir

Famciclovir and penciclovir (Fig. 33.5) are similar to acyclovir in structure, mechanism of action, therapeutic use, and physicochemical and pharmacokinetic properties. Famciclovir is an orally available prodrug of penciclovir and is indicated to treat viral infections caused by HSV, herpes labialis, and herpes zoster. It is also used off-label to treat VZV in patients with HIV. Penciclovir is used topically to treat herpes labialis.[28,34]

Mechanism of Action

The mechanism of action of famciclovir and penciclovir mirrors the mechanism of action of acyclovir with a few differences. Once administered, famciclovir undergoes two metabolic processes, hydrolysis of the two acetyl ester groups and oxidation of the C_6 carbon atom, to form penciclovir, a deoxyguanosine analogue. Similar to acyclovir, penciclovir is initially, and selectively, phosphorylated by viral thymidine kinase to produce penciclovir monophosphate. The human enzyme, guanosine monophosphate kinase, then converts it to penciclovir triphosphate. Penciclovir triphosphate is then incorporated into the viral DNA and causes immediate chain termination of the DNA strand. As shown in Figure 33.5, the structure of penciclovir contains a surrogate 3′-OH group; however, due to the flexibility of the alicyclic chain, it is unable to efficiently reside in the proper location in the viral polymerase enzyme. This prevents it from efficiently reacting with subsequent nucleotides resulting in the inhibition of further chain elongation.[34]

Resistance to penciclovir is identical to that seen in acyclovir. Thus, patients with mutations of the viral-encoded thymidine kinase will be unable to effectively activate penciclovir.

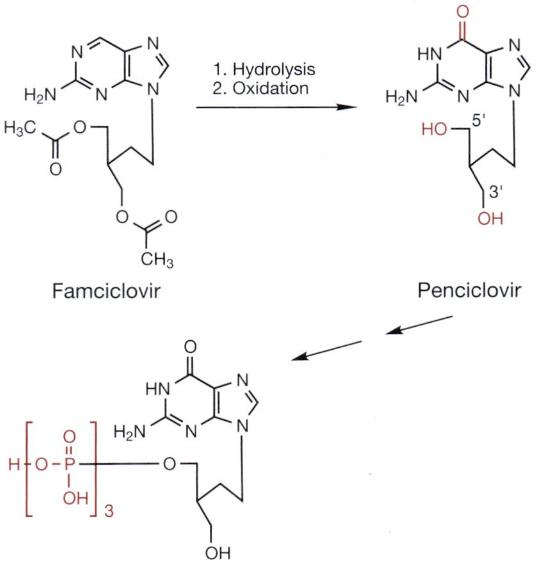

Figure 33.5 Metabolic activation of famciclovir and penciclovir.

Common Adverse Effects and Drug Interactions

Famciclovir is generally well tolerated with nausea, headache, diarrhea, and dysmenorrhea being the most common adverse effects. More serious adverse effects include thrombocytopenia, confusion, hallucinations, and nephrotoxicity. The topical application of penciclovir can cause mild erythema in about 50% of patients and headache in about 5% of patients. Drug interactions are uncommon for these two drugs.[27,28]

Receptor Binding and Structure-Activity Relationship

Similar to acyclo-GTP, penciclovir triphosphate structurally mimics dGTP and is able to bind to the viral DNA polymerase. The structure of penciclovir contains the three key structural features discussed for acyclovir: (a) a guanidine base, (b) a 5′-triphosphate, and (c) the lack of an available 3′-OH group. The main difference between acyclo-GTP and penciclovir is that acyclo-GTP lacks a 3′-OH group, while penciclovir does have a surrogate 3′-OH group. While this surrogate 3′-OH group could, in theory, link to a subsequent nucleotide, the flexibility of the alicyclic chain prevents any significant interactions.

Physicochemical and Pharmacokinetic Properties

Famciclovir and penciclovir are weak bases due to the presence of the substituted purine ring. The bioavailability of famciclovir is 77%, and its plasma protein binding is less than 20%. Famciclovir is rapidly metabolized to penciclovir by pathways that don't involve CYP450 enzymes. It is eliminated primarily in the urine (73%) with the remainder in the feces (23%). The half-life of famciclovir ranges from 2 to 4 hours. Similar to acyclovir and valacyclovir, its half-life is prolonged in patients with renal impairment.[26,28]

Trifluridine

Trifluridine is a synthetic analogue of deoxythymidine in which the methyl group at the C_5 position has been replaced with trifluoromethyl functional group. Trifluridine is used ophthalmically to treat herpes simplex keratitis. It is also used in combination with tipiracil for the treatment of metastatic colorectal cancer (see Chapter 36 for a discussion of this combination).[28,35,36]

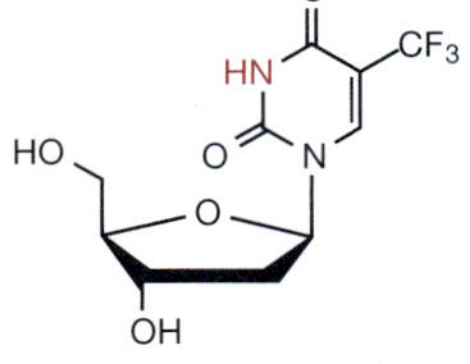

Trifluridine

Mechanism of Action

Within the viral particle, trifluridine is converted to both trifluridine monophosphate and trifluridine triphosphate. Trifluridine monophosphate inhibits thymidylate synthase and decreases the availability of deoxythymidine monophosphate (dTMP) for viral particles and inhibits replication. Trifluridine triphosphate can become incorporated into DNA. The trifluoro functional group is electron-withdrawing and enhances the acidity of the highlighted nitrogen atom. This results in an alteration of normal hydrogen bonding and base pairing. The ultimate effect is production of faulty mRNA and faulty viral proteins and enzymes.[35,36]

Common Adverse Effects and Drug Interactions

Common adverse effects of trifluridine are burning and stinging, which occur when administered ophthalmically, edema of the eyelids, local ocular hypersensitivity reactions, and other ocular effects. There are no known drug interactions for the ophthalmic administration of trifluridine.[28]

Receptor Binding and Structure-Activity Relationship

Trifluridine monophosphate and trifluridine triphosphate mimic dTMP and deoxythymidine triphosphate (dTTP). This structural similarity allows them to bind to the viral forms of thymidylate synthase and DNA polymerase. Trifluridine exhibits some selectivity for viral particles as compared to mammalian cells; however, this selectivity is not enough to allow systemic use for viral infections. The key structure-activity relationship (SAR) for trifluridine is the presence of an electron-withdrawing trifluoromethyl group instead of the normal methyl group present in thymidine. This alteration significantly enhances the acidity of the N_3 hydrogen atom of trifluridine as compared to thymidine ($pK_a = 9.96$). The predicted pK_a value for trifluridine is 7.95, indicating that a significant percentage of N_3 hydrogen atom will be ionized and disrupt base pairing and normal enzyme function.[26,35]

It should be noted that the structure of trifluridine contains a normal deoxyribose sugar, so unlike acyclovir and penciclovir, its mechanism of action does not involve immediate chain termination once it is incorporated into viral DNA.

Physicochemical and Pharmacokinetic Properties

Trifluridine is a weak acid and contains structural features that allow it to have significant water solubility such that it can be formulated in an aqueous solution. Trifluridine has a very short half-life, which necessitates frequent (every 2 hours) applications to treat ophthalmic infections. The major metabolite is a local base-catalyzed conversion of the trifluoromethyl group to a carboxylic acid. This metabolite is also formed in solution at a slightly alkaline pH; therefore, the commercial preparation is marketed as a buffered solution with a pH between 5.5 and 6.[28]

Docosanol

Docosanol (aka, behenyl alcohol) is a saturated C_{22} fatty alcohol that is used topically for the treatment of recurrent herpes simplex labialis infections (ie, cold sores and fever blisters).[26,28]

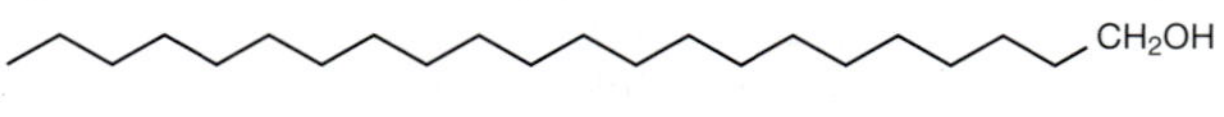

Docosanol (behenyl alcohol)

Mechanism of Action

Docosanol prevents viral entry into target cell by inhibiting the fusion between the human cell plasma membrane and the HSV envelope. This action prevents subsequent viral replication. Because docosanol does not inhibit any specific viral enzyme or protein, resistance to docosanol due to HSV mutations is unlikely.[26,37]

Common Adverse Effects and Drug Interactions

Docosanol is available as a 10% topical cream. It is applied 5 times daily to the lips or the face. Docosanol is generally well tolerated, and adverse effects are limited to application-site reactions. Docosanol should not be applied inside the mouth or in or near the eyes.[38]

Physicochemical and Pharmacokinetic Properties

Docosanol is highly lipid soluble and has a predicated log *P* value of 8.81 and easily penetrates through the layers of the skin. It is primarily oxidized to docosanoic acid, an endogenous component of cell membranes, especially in erythrocytes, brain, nerve myelin sheath, lung, and kidney.[26,38]

Antiviral Drugs to Treat Cytomegalovirus Infections

Ganciclovir and Valganciclovir

Ganciclovir and valganciclovir (Fig. 33.6) are structurally similar to acyclovir and valacyclovir in that valganciclovir is a valyl ester prodrug of ganciclovir, both drugs are synthetic analogues of deoxyguanosine, and both drugs have an acyclic chain instead of a ribose or deoxyribose sugar. Ganciclovir and valganciclovir are also structurally similar to famciclovir and penciclovir in that they contain a surrogate 3′-OH group. Both drugs are approved for the systemic use of CMV infections, and ganciclovir is approved for the topical treatment of herpes keratitis infections.[27,28] The main advantage of valganciclovir is that it can be administered orally, while ganciclovir must be administered IV.

Mechanism of Action

The mechanism of action of ganciclovir is extremely similar to those previously described for acyclovir and penciclovir. Ganciclovir is initially phosphorylated to ganciclovir triphosphate; however, it does not require a virus-specific thymidine

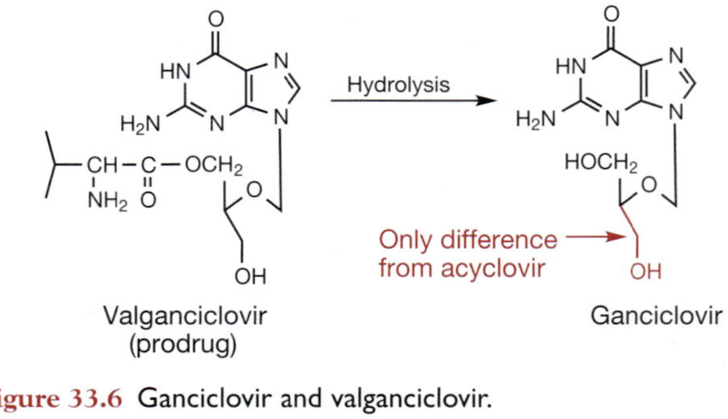

Figure 33.6 Ganciclovir and valganciclovir.

kinase for the initial phosphorylation. Once incorporated into CMV polymerase, it greatly decreases DNA polymerization due to the flexible nature of the acyclic surrogate 3′-OH group and the inability to effectively continue chain elongation. Ganciclovir has a higher affinity for CMV DNA polymerase as compared to human DNA polymerase and shows increased bioactivation in infected versus uninfected cells.[39,40]

Resistance is due to two mechanisms, a decreased phosphorylation to the active triphosphate and mutations in the viral DNA polymerase.

Common Adverse Effects and Drug Interactions

While ganciclovir is similar to acyclovir and penciclovir in terms of structure and mechanism, it is less selective for viral particles and thus can cause more serious adverse effects. The most serious adverse effects are hematologic toxicity, which can manifest as granulocytopenia, neutropenia, anemia, thrombocytopenia, and/or pancytopenia, and impairment of renal function. Other common, less severe adverse effects include anorexia, chills, diarrhea, fever, neuropathy, pruritis, sweating, and vomiting.[28,41]

Ganciclovir and zidovudine interact with one another, leading to a decreased concentration of ganciclovir and an increased concentration of zidovudine. Additionally, both of these drugs have the potential to cause neutropenia and anemia. Probenecid decreases the renal elimination of ganciclovir and increases its plasma concentration. If these two drugs are used in combination, a dosage reduction for ganciclovir may be required.[28,41]

Receptor Binding and Structure-Activity Relationship

Similar to acyclo-GTP and penciclovir triphosphate, ganciclovir triphosphate structurally mimics dGTP and is able to bind to the viral DNA polymerase. The structure of ganciclovir contains the three key structural features previously discussed for dGTP mimics: (a) a guanidine base, (b) a 5′-triphosphate, and (c) the presence of a flexible chain that decreases the availability of the surrogate 3′-OH group to continue DNA synthesis.

Physicochemical and Pharmacokinetic Properties

Ganciclovir is a weak base due to the presence of the substituted purine ring. It is highly water soluble and has poor oral absorption (<10%). Ganciclovir is not plasma protein bound to any significant extent, undergoes minimal metabolism, and is primarily eliminated (~90%) unchanged in the urine through glomerular filtration and active tubular secretion. Ganciclovir must be administered intravenously, and its half-life is 2.5 to 3.6 hours in patients with normal renal function. Dosage adjustments are required for patients with renal impairment.[26,28,41]

Similar to valacyclovir, valganciclovir is an amino acid ester prodrug of ganciclovir and is more basic due to the presence of the primary amine. The oral bioavailability of valganciclovir is approximately 60%, thus allowing for its oral use. It is rapidly converted to ganciclovir and has similar pharmacokinetic parameters.[26,28]

Cidofovir

Cidofovir is a structural analogue of cytidine monophosphate, in which the spacing of the surrogate 3′ and 5′ hydroxyl groups in the alicyclic ring is slightly closer than the alicyclic chains of acyclovir, penciclovir, and ganciclovir. Additionally, the structure of cidofovir contains a phosphonate functional group that is not present in any of the previous nucleotide mimics that have been discussed. Cidofovir is indicated for the treatment of CMV retinitis in patients with acquired immune deficiency syndrome (AIDS). It is also used off-label to treat HSV viral infections that are acyclovir-resistant.[26,28]

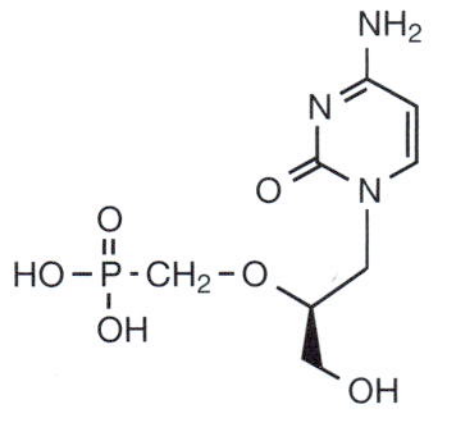

Cidofovir

Mechanism of Action

Cidofovir is phosphorylated to cidofovir diphosphate, a triphosphate analogue of deoxycytidine triphosphate (dCTP), by host cell enzymes. Since this activation occurs without viral nucleoside kinases, it is useful in treating patients who are resistant to ganciclovir and acyclovir. Similar to ganciclovir and the other dGTP analogues previously discussed, cidofovir diphosphate inhibits CMV DNA polymerase enzymes, is incorporated into growing DNA chains, and subsequently reduces the rate of viral DNA synthesis.[26,28,42]

Common Adverse Effects and Drug Interactions

The major toxicity seen with cidofovir is nephrotoxicity. Patients should avoid using other drugs with a nephrotoxic potential (eg, aminoglycosides, amphotericin B) unless therapeutic alternatives are not available. To avoid this adverse effect, cidofovir should be used in combination with probenecid, an organic acid transporter (OAT) inhibitor. Probenecid blocks the active tubular secretion of cidofovir, which decreases nephrotoxicity by decreasing the urine concentration and helps increase the duration of action by slowing its elimination. There are no major drug interactions beyond the beneficial use of OAT inhibitors.[28,43]

Receptor Binding and Structure-Activity Relationship

Cidofovir diphosphate mimics the structure of the naturally occurring dCTP and is competitively incorporated into viral DNA, where it significantly inhibits further polymerization. The structure of cidofovir contains the three key structural features previously discussed for nucleotide mimics: (a) a cytidine base, (b) a surrogate 5′-triphosphate that can be incorporated into viral DNA, and (c) the presence of a flexible chain that decreases the availability of the surrogate 3′-OH group to continue DNA synthesis.

Physicochemical and Pharmacokinetic Properties

The cytosine ring of cidofovir is weakly basic; however, the phosphonate functional group is a strong base that will be primarily ionized in all physiological environments. Cidofovir is highly water soluble, not orally absorbed, and administered intravenously once every 2 weeks. Cidofovir is not bound to plasma protein to any significant extent, and it does not undergo metabolism beyond phosphorylation to its active metabolite. It has a mean half-life elimination of 2.4 to 3.2 hours and is primarily eliminated in the urine.[26,28]

Foscarnet

Foscarnet, also known as phosphonoformic acid (PFA), is a stable analogue of PPi. It is approved for the treatment of CMV retinitis in patients with AIDS and acyclovir-resistant mucocutaneous HSV infection in patients who are immunocompromised.[26,28]

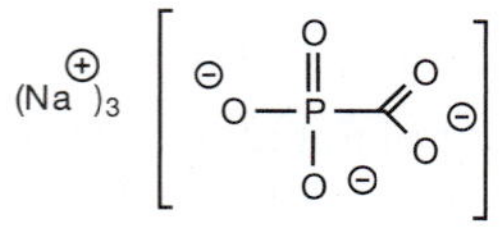

Foscarnet sodium

Mechanism of Action and Receptor Binding

Foscarnet binds to the PPi pocket of virus-specific DNA polymerases and RTs at concentrations that do not affect cellular (ie, human) polymerases. As previously described, DNA and RNA polymerase enzymes contain binding regions for the triphosphate portion of the nucleotide. Foscarnet mimics the terminal PPi that is released in the polymerase reaction, binds to this region in the polymerase binding site, and prevents further elongation (see Fig. 33.3). Unlike ganciclovir and other nucleoside analogues, foscarnet does not require activation by kinase or other enzymes.[44]

Common Adverse Effects and Drug Interactions

The most serious adverse effect that is seen with foscarnet is nephrotoxicity, which occurs in approximately 25% of patients. Other adverse effects include anemia, diarrhea, fever, granulocytopenia, nausea, and vomiting. Additionally, foscarnet can cause hypokalemia, hypocalcemia, hypomagnesemia, and hypophosphatemia. Foscarnet has no drug interactions; however, it should not be used in combination with other nephrotoxic drugs.[28]

Physicochemical and Pharmacokinetic Properties

Foscarnet is an acidic drug that will be ionized at almost all physiological environments. It is highly water soluble and not orally active. It is administered by IV infusion, is not metabolized, and is primarily eliminated through the urine. Its elimination half-life is between 3 and 4 hours.[26,28,44]

Letermovir

Letermovir is structurally unrelated to the nucleotides previously discussed. It is indicated for CMV prophylaxis in hematopoietic cell transplant recipients and kidney transplant recipients and is used both orally and via IV administration.[45]

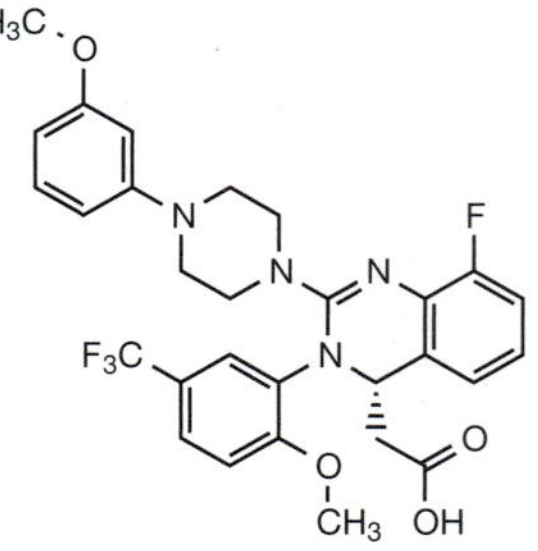

Letermovir

Mechanism of Action

Letermovir inhibits the CMV DNA terminase complex, which is required for viral DNA processing and packaging. Some viruses, including CMV, replicate their genetic material through the formation of concatemers, long continuous DNA strands that contain multiple copies of the same DNA sequence linked in series. By inhibiting the terminase complex, letermovir prevents the production of proper unit length genomes and interferes with virus maturation.[46,47]

Common Adverse Effects and Drug Interactions

The most serious adverse effects seen with letermovir were cardiac abnormalities, specifically fibrillation and tachycardia. Other common adverse effects are abdominal pain, cough, diarrhea, fatigue, headache, nausea, peripheral edema, and vomiting.

Letermovir is a substrate of organic anion-transporting polypeptide (OATP) 1B1/3. Coadministration with drugs that are inhibitors of OATP1B1/3 transporters may result in an increased plasma concentration of letermovir. Letermovir is an inhibitor of OATP1B1/3 transporters and may increase the plasma concentrations of co-administered OATP1B1/3 substrates. Letermovir is a moderate inhibitor of CYP3A and may increase the levels of other drugs that require this isozyme for normal metabolism.[28,45]

Physicochemical and Pharmacokinetic Properties

Letermovir is an acidic drug due to the presence of the carboxylic acid. This functional group will be primarily ionized at physiological pH. Letermovir is highly lipid soluble with a predicted log *P* value of 4.60 and is 99% plasma protein bound. Despite its high lipid solubility, it is primarily eliminated unchanged in the feces. A minor percentage undergoes glucuronide conjugation catalyzed by UDP-glucuronyltransferase (UGT) 1A1/1A3. Its elimination half-life is 12 hours, which allows for once-daily dosing.[26,28,45]

Maribavir

Maribavir bears some structural similarity to purine nucleosides but acts by a mechanism that is different from all of the other drugs used to treat CMV infections. It is indicated for the treatment of adults and pediatric patients with posttransplant CMV infection or a disease that is refractory to treatment with ganciclovir, valganciclovir, cidofovir, or foscarnet.[48,49]

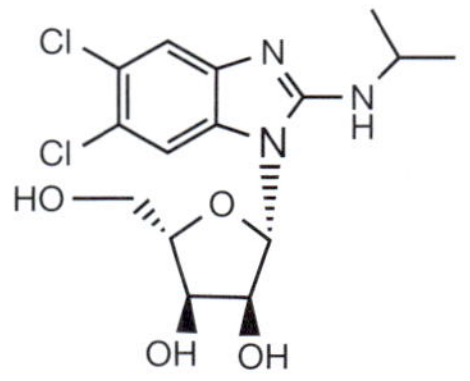

Maribavir

Mechanism of Action

Maribavir is a potent and completive inhibitor of the CMV UL97 protein kinase. Phosphorylation by this kinase is important for several functions that must occur during CMV replication. These include cell-cycle modulation and nuclear egress of newly formed viral particles, a process involving the translocation from the nucleus into the cytoplasm. Thus, inhibition of UL97 kinase provides an antiviral effect unique from ganciclovir, valganciclovir, cidofovir, or foscarnet and can be used in patients who are refractory to these drugs. Despite the fact that maribavir is structurally similar to purine nucleosides, studies have shown that the 5′-triphosphate has no significant effect on the incorporation of deoxynucleoside triphosphates by CMV DNA polymerase.[48,49]

Common Adverse Effects and Drug Interactions

The most common adverse effect seen with maribavir is some form of taste disturbances. Other common effects include diarrhea, fatigue, nausea, and vomiting.

Maribavir will mechanistically decrease the effectiveness of ganciclovir because UL97 kinase mediates the initial phosphorylation required for its conversion to the active ganciclovir triphosphate metabolite. Thus, these two drugs should not be used together. Maribavir is a substrate of CYP3A4, thus drugs that induce or inhibit this isozyme can potentially alter blood concentrations of maribavir. Maribavir is a weak inhibitor of CYP3A4 and an inhibitor of permeability glycoprotein (P-gp) and breast cancer–resistance protein (BCRP). It could potentially cause drug interactions, with other drugs requiring this enzyme and/or these proteins.[28,49]

Physicochemical and Pharmacokinetic Properties

Maribavir is a weakly basic drug due to the presence of the benzimidazole ring and will be primarily unionized at physiological pH. Maribavir is lipid soluble with a predicted log *P* value between 1.84 and 2.15. It is 98% plasma protein bound and is highly metabolized by CYP3A4 (major) and CYP1A2 (minor). Its primary metabolite is an inactive N-dealkylated metabolite. It is administered as an oral tablet, has a half-life of 4.3 hours, and is primarily eliminated in the urine.[26,28,49]

Influenza Viruses

Influenza viruses are significant causes of illness, hospitalization, and mortality in the United States and globally.[50] Major antigenic changes in influenza have led to worldwide epidemics that have resulted in millions of deaths. There are three types of influenza virus that infect humans: Influenza A, B, and C. Influenza A infects humans and other animal species (eg, birds, pigs) and is prone to substantial antigenic shifts due to reassortment or "mixing" of multiple influenza A strains. A good example of this is seen in the emergence of the 2009 hemagglutinin type 1 and neuraminidase type 1 (H1N1) "swine flu." This strain resulted from the reassortment of human, swine, and avian influenza viruses. Since this was a new influenza virus, individuals who were previously infected with influenza had no preexisting immunity to the new strain, allowing for a global pandemic.[51] Influenza B is less prone to major antigenic change but is nevertheless a major contributor to influenza cases and illness each year. Both Influenza A and B infections can induce severe illness and death. As such, current strains of Influenza A and B are included in the annual influenza vaccines. Influenza C causes only a mild illness similar to the common cold and is not included in annual flu vaccines. The remainder of this section will focus on Influenza A and B and the drugs to treat these infections.

Influenza viruses belong to the *Orthomyxoviridae* family, which includes enveloped, negative-sense RNA viruses. The viral envelope includes two viral glycoproteins: hemagglutinin (HA) and neuraminidase (NA). The nomenclature for Influenza A viruses is based upon the subtype of HA and NA (eg, H1N1, H3N2). HA is responsible for attachment to sialic acid on the host cell and for fusion with the cell membrane. HA is the major target of the neutralizing antibody response in the host and as such is the primary antigen in influenza vaccines. HA is subject to mutations in its amino acid sequence, allowing for selection of variants that can escape prior antibody responses and contribute to new outbreaks.[52] NA is best known for facilitating the exit of new viral particles from infected host cells, although NA may also contribute to early stages of the viral infection.[53] NA cleaves sialic acid to facilitate release of the viral particle during budding and removes sialic acid residues from HA to prevent aggregation of the newly made viral particles. Inhibitors of NA are the mainstay of anti-influenza therapy. All influenza viral particles also carry RDRP, which is necessary for transcribing the RNA genome upon entry into a host cell. The influenza RDRP includes an endonuclease domain that can be inhibited by the most recently approved class of anti-influenza agents, thereby offering an additional target for antiviral therapy.

Influenza virus spreads through airborne droplets or contact with contaminated surfaces. Its incubation period is relatively short, and symptoms manifest in 1 to 4 days. Transmission of the virus can occur 24 hours prior to symptom onset and extends for about 3 to 5 days in adults and up to 3 weeks in children.[54] Influenza infection is predominately restricted to the respiratory epithelium, and subsequent damage to the respiratory tract is driven by the replicating virus and the host immune response.[55] Typical symptoms include upper respiratory tract signs (eg, cough, sore throat, rhinitis), myalgia, headache, and fever. In children, GI symptoms (eg, diarrhea, vomiting) are also possible.[56] Antiviral therapy can reduce the duration and severity of influenza infections if administered less than 48 hours after symptom onset. Severe complications of influenza infection, such as pneumonia, secondary bacterial infections, myocarditis, and encephalitis, most often occur in vulnerable populations. Young children (age <5 years); older adults (age >65 years); pregnant patients; and individuals with chronic medical conditions such as diabetes, asthma, and obesity are most susceptible to severe infections.[57] Antiviral therapy is recommended for patients with severe complications regardless of time from symptom onset.[58]

Antiviral Drugs to Treat Influenza Infections

Neuraminidase Inhibitors

NA inhibitors are used to treat uncomplicated acute illness caused by influenza A or influenza B infections in patients who have been symptomatic for no more than 48 hours. They can also be used prophylactically to prevent infection in specific patient populations.

Role of Neuraminidase in Viral Infections

As discussed, the influenza virion structure includes an envelope that contains two viral surface glycoproteins, HA NA. While HA is important for viral binding to host cell receptors via a terminal sialic acid residue, NA removes the sialic acid from the surface glycoproteins. While these actions initially appear to be antagonistic to one another, the sequential actions of HA and NA allow the virus to establish and spread an infection within a human cell. It should be noted that sialic acid is a generic term for the *N*- or *O*-substituted derivatives of neuraminic acid. It is also commonly used as the name for the most common member of this group, *N*-acetylneuraminic acid.

The initial infection of a human host cell involves attachment of HA to sialic acid groups that are present on numerous glycoproteins on the host cell surface. The virus then moves from one sialic acid group to another until it finds the proper receptor to trigger endocytosis. The ability to move is provided by NA-catalyzed cleavage of the sialic group to which the virus was initially bound. Once the virus has entered the cell and replicated, new viral particles bud from the host cell membrane; however, the HA on these newly formed viral particles is initially attached to the host cell by sialic acid groups. The spread of infection then requires NA to cleave the sialic acid group and release the viral particle.[59-61]

Development, Mechanism of Action, and Structure-Activity Relationship

X-ray crystallography of NA has shown that while the amino acid sequence of NA from various viruses is considerably different, the sialic acid binding site is quite similar for type

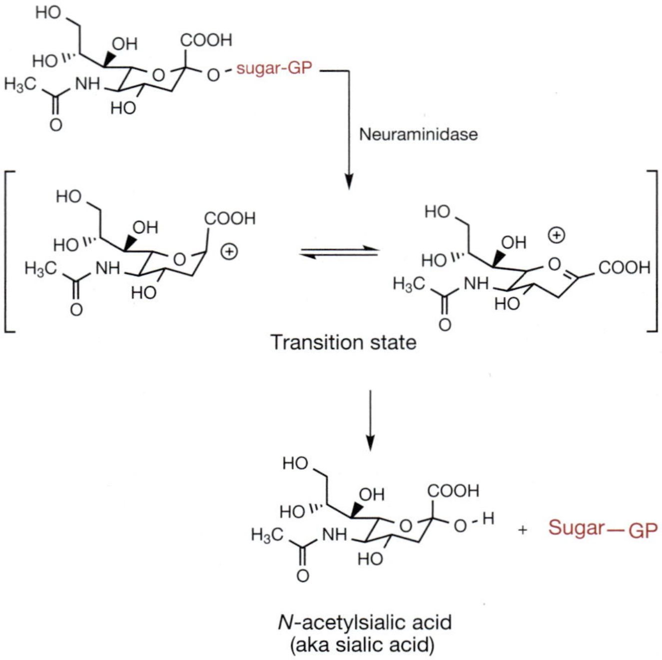

Figure 33.7 Neuraminidase-catalyzed removal of an N-acetylneuraminic acid residue from a glycoprotein chain. GP, glycoprotein; NA, neuraminidase.

A and B influenza viruses. In addition, it is believed that the hydrolysis of sialic acid proceeds through an oxonium cation–stabilized carbonium ion, as shown in Figure 33.7. Mimicking the transition state with novel carbocyclic derivatives of sialic acid led to the development of transition state–based inhibitors.[62] The first of these compounds, 2-deoxy-2,3-dehydro-*N*-acetylneuraminic acid (DANA, Fig. 33.8), was found to be an active NA inhibitor but lacked specificity for viral NA. Upon determination of the crystal structure of NA, more sophisticated measurements of the binding site for sialic acid lead initially to the development of zanamivir and later to oseltamivir and peramivir (Fig. 33.8).

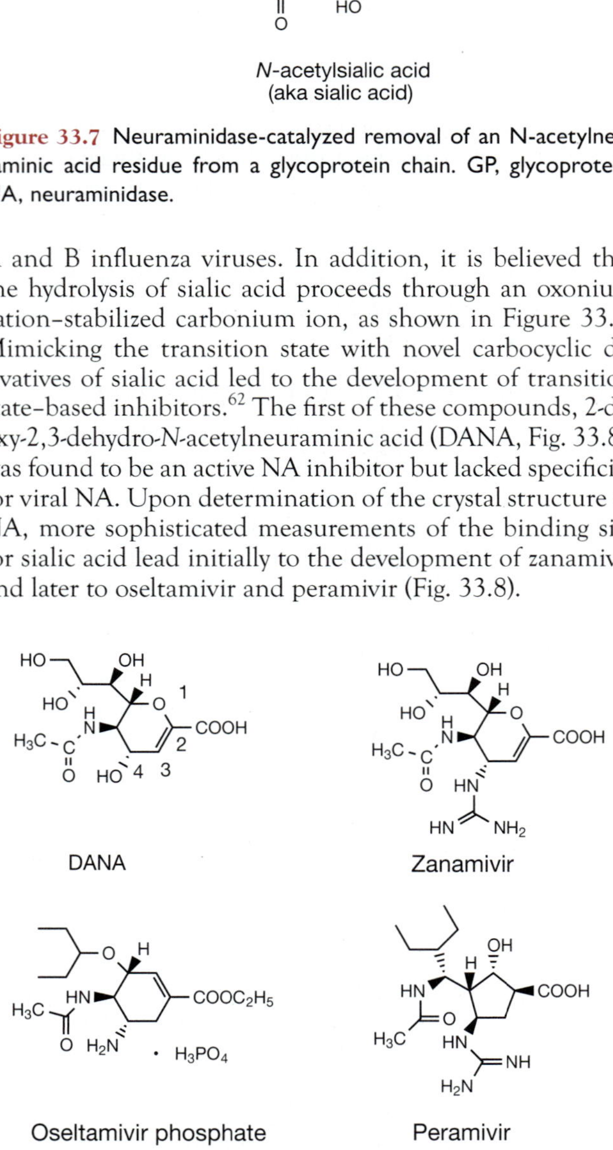

Figure 33.8 Sialic acid derivatives 2-deoxy-2,3-dehydro-*N*-acetylneuraminic acid (DANA), zanamivir, oseltamivir phosphate, and peramivir.

Crystallographic studies of DANA suggested that substitution of its 4-hydroxy group with basic functional groups should enhance binding. A 4-amino derivative of DANA was found to bind to a Glu119 residue in the receptor through a salt bridge, while a 4-guanidino derivative (zanamivir) was able to form both a salt bridge to the Glu119 residue and an ionic interaction with a glutamic acid at position 227. The result of these substitutions was a dramatic increase in binding capacity of the 4-amino and 4-guanidino derivatives to NA leading to effective competitive inhibition of the enzyme and zanamivir (see Fig. 33.8), the first US Food and Drug Administration (FDA)-approved NA inhibitor.

Further studies identified additional binding sites between NA and the C_5 acetamide group and the C_2 carboxylic acid in DANA, zanamivir, and other analogues as well as potential hydrophobic interactions with substituents at the C_6 position. SAR studies showed that maximum binding occurred to NA when the C_6 position was substituted with the 3-pentyloxy side chain, thereby leading to the development and approval of oseltamivir (see Fig. 33.8). Alterations of the size of the ring while maintaining the key functional groups for binding lead to the development of peramivir (see Fig. 33.8).[63]

Zanamivir, oseltamivir, and peramivir all exert their mechanism of action in treating influenza by mimicking the transition state of NA and inhibiting the enzyme. As described, NA is essential for both the initial infection of human cells in the respiratory tract as well as the subsequent spread of the infection. Due to the rapid spread of infection, in order for these NA inhibitors to produce a beneficial effect, they must be administered within 48 hours of the onset of symptoms.[28] Zanamivir and oseltamivir can also be used for the prophylaxis of influenza (A or B) infection.

Common Adverse Effects and Drug Interactions

The most common adverse effects seen with orally administered oseltamivir are nausea, vomiting, and headache, and the most serious adverse effect is bradycardia. Nausea and vomiting may be minimized if oseltamivir is taken with food. Zanamivir must be administered as an oral inhalation and can cause bronchospasm, sinusitis, sore throat, arthralgia, diarrhea, fever, and nausea. Zanamivir should not be used in patients with underlying airway disease. Peramivir must be administered IV and can cause diarrhea and neutropenia.[28,64] There are no significant drug interactions for any of these drugs.

Physiochemical and Pharmacokinetic Properties

Zanamivir and peramivir are amphoteric drugs, and the carboxylic acids and guanidine groups within their structures will be primarily ionized in most physiological environments. Both of these drugs are highly water soluble and are not orally absorbed to a significant extent. As mentioned earlier, zanamivir is administered as an oral inhalation, and peramivir is administered as a short IV infusion. Neither of these drugs undergoes any significant metabolism and is eliminated unchanged in the urine. The half-life of zanamivir is 2.5 to 5.1 hours allowing for bid dosing for 5 days, while the half-life of peramivir is approximately 20 hours allowing for a single IV infusion. Similar to oseltamivir, neither of these drugs is bound to plasma proteins to any significant extent.

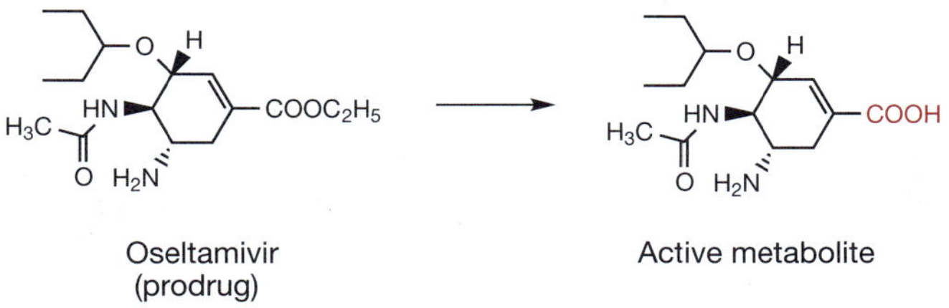

Figure 33.9 Metabolic activation of oseltamivir.

Oseltamivir is a prodrug that is hydrolyzed in vivo to produce oseltamivir carboxylate, its active metabolite (Fig. 33.9). The therapeutic advantage of the prodrug is that it provides a better water/lipid balance and allows for oral administration and absorption from the GI tract. In comparison, zanamivir has a log *P* value of approximately −3, while oseltamivir's log *P* is 1.3. Oseltamivir is a basic drug, while its active metabolite is amphoteric. Oseltamivir has an oral bioavailability of approximately 75% and a half-life of 1 to 3 hours as oseltamivir and 6 to 10 hours as oseltamivir carboxylate. Oseltamivir does not undergo any further metabolism once it is converted to oseltamivir carboxylate. Oseltamivir carboxylate is excreted primarily in the urine. Oseltamivir is administered once or twice daily depending on whether it is used prophylactically or to treat an active infection, respectively.[26,28,64]

Baloxavir Marvoxil

Baloxavir is a tripartite prodrug similar to those seen with angiotensin-receptor blockers (see Chapter 19) and cephalosporins (see Chapter 22). In vivo hydrolysis produces baloxavir, the active metabolite (Fig. 33.10). Similar to oseltamivir, the prodrug was designed to enhance the pharmacokinetic properties and oral absorption of baloxavir. Baloxavir is indicated for the treatment of acute uncomplicated influenza (A or B) infection in patients who have been symptomatic for no more than 48 hours. It is also indicated for prophylactic use in patients who had exposure to another individual with infection.

Mechanism of Action

The RNA polymerase complex in the influenza virus is a heterotrimer that is composed of three protein subunits: (1) polymerase acidic protein (PA), (2) polymerase basic

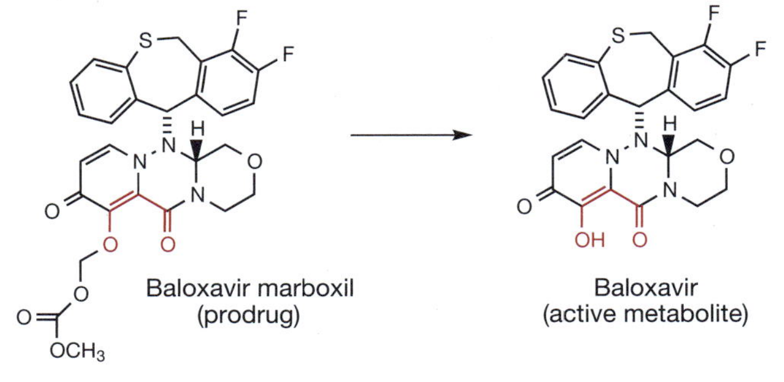

Figure 33.10 Metabolic activation of baloxavir marboxil.

protein 1 (PB1), and (3) polymerase basic protein 2 (PB2). Each of these subunits has a unique role in viral mRNA synthesis, and this polymerase complex is essential for viral gene transcription and replication. In the initial step, the PB2 subunit binds to the cap of host cellular pre-messenger RNA (pre-mRNA). This then allows the PA protein to cleave the capped pre-mRNA and provide an RNA primer required by the PB1 subunit to proceed with viral mRNA transcription. The endonuclease activity of the PA subunit is known as a "cap-snatching" process. Baloxavir selectively inhibits the PA protein, blocks the initiation of mRNA synthesis, and ultimately decreases the proliferation of the influenza virus.[65,66]

Resistance to baloxavir can occur if there is any alteration in the amino acid sequence of the PA protein.

Common Adverse Effects and Drug Interactions

Baloxavir is generally well tolerated with bronchitis, diarrhea, headache, nausea, and sinusitis occurring in a small percentage of patients. The coadministration of baloxavir with polyvalent cation–containing products such as antacids, dairy products, iron preparations, and multivitamins can decrease the absorption of baloxavir due to chelation of the cation with the highlighted portion of baloxavir, as shown in Figure 33.10.[28,40]

Receptor Binding and Structure-Activity Relationship

A key structural feature of baloxavir is the highlighted acidic functional group that is able to chelate Mn^{2+} in the active site of the PA endonuclease and inhibit the "cap-snatching" process. The development of baloxavir involved the screening of metal-chelating compounds, based on the successful rational design for HIV integrase inhibitors (discussed later in this chapter). Both the endonuclease portion of PA and the HIV integrase enzyme require a bicationic metal ion (Mg^{2+} for HIV integrase) in their active site, and the ability to bind to this metal has been shown to provide inhibitory activity.[65]

Physicochemical and Pharmacokinetic Properties

Baloxavir marboxil is a nonelectrolyte, while baloxavir, the active metabolite, has an acidic functional group that is similar to a β-dicarbonyl group. Baloxavir marboxil is almost completely converted to baloxavir via hydrolysis. Baloxavir is primarily metabolized by UGT1A3 to an inactive glucuronide metabolite. Metabolism by CYP3A4 is minor and produces an inactive sulfoxide. Baloxavir is approximately 93% plasma protein bound and has a half-life of 79 hours, which allows for single-dose therapy. Baloxavir and its metabolites are primarily excreted in the feces (80%).[26,28,67]

Amantadine and Rimantadine

Amantadine and rimantadine were approved for the treatment of influenza A infections; however, due to the development of resistance, the US Centers for Disease Control and Prevention (CDC) does not recommend treatment or prophylaxis of influenza A due to the high resistance levels.[68,69]

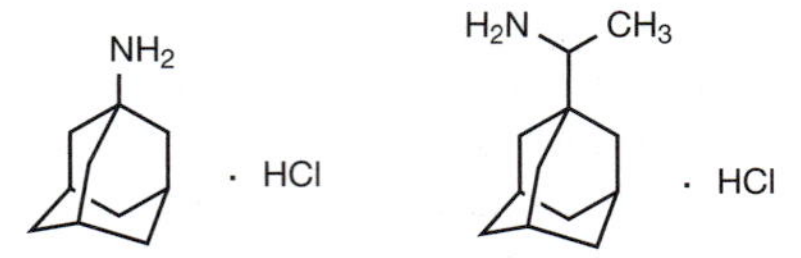

Amantadine Rimantadine

Amantadine and rimantadine are structurally similar to one another. Both drugs contain a tricyclic structure and a primary amine and are primarily ionized in all physiological environments. Rimantadine was developed to enhance the efficiency and decrease the adverse effects that are seen with amantadine. Both drugs exhibit similar mechanisms of action. They bind to the transmembrane domain of the viral M2 protein, a proton-selective ion channel. This binding interferes with the fusion of the viral particle with the target cell membrane and the subsequent uncoating of the virus and the release of the viral RNA into the human cell.[68,70]

Amantadine is also used to treat Parkinson disease by virtues of a second mechanism. Amantadine is a weak, noncompetitive antagonist of the N-methyl-D-aspartate (NMDA) receptor and increases dopamine release. Further discussion of the use of amantadine for Parkinson disease can be found in Chapter 10. Rimantadine is not used to treat Parkinson disease.

There are a number of adverse effects associated with amantadine including anxiety, constipation, dizziness, headache, insomnia, nausea, and orthostatic hypotension. Rimantadine is better tolerated and produces fewer adverse effects. The most common adverse effects seen with rimantadine are insomnia and nausea. Drug interactions are not normally seen with these two drugs when used to treat influenza A.[28]

Coronaviruses

Coronaviruses are a large family of enveloped, positive-sense RNA viruses. The coronaviruses are zoonotic in origin, meaning that the virus jumps from animals, typically bats or rodents, to humans.[71] Today, seven coronaviruses are associated with respiratory disease in humans. Four of these coronaviruses are relatively mild and are responsible for about 30% of common colds (eg, OC43, NL63, 229E, and HKU1). Since 2002, three highly pathogenic coronaviruses have emerged. Two of these deadly coronaviruses, SARS-CoV in 2002 and Middle Eastern respiratory syndrome coronavirus (MERS-CoV) in 2012, were limited to regional outbreaks.[72] However, in late 2019, SARS-CoV-2 was first detected in Wuhan, China, and subsequently became a worldwide pandemic. SARS-CoV-2 is responsible for causing coronavirus disease 19 (COVID-19), which varies from asymptomatic infections to severe and even fatal infections. Since the emergence of SARS-CoV-2, multiple approaches have been developed to control the spread and severity of COVID-19, including antiviral agents and vaccines.

At the time of writing, antiviral therapy is targeted to two SARS-CoV-2 proteins: RDRP and main protease (M^pro). As a positive-sense RNA virus, SARS-CoV-2 relies on RDRP for copying the RNA genome and transcription of subgenomic RNAs for translation of viral proteins.[73] SARS-CoV-2 also encodes for two polyproteins, which must undergo proteolytic processing to release the functional proteins. M^pro serves as the viral protease for SARS-CoV-2 and cleaves at least 11 sites in the polyprotein, ultimately leading to the generation of RDRP among other key viral proteins.[74] In addition to small-molecule drugs, monoclonal antibodies (mAbs) against the spike protein of SARS-CoV-2 were designed to prevent attachment of the virus to the host cell. While these mAbs are not currently recommended for active COVID-19 infections, the spike protein is the target of current vaccination strategies. As SARS-CoV-2 continues to evolve, it is likely that antiviral therapies will continue to be reviewed and modified to ensure coverage of current circulating strains.

SARS-CoV-2 is transmitted via respiratory droplets, which can be expelled through coughing, sneezing, or talking. Once infected, the incubation period varies widely but averages 5 days. Common symptoms include cough, loss of taste or smell, fever, myalgia, and rhinitis. Although many infections are asymptomatic or mild, COVID-19 can be severe or critical with the need for hospitalization.[75] More severe cases of COVID-19 can include pneumonia, acute respiratory distress syndrome (ARDS), cardiac injury, and kidney or liver injury. Hyperinflammation and dysregulated cytokine expression are observed in patients infected with COVID-19 with respiratory failure.[76] Older adult patients as well as those with diabetes, obesity, hypertension, or other chronic conditions have a greater risk for severe COVID-19 than younger and otherwise healthy patients. During pregnancy, SARS-CoV-2 infection is associated with greater maternal morbidity and mortality and increased risk of pregnancy loss and preterm birth. Although children are more likely to have asymptomatic infections or mild COVID-19, multisystem inflammatory syndrome in children (MIS-C) is a rare but life-threatening condition that can follow weeks after the infection. Importantly, vaccination reduces severe complications, hospitalizations, and mortality from COVID-19.

Antiviral Drugs to Treat COVID-19

Treatment of COVID-19 currently involves the use of three antiviral drugs and other supportive care.[77]

Nirmatrelvir and Ritonavir

The combination of nirmatrelvir and ritonavir (Paxlovid) is indicated to treat adult patients with mild-to-moderate COVID-19 infections who are at high risk for the progression to severe COVID-19. Both drugs serve a unique role in this combination. Nirmatrelvir is an inhibitor of a specific SARS-CoV-2 viral protease, and ritonavir prevents the metabolism of nirmatrelvir, thus increasing its concentrations.

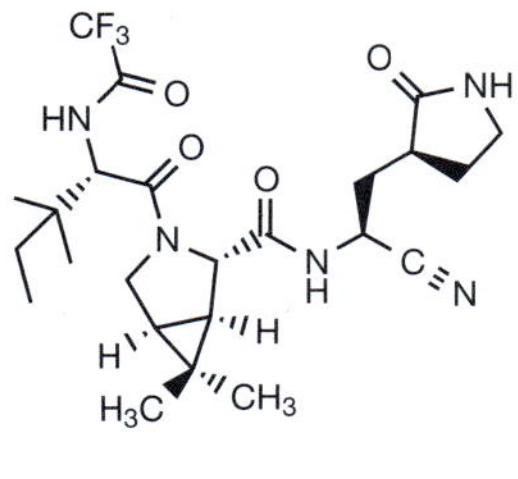

Nirmatrelvir

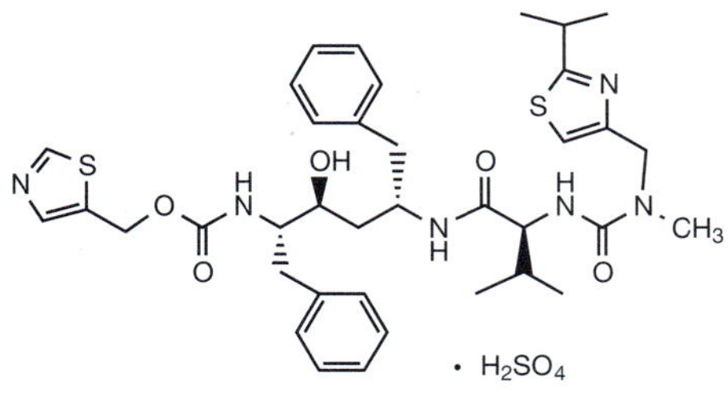

Ritonavir

Mechanism of Action

Nirmatrelvir is a peptidomimetic inhibitor of M^pro, a SARS-CoV-2 protease that is also referred to as 3C-like protease (3CL^pro) or nsp5 protease. Viral protease enzymes are unique in that they convert polypeptide chains into individual proteins. Human cells synthesize single proteins and do not rely on these types of protease enzymes. This provides selectivity for the viral particles as compared to human cells. Inhibition of SARS-CoV-2 M^pro renders it incapable of processing polyprotein precursors and prevents viral replication.[78]

Ritonavir does not bind to M^pro and does not have any direct antiviral activity against COVID-19 infections. Its purpose in this combination is to block the metabolism of nirmatrelvir and increase its plasma concentrations. Ritonavir is an RT inhibitor that was originally developed to treat HIV infections. Due to its toxicity and the development of more specific and less toxic RT inhibitors, ritonavir is now used in smaller, nontherapeutic doses as a pharmacokinetic enhancer. Specifically, it inhibits CYP3A4 and blocks the metabolism of other antiviral drugs that require this enzyme for metabolism. The overall result is a programmed drug interaction that leads to an enhancement in the plasma concentration and duration of action of other antiviral drugs.[79,80]

Common Adverse Effects and Drug Interactions

Overall, the adverse effects seen with the combination of nirmatrelvir and ritonavir are mild, with diarrhea, hypersensitivity reactions, and taste disturbance being the most common. Ritonavir is a strong CYP3A4 inhibitor and will decrease the metabolism of any drug that requires this isozyme. While ritonavir is used to create a beneficial drug interaction with nirmatrelvir and other antiviral drugs discussed later in this chapter, it will also increase the plasma concentrations and potential toxicity of other co-administered drugs. In many cases, ritonavir is contraindicated with other drugs requiring CYP3A4 for normal metabolism.[28]

Receptor Binding and Structure-Activity Relationship

As shown in Figure 33.11, the initial step in the cleavage of a viral polyprotein by M^{pro} involves two amino acids, cysteine and histidine. The histidine residue enhances the acidity and nucleophilicity of the cysteine sulfhydryl group, thereby resulting in an initial attack of the cysteine sulfhydryl ion on the labile polyprotein bond. Subsequent steps lead to the cleavage of this bond and the regeneration of the enzyme. Nirmatrelvir contains four amide bonds and a peptidomimetic structure. It is able to bind to M^{pro} and inhibit it due to the steric and electronic factors associated with its structure.[78]

Physicochemical and Pharmacokinetic Properties

Due to the presence of the electron-withdrawing nitrile group, the adjacent amide of nirmatrelvir is weakly acidic, with a predicted pK_a value of 7.1. It has a good balance between water and lipid solubility and has a log P value of 2.12. It is 69% plasma protein bound, and when it is combined with ritonavir, its metabolism is minimal. Nirmatrelvir is excreted in both the urine and the feces. If nirmatrelvir was used as monotherapy without ritonavir, it would be rapidly oxidized by CYP3A4 to one of the following inactive hydroxyl metabolites.[81]

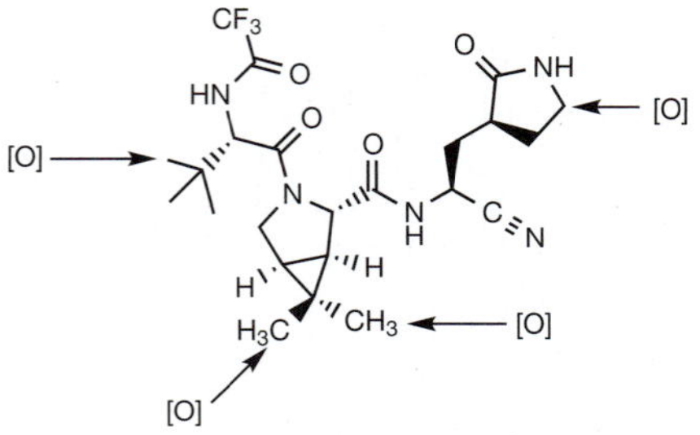

Sites of oxidation for nirmatrelvir

Ritonavir is a nonelectrolyte and has a predicted log P value of 4.24. Due to its high lipid solubility, ritonavir is 98% to 99% plasma protein bound. It is extensively metabolized by CYP3A4 (major) and CYP2D6 (minor). Thus, ritonavir is both a substrate for CYP3A4 and a strong inhibitor. It is primarily excreted in the feces, with a small amount in the urine.[26,28]

Molnupiravir

Molnupiravir is a cytidine analogue that is indicated for the treatment of adults (age >18 years) with mild-to-moderate COVID-19 who are at high risk for progression to severe COVID-19. Molnupiravir is not approved for hospitalized patients, for prophylactic use, or for more than 5 days of treatment.

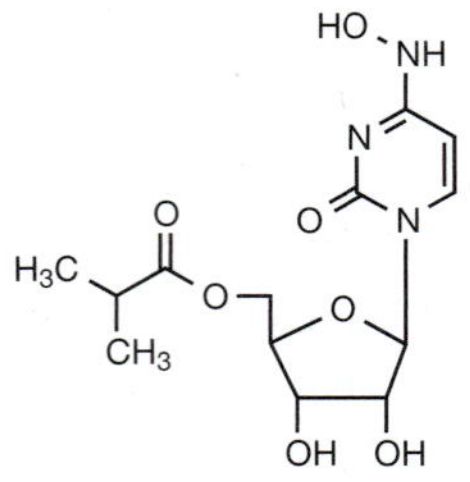

Molnupiravir (prodrug)

Mechanism of Action and Structure-Activity Relationship

Molnupiravir is a prodrug that is initially hydrolyzed to N^4-hydroxycytidine (NHC). NHC is then phosphorylated to its active triphosphate and is incorporated into SARS-CoV-2 RNA by the viral RNA polymerase. The presence of the N^4-hydroxy group alters normal C-G base pairing and results in an accumulation of errors in the viral genome, leading to inhibition of replication.[82,83]

Common Adverse Effects and Drug Interactions

Adverse effects with molnupiravir are generally mild. The most common adverse effects are diarrhea, dizziness, erythema, nausea, pruritus, rash, urticaria, and vomiting. Angioedema and hypersensitivity reactions can also occur. There are no known drug interactions.[28,83]

Physiochemical and Pharmacokinetic Properties

Molnupiravir is highly water soluble. The isobutyric acid prodrug enhances oral bioavailability and is readily hydrolyzed in vivo. The active triphosphate NHC does not undergo any significant metabolism nor is it significantly bound to plasma proteins. The elimination half-life is 3.3 hours, allowing twice-daily dosing.[26,28,83]

Remdesivir

Remdesivir is an adenosine analogue with a broad antiviral spectrum among RNA viruses. It is active against SARS-CoV-2, Ebola virus (EBOV), and MERS-CoV. It is indicated for the treatment of COVID-19 in adult and pediatric patients who require hospitalization as well as for the treatment of patients with mild-to-moderate COVID-19 who are at a high risk for progression to severe disease.[84,85]

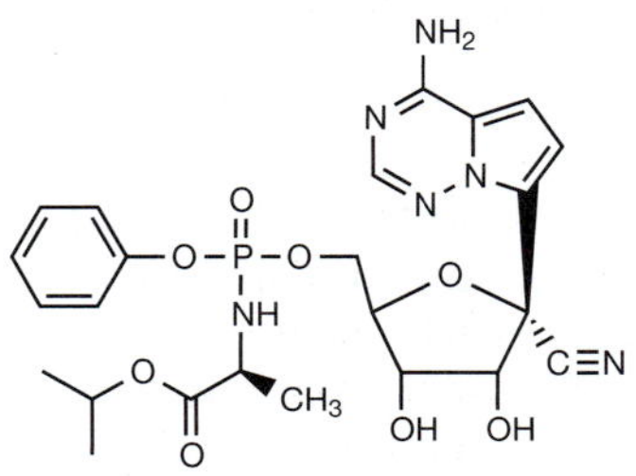

Remdesivir (prodrug)

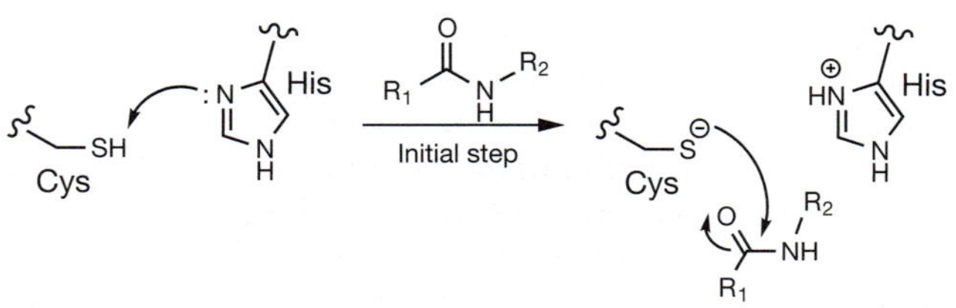

Figure 33.11 Initial step in M^{pro} cleave of a polyprotein.

Mechanism of Action and Structure-Activity Relationship

Remdesivir is a prodrug that is activated sequentially by the removal of the phenol, the isopropyl, and the phosphorylalanine groups. This is accomplished within the infected cell by either carboxyesterase 1 or cathepsin depending on the cell type and provides selectivity to infected cells as compared to simple ester prodrugs that can be hydrolyzed outside an infected cell. The resulting nucleoside is then phosphorylated to remdesivir triphosphate (RDV-TP). RDV-TP mimics adenosine triphosphate (ATP) and is incorporated into newly synthesized RNA chains by the SARS-CoV-2 RDRP. Studies have shown that once RDV-TP is incorporated into SARS-CoV-2, three additional nucleotides can be added; however, the C_1' nitrile sterically impairs the addition of the fourth nucleotide by clashing with Ser861 of the polymerase. This represents a translocation barrier that interferes with the entry of the next nucleotide and stalls viral RNA synthesis. Additionally, the presence of remdesivir compromises the efficiency of complementary base pairing and further inhibits viral RNA synthesis. The stalled state of RDRP may impair proofreading by the viral 3′-exonuclease. These actions may be due to the electron-withdrawing properties of the C_1' nitrile.[84,86]

Common Adverse Effects and Drug Interactions

The most common adverse effects seen with the use of remdesivir are increased serum glucose and decreased creatinine clearance. Other adverse effects are rash, nausea, decreased hemoglobin, lymphocytopenia, prolonged prothrombin time, increased aspartate aminotransferase (AST) and alanine aminotransferase (ALT), hypersensitivity reactions, and seizures. No major drug interactions are listed for remdesivir; however, since it can prolong prothrombin time, it may enhance the anticoagulant effects of warfarin.[28,84]

Physicochemical and Pharmacokinetic Properties

Remdesivir lacks any ionizable acidic or basic functional groups, has a log *P* value of 2.01, and is not orally absorbed. Prior to any metabolism, remdesivir is approximately 90% plasma protein bound; however, once converted to its active metabolites, it is no longer plasma protein bound. Remdesivir does not undergo any additional metabolism beyond the activation previously described. The half-life of remdesivir is 1 hour, but the half-life of its nucleoside metabolite is 27 hours. Remdesivir and its metabolites are primarily excreted in the urine.[26,84,87]

Monoclonal Antibodies

A number of mAbs have been approved by the FDA under the Emergency Use Authorization (EUA); however, they are no longer authorized to treat COVID-19 because subvariants of SARS-CoV-2 are not expected to be susceptible to these products.[75] In 2024, the mAb pemivibart was authorized as pre-exposure prophylaxis in patients who are immunocompromised.[88] Given that alterations and variations in these mAbs may eventually prove to be valuable, a brief discussion of the mechanism of action is provided here.

As part of its structure, SARS-CoV-2 contains a spike (or S) protein that is important for receptor recognition and cell membrane fusion. The spike protein is composed of two subunits, S1 and S2. The S1 subunit contains a receptor-binding domain that recognizes and binds to the angiotensin-converting enzyme 2 receptor that is located on the host cell. The S2 subunit mediates viral cell membrane fusion and entry of the virus into the cell. The original mAbs, casirivimab and imdevimab, bound to nonoverlapping epitopes of the S1 subunit of the spike protein and blocked the initial attachment of SARS-CoV-2 to the human angiotensin-converting enzyme 2. Variations of these original mAbs targeted other epitopes of the S1 subunit; however, mutations of the spike protein have mostly precluded their use.[75,89]

Respiratory Syncytial Virus

Respiratory syncytial virus (RSV) is a significant cause of respiratory disease, particularly in very young, older adult, and populations that are immunocompromised. RSV follows a seasonal pattern of infection with cases peaking in winter and early spring in the United States. Most children (~90%) are first infected by RSV by age 2, but immunity against the virus is not long-lasting and reinfection is common later in life. In healthy older children (age >5 years) and adults, RSV causes upper respiratory tract infections such as the common cold. In young children, RSV can present as bronchiolitis, which is a lower respiratory tract infection with obstruction of the small airways. Each year in the United States, RSV leads to over 2 million outpatient visits and 58,000 to 80,000 hospitalizations among young children.[90] RSV is increasingly realized as an important cause of illness in older adults as well, with estimates of 60,000 to 160,000 hospitalizations and 6,000 to 10,000 deaths in adults 65 years of age and older.[91,92] Supportive care is the mainstay of therapy for hospitalized patients with RSV infections, but antiviral agents are available to reduce the severity of RSV infections.[93]

Two RSV proteins are the focus of current therapeutic interventions: the fusion (F) protein and RDRP. The F protein is embedded in the viral envelope, where it fuses the RSV envelope and host cell membrane to facilitate viral entry. The F protein is found in two forms: a highly unstable prefusion state and a stable postfusion state. Neutralizing antibodies against RSV target a site in the F protein that is only accessible in the prefusion form.[94] As a negative-sense RNA virus, RSV also requires RDRP for replication of the viral genome and production of viral mRNAs. Although there are no currently available drugs that specifically inhibit RSV RDRP, its function can be inhibited by ribavirin, a broad-spectrum antiviral that produces a variety of effects on many RNA viruses.

Transmission of RSV occurs via respiratory droplets, with symptoms appearing about 4 to 6 days after initial infection. Infection is limited to the respiratory tract, where RSV infects epithelial cells, leading to cell death.[95] Although required for viral clearance, the immune response also contributes to disease through the production of inflammatory cytokines that enhance immune cell infiltration into the lung.[96] In infants, the small airways in the lung can become plugged by the resulting cellular debris and inflammatory infiltrates, leading to wheezing and respiratory distress. In older adults, the mechanisms of pathogenesis are less clear, but higher levels of inflammatory cytokines are associated with more severe disease in this age group.[97] Vaccine development for RSV has focused on strategies for both vulnerable age groups. Currently, maternal vaccination is recommended during pregnancy to provide sufficient maternal antibodies to the infant, and two RSV vaccines are also available for those 60 years of age or older.[98] All current RSV vaccines are designed to detect the prefusion form of the F protein.

Antiviral Drugs to Treat Respiratory Syncytial Virus Infections

Ribavirin

Ribavirin is a purine analogue in which the six-membered pyrimidine ring has been replaced with an amide. This provides flexibility that is not present in the naturally occurring purines. Ribavirin is a broad-spectrum antiviral that is used to treat both RSV infections and HCV infections. It is also effective in treating hepatitis E virus infections and viral hemorrhagic fever.[28]

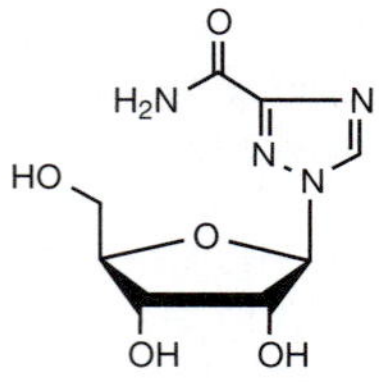

Ribavirin
(prodrug)

Mechanism of Action and Structure-Activity Relationship

Ribavirin has a number of mechanisms of action. As shown in Figure 33.12, ribavirin is able to mimic both adenosine and guanosine due to its flexibility about the amide side chain. Similar to other nucleoside analogues, ribavirin is a prodrug that must be phosphorylated to its active metabolites, ribavirin monophosphate (RMP) and ribavirin triphosphate (RTP). RMP and RTP inhibit a number of viral enzymes.

RMP is a potent, competitive inhibitor of inosine monophosphate dehydrogenase. Inhibition of this enzyme prevents the biosynthesis of GTP and lowers the concentration of GTP within the viral particle. RTP inhibits viral-specific RNA polymerase by mimicking GTP and ATP. RTP also inhibits the viral-specific mRNA capping enzymes, guanyl transferase and N^7-methyl transferase, by acting as a GTP substrate mimic. The viral mRNA cap provides protection from exonucleases and is required for the processing and translation of mRNA. Thus, inhibition of the capping enzymes decreases the formation of viral proteins and enzymes.[99,100]

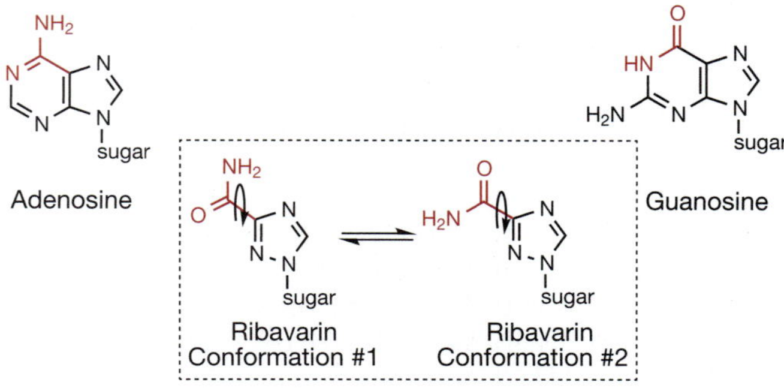

Figure 33.12 Ability of ribavirin to mimic both adenosine and guanosine.

Common Adverse Effects and Drug Interactions

While ribavirin can be used to treat RSV infections, it is most commonly used in combination with other drugs to treat HCV infections. Adverse effects listed in the literature are for these combinations, and it is difficult to separate which ones are caused by ribavirin. Adverse effects occurring in more than 10% of patients include fatigue, irritability, GI disorder, headache, rash, pruritus, musculoskeletal pain, insomnia, and decreased appetite. Ribavirin can cause an increase in myelotoxicity if used in combination with azathioprine, due to the inhibition of inosine monophosphate dehydrogenase, a major metabolizing enzyme required by azathioprine.[28]

Physicochemical and Pharmacokinetic Properties

Ribavirin lacks any ionizable acidic or basic functional groups; however, it is highly water soluble with a log *P* value of −1.9. It is orally absorbed and has a bioavailability of 64%. It is not plasma protein bound and does not undergo any additional metabolism beyond the activation previously described. The half-life of ribavirin is 120 hours, and it is primarily excreted in the urine.[26,28]

Nirsevimab and Palivizumab

Nirsevimab and palivizumab are mAbs that are indicated for the prevention of RSV in neonates, infants, and pediatric patients who are vulnerable to this infection.[28]

Nirsevimab is a recombinant human immunoglobulin G1 kappa (IgG1k) mAb that targets the highly conserved epitope site Ø on the prefusion form of the RSV F protein. As previously mentioned, the F protein is one of two glycoproteins on the RSV particle and is essential for the entry of the virus into the respiratory cells. Binding of nirsevimab to the F protein prevents the RSV particle from attaching to a human cell and blocks the spread of infection. Nirsevimab contains modifications of three amino acids in the highly conserved F_c region of the mAb. These modifications extend the serum half-life of nirsevimab, allowing it to be administered intramuscularly once per season. Nirsevimab is very well tolerated, with local injection-site reactions and rash being the main adverse effects (~1%). There are no significant drug interactions.[26,28,101,102]

Palivizumab is a humanized IgG1k mAb that is produced by recombinant DNA technology and binds to the antigenic A site of the F protein. It is composed of both human (95%) and murine (5%) sequences. Studies have shown that palivizumab neutralizes and inhibits the spread of RSV by preventing virus-to-cell and cell-to-cell fusion. Similar to nirsevimab, palivizumab is administered intramuscularly but must be given once monthly throughout each RSV season. The most common adverse effects seen with palivizumab are skin rash, fever, and antibody development.[26,28,103]

Hepatitis

Viral Hepatitis

Viral hepatitis is an inflammation of the liver induced by a virus infection. Almost all cases are due to one of the five hepatitis viruses. These are listed in Table 33.3 and are sequentially designated as hepatitis A virus through hepatitis E virus (HAV, HBV, HCV, HDV, and HEV). Although these viruses come from different virus families, all hepatitis viruses are capable of infecting hepatocytes, leading to cell death, inflammation, and liver damage. On occasion, disease can arise from hepatic infection with other viruses (eg, yellow fever virus, CMV, Epstein-Barr virus [EBV], and HSV). The hepatitis viruses present with similar symptoms during acute infection, including fever, nausea, vomiting, abdominal pain, and jaundice. Further laboratory testing is required to identify the specific virus in each case. The hepatitis viruses differ in their ability to establish chronic infections, with HBV and HCV as the most common causes. Chronic infection is associated with prolonged damage to the liver from the cytotoxic T cell response, cirrhosis, and the development of liver cancers, such as hepatocellular carcinoma (HCC). Hepatitis viruses account for more than half of liver cancer cases globally.[104] As such, prevention and treatment are key for protecting against both hepatitis and long-term liver disease.

In the United States, most cases of viral hepatitis are attributed to HAV, HBV, or HCV. In this section, the key features of each hepatitis virus are discussed.

Hepatitis A Virus

HAV is a nonenveloped, single-stranded RNA virus, and only one serotype of the virus exists. The viral particle is highly stable and can survive in contaminated water for extended periods, and under certain environmental conditions, it can persist for months.[105] Transmission occurs through the fecal-oral route, which can occur through ingestion of contaminated food or water, or via close person-to-person contact. Symptoms of acute infection appear more often in adults, whereas infections in children are more often asymptomatic. Recovery occurs in less than 2 months in most

Table 33.3 Hepatitis Viruses

Virus	Family	Genome	Transmission	Acute Infection	Chronic Infection	Vaccine
Hepatitis A virus (HAV)	*Picornaviridae*	Positive-sense RNA	Fecal-oral, sexual contact	Subclinical in children (70%) and some adults (30%)	No	Yes
Hepatitis B virus (HBV)	*Hepadnaviridae*	Single and double-stranded DNA	Contact with blood or other bodily fluids, perinatal transmission	Subclinical in children, symptomatic in some adults (~30%)	Common in newborns (90%), less common in adults (<5%)	Yes
Hepatitis C virus (HCV)	*Flaviviridae*	Positive-sense RNA	Contact with blood or other bodily fluids	Usually subclinical	Common in all ages (55%-85%)	No
Hepatitis D virus (HDV)	*Deltaviridae*	Negative-sense RNA	Contact with blood or other bodily fluids	Requires co-infection with HBV	Common with HBV superinfection	Vaccination for HBV protects against HDV
Hepatitis E virus (HEV)	*Hepeviridae*	Positive-sense RNA	Fecal-oral, consumption of contaminated meat	Mostly subclinical; symptomatic infections in young adults and pregnant patients	Rarely (eg, solid organ transplant)	Available in China only

cases, and chronic infection is not established. There are no antiviral agents for HAV, but immune globulin can be used for pre- and post-exposure prophylaxis. An effective vaccine has been available since 1995, but HAV remains hyperendemic in many developing countries.[106]

Hepatitis B Virus

HBV is an enveloped DNA virus that is part of the *Hepadnaviridae* family of viruses. Transmission occurs through contact with contaminated blood, sexual contact, or through perinatal transmission from the mother to the infant. After entering the bloodstream, HBV infects hepatocytes, leading to a cytotoxic immune response against the infected liver cells. In adults, 65% to 80% of infections are asymptomatic, and 90% to 95% of all patients have a complete recovery. Despite this, liver failure is possible during an acute infection, particularly in immunosuppressed patients. The severity of acute HBV infection is worsened by co-infection with HDV, although HDV does not cause liver disease independently. HBV can also establish chronic infections, especially in infants; 80% to 95% of infants and young children infected with HBV become chronic carriers and are at high risk of developing cirrhosis and HCC. An effective vaccine is available, but HBV still remains a major global health issue, causing over 1 million deaths per year.[107]

HBV possess an unusual genome that is partly double-stranded circular DNA. As part of its replication cycle, HBV uses a virally encoded RT enzyme to produce progeny DNA genomes from an RNA intermediate. As such, RT inhibitors that were first designed against HIV are also the mainstay of antiviral therapy against HBV.

Hepatitis C Virus

HCV is an enveloped, positive-stranded RNA virus from the *Flaviviridae* family. HCV is the most common blood-borne pathogen in the United States, and it is estimated that 57 million people are infected globally as of 2020.[108,109] It is transmitted through blood-to-blood contact, with injection drug use accounting for most new cases. HCV infects hepatocytes in the liver, which leads to cytotoxic T cell infiltration and immune-mediated death of the hepatocytes. Acute infections are usually asymptomatic with minor elevation of liver enzymes and a low incidence of jaundice. However, approximately 70% of patients with HCV develop chronic infections, and many are at risk of progressing to cirrhosis and HCC.[110] HCC is the second leading cause of cancer-related deaths globally, and 34% of HCC cases in the United States are attributed to HCV.[111]

At present, there is no vaccine available to prevent HCV infection; however, antiviral therapy can be effective for treating acute and chronic HCV depending on the genotype of the virus. A representation of the HCV genome is shown in Figure 33.13.[112] The genome consists of four major regions: a 5′ untranslated region, a region that codes for structural (S) proteins, a region that codes for nonstructural (NS) proteins, and a 3′ untranslated region. Structural proteins include the nucleocapsid and envelope glycoproteins. Key NS proteins are the NS3/4A protein, the NS5A protein, and the NS5B protein, as they serve as drug targets to treat patients with HCV infection. A further discussion of these NS proteins is provided later with the drugs that inhibit them.

Antiviral Drugs to Treat Hepatitis B Viral Infections

Current guidelines for the treatment of HBV infections list entecavir, tenofovir, and pegylated interferon alpha (PEG-IFN-α) as the preferred, first-line therapy. Alternate drugs that do not have as strong of a recommendation are adefovir, lamivudine, and telbivudine.[113] Tenofovir and lamivudine are also used to treat HIV infections and will be discussed later.

Pegylated Interferon alpha

Interferons consist of a mixture of small glycoproteins that exhibit species-specific antiviral activity and are classified as cytokines—biomolecules essential for cellular communication to trigger the immune system and eliminate invasive pathogens. They are active in extremely low concentrations.

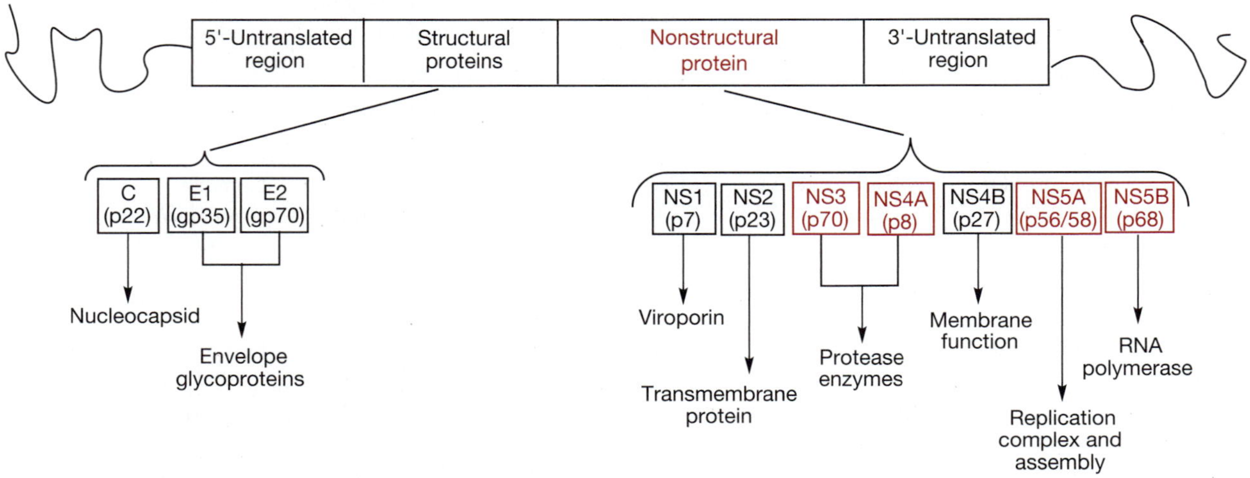

Figure 33.13 Proteins encoded by the hepatitis C virus (HCV) genome. Drug targets are highlighted in red.

The name, interferons, describes their ability to interfere with viral replication and assist the body in its efforts to defend viral infections. Human interferons are classified into three major types: alpha (α), beta (β), and gamma (γ). Interferon alpha is secreted by human leukocytes, interferon beta is secreted by human fibroblasts, and interferon gamma is secreted by lymphoid cells that have been exposed to a pre-sensitized antigen or have been stimulated to divide by mitogens. Interferon alpha and interferon beta are classified as type I interferons, and interferon gamma is classified as type II interferon. Interferon gamma is also called "immune" interferon. As compared with entecavir, tenofovir, adefovir, lamivudine, and telbivudine, PEG-IFN-α has a finite treatment duration and higher rates of seroconversion. The main disadvantage is the development of more prevalent adverse effects, leading to discontinuation of the drug.[114-116]

There are two commercially available forms of PEG-IFN-α, PEG-IFN-α2a, and PEG-IFN-α2b. These two forms differ in both the size and the nature of their respective polyethylene glycol (PEG) components. PEG-IFN-α2a is approved for the treatment of chronic HBV infections, essential thrombocythemia, and polycythemia vera. PEG-IFN-α2b is indicated for adjunct therapy in patients with melanoma. It is also used off-label for the treatment of HCV infections. The addition of PEG to interferon alpha increases the size of the interferon molecule, slows it absorption, decreases its degradation, prolongs its half-life, and enhances its duration of action.[28,117]

Mechanism of Action

The exact mechanism by which PEG-IFN-α acts to inhibit HBV replication is not totally understood; however, it does appear to involve both direct and indirect effects. PEG-IFN-α stimulates a number of non–virus-specific responses through the upregulation of specific genes. PEG-IFN-α has been shown to regulate gene expression and protein translation and inhibit HBV replication by decreasing RNA transcription. Additionally, PEG-IFN-α binds to surface receptors and activates both Janus-activated kinase (JAK) and tyrosine kinase. These initial phosphorylations trigger a cascade of events that eventually cause the transcription of mRNAs that encode human proteins that inhibit the transcription and translation of viral mRNA into required viral proteins and enzymes. These phosphorylation pathways are also involved in lipid metabolism, apoptosis, protein degradation, and inflammatory responses. PEG-IFN-α has also been shown to stimulate a number of immunologic effects, including the promotion of T-cell proliferation, prevention of T-cell apoptosis, and stimulation of natural killer cells.[116,118]

Common Adverse Effects and Drug Interactions

PEG-IFN-α has been shown to cause a number of adverse effects. Listed in Table 33.4 are those adverse effects that have an incidence in 10% of patients or more. PEG-IFN-α is known to be myelosuppressive and will have additive effects with other drugs with myelosuppressive activity. PEG-IFN-α is a weak inhibitor of CYP1A2 and could potentially cause drug interactions with other drugs requiring this isozyme.[28]

Table 33.4 Adverse Effects Associated With PEG-IFN-α

Central nervous system	Anxiety, depression, fatigue, fever, headache, insomnia, irritability, nervousness, pain, and rigor
Dermatologic	Alopecia, pruritus
Endocrine	Growth suppression
Gastrointestinal	Abdominal pain, anorexia, diarrhea, nausea, vomiting
Hematologic	Neutropenia
Local	Injection-site reaction
Metabolic	Increased serum ALT
Neuromuscular	Arthralgia, myalgia, weakness
Respiratory	Cough, flu-like symptoms

ALT, alanine aminotransferase; PEG-IFN-α, pegylated interferon alpha.

Physicochemical and Pharmacokinetic Properties

As mentioned earlier, the addition of polyethylene glycol units to IFN-α decreases its degradation and enhances its duration of action. This allows for a once-weekly dose given subcutaneously.[28]

Entecavir

Entecavir is a guanosine analogue in which the oxygen atom of deoxyribose has been replaced with a cyclopentane ring containing a methylidene group. Entecavir is indicated for the treatment of chronic HBV infection in adults and pediatric patients 2 years of age and older.

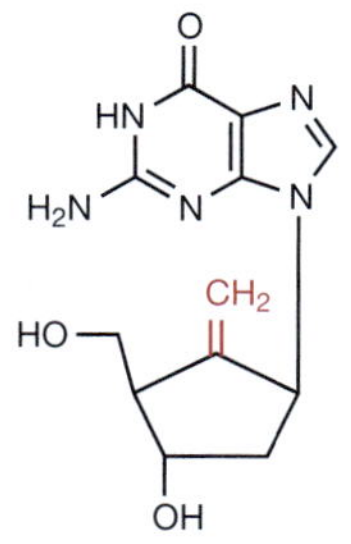

Entecavir
(prodrug)

Mechanism of Action and Structure-Activity Relationship

Entecavir is a prodrug that is phosphorylated by cellular kinases to its respective active triphosphate. Once activated, entecavir competitively competes with dGTP to inhibit three key steps required for the reverse transcription function of HBV polymerase. Inhibition of these steps suppresses HBV replication. Entecavir inhibits the (1) base priming of HBV, (2) reverse transcription of the negative strand from the pregenomic messenger RNA, and (3) synthesis of the positive strand of HBV DNA. Entecavir triphosphate is selective for HBV polymerase and does not interfere with human mitochondrial DNA synthesis. A key structural feature of entecavir is its methylidene group (highlighted in red). Entecavir triphosphate is able to be incorporated into HBV DNA; however, due to steric hindrance, it inhibits the polymerase.[119,120]

Common Adverse Effects and Drug Interactions

The most common adverse effects seen with entecavir are hematuria and an elevation in ALT levels. Other adverse effects, generally seen in less than 5% of patients, are skin rash, glycosuria, hyperglycemia, abdominal pain, diarrhea, dyspepsia, nausea, vomiting, headache, fatigue, and increased levels of serum lipase, creatinine, and bilirubin. There are no known drug interactions with entecavir; however, it should be administered 2 hours before or after a meal as food delays its absorption.[28]

Physicochemical and Pharmacokinetic Properties

Entecavir is water soluble with a log *P* value of −0.81. It has good oral bioavailability and is equally absorbed via tablets and solution. It is neither significantly bound to plasma proteins nor does it undergo any significant metabolism outside activation by kinase enzymes. It has a terminal half-life between 5 and 6 days and is primarily eliminated unchanged in the urine.[26,28,120]

Adefovir Dipivoxil

Adefovir dipivoxil is an adenosine analogue that is similar to acyclovir, penciclovir, ganciclovir, and cidofovir in that its structure has an acyclic chain instead of a ribose or deoxyribose sugar. Adefovir is indicated for the treatment of chronic HBV infection in patients at least 12 years old. Due to a high rate of resistance, the use of adefovir is relegated to second-line therapy.[28]

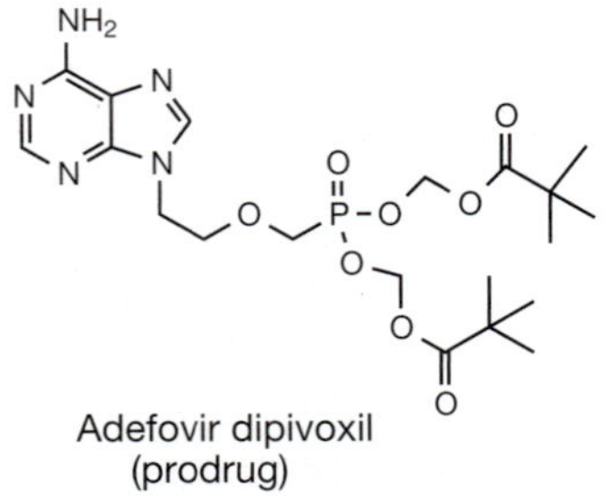

Mechanism of Action and Structure-Activity Relationship

Adefovir dipivoxil is a prodrug that must first undergo hydrolysis of its two pivoxil esters. The resulting drug, adefovir, then undergoes phosphorylation by cellular kinases to adefovir diphosphate, an alicyclic phosphonate that mimics ATP (Fig. 33.14). Adefovir diphosphate is then incorporated into HBV DNA and causes premature

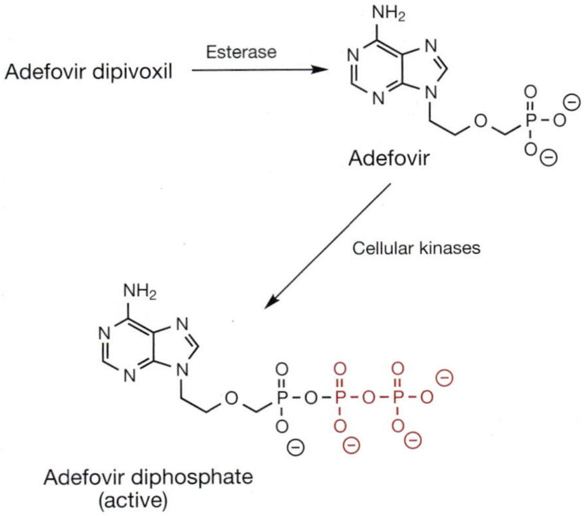

Figure 33.14 Activation of the prodrug adefovir dipivoxyl by esterase and cellular kinases.

termination of the chain due to the lack of a 3′-OH group. This premature termination of viral DNA synthesis is very similar to that discussed earlier in this chapter with acyclovir, penciclovir, ganciclovir, and cidofovir.[120,121] Resistance to adefovir has been shown to occur in approximately 6% of patients taking it for 2 to 3 years. Resistance is due to mutations in the HBV polymerase enzyme. Adefovir has been shown to be active against lamivudine-resistant HBV infections.

Common Adverse Effects and Drug Interactions

At the dose used to treat HBV infections, the adverse effects are very mild with dyspepsia and increased serum creatinine being the two most common reported adverse effects. Adefovir was originally developed to treat HIV infections; however, renal tubular dysfunction occurred at the higher dose required to treat HIV. These nephrotoxic adverse effects are not generally seen with the normal 10 mg once-daily doses used to treat HBV. Adefovir and its metabolites are substrates of OAT1/3. Other drugs that induce or inhibit these transporters could alter the renal elimination of adefovir.[28,120,121]

Physicochemical and Pharmacokinetic Properties

The dipivoxil esters enhance the overall lipid solubility of adefovir, thereby allowing this prodrug to have a 59% oral bioavailability. The drug is rapidly hydrolyzed and phosphorylated to its active diphosphate metabolite but does not undergo any further metabolism. Adefovir is minimally plasma protein bound and has an intracellular half-life of 18 hours, which allows for once-daily dosing, and is primarily eliminated in the urine.[26,28,120]

Telbivudine

Telbivudine is an analogue of thymidine in which the stereochemistry at the 3′ and 4′ positions of the deoxyribose sugar has been inverted. It is specific for HBV and is indicated for the treatment of chronic HBV infection.

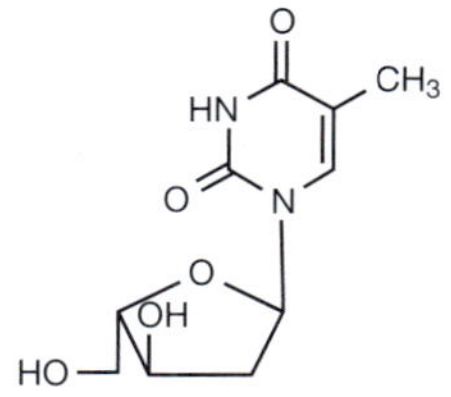

Telbivudine
(prodrug)

Mechanism of Action and Structure-Activity Relationship

Telbivudine is a prodrug that is converted by cellular kinases to telbivudine triphosphate. Once incorporated into viral DNA, it causes chain termination due to the altered stereochemistry of the 3′-OH group. This stereochemical inversion hinders its ability to effectively add the next nucleotide in the chain. HBV is an RT virus that requires two steps to convert a single-stranded RNA into a double-stranded DNA. The action of telbivudine is unique from lamivudine and other nucleosides in that its actions are primarily in the formation of the double-stranded DNA instead of the initial DNA-RNA intermediate. Telbivudine triphosphate is specific in that it does not inhibit human polymerases.[120,122]

Common Adverse Effects and Drug Interactions

Telbivudine can cause a number of adverse effects. The most common is an elevation of creatine phosphokinase (CPK) levels; however, this is transient and asymptomatic in most patients. Fatigue and headache are also common adverse effects, occurring in more than 10% of patients. Other adverse effects include abdominal pain, arthralgia, back pain, cough, diarrhea, dizziness, dyspepsia, fever, increased ALT and AST levels, insomnia, myalgia, nausea, neutropenia, pharyngolaryngeal pain, pruritis, and skin rash. Coadministration of PEG-IFN-α may enhance the incidence of peripheral neuropathy and should be avoided.[28]

Physicochemical and Pharmacokinetic Properties

Telbivudine is highly water soluble and is rapidly absorbed. The overall bioavailability is not known. It is neither plasma protein bound to any extent nor does it undergo any significant metabolism beyond its activation to the active triphosphate. Telbivudine has a terminal half-life elimination of 40 to 49 hours and is primarily eliminated in the urine.[28,120]

Antiviral Drugs to Treat Hepatitis C Viral Infections

Current guidelines for the treatment of HCV infections recommend the combination use of two or more inhibitors of specific NS HCV proteins with or without ribavirin. The specific proteins are NS3/4A, a protease that is responsible for cleaving the HCV polyprotein to produce specific proteins, NS5A, a protein that interacts with key viral components to regulate viral replication and assembly, and NS5B, an RNA-dependent RNA polymerase. Drugs that inhibit the NS HCV proteins are sometimes referred to as direct-acting antivirals (DAA) in order to distinguish them from the indirect-acting interferon that was previously, but no longer used, and ribavirin, which is not specific for HCV infections. The current recommended combinations as determined by the Infectious Diseases Society of America and the American Association for the Study of Liver Diseases are shown in Table 33.5. Also shown are combinations that were previously available but are no longer recommended.[123-125]

With the exception of sofosbuvir, an NS5B inhibitor, and ribavirin, all other drugs used to treat HCV infections are marketed as combination products. A summary of the available combinations is provided in Table 33.6.

Mechanism of Action and Structure-Activity Relationship

NS3/4A Inhibitors

The HCV NS3/4A protein is a serine protease that is essential for viral replication. Its function is to cleave the HCV polyprotein at four specific sites and generate the mature versions of NS3, NS4A, NS4B, NS5A, and NS5B proteins. The initial development of NS3/4A inhibitors focused on the use of linear peptidomimetics that contained a reactive ketoamide that occupied the cleavage site of the enzyme. The Ser139 responsible for catalyzing the polypeptide cleave forms a reversible bond with the electrophilic ketoamide. An example of this is shown in Figure 33.15 with boceprevir.[126]

While boceprevir, along with telaprevir and simeprevir, represents the first DAA drugs to treat HCV infections, they were voluntarily discontinued due to the development of drugs with better adverse drug reaction profiles and better therapeutic outcomes. Current NS3/4A inhibitors (Fig. 33.16) are structurally different from boceprevir in two aspects. The electrophilic ketoamide has been replaced with an acidic *N*-acylsulfonamide, and the linear peptidomimetic has been replaced by a macrocyclic peptidomimetic ring. These drugs act as competitive, reversible inhibitors of NS3/4A. Molecular modeling studies with glecaprevir revealed that the acidic functional *N*-acylsulfonamide group forms a key binding interaction with Lys136, and the bicyclic quinoxaline ring forms a cation-π interaction with His57. Additionally, van der Waals interactions with the hydrophobic regions of glecaprevir were noted. The interactions with glecaprevir are shown in Figure 33.16 and are also possible for the other NS3/4A inhibitors.[126,127]

HS5A Inhibitors

NS5A is one of the six NS proteins encoded in the single-stranded envelope of HCV RNA. NS5A consists of a 447-amino acid, zinc-binding phosphoprotein consisting of three domains connected by two linker regions. Once NS5A is cleaved from the HCV polyprotein, it has been shown to have multiple roles during replication. One is to interact with host cell membranes during virus replication. Its localization to membranes is followed by binding to the 3′-end of

Table 33.5 Recommended Combination Therapy for Adults With Hepatitis C Virus

Recommendations for Initial Therapy

Treatment-naïve without cirrhosis or with compensated cirrhosis

Recommended

Glecaprevir (NS3/4A inhibitor) + pibrentasvir (NS5A inhibitor)
Sofosbuvir (NS5B inhibitor) + velpatasvir (NS5A inhibitor)
Sofosbuvir (NS5B inhibitor) + ledipasvir (NS5A inhibitor)
Grazoprevir (NS3/4A inhibitor) + elbasvir (NS5A inhibitor)

Alternative

Sofosbuvir (NS5B inhibitor) + velpatasvir (NS5A inhibitor) + weight-based ribavirin
Sofosbuvir (NS5B inhibitor) + velpatasvir (NS5A inhibitor) + voxilaprevir (NS3/4A inhibitor)

Treatment-naïve with decompensated cirrhosis

Recommended

Sofosbuvir (NS5B inhibitor) + velpatasvir (NS5A inhibitor) with or without weight-based ribavirin
Sofosbuvir (NS5B inhibitor) + ledipasvir (NS5A inhibitor) with or without weight-based ribavirin

Recommendations for Retreatment in Patients With Prior Exposure

Recommended

Sofosbuvir (NS5B inhibitor) + velpatasvir (NS5A inhibitor) + voxilaprevir (NS3/4A inhibitor)
Sofosbuvir (NS5B inhibitor) + velpatasvir (NS5A inhibitor) + voxilaprevir (NS3/4A inhibitor) + weight-based ribavirin
Sofosbuvir (NS5B inhibitor) + velpatasvir (NS5A inhibitor) + weight-based ribavirin
Sofosbuvir (NS5B inhibitor) + glecaprevir (NS3/4A inhibitor) + pibrentasvir (NS5A inhibitor)
Sofosbuvir (NS5B inhibitor) + glecaprevir (NS3/4A inhibitor) + pibrentasvir (NS5A inhibitor) + weight-based ribavirin
Sofosbuvir (NS5B inhibitor) + ledipasvir (NS5A inhibitor) + weight-based ribavirin
Glecaprevir (NS3/4A inhibitor) + pibrentasvir (NS5A inhibitor)

Combinations No Longer Recommended

Ombitasvir (NS5A inhibitor), paritaprevir (NS3/4A inhibitor), and ritonavir
Ombitasvir (NS5A inhibitor), paritaprevir (NS3/4A inhibitor), ritonavir, and dasabuvir (NS5B inhibitor)

Table 33.6 Single and Combination NS Inhibitors to Treat Hepatitis C Virus Infections

Trade Name	Generic Names	Dosage Form and Strengths	Common Adverse Effects
Mavyret	Glecaprevir Pibrentasvir	Oral tablet: glecaprevir 100 mg/ pibrentasvir 40 mg	Fatigue, headache, and nausea
Zepatier	Elbasvir Grazoprevir	Oral tablet: elbasvir 50 mg/ grazoprevir 100 mg	Anemia, fatigue, headache, and nausea
Epclusa	Sofosbuvir Velpatasvir	Oral tablet: sofosbuvir 200 mg/ velpatasvir 50 mg; sofosbuvir 400 mg/ velpatasvir 100 mg	Anemia, diarrhea, fatigue, headache, insomnia, and nausea
Vosevi	Sofosbuvir Velpatasvir Voxilaprevir	Oral tablet: sofosbuvir 400 mg/velpatasvir 100 mg/voxilaprevir 100 mg	Diarrhea, fatigue, headache, increased serum bilirubin, and nausea
Harvoni	Ledipasvir Sofosbuvir	Oral tablet: ledipasvir 45 mg/ sofosbuvir 200 mg; ledipasvir 90 mg/ sofosbuvir 400 mg	Anemia, fatigue, headache, insomnia, and nausea
Sovaldi	Sofosbuvir	Oral tablet: 200 mg, 400 mg	Anemia, fatigue, headache, insomnia, and nausea
Viekira Pak	Ombitasvir Paritaprevir Ritonavir Dasabuvir	Oral tablet: ombitasvir 12.5 mg/ paritaprevir 75 mg/ritonavir 50 mg/ dasabuvir 250 mg	Anemia, asthenia, elevated ALT and bilirubin, fatigue, insomnia, nausea, pruritus, and skin reactions

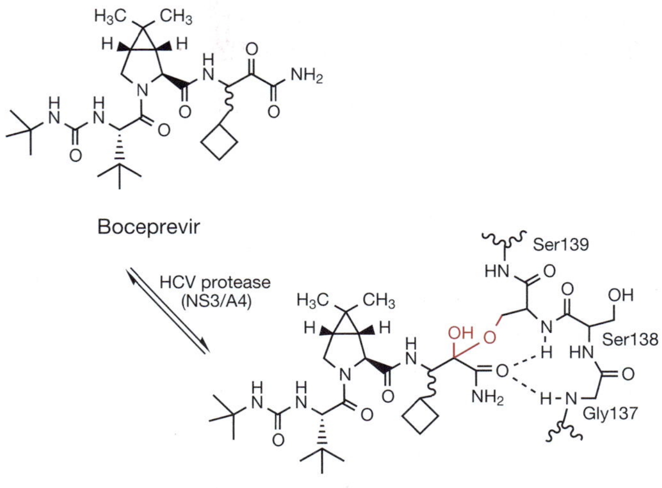

Figure 33.15 Representation of boceprevir reacting with the serine OH of hepatitis C virus (HCV) protease. This model is based on an x-ray co-crystal structure of telaprevir (discontinued from US market) bound to HCV NS3/4A protease complex.

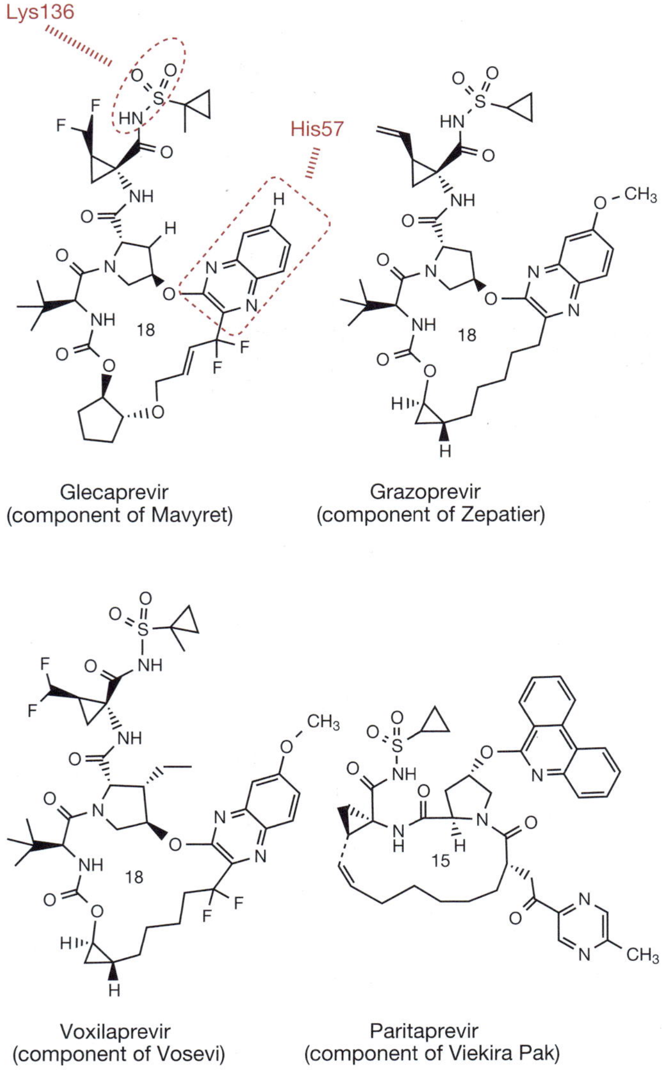

Figure 33.16 Inhibitors of hepatitis C virus (HCV) protease NS3/4a. Key binding interactions are shown for glecaprevir.

newly synthesized viral RNA and participation in genome replication. There are suggestions that NS5A may also play a role in the assembly and release of infectious HCV particles. Studies have shown that ledipasvir and ombitasvir bind to the NS5A protein to inhibit the development of HCV.

Key structural features that are required for binding and that are present in all NS5A inhibitors are a hydrophobic dimeric sequence located within the middle of the structure and a proline-valine-carbamate cap found at each end of the NS5A inhibitors (Fig. 33.17). Slight variations in the hydrophobic dimeric sequence as well as the proline-valine section are tolerated and allow the drug to bind to the HS5A protein.[128,129]

NS5B Inhibitors

NS5B is a viral RDRP that is essential for the viral particle to replicate. Currently two NS5B inhibitors are available: sofosbuvir and dasabuvir.

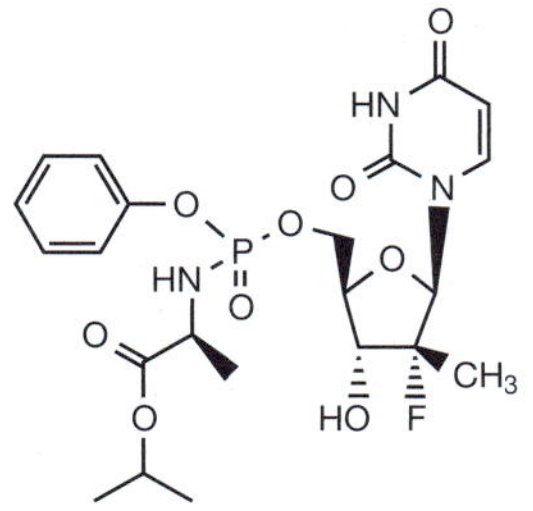

Sofosbuvir (Sovaldi)
(component of Epclusa,
Harvoni, Vosevi)
(prodrug)

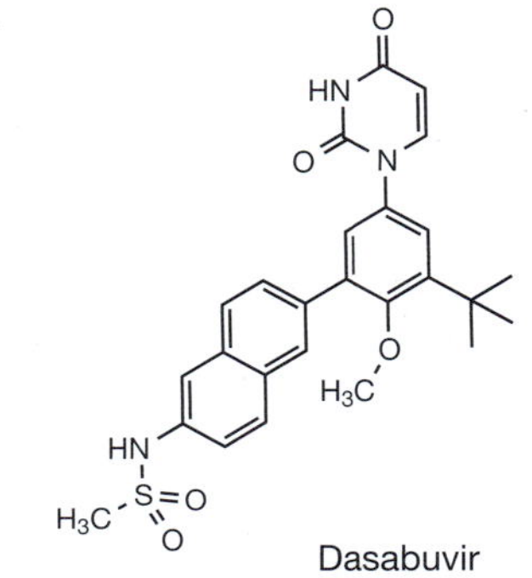

Dasabuvir
(component of
Viekira Pak)

Sofosbuvir is a prodrug that undergoes intracellular metabolism by multiple enzymes, including carboxylesterase 1, cathepisin A, uridine monophosphate-cytidine monophosphate kinase 1, and nucleoside diphosphate kinase, to form a uridine triphosphate analogue, which is shown in Figure 33.18. The resulting triphosphate can get incorporated into HCV RNA by the NS5B polymerase and acts as a chain terminator. The 2′-F group is electron-withdrawing and reduces the nucleophilicity of the 3′-OH group. Additionally, the 3-CH_3 group creates steric hindrance to further polymerization once incorporated into the HCV RNA.[130]

Dasabuvir is a nonnucleoside inhibitor of the HCV RDRP enzyme that binds to an allosteric site on the enzyme. This binding results in a conformational change in the enzyme that causes it to be nonfunctional. Dasabuvir has been designated as an NS5B-palm polymerase inhibitor. The palm domain contains the active site of the enzyme. A limitation of dasabuvir is that its binding site is poorly preserved across HCV genotypes.[131,132]

Common Adverse Effects and Drug Interactions

Since all NS3/4A inhibitors are used in combination with either an NS5A and/or an NS5B inhibitor, the adverse effects and drug interactions are due to the combined effects of all drugs in the combination. Anemia, fatigue, headache, and nausea appear to be the four most

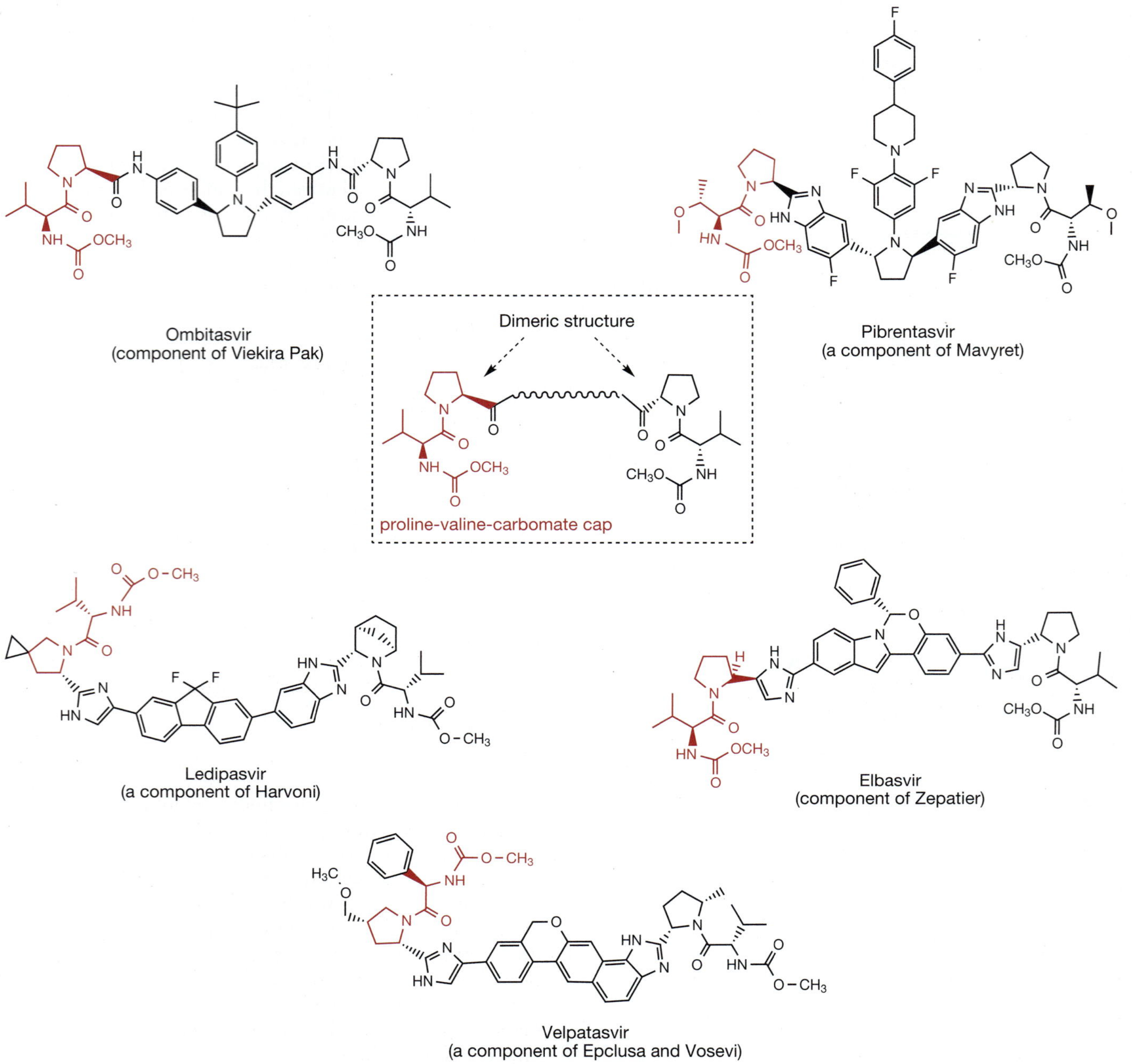

Figure 33.17 Inhibitors of hepatitis C virus (HCV) NS5A protein.

common adverse effects among all of the preparations. A list of common adverse effects for each preparation is provided in Table 33.6.[28]

Glecaprevir and Pibrentasvir

Glecaprevir and pibrentasvir are substrates of P-gp and/or BCRP, and glecaprevir is a substrate of OATP1B1/3. Coadministration of this combination with drugs that inhibit hepatic P-gp, BCRP, or OATP1B1/3 may increase the plasma concentrations of glecaprevir and/or pibrentasvir. Additionally, glecaprevir and pibrentasvir are inhibitors of the transport proteins mentioned earlier and may increase the plasma concentration of other drugs that require them for transport.[137]

Elbasvir and Grazoprevir

Grazoprevir is a substrate of OATP1B1/3 transporters, and both elbasvir and grazoprevir are substrates of CYP3A. Coadministration of grazoprevir with OATP1B1/3 inhibitors will significantly increase the plasma levels of grazoprevir. Coadministration with CYP3A inhibitors or inducers will increase or decrease plasma levels of these two drugs, respectively.[134]

Sofosbuvir

Sofosbuvir is a substrate of P-gp and BCRP; however, its active metabolite is not. Coadministration of sofosbuvir with P-gp inducers has been shown to decrease its absorption in the intestine.[135]

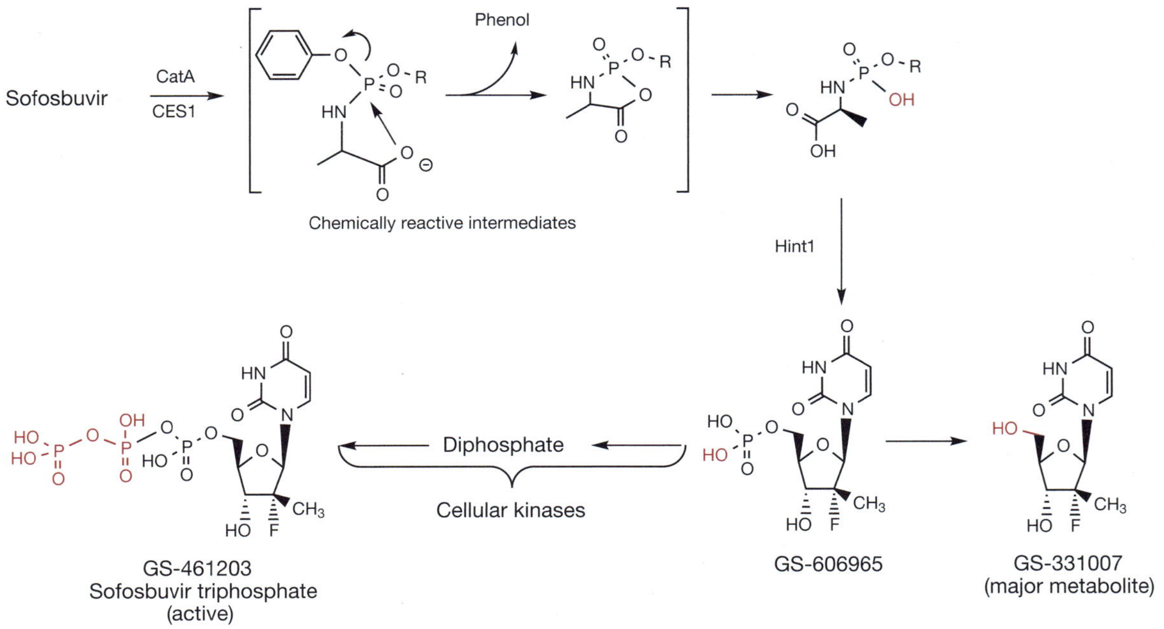

Figure 33.18 Metabolic activation of sofosbuvir to the active triphosphate form. This process is sequentially catalyzed by cathepsin A (CatA), carboxylesterase 1(CES1), and histidine triad nucleotide-binding protein 1 (HINT1). The intermediate constituent GS-606965 is inactivated by dephosphorylation or activated to the triphosphate by cellular kinases.

Sofosbuvir and Velpatasvir

Similar to sofosbuvir, velpatasvir is a substrate of P-gp and BCRP and should not be administered with P-gp inducers. Additionally, velpatasvir is an inhibitor of P-gp, BCRP, OATP1B1, OATP1B3, and OATP2B1. Coadministration of velpatasvir with drugs that require these transporters may increase their blood concentrations.[136]

Sofosbuvir, Velpatasvir, and Voxilaprevir

Drug interactions are similar to those seen with sofosbuvir alone and in combination with velpatasvir.[28]

Ledipasvir and Sofosbuvir

Ledipasvir is an inhibitor of P-gp and BCRP and may increase the intestinal absorption of other drugs that require these transporters. Similar to sofosbuvir, ledipasvir is a substrate of P-gp and BCRP and should not be administered with P-gp inducers.[28]

Ombitasvir, Paritaprevir, Ritonavir, and Dasabuvir

Paritaprevir is metabolized by the CYP3A4 isozyme, and dasabuvir is metabolized by the CYP2C8 isozyme. Therefore, other drugs inhibiting or inducing these isozymes have the potential to cause a drug interaction. Ritonavir is included in this combination to intentionally inhibit CYP3A4 and enhance the plasma levels of paritaprevir, similar to what was previously described with its combination with nirmatrelvir. Ombitasvir, paritaprevir, and dasabuvir are substrates of P-gp and BCRP. Paritaprevir is a substrate of OATP1B1 and OATP1B3. Other drugs affecting these transporters have the potential to cause drug interactions.[137]

Physicochemical and Pharmacokinetic Properties

The pharmacokinetic properties of NS inhibitors are provided in Table 33.7.[26,28,133-137] All of the NS3/4A protease inhibitors (PIs) contain a carbonyl group adjacent to their respective sulfonamide group. The carbonyl group enhances the acidity of the sulfonamide group, and the pK_a values for this functional group range from 3.74 to 3.8. As a result, this functional group will be ionized for all four of these inhibitors at physiologic pH. All of the NS5A protein inhibitors contain weakly basic functional groups. The structure of ombitasvir has an aromatic amine (pK_a = 2.16), while all of the other drugs in this class contain imidazole rings (pK_a ranging from 5.29 to 6.06) that will be primarily unionized at physiological pH. While the structures of the NS3/4A and NS5A inhibitors are similar to one another, respectively, the two NS5B polymerase inhibitors are structurally different. Dasabuvir contains an acidic sulfonamide functional group; however, since it is not adjacent to an electron-withdrawing group, as seen with the NS3/4A inhibitors, it is a weak acid (pK_a = 9.1) and is primarily unionized at physiological pH. The prodrug, sofosbuvir, is unionized at physiological pH; however, when converted to its active triphosphate metabolite, it is extensively ionized.

With the exception of sofosbuvir, all HCV NS inhibitors are highly lipid soluble and are extensively bound to plasma proteins. Despite the high lipid solubility, glecaprevir (an NS3/4A PI), ledipasvir, and pibrentasvir (NS5A inhibitors) undergo minimal to no metabolism and are primarily excreted unchanged. Sofosbuvir undergoes metabolic activation to its triphosphate, which is then primarily excreted in the urine. All other HCV NS inhibitors are primarily eliminated in the feces.

Table 33.7 Pharmacokinetic Properties of Hepatitis C Virus Nonstructural (NS) Inhibitors

Drug	Calculated Log *P*	Protein Binding (%)	Half-Life (h)	Metabolism	Major Route(s) of Elimination
NS3/4A Protease Inhibitors					
Glecaprevir	4.26	97.5	6	Minimal by CYP3A	Primarily fecal
Grazoprevir	3.26	98.8	31	Oxidative metabolism by CYP3A	Primarily fecal
Paritaprevir	3.5	97-98.6	5.5	Oxidative metabolism by CYP3A	Fecal (88%) Renal (8.8%)
Voxilaprevir	3.98	>99	33	Oxidative metabolism by CYP3A4 (major), CYP2C8, and CYP1A2 (minor)	Primarily biliary/ fecal
NS5A Protein Inhibitors					
Elbasvir	5.6	>99.9	24	Oxidative metabolism by CYP3A	Primarily fecal
Ledipasvir	5.98	>99.8	47	Minor, predominately eliminated unchanged	Fecal (87%) Renal (1%)
Ombitasvir	5.72	>99.9	21-25	Amide hydrolysis and oxidative metabolism	Fecal (90.2%) Renal (1.8%)
Pibrentasvir	5.95	>99.9	13	None	Primarily fecal
Velpatasvir	5.39	>99.5	15	Oxidative metabolism by CYP2B6, CYP2C8, and CYP3A4	Primarily fecal
NS5B Polymerase Inhibitors					
Dasabuvir	4.7	>99.5	5.5-6	Oxidative metabolism: CYP2C8 (major) and CYP3A4 (minor)	Fecal (94.4%) Renal (2%)
Sofosbuvir	1.63	61-65	0.4	Hydrolyzed and phosphorylated	Renal (80%) Fecal (14%) Respiratory (2.5%)

Human Immunodeficiency Virus

AIDS was first recognized in 1981, when a series of rare opportunistic infections appeared at unexpected rates in young homosexual men.[138] By 1983, HIV, a retrovirus that targets cells of the immune system, was identified as the cause of AIDS. Since that time, HIV had become a worldwide epidemic that continues to expand. It is estimated that there are 39 million people living with HIV across the globe as of 2022, of which 1.5 million are children under the age of 15 years. It was further estimated that 1.3 million new patients would be infected with HIV worldwide in 2022, with approximately 32,000 new infections in the United States. While these statistics appear to be bleak, the rate of new infections and the rate of AIDS-related deaths have both declined sharply. Annual deaths around the world due to AIDS-related complications have declined from a peak of 1.9 million in 2004 to 630,000 in 2022.[139] The reduction in new cases and AIDS-related deaths is due, in large part, to the success of highly active antiretroviral therapy (HAART). Although not curative for HIV, HAART effectively suppresses viral replication, preserves immune function, and prolongs the survival of patients infected with HIV.

HIV is part of the Lentivirus genus, which is associated with long incubation periods after acute infection. There are two main types of HIV: HIV-1 and HIV-2. Although both types share similar modes of transmission and can lead to immunosuppression, they only share 60% identity at the amino acid level.[140] HIV-1 is responsible for most HIV infections in the United States and globally. HIV-2 is less transmissible than HIV-1 and is endemic to West Africa, although cases are now found worldwide.[141] For the sake of this chapter, we will focus on HIV-1.

HIV-1 is an enveloped virus with two identical single-stranded RNA molecules within the viral particle, each of which contains information for only nine genes. The nine-step HIV infectious cycle is depicted in Figure 33.19 and begins when the viral envelope protein gp120 attaches to the CD4 receptor on host cells. CD4 is expressed on helper CD4 T cells and on monocytes/macrophages of the immune system, which explains the tropism of HIV for immune cells. After engaging CD4, gp120 undergoes a conformational change that allows it to attach to a co-receptor on the host cell (step 1). The co-receptors for HIV (CXCR4 or CCR5) are chemokine receptors that are widely expressed on human cells. Upon co-receptor binding, the viral gp41 protein inserts into the host cell membrane and fuses the viral

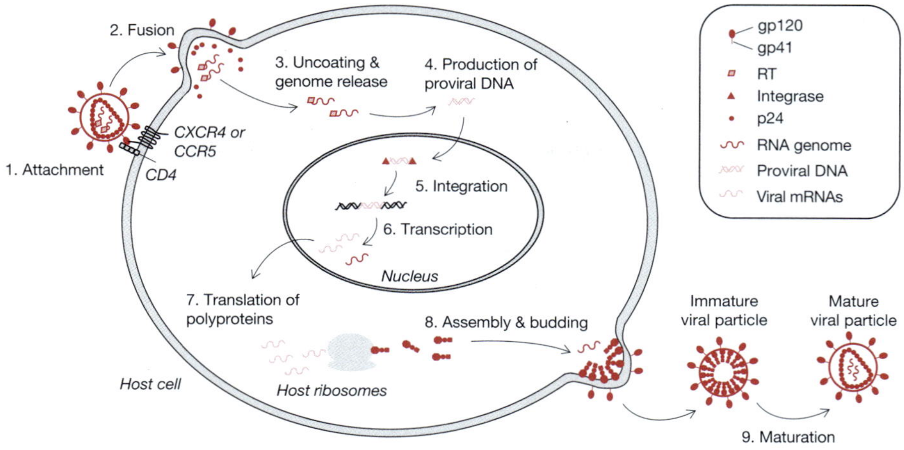

Figure 33.19 HIV infectious cycle. mRNA, messenger RNA; RT, reverse transcriptase.

envelope and cell membrane together, allowing for the viral capsid to enter the host cell (step 2). Following uncoating and genome release (step 3), the viral RNA genome serves as a substrate for RT, producing a proviral double-stranded DNA that is transported into the nucleus (step 4). The viral integrase enzyme then integrates (ie, incorporates) it into the host DNA (step 5). At this stage, the virus may enter a period of latency where the proviral DNA is not expressed. However, if the infected T cell is stimulated, the proviral DNA is transcribed and translated to produce new copies of the viral genome and polyproteins (steps 6 and 7). Similar to the positive-sense RNA viruses, the viral proteins are synthesized as large polyproteins, which assemble at the plasma membrane to allow budding of new viral particles (step 8). This initially produces an immature viral particle that is uninfectious. However, cleavage of the polyproteins by HIV protease produces the p24 protein and other viral proteins, allowing for assembly of the capsid, and formation of the mature, infectious virus (step 9). The HIV proteins and enzymes described here are targets of antiretroviral (ARV) agents.[142]

HIV-1 is transmitted by bodily fluids (eg, blood, semen, breastmilk). Sexual contact is the most common route of transmission, and an important risk factor is the use of nonsterile drug injections. Vertical transmission from the mother to the infant is also possible during delivery or breastfeeding, although HIV testing during pregnancy and antiretroviral therapy (ART) have greatly reduced perinatal transmission in the United States.[143] During acute HIV infection, viral titers are high, and symptoms are often nonspecific (eg, fever, fatigue, headache). A relatively long clinical latency follows, which can last several years. During this time, individuals may be asymptomatic, but viral replication persists, and the level of $CD4^+$ helper T cells steadily declines. Eventually, the patient's immune system becomes compromised, resulting in a variety of opportunistic infections and potentially meeting the criteria for AIDS. As discussed earlier, certain viral infections and conditions, such as CMV and Kaposi sarcoma, are of particular concern in patients with HIV experiencing immunosuppression.

Importantly, HAART has revolutionized the treatment of HIV and greatly reduced AIDS-related deaths. However, HIV remains a clinical challenge. The RT enzyme of HIV is highly error prone and makes mistakes transcribing the viral RNA genome, leading to mutations in the virus. These mutations can lead to drug resistance and/or evasion of the antibody response of the host. Thus, HIV vaccines, which ideally should induce the production of antibodies that recognize and bind to gp120, have not yet been effective. As will be discussed later, other viral processes, such as reverse transcription and proteolytic processing, are viable targets for small-molecule therapy.

Antiviral Drugs to Treat Human Immunodeficiency Virus Infections

In 1987, zidovudine became the first drug approved for the treatment of HIV infections. Since that time, over 30 individual drugs comprising six major classes have been approved. A timeline for the approval of HIV medications can be found at HIVinfo.NIH.gov.[144] The six major classes of HIV drugs are:

1. Nucleoside reverse transcriptase inhibitors (NRTIs)
2. Nonnucleoside reverse transcriptase inhibitors (NNRTIs)
3. Integrase strand transfer inhibitors (INSTIs)
4. PIs
5. Fusion and entry inhibitors
6. Capsid inhibitors

Current guidelines for the treatment of HIV infections in naïve and experienced patients consider individualized regimens that are based on the efficacy of the ARV regimen, potential adverse effects and drug interactions, dosing frequency, existing comorbid conditions, and known resistance or genetic factors.[145] ARV regimens for treatment-naïve patient generally consists of two NRTIs administered in combination with a third active ARV drug from one of three drug classes: an INSTI, an NNRTI, or a PI with a pharmacokinetic enhancer (also known as a booster). Specific recommended regimens are listed in the guidelines and are not repeated here, as they often change based on new developments and the introduction of new drugs.

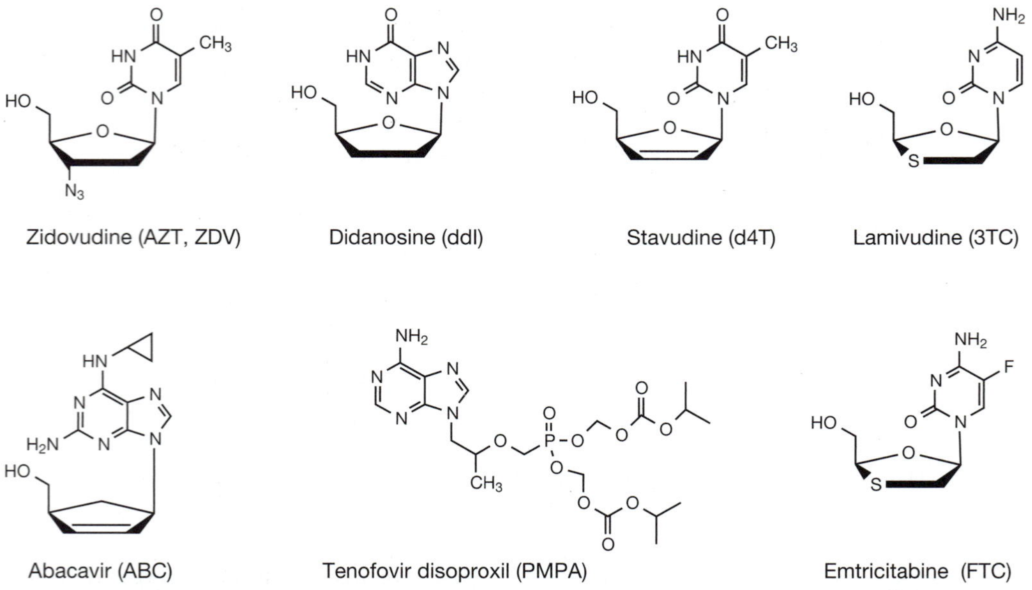

Figure 33.20 Nucleoside reverse transcriptase inhibitors (NRTIs).

Nucleoside Reverse Transcriptase Inhibitors

The seven currently available NRTIs are shown in Figure 33.20. All of these drugs are prodrugs that need to undergo phosphorylation in order to be converted to a tripeptide mimic of one of the four naturally occurring DNA nucleotides. Abacavir, didanosine, and tenofovir must undergo additional metabolic process to form their respective active triphosphates. A list of the active metabolites for all of the NRTIs and the nucleotides that they mimic can be found in Table 33.8. To avoid redundant or competitive therapy, it is essential that the two NRTIs used to treat HIV infections mimic different nucleotides (eg, lamivudine and tenofovir) and not the same nucleotide (eg, stavudine and zidovudine).[26,120,146,147]

Mechanism of Action and Structure-Activity Relationship

The mechanism of action of NRTIs is similar to that discussed earlier with acyclovir, penciclovir, ganciclovir, and cidofovir. While tenofovir contains an alicyclic phosphonate, all other NRTIs contain modified deoxyribose rings that lack a 3′-OH group. Zidovudine, stavudine, lamivudine, and emtricitabine can be directly converted to their respective triphosphates and incorporated into viral DNA by the HIV reverse transcription enzyme. Once present in viral DNA, the lack of the 3′-OH group will cause immediate viral DNA chain termination. All NRTIs inhibit RNA- and DNA-dependent DNA polymerase activities of RT.[26,28,120]

Didanosine, abacavir, and tenofovir require additional metabolism in order to form their active triphosphate metabolites but are ultimately incorporated into viral DNA and cause immediate viral DNA chain termination. Didanosine is an inosine analogue and can be converted to dideoxy-ATP through a normal endogenous biosynthetic pathway (Fig. 33.21).[15,120] Abacavir initially undergoes phosphorylation to abacavir monophosphate by adenosine phosphotransferase. This is then followed by a deamination catalyzed by a cytosolic enzyme to form carbovir monophosphate. The name of this intermediate comes from the presence of a carbocyclic ring instead of an altered deoxyribose ring. Subsequent phosphorylations provide the active carbovir triphosphate, a structural analogue of guanosine triphosphate (Fig. 33.22).[120,148] Tenofovir is available in two forms, a disoproxil diester shown in

Table 33.8 Active Metabolites and Mimics of Nucleoside Reverse Transcriptase Inhibitors

Drug and Abbreviations	Active Metabolite	Nucleotide Mimicked
Abacavir (ABC)	Carbovir triphosphate	dGTP
Didanosine (ddI)	Dideoxy-ATP (ddATP)	dATP
Emtricitabine (FTC)	3′-Thio-epi-fluoro-CTP	dCTP
Lamivudine (3TC)	3′-Thio-epi-CTP	dCTP
Stavudine (d4T)	Dehydro-dideoxy-TTP	dTTP
Tenofovir (PMPA)	Tenofovir diphosphate	dATP
Zidovudine (AZT, ZDV)	Deoxy-3′-aza-TTP	dTTP

dATP, deoxyadenosine triphosphate; dCTP, deoxycytidine triphosphate; dGTP, deoxyguanosine triphosphate; dTTP, deoxythymidine triphosphate

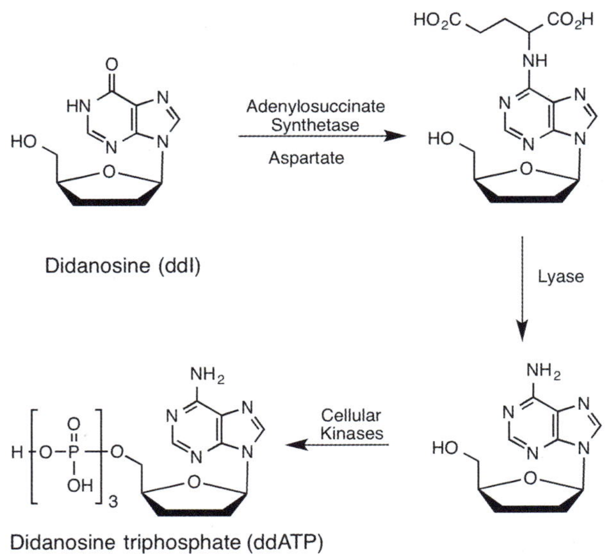

Figure 33.21 Bioactivation of didanosine.

Figure 33.20 and a phosphonoamidate ester identical to those present in remdesivir and sofosbuvir. The disoproxil diester is cleaved via plasma esterases, while the phosphonoamide ester requires multiple cellular enzymatic steps, as shown in Figure 33.18 with sofosbuvir. The resulting phosphonate is then phosphorylated to the active tenofovir diphosphate. The phosphonoamidate ester was developed to reduce adverse effects since its activation occurs in infected cells and not in the blood. This results in lower concentrations in the bloodstream, but higher concentrations within the infected cells.

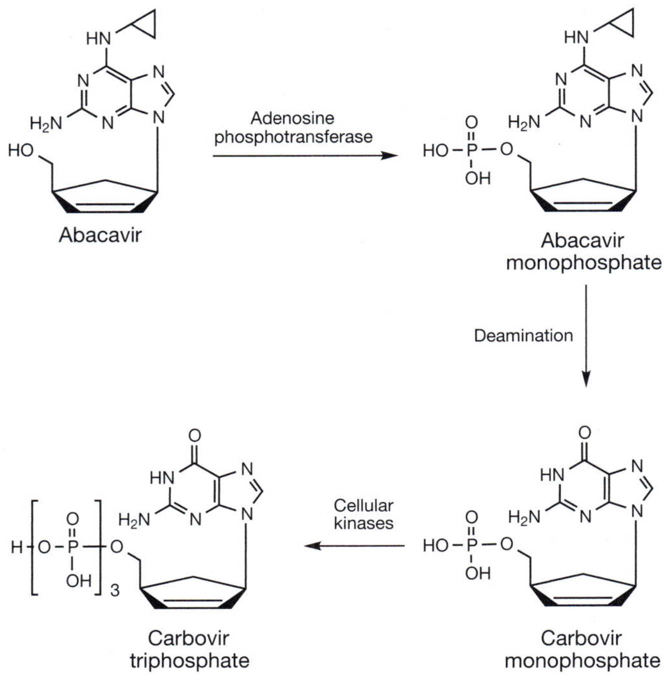

Figure 33.22 Bioactivation of abacavir.

Common Adverse Effects and Drug Interactions

A complete list of adverse effects for the NRTIs can be found in Table 33.9. Zidovudine, didanosine, stavudine, and zalcitabine were the first four NRTIs approved by the FDA and tend to have the most adverse effects. Dose-limiting toxicities for these drugs include myelosuppression for zidovudine and peripheral neuropathy for the other three drugs. Zalcitabine caused peripheral neuropathy in approximately 33% of patients and was discontinued in 2006. In contrast, emtricitabine, lamivudine, and tenofovir are well tolerated. The difference between these drugs can be attributed to their respective selectivity for human DNA polymerase-γ, a mitochondrial enzyme. Zidovudine, didanosine, and stavudine inhibit this enzyme, thereby resulting in anemia, granulocytopenia, myopathy, peripheral neuropathy, pancreatitis, and lactic acidosis. Lamivudine, emtricitabine, and tenofovir have a much lower affinity for DNA polymerase-γ and produce significantly less adverse effects.

Abacavir can cause a serious and potentially fatal hypersensitivity reactions, especially in patients who carry the HLA-B*5701 allele. Hypersensitivity reactions include fever, GI symptoms, malaise, rash and, on average, usually occur after 11 days. Prior to initiating therapy, all patients should be screened for the HLA-B*5701 allele. Abacavir is contraindicated in patients who test positive for the HLA-B*5701 allele and those with a prior hypersensitivity reaction to abacavir.

NRTIs are not metabolized by CYP450 enzymes and have relatively few drug interactions.[28,120,149]

Physicochemical and Pharmacokinetic Properties

The pharmacokinetic properties of the NRTIs can be found in Table 33.10. Due to the presence of their purine or pyrimidine rings, all NRTIs are weakly basic prior to metabolic activation. After activation to their respective triphosphates, these drugs are highly acidic. All these drugs are highly water soluble, have variable oral bioavailability, and are primarily or exclusively eliminated in the urine.[26,28]

Nonnucleoside Reverse Transcriptase Inhibitors

The six currently available NNRTIs are shown in Figure 33.23. This class of HIV medications can be subdivided into first- and second-generation drugs. Delavirdine, efavirenz, and nevirapine were approved in the mid- to late-1990s and are generally less sterically flexible than the second-generation drugs, etravirine (approved in 2008), rilpivirine (approved in 2011), and doravirine (approved in 2018).

Mechanism of Action and Structure-Activity Relationship

All NNRTIs bind to an allosteric site that is adjacent to the catalytic site within HIV-1 RT. This results in the inhibition of both RNA- and DNA-dependent polymerases and the synthesis of the viral complementary DNA (cDNA). Unlike NRTIs, NNRTIs neither require intracellular activation nor do they compete with normal nucleotides for bindings.

Table 33.9 Adverse Effects of Nucleoside Reverse Transcriptase Inhibitors (NRTIs) and Nonnucleoside Reverse Transcriptase Inhibitors (NNRTIs)

Drug	Adverse Effects
NRTIs	
Abacavir	Hypersensitivity reactions; increased risk of myocardial infarction
Didanosine	*Most common:* peripheral neuropathy, pancreatitis *Other adverse effects:* GI disturbances, insulin resistance, non-cirrhotic portal hypertension, optic neuritis and retinal changes
Emtricitabine	Well tolerated; hyperpigmentation of palms and soles
Lamivudine	Well tolerated
Stavudine	*Most common:* peripheral neuropathy *Other adverse effects:* diabetes, fatal lactic acidosis, hyperlipidemia, increased aminotransferase levels, pancreatitis
Tenofovir	Well tolerated; renal toxicity, decreased bone density and osteomalacia
Zidovudine	*Most common:* myelosuppression (neutropenia and anemia) *Other adverse effects:* diabetes, fatigue, headache, insomnia, malaise, nausea
NNRTIs	
Delavirdine	*Most common:* rash *Other adverse effects:* nausea, headache
Doravirine	Well tolerated; nausea, dizziness, abnormal dreams
Efavirenz	*Most common:* CNS effects (dizziness, abnormal dreams, headache, depression, suicidality, insomnia, somnolence) *Other adverse effects:* rash, QTc prolongation
Etravirine	Well tolerated; rash (including Stevens-Johnson syndrome)
Nevirapine	Rash (including Stevens-Johnson syndrome), hepatotoxicity (including hepatic failure), fever, nausea, headache
Rilpivirine	Depression, headache, skin rash, QTc prolongation

CNS, central nervous system; GI, gastrointestinal; QTc, corrected QT interval.

Table 33.10 Pharmacokinetic Properties of Nucleoside Reverse Transcriptase Inhibitors

Drug	Log *P*	Oral Bioavailability (%)	Half-Life (h)	Metabolism[a]	Route of Elimination
Abacavir	0.61	83-86	0.9-2.1	Alcohol dehydrogenase and glucuronide conjugation	Urine
Didanosine	–0.99	30-54	1-1.4	Purine metabolism to xanthine and uric acid	Urine
Emtricitabine	–0.3	75-93	10	Oxidation to sulfoxide; glucuronide conjugation	Urine (major) Feces (minor)
Lamivudine	–1.3	74-100	5-7	Oxidation to sulfoxide	Urine
Stavudine	–0.73	77-86	0.8-1.5	None	Urine
Tenofovir	–1.5	40-65	32	None	Urine
Zidovudine	–0.1	54-74	0.5-3	Glucuronide conjugation	Urine

[a]Metabolic processes listed do not include the bioactivation to triphosphates.

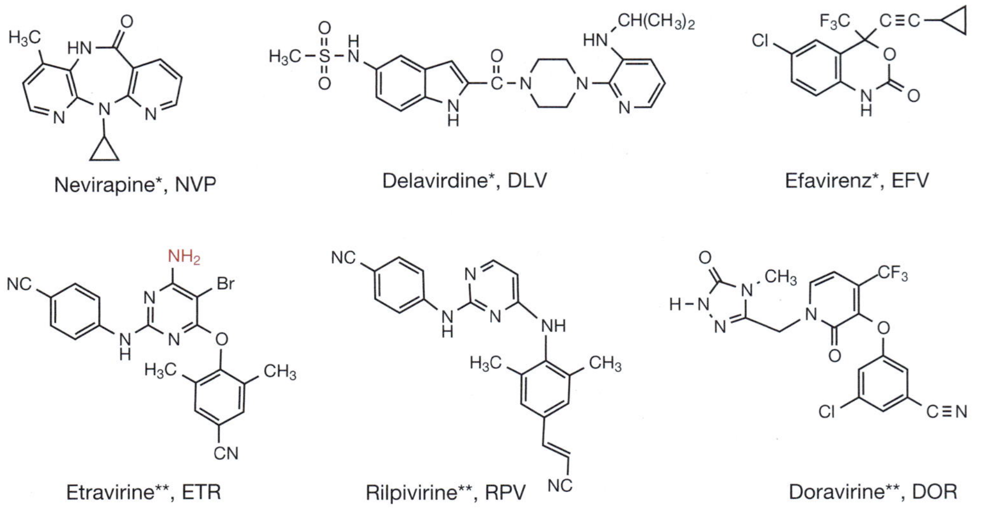

*1st Generation NNRTIs **2nd Generations NNRTIs

Figure 33.23 Nonnucleoside reverse transcriptase inhibitors (NNRTIs).

The NNRTIs do not inhibit HIV-2 RT, the human cellular DNA polymerases α, β, or the mitochondrial DNA polymerase γ. The specificity for HIV-1 RT is due to the presence of a unique hydrophobic binding pocket. Binding to this hydrophobic pocket causes a conformational change in HIV-1 RT and inhibits the enzyme. The NNRTIs have been proposed to assume a Y-shaped structure that allows π interactions with aromatic side chains of HIV RT residues located adjacent to the NNRTI-binding pocket.[150-155] An example of this is shown in Figure 33.24 with the binding of efavirenz. The cyclopropylethynyl group binds in a subpocket that contains the hydrophobic side chains of Tyr181, Tyr188, Trp229, and Phe227. Additionally, the benzoxazin-2-one ring system forms van der Waals and hydrophobic interactions with Leu100, Val106, and Tyr318. Finally, a key hydrogen bond is made with the mainchain carbonyl of Lys101 and the nitrogen atom.[156]

Resistance to the first-generation NNRTIs is thought to be due to mutations that occur near their binding sites on HIV-1 RT. The development of second-generation NNRTIs sought to overcome this resistance. As compared to the first-generation agents, the second-generation agents have a higher genetic barrier for initiating resistance and exhibit ARV activity against viral strains with reduced sensitivity to first-generation NNRTIs. This advantage has been attributed to the conformational flexibility about the central pyridine or pyridinone rings of these drugs and an increase ability to bind HIV RT.[157]

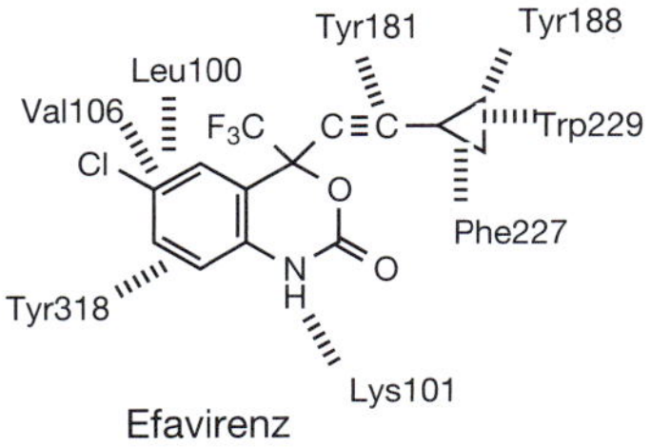

Figure 33.24 Binding interactions of efavirenz with the allosteric site of reverse transcriptase.

Common Adverse Effects and Drug Interactions

A complete list of adverse effects for the NNRTIs can be found in Table 33.9. Based on their efficacy and adverse effect profile, doravirine, efavirenz, and rilpivirine are the three currently recommended NNRTIs for initial use in combination with other ARV drugs. Of these three, doravirine is the best tolerated and exhibits the least number of adverse effects. A common adverse effect seen in all other NNRTIs is a skin rash. Efavirenz and rilpivirine can also prolong the corrected QT interval (QTc) interval, while efavirenz is known to cause a number of CNS effects. Nevirapine can cause severe hepatoxicity and is rarely used due to toxicity. Etravirine, while well tolerated, is not recommended as first-line therapy due to insufficient data in ART-naïve patients. Delavirdine is also well tolerated; however, it has shown inferior efficacy in treating HIV infections and must be dosed 3 times a day. All other NNRTIs can be dosed once daily, except for etravirine, which is dosed twice daily.[28,145,149]

Due to their lipophilic nature, all NNRTIs undergo oxidative metabolism with CYP450 isozymes and can either induce or inhibit these isozymes. As a result, drug interactions can occur when an NNRTI is used in combination with CYP450 inhibitors or inducers or with other drugs that require these isozymes for normal metabolism. Doravirine and rilpivirine are metabolized by CYP3A4 but do not inhibit or induce this isozyme. Efavirenz is primarily metabolized by CYP2B6 but is also a substrate for CYP3A4 and CYP2A6. Additionally, efavirenz is an inducer of CYP3A4, CYP2B6, and CYP2C19. Nevirapine is metabolized by CYP3A4 and CYP2D6 and also induces the activity of these isozymes. Delavirdine is primarily metabolized by CYP3A4 and is also a weak inhibitor of this isozyme. Etravirine is metabolized

Table 33.11 Pharmacokinetic Properties of Nonnucleoside Reverse Transcriptase Inhibitors

Drug	Log *P*	Protein Binding (%)	Oral Bioavailability (%)	Half-Life (h)	Metabolism[a]	Route of Elimination (%)
Delavirdine	2.77	98	85-100	5.8	Demethylation (major)	Urine (51) Feces (44)
Doravirine	3.51	76	64	15	Oxidation and rearrangement of triazole ring	Urine (major) Feces (minor)
Efavirenz	3.89	>99	42	40-55	Aromatic hydroxylation; glucuronide conjugation	Urine (34) Feces (61)
Etravirine	3.67	99.9	NA[b]	41 (±20)	Methyl and aromatic hydroxylation; glucuronide conjugation	Urine Feces (86, primarily unchanged)
Nevirapine	1.75	60	75-93	45	Methyl and aromatic hydroxylation; glucuronide conjugation	Urine (81) Feces (10)
Rilpivirine	3.8	99.7	NA	50	Methyl and aromatic hydroxylation; glucuronide conjugation	Urine (6) Feces (85)

[a]Specific CYP450 enzymes provided in text.
[b]Information not available.

by CYP3A4, CYP2C9, and CYP2C19 and also affects these isozymes. It is an inducer of CYP3A4 and an inhibitor of both CYP2C9 and CYP2C19.[28,145]

Coadministration of rilpivirine and delavirdine with drugs that increase gastric pH (eg, H_2 antagonists, proton pump inhibitors, antacids) can decrease the absorption of these two drugs. While the structure of etravirine is very similar to that of rilpivirine, its absorption is not dependent on gastric pH. The addition of a nitrogen atom (highlighted in red in Fig. 33.23) enhances the basicity of the pyrimidine ring and eliminates the pH-dependent absorption.

Physicochemical and Pharmacokinetic Properties

The pharmacokinetic properties of the NNRTIs can be found in Table 33.11.[26,28] Unlike the NRTIs, the NNRTIs are much more lipid soluble and, with the exception of etravirine, undergo extensive oxidative metabolism and glucuronide conjugation to form inactive metabolites. Interestingly, etravirine is significantly lipid soluble; however, it is primarily excreted unchanged. In contrast, nevirapine has the lowest lipid solubility, but it is significantly metabolized. The primary routes of metabolism for efavirenz, etravirine, nevirapine, and rilpivirine are aromatic and methyl oxidation followed by glucuronide conjugation. Doravirine undergoes oxidation and rearrangement of its triazole ring, and delavirdine undergoes N-dealkylation. Metabolic pathways of delavirdine, doravirine, efavirenz, and rilpivirine are shown in Figure 33.25. The metabolism of etravirine and nevirapine is omitted since etravirine is primarily excreted unchanged and nevirapine is rarely used due to toxicity.

Integrase Strand Transfer Inhibitors

Integrase, along with RT and protease, is one of three core enzymes encoded by the HIV genome. It is essential for successful integration of viral genetic material into the host genome and successful replication of the virus. INSTIs are drugs targeted to integrase, a viral enzyme that inserts the viral genome into the DNA of the host cell.[158] Strand integration is a critical step that occurs during retroviral replication, and thus inhibition of integrase prevents replication and prevents spread of the virus. Shown in Figure 33.26 are the five currently approved INSTIs. These drugs are structurally similar to one another, and all contain a β-dicarbonyl group (or analogue) that can chelate metals. Raltegravir, dolutegravir, and carbotegravir are available as individual drugs and in a variety of combinations, while elvitegravir is only available as a combination with cobicistat, emtricitabine, and tenofovir alafenamide (Genvoya), and bictegravir is only available as a combination with emtricitabine, and tenofovir alafenamide (Biktarvy).

Mechanism of Action and Structure-Activity Relationship

The mechanism of the integrase enzyme is shown in Figure 33.27. Following the production of viral cDNA by RT in the cytosol, it becomes part of a nucleoprotein complex known as the preintegration complex (PIC). The PIC is then transported to the nucleus in order for the viral cDNA to be integrated into cellular DNA. Prior to integration, the 3′-ends are modified, and the cleavage of a terminal 3′-GT dinucleotide sequence occurs on both

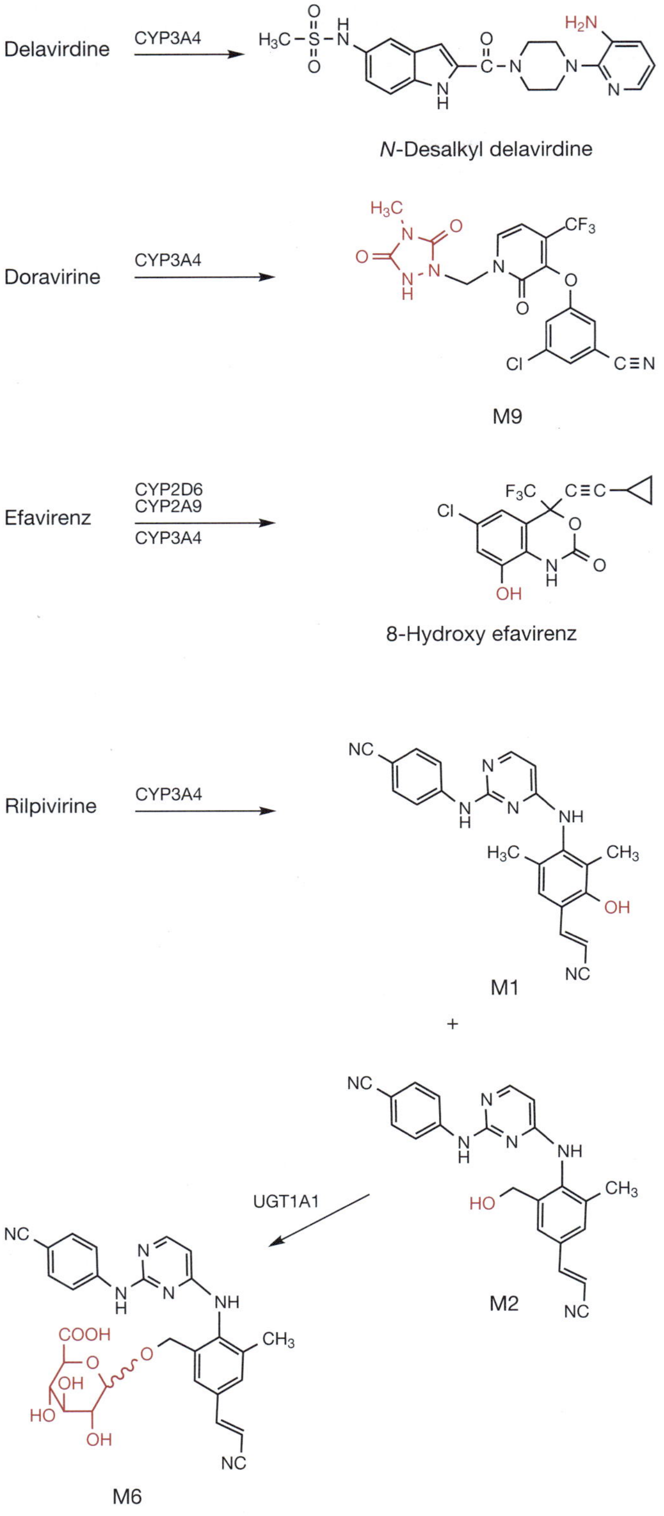

Figure 33.25 Metabolic pathways for nonnucleoside reverse transcriptase inhibitors (NNRTIs).

strands of the viral cDNA. Following this, the 3′-OH groups attack phosphodiester bonds on the host DNA, allowing the viral cDNA to become a permanent part of the host cellular DNA. Cellular enzymes, such as DNA ligase, are required to repair the cellular DNA and complete the integration process. HIV integrase is composed

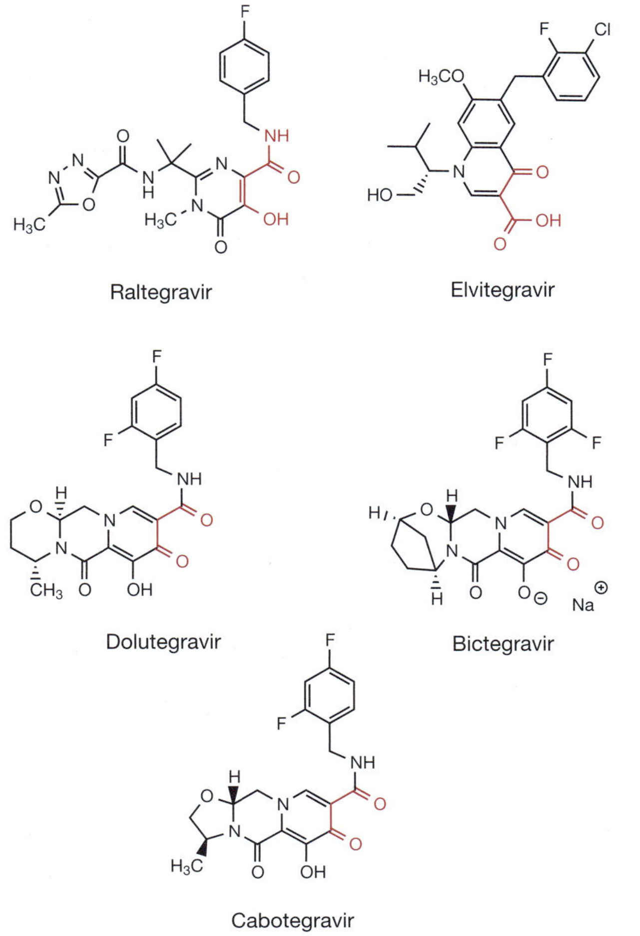

Figure 33.26 Integrase strand transfer inhibitors (INSTIs). The red highlight indicates the pharmacophore in INSTIs.

of three regions: an amino terminal domain, the catalytic core domain (CCD), and the carboxy-terminal domain. An essential part of the CCD is the presence of a metallic cationic cofactor, normally manganese (Mn^{2+}) or magnesium (Mg^{2+}), that binds to both the phosphate groups on DNA and either aspartate or glutamate residues within the CCD of the integrase enzyme.[159-161]

INSTIs interfere with the process described earlier by chelating a divalent cation at the CCD site of HIV integrase. This interaction is shown in Figure 33.28 with raltegravir; however, similar functional groups are present in all INSTIs (see Fig. 33.26). In this interaction, the INSTI binds to the integrase enzyme, prevents the enzyme from binding to viral cDNA, and prevents the integration of viral cDNA into cellular DNA. Coplanarity between the chelating groups improves their interaction with the metallic cationic cofactor.[159-161]

Common Adverse Effects and Drug Interactions

INSTIs are generally well tolerated, with most adverse effects occurring in less than 2% of patients. A summary of their major adverse effects is provided in Table 33.12. Bictegravir is only available as a combination product with emtricitabine and tenofovir alafenamide, and elvitegravir is only available as a combination product with cobicistat, emtricitabine,

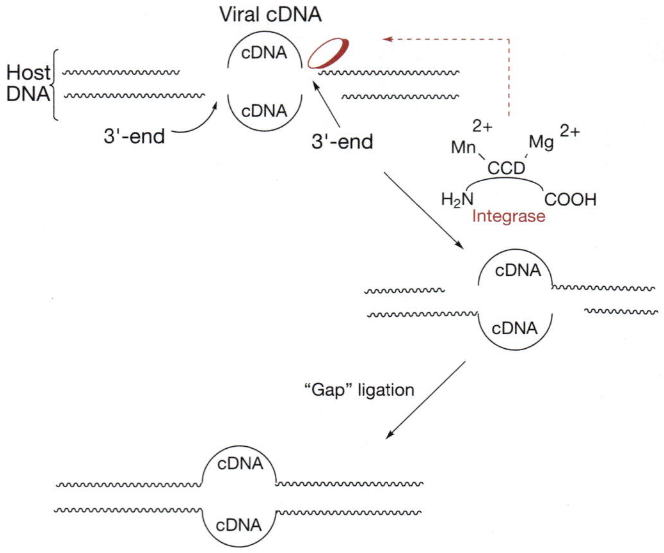

Figure 33.27 Integration of viral complementary DNA (cDNA) into host DNA through the action of integrase.

and either tenofovir alafenamide or tenofovir disoproxil fumarate. Therefore, the adverse effects of these combinations are a cumulative effect of all the drugs in combination.

Due to their ability to chelate metals, antacids, dairy products, iron preparations, and other medications that contain polyvalent cations will decrease the absorption of INSTIs if administered at the same time. In order to minimize this drug interaction, all medications containing polyvalent cations should be administered either 2 hours before an INSTI or 6 hours after.

Cabotegravir, dolutegravir, and raltegravir are primarily metabolized by UGT1A1, and if taken in combination with moderate-to-strong UGT1A1 inhibitors or inducers, will have their respective plasma concentrations increased or decreased, respectively. Bictegravir is a substrate for both CYP3A4 and UGT1A1 enzymes. Drugs that are strong inducers of both of these enzymes will substantially decrease the plasma levels of bictegravir. Strong CYP3A4 inhibitors will increase the plasma levels of bictegravir. Elvitegravir is primarily metabolized by CYP3A4 and is used in combination with cobicistat. Similar to ritonavir, previously discussed with nirmatrelvir and paritaprevir, cobicistat inhibits CYP3A4 and prevents the metabolism, increases the bioavailability, and extends the duration of action of elvitegravir. Both dolutegravir and bictegravir inhibit the renal

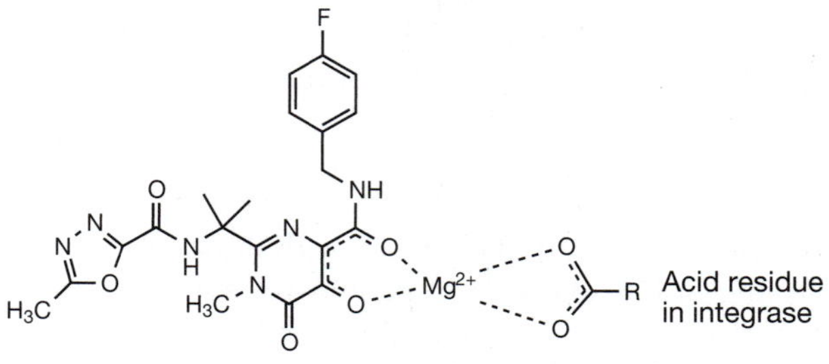

Figure 33.28 Chelation complex between raltegravir and integrase.

Table 33.12 Common Adverse Effects of Integrase Strand Transfer Inhibitors

Drug	Common Adverse Effects
Bictegravir (only available as combination product)	Diarrhea, elevated creatine phosphokinase, nausea, headache
Cabotegravir	IM: Induration at injection site, injection-site nodule, injection-site reaction Oral or IM: elevated creatine phosphokinase, headache
Dolutegravir	Elevated creatine phosphokinase, hyperglycemia, insomnia
Elvitegravir (only available as combination product)	Diarrhea, elevated creatine phosphokinase, hyperglycemia, nausea
Raltegravir	Diarrhea, elevated creatine phosphokinase, headache, insomnia, nausea, rash

IM, intramuscular.

organic cation transporter 2 (OCT2) and may increase the plasma levels of drugs that require this transporter.[26,28,149]

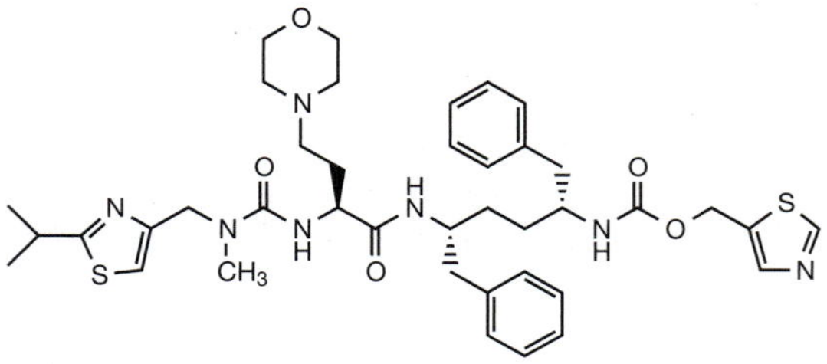

Physicochemical and Pharmacokinetic Properties

The pharmacokinetic properties of the INSTIs can be found in Table 33.13.[26,28] As shown in Figure 33.26, all INSTIs contain a β-dicarbonyl group (or analogue) and are acidic. The acidity varies among the INSTIs due to the presence of adjacent functional groups. The carboxylic acid seen in elvitegravir is the most acidic (pK_a = 5.97), with the β-dicarbonyl group of raltegravir being the second most acidic (pK_a = 7.02). These functional groups would be primarily ionized at a pH of 7.4. The acidic functional groups in the other INSTIs are much weaker (pK_a range = 9.8-10.1) and would be primarily unionized at a pH of 7.4. With the exception of raltegravir, all INSTIs are approximately 99% plasma protein bound. Elvitegravir is the most lipid soluble INSTI and is primarily metabolized by CYP3A4 oxidation, with glucuronide conjugation being a minor metabolic pathway. All other INSTIs primarily undergo glucuronide conjugation to inactive metabolites. Bictegravir and dolutegravir are also metabolized by CYP3A4 oxidation to a minor extent. The sites of glucuronide conjugation and CYP3A4 oxidation are shown in Figure 33.29.

Table 33.13 Pharmacokinetic Properties of Integrase Strand Transfer Inhibitors

Drug	Log *P*	Protein Binding (%)	Oral Bioavailability (%)	Half-Life (h)	Metabolism[a]	Route of Elimination (%)
Bictegravir	1.28	>99%	Rapid absorption	17.3	Glucuronide conjugation; aromatic oxidation	Feces (60.3) Urine (35)
Cabotegravir	1.04	>99%	Increased with high fat meal	41	Glucuronide conjugation	Feces (59, primarily unchanged) Urine (27)
Dolutegravir	0.98	>98.9	Increased with food	14	Glucuronide conjugation (major); benzylic oxidation	Feces (53, primarily unchanged) Urine (31)
Elvitegravir	3.66	99	Increased with food	8.7	Oxidative metabolism (major); glucuronide conjugation	Feces (~95%) Urine (~5)
Raltegravir	1.3	83	Increased with high fat meal	9	Glucuronide conjugation	Feces (51, primarily unchanged) Urine (32)

[a]The sites of glucuronide conjugation and CYP3A4 oxidation are shown in Figure 33.25.

With the exception of bictegravir, which can be taken with or without food, the oral bioavailability of INSTIs is increased if taken with food.

Protease Inhibitors

HIV protease was the second enzyme identified and pursued for the treatment of HIV infections. Its structure and function were determined in the late 1980s and early 1990s, and the first PI, saquinavir, was approved for treatment in 1995. Since then, a total of nine PIs have been approved by the FDA.

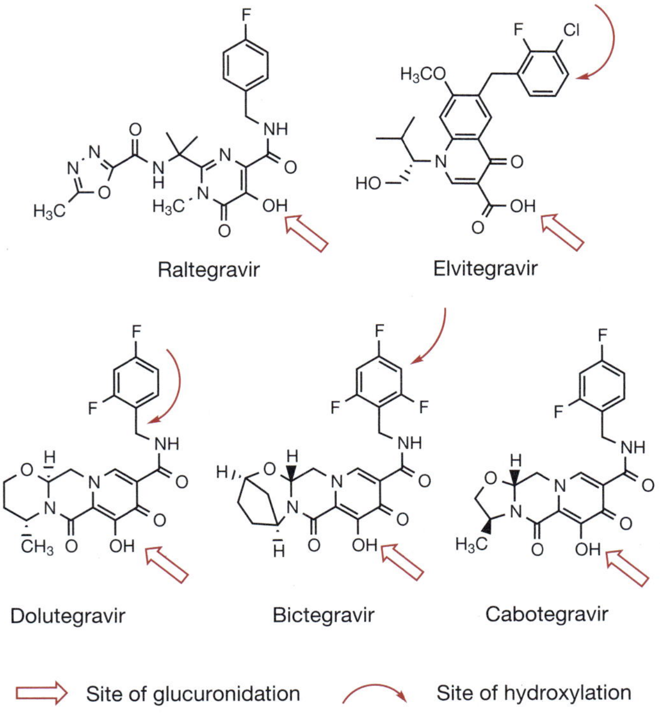

Figure 33.29 Metabolism of integrase inhibitors by UGT1A1 glucuronidation and CYP3A4 hydroxylation.

Mechanism of Action and Structure-Activity Relationship

During replication, the HIV genome produces polypeptide precursors, including gag and gag-pol, which must be cleaved in order for the immature viral particle to be converted to a mature viral particle. Along with RT, integrase, and RNase H, protease is originally produced as part of the gag-pol precursor polyprotein. During the maturation stage, which occurs after the viral particle leaves the infected host cell, autoprocessing of gag-pol releases the protease enzyme. Once released, protease is responsible for processing gag and gag-pol precursors into mature viral proteins and enzymes.[162-164]

Functional HIV protease exists as a dimer in which each monomer contains one of two conserved aspartic acid residues at the active site. There are several HIV protease cleavage sites on the polyprotein precursors, but the enzyme preferentially hydrolyzes the peptide bond on the amino terminal side of a proline.[165] Additionally, HIV protease prefers to have large hydrophobic amino acids such as phenylalanine and tyrosine on the opposite side of the scissile bond. As shown in Figure 33.30A, the amino acid R-groups flanking the scissile bond are sequentially designated P_1, P_2, and so forth on the amino terminus, and P_1', P_2', and so forth on the carboxyl terminus of the cleavage site.

The corresponding pockets on the enzyme that are responsible for binding the P groups of the substrate are sequentially termed S_1, S_2, S_1', S_2', and so forth. In the active site, a pair of aspartic acids (the Asp25 on each of the two subunits of the protein) work together to initially form a transition state, which subsequently collapses to cleave the peptide bond (Fig. 33.30B). Rationally designed PIs were

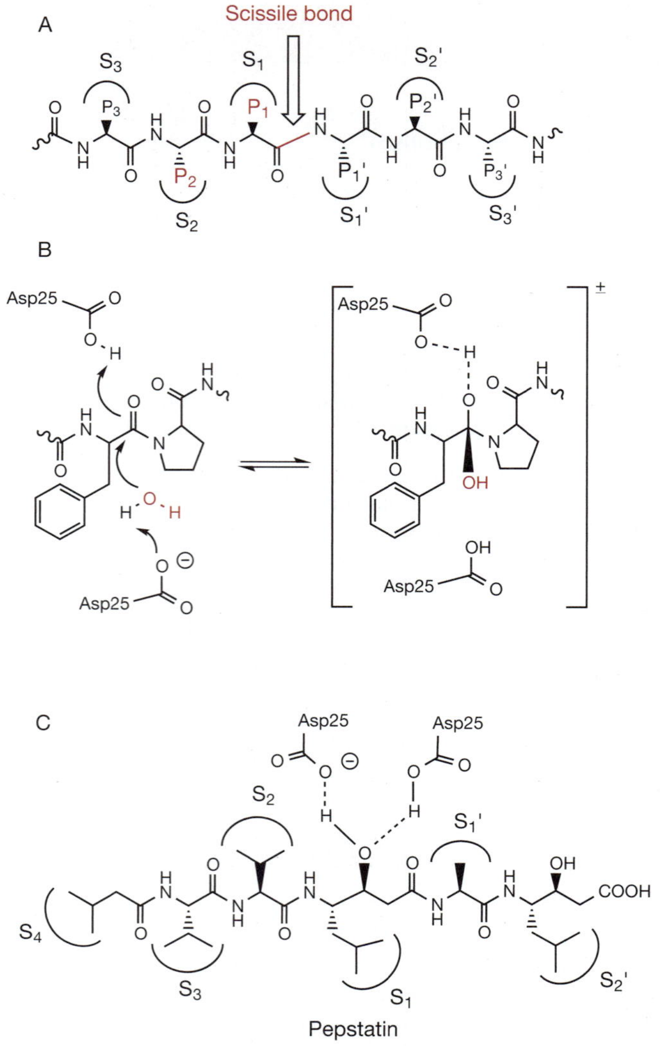

Figure 33.30 Design of transition-state analogue inhibitors of HIV protease. A. Nomenclature of amino acid side chains (P) and binding pockets (S) surrounding a protease cleavage site. B. Role of two Asp25 residues in formation of the hydrolytic transition state. C. Coordination of the Asp25 residues by the transition-state analogue pepstatin.

designed as transition-state mimics guided by the three-dimensional crystallographic analysis of the protein structure and mechanism. Figure 33.30C shows the PI pepstatin bound to the active site of HIV protease. Pepstatin is an inhibitor of all aspartic proteases but is used here to illustrate the mechanism by which transition-state analogues inhibit HIV protease.[166] Pepstatin contains an unnatural amino acid known as statine (Fig. 33.31), and its secondary hydroxyl group mimics the tetrahedral transition state that occurs during hydrolysis of the peptide bond.

While statine is a stable dipeptide mimic, it only contains one site of modification, the leucine side chain, and is not optimal for mimicking protease function. Thus, in the development of PIs, dipeptides mimicking hydroxyethylene and hydroxyethylamine (Fig. 33.31) were used.[167] Shown in Figure 33.32 are the structures of the nine currently available PIs. With the exception of tipranavir, the

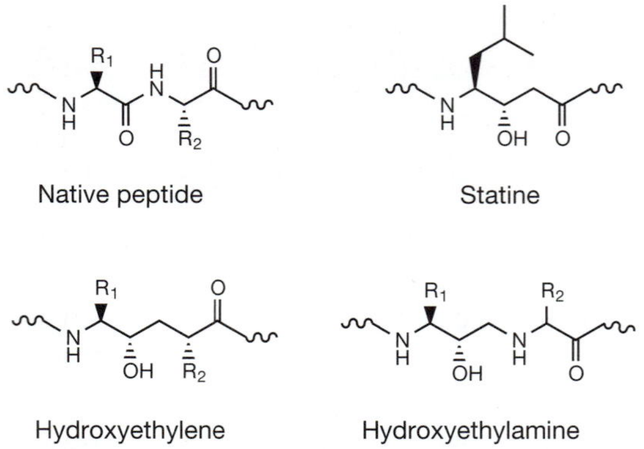

Figure 33.31 Transition-state mimics used in the design of human immunodeficiency virus (HIV) protease inhibitors.

structures of all PIs consist of a central secondary hydroxyl group flanked by phenylalanine or a phenylalanine analogue. This allows the PIs to act as stable substrate mimics and bind to HIV protease. The structures of nelfinavir and saquinavir also contain a bicyclic ring that loosely mimics proline. With the exception of tipranavir, all PIs can be classified as peptidomimetics; however, the peptide nature varies among the drugs. In Figure 33.32, Group A represents the three drugs that have a hydroxyethylene dipeptide mimic, and Group B represents the five drugs that have a hydroxyethylamine dipeptide mimic. The structural similarities of darunavir and fosamprenavir have also been highlighted. The only differences between these two drugs are the presence of a phosphate group in fosamprenavir and the substitution of a tetrahydrofuran ring in fosamprenavir with a bicyclic hexahydrofuro[2,3-*b*]furan ring in darunavir. Tipranavir is a structurally unique PI and does not contain either peptide mimic.

Resistance to PIs can occur due to mutations, and these mutations are classified as primary and secondary mutations. Primary mutations initially occur near the substrate-binding site of the enzyme and interfere with the binding of the PI to the viral protease. Secondary mutations occur away from the active site and may emerge subsequent to the primary mutations.[167] Due to its unique nonpeptide nature, tipranavir has been shown to be active against HIV infections that are resistant to other PIs.[168]

Common Adverse Effects and Drug Interactions

All PIs can cause the following adverse effects; however, the extent of these adverse effects varies among the drugs.

- Alteration of fat distribution
- Elevated liver enzymes (AST and ALT)
- GI effects: diarrhea, stool urgency
- Hepatotoxicity
- Hyperglycemia and increased insulin resistance
- Hyperlipidemia
- Increased bleeding in patients with hemophilia
- Increased risk of myocardial infarction

Additional adverse effects for each PI are provided in Table 33.14.[26,28,149] All PIs are metabolized by CYP3A4 and will have drug interactions with other drugs that are strong-to-moderate inhibitors or inducers of CYP3A4. As previously discussed with nirmatrelvir, ritonavir is poorly

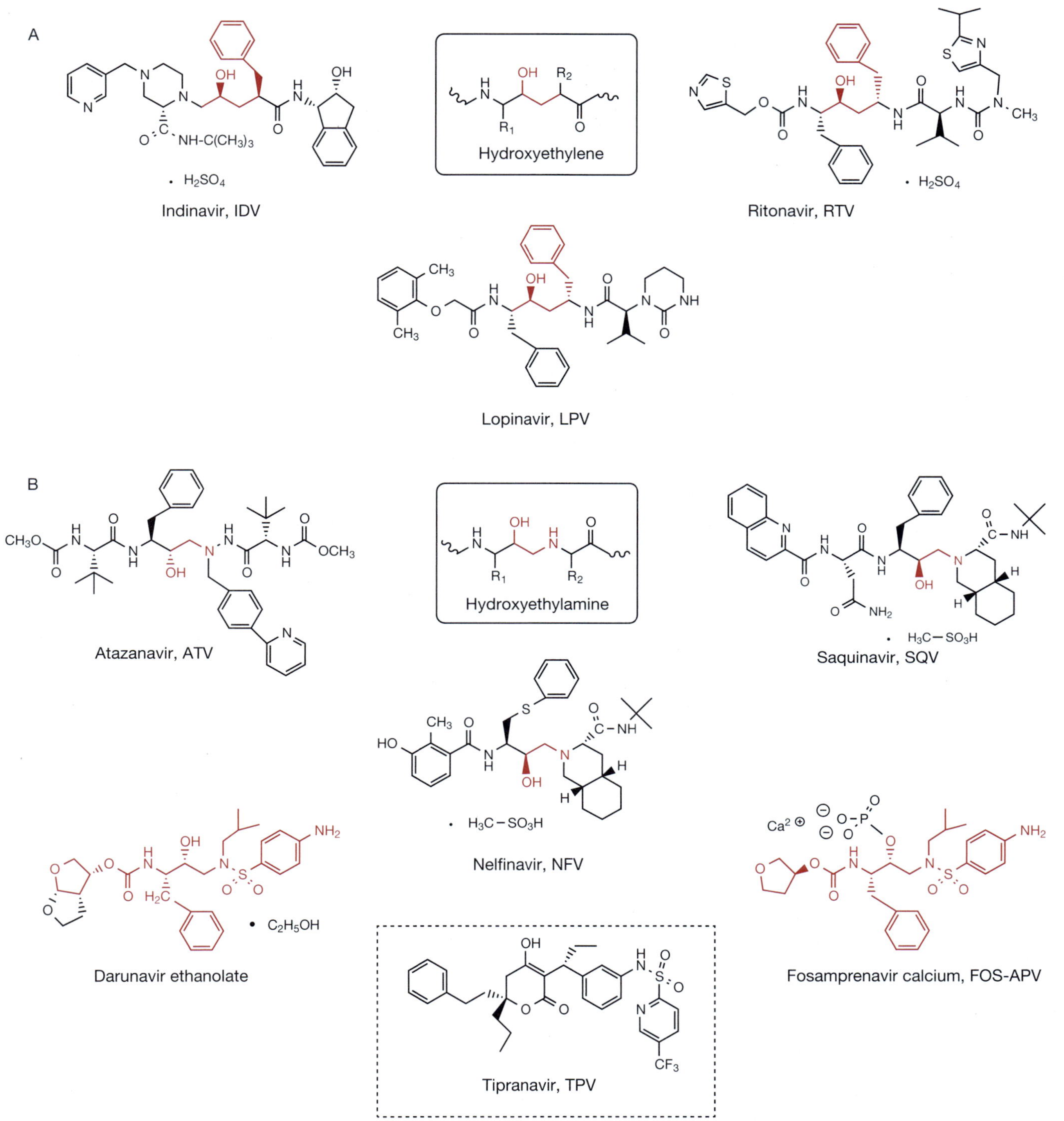

Figure 33.32 Human immunodeficiency virus (HIV) protease inhibitors.

tolerated if used at therapeutic doses; however, due to its ability to inhibit CYP3A4, it is currently used at subtherapeutic doses to inhibit CYP3A4 inactivation of other PIs. Currently, all PIs are used in combination with either ritonavir or cobicistat to prevent metabolism, increase duration, and therefore act as pharmacokinetic enhancers. With the exceptions of fosamprenavir and tipranavir, all PIs are strong inhibitors of CYP3A4 and will enhance the metabolism of other drugs that require this isozyme. Fosamprenavir is a moderate inhibitor of CYP3A4, and tipranavir is an inhibitor of CYP2D6 and UGT1A1 and could cause interactions with other drugs requiring these enzymes for normal metabolism.

Atazanavir requires an acidic gastric pH for optimal oral absorption. H_2 antagonists, proton pump inhibitors, and antacids will decrease oral absorption. If possible, H_2 antagonists and proton pump inhibitors should be avoided in patients taking atazanavir. Antacids can be used; however, they should be administered 1 to 2 hours before or 2 hours after taking atazanavir.

Table 33.14 Additional Adverse Effects of HIV Protease Inhibitors

Drug	Additional Adverse Effects
Atazanavir	Hyperbilirubinemia, rash, nephrolithiasis, cholelithiasis, and PR interval prolongation Comment: Less hyperlipidemia than other PIs
Darunavir	Rash Comment: Use in caution in patients with sulfa allergy
Fosamprenavir	Nephrolithiasis, perioral paresthesia, rash Comment: Use in caution in patients with sulfa allergy
Indinavir	Elevation of indirect bilirubin, nephrolithiasis, cholelithiasis, dry skin and mucous membranes, inflammation of the nail fold, and ingrown toenails. Comment: Recommend consumption of 1.5-2 L of water daily to decrease renal adverse effects.
Lopinavir	Headache, asthenia, pancreatitis, PR and QT interval prolongation Comment: Generally, well tolerated
Nelfinavir	Diarrhea Comment: Generally, well tolerated; however, is less potent than other PIs
Ritonavir	Hypertriglyceridemia, altered taste, paresthesia Comment: Based on low dose, adverse effects are mild
Saquinavir	Prolonged PR and QT interval prolongation Comment: Generally, well tolerated
Tipranavir	Abdominal pain, intracranial hemorrhage, severe hepatitis Comment: Use in caution in patients with sulfa allergy

HIV, human immunodeficiency virus; PI, protease inhibitor.

Physicochemical and Pharmacokinetic Properties

The pharmacokinetic properties of the PIs can be found in Table 33.15.[26,28] The PIs vary in their acidity and basicity. While most of these drugs will be unionized at physiological pH, the structures of nelfinavir (pK_a = 8.2) and saquinavir (pK_a = 8.5) contain tertiary amines that will be primarily ionized at physiological pH. The structure of indinavir also contains a tertiary amine; however, it is less basic (pK_a = 6.8). Additionally, the structure of tipranavir that contains a β-dicarbonyl (pK_a = 5.6) will also be primarily ionized at physiological pH. With the exceptions of atazanavir and indinavir, all PIs are at least 90% plasma protein bound. Fosamprenavir is the most water soluble PI; however, its active metabolite is 10-fold more lipid soluble. The highly lipid-soluble nature of the PIs is responsible for their extensive metabolism. In summary, aromatic oxidation, benzylic oxidation, alkyl oxidation, dealkylation, hydrolysis, and glucuronide conjugation comprised the major metabolic routes seen among the PIs. While nelfinavir and ritonavir are oxidized to active metabolites, all other metabolic processes lead to inactive metabolites.

Fusion and Entry Inhibitors

Prior to the establishment of an infection, the gp120 extracellular protein on the HIV particle viral must initially bind to the CD4 receptor on the host T lymphocyte. Following attachment, the viral envelope and the host cell membrane are fused, resulting in uncoating and the release of the viral components. Currently, there are four drugs, each with a unique mechanism, that inhibit this process.

Maraviroc

Maraviroc is a receptor antagonist for the chemokine co-receptor CCR5. It is approved for the treatment of CCR5-tropic HIV-1 infection in both adult and pediatric patients in combination with other ARV agents.

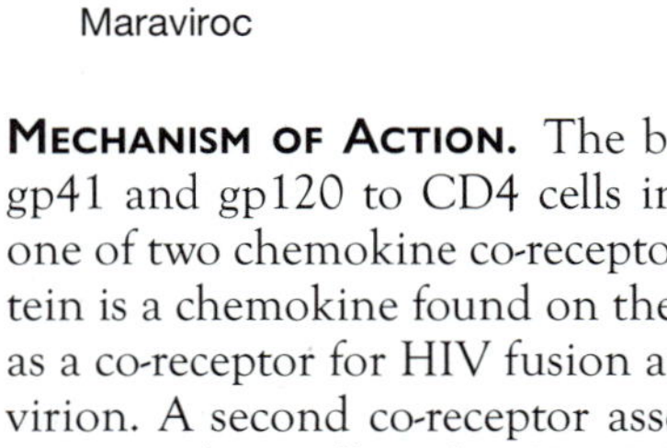
Maraviroc

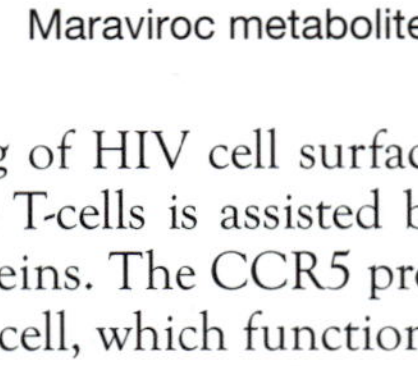
Maraviroc metabolite

Mechanism of Action. The binding of HIV cell surface gp41 and gp120 to CD4 cells in host T-cells is assisted by one of two chemokine co-receptor proteins. The CCR5 protein is a chemokine found on the host cell, which functions as a co-receptor for HIV fusion and penetration of the HIV virion. A second co-receptor associated with HIV penetration into host cells is the CXCR4 chemokine protein. It has been found that the majority of newly infected individuals contain CCR5-tropic infections.[169]

Table 33.15 Pharmacokinetic Properties of Human Immunodeficiency Virus Protease Inhibitors

Drug Name	Log *P*	Protein Binding (%)	Absorption with Meal	Half-life (h)	Metabolism	Route of Elimination (%)
Atazanavir	4.08	86	Increase	7	*Major:* Mono- and di-oxygenation *Minor:* Glucuronide conjugation; N-dealkylation; hydrolysis	Feces (79) Urine (13)
Darunavir	1.76	95	Increase	15	Hydrolysis; benzylic and aromatic oxidation; glucuronide conjugation	Feces (80) Urine (14)
Fosamprenavir Amprenavir	0.84 1.8	90	None	7.7	Hydrolyzed to amprenavir (active); oxidative metabolism; glucuronide conjugation	Feces (75) Urine (14)
Indinavir	3.26	60	Decrease	1.8	Oxidative metabolism; glucuronide conjugation	Feces (83) Urine (10)
Lopinavir	3.91	>98	Increased	6.9	Oxidative metabolism, primarily at the carbamate containing ring	Feces (83) Urine (10)
Nelfinavir	4.61	>98	Increase	3.5-5	Oxidation of *t*-butyl ring (active); aromatic hydroxylation	Feces (98)
Ritonavir	4.24	~99	Minimal	3-5	*Major:* Oxidation of isopropylthiazole (active) *Other:* Dealkylation, hydrolysis of carbamabate	Feces (34) Urine (5)
Saquinavir	4.04	98	None	1-2	Oxidized to mono- and di-hydroxyl metabolites	Feces (88) Urine (19)
Tipranavir	6.29	~99	None	5-6	Oxidative metabolism	Feces (92) Urine (4.5)

Maraviroc selectively binds to CCR5 inhibiting the binding of HIV to the CCR5~gp120/gp41 complex. As a result of this inhibition, HIV can initially bind to the host cell, but the fusion and penetration is prevented. Individuals with a genetic mutation in the *CCR5* gene (*CCR5-δ32*) may be unresponsive to maraviroc. Maraviroc is not effective on cells exhibiting CXCR4 co-receptors; therefore, a viral tropism assay is required, and the drug is not recommended for patients with dual/mixed or CXCR4-topic HIV infections.

Common Adverse Effects and Drug Interactions. The most common adverse effects are abdominal pain, cough, dizziness, fever, musculoskeletal symptoms, skin rash, and upper respiratory tract infections. Maraviroc requires CYP3A4 for metabolism; hence, drugs that induce or inhibit CYP3A4 will decrease or increase the plasma levels of maraviroc, respectively. Maraviroc is also a substrate for P-glycoprotein and will be affected by other drugs that alter its effects.

The dosing of maraviroc is dependent on the presence or absence of strong CYP3A4 inducers or inhibitors. The normal dose for patients taking other medications that do not induce or inhibit CYP3A is 300 mg po twice daily. The dose must be decreased by 50% to 150 mg po twice daily in patients taking other medications that inhibit CYP3A4, and the dose must be doubled to 600 mg po bid in patients taking other medications that induce CYP3A4.[170]

Physicochemical and Pharmacokinetic Properties. Maraviroc is a basic drug. The pK_a of the tertiary amine is 9.65, so maraviroc will be primarily ionized in all physiological environments. Its overall bioavailability is between 23% and 33%. Maraviroc is a substrate for CYP3A4 and is metabolized via N-dealkylation to the inactive metabolite shown earlier. It is 76% plasma protein bound and has an elimination half-life of 14 to 18 hours. It is excreted in the feces (76%) and urine (20%) with approximately 33% excreted as the unchanged drug.[26,28]

Fostemsavir

Fostemsavir is a prodrug that is initially hydrolyzed to its active metabolite, temsavir. Temsavir is an HIV attachment inhibitor that is currently indicated for treatment-experienced adults with multidrug-resistant HIV infection who have failed other HIV therapy due to either resistance, intolerance, or safety conditions.[28,171]

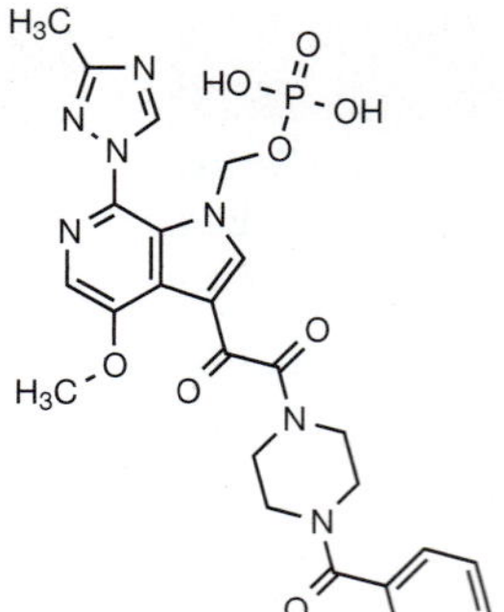

Fostemsavir (prodrug)

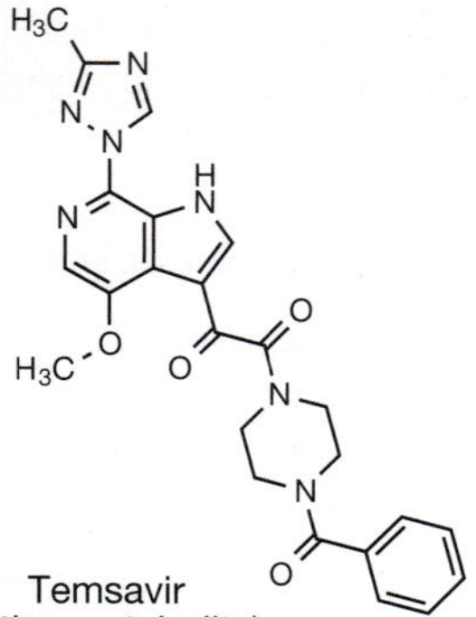

Temsavir (active metabolite)

Mechanism of Action. The active metabolite, temsavir, binds to the HIV envelope protein gp120 in close proximity to the gp120-CD4 binding site and prevents the required conformational change needed for the initial attachment of the viral particle and the host T cell. This prevents the first step in the infection of a host T cell. Temsavir can also inhibit gp120-dependent post-attachment steps required for viral entry into host cells.[26,171]

Common Adverse Effects and Drug Interactions. In general, fostemsavir is well tolerated, with nausea (10%) being the most common adverse effect. Other adverse effects occurring in 2% to 3% of patients are abdominal pain, diarrhea, dyspepsia, fatigue, headache, immune reconstitution inflammatory syndrome, rash, sleep disturbances, somnolence, and vomiting. Fostemsavir can also elevate laboratory levels, including liver enzyme (ALT and AST), creatinine, and direct bilirubin.

Fostemsavir can cause QTc prolongation at dosage levels higher than normally prescribed; however, coadministration of fostemsavir with other drugs that cause QTc prolongation may increase the risk of torsade de pointes. Fostemsavir is a substrate BCRP and CYP3A4. Drug interactions could occur due to inducers or inhibitors of CYP3A4 or other drugs affected by BCRP.[172]

Physicochemical and Pharmacokinetic Properties. Fostemsavir has a log *P* value of 0.64 and is highly water soluble. The phosphate prodrug enhances dissolution and increases its oral absorption. Temsavir, the active metabolite, is 88.4% plasma protein bound and has a half-life of 2 hours. Temsavir is excreted in the urine (51%) and feces (33%) primarily as metabolites. Temsavir is metabolized to inactive metabolites by CYP3A4-mediated N-dealkylation and hydrolysis of the terminal amide bond.[26,172]

Enfuvirtide

Enfuvirtide is a synthetic 36-amino acid peptide that is derived from the gp41 portion of the HIV glycoprotein envelope. It is used in combination with other ARV agents in HIV treatment–experienced patients.

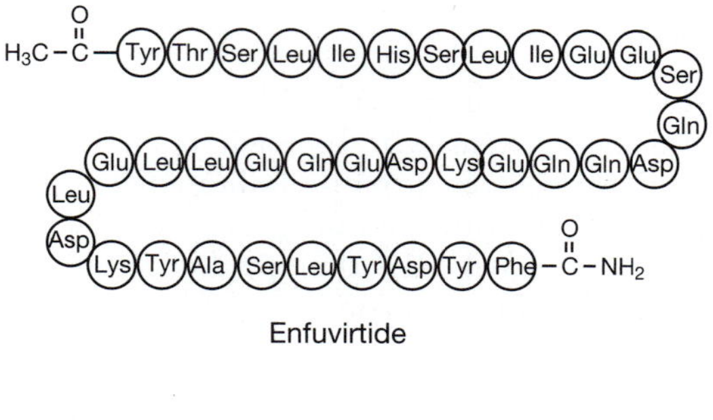

Enfuvirtide

Mechanism of Action. Enfuvirtide mimics an HR2 fragment of gp41, blocking the formation of a six-helix bundle structure, which is critical in the fusion of the HIV virion to a CD4-positive T lymphocyte. It specifically binds to the tryptophan-rich region of the gp41 protein. Normally, gp41 undergoes a conformational change following the binding of gp120 to CD4. The binding of enfuvirtide to gp41 prevents the subsequent fusion of the human and viral cells and blocks the entry of HIV particles into the T lymphocyte. Resistance to enfuvirtide can develop if the virus produces changes in a 10-amino acid domain between residues 36 and 45 in the gp41 HIV surface glycoprotein.[173,174]

Common Adverse Effects and Drug Interactions. Enfuvirtide is administered as a subcutaneous injection, and almost all patients experience an injection-site reaction (pain, erythema, pruritis), the severity of which varies among patients. Other common adverse effects include nausea, diarrhea, fatigue, and insomnia. Enfuvirtide has no clinically relevant drug interactions.[28]

Physicochemical and Pharmacokinetic Properties. Following subcutaneous injection into the abdomen, arm, or thigh, the absolute bioavailability is 84.3%. Enfuvirtide is 92% plasma protein bound and has a half-life between 3.2 and 4.4 hours. It is metabolized by peptidases and proteinases in the liver and kidney, and its amino acids can be either used or degraded.[28]

Ibalizumab

Ibalizumab is a recombinant humanized mAb that is reserved for use in treatment-experienced adults with multidrug-resistant HIV infection that is not responding to their current ARV regimen. It is used in combination with other ARV drugs.

Mechanism of Action. Ibalizumab prevents HIV particles from entering host T cells by binding to domain 2 of the CD4 receptor. Once bound, it interferes with post-attachment processes that are essential for the fusion of the viral particle and the human host cell. Specifically, it causes a conformational change that blocks the interaction of gp120 and HIV co-receptors CCR5 and CXCR4. While ibalizumab does not prevent the binding of HIV, its effects prevent viral entry and transmission. Since ibalizumab binds specifically to domain 2 of the CD4 receptor, it does not cause immunosuppression.[28,175]

Common Adverse Effects and Drug Interactions. Ibalizumab is administered via an IV infusion and is generally well tolerated. The most common adverse effects are diarrhea, dizziness, nausea, and rash. Similar to enfuvirtide, ibalizumab has no clinically relevant drug interactions.[28]

Physicochemical and Pharmacokinetic Properties. Ibalizumab has a half-life of 3 to 3.5 days and is metabolized by CD4 internalization.[26]

Capsid Inhibitor

Lenacapavir is the first HIV capsid protein to be approved by the FDA. It is indicated for use with other ARV drugs for the treatment of HIV infection in treatment-experienced adults with multidrug resistance to other medications.

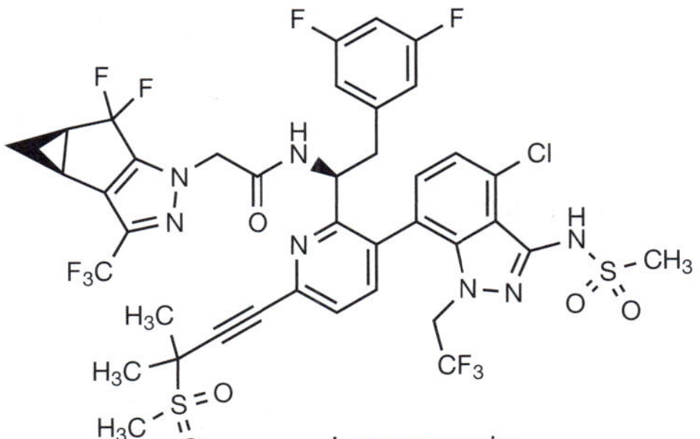

Lenacapavir

Mechanism of Action and Structure-Activity Relationship

Lenacapavir selectively inhibits multiple functions of the HIV capsid protein. The capsid protein is composed of hexamers and pentamers, each of which is composed of monomeric capsid proteins. The N- and C-terminal domains of the capsid monomers allow for specific interactions. Lenacapavir directly binds to the interface between capsid protein p24 subunits in hexamers. This binding inhibits the capsid-mediated nuclear uptake of HIV proviral DNA by interfering with two host proteins. In order for HIV to integrate with the host DNA, the capsid must be imported into the nucleus. To facilitate this, it uses the nuclear pore complex and two host proteins, cleavage and polyadenylation specificity factor subunit 6 (CPSF6), and nucleoporin 153 (Nup153). The difluorobenzyl ring of lenacapavir can overlap with tyrosine rings present in CPSF6 and Nup153 and occupy the same binding site. Since CPSF6 and Nup153 are essential for nuclear entry, the ability of lenacapavir to bind at this position inhibits these interactions and blocks capsid nuclear entry. Lenacapavir also interferes with normal gag-pol function and reduces the production of capsid protein subunits. Finally, it disrupts the rate of capsid subunit association, leading to malformed capsid subunits and an overall decrease in capsid core function.[28,176,177]

Common Adverse Effects and Drug Interactions. Lenacapavir is given both orally and subcutaneously. When given subcutaneously, the major adverse effect is an injection-site reaction. This occurs in 65% of the patients and can manifest as swelling, pain, erythema, nodule formation, induration, pruritus, and extravasation. The other common adverse effect is nausea.

Lenacapavir is a substrate of P-gp, UGT1A1, and CYP3A. Strong or moderate inhibitors or inducers of these proteins and enzymes could increase or decrease blood levels, respectively. Lenacapavir is a moderate inhibitor of CYP3A.[26,28]

Physicochemical and Pharmacokinetic Properties. Lenacapavir is an acidic drug. Its sulfonamide group has a pK_a of 6.7 and will be primarily ionized at physiological pH. Lenacapavir is also very lipid soluble and has a log *P* of 6.4. It is formulated and administered as its sodium salt. While the bioavailability of the subcutaneous injection is 100%, the bioavailability when given orally, either with or without food, is only 6% to 10%. It is at least 98.5% plasma protein bound and is extensively metabolized by CYP3A4 and UGT1A1. Metabolic pathways include N-dealkylation, amide hydrolysis, glucuronide conjugation, and glutathione conjugation.

Lenacapavir has a half-life of 10 to 12 days when given orally, and 8 to 12 weeks when given subcutaneously. It is primarily eliminated in the feces with less than 1% eliminated in the urine.[26,28]

CROFELEMER

Diarrhea is a common adverse effect of many of the drugs used to treat HIV infections. Crofelemer is a polymeric mixture of (+)-catechin, (−)-epicatechin, (+)-gallocatechin, and (−)-epigallocatechin monomer units and is indicated for the symptomatic relief of noninfectious diarrhea in adult patients with HIV/AIDS on ART. Crofelemer does not have antiviral properties but inhibits two chloride channels that regulate fluid secretion in the GI tract. Specifically, it inhibits the cyclic adenosine monophosphate (cAMP)-stimulated cystic fibrosis transmembrane conductance regulator (CFTR) chloride-ion channel and the calcium-activated chloride channels (CaCC) at the luminal membrane of enterocytes. Due to its ability to block chloride secretion and the accompanying water loss in diarrhea, crofelemer normalizes the flow of chloride and water in the GI tract. Crofelemer is given twice daily either with or without food.[28,178]

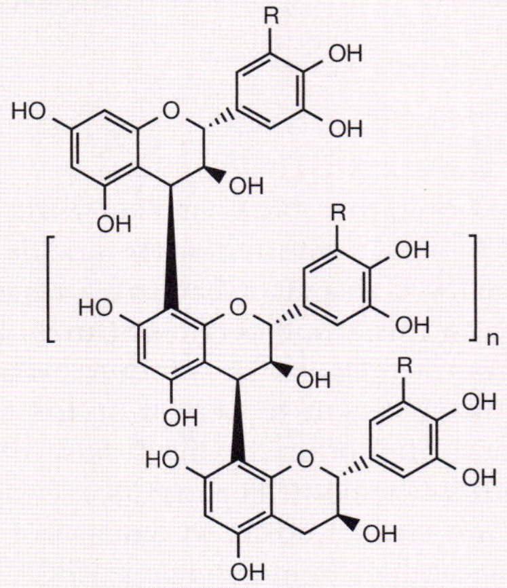

Crofelemer
(n = 1-28; R = H, OH)

Rare Viral Diseases

Smallpox

Smallpox is a devastating disease caused by the variola virus, a large double-stranded DNA virus from the *Poxviridae* family. Historic evidence suggests that smallpox has infected humans for over 3,000 years. In the 20th century alone, it was responsible for the deaths of approximately 500 million people across the globe.[179] However, after a remarkable vaccination campaign, the World Health Organization declared that smallpox was eliminated in 1980, making it the first infectious disease to earn that distinction.

Smallpox is predominately transmitted via the respiratory route among close contacts or in crowded conditions. After exposure, an incubation period of 7 to 17 days is followed by a sudden fever and headache. Approximately 1 day after the fever begins, a characteristic rash starts on the tongue and mouth and then spreads across the rest of the body, progressing to pustules after 6 to 8 days.[180] Mortality for smallpox is high (~30%), and survivors are often left with scars or disfigurement from the lesions.[181]

The last reported smallpox case in the United States was in 1949, and routine vaccination was halted in 1972. Today, it is estimated that less than half of the population in the United States has immunity to smallpox, leading to concerns about its use as an agent of bioterrorism. As such, the US Strategic National Stockpile stores smallpox vaccines and an antiviral therapy for those at high risk of disease and first responders in the event of variola release.[182]

Ebola Virus

EBOVs are among the most virulent viruses to infect humans. EBOV is a zoonotic disease and is endemic in Africa. It is believed that fruit bats are a reservoir for the virus.[183] After an initial spillover event in which EBOV is transferred from a fruit bat or another pathogenic host, transmission from person to person occurs through contact with blood and other bodily fluids. EBOV infects many cell types in the body. For instance, endothelial cells are killed by the virus, leading to damage of small blood vessels and subsequent hemorrhaging. EBOV also dysregulates the function of multiple immune cells (eg, B cells) and kills other immune cells via infection (eg, natural killer cells).[184] Ultimately, multi-organ failure can occur because of blood loss and disseminated intravascular coagulation. Case fatality rates from EBOV outbreaks vary by strain and setting (25%-90%), but the average is estimated at approximately 50%.[185]

There were 34 reported outbreaks of EBOV between 1976 and 2020, with most outbreaks occurring in Central and West Africa. The largest EBOV outbreak occurred in West Africa in 2014 to 2016. This outbreak spread to 10 countries and killed 11,325 people, 5% of whom were health care workers.[186] During this outbreak, 11 people were treated for EBOV in the United States, most of whom were infected outside the country. Studies of the humoral immune response in survivors showed the production of neutralizing antibodies against EBOV, highlighting the importance of a robust antibody response.[187] Small-molecule inhibitors are not available for EBOV, and supportive care (eg, electrolytes) is critical. Two mAb therapies were approved for EBOV in 2020. Inmazeb is a mix of three mAbs (atoltivimab, maftivimab, and odesivimab), and Ebanga (ansuvimab) is a single mAb derived from a survivor of a 1995 outbreak. Both mAbs target the surface glycoprotein of EBOV and prevent its attachment and entry into cells.[28]

Antiviral Drugs to Treat Rare Viral Infections

Tecovirimat

Tecovirimat is indicated for the treatment of human smallpox disease in adults and pediatric patients weighing at least 3 kg. It can be given either orally or IV. While it is the only approved treatment for smallpox viral disease, it is also effective against vaccinia, monkeypox, and cowpox as well as variola.[188]

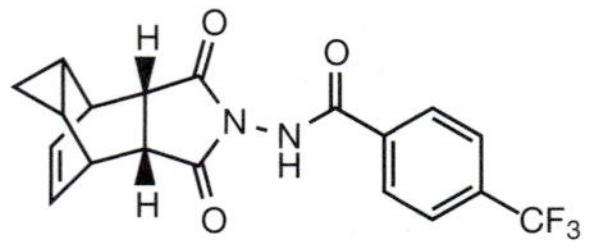

Tecovirimat

Mechanism of Action

Tecovirimat is highly specific for orthopoxviruses and targets the viral p37 protein, a highly conserved protein that has no homologs outside the *Orthopoxvirus* genus. Viral replication depends on the formation of infectious virion forms. One form of replication involves the formation of enveloped virions and a wrapping complex that is mediated by the viral p37 protein. The p37 protein interacts with the cellular Rab9 GTPase and tail-interacting protein 17 (TIP17), leading to the formation of a virus-specific wrapping complex for enveloped virions. Inhibition of p37 blocks the interaction with Rab9 and TIP47, prevents the formation of the wrapping complex, and inhibits the ability of the virus to form a viral envelope.[189,190]

Common Adverse Effects and Drug Interactions

Tecovirimat is administered IV and is well tolerated. The most common adverse effects are pain at the injection site and headache. Tecovirimat is a weak inhibitor of CYP2C19 and CYP2C8 and a weak inducer of CYP3A4. While drug interactions are possible if tecovirimat is taken with other drugs requiring these isozymes, the effects are predicted to be minimal. Since tecovirimat initially undergoes hydrolysis to inactive metabolites, drugs affecting UGT1A1 and UGT1A4 do not increase or decrease plasma levels of active drug.[28]

Pharmacokinetics

Following oral administration, tecovirimat is absorbed rapidly, achieves C_{max} within 6 hours, and has an elimination half-life of 20 hours. Tecovirimat is metabolized by initial hydrolysis of the amide bond and glucuronide conjugation of the resulting imide by UGT1A1 and UGT1A4. Approximately 95% of the dose is recovered primarily in the urine (73%) and feces (23%). The urinary excretion of the parent compound is minimal, with the glucuronide conjugate comprising the major elimination product.[26,28]

Structure Challenge

Shown below are the structures of five drugs that were discussed in this chapter. For each drug, provide the following information.

1. The specific viral infection(s) for which it is used.
2. From a structural evaluation, indicate if the drug is a prodrug or is active as drawn.
3. Highlight the key structural features of the drug that are required for its mechanism of action.

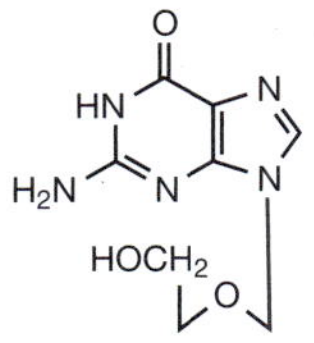

Acyclovir

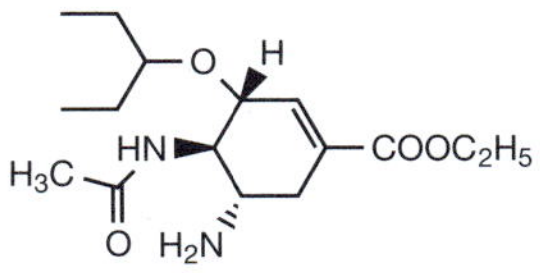

Oseltamivir

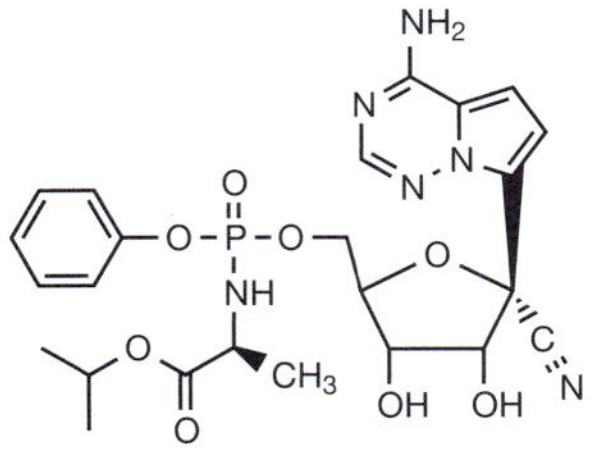

Remdesivir

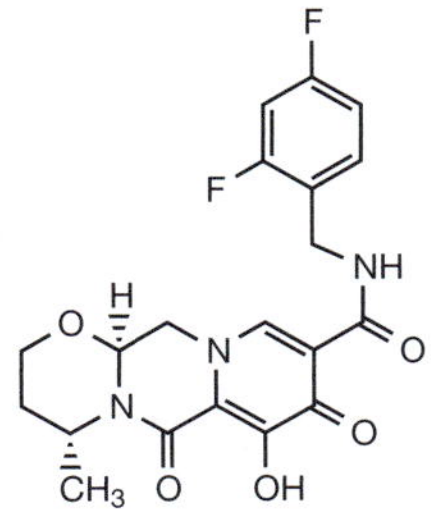

Dolutegravir

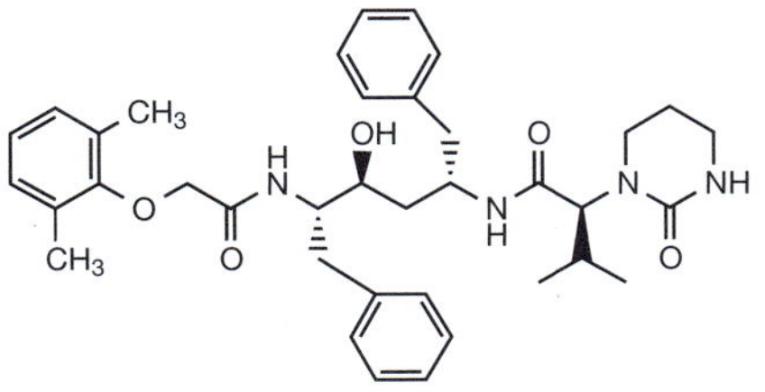

Lopinavir

Structure Challenge answers found immediately after References.

REFERENCES

1. Forni D, Cagliani R, Clerici M, et al. Disease-causing human viruses: novelty and legacy. *Trends Microbiol.* 2022;30:1232-1242.
2. Oldstone MBA. *Viruses, Plagues, and History.* 2nd ed. Oxford University Press; 2020.
3. Walker PJ, Siddell SG, Lefkowitz EJ, et al. Recent changes to virus taxonomy ratified by the International Committee on Taxonomy of Viruses (2022). *Arch Virol.* 2022;167:2429-2440.
4. Robbins AM. Why scientists should not name diseases based on location. Accessed May 2024. https://asm.org/articles/2021/may/why-scientists-should-not-name-diseases-after-plac#:~:text
5. Rampersad S, Tennant P. Replication and expression strategies of viruses. In: Tennant P, Fermin G, Foster JE, eds. *Viruses: Molecular Biology, Host Interactions and Applications to Biotechnology.* Academic Press; 2018:55-82.
6. Koonin EV, Krupovic M, Yutin N. Evolution of double-stranded DNA viruses of eukaryotes: from bacteriophages to transposons to giant viruses. *Ann N Y Acad Sci.* 2015;1341:10-24.
7. Abbas AA, Taylor LJ, Dothard MI, et al. Redondoviridae, a family of small, circular DNA viruses of the human oro-respiratory tract associated with periodontitis and critical illness. *Cell Host Microbe.* 2019;26:297.
8. Kerr SL, Mathew C, Ghildyal R. Rhinovirus and cell death. *Viruses.* 2021;13:629.
9. De Clercq E. Strategies in the design of antiviral drugs. *Nat Rev Drug Discov.* 2002;1:13-25.
10. Meganck, RM, Baric, RS. Developing therapeutic approaches for twenty-first-century emerging infectious viral diseases. *Nat Med.* 2021;27:401-410.
11. Thomson JM, Lamont IL. Nucleoside analogues as antibacterial agents. *Front Microbiol.* 2019;10:952.
12. Parker WB. Enzymology of purine and pyrimidine antimetabolites used in the treatment of cancer. *Chem Rev.* 2009;109:2880-2893.
13. Seley-Radtke KL, Yates MK. The evolution of nucleoside analogue antivirals: a review for chemists and non-chemists. Part 1: early structural modifications to the nucleoside scaffold. *Antivir Res.* 2018;154:66-86.
14. Harrold MW, Zavod RM. *Basic Concepts in Medicinal Chemistry.* 3rd ed. ASHP; 2023.
15. Nelson DL, Cox MM. *Lehninger Principles of Biochemistry.* 8th ed. Macmillan Learning; 2021:263-300.
16. Gatherer D, Depledge DP, Hartley CA, et al. ICTV virus taxonomy profile: *Herpesviridae* 2021. *J Gen Virol.* 2021;102.
17. Salsman J, Zimmerman N, Chen T, et al. Genome-wide screen of three herpesviruses for protein subcellular localization and alteration of PML nuclear bodies. *PLoS Pathog.* 2008;4:e1000100.
18. Grinde B. Herpesviruses: latency and reactivation–viral strategies and host response. *J Oral Microbiol.* 2013;5(1).
19. Lim F, Khalique H, Ventosa M, et al. Biosafety of gene therapy vectors derived from herpes simplex virus type 1. *Curr Gene Ther.* 2013;13:478-491
20. James C, Harfouche M, Welton NJ, et al. Herpes simplex virus: global infection prevalence and incidence estimates, 2016. *Bull World Health Organ.* 2020;98:315-329.
21. De Rose DU, Bompard S, Maddaloni C, et al. Neonatal herpes simplex virus infection: from the maternal infection to the child outcome. *J Med Virol.* 2023;95:e29024.
22. Zuhair M, Smit GSA, Wallis G, et al. Estimation of the worldwide seroprevalence of cytomegalovirus: a systematic review and meta-analysis. *Rev Med Virol.* 2019;29:e2034.
23. Dupont L, Reeves MB. Cytomegalovirus latency and reactivation: recent insights into an age old problem. *Rev Med Virol.* 2016;26:75-89.

24. Griffiths P, Reeves M. Pathogenesis of human cytomegalovirus in the immunocompromised host. *Nat Rev Microbiol.* 2021;19:759-773.
25. Centers for Disease Control and Prevention. Cytomegalovirus (CMV) and congenital CMV infection. Accessed May 2024. https://www.cdc.gov/cmv/congenital-infection.html
26. DrugBank Online (version 5.1.10, 2023). https://go.drugbank.com/drugs
27. Antiviral drugs for varicella-zoster virus and herpes simplex virus infections. *Med Lett Drugs Ther.* 2018;60:153-157.
28. UpToDate Lexicomp: Evidence-Based Drug Referential Content for Teams. Wolters Kluwer. Accessed October 2023. https://www.wolterskluwer.com/en/solutions/lexicomp
29. O'Brien JJ, Campoli-Richards DM. Acyclovir. An updated review of its antiviral activity, pharmacokinetic properties and therapeutic efficacy. *Drugs.* 1989;37:233-309.
30. King DH. History, pharmacokinetics, and pharmacology of acyclovir. *J Am Acad Dermatol.* 1988;18:176-179.
31. Elion GB, Furman PA, Fyfe JA, et al. Selectivity of action of an antiherpetic agent, 9-(2-hydroxyethoxymethyl) guanine. *Proc Natl Acad Sci U S A.* 1977;74:5716-5720.
32. Schalkwijk HH, Snoeck R, Andrei G. Acyclovir resistance in herpes simplex viruses: prevalence and therapeutic alternatives. *Biochem Pharmacol.* 2022:205:115322.
33. Perry CM, Faulds D. Valaciclovir. A review of its antiviral activity, pharmacokinetic properties and therapeutic efficacy in herpesvirus infections. *Drugs.* 1996;52:754-772.
34. De Clercq E, Field HJ. Antiviral prodrugs—the development of successful prodrug strategies for antiviral chemotherapy. *Br J Pharmacol.* 2006;147:1-11.
35. Carmine AA, Brogden RN, Heel RC, et al. Trifluridine: a review of its antiviral activity and therapeutic use in the topical treatment of viral eye infections. *Drugs.* 1982;23:329-353.
36. Kish T, Uppal P. Trifluridine/tipiracil (*Lonsurf*) for the treatment of metastatic colorectal cancer. *P T.* 2016;41:314-325.
37. Katz DH, Marcelletti JF, Khalil MH, et al. Antiviral activity of 1-docosanol, an inhibitor of lipid-enveloped viruses including herpes simplex. *Proc Natl Acad Sci U S A.* 1991;88:10825-10829.
38. GlaxoSmithKline Consumer Healthcare Inc. Docosanol prescribing information. Accessed October 2023. https://pdf.hres.ca/dpd_pm/00023035.PDF
39. Fletcher CV, Balfour HH Jr. Evaluation of ganciclovir for cytomegalovirus disease. *DICP.* 1989;23:5-12.
40. Matthews T, Boehme R. Antiviral activity and mechanism of action of ganciclovir. *Rev Infect Dis.* 1988;10:S490-S494.
41. Exela. Ganciclovir prescribing information. Accessed October 2023. www.accessdata.fda.gov/drugsatfda_docs/label/2017/209347lbl.pdf
42. Hitchcock MJM, Jaffe HS, Martin JC, Stagg RJ. Cidofovir, a new agent with potent anti-herpesvirus activity. *Antivir Chem Chemother.* 1996;7:115-127.
43. Gilead Sciences. Cidofovir prescribing information. Accessed October 2023. www.accessdata.fda.gov/drugsatfda_docs/label/1999/020638s003lbl.pdf
44. Chrisp P, Clissold SP. Foscarnet. A review of its antiviral activity, pharmacokinetic properties and therapeutic use in immunocompromised patients with cytomegalovirus retinitis. *Drugs.* 1991;41:104-129.
45. Merck & Co., Inc. Letermovir prescribing information. Accessed October 2023. https://www.merck.com/product/usa/pi_circulars/p/prevymis/prevymis_pi.pdf
46. Lischka P, Hewlett G, Wunberg T, et al. In vitro and in vivo activities of the novel anticytomegalovirus compound AIC246. *Antimicrob Agents Chemother.* 2010;54:1290-1297.
47. Ligat G, Cazal R, Hantz S, et al. The human cytomegalovirus terminase complex as an antiviral target: a close-up view. *FEMS Microbiol Rev.* 2018;42:137-145.
48. Choul S, Ercolani RJ, Derakhchan K. Antiviral activity of maribavir in combination with other drugs active against human cytomegalovirus. *Antiviral Res.* 2018;157:128-133.
49. Takeda Pharmaceuticals U.S.A. Maribavir prescribing information. Accessed October, 2023. https://www.accessdata.fda.gov/drugsatfda_docs/label/2021/215596lbl.pdf
50. GBD 2017 Influenza Collaborators. Mortality, morbidity, and hospitalizations due to influenza lower respiratory tract infections, 2017: an analysis for the Global Burden of Disease Study 2017. *Lancet Respir Med.* 2019;7:69-89.
51. Novel Swine-Origin Influenza A (H1N1) Virus Investigation Team. Emergence of a novel swine-origin influenza A (H1N1) virus in humans. *N Engl J Med.* 2009;360:2605-2615.
52. Knossow M, Skehel JJ. Variation and infectivity neutralization in influenza. *Immunology.* 2006;119:1-7.
53. Su B, Wurtzer S, Rameix-Welti MA, et al. Enhancement of the influenza A hemagglutinin (HA)-mediated cell-cell fusion and virus entry by the viral neuraminidase (NA). *PLoS One.* 2009;4:e8495.
54. Bridges CB, Kuehnert MJ, Hall CB. Transmission of influenza: implications for control in health care settings. *Clin Infect Dis.* 2003;37:1094-1101.
55. Kalil AC, Thomas PG. Influenza virus-related critical illness: pathophysiology and epidemiology. *Crit Care.* 2019;23:258.
56. Dilantika C, Sedyaningsih ER, Kasper MR, et al. Influenza virus infection among pediatric patients reporting diarrhea and influenza-like illness. *BMC Infect Dis.* 2010;10:3.
57. Uyeki TM. High-risk groups for influenza complications. *JAMA.* 2020;324:2334.
58. Uyeki TM, Bernstein HH, Bradley JS, et al. Clinical practice guidelines by the Infectious Diseases Society of America: 2018 Update on diagnosis, treatment, chemoprophylaxis, and institutional outbreak management of seasonal influenza. *Clin Infect Dis.* 2019;68:895-902.
59. Brooks GF, Butel JS, Morse SA, et al. *Jawetz, Melnick and Adelberg's Medical Microbiology.* 23rd ed. McGraw-Hill Companies; 2004.
60. Calfee DP, Hayden FG. New approaches to influenza chemotherapy. Neuraminidase inhibitors. *Drugs.* 1998;56:537-553.
61. Dou D, Revol R, Östbye H, et al. Influenza A virus cell entry, replication, virion assembly and movement. *Front Immunol.* 2018;9:1581.
62. Kim CU, Lew W, Williams MA, et al. Influenza neuraminidase inhibitors possessing a novel hydrophobic interaction in the enzyme active site: design, synthesis, and structural analysis of carbocyclic sialic acid analogues with potent anti-influenza activity. *J Am Chem Soc.* 1997;119:681-690.
63. Alame MM, Massaad E, Zaraket H. Peramivir: a novel intravenous neuraminidase inhibitor for treatment of acute influenza infections. *Front Microbiol.* 2016;7:450.
64. Antiviral drugs for influenza for 2022-2023. *Med Lett Drugs Ther.* 2022;64:185-90.
65. Dufrasne F. Baloxavir marboxil: an original new drug against influenza. *Pharmaceuticals.* 2022;15:28.
66. Noshi T, Kitano M, Taniguchi K, et al. In vitro characterization of baloxavir acid, a first-in-class cap-dependent endonuclease inhibitor of the influenza virus polymerase pa subunit. *Antiviral Res.* 2018;160:109-117.
67. Genentech USA, Inc. Baloxavir prescribing information. Accessed October 2023. https://www.accessdata.fda.gov/drugsatfda_docs/label/2018/210854s000lbl.pdf
68. Chang C, Ramphul K. Amantadine. In: *StatPearls* [Internet]. StatPearls Publishing; 2023.
69. Centers for Disease Control and Prevention. Antiviral dosage: guidance on the use of influenza antiviral agents. Accessed October 2023. https://www.cdc.gov/flu/professionals/antivirals/antiviral-dosage.htm
70. Vorobjev YN. An effective molecular blocker of ion channel of M2 protein as anti-influenza a drug. *J Biomol Struct Dyn.* 2021;39:2352-2363.
71. Holmes EC. COVID-19-lessons for zoonotic disease. *Science.* 2022;375:1114-1115.

72. da Costa VG, Moreli ML, Saivish MV. The emergence of SARS, MERS and novel SARS-2 coronaviruses in the 21st century. *Arch Virol.* 2020;165:1517-1526.
73. Parker MD, Lindsey BB, Leary, S, et al. Subgenomic RNA identification in SARS-CoV-2 genomic sequencing data. *Genome Res.* 2021; 31(4):645-658.
74. Jin Z, Du X, Xu Y, et al. Structure of M(pro) from SARS-CoV-2 and discovery of its inhibitors. *Nature.* 2020;582:289-293.
75. NIH Coronavirus disease 2019 (COVID-19) treatment guidelines. Accessed October 2023. https://www.covid19treatmentguidelines.nih.gov
76. Lamers MM, Haagmans BL. SARS-CoV-2 pathogenesis. *Nat Rev Microbiol.* 2022;20:270-284.
77. World Health Organization. Therapeutics and COVID 19: living guideline. Accessed October 2023. https://www.who.int/teams/health-care-readiness/covid-19/therapeutics
78. Marzi M, Vakil MK, Bahmanyar M, et al. Paxlovid: mechanism of action, synthesis, and in silico study. *Biomed Res Int.* 2022;2022:7341493.
79. Kotecha P, Light A, Checcucci E, et al. Repurposing of drugs for COVID-19: a systematic review and meta-analysis. *Panminerva Med.* 2022;64:96-114.
80. Hull MW, Montaner JS. Ritonavir-boosted protease inhibitors in HIV therapy. *Ann Med.* 2011;43:375-388.
81. Eng H, Dantonio AL, Kadar EP, et al. Disposition of nirmatrelvir, an orally bioavailable inhibitor of SARS-CoV-2 3C-like protease, across animals and humans. *Drug Metab Dispos.* 2022;50:576-590.
82. Kabinger F, Stiller C, Schmitzová J, et al. Mechanism of molnupiravir-induced SARS-CoV-2 mutagenesis. *Nat Struct Mol Biol.* 2021;28:740-746.
83. Merck & Co., Inc. Molnupiravir prescribing information. Accessed October 2023. https://www.fda.gov/media/155054/download
84. Gilead Sciences, Inc. Remdesivir prescribing information. Accessed October 2023. https://www.accessdata.fda.gov/drugsatfda_docs/label/2022/214787Orig1s010Lbl.pdf
85. Malin JJ, Suárez I, Priesner V, et al. Remdesivir against COVID-19 and other viral diseases. *Clin Microbiol Rev.* 2020;34:e00162-20.
86. Kokic G, Hillen H, Tegunov D, et al. Mechanism of SARS-CoV-2 polymerase stalling by remdesivir. *Nat Commun.* 2021;12:279.
87. Deb S, Reeves AA, Hopefl R, et al. ADME and pharmacokinetic properties of remdesivir: its drug interaction potential. *Pharmaceuticals.* 2021;14:655.
88. Invivyd, Inc. Pemivibart prescribing information. Accessed May 2024. https://www.fda.gov/media/177069/download
89. Huang Y, Yang C, Xu X-F, et al. Structural and functional properties of SARS-CoV-2 spike protein: potential antivirus drug development for COVID-19. *Acta Pharmacol Sin.* 2020;41:1141-1149.
90. McLaughlin JM, Khan F, Schmitt HJ, et al. Respiratory syncytial virus-associated hospitalization rates among us infants: a systematic review and meta-analysis. *J Infect Dis.* 2022;225:1100-1111.
91. Branche AR, Saiman L, Walsh EE, et al. Incidence of respiratory syncytial virus infection among hospitalized adults, 2017-2020. *Clin Infect Dis.* 2022;74:1004-1011.
92. Hansen CL, Chaves SS, Demont C, et al. Mortality associated with influenza and respiratory syncytial virus in the US, 1999-2018. *JAMA Netw Open.* 2022;5:e220527.
93. Jain H, Schweitzer JW, Justice NA. Respiratory syncytial virus infection in children. *StatPearls.* Accessed May 2024. https://www.ncbi.nlm.nih.gov/books/NBK459215
94. McLellan JS, Chen M, Leun, S, et al. Structure of RSV fusion glycoprotein trimer bound to a prefusion-specific neutralizing antibody. *Science.* 2013;340:1113-1117.
95. Simpson J, Loh Z, Ullah MA, et al. Respiratory syncytial virus infection promotes necroptosis and HMGB1 release by airway epithelial cells. *Am J Respir Crit Care Med.* 2020;201:1358-1371.
96. Miyairi I, DeVincenzo JP. Human genetic factors and respiratory syncytial virus disease severity. *Clin Microbiol Rev.* 2008;21:686-703.
97. Walsh EE, Peterson DR, Kalkanoglu AE, et al. Viral shedding and immune responses to respiratory syncytial virus infection in older adults. *J Infect Dis.* 2013;207:1424-1432.
98. Dieussaert I, Hyung JK, Luik S, et al. RSV prefusion F protein-based maternal vaccine—preterm birth and other outcomes. *N Engl J Med.* 2024;390:1009-1021.
99. Aljabr W, Touzelet O, Pollakis G, et al. Investigating the influence of ribavirin on human respiratory syncytial virus RNA synthesis by using a high-resolution transcriptome sequencing approach. *J Virol.* 2016;90:4876-4888.
100. Te HS, Randall G, Jensen DM. Mechanism of action of ribavirin in the treatment of chronic hepatitis C. *Gastroenterol Hepatol.* 2007;3:218-225.
101. Domachowske JB, Khan AA, Esser MT, et al. Safety, tolerability and pharmacokinetics of MEDI8897, an extended half-life single-dose respiratory syncytial virus prefusion F-targeting monoclonal antibody administered as a single dose to healthy preterm infants. *Pediatr Infect Dis J.* 2018;37:886-892.
102. Battles MB, Langedijk JP, Furmanova-Hollenstein P, et al. Molecular mechanism of respiratory syncytial virus fusion inhibitors. *Nat Chem Biol.* 2016;12:87-93.
103. Huang K, Incognito L, Cheng X, Ulbrandt ND, Wu H. Respiratory syncytial virus-neutralizing monoclonal antibodies motavizumab and palivizumab inhibit fusion. *J Virol.* 2010;84:8132-8140.
104. Maucort-Boulch D, de Martel C, Franceschi S, et al. Fraction and incidence of liver cancer attributable to hepatitis B and C viruses worldwide. *Int J Cancer.* 2018;142:2471-2477.
105. Nelson NP, Weng MK, Hofmeister MG, et al. Prevention of hepatitis A virus infection in the United States: recommendations of the Advisory Committee on Immunization Practices, 2020. *MMWR Recomm Rep.* 2020;69:1-38.
106. Cao G, Jing W, Liu J, et al. The global trends and regional differences in incidence and mortality of hepatitis A from 1990 to 2019 and implications for its prevention. *Hepatol Int.* 2021;15:1068-1082.
107. Stanaway JD, Flaxman AD, Naghavi M, et al. The global burden of viral hepatitis from 1990 to 2013: findings from the Global Burden of Disease Study 2013. *Lancet.* 2016;388:1081-1088.
108. Martinello M, Solomon SS, Terrault NA, et al. Hepatitis C. *Lancet.* 2023;402:1085-1096.
109. Brunner N, Bruggmann P. Trends of the global hepatitis c disease burden: strategies to achieve elimination. *J Prev Med Public Health.* 2021;54:251-258.
110. Thomas DL, Seeff LB. Natural history of hepatitis C. *Clin Liver Dis.* 2005;9:383-398.
111. Axley P, Ahmed Z, Ravi S, et al. Hepatitis C virus and hepatocellular carcinoma: a narrative review. *J Clin Transl Hepatol.* 2018;6:79-84.
112. Terrault NA, Lok ASF, McMahon BJ, et al. Update on prevention, diagnosis, and treatment of chronic hepatitis B: AASLD 2018 hepatitis B guidance. *Hepatology* 2018;67:1560-1599.
113. Pawlotsky JM. NS5A inhibitors in the treatment of hepatitis C. *J Hepatol.* 2013;59:375-382.
114. De Andrea M, Ravera R, Gioia D, et al. The interferon system: an overview, *Eur J Paediatr Neurol.* 2002;6:A41-A46.
115. Streuli M, Nagata S, Weissmann C. At least three human type alpha interferons: structure of alpha 2. *Science.* 1980;209:1343-1347.
116. Woo ASJ, Kwok R, Ahmed T. Alpha-interferon treatment in hepatitis B. *Ann Transl Med.* 2017;5:159.
117. Foster GR. Pegylated interferons for the treatment of chronic hepatitis C: pharmacological and clinical differences between peginterferon-alpha-2a and peginterferon-alpha-2b. *Drugs.* 2010;70:147-165.
118. Shuldiner SR, Gong L, Muir AJ, et al. PharmGKB summary: peginterferon-α pathway. *Pharmacogenet Genomics.* 2015;25:465-4674.
119. Clark DN, Tajwar R, Hu J, et al. The hepatitis B virus polymerase. *Enzymes.* 2021;50:195-226.
120. Paintsiland E, Cheng YC. Antiviral drugs. In: Schaechter M, ed. *Encyclopedia of Microbiology.* 3rd ed. Academic Press; 2009:223-257.
121. Dando T, Plosker G. Adefovir dipivoxil: a review of its use in chronic hepatitis B. *Drugs.* 2003;63:2215-2234.
122. Amarapurkar DN. Telbivudine: a new treatment for chronic hepatitis B. *World J Gastroenterol.* 2007;13:6150-6165.

123. Gu M, Rice CM. Structures of hepatitis C virus nonstructural proteins required for replicase assembly and function. *Curr Opin Virol.* 2013;3:129-136.
124. Bhattacharya D, Aronsohn A, Price J, et al. Hepatitis C guidance 2023 update: AASLD-IDSA recommendations for testing, managing, and treating hepatitis C virus infection. *Clin Infect Dis.* 2023:ciad319.
125. Naggie S, Muir AJ. Oral combination therapies for hepatitis C virus infection: successes, challenges, and unmet needs. *Annu Rev Med.* 2017;68:345-358.
126. Izquierdo L, Helle F, François C, et al. Simeprevir for the treatment of hepatitis C virus infection. *Pharmgenomics Pers Med.* 2014;7:241-249.
127. Timm J, Kosovrasti K, Henes M, et al. Molecular and structural mechanism of pan-genotypic HCV NS3/4A protease inhibition by glecaprevir. *ACS Chem Biol.* 2020:15:342-352.
128. Kohler JJ, Nettles JH, Amblard F, et al. Approaches to hepatitis C treatment and cure using NS5A inhibitors. *Infect Drug Resist.* 2014;7:41-56.
129. Ascher DB, Wielens J, Nero TL, et al. Potent hepatitis C inhibitors bind directly to NS5A and reduce its affinity for RNA. *Sci Rep.* 2014;4:4765.
130. Wang T, Babusis D, Park Y, et al. Species differences in liver accumulation and metabolism of nucleotide prodrugs of sofosbuvir. *Drug Metab Pharmacokinet.* 2020;35:334-340.
131. Trivella JP, Gutierrez J, Martin P. Dasabuvir: a new direct antiviral agent for the treatment of hepatitis C. *Expert Opin Pharmacother.* 2015;16:617-624.
132. Shen J, Serby M, Reed A, et al. Metabolism and disposition of hepatitis C polymerase inhibitor dasabuvir in humans. *Drug Metab Dispos.* 2016;44:1139-1147.
133. AbbVie Inc. Mavyret prescribing information. Accessed January 2024. https://www.rxabbvie.com/pdf/mavyret_pi.pdf
134. Merck Sharp & Dohme Corp. Zepatier prescribing information. Accessed January 2024. https://www.accessdata.fda.gov/drugsatfda_docs/label/2017/208261s002lbl.pdf
135. Gilead Sciences, Inc. Sofosbuvir prescribing information. Accessed January 2024. https://www.accessdata.fda.gov/drugsatfda_docs/label/2015/204671s002lbl.pdf
136. Gilead Sciences, Inc. Epclusa prescribing information. Accessed January 2024. https://www.accessdata.fda.gov/drugsatfda_docs/label/2016/208341s000lbl.pdf
137. AbbVie Inc. Viekira Pak prescribing information. Accessed January 2024. https://www.accessdata.fda.gov/drugsatfda_docs/label/2014/206619lbl.pdf
138. Sharp PM, Hahn BH. Origins of HIV and the AIDS pandemic. *Cold Spring Harb Perspect Med.* 2011;1:a006841.
139. Hiv.gov. The global HIV and AIDS epidemic. Accessed May 2024. https://www.hiv.gov/hiv-basics/overview/data-and-trends/global-statistics
140. Meissner ME, Talledge N, Mansky LM. Molecular biology and diversification of human retroviruses. *Front Virol.* 2022;2:872599.
141. Nyamweya S, Hegedus A, Jaye A, Rowland-Jones S, Flanagan KL, Macallan DC. Comparing HIV-1 and HIV-2 infection: lessons for viral immunopathogenesis. *Rev Med Virol.* 2013;23:221-240.
142. Bekker LG, Beyrer C, Mgodi N, et al. HIV infection. *Nat Rev Dis Primers.* 2023;9:42.
143. Irshad U, Mahdy H, Tonismae T. HIV in pregnancy. In: *StatPearls* [Internet]. StatPearls Publishing; 2024.
144. HIVinfo.NIH.gov. FDA approval of HIV medicines. Accessed February 2024. https://hivinfo.nih.gov/understanding-hiv/fact-sheets/fda-approved-hiv-medicines
145. U.S. Department of Health and Human Services Panel on Antiretroviral Guidelines for Adults and Adolescents. Guidelines for the use of antiretroviral agents in adults and adolescents with HIV. Accessed February 2024. https://clinicalinfo.hiv.gov/en/guidelines/adult-and-adolescent-arv
146. Mitsuya H. *Anti-HIV Nucleosides: Past, Present and Future.* Chapman and Hall; 1997.
147. Gorbach SL, Barlett JG, Blacklow NR. *Infectious Diseases.* W.B. Saunders Company; 1998.
148. Ray AS, Yang Z, Shi J, et al. Insights into the molecular mechanism of inhibition and drug resistance for HIV-1 RT with carbovir triphosphate. *Biochemistry.* 2002;41:5150-5162.
149. Drugs for HIV infection. Treatment guidelines. *Med Lett.* 2014;12:7-16.
150. Freimuth WW. Delavirdine mesylate, a potent non-nucleoside HIV-1 reverse transcriptase inhibitor. *Adv Exp Med Biol.* 1996;394:279-289.
151. Graul AI, Rabesseda X, Castaner J. Efavirenz. *Drugs Future.* 1998;23:133-141.
152. Schrijvers R. Etravirine for the treatment of HIV/AIDS. *Expert Opin Pharmacother.* 2013;14:1087-1096.
153. Ferretti F, Boffito M. Rilpivirine long-acting for the prevention and treatment of HIV infection. *Curr Opin HIV AIDS.* 2018;13:300-307.
154. Colombier MA, Molina JM. Doravirine: a review. *Curr Opin HIV AIDS.* 2018;13:308-314.
155. Srinivas RV, Fridland A. Human immunodeficiency viruses (Retroviridae), antiretroviral agents. In: Allan Granoff A, Webster RG, eds. *Encyclopedia of Virology.* 2nd ed. Elsevier; 1999:778-788.
156. Ren J, Milton J, Weaver KL, et al. Structural basis for the resilience of efavirenz (DMP-266) to drug resistance mutations in HIV-1 reverse transcriptase. *Structure.* 2000;8:1089-1094.
157. Lazerwith SE, Siegel D, McFadden RM, et al. New antiretrovirals for HIV and antivirals for HBV. In: Chackalamannil S, Rotella D, Ward SE, eds. *Comprehensive Medicinal Chemistry III.* Elsevier; 2017: 628-664.
158. Blanco JL, Whitlock G, Milinkovic A, et al. HIV integrase inhibitors: a new era in the treatment of HIV. *Expert Opin Pharmacother.* 2015;16:1313-1324.
159. Craigie R. The molecular biology of HIV integrase. *Future Virol.* 2012;7:679-686.
160. Mouscadet JF, Tchertanov L. Raltegravir: molecular basis of its mechanism of action. *Eur J Med Res.* 2009;14(suppl 3):5-16.
161. Lemke TL, Zito SW, Roche VF, et al. *Essentials of Foye's Principles of Medicinal Chemistry.* Wolters Kluwer; 2017:573-575.
162. Weber IT, Wang YF, Harrison RW. HIV protease: historical perspective and current research. *Viruses.* 2021;13:839.
163. Oroszlan S, Luftig RB. Retroviral proteinases. *Curr Top Microbiol Immunol.* 1990;157:153-185.
164. Konvalinka J, Kräusslich HG, Müller B. Retroviral proteases and their roles in virion maturation. *Virology.* 2015;479-480:403-417.
165. Bihani S, Das A, Prashar V, et al. X-ray structure of HIV-1 protease in situ product complex. *Proteins.* 2009;74:594-602.
166. Rich DH, Sun ET. Mechanism of inhibition of pepsin by pepstatin. Effect of inhibitor structure on dissociation constant and time-dependent inhibition. *Biochem Pharmacol.* 1980;29:2205-2212.
167. Ghosh AK, Osswald HL, Prato G. Recent progress in the development of HIV-1 protease inhibitors for the treatment of HIV/AIDS. *J Med Chem.* 2016;59:5172-5208.
168. Doyon L, Tremblay S, Bourgon L, et al. Selection and characterization of HIV-1 showing reduced susceptibility to the non-peptidic protease inhibitor tipranavir. *Antivir Res.* 2005;68:27-35.
169. Ray N. Maraviroc in the treatment of HIV infection. *Drug Des Devel Ther.* 2009;2:151-161.
170. Pfizer Labs. Maraviroc prescribing information. Accessed March 2024. https://www.accessdata.fda.gov/drugsatfda_docs/label/2007/022128lbl.pdf
171. Muccini C, Canetti D, Castagna A, et al. Efficacy and safety profile of fostemsavir for the treatment of people with human immunodeficiency virus-1 (HIV-1): current evidence and place in therapy. *Drug Des Devel Ther.* 2022;16:297-304.
172. ViiV Healthcare. Fostemsavir prescribing information. Accessed March 2024. https://www.accessdata.fda.gov/drugsatfda_docs/label/2020/212950s000lbl.pdf
173. Lalezari JP, Henry K, O'Hearn M, et al. Enfuvirtide, an HIV-1 fusion inhibitor, for drug-resistant HIV infection in north and south America. *N Engl J Med.* 2003;348:2175-2185.

174. Poveda E, Briz V, Soriano V. Enfuvirtide, the first fusion inhibitor to treat HIV infection. *AIDS Rev.* 2005;7:139-147.
175. Iacob SA, Iacob DG. Ibalizumab targeting CD4 receptors, an emerging molecule in HIV therapy. *Front Microbiol.* 2017;8:2323.
176. Zhuang S, Torbett BE. Interactions of HIV-1 capsid with host factors and their implications for developing novel therapeutics. *Viruses.* 2021;13:417.
177. Bester SM, Wei G, Zhao H, et al. Structural and mechanistic bases for a potent HIV-1 capsid inhibitor. *Science.* 2020;370:360-364.
178. Patel TS, Crutchley RD, Tucker AM, et al. Crofelemer for the treatment of chronic diarrhea in patients living with HIV/AIDS. *HIV AIDS (Auckl).* 2013;5:153-162.
179. Riedel S. Edward Jenner and the history of smallpox and vaccination. *Proc (Bayl Univ Med Cent).* 2005;18:21-25.
180. Breman JG, Henderson DA. Diagnosis and management of smallpox. *N Engl J Med.* 2002;346(17):1300-1308.
181. World Health Organization. Smallpox. Accessed May 2024. https://www.who.int/teams/health-product-policy-and-standards/standards-and-specifications/norms-and-standards/vaccine-standardization/smallpox
182. Petersen BW, Damon IK, Pertowski CA, et al. Clinical guidance for smallpox vaccine use in a postevent vaccination program. *MMWR Recomm Rep.* 2015;64:1-26.
183. Koch LK, Cunze S, Kochmann J, Klimpel S. Bats as putative Zaire ebolavirus reservoir hosts and their habitat suitability in Africa. *Sci Rep.* 2020;10:14268.
184. Falasca L, Agrati C, Petrosillo N, et al. Molecular mechanisms of Ebola virus pathogenesis: focus on cell death. *Cell Death Differ.* 2015;22:1250-1259.
185. Jacob ST, Crozier I, Fischer WA, et al. Ebola virus disease. *Nat Rev Dis Primers.* 2020;6:13.
186. Bosa HK, Kamara N, Aragaw M, et al. The west Africa Ebola virus disease outbreak: 10 years on. *Lancet Glob Health.* 2024;12(186):e1081-e1083.
187. Gunn BM, Roy V, Karim MM, et al. Survivors of Ebola virus disease develop polyfunctional antibody responses. *J Infect Dis.* 2020;221:156-161.
188. Yang G, Pevear DC, Davies MH, et al. An orally bioavailable antipoxvirus compound(ST-246) inhibits extracellular virus formation and protects mice from lethal orthopoxvirus challenge. *J Virol.* 2005;79:13139-13149.
189. Grosenbach DW, Jordan R, Hruby DE. Development of the small-molecule antiviral ST-246 as a smallpox therapeutic. *Future Virol.* 2011;6:653-671.
190. Jordan R, Leeds JM, Tyavanagimatt S, et al. Development of ST-246® for treatment of poxvirus infections. *Viruses.* 2010;2:2409-2435.

Structure Challenge Answers

1. Viral infections
   A. Acyclovir is used to treat HSV, CMV, and VZV infections.
   B. Oseltamivir is used to treat influenza A and influenza B infections.
   C. Remdesivir is used to treat COVID-19 infections.
   D. Dolutegravir is used to treat HIV infections.
   E. Lopinavir is used to treat HIV infections.
2. Prodrug or not.
   A. Acyclovir is a prodrug. All drugs mimicking naturally occurring purines or pyrimidines must be in their nucleotide form in order to produce an effect. Acyclovir is a nucleoside, lacks the triphosphate sequence required to be incorporated into viral DNA, and thus is a prodrug.
   B. Oseltamivir is a prodrug. An active NA inhibitor drug must have a carboxylic acid present in its structure. The ethyl ester present in the structure of oseltamivir must be hydrolyzed in order for it to be active.
   C. Remdesivir is a prodrug. Similar to acyclovir, it needs to be converted to its triphosphate in order to be incorporated into COVID-19 RNA.
   D. Dolutegravir is not a prodrug and is an active drug.
   E. Lopinavir is not a prodrug and is an active drug.
3. Key structural features.
   A. Acyclovir lacks a 3′-OH group. Once it is incorporated into viral DNA, it will cause immediate termination since the nucleophilic 3′-OH group required for the subsequent addition is missing.
   B. The overall structure of oseltamivir is similar to sialic acid, mimics the transition state of NA, and inhibits the enzyme.
   C. The C_1' nitrile sterically impairs the addition of the fourth nucleotide and stalls viral RNA synthesis. Additionally, the C_1' nitrile compromises the efficiency of complementary base pairing most likely due to its electron-withdrawing properties.
   D. The β-dicarbonyl group in dolutegravir and all INSTIs chelate a divalent cation within the HIV integrase enzyme. This interaction prevents the integration of viral cDNA into cellular DNA.
   E. The structure of lopinavir contains a hydroxyethylene dipeptide mimic that allows lopinavir to act as stable substrate mimic. The secondary hydroxyl group and the adjacent phenylalanine side chain mimic the transition state of hydrolysis. This enables them to bind to HIV protease and cause inhibition.

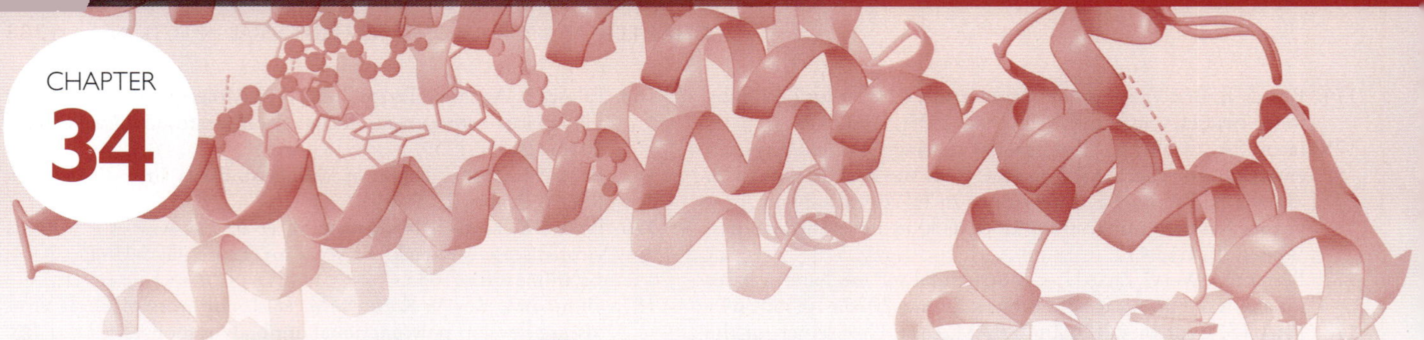

CHAPTER

34

Drugs Used to Treat Fungal Infections

Kimberly Beck

Drugs covered in this chapter:

POLYENES
- Amphotericin B
- Natamycin
- Nystatin

SQUALENE EPOXIDASE INHIBITORS

ALLYLAMINES
- Butenafine
- Naftifine
- Terbinafine

THIOCARBAMATE
- Tolnaftate

AZOLES

IMIDAZOLES
- Butoconazole
- Clotrimazole
- Econazole
- Ketoconazole
- Luliconazole
- Miconazole
- Oxiconazole
- Sertaconazole
- Sulconazole
- Tioconazole

TRIAZOLES
- Efinaconazole
- Fluconazole
- Isavuconazole
- Itraconazole
- Posaconazole
- Terconazole
- Voriconazole

TETRAZOLE
- Oteseconazole

ECHINOCANDINS
- Anidulafungin
- Caspofungin
- Micafungin
- Rezafungin

TRITERPENOID
- Ibrexafungerp

MISCELLANEOUS
- Ciclopirox
- Flucytosine
- Griseofulvin
- Tavaborole
- Undecylenic acid

Abbreviations

5-FdUMP 5-fluorodeoxyuridine monophosphate
5-FU 5-fluorouracil
ABC ATP-binding cassette
ABLC AmB lipid complex
AmB amphotericin B
ARDS acute respiratory distress syndrome
BBB blood-brain barrier
CAmB encochleated AmB
cLogP calculated log P; partition coefficient
CNS central nervous system
COMT catechol-*O*-methyltransferase
CoQ coenzyme Q, ubiquinone
CrCl creatinine clearance
CSF cerebrospinal fluid
CYP450 cytochrome P450
DDI drug-drug interaction
DHODH dihydroorotate dehydrogenase
FDA U.S. Food and Drug Administration
FMN flavin mononucleotide
FMNH2 dihydroflavin mononucleotide
GPI glycosylphosphatidylinositol
IC_{50} inhibitory concentration
IV intravenous
K_d dissociation constant
LeuRS leucyl-transfer RNA synthetase
Mdr1 multidrug resistance 1
MFS major facilitator superfamily
MIC minimum inhibitory concentration
MW molecular weight
OAT organic cation transporter
OTC over-the-counter
PCP *Pneumocystis* pneumonia
P-gp P-glycoprotein
spp. multiple species
SUBA super bioavailability
$t_{1/2}$ half-life
UDP uridine diphosphate
WHO World Health Organization

CLINICAL SIGNIFICANCE

Treating systemic fungal infections is challenging, and choosing the optimal antifungal agent is paramount for safe and successful clinical outcomes. However, doing so requires a strong understanding of an antifungal agent's medicinal chemistry and pharmacologic properties. Amphotericin B (AmB) deoxycholate's clinical use is limited by both infusion-related reactions and nephrotoxicity. Lipid formulations of AmB reduced these toxicities and offered a more tolerable treatment option. An encochleated form of AmB is entering phase III clinical trials, which may offer an oral formulation for the first time. Triazole antifungals have the broadest therapeutic use owing to their oral and intravenous (IV) dosage forms. However, these agents possess varying clinical utility and off-target effects that need to be considered. Oteseconazole, a tetrazole, may produce less off-target effects and offer a clinical advantage over current triazole options. Echinocandins have fewer off-target effects compared to triazoles, but they require daily IV administration. Rezafungin has once-weekly IV administration, which may improve transitions of care. Ibrexafungerp is a triterpenoid compound that is mechanistically similar to echinocandins but can be given orally, which may further improve patient care. These are just a small sampling of how medicinal chemistry changes impact the current and future clinical utility of antifungal agents. Therefore, a complete understanding of these concepts is vital to clinical decision-making and optimal patient outcomes, particularly as new and improved agents are entering the clinical arena.

Jarrett R. Amsden, PharmD

INTRODUCTION

Immunocompetent humans generally can ward off invading fungal pathogens with little difficulty; therefore, the demand for improvements in antifungal therapy had been low until recent decades. A dramatic increase in immunocompromised patients, due in part to medical advances, has led to a similarly dramatic increase in potentially lethal invasive fungal infections. The increased use of powerful immunosuppressive drugs for solid organ and stem cell transplantation, cancer chemotherapy, and for the treatment of autoimmune and inflammatory disorders, has resulted in an increased incidence of life-threatening fungal infections and a corresponding increase in demand for new drugs to treat these infections.[1] Diabetes, chronic obstructive pulmonary disease, and critically ill patients in the intensive care unit, including those with COVID-19 infection, are also among those at increased risk for fungal infections.[2-5] Furthermore, acquired resistance to existing antifungal agents and the emergence of new and intrinsically highly drug-resistant, fungal pathogens are increasing, requiring an increased arsenal of antifungal drugs.[6] The number of effective antifungal agents available is quite small compared to that available to treat bacterial infections, but research in this area is active. Several new agents have been introduced in the last few years, but more are needed, including antifungal drugs active against new targets and against pathogenic fungal species resistant to antifungal drugs currently available.[7,8]

EPIDEMIOLOGY AND ECONOMIC IMPACT OF FUNGAL INFECTIONS

The most recent data estimate that approximately 6.55 million new invasive fungal infections are diagnosed each year worldwide.[9] These fungal infections are directly responsible for an estimated 2.55 million deaths annually. The leading cause of the total global annual incidence of invasive fungal infections is invasive aspergillosis (32%), followed by chronic pulmonary aspergillosis (28%) and the combined occurrence of candidemia and invasive candidiasis (24%).[9]

Among all inpatient visits in the United States in 2018, approximately 666,235 included a fungal infection diagnosis.[2] Of the 666,235 inpatient fungal infections, approximately 29,335 cases had fungal infections listed as the primary cause of hospital admission (4%).[2] The majority of hospital admissions for fungal infections as the primary cause were for candidiasis (~15,890 cases, 54%), mostly noninvasive (~10,905 cases, 37%). Invasive candidiasis as the primary diagnosis (4,880, 17%) was the next highest cause, following by aspergillosis (2,480, 8.44%), invasive aspergillosis (1,545, 5.26%), and coccidioidomycosis (2,265, 7.7%).

The risk of death among inpatients with a fungal diagnosis is higher.[2] In 2018, patients diagnosed with mucormycosis exhibited the highest mortality rate (18.61%), followed by those with invasive candidiasis (16.97%), pneumocystosis (12.85%), and invasive aspergillosis (12.64%).[2] In the first 2 years of the COVID-19 pandemic (2020-2021), there was an increase in fungal deaths in the United States.[10] Of the deaths associated with fungal infections during this time, 21.9% were associated with COVID-19.[10] *Candida* and *Aspergillus* were involved in a higher percentage of COVID-19-associated fungal deaths than in non–COVID-19-associated fungal deaths.[10] This further supports COVID-19 as a risk factor for invasive candidiasis and invasive aspergillosis.

Total health care costs for inpatient visits where any fungal infections were diagnosed were $37.7 billion in 2018 in the United States.[2] When the primary diagnosis for inpatient visit was fungal infection, the total health care costs were $1.4 billion. Inpatient health care costs for patients with a fungal infection diagnosis are twice as high as for inpatients without a fungal infection.[2] In 2018, an estimated 6.6 million additional fungal infections were diagnosed during outpatient visits, primarily comprising dermatophytic infections, followed by noninvasive candidiasis.[2] It is estimated that the direct medical costs for fungal diseases in the United States in 2019 were nearly $7.5 billion.[11]

Fungal Diseases

The fungal kingdom includes yeasts, molds, rusts, and mushrooms. Most fungi are saprophytic, which means they live on dead organic matter in the soil or on decaying leaves or wood. Few fungi cause disease in humans (Table 34.1), and those that do can be limited to superficial topical infections, systemic, or both. A few of these fungi can cause opportunistic infections if they are introduced into a human through wounds or by inhalation. Some of these infections can be fatal. There are relatively few obligate animal parasites (ie, microorganisms that can only live on mammalian hosts) among the fungi, although *Candida albicans* is commonly found as part of the normal flora of the gastrointestinal (GI) tract and vagina. The obligatory parasites are limited to dermatophytes that have evolved to live on/in the keratin-containing hair, skin, and nails of mammals, where they cause diseases such as athlete's foot. A detailed description of fungal infections is beyond the scope of this chapter, but comprehensive textbooks and literature reviews are available.[12-18]

Most fungal infections are caused primarily by various yeasts and molds. Yeasts, such as the opportunistic pathogen *C. albicans*, typically grow as single oval cells and reproduce by budding. *C. albicans* and several other pathogenic yeasts also can grow in multicellular chains called hyphae. Infection sites may contain both yeast and hyphal forms of the microorganism. Molds, such as *Trichophyton rubrum*, one of the causative agents of ringworm, grow in clusters of hyphae called a mycelium. All fungi produce spores, which may be transported by direct contact or through the air. Although most topical fungal infections are readily treated, the incidence of life-threatening systemic fungal infections, including those caused by yeasts such as *C. albicans* and molds such as *Aspergillus fumigatus*, is increasing, and mortality is high.[3]

Table 34.1 Common Infectious Fungal Organisms

Disease State	Common Organisms	Topical/Systemic
Dermatomycosis: • Tinea capitis • Tinea pedis (athlete's foot) • Tinea cruris (jock itch) • Tinea unguium (nail infection) • Tinea corporis (ringworm)	*Epidermophyton* *Microsporum* *Trichophyton rubrum* *Trichophyton mentagrophytes*	Topical
Aspergillosis	*Aspergillus fumigatus* *Aspergillus flavus* *Aspergillus niger* *Aspergillus terreus*	Systemic
Blastomycosis	*Blastomyces dermatitidis*	Systemic
Candidiasis	*Candida albicans* *Candida auris* *Candida parapsilosis* *Candida tropicalis* *Nakaseomyces glabrata (Candida glabrata)* *Pichia kudriavzevii (Candida krusei)*	Topical/systemic
Coccidioidomycosis	*Coccidioides immitis* *Coccidioides posadasii*	Systemic
Cryptococcosis	*Cryptococcus neoformans*	Systemic
Histoplasmosis	*Histoplasma capsulatum*	Systemic
Mucormycosis	*Rhizopus, Mucor, Lichtheimia*	Topical/systemic
Pneumocystosis	*Pneumocystis jirovecii*	Systemic

Dermatophytes

Dermatophytes are fungi causing infections of the skin, hair, and nails.[19] Dermatophytes obtain nutrients from attacking the cross-linked structural protein keratin, which other fungi cannot use as a food source. Dermatophytic infections, known as tinea, are caused by species of three genera (*Trichophyton*, *Microsporum*, and *Epidermophyton*) and are named for the site of infection rather than for the causative organism. Tinea capitis is a fungal infection of the hair and scalp. Tinea pedis refers to infections of the feet, including athlete's foot, tinea manuum to fungal infection of the hands, tinea cruris to infection of the groin (jock itch), tinea unguium to infection of the fingernails or toenails, and tinea corporis to infection of the torso. Tinea corporis is more commonly known as ringworm even though it is not caused by a parasitic worm, but rather is named for the ringlike appearance of this fungal infection of the skin. Athlete's foot may be an infection involving several different fungi, including yeasts. Tinea unguium, the most common type of onychomycosis, is most often caused by the dermatophytes *Trichophyton rubrum and T. mentagrophytes*. Approximately 10% or more of the cases of onychomycosis are caused by non-dermatophyte molds and *Candida* spp.[20] Whether of the fingernails or toenails, onychomycosis can be particularly difficult to treat because the fungi invade the nail bed and nail matrix, areas which are difficult for drugs to reach. Topical drugs face the additional challenge of effectively penetrating the hardened nail plate to get to the site of infection. Appropriate drug therapy prevents the fungus from spreading to the newly formed nail. With some drug regimens, the infection is not cured until an entirely new, fungus-free nail has grown in. Due to slow nail growth, this takes months, requiring a lengthy drug regimen, and patient compliance can be a problem.

Yeasts

The most common cause of yeast infections is *C. albicans*, which is part of the normal flora in a significant portion of the population where it resides in the oropharynx, GI tract, vagina, and surrounding skin.[21] It is the principal cause of vaginal yeast infections and oral yeast infections (thrush). These commonly occur in mucosal tissue when the normal population of flora has been disturbed by treatment of a bacterial infection with an antibiotic or when growth conditions are changed by hormonal fluctuations, such as occur in pregnancy. *C. albicans* can cause infections of the skin and nails, although the latter are not common. In persons with healthy immune systems, *Candida* infections are limited to superficial infections of the skin and mucosa. In persons with impaired immune systems, however, *C. albicans* may also cause invasive infections, which can be fatal. Several other *Candida* spp. are clinically significant pathogens, including *C. tropicalis*, *C. krusei* (now known as *Pichia kudriavzevii* but still referred to as *C. krusei* clinically), *C. parapsilosis*, and *C. glabrata* (now known as *Nakaseomyces glabrata* but still referred to as *C. glabrata* clinically). *C. auris* is the newest *Candida* spp. of concern in humans.[21] It is classified as critical on the World Health Organization (WHO) Fungal Priority Pathogens List.[22,23] These non–*albicans Candida* spp. are more resistant to current antifungal therapy than *C. albicans*.

Cryptococcus neoformans is a yeast commonly found in certain bird droppings, particularly pigeon droppings.[24] When dust contaminated with spores is inhaled by persons with a competent immune system, the organism may be asymptomatic or cause a minor self-limiting lung infection. Such infections frequently are mistaken for a cold, and medical treatment is not sought. In immunocompromised persons, however, pulmonary cryptococcosis can escalate to fungal pneumonia with acute respiratory distress syndrome (ARDS). Furthermore, in immunocompromised individuals, the organism can be carried by the circulatory system from the lungs to the central nervous system (CNS) causing cryptococcal meningitis[18] or to the skin causing cutaneous cryptococcal infections.[24]

Although most yeast infections are caused by various species of *Candida* or *Cryptococcus*, other yeasts also can cause infections in humans, including *Malassezia furfur*, *Trichosporon asahii*, and *Magnusiomyces capitatus*.[25] These infections are relatively rare and are difficult to treat. A yeast-like opportunistic fungal pathogen, *Pneumocystis jirovecii*, targets exclusively the lungs of immunocompromised humans causing *Pneumocystis* pneumonia (PCP) in patients with low $CD4^+$ T lymphocytes or B cells.[26] This includes patients with HIV, in which the risk of PCP is on the decline due to increasing use of antiretroviral therapy.[27] PCP is increasingly observed in patients without HIV, including those who have undergone solid organ transplants.[26,28] *P. jirovecii* is not responsive to antifungal drugs. The treatment of choice for PCP is trimethoprim/sulfamethoxazole (see Chapter 32). Alternative treatments for PCP include the antiprotozoal drug pentamidine (see Chapter 35).

Molds

Aspergillus species are found worldwide and are virtually ubiquitous in the environment.[14,29,30] The most common *Aspergillus* species causing human disease, including invasive aspergillosis, is *A. fumigatus*.[14,29,30] Other important pathogenic *Aspergillus* species include *A. flavus*, *A. niger*, and *A. terreus*. Because *Aspergillus* spores are small and hydrophobic, they are easily dispersed, and inhalation is the most common route of inoculation, where they can colonize the lung and sinuses.[14,30] Cutaneous infection through wounds, burns, and the eye can also occur. Aspergillosis of the lungs may be contained, but invasive aspergillosis, also called invasive pulmonary aspergillosis, has a high mortality rate. Invasive aspergillosis is associated with severely immunocompromised individuals, such as those undergoing solid organ transplant, hematopoietic stem cell transplant, or cancer chemotherapy.[14,29] Admittance into the intensive care unit and COVID-19 infection are among the risk factors for invasive aspergillosis.

Mucormycosis is the term used to describe infections caused by the genera in the fungal order Mucorales.[15,31] The pathogenic species are opportunistic filamentous fungi. The most common infectious species are from the genera *Rhizopus*, *Mucor*, and *Lichtheimia*.[31] As with several other opportunistic fungal pathogens, these soil microorganisms generally are harmless to those with a competent immune system but can cause rapidly developing, fatal infections in an immunosuppressed patient. Diabetes is a risk factor for rhino-orbital-cerebral mucormycosis.[15,31] These organisms can infect the sinus cavity, from which they spread rapidly to the CNS.

Thermally Dimorphic Fungi

Thermally dimorphic fungi are saprophytes that grow as a mold form at room temperature and as a yeast form in a human host at 37 °C.[32-34] The most common infectious agents are *Blastomyces dermatitidis*, *Coccidioides immitis*, and *Histoplasma capsulatum*, the causative agents of blastomycosis, coccidioidomycosis, and histoplasmosis, respectively. These organisms live in soil and cause disease through inhalation of contaminated dust. The resulting lung infections are often mild and self-limiting, but they may progress to a serious lung infection. The circulatory system may transport the organisms to other tissues, where the resulting systemic infection may be fatal. In the United States, *B. dermatitidis* is endemic to Midwestern, South Central, and Southeastern states in areas around the Ohio and Mississippi River valleys as well as the Great Lakes and St. Lawrence River areas.[17,32] *C. immitis* is endemic to the dry areas of the Southwestern

United States.[16,33] It is particularly prevalent in the San Joaquin Valley of California and has been called "valley fever." *H. capsulatum* is endemic to the Mississippi and Ohio River valleys of the United States. Histoplasmosis is the most prevalent of the endemic mycoses in the United States.[34,35] Cases of dimorphic mycoses are now frequently diagnosed beyond their historically defined geographic boundaries.[35]

Biochemical Targets of Antifungal Chemotherapy

Antifungal chemotherapy depends on biochemical differences between fungi and mammals.[36] Unlike bacteria, which are prokaryotes, both fungi and mammals are eukaryotes, and the biochemical differences between them are not as great. At the cellular level, the greatest difference between fungal cells and mammalian cells is that fungal cells have cell walls, whereas mammalian cells do not. The fungal cell wall is a logical target for drugs, which would be expected to be potent antifungals yet have little human toxicity.[37] However, only a few potent inhibitors of fungal cell wall biosynthesis have become available for clinical use, and all direct their activity toward the same target.[36-38] Other targets for antifungal agents include inhibitors of DNA biosynthesis, disruption of mitotic spindles, and general interference with intermediary metabolism. The difference between fungal and mammalian cells that is most widely exploited, however, is that the cell membranes of fungi and mammals contain different sterols. Mammalian cell membranes contain cholesterol as the sterol component, whereas fungi contain ergosterol.[39] Ergosterol plays a critical role in fungal cell membrane fluidity, permeability, and essential cellular processes.[40]

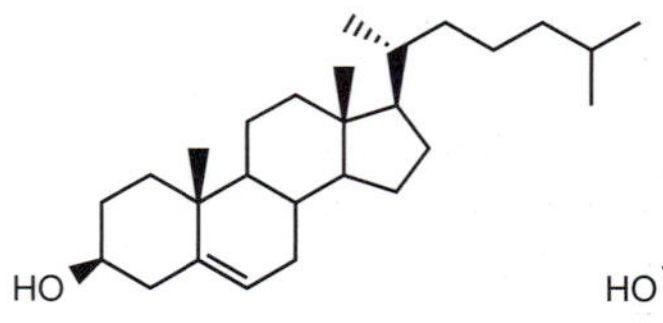

Cholesterol

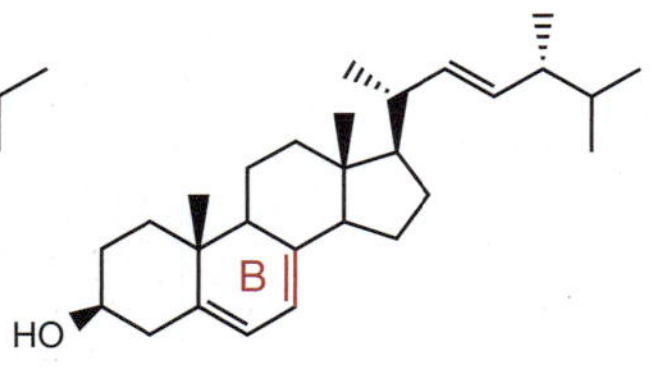

Ergosterol

Although the two sterols are quite similar, the side chains are slightly different, and, when three-dimensional models are constructed, the ring system of ergosterol is slightly flatter because of the additional double bond in the B ring. Nevertheless, this difference in sterol components provides the biochemical basis of selective toxicity for most of the currently available antifungal drugs.

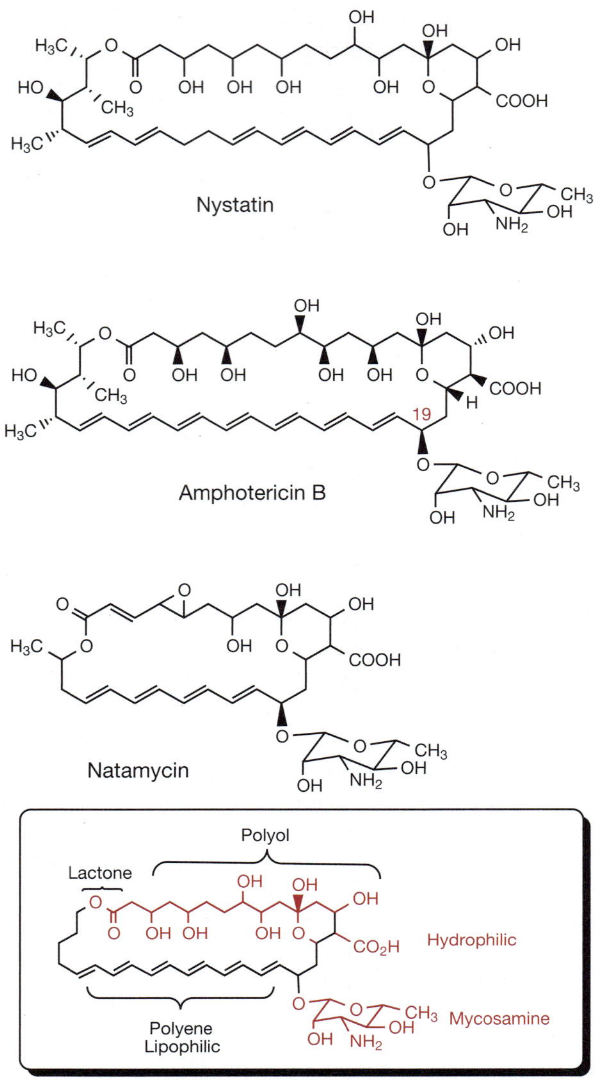

Figure 34.1 Commercially available polyenes. Box indicates chemical features of this class of antifungal agents.

Polyenes: Nystatin, Amphotericin B, and Natamycin

Before the mid-1950s, no reliable treatments existed for the few cases of deep-seated, highly lethal, systemic fungal infections that did occur. The discovery of the polyene antifungal agents (Fig. 34.1) provided a breakthrough and the first drug found to be effective against invasive (systemic) fungal infections.[41]

The polyenes are large macrocyclic lactones (macrolides) with distinct hydrophilic and lipophilic regions. The hydrophilic region contains a series of alcohols (the polyol area), a carboxylic acid, and a sugar glycosidically linked to the macrolide ring. In the natural product antifungal polyenes, the sugar moiety is the amino-containing mycosamine, which is critical for antifungal activity. Polyene derivatives devoid of mycosamine at C19 have no antifungal activity.[42] The antifungal polyenes are amphoteric, having both an acidic group and a basic group, and they are poorly water soluble. The lipophilic region contains a chromophore of four to seven conjugated double bonds (the polyene). The number of conjugated double bonds correlates directly with antifungal activity in vitro and inversely with the degree of toxicity to mammalian cells. AmB, which possesses seven conjugated double bonds, has approximately 10-fold more

Table 34.2 Polyene Formulations

Generic Name	Trade Name	Dosage Form
Nystatin	Generic, Kaylesta, Nyamyc, Nystop	Oral: suspension, tablet Topical: cream, ointment, powder
Natamycin	Natacyn	Ophthalmic suspension
Amphotericin B (deoxycholate)	Generic	Powder for solution for injection
Amphotericin B lipid complex (ABLC)	Abelcet	Suspension for injection
Amphotericin B liposomal (LAmB)	Generic, AmBisome	Powder for suspension for injection

potent antifungal activity than polyenes with four or five conjugated double bonds.[41] It is also the only polyene antifungal that may be used systemically (Table 34.2).[41]

Polyene Mechanism of Action

The ability of the polyenes to bind to the fungal sterol ergosterol is key to their antifungal activity.[42] The higher affinity of the polyenes for ergosterol over cholesterol is the basis for their greater toxicity to fungal cells.[43,44] Forming aggregates outside fungal cell membranes, the polyenes exert their antifungal activity by extracting ergosterol from the cell membrane through a "sterol sponge" mechanism, which ultimately leads to fungal cell death (Fig. 34.2).[45,46] The selectivity of polyenes to bind to ergosterol over cholesterol is not absolute. Cholesterol binding by AmB leads to adverse effects.

Specific Drugs

Nystatin (See Fig. 34.1). Nystatin is a conjugated tetraene isolated from cultures of the bacterium *Streptomyces noursei* in 1950.[41] Nystatin is a topical antifungal against a wide variety of organisms and is available in a variety of creams, ointments, and topical powders. Nystatin is too toxic to be used systemically, but because very little drug is absorbed following oral administration, it may be administered by mouth to treat fungal infections of the mouth and GI tract.[47,48]

Amphotericin B (See Fig. 34.1). AmB is isolated from *Streptomyces nodosus* and was initially approved by the U.S. Food and Drug Administration (FDA) in 1959.[41] As a heptane, it has low enough toxicity to mammalian cells to permit IV administration. To overcome its water insolubility, AmB is formulated with sodium deoxycholate to form a colloidal dispersion when reconstituted, which is suitable for injection.[49] Upon administration, the drug rapidly dissociates from deoxycholate and binds to plasma lipoproteins.[50] AmB is nevertheless a very toxic drug and must be used with caution.[50,51] Its adverse effects include anemia, thrombophlebitis, and infusion-related reactions, such as fever, chills, rigors, nausea, vomiting, and headache. Dose-dependent severe kidney toxicity limits use of AmB. The kidney toxicity

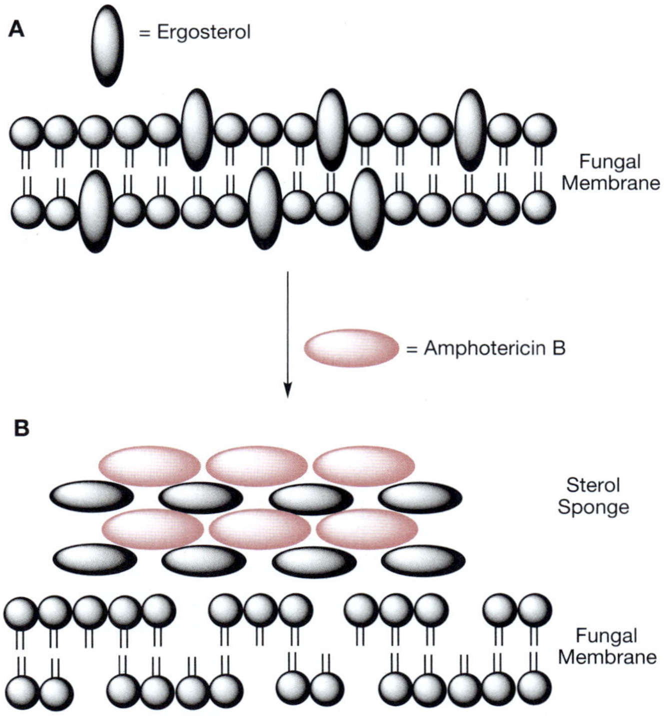

Figure 34.2 Mechanism of action of amphotericin B and polyene antifungals. A. Normal fungal cell membrane with ergosterol embedded within the membrane. B. Fungal cell membrane in the presence of amphotericin B. Amphotericin B forms extramembranous aggregates outside the fungal membrane and extracts ergosterol from the fungal membrane acting as a "sterol sponge". The extraction of ergosterol from the fungal cell membrane is fungicidal. (Modified from Anderson TM, Clay MC, Cioffi AG, et al. Amphotericin B forms an extramembranous and fungicidal sterol sponge. *Nat Chem Biol.* 2014;10:400-406.)

is attributed to a sterol sponge mechanism wherein AmB forms extramembranous aggregates on kidney cells extracting cholesterol from renal cell membranes.[52] Despite its toxicity, AmB and its lipid formulations (see later) continue to be used for many systemic, life-threatening fungal infections due to its broad spectrum of antifungal activity and infrequent resistance.[13-15,18] The drug, in all formulations, distributes to the brain to a limited extent, but it achieves sufficient antifungal concentrations.[53,54] AmB can be administered intrathecally for the treatment of fungal infections of the CNS.[55,56]

The nephrotoxicity of conventional AmB was a serious drawback to the use of this drug upon its introduction. Lipid formulations of AmB have dramatically decreased the toxicity of the drug, which permits higher plasma levels to be employed (Table 34.2).[51] The two commercially available products are AmB lipid complex (ABLC), composed of AmB complexed with two synthetic phospholipids (L-α-dimyristoyl phosphatidylcholine and L-α-dimyristoyl phosphatidylglycerol), and a liposomal encapsulation product.

Altered distribution is clearly a factor by which the lipid formulations decrease nephrotoxicity.[51] Because the blood vessels at the site of fungal infection are more permeable than those of normal tissue, the large, suspended particles of the lipid formulations can penetrate the site of infection more readily than they can penetrate healthy tissue. The result is selective delivery of AmB to the site of infection. Some evidence also indicates that the lipid formulations transfer AmB to ergosterol-containing fungal cells more efficiently than to cholesterol-containing mammalian cells.[57]

NATAMYCIN (SEE FIG. 34.1). Natamycin, a tetraene, is available as a 5% ophthalmic suspension applied topically for the treatment of fungal infections of the eye (Table 34.2).

ORAL AMPHOTERICIN B FORMULATION UNDER INVESTIGATION

Encochleated AmB (CAmB, MT2203) is under clinical evaluation as an oral dosage form of AmB. A cochleate is a lipid nanocrystal wherein AmB is incorporated into a lipid bilayer sheet formed with phosphatidylserine and calcium that is spiraled into a tight tube protecting AmB molecules within.[58-60] Upon oral administration, the CAmB is phagocytosed into macrophages and reticuloendothelial cells, which deliver it to the site of the fungal infection. The low intracellular calcium concentration of the macrophage causes the cochleate to unfurl as calcium moves out and AmB is released to fungal cells. Because AmB is sequestered either in the cochleate or inside the target fungal cell, toxicity should be decreased compared to the intravenous formulations. Phase I and II trials of MT2203 have been completed and results look promising.[59,60]

RENAL-SPARING AMPHOTERICIN B DERIVATIVE UNDER INVESTIGATION

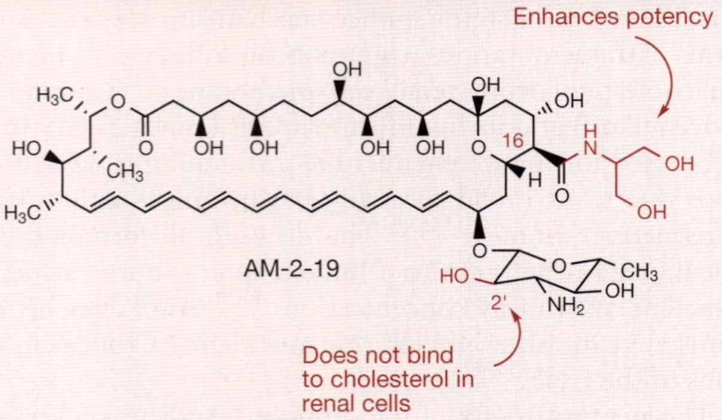

AmB-induced nephrotoxicity is caused by aggregates of AmB extracting cholesterol from renal cell membranes. While the mycosamine sugar of AmB is necessary for ergosterol binding, the C2′-OH group is not.[61] However, the AmB C2′-OH is critical for binding to cholesterol. Epimerization of the C2′-OH of AmB resulted in a compound that selectively binds to ergosterol and does not bind to cholesterol.[52] The polyene of AmB may form π-π stacking interactions with the diene in the B ring of ergosterol, which is lacking in cholesterol. While more selective for ergosterol, the C2′-OH epimerization derivative has less potent antifungal activity due to slower extraction of ergosterol from fungal cell membranes. The antifungal activity of the AmB C2′-OH epimer was enhanced by converting the carboxylic acid at C16 to a nonionizable amide of 2-amino-1,3-propanediol (serinol) to afford the non-amphoteric compound AM-2-19.[52] AM-2-19 extracts ergosterol more quickly than AmB and it selectively binds to ergosterol only, rendering it nontoxic to renal cells. AM-2-19 demonstrates that it is possible to synthesize polyene antifungals that lack nephrotoxicity.

Ergosterol Biosynthesis Inhibitors

A schematic of fungal ergosterol biosynthesis starting from squalene, which occurs in the endoplasmic reticulum, is shown in Figure 34.3. The biosynthetic pathway has been simplified to emphasize steps important to the action of currently employed antifungal drugs.[39,40] The hydrocarbon squalene is converted to squalene epoxide by the enzyme squalene epoxidase, also called Erg1 (encoded by the *ERG1* gene). Squalene epoxide, the last nonsteroidal precursor to both ergosterol and cholesterol, is then cyclized to lanosterol, the first steroid in the pathway. The steps involved in converting the side chain of lanosterol to the side chain of ergosterol and in the removal of the geminal dimethyl groups on position 4 are not shown, because none of these reactions is targeted by clinically employed antifungal agents.

A key step in the conversion of lanosterol to both cholesterol and ergosterol is removal of the 14α-methyl group. This reaction is carried out by a cytochrome P450 (CYP450) enzyme, sterol 14α-demethylase, CYP51, also known as Erg11 (encoded by the *ERG11* gene) in fungi.[39,40] The mechanism of this reaction involves three successive hydroxylations of the 14α-methyl group, sequentially converting it into the alcohol, aldehyde, and carboxylic acid oxidation states (Fig. 34.4).[62] The methyl group is eliminated as formic acid to afford a double bond between C14 and C15 of the D ring. This enzyme is the primary target of the azole antifungal agents discussed later.

Eventually, either before or after modification of the side chain, the Δ14 double bond is reduced by a sterol C-14 reductase (Erg24) to form a *trans* ring juncture between the C and D rings. Several steps later, the double bond between C8 and C9 is isomerized to a Δ7 double bond by the enzyme sterol C-8 isomerase (Erg2), and the C5 double bond is introduced to the B ring by sterol C-5 desaturase (Erg3) to form the diene in ring B found in ergosterol but not in cholesterol. Many of the steps are identical to those involved in mammalian cholesterol biosynthesis, and the basis for selective toxicity to fungal cells will be discussed under the specific agents.

Squalene Epoxidase Inhibitors

Squalene epoxidase inhibitors include a group of drugs generally known as allylamines[63] and one thiocarbamate derivative, tolnaftate[64] (Fig. 34.5). The allylamines include naftifine, terbinafine, and butenafine. The benzyl group of butenafine can be considered bioisosteric with the allyl group of naftifine and terbinafine. These drugs have a more limited spectrum

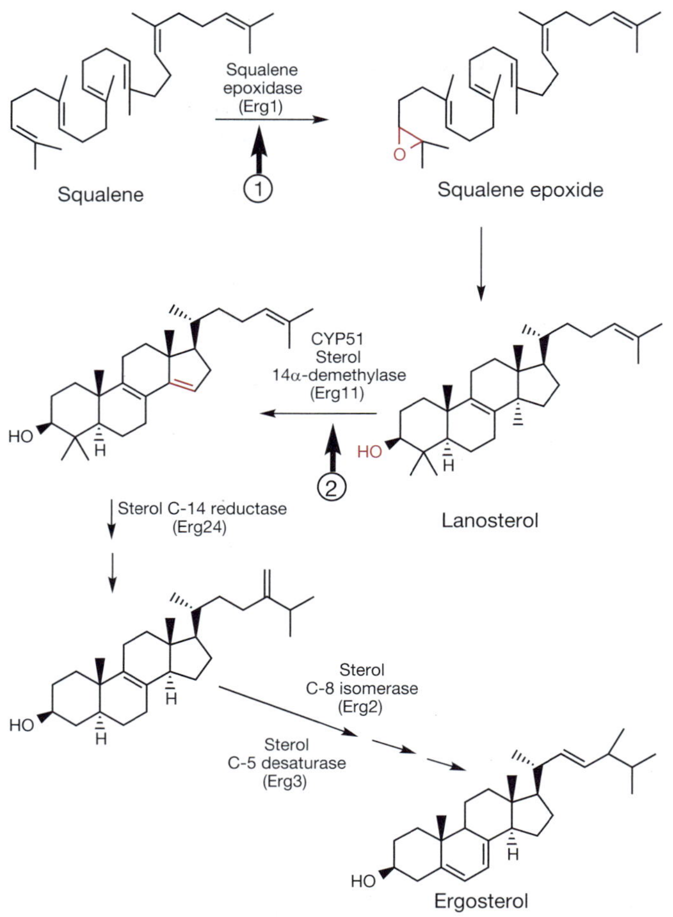

Figure 34.3 Key steps in the biosynthesis of ergosterol in the yeast *Saccharomyces cerevisiae*. Enzymatic steps known to be the site of action of currently employed antifungal agents are indicated by a heavy black arrow and a number. Squalene epoxidase inhibitors act at Site 1. Azole antifungals act at Site 2.

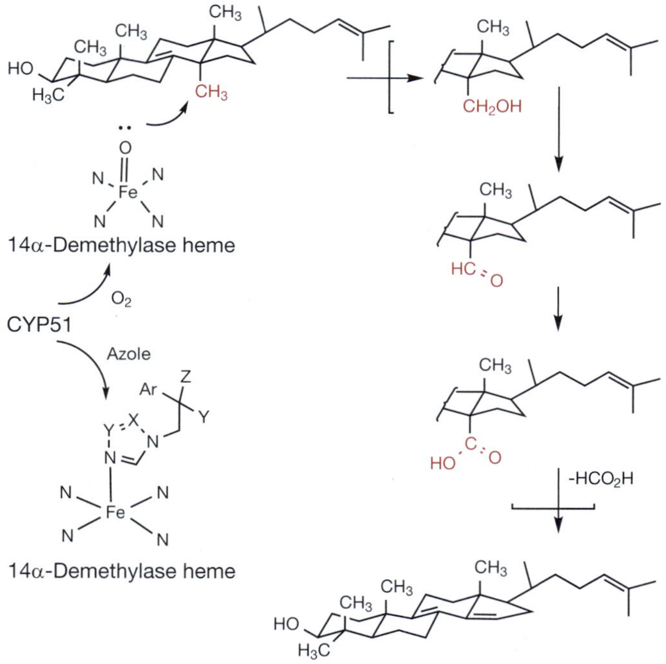

Figure 34.4 Demethylation of the 14α-methyl group from lanosterol via the CYP450 enzyme sterol 14α-demethylase, CYP51 (Erg11). Three successive heme-catalyzed insertions of activated oxygen into the 14α-methyl group, which raises the oxidation state of the methyl group to a carboxylic acid, result in the removal of the 14α-methyl group as formic acid. The azole antifungals bind to CYP51 through the basic nitrogen atom of the azole, preventing oxygen transfer.

of activity than the azole antifungals and are effective only against dermatophytes. Therefore, they are employed in the treatment of fungal infections of the skin and nails.[19,20]

Mechanism of Action. All the drugs in Figure 34.5 act through noncompetitive inhibition of the enzyme squalene epoxidase (Fig. 34.3, Site 1). Inhibition of this enzyme has two effects, both of which appear to be involved in the fungicidal mechanism of this class.[63-65] First, inhibition of squalene epoxidase results in an ergosterol deficiency within the fungal cell membrane, disturbing cell membrane function and processes. Second, and likely more important, inhibition of squalene epoxidase results in accumulation of squalene, which is toxic when present in abnormally high amounts. Squalene epoxidase is also involved in cholesterol biosynthesis in mammals. However, the squalene epoxidase inhibitors are much more selective for fungal squalene epoxidase than the corresponding enzyme in mammals. For example, terbinafine has a *Ki* of 0.03 μM for squalene epoxidase from *C. albicans* compared to 77 μM for the same enzyme from rat liver, demonstrating the tremendous selectivity for fungal squalene epoxidase.[65] High terbinafine selectivity for *T. rubrum* squalene epoxidase over the mammalian enzyme is also observed.[66]

Specific Drugs

Naftifine (See Fig. 34.5). Naftifine was the first allylamine to be discovered and marketed.[63] It undergoes extensive first-pass metabolism, precluding its oral activity; consequently, it is only available in topical cream and gel formulations.[67,68] The widest use of naftifine is against various tinea infections of the skin.

Butenafine (See Fig. 34.5). Butenafine, like naftifine, is only available topically. It is formulated as a cream for the treatment of dermatophytic infections.[19]

Terbinafine (See Fig. 34.5). Terbinafine is available in both topical (cream, gel, spray) and oral[68] dosage forms and is effective against a variety of dermatophytic infections when employed topically or systemically.[19] A unique property of oral terbinafine is its effectiveness in the treatment of onychomycoses (nail infections).[69,70] Given orally, the highly lipophilic drug (calculated log P [cLogP] 5.6)[71] redistributes from the plasma into the nail bed and nail matrix, then into the nail itself, where the infection resides,[72] making terbinafine superior to other agents for treating this type of infection. The treatment duration for onychomycosis with daily oral terbinafine is 6 weeks for fingernail infections and 12 weeks for toenail infections.[20,69] Terbinafine is extensively metabolized by seven CYP450 enzymes, including CYP1A2, CYP2B6, CYP2C8, CYP2C9, CYP2C19, CYP2D6, and CYP3A4.[73,74] The multiple pathways of terbinafine metabolism make inhibition of any one isoform unlikely to affect

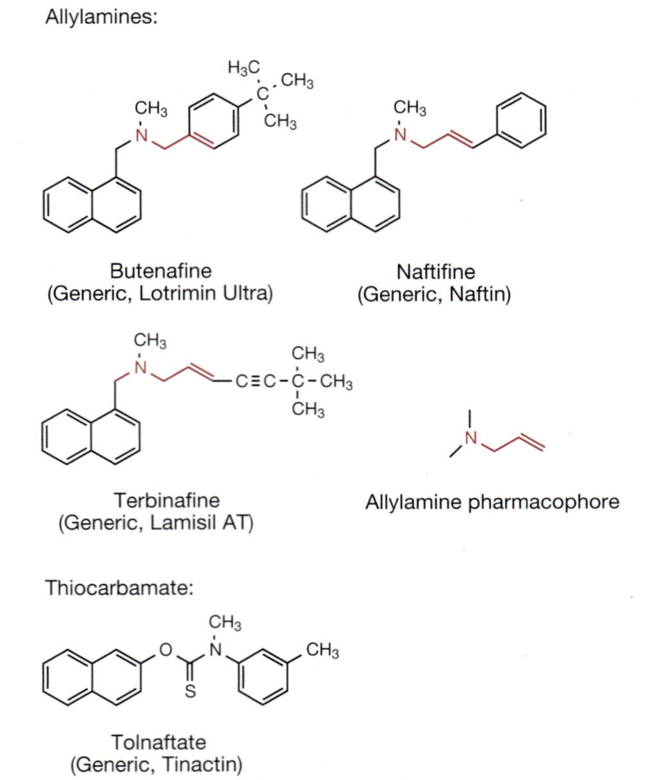

Figure 34.5 Squalene epoxidase inhibitors. Allylamines butenafine and naftifine are for topical use only, while terbinafine may be used topically or systemically. The thiocarbamate tolnaftate is for topical use only.

the overall clearance of the drug. Drugs that inhibit several CYP450 enzymes, such as cimetidine, can increase terbinafine plasma levels. Conversely, rifampin, an inducer of multiple CYP450 enzymes, can reduce terbinafine plasma levels. Terbinafine is a strong inhibitor of CYP2D6 and, when used systemically, it can have significant interactions with drugs that are metabolized by this enzyme, including desipramine, selective serotonin reuptake inhibitors, and certain β-blockers.[75] Oral terbinafine is associated with rare severe liver toxicity.[76] A reactive aldehyde metabolite, TBF-A, possible via three pathways involving *N*-demethylation of terbinafine, has been proposed as a mechanism leading to terbinafine-induced liver toxicity.[74,76]

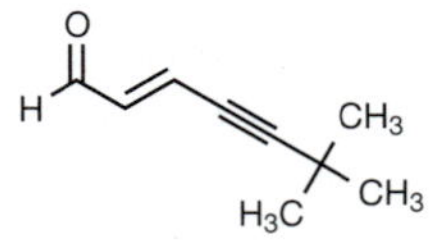

TBF-A

Two isoforms, CYP2C9 and CYP3A4, account for 80% of TBF-A formation from terbinafine.[74] TBF-A can form a reversible glutathione conjugate via a 1,6-Michael addition, which is the major glutathione conjugate.[76] Glutathione conjugation is also possible via 1,4-Michael addition. This indicates that TBF-A is a reactive metabolite.

Tolnaftate (See Fig. 34.5). Tolnaftate, a thiocarbamate derivative, is an old drug that was used topically to treat dermatophytic infections for years before its mechanism was discovered to be the same as that of allylamines, inhibition of squalene epoxidase.[64] Tolnaftate is available in a wide variety of over-the-counter (OTC) antifungal topical formulations, including cream, emulsion, gel, powder, solution, and powder spray products, for treating athlete's foot, jock itch, and ringworm.

Azoles—Imidazoles, Triazoles, and a Tetrazole

The characteristic chemical feature of azoles, from which their name is derived, is the presence of a five-membered aromatic ring containing two to four nitrogen atoms. Imidazole rings have two nitrogens, triazoles have three, and tetrazoles have four. In all cases, the azole ring is attached through N1 to a side chain containing at least one aromatic ring.

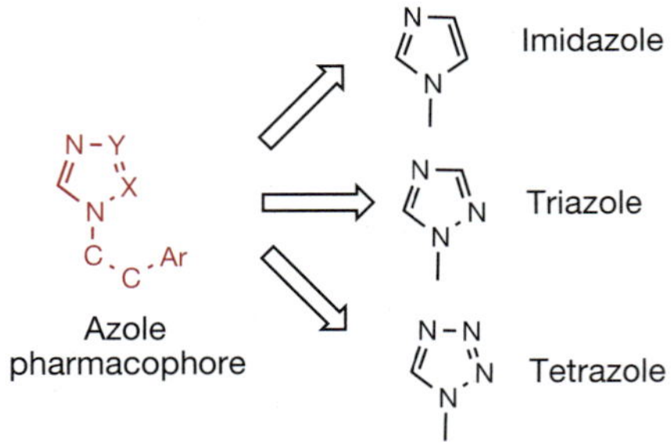

Azole antifungal agents are the largest class of antimycotics available today, with more than 27 drugs on the market in the Unites States or other countries and more than 20 in various stages of clinical development.[77] The antifungal imidazoles (Fig. 34.6) are primarily used topically to treat superficial dermatophytic and yeast infections.

The antifungal triazoles (Fig. 34.7) are administered orally for the treatment of systemic fungal infections, or topically against dermatophytes or vulvovaginal candidiasis. The tetrazole, oteseconazole, will be presented and discussed later in the chapter. The oral bioavailability of some azoles, in contrast to AmB, combined with their generally broad spectrum of activity and lack of nephrotoxicity, has led to their widespread use in treating a variety of serious fungal infections supplanting the use of AmB in most.

MECHANISM OF ACTION. All antifungal azoles act by inhibiting ergosterol biosynthesis through inhibition of the sterol 14α-demethylase, CYP51, discussed earlier under ergosterol biosynthesis (see Fig. 34.3, Site 2). Within the azole antifungals, it is the N3 atom of the imidazole or the N4 of the triazole or tetrazole rings, which forms a bond with the heme iron of the CYP450 prosthetic group in the position normally occupied by the activated oxygen (see Fig. 34.4). The remainder of the azole antifungal forms noncovalent interactions with the apoprotein in a manner that determines the relative selectivity of the drug for the fungal 14α-demethylase versus other CYP450 enzymes.

Inhibition of 14α-demethylase results in decreased fungal ergosterol content. Furthermore, when 14α-demethylase is inhibited, an alternate pathway for lanosterol is activated, involving Erg3, which leads to accumulation of the toxic 14α-methyl sterol 14α-methylergosta-8,24(28)-dien-3β,6α-diol (Fig. 34.8).[40,78,79] Together, these effects lead to fungal cell death.

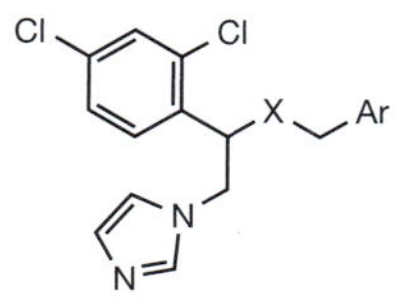

Generic Name	Tradename	X	Ar
Econazole	Generic, Econasil, Ecoza	O	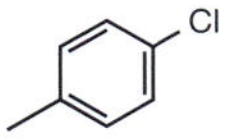
Miconazole	Generic, Azolen, Baza, Desenex, Fungoid, Micatin, Micotrin, Mycozyl, Monistat, Oravig, Zeosorb	O	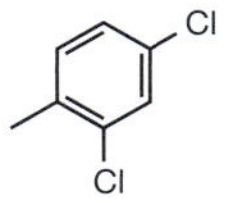
Oxiconazole	Generic, Oxistat	=N-O	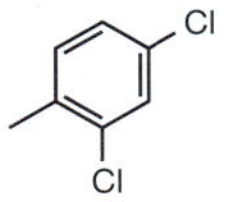
Sertaconazole	Ertaczo	O	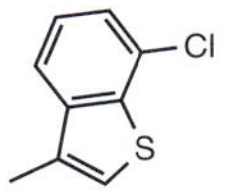
Sulconazole	Generic, Exelderm	S	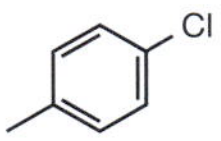
Tioconazole	Generic, Vagistat	O	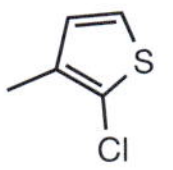

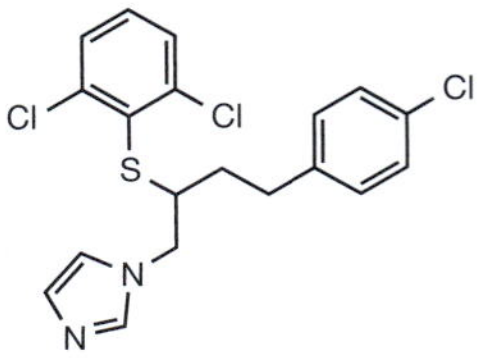

Butoconazole
(Gynazole)

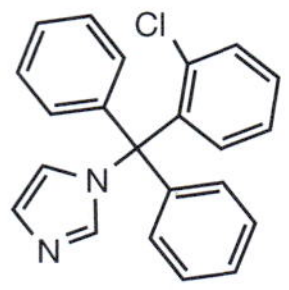

Clotrimazole
(Generic, Alevazol, Gyne-Lotrimin, Votriza)

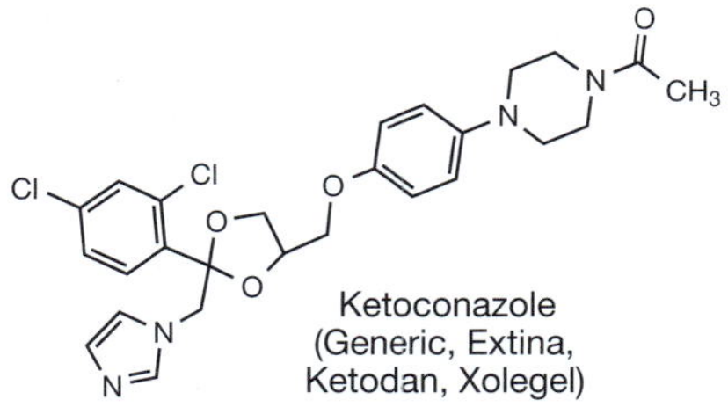

Ketoconazole
(Generic, Extina, Ketodan, Xolegel)

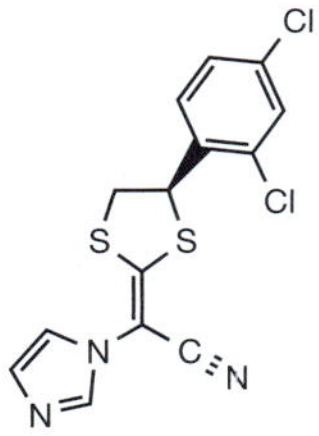

Luliconazole
(Generic, Luzu)

Figure 34.6 Imidazole antifungal agents. All imidazole antifungals are used topically except ketoconazole, which is available in both a topical and systemic dosage form.

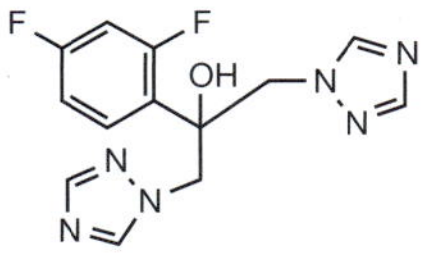

Fluconazole
(Generic, Diflucan)

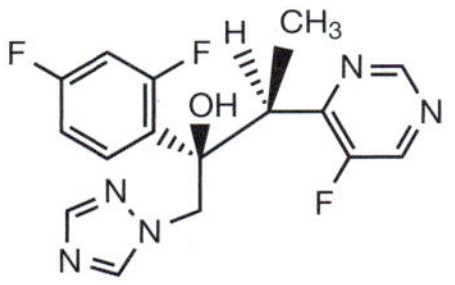

Voriconazole
(Generic, Vfend)

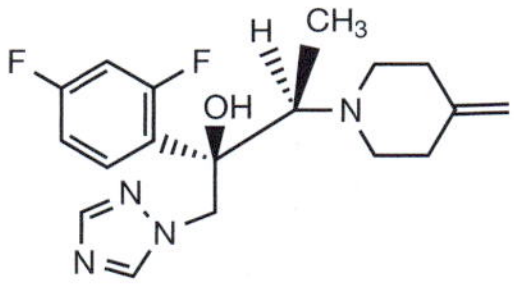

Efinaconazole
(Jublia)

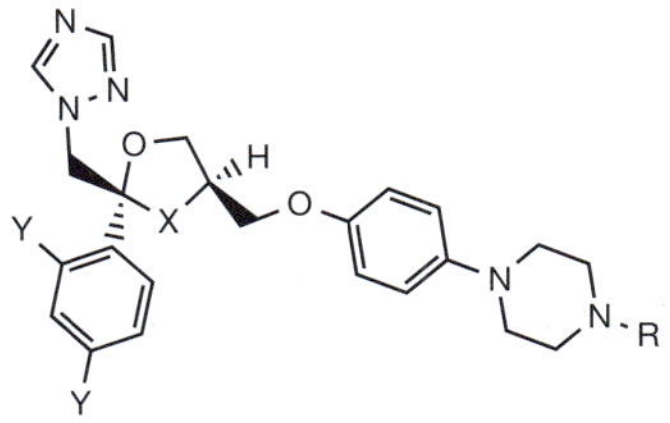

Itraconazole
(Generic, Sporanox, Tolsura)

X=O, Y = Cl, R = 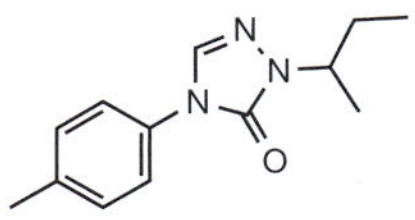

Posaconazole
(Generic, Noxafil)

X=CH$_2$, Y = F, R = 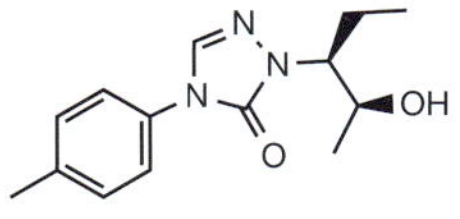

Terconazole
(Generic)

X=O, Y = Cl, R = 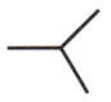

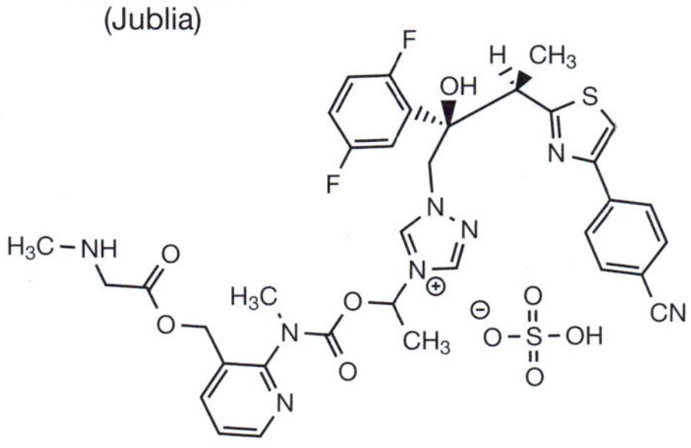

Isavuconazonium sulfate
(Cresemba)

Plasma esterases

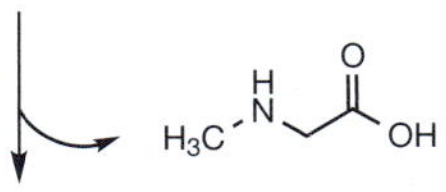

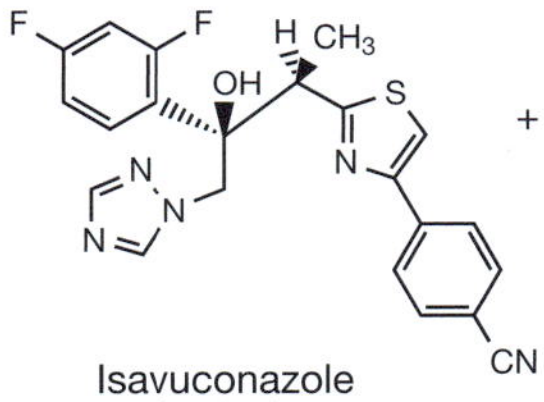

Isavuconazole
(active)

+

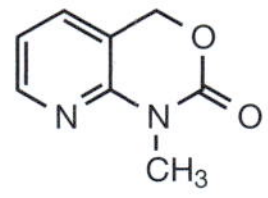

BAL 8728
(inactive)

+

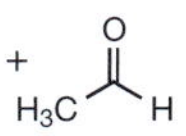

Figure 34.7 Triazole antifungal agents. While efinaconazole and terconazole are used topically, the remaining triazoles are used systemically.

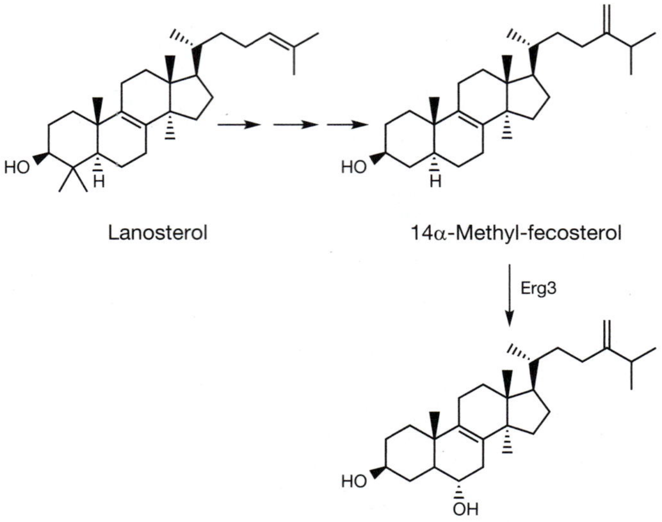

Figure 34.8 Alternate pathway for lanosterol under 14α-demethylase (CYP51, Erg11) inhibition. When 14α-demethylase is inhibited, lanosterol is shunted to the formation of 14α-methylergosta-8,24(28)-dien-3β,6α-diol, which is toxic to fungal cells.

Biosynthesis of the mammalian membrane sterol cholesterol also employs a CYP450 14α-demethylase, but 14α-methyl sterols do not accumulate in human cell membranes during azole antifungal therapy due to species-specific enzyme inhibition. For example, the inhibitory concentration (IC_{50}) for ketoconazole against the CYP51 from C. *albicans* is 0.064 μM versus 0.43 μM for human CYP51.[80] Ketoconazole shows a selectivity ratio for human CYP51 to C. *albicans* CYP51 of 7. In comparison, the human CYP51/C. *albicans* CYP51 selectivity ratio for itraconazole is 769.[80] The higher ratio indicates a greater selectivity for the fungal CYP51 over the human enzyme. However, many of the azole antifungal drugs used systemically are inhibitors or substrates for other mammalian CYP450 enzymes (Table 34.3).

The early azole antifungal drugs were all either extensively and rapidly degraded by first-pass metabolism or too toxic for systemic use. As a result, only those drugs with reduced or slow first-pass metabolism (ketoconazole, fluconazole, itraconazole, voriconazole, posaconazole, isavuconazole, and oteseconazole) are used systemically. The other azoles are available in a variety of creams and ointments for topical treatments of dermatophytic infections, and intravaginal use for vaginal yeast infections.

There are two topical triazole antifungals, terconazole and efinaconazole (see Fig. 34.7). Terconazole, the first triazole antifungal drug commercially available for use in humans,[81] is available as a vaginal cream and vaginal suppository for the treatment of vulvovaginal candidiasis. The triazole efinaconazole is the only azole to be employed topically in the treatment of onychomycosis.[82] It is formulated as a 10% solution applied topically to the infected nail. The antifungal activity resides almost exclusively in the *R*,*R*-diastereomer.[83] The low affinity of efinaconazole for the nail protein keratin is thought to be a significant factor in the drug's effectiveness versus other topical antimycotics.[84]

Table 34.3 Drug-Drug Interaction Potential of Azole Antifungals

Azole Antifungal	CYP Inhibitor	CYP Substrate	Transporter Protein Inhibitor	Drug-Drug Interactions
Ketoconazole	2C8 (weak) 2C19 (weak) 3A4 (strong)	3A4	P-gp	Yes
Fluconazole	2C9 (moderate) 2C19 (strong) 3A4 (moderate)	Low CYP metabolism	No	Yes
Itraconazole	3A4 (strong)	3A4	P-gp	Yes
Voriconazole	2C9 (weak) 2C19 (moderate) 3A4 (strong)	2C9, 2C19, 3A4	No	Yes
Posaconazole	3A4 (strong)	Low CYP metabolism[a]	P-gp	Yes
Isavuconazole	3A4 (moderate) CYP2D6 (weak inducer)	3A4	P-gp, OCT1, OCT2	Yes
Oteseconazole	None	Does not undergo significant metabolism	BCRP	Lower potential

BCRP, breast cancer resistance protein; OCT, organic cation transporter; P-gp, P-glycoprotein.
[a]Posaconazole is a substrate of UGT1A4.
Data from *Lexi-Drugs*. UpToDate Lexidrug. UpToDate Inc. Accessed April 22, 2024. https://online.lexi.com

Specific Azole Drugs Used Systemically

Ketoconazole (See Fig. 34.6). Ketoconazole, an imidazole, was the first orally active antifungal azole to be discovered and has been widely studied and employed for the treatment of systemic fungal infections, primarily candidiasis. Ketoconazole has little effect on *Aspergillus* or *Cryptococcus* spp. Ketoconazole is highly dependent on low stomach pH for dissolution and absorption, and antacids or drugs that raise stomach pH will lower the bioavailability of ketoconazole. Although ketoconazole has been available for decades, its metabolism in humans is not entirely clear. It is extensively metabolized primarily by CYP3A4.[85-87] Nineteen metabolites of ketoconazole have been identified in human liver microsomes and hepatocytes.[86,87] The package insert for oral ketoconazole has a boxed warning indicating it may cause severe hepatotoxicity that may be fatal.[85] Ketoconazole-induced hepatotoxicity is proposed to involve the *N*-deacetyl ketoconazole metabolite and subsequent oxidative metabolism forming reactive intermediates including a dialdehyde metabolite (Fig. 34.9).[88,89] The metabolic pathway from ketoconazole to the dialdehyde metabolite is not CYP mediated, but rather involves arylacetamide deacetylase and flavin monooxygenases.[88,89]

Not only is ketoconazole a substrate of CYP3A4, it is a powerful inhibitor of human CYP3A4 and, consequently, it has many drug-drug interactions (DDIs).[90] Ketoconazole is also a weak inhibitor of CYP2C8 and 2C19.

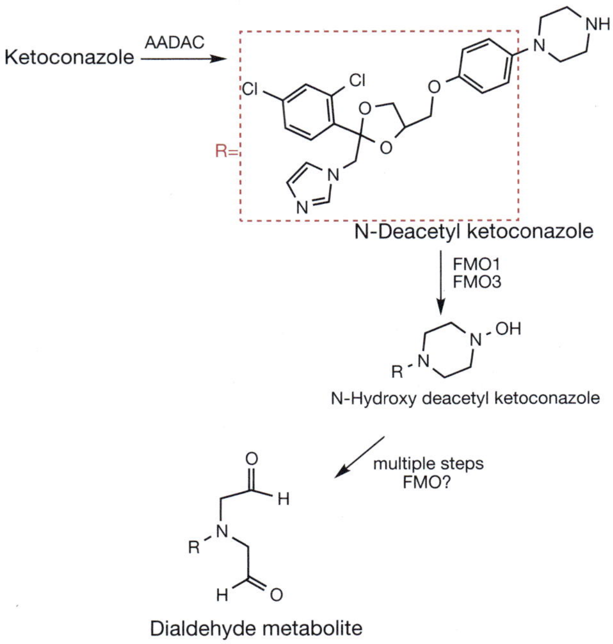

Figure 34.9 Proposed ketoconazole metabolic pathway forming reactive metabolites leading to hepatotoxicity. AADAC, arylacetamide deacetylase; FMO, flavin-containing monooxygenase. (Modified from Rodriguez RJ, Proteau PJ, Marquez BL, Hetherington CL, Buckholz CJ, O'Connell KL. Flavin-containing monooxygenase-mediated metabolism of N-deacetyl ketoconazole by rat hepatic microsomes. *Drug Metab Dispos*. 1999;27[8]:880-886; Fukami T, Iida A, Konishi K, Nakajima M. Human arylacetamide deacetylase hydrolyzes ketoconazole to trigger hepatocellular toxicity. *Biochem Pharmacol*. 2016;116:153-161.)

Ketoconazole inhibits steroidogenesis via inhibition of CYP11A1, CYP17A1, CYP11B1, and CYP11B1 and is used off-label for the treatment of Cushing syndrome.[91] While ketoconazole is marketed as the racemic mixture for antifungal use, the steroidogenic inhibitory activity is nearly exclusively in the 2S,4R isomer, levoketoconazole. Levoketoconazole is FDA approved for the treatment of Cushing syndrome.[92]

With the availability of more effective systemic agents, ketoconazole's clinical use has generally been restricted to topical applications in a variety of dosage forms, including cream, foam, gel, and shampoo.

Itraconazole (See Fig. 34.7). Itraconazole and fluconazole were the first triazole antifungals introduced into clinical use.[93] Itraconazole is a triazole derivative of ketoconazole with a more elaborate phenyl piperazine side chain. Itraconazole's oral bioavailability is variable, it is increased by food and influenced by stomach pH. A strongly acidic pH is required for dissolution and good absorption, similar to ketoconazole.[94] The oral bioavailability of the oral capsule formulation is approximately 55% and improved with acidic gastric pH and food. Concomitant use of drugs that raise gastric pH, including proton pump inhibitors, histamine H_2 receptor antagonists, and antacids, decreases oral absorption of itraconazole. Due to its poor solubility, the oral solution is formulated with the addition of a solubilizer, hydroxypropyl-β-cyclodextrin, which improves oral bioavailability to almost 80%.[94] To improve oral bioavailability and decrease variability, a *super bioavailability* (SUBA) itraconazole formulation (Tolsura) was developed as an oral capsule.[95] The SUBA-itraconazole formulation is a solid dispersion of the drug in a pH-dependent polymeric matrix that is insoluble in the acidic pH of the stomach and is released in the small intestine where it has enhanced dissolution and absorption.[95] The SUBA-itraconazole formulation has a relative bioavailability of 173% compared to conventional itraconazole, and the bioavailability is less variable.[95]

Itraconazole is extensively metabolized by CYP3A4 following oral administration (Fig. 34.10). The most notable metabolite is the ω-1 hydroxylation product, hydroxyitraconazole, an active metabolite.[96] The antifungal activity of hydroxyitraconazole is similar to itraconazole and the plasma levels are higher than the parent compound.[96] Like ketoconazole, itraconazole has been demonstrated to be a strong inhibitor of CYP3A4 and P-glycoprotein (P-gp).[96] Consequently, the risk is high for potentially serious DDIs with itraconazole and drugs metabolized by CYP3A4 or drugs that are P-gp substrates. The antifungal spectrum of itraconazole includes most *Candida* spp., requiring higher minimum inhibitory concentrations (MICs) for *C. glabrata*, *C. krusei*, *C. neoformans*, and thermally dimorphic molds.[94] It also has some activity against molds such as *A. fumigatus*, but not against species in the Mucorales order. Itraconazole is large (molecular weight [MW] 705 Da), is a P-gp substrate, and achieves low levels in the cerebrospinal fluid (CSF); therefore, it is generally ineffective for the treatment of fungal infections in the CNS, except for CNS histoplasmosis in which it is included in treatment guidelines.[18,97-99] The clinical utility of itraconazole in CNS histoplasmosis may be due to the drug achieving higher concentrations in brain tissue over CSF and its low MIC against *Histoplasma*.[97]

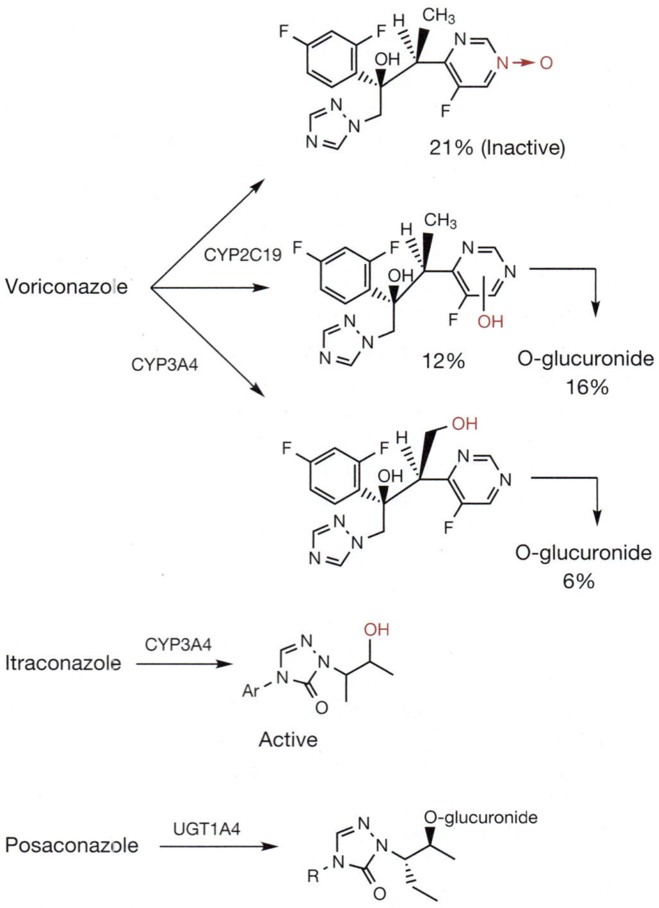

Figure 34.10 Major metabolic products formed from metabolism of systemic azoles.

Fluconazole (See Fig. 34.7). Fluconazole was introduced at the same time as itraconazole. Fluconazole is not extensively metabolized and is mostly excreted unchanged.[100] Fluconazole is small (MW 306 Da) and more hydrophilic (cLogP 0.4) compared to itraconazole (cLogP 5.7).[101,102] Consequently, a major advantage of fluconazole over itraconazole is that it can cross the blood-brain barrier (BBB) and achieves high concentrations in the CSF.[103] Fluconazole also differs in that it is not only a moderate inhibitor of CYP3A4, but also moderate inhibitor of CYP2C9 and a strong inhibitor of CYP2C19.[104]

The antifungal spectrum of fluconazole includes most yeasts, including *C. neoformans*, although not *C. krusei*.[94] It has variable activity against thermally dimorphic fungi, and is generally not used for these infections, but it does not have activity against molds, such as *A. fumigatus*.[94] Fluconazole resistance is increasing. *Candida* spp. mechanisms of resistance to fluconazole and other azole antifungals include alteration of the azole target Erg11 (14α-demethylase, CYP51), overexpression of Erg11, upregulation of azole-targeting efflux pumps, and loss-of-function mutations to *ERG3*. *ERG3* is the gene that encodes the sterol C-5 desaturase responsible for forming the fungal toxin 14α-methylergosta-8,24(28)-dien-3β,6α-diol upon azole-induced inhibition of Erg11 (see Fig. 34.8).[105,106]

A common mechanism of azole resistance in *C. albicans* is *ERG11* mutations, leading to amino acid substitution in Erg11, which results in lower affinity of the azole drug to the fungal 14α-demethylase.[105,106] The most common mechanism of resistance to *C. auris*, in which the majority of isolates are fluconazole resistant, is *ERG11* mutation.[107] A mechanism of overexpression of Erg11 in *C. albicans* is a gain-of-function mutation in *UPC2*.[105,106] *UPC2* encodes the transcriptional activator, Upc2, which causes overexpression of *Erg11* genes, leading to a reduction of fluconazole susceptibility. Overexpression of azole efflux pumps is a resistance mechanism employed by several *Candida* spp. Overexpression of ATP-binding cassette (ABC) transporters, Cdr1 and Cdr2, occurs in resistant strains of *C. albicans* and *C. glabrata*. The overexpression of ABC transporter Snq2 plays a role in *C. glabrata* azole resistance. The major facilitator superfamily (MFS) transporter multidrug resistance 1 (Mdr1) efflux pump may also be overexpressed in fluconazole-resistant *C. albicans*.[105] Expression of other efflux pumps is involved in *Candida* spp. resistance to azoles. Loss-of-function mutations in *ERG3* by *C. albicans* blocks the accumulation of 14α-methylergosta-8,24(28)-dien-3β,6α-diol, which is toxic to the fungal cell, and leads to an increase in concentration of 14α-methylfecosterol incorporated into the fungal cell membrane. *Candida* spp. can grow and replicate in the presence of 14α-methylfecosterol, rendering the yeast resistant to the Erg11 inhibition of azole antifungals.

Voriconazole (See Fig. 34.7). Voriconazole is an analog of fluconazole that was developed to increase the potency and spectrum of activity of fluconazole.[108,109] Introducing a methyl group to the methylene group adjacent to one of the triazole rings in fluconazole by 10-fold to 14α-demethylase in *A. fumigatus*.[108,109] Subsequently, replacing a triazole ring with a pyrimidine ring increased the potency against *A. fumigatus* further and adding a 5-fluoro group to the pyrimidine ring enhanced efficacy.[109] The activity is nearly exclusively in the 2R,3S enantiomer.[109] Voriconazole has a broad range of antifungal activity against yeasts, molds, and thermally dimorphic fungi.[14,94] Its spectrum includes *Aspergillus*, most *Candida* spp., even some fluconazole-resistant *C. glabrata* strains, *Cryptococcus*, as well as other molds such as *Fusarium* species and some *Scedosporium* spp.[14,94,109] Voriconazole is orally absorbed and, like fluconazole, penetrates the BBB.[110] Voriconazole is extensively metabolized by CYP450 enzymes (see Fig. 34.10), primarily by CYP2C19 to the N-oxide and fluoropyrimidine hydroxylated products.[111-113] CYP3A4, FMO1, and FMO3 also play a role in metabolism to the N-oxide metabolite but to a lower extent.[114] CYP3A4 is responsible for the hydroxylation of the methyl group.[114] Voriconazole exhibits nonlinear, saturable kinetics, and because CYP2C19 exhibits genetic polymorphism, plasma levels can be higher in poor metabolizers versus extensive metabolizers.[110,115] Adverse effects unique to voriconazole include visual disturbances and a photosensitivity skin rash.[94,110] Furthermore, voriconazole is a moderate inhibitor of CYP2C19, a weak inhibitor of CYP2C9, and a strong inhibitor of CYP3A4, leading to many drug interactions.[116]

Voriconazole is available as an oral tablet, powder for oral suspension, and solution for injection. Voriconazole is poorly water soluble; therefore, the solution for injection requires the solubilizing agent sulfobutylether β-cyclodextrin sodium.[94,117] Sulfobutylether β-cyclodextrin can accumulate in patients with decreased kidney function (creatinine clearance [CrCl] <50 mL/min).[117]

Posaconazole (See Fig. 34.7). Posaconazole has a wide spectrum of activity compared to other azoles, particularly against *Aspergillus* and other increasingly common nosocomial infections resistant to treatment by other antifungal drugs, including other molds such as Mucorales, *Fusarium* spp., and some activity against *Scedosporium* spp.[94,118] It also has activity against a wide range of *Candida* spp. and *Cryptococcus*, as well as thermally dimorphic fungi.[94] *Aspergillus* resistance to azole antifungals has been attributed to the unique presence in *Aspergillus* of two distinct 14α-demethylases CYP51A and CYP51B.[119] *Aspergillus CYP51A* gene mutation is the most common resistance mechanism. The most frequent mutations are TR_{34}/L98H and TR_{46}/Y121F/T289A causing resistance to itraconazole and voriconazole, respectively.[107] TR_{34}/L98H involves both inclusion of a 34-base-pair tandem repeat sequence in the promoter region in *CYP51A* and substitution of leucine to histidine at amino acid 98 in the CYP51A protein.[107,120] TR_{46}/Y121F/T289A also involves the inclusion of a tandem repeat sequence in the *CYP51A* promoter region, albeit a 46-base-pair sequence. Additionally, two amino acid mutations at positions 121 and 289 in the CYP51A protein occur with this second common mutation.[107,120] These mutations result in upregulation of gene transcription via the insertion of the tandem repeat sequence, while the azole binding site is modified with the amino acid substitutions resulting in decreased affinity of drug.[107,120] Although resistance to posaconazole exists, it retains activity in some azole-resistant isolates.[118]

Posaconazole is metabolized primarily by phase II glucuronide conjugation via UGT1A4 (see Fig. 34.10).[121] It is a strong inhibitor of CYP3A4.[118] It both inhibits P-gp and is a substrate for P-gp.[118,122] Posaconazole is structurally similar to itraconazole; the main difference is that it contains a tetrahydrofuran ring in place of the dioxolane ring. Posaconazole is available as an oral gastro-resistant tablet, oral suspension, delayed-release powder for oral suspension, and a solution for injection. The oral suspension is associated with erratic absorption affected by food and pH.[123] The ketoconazole-like azole antifungals all have poor solubility due to their large size and weakly basic nature. The problems with the oral suspension led to the gastro-resistant tablet and delayed-release powder for oral suspension, which are formulated to release the drug in the small intestine circumventing the effect of pH on absorption.[118] Food does increase the absorption of the oral formulations.[118,124] Like voriconazole, the posaconazole solution for injection requires the solubilizer sulfobutylether β-cyclodextrin sodium, which can accumulate in patients with CrCl less than 50 mL/min.[124] Posaconazole has poor penetration into the CNS.[94,118]

Isavuconazonium Sulfate and Isavuconazole. The clever triazolium salt prodrug isavuconazonium sulfate and its active metabolite isavuconazole (see Fig. 34.7) are novel triazoles for systemic use.[125] Isavuconazole has poor solubility; therefore, the water-soluble prodrug was designed.[125] Unlike the parental forms of voriconazole and posaconazole, the prodrug isavuconazonium is available as a water-soluble injectable formulation that does not require the addition of sulfobutylether β-cyclodextrin sodium to facilitate solubility.[126] Isavuconazonium sulfate is also available as capsules for oral administration. The prodrug is rapidly converted to the active form, isavuconazole, by plasma esterases.[126] Isavuconazole is slowly but thoroughly further metabolized by CYP3A4/5 to a variety of inactive oxidized products (not shown), which are conjugated as glucuronides.[126]

Isavuconazole is a derivative of voriconazole in which the 2,4-difluorophenyl group is replaced with a 2,5-difluorophenyl group and the 5-fluoropyrimidine ring is replaced with a 4-(*p*-cyanophenyl)thiazole ring.[125] Isavuconazole is an extended-spectrum azole antifungal with antifungal activity ranging from yeasts to molds, including *Aspergillus* spp., Mucorales, *Fusarium* spp., and some *Scedosporium* spp.[94,127] It also has activity against thermally dimorphic fungi.[127] As a relatively small fluconazole-like structure, isavuconazole achieves clinically useful activity for at least some CNS infections, including Mucorales, *Aspergillus* spp., and *Cryptococcus* spp.[128] Isavuconazole is a moderate inhibitor of CYP3A4 and a CYP2D6 weak inducer.[129] It also inhibits P-gp, organic cation transporter (OCT)1 and OCT2.[129] While all other azole antifungals prolong the QTc interval, isavuconazole shortens the QTc interval by 5 msec.[128]

Oteseconazole

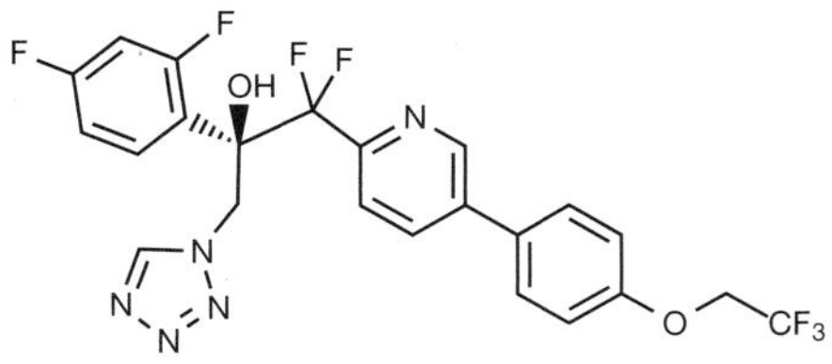

Oteseconazole
(Vivjoa)

Oteseconazole is the newest oral azole antifungal drug and the first to possess a tetrazole ring. It is a derivative of voriconazole. The goal in designing oteseconazole was to find a group that would bind to the iron of the heme prosthetic group in fungal CYP51 less avidly so that the drug would not bind to human CYP enzymes.[130] This would require potency-enhancing modifications in the rest of the molecule to compensate for the decreased binding to the heme iron. The tetrazole replacement of the triazole ring was chosen due to its decreased basicity ($pK_a = 1.1$) compared to the tetrazole ring ($pK_a = 2.3$), which would decrease the affinity for iron.[130] Potency to fungal CYP51 increased by replacing the methyl group and the fluoropyrimidine ring in the side chain of voriconazole. The side chain in oteseconazole includes a metabolically resistant gem-difluoro linker[131] bound to the 2-position of a pyridine substituted with a *para*-trifluoroethylether phenyl group at the 5-position.[130] Oteseconazole interacts with 22 amino acids in C. *albicans* CYP51.[62] The 2,5-substituted pyridine of oteseconazole forms a π-stacking interaction with a conserved Tyr118 residue in the *C. albicans* CYP51 active site. Furthermore, the ether group forms a H-bond with His377 in the binding region.[62] The His377 residue is conserved in CYP51 in all *Candida* spp., which confers high potency of oteseconazole against *C. glabrata* and *C. krusei*, which are intrinsically resistant to fluconazole.[62]

Oteseconazole has high affinity for *C. albicans* CYP51 with a dissociation constant (K_d) ≤ 39 nM.[132] There is no detectable binding affinity of oteseconazole to human CYP51 in concentrations up to 86 μM, demonstrating a more than 2,000-fold selectivity for the yeast enzyme over the human enzyme.[132] Oteseconazole does not inhibit human drug metabolizing enzymes with a CYPC29 IC_{50} = 99 μM, CYP2C19 IC_{50} = 72 μM, and CYP3A4 IC_{50} = 65 μM.[132] This is in contrast to other azole antifungals, for example, itraconazole is a strong CYP3A4 inhibitor with an IC_{50} = 0.8 μM.[132] Oteseconazole does inhibit the breast cancer–resistant protein.[133] Oteseconazole does not undergo significant metabolism.[130] It is indicated for the treatment of recurrent vulvovaginal candidiasis in postmenopausal women or those who are permanently infertile.[133] It is contraindicated in females of reproductive potential and in pregnant and lactating women because it is teratogenic in animals. The half-life of oteseconazole is approximately 138 days; therefore, it remains in the body for nearly 2 years.[133] The long half-life also enables initial once-a-day dosing, followed by once-a-week dosing.

INHALED TRIAZOLE ANTIFUNGAL UNDER INVESTIGATION

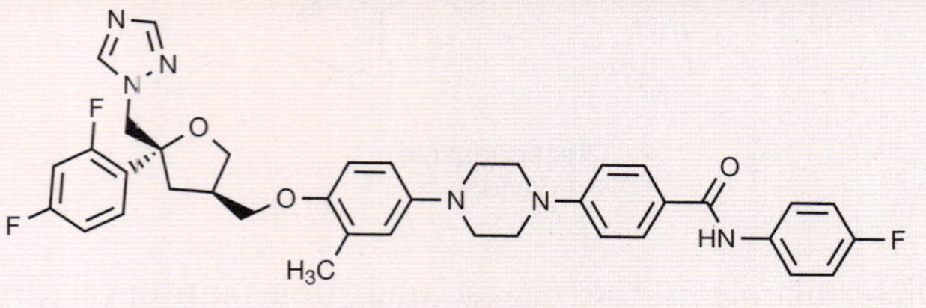

Opelconazole

Opelconazole (PC945) is an inhaled triazole antifungal under investigation for the treatment of invasive pulmonary aspergillosis.[134] Additionally, it has been shown to have in vitro activity against *Candida* spp., including *C. glabrata*, *C. krusei*, and *C. neoformans*, among other fungal pathogens.[135] It was designed for inhaled administration to achieve high antifungal levels in the lung with minimal systemic effects. While it is a potent inhibitor of CYP3A4 in vitro, the low systemic absorption (mean plasma C_{max} of 951 pg/mL after 7 days of once-daily 5-mg dosing) precludes CYP3A4 inhibition in vivo.[136] Consequently, inhaled opelconazole is expected to have a lower potential for DDIs and other adverse effects compared to oral azole antifungals. Opelconazole is formulated as an aqueous suspension to be used with commercially available nebulizers with once-a-day dosing. It is currently being evaluated in a phase III trial in combination with a systemic antifungal drug.[137]

Inhibitors of Cell Wall Biosynthesis

The most notable difference between fungal and mammalian cells is that fungi have a cell wall and mammals do not; therefore, drugs interfering with cell wall biosynthesis would be expected to be relatively nontoxic to mammals. Such drugs have been the foundation of antibacterial therapy since the discovery of penicillin and the development of dozens of effective β-lactam antibiotics, including penicillins, cephalosporins, carbapenems, and a monobactam. However, only a few drugs affecting fungal cell wall biosynthesis have become available, the echinocandins and one triterpenoid. Echinocandins (see Fig. 34.11), a group of cyclic peptides with long lipophilic side chains, sometimes called lipopeptides, are the main group of fungal cell wall inhibitors. Ibrexafungerp is a first-in-class triterpenoid antifungal.

Cell Wall Inhibitor Mechanism of Action

Echinocandins interfere with cell wall biosynthesis through inhibition of the enzyme β-1,3-glucan synthase. β-1,3-D-Glucan is an important polymer component of most fungal cell walls, serving as an anchor to other cell wall components.[36] It is synthesized by the enzyme β-1,3-glucan synthase, which is a transmembrane catalytic protein, called Fks, encoded primarily by *FKS1* and *FKS2* genes.[138] Echinocandins inhibit β-1,3-glucan synthesis by noncompetitive binding to Fks.[138] The subsequent reduction in the β-1,3-D-glucan content weakens the cell wall, leaving the fungal cell susceptible to osmotic imbalances and leading to rupture of the fungal cell.[36]

The triterpenoid antifungal ibrexafungerp is an oral β-1,3-glucan synthase inhibitor.[139] Ibrexafungerp is also a noncompetitive inhibitor of β-1,3-glucan synthase via binding to Fks. The binding sites of echinocandins and ibrexafungerp on Fks only partially overlap, rendering ibrexafungerp active against some echinocandin-resistant fungal pathogens.[139]

Echinocandins

Four semisynthetic echinocandins have been approved for use in treating life-threatening systemic fungal infections, caspofungin, micafungin, anidulafungin, and rezafungin (Fig. 34.11).[36] These are effective against a variety of *Candida* species, including those proven to be resistant to other agents. They have fungistatic activity against some *Aspergillus* spp., but lack activity against other molds.[94,140,141] The echinocandins do not have activity against *C. neoformans*, nor do they have activity against thermally dimorphic fungi. None of these drugs is orally active, and all must be administered by IV infusion. Due to their large size, all have MW over 1,000 Da, and they have low penetration into the CNS.

Caspofungin is metabolized by hydrolysis of the hexapeptide ring at the aminal of the ornithine residue followed by an interesting cyclization to form a five-membered cyclic hemiaminal, M0, involving the loss of ethylenediamine (Fig. 34.12).[142] M0 undergoes further hydrolysis to liberate the 3,4-dihydroxy-L-homotyrosine residue followed by *N*-acetylation to M2.[142] Caspofungin undergoes slow clearance.[142] At 24 hours after IV administration, caspofungin is the main circulating component in the plasma. After 5 days,

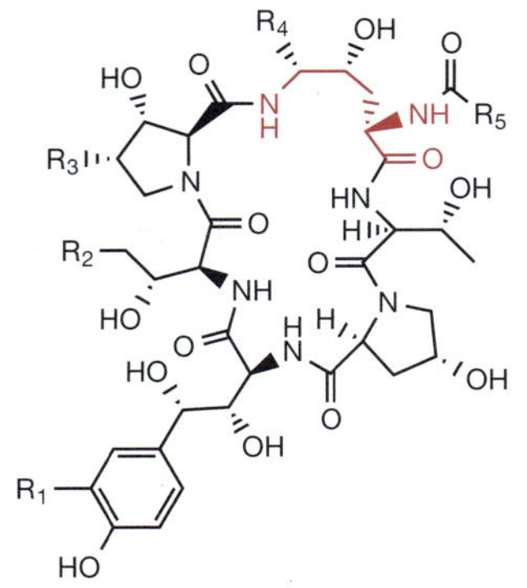

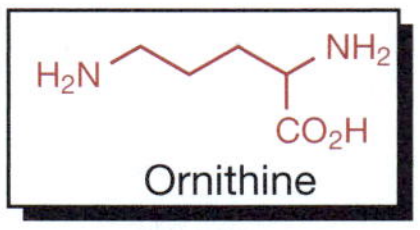

Drug	R_1	R_2	R_3	R_4	R_5
Caspofungin (Cancidas)	H	CH_2NH_2	H	$NHCH_2CH_2NH_2$	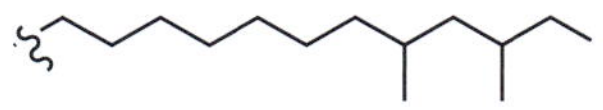
Micafungin (Mycamine)	OSO_3H	$CONH_2$	CH_3	OH	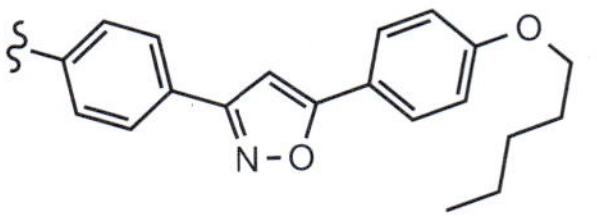
Anidulafungin (Eraxis)	H	H	CH_3	OH	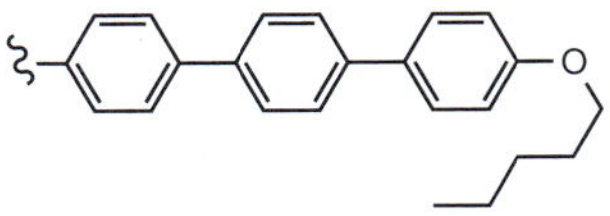
Rezafungin (Rezzayo)	H	H	CH_3	$OCH_2CH_2\overset{\oplus}{N}(CH_3)_3$	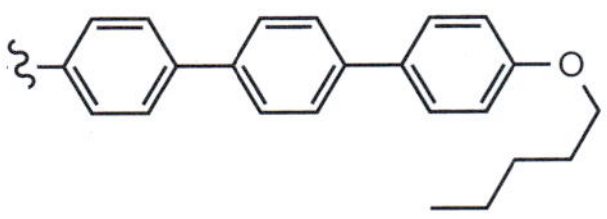

Figure 34.11 Echinocandins.

caspofungin decreases in the plasma, and M0 becomes the major plasma metabolite. Caspofungin is the main urinary metabolite at 24 hours after IV administration. After 16 days postdose, however, the major cumulative metabolite in the urine is M2.

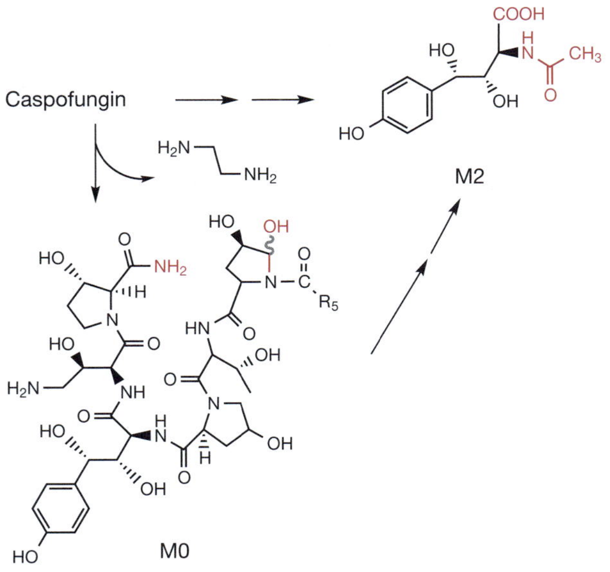

Figure 34.12 Metabolic products formed from caspofungin.

Micafungin is metabolized by a sulfotransferase and by catechol-O-methyltransferase (COMT).[143,144] Anidulafungin does not appear to be actively metabolized but rather slowly degrades.[145,146] Rezafungin is also very slowly eliminated.[147] Unchanged drug is the main circulating component in plasma.[147] Fecal excretion of unchanged drug is the main route of elimination. Low levels of various metabolites, formed from hydroxylation of the pentyl group, circulate in the plasma and are eliminated in the urine. After 17 days of an IV dose of [^{14}C]-rezafungin, only 52% of cumulative radioactivity was recovered (38% in feces, 14% in urine), indicating the very slow elimination.[147] Echinocandins have limited or no hepatic metabolism, they neither inhibit nor induce CYP enzymes, and they are neither substrates nor inhibitors of P-pg, which greatly limits DDIs.[145,148,149]

The half-lives of caspofungin ($t_{1/2}$ = 9-11 hours), micafungin ($t_{1/2}$ = 10-17 hours), and anidulafungin ($t_{1/2}$ = 24 hours) enable once-daily dosing.[38,140,145] Rezafungin is a choline-containing hemiaminal ether derivative of anidulafungin. This modification affords rezafungin with a much longer half-life of approximately 80 hours after the first dose and approximately 150 hours after the second or third dose, enabling once-weekly dosing.[150]

Echinocandin resistance occurs via mutations in the Fks protein in three conserved "hotspot" regions.[151] For example, the most frequent mutations in echinocandin-resistant

C. *albicans* include F641S (Phe at residue 641 is substituted with Ser) and S645P (Ser at residue 645 is substituted with Pro), both located within hotspot 1.[138,151] Fks mutations may interfere with echinocandin binding to Fks.[139,151] Other mechanisms may be involved in Fks mutations leading to echinocandin resistance.[151]

Triterpenoid—Ibrexafungerp

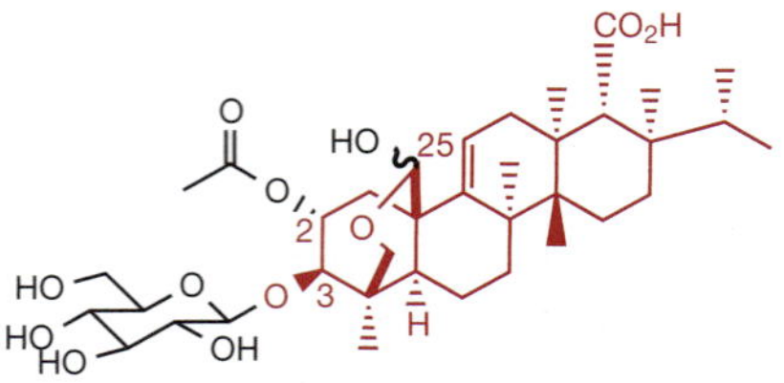

Lead compound: Enfumafungin
a triterpene glycoside isolated from
the fermentation of a *Hormonema* species

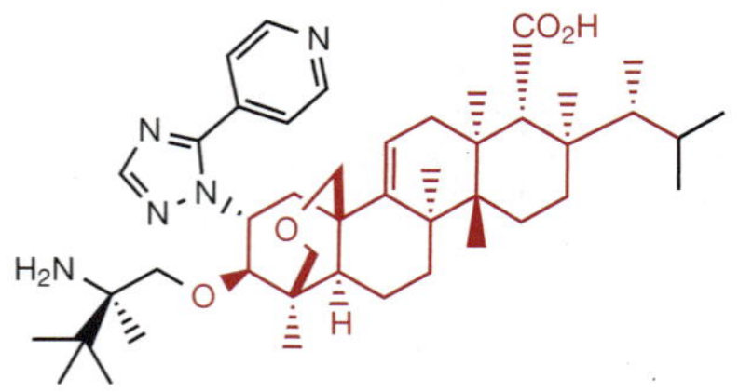

Ibrexafungerp
(Brexafemme)

Ibrexafungerp is a semisynthetic triterpene derivative of the natural product enfumafungin, identified in a screen of extracts of a *Hormonema* species.[152] Ibrexafungerp was designed to have improved oral efficacy over enfumafungin. This was achieved by replacing the acetoxy group at C2 of enfumafungin with a pyridyltriazole group, replacing the glycoside at C3 with an amino ether possessing a *t*-butyl group, and simplifying the C25 bridging hemiacetal to an ether.[153]

Similar to the echinocandins, ibrexafungerp has fungicidal activity against *Candida* spp., and it is fungistatic against *Aspergillus* spp.[154] Ibrexafungerp has demonstrated in vitro activity against *C. auris* and *C. glabrata*, including azole- and echinocandin-resistant isolates.[154-156] Among ibrexafungerp-resistant *C. glabrata* isolates, the majority possess a mutation in the *FKS2* gene.[157] Ibrexafungerp is active against *C. glabrata* strains with *FKS2* mutations conferring echinocandin resistance, most notably at hotspot position Ser663 in Fks2 and Ser629 in Fks1.[157]

Ibrexafungerp is a substrate for CYP3A4. It undergoes hydroxylation to an inactive metabolite, the structure of which has not been published, followed by glucuronidation and sulfonation of the hydroxyl metabolite.[154,158] About 90% is eliminated in the feces with approximately 51% unchanged. A minor amount is eliminated in the urine.[154] Ibrexafungerp is an inhibitor of CYP2C8, CYP3A4, P-gp, and OATP1B3.[154,158] It is a substrate for P-gp.[154,158] It has little distribution to the CNS.[154] It has a boxed warning that it may cause fetal harm, and it is contraindicated in pregnancy. Therefore, women of reproductive age should use contraception during treatment.

The half-life of ibrexafungerp is approximately 20 hours.[158] It is administered as an oral tablet every 12 hours for 1 day (two doses) for the treatment of vulvovaginal candidiasis and the reduction in the incidence of recurrent vulvovaginal candidiasis.

FOSMANOGEPIX/MANOGEPIX: TARGETING A NOVEL CELL WALL PATHWAY

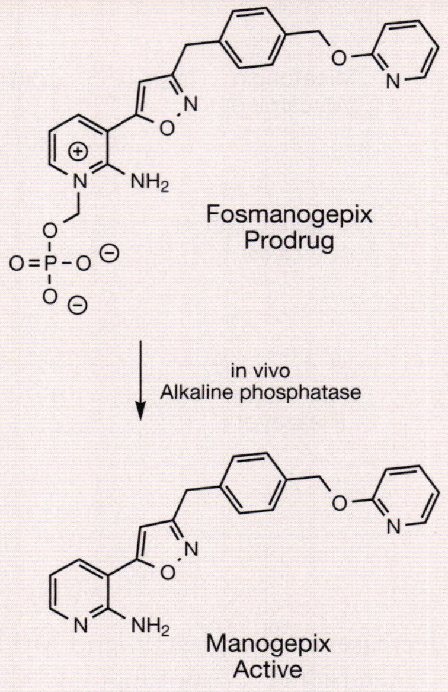

Fosmanogepix is a water-soluble prodrug, in formulations for IV and oral administration, of the active antifungal drug manogepix. Manogepix inhibits the fungal enzyme glycosylphosphatidylinositol (GPI)-anchored wall transfer protein 1, Gwt1, in the endoplasmic reticulum.[159,160] This impairs localization of essential cell wall mannoproteins, thereby compromising cell wall integrity.[159,160] The reduction of mannoprotein cell wall content also decreases fungal adhesion to host cells and pathogenicity. Manogepix has a broad spectrum of antifungal activity in vitro against yeasts and molds, including some azole-, echinocandin-, and AmB-resistant pathogens.[159,160] It has activity against a wide range of *Candida* spp., including *C. auris*, but not *C. krusei*, and *C. neoformans*. It also has antifungal activity against a wide range of molds, including *Aspergillus* spp., *Fusarium* spp., and *Scedosporium* spp. Manogepix has the added benefit of penetrating the CNS.[160]

Fosmanogepix has high oral bioavailability (>90%) and complete conversion to manogepix, making consistent conversion from IV to oral dosage forms.[160] The half-life of manogepix ranges from approximately 48 to 75 hours.[160] It is under phase III investigation in the treatment of adults with candidemia and/or invasive candidiasis.[161]

Miscellaneous Antifungals Acting Through Other Mechanisms

Ciclopirox

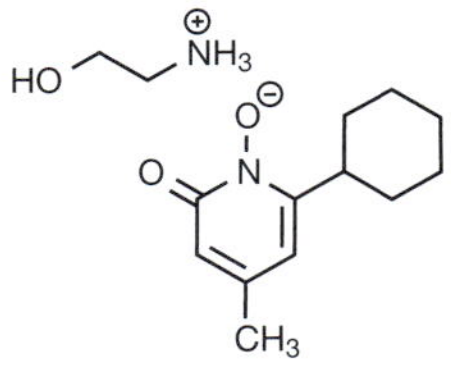

Ciclopirox olamine
(Generic, Ciclodan, Loprox)

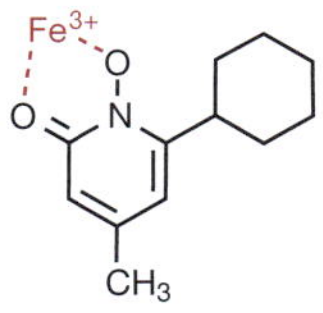

Chelation with polyvalent
metal cations

Ciclopirox is a hydroxylated pyridinone that is employed for superficial dermatophytic infections, including onychomycosis. The mechanism of action of ciclopirox is poorly understood but likely involves interference with many biochemical pathways through chelation of polyvalent cations, such as Fe^{3+}, which causes inhibition of several metal-dependent enzymes within the fungal cell.[162] Ciclopirox has been available for many years in a variety of topical dosage forms, including a cream, gel, shampoo, suspension, and a formulation of an 8% nail lacquer for treating onychomycosis.[163]

Flucytosine

Flucytosine is a powerful antifungal agent used in the treatment of serious systemic fungal infections, such as *C. neoformans* and *Candida* spp.

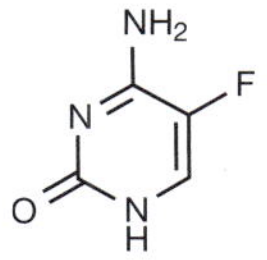

Flucytosine
(Generic, Ancobon)

Flucytosine itself is not cytotoxic; it is a prodrug that is taken up by fungi by cytosine permease located in the fungal cell membrane. Once inside the fungal cell, it is metabolized to 5-fluorouracil (5-FU) by fungal cytidine deaminase (Fig. 34.13).[164] 5-FU is then converted to 5-fluorodeoxyuridine monophosphate (5-FdUMP), a thymidylate synthase inhibitor that results in inhibition of DNA synthesis. 5-FU is also converted into 5-fluorouridine triphosphate, which is erroneously incorporated into fungal RNA and blocks protein synthesis. Both actions are important for the antifungal activity of flucytosine. 5-FU is cytotoxic, and is employed in cancer chemotherapy (see Chapter 36). Human cells do not contain cytosine deaminase and therefore do not convert flucytosine to 5-FU. Some intestinal microflora, however, do convert the drug to 5-FU, so human toxicity can result from this metabolism.[164] Resistance rapidly develops to flucytosine when used alone, so it is almost always used in conjunction with AmB. Use of flucytosine has declined since the discovery of fluconazole.

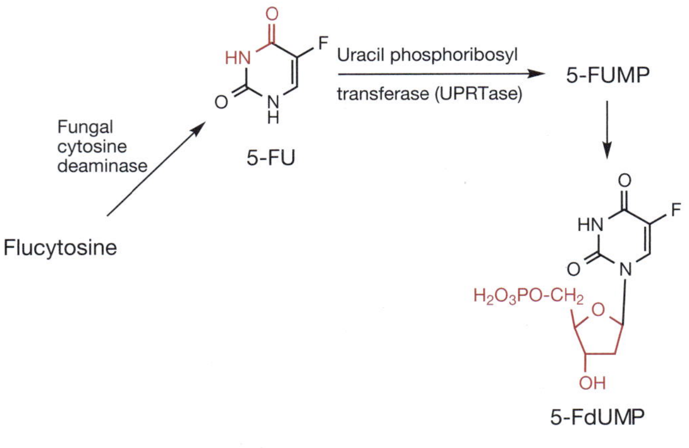

Figure 34.13 Metabolic activation of flucytosine by deamination, conjugation with ribosyl phosphate to 5-fluorouracil monophosphate (5-FUMP), followed by conversion to the active thymidylate synthase inhibitor 5-fluorodeoxyuridine monophosphate (5-FdUMP).

DIHYDROOROTATE DEHYDROGENASE INHIBITOR UNDER INVESTIGATION: OLOROFIM

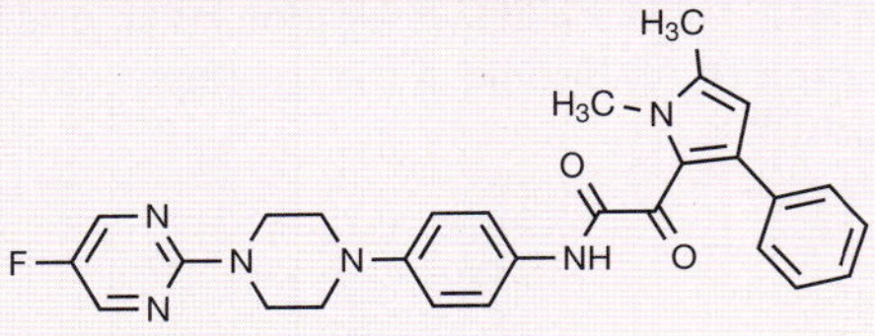

Olorofim

Olorofim is a reversible inhibitor of dihydroorotate dehydrogenase (DHODH), in select molds and thermally dimorphic fungi.[165,166] DHODH, encoded by the *PyrE* gene in *A. fumigatus*, is a critical mitochondrial enzyme for de novo pyrimidine biosynthesis; therefore, inhibiting this fungal enzyme halts DNA and RNA synthesis.[165] Furthermore, DHODH is essential for synthesizing precursors to lipid and carbohydrate metabolism, such as uridine diphosphate (UDP)-glucose, necessary for the production of β-1,3-glucan, a critical component of the cell wall. DHODH, bound to the cofactors flavin mononucleotide (FMN) and ubiquinone (coenzyme Q, CoQ), catalyzes the conversion of dihydroorotate to orotate. Olorofim was designed from a lead compound identified from a large library of small molecules screened for in vitro activity against *A. fumigatus*. It is representative of a class of compounds described as orotomides, named after the dihydroorotate-based mechanism of action and the α-ketoamide structural feature.[165]

Olorofim binds to a hydrophobic region of DHODH described as the "quinone channel," where CoQ enters the enzyme from the inner mitochondrial membrane.[165] Olorofim blocks the reoxidation of the dihydroflavin mononucleotide (FMNH2) cofactor by competitively inhibiting CoQ binding to DHODH, thereby preventing the synthesis of orotate. Olorofim is over 2,200 times more potent against *A. fumigatus* DHODH over the human enzyme.[165]

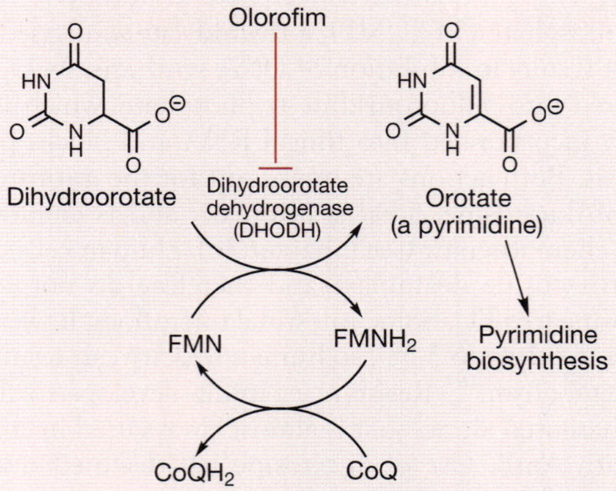

Olorofim has a unique spectrum in that it exhibits no activity against yeasts. The antifungal activity is targeted against *Aspergillus* spp., *Scedosporium* spp., some *Fusarium* spp., and thermally dimorphic fungi.[165,166] This is due to interspecies variations in the shape of the quinone channel of DHODH.[165] Due to the mechanism of action, olorofim has activity against the common azole-resistant *A. fumigatus* strain carrying the *CYP51A* TR_{34}/L98H mutation. Olorofim is under phase III investigation, as an oral tablet, in comparison to AmBisome in the treatment of invasive aspergillosis.[167]

Griseofulvin

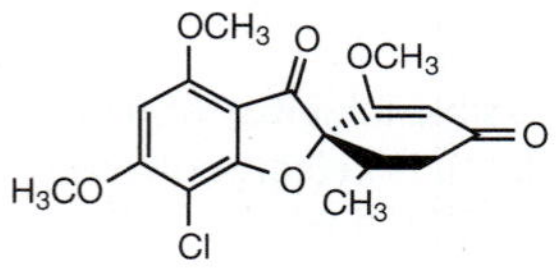

Griseofulvin

Griseofulvin is an antifungal antibiotic originally isolated from *Penicillium griseofulvum.*[168] It is used orally to treat superficial fungal infections caused by dermatophytes. It does not penetrate skin or nails if used topically. When given orally, however, griseofulvin in the blood becomes incorporated into keratin precursor cells and, ultimately, into keratin, which cannot then support fungal growth. The infection is cured when the diseased tissue is replaced by new uninfected tissue, which can take months for nails. The antifungal effects of griseofulvin are attributed to its antimitotic effects, which disrupt the function of the mitotic spindle, thereby inhibiting cell division. Other agents have mostly replaced griseofulvin in the United States in the treatment of onychomycosis,[20,70] although griseofulvin is first-line therapy in the treatment of tinea capitis in children.[169,170]

Tavaborole

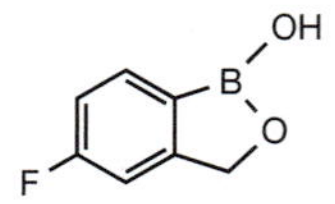

Tavaborole (Kerydin)

Tavaborole, an uncommon benzoxaborole-containing drug, inhibits a unique antifungal target for the treatment of onychomycosis.[171-173] It is a noncompetitive inhibitor of fungal leucyl-transfer RNA synthetase (LeuRS). Tavaborole inhibits LeuRS by forming a stable adduct between the boron atom and the 2′- and 3′-hydroxyl groups on the 3′-terminal adenosine residue of uncharged leucine transfer RNA within the LeuRS editing active site (Fig. 34.14). The resultant spiroborate adduct is trapped in the editing active site of LeuRS, thereby blocking protein synthesis.[172,173] Tavaborole has excellent penetration of human nails when applied topically as a solution.[174,175]

Undecylenic Acid

$$H_2C{=}CH(CH_2)_8COOH$$

Undecylenic acid

Undecylenic acid is employed, frequently as the zinc salt, in OTC preparations for topical treatment of infections by dermatophytes.[176] Undecylenic acid is fungistatic and acts through a nonspecific interaction with components in the fungal cell membrane.

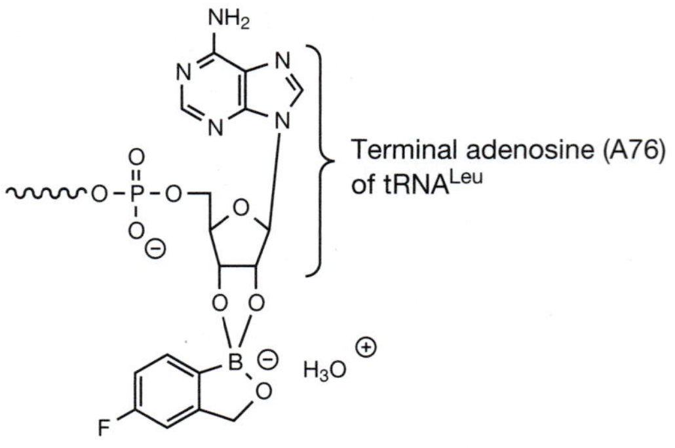

Figure 34.14 Binding between tavaborole and uncharged leucine transfer RNA in the editing active site of leucyl-transfer RNA synthetase (LeuRS).

Structure Challenge

1. Which of the following is a prodrug? Select all that apply.

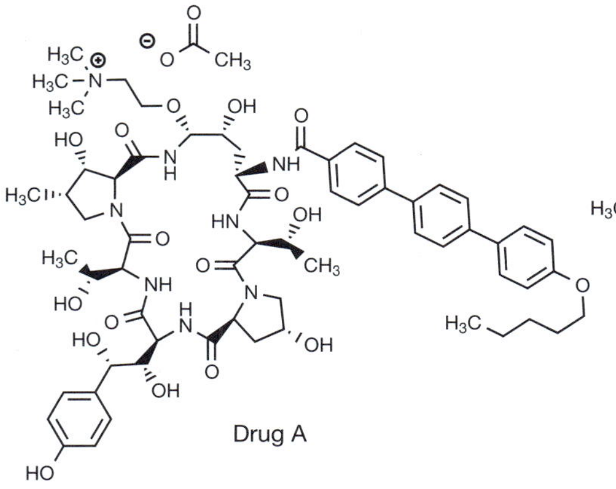

Drug A

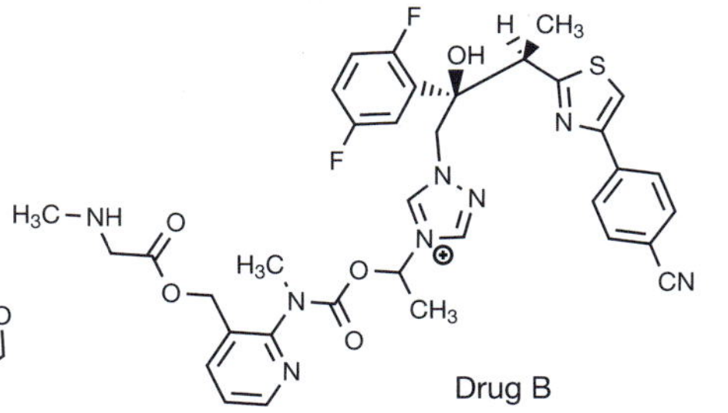

Drug B

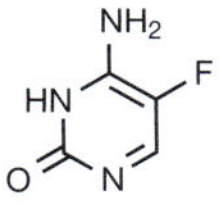

Drug C

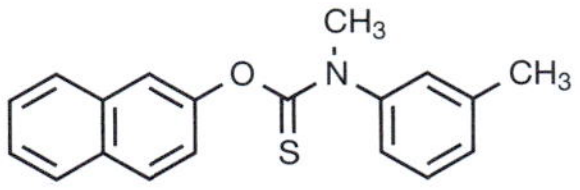

Drug D

2. Which of the following inhibits fungal cell wall biosynthesis? Select all that apply.

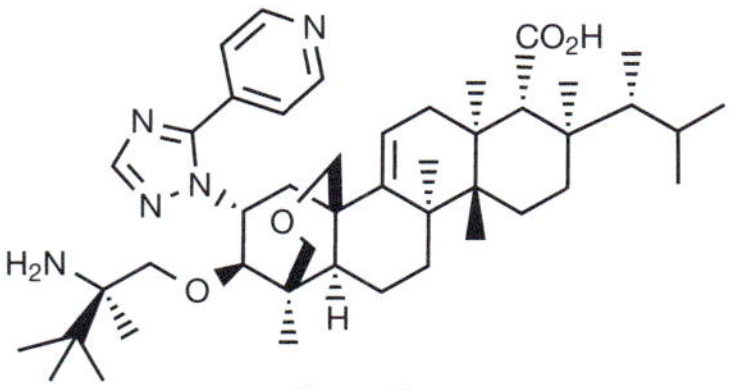

Drug A

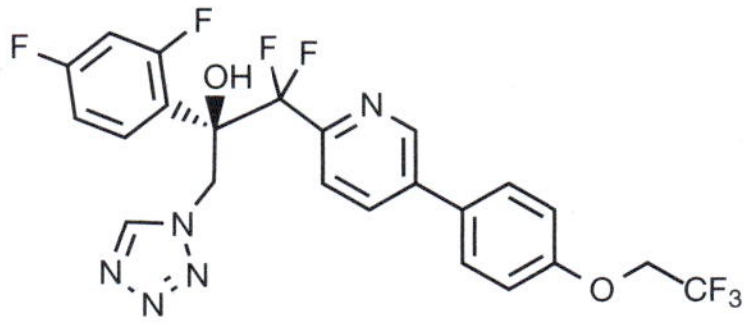

Drug B

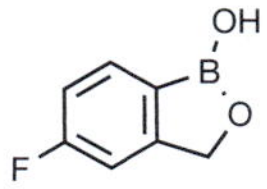

Drug C

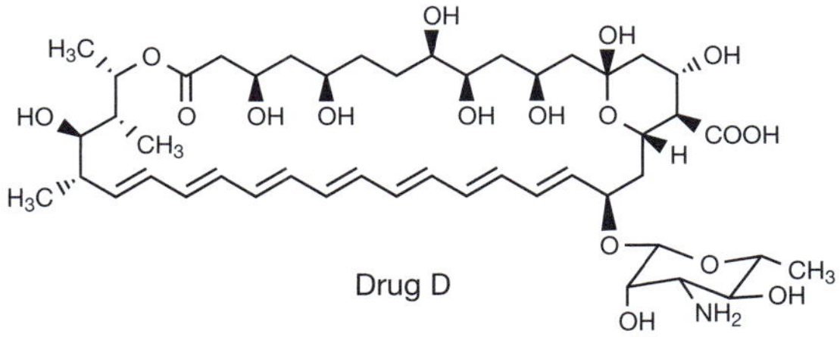

Drug D

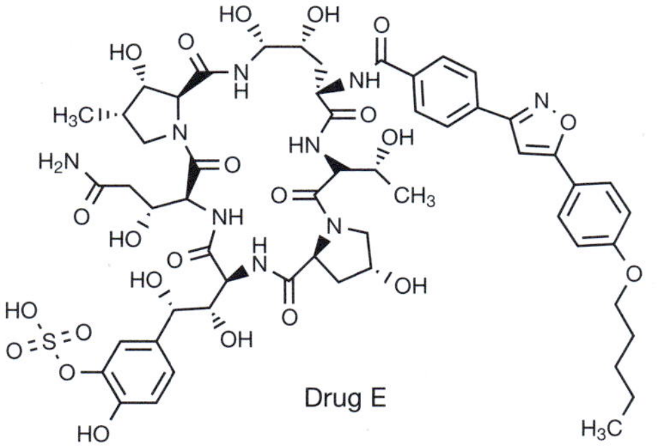

Drug E

3. For each of the following drugs, indicate whether it is topical or systemic.

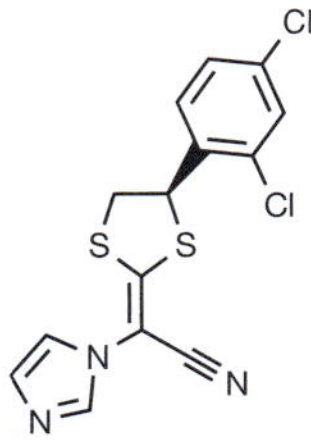

Drug A

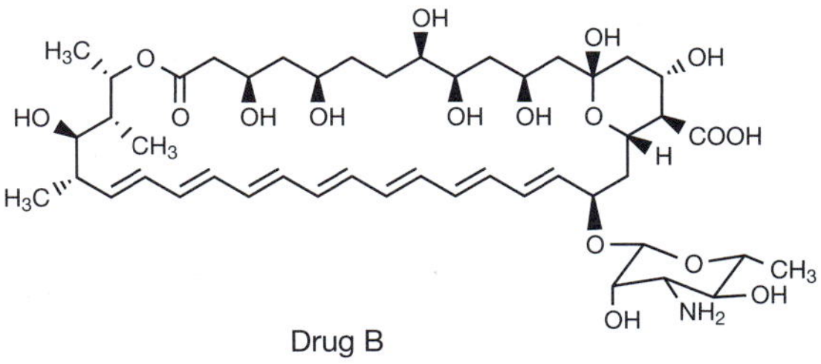

Drug B

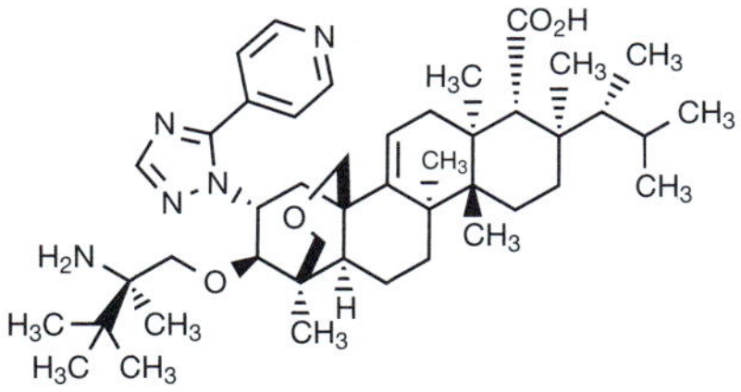

Drug C

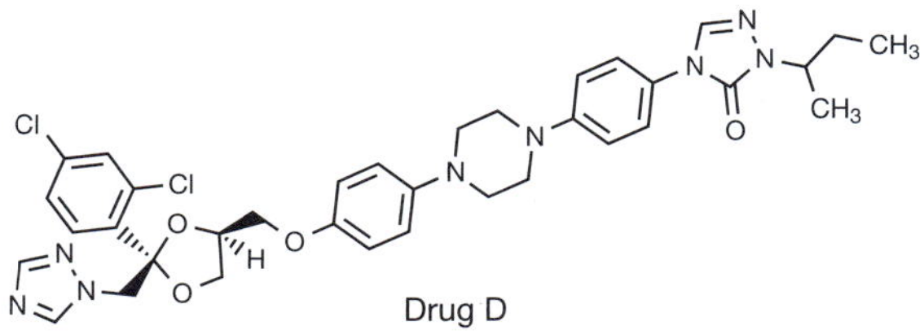

Drug D

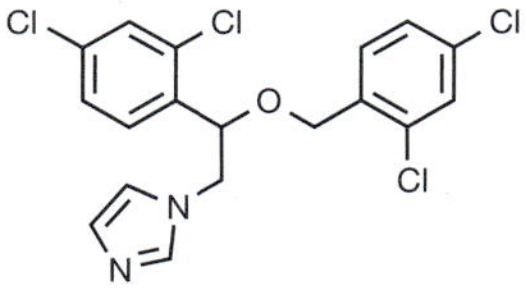

Drug E

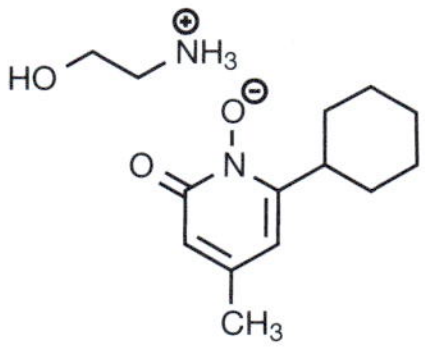

Drug F

Structure Challenge answers found immediately after References.

ACKNOWLEDGMENT

The author wishes to acknowledge the work of Robert K. Griffith, PhD, who authored content within this chapter in the 8th edition of this text.

REFERENCES

1. Jenks JD, Cornely, OA, Chen SCA, et al. Breakthrough invasive fungal infections: who is at risk? *Mycoses*. 2020;63(10):1021-1032.
2. Rayens E, Norris KA. Prevalence and healthcare burden of fungal infections in the United States, 2018. *Open Forum Infect Dis*. 2022;19(1):ofab593.
3. Rodrigues CF, Rodrigues ME, Henriques M. *Candida* sp. infections in patients with diabetes mellitus. *J Clin Med*. 2019;8(1):76.
4. Sung AH, Martin S, Phan B, et al. Patient characteristics and risk factors in invasive mold infections: comparison from a systematic review and database analysis. *Clinicoecon Outcomes Res*. 2021;13:593-602.
5. Hoenigl M, Seidel D, Sprute R, et al. COVID-19-associated fungal infections. *Nat Microbiol*. 2022;7(8):1127-1140.
6. Gow NAR, Johnson C, Berman J, et al. The importance of antimicrobial resistance in medical mycology. *Nat Commun*. 2022; 13(1):5352.
7. Puumala E, Fallah S, Robbins N, Cowen LE. Advancements and challenges in antifungal therapeutic development. *Clin Microbiol Rev*. 2024;37(1):e0014223.
8. Hoenigl M, Sprute R, Arastehfar A, et al. Invasive candidiasis: investigational drugs in the clinical development pipeline and mechanisms of action. *Expert Opin Investig Drugs*. 2022;31(8):795-812.
9. Denning DW. Global incidence and mortality of severe fungal disease. *Lancet Infect Dis*. 2024;24(7):e428-e438. doi:10.1016/S1473-3099(23)00692-8
10. Gold JAW, Ahmad FB, Cisewski JA, et al. Increased deaths from fungal infections during the coronavirus disease 2019 pandemic—national vital statistics system, United States, January 2020-December 2021. *Clin Infect Dis*. 2023;76(3):e255-e262.
11. Benedict K, Whitham HK, Jackson BR. Economic burden of fungal diseases in the United States. *Open Forum Infect Dis*. 2022;9(4):ofac097.
12. Hospenthal DR, Rinaldi MG, Walsh TJ, eds. *Diagnosis and Treatment of Fungal Infections*. 3rd ed. Springer; 2023.
13. McCarty TP, White CM, Pappas PG. Candidemia and invasive candidiasis. *Infect Dis Clin North Am*. 2021;35:389-413.
14. Thompson GR III, Young JH. Aspergillus infections. *N Engl J Med*. 2021;385(16):1496-1509.
15. Steinbrink JM, Miceli MH. Clinical review of mucormycosis. *Infect Dis Clin North Am*. 2021;35(2):435-452.
16. Galgiani JN, Kauffman CA. Coccidioidomycosis and histoplasmosis in immunocompetent persons. *N Engl J Med*. 2024;390(6):536-547.
17. Linder KA, Kauffman CA, Miceli MH. Blastomycosis: a review of mycological and clinical aspects. *J Fungi (Basel)*. 2023;9(1):117.
18. Nathan CL, Emmert BE, Nelson E, Berger JR. CNS fungal infections: a review. *J Neurol Sci*. 2021;422:117325.
19. González GM, Bonifaz A. Dermatophytosis (tinea) and other superficial fungal infections. In: Hospenthal DR, Rinaldi MG, Walsh TJ, eds. *Diagnosis and Treatment of Fungal Infections*. 3rd ed. Springer; 2023:351-367.
20. Falotico JM, Lipner SR. Updated perspectives on the diagnosis and management of onychomycosis. *Clin Cosmet Investig Dermatol*. 2022;15:1933-1957.
21. Ostrosky-Zeichner L, Sobel JD. Candidiasis. In: Hospenthal DR, Rinaldi MG, Walsh TJ, eds. *Diagnosis and Treatment of Fungal Infections*. 3rd ed. Springer; 2023:151-166.
22. Sharma C, Kadosh D. Perspective on the origin, resistance, and spread of the emerging human fungal pathogen *Candida auris*. *PLoS Pathog*. 2023;19(3):e1011190.
23. Rodrigues ML, Nosanchuk JD. Recognition of fungal priority pathogens: what next? *PLoS Negl Trop Dis*. 2023;17(3):e0011136.
24. Maziarz EK, Perfect JR. Cryptococcosis. In: Hospenthal DR, Rinaldi MG, Walsh TJ, eds. *Diagnosis and Treatment of Fungal Infections*. 3rd ed. Springer; 2023:245-265.
25. Colombo RE, Vazquez JA. Infections due to non-candidal yeasts. In: Hospenthal DR, Rinaldi MG, Walsh TJ, eds. *Diagnosis and Treatment of Fungal Infections*. 3rd ed. Springer; 2023:167-182.
26. Wright TW, Gigliotti F. Pneumocystosis. In: Hospenthal DR, Rinaldi MG, Walsh TJ, eds. *Diagnosis and Treatment of Fungal Infections*. 3rd ed. Springer; 2023:237-243.
27. Rayens E, Norris KA, Cordero JF. Mortality trends in risk conditions and invasive mycotic disease in the United States, 1999-2018. *Clin Infect Dis*. 2022;74(2):309-318.
28. Azar MM, Cohen E, Ma L, et al. Genetic and epidemiologic analyses of an outbreak of *Pneumocystis jirovecii* pneumonia among kidney transplant recipients in the United States. *Clin Infect Dis*. 2022;74(4):639-647.
29. Boucher HW, Patterson TF. Aspergillosis. In: Hospenthal DR, Rinaldi MG, Walsh TJ, eds. *Diagnosis and Treatment of Fungal Infections*. 3rd ed. Springer; 2023:183-195.
30. Arastehfar A, Carvalho A, Houbraken J, et al. *Aspergillus fumigatus* and aspergillosis: from basics to clinics. *Stud Mycol*. 2021;100(1):100115.
31. Antachopoulos C, Petraitiene R, Roilides E, Walsh TJ. Mucormycosis. In: Hospenthal DR, Rinaldi MG, Walsh TJ, eds. *Diagnosis and Treatment of Fungal Infections*. 3rd ed. Springer; 2023:221-235.
32. Sullivan DC, Nolan RL III. Blastomycosis. In: Hospenthal DR, Rinaldi MG, Walsh TJ, eds. *Diagnosis and Treatment of Fungal Infections*. 3rd ed. Springer; 2023:267-277.
33. Heidari A, Kuran R, Johnson R. Coccidioidomycosis. In: Hospenthal DR, Rinaldi MG, Walsh TJ, eds. *Diagnosis and Treatment of Fungal Infections*. 3rd ed. Springer; 2023:279-293.
34. Abdallah W, Hage C. Histoplasmosis. In: Hospenthal DR, Rinaldi MG, Walsh TJ, eds. *Diagnosis and Treatment of Fungal Infections*. 3rd ed. Springer; 2023:303-311.
35. Mazi PB, Sahrmann JM, Olsen MA, et al. The geographic distribution of dimorphic mycoses in the United States for the modern era. *Clin Infect Dis*. 2023;76(7):1295-1301.
36. Zhou Y, Reynolds TB. Innovations in antifungal drug discovery among cell envelope synthesis enzymes through structural insights. *J Fungi (Basel)*. 2024;10(3):171.
37. Gow NAR, Lenardon MD. Architecture of the dynamic fungal cell wall. *Nat Rev Microbiol*. 2023;21(4):248-259.
38. Szymański M, Chmielewska S, Czyżewska U, Malinowska M, Tylicki A. Echinocandins—structure, mechanism of action and use in antifungal therapy. *J Enzyme Inhib Med Chem*. 2022;37(1):876-894.
39. Dhingra S, Cramer RA. Regulation of sterol biosynthesis in the human fungal pathogen *Aspergillus fumigatus*: opportunities for therapeutic development. *Front Microbiol*. 2017;8:92.
40. Jordá T, Puig S. Regulation of ergosterol biosynthesis in *Saccharomyces cerevisiae*. *Genes (Basel)*. 2020;11(7):795.
41. Hamilton-Miller JM. Chemistry and biology of the polyene macrolide antibiotics. *Bacteriol Rev*. 1973;37:166-196.
42. Gray KC, Palacios DS, Dailey I, et al. Amphotericin primarily kills yeast by simply binding to ergosterol. *Proc Natl Acad Sci U S A*. 2012;109(7):2234-2239.
43. Kotler-Brajtburg J, Price HD, Medoff G, Schlessinger D, Kobayashi GS. Molecular basis for the selective toxicity of amphotericin B for yeast and filipin for animal cells. *Antimicrob Agents Chemother*. 1974;5(4):377-382.
44. Neumann A, Baginski M, Czub J. How do sterols determine the antifungal activity of amphotericin B? Free energy of binding between the drug and its membrane targets. *J Am Chem Soc*. 2010;132(51):18266-18272.
45. Anderson TM, Clay MC, Cioffi AG, et al. Amphotericin forms an extramembranous and fungicidal sterol sponge. *Nat Chem Biol*. 2014;10:400-406.

46. Guo X, Zhang J, Li X, et al. Sterol sponge mechanism is conserved for glycosylated polyene macrolides. *ACS Cent Sci.* 2021;7(5):781-791.
47. Pappas PG, Kauffman CA, Andes DR, et al. Clinical practice guideline for the management of candidiasis: 2016 update by the Infectious Diseases Society of America. *Clin Infect Dis.* 2016;62(4):e1-e50.
48. Hellstein JW, Marek CL. Candidiasis: red and white manifestations in the oral cavity. *Head Neck Pathol.* 2019;13(1):25-32.
49. Amphotericin B. Package insert. XGen Pharmaceuticals; Revised January 2022. Accessed April 14, 2024. https://dailymed.nlm.nih.gov/dailymed/drugInfo.cfm?setid=a0a54943-9ce4-4f3e-b681-a1a9144c16ce
50. Hamill RJ. Amphotericin B formulations: a comparative review of efficacy and toxicity. *Drugs.* 2013;73(9):919-934.
51. Laniado-Laborín R, Cabrales-Vargas MN. Amphotericin B: side effects and toxicity. *Rev Iberoam Micol.* 2009;26(4):223-227.
52. Maji A, Soutar CP, Zhang J, et al. Tuning sterol extraction kinetics yields a renal-sparing polyene antifungal. *Nature.* 2023;623(7989):1079-1085.
53. McCarthy M, Rosengart A, Schuetz AN, Kontoyiannis DP, Walsh TJ. Mold infections of the central nervous system. *N Engl J Med.* 2014;371(2):150-160.
54. Groll AH, Rijnders BJA, Walsh TJ, Adler-Moore J, Lewis RE, Brüggemann RJM. Clinical pharmacokinetics, pharmacodynamics, safety and efficacy of liposomal amphotericin B. *Clin Infect Dis.* 2019;68(suppl 4):S260-S274.
55. Ho J, Fowler P, Heidari A, Johnson RH. Intrathecal amphotericin B: a 60-year experience in treating coccidioidal meningitis. *Clin Infect Dis.* 2017;64(4):519-524.
56. Nailor MD, Goodlet KJ, Gonzalez O, Haller JT. Early experiences with intrathecal administration of amphotericin B liposomal formulation at a neurosurgical center. *CNS Drugs.* 2024;38(3):225-229.
57. Slain D. Lipid-based amphotericin B for the treatment of fungal infections. *Pharmacotherapy.* 1999;19(3):306-323.
58. Faustino C, Pinheiro L. Lipid systems for the delivery of amphotericin B in antifungal therapy. *Pharmaceutics.* 2020;12(1):29.
59. Skipper CP, Atukunda M, Stadelman A, et al. Phase I EnACT trial of the safety and tolerability of a novel oral formulation of amphotericin B. *Antimicrob Agents Chemother.* 2020;64(10):e00838-20.
60. Boulware DR, Atukunda M, Kagimu E, et al. Oral lipid nanocrystal amphotericin B for cryptococcal meningitis: a randomized clinical trial. *Clin Infect Dis.* 2023;77(12):1659-1667.
61. Wilcock BC, Endo MM, Uno BE, Burke MD. C2′-OH of amphotericin B plays an important role in binding the primary sterol of human cells but not yeast cells. *J Am Chem Soc.* 2013;135(23):8488-8491.
62. Hargrove TY, Friggeri L, Wawrzak Z, et al. Structural analyses of *Candida albicans* sterol 14α-demethylase complexed with azole drugs address the molecular basis of azole-mediated inhibition of fungal sterol biosynthesis. *J Biol Chem.* 2017;292(16):6728-6743.
63. Petranyi G, Ryder NS, Stütz A. Allylamine derivatives: new class of synthetic antifungal agents inhibiting fungal squalene epoxidase. *Science.* 1984;224(4654):1239-1241.
64. Barrett-Bee KJ, Lane AC, Turner RW. The mode of antifungal action of tolnaftate. *J Med Vet Mycol.* 1986;24(2):155-160.
65. Ryder NS. The mechanism of action of terbinafine. *Clin Exp Dermatol.* 1989;14(2):98-100.
66. Favre B, Ryder NS. Differential inhibition of fungal and mammalian squalene epoxidases by the benzylamine SDZ SBA 586 in comparison with the allylamine terbinafine. *Arch Biochem Biophys.* 1997;340(2):265-269.
67. Schatz F, Haberl H, Battig F, et al. Major routes of naftifine biotransformation in laboratory animals and man. *Arzneimittelforschung.* 1986;36(2):248-255.
68. Stütz A, Petranyi G. Synthesis and antifungal activity of (E)-N-(6,6-dimethyl-2-hepten-4-ynyl)-N-methyl-1-naphthalenemethanamine (SF 86-327) and related allylamine derivatives with enhanced oral activity. *J Med Chem.* 1984;27(12):1539-1543.
69. Frazier WT, Santiago-Delgado ZM, Stupka KC 2nd. Onychomycosis: rapid evidence review. *Am Fam Physician.* 2021;104(4):359-367.
70. Kreijkamp-Kaspers S, Hawke K, Guo L, et al. Oral antifungal medication for toenail onychomycosis. *Cochrane Database Syst Rev.* 2017;7(7):CD010031.
71. Finlay AY. Pharmacokinetics of terbinafine in the nail. *Br J Dermatol.* 1992;126(suppl 39):28-32.
72. National Center for Biotechnology Information. PubChem compound summary for CID 1549008, Terbinafine. Accessed April 21, 2024. https://pubchem.ncbi.nlm.nih.gov/compound/Terbinafine
73. Vickers AE, Sinclair JR, Zollinger M, et al. Multiple cytochrome P-450s involved in the metabolism of terbinafine suggest a limited potential for drug-drug interactions. *Drug Metab Dispos.* 1999;27(9):1029-1038.
74. Barnette DA, Davis MA, Flynn N, Pidugu AS, Swamidass SJ, Miller GP. Comprehensive kinetic and modeling analyses revealed CYP2C9 and 3A4 determine terbinafine metabolic clearance and bioactivation. *Biochem Pharmacol.* 2019;170:113661.
75. Gupta AK, Versteeg SG, Shear NH. Common drug-drug interactions in antifungal treatments for superficial fungal infections. *Expert Opin Drug Metab Toxicol.* 2018;14(4):387-398.
76. Iverson SL, Uetrecht JP. Identification of a reactive metabolite of terbinafine: insights into terbinafine-induced hepatotoxicity. *Chem Res Toxicol.* 2001;14(2):175-181.
77. Shafiei M, Peyton L, Hashemzadeh M, Foroumadi A. History of the development of antifungal azoles: a review on structures, SAR, and mechanism of action. *Bioorg Chem.* 2020;104:104240.
78. Bhattacharya S, Esquivel BD, White TC. Overexpression or deletion of ergosterol biosynthesis genes alters doubling time, response to stress agents, and drug susceptibility in *Saccharomyces cerevisiae*. *mBio.* 2018;9(4):e01291-18.
79. Kelly SL, Lamb DC, Kelly DE, et al. Resistance to fluconazole and cross-resistance to amphotericin B in *Candida albicans* from AIDS patients caused by defective sterol $\Delta^{5,6}$-desaturation. *FEBS Lett.* 1997;400(1):80-82.
80. Trösken ER, Adamska M, Arand M, et al. Comparison of lanosterol-14α-demethylase (CYP51) of human and *Candida albicans* for inhibition by different antifungal azoles. *Toxicology.* 2006;228(1):24-32.
81. Heeres J, Hendrickx R, Van Cutsem J. Antimycotic azoles. 6. Synthesis and antifungal properties of terconazole, a novel triazole ketal. *J Med Chem.* 1983;26(4):611-613.
82. Elewski BE, Rich P, Pollak R, et al. Efinaconazole 10% solution in the treatment of toenail onychomycosis: two phase III multicenter, randomized, double-blind studies [published correction appears in *J Am Acad Dermatol.* 2014 Feb;70(2):399]. *J Am Acad Dermatol.* 2013;68(4):600-608.
83. Ogura H, Kobayashi H, Nagai K, et al. Synthesis and antifungal activities of (2R,3R)-2-aryl-1-azolyl-3-(substituted amino)-2-butanol derivatives as topical antifungal agents. *Chem Pharm Bull (Tokyo).* 1999;47(10):1417-1425.
84. Sugiura K, Sugimoto N, Hosaka S, et al. The low keratin affinity of efinaconazole contributes to its nail penetration and fungicidal activity in topical onychomycosis treatment. *Antimicrob Agents Chemother.* 2014;58(7):3837-3842.
85. Ketoconazole. Package insert. Taro Pharmaceuticals; Revised September 2023. Accessed April 23, 2024. https://dailymed.nlm.nih.gov/dailymed/drugInfo.cfm?setid=8ca815a8-bccb-4ee2-a042-922373329cae
86. Fitch WL, Tran T, Young M, Liu L, Chen Y. Revisiting the metabolism of ketoconazole using accurate mass. *Drug Metab Lett.* 2009;3(3):191-198.
87. Kim JH, Choi WG, Lee S, Lee HS. Revisiting the metabolism and bioactivation of ketoconazole in human and mouse using liquid chromatography-mass spectrometry-based metabolomics. *Int J Mol Sci.* 2017;18(3):621.
88. Rodriguez RJ, Proteau PJ, Marquez BL, Hetherington CL, Buckholz CJ, O'Connell KL. Flavin-containing monooxygenase-mediated

metabolism of N-deacetyl ketoconazole by rat hepatic microsomes. *Drug Metab Dispos.* 1999;27(8):880-886.
89. Fukami T, Iida A, Konishi K, Nakajima M. Human arylacetamide deacetylase hydrolyzes ketoconazole to trigger hepatocellular toxicity. *Biochem Pharmacol.* 2016;116:153-161.
90. Ketoconazole. Lexi-Drugs. UpToDate Lexidrug. UpToDate Inc. Accessed April 22, 2024. https://online.lexi.com
91. Fleseriu M, Auchus RJ, Pivonello R, Salvatori R, Zacharieva S, Biller BMK. Levoketoconazole: a novel treatment for endogenous Cushing's syndrome. *Expert Rev Endocrinol Metab.* 2021;16(4):159-174.
92. Recorlev. Package insert. Xeris Pharmaceuticals; Revised June 2023. Accessed April 24, 2024. https://dailymed.nlm.nih.gov/dailymed/drugInfo.cfm?setid=d4c5fead-bc4a-fb02-e053-2a95a90ae4fc
93. Warnock DW. Itraconazole and fluconazole: new drugs for deep fungal infection. *J Antimicrob Chemother.* 1989;24(3):275-277.
94. Nett JE, Andes DR. Antifungal agents: spectrum of activity, pharmacology, and clinical indications. *Infect Dis Clin North Am.* 2016;30(1):51-83.
95. Lindsay J, Mudge S, Thompson GR 3rd. Effects of food and omeprazole on a novel formulation of super bioavailability itraconazole in healthy subjects. *Antimicrob Agents Chemother.* 2018;62(12):e01723-18.
96. Poirier JM, Cheymol G. Optimisation of itraconazole therapy using target drug concentrations. *Clin Pharmacokinet.* 1998;35(6):461-473.
97. Stott KE, Hope W. Pharmacokinetics-pharmacodynamics of antifungal agents in the central nervous system. *Expert Opin Drug Metab Toxicol.* 2018;14(8):803-815.
98. Panel on Guidelines for the Prevention and Treatment of Opportunistic Infections in Adults and Adolescents with HIV. *Guidelines for the Prevention and Treatment of Opportunistic Infections in Adults and Adolescents with HIV: Histoplasmosis.* National Institutes of Health, Centers for Disease Control and Prevention, HIV Medicine Association, and Infectious Diseases Society of America; January 10, 2024. Accessed April 27, 2024. https://clinicalinfo.hiv.gov/en/guidelines/hiv-clinical-guidelines-adult-and-adolescent-opportunistic-infections/histoplasmosis?view=full
99. Miller R, Assi M; AST Infectious Diseases Community of Practice. Endemic fungal infections in solid organ transplant recipients—guidelines from the American Society of Transplantation Infectious Diseases Community of Practice. *Clin Transplant.* 2019;33(9):e13553.
100. Brammer KW, Coakley AJ, Jezequel SG, Tarbit MH. The disposition and metabolism of [14C]fluconazole in humans. *Drug Metab Dispos.* 1991;19(4):764-767.
101. National Center for Biotechnology Information. PubChem compound summary for CID 3365, Fluconazole. Accessed April 27, 2024. https://pubchem.ncbi.nlm.nih.gov/compound/Fluconazole
102. National Center for Biotechnology Information. PubChem compound summary for CID 55283, Itraconazole. Accessed April 27, 2024. https://pubchem.ncbi.nlm.nih.gov/compound/Itraconazole
103. Brammer KW, Farrow PR, Faulkner JK. Pharmacokinetics and tissue penetration of fluconazole in humans. *Rev Infect Dis.* 1990;12(suppl 3):S318-S326.
104. Fluconazole. Lexi-Drugs. UpToDate Lexidrug. UpToDate Inc. Accessed April 22, 2024. https://online.lexi.com
105. Lee Y, Puumala E, Robbins N, Cowen LE. Antifungal drug resistance: molecular mechanisms in *Candida albicans* and beyond. *Chem Rev.* 2021;121(6):3390-3411.
106. Nishimoto AT, Sharma C, Rogers PD. Molecular and genetic basis of azole antifungal resistance in the opportunistic pathogenic fungus *Candida albicans*. *J Antimicrob Chemother.* 2020;75(2):257-270.
107. Lockhart SR, Chowdhary A, Gold JAW. The rapid emergence of antifungal-resistant human-pathogenic fungi. *Nat Rev Microbiol.* 2023;21(12):818-832.
108. Sabo JA, Abdel-Rahman SM. Voriconazole: a new triazole antifungal. *Ann Pharmacother.* 2000;34(9):1032-1043.
109. Dickinson RP, Bell AS, Hitchcock CA, Narayanaswami S. Novel antifungal 2-aryl-1-(1*H*-1,2,4-triazol-1-yl)butan-2-ol derivatives with high activity against *Aspergillus fumigatus*. *Bioorg Med Chem Lett.* 1996;6(16):2031-2036.
110. Theuretzbacher U, Ihle F, Derendorf H. Pharmacokinetic/pharmacodynamic profile of voriconazole. *Clin Pharmacokinet.* 2006;45(7):649-663.
111. Roffey SJ, Cole S, Comby P, et al. The disposition of voriconazole in mouse, rat, rabbit, guinea pig, dog, and human. *Drug Metab Dispos.* 2003;31(6):731-741.
112. Hyland R, Jones BC, Smith DA. Identification of the cytochrome P450 enzymes involved in the N-oxidation of voriconazole. *Drug Metab Dispos.* 2003;31(5):540-547.
113. Murayama N, Imai N, Nakane T, Shimizu M, Yamazaki H. Roles of CYP3A4 and CYP2C19 in methyl hydroxylated and N-oxidized metabolite formation from voriconazole, a new antifungal agent, in human liver microsomes. *Biochem Pharmacol.* 2007;73(12):2020-2026.
114. Yanni SB, Annaert PP, Augustijns P, et al. Role of flavin-containing monooxygenase in oxidative metabolism of voriconazole by human liver microsomes. *Drug Metab Dispos.* 2008;36(6):1119-1125.
115. Moriyama B, Obeng AO, Barbarino J, et al. Clinical Pharmacogenetics Implementation Consortium (CPIC) guidelines for CYP2C19 and voriconazole therapy [published correction appears in *Clin Pharmacol Ther.* 2018 Feb;103(2):349]. *Clin Pharmacol Ther.* 2017;102(1):45-51.
116. Voriconazole. Lexi-Drugs. UpToDate Lexidrug. UpToDate Inc. Accessed April 22, 2024. https://online.lexi.com
117. Voriconazole. Package insert. Fresenius Kabi USA; Revised February 2024. Accessed April 28, 2024. https://dailymed.nlm.nih.gov/dailymed/drugInfo.cfm?setid=25eb8d91-5abd-4fdb-a331-dacc960a95d9
118. Chen L, Krekels EHJ, Verweij PE, Buil JB, Knibbe CAJ, Brüggemann RJM. Pharmacokinetics and pharmacodynamics of posaconazole. *Drugs.* 2020;80(7):671-695.
119. Warrilow AG, Melo N, Martel CM, et al. Expression, purification, and characterization of *Aspergillus fumigatus* sterol 14-alpha demethylase (CYP51) isoenzymes A and B. *Antimicrob Agents Chemother.* 2010;54(10):4225-4234.
120. Nywening AV, Rybak JM, Rogers PD, Fortwendel JR. Mechanisms of triazole resistance in *Aspergillus fumigatus*. *Environ Microbiol.* 2020;22(12):4934-4952.
121. Ghosal A, Hapangama N, Yuan Y, et al. Identification of human UDP-glucuronosyltransferase enzyme(s) responsible for the glucuronidation of posaconazole (Noxafil). *Drug Metab Dispos.* 2004;32(2):267-271.
122. Posaconazole. Lexi-Drugs. UpToDate Lexidrug. Accessed April 22, 2024. UpToDate Inc. https://online.lexi.com
123. Krishna G, Moton A, Ma L, Medlock MM, McLeod J. Pharmacokinetics and absorption of posaconazole oral suspension under various gastric conditions in healthy volunteers. *Antimicrob Agents Chemother.* 2009;53(3):958-966.
124. Noxafil. Package insert. Merck Sharp & Dohme; Revised October 2023. Accessed April 28, 2024. https://dailymed.nlm.nih.gov/dailymed/drugInfo.cfm?setid=b073b082-7b57-4423-8c06-4fd4263d6f84
125. Ohwada J, Tsukazaki M, Hayase T, et al. Design, synthesis and antifungal activity of a novel water soluble prodrug of antifungal triazole. *Bioorg Med Chem Lett.* 2003;13(2):191-196.
126. Cresemba. Package insert. Astellas Pharma US; Revised December 2023. Accessed April 28, 2024. https://dailymed.nlm.nih.gov/dailymed/drugInfo.cfm?setid=8f7f73b8-586a-4df0-935f-fecd4696c16c
127. Lewis JS 2nd, Wiederhold NP, Hakki M, Thompson GR 3rd. New perspectives on antimicrobial agents: isavuconazole. *Antimicrob Agents Chemother.* 2022;66(9):e0017722.

128. Schwartz S, Cornely OA, Hamed K, et al. Isavuconazole for the treatment of patients with invasive fungal diseases involving the central nervous system. *Med Mycol.* 2020;58(4):417-424.
129. Isavuconazonium sulfate. Lexi-Drugs. UpToDate Lexidrug. UpToDate Inc. Accessed April 22, 2024. https://online.lexi.com
130. Hoekstra WJ, Garvey EP, Moore WR, Rafferty SW, Yates CM, Schotzinger RJ. Design and optimization of highly-selective fungal CYP51 inhibitors. *Bioorg Med Chem Lett.* 2014; 24(15):3455-3458.
131. Eto H, Kaneko Y, Sakamoto T. New antifungal 1,2,4-triazoles with difluoro(heteroaryl)methyl moiety. *Chem Pharm Bull (Tokyo).* 2000;48(7):982-990.
132. Warrilow AG, Hull CM, Parker JE, et al. The clinical candidate VT-1161 is a highly potent inhibitor of *Candida albicans* CYP51 but fails to bind the human enzyme. *Antimicrob Agents Chemother.* 2014;58(12):7121-7127.
133. Vivjoa. Package insert. Mycovia Pharmaceuticals; Revised July 2022. Accessed April 28, 2024. https://dailymed.nlm.nih.gov/dailymed/drugInfo.cfm?setid=e21d5008-800e-4417-927f-14340341865f
134. Murray A, Cass L, Ito K, et al. PC945, a novel inhaled antifungal agent, for the treatment of respiratory fungal infections. *J Fungi (Basel).* 2020;6(4):373.
135. Colley T, Alanio A, Kelly SL, et al. In vitro and in vivo antifungal profile of a novel and long-acting inhaled azole, PC945, on *Aspergillus fumigatus* infection. *Antimicrob Agents Chemother.* 2017;61(5):e02280-16.
136. Cass L, Murray A, Davis A, et al. Safety and nonclinical and clinical pharmacokinetics of PC945, a novel inhaled triazole antifungal agent. *Pharmacol Res Perspect.* 2021;9(1):e00690.
137. Safety and efficacy of PC945 (opelconazole) in combination with other antifungal therapy for the treatment of refractory invasive pulmonary aspergillosis (OPERA-T Study). ClinicalTrials.gov identifier: NCT05238116. Updated March 18, 2024. Accessed April 29, 2024. https://clinicaltrials.gov/study/NCT05238116
138. Perlin DS. Mechanisms of echinocandin antifungal drug resistance. *Ann N Y Acad Sci.* 2015;1354(1):1-11.
139. Kumar V, Huang J, Dong Y, Hao GF. Targeting Fks1 proteins for novel antifungal drug discovery. *Trends Pharmacol Sci.* 2024; 45(4):366-384.
140. Liu W, Yuan L, Wang S. Recent progress in the discovery of antifungal agents targeting the cell wall. *J Med Chem.* 2020;63(21): 12429-12459.
141. James KD, Laudeman CP, Malkar NB, Krishnan R, Polowy K. Structure-activity relationships of a series of echinocandins and the discovery of CD101, a highly stable and soluble echinocandin with distinctive pharmacokinetic properties. *Antimicrob Agents Chemother.* 2017;61(2):e01541-16.
142. Balani SK, Xu X, Arison BH, et al. Metabolites of caspofungin acetate, a potent antifungal agent, in human plasma and urine. *Drug Metab Dispos.* 2000;28(11):1274-1278.
143. Hebert MF, Smith HE, Marbury TC, et al. Pharmacokinetics of micafungin in healthy volunteers, volunteers with moderate liver disease, and volunteers with renal dysfunction. *J Clin Pharmacol.* 2005;45(10):1145-1152.
144. Micafungin. Package insert. Apotex; Revised July 2023. Accessed May 1, 2024. https://dailymed.nlm.nih.gov/dailymed/drugInfo.cfm?setid=e0f728eb-cb52-5629-e92a-e10260d7687e
145. Damle BD, Dowell JA, Walsky RL, Weber GL, Stogniew M, Inskeep PB. In vitro and in vivo studies to characterize the clearance mechanism and potential cytochrome P450 interactions of anidulafungin. *Antimicrob Agents Chemother.* 2009;53(3):1149-1156.
146. Eraxis. Package insert. Roerig; Revised February 2024. Accessed May 1, 2024. https://dailymed.nlm.nih.gov/dailymed/drugInfo.cfm?setid=d138ab10-1ed9-44be-8d81-49dda1e434ac
147. Ong V, Wills S, Watson D, Sandison T, Flanagan S. Metabolism, excretion, and mass balance of [14C]-rezafungin in animals and humans. *Antimicrob Agents Chemother.* 2022;66(1):e0139021.
148. Chen SC, Slavin MA, Sorrell TC. Echinocandin antifungal drugs in fungal infections: a comparison [published correction appears in *Drugs.* 2011 Jan 22;71(2):253]. *Drugs.* 2011;71(1):11-41.
149. Flanagan S, Walker H, Ong V, Sandison T. Absence of clinically meaningful drug-drug interactions with rezafungin: outcome of investigations. *Microbiol Spectr.* 2023;11(3):e0133923.
150. Sandison T, Ong V, Lee J, Thye D. Safety and pharmacokinetics of CD101 IV, a novel echinocandin, in healthy adults. *Antimicrob Agents Chemother.* 2017;61(2):e01627-16.
151. Hu X, Yang P, Chai C, et al. Structural and mechanistic insights into fungal β-1,3-glucan synthase FKS1. *Nature.* 2023;616(7955):190-198.
152. Peláez F, Cabello A, Platas G, et al. The discovery of enfumafungin, a novel antifungal compound produced by an endophytic *Hormonema* species biological activity and taxonomy of the producing organisms. *Syst Appl Microbiol.* 2000;23(3): 333-343.
153. Apgar JM, Wilkening RR, Parker DL Jr, et al. Ibrexafungerp: an orally active β-1,3-glucan synthesis inhibitor. *Bioorg Med Chem Lett.* 2021;32:127661.
154. Jallow S, Govender NP. Ibrexafungerp: a first-in-class oral triterpenoid glucan synthase inhibitor. *J Fungi (Basel).* 2021;7(3):163.
155. Arendrup MC, Jørgensen KM, Hare RK, Chowdhary A. In vitro activity of ibrexafungerp (SCY-078) against *Candida auris* isolates as determined by EUCAST methodology and comparison with activity against *C. albicans* and *C. glabrata* and with the activities of six comparator agents. *Antimicrob Agents Chemother.* 2020;64(3):e02136-19.
156. Ghannoum M, Arendrup MC, Chaturvedi VP, et al. Ibrexafungerp: a novel oral triterpenoid antifungal in development for the treatment of *Candida auris* infections. *Antibiotics (Basel).* 2020;9(9):539.
157. Jiménez-Ortigosa C, Perez WB, Angulo D, Borroto-Esoda K, Perlin DS. De novo acquisition of resistance to SCY-078 in *Candida glabrata* involves FKS mutations that both overlap and are distinct from those conferring echinocandin resistance. *Antimicrob Agents Chemother.* 2017;61(9):e00833-17.
158. Brexafemme. Package insert. Scynexis; Revised December 2023. Accessed May 2, 2024. https://dailymed.nlm.nih.gov/dailymed/drugInfo.cfm?setid=c33be3a1-c4fd-512c-e053-2995a90a63eb
159. Shaw KJ, Ibrahim AS. Fosmanogepix: a review of the first-in-class broad spectrum agent for the treatment of invasive fungal infections. *J Fungi (Basel).* 2020;6(4):239.
160. Hodges MR, Ople E, Wedel P, et al. Safety and pharmacokinetics of intravenous and oral fosmanogepix, a first-in-class antifungal agent, in healthy volunteers. *Antimicrob Agents Chemother.* 2023;67(4):e0162322.
161. A phase 3 efficacy and safety study of fosmanogepix for the treatment of adult participants with candidemia and/or invasive candidiasis. ClinicalTrials.gov identifier: NCT05421858. Updated April 24, 2024. Accessed May 3, 2024. https://clinicaltrials.gov/study/NCT05421858
162. Subissi A, Monti D, Togni G, Mailland F. Ciclopirox: recent nonclinical and clinical data relevant to its use as a topical antimycotic agent. *Drugs.* 2010;70(16):2133-2152.
163. Ciclodan. Package insert. Medimetriks Pharmaceuticals; Revised December 2020. Accessed May 1, 2024. https://dailymed.nlm.nih.gov/dailymed/drugInfo.cfm?setid=246676e5-60a0-41dc-b665-30d5e670b426
164. Sigera LSM, Denning DW. Flucytosine and its clinical usage. *Ther Adv Infect Dis.* 2023;10:20499361231161387.
165. Oliver JD, Sibley GEM, Beckmann N, et al. F901318 represents a novel class of antifungal drug that inhibits dihydroorotate dehydrogenase. *Proc Natl Acad Sci U S A.* 2016;113(45): 12809-12814.
166. Wiederhold NP. Pharmacodynamics, mechanisms of action and resistance, and spectrum of activity of new antifungal agents. *J Fungi (Basel).* 2022;8(8):857.

167. Olorofim Aspergillus Infection Study (OASIS). ClinicalTrials.gov identifier: NCT05101187. Updated April 17, 2024. Accessed May 3, 2024. https://clinicaltrials.gov/study/NCT05101187
168. Petersen AB, Rønnest MH, Larsen TO, Clausen MH. The chemistry of griseofulvin. *Chem Rev.* 2014;114(24):12088-12107.
169. Gupta AK, Mays RR, Versteeg SG, et al. Tinea capitis in children: a systematic review of management. *J Eur Acad Dermatol Venereol.* 2018;32(12):2264-2274.
170. Griseofulvin. Package insert. Chartwell RX; Revised December 2022. Accessed May 1, 2024. https://dailymed.nlm.nih.gov/dailymed/drugInfo.cfm?setid=9f7e4ecf-f992-42c5-81ea-91e6587b22a5
171. Baker SJ, Zhang YK, Akama T, et al. Discovery of a new boron-containing antifungal agent, 5-fluoro-1,3-dihydro-1-hydroxy-2,1-benzoxaborole (AN2690), for the potential treatment of onychomycosis. *J Med Chem.* 2006;49(15):4447-4450.
172. Rock FL, Mao W, Yaremchuk A, et al. An antifungal agent inhibits an aminoacyl-tRNA synthetase by trapping tRNA in the editing site. *Science.* 2007;316(5832):1759-1761.
173. Seiradake E, Mao W, Hernandez V, et al. Crystal structures of the human and fungal cytosolic Leucyl-tRNA synthetase editing domains: a structural basis for the rational design of antifungal benzoxaboroles. *J Mol Biol.* 2009;390(2):196-207.
174. Hui X, Baker SJ, Wester RC, et al. In vitro penetration of a novel oxaborole antifungal (AN2690) into the human nail plate. *J Pharm Sci.* 2007;96(10):2622-2631.
175. Coronado D, Merchant T, Chanda S, Zane LT. In vitro nail penetration and antifungal activity of tavaborole, a boron-based pharmaceutical. *J Drugs Dermatol.* 2015;14(6):609-614.
176. Rossi A, Martins MP, Bitencourt TA, et al. Reassessing the use of undecanoic acid as a therapeutic strategy for treating fungal infections. *Mycopathologia.* 2021;186(3):327-340.

Structure Challenge Answers

1. B and C
2. A and E
3. A. topical; B. systemic; C. systemic; D. systemic; E. topical; F. topical

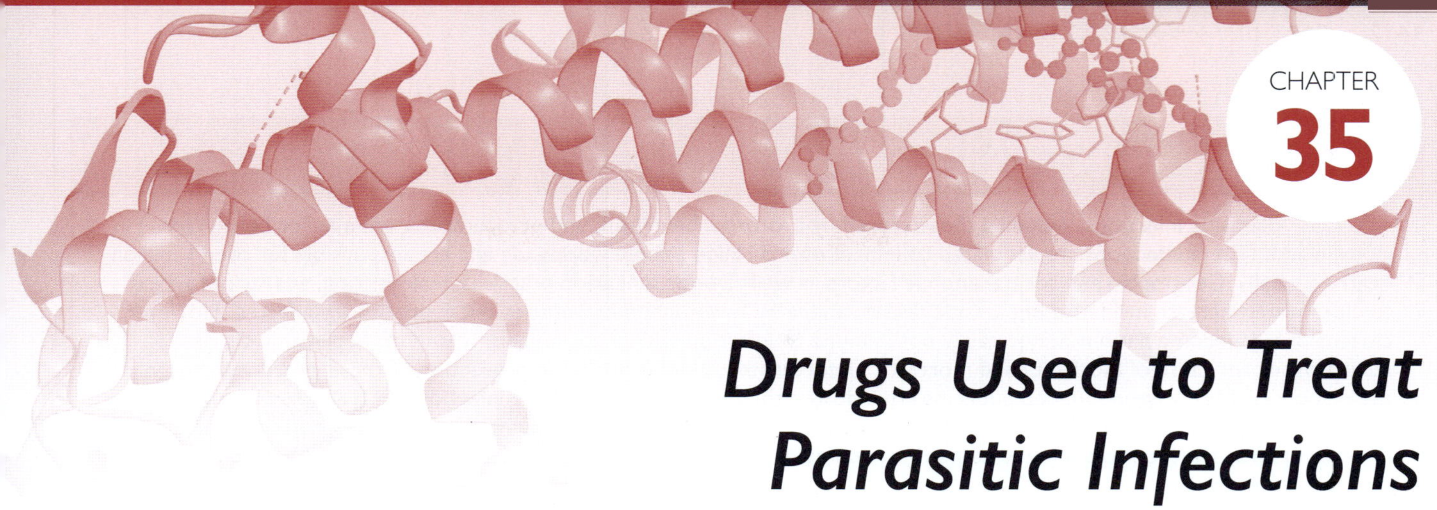

CHAPTER 35

Drugs Used to Treat Parasitic Infections

Kirk E. Hevener and Bob M. Moore II

Drugs covered in this chapter

Treatment of amebiasis, giardiasis, and trichomoniasis
- Metronidazole
- Nitazoxanide
- Paromomycin
- Tinidazole

Treatment of trypanosomiasis
- Benznidazole
- Eflornithine
- Fexinidazole
- Melarsoprol
- Nifurtimox
- Pentamidine isethionate
- Suramin sodium

Treatment of leishmaniasis
- Amphotericin B
- Miltefosine
- Sodium stibogluconate

Treatment of toxoplasmosis
- Clindamycin
- Pyrimethamine
- Spiramycin
- Sulfadiazine

Treatment of malaria
- Artemisinins (artemether, artesunate, dihydroartemisinin)
- Atovaquone-proguanil
- Chloroquine
- Lumefantrine
- Mefloquine
- Piperaquine
- Primaquine
- Quinine
- Tafenoquine

Treatment of helminth infections
- Albendazole
- Ivermectin
- Mebendazole
- Moxidectin
- Praziquantel
- Pyrantel pamoate
- Triclabendazole

Treatment of scabies and pediculosis
- Crotamiton
- Ivermectin
- Malathion
- Permethrin
- Pyrethrum
- Spinosad

Abbreviations

ABD amphotericin B deoxycholate
AChE acetylcholinesterase
ACT artemisinin-based combination therapy
ATP adenosine 5′-triphosphate
BBB blood-brain barrier
CDC US Centers for Disease Control and Prevention
CNS central nervous system
DDT dichlorodiphenyltrichlorethane
DHFR dihydrofolate reductase
DNA deoxyribonucleic acid
FDA US Food and Drug Administration
G6PD glucose-6-phosphate dehydrogenase
GABA γ-aminobutyric acid
GI gastrointestinal
HIV human immunodeficiency virus
HM 2-hydroxymethylmetronidazole
IV intravenous
IVM ivermectin
nAChRs nicotinic acetylcholine receptors
NAD nicotinamide adenine dinucleotide
NADH nicotinamide adenine dinucleotide plus hydrogen
NPIs neglected parasitic infections
NTZ nitazoxanide
ODC ornithine decarboxylase
OTC over the counter
OYE old yellow enzyme (a prostaglandin $F_{2\alpha}$ synthase)
PABA *p*-aminobenzoic acid
PCP *Pneumocystis jirovecii* pneumonia
PfATP6 *Plasmodium falciparum*
PFOR pyruvate:ferredoxin oxidoreductase
PZQ praziquantel
RBC red blood cell
RNA ribonucleic acid
ROS reactive oxygen species
TIZ tizoxanide
TRPV4 transient receptor potential vanilloid 4
US United States
WHO World Health Organization

CLINICAL SIGNIFICANCE

Parasitic infections, including those caused by protozoa, helminths, and ectoparasites, are a major burden for global health. These infections are estimated to impact over 3 billion people worldwide and are responsible for over 1 million deaths annually. Geographic and socioeconomic factors as well as poor sanitation practices, malnutrition, and lack of access to clean water increase incidence of parasitic disease and leave lower-income countries disproportionally affected. However, citizens of high-income nations are certainly not immune to infection with these organisms, and many parasitic diseases remain a significant cause of morbidity and mortality. Unfortunately, identification and prevention of these infections is largely the responsibility of a poorly funded public health industry, thus management of these infections with antiparasitic medications is vital. Antiparasitic medications comprise several drug classes targeting a broad range of diseases caused by parasites. Pharmacists play a pivotal role in understanding the complex mechanisms of action, adverse effect profiles, and required monitoring for these agents.

Treatment of parasitic diseases remains challenging, as they are caused by a wide variety of organisms often with complex life cycles and sophisticated mechanisms to evade the host immune response. Historically, medicinal chemistry has been especially important in the treatment of these infections as many currently used antiparasitic medications were originally developed for other indications and identified as prospective antiparasitic chemotherapeutics based on their chemical structures. Similarly to antimicrobial resistance, antiparasitic resistance is a growing concern to global health and has limited available treatment options for parasitic diseases. Extensive knowledge of drug chemical structure-activity relationship can be utilized to optimize medication therapy as well as develop new antiparasitic agents by bypassing known mechanisms of resistance and targeting newly discovered biochemical pathways. These principles can be exercised to inform treatment decisions and ultimately enhance patient care.

Lindey Lane, PharmD

INTRODUCTION

The antiparasitic agents covered in this chapter include those drugs used to treat what the World Health Organization (WHO) calls "vector-transmitted infectious diseases." The vectors commonly referred to are mosquitoes, sandflies, ticks, triatomine bugs, tsetse flies, fleas, black flies, aquatic snails, and lice. This chapter discusses drugs used to treat the following disease-producing organisms: protozoa (responsible for amebiasis, giardiasis, trichomoniasis, leishmaniasis, malaria), helminths (responsible for intestinal worm infections and systemic infections such as schistosomiasis and onchocerciasis), and ectoparasites (responsible for scabies, pediculosis, chiggers, and bedbugs [Cimicidae family]). It should be noted that the US Centers for Disease Control and Prevention (CDC) has targeted for surveillance, prevention, and treatment five neglected parasitic infections (NPIs), which include Chagas disease (transmitted by a blood-sucking triatomine), cysticercosis and toxocariasis (infections associated with helminths), and toxoplasmosis and trichomoniasis (infections caused by protozoans).

PROTOZOAL INFECTIONS

Types of Protozoal Infections

Amebiasis

Amebiasis (Table 35.1) is a disease of the large intestine caused by *Entamoeba histolytica*. The disease occurs mainly in the tropics, but it is also seen in temperate climates. Amebiasis can be carried without significant symptoms, or it can lead to severe, life-threatening dysentery. The organism exists in one of two forms: the motile trophozoite form or the dormant cyst form. The trophozoite form is found in the intestine or in the wall of the colon and can be expelled from the body with the feces. The cyst form is encased by a chitinous wall that protects the organism from the environment, including chlorine used in water purification; thus, the organism can be transmitted through contaminated water and foods.

The cyst form is responsible for transmission of the disease. Direct person-to-person contact spreads the cyst form and is commonly associated with living conditions in which poor personal hygiene, poor sanitation, poverty, and ignorance of sound public health practices exist. The hosts can be rendered susceptible to infection by preexisting conditions, such as protein malnutrition, pregnancy, human immunodeficiency virus (HIV) infection, or high carbohydrate intake. Under these conditions, the organism is capable of invading body tissue. The protozoal invasion is not well understood, but it does appear to involve the processes indicated in Table 35.1. Symptoms can range from intermittent diarrhea (foul-smelling loose/watery stools) to tenderness and enlargement of the liver (with the extraintestinal form) to acute amebic dysentery. Some patients may experience no symptoms.

Giardiasis

Giardiasis (see Table 35.1) is a disease that shows considerable similarity to amebiasis. It is caused by *Giardia lamblia*, an organism that can be found in the duodenum and jejunum. The organism exists in a motile trophozoite form and an infectious cyst form. The cyst form can be deposited in water (lives up to 2 months), and the contaminated water can

Table 35.1 Diseases Associated with Protozoal Infections and Their Characteristics

Disease	Organism	Life Stages	Infected Organ, Cells	Transmitter
Amebiasis	*Entamoeba histolytica*	Cyst, trophozoite	Intestine, liver	Contaminated food/ water
Giardiasis	*Giardia lamblia*	Cyst, trophozoite	Intestine, liver	Contaminated water
Trichomoniasis	*Trichomonas vaginalis*	Trophozoite	Vagina, urethra, prostate	Sexual contact
Trypanosomiasis				
Sleeping sickness	*Trypanosoma brucei*	Trypomastigote;	Central nervous system (CNS)	Tsetse fly
Chagas disease	*Trypanosoma cruzi*	Trypomastigote, amastigote	Heart	Reduviid bug
Leishmaniasis	*Leishmania* spp.	Promastigote, amastigote	Skin, systemic	Female sandflies
Toxoplasmosis	*Toxoplasma gondii*	Tachyzoites, bradyzoites	Spleen, liver, lungs, lymphoid tissue, blood, CNS, amniotic fluid	Contaminated food/ water, cat feces
Malaria	*Plasmodium* spp.	Sporozoite, merozoite, trophozoite, gametes	Liver, red blood cells	Anopheles mosquito

then be ingested by the human. The trophozoite, if expelled from the gastrointestinal (GI) tract, normally will not survive. *G. lamblia* is the single most common cause of waterborne diarrhea in the United States. Giardiasis is a common disease among campers who drink water from contaminated streams. It also can be spread between family members, children in day care centers, and dogs and their owners. The organism can attach to the mucosal wall via a ventral sucking disk and, similar to amebiasis, the patient can be asymptomatic or develop watery diarrhea, abdominal cramps, distention and flatulence, anorexia, nausea, and vomiting. Usually, the condition is self-limiting in 1 to 4 weeks.

Trichomoniasis

Trichomoniasis (see Table 35.1) is a protozoal infection caused by *Trichomonas vaginalis*, which exists only in a trophozoite form. The organs most commonly involved in the infection include the vagina, urethra, and prostate; thus, the disease is considered to be a venereal infection. Sexual contact transmits the condition, and it is estimated that trichomoniasis affects 180 million individuals worldwide. Infections in the male can be asymptomatic, whereas in the female, the symptoms can consist of vaginitis, profuse and foul-smelling discharge, burning and soreness on urination, and vulvar itching. Diagnosis is based on microscopic identification of the organism in fluids from the vagina, prostate, or urethra.

ORGANISMS THAT COMMONLY CAUSE VAGINITIS

Vaginitis can also be caused by *Haemophilus vaginalis* (bacteria) or *Candida albicans* (fungus), which are treated differently from the protozoal infection.

Tritryps

Three protozoan pathogens that belong to the family Trypanosomatidae are Leishmania major, which is responsible for leishmaniasis; *Trypanosoma brucei*, which is responsible for African trypanosomiasis (African sleeping sickness); and *Trypanosoma cruzi*, which is the responsible organism for Chagas disease (see Table 35.1). Referred to as the "tritryps," these eukaryotic organisms share characteristic subcellular structures of a kinetoplast (a network of circular DNA [deoxyribonucleic acid]) and glycosomes (an organelle containing glycolytic enzymes), are unicellular motile protozoa, are transmitted by various insect vectors, and infect mammalian hosts. The genomes of tritryps have recently been reported.[1-3] Together, they infect hundreds of millions of people annually.

TRYPANOSOMIASIS. There are two distinct forms of trypanosomiasis (see Table 35.1): Chagas disease and African sleeping sickness.[4]

Chagas Disease. Chagas disease, also known as American trypanosomiasis, is caused by the parasitic protozoa *Trypanosoma cruzi* and is found only in the Americas, primarily in Brazil but also in the southern United States. The protozoan lives in mammals and is spread by the blood-sucking insect known as the reduviid bug, assassin bug, or kissing bug. The insect becomes infected by drawing blood from an infected mammal and releases the protozoa with discharged feces. The pathogen then enters the new host through breaks in the skin. Inflammatory lesions are seen at the site of entry. The disease also can be spread through transfusion with contaminated blood. Signs of initial infection can include malaise, fever, anorexia, and skin edema at the site where the protozoa entered the host. The disease can invade the heart, where after decades of infection with chronic Chagas disease, the patient can experience an infection-associated heart attack. It is estimated that 6 million persons living in the Americas have Chagas disease, including an estimated 240,000 to 350,000 US residents of Latin American origin.[5]

African Trypanosomiasis. African trypanosomiasis, or sleeping sickness, is caused by several subspecies of *Trypanosoma brucei* (*T. brucei* rhodesiense [east African sleeping sickness] and *T. brucei* gambiense [west African sleeping sickness]). In this case, the blood-sucking tsetse fly bites the infected animal. The protozoa, initially present in the gut of the vector, appear in the salivary gland for inoculation during the subsequent biting of a human. It is estimated that some 50 million people are at risk of African sleeping sickness, with 300,000 to 500,000 cases occurring in sub-Saharan Africa each year.[6]

The infection progresses through two stages. Stage I can present as fever and elevated temperatures lasting several days; hematologic and immunologic changes occur during this stage. Stage II occurs after the organism enters the central nervous system (CNS) and can involve symptoms suggesting the disease name—daytime somnolence, loss of spontaneity, halting speech, listless gaze, and extrapyramidal signs (eg, tremors and choreiform movements). A breakdown of neurological function leading to coma and death can occur. Death can occur within weeks if untreated (*T. brucei rhodesiense*) or only after several years (*T. brucei gambiense*). It should be noted that the sole source of energy for the trypanosomal organism is glycolysis, which in turn can account for the hypoglycemia seen in the host. In addition, the migration of the organism into the CNS can be associated with the organism's search for a rich source of available glucose.

LEISHMANIASIS. Leishmaniasis is a disease caused by a number of protozoa in the genus *Leishmania*. The protozoa can be harbored in diseased rodents, canines, and various other mammals. Once transmitted from the infected mammal to man by bites from female sandflies of the genus Phlebotomus, it then appears in one of four major clinical syndromes: visceral leishmaniasis, cutaneous leishmaniasis, mucocutaneous leishmaniasis, or diffuse cutaneous leishmaniasis. The sandfly, the vector involved in spreading the disease, breeds in warm, humid climates; thus, the disease is more common in the tropics. As many as 12 million individuals, worldwide are infected by this organism with an estimate of 600,000 to 1,000,000 new cases annually.[7]

The visceral leishmaniasis, also known as kala azar (black fever), is caused by *Leishmania donovani*. This form of the disease is systemic and is characterized in patients by fever (typically nocturnal), diarrhea, cough, and enlarged liver and spleen. The skin of the patient can become darkened. Without treatment, death can occur in 20 months and is commonly associated with diarrhea, superinfections, or GI hemorrhage. Visceral leishmaniasis is most commonly found in India and Sudan.

Both cutaneous and mucocutaneous leishmaniasis are characterized by single or multiple localized lesions. These slow-healing and painful ulcers can lead to secondary bacterial infections. The Old World cutaneous leishmaniasis is caused by *Leishmania tropica*, which is found most commonly in children and young adults in regions bordering the Mediterranean, the Middle East, Southern Russia, and India. Leishmania major is endemic to desert areas in Africa, the Middle East, and Russia, whereas *Leishmania aethiopica* is found in the Kenyan highlands and Ethiopia. The New World disease caused by *Leishmania peruviana, Leishmania braziliensis*, and *Leishmania panamensis* is found in South and Central America, whereas *Leishmania mexicana* can be endemic to southcentral Texas. The incubation period for cutaneous leishmaniasis ranges from a few weeks to several months. The slow-healing lesions can be seen on the skin in various regions of the body depending on the specific strain of organism. Usually, these conditions exhibit spontaneous healing, but this also can occur over an extended period of time (1-2 years).

Malaria

The infected female Anopheles mosquito transmits malaria (see Table 35.1). The specific protozoan organisms causing malaria are from the genus *Plasmodium*. Only five of approximately 100 species cause malaria in humans. The remaining species affect birds, monkeys, livestock, rodents, and reptiles. The five species that affect humans are *P. falciparum, P. vivax, P. malariae, P. ovale*, and *P. knowlesi*. Concurrent infections by more than one of these species are seen in endemically affected regions of the world. Such multiple infections further complicate patient management and the choice of treatment regimens. In 2022, there were an estimated 249 million cases of malaria in 85 malaria-endemic countries resulting in 608,000 deaths.[8] Approximately 75% of total malaria deaths occur in children under the age of 5 years.

Although this disease is found primarily in the tropics and subtropics, it has been observed far beyond these boundaries. Malaria was almost completely eradicated from the United States between 1947 and 1951 through the use of the insecticide DDT (dichloro-diphenyl-trichloroethane), which destroys the insect vector; however, recent endemic cases in parts of the United States have been linked to local *Anopheles* mosquitoes.[9] In 1955, the WHO launched the Global Malaria Eradication Program. The program intended to eradicate the disease worldwide through the use of DDT and disease treatment with chloroquine, but due to the development of DDT-resistant *Anopheles* mosquitoes, drug-resistant plasmodium, and political resistance, WHO abandoned its program in 1972. Recently, there has been an increased global interest in addressing the disease through the use of preventative measures, development of multidrug treatments, and the development of malaria vaccinations. The first malaria vaccine began its use in 2021, and there are currently two vaccines used for prevention of malaria in children living in endemic areas.

While malaria has been nearly eradicated in most temperate-zone countries, between 2,000 and 2,500 cases are documented annually in US citizens returning from travel abroad. Today, malaria is found in most countries of Africa, Central and South America, and Southeast Asia, with Africa accounting for 94% of cases globally. According to the WHO, the global incidence of malaria has been declining since 2000.[8] Malarial infection can cause anemia, pulmonary edema, renal failure; jaundice; shock; cerebral malaria; and, if not treated in a timely manner, even death.

Types of Malaria. Malarial infections are known according to the species of the parasite involved.

Plasmodium falciparum. Infection with *Plasmodium falciparum* has an incubation period (time from mosquito bite to clinical symptoms) of 1 to 3 weeks (average, 12 days). The *P. falciparum* life cycle in humans begins with the bite of an infected female mosquito. The parasites in the sporozoite stage enter the circulatory system, through which they can reach the liver in approximately 1 hour. These organisms grow and multiply 30,000- to 40,000-fold by asexual division within liver cells in 5 to 7 days. Then, as merozoites, they leave the liver to reenter the bloodstream and invade the erythrocytes, or red blood cells (RBCs), where they continue to grow and multiply further for 1 to 3 days. Specific receptors on the surface of the erythrocytes serve as binding sites for the merozoite. These infected RBCs rupture, releasing merozoites in intervals of approximately 48 hours. Chemicals released by the ruptured cells in turn cause activation and release of additional substances associated with the patient's symptoms. The clinical symptoms include chills, fever, sweating, headaches, fatigue, anorexia, nausea, vomiting, and diarrhea.

Some of the released merozoites are sequestered in vital organs (brain and heart), where they continue to grow. Recurrence of the clinical symptoms on alternate days leads to the terminology of tertian malaria. The *P. falciparum* parasite also can cause RBCs to clump and adhere to the wall of blood vessels. Such a phenomenon has been known to cause partial obstruction and, sometimes, restriction of the blood flow to vital organs like the brain, liver, and kidneys. Reinfection of RBCs can occur, allowing further multiplication and re-manifestation of the malaria symptoms. Some merozoites develop into male and female sexual forms, called gametocytes, which can then be acquired by the female mosquito after biting the infected human. Gametocytes mature in the mosquito's stomach to form zygotes. Growth of the zygotes leads to the formation of oocysts (spherical structures located on the outside wall of the stomach). Sporozoites develop from the oocysts, are released into the body cavity of the mosquito, and migrate to the salivary gland of the insect, from which they can be transmitted to another human following a mosquito bite. The life cycle of the malaria parasites is shown in Figure 35.1. The genome of the *P. falciparum* and that of the *Anopheles* mosquito are now known and are expected to provide potential new avenues for drug development. Genome information is also expected to give insight regarding the mechanisms of resistance and improve drug treatment.

Plasmodium vivax. *Plasmodium vivax* (benign tertian) is the most prevalent form of malaria. It has an incubation period of 1 to 4 weeks (average, 2 weeks). This form of malaria can cause spleen rupture and anemia. Relapses (renewed manifestations of erythrocytic infection) can occur. This results from the periodic release of dormant parasites (hypnozoites) from the liver cells. The erythrocytic forms generally are considered to be susceptible to treatment.

Plasmodium malariae. *Plasmodium malariae* is responsible for quartan malaria. It has an incubation period of 2 to 4 weeks (average, 3 weeks). The asexual cycle occurs every 72 hours. In addition to the usual symptoms, this form also causes nephritis. This is the mildest form of malaria and does not relapse. The RBC infection associated with *P. malariae* can last for many years, and the organism is quite unlikely to become resistant.

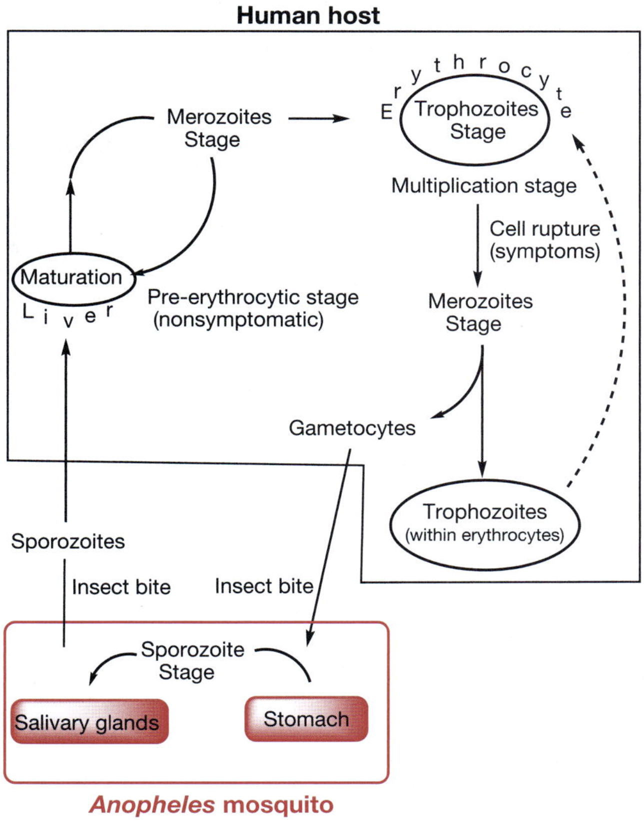

Figure 35.1 Life cycle of malarial protozoa.

Plasmodium ovale. Infection with *Plasmodium ovale* has an incubation period of 9 to 18 days (average, 14 days). Relapses have been known to occur in individuals infected with this plasmodium. The relapse can be indicative of ovale tertian malaria and is associated with the ability of the organism to lay dormant (hypnozoites) in hepatic tissue for extended periods of time.

General Approaches to Antimalarial Chemotherapy. Generally, antimalarial drugs are classified by the life cycle stage (see Fig. 35.1) that the drugs are effective against, although they can be also classified by their structural type. Listed next are the theoretical approaches through which drugs can intervene to destroy the organism. Currently, the majority of drugs act upon the intracellular erythrocytic form of the disease. It should be noted that some antimalarials can be effective against more than one form of the organism while others may be species specific.

Tissue Schizonticides. These drugs eradicate the exoerythrocytic liver-tissue stages of the plasmodium parasite, which prevents the parasite's entry into the blood. Drugs of this type are useful for prophylaxis. Some tissue schizonticides can act on the long-lived tissue form (hypnozoites of *P. vivax* and *P. ovale*) and, thus, can prevent relapses.

Blood Schizonticides. These drugs destroy the erythrocytic stages of parasites and can cure cases of falciparum malaria or suppress relapses. This is the easiest phase to treat because drug delivery into the bloodstream can be accomplished rapidly.

Gametocytocides. Agents of this type kill the sexual forms of the plasmodia (gametocytes), which are transmittable to the Anopheles mosquito, thereby preventing transmission of the disease.

Sporontocides (Sporozooiticides). These drugs act against sporozoites and are capable of killing these organisms as soon as they enter the bloodstream following a mosquito bite.

Despite the history of malaria, the epidemiology and clinical features of the disease are not that well documented. In many parts of Africa, the diagnosis of the disease is not routinely performed, and therefore, the success of prevention efforts and treatment cannot be known. For more details on these difficulties, the reader is directed to an excellent review by Greenwood et al.[10]

General Approaches to Protozoal Therapy

Amebiasis and Giardiasis

Amebiasis and giardiasis infections usually occur by consumption of contaminated drinking water and food. Preventative measures including drinking bottled water, boiling, or disinfecting the water, and sanitary food preparation and storage are integral to the prevention of these diseases. Additionally, improvements in personal hygiene and general sanitation are beneficial in limiting transmission of *Entamoeba histolytica* and *Giardia duodenalis,* the infective entities causing amebiasis and giardiasis, respectively.

Trypanosomiasis, Leishmaniasis, and Malaria

The insect-borne protozoal infections trypanosomiasis, leishmaniasis, and malaria are endemic in many parts of the tropical and subtropical regions. Protozoans in these families have multiple host species, thus limiting the efficacy of insect eradication strategies that cannot destroy reservoirs of the diseases. Visitors to regions with endemic infections can limit exposure using insect repellents and protective clothing. Malaria chemoprophylaxis can be used for travelers visiting endemic regions; the choice of agent is dependent on the destination, season, duration of stay, and local living conditions.[11] For populations living in these areas, early detection and drug therapy is the method of treatment.

Drug Therapy for Protozoal Infections

Treatment of Amebiasis, Giardiasis, and Trichomoniasis

METRONIDAZOLE (FLAGYL, GENERIC FORMS)

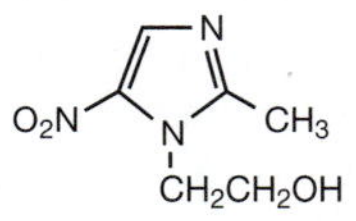

Metronidazole

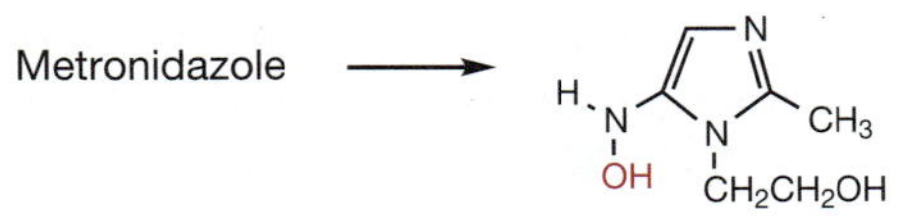

Figure 35.2 Anaerobic metabolic activation of metronidazole.

Metronidazole is a synthetic analogue of azomycin, an antibiotic first isolated from *Streptomyces eurocidicus* in 1953.[12] Metronidazole was initially introduced for the treatment of vaginal infections caused by *T. vaginalis* but has since been shown to be effective for treatment of amebiasis, giardiasis, and anaerobic bacterial infections, including *Clostridioides difficile*.

Mechanism of Action. Metronidazole is a prodrug that exploits unique energy-producing pathways in anerobic microorganisms. The predominate pathways for anaerobes are fermentative and glycolytic, which use pyruvate:ferredoxin oxidoreductase (PFOR) as a component of electron transport.[13,14] Capture of an electron from PFOR by the nitro group in metronidazole is proposed to activate the drug causing cytotoxicity via two potential pathways. The drug's mechanism involves reduction of the nitro group to a hydroxylamine, as shown in Figure 35.2, then imidazole ring fission and generation of reactive hydroxyethyl oxamic acid and acetamide that can damage DNA, proteins, and membranes. The second pathway was discussed by DoCampo,[15] reporting that nitroaryl compounds (nitroimidazoles, metronidazole; nitrofurans, nifurtimox) are reduced to nitro radical anions, which in turn react with oxygen to regenerate the nitroaryl and the superoxide radical anion (Fig. 35.3). Further reduction of superoxide radical anion leads to hydrogen peroxide, and homolytic cleavage of the latter leads to hydroxyl radical formation. Superoxide radical anion, hydrogen peroxide, and hydroxyl radicals are referred to as reactive oxygen species

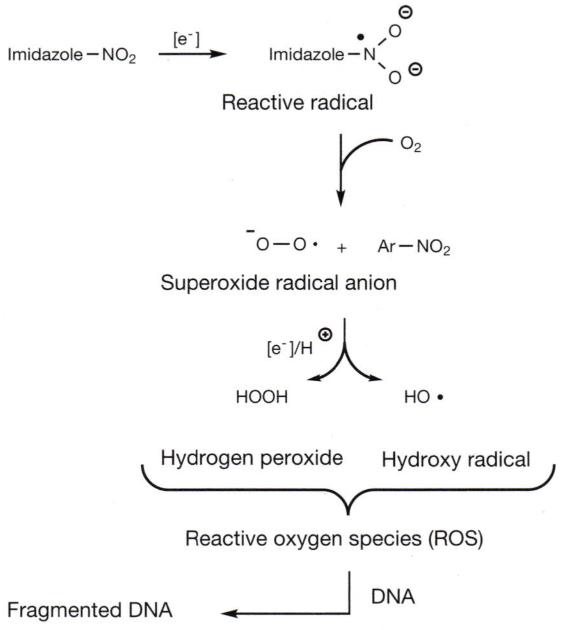

Figure 35.3 Formation of reactive oxygen species (ROS) from nitroimidazole compounds.

(ROS) and are the reactive substances that are implicated in damage to critical cellular components of the parasite.

Metabolism. Liver metabolism of metronidazole leads to two major metabolites: hydroxylation of the 2-methyl group to 2-hydroxymethylmetronidazole (HM) and its oxidation to metronidazole acetic acid.[16] The HM metabolite possess approximately 65% of the activity of the parent drug, while the acid metabolite possesses approximately 5%.[17] Glucuronide and sulfate conjugates of HM are also found in the urine.[18] In addition, a small amount of metronidazole is oxidized to acetamide, a known carcinogen in rats but not in humans, and to the oxalate derivative shown in Figure 35.4.[19]

Pharmacokinetics. Metronidazole is available in a variety of dosage forms, including IV, oral, topical, rectal, and vaginal suppositories.[20] The bioavailability of metronidazole is nearly 100% when administered orally but is significantly less when administered via the rectal (67%-82%) or the vaginal (19%-56%) routes. The drug is not bound to plasma protein and distributed fairly uniform throughout the body, including breast milk.[21]

Therapeutic Application. Metronidazole is considered to be the drug of choice for treatment of the protozoal infections amebiasis (intestinal and extraintestinal), giardiasis, and trichomoniasis.[13] Previously recommended for treatment of C. *difficile* infection, it is now considered a third-line agent for this infection.[22] It is also used in combination is a first-line therapy for *Helicobacter pylori* infections.[23] The common side effects exhibited with metronidazole include abdominal distress, a metallic taste, and a disulfiram-like effect if taken with alcohol. The drug is reported to be carcinogenic in mice, possibly related to the metabolite acetamide, and as a result should not be used during the first trimester of pregnancy.

Tinidazole (Tindamax)

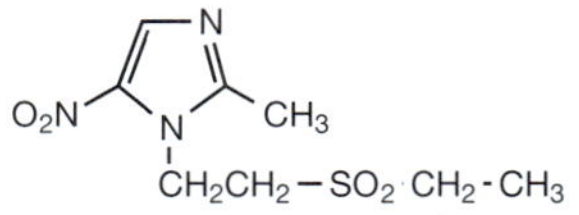

Tinidazole

Tinidazole has been approved by the US Food and Drug Administration (FDA) for the treatment of amebiasis, giardiasis, and trichomoniasis. Additionally, it is also an alternative to metronidazole in the quadruple therapy for *H. pylori* infections,[23] although it is not approved for this use. The drug is rapidly and completely absorbed following oral administration and can be administered with food to reduce GI disturbance. Tinidazole has a mechanism of action that parallels that of metronidazole, as well as a similar metabolic pathway leading to hydroxylation at the 2-methyl group catalyzed by CYP3A4. Tinidazole appears to mimic the actions of metronidazole, although there are reports that it is effective against some protozoa that are resistant to metronidazole.

Nitazoxanide (Alinia)

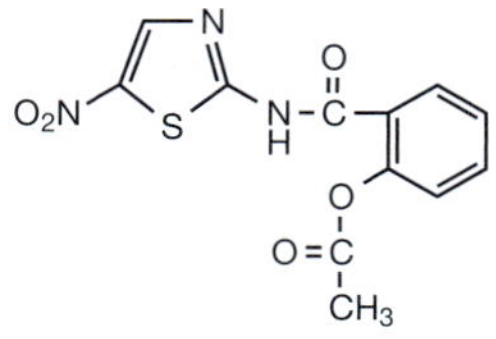

Nitazoxanide

Nitazoxanide (NTZ) is a nitro-thiazole prodrug originally approved for the treatment of diarrhea associated with giardiasis in children aged 1 to 11 years. Subsequent approval was granted for the treatment of diarrhea caused by cryptosporidiosis in patients with AIDS. This protozoal infection is caused by *Cryptosporidium parvum*, and while uncommon in healthy individuals, the infection (such as HIV infections) can be life-threatening in patients with immunosuppression.

Mechanism of Action. Activation of NTZ occurs by metabolic cleavage of the acetyl group yielding the drug tizoxanide (TIZ) (Fig. 35.5).[10] TIZ is further reduced via a four-electron reduction of the 5-nitro group giving various short-lived intermediates (eg, hydroxylamine derivative), which represent the active forms of NTZ. Whereas these intermediates would suggest that NTZ has the same

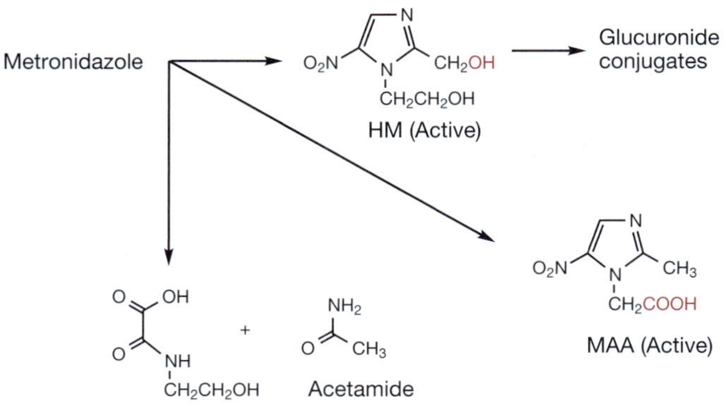

Figure 35.4 Hepatic metabolism of metronidazole. HM, 2-hydroxymethylmetronidazole; MAA, metronidazole acetic acid.

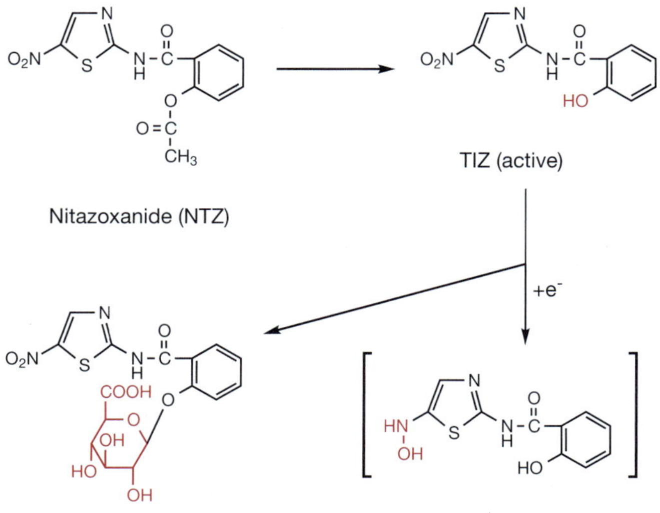

Figure 35.5 Metabolic activation of nitazoxanide. TIZ, tizoxanide.

mechanism of action as metronidazole, in fact the drug inhibits PFOR, the same enzyme that activates metronidazole. The cytotoxic mechanism is disruption of the bioenergetics of these organisms, and not DNA fragmentation observed with nitroimidazoles, thus NTZ is not considered to be mutagenic. Additional metabolites of TIZ include the glucuronide, which shows some biological activity, and an aromatic hydroxylation product (Fig. 35.5). A more recent study suggests that NTZ may act on an ion channel via its action on the *avr-14* gene.[24]

Pharmacokinetics. NTZ is available as a powder that is reconstituted and dispensed as an oral suspension and as a tablet. The product can be taken with food and is well absorbed from the GI tract. It is rapidly metabolized with elimination products appearing in the urine and feces. The only identified products in the plasma are TIZ and its glucuronide.[25]

Therapeutic Application. NTZ (powder) was previously approved for treatment of pediatric patients with *G. lamblia*, and it is now approved in tablet form for diarrhea caused by this organism in adults and children over age 12. The drug also possesses activity against *Cryptosporidium parvum* as well as the protozoa *Entamoeba histolytica* and *T. vaginalis*; the bacteria *H. pylori* and *Clostridium perfringens*; and various helminths, including *Ascaris lumbricoides*, *Enterobius vermicularis*, *Ancylostoma doudenale*, and *Strongyloides stercoralis*.[26,27]

PAROMOMYCIN

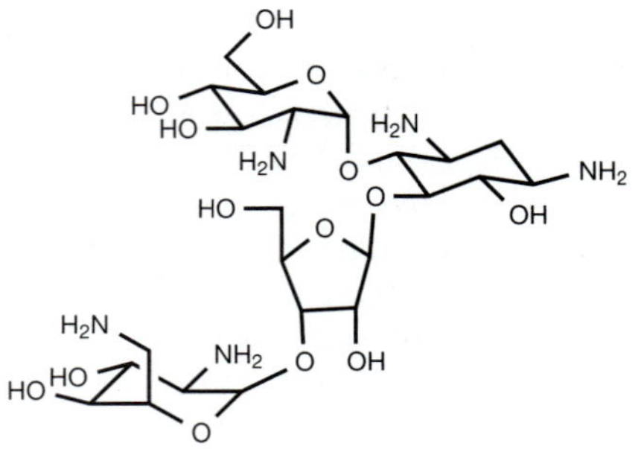

Paromomycin

Paromomycin is an aminoglycoside antibiotic used to treat luminal (intestinal) amebiasis and as an alternative agent for giardiasis. The drug is poorly absorbed and used to clear luminal colonization after treatment with nitroimidazoles (eg, metronidazole) or related drugs. Paromomycin binds to the 16S ribosomal RNA, leading to interference resulting in errors in amino acid addition and termination of translation.

The drug is dosed at 25 to 35 mg/kg/d, by mouth, in three divided daily doses for 7 days for amebiasis. As an alternative agent for giardiasis, the drug is dosed at 10 mg/kg by mouth 3 times daily for 5 to 7 days. Because paromomycin is poorly absorbed, adverse effects are minimal and primarily GI related (nausea, diarrhea, and abdominal cramps). In rare cases of concomitant inflammatory bowel disease, some drug can be absorbed systemically and result in ototoxicity and nephrotoxicity.

Treatment of Trypanosomiasis

SURAMIN SODIUM

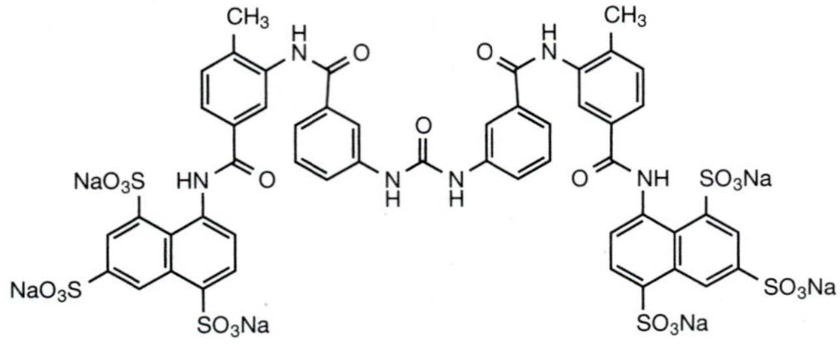

Suramin sodium

Paul Ehrlich first discovered that the aniline dyes trypan red and trypan blue were effective in treating trypanosomiasis in animal models but not in humans.[28] Bayer built on this discovery, resulting in the introduction of suramin, a bis-hexa-sulfonated-naphthylurea, as a therapy for the treatment of first-stage African trypanosomiasis (sleeping sickness) in the 1920. Suramin (available from the CDC) is still considered to be the drug of choice for treatment of non-CNS-associated African trypanosomiasis.

Mechanism of Action. The mechanism of action of suramin is unproven, but the drug is known to have a high affinity for binding to a number of critical enzymes in the pathogen. Among the enzymes to which suramin has been shown to bind are several dehydrogenases and kinases.[29] Suramin has been shown to be an inhibitor of dihydrofolate reductase (DHFR), a crucial enzyme in folate metabolism, and thymidine kinase. In addition, suramin is an inhibitor of glycolytic enzymes in *Trypanosoma brucei*, with binding constants much lower than those seen in mammalian cells. Inhibition of glycolysis would be expected to block energy sources of the pathogen, leading to lysis. More recently it has been proposed that the mechanism of action of suramin involves binding to RuvB-like DNA helicase.[30] Whether one or more of these inhibitor actions represent the toxic action of suramin on the pathogen remains an open question.

Pharmacokinetics. Suramin sodium is a water-soluble compound that is poorly absorbed via oral administration and must be administered IV in multiple injections. Because of its highly ionic nature, suramin will not cross the blood-brain barrier (BBB) and, therefore, is ineffective for the treatment of trypanosomal infections that reach the CNS. Although suramin is tightly bound to serum albumin (~98%), the drug is preferentially absorbed by trypanosomes through a receptor-mediated endocytosis of serum protein. Additionally, suramin has value as a prophylactic drug because the drug remains in the bloodstream for an extended period of time ($t_{1/2}$ ~50 days).

Therapeutic Application. Suramin sodium is effective against East African trypanosomiasis, but it has limited value against West African trypanosomiasis. As indicated, the drug will not enter the CNS and thus is only useful for treatment of initial stages of the disease. The drug exhibits a wide variety of side effects, which can be severe in debilitated individuals and includes nausea, vomiting, and fatigue.

PENTAMIDINE ISETHIONATE (PENTAM, NEBUPENT)

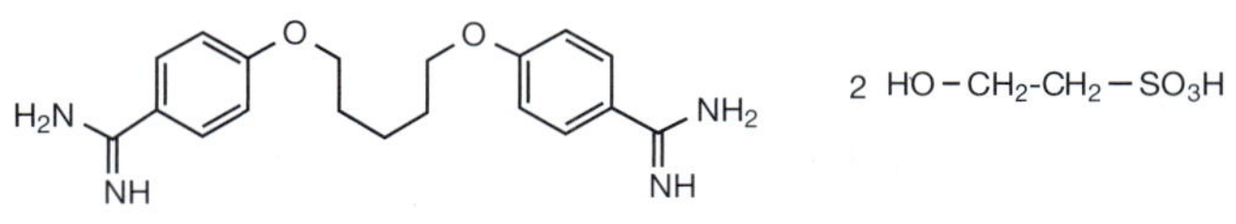

Pentamidine isethionate

First introduced as a therapy for trypanosomiasis in 1937, pentamidine is now used in a variety of protozoal and fungal infections and finds use in the treatment of trypanosomiasis, leishmaniasis, and *Pneumocystis jirovecii* pneumoniae (PCP). The drug is primarily used for treatment of PCP. When used for trypanosomiasis, pentamidine is only effective against *T. brucei* rhodesiense (East African sleeping sickness) and, even then, only during the early stage of the disease because the drug does not readily cross the BBB.

Mechanism of Action. Several biochemical actions have been reported for pentamidine. The drug has been shown to bind to DNA through hydrogen-bonding of the amidine protons with the adenine-thymine–rich regions of DNA. More specifically, pentamidine binds to the N-3 of two adenines separated by four to five base pairs forming interstrand cross-bonding.[31] In addition to, and possibly separate from this action, pentamidine appears to be a potent inhibitor of type II topoisomerase of cyclic mitochondrial DNA (kinetoplast DNA) of the trypanosomal parasite.[32] This inhibition leads to double-stand breaks and linearization of the DNA. The relationship between binding to specific regions of the DNA and inhibition of topoisomerase is unclear. In the case of *T. brucei*, resistant strains are common. It is thought that resistance develops through an inability of the drug to reach the mitochondrial DNA.[33] Transport into the mitochondria is a carrier-mediated process which is absent in the resistant strains.

EFLORNITHINE

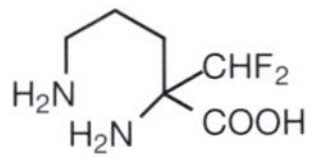

Eflornithine

Metcalf et al reported the synthesis of eflornithine in 1978.[34] Their interest arose from the desire to prepare ornithine decarboxylase (ODC) inhibitors as tools for studying the role of polyamines as regulators of growth processes. ODC catalyzes the conversion of ornithine to putrescine (1,4-diaminobutane), which in turn leads to the formation of the polyamines spermine and spermidine. It was not until 1980 that Bacchi et al demonstrated the potential of eflornithine in the treatment of trypanosomiasis.[35] In December 2023, the US FDA–approved eflornithine for treatment of neuroblastoma in adult and pediatric patients.

Mechanism of Action. Difluoromethyl ornithine is a suicide-substrate inhibitor of ODC, a pyridoxal phosphate-dependent enzyme, as shown in Figure 35.6. Evidence suggests that cysteine-360 in ODC is the site of eflornithine alkylation.[36] Alkylation of ODC blocks the synthesis of putrescine, which is the rate-determining step in the synthesis of polyamines. Mammalian ODC can also be inhibited, but because the turnover of ODC is so rapid in mammals, eflornithine does not produce serious side effects.

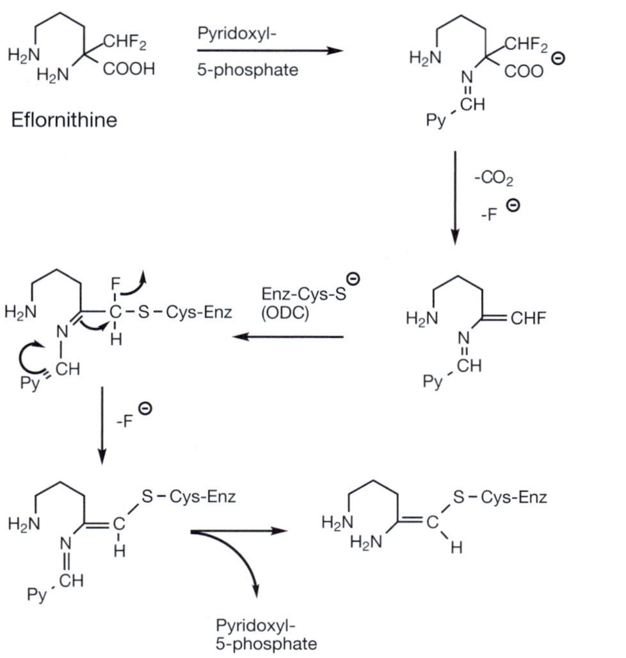

Figure 35.6 Inhibition of ornithine decarboxylase (Enz-Cys-SH) by eflornithine.

Pharmacokinetics. Eflornithine can be administered either intravenously or orally, though the IV formulation is no longer available in the United States. The zwitterionic nature of the drug (an amino acid) limits oral bioavailability. IV administration requires large and frequent dosing. The drug does not bind to plasma protein and enters the CNS readily, likely via an amino acid transport system. As a result, the drug can be used for both early and late stages of trypanosomiasis.

Therapeutic Application. Eflornithine is indicated for the treatment of West African trypanosomiasis caused by *Trypanosoma brucei gambiense* but has proven to be ineffective against East African trypanosomiasis. The cause of this ineffectiveness remains a mystery, although evidence suggests that endogenous ornithine plus increased activity of *S*-adenosylmethionine decarboxylase allow sufficient synthesis of spermidine and spermine to support cell division. Thus, resistance arises from bypassing ODC for de novo synthesis of ornithine.[37] Side effects reported for eflornithine consist of anemia, diarrhea, and leukopenia.

NIFURTIMOX (LAMPIT)

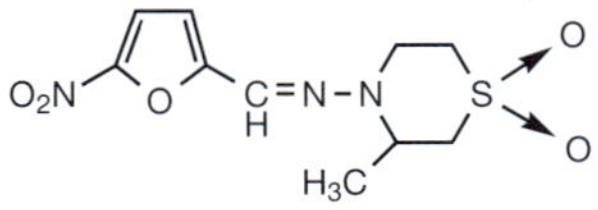

Nifurtimox

Nifurtimox is a nitroaryl compound that has proven to be useful as a drug for the treatment of trypanosomiasis and one of the two drugs approved for the treatment of Chagas disease. The CDC estimates that 8 million individuals in the Americas have Chagas disease, and more than 300 thousand with *T. cruzi* infection live in the United States.

Mechanism of Action. Nifurtimox is thought to undergo reduction, similar to that of metronidazole, followed by oxidation and generation of ROS such as the superoxide radical anion, hydrogen peroxide, and hydroxyl radical (see Fig. 35.3).[15] These species are potent oxidants, producing oxidative stress that can induce damage to DNA and affect cellular membranes via lipid oxidation. In addition, Henderson et al have reported that nifurtimox inhibits trypanothione reductase reducing trypanothione formation by 93%.[38] Trypanothione reductase is a critical protective enzyme found uniquely in trypanosomal parasites.

Therapeutic Application. Nifurtimox is the drug of choice for the treatment of acute Chagas disease. The drug is not effective for the chronic stages of the disease. In the acute stage, the drug has an 80% cure rate. Side effects of the drug include hypersensitivity reactions, GI complications (nausea and vomiting), myalgia, and weakness.

Benznidazole

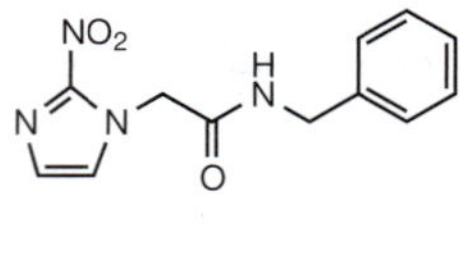

Benznidazole

Benznidazole is the first drug approved for treatment of Chagas disease in the United States for pediatric patients aged 2 to 12 years. Like nifurtimox, it is effective against the circulating form of *T. cruzi* during the acute phase of the disease, but also like nifurtimox, it is ineffective during the chronic stage of the disease.

Mechanism of Action. The mechanism of action of benznidazole remains under investigation. Studies suggest that benznidazole may partially catalyze the formation of ROS through the action of type I nitroreductase, leading to cell death (Fig. 35.7). Additionally, it has been proposed that benznidazole undergoes metabolic activation via a protozoal prostaglandin $F_{2\alpha}$ synthase referred to as old yellow enzyme (OYE), leading to the formation of glyoxal, which, in turn, forms an adduct with the guanosine of DNA that results in genetic damage and cell death.[39]

Therapeutic Application. Benznidazole, like nifurtimox, is only of value for the treatment of acute Chagas disease. The drug is not effective for the chronic stages of the disease, and is administered orally in a tablet form.

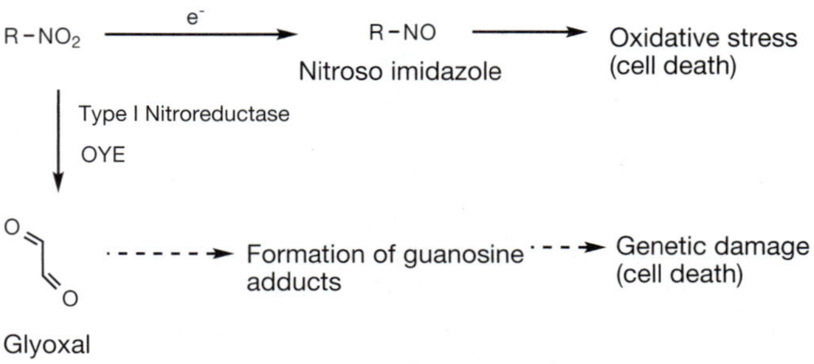

Figure 35.7 Proposed mechanism of action of benznidazole. OYE, old yellow enzyme (a prostaglandin F2α synthase).

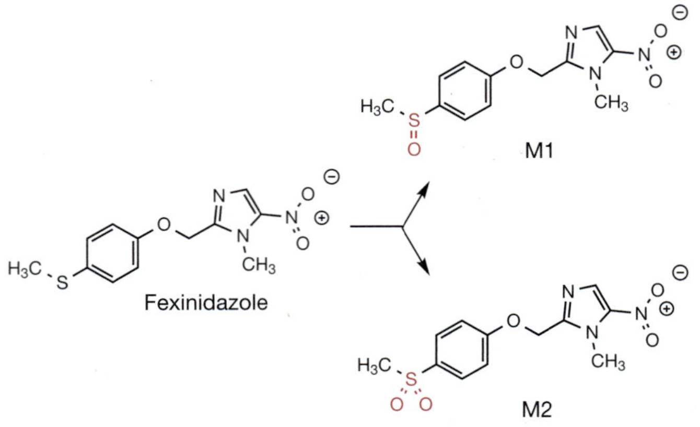

Figure 35.8 Fexinidazole metabolism.

Adverse Effects. A number of serious adverse effects have been reported, including the potential for genotoxicity, carcinogenicity, and mutagenicity. Additionally, hypersensitivity skin reactions, manifestations of bone marrow depression, and peripheral neuropathy may occur. The drug should not be administered with disulfiram.

Fexinidazole. Fexinidazole was approved by the FDA in 2021 for the treatment of first and second stage *T. brucei gambiense* infections (Fig. 35.8).[40] The drug benefits from the ability to be taken orally but is less effective than nifurtimox with eflornithine.[41] It has been evaluated for the treatment of Chagas disease but was found to be ineffective as a monotherapy.[42]

Mechanism of Action. Fexinidazole, the sulfoxide M1 metabolite, and the sulfone M2 metabolite (Fig. 35.8) possess antitrypanosomal activity.[43] The parent drug and metabolites are prodrugs that undergo activation via a type I nitroreductase, yielding reactive metabolites.[44] Although the exact chemical species responsible for toxicity have yet to be identified, it is thought that ROS generation analogous to nifurtimox and metronidazole is responsible.

Therapeutic Application. Fexinidazole is administered orally over 10 days in a tablet form and must be taken with food. The drug is effective against early- and late-stage *T. brucei* infections and is the first-line treatment for early-stage infections without CNS involvement.

Adverse Effects. Several adverse effects have been reported, including nausea, vomiting, asthenia, and adverse neuropsychiatric reactions. A prolonged QT interval and neutropenia has been observed in some patients.[45]

Melarsoprol (Arsobal)

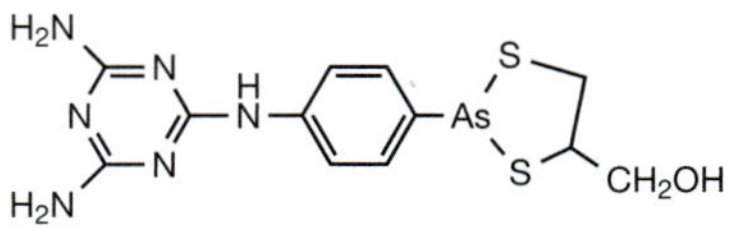

Melarsoprol

Knowingly or unknowingly, arsenic-containing drugs have been used for treatment of parasitic conditions for thousands of years. In the late 1800s and early 1900s, Paul Ehrlich introduced the use of trivalent arsenicals. Melarsoprol (available from the CDC), an organo-arsenical, came into use in the late 1940s, and it remains a first-choice drug in

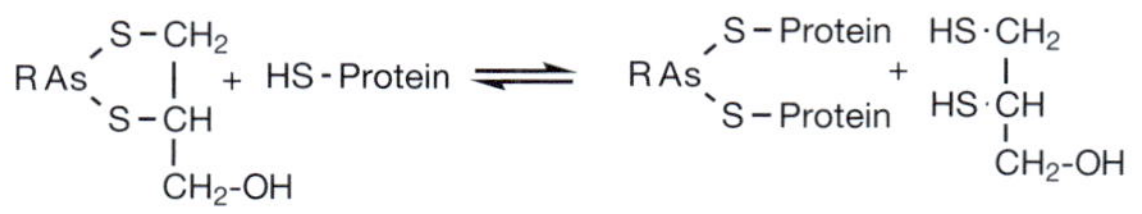

Figure 35.9 Mechanism of action of trivalent arsenic compounds with *Trypanosoma* organism.

the treatment of late-stage African trypanosomiasis (*T. brucei rhodesiense*). Until 1990, it was also the only treatment for late-stage sleeping sickness.

Mechanism of Action. It is known that trivalent arsenic reacts rapidly and reversibly with sulfhydryl-containing proteins, as shown in Figure 35.9. It is believed that the enzyme with which melarsoprol reacts is involved in glycolysis, and as a result, inhibition of pyruvate kinase occurs. It is argued, however, that the inhibition cannot occur at pyruvate kinase but rather at a step before the pyruvate kinase. More recently, Fairlamb et al proposed a mechanism of action wherein melarsoprol is oxidized to melarsen oxide, which then forms a stable complex with trypanothione reductase via interactions with cysteine sulfhydryl in the enzyme (Fig. 35.10).[46] Supportive of this mechanism is the synergistic action of melarsoprol with eflornithine, two drugs that produce sequential blockage of the synthesis of trypanothione.

Pharmacokinetics. Melarsoprol is administered intravenously in multiple doses and multiple sessions. Its major metabolite in humans is the lipophilic melarsen oxide, which can penetrate into the CNS. This metabolite apparently is responsible for the protein-binding characteristic for melarsoprol.

Therapeutic Application. Melarsoprol is now considered last-line treatment of late-stage trypanosomiasis (*T. brucei gambiense*) and is used only if the other therapies are not available. Because the drug has the potential for serious nervous system toxicities (eg, convulsions, acute cerebral edema, and coma), it is usually administered in a hospital setting with supervision. An additional problem with melarsoprol is the development of resistance by the parasite.

Treatment of Leishmaniasis

Sodium Stibogluconate

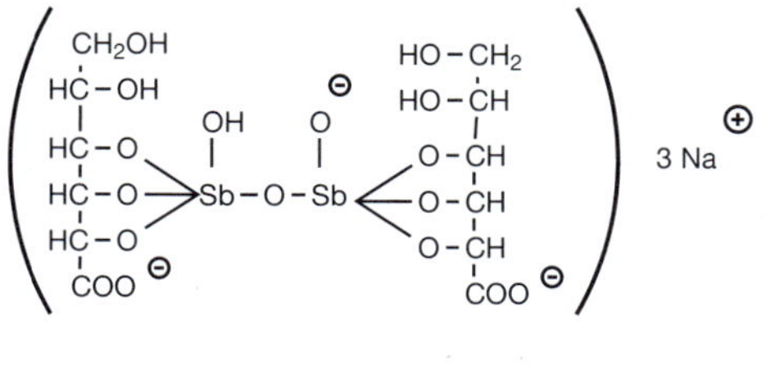

Sodium stibogluconate

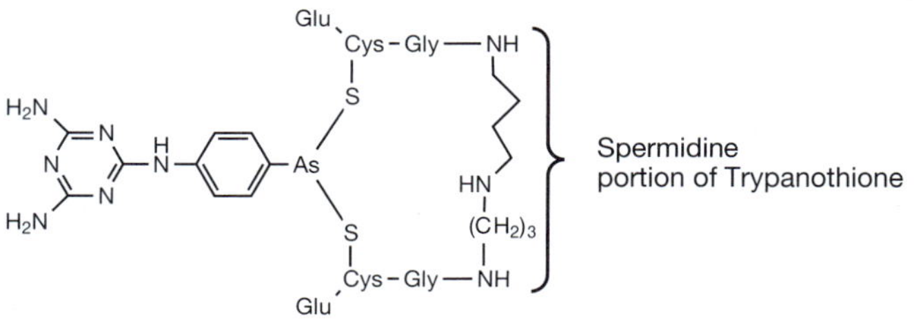

Figure 35.10 Structure of melarsoprol trypanothione complex.

Leishmaniasis was first described in the medical literature by Deishman and Donovan in 1903, and shortly after that, antimony-based drugs were introduced as therapeutic agents to treat this disease.[47] The drug is a water-soluble preparation that is administered intramuscularly or intravenously. Pentavalent antimony compounds are thought to inhibit bioenergetic processes in the pathogen, with catabolism of glucose and inhibition of glycolytic enzymes being the primary mechanism of action (glucose catabolism is 86%-94% inhibited). This in turn results in inhibition of adenosine triphosphate (ATP)/guanosine triphosphate formation.

Sodium stibogluconate (available from the CDC, or meglumine antimonate, another pentavalent antimony agent) is used for the treatment of cutaneous, mucocutaneous, and visceral leishmaniasis. The recommended dose is 20 mg antimony/kg/d, not to exceed 850 mg antimony/d. A number of other drugs have been reported to be effective in the treatment of leishmaniasis, including pentamidine, amphotericin B, paromomycin, alkyl phosphocholine analogues, rifampin, and ketoconazole.[48,49]

Miltefosine (Impavido)

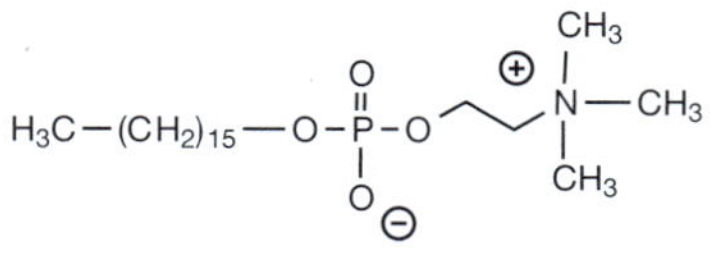

Miltefosine

Miltefosine is an orally active drug approved by the FDA for adults and adolescents aged 12 years and older. It is effective against cutaneous and visceral forms of leishmaniasis. This drug is especially important since the only other drugs available are sodium stibogluconate and amphotericin B (visceral leishmaniasis), which are administered parenterally, thus limiting their utility, and have a high potential for toxicities. Miltefosine has been reported to exhibit activity in vitro against a broad range of leishmanial strains.[50]

Mechanism of Action. Several mechanisms have been proposed to account for miltefosine's anti-leishmanial activity; however, the precise mechanism remains unknown. The fact that the drug is effective against the promastigote and amastigote stages suggests several mechanisms of therapeutic action.[51] Miltefosine has been demonstrated to inhibit cytochrome c oxidase causing the death of the organism, possibly due to reduced intracellular ATP synthesis and oxygen consumption.[52] In addition, the drug may inhibit phosphatidylcholine synthesis via inhibition of phosphatidylethanolamine *N*-methyltransferase.[53] Recent work has demonstrated that miltefosine can increase accumulation of intracellular Ca^{2+} via opening sphingosine-activated plasma membrane Ca^{2+} channels in the parasite.[54]

Pharmacokinetics. The drug is well absorbed via the oral route and well distributed with a half-life of 6 to 8 days.[55] Miltefosine is highly bound to serum albumin and lipoproteins with a preference for albumin (~97%).[56]

Adverse Effects. Miltefosine is contraindicated in pregnant women since it has been reported to cause fetal death and teratogenicity in animals. Reduced fertility and testicular atrophy have been reported in male rats. Other adverse effects reported include decreased appetite and headaches, GI disorders, edema, jaundice, and seizures.

Liposomal Amphotericin B (AmBisome). Amphotericin B deoxycholate (ABD) was originally approved to treat severe fungal infections (see Chapter 34) and was later reformulated into liposomal preparations to reduce the dose-limiting toxicity of ABD. AmBisome (LAMB), which is a liposomal formulation consisting of phospholipids and cholesterol, was approved by the FDA in 1997 for the treatment of visceral leishmaniasis.

Mechanism of Action. The predominant mechanism of anti-leishmanial activity is binding to ergosterol, analogous to that of fungi.[57] Tetramer and octamer accumulation in the lipid membrane forms pores that allow the extravasation of electrolytes, proton influx, and cell death. Destabilizing the phospholipid bilayer and oxidative stress have also been implicated in the activity of Amphotericin B.

Treatment of Toxoplasmosis

Toxoplasmosis is a parasitic infection resulting from ingestion of *Toxoplasma gondii* on undercooked cooked meats (particularly pork and lamb) or cat feces. According to the CDC, toxoplasmosis is the leading cause of foodborne illness–related deaths[58]; however, healthy individuals normally recover from infection without treatment. Patients with a compromised immune system, pregnant women, infants, and newborns may require treatment consisting of pyrimethamine or a combination with other drugs. Combination therapies are the gold standard particularly in treating ocular and encephalitic toxoplasmosis, a common pathology in patients with compromised immune system.

Pyrimethamine (Daraprim)

Mechanism of Action. Pyrimethamine is a competitive inhibitor of the enzyme dihydrofolate reductase (DHFR). The drug blocks the conversion of dihydrofolate to tetrahydrofolic acid. Tetrahydrofolic acid is essential for the de novo synthesis nucleic acid, thus inhibition of DHFR results in downstream blockade of RNA (ribonucleic acid) and DNA synthesis, inhibition of cell division, and parasite death.

Pharmacokinetics. Pyrimethamine is well absorbed, with an oral bioavailability greater than 90% and high protein binding (85%-90%).[59] Peak plasma concentrations occur between 2 and 6 hours, with a half-life of approximately 96 hours.

Therapeutic Application. In combination with sulfadiazine or clindamycin (see upcoming sections), pyrimethamine is the first-line treatment for toxoplasmosis.[60] Bone marrow suppression can occur from pyrimethamine administration, which can be addressed by the addition of folinic acid (leucovorin).

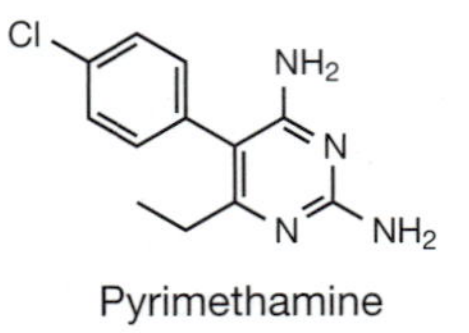

Pyrimethamine

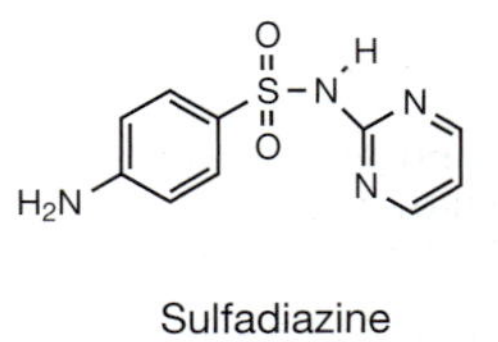

Sulfadiazine

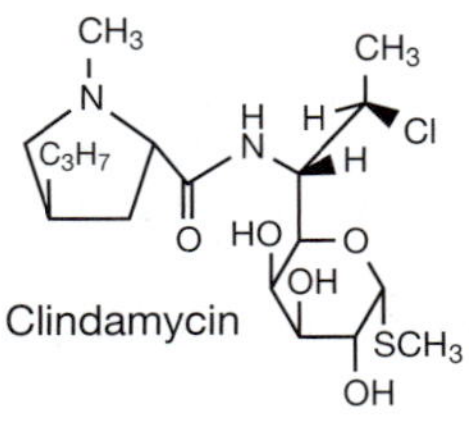

Clindamycin

Sulfadiazine. Sulfadiazine is a sulfonamide antibiotic (see Chapter 32) used in combination with pyrimethamine to treat toxoplasmosis. This is considered the gold standard for the treatment of toxoplasmosis in humans.

Mechanism of Action. Sulfadiazine is a competitive inhibitor of the enzyme dihydropteroate synthetase, which produces dihydropteroic acid and is the initiating step in the tetrahydrofolate biosynthesis pathway. Thus, the combination of sulfadiazine and pyrimethamine blocks two steps in the pathway required for the de novo synthesis of tetrahydrofolate. Ultimately, purine and pyrimidine nucleic acid synthesis is blocked, leading to inhibition of cell division.

Pharmacokinetics. Sulfadiazine is well absorbed, with a bioavailability between 73% and 78%.[61] Peak plasma concentrations occur at 7 hours, with an average half-life of 15 hours.[62]

Clindamycin (Cleocin). Clindamycin is an antibacterial agent (see Chapter 32) that is used as an alternative to sulfadiazine in combination with pyrimethamine for patients sensitive to sulfa drugs.

Mechanism of Action. The mechanism of action of clindamycin against toxoplasmosis is unclear but may involve inhibition of protein synthesis in the mitochondria or cytoplasm.[63] This may involve binding to the parasite's equivalent of the 50S ribosome, as known for the drug's bacteriostatic activity.

Pharmacokinetics. Clindamycin is well absorbed, with a bioavailability of 93%, peak concentrations at 45 minutes, and half-life of 2.3 hours.[64]

Spiramycin

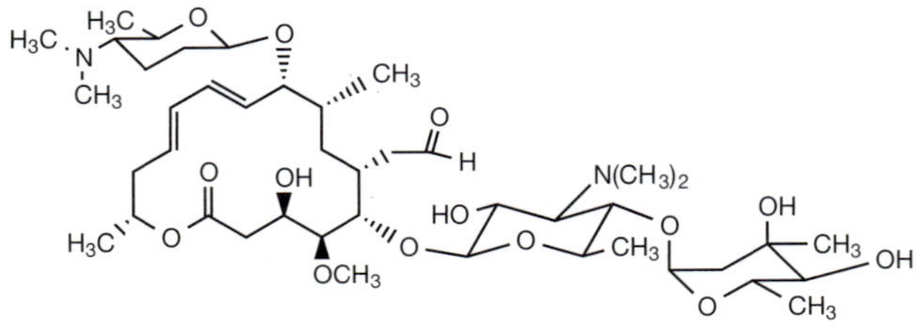

Spiramycin

Spiramycin is a macrolide antibiotic approved for use in Europe, Canada, and Mexico and is available with special permission from the FDA to prevent fetal transmission of toxoplasmosis. The vertical fetal transmission rate of toxoplasmosis in the first trimester is approximately 6%, versus 60% to 80% at 36 weeks, thus early treatment can prevent lifelong consequences of fetal infection.[65] The drug does not cross the placental barrier and is administered throughout pregnancy.

Mechanism of Action. Spiramycin binds to the 50S ribosome in bacteria, and it is proposed that a similar mechanism is operative in toxoplasmosis activity.

Therapeutic Application. Early administration of spiramycin can reduce the risk of placental transfer by 60%. The drug is taken orally every 8 hours for a total of 3 g/d.[66]

Treatment of Malaria

Historical Background

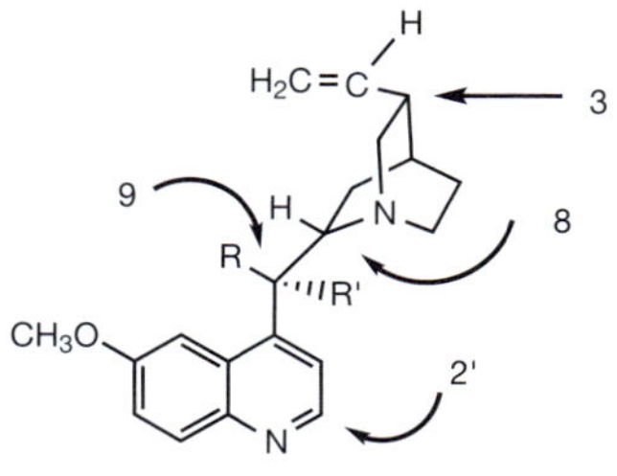

Quinine (R = OH, R' = H)
Quinidine (R = H, R' = OH)

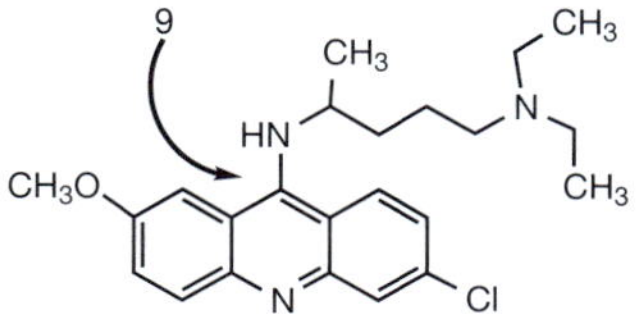

Quinacrine

Quinine was the first known antimalarial. It is a 4-quinoline-methanol derivative bearing a substituted quinuclidine ring. The use of quinine in Europe began in the 17th century, after the Incas of Peru informed the Spanish Jesuits about the antimalarial properties of the bark of an evergreen mountain tree they called quinquina (later called cinchona, after Dona Franciscoa Henriquez de Ribera [1576-1639], Countess of Chinchon and wife of the Peruvian Viceroy). The bark, when made into an aqueous solution, was capable of curing most forms of malaria. It was listed in the London Pharmacopeia of 1677. The alkaloid derived from the bark, quinine, was isolated in the mid-1820s. Quinine, a very bitter substance, has been used by millions of malaria sufferers. Quinine, in combination with other agents, is now considered a third-line agent in the treatment of chloroquine-resistant strains of malarial infection. Quinidine, the C-9 stereoisomer of quinine, is also possesses antimalarial activity, but suffers from the fact that it is considerably more cardiotoxic than quinine. It was previously used to treat severe malarial infections but is no longer recommended. Quinidine is now used solely as an antiarrhythmic agent.

A second class of chemicals that played a role in the development of synthetic antimalarials is the 9-aminoacridines. 9-aminoacridine was known to exhibit antibacterial activity, whereas a derivative of 9-aminoacridine synthesized in 1934, quinacrine, was found to possess weak antimalarial activity. With the beginning of World War II and concern about an interruption in the supply of cinchona bark from the East Indies, a massive effort was begun to search for synthetic alternatives to quinine and to develop more effective antimalarial agents than quinacrine. With a basic understanding of the structure-activity relationship of quinine (see next section) and the chemical similarities seen with quinacrine, it is easy to visualize the relationship between these agents and the synthetic antimalarials (Fig. 35.11).

A third class of chemicals, which today represents the first-line standard treatment of malaria, is the artemisinins and the semisynthetic derivatives of this natural product. Artemisinin was first isolated over 2,000 years ago from the sweet wormwood or annual wormwood plant qing hao (*Artemisia annua*). This natural product was used as an herbal medicine through the Chinese culture and was used for the treatment of malaria in the late 1500s. Major developments in the chemistry of artemisinin were not reported until the 1970s, which lead to the development of semisynthetic analogues. The 2015 Nobel Prize in Physiology and Medicine was awarded to Tu Youyou for her contributions to the development of artemisinins and their use in treating malaria. Today, artemisinin-based combination therapy (ACT), utilizing artemether, artesunate, and dihydroartemisinin, serves as the main stay of antimalarial treatments (Fig. 35.12).

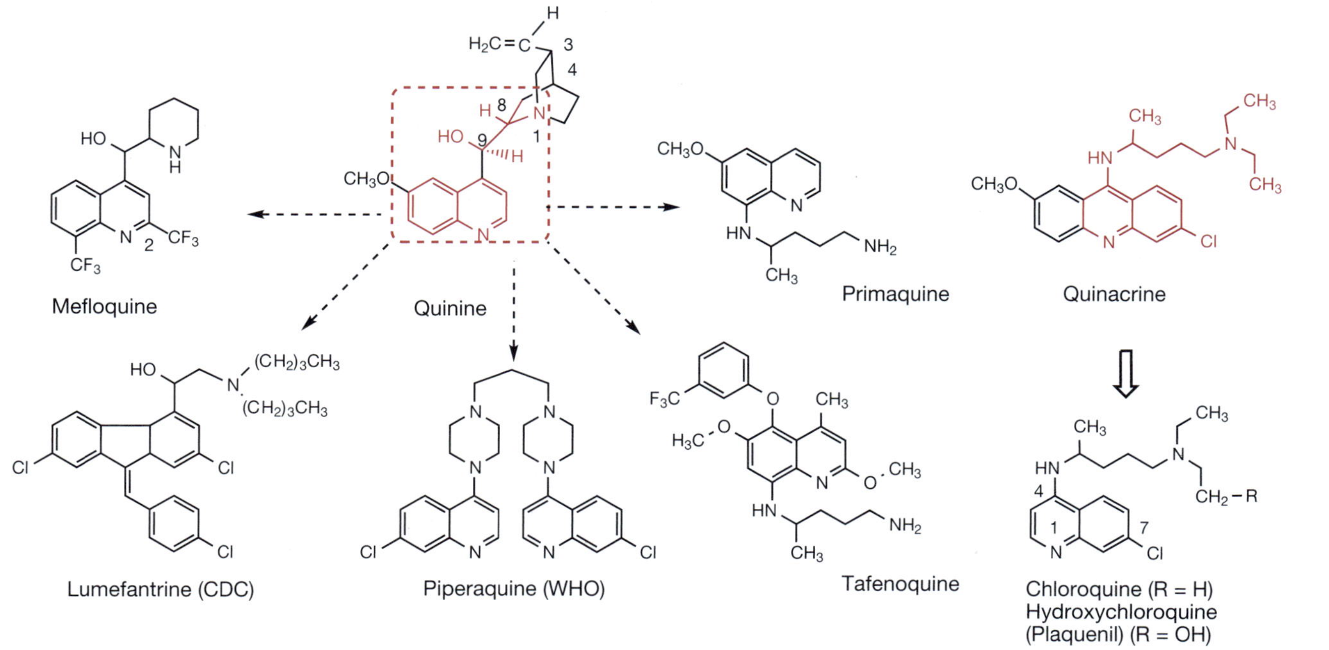

Figure 35.11 Structure similarity between the lead antimalarials (quinine and quinacrine) and the available antimalarials. CDC, Center for Disease Control; WHO, World Health Organization.

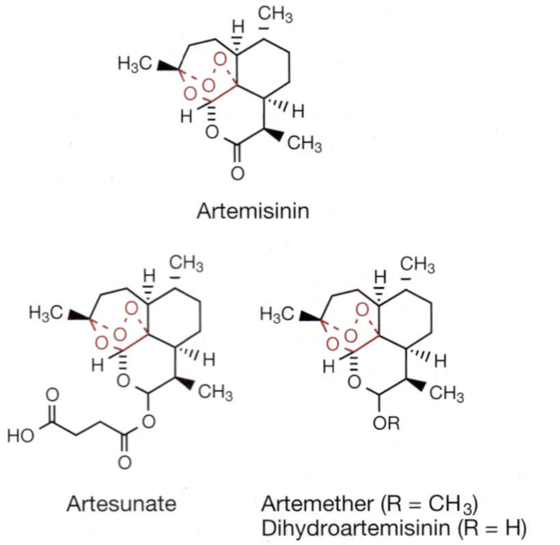

Figure 35.12 Structures of artemisinin and artemisinin derivatives.

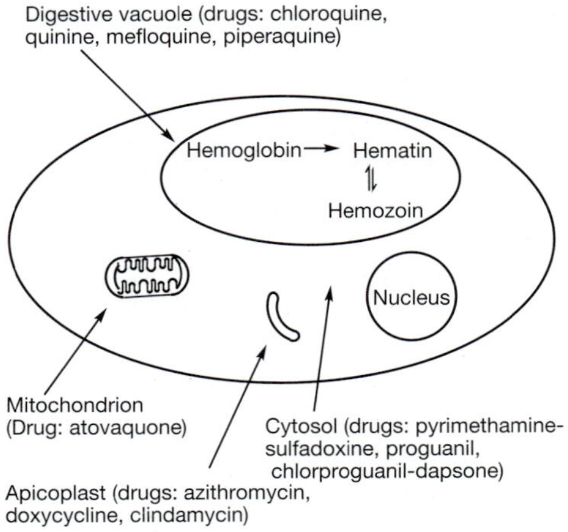

Figure 35.13 Plasmodium parasite cell as present within the erythrocyte and sites of drug action.

4-Substituted Quinolines. Six compounds can be considered within this class of drugs: quinine, chloroquine, and hydroxychloroquine, mefloquine, lumefantrine, and piperaquine. These compounds not only share a structural similarity but are also thought to have similar mechanisms of action, are effective on the same stage of the parasite, and share similar mechanisms of resistance.

General Properties

Mechanism of Action. The mechanism of action of chloroquine has been studied in depth, and the results of these studies have been assumed to be applicable to the other 4-substituted quinolines.[67] Various mechanisms of actions have been offered to explain the action of this class of drugs, including the DNA intercalation mechanism, the weak base hypothesis, and the ferriprotoporphyrin hypothesis.[68,69] Recently, an additional mode of action was proposed for quinine and mefloquine that involved their inhibition of the enzyme purine nucleoside phosphorylase.[70] This enzyme plays a role in the salvage and recycling of purines, suggesting these quinolines may interfere with nucleic acid production. The present understanding about the mechanism of action would appear to utilize various aspects of each of these mechanisms.

It is known that hemoglobin is transported into the food vacuoles of the plasmodium (Figs. 35.13 and 35.14), where digestion of the hemoglobin supplies the organism with a source of amino acids. One of the products of this digestion is a free heme called hematin. Hematin is toxic to the plasmodium cell, but it has been demonstrated that within the plasmodium vacuole the organism is capable of converting the hematin to nontoxic hemozoin. While it was initially thought that hemozoin was a polymeric form of hematin, it is now thought that the detoxification occurs through biocrystallization.[71,72] The dimeric hemozoin as a biocrystal is insoluble and chemically inert and, therefore, has no biologic effect on the plasmodium. The quinolines bind to hematin through a drug-heme complex, in which the aromatic quinoline ring binds via π-stacking to the porphyrin nucleus.[73] This drug-heme complex blocks further biocrystallization. The result of this complexation is that newly formed, free toxic hematin is now present, which leads to the death of the plasmodium. Additionally, since heme is not a component of plasmodium, it appears unlikely that the organism will be capable of developing a resistance mechanism to this type of activity. The accumulation of the 4-substituted quinolines in the acidic food vacuoles (pH 4.8-5.2) is based on the fact that these drugs are weak bases, as indicated by their pK_a values. The extracellular fluid of the parasite is at pH 7.4, and as a result, the weak base will move toward the more acidic pH of the vacuoles, reaching concentrations hundreds of times those in the plasma. Additionally, the binding of the quinoline to the heme draws additional quantities into the vacuole.

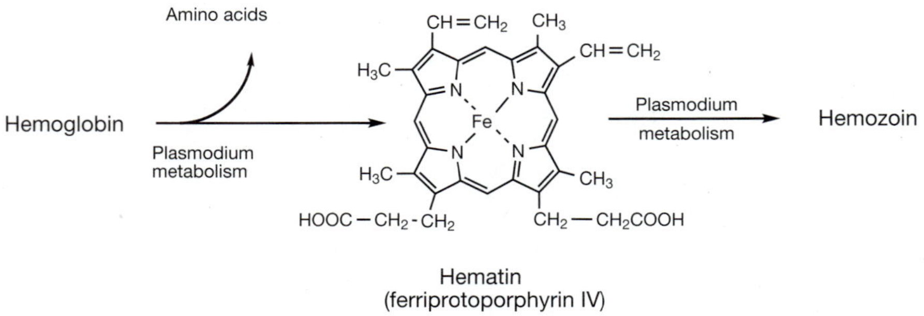

Figure 35.14 Proteolytic degradation of hemoglobin by the plasmodium organism to the potentially toxic hematin and then to the nontoxic dimers hemozoin.

Mechanism of Resistance. A limiting factor for many antimalarial drugs is the development of resistant strains of plasmodium. It should be noted that resistance differs from region to region, and, in some cases, a resistant strain can develop to a particular drug without that drug ever having been introduced to the region (possible cross-resistance). The development of resistance is thought to be due to a spontaneous gene mutation. Several mechanisms of resistance appear to be operating.[69] One of these mechanisms is based on the *Plasmodium falciparum* chloroquine-resistance transporter (PfCRT) mechanism, which is sufficient and necessary to impart resistance.[74] A gene encodes for a transmembrane transporter protein found in the membrane of the food vacuole. Multiple mutations within a specific region of this gene result in reduced accumulation of chloroquine, resulting from the increased efflux of the drug. Additionally, P-glycoprotein and other transporters may be involved in resistance, including the transporter known as *P. falciparum* multidrug resistance-associated protein (PfMRP).

Pharmacokinetics. In general, the quinolines are well absorbed via the oral route, with the exception of the fat-soluble drugs (eg, lumefantrine and piperaquine), and have similar pharmacokinetic properties (Table 35.2).

Therapeutic Application. The 4-substituted quinolines are referred to as rapidly acting blood schizonticides, with activity against plasmodium in the erythrocytic stage. Chloroquine is the drug of choice for use in non-resistant strains, but unfortunately, the incidence of chloroquine-resistant strains is common today. The spread of chloroquine resistance has reached most areas of the world where malaria is endemic. In addition, multidrug-resistant and cross-resistant strains of plasmodium are now common. The drug of choice for the treatment of malaria caused by chloroquine-resistant strains of *P. falciparum*, *P. ovale*, and *P. vivax* is the artemether-lumefantrine combination (Coartem, discussed later) (Table 35.3). Of interest is the observation that after years of non-use of chloroquine, a reemergence of chloroquine-sensitive parasites has been found.

Antimalarial drugs can also be used for prophylaxis of malaria. Two types of prophylaxis are possible: causal and suppressive. The former prevents the establishment of hepatic forms of the parasite, whereas the latter eradicates the erythrocytic parasites but has no effect on the hepatic forms. Agents used for causal prophylaxis must be continued for 7 days after leaving the endemic area, while agents used for suppressive prophylaxis must be continued for 4 weeks after leaving the endemic area. The primary agent currently recommended for causal prophylaxis in all malaria-endemic areas is the atovaquone-proguanil combination (Malarone; discussed later), which is effective for causal prophylaxis. The 4-substituted quinolines, chloroquine and hydroxychloroquine, can be used for suppressive prophylaxis in areas with chloroquine-sensitive strains.

Quinine. Quinine (see Fig. 35.11) is the most prevalent alkaloid present in the bark extracts (~5%) of cinchona. Four stereochemical centers exist in the molecule (at C-3, C-4, C-8, and C-9). Quinine (absolute configuration of 3R:4S:8S:9R), quinidine (absolute configuration of 3R:4S:8R:9S), and their enantiomers all have antimalarial activity, whereas their diastereomeric C-9 epimers (ie, the epi-series having either 3R:4S:8R:9R or 3R:4S:8S:9S configurations) are inactive. Modification of the secondary alcohol at C-9, through oxidation, esterification, or similar processes, diminishes activity. The quinuclidine portion is not necessary for activity; however, an alkyl tertiary amine moiety substituted at C-9 is important.

Quinine is metabolized in the liver to the 2′-hydroxy derivative, followed by additional hydroxylation on the quinuclidine ring, with the 2,2′-dihydroxy derivative as the major metabolite. This metabolite has low antimalarial activity and is rapidly excreted. The metabolizing enzyme of quinine is CYP3A4. As quinine, in combination with other drugs, is still an alternative agent for treatment of chloroquine-resistant malaria, the potential for drug interactions based on the many known substrates for CYP3A4 is of concern.[75]

A quinine overdose causes tinnitus and visual disturbances; these side effects disappear on discontinuation of the drug. Quinine also can cause premature contractions during the late stages of pregnancy. Although quinine is suitable for parenteral administration, this route is considered to be hazardous because of its ability to cause hemolysis. Quinidine, the (+)-enantiomer of quinine, has been shown

Table 35.2 Pharmacokinetics of Quinoline Antimalarials

Generic Name	Protein Binding	Bioavailability	Half-Life (d)	Route of Excretion
Chloroquine	~55%	75%	3-5	Urine/feces
Hydroxychloroquine	~40%	~70%	~40	Urine/feces
Lumefantrine	99%	Low (5%-11%)	3-6	Feces
Mefloquine	~98%	~85%	20 (median)	Feces
Piperaquine	97%	Not reported	20-30	Urine
Primaquine	~20%	~96%	~7 h	Urine
Quinine	69%-92%	76%-88%	~0.5	Urine
Tafenoquine	>99%	Not reported	~15	Feces

Table 35.3 Guidelines for Adult Treatment of Malaria in the United States[a]

Clinical Diagnosis	Sensitivity	Drug Recommendation
Uncomplicated malaria *Plasmodium falciparum*	Chloroquine sensitive	a. Chloroquine phosphate; or Hydroxychloroquine
	Chloroquine resistant or unknown	a. Artemether-lumefantrine b. Atovaquone-proguanil c. Quinine sulfate + one of the following: 1. Doxycycline 2. Tetracycline 3. Clindamycin d. Mefloquine
Uncomplicated malaria *P. vivax* or *P. ovale*	Chloroquine sensitive	a. Chloroquine phosphate; or Hydroxychloroquine AND 1. Primaquine phosphate; or 2. Tafenoquine
Uncomplicated malaria *P. vivax* or *P. ovale*	Chloroquine resistant	a. Artemether-lumefantrine b. Atovaquone-proguanil c. Quinine sulfate + one of the following: 1. Doxycycline 2. Tetracycline 3. Clindamycin d. Mefloquine AND 1. Primaquine phosphate
Uncomplicated malaria *P. malariae, P. knowlesi*[b]	Chloroquine sensitive	a. Chloroquine phosphate; or Hydroxychloroquine b. Artemether-lumefantrine c. Atovaquone-proguanil d. Quinine sulfate + one of the following: 1. Doxycycline 2. Tetracycline 3. Clindamycin e. Mefloquine
Severe malaria	Chloroquine sensitive/resistant	a. IV artesunate PLUS 1. Artemether-lumefantrine; or 2. Atovaquone-proguanil; or 3. Quinine sulfate; or 4. Mefloquine

[a]Information taken from the CDC Guideline for Treatment of Malaria in the United States. Updated June 28, 2023. For more details including infectious region and dosing go to: https://www.cdc.gov/malaria/resources/pdf/Malaria_Treatment_Table_202306.pdf

[b]There has been no widespread occurrence of chloroquine resistance in *P. malariae* and *P. knowlesi* species.

to be more effective in combating the disease, but as it has undesirable cardiac side effects, and with the advent of ACT, it is no longer recommended for treatment of malaria.

Chloroquine, Hydroxychloroquine. Chloroquine (see Fig. 35.11) is the most effective of the hundreds of 4-aminoquinolines synthesized and tested during World War II as potential antimalarials. Structure-activity relationships (SARs) demonstrated that the chloro at the 8-position increased activity, whereas alkylation at C-3 and C-8 diminished activity. The replacement of one of its *N*-ethyl groups with a hydroxyethyl produced hydroxychloroquine, a compound with reduced toxicity that is rarely used today except in cases of rheumatoid arthritis. Chloroquine is commonly administered as the racemic mixture because little is gained by using the individual isomers, which are more costly to produce. The drug is well absorbed from the GI tract and distributed to many tissues, where it is tightly bound and slowly eliminated (Table 35.2). The drug is metabolized by N-dealkylation by CYP2D6 and CYP3A4 isoforms.

Chloroquine is an excellent suppressive agent for treating acute attacks of malaria caused by susceptible *P. falciparum*, *P. vivax*, and *P. ovale*. The drug is also effective for cure and as a suppressive prophylactic for *Plasmodium malariae* and *Plasmodium knowlesi*. Chloroquine is a safe drug, with toxicity occurring only at high doses of medication or if the drug is administered too rapidly via parenteral routes. With oral administration, the side effects primarily are GI upset, mild headache, visual disturbances, and urticaria.

Mefloquine. Mefloquine (see Fig. 35.11), which was synthesized with the intent of blocking the site of metabolism in quinine with the chemically stable CF_3 group, exists as four optical isomers of nearly equal activity.[76] This agent showed initial activity against chloroquine-resistant strains of plasmodium; however resistance, believed to be due to PfMRP-mediated drug transport, is now common, and mefloquine is now a recommended fourth-line agent for treatment of chloroquine-resistant *P. falciparum*, *P. vivax*, and *P. ovale* and fifth-line agent for *P. malariae* and *P. knowlesi*. Mefloquine is slowly metabolized through CYP3A4 oxidation to its major inactive metabolite, carboxy-mefloquine (Fig. 35.15). Most of the parent drug is excreted unchanged into the urine. Coadministration with CYP3A4 inhibitors (eg, clarithromycin, itraconazole) will increase the area under the curve for mefloquine by inhibiting its metabolism to carboxy-mefloquine. Mefloquine is only available in an oral dosage form, which is well absorbed. The presence of food in the GI tract affects the pharmacokinetic properties of the drug, usually enhancing absorption. The lipophilic nature of the drug accounts for the extensive tissue binding and low clearance of total drug, although the drug does not accumulate after prolonged administration. The drug has a high affinity for erythrocyte membranes.

The incidence of side effects with mefloquine is considered to be high. The effects are classified as neuropsychiatric, GI, dermatologic, and cardiovascular. The neuropsychiatric effects can be serious (eg, suicidal tendencies or seizures) or minor (eg, dizziness, vertigo, ataxia, and headaches). GI side effects included nausea, vomiting, and diarrhea, whereas the dermatologic effects include rash, pruritus, and urticaria. Finally, cardiovascular side effects can include bradycardia, arrhythmias, and extrasystoles.

Lumefantrine. Lumefantrine (see Fig. 35.11), an effective erythrocytic schizonticide, has been reported to exhibit antimalarial activity when combined with artemether in the treatment of multidrug-resistant *P. falciparum*. The drug is used only in combination with artemether (artemisinin-based combination therapies [ACTs]), in which a synergistic effect has been noted (see later). Lumefantrine has a long half-life of 3 to 6 days, which makes it ideal for combination with the short half-life artemisinins. The drug is quite lipophilic, and a diet rich in fat increases the bioavailability of the drug. Unfortunately, many patients suffering from malaria do not tolerate food, and therefore the bioavailability of lumefantrine can be low. No evidence of cardiotoxicity has been reported with this combination, which offers promise for successful treatment of resistant organisms. The artemether-lumefantrine combination (Coartem) is now the recommended first-line choice for treatment of chloroquine-resistant *P. falciparum*, *P. vivax*, and *P. ovale*, and second-line for treatment of *P. malariae* and *P. knowlesi*.

Piperaquine. Piperaquine (see Fig. 35.11) was developed in the 1960s but did not find significant use until the 1990s. With the development of chloroquine-resistant strains, piperaquine gained importance especially when used in combination with dihydroartemisinin. As with other quinolines, the drug enters the food vacuole of the plasmodium, where it is suggested to have a mechanism of action similar to the other 4-quinolines. It is not available for use in the United States, but is available in other countries for treatment of uncomplicated malaria as an alternative to chloroquine. The long half-life combined with a shorter acting artemisinin has been useful in combination therapy.[77,78] Metabolism has been reported to involve oxidation to the carboxylic acid (Fig. 35.16).

8-Aminoquinolines

Therapeutic Application. The 8-aminoquinoline agents, primaquine and tafenoquine, are active against the primary and latent tissue or hepatic stages of *Plasmodium* infection (see Fig. 35.11). They are not active against the erythrocytic stage of infection but do possess gametocidal activity against all plasmodium strains.

Primaquine

Therapeutic Application. Primaquine (see Fig. 35.11) is primarily used as add-on therapy with chloroquine in chloroquine-sensitive *P. vivax* and *P. ovale* strains, and with other agents (eg, artemether-lumefantrine) in chloroquine-resistant *P. vivax* and *P. ovale* strains, to prevent malaria relapse. Primaquine is also used as an alternative prophylactic agent to prevent *P. vivax* infection. A major problem with primaquine is its short half-life (see Table 35.2) and the fact that it cannot be given for long-term treatment because of potential toxicity and sensitization. The sensitivity appears most commonly in individuals who have glucose-6-phosphate dehydrogenase deficiency (G6PD). In these cases, hemolytic anemia can develop. Primaquine too cannot be given to pregnant women.

Mechanism of Action. The mechanism of action of the 8-aminoquinolines is unknown, but primaquine can generate ROS via an autoxidation of the 8-amino group. The formation of a radical anion at the 8-amino group has been proposed by Augusto et al.[79] As a result, cell-destructive oxidants, such as hydrogen peroxide, superoxide, and hydroxyl radical, can be formed, as shown in Figure 35.3, leading to oxidative damage to critical cellular components of the organism.

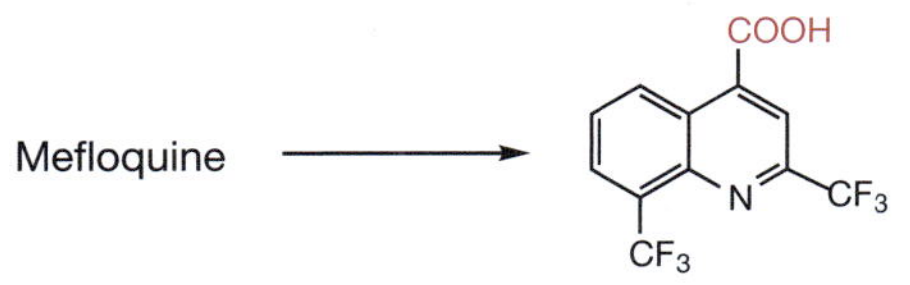

Figure 35.15 *Plasmodium falciparum* metabolism of mefloquine.

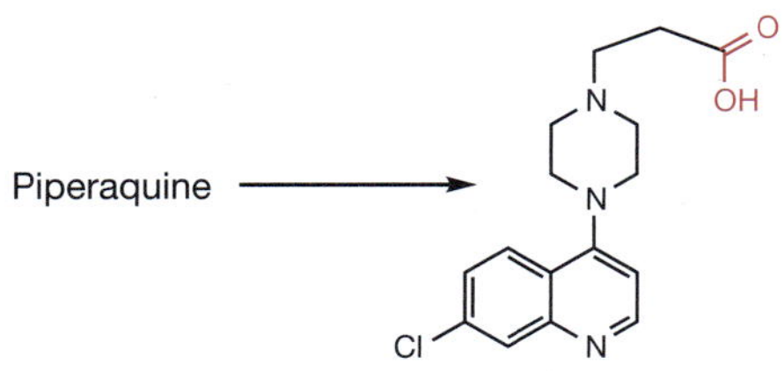

Figure 35.16 Metabolism of piperaquine.

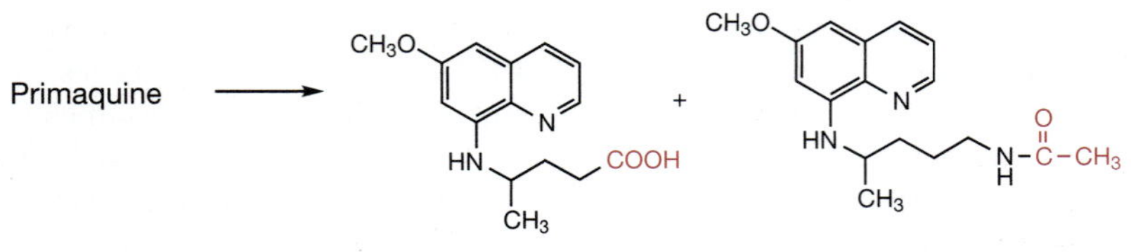

Carboxyprimaquine N-Acetylprimaquine

Figure 35.17 Metabolism of primaquine.

Metabolism. Primaquine is almost completely metabolized by CYP3A4 (99%), with the primary metabolite being carboxy-primaquine (Fig. 35.17).[80] Trace amounts of N-acetyl-primaquine plus aromatic hydroxylation and conjugation metabolites have also been reported.

Tafenoquine (Krintafel)

Therapeutic Application. Approved for use in the United States in 2018, this 8-aminoquinoline (see Fig. 35.11) is used as an alternative to primaquine for prevention of malaria relapse in *P. vivax* and *P. ovale* infections. While the 4-aminoquinolines are effective against the blood stage (erythrocytic stage) of the disease, the 8-aminoquinolines (primaquine and tafenoquine) are active against the hypnozoites (liver stage). A distinct advantage of this agent over primaquine is the long half-life (~2 weeks; see Table 35.2), which allows for single dose administration. The drug should still be avoided in patients with G6PD due to the risk of hemolytic anemia and should not be used in pregnant women. It is also contraindicated in patients with psychoses or psychotic symptoms. Tafenoquine's bioavailability can be improved if administered with a high-fat meal, and the drug is reported to exhibit high protein binding (>99.5%). This, combined with the slow metabolic activation, may account for the long half-life.

Mechanism of Action. Tafenoquine has shed additional light on the mechanism of action of the 8-aminoquinolines. Tafenoquine is considered a prodrug, which requires metabolism by CYP2D6 to produce the active tafenoquine 5,6-quinone (Fig. 35.18), a source of ROS.[81,82]

ATOVAQUONE-PROGUANIL (MALARONE)

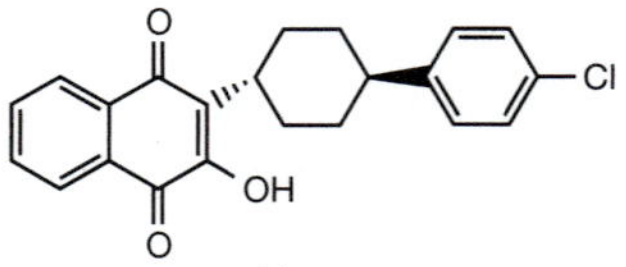

Atovaquone

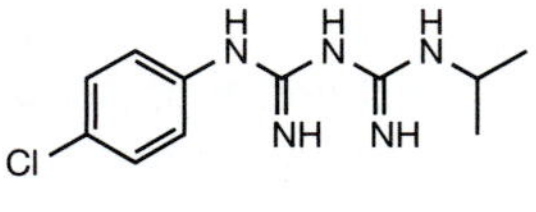

Proguanil

Atovaquone was originally developed as an antimalarial, but because of the high failure rate (~30%), it is not prescribed as a single chemical entity but rather is used to treat pneumocystis (see Chapter 34). More recently, however, atovaquone has been combined with proguanil as an effective prophylactic and therapeutic antimalarial.[74] The two drugs together exhibit synergy in which proguanil reduces the effective concentration of atovaquone needed to damage the mitochondrial membrane. In turn, atovaquone increases the effectiveness of proguanil but not its active metabolite (for the mechanism of action of atovaquone, see Chapter 34). Proguanil was developed decades earlier as a folic acid antagonist and functions as a prodrug. The active form of proguanil is cycloguanil (Fig. 35.19), which acts as a DHFR inhibitor. The action of this combination occurs at two distinct locations. Atovaquone is active within the mitochondrion of the plasmodium, while the proguanil acts as an antifolate in the cytosol (see Fig. 35.13). Because both atovaquone and proguanil have causal prophylactic activity, the combination is recommended as a first choice for malaria prevention in travelers.

Resistance to atovaquone used as a monotherapy might have been associated with the pharmacokinetics of the drug. Atovaquone is quite lipophilic and has slow uptake, resulting in the pathogen experiencing low concentrations of the drug over an extended period of time, both of which encourage the development of resistance. A single point mutation appears to be sufficient for resistance.[83] To date, few cases of resistance to the combination have been reported, primarily due to mutations in the DHFR gene and in the cytochrome b gene.[84,85]

ARTEMISININS. The most recent additions to the drug therapy for malaria are artemisinin and its derivatives (see Fig. 35.12).[86-89] Isolated from Artemisia annua (qinghao,

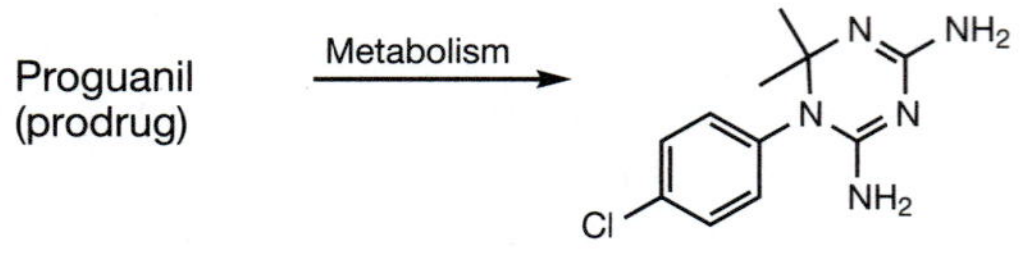

Cycloguanil

Figure 35.19 Activation of proguanil leading to cycloguanil.

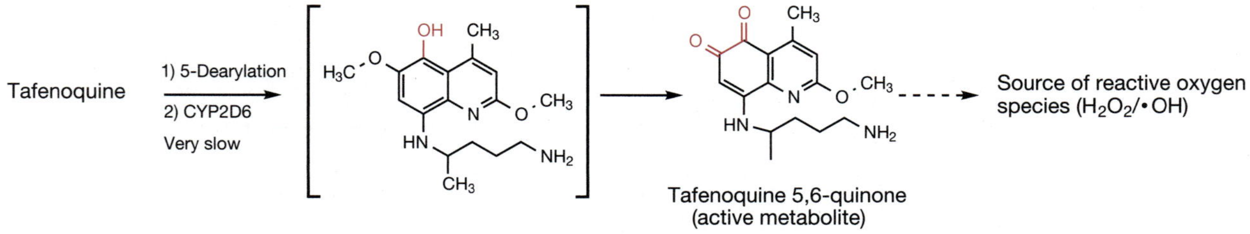

Figure 35.18 Metabolic activation of tafenoquine.

sweetworm wood), this material has been used by Chinese herbalists since 168 BC. Artemisinin and the synthetic and semisynthetic derivatives, artemether, arteether, artesunate, and dihydroartemisinin, are active by virtue of the endoperoxide. The artemisinin derivatives are built upon the 1,2,4-trioxane ring system (highlighted in red in the following figure). The recommendation for treating malaria with artemisinins is that these drugs should not be used individually but rather in combination with at least one other effective medication with a different mechanism of action.

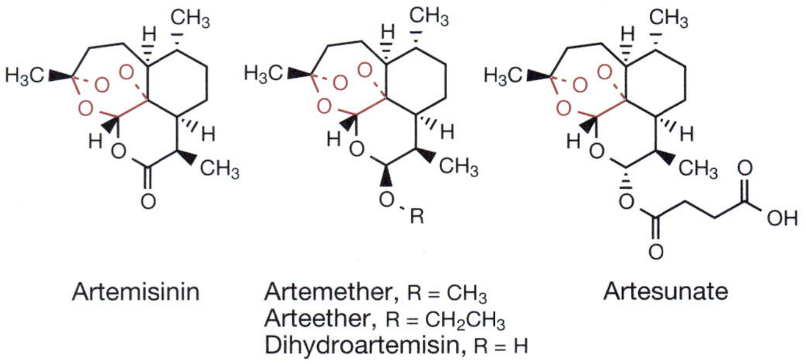

Mechanism of Action. Two mechanisms have been suggested to account for the antimalarial action of the artemisinins. In the first mechanism, the artemisinins appear to kill the parasite by a free radical mechanism; not by the generation of ROS but rather by virtue of a free radical associated with the endoperoxide, possibly involving a carbon radical. It is proposed that the heme in the form of hemazoin within the digestive vacuole is a source of Fe^{2+}, which reacts with the peroxide to generate an oxy radical and Fe^{3+}.[90] A carbon radical is formed from the oxy radical, which is then lethal to the plasmodium within the erythrocyte. The second mechanism suggests endoperoxide activation via an iron-dependent mechanism, but the activated artemisinins target sarcoplasmic/endoplasmic reticulum Ca^{2+}-ATPase of the *Plasmodium falciparum* (PfATP6), altering calcium stores.[91,92] The artemisinins actually can form covalent adducts to specific membrane-associated proteins after concentrating in infected erythrocytes.

Pharmacokinetics. The artemisinins are hydrophobic in nature with the exception of artesunate, which is available as a water-soluble hemi-succinate salt, and are partitioned into the membrane of the plasmodium. The artemisinin derivatives are available in various dosage forms, including oral tablets, intramuscular injectables, and rectal suppositories (outside the United States). Artemether and dihydroartemisinin are highly bound to plasma protein (93%-95%) with rapid elimination ($t_{1/2}$ 1-5 hour). Artesunate is rapidly metabolized (~2 minutes via esterases) to dihydroartemisinin as is artemether via CYP3A4 and, to a lesser extent, by other cytochromes (Fig. 35.20).

Therapeutic Application. The artemisinins have gametocytocidal activity and activity against all asexual stages of the parasites. These agents are short acting with short half-lives and thus should not be used for malaria prophylaxis. Currently, the combination product artemether-lumefantrine (Coartem) is recommended for first-line therapy of chloroquine-resistant *P. falciparum*, *P. vivax*, and *P. ovale* and second-line for *P. malariae* and *P. knowlesi* (see Table 35.3). The injectable artesunate is considered first-line treatment for severe malaria infection. Artemisinins should not be used in pregnant women due to reports of embryo malformations in animals. Little or no resistance has been reported, with the drugs rapidly clearing the blood of parasites. The combination artemether-lumefantrine and injectable artesunate are available in the United States; a variety of other combination formulations are available worldwide (Table 35.4). Combination therapy has the goal of reducing resistance with the hope for synergism and, when combined with longer acting drugs, an improved therapy.

Common adverse effects include hypersensitivity reactions, GI disturbance, dizziness, and elevated liver enzymes. The use of the artemisinins and artemisinin derivatives in other parasitic infections has received recent attention.[93-96] Specifically, several derivatives of artemisinin exhibited

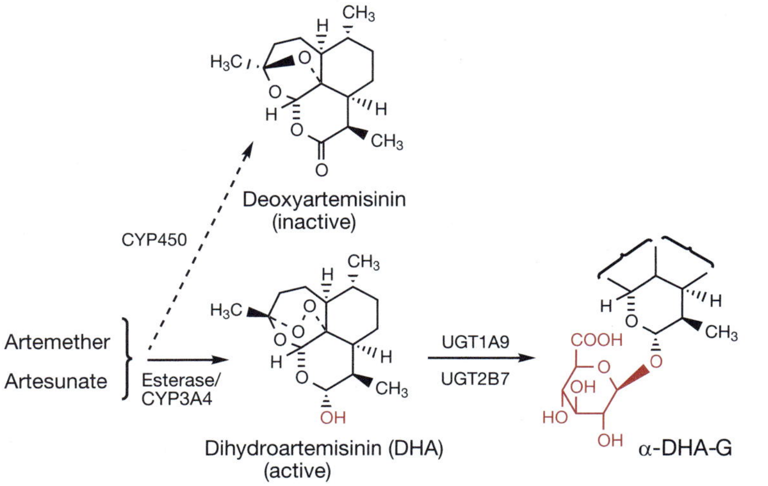

Figure 35.20 Metabolism of artemisinins.

Table 35.4 Artemisinins Used in Artemisinin-Based Combination Therapy (ACT)

Artemisinin	Second Component of ACT	Trade Name/ Alternative Name
Artemether	Lumefantrine	Coartem[a]
Artesunate	Amodiaquine	ASAQ
Artesunate	Mefloquine	ASMQ
Artesunate	Pyronaridine	Pyramax
Artesunate	Sulfadoxine/ Pyrimethamine	Ariplus or Amalar plus
Dihyroartemisinin	Piperaquine	Eurartesim

[a]The only FDA-approved combination artemisinin in the United States.

activity as anti-leishmanial agents, in treatment of schistosomiasis, and in treatment of trypanosomiasis. Combinations of artesunate-sulfadoxine-pyrimethamine and artemether-lumefantrine are effective against *S. mansoni*, and artemisinin was reported to show activity against *T. rhodesiense*, *T. cruzi*, and *L. donovani* in vitro.

Antibiotic Agents

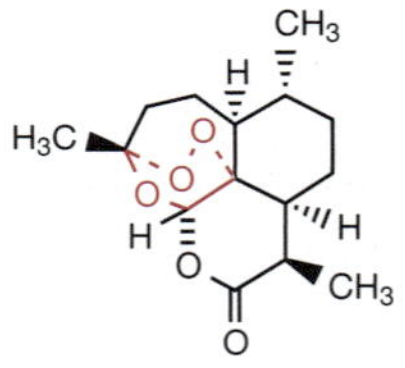

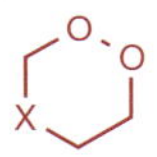

Core nucleus of the artemisinins
1,2,4-Trioxane (X = O)
1,2-Dioxane ($X = CH_2$) rings

Several antibiotics have proven useful in the treatment of malaria. They can be used alone as prophylaxis or in combination with quinine as treatment measures. Antibiotics currently recommended in combination with quinine for treatment of malaria are doxycycline, tetracycline, and clindamycin. Doxycycline is also a recommended agent for prophylaxis of malaria when traveling to endemic countries. Their mechanisms of action are the same as those seen when treating a bacterial infection and involve interference in protein synthesis (see Chapter 32). What is unique about the use of the antibiotics in malaria is the site of action. The antibiotics affect protein synthesis within the apicoplast (see Fig. 35.13). The apicoplast is an organelle found in most Apicomplexa (a group of eukaryotic microorganisms that include *Plasmodium*). The apicoplast is a non-photosynthesizing plastid with undefined function, although it does contain tRNAs, rRNAs, RNA polymerases, and ribosomal protein and is essential to the parasite's survival. Interference with protein synthesis blocks replication of the apicoplast organelle and prevents a second replication of the life cycle of the plasmodium and thus the prophylactic action. Limitations on the use of doxycycline include children and pregnant women, two major groups of patients with malaria, which explain the recommended use of clindamycin in these populations.

Clinical Application of Antimalarials. The treatment of malaria in children and adults as defined by WHO requires an integrated approach involving prompt treatment with effective drugs. Over the years, drug therapy has gone from monotherapy with quinolines to the use of ACT today. The treatment of uncomplicated malaria requires the cure of the infection as rapidly as possible, while the goal for severe malaria is to prevent death. In addition, it is important to use preventive therapy in healthy people when traveling to endemic regions. The goal of treatment is to eliminate the parasite from the blood, and for this, WHO recommends ACT for uncomplicated *P. falciparum* malaria. The ACT drugs should be active against the erythrocytic form of the disease. Activity against the gamete form of the disease is also important to prevent the spread of the disease. The site of activity for the presented drugs is shown in Table 35.5. For a detailed review of the disease and its treatment, the reader is referred to the WHO Guidelines for Malaria, November 2024 (available at https://www.who.int/publications/i/item/guidelines-for-malaria).

Helminth Infections

Helminthiasis, or worm infestation, is one of the most prevalent diseases—and one of the most serious public

Table 35.5 Site of Action of Antimalarial Drugs

Drug/Drug Class	Site of Action		
	Liver	Erythrocyte	Gametocyte
Artemisinins		√	√
Chloroquine		√	
Hydroxychloroquine		√	
Lumefantrine		√	
Mefloquine		√	
Quinine		√	√ [a]
Piperaquine		√	
Primaquine	√		√
Tafenoquine	√		√

[a]Gametocidal versus *P. vivax* and *P. malariae* but not against *P. falciparum*.

health problems—in the world. Many worms are parasitic in humans and cause serious complications. It is estimated that 1.5 billion people are infected with at least one species of parasitic worm.[97] It is interesting to note that helminths differ from many other parasites in that these organisms multiply outside the definitive host and have the unique ability to evade host immune defenses for reasons that are not fully understood. As a result, helminth infections tend to be chronic, potentially lasting for the entire lifetime of the host. Interested readers are directed to a classic review of helminth infections published by Maizels et al.[98]

Helminths that infect human hosts are divided into two categories, or phyla: platyhelminths (flatworms) and aschelminths or nematodes (roundworms). The nematode class includes helminths common to the United States: roundworm, hookworm, pinworm, and whipworm. These worms are cylindrical in shape, with significant variations in size, proportion, and structure. The flatworms include the classes cestode (tapeworms) and trematode (flukes or schistosomes). A list of common human helminths is shown in Table 35.6.

Nematode Infections

Ancylostomiasis or Hookworm Infection

The two most widespread types of hookworm in humans are the American hookworm (*Necator americanus*) and the "Old World" hookworm (*Ancylostoma doudenale*). The life cycles of both are similar. The larvae are found in the soil and are transmitted either by penetrating the skin or by getting ingested orally. The circulatory system transports the larvae via the respiratory tree to the digestive tract, where they mature and live for 9 to 15 years if left untreated. These worms feed on intestinal tissue and blood. Infestations cause pulmonary lesions, skin reactions, intestinal ulceration, and anemia. The worms are most prevalent in regions of the world with temperatures of 23 °C to 33 °C, abundant rainfall, and well-drained, sandy soil.

Enterobiasis or Pinworm Infection (Enterobius vermicularis)

These worms are widespread in temperate zones and are a common infestation of households and institutions. The pinworm lives in the lumen of the GI tract, attaching itself by the mouth to the mucosa of the cecum. Mature worms reach a size of 10 mm. The female migrates to the rectum, usually at night, to deposit her eggs. This event is noted by the symptom of perianal pruritus. The eggs infect fingers and contaminate nightclothes and bed linen, where they remain infective for up to 3 weeks. Eggs resist drying and can be inhaled with household dust to continue the life cycle. Detection of the worm in the perianal region can be accomplished by means of a cellophane tape swabbed in the perianal region in the evening. The worms can be visible with the

Table 35.6 Human Infection Helminths

Common Name	Phylum/Latin Name	Diseases	Location in Host
Roundworms	**Nematode**		
Hookworm	*Nector americanus*	Ancylostomiasis	Digestive tract
Hookworm	*Ancylostoma doudenale*	Ancylostomiasis	Digestive tract
Pinworm	*Enterobius vermicularis*	Enterobiasis	Digestive tract
Roundworm	*Ascaris lumbricoides*	Ascariasis	Small intestine
Whipworm	*Trichuris trichiura*	Trichuriasis	Intestinal wall
Eyeworm	*Trichinella spiralis*	Trichuriasis	Intestinal wall
River blindness	*Mansonella streptocerca*[a]	Filariasis	Subcutaneous layer
Timor filariasis	*Onchocerca volvulus*	Onchocerciasis	Dermis
	Wuchereria bancrofti	Elephantiasis	Lymphatic-dwelling
	Brugia malayi	Elephantiasis	Lymphatic-dwelling
	Brugia timori	Elephantiasis	Lymphatic-dwelling
Flatworms	**Cestode**		
Beef tapeworm	*Taenia saginata*	Taeniasis	Digestive tract
Pork tapeworm	*Taenia solium*	Cysticercosis	Digestive tract
Dwarf tapeworm	*Hymenolepis nana*		Digestive tract
Fish tapeworm	*Diphyllobothrium latum*		Digestive tract
	Trematode		
Blood fluke	*Schistosoma haematobium*	Schistosomiasis	Urinary bladder
Blood fluke	*Schistosoma mansoni*	Schistosomiasis	Blood vessels of GI tract
Blood fluke	*Schistosoma japonicum*	Schistosomiasis	Blood vessels of GI tract

[a]*M. streptocerca*, *O. volvulus*, *W. bancrofti*, *B. malayi*, and *B. timori* are commonly referred to as lymphatic-dwelling filariae. An early stage of these parasites is the microfilariae stage.

naked eye. The eggs can be collected similarly but can only be seen under a microscope.

Ascariasis or Roundworm Infections (Ascaris lumbricoides)

These roundworms are common in developing countries, with the adult roundworm reaching 25 to 30 cm in length and lodging in the small intestine. Some infections are without symptoms, but abdominal discomfort and pain are common with heavy infestation. Roundworm eggs are released into the soil, where they incubate and remain viable for up to 6 years. When the egg is ingested, the larvae are released in the small intestine, penetrate the intestinal walls, and are carried via the blood to the lungs. The pulmonary phase of the disease lasts approximately 10 days, with the larvae passing through the bronchioles, bronchi, and trachea before getting swallowed and returning to the small intestine. Some patients have reported adult worms exiting the esophagus through the oral cavity, and it is not unusual for live ascaris to be expelled with a bowel movement. Poor or absent sanitary facilities expose the population to infestation through contaminated foods and beverages.

Trichuriasis or Whipworm Infections (Trichuris trichiura)

Infections by this parasite are caused by swallowing eggs from contaminated foods and beverages. The eggs are passed with the feces from an infected individual. These eggs can live in the soil for many years. The ingested eggs hatch in the small intestine, and the larvae embed in the intestinal wall. The worms then migrate to the large intestine, where they mature. Adult worms, which reach approximately 5 cm in length, thread their bodies into the epithelium of the colon. They feed on tissue fluids and blood. Infections from this worm cause symptoms of irritation and inflammation of the colonic mucosa, abdominal pain, diarrhea, and distention. Infections can last 5 years or more if not treated. Whipworm infections are commonly seen in individuals returning from visits to the subtropics and are more common in rural areas of the southeastern United States.

Trichinosis or Trichina Infection (Trichinella spiralis)

Trichinella spiralis produces an infection that can be both intestinal and systemic. The worm is found in muscle meat, where the organism exists as an encysted larva. Traditionally, the worm has been associated with domestic pork that feeds on untreated garbage. More recently, outbreaks have occurred in individuals eating infected game, such as wild boar, bear, or walrus. Trichinosis infections are more likely to occur after consumption of homemade pork or wild game sausages. After ingestion, the larvae are released from the cyst form and then migrate into the intestinal mucosa. After maturation and reproduction, the newly released larvae penetrate the mucosal lining and are distributed throughout the body, where they enter skeletal muscle. During the adult intestinal stage, diarrhea, abdominal pain, and nausea are the most common symptoms, whereas the muscular form of the disease has symptoms that can include muscle pain and tenderness, edema, conjunctivitis, and weakness.

Filariasis

The term "filariasis" denotes infections with any of the human-disease causing Filarioidea. Filariasis can be categorized into three groups: lymphatic filariasis caused by *Wuchereria bancrofti*, *Brugia malayi*, and *Brugia timori*; subcutaneous filariasis caused by *Mansonella streptocerca*, *Loa loa*, and *Onchocerca volvulus*; and cavity filariasis caused by *Mansonella perstans* and *Mansonella ozzardi*. Elephantiasis tropica, caused by *W. bancrofti*, is a common type of lymphatic filariasis. *Loa Loa* and *O. volvulus* are referred to as the eyeworm and river blindness worm, respectively, and cause subcutaneous filariasis. *M. perstans* and *M. ozzardi* infect the abdominal cavity. These parasites vary in length from 6 cm for *Brugia* to 50 cm for *Onchocerca*. The incubation periods also vary from 2 months for brugian to 12 months for bancroftian filaria. It is estimated that 400 million persons are infected with human filarial parasites. Depending on the specific organism, various intermediate hosts are involved in spreading the infection. Mosquitoes are involved with the spread of *W. bancrofti*, *B. malayi*, and *B. timori*, whereas the female blackfly spreads river blindness. The larvae released by the female filaria are referred to as microfilariae and can commonly be found in the lymphatics.

Cestode and Trematode Infections

Cysticercosis or Tapeworm Infection

Helminths of this class that are of concern as potential parasites in humans include the following:

Beef Tapeworm (*Taenia saginata*). This worm is found worldwide and infects people who eat undercooked beef. The worm reaches a length of 4 to 10 m, and it contains approximately 100 segments/m. Each of these segments contains its own reproductive organs.

Pork Tapeworm (*Taenia solium*). Pork tapeworms sometimes are called bladder worms and occasionally are found in uncooked pork. The worm attaches itself to the intestinal wall of the human host. The adult worm reaches 2 to 3 m in length and, if untreated, survives in the host for many years.

Dwarf Tapeworm (*Hymenolepis nana*). This infection is transmitted directly from one human to another without an intermediate host. *Hymenolepis nana* reaches only 3 to 4 cm in length. It is found in temperate zones, and children are most frequently infected.

Fish Tapeworm (*Diphyllobothrium latum*). The fish tapeworm can reach a length of 10 m and contains approximately 400 segments/m. These tapeworms attach themselves to the intestinal wall and rob the host of nutrients. They especially absorb vitamin B_{12} and folic acid. Depletion of these critical nutrients, especially vitamin B_{12}, can lead to pernicious anemia. Tapeworm eggs are passed in the patient's feces, and contamination of food and drink can result in transmission of the infection.

Schistosomiasis or Blood Flukes

Three primary trematode species cause schistosomiasis in humans: *Schistosoma haematobium*, *Schistosoma mansoni*, and *Schistosoma japonicum*. Infections result from the penetration of normal skin by living (free-swimming) cercaria (the name given to the infectious stage of the parasite) with the aid of secreted enzymes. The cercariae develop to preadult forms in the lungs and skin. Then, these parasites travel in pairs via the bloodstream and invade various tissues. The adult worm reaches approximately 2 cm in length. The female deposits her eggs near the capillary beds, where granulomas form. Some of the eggs will move into the lumen of the intestines, bladder, or ureters and are released into the environmental surroundings, where the parasite will seek out the intermediate snail vector. Asexual reproduction occurs in the snail. After a period of time, the cercariae are again released from the snail to continue the cycle.

Patients might experience headache, fatigue, fever, and GI disturbances during the initial stages of the disease. Hepatic fibrosis and ascites occur during later stages. Untreated patients can harbor as many as 100 pairs of worms. Untreated worms can live 5 to 10 years within the host. As many as 250 million persons worldwide are estimated to be infected with schistosomes. Depending on the species of schistosome, the disease is found in parts of South America, the Caribbean Islands, Africa, and the Middle East.

Drug Therapy for Helminth Infections

Helminths represent a biologically diverse group of parasitic organisms differing in size, life cycle, site of infection (local and systemic), and susceptibility to chemotherapy.[99] With such variation in infectious organisms, it is not surprising that the drugs used to control helminth infections also represent a varied group of chemical classes.

Benzimidazoles

The benzimidazoles are a broad-spectrum group of drugs discovered in the 1960s with activity against GI helminths. Several thousand benzimidazoles have been synthesized and screened for anthelmintic activity, with albendazole, mebendazole, and triclabendazole representing the only benzimidazoles marketed in the United States today and included on the WHO 2023 essential medicines list (Fig. 35.21). The development and chemistry of this class of agents have been reviewed by Townsend and Wise.[100]

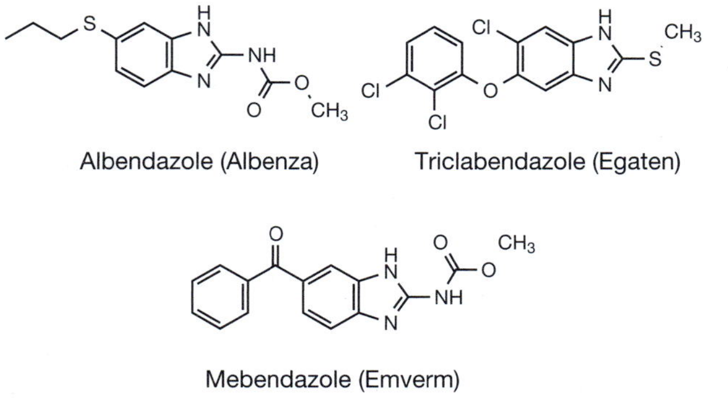

Figure 35.21 US marketed and World Health Organization listed benzimidazole anthelmintics.

Mechanism of Action. Two mechanisms have been proposed to account for the action of the benzimidazoles. Fumarate reductase is an important enzyme in helminths that is involved in oxidation of nicotinamide adenine dinucleotide plus hydrogen (NADH) to nicotinamide adenine dinucleotide (NAD). The benzimidazoles are capable of inhibiting fumarate reductase.[101] Inhibition of fumarate reductase ultimately uncouples oxidative phosphorylation, which is important in ATP production. A second mechanism, and probably the primary action of the benzimidazoles, is associated with their ability to bind to the protein tubulin and, thus, prevent tubulin polymerization to microtubules.[102,103] Tubulin is a dimeric protein that is in dynamic equilibrium with the polymeric microtubules. Binding to the tubulin prevents the self-association of tubulin subunits and creates a "capping" of the microtubule at the associating or polymerizing end. The microtubule continues to dissociate or erode from the opposite end, with a net loss of microtubule length. What is interesting is the unique selectivity of the benzimidazoles. Benzimidazole can also bind to mammalian tubulin, but when used as anthelmintics, these drugs are destructive to the helminth with minimal toxicity to the host. It has been suggested that the selectivity is associated with differing pharmacokinetics between binding to the two different tubulin proteins.

Metabolism. The benzimidazoles have limited water solubility and, as a result, are poorly absorbed from the GI tract (a fatty meal will increase absorption). Poor absorption can be beneficial for the drugs that are used primarily to treat intestinal helminths. To the extent that the drugs are absorbed, they undergo rapid metabolism in the liver and are excreted in the bile (Fig. 35.22).[104,105] In most cases, the parent compound is rapidly and nearly completely metabolized, with predominance of oxidative and hydrolytic processes. The phase 1 oxidative reaction commonly is a cytochrome P450–catalyzed reaction, which can then be followed by a phase 2 conjugation.

The presence of a thioether substituent at the 5-position of albendazole increases the likelihood of sulfur oxidation. The initial metabolite, albendazole sulfoxide, is a potent anthelmintic. This initial oxidation is catalyzed principally (70%) by CYP3A4 and CYP1A2, and 30% is metabolized by flavin-containing monooxygenase, giving rise to a compound that is bound to plasma protein. This intermediate has an expanded utility in that it has been shown to be active against the hydatid cyst found in echinococciasis, a tapeworm disease.[106] Further oxidation by cytochrome P450 leads to the inactive sulfone. Additional metabolic biotransformation of the sulfone has been reported, including carbamate hydrolysis to the amine and oxidation of the 5-propyl side chain. These reactions occur only to a minor extent.

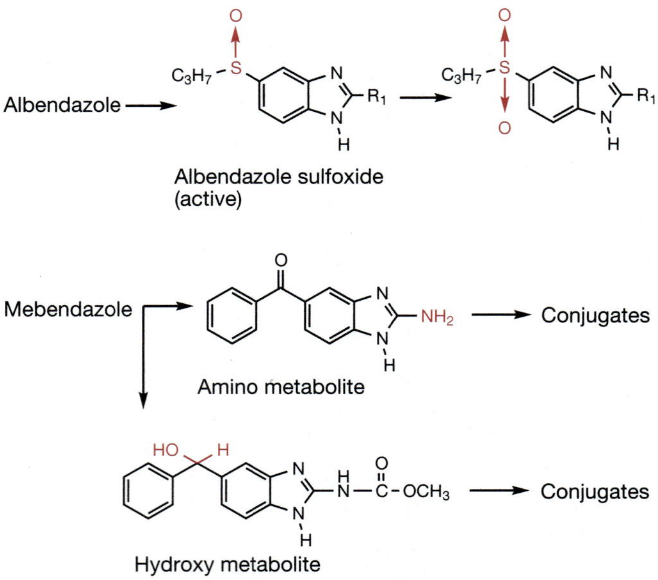

Figure 35.22 Metabolism of benzimidazoles.

Metabolism of mebendazole occurs primarily by reduction of the 5-carbonyl to a secondary alcohol, which increases the water solubility of this compound. An additional phase 1 metabolite resulting from carbamate hydrolysis has been reported as well. Both the secondary alcohol and the amine are readily conjugated (a phase 2 reaction). Evidence would suggest that the anthelmintic activity of mebendazole resides in the parent drug and not in the metabolites.

Like the other benzimidazole agents, food increases the oral absorption of triclabendazole, and the drug undergoes extensive first-pass metabolism in the liver. Similar to albendazole, triclabendazole is initially metabolized at the thio-ether to an active sulfoxide metabolite, in this case primarily by CYP1A2.[107] The sulfoxide is further metabolized by CYP2C9 to an inactive sulfone metabolite. Both the active and inactive metabolites of triclabendazole are highly protein bound (>99%).

Therapeutic Application. As indicated in Table 35.7, mebendazole and albendazole have a wide spectrum of activity against intestinal nematodes. The drugs are useful and effective against mixed infections. The adverse reactions are commonly

Table 35.7 Therapeutic Application of Anthelmintics for Specific Helminth Infections

	MBZ	ABZ	IVM	PZQ	PYR
Nematodes (roundworms)					
Necator americanus	✓	✓			
Ancylostoma doudenale	✓	✓			✓
Enterobius vermicularis	✓	✓	✓		✓
Ascaris lumbricoides	✓	✓	✓		✓
Trichuris trichiura	✓	✓	✓		
Trichinella spiralis	✓	✓			
Wuchereria bancrofti			✓		
Brugia malayi			✓		
Brugia timori					
Loa Loa		✓			
Onchocerca volvulus		✓	✓		
Cestodes (tapeworms)					
Taenia saginata	✓	✓		✓	
Taenia solium	✓	✓		✓	
Hymenolepis nana	✓			✓	
Diphyllobothrium latum				✓	
Trematodes (flukes)					
Schistosoma haematobium				✓	
Schistosoma mansoni				✓	
Schistosoma japonicum				✓	

ABZ, albendazole; IVM, ivermectin; MBZ, mebendazole; PP, pyrantel; PZQ, praziquantel.

GI in nature (nausea, vomiting, and diarrhea). Both drugs have been reported to be teratogenic in rats and, therefore, should not be used during the first trimester of pregnancy. Triclabendazole has a significantly more narrow-spectrum of activity and has limited activity against nematodes, cestodes, and most trematodes. It is highly specific for the trematode Fasciola and Paragonimus species, which are liver and lung flukes that cause fascioliasis and paragonimiasis, respectively.

Macrocyclic Lactones

Avermectins and milbemycins are two subfamilies of 16-membered macrocyclic lactone compounds derived from *Streptomyces* spp. They have broad-spectrum endoparasitic activity against nematodes and ectoparasitic activity against arthropods.[108] The two chemical series differ by the presence of a disaccharide group at the 13-position of avermectins that is absent in the milbemycin family. The two subfamilies are mechanistically similar in that they have high binding affinity for invertebrate glutamate-gated chloride channels, which can interfere with neurotransmission and muscle action in the target species.[109] The clinically marketed agents, ivermectin (IVM) and moxidectin, are used with relative safety in mammals because glutamate-gated chloride channels are found only in the CNS of mammals, and these agents do not penetrate the BBB. Additionally, they have low affinity for other mammalian ligand-gated ion channels. Though they possess a similar mechanism of action, because of the structural differences between the two subfamilies, they have significantly different pharmacokinetic and pharmacodynamic parameters and toxicity profiles.

IVERMECTIN (STROMECTOL)

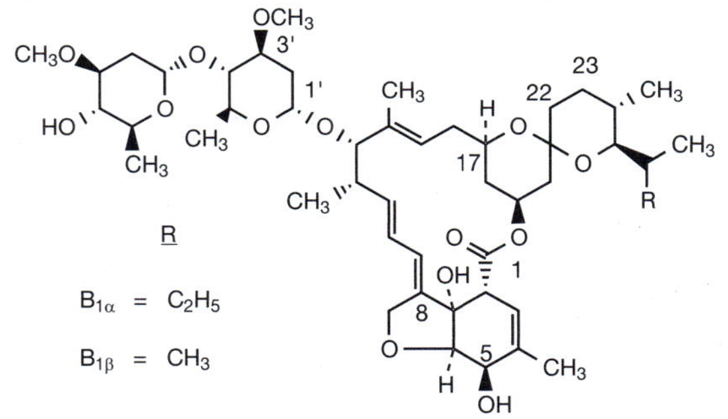

Ivermectin

Extracted from the soil actinomycete *Streptomyces avermitilis*, the natural avermectins are 16-membered macrocyclic lactones, which are 80:20 mixtures of avermectin $B_1\alpha$ and $B_1\beta$, respectively, and used under the generic name abamectin. As such the product is used for the control of various insects, mite pests, fire ants, and as a veterinary anthelmintic. Reduction of the $C_{22\text{-}23}$ double bond gives rise to IVM, which is an 80:20 mixture of dihydroavermectin $B_1\alpha$ and $B_1\beta$, respectively. The natural avermectins have minimal biological activity, but IVM has proven to be quite beneficial in the treatment of various nematode and ectoparasitic infections.

Mechanism of Action. The mechanism of action of IVM has been extensively investigated, and several theories have been published.[99,110,111] It is currently believed that the primary mechanism of action is an indirect action in which motility of microfilaria is reduced, which in turn allows cytotoxic cells of the host to adhere to the parasite, resulting in elimination from the host. This action can occur by virtue of the ability of IVM to act either as an inducer of chloride ion influx, or as a γ-aminobutyric acid (GABA) agonist, leading to hyperpolarization and muscle paralysis. The chloride ion influx appears to be the more plausible mechanism.[112] It has been shown that IVM binds irreversibly to an allosteric site on the glutamate-gated chloride channel of the nematode *Haemonchus contortus*, in which the channel is in an open conformation. The binding then remains locked in the open conformation, allowing ions to cross the membrane, leading to the paralytic action of IVM.[113] The result of this action is a rapid decrease in microfilarial concentrations.

Metabolism. IVM is rapidly absorbed, bound to plasma protein, and excreted in the urine or feces either unchanged or as the 3′-O-demethyl-22,23-dihydroavermectin $B_{1\alpha}$ or dihydroavermectin $B_1\alpha$ monosaccharide metabolites. The absorption of IVM is significantly affected by the presence of alcohol. Administration of IVM as an alcoholic solution can result in as much as a 100% increase in absorption. IVM, and other macrocyclic lactones, are actively transported by efflux proteins in mammals and in parasite cell membranes, and this is believed to significantly contribute to drug elimination.[114]

Therapeutic Application. Although IVM has activity against a variety of microfilaria, including *W. bancrofti*, *B. malayi*, *Loa loa*, and *M. ozzardi* as well as activity against *Strongyloides stercoralis*, the drug is used primarily in the treatment of onchocerciasis (African river blindness) caused by *O. volvulus*. It is estimated that at least 20 million people are affected by this condition, and an additional 123 million are at risk of the infection. The drug is effective against both the eyeworm as well as skin infections of *O. volvulus*. IVM has the distinct advantage over the previously available diethylcarbamazine (now discontinued in the United States) in that it has far less likelihood of causing the potentially fatal anaphylactic reaction (Mazzotti reaction), it can be dosed infrequently, and it can be used for mass treatment programs. The current CDC recommendation is a 150 to 200 μg/kg administered every 6 months for the life span of the adult worms (10-15 years). WHO guidelines state IVM should be administered "at least once yearly" for 10 to 15 years. A special caution with IVM is that it can cause acute encephalopathy when administered to a patient co-infected with *Loa Loa*. Treatment strategies must be adjusted in these cases. In addition to the systemic formulations for onchocerciasis, two topical dosage forms of IVM are available for the treatment of head lice (Sklice) and rosacea lesions (Soolantra; discussed later).

MOXIDECTIN

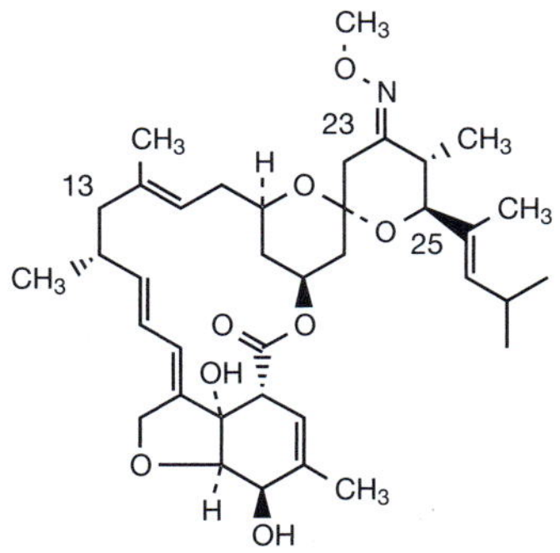

Moxidectin

Moxidectin, a non-glycosylated milbemycin-derivative, was approved in the United States in 2018 for treatment of patients aged 12 years and older with onchocerciasis (river blindness) due to *O. volvulus*. The drug is a semisynthetic derivative of nemadectin, a fermentation-derived milbemycin agent. In addition to the absence of a C_{13} disaccharide, moxidectin differs from IVM by the presence of a methoxime group at C_{23} and a substituted olefinic side chain at C_{25}. Like IVM, the drug is effective against the microfilaria and not effective against the adult form of the worm. The mechanism of action of moxidectin is reported to be the same as IVM activation of glutamate-gated chloride ion channels, leading to nerve and muscle interference. However, reports of moxidectin activity against IVM-resistant strains of *C. elegans*, and the effective use of this agent against IVM-resistant parasites, have led to some theories of binding site differences.[115] Moxidectin is also reported to have decreased Pgp-mediated efflux, relative to IVM, which may also affect its activity against resistant parasites. The adverse effect profiles differ between the two agents, with moxidectin having a lower incidence of neurotoxicity compared to IVM,[116] but a higher incidence of orthostatic hypotension and elevated bilirubin. Similar to IVM, there is a risk of acute encephalopathy when the drug is administered to a patient co-infected with *Loa loa*.

Metabolism. Moxidectin is highly lipophilic and distributes into adipose tissues following oral absorption, resulting in a high volume of distribution. The result is a depot-like release of the drug for several months following administration. Moxidectin has a longer half-life and larger volume of distribution compared to IVM. Moxidectin is not acted upon by CYP enzymes and is primarily eliminated unchanged in the feces.

Therapeutic Application. Moxidectin is administered as a single 8-mg dose (four 2-mg tablets), with or without food. Patients should be cautioned that they may have flu-like symptoms (malaise, myalgia, headache) during the first week after treatment. Other side effects may include tachycardia, hypotension, and pruritus. Because moxidectin does not kill adult *O. volvulus* parasites, follow-up with physician is advised and annual or biannual dosing, similar to IVM, for the life span of the adult worm will likely be necessary. Moxidectin is currently under evaluation for treatment of ectoparasitic infections but is not currently approved for this use.

Praziquantel (Biltricide)

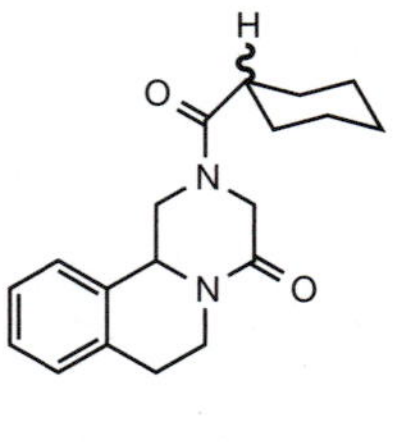

Praziquantel
(Biltricide)

Praziquantel (PZQ) is a tetrahydro-isoquinoline derivative, with most of the biological activity found in the *R*-enantiomer (levo), though the drug is marketed as a racemic mixture. The compound has no activity against nematodes, but it is highly effective against cestodes and trematodes.

Mechanism of Action. More than one mechanism of action can exist for PZQ, depending on the type of parasite being treated. The mechanism of action appears to involve Ca^{2+} redistribution, either directly or indirectly.[117,118] In the case of helminths found in the lumen of the host (cestode infection), the drug leads to muscle contraction and paralysis, leading in turn to worm expulsion. Additionally, PZQ has been shown to inhibit phosphoinositide metabolism, which, by an undetermined mechanism, leads to the worm paralysis.[119] With intravascular-dwelling schistosomes, PZQ leads to drug-induced damage of the tegument of the worm. As a result, antigens in the helminth are subject to attack by immune antibodies of the host.[117,120] An antigen-antibody immunological reaction leads to the death of the parasite. Finally, PZQ affects glycogen content and energy metabolism.[121,122]

Metabolism. Praziquantel is rapidly absorbed (~80%) following oral administration and undergoes extensive hepatic first-pass metabolism. The drug is primarily eliminated in the urine as metabolites. The metabolites are either less active or inactive and consist of hydroxylated compounds. In the serum, the major metabolite appears to be the mono-hydroxylated 4-hydroxy-cyclohexylcarboxylate, whereas in the urine 50%-60% of the initial PZQ exists as di-hydroxylated products and drug conjugates (Fig. 35.23).[123] The metabolism of praziquantel appear to be stereospecific, with the *R*-isomer being primarily metabolized by CYP1A2 and CYP 2C19 and the *S*-isomer being metabolized by CYP2C19 and CYP3A4.[124] The more active *R*-isomer is cleared 2.5 times faster than the less active *S*-isomer.

Therapeutic Application. Praziquantel is active against a broad range of cestodes and trematodes and is the drug of choice for treatment of tapeworm infections (cestodes), schistosomiasis, and infections caused by liver flukes (trematodes). The drug is stage specific, with activity against the invasive stages. This includes the cercariae and young schistosomula and the mature worms but not the liver stages. The drug has a bitter taste (attributed to the less active *S*-isomer) and, therefore, should not be chewed. The side effects usually are not severe and consist of abdominal discomfort (pain and diarrhea). Mounting evidence suggests that resistance can become a significant problem.[125]

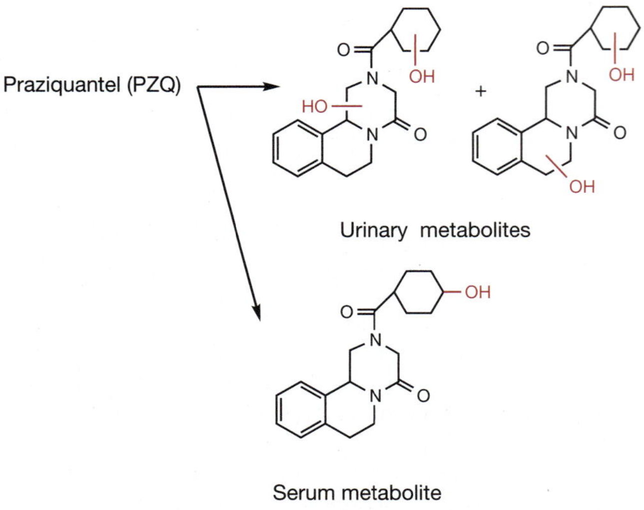

Figure 35.23 Metabolism of praziquantel (PZQ).

Pyrantel Pamoate

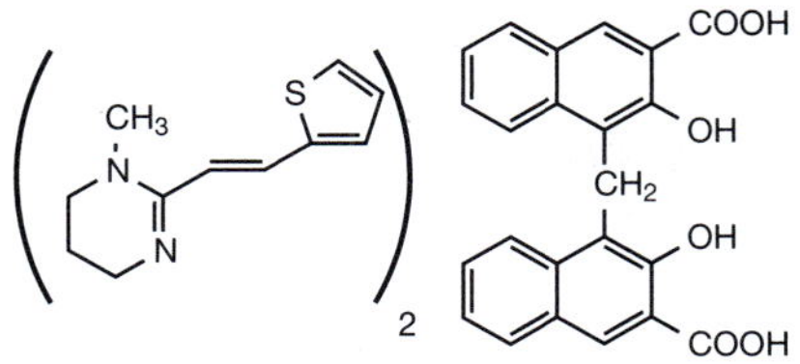

Pyrantel pamoate

Pyrantel was first reported for its anthelmintic activity in 1966.[126] Although it has activity against most intestinal roundworm infections, it is considered to be the drug of choice in the treatment of pinworms (enterobiasis). The drug is used as the pamoate salt, which is quite insoluble and, as a result, is not readily absorbed. This property improves the usefulness of the drug for treatment of intestinal helminths. In addition to its value in treating enterobiasis, the drug is effective for hookworm and roundworm (ascariasis) infections.

Mechanism of Action. Pyrantel acts as a depolarizing neuromuscular blocking agent that activates nicotinic receptors and inhibits cholinesterase, leading to worm paralysis.

Therapeutic Applications. Pyrantel pamoate is effective in the treatment of roundworm infections and is considered the drug of choice for treatment of pinworm infections (*Enterobius vermicularis*), as indicated in Table 35.7). The drug should not be used if *Trichuris* (whipworm) is suspected; in this case, mono- or combination therapy with the investigational oxantel pamoate is recommended (see Oxantel).

OXANTEL

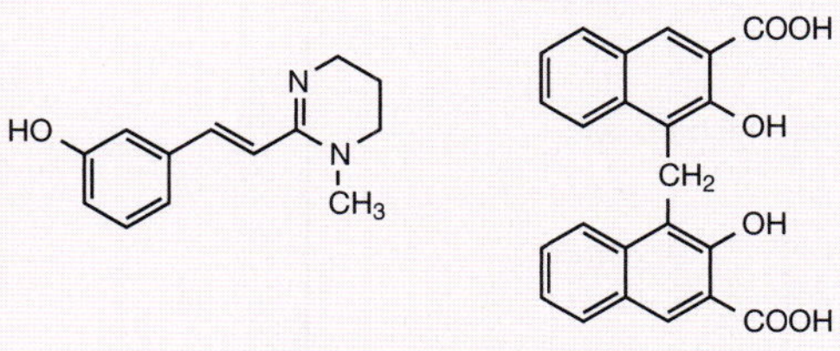

Oxantel pamoate

Oxantel, as the pamoate salt, is currently under development as monotherapy and in combination with albendazole for treatment of *Trichuris trichiura* (whipworm) infection.[127] Similar to pyrantel, the pamoate salt of this compound serves to decrease the solubility of the compound, thus signficantly decreasing the amount of the drug absorbed systemically and minimizing adverse effects related to the drug's binding to human nicotinic receptors. Like pyrantel, oxantel is a tetrahydropyrimidine derivative, but with an *m*-phenol group substituted for the pyrantel's thiophene ring. These chemical differences affect the pharmacology of oxantel, which preferentially binds to the N-subtype nicotinic receptor, while pyrantel binds preferentially to the L-subtype. For this reason, combination of oxantel with other anthelmintics, including pyrantel, results in high efficacy against a wide range of intestinal helminths.

ADDITIONAL WHO ESSENTIAL LIST ANTHELMINTICS

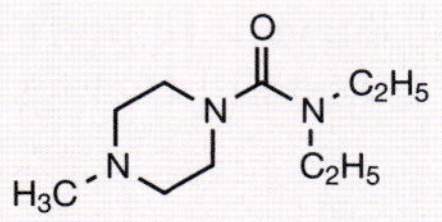

Diethylcarbamazine

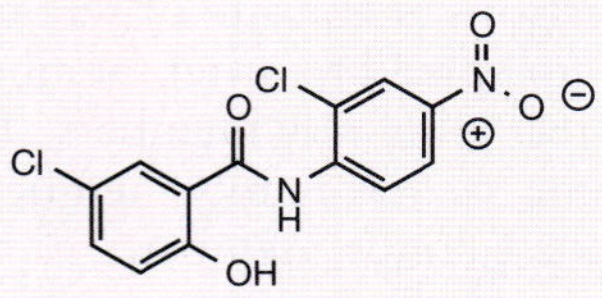

Niclosamide

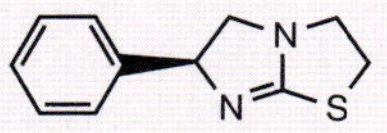

Levamisole

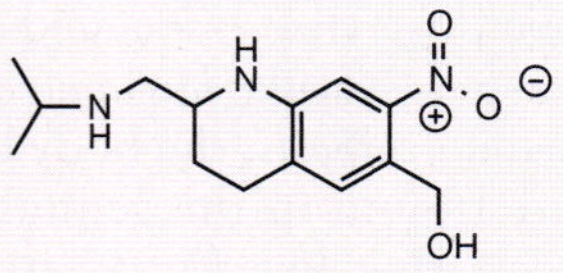

Oxamniquine

These agents are no longer marketed for clinical use in the United States but continue to be listed in the WHO Model List of Essential Medicines—23rd List (2023). Diethylcarbamazine (formulated as the citrate salt) is used for treatment of filariasis, niclosamide is an intestinal anthelmintic with activity against tapeworms, oxamniquine is listed as a complementary agent (for use when praziquantel fails) for treatment of schistosomiasis, and levamisole is an intestinal anthelmintic with activity against *A. lumbricoides* (roundworm) and *A. duodenale* (hookworm).

Ectoparasitic Infections

Three parasitic organisms that cause common topical infections are *Sarcoptes scabiei*, which is responsible for scabies, *Pediculus humanus*, subspecies of which are responsible for lice infections, and *Cimex lectularius* the common bedbug, which is an insect living exclusively on the blood of warm-blooded animals. This latter organism has shown a recent reemergence, and while its bite is normally not responsible for a primary or secondary infection, the topical irritation and the social implications can be quite disturbing to the patient. The only treatment of bedbug infestation is the use of antipruritic and the hiring of a professional exterminator.

Scabies

Scabies, sometimes referred to as the "7-year itch," is a condition caused by *Sarcoptes scabiei*, or the itch mite. The condition is commonly spread by direct, person-to-person contact, although the organism is capable of living for 2 to 3 days in clothing, bedding, or house dust. Sharing of clothing is a common means whereby the condition spreads. The organism burrows into the epidermis, usually in the folds of the skin of the fingers, the elbows, female breast, penis, scrotum, and buttocks. The female parasite lays eggs in the skin, which then hatch and mature to adults. The itch mite can live for 30 to 60 days. The infections are most common in children, but they can also be found in adults in institutional settings. The primary symptom of severe itching can foster secondary infections at the site of scratching. Because of the potential for spread to other members of a family, it is common to treat all family members. This will prevent reinfection from a second family member after successful therapy of the first family member.

Lice

Pediculosis (lice associated disease) is caused by any of the parasites *Pediculus humanus capitis*, the head louse; *Pediculus humanus corporis*, the body louse; or *Pthirus pubis*, the crab louse (found in the genital area). Lice are blood-sucking insects that live for 30 to 40 days on the body of the host. The organisms reproduce, and the female lays her eggs, the nits, which become attached to hair. The nits are white in color and hatch in 8 to 10 days. For the parasite to live, it must feed on blood, which it sucks through punctures in the skin. A hypersensitivity reaction occurs at these puncture sites, which then leads to pruritus, host scratching, and possible secondary infection. In addition to the scalp and skin, the eyebrows, eyelids, and beard can become sites of infection. The transfer of infection can occur through person-to-person contact and from infected clothing, on which the organism can survive for up to 1 week. The sharing of clothing is a common means for the spread of body lice. Head lice are quite common among children in grade school, whereas crab lice are common among individuals who are sexually active. Treatment of family members is recommended, and clothing and bed linens should be removed and washed in hot water.

Drug Therapy for Scabies and Pediculosis

Pyrethrum and Pyrethroids

The naturally occurring pyrethrums have been used as insecticides since the 1800s. These compounds are extracted from the flowering portion of the Chrysanthemum plant. The flowers produced in Kenya have, on average, 1.3% pyrethrins. These pyrethrum extracts have been a major agricultural product for that country.

CHEMISTRY. The Chrysanthemum extract is a mixture of alcohols and esters, including chrysanthemic and pyrethric acids (Fig. 35.24). The esters are prone to hydrolysis and oxidation and, as a result, should be stored in the cold and protected from light. Because of the prohibitive cost, limited availability, and rapid degradation, the natural pyrethrum mixture has limited utility today and is found in only a few over-the-counter (OTC) products. In products using

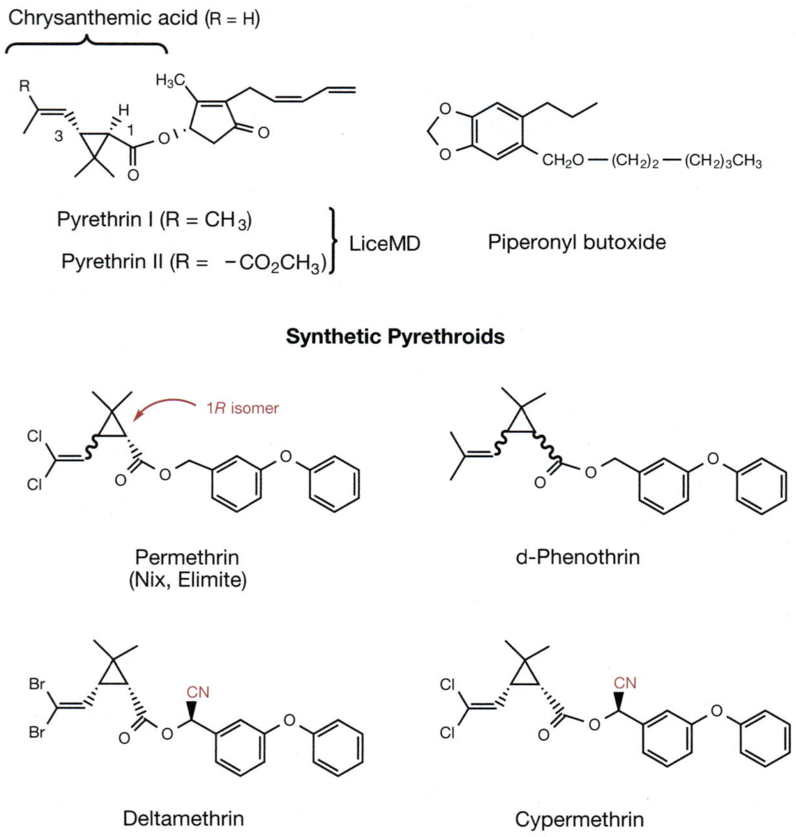

Figure 35.24 Structures of the naturally occurring pyrethrins, the synergist piperonyl butoxide, and the pyrethroid derivatives.

pyrethrums, piperonyl butoxide is commonly added as a synergist to reduce insect metabolism. Synthetic derivatives, known as pyrethroids, have mostly replaced pyrethrins in clinical use. The pyrethroids have the same mechanism of action as pyrethrum.

Mechanism of Action. The pyrethrins and pyrethroids are nerve membrane sodium channel toxins that do not affect potassium channels.[128-131] The compounds bind to specific sodium channel proteins and slow the rate of inactivation of the sodium current elicited by membrane depolarization and, as a result, prolong the open time of the sodium channel. At low concentrations, the pyrethroids produce repetitive action potentials and neuron firing; at high concentrations, the nerve membrane is depolarized completely, and excitation is blocked.

The receptor interaction of the pyrethrums with the sodium channel complex is stereospecific and dependent on the stereochemistry of the cyclopropane ring. In the case of the pyrethroids, the most active isomers are the 1*R*,3*S*-*trans* and 1*R*,3*R*-*cis* stereoisomers. The 1*S*,3*S*-*cis* and 1*S*,3*R*-*trans* stereoisomers are inactive and can actually be antagonistic to the action of the 1*R* stereoisomers.

Metabolism. A property that enhances the usefulness of the pyrethroids is that these compounds are highly toxic to the ectoparasites but relatively nontoxic to mammals if absorbed. The apparent lack of toxicity is associated with the rapid metabolism of these drugs through hydrolysis and/or oxidation.[132,133] The rapid breakdown of these agents also accounts for their low persistence in the environment.

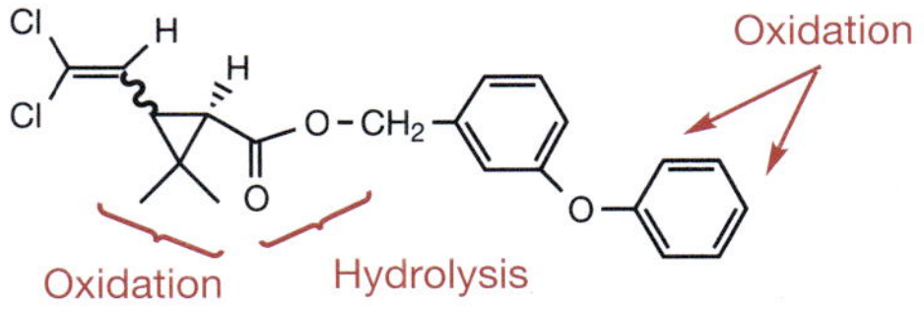

Permethrin

Therapeutic Application

Permethrin (Nix, Elimite)

Permethrin, because of its increased stability and its synthetic availability, is not used with a synergist. The compound is used in a 1% lotion for the treatment of pediculosis capitis and in a 5% cream as a scabicide. The 5% cream is a prescription product while the 1% lotion is available OTC. The permethrins are meant to kill the scabies mite and eggs.

The pyrethroids are also commonly found in OTC backyard insecticides and agricultural and veterinary products. These pyrethroids are divided into two classes depending on the absence (type I: permethrin, d-phenothrin) or presence (type II: cypermethrin, deltamethrin) of a cyano group. The type II products are the more potent insecticides.[134]

Crotamiton (Crotan, Eurax)

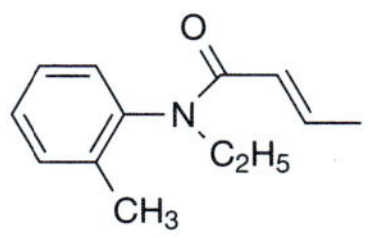

Crotamiton

Crotamiton is available as a 10% lotion for the treatment of scabies, although it is less effective than pyrethrins or permethrin.[135,136] Crotamiton is reported to inhibit the transient receptor potential vanilloid 4 (TRPV4) channel, which is believed to contribute to a favorable anti-itch property of the drug.[137] The anti-scabies mechanism of action of crotamiton remains unknown. Following an initial shower or bath, crotamiton is applied 2 to 3 times, from the chin to the toes (including "folds and creases"), with a 24-hour period between applications. Patients should be counseled to shower no sooner than 48 hours after the last application. Because of the recommendation for repeated applications versus permethrin, which typically requires a single application, poor patient compliance can reduce the drug's effectiveness. Crotamiton is now considered a second-line agent for treatment of scabies.

Malathion (Ovide)

Malathion is an organophosphate insecticide that is used commercially as an agricultural pesticide and medically for treatment of head lice. Malathion has relatively low toxicity in humans compared to insects. Its insecticidal properties are believed to be due to the conversion of malathion to malaoxon, a more potent inhibitor of acetylcholinesterase (AChE), in insects.

Mechanism of Action. Malathion is an irreversible inhibitor of AChE. In insects, malathion, a weak AChE inhibitor, is rapidly oxidized to malaoxon (Fig. 35.25), a strong AChE inhibitor and the ethyl ester is slowly hydrolyzed. In contrast, in mammals the ethyl ester hydrolysis occurs quickly, yielding an inactive metabolite, while the activating oxidation reaction occurs slowly. The carboxylesterase that detoxifies malathion is prominent in mammals, but only sporadically present in insects.[138]

Therapeutic Application. Malathion is considered a second-line agent for the treatment of head lice in patients aged 6 years or older. The use of this drug is limited by toxicity concerns and reports of resistance. Though

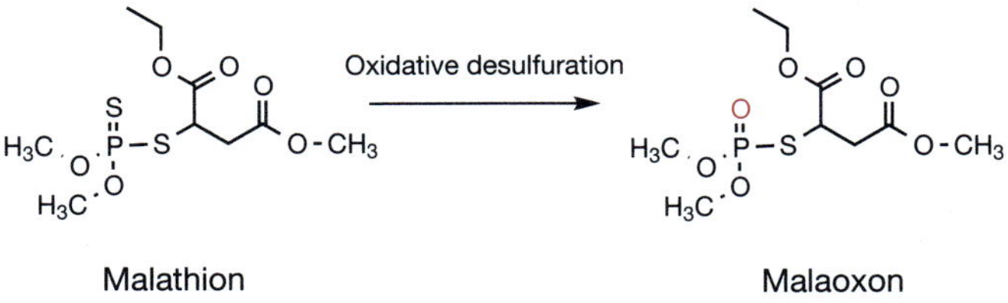

Figure 35.25 Oxidative desulfuration of malathion.

malathion is a weak inhibitor of AChE, a portion of topically administered drug can be absorbed, particularly in neonates and infants as their scalps are more permeable and can result in systemic effects. For this reason, the drug is contraindicated for use children younger than age 2 years. Signs of toxicity include increased cholinergic activity: salivation, sweating, GI motility, and bradycardia. Malathion lotion is prepared in a 78% isopropyl alcohol vehicle, which makes the lotion flammable. Patients should be counseled to avoid open flames or electric heat sources, such as hair dryers and electric curlers, after application of the lotion to their hair. Skin irritation is the most common adverse effect.

Spinosad (Natroba)

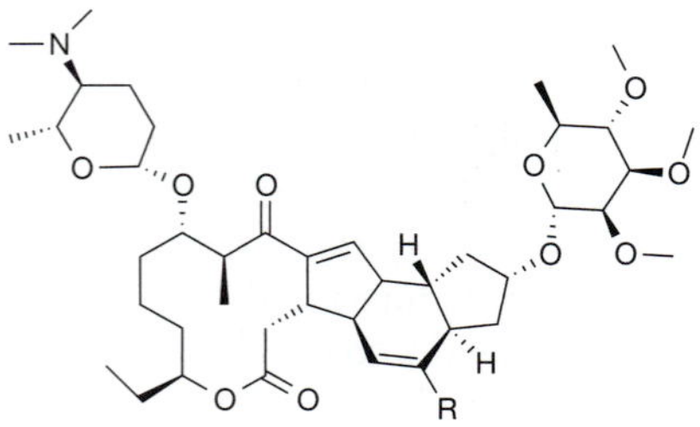

Spinosad (Natroba)

(Spinosyn A: R = H, Spinosyn D: R = CH_3)

Spinosad is a naturally occurring 12-member macrolide consisting of a mixture of spinosyn A and D produced by the bacterium *Saccharopholyspora spinose*, a member of the actinomycete family. The product was a serendipitous discovery isolated from a soil sample found in an abandoned rum distillery on a Caribbean island, by an employee of Eli Lilly. The mixture has a broad spectrum of activity and was approved for agricultural use by the Environmental Protection Agency in 1995 and by the FDA for treatment of head lice in 2011.[139]

Mechanism of Action. The mechanism of action has been investigated and found to lead to death of the insect via rapid excitation of the insect's nervous system. Spinosad is an insecticide by virtue of its ability to act as an agonist at the nicotinic acetylcholine receptors (nAChRs) and more specifically at the Da6 subunit.[140-142] Thus, spinosad has a novel mechanism of action compared to other insecticides. The results are that spinosad creates prolonged hyperexcitation of the CNS of the insects and eventually paralysis and death of the organism. It has also been suggested that the drug may function as an antagonist at GABA receptors.

Therapeutic Application. The product is available as a 0.9% topical suspension, which is applied to a dry scalp and hair for a period of 10 minutes and then rinsed with water. Because spinosad has ovicidal activity, nit combing is not required. Studies would suggest that spinosad, which requires a single treatment, is more effective (~80%) than permethrin (~45%) especially after a single treatment. Fewer topical adverse events were noted with spinosad versus permethrin, and presently resistance, a growing problem with the permethrin, has not been reported for spinosad.[140,141]

Ivermectin (Sklice)

As indicated earlier, IVM in the form of a topical lotion is approved for the treatment of head lice. IVM binds to glutamate and GABA-gated chloride ion channels and, as a result, leads to parasite paralysis and death. The drug can be used without nit combing, and although it does not kill nits, the nits die following hatching since the nymphs are unable to feed due to the paralysis of mouthparts caused by the IVM. Minimal absorption of the drug is found following topical application, and few dermatological adverse effects have been reported. Table 35.8 summarizes the currently available topical treatments for head lice.

Acknowledgment

This chapter is based on the 8th edition chapter written by Dr Thomas L. Lemke. The authors gratefully acknowledge the previous work of Dr Lemke.

Table 35.8 Summary of Head Lice Treatment

Drug	Formulation	Rx or Over the Counter (OTC)	Ovicidal?	Pediatric Use
Pyrethrins (Rid)	Shampoo[a]	OTC	No	2 y or older
Permethrin (Nix)	1% lotion	OTC	Yes[b]	2 mo or older
Malathion (Ovide)	0.5% lotion	Rx	Yes[c]	6 y or older
Spinosad (Natroba)	0.9% suspension	Rx	Yes	6 mo or older
Ivermectin (Sklice)	0.5% lotion	OTC	No[d]	6 mo or older

[a]0.33% pyrethrum extract, 4% piperonyl butoxide.
[b]Yes according to mfr., but only partially per literature. Recommend a second treatment if live lice are present on day 9 (per CDC).
[c]Malathion is "partially ovicidal" (kills some lice eggs). A second treatment is recommended if live lice are still present 7 to 9 days after treatment.
[d]Ivermectin is technically not ovicidal, but it does prevent newly hatched lice (nymphs) from surviving; thus, in most cases, a second treatment is not required.

Structure Challenge

Using the structures provided in the following figure, answer the following questions related to the appropriate selection and patient counseling on drug therapy:

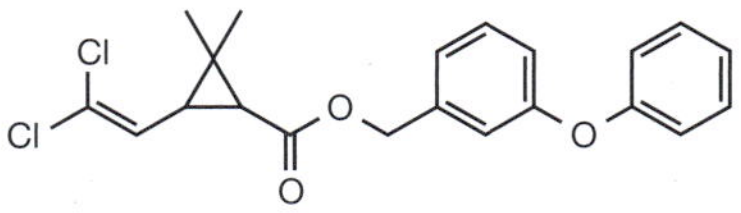

Compound I

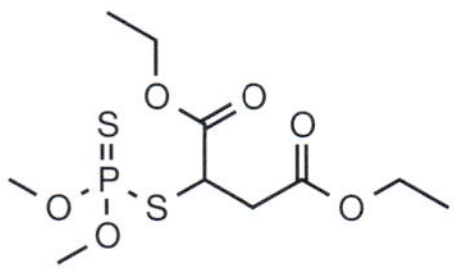

Compound II

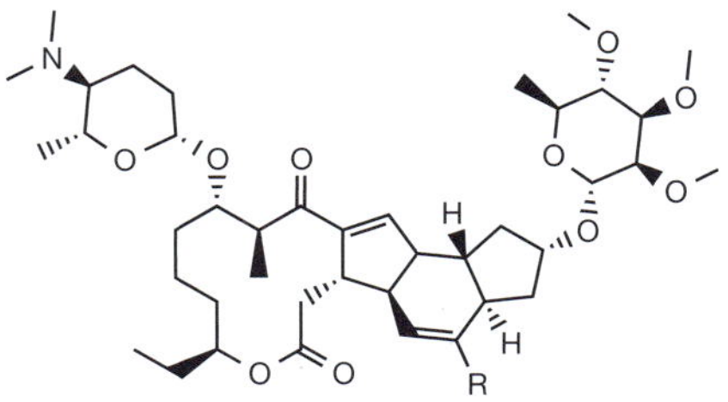

Compound III

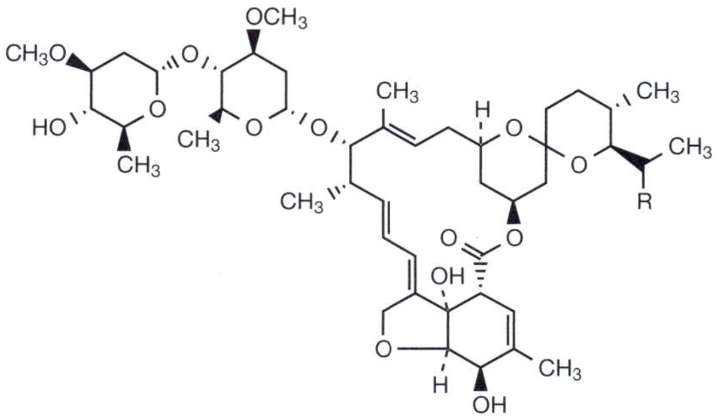

Compound IV

1. Which pediculicide agent would be most effective over-the-counter (OTC) option for treatment of head lice?
2. What patient counseling points should be covered with these agents when they are dispensed by a pharmacist?

Structure Challenge answers found immediately after References.

REFERENCES

1. El-Sayed NM, Myler PJ, Blandin G, et al. Comparative genomics of trypanosomatid parasitic protozoa. *Science*. 2005;309:404-409.
2. El-Sayed NM, Myler PJ, Bartholomeu DC, et al. The genome sequence of *Trypanosoma cruzi*, etiologic agent of Chagas disease. *Science*. 2005;309:409-415.
3. Berriman M, Ghedin E, Hertz-Fowler C, et al. The genome of the African trypanosome Trypanosoma brucei. *Science*. 2005; 309:416-422.
4. Barrett MP, Burchmore RJS, Stich A, et al. The trypanosomiases. *Lancet*. 2003;362:1469-1480.
5. Irish A, Whitman JD, Clark EH, Marcus R, Bern C. Updated estimates and mapping for prevalence of chagas disease among adults, United States. *Emerg Infect Dis*. 2022;28:1313-1320.
6. Bouteille B, Oukem O, Bisser S, Dumas M. Treatment perspectives for human African trypanosomiasis. *Fundam Clin Pharmacol*. 2003;17:171-181.
7. Leishmaniasis in high-burden countries: an epidemiological update based on data reported in 2014. *Wkly Epidemiol Rec*. 2016; 91:287-296.
8. Venkatesan P. The 2023 WHO World malaria report. *Lancet Microbe*. 2024;5:e214.
9. Dye-Braumuller KC, Kanyangarara M. Malaria in the USA: how vulnerable are we to future outbreaks? *Curr Trop Med Rep*. 2021;8:43-51.
10. Greenwood BM, Fidock DA, Kyle DE, et al. Malaria: progress, perils, and prospects for eradication. *J Clin Invest*. 2008;118:1266-1276.
11. Lalloo DG, Hill DR. Preventing malaria in travellers. *BMJ*. 2008;336:1362-1366.
12. Maeda K, Osato T, Umezawa H. A new antibiotic, azomycin. *J Antibiot (Tokyo)*. 1953;6:182.
13. Dingsdag SA, Hunter N. Metronidazole: an update on metabolism, structure-cytotoxicity and resistance mechanisms. *J Antimicrob Chemother*. 2018;73:265-279.
14. Samuelson J. Why metronidazole is active against both bacteria and parasites. *Antimicrob Agents Chemother*. 1999;43:1533-1541.
15. Docampo R. Sensitivity of parasites to free radical damage by antiparasitic drugs. *Chem Biol Interact*. 1990;73:1-27.
16. Stambaugh JE, Feo LG, Manthei RW. The isolation and identification of the urinary oxidative metabolites of metronidazole in man. *J Pharmacol Exp Ther*. 1968;161:373-381.
17. Haller I. In vitro activity of the two principal oxidative metabolites of metronidazole against Bacteroides fragilis and related species. *Antimicrob Agents Chemother*. 1982;22:165-166.
18. Ralph ED. Clinical pharmacokinetics of metronidazole. *Clin Pharmacokinet*. 1983;8:43-62.
19. Kock RL, Beaulieu BB Jr, Chrystal EJ, Goldman P. A metronidazole metabolite in human urine and its risk. *Science*. 1981; 211:398-400.
20. Lau AH, Lam NP, Piscitelli SC, Wilkes L, Danziger LH. Clinical pharmacokinetics of metronidazole and other nitroimidazole anti-infectives. *Clin Pharmacokinet*. 1992;23:328-364.
21. Lamp KC, Freeman CD, Klutman, NE, Lacy MK. Pharmacokinetics and pharmacodynamics of the nitroimidazole antimicrobials. *Clin Pharmacokinet*. 1999;36:353-373.
22. Johnson S, Lavergne V, Skinner AM, et al. Clinical Practice Guideline by the Infectious Diseases Society of America (IDSA) and Society for Healthcare Epidemiology of America (SHEA): 2021 focused update guidelines on management of *Clostridioides difficile* infection in adults. *Clin Infect Dis*. 2021;73:e1029-e1044.
23. Chey WD, Leontiadis GI, Howden CW, Moss SF. ACG clinical guideline: treatment of *Helicobacter pylori* infection. *Am J Gastroenterol*. 2017;112:212-239.

24. Somvanshi VS, Ellis BL, Hu Y, Aroian RV. Nitazoxanide: nematicidal mode of action and drug combination studies. *Mol Biochem Parasitol.* 2014;193:1-8.
25. Stockis A, De Bruyn S, Gengler C, Rosillon D. Nitazoxanide pharmacokinetics and tolerability in man during 7 days dosing with 0.5 g and 1 g b.i.d. *Int J Clin Pharmacol Ther.* 2002;40:221-227.
26. Abaza H, El-Zayadi AR, Kabil SM, Rizk H. Nitazoxanide in the treatment of patients with intestinal protozoan and helminthic infections: a report on 546 patients in egypt. *Curr Ther Res.* 1998; 59:116-121.
27. Anderson VR, Curran MP. Nitazoxanide: a review of its use in the treatment of gastrointestinal infections. *Drugs.* 2007;67: 1947-1967.
28. Wainwright M. Dyes, trypanosomiasis and DNA: a historical and critical review. *Biotech Histochem.* 2010;85:341-354.
29. Wiedemar N, Hauser DA, Maser P. 100 years of suramin. *Antimicrob Agents Chemother.* 2020;64:e01168-19.
30. Albisetti A, Halg S, Zoltner M, Maser P, Wiedemar N. Suramin action in African trypanosomes involves a RuvB-like DNA helicase. *Int J Parasitol Drugs Drug Resist.* 2023;23:44-53.
31. Edwards KJ, Jenkins TC, Neidle S. Crystal structure of a pentamidine-oligonucleotide complex: implications for DNA-binding properties. *Biochemistry.* 1992;31:7104-7109.
32. Shapiro TA, Englund PT. Selective cleavage of kinetoplast DNA minicircles promoted by antitrypanosomal drugs. *Proc Natl Acad Sci U S A.* 1990;87:950-954.
33. Dykstra CC, Tidwell RR. Inhibition of topoisomerases from *Pneumocystis carinii* by aromatic dicationic molecules. *J Protozool.* 1991;38:78S-81S.
34. Metcalf BW, Bey P, Danzin C, Jung MJ, Casara P, Vevert JP. Catalytic irreversible inhibition of mammalian ornithine decarboxylase (E.C.4.1.1.17) by substrate and product analogs. *J Am Chem Soc.* 1978;100:2551-2553.
35. Bacchi CJ, Nathan HC, Hutner SH, McCann PP, Sjoerdsma A. Polyamine metabolism: a potential therapeutic target in trypanosomes. *Science.* 1980;210:332-334.
36. Poulin R, Lu L, Ackermann B, Bey P, Pegg AE. Mechanism of the irreversible inactivation of mouse ornithine decarboxylase by alpha-difluoromethylornithine. Characterization of sequences at the inhibitor and coenzyme binding sites. *J Biol Chem.* 1992;267:150-158.
37. Bacchi CJ, Garofalo J, Ciminelli M, et al. Resistance to DL-alpha-difluoromethylornithine by clinical isolates of Trypanosoma brucei rhodesiense. Role of S-adenosylmethionine. *Biochem Pharmacol.* 1993;46:471-481.
38. Henderson GB, Ulrich P, Fairlamb AH, et al. "Subversive" substrates for the enzyme trypanothione disulfide reductase: alternative approach to chemotherapy of Chagas disease. *Proc Natl Acad Sci U S A.* 1988;85:5374-5378.
39. Garcia-Huertas P, Mejia-Jaramillo AM, Machado CR, Guimaraes AC, Triana-Chavez O. Prostaglandin F2α synthase in *Trypanosoma cruzi* plays critical roles in oxidative stress and susceptibility to benznidazole. *R Soc Open Sci.* 2017;4:170773.
40. Deeks ED. Fexinidazole: first global approval. *Drugs.* 2019;79: 215-220.
41. Tarral A, Blesson S, Mordt OV, et al. Determination of an optimal dosing regimen for fexinidazole, a novel oral drug for the treatment of human African trypanosomiasis: first-in-human studies. *Clin Pharmacokinet.* 2014;53:565-580.
42. Pinazo MJ, Forsyth C, Losada I, et al. Efficacy and safety of fexinidazole for treatment of chronic indeterminate Chagas disease (FEXI-12): a multicentre, randomised, double-blind, phase 2 trial. *Lancet Infect Dis.* 2024;24:395-403.
43. Torreele E, Trunz BB, Tweats D, et al. Fexinidazole—a new oral nitroimidazole drug candidate entering clinical development for the treatment of sleeping sickness. *PLoS Negl Trop Dis.* 2010;4:e923.
44. Wyllie S, Foth BJ, Kelner A, Sokolova AY, Berriman M, Fairlamb AH. Nitroheterocyclic drug resistance mechanisms in *Trypanosoma brucei*. *J Antimicrob Chemother.* 2016;71:625-634.
45. WHO interim guidelines for the treatment of gambiense human African trypanosomiasis. World Health Organization; 2019. https://www.who.int/publications/i/item/9789241550567
46. Fairlamb AH, Henderson GB, Cerami A. Trypanothione is the primary target for arsenical drugs against African trypanosomes. *Proc Natl Acad Sci U S A.* 1989;86:2607-2611.
47. Berman JD. Chemotherapy for leishmaniasis: biochemical mechanisms, clinical efficacy, and future strategies. *Rev Infect Dis.* 1988;10: 560-586.
48. Cook GC. Leishmaniasis: some recent developments in chemotherapy. *J Antimicrob Chemother.* 1993;31:327-330.
49. Singh S, Sivakumar R. Challenges and new discoveries in the treatment of leishmaniasis. *J Infect Chemother.* 2004;10:307-315.
50. Dorlo TP, Balasegaram M, Beijnen JH, de Vries PJ. Miltefosine: a review of its pharmacology and therapeutic efficacy in the treatment of leishmaniasis. *J Antimicrob Chemother.* 2012;67:2576-2597.
51. Escobar P, Matu S, Marques C, Croft SL. Sensitivities of Leishmania species to hexadecylphosphocholine (miltefosine), ET-18-OCH(3) (edelfosine) and amphotericin B. *Acta Trop.* 2002;81: 151-157.
52. Luque-Ortega JR, Rivas L. Miltefosine (hexadecylphosphocholine) inhibits cytochrome c oxidase in *Leishmania donovani* promastigotes. *Antimicrob Agents Chemother.* 2007;51:1327-1332.
53. Rakotomanga M, Blanc S, Gaudin K, Chaminade P, Loiseau PM. Miltefosine affects lipid metabolism in *Leishmania donovani* promastigotes. *Antimicrob Agents Chemother.* 2007;51:1425-1430.
54. Pinto-Martinez AK, Rodriguez-Duran J, Serrano-Martin X, Hernandez-Rodriguez V, Benaim G. Mechanism of action of miltefosine on *Leishmania donovani* involves the impairment of acidocalcisome function and the activation of the sphingosine-dependent plasma membrane Ca^{2+} channel. *Antimicrob Agents Chemother.* 2018;62:e01614-17.
55. Dorlo TP, van Thiel PPAM, Huitema ADR, et al. Pharmacokinetics of miltefosine in Old World cutaneous leishmaniasis patients. *Antimicrob Agents Chemother.* 2008;52:2855-2860.
56. Kotting J, Marschner NW, Neumuller W, Unger C, Eibl H. Hexadecylphosphocholine and octadecyl-methyl-glycero-3-phosphocholine: a comparison of hemolytic activity, serum binding and tissue distribution. *Prog Exp Tumor Res.* 1992;34:131-142.
57. Frezard F, Aguiar MMG, Ferreira LAM, et al. Liposomal amphotericin B for treatment of leishmaniasis: from the identification of critical physicochemical attributes to the design of effective topical and oral formulations. *Pharmaceutics.* 2022;15:99.
58. Parasites - Toxoplasmosis (Toxoplasma Infection). U.S. Centers for Disease Control; 2023. Accessed March 14, 2024. https://www.cdc.gov/parasites/toxoplasmosis/index.html
59. Nyunt MM, Adam I, Kayentao K, et al. Pharmacokinetics of sulfadoxine and pyrimethamine in intermittent preventive treatment of malaria in pregnancy. *Clin Pharmacol Ther.* 2010;87:226-234.
60. Montoya JG, Boothroyd JC, Kovacs JA. Toxoplasma gondii. In: Bennett JE, Dolin R, Blaser MJ, eds. *Mandell, Douglas, and Bennett's Principles and Practice of Infectious Diseases.* Elsevier, Inc; 2020: 3355-3387.
61. Ritschel WA, Ritschel G, Buncher CR, Rotmensch J. Study on bioavailability of sulfadiazine tablets in man. *Drug Intell Clin Pharm.* 1976;10:402-408.
62. Mannisto P, Tuomisto J, Saris NE, Lehtinen T. Pharmacokinetic studies with trimethoprim and different doses of sulfadiazine in healthy human subjects. *Chemotherapy.* 1973;19:289-298.
63. Pfefferkorn ER, Nothnagel RF, Borotz SE. Parasiticidal effect of clindamycin on Toxoplasma gondii grown in cultured cells and selection of a drug-resistant mutant. *Antimicrob Agents Chemother.* 1992;36:1091-1096.
64. Mazur D, Schug BS, Evers G, et al. Bioavailability and selected pharmacokinetic parameters of clindamycin hydrochloride after administration of a new 600 mg tablet formulation. *Int J Clin Pharmacol Ther.* 1999;37:386-392.
65. Dunn D, Wallon M, Peyron F, Petersen E, Peckham C, Gilbert R. Mother-to-child transmission of toxoplasmosis: risk estimates for clinical counselling. *Lancet.* 1999;353:1829-1833.
66. Montoya JG, Remington JS. Management of *Toxoplasma gondii* infection during pregnancy. *Clin Infect Dis.* 2008;47:554-566.
67. Ward SA. Mechanisms of chloroquine resistance in malarial chemotherapy. *Trends Pharmacol Sci.* 1988;9:241-246.

68. Tripathy S, Dassarma B, Roy S, Chabalala H, Matsabisa MG. A review on possible modes of action of chloroquine/hydroxychloroquine: repurposing against SAR-CoV-2 (COVID-19) pandemic. *Int J Antimicrob Agents*. 2020;56:106028.
69. Foley M, Tilley L. Quinoline antimalarials: mechanisms of action and resistance and prospects for new agents. *Pharmacol Ther*. 1998;79:55-87.
70. Dziekan JM, Yu H, Chen D, et al. Identifying purine nucleoside phosphorylase as the target of quinine using cellular thermal shift assay. *Sci Transl Med*. 2019;11:eaau3174.
71. Hempelmann E. Hemozoin biocrystallization in *Plasmodium falciparum* and the antimalarial activity of crystallization inhibitors. *Parasitol Res*. 2007;100:671-676.
72. Kurosawa Y, Dorn A, Kitsuji-Shirane M, et al. Hematin polymerization assay as a high-throughput screen for identification of new antimalarial pharmacophores. *Antimicrob Agents Chemother*. 2000; 44:2638-2644.
73. Sullivan DJ Jr, Gluzman IY, Russell DG, Goldberg DE. On the molecular mechanism of chloroquine's antimalarial action. *Proc Natl Acad Sci U S A*. 1996;93:11865-11870.
74. Arav-Boger R, Shapiro TA. Molecular mechanisms of resistance in antimalarial chemotherapy: the unmet challenge. *Annu Rev Pharmacol Toxicol*. 2005;45:565-585.
75. Zhao XJ, Ishizaki T. Metabolic interactions of selected antimalarial and non-antimalarial drugs with the major pathway (3-hydroxylation) of quinine in human liver microsomes. *Br J Clin Pharmacol*. 1997;44:505-511.
76. Palmer KJ, Holliday SM, Brogden RN. Mefloquine. A review of its antimalarial activity, pharmacokinetic properties and therapeutic efficacy. *Drugs*. 1993;45:430-475.
77. Davis TM, Hung TY, Sim IK, Karunajeewa HA, Ilett KF. Piperaquine: a resurgent antimalarial drug. *Drugs*. 2005;65:75-87.
78. Tarning J, Lindegardh N, Sandberg S, Day NJP, White NJ, Ashton M. Pharmacokinetics and metabolism of the antimalarial piperaquine after intravenous and oral single doses to the rat. *J Pharm Sci*. 2008;97:3400-3410.
79. Augusto O, Schreiber J, Mason RP. Direct ESR detection of a free radical intermediate during the peroxidase-catalyzed oxidation of the antimalarial drug primaquine. *Biochem Pharmacol*. 1988;37:2791-2797.
80. Mihaly GW, Ward SA, Edwards G, Orme ML, Breckenridge AM. Pharmacokinetics of primaquine in man: identification of the carboxylic acid derivative as a major plasma metabolite. *Br J Clin Pharmacol*. 1984;17:441-446.
81. Ebstie YA, Abay SM, Tadesse WT, Ejigu DA. Tafenoquine and its potential in the treatment and relapse prevention of *Plasmodium vivax* malaria: the evidence to date. *Drug Des Devel Ther*. 2016;10:2387-2399.
82. Vuong C, Xie LH, Potter BMJ. Differential cytochrome P450 2D metabolism alters tafenoquine pharmacokinetics. *Antimicrob Agents Chemother*. 2015;59:3864-3869.
83. Olliaro P. Mode of action and mechanisms of resistance for antimalarial drugs. *Pharmacol Ther*. 2001;89:207-219.
84. Cottrell G, Musset L, Hubert V, et al. Emergence of resistance to atovaquone-proguanil in malaria parasites: insights from computational modeling and clinical case reports. *Antimicrob Agents Chemother*. 2014;58:4504-4514.
85. Massamba L, Madamet M, Benoit N, et al. Late clinical failure associated with cytochrome b codon 268 mutation during treatment of falciparum malaria with atovaquone-proguanil in traveller returning from Congo. *Malar J*. 2020;19:37.
86. Cumming JN, Ploypradith P, Posner GH. Antimalarial activity of artemisinin (qinghaosu) and related trioxanes: mechanism(s) of action. *Adv Pharmacol*. 1997;37:253-297.
87. Meshnick SR, Taylor TE, Kamchonwongpaisan S. Artemisinin and the antimalarial endoperoxides: from herbal remedy to targeted chemotherapy. *Microbiol Rev*. 1996;60:301-315.
88. Posner GH, Cumming JN, Woo SH, Ploypradith P, Xie S, Shapiro TA. Orally active antimalarial 3-substituted trioxanes: new synthetic methodology and biological evaluation. *J Med Chem*. 1998; 41:940-951.
89. Cumming JN, Wang D, Park SB, Shapiro TA, Posner GH. Design, synthesis, derivatization, and structure-activity relationships of simplified, tricyclic, 1,2,4-trioxane alcohol analogues of the antimalarial artemisinin. *J Med Chem*. 1998;41:952-964.
90. Meshnick SR. The mode of action of antimalarial endoperoxides. *Trans R Soc Trop Med Hyg*. 1994;88(suppl 1):S31-S32.
91. Eckstein-Ludwig U, Webb RJ, Van Goethem IDA, et al. Artemisinins target the SERCA of Plasmodium falciparum. *Nature*. 2003;424:957-961.
92. Yue L, Pan Y, Wang J, et al. Design, synthesis, and antitumor activities of isomers of artemisinin dimer derivatives. *Chem Biodivers*. 2023;20:e202300615.
93. Hencken CB, Kalinda AS, D'Angelo JG. The anti-infective and anti-cancer properties of artemisinin and its derivatives. In: Macor JE, ed. *Annual Reports in Medicinal Chemistry*. Vol 44. Academic Press; 2009:359-378.
94. Verma A, Ghosh S, Salotra P, Singh R. Artemisinin-resistant Leishmania parasite modulates host cell defense mechanism and exhibits altered expression of unfolded protein response genes. *Parasitol Res*. 2019;118:2705-2713.
95. Perez del Villar L, Burguillo FJ, Lopez-Aban J, Muro A. Systematic review and meta-analysis of artemisinin based therapies for the treatment and prevention of schistosomiasis. *PLoS One*. 2012;7:e45867.
96. Naß J, Efferth T. The activity of *Artemisia* spp. and their constituents against Trypanosomiasis. *Phytomedicine*. 2018;47:184-191.
97. Lustigman S, Prichard RK, Gazzinelli A, et al. A research agenda for helminth diseases of humans: the problem of helminthiases. *PLoS Negl Trop Dis*. 2012;6:e1582.
98. Maizels RM, Bundy DA, Selkirk ME, Smith DF, Anderson RM. Immunological modulation and evasion by helminth parasites in human populations. *Nature*. 1993;365:797-805.
99. de Silva N, Guyatt H, Bundy D. Anthelmintics. A comparative review of their clinical pharmacology. *Drugs*. 1997;53:769-788.
100. Townsend LB, Wise DS. The synthesis and chemistry of certain anthelmintic benzimidazoles. *Parasitol Today*. 1990;6:107-112.
101. Prichard RK. Mode of action of the anthelminthic thiabendazole in *Haemonchus contortus*. *Nature*. 1970;228:684-645.
102. Friedman PA, Platzer EG. Interaction of anthelmintic benzimidazoles and benzimidazole derivatives with bovine brain tubulin. *Biochim Biophys Acta*. 1978;544:605-614.
103. Lacey E. Mode of action of benzimidazoles. *Parasitol Today*. 1990;6: 112-115.
104. Braithwaite PA, Roberts MS, Allan RJ, Watson TR. Clinical pharmacokinetics of high dose mebendazole in patients treated for cystic hydatid disease. *Eur J Clin Pharmacol*. 1982;22:161-169.
105. Gottschall DW, Theodorides VJ, Wang R. The metabolism of benzimidazole anthelmintics. *Parasitol Today*. 1990;6:115-124.
106. Marriner SE, Morris DL, Dickson B, Bogan JA. Pharmacokinetics of albendazole in man. *Eur J Clin Pharmacol*. 1986;30:705-708.
107. Novartis Pharmaceuticals Corp. Egaten (triclabendazole) [package insert]. U.S. Food and Drug Administration. Accessed April 15, 2024. Revised February 2019. www.accessdata.fda.gov/drugsatfda_docs/label/2019/208711s000lbl.pdf
108. Prichard R, Menez C, Lespine A. Moxidectin and the avermectins: consanguinity but not identity. *Int J Parasitol Drugs Drug Resist*. 2012;2:134-153.
109. Bloomquist JR. Chloride channels as tools for developing selective insecticides. *Arch Insect Biochem Physiol*. 2003;54:145-156.
110. Goa KL, McTavish D, Clissold SP. Ivermectin. A review of its antifilarial activity, pharmacokinetic properties and clinical efficacy in onchocerciasis. *Drugs*. 1991;42:640-658.
111. Martin RJ, Robertson AP, Choudhary S. Ivermectin: an anthelmintic, an insecticide, and much more. *Trends Parasitol*. 2021;37:48-64.
112. Ottesen EA, Campbell WC. Ivermectin in human medicine. *J Antimicrob Chemother*. 1994;34:195-203.
113. Forrester SG, Beech RN, Prichard RK. Agonist enhacement of macrocyclic lactone activity at a glutamate-gated chloride channel subunit from *Haemonchus contortus*. *Biochem Pharmacol*. 2004;67:1019-1024.

114. Lespine A, Alvinerie M, Vercruysse J, Prichard RK, Geldhof P. ABC transporter modulation: a strategy to enhance the activity of macrocyclic lactone anthelmintics. *Trends Parasitol.* 2008;24:293-298.
115. Ardelli BF, Stitt LE, Tompkins JB, Prichard RK. A comparison of the effects of ivermectin and moxidectin on the nematode Caenorhabditis elegans. *Vet Parasitol.* 2009;165:96-108.
116. Menez C, Sutra JF, Prichard R, Lespine A. Relative neurotoxicity of ivermectin and moxidectin in Mdr1ab (-/-) mice and effects on mammalian GABA(A) channel activity. *PLoS Negl Trop Dis.* 2012;6:e1883.
117. Xiao SH, Catto BA, Webster LT Jr. Effects of praziquantel on different developmental stages of Schistosoma mansoni in vitro and in vivo. *J Infect Dis.* 1985;151:1130-1137.
118. Xiao SH, Friedman PA, Catto BA, Webster LT Jr. Praziquantel-induced vesicle formation in the tegument of male Schistosoma mansoni is calcium dependent. *J Parasitol.* 1984;70:177-179.
119. Wiest PM, Li Y, Olds GR, Bowen WD. Inhibition of phosphoinositide turnover by praziquantel in Schistosoma mansoni. *J Parasitol.* 1992;78:753-755.
120. Fallon PG, Cooper RO, Probert AJ, Doenhoff MJ. Immune-dependent chemotherapy of schistosomiasis. *Parasitology.* 1992; 105:S41-S48.
121. Utzinger J, Keiser J, Shuhua X, Tanner M, Singer BH. Combination chemotherapy of schistosomiasis in laboratory studies and clinical trials. *Antimicrob Agents Chemother.* 2003;47:1487-1495.
122. Cioli D, Pica-Mattoccia L, Archer S. Antischistosomal drugs: past, present...and future? *Pharmacol Ther.* 1995;68:35-85.
123. Bühring KU, Diekmann HW, Müller H, Garbe A, Nowak H. Metabolism of praziquantel in man. *Eur J Drug Metab Pharmacokinet.* 1978;3:179-190.
124. Kapungu NN, Li X, Nhachi C, Masimirembwa C, Thelingwani RS. In vitro and in vivo human metabolism and pharmacokinetics of *S*- and *R*-praziquantel. *Pharmacol Res Perspect.* 2020;8:e00618.
125. Wang W, Wang L, Liang YS. Susceptibility or resistance of praziquantel in human schistosomiasis: a review. *Parasitol Res.* 2012;111:1871-1877.
126. Austin WC, Courtney W, Danilewicz JC, et al. Pyrantel tartrate, a new anthelmintic effective against infections of domestic animals. *Nature.* 1966;212:1273-1274.
127. Palmeirim MS, Specht S, Scandale I, et al. Preclinical and clinical characteristics of the trichuricidal drug oxantel pamoate and clinical development plans: a review. *Drugs.* 2021;81:907-921.
128. Narahashi T. Nerve membrane ionic channels as the primary target of pyrethroids. *Neurotoxicology.* 1985;6:3-22.
129. Vijverberg HP, de Weille JR. The interaction of pyrethroids with voltage-dependent Na channels. *Neurotoxicology.* 1985;6:23-34.
130. Soderlund DM. Pyrethroid-receptor interactions: stereospecific binding and effects on sodium channels in mouse brain preparations. *Neurotoxicology.* 1985;6:35-46.
131. Lombet A, Mourre C, Lazdunski M. Interaction of insecticides of the pyrethroid family with specific binding sites on the voltage-dependent sodium channel from mammalian brain. *Brain Res.* 1988;459:44-53.
132. Soderlund DM. Metabolic considerations in pyrethroid design. *Xenobiotica.* 1992;22:1185-1194.
133. Ruzo LO, Casida JE. Metabolism and toxicology of pyrethroids with dihalovinyl substituents. *Environ Health Perspect.* 1977;21:285-292.
134. Anand SS, Bruckner JV, Haines WT, et al. Characterization of deltamethrin metabolism by rat plasma and liver microsomes. *Toxicol Appl Pharmacol.* 2006;212:156-166.
135. Taplin D, Meinking TL, Chen JA, Sanchez R. Comparison of crotamiton 10% cream (Eurax) and permethrin 5% cream (Elimite) for the treatment of scabies in children. *Pediatr Dermatol.* 1990;7:67-73.
136. Amer M, el-Gharib I. Permethrin versus crotamiton and lindane in the treatment of scabies. *Int J Dermatol.* 1992;31:357-358.
137. Kittaka H, Yamanoi Y, Tominaga M. Transient receptor potential vanilloid 4 (TRPV4) channel as a target of crotamiton and its bimodal effects. *Pflugers Arch.* 2017;469:1313-1323.
138. Gaines TB. Acute toxicity of pesticides. *Toxicol Appl Pharmacol.* 1969;14:515-534.
139. Stough D, Shellabarger S, Quiring J, Gabrielsen AA Jr. Efficacy and safety of spinosad and permethrin creme rinses for pediculosis capitis (head lice). *Pediatrics.* 2009;124:e389-e395.
140. Salgado VL. Studies on the mode of action of spinosad: insect symptoms and physiological correlates. *Pestic Biochem Physiol.* 1998;60:91-102.
141. Salgado VL, Sheets JJ, Watson GB, Schmidt AL. Studies on the mode of action of spinosad: the internal effective concentration and the concentration dependence of neural excitation. *Pestic Biochem Physiol.* 1998;60:103-110.
142. Snyder DE, Meyer J, Zimmermann AG, et al. Preliminary studies on the effectiveness of the novel pulicide, spinosad, for the treatment and control of fleas on dogs. *Vet Parasitol.* 2007;150:345-351.

Structure Challenge Answers

1. Of the agents shown, Compound I, permethrin, and Compound IV, ivermectin (IVM), are available over the counter (OTC) for treatment of head lice. Permethrin possesses a similar mechanism of action as a related OTC agent, pyrethrins (Rid). The Pharmacist should note differences in the products' approval age for pediatric use, with permethrin being approved for use in children aged 2 months and older, while IVM is approved for children aged 6 months and older. The pharmacist should also be aware that there is a high resistance rate in head lice to permethrin, approaching 75% in some areas of the United States. This can result in treatment failure, even with repeated application. Depending on the local resistance rates, Pharmacists may need to consider suggesting either OTC IVM, or one of the agents available by prescription. The local health department is often a good source of information for head lice resistance rates.
2. Key counseling points for any head lice treatment are whether second application of the product is needed and whether the patient should use a nit comb to remove lice eggs following treatment. Both of these points typically depend on whether the agents possess ovicidal activity. Of the agents shown, both Compound III, spinosad (Natroba), and Compound IV, IVM (Sklice), do not generally require a second treatment application. Spinosad possesses ovicidal activity and IVM, while not technically ovicidal, has insecticidal activity against newly hatched lice (nymphs). According to their manufacturers, nit combing is not required for both these agents, though the pharmacist may consider counseling the patient or parents to purchase a special nit comb or use a fine-tooth comb to remove dead lice and nits. Permethrin and malathion are only partially ovicidal; hence, second treatment applications approximately 7 to 10 days after the initial treatment are currently recommended for both agents to kill newly hatched lice, and nit combing is typically required. Additional counseling points for malathion include cautioning the patient that they may notice the drug to possess a bad odor and to avoid the use of curling irons or hair dryers after applying due to the highly flammable formulation.

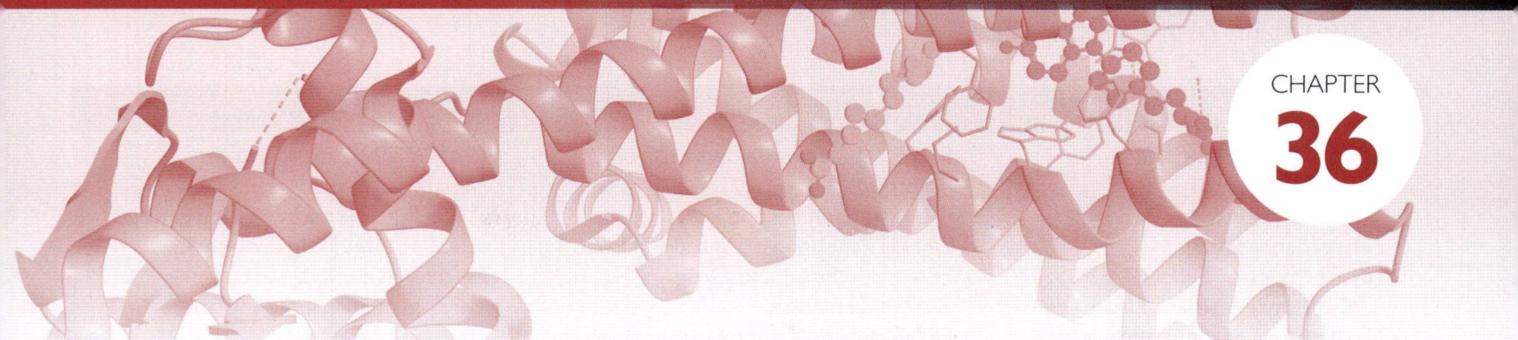

CHAPTER 36

Drugs Used to Treat Neoplastic Diseases—Classical Chemotherapy

Sushma Ramsinghani, Sonali Kurup, and Victoria F. Roche

Drugs covered in this chapter:

TOPOISOMERASE POISONS

CAMPTOTHECINS
- Irinotecan
- Topotecan

EPIPODOPHYLLOTOXINS
- Etoposide
- Teniposide

ANTHRACYCLINES AND ANTHRACENEDIONES
- Aldoxorubicin
- Daunorubicin
- Doxorubicin
- Epirubicin
- Idarubicin
- Mitoxantrone
- Valrubicin

MITOSIS INHIBITORS
- Cabazitaxel
- Docetaxel
- Eribulin
- Ixabepilone
- Paclitaxel
- Vinblastine
- Vincristine
- Vinorelbine

ANTIMETABOLITES

PURINE ANTAGONISTS
- Mercaptopurine
- Thioguanine

PYRIMIDINE ANTAGONISTS
- Capecitabine
- Floxuridine
- Fluorouracil

ANTIFOLATES
- Methotrexate
- Pemetrexed
- Pralatrexate

DNA POLYMERASE INHIBITORS
- Cladribine
- Clofarabine
- Cytarabine
- Fludarabine
- Gemcitabine
- Trifluridine/tipiracil

DNA METHYLTRANSFERASE INHIBITORS
- Azacitidine
- Decitabine
- Nelarabine

MISCELLANEOUS ANTIMETABOLITES
- Hydroxyurea
- Pentostatin

DNA-CROSSLINKING AGENTS

NITROGEN MUSTARDS
- Bendamustine
- Chlorambucil
- Cyclophosphamide
- Ifosfamide
- Mechlorethamine
- Melphalan
- Thiotepa

TRIAZENES AND PROCARBAZINE
- Dacarbazine
- Procarbazine
- Temozolomide

NITROSOUREAS
- Carmustine
- Lomustine
- Streptozocin

ORGANOPLATINUM COMPLEXES
- Carboplatin
- Cisplatin
- Oxaliplatin

MISCELLANEOUS DNA ALKYLATORS
- Busulfan

HORMONE-BASED ANTINEOPLASTIC AGENTS (REPRESENTATIVE)

AROMATASE INHIBITORS
- Anastrozole

ANTIESTROGENS
- Tamoxifen

ANTIANDROGENS
- Enzalutamide

GONADOTROPIN-RELEASING HORMONE MODULATORS
- Leuprolide
- Relugolix

MISCELLANEOUS ANTICANCER AGENTS
- Arsenic trioxide
- Asparaginase
- Bexarotene
- Bleomycin
- Dactinomycin
- Lurbinectedin
- Mitomycin
- Mitotane
- Trabectedin
- Tretinoin

Abbreviations

7,8-DHF 7,8-dihydrofolate
5-FU 5-fluorouracil
17β-HSD 17β-hydroxysteroid dehydrogenase
5,10-methylene THF 5,10-methylenetetrahydrofolate
6TGNs 6-thioguanine nucleotides
ABC adenosine triphosphate–binding cassette
ADC antibody-drug conjugate
AIC aminoimidazole-4-carboxamide
AKR aldo-keto reductase
ALL acute lymphoblastic leukemia
AML acute myeloid leukemia
AMP adenosine monophosphate
APL acute promyelocytic leukemia
ATP adenosine triphosphate
AUC area under the plasma concentration curve
BBB blood-brain barrier
BCG bacille Calmette-Guérin
BCRP breast cancer–resistance protein
CBR carbonyl reductase
CLL chronic lymphocytic leukemia
C_{max} maximum plasma concentration
CML chronic myelogenous leukemia
CNS central nervous system
CNU chloroethyl-containing nitrosourea
CRPC castration-resistant prostate cancer
CYP cytochrome P450
DACH diaminocyclohexane
DAMPA 4-deoxy-4-amino-N^{10}-methylpteroic acid
DCIS ductal carcinoma in situ
DDI drug-drug interaction
DHF dihydrofolate
DHFR dihydrofolate reductase
DNMT DNA methyltransferase
DPD dihydropyrimidine dehydrogenase
dTMP deoxythymidine monophosphate
dUMP deoxyuridine monophosphate
ECG electrocardiogram
EGCG epigallocatechin-3-gallate
EGF epidermal growth factor
EGFR epidermal growth factor receptor
ER, estrogen receptor
FAN1 Fanconi-associated nuclease 1
FDA U.S. Food and Drug Administration
FPGS folylpolyglutamate synthase
FSH follicle-stimulating hormone
FU fluorouracil
GAR glycinamide ribonucleotide
G-CSF granulocyte colony–stimulating factor
GFR glomerular filtration rate
GI gastrointestinal
GMP guanosine monophosphate
GnRH gonadotropin-releasing hormone
GnRH-R gonadotropin-releasing hormone receptor
GSH reduced glutathione
GTP guanosine triphosphate
HGPRT hypoxanthine-guanine phosphoribosyl transferase
HPV human papillomavirus
IM intramuscular
IMPDH inosine monophosphate dehydrogenase
ITP inosine triphosphate
ITPA inosine triphosphate pyrophosphatase
IV intravenous
LBL lymphoblastic lymphoma
LH luteinizing hormone
MAb monoclonal antibody
MAP microtubule-associated protein
MBC metastatic breast cancer
MDR multidrug resistance
miRNA microRNA
MLL mixed lineage leukemia
MMR mismatch repair
mRNA messenger RNA
MRP multidrug resistance–associated proteins
MTIC 3-methyl-(triazen-1-yl) imidazole-4-carboxamide
NAD(P)H nicotinamide adenine dinucleotide (phosphate) reduced
ncRNA noncoding RNA
NER nucleotide excision repair
NHL non-Hodgkin lymphoma
NSAIDs nonsteroidal anti-inflammatory drugs
NSCLC non–small cell lung cancer
NUDT15 nudix hydrolase 15
OS overall survival
PCFT proton-coupled folate transporter
PDGF platelet-derived growth factor
PFS progression-free survival
P-gp P-glycoprotein
Ph Philadelphia chromosome
PM poor metabolizer
PML promyelocytic gene
PSA prostate-specific antigen
RARG retinoid acid receptor γ
RARα retinoic acid receptor α
RFC1 reduced-folate carrier 1
RNAi RNA interference
ROS reactive oxygen species
SAM S-adenosylmethionine
SC subcutaneous
SCLC small cell lung cancer
SERM selective estrogen receptor modulator
SHMT serine hydroxymethyltransferase
SNP single nucleotide polymorphism
SPARC secreted *p*rotein *a*cidic and *r*ich in *c*ysteine
SPF sun protection factor
SSB single-strand breaks
SSBR single-strand break repair
STS soft tissue sarcoma
T-A thymine-adenine
TGN thioguanine nucleotide
TdGDP/TdGTP thio-deoxyguanosine-5′-di/triphosphate
TGTP thioguanosine triphosphate
THF tetrahydrofolate
TKI tyrosine kinase inhibitor
TopI topoisomerase type I
TopIIα topoisomerase type IIα
TPMT thiopurine methyl transferase
TS thymidylate synthase
VEGF vascular endothelial growth factor

CLINICAL SIGNIFICANCE

Doxorubicin is a versatile anticancer medication commonly known as the "red devil" for its brilliant red color, which is the result of extensive conjugation in its chemical structure. Patients should be counseled that the medication can color body fluids, such as sweat and urine, for approximately 48 hours after administration, and that this change is not caused by blood in the urine or other body fluids. More concerning is its lifetime dose dependent and potentially irreversible cardiotoxicity, the result of a long-lived "rubicinol" metabolite that sequesters in the myocardium. Clinicians will usually be conservative and avoid anthracycline in a new cancer diagnosis use, when efficacious alternatives exist, if the patient may have been previously exposed to these agents.

Bradi L. Frei, PharmD, MSc, BCPS, BCOP

CANCER

"*You gain strength, courage, and confidence by every experience in which you really stop to look fear in the face*" (Eleanor Roosevelt)

Eleanor Roosevelt's inspiring words are appropriate to this chapter's content, as the thought or confirmation of a cancer diagnosis is something that can strike fear in the hearts and minds of many.[1] Carcinophobia can run the gamut, from prognosis and longevity-related anxieties about the well-recognized adverse effects of classical chemotherapy to concerns about the impact on the emotional and financial well-being of loved ones. However, by looking fear in the face through scientifically grounded information and engaged partnerships with providers, patients and their families can find the strength and courage needed to make personalized care decisions, along with confidence in the potential of their choices to promote quality and extend the quantity of life.

Public Health Considerations

Despite a steady decline in cancer-related mortality over approximately three decades, this constellation of diseases continues to be the second leading cause of death in the United States.[2] Cronin et al[3] report that the overall incidence of cancer in the United States from 2014 to 2018 was 457.5 per 100,000 population, and cancer mortality from 2015 to 2019 was 152.4 per 100,000. The American Cancer Society makes annual projections for the number of new cancer cases and cancer-related deaths based on data from preceding years. In 2024, it was expected that there would be 2,001,140 new cases and 611,720 deaths from cancer in the United States. For males, prostate, lung, and colorectal cancers are the top three for new cases, while, in females, breast, lung, and colorectal cancers are at the top of the list. In both sexes, lung cancer is the leading cause of cancer-related mortality.[4]

Age, race/ethnicity, poverty, and access to health care resources for screening and treatment also impact cancer incidence and mortality risk, often in interconnected ways.[2,3] Regarding ethnicity, cancer mortality is significantly higher in American Indian/Alaska Native and Black populations compared to White populations, even when incident rates are lower, pointing to therapeutic inequities that demand the action-oriented attention of clinical practice and research communities.[2,3,5,6]

On the positive side, survival rates have been steadily increasing in many neoplastic disorders, in part due to routine screening protocols (eg, mammography, prostate-specific antigen [PSA], colonoscopy) and resultant early detection, risk attenuation (eg, smoking cessation), and the exploding development and availability of targeted small molecule-based therapies and immunotherapies (see Chapter 37).[3,5,6] The risk of developing cancers associated with diabetes, inactivity, and/or obesity (eg, pancreatic, thyroid, liver, and kidney) is still problematic but could conceivably be lowered through a "culture shift" that includes focused public health education and sustained personal commitments to behaviors and practices that promote overall health and wellness.[3,6]

As of January 1, 2019, there were approximately 16.9 million US citizens living with a cancer diagnosis, and that number is expected to climb to 22.2 million by 2030.[7] Garner et al[6] have projected that, from 2020 to 2040, a 29.5% increase in US yearly cancer diagnoses will exceed the anticipated 12.3% growth in population. Older adults and people of color are expected to be disproportionately impacted. As these authors state, "The burden of disease will remain substantial" into the foreseeable future.

Economic Considerations

Economically, the impact of active treatment and chronic disease management on individuals, families, and communities can be staggering. Yabroff et al[8] confirm that cancer is one of the most financially burdensome diseases and that the cost of care is rising due to the diverse array of expensive new treatment options and advances in diagnostics. In 2019, the national economic impact on patients, including out-of-pocket and time costs, was estimated at $21.1 billion. Out-of-pocket expense (including prescription drugs) varies with diagnosis and stage but is generally highest when therapy is initiated (and co-pays are steep) and in the terminal phase of life. The authors evaluated cost data for Medicare eligible and younger patient cohorts and warned of the risk of financial hardship leading to treatment delays or termination when patients are uninsured or underinsured.[8]

In addition to direct medical care and prescription drug expenses, patients with cancer and their families can incur additional costs related to adverse effects, support therapy, mental health services, childcare, transportation and caregiving expenses, cosmetic support, and lost wages. For myriad reasons, the importance of cancer prevention through healthy lifestyle choices and routine screenings that detect early-stage diseases that may require less aggressive (and less costly) therapy cannot be overstated.[9]

Etiology

Healthy cells are under strict biochemical control for growth and differentiation. Cells divide and proliferate under the influence of various growth stimulators and are subject to arrested growth (senescence) and programmed cell death (apoptosis). In cancer, these regulatory processes have gone awry, and cells grow and divide uncontrollably, consuming energy and losing both structure and function. Rampant cell division is accompanied by disabled cell death processes, leading first to cellular immortality and, eventually, to genetic instability.[10,11]

The causes of cancer are many and varied, including chemical, environmental, viral, and mutagenic etiologies. Proto-oncogenes and tumor-suppressor genes play an important role in normal cell differentiation and proliferation. Mutation in these genes can push cell proliferation into overdrive.[10,11] As cancer progresses, cellular proliferation leads to augmented invasion of the primary site and migration to new tissues through the bloodstream or lymphatic system in a process called metastasis.[11] Staging is an essential prerequisite for the prediction of prognosis and the identification of the most appropriate treatment plan and dosing regimen. Taking into consideration the tumor mass size, extent of lymph node involvement, and the presence/absence of distant metastases, a comprehensive staging scale has been developed that ranges from I (localized) to IV (metastatic). The intermediate disease severity stages indicate local (stage II) or regional (stage III) tissue invasion.[11]

Many cancers have the ability to generate new blood vessels (angiogenesis) to ensure an ongoing supply of essential nutrients and to provide an escape route for meandering cells to travel to distant sites and initiate metastatic disease. Vascular endothelial growth factor (VEGF) and platelet-derived growth factor (PDGF) promote angiogenesis and serve as the molecular targets of some protein kinase inhibitor antineoplastic agents (see Chapter 37). Fortunately, there are many opportunities within the metastatic cascade for the body to mount an immunologic defense designed to destroy the would-be invaders.

Environmental carcinogens are all around us (Table 36.1),[12] but individuals can protect themselves from exposure through smoking cessation, low (or no) alcohol consumption, using high-SPF (sun protection factor) sunscreens, eating foods low in fat but rich in carotenoids, vitamins A and C, folate, selenium, and/or fiber, and vaccinating against human papillomavirus (HPV).

Table 36.1 Some Environmental and Viral Carcinogens and Cancer Types

Carcinogen	Cancer Type
Tobacco	Lung, oral, bladder, pancreatic, stomach, and renal cancer
Alcohol	Liver, rectal, and breast cancer
Ionizing and ultraviolet radiation	Leukemia, breast, thyroid, lung, and skin cancer
Halogenated compounds	Bladder cancer
Radon	Lung cancer
Hepatitis B, C virus	Hepatocellular carcinoma
Human papillomavirus (HPV)	Cervical, skin, and anogenital cancer

Historical Evolution of Cancer Chemotherapy[13,14]

In the 1940s, cortisone and prednisone were among the first nonmetallic therapeutic agents to show benefit in the treatment of cancer (acute leukemia). In the same decade, the retrospective recognition that World War I soldiers exposed to sulfur mustard gas suffered from damaged lymphoid tissue and bone marrow led to the development of cytotoxic nitrogen mustards for the treatment of lymphoma. Conjugating aromatic rings with the mustard nitrogen led to less reactive agents that were orally active and less systemically toxic. More recently, the oxazaphosphorine-based prodrug mustards cyclophosphamide and ifosfamide have enjoyed widespread clinical use in the treatment of hematologic cancers, and testicular cancer and pediatric solid tumors, respectively.

The discovery in 1940 that *p*-aminobenzenesulfonamide (sulfanilamide) inhibited the bacterial synthesis of folic acid and was effective against streptococcal infections ushered in the era of antimetabolite chemotherapy. Antifolate antineoplastics, which were shown to be effective in combating childhood leukemias, were developed in the late 1940s. Antimetabolites based on the structures of endogenous purine and pyrimidine bases followed in the mid to late 1950s. Perhaps the most exciting discovery in this regard was the recognition that a very simple analog of the endogenous pyrimidine uracil (5-fluorouracil [5-FU]) was a potent inhibitor of deoxythymidine monophosphate (dTMP) biosynthesis and that inhibiting the production of this essential nucleotide produced positive results in patients suffering from colon, stomach, pancreatic, and breast cancers. Antimetabolites that target DNA polymerase (eg, gemcitabine) were first conceptualized and synthesized in the late 1950s and have found use in a variety of solid tumor and hematologic cancers.

The antibiotic antineoplastics came into clinical utility when the highly toxic actinomycin (discovered in the 1940s) was found to be effective in the treatment of human testicular cancer and uterine choriocarcinoma. In the 1960s, other natural anticancer antibiotics, such as bleomycin, were subsequently found to be active against various hematologic cancers and solid tumors, which led to the development of semisynthetic analogs with both high potency and wider margins of safety. The antimitotic vinca alkaloids, vincristine and vinblastine, were shown to have activity against Hodgkin disease and acute lymphoblastic leukemia (ALL) around the same time that the antibiotic antineoplastics were being developed.

Cancer chemotherapy appeared to come full circle since the "metal-intense renaissance" with the introduction of organometallic platinum complexes in the early 1970s. The fortuitous discovery of organoplatinum complexes in the treatment of cancer is attributed to Dr. Barnett Rosenberg, who was studying the impact of electromagnetic radiation on bacterial cell growth using platinum electrodes.[15] He followed up on the astute observation that the bacteria exposed to the electrodes experienced profound changes in cellular structure, which ultimately were attributed to the in situ generation of cisplatin, the first organoplatinum complex to be marketed. Subsequent additions to the organoplatinum complex family were designed to either attenuate use-limiting toxicity (carboplatin) or overcome cisplatin resistance (oxaliplatin). In addition to organometallics, the efficacy of sex hormones and hormone antagonists in fighting hormone-dependent cancers (eg, estrogen receptor [ER]–positive breast cancer or prostate cancer, see Chapter 25) and the advent of therapeutic biologic response modifiers with direct antiproliferative effects (eg, interferons) have added significantly to the therapeutic options available to providers and the patients for whom they care.

The late 1990s saw the ground-breaking introduction of tyrosine kinase inhibitors (TKIs) to the chemotherapeutic war chest, which ushered in a new era of targeted cancer chemotherapy (see Chapter 37).[16] Targeted therapies often provide safer and more effective treatment options compared to the classical/traditional chemotherapeutic agents discussed in this chapter. The recognition in 1960 that a mutant chromosome known as BCR-ABL (or the Philadelphia chromosome [Ph]) appeared consistently in the cells of patients with chronic myelogenous leukemia (CML) represented the first time a chromosomal aberration had been directly linked to a neoplastic disorder. The product of this abbreviated chromosome, the Bcr-Abl protein, is an unregulated tyrosine kinase that promotes cellular proliferation at the expense of apoptosis. Imatinib, the first rationally designed drug in the TKI class,[17] was made available in 2001 and dramatically changed the treatment and clinical outcome of Ph+ leukemias. Although imatinib selectively targets the Bcr-Abl protein, inhibitors with selectivity for a multitude of other cancer-promoting kinases soon followed. Several monoclonal antibodies (MAbs) targeted to tumor cell antigens or proteins critical to cellular proliferation (eg, human epidermal growth factor [EGF], VEGF, tyrosine kinase, and proteasomes) have also found their way to the US market (see Chapter 37).

Molecules derived from plant or marine animal sources have also demonstrated value either as cytotoxic chemotherapeutic agents themselves or as synthetic springboards to anticancer drugs that can be readily produced in the laboratory.[13] Prime examples of anticancer drugs or precursors found in plants include paclitaxel and its precursor 10-deacetylbaccatin III, the vinca alkaloids vincristine and vinblastine, podophyllotoxin (precursor to the epipodophyllotoxins etoposide and teniposide), and camptothecin (precursor to topotecan and irinotecan). Sea sponges have added cytarabine and eribulin to the array of available therapeutic options.

General Principles of Cancer Chemotherapy[18-21]

The advent of cancer therapy began with drugs that target the cell cycle to cause cytotoxic effects of cell death (apoptosis). These nonselective drugs are now considered in the realm of classical chemotherapy, with newer, target-specific drugs prominent in contemporary drug design, discovery, and development. Although the cytotoxic agents are "older" drugs, they continue to have an invaluable place in cancer chemotherapy.

Cell division in normal cells occurs in a controlled manner. When like cells come in contact with each other, further cell division is inhibited (contact inhibition), and the cells become quiescent in the G_0 phase until cell division is needed again to sustain life. In contrast, due to some malignant transformations, cancer cells divide more frequently and in an uncontrolled manner. To maintain this pace of cell division, cancer cells have an accelerated activity of nucleotide synthesis, DNA replication, and RNA and protein synthesis. The cytotoxic drugs target and hinder these activities in a variety of ways, such as mimicking a metabolite and inhibiting cellular nucleotide synthesis, inserting into DNA or RNA to interfere with the nucleic acid synthesis, interfering with topoisomerase function of relieving DNA supercoils, modifying DNA structure through alkylation or cross-linking, or interfering with the mitotic phase of the cell cycle. The severity of these interferences and an inability to overcome them cause the cancer cells to undergo apoptosis.

The difference between the rapid cell division of cancer cells and the slower division of normal cells provides some measure of selectivity for the cytotoxic drugs, although it is not as distinct as that seen for antibiotics used against microbial infections. This is partly because the cancer cells originate from a normal cell where some cellular features or activities have gone awry (eg, mutated genes). However, cell morphology or biochemical processes in the cancer cell are not different enough to allow for the drug to bind to an exclusive target. The cytotoxic drugs, ideally go after the rapid cell division of cancer cells sparing the normal cells that are quiescent. Unfortunately, certain normal cells that undergo rapid proliferation, such as those of the blood (produced in bone marrow), hair follicles, and mucosa of the mouth and digestive tract, also come under attack. Thus, myelosuppression (with increased risk of infection, anemia, or bleeding), hair loss, and nausea/vomiting are common adverse effects associated with cytotoxic drugs. These adverse effects are generally reversible and resolve with the withdrawal of chemotherapy. However, other adverse effects such as cardiotoxicity or neurotoxicity associated with some cytotoxic drugs can be chronic and irreversible in nature.

When the cytotoxic drugs target a single feature of the cell cycle, they can be described as cell cycle specific (eg, antimetabolites target the S phase, while antimitotic taxanes target the M phase). Cell cycle–nonspecific agents produce their effect in any phase of the cell cycle including the G_0 phase (eg,

DNA-alkylating drugs). Not all cancer cells will die with just one round of treatment, and the cells that are not killed will continue to proliferate. For this reason, several rounds of chemotherapy are given in an attempt to achieve remission. Chemotherapy regimens are often designed with periods of rest between rounds of chemotherapy to allow normal cells to recover from the toxic effects of drugs. Further, chemotherapy regimens often include a combination of drugs to attack the cancer cells through different mechanistic targets to minimize the development of resistance to treatment and sometimes allow for a reduction in drug doses. Finally, cytotoxic drugs can be used in different settings for their chemotherapeutic effect. In induction therapy, they constitute the primary treatment and are considered the best option for the cancer. In neoadjuvant therapy, they are used to shrink the size of a tumor for a better surgical or radiation outcome, and in adjuvant therapy, they are utilized after primary surgery or radiation treatment to eliminate any remaining cancer cells and decrease the chance of a relapse.

Resistance to Cancer Chemotherapy

Unfortunately, cancer cells do not always succumb to chemotherapeutic intervention but, rather, can "fight back" in an attempt to retain immortality. Some cancer cells acquire resistance to anticancer drugs by downregulating enzymes and carriers essential for drug transport, for the activation of antineoplastic prodrugs, or by upregulating the enzymes inhibited by the drug. Other mechanisms of cancer cell retaliation include downregulation of target enzymes or antigens, activation of kinase-associated biochemical pathways, altered drug uptake, activation of cellular repair pathways, apoptosis inhibition, and upregulated drug efflux mechanisms. Efflux proteins involved in cancer chemotherapy resistance include classic multidrug resistance (MDR, eg, P-glycoprotein [P-gp]) and multidrug resistance–associated proteins (MRP).[22]

It has been estimated that up to 90% of cancer-related deaths can be linked in some way to intrinsic (phenotype-related) or acquired resistance to therapy,[23] and the identification and development of compounds that combat acquired resistance is an active area of research. Fortunately, in addition to chemotherapeutic agents and precursors, Mother Nature's medicine cabinet is known to house molecules with this desirable property,[24] underscoring the need to actively preserve the world's natural resources for generations to come.

Therapeutic Classes of Anticancer Drugs

The remainder of this chapter will focus on the cytotoxic drugs that either enjoy widespread clinical use or are considered first- or second-line therapy in very specific indications with narrowly defined patient populations.

Topoisomerase Poisons

Topoisomerases are enzymes that control the degree of DNA supercoiling and, in so doing, maintain proper DNA structure during replication and transcription.[25] Type I topoisomerase (topI) cleaves one strand of the DNA, allows the other strand to pass through it, and then rejoins the cleaved DNA strand. Type II topoisomerase (topII) cleaves both strands of the DNA, allows the passage of another double-stranded DNA segment through the cleavage, and then rejoins the cleaved DNA.[26] The cleaving and rejoining (religation) of DNA by topI and topII increases or decreases supercoiling by one and two twists, respectively.[27] The α and β isoforms of topII differ in their cellular expression. While topIIβ is expressed in all cells, topIIα is expressed mostly in rapidly proliferating cells with maximum expression occurring in the S and G_2 phases.[28] Many cancer cells have an increased expression or activity of topI or topIIα making these enzymes a target for cancer therapy. Antineoplastic agents that function as topoisomerase poisons allow the DNA cleavage reaction to occur but inhibit the DNA rejoining activity of the enzymes, leaving the DNA irreversibly damaged and unable to replicate. The "poisoning" effect manifests wherein the topoisomerase becomes a "toxic enzyme" that fragments the DNA leading to cell death.[27,29]

Three chemically distinct classes of anticancer agents can be classified as topoisomerase poisons: camptothecins, epipodophyllotoxins, and anthracyclines and related anthracenediones. The common feature in the mechanism of action of all three classes is the stabilization of the drug-topoisomerase-DNA ternary complex, which prevents DNA replication or transcription.

Camptothecins

Mechanism of Action. Camptothecins are chiral, extensively conjugated pentacyclic lactones (Fig. 36.1). The biologic target of camptothecins is topI. The binding of camptothecins occurs in such a way as to stabilize a covalent DNA-topoisomerase bond at the point of single-strand breakage (Tyr723 on the human enzyme) but sterically prevent the topI Lys532 residue from catalyzing the DNA religation reaction.[30,31] The binding pocket, located within the DNA strand, is revealed only after the normal DNA cleavage has occurred, explaining why these poisons preferentially bind to the enzyme–DNA complex rather than to the DNA or enzyme by itself. This stable ternary complex neither allows for the rejoining of cleaved DNA nor for the dissociation of topI from the DNA. When the replication fork encounters the ternary complex, shear stress induces a double-stranded DNA break, killing the cell.[32] Camptothecins are most toxic to cells undergoing active DNA replication and cell division (ie, they are S-G_2 phase specific).[32]

The flat camptothecin ring system intercalates into DNA at the site of cleavage, mimicking a DNA base pair.[31] The crystal structures of human ternary complexes involving the parent alkaloid, camptothecin (the water-insoluble natural product), and the semisynthetic analog, topotecan, have been determined, and important drug-protein interacting entities are noted in Table 36.2.[30,31,33] The C_7, C_9, and/or C_{10} substituents of the marketed compounds, which project into the major groove of DNA, do not hinder binding and may actually enhance it through hydrophobic and/or H-bonding interactions.[34] Position 7 is viewed as the most favorable for activity-enhancing modifications, as the

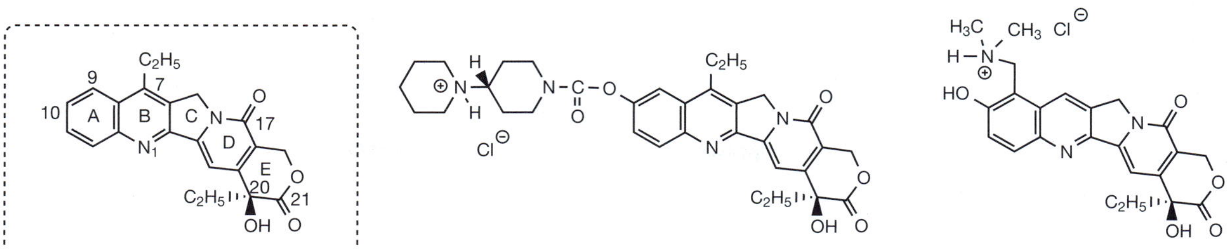

Camptothecin (water insoluble natural product)

Irinotecan hydrochloride (Camptosar, Onivyde)

Topotecan hydrochloride (Hycamtin)

Figure 36.1 Camptothecin topoisomerase I (TopI) poisons.

topI region accommodating substituents at this position is spacious.[35]

Proposed camptothecin resistance mechanisms are similar to those operational in many other classes of cytotoxic antineoplastic drugs, including downregulation or mutation of the target enzyme and cellular efflux. Breast cancer-resistance protein (BCRP) and MRPs, MAP-2 (microtubule-associated protein-2) and MAP-3 (rather than P-gp), have been suggested as resistance mediators. Another resistance mechanism at play could be the exposure of single-strand breaks (SSB) that trigger single-strand break repair (SSBR) processes following proteasomal destruction of topI.[36] TopI degradation in diseased cells is distinct from enzyme processing in healthy cells, and the extent of topI-Ser10 phosphorylation in tumors appears directly related to the rate of ubiquitin tagging, proteasome-mediated destruction, and camptothecin resistance.[37]

Chemistry. The parent camptothecin alkaloid, isolated from the bark of *Camptotheca acuminata* (the Chinese xi shu or "happy tree"),[32,38] has antitumor activity, but its limited water solubility necessitated delivery as the sodium salt of the significantly less active hydrolyzed lactone. Lactonization of the hydroxy acid in acidic urine is significant, and elevated levels of active intact alkaloids in the kidney accounted for the hemorrhagic cystitis induced by this compound. For these reasons, the development of this natural product as a chemotherapeutic agent was abandoned in the 1970s.[32] It would take another two decades before the currently available agents, irinotecan and topotecan, received U.S. Food and Drug Administration (FDA) approval.

Table 36.2 Topotecan Topoisomerase I Interactions

Topotecan Functional Group	Topoisomerase I Residue
Pyridine N_1	Arg364
C_{10}-OH	Enzyme-associated water (H-bond)
C_{17}-pyridone carbonyl	Asn722
C_{20}-OH	Asp533 (H-bond)
C_{21}-lactone carbonyl	Tyr723-phosphate, Lys532

While camptothecin's quinoline ring system is primarily unsubstituted, the currently marketed analogs have a basic side chain incorporated at either C_9 (topotecan) or C_{10} (irinotecan), allowing the formation of water-soluble salts of the intact semisynthetic alkaloid. At a pH of 7.4, the active lactone exists in equilibrium with the hydroxy acid hydrolysis product, with the direction dictated by the extent of binding to serum albumin. The preferential protein binding of the lactone, which occurs with irinotecan, shifts the equilibrium to favor the production of the more active lactone, thus enhancing potency.

While only two camptothecin analogs are available clinically, there is an interest in mining this structural prototype for novel agents of therapeutic value. A quantitative study on camptothecin structure-property relationships has been published,[39] along with reviews summarizing the current literature on the chemical and pharmacologic activities of both well-known and new entities.[32,34,40]

Specific Drugs

Irinotecan Hydrochloride

Conventional Formulation. In combination with 5-FU and leucovorin, irinotecan is considered first-line therapy in the treatment of metastatic colorectal cancer and can be used as second-line therapy in 5-FU-resistant patients. With a 22% increase in 1-year survival in 5-FU refractory disease (monotherapy), and overall survival (OS) beyond 30 months when combined with 5-FU/leucovorin/oxaliplatin/bevacizumab in clinical trials, irinotecan is a major player in colorectal cancer chemotherapy.[41] Fortunately, no significant drug-drug interactions (DDIs) with commonly coadministered chemotherapeutic agents have been noted.[42]

Given intravenously (IV) at a usual initial dose of 125 mg/m^2, conventional irinotecan is slowly bioactivated in the liver through hydrolysis of the C_{10}-carbamate ester. The metabolite, known as SN-38, is 100 to 1,000 times more active than the parent drug (Fig. 36.2). The organic anion transporter, OATP1B1, facilitates hepatic uptake of irinotecan, and the primary activating enzyme is the saturable carboxylesterase CES2. Butyrylcholinesterase can also activate irinotecan in plasma.[42] Levels of SN-38 are 50 to 100 times lower than the parent drug, but preferential protein binding of the lactone (95%) permits significant plasma levels of SN-38 compared to the less active hydroxy acid metabolite. There is significant individual variability in kinetics and clearance for irinotecan (30%) and SN-38 (80%), and an SN-38 terminal half-life of between 6 and 32 hours has been reported (compared

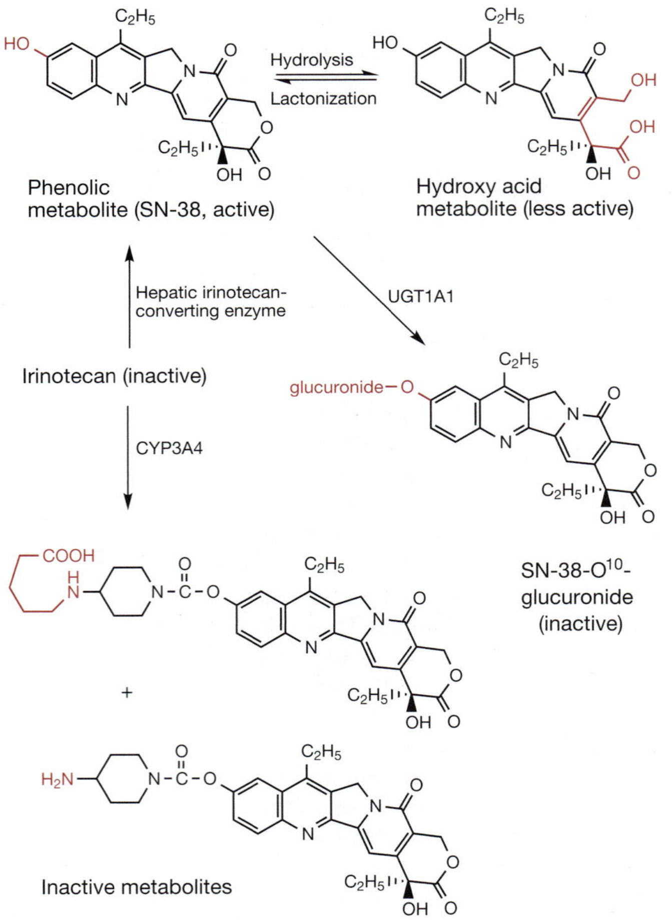

Figure 36.2 Irinotecan metabolism.

to 5-18 hours for the prodrug).[41,42] The cytochrome P450 (CYP) isozyme CYP3A4 cleaves the terminal piperidine ring through oxidation at the α-carbons, which is followed by hydrolysis of the resultant amides to inactive metabolites. Drug-induced toxicity can be exacerbated if strong CYP3A4 inhibitors are coadministered. Prior to elimination, irinotecan is glucuronidated by UGT1A1 or sulfonated at the C_{10} phenol. Elimination of the parent drug and all metabolites except SN-38 glucuronide is predominantly fecal (66%), and biliary excretion is facilitated by adenosine triphosphate (ATP)–binding cassette (ABC) transporter proteins.[41,42]

Diarrhea is a hallmark irinotecan adverse effect, potentially exacerbated by coadministered 5-FU. Acute episodes that can begin during drug administration are attributed to acetylcholinesterase inhibition. Pretreatment with an anticholinergic agent (eg, atropine) can effectively address this toxicity and help patients avoid "cholinergic syndrome," a collection of effects that include abdominal pain, sweating, blurred vision, and less commonly, bradycardia. The delayed diarrhea that occurs approximately 7 to 10 days post-administration is attributed to drug-induced mucosal damage. It is dose limiting, potentially fatal, and the primary impetus behind a boxed warning. Vigorous loperamide therapy should be instituted at the first sign of symptoms, and fluid, electrolytes, and antibiotics should be administered as needed. Camptothecins are also myelosuppressive, and neutropenia (also potentially worsened by 5-FU) can be severe, particularly in females and patients with elevated bilirubin levels or prolonged systemic exposure to SN-38.[42] Extensive biotransformation also demands cautious use of irinotecan in patients with hepatic dysfunction. Prophylactic antiemetic therapy should be given at least 30 minutes before the administration of irinotecan to minimize the nausea and vomiting associated with this anticancer agent.

Some patients may be pharmacogenetically predisposed to serious camptothecin-induced toxicity. Variations in the expression of genes involved in the inactivating glucuronidation of irinotecan, specifically overexpression of the low activity UGT*1A1*6* and UGT*1A1*28* alleles more common in Asian and White populations, respectively, are deemed responsible. Doses must be decreased in patients homozygous (eg, UGT*1A1*28/*28*, **6/*6*) or double heterozygous (eg, UGT*1A1*6/*28*) for these poor metabolizer (PM) alleles to circumvent life-threatening neutropenia and diarrhea. Dose reduction by at least one dose level is recommended and precise dose reduction guidelines are available.[42,43] While not yet standard procedure, genotyping prior to initiating therapy can more safely and effectively individualize therapy in at-risk individuals.[41,44,45]

Liposomal Formulation. A pegylated nanoliposomal formulation of irinotecan is marketed as Onivyde for use in combination with 5-FU/leucovorin in patients with metastatic pancreatic adenocarcinoma who have relapsed after gemcitabine (DNA polymerase inhibitor) therapy.[46] The usual starting dose of 70 mg/m^2 should be reduced to 50 mg/m^2 in UGT*1A1*28/*28* carriers and slowly increased as tolerated. As with most liposomal formulations, the drug is stable in circulation and is preferentially taken up and retained for a longer time in the tumor cell. This results in a more potent therapeutic effect with fewer adverse reactions, although the boxed warning for life-threatening neutropenia and diarrhea noted for the conventional formulation still applies. The elimination $t_{1/2}$ of liposomal irinotecan and SN-38 is approximately 26 and 68 hours, respectively, significantly longer than the half-lives of these entities after conventional IV administration (6-12 hours for irinotecan and 10-20 hours for SN-38).[43] Binding to serum proteins is blocked by the polyethylene glycol attached to the liposomal surface.

Clinical trials have documented the value of liposomal irinotecan in prolonging median OS, progression-free survival (PFS), and objective response rate in metastatic pancreatic adenocarcinoma compared to 5-FU/leucovorin alone.[46] A combination therapy of nanoliposomal irinotecan, 5-FU/leucovorin, and oxaliplatin (Nalirifox) was approved in 2024 as a first-line treatment for metastatic pancreatic adenocarcinoma.[47] As with conventional IV irinotecan, pretreatment with antiemetic and anticholinergic medications prior to infusion is advised.

A targeted therapy, sacituzumab govitecan-hziy, is an antibody-drug conjugate (ADC) of a humanized MAb hRS7 and SN-38 approved in 2023 (see Chapter 37) for refractory, metastatic triple-negative breast cancer.[43,48]

Topotecan[43,49]. This active camptothecin analog is used by the IV route in the treatment of ovarian, cervical, and small cell lung cancer (SCLC) that has either not responded to or relapsed after first-line therapy. An oral dosage form is available for use in relapsed SCLC. The drug carries a boxed warning for myelosuppression, particularly neutropenia, which precludes combination therapy with other bone marrow-suppressing drugs. Thrombocytopenia and anemia occur in approximately one-third of treated patients.

When administered IV, topotecan is commonly infused in doses of 1.5 mg/m^2 for 5 consecutive days of a 21-day cycle in ovarian and SCLC, and at 0.75 mg/m^2 on days 1 to 3 of a 21-day cycle in recurrent/resistant cervical cancer. Schedules that call for 5 consecutive days of administration can result in serious mucositis and diarrhea. For the oral formulation, the appropriate number of 1 and 0.25 mg capsules is administered to provide a final dose of 2.3 mg/m^2 (rounded to the nearest 0.25 mg). Oral absorption is rapid, and bioavailability approaches 40%.

Topotecan elimination is biphasic with a terminal half-life of 2 to 3 hours after IV administration. Plasma clearance is approximately 24% higher in males, but pharmacokinetic behavior after oral administration appears gender independent. Lactone hydrolysis is rapid, reversible, and pH dependent, and binding to serum proteins is limited to approximately 35%. CYP3A4-mediated N-dealkylation to mono- and di-dealkylated metabolites occurs to a limited extent, and the O-glucuronides that form at multiple points along the metabolic path are excreted via the kidney (Fig. 36.3). Extensive renal clearance demands dosage adjustment in patients with kidney disease.

Because both topotecan and irinotecan are metabolized by CYP3A4, coadministration of strong CYP3A4 inducers and inhibitors should be avoided. It has been reported that Asian patients have greater topotecan exposure than White patients with similar renal function, and the possibility of a genetic difference in the ABCG2 transporter (specifically, the potential for a Q141K mutant in Asians that can increase oral bioavailability) was proposed.[50] The total topotecan exposure difference in patients with normal renal function is 30% and rises to 60% to 70% in moderate-to-severe impairment. Unlike irinotecan, no correlation of topotecan toxicity to UGT1A1 polymorphism has been reported thus far.

There is no topotecan liposomal formulation currently marketed, in part because of difficulties with low encapsulation efficiency and rapid plasma clearance, although explorations to address these challenges are ongoing.[50-52] Nanotechnology approaches to topotecan delivery are also being actively investigated.[53,54]

Epipodophyllotoxins

The epipodophyllotoxins (Fig. 36.4) are semisynthetic glycosidic derivatives of podophyllotoxin, the major component of the resinous podophyllin isolated from the dried roots of the American mandrake or mayapple plant (*Podophyllum peltatum*). Although these compounds are capable of binding to tubulin and inhibiting mitosis, their primary mechanism of antineoplastic action is topIIα poisoning, a mechanism that they share with anthracyclines (see next section). TopIIα cleaves double-stranded DNA via a transesterification reaction involving a topoisomerase Tyr residue and the 5′-phosphate of the 3′,5′-phosphodiester bond. After strand passage, the enzyme religates the cleaved DNA by reverse transesterification aided by ATP binding and hydrolysis.[55] TopIIα has two distinct DNA-independent binding sites for the epipodophyllotoxins, one within the catalytic domain and a second within the N-terminal ATP-binding domain.[56] Once bound, the toxins stabilize the ternary complex and inhibit DNA resealing. The DNA-topoisomerase fragments accumulate in the cell, ultimately resulting in apoptosis. The RNA transcription processes are also disrupted by the interaction of epipodophyllotoxins with topIIα.

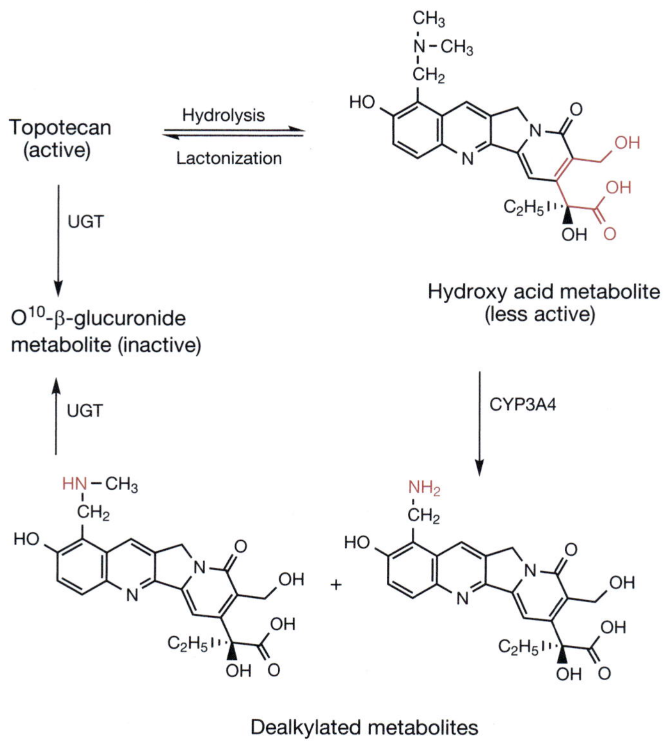

Figure 36.3 Topotecan metabolism.

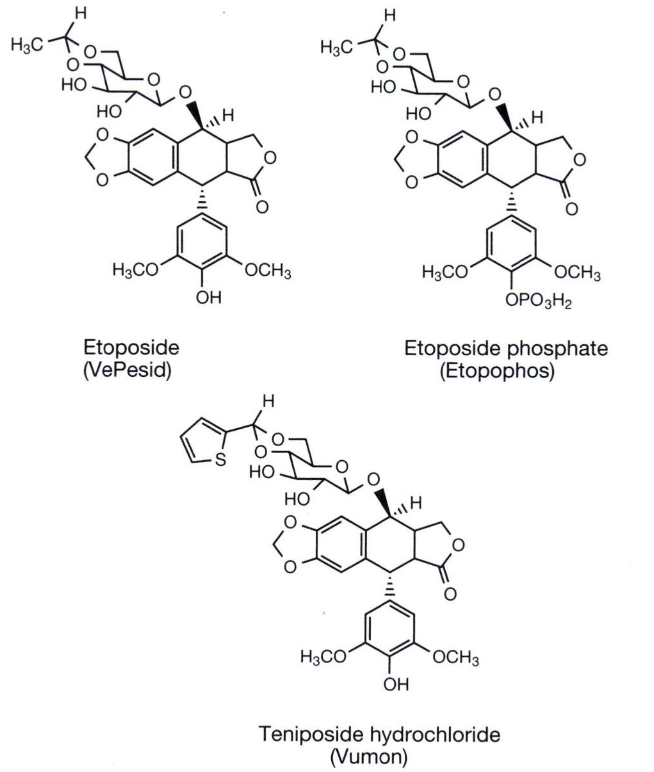

Figure 36.4 Epipodophyllotoxin topoisomerase IIα (TopIIα) poisons.

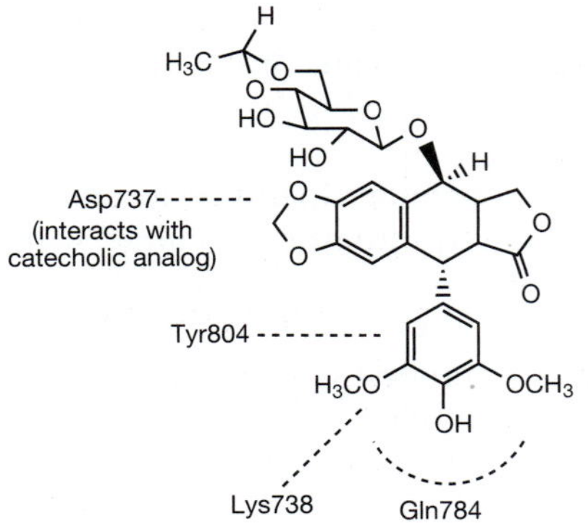

Figure 36.5 Proposed etoposide-TopIIα binding interactions.

The epipodophyllotoxin binding site has been probed with a carbene-generating diazirine photoaffinity label,[57] and a virtual library of 143 epipodophyllotoxin derivatives has been docked to a three-dimensional human topIIα receptor model to identify key drug–enzyme interactions (Fig. 36.5).[58] An X-ray crystal of two etoposide molecules bound in a ternary complex with cleaved DNA and topIIβ (an isoform found in myocardium) has been solved, documenting that the area that binds the glycoside moiety of epipodophyllotoxins is unhindered.[59]

Epipodophyllotoxins are cell cycle specific and have their most devastating impact on cells in the S or early G_2 phase. For this reason, doses are divided and administered over several days. Resistance is multifaceted and involves downregulation of topIIα, attenuation of enzymatic activity levels, development of novel DNA repair mechanisms, and P-gp–mediated cellular efflux.

CHEMISTRY. Structurally, the two marketed epipodophyllotoxins, etoposide and teniposide, differ only in the nature of one β-D-glucopyranosyl substituent (methyl or thienyl, respectively). Both are highly water insoluble, but teniposide's higher lipophilicity facilitates cellular uptake and results in a 10-fold enhancement of potency. The need for solubility enhancers, such as polysorbate 80 (Tween, etoposide) or polyoxyethylated castor oil (Kolliphor EL, teniposide), in IV formulations puts patients at risk for hypersensitivity reactions that can manifest as hypotension and thrombophlebitis. Antihistamines and corticosteroids are often coadministered to minimize this toxic liability. A water-soluble phosphate ester analog of etoposide can be administered in standard aqueous vehicles, permitting higher doses than the oil-modified formulations would allow. The phosphate ester is rapidly cleaved to the free alcohol in the bloodstream.

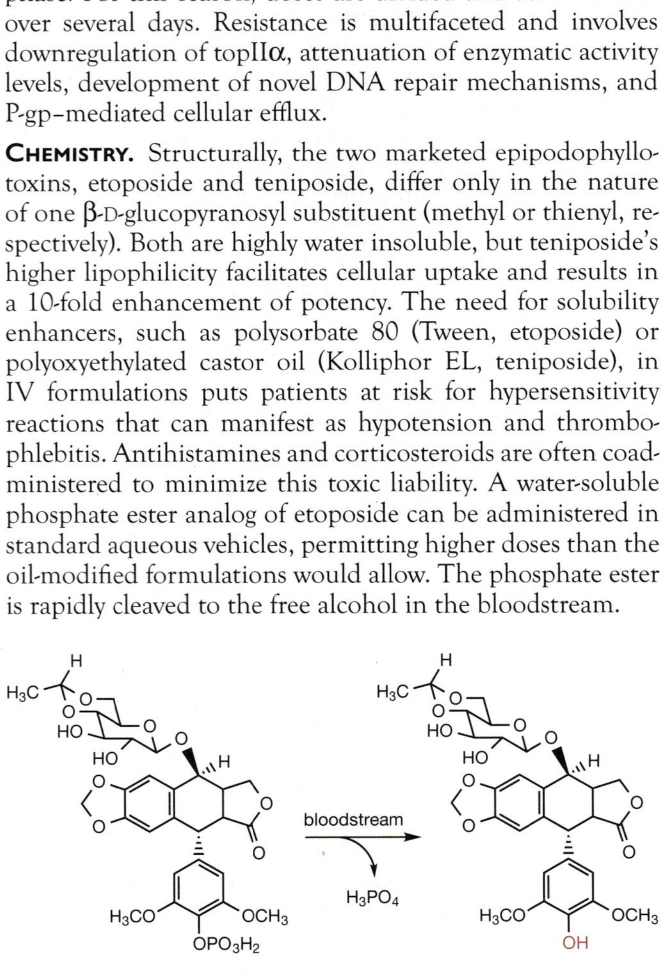

Etoposide phosphate Etoposide

METABOLISM. Epipodophyllotoxins are subject to metabolic transformation before renal and biliary elimination (Fig. 36.6). Etoposide is stable enough for oral administration, although a dose approximately twice that of the IV formulation must be administered.[43] Teniposide is more extensively metabolized, presumably due to its enhanced ability to penetrate hepatocytes, and no oral dosage form is marketed. Both drugs undergo lactone hydrolysis to generate the inactive hydroxy acid as the major metabolite, but the parent drugs can also be transformed by CYP3A4-catalyzed O-demethylation and phase 2 glucuronide or sulfate conjugation. Phase 2 metabolism accounts for between 5% and 22% of the dose. Clinically significant interactions between epipodophyllotoxins and CYP3A4 inducers have been documented, and coadministration can enhance antineoplastic drug clearance by as much as 77%. Conversely, CYP3A4 inhibitors can decrease clearance, leading to unwanted toxicity.

Both etoposide and teniposide carry a boxed warning for severe myelosuppression that can result in infection (leukopenia) or hemorrhage (thrombocytopenia). Teniposide's warning extends to hypersensitivity due to the need for the more problematic solubilizer, Kolliphor EL. The catechol metabolite can oxidize to a reactive orthoquinone, and both have been proposed to promote topoisomerase-mediated DNA cleavage, potentially enhancing the risk of the translocations that result in therapy-induced acute myeloid leukemia (AML) in children treated with these drugs.[60]

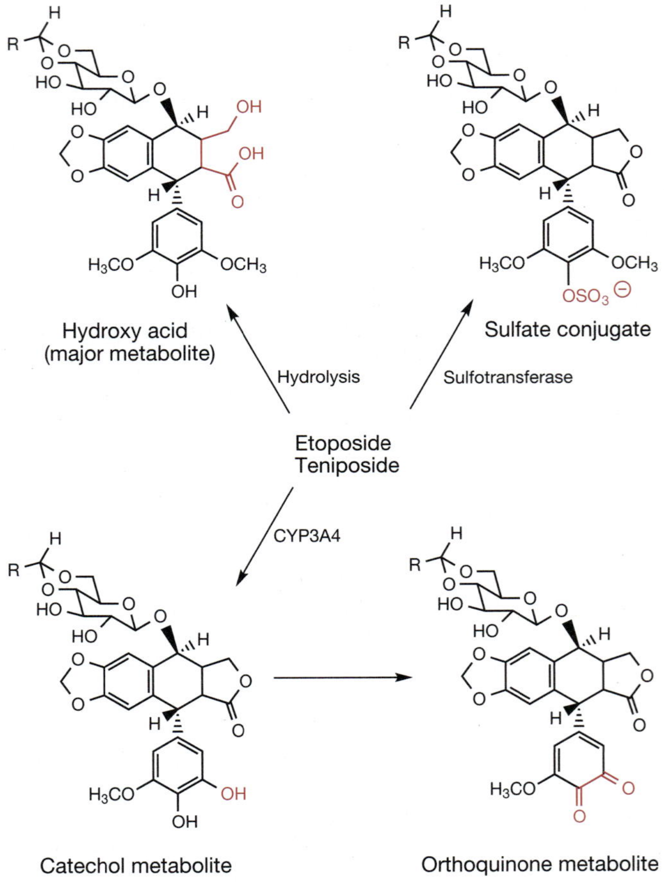

Figure 36.6 Epipodophyllotoxin metabolism.

While the orthoquinone can be detoxified with reduced glutathione (GSH),[61] endogenous supplies of this electrophilic scavenger are limited. Epipodophyllotoxin-induced leukemia occurs in 2% to 12% of patients and is believed to result from translocation of the MLL (mixed lineage leukemia) gene at chromosome band 11q23. The mean latency period of 2 years is shorter than the 5- to 7-year latency for leukemia induced by DNA alkylators, and the drug-induced cancer is often resistant to standard treatment, including bone marrow transplantation.[62] Another serious adverse effect is dose-limiting mucositis. Alopecia is common, and nausea and vomiting, most noticeable with the oral dosage form, are generally mild.

Specific Drugs

Etoposide. Etoposide and etoposide phosphate ester are used IV in combination with an organoplatinum agent (cisplatin, carboplatin) in the treatment of SCLC, and in combination with other agents in refractory testicular cancer. The dose of both runs from 35 to 50 mg/m^2 depending on whether a 5- or 4-day administration per cycle regimen is prescribed. Even though etoposide requires an oil-based solubilizer, it is the more commonly used drug. This preference is most likely due to a decreased cost, as compared to the prodrug, and the ability of a corticosteroid/antihistamine pretreatment to minimize the polysorbate 80-induced hypersensitivity reaction. The phosphate ester would be a viable choice in patients who do exhibit hypersensitivity to etoposide despite pretreatment. The oral formulation is reserved for patients with lung cancer. Oral bioavailability is concentration dependent and runs approximately 50% for the 50-mg capsule. Doses twice the IV dose (rounded to the nearest 50 mg) are administered.

Etoposide is approximately 97% protein bound, undergoes biphasic elimination, and has a terminal half-life of 4 to 11 hours. Approximately 56% of a dose is eliminated via the kidneys, and the remainder is excreted in feces. The drug should be used with caution in patients with renal impairment or liver disease that impacts protein-binding sites (eg, hyperbilirubinemia). Specifically, doses should be decreased in patients with creatinine clearance of 50 mL/min or less or bilirubin levels of more than 1.5 mg/dL. Organoplatinum anticancer agents decrease etoposide clearance, especially in children. If used in combination, administration must be separated by at least 2 days. The list of drugs interacting with etoposide via metabolic or other mechanisms is extensive.

Teniposide. Teniposide is used in combination with other agents for the treatment of refractory childhood ALL. The common dose is 165 mg/m^2 twice weekly. Compared to etoposide, it is more highly protein bound (>99%), more extensively metabolized, more slowly cleared (terminal half-life of 5-40 hours), and less dependent on renal elimination (10%-21%). The lack of oral bioavailability precludes the marketing of an oral dosage form, and no phosphate ester prodrug formulations are available. The hypersensitivity risk from Kolliphor EL is significant, and, although normally controlled with pretreatment, patients should be closely observed throughout the infusion. The infusion is given over the course of 0.5 to 1 hour to avoid a drop in blood pressure.[43]

Exposure to heparin can cause teniposide to precipitate, so lines must be thoroughly flushed before and after teniposide administration. The drug can also spontaneously precipitate, particularly if solutions are over agitated, and patients receiving prolonged infusions should be monitored for blockage of access catheters.

Anthracyclines and Anthracenediones

Anthracycline antineoplastics are very closely related to tetracycline antibacterials. Structurally, they are glycosides and contain a sugar portion (L-daunosamine) and a nonsugar (aglycone) organic portion. The aglycone moiety of anthracyclines is referred to as the anthracyclinone or anthraquinone.

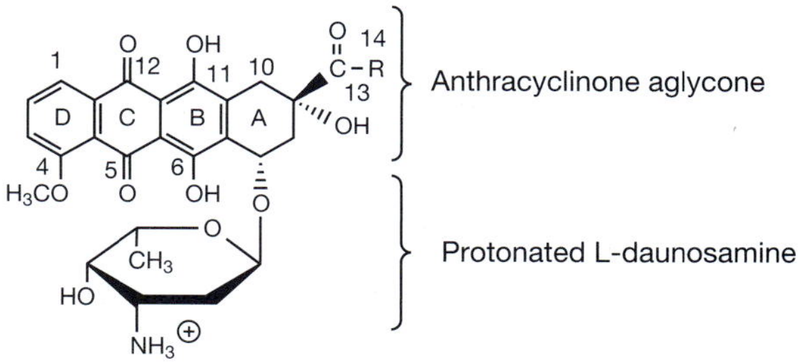

Mechanism of Action. TopIIα, the topII isoform that predominates in rapidly dividing cells, is the molecular target for anthracycline anticancer agents.[28] Like the poisons discussed earlier, they stabilize the ternary drug-enzyme-DNA complex, allowing DNA to be cut and covalently linked to the conserved Tyr residue. However, by inhibiting proper alignment of the cleaved DNA segments, they inhibit the resealing reaction. The aromatic portion of the anthracyclinone and the daunosamine sugar bind to DNA, with the anthracyclinone A ring bridging the gap between DNA and enzyme.[63] The site of DNA cleavage contains an essential thymine-adenine (T-A) dinucleotide, and a small number of anthracycline-induced DNA breaks here results in a high level of cell death.[64]

Chemistry. DNA intercalation by rings B, C, and D of the anthracyclinone initiates antineoplastic action.[65] The planar aromatic structure orients perpendicular to the long axis of DNA, and the complex is stabilized through π-stacking and other affinity-enhancing interactions. Ring A and the amino sugar bind into the minor groove of the DNA, projecting from the helix to interact with TopIIα, thus stabilizing the ternary complex.[66] A study that docked doxorubicin in a modeled DNA "postcleavage" intercalation site proposed highly efficacious H-bonds between topIIα Ser740 and the C_5 quinone oxygen (ring C), Thr744 and the C_4-OCH_3 (ring D), and a DNA thymidine residue and the C_9-OH (ring A).[65] If present, a C_{14}-OH should H-bond with the carbonyl oxygen of another DNA thymidine residue (Fig. 36.7). Although the C_4-OCH_3 helps hold the drug to its target enzyme, its removal increases planarity, facilitates intercalation, and directs daunosamine binding to better stabilize the ternary cleavable complex, thus increasing antineoplastic potency.[67]

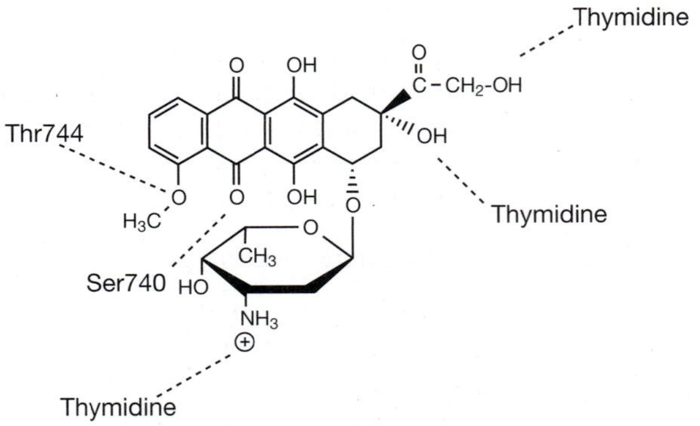

Figure 36.7 Proposed interaction between doxorubicin, DNA, and topoisomerase IIα.

Daunosamine binds in the DNA minor groove at the interface with topIIα and orchestrates DNA intercalation and the overall poisoning process.[67] The aforementioned molecular modeling study suggested that the cationic 3′-amino group binds with high affinity to the carbonyl oxygen of a DNA thymidine residue when in the naturally occurring α-configuration. In the epimerized β-configuration, the distance between these two moieties increases and unfavorable steric interactions with other DNA residues occur, yet cytotoxic potency increases. Antitumor activity of anthracyclines is thought to be related more to the proper positioning and stabilization of the drug within the cleavable ternary complex than to the actual drug affinity for DNA.[67] The daunosamine 3′-amino group is in the natural α-configuration in all marketed anthracycline antineoplastics.

Resistance to anthracycline chemotherapy can be intrinsic or acquired. Major resistance mechanisms include: (1) compromised drug transport across cell membranes due to active efflux via P-gp and MRP transporters, (2) changes in tumor cell responsiveness to apoptotic triggers, including loss or mutation of tumor-suppressor p53 protein or induction of DNA repair, (3) alterations in topIIα expression and activity, and (4) augmented biochemical defenses against anthracycline-induced oxidative stress, such as upregulation of superoxide dismutase or increased production of glutathione.[68,69] Many of these resistance mechanisms are aided by upregulated metabolic pathways such as glycolysis, pentose phosphate pathways, or nucleotide biosynthesis in the cancer cells.[70] There is growing evidence that upregulation of the reductase enzymes that convert anthracyclines to their less active or inactive secondary alcohol (rubicinol) metabolites is a potential mechanism of acquired resistance.[71] The reason for the reduction in cytotoxic activity is 3-fold: In addition to having a lower DNA binding potential, rubicinols can be retained in lysosomes and are more vigorously effluxed from tumor cells by P-gp. As noted later, rubicinols concentrate in myocardial tissue and mediate the chronic cardiac toxicity that is the major use-limiting adverse effect of these drugs. Therefore, inhibiting these enzymes could conceivably help prevent/reverse resistance and could potentially protect against myocardial damage.[72]

Interestingly, the polyphenol epigallocatechin-3-gallate (EGCG, found in green tea) has been shown to inhibit cellular efflux of the anthracycline doxorubicin[73,74] and to sensitize doxorubicin-treated/resistant human colon carcinoma cells.[75] Moreover, it may provide some protection from doxorubicin-induced inflammation and cardiotoxicity.[76,77]

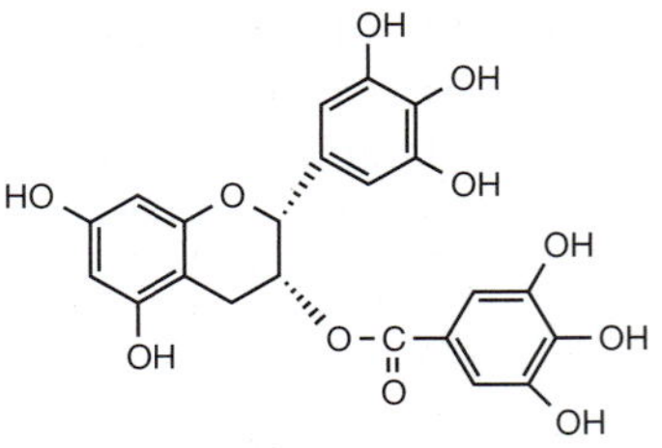

Epigallocatechin 3-gallate
(EGCG from Green tea)

Chemical Mechanism of Cardiotoxicity. Anthracycline drugs have a propensity to cause cardiotoxicity that can be acute or chronic in nature. Acute toxicity is observed as transient and reversible asymptomatic left ventricular dysfunction. It occurs in less than 1% of patients and generally manifests within 14 days following drug administration. Chronic cardiotoxicity has a 9% incidence and is characterized by the signs and symptoms of heart failure. It is irreversible and may have an early or late onset. Early onset chronic cardiotoxicity presents within 1 year of treatment and occurs more frequently than late onset toxicity, which has a median onset of 7 years posttreatment.[78] Notably, the risk of developing anthracycline-induced cardiotoxicity increases with increasing cumulative dose, from about 5% at 400 mg/m^2 to as high as 48% at 700 mg/m^2.[79]

Acute Toxicity. The traditional and potentially still relevant mechanism, particularly in the early phase of acute toxicity, is the formation of reactive oxygen species (ROS). The myocardium requires a continuously high level of energy supplied through mitochondrial oxidative phosphorylation. The quinone ring of anthracyclines undergoes a one-electron reduction by nicotinamide adenine dinucleotide (phosphate) reduced (NAD(P)H) oxidoreductase to hydroquinone via a semiquinone radical intermediate. In the oxygen-rich environment of

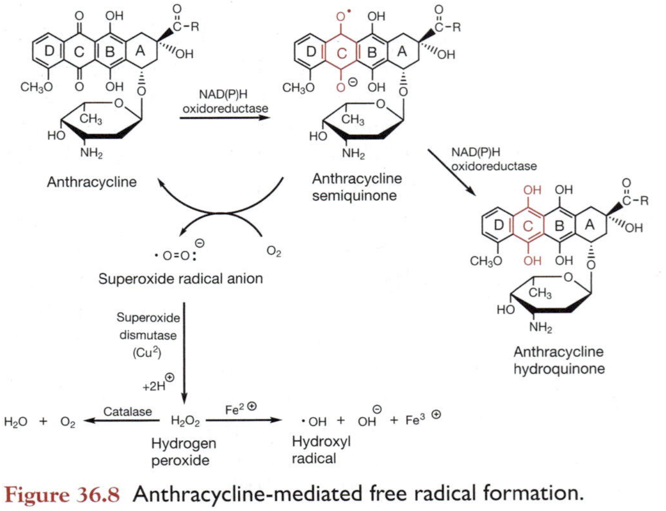

Figure 36.8 Anthracycline-mediated free radical formation.

mitochondria, the semiquinone autooxidizes to form the parent anthracycline and the superoxide radical anion (Fig. 36.8). This ROS rapidly generates hydrogen peroxide (H_2O_2) in a Cu^{2+}-dependent process that requires superoxide dismutase and protons.[80]

The fate of H_2O_2 dictates the degree of acute myotoxicity observed from the anthracycline. In the presence of catalase, H_2O_2 is rapidly converted to water and oxygen. However, in the absence of catalase and in the presence of ferrous ion (Fe^{2+}), the highly damaging hydroxyl radical is generated via the Fenton reaction[81] (Fig. 36.8). Anthracyclines chelate strongly with di- and trivalent cations, including intracellular Fe^{3+}, which can be reduced to Fe^{2+} enzymatically or via auto-reduction if the C_{13} substituent is CH_2OH.[82-84] Therefore, the ready availability of the iron needed to generate hydroxyl radicals from H_2O_2 is essentially guaranteed.

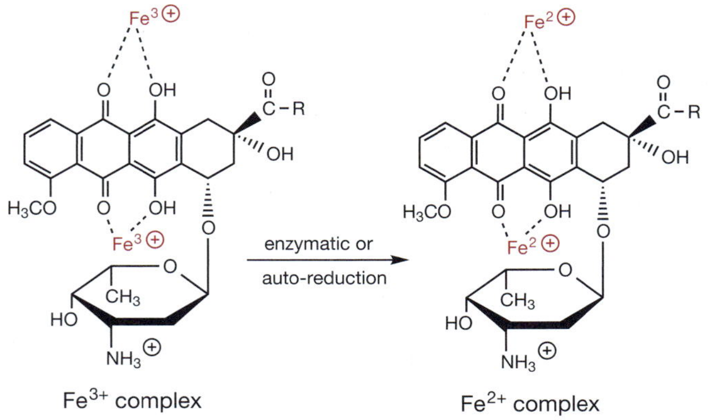

Hydroxyl radicals promote SSB in DNA and could conceivably augment the cytotoxic action of anthracyclines; however, this is uncommon in tumor cells at standard antineoplastic doses.[64] In contrast, hydroxyl radicals are readily generated in the myocardium because cardiac tissue does not contain significant amounts of catalase and other relevant cytoprotective enzymes.[85] When H_2O_2 forms in the myocardium, it has no choice but to go down the Fenton pathway.

Cardiac toxicity is the major use-limiting side effect of anthracyclines, but coadministration of dexrazoxane (an antioxidant and iron chelator) has been shown to lower its incidence when used with the C_{13}-CH_2OH substituted anthracyclines doxorubicin and epirubicin.[86,87] As discussed later, dexrazoxane's mechanism of cardioprotective action likely lies outside of its iron-chelating ability.

Chronic (Delayed) Cardiotoxicity. Rubicinol metabolites are believed to be responsible for the more life-threatening chronic cardiotoxicity that some patients experience. The C_{13}-carbonyl is reduced via a two-electron mechanism to a usually less active[88,89] or inactive[84] rubicinol via cytosolic aldo-keto reductase (AKR1C3) and carbonyl reductase (CBR1) enzymes[72] (Fig. 36.9). Before excretion, anthracyclines can be further metabolized via hydrolytic or reductive deglycosidation to their 7-hydroxy or 7-deoxy aglycones, respectively, followed by O-dealkylation of the C_4 methoxy ether (if present) and conjugation with either glucuronic acid or sulfate. The aglycones may also have cardiotoxic properties.[84,90]

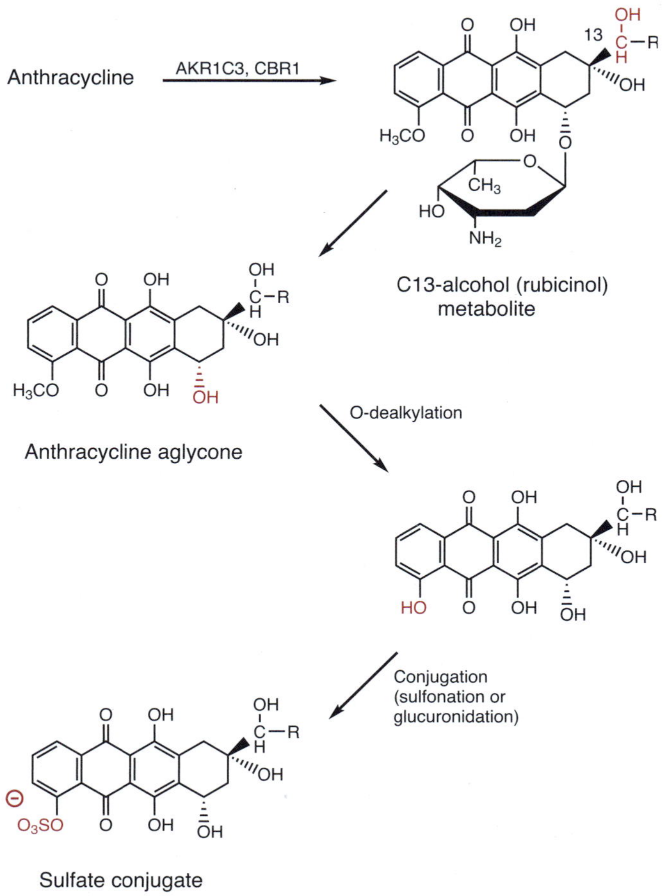

Figure 36.9 Anthracycline metabolism. AKR, aldo-keto reductase; CBR, carbonyl reductase.

The larger the C_{13}-substituent the slower the AKR/CBR-catalyzed reduction reaction, and the longer the duration of cytotoxic activity. C_{13}-substituents found on the marketed anthracyclines include CH_3 (daunorubicin and idarubicin) and CH_2OH (doxorubicin and epirubicin).

Rubicinol metabolites concentrate in cardiomyocytes and induce profound increases in intracellular calcium concentrations through a variety of mechanisms, which can include: (1) prolonged inhibition of calcium loading, (2) inhibition of Ca^{2+}, Mg^{2+}-ATPase and stimulation of vesicular calcium release in the sarcoplasmic reticulum, and (3) inhibition of Na^+/K^+-ATPase in the sarcolemma.[72] The synthesis of sarcomeric proteins essential to cardiomyocyte integrity is also impaired.[90,91] As a result, myocardial contractility is compromised, and the myopathy presents as severe congestive heart failure involving systolic and diastolic dysfunction.

TopIIβ, the predominant topII isoform in quiescent cells, is the only isoform found in the myocardium, and a critical role for this protein in anthracycline-induced cardiotoxicity has been proposed.[92] Anthracycline binding to myocardial topIIβ disrupts mitochondrial function, initiates DNA double-strand breaks, stimulates p53-induced apoptosis in cardiomyocytes, and may facilitate formation of ROS.[93] Studies in mice genetically engineered to be topIIβ deficient were resistant to anthracycline-induced cardiac toxicity. A small, isolated study found patients sensitive to anthracycline-induced cardiac effects had significantly higher peripheral blood leukocyte levels of topIIβ than resistant patients.[93] TopIIβ is currently viewed as a highly significant (and likely a primary) mediator of anthracycline-related cardiotoxicity.

Although the acute and chronic phases of anthracycline-induced cardiomyopathy appear metabolically distinct, a unifying hypothesis suggests that induction of ROS-mediated oxidative stress may upregulate AKR, thereby facilitating the development of rubicinol-induced chronic cardiotoxicity.[84] It is also thought that rubicinol metabolites can generate ROS, and that acute toxicity (eg, left ventricular systolic dysfunction) from "real-time" drug exposure can predispose patients to worsening myopathy over time.[90]

Clinical Aspects. Fortunately, acute anthracycline-induced cardiotoxicity is generally self-limiting. It commonly manifests during or a few weeks after therapy and often presents as disturbances in electrocardiogram (ECG), cardiac rhythm, and ventricular function. Symptoms commonly resolve within 1 week, although the caution about early damage predisposing to chronic pathology must be noted.[90,94] Evaluation of troponin levels as a biomarker for detecting cardiotoxicity during anthracycline chemotherapy has been suggested.[95]

In contrast, rubicinols form long-lived reservoirs of cardiotoxic within the myocardium,[90] and chronic anthracycline-induced heart failure can manifest without warning years (even decades) after therapy concludes. It is often unresponsive to therapeutic intervention, and more than half of the patients so diagnosed die within 2 years.[84,94] Elevated risk occurs with high cumulative doses, age extremes, genetic polymorphisms impacting ROS production, rubicinol formation and/or anthracycline transport, coadministration of other cardiotoxic drugs, and underlying cardiovascular disease.[90,96] Female and Black populations are at risk for increased incidence or severity of drug-induced cardiomyopathy.[93,97] Because toxicity is dose dependent,[92] dosage adjustments must be made in patients with liver dysfunction who cannot adequately metabolize and clear anthracyclines to avoid life-threatening toxicity. Additionally, cardiotoxicity may be enhanced by other drugs in a chemotherapy regimen such as trastuzumab. This mAb is used in combination with anthracycline for breast cancer and can interfere with myocyte survival pathways.[95]

To reduce anthracycline-induced toxicity, genetic testing for UGT1A6*4 and retinoid acid receptor γ (RARG) may be considered in pediatric patients prior to treatment. The UGT1A6*4 carriers have a reduced glucuronidating activity and a consequent reduced clearance of the cardiotoxic anthracycline metabolites.[98] RARG has been shown to repress the expression of topIIβ, the target enzyme for chronic cardiotoxicity. Carriers of the RARG rs2229774 A (S247L) variant expressed higher levels of topIIβ because of the removal of repressive effect of RARG.[99] While these cardioprotecting precautions appear scientifically sound, the overall quality of the evidence of positive clinical outcomes is poor. Due to lack of evidence, similar testing is not recommended in adult patients at present.

Dexrazoxane. As noted, coadministration of dexrazoxane, an antioxidant and prodrug iron-chelating agent, can attenuate anthracycline-induced cardiotoxicity (including chronic, delayed heart failure) from the C_{13}-CH_2OH substituted anthracyclines, doxorubicin and epirubicin, in both adults and children. The level of protection has been estimated at 80%.[90,96] Dexrazoxane readily enters cells and is hydrolyzed to the active Fe^{2+} and Fe^{3+} chelating form ADR-925. It is administered IV 30 minutes prior to the anthracycline to allow distribution to cells where it will be needed. Although the affinity of ADR-925 for iron surpasses that of doxorubicin, chelation-independent mechanisms for cardioprotection by dexrazoxane have been proposed, including altering topIIβ-configuration in a way that inhibits anthracycline binding and inducing transient topIIβ depletion.[84,93,96,100] The facts that: (1) other iron chelators and free radical scavengers are ineffective in providing cardioprotection, (2) inhibition of dexrazoxane hydrolysis does not abolish its cardioprotective effect, and (3) direct application of ADR-925 to cardiomyocytes does not protect against anthracycline-induced damage lend strong support to these alternative mechanisms of action and to the dexrazoxane parent structure as the active entity.[96]

Per current guidelines, dexrazoxane may be administered to prevent cardiotoxicity in patients receiving high-dose anthracyclines (eg, doxorubicin ≥250 mg/m^2 or epirubicin ≥600 mg/m^2). The dexrazoxane-to-doxorubicin ratio is 10:1, and doxorubicin must be administered within 30 minutes of dexrazoxane infusion.[43] Dexrazoxane can also be used to attenuate serious tissue injury following accidental anthracycline extravasation.[101] For this indication, it is administered IV once daily for 3 days, beginning within 6 hours of the extravasation incident.

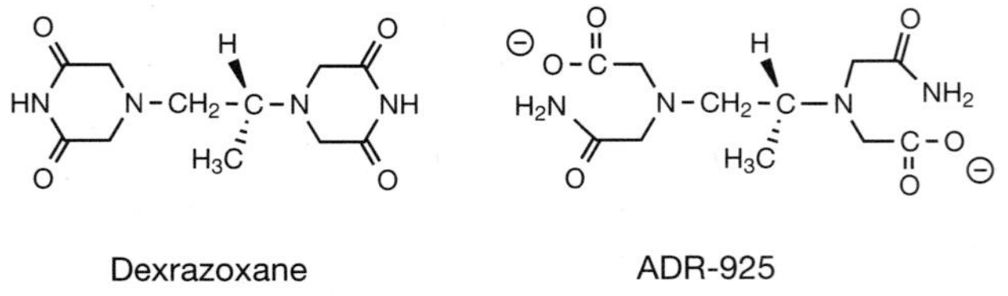

In addition to dexrazoxane administration, other suggested strategies for attenuating anthracycline-induced cardiomyopathy include limiting the cumulative (lifetime) dose, administering the anthracycline by continuous infusion and in divided doses (vs bolus administration), and electing liposomal formulations when appropriate.[93] Fortifying mitochondrial function with coenzyme Q or other natural products may also prove beneficial.[102,103] Ongoing clinical trials with structurally modified anthracyclines that spare the TopIIβ in cardiomyocytes, coupled with liposomal-facilitated delivery, may yield promising anthracycline drugs with low cardiotoxicity.[104]

OTHER TOXICITIES. In addition to cardiac toxicity, all anthracycline antineoplastics can cause severe myelosuppression (especially leukocytopenia) as well as moderate-to-severe nausea and vomiting, mucositis leading to hemorrhage and potentially fatal infection, and alopecia. Boxed warnings for these life-threatening adverse effects are applicable to all anthracyclines. Side effects are dose dependent.

Most of the anthracyclines are orally inactive and must be given by IV injection. They are highly necrotic to skin, and extravasation can cause severe blistering and ulceration that may require skin excision followed by plastic surgery. The anthracyclines contain photosensitive phenolic groups that must be protected from light and air. The highly conjugated structure imparts a reddish-orange color to these compounds (implied in the name "rubicin"), which is maintained when these compounds are excreted in the urine.

Specific Drugs. The structures of the currently marketed anthracycline anticancer agents and a related anthracenedione are provided in Figure 36.10.

Doxorubicin Hydrochloride. Doxorubicin is used either alone or in combination therapy to treat a wide range of neoplastic disorders, including hematologic cancers and solid tumors in breast, ovary, stomach, bladder, and thyroid gland. In addition to cardiomyopathy and myelosuppression, the boxed warning advises on the dangers of extravasation and the risk of secondary AML.[43]

The C_{13} substituent of doxorubicin is hydroxymethyl, which retards the action of cytosolic reductase and slows conversion to the less active and chronically cardiotoxic doxorubicinol. This contributes to the longer duration of action compared to analogs that have CH_3 at this position (eg, daunorubicin). It is given IV in starting doses that range from 25 to 75 mg/m^2, and cumulative doses above 550 mg/m^2 are associated with an elevated risk of cardiac toxicity. As noted, doses are decreased in hepatic impairment, and the cardioprotectant dexrazoxane should be coadministered when cumulative doses reach 250 mg/m^2.

Doxorubicin is highly lipophilic and concentrates in the liver, lymph nodes, muscle, bone marrow, fat, and skin. Elimination is triphasic, and the drug has a terminal half-life of 20 to 48 hours. It is 75% protein bound. Most of the administered dose is excreted in the feces, approximately half of it is unchanged.[43]

A pegylated nano-liposomal formulation of doxorubicin, marketed as Doxil, is used in the treatment of AIDS-related Kaposi sarcoma, refractory multiple myeloma (in combination with bortezomib), and organoplatinum-resistant ovarian cancer.[93] Liposomes are taken up selectively into tumor cells, presumably due to their persistence in the bloodstream and enhanced permeability of tumor vascular membranes. In liposomal form, the drug is protected against enzymes that generate cardiotoxic metabolites and is less likely to concentrate in the heart.[105] However, because this form of the drug can still induce potentially fatal congestive heart failure, all precautions outlined for the use of doxorubicin should be taken, and the boxed warning for conventional doxorubicin applies.

The pegylation extends the half-life of Doxil to approximately 55 hours, and it is administered in doses ranging from 20 to 50 mg/m^2 every 3 to 4 weeks. The area under the plasma concentration curve (AUC) of the liposomal formulation is approximately 3 times that of the free drug formulation. It is cleared more slowly than conventional doxorubicin and generates very little of the doxorubicinol metabolite.[106] Significant adverse effects have occurred when the liposomal formulation is erroneously dispensed, so pharmacists must be vigilant when interpreting therapeutic orders.

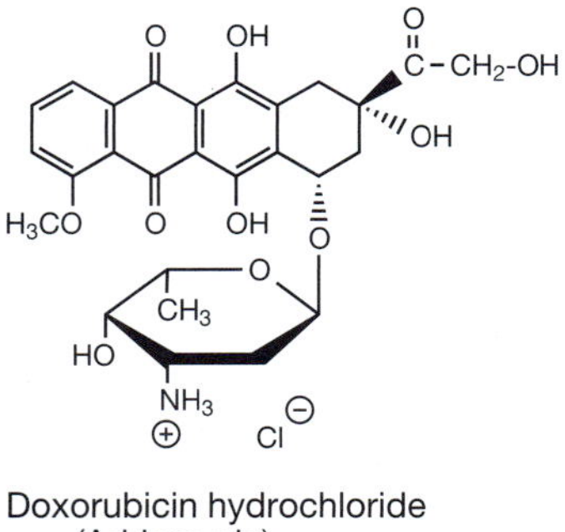

Doxorubicin hydrochloride
(Adriamycin)

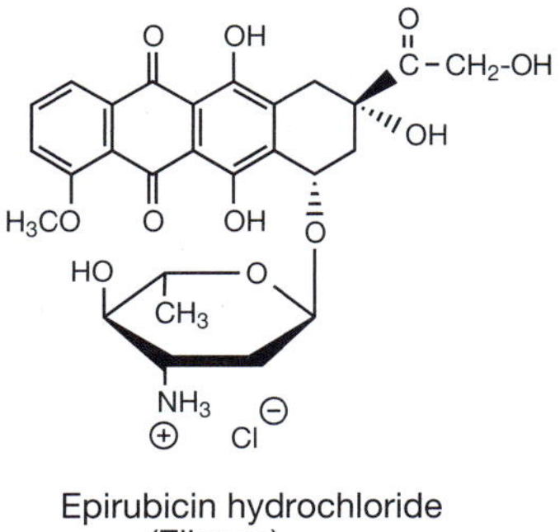

Epirubicin hydrochloride
(Ellence)

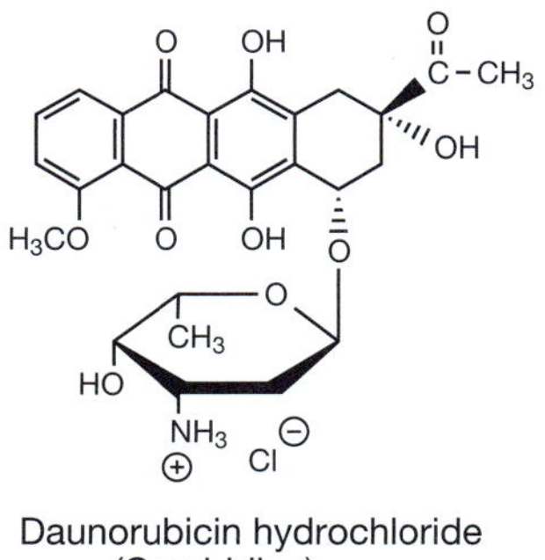

Daunorubicin hydrochloride
(Cerubidine)

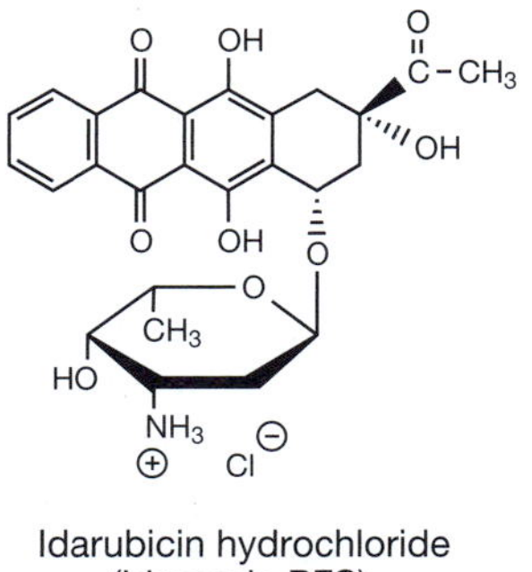

Idarubicin hydrochloride
(Idamycin PFS)

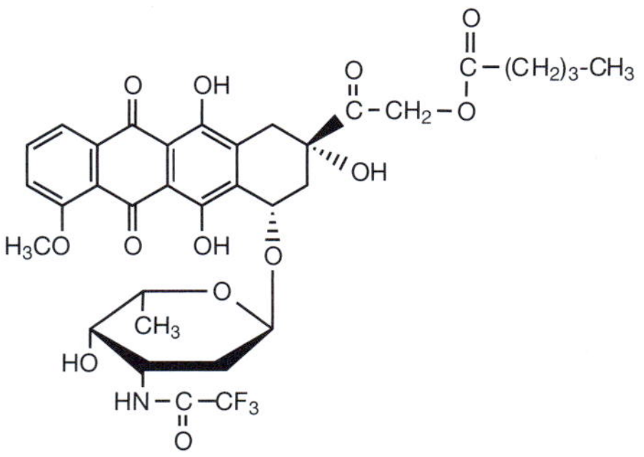

Valrubicin
(Valstar)

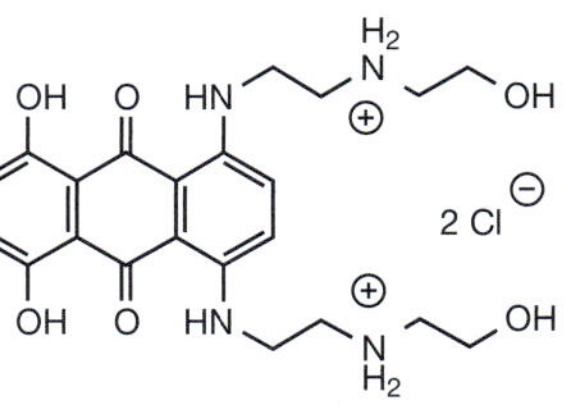

Mitoxantrone hydrochloride
(Novantrone)

Figure 36.10 Anthracycline and related anticancer agents.

ALDOXORUBICIN: AN INVESTIGATIONAL ANTHRACYCLINE PRODRUG

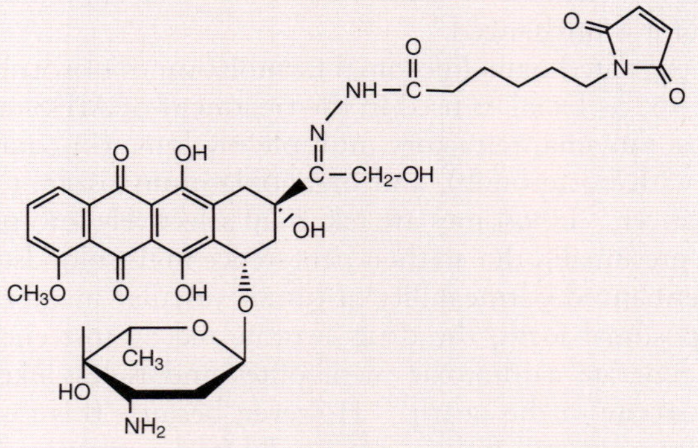

Aldoxorubicin

Aldoxorubicin is a doxorubicin prodrug that takes full chemical advantage of (1) an accessible Cys34 residue on serum albumin, (2) the propensity of tumors to accumulate macromolecules, and (3) the acidic pH of the hypoxic tumor cell. Equipped with a sterically unhindered Michael-alkylating maleimido moiety that specifically reacts with sulfhydryl (thiol) groups at physiologic pH, aldoxorubicin is attacked by Cys34 within minutes of IV administration. The covalent complex is transported throughout the bloodstream and drawn into the highly permeable tumor cells, where the acidic environment catalyzes the hydrolysis of the hydrazone linker and achieves targeted delivery of doxorubicin exactly where it is needed.[107]

Pharmacokinetic studies have confirmed that all but a small fraction of aldoxorubicin is securely tethered to circulating albumin, and serum concentrations of free doxorubicin and the highly cardiotoxic doxorubicinol metabolite are minimal. Neutropenia can be effectively managed with concomitant granulocyte colony–stimulating factor (G-CSF) therapy. Fatigue and mucositis are common adverse effects, but alopecia is less frequently observed than with doxorubicin.[108-110]

Phase II and III clinical trials comparing aldoxorubicin to free doxorubicin or oncologist's choice of therapy in advanced or metastatic soft tissue sarcoma (STS) documented superior median PFS and overall response outcomes for the prodrug.[108-110] The prevailing clinical opinion is that aldoxorubicin provides a significant therapeutic and safety advantage over doxorubicin as first-line therapy in advanced, relapsed, or refractory STS. To this effect, aldoxorubicin received orphan drug designation for STS treatment in 2017.

Epirubicin Hydrochloride. This stereoisomer of doxorubicin has the 4′-hydroxy group of the daunosamine sugar oriented in the unnatural β-position. This configurational change has a major impact on the pharmacodynamics and pharmacokinetic properties. The higher starting dose of 100 to 120 mg/m^2 for epirubicin in breast cancer (its only indication) compared to doxorubicin's single agent dose of 60 to 75 mg/m^2 indicates a less potent topIIα-inhibiting action. Although excretion is primarily biliary, dose reduction in severe renal impairment, as well as in hepatic dysfunction, is warranted.

Epirubicin is reduced to the C_{13} alcohol (epirubicinol) to a much lower (60%) extent than doxorubicin, preferentially generating the reduced aglycone doxorubicinolone that is more easily eliminated. The rate of C_4-glucuronidation of the O-dealkylated phenol is faster than that of doxorubicin, and the terminal half-life of 33 hours is shorter. Because it is readily trapped in lysosomes and other acidic organelles, it is not highly susceptible to ROS-generating one-electron oxidation. The overall cardiotoxicity has been estimated at 30% lower than doxorubicin. However, the margin of safety is mitigated by epirubicin's greater propensity to accumulate in myocardiocytes.[84,90,111] Other adverse effects and precautions are as outlined for doxorubicin.

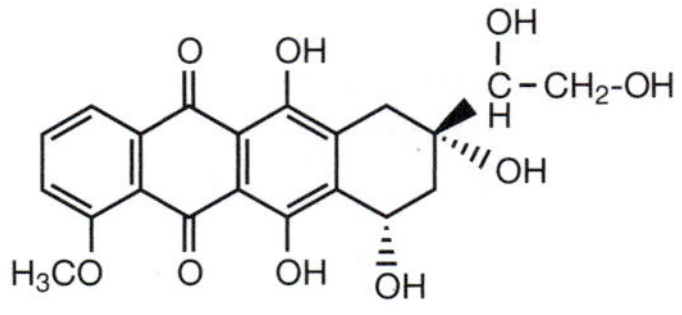

Doxorubicinolone

Daunorubicin Hydrochloride. The absence of the OH group at C_{14} in daunorubicin results in a faster conversion to the less active and chronically cardiotoxic duanorubicinol compared to CH_2OH-substituted anthracyclines such as doxorubicin. The 18.5-hour terminal half-life is approximately half that of doxorubicin, and the terminal half-life of the daunorubicinol metabolite is 27 hours. Excretion is approximately 40% biliary and 25% urinary. Daunorubicin is administered IV at a dose of 45 mg/m^2 for the treatment of lymphocytic leukemia and AML. The toxicity and side effect profile of this anthracycline is similar to that of doxorubicin, and all previously identified precautions apply.[43] In a liposomal formulation of daunorubicin and cytarabine, the terminal half-life of the anthracycline is extended to 31.5 hours.

Idarubicin Hydrochloride. Idarubicin is the 4-desmethoxy analog of daunorubicin, which facilitates intercalation between DNA base pairs. In turn, this orients the daunosamine sugar in the minor groove in a way that better stabilizes the ternary complex for the DNA cleavage reaction.[67] The loss of the 4-methoxy moiety also makes this compound more lipophilic than other anthracyclines, resulting in better penetration into tumor cells.

Idarubicin is reduced to idarubicinol, which, unlike other rubicinols, is as active an antitumor agent as the parent drug.[72,89] Importantly, idarubicin has limited affinity for P-gp (a major anthracycline resistance mechanism), although the idarubicinol metabolite is still actively effluxed from tumor cells.[72] The elimination half-lives of idarubicin and idarubicinol are 22 and 45 hours, respectively.

Idarubicin's primary indication is AML, and it is administered in combination with other cytotoxic agents at a dose of 10 to 12 mg/m^2 (much lower than other anthracyclines). Its higher potency can be attributed to its four previously highlighted pharmacodynamics and pharmacokinetic distinctions: (1) better DNA intercalation, (2) more effective tumor cell penetration, (3) resistance to P-gp efflux, and (4) an equally cytotoxic idarubicinol metabolite. In addition, the lack of the C_4-methoxy means no O-dealkylation and no phenolic conjugation with glucuronic acid. The major metabolite is idarubicinol, and, like other anthracyclines, excretion is predominantly fecal with a lesser dependence on renal elimination.

Some authors have shown that idarubicin is transported into cardiac tissue via a saturable transporter and that coadministration of methylxanthines (eg, caffeine) can increase both myocardial drug concentrations and the risk of idarubicin-induced cardiotoxicity.[112]

Valrubicin. Chemically, valrubicin differs from doxorubicin by the addition of a carbon-rich C_{14}-valerate ester and a nonionizable 3′-trifluoroacetamide moiety. After solubilizing with Kolliphor EL, the drug is instilled intervesically in the treatment of bacille Calmette-Guérin (BCG)-refractory carcinoma in situ of the bladder.[113] Its high lipophilicity effectively traps it at the site of action, so therapy can be considered local.

Valrubicin is not a doxorubicin prodrug; the trifluoroacetamide and valerate ester remain intact within the bladder. The drug should not be given to patients with compromised bladder wall integrity, as it can reach the bloodstream and hydrolyze to doxorubicin, initiating serious toxicity that would not otherwise manifest. Its primary mechanism is cell chromosomal damage and cell cycle arrest through the inhibition of DNA synthesis.[114] Although having limited use, valrubicin is a viable option for patients who are unwilling or unfit for radial cystectomy.[115]

Mitoxantrone Hydrochloride. Chemically, mitoxantrone is classified as an anthracenedione. The cationic sidechain amines bind to the anionic phosphate residue of the DNA backbone in the same fashion that the anthracycline cationic amino group is believed to do. The anthracenedione ring system intercalates DNA to initiate topIIα inhibition, but the enhanced stability of the quinone ring (possibly through an increased potential for intramolecular hydrogen bonding) results in an 8-fold lower ability to chelate Fe^{3+}.[83] This limits the formation of highly toxic ROS. In addition, there is no rubicinol to induce chronic toxicity.

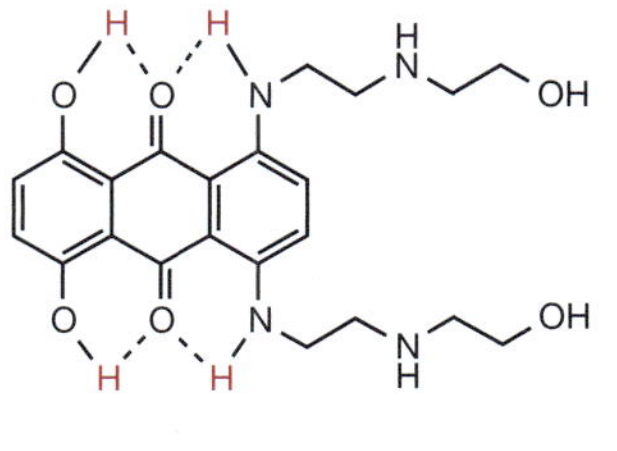

Mitoxantrone

The chance of cardiac toxicity from mitoxantrone is significantly decreased compared to true anthracyclines, although patients, particularly those who have previously received anthracycline therapy, are still at risk. While the symptoms mimic anthracycline-induced toxicity, the mechanism is unknown and cardioprotection therapy is not available. The drug carries a maximum lifetime cumulative dose of 140 mg/m^2.[116] It is also myelosuppressive, but nonhematologic toxicities are less serious than observed with anthracyclines.

The major mitoxantrone metabolites are mono- and dicarboxylic acid products of N-dealkylation and CYP oxidation, and they are inactive and excreted as glucuronide conjugates in the urine (along with 65% unchanged drug) with a median half-life of elimination of 75 hours. A naphthoquinoxaline metabolite also forms that retains cytotoxic action and has been found to be less cardiotoxic than mitoxantrone in isolated differentiated H9c2 cells. Consideration of the development of this metabolite as a potential anti-cancer drug has been encouraged.[116]

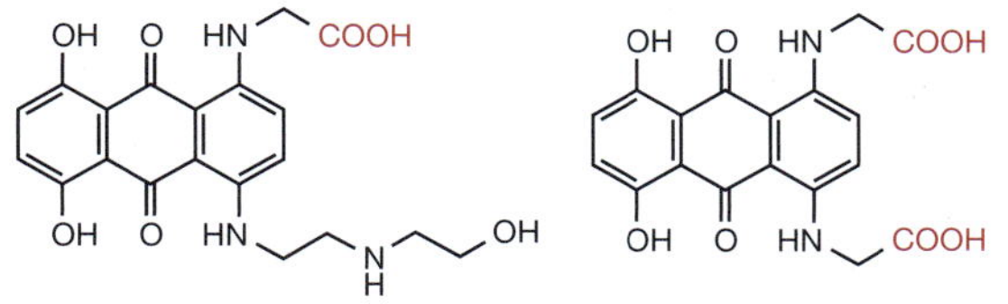

Mitoxantrone mono- and dicarboxylic acid metabolites (inactive)

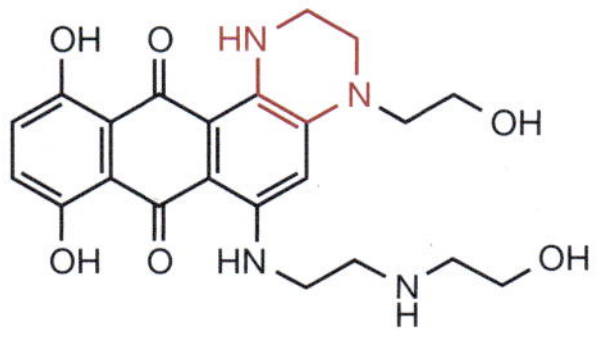

Naphthoquinoxaline metabolite (active)

Mitoxantrone is used with other agents during the initial treatment of acute nonlymphocytic leukemia and castration-resistant prostate cancer (CRPC). In contrast to the "fire engine red" color of the anthracyclines, the conjugated anthracenedione is a vibrant blue, a color that can be apparent in urine and the whites of the eyes.

Mitosis Inhibitors

The mitotic process depends on the structural and functional viability of microtubules, which are polymeric heterodimers consisting of α- and β-tubulin. These distinct but nearly identical 50-kDa proteins lie adjacent to one another and roll up to form an open, pipelike cylinder akin to a hollow peppermint candy stick. A γ-tubulin protein is found at the organizational center of the microtubule and helps initiate the polymerization process.

During cell division, microtubules undergo periods of structural growth and erosion known as "dynamic instability." The proteins alternatively polymerize or depolymerize through guanosine triphosphate (GTP) and Ca^{2+}-dependent processes, respectively. Polymerization causes lengthening of microtubule by adding tubulin dimers more rapidly to the (+) end where the GTP is still intact (GTP cap). Depolymerization results in microtubule shortening due to depletion of tubulin dimer and loss of the GTP cap.[117] This rapid polymerization-depolymerization required for cell division and facilitated by MAPs allows for the formation of the mitotic spindle and the

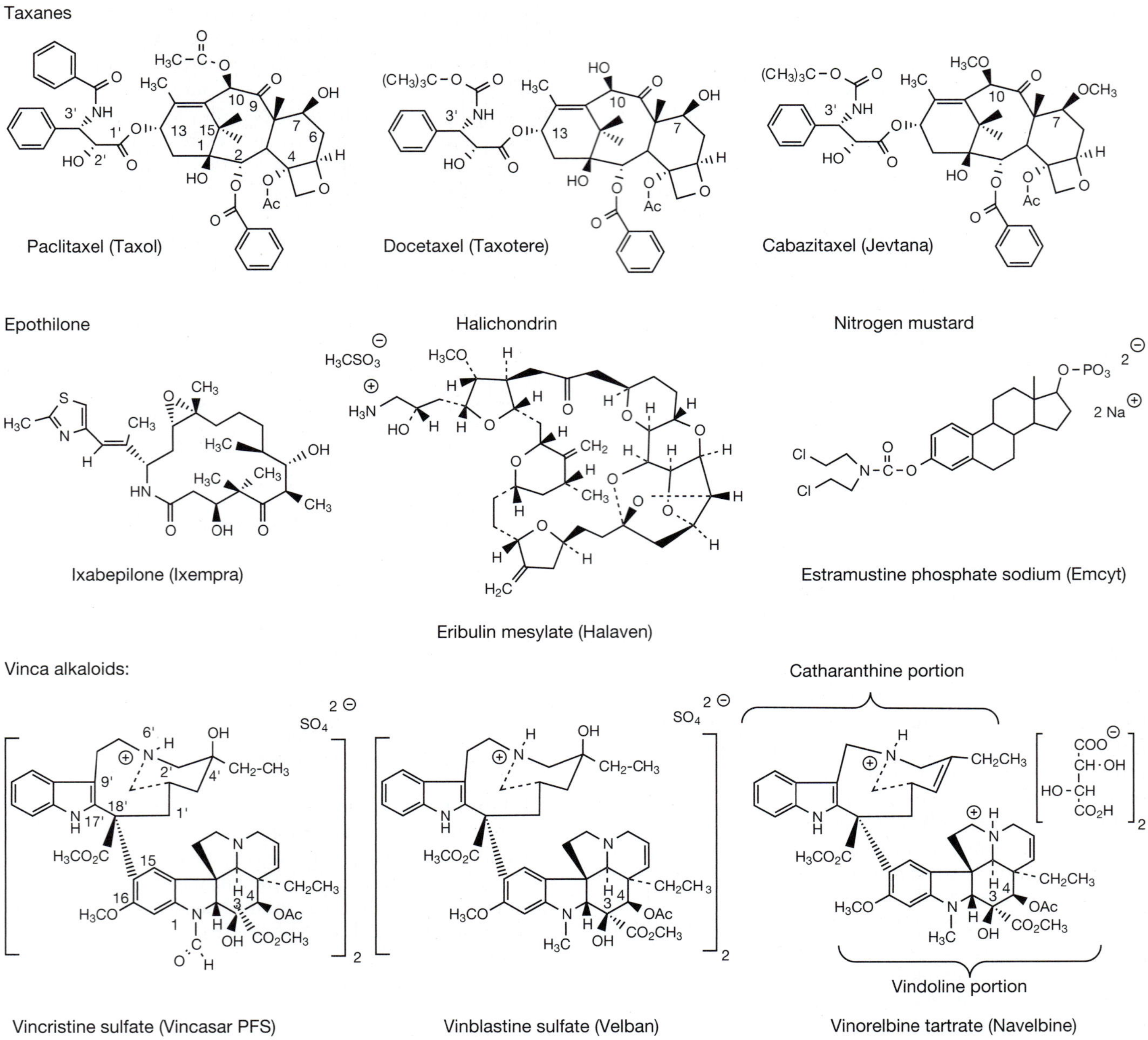

Figure 36.11 Mitosis inhibitors.

attachment of chromosomes to it, followed by pulling away of the sister chromatids toward the opposite ends of the cell. Inhibiting the essential hyperdynamic changes in microtubular structure results in mitotic arrest and apoptosis.[118]

Two general chemical classes of mitosis inhibitors have historically been marketed for the treatment of cancer: taxanes and vinca alkaloids (Fig. 36.11). Although they act through opposing mechanisms of inhibiting microtubule depolymerization and polymerization, respectively, the resultant effect of each is the stabilization of microtubule structure that causes mitotic arrest of the cell cycle.[119] The epothilone (ixabepilone) and halichondrin B (eribulin) have limited use at present. These mitosis inhibitor drugs bind to specific locations on the microtubule that either prevents microtubule erosion (taxane and epothilone) or prevents microtubule lengthening (vinca alkaloids and halichondrin B). Estramustine, an estrogen-based nitrogen mustard-like carbamate that stabilizes microtubule dynamics,[120,121] is no longer recommended for use in metastatic CRPC (its only original indication) due to a lack of clinical benefit.[43] In general, mitosis inhibitors are associated with neurotoxicity/neuropathy due to the high concentration of microtubules in the neurons that are targeted by these drugs.

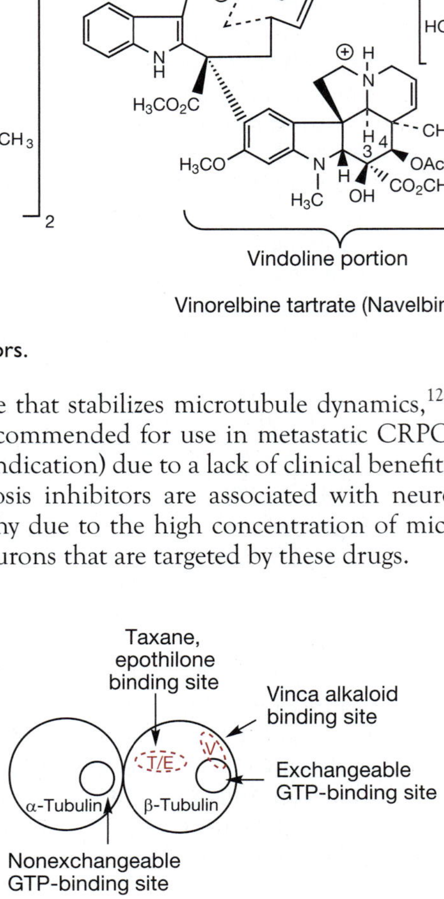

Taxanes

Mechanism of Action. Antineoplastic taxanes were originally isolated from the bark of the Pacific yew (*Taxus brevifolia*) but are now produced semisynthetically from an inactive natural precursor (10-deacetylbaccatin III) found in the leaves of the European yew (*Taxus baccata*), a renewable resource. Taxanes bind to polymerized β-tubulin at a specific hydrophobic receptor site comprising the 31 N-terminal residues located deep within the tubular lumen.[122] At standard therapeutic doses, binding promotes a stable tubulin conformation similar to that of the GTP-bound protein, rendering the microtubules prone to further polymerization and resistant to erosion. Dynamic instability is disrupted, the mitotic spindle does not form, and microtubules collapse into dense aberrant structures known as asters. In other words, mitosis stops, and the cell dies.

Cellular efflux by P-gp is a major mechanism of taxane resistance, as is β-tubulin mutation and overexpression of another isotype, βIII-tubulin.[123-125] Some other resistance mechanisms that have been identified are "mitotic slippage," wherein taxane-treated cells may remain in prolonged mitosis and then progress into the G1 phase without cell division,[126] microRNA (miRNA)-induced synthesis of aberrant proteins, and overproduction of the calcium-binding protein sorcin that helps the cancer cells evade apoptosis.[127]

Chemistry. Diterpenoid taxanes consist of a 15-membered tricyclic taxane ring system (tricyclo[9.3.1.0]pentadecane) fused to an oxetane ring and contain an esterified β-phenylisoserine side chain at C_{13}. As shown in Figure 36.11, the three-marketed taxane antineoplastics differ in substitution pattern at C_{13} (benzamido or *t*-butoxycarboxamido), C_{10} (secondary alcohol, acetate ester, or methoxy ether), and/or C_7 (secondary alcohol or methoxy ether). The taxane ring system is conceptualized as having two parts. The northern part, comprising the C_7, C_9, and C_{10} positions, ensures the proper orientation of critical functional groups, including the C_{13}-isoserine side chain and its substituent groups. The southern part, consisting of C_{14}, C_1, C_2, C_4, and the oxetane ring, plays a critical role in receptor binding. The free $C_{2'}$-hydroxyl, in particular, is essential to taxane antimitotic action.[128-130]

The key taxane-tubulin-binding interactions are identified in Table 36.3 using paclitaxel as the ligand.[131,132] Paclitaxel interacts in a folded ("T" or "butterfly") conformation that places the C_2-benzoyloxy and $C_{3'}$-benzamido groups in proximity of each other.[129,132,133] Their independent intermolecular engagement with a critical β-tubulin His-residue perfectly positioned between them keeps them from interacting with one another. The oxetane ring, although capable of hydrogen bonding with receptor residues, is believed to serve a more critical role in properly orienting the C_4-acetoxy moiety for interaction within its hydrophobic-binding pocket.[131,130] The C_1-OH also promotes conformational stability through intramolecular interaction with the carbonyl oxygen of the C_2 benzoyloxy moiety.[129] The areas of the paclitaxel structure where steric influences are most critical to receptor binding have been identified.[128]

Table 36.3 Paclitaxel-β-Tubulin-Binding Interactions

Paclitaxel Functional Group	β-Tubulin-Binding Residues	Interaction
C_2-benzoyloxy phenyl	Leu217, Leu219, His229, Leu230	Hydrophobic
C_2-benzoyloxy carbonyl	Arg278	Hydrogen bond
$C_{3'}$-benzamido NH	Asp26	Hydrogen bond
$C_{3'}$-benzamido carbonyl	His229	Hydrogen bond
$C_{3'}$-phenyl	Ala233, Ser236, Phe272	Hydrophobic
C_4-acetoxy	Leu217, Leu230, Phe272, Leu275	Hydrophobic
C_7-OH	Thr276, Ser277, Arg278	Hydrogen bond
C_{12}-CH_3	Leu217, Leu230, Phe272, Leu275	Hydrophobic
$C_{2'}$-OH	Arg369, Gly370 (NH)	Hydrogen bond
$C_{3'}$-carbonyl	Gly370 (NH)	Hydrogen bond
Oxetane oxygen	Thr276 (NH)	Hydrogen bond

From Maccari L, Manetti F, Corelli F, et al. 3D QSAR studies for the β-tubulin binding site of microtubule-stabilizing anticancer agents (MSAAs). A pseudoreceptor model for taxanes based on the experimental structure of tubulin. *Il Farmaco*. 2003;58:659-668; Gueritte F. General and recent aspects of the chemistry and structure-activity relationships of taxoids. *Curr Pharm Des*. 2001;7:1229-1249.

Metabolism. The taxanes are metabolized to significantly less cytotoxic metabolites by CYP enzymes (Fig. 36.12). In humans, CYP2C8 converts paclitaxel to 6α-hydroxypaclitaxel, the major metabolite, which is 30-fold less active than the parent structure.[134] Patients carrying CYP2C8*3 may have an increased metabolism of paclitaxel with shorter systemic exposure.[135] CYP3A4 mediates the formation of additional minor *p*-hydroxylated metabolites of the phenyl and benzoyloxy moieties at $C_{3'}$ and C_2, respectively, and the 10-desacetyl metabolite has been documented in plasma.[136,137]

Docetaxel is oxidized exclusively by CYP3A4/5, with CYP3A4 having a 10-fold higher affinity for the drug than CYP3A5. The major metabolite, known as hydroxydocetaxel, is the hydroxymethyl derivative of the 3′-*t*-butoxycarboxamide side chain.[134] Hydroxydocetaxel can be further oxidized and cyclized to oxazolidinedione and diastereomeric hydroxyoxazolidinone metabolites prior to excretion. The oxazolidinedione has been linked to edema and weight gain that are problematic adverse effects of docetaxel.[138]

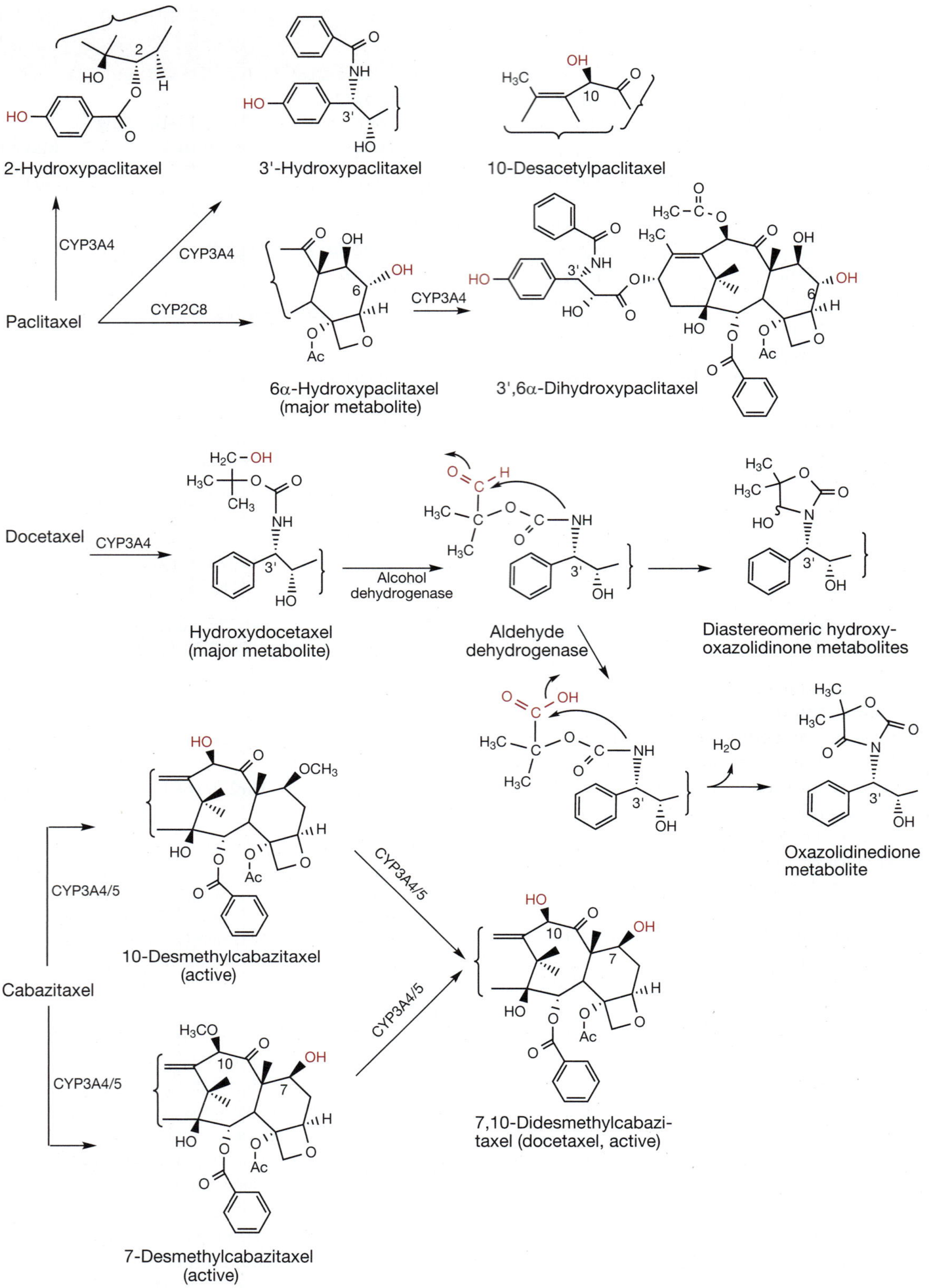

Figure 36.12 Taxane metabolism.

Cabazitaxel is metabolized predominantly (80%-90%) by CYP3A4/5, with CYP2C8 taking on a minor biotransformation role. Three active metabolites (including docetaxel) result from O-demethylation at C_7 and/or C_{10}. The elimination of taxanes is predominantly biliary.

The C_{13} side chain is believed to guide the positioning of taxanes within the catalytic site of CYP enzymes. Specifically, the 3′-phenyl of paclitaxel has been proposed to properly orient C_6 for hydroxylation through π-stacking interactions with CYP2C8 active site residues while decreasing affinity for CYP3A4-binding groups. The hydrophobic character of the 10-acetoxy group, found in paclitaxel, enhances CYP-mediated hydroxylation 2- to 5-fold by facilitating substrate binding and/or augmenting catalytic capability. Both isoforms are impacted by the presence of this ester, often to the same extent.[134]

Epothilones

CHEMISTRY. Low water solubility is a significant drawback to the therapeutic utility of the taxanes. This is particularly true of paclitaxel, which has a more lipophilic acetate moiety at C_{10} compared to docetaxel's polar hydroxyl group. Paclitaxel is administered in a vehicle of 50% alcohol/50% Kolliphor EL, which can lead to an enhanced risk of hypersensitivity reactions (dyspnea, hypotension, angioedema, and urticaria) in patients not pretreated with H_1 and H_2 antagonists and dexamethasone. As noted previously, high P-gp-mediated cellular efflux of paclitaxel and docetaxel can result in drug resistance.

To overcome these problems, epothilones, 16-membered macrolides structurally unrelated to the taxanes but with functional groups properly positioned to mimic critical tubulin-binding groups, have been investigated for use in a variety of solid tumor and hematologic cancers (Fig. 36.13). Epothilone B binds with high affinity to the taxane-binding site on polymerized β-tubulin and acts through the same cytotoxic mechanism (microtubule polymerization and stabilization).[139] In addition to enhanced water solubility and a lack of P-gp affinity, epothilone B is more efficiently produced through fermentation with the myxobacterium *Sorangium cellulosum* and has a higher antineoplastic potency.[132,140,141] The lactam analog ixabepilone has a comparable anticancer activity with an even higher water solubility and better in vivo and in vitro stability[139] (Fig. 36.14). The story of the discovery and subsequent development of this lactam as the lead compound in the search for a paclitaxel alternative makes for interesting reading.[142]

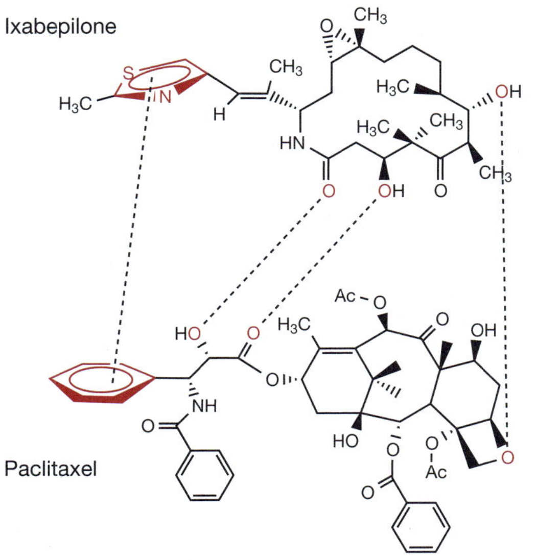

Figure 36.13 Complementary ixabepilone and paclitaxel functional groups.

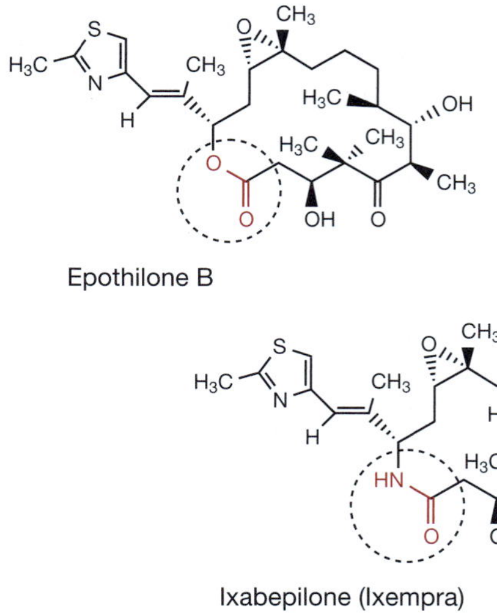

Figure 36.14 Epothilones.

Epothilones and taxanes bind to a shared tubulin-binding site in distinct ways.[124,143,144] A comparison of the crystal structures of tubulin-bound epothilone A (the 12-desmethyl derivative of epothilone B) and paclitaxel documented that the smaller macrolide fills only about half the binding site volume of the larger taxane ligand. The binding site is plastic, and residues adjust their sidechain conformations to accommodate either drug. Despite being surrounded by identical tubulin residues, the only common binding interaction is a hydrogen bond between Arg282 and the 7-OH group of taxanes and epothilones,[143] although the relevance of this interaction to epothilone affinity has been questioned.[144]

Although epothilone B is nearly identical in structure to epothilone A, it binds to β-tubulin via a distinct mode. Molecular dynamics simulations with the native protein complexed with epothilone B have identified key binding interactions (Fig. 36.15), while studies with selected mutant proteins revealed mechanisms of epothilone resistance. Specifically, T274I, R282Q, and Q292E mutations alter the protein's M-loop conformation, disrupting important polar interactions with the ligand that decrease β-tubulin affinity. Gln292 does not bind directly to epothilone B, but it does assure favorable interactions between tubulin dimers important to microtubule formation. Mutation of Gln292 to anionic Glu produces the most profound resistance of any of the mutants studied. Phe270 engages in a critical

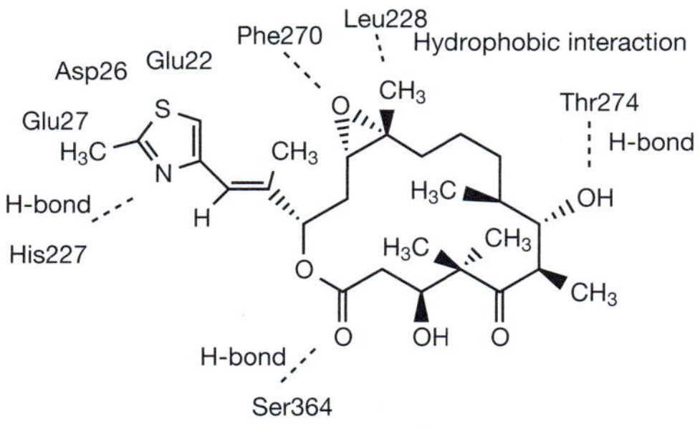

Figure 36.15 Epothilone B-β-tubulin interactions.

interaction with the epoxide oxygen of epothilone B. While mutation to Val (F270V) also significantly decreases ligand affinity, the impact on resistance was the lowest of the four mutants.[144]

Specific Drugs

PACLITAXEL. Paclitaxel is claimed to be "one of the most successful drugs ever used in cancer chemotherapy"[145] and also the "best-selling."[129] It is available in conventional injection (Taxol) and albumin-bound nanoparticle (Abraxane) formulations.

Conventional Injection. Paclitaxel conventional injection is indicated for IV use in combination with cisplatin as first-line therapy for advanced ovarian and non–small cell lung cancer (NSCLC). It is also used alone or in combination with the fluorouracil (FU) prodrug capecitabine in anthracycline-resistant metastatic breast cancer (MBC). Paclitaxel's ability to upregulate thymidine phosphorylase, one of capecitabine's activating enzymes, is the rationale behind the combination therapy.[146]

The Kolliphor EL-solubilized drug is infused in doses of 135 to 175 mg/m^2, most commonly over 3 hours, and can be passed through an in-line, 0.22-μm filter to reduce vehicle-related cloudiness. In addition to hypersensitivity reactions (generally kept at bay by antihistamine/corticosteroid pretreatment), the major use-limiting adverse effect of paclitaxel is dose-dependent myelosuppression, particularly neutropenia, and first doses might need to be decreased in patients with hepatic dysfunction. Subsequent dose reductions, if any, should be tailored to individual responses. The drug should not be given to patients who have baseline neutrophil counts below 1,500 cells/mm^3. The drug carries a boxed warning for both of these serious toxicity risks.[43]

Peripheral sensory neuropathy is a frequently observed adverse effect. This toxicity is cumulative, and, while usually reversible, it can progress to become painful and permanent. Kolliphor EL is known to potentiate the myelosuppressive and neurotoxic adverse effects of this agent.[147] Gastrointestinal (GI) disturbances are common, and alopecia is essentially a given. The drug can severely irritate skin, and hyaluronidase should be administered IV or subcutaneously (SC) if extravasation occurs. Paclitaxel can cause fetal harm and carries a high risk of intrauterine mortality. Both male and female patients are advised not to attempt conception while on this drug. Due caution should be observed when coadministering paclitaxel with drugs that inhibit or compete for metabolizing enzymes, particularly CYP2C8 (eg, 17α-ethinylestradiol and diazepam).

As noted, paclitaxel resistance is mediated primarily through P-gp and βIII-tubulin overexpression. Regarding the latter, it is proposed that the exchange of Ala for Ser at position 277 in βIII-tubulin disrupts the critical H-bond with the C_7-OH, resulting in a loss of affinity.[124]

Albumin-Bound Nanoformulation. Albumin-bound paclitaxel nanoparticles (Abraxane; sometimes referred to as nab-paclitaxel) are administered IV in the same disease states as the conventional injection, although pancreatic carcinoma replaces advanced ovarian cancer as an indication. The boxed warning accompanying this formulation relates to the severe myelosuppression (primarily neutropenia) and cautions against interchanging it with the conventional injection. The colloidal suspension of paclitaxel nanoparticles contains 3% to 4% albumin, which surrounds and solubilizes the drug, eliminating the need for Kolliphor EL. Infusion times drop to 30 minutes, and disease-specific doses of 100 to 260 mg/m^2 are employed.

In addition to the naturally high permeability and impaired lymphatic drainage of neovascularized tumors, targeted delivery to malignant cells is facilitated by active transport of the nanoparticles secondary to albumin binding to gp60 receptors found on the surface of tumor vascular endothelial cells. Binding activates a membrane protein called caveolin-1, which stimulates the formation of vesicles (or caveolae) that accumulate drug-bound albumin and traverse the endothelial cell, ultimately depositing in the interstitial space. Many tumor cells (including NSCLC and pancreatic and ovarian cancer cells) overexpress an albumin-binding glycoprotein known as SPARC (*s*ecreted *p*rotein *a*cidic and *r*ich in *c*ysteine). The binding of albumin to SPARC allows for internalization of paclitaxel and it makes its way to the nucleus (its site of action).[147,148]

The literature is replete with reports of Abraxane trials in various cancers, often in combination with other drugs. In NSCLC, a multinational phase III trial in patients with advanced disease showed nab-paclitaxel to provide PFS and OS outcomes statistically equivalent to conventional paclitaxel, while providing a statistically significant increase in overall response rate, particularly among patients with squamous cell pathology.[147] A lower frequency of neuropathy was noted in the nab-paclitaxel arm of the study, possibly due to the absence of Kolliphor EL. Still, it has been reported that the overall response rate elicited by Abraxane is 21%, which has fueled the ongoing quest for novel paclitaxel delivery systems that retain all of nab-paclitaxel's clinical advantages and improve upon its therapeutic efficacy.[145] Nanoformulations of paclitaxel in liposomal and micelle-based delivery systems are available in many countries.[149]

DOCETAXEL. The indications for docetaxel include cancers of the breast, prostate, and head/neck as well as NSCLC and gastric adenocarcinoma. It has greater water solubility than paclitaxel due to the unesterified C_{10}-OH group, and it is formulated with polysorbate 80 (Tween) rather than with Kolliphor EL. Hypersensitivity reactions, while less likely, are still possible, and all patients should receive antihistamine/corticosteroid premedication. In addition to neutropenia and teratogenicity, this taxane can induce significant fluid retention, and 2-kg weight gains are not uncommon. As noted previously, fluid retention has been associated with the cyclized oxazolidinedione metabolite (see Fig. 36.12). A significant association between ABCB1 polymorphism with risk of hematologic toxicity (C3435T) and fluid retention (G2677T) was also found.[150] A boxed warning advises about hypersensitivity, edema, myelosuppression, and use in patients with significant liver impairment. Notably, alopecia, which is reversible with most cytotoxic drugs, can be permanent with high-dose docetaxel (cumulative dose 400 mg/m^2). Scalp cooling with a hypothermia gel cap while receiving docetaxel can prevent this adverse effect.[151] While uncommon, treatment-related deaths from sepsis have also been reported.

DDIs have been noted when docetaxel is coadministered with drugs that inhibit or compete for CYP3A4 enzymes.[152] Like paclitaxel, docetaxel is a P-gp substrate, and strict attention must be paid when drugs that bind to or inhibit this efflux protein are a part of the patient's therapeutic regimen.

CABAZITAXEL. Although currently less widely used than paclitaxel or docetaxel, cabazitaxel has some unique activities and advantages that deserve mention.

The 7,10-dimethoxy ether moieties of cabazitaxel dramatically lower affinity for P-gp, resulting in sustained retention in tumor cells (twice that of docetaxel) and efficacy in docetaxel-resistant cell lines where resistance is due to P-gp overexpression.[123,153] It is currently approved for use only in metastatic CRPC that has progressed despite docetaxel therapy. A recent meta-analysis comparing the efficacy of cabazitaxel against other CRPC therapies (including docetaxel, both in combination with prednisolone) identified cabazitaxel as the most suitable agent in this disease due to equitable or superior efficacy as evaluated by PFS, OS, and PSA attenuation.[154] In addition, cabazitaxel was viewed as having a better overall margin of safety. Other studies comparing these two taxanes have reported similar findings and claim that their different adverse effect profiles may help practitioners optimize safety and quality of life for individual patients.[155]

Neutropenia is the most problematic dose-limiting reaction of cabazitaxel, although its incidence and severity are no worse than those observed with other taxanes. It does not promote the fluid retention commonly observed with docetaxel. Peripheral neuropathy can be persistent, although some studies have claimed the incidence of this adverse effect is low.[156] The relatively high incidence of diarrhea (up to 47%) may be explained by the accumulation of the drug in enterocytes, cells that constitutively express P-gp and, therefore, actively evict other taxanes. The use of the recommended starting dose of 20 mg/m^2 has been associated with fewer adverse effects than the upper limit dose of 25 mg/m^2. Importantly, the lower dose demonstrated noninferiority efficacy.[156] Administration is via a 1-hour IV infusion once every 3 weeks.

Despite the conversion of the two secondary alcohols to more lipophilic ethers, cabazitaxel's aqueous solubility is similar to that of docetaxel. Like docetaxel, it is formulated with polysorbate 80 rather than the more hypersensitivity-inducing Kolliphor EL. It is administered by IV infusion in doses of 25 mg/m^2 every 3 weeks, and a boxed warning cautions about hypersensitivity and neutropenia.[43]

IXABEPILONE. The epothilone ixabepilone is used in combination with the thymidylate synthesis inhibitor capecitabine in anthracycline- and/or taxane-resistant advanced breast cancer or MBC, or when these alternative drugs are contraindicated. Like cabazitaxel, it retains activity in tumors overexpressing P-gp, although the literature differs on the issue of efficacy in βIII-tubulin expressing cells.[124,139] The lactam moiety provides stability to carboxyesterase-catalyzed hydrolysis, but the drug is extensively metabolized by CYP3A4 to over 30 inactive metabolites prior to predominately fecal excretion.[139] DDIs with CYP3A4 substrates, inducers, or inhibitors have been reported, and dosage adjustments may be warranted if coadministration cannot be avoided. Dose reductions are also required in patients with compromised hepatic function. A boxed warning cautions against administration to patients with elevated liver enzymes and/or bilirubin due to an increased risk of neutropenia-associated fatalities.[43]

Some phase II clinical trials have shown overall response rates to this agent as high as 57% in patients with previously untreated breast cancer and up to 30% in patients who had been heavily pretreated.[157] Ixabepilone-capecitabine combination therapy provides superior outcomes compared to capecitabine monotherapy but with a higher risk of adverse cardiac events, including ischemia and ventricular dysfunction. Ixabepilone is less effective than paclitaxel in advancing PFS and OS, but essentially equivalent in efficacy and safety to eribulin, a synthetic analog of a marine-derived natural product (halichondrin B) also used in the treatment of MBC (see next).[158]

Like cabazitaxel, ixabepilone's serious use-limiting adverse effects include peripheral neuropathy and neutropenia. Diarrhea can occur, likely due to the retention of drug in enterocytes, but the incidence with monotherapy (22%) is less than half that of cabazitaxel. Like paclitaxel, it uses Kolliphor EL for solubilization, so prophylactic premedication to protect against hypersensitivity reactions is required. The most common IV dosage regimen is 40 mg/m^2 administered over 3 hours every third week. This regimen increases the overall response rate compared to once-weekly dosing but with an elevated incidence of peripheral neuropathy. The once-weekly regimen may be valuable in patients in whom neutropenia risk must be minimized. Diarrhea incidence between the two regimens is similar.[158]

Vinca Alkaloids

MECHANISM OF ACTION. Several alkaloids found naturally in *Catharanthus roseus* (periwinkle) have potent antimitotic activity. In contrast to taxanes and epothilones, vinca alkaloids halt cell division by inhibiting microtubule polymerization. They bind to a single high-affinity β-tubulin site at the interface of two heterodimers within the tubular lumen near the GTP-binding site on the (+) end of the tubules. Once bound, these alkaloids prevent the uptake of the GTP essential to tubule elongation.[159] Simultaneous binding to the α- and β-tubulin results in protein cross-linking, which promotes a stabilized protofilament structure.[160] Inhibition of microtubule elongation occurs at substoichiometric concentrations, at which alkaloid occupation of only 1% to 2% of the total number of high-affinity sites can result in up to a 50% inhibition of microtubule assembly.[161,162] At high concentrations, when alkaloid binding to high-affinity sites becomes stoichiometric and lower-affinity binding sites on the tubule wall are also occupied, microtubular depolymerization is stimulated, leading to the exposure of additional alkaloidal-binding sites and resulting in dramatic changes in microtubular conformation. Spiral aggregates, protofilaments, and highly structured crystals form, and the mitotic spindle ultimately disintegrates.[146,163] The loss of the directing mitotic spindle promotes chromosome "clumping" in unnatural shapes (balls and stars), leading to cell death. Other nonmitotic toxicities related to the microtubule-disrupting action of vinca alkaloids include inhibition of axonal transport and secretory processes, and disturbances in platelet structure and function.[161]

The mutant *p53* oncogene is associated with resistance to vinca alkaloid-induced cytotoxicity due to its augmentation of MAP-4-mediated microtubulin polymerization, which counteracts the depolymerizing mechanism of the alkaloids. In addition, the mutant oncogene causes the overexpression of a cytosolic protein, stathmin, which in its phosphorylated state prevents the cells from entering mitosis. Finally, *p53* upregulates the MRP-1 efflux protein that ejects vinca alkaloids from cells. It has been suggested that establishing a patient's *p53* phenotype could better predict the anticipated susceptibility to various mitosis inhibitor antineoplastic therapy options.[164]

CHEMISTRY. The vinca alkaloids are complex structures composed of two polycyclic segments, catharanthine and vindoline (see Fig. 36.11), both of which are essential for high-affinity tubulin binding. Of the three-marketed vinca-based mitosis inhibitors, two are natural products (vincristine and vinblastine), and one is a semisynthetic alkaloid derivative (vinorelbine). Vincristine and vinblastine have the highest and lowest tubulin affinity, respectively.[162]

Molecular simulation and docking studies with crystal structures of tubulin and vinblastine have allowed for the identification of potential tubulin-binding modes and suggested specific drug–tubulin interactions.[165,166] Chi et al[165] have proposed a "double faces sticking mechanism," where the polar functional groups of the catharanthine and vindoline moieties (the two "faces") seek out identical polar/charged residues on the dimerized tubulin, including residues within the 178 to 226 range on β-tubulin and 326 to 336 on α-tubulin. The point of difference in the binding options is the replacement of an α-tubulin Lys352 in the catharanthine mode by a β-tubulin Lys176 in the vindoline approach.

The three available vinca structures differ in the length of the alkyl chain bridging positions 6′ and 9′ of the catharanthine moiety (methylene or ethylene), in the substituents at position 4′ (olefin or tertiary alcohol), and in the vindoline indole nitrogen substituent (methyl or formyl). Although subtle, these structural changes lead to significant differences in clinical spectrum, potency, and toxicity. For example, vincristine's relative lack of bone marrow toxicity at standard therapeutic doses makes it popular in combination therapy with more myelosuppressive anticancer agents, whereas vinblastine's relative lack of neurotoxicity permits its coadministration with cisplatin. It is known that acetylation of either hydroxyl group destroys antineoplastic action, and reduction of the vindoline olefinic linkage greatly attenuates activity. The C_{18}′-methoxycarbonyl and the stereochemistry at positions 18′ and 2′ are believed to be critical to activity, as is the dihedral angle involving carbons 17′, 18′, 15, and 16 that connects the catharanthine and vindoline moieties of the alkaloids.[165-167]

Because vinca alkaloids enter cells by passive diffusion, unbound vinorelbine and vinblastine (being more lipophilic than vincristine) may be more extensively taken up into tissues. Vincristine, however, is cleared more slowly from the system and has the longest terminal half-life of the three agents, resulting in a more prolonged tumor cell exposure. Like paclitaxel and docetaxel, resistance is mediated, in part, through P-gp.

Vinca alkaloids undergo O_4-deacetylation to yield metabolites that are equipotent to or more active than the parent drug. They are also subject to extensive CYP3A4/5-mediated metabolism before biliary excretion.[168-173] Vincristine alone is selectively metabolized by the 3A5 isoform.[170] About 35 metabolites of vinblastine have been identified.[174] A representative hydrolyzed metabolite of vinblastine and the major CYP3A-generated metabolites of the other vinca alkaloids are shown in Figure 36.16. As CYP metabolism is inactivating and CYP3A overexpression has been noted in human tumors, it has been proposed that CYP3A enzymes could contribute to vinca alkaloid resistance.[172]

SPECIFIC DRUGS. Vinca alkaloids contain two ionizable nitrogen atoms and are marketed as water-soluble salts. No oil-based solubilizers are required for IV administration.

Vincristine Sulfate. Vincristine is employed in many hematologic malignancies and is a common choice in pediatric and adult ALL. It is also given in Wilms tumor (an almost exclusively pediatric renal cancer), rhabdomyosarcoma, and neuroblastoma. The drug is given by IV infusion over 5 to 10 minutes using a minibag, via a 1-minute IV push or, less commonly, infused over 24 hours. Continuous infusion may result in more pronounced toxicity, and the drug is fatal if administered by the intrathecal route. A liposomal formulation, marketed as Marqibo, is available to treat relapsed ALL. As with the liposomal anticancer agents discussed previously, this formulation is not interchangeable with the conventional IV dosage form. The urinary elimination half-life of liposomal vincristine is approximately 45 hours.

Elimination of conventional vincristine is triphasic, with the first phase (5 minutes) representing rapid uptake into tissues and the terminal phase (85 hours) representing release back to the plasma from tubulin-containing cells. Since the drug is extensively metabolized by O_4-deacetylation and selective CYP3A5-catalyzed oxidation in the liver, patients with hepatic dysfunction are at an increased risk for toxicity, and dosage reductions should be considered.

The most significant dose-limiting adverse effect is peripheral neuropathy, which initially manifests as numbness and painful paresthesias in the extremities and progresses to muscular pain, severe weakness, and loss of coordination. White children receiving vincristine experience a higher level of drug-induced neurotoxicity compared to African American pediatric patients. The significantly higher incidence of the rapidly metabolizing *CYP3A5*1* allele phenotype in the latter population (75% vs 19%) may explain the toxicity difference.[171] Patients can also experience constipation secondary to intestinal neurotoxicity, which may require treatment with cathartics. Myelosuppression is not particularly problematic because it occurs at doses higher than those that can be tolerated.

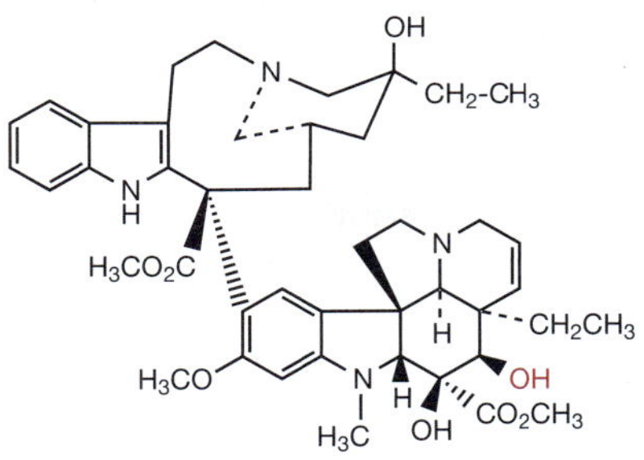

Deacetylvinblastine (active)

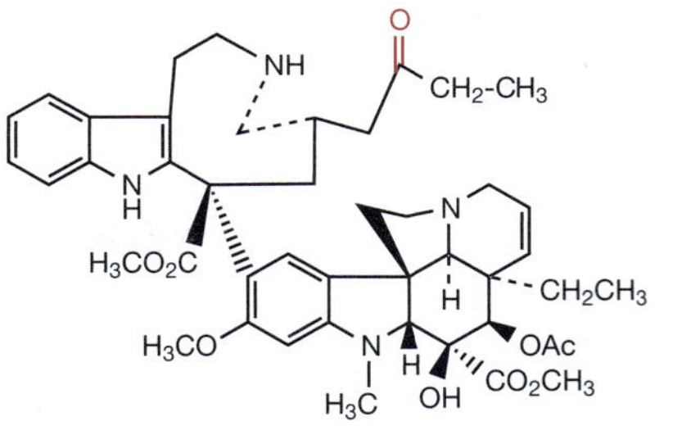

Vincristine M1 metabolite (inactive)

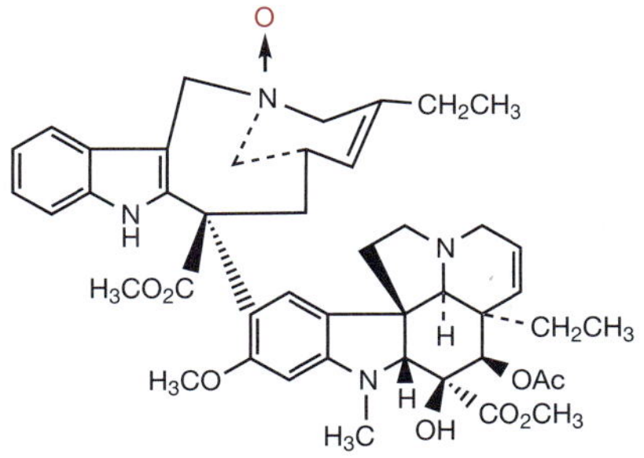

Vinorelbine N-oxide metabolite (inactive)

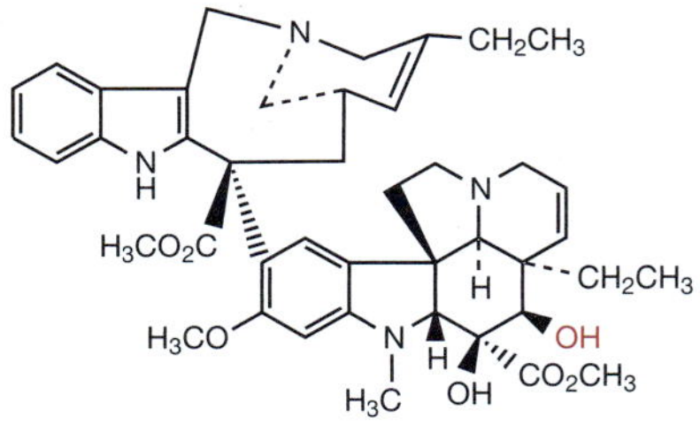

Deacetylvinorelbine (active)

Figure 36.16 Major metabolites of vinca alkaloids.

All vinca alkaloids are severe vesicants that can induce necrosis, cellulitis, and/or thrombophlebitis. Proper needle placement before administration should be assured to eliminate the risk of extravasation. Unlike the tissue damage caused by the vesicant action of nitrogen mustards (discussed later) and anthracyclines, cold exacerbates tissue destruction. If extravasation occurs, apply heat for 1 hour 4 times a day for 3 to 5 days, coupled with local hyaluronidase injections. Vincristine and vinblastine carry boxed warnings for extravasation risk and appropriate administration routes.

Vinblastine Sulfate. Vinblastine is used as palliative therapy in hematologic malignancies and has found utility in the treatment of advanced testicular carcinoma (often in combination with bleomycin), advanced mycosis fungoides, and Kaposi sarcoma. Leukopenia is the dose-limiting adverse effect, and the dose should be cut in half for patients with serum bilirubin levels between 3 and 5 mg/dL. Patients with serum bilirubin above 5 mg/dL should not receive vinblastine. The drug-related impact on erythrocyte and thrombocyte levels is usually insignificant.

Short IV infusions through a minibag are the preferred administration route, but 1-minute infusions into a free-flowing IV line are allowed. Prolonged infusion (>0.5-1 hour) increases the risk of extravasation. The initial elimination half-life of 3.7 minutes is similar to vincristine, but the 25-hour terminal half-life is significantly shorter. Since CYP3A metabolism is not specific for the 3A5 isoform, pharmacogenetic-related variability in efficacy and safety is of no concern.

Vinorelbine Tartrate. Vinorelbine is used alone or in combination with cisplatin for first-line treatment of NSCLC. It is administered by IV push or rapid bolus over 6 to 10 minutes. Administration over a longer time period can result in phlebitis and injection pain. As with the other drugs in this class, intrathecal administration is fatal.

Vinorelbine's initial phase elimination half-life is on par with that of vincristine and vinblastine, and the terminal half-life is between 28 and 44 hours. Although dose-limiting granulocytopenia is the major adverse effect (and myelosuppression the reason behind its boxed warning), potentially fatal interstitial pulmonary changes have been noted. Patients with symptoms of respiratory distress should be promptly evaluated. As with all vinca alkaloids, elimination is primarily biliary, and dosage reduction should be considered in patients with liver dysfunction. Deacetylvinorelbine is the predominant human metabolite. While active, its serum concentration is minimal. Both CYP3A4 and 3A5 are involved in inactivating metabolism so the pharmacogenetic-based impact of higher or lower 3A5 activity on tumor response or rate/severity of adverse effects is not significant.

Halichondrins

Halichondrin B is a chemical found in *Halichondria okadai*, a rare Japanese sea sponge. This structure and its therapeutically active macrolide component known as eribulin destabilize microtubules by interfering with the elongation phase of dynamic instability, inhibiting polymerization without any direct impact on erosion.[175] The interaction of these two large molecules with β-tubulin has been modeled.[176] Their binding site is within the vinca alkaloid domain on the ends of β-tubulin, approximately 16 Å from vinblastine's binding site, and they serve as competitive inhibitors of vinblastine binding. Eribulin's affinity for this binding site is 3 times higher than that of halichondrin B. Five hydrogen bonds involving O_3, O_7, O_{11}, and N_1 are particularly crucial to eribulin-tubulin binding.

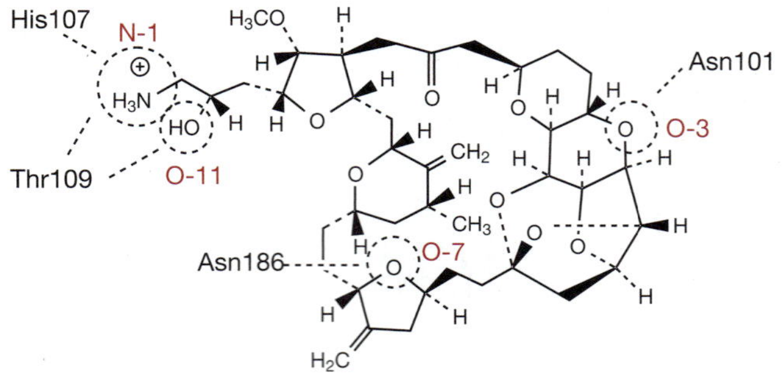

Eribulin-tubulin interactions

Eribulin Mesylate. Eribulin mesylate is indicated in patients with MBC who have received at least two prior regimens that included a taxane and an anthracycline. Phase III trials comparing eribulin to the physician's choice of alternative chemotherapy have documented significant improvement in median OS and objective response rate; PFS was also augmented.[177] As noted earlier, one clinical trial found eribulin's efficacy to be equivalent to ixabepilone.[158]

Like vinca alkaloids, eribulin contains a basic amino nitrogen that readily protonates at physiologic pH. The water-soluble mesylate salt can be reconstituted in sterile water and administered directly or diluted with normal saline. Eribulin is administered by IV infusion over 2 to 5 minutes, and patients seem to do better when the drug is given on days 1 and 8 of a 21-day cycle than on days 1, 8, and 15 of a 28-day cycle.[178] Serious side effects include myelosuppression (specifically neutropenia and anemia), constipation, and peripheral neuropathy (the most common cause of drug discontinuation). Many patients experience fatigue. QT-interval prolongation can sometimes occur on day 8 (but not on day 1) of eribulin therapy. The effect can be additive with other drugs that also prolong the QT interval.[43] Eribulin is not significantly metabolized, and the risk of DDIs with CYP substrates, inhibitors, or inducers is insignificant.[175] Fecal excretion of unchanged drug predominates.

Antimetabolites

Many antimetabolites stop de novo DNA biosynthesis by inhibiting the formation of the nucleotides that make up these life-sustaining polymers. The rate-limiting enzymes of nucleotide biosynthesis are the primary targets for the antimetabolites since inhibition of these key enzymes is the most efficient way to shut down any biochemical reaction sequence. Other enzymes required in DNA biosynthesis can be inhibited, or chain elongation can be arrested through the incorporation of false nucleotides into the growing DNA strand.

The antimetabolites serve as false substrates for critical nucleotide biosynthesis or polymerizing enzymes. These enzyme inhibitors are designed to structurally mimic the normal (endogenous) substrate. Antimetabolites can bind irreversibly or pseudoirreversibly to their target enzyme(s) and shut down enzyme activity. If the building block nucleotides cannot be synthesized or DNA polymerization is blocked, then DNA synthesis (and tumor growth) is stopped dead in its tracks.

Many antimetabolite antineoplastics are categorized by the class of nucleotide they inhibit. Purine antagonists inhibit the synthesis of adenosine monophosphate (AMP) and guanosine monophosphate (GMP), while pyrimidine antagonists stop the production of dTMP. Antifolates shut down purine and pyrimidine biosynthesis pathways since folate cofactors are essential to both. DNA polymerase inhibitors are nucleotide mimics that, when added to a growing DNA chain, halt further chain elongation. The structures of the anticancer antimetabolites are provided in Figure 36.17.

Purine Antagonists

AMP and GMP Biosynthesis. Purine antagonists that inhibit the de novo biosynthesis of AMP and GMP target the rate-limiting enzyme amidophosphoribosyltransferase, also known as glutamine-5-phosphoribosylpyrophosphate amidotransferase (Fig. 36.18). The rate-limiting step is the first of the purine biosynthetic pathway; if that step is inhibited no other step can proceed. Since the rate-limiting transferase enzyme works on a phosphorylated ribose substrate, no enzyme in the sequence will function without its presence. The formylation reaction catalyzed by glycinamide ribonucleotide (GAR) formyltransferase requires the one-carbon-donating 10-formyltetrahydrofolate and can be inhibited by the antifolates methotrexate and pemetrexed (discussed next).

Chemistry. Mercaptopurine and thioguanine are the two 6-thiol purine antagonists currently marketed (Fig. 36.17). They are prodrugs and must be converted to ribonucleotides by hypoxanthine-guanine phosphoribosyltransferase (HGPRT) before they can exert their cytotoxic actions (Fig. 36.19). Thioinosine-5′-monophosphate and its S-methylated metabolite halt AMP and GMP biosynthesis by inhibiting amidophosphoribosyltransferase (the rate-limiting enzyme of de novo purine biosynthesis) and inosine monophosphate dehydrogenase (IMPDH, the enzyme that generates xanthylic acid from inosinic acid later in the pathway). A second mechanism, believed to be the more therapeutically important one for both thiopurines, involves the incorporation of thioguanine triphosphate deoxyribo- and ribonucleotides (generally referred to as 6-thioguanine nucleotides or 6TGNs) generated within the tumor cell into DNA and RNA, respectively.[179,180] This illicit substitution causes structural changes in DNA, activates the DNA mismatch repair (MMR) system, and induces apoptosis.[181]

As alluded to, thiopurines are metabolized by S-methylation via the polymorphic enzyme thiopurine methyl transferase (TPMT) with S-adenosylmethionine (SAM) serving as a cofactor. The 6-methylthioinosine-5′-monophosphate metabolite (also known as 6-methylthioinosinic acid) is a potent inhibitor of the amidophosphoribosyltransferase enzyme and can contribute to the cytotoxic action of the parent nucleotide (Fig. 36.19). However, since the primary therapeutic mechanism of thiopurines is cell cycle arrest and apoptosis secondary to the incorporation of 6TGNs into DNA, methylation is viewed as detracting from therapeutic efficacy.[180,182] In contrast to 6-methylthioinosine-5′-monophosphate, little

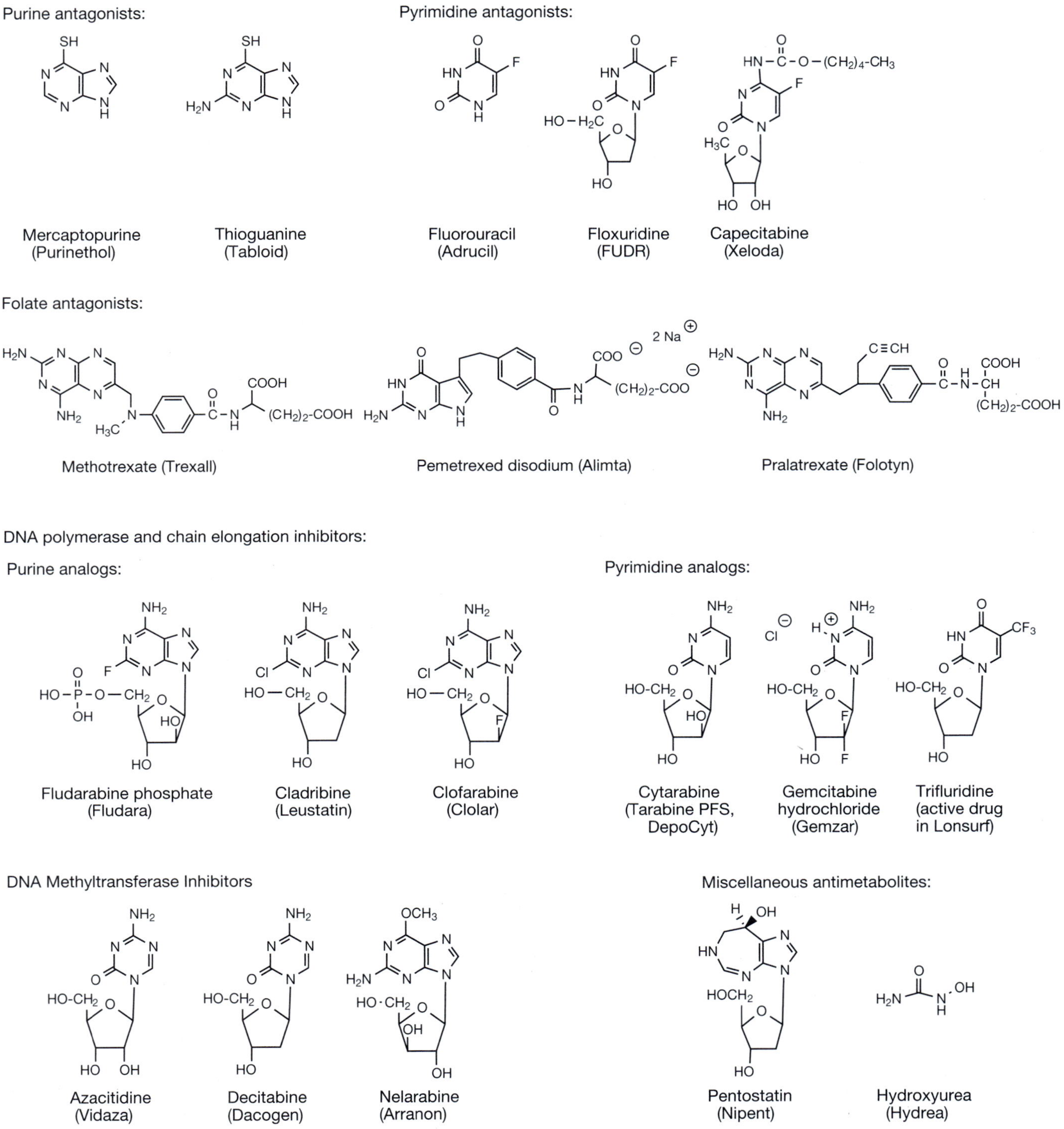

Figure 36.17 Antimetabolites.

or no 6-methylthioguanosine-5′-monophosphate (6-methylthioguanylic acid) is produced inside the cell.[183,184] The thiopurine bases can also be methylated by TPMT, but these metabolites do not react with HGPRT and remain permanently inactive, a fact the drug manufacturers take into consideration when establishing dosing regimens.

TPMT is polymorphic, and the *3, *3A, *3B, and *3C alleles are associated with only about 10% of wild-type (normal) enzyme activity.[180] Patients who are poor TPMT metabolizers (PMs) (~10% of Whites but also evident in other races) will not experience inactivating methylation of the prodrug structure and will generate more of the active 6-thioinosinic/thioguanylic acid per dose than patients with normal or excessive levels of the enzyme. The TPMT genotype of patients should be assessed before initiating thiopurine therapy because PMs are at a high risk of life-threatening myelosuppression and serious infection from elevated levels of 6TGNs, even when standard doses are administered.[180,182,183] In addition,

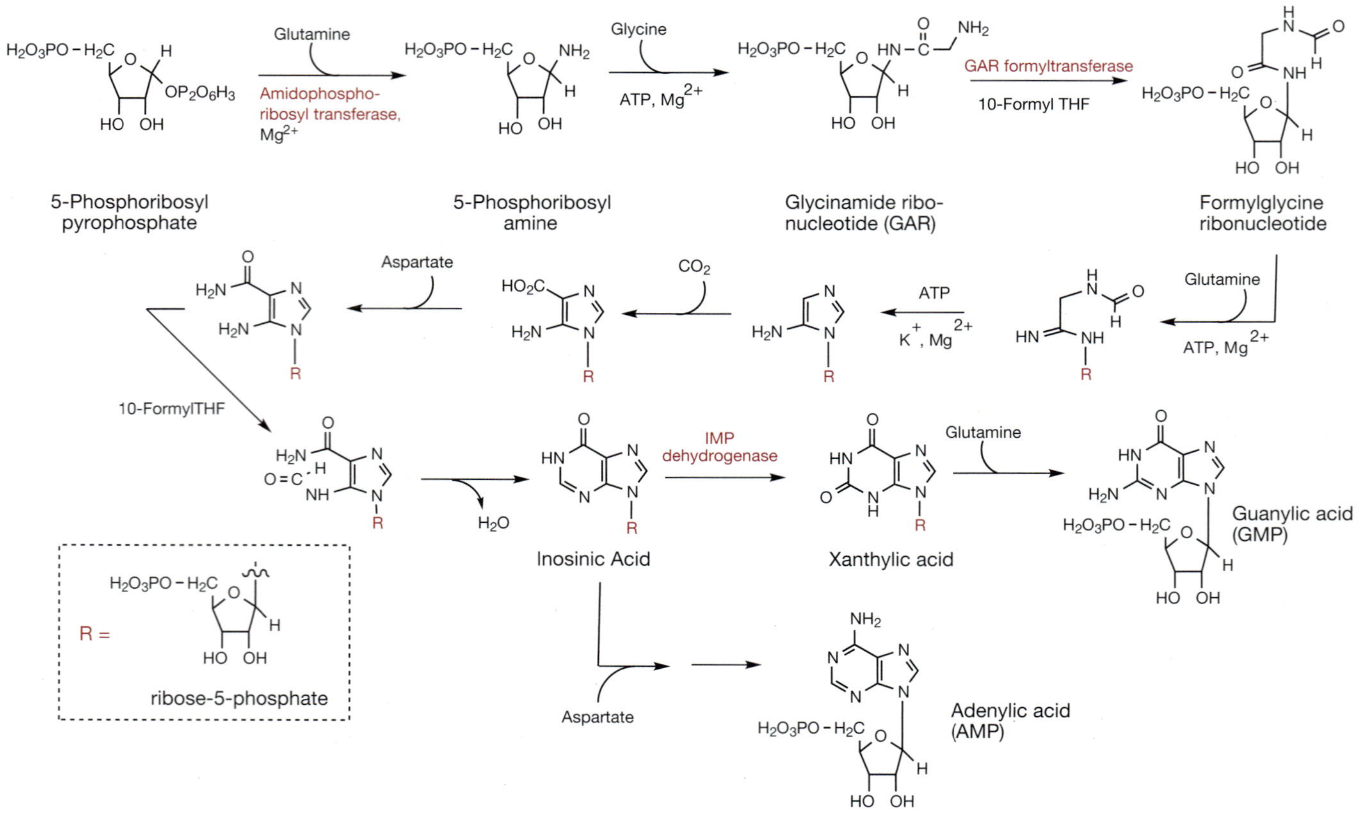

Figure 36.18 Biosynthesis of purine nucleotides.

the accumulation of mutagenic thiopurine-based ribonucleotides and their incorporation into DNA puts these patients at higher risk for secondary malignancies.[182,184] Thiopurines can still be used in TPMT PMs, but the dose should be significantly decreased in accordance with published guidelines[43] and white blood cell counts monitored vigilantly. Mercaptopurine appears to be more highly impacted by the TPMT genotype than thioguanine.[185]

On the flip side, extensive TPMT metabolizers, who represent up to 90% of patients on thiopurine therapy, will form lower amounts of apoptotic 6TGNs potentially leading to treatment failure and relapse. Higher doses of mercaptopurine are required in these patients.[186] Coupled to that, in the case of mercaptopurine, the molecules of ribonucleotide generated will be methylated very rapidly to 6-methylthioinosinic acid, and this can predispose to drug-induced hepatotoxicity.[180,182,183] In contrast, extensive TPMT metabolizers show a decreased sensitivity to thioguanine because there is no compensatory increase in the formation of methylated ribonucleotide to offset the decreased production of 6-thioguanylic acid.[184]

It is claimed that approximately 70% of patients who experience adverse effects from thiopurines have normal TPMT levels, so TPMT genetic testing (as important as it is) is not a panacea.[180] Yet another genetic variation that has a strong association with hematologic toxicity is *NUDT15*, a gene that encodes for a nucleotide diphosphatase protein nudix hydrolase 15. The NUDT15 protein enzymatically converts cytotoxic thioguanosine triphosphate (TGTP) and thiodeoxyguanosine triphosphate (TdGTP) to monophosphates.[187] Carriers of *NUDT15*3* and *NUDT15*2* produce NUDT15 protein that is devoid of activity, thus increasing exposure to cytotoxic TGTP and TdGTP. Dose reduction to less than 10% in PMs and 30% to 80% of the normal dose in intermediate metabolizers is recommended. The NUDT15*3 variant is most common in Asian populations.[188,189]

Similarly, genes that encode for inosine triphosphate pyrophosphatase (ITPA) are also known to impact the metabolic and toxicity profiles of mercaptopurine. ITPA normally converts inosine triphosphate (ITP) to the monophosphate and, in so doing, advances AMP and GMP biosynthesis. However, it also hydrolyzes 6-mercaptopurine triphosphate to the monophosphate.[182] The ITPA 94C>A variant expresses ITPA that has half the activity of the wild-type enzyme, causing a buildup of the toxic thioinosine triphosphate metabolite. Carriers of this variant appear to be at significantly higher risk for the development of mercaptopurine-induced febrile neutropenia even after TPMT genotype-based dosage adjustment.[190-192] Other potential pharmacogenetic-based influences on thiopurine drug disposition in children have been proposed.[182,193]

Xanthine oxidase competes with TPMT for mercaptopurine and converts it to inactive 6-thiouric acid, which is excreted in the urine (Fig. 36.19).[194] 6-Thioinosinic acid is also subject to metabolism via the xanthine oxidase pathway, ultimately forming the same inactive metabolite. Allopurinol, which inhibits xanthine oxidase and increases levels of active 6-thioinosinic acid, can be coadministered with mercaptopurine to increase the duration of action and antineoplastic potency. However, the mercaptopurine dose must be cut to 25% to 33% of the standard dose to avoid serious toxicity.[43,179]

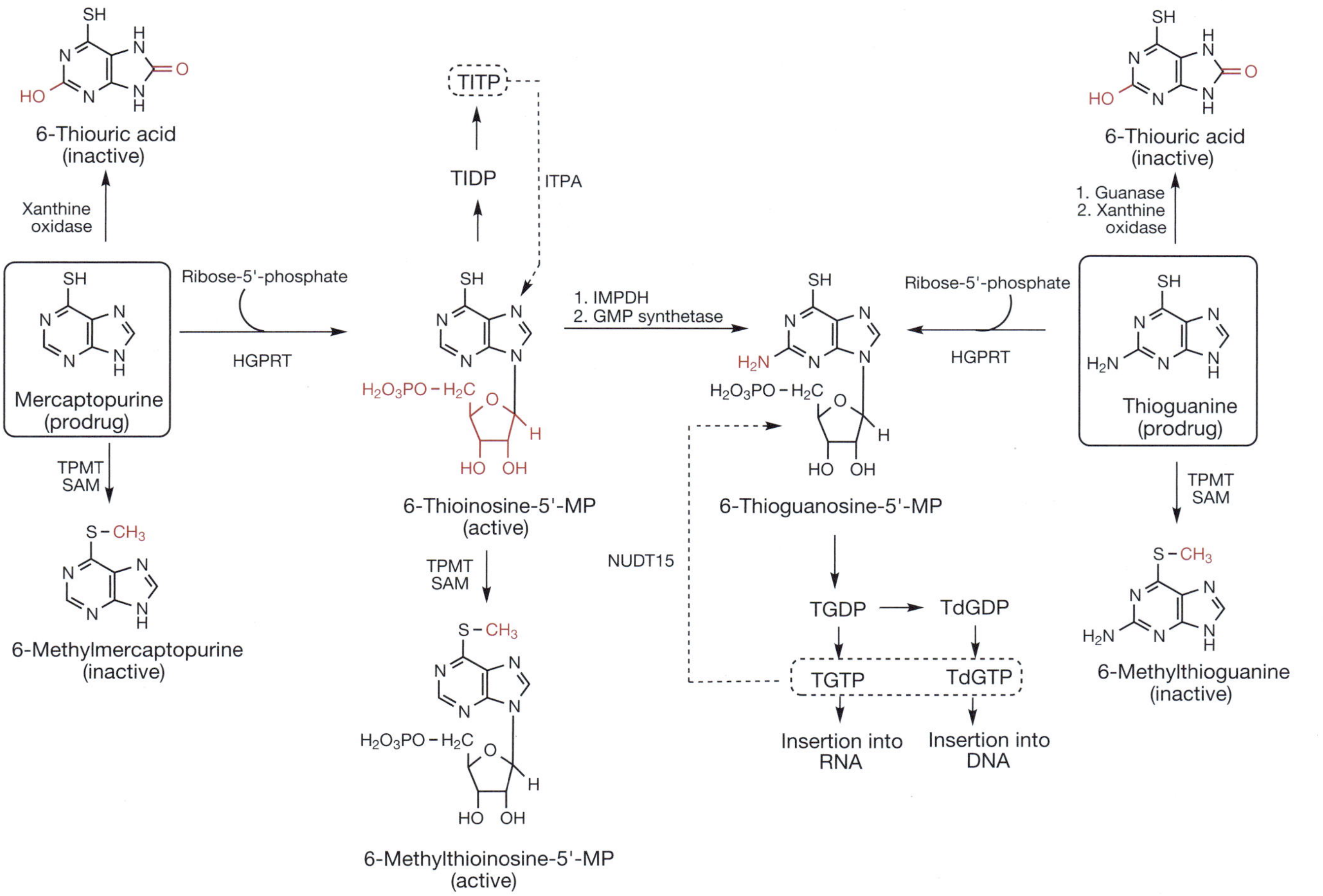

Figure 36.19 Thiopurine metabolism leading to activation and inactivation. HGPRT, hypoxanthine-guanine phosphoribosyl transferase; IMPDH, inosine monophosphate dehydrogenase; ITPA, inosine triphosphate pyrophosphatase; NUDT15, Nudix hydrolase 15; SAM, *S*-adenosylmethionine; TdGDP/TdGTP, 6-thiodeoxyguanosine-5′-di/triphosphate; TGDP/TGTP, 6-thioguanosine-5′-di/triphosphate; TIDP/TITP, 6-thioinosine-5′-di/triphosphate; TPMT, thiopurine methyltransferase.

There are literature reports of children with ALL who experienced use-limiting hepato- or pancreatic toxicity on standard mercaptopurine doses but who were able to continue treatment on a much lower dose (commonly 33% of normal) when this combination therapy strategy was employed.[186,195] In contrast to mercaptopurine, allopurinol does not produce the same level of increase in thioguanine availability and, therefore, is not used as a cotherapy with thioguanine.

Specific Drugs

Mercaptopurine. Mercaptopurine (see Fig. 36.17) is used in the treatment of ALL, and its role in maintenance therapy is believed to have contributed to the 90% OS rate in children with this malignancy.[195] It is available in an oral dosage form, but absorption can be erratic and is reduced by the presence of food. The usual daily dose is 1.5 to 2.5 mg/kg (50-75 mg/m^2) in adults and children, with appropriate adjustment if excessive leukopenia, thrombocytopenia, or anemia is noted. Dosage adjustments should be considered in the face of renal or hepatic impairment. In addition to myelosuppression, immunosuppression and GI distress are common. High levels of methylated metabolites can induce potentially fatal hepatotoxicity requiring drug discontinuation. As noted previously, coadministration of allopurinol allows a significantly lower effective dose of mercaptopurine, potentially permitting continuation of therapy after recovery from drug-induced toxicity.

Resistance to mercaptopurine (and thioguanine) therapy involves deficiency in the activating HGPRT enzyme, increases in alkaline phosphatase, TPMT extensive metabolizer phenotype, and attenuated active uptake via nucleoside transporters.[196,197]

Thioguanine. Thioguanine (see Fig. 37.17) is administered orally at a daily dose of 2 mg/kg in the acute treatment of AML. Its value when added to other antineoplastic agents has been questioned,[179] and it is not recommended for maintenance therapy due to a high risk of hepatotoxicity.[43] Like mercaptopurine, absorption is incomplete and variable, and the toxicities are qualitatively similar. The risk of secondary malignancies may be greater since 6-thioguanylate is not an effective inhibitor of the amidotransferase enzyme and acts almost exclusively through the DNA/RNA incorporation of false guanine nucleotides.

Pyrimidine Antagonists

dTMP Biosynthesis. Looked at simply, dTMP is produced via C_5-methylation of deoxyuridine monophosphate (dUMP).

The rate-limiting enzyme of the dTMP synthetic pathway is the cysteine-containing thymidylate synthase (TS), with 5,10-methylenetetrahydrofolate (5,10-methylene THF) serving as the methyl-donating cofactor. All dTMP synthesis inhibitors will inhibit TS either directly or indirectly, and this will result in a "thymineless death" in actively dividing cells. Without dTMP and its deoxythymidine triphosphate metabolite, DNA will fragment, and the cell will die.[198] An examination of the different steps in the conversion of dUMP to dTMP (Fig. 36.20) will facilitate understanding of how the pyrimidine antagonist drugs work.

Chemistry. The TS enzyme is a large homodimer and the active site–binding motifs for both substrate and cofactor are highly conserved regardless of source.[199] The noncovalent binding of substrate and cofactor promotes a conformational change in TS that properly orients all key functional groups for the reaction to occur.[200] The dUMP substrate binds to TS first, quickly followed by 5,10-methylene THF cofactor binding. In this loosely bound noncovalent ternary complex, the pteridine ring of the cofactor is stacked directly above the pyrimidine ring of dUMP while the *p*-aminobenzoic acid-glutamate tail projects upward.[201,202] As the TS adopts the required closed conformation, a slow opening of the 5,10-imidazolidine ring and N_{10} protonation of the cofactor produces the reactive N_5-iminium ion, **1** (see Fig. 36.20). The sulfhydryl moiety of synthase Cys195, as the thiolate anion, launches a nucleophilic attack on the highly electrophilic C_6 of dUMP, forming a covalent bond. The bond that breaks, as a result, is the 5,6-double bond of dUMP, and the substrate rearranges into a $C_{4,5}$-enolate, **2**.[203] The subsequent attack by the enolate on the δ^+ methylene group of the N_5-iminium ion results in a covalent ternary complex, **3**, of the enzyme, substrate, and cofactor.[204] Base-mediated abstraction of the substrate C_5-H, (possibly by TS Tyr94 or water molecules associated with it)[203,205] and release of cofactor N_5-methylene dissociate the ternary complex into an intermediate, **4**, with an exocyclic methylene group at C_5. The electron-enriched cofactor N_5 formed through ternary complex breakdown was transiently protonated, but proton abstraction by base results in the generation of a 5,6-double bond with subsequent displacement of the C_6-H as hydride (H^-). The liberated hydride attacks the δ^+ methylene group, converting it to methyl, which restores the 5,6-pyrimidine double bond in the product (dTMP) and regenerates TS. The 7,8-dihydrofolate (7,8-DHF) prodced as a reaction by-product is reduced to tetrahydrofolate (THF) by dihydrofolate reductase (DHFR) and NADPH. Finally, THF is converted to the 5,10-methylene THF cofactor through the action of serine hydroxymethyltransferase (SHMT) and pyridoxyl phosphate (vitamin B_6). With the enzyme and cofactor regenerated, the cell is ready to synthesize another molecule of dTMP utilizing stored dUMP. This happens at a normal pace in healthy cells and at an uncontrolled rate in cancer cells.

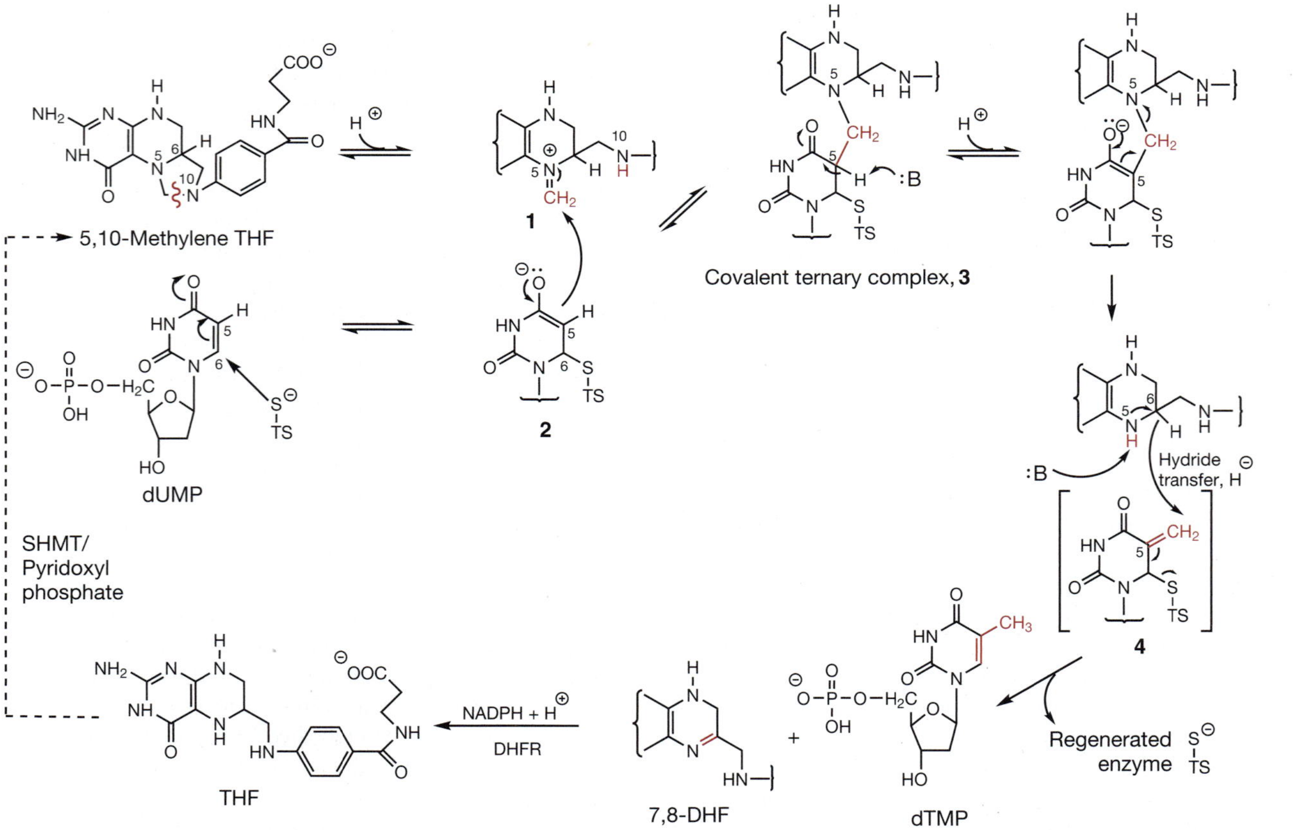

Figure 36.20 Synthesis of deoxythymidine monophosphate (dTMP). DHF, dihydrofolate; DHFR, dihydrofolate reductase; dUMP, deoxyuridine monophosphate; SHMT, serine hydroxymethyl transferase; THF, tetrahydrofolate; TS, thymidylate synthase.

Specific Drugs: Pyrimidine Analogs

Fluorouracil. This fluorinated pyrimidine prodrug must be converted to its deoxyribonucleotide before it will be recognized by TS (Fig. 36.21). The active form differs from the endogenous substrate only by the presence of the 5-F group, which holds the key to the DNA biosynthesis inhibiting action of this drug. The C_6 position of the false substrate is significantly more δ^+ than normal due to the strong electron-withdrawing effect of the adjacent C_5-fluorine. This greatly increases the rate of attack by TS Cys195, resulting in a very fast formation of a fluorinated ternary complex (Fig. 36.22). The small size of the fluorine atom assures no steric hindrance to the formation of this false complex.

The next step in the pathway requires the abstraction of the C_5-F by the enzymatic base (TS Tyr94 or associated water molecules). However, due to the high bond strength, the C–F bond is stable to cleavage, and the fluoro group cannot be abstracted.[206] The ternary complex cannot progress further, no thymidine-based product is formed, no folate cofactor is released, and most importantly, the rate-limiting TS enzyme is not regenerated. With TS directly and irreversibly inhibited, dTMP and thereby dTTP can no longer be synthesized. DNA synthesis or repair cannot occur, and the cell will die.

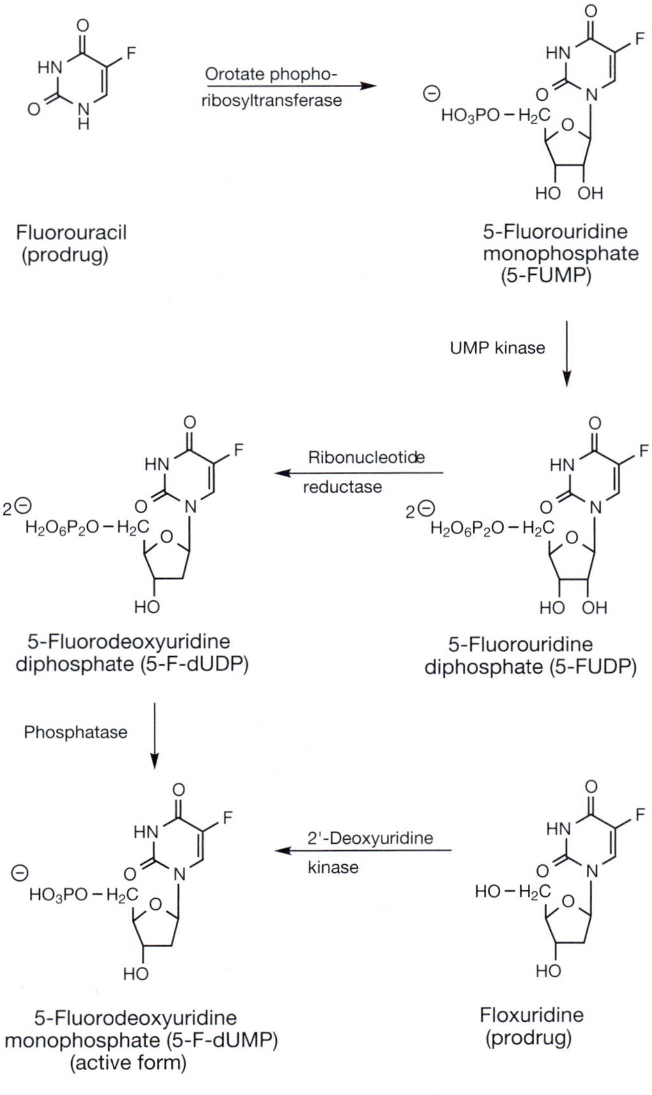

Figure 36.21 Activation of fluorouracil and floxuridine.

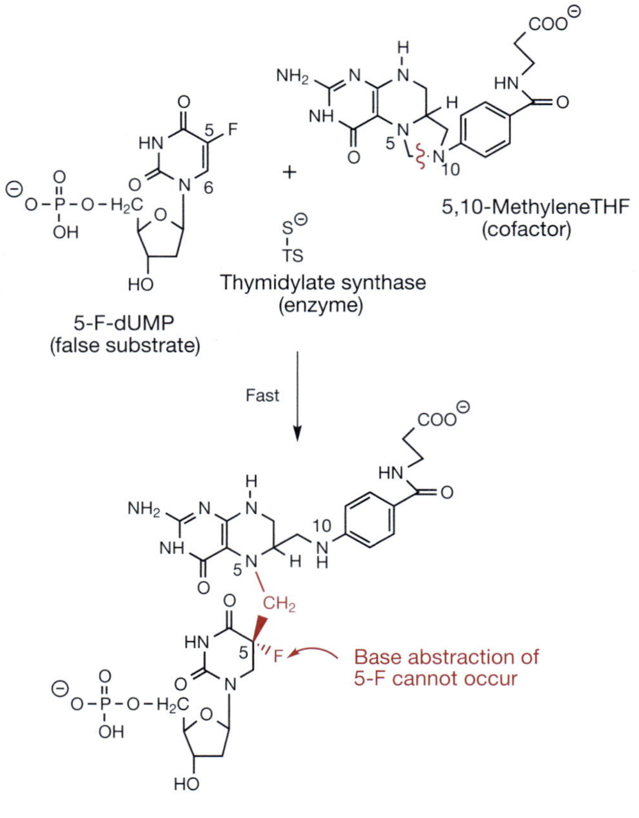

Figure 36.22 Mechanism of action of fluorouracil.

Importantly, a secondary mechanism of therapeutic FU toxicity is the incorporation of the false triphosphorylated ribonucleotide (5-F-UTP) into RNA, a chemical deal breaker for RNA viability.[207] Therefore, fluorinated uracil antimetabolites inhibit the biosynthesis of both DNA and RNA.

The antitumor efficacy of FU is dependent upon the availability of the cofactor 5,10-methylene THF to form the ternary complex. Low cofactor concentration causes dissociation of the ternary complex. To overcome this negative consequence, 5-formyltetrahydrofolate (leucovorin) may be coadministered with FU. Through intracellular conversions, the leucovorin is converted to 5,10-methylene THF, increasing the cofactor pool. This stabilizes the binding of 5-fluorodeoxyruridine monophosphate (5-FdUMP) to TS in the ternary complex, potentiating the cytotoxic effect of FU (Fig. 36.23).[208,209]

FU is administered IV in the palliative treatment of colorectal, breast, stomach, and pancreatic cancers with disease state-dependent doses and regimens. It is rapidly cleared from the bloodstream, and although up to 20% of a dose is excreted unchanged in the urine, most undergoes hepatic catabolism via a series of enzymes that includes the polymorphic dihydropyrimidine dehydrogenase (DPD) (Fig. 36.24). Approximately 5% of the population genetically deficient in this enzyme will experience a more pronounced effect from this drug and are at significant risk for use-limiting or life-threatening toxicity unless doses are appropriately adjusted.[210] Dose adjustment guidelines are available for

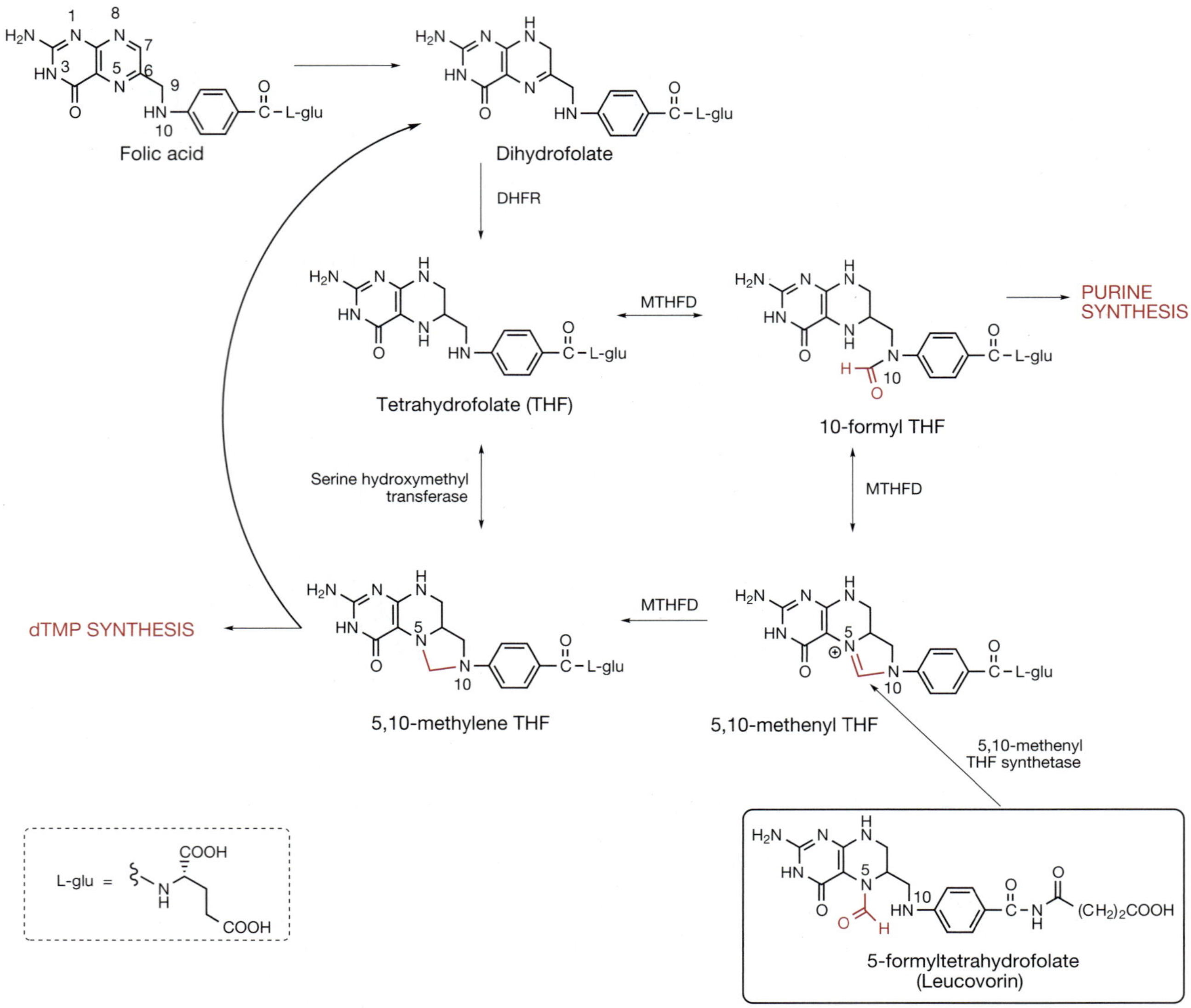

Figure 36.23 Leucovorin and interconversion of tetrahydrofolate cofactors. DHFR, dihydrofolate reductase; MTHFD, methylene tetrahydrofolate dehydrogenase.

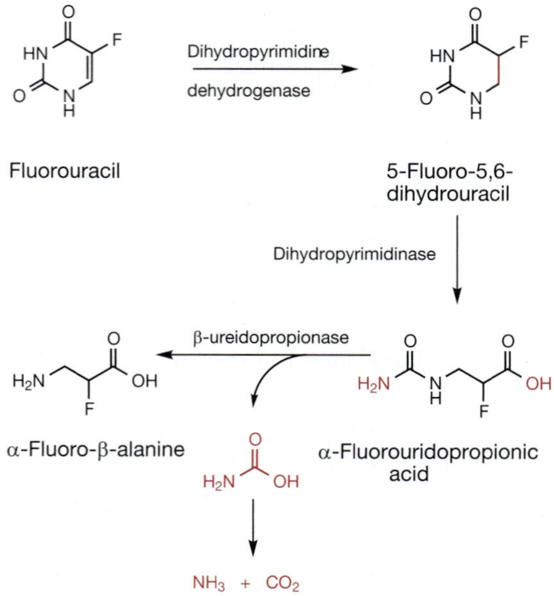

Figure 36.24 Fluorouracil metabolism.

various DPD genotypes.[211] Neutropenia, neurotoxicity, diarrhea, mucositis, and cardiotoxicity are the most common adverse effects. Topical FU cream (5%) is used for basal cell carcinoma if multiple lesions are present or if lesions are at difficult treatment sites.

It has been estimated that between 40% and 60% of patients who experience severe toxicity from FU are DPD deficient.[212] The incidence of DPD deficiency in African American populations is 3-fold higher than in White populations, and Black women have a 3-fold higher incidence of DPD deficiency than Black men.[212] A simple "bedside" mechanism of determining DPD phenotype based on the serum dihydrouracil:uracil ratio has been reported (ratio <4 indicating a PM phenotype).[213] FU dose in patients who are PM being treated for digestive tract cancers was decreased by an average of 35%, which retained therapeutic efficacy while significantly decreasing the incidence of serious toxicity.

The efficacy of uridine triacetate (Vistogard, a uridine prodrug) as an antidote for FU or capecitabine (discussed later) toxicity due to overdose or DPD deficiency is documented. Regardless of the toxicity mechanism, the uridine generated by the hydrolysis of uridine triacetate competes with FU for access to target enzymes and prevents cellular damage and destruction.[207] In animal studies designed to mimic clinical toxicity, the greatest protection benefit was observed when uridine triacetate was administered within 24 hours of the last dose of antimetabolite.[214]

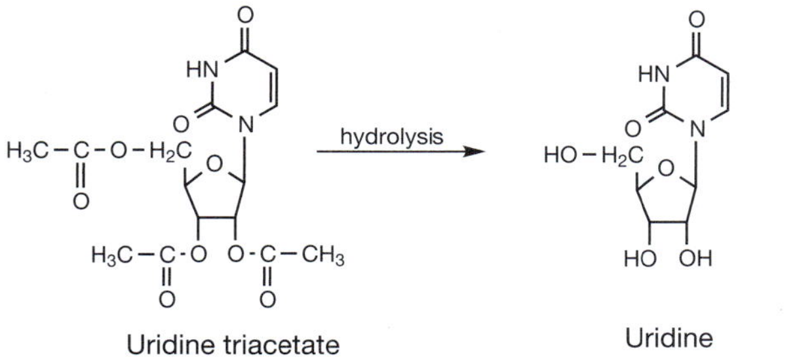

In patients with normal DPD activity, dosage adjustments are usually not required in hepatic or renal dysfunction. Major toxicities are related to bone marrow depression, stomatitis/esophagopharyngitis, and potential GI ulceration. Nausea and vomiting are common.

Solutions of FU are light sensitive, but discolored products that have been properly stored and protected from light are still safe to use.

Floxuridine. This deoxyribonucleoside prodrug is bioconverted via 2′-deoxyuridine kinase-mediated phosphorylation to the same active 5-fluoro-dUMP structure generated in the multistep biotransformation of FU (see Fig. 36.21). It is given by intra-arterial infusion for the palliative treatment of GI adenocarcinoma that has metastasized to the liver and that cannot be managed surgically. Because floxuridine does not generate FU, its kinetic profile is not impacted by DPD pharmacogenetic status.

Capecitabine. Although capecitabine is a carbamylated analog of cytidine, the drug actually is another 5-fluoro-dUMP prodrug (Fig. 36.25). Given orally, it is extensively metabolized to FU, which is then converted to the active fluorinated deoxyribonucleotide as previously described. Thymidine phosphorylase, an enzyme involved in this biotransformation, is much more active in tumor cells than in normal tissue, which improves the tumor-selective generation of FU. Levels of active drug in the tumor can be up to 3.5-fold higher than in surrounding tissue, leading to a lower incidence of adverse effects compared to FU therapy.[215] Because capecitabine is biotransformed to FU, it follows the same catabolic and elimination pathways reported for FU (see Figs. 36.21 and 36.24). Doses should be decreased by 25% in moderate renal impairment, and the caution relative to the augmented risk of toxicity in patients with DPD deficiency applies.

Capecitabine is currently indicated for use as first-line therapy in patients with colorectal cancer. It is also used alone or in combination with docetaxel in patients with MBC who have experienced disease progression or recurrence after anthracycline therapy. Capecitabine is also approved for use in several other malignancies in combination with kinase inhibitors, DNA-crosslinking antineoplastics, mitosis inhibitors, and MAbs. Given twice daily in tablet form or as an extemporaneous oral solution, the total daily dose is calculated based on patient body surface area and is taken 30 minutes after eating to avoid food-induced decreases in absorption. In addition to bone marrow suppression, nausea, and vomiting, the drug can induce severe diarrhea and a potentially disabling disorder termed "hand-and-foot syndrome" (palmar-plantar erythrodysesthesia). As noted, since capecitabine acts through the generation of 5-FU, uridine triacetate can be used to reduce toxicity in overdose or in DPD PMs.

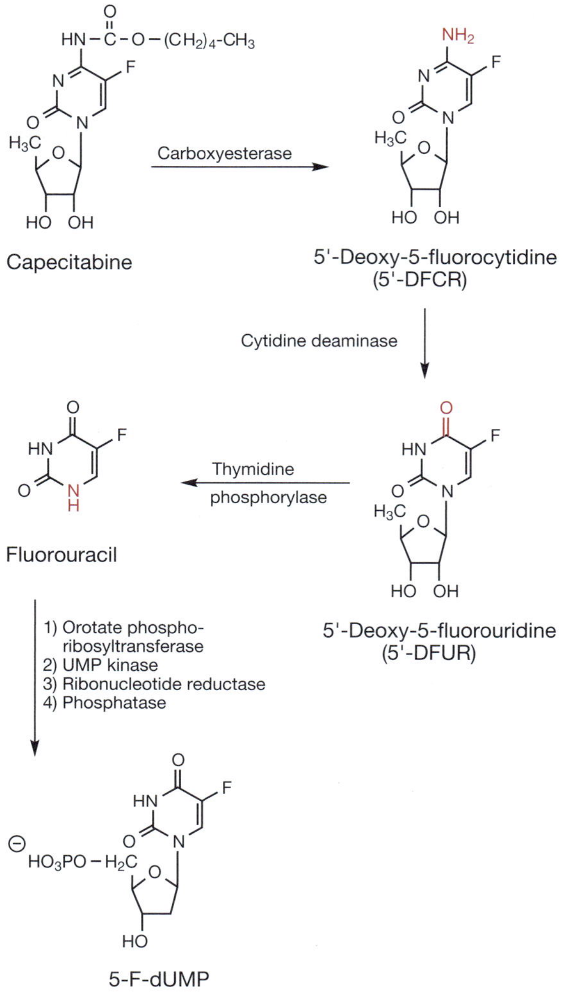

Figure 36.25 Capecitabine activation.

Capecitabine inhibits CYP2C9 and, along with competition for serum protein-binding sites, results in clinically significant DDIs with both warfarin and phenytoin. The interaction with warfarin carries a boxed warning, as it can result in potentially fatal bleeding episodes that appear within days of combination therapy or can be delayed up to 1 month after discontinuation of capecitabine therapy.

Specific Drugs: Antifolates

Methotrexate. Methotrexate (see Fig. 36.17) is a folic acid antagonist structurally designed to compete successfully with 7,8-DHF for the DHFR enzyme. The direct inhibition of DHFR causes cellular levels of 7,8-DHF to rise, which in turn results in feedback (indirect) inhibition of TS. Methotrexate also inhibits GAR formyltransferase, a key enzyme in the synthesis of purine nucleotides (see Fig. 36.18). Newer mechanisms of action have emerged for methotrexate when used in immunopathologies such as rheumatoid arthritis or psoriasis.[216,217]

Methotrexate's C_4-NH_2 substituent and the fully aromatic pteridine ring system hold the key to its DHFR-inhibiting action. It has been proposed that the N_5 position of endogenous DHF is protonated by Glu30 of DHFR[218] and, in cationic form, binds to DHFR Asp27 (see Fig. 36.26). N_5 is the strongest base in the DHF structure, in part due to the attenuating impact of the C_4 carbonyl on N_1 electron density. Additional affinity-enhancing interactions between enzyme and substrate have been identified.[219-221] Once bound, the substrate's 5,6-double bond is positioned close to the NADPH cofactor so that the transfer of hydride can proceed.

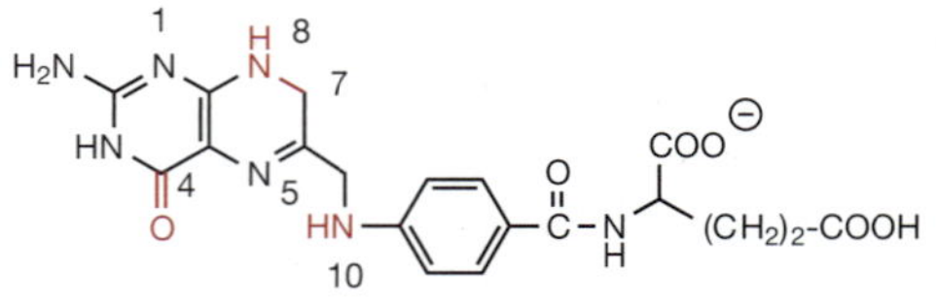

7,8-Dihydrofolate

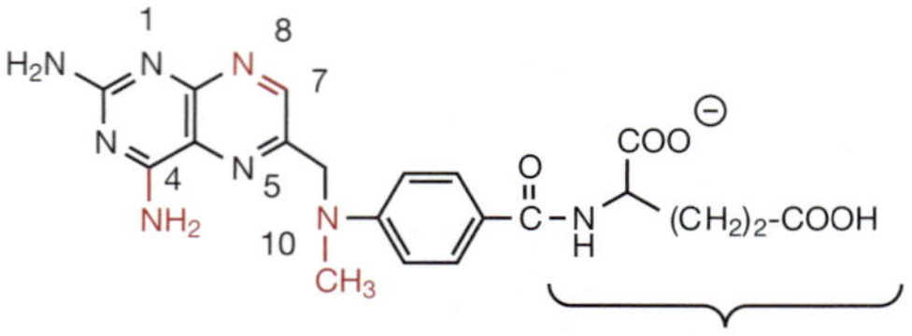

Methotrexate Glutamate tail

In contrast, the C_4-NH_2 substituent of methotrexate enriches electron density at N_1 through π-electron donation, increasing its basic character between 10- and 1,000-fold and promoting protonation by Glu30 at the expense of N_5. Because N_1 and N_5 are across the pteridine ring from one another, the interaction of N_1 with the DHFR Asp27 will effectively stand the false substrate "on its head" relative to the orientation of 7,8-DHF (Fig. 36.26).[221,222] In this flipped orientation with the 5,6-double bond of methotrexate 180° away from the bound NADPH cofactor, and stabilized by the fully aromatic pteridine ring, the possibility for reduction of the 5,6-double bond is eliminated.[219] The DHFR enzyme will be pseudoirreversibly bound to the methotrexate molecule it cannot reduce, which ties up the DHFR enzyme and prevents the conversion of DHF to THF. In turn, this halts the synthesis of the 5,10-methylene THF cofactor required for dTMP biosynthesis and causes feedback inhibition of the TS enzyme. The cell will die a "thymineless death."

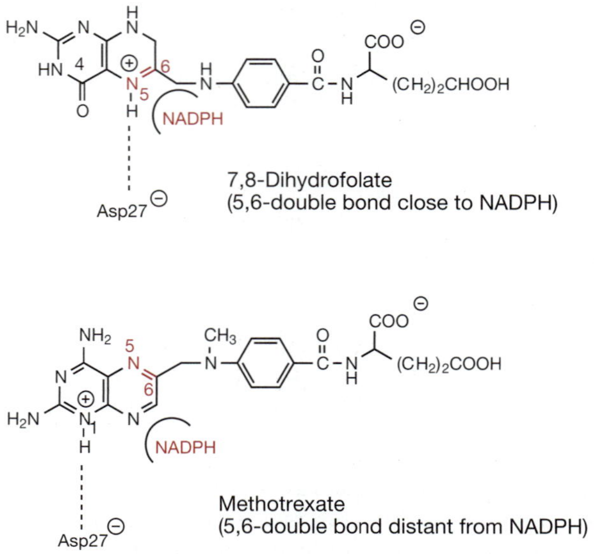

Figure 36.26 Flipped orientation of methotrexate at dihydrofolate reductase.

Methotrexate is given orally in the treatment of ALL, breast, head and neck, and various lung cancers as well as in non-Hodgkin lymphoma (NHL). The sodium salt form is also marketed for IV, intramuscular (IM), intra-arterial, or intrathecal injection. Oral absorption is dose dependent and peaks at 80 mg/m^2 due to site saturation. For intrathecal administration and high-dose therapy, the formulation should be free of preservatives (benzyl alcohol) to avoid "gasping syndrome" toxicity.

The monoglutamate tail of methotrexate permits active transport into cells via a reduced-folate carrier (RFC1), a transporter extensively expressed on tumor cell membranes. It then subsequently undergoes intracellular folylpolyglutamate synthase (FPGS)-catalyzed polyglutamation. This process adds several anionic carboxylate groups to the molecule and traps the drug at the site of action.[223] Polyglutamation is more efficient in tumor cells than in healthy cells, which promotes the selective toxicity of this drug.[224] The polyglutamated drug will be hydrolyzed back to the parent structure by γ-glutamyl hydrolase before renal elimination. Up to 90% of an administered dose is excreted unchanged in the urine within 24 hours.

Several boxed warnings have been issued for methotrexate use.[43] Toxicity occurs if the drug is allowed to accumulate in ascites and pleural effusions and/or when renal excretion is impaired by kidney disease. Methotrexate-induced lung disease is a particularly critical problem because it arises at any time and at any dose and can be fatal. Severe GI adverse effects, including ulcerative stomatitis and hemorrhagic enteritis leading to intestinal perforation, can also occur. Potentially fatal skin reactions are a risk as well. Methotrexate and its aldehyde oxidase-generated 7-hydroxy metabolite (which has a 3- to 5-fold lower water solubility) can precipitate in the renal tubule, causing damaging crystal nephropathy (crystalluria). The drug should not be given to patients unless their urinary pH is at or above 7.5. Additionally, vigorous hydration, along with parenteral and/or enteral administered urinary alkalinizing agents, should be instituted if doses 1,000 mg/m^2 or more are used.[225,226] Concomitant use of nonsteroidal anti-inflammatory drugs (NSAIDs) or proton-pump inhibitors may reduce drug excretion leading to toxic levels. Methotrexate can cause embryo-fetal toxicity and should not be given to women who are pregnant or planning to become pregnant.

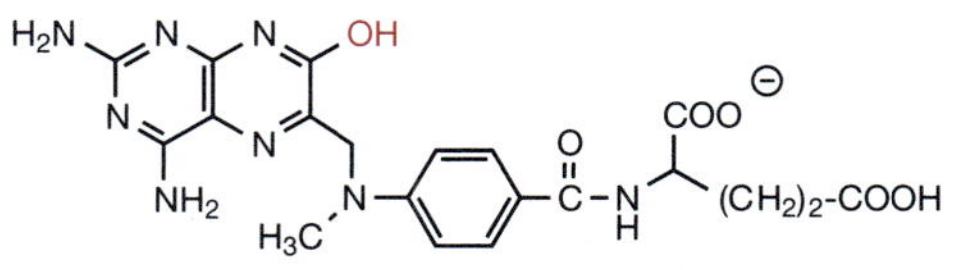

7-hydroxymethotrexate

If severe methotrexate toxicity occurs, reduced-folate replacement therapy with leucovorin must be initiated as soon as possible. Leucovorin generates the folate cofactors needed by DHFR and GAR formyltransferase to ensure the continued synthesis of pyrimidine and purine nucleotides in healthy cells, without having to undergo reduction by DHFR (see Fig. 36.23). "Leucovorin rescue" is often given prophylactically 24 hours after the start of high-dose methotrexate therapy.[226,227] Glucarpidase, a recombinant enzyme that rapidly hydrolyzes methotrexate to the nontoxic 4-deoxy-4-amino-N^{10}-methylpteroic acid (DAMPA) and glutamic acid, can prevent high-dose methotrexate-induced acute kidney injury if administered within 48 to 60 hours.[228]

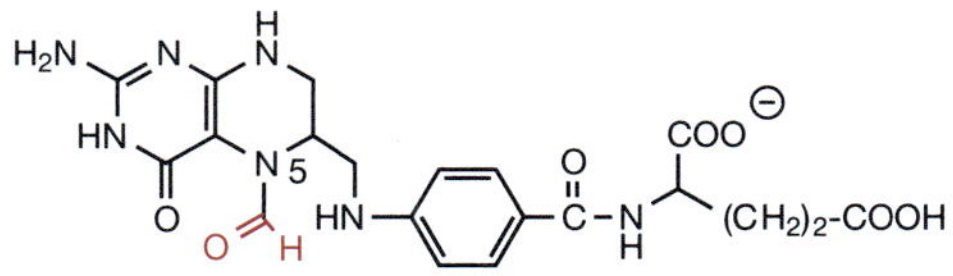

5-Formyltetrahydrofolate
(Leucovorin)

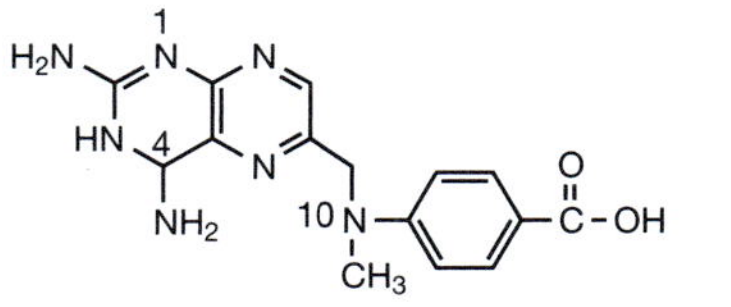

4-Deoxy-4-amino-N^{10}-methylpteroic acid
(DAMPA)

Cancer cells can become resistant to methotrexate over time. Acquired resistance mechanisms include increased expression of DHFR and other enzyme targets, impaired RFC1-mediated transport, active cellular efflux by P-gp, and/or attenuated intracellular polyglutamation.[223]

Pemetrexed Disodium. Pemetrexed (see Fig. 36.17) is a multitarget antifolate administered IV in combination with an organoplatinum agent for the treatment of advanced or metastatic nonsquamous NSCLC[229] and malignant pleural mesothelioma. In addition to DHFR, polyglutamated pemetrexed (but not the monoglutamated parent) binds tightly to TS and, to a lesser extent, GAR formyltransferase.[230-233] Since intracellular polyglutamation of pemetrexed is so efficient, this drug realizes a significant portion of its potent anticancer activity through the inhibition of these two enzymes. In fact, TS is considered its primary target.

Pemetrexed's affinity for RFC1 is approximately twice that of methotrexate.[230] While methotrexate transport reaches a plateau after a relatively short drug exposure time, pemetrexed uptake continues to increase for a prolonged period, resulting in significantly more drug being ferried into the tumor cell over time.[230] If RFC1 transport is impaired, pemetrexed is transported intracellularly by proton-coupled folate transporter (PCFT). PCFT is found in a majority of solid tumor cell lines, and the affinity of pemetrexed for this carrier is approximately 20 times that of methotrexate.[230]

The K_m of pemetrexed for FPGS is 100-fold lower than methotrexate, and this higher affinity results in more polyglutamated drug being rapidly generated and trapped inside the cancer cell.[230] Tetra- and pentaglutamates predominate. Both mono- and polyglutamated forms of pemetrexed are capable of inhibiting DHFR, and they do so with comparable activity.[231,234] Unlike methotrexate, pemetrexed does not distribute centrally to any significant extent.[234] It is minimally metabolized and up to 90% is excreted unchanged in urine.[229,235] As noted earlier, pemetrexed is used in combination with an organometallic, most commonly cisplatin.[231] A synergistic effect with gemcitabine, a DNA polymerase inhibitor, in the treatment of patients with lung cancer has also been noted as long as gemcitabine is administered immediately prior to the antifolate.[234]

Patients on pemetrexed must take folic acid (commonly 400 μg daily) and vitamin B_{12} (1 mg IM on an established schedule) to reduce the risk of bone marrow suppression (neutropenia, thrombocytopenia, and anemia) and use-limiting GI adverse effects such as mucositis and stomatitis. A 3-day course of corticosteroid therapy beginning the day before pemetrexed can reduce the risk of drug-induced skin rash.[43] Antiemetic therapy to proactively combat drug-induced nausea and vomiting is also warranted.[234] Pemetrexed has a half-life of 3.5 hours and is excreted primarily unchanged via the kidneys.

Resistance to pemetrexed is mediated predominantly through a decrease in FPGS activity, enhanced hydrolysis of pemetrexed polyglutamates via γ-glutamyl hydrolase, and upregulation of the TS target.[231,235] In contrast to methotrexate, downregulation of RFC1 is not involved in acquired resistance to pemetrexed as long as PCFT is functioning.[230] Likewise, upregulation of DHFR is not a pemetrexed resistance mechanism since DHFR is not a primary target of this antifolate.

In addition to the level of TS expression, differences in ABCC11 transporters may be an important predictor of sensitivity to pemetrexed chemotherapy.[236] In the ABCC11 single nucleotide polymorphism (SNP) G538A, the A/A variant (unlike the G/G or G/A) does not promote pemetrexed efflux from the cancer cell. ABCC11 genotype also impacts the nature of earwax, and it has been noted that East Asians (80%-95% of whom express the A/A variant and have dry earwax) are particularly responsive to pemetrexed-cisplatin chemotherapy. Patients expressing the other ABCC11 variants would be at risk for pemetrexed resistance due to excessive drug efflux.

Pralatrexate. Pralatrexate (see Fig. 36.17) is a 10-deaza analog of methotrexate where the chiral carbon atom replacing N_{10} has been substituted with a propargyl moiety. This structural alteration results in a significantly enhanced tumor cell uptake via RFC1.[237] The rate of active transport of pralatrexate by RFC1 has been measured at approximately 10 to 14 times that of methotrexate. In addition, pralatrexate is polyglutamated by FPGS at a rate that is comparable to pemetrexed and 10-fold higher than methotrexate.[238,239] This translates to more active drug inside the tumor cell for a longer period of time.

Unlike pemetrexed, which is also more extensively polyglutamated than methotrexate, pralatrexate's primary antineoplastic enzymatic target is DHFR. Although it interacts with and inhibits the isolated DHFR enzyme 2- to 3-fold less vigorously than methotrexate (K_i apparent = 26 and 45 nmol/L, respectively), the RFC1 cellular influx and FPGS polyglutamation first-order rate constants (V_{max}/K_m) are 12- and 10-fold greater, respectively.[240] Higher concentrations of active polyglutamated drug trapped within the cell provide a more potent DHFR inhibitory effect compared to methotrexate and a greater antitumor response than either methotrexate or pemetrexed.[237,240]

Like pemetrexed, pralatrexate is not significantly metabolized and is excreted in both urine and feces. The marketed product is a racemic mixture, and the two isomers have differing volumes of distribution (37 vs 105 L for the *R* and *S* isomers, respectively).

Pralatrexate is currently used exclusively in peripheral T-cell lymphoma,[241] although it might eventually find use in other cancers (eg, NSCLC, NHL). Some patients with T-cell lymphoma treated with pralatrexate have achieved complete remission.[242] Dosing is based on body surface area in order to standardize exposure to active drug. When used in combination with gemcitabine, the synergistic apoptotic effect is maximized when the antifolate is administered before the polymerase inhibitor.[240] Pralatrexate is not effective against B-cell lymphoma.[238] Unlike methotrexate, acquired resistance is believed to be more highly dependent on reduced RFC1 expression than on an increased expression of DHFR.[243]

As with other antifolates, patients on pralatrexate should receive daily folic acid supplementation and vitamin B_{12} to reduce the risk of mucositis/stomatitis and bone marrow suppression. Whereas the latter adverse effect is viewed as a minor risk,[240] mucositis has been termed the major dose-limiting adverse reaction. Folic acid/vitamin B_{12} normalizes levels of methylmalonic acid, which decreases mucositis risk without compromising antineoplastic activity.[244] Mucositis generally occurs early in therapy (eg, in the first cycle), so gradual dose escalation can potentially minimize risk, as can concomitant oral leucovorin prophylaxis (15 mg daily other than the day before or after, and of pralatrexate therapy). Unlike methotrexate, pralatrexate's efficacy is not negatively impacted by leucovorin, an advantage likely due to pralatrexate's very rapid and extensive intracellular transport via RCF1.[239]

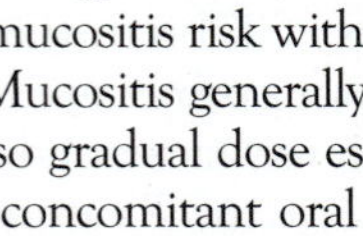

Methylmalonic acid

DNA Polymerase/DNA Chain Elongation Inhibitors

MECHANISM OF ACTION. Six halogenated and/or ribose-modified DNA nucleoside and nucleotide analogs are marketed for the treatment of a wide variety of hematologic cancers and solid tumors (see Fig. 36.17). These agents have complex and multifaceted mechanisms, but all include inhibition of DNA polymerase and/or DNA chain elongation among their actions. The nucleosides are actively transported into tumor cells and tumors deficient in these transporters will be resistant to this class of drugs. Once inside the cell, the drugs are converted to the triphosphorylated nucleotides by specific kinases and subsequently incorporated into the growing DNA chain, thus arresting further elongation. This causes stalling at the replication fork and induces apoptosis. Moreover, many of these drugs in their nucleotide form also inhibit ribonucleotide reductase, halting the conversion of ribonucleotides to deoxyribonucleotides required for DNA synthesis, thus adding to the cytotoxic effect.[245,246]

Structural differences among the nucleoside analog drugs make for subtle differences in the overall inhibition of DNA polymerase and/or DNA chain elongation. In cytarabine and fludarabine, the epimeric 2′-OH of the arabinose sugar hinders the conformational change required in DNA polymerase to complete the addition of the false nucleotide.[247] The trifluoromethyl group in trifluridine prevents base pairing and interferes with DNA replication.[248] In gemcitabine, the substitution at 2′ (fluorine is no larger than hydrogen) does not impact the incorporation of the false nucleotide at the 3′-OH of the last nucleotide in the DNA chain (Fig. 36.27).

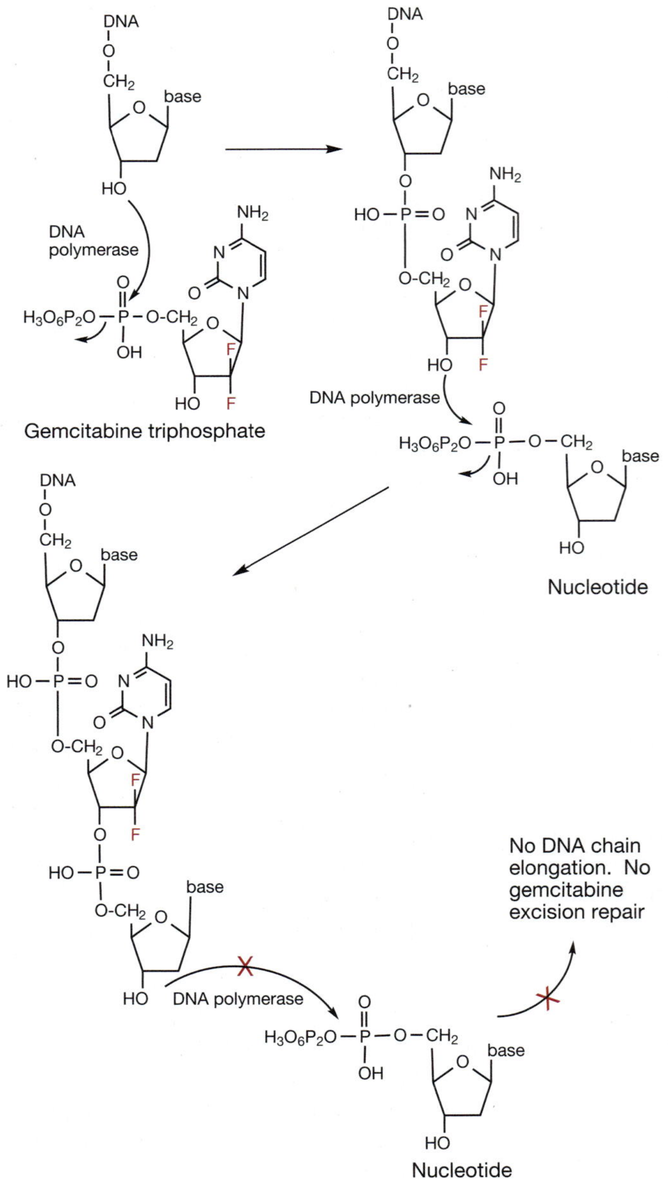

Figure 36.27 Gemcitabine triphosphate inhibition of DNA polymerase.

One more nucleotide can be added to the incorporated gemcitabine.[249] However, when it's time to add the next nucleotide, in a "masked chain termination," the highly electronegative 2′-fluorine atoms inhibit the polymerase enzyme and chain elongation stops. While DNA polymerase has "proofreading" capabilities and can correct the misincorporation of a wrong nucleotide, the false nucleotide looks so much like the expected dCTP that it is not recognized by this "seek and repair" enzyme machinery.[249,250]

With the exception of trifluridine, all drugs in this pharmacologic class are administered IV. They are excreted predominantly via the kidneys and induce myelosuppression as their major use-limiting adverse effect. Resistance can involve aberrations in the expression of metabolizing enzymes as well as of transporting and effluxing proteins. Some in vitro evidence points to the loss of functional nucleoside transporter proteins (specifically hENT1/SLC29A1) and deoxycytidine kinase enzymes as the primary causes of acquired resistance to DNA polymerase inhibitors.[251] Many drugs in this class are available in combination with other antineoplastic drugs.

Specific Drugs

Fludarabine, Cladribine, and Clofarabine. These 3-halogenated adenosine-based nucleosides (see Fig. 36.17) undergo conversion to the active triphosphate nucleotides after facilitated transport into tumor cells. All are initially phosphorylated by deoxycytidine kinase, and cells with high levels of this enzyme should respond well to these agents. Mono- and diphosphate kinases complete the metabolic conversion to the active form. The C_2-halogen renders the molecules relatively resistant to the degradative action of adenosine deaminase, and a significant fraction of the dose is eliminated unchanged in urine.

Fludarabine, an arabinoside, is marketed as the monophosphate nucleotide to enhance water solubility for IV administration, but this group is cleaved rapidly in the bloodstream, allowing the free nucleoside to take advantage of the nucleoside-specific transporting proteins.

Cladribine is indicated in the treatment of hairy cell leukemia, whereas fludarabine phosphate is used in refractory/progressive chronic lymphocytic leukemia (CLL). In addition to myelosuppression, fludarabine can induce hemolytic anemia, along with severe central nervous system (CNS) toxicity when used in high doses, and this has resulted in a boxed warning. The warning also cautions on the high incidence of fatal pulmonary toxicity when fludarabine phosphate is used in combination with pentostatin and is therefore not recommended. The boxed warning for cladribine is focused on myelosuppression, neurotoxicity, and nephrotoxicity.

Clofarabine is used in patients 21 years or younger with relapsed/refractory ALL who have failed at least two previous regimens. In addition to inhibiting DNA chain elongation, this drug also inhibits ribonucleotide reductase (required for the conversion of ribonucleotides to deoxyribonucleotides) and facilitates the release of proapoptotic proteins from mitochondria. The rapid attenuation of leukemia cells after administration of this agent can result in a condition known as tumor lysis syndrome, and respiratory and cardiac toxicities can occur secondary to cytokine release. Toxicity can progress to potentially fatal capillary leak syndrome and organ failure, and patients should receive IV fluids for the entire 5-day course of therapy to minimize the risk of serious adverse events. Despite these serious toxicities, this DNA polymerase inhibitor carries no boxed warning.

Cytarabine, Gemcitabine, and Trifluridine. All of these pyrimidine-based anticancer agents (see Fig. 36.17) undergo initial phosphorylation by deoxycytidine kinase (cytarabine, gemcitabine) or thymidine kinase (trifluridine) to the monophosphate with subsequent phosphorylation catalyzed by pyrimidine monophosphate and diphosphate kinases. Cytarabine, an arabinoside, is catabolized by cytidine and deoxycytidylate (deoxycytidine monophosphate or dCMP) deaminases to inactive uracil analogs (Fig. 36.28). The significantly longer half-life of gemcitabine (19 hours) compared to conventional cytarabine (3.6 hours) is due to the inhibitory action of the difluorodeoxycytidine triphosphate metabolite on the dCMP deaminase enzyme.[215] Gemcitabine elimination is gender dependent, with women having the greater risk for toxicity due to lower renal clearance.

Gemcitabine is indicated in the treatment of breast, pancreatic, and NSCLCs. Cytarabine, which can be administered SC and intrathecally as well as IV, is used in the treatment of various leukemias. A liposomal formulation of cytarabine is available for the treatment of lymphomatous meningitis.

Trifluridine, the only orally administered DNA polymerase inhibitor, is highly vulnerable to the inactivating enzyme thymidine phosphorylase, which cleaves the deoxyribose moiety from the trifluorothymidine base. Although this reaction occurs rapidly and extensively via prehepatic (gut) and first-pass metabolism, therapeutic utility is assured because the marketed product also contains the thymidine

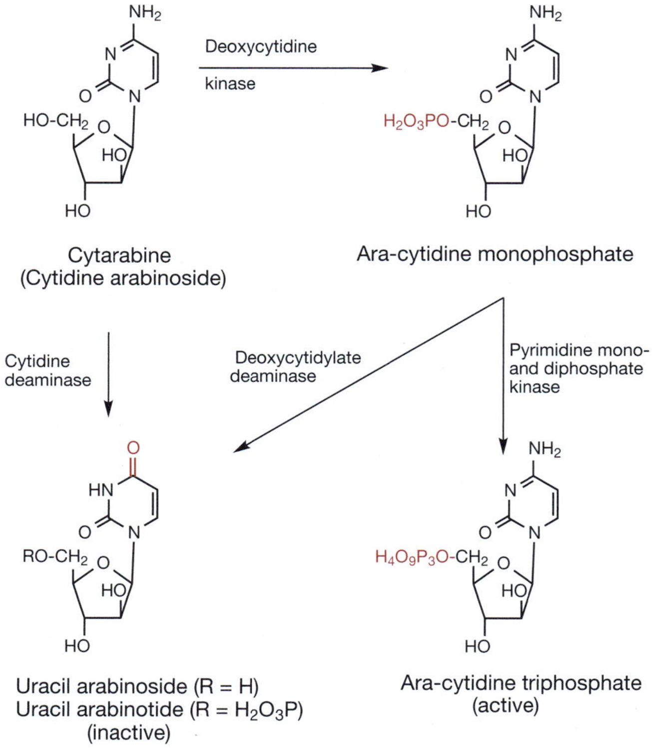

Figure 36.28 Cytarabine metabolism.

phosphorylase inhibitor tipiracil hydrochloride in a 2:1 molar ratio (trifluridine/tipiracil). When administered orally in combination with tipiracil, trifluridine's AUC increases by 100-fold, and the maximum plasma concentration (C_{max}) is over 70-fold higher compared to trifluridine alone. Tipiracil itself is not extensively absorbed from the GI tract.[252]

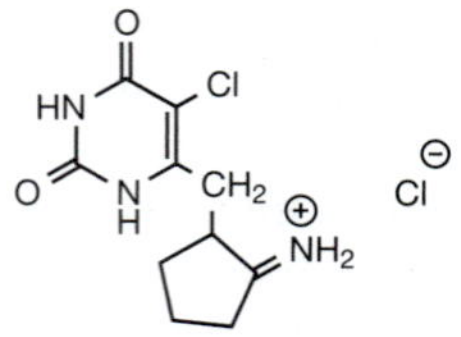

Tipiracil hydrochloride

Trifluridine is used in metastatic colon cancer refractory to first-line cytotoxic and targeted chemotherapies from several chemical/pharmacologic classes. In addition to DNA polymerase inhibition by trifluridine triphosphate, the monophosphorylated nucleotide inhibits TS, binding directly to Tyr146 within the active site.[245] Trifluridine is claimed to be tumoristatic, rather than tumoricidal, with modest PFS and OS benefits, supporting the ongoing search for response enhancing co-therapies and predictive biomarkers.[252,253] Neutropenia, leukopenia, anemia, thrombocytopenia, and GI distress are the major adverse effects, with myelosuppression being dose limiting. Neutropenia of grade 3 or higher during any cycle of trifluridine therapy has been associated with better survival outcomes.[253,254] The drug is administered twice daily within 1 hour after morning and evening meals to enhance tolerability.[255]

DNA Methyltransferase Inhibitors

Mechanism of Action. Three nucleic acid–based chemotherapeutic agents, azacitidine, decitabine, and nelarabine (see Fig. 36.17), block abnormal cellular proliferation by inhibiting DNA methylation on genes responsible for differentiation and growth. Aberrant epigenetic DNA methylation in cancer most commonly occurs at C_5 of cytidine nucleotides that precede guanylate residues (CpG dinucleotides or "islands") and results in tumor-suppressor-, apoptosis-, and DNA-repair-related gene silencing and overall genomic instability.[256-259] SAM serves as the methyl donor. The hypomethylation effect of these agents, mediated through the inhibition of DNA methyltransferase (DNMT) subtype 1, can sometimes restore normal gene function while selectively killing cells that have stopped responding to the body's cellular proliferation control processes. A review of decitabine's impact on gene expression proposes a multifaceted mechanism involving the activation of genes beyond those influencing DNA methylation.[259]

All of the marketed DNMT inhibitors are nucleosides that, once actively transported and converted to triphosphate nucleotides inside the cell, are mistakenly incorporated into DNA in lieu of their cytidine or guanine nucleotide counterparts. Interaction of the false nucleotide with DNMT1 results in covalent bond formation that irreversibly inhibits the enzyme, which is followed by destruction via proteasomal cleavage.[258,260] The therapeutic effect manifests slowly over several drug administration cycles, and only between 30% and 40% of eligible patients respond.[258] Research in this area has branched out into nonnucleoside small molecules that mimic SAM and oligonucleotides that mimic DNA and RNA, but more work is needed to identify novel DNMT inhibitors with both high therapeutic efficacy and selectivity.[257]

Chemistry. The nucleoside-based DNMT inhibitors hydrolyze in aqueous solution and must be administered soon after the dose is constituted. Their vulnerability to deaminase enzymes explains their short elimination half-lives of less than or equal to 4 hours.[257,258] Nelarabine will be O-demethylated to ara-G by adenosine deaminase prior to phosphorylation and DNA incorporation[261] and can be further metabolized to guanine, xanthine, and uric acid. Anemia, neutropenia, and thrombocytopenia are among the most common side effects of this class of drugs, and low-grade GI disturbances are frequent.

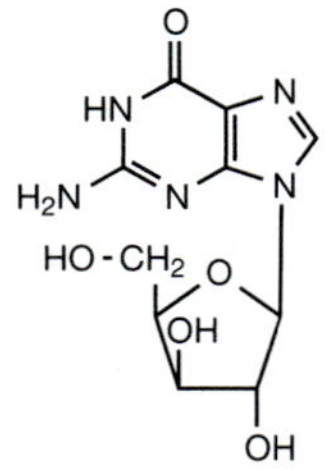

Ara-G

Specific Drugs

Azacitidine and Decitabine. Decitabine is the deoxyribonucleoside analog of azacitidine. Decitabine is phosphorylated by deoxycytidine kinase and, in triphosphorylated nucleotide form, incorporated exclusively into DNA.[262] In contrast, azacitidine is phosphorylated by uridine-cytidine kinase. At the diphosphate stage of azacitidine activation, up to 20% will be converted to decitabine diphosphate via ribonucleotide reductase and, after conversion to the triphosphate, will inhibit DNMT1 as described earlier. The remainder of the azacitidine diphosphate metabolite will add a final phosphate residue and be incorporated into RNA, where it interferes with the synthesis of messenger RNA (mRNA) and proteins (Fig. 36.29).[256,258,260,262] Given the significant difference in pharmacodynamics, it may not be surprising that in vitro studies have demonstrated no cross-resistance between the two structurally related agents.[262]

Azacitidine may be given IV, SC, or orally, while decitabine is given IV for the treatment of myelodysplastic syndrome, a disorder of blood-forming stem cells known to express a hypermethylated *p5*(INK*4B*) gene and which can progress to AML.[256] The absolute bioavailability of SC-administered azacitidine is approximately 89%, and administration by this route results in twice the half-life achieved after IV administration.[257,258,262] Oral azacitidine should not be interchanged with the IV or SC formulations. The low oral bioavailability of decitabine precludes administration via this route unless the cytidine deaminase inhibitor cedazuridine is coadministered.[258]

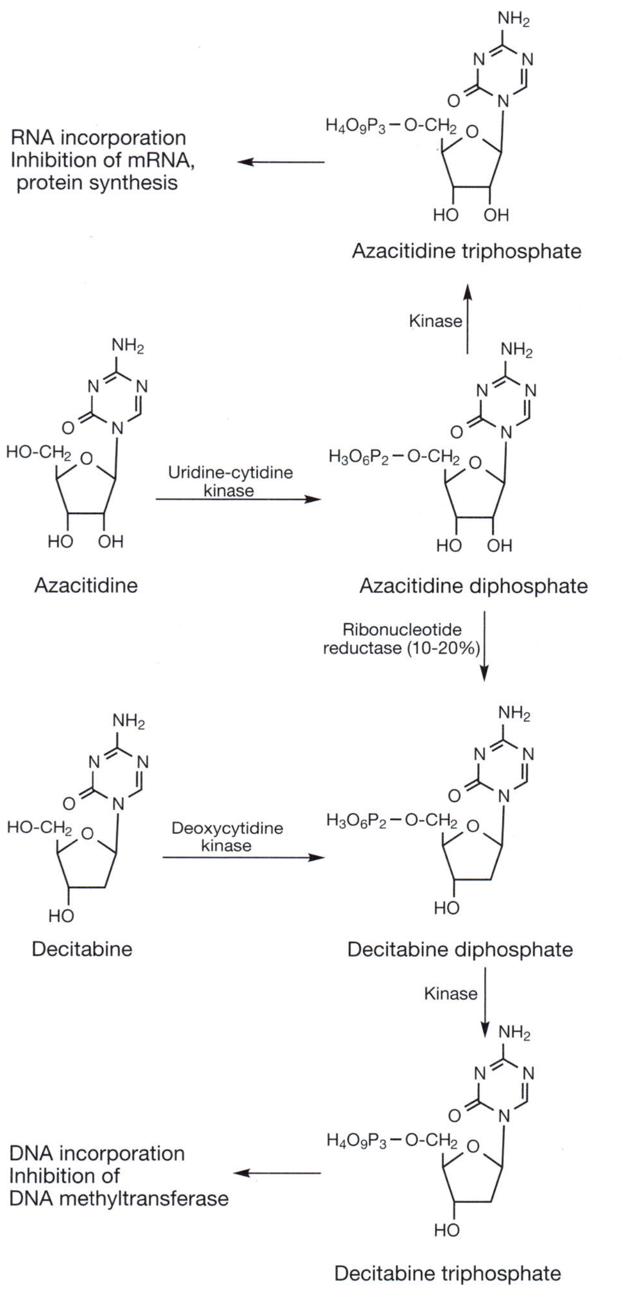

Figure 36.29 Azacitidine and decitabine metabolism and mechanism.

Both azacitidine and decitabine are resistant to CYP and phase 2 conjugating enzymes but are inactivated via cytidine deaminase and/or nonenzymatic hydrolysis.[43,262] Unchanged azacitidine and its metabolites are excreted in urine, but the excretion profile of decitabine is currently unknown.

Patients on either azacitidine or decitabine should be monitored for hematologic and renal toxicities. Both drugs are known to cause fetal harm, and patients should be actively counseled to take appropriate reproductive precautions.[43] Resistance related to genetic adaptations and instability is, unfortunately, commonly encountered.[256] As with so many other anticancer drugs, the search is on for predictive biomarkers to facilitate the identification of patients most likely to respond favorably to these agents.[256,262]

Nelarabine. Nelarabine (see Fig. 36.17) is considered a third-line treatment for T-cell ALL or lymphoma. It is rapidly and efficiently converted to ara-G in the bloodstream, and then selectively accumulates in malignant T cells for phosphorylation and DNA incorporation.[261] It is administered by IV infusion over 1 or 2 hours in pediatric and adult patients, respectively. The drug can induce severe and potentially irreversible neurologic symptoms including convulsions, severe central depression, and peripheral neuropathy that can mimic Guillain-Barré syndrome and carries a boxed warning as a result. These adverse effects are dose limiting, but there is early evidence that administration via 24-hour continuous infusion might attenuate these serious toxicities.[261] As noted, nelarabine can be metabolized to uric acid. Along with hydration and urine basification, allopurinol (a xanthine oxidase inhibitor) can be given prophylactically to minimize the risk of nelarabine-induced hyperuricemia.

Miscellaneous Antimetabolites

The antimetabolites described below are less widely used than those discussed earlier and are included in Figure 36.17.

Specific Drugs

Hydroxyurea. Hydroxyurea, a drug with a 100-plus year history, blocks the synthesis of DNA by trapping a tyrosyl free radical species at the catalytic site of ribonucleotide reductase, thereby inhibiting the enzyme that converts ribonucleotide diphosphates into their corresponding deoxyribonucleotides. It is used orally for the treatment of resistant CML and as an adjunct to radiation in the treatment of squamous cell head and neck cancer. Hydroxyurea increases the effectiveness of radiation therapy through its selective toxicity to cells in the radiation-resistant S phase and by stalling the cell cycle in the G_1 stage, in which radiation therapy does the greatest damage. In addition, hydroxyurea thwarts the normal damage repair mechanisms of surviving cells. A review of its chemical, pharmacologic, metabolic, and therapeutic properties has been published.[263]

Hydroxyurea has excellent oral bioavailability (80%-100%), and serum levels peak within 2 hours of administration. If a positive response is noted within 6 weeks, toxicities are mostly mild enough to permit long-term or indefinite therapy on either a daily or every-3-day basis. Mucositis risk is augmented with high-dose therapy (≥75 mg/kg/d).[264] Leukopenia and, less commonly, thrombocytopenia and/or anemia are the most serious adverse effects, and the drug carries a boxed warning for severe myelosuppression and the induction of secondary malignancies. Excretion of the unchanged drug and the urea metabolite is via the kidneys. The carbon dioxide produced as a by-product of hydroxyurea metabolism is excreted in the expired air.

Pentostatin. Pentostatin is a ring-expanded purine ribonucleoside that inhibits adenosine deaminase and is primarily used in the treatment of hairy cell leukemia. The elevated levels of dATP that result from inhibition of this degradative enzyme inhibit the action of ribonucleotide reductase, thus halting DNA synthesis within the tumor cell. When used in CLL, some authors claim that pentostatin offers a therapeutic efficacy comparable to fludarabine but with a lower risk of toxicity.[265,266] The combination of pentostatin and fludarabine in this disease state has resulted in fatal pulmonary toxicity, which prompted the issuance of a boxed warning.[43]

Several phase II clinical trials conducted in a total of 288 patients with progressive, treatment naïve CLL that employed pentostatin-based chemoimmunotherapy documented overall response rates of more than 90%, a complete remission rate of 41%, an approximately 10-year median OS, and a median treatment-free survival of almost 4 years.[266]

DNA-Alkylating and Crosslinking Agents

The primary target of DNA-alkylating and crosslinking agents is the actively dividing DNA molecule. The DNA cross-linkers are extremely reactive electrophilic structures. The nucleophilic groups on various DNA bases (particularly, but not exclusively, the N_7 of guanine) readily attack the electrophilic drug, resulting in irreversible alkylation or complexation of the DNA base.

Some DNA-alkylating agents, such as nitrogen mustards and nitrosoureas, are bifunctional, meaning that one molecule of the drug can bind two distinct DNA bases. Most commonly, the alkylated bases are on different DNA molecules, and interstrand DNA cross-linking through two guanine N_7 atoms results. Cell cycle arrest and apoptosis follow as the cell tries unsuccessfully to repair the chemical insult. The DNA-alkylating antineoplastics are not cell cycle specific, but they are more toxic to cells in the late G_1 or S phases of the cycle. This is the time when DNA is unwinding and exposing its nucleotides, increasing the chance that vulnerable DNA functional groups will encounter the electrophilic antineoplastic drug and launch the nucleophilic attack that leads to its own destruction. The DNA alkylators have a great capacity for inducing both mutagenesis and carcinogenesis.

Organoplatinum complexes also crosslink DNA, and many do so by binding to adjacent guanine nucleotides on the same strand of DNA, forming diguanosine dinucleotides. This leads to intrastrand DNA cross-linking. The anionic phosphate group on a second strand of DNA stabilizes the drug-DNA complex and makes the damage to DNA replication irreversible. Some organoplatinum agents also damage DNA through interstrand cross-linking. The DNA-alkylating and crosslinking antineoplastics are shown in Figure 36.30. Those that enjoy the most widespread clinical use are described under "Specific Drugs" sections.

Nitrogen Mustards and Aziridine-Mediated Alkylators

Nitrogen mustards are bis(β-haloalkyl)amines. The term "bis" means two, and the "halo" (short for halogen) in the nomenclature is invariably chlorine. The two chlorine atoms dramatically decrease the basic strength of the amino nitrogen through a strong negative inductive effect. As a result, the unionized conjugate of these drugs predominates at physiologic pH. This is intentional because it is the lone pair of electrons on the unionized amine that allows for the formation of the highly electrophilic aziridinium ion, which is the reactive DNA-destroying intermediate generated by all true mustards.

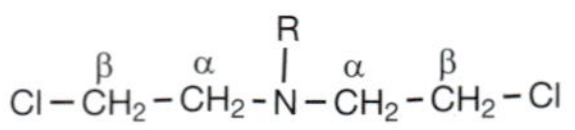

Bis-β-haloalkylamine

Mechanism of Action. The mechanism of action of the nitrogen mustards is depicted in Figure 36.31.[267,268] In step 1, the lone pair of electrons on the unionized amine conducts an intramolecular nucleophilic attack at the β-carbon of the nitrogen mustard, displacing a chloride anion and forming the highly electrophilic aziridinium ion intermediate. The carbon atoms of this strained quaternary amine are highly electrophilic due to the strong negative inductive effect of the cationic nitrogen.

In step 2, a DNA nucleophile conducts an intermolecular nucleophilic attack, which breaks the aziridine ring and alkylates DNA. Although guanine is the preferred nucleic acid base involved, the less nucleophilic adenine is also known to react.[268] Of critical importance is the fact that the lone pair of electrons on the mustard nitrogen is regenerated when the aziridine ring cleaves.

Steps 3 and 4 are simply repetitions of steps 1 and 2, respectively, involving the second arm of the mustard and a second molecule of DNA. Ultimately, two molecules of DNA will be crosslinked through the carbon atoms of what was once the nitrogen mustard. Tethered together, the DNA strands cannot separate nor replicate, so transcription of DNA to RNA is halted. In an attempt to liberate the DNA from the mustard's covalent stranglehold, hydrolytic depurination (step 5) cleaves the bound guanine residues from the DNA strand. However, the DNA released from this mustard trap is damaged and unable to replicate, which inevitably results in cell death. If this is happening in a tumor cell, the therapeutic goal has been accomplished. If it is happening in a healthy cell, particularly one with a short half-life, the patient may experience adverse effects that can be use-limiting.

Chemistry. The structure of nitrogen mustards differs only in the nature of the third group (R) attached to the amino nitrogen. This group, which can be either aliphatic or aromatic, is the prime determinant of chemical reactivity, oral bioavailability, and the nature and extent of adverse effects.

An aliphatic nitrogen substituent (eg, CH_3) will release electrons to the amine through σ bonds. This electronic enrichment enhances the nucleophilic character of the lone pair of electrons and increases the speed at which the δ^+ β-carbon of the mustard will be attacked. Whether in a tumor cell or a healthy cell, as soon as the aziridinium ion forms, it will react with unpaired DNA and/or other cellular nucleophiles, such as electron-rich SH, OH, and NH groups of amino acids on enzymes or membrane-bound receptors.[268] The aqueous environment of the body can also react with the aziridinium ion and inactivate it. The intra- and intermolecular reactions designated as steps 1 through 4 in Figure 36.31 happen rapidly, so little opportunity exists for tissue or cell specificity. This results in a significant risk of serious adverse effects and use-limiting toxicity.

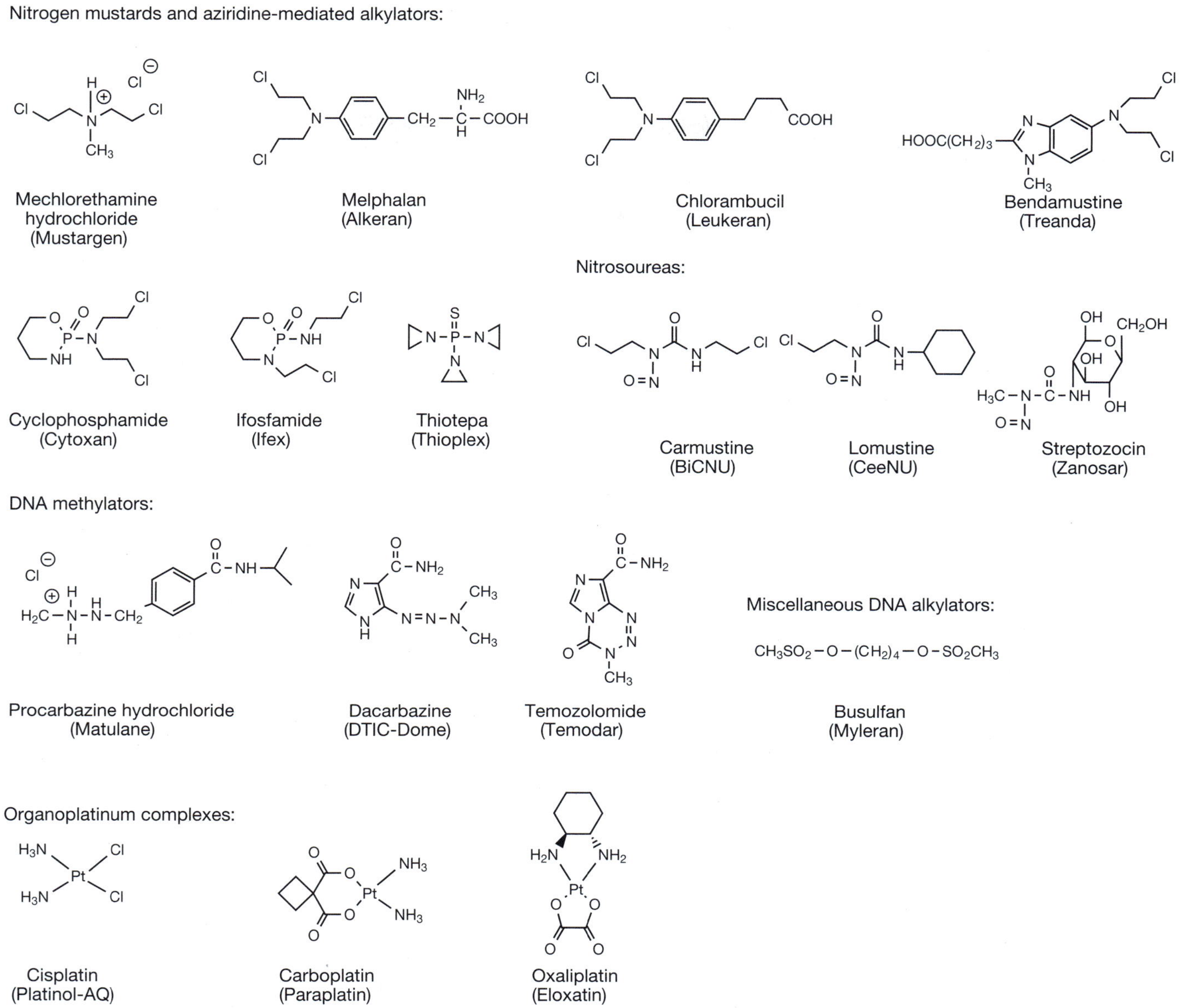

Figure 36.30 DNA-alkylating and crosslinking agents.

Conversely, an adjacent aromatic ring that is conjugated with the mustard nitrogen will stabilize the lone pair of electrons through resonance. Resonance delocalization significantly slows the rate of intramolecular nucleophilic attack, aziridinium ion formation, and DNA alkylation. Aromatic mustards have a reactivity sufficiently controlled to permit oral administration and attenuate the severity of adverse effects. The higher stability also provides the chance for enhanced tissue selectivity by giving the intact mustard time to reach malignant cells before generating the cytotoxic aziridinium ion.

Nitrogen mustards can decompose in aqueous media through the formation of the inactive dehalogenated diol shown in Figure 36.32. Both the mustard nitrogen (pathway a) and the oxygen of water (pathway b) can act as nucleophiles to advance this degradative process. The decomposition reactions can be inhibited if the nucleophilic character of these atoms is eliminated through protonation, so buffering solutions to an acidic pH (eg, 3-5) helps to enhance stability in aqueous solution.

Specific Drugs.

Mechlorethamine Hydrochloride. Mechlorethamine (see Fig. 36.30) was the first alkylating agent developed and is the only aliphatic nitrogen mustard currently on the US market. The drug is available as a topical gel (0.02% mechlorethamine HCl) for the treatment of mycosis fungoides–type cutaneous T-cell lymphoma. There is no systemic absorption of the drug, thus avoiding drug interactions.[269] Dermatitis and other skin-related adverse effects may occur. Mechlorethamine for IV administration is no longer marketed.

Chlorambucil and Melphalan. Chlorambucil (see Fig. 36.30) is one of three aromatic nitrogen mustards with a resonance-stabilized amine that results in oral activity. The drug is active intact and also undergoes β-oxidation to provide an active phenylacetic acid mustard metabolite

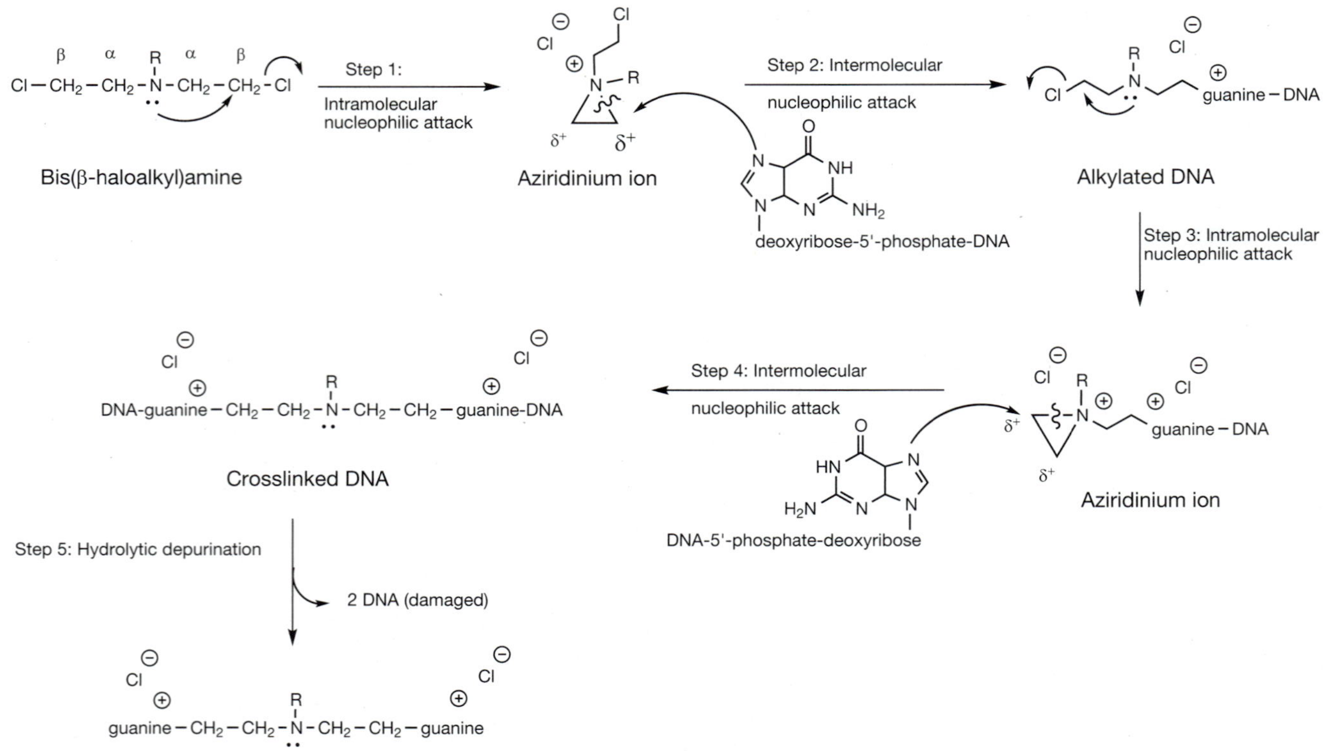

Figure 36.31 DNA destruction through nitrogen mustard–mediated alkylation.

which is responsible for some of the observed antineoplastic activity. There is a reduced incidence of nausea and vomiting, but patients still experience myelosuppression severe enough to carry a boxed warning. It is also mutagenic, teratogenic, and carcinogenic; it can induce nonlymphocytic leukemia, although secondary malignancies are considered rare events.[270] It is administered in tablet form in doses ranging from 0.1 to 0.2 mg/kg/d for the management of CLL, NHL, and Hodgkin lymphoma. Patients with Hodgkin disease generally require doses on the high end of this range. Absorption is over 70% and, although decreased by the presence of food, regimens do not demand an empty stomach. C_{max} is achieved within an hour, and the drug is extensively bound to serum protein. Elimination of inactive mono- and dihydroxy spontaneous hydrolysis products[271] of both the parent drug and phenylacetic acid metabolite is primarily via the urine.[43]

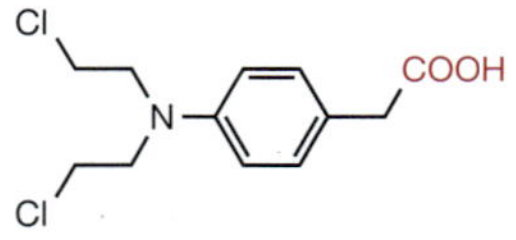

Phenylacetic acid mustard (active chlorambucil metabolite)

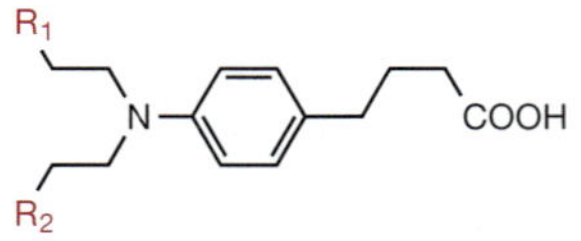

Inactive chlorambucil hydrolysis products
(R_1= OH, R_2 = Cl [monohydroxy])
(R_1 = R_2 = OH [dihydroxy])

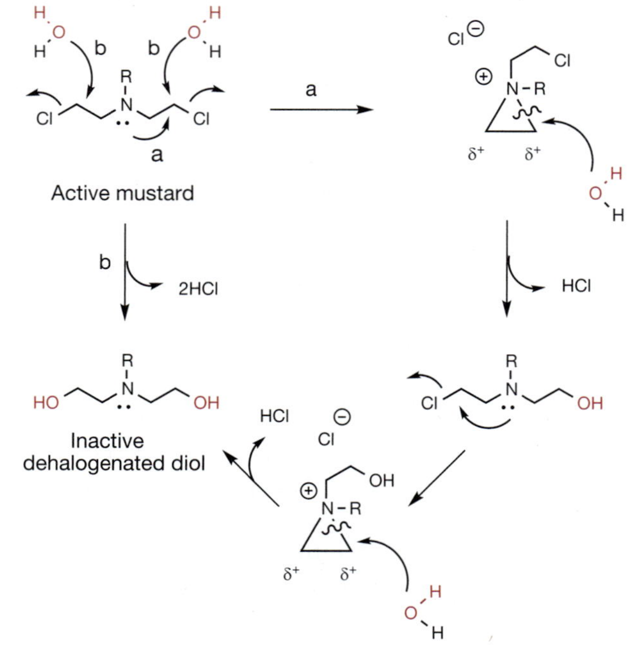

Figure 36.32 Aqueous decomposition of nitrogen mustards.

A structurally similar aromatic mustard, melphalan, is used primarily in the treatment of multiple myeloma. L-Phe was purposefully incorporated into this antineoplastic to promote active transport into tumor cells; however, studies indicate that melphalan enters cells through facilitated diffusion rather than by active transport.[272]

Bendamustine Hydrochloride. Bendamustine, an antineoplastic "old timer" first synthesized in 1963, is the N-methylbenzimidazole analog of chlorambucil (see Fig. 36.30). The incorporation of this purine-like aromatic ring was purposefully done to promote an antimetabolite mechanism in addition to DNA alkylation. DNA damage is more extensive and less repairable than that induced by other aromatic alkylating agents,[273] and the drug is unique in its ability to stimulate *p21* and *p53*-induced apoptosis, S-phase cell cycle arrest, and "mitotic catastrophe."[274] The risk of acquired resistance and cross-resistance via the upregulation of alkylguanyl transferase appears lower than with other DNA alkylators.[273,275]

Unlike chlorambucil, bendamustine is given only IV on days 1 and 2 of a 21-day (NHL) or 28-day (CLL) cycle. The dose in these disease states is commonly 100 and 120 mg/m^2, respectively, and it can be given alone or in combination with other antineoplastic agents (eg, the anti-CD20 MAbs rituximab or obinutuzumab). It has a rapid attenuating effect on lymphocyte count and lymphadenopathy and may be valuable as a debulking agent prior to treatment with targeted therapies.[273]

Compared to chlorambucil, bendamustine therapy in CLL results in higher response rates but at the cost of an increased risk of infection.[270] Myelosuppression, hypersensitivity/anaphylaxis, and skin reactions have also been noted with its use, along with fatigue, anticholinergic actions, and delayed nausea. Despite this, the long-term safety of bendamustine in both CLL and NHL is generally viewed as acceptable.[276] Pretreatment with antihistamines and corticosteroids can help minimize infusion reactions, a major cause of drug discontinuation. Like chlorambucil, it is viewed as a viable alternative in older adult and/or frail patients unable to withstand more aggressive chemotherapy regimens.[273]

Bendamustine undergoes minor CYP1A2-catalyzed N-demethylation and γ-hydroxylation.[273] While active, these metabolites are clinically insignificant, and the drug is eliminated almost exclusively (90%) in feces. There is currently no evidence of serious metabolism-based interactions or toxicities associated with bendamustine.

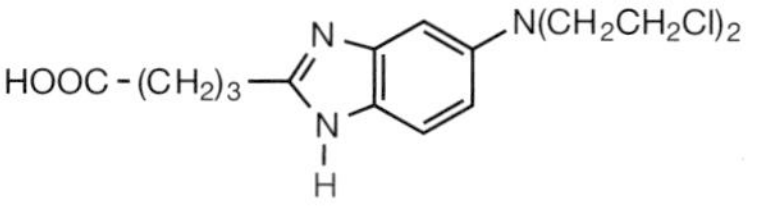

N-Desmethylbendamustine

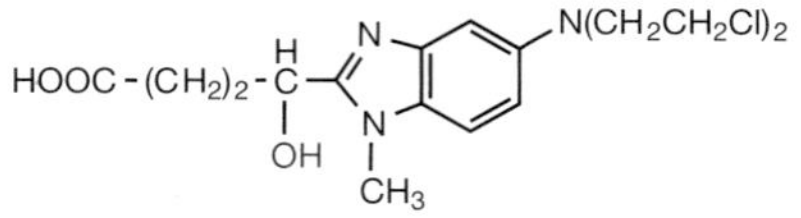

γ–Hydroxybendamustine

(Bendamustine metabolites)

Cyclophosphamide. Cyclophosphamide (see Fig. 36.30) is a chiral prodrug requiring activation by metabolic and nonenzymatic processes (Fig. 36.33).[277] The initial metabolic step is mediated primarily by CYP2B6 (and, to a lesser extent, by CYP3A4 and CYP2C isoforms) and involves regioselective hydroxylation at C_4 of the oxazaphosphorine ring to generate a carbinolamine.[277,278] This hydroxylation reaction must occur before the molecule will be transported into cells, and approximately 90% of an administered dose will be appropriately converted.[277] CYP3A4 and CYP2B6 stereospecifically catalyze an inactivating N-dechloroethylation reaction on the *R* and *S* isomers, respectively, which yields highly nephrotoxic and neurotoxic chloroacetaldehyde.[277,278] Chloroacetaldehyde toxicity is accompanied by GSH depletion, indicating that (as expected) this electrophilic by-product alkylates Cys residues of critical cell proteins.[279] Alkylation of Lys, adenosine, and cytidine residues is also possible.

The CYP-generated carbinolamine undergoes nonenzymatic, reversible cleavage to provide the aldophosphamide tautomer, either in the bloodstream or inside cells.[280,281] Acrolein, a highly reactive α,β-unsaturated aldehyde, is cleaved from aldophosphamide via intracellular spontaneous β-elimination,

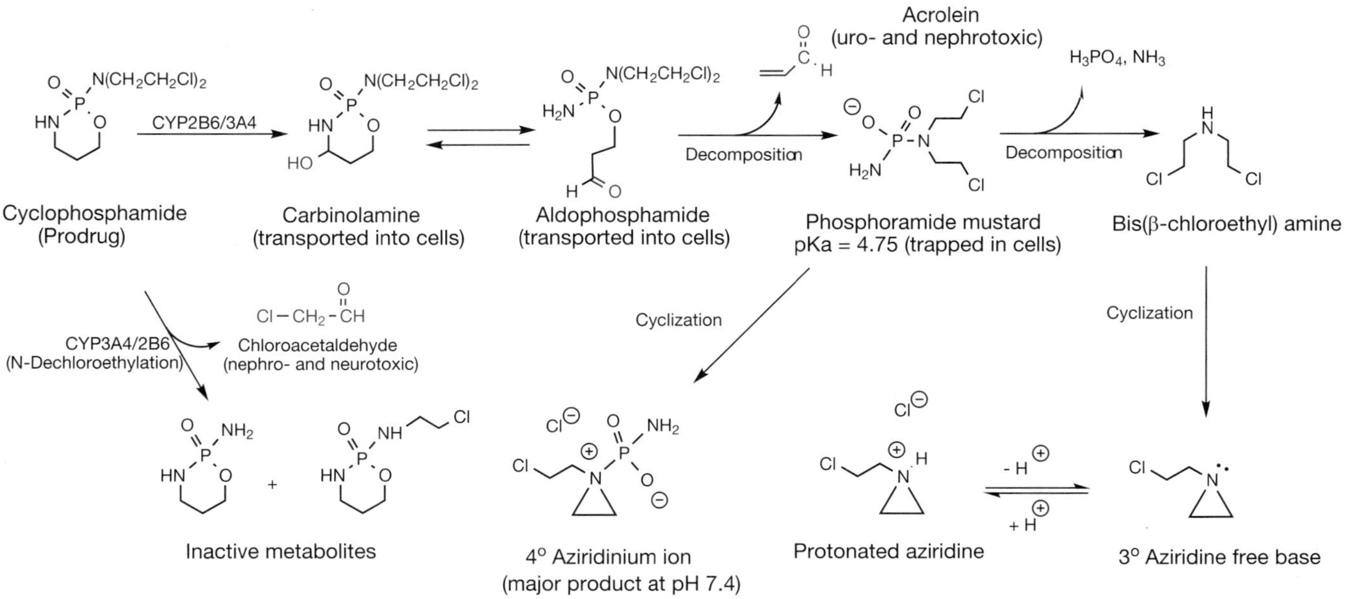

Figure 36.33 Cyclophosphamide metabolism.

generating phosphoramide mustard. With a pK_a of 4.75, the mustard will be persistently anionic at intracellular pH and trapped inside the cell.

The fate of phosphoramide mustard is varied. Most cyclizes to the quaternary aziridinium ion, which alkylates DNA in the manner of all mustards. Some of it decomposes, losing phosphoric acid and ammonia. This leaves the secondary bis(β-chloroethyl)amine mustard, which cyclizes to form a tertiary aziridine species. The free tertiary aziridine will protonate at intracellular pH to provide the cationic conjugate acid, and the carbon atoms of both conjugates are still sufficiently δ^+ to attract DNA nucleophiles, albeit less vigorously than the permanently cationic quaternary amine. The net result is DNA alkylation and cell death. Oxidation of oxazaphosphorine intermediates along the metabolic pathway by cytosolic alcohol or aldehyde dehydrogenase is inactivating.[277,280]

The need for metabolic activation in the liver means lowered GI toxicity and less nonspecific toxicity for cyclophosphamide as compared with other DNA-alkylating agents, but cyclophosphamide is not without its toxic effects. Acrolein, generated during the decomposition of aldophosphamide, is a very electrophilic and highly reactive species, and it causes extensive damage to cells of the kidney and bladder. While acrolein can be produced in the kidney via CYP3A4-mediated metabolism, it is predominantly generated in the liver, where it readily conjugates with GSH (Fig. 36.34).[282,283] However, when the acrolein-GSH or mercapturic acid (*N*-acetylcysteine) conjugate is delivered to the bladder for excretion, the conjugate can cause direct toxicity or cleave to release electrophilic acrolein to the cells.[282] Without additional GSH to re-scavenge liberated toxin, the acrolein will be attacked at its δ^+ terminus by the nucleophilic -SH of bladder cell Cys residues (Fig. 36.34). More complex biochemical cascades involving the generation of ROS, increased levels of preoxynitrite, and subsequent lipid peroxidation also contribute to the observed urotoxicity.[277,284] Physiologic results can include severe hemorrhage that can progress to sclerosis and fibrosis. Secondary bladder cancer that can develop years after treatment completion is a dose-dependent liability, and patients with ovarian cancer who are administered cyclophosphamide have a 4-fold increased risk for this diagnosis.[285] Acrolein also damages the nephron, particularly when used in high doses, in children, in patients with only one kidney, or when coadministered with other nephrotoxic agents (eg, cisplatin).

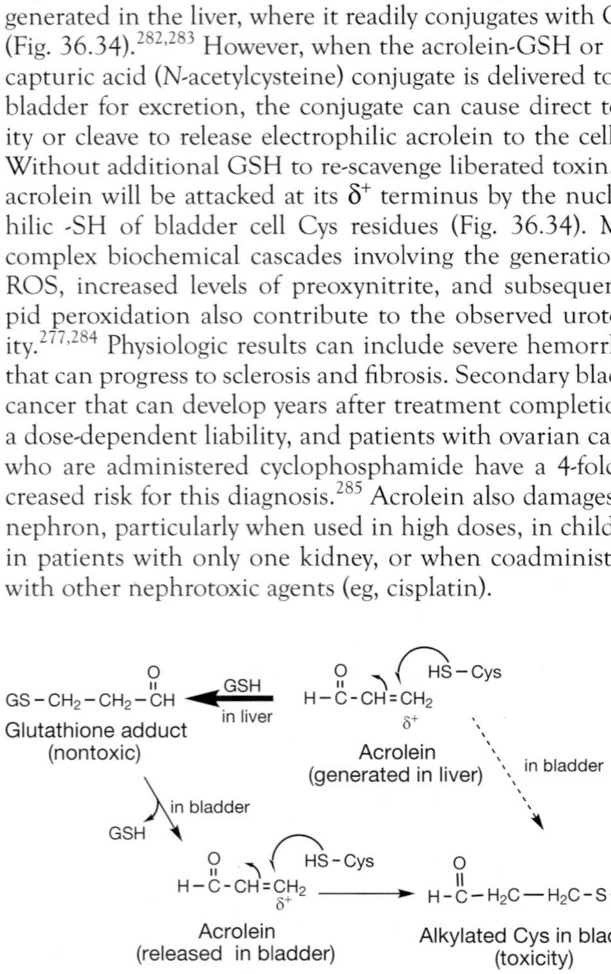

Figure 36.34 Glutathione conjugation with acrolein.

To minimize the risk of acrolein-induced hemorrhagic cystitis (a known risk factor for delayed secondary malignancies), administer the drug during daylight hours, force fluids to prompt frequent voiding, and consider bladder irrigation. Mesna (Mesnex) is available as adjuvant therapy in case of overt toxicity or as a prophylactic protectant. A sulfhydryl reagent, mesna, is transported in the bloodstream as the inactive disulfide (dimesna) and reduced by glutathione dehydrogenase to the reactive sulfhydryl in the proximal tubules.[284] After delivery to the bladder, the SH group competes with Cys residues for the alkylating acrolein, as shown in Figure 36.35. Many investigators have sought alternatives to mesna as prophylaxis against hemorrhagic cystitis, but most potential substitutes had fatal flaws, and none provided superior protection.[284]

Mesna concentrates in the bladder and will prevent damage to those cells. It does not concentrate to any appreciable extent in the nephron and, therefore, is not good protection against acrolein-induced nephrotoxicity. It also does little to spare the kidney and nerve cells from chloroacetaldehyde, the other toxic by-product of cyclophosphamide metabolism.[286] Fortunately, only about 10% of a standard dose of cyclophosphamide undergoes the dechloroethylation reaction, and most of the chloroacetaldehyde generated can be scavenged by GSH. Since the competing hydroxylation reaction is saturable, this percentage can rise if higher doses are used.[278]

Cyclophosphamide is most commonly used in combination with other antineoplastic agents to treat a wide range of neoplasms, including leukemias, lymphomas, multiple myeloma, ovarian adenocarcinoma, and breast cancer. It is metabolized in the liver and eliminated via the kidney, with approximately 10% to 20% of a given dose being excreted unchanged. While the parent drug is only 20% protein bound, some metabolites show up to 3 times the affinity for serum protein.

When given IV, initial divided doses of 40 to 50 mg/kg administered over 2 to 5 days are usual. Doses should be reduced by one-third to one-half in patients with myelosuppression (leukopenia), and a 25% reduction considered if creatinine clearance falls below 10 mL/min or serum bilirubin is between 3.1 and 5 mg/dL.[43] The drug is also administered in capsule form in some hematologic malignancies (1-5 mg/kg/d). When used in lower doses (1-3 mg/kg/d), a significant component of the anticancer activity has been

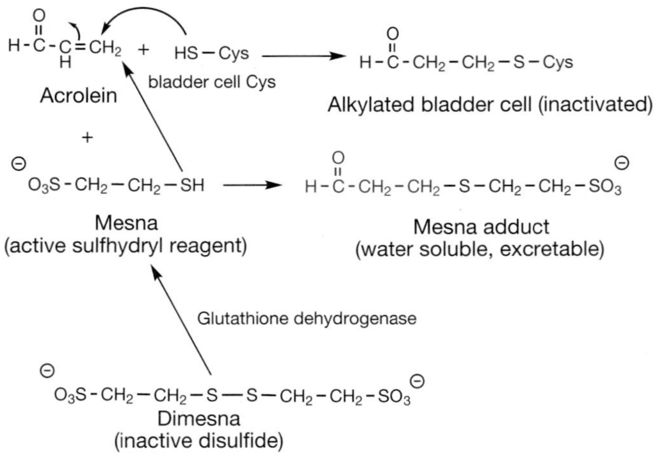

Figure 36.35 Acrolein detoxification by mesna.

proposed to be mediated by regulatory T-cell depletion and concomitant effector T-cell activation.[280] Significant stereochemistry-based variations in the metabolic, enzyme inhibition, excretion, and toxicity profiles of cyclophosphamide and related oxazaphosphorine antineoplastic agents have been described in the literature.[277,281]

Ifosfamide. Ifosfamide, a cyclophosphamide analog, has the two arms of the mustard on different nitrogen atoms (see Fig. 36.30). It also requires metabolic activation (Fig. 36.36), but this time, it is the CYP3A4 isoform that converts the majority of the dose to the carbinolamine, with CYP2B6 taking on a minor supporting role.[287] Because ifosfamide has a lower affinity for the hydroxylating CYP3A4 and CYP2B6 enzymes, presumably as a result of steric hindrance, bioactivation proceeds at a slower rate.[288] Doses 3- to 4-fold higher than cyclophosphamide are required to achieve the same antineoplastic result.

Unlike cyclophosphamide, dechloroethylation is a significant metabolic pathway for ifosfamide, and up to 60% of a standard dose will undergo this toxicity-inducing biotransformation.[277,289] CYP3A4/3A5 catalyzes approximately 70% of ifosfamide dechloroethylation, with CYP2B6 taking care of the remainder.[278] Ultimately, both chloroalkyl groups are lost before the compound is excreted. So much chloroacetaldehyde is generated that endogenous GSH (available in limited quantities) is overwhelmed. Because ifosfamide is selectively taken up by the proximal tubules, this reaction can generate chloroacetaldehyde directly in the nephron, contributing to a significantly higher nephrotoxicity that can result in glomerular and renal tubular failure.[288,290] Chloroacetaldehyde also produces neurotoxicity which is most commonly central in origin (eg, mental status dysfunction, seizures) and, in severe forms, can progress to coma and death.

Because acrolein is generated during the bioactivation of ifosfamide, the same precautions against hemorrhagic cystitis that were outlined for cyclophosphamide must be taken: hydrate well, irrigate thoroughly, and administer mesna prophylactically. Ifosfamide is more water soluble than cyclophosphamide and will concentrate in the renal system. In addition, since higher doses must be administered to achieve the same degree of antineoplastic action, more molecules of nephro- and urotoxic acrolein will be produced. It is claimed that some urothelial and mucosal damage will occur even with standard prophylactic doses of mesna.[284]

As stated, mesna will not prevent chloroacetaldehyde-induced nephro- and neurotoxicity. However, strategies for successfully treating pediatric patients at risk for ifosfamide-induced nephrotoxicity with N-acetylcysteine (Mucomyst) have been published,[291] and the approach has been supported by the work of others (Fig. 36.37).[292] While N-acetylcysteine is not yet a standard of care in pediatric patients receiving ifosfamide, it is certainly possible that it may at some point be included in the treatment protocol, and it could also be a legitimate therapeutic approach to adult patients at risk for serious nephrotoxicity secondary to ifosfamide therapy. Because N-acetylcysteine does not penetrate the blood-brain barrier (BBB), it would be of little value in central neurotoxicity prophylaxis.[277]

Ifosfamide is currently used in combination with other antineoplastics as third-line therapy in testicular cancer, although it has also shown activity in a number of other solid tumors and hematologic malignancies. For its primary indication, 1.2 g/m^2 is administered IV for 5 consecutive days and, if tolerated, repeated every 3 weeks. In addition to the acrolein- and chloroacetaldehyde-related toxicities discussed earlier, the drug carries a boxed warning for severe myelosuppression leading to potentially fatal infections. It does not bind to serum protein, and as much as 18% (low dose) and 61% (high dose) can be excreted unchanged in urine.[43] Ifosfamide in combination with cisplatin will exacerbate nephrotoxicity.

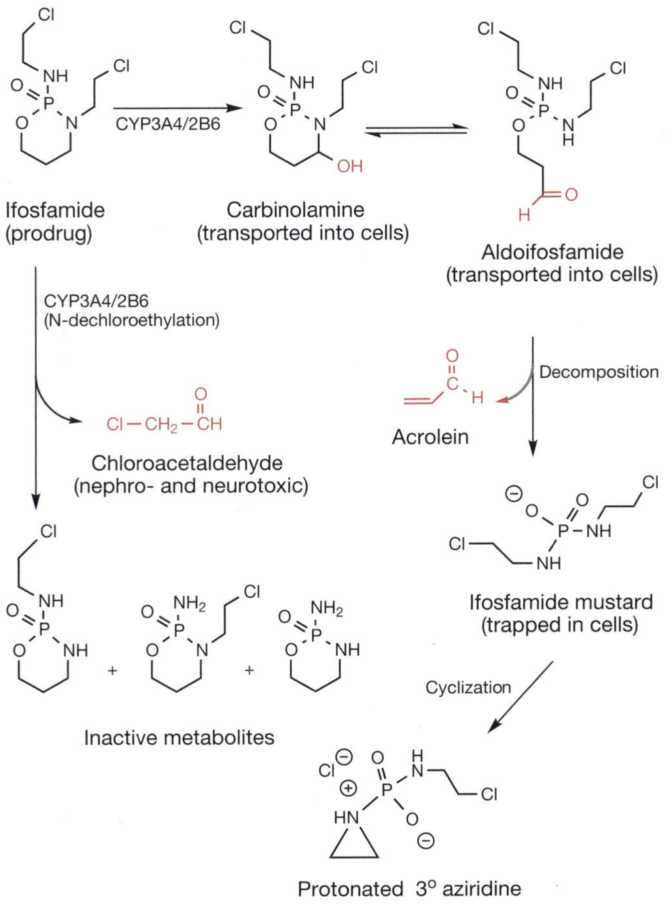

Figure 36.36 Ifosfamide metabolism.

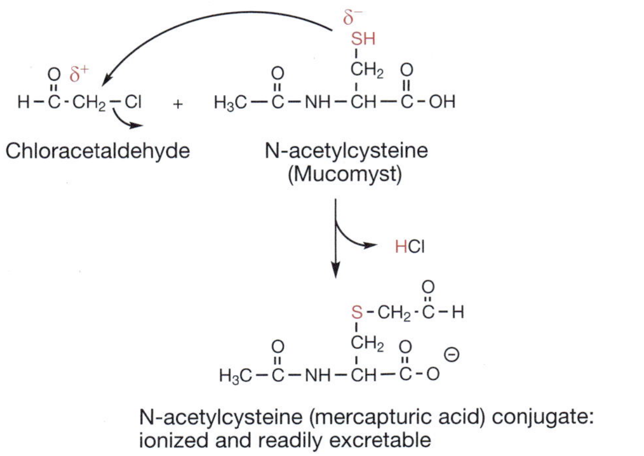

Figure 36.37 Chloroacetaldehyde detoxification by N-acetylcysteine.

DNA Methylators: Triazenes and Procarbazine

The triazenes (temozolomide and dacarbazine) and procarbazine act by different mechanisms, but they both exert an antineoplastic effect through the O^6-methylation of guanine nucleotides (see Fig. 36.30). O^6-Methylguanine pairs preferentially with thymine, and these "mispairings" prompt point mutations during subsequent DNA replication cycles and trigger cell destruction through the activation of the normal post-replication MMR system. Patients who are able to repair this damage through the action of O^6-alkylguanine-DNA-alkyltransferase, which transfers the offending CH_3 group to Cys145 on the alkyltransferase protein, will exhibit resistance to these agents, whereas those who underexpress this protein should respond well.[293,294] Since the alkyltransferase is irreversibly inactivated in the DNA rescue process, enzyme depletion with subsequent loss of DNA repair capability is a significant risk.

The triazenes methylate DNA guanine via diazomethane and/or methyl carbocation generated in situ. Although temozolomide is converted to the diazomethane precursor 3-methyl-(triazen-l-yl)imidazole-4-carboxamide (MTIC) through nonenzymatic mechanisms, the conversion of dacarbazine to MTIC depends on the action of CYP1A1 and CYP1A2 enzymes, with a smaller contribution by CYP2E1 (Fig. 36.38).[293,295-298] The O^6 and N^7 positions of guanine are the most vulnerable to triazene methylation.

In contrast, procarbazine metabolism involves CYP1A and CYP2B enzymes,[295] and DNA alkylation operates through a free radical mechanism (Fig. 36.39). The major degradation pathway involves benzylic oxidation of azoprocarbazine, producing methylhydrazine that generates a methyl radical through an unstable diazene intermediate.[299,300] In addition to O^6, the reactive methyl radical formed can alkylate the C^8 and N^7 positions of guanine.

Specific Drugs

Temozolomide. This imidazolotetrazine derivative is the most widely used agent within the DNA methylator class of antineoplastics. It is administered IV or in capsule form for the treatment of glioblastoma multiforme, a brain cancer with a dire prognosis, and in patients with anaplastic astrocytoma who have not responded to procarbazine or nitrosoureas (see below). The dosing for both routes is identical and based on body surface area. Oral absorption is rapid and complete, although decreased by food. Administration on an empty stomach also attenuates drug-induced nausea and vomiting.

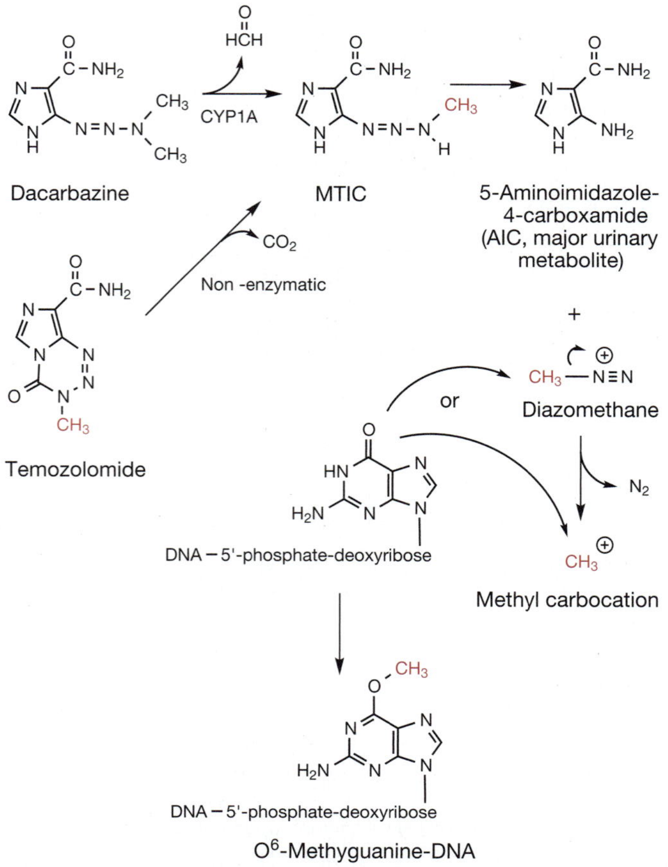

Figure 36.38 Metabolic activation of triazenes.

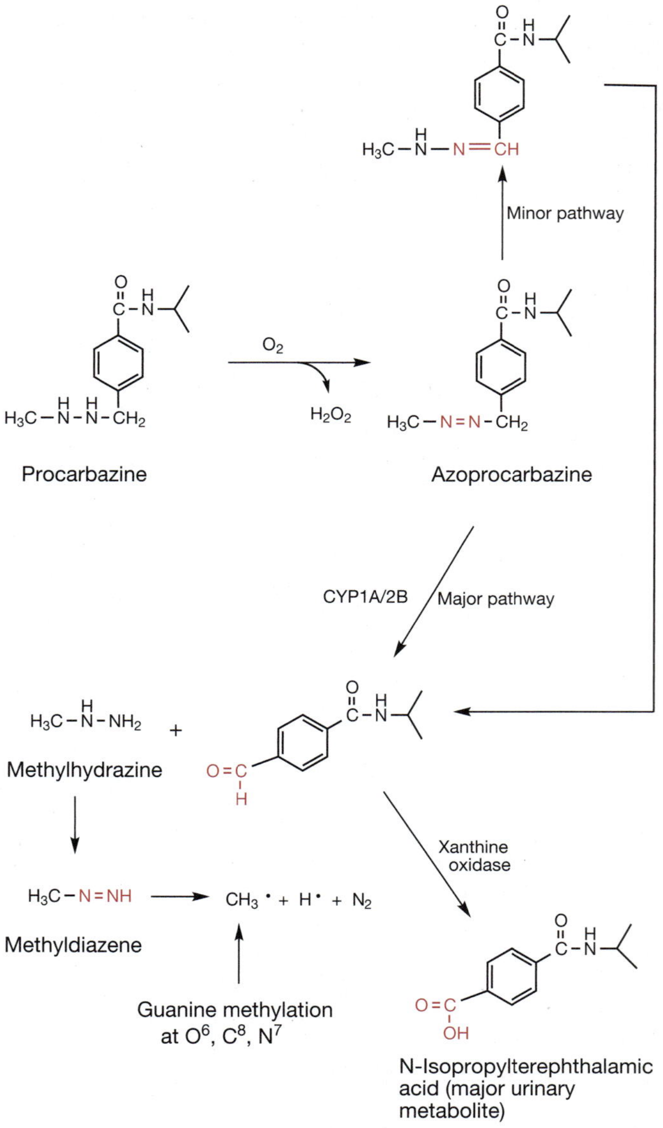

Figure 36.39 Procarbazine metabolism and mechanism of action.

While CYP enzymes are not extensively involved in temozolomide metabolism, less than 6% of the drug is excreted unchanged in the urine. Women clear the drug less effectively than men and have a higher incidence of severe neutropenia and thrombocytopenia in the initial therapy cycle. Myelosuppression is the most significant adverse effect.

Resistance to temozolomide primarily involves drug-induced damage reversal by overexpressed O^6-methylguanine-DNMT.[301] Disappointingly, inhibitors of this DNA repair enzyme, while effective in augmenting temozolomide activity in tumor cells that overexpress the methyltransferase, have shown unacceptably high myelotoxicity in clinical trials.[302] Other potential mechanisms of resistance are currently being explored, including overexpression of the base excision repair protein methylpurine-N-glycosylase, epidermal growth factor receptor (EGFR) upregulation, and drug-induced genetic alterations (eg, *p53*) that favor tumor cell survival. Challenges to the development of therapeutically viable resistance inhibitors include assurance of efficacy in multifaceted resistance systems and the ability to cross the BBB.[293,302] Inhibition of specific mRNA through a strategy termed RNA interference (RNAi) may hold promise in keeping glioblastoma cells responsive to the lethal effects of temozolomide.[303]

Dacarbazine. This DNA-methylating agent is administered IV as a single agent in the treatment of metastatic malignant melanoma and in combination with other agents in the treatment of stage III and IV Hodgkin lymphoma. Approximately 40% of the drug is excreted unchanged, but both the 5-aminoimidazole-4-carboxamide (AIC, formed through the action of CYP1A enzymes) and the carboxylic acid (AIC hydrolysis product) are major urinary metabolites (see Fig. 36.38). Leukopenia and thrombocytopenia are the most common adverse effects and can be fatal. Patients are also at risk for hepatotoxicity, including hepatocellular necrosis, and the drug carries a boxed warning for all of these serious potential toxicities.

The advent of effective and less toxic targeted and immunotherapies for the first- and second-line treatment of dacarbazine's primary indications have diminished this agent's importance in contemporary chemotherapy.

Procarbazine. This methyl radical generator is used primarily in the treatment of Hodgkin disease. It is administered as part of a multidrug regimen that includes a nitrogen mustard (cyclophosphamide), a mitosis inhibitor (vincristine), and prednisone. It is administered as a capsule and is absorbed well after oral administration. Procarbazine is extensively metabolized in the liver, and 70% of an administered dose is excreted in the urine as N-isopropylterephthalamic acid (see Fig. 36.39). In addition to methylating DNA guanine residues, it is proposed to inhibit the de novo synthesis of proteins and nucleic acids.

Procarbazine inhibits monoamine oxidase, leading to several significant and potentially fatal DDIs and drug-food interactions. Facial flushing and other disulfiram-like symptoms are noted when alcohol is concomitantly consumed because the drug also inhibits enzymes involved in ethanol metabolism.

Miscellaneous DNA Alkylators

Busulfan. Chemically busulfan is an alkylsulfonate with a butyl chain linked to two methane sulfonate groups. It is a bifunctional alkylating agent where one or both methylsulfonate ester moieties can be displaced by the nucleophilic N^7 of guanine leading to monoalkylated or crosslinked DNA (Fig. 36.40). Intrastrand DNA cross-linking occurs more readily than interstrand cross-linking with adducts observed at 5′-GA-3′ and 5′-GG-3′ sequences.[304-306]

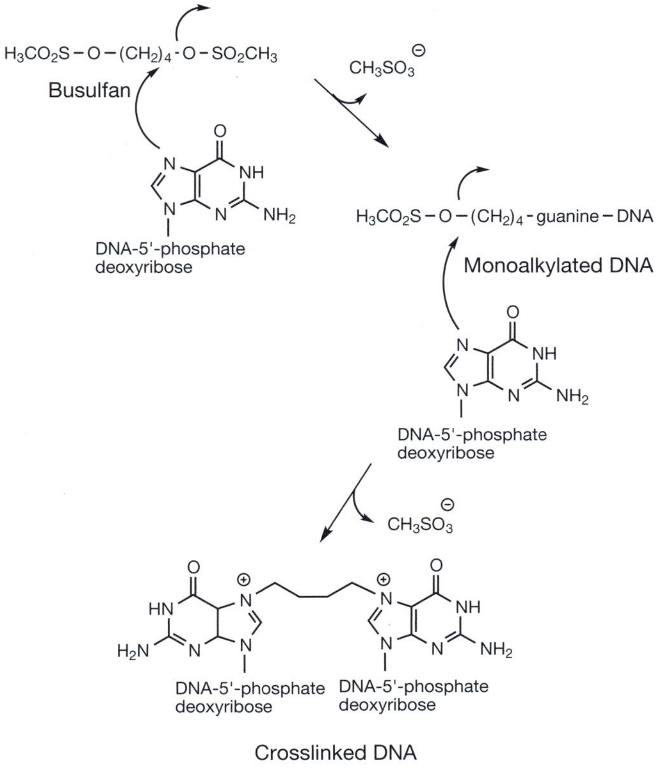

Figure 36.40 Busulfan-mediated DNA alkylation.

Busulfan is used in the treatment of CML and can be administered orally or by IV infusion. Serious bone marrow toxicity and myelosuppression are possible, and recovery from busulfan pancytopenia can take up to 4 years. Other toxicities include seizures, veno-occlusive disease, and pulmonary toxicity.[307] Concurrent administration with itraconazole antifungal can reduce busulfan clearance and may require dose reduction.

Nitrosoureas

The chloroethyl-containing nitrosoureas (CNUs) are unstable structures that decompose readily in the aqueous environment of the cell to generate electrophilic chloroethyl- and hydroxyethyl carbocations that target both the N^7 and O^6 positions of guanine (Figs. 36.41 and 36.42). The N^7 atom of guanine is the most commonly alkylated atom, although all DNA bases are vulnerable. The N^7-hydroxyethyl analog could be envisioned to form directly from the chloroethylated guanine, but hydrolysis is known to be sluggish. Rather, direct N^7-hydroxyethylation has been proposed, as has "progressive alkylation," where rearrangements transfer the chloroethyl or hydroxyethyl group to various positions on the DNA base.[308] Pyrimidine bases are consistently alkylated at N^3. DNA alkylation by CNUs results in apoptosis and necrosis in the impacted cell.[309]

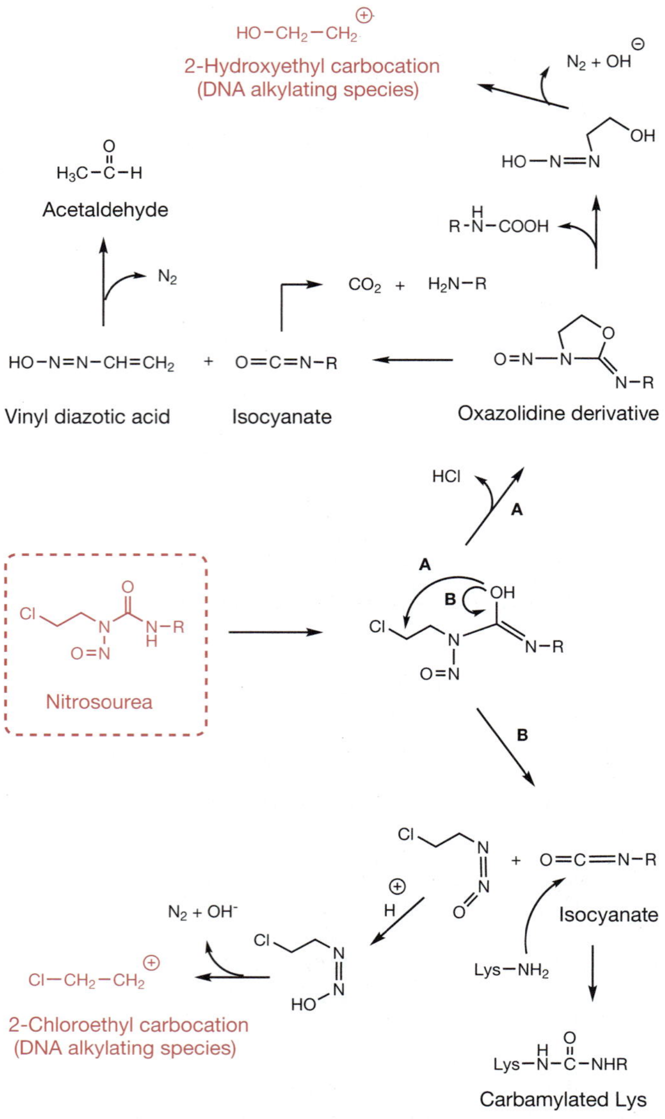

Figure 36.41 Nitrosourea decomposition to cytotoxic electrophiles.

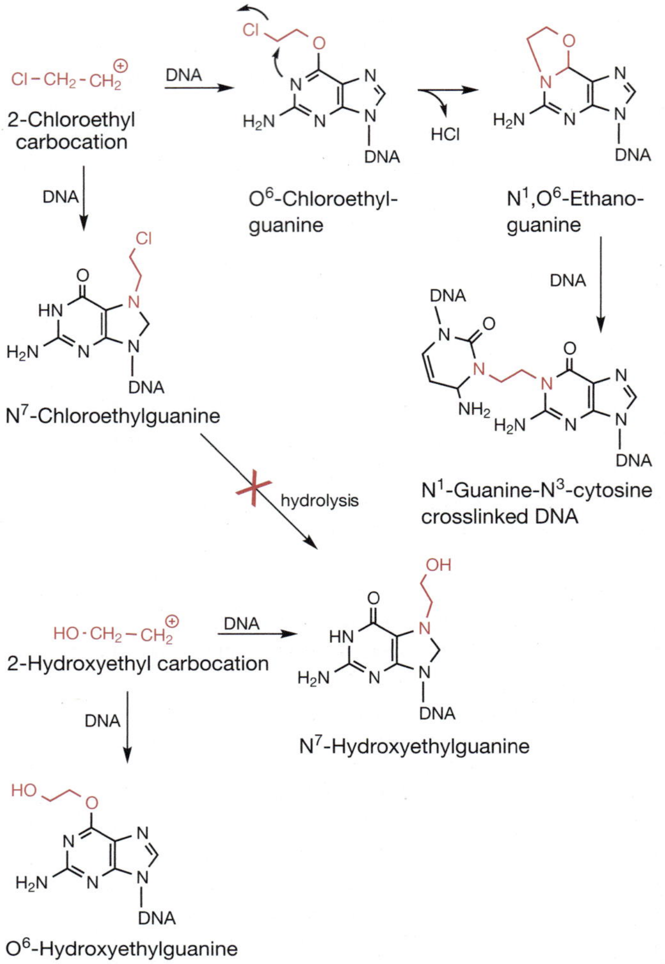

Figure 36.42 DNA alkylation and cross-linking by 2-chloroethyl carbocation and 2-hydroxyethyl carbocation.

While less commonly generated, O^6-chloroethylguanine is particularly unstable and spontaneously cyclizes to form N^1,O^6-ethanoguanine that covalently links via the purine's N^1 position to a complementary cytosine residue through the pyrimidine's N^3 position (see Fig. 36.42).[308-310] In contrast, the stable O^6-hydroxyethyl analog does not cyclize but is presumed to mismatch during DNA replication and transcription, stimulating mutagenesis.[308] While base alkylation with or without subsequent cyclization is toxic, the more interstrand crosslinks generated the more lethal cellular response; 20 to 40 crosslinks normally result in cell death if repair mechanisms are absent or ineffective.[309]

Resistance to CNU chemotherapy is known to involve O^6-alkylguanine-DNA alkyltransferase, the same enzyme that thwarts the cytotoxic action of triazenes and procarbazine. Transfer of the aberrant alkyl moiety to Cys145 is the common mechanism.[308,309] Interstrand crosslinks can also be reversed by nucleotide excision repair (NER) proteins, and Fanconi-associated nuclease 1 (FAN1) has also been proposed to play a DNA restorative role.[309] Drug sequestration by neuroprotective metallothionein proteins may also be involved in CNU resistance.[311]

Specific Drugs

Carmustine and Lomustine. Carmustine and lomustine (see Fig. 36.30) are both highly lipophilic CNUs marketed for use in brain tumors and Hodgkin disease.[309] Carmustine has also shown value in the treatment of NHL and multiple myeloma, and it is given IV or incorporated into biodegradable wafers that are implanted directly into the CNS after tumor resection. The high lipophilicity of carmustine precludes a totally aqueous IV formulation, and the drug is administered in 10% ethanol. Although carmustine degrades within 15 minutes of IV administration, lomustine is stable enough for oral use and is marketed in capsule form. Excretion of both drugs is predominantly via the urine, although any CO_2 generated from decomposition will be exhaled. Carmustine can decompose in vitro if exposed to temperatures around 90 °F. Pure carmustine is a low-melting solid, but the decomposed product is an oil and, therefore, readily detected. Vials of carmustine that appear oily should be discarded.

Combination therapy with dacarbazine pretreatment has been proposed to deplete O^6-alkylguanine-DNA alkyltransferase, thus enhancing sensitivity to CNUs in tumors overexpressing the resistance-promoting enzyme. Dacarbazine and lomustine coadministration in glioblastoma multiforme has resulted in greater disease stability compared to dacarbazine alone. Small molecule inhibitors of the alkyltransferase, including the thiol scavenger disulfiram, are also being investigated as possible adjuncts to CNU chemotherapy.[309]

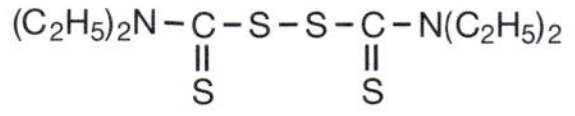

Disulfiram

Both carmustine and lomustine can induce thrombocytopenia and leukopenia, leading to hemorrhage and massive infection, and the drugs carry boxed warnings for these toxicities. Acute and delayed pulmonary toxicity is also a risk with carmustine (boxed warning). Pulmonary toxicity is dose related, and individuals who received the drug in childhood or early adolescence are at higher risk for the potentially fatal delayed reaction. The grand mal seizures that are possible with the wafer formulation of carmustine appear to result from the wafer itself, rather than from the nitrosourea.

Organoplatinum Complexes

MECHANISM OF ACTION. Organoplatinum antineoplastic agents contain an electron-deficient metal atom that acts as a magnet for electron-rich DNA nucleophiles. Like nitrogen mustards, organoplatinum complexes are bifunctional and can accept electrons from two DNA nucleophiles. Intrastrand crosslinks most frequently occur between adjacent guanine residues referred to as diguanosine dinucleotides (60%-65%) or adjacent guanine and adenine residues (25%-30%).[312] Interstrand cross-linking, which occurs much less frequently (1%-3%), usually involves guanine and adenine bases.[313]

CHEMISTRY. All currently marketed organoplatinum anticancer agents are Pt(II) complexes with square planar geometry. Platinum is inherently electron deficient, but the net charge on the organometallic complex is zero due to the contribution of electrons by two of the four ligands bound to the parent structure. Most commonly, the electron-donating ligand is chloride. Before reacting with DNA, the electron-donating ligands are displaced through nucleophilic attack by cellular water. When the displaced ligands are chloride anions (eg, cisplatin), the chloride-poor environment of the tumor cell facilitates the process, driving the generation of the active, cytotoxic hydrated forms (Fig. 36.43). Since the original ligands leave the metal with their electrons, the hydrated organoplatinum molecule has a net positive charge.

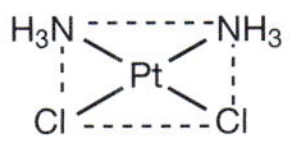

Cisplatin (square planar geometry)

The hydrated Pt analogs are readily attacked by DNA nucleophiles (eg, the N^7 of adjacent guanine residues) due to the net positive charge that has been regained on the Pt atom (see Fig. 36.43). The DNA bases coordinate with the Pt, and in the *cis* configuration, DNA repair mechanisms are unable to permanently correct the damage. The net

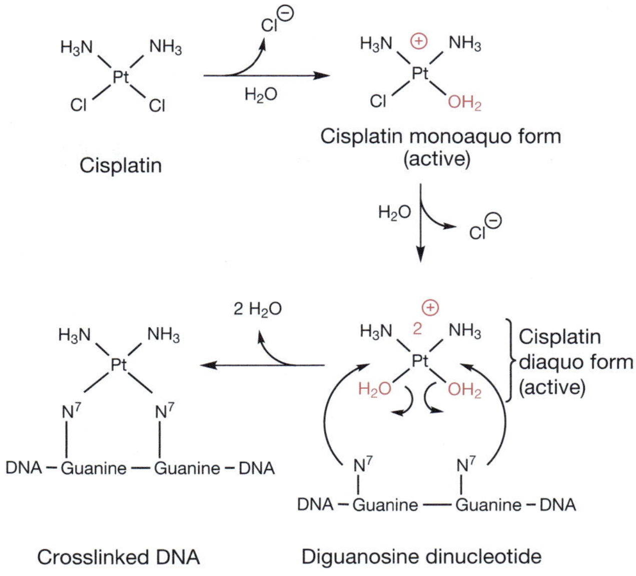

Figure 36.43 **Cisplatin activation and DNA cross-linking.**

result is a major change in DNA conformation such that base pairs that normally engage in hydrogen bond formation are not permitted to interact. The two amine ligands of the complex are bound irreversibly to the Pt atom through very strong coordinate covalent bonds. They cannot be displaced by DNA nucleophiles, but they do stabilize the crosslinked DNA-Pt complex by forming strong ion-dipole bonds with the anionic phosphate residues on DNA. The DNA distortion prompts a futile cycle of damage recognition and repair before succumbing to cell cycle arrest and apoptosis. In contrast to cisplatin, the leaving ligand in carboplatin and oxaliplatin is chelated, making it more stable to aquation.[314]

SPECIFIC DRUGS

Cisplatin. The simplest of the organometallic antineoplastic agents, cisplatin (see Fig. 36.30), is used IV in the treatment of metastatic testicular and ovarian cancer and advanced bladder cancer. It is rapidly hydrated, resulting in a short plasma half-life of less than 30 minutes. It is eliminated predominantly via the kidney, but approximately 10% of a given dose undergoes biliary excretion. It is highly nephrotoxic and can cause significant damage to the renal tubules, especially in patients with preexisting kidney disease or who are concurrently receiving other nephrotoxic drugs (eg, cyclophosphamide or ifosfamide). Dosages should be reduced in any of these situations. Clearance decreases with chronic therapy, and toxicities can manifest at a later date.

To proactively protect against kidney damage, patients should be aggressively hydrated with chloride-containing solutions, and potassium and magnesium supplementation should be initiated. Mannitol diuretics can be administered to promote continuous excretion of the drug and its hydrated analogs.[315,316] Sodium thiosulfate and amifostine, a thiol-generating prodrug bioactivated by alkaline phosphatase, have been employed to neutralize cisplatin (Fig. 36.44). However, with lower-dose cisplatin regimens, these are no longer required.

Cisplatin carries a boxed warning for many serious toxicities. In addition to cumulative nephrotoxicity, myelosuppression is common. Cisplatin is also a very severe emetogen, and

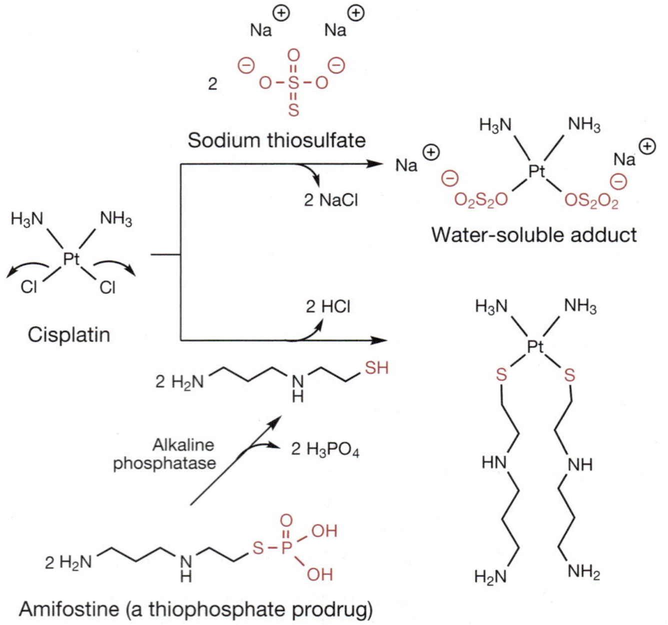

Figure 36.44 Cisplatin inactivation by sodium thiosulfate and amifostine.

vomiting almost always occurs unless antiemetic therapy is coadministered. Hypersensitivity reactions can occur within minutes of administration and can result in a respiratory and/or cardiovascular emergency; epinephrine, corticosteroids, and/or antihistamines should be at hand for immediate administration in the event of anaphylaxis. Ototoxicity that can lead to irreversible hearing loss can also occur with cisplatin use. The ototoxicity is related to a high cochlear uptake of cisplatin with subsequent destruction of sensory hair cells by ROS that can be generated by this drug.[317] High-frequency hearing is the first to be impacted.[318]

Resistance to cisplatin therapy can be intrinsic in colorectal, prostate, and lung cancer, or acquired after multiple courses of therapy (eg, in ovarian cancer).[319] Resistance is mediated through several distinct mechanisms, including: (1) compromised carrier-mediated cellular transport via the copper-transporting protein CTR1; (2) enhanced intracellular inactivation through drug trapping in vesicles; (3) drug inactivation through conjugation to Cys and/or Met-containing GSH and metallothionein proteins; (4) uncontrolled expression of noncoding RNA (ncRNA); (5) cellular efflux by P-type ATP 7A/7B, MDR, and (possibly) P-gp proteins; and (6) increased DNA repair and/or tolerance to cisplatin-induced DNA damage.[319,320] Regarding the latter mechanism, cisplatin damage can be successfully repaired by NER proteins, which remove platinum-damaged segments from the DNA, and these proteins are often upregulated in cisplatin-resistant tumors. Cisplatin-DNA (and carboplatin-DNA, discussed later) adducts are also recognized by MMR proteins. The downregulation of MMR in cisplatin and carboplatin-treated cancer cells induces resistance through the loss of an apoptotic response that normally follows several ill-fated attempts to repair organoplatinum-induced damage.[319] Testicular tumors are particularly responsive to cisplatin due to their inherent deficiency in DNA repair processes.

Cisplatin is administered IV in accordance with disease-specific regimens. It is a vesicant in high doses and can blister skin. Extravasation should be managed with IV and SC sodium thiosulfate (see Fig. 36.44) and the affected limb elevated. Cisplatin and the other organoplatinum anticancer agents react with aluminum and cannot be administered through aluminum-containing needles. The drug is photosensitive, is packaged in amber bottles, and must be protected from light.[43]

Carboplatin. Carboplatin (see Fig. 36.30) forms the same cytotoxic hydrated intermediate as cisplatin but does so at a 10-fold slower rate, making it a 20- to 40-fold less potent chemotherapeutic agent.[320] The ultimate damage done to cells as a result of carboplatin use approaches that of cisplatin, but the adverse effect profile is significantly milder. Suppression of platelets and white blood cells is the most significant toxic reaction, and nonhematologic toxicities (eg, emesis, nephrotoxicity, and ototoxicity) are rare. The plasma half-life of carboplatin is 3 hours, and the drug is less extensively bound to serum proteins than cisplatin. Excretion is still predominantly renal, however, and doses must be reduced in patients with kidney disease.

Carboplatin is only approved for use in the treatment of advanced ovarian cancer and is dose-personalized using target AUC and patient glomerular filtration rate (GFR) to minimize thrombocytopenia.[321] It can be used as a single agent or in combination with the mitosis inhibitors docetaxel or paclitaxel or with the antimetabolite gemcitabine. Off-label uses for carboplatin include combination therapy in a myriad of solid and hematologic malignancies (including NSCLC, head and neck cancer, and GI and reproductive tract cancers), in which it has been shown to be a reasonable and often less toxic alternative to cisplatin.[322,323]

Oxaliplatin. This Pt(II) complex loses its oxalate dianion ($^-$OOC-COO$^-$) in vivo and forms the mono- and dihydrated diaminocyclohexane (DACH) platinum analogs shown in Figure 36.45. The *trans*-(*R*,*R*)-DACH structure serves as the carrier for the cytotoxic hydrated platinum and extends into the major groove of DNA where the DNA-Pt complex forms.[324] Hydrophobic DNA intrusion is believed to contribute to the cytotoxicity of this organometallic. Oxaliplatin engages primarily in intrastrand cross-linking with diguanosine dinucleotides, adjacent A-G nucleotides, and

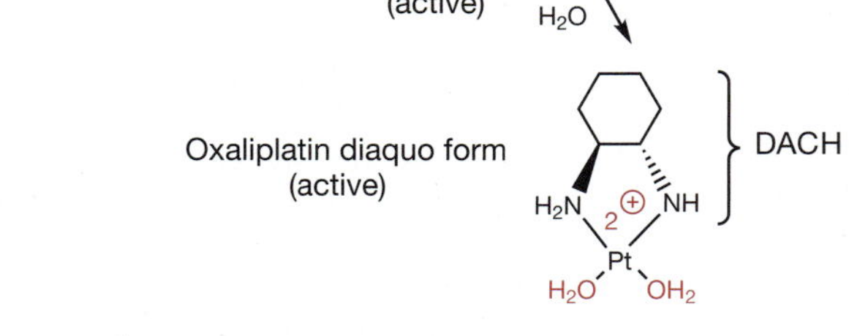

Figure 36.45 Activation of oxaliplatin.

guanines that are separated by one nucleotide (G-X-G). Interstrand cross-linking, although less common, also occurs.

The adduct formed between oxaliplatin and DNA diguanosine dinucleotides is conformationally distinct from the adduct formed with cisplatin or carboplatin. Specifically, whereas the cisplatin diguanosine dinucleotide adduct bends the DNA by 60° to 80° and presents a relatively wide minor groove, the oxaliplatin adduct produces a 31° bend with a comparatively narrow minor groove.[325] This distinct oxaliplatin conformation is believed to result from the steric impact of the (*R*,*R*)-DACH carrier, which permits the *cis*-NH_3 moieties to hydrogen bond with a guanine-O^6, a bond that the inactive (*S*,*S*)-isomer cannot make.[326] The conformation of the oxaliplatin-DNA adduct is much less likely to be recognized by MMR proteins, and the effectiveness of oxaliplatin in MMR-deficient cells is, at least in part, responsible for the lack of resistance that has plagued cisplatin and carboplatin.[327,328] Oxaliplatin is also less dependent on the copper-transporting protein CTR1 for intracellular access and often retains activity in patients who are no longer responding to the first-generation organoplatinum agents. It is significantly less mutagenic, nephrotoxic, hematotoxic, and ototoxic than cisplatin. Excretion is via the kidney. Oxaliplatin decomposes in alkaline media and should not be coadministered with drugs that will increase the pH of the IV solution.

Oxaliplatin is used in the treatment of metastatic colon or rectal cancer in combination with FU/leucovorin (FOLFOX regimen). The usual adult dose is 85 mg/m^2 infused over 2 hours to minimize hypersensitivity risk (the reason for Oxaliplatin boxed warning), repeating every 2 weeks. Literature suggests that faster infusion rates of 1 $mg/m^2/min$ can be used to expedite drug delivery without increasing the hypersensitivity reaction risk.[329] Pulmonary fibrosis and anaphylaxis can be life threatening, and dose- and/or use-liming peripheral sensory neuropathy that can become permanent and painful significantly impacts patient quality of life. The acute neuropathy that occurs in up to 98% of oxaliplatin-treated patients is reversible. Chronic neuropathy (often with negative functional consequences) will manifest in approximately 15% of patients who receive cumulative doses of 780 to 850 mg/m^2.[330] Neuropathy has been attributed to the chelation of intracellular Ca^{2+} by the oxalate dianion that is displaced from the parent drug by water, which disrupts the function of calcium-gated ion channels in sensory nerve cells.[331]

Patients at risk of chemotherapy-induced neurotoxicity are given oxaliplatin at a slower infusion rate, and those with persistent neuropathy are given a holiday from oxaliplatin, with therapy resuming when benefits outweigh risks. All patients should avoid exposure to cold, which exacerbates neuropathic pain. A meta-analysis of therapeutic intervention with Ca^{2+}/Mg^{2+} infusion, glutathione, N-acetylcysteine, n-3 polyunsaturated fatty acids, or herbal products (AC591 and guilongtongluofang) found that each had the potential to prevent oxaliplatin-induced peripheral neuropathy.[332] Studies exploring the impact of pharmacogenetics on patient response to therapy that includes oxaliplatin are being reported, and exploitation of genetic differences in the expression of various repair proteins, growth factors, and metabolizing enzymes may ultimately allow the tailoring of oxaliplatin therapy based on an individual's pharmacogenetic profile.[327,333,334]

Hormone-Based Antineoplastic Agents (Representative)

Structures that modulate the activity of estrogen and androgen receptors or influence levels of circulating hormones that can impact steroid-dependent tumors are available as antineoplastic agents. These therapeutic entities are discussed in detail in Chapter 25, but one representative molecule from each pharmacologic class is highlighted in Figure 36.46.

Aromatase Inhibitors

Aromatase inhibitors are used in the treatment of postmenopausal ER+ breast cancer, as adjuvant (early), first-line (locally advanced or metastatic), and/or alternate (disease that has progressed on estrogen antagonists) therapy. In postmenopausal women, estrogen is biosynthesized in the breast via the oxidation of androstenedione. The catalyzing enzyme is CYP19A1 (aromatase), and the estrogen generated in situ fuels the progression of HR+ breast cancers. Of the three currently marketed aromatase inhibitors, exemestane is an irreversible steroidal inhibitor, and anastrozole and letrozole are nonsteroidal reversible inhibitors. The reversible inhibitors enjoy widespread clinical use.

ANASTROZOLE.[43,335] Anastrozole (see Fig. 36.46) binds competitively and selectively to the heme moiety of the aromatase enzyme, interfering with its oxidizing potential. As a result, cellular levels of estrone, the product of androstenedione

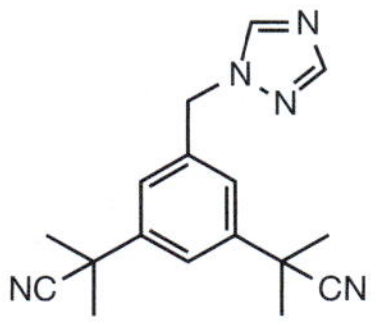

Anastrozole (Arimidex)

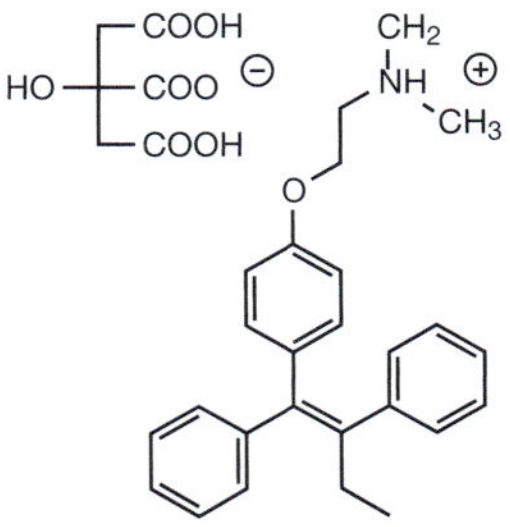

Tamoxifen citrate

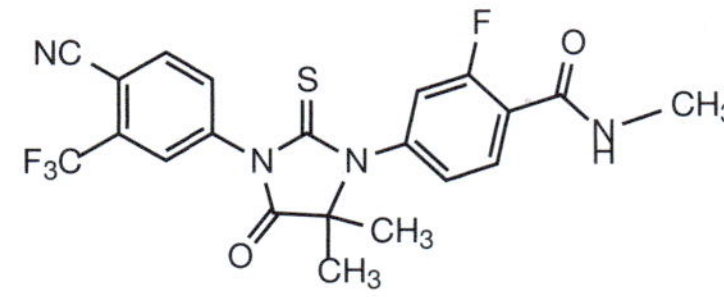

Enzalutamide (Xtandi)

PyroGlu—His—Trp—Ser—Tyr—Gly—*D*-Leu—Arg—Pro—NH_2 • $H_3C\cdot COOH$

Leuprolide acetate (Lupron)

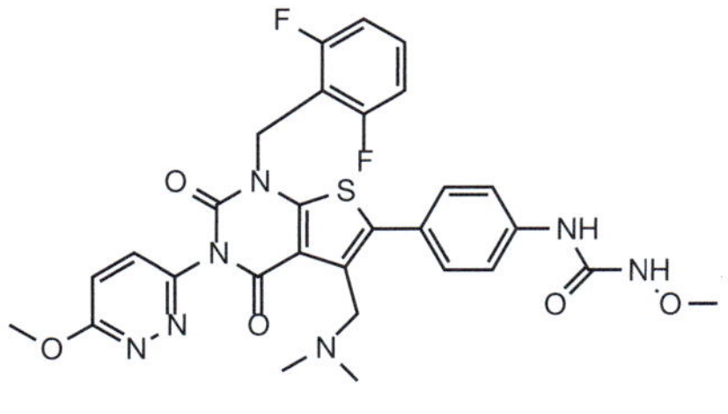

Relugolix (Orgovyx)

Figure 36.46 Representative hormone-based antineoplastic agents.

oxidation, fall up to 85%. This leads to a significant decrease in the production of estradiol, the most potent receptor estrogen. The reversible conversion of estrone to estradiol is generated by 17β-hydroxysteroid dehydrogenase (17β-HSD). Recent work has identified that anastrozole, but not exemestane or letrozole, binds to ERα and causes its degradation and that estradiol adds to this effect by downregulating ERα expression. This novel mechanism may have therapeutic potential in aromatase inhibitor-resistant breast cancer.[336]

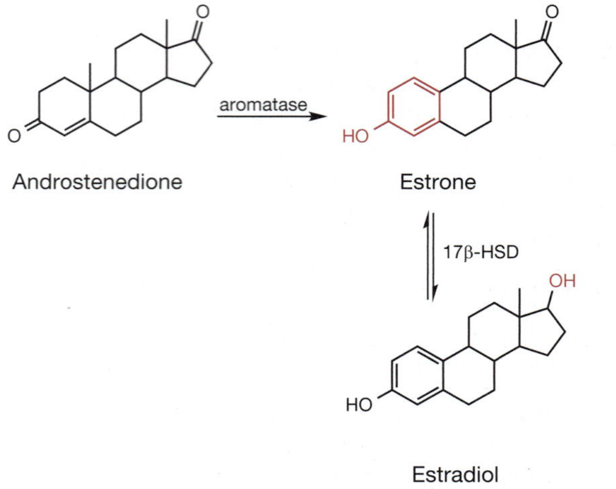

Anastrozole has demonstrated efficacy in all of the aforementioned clinical situations, and one 1-mg tablet is administered once daily. While it can be administered without regard to food, absorption is faster (but no less extensive) on an empty stomach. A 70% reduction in estrogen levels is achieved within 1 day, with an additional 10% reduction after 2 weeks of therapy. The drug undergoes aromatic hydroxylation at C_4, methyl hydroxylation at the cyanopropyl moiety, and N-dealkylation to release the primary inactive metabolite, triazole.[337] Glucuronide conjugates are excreted primarily in urine.

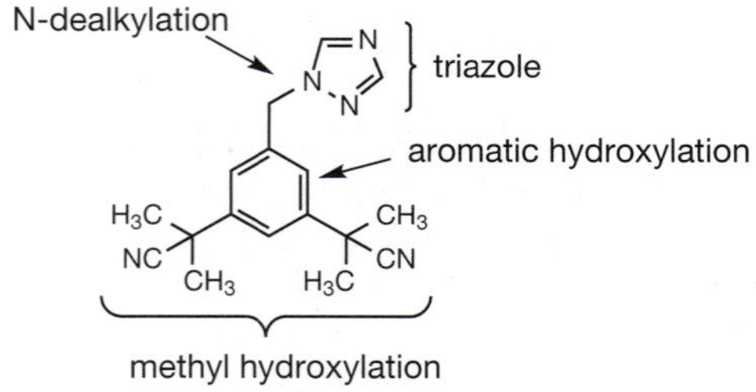

Anastrozole Phase 1 metabolism

Antiestrogens

The antiestrogens used in the treatment of breast cancer often exhibit tissue-specific action at ERs, blocking hormone binding in breast and reproductive organs while displaying agonist actions in other tissues (eg, uterus, bone). These dual-acting agents are more accurately referred to as selective estrogen receptor modulators or SERMs. The 3-fold structural requirements for ER blockade by SERMs include: (1) three aromatic (phenyl) rings with a strictly maintained three-dimensional structure, (2) a *cis* ring that bears a potentially cationic amine moiety linked through an alkyl ether group, and (3) a phenol-bearing *trans* ring, where the OH (or isostere) is either a component of the parent drug or generated via metabolism. The binding of SERMs to the ER has been well characterized (see Chapter 25). One anticancer agent in this pharmacologic class, fulvestrant, is a pure antiestrogen and decreases cellular levels of the receptor protein through degradation.

Tamoxifen Citrate.[43,338] It is hard to overestimate the positive therapeutic benefit of the relatively simple molecule tamoxifen (see Fig. 36.46). It has been termed "ground-breaking" and "pioneering" in that it introduced the SERM pharmacologic concept and ushered in the era of targeted breast cancer treatment and prevention therapy. This drug has saved countless lives with few use-limiting adverse effects. Unlike many targeted cancer therapies, it is inexpensive and, therefore, accessible to essentially all patients worldwide. Its indications range from disease prevention in high-risk patients to early-advanced breast cancer to ductal carcinoma in situ (DCIS). A boxed warning on potentially fatal uterine malignancies (adenocarcinoma and sarcoma) and cardiovascular events, including stroke and pulmonary embolism, applies to patients with high-risk breast cancer, those with DCIS, and/or coadministration with cytotoxic therapies.

Therapeutic action is realized through two major metabolites of isomerically pure Z (*trans*) tamoxifen, both of which have the essential phenolic OH generated through CYP2D6 metabolism. The CYP3A4-generated desmethyl metabolite is only active if 2D6-catalyzed *p*-hydroxylation has occurred. Patients who are 2D6 intermediate or poor metabolizers may see little or no clinical benefit from tamoxifen, and the concomitant use of drugs that inhibit this isoform should be avoided.

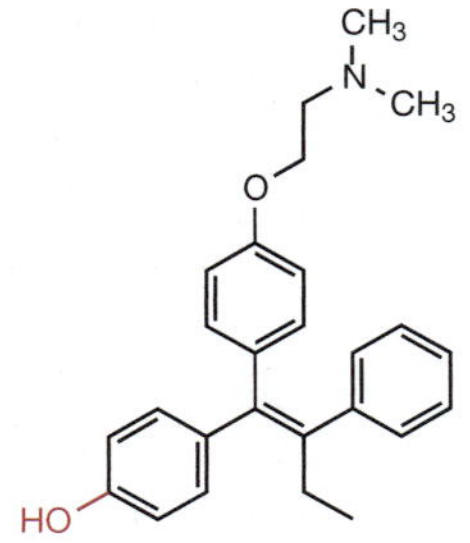

4-hydroxytamoxifen (active)

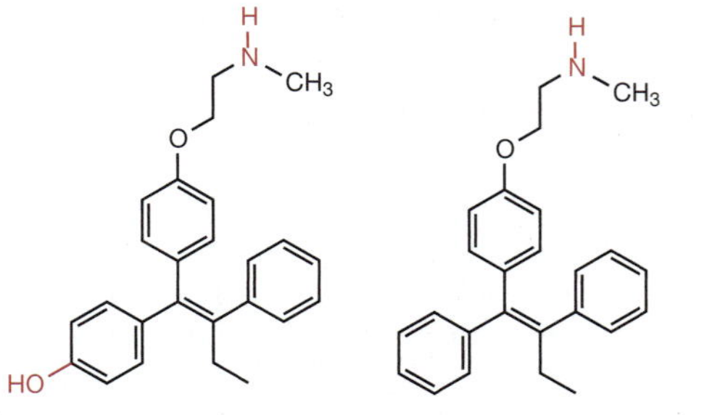

N-desmethyl-4-hydroxytamoxifen (active)   N-desmethyltamoxifen (inactive)

The usual dosage regimen of tamoxifen is 20 to 40 mg/d for 5 years, with the higher doses being used in metastatic disease. The drug is administered in tablet form and concentrates in the breast (antiestrogen action) and uterus/endometrium (estrogen agonist action). It is highly protein bound, and the half-life of the parent drug and desmethyl metabolite ranges from 1 to 2 weeks, respectively. Extensive enterohepatic cycling occurs, and excretion is predominantly fecal. The significant risk of metabolic and other DDIs warrants vigilant monitoring by the pharmacist.

Antiandrogens

Compounds that antagonize or otherwise disrupt the function of androgen receptors have value in CRPC, a disease characterized by dysregulated androgen receptor signaling with subsequent loss of the homeostatic balance between cellular proliferation and apoptosis. Antiandrogens are used when disease progression is realized or anticipated despite androgen deprivation therapy (see Gonadotropin-Releasing Hormone Modulators discussion) or testicular removal (orchidectomy). While the prognosis for CRPC is poor, early use of selected agents (ie, with androgen deprivation or surgical castration) may delay progression and/or metastasis.

Structural requirements for high-affinity androgen receptor binding of these antagonists include an aniline ring substituted with an electron-withdrawing group at the *m*- and *p*-positions (eg, CF_3 and CN or NO_2, respectively), and a propanamide moiety (often cyclic) that may serve as a bridge between the aniline core and a second aromatic ring. The common interactions of antiandrogens with key ligand-binding domain residues have been identified (see Chapter 25).

ENZALUTAMIDE.[43,339] Enzalutamide (see Fig. 36.46), a second-generation pure antiandrogen, meets the structural requirements for an androgen receptor antagonist. In addition to blocking testosterone/dihydrotestosterone binding to the cytoplasmic receptor, it also inhibits translocation of the occupied receptor dimer to the nucleus (where it would normally regulate DNA transcription) and interferes with the binding of any nuclear receptor dimers with the androgen response elements of DNA. These latter actions are important, as CRPC is often characterized by androgen receptor overexpression secondary to gene amplification, which provides a greater opportunity for androgen receptor signaling that can drive tumor growth.

Enzalutamide is marketed as 40-mg capsules, and the usual dose is four capsules (160 mg) taken at once at a consistent time of day. Absorption is rapid and food independent, and peak plasma levels are achieved within 3 hours (most commonly by 1 hour). An active N-desmethyl metabolite is generated by CYP2C8, and the parent drug and metabolite have half-lives of 5.8 and 7.8 to 8.6 days, respectively. Urinary excretion predominates.

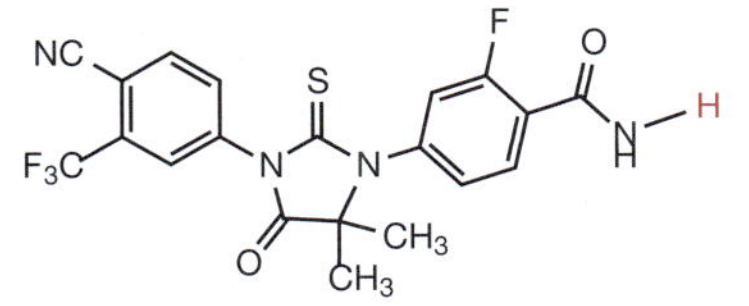

Desmethylenzalutamide (active metabolite)

Resistance to enzalutamide can occur through multiple mechanisms, with androgen receptor aberrations such as reactivation, splice variants, and mutations being most common.[340] Drug-associated seizures requiring enzalutamide discontinuation have been noted in patients with predisposing risk factors.

Gonadotropin-Releasing Hormone Modulators

Two types of gonadotropin-releasing hormone (GnRH) modulators, the GnRH agonists and the GnRH receptor (GnRH-R) antagonists, are available for advanced prostate cancer therapy. Both reduce testosterone levels to below castration levels, albeit through opposing mechanisms. GnRH agonists (eg, leuprolide) initially stimulate the release of luteinizing hormone (LH) and follicle-stimulating hormone (FSH) from the anterior pituitary, promoting steroidogenesis. The unrelenting agonism of the GnRH-R induces a profound desensitization due to the negative feedback inhibition of the hypothalamus by the high serum concentrations of sex steroids. This results in GnRH-R downregulation and a profound decrease in testicular steroid production. In contrast, the GnRH-R antagonists (eg, degarelix and relugolix) directly compete with the endogenous GnRH for receptor binding in the anterior pituitary, reducing LH and FSH levels, thereby inhibiting steroidogenesis. Through both approaches, testicular biosynthesis of androgens is essentially halted, and testosterone levels drop below castration levels, delaying progression to CRPC.

LEUPROLIDE ACETATE.[43,341] Leuprolide acetate (see Fig. 36.46), a potent GnRH agonist, has been used to induce androgen deficiency in prostate cancer for over three decades. The drug is a decapeptide and commonly administered IM. The delivery system (microsphere or biodegradable polymer) generates a depot that provides continuous release of the high affinity and metabolically stable GnRH-mimetic leuprolide. Concentrations are available to deliver the drug anywhere from 1 to 6 months, but formulations should not be used in combination nor fractionated. During the initial steroidogenesis stage, patients can experience tumor exacerbation, bone pain, hematuria, and neuropathy, but these adverse effects usually subside as testosterone biosynthesis attenuates. Once testosterone levels drop, gynecomastia, breast pain, and hot flashes can be problematic. Leuprolide prolongs the QT interval and can lead to life-threatening arrhythmia if other drugs with this effect are coadministered. Seizures have also been noted with leuprolide use, and depressive symptoms can worsen.

The major leuprolide metabolite is an inactive pentapeptide (M1) generated by peptidase enzymes.

RELUGOLIX.[43,342] Relugolix (see Fig. 36.46) is a nonpeptide, small molecule GnRH-R antagonist for advanced prostate cancer. It is the first GnRH modulator available in oral form, although its bioavailability is low (12%). Relugolix is a substrate of P-gp and is metabolized by CYP3A4/5 and CYP2C8. Concomitant therapy with inhibitors or inducers of these enzymes should be avoided to prevent DDIs. The drug is dosed at 360 mg on day 1 and 120 mg daily thereafter. Hot flashes are the most common adverse effect, followed by fatigue, constipation/diarrhea, and arthralgia. Relugolix is less cardiotoxic than leuprolide, and 95% to 97% of male patients achieved lower serum testosterone levels compared to 57% to 89% on leuprolide.[343]

Miscellaneous Antineoplastic Agents

The anticancer agents included in this section are "one-of-a-kind" structures that do not fit neatly into other antineoplastic drug classes. Newer drugs and those that are more commonly used clinically are described later. Drugs that are less commonly used are summarized in Table 36.4.

Table 36.4 Selected Therapeutic Properties of Miscellaneous Anticancer Agents

Anticancer Agent	Mechanism	Indication	Administration Route	Metabolism/ Metabolizing Enzymes	Boxed Warning
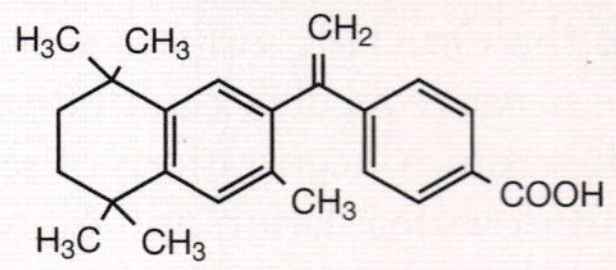 Bexarotene (Targretin)	Retinoid X receptor agonist	Cutaneous T-cell lymphoma	po, topical	3A4, glucuronidation	Teratogenic
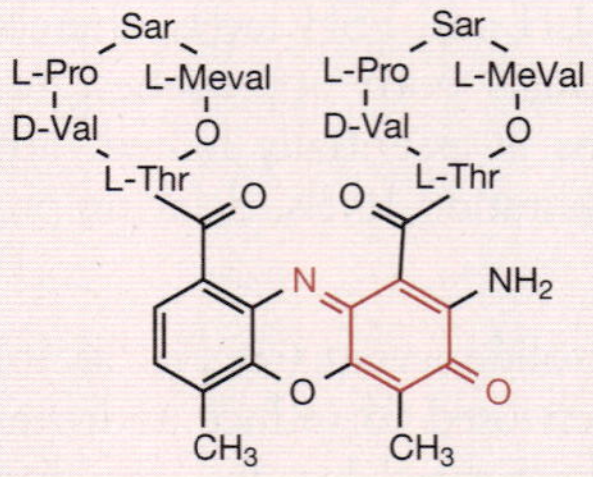 Dactinomycin (Cosmegen)	DNA intercalation	Ewing sarcoma, Wilms tumor, childhood rhabdosarcoma, testicular cancer	IV	Negligible metabolism	Teratogenic, mutagenic, carcinogenic, corrosive
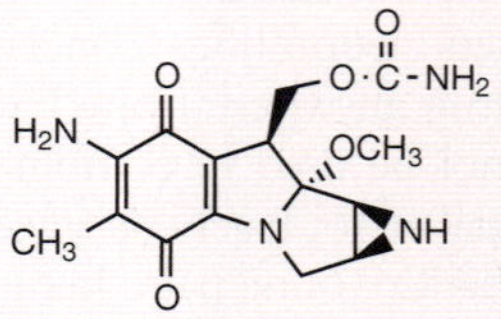 Mitomycin (Mutamycin)	DNA alkylation	Gastric cancer, pancreatic cancer	IV	NQO1 reductase, NADPH/CYP450 reductase	Myelotoxicity, hemolytic uremic syndrome
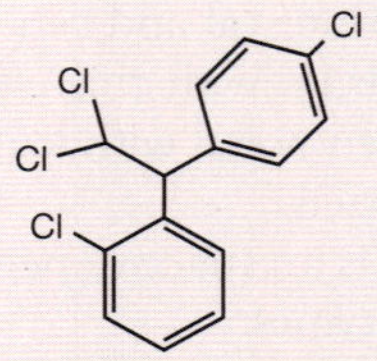 Mitotane (Lysodren)	Adrenolytic	Adrenocortical carcinoma	po	Unknown	Adrenal crisis
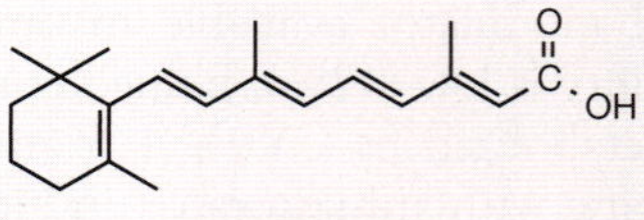 Tretinoin (all-*trans*-Retinoic acid)	APL proliferation inhibitor and differentiation inducer	Remission induction	po	CYP	Teratogenic, leukocytosis, retinoic acid-differentiation syndrome

APL, acute promyelocytic leukemia; IV, intravenous; po, oral.

Specific Drugs

Arsenic Trioxide. The toxic effects of arsenic, a name derived from the Greek word for "potent," have been recognized for millennia.[344,345] Arsenic trioxide (As_2O_3, the "King of Poisons")[346] is an odorless and tasteless toxin well known in ancient Chinese medicine. It was originally introduced into Western medicine in the late 19th century for the treatment of leukemia, subsequently falling out of favor as newer chemotherapeutic and radiation-based approaches to care became available. The drug experienced a pharmacotherapeutic renaissance in the late 20th century, and it is currently used IV to induce remission in patients with acute promyelocytic leukemia (APL).[345,346] APL is characterized by the reciprocal translocation of chromosomes 15 and 17, resulting in the abnormal joining of the promyelocytic gene (PML) and retinoic acid receptor α (RARα) gene which produces a PML-RARα fusion protein.[347] This, in turn, results in the generation of immature leukemia cells, differentiation arrest, and the induction of serious/fatal hemorrhagic and other coagulation-related disorders. As_2O_3 induces remission in patients with APL through the destruction of the offending fusion protein, promotion of promyelocyte differentiation, and stimulation of apoptosis in malignant cells. One documented chemical apoptotic mechanism is the inhibition of intracellular catalase and glutathione peroxidase, with the resultant accumulation of the free radical precursor H_2O_2. Another is the downregulation of the antiapoptotic protein Bcl-2.[344]

The pentavalent As(V) in the parent drug is rapidly reduced to the active trivalent As(III) by arsenate reductase. Along with oncogenic, antiangiogenesis, and cytokine signaling pathway mechanisms yet to be fully elucidated, As(III) is known to generate ROS in mitochondria that damage DNA and stimulate apoptosis.[345] Prior to urinary excretion, As(III) is methylated to mono- and dimethylarsinic acid. Although As_2O_3 is usually well tolerated, the possibility of QT-interval prolongation, torsades de pointes, and complete atrioventricular block demands an assessment of serum electrolytes (particularly magnesium and potassium) prior to the initiation of therapy. APL differentiation syndrome (also known as retinoic acid syndrome and characterized by pleural/pericardial/pulmonary infiltrates or effusions, dyspnea, weight gain, and fatigue) responds to corticosteroid intervention. Reversible hepatotoxicity has also been noted, and the strong emetogenic potential of As_2O_3 warrants coadministration of drugs to control nausea and vomiting. A remarkable feature of As_2O_3 is its freedom from causing bone marrow suppression.[348]

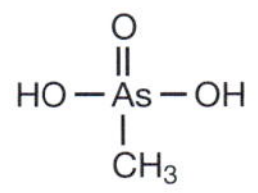

Monomethylarsonic acid

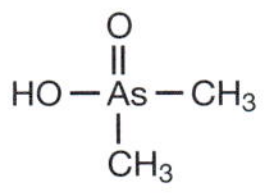

Dimethylarsonic acid

The rapid clearance of As(III) and its methylated metabolites from the blood precludes As_2O_3 use in solid tumors, although studies in multiple solid tumor cell lines document efficacy. Strategies to harness the power of this ancient toxin in treating solid malignancies without increasing the dose to intolerable levels have included combination therapy with GSH-depleting agents and encapsulation in nanoparticles, liposomes, and polymersomes.[345,346] Clinical trials are ongoing and preliminary findings are encouraging.

A review of the evolution of arsenic as the agent of choice for medieval "professional poisoners" during the renaissance to a valued antineoplastic used to prolong life is well worth the read for pharmacy professionals and history enthusiasts alike.[345]

Bleomycin Sulfate. The commercially available bleomycin drug product is a mixture of naturally occurring glycopeptides, predominantly bleomycin A_2. Through DNA intercalation in guanine-rich regions, the aromatic bithiazole ring system (in partnership with the pyrimidine ring on the opposite side of the structure) positions bleomycin for DNA destruction via cytotoxic free radicals.[349] The disaccharide, polyamine, imidazole, and pyrimidine structures are very electron rich and readily chelate intracellular Fe^{2+}. Once chelated, Fe^{2+} is oxidized to Fe^{3+} with a concomitant reduction of bound oxygen and the release of the highly reactive and cytotoxic hydroxyl radical (Fig. 36.47). The ferric hydroperoxide bleomycin complex is considered the cytotoxic form responsible for both single- and double-stranded DNA breaks.[350] Through the direct abstraction of a hydrogen atom from 4′ of a deoxyribose, a free radical is generated that subsequently decomposes to a DNA-destroying 4′-hydroperoxide. A highly electrophilic pyrimidine base propenal that inactivates essential cellular proteins via Cys alkylation is also produced. Reduced GSH is proposed to serve a protective role by acting as propenal

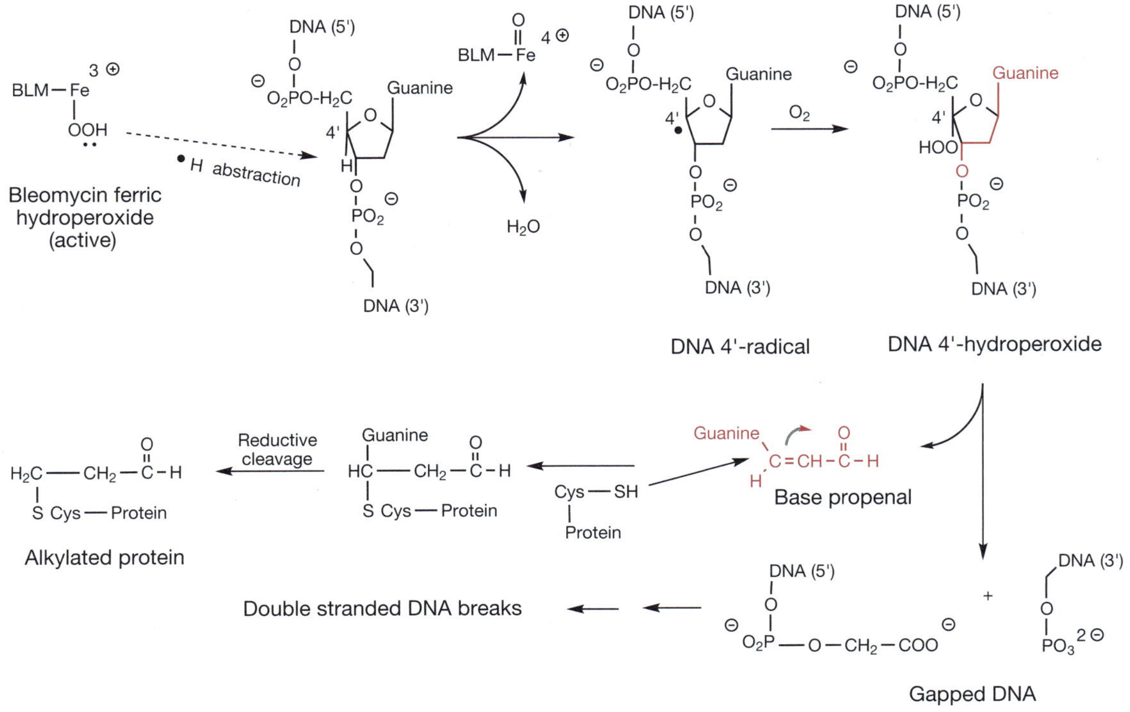

Figure 36.47 Mechanism of bleomycin-induced damage of DNA and proteins.

scavenger and, until depleted, saves cellular proteins from alkylation.[349,351] A review of the multifaceted mechanisms of bleomycin-induced DNA/chromosomal damage and damage repair has been published.[352]

Bleomycin is a natural product isolated from *Streptomyces verticillus*. It is naturally chelated with Cu^{2+}, which must be removed via catalytic reduction before marketing. This increases the cost of the drug but is essential to the liberation of critical bleomycin functional groups for chelation with intracellular Fe^{2+}.

The action of bleomycin is terminated through the action of bleomycin hydrolase, a cytosolic aminopeptidase that cleaves the terminal amide moiety to form the inactive carboxylate metabolite (Fig. 36.48). The metabolic conversion of the electron-withdrawing amide to an electron-donating carboxylate increases the pK_a of the α-amino group, greatly enhances its ionization, and removes its interaction with DNA in its unionized form. After hydrolysis, the ratio of ionized to unionized amine increases approximately 126-fold, destroying DNA affinity and leading to the loss of therapeutic action. Drug destruction via the bleomycin hydrolase pathway is rapid, and tumors will be resistant to bleomycin if they contain high concentrations of the enzyme. Conversely, tumors that are poor in bleomycin hydrolase (eg, squamous cell carcinoma) respond well to this agent.

Bleomycin hydrolase is found in all tissues except the skin and lungs. Approximately 10% of patients who are administered bleomycin will experience potentially fatal pulmonary fibrosis, which can occur during therapy or several months following termination of therapy, often without warning. The copper-complexing agent, tetrathiomolybdate, may reduce the risk of bleomycin-induced fibrosis by inhibiting the action of copper-dependent inflammatory cytokines.[353]

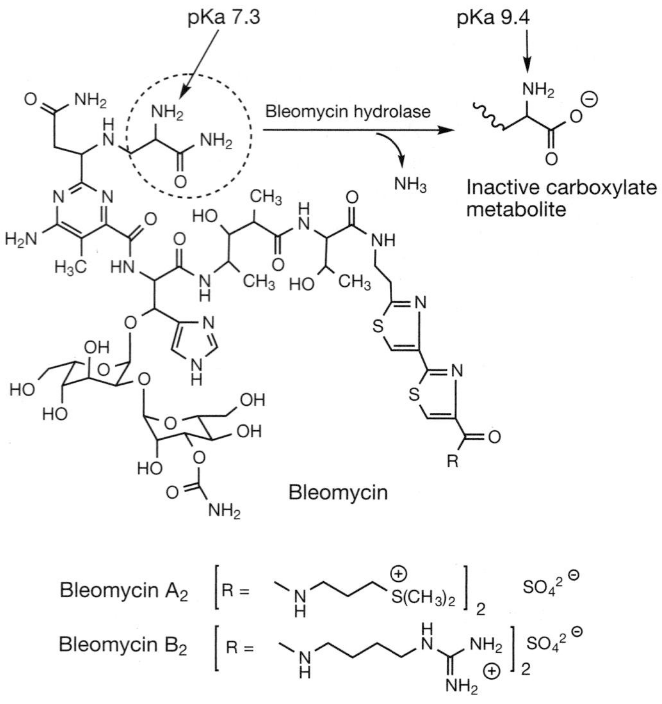

Figure 36.48 Bleomycin hydrolase–mediated inactivation of bleomycin.

Inhibitors of the N-terminal catalytic site of angiotensin-converting enzyme (eg, N-acetyl-Ser-Asp-Lys-Pro or AcSDKP) have also shown a protective effect.[354] Erythema and hyperpigmentation are common cutaneous adverse effects of bleomycin therapy.

Bleomycin is used IV in the palliative treatment of squamous cell head and neck cancers, testicular and other genital carcinomas, and Hodgkin lymphoma. It is excreted via the kidneys, and serum concentrations of active drugs are increased in patients with renal disease. The elimination half-life can rise from 2 to 4 hours to more than 20 hours in renal failure, resulting in significant toxicity, especially pulmonary toxicity. Dosage adjustments are warranted. Unlike many antineoplastic agents, bleomycin does not suppress the bone marrow,[352] and it is often given in combination with compounds that do so that the dose of all drugs can be optimized. Nausea and vomiting are also relatively mild, but approximately 1% of patients with lymphoma who are treated with bleomycin will experience an immediate or delayed severe idiosyncratic reaction that mimics anaphylaxis.

TRABECTEDIN. Trabectedin, a tri-tetrahydroisoquinoline-containing alkaloid derived from the marine tunicate *Ecteinascidia turbinata* (Fig. 36.49), is indicated in unresectable, metastatic, refractory STS (liposarcoma and leiomyosarcoma; the "L-sarcomas"). Treatment of this rare cancer is challenged by more than 50 to 60 histologic subtypes that exist, and prognosis after first-line chemotherapy with doxorubicin (alone or with ifosfamide) is dismal.[355,356] The availability in 2015 of this naturally occurring chemotherapy, which has demonstrated value in anthracycline- and nitrogen mustard-resistant tumors, provided a new option to patients who previously had very few. It is proposed to act by several mechanisms, including the alkylation of guanine N^2 within a CGG-rich region of the minor groove. This binding leads to DNA double-strand cleavage and, through simultaneous interaction with nearby proteins, RNA polymerase II degradation, and transcription inhibition via a NER-dependent process. The cell cycle is arrested in the G2-M phase and apoptosis results. Trabectedin also interferes with oncogenic transcription factor FUS-CHOP function in liposarcomas, which promotes normalizing adipocyte differentiation. Of prime importance to its mechanism is the attenuation of inflammation and angiogenesis through selective interference with monocytes and macrophages within the tumor microenvironment.[355-357]

Trabectedin is administered via 24-hour continuous IV infusion through a central venous catheter in a usual dose of 1.5 mg/m^2. While efficacy is slightly superior in patients with L-sarcoma versus unselected disease, use in all STS subtypes is feasible, particularly if tumor burden is manageable and disease stabilization with a positive quality of life is the objective.[357] Combination therapy with doxorubicin may provide a response advantage and is being explored.[356]

Trabectedin is 94% to 98% protein bound, rapidly converted to many metabolites (Fig. 36.49), and eliminated in feces.[358] The terminal half-life is long at approximately 7.5 days. As multiple CYP isoforms (including 3A4) are presumed to be involved in the complex metabolic pathway of

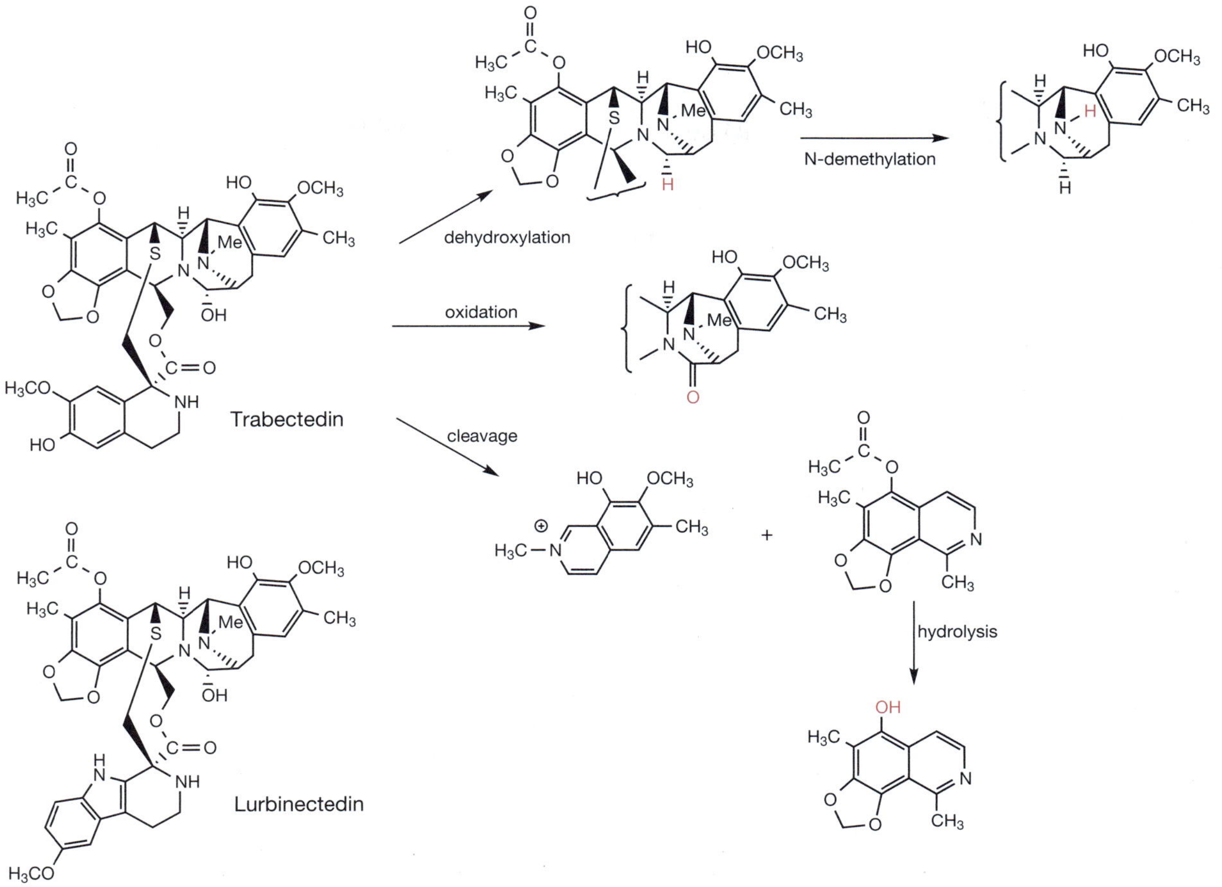

Figure 36.49 Proposed trabectedin metabolism and lurbinectedin.

trabectedin, coadministration with CYP inhibitors or enhancers should be undertaken with caution.[358] The most commonly observed adverse effects are myelosuppression (neutropenia, thrombocytopenia), GI distress, and hepatic enzyme elevation.[356]

LURBINECTEDIN.[43,359] Lurbinectedin (Fig 36.49) has the same pentacyclic structure as trabectedin but with a tetrahydro-β-carboline replacing tetrahydroisoquinoline as the additional ring. It mimics trabectedin in its antineoplastic activity and is currently approved for metastatic SCLC when the disease has progressed after organoplatinum therapy.

Lurbinectedin is administered IV in a 3.2 mg/m^2 dose once every 21 days until disease progression or drug intolerability. It is primarily metabolized by CYP3A4, and caution is warranted if concomitant therapy with CYP3A4 inhibitors or inducers is needed. It is 99% bound to both albumin and α-1-glycoprotein and excreted mostly through feces with an elimination half-life of 15 hours. Adverse effects of significance include bone marrow suppression and GI and hepatic toxicity.

ASPARAGINASE. Asparaginase is an essential component of the chemotherapy regimen for ALL and lymphoblastic lymphoma (LBL). Many leukemic and lymphoblastic cells rely on an exogenous supply of L-asparagine for protein synthesis because they lack L-asparagine synthetase. Reducing plasma asparagine levels by the enzyme L-asparaginase depletes cells of the exogenous asparaginase and signals cells into apoptosis.[360] The tetrameric L-asparaginase has four active sites, each located as two adjacent subunits. Threonine in the active site conducts a nucleophilic attack on the electrophilic carbonyl carbon of the asparagine amide side chain, releasing the amide NH_2 as ammonia. Subsequent hydrolysis of the enzyme-substrate ester bond generates the carboxylate side chain of aspartate (Fig. 36.50).[361]

Currently, three L-asparaginase formulations are available: One is the short-acting recombinant *Erwinia chrysanthemi* asparaginase (half-life 15 hours), and the other two

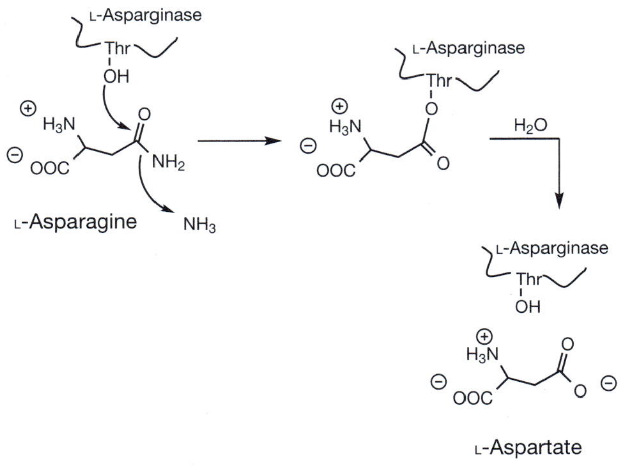

Figure 36.50 Conversion of L-asparagine to L-aspartate by L-asparaginase.

are long-acting pegylated asparaginases (pegaspargase and calaspargase, half-life 5-12 days and 13-17 days, respectively). The half-life of L-asparaginase in all formulations decreases with production of anti-asparaginase antibodies. Hypersensitive reactions ranging from transient erythema to anaphylaxis can occur. Pancreatitis, hemorrhage, and hepatotoxicity are other adverse effects. The recombinant formulation is administered IM, while the pegylated formulation may be administered IM or IV. Asparaginase administration before or concurrent with other cytotoxic drugs may decrease cell replication and diminish the desired cytotoxic outcome.

Structure Challenge

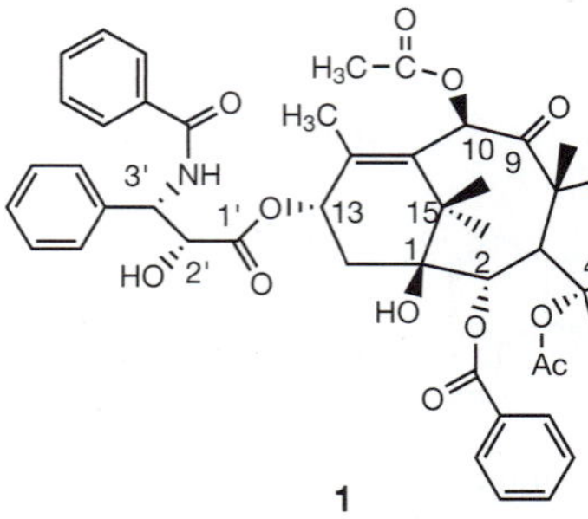

1

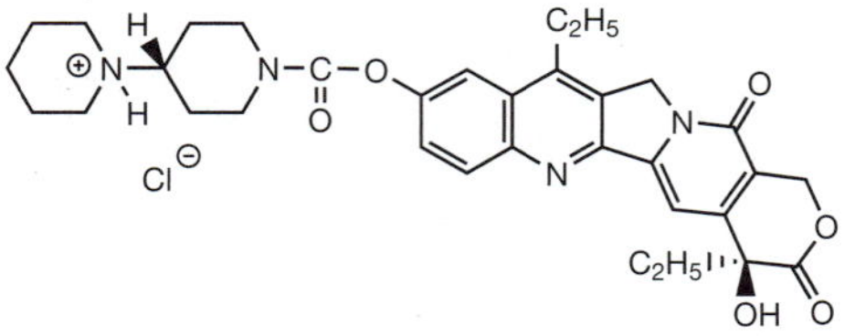

2

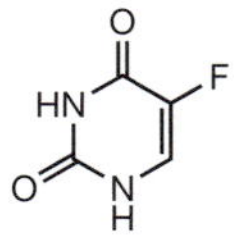

3

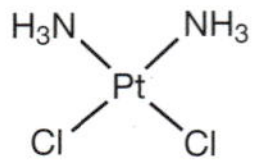

4

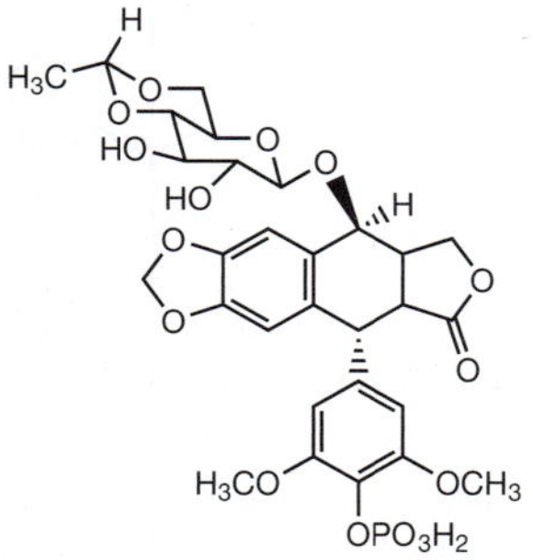

5

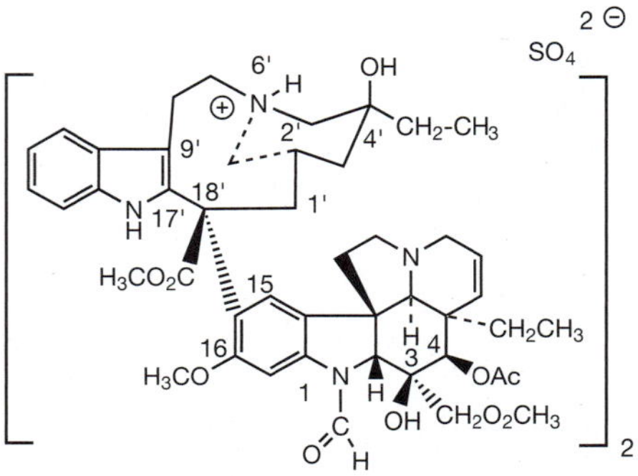

6

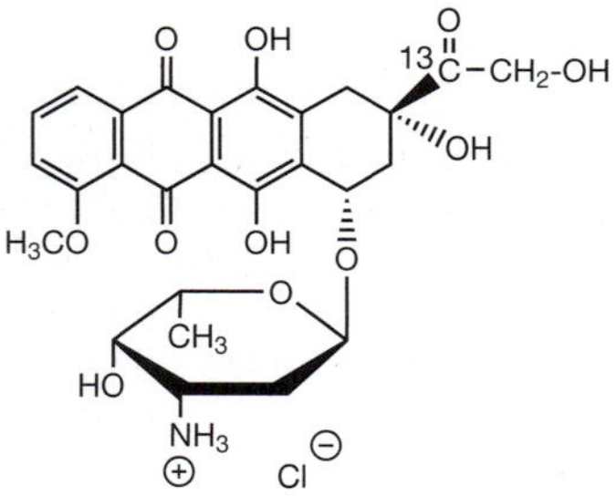

7

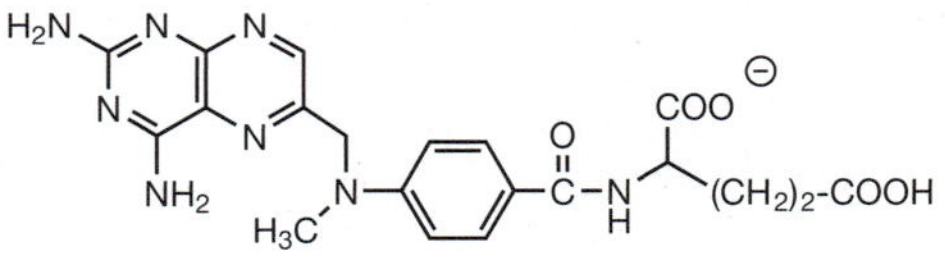

8

Classical chemotherapeutic drugs act via a multitude of chemically complex mechanisms, and agents within a mechanistic class commonly have rationally designed structural differences that permit optimization of therapy for individual patients. Using your knowledge of cytotoxic mechanisms and structure activity relationships (SARs), evaluate the structures of the eight commonly utilized antineoplastic drugs and answer the questions that follow.

1. Identify all antineoplastic drugs that act by each of the mechanisms listed.
   a. Prevents the hyperdynamic changes in microtubules
   b. Inhibits nucleotide biosynthesis enzymes by masquerading as an endogenous substrate
   c. Interferes with topoisomerase activity
   d. Crosslinks DNA
2. What structural feature of antineoplastic drug 2 makes it water soluble? What is the active form of the drug, and how is it generated?

3. What physicochemical property and structural feature of antineoplastic drug 1 makes it necessary to use Kolliphor EL for drug solubilization? What is a therapeutic challenge associated with this vehicle?
4. For antineoplastic drug structure 7, match the structural features (a-c) to the drug effect (1-3).

a. Conjugated double bonds	1. Delayed and chronic cardiotoxicity
b. *p*-Quinone structure	2. Red-colored urine
c. Reduction at C_{13}	3. Acute cardiotoxicity

5. What is the role of the phosphate in antineoplastic drug structure 5?
   a. It acts as a substrate for kinases.
   b. It makes the drug water soluble.
   c. It maintains the stereochemistry of the drug.
   d. It prevents rapid hydrolysis of the drug.
6. What is the common chemical name of leucovorin? Which two antineoplastic drugs benefit from leucovorin administration, and what is its function in each case?
7. Explain the structural change that traps antineoplastic drug 8 inside the tumor cell.
8. Which of the antineoplastic drugs undergo lactone hydrolysis? How does the activity of the metabolite compare to that of the parent drug?
9. What reactive species is generated from antineoplastic drug 4, and how does it produce a cytotoxic effect?

Structure Challenge answers found immediately after References.

REFERENCES

1. Begley M. How to stop the fear of cancer in its tracks. Updated 2019. Accessed October 25, 2023. https://www.mskcc.org/news/how-stop-fear-cancer-its-tracks
2. Siegel RL, Miller KD, Wagle NS, et al. Cancer statistics, 2023. *CA Cancer J Clin.* 2023;73:17-48.
3. Cronin KA, Scott S, Firth AU, et al. Annual report to the nation on the status of cancer, part 1: National cancer statistics. *Cancer.* 2022;128:4251-4284.
4. Siegel RL, Giaquinto AN, Jemal A. Cancer statistics, 2024. *CA Cancer J Clin.* 2024;74:12-49.
5. Giaquinto AN, Miller KD, Tossas KY, et al. Cancer statistics for African American/black people 2022. *CA Cancer J Clin.* 2022;72:202-229.
6. Garner WB, Smith BD, Ludmir EB, et al. Predicting future cancer incidence by age, race, ethnicity, and sex. *J Geriatr Oncol.* 2023;14:101393.
7. National Cancer Institute. Cancer statistics. Updated 2020. Accessed October 25, 2023. https://www.cancer.gov/about-cancer/understanding/statistics
8. Yabroff KR, Mariotto A, Tangka F, et al. Annual report to the nation on the status of cancer, part 2: patient economic burden associated with cancer care. *J Natl Cancer Inst.* 2021;113:1670-1682.
9. Singleterry J. The cost of cancer-addressing patient costs. American Chemical Society cancer action network web site. Accessed October 25, 2023. https://www.fightcancer.org/sites/default/files/Costs%20of%20Cancer%20-%20Final%20Web.pdf
10. Kontomanolis EN, Koutras A, Syllaios A, et al. Role of oncogenes and tumor-suppressor genes in carcinogenesis: a review. *Anticancer Res.* 2020;40:6009-6015.
11. Cordes LM, Cuellar S. Cancer: the disease and treatment. In: DiPiro JT, Yee GC, Haines ST, et al, eds. *DiPiro's Pharmacotherapy: A Pathophysiologic Approach.* 12th ed. McGraw Hill; 2023.
12. Belpomme D, Irigaray P, Hardell L, et al. The multitude and diversity of environmental carcinogens. *Environ Res.* 2007;105:414-429.
13. Masood I, Kiani MH, Ahmad M, et al. Major contributions towards finding a cure for cancer through chemotherapy: a historical review. *Tumori.* 2016;102:6-17.
14. Burchenal JH. The historical development of cancer chemotherapy. *Semin Oncol.* 1977;4:135-146.
15. Rosenberg B, Van Camp L, Krigas T. Inhibition of cell division in *Escherichia coli* by electrolysis products from a platinum electrode. *Nature.* 1965;205:698-699.
16. Johnson LN. Protein kinase inhibitors: contributions from structure to clinical compounds. *Q Rev Biophys.* 2009;42:1-40.
17. Druker BJ, Talpaz M, Resta DJ, et al. Efficacy and safety of a specific inhibitor of the BCR-ABL tyrosine kinase in chronic myeloid leukemia. *N Engl J Med.* 2001;344:1031-1037.
18. Makin G. Principles of chemotherapy. *Paediatr Child Health.* 2018;28:183-188.
19. Ricevuto E, Bruera G, Marchetti P. General principles of chemotherapy. *Eur Rev Med Pharmacol Sci.* 2010;14:269-271.
20. Kaur S, Mayanglambam P, Bajwan D, et al. Chemotherapy and its adverse effects—a systematic review. *Int J Nur Edu Res.* 2022;10:399-402.
21. Brianna, Lee SH. Chemotherapy: how to reduce its adverse effects while maintaining the potency? *Med Oncol.* 2023;40:88.
22. Nikolaou M, Pavlopoulou A, Georgakilas AG, et al. The challenge of drug resistance in cancer treatment: a current overview. *Clin Exp Metastasis.* 2018;35:309-318.
23. Yuan R, Hou Y, Sun W, et al. Natural products to prevent drug resistance in cancer chemotherapy: a review. *Ann N Y Acad Sci.* 2017;1401:19-27.
24. Kumar A, Jaitak V. Natural products as multidrug resistance modulators in cancer. *Eur J Med Chem.* 2019;176:268-291.
25. Buzun K, Bielawska A, Bielawski K, et al. DNA topoisomerases as molecular targets for anticancer drugs. *J Enzyme Inhib Med Chem.* 2020;35:1781-1799.
26. Pommier Y, Nussenzweig A, Takeda S, et al. Human topoisomerases and their roles in genome stability and organization. *Nat Rev Mol Cell Biol.* 2022;23:407-427.
27. Mastrangelo S, Attina G, Triarico S, et al. The DNA-topoisomerase inhibitors in cancer therapy. *Biomed Pharmacol J.* 2022;15:553-562.
28. Marinello J, Delcuratolo M, Capranico G. Anthracyclines as topoisomerase II poisons: from early studies to new perspectives. *Int J Mol Sci.* 2018;19:3480.
29. Ketron AC, Osheroff N. Phytochemicals as anticancer and chemopreventive topoisomerase II poisons. *Phytochem Rev.* 2014;13:19-35.
30. Mancini G, D'Annessa I, Coletta A, et al. Structural and dynamical effects induced by the anticancer drug topotecan on the human topoisomerase I–DNA complex. *PLoS One.* 2010;5:e10934.
31. Staker BL, Hjerrild K, Feese MD, et al. The mechanism of topoisomerase I poisoning by a camptothecin analog. *Proc Natl Acad Sci U S A.* 2002;99:15387-15392.
32. Li F, Jiang T, Li Q, et al. Camptothecin (CPT) and its derivatives are known to target topoisomerase I (Top1) as their mechanism of action: did we miss something in CPT analogue molecular targets for treating human disease such as cancer? *Am J Cancer Res.* 2017;7:2350.

33. Staker BL, Feese MD, Cushman M, et al. Structures of three classes of anticancer agents bound to the human topoisomerase I—DNA covalent complex. *J Med Chem.* 2005;48:2336-2345.
34. Liu Y, Li W, Morris-Natschke SL, et al. Perspectives on biologically active camptothecin derivatives. *Med Res Rev.* 2015;35:753-789.
35. Liu W, Zhu L, Guo W, et al. Synthesis and biological evaluation of novel 7-acyl homocamptothecins as Topoisomerase I inhibitors. *Eur J Med Chem.* 2011;46:2408-2414.
36. Mei C, Lei L, Tan L, et al. The role of single strand break repair pathways in cellular responses to camptothecin induced DNA damage. *Biomed Pharmacother.* 2020;125:109875.
37. Ando K, Shah AK, Sachdev V, et al. Camptothecin resistance is determined by the regulation of topoisomerase I degradation mediated by ubiquitin proteasome pathway. *Oncotarget.* 2017;8:43733-43751.
38. Kirschbaum M. A comeback for camptothecins? *Leuk Lymphoma.* 2009;50:1914-1915.
39. Xu C, Barchet TM, Mager DE. Quantitative structure-property relationships of camptothecins in humans. *Cancer Chemother Pharmacol.* 2009;65:325-333.
40. Wang X, Zhuang Y, Wang Y, et al. The recent developments of camptothecin and its derivatives as potential anti-tumor agents. *Eur J Med Chem.* 2023;260:115710.
41. Fujita K, Kubota Y, Ishida H, et al. Irinotecan, a key chemotherapeutic drug for metastatic colorectal cancer. *World J Gastroenterol.* 2015;21:12234-12248.
42. de Man FM, Goey AK, van Schaik RH, et al. Individualization of irinotecan treatment: a review of pharmacokinetics, pharmacodynamics, and pharmacogenetics. *Clin Pharmacokinet.* 2018;57: 1229-1254.
43. Facts & Comparisons eAnswers [database online].
44. Takano M, Sugiyama T. UGT1A1 polymorphisms in cancer: impact on irinotecan treatment. *Pharmacogenomics Pers Med.* 2017;10: 61-68.
45. Karas S, Innocenti F. All you need to know about UGT1A1 genetic testing for patients treated with irinotecan: a practitioner-friendly guide. *JCO Oncol Pract.* 2022;18:270-277.
46. Lamb YN, Scott LJ. Liposomal irinotecan: a review in metastatic pancreatic adenocarcinoma. *Drugs.* 2017;77:785-792.
47. Nevala-Plagemann C, Garrido-Laguna I. NALIRIFOX for metastatic pancreatic adenocarcinoma: hope or hype? *Nat Rev Clin Oncol.* 2024;21:1567-568.
48. Seligson JM, Patron AM, Berger MJ, et al. Sacituzumab govitecan-hziy: an antibody-drug conjugate for the treatment of refractory, metastatic, triple-negative breast cancer. *Ann Pharmacother.* 2021;55:921-931.
49. Hycamtin (topotecan) for injection. Updated 2015. https://www.novartis.com/us-en/sites/novartis_us/files/hycamtin_inj.pdf
50. Devriese LA, Witteveen PE, Mergui-Roelvink M, et al. Pharmacodynamics and pharmacokinetics of oral topotecan in patients with advanced solid tumours and impaired renal function. *Br J Clin Pharmacol.* 2015;80:253-266.
51. Saraf S, Jain A, Hurkat P, et al. Topotecan liposomes: a visit from a molecular to a therapeutic platform. *Crit Rev Ther Drug Syst.* 2016;33:401-432.
52. Jain A, Jain SK. Multipronged, strategic delivery of paclitaxel-topotecan using engineered liposomes to ovarian cancer. *Drug Dev Ind Pharm.* 2016;42:136-149.
53. Padhi S, Kapoor R, Verma D, et al. Formulation and optimization of topotecan nanoparticles: in vitro characterization, cytotoxicity, cellular uptake and pharmacokinetic outcomes. *J Photochem Photobiol B.* 2018;183:222-232.
54. Alshammari MK, Alghazwni MK, Alharbi AS, et al. Nanoplatform for the delivery of topotecan in the cancer milieu: an appraisal of its therapeutic efficacy. *Cancers.* 2022;15:65.
55. Meresse P, Dechaux E, Monneret C, et al. Etoposide: discovery and medicinal chemistry. *Curr Med Chem.* 2004;11:2443-2466.
56. Vilain N, Tsai-Pflugfelder M, Benoit A, et al. Modulation of drug sensitivity in yeast cells by the ATP-binding domain of human DNA topoisomerase IIalpha. *Nucleic Acids Res.* 2003;31:5714-5722.
57. Chee GL, Yalowich JC, Bodner A, et al. A diazirine-based photoaffinity etoposide probe for labeling topoisomerase II. *Bioorg Med Chem.* 2010;18:830-838.
58. Naik PK, Dubey A, Soni K, et al. The binding modes and binding affinities of epipodophyllotoxin derivatives with human topoisomerase IIα. *J Mol Graph Model.* 2010;29:546-564.
59. Yadav AA, Chee G, Wu X, et al. Structure-based design, synthesis, and biological testing of piperazine-linked *bis*-epipodophyllotoxin etoposide analogs. *Bioorg Med Chem.* 2015;23:3542-3551.
60. Zhang W, Gou P, Dupret J, et al. Etoposide, an anticancer drug involved in therapy-related secondary leukemia: enzymes at play. *Transl Oncol.* 2021;14:101169.
61. Mans D, Lafleur M, Westmijze IR, et al. Reactions of glutathione with the catechol, the ortho quinone, and the semi-quinone free radical of etoposide. Consequences for DNA inactivation. *Biochem Pharmacol.* 1992;43:1761-1768.
62. Felix CA. Secondary leukemias induced by topoisomerase-targeted drugs. *Biochim Biophys Acta.* 1998;1400:233-255.
63. Pommier Y, Leo E, Zhang HL, et al. DNA topoisomerases and their poisoning by anticancer and antibacterial drugs. *Chem Biol Rev.* 2010;17:421-433.
64. Gerwirtz DA. A critical evaluation of the mechanisms of action proposed for the antitumor effects of the anthracycline antibiotics adriamycin and daunorubicin. *Biochem Pharmacol.* 1999;57:727-741.
65. Dal Ben D, Palumbo M, Zagotto G, et al. DNA topoisomerase II structures and anthracycline activity: insights into ternary complex formation. *Curr Pharm Des.* 2007;13:2766-2780.
66. Martins-Teixeira MB, Carvalho I. Antitumour anthracyclines: progress and perspectives. *ChemMedChem.* 2020;15:933-948.
67. Zunino F, Pratesi G, Perego P. Role of the sugar moiety in the pharmacological activity of anthracyclines: development of a novel series of disaccharide analogs. *Biochem Pharmacol.* 2001;61: 933-938.
68. Chien AJ, Moasser MM. Cellular mechanisms of resistance against taxanes and anthracyclines in cancer: intrinsic and acquired. *Semin Oncol.* 2008;35(suppl 2):S1-S14.
69. Shandilya M, Sharma S, Das PP, et al. Molecular-level understanding of the anticancer action mechanism of anthracyclines. In: Arnouk H, Hassan B, eds. *Advances in Precision Medicine Oncology.* IntechOpen; 2020:11-21.
70. Capelôa T, Benyahia Z, Zampieri LX, et al. Metabolic and non-metabolic pathways that control cancer resistance to anthracyclines. *Semin Cell Dev Biol.* 2020;98:181-191.
71. Penning TM, Jonnalagadda S, Trippier PC, et al. Aldo-keto reductases and cancer drug resistance. *Pharmacol Rev.* 2021;73:1150-1171.
72. Piska K, Koczurkiewicz P, Bucki A, et al. Metabolic carbonyl reduction of anthracyclines - role in cardiotoxicity and cancer resistance. Reducing enzymes as putative targets for novel cardioprotective and chemosensitizing agents. *Invest New Drugs.* 2017;35:375-385.
73. Mei Y, Qian F, Wei M, et al. Reversal of cancer by green tea polyphenols. *J Pharm Pharmacol.* 2004;56:1307-1314.
74. Sadzuka Y, Sugiyama T, Sonobe T. Efficacies of tea components on doxorubicin induced antitumor activity and reversal of multidrug resistance. *Toxicol Lett.* 2000;114:155-162.
75. Stammler G, Volm M. Green tea catechins (EGCG and EGC) have modulating effects on the activity of doxorubicin in drug resistant cell lines. *Anticancer Drugs.* 1997;8:265-268.
76. Fabbri R, Macciocca M, Vicenti R, et al. Epigallocatechin-3-gallate inhibits doxorubicin-induced inflammation on human ovarian tissue. *Biosci Rep.* 2019;39:BSR20181424.
77. Yao Y, Liu X, Li W, et al. (−)-Epigallocatechin-3-gallate alleviates doxorubicin-induced cardiotoxicity in sarcoma 180 tumor-bearing mice. *Life Sci.* 2017;180:151-159.
78. Ferrera A, Fiorentini V, Reale S, et al. Anthracyclines-induced cardiac dysfunction: what every clinician should know. *Rev Cardiovasc Med.* 2023;24:148.
79. Huang J, Wu R, Chen L, et al. Understanding anthracycline cardiotoxicity from mitochondrial aspect. *Front Pharmacol.* 2022;13:811406.

80. Narezkina A, Narayan HK, Zemljic-Harpf AE. Molecular mechanisms of anthracycline cardiovascular toxicity. *Clin Sci.* 2021;135:1311-1332.
81. Sawicki KT, Sala V, Prever L, et al. Preventing and treating anthracycline cardiotoxicity: new insights. *Annu Rev Pharmacol Toxicol.* 2021;61:309-332.
82. Malisza KL, Hasinhoff BB. Production of hydroxyl radical by iron(III)—anthraquinone complexes through self-reduction and through reductive activation by the xanthine oxidase/hypoxanthine system. *Arch Biochem Biophys.* 1995;1:51-60.
83. Hasinhoff BB, Wu X, Patel D, et al. Mechanisms of action and reduced cardiotoxicity of pixantrone: a topoisomerase II targeting agents with cellular selectivity for the topoisomerase IIa isoform. *J Pharmacol Exp Ther.* 2016;356:397-409.
84. Mordente A, Meucci E, Silvestrini GE, et al. New developments in anthracycline-induced cardiotoxicity. *Curr Med Chem.* 2009;16:1656-1672.
85. Lothstein L, Israel M, Sweatman TW. Anthracycline drug targeting: cytoplasmic versus nuclear-a fork in the road. *Drug Res Updates.* 2001;4:169-177.
86. Swain SM, Vici P. The current and future role of dexrazoxane as a cardioprotectant in anthracycline treatment: expert panel review. *J Cancer Res Clin Oncol.* 2004;130:1-7.
87. Malisza KL, Hasinhoff BB. Inhibition of anthracycline semiquinone formation by ICRF-187 (dexrazoxane) in cells. *Free Radic Biol Med.* 1996;20:905-914.
88. Kassner N, Huse K, Martin HJ, et al. Carbonyl reductase 1 is a predominant doxorubicin reductase in human liver. *Drug Metab Dispos.* 2008;36:2113-2120.
89. Yamashita T, Fukushima T, Ueda T. Pharmacokinetic self-potentiation of idarubicin by induction of anthracycline carbonyl reducing enzymes. *Leuk Lymphoma.* 2008;49:809-814.
90. Mele D, Nardozza M, Spallarossa P, et al. Current views on anthracycline cardiotoxicity. *Heart Fail Rev.* 2016;21:621-634.
91. Giesberg CA, Sawyer DB. Mechanisms of anthracycline cardiotoxicity and strategies to decrease cardiac damage. *Curr Hypertens Rep.* 2010;12:404-410.
92. Vejpongsa P, Yeh E. Topoisomerase 2b; a promising molecular target for primary prevention of anthracycline-induced cardiotoxicity. *Clin Pharmacol Ther.* 2014;95:45-52.
93. Vejpongsa P, Yeh E. Prevention of anthracycline-induced cardiotoxicity. *J Am Coll Cardiol.* 2014;64:938-945.
94. Tahover E, Patil YP, Gabizon AA. Emerging delivery systems to reduce doxorubicin cardiotoxicity and improve therapeutic index: focus on liposomes. *Anticancer Drugs.* 2014;26:241-258.
95. Cardinale D, Iacopo F, Cipolla CM. Cardiotoxicity of anthracyclines. *Front Cardiovasc Med.* 2020;7:26.
96. Deng S, Yan T, Jendrny C, et al. Dexrazoxane may prevent doxorubicin-induced DNA damage via depleting both topoisomerase II isoforms. *BMC Cancer.* 2014;14:842.
97. Hasan S, Dinh K, Lombardo F, et al. Doxorubicin cardiotoxicity in African Americans. *J Natl Med Assoc.* 2004;96:196-199.
98. Linschoten M, Teske AJ, Cramer MJ, et al. Chemotherapy-related cardiac dysfunction: a systematic review of genetic variants modulating individual risk. *Circ Genom Precis Med.* 2018;11:e001753.
99. Aminkeng F, Bhavsar AP, Visscher H, et al. A coding variant in RARG confers susceptibility to anthracycline-induced cardiotoxicity in childhood cancer. *Nat Genet.* 2015;47:1079-1084.
100. Lyu YL, Kerrigan JE, Lin CP, et al. Topoisomerase IIbeta mediated DNA double-strand breaks: implications in doxorubicin cardiotoxicity and prevention by dexrazoxane. *Cancer Res.* 2007; 67:8839-8846.
101. Hasinoff BB. The use of dexrazoxane for the prevention of anthracycline extravasation injury. *Expert Opin Invest Drugs.* 2008; 17:217-223.
102. Kalyanaraman B. Teaching the basics of the mechanism of doxorubicin-induced cardiotoxicity: have we been barking up the wrong tree? *Redox Biol.* 2020;29:101394.
103. Varela-López A, Battino M, Navarro-Hortal MD, et al. An update on the mechanisms related to cell death and toxicity of doxorubicin and the protective role of nutrients. *Food Chem Toxicol.* 2019;134:110834.
104. Dempke WCM, Zielinski R, Winkler C, et al. Anthracycline-induced cardiotoxicity—are we about to clear this hurdle? *Eur J Cancer.* 2023;185:94-104.
105. Waterhouse DN, Tardi PG, Mayer LD, et al. A comparison of liposomal formulations of doxorubicin with drug administered in free form: changing toxicity profiles. *Drug Saf.* 2001;24:903-920.
106. Makwana V, Karanjia J, Haselhorst T, et al. Liposomal doxorubicin as targeted delivery platform: current trends in surface functionalization. *Int J Pharm.* 2021;593:120117.
107. Kratz F, Warnecke A, Scheuermann K, et al. Probing the cysteine-34 position of endogenous serum albumin with thiol-binding doxorubicin derivatives. Improved efficacy of an acid-sensitive doxorubicin derivative with specific albumin-binding properties compared to that of the parent compound. *J Med Chem.* 2002;45:5523-5533,
108. Gong J, Yan J, Forscher C, et al. Aldoxorubicin: a tumor-targeted doxorubicin conjugate for relapsed or refractory soft tissue sarcomas. *Drug Des Devel Ther.* 2018;12:777-786.
109. Sachdev E, Sachdev D, Mita M. Aldoxorubicin for the treatment of soft tissue sarcoma. *Expert Opin Invest Drugs.* 2017;26:1175-1179.
110. Seetharam M, Kolla KR, Ganjoo KN. Aldoxorubicin therapy for the treatment of patients with advanced soft tissue sarcoma. *Future Oncol.* 2018;14:2323-2333.
111. Salvatorelli E, Menna P, Lusini M, et al. Doxorubicinolone formation and efflux: a salvage pathway against epirubicin accumulation in human heart. *J Pharmacol Exp Ther.* 2009;329:175-184.
112. Kang W, Weiss M. Caffeine enhances the myocardial uptake of idarubicin but reverses its negative inotropic effect. *Naunyn Schmiedelbergs Arch Pharmacol.* 2003;367:151-155.
113. Sharma P, Zarger-Shoshtari K, Sexton WJ, et al. Valrubicin in refractory non-muscle invasive bladder cancer. *Expert Rev Anticancer Ther.* 2015;15:1379-1389.
114. Grossman HB, O'Donnell MA, Cookson MS, et al. Bacillus Calmette-Guerin failures and beyond: contemporary management of non-muscle invasive bladder cancer. *Rev Urol.* 2008;10:281-289.
115. New treatment options emerging for patients with refractory NMIBC. Accessed November 14, 2023. https://www.auadailynews.org/aua-2022/article/22235971/new-treatment-options-emerging-for-patients-with-refractory-nmibc
116. Reis-Mendes A, Gomes AS, Carvalho RA, et al. Naphthoquinoxaline metabolite of mitoxantrone is less cardiotoxic than the parent compound and it can be a more cardiosafe drug in anticancer therapy. *Arch Toxicol.* 2017;91:1871-1890.
117. Akhmanova A, Steinmetz MO. Control of microtubule organization and dynamics: two ends in the limelight. *Nat Rev Mol Cell Biol.* 2015;16:711-726.
118. Mosca L, Ilari A, Fazi F, et al. Taxanes in cancer treatment: activity, chemoresistance and its overcoming. *Drug Resist Updat.* 2021;54:100742.
119. Dumontet C, Jordan MA. Microtubule-binding agents: a dynamic field of cancer therapeutics. *Nat Rev Drug Discov.* 2010; 9:790-803.
120. Panda D, Miller HP, Islam K, et al. Stabilization of microtubule dynamics by estramustine by binding to a novel site in tubulin: a possible mechanistic basis for its antitumor action. *Proc Natl Acad Sci USA.* 1997;94:10560-10564.
121. Mojsilovic SS, Mojsilovic S, Bjelica S, et al. Estramustine phosphate inhibits TGF-β-induced mouse macrophage migration and urokinase-type plasminogen activator production. *Anal Cell Pathol (Amst).* 2018;2018:3134102.
122. Yue QX, Liu X, Guo DA. Microtubule-binding natural products for cancer therapy. *Planta Med.* 2010;76:1037-1043.
123. Duran GE, Derdau V, Weitz D, et al. Cabazitaxel is more active than first generation taxanes in ABCB1(+) cell lines due to its

reduced affinity for P-glycoprotein. *Cancer Chemother Pharmacol.* 2018;81:1095-1103.
124. Lopus M, Smiyun G, Miller H, et al. Mechanism of action of ixabepilone and its interaction with the bIII-tubulin isotype. *Cancer Chemother Pharmacol.* 2015;76:1013-1024.
125. Maloney SM, Hoover CA, Morejon-Lasso LV, et al. Mechanisms of taxane resistance. *Cancers.* 2020;12:3323.
126. Rodrigues-Ferreira S, Moindjie H, Haykal MM, et al. Predicting and overcoming taxane chemoresistance. *Trends Mol Med.* 2021;27:138-151.
127. Krause W. Resistance to anti-tubulin agents: from vinca alkaloids to epothilones. *Cancer Drug Resist.* 2019;2:82-106.
128. Islam MN, Song Y, Iskander MN. Investigation of structural requirements of anticancer activity at the paclitaxel/tubulin binding site using CoMFA and CoMSIA. *J Mol Graph Model.* 2003;21:263-272.
129. Maccari L, Manetti F, Corelli F, et al. 3D QSAR studies for the β-tubulin binding site of microtubule-stabilizing anticancer agents (MSAAs). A pseudoreceptor model for taxanes based on the experimental structure of tubulin. *Il Farmaco.* 2003;58:659-668.
130. Gueritte F. General and recent aspects of the chemistry and structure activity relationships of taxoids. *Curr Pharm Des.* 2001;7:1229-1249.
131. Manetti F, Forli S, Maccari L, et al. 3D QSAR studies of the interaction between β-tubulin and microtubule stabilizing antimitotic agents (MSAA): a combined pharmacophore generation and pseudoreceptor modeling approach applied to taxanes and epothilones. *Farmaco.* 2003;58:357-361.
132. Manetti F, Maccari L, Corelli F, et al. 3D QSAR models of interactions between β-tubulin and microtubule stabilizing antimitotic agents (MSAA): a survey on taxanes and epothilones. *Curr Topics Med Chem.* 2004;4:203-217.
133. Yang Y, Alcaraz AA, Snyder JP. The tubulin-bound conformation of paclitaxel: T-taxol vs. "PTX-NY". *J Natl Prod.* 2009;72:422-429.
134. Cresteil T, Monsarrat B, DuBois J, et al. Regioselective metabolism of taxoids by human CYP3A4 and 2C8: structure-activity relationship. *Drug Metab Dispos.* 2002;39:438-445.
135. Marcath LA, Kidwell KM, Robinson AC, et al. Patients carrying CYP2C8* 3 have shorter systemic paclitaxel exposure. *Pharmacogenomics.* 2019;20:95-104.
136. Zhang W, Dutschman GE, Li X, et al. Quantitation of paclitaxel and its two major metabolites using a liquid chromatography–electrospray ionization tandem mass spectrometry. *J Chromatogr B.* 2011;879:2018-2022.
137. Yamaguchi H, Fujikawa A, Ito H, et al. Quantitative determination of paclitaxel and its metabolites, 6α-hydroxypaclitaxel and p-3′-hydroxypaclitaxel, in human plasma using column-switching liquid chromatography/tandem mass spectrometry. *Biomed Chromatogr.* 2013;27:539-544.
138. Rosing H, Lustig V, Van Warmerdam L, et al. Pharmacokinetics and metabolism of docetaxel administered as a 1-h intravenous infusion. *Cancer Chemother Pharmacol.* 2000;45:213-218.
139. De Luca A, D'Alessio A, Maiello MR, et al. Evaluation of the pharmacokinetics of ixabepilone for the treatment of breast cancer. *Expert Opin Drug Metab Toxicol.* 2015;11:1177-1185.
140. Altmann K. Epothilone B and its analogs: a new family of anticancer agents. *Mini Rev Med Chem.* 2003;3:149-158.
141. Buey RM, Diaz JF, Andreu JM, et al. Interaction of epothilone analogs with the paclitaxel binding site: relationship between binding affinity, microtubule stabilization, and cytotoxicity. *Chem Biol Rev.* 2004;11:225-236.
142. Hunt JT. Discovery of ixabepilone. *Mol Cancer Ther.* 2009;8:275-281.
143. Heinz DW, Schubert W, Hofle G. Much anticipated—the bioactive conformation of epothilone and its binding to tubulin. *Angew Chem Int Ed.* 2005;44:1298-1301.
144. Navarrete KR, Alderete JB, Jimenez VA. Structural basis for drug resistance conferred by b tubulin mutations: a molecular modeling study on native and mutated tubulin complexes with epothilone B. *J Biomol Struct Dyn.* 2015;33:2530-2540.
145. Wang F, Porter M, Konstantopoulos A, et al. Preclinical development of drug delivery systems for paclitaxel-based cancer chemotherapy. *J Control Release.* 2017;267:100-118.
146. Hait WN, Rubin E, Goodin S. Tubulin-targeting agents. In: Giaconne G, Schilsky R, Sondel P, eds. *Cancer Chemotherapy and Biological Response Modifiers.* Elsevier B.V.; 2003:41-67.
147. Gupta N, Hatoum H, Dy GK. First line treatment of advanced non-small cell lung cancer—specific focus on albumin bound paclitaxel. *Int J Nanomedicine.* 2014;9:209-221.
148. Spada A, Emami J, Tuszynski JA, et al. The uniqueness of albumin as a carrier in nanodrug delivery. *Mol Pharm.* 2021;18:1862-1894.
149. Bernabeu E, Cagel M, Lagomarsino E, et al. Paclitaxel: what has been done and the challenges remain ahead. *Int J Pharm.* 2017;526:474-495.
150. Yan M, Fan X, Si H, et al. Association between gene polymorphism and adverse effects in cancer patients receiving docetaxel treatment: a meta-analysis. *Cancer Chemother Pharmacol.* 2022;89:173-181.
151. Martín M, de la Torre-Montero JC, López-Tarruella S, et al. Persistent major alopecia following adjuvant docetaxel for breast cancer: incidence, characteristics, and prevention with scalp cooling. *Breast Cancer Res Treat.* 2018;171:627-634.
152. Engles FK, Ten-Tije AJ, Baker SD, et al. Effect of cytochrome P450 3A4 inhibition on the pharmacokinetics of docetaxel. *Clin Pharmacol Ther.* 2004;75:448-454.
153. Mita AC, Denis LJ, Rowinsky EK, et al. Phase I and pharmacokinetic study of XRP6258 (RPR 116258A), a novel taxane, administered as a 1-hour infusion every 3 weeks in patients with advanced solid tumors. *Clin Cancer Res.* 2009;15:723-730.
154. Song P, Huang C, Wang Y. The efficacy and safety comparison of docetaxel, cabazitaxel, estramustine, and mitoxantrone for castration-resistant prostate cancer: a network meta-analysis. *Int J Surg.* 2018;56:133-140.
155. Oudard S, Kizazi K, Sengelov L, et al. Cabazitaxel vs. docetaxel as first-line therapy for patients with metastatic castration-resistant prostate cancer: a randomized phase III trial-FIRSTANA. *J Clin Oncol.* 2017;35:3189-3197.
156. Eisenberger M, Hardy-Bessard AC, Kim CS, et al. Phase III study comparing a reduced dose of cabazitaxel (20 mg/m^2) and the currently approved dose (25 mg/m^2) in postdocetaxel patients with metastatic castration-resistant prostate cancer-PROSELICA. *J Clin Oncol.* 2017;35:3198-3206.
157. Donovan D, Vahdat LT. Epothilones: clinical update and future directions. *Oncology.* 2008;22:408-416.
158. Li J, Ren J, Sun W. Systematic review of ixabepilone for treating metastatic breast cancer. *Breast Cancer.* 2017;24:171-179.
159. Pellegrini F, Budman DR. Review: tubulin function, actions of antitubulin drugs, and new drug development. *Cancer Invest.* 2005;23:264-273.
160. Gigant B, Wang C, Ravelli R, et al. Structural basis for the regulation of tubulin by vinblastine. *Nature.* 2005;435:519-522.
161. Beck WT, Cass CE, Houghton PJ. Microtubule-targeting anticancer drugs derived from plants and microbes: vinca alkaloids, taxanes and epothiolones. In: Bast RJ, Kufe DW, Pollock RE, et al., eds. *Cancer Medicine.* Vol 5. BC Decker, Inc.; 2003.
162. Islam MN, Iskander MN. Microtubulin binding sites as target for developing anticancer agents. *Mini Rev Med Chem.* 2004;4:1077-1104.
163. Martino E, Casamassima G, Castiglione S, et al. Vinca alkaloids and analogues as anti-cancer agents: looking back, peering ahead. *Bioorg Med Chem Lett.* 2018;28:2816-2826.
164. Hait WN, Yang J. The individualization of cancer therapy: the unexpected role of p53. *Trans Am Clin Climatol Assoc.* 2006;117:85.

165. Chi S, Xie W, Zhang J, et al. Theoretical insight into the structural mechanism for the binding of vinblastine with tubulin. *J Biomol Struct Dyn.* 2015;33:2234-2254.
166. Kelly EB, Tuszynski JA, Klobukowski M. QM and QM/MD simulations of the Vinca alkaloids docked to tubulin. *J Mol Graph Model.* 2011;30:50-66.
167. Chabner BA, Ryan DP, Paz-Ares L, et al. Antineoplastic agents. In: Hardman JG, Limbird LE, eds. *Goodman & Gilman's The Pharmacological Basis of Therapeutics.* 10th ed. McGraw Hill; 2001.
168. Beulz-Riche D, Grude P, Puozzo C, et al. Characterization of human cytochrome P450 isoenzymes involved in the metabolism of vinorelbine. *Fundam Clin Pharmacol.* 2005;19:545-553.
169. Egbelakin A, Ferguson MJ, MacGill EA. Increased risk of vincristine neurotoxicity associated with low CYP3A5 expression genotype in children with acute lymphoblastic leukemia. *Pediatr Blood Cancer.* 2011;56:361-367.
170. Dennison JB, Mohutsky MA, Barbuch RJ, et al. Apparent high CYP3A5 expression is required for significant metabolism of vincristine by human cryopreserved hepatocytes. *J Pharmacol Exp Ther.* 2008;327:248-257.
171. Topletz AR, Dennison JB, Barbuch RJ, et al. The relative contributions of CYP3A4 and CYP3A5 to the metabolism of vinorelbine. *Drug Metab Dispos.* 2013;41:1651-1661.
172. Yao D, Ding S, Burchell B, et al. Detoxication of vinca alkaloids by human P450 CYP3A4-mediated metabolism: implications for the development of drug resistance. *J Pharmacol Exp Ther.* 2000;294:387-395.
173. Sangkuhl K. Vinka alkaloid pathway, pharmacokinetics. 2012. https://www.pharmgkb.org/pathway/PA150981002
174. Chagas CM, Alisaraie L. Metabolites of vinca alkaloid vinblastine: tubulin binding and activation of nausea-associated receptors. *ACS Omega.* 2019;4:9784-9799.
175. Preston JN, Trivedi MV. Eribulin: a novel cytotoxic chemotherapy agent. *Ann Pharmacother.* 2012;46:802-810.
176. Bai R, Nguyen TL, Burnett JC, et al. Interactions of halichondrin B and eribulin with tubulin. *J Chem Inf Model.* 2011; 51:1393-1404.
177. Jain S, Cigler T. Eribulin mesylate in the treatment of metastatic breast cancer. *Biologics.* 2012;6:21-29.
178. Vahdat LT, Pruitt B, Fabian CJ, et al. Phase II study of eribulin mesylate, a Halichondrin B analog, in patients with metastatic breast cancer previously treated with an anthracycline and a taxane. *J Clin Oncol.* 2009;27:2954-2961.
179. Gerson SL, Caimi PF, William BM, et al. Pharmacology and molecular mechanisms of antineoplastic agents for hematologic malignancies. In: Hoffman R, Benz E, Silberstein LB, et al, eds. *Hematology: Basic Principles and Practice.* 7th ed. Elsevier; 2018.
180. Asadov C, Aliyeva G, Mustafayeva K. Thiopurine S-methyltransferase as a pharmacogenetic biomarker: significance of testing and review of major methods. *Cardiovasc Hematol Agents Med Chem.* 2017; 15:23-30.
181. Coulthard SA, McGarrity S, Sahota K, et al. Three faces of mercaptopurine cytotoxicity in vitro: methylation, nucleotide homeostasis, and deoxythioguanosine in DNA. *Drug Metab Disposition.* 2018;46:1191-1199.
182. de Beaumais TA, Jacqz-Aigrain E. Pharmacogenetic determinants of mercaptopurine disposition in children with acute lymphoblastic leukemia. *Eur J Clin Pharmacol.* 2012;68:1233-1242.
183. Cara CJ, Pena AS, Sans M, et al. Reviewing the mechanism of action of thiopurine drugs: towards a new paradigm in clinical practice. *Med Sci Mont.* 2004;10:247-254.
184. Coulthard SA, Hogarth LA, Little M, et al. The effect of thiopurine methyltransferase expression on sensitivity to thiopurine drugs. *Mol Pharmacol.* 2002;62:102-109.
185. Hartford C, Vasquez E, Schwab M, et al. Differential effects of targeted disruption of thiopurine methyltransferase on mercaptopurine and thioguanine pharmacodynamics. *Cancer Res.* 2007;67:4965-4972.
186. Giamanco NM, Cunningham BS, Klein LS, et al. Allopurinol use during maintenance therapy for acute lymphoblastic leukemia avoids mercaptopurine-related hepatotoxicity. *J Pediatr Hematol Oncol.* 2016;38:147-151.
187. Moyer AM. NUDT15: a bench to bedside success story. *Clin Biochem.* 2021;92:1-8.
188. Khaeso K, Komvilaisak P, Chainansamit S, et al. NUDT15 is a key genetic factor for prediction of hematotoxicity in pediatric patients who received a standard low dosage regimen of 6-mercaptopurine. *Drug Metab Pharmacokinet.* 2022;43:100436.
189. Relling MV, Schwab M, Whirl-Carrillo M, et al. Clinical pharmacogenetics implementation consortium guideline for thiopurine dosing based on TPMT and NUDT 15 genotypes: 2018 update. *Clin Pharmacol Ther.* 2019;105:1095-1105.
190. Marsh S, Booven DJ. The increasing complexity of mercaptopurine pharmacogenomics. *Clin Pharmacol Ther.* 2009;85:139-141.
191. Stocco G, Cheok MH, Crews KR, et al. Genetic polymorphism of inositol triphosphate pyrophosphatase is a determinant of mercaptopurine metabolism and toxicity during treatment for lymphoblastic leukemia. *Clin Pharmacol Ther.* 2009;85:164-172.
192. Lee Y, Jang EJ, Yoon H, et al. Effect of ITPA polymorphism on adverse drug reactions of 6-mercaptopurine in pediatric patients with acute lymphoblastic leukemia: a systematic review and meta-analysis. *Pharmaceuticals.* 2022;15:416.
193. Franca R, Zudeh G, Pagarin S, et al. Pharmacogenetics of thiopurines. *Cancer Drug Resist.* 2019;2:256-270.
194. Coulthard S, Hogarth L. The thiopurines: an update. *Invest New Drugs.* 2005;23:523-532.
195. Zerra P, Bergsagel J, Keller FG, et al. Maintenance treatment with low-dose mercaptopurine in combination with allopurinol in children with acute lymphoblastic leukemia and mercaptopurine-induced pancreatitis. *Pediatr Blood Cancer.* 2016;63:712-715.
196. Fotoohi AK, M L, Peterson C, et al. Impaired transport as a mechanism of resistance to thiopurines in human T-lymphoblastic leukemia cells. *Nucleosides Nucleotides Nucleic Acids.* 2006;25: 1039-1044.
197. Saif MW, Chu E. Antimetabolites. In: DeVita VT, Lawrence TB, Rosenberg SA, eds. *DeVita, Hellman and Rosenberg's Cancer: Principles & Practice of Oncology.* 10th ed. Wolters Kluwer; 2015.
198. Khodursky A, Guzmán EC, Hanawalt PC. Thymineless death lives on: new insights into a classic phenomenon. *Annu Rev Microbiol.* 2015;69:247-263.
199. Guliana S, Polkinghorne I, Smith GA, et al. Macropodid herpesvirus 1 encodes genes for both thymidylate synthase and ICP34.5. *Virus Genes.* 2002;24:207-213.
200. Jarmula A, Fraczyk T, Cieplak P, et al. Mechanism of influence of phosphorylation on serine 124 on a decrease of catalytic activity of human thymidylate synthase. *Bioorg Med Chem.* 2010;18:3361-3370.
201. Pozzi C, Ferrari S, Luciani R, et al. Structural comparison of enterococcus faecalis and human thymidylate synthase complexes with the substrate dUMP and its analogue FdUMP provides hints about enzyme conformational variabilities. *Molecules.* 2019;24:1257.
202. Stroud RM, Finer-Moore JS. Conformational dynamics along an enzymatic reaction pathway: thymidylate synthase, "the movie". *Biochemistry.* 2003;42:239-247.
203. Hyatt DC, Maley F, Montfort WR. Use of strain in a stereospecific catalytic mechanism: crystal structures of *Escherichia coli* thymidylate synthase bound to FdUMP and methylenetetrahydrofolate. *Biochemistry.* 1997;36:4585-4594.
204. Gibson LM, Celeste LR, Lovelace LL, et al. Structures of human thymidylate synthase R163K with dUMP, FdUMP and glutathione show asymmetric ligand binding. *Acta Crystallogr Sect D Biol Crystallogr.* 2011;D67:60-66.
205. Ghosh AK, Islam Z, Krueger J, et al. The general base in the thymidylate synthase catalyzed proton abstraction. *Phys Chem Chem Phys.* 2015;17:30867-30875.

206. Cavaliere A, Probst KC, Westwell AD, et al. Fluorinated nucleosides as an important class of anticancer and antiviral agents. *Future Med Chem.* 2017;9:1809-1833.
207. Ma WW, Saif MW, El-Rayes BF, et al. Emergency use of uridine triacetate for the prevention and treatment of life-threatening 5-flurouracil and capecitabine toxicity. *Cancer.* 2017;123:345-356.
208. Tsujimoto H, Tsukioka S, Ono S, et al. Effect of leucovorin on the antitumor efficacy of the 5-FU prodrug, tegafur-uracil, in human colorectal cancer xenografts with various expression levels of thymidylate synthase. *Oncol Lett.* 2010;1:973-980.
209. Jolivet J. Role of leucovorin dosing and administration schedule. *Eur J Cancer.* 1995;31:1311-1315.
210. Lee A, Ezzeldin H, Fourie J, et al. Dihydropyrimidine dehydrogenase deficiency: impact of pharmacogenetics on 5-fluorouracil therapy. *Virchows Arch.* 2004;2:527-532.
211. Amstutz U, Henricks LM, Offer SM, et al. Clinical Pharmacogenetics Implementation Consortium (CPIC) guideline for dihydropyrimidine dehydrogenase genotype and fluoropyrimidine dosing: 2017 update. *Clin Pharmacol Ther.* 2018;103:210-216.
212. Mattison LK, Fourie J, Desmond RA, et al. Increased prevalence of dihydropyrimidine dehydrogenase deficiency in African-Americans compared to Caucasians. *Cancer Ther Clin.* 2006;12:5491-5495.
213. Launay M, Dahan L, Duval M, et al. Beating the odds: efficacy and toxicity of dihydropyrimidine dehydrogenase-driven adaptive dosing of 5-FU in patients with digestive cancer. *Br J Clin Pharmacol.* 2016;81:124-130.
214. Garcia R, Saydoff JA, Bamat MK, et al. Prompt treatment with uridine triacetate improves survival and reduces toxicity due to fluorouracil and capecitabine overdose or dihydropyrimidine dehydrogenase deficiency. *Toxicol Appl Pharmacol.* 2018;353:67-73.
215. Kummar S, Noronha V, Chu E. Antimetabolites. In: DeVita VJ, Hellman S, Rosenberg SA, eds. *Cancer: Principles and Practice of Oncology.* 7th ed. Lippincott Williams & Wilkins; 2005.
216. Koźmiński P, Halik PK, Chesori R, et al. Overview of dual-acting drug methotrexate in different neurological diseases, autoimmune pathologies and cancers. *Int J Mol Sci.* 2020;21:3483.
217. Cronstein BN, Aune TM. Methotrexate and its mechanisms of action in inflammatory arthritis. *Nat Rev Rheumatol.* 2020;16:145-154.
218. Dummins PL, Gready JE. Energetically most likely substrate and active-site protonation sites and pathways in the catalytic mechanism of dihydrofolate reductase. *J Am Chem Soc.* 2001;123:3418-3428.
219. Cannon WR, Garrison BJ, Benkovic SJ. Consideration of the pH-dependent inhibition of dihydrofolate reductase by methotrexate. *J Mol Biol.* 1997;271:656-668.
220. Cody V, Luft JR, Ciszak E, et al. Crystal structure determination at 2.3 angstrom of recombinant human dihydrofolate reductase ternary complex with NADPH and methotrexate-γ-tetrazole. *Anticancer Drug Des.* 1992;7:483-491.
221. Klon AE, Heroux A, Ross LJ, et al. Atomic structures of human dihydrofolate reductase complexed with NADPH and two lipophilic antifolates at 1.09 angstrom and 1.05 angstrom resolution. *J Mol Biol.* 2002;320:677-693.
222. Meiering EM, Li H, Delcamp TJ, et al. Contributions of tryptophan 24 and glutamate 30 to binding long-lived water molecules in the ternary complex of human dihydrofolate reductase with methotrexate and NADPH studies by site directed mutagenesis and nuclear magnetic resonance spectroscopy. *J Mol Biol.* 1995;241:309-325.
223. Wojtuszkiewicz A, Peters GJ, van Woerden NL, et al. Methotrexate resistance in relation to treatment outcome in childhood acute lymphoblastic leukemia. *J Hematol Oncol.* 2015;8:61.
224. Visentin M, Unal ES, Zhao R, et al. The membrane transport and polyglutamation of pralatrexate: a new generation dihydrofolate reductase inhibitor. *Cancer Chemother Pharmacol.* 2013;72:597-606.
225. Rouch JA, Burton B, Dabb A, et al. Comparison of enteral and parenteral methods of urine alkalinization in patients receiving high-dose methotrexate. *J Oncol Pharm Pract.* 2017;23:3-9.
226. Zelcer S, Kellick M, Wexler LH, et al. The Memorial Sloan Kettering Cancer Center experience with outpatient administration of high dose methotrexate with leucovorin rescue. *Pediatr Blood Cancer.* 2008;50:1176-1180.
227. Flombaum CD, Meyers PA. High dose leucovorin as sole therapy for methotrexate toxicity. *J Clin Oncol.* 1999;17:1589-1594.
228. Ramsey LB, Balis FM, O'Brien MM, et al. Consensus guideline for use of glucarpidase in patients with high-dose methotrexate induced acute kidney injury and delayed methotrexate clearance. *Oncologist.* 2018;23:52-61.
229. Perez-Moreno MA, Galvan-Banqueri M, Flores-Moreno S, et al. Systematic review of efficacy and safety of pemetrexed in non-small-cell-lung cancer. *Int J Clin Pharm.* 2014;36:476-487.
230. Chattopadhyay S, Moran RG, Goldman DI. Pemetrexed: biochemical and cellular pharmacology, mechanisms, and clinical applications. *Mol Cancer Ther.* 2007;6:404-417.
231. Joerger M, Omlin A, Cerny T, et al. The role of pemetrexed in advanced non small-cell lung cancer: special focus on pharmacology and mechanism of action. *Curr Drug Topics.* 2010;11:37-47.
232. Mendelsohn LG, Shih C, Chen VJ, et al. Enzyme inhibition, polyglutamation and the effect of LY231514 (MTA) on purine biosynthesis. *Semin Oncol.* 1999;26(suppl 6):42-47.
233. Sayre PH, Finer-Moore JS, Fritz TA, et al. Multi-targeted antifolates aimed at avoiding drug resistance form covalent closed inhibitory complexes with human and *Escherichia coli* thymidylate synthases. *J Mol Biol.* 2001;313:813-829.
234. Villela LR, Stanford BL, Shah SR. Pemetrexed, a novel antifolate therapeutic alternative for cancer chemotherapy. *Pharmacotherapy.* 2006;26:641-654.
235. Liu Y, Yin T, Zhou R, et al. Expression of thymidylate synthase predicts clinical outcomes of pemetrexed-containing chemotherapy for non-small-cell lung cancer: a systematic review and meta-analysis. *Cancer Chemother Pharmacol.* 2013;72:1125-1132.
236. Uemura T, Oguri T, Ozasa H, et al. ABCC11/MRP8 confers pemetrexed resistance in lung cancer. *Cancer Sci.* 2010;101:2404-2410.
237. Izbicka E, Diaz A, Streeper R, et al. Distinct mechanistic activity profile of pralatrexate in comparison to other antifolates in in vitro and in vivo models of human cancers. *Cancer Chemother Pharmacol.* 2009;64:993-999.
238. O'Connor OA. Pralatrexate: an emerging new agent with activity in T-cell lymphoma. *Curr Opin Oncol.* 2006;18:591-597.
239. O'Connor OA, Amengual J, Colbourn D, et al. Pralatrexate: a comprehensive update on pharmacology, clinical activity and strategies to optimize use. *Leuk Lymphoma.* 2017;58:2548-2557.
240. Molina JR. Pralatrexate, a dihydrofolate reductase inhibitor for the potential treatment of several malignancies. *IDrugs.* 2008;11:508-521.
241. Rueda A, Casanova M, Quero C, et al. Pralatrexate, a new hope for aggressive T-cell lymphoma? *Clin Transl Oncol.* 2009;11:215-220.
242. O'Connor OA, Hamlin PA, Portlock C, et al. Pralatrexate, a novel class of antifol with high affinity for the reduced folate carrier-type 1, produces marked complete and durable remissions in a diversity of chemotherapy refractor cases of T-cell lymphoma. *Br J Haematol.* 2007;139:425-428.
243. Serova M, Bieche I, Sablin MP, et al. Single agent and combination studies of pralatrexate and molecular correlates of sensitivity. *Br J Cancer.* 2011;104:272-280.
244. Mould DR, Sweeney K, Duffull SB, et al. A population pharmacokinetic and pharmacodynamic evaluation of pralatrexate in patients with relapsed or refractory non-Hodgkin's or Hodgkin's lymphoma. *Clin Pharmacol Ther.* 2008;86:190-196.
245. Weinberg BA, Marshall JL, Salem ME. Trifluridine/tipiracil and regorafenib: new weapons in the war against metastatic colorectal cancer. *Clin Adv Hematol Oncol.* 2016;14:630-639.

246. Berdis AJ. Inhibiting DNA polymerases as a therapeutic intervention against cancer. *Front Mol Biosci*. 2017;4:78.
247. Berdis AJ. DNA polymerases as therapeutic targets. *Biochemistry*. 2008;47:8253-8260.
248. Talaat W, Kaddah MMY, Keshk RM. Selective sensing of the nucleoside analogue, trifluridine and tipiracil in dosage form and biological matrices. *Talanta*. 2022;238:123009. doi:10.1016/j.talanta.2021.123009
249. Plunkett W, Huang P, Xu YZ, et al. Gemcitabine: metabolism, mechanism of action, and self-potentiation. *Semin Oncol*. 1995;22:3-10.
250. Galmarini CM, Mackey JR, Dumontet C. Nucleoside analogues: mechanisms of drug resistance and reversal strategies. *Leukemia*. 2001;15:875-890.
251. Cai J, Damaraju VL, Grouix N, et al. Two distinct molecular mechanisms underlying cytarabine resistance in human leukemic cells. *Cancer Res*. 2008;68:2349-2357.
252. van der Velden DL, Opdam FL, Voest EE. TAS-102 for treatment of advanced colorectal cancers that are no longer responding to other therapies. *Clin Cancer Res*. 2016;22:2835-2839.
253. Puthiamadathil JM, Weinberg BA. Emerging combination therapies for metastatic colorectal cancer-impact of trifluridine/tipiracil. *Cancer Manag Res*. 2017;9:461-469.
254. Lee JL, Chu E. Adherence, dosing, and managing toxicities with trifluridine/tipiracil (TAS-102). *Clin Colorectal Cancer*. 2017;16:85-92.
255. White T, Larson H, Minnella A, et al. Metastatic colorectal cancer. *Clin J Oncol Nurs*. 2017;21:E30-E37.
256. Fakih RE, Komrokji R, Shaheen M, et al. Azacitidine use for myeloid neoplasms. *Clin Lymphoma Myeloma Leuk*. 2018;18:e147-e155.
257. Xu P, Hu G, Luo C, et al. DNA methyltransferase inhibitors: an updated patent review (2012-2015). *Expert Opin Ther Pat*. 2016;26:1017-1030.
258. Bohl SR, Bullinger L, Rucker FG. Epigenetic therapy: azacytidine and decitabine in acute myeloid leukemia. *Expert Rev Hematol*. 2018;11:361-371.
259. Seelan RS, Mukhopadhyay P, Piasano MM, et al. Effects of 5-aza-2′-deoxycytidine (decitabine) on gene expression. *Drug Metab Rev*. 2018;50:193-207.
260. Anders NM, Liu J, Wanjiku T, et al. Simultaneous quantitative determination of 5-aza-2′-deoxycytidine genomic incorporation and DNA methylation by liquid chromatography tandem mass spectrometry as exposure-response measures of nucleoside analog DNA methyltransferase inhibitors. *J Chromatogr B*. 2016;1022:38-45.
261. Kadia TM, Gandhi V. Nelarabine in the treatment of pediatric and adult patients with T-cell acute lymphoblastic leukemia and lymphoma. *Expert Rev Hematol*. 2017;10:1-8.
262. Scott LJ. Azacitidine: a review in myelodysplastic syndromes and acute myeloid leukaemia. *Drugs*. 2016;76:889-900.
263. Kovacic P. Hydroxyurea (therapeutics and mechanism): metabolism, carbamoyl nitroso, nitroxyl, radicals, cell signaling and clinical applications. *Med Hypotheses*. 2011;76:24-31.
264. Trepte ML, Auten JJ, Clark SM, et al. Dose related mucositic with hydroxyurea for cytoreduction in acute myeloid leukemia. *J Oncol Pharm Pract*. 2019;25:801-805.
265. Lamanna N, Kay NE. Pentostatin treatment combinations in chronic lymphocytic leukemia. *Clin Adv Hematol Oncol*. 2009;7:386-392.
266. Kay NE, LaPlant BR, Pettinger AM, et al. Cumulative experience and long term follow-up of pentostatin-based chemoimmunotherapy trials for patients with chronic lymphocytic leukemia. *Expert Rev Hematol*. 2018;11:337-349.
267. Ludeman SM. The chemistry of the metabolites of cyclophosphamide. *Curr Pharm Des*. 1999;5:627-643.
268. Larranaga O, de Cozar A, Cossio FP. Mono- and di-alkylation process of DNA bases by nitrogen mustard mechlorethamine. *Chem Phys Chem*. 2017;18:3390-3401.
269. Querfeld C, Geskin LJ, Kim EJ, et al. Lack of systemic absorption of topical mechlorethamine gel in patients with mycosis fungoides cutaneous T-cell lymphoma. *J Invest Dermatol*. 2021;141:1601.
270. Vidal L, Gurion R, Ram R, et al. Chlorambucil for the treatment of patients with chronic lymphocytic leukemia (CLL)—a systematic review and meta-analysis of randomized trials. *Leuk Lymphoma*. 2016;57:2047-2057.
271. Dulik DM, Colvin OM, Fenselau C. Characterization of glutathione conjugates of chlorambucil by fast atom bombardment and thermospray liquid chromatography/mass spectrometry. *Biomed Environ Mass Spectrom*. 1990;19:248-252.
272. Goldenberg GJ, Lee M, Lam HY, et al. Evidence for carrier-mediated transport of melphalan by L5178Y lymphoblasts in vitro. *Cancer Res*. 1977;37:755-760.
273. Al-Sawaf O, Cramer P, Goede V, et al. Bendamustine and its role in the treatment of unfit patients with chronic lymphocytic leukemia: a perspective review. *Ther Adv Hematol*. 2017;8:197-205.
274. Tageja N, Nagi J. Bendamustine: something old, something new. *Cancer Chemother Pharmacol*. 2010;66:413-423.
275. Montillo M, Ricci F, Tedeschi A, et al. Bendamustine: new perspective for an old drug in lymphoproliferative disorders. *Expert Rev Hematol*. 2010;3:131-148.
276. Martin P, Barr PM, James L, et al. Long-term safety experience with bendamustine for injection in a real-world setting. *Expert Opin Drug Saf*. 2017;16:647-650.
277. Giraud B, Herbert G, Deroussent A, et al. Oxazaphosphorines: new therapeutic strategies for an old class of drugs. *Expert Opin Drug Metab Toxicol*. 2010;6:919-938.
278. Huang A, Roy P, Waxman DJ. Role of human liver microsomal CYP3A4 and CYP2B6 in catalyzing N-dechloroethylation of cyclophosphamide and ifosfamide. *Biochem Pharmacol*. 2000;59:961-972.
279. Lind MJ, McGown AT, Hadfield JA, et al. The effect of ifosfamide and its metabolites on intracellular glutathione levels in vitro and in vivo. *Biochem Pharmacol*. 1989;38:1835-1840.
280. Madondo MT, Quinn M, Plebanski M. Low dose cyclophosphamide: mechanisms of T cell modulation. *Cancer Treat Rev*. 2016;42:3-9.
281. Voelcker G. The mechanism of action of cyclophosphamide and its consequences for the development of a new generation of oxazaphosphorine cytostatics. *Scientia Pharmaceutica*. 2020;88:42.
282. Ramu K, Fraiser LH, Mamiya B, et al. Acrolein mercapturates: synthesis, characterization and assessment of their role in the bladder toxicity of cyclophosphamide. *Chem Res Toxicol*. 1995;8:515-524.
283. Ramu K, Perry CS, Ahmed T, et al. Studies on the basis for the toxicity of acrolein mercapturates. *Toxicol Appl Pharmacol*. 1996;140:487-498.
284. Matz EL, Hsieh MH. Review of advances in uroprotective agents for cyclophosphamide-and ifosfanide-induced hemorrhagic cystitis. *Urology*. 2017;100:16-19.
285. Sannu A, Radha R, Mathews A, et al. Ifosfamide-induced malignancy of ureter and bladder. *Cureus*. 2017;9:e1594.
286. Springate JE. Ifosfamide metabolite chloroacetaldehyde causes renal dysfunction in vivo. *J Appl Toxicol*. 1997;17:75-79.
287. Roy P, Yu LJ, Crespi CL, et al. Development of a substrate-activity based approach to identify the major human liver P-450 catalysts of cyclophosphamide and ifosfamide activation based on cDNA-expressed activities and liver microsomal P-450 profiles. *Drug Metab Dispos*. 1999;27:655-666.
288. Woodland D, Ito S, Granvil CP, et al. Evidence of renal metabolism of ifosfamide to nephrotoxic metabolites. *Life Sci*. 2000;68:109-117.
289. Storme T, Deroussent A, Mercier L, et al. New ifosfamide analogs designed for lower associated neurotoxicity and nephrotoxicity with modified alkylating kinetics leading to enhanced in vitro anticancer activity. *J Pharmacol Exp Ther*. 2009;328:598-609.
290. Sprangers B, Lapman S. The growing pains of ifosfamide. *Clinical Kidney Journal*. 2020;13:500-503.

291. Hanly LN, Chen N, Aleksa K, et al. N-acetylcysteine as a novel prophylactic treatment for ifosfamide-induced nephrotoxicity in children: translational pharmacokinetics. *J Clin Pharmacol.* 2012;52:55-64.
292. El-Din A, El-Sisi E, El-Syaad ME, et al. Protective effects of alpha lipoic acid versus N-acetylcysteine on ifosfamide-induced nephrotoxicity. *Toxicol Ind Health.* 2015;31:97-107.
293. Syro LV, Rotondo F, Camargo M, et al. Temozolomide and pituitary tumors: current understanding, unresolved issues, and future directions. *Front Endocrinol.* 2018;9:318.
294. Kaina B. Temozolomide, procarbazine and nitrosoureas in the therapy of malignant gliomas: update of mechanisms, drug resistance and therapeutic implications. *J Clin Med.* 2023;12:7442.
295. Patterson LH, Murray GI. Tumour cytochrome P450 and drug activation. *Curr Pharm Des.* 2002;8:1335-1347.
296. Yamagata S, Ohmori S, Suzuki N, et al. Metabolism of dacarbazine by rat liver microsomes: contribution of CYP1A enzymes to dacarbazine N-demethylation. *Drug Metab Dispos.* 1998;26: 379-382.
297. Friedman HS, Kerby T, Calvert H. Temozolomide and treatment of malignant glioma. *Clin Cancer Res.* 2000;6:2585-2597.
298. Saleem A, Brown GD, Brady F, et al. Metabolic activation of temozolomide measured in vivo using positron emission tomography. *Cancer Res.* 2003;63:2409-2415.
299. Moloney SJ, Prough RA. Studies on the pathway of methane formation from procarbazine, a 2-methylbenzylhydrazine derivative, by rat liver microsomes. *Arch Biochem Biophys.* 1983;221:577-584.
300. Moloney SJ, Wiebkin P, Cummings SW, et al. Metabolic activation of the terminal N-methyl group of N-isopropyl-alpha-(2-methylhydrazino)-p-toluamide hydrochloride (procarbazine). *Carcinogenesis.* 1985;6:397-401.
301. Jiang G, Jiang A, Xin Y, et al. Progression of O6-methylguanine-DNA methyltransferase and temozolomide resistance in cancer research. *Mol Biol Rep.* 2014;41:6659-6665.
302. Messaoudi K, Clavreul A, Lagarce F. Toward an effective strategy in glioblastoma treatment. Part I: resistance mechanisms and strategies to overcome resistance of glioblastoma to temozolomide. *Drug Discov Today.* 2015;20:899-905.
303. Messaoudi K, Clavreul A, Lagarce F. Toward an effective strategy in glioblastoma treatment. Part II: RNA interference as a promising way to sensitize glioblastomas to temozolomide. *Drug Discov Today.* 2015;20:772-779.
304. Ponti M, Souhami RL, Fox BW, et al. DNA interstrand crosslinking and sequence selectivity of dimethanesulphonates. *Br J Cancer.* 1991;63:743-747.
305. Tong WP, Ludlum DB. Crosslinking of DNA by busulfan Formation of diguanyl derivatives. *Biochim Biophys Acta.* 1980;608:174-181.
306. Iwamoto T, Hiraku Y, Oikawa S, et al. DNA intrastrand crosslink at the 5′-GA-3′ sequence formed by busulfan and its role in the cytotoxic effect. *Cancer Sci.* 2004;95:454-458.
307. Westerhof GR, Ploemacher RE, Boudewijn A, et al. Comparison of different busulfan analogues for depletion of hematopoietic stem cells and promotion of donor-type chimerism in murine bone marrow transplant recipients. *Cancer Res.* 2000; 60:5470-5478.
308. Ludlum DB. DNA alkylation by the haloethylnitrosoureas: nature of modifications produced and their enzymatic repair or removal. *Mut Res.* 1990;233:117-126.
309. Nikolova T, Roos WP, Kramer OH, et al. Chloroethylating nitrosoureas in cancer therapy: DNA damage, repair and cell death signaling. *Biochim Biophys Acta.* 2017;1868:29-39.
310. Eisenbrand G, Muller N, Denkel E, et al. DNA adducts and DNA damage by antineoplastic and carcinogenic N-nitrosocompounds. *J Cancer Res Clin Oncol.* 1986;112:196-204.
311. Bacolod MD, Fehdrau R, Johnson SP, et al. BCNU sequestration by metallothioneins may contribute to resistance in a medulloblastoma cell line. *Cancer Chemother Pharmacol.* 2009;63:753-758.
312. Teicher B. Newer cytotoxic agents: attacking cancer broadly. *Clin Cancer Res.* 2008;24:1610-1617.
313. Chaney SG, Campbell SL, Bassett E, et al. Recognition and processing of cisplatin- and oxaliplatin-DNA adducts. *Crit Rev Oncol.* 2005;53:3-11.
314. Zhang C, Xu C, Gao X, et al. Platinum-based drugs for cancer therapy and anti-tumor strategies. *Theranostics.* 2022;12:2115-2132.
315. Duffy EA, Fitzgerald W, Boyle K, et al. Nephrotoxicity: evidence in patients receiving cisplatin therapy. *Clin J Oncol Nurs.* 2018;22:175-183.
316. Crona DJ, Faso A, Nishijima TF, et al. A systematic review of strategies to prevent cisplatin-induced nephrotoxicity. *Oncologist.* 2017;22:609-619.
317. Sheth S, Mukherjea D, Rybak LP, et al. Mechanisms of cisplatin-induced ototoxicity and otoprotection. *Front Cell Neurosci.* 2017;11:338.
318. Gurney JG, Bass JK, Onar-Thomas A, et al. Evaluation of amifostine for protection against cisplatin-induced serious hearing loss in children treated for average-risk or high-risk medulloblastoma. *Neuro Oncol.* 2014;16:848-855.
319. Hu Y, Zhu QN, Deng JL, et al. Emerging role of non-coding RNAs in cisplatin resistance. *Onco Targets Ther.* 2018;11:3185-3194.
320. Kelland L. The resurgence of platinum-based cancer chemotherapy. *Nat Rev Clin Oncol.* 2007;7:573-584.
321. Calvert H. The clinical development of carboplatin—a personal perspective. *Inorg Chim Acta.* 2019;498:118987.
322. Aguiar PJ, Tadokoro H, daSilva GF, et al. Definitive chemoradiotherapy for squamous head and neck cancer: cisplatin vs. carboplatin? A meta-analysis. *Future Oncol.* 2016;12:2755-2764.
323. Ho GY, Woodward N, Coward J. Cisplatin versus carboplatin: comparative review of therapeutic management in solid malignancies. *Crit Rev Oncol.* 2016;102:37-46.
324. Mishima M, Samimi G, Kondo A, et al. The cellular pharmacology of oxaliplatin resistance. *Eur J Cancer.* 2002;38:1405-1412.
325. Chaney SG, Campbell SL, Temple B, et al. Protein interactions with platinum-DNA adducts: from structure to function. *J Inorg Biochem.* 2004;98:1551-1559.
326. Barnes KR, Lippard SJ. Cisplatin and related anticancer drugs: recent advances and insights. *Met Ions Biol Syst.* 2004;42:143-177.
327. Kweekel DM, Gelderblom H, Guchelaar H. Pharmacology of oxaliplatin and the use of pharmacogenomics to individualize therapy. *Cancer Treat Rev.* 2005;31:90-105.
328. McKeage MJ. New-generation platinum drugs in the treatment of cisplatin-resistant cancers. *Expert Opin Invest Drugs.* 2005;14:1033-1046.
329. Cercek A, Park V, Yaeger R, et al. Faster FOLFOX: oxaliplatin can be safely infused at a rate of 1 $mg/m^2/min$. *J Oncol Pract.* 2016;12:548.
330. Wen F, Zhou Y, Wang W, et al. Ca/Mg infusions for the prevention of oxaliplatin-related neuropathy in patients with colorectal cancer: a meta analysis. *Ann Oncol.* 2013;24:171-178.
331. Grolleau F, Gamelin L, Boisdron-Celle M, et al. A possible explanation for a neurotoxic effect of the anticancer agent oxaliplatin on neuronal voltage-gated sodium channels. *J Neurophysiol.* 2001;85:2293-2297.
332. Peng S, Ying AF, Chan NJH, et al. Prevention of oxaliplatin-induced peripheral neuropathy: a systematic review and meta-analysis. *Front Oncol.* 2022;12:731223.
333. Shahnam A, Ridha Z, Wiese MD, et al. Pharmacogenetic and ethnicity influence on oxaliplatin therapy for colorectal cancer: a meta-analysis. *Pharmacogenomics.* 2016;17:1725-1732.
334. Suenaga M, Schirripa M, Cao S, et al. Clinical significance of enterocyte-specific gene polymorphisms as candidate markers of oxaliplatin-based treatment for metastatic colorectal cancer. *Pharmacogenomics J.* 2021;21:285-295.
335. Barros-Oliveira MdC, Costa-Silva DR, Andrade DBd, et al. Use of anastrozole in the chemoprevention and treatment of breast cancer: a literature review. *Revista da Associação Médica Brasileira.* 2017;63:371-378.

336. Cairns J, Ingle JN, Dudenkov TM, et al. Pharmacogenomics of aromatase inhibitors in postmenopausal breast cancer and additional mechanisms of anastrozole action. *JCI Insight*. 2020;5:e137571.
337. Kamdem LK, Liu Y, Stearns V, et al. In vitro and in vivo oxidative metabolism and glucuronidation of anastrozole. *Br J Clin Pharmacol*. 2010;70:854-869.
338. Shagufta IA. Tamoxifen a pioneering drug: an update on the therapeutic potential of tamoxifen derivatives. *Eur J Med Chem*. 2018;143:515-531.
339. Schalken J, Fitzpatrick JM. Enzalutamide: targeting the androgen signalling pathway in metastatic castration-resistant prostate cancer. *BJU Int*. 2016;117:215-225.
340. Wang Y, Chen J, Wu Z, et al. Mechanisms of enzalutamide resistance in castration-resistant prostate cancer and therapeutic strategies to overcome it. *Br J Pharmacol*. 2021;178:239-261.
341. Hoda MR, Kramer MW, Merseburger AS, et al. Androgen deprivation therapy with Leuprolide acetate for treatment of advanced prostate cancer. *Expert Opin Pharmacother*. 2017;18:105-113.
342. Shirley M. Relugolix: a review in advanced prostate cancer. *Target Oncol*. 2023;18:295-302.
343. Shore ND, Sutton J. Plain language summary of the HERO study comparing relugolix with leuprolide for men with advanced prostate cancer. *Future Oncol*. 2022;18:2575-2584.
344. Bairey O, Vanichkin A, Shpilberg O. Arsenic-trioxide-induced apoptosis of chronic lymphocytic leukemia cells. *J Biol Inorg Chem*. 2010;32:e77-e85.
345. Hoonjan M, Jadhav V, Bhatt P. Arsenic trioxide: insights into its evolution to an anticancer agent. *J Biol Inorg Chem*. 2018;23:313-329.
346. Akhtar A, Wang SX, Ghali L, et al. Recent advances in arsenic trioxide encapsulated nanoparticles as drug delivery agents to solid cancers. *J Biomed Res*. 2017;31:177-188.
347. Leu L, Mohassel L. Arsenic trioxide as first-line treatment for acute promyelocytic leukemia. *Am J Health Syst Pharm*. 2009;66:1913-1918.
348. Mirzaei A, Zareian Baghdadabad L, Khorrami MH, et al. Arsenic trioxide; a novel therapeutic agent for prostate and bladder cancers. *Transl Res Urol*. 2019;1:1-7.
349. Chen J, Stubbe J. Bleomycins: towards better therapeutics. *Nat Rev Cancer*. 2005;5:102-112.
350. Chow MS, Liu LV, Soloman EI. Further insights into the mechanism of the reaction of activated bleomycin with DNA. *Proc Natl Acad Sci*. 2008;105:13241-13245.
351. Grollman AP, Takeshita M, Pillai KMR, et al. Origin and cytotoxic properties of base propenals derived from DNA. *Cancer Res*. 1985;45:1127-1131.
352. Bolzan AD, Bianchi MS. DNA and chromosome damage induced by bleomycin in mammalian cells: an update. *Mutat Res Rev Mutat Res*. 2018;775:51-62.
353. Brewer GJ, Dick R, Ullenbruch MR, et al. Inhibition of key cytokines by tetrathiomolybdate in the bleomycin model of pulmonary fibrosis. *J Inorg Biochem*. 2004;98:2160-2167.
354. Li P, Xiao HD, Xu J, et al. Angiotensin converting enzyme N-terminal inactivation alleviates bleomycin-induced lung injury. *Am J Pathol*. 2010;177:1113-1121.
355. Petek BJ, Loggers ET, Pollack SM, et al. Trabectedin in soft tissue sarcomas. *Mar Drugs*. 2015;13:974-983.
356. Desar IME, Constantinidou A, Kaal S, et al. Advanced soft-tissue sarcoma and treatment options: critical appraisal of trabectedin. *Cancer Manag Res*. 2016;8:95-104.
357. DeSanctis R, Marrari A, Santoro A. Trabectedin for the treatment of soft tissue sarcomas. *Exp Opin Pharmacother*. 2016;17:1569-1577.
358. Beumer JH, Rademaker-Lakhai JM, Rosing H, et al. Metabolism of trabectedin (ET-43, YondelisTM) in patients with advanced cancer. *Cancer Chemother Pharmacol*. 2007;59:825-837.
359. Santamaría Nuñez G, Robles CMG, Giraudon C, et al. Lurbinectedin specifically triggers the degradation of phosphorylated RNA polymerase II and the formation of DNA breaks in cancer cells. *Mol Cancer Ther*. 2016;15:2399-2412.
360. Lubkowski J, Wlodawer A. Structural and biochemical properties of L-asparaginase. *FEBS J*. 2021;288:4183-4209.
361. Batool T, Makky EA, Jalal M, et al. A comprehensive review on L-asparaginase and its applications. *Appl Biochem Biotechnol*. 2016;178:900-923.

Structure Challenge Answers

1. a. Antineoplastic drugs 1 (paclitaxel) and 6 (vincristine), b. antineoplastic drugs 3 (fluorouracil) and 8 (methotrexate [MTX]), c. antineoplastic drugs 2 (irinotecan), 5 (etoposide), and 7 (doxorubicin), d. antineoplastic drug 4 (cisplatin)
2. The basic side chain at C_{10} of antineoplastic drug 2 (irinotecan) will be cationic at physiologic pH, which promotes water solubility. The active metabolite of irinotecan is the phenolic SN-38 and is formed by the hydrolysis of the C_{10} carbamate ester by hepatic irinotecan converting enzyme (a carboxylesterase).
3. The highly lipophilic nature of antineoplastic drug 1 (paclitaxel) is augmented by the acetate group at C_{10}, making it necessary to use the oil-based solubilizer Kolliphor EL (polyoxyethylated castor oil). The vehicle consists of 50% ethanol and 50% Kolliphor EL. This solubilizer can cause a hypersensitivity reaction that can be managed by pretreatment with an antihistamine and a glucocorticoid.
4. a. 2, b. 3, c. 1
5. b
6. Leucovorin is 5-formyltetrahydrofolate (5-formyl THF, folinic acid). It is used with antineoplastic drugs 3 (5-fluorouracil [5-FU]) and 8 (MTX). In the case of 5-FU, leucovorin supplements the 5,10-methyleneTHF cofactor that stabilizes the binding of 5-FdUMP to thymidylate synthase, thus potentiating 5-FU's cytotoxic effect. In the case of MTX, leucovorin is given as a rescue therapy to supply the normal cells with THF cofactors required for purine and dTMP syntheses.
7. Antineoplastic drug 8 (MTX) undergoes polyglutamation inside the tumor cell. This causes a highly negatively charged structure that cannot cross the cell membrane and traps the drug inside the cell.
8. Antineoplastic drugs 2 (irinotecan) and 5 (etoposide phosphate) undergo lactone hydrolysis that causes ring opening to form the less active or inactive hydroxy acid metabolite.
9. The two reactive species of antineoplastic drug 4 (cisplatin) are the mono- and the di-aquo forms produced by nucleophilic attack by water and displacement of one or both chloride ligands. The nucleophilic N^7 of adjacent guanosine dinucleotides in DNA then conduct a nucleophilic attack at the electron-deficient platinum atom of the reactive species. In the case of the di-aquo intermediate, intrastrand DNA cross-linking results.

CHAPTER
37

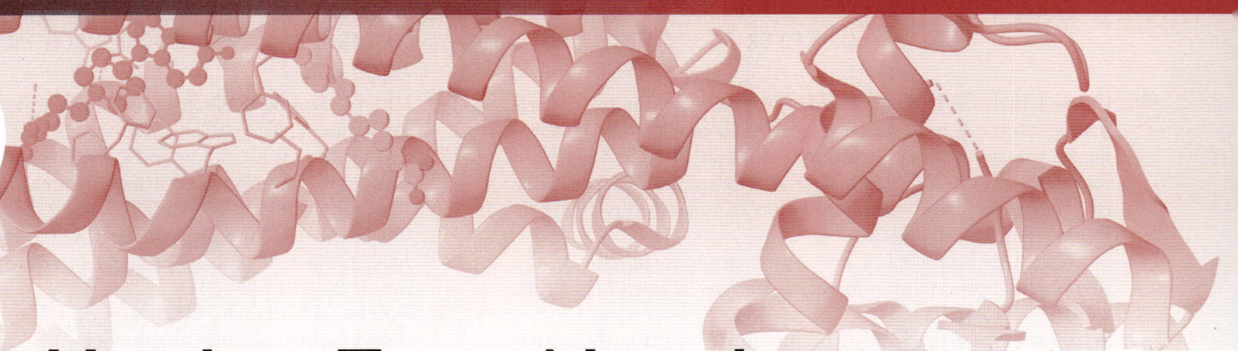

Drugs Used to Treat Neoplastic Diseases: Targeted Therapy

Sonali Kurup, Sushma Ramsinghani, and Victoria F. Roche

Drugs covered or mentioned in this chapter:

TARGETED THERAPIES

KINASE INHIBITORS

AKT INHIBITORS
- Capivasertib

ALK INHIBITORS
- Alectinib
- Brigatinib
- Ceritinib
- Crizotinib
- Lorlatinib

BCR-ABL INHIBITORS
- Asciminib
- Bosutinib
- Dasatinib
- Imatinib
- Nilotinib
- Ponatinib

CHECKPOINT KINASE (CDK4/6) INHIBITORS
- Abemaciclib
- Palbociclib
- Ribociclib

FGFR INHIBITORS
- Erdafitinib
- Futibatinib
- Infigratinib
- Pemigatinib

JAK INHIBITORS
- Fedratinib
- Momelotinib
- Pacritinib
- Ruxolitinib

mBRAF INHIBITORS
- Dabrafenib
- Encorafenib
- Vemurafenib

MEK INHIBITORS
- Binimetinib
- Cobimetinib
- Selumetinib
- Trametinib

mEGFR/HER2 INHIBITORS
- Afatinib
- Dacomitinib
- Erlotinib
- Gefitinib
- Osimertinib

mFLT3 INHIBITORS
- Gilteritinib
- Midostaurin
- Quizartinib

mKRAS INHIBITORS
- Adagrasib
- Sotorasib

mTOR INHIBITORS
- Everolimus
- Temsirolimus

NTRK/ROS/RET INHIBITORS
- Entrectinib
- Larotrectinib
- Pralsetinib
- Repotrectinib
- Selpercatinib

PDGFRα/KIT INHIBITORS
- Avapritinib
- Ripretinib

PI3Kδ/γ INHIBITORS
- Duvelisib
- Idelalisib
- Umbralisib

PI3KCα INHIBITORS
- Alpelisib

VEGFR INHIBITORS
- Axitinib
- Fruquintinib
- Lenvatinib
- Pazopanib
- Regorafenib
- Sorafenib
- Sunitinib

NONKINASE INHIBITORS

BCL-2 INHIBITORS
- Venetoclax

EXPORTIN INHIBITORS
- Selinexor

EZH2 INHIBITORS
- Tazemetostat

HEDGEHOG SIGNALING INHIBITORS
- Glasdegib

HDAC INHIBITORS
- Belinostat
- Romidepsin
- Vorinostat

IMMUNOMODULATORS
- Lenalidomide
- Pomalidomide
- Thalidomide

mIDH INHIBITORS
- Enasidenib
- Ivosidenib
- Olutasidenib

PARP INHIBITORS
- Niraparib
- Olaparib
- Rucaparib
- Talazoparib

PROTEASOME INHIBITORS
- Bortezomib

Drugs covered or mentioned in this chapter:—continued

- Carfilzomib
- Ixazomib

RETINOIC ACID RECEPTOR LIGANDS

- Tretinoin

BIOLOGICS

THERAPEUTIC MONOCLONAL ANTIBODIES

- Alemtuzumab
- Bevacizumab
- Cetuximab
- Daratumumab
- Dinutuximab
- Elotuzumab
- Isatuximab
- Motixafortide
- Necitumumab
- Obinutuzumab
- Ofatumumab
- Olaratumab
- Panitumumab
- Pertuzumab
- Ramucirumab
- Rituximab
- Trastuzumab

IMMUNE CHECKPOINT INHIBITORS

- Atezolizumab
- Avelumab
- Cemiplimab
- Dostarlimab
- Durvalumab
- Ipilimumab
- Nivolumab

BISPECIFIC ANTIBODIES

- Amivantamab
- Blinatumomab

ANTIBODY-DRUG CONJUGATES

- Ado-trastuzumab emtansine
- Brentuximab vedotin
- Enfortumab vedotin
- Fam-trastuzumab deruxtecan
- Gemtuzumab ozogamicin
- Inotuzumab ozogamicin
- Loncastuximab tesirine
- Mirvetuximab soravtansine
- Polatuzumab vedotin
- Sacituzumab govitecan
- Tisotumab vedotin

CHIMERIC ANTIGEN RECEPTOR T-CELL IMMUNOTHERAPEUTICS

- Axicabtagene ciloleucel
- Sipuleucel-T
- Tisagenlecleucel

RADIOIMMUNOCONJUGATES

- ^{177}Lu vipivotide tetraxetan
- ^{90}Y Ibritumomab tiuxetan

Abbreviations

ABL Abelson
ACVR1 activin A receptor type 1
ADCC antibody-dependent cellular cytotoxicity
AKT protein kinase B
ALK anaplastic lymphoma kinase
ALL acute lymphoid leukemia
AML acute myeloid leukemia
APL acute promyelocytic leukemia
ATP adenosine triphosphate
AUC area under the concentration curve
BAK BCL-2 antagonist killer 1
BAX BCL-2–associated X protein
BBB blood-brain barrier
BCL-2 B-cell lymphoma-2
BCR B-cell receptor
BCR-ABL breakpoint cluster region/Abelson tyrosine kinase
BCRP breast cancer resistance protein
BH BCL-2 homology
BIM BCL-2 interacting mediator of cell death
BRAF/B-Raf B-rapidly accelerated fibrosarcoma
BRCA1 breast cancer gene 1
BRCA2 breast cancer gene 2
BTK Bruton tyrosine kinase
CAR-T chimeric antigen receptor T-cell
CD cluster of differentiation
CDK cyclin-dependent kinase
CLL chronic lymphocytic leukemia
CML chronic myelogenous leukemia
CNS central nervous system
CRC colorectal cancer
CSK C-terminal Src kinase
CTLA-4 cytotoxic T-lymphocyte–associated antigen-4
CXCR4 chemokine receptor 4
CXCL12 chemokine ligand 12
CYP cytochrome P450
DCE discrete choice experiments
DDI drug-drug interaction
DFG aspartate, phenylalanine, glycine
dMMR deficient mismatch repair system
EGFR epidermal growth factor receptor
EGFR-TKI epidermal growth factor receptor tyrosine kinase inhibitor
EML4 echinoderm microtubule–associated protein-like 4
ERK extracellular signal–regulated kinase
EZH2 enhancer of zeste homolog 2
FDA U.S. Food and Drug Administration
FGFR fibroblast growth factor receptor kinase
FLT3 FMS-like tyrosine kinase 3
FLT3-ITD FMS-like tyrosine kinase 3 internal tandem duplication
FR folate receptor
GP glycoprotein
HAT histone acetyltransferase
HCC hepatocellular carcinoma
HDAC histone deacetylase
HER human epidermal growth factor receptor kinase
HER2 human epidermal growth factor receptor kinase 2
HER2-TKI human epidermal growth factor receptor kinase 2 tyrosine kinase inhibitor
HR hormone receptor
IDH isocitrate dehydrogenase
IκB inhibitor of nuclear factor kappa B
IMiD immunomodulatory drug
ITD internal tandem duplication
IV intravenous
JAK Janus kinase
Kit stem cell factor receptor tyrosine kinase
KRAS Kirsten rat sarcoma
mAb monoclonal antibody
MAPK mitogen-activated protein kinase
mBRAF mutant B-rapidly accelerated fibrosarcoma
mBRCA mutant breast cancer resistance gene
MCL mantle cell lymphoma
mEGFR mutant epidermal growth factor receptor kinase
MEK mitogen-activated protein kinase kinase
MET hepatocyte growth factor receptor kinase

mEZH2 mutant enhancer of zeste homolog 2
mFLT3 mutant FMS-like tyrosine kinase 3
mKRAS mutant Kirsten rat sarcoma
MM multiple myeloma
MMR mismatch repair
MPN myeloproliferative neoplasms
mTOR mammalian target of rapamycin
NF-κB nuclear factor kappa B
NGS next-generation sequencing
NPM nucleophosmin
NRAS neuroblastoma rat sarcoma
NRTK nonreceptor tyrosine kinase
NSCLC non–small cell lung cancer
NTRK neurotrophic receptor tyrosine kinase
OCT organic cation transporter
OS overall survival
PARP poly(ADP-ribose) polymerase
PCFT proton-coupled folate transporter
PDGFR platelet-derived growth factor receptor
PD-1 programmed death protein 1
PD-L1 programmed death ligand 1
PFS progression-free survival
Pgp P-glycoprotein
PI3K phosphatidylinositol 3 kinase
PLC phospholipase C
POI protein of interest
PROTAC proteolysis targeting chimera
PTEN phosphatase and tensin homolog deleted on chromosome 10
RAF rapidly accelerated fibrosarcoma
RAS rat sarcoma
Rb retinoblastoma
RCC renal cell carcinoma
REMS Risk Evaluation and Mitigation Strategy
RET REarranged during Transfection
RFC reduced folate carrier
ROS1 ROS proto-oncogene 1, receptor tyrosine kinase
RTK receptor tyrosine kinase
SAM S-adenosylmethionine
SC subcutaneous
SMO smoothened
SRC Src kinase, nonreceptor kinase
STAT signal transducer and activator of transcription
$T_{1/2}$ elimination half-life
TK tyrosine kinase
TKI tyrosine kinase inhibitor
T_{max} time to peak plasma concentration
TRK tropomyosin receptor tyrosine kinase
VEGFR vascular endothelial growth factor receptor kinase
wt wild-type

CLINICAL SIGNIFICANCE

Treatment selection for targeted therapies is guided through the utilization of next-generation sequencing (NGS) for the majority of patients with metastatic or advanced cancers. It is not only important to ensure that the right drug is being prescribed for the right patient, but also that the right drug is being prescribed for the right molecular target. Currently, the U.S. Food and Drug Administration (FDA) approvals for targeted therapies are subject to selective genetic alterations in specific tumor types, and some have been granted biomarker-dependent histology-agnostic approval. Many institutions have implemented Molecular Tumor Boards (MTBs) comprising a multidisciplinary team of medical oncologists, surgeons, genetic counselors, pharmacists, pathologists, radiologists, and scientists to assist in the interpretation of NGS reports, make recommendations for targeted therapies, and/or identify candidates for enrollment into clinical trials. For patients who qualify for an oral targeted agent, comprehensive patient and caregiver education should be provided by the pharmacist that includes potentially use-limiting adverse effects predictable from their structure-dependent mechanism, as well as drug-drug and drug-food interactions, and the importance of adherence. Health care providers need to remain vigilant in providing coordinated care for every patient so that the promise of improved outcomes and lower toxicity with these rationally designed targeted therapies can be realized.

Claire Saadeh, PharmD

Contemporary Directions and Developments in Cancer Therapy

The introduction to Chapter 36 (Classical Chemotherapy) provided an overview of cancer's public health and economic burdens, disease etiology, a historical overview of anticancer drug development, and common mechanisms of drug resistance. Readers are encouraged to consult that introduction for important background to the targeted agents discussed in this chapter.

Targeted Therapy

Personalized or precision medicine in the treatment of neoplastic disease involves the use of gene-directed or antibody-directed prodrugs, kinase and other enzyme inhibitors that target molecular determinants of selected cancers identified through genetic screening, and monoclonal antibody (mAb)-based therapies.[1] This antineoplastic "hot topic" has been the focus of intense research and dedicated issues of cancer-related journals.[2] One goal of targeted cancer therapy is to avoid use-limiting, nonspecific toxicity inherent in cytotoxic chemotherapy by selectively directing drugs to the genes or proteins that mediate uncontrolled growth within cancer cells. Targeted cancer therapy comes with its own set of specific toxicities and adverse effects, but they are generally better tolerated than the classic chemotherapy drugs discussed in Chapter 36.

Small molecule enzyme inhibitors are the most utilized drugs in the targeted therapy arsenal, and they have varying levels of selectivity for potential therapeutic targets. The less selective (promiscuous) inhibitors bind to multiple targets, and their use does not generally require individualized genetic mapping of the tumor. Selective and specific inhibitors bind to a select few or a single target, respectively, and are more commonly employed once a predictive biomarker indicating responsiveness is identified.[3] Clearly, the more selective/specific an inhibitor, the less likely it is to induce adverse effects through inhibition of unintended targets.

The excitement over the therapeutic value of this more neoplasm-specific approach is evidenced by the fact that, from 2000 to 2014, 79.5% of new cancer drugs approved by the FDA were targeted therapeutic agents.[4] The pace of their design, development, and approval has remained vigorous; since imatinib, the first tyrosine kinase inhibitor (TKI), hit the market at the turn of the century, the number of targeted cancer therapeutics approved by the FDA has far exceeded the approval of cytotoxic classic antineoplastic drugs. In 2020, 43 drugs directed toward protein kinases and other enzymatic targets were available in the United States.[3] In 2021, 10 novel targeted drugs were approved for the treatment of a variety of neoplastic diseases, and another 10 marketed agents received supplemental approval for expanded indications or adjuvant (post-therapy) or neoadjuvant (presurgery) administration.[5] In addition to small molecule and biologics (including immunotherapy), other novel approaches to selectively obliterating cancer cells include nanocarrier delivery systems[6,7] and biosimilars.[8,9] In 2023, 13 out of 55 new drugs approved were for cancer, which included six small molecule kinase inhibitors, six biologics, and one hormonal agent.

In reviewing the significant progress made over the first two decades of targeted cancer therapy development, Bedard et al[3] also cite challenges to further advancement, including yet unknown or overly responsive targets, time-intensive (and, for severely ill patients, time-sensitive) biomarker screening processes, shortened efficacy due to the development of resistance, and a dearth of successful combination inhibitor therapies. They underscore the urgency in developing "next-generation" inhibitors that expand (vs duplicate) the positive therapeutic impact of these drugs and highlight ongoing efforts and opportunities that should help make that goal a reality.

In 2023, Jiang et al[10] published a comprehensive review of studies measuring patients' targeted therapy preferences through an evaluation of discrete choice experiments (DCE), a relatively new tool. They report that patients treated with targeted therapies put the greatest emphasis on efficacy measures, especially overall survival (OS), followed by cost. Less important were drug administration processes, including treatment regimens. Patients were willing to assume an average personal financial burden of $716 and $561 for a 1-month gain in OS and progression-free survival (PFS), respectively, which translates to an annual out-of-pocket cost of $8,592 (OS) and $6,732 (PFS). Willingness to shoulder these costs is inversely related to the anticipated survival rate of the diagnosed cancer and is anticipated to be directly related to patient income. As the patient is the ultimate driver of what therapeutic plans will be accepted and implemented, their opinions are paramount, and the authors offer several important suggestions to increase the reliability, validity, and utility of future DCE studies.

The introduction to Chapter 36 started with a quote by Eleanor Roosevelt about gaining strength, courage, and confidence by staring fear in the face and relating that concept to patients living with cancer. The era of targeted cancer therapy that began with the introduction of imatinib has made it easier for patients with cancer treated with these novel agents to "not blink first" in the face of their diagnosis. The important take-home message from contemporary cancer treatment literature is that, with intense and sustained attention being focused on scientifically grounded approaches to targeted therapy, the future holds great promise for safer and more effective therapeutic options that can offer real hope for enhanced longevity with a good quality of life.

PRECISION ONCOLOGY

The introduction of TKIs,[11] specifically imatinib,[12] was stimulated by the groundbreaking recognition that a mutant chromosome known as breakpoint cluster region/Abelson tyrosine kinase (BCR-ABL), or the Philadelphia (Ph) chromosome, appeared consistently in the cells of patients with chronic myelogenous leukemia (CML). The product of this aberrant chromosome, the BCR-ABL protein, is an unregulated tyrosine kinase (TK) that promotes cellular proliferation at the expense of apoptosis. Ongoing advances in genetics and molecular biology have led to the identification of other specific processes that are either uniquely dysfunctional within the cancer cell or overexpressed in the cancer cells over normal cells.[13,14] Molecular determinants of these dysfunctional carcinogenic pathways can now be identified through genetic screening as biomarkers and include receptor overexpression, persistent activation of intracellular signaling pathways, epigenetic processes, increased tumor vascularity, DNA repair defects, suppressed apoptotic pathways, and immune escape mechanisms. Precision oncology matches anticancer therapy to the biochemical characterization of tumors achieved through patient genomic profiling.[15,16] The treatment plan is tailored to include drugs that inhibit patient-specific oncogenic drivers, bypassing those that would not only be less effective but also more nonselectively toxic.

The explosion of new targeted drugs was propelled by the rapidly expanding knowledge of cancer biology and the ability to analyze cancer genome alterations in thousands of patient samples, leading to a better understanding of the molecular evolution of cancer.[4,17-20] New insights include (1) oncogene addiction (discussed later) that makes cancers particularly susceptible to inhibitors of specific dysfunctional pathways that sustain neoplastic cells and (2) biomarker proteins that can be prognostic (telling clinicians whom to treat), predictive (informing clinicians on how to treat),[21] and/or inform on the likelihood of acquired resistance to therapy. Neoplasms once thought to be uniform in nature can now be distinguished into subtypes based on defining molecular properties.[22]

The FDA has approved tests that must be administered for the detection of patient-specific oncogenic drivers prior to initiating targeted therapies and immunotherapies. For example, molecular screening can detect the presence of oncogenic drivers, allowing tumors to be classified as positive or negative for a mutant (m) form of epidermal growth factor receptor kinase (mEGFR), Kirsten rat sarcoma (mKRAS) or B-rapidly accelerated fibrosarcoma (mBRAF). Cancers that are positive for these markers have been effectively and safely treated with anticancer drugs developed to specifically inhibit these dysfunctional pathways. In addition, non–small cell lung cancer (NSCLC) could express oncogenic mEGFR or be dependent on the oncofusion protein, anaplastic lymphoma kinase-echinoderm microtubule–associated protein-like 4 (ALK-EML4) for cell proliferation and tumor growth.[22] The mEGFR kinase inhibitors are effective treatments for patients with NSCLC with mEGFR+ status. Among patients with mEGFR+ NSCLC, those with EGFR exon 19 deletions (ex19del) are more responsive to anti-EGFR-targeted therapies than those with L858R EGFR exon 21 mutations. This example underscores how molecular screening can reveal oncogenic drivers that dictate therapeutic choices for a more rationally designed treatment plan.[19,23,24]

The keen interest in discovering newer and reliable oncogenic drivers and prognostic biomarkers and exploiting them for therapeutic benefit has resulted in an array of medicinal agents and tools being approved under precision oncology, which has changed the treatment paradigm for solid tumors and hematologic malignancies.[1,2,25-32] Tables 37.1 through 37.3 list the targeted therapies, and Table 37.4 lists

Table 37.1 Selected Therapeutic Parameters of Oncofusion Protein Signaling Inhibitors Based on Biomarker Screening

Drug	Biomarker	Indications	Trade Name	Type
BCR-ABL Inhibitors				
Asciminib	Ph+ (T315I BCR-ABL)	Imatinib-resistant Ph+ CML Effective in T315I mutants	Scemblix	Kinase inhibitor
Bosutinib	Ph+	Imatinib-resistant Ph+ CML Not effective in T315I mutants	Bosulif	Kinase inhibitor
Dasatinib	Ph+	Imatinib-resistant Ph+ CML, ALL Not effective in T315I mutants	Sprycel	Kinase inhibitor
Imatinib	Ph+	Ph+ CML, ALL GIST Not effective in T315I mutants	Gleevec	Kinase inhibitor
Nilotinib	Ph+	Imatinib-resistant Ph+ CML Not effective in T315I mutants	Tasigna	Kinase inhibitor
Ponatinib	Ph+ (T315I BCR-ABL)	Imatinib-resistant Ph+ CML, ALL Effective in T315I mutants	Iclusig	Kinase inhibitor
ALK Inhibitors				
Alectinib	ALK rearrangement	ALK+ NSCLC	Alecensa	Kinase inhibitor
Brigatinib	ALK rearrangement	ALK+ NSCLC	Alunbrig	Kinase inhibitor
Ceritinib	ALK rearrangement	ALK+ NSCLC	Zykada	Kinase inhibitor
Lorlatinib	ALK rearrangement	ALK+ NSCLC	Lorbrena	Kinase inhibitor
ROS1/NTRK/RET Inhibitors				
Entrectinib	ROS1 rearrangement	ROS1+ NSCLC	Rozlytrek	Kinase inhibitor
Larotrectinib	NTRK rearrangement$^+$	NTRK+ tumors	Vitrakvi	Kinase inhibitor
Pralsetinib	RET fusion	RET+ NSCLC, thyroid cancer, and solid tumors	Gavreto	Kinase inhibitor
Repotrectinib	ROS1 rearrangement	ROS1+ NSCLC	Augtyro	Kinase inhibitor
Selpercatinib	RET fusion	RET+ NSCLC, thyroid cancer, and solid tumors	Retevmo	Kinase inhibitor

ALK, anaplastic lymphoma kinase; ALL, acute lymphoid leukemia; AML, acute myeloid leukemia; BCR-ABL, breakpoint cluster region/Abelson tyrosine kinase; CML, chronic myelogenous leukemia; NSCLC, non–small cell lung cancer; NTRK, neurotrophic receptor kinase; Ph$^+$, Philadelphia chromosome-positive; RET, REarranged during Transfection; ROS1, proto-oncogene 1, receptor tyrosine kinase.

Table 37.2 Selected Therapeutic Parameters for RAS/RAF/MEK Pathway Inhibitors Based on Biomarker Screening

Drug	Biomarker	Indications	Trade Name	Type
EGFR/HER2 Inhibitors				
Afatinib	del19 EGFR, L858R EGFR, T790M EGFR, wtKRAS	del19 EGFR+ NSCLC, L858R EGFR+ NSCLC	Gilotrif	Kinase inhibitor
Dacomitinib	del19EGFR, L858R EGFR	NSCLC	Vizimpro	Kinase inhibitor
Erlotinib	del19 EGFR, L858R EGFR, wtKRAS	del19 EGFR+ NSCLC, L858R EGFR+ NSCLC, Pancreatic cancer	Tarceva	Kinase inhibitor
Gefitinib	del19 EGFR, L858R EGFR, wtKRAS	del19 EGFR+ NSCLC, L858R EGFR+ NSCLC	Iressa	Kinase inhibitor
Lapatinib	HER2	HER2+ BC	Tykerb	Kinase inhibitor
Neratinib	HER2	HER2+ BC	Nerlynx	Kinase inhibitor
Osimertinib	del19 EGFR, L858R EGFR, wtKRAS T790M EGFR, wtKRAS	del19 EGFR+, wtKRAS+ NSCLC L858R EGFR+, wtKRAS+ NSCLC, T790M EGFR+, wtKRAS+ NSCLC	Tagrisso	Kinase inhibitor
Tucatinib	HER2+ HER2+/wtKRAS	HER2+ breast cancer HER2+/wtKRAS CRC	Tukysa	Kinase inhibitor
mKRAS Inhibitors				
Adagrasib	KRAS G12C	KRAS G12C+ NSCLC	Krazati	Nonkinase inhibitor
Sotorasib	KRAS G12C	KRAS G12C+ NSCLC	Lumakras	Nonkinase inhibitor
mBRAF/MEK Inhibitors				
Dabrafenib/ trametinib	BRAF V600E, BRAF V600K	BRAF V600E CRC, BRAF V600E NSCLC, BRAF V600E melanoma, BRAF V600K melanoma BRAF V600E glioma in combination with trametinib	Tafinlar/ Mekinist	Kinase inhibitor
Encorafenib/ binimetinib	BRAF V600E, BRAF V600K	BRAF V600E CRC, BRAF V600E NSCLC, BRAF V600E/V600K melanoma	Braftovi	Kinase inhibitor
Vemurafenib/ cobimetinib	BRAF V600E, BRAF V600K	BRAF V600E melanoma BRAF V600K melanoma In combination with cobimetinib	Zelboraf/ Cotellic	Kinase inhibitor
PI3K/AKT/mTOR Pathway Inhibitors				
Alpelisib	HR positive, HER2 negative, PIK3CA mutated	In combination with fulvestrant for HR-positive, HER2-negative, PIK3CA-mutated breast cancer	Piqray	Kinase inhibitor
Capivasertib	HR positive, HER2 negative, PIK3CA, AKT1, and/or PTEN altered	In combination with fulvestrant for HR-positive, HER2-negative, PIK3CA, AKT1, and/or PTEN-altered breast cancer	Truqap	Kinase inhibitor
Duvelisib	No biomarker (Target = PI3Kδ)	CLL, small lymphocytic lymphoma,	Copiktra	Kinase inhibitor

(continued)

Table 37.2 Selected Therapeutic Parameters for RAS/RAF/MEK Pathway Inhibitors Based on Biomarker Screening (*continued*)

Drug	Biomarker	Indications	Trade Name	Type
Everolimus	No biomarker (Target = mTOR)	Advanced RCC HR positive, HER2 negative Advanced BC neuroendocrine tumors	Afinitor	Kinase inhibitor
Idelalisib	No biomarker (Target = PI3Kδ)	CLL SLL Follicular B-cell non-Hodgkin lymphoma	Zydelig	Kinase inhibitor
Temsirolimus	No biomarker (Target = mTOR)	Advanced RCC	Torisel	Kinase inhibitor
BTK Inhibitors				
Acalabrutinib	None	MCL (previously treated)	Calquence	Kinase inhibitor
Ibrutinib	None	Refractory CLL, SLL	Imbruvica	Kinase inhibitor
Pirtobrutinib	None	CLL, mantle cell lymphoma	Jaypirca	Kinase inhibitor
Zanubrutinib	None	CLL, mantle cell lymphoma, marginal zone lymphoma, Waldenström macroglobulinemia	Brukinsa	Kinase inhibitor
NF-κB Pathway Inhibitors				
Immunomodulatory Drugs				
Lenalidomide	None Target: multiple MOA, indirect NF-κB inhibition	MM	Revlimid	Nonkinase inhibitor
Pomalidomide	None Target: multiple MOA, indirect NF-κB inhibition	MM	Pomalyst	Nonkinase inhibitor
Thalidomide	None Target: multiple MOA, indirect NF-κB inhibition	MM	Thalomid	Nonkinase inhibitor
Proteasome Inhibitors				
Bortezomib	None Target: Proteasome	MM	Velcade	Nonkinase inhibitor
Carfilzomib	None Target: Proteasome	MM	Kyprolis	Nonkinase inhibitor
Ixazomib	None Target: Proteasome	MM	Ninlaro	Nonkinase inhibitor
Apoptosis Inducers				
Venetoclax	None Target: BCL-2	AML, CLL	Venclexta	Nonkinase inhibitor
Inhibitors of Dysfunctional Myeloproliferative Processes				
mFLT3 Inhibitors				
Gilteritinib	mFLT3	mFLT3+ AML	Xospata	Kinase inhibitor

Table 37.2 Selected Therapeutic Parameters for RAS/RAF/MEK Pathway Inhibitors Based on Biomarker Screening (*continued*)

Drug	Biomarker	Indications	Trade Name	Type
Midostaurin	mFLT3	mFLT3+ AML	Rydapt	Kinase inhibitor
Quizartinib	FLT3-ITD	FLT3-ITD+ AML	Vanflyta	Kinase inhibitor
JAK Inhibitors				
Fedratinib	None	Myelofibrosis	Inrebic	Kinase inhibitor
Pacritinib	None	Myelofibrosis	Vonjo	Kinase inhibitor
Ruxolitinib	None	Myeloproliferative neoplasms (myelofibrosis, polycythemia vera)	Jakafi	Kinase inhibitor
Mutant Isocitrate Dehydrogenase (mIDH) Inhibitors				
Enasidenib	mIDH2	mIDH2+ AML	Idhifa	Kinase inhibitor
Ivosidenib	mIDH1	mIDH1+ AML, myelodysplastic syndrome, cholangiocarcinoma	Tibsovo	Kinase inhibitor
Olutasidenib	mIDH1	mIDH1+ AML	Rezlidhia	Kinase inhibitor
Other Myeloproliferative Inhibitors				
Glasdegib	No biomarker (Target = SMO/hedgehog signaling)	AML	Daurismo	Nonkinase inhibitor
Tretinoin	*t*(15;17)	APL	ATRA	Nonkinase inhibitor

AKT, protein kinase B; AML, acute myeloid leukemia; APL, acute promyelocytic leukemia; ATRA, all-*trans* retinoic acid; BC, breast cancer; BCL-2, B-cell lymphoma-2; BRAF, B-rapidly accelerated fibrosarcoma; BTK, Bruton tyrosine kinase; CLL, chronic lymphocytic leukemia; CRC, colorectal cancer; EGFR, epidermal growth factor receptor kinase; FLT3-ITD, FMS-like tyrosine kinase 3 internal tandem duplication; HER2, human epidermal growth factor 2; HR, hormone receptor; MCL, mantle cell lymphoma; MEK, mitogen-activated protein kinase kinase; mFLT3, mutant FMS-like tyrosine kinase 3; mIDH1, mutant isocitrate dehydrogenase 1; mIDH2, mutant isocitrate dehydrogenase 2; MM, multiple myeloma; MOA, mechanism of action; mTOR, mammalian target of rapamycin; NF-κB, nuclear factor kappa B; NSCLC, non–small cell lung cancer; PI3K, phosphatidylinositol 3 kinase; PTEN, phosphatase and tensin homolog deleted on chromosome 10; RCC, renal cell carcinoma; SLL, small lymphocytic lymphoma; SMO, Smoothened; wtKRAS, wild-type Kirsten rat sarcoma.

Table 37.3 Selected Therapeutic Parameters for Miscellaneous Targeted Therapies Based on Biomarker Screening

Drug	Biomarker	Indications	Trade Name	Type
VEGFR Inhibitors				
Axitinib	None	Advanced RCC	Inlyta	Kinase inhibitor
Fruquintinib	None	Metastatic CRC	Fruzaqla	Kinase inhibitor
Lenvatinib	None	Advanced RCC Iodine-refractory differentiated TC	Lenvima	Kinase inhibitor
Pazopanib	None	Advanced RCC Advanced soft tissue sarcoma	Votrient	Kinase inhibitor

(*continued*)

Table 37.3 Selected Therapeutic Parameters for Miscellaneous Targeted Therapies Based on Biomarker Screening (*continued*)

Drug	Biomarker	Indications	Trade Name	Type
Regorafenib	None	GIST Metastatic CRC HCC	Stivarga	Kinase inhibitor
Sorafenib	None	Advanced RCC TC HCC	Nexavar	Kinase inhibitor
Sunitinib	None	Advanced RCC Advanced pancreatic NET Imatinib-resistant GIST	Sutent	Kinase inhibitor
Tivozanib	None	RCC	Fotivda	Kinase inhibitor
FGFR Inhibitors				
Erdafitinib	Altered FGFR2/FGFR3	Urothelial carcinoma	Balversa	Kinase inhibitor
Futibatinib	pan-FGFR inhibitor	FGFR2+ cholangiocarcinoma	Truseltiq	Kinase inhibitor
Infigratinib	pan-FGFR inhibitor	FGFR2+ cholangiocarcinoma	Lytgobi	Kinase inhibitor
Pemigatinib	Altered FGFR2; altered FGFR1	FGFR1+ myeloid/lymphoid cancers FGFR2+ cholangiocarcinoma	Pemazyre	Kinase inhibitor
PDGFRα/Kit Inhibitors				
Avapritinib	PDGFRα exon 18 PDGFRα D842V	PDGFRα exon 18 or PDGFRα D842V+ GIST	Ayvakit	Kinase inhibitor
Ripretinib	No biomarker (Target = PDGFR)	GIST	Qinlock	Kinase inhibitor
CDK4/6 Inhibitors				
Abemaciclib	HR positive, HER2 negative	In combination with fulvestrant or aromatase inhibitors for HR-positive, HER2-negative breast cancer	Verzenio	Kinase inhibitor
Palbociclib	HR positive, HER2 negative	In combination with fulvestrant or aromatase inhibitors for HR-positive, HER2-negative breast cancer	Ibrance	Kinase inhibitor
Ribociclib	HR positive, HER2 negative	In combination with fulvestrant or aromatase inhibitors for HR-positive, HER2-negative breast cancer	Kisqali	Kinase inhibitor
Trilaciclib	None	Supportive care for platinum, etoposide, or topotecan-induced myelosuppression in small cell lung cancer	Cosela	Kinase inhibitor
HDAC/EZH2 Inhibitors				
Romidepsin	No biomarker (Target = HDAC)	Cutaneous T-cell lymphoma	Istodex	Nonkinase inhibitor
Tazemetostat	mEZH2	Follicular lymphoma	Tazverik	Nonkinase inhibitor
Vorinostat	No biomarker (Target = HDAC)	Cutaneous T-cell lymphoma	Zolinza	Nonkinase inhibitor
PARP Inhibitors				
Niraparib	mBRCA positive, HER2 negative; HR positive	mBRCA-positive, HER2-negative breast cancer; HR-positive prostate cancer	Zejula	Nonkinase inhibitor

Table 37.3 Selected Therapeutic Parameters for Miscellaneous Targeted Therapies Based on Biomarker Screening (*continued*)

Drug	Biomarker	Indications	Trade Name	Type
Olaparib	mBRCA positive, HER2 negative; HR positive	mBRCA-positive, HER2-negative breast cancer; HR-positive prostate cancer	Lynparza	Nonkinase inhibitor
Rucaparib	mBRCA positive, HER2 negative; HR positive	mBRCA-positive, HER2-negative breast cancer; HR-positive prostate cancer	Rubraca	Nonkinase inhibitor
Talazoparib	mBRCA positive, HER2 negative; HR positive	mBRCA-positive, HER2-negative breast cancer; HR-positive prostate cancer	Talzenna	Nonkinase inhibitor

CDK, cyclin-dependent kinase; CRC, colorectal cancer; FGFR, fibroblast growth factor receptor kinases; GIST, gastrointestinal stromal tumor; HCC, hepatocellular carcinoma; HDAC, histone deacetylase; HER2, human epidermal growth factor 2; HR, hormone receptor; KIT, stem cell factor receptor tyrosine kinase; mBRCA, mutant breast cancer resistance gene; mEZH2, mutant enhancer of zeste homolog 2; NET, neuroendocrine tumors; PARP, poly(ADP-ribose) polymerase; PDGFRα, platelet-derived growth factor receptor α; RCC, renal cell carcinoma; TC, thyroid carcinoma, VEGFR, vascular endothelial growth factor receptor kinase.

Table 37.4 U.S. Food and Drug Administration–Approved Cancer Biologics and Immunotherapies

Drug	Type	Antibody Type	Antigenic Target/ Biomarker	Indications
Alemtuzumab	mAb	Humanized	CD52	B-cell CLL
Bevacizumab	mAb	Humanized	VEGF	Metastatic/recurrent/progressive cervical, colorectal, ovarian, glioblastoma, non-squamous NSCLC, renal cell cancers
Cetuximab	mAb	Human/mouse chimeric	EGFR	Metastatic/recurrent colorectal, head and neck squamous cell carcinoma
Daratumumab	mAb	Human	CD38	Relapsed/refractory multiple myeloma
Dinutuximab	mAb	Human/mouse chimeric	GD2	Neuroblastoma
Elotuzumab	mAb	Humanized	SLAMF7	Relapsed/refractory multiple myeloma
Isatuximab	mAb	Mouse/human chimeric	CD38	MM
Necitumumab	mAb	Human	EGFR	Metastatic squamous NSCLC
Obinutuzumab	mAb	Humanized	CD20	Previously untreated CLL, previously untreated or relapsed/refractory follicular lymphoma
Ofatumumab	mAb	Human	CD20	Relapsed, refractory, or previously untreated CLL
Olaratumab	mAb	Human	PDGFRα	Soft tissue sarcoma
Panitumumab	mAb	Human	EGFR	Metastatic colorectal cancer
Pertuzumab	mAb	Humanized	HER2	Early or metastatic HER2+ breast cancer
Ramucirumab	mAb	Human	VEGFR2	Advanced/metastatic NSCLC, colorectal, gastric cancers
Rituximab	mAb	Mouse/human chimeric	CD20	CLL, NHL, previously untreated diffuse large B-cell lymphoma (with recombinant human hyaluronidase), follicular lymphoma (with recombinant human hyaluronidase)

(*continued*)

Table 37.4 U.S. Food and Drug Administration–Approved Cancer Biologics and Immunotherapies (*continued*)

Drug	Type	Antibody Type	Antigenic Target/ Biomarker	Indications
Trastuzumab	mAb	Humanized	HER2	HER2+ MBC and gastric cancer
Immune Checkpoint Inhibitors				
Atezolizumab	Immune checkpoint inhibitor (mAb)	Humanized	PD-L1	Metastatic NSCLC, advanced/metastatic urothelial carcinoma
Avelumab	Immune checkpoint inhibitor (mAb)	Human	PD-L1	Metastatic Merkel cell carcinoma, advanced/metastatic urothelial carcinoma
Cemiplimab	Immune checkpoint inhibitor (mAb)	Human	PD-1	NSCLC, BCC, cutaneous squamous cell carcinoma
Dostarlimab	Immune checkpoint inhibitor (mAb)	Human	PD-1	mismatch repair deficient (dMMR) cancers
Durvalumab	Immune checkpoint inhibitor (mAb)	Human	PD-L1	Unresectable NSCLC, advanced/metastatic urothelial carcinoma
Ipilimumab	Immune checkpoint inhibitor (mAb)	Human	CTLA-4	Unresectable/metastatic melanoma
Nivolumab	Immune checkpoint inhibitor (mAb)	Human	PD-1	Metastatic/recurrent/progressive NSCLC, colorectal, squamous cell head and neck and renal cell cancers, Hodgkin lymphoma, urothelial carcinoma, hepatocellular carcinoma, melanoma
Pembrolizumab	Immune checkpoint inhibitor (mAb)	Human	PD-1	Metastatic/recurrent/progressive NSCLC, colorectal, squamous cell head and neck and renal cell cancers, Hodgkin lymphoma, urothelial carcinoma, hepatocellular carcinoma, melanoma
Bispecific Antibodies				
Amivantamab	Bispecific antibody (mAb)	Humanized	EGFR exon 20, MET	Exon 20–positive NSCLC
Blinatumomab	Bispecific antibody (mAb)	Mouse	CD19, CD3	Relapsed/refractory ALL
Antibody-Drug Conjugates (ADCs)				
Ado-trastuzumab emtansine	ADC	Humanized, conjugated with DM1 (maytansine-based mitosis inhibitor)	HER2	HER2+ MBC
Brentuximab vedotin	ADC	Human/mouse chimeric, conjugated with monomethylauristatin E (mitosis inhibitor)	CD30	Primary or systemic anaplastic large cell lymphoma, relapsed/refractory HL
Enfortumab vedotin	ADC	Humanized, conjugated with monomethylauristatin E (mitosis inhibitor)	Nectin	Urothelial cancer
Fam-trastuzumab deruxtecan	ADC	Humanized, conjugated with deruxtecan (irinotecan-based DNA topoisomerase inhibitor)	HER2	HER2+ MBC

Table 37.4 U.S. Food and Drug Administration–Approved Cancer Biologics and Immunotherapies (*continued*)

Drug	Type	Antibody Type	Antigenic Target/ Biomarker	Indications
Gemtuzumab ozogamicin	ADC	Humanized, conjugated with calicheamicin derivative (DNA strand cleavage inducer)	CD33	AML
Inotuzumab ozogamicin	ADC	Humanized, conjugated with calicheamicin derivative (DNA strand cleavage inducer)	CD22	Relapsed/refractory ALL
Loncastuximab tesirine	ADC	Mouse/human chimeric conjugated with SG3199 (alkylating agent/DNA crosslinker)	CD19	Relapsed/refractory large B-cell lymphoma
Mirvetuximab soravtansine	ADC	Mouse/human chimeric, conjugated with soravtansine (maytansine-based antimitotic agent)	FRα	FRα+ ovarian, fallopian tube, and primary peritoneal cancer
Polatuzumab vedotin	ADC	Humanized, conjugated with monomethylauristatin E (mitosis inhibitor)	CD79b	Previously treated, relapsed/refractory DLBCL
Sacituzumab govitecan	ADC	Humanized conjugated with govitecan (irinotecan-based DNA topoisomerase inhibitor)	TROP2	Advanced, metastatic breast cancer or urothelial cancer
Tisotumab vedotin	ADC	Humanized, conjugated with monomethylauristatin E (mitosis inhibitor)	Tissue factor	Urothelial cancer
CAR-T Cell Therapy				
Axicabtagene ciloleucel	CAR-T cell	Modified T cells	CD19	Relapsed/refractory DLBCL, FL
Sipuleucel-T	CAR-T cell	Modified T cells	Prostatic acid phosphatase (PAP)	Prostate cancer
Tisagenlecleucel	CAR-T cell	Modified T cells	CD19	Relapsed/refractory ALL, DLBCL, FL
Radioimmunoconjugates				
Lu^{33} vipivotide tetraxetan	Radioimmunoconjugate	PSMA binder chelated with ^{177}Lu (β-emitting isotope)	PSMA	PSMA-positive metastatic castration-resistant prostate cancer
^{90}Y ibritumomab tiuxetan	Radioimmunoconjugate	Mouse, chelated with ^{90}Y (β-emitting isotope)	CD20	Relapsed/refractory NHL

ADC, antibody-drug conjugate; ALL, acute lymphoblastic leukemia; AML, acute myeloid leukemia; BCC, basal cell carcinoma; CAR, chimeric antigen receptor; CD, cluster of differentiation; CLL, chronic lymphocytic leukemia; CTLA-4, cytotoxic T-lymphocyte–associated antigen-4; DLBCL, diffuse large B-cell lymphoma; EGFR, epidermal growth factor receptor kinase; FL, follicular lymphoma; FRα, folate receptor α; HER2, human epidermal growth factor receptor 2; HL, Hodgkin lymphoma; mAb, monoclonal antibody; MBC, metastatic breast cancer; MM, multiple myeloma; NHL, non-Hodgkin lymphoma; NSCLC, non-small cell lung cancer; PD-1, programmed death protein 1; PD-L1, programmed death ligand 1; PSMA, prostate-specific membrane antigen; SLAMF7, signaling lymphocytic activation molecule family member 7; VEGFR, vascular endothelial growth factor receptor kinase.

the immunotherapies with approved indications following confirmation of oncogenic drivers as predictive biomarkers through genetic testing.

To gain an appreciation for the diverse classes of targeted therapies and immunotherapies available under precision oncology, it is vital to understand the process of carcinogenesis and the dysfunctional pathways that drive tumor growth and metastases. This chapter describes these processes and reviews the varied pharmacologic and chemical classes of targeted therapies, including kinase inhibitors and nonkinase enzyme inhibitors. The pharmacodynamic (mechanisms of action, adverse effects, toxicity, and resistance profiles) and pharmacokinetic properties (absorption, distribution, metabolism, excretion profile) are discussed in the subsequent sections.

Carcinogenesis and Oncogenic Drivers

Cell homeostasis is tightly regulated through processes of cell division, growth, repair, and death.[34] Normal cells progress through phases of the cell cycle and undergo cell division in a tightly regulated manner.[35] In normal physiology, aberrant or dysfunctional cells are enzymatically repaired (eg, with mismatch repair [MMR] enzymes). Cell death and survival is also tightly regulated by extrinsic apoptotic and intrinsic pathways. Proapoptotic and antiapoptotic proteins are expressed or repressed based on a need to activate cell survival or trigger cell death.[36]

Cancer or malignancy arises from a single abnormal cell that continues to divide indefinitely. Cancer cells are characterized by dysregulated cell homeostasis associated with uncontrolled cell division and growth, dysfunctional repair systems, and avoidance of cell death mechanisms (Fig. 37.1). A solid mass (tumor) may result from uncontrolled cell proliferation and tissue growth. The most common type of solid tumor is an adenocarcinoma, which starts in the epithelial cells of the secretory glands of the lung, colon, esophagus, stomach, breast, prostate gland, or pancreas that normally secrete substances important to their function, such as mucus or digestive juices.[37] Hematologic malignancies are associated with blood and lymphoid tissue and are categorized as lymphomas (characterized by abnormal B and T lymphocytes), lymphoid leukemias (characterized by abnormal B and T lymphoblasts), myeloid leukemias (characterized by abnormal myeloblasts), and multiple myeloma (MM; characterized by abnormal plasma cells). Carcinogenesis is characterized by four phases, initiation, promotion, malignant conversion, and progression.

Oncogene Addiction and Cancer Initiation

Initiation of carcinogenesis in a normal cell is caused by exposure to a carcinogen or through activation of a mutant gene (oncogene). Some of the aberrant processes that are unique to cancer cells include altered enzyme or receptor pathways that control cell division. The altered pathway becomes the primary pathway for cell proliferation, with reduced contributions from pathways operational in healthy cells, a condition termed ***oncogene addiction***.[38-41] As a consequence, the cancer cell expressing the mutant enzyme demonstrates uncontrolled cell division, resulting in continuous tumor growth. Oncogene addiction is characterized by a genetic alteration through point mutations such as mEGFR in NSCLC or mBRAF in melanoma.

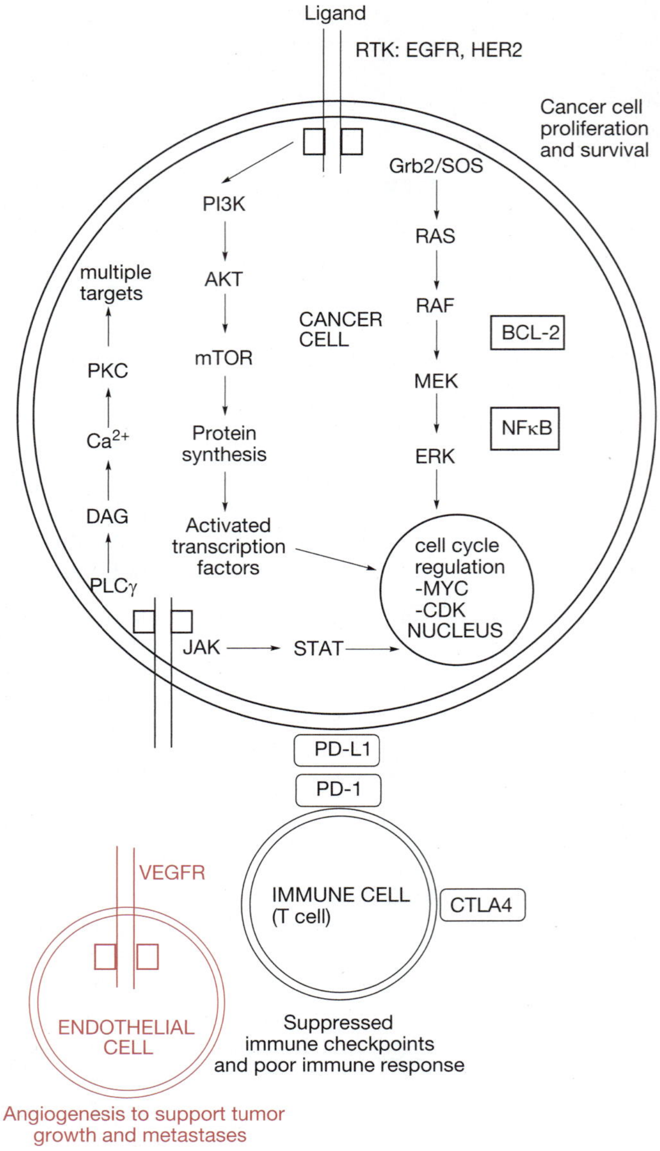

Figure 37.1 Dysfunctional molecular pathways in cancer. AKT, protein kinase B; BCL-2, B-cell lymphoma-2; CDK, cyclin-dependent kinase; CTLA4, cytotoxic T-lymphocyte–associated antigen-4; DAG, diacylglycerol; EGFR, epidermal growth factor receptor; Grb2, growth factor receptor-bound protein 2; HER2, human epidermal growth factor 2; JAK, Janus kinase; MEK, mitogen-activated protein kinase kinase; mTOR, mammalian target of rapamycin; NF-κB, nuclear factor kappa B; PD-1, programmed death protein 1; PD-L1, programmed death ligand 1; PKC, protein kinase C; PI3K, phosphatidylinositol 3 kinase; PLC, phospholipase C; RAF, rapidly accelerated fibrosarcoma; RAS, rat sarcoma; RTK, receptor tyrosine kinase; SOS, son of sevenless; STAT, signal transducer and activator of transcription; VEGFR, vascular endothelial growth factor receptor kinase.

It may also be characterized by receptor overexpression such as human epidermal growth factor receptor kinase 2 (HER2) overexpression in breast cancer. Oncogene addiction is also characterized by chromosomal rearrangements that result in the expression of constitutively active aberrant fusion oncoproteins such as BCR-ABL kinase in CML. The oncogenes commit the cell to becoming malignant and drive several processes critical to the development of cancer. Key oncogenic drivers are shown in Tables 37.1 through 37.4 and Figure 37.1.

Genetic Instability, Inactivation of Tumor Suppression, Dysfunction in Immune Surveillance, and Cancer Promotion

Clonal expansion and proliferation of an initiated cell is characterized by the inactivation of tumor suppressor genes.[42,43] Breast cancer gene 1 (*BRCA1*) and breast cancer gene 2 (*BRCA2*) are involved in DNA repair and maintain the integrity of DNA. Mutations in BRCA inhibit DNA repair and allow for proliferation of abnormal cells.[44,45] Breast cancer cells are characterized by dysfunctional repair enzymes arising from mutant breast cancer resistance genes (mBRCAs).[46,47] Dysfunction in the phosphatase and tensin homolog deleted on chromosome 10 (PTEN) suppressor gene increases the risk of melanoma and lung and prostate cancer.

Epigenetic changes such as hypermethylation of DNA bases and decreased histone acetylation reduce the expression of proapoptotic proteins and are seen in the promotional phase of hematologic malignancies.[48,49] Abnormal cells overexpress enzymes such as histone deacetylases (HDACs) that drive these processes. Genetic abnormalities such as chromosomal instability and deficient MMR (dMMR) are seen in colorectal cancers (CRCs).[50-52]

The immune system is the body's natural defense and eradicates abnormal cells. However, precancerous cells express receptors that reduce susceptibility to immune-mediated cell death.[53,54] The programmed death protein 1/programmed death ligand 1 (PD-1/PD-L1) are examples of immunosuppressive receptors that allow for unregulated cell survival and avoidance of immune-mediated clearance.[55-57]

Malignant Conversion, Tumor Progression, and Metastases

Genetic changes over 5 to 20 years cause an irreversible conversion of a precancerous cell to a cancer cell fully equipped to compete with and outlast the body's normal cellular processes.[58,59] Cancer cells express proteins and enzymes that support and sustain accelerated tumor growth (see Fig. 37.1). Progression to a tumor is characterized by uncontrolled cell proliferation, tissue invasion, and distant metastasis. Cancer cells progress through the cell cycle despite their biochemical irregularities. This is due to breakdowns in normal cell cycle checkpoints designed to regulate cell division, dysfunctions such as deficiency in the retinoblastoma (Rb) protein, and/or overexpression of cyclin-dependent kinases (CDKs).

Cancer cells are also characterized by an imbalance in pro- and antiapoptotic proteins due to dysfunctional apoptotic signaling. For example, B-cell lymphoma-2 (BCL-2) overexpression in hematologic malignancies leads to prolonged survival and avoidance of cell death.[60,61] Cancer cells develop replicative immortality due to mutations in telomerase enzymes that allow telomeres to remain long enough to continually support cell division. Mutations in telomerases are associated with melanoma, an aggressive form of skin cancer.[62] Angiogenesis is the process of formation of new blood vessels from existing tumor vasculature.[63-65] The new blood vessels are used to secure additional nutrients and provide avenues for the tumor to grow locally as well as metastasize to sites distal from the primary tumor. Vascular endothelial growth factor receptor kinase (VEGFR) drives angiogenesis and plays a key role in tumor growth and metastases (see Fig. 37.1).

Compared to healthy cells, malignant cells have altered glucose, amino acid, and fatty acid metabolism. For example, cancers such as acute lymphoid leukemia (ALL) are more highly dependent on aerobic glycolysis without a concomitant increase in reliance on oxidative phosphorylation (the Warburg effect) to convert almost all glucose to lactate even in the presence of oxygen.[66] A variation in the tricarboxylic acid (TCA) cycle and generation of oncometabolites that inhibit myeloblast differentiation is observed in acute myeloid leukemia (AML).[67]

Cancer cells further express proteins that allow for their proliferation at the expense of healthy cells, resulting in parasitic colonization of the tissue or organ.[68-70] Cancer cells express inflammatory mediators that preferentially allow cancer cell survival while destroying normal cells.[68] The transcription factor nuclear factor kappa B (NF-κB) is activated in MM and drives myeloma cell survival, inflammatory response, immune response, and angiogenesis.[69,70] The biologic hallmarks of cancer include avoidance of growth suppressors, evading immune-mediated cell death, replicative immortality, tumor-promoting inflammation, persistent proliferative signaling, deregulated cellular energetics, resisting cell death, genome instability, increased angiogenesis, and activated pathways for invasion and metastases.[71,72]

The subsequent sections of this chapter describe the varied classes of targeted therapies and cancer biologics and correlate their mechanism of action to the dysfunctional molecular pathways described earlier. Drugs have been grouped by chemical class, pharmacologic class, mechanism of action, and routes of administration. Specific targeted therapies and biologics approved for the treatment of cancer is discussed in terms of the structural relevance related to mechanism, resistance, adverse effects, and pharmacokinetic profiles.

Targeted Therapies and Cancer Immunotherapies

Targeted therapies and immunotherapies have clearly changed the face of cancer chemotherapy.[1,2,25-32] They can sidestep the sometimes use-limiting nonspecific toxicity inherent in classic chemotherapy and are generally better tolerated.[73,74] However, targeted therapies and biologics come with their own set of specific toxicities and adverse effects which, while often reversible, necessitate supportive care.

Small molecule–targeted therapies have varying levels of selectivity for molecular targets, which impact their adverse effect profile.[74] For example, based on the role of phosphatidylinositol 3 kinase (PI3K) in glucose metabolism, hyperglycemia is an on-target mechanistic adverse effect of PI3K inhibitors. Adverse effects of cancer biologics are related to their composition and mechanistic effects on immune system activation.[75]

The targeted therapies are administered for long periods of time and present unique challenges. Both efficacy and tolerability are key considerations in treatment choice with targeted therapies.[76] Among these challenges are (1) acquired resistance secondary to gene mutation, with expression of proteins that no longer bind or respond to drug,[77-79] and (2) risk of clinically significant drug-drug interactions (DDIs) with cytochrome P450 (CYP) and/or P-glycoprotein (Pgp) inhibitors and inducers, as well as with drugs that raise gastric pH (eg, proton-pump inhibitors [PPIs], H_2 antagonists) and food.[80-82] CYP3A4, which metabolizes the greatest number of clinically relevant drugs, is the most problematic isoform involved in serious and/or life-threatening DDIs with kinase inhibitors.

Targeted therapies and immunotherapies have been chemically classified into small molecules and biologics and can be correlated to the routes of administration. Small molecule–targeted therapies are predominantly administered orally as tablets and capsules. Cancer immunotherapies are often administered intravenously (IV) but can also be given topically in skin cancer and by instillation in bladder cancer. Targeted therapies can be further stratified pharmacologically as kinase inhibitors and nonkinase inhibitors based on their mechanism of action.[1,2,25-28] Tables 37.1 through 37.3 list the targeted therapies classified as kinase and nonkinase inhibitors together with corresponding indications and approved biomarkers. The chemical class, source, molecular target, and therapeutic indications of marketed agents are provided in Table 37.4.

Kinase Inhibitors

Kinase Families

Kinases catalyze the phosphorylation of amino acid residues on substrate proteins using adenosine triphosphate (ATP) and are classified by their target residue (eg, TK, serine/threonine kinase, or lipid kinase).[78] TKs may be further classified as receptor tyrosine kinases (RTKs) and nonreceptor tyrosine kinases (NRTKs). The RTKs have an extracellular domain, a transmembrane domain, and an intracellular domain and include EGFR, HER2, and fibroblast growth factor receptor kinase (FGFR). The kinase catalytic site is present on the intracellular domain. Activation of RTK involves binding of growth factors, receptor dimerization, and activation of intracellular signaling. The NRTKs are cytosolic and include fusion oncoproteins, ALK-EML4, and BCR-ABL kinase. Lipid kinases phosphorylate membrane-associated proteins. PI3K is a therapeutically relevant lipid kinase that is frequently mutated in varied cancers and drives tumor growth through activation of the PI3K/protein kinase B (AKT)/mammalian target of rapamycin (mTOR) pathway.[79-81]

The kinase-catalyzed phosphorylation of a single protein in a kinase signaling cascade can activate the entire pathway.[80-83] Kinase signaling cascades are a very complex series of enzymatic processes involving a multitude of cell sustaining players, many of which serve as antineoplastic therapeutic targets.[79] Once a substrate protein is phosphorylated, it is active and, in turn, phosphorylates and activates the next protein in the sequence. This continues through a downstream signaling cascade of kinases that finally activate processes that support cell division and growth. Several examples of this are described later and shown in Figure 37.1. Activated RTKs will, in turn, activate the rat sarcoma (RAS)/rapidly accelerated fibrosarcoma (RAF)/mitogen-activated protein kinase kinase (MEK)/extracellular signal–regulated kinase (ERK) signaling pathway that controls cell growth, proliferation, and survival.[83] The BRAF kinase is one component of the RAS/RAF/MEK/ERK signaling cascade. Activated BRAF phosphorylates and activates MEK, which, in turn, phosphorylates and activates ERK, resulting in increased cell proliferation. Persistent signaling through dysfunctional kinases in the RTK/RAS/RAF/MEK/ERK pathway, PI3K/AKT/mTOR pathway, and/or Janus kinase (JAK)/signal transducer and activator of transcription (STAT) pathways and other signaling pathways drive cancer cell proliferation through constitutively activated kinases and signaling molecules.

Based on their role in inhibiting pathways required for normal cell proliferation and survival, kinase inhibitors do not kill cells but, rather, produce a cytostatic effect that prevents tumor growth. A reduction in tumor burden is not immediately seen with cytostatic agents.[84,85] This is a major difference in the mechanism of action for targeted therapies (including kinase inhibitors) compared to classic chemotherapeutic agents. Classic chemotherapy is predominantly cytotoxic/cytocidal, although cytostatic effects are observed in apoptosis-resistant cells. Cytostatic cells are usually cleared by homeostatic processes; however, reports have shown that treatment-induced cytostatic cancer cells could create a reservoir for resistant clones to develop, leading to relapse.

Chemical and Pharmacologic Classes

All kinases utilize ATP as the phosphate source and catalyze reactions between two entities, ATP and the substrate protein.[65,86-89] Thus, kinases have binding sites for both ATP and the substrate protein. The ATP pocket of kinases is made up of the adenine region, hinge region, ribose pocket, phosphate-binding region, solvent-exposed region, hydrophobic region I at the back of the ATP site, and a narrow hydrophobic region II by the hinge region toward the front of the ATP site (Fig. 37.2).[65,86-89] Most kinases also have a key amino acid residue termed the *gatekeeper* that controls access to hydrophobic region I. ATP occupies the adenine region, hinge region, ribose pocket, and phosphate-binding region. The kinases have two lobes, the N-terminal and C-terminal lobes that are linked by a flexible hinge. A deep cleft is found at the interface of the

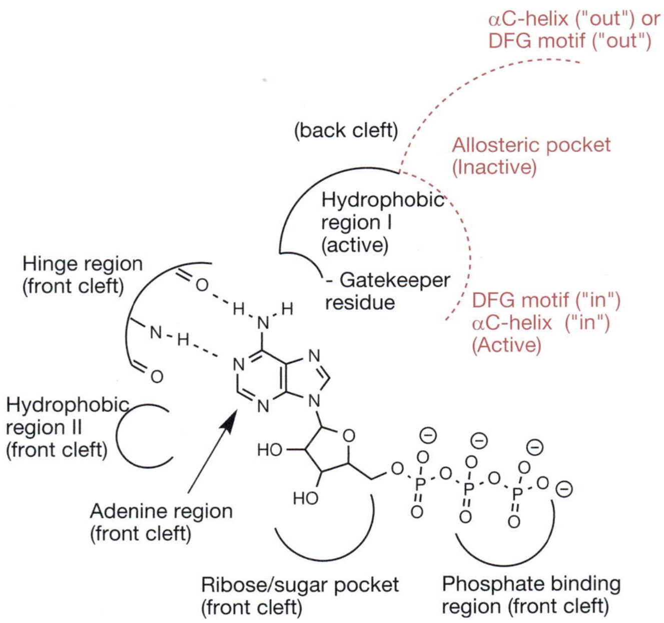

Figure 37.2 Binding pocket of kinases. DFG, aspartate, phenylalanine, glycine.

kinase lobes that creates the active site pocket where ATP and the substrate protein bind. Activation of the kinase is controlled by multiple regulatory elements, including the position of the kinase aspartate, phenylalanine, glycine (DFG) motif; the position of the αC-helix, access to Mg^{2+} in the ATP site; the phospho-acceptor site or activation segment comprising the flexible activation loop (α-loop) adjacent to DFG; and a glycine-proline–rich loop (P-loop). Following dimerization, the ATP catalytic site exists in an active conformation that allows phosphorylation. The active conformation of kinases is a tightly closed conformation formed from an "in" conformation of the DFG motif and αC-helix. The inactive conformation of kinases has a larger back pocket and an extended or open conformation formed from an "out" conformation of the DFG motif and/or αC-helix.

Most FDA-approved kinase inhibitors are competitive inhibitors and bind directly to the ATP pocket. In recent years, allosteric kinase inhibitors have been identified. These inhibitors bind outside the ATP pocket and induce conformational changes that disrupt kinase activation. Most marketed inhibitors bind to the kinase in one of six distinct ways (types I-VI as described next and shown in Fig. 37.3).[65,86-88]

Kinase Inhibitor–Binding Modes

Type I Inhibitors. Type I kinase inhibitors (eg, erlotinib) compete with ATP and bind to the enzyme in its active form. In general, type I inhibitors will contain a heteroaromatic ring that directly competes with ATP for access to the adenine-binding domain of the hinge region. Lipophilic and hydrogen bonding functional groups attached to the heteroaromatic system insert into hydrophobic pockets adjacent to the adenine pocket, enhancing affinity. Many contain polar functional groups that extend into the solvent interface.

Type II Inhibitors. Type II kinase inhibitors (eg, lapatinib, imatinib) bind to the inactive kinase conformer, which differs from the active form in the outward versus inward orientation of the DFG motif. These molecules access the type I–binding area using many of the structural elements found on type I inhibitors and incorporate long side chains that further extend into the allosteric back pocket. The type II inhibitors span the ATP-binding site and the adjacent allosteric back pocket.

Type III Inhibitors. Type III kinase inhibitors (eg, trametinib) do not compete with ATP and fit into a binding pocket

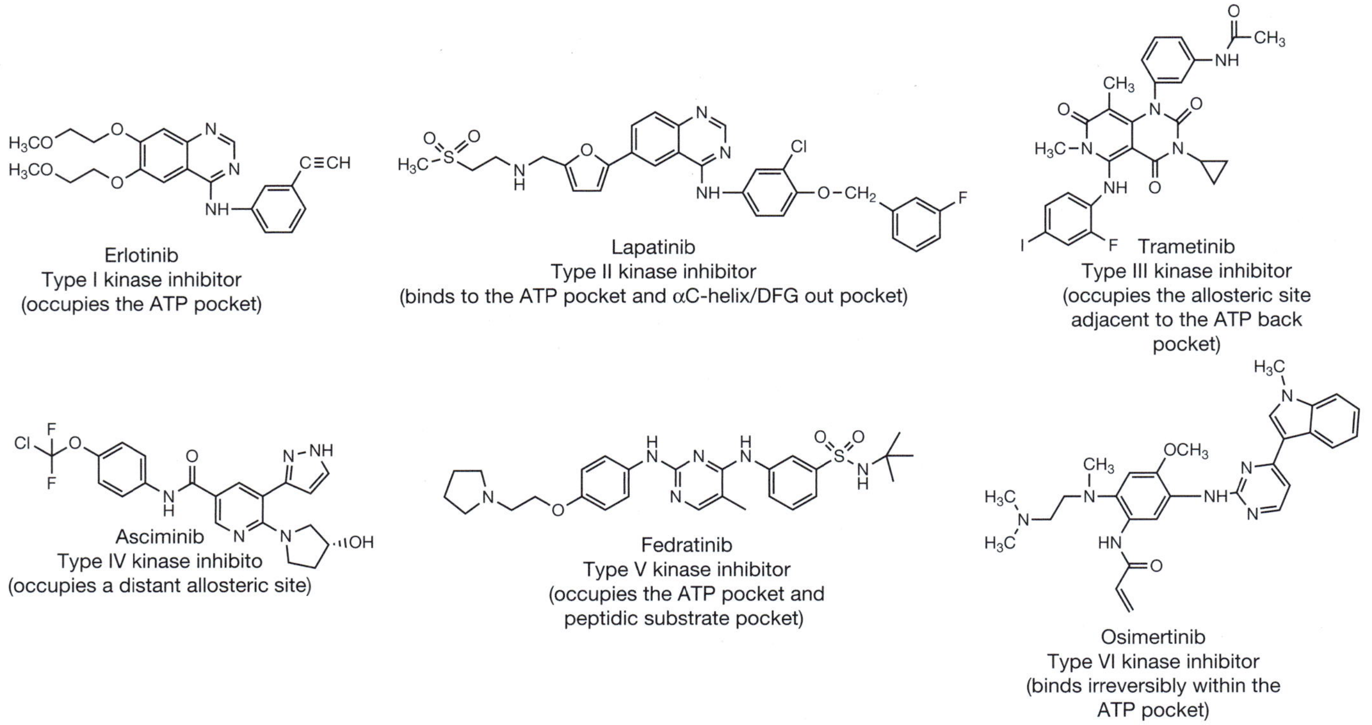

Figure 37.3 Representative inhibitors of the six modes of kinase binding. ATP, adenosine triphosphate; DFG, aspartate, phenylalanine, glycine.

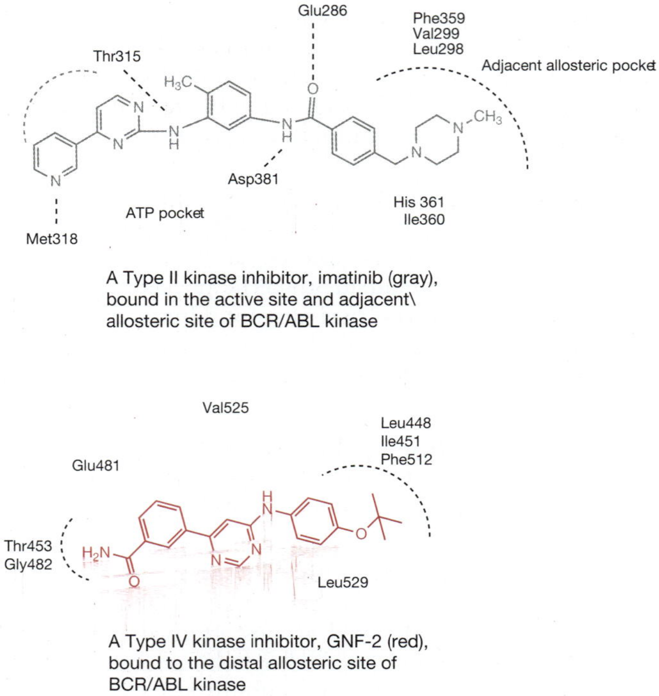

Figure 37.4 Types II and IV inhibitor bound within BCR-ABL kinase. ATP, adenosine triphosphate; BCR-ABL, breakpoint cluster region/ Abelson tyrosine kinase.

adjacent to the active site (allosteric binding). Hydrophobic, π stacking, and hydrogen-bonding are essential for inhibitor affinity and potency. In addition, with ATP bound in the adjacent pocket, electrostatic interactions between the inhibitor and the anionic terminal phosphate of ATP, and/or charged or polar residues lining the catalytic site, are often possible.

Type IV Inhibitors. Type IV kinase inhibitors seek out an allosteric binding site that is distant from the ATP-binding site. Since they bind at a distance from the adenine pocket, type IV inhibitors do not have any significant interactions with ATP.[11,86,87] The BCR-ABL kinase inhibitors GNF-2 (investigational) and asciminib (approved in 2021) are examples of type IV ligands. Imatinib, a type II inhibitor that occupies the active site and an adjacent allosteric pocket, and GNF-2, a type IV inhibitor that occupies a distal allosteric pocket, are shown bound to BCR-ABL kinase in Figure 37.4.

Type V Inhibitor. Type V kinase inhibitors are bisubstrate ligands that span both substrate-binding sites, the ATP pocket, and the peptidic substrate pocket (Fig. 37.5).[86,88] The multikinase inhibitor fedratinib has been suggested to bind to target enzymes as a bisubstrate inhibitor.

Type VI Inhibitors. Type VI inhibitors (eg, osimertinib) are irreversible ligands that form covalent bonds within the ATP pocket. These electrophilic kinase inhibitors contain a Michael-alkylating moiety that allows them to act irreversibly through covalent bond formation with a nucleophilic cysteine residue that flanks the ATP-binding site (see Fig. 37.5 and 37.6).

Structural Elements. Kinase inhibitors can also be classified based on their heterocyclic scaffolds, which may be monocyclic (eg, osimertinib, imatinib) or contain two fused rings (eg, gefitinib, neratinib, alectinib) (Fig. 37.6). Intramolecular hydrogen bonding can be intentionally embedded within the inhibitor structures to stabilize bioactive conformations. While uncommon, larger heteroaromatic scaffolds, including macrocycles, can also be employed.[87] Macrocyclic kinase inhibitors (eg, lorlatinib) bind to the ATP-binding pocket (type I) and include 12-membered rings.[90,91] Other natural product macrocyclic-targeted therapies are known (eg, everolimus, an mTOR inhibitor), but they are not classified as macrocyclic kinase inhibitors. Kinase inhibitors have a balance of lipophilic and hydrophilic groups to allow for oral bioavailability.[1,2,25-28] Lipophilic functional groups are necessary for hydrophobic interactions within the ATP pocket. Polar functional groups engage in hydrogen bonding interactions with residues within the hinge region. In addition, almost all kinase inhibitors include an ionizable functional group oriented toward the enzyme's solvent interface, which confers water solubility to balance the inhibitor's hydrophobicity.

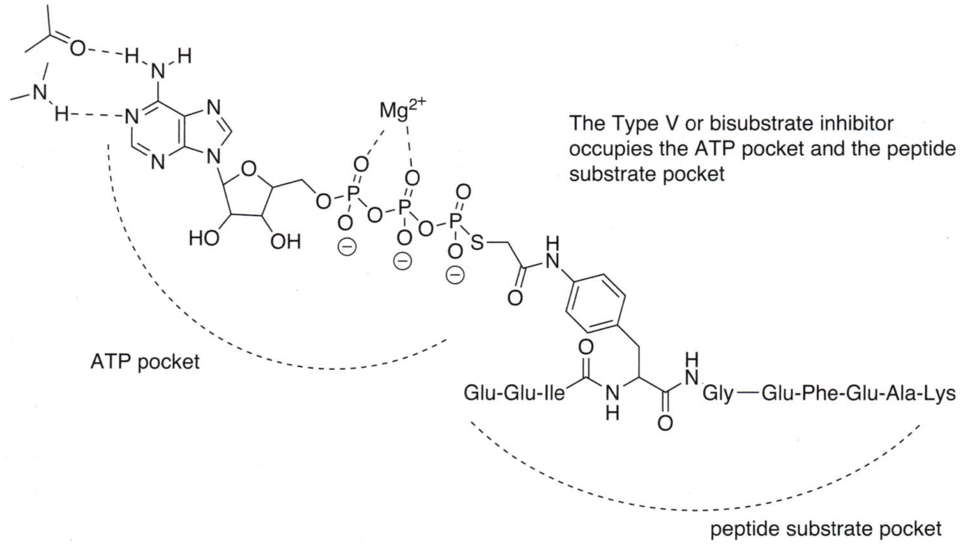

Figure 37.5 Type V inhibitor bound within SRC kinase. ATP, adenosine triphosphate.

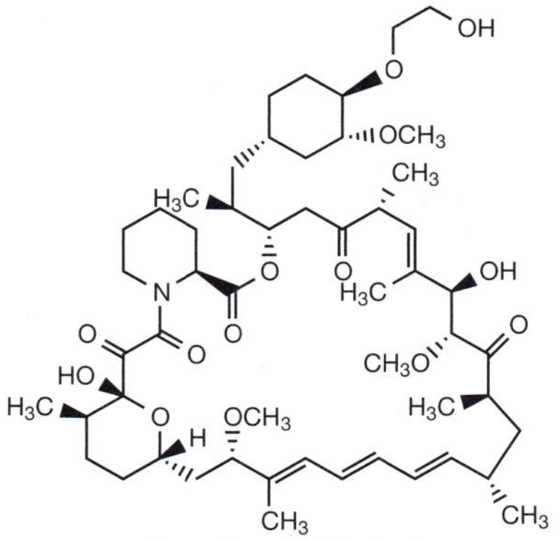

Everolimus (Afinitor)
Macrolide (natural product derivative)

Pharmacokinetics and Metabolism-Based Drug-Drug Interactions

Tables 37.5 through 37.7 list the pharmacokinetic properties of kinase inhibitors, including dosage form, time to peak plasma concentration (T_{max}), elimination half-life ($T_{1/2}$), protein binding, and route of administration. All kinase inhibitors are orally bioavailable, although the rate and extent of absorption can vary based on the presence or absence of food.[92-94] To maximize absorption, patients must be counseled on whether to take their medication in a fed or fasted state. Kinase inhibitors typically show high plasma protein binding, which leads to a prolonged presence in the body and possibly decreased availability at the site of action.[92-94] The drugs have elimination half-lives of 12 to 24 hours, and most require once-daily oral administration.

An acidic pH is necessary for the absorption of some kinase inhibitors. An increase in gastric pH due to concurrent administration of PPIs resulting in achlorhydria has caused a decrease in the absorption of some TKIs (eg, neratinib; Fig. 37.6), which compromises efficacy.[95] Coadministration of antacids, H_2 antagonists, or PPIs with TKIs should be separated by at least 2 hours or, ideally, avoided altogether. Conversely, drinking acidic beverages such as cola with TKIs, dasatinib, or erlotinib has resulted in increased absorption of the inhibitor, even when PPIs were coadministered.[96]

The TKIs are commonly metabolized by CYP3A4. The metabolism for dasatinib, a member of the BCR-ABL inhibitor class, is shown in Figure 37.7. All phase I metabolites retain activity, but since they represent only 5% of the area under the concentration curve (AUC), their clinical relevance is questionable. Of potential importance to dasatinib's toxicity profile is the ability of the CYP-generated *p*-hydroxylated metabolite to oxidize to a potentially

Table 37.5 Mechanism of Action and Selected Pharmacokinetic Properties for Therapies Targeting Oncofusion Drivers

Drug	MOA	Dosage Form	T_{max} (h)	$T_{1/2}$ (h)	Protein Binding (%)	Administration
ALK Inhibitors						
Alectinib	ALK-EML4 inhibitor	Capsule	4	33	>99	Oral, administer with food
Brigatinib	ALK-EML4 inhibitor	Tablet	1-4	25	66	Oral, food independent
Ceritinib	ALK-EML4 inhibitor	Capsule	4-6	41 (fasted)	97	Oral, administer with food
Crizotinib	ALK-EML4 inhibitor	Capsule	4-6	42	91	Oral, food independent
Lorlatinib	ALK-EML4 inhibitor	Tablet	0.5-4	24	66	Oral, food independent
BCR-ABL Kinase Inhibitors						
Asciminib	T315I BCR-ABL inhibitor	Tablet	2-3	5.5	97	Oral, administer on empty stomach
Bosutinib	BCR-ABL inhibitor	Tablet	6	22-27	94	Oral, administer with food
Dasatinib	BCR-ABL inhibitor	Tablet	0.5-6	3-5	96	Oral, food independent
Imatinib	BCR-ABL inhibitor	Tablet	2-4	18	95	Oral, administer with food
Nilotinib	BCR-ABL inhibitor	Capsule	3	17	98	Oral, administer on empty stomach
Ponatinib	T315I BCR-ABL inhibitor	Tablet	≤6	12-66	<99	Oral, food independent

ALK, anaplastic lymphoma kinase; ALL, acute lymphoid leukemia; AML, acute myeloid leukemia; BCR-ABL, breakpoint cluster region/Abelson tyrosine kinase; EML4, echinoderm microtubule–associated protein; MOA, mechanism of action; $T_{1/2}$, elimination half-life; T_{max}, time to peak plasma concentration.

Table 37.6 Mechanism of Action and Selected Pharmacokinetic Properties of Therapies Targeting Signaling Pathways

Drug	MOA	Dosage Form	T_{max} (h)	$T_{1/2}$ (h)	Protein Binding (%)	Administration
BCL2 Inhibitors						
Venetoclax	Apoptosis inducer	Tablet	5-8	26	>99	Administer with food
BRAF/MEK Inhibitors						
Binimetinib	MEK inhibitor (RAS/RAF/MEK pathway)	Tablet	1-2	3-4	97	Oral, food independent
Cobimetinib	MEK inhibitor (RAS/RAF/MEK pathway)	Tablet	2.4	44	46	Oral, food independent
Dabrafenib	BRAF inhibitor V600E/V600K (RAS/RAF/MEK pathway)	Capsule, tablet	2	8 (parent)	>99	Administer on empty stomach
Encorafenib	BRAF inhibitor V600E/V600K (RAS/RAF/MEK pathway)	Capsule	2	4	86	Oral, food independent
Trametinib	MEK inhibitor (RAS/RAF/MEK pathway)	Solution/tablet	1.5	4-5 d	97	Administer on empty stomach
Vemurafenib	BRAF inhibitor V600E/V600K (RAS/RAF/MEK pathway)	Tablet	3	57	>99	Oral, food independent, administer doses 12 h apart
BTK Inhibitors						
Acalabrutinib	BTK inhibitor (B-cell signaling pathway)	Capsule	0.75	0.6-2.8	97.5	Oral, food independent
Ibrutinib	BTK inhibitor (B-cell signaling pathway)	Tablet, capsule	1-2 (fasted) 4 (fed)	4-6	97	Oral, food independent
Pirtobrutinib	BTK inhibitor (B-cell signaling pathway)	Tablet	2	19	96	Oral, food independent
Zanubrutinib	BTK inhibitor (B-cell signaling pathway)	Capsule	2	2-4	94	Oral, food independent
EGFR/HER2 Inhibitors						
Afatinib	mEGFR inhibitor (RAS/RAF/MEK pathway inhibitor)	Tablet	2-5	37	95	Administer on empty stomach
Dacomitinib	mEGFR inhibitor (RAS/RAF/MEK pathway)	Tablet	2-24 (~ 6)	70	98	Oral, food independent
Erlotinib	mEGFR inhibitor (RAS/RAF/MEK pathway inhibitor)	Tablet	4	36	93	Administer on empty stomach
Gefitinib	mEGFR inhibitor (RAS/RAF/MEK pathway inhibitor)	Tablet	3-7	48	90	Oral, food independent
Lapatinib	HER2 inhibitor (RAS/RAF/MEK pathway)	Tablet	4	24	>99	Administer on empty stomach
Neratinib	HER2 inhibitor (RAS/RAF/MEK pathway)	Tablet	2-8	7-17	>99	Administer with food
Osimertinib	mEGFR inhibitor (RAS/RAF/MEK pathway)	Tablet	3-24	48	95	Oral, food independent

Table 37.6 Mechanism of Action and Selected Pharmacokinetic Properties of Therapies Targeting Signaling Pathways (*continued*)

Drug	MOA	Dosage Form	T_{max} (h)	$T_{1/2}$ (h)	Protein Binding (%)	Administration
JAK Inhibitors						
Ruxolitinib	JAK2 inhibitor	Tablet	1-2	3	97	Oral, food independent
Fedratinib	mFLT3/JAK2 inhibitor	Capsule	2-4	114 (41)	>92	Oral, food independent
Pacritinib	mFLT3/JAK2 inhibitor	Capsule	4-5	28	99	Oral, food independent
mFLT3 Inhibitors						
Gilteritinib	mFLT3 inhibitor	Tablet	4-6	113	94	Oral, food independent
Midostaurin	mFLT3 inhibitor	Capsule	1-3 (fasted) 2.5-3 (fed)	21	>99.8	Administer with food
Quizartinib	mFLT3 inhibitor	Tablet	2-8	81	>99	Oral, food independent
mIDH Inhibitors						
Enasidenib	mIDH inhibitor	Tablet	4	8 d	98	Oral, food independent
Ivosidenib	mIDH inhibitor	Tablet	3	58	92-96	Oral, food independent
Olutasidenib	mIDH inhibitor	Capsule	4	67	93	Oral, administer on empty stomach, avoid food 2 h prior and 1 h after taking the drug
mKRAS Inhibitors						
Adagrasib	mKRAS inhibitor (RAS/RAF/MEK pathway)	Tablet	6	23	98	Oral, food independent
Sotorasib	mKRAS inhibitor (RAS/RAF/MEK pathway)	Tablet	1	5	89	Oral, food independent
NF-κB Pathway Inhibitors						
Bortezomib	Inhibit IκB degradation (NF-κB pathway)	IV, SC	N/A	9-15	83	IV, SC (pH 2-6.5)
Carfilzomib	Inhibit IκB degradation (NF-κB pathway)	IV	N/A	<1	97	IV (pH 3.5)
Ixazomib	Inhibit IκB degradation (NF-κB pathway)	Capsule	1	9.5 d	99	Oral, food independent
Lenalidomide	Multitargeted indirect inhibition of NF-κB (NF-κB pathway)	Capsule	0.5-6	3-5	30	Oral, food independent
Pomalidomide	Multitargeted indirect inhibition of NF-κB (NF-κB pathway)	Capsule	2-3	7-8	12-44	Oral, food independent
Thalidomide	Multitargeted indirect inhibition of NF-κB (NF-κB pathway)	Capsule	2-5	5-7	55-66	Administer at bedtime following the evening meal
PI3K/AKT/mTOR Pathway Inhibitors						
Alpelisib	PI3Kα inhibitor (PI3K/AKT/mTOR pathway)	Tablet	2-4	8-9	89	Oral, food independent
Capivasertib	AKT inhibitor (PI3K/AKT/mTOR pathway)	Tablet	1-2	8-9	22	Oral, food independent

(continued)

Table 37.6 Mechanism of Action and Selected Pharmacokinetic Properties of Therapies Targeting Signaling Pathways (*continued*)

Drug	MOA	Dosage Form	T_{max} (h)	$T_{1/2}$ (h)	Protein Binding (%)	Administration
Duvelisib	PI3Kδ/γ inhibitor (PI3K/AKT/mTOR pathway)	Capsule	1-2	4-5	>98	Oral, food independent
Everolimus	mTOR inhibitor (PI3K/AKT/mTOR pathway)	Tablet	1-2	30	74	Oral, food independent
Idelalisib	PI3Kδ/γ inhibitor (PI3K/AKT/mTOR pathway)	Tablet	1.5	8.2	≥84	Oral, food independent
Temsirolimus	mTOR inhibitor (PI3K/AKT/mTOR pathway)	IV	0.5-2	17	N/A	IV, administer using non-DEHP tubing
Retinoic Acid Receptor Binder						
Tretinoin	RAR binder (inhibits RAR/RXR interactions)	Capsule	1-2	0.5-2	>95	Oral, food independent

AKT, protein kinase B; AML, acute myeloid leukemia; APL, acute promyelocytic leukemia; ATRA, all-*trans* retinoic acid; BC, breast cancer; BCL-2, B-cell lymphoma-2; BRAF, B-rapidly accelerated fibrosarcoma; BTK, Bruton tyrosine kinase; CLL, chronic lymphocytic leukemia; CRC, colorectal cancer; DEHP, diethylhexyl phthalate; EGFR, epidermal growth factor receptor kinase; FLT3-ITD, FMS-like tyrosine kinase 3 internal tandem duplication; HER2, human epidermal growth factor 2; HR, hormone receptor; IV, intravenous; JAK, Janus kinase; MCL, mantle cell lymphoma; mFLT3, mutant FMS-like tyrosine kinase 3; mIDH1, mutant isocitrate dehydrogenase 1; mIDH2, mutant isocitrate dehydrogenase 2; MM, multiple myeloma; MOA, mechanism of action; mTOR, mammalian target of rapamycin; NF-κB, nuclear factor kappa B; NSCLC, non–small cell lung cancer; PI3K, phosphatidylinositol 3 kinase; PTEN, phosphatase and tensin homolog deleted on chromosome 10; RAR, retinoic acid receptor; SLL, small lymphocytic lymphoma; SMO, Smoothened; $T_{1/2}$, elimination half-life; T_{max}, time to peak plasma concentration; wtKRAS, wild-type Kirsten rat sarcoma.

Table 37.7 Mechanism of Action and Selected Pharmacokinetic Properties for Angiogenesis Inhibitors and Checkpoint Kinase Inhibitors

Drug	MOA	Dosage Form	T_{max} (h)	$T_{1/2}$ (h)	Protein Binding (%)	Administration
CDK4/6 Inhibitors						
Abemaciclib	CDK4/6 inhibitor	Tablet	8	18.3	96	Oral, food independent
Palbociclib	CDK4/6 inhibitor	Tablet/capsule	6-12	29	85	Oral, food independent
Ribociclib	CDK4/6 inhibitor	Tablet	1-4	30-55	70	Oral, food independent
Trilaciclib	CDK4/6 inhibitor	IV	NA	14	69	IV, administer 4 h prior to the start of chemotherapy
FGFR Inhibitors						
Erdafitinib	FGFR inhibitor	Tablet	2-6	59	99	Oral, food independent
Futibatinib	FGFR inhibitor	Tablet	2	2.9	95	Oral, food independent
Infigratinib	FGFR inhibitor	Capsule	6	33.5	97	Administer on empty stomach, avoid or space from proton-pump inhibitors, H_2 antagonists and antacids
Pemigatinib	FGFR inhibitor	Tablet	1	15	91	Oral, food independent
PDGFRα/Kit Inhibitors						
Avapritinib	PDGFRα/Kit inhibitor	Tablet	2-4	32-57	99	Administer on empty stomach
Ripretinib	PDGFRα inhibitor	Tablet	4	15	>99	Oral, food independent

Table 37.7 Mechanism of Action and Selected Pharmacokinetic Properties for Angiogenesis Inhibitors and Checkpoint Kinase Inhibitors (*continued*)

Drug	MOA	Dosage Form	T_{max} (h)	$T_{1/2}$ (h)	Protein Binding (%)	Administration
VEGFR Inhibitors						
Axitinib	Multitargeted VEGFR inhibitor	Tablet	2.5-4	2.5-6.1	>99	Oral, food independent
Fruquintinib	Multitargeted VEGFR inhibitor	Capsule	2	42	95	Oral, food independent
Lenvatinib	Multitargeted VEGFR inhibitor	Capsule	1-4	28	98-99	Oral, food independent
Pazopanib	Multitargeted VEGFR inhibitor	Tablet	2-4	31	>99	Administer on empty stomach
Regorafenib	Multitargeted VEGFR inhibitor	Tablet	4	28	99.5	Administer with food (low fat)
Sorafenib	Multitargeted VEGFR inhibitor	Tablet	3	25-48	99.5	Administer on empty stomach
Sunitinib	Multitargeted VEGFR inhibitor	Capsule	6-12	40-60	95	Oral, food independent
Tivozanib	Multitargeted VEGFR inhibitor	Capsule	111	10	>99	Oral, food independent

CDK, cyclin-dependent kinase; FGFR, fibroblast growth factor receptor kinase; KIT, stem cell factor receptor tyrosine kinase; MOA, mechanism of action; PDGFRα, platelet-derived growth factor receptor kinase α; $T_{1/2}$, elimination half-life; T_{max}, time to peak plasma concentration; VEGFR, vascular endothelial growth factor receptor kinase.

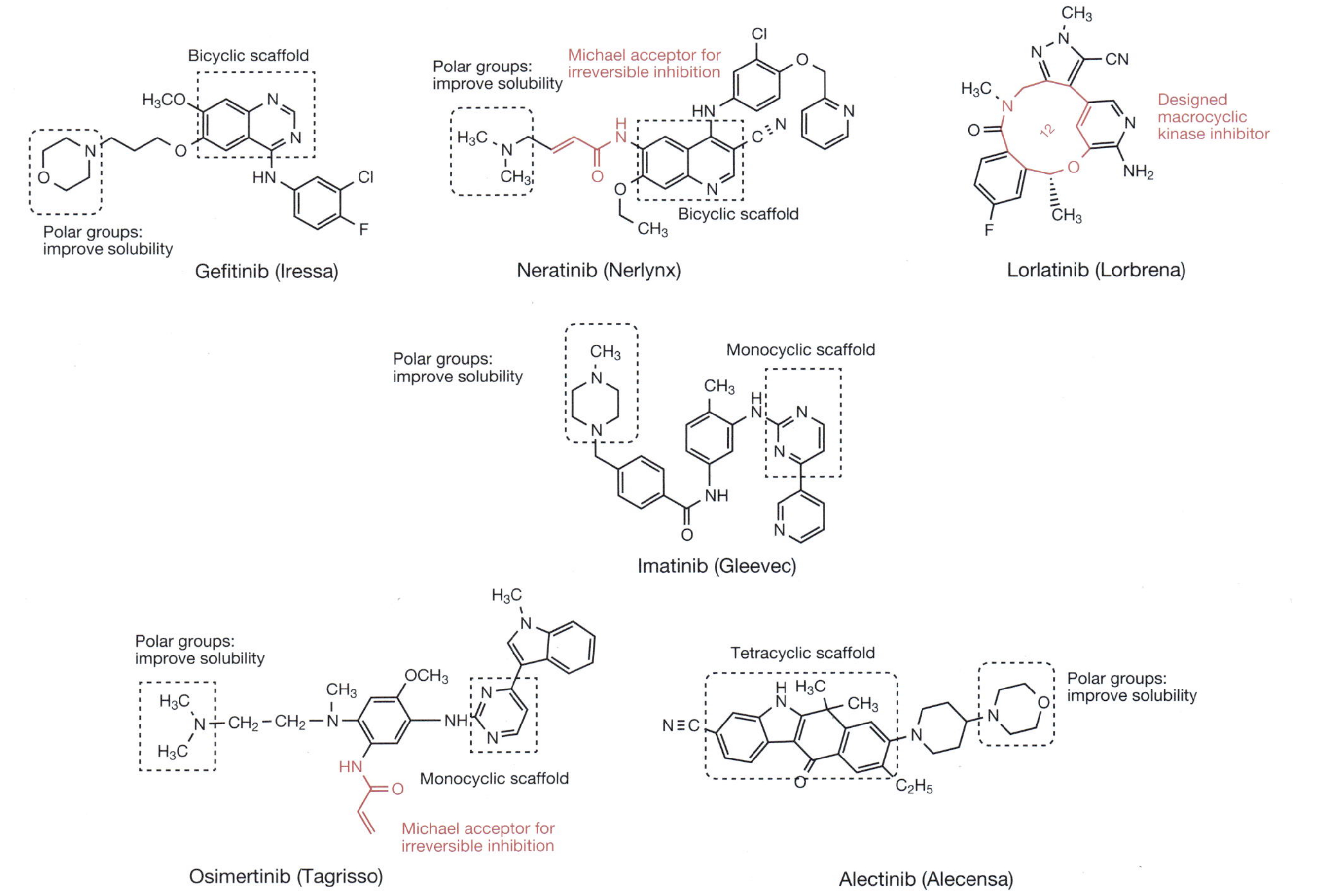

Figure 37.6 Structural elements of kinase inhibitors.

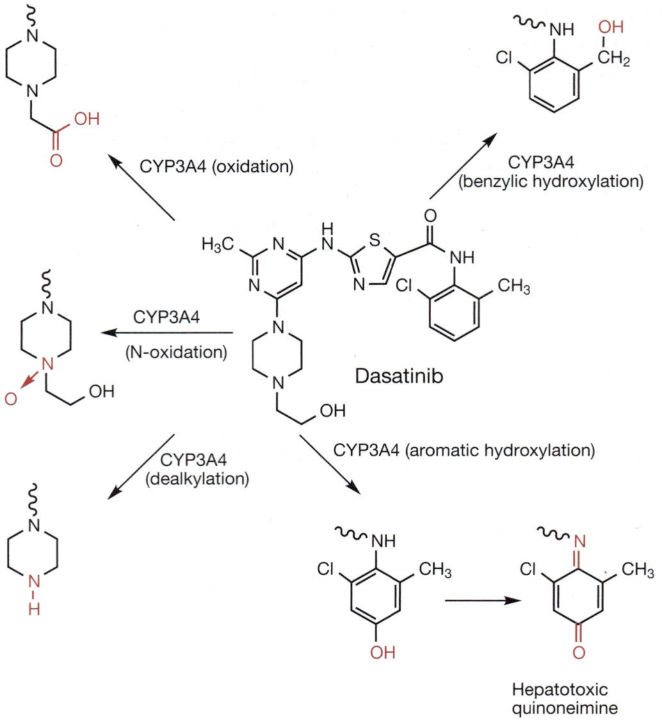

Figure 37.7 Dasatinib metabolism.

hepatotoxic quinoneimine, a property this TKI shares with several others that contain an aniline moiety vulnerable to CYP-mediated *p*-hydroxylation.[97-99] Hepatotoxicity results when the highly electrophilic quinoneimine metabolite is attacked by powerful nucleophiles (eg, SH groups of Cys residues) found on hepatocytes cell membranes.

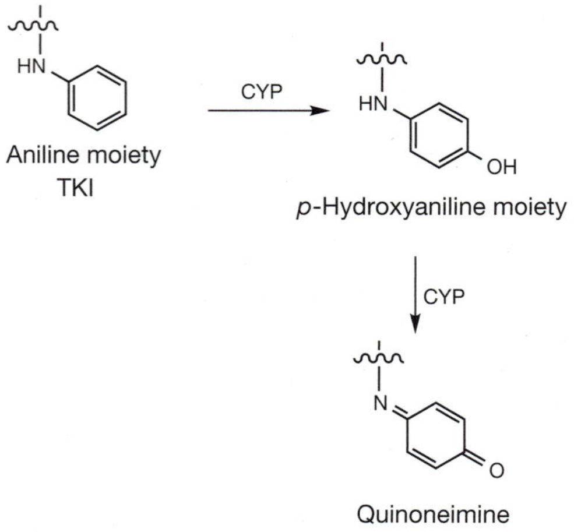

Some (but not all) aniline-containing TKIs where the *p*-position is blocked by a halogen can undergo oxidative dehalogenation followed by hydroxylation to the labile *p*-hydroxyaniline (eg, gefitinib; see Fig. 37.6).[98] The *o*-Cl group increases the electrophilic character of the resultant quinoneimine, making it more vulnerable to attack by reduced glutathione (GSH), and after stores of that scavenger are exhausted, cell nucleophiles (eg, Cys residues).

Several TKIs generate active metabolites that contribute to adverse effects or unpredictable pharmacokinetics (Fig. 37.8). The generation of active metabolites also allows for the once-daily dosing seen for the kinase inhibitor drug class.

The CYP-mediated metabolism for kinase inhibitors leads to a high risk of DDIs with 3A4 substrates, inducers, and inhibitors, including grapefruit juice. Many TKIs inhibit one or more CYP isoforms,[92-94] and the concomitant use of strong CYP inhibitors or inducers can lead to increased adverse effects from both agents. Caution against coadministration of drugs and foods that strongly impact CYP3A4 activity is necessary, and dose adjustments are required if coadministration cannot be avoided.[92-94] Grapefruit juice must be avoided with the kinase inhibitor, cobimetinib, and therapy modifications are needed for erlotinib. In addition to grapefruit juice, consumption of Seville oranges and juice (which contain naringin, one of the intestinal CYP3A4-inhibiting compounds in grapefruit) is contraindicated. The TKIs may also be substrates or inhibitors of cellular efflux pumps like Pgp and breast cancer resistance protein (BCRP) that can impact their therapeutic effects. Gefitinib is a Pgp substrate, and this transporter is believed to play a role in resistance.[92-94] All TKIs are excreted predominantly in the feces.

Adverse Effects

Most adverse effects of kinase inhibitors are mild in comparison to classic chemotherapy on account of their cytostatic effects.[73,74] The mild adverse effects include diarrhea, skin rash, gastrointestinal (GI) disturbances, fever, and fatigue. However, serious adverse effects may also be seen. These adverse effects may be due to the inhibition of the wild-type (wt)/nononcogenic kinases and corresponding function or may be due to on-target mechanistic adverse effects. Examples of serious mechanism-based adverse effects include QT prolongation for HER2 inhibitors, bradycardia for ALK inhibitors, acneiform skin rash for EGFR inhibitors due to effects on wtEGFR, and hypertension for VEGFR2 inhibitors. Metabolism-based adverse effects may be related to the formation of hepatotoxic metabolites as described earlier and/or by inhibiting the metabolism of coadministered CYP-dependent drugs. The EGFR inhibitors are associated with a risk of hepatotoxicity and produce the hepatotoxic quinoneimine metabolite under the actions of CYP3A4. Nonselective action of kinase inhibitors on off-target kinases can also lead to unwanted toxicity, all of which can be exacerbated based on the patient general health status, as well as specific cardiac, respiratory, renal, or hepatic function. Adverse effects and boxed warnings for kinase inhibitors are detailed in Tables 37.8 and 37.9.

Selectivity and Resistance

All kinase enzymes utilize ATP as their phosphate-donating substrate. Consequently, significant sequence homology has been observed among kinases, and a recurring challenge for kinase inhibitors has been selectivity for the target kinase over the human kinome.[73,74] Kinase inhibitors also suffer from challenges of acquired resistance.[78,79] Resistance to kinase inhibitors is multifaceted, with predominant resistance pathways mediated through affinity-attenuating mutations or conformational changes in the kinase enzyme.

A key contributor toward the development of resistance is a gatekeeper mutation that alters inhibitor binding in the kinase active site.[100] A gatekeeper mutation may involve replacing a smaller amino acid with a bulkier residue that sterically hinders inhibitor binding. Alternatively, the gatekeeper mutation may induce a conformational change that favors the binding of the ATP substrate over ATP-competitive inhibitors within the kinase. Lastly, gatekeeper mutations may stimulate the development of a hydrophobic spine that leads to a smaller and a more closed inactive conformation that precludes inhibitor binding. Additional resistance mechanisms include upregulation of parallel pathways that accomplish the biochemical goals of the inhibited kinase, epigenetic modification of the tumor cell's phenotype, and negative influences on inhibitor pharmacokinetics or metabolic stability.[46]

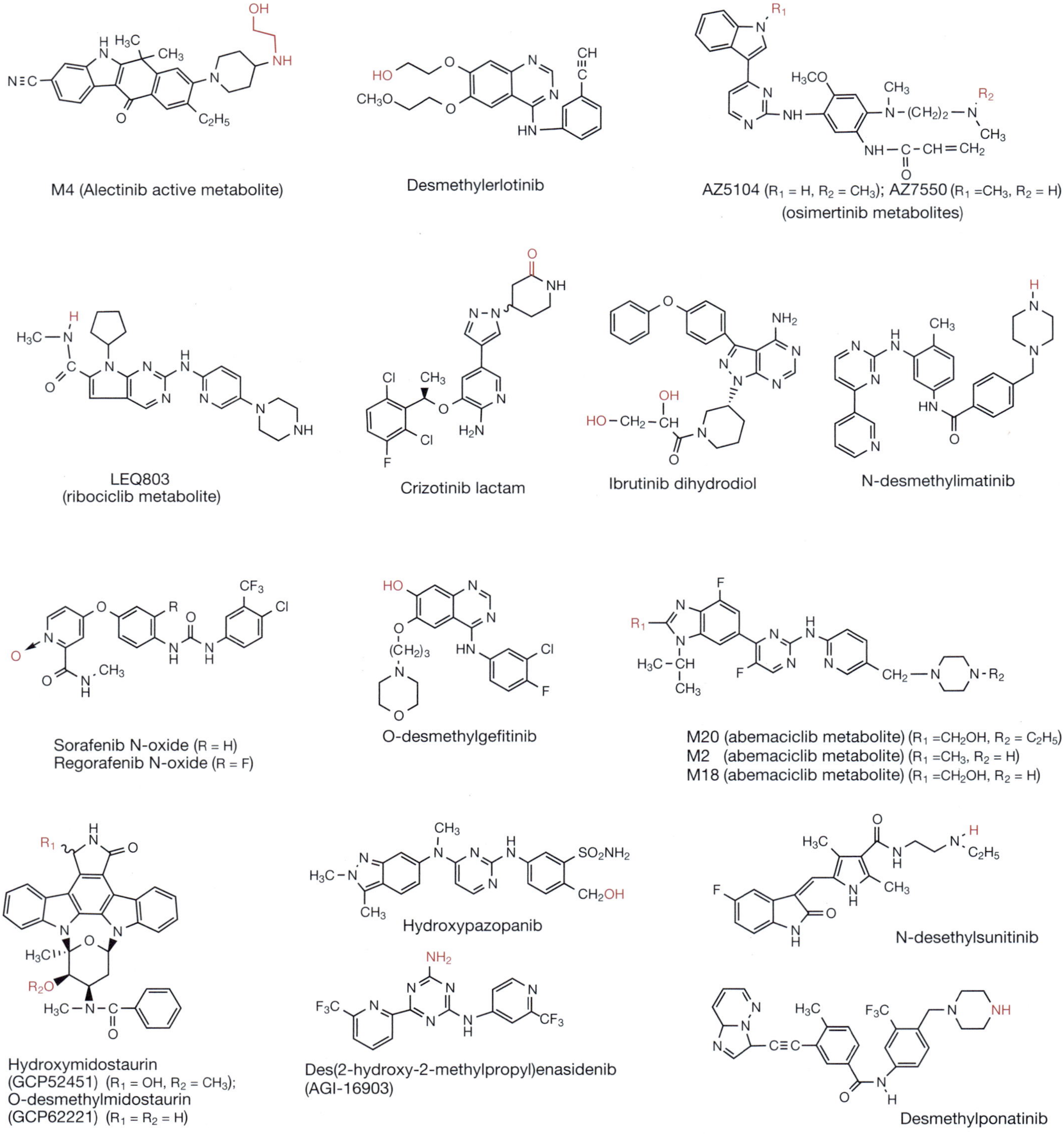

Figure 37.8 Active metabolites of kinase inhibitors (part A)

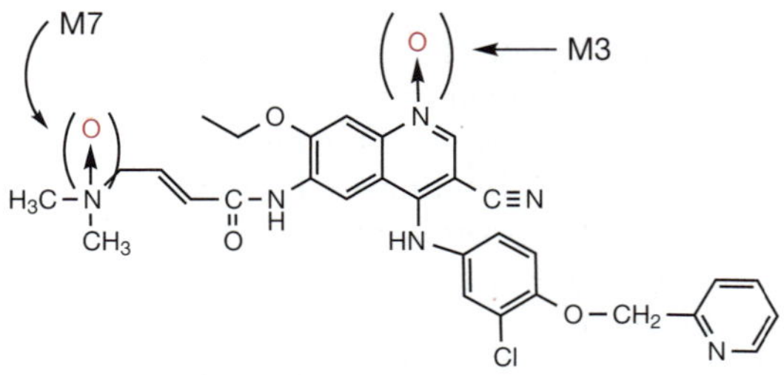

Neratinib N-oxide metabolites (M3 & M7)

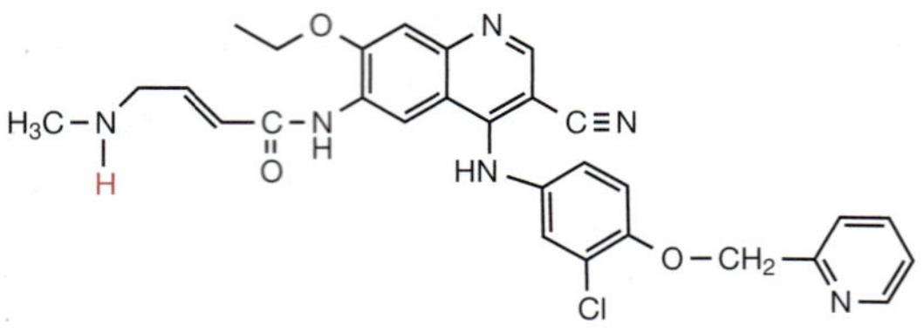

Desmethylneratinib (M6)

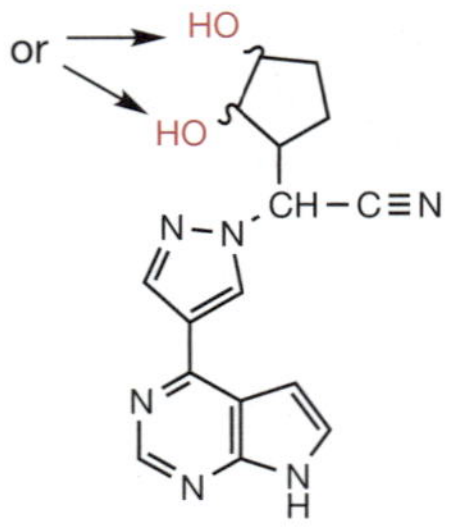

2-Hydroxyruxolitinib
3-Hydroxyruxolitinib

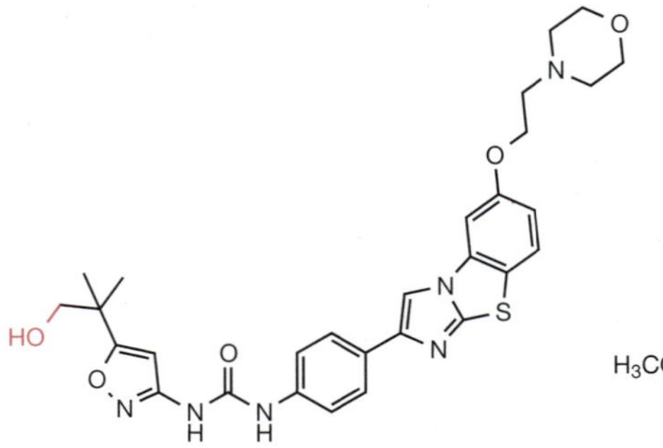

Quizartinib metabolite
(AC886)

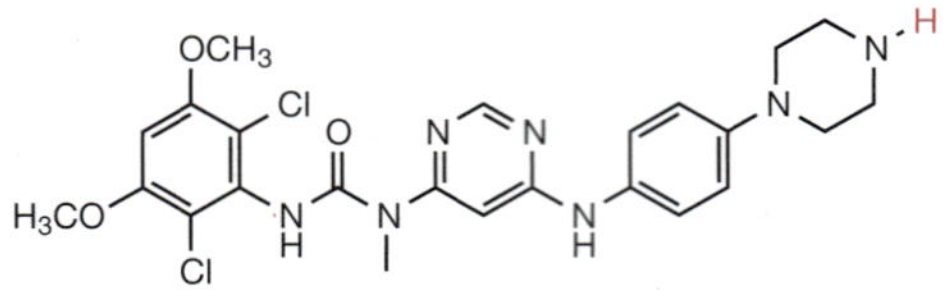

Infigratinib metabolite
(BHS697)

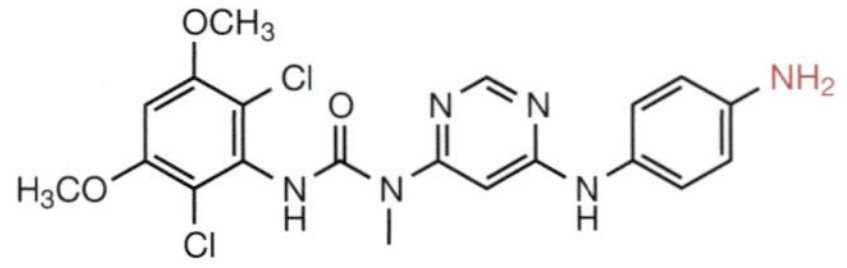

Infigratinib metabolite
(CQM157)

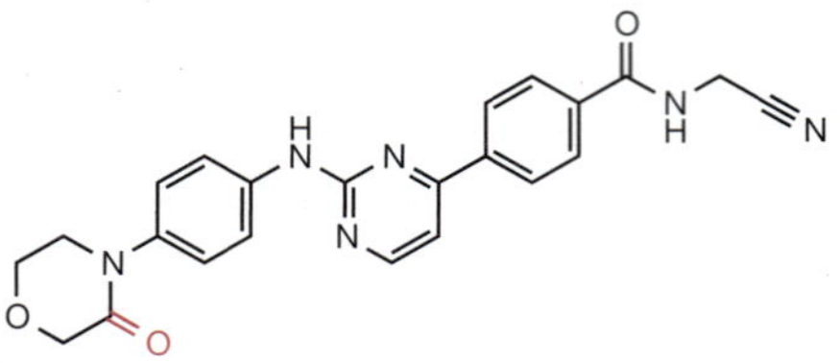

Momelotinib metabolite (morpholino lactam M21)

Figure 37.8 Active metabolites of kinase inhibitors (part B)

Table 37.8 Drug Class–Specific Adverse Effects for Targeted Therapies

Drug Class	Adverse Effects
ALK inhibitors	Bradycardia, edema, constipation, anemia, hyperbilirubinemia, elevated creatinine levels, cognitive dysfunction
AKT inhibitors	Hyperglycemia, increased serum triglycerides, hypokalemia, hypocalcemia, neutropenia, skin rash, diarrhea
BCL-2 inhibitors	Tumor lysis syndrome, neutropenia, thrombocytopenia, electrolyte imbalance (hypocalcemia, hyperkalemia, hypophosphatemia), infection risk
BCR-ABL kinase inhibitors	Myelosuppression, cardiovascular complications (QT prolongation, heart failure), hepatotoxicity, pancreatitis, arterial thrombosis
BRAF/MEK inhibitors	Alopecia, hyperkeratosis, cutaneous secondary malignancies, diarrhea, arthralgia, increased serum creatinine, hyperglycemia
BTK inhibitors	Heart failure, atrial flutter, neutropenia, thrombocytopenia, anemia, infection risk, hemorrhage risk, hypertension, secondary malignancies
CDK4/6 inhibitors	Transient neutropenia, decreased WBC, lymphocytopenia, anemia, abdominal pain, elevated liver enzymes, infection risk

Table 37.8 Drug Class–Specific Adverse Effects for Targeted Therapies (*continued*)

Drug Class	Adverse Effects
FGFR-TKIs	Nail bed disorders, hyperphosphatemia, vision disturbances, PPE, alopecia, anemia, increased hepatic enzymes, diarrhea, constipation, stomatitis, electrolyte disturbances
HDAC inhibitors	Severe diarrhea, myelosuppression, cardiovascular toxicities (arrhythmia, peripheral edema), infection risk, electrolyte abnormalities
HER2-TKIs	Severe diarrhea, hepatotoxicity, PPE
Immunomodulators	Venous thromboembolism, neutropenia, thrombocytopenia, embryo-fetal toxicity (birth defects)
JAK2 inhibitors	Headache, dizziness and bruising, encephalopathy, anemia, thrombocytopenia, neutropenia, infection, diarrhea
mEGFR-TKIs	Skin rash, cough, interstitial lung disease, elevated liver enzymes, anemia, diarrhea
mFLT3-TKIs	Differentiation syndrome, arthralgia, dyspnea, infection risk, edema, diarrhea, electrolyte abnormalities
mIDH inhibitors	Differentiation syndrome, hypocalcemia, hypokalemia, hepatotoxicity (increased serum bilirubin), diarrhea
mKRAS inhibitors	Skin rash, edema, anemia, proteinuria, elevated liver enzymes, musculoskeletal pain, diarrhea
PARP inhibitors	Myelosuppression, alopecia, edema
PDGFRα/Kit inhibitors	Edema, alopecia, cutaneous malignancy, wound healing complications, CNS effects (cognitive defects), GI, endocrine and metabolic disturbances
PI3K inhibitors	Hyperglycemia, edema, alopecia, lymphocytopenia, hepatotoxicity (elevated liver enzymes), pneumonia, neutropenia, increased creatinine levels, severe diarrhea, skin rash
Proteasome inhibitors	Peripheral neuropathy, constipation, neutropenia, thrombocytopenia
Tretinoin	Differentiation syndrome, leukocytosis, dyspnea
VEGFR-TKIs	Wound healing complications, hypertension, PPE, proteinuria, thromboembolic events, increased creatinine levels

AKT, protein kinase B; ALK, anaplastic lymphoma kinase; BCL-2, B-cell lymphoma-2; BCR-ABL, breakpoint cluster region/Abelson tyrosine kinase; BRAF, B-rapidly accelerated fibrosarcoma; BTK, Bruton tyrosine kinase; CDK, cyclin-dependent kinase; HDAC, histone deacetylase; HER2, human epidermal growth factor 2; JAK, Janus kinase; mFLT3, mutant FMS-like tyrosine kinase 3; MEK, mitogen-activated protein kinase kinase; mIDH, mutant isocitrate dehydrogenase; mKRAS, mutant Kirsten rat sarcoma; PDGFRα, platelet-derived growth factor receptor kinase α; PI3K, phosphatidylinositol 3 kinase; PPE, palmar-plantar erythrodysesthesia; TKI, tyrosine kinase inhibitor; VEGFR, vascular endothelial growth factor receptor kinase; WBC, white blood cell.

Drug design strategies developed with the goal of minimizing resistance and maximizing target selectivity of kinase inhibitors include targeting new regions of the kinase domain and exploring novel binding interactions within the ATP-binding pocket.

Nonkinase Inhibitors

The nonkinase inhibitor therapeutic class refers to drugs that inhibit specific oncogenic drivers that are not classified biochemically as kinases. Like kinase signaling systems, various nonkinase molecular pathways are implicated in cancer.

Apoptosis, a natural phenomenon, is regulated through proapoptotic and antiapoptotic proteins in the BCL-2 protein family.[37] The BCL-2 protein family is a master regulator of the intrinsic apoptotic signaling pathway and incorporates BCL-2 homology (BH) domains BH1, BH2 and BH3, the latter of which is strictly proapoptotic. The proapoptotic proteins in this family include BCL-2–interacting mediator of cell death (BIM), BCL-2–associated X protein (BAX), and BCL-2 antagonist killer 1 (BAK), while the protein BCL-2 is antiapoptotic. The proapoptotic proteins BIM, BAX, and BAK bind through their BH3 domain to the prosurvival and antiapoptotic protein BCL-2, neutralize it, and initiate programmed cell death as part of healthy cell homeostasis. Dysfunction in BCL-2–mediated apoptotic signaling, where neutralization of BCL-2 does not occur, causes persistent antiapoptotic signaling and increased cancer cell survival.

The transcription factor, NF-κB is another key player in the development of varied cancers.[69,70] NF-κB is an apex regulator of the tumor microenvironment that helps cancer cells avoid immune system–orchestrated destruction, creates an inflammatory environment that allows cancer cells to flourish at the expense of normal cells, and supports tumor angiogenesis. It is a major oncogenic driver for B- and T-cell malignancies, including MM. Enzymes such as HDAC that induce epigenetic modifications, and DNA repair enzymes such as poly(ADP-ribose) polymerase (PARP), are also

Table 37.9 Boxed Warnings for Targeted Therapies

Drug	Boxed Warnings
Duvelisib	Fatal toxicities: infections, colitis/diarrhea, pneumonitis, cutaneous reactions
Enasidenib	Differentiation syndrome
Fedratinib	Encephalopathy
Gilteritinib	Differentiation syndrome
Glasdegib	Embryo/fetal toxicity
Idelalisib	Potentially fatal hepatotoxicity, diarrhea, pneumonitis, infection and intestinal perforation
Ivosidenib	Differentiation syndrome
Lapatinib	Potentially fatal hepatotoxicity
Lenalidomide	Pregnancy, thromboembolic events
Nilotinib	QT-interval prolongation leading to sudden death
Olutasidenib	Differentiation syndrome
Pazopanib	Potentially fatal hepatotoxicity
Pomalidomide	Pregnancy, thromboembolic events
Ponatinib	Vascular occlusion, heart failure, hepatotoxicity, venous thromboembolism
Quizartinib	QT prolongation
Regorafenib	Potentially fatal hepatotoxicity
Sunitinib	Potentially fatal hepatotoxicity
Thalidomide	Pregnancy, thromboembolic events
Tretinoin	Differentiation syndrome, leukocytosis, pregnancy

nonkinase targets for therapeutic intervention in selected cancers. Likewise, the GTPase enzymes that phosphorylate signaling proteins using guanosine triphosphate (GTP) instead of ATP have been classified under non–kinase-targeted therapies. An example of a GTPase and nonkinase molecular target is mKRAS.

The chemical classes of non–kinase-targeted therapies are diverse and include metal chelators such as boronic acid (proteasome inhibitors), hydroxamic acid (HDAC inhibitors), and nicotinamide adenine dinucleotide (NAD^+) mimetics (PARP inhibitors) (Fig. 37.9). Non–kinase-targeted therapies range from orally bioavailable small molecules, such as lenalidomide, olaparib, and vorinostat, to large peptides and injectable drugs such as carfilzomib and romidepsin.[37,40,70] The small molecule non–kinase-targeted therapies share many pharmacokinetic and adverse effect similarities with their kinase inhibitor counterparts. Detailed information

TARGETED THERAPY DRUG NOMENCLATURE

Most kinase inhibitors (eg, mEGFR, HER2, BCR-ABL, ROS proto-oncogene 1 [ROS1], mutant FMS-like tyrosine kinase 3 [mFLT3], JAK, VEGFR, FGFR, PDGFR) include the suffix: inib

Kinase inhibitors with expanded or unique suffixes:

- NTRK inhibitors: trectinib
- BRAF inhibitors: rafenib
- MEK inhibitors: metinib
- PI3K inhibitors: lisib
- mTOR: rolimus
- BTK: brutinib
- CDK: ciclib
- HDAC (hydroxamic acid), enhancer of zeste homolog 2 (EZH2) inhibitors: stat

Nonkinase inhibitors:

- mKRAS inhibitors: rasib
- NF-κB: lidomide
- Proteasome inhibitors: zomib

on chemical and pharmacologic classes, biomarker screening, pharmacokinetic properties, and adverse effect profiles for each subclass within non–kinase-targeted therapies are discussed later and listed in Tables 37.1 through 37.3 and 37.5 through 37.9.

Cancer Biologics

Cancer immunotherapies, also referred to as cancer biologics, include drugs that activate the immune system to drive immune-mediated cancer cell death. The body's own immunochemical surveillance and defense mechanisms are called into play when primary or metastatic neoplastic cells threaten, and immunotherapy bolsters this self-preservation response by activating T lymphocytes designed to destroy invading cancer cells.

Recent years have witnessed a significant increase in approvals of novel cancer immunotherapies. The following discussion focuses on the different classes of cancer immunotherapies and categorizes them based on mechanism of action, chemistry, adverse effect profiles, and therapeutic subclasses. The therapeutic subclasses of cancer biologics, biomarker screening, and therapeutic indications are shown in Table 37.4. Additional details on the chemical properties of cancer biologics can be found in Chapter 38.

Mechanism of Action

All cancer biologics include a mAb as their key component. The mAbs target antigens located on cell surface receptors,[28-32] leading to natural killer cell–mediated destruction of those cells in a process called antibody-dependent cellular cytotoxicity (ADCC). The release of perforin and granzymes from cytoplasmic granules into the cytoplasm of the antibody-bound cell triggers cell lysis. Another potential mechanism of cancer cell destruction

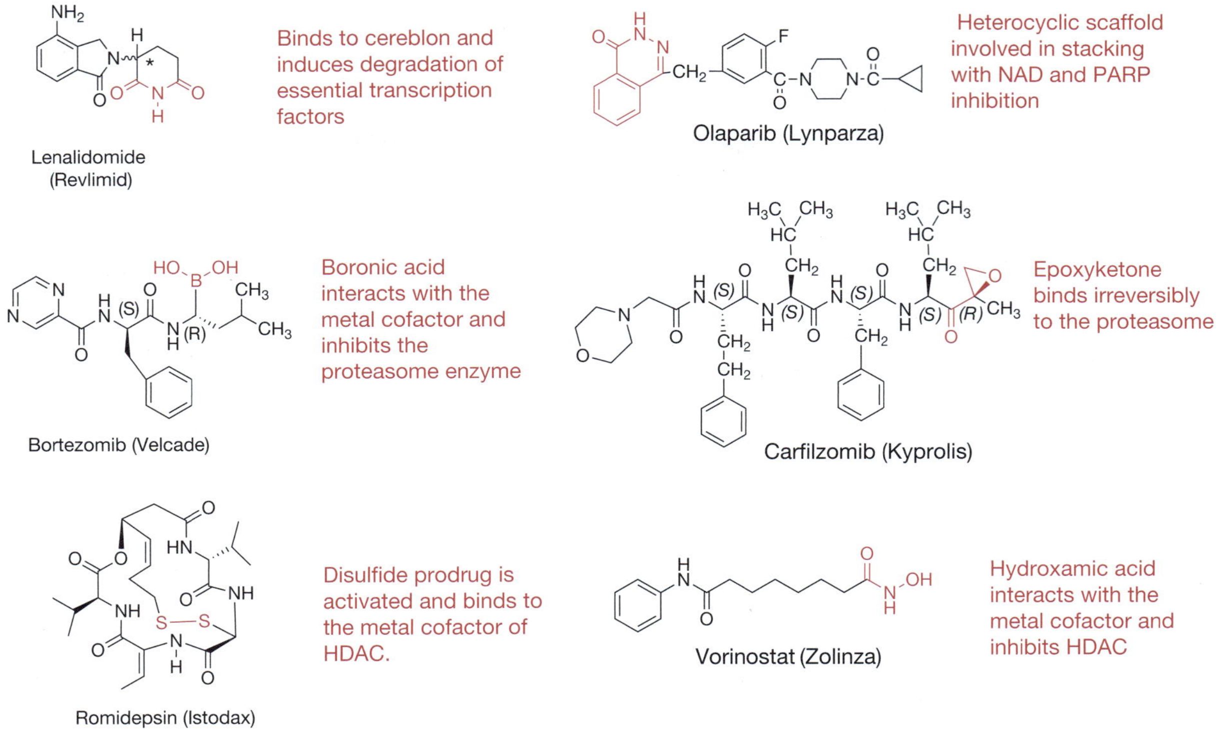

Figure 37.9 Structural elements of nonkinase inhibitors. HDAC, histone deacetylase; PARP, poly(ADP-ribose) polymerase.

involves simply blocking endogenous ligands from binding to the cell surface receptor, which inhibits their function. For example, cetuximab binds to the extracellular domain of EGFR, blocking normal EGFR activation and downstream signaling cascades. In a mechanistic twist, bevacizumab, binds to the growth factor VEGF (the endogenous ligand for VEGFR), preventing it from binding to VEGFR and thereby inhibits angiogenesis.

Immune cells (T cells) may express cell surface receptors that suppress both recognition of abnormal cancer cells and T-cell–mediated cell death. The mAbs bind to these immune cell surface receptors and reactivate immune cell function and surveillance. Pembrolizumab functions in this way, binding to PD-1 receptors expressed on the surface of T cells and restoring T-cell–mediated cell death. Lastly, mAbs conjugated to classic chemotherapeutic agents have been approved as biologics that specifically deliver cytotoxic agents to their target cancer cells. Without the antibody "homing device," the chemotherapeutic would penetrate and destroy healthy cells it encounters on its way to the tumor, leading to potentially severe adverse effects (see Chapter 36). The HER2-targeted antibody-drug conjugate, ado-trastuzumab emtansine, uses the HER2-targeted mAb trastuzumab for the breast cancer cell–specific delivery of the antimitotic agent, emtansine.

Chemical and Pharmacologic Classes

The mAbs are B-cell–derived immunoglobulins (Igs) with a molecular mass of more than 100 kDa. Chimeric mAbs end with a "ximab" suffix and are produced by a fusion of human constant (Fc) and mouse variable (Fv) domains. Humanized mAbs end with a "zumab" suffix and are produced by the insertion of nonhuman antigen–binding regions into a human IgG protein scaffold. The mAbs that are entirely human in origin are termed *human* and end with a "mumab" suffix. mAbs differ in their immunogenicity and corresponding adverse effect profile based on the source of origin.

Antibody (IgG1) elements that are relevant for use in cancer treatment include Fab and Fc domains. All mAbs bind to the cancer cell surface receptor through the Fab domain and to immune cells through the Fc domain. Binding through the Fc domain drives ADCC.

Cancer biologics have been developed for EGFR+, and HER2+, and VEGFR+ solid tumors and surface receptors that are common in hematologic malignancies such as cluster of differentiation (CD) including CD38, CD22, CD33, CD52, and signaling lymphocytic activation molecule family member 7 (SLAMF7). In addition to "simple" or pure mAbs, innovative subclasses of these therapeutic proteins have been developed to both broaden their mechanistic approach and enhance clinical utility in treatment-resistant cancers.[100-103] The strategies described later may be effective as monotherapy, although many will likely be used in combination, either with other immunotherapies or with traditional cytotoxic chemotherapy or radiotherapy.

Bispecific Antibodies. Bispecific antibodies that bind to two different surface antigens allow for multitargeted suppression of the cancer cell. A recent example is amivantamab, a dual-targeted mAb that binds to the extracellular domains of the RTKs, EGFR (with exon 20 mutations) and MET. Amivantamab is the only approved therapeutic option for exon 20 EGFR+ NSCLC.

Immune Checkpoint Inhibitors. The immune checkpoint inhibitors, also termed checkpoint-blockade therapy, target immune cells to undo the cancer's inhibitory damage to normal immune response pathways. Immune checkpoint inhibitors overcome cytotoxic T-lymphocyte–associated antigen-4 (CTLA-4)-mediated blockade or the PD-1/PD-L1 interaction-mediated suppression of the immune response. They have been successfully incorporated in the management of varied cancers including melanoma, breast, prostate, kidney, lung, and hematologic malignancy following biomarker screening. The drugs are well tolerated and adverse effects are generally mild; however, sudden and major organ dysfunction may occur. This is rare but life-threatening and must be immediately managed. Serious adverse effects include colitis, pneumonitis, and hepatitis, among other inflammatory conditions, causing the immune checkpoint inhibitors to sometimes be referred to as the "itis" drugs.

Antibody-Drug Conjugates and Radioimmunoconjugates. Conjugation allows the delivery of two entities (antibody and drug/toxin/nuclide) to the tumor that act synergistically, and the use of humanized and fully human antibodies has attenuated the immunogenicity that was a therapeutic deal-breaker with previously employed murine antibodies. In addition to being tumor specific or selective, the target antigen should be readily internalized when bound to the antibody in order to transport the cytotoxic entity to intracellular sites of action. Several different types of cytotoxic molecules have been utilized in the development of conjugated drugs, including cytotoxic drugs (eg, irinotecan), transporters (eg, folate receptor α [FRα]), and radionuclides (eg, ^{131}I, ^{90}Y).

The chemical linker that connects the cytotoxic drug and antibody is critical to the action of the conjugate, as it must (1) ensure stability in the bloodstream until the target cell is reached, (2) allow penetration of the conjugate into tumor vasculature, and (3) release the toxin in tumor lysosomes or endosomes, either through hydrolysis or through reduction (cleavable linkers) or degradation (noncleavable linkers). The drugs selected for conjugation must be stable in the acidic environment of the drug-liberating organelle and potent in subnanomolar concentrations since only a few conjugates (1%-2% of the administered dose) reach their intended target. The cytotoxic payload should be high enough to ensure maximum drug delivery to the tumor, but not so high as to negatively impact the stability and pharmacokinetic properties of the conjugate. The most common classes of antineoplastic drugs used to generate therapeutic antibody conjugates include mitosis inhibitors (eg, monomethylauristatin E) and DNA toxins (eg, calicheamicin).

Ado-trastuzumab emtansine (Kadcyla)

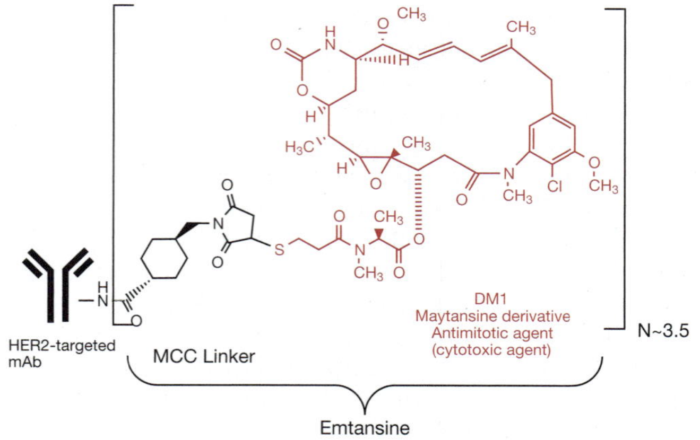

Brentuximab vedotin (Adcetris)-MAb CAc10 - CD30-directed, N ~4

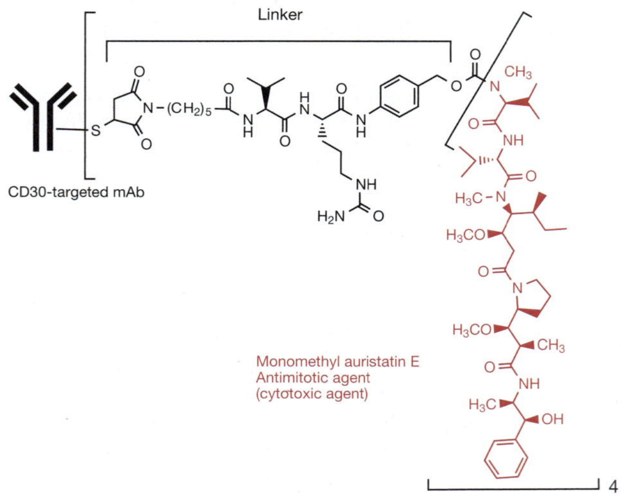

Fam-trastuzumab deruxtecan-NXKI (Enhertu)

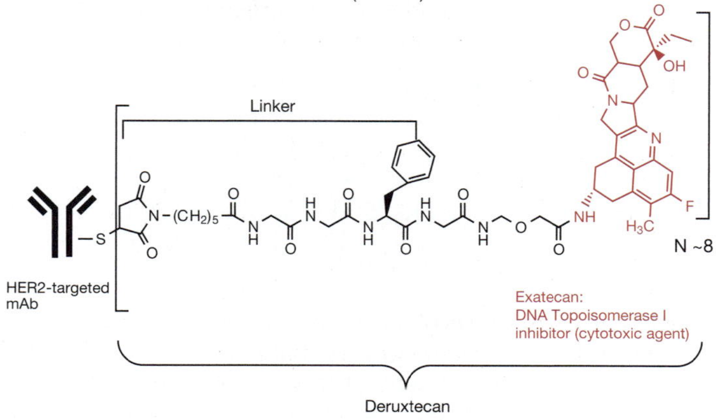

Inotuzumab ozogamicin (Besponsa)

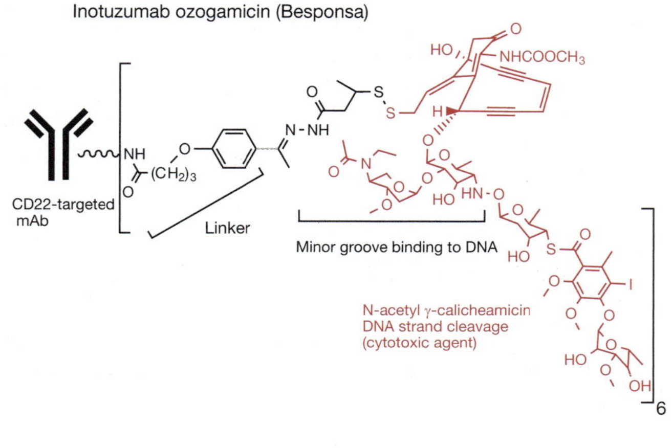

Chimeric Antigen Receptor T-Cell Therapy. In chimeric antigen receptor T-cell (CAR-T) therapy, patient-derived T cells are genetically manipulated to fuse an antibody that targets the CD19 antigen expressed by the patient's leukemia cells. Upon binding to the target antigen after reinfusion, modified CAR-T proliferation with release of cancer cell annihilating cytokines occurs. The CAR-T therapies have improved survival outcomes; however, they are associated with high costs of administration and significant life-threatening toxicities. Tisagenlecleucel is an example of CAR-T therapy approved for refractory or relapsing ALL in patients up to age 25 years. Anticipated toxicities from tisagenlecleucel include cytokine release syndrome (boxed warning), which can induce adverse effects ranging from mild to fatal, neurologic damage, infection, hepatotoxicity, and destruction of healthy cells expressing the target antigen. In one multicenter global phase II clinical trial involving 75 patients with relapsed or refractory ALL on tisagenlecleucel, serious drug-related toxicity occurred in 73%, with 77% experiencing symptoms of cytokine release syndrome and 40% experiencing neurologic toxicity (eg, encephalopathy, confusion). Due to the potential for serious or fatal toxicity, tisagenlecleucel can only be administered in certified health centers under a Risk Evaluation and Mitigation Strategy (REMS) program.

Adverse Effects and Pharmacokinetics

As large proteins, mAbs cannot passively penetrate cell membranes, nor are they actively transported intracellularly. Based on their target-specific action on the outside of the cell, mAbs have mild adverse effects, the most common of which include infusion-related reactions, hypersensitivity reactions based on the source of the mAb, and increased infection risk. Mechanistic adverse effects may also be observed. For example, a skin rash is a common adverse effect for EGFR-targeting mAbs and is consistent with inhibition of EGFR distributed in the skin. This reaction is also observed with EGFR-TKIs. Rare but serious and life-threatening adverse effects are possible, such as an increase in the incidence of autoimmune reactions and possible major organ dysfunction such as hepatotoxicity, pulmonary toxicity, thrombocytopenia, and cardiotoxicity. As a result, REMS certification is required for providers administering certain cancer biologics.

Cancer immunotherapies target tumor cells by binding to specific antigens expressed on the cancer cell's surface, which shuts down signaling pathways and triggers ADCC. They are mostly administered as injectables, IV or subcutaneous (SC), have long half-lives of days to weeks permitting less frequent dosing, and may be eliminated unchanged.

Drug Classes Based on Dysfunctional Pathways and Molecular Targets

The subsequent section focuses on targeted therapies organized by dysfunctional signaling pathways and miscellaneous oncogenic drivers.

Signaling Pathway Inhibitors

Inhibitors of Oncofusion Protein–Mediated Signaling

Rearrangements and gene fusions have resulted in oncofusion protein kinases being expressed exclusively in cancer cells that drive tumorigenic processes. The mechanism of action and pharmacokinetic properties of targeted therapies inhibiting oncofusion drivers are shown in Table 37.5.

BCR-ABL Kinase Inhibitors. Shown in Figure 37.10 are the six currently available BCR-ABL kinase inhibitors: asciminib, bosutinib, dasatinib, imatinib, nilotinib, and ponatinib. A frequent occurrence in ALL and CML is the presence of the Ph chromosome or oncogene (t 9,22) formed by the translocation of the long arms of chromosomes 9 (ABL locus) and 22 (BCR regions).[41] Transcription of the Ph chromosome produces the fusion oncoprotein, BCR-ABL kinase. The BCR-ABL kinase is an exclusively cytosolic non-RTK. It is constitutively active (always ON and signaling cell division) and feeds the RAS/RAF/MEK/ERK, JAK/STAT, and PI3K/AKT pathways (Fig. 37.1) that support uncontrolled proliferation and clonal expansion, leading to Ph+ ALL and Ph+ CML. The BCR-ABL TKIs were the first kinase inhibitors to be introduced, and they literally transformed the course of CML therapy.[100] The BCR-ABL kinase inhibitors have their greatest effect in the initial (chronic) phase of Ph+ CML, when the malignant cells are proliferating slowly. These inhibitors have also been approved for Ph+ ALL.

The BCR-ABL TKIs are reversible inhibitors that vary in their binding interactions within the kinase pocket.[94,103-121] Imatinib was the first TKI approved and the springboard to the multitude of TKIs currently on the U.S. market. It is a reversible, ATP-competitive BCR-ABL kinase inhibitor that binds to the extended, inactive conformation of BCR-ABL. Referred to as a "wonder drug" for its impact on patient care and practitioner understanding of molecular mechanisms of cancer, its ability to induce complete hematologic and cytogenetic responses has led to significant increases in survival and quality of life.[105-107] However, patients treated with imatinib develop resistance within 12 months of initiating therapy, and some become intolerant to the drug.

The residues Met290, Leu301, His361, and Phe382 make up the hydrophobic spine of the kinase, with Phe382 belonging to the catalytic triad DFG involved in kinase activation. The hydrophobic spine is a highly conserved network of interactions characteristic of the active kinase conformation. A primary mechanism of resistance includes point mutations within the BCR-ABL kinase. The mutation T315I BCR-ABL, where the gatekeeper residue Thr315 is changed to Ile, blocks the entrance of a BCR-ABL kinase inhibitor into the hydrophobic back pocket but still allows ATP to bind, thus maintaining the kinase activity but preventing inhibitor binding. A secondary mechanism of resistance includes redundant signaling through transduction pathways, such as SRC, PI3K, KRAS, JAK2, and MEK. In

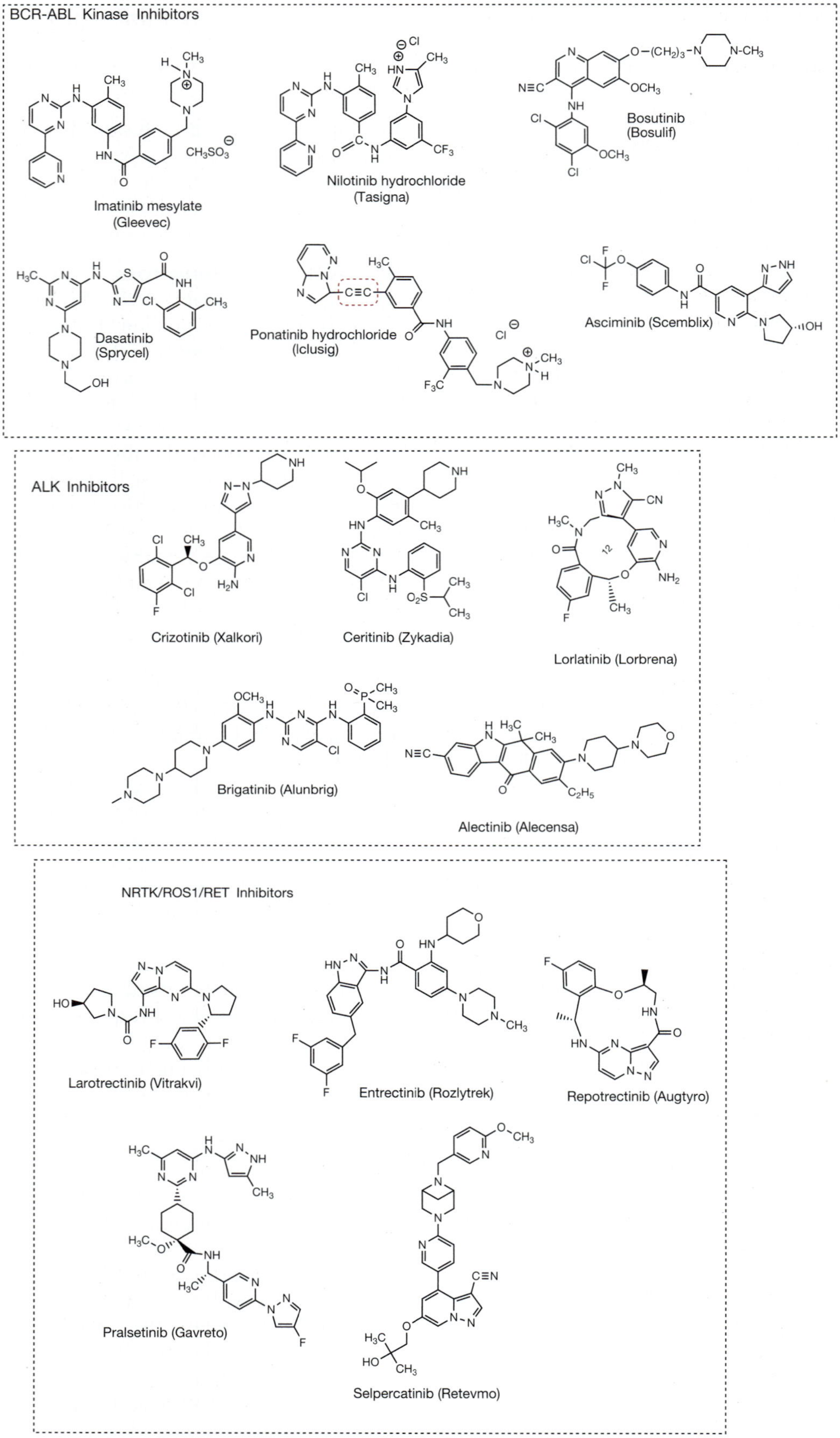

Figure 37.10 Oncofusion protein signaling inhibitors. ALK, anaplastic lymphoma kinase; NRTK, neurotrophic receptor kinase; RET, REarranged during Transfection; ROS1, proto-oncogene 1, receptor tyrosine kinase.

addition, low levels of the cellular influx pump for imatinib through the organic cation transporter-1 (OCT1) reduces the intracellular availability of effective levels of imatinib for BCR-ABL inhibition.[104]

The development of second- (nilotinib, dasatinib, and bosutinib) and third-generation (ponatinib) BCR-ABL TKIs was pursued to ensure efficacy in imatinib-resistant CML.[109-120] Asciminib is the latest addition to the approved BCR-ABL kinase inhibitors.[121-124] Asciminib is a first-in-class allosteric inhibitor of BCR-ABL kinase that has been approved for Ph+ CML previously treated with two or more TKIs and/or which harbors a T315I mutation.[125]

Chemistry. BCR-ABL kinases can adopt the active "DFG-in" conformation or the inactive "DFG-out" conformation.[56] In the inactive conformation, the DFG motif is out and the aspartate residue at the beginning of the activation loop is rotated out of the active site and thus is no longer able to coordinate the Mg^{2+} ion necessary for the transfer of the phosphate in the kinase catalytic reaction.

Imatinib, nilotinib, and ponatinib are type II kinase inhibitors that bind to the ATP pocket and the adjacent hydrophobic pocket in the inactive conformation (see Fig. 37.8). Ponatinib has been referred to as a pan-TKI[110-114] and is reserved for patients with Ph+ CML or ALL, who have failed or progressed on at least two first-line TKIs, or those who have accelerated or blast-phase disease.

The *o*-methyl substituent found on imatinib and nilotinib confers selectivity for the cytosolic BCR-ABL protein in its inactive conformation, although the benzamide moiety permits some inhibition of platelet-derived growth factor receptor (PDGFR) kinase. It is the PDGFR-related component of the activity profile that is believed responsible for the fluid retention induced by these two TKIs. These agents also contain a pyridyl substituent at C_4 of the pyrimidine ring, which enhances affinity through H bonding with the amide NH of Met318 within the hinge region (see Fig. 37.11). The amide moiety, inverted in nilotinib compared to imatinib, forms H bonds with Glu286 and Asp381.[105-107,109] Another H bond is formed between gatekeeper Thr315 and the NH group connecting the pyrimidine and phenyl rings. Thus, nilotinib and imatinib are ineffective in T315I mutations.

The [(piperazinyl)methyl]phenyl moiety of imatinib seeks out the DFG-out pocket in the inactive conformation, where the cationic piperazine nitrogen atom interacts with the backbone of His361 and Ile360. Nilotinib's trifluoromethylated imidazole-phenyl group allows for tighter binding deeper within this site. The affinity-enhancing hydrophobic interactions with Leu298, Val299, and Phe359 are, in part, responsible for nilotinib's 10- to 50-fold increase in TK-inhibiting potency compared to imatinib. The methylimidazole moiety in nilotinib also augments affinity through hydrophobic interactions with Leu285, Glu286, and Val289, while leaving the basic nitrogen exposed to the aqueous environment.

Bosutinib and dasatinib demonstrate a preference for type I kinase inhibition and bind exclusively to the ATP pocket.[105,107-112] Although dasatinib contains a pyrimidine ring, this moiety does not bind in the hinge region as the pyrimidine rings of imatinib and nilotinib do. Rather, a

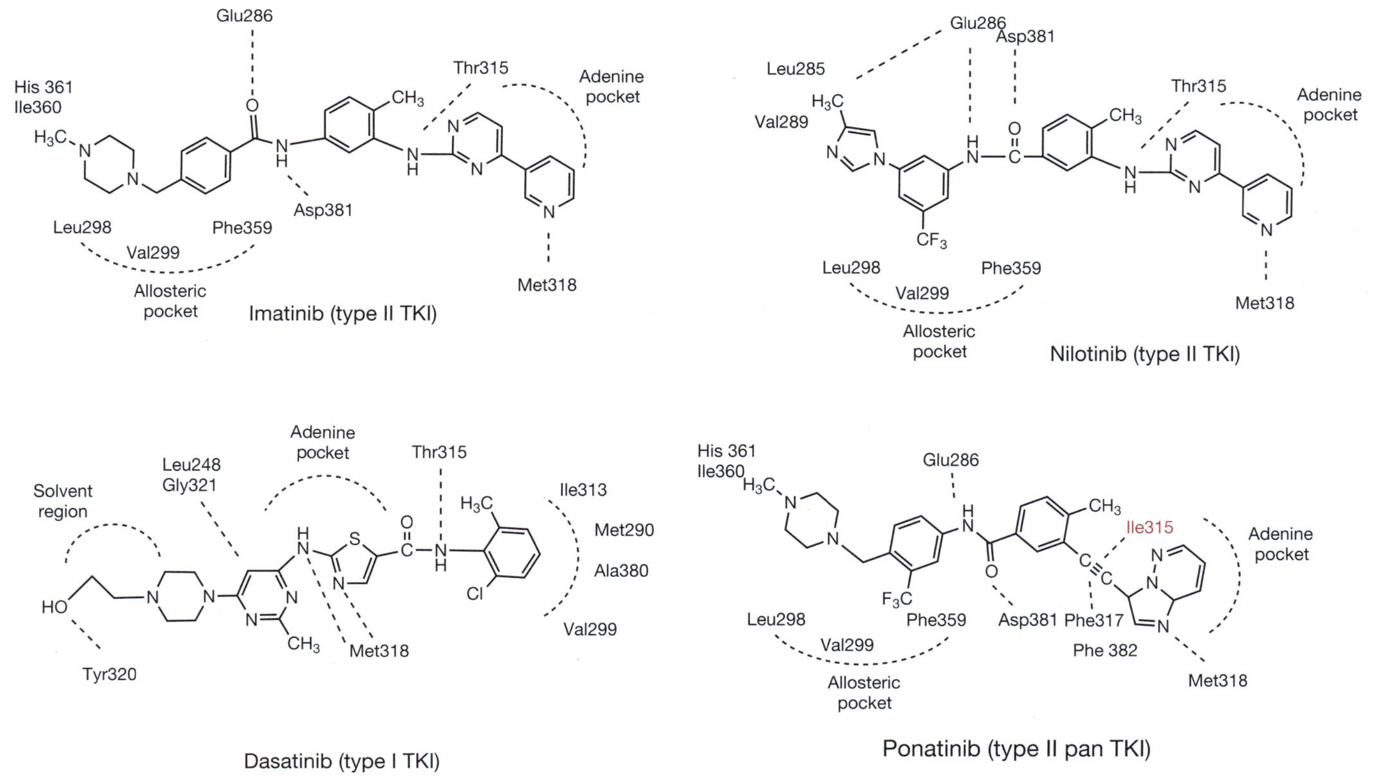

Figure 37.11 Binding interactions for ATP-competitive BCR-ABL kinase inhibitors. ATP, adenosine triphosphate; BCR-ABL, breakpoint cluster region/Abelson tyrosine kinase; TKI, tyrosine kinase inhibitor.

critical hydrogen bond forms between the thiazole nitrogen atom of the aminothiazole and the amide NH of Met318. The carbonyl oxygen atom of Met318 also binds to the hydrogen of the amino group connecting the thiazole and pyrimidine rings. A third hydrogen bond between the drug's amide nitrogen and the hydroxyl group of gatekeeper residue Thr315 not only ensures high affinity for the active (DFG-in) state of the kinase but also causes the drug to fall prey to T315I-induced resistance. Dasatinib's ability to bind to the active kinase conformation has been attributed to the fact that it does not insert into the hydrophobic pocket containing Phe382, as the substituted benzyl moiety of imatinib does. The preference for type I inhibition is driven by stabilization of the hydrophobic spine upon dasatinib binding.

The quinoline nitrogen atom of bosutinib (see Fig. 37.11) forms a crucial bond with the amide moiety of Met318.[110-114] The sterically unobtrusive nitrile and the aniline nitrogen atom that bridges the quinoline and chlorinated phenyl rings bind within separate hydrophobic pockets adjacent to Thr315, providing a bound kinase conformation distinct from that formed with dasatinib. Bosutinib has a similar resistance profile to dasatinib. Dasatinib and bosutinib demonstrate dual SRC and BCR-ABL inhibition and are effective in imatinib-resistant tumors but are ineffective in T315I imatinib-resistant mutants. Dasatinib has additional effects on stem cell factor receptor tyrosine kinase (Kit) and PDGFR as well.

Ponatinib is a type II BCR-ABL kinase inhibitor and is effective in the T315I imatinib-resistant mutant.[115,119,120] Ponatinib adopts an extended mode of binding with the alkyne moiety (see Fig. 37.11), providing a short, rigid, and narrow linker that orients the N-aryl benzamide moiety toward hydrophobic region I while avoiding steric clashes with Ile315 of imatinib-resistant T315I BCR/ABL mutants. The alkyne moiety forms van der Waals interactions with Ile315, Phe317 and Phe382. Consistent with all kinase inhibitors, the BCR-ABL TKIs include ionizable functional groups such as the N-methyl piperazine seen in imatinib, bosutinib, and ponatinib that are solvent exposed and allow for improved water solubility.

Asciminib (see Fig. 37.10) is noncompetitive with ATP and binds to an allosteric myristate pocket similar to GNF-2 (see Fig. 37.4) and has, therefore, been classified as a TKI specifically targeting the Abl myristoyl pocket (STAMP).[122,123] Myristic acid, also known as tetradecanoic acid, is a C_{14} saturated fatty acid that has been suggested to have an inhibitory role in the autoregulation of ABL. The myristoyl group binds to an internal "myristate-binding pocket" in the C-lobe of the ABL kinase domain and induces an inactive state. Asciminib induces a similar inactive conformation on binding to the myristoyl pocket.[123] Asciminib is a highly selective, reversible BCR-ABL kinase inhibitor and does not inhibit a panel of over 60 recombinant kinases, including SRC kinase, when tested at concentrations <10 μM. It is also inactive against G protein coupled receptors (GPCRs), ion channels, nuclear receptors, and transporters. In a phase 3, open-label, randomized study, asciminib was compared to bosutinib in CML after previous treatment with at least two TKIs and demonstrated superior efficacy, with a major molecular response rate at week 24 of 25.5% for asciminib versus 13.2% for bosutinib.[124] In addition, asciminib was associated with fewer grade 3 adverse events (50.6% vs >60%) and fewer adverse events leading to treatment discontinuation (5.8% vs 21.1%).

Pharmacokinetics. The oral bioavailability of BCR-ABL kinase inhibitors is compromised by poor absorption and rapid first-pass CYP3A4-mediated biotransformation (see Table 37.5).[110] In addition to screening for tumor markers and genomic profiles, individual drug pharmacokinetic parameters, overall patient health status, and preexisting conditions are key considerations prior to initiating therapy. While the drugs discussed earlier are classified as BCR-ABL TKIs, their spectrum of action is actually broader, commonly also blocking Src, Kit, and/or PDGFR. Imatinib's approved indications have now been expanded to include GI stromal tumors expressing Kit and myeloproliferative disorders that overexpress PDGFRβ.

Adverse Effects. All BCR-ABL inhibitors are associated with significant myelosuppression and fatigue.[110,113,115] Additional serious adverse reactions associated with imatinib include cardiovascular complications, diarrhea, fluid retention, nausea, and rash. Nilotinib is significantly more potent than imatinib, but on the downside, its use is associated with life-threatening toxicities, including elevated bilirubin and lipase, hypokalemia, hypophosphatemia, increased transaminases, myelosuppression, rash, and cardiotoxicity manifesting as QT prolongation. The QT-interval prolongation in nilotinib can progress to torsades de pointes and sudden death. The risk of potentially fatal myocardial toxicity is elevated if the drug is taken with potent CYP3A4 inhibitors, and the dose should be halved if coadministration with CYP3A4 inhibitors is required. Typical adverse reactions for dasatinib include diarrhea, fluid retention, myelosuppression, rash, and QT prolongation. Unlike nilotinib, there is no boxed warning related to QT-interval prolongation, but the potential of dasatinib to exacerbate the toxicity of other agents should not be ruled out.

A major advantage claimed for bosutinib over other BCR-ABL TKIs is an improved safety profile; the risk of edema, cardiovascular toxicity, and electrolyte imbalance that can lead to muscle cramping is comparatively low.[113] Typical adverse reactions for bosutinib include diarrhea, nausea, myelosuppression, hemorrhage, vomiting, abdominal pain, rash, and anemia.

Ponatinib is a third-generation type II BCR-ABL TKI with affinity for the broadest range of kinases among all BCR-ABL TKIs. It is among the most toxic of the BCR-ABL TKIs, with adverse effects including arterial thrombosis, hepatotoxicity, hypertension, heart failure, pancreatitis, cardiac arrhythmia, and myelosuppression. In fact, the risk of arterial and venous occlusions prompted a temporary suspension of U.S. marketing in 2013 before the drug was reintroduced with a restricted indication limited to patients with T315I mutation or for whom no other TKI was indicated. Ponatinib carries a boxed warning related to life-threatening arterial occlusive events, venous thromboembolism (VTE), heart failure, and hepatotoxity.[126] Hypertension can occur in up to 74% of patients taking this drug.

The most common adverse reactions for asciminib include upper respiratory tract infections, musculoskeletal pain, fatigue, nausea, rash, and diarrhea.[121,127] Serious adverse effects include myelosuppression, pancreatic toxicity, hypertension, and hypersensitivity reactions. Decreased platelet count, increased triglycerides, decreased neutrophil count, decreased hemoglobin, increased creatine kinase, increased alanine aminotransferase, lipase, and amylase have also been observed.

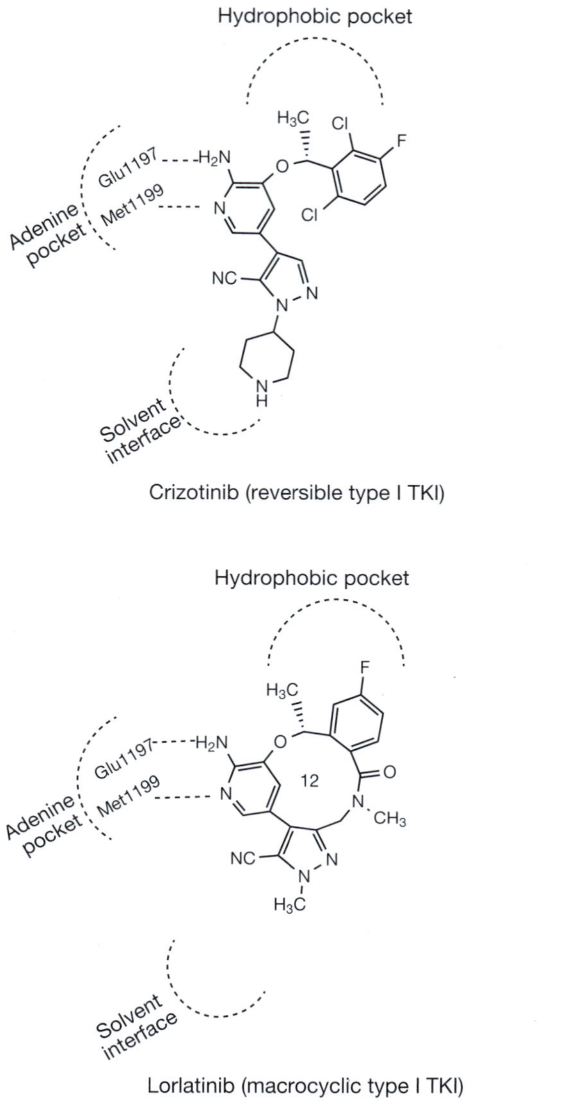

Figure 37.12 Binding interactions for ALK inhibitors. ALK, anaplastic lymphoma kinase; TKI, tyrosine kinase inhibitor.

ALK Inhibitors. Shown in Figure 37.10 are the five currently available ALK inhibitors: alectinib, brigatinib, ceritinib, crizotinib, and lorlatinib. ALK belongs to the insulin receptor superfamily.[128] The physiologic purpose of ALK is not fully understood, but it is suggested to have a role in the normal development of the central (CNS) and peripheral nervous systems. The oncofusion protein ALK-nucleophosmin (NPM) was isolated in an anaplastic large cell lymphoma (ALCL) cell line with a *t*(2;5) chromosomal rearrangement. Aberrant neoplastic cells also express ALK fused with EML4. The oncogenic ALK-EML4 and ALK-NPM fusion proteins are constitutively active, ligand-independent and trigger downstream signaling cascades such as the PI3K/AKT/mTOR or RAS/RAF/MEK/ERK pathway, resulting in cancer cell proliferation (see Fig. 37.1). The ALK inhibitors shut down signaling cascades activated by the ALK fusion oncoproteins and inhibit cancer cell proliferation and tumor growth. The ALK inhibitors are effective in ALK+ tumors and have been approved for ALK+ NSCLC that expresses ALK-EML4 (see Table 37.1).

Crizotinib was the first FDA-approved ALK inhibitor and is classified as a first-generation inhibitor. The limited efficacy of crizotinib led to the development of second-generation ALK inhibitors ceritinib, brigatinib, and alectinib, and a third-generation inhibitor, lorlatinib, with improved CNS distribution and efficacy in crizotinib-resistant cancers.[129-140] Lorlatinib is a macrocyclic ALK inhibitor that was approved for ALK+ NSCLC following progression on crizotinib, ceritinib, or alectinib.[141-149] Lorlatinib is effective against L1196M-, C1156Y-, and G1202R-resistant mutants. None of the ALK inhibitors are effective against the double-mutant G1202R/L1196M ALK.[150,151] Redundant signaling through the hepatocyte growth factor (HGF)/Met pathway and the EGFR pathway contributes to this resistance.

Chemistry. The ALK inhibitors are type I kinase inhibitors that seek out hinge region residues in the ATP-binding pocket and insert lipophilic moieties into adjacent hydrophobic pockets (Fig. 37.12).[141] Cocrystal structures have demonstrated key binding site interactions with the adenine region, hinge region, hydrophobic pocket, and residues near the solvent interface.[128,133,138] Crizotinib occupies the front pocket of the ATP-binding site in the active "DFG-in" conformation and interacts through hydrogen bonds with Glu1197 and Met1199 of the hinge region; however, resistance develops rapidly.[128,129] The most common resistance-promoting mutations include a gatekeeper leucine to methionine at position 1196 (L1196M), cysteine to tyrosine at position 1156 (C1156Y), and glycine to arginine at 1202 (G1202R).[130] In addition, patients with ALK+ NSCLC relapse due to brain metastases. ALK inhibitors, including crizotinib, are ineffective in treating these brain tumors because they are substrates for Pgp efflux pumps in capillary epithelial cells in the blood-brain barrier (BBB) and are readily effluxed from the CNS.

Ceritinib includes an aminopyridine core scaffold that binds to the adenine region of the ATP pocket and forms two H bonds with the hinge region residues Met1199. The piperidine ring forms a salt bridge with Glu1210. The isopropoxy group can form favorable interactions with Arg1120 and Glu1132. Ceritinib is effective against the L1196M mutant.

Brigatinib is a dimethylphosphine oxide (DMPO)-substituted-2-aminopyrimidine–based ALK inhibitor. In addition to ALK, brigatinib also inhibits mEGFR, ROS1, insulin-like growth factor-1 receptor (IGF-1R), and FLT3. Interactions are observed for the methoxy group with Leu1198, the C_5-chlorine atom with Leu1196, and the DMPO moiety with the DFG motif.[133] The DMPO moiety acts as a H bond acceptor and stabilizes a U-shaped conformation for brigatinib through intramolecular interactions. It is a first-line agent for ALK+ NSCLC that retains efficacy in the face of L1196M and C1156Y mutations.[133-135] Like crizotinib, it has affinity for related kinases (albeit with higher IC_{50} values), including ROS1, FLT3, and the EGFR T790M (threonine-to-methionine mutation) mutant. The unique phosphine oxide moiety's ability to engage in strong inter- and intramolecular hydrogen bonding is believed to be responsible for the high ALK selectivity, as well as brigatinib's beneficial pharmacokinetic profile. For example, the higher polarity of the DMPO moiety, compared to the isopropylsulfone group of certinib, results in significantly lower binding to serum proteins.[133-136]

Alectinib includes a tetracyclic benzo[*b*]carbazolone scaffold that adopts a planar conformation where the carbonyl and cyano groups form favorable H bond interactions with Met1199 and Lys1150.[137] Alectinib is effective against tumors with brain metastases due to the increased permeability across the BBB compared to crizotinib and effective against crizotinib-refractory tumors harboring the L1196M and C1156Y ALK mutants.

Macrocyclization restricts the flexibility of lorlatinib and was utilized to adopt a bioactive conformation without the entropic penalty.[141-146] The rigid macrocycle occupies the adenine-binding site. The common aminopyridine cores of crizotinib and lorlatinib interact through hydrogen bonds with residues Glu1197, Leu1198, and Met1199 of the hinge region (see Fig. 37.12).[146] The fluorophenyl group is common to crizotinib and lorlatinib and lies close to the edge of the type I pocket and the DFG motif with similar interactions with Val1130, Lys1150, Asn1256, and Asp1270. The pyrazole moiety common to both crizotinib and lorlatinib binds between Leu1122 and Gly1202. Crizotinib's pyrazole is piperidine substituted and solvent exposed with interactions with Gly1123, Ala1200, and Ser1206 in the front pocket area. Lorlatinib's pyrazole moiety was optimized as a 2-methylpyrazole-3-carbonitrile, allowing interactions with Arg1120 and Glu1132. While the core scaffolds of crizotinib and lorlatinib have similar kinase-binding modes, the incorporation of the macrocycle allows for different activity profiles. Lorlatinib is effective against L1196M, C1156Y, and G1202R crizotinib-resistant mutants.

Pharmacokinetics. All currently marketed ALK inhibitors are metabolized by CYP3A4. Slightly over half of the crizotinib dose is excreted unchanged in feces, potentially representing unabsorbed drug. CYP3A4- and CYP2C8-catalyzed N-demethylation and Cys conjugation represent the two major brigatinib metabolic routes. Unchanged brigatinib and the unidentified 3-fold less active primary metabolite account for 92% and 3.5% of the circulating drug, respectively. In addition to being biotransformed by CYP3A4, brigatinib can induce this isoform.[72] Given the risk of serious adverse effects when blood levels rise (including pulmonary toxicity, hypertension, and visual disturbances), coadministration with strong CYP3A4 inhibitors should be avoided.[72] The major alectinib metabolite is the CYP3A4-generated morpholine ring-opened structure shown as M4 in Figure 37.8. Although present in plasma at concentrations less than the parent drug (5.8% vs 84%), it retains activity comparable to the parent and contributes to the therapeutic response elicited by alectinib.[138] Lorlatinib displays optimal pharmacokinetic properties for CNS penetration and is effective for metastatic brain cancers. In addition, lorlatinib is not a Pgp substrate and demonstrates excellent CNS retention.[149,152] Lorlatinib undergoes phase I oxidation and phase II glucuronidation catalyzed primarily by CYP3A4 and UGT1A4, respectively, with minor involvement from CYP2C8, CYP2C19, CYP3A5, and UGT1A3. The parent drug is a moderate inducer of CYP3A and a weak inducer of UGT1A. As is typical for most kinase inhibitors, the concomitant use of lorlatinib with strong CYP inducers or inhibitors could alter the therapeutic efficacy. In particular, the concomitant use of lorlatinib with strong CYP3A4/5 inducers is contraindicated, and a dose reduction is recommended with strong CYP3A4 inhibitors. Lorlatinib undergoes renal (48% with 9% unchanged) and biliary excretion (41% with 1% unchanged), and dose reductions are recommended for patients with severe renal impairment.

Adverse Effects. The most common adverse effects associated with ALK inhibitors include vision disturbances, nausea and diarrhea, hypercholesterolemia, increased triglycerides, edema, and elevated liver enzymes.[153,154] Vision disturbances are as high as 70% for crizotinib, while lorlatinib has the highest incidence of hypercholesterolemia and hypertriglyceridemia. Peripheral edema is possible for both alectinib and lorlatinib. Due to their CNS penetration capability, lorlatinib and alectinib also display central adverse events such as cognitive defects (memory impairment and amnesia) and behavioral changes (irritability, anxiety, depression). The ALK inhibitors may also induce adverse effects such as cardiovascular toxicity presenting as bradycardia. Newer generations of ALK inhibitors are being pursued to improve upon the problematic resistance and adverse effect profile of currently available ALK inhibitors.

ROS1/TRK Inhibitors. There is a significant overlap between ALK and c-ros oncogene 1 (ROS1). ROS1 is a fusion oncoprotein with RTK activity.[155,156] The most frequent fusion is CD74-ROS1 that represents 44% of cases. It belongs to the insulin receptor family and promotes the PI3K/AKT/mTOR and RAS/RAF/MAPK (mitogen-activated protein kinase) pathways leading to cancer cell proliferation and tumor growth. Crizotinib, grouped with the ALK inhibitors in Figure 37.10, demonstrated ROS1 inhibition and was approved for ROS1+ cancers; however, resistance developed rapidly due to ROS1 mutations, including D2033N, G2032R, and L2026M.[128,144,148,157] Clinical studies documented effectiveness against crizotinib-resistant ROS1+ cancers that did not contain the G2032R mutation.

Chromosomal rearrangements involving fusions of neurotrophic receptor tyrosine kinase (*NTRK*) genes result in constitutively active tropomyosin receptor tyrosine kinases (TRKs) that drive cancer cell proliferation and survival.[33,158-166] There are three types of TRKs, TRKA, TRKB, and TRKC, that serve as oncogenic drivers in pediatric gliomas, thyroid cancer, lung cancer, glioblastoma, and CRC. Three inhibitors, entrectinib, larotrectinib, and repotrectinib, are approved for NTRK+ solid tumors and can be recognized by their "trectinib" suffix (see Fig. 37.7). Entrectinib is a potent, orally available, pan-TRK, ROS1, and ALK inhibitor with good CNS penetration.[161,162] Based on its mechanism of action as a pan-TRK inhibitor, entrectinib has been approved for solid tumors with *NTRK* gene fusions. It has also been approved for ROS1+ NSCLC but is not effective against crizotinib-resistant ROS1 mutations D2033N, G2032R, and L2026M.[163,164] Larotrectinib is an ATP-competitive, type II kinase inhibitor with pan-TRK activity.[165] It is a selective TRK inhibitor with over 1,000-fold selectivity for TRK relative to other kinases and has been approved for cancers with *NTRK* gene fusions. Larotrectinib is not effective in those with TKA G595R mutations. Resistance to this inhibitor has also developed due to G623R, G696A, and F617L TRKC mutations.[166] Repotrectinib is a second-generation TRK inhibitor that is a macrocyclic, conformationally restricted analog of entrectinib.[166,33] Repotrectinib retains activity against ROS1 mutations, including G2032R, and TRK mutations. Repotrectinib has been approved for advanced/metastatic ROS1+ NSCLC, including crizotinib-resistant NSCLC expressing G2032R ROS1 mutations. Repotrectinib is effective against tumors with *NTRK* fusions, including entrectinib-resistant tumors.[166,33]

Chemistry. The NTRK inhibitors include a pyrazolo [1,5-*a*]pyrimidine core scaffold and bind to the DFG-in, active conformation of TRK. Entrectinib binds to all TRKs in a type I, ATP-competitive mode, with interactions observed only in the front cleft.[162] The macrocyclic core in repotrectinib was incorporated to limit steric clashes with resistance mutations within the ATP pocket because of the more compact binding interface.[166,33] The macrocycle allows for improved selectivity against ROS1, TRKA, TRKB, TRKC, and mutant TRK compared to other mutant and nonmutant kinases in the human kinome. Repotrectinib is more potent as a ROS1 inhibitor as compared to crizotinib, with activity against ALK and TRK receptors. Crystal structures for repotrectinib binding with the resistant mutant G595R TRKA showed that the macrocycle maintained its key hinge region and hydrophobic pocket interactions while forming a new hydrogen bond with the side chain of Arg595. A similar interaction is expected within G2032R ROS1.

Pharmacokinetics. All marketed ROS1/TRK inhibitors undergo CYP3A4-mediated metabolism and may be administered orally. Consistent with other kinase inhibitors, coadministration of CYP3A4 inhibitors, inducers, and substrates must be avoided.

Adverse Effects. Common adverse effects for TRK inhibitors are mechanistic and based on the physiologic role of TRK in CNS function (dizziness, delirium), balance (gait disturbances), pain (neuropathy, withdrawal pain), and appetite control (weight gain).[161,163,165] Adverse effects for entrectinib include fatigue, dysgeusia (loss of taste), nausea, dizziness, cognitive impairment, and vision disorders. Serious adverse effects including congestive heart failure have been reported. Dose reductions can sometimes be sufficient to manage entrectinib's toxicity, but treatment discontinuation may be required in severe toxicity. Larotrectinib shows a better adverse effect profile compared to entrectinib, and cardiovascular complications and vision disturbances are not observed.[165] Common adverse effects include fatigue, dizziness, cough, nausea/vomiting, and elevated liver enzymes that can potentially lead to hepatotoxicity. Peripheral neuropathy, including paresthesia, is possible, and patients are advised against driving or operating heavy machinery if they experience central neurotoxic symptoms. Toxicity is reversed by dose adjustments or discontinuation of the drug. Adverse effects for repotrectinib are mild.

Targeted Therapies for RET Rearrangements. The REarranged during Transfection kinase (RET) is constitutively active due to RET mutations and gene fusions that trigger downstream signaling cascades that support tumor growth.[167] RET plays an aggressive role in the progression of medullary thyroid cancer (MTC).[168] Alectinib, an ALK inhibitor discussed, also inhibits RET. Additional multitargeted small molecule inhibitors sorafenib and lenvatinib have been approved for use in tumors with RET rearrangements; however, these drugs have significant toxicities based on their effects on VEGFR2 or kinase domain receptor (KDR).[169,170] Efforts made to improve the selectivity for RET while reducing the effects on KDR led to the development of selpercatinib and pralsetinib (see Fig. 37.10). These two inhibitors demonstrate higher efficacy, RET selectivity, improved pharmacokinetic properties, and fewer off-target interactions as compared to previously marketed multitargeted kinase inhibitors. Pralsetinib and selpercatinib are approved in the treatment of RET-mutant and RET fusion–positive cancers, including RET+ NSCLC and refractory MTC harboring RET gene fusions. Selpercatinib inhibits wtRET, multiple mutated RET isoforms, VEGFR1 and VEGFR3, and FGFR1, FGFR2, and FGFR3. Pralsetinib, a multitargeted kinase inhibitor, inhibits DDR1, TRKC, FLT3, JAK1-2, TRKA, VEGFR2, PDGFRβ, and FGFR1.

Chemistry. Selpercatinib and pralsetinib are ATP-competitive inhibitors that incorporate hydrogen bonding with Ala807, Tyr806, and Glu805 of the hinge region and hydrophobic interactions with Gly736, Val738, Ala756, Lys737, Lys758, and Leu730 in the hydrophobic back pocket II (Fig. 37.13).[167,168] While these molecules bind to the front and back pocket of RET, they have a unique mode of binding

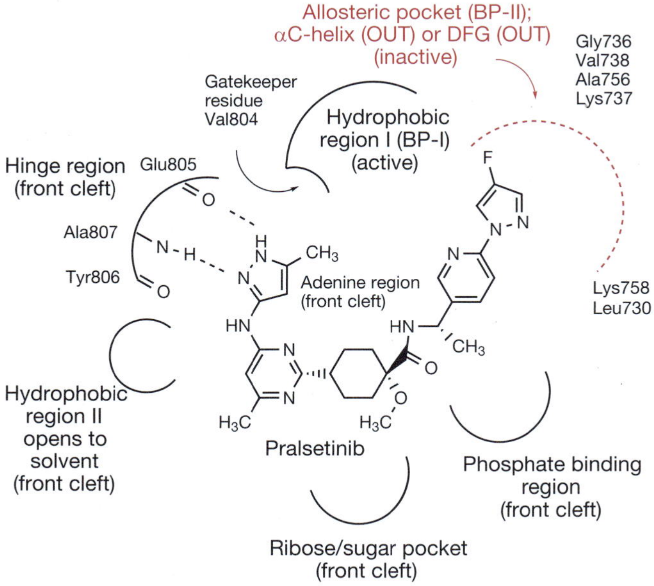

Figure 37.13 Binding interactions for pralsetinib within RET. BP-II, back pocket II; DFG, aspartate, phenylalanine, glycine; RET, REarranged during Transfection.

where they do not go through gatekeeper residue Val804 across back pocket I to access back pocket II. Instead, they wrap around the gatekeeper to access hydrophobic region II. The aminopyrimidinyl and methylaminopyrazole rings of pralsetinib and pyrazolopyridine rings of selpercatinib occupy the adenine pocket. Acquired mutations in the hinge region and adenine pocket contribute more to resistance than gatekeeper mutations. Resistant mutations include point mutations at Gly810 (G810R, G810S, G810C, G810V) and Tyr806 (Y806C, Y806N) that sterically clash with the aminopyrimidinyl and methylaminopyrazole moieties of pralsetinib and the pyrazolopyridine ring of selpercatinib.

Pharmacokinetics. Both pralsetinib and selpercatinib are metabolized by CYP3A4 and CYP2C8.[103] Moderate and strong CYP inducers and inhibitors must be avoided. The RET inhibitors demonstrate pH-dependent absorption and must be given on an empty stomach when gastric acidity is highest. Food and antacids should be appropriately spaced so as not to interfere with absorption. In addition, PPIs and H_2 antagonists should be avoided.

Adverse Effects. Selpercatinib and pralsetinib are more selective for RET kinase over other kinases in the kinome. They have a better adverse effect profile compared to other multitargeted kinase inhibitors; however, adverse effects mediated through EGFR and VEGFR may still be observed with pralsetinib. These include hypertension, cutaneous toxicities, hepatotoxicity, and wound healing complications.[170,171] Hematologic toxicities, a risk of hemorrhage, tumor lysis syndrome, hypertension, fatigue, and edema may also be seen. Pralsetinib is associated with a higher incidence of interstitial lung disease compared to selpercatinib. Selpercatinib does not inhibit KDR or VEGFR2 but is associated with an increased risk of QT prolongation.

RAS/RAF/MEK/ERK Pathway Inhibitors

Mutations or overexpression of members of the RAS/RAF/MEK/ERK pathway have resulted in tumor growth and disease progression. The aberrant molecular targets in the RAS/RAF/MEK/ERK pathway include EGFR, HER2, mKRAS, mBRAF, and MEK.

EGFR-TKIs. The EGFR kinase feeds the RAS/RAF/MEK and PI3K/AKT/mTOR pathways (see Fig. 37.1).[172] mEGFR is a key oncogenic driver for NSCLC that expresses activating mutations that trigger downstream signaling cascades to promote tumor growth and metastasis.[173-176] The most common activating mutations are deletions in exon 19 (del19 EGFR) EGFR and a leucine-to-arginine mutation in exon 21 (L858R EGFR) that result in a permanently activated state that drives persistent mEGFR-mediated signaling. These aberrant mutations are absent in noncancerous wtEGFR.

The EGFR kinase is a RTK that has an extracellular domain, transmembrane domain, and intracellular domain. The intracellular domain houses the kinase catalytic site and ATP pocket. EGFR kinase binds to ATP and phosphorylates substrate proteins that trigger downstream signaling through the RAS/RAF/MEK and PI3K/AKT pathways to promote cancer cell proliferation. EGFR-TKIs (Fig. 37.14) are used in the first-line treatment of mEGFR-driven NSCLC.

Erlotinib and gefitinib are first-generation EGFR-TKIs approved in the early 2000s. Afatinib and dacomitinib are second-generation EGFR-TKIs, and osimertinib is a third-generation EGFR-TKI approved for mEGFR-positive NSCLC. Osimertinib was approved in 2017 based on the AURA3 trial for T790M EGFR+ NSCLC detected by an FDA-approved liquid biopsy companion diagnostic test (cobas EGFR mutant 2).[176,177] It was initially recommended as a second-line agent for patients with T790M EGFR+ NSCLC after disease progression on erlotinib, gefitinib, afatinib, or dacomitinib. Osimertinib retains activity against del19 EGFR and L858R EGFR and has subsequently been approved for additional indications including first-line treatment of patients with NSCLC with confirmed del19EGFR+ or L858R EGFR+ status (FLAURA trial), for adjuvant therapy of patients with NSCLC with confirmed del19EGFR+ or L858R EGFR+ status following tumor resection (ADAURA trial), and in combination with platinum-based chemotherapy for patients with NSCLC with confirmed del19 EGFR+ or L858R EGFR+ status (FLAURA 2 trial).[178-181]

Resistance to EGFR-TKIs involves activation of redundant oncogenic signaling mediated through MET, IGF-1R, HER3, and MEK; mutations in KRAS; and epithelial-to-mesenchymal transformation of NSCLC cells. Resistance to osimertinib has been reported based on a cysteine797-to-serine (C797S) mutation.[182-184] Several drug discovery programs are focused on developing molecules to treat osimertinib-resistant cancers, including an investigation of reversible type II inhibitors with extensive front cleft binders (BLU945) and allosteric type III EGFR-TKIs.

Patients with mutations in KRAS do not respond well to any of the EGFR-TKIs due to persistent signaling downstream of KRAS, regardless of mEGFR inhibition.[185,186] Thus, in addition to detecting mEGFR prior to initiating therapy, a wtKRAS status must also be detected in patients with NSCLC for EGFR-TKIs to be effective.

The first-, second-, and third-generation EGFR-TKIs are ineffective in cancers expressing EGFR with exon 20 mutations.[187,188] Mobocertinib (see Fig. 37.14) was approved as a small molecule inhibitor of EGFR with exon 20 mutations; however, it was voluntarily withdrawn by Takeda based on failure to meet the primary outcome of superior PFS compared to platinum therapy among patients enrolled in the phase 3 EXCLAIM trial. Amivantamab, a bispecific antibody that binds to both MET and exon 20 EGFR, is currently the only approved drug for exon 20 EGFR+ NSCLC.

Chemistry. The EGFR-TKIs erlotinib, gefitinib, afatinib, and dacomitinib contain a 4-anilinoquinazoline pharmacophore with an oxygen-containing substituent at C_6 or C_7.[189] An electron-withdrawing substituent at position 3′ of the aniline phenyl ring provides high selectivity for EGFR kinase. The 4′ position may remain unsubstituted (erlotinib) or may be modified with a very small substituent, such as fluorine (gefitinib, afatinib, and dacomitinib). Erlotinib

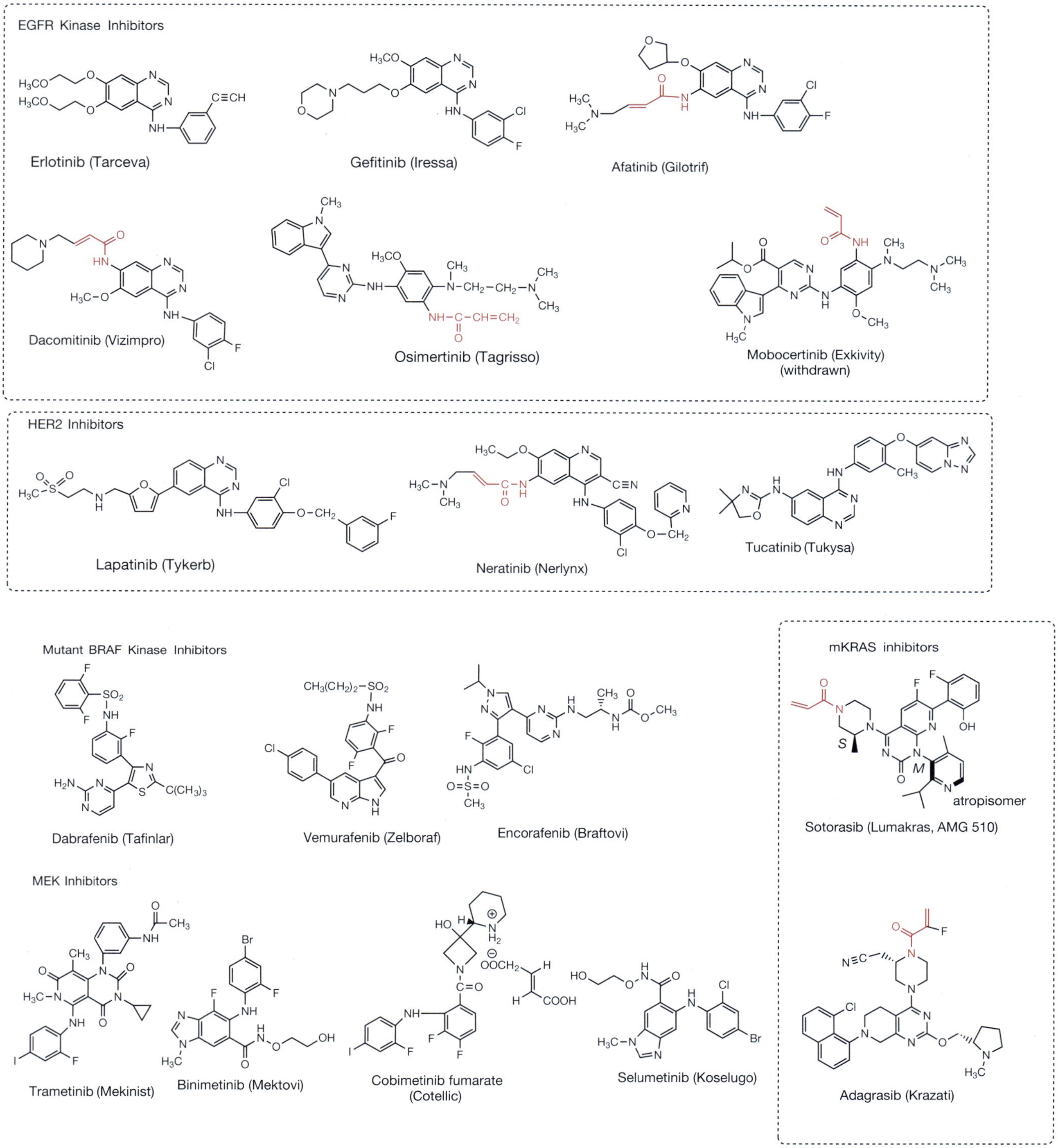

Figure 37.14 RAS/RAF/MEK/ERK inhibitors. BRAF, B-rapidly accelerated fibrosarcoma; EGFR, epidermal growth factor receptor; HER2, human epidermal growth factor 2; mKRAS, mutant Kirsten rat sarcoma; MEK, mitogen-activated protein kinase kinase; RAF, rapidly accelerated fibrosarcoma; RAS, rat sarcoma.

and gefitinib are quintessential type I TKIs, with the *m*-substituted phenyl ring of the anilino moiety enhancing affinity through binding with hydrophobic pocket residues of the active (open) enzyme. The H bonds formed between the quinazoline nitrogen atoms and hinge residues Met793 (N_1) and Thr790 (N_3) are crucial to activity (Fig. 37.15). The halogenated and acetylene-substituted phenyl rings of gefitinib and erlotinib, respectively, are maintained at a 42° angle relative to the quinazoline ring and, in this orientation, bind well in the hydrophobic pocket near Thr790.

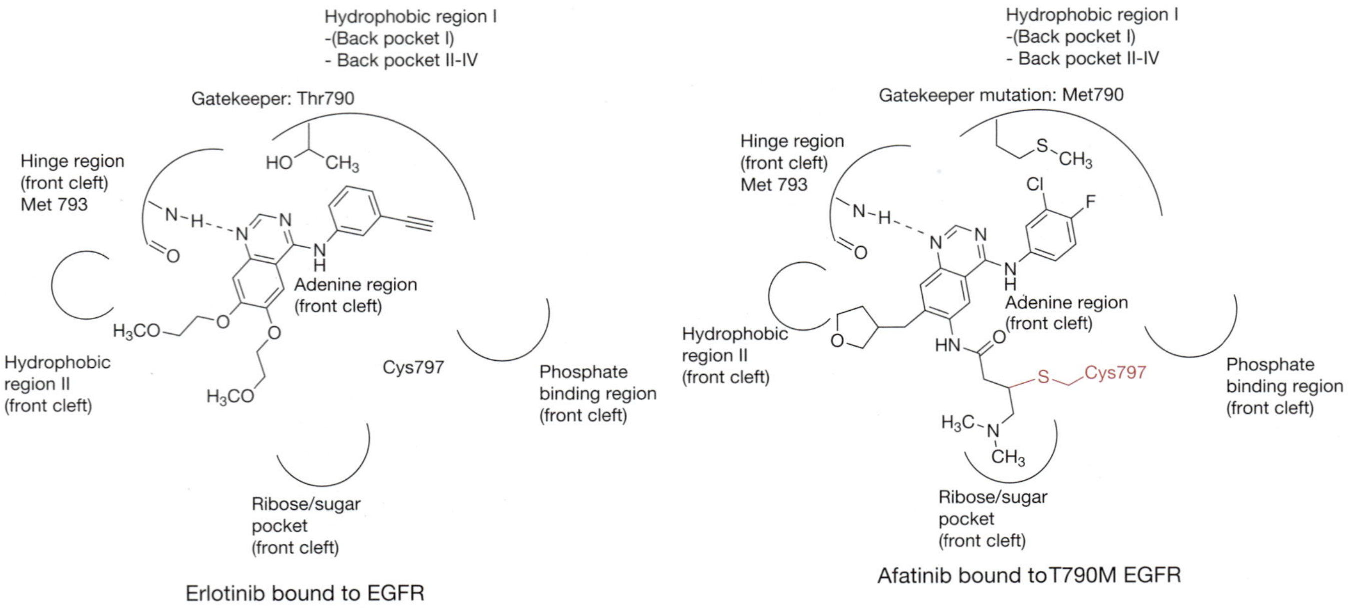

Figure 37.15 Binding interactions for erlotinib and afatinib within EGFR. EGFR, epidermal growth factor receptor.

The efficacy of the first-generation EGFR-TKIs erlotinib and gefitinib is short-lived and resistance develops due to a gatekeeper T790M in the ATP pocket.[190,191] The T790M EGFR mutation contributes to 60% of the resistant cases. Unlike the acquired BCR-ABL kinase resistance, which was predominantly steric in nature, an unfavorable TKI/ATP-binding affinity ratio in the T790M mutant has been proposed to explain acquired resistance to EGFR-TKIs. The T790M mutation stabilizes the active conformation due to interactions with Met766, Leu777, and the DFG motif of EGFR. A change in the EGFR conformation induced by a T790M mutation results in an increase in binding affinity for ATP over the EGFR-TKIs, erlotinib and gefitinib.

The T790M EGFR mutant enzyme has enhanced affinity for the endogenous ATP substrate such that reversible mEGFR inhibitors cannot effectively compete with ATP at safe therapeutic doses. One approach to overcoming this resistance was the development of irreversibly acting inhibitors. As noted previously, a unique Cys797 residue is located at the edge of the ATP-binding domain, and electrophilic TKIs capable of irreversibly inactivating the protein through covalent bond formation showed promise in inhibiting the T790M EGFR mutant.[192,193] The SH group of Cys797 is positioned to conduct a nucleophilic attack at the electrophilic terminal carbon of the acrylamide moiety, highlighted in red in Figure 37.14. An example of an irreversible bond between afatinib and EGFR is shown in Figure 37.15.

Pharmacokinetics. The EGFR-TKIs are metabolized primarily by CYP3A4.[194,195] Osimertinib undergoes a CYP3A4-mediated N-dealkylation at the indole and terminal amine moieties, generating two active metabolites, AZ5104 and AZ7550 (see Fig. 37.8). AZ7550 retains both the potency and desired selectivity of the parent drug. AZ5104 is 8 times more potent than osimertinib in inhibiting mEGFR; however, it lacks selectivity and is 15 times more potent for wtEGFR compared to osimertinib.

The EGFR-TKIs impact efflux pumps. Osimertinib is a Pgp substrate, but not an OCT1 substrate. It inhibits BCRP. Osimertinib is able to penetrate the BBB and is effective in mEGFR+ NSCLC with brain metastases. Afatinib is a substrate and mild inhibitor of Pgp and BCRP. There is an increased risk of afatinib-induced hepatotoxicity due, in part, to the formation of an electrophilic quinoneimine from a CYP3A4- and CYP1A1-generated phenolic metabolite.

Adverse Effects. The most common adverse effects for EGFR-TKIs include skin rash, fatigue, nail bed disorders, diarrhea, and dry skin.[196] The most serious adverse effects include interstitial lung disease and pneumonitis. The adverse effect profile, while qualitatively similar to other EGFR-TKIs, is of lower frequency and severity in osimertinib due to its high selectivity for mEGFR over wtEGFR.

A maculopapular rash commonly induced by EGFR-TKIs has been correlated to wtEGFR inhibition and worsens when exposed to sunlight.

HER2-TKIs. The overexpression of HER2 is a classic feature of breast cancer and colon cancer.[197] HER2 is an RTK, and HER2-TKIs targeting the intracellular kinase domain, as well as biologics for the extracellular domain, have been developed.[96,198-209] The biologics approved for HER2+ cancers include mAbs trastuzumab and pertuzumab, and ADCs fam-trastuzumab deruxtecan and ado-trastuzumab emtansine. The HER2-TKIs lapatinib, neratinib, and tucatinib are ATP-competitive inhibitors that bind to the intracellular HER2 kinase catalytic site (see Fig. 37.14).[198,199]

The kinases EGFR (HER1) and HER2 belong to the HER family of closely related membrane-bound TKs. The EGFR-TKI, afatinib, discussed earlier, also has activity against HER2. Lapatinib and neratinib are dual EGFR/HER2 inhibitors,[199,200] while tucatinib is selective for HER2 and displays minimal EGFR binding.[201] Neratinib has been approved in combination with the antimetabolite capecitabine (Chapter 36) for patients with advanced HER2+ breast cancer who have received two or more prior anti–HER2-based regimens based on the NALA trial.[205] As a mAb biologic, trastuzumab binds to the extracellular domain; hence, it can be coadministered with neratinib in the treatment of HER2+ breast cancer. Tucatinib has been approved in combination with trastuzumab and capecitabine for HER2+ breast cancer, and in combination with trastuzumab for patients with wtKRAS, HER2+ CRC who have received one or more prior anti–HER2-based regimens based on the HER2 CLIMB trial.[206]

Chemistry. The HER2-TKIs were developed by increasing the size of the 4-substituent of the quinazoline or quinoline ring of EGFR-TKIs, which allows for the binding to the inactive HER2 conformation (type II binding). The quinazoline ring of lapatinib binds with residues in the hinge region of the ATP-binding domain (adenine pocket). Lapatinib's 2-furanyl substitution extends out into the aqueous environment. The *m*-fluorobenzyloxyanilino moiety binds within a lipophilic pocket of the HER2. Tucatinib's structure also includes an anilinoquinazoline scaffold that binds to the adenine region of the ATP pocket and forms a hydrogen bond with Met801 of the hinge region, a function served by neratinib's anilinoquinoline ring system.

A cysteine residue (Cys805) is found within the ATP-binding domain of HER2 at a similar position as Cys797 of EGFR. Similar to EGFR-TKIs, covalent interactions between appropriately substituted TKIs and the Cys805 were explored for the development of irreversible HER2 inhibitors.[200] Neratinib is an irreversible HER2 inhibitor that contains an electrophilic acrylamide that forms a covalent bond with Cys805 in HER2 in the manner described earlier. Neratinib is co-classified as a type II and VI EGFR inhibitor owing to its ability to bind in the active site of that kinase and extend into the back pocket allosteric site, while also forming a covalent bond with HER2.

Similar to lapatinib, tucatinib lacks an acrylamide and is a reversible inhibitor; however, unlike the other drugs in this class, it has significantly improved selectivity for HER2 over EGFR. Tucatinib incorporates a bulky triazolopyridine *p*-anilino substituent instead of the planar single-ring aromatic substituents found in neratinib and lapatinib. The triazolopyridine substituent occupies the allosteric pocket in the back cleft of HER2 and sterically hinders binding to other kinases, including EGFR.

Pharmacokinetics. The HER2-TKIs are metabolized extensively by CYP enzymes and are associated with a risk of DDIs with CYP inducers, inhibitors, and substrates.[96,203] DDIs and drug-food interactions are relevant with the HER2-TKIs because of significant CYP-mediated metabolism by several isoforms. Tucatinib is predominately biotransformed by CYP2C8, which is a minor metabolizing enzyme for lapatinib (as is CYP2C19). CYP3A4/5 are the dominant isoforms in lapatinib and neratinib metabolism.

Adverse Effects. Diarrhea is the most common adverse effect of HER2 inhibitors and requires management with antidiarrheals, such as loperamide (Chapter 16).[96] Elevated liver enzymes and hepatotoxicity may also be seen with all agents, while nausea and palmar plantar erythrodyesthesia are more commonly observed with tucatinib. Cardiotoxicity is an adverse effect observed for the HER2-targeted mAb trastuzumab; however, this risk is not associated with HER2-TKIs.

mKRAS Inhibitors. The RAS viral oncogene homolog enzymes are small GTPases that are activated on binding GTP.[210] This results in the activation of downstream signaling through the RAS/RAF/MEK/ERK and RAS/PI3K/AKT pathways. The RAS enzymes are classified as HRAS, NRAS, and KRAS. Mutations occur in RAS GTPases that contribute to a hyperexcited state with increased signaling down the RAS/MEK/ERK pathway. An oncogenic alteration in the KRAS gene leading to mKRAS is the most frequent in pancreatic cancer, CRC, and lung cancer, while mutated HRAS is the most common in dermatologic and head and neck cancers. NRAS mutations are often detected in hematologic malignancies. Inhibitors of mRAS-mediated signaling decrease cancer progression.

The mutations in KRAS typically occur at wt position 12 and include a glycine to cysteine (G12C), valine (G12V) or aspartate (G12D) mutation. These mutations prevent hydrolysis of KRAS-bound GTP, leading to a permanently activated mKRAS and persistent signaling that drives cell proliferation and tumor growth. The distribution of KRAS mutations varies among cancers, with KRAS (G12C) being expressed in 41% of lung adenocarcinoma, the most common histologic subtype of NSCLC.[211] The KRAS G12D and G12V are more common mutants in CRC and pancreatic ductal adenocarcinoma.

The RAS enzymes have a catalytic GTP-binding site and allosteric pockets termed switch region I and II, which control binding to effector proteins son of sevenless (SOS), RAF, and PI3K.[212] Small molecules that are GTP competitive were explored as inhibitors; however, the high binding affinity of RAS proteins for GTP made this approach particularly challenging. A second approach involved inhibitor binding to the allosteric pockets in the switch regions to force an inactive conformation, disrupting the interaction of KRAS with effector proteins. However, the small size of the allosteric pocket in the switch regions, along with the shallow surface and high flexibility of KRAS made it difficult to develop allosteric inhibitors. For decades, mKRAS was considered an undruggable target until the approval of sotorasib and adagrasib (see Fig. 37.14) for advanced NSCLC with KRAS G12C mutations.[213-218] Sotorasib was approved in 2021, followed by adagrasib in 2022. The approvals were based on improved overall response rate (ORR) and duration of response (DR). The PFS reported for sotorasib and adagrasib is 6.8 and 8.5 months, respectively.

Chemistry. Sotorasib and adagrasib are irreversible inhibitors that target Cys12 in the allosteric pocket of the KRAS G12C mutant. Both drugs include a piperazinyl acrylamide as an electrophilic warhead to form a covalent bond with Cys12 in the inactive, GDP-bound state of KRAS G12C. The pyridopyrimidinone core of sotorasib orients the reactive acrylamide toward Cys12. In addition, sotorasib includes a configurationally stable M atropisomer, an axially chiral biaryl moiety that allows for the optimal orientation of the isopropylmethylpyridine substituent for interaction with His95 and Tyr96 in the allosteric pocket, inducing a 10-fold improvement in potency.

Point mutations in KRAS at G12C and redundant signaling through effectors downstream of mKRAS are a common mechanism of resistance. Clinical trials are ongoing for mKRAS inhibitors in combination with inhibitors of upstream or downstream targets in the RAS/RAF/MEK/ERK pathway. Drug discovery efforts are also underway to continue the development of mKRAS inhibitors effective against additional mutants, such as G12V and G12D.

Pharmacokinetics. Both mKRAS inhibitors are orally administered and metabolized by CYP enzymes. Sotorasib and adagrasib are metabolized predominantly by CYP3A4. Sotorasib is also a Pgp substrate, while adagrasib is vulnerable to ATP-binding cassette subfamily B member 1 (ABCB1)-mediated efflux. Strong CYP3A4 and Pgp substrates, inducers, and inhibitors must be avoided. Both drugs demonstrate food-independent absorption, but sotorasib administration must be appropriately spaced from gastric pH-raising antacids and PPIs.

Adverse Effects. The adverse effects commonly observed for mKRAS inhibitors include diarrhea, hepatic toxicities, and fatigue. The adverse effects are typically mild to moderate in severity and can be managed with dose modification and monitoring. The rare but severe adverse effects include interstitial lung disease and hepatotoxicity.

mBRAF Inhibitors. Oncogenic mutations have been described for BRAF that are key drivers of melanoma (>50%), CRC (5%-10%), thyroid carcinomas (25%-45%), and hairy cell leukemia (~100%). The most common mutations that represent 90% of BRAF-driven cancers include the replacement of valine with a polar anionic glutamate (BRAF V600E) or a cationic lysine residue (BRAF V600K).[219,220] The BRAF oncogenic mutations render BRAF constitutively active and insensitive to negative feedback through ERK.

Several molecules have been investigated as BRAF inhibitors. Sorafenib is a first-generation, type I (αC-helix-in/DFG-in) multitargeted nonselective kinase inhibitor that targets wtBRAF, mBRAF (V600E/V600K), CRAF, VEGFR1, VEGFR2, VEGFR3, PDGFR, KIT, FLT3, and RET. Based on the nonselective effects, sorafenib is associated with significant adverse effects, which limit therapeutic utility. The second-generation BRAF inhibitors, vemurafenib, dabrafenib, and encorafenib (see Fig. 37.14) are selective for mBRAF (V600E/V600K) with minimal effects on wtBRAF. Dabrafenib, vemurafenib, and encorafenib have been approved for BRAF V600E or V600K melanoma, thyroid cancer, NSCLC, gliomas, and CRC.

Chemistry. Vemurafenib, dabrafenib, and encorafenib are type $I^{1/2}$ (αC-helix-out/DGF-in) inhibitors that bind in the ATP pocket and αC-helix-out pocket of inactive mBRAF.[221] The second-generation BRAF kinase inhibitors are similar in that they all include an acidic sulfonamide moiety as the pharmacophore that binds to Lys483 through an ionic bond. The sulfonamides are conjugated with electron-withdrawing halogenated rings, which promote dissociation to the anionic conjugate for binding to the cationic Lys. The pyrrolopyridine in vemurafenib and aminopyrimidine in dabrafenib and encorafenib occupy the adenine region and access the hinge region, placing the difluorinated (vemurafenib) or monofluorinated (dabrafenib, encorafenib) ring in the adjacent hydrophobic pocket. The binding interactions of dabrafenib are illustrated in Figure 37.16. The sulfonamide moiety with its attached fluorinated phenyl ring in dabrafenib interacts with the regulatory Phe595 of the DFG motif. The thiazole ring binds within the domain that normally accommodates the ribose of the nucleotide substrate. Vemurafenib mimics a similar binding mode, and the *p*-chlorophenyl moiety of vemurafenib is solvent exposed. The BRAF inhibitors bind to BRAF monomers and do not bind to activated dimers due to a steric clash.

BRAF monotherapy is not sufficient to completely disrupt RAS/RAF/MEK/ERK pathway–mediated cell proliferation.[222] While mBRAF inhibitors block the action of the V600E mutant, they activate wtBRAF and, in turn, trigger ERK phosphorylation. In the presence of mBRAF, dimerization of wtBRAF occurs in normal (noncancerous) cells and induces wtBRAF-mediated signaling that can lead to secondary malignancies, including skin lesions, squamous cell carcinomas, and gastric and colonic polyps.[219] Another unusual occurrence is the paradoxical homo- or heterodimerization and reactivation of the MAPK signaling pathway.[223] Acquired resistance to mBRAF inhibitors due to reactivation of the RAF/MEK/ERK/MAPK normally develops within a year.

MEK Inhibitors. Approaches to providing a more sustained therapeutic response for mBRAF kinase inhibitors include combination therapy with MEK inhibitors that work immediately downstream of BRAF.[223-227] The MEK kinases, MEK1 and MEK2, are mitogen-activated protein kinases with dual specificity to phosphorylate serine/threonine and tyrosine residues in the activation loop of ERK1 and ERK2. Four MEK inhibitors, trametinib, binimetinib, selumetinib, and cobimetinib (see Fig. 37.14), have been approved for use in specific types of cancer. The MEK

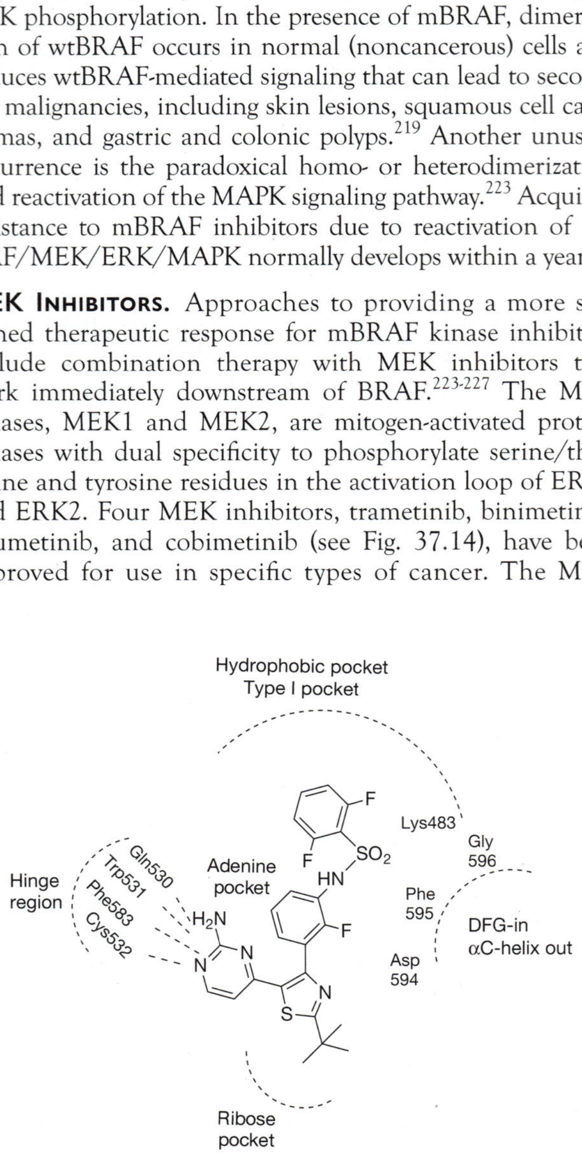

Figure 37.16 Binding interactions for dabrafenib within V600E BRAF. BRAF, B-rapidly accelerated fibrosarcoma.

inhibitors are highly effective in combination with mBRAF inhibitors. Several combinations of mBRAF and MEK inhibitors have been approved, including vemurafenib/cobimetinib and encorafenib/binimetinib for BRAF V600E/V600K melanoma, and dabrafenib/trametinib for BRAF V600E/V600K melanoma and NSCLC. Selumetinib is an approved targeted therapy for plexiform neurofibromas with mutated *NF1* in pediatric patients. Mutated NF1 leads to an overactive RAS/RAF/MAP/ERK pathway. Selumetinib shuts off this pathway by inhibiting MEK.

Chemistry. The X-ray crystal structures for approved MEK inhibitors have demonstrated that they bind to the allosteric site of the kinase in an inactive conformation.[228] Binding to the allosteric pocket instead of the ATP pocket improves selectivity for MEK. In contrast to asciminib, a type IV BCR-ABL kinase inhibitor that binds to an allosteric site remotes from the ATP pocket, the MEK inhibitors bind to an allosteric pocket that is adjacent to the ATP active site and are classified as type III kinase inhibitors (allosteric and ATP noncompetitive). Selumetinib, binimetinib, cobimetinib, and trametinib bind to the BRAF/MEK complex and not to the uncomplexed, active MEK. The inhibitors bind in an elongated preformed pocket. The crystal structure of trametinib bound to BRAF/MEK shows the MEK inhibitor inserting an aromatic group, typically a 4-bromo-2-fluorophenyl or 4-iodo-2-fluorophenyl into a lipophilic site at the back of the inhibitor-binding pocket and forming a hydrogen bond between an inhibitor carbonyl group (eg, of the pyrimidopyridine scaffold of trametinib) with the main-chain amide of Ser212 in the MEK activation segment (Fig. 37.17). Selumetinib and binimetinib contain a polar 2-hydroxyethoxy arm, which forms hydrogen bonds

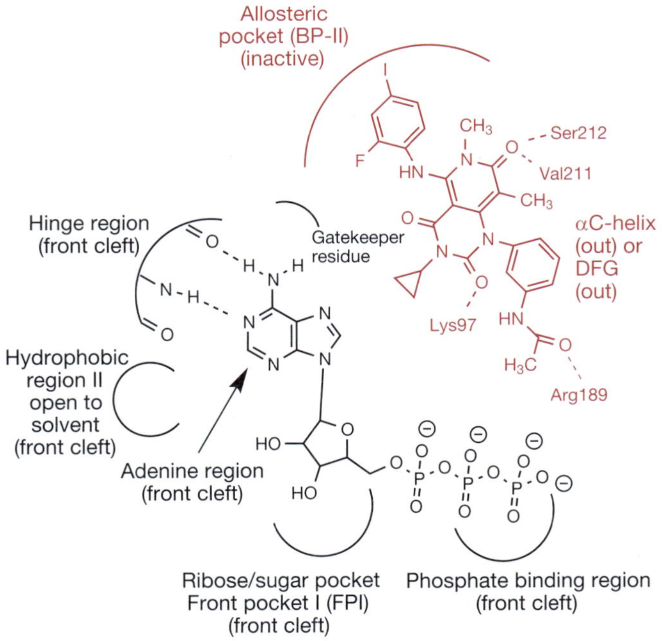

Figure 37.17 Binding interactions for trametinib, a type III kinase inhibitor in the allosteric pocket Of MEK with ATP bound within the active site. ATP, adenosine triphosphate; BP-II, back pocket II; DFG, aspartate, phenylalanine, glycine.

with phosphate oxygen of ATP. The MEK inhibitors, trametinib and cobimetinib, include additional substituents that form hydrophobic interactions and polar interactions within MEK.

Pharmacokinetics. The pharmacokinetic properties of BRAF/MEK inhibitors are provided in Table 37.6.[229-233] Redundant signaling through PI3K/AKT/mTOR pathway and alternate targets can contribute to resistance. Thus, newer agents continue to be developed to improve resistance and adverse effect profiles.

Adverse Effects. The most common adverse effects with BRAF/MEK combination therapy include mild fatigue, nausea, diarrhea, and abdominal pain.[234-236] Severe adverse effects include cardiotoxicity, hemorrhage, hyperglycemia, secondary skin malignancies, and ocular toxicities. The BRAF/MEK inhibitors are associated with a risk of cardiovascular toxicities presenting as heart failure, arrhythmia, and hypertension. The MAPK pathway is suggested to be cardioprotective, and its inhibition with mBRAF and MEK inhibitors could interfere with that protection. The mBRAF and MEK inhibitors also have effects on the renin-angiotensin pathway and cause an increase in blood pressure. The MEK inhibitors are associated with ocular toxicity that is linked to their mechanism of action. The two most common and sight-threatening events include retinal vein occlusion and subretinal fluid accumulation. Ophthalmic examinations at regular intervals during therapy are recommended. As noted, mBRAF inhibitors stimulate wtBRAF in normal (noncancerous) cells, leading to secondary malignancies including skin lesions, squamous cell carcinomas, and gastric and colonic polyps.

Inhibitors of the PI3K/AKT/mTOR Pathway

The PI3Ks are signal transducing lipid kinases that mediate key cellular functions in cancer and immunity.[81-83] PI3K incorporates a catalytic subunit (p110 with α, β, γ, or δ subtypes) and an inhibitory p85 subunit. The PI3Ks phosphorylate phosphatidylinositol bisphosphate (PIP2) to generate the second messenger inositol triphosphate (IP3), which, in turn, phosphorylates downstream effectors that support cell proliferation. Dysfunction of the tumor suppressor PTEN leads to unchecked signaling through the PI3K/AKT/mTOR pathway, increased cellular proliferation, and cancer. PI3Ks are divided into three classes (I, II, and III) based on substrate specificity and regulatory subunits.[237-239] Class I PI3Ks include two groups: class IA, made up of PI3Kα, PI3Kβ, and PI3Kδ, and class IB, which contains only one member, PI3Kγ. While class IA PI3Ks are predominantly activated by RTK signaling, PI3Kγ is activated primarily by G protein coupled receptors. Mutations or amplifications of genes encoding RTKs, RAS, p110 catalytic subunit of PI3Ks, and AKT and the loss or inactivation of functional mutation of PTEN tumor suppressor lead to continued activation of the PI3K/AKT/mTOR signaling cascade and tumor growth.

PI3Kγ/δ Inhibitors. Hyperactive PI3Kγ- and PI3Kδ-mediated signaling has been observed in lymphomas, where they reduce differentiation, migration, and increase survival of B and T cells.[240] PI3Kγ is expressed in T cells, and PI3Kδ is expressed in B cells. Several PI3K inhibitors have been approved over the past decade, starting in 2014 with idelalisib,

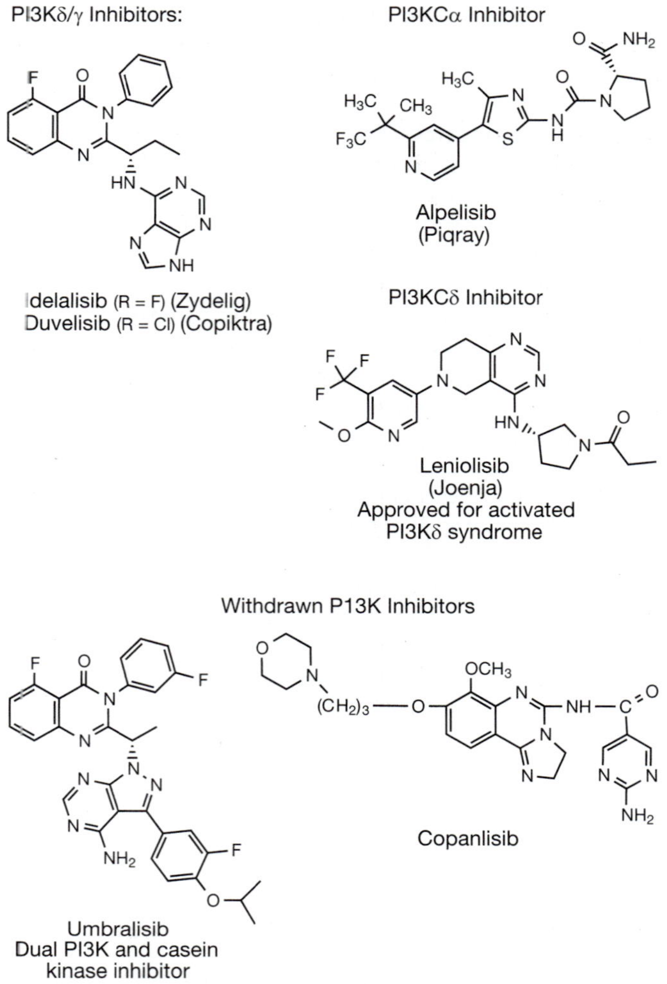

Figure 37.18 PI3K inhibitors. PI3K, phosphatidylinositol 3 kinase.

a PI3Kδ inhibitor (Fig. 37.18).[241-244] The second molecule in the class to be marketed, copanlisib, is a "pan PI3K" inhibitor with a preference for the α and δ subtypes.[245-247] Duvelisib, a dual PI3Kδ/γ was approved in 2018, and umbralisib, a PI3Kδ and casein kinase 1 epsilon (CK1ε) inhibitor, was approved in 2021, although withdrawn shortly thereafter.[248]

While PI3K is one of the most prevalent biomarkers in cancer, targeted therapy with PI3K inhibitors has been unlike typical TKI therapy. PI3K inhibitors have a limited therapeutic window due to on-target, off-tumor mechanistic adverse effects that prohibit the continuous dosing allowed with other TKIs. In particular, hyperglycemia and hyperinsulinemia are major dose-limiting toxicities that require supportive care with metformin and/or other antidiabetics, or interruption in therapy. Although the PI3K inhibitor drug class has faced several challenges in oncology, they show promise in other diseases, including rare diseases. Leniolisib, a PI3Kδ inhibitor, has been approved as a first-in-class targeted therapy for activated PI3Kδ syndrome in young adults, a condition that leaves them highly vulnerable to respiratory infections.

Chemistry. Idelalisib is a type II kinase inhibitor that binds within the active site and neighboring allosteric pocket. Idelalisib's purine core binds via hydrogen bonds to the peptidic backbone of Val828 and Glu826 of the hinge region of the ATP active site pocket. The fluorinated quinazolinone aromatic system induces an inactive conformation with access to a hydrophobic allosteric pocket and fits tightly within it. The phenyl substituent makes additional hydrophobic interactions. Idelalisib adopts a "propeller conformation," in which the two aromatic moieties are oriented at the right angles to one another.

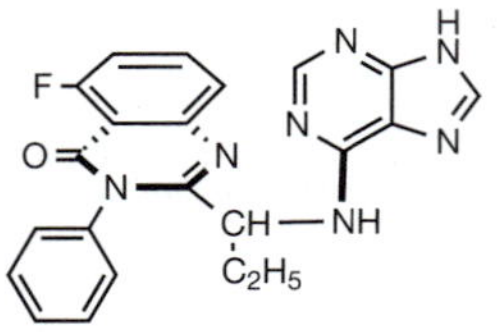

Idelalisib (propeller conformation)

Pharmacokinetics. Aldehyde oxidase is the primary metabolizing enzyme of idelalisib, generating the inactive circulating imidazolinone metabolite GS-563117. CYP3A4 plays a relatively minor role in idelalisib metabolism (19%), as does phase II glucuronidation (7%). None of these minor metabolites are found in plasma. Duvelisib is primarily metabolized via CYP3A4.

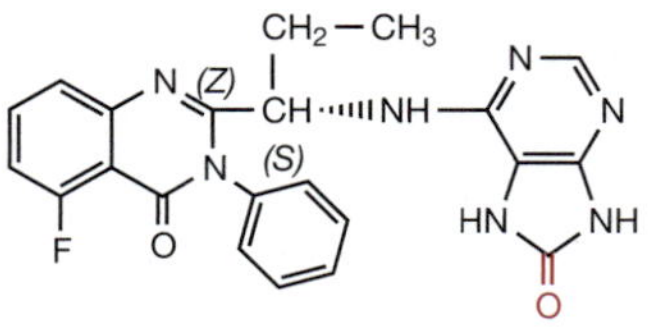

GS-563117 (Idelalisib inactive metabolite)

Adverse Effects. The PI3Kγ/δ inhibitors approved for hematologic malignancies are plagued by mechanism-dependent and mechanism-independent toxicities that have led to drug withdrawals.[249,250] The expression and function of PI3Ks pose challenges with increased toxicity. PI3Kα and PI3Kβ are ubiquitously expressed in the body. PI3Kδ and PI3Kγ are found in normal blood–based immune cells, and inhibition leads to serious risks of immunosuppression and infection, including from cytomegalovirus and *Pneumocystis jirovecii*. PI3Kδ not only drives oncogenesis in B and T cells but also plays a role in normal physiologic functioning. PI3K is involved in insulin signaling and glucose metabolism in the liver and muscles. Inhibition of the PI3K/AKT/mTOR pathway in these tissues impairs insulin signaling, leads to insulin resistance, and induces hyperglycemia and hyperinsulinemia. PI3Kβ is associated with platelet activation. GI toxicities (colitis and diarrhea), hematologic toxicities (neutropenia, thrombocytopenia), pulmonary toxicity and pneumonitis, and cutaneous reactions are also observed.

These mechanistic adverse effects prevent PI3K inhibitors from being dosed at high enough concentrations to fully suppress PI3K signaling in the tumor, leading to suboptimal clinical efficacies. This has resulted in boxed warnings associated with their use, and they are distributed through the REMS program. Idelalisib has boxed warnings for hepatotoxicity, diarrhea or colitis, infection risk, intestinal perforation, and pneumonitis. Duvelisib is associated with a boxed warning of serious adverse effects, including infections, diarrhea or colitis, skin reactions, and pneumonitis. Copanlisib, the dual PI3Kδ/γ inhibitor, was approved for IV administration in relapsed follicular lymphoma in 2017; however, it was voluntarily withdrawn based on failure to meet therapeutic outcomes in the CHRONOS-4 clinical trial compared to conventional therapy. As previously noted, the FDA approval of umbralisib was withdrawn due to safety concerns and an increased risk of death from the UNITY-CLL clinical trial.[251]

PI3KCα Inhibitor. The activating mutation of PI3KCα is the second most frequent in human cancers, including breast, colon, head, and neck squamous cell carcinoma and uterine and endometrial cancers.[252] The mutations E542K, E545K, and H1047R change the conformation of PI3KCα and trigger uncontrolled proliferation. Approximately 30% of advanced HR positive, HER2 negative breast cancers harbor an activating PIK3Cα mutation. Alpelisib (see Fig. 37.18) is a reversible ATP-competitive inhibitor of mutated PI3KCα.[253,254] PIK3Cα mutant breast cancers are particularly sensitive to PI3KCα inhibition; however, inhibition of mutant PI3Kα results in an increase in ER transcription in breast cells.[255] Fulvestrant, a selective ER downregulator, counteracts breast cell proliferation induced by mutant PI3Kα inhibition, justifying combination therapy. Alpelisib has been approved in combination with fulvestrant for the treatment of advanced or metastatic breast cancer in postmenopausal women and men with HR positive, HER2 negative disease.

Alpelisib tablets are administrated daily with food. Absorption is rapid (T_{max} ~ 2 hours), and the extent is estimated to be ~56%, with the drug appearing in plasma and red blood cells (RBCs). The drug is highly bound to plasma protein (89%).[256]

Alpelisib is relatively stable in GI fluid but undergoes hydrolytic metabolism to an inactive metabolite (M4) through the action of several enzymes, including amidase, carbox-ylesterase, and cholinesterases. A significant amount (~38%) of the parent compound is excreted unchanged, appearing primarily in feces and, to a lesser extent, in urine. Minor metabolism involving CYP3A4 occurs, but not enough to cause clinically relevant DDIs with CYP inhibitors or inducers. Alpelisib is associated with severe hyperglycemia, and dose adjustments, antidiabetic medications, and/or other modifications in therapy may be needed.[257] Alpelisib under the brand name Vijoice is also approved for PI3KCα overgrowth spectrum disease, a congenital condition that causes asymmetrical malformations in the brain, limbs, torso, and face.

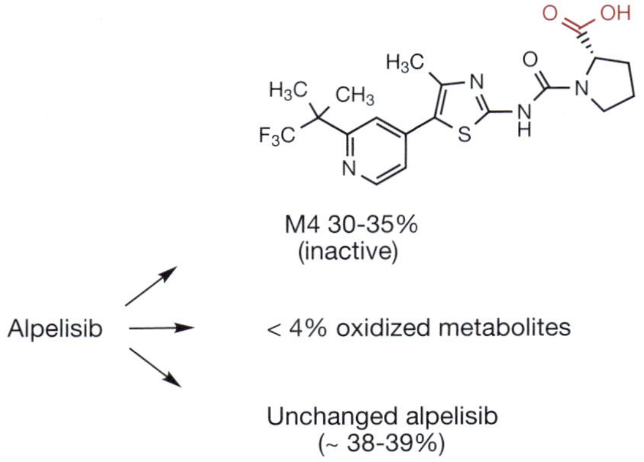

AKT Inhibitors. The serine/threonine kinase, AKT, is found downstream of PI3K and is activated by IP3 generated following PI3K activation. This, in turn, triggers downstream signaling that supports cancer cell proliferation. Three AKT isoforms, AKT1, AKT2, and AKT3, have been identified with high sequence homology. AKT1 and AKT2 have been implicated in cancer.[81,83]

Hyperactivation of the PI3K/AKT/mTOR pathway is observed in several cancers, and an AKT1 (E17K) mutant has been identified in patients with HR+ breast cancer.[257] Capivasertib, a pyrrolo[2,3-*d*]pyrimidine-containing structure, is a type I first-in-class pan-AKT inhibitor approved for use in combination with fulvestrant for advanced hormone-dependent, HER2-negative, PIK3CA, AKT1, and/or PTEN-altered breast cancer.

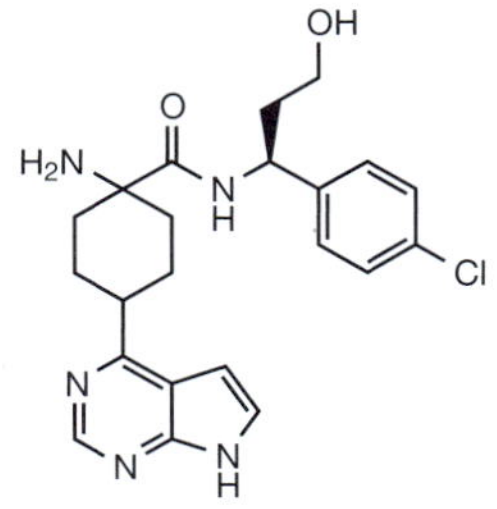

Capivasertib
(Truqap)

Similar to alpelisib, capivasertib is administered in combination with fulvestrant after confirmation of altered PIK3CA/AKT1/PTEN status.[258-260] In the CAPItello-291 trial that compared a combination of capivasertib and fulvestrant to fulvestrant alone in patients with HR positive breast cancer, the capivasertib/fulvestrant combination showed longer PFS.[258,259] Diarrhea, skin rash, and hyperglycemia were the main dose-limiting toxicities. The incidence of hyperglycemia was much lower than observed for the alpelisib and fulvestrant combination in the SOLAR trial, which has been attributed to the intermittent dosing schedule used for the capivasertib/fulvestrant combination. Capivasertib does not demonstrate significant plasma protein binding (22%) and has low oral bioavailability (29%). It undergoes significant CYP3A4 and UGT2B7-mediated metabolism and is associated with significant CYP3A-mediated DDIs.

mTOR Inhibitors. The systems and tissues most commonly impacted by PI3K/AKT/mTOR dysregulation are neuroendocrine, kidney, and breast.[261] mTOR is a component of the PI3K/AKT/mTOR signaling pathway and, like the pathways discussed previously, is intimately involved in regulating cellular homeostasis. When activated, mTOR phosphorylates kinases that ultimately result in the de novo synthesis of proteins (including VEGF) that stimulate angiogenesis and promote cellular growth. The two marketed mTOR inhibitors, everolimus and temsirolimus (Fig. 37.19), are O_{13} analogs of rapamycin (also known as sirolimus), an antibiotic isolated from soil.[262] Cell growth with mTOR inhibitors is arrested at the G1 phase, and inhibition of hypoxia-inducible factors (HIFs) resulting from mTOR blockade halts angiogenesis by attenuating levels of VEGF and PDGF.

Everolimus and temsirolimus have been approved for advanced renal cell carcinoma (RCC).[263] Everolimus in

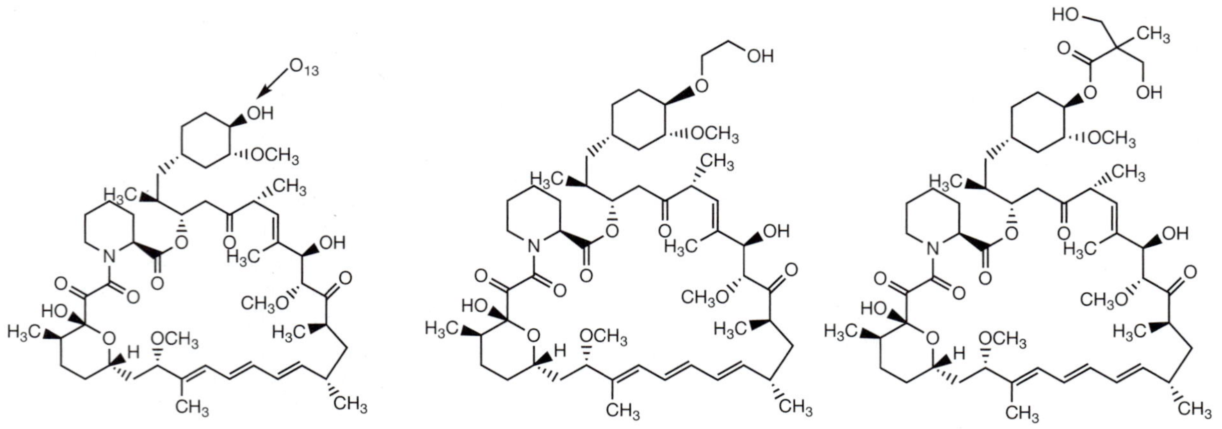

Rapamycin (Sirolimus) | Everolimus (Afinitor) | Temsirolimus (Torisel)

Figure 37.19 mTOR inhibitors. mTOR, mammalian target of rapamycin.

combination with exemestane is approved for use following sunitinib (or sorafenib) failure in HR-positive, HER2-negative breast cancer that is resistant to the aromatase inhibitors, letrozole and anastrazole (Chapters 25 and 36). Everolimus is also used in tuberous sclerosis complex, a rare disease characterized by multiple benign tumors.

The *mTOR* gene is vulnerable to mutation, leading to changes in the kinase structure that induce mTOR inhibitor resistance. Alterations in the rate of phosphorylation of the S6K1 protein, which happens after normal mTOR activation, is another harbinger of resistance, as it indicates tumor-driven "workarounds" of normal signaling pathways. A multitude of other resistance mechanisms, including "survival-promoting signaling feedback loops," have been identified.

Chemistry. The kinase domain of the mTOR protein resides in the C-terminal area, with a 100-residue macrolide-binding domain (known as FKBP12-FRB) located close to its N-terminal side.[261] The ATP-binding hinge region common to all kinases joins the C- and N-terminal lobes. mTOR forms two complexes (mTORC1 and mTORC2) that serve distinct functions, regulating cell growth and promoting cell survival, respectively. Rapamycin binds tightly to FKBP12-FRB and, by burrowing into a deep "gap" between these proteins, promotes an interaction that is not observed in the absence of the macrolide. This inhibits the ability of the kinase to function. The van der Waals interactions with a number of Tyr, Phe, and Trp residues in the FKBP12 domain, along with H bonds with Asp and Tyr side chains, promote high-affinity binding between inhibitor and enzyme. Hydrophobic interactions between the carbon-rich macrolide and the kinase are known to occur and are the only interactions believed to form with the FRB domain. Rapamycin is 92% buried when bound to these two mTOR domains.

The mTOR inhibitors bind to the allosteric FKBP12-FRB domain of mTORC1, which is adjacent to the catalytic ATP-binding domain.[262-264] The mTOR inhibitors sirolimus, everolimus, and temsirolimus could be categorized as type IV inhibitors (those that bind distal to the ATP site); however, it should be noted that they bind first to FKBP12, which then binds mTOR. This results in an inhibition of catalysis. The mTOR inhibitors do not directly bind to mTOR itself. Once bound through FKBP12, they prevent a regulatory protein known as regulatory-associated protein of mTOR, or "raptor," from binding to the complex.

Pharmacokinetics. Everolimus is orally active and available in tablet and soluble tablet forms. Temsirolimus is used IV in the treatment of advanced RCC.[265,266] The drug has no ionizable functional groups and must be solubilized for IV administration with polysorbate 80 (Tween). Both everolimus and temsirolimus undergo CYP3A4-catalyzed hydroxylation, dealkylation, and N-oxidation reactions (along with lactone cleavage), and coadministration of strong CYP3A4 inhibitors and inducers must be avoided. Temsirolimus is also hydrolyzed to sirolimus (rapamycin), which retains the activity of the parent and has a significantly longer elimination half-life (55 vs 17 hours). None of the other metabolites retain therapeutically relevant activity.

Adverse Effects. In addition to other commonly observed kinase inhibitor adverse effects (eg, fatigue, rash, GI distress), everolimus is immunosuppressive, explaining its use in renal transplantation for rejection prophylaxis. Temsirolimus must be solubilized for IV administration with polysorbate 80. Since this can induce a hypersensitivity reaction that can manifest as hypotension and breathing difficulties, patients must be pretreated with an H_1 antagonist (eg, diphenhydramine) before each administration. Drug discontinuation and supportive therapy are required in the event of a hypersensitivity reaction. Patients on temsirolimus can experience mechanism-related hyperglycemia and potentially severe elevations in serum cholesterol and triglycerides.

Bruton Tyrosine Kinase Inhibitors. The nonreceptor Bruton tyrosine kinase (BTK) is essential to proper B-lymphocyte development and B-cell receptor (BCR) signaling and is expressed by a gene associated with the X chromosome.[266] It was named for U.S. Navy pediatrician Ogden Bruton, who first described an X-linked immunodeficiency syndrome caused by mutations in the *BTK* gene. BTK is activated downstream of the BCR in B lymphocytes.[267] Under normal circumstances, BTK phosphorylates phospholipase Cγ2 (PLCγ2), mobilizing Ca^{2+} and activating several signaling cascades, including mammalian PI3K/AKT/mTOR that is critical to B-cell homeostasis. Hyperactive BTK drives B-cell signaling and proliferation, leading to lymphoid malignancies such as lymphomas and lymphoid leukemias.[82] Importantly, BTK inhibition spares T cells since the protein is not found there, thus also sparing the patient's immune function.

Ibrutinib, the first BTK inhibitor, was followed by second-generation acalabrutinib and zanubrutinib and, in 2023, by pirtobrutinib, a third-generation inhibitor (Fig. 37.20).[268-272] Ibrutinib is a potent BTK inhibitor; however, it has modest selectivity and inhibits EGFR, HER2, HER4, C-terminal Src kinase (CSK), JAK3, and interleukin-2–inducible T-cell kinase (ITK). The second-generation agents are much more selective, leading to fewer adverse effects. Efficacy of the three irreversible BTK inhibitors is short-lived.[273] Resistance occurs primarily through a C481S mutation, which destroys the ability of the enzyme to attack the electrophilic acrylamide or butynamide moiety. Approximately 50% of patients with Waldenström macroglobulinemia have BTK C481S mutations at progression. A similar mutation (C797S) was previously described for the irreversibly acting osimertinib. Alternate mechanisms of resistance, such as T316A and R665W PLCγ2 mutants, are also observed for BTK inhibitors. Pirtobrutinib is the latest addition to the BTK class of targeted anticancer therapies. It is a reversible BTK inhibitor and is capable of binding to both BTK and the C481S mutant, providing an advantage over previous BTK inhibitors.[272,274]

BTK inhibitors have changed the treatment paradigm for B-cell malignancies from chemoimmunotherapy to targeted therapy and are the current standard of care. The irreversible BTK inhibitors, ibrutinib, acalabrutinib, and

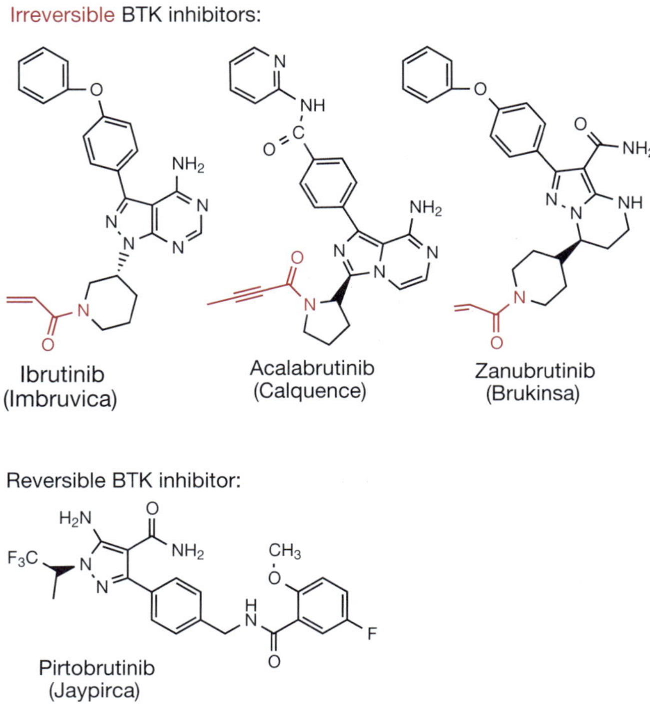

Figure 37.20 BTK inhibitors. BTK, Bruton tyrosine kinase.

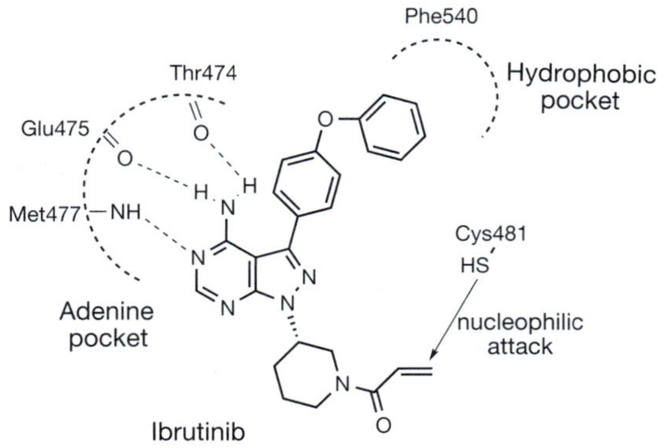

Figure 37.21 Binding interactions for ibrutinib.

zanubrutinib, are approved for use in several BCLs and leukemias including chronic lymphocytic leukemia (CLL) and mantle cell lymphoma (MCL), although the development of C481S mutation can lead to an insufficient response. Pirtobrutinib is reserved for relapsed or refractory lymphocytic leukemia and MCL after progression on at least two lines of systemic therapy, including a BTK and BCL-2 inhibitor.

Chemistry. Binding interactions for ibrutinib within BTK are shown in Figure 37.21. The ATP pocket of BTK includes a Cys481 residue similar to EGFR and HER2.[267] The first- and second-generation BTK inhibitors include the now familiar electrophilic acrylamide (or analogous butynamide) substituent that can form a covalent bond with Cys481 in a manner similar to the irreversible alkylation mechanisms of the EGFR-TKIs afatinib and osimertinib, and the HER2-TKI neratinib.[269,270] Hydrogen bonding interactions are observed with the backbone of Thr474, Glu475, and Met477 of the hinge region, and hydrophobic interactions are seen with Phe540.[271]

Pirtobrutinib binds reversibly to the ATP pocket and forces a closed, inactive kinase conformation. The molecule forms three hydrogen bonds with the backbone of Glu475 and Met477 in the hinge region and demonstrates additional binding in the pocket through hydrogen bonds with Lys430 and Asp539, and an edge-to-face π stacking interaction with Phe540. Pirtobrutinib exploits different regions of the pocket allowing for activity in C481S BTK that is resistant to irreversible BTK inhibitors. Instead, pirtobrutinib extends further into the back pocket toward the activation loop and αC-helix.

Pharmacokinetics. The BTK inhibitors are administered orally and predominantly metabolized by CYP3A4 and glucuronidation.[268] Clinically significant drug interactions between the approved BTK inhibitors and CYP3A inhibitors or inducers have been observed. Acalabrutinib also undergoes minor glutathione conjugation and amide hydrolysis. Raising the gastric pH decreases the absorption of acalabrutinib capsules (but not the film-coated tablets), and coadministration with PPIs should be avoided. Zanubrutinib is rapidly absorbed after oral administration. The $T_{1/2}$ is ~2 to 4 hours, and T_{max} is 2 hours. Pirtobrutinib has good oral bioavailability (86%),[275] a high plasma protein binding (96%), and a half-life of 19 hours, which is significantly longer than other BTKs. Only 28% of the drug is eliminated unchanged, and UGT1A8 and UGT1A9 are both involved in its phase II metabolism.

Adverse Effects. Mild adverse effects, including GI distress, rash, and headache, are observed for all BTK inhibitors.[271,276] More serious adverse effects, such as an increased risk of infections, bleeding risk, and cardiotoxicity, are also observed, especially with ibrutinib. The most frequent infections are aspergillosis and *P. jirovecii* infections. BTK is involved in platelet activation through GP VI signaling. BTK inhibition blocks GP VI–mediated platelet aggregation, which explains the bleeding risk, including intracranial hemorrhage. Cardiovascular adverse effects often manifest as atrial fibrillation caused by inhibition of CSK expressed in heart tissue.[277] Additional cardiomyopathies are seen due to the presence of HER2 and HER4 in cardiomyocytes. Variability in the incidence of this adverse effect is observed among BTK inhibitors depending on their impact on CSK. As noted earlier, the more selective second-generation agents are associated with a lower risk of serious adverse reactions than ibrutinib. A risk of secondary malignancies has also been reported.

Inhibitors of NF-κB Pathway–Mediated Inflammation

NF-κB is a master regulator of the inflammatory tumor microenvironment that supports the progression of MM and other B-cell malignancies. Two broad classes of non–kinase-targeted therapies, immunomodulators and proteasome inhibitors, that directly or indirectly suppress NF-κB–mediated inflammatory signaling have been approved. These drugs are used in combination with dexamethasone, a corticosteroid that also inhibits the inflammatory tumor microenvironment in MM and has led to complete remission.

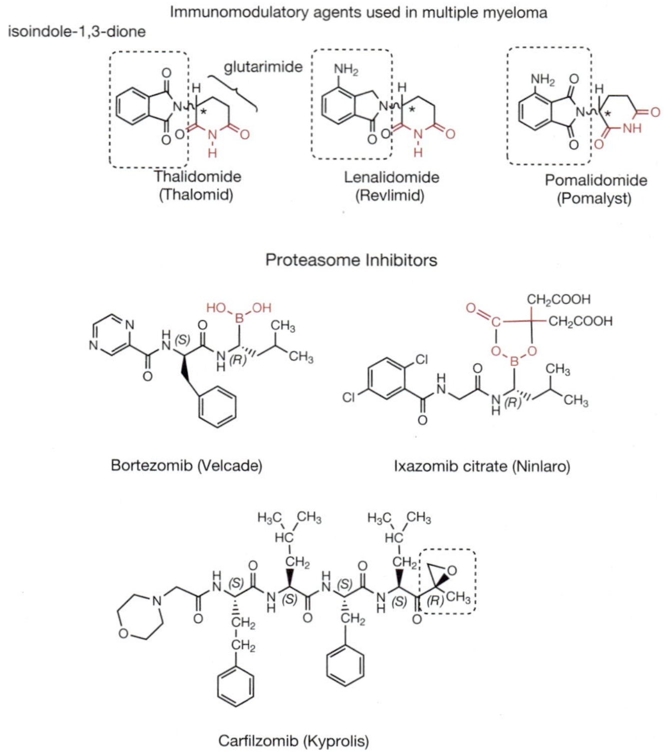

Figure 37.22 Nuclear factor kappa B pathway inhibitors.

IMMUNOMODULATORS. Anyone of the "baby boomer" or World War II generation will recognize the name of the drug thalidomide (Fig. 37.22) because it induced perhaps the most well-known incident of drug-associated birth defects. Used in the late 1950s and early 1960s as an antiemetic and sedative in pregnancy, more than 10,000 European children were born with flipper-like arms and legs, a condition called phocomelia, or "seal limb."[278] Although not licensed in the United States during those years, the drug was banned by the FDA until 1997. However, thalidomide has since demonstrated antiproliferative and proapoptotic actions in cancer cells with unique clinical benefits in MM. This led to thalidomide being approved for very cautious use in MM as an immunomodulatory drug (IMiD).[279]

IMiDs work through multiple mechanisms of action.[69,280,281] In addition to arresting uncontrolled cell growth, thalidomide and its analogs deny MM cells access to bone marrow stromal cells and various growth factors needed for tumor cell survival and increase circulating levels of natural killer cells interleukin (IL)-2 and interferon-γ. This triggers T-cell–mediated cell cytotoxicity and augments the immune response. The IMiDs indirectly inhibit the NF-κB pathway by blocking tumor necrosis factor α (TNFα) and IL-1β signals and activating inhibitor of nuclear factor-κB (IκB) kinase (IKK). They also bind to the protein cereblon and activate the E3 ubiquitin ligase complex. Lenalidomide induces the ubiquitination and proteolytic degradation of substrate proteins Ikaros (IKZF1) and Ailos (IKZF3) that are crucial for the survival of myeloma cells.[282] Proteolytic degradation of IKZF1 and IKZF3 triggers myeloma cell death.

IMiDs are contraindicated in pregnancy. Boxed warnings mandate that female patients capable of becoming pregnant document they are not pregnant for 2 months prior to beginning therapy and either use two contraceptive methods or opt for total abstinence during, and for 1 month following, therapy. During and for 1 month following therapy, male patients must use condoms during intercourse with those capable of childbearing. These drugs are only available through the appropriate restricted distribution (REMS) program. Lenalidomide and pomalidomide, as more potent and less toxic immunomodulatory analogs, have effectively taken thalidomide's therapeutic place.[283-285] Pomalidomide is the most potent immunomodulator of the three substituted isoindolinones and is indicated for patients who have progressed on lenalidomide/bortezomib and at least one other therapy.

Chemistry. Lenalidomide and pomalidomide are thalidomide analogs used as IMiDs in the treatment of MM. All are dioxopiperidin-3-yl-(glutar*imide*) substituted isoindolinones; thalidomide and pomalidomide have the isoindoline-1,3-dione (phthalimide) structure, and lenalidomide and pomalidomide are aniline derivatives. Thalidomide was used in pregnancy due to its sedative actions. However, the sedative and later identified teratogenic actions of chiral thalidomide are mediated by different stereoisomers. The in vivo inversion of the therapeutic *R*-isomer to its cytotoxic *S*-enantiomer led to the birth defects and prohibits the use of thalidomide in those who were or could become pregnant. Lenalidomide and pomalidomide are also marketed as racemic mixtures of the *R*- and *S*-enantiomers, and as in thalidomide, chiral inversion also occurs in vivo.

Pharmacokinetics. As previously noted, lenalidomide is marketed as the racemic mixture, and chiral inversion converts 5% of the *R*-isomer to *S* within an hour after administration.[286,287] Slow nonenzymatic hydrolysis of the glutarimide ring occurs, but CYP2C19-catalyzed oxidation (5-hydroxylation) and phase II N-acetylation (at the primary aromatic NH_2) is minimal, as is the risk of kinetics-related DDIs. The drug is excreted essentially unchanged. In contrast, pomalidomide is extensively metabolized, primarily by CYP1A2 and CYP3A4, and only about 10% is excreted as the parent drug. Phase II glucuronic acid conjugation and *N*-acetylation commonly precede renal elimination.

Adverse Effects. In addition to teratogenicity, the use of IMiDs in MM is associated with adverse effects and boxed warnings. Lenalidomide's and pomalidomide's adverse effect profiles are milder than thalidomide's, but significant venous thromboembolic (deep vein thrombosis, pulmonary embolism) and hematologic events (thrombocytopenia and neutropenia) can still occur, leading to boxed warnings for embryo-fetal toxicity, venous and arterial thromboembolism, and hematologic toxicities.[69,281-284] Additional adverse effects include rash and constipation.

Proteasome Inhibitors. Facilitated by ubiquitin tagging, proteasomes selectively clear cells of cytoplasmic regulatory proteins by cleaving them into short peptides.[288] The 26S proteasome serves as the recognition site for ubiquitinated proteins tagged for degradation. Through the action of an ATP-dependent 19S regulatory unit, these ubiquitinylated proteins are transferred to the 20S "core particle" proteolytic domain (a chamber from which there is no escape) for destruction.[289,290] The β-OH group of the N-terminal threonine residue (Thr1) serves as the proteolytic nucleophile responsible for peptide bond cleavage. The abnormal plasma cells in MM produce large amounts of Igs and are dependent on proteasomes to clear the excess protein and maintain cell viability and function. Inhibition of this homeostatic process through the blockade of the 20S proteasome induces apoptosis via a build-up of aged or conformationally altered proteins.[288-290] A secondary mechanism involves the inhibition of the proteasomal degradation of IκB in MM cells with indirect effects on NF-κB.[291] The IκB protein complexes with NF-κB in the cytosol and prevents activation of the NF-κB pathway, inhibiting NF-κB's inflammatory effects. Inhibition of the proteasomal degradation of IκB in MM cells results in increased levels of complexed NF-κB and suppresses the NF-κB–mediated pro-inflammatory and prosurvival effects.

Bortezomib, ixazomib, and carfilzomib are proteasome inhibitors that have been approved for MM (see Fig. 37.22).[292] The proteasome inhibitors used in combination with IMiDs and corticosteroids are the backbone of MM treatment. Proteasome inhibitors inhibit the 20S proteasome and impair homeostatic clearance of cellular proteins "whose time has come." This induces fatal endoplasmic reticular stress by rendering the malignant cells incapable of managing the high amounts of mis-folded Ig produced. Apoptosis results. As with many targeted therapies, resistance can manifest. Bortezomib resistance has been the most intensely studied, and point mutations in the β5 subunit gene (eg, A40T, A50V), altered expression of β5 ubiquitin-proteasome pathway proteins, induction of homeostatic heat shock (cell repair) proteins, and Pgp upregulation have all been implicated.[293]

Chemistry. Bortezomib, ixazomib, and carfilzomib are peptidic and interact with residues within the proteolytic domain [the trypsin- (β2) and caspase-like (β1) sites] of the 20S proteasome.[291,294,295] The proteolytic site houses a catalytic zinc ion, and the proteasome inhibitors include functional groups that interact with zinc. The dipeptide proteasome inhibitors, bortezomib and ixazomib, bind reversibly to the zinc through a boronic acid moiety. Ixazomib is a boronate ester prodrug that is activated to the corresponding boronic acid when exposed to an aqueous environment.[290] The crystal structure of the bortezomib-20S proteasome complex from yeast has been reported, and specific drug-proteasome interactions with the chymotrypsin-like site (also known as the β5 subunit) have been identified.[294] The phenylmethyl moiety of the Phe component of the dipeptide inserts into a proteasome pocket but does not interact with the protein, so its loss in ixazomib is tolerated. Ixazomib has chlorine atoms in the same relative position as bortezomib's pyrazine nitrogen atoms. Since Asp114 is proposed to interact in free acid form with one unionized bortezomib pyrazine nitrogen, an electron-rich chlorine can serve the same binding function. The boronic acid moiety is essential to the proteasome-specific action of the reversible inhibitors, as CYP-mediated deboronation of bortezomib yields an inactive metabolite.

Carfilzomib is an epoxyketone that forms a covalent bond within the 20S proteasome and induces irreversible 20S proteasome inhibition. The human 20S proteasome bound to the irreversible proteasome inhibitor carfilzomib has been crystallized.[295] Unlike bortezomib and ixazomib, this inhibitor shows high selectivity for the chymotrypsin-like (β5) site [vs the trypsin- (β2) and caspase-like (β1) sites] of constitutive proteasomes. The nucleophilic β-OH of a threonine residue within the proteasome active site attacks the electrophilic epoxyketone of carfilzomib at the carbonyl carbon. The electron-deficient oxirane carbon alkylates the terminal NH_2, forming an adduct where the drug and enzyme are covalently joined through a newly generated morpholine ring. Like the phenylmethyl of bortezomib, the morpholine ring on the N-terminal end of the parent drug does not bind to any proteasome residues.

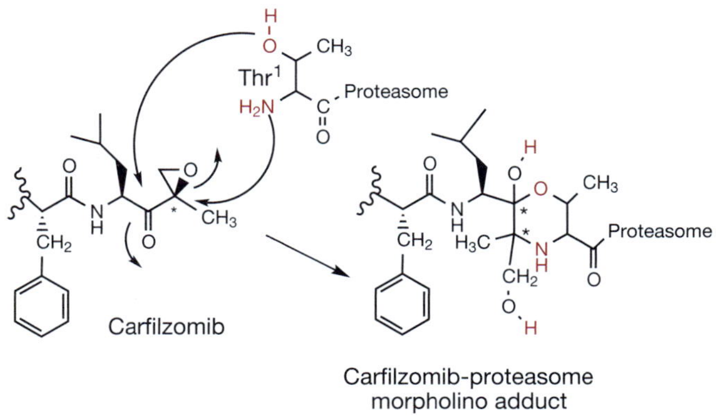

Pharmacokinetics. Bortezomib is administered IV or SC as first-line therapy in MM.[292,296] Following inactivating deboronization, bortezomib is hydroxylated at various positions prior to excretion. The CYP isoforms involved in this biotransformation include primarily CYP3A4 and CYP2C19, although the 1A2 and 2D6 are also involved to a minor extent. Ixazomib is an orally active analog of bortezomib used in combination with lenalidomide and dexamethasone in patients with MM who have progressed on at least one prior therapy. The hydrolytic activation of ixazomib citrate is shown below. Compared to bortezomib, the maximum plasma concentration of ixazomib is 19 times greater, the AUC slightly more than 2 times higher, and protein binding more extensive (99% vs 83%).

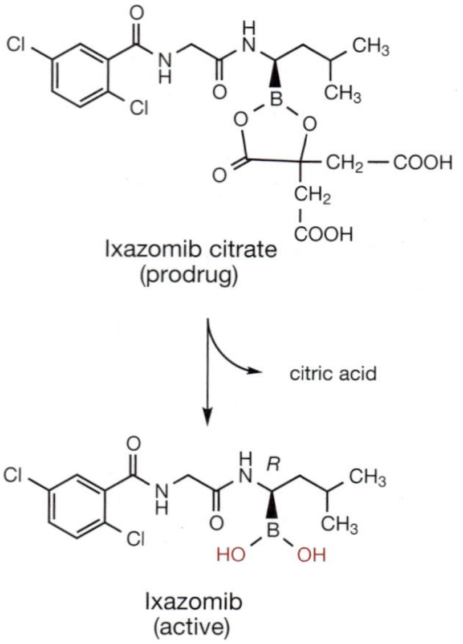

Carfilzomib is administered IV and dosed in accordance with the patient's body surface area and the prescribed regimen.[297] It is used in refractory/relapsed disease either as monotherapy or in combination with lenalidomide and/or dexamethasone and has demonstrated positive response and survival outcomes in patients unresponsive or intolerant to bortezomib and lenalidomide. Carfilzomib has a short plasma half-life due to covalent bonding to the β5 site of the 20S proteasome. Carfilzomib is not metabolized to any appreciable extent by CYP enzymes but is extensively transformed by peptidase-catalyzed cleavage and epoxide hydrolysis prior to excretion.

Adverse Effects. Proteasome inhibitors cause myelosuppression leading to neutropenia and thrombocytopenia and can induce serious peripheral neuropathy.[296] In addition to GI distress, serious cardiac and pulmonary complications have also been reported, including left ventricular ejection fraction dysfunction, arrhythmia, and acute respiratory distress syndrome.[298] Peripheral neuropathy is a dose-limiting toxicity for bortezomib; however, this is less problematic with carfilzomib and ixazomib.[296,299]

Apoptosis Pathway Modulators

BCL-2 Inhibitors. Apoptosis is maintained through interactions between proapoptotic and antiapoptotic proteins.[300] The BCL-2 protein is an antiapoptotic protein and a master regulator of the intrinsic apoptotic signaling pathway. The BCL-2 protein contains BH1 and BH2 domains. The proapoptotic proteins include BIM, BAX, and BID and contain a BH3 domain. The BH3-only proteins initiate programmed cell death in response to stress by binding to prosurvival/antiapoptotic proteins or by activating the effectors of apoptosis. The proapoptotic proteins BIM, BAX, and BID bind to and neutralize BCL-2. The BIM/BCL-2 interaction promotes apoptosis and triggers cell death.

In CLL, the BCL-2 protein is overexpressed, and cancer cells become dependent on it for their survival.[301] The overexpression of BCL-2 inhibits apoptosis and promotes cellular survival and leukemic cell accumulation. Characterization of the functions and structural interactions between proapoptotic and prosurvival BCL-2 family members led to the development of small molecules as BH3 mimetics that kill cancer cells by targeting prosurvival BCL-2 members. The BCL-2 inhibitor venetoclax is approved for CLL.[302,303] Venetoclax binds directly to the BCL-2 protein in the manner of BH3 and liberates the apoptotic BAX and BAK proteins that restore cancer cell mortality. Binding interactions of importance include hydrophobic tethering through the *p*-chlorophenyl and dimethylcyclohexene rings, as well as an electrostatic interaction between an anionic center on venetoclax (potentially the sulfonylbenzamide moiety) and cationic Arg103 of the protein. Venetoclax's reduced affinity for a related antiapoptotic protein ($BCL\text{-}X_L$) decreases the potential for thrombocytopenia, which plagued a precursor BCL-2 inhibitor, navitoclax.[304,305]

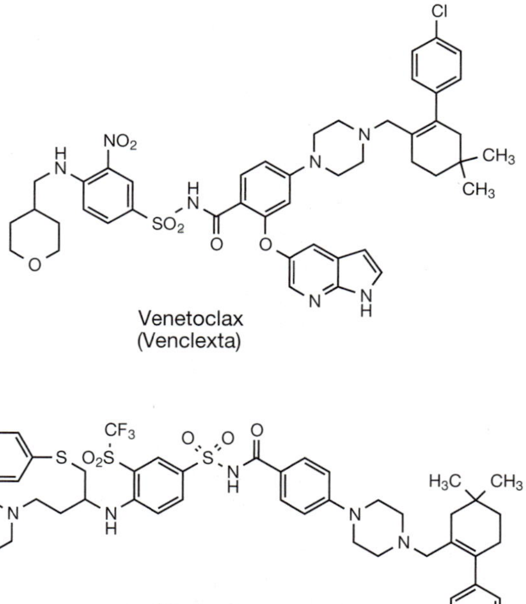

Venetoclax
(Venclexta)

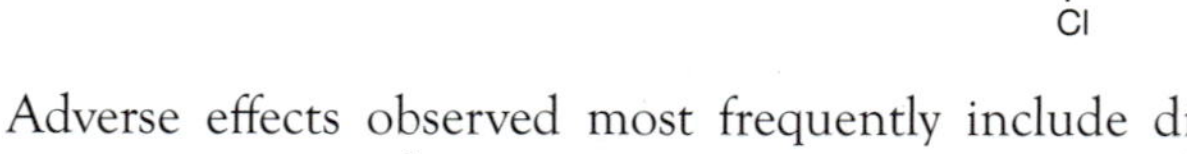

Navitoclax
(not approved)

Adverse effects observed most frequently include diarrhea, neutropenia, fatigue, upper respiratory tract infections, and cough. The risk of potentially fatal tumor lysis syndrome can be lessened by incrementally increasing the daily dose from 20 mg (initial) to 400 mg (maintenance) over 5 weeks in accordance with a recommended schedule.

The half-life of venetoclax runs between 19 and 26 hours, and the T_{max} is 6 to 8 hours. It is strongly plasma protein bound.

CYP3A4 hydroxylation at position 6 of the cyclohexene ring followed by cyclization generates a significantly less active metabolite that represents 30% of total drug concentration at the 400 mg maintenance dose. The route of elimination is almost exclusively biliary, with 21% of the drug being excreted unchanged in feces. Venetoclax is also a Pgp substrate, and the coadministration of CYP3A4 inducers or inhibitors, as well as Pgp inhibitors, should be avoided.

Inhibitors of Myeloid Differentiation Pathways

The hematologic malignancy, AML, is characterized by abnormal proliferation and accumulation of immature myeloblasts in the bone marrow, peripheral blood, and other tissues. Poorly differentiated myeloblasts can interfere with normal hematopoietic processes, thus leading to severe infections, anemia, and hemorrhage.[306] Dysfunctional enzymes have been known to drive abnormal myeloblast proliferation and accumulation. Mutations in FLT3, isocitrate dehydrogenase (IDH), and hyperactive JAK have been associated with myeloproliferative disease, including AML.[306,307] Altered retinoic acid receptor (RAR) has been associated with acute promyelocytic leukemia (APL) and is known to be a precursor to AML. Myeloproliferative diseases are characterized by dysfunctional pathways that support the proliferation of aberrant mature blood cells. A common type of myeloproliferative disorder is polycythemia vera, which is characterized by abnormal RBCs and effectively treated by JAK2 inhibitors. Targeted therapies that inhibit aberrant myeloid differentiation are shown in Figure 37.23.

FLT3-TKIs. The kinase FLT3 is necessary for the survival, proliferation, and differentiation of hematopoietic stem cells.[306-308] The FLT3 kinase is a RTK that shares sequence homology with Kit, c-Fms, and PDGFR. The binding of a ligand to the extracellular domain of FLT3 results in receptor dimerization and autophosphorylation of tyrosine residues in the intracellular domain, which, in turn, activate the JAK/STAT, RAS/MAPK/MEK/ERK, and PI3K/AKT/mTOR pathways that support proliferation and survival.[307-309] Mutations in the *FLT3* gene result in mFLT3 with internal tandem duplications in the juxtamembrane domain (FLT3-ITD) or point mutations or deletion in the tyrosine kinase domain (FLT3-TKD).[310] Both FLT3-ITD and FLT3-TKD mutations are constitutively active and induce ligand-independent activation of downstream pathways that lead to AML. Approximately 30% of patients with AML harbor mFLT3 as an oncogenic driver.

Several multitargeted kinase inhibitors such as sorafenib and sunitinib have been investigated as mFLT3-TKIs based on sequence homology with Kit and PDGFR.[311,312] There are currently three approved mFLT3 inhibitors, midostaurin, gilteritinib, and quizartinib (see Fig. 37.23).[313] The mFLT3-TKIs reduce proliferation of abnormal myeloblasts and promote differentiation and maturation of abnormal myeloblasts in mature white blood cells. These effects allow for the regression of AML and blood counts to return to normal.

Midostaurin is a first-generation mFLT3 inhibitor approved for mFLT3+ AML in combination with cytarabine and daunorubicin. In addition to mFLT3, midostaurin is also an inhibitor of many other kinases, including protein kinase C (PKC), VEGFR, PDGFR, Kit, and others. Its broad spectrum has resulted in its classification as a multitargeted kinase inhibitor in drug information resources. In going from the first- to second-generation mFLT3-TKIs, the therapeutic efficacy and selectivity profile has improved. While midostaurin is a multitargeted kinase inhibitor, gilteritinib and quizartinib are more selective. Gilteritinib is a second-generation mFLT3-TKI with a more complete and selective inhibition of mFLT3 compared to midostaurin due to its ability to promote myeloblast differentiation to mature white blood cells in addition to inhibiting abnormal proliferation. Gilteritinib also demonstrates inhibition of AXL and is approved for use in refractory or relapsed mFLT3+ AML. Quizartinib, a second-generation agent, is approved in combination with anthracyclines and cytarabine for newly diagnosed mFLT3$^+$ AML, including in older adults.[314] It is mutant selective, inhibiting only FLT3-ITD and not FLT3-TKD, and is approved only for FLT3-ITD+ AML.

The second-generation mFLT3 inhibitors can be used at lower doses and produce a more robust clinical response due to not only inhibiting mFLT3-mediated myeloblast proliferation but also promoting myeloblast differentiation. Resistance to mFLT3 inhibitors has involved development of acquired FLT3 resistance mutations and redundant signaling mediated through RAS and proviral integration site for Moloney murine leukemia virus (Pim) kinase.[315]

Chemistry. The approved mFLT3-TKIs, midostaurin and gilteritinib, are reversible type I inhibitors that bind to the active conformation of mFLT3 in a closed, DFG-in conformation.[316] Midostaurin, a complex multiple fused ring system, is the N-benzoyl derivative of staurosporine, an alkaloid produced by *Streptomyces staurosporeus*. Gilteritinib is a smaller structure that includes an anilinopyrimidine scaffold.

Quizartinib includes a tricyclic imidazobenzothiazole core scaffold. It is a type II inhibitor that binds to the extended, inactive, DFG-out conformation of mFLT3. The DFG-out pocket is only accessible in the FLT3-ITD mutant and cannot be accessed in the TKD mutant. Hence, quizartinib is approved only for AML expressing FLT3-ITD. Key interactions for quizartinib in the pocket have included binding of the core imidazobenzothiazole scaffold within the adenine region, with hydrogen bonds to the hinge region. Interestingly, a π stacking interaction is observed with Tyr693 of the hinge region. A weak bond is suggested between Cys694 and the sulfur atom of the imidazobenzothiazole. The urea moiety forms key hydrogen bonds with Glu661 and Asp829, while the phenyl ring forms stacking interactions with the gatekeeper Phe691 and the Phe830 of the DFG motif in the back pocket. The tert-butyl substitution of the isoxazole ring occupies a hydrophobic pocket in the back cleft and interacts with Met664, Met665, Leu802, and Ile827. The morpholinoethoxy moiety is oriented toward solvent and does

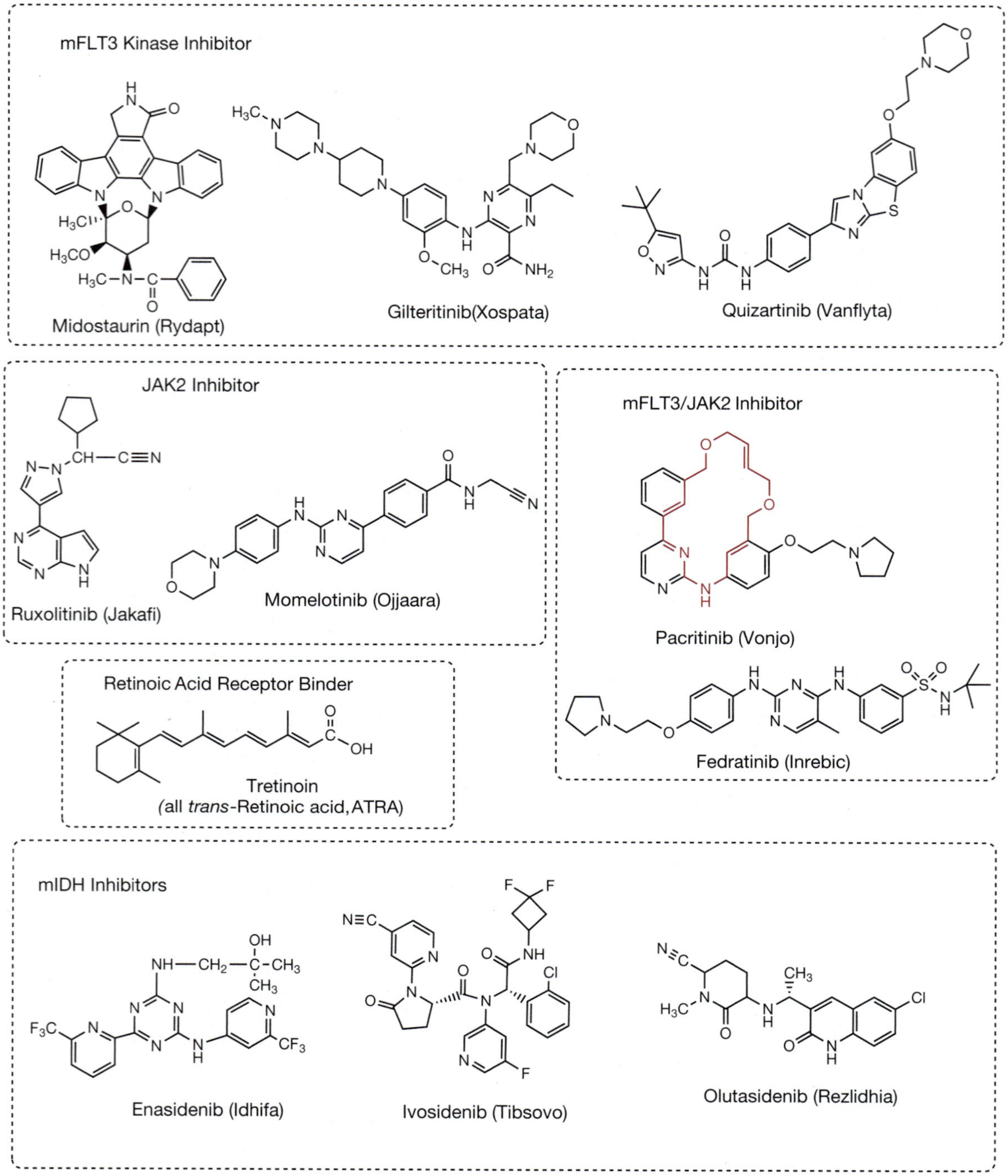

Figure 37.23 Myeloid differentiation pathway inhibitors. JAK2, Janus kinase 2; mFLT3, mutant FMS-like tyrosine kinase 3; mIDH, mutant isocitrate dehydrogenase.

not contribute to the potency of the drug; it is incorporated primarily to improve water solubility.

Pharmacokinetics. Midostaurin is orally administered. Once absorbed from the GI tract, it is bound to α-1 acidic glycoprotein (GP) for transport in the plasma. It is extensively metabolized via CYP3A4.[317] Two active FLT3 kinase and spleen tyrosine kinase (SYK)-inhibiting metabolites are produced; the epimeric mixture of the 7-hydroxy derivative (CGP52421) and the O-demethylation product (CGP62221). CGP62221 is equipotent with the parent as an inhibitor of FLT3-ITD–dependent cell proliferation while CGP52421 is approximately 10-fold less active. CGP52421 has a long terminal elimination half-life (~36 days) likely associated with protein binding. Clinically relevant DDIs are anticipated if midostaurin is coadministered with moderate to strong CYP3A4 inhibitor or inducers.

Gilteritinib is available in 40 mg tablets and is dosed at 120 mg once daily.[318] The drug has high oral bioavailability, high plasma protein binding, and a half-life of 113 hours. It is predominantly metabolized by CYP3A4 via N-dealkylation and oxidation reactions. Quizartinib is dosed orally, has a high oral bioavailability (71%), and is highly plasma protein bound (>99%).[319] The drug is extensively metabolized predominantly by CYP3A4 to the active metabolite AC886 (see Fig. 37.8). The half-life of quizartinib is 81 hours, while that of AC886 is 136 hours. The drug undergoes predominantly fecal elimination (76%).

Adverse Effects. The most common adverse effects for the mFLT3-TKIs include nausea, vomiting, and diarrhea. Additional adverse effects include fatigue, edema, electrolyte imbalances, and arthralgia.[304-306] Serious adverse effects of febrile neutropenia and pulmonary toxicity (specifically interstitial lung disease) may be observed.[316] Neutropenia is suggested to be caused by Kit and VEGFR inhibition in hematopoietic stem cells due to similarity in the binding pockets for Kit, VEGFR, and mFLT3. Drug-induced neutropenia poses a risk for fungal infections, and antifungal prophylaxis typically accompanies mFLT3-TKI therapy. The first-generation midostaurin has greater off-target adverse effects compared to the more selective later generation gilteritinib and quizartinib.[320] Gilteritinib is associated with an increased risk of differentiation syndrome, an oncologic emergency characterized by a severe immune response that can progress to multiorgan failure on account of excessive production of cytokines and inflammatory substances by abnormal myeloblasts. This has resulted in a boxed warning. QT prolongation for quizartinib may progress to torsades de pointes and cardiac arrest.[314] This has resulted in a boxed warning and distribution through the REMS program.

Janus-Associated Kinase Inhibitors. The JAKs are a family of NRTKs (JAK1, JAK2, JAK3), and nonreceptor tyrosine kinase 2 (TYK2).[83] They associate with the cytoplasmic end of cytokine receptors and mediate signals that impact hematopoiesis and immune function. Integral to the action of JAK are the STAT proteins. JAK enzymes phosphorylate STAT, which then translocate from the cytosol to the nucleus where they activate gene transcription processes, leading to angiogenesis and immunosuppression. Dysregulation in JAK has been associated with the initiation and progression of hematologic cancers.[321] Point mutations, specifically JAK2 V617F, results in a "supercharged" kinase and have been linked to myeloproliferative neoplasms (MPN), such as polycythemia vera and myelofibrosis. The JAK2 V617F mutation is the primary TK contributing to MPN pathology and results from a guanine-to-thymine nucleotide shift at position 1849 in the JAK2 gene (G1849T).[322]

Several pan and selective JAK inhibitors are clinically used in myelofibrosis.[322-326] Treatments for myelofibrosis are not driven by molecular markers but are made based on symptom burden. Tofacitinib, baricitinib, and upadacitinib that work primarily through JAK1 inhibition but also inhibit JAK2/3 have also been approved for rheumatoid arthritis. Approved JAK2 inhibitors include ruxolitinib, fedratinib, and pacritinib (see Fig. 37.23), with fedratinib and pacritinib working through a dual JAK2/FLT3 inhibitory mechanism.[325,326] Genetic mutations in FLT3 and JAK2 are mutually exclusive in MPN; however, both mutations are individually associated with AML. Dual JAK2/FLT3 inhibitors approved for myelofibrosis are also being investigated in AML. Momelotinib (see Fig. 37.23) is a wt JAK1/JAK2 and mutant JAK2V617F inhibitor that also works as an activin A receptor type 1 (ACVR1) inhibitor.[327] ACVR1 is a transmembrane kinase receptor belonging to bone morphogenic protein receptors (BMPs) that plays a role in iron homeostasis. Inhibition of ACVR1 increases the availability of iron for erythropoiesis and increases RBC production.

Chemistry. Ruxolitinib is an ATP-competitive, type I JAK2 inhibitor that interacts with hinge region residues Leu932 and Glu930 through the N_1 (pyrimidine) and N_7 (pyrrole) substituents.[325,328,329] Fedratinib is a dual JAK2/mFlt3 kinase inhibitor with a dianilinopyrimidine core that also works as an inhibitor of BRD4, a BET enzyme. Two crystal structures have been solved for fedratinib with JAK2, providing speculative modes of binding. Fedratinib was reported to bind in a type V mode with the full-length enzyme acting as a bisubstrate that spans the ATP pockets and peptidic substrate pockets of the kinase catalytic site.[330] However, with a truncated enzyme, fedratinib was shown to occupy the DFG-in, closed conformation of JAK2 and was suggested to be a type I ATP-competitive inhibitor.[331] A docking study of fedratinib with a previously reported crystal structure of mFLT3 also showed a similar ATP-competitive, type I mode of binding, similar to that seen with truncated JAK2.[332]

Pacritinib is a macrocyclic JAK2/FLT3 inhibitor with activity against kinases JAK2 and mutated V617F JAK2. It also inhibits FLT3, interleukin-1 receptor–associated kinase-1 (IRAK1), activin A receptor, type 1/activin receptor like kinase 2 (ACVR1/ALK2).[326] Pacritinib is selective for JAK2 over JAK3 and JAK1 at clinically relevant concentrations. While both pacritinib and ruxolitinib are JAK2 selective, in patients with myelofibrosis and thrombocytopenia, including those with prior anti-JAK therapy, pacritinib twice daily was more effective than ruxolitinib in reducing total symptom scores and in inducing spleen volume reduction that are characteristic features of myelofibrosis.[326]

Pacritinib's novel macrocyclic structure, highlighted in Figure 37.23, was generated by connecting the open ends of a substituted anilinopyrimidine motif.[333] The linker length was optimized to eight atoms and incorporated dibenzylic ether linkers. The incorporation of the macrocycle improved potency for JAK2 and FLT3 while maintaining selectivity for target kinases. An *N*-pyrrolidinylethoxy substituent was incorporated to improve water solubility and was found to interact with the JAK2 side chain of Ser936.

Pharmacokinetics. The JAK2 inhibitors are extensively metabolized by CYP3A4 enzymes and may produce active metabolites. Coadministration of JAK2 inhibitors with CYP3A4 inhibitors or inducers should be undertaken only with careful monitoring, and strong CYP3A4 inhibitor co-therapy should be avoided. Ruxolitinib is rapidly and almost completely absorbed after oral administration.[334] The half-life is short (3 hours) due to oxidative metabolism primarily catalyzed by CYP3A4 and, to a lesser extent, by CYP2C9. Ruxolitinib represents the major component (~50%) in the plasma, and active isomeric metabolites contributing 18% to the therapeutic action result from cyclopentane hydroxylation at position 2 or 3. Pacritinib is given orally and has high plasma protein binding. The half-life of the drug is approximately 28 hours, and it undergoes extensive CYP3A4-mediated metabolism.[326] Pacritinib has been suggested to have an increased risk of QT prolongation. Momelotinib is extensively metabolized by a variety of CYP enzymes, including 3A4 (36%), 2C8 (19%), 2C9 (17%), 2C19 (19%), and 1A2 (9%). An active metabolite formed by CYP- and aldehyde oxidase–catalyzed oxidation of the morpholine ring to a lactone (M21) retains ~40% of the pharmacologic activity of momelotinib (see Fig. 37.8).[335]

Adverse Effects. Anemia, neutropenia, and thrombocytopenia are mechanistic adverse effects of JAK2 inhibition. Close monitoring of the blood count during the initial phase of therapy is recommended. There is an increase in infection risk for JAK2 inhibitors. A reactivation of shingles is common, and patients must be prophylactically vaccinated. Headache, dizziness, and bruising may also be observed. Wernicke encephalopathy was reported in clinical trials for fedratinib and is a boxed warning for this inhibitor, with inhibition in thiamine uptake suggested as a possible mechanism.[336] Thiamine supplementation could reduce this risk. The FLT3-mediated adverse effects of fedratinib include nausea, vomiting, and diarrhea and must be managed.

MUTANT IDH1/2 INHIBITORS. IDH2, an $NADP^+$-dependent enzyme active in the TCA cycle, converts isocitrate to α-ketoglutarate and generates NADPH and, in so doing, promotes mitochondrial oxidative respiration.[337] Mutations in mitochondrial IDH2 or its cytosolic isozyme IDH1 (collectively referred to as mIDH1/2) are found in approximately 20% of patients diagnosed with AML and drive the neoplastic process. Oncogenic IDH1 mutations occur at the highly conserved Arg132 (R132H, R132C) while, at IDH2, positions 172 and 140 are involved (R172K, R140Q). The guanidinium moiety of the Arg residues in the wt enzyme stabilizes β-carboxyl addition in the interconversion of isocitrate and α-ketoglutarate in IDH, so IDH mutants are unable to convert isocitrate to α-ketoglutarate.[338] Instead, IDH mutants catalyze the conversion of α-ketoglutarate to 2-hydroxyglutarate (2-HG) as shown. IDH enzymes normally exist as homodimers, and mIDH enzymes retain the ability to dimerize with wt proteins, which, in the case of IDH1 mutants, has been proposed to facilitate reduction of α-ketoglutarate to 2-HG. The 2-HG accumulates in the cancer cell at concentrations over 100 times normal levels and serves as an oncometabolite by hypermethylating DNA and histones, inhibiting cellular differentiation, and dysregulating homeostatic biochemical pathways.[339] The epigenetic signature of IDH1/2 mutants in AML involves cytosine 5-methylation throughout the genome.

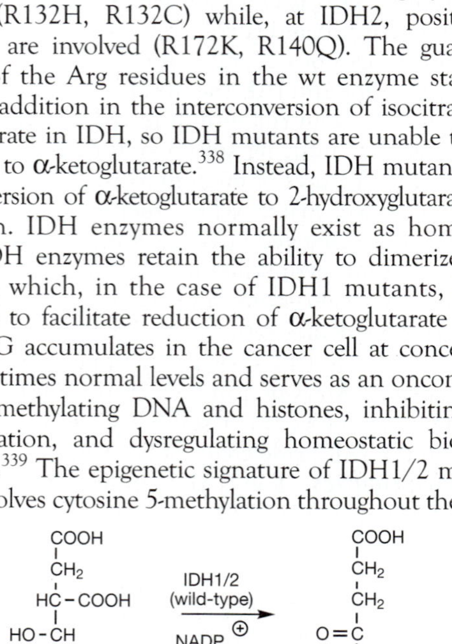

Three mIDH inhibitors, enasidenib, ivosidenib, and olutasidenib (see Fig. 37.23), have been approved to date.[340-342] Enasidenib works primarily as a mIDH2 inhibitor, while ivosidenib and olutasidenib work as mIDH1 inhibitors. By inhibiting mIDH, these drugs promote myeloblast differentiation and are effective in the treatment of AML. Enasidenib has been approved for relapsed/refractory AML with IDH2 mutations. In an open-label, randomized, phase 3 trial that compared enasidenib with conventional care regimens in patients aged 60 years and above with late-stage, mIDH2-relapsed/refractory AML and prior AML-directed therapies, enasidenib showed improved outcomes, including improvement in event-free survival and ORR.[340] Ivosidenib is used orally in the treatment of relapsed/refractory AML in patients expressing mIDH1. The DR was 8.2 months with OS of 8.8 months.[341] It has also been approved as either monotherapy and in combination with cytarabine for the treatment of relapsed/refractory AML with IDH1 mutations. Olutasidenib is a potent, oral, brain-penetrable mIDH1 inhibitor that has been approved for patients with relapsed and refractory AML with mIDH1 mutations. The DR was 25.9 months with OS of 11.6 months.[342]

Chemistry. The nitrogen atoms of enasidenib's heteroaromatic triazine ring are weakly basic and remain predominantly unionized at physiologic pH, allowing binding to the divalent cation-binding region at the juncture of the IDH2 dimer.[343] This forces an open protein conformation, which lowers affinity for $NADP^+$ and inhibits function. The affinity for mIDH2 is 40 times that of wtIDH, promoting tumor selectivity. Ivosidenib incorporates a phenylglycine scaffold and is an allosteric inhibitor of mIDH1 that locks mIDH1 in an inactive conformation, preventing the formation of 2-HG.

Olutasidenib is also an allosteric mIDH inhibitor that binds in the hydrophobic allosteric pocket and stabilizes an inactive conformation of the dehydrogenase (Fig. 37.24).[344] Olutasidenib incorporates a quinolinone scaffold and binds to mIDH in a unique 2:1 stoichiometry. In a recent study, the crystal structure of mIDH1 used was a dimer with one molecule of olutasidenib bound to the allosteric pocket near the dimer interface within each monomer of IDH1. The interactions for olutasidenib within mIDH1 are shown in Figure 37.24. The quinoline lactam in the crystallized ligand forms hydrogen bonds with the side chains of Arg109 and Asp279. The nitrile substitution on the pyridinone

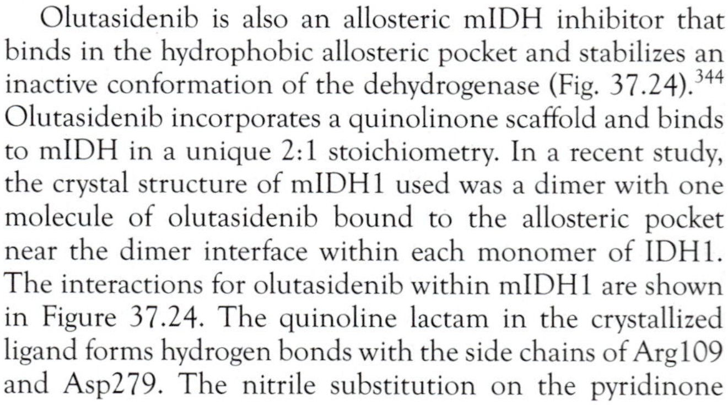

Figure 37.24 Binding interactions for olutasidenib within the allosteric pocket of mutant isocitrate dehydrogenase 1.

interacts through a hydrogen bond with the backbone NH of Leu120, and the linker secondary amine (NH) forms a hydrogen bond with the carbonyl oxygen of Ile128.

In preclinical studies, olutasidenib was shown to be effective in the ivosidenib-resistant R132C/S280F and R132H/S280F mutants. Olutasidenib's durable response and possible efficacy in the resistant S280F mutant have been attributed to its 2:1 binding stoichiometry to mIDH1. Ivosidenib, on the other hand, binds the mutant enzyme in a 1:1 stoichiometry.

Pharmacokinetics. All mIDH inhibitors may be given orally and are metabolized by CYP3A4.[340-342] N-Dealkylation by a wide variety of CYP isoforms generates an active metabolite of enasidenib, AGI-16903 (Fig. 37.8), which accounts for 10% of the circulating drug concentration.[345] Both the parent drug and metabolite are highly protein bound. Several glucuronidating isoforms are involved in phase II metabolism, and biliary excretion predominates over renal (89% vs 11%). No significant DDIs have been reported. Ivosidenib is rapidly absorbed and has a prolonged half-life of 3 to 6 days. While CYP3A4 is known to play a metabolic role, the parent drug is excreted predominantly unchanged in feces. Olutasidenib is also metabolized predominantly by CYP3A4 (with minor contributions from several other isoforms) and may undergo interactions with CYP3A4 inducers.[342] N-Dealkylation, demethylation, oxidative deamination, oxidation, and UDP-catalyzed phase II glucuronidation are common reactions. The drug has high oral bioavailability, high plasma protein binding, and a half-life of 65 hours.

Adverse Effects. Hyperbilirubinemia and nausea were among the most common adverse effects experienced by patients on enasidenib, although some experienced tumor lysis syndrome characterized by altered levels of serum electrolytes and nitrogenous compounds released by destroyed cells.[340-342] QT-interval prolongation, leukocytosis, fatigue, rash, GI distress, and respiratory events (eg, dyspnea, cough) are among the more serious adverse effects of enasidenib. Ivosidenib carries a boxed warning for QTc-interval prolongation and may require monitoring and dose adjustments. Typical adverse effects associated with olutasidenib include hepatotoxicity and high liver enzymes, high uric acid levels. The most serious mechanism-related toxicity among mIDH inhibitors is differentiation syndrome, and all of these agents carry a boxed warning for this potentially fatal adverse event. Additional adverse effects for this class include diarrhea and electrolyte imbalances.

TRETINOIN. APL, a subclass of AML, is characterized by a translocation between chromosomes 15 and 17 producing an aberrant fusion gene termed *altered retinoic acid receptor* (RAR).[346] In the presence of RAR, promyelocytes fail to differentiate and tend to accumulate. Tretinoin (see Fig. 37.23) binds to the altered RAR and induces an RAR-RXR (retinoid X receptor) dimer that binds to DNA and induces transcription of genes that promote maturation of promyelocytes.

Tretinoin is a vitamin A analog and is marketed as a single geometric isomer, all-*trans* retinoic acid (ATRA). The drug is administered orally and is associated with adverse effects similar to vitamin A intoxication. Tretinoin has a boxed warning for differentiation syndrome similar to differentiation promoters, mFLT3 inhibitors, and mIDH inhibitors.

Miscellaneous Targeted Therapies

The remaining targeted therapies discussed in this chapter have diverse mechanisms of action, including inhibition of angiogenesis (VEGFR, FGFR, and PDGFR inhibitors), cell cycle progression (CDK4/6 inhibitors), epigenetic modification (HDAC and EZH2 inhibitors), DNA repair (PARP inhibitors), exportin inhibition, inhibition of hedgehog signaling, and hematopoietic stem cell mobilization.

Angiogenesis Inhibitors

VEGFR-TKIs. Angiogenesis is a complex process involving the proliferation and subsequent migration of endothelial cells, resulting in new blood vessel formation.[347] This process is finely regulated by diverse endogenous pro- and antiangiogenic factors and normally occurs during embryonic development and wound healing. The VEGFR family includes VEGFR1 (FLT1), VEGFR2 (KDR), and VEGFR3 (FLT4).[348] The RTK VEGFR2 is produced in endothelial cells and is the most significant controller of angiogenic factors involved in tumor angiogenesis and lymphangiogenesis. Lymphangiogenesis is the process by which new lymphatic vessels are formed from existing lymphatic vasculature. Binding of the growth factor, VEGF to VEGFR, triggers endothelial cell proliferation, migration, and survival through activation of varied pathways. Both mAbs and small molecule inhibitors targeting the VEGF/VEGFR axis have been approved.[349] The approved small molecule VEGFR inhibitors bind to the intracellular kinase domain and include sorafenib, sunitinib, pazopanib, regorafenib, axitinib, lenvatinib, cabozantinib, tivozanib, and fruquintinib (Fig. 37.25).[350-360] Most VEGFR inhibitors are multitargeted and inhibit additional angiogenic kinases, such as FGFR, KIT and PDGFRβ. Fruquintinib is the most recent VEGFR kinase inhibitor to be approved (2024). It is highly selective with actions only on VEGFR1, VEGFR2, and VEGFR3 in the human kinome.[360] Fruquintinib has been approved for use in the treatment of metastatic CRC in adults who have been previously treated with fluoropyrimidine-, oxaliplatin-, and irinotecan-based chemotherapy (Chapter 36), an anti-VEGF therapy, and an anti-EGFR therapy with wtKRAS status. In the phase 3 FRESCA trial, fruquintinib showed an improvement in both PFS and OS among treated patients versus placebo.

Chemistry. The VEGFR inhibitors include key chemical scaffolds that anchor the molecule through hydrogen bonding, including urea in sorafenib, regorafenib, lenvatinib and tivozanib, and an amide in sunitinib and cabozantinib.[349-358] Sorafenib and regorafenib differ by an aryl fluorine substituent. Pazopanib and axitinib share a heterocyclic indazole structure, while fruquintinib, tivozanib, lenvatinib, and cabozantinib all incorporate a 7-methoxyquinoline and sunitinib incorporates an oxindole. The VEGFR inhibitors can bind to both the active and inactive conformations of VEGFR. Most small molecule VEGFR kinase inhibitors are typically type I 1/2 or type II inhibitors with binding modes

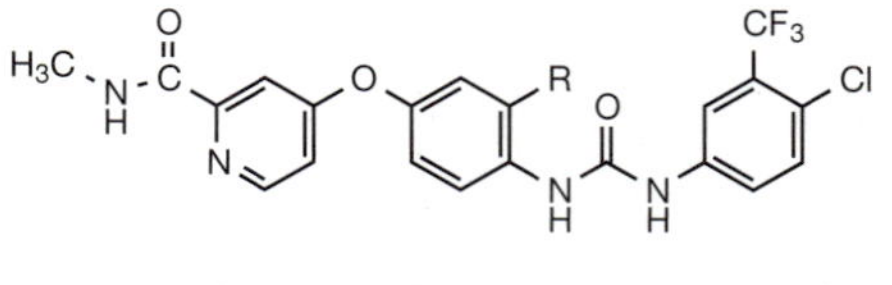

Sorafenib (R = H) (Nexavar)
Regorafenib (R = F) (Stivarga)

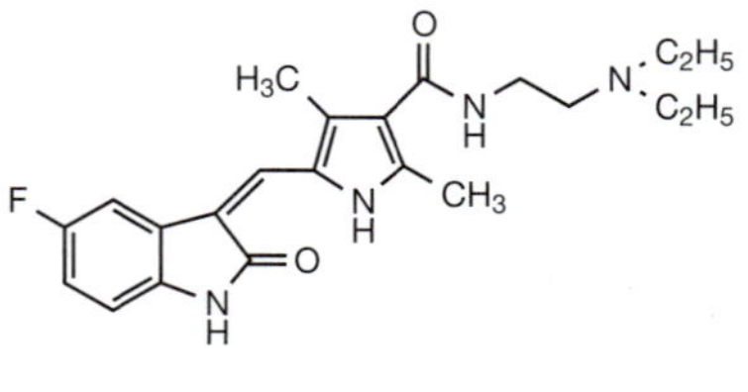

Sunitinib malate
(Sutent)

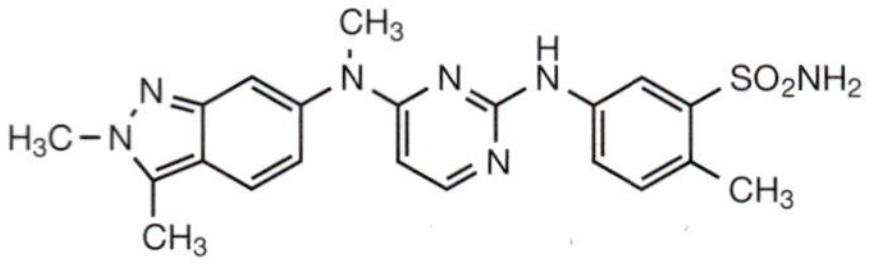

Pazopanib hydrochloride
(Votrient)

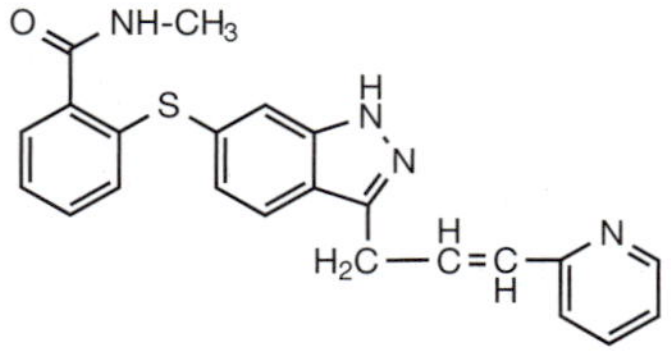

Axitinib
(Inlyta)

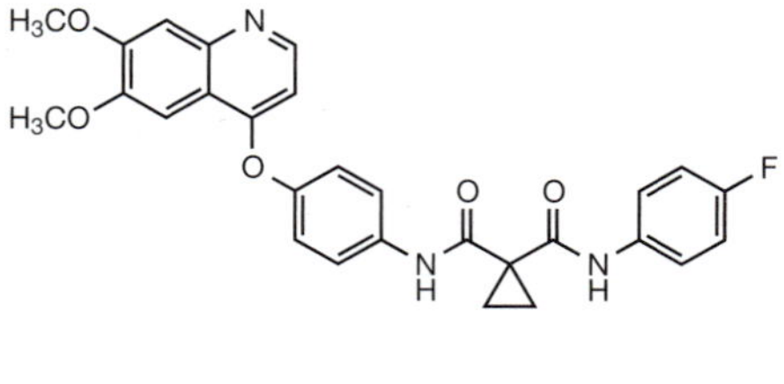

Cabozantinib maleate
(Exelixis)

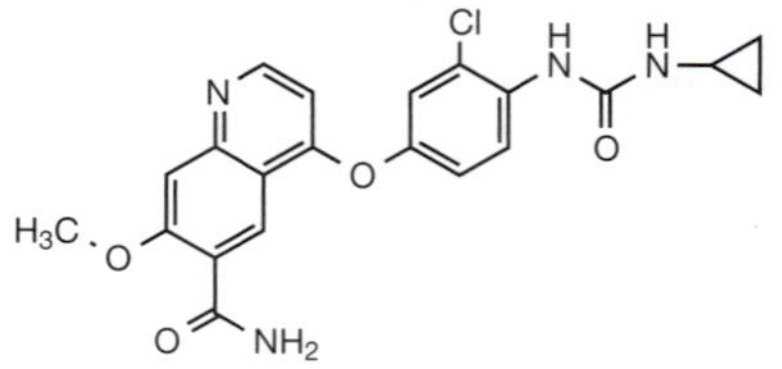

Lenvatinib mesylate
(Lenvima)

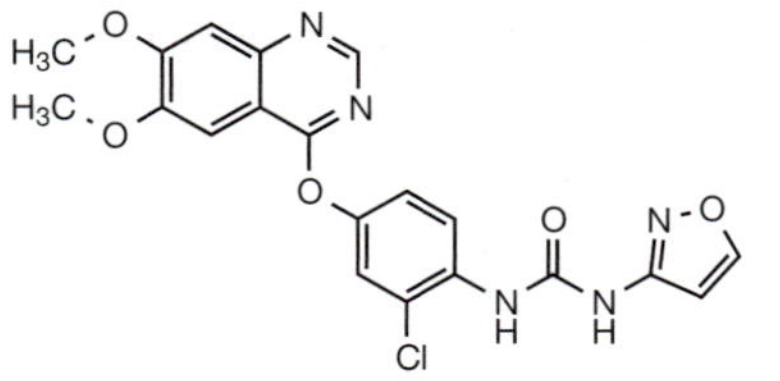

Tivozanib
(Fotivda)

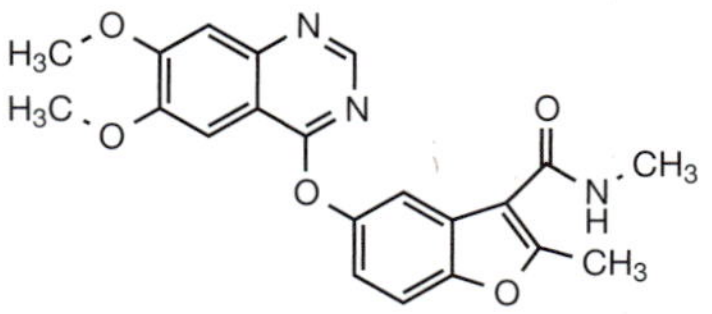

Fruquintinib
(Fruzaqia)

Figure 37.25 Vascular endothelial growth factor receptor kinase inhibitors.

that span the ATP pocket and extend into the allosteric pocket (αC-helix-out or DFG-out) in the back cleft.

Sunitinib, sorafenib, regorafenib, tivozanib, and pazopanib are multitargeted kinase inhibitors and suffer from poor selectivity across the kinome. The poor selectivity results in increased toxicities. Efforts over the past decade have focused on improving the selectivity of VEGFR inhibitors to improve therapeutic efficacy and limit toxicity, which makes the release of the highly selective fruquintinib an exciting chemical and welcome therapeutic breakthrough.

Pharmacokinetics. The pharmacokinetic properties for VEGFR inhibitors are included in Table 37.7. The VEGFR inhibitors are primarily metabolized by CYP3A4. Active metabolites for VEGFR inhibitors such as hydroxypazopanib, sorafenib and regorafenib N-oxides, and desethylsunitinib are shown in Figure 37.8.

Adverse Effects. Typical adverse effects for the VEGFR-TKIs include wound healing complications, hypertension, thromboembolic events, diarrhea, and skin reactions.[349-362] Nail bed toxicities and nephrotoxicity may also be seen. The adverse effects are most problematic with the multitargeted inhibitors. The VEGFR2 inhibitors are extensively metabolized by CYPs and produce several active metabolites.[363,364]

FGFR Inhibitors. The FGFR family comprises four highly conserved RTKs, FGFR1, FGFR2, FGFR3, and FGFR4, that sustain cell growth.[365] Dysregulated FGFR signaling has been associated with cancers, including FGFR overexpression in gastric cancer and hepatocellular carcinoma (HCC). Specifically, FGFR4 is a key player in HCC. Mutations in FGFR are seen in bladder cancers and myelomas.

The structures of the four approved FGFR inhibitors are shown in Figure 37.26. Erdafitinib is a first-in-class FGFR inhibitor approved for urothelial carcinoma.[366,367] Erdafitinib inhibits FGFR1-4 and inhibits RET, CSF1R, PDGFRα, PDGFRβ, FLT4, KIT, and VEGFR2. Pemigatinib is an FGFR1, FGFR2, and FGFR3 inhibitor that was approved for FGFR2-driven cholangiocarcinoma and myelomas.[368] Infigratinib and futibatinib are pan-FGFR (FGFR1-4) inhibitors approved for FGFR2-driven cholangiocarcinoma.[369]

Chemistry. A cysteine residue at position 552 in the hinge region of the ATP pocket has been observed in FGFR4.[367] Covalent interactions with Cys552 have been exploited to improve selectivity, including futibatinib's irreversible FGFR4 binding through the now familiar acrylamide-driven Cys552 alkylation reaction. An X-ray crystal structure of FGFR4 and futibatinib revealed that the aminoquinazoline core formed two hydrogen bonds with the hinge region Ala553 while the acrylamide (see Fig. 37.26) successfully formed the intended covalent bond with Cys552.[370] Futibatinib is a potent FGFR4 inhibitor; however, it is not selective for FGFR4 over FGFR1, FGFR2, and FGFR3 due to the noncovalent accommodation across all FGFR pockets.[371,372] Multitargeted FGFR inhibitors are associated with significant adverse effects. Newer analogs with bulkier side chains that sterically prevent FGFR1-3

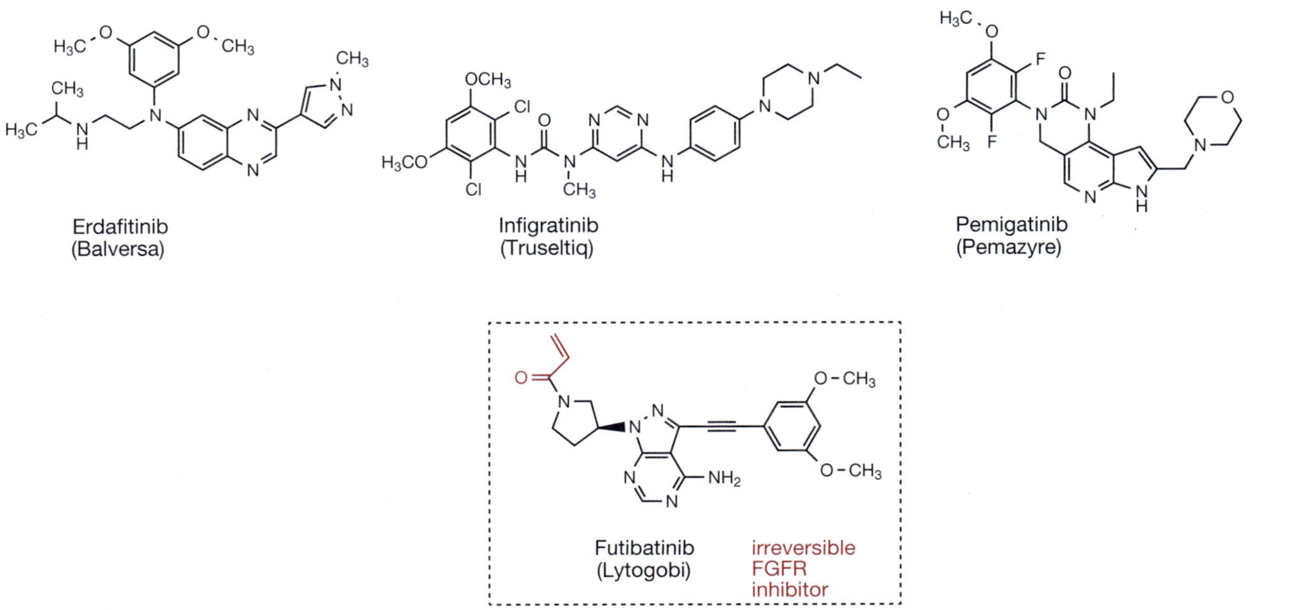

Figure 37.26 FGFR inhibitors. FGFR, fibroblast growth factor receptor.

binding are being pursued to reduce toxicity and optimize FGFR4 selectivity.

Pharmacokinetics. Pharmacokinetic properties for FGFR inhibitors are included in Table 37.7. The FGFR inhibitors are primarily metabolized by CYP3A4. Infigratinib produces two active metabolites, BHS697 and CQM157, that account for up to approximately 30% and 10% of infigratinib's activity, respectively (see Fig. 37.8).[369]

Adverse Effects. Dermatologic adverse effects are the most common class effect seen for FGFR inhibitors.[373] These present as brittle nails, stomatitis (mouth sores), and hand-foot syndrome. Hyperphosphatemia is observed due to on-target FGFR1 inhibition that induces renal wasting and interferes with GI absorption. Diarrhea due to FGFR4 inhibition is also observed. Ocular disturbances are commonly observed in patients, although the mechanism for this is unclear.

PDGFRα/Kit Inhibitors. The proto-oncogene *c-kit* encodes Kit, an RTK that binds to stem cell factor and has essential roles in fertility, cell proliferation, and survival.[374] Kit aberrations, either overexpression or mutations such as D816V, have been implicated in many cancers, including GI stromal tumors, mastocytosis, AML, and breast, thyroid, and CRC. As noted earlier, imatinib was originally approved for use in Ph+ CML but was later found to also inhibit Kit and is effective in Kit-positive GI stromal tumors. Subsequently, other multitargeted kinase inhibitors that demonstrated Kit inhibition, such as sunitinib, sorafenib, dasatinib, regorafenib, nilotinib, and tivozanib, have also been developed. The most recent approvals include avapritinib and ripretinib (Fig. 37.27) that block PDGFRα and Kit mutants that inhibit Kit and PDGFRα-mediated cell signaling cascades.[375,376] Pharmacokinetic properties adverse effects for Kit/PDGFRα inhibitors are included in Tables 37.7 and 37.8.

Cell Cycle Targeted Therapies

Cyclin-Dependent Kinase Inhibitors. Overactivation of checkpoint kinases supports uncontrolled cell proliferation. Checkpoint kinase inhibitors have shown benefit in inhibiting cell cycle progression and inhibiting uncontrolled cell division. The CDKs are a family of over 20 serine/threonine protein kinases that modulate intracellular signaling during cell cycle progression and are referred to as checkpoint kinases.[377] Aberrant CDK activities, particularly CDK2, CDK4, and CDK6, are associated with carcinogenic transformations, including breast cancer initiation and invasive progression.

The Rb protein plays a central role in placing a brake on progression through the cell cycle until the DNA synthetic machinery is ready for progression through to the S phase.[378,379] Once no anomalies are determined, phosphorylation of Rb by CDKs inactivates the Rb protein–induced

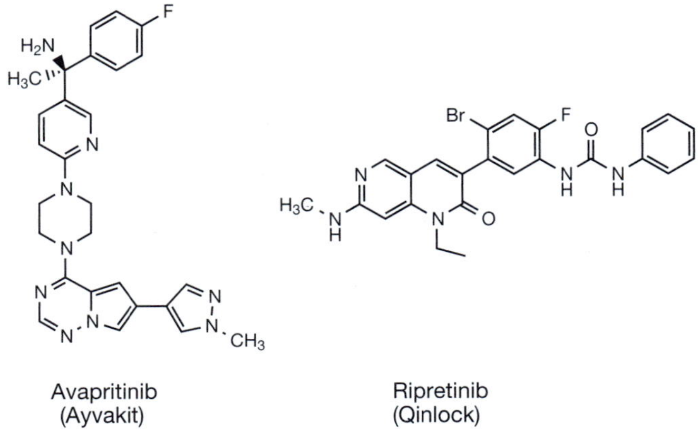

Figure 37.27 PDGFRα/Kit inhibitors. PDGFR, platelet-derived growth factor receptor α.

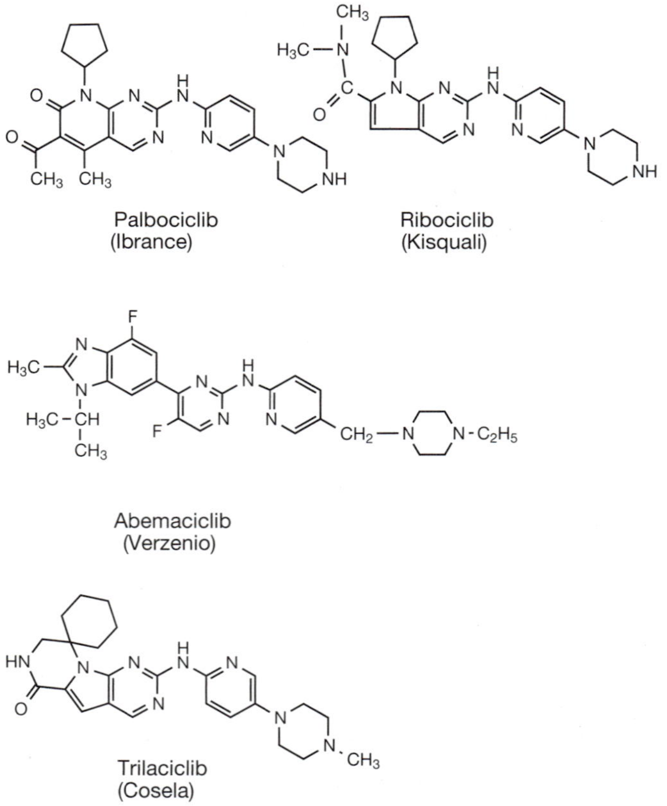

Figure 37.28 CDK inhibitors. CDK, cyclin-dependent kinase.

stop. If the cell determines that it is not ready to move ahead with DNA replication, the CDKs are not activated and Rb remains unphosphorylated. Thus, CDKs are involved in the progression from the G1 to S phase of the cell cycle. CDKs are overexpressed and active in cancer cells and cause increased phosphorylation of the Rb protein in the cell cycle, abolishing the Rb-induced brake and allowing continued cell cycle progression. Inhibition of CDKs maintains Rb in the unphosphorylated state, causing G1 arrest.

Four CDK4/6 inhibitors (Fig. 37.28) have been approved within a 6-year timespan: palbociclib (2015), ribociclib (2017), abemaciclib (2018), and trilaciclib (2021).[380-382] The typical predictive biomarker for CDK4/6 inhibitor benefit is HR positive status.[383-385] The CDK4/6 inhibitors are particularly effective in cancer cells with functional retinoblastoma (Rb+) levels.[386] Abemaciclib is approved for use either as monotherapy or in combination with anti-estrogen therapy (fulvestrant or an aromatase inhibitor) for HR positive, HER2 negative breast cancer, including in the adjuvant setting based on outcomes of the monarchE trial.[387] Palbociclib and ribociclib share this indication but only in combination with the aforementioned anti-estrogens. Palbociclib has similar affinities for CDK4 and CDK6, while ribociclib and abemaciclib preferentially bind to CDK4 over CDK6. Abemaciclib is the most potent and selective CDK4 inhibitor and is given continuously, while palbociclib and ribociclib are dosed on an intermittent schedule. Trilaciclib, a CDK4/6 inhibitor, was approved in the supportive care of bone marrow suppression and not as an anticancer agent.[388]

Chemistry. Like all kinases, the CDKs include an ATP pocket made up of a hinge region, adenine region, ribose pocket, phosphate-binding region and hydrophobic pockets.[389,390] The CDK4/6 inhibitors interact with Val101, His101, and Asp163 in the hinge region. Planar heterocycles bind to the adenine region. Interactions are observed between the CDK6 inhibitors and the gatekeeper residue Phe98. Hydrogen bonding interactions are observed with Thr107 (Thr99 or Thr102 in CDK4) near the phosphate-binding region and solvent interface. SAR studies demonstrated the importance of a cationic moiety (eg, piperazine) in improving CDK4/6 selectivity. The cationic moiety is positioned to form an affinity-enhancing ionic bond with the Asp104 residue in CDK4/6 while repelling the cationic Lys reside found on other CDKs (eg, CDK1/2). Additional selectivity for CDK4/6 over other kinases is achieved by exploiting interactions with His101.

Pharmacokinetics. All four CDK4/6 inhibitors are vulnerable to CYP3A4-catalyzed metabolism. Ribociclib is metabolized to the active metabolite, LEQ803. Abemaciclib produces multiple clinically relevant active metabolites, M2, M18, and M20 (see Fig. 37.8).[391-393] Selected pharmacokinetic properties appear in Table 37.7.

Adverse Effects. Fatigue, GI distress, rash, and alopecia are common adverse effects of all CDK4/6 inhibitors. The drug class may also induce rare but serious adverse effects, such as myelosuppression, interstitial lung disease presenting as cough and respiratory distress, VTE, and hepatotoxicity.[390,394] Myelosuppression, including anemia, leukocytopenia, neutropenia, and lymphopenia, can be exacerbated with CDK4/6 use after radiation in patients with breast cancer. A decrease in the incidence of neutropenia is observed for CDK4 over CDK4/6 inhibitors. The risk of VTE may be worsened if used in combination with aromatase inhibitors and the selective estrogen receptor modulator (SERM) tamoxifen. Diarrhea and electrolyte imbalances are observed for abemaciclib, while ribociclib is specifically associated with QT prolongation and hepatotoxicity.

Inhibitors of Epigenetic Modifications

Epigenetic modifications, such as the post-translational alteration of histones through acetylation and methylation, control gene regulation. Aberrant histone methylation or acetylation inhibits tumor suppressor gene expression and has been observed in several malignancies. Inhibitors of epigenetic modifiers have added benefit when used in combination with other anticancer agents.

HISTONE DEACETYLASE INHIBITORS. Histones are highly basic, Lys-rich proteins that process DNA into nucleosomes required for chromatin formation.[395] The histone acetyltransferases (HATs) catalyze the forward acetylation reaction, and HDACs catalyze the reverse deacetylation reaction of lysine residues on histones. Lysine acetylation by HAT reduces the basicity of the Lys terminal amine. This leads to a more open chromatin conformation for acetylated histones, allowing transcription factors to more readily access DNA and initiate RNA synthesis. Some of the proteins expressed include apoptotic proteins and repair enzymes.

Histone deacetylation by HDAC results in a closed chromatin conformation that is tightly bound to histones, leading to gene silencing and a reduced expression of proteins. The overexpression of HDACs has been observed in multiple cancers, particularly hematologic malignancies, resulting in continued cell cycle progression and uncontrolled proliferation.[396] DNA repair genes are silenced through HDAC, increasing the survival of abnormal cells and progression to cancer. Halting the HDAC-catalyzed deacetylation reaction with HDAC inhibitors keeps the chromatin in a relaxed conformation and allows gene expression of tumor suppressors and repair enzymes.

In humans, there are 18 HDACs that fall into two families based on their catalytic mechanism.[397] Eleven of the HDACs are zinc-dependent metalloenzymes named HDAC1-11 that hydrolyze the amide bond of acetylated Lys using water as a nucleophile. The remaining seven are termed sirtuins 1 through 7 and employ NAD^+ as a cofactor to transfer the acetyl group cleaved from Lys to the C_2 position of the ribose sugar. Although both enzyme families perform the same chemical reaction of deacetylating histones, the term HDAC usually refers to the zinc-dependent enzymes, and sirtuins refer to the NAD^+-dependent enzymes.

The structures of HDAC inhibitors are shown in Figure 37.29. Vorinostat became the first HDAC inhibitor to receive FDA approval in 2006 for the treatment of cutaneous T-cell lymphoma. Vorinostat includes a hydroxamic acid core scaffold. In parallel, the natural product, romidepsin, was discovered based on observed HDAC inhibition. Romidepsin, vorinostat, and belinostat are approved for the treatment of T-cell lymphoma. Panobinostat was indicated in combination with bortezomib and dexamethasone for relapsed/refractory MM; however, it has been voluntarily withdrawn.[92,398-401]

Crystal structures for HDAC have shown a long and narrow active site with a zinc ion located deep at one end of the pocket (Fig. 37.30).[395] The HDAC inhibitors include a zinc chelator, a hydrophobic linker, and a hydrophobic cap. The hydroxamic acid anion in vorinostat, belinostat, and panobinostat serves as the Zn-chelating entity, and the long, slender hydrocarbon chain allows these drugs to dangle the zinc chelator (cation magnet) into the tube-like "fishing hole" that shelters the Zn^{2+} ion.[399] The aromatic moiety at the opposite end of the structure caps the entrance to the tubular pocket, ensuring effective inhibition of the cofactor. The hydrophobic linker makes interactions within the pocket while the hydrophobic cap binds at the front end of the pocket. Romidepsin is a disulfide prodrug that is reduced in vivo to the active sulfhydryl that chelates with zinc in the HDAC pocket. The HDAC inhibitors are chemically classified as hydroxamic acids or depsipeptides. The depsipeptide HDAC inhibitors have a "depsin" suffix and include peptide scaffolds where one or more amide bonds have been replaced by an ester. The HDAC inhibitors are identified by the "stat" suffix if they include the hydroxamic acid pharmacophore. Vorinostat and panobinostat are oral medications, while romidepsin and belinostat are administered by IV infusion.

Resistance to the HDAC inhibitors involves BCL-2 overexpression, leading to limited therapeutic success.[395,401,402]

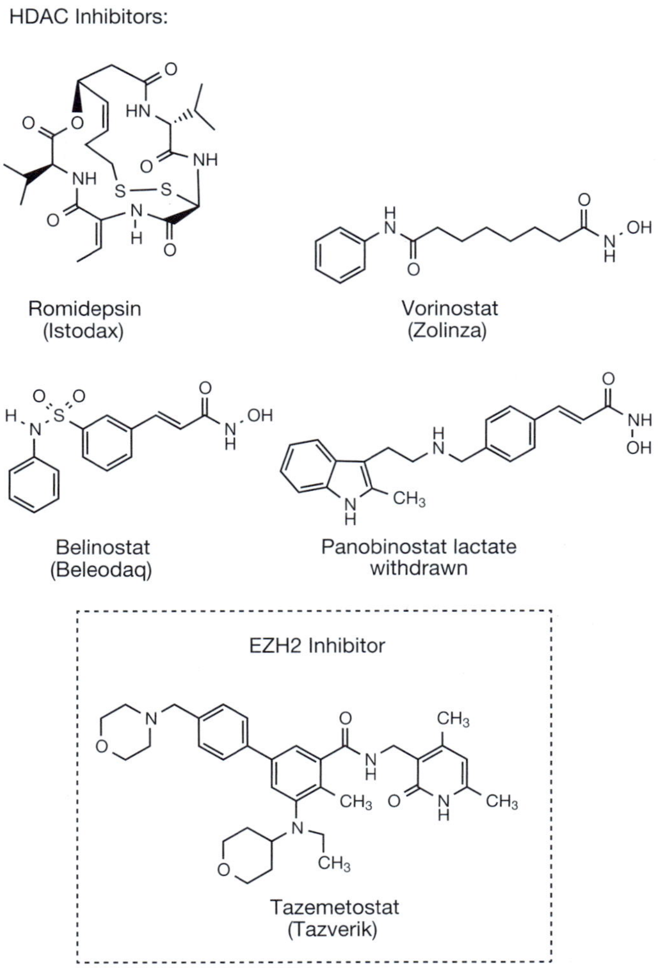

Figure 37.29 HDAC and EZH2 inhibitors. HDAC, histone deacetylase; EZH2, enhancer of zeste homolog 2.

The HDACs are highly conserved and share sequential similarity among HDAC classes. Inhibition of multiple HDAC isoforms and off-target effects has resulted in mechanistic hematologic and cardiovascular toxicities. Concerns have been raised about the clinical use of HDAC inhibitors, as they display rapid clearance and serious toxicities through nontarget inhibition.[403] In addition, while effective in hematologic malignancies, the HDAC inhibitors are not effective in solid tumors. Newer HDAC inhibitors with better therapeutic profiles are needed.

Inhibitors for Enhancers of Zeste Homolog 2. Methylation of lysine residues on histone proteins relaxes the chromatin conformation allowing gene expression, including the expression of tumor suppressor genes.[404] Aberrant histone

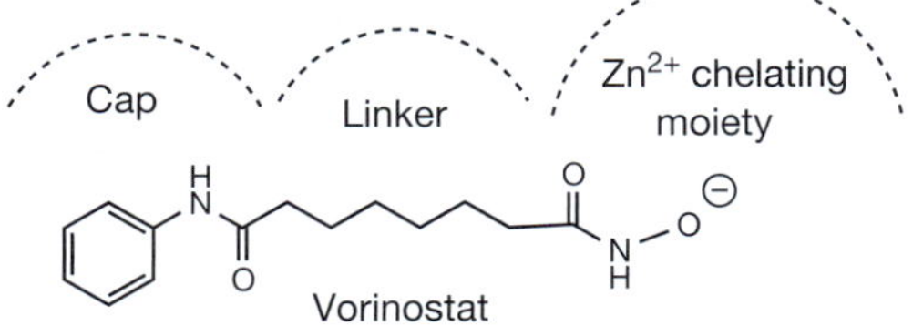

Figure 37.30 Histone deacetylase inhibitor pharmacophore.

methylation inhibits tumor suppressor gene expression and has been observed in several malignancies. The EZH2 is a histone methyltransferase that catalyzes the methylation of lysine residues on histone proteins. The EZH2 enzyme uses *S*-adenosylmethionine (SAM) as the methyl source. Mutations in EZH2 have enhanced enzymatic activity and have also been observed in hematologic malignancies. Follicular lymphoma displays EZH2 gain-of-function mutations including Y646X and A687V that lead to histone trimethylation. Sarcomas that harbor mutations in the switch/sucrose nonfermentable complex are dependent on EZH2 for methylation.

Tazemetostat is a first-in-class EZH2 inhibitor (Fig. 37.29).[405,406] It is an oral drug that was approved in 2020 for patients with epithelioid sarcoma, a rare soft tissue cancer that often occurs in young adults. Tazemetostat has also been approved for relapsed or refractory EZH2 mutation-positive follicular lymphoma. The catalytic site resides in the C-terminal SET domain of EZH2. Tazemetostat incorporates a pyridone motif that is essential for binding. Replacement or substitution of the pyridone results in decreased potency. Crystal structure analysis has shown that the pyridone moiety partially overlays the cofactor SAM site and supports a SAM-competitive mechanism of EZH2 inhibition.

The adverse effects of tazemetostat are generally mild and include pain, fatigue, nausea, decreased appetite, vomiting, and GI disturbances. An increased risk of secondary malignancies including lymphoma, myelodysplastic syndrome, and leukemia is possible due to increased gene expression. A longer duration of treatment with tazemetostat and correspondingly prolonged loss of function of EZH2 increase the risk of secondary malignancies.[407]

Inhibitors of DNA Repair

PARP Inhibitors. Single- or double-stranded breaks in DNA can occur during cell growth because of various exogenous or endogenous factors.[408] The cells utilize varied DNA repair systems for the detection and repair of damaged DNA in order to maintain the integrity and stability of genetic information. *BRCA1* and *BRCA2* are tumor suppressor genes. Proteins expressed by *BRCA1* and *BRCA2* facilitate DNA repair through homologous recombination repair and maintain genomic integrity. Mutations in *BRCA* reduce the tumor suppressor function, making them susceptible to progression toward breast and ovarian cancer. Cells with mBRCA become entirely dependent on non-*BRCA* DNA repair pathways to maintain their integrity and support tumorigenic processes.

The PARP enzymes play essential roles in DNA repair in mBRCA-positive tumors. In the presence of PARP inhibitors, cancer cells expressing mBRCA are incapable of repairing damaged DNA. The loss of PARP or *BRCA* activity due to mutations can independently be tolerated; however, the simultaneous inhibition of PARP and dysfunction of mutant *BRCA* cannot be tolerated and has devastating effects on the cell.[409] The combination of PARP inhibition and *BRCA* mutation results in cancer cell death and is termed *synthetic lethality*.

The PARP inhibitors are also highly effective in combination with classic agents temozolomide and topoisomerase inhibitors (see Chapter 36). Combination therapy of PARP1

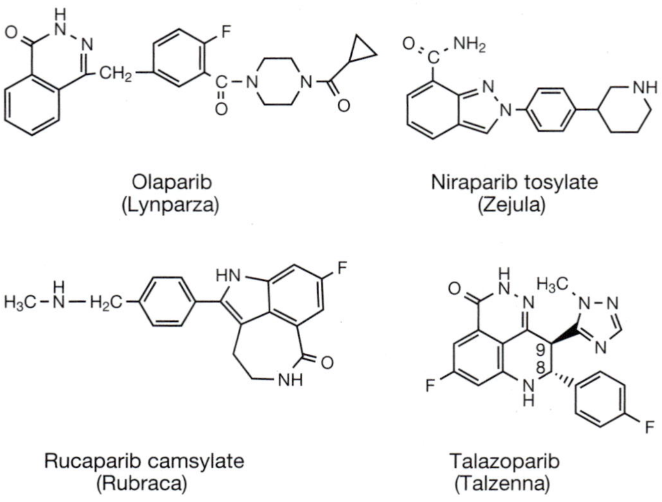

Figure 37.31 Poly(ADP-ribose) polymerase inhibitors.

inhibitors with DNA topoisomerase inhibitors prevents DNA repair and improves efficacy of the topoisomerase inhibitors. Olaparib, niraparib, rucaparib, and talazoparib are PARP inhibitors approved for mBRCA-positive breast, prostate, pancreatic, and ovarian cancers (Fig. 37.31).[407-411] Talazoparib is the most potent PARP inhibitor approved to date and demonstrates PARP1 and PARP2 inhibition.

Chemistry. The PARP enzymes bind to DNA single-strand breaks, catalyze poly-ADP ribosylation (PARylation), and repair DNA damage via base excision repair.[410] The PARP enzyme consists of three domains: the N-terminal DNA-binding domain, the automodification domain, and the C-terminal catalytic domain. The DNA-binding domain includes three zinc fingers that are involved in recognition of DNA strand breaks and binding. The catalytic domain includes an NAD^+-binding site and a catalytic site for the synthesis and transfer of PARP. The PARP enzyme binds to DNA via a zinc finger, cleaves NAD^+ into nicotinamide and ADP-ribose, and catalyzes PAR transfer from NAD^+ onto acceptor DNA repair proteins.

Olaparib, niraparib, rucaparib, and talazoparib are substrate-competitive PARP inhibitors that mimic the nicotinamide component of the NAD^+ substrate and bind to the NAD^+ and PAR sites of the catalytic domain of PARP (Fig. 37.32).[411-416] The benzamide moiety binds to the nicotinamide-binding domain on PARP, and the optimal *s-trans* conformation is promoted through incorporation into a ring (olaparib, rucaparib) or via an intramolecular H bond (niraparib). Talazoparib incorporates a tetrahydropyridophthalazinone core with disubstitution at the 8 and 9 positions and binds with distinct stereospecificity to PARP.[409,417] The *trans* (*8S,9R*) stereoisomer is a highly potent PARP inhibitor.

Pharmacokinetics. Olaparib and rucaparib are administered orally twice a day, while niraparib and talazoparib are administered orally once a day.[417] Talazoparib is administered in 1-mg doses, which is significantly lower than the 200- to 600-mg twice-daily doses of olaparib and rucaparib. The low dose is attributed to both the tight binding of the *8S,9R* (*trans*) isomer within the PARP catalytic site and minimal hepatic metabolism. Talazoparib is also minimally metabolized prior to excretion. Olaparib is biotransformed by CYP3A4

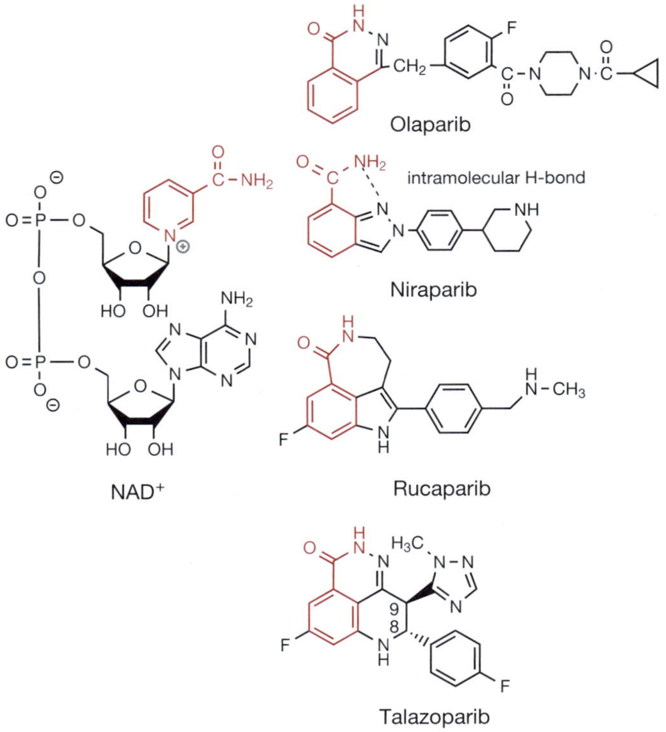

Figure 37.32 Poly(ADP-ribose) polymerase inhibitors with π stacking moieties of drugs and NAD^+ shown in red. NAD^+, nicotinamide adenine dinucleotide.

and CYP1A1 hydroxylations, and rucaparib by CYP2D6 oxidation, followed by phase II glucuronide or sulfate conjugation for both drugs. Niraparib is similar to talozaparib with the once-daily dosing and is also not metabolized by CYPs. It is metabolized predominantly by carboxylesterase to the inactive carboxylic acid, which is excreted as the glucuronide conjugate. Niraparib, in contrast to talozaparib, requires 200- to 300-mg doses. Based on the CYP-mediated metabolism, olaparib and rucaparib have a high risk for DDIs. A lower risk of DDI is observed for niraparib, and a minimal risk is seen for talazoparib. Most approved PARP inhibitors are Pgp substrates and suffer from poor CNS penetration due to Pgp efflux. Niraparib, the exception, retains efficacy in patients with brain metastases.

Adverse Effects. The most common adverse reactions for PARP inhibitors include fatigue, nausea, alopecia, and headaches.[418] Niraparib has also been associated with peripheral edema, rash, and hypertension. More serious adverse effects of PARP inhibitors include myelosuppression (anemia, neutropenia, and thrombocytopenia), teratogenicity, and an increased risk of secondary malignancy, specifically AML and myelodysplastic syndrome.

Exportin Inhibitor

Specialized proteins, importins and exportins located in the nuclear pore complex, play an important role in regulating transport of proteins and RNA across the nuclear envelope. The nuclear export protein exportin-1 (XPO1) (also known as chromosome maintenance protein 1) binds messenger RNA (mRNA) and other tumor suppressor proteins and transports them out of the nucleus and into the cytoplasm. In certain cancer cells, XPO1 is overexpressed, and XPO1-mediated transport is accelerated to meet the increased cellular needs for proliferation. Selinexor is a first-in-class inhibitor of XPO1.[419,420] Selinexor forms a covalent bond with the exportin protein and inhibits XPO1-mediated transport in a slowly reversible manner, resulting in accumulation of tumor suppressor proteins, which induces apoptosis. Selinexor is approved for the treatment of relapsed/refractory diffuse large B-cell lymphoma (DLBCL) and is approved in combination with bortezomib and dexamethasone for MM. Selinexor is administered orally and metabolized by CYP3A4 followed by phase II glucuronidation and glutathione conjugation. Adverse effects include nausea and fatigue. Serious adverse effects include thrombocytopenia and hyponatremia.

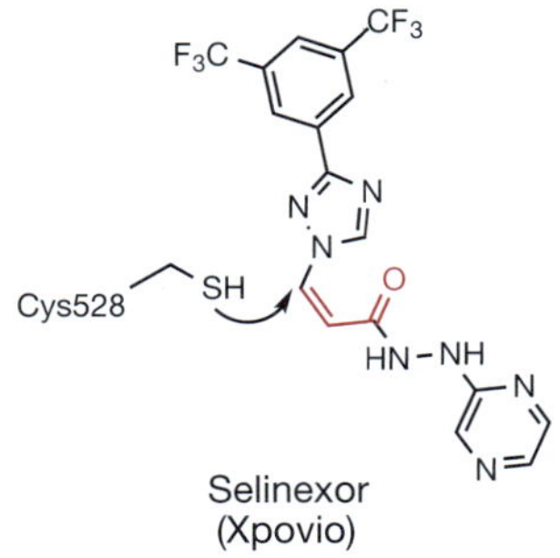

Hedgehog Signaling Pathway Inhibitors

The hedgehog signaling cascade plays a role in embryonic development. It is minimally expressed in mature adults but is functional in cancers such as hematologic malignancies and basal cell carcinoma (BCC). Thus, inhibitors of the hedgehog signaling cascade have been pursued among targeted therapies (Fig. 37.33). Vismodegib was approved in 2012 for the treatment of BCC.[421] Glasdegib was approved in 2018 for use in combination with the antimetabolite, cytarabine, for patients with AML who are at least age 75 years and unable to receive intensive induction chemotherapy.[422] Both drugs work by inhibiting the hedgehog signaling cascade that plays a role in cancer cell proliferation. They bind to Smoothened (SMO), a receptor in the hedgehog signaling cascade, and shut off the signaling cascade, thereby inhibiting the proliferation of cancer cells, hematopoietic stem cells in AML, and basal cells in BCC. The adverse effects of both drugs are generally mild; however, they are associated with a boxed warning of embryo-fetal toxicity owing to the role of the hedgehog signaling cascade in embryonic development. Reproductive counseling for both men and women, and confirming nonpregnant status prior to initiating therapy in female patients, is required before these drugs can be administered.

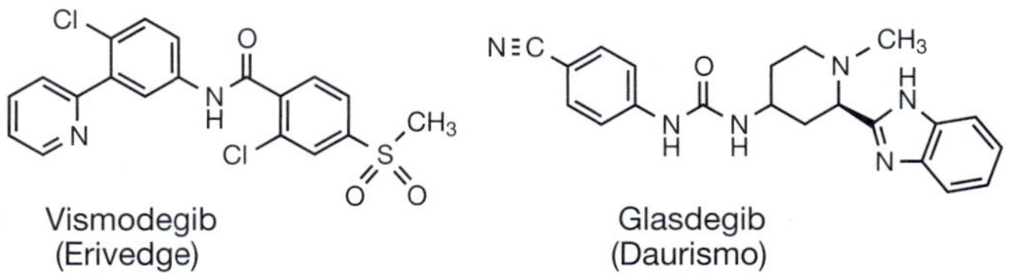

Figure 37.33 Hedgehog signaling inhibitors.

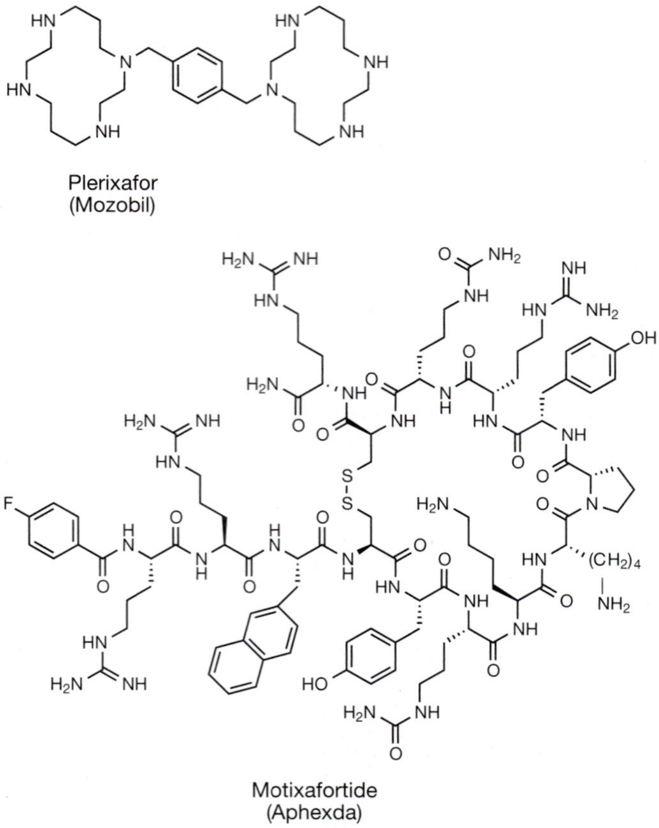

Figure 37.34 C-X-C motif chemokine receptor 4 inhibitors.

CXCR4 Inhibitors

The C-X-C motif chemokine ligand 12 (CXCL12), also referred to as stromal cell–derived factor 1 (SDF-1), and its receptor C-X-C motif chemokine receptor 4 (CXCR4) are expressed in several cell types, including hematopoietic stem cells.[423] Hematopoietic stem cells are maintained within the bone marrow via multiple anchors, including the CXCL12/CXCR4 complex. Disruption of CXCL12/CXCR4 releases stem cells to the peripheral blood.

The CXCR4 inhibitors, motixafortide and plerixafor, have demonstrated benefits as hematopoietic stem cell mobilizers (Fig. 37.34). Motixafortide is a second-generation CXCR4 inhibitor, the first-generation being plerixafor. Motixafortide is a selective CXCR4 inhibitor and incorporates six cationic residues that interact ionically with acidic CXCR4 residues, while the bulky side chains of motixafortide sterically hinder the adoption of the active CXCR4 conformation.[424] Motixafortide has been approved for use in combination with filgrastim for autologous transplantation in patients with MM. Motixafortide has a longer duration of action (>72 hours) compared to plerixafor (4-18 hours) and causes a greater mobilization of hematopoietic stem cells in an indirect comparison to plerixafor.[425] Both agents are given by SC injection.

Investigational Targeted Therapies

Targeted Protein Degraders

Targeted protein degradation is a novel approach being used for the development of unique targeted therapies that harness the physiologic proteasomal degradation machinery.[426,427] This approach utilizes heterobifunctional molecules termed proteolysis targeting chimeras (PROTACs). A PROTAC includes a targeted therapy as the first ligand that binds to the protein of interest (POI). The targeted therapy is linked to a second ligand that binds to an E3 ubiquitin ligase and activates the ubiquitin-proteasome system. Simultaneous binding of the PROTAC to the POI and the ligase induces ubiquitylation of the POI. The POI is tagged for degradation by the ubiquitin-proteasome system. The PROTACs are intended to degrade the oncogenic driver proteins and thereby shut down the processes that drive tumor growth and progression. Typical POIs include oncogenic drivers, such as kinases, surface receptors, and epigenetic modifiers.[428-431] The E3 ubiquitin ligases have included cereblon, von Hippel-Lindau, and inhibitors of apoptosis proteins. Both POIs and E3 ubiquitin ligases have been targeted by small molecule ligands that are connected through linkers of varied lengths.

ALK-targeted PROTACs have been developed, as shown in Figure 37.35. The ALK inhibitor, alectinib, has been linked to the immunomodulator, pomalidomide. The alectinib fragment of the PROTAC binds to ALK, the POI, and pomalidomide binds to the E3 ubiquitin ligase, cereblon. The ALK-bound pomalidomide fragment of the PROTAC activates proteolytic degradation of ALK. As noted earlier, the PROTACs cause degradation of key oncogenic drivers and utilize targeted therapies for tumor-specific degradation. However, a challenge on the path to drug approval is the possibility of binding to off-target hits, bioavailability and toxicity to healthy cells.

Tumor Transporter Targeted Delivery

Anticancer agents that utilize tumor-specific transporters have been developed to achieve tumor-specific delivery.[432-434] Normal cells utilize reduced folate carrier (RFC) for folate uptake.[432] Tumors preferentially express and utilize FRs and proton-coupled folate transporter (PCFT) over RFC for folate uptake.[432] Mirvetuximab soravtansine is an approved antibody-drug conjugate targeting FRα for tumor-specific delivery of soravtansine, an antimitotic agent.[433] Novel antifolates are also being investigated as tumor-targeted cytotoxic agents that are taken up selectively by FRα or PCFT expressed in tumor cells while sparing normal cells.[434,435]

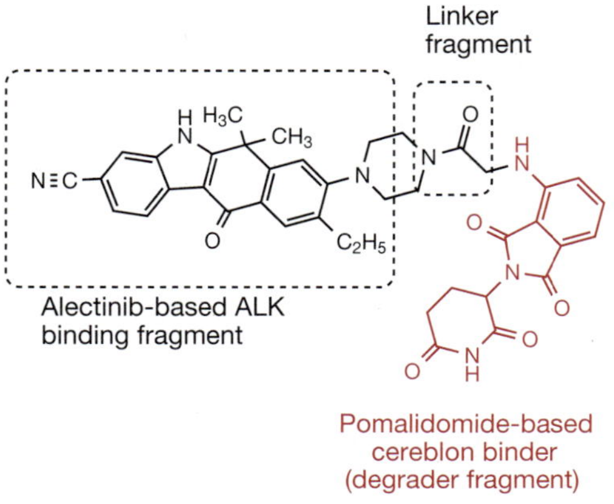

Figure 37.35 ALK-targeted PROTAC. ALK, anaplastic lymphoma kinase; PROTAC, proteolysis targeting chimera.

SUMMARY

Significant advancements in targeted therapy drug discovery have been made, leading to multiple drug approvals annually. Two design strategies have been particularly successful and include the development of covalent inhibitors and macrocyclization. The formation of a covalent bond to a cysteine residue in the active site of kinases for irreversible kinase inhibition has been applied to mEGFR, HER2, BTK, and, most recently, to FGFR, leading to 12 irreversible kinase inhibitors being approved thus far. Irreversible kinase inhibition has helped overcome resistance due to gatekeeper mutations such as T790M in EGFR and V561M in FGFR. The incorporation of a covalent bond has improved selectivity for target kinases, and the high binding affinity has allowed for the drug to be used at low concentrations. Macrocyclization efforts have focused on locking the molecule in its bioactive conformation that has translated to improved potencies, lower doses used, improved selectivity for target kinases, and increased CNS distribution. A combination approach among targeted therapies has also been successful. The combination of mBRAF and MEK inhibitors has been successful for CRC and melanoma. Improved outcomes have also been possible based on a combination of biologics and targeted therapies. Trastuzumab and lapatinib are effective for $HER2^+$ breast cancer in combination. Irreversible inhibitors have also been successful among non–kinase-targeted therapies, such mKRAS and XPO1. Previously undruggable targets such as mKRAS are no longer considered undruggable. Two currently approved drugs are on the market for mKRAS. More recently, the cancer biologics are gaining momentum and many PROTAC-based targeted therapies are also being clinically investigated.

Biomarker screening prior to initiating treatment with targeted therapy has improved therapeutic outcomes and quality of life. Targeted therapies based on patient-specific tumor markers have more manageable side-effect profile compared to classic chemotherapy. The oral route of administration and prolonged duration of therapy with targeted therapies require that pharmacists in community, specialty, and hospital pharmacies are trained appropriately to assist physicians and guide patients in the in-patient and outpatient settings to achieve optimal treatment outcomes.

Targeted Cancer Therapy Comprehension Questions

1. Osimertinib is classified as a type VI mEGFR inhibitor. Identify the functional group that allows for its classification as a type VI inhibitor.

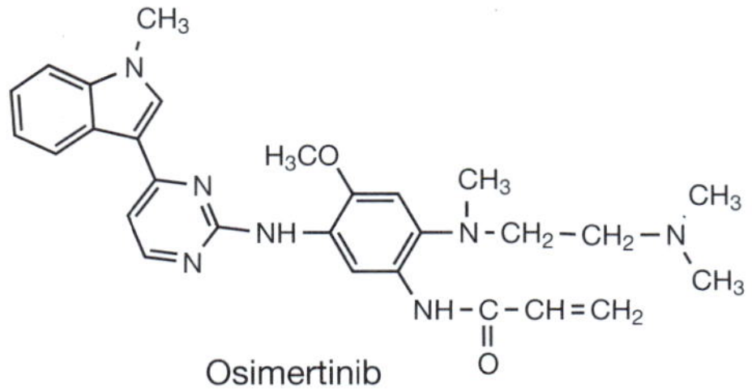

Osimertinib

2. Identify the amino acid within the ATP pocket of mEGFR that allows for osimertinib's classification as a type VI inhibitor.

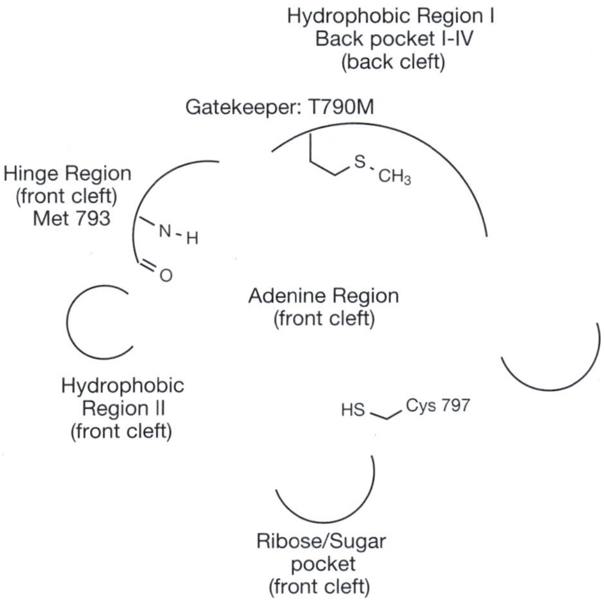

The ATP pocket of mutant EGFR

Targeted Cancer Therapy Comprehension Questions (continued)

3. A patient has been diagnosed with EGFR+ NSCLC and will be initiated on osimertinib. Which of the following could be possible reasons to **initiate** osimertinib? Select ALL that apply.
   A. wtKRAS-positive cancer
   B. mKRAS-positive cancer
   C. Detection of a T790M EGFR mutation
   D. Detection of a C797S EGFR mutation
   E. Detection of a L858R EGFR mutation
4. What is the role of the boxed functional group in lapatinib?

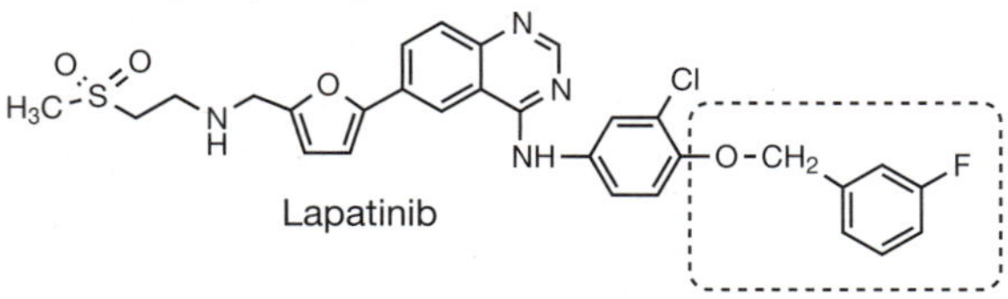

Lapatinib

5. Compare and contrast the drug pairs drawn below in terms of pharmacologic class, structural features impacting activity, mechanism of action, route of administration, and clinical application.

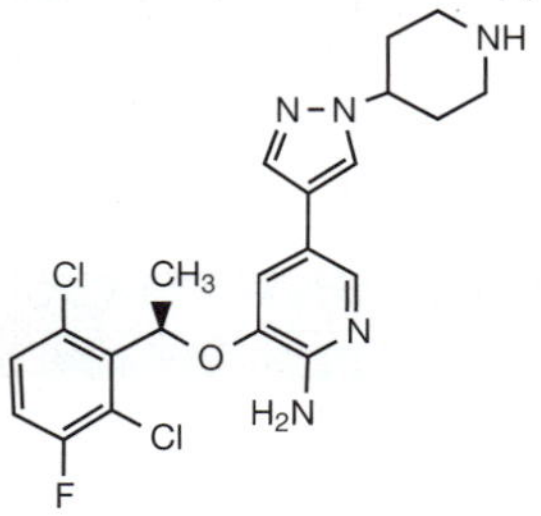

Crizotinib

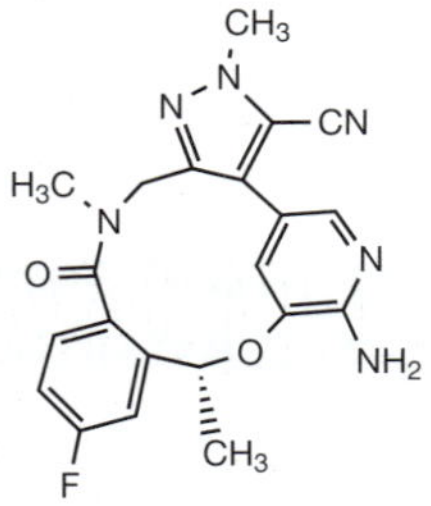

Lorlatinib

6. Compare and contrast the drug pair shown below in terms of pharmacologic class, structural features impacting activity, mechanism of action, route of administration, and clinical application.

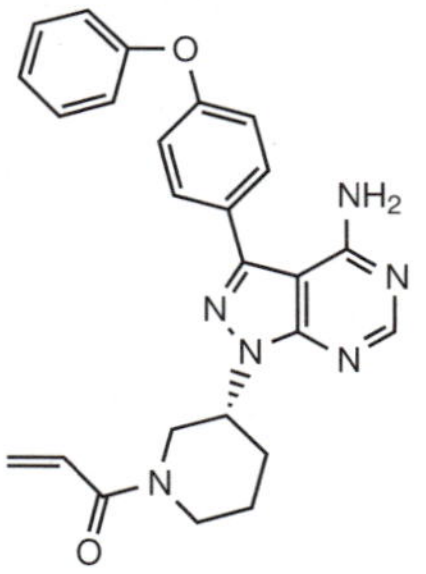

Ibrutinib

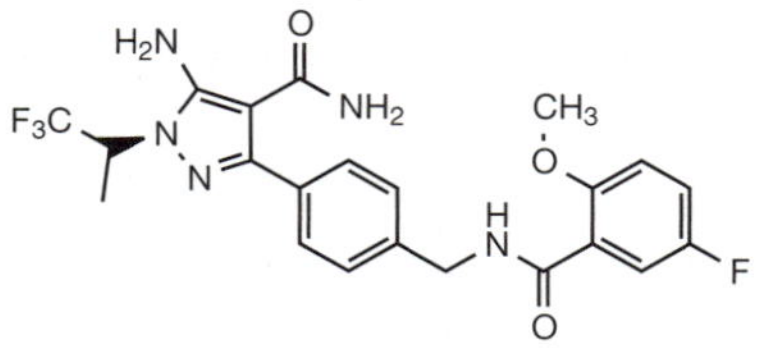

Pirtobrutinib

7. Which of the three proteasome inhibitors shown below may be given orally?

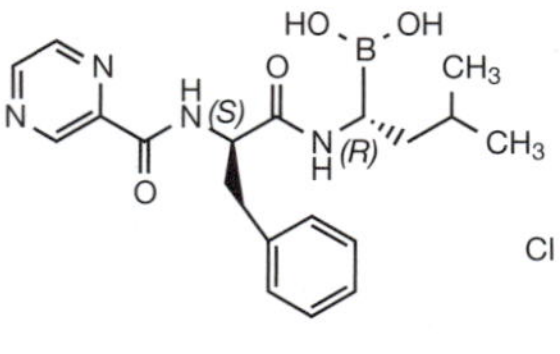

A

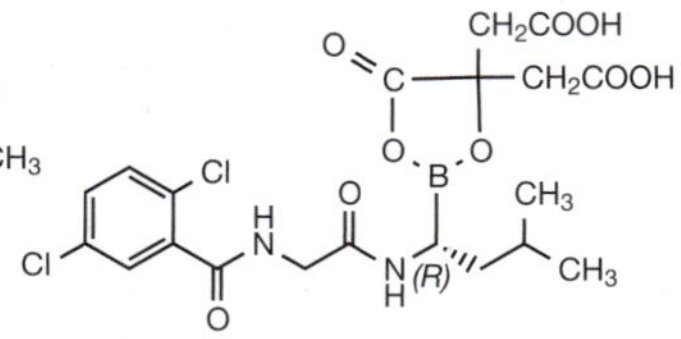

B

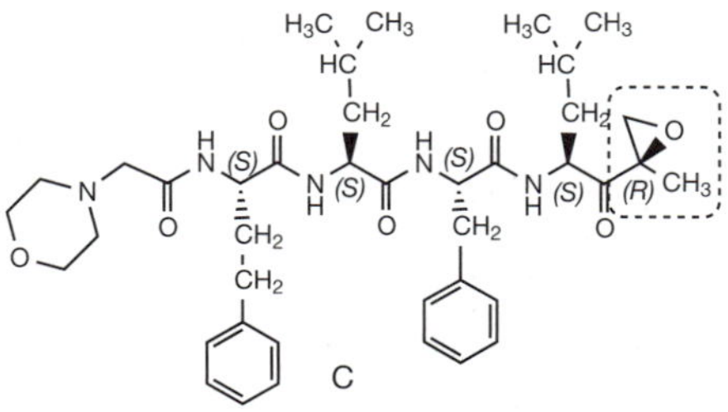

C

Answers found immediately after References.

REFERENCES

1. Bao J, Qiao L. New developments on cancer chemotherapy: multi-faceted issues in targeted cancer therapy. *Cancer Lett.* 2017;387:1-2.
2. Abdelmoez A, Coraca-Huber DC, Thurner GC, et al. New developments on targeted cancer chemotherapy. *Cancer Lett Special Issue.* 2017;387:1-126.
3. Bedard P, Hyman D, Davids M, et al. Small molecules, big impact: 20 years of targeted therapy in oncology. *Lancet.* 2020;395:1078-1088.
4. Perez-Herrero E, Fernandez-Medarde A. Advanced targeted therapies in cancer: drug nanocarriers, the future of chemotherapy. *Eur J Pharm Biopharm.* 2015;93:52-79.
5. Kandemir E. Review of novel and supplemental approvals of targeted cancer drugs by the Food and Drug Administration in 2021. *J Oncol Pharm Practice.* 2023;29(1):191-207.
6. Kabil M, Badary O, Bier F, et al. A comprehensive review on lipid nanocarrier systems for cancer treatment: fabrication, future prospects and clinical trials. *J Liposome Res.* 2024;34:135-177.
7. Almalki W. An up-to-date review on protein-based nanocarriers in the management of cancer. *Curr Drug Deliv.* 2024;21:509-524.
8. Rugo H, Linton K, Cervi P, et al. A clinician's guide to biosimilars in oncology. *Cancer Treat Rev.* 2016;46:73-79.
9. Liu Y. Utilizing oncology biosimilars to minimize the economic burden associated with cancer treatment: managed care considerations. *Am J Manag Care.* 2021;27(suppl 14).
10. Jiang S, Ren R, Gu Y, et al. Patient preferences in targeted pharmacotherapy for cancers: a systematic review of discrete choice experiments. *Pharmacoeconomics.* 2023;41:43-57.
11. Johnson L. Protein kinase inhibitors: contributions from structure to clinical compounds. *Q Rev Biophys.* 2009;42:1-40.
12. Drucker B, Talpaz M, Resta D, et al. Efficacy and safety of a specific inhibitor of the BRC-ABL tyrosine kinase in chronic myeloid leukemia. *N Engl J Med.* 2001;344:1031-1037.
13. Chakravarty D, Johnson A, Sklar J, et al. Somatic genomic testing in patients with metastatic or advanced cancer: ASCO provisional clinical opinion. *J Clin Oncol.* 2022;40:1231-1258.
14. Liu S, Zheng B, Sheng Y, et al. Identification of cancer dysfunctional subpathways by integrating DNA methylation, copy number variation, and gene-expression data. *Front Genet.* 2019;10:441.
15. Tomasik B, Garbicz F, Braun M, et al. Heterogeneity in precision oncology. *Camb Prism Precis Med.* 2024;2:e2.
16. Yu L, Webster K. Cancer pharmacogenomics: challenges, promises, and its application to cancer drug discovery. In: Thiagalingam S, ed. *Systems Biology of Cancer.* Cambridge University Press; 2015: 499-517.
17. Vivot A, Boutron I, Ravaud P, et al. Guidance for pharmacogenomic biomarker testing in labels of FDA-approved drugs. *Genet Med.* 2015;9:733-738.
18. Vivot A, Boutron I, Béraud-Chaulet G, et al. Evidence for treatment-by-biomarker interaction for FDA-approved oncology drugs with required pharmacogenomic biomarker testing. *Sci Rep.* 2017;7:6882.
19. Lee M, Abu Rous F, Borczuk A, et al. *Targeting Oncogenic Driver Mutations in Lung Cancer.* Cambridge University Press; 2023.
20. Jørgensen JT. A paradigm shift in biomarker guided oncology drug development. *Ann Transl Med.* 2019;7(7):148.
21. Bosman F, True L. Prognostic biomarkers: an introduction. *Virchows Arch.* 2014;464:253-256.
22. Kumar M, Ernani V, Owonikoko T. Biomarkers and targeted systemic therapies in advanced non-small cell lung cancer. *Mol Aspects Med.* 2015;45:55-66.
23. Reckamp KL. Molecular targets beyond the big 3. *Thorac Surg Clin.* 2020;30:157-164.
24. Steuer C, Ramalingam S. Targeting EGFR in lung cancer: lessons learned and future perspectives. *Mol Aspects Med.* 2015;45:67-73.
25. Padma V. An overview of targeted cancer chemotherapy. *BioMed.* 2015;5:1-6.
26. Baudino T. Targeted cancer therapy: the next generation of cancer treatment. *Curr Drug Discov Technol.* 2015;12:3-20.
27. Conde-Estevez D. Targeted cancer therapy: interactions with other medicines. *Clin Transl Oncol.* 2017;19:21-30.
28. Farkona S, Diamandis E, Blasutig I. Cancer immunotherapy: the beginning of the end of cancer? *BMC Med.* 2016;14:73.
29. Meiliana A, Dewi N, Wijaya A. Cancer immunotherapy: a review. *Indones Biomed J.* 2016;8:1-20.
30. Nasiri H, Valedkarimi Z, Aghebati-Maleki L, et al. Antibody-drug conjugates: promising and efficient tools for targeted cancer therapy. *J Cell Physiol.* 2018;233:6441-6457.
31. Diamantis N, Banerji Y. Antibody-drug conjugates—an emerging class of cancer treatment. *Br J Cancer.* 2016;114:362-367.
32. Smaglo B, Aldeghaither D, Weiner L. The development of immunoconjugates for targeted cancer therapy. *Nat Rev Clin Oncol.* 2014;11:637-648.
33. Drilon A, Ou SHI, Cho BC, et al. Repotrectinib (TPX-0005) is a next-generation ROS1/TRK/ALK inhibitor that potently inhibits ROS1/TRK/ALK solvent-front mutations. *Cancer Discov.* 2018;8(10):1227-1236.
34. Garraway LA, Weir BA, Zhao X, et al. "Lineage addiction" in human cancer: lessons from integrated genomics. *Cold Spring Harb Symp Quant Biol.* 2005:70;25-34.
35. Luo J, Solimini NL, Elledge SJ. Principles of cancer therapy: oncogene and non-oncogene addiction. *Cell.* 2009;136;823-837.
36. Sharma SV, Settleman J. Oncogene addiction: setting the stage for molecularly targeted cancer therapy. *Genes Dev.* 2007;21,3214-3231.
37. Vogler M. Targeting BCL2-proteins for the treatment of solid tumours. *Adv Med.* 2014;2014:943648.
38. Weinstein IB, Joe A. Oncogene addiction. *Cancer Res.* 2008;68:3077-3080.
39. Latysheva NS, Babu MM. Molecular signatures of fusion proteins in cancer. *ACS Pharmacol Transl Sci.* 2019;2:122-133.
40. Balmain A, Brown K. Oncogene activation in chemical carcinogenesis. *Adv Cancer Res.* 1988;51:147-182.
41. Koretzky GA. The legacy of the Philadelphia chromosome. *J Clin Invest.* 2007;117(8):2030-2032.
42. Narod SA, Salmena L. BRCA1 and BRCA2 mutations and breast cancer. *Discov Med.* 2011;12(66):445-453.
43. Smith KL, Isaacs C. BRCA mutation testing in determining breast cancer therapy. *Cancer J.* 2011;17(6):492-499.
44. Birkbak NJ, Kochupurakkal B, Izarzugaza JM, et al. Tumor mutation burden forecasts outcome in ovarian cancer with BRCA1 or BRCA2 mutations. *PLoS One.* 2013;8(11):e80023.
45. Lorusso D, Tripodi E, Maltese G, et al. Spotlight on olaparib in the treatment of BRCA-mutated ovarian cancer: design, development and place in therapy. *Drug Des Devel Ther.* 2018;12:1501-1509.
46. Mas-Ponte D, McCullough M, Supek F. Spectrum of DNA mismatch repair failures viewed through the lens of cancer genomics and implications for therapy. *Clin Sci (Lond).* 2022; 136(5):383-404.
47. Hua H, He W, Chen N, et al. Genomic and transcriptomic analysis of MSI-H colorectal cancer patients with targetable alterations identifies clinical implications for immunotherapy. *Front Immunol.* 2023;13:974793.
48. Walton E. On the road to epigenetic therapy. *Biomed J.* 2016;39: 161-165.
49. Bradbury J. Human epigenome project—up and running. *PLoS Biol.* 2003;1(3):e82.
50. Esteller M. The necessity of a human epigenome project. *Carcinogenesis.* 2006;27:1121-1125.
51. Jones P, Archer T, Baylin S. Moving AHEAD with an international human epigenome project. *Nature.* 2008;454:711-715.
52. Mulet-Margalef N, Linares J, Badia-Ramentol J, et al. Challenges and therapeutic opportunities in the dmmr/msi-h colorectal cancer landscape. *Cancers.* 2023;15:1022.
53. Leach DR, Krummel MF, Allison JP. Enhancement of antitumor immunity by CTLA-4 blockade. *Science.* 1996;271:1734-1736.
54. Sharma P, Allison JP. Immune checkpoint targeting in cancer therapy: toward combination strategies with curative potential. *Cell.* 2015;161(2):205-214.

55. Hodi FS, O'Day SJ, McDermott DF, et al. Improved survival with ipilimumab in patients with metastatic melanoma. *N Engl J Med.* 2010;363(8):711-723.
56. Robert C, Schachter J, Long GV, et al. Pembrolizumab versus ipilimumab in advanced melanoma. *N Engl J Med.* 2015;372(26):2521-2532.
57. Topalian SL, Hodi FS, Brahmer JR, et al. Safety, activity, and immune correlates of anti-PD-1 antibody in cancer. *N Engl J Med.* 2012;366(26):2443-2454.
58. Hanahan D. Hallmarks of cancer: new dimensions. *Cancer Discov.* 2022;12:31-46.
59. Hanahan D, Weinberg RA. The hallmarks of cancer. *Cell.* 2000;100:57-70.
60. D'Aguanno S, Del Bufalo D. Inhibition of anti-apoptotic Bcl-2 proteins in preclinical and clinical studies: current overview in cancer. *Cells.* 2020;9(5):1287.
61. Qian S, Wei Z, Yang W, et al. The role of BCL-2 family proteins in regulating apoptosis and cancer therapy. *Front Oncol.* 2022;12:985363.
62. Bajaj S, Kumar MS, Peters GJ, et al. Targeting telomerase for its advent in cancer therapeutics. *Med Res Rev.* 2020;40(5):1871-1919.
63. Dudley AC, Griffioen AW. Pathological angiogenesis: mechanisms and therapeutic strategies. *Angiogenesis.* 2023;26(3):313-347.
64. Folkman J. Tumor angiogenesis: therapeutic implications. *N Engl J Med.* 1971;285(21):1182-1186.
65. Ferguson FM, Gray NS. Kinase inhibitors: the road ahead. *Nat Rev Drug Discov.* 2018;17(5):353-377.
66. Poliakova M, Aebersold D, Zimmer Y, et al. The relevance of tyrosine kinase inhibitors for global metabolic pathways in cancer. *Mol Cancer.* 2018;17(1):27.
67. Alshiekh Nasany R, de la Fuente MI. Therapies for IDH-mutant gliomas. *Curr Neurol Neurosci Rep.* 2023;23(5):225-233.
68. Boedtkjer E, Pedersen SF. The acidic tumor microenvironment as a driver of cancer. *Annu Rev Physiol.* 2020;82:103-126.
69. Vrábel D, Pour L, Ševčíková S. The impact of NF-κB signaling on pathogenesis and current treatment strategies in multiple myeloma. *Blood Rev.* 2019;34:56-66.
70. Yu H, Lin L, Zhang Z, et al. Targeting NF-κB pathway for the therapy of diseases: mechanism and clinical study. *Sig Transduct Target Ther.* 2020;5:209.
71. Martínez-Jiménez F, Muiños F, Sentís I, et al. A compendium of mutational cancer driver genes. *Nat Rev Cancer.* 2020;20(10):555-572.
72. Hanahan D, Weinberg RA. Hallmarks of cancer: the next generation. *Cell.* 2011;144:646-647.
73. Tanramluk D, Schreyer A, Pitt WR, et al. On the origins of enzyme inhibitor selectivity and promiscuity: a case study of protein kinase binding to staurosporine. *Chem Biol Drug Des.* 2009;74(1):16-24.
74. Shyam Sunder S, Sharma UC, Pokharel S. Adverse effects of tyrosine kinase inhibitors in cancer therapy: pathophysiology, mechanisms and clinical management. *Sig Transduct Target Ther.* 2023;8:262.
75. Schneider BJ, Naidoo J, Santomasso BD, et al. Management of immune-related adverse events in patients treated with immune checkpoint inhibitor therapy: ASCO guideline update. *J Clin Oncol.* 2021;39(36):4073-4126.
76. Buchler T, Poprach A. Planned discontinuation of tyrosine kinase inhibitor therapy in metastatic renal cell carcinoma: lessons for the era of immunotherapy. *Target Oncol.* 2024;19:175-180.
77. Aldea M, André F, Marabelle A, et al. Overcoming resistance to tumor-targeted and immune-targeted therapies. *Cancer Discov.* 2021;11(4):874-899.
78. Wu D, Wang DC, Cheng Y, et al. Roles of tumor heterogeneity in the development of drug resistance: a call for precision therapy. *Semin Cancer Biol.* 2017;42:13-19.
79. Li X, Li M, Huang M, et al. The multi-molecular mechanisms of tumor-targeted drug resistance in precision medicine. *Biomed Pharmacother.* 2022;150:113064.
80. Santarpia L, Lippman SM, El-Naggar AK. Targeting the MAPK-RAS-RAF signaling pathway in cancer therapy. *Expert Opin Ther Targets.* 2012;16(1):103-119.
81. Porta C, Paglino C, Mosca A. Targeting PI3K/Akt/mTOR signaling in cancer. *Front Oncol.* 2014;4:64.
82. Corneth OBJ, Klein Wolterink RGJ, Hendriks RW. BTK signaling in B cell differentiation and autoimmunity. *Curr Top Microbiol Immunol.* 2016;393:67-105.
83. Owen KL, Brockwell NK, Parker BS. JAK-STAT signaling: a double-edged sword of immune regulation and cancer progression. *Cancers (Basel).* 2019;11(12):2002.
84. Anttila JV, Shubin M, Cairns J, et al. Contrasting the impact of cytotoxic and cytostatic drug therapies on tumour progression. *PLoS Comput Biol.* 2019;15(11):e1007493.
85. Kim PY, Leung CT. Therapeutic potentials and challenges of cytostatic persister cancer cells. *Oncotarget.* 2023;14:944-945.
86. Kurup S, Sakharkar P. Three-dimensional visualization of kinase inhibitors as therapeutically relevant examples to reinforce types of enzyme inhibitors. *J Chem Educ.* 2019;96(2):296-303.
87. Zhao Z, Wu H, Wang L, et al. Exploration of type II binding mode: a privileged approach for kinase inhibitor focused drug discovery? *ACS Chem Biol.* 2014;9:1230-1241.
88. Levinson NM, Kuchment O, Shen K, et al. A Src-like inactive conformation in the Abl tyrosine kinase domain. *PLoS Biol.* 2006;4(5):e144.
89. Roskoski R Jr. Classification of small molecule protein kinase inhibitors based upon the structures of their drug-enzyme complexes. *Pharmacol Res.* 2016;103:26-48.
90. Amrhein JA, Knapp S, Hanke T. Synthetic opportunities and challenges for macrocyclic kinase inhibitors. *J Med Chem.* 2021;64(12):7991-8009.
91. Cohen P, Cross D, Jänne PA. Kinase drug discovery 20 years after imatinib: progress and future directions. *Nat Rev Drug Discov.* 2021;20:551-569.
92. Facts & Comparisons [database online].
93. Van Erp N, Gelderblom H, Guchelaar H-J. Clinical pharmacokinetics of tyrosine kinase inhibitors. *Cancer Treat Rev.* 2009;35:692-706.
94. Duckett D, Cameron M. Metabolism considerations for kinase inhibitors in cancer treatment. *Expert Opin.* 2010;6:1775-1793.
95. Cross D, Ashton S, Ghiorghiu S, et al. AZD9291, an irreversible EGFR TKI, overcomes T790M-mediated resistance to EGFR inhibitors in lung cancer. *Cancer Discov.* 2014;4:1046-1061.
96. Kourie H, Chaix M, Gombos A, et al. Pharmacodynamics, pharmacokinetics and clinical efficacy of neratinib in HER2-positive breast cancer and breast cancer with HER2 mutations. *Expert Opin Drug Metab Toxicol.* 2016;12:947-957.
97. Knoebel RW, Larson RA. Pepsi® or Coke®? Influence of acid on dasatinib absorption. *J Oncol Pharm Pract.* 2018;24(2):156-158.
98. Li X, Kamenecka T, Cameron M. Bioactivation of the epidermal growth factor receptor inhibitor gefitinib: implications for pulmonary and hepatic toxicities. *Chem Res Toxicol.* 2009;22:1736-1742.
99. Wind S, Schnell D, Ebner T, et al. Clinical pharmacokinetics and pharmacodynamics of afatinib. *Clin Pharmacokinet.* 2017;56:235-250.
100. Zhou Y, Xiang S, Yang F, et al. Targeting gatekeeper mutations for kinase drug discovery. *J Med Chem.* 2022;65(23):15540-15558.
101. Cha JH, Chan LC, Song MS, et al. New approaches on cancer immunotherapy. *Cold Spring Harb Perspect Med.* 2020;10(8):a036863.
102. Pan C, Liu H, Robins E, et al. Next-generation immuno-oncology agents: current momentum shifts in cancer immunotherapy. *J Hematol Oncol.* 2020;13(1):29.
103. https://www.fda.gov/drugs/novel-drug-approvals-fda/novel-drug-approvals-2023
104. Suttorp M, Bornhauser M, Metzler M, et al. Pharmacology and pharmacokinetics of imatinib in pediatric patients. *Clin Pharmacol.* 2018;11:219-231.
105. Zheng Q, Wu P, Yu Q, et al. ABCB1 polymorphisms predict imatinib response in chronic myeloid leukemia patients: a systematic review and meta-analysis. *Pharmacogenomics J.* 2015;15:127-134.
106. Muller B. Imatinib and its successors: how modern chemistry has changed drug development. *Curr Pharm Des.* 2009;15:120-133.

107. Deininger M, Druker B. Specific targeted therapy of chronic myelogenous leukemia with imatinib. *Pharmacol Rev.* 2003;55:401-422.
108. Schenone S, Bruno O, Radi M, et al. New insights into small-molecule inhibitors of Bcr-Abl. *Med Res Rev.* 2009;31:1-41.
109. Weisberg E, Manley P, Breitenstein W, et al. Characterization of AMN107, a selective inhibitor of native and mutant Bcr-Abl. *Cancer Cell.* 2005;7:129-141.
110. Jarkowski AI, Sweeny R. Nilotinib: a new tyrosine kinase inhibitor for the treatment of chronic myelogenous leukemia. *Pharmacotherapy.* 2008;28:1374-1382.
111. Keskin D, Sadri S, Eskazan A. Dasatinib for the treatment of chronic myeloid leukemia: patient selection and special considerations. *Drug Des Devel Ther.* 2016;10:3355-3361.
112. Ault P, Rose J, Nodzon L, et al. Bosutinib therapy in patients with chronic myeloid leukemia: practical considerations for management of side effects. *J Adv Pract Oncol.* 2016;7:160-175.
113. Kong G, Kim A, Hill B, et al. The safety of bosutinib for the treatment of chronic myeloid leukemia. *Expert Opin Drug Saf.* 2017;16:1203-1209.
114. Tokarski J, Newitt J, Chang C, et al. The structure of dasatinib (BMS-354825) bound to activated Abl kinase domain elucidates its inhibitory activity against imatinib-resistant Abl mutants. *Cancer Res.* 2006;66:5790-5797.
115. Signorovitch J, Ayyagari R, Reichmann W, et al. Major molecular response during the first year of dasatinib, imatinib or nilotinib treatment for newly diagnosed chronic myeloid leukemia; a network meta-analysis. *Cancer Treat Rev.* 2014;40:285-292.
116. Iqbal N, Iqbal N. Imatinib: a breakthrough of targeted therapy in cancer. *Chemother Res Pract.* 2014;2014:e357027.
117. Chen R, Chen B. The role of dasatinib in the management of chronic myeloid leukemia. *Drug Des Devel Ther.* 2015;9:773-779.
118. Huang W-S, Metcalf C, Sundaramoorthi R, et al. Discovery of 3-[2-(imidazo[1,2-b]pyridazin-3-yl)ethynyl]-4-methyl-N-{4-[(4-methylpiperazin-1-yl)-methyl]-3-(trifluoromethyl)phenyl}benzamide (AP24534), a potent, orally active pan-inhibitor of breakpoint cluster region-abelson (BCR-ABL) kinase including the T315I gatekeeper mutant. *J Med Chem.* 2010;53:4701-4719.
119. Shamroe C, Comeau J. Ponatinib: a new tyrosine kinase inhibitor for the treatment of chromic myeloid leukemia and Philadelphia chromosome-positive acute lymphoblastic leukemia. *Ann Pharmacol.* 2013;47:1540-1546.
120. Massaro F, Molica M, Breccia M. Ponatinib: a review of efficacy and safety. *Curr Cancer Drug Targets.* 2017;17:1-10.
121. Gainor J, Chabner B. Ponatinib: accelerated disapproval. *Oncologist.* 2015;20:847-848.
122. Schoepfer J, Jahnke W, Berellini G, et al. Discovery of asciminib (ABL001), an allosteric inhibitor of the tyrosine kinase activity of BCR-ABL1. *J Med Chem.* 2018;61(18):8120-8135.
123. Jones JK, Thompson EM. Allosteric inhibition of ABL Kinases: therapeutic potential in cancer. *Mol Cancer Ther.* 2020;19(9):1763-1769.
124. Réa D, Mauro MJ, Boquimpani C, et al. A phase 3, open-label, randomized study of asciminib, a STAMP inhibitor, vs bosutinib in CML after 2 or more prior TKIs. *Blood.* 2021;138(21):2031-2041.
125. Teng M, Luskin MR, Cowan-Jacob SW, et al. The dawn of allosteric BCR-ABL1 drugs: from a phenotypic screening hit to an approved drug. *J Med Chem.* 2022;65(11):7581-7594.
126. Pulte ED, Chen H, Price LSL, et al. FDA Approval summary: revised indication and dosing regimen for ponatinib based on the results of the OPTIC trial. *Oncologist.* 2022;27(2):149-157.
127. Tesileanu CMS, Michaleas S, Gonzalo Ruiz R, et al. The EMA assessment of asciminib for the treatment of adult patients with Philadelphia chromosome-positive chronic myeloid leukemia in chronic phase who were previously treated with at least two tyrosine kinase inhibitors. *Oncologist.* 2023;28(7):628-632.
128. Kong X, Pan P, Sun H, et al. Drug discovery targeting anaplastic lymphoma kinase (ALK). *J Med Chem.* 2019;62(24):10927-10954.
129. Epstein LF, Chen H, Emkey R, et al. The R1275Q neuroblastoma mutant and certain ATP-competitive inhibitors stabilize alternative activation loop conformations of anaplastic lymphoma kinase. *J Biol Chem.* 2012;287(44):37447-37457.
130. Katayama R. Drug resistance in anaplastic lymphoma kinase-rearranged lung cancer. *Cancer Sci.* 2017;109:572-580.
131. Huang Q, Johnson TW, Bailey S, et al. Design of potent and selective inhibitors to overcome clinical anaplastic lymphoma kinase mutations resistant to crizotinib. *J Med Chem.* 2014;57(4):1170-1187.
132. De Pas T, Pala L, Catania C, et al. Molecular and clinical features of second-generation anaplastic lymphoma kinase inhibitors. *Future Oncol.* 2017;13:2629-2644.
133. Friboulet L, Li N, Katayama R, et al. The ALK inhibitor ceritinib overcomes crizotinib resistance in non-small cell lung cancer. *Cancer Discov.* 2014;4:662-673.
134. Mezquita L, Planchard D. The role of brigatinib in crizotinib-resistant non-small cell lung cancer. *Cancer Manag Res.* 2018;10:123-130.
135. Jain R, Chen H. Spotlight on brigatinib and its potential in the treatment of patients with metastatic ALK-positive non-small cell lung cancer who are resistant or intolerant to crizotinib. *Lung Cancer Targ Ther.* 2017;8:169-177.
136. Huang WS, Liu S, Zou D, et al. Discovery of brigatinib (AP26113), a phosphine oxide-containing, potent, orally active inhibitor of anaplastic lymphoma kinase. *J Med Chem.* 2016;59(10):4948-4964.
137. Gadgeel S. The use of alectinib in the first-line treatment of anaplastic lymphoma kinase-positive non-small-cell lung cancer. *Future Oncol.* 2018;14:1875-1882.
138. Sato-Nakai M, Kawashima K, Nakagawa T, et al. Metabolites of alectinib in human: their identification and pharmacological activity. *Heliyon.* 2017;3:e00354.
139. Samacá-Samacá D, Prieto-Pinto L, Peréz AY, et al. Alectinib for treating patients with metastatic ALK-positive NSCLC: systematic review and network metanalysis. *Lung Cancer Manag.* 2023;12(2):LMT59.
140. Hatcher JM, Bahcall M, Choi HG, et al. Discovery of inhibitors that overcome the G1202R anaplastic lymphoma kinase resistance mutation. *J Med Chem.* 2015;58(23):9296-9308.
141. Chen C, He Z, Xie D, et al. Molecular mechanism behind the resistance of the G1202R-mutated anaplastic lymphoma kinase to the approved drug ceritinib. *J Phys Chem B.* 2018;122(17):4680-4692.
142. Siblini L, Schott R, Trensz P, et al. Primary resistance to ALK inhibitors in KLC1/ALK-rearranged pleural metastatic lung adenocarcinoma: a case report. *Transl Lung Cancer Res.* 2023;12:2342-2346.
143. Basit S, Ashraf Z, Lee K, et al. First macrocyclic 3rd-generation ALK inhibitor for treatment of ALK/ROS1 cancer: clinical and designing strategy update of lorlatinib. *Eur J Med Chem.* 2017;134:348-356.
144. Shiba-Ishii A, Johnson TW, Dagogo-Jack I, et al. Analysis of lorlatinib analogs reveals a roadmap for targeting diverse compound resistance mutations in ALK-positive lung cancer. *Nat Cancer.* 2022;3(6):710-722.
145. Garcia Jimenez D, Poongavanam V, Kihlberg J. Macrocycles in drug discovery—learning from the past for the future. *J Med Chem.* 2023;66(8):5377-5396.
146. Zhao Z, Bourne PE. Rigid scaffolds are promising for designing macrocyclic kinase inhibitors. *ACS Pharmacol Transl Sci.* 2023;6(8):1182-1191.
147. Shaw AT, Friboulet L, Leshchiner I, et al. Resensitization to crizotinib by the lorlatinib alk resistance mutation L1198F. *N Engl J Med.* 2016;374(1):54-61.
148. Gil M, Knetki-Wróblewska M, Niziński P, et al. Effectiveness of ALK inhibitors in treatment of CNS metastases in NSCLC patients. *Ann Med.* 2023;55(1):1018-1028.
149. Fabbri L, Di Federico A, Astore M, et al. From development to place in therapy of lorlatinib for the treatment of ALK and ROS1 rearranged non-small cell lung cancer (NSCLC). *Diagnostics.* 2023;14(1):48.
150. He L, Dar AC. Targeting drug-resistant mutations in ALK. *Nat Cancer.* 2022;3(6):659-661.

151. Cooper AJ, Sequist LV, Lin JJ. Third-generation EGFR and ALK inhibitors: mechanisms of resistance and management. *Nat Rev Clin Oncol*. 2022;19(8):499-514.
152. Chen J, O'Gorman MT, James LP, et al. Pharmacokinetics of lorlatinib after single and multiple dosing in patients with anaplastic lymphoma kinase (ALK)-positive non-small cell lung cancer: results from a global phase I/II study. *Clin Pharmacokinet*. 2021;60(10):1313-1324.
153. Luo Y, Zhang Z, Guo X, et al. Comparative safety of anaplastic lymphoma kinase tyrosine kinase inhibitors in advanced anaplastic lymphoma kinase-mutated non-small cell lung cancer: systematic review and network meta-analysis. *Lung Cancer*. 2023;184:107319.
154. Sisi M, Fusaroli M, De Giglio A, et al. Psychiatric adverse reactions to anaplastic lymphoma kinase inhibitors in non-small-cell lung cancer: analysis of spontaneous reports submitted to the FDA adverse event reporting system. *Target Oncol*. 2022;17(1):43-51.
155. Killock D. Lorlatinib in ROS1-positive NSCLC. *Nat Rev Clin Oncol*. 2020;17(1):7.
156. Panda GS, Noronha V, Shetty O, et al. ROS1-positive non-small-cell lung cancer. *Cancer Res Stat Treat*. 2022;5(3):544.
157. Solomon BJ, Bauer TM, Mok TSK, et al. Efficacy and safety of first-line lorlatinib versus crizotinib in patients with advanced, ALK-positive non-small-cell lung cancer: updated analysis of data from the phase 3, randomised, open-label CROWN study. *Lancet Respir Med*. 2023;11(4):354-366.
158. Yan W, Lakkaniga NR, Carlomagno F, et al. Insights into current tropomyosin receptor kinase (TRK) inhibitors: development and clinical application. *J Med Chem*. 2019;62(4):1731-1760.
159. Vaishnavi A, Le AT, Doebele RC. TRKing down an old oncogene in a new era of targeted therapy. *Cancer Discov*. 2015;5(1):25-34.
160. Shah N, Lankerovich M, Lee H, et al. Exploration of the gene fusion landscape of glioblastoma using transcriptome sequencing and copy number data. *BMC Genomics*. 2013;14(1):818.
161. Sehgal K, Piper-Vallillo AJ, Viray H, et al. Cases of ROS1-rearranged lung cancer: when to use crizotinib, entrectinib, lorlatinib, and beyond? *Precis Cancer Med*. 2020;3:17.
162. Menichincheri M, Ardini E, Magnaghi P, et al. Discovery of entrectinib: a new 3-aminoindazole as a potent anaplastic lymphoma kinase (ALK), c-ros oncogene 1 kinase (ROS1), and pan-tropomyosin receptor kinases (Pan-TRKs) inhibitor. *J Med Chem*. 2016;59(7):3392-3408.
163. Doebele RC, Drilon A, Paz-Ares L, et al. Entrectinib in patients with advanced or metastatic NTRK fusion-positive solid tumours: integrated analysis of three phase 1-2 trials. *Lancet Oncol*. 2020;21(2):271-282.
164. Ardini E, Menichincheri M, Banfi P, et al. Entrectinib, a pan-TRK, ROS1, and ALK inhibitor with activity in multiple molecularly defined cancer indications. *Mol Cancer Ther*. 2016;15(4):628-639.
165. Drilon A, Laetsch TW, Kummar S, et al. Efficacy of larotrectinib in TRK fusion-positive cancers in adults and children. *N Engl J Med*. 2018;378(8):731-739.
166. Murray BW, Rogers E, Zhai D, et al. Molecular characteristics of repotrectinib that enable potent inhibition of TRK fusion proteins and resistant mutations. *Mol Cancer Ther*. 2021;20(12):2446-2456.
167. Saha D, Ryan KR, Lakkaniga NR, et al. Targeting rearranged during transfection in cancer: a perspective on small-molecule inhibitors and their clinical development. *J Med Chem*. 2021;64(16):11747-11773.
168. La Monica G, Pizzolanti G, Baiamonte C, et al. Design and synthesis of novel thieno[3,2-c]quinoline compounds with antiproliferative activity on ret-dependent medullary thyroid cancer cells. *ACS Omega*. 2023;8(38):34640-34649.
169. Subbiah V, Shen T, Terzyan SS, et al. Structural basis of acquired resistance to selpercatinib and pralsetinib mediated by non-gatekeeper RET mutations. *Ann Oncol*. 2021;32(2):261-268.
170. Mathison CJN, Yang Y, Nelson J, et al. Antitarget selectivity and tolerability of novel pyrrolo[2,3-*d*]pyrimidine RET inhibitors. *ACS Med Chem Lett*. 2021;12(12):1912-1919.
171. Nardo M, Gouda MA, Nelson BE, et al. Strategies for mitigating adverse events related to selective RET inhibitors in patients with RET-altered cancers. *Cell Rep Med*. 2023;4(12):101332.
172. Yarden Y, Sliwkowski M. Untangling the ErbB signalling network. *Nat Rev Mol Cell Biol*. 2001;2:127-137.
173. Ciardiello F, Tortora G. A novel approach in the treatment of cancer: targeting the epidermal growth factor receptor. *Clin Cancer Res*. 2001;7:2958-2970.
174. Niggenaber J, Hardick J, Lategahn J, et al. Structure defines function: clinically relevant mutations in ErbB kinases: miniperspective. *J Med Chem*. 2020;63(1):40-51.
175. Sordella R, Bell DW, Haber DA, et al. Gefitinib-sensitizing EGFR mutations in lung cancer activate anti-apoptotic pathways. *Science*. 2004;305:1163-1167.
176. Mok TS, Wu Y-L, Ahn M-J, et al. Osimertinib or platinum-pemetrexed in EGFR T790M-positive lung cancer. *N Engl J Med*. 2017;376(7):629-640.
177. John T, Akamatsu H, Delmonte A, et al. EGFR mutation analysis for prospective patient selection in AURA3 phase III trial of osimertinib versus platinum-pemetrexed in patients with EGFR T790M-positive advanced non-small-cell lung cancer. *Lung Cancer*. 2018;126:133-138.
178. Soria JC, Ohe Y, Vansteenkiste J, et al. Osimertinib in untreated EGFR-mutated advanced non-small-cell lung cancer. *N Engl J Med*. 2018;378(2):113-125.
179. Ramalingam SS, Yang JCH, Lee CK, et al. Osimertinib as first-line treatment of EGFR mutation-positive advanced non-small-cell lung cancer. *J Clin Oncol*. 2018;36(9):841-849.
180. Herbst RS, Wu YL, John T, et al. Adjuvant osimertinib for resected EGFR-mutated stage IB-IIIA non-small-cell lung cancer: updated results from the phase III randomized ADAURA trial. *J Clin Oncol*. 2023;41(10):1830-1840.
181. Asahina H, Tanaka K, Morita S, et al. A phase II study of osimertinib combined with platinum plus pemetrexed in patients with EGFR-mutated advanced non-small-cell lung cancer: the OPAL study (NEJ032C/LOGIK1801). *Clin Lung Cancer*. 2021;22(2):147-151.
182. Fu K, Xie F, Wang F, et al. Therapeutic strategies for EGFR-mutated non-small cell lung cancer patients with osimertinib resistance. *J Hematol Oncol*. 2022;15(1):173.
183. Chen L, Fu W, Zheng L, et al. Recent Progress of small-molecule epidermal growth factor receptor (EGFR) inhibitors against C797S resistance in non-small-cell lung cancer. *J Med Chem*. 2018;61:4290-4300.
184. Lategahn J, Keul M, Klövekorn P, et al. Inhibition of osimertinib-resistant epidermal growth factor receptor EGFR-T790M/C797S. *Chem Sci*. 2019;10(46):10789-10801.
185. Zhang SM, Zhu QG, Ding XX, et al. Prognostic value of EGFR and KRAS in resected non-small cell lung cancer: a systematic review and meta-analysis. *Cancer Manag Res*. 2018;10:3393-3404.
186. Cancer Genome Atlas Research Network. Comprehensive molecular profiling of lung adenocarcinoma. *Nature*. 2014;511:543-550.
187. Zeng Y, Yu D, Tian W, et al. Resistance mechanisms to osimertinib and emerging therapeutic strategies in nonsmall cell lung cancer. *Curr Opin Oncol*. 2022;34(1):54-65.
188. Chen H, Hu S, Patterson AV, et al. Structural mechanism and inhibitors targeting EGFR exon 20 insertion (Ex20ins) mutations. *J Med Chem*. 2023;66(17):11656-11671.
189. Stamos J, Sliwkowski M, Eigenbrot C. Structure of the epidermal growth factor receptor kinase domain alone and in complex with a 4-anilinoquinazoline inhibitor. *J Biol Chem*. 2002;277:46265-46272.
190. Chong CR, James PA. The quest to overcome resistance to EGFR-targeted therapies in cancer. *Nat Med*. 2013;19:1389-1400.

191. Yun CH, Mengwadder KE, Toms AV, et al. The T790M mutation in EGFR kinase causes drug resistance by increasing the affinity for ATP. *Proc Natl Acad Sci U S A*. 2008;105:2070-2075.
192. Solea F, Dahl G, Zoephel A, et al. Target binding properties and cellular activity of afatinib (BIBW 2992), an irreversible ErbB family blocker. *J Pharmacol Exp Ther*. 2012;343:342-350.
193. Reed JE, Smaill JB. The discovery of dacomitinib, a potent irreversible EGFR inhibitor. In: *Comprehensive Accounts of Pharmaceutical Research and Development: From Discovery to Late-Stage Process Development Volume 1*. Vol 1239. ACS Symposium Series. American Chemical Society; 2016:207-233.
194. Vishwanathan K, So K, Thomas K, et al. Absolute bioavailability of osimertinib in healthy adults. *Clin Pharmacol Drug Dev*. 2019;8(2):198-207.
195. Han M, Zhang X, Ye Z, et al. Effects of CYP2D6 genetic polymorphism and drug interaction on the metabolism of dacomitinib. *Chem Res Toxicol*. 2022;35(2):265-274.
196. Hoyt KW, Urul DA, Ogboo BC, et al. Pitfalls and considerations in determining the potency and mutant selectivity of covalent epidermal growth factor receptor inhibitors. *J Med Chem*. 2024;67(1):2-16.
197. Dorta-Suárez M, de Miguel M, Amor-Carro O, et al. The state of the art of EGFR exon 20 insertions in non-small cell lung cancer: diagnosis and future perspectives. *Cancer Treat Rev*. 2023;124:102671.
198. Salkeni MA, Rizvi W, Hein K, et al. New perspectives, therapies, and challenges for metastatic HER2-positive breast cancer. *Breast Cancer*. 2021;13:539-557.
199. Elwaie TA, Abbas SE, Aly EI, et al. HER2 kinase-targeted breast cancer therapy: design, synthesis, and *in vitro* and *in vivo* evaluation of novel lapatinib congeners as selective and potent HER2 inhibitors with favorable metabolic stability. *J Med Chem*. 2020;63(24):15906-15945.
200. Tiwari S, Mishra P, Abraham J. Neratinib, a novel HER2-targeted tyrosine kinase inhibitor. *Clin Breast Cancer*. 2016;5:344-348.
201. Li D, Tu Y, Jin K, et al. Discovery of SPH5030, a selective, potent, and irreversible tyrosine kinase inhibitor for HER2-amplified and HER2-mutant cancer treatment. *J Med Chem*. 2022;65(7):5334-5354.
202. D'Amato V, Raimondo L, Formisano L, et al. Mechanisms of lapatinib resistance in HER2-driven breast cancer. *Cancer Treat Rev*. 2015;41:377-388.
203. Shi H, Zhang W, Zhi Q, et al. Lapatinib resistance in $HER2^+$ cancers: latest findings and new concepts on molecular mechanisms. *Tumor Biol*. 2016;37:15411-15431.
204. Kourie H, El Rassy E, Clatot F, et al. Emerging treatments for HER2-positive early stage breast cancer: focus on neratinib. *Onco Targets Ther*. 2017;10:3363-3372.
205. Curigliano G, Mueller V, Borges V, et al. Tucatinib versus placebo added to trastuzumab and capecitabine for patients with pretreated $HER2^+$ metastatic breast cancer with and without brain metastases (HER2CLIMB): final overall survival analysis. *Ann Oncol*. 2022;33(3):321-329.
206. Saura C, Oliveira M, Feng YH, et al. Neratinib plus capecitabine versus lapatinib plus capecitabine in HER2-positive metastatic breast cancer previously treated with ≥ 2 HER2-directed regimens: phase III NALA trial. *J Clin Oncol*. 2020;38(27):3138-3149.
207. Criscitiello C, Corti C, De Laurentiis M, et al. Tucatinib's journey from clinical development to clinical practice: new horizons for HER2-positive metastatic disease and promising prospects for brain metastatic spread. *Cancer Treat Rev*. 2023;120:102618.
208. Jm L, Rv C. Ado-trastuzumab Emtansine (T-DM1): an antibody-drug conjugate (ADC) for HER2-positive breast cancer. *J Med Chem*. 2014;57(16):6949-6964.
209. Brazel D, Nagasaka M. The development of amivantamab for the treatment of non-small cell lung cancer. *Respir Res*. 2023; 24(1):256.
210. Hackshaw MD, Danysh HE, Singh J, et al. Incidence of pneumonitis/interstitial lung disease induced by HER2-targeting therapy for HER2-positive metastatic breast cancer. *Breast Cancer Res Treat*. 2020;183(1):23-39.
211. Zheng Q, Peacock DM, Shokat KM. Drugging the next undruggable KRAS allele-Gly12Asp. *J Med Chem*. 2022;65(4):3119-3122.
212. Huestis MP, Dela Cruz D, DiPasquale AG, et al. Targeting KRAS mutant cancers via combination treatment: discovery of a 5-fluoro-4-(3 *h*)-quinazolinone aryl urea pan-RAF kinase inhibitor. *J Med Chem*. 2021;64(7):3940-3955.
213. Murray JI, Zhang L, Simon A, et al. Kinetic and mechanistic investigations to enable a key Suzuki coupling for sotorasib manufacture—what a difference a base makes. *Org Process Res Dev*. 2023;27(1):198-205.
214. Chen H, Smaill JB, Liu T, et al. Small-molecule inhibitors directly targeting KRAS as anticancer therapeutics. *J Med Chem*. 2020;63(23):14404-14424.
215. Fell JB, Fischer JP, Baer BR, et al. Identification of the clinical development candidate MRTX849, a covalent $KRAS^{G12C}$ inhibitor for the treatment of cancer. *J Med Chem*. 2020;63(13):6679-6693.
216. Zhu C, Guan X, Zhang X, et al. Targeting KRAS mutant cancers: from druggable therapy to drug resistance. *Mol Cancer*. 2022;21(1):159.
217. Santarpia M, Ciappina G, Spagnolo CC, et al. Targeted therapies for KRAS-mutant non-small cell lung cancer: from preclinical studies to clinical development-a narrative review. *Transl Lung Cancer Res*. 2023;12(2):346-368.
218. Zhang J, Johnson M, Barve M, et al. Practical guidance for the management of adverse events in patients with KRASG12C-mutated non-small cell lung cancer receiving adagrasib. *Oncologist*. 2023;28(4):287-296.
219. Singh AK, Sonawane P, Kumar A, et al. Challenges and opportunities in the crusade of BRAF inhibitors: from 2002 to 2022. *ACS Omega*. 2023;8(31):27819-27844.
220. Cabanillas M, Patel A, Danysh B, et al. BRAF inhibitors: experience in thyroid cancer and general review of toxicity. *Horm Cancer*. 2015;6:21-36.
221. Subbiah V, Kreitman R, Wainberg Z, et al. Dabrafenib and trametinib treatment in patients with locally advanced or metastatic BRAF V600E-mutant anaplastic thyroid cancer. *J Clin Oncol*. 2018;36:7-13.
222. Agianian B, Gavathiotis E. Current insights of BRAF inhibitors in cancer. *J Med Chem*. 2018;61(14):5775-5793.
223. Griffin M, Scotto D, Josephs D, et al. BRAF inhibitors: resistance and the promise of combination treatments for melanoma. *Oncotarget*. 2017;8:78174-78192.
224. Arozarena I, Wellbrock C. Overcoming resistance to BRAF inhibitors. *Ann Transl Med*. 2017;5:387.
225. Gibney GT, Messina JL, Fedorenko IV, Sondak VK, Smalley KSM. Paradoxical oncogenesis—the long-term effects of BRAF inhibition in melanoma. *Nat Rev Clin Oncol*. 2013;10(7):390-399.
226. Roskoski R Jr. Allosteric MEK1/2 inhibitors including cobimetinib and trametinib in the treatment of cutaneous melanomas. *Pharmacol Res*. 2017;117:20-31.
227. Weart T, Miller K, Simone C II. Spotlight on dabrafenib/trametinib in the treatment on non-small cell lung cancer: place in therapy. *Cancer Manag Res*. 2018;10:647-652.
228. Gonzalez-Del Pino GL, Li K, Park E, et al. Allosteric MEK inhibitors act on BRAF/MEK complexes to block MEK activation. *Proc Natl Acad Sci U S A*. 2021;118(36):e2107207118.
229. Goldinger S, Rinderknecht J, Dummer R, et al. A single-dose mass balance and metabolite-profiling study of vemurafenib in patients with metastatic melanoma. *Pharmacol Res Perspect*. 2015;3:e00113.
230. Bershas D, Ouellet D, Mamaril-Fishman D, et al. Metabolism and disposition of oral dabrafenib in cancer patients: proposed participation of aryl nitrogen in carbon-carbon bond cleavage via decarboxylation following enzymatic oxidation. *Drug Metab Dispos*. 2013;41:2215-2224.

231. Takahashi R, Choo E, Ma S, et al. Absorption, metabolism, excretion and the contribution of intestinal metabolism to the oral disposition of [14C] cobimetinib, a MEK inhibitor, in humans. *Drug Metab Dispos.* 2015;44:28-39.
232. Campagne O, Yeo KK, Fangusaro J, et al. Clinical pharmacokinetics and pharmacodynamics of selumetinib. *Clin Pharmacokinet.* 2021;60(3):283-303.
233. Piscitelli J, Hens B, Tomaszewska I, et al. Effect of food and a proton-pump inhibitor on the absorption of encorafenib: an *in vivo—in vitro—in silico* approach. *Mol Pharmaceutics.* 2023;20(5):2589-2599.
234. Wahid M, Jawed A, Mandal R, et al. Recent developments and obstacles in the treatment of melanoma with BRAF and MET inhibitors. *Crit Rev Oncol Hematol.* 2018;125:84-88.
235. Mincu RI, Mahabadi AA, Michel L, et al. Cardiovascular adverse events associated with BRAF and MEK inhibitors: a systematic review and meta-analysis. *JAMA Netw Open.* 2019;2(8):e198890.
236. Garutti M, Bergnach M, Polesel J, et al. BRAF and MEK inhibitors and their toxicities: a meta-analysis. *Cancers (Basel).* 2022;15(1):141.
237. Garces AE, Stocks MJ. Class 1 PI3K clinical candidates and recent inhibitor design strategies: a medicinal chemistry perspective. *J Med Chem.* 2019;62(10):4815-4850.
238. Kandoth C, McLellan MD, Vandin F, et al. Mutational landscape and significance across 12 major cancer types. *Nature.* 2013;502(7471):333-339.
239. Huang J, Chen L, Wu J, et al. Targeting the PI3K/AKT/mTOR signaling pathway in the treatment of human diseases: current status, trends, and solutions. *J Med Chem.* 2022;65(24):16033-16061.
240. Berndt A, Miller S, Williams O, et al. The p110d crystal structure uncovers mechanisms for selectivity and potency of novel PI3K inhibitors. *Nat Chem Biol.* 2010;6:117-124.
241. Shah A, Mangaonkar A. Idelalisib: a novel PI3Kd inhibitor for chronic lymphocytic leukemia. *Ann Pharmacother.* 2015;49:1162-1170.
242. Cheah C, Fowler N. Idelalisib in the management of lymphoma. *Blood.* 2016;128:331-336.
243. Ramanathan S, Jin F, Sharma S, et al. Clinical pharmacokinetic and pharmacodynamic profile of idelalisib. *Clin Pharmacokinet.* 2016;55:33-45.
244. Zhao W, Qiu Y, Kong D. Class I phosphatidylinositol 3-kinase inhibitors for cancer therapy. *Acta Pharm Sin B.* 2017;7:27-37.
245. Scott W, Hentemann M, Rowley R, et al. Discovery and SAR of novel 2,3-dihydroimidazo[1,2-c]-quinazoline PI3K inhibitors: identification of copanlisib (BAY 80-6946). *Chem Med Chem.* 2016;11:1517-1530.
246. Matasar MJ, Dreyling M, Leppä S, et al. Feasibility of combining the phosphatidylinositol 3-kinase inhibitor copanlisib with rituximab-based immunochemotherapy in patients with relapsed indolent b-cell lymphoma. *Clin Lymphoma Myeloma Leuk.* 2021;21(11):e886-e894.
247. Dreyling M, Santoro A, Mollica L, et al. Phosphatidylinositol 3-kinase inhibition by copanlisib in relapsed or refractor indolent lymphoma. *J Clin Oncol.* 2017;35:3898-3905.
248. Gerish M, Schwarz T, Lang D, et al. Pharmacokinetics of intravenous pan-class I phosphatidylinositol 3-kinase (PI3K) inhibitor [14C]copanlisib (BAY 80-6946) in a mass balance study in healthy male volunteers. *Cancer Chemother Pharmacol.* 2017;80:535-544.
249. Yu M, Chen J, Xu Z, et al. Development and safety of PI3K inhibitors in cancer. *Arch Toxicol.* 2023;97(3):635-650.
250. Bou Zeid N, Yazbeck V. PI3K inhibitors in NHL and CLL: an unfulfilled promise. *Blood Lymphat Cancer.* 2023;13:1-12.
251. Gribben JG, Jurczak W, Jacobs RW, et al. Umbralisib plus ublituximab (U2) is superior to obinutuzumab plus chlorambucil (O+Chl) in patients with treatment naïve (TN) and relapsed/refractory (R/R) chronic lymphocytic leukemia (CLL): results from the Phase 3 Unity-Cll Study. *Blood.* 2020;136(suppl 1):37-39.
252. Arafeh R, Samuels Y. PIK3CA in cancer: the past 30 years. *Semin Cancer Biol.* 2019;59:36-49.
253. Furet P, Guagnano V, Fairhurst RA, et al. Discovery of NVP-BYL719 a potent and selective phosphatidylinositol-3 kinase alpha inhibitor selected for clinical evaluation. *Bioorg Med Chem Lett.* 2013;23(13):3741-3748.
254. André F, Ciruelos E, Rubovszky G, et al. Alpelisib for PIK3CA-mutated, hormone receptor-positive advanced breast cancer. *N Engl J Med.* 2019;380(20):1929-1940.
255. André F, Ciruelos EM, Juric D, et al. Alpelisib plus fulvestrant for PIK3CA-mutated, hormone receptor-positive, human epidermal growth factor receptor-2-negative advanced breast cancer: final overall survival results from SOLAR-1. *Ann Oncol.* 2021;32(2):208-217.
256. Royer B, Kaderbhaï CG, Schmitt A. Pharmacokinetics and pharmacodynamic of alpelisib. *Clin Pharmacokinet.* 2023;62(1):45-53.
257. Tau S, Miller TW. Alpelisib efficacy without cherry-PI3King mutations. *Clin Cancer Res.* 2023;29(6):989-990.
258. Addie M, Ballard P, Buttar D, et al. Discovery of 4-amino-N-[(1S)-1-(4-chlorophenyl)-3-hydroxypropyl]-1-(7H-pyrrolo[2,3-d]pyrimidin-4-yl)piperidine-4-carboxamide (AZD5363), an orally bioavailable, potent inhibitor of Akt kinases. *J Med Chem.* 2013;56(5):2059-2073.
259. Turner NC, Oliveira M, Howell SJ, et al. Capivasertib in hormone receptor-positive advanced breast cancer. *N Engl J Med.* 2023;388(22):2058-2070.
260. Howell SJ, Casbard A, Carucci M, et al. Fulvestrant plus capivasertib versus placebo after relapse or progression on an aromatase inhibitor in metastatic, oestrogen receptor-positive, HER2-negative breast cancer (FAKTION): overall survival, updated progression-free survival, and expanded biomarker analysis from a randomised, phase 2 trial. *Lancet Oncol.* 2022;23(7):851-864.
261. Lin T, Leung C, Nguyen K, et al. Mammalian target of rapamycin (mTOR) inhibitors in solid tumors. *Clin Pharmacist.* 2016;8:3.
262. Saran U, Foti M, Dufour J-F. Cellular and molecular effects of the mTOR inhibitor everolimus. *Clin Sci.* 2015;129:895-914.
263. Zollinger M, Sayer C, Dannecker R, et al. The macrolide everolimus forms an unusual metabolite in animals and humans: identification of a phosphocholine ester. *Drug Metab Dispos.* 2008;36:1457-1460.
264. Huang Z, Wu Y, Zhou X, et al. Clinical efficacy of mTOR inhibitors in solid tumors: a systematic review. *Future Oncol.* 2015;11:1687-1699.
265. Boni J, Hug B, Leister C, et al. Intravenous temsirolimus in cancer patients: clinical pharmacology and dosing considerations. *Sem Oncol.* 2007;36:S18-S25.
266. Cai P, Tsao R, Ruppen M. In vitro metabolic study of temsirolimus: preparation, isolation and identification of the metabolites. *Drug Metab Dispos.* 2007;35:1554-1563.
267. Ahn IE, Brown JR. Targeting Bruton's tyrosine kinase in CLL. *Front Immunol.* 2021;12:687458.
268. Shirley M. Bruton Tyrosine kinase inhibitors in B-cell malignancies: their use and differential features. *Target Oncol.* 2022;17(1):69-84.
269. Brown JR. How I treat CLL patients with ibrutinib. *Blood.* 2018;131(4):379-386.
270. Rhodes JM, Mato AR. Zanubrutinib (BGB-3111), a second-generation selective covalent inhibitor of Bruton's tyrosine kinase and its utility in treating chronic lymphocytic leukemia. *Drug Des Devel Ther.* 2021;15:919-926.
271. Estupiñán HY, Berglöf A, Zain R, et al. Comparative analysis of BTK inhibitors and mechanisms underlying adverse effects. *Front Cell Dev Biol.* 2021;9:630942.
272. Thompson PA, Tam CS. Pirtobrutinib: a new hope for patients with BTK inhibitor-refractory lymphoproliferative disorders. *Blood.* 2023;141(26):3137-3142.
273. Stephens DM, Byrd JC. Resistance to Bruton tyrosine kinase inhibitors: the Achilles heel of their success story in lymphoid malignancies. *Blood.* 2021;138(13):1099-1109.

274. Pal D, Vann KR, Joshi S, et al. The BTK/PI3K/BRD4 axis inhibitor SRX3262 overcomes Ibrutinib resistance in mantle cell lymphoma. *iScience*. 2021;24(9):102931.
275. Mato AR, Shah NN, Jurczak W, et al. Pirtobrutinib in relapsed or refractory B-cell malignancies (BRUIN): a phase 1/2 study. *Lancet*. 2021;397(10277):892-901.
276. Sharma S, Pepin X, Burri H, et al. New acalabrutinib formulation enables co-administration with proton pump inhibitors and dosing in patients unable to swallow capsules (ELEVATE-PLUS). *Blood*. 2021;138(suppl 1):4365.
277. Xiao L, Salem JE, Clauss S, et al. Ibrutinib-mediated atrial fibrillation attributable to inhibition of C-terminal Src kinase. *Circulation*. 2020;142(25):2443-2455.
278. Lecutier M. Phocomelia and internal defects due to thalidomide. *Br Med J*. 1962;2:1147-1148.
279. Amare GG, Meharie BG, Belayneh YM. A drug repositioning success: the repositioned therapeutic applications and mechanisms of action of thalidomide. *J Oncol Pharm Pract*. 2021;27(3):673-678.
280. Copur M, Rose M, Gettinger S. Miscellaneous chemotherapeutic agents. In: DeVita VJ, Lawrence T, Rosenberg S, eds. *Cancer: Principles and Practice of Oncology*. 8th ed. Lippincott Williams & Wilkins; 2008:490-495.
281. Cavello F, Boccadoro M, Palumbo A. Review of thalidomide in the treatment of newly diagnosed multiple myeloma. *Ther Clin Risk Manag*. 2007;3:543-552.
282. Lu G, Middleton RE, Sun H, et al. The myeloma drug lenalidomide promotes the cereblon-dependent destruction of Ikaros proteins. *Science*. 2014;343(6168):305-309.
283. Chen N, Zhou S, Palmisano M. Clinical pharmacokinetics and pharmacodynamics of lenalidomide. *Clin Pharmcokinet*. 2017;56:139-152.
284. Hanaizi Z, Flores B, Hemmings R, et al. The European medicines agency review of pomalidomide in combination with low-dose dexamethasone for the treatment of adult patients with multiple myeloma: summary of the scientific assessment of the committee for medicinal products for human use. *Oncologist*. 2015;20:329-334.
285. Touzeau C, Moreau P. Pomalidomide in the management of relapsed multiple myeloma. *Future Oncol*. 2016;12:1975-1983.
286. Hoffman M, Kasserra C, Reyes J, et al. Absorption, metabolism and excretion of [^{14}C]pomalidomide in humans following oral administration. *Cancer Chemother Pharmacol*. 2013;71:489-501.
287. Chowdhury G, Shibata N, Yamakazi H, et al. Human cytochrome P450 oxidation of 5-hydroxythalidomide and pomalidomide, an amino analogue of thalidomide. *Chem Res Toxicol*. 2014;27:147-156.
288. Noonan K, Colson K. Immunomodulatory agents and proteasome inhibitors in the treatment of multiple myeloma. *Sem Oncol*. 2017;33:279-291.
289. Vandross A. Proteasome inhibitor-based therapy for treatment of newly diagnosed multiple myeloma. *Sem Oncol*. 2017;44:381-384.
290. Brayer J, Baz R. The potential of ixazomib, a second-generation proteasome inhibitor, in the treatment of multiple myeloma. *Ther Adv Hematol*. 2017;8:209-220.
291. Israël A. The IKK complex, a central regulator of NF-kappaB activation. *Cold Spring Harb Perspect Biol*. 2010;2:a000158.
292. Scalzulli E, Grammatico S, Vozella F, et al. Proteasome inhibitors for the treatment of multiple myeloma. *Expert Opin Pharmacother*. 2018;19:375-386.
293. Wallington-Beddoe C, Sobieraj-Teague M, Kuss B, et al. Resistance to proteasome inhibitors and other targeted therapies in myeloma. *Br J Haematol*. 2018;182:11-28.
294. Groll M, Berkers C, Ploegh H, et al. Crystal structure of the boronic acid-based proteasome inhibitor bortezomib in complex with the yeast 20S proteasome. *Structure*. 2006;14:451-456.
295. Harshbarger W, Miller C, Diedrich C, et al. Crystal structure of the human 20S proteasome in complex with carfilzomib. *Structure*. 2015;23:418-424.
296. Selvy M, Kerckhove N, Pereira B, et al. Prevalence of chemotherapy-induced peripheral neuropathy in multiple myeloma patients and its impact on quality of life: a single center cross-sectional study. *Front Pharmacol*. 2021;12:637593.
297. Yago MR, Mehta K, Bose M, et al. Mechanistic pharmacokinetic/pharmacodynamic modeling in support of a patient-convenient, longer dosing interval for carfilzomib, a covalent inhibitor of the proteasome. *Clin Pharmacokinet*. 2023;62(5):779-788.
298. Georgiopoulos G, Makris N, Laina A, et al. Cardiovascular toxicity of proteasome inhibitors: underlying mechanisms and management strategies: JACC: cardioOncology state-of-the-art review. *JACC CardioOncol*. 2023;5(1):1-21.
299. Muz B, Ghazarian RN, Ou M, et al. Spotlight on ixazomib: potential in the treatment of multiple myeloma. *Drug Des Devel Ther*. 2016;10:217-226.
300. Pullarkat V, Newman E. BCL2 inhibition by venetoclax: targeting the Achilles' heel of the acute myeloid leukemia stem cell? *Cancer Discov*. 2016;6:1082-1083.
301. Anderson M, Deng J, Seymour J, et al. The BCL2 selective inhibitor venetoclax induces rapid onset apoptosis of CLL cells in patients via a TP43-independent mechanism. *Blood*. 2016;127:3215-3224.
302. Cang S, Iragavarapu C, Savooji J, et al. ABT-199 (venetoclax) and BCL-2 inhibitors in clinical development. *J Hematol Oncol*. 2015;8:129.
303. King A, Peterson T, Horvat T, et al. Venetoclax: a first-in-class oral BCL-2 inhibitor for the management of lymphoid malignancies. *Ann Pharmacother*. 2017;51:410-416.
304. Stilgenbauer S, Eichhorst B, Schetelig J, et al. Venetoclax in relapsed or refractory chronic lymphocytic leukaemia with 17p deletion: a mutlicentre, open-label, phase 2 study. *Lancet Oncol*. 2016;17:768-778.
305. *Pharmacological Reviews (Venetoclax)*. U.S. Food and Drug Administration; Center for Drug Evaluation and Research; 2016.
306. Döhner H, Weisdorf DJ, Bloomfield CD. Acute myeloid leukemia. *N Engl J Med*. 2015;373(12):1136-1152.
307. Sexauer A, Perl A, Yang X, et al. Terminal myeloid differentiation in vivo is induced by FLT3 inhibition in FLT3/ITD AML. *Blood*. 2012;120(20):4205-4214.
308. Passamonti F, Mora B. Myelofibrosis. *Blood*. 2023;141(16):1954-1970.
309. Ikeda K, Ueda K. Gaining MOMENTUM against anaemic myelofibrosis. *Lancet*. 2023;401(10373):248-249.
310. Staudt D, Murray HC, McLachlan T, et al. Targeting oncogenic signaling in mutant FLT3 acute myeloid leukemia: the path to least resistance. *Int J Mol Sci*. 2018;19(10):3198.
311. Ambinder AJ, Levis M. Potential targeting of FLT3 acute myeloid leukemia. *Haematologica*. 2021;106(3):671-681.
312. Zhong Y, Qiu RZ, Sun SL, et al. Small-molecule Fms-like tyrosine kinase 3 inhibitors: an attractive and efficient method for the treatment of acute myeloid leukemia. *J Med Chem*. 2020;63(21):12403-12428.
313. Weis TM, Marini BL, Bixby DL, et al. Clinical considerations for the use of FLT3 inhibitors in acute myeloid leukemia. *Crit Rev Oncol Hematol*. 2019;141:125-138.
314. Cortes JE, Khaled S, Martinelli G, et al. Quizartinib versus salvage chemotherapy in relapsed or refractory FLT3-ITD acute myeloid leukaemia (QuANTUM-R): a multicentre, randomised, controlled, open-label, phase 3 trial. *Lancet Oncol*. 2019;20(7):984-997.
315. Desikan SP, Daver N, DiNardo C, et al. Resistance to targeted therapies: delving into FLT3 and IDH. *Blood Cancer J*. 2022;12(6):1-8.
316. Novatcheva ED, Anouty Y, Saunders I, et al. FMS-like tyrosine kinase 3 inhibitors for the treatment of acute myeloid leukemia. *Clin Lymphoma Myeloma Leuk*. 2022;22(3):e161-e184.
317. He H, Tran P, Gu H, et al. Midostaurin, a novel protein kinase inhibitor for the treatment of acute myelogenous leukemia: insights from human absorption, metabolism, and excretion studies of a BDDCS II drug. *Drug Metab Dispos*. 2017;45(5):540-555.

318. Marconi G, Giannini MB, Bagnato G, et al. The safety profile of FLT3 inhibitors in the treatment of newly diagnosed or relapsed/refractory acute myeloid leukemia. *Expert Opin Drug Saf.* 2021;20(7):791-799.
319. Aikawa T, Togashi N, Iwanaga K, et al. Quizartinib, a selective FLT3 inhibitor, maintains antileukemic activity in preclinical models of RAS-mediated midostaurin-resistant acute myeloid leukemia cells. *Oncotarget.* 2020;11(11):943.
320. Cerchione C, Peleteiro Raíndo A, Mosquera Orgueira A, et al. Safety of FLT3 inhibitors in patients with acute myeloid leukemia. *Expert Rev Hematol.* 2021;14(9):851-865.
321. Senkevitch E, Durum S. The promise of Janus kinase inhibitors in the treatment of hematologic malignancies. *Cytokine.* 2017;98:33-41.
322. Delhommeau F, Dupont S, Tonetti C, et al. Evidence that the JAK2 G1849T (V617F) mutation occurs in a lymphomyeloid progenitor in polycythemia vera and idiopathic myelofibrosis. *Blood.* 2007;109:71-77.
323. Wade R, Hodgson R, Biswas M, et al. A review of ruxolitinib for the treatment of myelofibrosis: a critique of the evidence. *Pharmacoeconomics.* 2017;35:203-213.
324. McKeage K. Ruxolitinib: a review in polycythaemia vera. *Drugs.* 2015;75:1773-1781.
325. Shen P, Wang Y, Jia X, et al. Dual-target Janus kinase (JAK) inhibitors: comprehensive review on the JAK-based strategies for treating solid or hematologic malignancies and immune-related diseases. *Eur J Med Chem.* 2022;239:114551.
326. Mascarenhas J, Hoffman R, Talpaz M, et al. Pacritinib vs best available therapy, including ruxolitinib, in patients with myelofibrosis: a randomized clinical trial. *JAMA Oncol.* 2018;4(5):652-659.
327. Bassiony S, Harrison CN, McLornan DP. Evaluating the safety, efficacy, and therapeutic potential of momelotinib in the treatment of intermediate/high-risk myelofibrosis: evidence to date. *Ther Clin Risk Manag.* 2020;16:889-901.
328. Newton AS, Deiana L, Puleo DE, et al. JAK2 JH2 fluorescence polarization assay and crystal structures for complexes with three small molecules. *ACS Med Chem Lett.* 2017;8(6):614-617.
329. Wang Z, Cai J, Cheng J, et al. FLT3 inhibitors in acute myeloid leukemia: challenges and recent developments in overcoming resistance. *J Med Chem.* 2021;64(6):2878-2900.
330. Kesarwani M, Huber E, Kincaid Z, et al. Targeting substrate-site in Jak2 kinase prevents emergence of genetic resistance. *Sci Rep.* 2015;5:14538.
331. Davis RR, Li B, Yun SY, et al. Structural insights into JAK2 inhibition by ruxolitinib, fedratinib, and derivatives thereof. *J Med Chem.* 2021;64(4):2228-2241.
332. Ciceri P, Müller S, O'Mahony A, et al. Dual kinase-bromodomain inhibitors for rationally designed polypharmacology. *Nat Chem Biol.* 2014;10(4):305-312.
333. William AD, Lee ACH, Blanchard S, et al. Discovery of the macrocycle 11-(2-pyrrolidin-1-yl-ethoxy)-14,19-dioxa-5,7,26-triaza-tetracyclo[19.3.1.1(2,6).1(8,12)]heptacosa-1(25),2(26),3,5,8,10,12(27),16,21,23-decaene (sb1518), a potent Janus kinase 2/Fms-like tyrosine kinase-3 (JAK2/FLT3) inhibitor for the treatment of myelofibrosis and lymphoma. *J Med Chem.* 2011;54(13):4638-4658.
334. Shilling A, Nedza F, Emm T, et al. Metabolism, excretion and pharmacokinetics of [^{14}C]INCB018424, a selective Janus tyrosine kinase 1/2 inhibitor in humans. *Drug Metab Dispos.* 2010;38:2023-2031.
335. Xin Y, Kawashima J, Weng W, et al. Pharmacokinetics and safety of momelotinib in subjects with hepatic or renal impairment. *J Clin Pharmacol.* 2018;58(4):522-532.
336. Zhang Q, Zhang Y, Diamond S, et al. The Janus kinase 2 inhibitor fedratinib inhibits thiamine uptake: a putative mechanism for the onset of Wernicke's encephalopathy. *Drug Metab Dispos.* 2014;42(10):1656-1662.
337. Buege M, DiPippo A, DiNardo C. Evolving treatment strategies for elderly leukemia patients with IDH mutations. *Cancers (Basel).* 2018;10(6):187.
338. Popovici-Muller J, Saunders JO, Salituro FG, et al. Discovery of the first potent inhibitors of mutant IDH1 that lower tumor 2-HG in vivo. *ACS Med Chem Lett.* 2012;3(10):850-855.
339. Gross S, Cairns RA, Minden MD, et al. Cancer-associated metabolite 2-hydroxyglutarate accumulates in acute myelogenous leukemia with isocitrate dehydrogenase 1 and 2 mutations. *J Exp Med.* 2010;207(2):339-344.
340. Fan B, Chen Y, Yin F, et al. Pharmacokinetic/pharmacodynamic evaluation of ivosidenib or enasidenib combined with intensive induction and consolidation chemotherapy in patients with newly diagnosed IDH1/2-mutant acute myeloid leukemia. *Clin Pharmacol Drug Dev.* 2022;11:429-441.
341. DiNardo CD, Stein EM, de Botton S, et al. Durable remissions with ivosidenib in IDH1-mutated relapsed or refractory AML. *N Engl J Med.* 2018;378(25):2386-2398.
342. de Botton S, Fenaux P, Yee K, et al. Olutasidenib (FT-2102) induces durable complete remissions in patients with relapsed or refractory IDH1-mutated AML. *Blood Adv.* 2023;7(13):3117-3127.
343. Liu S, Abboud M, Mikhailov V, et al. Differentiating inhibition selectivity and binding affinity of isocitrate dehydrogenase 1 variant inhibitors. *J Med Chem.* 2023;66:5279-5288.
344. Caravella JA, Lin J, Diebold RB, et al. Structure-based design and identification of FT-2102 (olutasidenib), a potent mutant-selective IDH1 inhibitor. *J Med Chem.* 2020;63(4):1612-1623.
345. Li Y, Liu L, Gomez D, et al. Pharmacokinetics and safety of enasidenib following single oral doses in Japanese and Caucasian subjects. *Pharmacol Res Perspect.* 2018;6(6):e00436.
346. Liang B, Zheng Z, Shi Y, et al. Maintenance therapy with all-trans retinoic acid and arsenic trioxide improves relapse-free survival in adults with low- to intermediate-risk acute promyelocytic leukemia who have achieved complete remission after consolidation therapy. *Onco Targ Ther.* 2017;10:2305-2313.
347. Musumeci F, Radi M, Brullo C, et al. Vascular endothelial growth factor (VEGF) receptors: drugs and new inhibitors. *J Med Chem.* 2012;55(24):10797-10822.
348. Cheng K, Liu CF, Rao GW. Anti-angiogenic agents: a review on vascular endothelial growth factor receptor-2 (VEGFR-2) inhibitors. *Curr Med Chem.* 2021;28(13):2540-2564.
349. Mabeta P, Steenkamp V. The VEGF/VEGFR axis revisited: implications for cancer therapy. *Int J Mol Sci.* 2022;23(24):15585.
350. Iacovelli R, Verri E, Rocca M, et al. Is there still a role for sorafenib in metastatic renal carcinoma? A systematic review and meta-analysis of the effectiveness of sorafenib over other targeted agents. *Crit Rev Oncol Hematol.* 2016;99:324-331.
351. Keating G. Sorafenib: a review in hepatocellular carcinoma. *Target Oncol.* 2017;12:243-253.
352. Cella D, Beaumont J. Pazopanib in the treatment of advanced renal cell carcinoma. *Ther Adv Urol.* 2016;8:61-69.
353. Bellesoeur A, Carton E, Alexandre J, et al. Axitinib in the treatment of renal cell carcinoma: design, development, and place in therapy. *Drug Des Devel Ther.* 2017;11:2801-2811.
354. De Lisi D, De Giorgi U, Lolli C, et al. Lenvatinib in the management of metastatic renal cell carcinoma: a promising combination therapy? *Expert Opin Drug Metab Toxicol.* 2018;14:461-467.
355. Keating G. Axitinib: a review in advanced renal cell carcinoma. *Drugs.* 2015;75:1903-1913.
356. Faivre S, Noccoli P, Castellano D, et al. Sunitinib in pancreatic neuroendocrine tumors: updated progression-free survival and final overall survival from a phase III randomized study. *Ann Oncol.* 2017;28:339-343.
357. Skarderud M, Polk A, Kjeldgaard K, et al. Efficacy and safety of regorafenib in the treatment of metastatic colorectal cancer: a systematic review. *Cancer Treat Rev.* 2018;62:61-73.
358. Cowey L. Profile of tivozanib and its potential for the treatment of advanced renal cell carcinoma. *Drug Des Devel Ther.* 2013;7:519-527.
359. Lightfoot HL, Goldberg FW, Sedelmeier J. Evolution of small molecule kinase drugs. *ACS Med Chem Lett.* 2019;10(2):153-160.

360. Sun Q, Zhou J, Zhang Z, et al. Discovery of fruquintinib, a potent and highly selective small molecule inhibitor of VEGFR 1, 2, 3 tyrosine kinases for cancer therapy. *Cancer Biol Ther.* 2014;15(12):1635-1645.
361. Carlisle B, Demko N, Freeman G, et al. Benefit, risk, and outcomes in drug development: a systematic review of sunitinib. *J Natl Cancer Inst.* 2016;108:djv292.
362. Qin F, Yu H, Bai J. Safety and toxicity of axitinib and sorafenib monotherapy for patients with renal cell carcinoma: a meta-analysis. *J Biomed Res.* 2018;32:30-38.
363. Lacy S, Hsu B, Miles D, et al. Metabolism and disposition of cabozantinib in healthy male volunteers and pharmacologic characterization of its major metabolites. *Drug Metab Dispos.* 2015;43:1190-1207.
364. Gerish M, Hafner F-T, Lang D, et al. Mass balance, metabolic disposition, and pharmacokinetics of a single oral dose of regorafenib in healthy human subjects. *Cancer Chemother Pharmacol.* 2018;81:195-206.
365. Shvartsbart A, Roach JJ, Witten MR, et al. Discovery of potent and selective inhibitors of wild-type and gatekeeper mutant fibroblast growth factor receptor (FGFR) 2/3. *J Med Chem.* 2022;65(22):15433-15442.
366. Lu X, Chen H, Patterson AV, Smaill JB, Ding K. Fibroblast growth factor receptor 4 (FGFR4) selective inhibitors as hepatocellular carcinoma therapy: advances and prospects. *J Med Chem.* 2019;62(6):2905-2915.
367. Loriot Y, Necchi A, Park SH, et al. Erdafitinib in locally advanced or metastatic urothelial carcinoma. *N Engl J Med.* 2019;381(4):338-348.
368. Yu J, Mahipal A, Kim R. Targeted therapy for advanced or metastatic cholangiocarcinoma: focus on the clinical potential of infigratinib. *Onco Targets Ther.* 2021;14:5145-5160.
369. Abou-Alfa GK, Sahai V, Hollebecque A, et al. Pemigatinib for previously treated, locally advanced or metastatic cholangiocarcinoma: a multicentre, open-label, phase 2 study. *Lancet Oncol.* 2020;21(5):671-684.
370. Sootome H, Fujita H, Ito K, et al. Futibatinib is a novel irreversible FGFR 1-4 inhibitor that shows selective antitumor activity against FGFR-deregulated tumors. *Cancer Res.* 2020;80(22):4986-4997.
371. Ito S, Otsuki S, Ohsawa H, et al. Discovery of futibatinib: the first covalent FGFR kinase inhibitor in clinical use. *ACS Med Chem Lett.* 2023;14(4):396-404.
372. Kalyukina M, Yosaatmadja Y, Middleditch MJ, et al. TAS-120 cancer target binding: defining reactivity and revealing the first fibroblast growth factor receptor 1 (FGFR1) irreversible structure. *ChemMedChem.* 2019;14(4):494-500.
373. Subbiah V, Verstovsek S. Clinical development and management of adverse events associated with FGFR inhibitors. *Cell Rep Med.* 2023;4(10):101204.
374. Lu Y, Mao F, Li X, et al. Discovery of potent, selective stem cell factor receptor/platelet derived growth factor receptor alpha (c-KIT/PDGFRα) dual inhibitor for the treatment of imatinib-resistant gastrointestinal stromal tumors (GISTs). *J Med Chem.* 2017;60(12):5099-5119.
375. Gebreyohannes YK, Wozniak A, Zhai ME, et al. Robust activity of avapritinib, potent and highly selective inhibitor of mutated KIT, in patient-derived xenograft models of gastrointestinal stromal tumors. *Clin Cancer Res.* 2019;25(2):609-618.
376. Blay JY, Serrano C, Heinrich MC, et al. Ripretinib in patients with advanced gastrointestinal stromal tumours (INVICTUS): a double-blind, randomised, placebo-controlled, phase 3 trial. *Lancet Oncol.* 2020;21(7):923-934.
377. Bilgin B, Sendur M, Sdede D, et al. A current and comprehensive review of cyclin-dependent kinase inhibitors for the treatment of metastatic breast cancer. *Curr Med Res Opin.* 2017;33:1559-1569.
378. Knudsen ES, Pruitt SC, Hershberger PA, et al. Cell cycle and beyond: exploiting new RB1 controlled mechanisms for cancer therapy. *Trends Cancer.* 2019;5(5):308-324.
379. Knudsen ES, Witkiewicz AK, Rubin SM. Cancer takes many paths through G1/S. *Trends Cell Biol.* 2024;34(8):636-645.
380. Li T, Tianwei W, Zuo M, et al. Recent progress of cyclin-dependent kinase inhibitors as potential anticancer agents. *Future Med Chem.* 2016;8:2047-2076.
381. Xu H, Yu S, Liu Q, et al. Recent advances of highly selective CDK4/6 inhibitors in breast cancer. *J Hematol Oncol.* 2017;10:97.
382. Kwapisz D. Cyclin-dependent kinase 4/6 inhibitors in breast cancer: palbociclib, ribocicilb, and abemaciclib. *Breast Cancer Res.* 2017;166:41-54.
383. Tripathy D, Im SA, Colleoni M, et al. Ribociclib plus endocrine therapy for premenopausal women with hormone-receptor-positive, advanced breast cancer (MONALEESA-7): a randomised phase 3 trial. *Lancet Oncol.* 2018;19(7):904-915.
384. Cristofanilli M, Turner NC, Bondarenko I, et al. Fulvestrant plus palbociclib versus fulvestrant plus placebo for treatment of hormone-receptor-positive, HER2-negative metastatic breast cancer that progressed on previous endocrine therapy (PALOMA-3): final analysis of the multicentre, double-blind, phase 3 randomised controlled trial. *Lancet Oncol.* 2016;17(4):425-439.
385. Slamon DJ, Fasching PA, Hurvitz S, et al. Rationale and trial design of NATALEE: a Phase III trial of adjuvant ribociclib + endocrine therapy versus endocrine therapy alone in patients with $HR^+/HER2^-$ early breast cancer. *Ther Adv Med Oncol.* 2023;15:17588359231178125.
386. Condorelli R, Spring L, O'Shaughnessy J, et al. Polyclonal RB1 mutations and acquired resistance to CDK 4/6 inhibitors in patients with metastatic breast cancer. *Ann Oncol.* 2018;29(3):640-645.
387. Johnston SRD, Harbeck N, Hegg R, et al. Abemaciclib combined with endocrine therapy for the adjuvant treatment of HR^+, $HER2^-$, node-positive, high-risk, early breast cancer (monarchE). *J Clin Oncol.* 2020;38(34):3987-3998.
388. Tan AR, Wright GS, Thummala AR, et al. Trilaciclib prior to chemotherapy in patients with metastatic triple-negative breast cancer: final efficacy and subgroup analysis from a randomized phase II study. *Clin Cancer Res.* 2022;28(4):629-636.
389. Shi Z, Tian L, Qiang T, et al. From structure modification to drug launch: a systematic review of the ongoing development of cyclin-dependent kinase inhibitors for multiple cancer therapy. *J Med Chem.* 2022;65(9):6390-6418.
390. Chen P, Lee NV, Hu W, et al. Spectrum and degree of CDK drug interactions predicts clinical performance. *Mol Cancer Ther.* 2016;15(10):2273-2281.
391. Yu Y, Loi C-M, Hoffman J, et al. Physiologically based pharmacokinetic modeling of palbociclib. *J Clin Pharmacol.* 2017;57:173-184.
392. Curigliano G, Criscitiello C, Esposito A, et al. Pharmacokinetic drug evaluation of ribociclib for the treatment of metastatic hormone-positive breast cancer. *Expert Opin Drug Metab Toxicol.* 2017;13:575-581.
393. Martínez-Chávez A, Tibben MM, de Jong KA, et al. Simultaneous quantification of abemaciclib and its active metabolites in human and mouse plasma by UHPLC-MS/MS. *J Pharm Biomed Anal.* 2021;5:114225.
394. Pavlovic D, Niciforovic D, Papic D, et al. CDK4/6 inhibitors: basics, pros, and major cons in breast cancer treatment with specific regard to cardiotoxicity—a narrative review. *Ther Adv Med Oncol.* 2023;15:17588359231205848.
395. Ho TCS, Chan AHY, Ganesan A. Thirty years of HDAC inhibitors: 2020 insight and hindsight. *J Med Chem.* 2020;63(21):12460-12484.

396. Mukherjee A, Zamani F, Suzuki T. Evolution of slow-binding inhibitors targeting histone deacetylase isoforms. *J Med Chem*. 2023;66(17):11672-11700.
397. Sultana F, Manasa K, Shaik S, et al. Zinc dependent histone deacetylase inhibitors in cancer chemotherapy: recent update. *Curr Med Chem*. 2018;25:1-66.
398. McGraw A. Romidepsin for the treatment of T-cell lymphomas. *Am J Health-Syst Pharm*. 2013;70:1115-1122.
399. Geurs S, Clarisse D, De Bosscher K, et al. The zinc-binding group effect: lessons from non-hydroxamic acid vorinostat analogs. *J Med Chem*. 2023;66(12):7698-7729.
400. Cheng T, Grasse L, Shah J, et al. Panobinostat, a pan-histone deacetylase inhibitor: rationale for and application to treatment of multiple myeloma. *Drugs Today*. 2015;51:491-504.
401. Newbold A, Lindemann R, Cluse L, et al. Characterisation of the novel apoptotic and therapeutic activities of the histone deacetylase inhibitor romidepsin. *Mol Cancer Ther*. 2008;7:1066-1079.
402. Clive S, Woo M, Nydam T, et al. Characterizing the disposition, metabolism, and excretion of an orally active pan-deacetylase inhibitor, panobinostat, via trace radiolabeled 14C material in advanced cancer patients. *Cancer Chemother Pharmacol*. 2012;70:513-522.
403. Rana Z, Diermeier S, Hanif M, et al. Understanding failure and improving treatment using HDAC inhibitors for prostate cancer. *Biomedicines*. 2020;8(2):22.
404. Kuntz KW, Campbell JE, Keilhack H, et al. The importance of being me: magic methyls, methyltransferase inhibitors, and the discovery of tazemetostat. *J Med Chem*. 2016;59(4):1556-1564.
405. Straining R, Eighmy W. Tazemetostat: EZH2 inhibitor. *J Adv Pract Oncol*. 2022;13(2):158-163.
406. Liang R, Tomita D, Sasaki Y, et al. A chemical strategy toward novel brain-penetrant ezh2 inhibitors. *ACS Med Chem Lett*. 2022;13(3):377-387.
407. Khanna A, Côté A, Arora S, et al. Design, synthesis, and pharmacological evaluation of second generation EZH2 inhibitors with long residence time. *ACS Med Chem Lett*. 2020;11(6):1205-1212.
408. Liu F, Chen J, Li X, et al. Advances in development of selective antitumor inhibitors that target PARP-1. *J Med Chem*. 2023;66(24):16464-16483.
409. Zhang J, Gao Y, Zhang Z, et al. Multi-therapies based on PARP inhibition: potential therapeutic approaches for cancer treatment. *J Med Chem*. 2022;65(24):16099-16127.
410. Canan S, Maegley K, Curtin N. Strategies employed for the development of PARP inhibitors. In: Tulin AV, ed. *Poly(ADP-Ribose) Polymerase: Methods and Protocols*. Vol 1608. Humana Press; 2017:271-297.
411. Scarpelli R, Boueres J, Cerratani M, et al. Synthesis and biological evaluation of substituted 2-phenyl-2H-indazole-7-carboxamides as potent poly(ADP-ribose)polymerase (PARP) inhibitors. *Bioorg Med Chem Lett*. 2010;20:488-492.
412. Chen Y, Du H. The promising PARP inhibitors in ovarian cancer therapy: from olaparib to others. *Biomed Pharmacother*. 2018;99:552-560.
413. Munroe M, Kolesar J. Olaparib for the treatment of BRAC-mutated advanced ovarian cancer. *Am J Health Syst Pharm*. 2016;73:1037-1041.
414. Musella A, Bardhi E, Marchetti C. Rucaparib: an emerging PARP inhibitor for treatment of recurrent ovarian cancer. *Cancer Treat Rev*. 2018;66:7-14.
415. Dockery L, Gunderson C, Moore K. Rucaparib: the past, present and future of a newly approved PARP inhibitor for ovarian cancer. *Onco Targets Ther*. 2017;10:3029-3037.
416. Ethier J-L, Lheureux S, Oza A. The role of niraparib for the treatment of ovarian cancer. *Future Oncol*. 2018;14(25):2565-2577.
417. Luo Y, Cheng Y, Wu C, et al. Pharmacokinetics, safety, and antitumor activity of talazoparib monotherapy in Chinese patients with advanced solid tumors. *Invest New Drugs*. 2023;41(3):503-511.
418. Bruin MAC, Sonke GS, Beijnen JH, et al. Pharmacokinetics and pharmacodynamics of PARP inhibitors in oncology. *Clin Pharmacokinet*. 2022;61(12):1649.
419. Abdul Razak AR, Mau-Soerensen M, Gabrail NY, et al. First-in-class, first-in-human phase I study of selinexor, a selective inhibitor of nuclear export, in patients with advanced solid tumors. *J Clin Oncol*. 2016;34(34):4142-4150.
420. Mo CC, Yee AJ, Midha S, et al. Selinexor: targeting a novel pathway in multiple myeloma. *eJHaem*. 2023;4(3):792-810.
421. Bakshi A, Chaudhary SC, Rana M, et al. Basal cell carcinoma pathogenesis and therapy involving hedgehog signaling and beyond. *Mol Carcinog*. 2017;56(12):2543-2557.
422. Heuser M, Smith BD, Fiedler W, et al. Clinical benefit of glasdegib plus low-dose cytarabine in patients with de novo and secondary acute myeloid leukemia: long-term analysis of a phase II randomized trial. *Ann Hematol*. 2021;100(5):1181-1194.
423. Bockorny B, Semenisty V, Macarulla T, et al. BL-8040, a CXCR4 antagonist, in combination with pembrolizumab and chemotherapy for pancreatic cancer: the COMBAT trial. *Nat Med*. 2020;26(6):878-885.
424. Crees ZD, Rettig MP, Jayasinghe RG, et al. Motixafortide and G-CSF to mobilize hematopoietic stem cells for autologous transplantation in multiple myeloma: a randomized phase 3 trial. *Nat Med*. 2023;29(4):869-879.
425. Rebolledo-Bustillo M, Garcia-Gomez D, Dávila EM, et al. Structural basis of the binding mode of the antineoplastic compound motixafortide (BL-8040) in the CXCR4 chemokine receptor. *Int J Mol Sci*. 2023;24(5):4393.
426. Patel U, Smalley JP, Hodgkinson JT. PROTAC chemical probes for histone deacetylase enzymes. *RSC Chem Biol*. 2023;4(9):623-634.
427. Békés M, Langley DR, Crews CM. PROTAC targeted protein degraders: the past is prologue. *Nat Rev Drug Discov*. 2022;21(3):181-200.
428. Kargbo RB. PROTAC: harnessing targeted chimeras for selective BCL-2 degradation in cancer treatment. *ACS Med Chem Lett*. 2023;14(5):541-542.
429. Conway SJ. Bifunctional molecules beyond PROTACs. *J Med Chem*. 2020;63(6):2802-2806.
430. Zhou Z, Zhou G, Zhou C, et al. Discovery of a potent, cooperative, and selective SOS1 PROTAC ZZ151 with in vivo antitumor efficacy in KRAS-mutant cancers. *J Med Chem*. 2023;66(6):4197-4214.
431. Zhao HY, Wang HP, Mao YZ, et al. Discovery of potent PROTACs targeting EGFR mutants through the optimization of covalent EGFR ligands. *J Med Chem*. 2022;65(6):4709-4726.
432. Xia W, Low PS. Folate-targeted therapies for cancer. *J Med Chem*. 2010;53(19):6811-6824.
433. Matulonis UA, Lorusso D, Oaknin A, et al. Efficacy and safety of mirvetuximab soravtansine in patients with platinum-resistant ovarian cancer with high folate receptor alpha expression: results from the SORAYA study. *J Clin Oncol*. 2023;41(13):2436-2445.
434. Ravindra M, Wilson MR, Tong N, et al. Fluorine-substituted pyrrolo[2,3- d]pyrimidine analogues with tumor targeting via cellular uptake by folate receptor α and the proton-coupled folate transporter and inhibition of de novo purine nucleotide biosynthesis. *J Med Chem*. 2018;61(9):4228-4248.
435. O'Connor C, Wallace-Povirk A, Ning C, et al. Folate transporter dynamics and therapy with classic and tumor-targeted antifolates. *Sci Rep*. 2021;11(1):6389.

Answers to Targeted Cancer Therapy Comprehension Questions

1. Type VI kinase inhibitors bind irreversibly to the kinase enzyme. Type VI inhibitors include a Michael acceptor (electrophile) as part of their structure that interacts with a nucleophilic side chain of an amino acid (eg, Cys) in the enzyme pocket. Osimertinib's acrylamide moiety is a strong electrophile and serves as a Michael acceptor for the electrons donated by Cys797 of EGFR kinase.

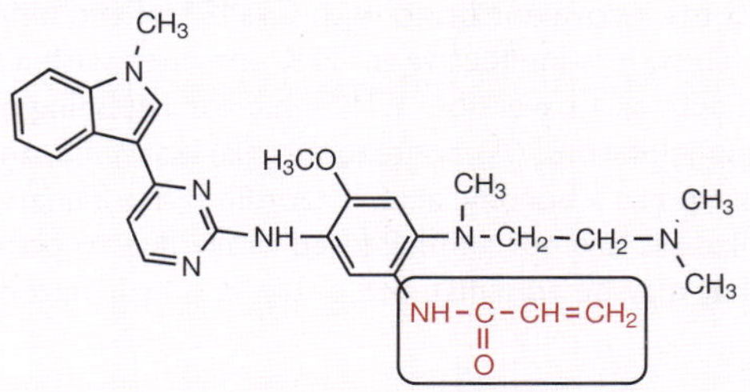

Osimertinib
(Tagrisso)

2. As noted, osimertinib binds covalently to Cys797 of the target EGFR kinase.

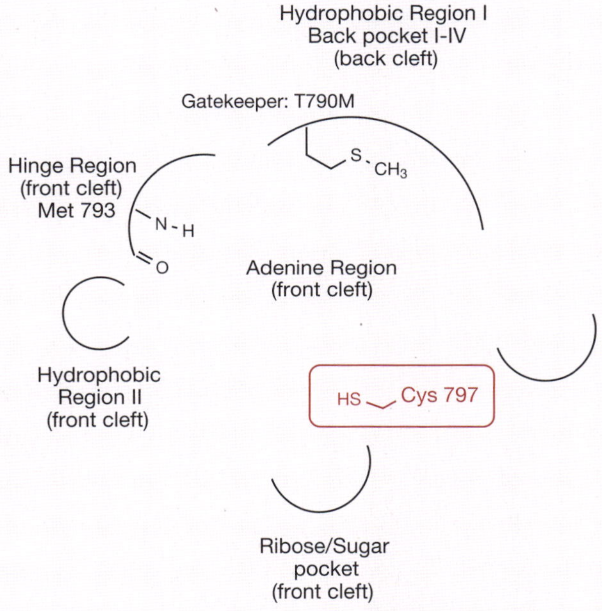

The ATP pocket of mutant EGFR

3. The patient must be screened prior to initiating osimertinib and must show the following
   A, C and E are correct. Osimertinib can bind covalently to oncogenic EGFR including del19 EGFR and L858R EGFR in a type VI mode of binding. Osimertinib binds irreversibly to Cys797 within oncogenic EGFR. Osimertinib does not bind to Thr790 and retains its efficacy in tumors that express a T790M mutation. However, mutation of Cys797 to Ser797 will prevent the formation of a covalent bond, weaken osimertinib's binding to EGFR, and produce a weaker therapeutic response. Hence, osimertinib is ineffective in tumors expressing the C797S mutatio EGFR is upstream of wtKRAS in the RAS/RAF/MEK pathway. By inhibiting EGFR upstream of KRAS, osimertinib is capable of effectively shutting off the RAS/RAF/MEK signaling pathway that drives tumor growth. Osimertinib is thus effective in wtKRAS tumors. However, mutations in KRAS activate the RAS/RAF/MEK pathway downstream of EGFR. The EGFR inhibition by osimertinib upstream in the RAS/RAF/MEK pathway is overridden by mKRAS, and continued signaling pathway activation drives tumor growth. Hence, osimertinib is effective in inhibiting wt-KRAS expressing tumors, but not mKRAS expressing tumors.
4. The boxed functional group in lapatinib allows for binding within the Cα-helix-out pocket of EGFR and HER2 and permits a type II mode of binding as a kinase inhibitor.
5. Crizotinib and lorlatinib are ALK inhibitors. Crizotinib is ineffective in ALK+ NSCLC lung cancer with brain metastases since it is a substrate for Pgp efflux. It also develops resistance due to multiple resistant mutations, including L1196M, C1156Y, and G1202R. Lorlatinib is a macrocyclic kinase inhibitor. On account of being macrocyclic, it

Answers to Targeted Cancer Therapy Comprehension Questions (continued)

is accommodated and retains efficacy against drug-resistant L1196M, C1156Y, and G1202R mutants. In addition, the macrocyclic core prevents efflux via Pgp efflux pumps, and lorlatinib is effective in ALK+ NSCLC with brain metastases.

6. Ibrutinib and pirtobrutinib are oral BTK inhibitors with clinical applications in hematologic malignancies. Ibrutinib is an irreversible BTK inhibitor and forms a covalent bond with Cys481 of the kinase, a reaction allowed by its electrophilic acrylamide functional group. Thus, it is ineffective in BTK enzymes with a C481S mutation. Pirtobrutinib lacks an acrylamide functional group and acts as a reversible BTK inhibitor retaining efficacy in C481S BTK.
7. The structures show the proteasome inhibitors: (A) bortezomib, (B) ixazomib, and (C) carfilzomib. Among these structures, bortezomib is chemically classified as a boronic acid, ixazomib is a boronate ester, and carfilzomib is a peptidic epoxyketone. Bortezomib and carfilzomib are not administered orally due to poor oral stability and bioavailability. Ixazomib is a boronate ester prodrug that may be administered orally. It is hydrolyzed to boronic acid in vivo.

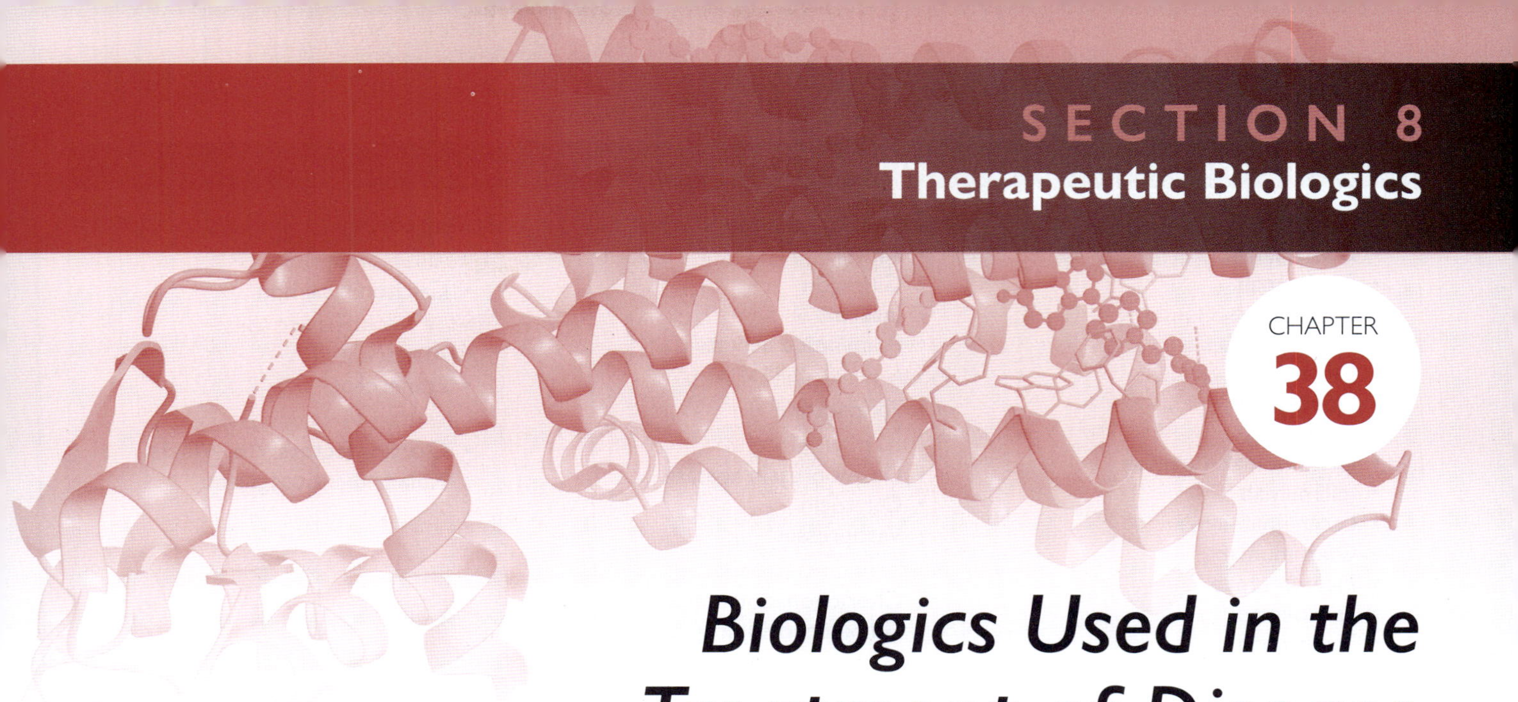

SECTION 8

Therapeutic Biologics

CHAPTER 38

Biologics Used in the Treatment of Disease

Vijaya L. Korlipara and Tanaji T. Talele

Drugs covered in this chapter:

ADRENOCORTICOTROPIC HORMONES
- Adrenocorticotropic hormone
- Cosyntropin

ANTIBODY-DRUG CONJUGATES
- Ado-trastuzumab emtansine
- Brentuximab vedotin
- Enfortumab vedotin
- Gemtuzumab ozogamicin
- Inotuzumab ozogamicin
- Loncastuximab tesirine
- Mirvetuximab soravtansine
- Polatuzumab vedotin
- Sacituzumab govitecan
- Tisotumab vedotin
- Trastuzumab deruxtecan

ANTISENSE OLIGONUCLEOTIDES INCLUDING SIRNA
- Casimersen
- Givosiran
- Golodirsen
- Inclisiran
- Inotersen
- Lumasiran
- Nusinersen
- Patisiran
- Vutrisiran

CYTOKINES
- Anakinra
- Interferon alpha
- Interferon beta
- Interferon gamma
- Interleukin-1
- Interleukin-2/aldesleukin
- Interleukin-2 fusion protein
- Rilonacept

ENZYMES

TISSUE PLASMINOGEN ACTIVATORS
- Alteplase
- Reteplase
- Tenecteplase

DORNASE A

FUSION PROTEINS
- Tagraxofusp

ENZYME-REPLACEMENT THERAPY
- Alglucosidase α
- Idursulfase
- Imiglucerase

GONADOTROPINS
- Follitropin α
- Follitropin β
- Menotropins

GONADOTROPIN-RELEASING HORMONE AGONISTS AND ANTAGONISTS
- Cetrorelix acetate
- Degarelix acetate
- Ganirelix acetate
- Goserelin acetate
- Histrelin acetate
- Leuprolide acetate
- Leuprolide camsylate
- Nafarelin acetate
- Triptorelin pamoate

GROWTH HORMONES
- Becaplermin
- Pegvisomant
- Somapacitan
- Somatropin

HEMATOPOIETIC GROWTH FACTORS
- Erythropoietin (epoetin α)
- Filgrastim
- Sargramostim

MISCELLANEOUS PEPTIDIC DRUGS
- Linaclotide
- Pegcetacoplan
- Plecanatide
- Semaglutide
- Teduglutide
- Terlipressin
- Tirzepatide
- Voclosporin

MONOCLONAL ANTIBODIES
- Aducanumab
- Basiliximab
- Belimumab
- Benralizumab
- Bevacizumab
- Blinatumomab
- Brolucizumab
- Canakinumab
- Certolizumab pegol
- Crizanlizumab
- Denosumab

Drugs covered in this chapter:—continued

- Donanemab
- Dostarlimab
- Eculizumab
- Emicizumab
- Eptinezumab
- Evinacumab
- Golimumab
- Ibalizumab
- Ibritumomab tiuxetan
- Ipilimumab
- Lecanemab-irmb
- Ofatumumab
- Panitumumab
- Spesolimab
- Teplizumab
- Teprotumumab
- Trastuzumab
- Ublituximab

PANCREATIC HORMONES
- Amylin
- Glucagon
- Insulin
- Pramlintide acetate

PARATHYROID HORMONES
- Teriparatide

PITUITARY HORMONES
- Desmopressin acetate
- Oxytocin
- Vasopressin

PLACENTAL HORMONES
- Choriogonadotropin α
- Human chorionic gonadotropin

SOMATOSTATINS
- Indium pentetreotide
- Octreotide acetate

THYROTROPIN

THYROID HORMONES
- Calcitonin salmon

TUMOR NECROSIS FACTORS
- Abatacept
- Etanercept

OTHER GROWTH FACTORS
- Clotting factors VIIa, VIII, IX, XIIIa and anticoagulant

Abbreviations

111In indium-111
2′-MOE 2′-*O*-2-methoxyethyl
Aβ amyloid beta
ACTH adrenocorticotropic hormone
AD Alzheimer disease
ADC antibody-drug conjugate
ADCC antibody-dependent cell-mediated cytotoxicity
AEEA amino(ethoxyethoxy)acetic acid
AIDS acquired immunodeficiency syndrome
ALAS1 aminolevulinate synthase 1
ALCL anaplastic large cell leukemia
ALL acute lymphoblastic leukemia
AMD age-related macular degeneration
AML acute myeloid leukemia
ANGPTL3 angiopoietin-like protein 3
ARIA amyloid-related imaging abnormalities
ARIA-H amyloid-related imaging abnormalities hemosiderin deposition
ART assisted reproductive therapy
ASCT autologous stem cell transplant
ASO antisense oligonucleotide
BAFF B cell–activating factor
BiTE bispecific T-cell engaging
BPDCN blastic plasmacytoid dendritic cell neoplasm
cDNA complementary DNA
CF cystic fibrosis
CFTR cystic fibrosis transmembrane conductance regulator
cGMP cyclic guanosine monophosphate
CGRP calcitonin gene–related peptide
CHO Chinese hamster ovary
CIC chronic idiopathic constipation
CLL chronic lymphocytic leukemia
CMV cytomegalovirus
CNS Central nervous system
CRF corticotropin-releasing factor
CSF colony-stimulating factor
CT calcitonin
CTCL cutaneous T-cell lymphoma
CTLA-4 cytotoxic T-lymphocyte–associated antigen-4
DAR drug-antibody ratio
DDAVP desamino-D-arginine vasopressin
DM diabetes mellitus
DMARD disease-modifying antirheumatic drug
DMD Duchenne muscular dystrophy
dMMR DNA mismatch repair
DPP-IV dipeptidyl peptidase IV
DT diphtheria toxin
DTPA diethylenetriaminepentaacetic acid
EGF epidermal growth factor
EGFR epidermal growth factor receptor
EPO erythropoietin
ERT enzyme-replacement therapy
Fab functional human antibody
Fc fragment crystallizable
FDA US Food and Drug Administration
FIXα activated factor IX
FRα folate receptor α
FSH follicle-stimulating hormone
FVIII Factor VIII
FX factor X
FXa activated factor X
GAG glycosaminoglycan
GalNAc *N*-acetylgalactosamine
GC-C guanylyl cyclase C
G-CSF granulocyte colony-stimulating factor
GH growth hormone
GI gastrointestinal
GIP glucose-dependent insulinotropic polypeptide
GIPR gastric inhibitory polypeptide receptor
GLP-1 glucagon-like peptide-1
GLP-1R glucagon-like peptide-1 receptor
GLP-2 glucagon-like peptide-2
GM-CSF granulocyte-macrophage colony-stimulating factor
GnRH gonadotropin-releasing hormone
GPP generalized pustular psoriasis
HAMA human anti-mouse antibody
hCG human chorionic gonadotropin

Abbreviations—continued

hCRF human corticotropin-releasing factor
HER2 human epidermal growth factor receptor 2
hGH human growth hormone
HIV human immunodeficiency virus
HIV-1 human immunodeficiency virus type 1
hnRNPs heterogeneous nuclear ribonucleoproteins
HoFH homozygous familial hypercholesterolemia
HP hepatic porphyria
HR hormone receptor
IBS-C irritable bowel syndrome accompanied by constipation
IFN interferon
IGF-1 insulin-like growth factor 1
IGF-1R insulin-like growth factor-1 receptor
IgG4 immunoglobulin class G subtype 4
IgG immunoglobulin G
IL interleukin
IL-1 interleukin 1
IL-5Rα human interleukin-5 receptor
IM intramuscularly
InO inotuzumab ozogamicin
IRR infusion-related reaction
IV intravenous
IVF in vitro fertilization
LDL-C low-density lipoprotein-cholesterol
LH luteinizing hormone
LN lupus nephritis
MAb monoclonal antibody
MAPK mitogen-activated protein kinase
M-CSF macrophage colony-stimulating factor
mc-vc-PAB maleimidocaproyl-valine-citrulline-*para*-aminobenzyloxycarbonyl
MMAE monomethyl auristatin E
MPS mucopolysaccharidosis
mRNA messenger RNA
MS multiple sclerosis
MTX methotrexate
MW molecular weight
NHL non-Hodgkin lymphoma
NLRP-3 nucleotide-binding domain, leucine-rich family, pyrin domain-containing-3
oCRF sheep corticotropin-releasing factor
PCSK9 proprotein convertase subtilisin kexin type 9
PD-1 programmed cell death protein 1
PDC peptide-drug conjugate
PDGF platelet-derived growth factor
PD-L1 programmed death-ligand 1
PD-L2 programmed death-ligand 2
PEG polyethylene glycol
PET positron emission tomography
PH1 primary hyperoxaluria type 1
PI3K phosphatidylinositol 3-kinase
PMO phosphorodiamidate morpholino oligomer
PNH paroxysmal nocturnal hemoglobinuria
PTH parathyroid hormone
RA rheumatoid arthritis
RANK receptor activator of nuclear factor-κB
RANKL receptor activator of nuclear factor-κB ligand
RBC red blood cell
rDNA recombinant DNA
rH recombinant human
rHuEPO-α recombinant human erythropoietin alfa
RNAi RNA interference
SBS short-bowel syndrome
SC subcutaneous
siRNAs small interfering RNAs
SLE systemic lupus erythematosus
SMA spinal muscular atrophy
SMN survival motor neuron
STS soft tissue sarcoma
T1D type 1 diabetes
TF-011 tissue factor-011
TNF tumor necrosis factor
t-PA tissue-type plasminogen activator
TPN total parenteral nutrition
Trp9Me 1-methyl-L-tryptophan
TTR transthyretin
VEGF vascular endothelial growth factor
VEGFR vascular endothelial growth factor receptor
VIP vasoactive intestinal peptide
VOC vaso-occlusive crisis

CLINICAL SIGNIFICANCE

The discovery and development of biologic drugs, particularly antibody-drug conjugates (ADCs), driven by medicinal chemistry, have significantly advanced the treatment landscape for various cancers. The medicinal chemistry of ADCs involves optimizing the linkers that attach the cytotoxic drugs (payload) to the antibodies.[1] These linkers, when stable in circulation, release the drug inside the target cell. This offers a targeted approach, delivering cytotoxic drugs directly to cancer cells, thereby minimizing damage to healthy tissues, improving efficacy, and reducing systemic toxicity. The clinical significance of ADCs is underscored by their potential to improve patient outcomes, offering enhanced efficacy and reduced side effects compared to traditional chemotherapy. Furthermore, the precision and specificity of biologic agents are crucial in drug selection in the treatment of cancers with limited therapeutic options, making them a vital component of personalized medicine.

Danielle Ezzo, PharmD

INTRODUCTION

Banting et al demonstrated more than a century ago that pancreatic extract markedly reduces blood sugar, even to normal levels, with relatively low toxicity in human diabetes mellitus (DM).[2] The internal secretion of pancreas that was responsible for this miraculous achievement was the 51-amino acid peptide hormone insulin. Animal-derived insulin became the first commercially available peptide drug in 1923, and with the introduction of human insulin in 1982, it achieved the distinction of being the first recombinant drug. The perception that the disadvantages of peptide drugs far outweigh their advantages led to their loss of prominence in clinical development. However, rapid biotechnological advances toward the end of the 20th century resulted in a renaissance of peptidic drugs. Currently, more than 100 peptide drugs are approved for human use worldwide.[3] In addition, an estimated 90 peptidic drugs are currently undergoing different phases of clinical trials.[3]

Recombinant therapeutic proteins (including antibodies, enzymes, fusion proteins, coagulation factors, and cytokines) provide interventions for some of the most intractable diseases and, in addition, find applications as diagnostic tools. An estimated 350 protein therapeutic agents are approved,[4] and several others are currently being evaluated in different phases of clinical trials. Protein therapeutics include antibody-drug conjugates (ADCs), peptide-drug conjugates (PDCs), monoclonal antibodies (MAbs), vaccines, enzymes, natural/recombinant cytokines, and interferons.

Peptide and protein therapeutics elicit a high degree of specificity toward molecular targets and are attractive because of their low toxicity. More than 450 peptide[3] and protein[4] therapeutics have been approved for the treatment of neoplastic and infectious diseases as well as a range of disorders that include metabolic, hematologic, immunologic, neurologic, genetic, bone, cardiac, eye, neurologic, respiratory, malabsorption, and hormonal disorders.[5]

THERAPEUTIC PEPTIDE AND PROTEIN DRUGS

The following sections introduce a variety of peptide and protein hormones, both natural and synthetic, and their recombinant analogues that are commercially available for the treatment of various diseases. The peptide hormones are obtained synthetically from natural sources or via genetic engineering. They are categorized, for the most part, according to their endocrine organ of origin.

Recombinant DNA (rDNA) technology provides a powerful tool for new pharmaceutical product development and production. Biotechnology-produced medicinal agents discussed in this chapter include hormones, enzymes, cytokines, hematopoietic growth factors, other growth factors, blood clotting factors and anticoagulants, vaccines, MAbs, ADCs, and PDCs. Some MAb-based in-home test kits are summarized in Chapter 5 (Table 5.3), and US Food and Drug Administration (FDA)-approved MAb therapeutic agents are discussed later in this chapter.

Peptide and Protein Hormones and Analogues

Hormones of Hypothalamic Origin

The hypothalamus, a relatively small organ located in the brain and responsible for thermoregulation and other functions, is the secretory source for several peptide hormones that are transported to the pituitary gland situated immediately below it. These hormones regulate the synthesis of other peptide hormones produced by the anterior pituitary (adenohypophysis) and are thus called releasing hormones, releasing factors, or inhibitory factors. The release of these hypothalamic hormones is regulated via cholinergic and dopaminergic stimuli from higher brain centers, and their synthesis and release are controlled by feedback mechanisms from their target organs.

GONADOTROPIN-RELEASING HORMONE. Gonadotropin-releasing hormone (GnRH) is a decapeptide (Fig. 38.1) that causes the release of the gonadotropins luteinizing hormone (LH) and follicle-stimulating hormone (FSH) from the anterior pituitary gland but not in equal amounts. Therefore,

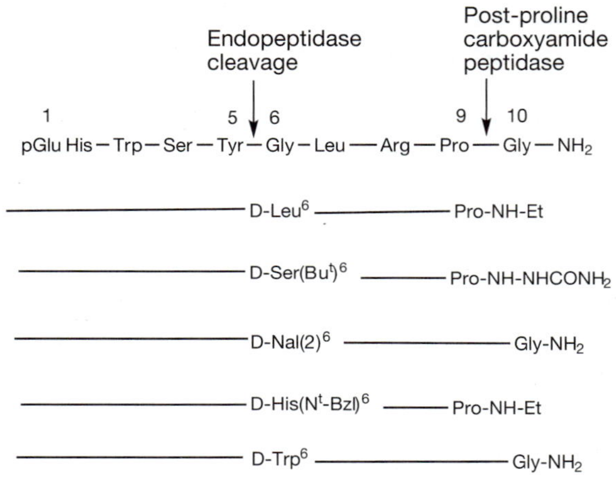

Drug	Trade Name
GnRH	
Leuprolide acetate	Eligard, Lupron, Fensolvi
Leuprolide mesylate	Camcevi
Goserelin acetate	Zoladex
Nafarelin acetate	Synarel
Histrelin acetate	Supprelin
Triptorelin pamoate	Trelstar LA and Depot

Figure 38.1 GnRH-based drugs that are commercially available. Note that leuprolide, goserelin, nafarelin, histrelin, and triptorelin are all superagonists and contain a D-amino acid in place of Gly6 and that three of the five are missing the C-terminal Gly (the line indicates an identical sequence of amino acids). But, *t*-butyl; D-Nal(2), D-3-(2-naphthyl)alanine; Nt-Bzl, 1-benzyl-D-histamine; pGlu, pyroglutamic acid.

GnRH is closely involved in the control of both male and female reproduction. Medicinal chemists have capitalized on the relatively simple decapeptide structure of GnRH by preparing several analogues as potential fertility and antifertility agents, some of which are commercially available. It is known that GnRH can be degraded by enzymatic cleavage between Tyr5-Gly6 and Pro9-Gly10. Structure-activity relationship studies of GnRH analogues have shown that when Gly6 is replaced with certain hydrophobic D-amino acids, as well as with changes in the peptide C-terminus, they generally are less susceptible to proteolytic enzymes, resulting in a longer duration of action. For that reason, they are referred to as superagonists.

In physiologic doses, GnRH agonists can induce ovulation and spermatogenesis by increasing LH and FSH levels and the resulting sex steroid levels, as does the normal hormone. In larger pharmacologic (therapeutic) doses, GnRH agonists, especially the superagonists, block implantation of the fertilized egg, cause luteolysis of the corpus luteum, and can act as postcoital contraceptive agents (although they are not approved for this latter use). This "paradoxical" antifertility effect seen with the superagonists has been attributed to the fact that GnRH must be administered in a low-dose, pulsatile manner that mimics natural hypothalamic GnRH release for it to be therapeutically effective as a fertility agent. When GnRH or a superagonist is administered in pharmacologic doses each day, LH and FSH levels will initially rise but then begin to fall after a few days because of target tissue desensitization/downregulation of pituitary GnRH receptors. The continued use of these agents in a nonpulsatile manner will result in a drastic drop of the gonadal steroid levels to near castrate levels in both men and women, thereby giving rise to their use in conditions such as precocious puberty, endometriosis, and advanced metastatic breast and prostate carcinoma. Typically, the GnRH superagonists take approximately 2 weeks to finally desensitize the GnRH receptors. During this time, there is a transient rise in LH and FSH levels, which often results in an initial "flare-up" of the original symptoms.

The following discussion is focused on the medicinal chemistry and medical use of the commercially available GnRH analogues.[6-8]

Specific Drugs

Leuprolide Acetate (Lupron, Eligard, Fensolvi). Leuprolide acetate, a synthetic nonapeptide analogue of GnRH that possesses greater potency than the natural hormone, is a commercially available superagonist. Leuprolide acetate contains substitutions that hinder enzymatic degradation, D-Leu and NH-Et in place of Gly6 and Gly10-NH_2, respectively (see Fig. 38.1). Leuprolide acetate exhibits 15-fold higher potency than natural GnRH. When given continuously and in therapeutic doses, leuprolide acetate inhibits LH and FSH secretion by desensitizing/downregulating the GnRH receptors, as discussed previously. After an initial stimulation, chronic administration of leuprolide acetate results in suppression of ovarian and testicular steroidogenesis. In premenopausal women, estrogens are reduced to postmenopausal levels; in men, testosterone is reduced to castrate levels.[9]

Leuprolide acetate is administered by daily injections or as depot injections that can be given once every 1 to 6 months as a palliative treatment in advanced prostatic carcinoma (as an alternative to orchiectomy, see Chapters 25 and 36). Because dihydrotestosterone, a metabolite of testosterone, can stimulate the growth of prostate cancer, the ability of leuprolide acetate to bring testosterone to near castrate levels is responsible for its use as a palliative in advanced disease. The addition of a nonpeptidic antiandrogen, such as flutamide or bicalutamide, to the leuprolide acetate regimen inhibits adrenal and testicular synthesized androgens from binding to, or being taken up by, target prostate cancer tissue. This combination therapy helps control the initial flare-up by blocking all sources of androgen and is referred to as maximal androgen blockade.

Leuprolide acetate, in monthly and every-3-month depot formulations, is useful in treating women diagnosed with endometriosis, but not for longer than 6 months because of the chance of developing osteoporosis. Because estrogens stimulate the growth of endometrial tissue, the ability of this drug to drastically reduce estrogen levels suggests its beneficial effect in treating endometriosis.

Central precocious puberty that is idiopathic- or gonadotropin-dependent can cause the development of secondary sexual characteristics in female children before age 8 and in male children before age 9. In addition to the psychological and physiologic changes that occur because of entering puberty too early, there is the risk of children failing to reach their full adult height. Therefore, leuprolide acetate's ability to suppress LH and sex steroid levels (testosterone and estradiol) to prepubertal levels is the reason that leuprolide acetate is approved for treating children with this disease. Use of this drug in a child with precocious puberty will slow or stop that child's secondary sexual development, slow linear growth, and skeletal maturation, and, in girls, bring about the cessation of menstruation.

Uterine leiomyomas (fibroids), which are benign neoplasms derived from smooth muscle, can cause excessive vaginal bleeding, which may lead to anemia. Leuprolide acetate, concomitant with iron therapy, is used in treating the anemia that arises from uterine leiomyoma. The decrease in the formation of the steroid sex hormones reduces fibroid and uterine volume, produces relief in the clinical symptoms (pelvic pain), and stops the excessive vaginal bleeding, thus correcting the anemia.

Leuprolide Mesylate (Camcevi). Leuprolide mesylate, a subcutaneous (SC) depot formulation, was approved for the treatment of patients with advanced prostate cancer.[10]

Goserelin Acetate (Zoladex). Goserelin acetate, like leuprolide acetate, is a synthetic superagonist nonapeptide analogue of GnRH that demonstrates greater potency than the natural hormone. It contains D-Ser (*tert*-butyl) and NH—$NHCONH_2$ in place of Gly6 and Gly10—NH_2, respectively (see Fig. 38.1). That is, the C-terminal modification simply has an —NH— substituting for the —CH_2— of glycine, and like the C-terminal change in leuprolide acetate, this inhibits its enzymatic degradation of the peptide by the postproline carboxyamide peptidase.

Goserelin acetate is available in the form of a small solid pellet that is administered as an SC implant for the palliative treatment of advanced metastatic breast cancer in pre- and perimenopausal women or, similarly, as a palliative in advanced prostatic cancer. The rationale for this superagonist's use is its ability to bring the levels of estradiol or testosterone to near-castrate levels, thus slowing the progression of breast or prostate carcinoma, respectively. Additionally, goserelin acetate is approved for the treatment of endometriosis for up to 6 months.

Goserelin acetate is also used in combination with antiandrogen flutamide for shrinking prostate carcinoma before radiation therapy. This maximal androgen blockade combination is used when the prostate carcinoma has been staged as locally confined to the prostate gland, with one or both lobes, as well as the seminal vesicles, involved. The treatment should start 8 weeks before radiation treatment begins and be continued throughout the radiation therapy.

Furthermore, patients who are to undergo hysterectomy for menorrhagia (heavy menstrual bleeding) can benefit from pretreatment with goserelin acetate because it is able to induce endometrial thinning. This thinning of the endometrium improves the operating environment by causing less intrauterine bleeding, increases postoperative amenorrhea, and decreases dysmenorrhea following surgery.

Nafarelin Acetate (Synarel). Nafarelin acetate, another synthetic superagonist decapeptide analogue of GnRH, contains D-Nal(2) 6 [Nal = 3-(2-naphthyl)-Ala] in place of Gly6, but the C-terminal Gly10–NH_2 is identical with natural GnRH (Fig. 38.1). Nafarelin acetate is available as a 0.2% nasal spray for the relief of endometriosis. Estrogen is needed for the growth of endometrial tissue; thus, decreased estrogen leads to shrinkage of errant endometrial tissue. The observed adverse effects of nafarelin acetate are related to falling estrogen levels and include decreased libido, amenorrhea, hot flashes, and vaginal dryness. When used consistently, nafarelin acetate will inhibit ovulation and stop menstruation.

Nafarelin acetate is also used in male and female children for the treatment of central precocious puberty. By suppressing the release of LH, the estradiol or testosterone levels fall to prepubertal levels; early secondary sexual development is arrested; linear growth and skeletal maturation are slowed; and in girls, menstruation stops.

Histrelin Acetate (Supprelin). Histrelin acetate, a superagonist analogue of GnRH, contains D-His(N1-Bzl)6 in place of Gly6, and the C-terminus is identical to leuprolide acetate namely, NH–Et in place of Gly10–NH_2 (Fig. 38.1). This GnRH analogue is commercially available in the form of an implantable device (SC in the upper arm) that slowly releases the drug over a 12-month period, resulting in decreased testicular steroidogenesis. It is used for the palliative treatment of advanced prostate cancer.

Triptorelin Pamoate (Trelstar). Triptorelin pamoate is another superagonist analogue of GnRH that, like nafarelin acetate, contains only a single amino acid substitution (D-Trp6 for Gly6) when compared to the natural hormone (see Fig. 38.1). As described earlier, the treatment of advanced prostate cancer involves reduction of serum testosterone to very low levels, which can be achieved surgically by orchiectomy. When this surgical method is unacceptable to the patient, an alternative approach is "chemical castration," which can be achieved by use of estrogen therapy, leuprolide, goserelin or histrelin acetates, or triptorelin pamoate. This product is available for intramuscular (IM) depot injection (monthly or every 3 months), and treatment drops serum testosterone concentrations to a level generally seen in surgically castrated men.

Ganirelix Acetate (Fyremadel, Ganirelix). Ganirelix acetate is an analogue of GnRH with substitutions at residues 1, 2, 3, 6, 8, and 10 (Fig. 38.2).[11] It is not a superagonist but, rather, is a synthetic decapeptide with high antagonist activity and the first GnRH antagonist to be marketed. It is approved for the suppression of LH surges in women who are undergoing ovarian hyperstimulation fertility treatment; LH surges normally promote ovulation. The therapeutic goal of this drug is to significantly reduce the number of medication days necessary to suppress the LH surge, thereby maintaining eggs in the ovaries. In vitro fertilization (IVF) treatment cycles were historically initiated by the administration of leuprolide acetate to suppress the premature release of LH. This inhibits ovulation so that the eggs remain available for retrieval by a fertility specialist. For this purpose, leuprolide acetate is usually injected for as many as 26 days. Clinical studies have shown that ganirelix acetate can shut down the LH surge with only 5 days of treatment, that the suppression of LH is more pronounced than that induced by FSH, and that the shorter treatment time minimizes unpleasant side effects, such as hot flashes and headaches.

Cetrorelix Acetate (Cetrotide). Cetrorelix acetate[12] is an analogue of GnRH with amino acid substitutions at residues 1, 2, 3, 6, and 10 and differing from ganirelix at amino acids

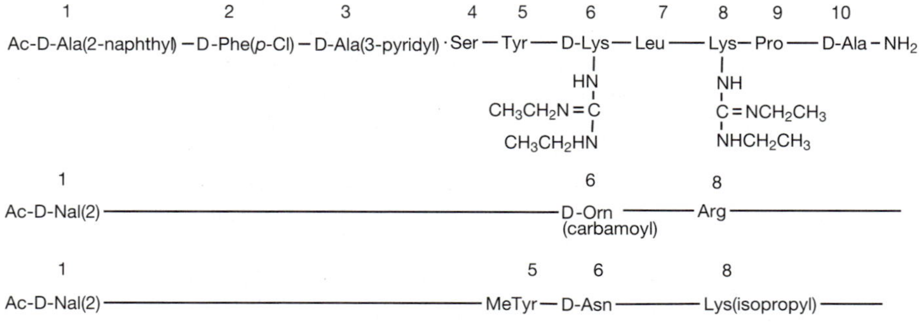

Drug	Trade Name
Ganirelix acetate	Fyremadel
Cetrorelix acetate	Cetrotide
Abarelix	Plenaxis

Figure 38.2 Gonadotropin-releasing hormone receptor antagonists. Ac-D-Nal(2), *N*-acetyl-D-2-naphthylalanine; D-Aph(hor), 4-dihydroorotoylamino-D-phenylalanine; D-Aph(ur), 4-ureido-D-phenylalanine; D-Orn(carbamoyl), D-ornithine.

1, 6, and 8 (see Fig. 38.2). These substitutions are synthetic, non–DNA-directed amino acids and, like ganirelix acetate, impart GnRH antagonist activity to cetrorelix acetate. This drug is also marketed for use in women undergoing assisted reproductive therapy (ART) procedures, in which it is necessary to control their LH surge. This allows the follicles to develop to a size, as determined by ultrasound, which increases the success of timed insemination and oocyte retrieval for IVF. Like ganirelix acetate, cetrorelix acetate has an advantage over GnRH agonists such as leuprolide acetate because it reduces the fertility therapy cycle to days rather than weeks.

Degarelix acetate (Firmagon). Degarelix acetate is an analogue of GnRH with amino acid substitutions at residues 1, 2, 3, 5, 6, 8, and 10 (see Fig. 38.2). These substitutions are synthetic, non–DNA-directed amino acids and, like ganirelix acetate, impart competitive and reversible GnRH antagonist activity, leading to suppression of LH release from the pituitary gland. Degarelix acetate is indicated for treatment of patients with advanced prostate cancer (see Chapters 25 and 36).[13] Like the superagonists, degarelix affords a drop in testosterone to castrate levels. Degarelix does not, however, produce the initial rise in testosterone levels and the resulting flare-up of symptoms often seen with the superagonists. Relative to its predecessors, degarelix has increased aqueous solubility due to the presence of unnatural amino acids at positions 5 and 6 with polar dihydropyrimidinedione carboxamide and urea moieties that have extensive hydrogen-bonding capabilities. Replacement of Arg8 by (Nε-isopropyl)Lys minimizes the histamine-releasing properties, an unwanted side effect with other GnRH antagonists.

SOMATOSTATINS. Somatostatin is a cyclic 14-amino acid peptide that was first isolated by Guillemin in 1973 and is probably the most thoroughly investigated and most important of the inhibitory factors produced by the hypothalamus (Fig. 38.3).[14] The principal activity of somatostatin is inhibition of the release of growth hormone (GH) from the anterior pituitary. Too much GH, as in pituitary tumors, causes acromegaly, a form of gigantism. Conversely, too little

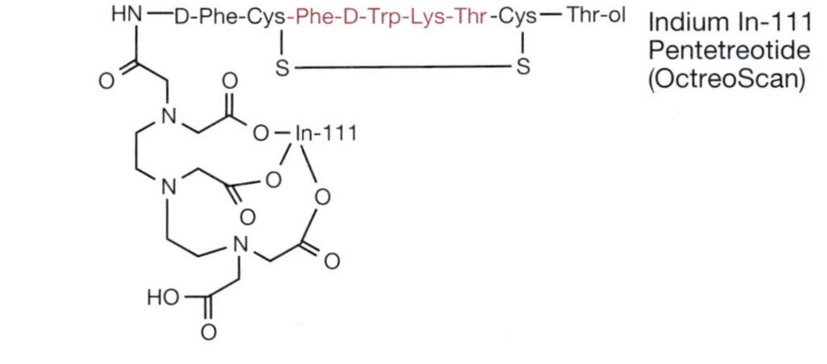

Figure 38.3 Somatostatin and its analogues.

GH leads to dwarfism. Somatostatin has also been found in the pancreas and the gastrointestinal (GI) tract, where it inhibits the secretion of both insulin and glucagon from the pancreas, as well as the secretion of a variety of intestinal peptides (eg, gastrin, secretin, pepsin, and renin). The short half-life of somatostatin, which is less than 3 minutes, has precluded its use as a therapeutic agent. Consequently, many derivatives of somatostatin were developed to increase duration of action and/or to enhance the selectivity profile. The culmination of these structure-activity relationship studies was the development of octreotide acetate.

Specific Drugs

Octreotide Acetate (Sandostatin). Octreotide acetate, a long-acting octapeptide analogue of somatostatin, has a half-life of approximately 100 minutes. A comparison of the primary structures of octreotide and somatostatin suggests little similarity, but studies have shown that the essential fragment for its activity was the tetrapeptide Phe7-Trp8-Lys9-Thr10 (see Fig. 38.3). These studies helped in the design of the potent drug now known as octreotide acetate, which incorporates D-Trp in the essential tetrapeptide segment.[15] This drug suppresses the secretion of gastroenteropancreatic peptides, such as gastrin, vasoactive intestinal peptide (VIP), insulin, and glucagon, as well as pituitary GH. Furthermore, it is more potent than natural somatostatin in inhibiting the release of glucagon, insulin, and GH.

Octreotide acetate is used by SC injection in the palliative treatment of metastatic carcinoid tumors, which are tumors of the endocrine system, GI tract, and lung. It is also used in the palliative management of VIP-secreting tumors (VIPomas, usually pancreatic tumors). Patients with VIPomas have profuse, watery diarrhea syndrome, and octreotide acetate can help by decreasing the release of damaging intestinal tumor cell secretions. Octreotide also helps reduce hypokalemia by correcting electrolyte imbalances.

Octreotide acetate can decrease the secretion of GH from the pituitary and is used in patients with acromegaly who are unresponsive to pituitary radiation therapy or surgery. It is used in the treatment of acromegaly because it reduces the blood levels of both GH and insulin-like growth factor 1 (IGF-1). The long-acting repository form of octreotide acetate is administered as monthly depot injections for all the indications mentioned earlier. Octreotide acetate (Mycapssa), a delayed-release capsule, was approved in 2020 for the long-term maintenance treatment of acromegaly.

Octreotide for intravenous (IV) injection is used for the treatment of acute bleeding from esophageal varices. Variceal bleeding occurs in about half the patients with cirrhosis of the liver and is responsible for about one-third of deaths in these patients. Octreotide is a potent vasoconstrictor that reduces portal and collateral blood flow by constricting visceral vessels, which leads to reduced portal blood pressure and decreased bleeding.

Indium-111 Pentetreotide (OctreoScan). Somatostatin receptors have a broad distribution in normal tissue, as well as in a variety of human malignancies (eg, small-cell lung, brain, breast, pituitary, and endocrine pancreatic cancers). For this reason, octreotide, which binds to somatostatin receptors, was converted to a radionuclide-containing peptide by reacting the amino terminus with an active ester of diethylenetriaminepentaacetic acid (DTPA) to give DTPA-octreotide and then chelated to the radionuclide indium-111 (111In) (see Fig. 38.3). This radiopharmaceutical, marketed as OctreoScan, is used as a diagnostic agent for the early detection and localization of small tumors and their metastases, especially tumors that originate from neuroendocrine cells.[16] Administration of this diagnostic agent in total parenteral nutrition (TPN) admixtures or injection into TPN IV administration lines may lead to the formation of a complex glycosyl octreotide conjugate and is contraindicated.

Hormones Originating in the Anterior Lobe of the Pituitary Gland

The pituitary, located just below the hypothalamus, is a small gland that can be divided into an anterior and a posterior lobe. This gland is responsible for the secretion of several important peptide hormones, two of which are released by the posterior lobe (oxytocin and vasopressin). The remaining anterior pituitary peptide hormones control important functions such as growth, reproduction, metabolic and ion balance, as well as several other functions.

Growth Hormone. Human GH(hGH), a 191-amino acid protein with a molecular weight (MW) of 22 kDa, is roughly spherical with a hydrophobic interior. GH is secreted by the anterior pituitary in response to the liberation of GH-releasing factor from the hypothalamus. This contrasts with somatostatin, which inhibits the release of GH. The primary function of GH is to promote skeletal growth. When GH is absent during childhood, or if there is an inadequate supply, dwarfism results. Before 1985, children of short stature were sometimes treated with hGH of pituitary origin, which was obtained from cadavers, but hGH of natural origin was discontinued in 1985 by the FDA when several young adults who had received hGH died. Their deaths were attributed to contaminated hGH, and the contaminant was later found to be an infective agent, known as a prion, that causes Creutzfeldt-Jakob disease, a rare and fatal neurodegenerative disease.[17] Naturally occurring hGH has been replaced by the product that is derived from rDNA methodology.

Specific Drugs

Somatropin (Genotropin, Humatrope, Norditropin, Nutropin, Omnitrope, Saizen, Serostim, Zomacton). Somatropin, which is an hGH prepared by rDNA procedures, contains the identical sequence of 191 amino acids as the natural hormone. Several of these products are indicated for the long-term treatment of children who fail to grow because of inadequate secretion of endogenous GH and for growth problems associated with chronic renal failure.[18] Even adults who are diagnosed with GH deficiency, which can arise because of pituitary or hypothalamic disease, surgery, radiation therapy, or other reasons, can benefit from hGH replacement therapy. Turner syndrome, a genetic disease in which there is a complete or partial absence of one of the two X chromosomes in female children, causes short stature, as one of its many symptoms. Female children with Turner syndrome can benefit from the use of Humatrope, Norditropin, or Nutropin during their growth years. A long-acting dosage form of somatotropin is approved for use in children with Prader-Willi syndrome, a rare genetic disorder that causes short stature, an involuntary, continuous urge to eat that is life-long and may be life-threatening, low muscle tone, and cognitive disorders. The formulation was designed to reduce the frequency of injections to once or twice a month by encapsulating the agent in biodegradable microspheres.

The anabolic properties of hGH are the basis for the orphan drug use of several of these recombinant products. hGH (Serostim) is used in acquired immunodeficiency syndrome (AIDS)-associated catabolism or weight loss, in cachexia resulting from AIDS, and as an anabolic agent in patients with severe burns.

Pegvisomant (Somavert). This recombinant product contains 191 amino acid residues, the same number as in GH, but there are substitutions at residues 18, 21, 120, 167, 168, 171, 172, 174, and 179. This product is covalently linked to several polyethylene glycol (PEG) molecules, and the PEGylated protein becomes a GH receptor antagonist. As such, pegvisomant binds to the GH receptor and blocks endogenous GH from binding. The result is a blocking of the GH-stimulated overproduction of IGF-1 that contributes to the disabling symptoms and long-term health problems associated with acromegaly.[19]

Somapacitan-beco (Sogroya). Somapacitan is a conjugate of hGH with albumin ligand, approved in 2020 for the replacement of endogenous GH in adults with GH deficiency as a once-weekly injection.[20] It is an analogue of hGH with a single substitution in the amino acid backbone (L101C) to which an albumin-binding moiety has been attached. The albumin-binding moiety (side chain) consists of an albumin binder and a hydrophilic spacer attached to position 101 of the protein. The protein part consists of 191 amino acids. Somapacitan-beco is produced in *Escherichia coli* by rDNA technology. Somapacitan-beco binds to a dimeric GH receptor in the cell membrane of target cells, resulting in intracellular signal transduction and a host of pharmacodynamic effects. Some of these pharmacodynamic effects are primarily mediated by IGF-1 produced in the liver, while others are primarily a consequence of the direct effects of somapacitan-beco.

Gonadotropins. The gonadotropins FSH and LH are large glycoproteins released by the anterior pituitary upon stimulation by GnRH produced in the hypothalamus. Both FSH and LH consist of two noncovalently associated α and β subunits. The α subunits contain 92 amino acids and are identical in both hormones, whereas the β subunit consists of 121 amino acids in LH and 111 amino acids in FSH. As the β subunit structures are dissimilar,[21] they are responsible for each hormone's bioactivity and rate of degradation (biologic half-life of LH is 20 min, which is shorter than that of FSH's 3-4 hours).

Both LH and FSH are referred to as gonadotropins because they act on the male and female gonads, which results in the production of the sex steroids testosterone and estradiol, respectively. FSH is a 34-kDa glycoprotein (~14% carbohydrate), and LH is a 26-kDa glycoprotein. In women, FSH and LH act in concert in regulating ovarian function;

egg maturation and estradiol secretion are stimulated by FSH, while ovulation, transformation of the ruptured follicle into the corpus luteum, and progesterone secretion are LH-mediated actions. In men, spermatogenesis is dependent on these two hormones. FSH stimulates the maturation of sperm in the testes, while LH enables the testicular secretion of testosterone.

Male infertility is generally caused by the quality and/or quantity of the sperm produced. Female infertility, however, may be caused by several factors, such as the inability to produce an egg, to ovulate, to achieve fertilization, and for implantation of the fertilized ovum in the uterus. Several of the commercially available gonadotropins can help in enhancing both male and female fertility, as discussed later.

Specific Drugs

Menotropins (Menopur). Menotropins are natural products obtained from the urine of postmenopausal women and then biologically standardized (international units) for FSH and LH activities in an approximate ratio of 1:1. Menotropins are used in men with primary (hypothalamic) or secondary (pituitary) hypogonadism to stimulate spermatogenesis. Patients must have been treated previously with human chorionic gonadotropin (hCG; a peptide hormone of placental origin that has activity very similar to LH, as discussed later) to effect masculinization through increased testosterone production. Menotropins and hCG are given sequentially for the purposes of inducing ovulation in women with either hypothalamic or pituitary hormonal dysfunction. The menotropins are given for 7 to 12 days, and after clinical evaluation (via ultrasound) indicates the presence of a mature follicle, a single dose of hCG is given to simulate the typical LH surge that normally triggers ovulation. Also, women use the combination of menotropins and hCG to promote the development of multiple follicles when they are participating in an IVF program requiring the recruitment of follicles.

Follitropins. Follitropins are hormonal products that consist entirely of FSH and are used to stimulate ovarian follicle growth in women who do not have primary ovarian failure. In the absence of an adequate endogenous LH surge, hCG must be given following the use of follitropins to stimulate ovulation.

Follitropin α (Gonal-F, Gonal-F RFF, Gonal-F RFF Pen). Follitropin α is a human FSH preparation of rDNA origin. Because FSH is a glycoprotein, alterations in the carbohydrate side chain attachments afford different isoforms, which leads to different pharmacokinetic and pharmacodynamic properties. Because it is of recombinant origin and not isolated from the urine, it is free of any additional substances, such as urinary proteins and LH.

Follitropin α is marketed for promoting the development of multiple follicles, which can then be induced to ovulate, via hCG administration, so that the oocytes can be collected for IVF. It is also used in women who wish to become pregnant and are anovulatory because of polycystic ovary syndrome, in whom it can enhance follicle maturation before hCG administration for final ovulation.

Men with infertility can also benefit from therapy with follitropin α if their infertility is related to hypothalamic or pituitary hormonal dysfunction and not primary testicular failure because it induces spermatogenesis. Just as with therapy using menotropins, pretreatment with hCG is performed for 3 months to achieve serum testosterone levels within the normal range before hCG and follitropin α therapy.

Follitropin β (Follistim AQ). Follitropin β is a human FSH preparation of rDNA origin that differs chemically from natural FSH and follitropin α only by slight changes in the composition of the carbohydrate side chains. In fact, the primary and tertiary structures of both follitropins α and β are indistinguishable from those of natural human FSH. Furthermore, bioassays and physiochemical studies indicate that follitropins α and β are indistinguishable from each other. Therefore, follitropin β is approved for the same indications as follitropin α.

ADRENOCORTICOTROPIC HORMONE (ACTHAR GEL). The anterior pituitary, under the influence of the hypothalamic hormone human corticotropin-releasing factor (hCRF), releases adrenocorticotropic hormone (ACTH), a single-chain peptide of 39 amino acids (also known as corticotropin). The sequence of 24 amino acid residues beginning from the amino terminus contains all the biologic activity of the parent. The remaining 15 C-terminal residues confer species specificity, as well as enhance the stability of ACTH toward proteolytic cleavage. Amino acids 1 to 24, which are critical for ACTH activity, are identical in humans, pigs, sheep, and cattle, whereas these species differ only slightly from each other in the final 15 amino acids. The main action of ACTH on the adrenal cortex involves the release of the glucocorticoid hormone hydrocortisone and the mineralocorticoid hormone aldosterone.

Commercial ACTH is obtained from natural sources and is available in 16% gelatin (repository gel) to prolong its release after SC or IM injection. ACTH has both anti-inflammatory and immunosuppressant properties, which contributes to its use in the treatment of acute exacerbations of multiple sclerosis (MS).

COSYNTROPIN (CORTROSYN). Cosyntropin is a synthetic polypeptide consisting of amino acids 1 through 24 of human ACTH that are required for full biologic activity. Since it is of synthetic origin, it is less allergenic than ACTH of natural origin. Cosyntropin is used as a diagnostic agent in the screening of patients suspected of having adrenocortical insufficiency.

THYROTROPIN ALFA (THYROGEN). Thyroid-stimulating hormone (thyrotropin) is a 28- to 30-kDa glycoprotein secreted by the anterior lobe of the pituitary gland that is necessary for the growth and function of the thyroid. A recombinant thyrotropin α useful for the detection and treatment of thyroid cancer was approved by the FDA in 1998.

Hormones Released from the Posterior Lobe of the Pituitary Gland

As previously discussed, the pituitary gland is responsible for the secretion of several peptide hormones, only two of which are released by the posterior lobe. In fact, these two hormones, oxytocin and vasopressin, are synthesized in neurons originating in the hypothalamus and are transported to the posterior pituitary for storage until release is required.

Oxytocin (Pitocin). Oxytocin is a cyclic nonapeptide hormone and neurotransmitter containing a 20-membered tocin ring (from Cys1 to Cys6) and an acyclic tripeptide tail (from Pro7 to $GlyNH_2$9). Like somatostatin, it contains a large ring that includes a disulfide bridge (Fig. 38.4). Oxytocin has uterotonic action, contracting the muscles of the uterus during gestation, and plays an important role in milk ejection. Exogenous oxytocin is most commonly used for induction of labor, wherein it improves uterine contractions to achieve early vaginal delivery for reasons of fetal or maternal well-being (eg, preeclampsia, Rh factor problems, pregnancy that has exceeded 42 weeks). It also finds use following delivery of the placenta because it promotes contraction and vasoconstriction and helps control postpartum bleeding.

Vasopressin (Vasostrict). Human vasopressin, or Arg-vasopressin, is chemically very similar to oxytocin and, therefore, sometimes is referred to as (Phe3, Arg8) oxytocin (see Fig. 38.4). The physiologic role of vasopressin is the regulation of water reabsorption in the renal tubules and, thus, it is often referred to as the antidiuretic hormone. In high doses, vasopressin promotes the contraction of arterioles and capillaries, resulting in an increase in blood pressure (thus the name vasopressin). An inadequate output of pituitary antidiuretic hormone can cause diabetes insipidus, which is characterized by the chronic excretion of large amounts of pale urine and results in dehydration and extreme thirst.

Desmopressin Acetate (Nocdurna). Desmopressin, as its acetate salt, is a synthetic analogue of vasopressin in which the N-terminal Cys is devoid of its α-amino function (1-desamino) and where Arg8 is present as its D-isomer

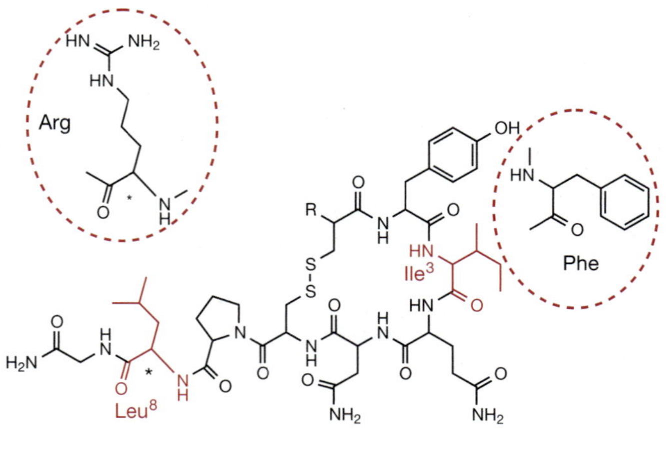

Oxytocin, [R = NH_2, *S]
(Pitocin)

Vasopressin, [R = NH_2, *S], replace Ile^3 with Phe^3 and Leu^8 with Arg^8
(Vasostrict)

Desmopressin, [R = H, *R], replace Ile^3 with Phe^3 and Leu^8 with Arg^8
(Nocdurna)

Figure 38.4 Structural relationship between oxytocin, vasopressin, and desmopressin.

(D-Arg8), thus abbreviated as DDAVP (see Fig. 38.4). The presence of D-Arg and the absence of the N-terminal amine in the desmopressin structure have contributed to its increased half-life, and it is available for oral, parenteral, or nasal use. It is used by all three of these routes to prevent or control polydipsia (excessive thirst), polyuria, and dehydration of patients with diabetes insipidus caused by a deficiency of vasopressin. It has also been approved for the treatment of nocturnal enuresis (bedwetting), which is believed to be caused by an absence of the normal nighttime rise in vasopressin levels.

Desmopressin is known to cause an increase in both plasma factor VIII (antihemophilic factor) and plasminogen activator. Therefore, it is approved by the FDA for use, parenterally and nasally, in reducing spontaneous or trauma-induced bleeding episodes in patients with hemophilia A and type I von Willebrand disease, provided that their plasma factor VIII activity is greater than 5%.

Hormones of Placental Origin

If, after ovulation occurs in women, the liberated ovum is fertilized and then implants in the endometrium, the resulting placenta that forms between mother and fetus begins to release hCG, the function of which is to maintain and prolong the life of the ovarian corpus luteum. The corpus luteum is important for the continued production of progesterone. Progesterone is especially important because it prepares the uterus for pregnancy and helps in the maintenance of the placenta. hCG begins to appear in the maternal bloodstream and urine shortly after conception and implantation of the fertilized ovum. As a result of this early release of hCG, its detection in the urine forms the basis for the home pregnancy kits that have become so popular in the early detection of pregnancy.

Human Chorionic Gonadotropin (Novarel, Pregnyl). Placental hCG is a complex protein that consists of an α and β subunit. The α subunit consists of 92 amino acids that are identical in sequence with those found in both LH and FSH, whereas the β subunit contains 145 amino acids and is responsible for its biologic specificity. The biologic actions of hCG closely resemble those of LH, but the former has a longer half-life and minimal FSH activity.

Like LH, hCG stimulates the production of testosterone by the testes; therefore, it is used in treating male hypogonadism and to stimulate testicular descent in prepubertal cryptorchidism in young male children aged 4 to 9 years. In treating infertility caused by pituitary dysfunction, hCG, in combination with menotropins (as previously discussed) or clomiphene, can induce ovulation and pregnancy in anovulatory women. This hCG, which is of natural origin, is purified from the urine of pregnant women.

Choriogonadotropin a (Ovidrel). Choriogonadotropin α is obtained by rDNA technology and is biologically and chemically identical to hCG of natural origin. Like hCG of natural origin, it is used for inducing ovulation in women with anovulatory infertility. Following proper pretreatment with a GnRH antagonist or superagonist to desensitize the pituitary, women participating in ART are treated with a follicle-stimulating agent (eg, menotropins) to affect the final maturation of the follicles within the ovaries. Ultrasonograms are used to determine proper follicle maturation before the administration of choriogonadotropin α to induce ovulation. A distinct advantage of this product is that it can be self-administered by the patient via SC injection.

Hormone of Parathyroid Origin

The four parathyroid glands exist as two pairs, one pair of which is embedded on the back surface of each of the two lobes of the thyroid gland. These very small glands are responsible for the secretion of parathyroid hormone (PTH), the action of which is the regulation of both calcium and phosphate metabolism within bone and kidney. In humans, the Ca^{2+} concentration is carefully regulated, and when it falls below homeostatic levels, the parathyroid glands secrete PTH, an 84-amino acid, single-chain protein. Depending on whether exogenous PTH is administered intermittently or continuously, it can stimulate bone formation (osteoblastic activity) or breakdown (osteoclastic activity or resorption), respectively.

TERIPARATIDE (FORTEO). Teriparatide, a polypeptide prepared by rDNA techniques, consists of the first 34 amino acids from the N-terminal end of PTH. It has been shown to contain all the structural requirements for the full biologic activity of PTH. When teriparatide is administered daily by SC injection, it stimulates osteoblastic activity at the expense of osteoclastic activity, and this enhances bone formation. This is the basis for teriparatide's use in treating high-risk patients in danger of bone fracture resulting from osteoporosis, men with primary or hypogonadal osteoporosis, and women with postmenopausal osteoporosis.[22] It carries a Boxed Warning for increased risk of osteosarcoma.

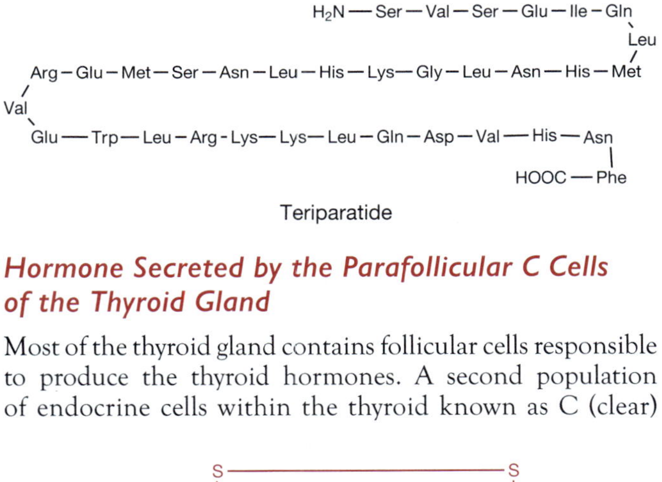

Teriparatide

Hormone Secreted by the Parafollicular C Cells of the Thyroid Gland

Most of the thyroid gland contains follicular cells responsible to produce the thyroid hormones. A second population of endocrine cells within the thyroid known as C (clear) cells, or parafollicular cells, produce the hormone calcitonin (CT), which has an opposing action to that of PTH in that it decreases the Ca^{2+} concentration in body fluids. It accomplishes this by inhibiting the activity of osteoclasts (ie, decreasing Ca^{2+} release from bone by inhibiting bone resorption). The actual biosynthesis and release of CT is regulated by the concentration of Ca^{2+} in plasma; when it is high, CT secretion increases.

SALMON CALCITONIN (MIACALCIN). CT is a single-chain polypeptide consisting of 32 amino acids (Fig. 38.5). CTs obtained from different species are identical at seven of the first nine amino acids, contain Gly at position 28, and all terminate with Pro–NH_2. The C-terminal Pro amide (Pro–NH_2) is very important for the biologic function of CT, as is the disulfide bridge between Cys amino acids at positions 1 and 7. In contrast, the amino acids from 10 to 27 can be varied and seem to influence CT's potency, as well as its duration of action. Salmon CT differs from human CT at 16 amino acids.

Only salmon CT is commercially available for medical use because, on a weight basis, it is approximately 45-fold more potent than human CT. Salmon CT, in parenteral form, is approved for treating Paget disease of bone (generally seen in older persons; involves increased bone resorption and softening of bones), postmenopausal osteoporosis, and hypercalcemia of malignancy (multiple myeloma or advanced breast carcinoma). Salmon CT is also available in a nasal spray formulation, which is used exclusively in the treatment of postmenopausal osteoporosis (see Chapter 27).

Hormones of Endocrine Pancreatic Origin

The exocrine pancreas consists mostly (~99%) of gland cells known as pancreatic acini, which are responsible for secreting several digestive enzymes. The endocrine pancreas, or the remaining 1% of the gland, consists of a group of cells known as pancreatic islets or islets of Langerhans. Each of these islets consists of four distinct cell types, designated as α, β, γ, and δ cells. The α cells secrete glucagon, the β cells secrete insulin and amylin, the δ cells secrete a peptide that is identical to somatostatin of hypothalamic origin, and the γ cells secrete pancreatic polypeptide, of which little concerning its physiologic action is known. Insulin, glucagon, and somatostatin are essential in regulating carbohydrate, lipid, and amino acid metabolism. Insulin is

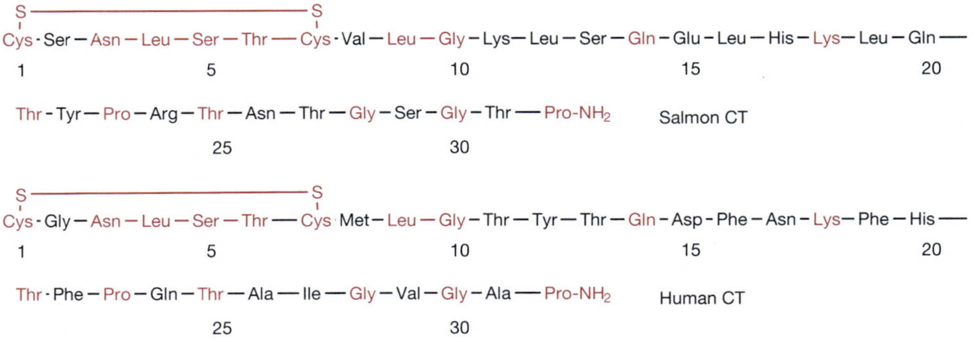

Figure 38.5 Primary structures of salmon and human calcitonin (CT). Similarities are highlighted in red.

responsible for promoting the storage of glucose as glycogen and effecting hypoglycemia, whereas glucagon mobilizes glucose from its glycogen stores and causes hyperglycemia. The primary action of somatostatin of hypothalamic origin is to inhibit the release of GH from the pituitary, but pancreatic somatostatin suppresses the production of both insulin and glucagon. Amylin, which is co-secreted with insulin from the β cells, has physiologic actions that include slowing of gastric emptying, suppression of postprandial glucagon secretion, reduction of food intake, and inhibition of the secretion of both stomach acid and pancreatic digestive enzymes.

Specific Drugs

Insulin. Insulin has anabolic properties that include the stimulation of both skeletal muscle and liver cells to incorporate glucose and convert it to glycogen, to synthesize proteins from amino acids in the blood, and to act on fat cells to enhance their uptake of glucose and the synthesis of fat. In short, insulin encourages anabolism rather than catabolism because it promotes the synthesis of glycogen, proteins, and lipids. A deficiency of insulin, which characterizes the disease DM, causes extreme changes in the entire metabolic pattern of individuals with the disease (see Chapter 22). Patients with DM often demonstrate elevated blood glucose levels, excess glucose in the urine, and failure to properly use carbohydrate and lipids. Untreated DM can be fatal. Even when treated, however, there can be numerous circulatory and renal complications, and some metabolic abnormalities may lead to blindness (diabetic retinopathy).

The human insulin molecule, consisting of 51 amino acids, has the structural characteristics of a large protein yet is only the size of a polypeptide. Two disulfide bonds (CysA7 to CysB7 and CysA20 to CysB19) link two polypeptide chains, with the A-chain consisting of 21 amino acids and the B-chain consisting of 30 amino acids. An additional disulfide loop is found in the A-chain between CysA6 and CysA11.

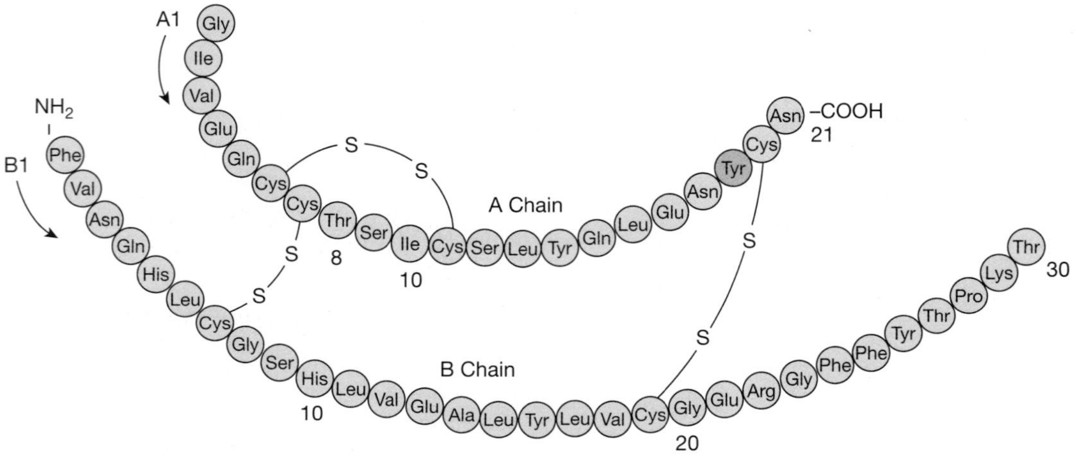

Primary structure of human insulin chains A and B

The primary sequences of insulin from several species are known, and porcine insulin is the closest to that of humans. Their A-chains are identical, and they differ only in their B-chains, with Ala30 (porcine) in place of Thr30 (human). Human and bovine insulin differ in each chain, with Ala8 and Val10 in the A-chain (bovine) and Ala30 in the B-chain (bovine). Recombinant insulin, approved in 1982 for the treatment of insulin-dependent diabetes, is the first FDA-approved rDNA drug. The biotechnology-derived insulin has several advantages over insulin derived from animal sources: (1) It has potentially fewer serious immune reactions, (2) it is pyrogen free, (3) it is not contaminated with other peptide hormones (eg, glucagon, somatostatin, proinsulin), and (4) it can be produced in large amounts.

Human insulin of rDNA origin is available commercially as Humulin, Novolin, and several analogues, and they are classified based on their duration of action.[23] The Humulin and Novolin products are produced using genetically modified strains of two different microorganisms. Humulin is prepared using recombinant *E. coli* bacteria. The pharmaceutical preparation is reported to contain less than 4 ppm of immunoreactive bacterial polypeptides that act as possible contaminants. Baker yeast (*Saccharomyces cerevisiae*) serves as the recombinant organism to produce Novolin.

Studies in animals, healthy adults, and patients with type 1 DM have shown human insulin to have pharmacologic effects identical to those of purified porcine insulin. A comparable pharmacokinetic profile has also been shown. Human insulin, however, administered IM or IV may have a slightly faster onset and slightly shorter duration of action when compared with purified porcine insulin in patients with diabetes. The usual precautions concerning toxic potentials observed with insulin of animal origin should be followed with rDNA human insulin. As would be expected, the recombinant product has been shown to be less immunogenic than nonhuman insulins.

Insulin remains the only treatment option for type 1 diabetes (T1D) and is still widely used to treat patients with type 2 diabetes (T2D) who do not respond adequately to other pharmacotherapies. rDNA technology has led to the development of insulin analogues that have greater utility in certain situations and may more closely resemble the normal diurnal pattern of insulin secretion. The newly engineered analogues have specific amino acid sequence modifications that improve absorption properties and biologic profiles. Insulin lispro (Humalog) has a more rapid onset and shorter duration of action than regular human insulin. Unlike regular insulin that must be injected 30 to 60 minutes before a meal, recombinant insulin lispro is effective when injected 15 minutes before a meal. The analogue differs from natural human insulin because the B-chain amino acids B28 Pro and B29 Lys are exchanged. Insulin aspart (Novolog), which is homologous with human insulin except for the single amino acid substitution of Asp for Pro at B28, is effective when injected 5-10 minutes before a meal. An ultra-long-acting agent, insulin glargine (Lantus, Toujeo) differs from human insulin in that the amino acid Asn at residue A21 is replaced by Gly, and two Arg residues are added to the C-terminus of the B chain. When administered SC, insulin glargine has a duration of action up to 24 to 48 hours. This change in action profile resulted from structural modifications that enhance the product's basicity, thus causing the product to precipitate at neutral pH post injection and increasing its duration of action.

Glucagon (GlucaGen). Glucagon, a 29-amino acid, straight-chain polypeptide of α-cell pancreatic origin, triggers liver glycogenolysis and gluconeogenesis, thereby elevating glucose levels. The principal action of glucagon is the liver-mediated release into the blood of abnormally high concentrations of glucose, which causes hyperglycemia. This means that glucagon influences blood glucose levels that is the opposite of insulin.[24]

Glucagon of rDNA origin is now available. Replacing the bovine product with the rDNA-derived drug would eliminate the risk of acquiring bovine spongiform encephalopathy from glucagon therapy. Human glucagon of rDNA origin is marketed for the treatment of severe hypoglycemic reactions in patients with diabetes, as can occur when there is an overdose of insulin. In patients with T1D, the increase in glucose resulting from glucagon administration may not be sufficient, and supplemental carbohydrates may need to be administered quickly, especially in children.

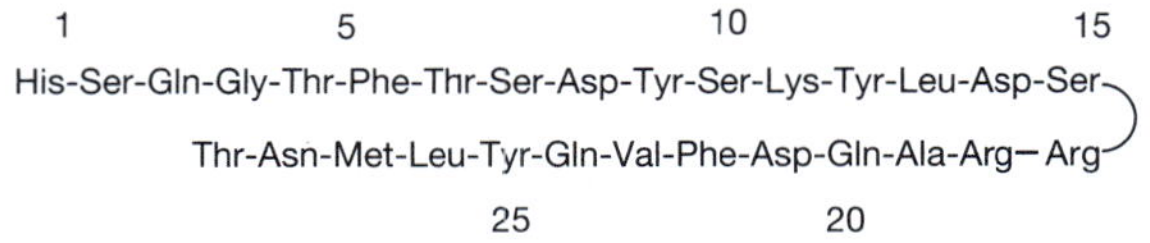

Amino acid sequence of glucagon

Pramlintide Acetate (SymlinPen). Pramlintide acetate is a synthetic analogue of amylin with Pro substitutions at amino acids 25, 28, and 29 (Fig. 38.6). These substitutions change its physical properties such that it can be formulated for SC injection. When pramlintide is used in combination with insulin, it slows gastric emptying, lowers blood glucose levels after meals, and affords a feeling of fullness that leads to decreased caloric intake and the potential for weight loss. Pramlintide has been approved for use in adults with T1D or T2D as an adjunct to insulin.[25]

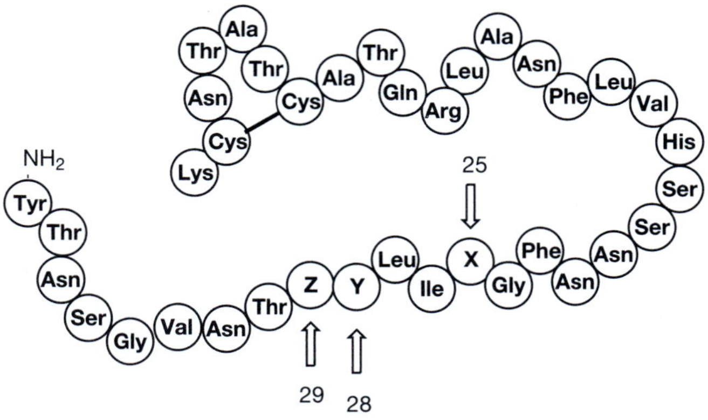

Amylin (human) X = Ala, Y = Z = Ser

Pramlintide (Symlin) X = Y = Z = Pro

Figure 38.6 Amino acid sequence of amylin and pramlintide.

Miscellaneous Peptidic Drugs

Specific Drugs

Linaclotide (Linzess). Linaclotide is a first-in-class, orally administered, locally acting, and minimally absorbed 14-amino acid peptide approved by the FDA in 2012 for the treatment of pain associated with irritable bowel syndrome accompanied by constipation (IBS-C) and for the treatment of chronic idiopathic constipation (CIC) (Fig. 38.7). Linaclotide achieves significant improvement in complete spontaneous bowel movements, abdominal pain, and other abdominal symptoms.

Linaclotide is a structural analogue of various naturally occurring guanylyl cyclase C (GC-C) agonists, including heat-stable bacterial enterotoxins produced by *E. coli*,

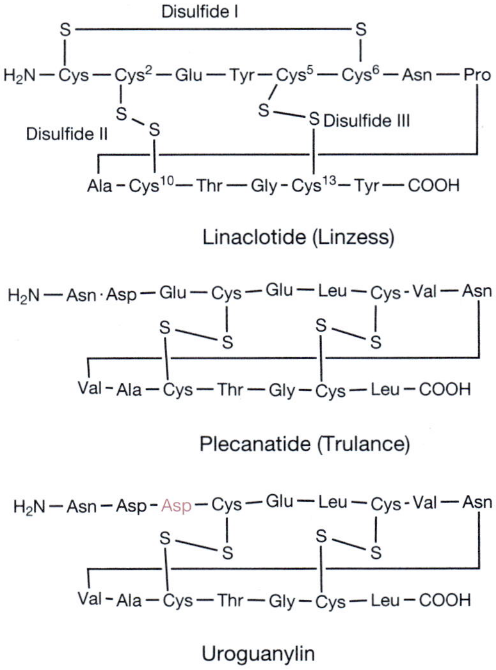

Figure 38.7 Amino acid sequences of guanylyl cyclase C agonists. Plecanatide contains Glu3 in place of Asp3 of uroguanylin.

Klebsiella spp., and *Yersinia enterocolitica*, which have the same 14-amino acid core, but in one case contains an additional pentapeptide sequence (Asn-Cys-Cys-Asn-Tyr-) attached to the N-terminal sequence of linaclotide. The heat-stable enterotoxins are responsible for the severe diarrhea produced by these organisms due to their agonist action at GC-C receptors. The intrachain disulfide bonds are required for activity, as well as for the reported stability toward acid and pepsin. Disulfide bonds II and III are essential for activity (see Fig. 38.7). Linaclotide is relatively stable to gastric acid and is metabolized by carboxypeptidase A to a 13-amino acid peptide with removal of the C-terminal Tyr to an active metabolite, while remaining stable to further metabolism by pepsin. Linaclotide and its active metabolite mimic the actions of the endogenous intestinal peptides guanylin (15 amino acids) and uroguanylin (16 amino acids) by activating GC-C on the intestinal epithelium. Activation of GC-C leads to increased intra- and extracellular levels of cyclic guanosine monophosphate (cGMP) and activation of the cystic fibrosis transmembrane conductance regulator (CFTR) ion channel, resulting in increased levels of bicarbonate, chloride ions, and water in the intestinal lumen and accelerated GI transit.

The most common adverse reactions include diarrhea, abdominal pain, flatulence, and abdominal distension. It carries a Boxed Warning for pediatric use and is contraindicated in pediatric patients up to the age of 6 years.[26-28]

PLECANATIDE (TRULANCE). Plecanatide is a newer GC-C agonist and the first uroguanylin analogue approved by the FDA in 2017 for the treatment of CIC (see Fig. 38.7).[27] It has also been used for the treatment of IBS-C. Although it is a peptidic drug, its site of action is in the upper GI tract, and thus, it is orally active. It has minimal systemic exposure upon oral administration and can be administered with or without food.

TEDUGLUTIDE (GATTEX). Teduglutide is a glucagon-like peptide-2 (GLP-2) agonist approved in 2012 for the treatment of adult patients with short-bowel syndrome (SBS) who are dependent on parenteral nutrition. SBS is a rare and potentially life-threatening condition in which nutrients are not properly absorbed because a large part of the small intestine is missing or has been surgically removed. GLP-2 is a 33-amino acid endogenous peptide hormone located at the carboxy terminus of proglucagon and secreted by intestinal enteroendocrine L-cells in the small and large intestines. GLP-2 helps compensate for a loss of absorptive and digestive capacity associated with SBS. Teduglutide was designed to be resistant to degradation by dipeptidyl peptidase IV (DPP-IV) by replacing Ala at position 2 of the N-terminus with Gly and is manufactured using rDNA technology.[28]

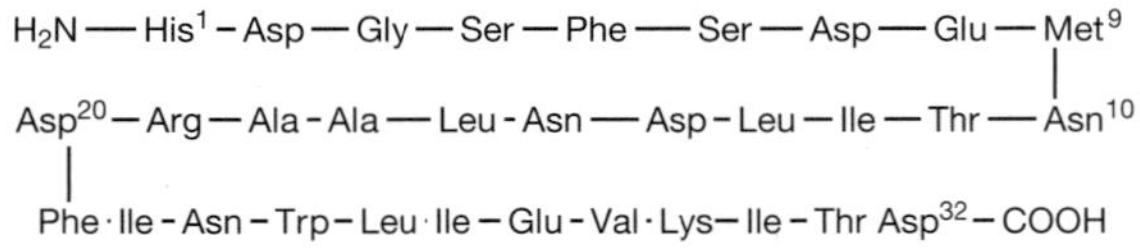

Teduglutide

PEGCETACOPLAN (EMPAVELI). Pegcetacoplan is a complement C3 inhibitor indicated for the treatment of adult patients with paroxysmal nocturnal hemoglobinuria (PNH). PNH is caused by mutations in the *phosphatidylinositol N-acetylglucosaminyltransferase subunit* A gene. Pegcetacoplan is a symmetrical molecule composed of two identical pentadecapeptides covalently bound to the ends of a linear 40-kDa PEG molecule. The peptide portions of pegcetacoplan contain 1-methyl-L-tryptophan (Trp9Me) in position 4 and amino(ethoxyethoxy)acetic acid (AEEA) in position 14.[29] Pegcetacoplan is derived from the compstatin family of structurally related cyclic peptides that disrupt the complement system at the proximal juncture.

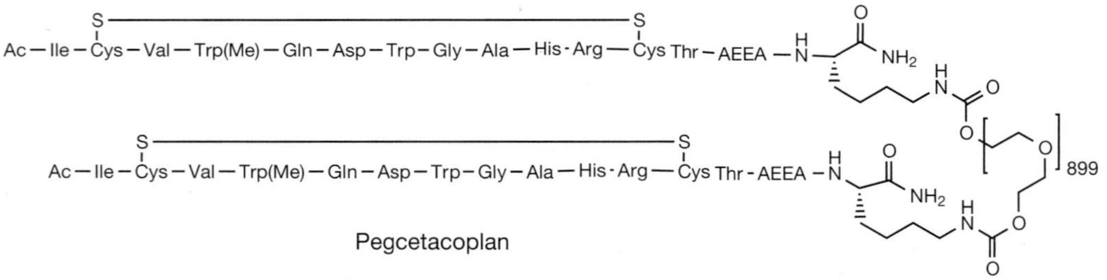

Pegcetacoplan

VOCLOSPORIN (LUPKYNIS). Voclosporin, a calcineurin-inhibitory immunosuppressant, is indicated in combination with a background immunosuppressive therapy regimen for the treatment of adult patients with active lupus nephritis (LN). LN is a common manifestation of systemic lupus erythematosus (SLE). About 40% of patients with SLE develop LN. Voclosporin is a cyclic undecapeptide that binds cyclophilin A in T cells and thereby inhibits calcineurin activity and exerts immunosuppressant activity.[30] Most common adverse effects include nephrotoxicity, hypertension, neurotoxicity, hyperkalemia, hypermagnesemia, diarrhea, headache, alopecia, and nausea.

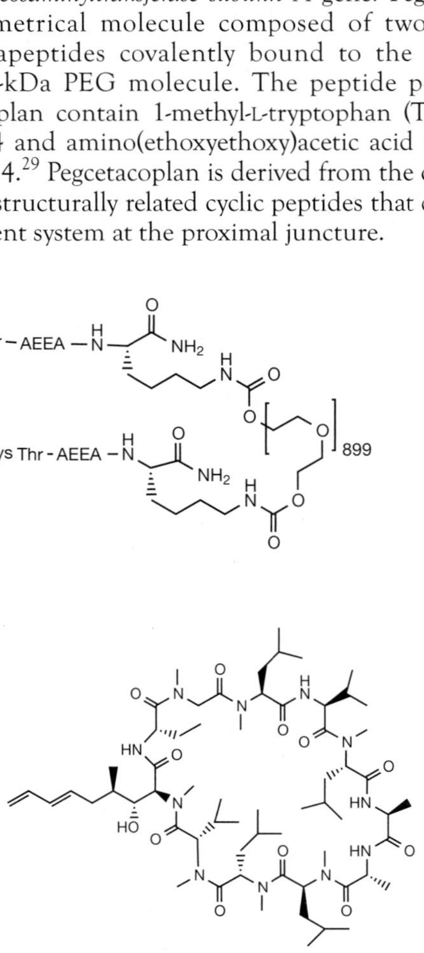

Voclosporin

TIRZEPATIDE (MOUNJARO, ZEPBOUND). Tirzepatide is a glucose-dependent insulinotropic polypeptide (GIP) receptor and glucagon-like peptide-1 (GLP-1) receptor agonist indicated as an adjunct to a reduced-calorie diet and increased physical activity for chronic weight management in adults. Gastric inhibitory polypeptide receptor (GIPR) agonists and glucagon-like peptide-1 receptor (GLP-1R) agonists synergistically improve insulin secretion and glycemic control and promote weight loss in patients with T2D patients. Structurally, tirzepatide is a 39-amino acid linear peptide composed of the bioreactive peptide sequence of GLP-1 and GIP attached to a C20 fatty di-acid that binds albumin and prolongs half-life.[31]

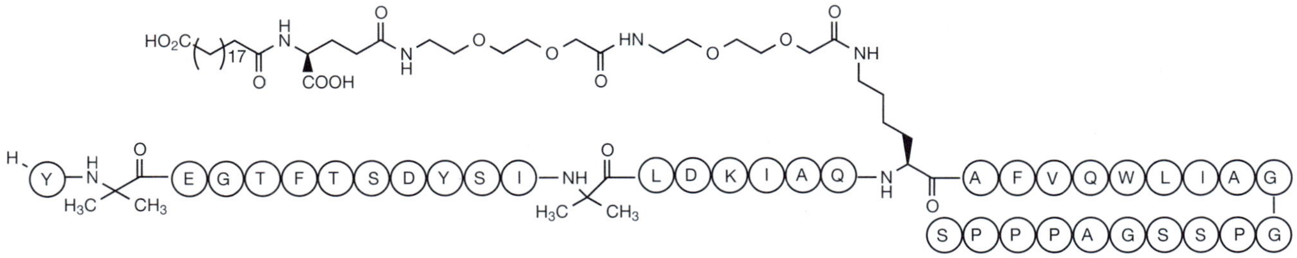

Tirzepatide

TERLIPRESSIN (TERLIVAZ). Terlipressin is a synthetic vasopressin receptor agonist indicated to improve kidney function in adults with hepatorenal syndrome, with rapid reduction in kidney function. It is a 12-amino acid peptide with the chemical name *N*-[*N*-(*N*-glycyl-glycyl)glycyl]-8-L-lysine vasopressin.[32] It differs from vasopressin in the substitution of lysine for arginine at position 8 of endogenous vasopressin and the addition of three glycyl residues at the amino terminus. Terlipressin has twice the selectivity for vasopressin V_1 receptors versus V_2 receptors. In addition to having pharmacologic activity on its own, terlipressin is converted by endopeptidases in vivo into the active lysine-vasopressin. Most common adverse effects include abdominal pain, nausea, respiratory failure, diarrhea, and dyspnea.

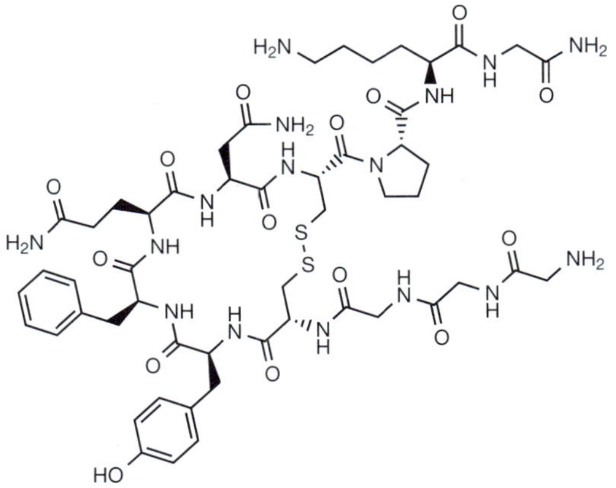

Terlipressin

SEMAGLUTIDE (OZEMPIC, WEGOVY, RYBELSUS). Since the discovery of the first GLP-1R agonist, exendin-4, a 39-amino acid peptide from saliva extracts of the Gila monster, and subsequent cloning of GLP-1R in 1992, there have been intense efforts to design GLP-1 receptor agonists. FDA approved the injectable drugs exenatide (Byetta) in 2005, dulaglutide (Trulicity) in 2014, and semaglutide (Ozempic) in 2017. Semaglutide is a GLP-1 analogue in which Lys26 is modified with a hydrophilic spacer and a C18 di-acid to enable once-weekly injection. It is available as an adjunct to diet and exercise to improve glycemic control in adults with T2D. As a group, GLP-1 agonists have transformed the T2D treatment, and more recently weight loss management. Innovation in GLP-1 therapy has continued, and a major outcome was the introduction of orally administered GLP-1R agonist drugs. Semaglutide, combined with the gastric absorption enhancer compound, sodium *N*-(8-[2-hydroxybenzoyl]amino)caprylate, is available as Rybelsus, for once-daily oral administration.[33]

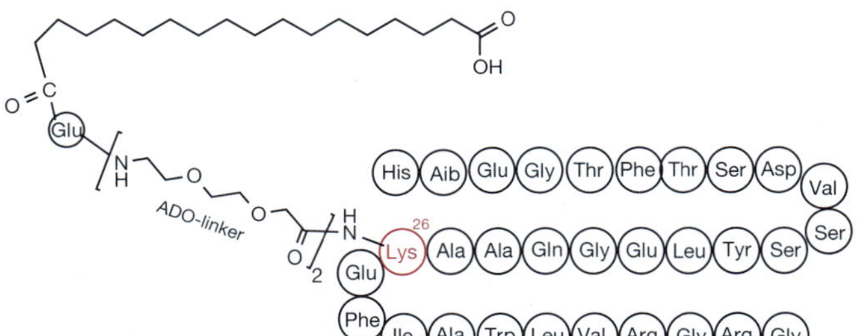

Semaglutide (Ozempic)

Enzymes

Tissue-Type Plasminogen Activator

The fibrinolytic system is activated in response to the presence of an intracellular thrombus or clot. The process of clot dissolution is initiated by the conversion of plasminogen to plasmin. Plasminogen activation is catalyzed by two endogenous and highly specific serine proteases, urokinase-type plasminogen activator and tissue-type plasminogen activator (t-PA).

The mature human t-PA (alteplase) is a glycoprotein consisting of a single chain of 527 amino acids. Its MW is approximately 70 kDa. Human t-PA contains 35 Cys residues assigned to 17 disulfide bonds. A serine protease domain of approximately 270 amino acids is located at the carboxy-terminal end of this protein. A fibronectin "finger" domain, two kringle domains, and an epidermal growth factor domain are also present. The t-PA protease domain is approximately 35% to 40% homologous with typical serine proteases, such as bovine trypsin and chymotrypsin.

Mammalian cells produce two t-PA variants of N-linked glycosylation, type 1 (at Asn117, 184, and 448) and type 2 (only at Asn117 and 448). The rate of fibrin-dependent plasminogen activation is 2- to 3-fold faster for type 2 compared with type 1. The complementary DNA (cDNA) obtained from a human melanoma cell line was expressed in Chinese hamster ovary (CHO) cells to achieve a glycosylated protein identical to the natural protein. Protein engineering studies have produced variant t-PA molecules with modified pharmacokinetics, affinity for fibrin, catalytic activity, and side effects.

Three rDNA thrombolytic agents are approved in the United States.[34] The first is alteplase, an enzyme equivalent to human t-PA. It is indicated for the treatment of acute myocardial infarction (administered as a bolus), acute massive pulmonary embolism (administered by IV infusion), and ischemic stroke. It is the first fibrin-selective thrombolytic agent preferentially activating fibrinogen bound to fibrin. Thus, the thrombolytic effect is localized to a blood clot and avoids systemic activation of fibrinogen, thereby preventing bleeding elsewhere in the body. Alteplase is rapidly cleared from circulating plasma, with 50% cleared within 5 minutes after termination of infusion.

The second agent, reteplase, is a recombinant, nonglycosylated deletion mutation of human t-PA containing 355 of 527 amino acids of native t-PA. The drug is indicated for acute myocardial infarction and is given as a 10 U + 10 U double bolus.

The most recent addition to the marketed rDNA-derived t-PAs is tenecteplase. This recombinant protein contains three modifications from natural human t-PA. In the kringle 1 domain of natural t-PA, Thr103 is replaced by Asn; the kringle 1 domain Asn117 is replaced by Gln; and in the protease domain, four amino acids (Lys, His, and two Arg residues) are replaced by four Ala residues. The drug is indicated for acute myocardial infarction. Bleeding at the injection site is similar to that with alteplase, but there is a reduction in noncerebral bleeding complications. It is administered as a single, 5-second bolus.

DNase—Dornase α (Pulmozyme)

According to the Cystic Fibrosis Foundation, cystic fibrosis (CF) is the most common fatal genetic disorder, afflicting approximately 30,000 patients in the United States. Breakthrough treatments have increased the median survival age to close to 40 years. Patients with CF develop thick mucus secretions and have severe, frequent lung infections. Studies during the 1950s and 1960s determined that CF-related secretions in the lungs contained large amounts of DNA. Mucous-thickening DNA release resulted from an inflammatory response and ensuing white blood cell death. The enzyme DNase I specifically cleaves extracellular DNA, such as that found in the mucous secretion of patients with CF and has no effect on the DNA of intact cells. The FDA has approved a recombinant human (rH) DNase.

The enzyme DNase I is a glycoprotein containing 260 amino acids with an approximate MW of 37 kDa. The recombinant protein is expressed by genetically engineered CHO cells encoding for the native enzyme, although DNase I was not purified or sequenced from human sources at the time. A degenerate sequence, based on the sequence of bovine DNase (263 amino acids), was used to synthesize probes, and screen a human pancreatic DNA library. The primary amino acid sequence of rhDNase is identical to native human DNase I.

The only FDA-approved DNase product, dornase α (inhalation solution), has been developed as a therapeutic agent for the management of CF. It is administered by nebulizer aerosol delivery systems.

Dornase α[35] is indicated for daily administration in conjunction with standard CF therapies to reduce the frequency of respiratory infections requiring parenteral antibiotics to improve pulmonary function. The breakdown of DNA in infected sputum results in improved airflow in the lung and reduced risk of bacterial infection. Although effective for the management of the respiratory symptoms of CF, dornase α is not a replacement for antibiotics, bronchodilators, and daily physical therapy. This product also finds application in treating chronic bronchitis.

Enzyme-Replacement Therapy

Enzyme-replacement therapy (ERT) is available for many of the lysosomal storage diseases, including Gaucher disease, Fabry disease, Pompe disease, mucopolysaccharidosis (MPS) type I (Hurler, Scheie, and Hurler/Scheie syndromes), MPS II (Hunter syndrome), and MPS VI (Maroteaux-Lamy syndrome).[36] The most frequent drug-related adverse events of ERT are infusion-related reactions (IRRs). Antibodies formed against infused enzymes are usually of the immunoglobulin G (IgG) serotype. Signs and symptoms of IRRs can include cutaneous reactions, pyrexia, headache, and hypertension. The precise relationship between antibody formation and occurrence of IRRs is unclear. Not all IRRs are antibody mediated, and not all patients who develop antibodies develop IRRs.[36]

Imiglucerase (Cerezyme)

Type 1 Gaucher disease, the most common form, is an inherited disorder. Fewer than 1 in 40,000 people in the general population have Gaucher disease. Patients with the disease lack the normal form of the enzyme glucocerebrosidase. They cannot break down glucocerebroside, leading to its accumulation within the lysosomes. This leads to the poor functioning of macrophages and an accumulation of "Gaucher cells" in the spleen, liver, and bone marrow. Imiglucerase is an analogue of glucocerebrosidase produced by rDNA technology using mammalian cell culture system. The drug is a monomeric glycoprotein consisting of 497 amino acids (MW ~60 kDa), with four N-linked glycosylation sites, and differs from the human placental glucocerebrosidase by one amino acid (His replaces Arg at position 495). Imiglucerase carries out the normal function of the missing enzyme and has been shown to be safe in long-term safety studies.[37]

Alglucosidase α (Lumizyme)

Pompe disease, a rare genetic disorder affecting nearly one in every 40,000 births, is caused by the mutation in a gene that makes the α-glucosidase enzyme. It was the first disease to be identified as a lysosomal storage disorder. α-Glucosidase enzyme is responsible for the breakdown of glycogen to glucose. The lack of degradation results in the accumulation of glycogen in lysosomes in all tissues, most notably in skeletal and cardiac muscles. The disease is characterized as early-onset or late-onset Pompe disease based on age at the time of onset. Severe α-glucosidase deficiency manifests during infancy with rapidly progressing muscle weakness, hypotonia, and cardiomyopathy and eventually lethal muscle disorder. As with other lysosomal storage disorders, ERT is the patient's only hope.

Alglucosidase α drug (Lumizyme) was approved by the FDA in 2010 for patients aged 8 years and older with late-onset (noninfantile) Pompe disease.[38] Alglucosidase α is an rH enzyme produced by transfected CHO cells as a 110-kDa precursor that targets lysosomes via the mannose-6-phosphate receptor. Following endocytosis, the enzyme is transformed to its mature 76-kDa form that restores glycogen processing and reverses accumulation. Alglucosidase α therapy has been shown to improve cardiac and muscle function.

Idursulfase (Elaprase)

MPS II (Hunter syndrome), a disease with an incidence of approximately 1 in 162,000 births, is caused by the deficiency of the lysosomal enzyme iduronate-2-sulfatase. This enzyme is responsible for a crucial step in the degradation of two glycosaminoglycans (GAGs), dermatan sulfate and heparin sulfate, in the lysosomes of various cells. Iduronate-2-sulfatase deficiency causes an accumulation of GAGs in tissue, and the patient's only recourse is ERT. The clinical manifestations of this deficiency are short stature, joint stiffness, harsh facial features, hepatosplenomegaly, and progressive intellectual disability. Recombinant iduronate-2-sulfatase has been available in the United States since 2006. It is produced from HT-1080 cells for proper translational attachment of N-linked oligosaccharides and the crucial mannose-6-phosphate groups as the targeting phosphate into lysosomes.[39] In addition to being fully glycosylated with eight mannose-6-phosphate groups, the enzyme possesses sialylated moieties that improve its stability in circulation. For full activity, Cys59 must undergo modification to formylglycine.

Cytokines

Cytokines communicate in a dynamic cellular network during an immune/inflammatory response to an antigen. Lymphokine and monokine are the terms used for a cytokine derived from lymphocytes and macrophages, respectively. Chemokines are a group of at least 25 structurally homologous, low-MW cytokines that stimulate leukocyte movement and regulate the migration of leukocytes from the blood to tissues. Cytokines, usually released and targeted to produce a localized effect, regulate the growth, differentiation, and activation of the hematopoietic cells responsible for the maintenance of the immune response. A wide array of glycoproteins, including interferons, interleukins (ILs), hematopoietic growth factors, and tumor necrosis factors (TNFs), are cytokines. Cytokines can only act on target cells that express receptors for that cytokine. There are five families of cytokine receptor proteins: class I cytokine receptors, class II cytokine receptors, TNF receptors, chemokine receptors, and immunoglobulin superfamily receptors (Table 38.1).[40]

Interferons

The interferons are a family of cytokines discovered in the late 1950s with broad-spectrum antiviral and potential anticancer activity, making them biologic response modifiers. Biotherapy (therapeutic use of any substance of biologic origin) of cancer is different than standard cytotoxic chemotherapy. That is, biotherapeutic agents belong to a group of compounds that enhance normal immune interactions (therefore, they are also immunomodulators) with cells in a specific or nonspecific fashion. Chemotherapeutics interact directly with the cancer cells themselves.

Three types of naturally occurring interferons have been found in small quantities: leukocyte interferon (IFN-α), produced by lymphocytes and macrophages; fibroblast interferon (IFN-β), produced by fibroblasts, epithelial cells, and macrophages; and immune interferon (IFN-γ), synthesized by $CD4^+$, $CD8^+$, and natural killer lymphocytes. Both IFN-α and IFN-β, also known as type I interferons, exhibit approximately 30% primary sequence homology but no structural similarity to IFN-γ, a type II interferon. All three are glycoproteins. Previously only available in low yields by chemical synthesis or isolation, several rDNA interferon pharmaceuticals now have been marketed in the United States, including three IFN-α products, two IFN-β agents, and an IFN-γ drug.

Interferon-Alpha. At least 24 different human genes producing 16 distinct mature IFN-α molecules with slight structural variations are known. Human IFN-α proteins generally are composed of either 165 or 166 amino acids.

Table 38.1 Five Families of Cytokine Receptors and Some Ligands

Receptor Families	Ligands
Class I cytokine receptors	IL-2, IL-7, IL-9, IL-11, IL-13, IL-15, GM-CSF, G-CSF
Class II cytokine receptors	INF-α, INF-β, INF-γ
Tumor necrosis factor receptors	TNF-α, TNF-β, CD30, CD40, FAS
Chemokine receptors	IL-8, RANTES, MIP-1, PF-4, MCAF
Immunoglobulin superfamily receptors	IL-1, M-CSF

G-CSF, granulocyte colony-stimulating factor; GM-CSF, granulocyte-macrophage colony-stimulating factor; IL-1, 2, 7, 8, 9, 11, 13, 15, interleukin 1, 2, 7, 8, 9, 11, 13, 15; INF-α, β, γ, interferon alpha, beta, gamma; MCAF, monocyte chemotactic and activating factor; M-CSF, macrophage colony-stimulating factor; TNF-α, β, tumor necrosis factor alpha, beta.

The two primary subtypes, IFN-α2a (Pegasys) and IFN-α2b (Ropeginterferon alfa-2b-njft), both contain 165 amino acids, differing only at position 23, with IFN-α2a containing an Lys residue and IFN-α2b an Arg residue at this position. Although cultures of genetically modified *E. coli* produce two recombinant FDA-approved IFN-α products, IFN-α2a and IFN-α2b, their method of purification differs. Purification of IFN-α2a includes affinity chromatography using a murine MAb, whereas that of IFN-α2b does not.

Interferon-alpha possesses complex antiviral, antineoplastic, and immunomodulating activities. Although the precise mechanism of action of IFN-α is not known, it is believed to interact with cell surface receptors to produce biologic effects. The actions appear to result from a complex cascade of biologic modulation and pharmacologic effects that include the modulation of host immune responses, cellular antiproliferative effects, cell differentiation, transcription, and translation processes, and reduction of oncogene expression. Interferon-alpha is filtered through the glomeruli in the kidney and undergoes rapid proteolytic degradation during tubular reabsorption.

Consensus Interferon (IFN Alfacon-1). Hepatitis C infection results in a chronic disease state in 50% to 70% of cases and is now the most important known cause of chronic liver disease. Following the acute phase, as many as 80% of patients may progress to the chronic phase of the infectious disease. An estimated 20% of patients with a chronic form of the disease progress to cirrhosis. The only agents shown to be effective in the treatment of hepatitis C are interferons. A unique recombinant molecule, a consensus IFN, known as IFN alfacon-1, has been approved for the treatment of chronic hepatitis C infection. It is a 19.5-kDa recombinant protein produced in *E. coli* and contains 166 amino acids in a relationship in which each amino acid position in the molecule contains the most commonly occurring amino acid among all the natural IFN-α subtypes. IFN alfacon-1 exhibits 5- to 10-fold higher biologic activity when compared to either IFN-α2a or IFN-α2b.

Interferon-Beta. Normally produced by fibroblasts, human IFN-β was first cloned and expressed in 1980; however, its instability made it unsuitable for clinical use. The more stable recombinant IFN-β1b (Betaseron), a 165-amino acid analogue of human IFN-β, differs from the native protein with a Ser residue substituted for Cys at position 17. The highly purified rDNA technology–derived product has an MW of 18.5 kDa. It is produced in a recombinant *E. coli*. Approved in 1993 by the FDA, IFN-β1b is indicated for the treatment of patients with exacerbating-remitting MS. A vial of recombinant IFN-β1b contains 0.3 mg of protein with dextrose and human albumin as stabilizers. The exact mechanism of action of IFN-β1b is not known. Its immunomodulating effects, however, may benefit patients with MS by decreasing the levels of endogenous IFN-γ. Levels of IFN-γ are believed to rise before and during acute attacks in patients with MS.

Whereas IFN-β1b of rDNA origin was the first to the market, IFN-β1a (Avonex, Rebif, Plegridy) also is now available. IFN-β1a is produced in mammalian cells and has the same amino acid sequence and carbohydrate side chain as natural IFN-β. Recombinant IFN-β1a is administered to patients once weekly by IM injection. This differs from the SC administration every other day of rDNA-produced IFN-β1b.

Interferon-Gamma. Human IFN-γ[41] is a single-chain glycoprotein with an MW of approximately 15.5 kDa. The cytokine mainly exists as a noncovalent dimer of differentially glycosylated chains in solution in vivo. Glycosylation does not appear to be necessary for biologic activity. The 140-amino acid IFN-γ1b (Actimmune) is produced by fermentation of a recombinant *E. coli*. IFN-γ1b was approved in 1990 by the FDA.

IFN-γ1b possesses biologic activity identical to the natural human IFN-γ derived from lymphoid cells. Although all the IFNs share certain biologic effects, IFN-γ differs distinctly from IFN-α and IFN-β by its potent capacity to activate phagocytes involved in host defense. These activating effects include the ability to enhance the production of toxic oxygen metabolites within phagocytes, resulting in a more efficient killing of various microorganisms. This activity is the basis for the use of IFN-γ1b in the management of chronic granulomatous disease. Chronic granulomatous disease is a group of rare X-linked or autosomal genetic disorders of the phagocytic oxygen metabolite–generating system, leaving patients susceptible to severe infections. The drug extends the time that patients spend without being hospitalized for infectious episodes. Investigational applications of IFN-γ include the treatment of renal cell carcinoma, small-cell lung cancer, infectious disease, trauma, atopic dermatitis, asthma, allergies, rheumatoid arthritis (RA), and venereal warts.[42]

Interleukins

ILs are cytokines involved in immune cell communication. Synthesized by monocytes, macrophages, and lymphocytes, ILs serve as soluble messengers between leukocytes. Currently, at least 18 ILs have been observed. One of the most studied cytokines is IL-2, originally called T-cell growth factor because of its ability to stimulate growth of T lymphocytes.

Interleukin 1. Interleukin 1 (IL-1) is a major inflammatory mediator and exists in two forms: IL-1α and IL-1β. Each form is a product of two separate genes, but the two are related to each other structurally at a three-dimensional level. IL-1β is a systemic, hormone-like mediator intended to be released from cells, whereas IL-1α is primarily a regulator of intracellular events and mediator of local inflammation. The recombinant protein anakinra, which is an IL-1 receptor antagonist, and the fusion protein rilonacept, which blocks the excessive IL-1β signaling, are commercially available, which are described in the next section.[43,44]

Anakinra (Kineret). RA is a chronic, inflammatory disease affecting synovial joints. Patients with persistent, active disease are traditionally treated with disease-modifying antirheumatic drugs (DMARDs). IL-1 receptor antagonist is an endogenous cytokine that blocks the binding of proinflammatory cytokine IL-1 to its receptor, thereby balancing the cartilage destruction and bone resorption mediated by IL-1.

Anakinra is the first rH IL-1 receptor antagonist and differs from the native human protein in that it is not glycosylated and has an additional N-terminal Met residue (rmetHuIL-1 receptor antagonist). Anakinra, a 17.3-kDa recombinant protein expressed in *E. coli*, was approved in 2001 for treating the signs and symptoms and the joint-destructive components of RA.[43-45] However, the challenge for anakinra for occupying the large number of IL-1 receptors is formidable, as these receptors are expressed on all cells except red blood cells (RBCs). Moreover, anakinra is rapidly excreted by the kidney, and blood levels are low after 24 hours. IL-1 receptors are also readily generated each day, necessitating a daily SC injection.

Rilonacept (Arcalyst). Cryopyrin-associated periodic syndromes are inherited disorders caused by mutations in the nucleotide-binding domain, leucine-rich family, pyrin domain-containing-3 (*NLRP-3*) gene, which encodes the protein cryopyrin. Cryopyrin regulates the protease caspase-1 and controls activation of IL-1β. Mutations in the *NLRP-3* (nucleotide-binding domain, leucine-rich family, pyrin domain-containing-3) gene can cause an overactive inflammasome, resulting in excessive levels of activated IL-1β, which causes inflammation, joint pain, rash or skin lesions, fever and chills, eye redness or pain, and fatigue. Rilonacept is a 252-kDa recombinant fusion protein produced in CHO cells and approved by the FDA in 2008 for the long-term treatment of familial cold autoinflammatory syndrome and Muckle-Wells syndrome. These two cryopyrin-associated periodic syndromes are extremely rare, affecting approximately 300 people in the United States.

Rilonacept's mechanism of intervention involves blockade of excessive IL-1β signaling.[43,44,46] Rilonacept combines the extracellular binding domains of the human IL-1 receptor component and IL-1 receptor accessory protein in a single chain, with two of these chains joined to the fragment crystallizable (Fc) portion of human IgG, creating a dimeric molecule. Rilonacept serves as an effective soluble IL-1β sink or trap, since the coupled receptor components bind IL-1β with higher affinity than either individual receptor. It exerts its effects through a multicomponent receptor system and is more effective than drugs that target only one of the components, such as the IL-1 receptor antagonist anakinra. With its weekly SC dosing regimen, rilonacept may have better patient compliance than anakinra.

Concomitant administration of other IL-1 blockers and anti-TNF-α agents has been associated with an increased risk of serious infection and neutropenia. Because IL-1 blockade may interfere with the immune response to infections, patients should not initiate rilonacept with an existing infection. Patients with chronic inflammation tend to have suppressed formation of CYP450 enzymes. Treatment with rilonacept is expected to normalize CYP450 distribution, so plasma levels of co-administered drugs that are CYP450 substrates with narrow therapeutic indexes should be carefully monitored for potential dose modification.

INTERLEUKIN-2. Human IL-2 is a 133-amino acid, 15.4-kDa protein that is O-glycosylated at a Thr in position 3. An intramolecular disulfide bond between Cys58 and Cys105 is essential for biologic activity. A recombinant version of IL-2 is marketed as aldesleukin, as described next.[47,48]

Aldesleukin (Proleukin). Aldesleukin differs from the native protein by the absence of glycosylation, a lack of the N-terminal Ala residue at position 1 (132 amino acids), and the replacement of Cys with Ser at position 125 of the primary sequence. Sequence changes were accomplished by site-directed mutagenesis to the IL-2 gene before cloning and expression. Aldesleukin exists as noncovalent microaggregates with an average size of 27 recombinant IL-2 molecules. The recombinant drug possesses the biologic activity of the native protein.

Aldesleukin is used in cancer biotherapy as a biologic response modifier for the treatment of metastatic renal cell carcinoma and metastatic melanoma. Side effects are the major dose-limiting factor because aldesleukin is an extremely toxic drug. Aldesleukin should be restricted to patients with normal cardiac and pulmonary functions and administered in a hospital setting under the supervision of a qualified physician experienced in the use of anticancer agents.

INTERLEUKIN-2 FUSION PROTEIN. Using ligation chemistry approaches during the preparation of recombinant proteins, researchers have created biologically active molecules that combine the activities of two individual proteins into "fusion molecules." These fusion technologies hold promise for developing custom molecules expressing a wide variety of dual activities.

Denileukin Diftitox-cxdl (Lymphir). Denileukin Diftitox (Ontak), a recombinant fusion protein of diphtheria toxin (DT) and human IL-2, was voluntarily withdrawn in 2014 due to manufacturing challenges. Consequently, Denileukin Diftitox-cxdl was developed using a refined manufacturing process that exhibited an increased percentage of protein monomer species and decreased levels of misfolded protein and protein aggregates.[49] The FDA has set a date of August 13, 2024, for approval to treat patients with relapsed or refractory cutaneous T-cell lymphoma (CTCL). CTCL is a general term for a group of low-grade, non-Hodgkin lymphomas (NHLs) affecting approximately 1,000 new patients per year. Malignant T cells manifest initially in the skin. Over time, there is systemic involvement. For many patients, CTCL is a persistent, disfiguring, and debilitating disease that requires multiple treatments. Malignant CTCL cells express one or more of the components of the IL-2 receptor. The fusion protein binds to IL-2 receptors on neoplastic T cells and is internalized via receptor-mediated endocytosis, delivering DT directly to kill the CTCL target. Men are twice as likely as women to have the disease.

Tumor Necrosis Factor

TNFs, a family of cytokines produced mainly by activated mononuclear phagocytes, have both beneficial and potentially harmful effects, mediating cytotoxic and inflammatory reactions. The TNFs are endogenous pyrogens capable of inducing chills, fever, and other flu-like symptoms. TNF-α, also called cachectin (and commonly referred to as TNF), and TNF-β, also called lymphotoxin, both bind to the same receptor and induce similar biologic activities. Biologic effects of TNF-α include selective toxicity against a range of tumor cells, mediation of septic shock, activation of elements of the immune system in response to Gram-negative bacteria, and induction/regulation of inflammation. rDNA-derived TNF-α has been studied extensively, but it has not been developed into a useful drug.

ETANERCEPT (ENBREL). Etanercept is an rDNA-produced fusion protein that binds specifically to TNF and blocks its interaction with cell surface TNF receptors.[50,51] It is indicated for the treatment of moderate-to-severe active RA in adults and for juvenile RA in patients who have had an inadequate response to one or more DMARDs. It is a genetically engineered protein that includes two components. The extracellular, ligand-binding portion (p75) of the human TNF receptor is linked as a fusion protein to the Fc portion of the human IgG1 antibody. Each etanercept molecule binds specifically to two TNF molecules found in the synovial fluid of patients with RA, blocking the interaction of TNF with the TNF receptor. The drug inhibits both TNF-α and TNF-β. The Fc portion of the fusion protein helps clear the etanercept-TNF complex from the body.

ABATACEPT (ORENCIA). With the recognition that T cells play a central role in the pathogenesis of RA, abatacept has been developed as a novel, rational approach to interfere with the upstream effector of inflammation. This drug has the potential to meet the needs of patients who fail to respond adequately to existing therapy using traditional DMARDs such as methotrexate (MTX) or TNF-blocking agents. Abatacept is a soluble 92-kDa human fusion protein approved for the treatment of RA as a new class of DMARDs.[52] Structurally, abatacept consists of a fusion between the extracellular domain of human cytotoxic T-lymphocyte–associated antigen-4 (CTLA-4) linked to the modified Fc portion of human IgG1. Abatacept selectively modulates the CD80/CD86:CD28 costimulatory signal required for full T-cell activation. By targeting the activation of T cells, an upstream event in the immune cascade that underlies RA, abatacept has the potential to impact multiple downstream aspects of RA immunogenesis, such as the production of cytokines, autoantibodies, and inflammatory proteins. The immunoglobulin portion of the abatacept serves as a handle to facilitate purification of the protein produced by rDNA technology in a mammalian cell expression system. It also enhances the solubility and serum half-life of the fusion protein. The serum half-life of 14.7 days is independent of dose, and rate of elimination remains constant, supporting the lack of antidrug antibody generation.

Abatacept was found to be well tolerated for up to 7 years of exposure in patients with RA who had an inadequate response to MTX or other traditional DMARDs or who failed to respond to treatment with anti-TNF agents.[53] The potential for increased risk of infection is an important safety concern in patients with RA receiving biologic therapies. During abatacept treatment, live vaccinations should be avoided because the drug may diminish the effectiveness of some immunizations, and anti-TNF agents should be avoided due to risk of infections.

Miscellaneous Fusion Protein

Fusion proteins are a novel class of biomolecules with multifunctional properties. They are obtained by fusing two or more protein domains together using a linker resulting in a fusion protein that may possess distinct functions derived from each of their component moieties. Several fusion protein drugs have been approved by the FDA and include TNF/Fc-IgG1 (Enbrel), IL-2/DT (Lymphir), cytotoxic T-lymphocyte antigen-4/Fc-IgG1 (Orencia), leukocyte function antigen-3/Fc-IgG1 (Amevive), IL-1 receptor extracellular domain/Fc-IgG1 (Arcalyst), and thrombopoietin/Fc-IgG1 (Nplate).[54]

Specific Drugs

TAGRAXOFUSP (ELZONRIS). Tagraxofusp, a CD123-directed cytotoxin, is a 57-kDa fusion protein composed of a rH IL-3 and truncated DT that inhibits protein synthesis and causes cell death in CD123-expressing cells.[55] It is constructed by rDNA technology and produced in *E. coli* cells. Tagraxofusp is approved for the treatment of blastic plasmacytoid dendritic cell neoplasm (BPDCN) in adults and in pediatric patients aged 2 years and older. CD123 is overexpressed on several types of hematologic cancer cells, including BPDCN cells, and expressed at a low level on normal hematopoietic cells, which makes it a suitable target for treatment. Upon binding to CD123, tagraxofusp is internalized, and the toxin payload is released which inhibits protein synthesis triggering apoptosis. Most common adverse reactions (incidence >30%) are capillary leak syndrome, nausea, fatigue, peripheral edema, pyrexia, and weight increase.

Hematopoietic Growth Factors

Hematopoiesis is the complex series of events involved in the formation, proliferation, differentiation, and activation of RBCs, white blood cells, and platelets. Hematopoietic growth factors are cytokines that regulate these events. Investigators have identified and cloned at least 20 factors, including IL-3 (or multi–colony-stimulating factor [CSF]), IL-4, IL-5, IL-6, IL-7, erythropoietin (EPO), granulocyte-macrophage colony-stimulating factor (GM-CSF), granulocyte colony-stimulating factor (G-CSF), macrophage colony-stimulating factor (M-CSF), and stem cell factor. Figure 38.8 summarizes the elaborate hematopoietic cascade. All blood cells originate within the bone marrow from a single class of pluripotent stem cells. In response to various external and internal stimuli, regulated by hematopoietic growth factors, stem cells give rise to additional new stem cells (self-renewal) and differentiate into mature, specialized blood cells.

ERYTHROPOIETIN—EPOETIN A (EPOGEN, PROCRIT). EPO,[56-58] a glycoprotein with an MW of 30 to 34 kDa produced by the kidney, stimulates the division and differentiation of erythroid progenitors in the bone marrow, increasing the production of RBCs. Epoetin α (sometimes called rH erythropoietin alfa [rHuEPO-α]), a recombinant EPO prepared from cultures of genetically engineered mammalian CHO cells, consists of the identical 165-amino acid sequence of endogenous EPO. The MW is approximately 30.4 kDa.

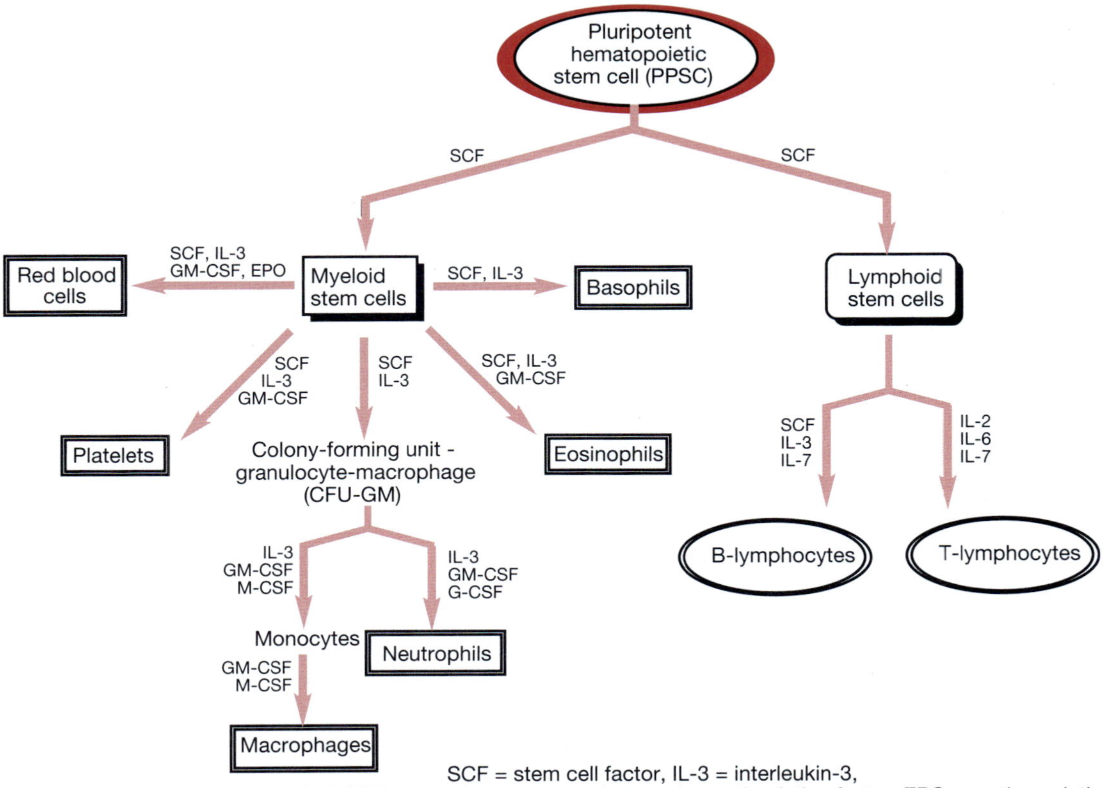

SCF = stem cell factor, IL-3 = interleukin-3,
GM-CSF = granulocyte-macrophage colony-stimulating factor, EPO = erythropoietin,
G-CSF = granulocyte colony-stimulating factor, M-CSF = macrophage colony-stimulating factor.

Figure 38.8 Schematic overview of hematopoiesis.

The protein contains two disulfide bonds (linking Cys residues 7 with 161 and 29 with 33) and four sites of glycosylation (one O-site and three N-sites); the disulfide bonds and glycosylation are necessary for the hormone's biologic activity. Deglycosylated natural EPO and bacterial-derived EPO (without glycosylation) have greatly decreased in vivo activity, although in vitro activity is largely conserved. The sugars may play a role in thermal stability or the prevention of aggregation in vivo.

The marketed products are formulated as a sterile, colorless, preservative-free liquid for IV or SC administration. Epoetin α is indicated for the treatment of various anemias. Epoetin α also represents a major scientific advance in the treatment of patients with chronic renal failure, serving as replacement therapy for inadequate production of endogenous EPO by failing kidneys. Epoetin α may decrease the need for infusions in dialysis patients. By several mechanisms related to elevating the erythroid progenitor cell pool, epoetin α increases the production of RBCs.

The manufacturer's full prescribing information should be consulted for dosing regimens because the dose is titrated individually to maintain the patient's target hematocrit. The circulating half-life is 4 to 13 hours in patients with chronic renal failure. Peak serum levels are achieved within 5 to 24 hours following SC administration.

Colony-Stimulating Factors. The CSFs are glycoprotein cytokines that promote progenitor proliferation, differentiation, and some functional activation. The name "colony-stimulating factor" results from the fact that these proteins often are assayed by their ability to stimulate the formation of cell colonies in bone marrow cultures. The names added to "CSF" reflect the types of cell colonies that arise in these assays.

Granulocyte Colony-Stimulating Factor—Filgrastim (Neupogen), Tbo-Filgrastim (Granix), Filgrastim-aafi (Nivestym), Filgrastim-ayow (Releuko), and Filgrastim-sndz (Zarxio). rDNA-derived G-CSF,[59-62] or filgrastim, was approved by the FDA in 1991 to decrease the incidence of infection in patients with nonmyeloid malignancies who are receiving myelosuppressive anticancer drugs. Filgrastim is a 175-amino acid, single-chain protein with an MW of 18.8 kDa. Filgrastim, produced by a recombinant bacterium, differs from the endogenous human protein by the addition of a Met at the N-terminus (recombinant methionyl G-CSF is sometimes called r-metHuG-CSF) and the lack of glycosylation. Glycosylation, however, does not appear to be necessary for biologic activity.

Filgrastrim is administered by IV infusion or by SC injection or infusion. The drug is rapidly absorbed, with peak serum concentrations reached in 4 to 5 hours. The elimination half-life is approximately 3.5 hours.

Filgrastim is selective for the neutrophil lineage type of white blood cells, whereas GM-CSF is multilineage, stimulating progenitors of neutrophils, monocytes, basophils, and eosinophils. The drug reduces the period of neutropenia, the number of infections, and the number of days the patient is on antibiotics. Filgrastim generally is well tolerated, with medullary bone pain being the most frequently encountered side effect.

Granulocyte-Macrophage Colony-Stimulating Factor —Sargramostim (Leukine). GM-CSF[59-62] has been produced by rDNA technology in the yeast *S. cerevisiae*. Sargramostim is a glycoprotein of 127 amino acids, differing from the endogenous human GM-CSF by substituting Leu at position 23. Also, the glycosylation pattern may differ from that of the native protein.

The various cellular responses such as division, maturation, and activation are induced through the binding of GM-CSF to specific receptors expressed on the surface of target cells.[63] On 2-hour IV infusion, the initial α half-life is 12-17 minutes, followed by a slower decrease (β half-life) of 2 hours.

Other Growth Factors

Becaplermin (Regranex). Growth factors are cytokines responsible for regulating cell proliferation, differentiation, and function. They act as intercellular signals. Each cell type's response is specific for each growth factor and differs from growth factor to growth factor. Platelet-derived growth factor (PDGF) is an endogenous growth-promoting protein that is released from cells involved in the healing process and is evident at the cell proliferation stage of a healing open wound. An rH PDGF B homodimer has been produced from genetically engineered *S. cerevisiae* cells. Becaplermin is the B-chain of the PDGF B protein. Thus, becaplermin is also referred to as rHPDGF-BB. The 25-kDa protein is formulated into a gel that mimics natural PDGF when applied to diabetic foot ulcers.

Clotting Factor VIIa, VIII, IX, XIIIa, and Anticoagulant. Factor VIIa, a recombinant product, is the activated form of factor VII used for the treatment of patients with hemophilia A or B. Antihemophilic factor, or factor VIII, is required for the transformation of prothrombin (factor II) to thrombin by the intrinsic clotting pathway. Hemophilia A, a lifelong bleeding disorder, results from a deficiency of factor VIII. Conventional biotherapy for the treatment of hemophilia A includes protein concentrates from human plasma collected by transfusion services or commercial organizations. Therefore, the concentrates may contain other native human proteins and microorganisms, such as viruses (eg, human immunodeficiency virus [HIV] and hepatitis) derived from infected blood.

Four versions of recombinant factor VIII that are highly purified and microorganism-free proteins are now available. All four therapeutic proteins are produced by the insertion of cDNA encoding for the entire factor VIII protein into mammalian cells. The mature, heavily glycosylated protein is composed of 2,332 amino acids (293 kDa) and contains sulfate groups. Stability of the large protein is a concern because of degradation by proteases. The products have proved to be safe and effective for reducing bleeding time in patients. There is the possibility, however, of induction of inhibitors in previously untreated patients.

Hemophilia B results when a patient is deficient in specific clotting factor IX. It affects men primarily and makes up approximately 15% of all hemophilia cases. An rH factor IX is now available.

Factor XIIIa, an active form of coagulation factor XIII, catalyzes the formation of γ-glutamyl-ε-lysine cross-links between fibrin units and, thus, increases the elasticity of the clot network. It is used for the treatment of bleeding disorders.

Surgeons have used medicinal leeches (*Hirudo medicinalis*) for years to prevent thrombosis in fine vessels of reattached digits. Hirudin is the potent, specific thrombin inhibitor isolated from the leech.

Monoclonal Antibody Therapeutic Agents

Hybridoma technology and advanced antibody engineering has led to the design of an increasing number of site-directed therapeutic agents for the treatment and prevention of transplant rejection, therapy in RA, treatment of NHL, and other indications. These products are examples of murine (eg, tositumomab), chimeric (eg, cetuximab), human (eg, panitumumab), and humanized (eg, trastuzumab) MAbs, and they represent significant advances in pharmacotherapy. Murine MAbs are derived from mice. Chimeric MAbs contain 65% to 90% human protein that is fused with the murine antibody variable region, which allows for functional complement activation and antibody-dependent cell-mediated cytotoxicity (ADCC) in humans. Variations of chimeric MAbs, such as partially humanized and de-immunized MAbs, are 95% human protein, and are composed of a few critical residues involved in the antigen-binding site from the murine antibody or modified murine variable domains containing nonimmunogenic amino acid sequences, respectively. To prevent any human anti-mouse antibody (HAMA) response, fully humanized MAbs containing only human protein sequences have been developed from mice that have had human immunoglobulin genes placed in their genome.

Therapeutic MAbs (see Table 38.2) can be divided into three main classes, based on their mechanism of action: (1) MAbs as directed targeted therapy; these MAbs either block or stimulate a particular cell membrane molecule (eg, growth factor signal receptor) or ligand (vascular endothelial growth factor [VEGF]), thereby inhibiting tumor growth or activating effector cells; (2) cytotoxicity by chaperoning cytotoxic molecules (immunoconjugates); these MAbs are conjugated to various cytotoxic molecules/atoms including chemotherapeutic drugs, radioisotopes such as yttrium-90, cellular toxins such as DT, or biologic agents such as IFN; and (3) modulating an immunologic mechanism; these MAbs exert their cytotoxic effects by ADCC or complement-dependent cytotoxicity.

Specific Drugs

Trastuzumab (Herceptin, Trazimera, Kanjinti, Ogivri, Ontruzant). Advances in the understanding of tumor pathobiology and molecular biology have facilitated the development of targeted therapies in breast cancer. ErbB2

Table 38.2 US Food and Drug Administration–Approved Monoclonal Antibody (MAb) Therapeutic Agents

Generic Name	Trade Name	MAb Type	Indication
Adalimumab	Humira	Fully human	Rheumatoid arthritis
Aducanumab	Aduhelm	Fully human	Alzheimer disease
Alemtuzumab	Campath	Humanized	B-cell chronic lymphocytic leukemia
Amivantamab	Rybrevant	Fully human	Anticancer
Anifrolumab	Saphnelo	Fully human	Systemic lupus erythematosus (SLE)
Ansuvimab	Ebanga	Fully human	Ebola virus infection
Atezolizumab	Tecentriq	Humanized	Urothelial carcinoma (PD-1/PD-L1 inhibitor)
Avelumab	Bavencio	Fully human	PD-1/PD-L1 inhibitor approved for metastatic Merkel cell carcinoma
Basiliximab	Simulect	Chimeric	Prevention of transplant rejection
Belimumab	Benlysta	Fully human	SLE plus standard therapy
Benralizumab	Fasenra	Humanized	Asthma
Bevacizumab	Avastin	Humanized	Metastatic colorectal cancer
Bezlotoxumab	Zinplava	Fully human	Prevent *Clostridioides difficile* reinfection (CDI)
Blinatumomab	Blincyto	Mouse	Acute lymphoblastic leukemia (ALL)
Brodalumab	Siliq	Fully human	Moderate-to-severe plaque psoriasis
Brolucizumab	Beovu	Humanized	Wet macular degeneration, humanized single chain antibody
Burosumab	Crysvita	Fully human	X-linked hypophosphatemia
Canakinumab	Ilaris	Fully human	Cryopyrin-associated periodic syndromes and Muckle-Wells syndrome
Cemiplimab	Libtayo	Humanized	Anticancer (metastatic or locally advanced cutaneous squamous cell carcinoma)
Certolizumab pegol	Cimzia	Humanized	Crohn disease
Cetuximab	Erbitux	Chimeric	Colorectal cancer
Crizanlizumab	Adakveo	Humanized	Sickle cell disease
Daratumumab	Darzalex	Fully human	Multiple myeloma (IgG1κ)
Denosumab	Prolia	Fully human	Postmenopausal osteoporosis
Dinutuximab	Unituxin	Chimeric	Neuroblastoma
Donanemab	Kisunla	Humanized	Alzheimer disease
Dostarlimab	Jemperli	Humanized	Endometrial anticancer
Dupilumab	Dupixent	Humanized	Severe atopic dermatitis (eczema)
Durvalumab	Imfinzi	Humanized	Locally advanced or metastatic urothelial carcinoma
Eculizumab	Soliris	Fully human	Paroxysmal nocturnal hemoglobinuria
Elotuzumab	Empliciti	Humanized	Multiple myeloma
Emicizumab	Hemlibra	Humanized	Hemophilia A
Eptinezumab	Vyepti	Humanized	Migraine prevention
Erenumab	Aimovig	Fully human	Migraine prevention

(continued)

Table 38.2 US Food and Drug Administration–Approved Monoclonal Antibody (MAb) Therapeutic Agents (*continued*)

Generic Name	Trade Name	MAb Type	Indication
Etanercept	Enbrel	Fusion MAb	Rheumatoid and psoriatic arthritis and ankylosing spondylitis
Evinacumab	Evkeeza	Fully human	Homozygous familial hypercholesterolemia
Evolocumab	Repatha	Fully human	Hypercholesterolemia
Faricimab	Vabysmo	Fully human	Wet age-related macular degeneration and diabetic macular edema
Fremanezumab	Ajovy	Humanized	Migraine prevention
Galcanezumab	Emgality	Humanized	Migraine prevention
Gemtuzumab	Mylotarg	Fusion MAb	Treatment of CD33-positive acute myeloid leukemia
Golimumab	Simponi	Fully human	Rheumatoid and psoriatic arthritis and ankylosing spondylitis
Guselkumab	Tremfya	Humanized	Psoriasis
Ibalizumab	Trogarzo	Humanized	HIV-1 infection
Ibritumomab tiuxetan	Zevalin	Murine	Non-Hodgkin lymphoma
Idarucizumab	Praxbind	Humanized	Reverses anticoagulant effects of dabigatran
Inebilizumab	Uplizna	Humanized	Neuromyelitis optica spectrum disorder
Infliximab	Remicade	Chimeric	Crohn disease
Ipilimumab	Yervoy	Fully human	Late-stage melanoma
Isatuximab	Sarclisa	Humanized	Multiple myeloma
Ixekizumab	Taltz	Humanized	Moderate to severe plaque psoriasis
Lanadelumab	Takhzyro	Fully human	Hereditary angioedema
Lecanemab	Leqembi	Humanized	Alzheimer disease
Margetuximab	Margenza	Chimeric	HER2-positive breast cancer
Mepolizumab	Nucala	Humanized	Severe eosinophilic asthma
Mosunetuzumab	Lunsumio	Fully human	Relapsed or refractory follicular lymphoma
Natalizumab	Tysabri	Humanized	Multiple sclerosis
Naxitamab	Danyelza	Humanized	Neuroblastoma
Necitumumab	Portrazza	Fully human	Metastatic squamous non–small-cell lung cancer (NSCLC)
Nivolumab	Opdivo	Fully human	Metastatic melanoma and NSCLC
Nivolumab and Relatlimab	Opdualag	Fully human	Unresectable or metastatic melanoma
Obiltoxaximab	Anthim	Chimeric	Inhalational anthrax (in combination with appropriate antibacterial drugs)
Obinutuzumab	Gazyva	Humanized	Chronic lymphocytic leukemia (in combination with chlorambucil)
Ocrelizumab	Ocrevus	Humanized	Multiple sclerosis
Ofatumumab	Arzerra	Fully human	Chronic lymphocytic leukemia
Palivizumab	Synagis	Humanized	Respiratory syncytial virus prophylaxis
Panitumumab	Vectibix	Fully human	First- or second-line treatment of metastatic colorectal cancer
Pembrolizumab	Keytruda	Humanized	Advanced or unresectable melanoma and treatment of non–small-cell lung cancer

Table 38.2 US Food and Drug Administration–Approved Monoclonal Antibody (MAb) Therapeutic Agents (*continued*)

Generic Name	Trade Name	MAb Type	Indication
Pertuzumab	Perjeta	Humanized	HER2-positive metastatic breast cancer
Ramucirumab	Cyramza	Fully human	Advanced or metastatic stomach or gastroesophageal junction cancer
Ranibizumab	Lucentis	Fully human	Neovascular age-related macular degeneration
Ravulizumab	Ultomiris	Humanized	Antianemic
REGN-EB3	Inmazeb	Fully human	Ebola virus infection; cocktail of three fully human MAbs
Reslizumab	Cinqair	Humanized	Maintenance treatment of severe asthma
Rituximab	Rituxan	Chimeric	B-cell non-Hodgkin lymphoma
Romosozumab	Evenity	Humanized	Musculoskeletal disease, osteoporosis
Sarilumab	Kevzara	Fully human	Rheumatoid arthritis
Secukinumab	Cosentyx	Fully human	Rheumatoid arthritis, ankylosing spondylitis, plaque psoriasis
Siltuximab	Sylvant	Chimeric	Multicentric Castleman disease (MCD) patients who are HIV negative
Spesolimab	Spevigo	Humanized	Generalized postular psoriasis
Sutimlimab	Enjaymo	Humanized	Cold agglutinin disease
Tafasitamab	Monjuvi	Humanized	Relapsed or refractory diffuse large B-cell lymphoma
Teclistamab	Tecvayli	Humanized	Relapsed and refractory multiple myeloma
Teplizumab	Tzield	Humanized	Type 1 diabetes
Teprotumumab	Tepezza	Humanized	Thyroid eye disease
Tezepelumab	Tezspire	Fully human	Asthma
Tildrakizumab	Ilumya	Humanized	Psoriasis
Tralokinumab	Adbry	Fully human	Atopic dermatitis
Trastuzumab	Herceptin	Humanized	Refractory breast cancer
Tremelimumab	Imjudo	Fully human	Unresectable hepatocellular carcinoma
Ublituximab	Briumvi	Chimeric	Relapsing multiple sclerosis
Ustekinumab	Stelara	Fully human	Moderate to severe psoriasis
Vedolizumab	Entyvio	Humanized	Moderate to severe ulcerative colitis or Crohn disease

HER-2, human epidermal growth factor receptor 2; PD-1, programmed cell death protein 1; PD-L1, programmed death-ligand 1; PD-L2, programmed death-ligand 2.

(or human epidermal growth factor receptor 2 [HER2]) is a transmembrane tyrosine kinase receptor that belongs to the epidermal growth factor receptor (EGFR) family. HER2 protein overexpression is observed in approximately 30% of primary breast cancers. Activated erbB2s stimulate many intracellular signaling pathways, mainly the mitogen-activated protein kinase (MAPK) and the phosphatidylinositol 3-kinase (PI3K)-Akt pathways. In 1998, trastuzumab was approved by the FDA for clinical use largely based on a randomized clinical trial that compared cytotoxic chemotherapy alone with chemotherapy plus trastuzumab as a front-line treatment for patients with erbB2-overexpressing metastatic breast cancer.[64]

Trastuzumab is a recombinant humanized anti-erbB2 MAb that binds the extracellular domain of the erbB2 receptor and blocks intracellular signaling. Both cytostatic and cytotoxic mechanisms of action of trastuzumab were identified in preclinical studies. In vitro, downregulation of erbB2 disrupts receptor dimerization and signaling through the downstream PI3K cascade. It effectively prevents cell proliferation of the erbB2-overexpressing breast cancer SK-BR-3 cell line.

Trastuzumab is administered as single agent in women with erbB2-overexpressing metastatic breast cancer, including those who have progressed after chemotherapy.[64]

Bevacizumab (Avastin, Mvasi, Zirabev, Alymsys, Vegzelma). Angiogenesis, the process of developing new blood vessels from existing ones, is critical for tumor cell growth, survival, invasion, and metastasis. Numerous growth factors work in the tumor microenvironment to promote angiogenesis. Of these, VEGF may be among the most important, based on its specificity as an endothelial cell mitogen and the ability of many tumor types to produce it in physiologically relevant quantities. Oncogenic activation, loss of tumor suppressor factors, and tumor hypoxia lead to the upregulation of VEGF production. There are four isoforms of VEGF (A, B, C, and D) and three types of VEGF receptors (VEGFRs). Once produced, VEGF-A binds to two tyrosine kinase receptors, termed VEGFR-1 and VEGFR-2, which are predominantly located on the surface of vascular endothelial cells. VEGFR-2 appears to be the more important of the two receptors for mediating the angiogenic effects of VEGF, whereas VEGFR-1 may be a decoy receptor that modulates the amount of VEGF available for binding to VEGFR-2. VEGF and its receptors have emerged as anticancer targets based on their central and specific role in angiogenesis. In principle, VEGF-targeted therapy may inhibit tumor growth by blocking new vessel growth. Bevacizumab was approved in 2004 for the treatment of metastatic colorectal cancer in combination with fluorouracil-based chemotherapy.[65]

Bevacizumab, a 149-kDa recombinant humanized monoclonal IgG1 antibody (93% human, 7% murine sequences) directed against VEGF-A, is believed to globally prevent the binding of all VEGF isoforms to all VEGFRs. Bevacizumab is composed of two identical light chains (214 amino acids) and two heavy chains (453 amino acids) and is produced in a CHO cell expression system.[65] It carries a Boxed Warning for GI perforation, surgery and wound healing complications, and hemorrhage.

Panitumumab (Vectibix). EGFR, a transmembrane cell surface glycoprotein belonging to the subfamily of type I tyrosine kinase receptors, is overexpressed in certain human cancers, including colon and rectum cancers. The binding of ligands such as EGF and transforming growth factor-α to EGFR triggers autophosphorylation and internalization of EGFR, thereby activating various signaling pathways involved in proliferation, angiogenesis, inhibition of apoptosis, and metastasis.

Panitumumab is a 147-kDa recombinant, fully human IgG2 anti-EGFR MAb produced in genetically engineered mammalian CHO cells. Panitumumab was discovered using Abgenix's XenoMouse technology and was approved by the FDA in 2006.[66] Proposed mechanisms explaining the antitumor activity of panitumumab include downregulation of EGFR expression resulting from receptor internalization, induction of apoptosis via inhibition of EGFR signaling pathways and induction of cell cycle arrest, induction of autophagy, and inhibition of angiogenesis.

Panitumumab is used in combination with chemotherapy for the treatment of metastatic colorectal cancer or as monotherapy for the treatment of chemotherapy-refractory metastatic colorectal cancer in patients with wild-type rather than mutant *K-ras* tumors. *K-ras* protein is a membrane-bound G protein and is activated by receptor tyrosine kinases and is found to be mutated in 30% to 40% of colorectal cancer patients.[67,68] Panitumumab has an acceptable tolerability profile when administered as monotherapy or in combination with chemotherapy. It is associated with dermatologic toxicity, which is a characteristic of EGFR inhibitors.

Ofatumumab (Arzerra, Kesimpta). Chronic lymphocytic leukemia (CLL) is the most common adult leukemia and one of the most common malignant lymphoid diseases. Based on American Cancer Society's 2024 estimates, leukemia accounts for approximately 63,000 new cases and more than 23,000 deaths in the United States. CLL accounts for approximately 21,000 new cases with more than 4,400 deaths. CLL cells are malignant B cells that have low surface expression levels of CD20 molecules. B cells normally protect the body from invading pathogens by developing into plasma cells, which make antibodies. These antibodies directly inactivate pathogens or attach to pathogens to prepare them for destruction by other white blood cells. Ofatumumab received accelerated approval in 2009 for the treatment of patients with CLL refractory to fludarabine and alemtuzumab.

Ofatumumab is a fully human 149-kDa IgG1κ anti-CD20 MAb generated via transgenic mouse and hybridoma technology and is produced in a recombinant murine cell line (NS0), using standard mammalian cell culture and purification technologies.[69] Ofatumumab binds specifically to both the small and large extracellular loops of the CD20 molecule. Ofatumumab is highly potent in lysing B cells, which is presumably due to its binding to the membrane-proximal, small extracellular loop of the target CD20 protein and its slow release from the target molecule.[70] As with other human MAbs, ofatumumab induces both ADCC and complement-dependent cytotoxicity. It carries a boxed warning for severe allergic reactions and/or anaphylaxis and prolonged and severe cytopenia.

Ibritumomab Tiuxetan (Zevalin). Radioimmuno-therapy is an innovative form of cancer therapy, combining an MAb against a specific target antigen with a source of radiation such as a radioisotope. Technical advances have made it possible to link radionuclides such as yttrium-90 (^{90}Y) to MAbs specifically to target radiation to lymphoma cells. Yttrium-90 is a β-emitting radionuclide that delivers 90% of its radiation (2.3 MeV) over a mean path length of 5 mm and has a half-life of 64 hours. These characteristics are particularly advantageous for treating bulky, poorly vascularized tumors and tumors with heterogeneous antigen expression. Ibritumomab tiuxetan therapeutic regimen became the first radioimmunotherapy approved by the FDA in 2002 for the treatment of NHL. Based on American Cancer Society's 2024 estimates, more than 80,000 new cases of NHL will be diagnosed in the United States and will account for nearly 21,000 deaths.

Ibritumomab tiuxetan, a 148-kDa radioimmunoconjugate, is a short-course therapy that uses immunobiologic and radiolytic mechanisms of action to destroy both dividing and nondividing tumor cells. Ibritumomab is a murine IgG1κ MAb produced in CHO cells. It is directed against the CD20 antigen found on the surface of malignant B lymphocytes in patients with B-cell NHL, as well as on normal mature B lymphocytes. Tiuxetan, *N*-{2-[Bis(carboxymethyl)amino]-3-(4-isothiocyanatophenyl)propyl}-*N*-{2-[bis(carboxymethyl)amino]propyl}glycine, forms a stable covalent thiourea-type linkage with the Lys and Arg residues of the antibody and can chelate a radionuclide via its carboxyl groups (Fig. 38.9). Ibritumomab tiuxetan can chelate indium-111 (^{111}In) for imaging or ^{90}Y for therapy. Thus, the antibody specifically targets radiation to CD20-positive cells while sparing normal nonlymphoid cells.

Ibritumomab tiuxetan is indicated for the treatment of patients with relapsed or refractory, low-grade, follicular, or transformed B-cell NHL, including patients with rituximab-refractory follicular NHL. After ^{90}Y Zevalin enters the bloodstream, the MAb ibritumomab recognizes and attaches to the CD20 antigen, allowing β radiation emitted by the ^{90}Y isotope to penetrate and damage the B cell, as well as neighboring cells.[71] It carries a Boxed Warning of acute infusion reactions, severe cutaneous and mucocutaneous reactions, and prolonged and severe cytopenia.

Canakinumab (Ilaris). Canakinumab was approved in 2009 for the treatment of cryopyrin-associated periodic syndromes, known as familial cold autoinflammatory syndrome and Muckle-Wells syndrome, in patients 4 years of age and older. The two syndromes are serious inherited autoimmune inflammatory disorders that are believed to result from cryopyrin-activated overproduction of IL-1β.

Canakinumab is a 150 kDa, fully human, IgG1 anti–IL-1β MAb produced in mouse hybridoma Sp2/0-Ag14 cell line by rDNA technology.[72] Compared to other drugs targeting IL-1β, such as anakinra and rilonacept, canakinumab possesses a less frequent dosing regimen and instigates fewer injection-site reactions. Because IL-1β suppression can hinder the immune response, the labeling recommends that patients receive all recommended vaccinations before starting canakinumab therapy. No live vaccines should be administered during treatment with canakinumab, and patients should be tested for latent tuberculosis before receiving the drug. Similar to rilonacept, the labeling warns against the concomitant administration of canakinumab and TNF inhibitors, and therapeutic monitoring is recommended with concurrent administration of drugs that interact with the CYP450 system.

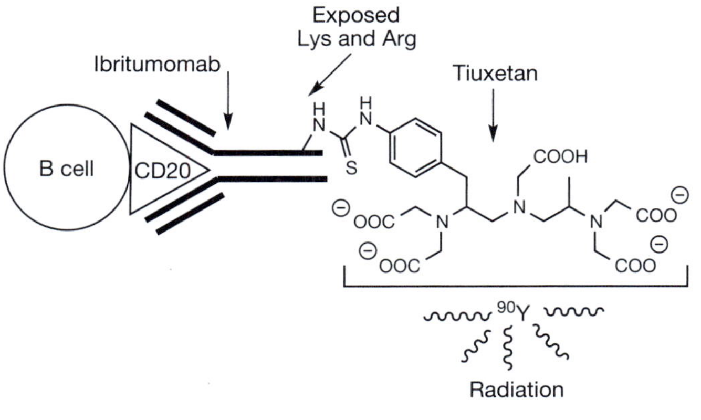

Figure 38.9 Structure of ibritumomab tiuxetan radioimmunoconjugate monoclonal antibody (MAb) and its binding to the target CD20 on the surface of the B cell.

Certolizumab Pegol (Cimzia). Crohn disease is an immunologically mediated chronic relapsing inflammatory bowel disease that can potentially affect the entire GI tract, but most commonly occurs in the terminal ileum and colon. Active Crohn disease is associated with excessive levels of proinflammatory cytokines, including TNF-α. The incidence is on the rise in both developing and developed countries, with the rate in North America among the highest at 6 to 23 cases per 100,000 person-years.[73]

Certolizumab pegol is a TNF-α blocker approved for the treatment of moderate-to-severe Crohn disease.[74,75] It is specifically indicated for reducing signs and symptoms and maintaining clinical response in adult patients who have had an inadequate response to conventional therapy. Certolizumab pegol is a 91-kDa humanized antibody fragment antigen-binding (Fab) that is manufactured in *E. coli*, purified, and conjugated to PEG. The addition of the PEG moiety significantly enhances the plasma half-life of the antibody, allowing for less frequent dosing.

Certolizumab is the third anti-TNF-α biologic to be marketed for Crohn disease behind infliximab and adalimumab, and it has a higher affinity than either of these drugs for TNF-α. Unlike the full-length infliximab and adalimumab antibodies, certolizumab pegol does not contain an Fc region and, therefore, does not induce complement activation, antibody-dependent cellular cytotoxicity, or apoptosis in vitro. As with other TNF-α inhibitors, the drug is associated with an increased risk of opportunistic infections and malignancy, and it carries a Boxed Warning for the risk of serious infections such as histoplasmosis.

Golimumab (Simponi). The proinflammatory cytokine TNF-α has been implicated as the primary mediator of articular inflammation in diseases such as RA, psoriatic arthritis, and ankylosing spondylitis. Targeting TNF-α has been a successful strategy in the intervention of a range of immunoinflammatory disorders. Golimumab is a 150-kDa, fully human, IgG1 anti-TNF MAb produced in murine Sp2/0 cell line. It was approved by the FDA in 2009.[76] Golimumab binds to both soluble and transmembrane forms of TNF-α, is the first once-monthly SC agent to enter the market, and is currently approved for the treatment of RA and psoriatic arthritis in combination with MTX and for treatment of ankylosing spondylitis. The drug is administered as an SC injection once a month. Live vaccines should not be administered while being treated with golimumab. The drug carries a Boxed Warning regarding the risk of serious infections including tuberculosis and invasive fungal infections, such as histoplasmosis. Furthermore, patients are also warned that lymphoma and other malignancies, some fatal, have been reported in children and adolescent patients treated with TNF blockers.

Eculizumab (Soliris). PNH is a clonal hematopoietic stem cell disorder that is characterized by the production of abnormal RBCs. Eculizumab, a fully humanized anti-CD5 MAb with an approximate MW of 148 kDa, is used for the treatment of patients with PNH to reduce hemolysis.[77,78] It is the first therapy to be introduced for this rare and life-threatening form of hemolytic anemia. Eculizumab is effective in controlling serum hemolytic activity and has been granted orphan drug status from both the FDA and European regulatory agencies. The drug carries a Boxed Warning for the potential increased risk of meningococcal infections and requires patients to receive a meningococcal vaccine at least 2 weeks prior to receiving the first dose of eculizumab.

Denosumab (Prolia, Xgeva). Osteoporosis is a chronic, debilitating disease in which the bones become porous and break easily. Approximately 10 million people in the United States are estimated to have osteoporosis, and almost 43 million Americans are estimated to have low bone mass, placing them at increased risk for osteoporosis.[79] Receptor activator of nuclear factor-κB ligand (RANKL) is a protein expressed by osteoblasts and bone-lining cells that bind to receptor activator of nuclear factor-κB (RANK) receptors on osteoclast and osteoclast precursors. The RANKL/RANK complex stimulates osteoclast precursors to mature to osteoclasts and increases osteoclast activity on bone resorption. After menopause, as estrogen levels drop, RANKL levels increase. Denosumab, a 147-kDa fully human MAb produced in genetically engineered mammalian CHO cells, is specific for RANKL and was approved by the FDA in 2010 for the treatment of postmenopausal osteoporosis in women (see Chapter 27). By inhibiting RANKL, denosumab inhibits osteoclast-mediated bone resorption. Denosumab has been shown to increase bone mineral density and decrease fracture risk in postmenopausal women with osteoporosis.

Blinatumomab (Blincyto). Blinatumomab is a constructed MAb approved in 2014 for the treatment of acute lymphoblastic leukemia (ALL) in patients with Philadelphia chromosome–negative B-cell precursor ALL (Fig. 38.10). It is a bioengineered bispecific T-cell engaging (BiTE) antibody, which is expected to engage polyclonal T cells and CD19-expressing B cells common in most cases of ALL. It is responsible for bringing T cells close to malignant B cells to potentiate T cell–induced cytotoxicity toward the malignant cells. This is a result of its binding to the CD3 site on T cells and CD19 site of the B cells.

Blinatumomab, a nonglycosylated 55-kDa MAb, is administered as a single-cycle continuous IV infusion for 4 weeks and may be followed by multiple cycles at increased drug concentration. The drug has a mean half-life of 1.25 hours.

Adverse effects include life-threatening cytokine-release syndrome (fever, chills, hypotension, and shortness of breath) for which the preadministration of dexamethasone may prove valuable. Leukopenia and hypogammaglobulinemia have been reported in a high number of patients (~70%) leading to an increased risk of infection. Central nervous system (CNS) events including seizures and confusion have also been reported.[80] It carries a Boxed Warning for cytokine release syndrome and neurologic toxicities.

Aducanumab (Aduhelm). Aducanumab is a 146-kDa rH IgG1κ MAb directed against aggregated soluble and insoluble forms of amyloid beta (Aβ) and is expressed in the CHO cell line.[81] Aducanumab was approved in 2021 for the treatment of Alzheimer disease (AD). AD is a progressive neurodegenerative disorder characterized by the presence of amyloid plaques composed primarily of Aβ. Treatment with Aducanumab should be initiated in patients with mild dementia stage of disease. No safety or effectiveness data on initiating treatment at earlier or later stages of the disease were studied. In clinical trials, aducanumab was found to reduce Aβ plaque levels compared to placebo based on the positron emission tomography (PET) imaging studies. Enhanced clinical vigilance for amyloid-related imaging abnormalities (ARIA) and ARIA-hemosiderin deposition (ARIA-H) is recommended. Most common adverse effects compared to placebo are ARIA-edema, headache, ARIA-H microhemorrhage, ARIA-H superficial siderosis, and fall.

Benralizumab (Fasenra). Benralizumab is a 150-kDa recombinant humanized IgG1κ MAb expressed in CHO cells deficient in α-1,6-fucosyltransferase.[82] It is an afucosylated MAb (Fc region of antibody is devoid of any fucose sugar units) that binds directly to the α subunit of human interleukin-5 receptor (IL-5Rα) and is indicated for the add-on maintenance treatment of patients with severe asthma aged 12 years and older and with an eosinophilic phenotype. Eosinophilic asthma, which accounts for

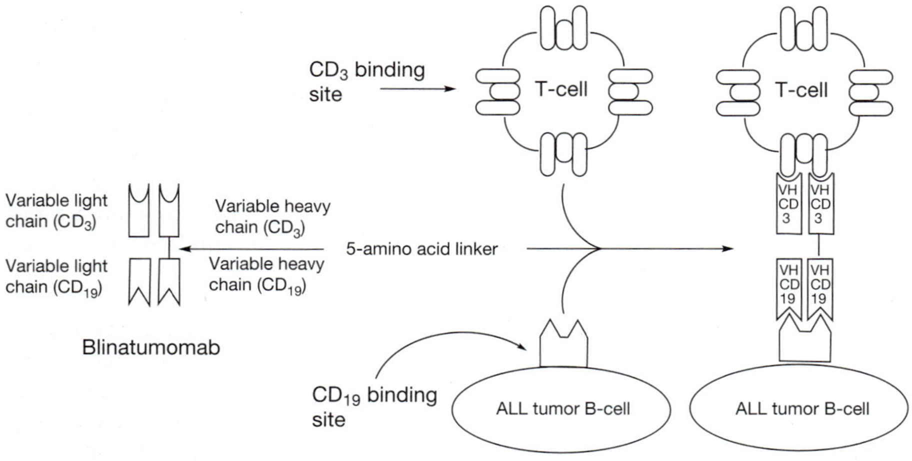

Figure 38.10 Mechanism of action of blinatumomab in which the drug binds to T cells and the ALL tumor B cell to initiate cytotoxic response.

40% to 50% of patients with asthma, is a condition with frequent exacerbations requiring hospital or emergency interventional care and may lead to death. Benralizumab, an antagonist of IL-5Rα, reduces eosinophils through ADCC. Most common adverse reactions of benralizumab include headache and pharyngitis.

BROLUCIZUMAB (BEOVU). Brolucizumab is a humanized single-chain Fv (scFv) antibody fragment produced by *E. coli* expression system.[83] It is obtained by grafting the complementarity-determining regions of an anti-VEGF-A antibody to a human single-chain-antibody scaffold, resulting in a 26-kDa protein. It is indicated for neovascular (wet) age-related macular degeneration (AMD) and administered by intravitreal injection. AMD is a chronic, degenerative eye disease caused by an excess of VEGF, which promotes the growth of abnormal, leaky blood vessels under the macula, the area of the retina responsible for sharp, central vision. Symptoms include blurred or lost vision in the center of the visual field. By inhibiting VEGF-A isoforms (VEGF110, VEGF121, and VEGF165), brolucizumab suppresses endothelial cell proliferation, neovascularization, and vascular permeability. Due to its small size and high solubility, brolucizumab can be formulated at a 10- to 20-fold higher molarity than existing anti-VEGF wet AMD therapies, enabling the delivery of more active drug molecules per injection. The small molecular size of brolucizumab also leads to better penetration in the eye and faster systemic clearance, and thus lower systemic exposure, relative to current antibody-based wet AMD treatments. Adverse reactions of brolucizumab include blurred vision, cataract, conjunctival hemorrhage, eye pain, and vitreal floaters.

CRIZANLIZUMAB (ADAKVEO). Crizanlizumab is a 146-kDa humanized IgG2κ MAb produced using rDNA technology in the CHO cells.[84] Crizanlizumab is a first-in-class anti-P-selectin MAb approved for vaso-occlusive crisis (VOC) associated with sickle cell disease in adults and pediatric patients aged 16 years and older. The pathophysiology of VOCs is thought to involve adhesive interactions between hemoglobin S-containing erythrocytes and activated endothelial cells, leukocytes, and platelets. P-selectin, a cell-adhesion protein expressed on activated platelets and endothelial cells, plays a central role in this process. Sickle cell disease is one of the most common inherited diseases, with an estimated 300,000 to 400,000 children born worldwide annually with it.[85] Sickle cell disease is caused by a single point mutation in the gene encoding the β-globin hemoglobin subunit. The mutation produces RBCs that assume a rigid, sickle-like shape and are impaired in their function, leading to health complications. The altered RBCs can subsequently obstruct vasculature circulation by making adhesive interactions with the endothelium, which leads to episodes of pain, hemolytic anemia, irreversible organ injury, and in extreme cases early mortality. Crizanlizumab reduces adhesion of sickle cell RBCs, platelets, and leukocytes to the endothelium by blocking P-selectin. Common adverse reactions include nausea, arthralgia, back pain, and pyrexia.

DOSTARLIMAB (JEMPERLI). Dostarlimab is a 144-kDa humanized immunoglobulin class G subtype 4 (IgG4) MAb produced in the CHO cells.[86] It is a programmed cell death protein 1 (PD-1) antagonist approved for the treatment of adult patients with DNA mismatch repair (dMMR) deficient recurrent or advanced endometrial cancer that has progressed during or following treatment with a platinum-based regimen. Endometrial cancer is the fifth most common cancer among women and is the most common female reproductive system cancer. PD-1 is a receptor that is predominantly expressed by T cells and plays critical roles in immune system regulation, cancer immunology, and autoimmune pathology. On activated T cells, interaction of PD-1 with its ligands, programmed death-ligand 1 (PD-L1) and programmed death-ligand 2 (PD-L2), downregulates the immune response and enables an immune-escape mechanism employed by tumors to avoid apoptosis. The endometrial cancer dMMR subtype is deficient in mismatch repair mechanisms and has been shown to exhibit a high prevalence of PD-L1 expression. Dostarlimab potently binds to PD-1 and thereby blocks the interaction of both PD-L1 and PD-L2 with the PD-1 receptor. Most common adverse effects are fatigue/asthenia, nausea, diarrhea, anemia, and constipation.

EMICIZUMAB (HEMLIBRA). Emicizumab is a 146-kDa humanized IgG4 MAb produced in CHO cells. It is a first-in-class bispecific antibody indicated for routine prophylaxis to prevent or reduce the frequency of bleeding episodes in adult as well as in newborn and older pediatric patients with hemophilia A (congenital factor VIII deficiency) with or without factor VIII.[87] Emicizumab bridges activated factor IX (FIXa) and factor X (FX) replacing the function of missing activated factor VIII with resultant downstream thrombin generation and activation of the coagulation cascade. Hemophilia A is inherited as an X-linked recessive bleeding disorder characterized by a lifelong bleeding diathesis due to deficiency of factor VIII. Based on US Centers for Disease Control and Prevention's estimate, hemophilia affects more than 400,000 people worldwide, predominantly men. Such dual binding positions the two proteins in a manner that enables FIXa to transform FX from its zymogen state into activated factor X (FXa) protein. In this manner, emicizumab duplicates the function of Factor VIII (FVIII) and thereby enables the coagulation cascade to proceed, ultimately resulting in the production of thrombin. However, the specific details of emicizumab interactions with FIXa and FX are not identical to those of FVIII. Importantly, emicizumab has no structural relationship or sequence homology to FVIII and thus does not induce anti-FVIII antibodies. Emicizumab was identified from a broad screening and optimization effort that evaluated approximately 40,000 bispecific IgG antibodies for their ability to properly bind and position FIXa and FX. Most common adverse reactions of emicizumab are injection-site reactions, headache, and arthralgia.

EPTINEZUMAB (VYEPTI). Eptinezumab is a 143-kDa humanized IgG1κ MAb targeting calcitonin gene–related peptide (CGRP) that was approved for the preventative treatment of migraine in adults.[88] Migraine is a prevalent neurologic disorder that affects nearly 12% of the general population.[89] CGRP has emerged as an important antimigraine target, with evidence that it elicits nociceptive signaling pathways involved in migraine pathophysiology. Eptinezumab is a

CGRP antagonist that followed the approvals of erenumab, fremanezumab, and galcanezumab, all of which have similar properties, with the primary difference being route of administration, and they target CGRP receptor. Eptinezumab is administered IV, while the others are administered SC.

Evinacumab (Evkeeza). Evinacumab is a 146-kDa rH IgG4κ MAb targeting angiopoietin-like protein 3 (ANGPTL3) and is expressed in the CHO cell line.[90] It is approved as an adjunct to other low-density lipoprotein-cholesterol (LDL-C) lowering therapies for the treatment of adults and pediatric patients aged 5 years and older, with homozygous familial hypercholesterolemia (HoFH). HoFH is a rare, life-threatening genetic disorder attributable to loss-of-function mutation in both alleles of the low-density lipoprotein receptor gene and is characterized by abnormally high levels of LDL-C from birth. This leads to early-onset atherosclerosis and, ultimately, myocardial infarction and death if left untreated. ANGPTL3 inhibits lipoprotein lipase activity, the main enzyme responsible for hydrolysis of triglyceride-rich proteins, and patients with loss-of-function mutations in ANGPTL3 have lowered LDL-C levels. Thus, it was hypothesized that neutralizing ANGPTL3 with an MAb might provide therapeutic efficacy for reducing LDL-C in the context of HoFH. Evinacumab is a fully human MAb derived from humanized transgenic mice that binds to both human and murine ANGPTL3 in picomolar affinities. Most common adverse reactions include hypersensitivity reactions, nasopharyngitis, nausea, dizziness, extremity pain, and rhinorrhea.

Ibalizumab (Trogarzo). Ibalizumab is a 150-kDa humanized IgG4 MAb expressed in the murine NS0 cells.[91] It exhibits a unique mechanism of action as a CD4-directed post-attachment inhibitor of human immunodeficiency virus type 1 (HIV-1) and is indicated for use in combination with other antiretrovirals in heavily treatment-experienced adults with multidrug resistant HIV-1 infection failing their current antiretroviral regimen. HIV is the causative agent of AIDS, a disease that has attained global pandemic status. Ibalizumab binds to amino acid positions within domains 1 and 2 of the CD4 cell, which induces steric hindrance and prevents the conformational changes between gp120 and the CD4 cell to ultimately prevent viral fusion.

Spesolimab (Spevigo). Spesolimab is a 146-kDa humanized IgG1κ MAb with L234A and L235A mutations to eliminate effector function. It is an anti-IL-36R MAb produced in CHO cells and indicated for generalized pustular psoriasis (GPP) flares in adults.[92] Dysregulation of IL-36 signaling has a key role in GPP pathogenesis. GPP is a rare, severe autoinflammatory skin disorder with skin pustulation with or without systemic symptoms such as fever, pain, fatigue, general malaise, and arthritis. Genetic links have been identified between GPP and mutations in *IL36RN* gene encoding the anti-inflammatory cytokine IL-36R antagonist. Mutations affect stability of IL-36R antagonist and interaction with its receptor leading to enhanced production of inflammatory cytokines by keratinocytes. Spesolimab binds specifically to IL-36R and prevents its activation by cognate ligand (IL-36Rα, β, and γ), inhibiting downstream activation of pro-inflammatory and pro-fibrotic pathways.

Teplizumab (Tzield). Teplizumab is a 150-kDa humanized monoclonal IgG1κ produced in CHO cells. It is a CD3-targeting antibody indicated for T1D in adults and pediatric patients aged 8 years and older with stage 2 T1D to delay the onset of stage 3 T1D.[93] About 90% of childhood-onset diabetes and 10% of all diabetes cases in children and adolescents are attributed to T1D, the most frequent type of DM in this age group. T1D is characterized by autoimmune destruction of insulin-producing β cells in the pancreas, leading to hyperglycemia. Current treatment focuses on management of glycemic levels using exogenous insulin or insulin analogues, diet management, cell-based insulin delivery, and protection of endogenous β cells by immunomodulation. Treatment with immunomodulatory agents including anti-CD3, anti-CD20, CTLA-4, anti-CD2, anti-interleukin 1 (anti-IL-1), and TNF-α may allow for delayed onset of later stages of T1D. Autoreactive T cells mediate destruction of pancreatic β cells. Teplizumab binds CD3 on the surface of T cells and induces deactivation and transient depletion of T cells, thereby promoting induction of tolerance and protection of pancreatic β cells. Most common adverse reactions were lymphopenia, rash, leukopenia, and headache.

Teprotumumab (Tepezza). Teprotumumab is a 150-kDa humanized IgG1κ MAb produced in CHO cells. It was approved in 2020 as a first-in-class treatment for thyroid eye disease, also known as Graves eye disease.[94] Thyroid eye disease is a rare autoimmune condition that is caused when autoreactive antibodies target fibroblasts located in the muscle structure at the rear of the eye. This causes the local muscle and fat tissues to inflame, resulting in bulging of the eye (proptosis) and pressure on the optic nerve. Symptoms of thyroid disease include double vision, eye pain, light sensitivity, and difficulty closing the eyes. Insulin-like growth factor-1 receptor (IGF-1R) is overexpressed in thyroid eye disease, and IGF-1R signaling is known to drive cell proliferation and migration and the induction of proinflammatory factors. Teprotumumab recognizes IGF-1R and blocks binding of the IGF ligands, thereby inhibiting the activation and signaling of the receptor. Most common adverse effects include infections, muscle spasm, nausea, diarrhea, alopecia, and headache.

Ublituximab (Briumvi). Ublituximab received FDA approval in 2022 and is a 147-kDa chimeric mouse-human IgGκ antibody targeting CD20 on B cells.[95] It enhances ADCC and produces B-cell depletion. Ublituximab is indicated for the treatment of relapsing forms of MS, to include clinically isolated syndrome, relapsing-remitting disease, and active secondary progressive disease, in adults. MS is a chronic inflammatory neurodegenerative disease affecting the central nervous system and characterized by axon demyelination. An estimated 1 million people live with MS in the United States, and there are approximately 2.8 million patients worldwide. Relapsing MS is the most common type of MS, affecting 85% to 90% of patients. CD20 is a specific marker of B cells beyond the early immature stage. B cells contribute to the pathogenesis of MS through mechanisms including proinflammatory signaling and autoantibody production. Anti-CD20 antibodies such as ocrelizumab and ofatumumab that deplete B cells have been previously approved for the treatment of MS. Ublituximab binds CD20-positive B cells through an epitope distinct from those of other anti-CD20 antibodies and thereby promotes ADCC of B cells. Most common adverse reactions were infusion reactions and upper respiratory tract infections.

Lecanemab-irmb (Leqembi). Lecanemab-irmb is a 150-kDa recombinant humanized IgG1 MAb directed against aggregated soluble and insoluble forms of Aβ and is expressed in the CHO cell line. Lecanemab was approved in 2023 for the treatment of AD in patients with mild cognitive impairment or mild dementia stage of disease. Lecanemab was found to reduce markers of amyloid in early AD and resulted in moderately less decline in measures of cognition and function than placebo at 18 months but was associated with adverse events.[96] Enhanced clinical vigilance for ARIA is recommended. Most common adverse reactions associated with lecanemab were IRRs, ARIA-microhemorrhages, ARIA-edema, effusion, and headache.

Donanemab-azbt (Kisunla). Donanemab-azbt is a 145-kDa recombinant humanized IgG1 MAb directed against insoluble N-truncated pyroglutamate amyloid β to reduce amyloid β plaques. It is expressed in the CHO cell line. Donanemab-azbt was approved in July 2024 for the treatment of patients with AD with mild cognitive impairment or mild dementia stage of disease.[97,98] Most common adverse reactions associated with donanemab were ARIAs, hypersensitivity reactions, and IRRs.

Antibody-Drug Conjugates

The field of ADCs has exploded in the last two decades with the successful launching of a series of ADCs into the market and several more currently in clinical trials. The principles behind the design of new ADC therapeutics, including the linker technology and use of payloads to attach to an antibody directed toward an antigen expressed on a cell type of interest, are described in Chapter 5.

Specific Drugs

Brentuximab Vedotin (Adcetris). Brentuximab vedotin was approved by the FDA in 2011 for treatment of Hodgkin lymphoma in patients who have failed autologous stem cell transplant (ASCT) or ASCT-ineligible patients who have failed on at least two prior chemotherapy regimens, and for second-line treatment of systemic anaplastic large-cell leukemia (ALCL). Brentuximab vedotin (MW = 153 kDa) is a CD-30–directed ADC. It contains three components: (1) the chimeric IgG1 antibody cAC10 that binds to CD30 protein expressed on the cancer cell surface, (2) the microtubule-disrupting cytotoxic component, monomethyl auristatin E (MMAE), and (3) a protease-cleavable linker that covalently attaches MMAE to cAC10 (Fig. 38.11).[99,100] MMAE is a synthetic analogue of dolastatin-10 that is covalently linked to the chimeric CD30 antibody cAC10 at Cys residues by a Val-citrulline dipeptide linker that contains a self-immolative *p*-aminobenzyl carbamate spacer. The Val-citrulline dipeptide undergoes cleavage by lysosomal enzymes such as cathepsin B, which leads to self-immolation of

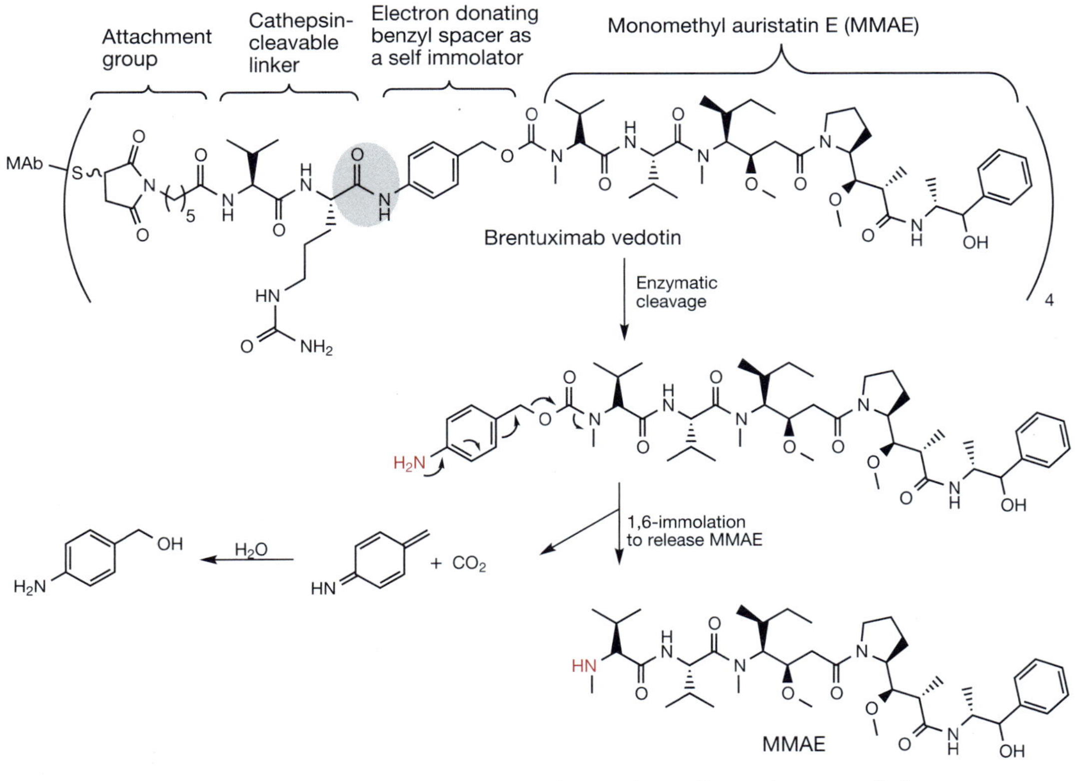

Figure 38.11 Structure of brentuximab vedotin and its self-immolative metabolism.

p-aminobenzyl carbamate and release of MMAE. Brentuximab vedotin has approximately four molecules of MMAE attached to each antibody molecule. The most common serious adverse effects include neutropenia, thrombocytopenia, anemia, and peripheral sensory and motor neuropathy. It is administered as an IV infusion. It carries a Boxed Warning of progressive multifocal leukoencephalopathy.

Ado-Trastuzumab Emtansine (Kadcyla). Ado-trastuzumab emtansine was approved by the FDA in 2013 for the treatment of patients with HER2-positive metastatic breast cancer who previously received trastuzumab and a taxane, separately or in combination.[101] Ado-trastuzumab emtansine is an HER2-targeted ADC that contains the humanized anti-HER2 IgG1, trastuzumab, covalently linked at Lys residues with the maytansinoid DM1 via a noncleavable thioether linker MCC (4-[*N*-maleimidomethyl] cyclohexane-1-carboxylate). Emtansine refers to the MCC-DM1 complex.[100] Ado-trastuzumab emtansine contains an average of 3.5 DM1 molecules per antibody. The antibody component of the ADC binds to HER2-positive tumor cell surface and undergoes subsequent internalization via receptor-mediated endocytosis and releases the active cytotoxic DM1 moiety upon proteolytic degradation in the lysosome. DM1 disrupts the microtubule assembly/disassembly dynamics to produce cell cycle arrest and, ultimately, tumor cell death.[102] The most common side effects include fatigue, nausea, musculoskeletal pain, hemorrhage, thrombocytopenia, increased transaminases, headache, and constipation. It is administered as an IV infusion.

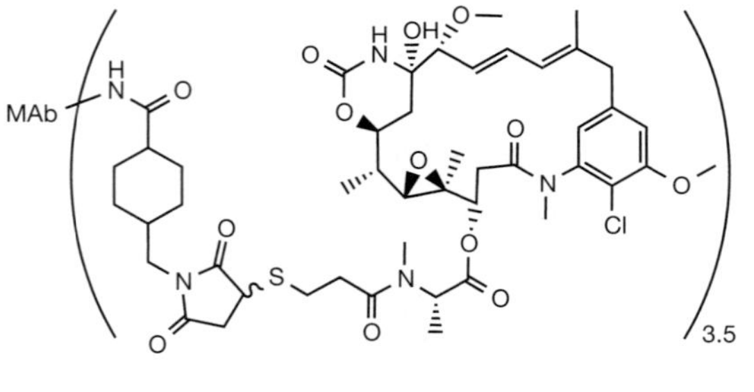

Ado-trastuzumab emtansine

Inotuzumab Ozogamicin (Besponsa). Inotuzumab ozogamicin (InO) was approved in 2017 for the treatment of adults with CD22-positive relapsed or refractory B-cell precursor ALL. It is a CD22-directed antibody-drug conjugate consisting of three components: (1) the recombinant humanized IgG4κ antibody inotuzumab, specific for human CD22, (2) *N*-acetyl-γ-calicheamicin that causes double-stranded DNA breaks, and (3) an acid-cleavable linker composed of the condensation product of 4-(4′-acetylphenoxy)-butanoic acid and 3-methyl-3-mercaptobutane hydrazide (known as dimethylhydrazide) that covalently attaches *N*-acetyl-γ-calicheamicin to inotuzumab.[100] Upon binding to CD22, InO internalizes into lysosomes where calicheamicin is released. Calicheamicin binds within the minor groove of DNA, which leads to double-stranded breaks and subsequent apoptosis as shown in Figure 38.12. InO has a MW of 160 kDa with approximately six molecules of calicheamicin derivative molecules attached to each antibody molecule. The most common adverse reactions are thrombocytopenia, neutropenia, infection, anemia, leukopenia, fatigue, hemorrhage, pyrexia, nausea, headache, febrile neutropenia, increased transaminases, abdominal pain, increased γ-glutamyltransferase, and hyperbilirubinemia. It is administered as an IV infusion.

Gemtuzumab Ozogamicin (Mylotarg). In 2017, the FDA-approved gemtuzumab ozogamicin for the treatment of adults with newly diagnosed acute myeloid leukemia (AML) who carry CD33 antigen–overexpressing tumors and patients aged 2 years and older with CD33-positive AML who have experienced a relapse or who are refractory to first-line therapy. It is an ADC composed of a CD33-directed MAb that is covalently linked to the highly cytotoxic DNA-strand breaking *N*-acetyl-γ-calicheamicin. The molecular mechanism of activation of this ADC is similar to that of InO.[100] Gemtuzumab ozogamicin contains an average of 2-3 moles of calicheamicin derivatives per mole of gemtuzumab. Common side effects include fever, infection, nausea, vomiting, bleeding, constipation, rash, headache, fever, thrombocytopenia, swelling in the mouth, and neutropenia. It is administered as an IV infusion. It carries a boxed warning for hepatotoxicity, including severe hepatic veno-occlusive disease.

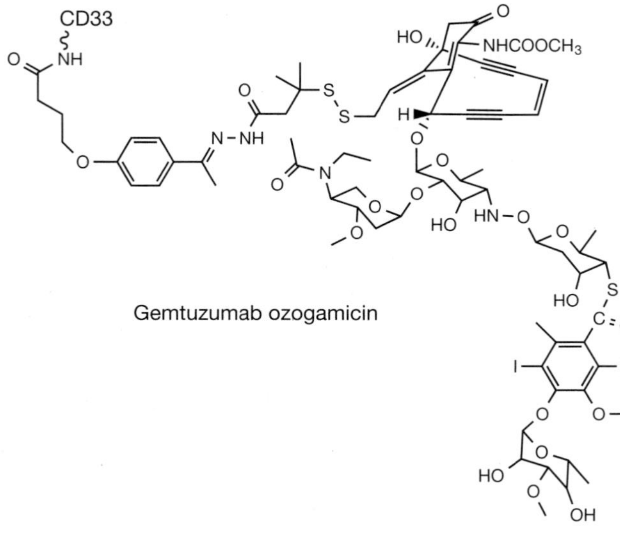

Gemtuzumab ozogamicin

Mirvetuximab soravtansine-gynx (Elahere). Mirvetuximab soravtansine-gynx is a first-in-class ADC targeting folate receptor α (FRα), approved for the treatment of FRα-positive platinum-resistant ovarian cancer.[103] It comprises an FRα-binding antibody, a cleavable glutathione-sensitive disulfide linker, and a potent microtubule inhibitor, the maytansinoid DM4. It binds to high-affinity FRα expressing tumor cells, internalizes, and is proteolytically cleaved to release DM4, which causes disruption of microtubule and apoptotic cell death.[104] It contains an average of 3.5 moles of maytansinoid DM4 per mole of mirvetuximab. The most common side effects include vision impairment, fatigue, abdominal pain, decreased lymphocytes, peripheral neuropathy, diarrhea, decreased neutrophils, and decreased hemoglobin. It carries a boxed warning for ocular toxicity.

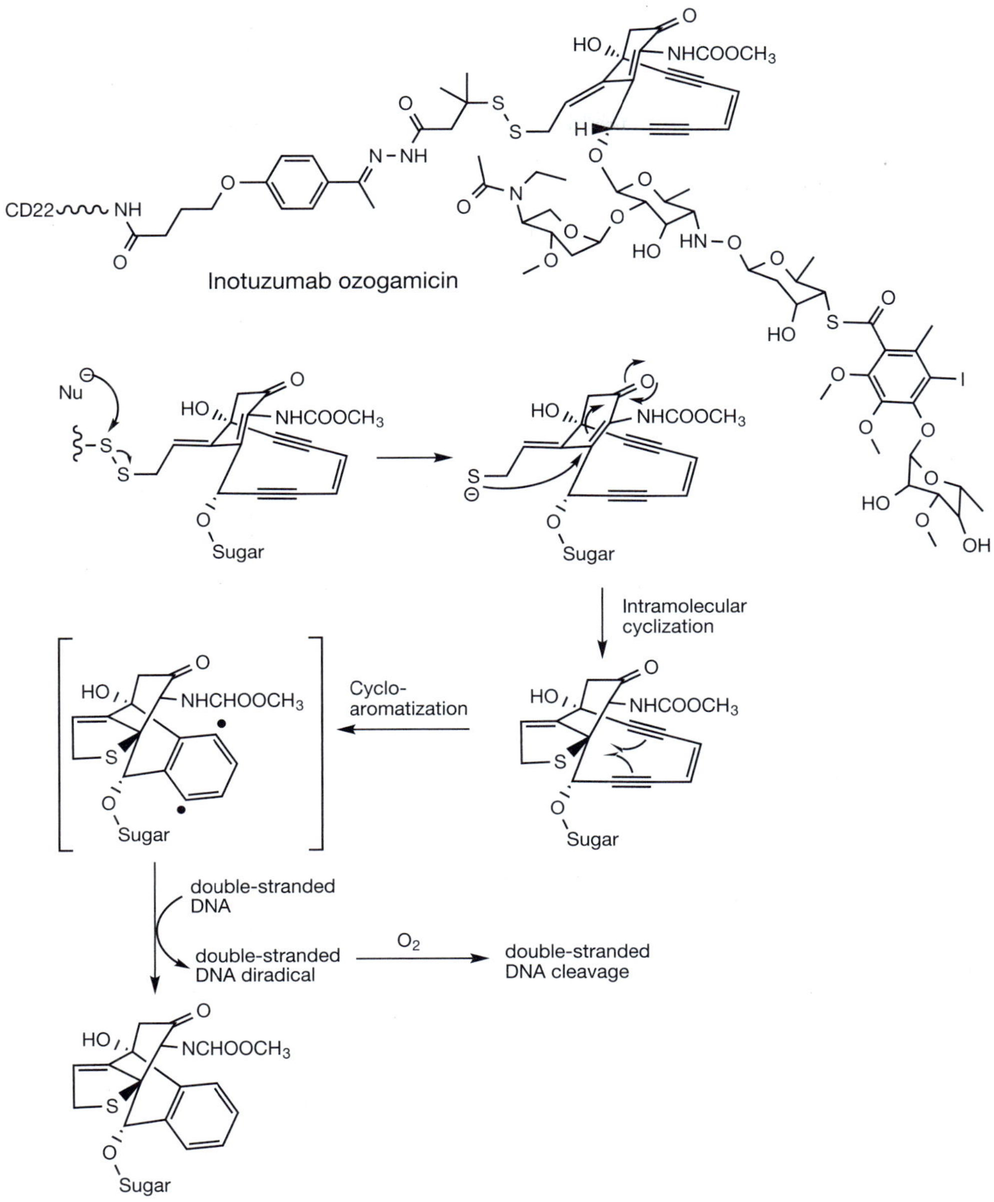

Figure 38.12 Structure of inotuzumab ozogamicin and molecular mechanism of DNA cleavage by calicheamicin.

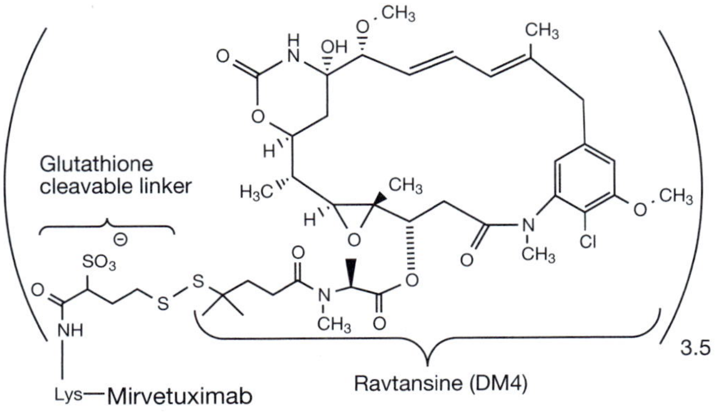

Mirvetuximab soravtansine-gynx

Tisotumab vedotin-tftv (Tivdak). Tisotumab vedotin-tftv involves conjugation of tissue factor (TF-011) targeted fully humanized MAb to microtubule-disrupting agent, MMAE via protease-cleavable linker. The anticancer activity of this ADC is due to its binding to TF-expressing cancer cells, followed by internalization of the ADC-TF complex, and release of microtubule disrupting agent, MMAE, via proteolytic cleavage. It is approved for the treatment of adult patients with recurrent or metastatic cervical cancer.[105] It contains an average of 4 moles of MMAE per mole of tisotumab. The most common side effects include ocular toxicity, peripheral neuropathy, pneumonitis, embryo-fetal toxicity, haptic impairment, and decreased hemoglobin, lymphocytes, and leukocytes. It carries a Boxed Warning for ocular toxicity.

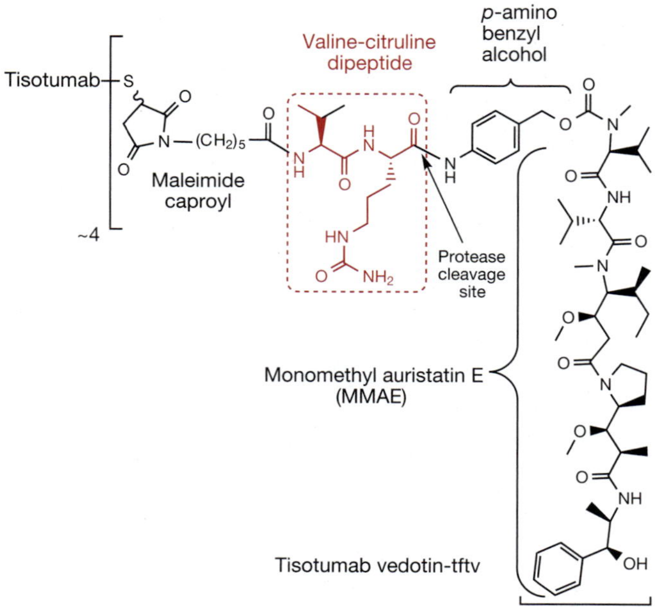

Tisotumab vedotin-tftv

Enfortumab vedotin-ejfv (Padcev). Enfortumab vedotin-ejfv is a Nectin-4-directed MAb conjugated to MMAE, a microtubule-disrupting agent, through a cleavable valine-citrulline dipeptide linker. Its structure is same as that of tisotumab vedotin, in which enfortumab replaces tisotumab. It binds to Nectin-4-expressing cells and undergoes internalization and proteolytic cleavage to release MMAE. MMAE induces cell cycle arrest and apoptotic cell death. It is approved for the treatment of adult patients with locally advanced or metastatic urothelial carcinoma.[106] Its drug-antibody ratio (DAR) is 3.8. The most common adverse reactions include skin reactions, hyperglycemia, pneumonitis, peripheral neuropathy, ocular disorders, and infusion site extravasation.

Polatuzumab vedotin-piiq (Polivy). Polatuzumab vedotin-piiq is composed of three components: (a) CD79b-directed humanized MAb, (b) MMAE, and (c) a protease-cleavable linker maleimidocaproyl-valine-citrulline-*para*-aminobenzyloxycarbonyl (mc-vc-PAB) that covalently links MMAE to the polatuzumab.[107] The ADC binds to B-cell-specific MAb, CD79b. Subsequently, it is internalized, and the linker is cleaved by lysosomal proteases to enable intracellular release of MMAE. Its structure is the same as that of tisotumab vedotin, in which polatuzumab replaces tisotumab. It is indicated in combination with bendamustine and a rituximab product for adult patients with relapsed or refractory diffuse B-cell lymphoma. It has a DAR of 3.5. The most common adverse reactions include peripheral neuropathy, myelosuppression, IRRs, opportunistic infections, progressive multifocal leukoencephalopathy, tumor lysis syndrome, embryo-fetal toxicity, and hepatotoxicity.

Loncastuximab tesirine-lpyl (Zynlonta). Loncastuximab tesirine-lpyl is a CD19-directed MAb conjugated to an alkylating agent (SG3199) through a protease-sensitive valine-alanine dipeptide linker. It is approved for the treatment of adult patients with relapsed or refractory large B-cell lymphoma.[108] Upon ADC binding to CD19 on the tumor cell surface, it undergoes internalization, protease-sensitive linker cleavage, and release of cytotoxic alkylating agent in tumor cells. The released drug then binds to the minor groove of the tumor cell DNA and forms cytotoxic DNA cross-links in a sequence selective manner. The cross-linked DNA leads to stalled replication forks, impeding cell division and tumor cells apoptosis. It contains an average of 2.3 moles of SG3199 per mole of loncastuximab. The most common side effects include myelosuppression, infections, cutaneous reactions, fluid retention, skin rash, fatigue, and joint pain.

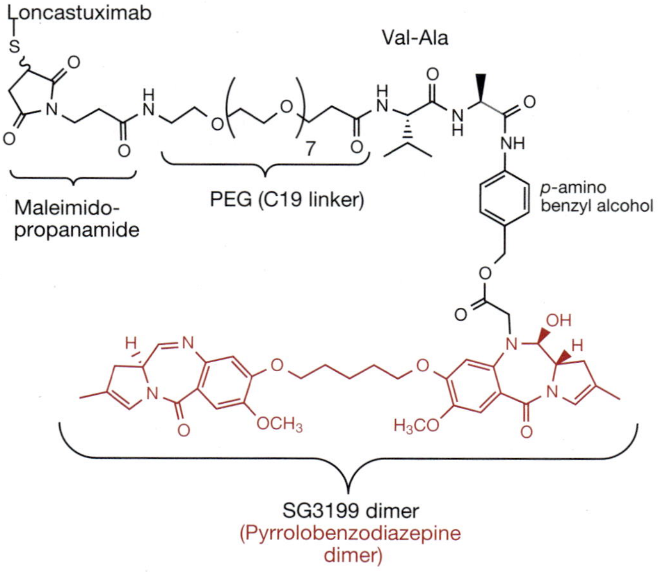

Loncastuximab tesirine-lpyl

Sacituzumab govitecan-hziy (Trodelvy). Sacituzumab govitecan-hziy is a Trop-2-directed MAb conjugated to a topoisomerase I inhibitor (SN-38) through a pH-dependent hydrolysable linker.[109] It is approved for the treatment of patients with hormone receptor (HR)-positive and HER2-negative breast cancer.[110] The ADC-Trop-2 complex formed on the surface of tumor cells undergoes internalization and hydrolytic cleavage in lysosomes to yield SN-38. SN-38 then enters the nucleus and induces DNA breaks and apoptosis. Unlike other ADCs, it has a DAR of approximately 8. The most common side effects include decreased leukocyte count, neutrophil count, hemoglobin, lymphocyte count, and diarrhea, nausea, and alopecia.

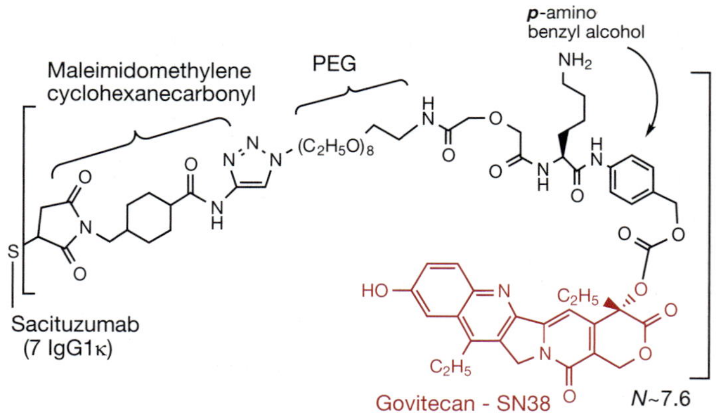

Sacituzumab govitecan-hziy

Fam-trastuzumab deruxtecan-nxki (Enhertu). Fam-trastuzumab deruxtecan-nxki contains humanized MAb, trastuzumab, covalently linked to deruxtecan. Deruxtecan contains a tetrapeptide (Gly-Gly-Phe-Gly)-based cleavable linker and the topoisomerase I inhibitor exatecan (DX-8951).[111] Fam-trastuzumab deruxtecan-nxki binds to HER2 on the tumor cell surface and undergoes internalization and intracellular cleavage by lysosomal enzymes to release exatecan, which causes DNA damage and apoptotic cell death. Its DAR ratio is 7.7. It is approved for adult patients with unresectable or metastatic HER2-low breast cancer. The most common adverse reactions include alopecia, anemia, nausea, fatigue, vomiting, constipation, decreased appetite, and musculoskeletal pain. It has a boxed warning of interstitial lung disease and embryo-fetal toxicity.

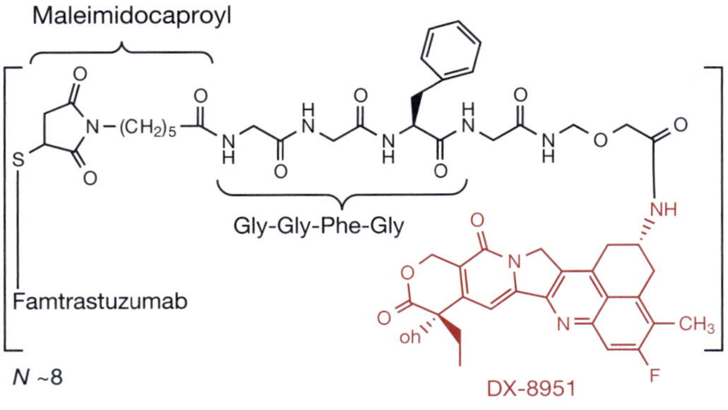

Fam-trastuzumab deruxtecan-nxki

Antisense Oligonucleotides

Antisense oligonucleotides (ASOs) are short oligonucleotides with an average length of 12 to 30 nucleotides that bind to RNA in a target-specific manner and subsequently modify protein expressions. The modulating mechanisms of these oligonucleotides include (1) binding to RNA and interference with its function without facilitating RNA degradation and (2) promotion of RNA degradation through endogenous enzymes. The key aspects of ASO design include structural modifications to maintain the ability to recognize target RNA by Watson-Crick base pairing, enhanced resistance toward nucleolytic degradation, wide distribution to tissues, and preferential localization in the cellular compartments that contain target RNA of interest. ASOs can be classified into three generations based on the chemical modifications. First generation ASOs contain modifications of the phosphodiester backbone and include groups such as the phosphorothioate, methylphosphonate, and phosphoramidate groups. Second-generation modifications include modification of the ribose sugar with an alkyl group and include 2′-O-methyl and 2′-O-methoxyethyl substitutions. Third-generation modifications are more heterogeneous. Common modifications include locked nucleic acids, corresponding to a methylene bridge connecting the 2′-oxygen and 4′-carbon, and phosphorodiamidate morpholino oligomers (PMO) in which the ribose is replaced by a morpholine moiety and the phosphodiester bond by a phosphorodiamidate bond.[112,113]

ASOs represent a new and highly promising class of drugs for personalized medicine and can be used to treat both rare and common diseases.[114] ASO-based therapeutics can also be used for individualized treatments, as is the case with milasen, an ASO developed for the treatment of Batten disease in a single patient.[115] FDA-approved drugs are summarized in Table 38.3,[116] and representative ASOs are discussed in the next section.

Specific Drugs

Nusinersen (Spinraza)

Nusinersen is approved for the treatment of pediatric and adult patients diagnosed with spinal muscular atrophy (SMA). SMA results from a genetic defect in the *SMN1*

Table 38.3 US Food and Drug Administration–Approved Antisense Oligonucleotide Therapeutic Agents

Generic Name	Trade Name	Size	Mechanism of Action	Target	Indication
Eteplirsen	Exondys51	30-mer	Splicing modulation	Exon51 of *DMD*	Duchenne muscular dystrophy
Nusinersen	Spinraza	18-mer	Splicing modulation	Exon 7 of *SMN2*	Spinal muscular atrophy
Inotersen	Tegsedi	20-mer	RNase H degradation	Transthyretin	Polyneuropathy caused by hereditary transthyretin-mediated (hATTR) amyloidosis
Golodirsen	Vyondys53	25-mer	Splicing modulation	Exon53 of *DMD*	Duchenne muscular dystrophy
Viltolarsen	Viltepso	21-mer	Splicing modulation	Exon53 of *DMD*	Duchenne muscular dystrophy
Casimersen	Amondys45	22-mer	Splicing modulation	Exon45 of *DMD*	Duchenne muscular dystrophy

gene located in chromosome 5q, leading to a deficiency of survival motor neuron (SMN) protein. Low levels of SMN protein lead to loss of function of neuronal cells in the anterior horn of the spinal cord, leading to muscular atrophy.

There are four classifications of the disease (SMA1-SMA4) related to the onset and severity of the condition. SMA1 (infantile—also known as Werdnig-Hoffmann disease) is nearly always fatal and is characterized by loss of motor neurons affecting many organs of the body. The respiratory system is especially affected leading to pneumonia and death. In patients with SMA, the *SMN1* gene is mutated such that it is not able to code correctly for the SMN protein. The reduced level of this critical protein ultimately leads to death of the motor neuron cells and a decrease in contractile activity. The *SMN2* gene can produce small amounts of SMN protein but, without exon 7 within the *SMN2* gene, the mRNA produces an SMN protein that is unstable and only displays partial functionality. Nusinersen directed to the *SMN2* gene promotes exon 7 retention via displacement of heterogeneous nuclear ribonucleoproteins (hnRNPs), which normally works to silence exon 7. Thus, it is expected to promote additional functional SMN protein to offset the loss of *SMN1* gene–producing SMN protein.

Nusinersen is administered as a single intrathecal bolus and has a long half-life of 4 to 6 months. It is metabolized by exonuclease, which hydrolyzes the 3′- to 5′ phosphodiester bonds. It is well-tolerated when administered intrathecally. The most common adverse effects consist of headache and backache.[117,118]

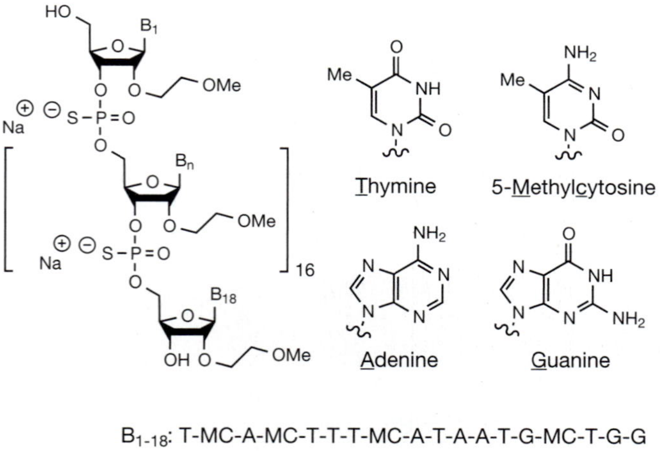

Nusinersen

Casimersen (Amondys 45)

Casimersen is a 22-mer PMO indicated for the treatment of Duchenne muscular dystrophy (DMD) in patients who have confirmed mutation of the *DMD* gene that is amenable to exon 45 skipping.[119] Based on National Human Genome Research Institute, DMD primarily affects men with an incidence of approximately 1 in 3,500 male births worldwide. PMOs are synthetic molecules in which the five-membered ribofuranosyl rings found in natural DNA and RNA are replaced by a six-membered morpholino ring. Each morpholino ring is linked through an uncharged phosphorodiamidate moiety rather than the negatively charged phosphate linkage that is present in natural DNA and RNA. Casimersen contains 22 linked subunits with a 5′ to 3′ end sequence of CAATGCCATCCTGGAGTTCCTG.

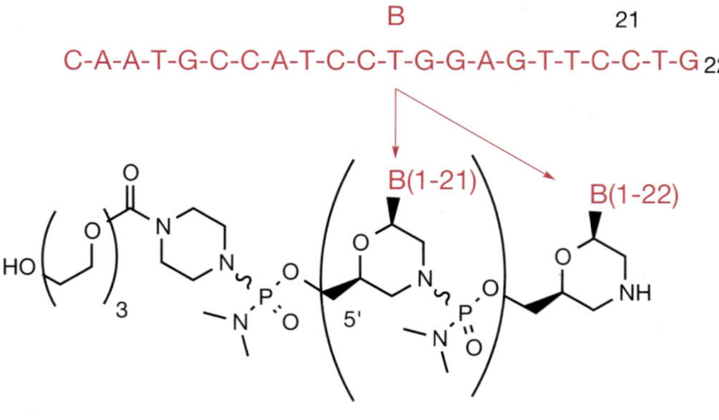

Casimersen

Golodirsen (Vyondys)

Golodirsen is an ASO indicated for the treatment of DMD in patients who have confirmed mutation of the *DMD* gene that is amenable to exon 53 skipping.[120] DMD is an X-linked recessive genetic disorder caused by mutations in the *DMD* gene, which encodes the dystrophin protein. Absence of appropriately functional dystrophin in muscle leads to progressive muscle wasting that is ultimately fatal in impacted patients. Golodirsen is an ASO of the PMO subclass.

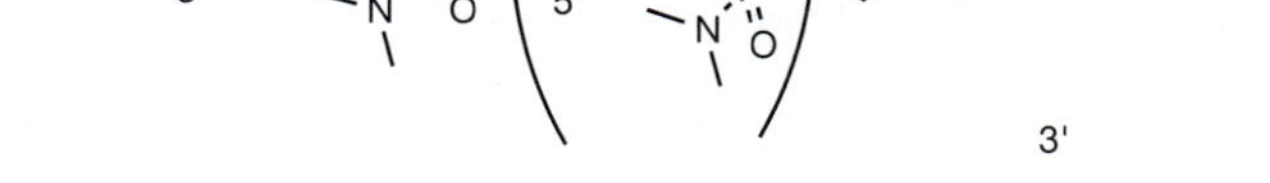

Golodirsen

Inotersen (Tegsedi)

Inotersen is a 2′-O-2-methoxyethyl (2′-MOE) phosphorothioate ASO that binds to transthyretin (TTR) mRNA. It causes degradation of transcripts via the RNase H pathway and thus blocks the production of TTR protein. It is approved for the treatment of polyneuropathy of hereditary TTR-mediated amyloidosis in adults.[121]

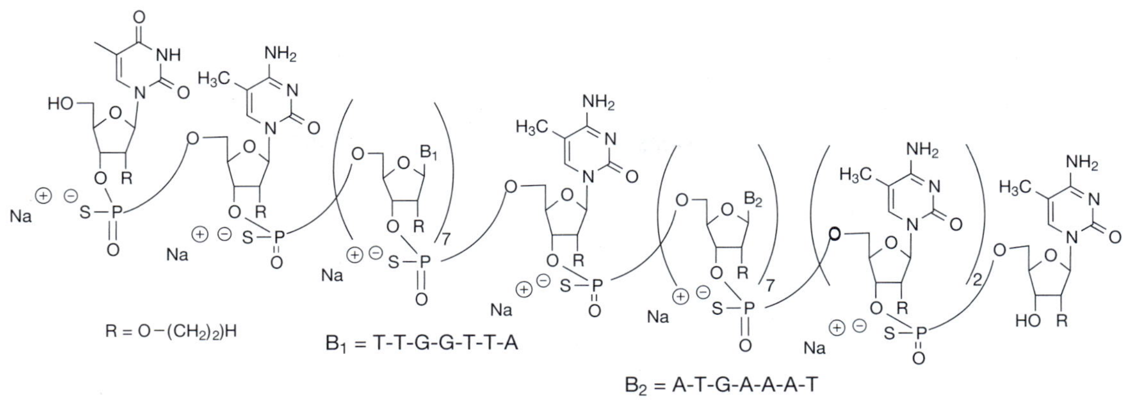

Inotersen

Small Interfering RNAs

Small interfering RNAs (siRNAs) have garnered substantial attention in precision medicine due to their shorter research and development timeline and broader therapeutic scope. siRNAs are nucleic acid-based drugs that treat disease by selectively silencing disease-related genes through sequence specific binding.[122] Four attractive features of siRNAs are: specificity in gene silencing, exceptional safety profile, remarkable efficiency, and unlimited number of potential targets. Currently approved siRNAs are used for the treatment of genetic disorders. Five siRNA-based drugs are FDA approved, and several others are in clinical trials.[123]

Specific Drugs

Lumasiran (Oxlumo)

Lumasiran (Fig. 38.13), an RNA interference (RNAi) therapeutic agent, is approved for the treatment of a rare genetic disease, primary hyperoxaluria type 1 (PH1).[124] In PH1, there is an overproduction of oxalate that can combine with calcium to cause kidney stones, nephrocalcinosis, kidney failure, and systemic oxalosis. Lumasiran is designed for selective uptake into hepatocytes. Lumasiran works by decreasing oxalate production via lowering glycolate oxidase enzyme levels. It does so by targeting the hydroxyacid oxidase 1 mRNA in hepatocytes through RNAi. The most common side effects include injection-site reaction and abdominal pain.

Givosiran (Givlaari)

Givosiran (see Fig. 38.13) is approved for adults with acute hepatic porphyria (HP).[125] HP is a genetic disorder manifested by the buildup of toxic porphyrin molecules during the production of heme. The buildup of porphyrin leads to severe pain and paralysis, respiratory failure, seizures, and mental status changes. Givosiran is an aminolevulinate synthase 1 (ALAS1)-directed siRNAs covalently linked to a ligand to enable specific delivery of siRNA to hepatocytes. Inside hepatocytes, it downregulates ALAS1 mRNA and blocks accumulation of neurotoxic δ-aminolevulinic acid and porphobilinogen involved in acute HP attacks. The most common side effects include injection site reactions and nausea.

Patisiran (Onpattro)

Patisiran, a small, double-stranded interfering RNA, is approved for the treatment of peripheral nerve disease caused by hereditary TTR-mediated amyloidosis in adult patients.[126] It interferes with RNA production of an abnormal form of TTR and thereby blocks the production of TTR. The most common side effects include IRRs such as nausea, back pain, abdominal pain, flushing, dyspnea, and headache.

Vutrisiran (Amvuttra)

Vutrisiran is a synthetic siRNA directed against TTR mRNA (see Fig. 38.13). It is approved for the treatment of adults with polyneuropathy of hereditary TTR-mediated amyloidosis.[127] The most common side effects include pain in extremities, joint pain, and trouble breathing.

Inclisiran (Leqvio)

Inclisiran is an siRNA directed to proprotein convertase subtilisin kexin type 9 (PCSK9) mRNA (see Fig. 38.13). It is indicated as an adjunct to diet and maximally tolerated statin therapy for the treatment of adults with heterozygous familial hypercholesterolemia or clinical atherosclerotic cardiovascular disease, who require additional lowering of LDL-C. Inclisiran contains a covalently linked ligand containing three *N*-acetylgalactosamine (GalNAc) residues to facilitate delivery to hepatocytes. With one exception, the 2′-ribose moieties of the inclisiran sodium are present as 2′-F or 2′-OMe ribonucleotides. In addition, six of the terminal phosphodiester backbones are present as phosphorothioate linkages. Inclisiran specifically binds to *N*-acetylgalactosamine

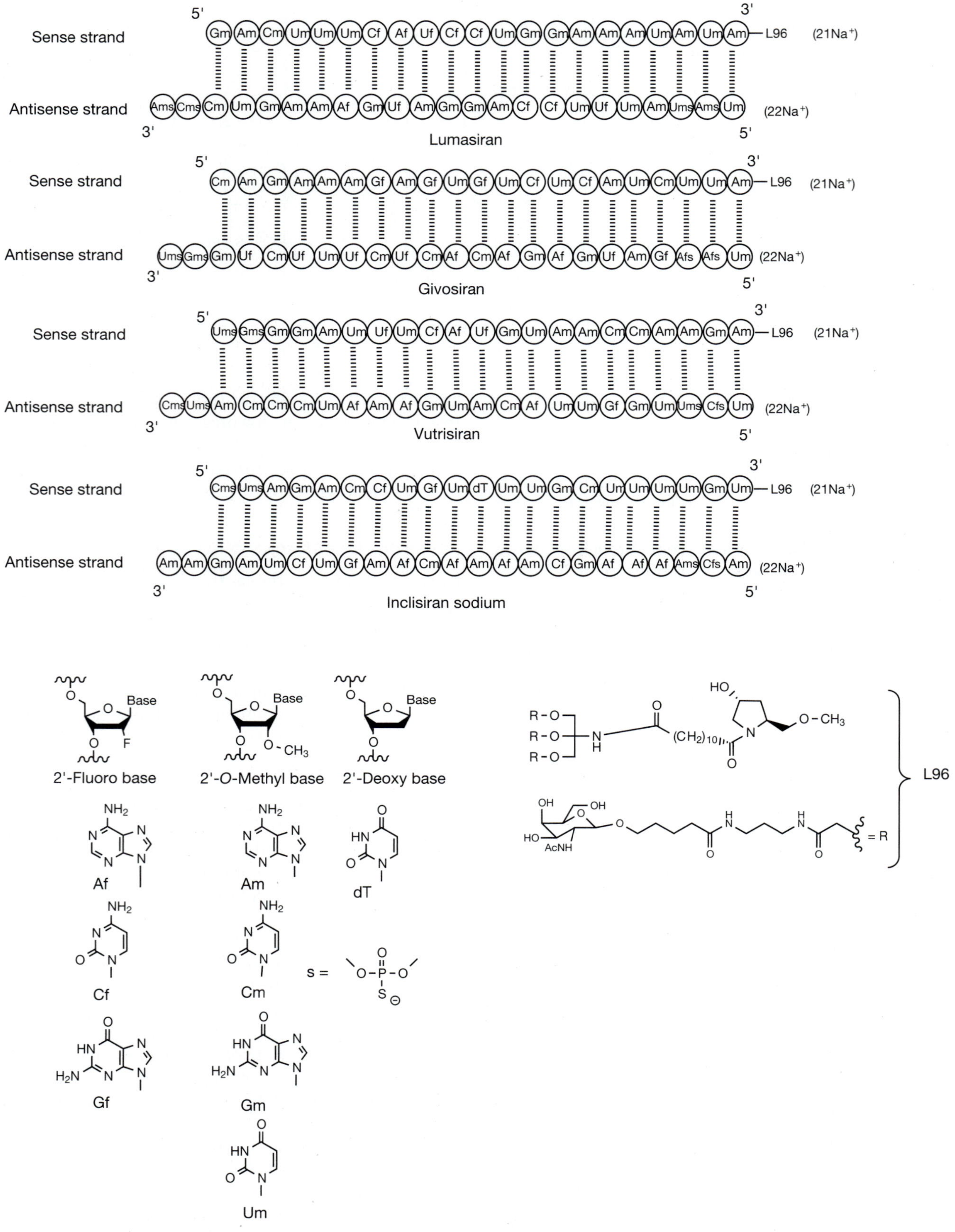

Figure 38.13 Structures of siRNAs.

and asialoglycoprotein receptor in hepatocytes, utilizes the RNAi mechanism, and directs catalytic breakdown of mRNA for PCSK9. This increases LDL-C receptor recycling and expression on the hepatocyte cell surface, which increases LDL-C uptake and lowers LDL-C levels in the circulation.[128]

Summary

The field of peptide and protein therapeutics has exploded in recent years, with advances in a vast array of technologies that facilitate the discovery of novel peptides and proteins, as well as their conjugates with small molecules. The synthesis of moderately long peptides (30-50 amino acids long) using modern solid-phase peptide synthesizer is now considered relatively routine. Various synthetic strategies and purification techniques have been developed for complicated peptides that are potent, efficient, innocuous, and affordable alternatives to small-molecule drugs. Advances in predicting and preventing the potential for peptides and proteins to elicit immunogenic responses, along with innovations in their formulation and delivery, have further stimulated growth in the peptide and protein therapeutics industry and now account for more than 17% of all FDA-approved drugs.[3] The number of drugs in this category will continue to increase, providing patients with innovative new treatments across a wide range of therapeutic areas. An area of particular interest and opportunity for medicinal chemists is the development of technologies to produce novel ADCs. ADCs combine the specificity of MAbs with the high cell-killing power of small cytotoxic molecules attached via a suitable linker. These revolutionary drug products hold the promise of targeting the disease while sparing the healthy tissue, bringing the concept of "magic bullet" closer to reality. siRNAs are emerging as a promising new category of macromolecular therapeutics with application prospects in treatment of various diseases. Development of siRNA delivery technologies for transporting them to different tissues such as brain, lung, muscle, and others will revolutionize therapeutic procedures and will be of great benefit in the future.[129]

Structure Challenge

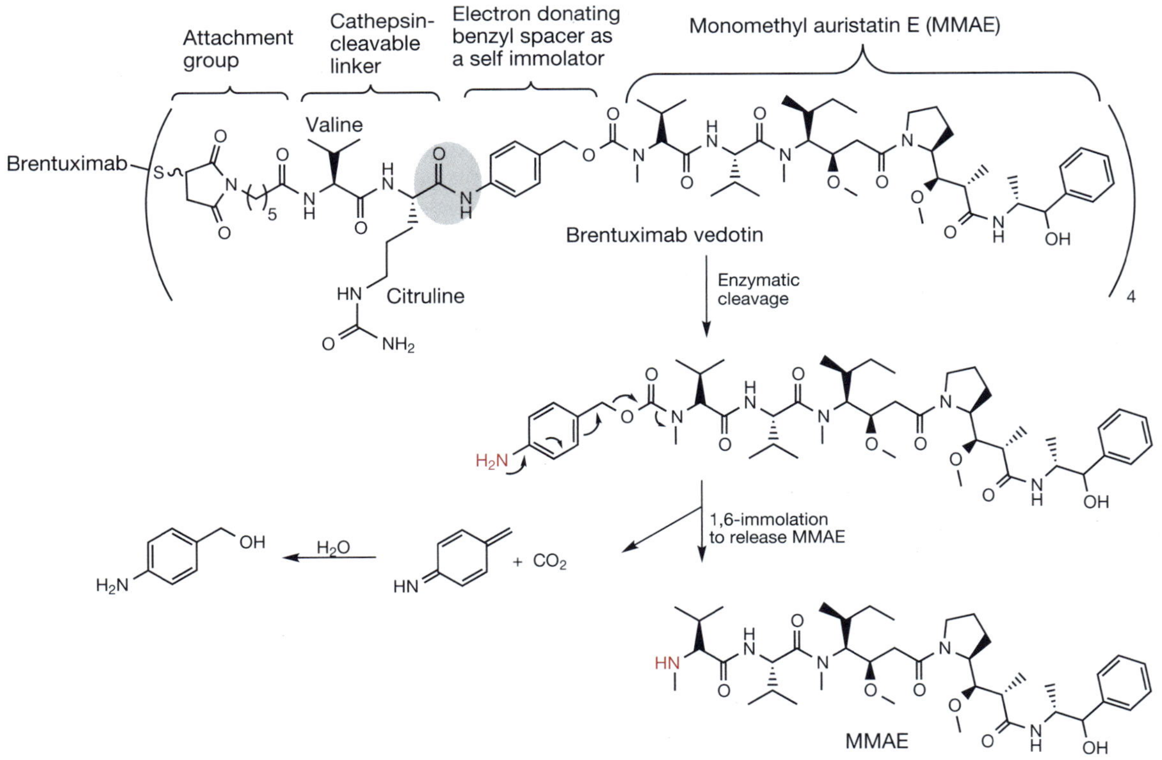

Conduct a structural analysis of the brentuximab vedotin.

1. What type of linker does brentuximab vedotin contain? Explain based on its structure.
2. Show the steps involved in the release of the active cytotoxic component MMAE. Explain based on cleavable linker.
3. What is the mechanism of MMAE cytotoxicity?

Structure Challenge Answers found immediately after References

REFERENCES

1. Lambert JM, Chari RVJ. Ado-trastuzumab Emtansine (T-DM1): an antibody–drug conjugate (ADC) for HER2-positive breast cancer. *J Med Chem*. 2014;57(16):6949-6964.
2. Banting FG, Best CH, Collip JB, Campbell WR, Fletcher AA. Pancreatic extracts in the treatment of diabetes mellitus. *Can Med Assoc J*. 1922;12(3):141-146.
3. Sharma K, Sharma KK, Sharma A, Jain R. Peptide-based drug discovery: current status and recent advances. *Drug Discov Today*. 2023;28(2):103464.
4. Ebrahimi SB, Samanta D. Engineering protein-based therapeutics through structural and chemical design. *Nat Commun*. 2023;14(1):2411.
5. Usmani SS, Bedi G, Samuel JS, et al. THPdb: database of FDA-approved peptide and protein therapeutics. *PLoS One*. 2017;12(7):e0181748.
6. Chengalvala MV, Pelletier JC, Kopf GS. GnRH agonists and antagonists in cancer therapy. *Curr Med Chem Anticancer Agents*. 2003;3(6):399-410.
7. Schally AV. Luteinizing hormone-releasing hormone analogues and hormone ablation for prostate cancer: state of the art. *BJU Int*. 2007;100(suppl 2):2-4.
8. Padula AM. GnRH analogues—agonists and antagonists. *Anim Reprod Sci*. 2005;88(1-2):115-126.
9. Wilson AC, Meethal SV, Bowen RL, Atwood CS. Leuprolide acetate: a drug of diverse clinical applications. *Expert Opin Investig Drugs*. 2007;16(11):1851-1863.
10. Shore N, Mincik I, DeGuenther M, et al. A phase 3, open-label, multicenter study of a 6-month pre-mixed depot formulation of leuprolide mesylate in advanced prostate cancer patients. *World J Urol*. 2020;38(1):111-119.
11. Nestor JJ Jr, Tahilramani R, Ho TL, McRae GI, Vickery BH. Potent, long-acting luteinizing hormone-releasing hormone antagonists containing new synthetic amino acids: *N,N′*-dialkyl-D-homoarginines. *J Med Chem*. 1988;31(1):65-72.
12. Reissmann T, Schally AV, Bouchard P, Riethmiiller H, Engel J. The LHRH antagonist cetrorelix: a review. *Hum Reprod Update*. 2000;6(4):322-331.
13. Klotz L. Degarelix acetate for the treatment of prostate cancer. *Drugs Today (Barc)*. 2009;45(10):725-730.
14. Brazeau P, Vale W, Burgus R, et al. Hypothalamic polypeptide that inhibits the secretion of immunoreactive pituitary growth hormone. *Science*. 1973;179(4068):77-79.
15. Bauer W, Briner U, Doepfner W, et al. SMS 201-995: a very potent and selective octapeptide analogue of somatostatin with prolonged action. *Life Sci*. 1982;31(11):1133-1140.
16. Olsen JO, Pozderac RV, Hinkle G, et al. Somatostatin receptor imaging of neuroendocrine tumors with indium-111 pentetreotide (Octreoscan). *Semin Nucl Med*. 1995;25(3):251-261.
17. Hintz RL. Untoward events in patients treated with growth hormone in the USA. *Horm Res*. 1992;38(suppl 1):44-49.
18. Cazares-Delgadillo J, Ganem-Rondero A, Kalia YN. Human growth hormone: new delivery systems, alternative routes of administration, and their pharmacological relevance. *Eur J Pharm Biopharm*. 2011;78(2):278-288.
19. Tritos NA, Biller BM. Pegvisomant: a growth hormone receptor antagonist used in the treatment of acromegaly. *Pituitary*. 2017;20(1):129-135.
20. Zaragoza F. Non-covalent albumin ligands in FDA-approved therapeutic peptides and proteins. *J Med Chem*. 2023;66(6):3656-3663.
21. Combarnous Y. Molecular basis of the specificity of binding of glycoprotein hormones to their receptors. *Endocr Rev*. 1992;13(4):670-691.
22. Jiang Y, Zhao JJ, Mitlak BH, Wang O, Genant HK, Eriksen EF. Recombinant human parathyroid hormone (1-34) [teriparatide] improves both cortical and cancellous bone structure. *J Bone Miner Res*. 2003;18(11):1932-1941.
23. Jin X, Zhu DD, Chen BZ, Ashfaq M, Guo XD. Insulin delivery systems combined with microneedle technology. *Adv Drug Deliv Rev*. 2018;127:119-137.
24. Ceriello A, Genovese S, Mannucci E, Gronda E. Glucagon and heart in type 2 diabetes: new perspectives. *Cardiovasc Diabetol*. 2016;15(1):123.
25. Edelman S, Maier H, Wilhelm K. Pramlintide in the treatment of diabetes mellitus. *BioDrugs*. 2008;22(6):375-386.
26. McWilliams V, Whiteside G, McKeage K. Linaclotide: first global approval. *Drugs*. 2012;72(16):2167-2175.
27. Pitari GM. Pharmacology and clinical potential of guanylyl cyclase C agonists in the treatment of ulcerative colitis. *Drug Des Devel Ther*. 2013;7:351-360.
28. Fretzen A. Peptide therapeutics for the treatment of gastrointestinal disorders. *Bioorg Med Chem*. 2018;26(10):2863-2872.
29. Hoy SM. Pegcetacoplan: first approval. *Drugs*. 2021;81(12):1423-1430.
30. Kale A, Shelke V, Lei Y, Gaikwad AB, Anders HJ. Voclosporin: unique chemistry, pharmacology and toxicity profile, and possible options for implementation into the management of lupus nephritis. *Cells*. 2023;12(20):2440.
31. Syed YY. Tirzepatide: first approval. *Drugs*. 2022;82(11):1213-1220.
32. Jamil K, Pappas SC, Devarakonda KR. In vitro binding and receptor-mediated activity of terlipressin at vasopressin receptors V(1) and V(2). *J Exp Pharmacol*. 2018;10:1-7.
33. Fields T, Woerly EM, Bell MG, Sloop KW, Ho JD. Advances toward an oral non-peptide agonist of the GLP-1 receptor. In: Rudolph J, Bronson JJ, eds. *2023 Medicinal Chemistry Reviews*. Vol 58. MEDI, Inc. Published by American Chemical Society; 2023:107-132.
34. Higgins DL, Bennett WF. Tissue plasminogen activator: the biochemistry and pharmacology of variants produced by mutagenesis. *Annu Rev Pharmacol Toxicol*. 1990;30:91-121.
35. Wagener JS, Kupfer O. Dornase alfa (Pulmozyme). *Curr Opin Pulm Med*. 2012;18(6):609-614.
36. Burton BK, Whiteman DA. Incidence and timing of infusion-related reactions in patients with mucopolysaccharidosis type II (Hunter syndrome) on idursulfase therapy in the real-world setting: a perspective from the Hunter Outcome Survey (HOS). *Mol Genet Metab*. 2011;103(2):113-120.
37. Starzyk K, Richards S, Yee J, Smith SE, Kingma W. The long-term international safety experience of imiglucerase therapy for Gaucher disease. *Mol Genet Metab*. 2007;90(2):157-163.
38. van der Ploeg AT, Clemens PR, Corzo D, et al. A randomized study of alglucosidase alfa in late-onset Pompe's disease. *New Engl J Med*. 2010;362(15):1396-1406.
39. Hegde S, Schmidt M. Idursulfase. In: Macor JE, ed. *Annual Reports in Medicinal Chemistry*. Vol 42. Academic Press; 2007:520-522.
40. Deckers J, Anbergen T, Hokke AM, et al. Engineering cytokine therapeutics. *Nat Rev Bioeng*. 2023;1(4):286-303.
41. Gauthier T, Chen W. IFN-γ and TGF-β, crucial players in immune responses: a tribute to Howard Young. *J Interferon Cytokine Res*. 2022;42(12):643-654.
42. Miller CH, Maher SG, Young HA. Clinical use of interferon-gamma. *Ann N Y Acad Sci*. 2009;1182:69-79.
43. Molto A, Olive A. Anti-IL-1 molecules: new comers and new indications. *Joint Bone Spine*. 2010;77(2):102-107.
44. Hoffman HM. Therapy of autoinflammatory syndromes. *J Allergy Clin Immunol*. 2009;124(6):1129-1138; quiz 1139-1140.
45. Bernardelli P, Gaudilliere B, Vergne F. Anakinra. In: Doherty AM, ed. *Annual Reports in Medicinal Chemistry*. Vol 37. Academic Press; 2002:261.
46. Hegde S, Schmidt M. Rilonacept (genetic autoinflammatory syndromes). In: Macor JE, ed. *Annual Reports in Medicinal Chemistry*. Vol 44. Academic Press; 2009:615-616.
47. Arenas-Ramirez N, Woytschak J, Boyman O. Interleukin-2: biology, design and application. *Trends Immunol*. 2015;36(12):763-777.
48. Conrad A. Interleukin-2—where are we going? *J Assoc Nurses AIDS Care*. 2003;14(6):83-88.

49. Foss FM, Kim YH, Prince HMM, et al. Efficacy and safety of E7777 (improved purity Denileukin diftitox [ONTAK]) in patients with relapsed or refractory cutaneous T-cell lymphoma: results from pivotal study 302. *Blood*. 2022;140(suppl 1):1491-1492.
50. Hoy SM, Scott LJ. Etanercept: a review of its use in the management of ankylosing spondylitis and psoriatic arthritis. *Drugs*. 2007;67(17):2609-2633.
51. Newton RC, Decicco CP. Therapeutic potential and strategies for inhibiting tumor necrosis factor-alpha. *J Med Chem*. 1999;42(13):2295-2314.
52. Kaine JL. Abatacept for the treatment of rheumatoid arthritis: a review. *Curr Ther Res Clin Exp*. 2007;68(6):379-399.
53. Khraishi M, Russell A, Olszynski WP. Safety profile of abatacept in rheumatoid arthritis: a review. *Clin Ther*. 2010;32(11):1855-1870.
54. Chen X, Zaro JL, Shen WC. Fusion protein linkers: property, design and functionality. *Adv Drug Deliv Rev*. 2013;65(10):1357-1369.
55. Jen EY, Gao X, Li L, et al. FDA approval summary: tagraxofusp-erzs for treatment of blastic plasmacytoid dendritic cell neoplasm. *Clin Cancer Res*. 2020;26(3):532-536.
56. Faulds D, Sorkin EM. Epoetin (recombinant human erythropoietin). A review of its pharmacodynamic and pharmacokinetic properties and therapeutic potential in anaemia and the stimulation of erythropoiesis. *Drugs*. 1989;38(6):863-899.
57. Graber SE, Krantz SB. Erythropoietin: biology and clinical use. *Hematol Oncol Clin North Am*. 1989;3(3):369-400.
58. Mertelsmann R. Hematopoietins: biology, pathophysiology, and potential as therapeutic agents. *Ann Oncol*. 1991;2(4):251-263.
59. Blackwell S, Crawford J. Colony-stimulating factors: clinical applications. *Pharmacotherapy*. 1992;12(2 pt 2):20S-31S.
60. Lieschke GJ, Burgess AW. Granulocyte colony-stimulating factor and granulocyte-macrophage colony-stimulating factor (1). *N Engl J Med*. 1992;327(1):28-35.
61. Petros WP. Pharmacokinetics and administration of colony-stimulating factors. *Pharmacotherapy*. 1992;12(2 pt 2):32S-38S.
62. Smith SP, Yee GC. Hematopoiesis. *Pharmacotherapy*. 1992;12(2 pt 2):11S-19S.
63. Park LS, Friend D, Gillis S, Urdal DL. Characterization of the cell surface receptor for human granulocyte/macrophage colony-stimulating factor. *J Exp Med*. 1986;164(1):251-262.
64. Bernard-Marty C, Lebrun F, Awada A, Piccart MJ. Monoclonal antibody-based targeted therapy in breast cancer: current status and future directions. *Drugs*. 2006;66(12):1577-1591.
65. Press MF, Lenz HJ. EGFR, HER2 and VEGF pathways: validated targets for cancer treatment. *Drugs*. 2007;67(14):2045-2075.
66. Keating GM. Panitumumab: a review of its use in metastatic colorectal cancer. *Drugs*. 2010;70(8):1059-1078.
67. Gaedcke J, Grade M, Jung K, et al. KRAS and BRAF mutations in patients with rectal cancer treated with preoperative chemoradiotherapy. *Radiother Oncol*. 2010;94(1):76-81.
68. Castagnola P, Giaretti W. Mutant KRAS, chromosomal instability and prognosis in colorectal cancer. *Biochim Biophys Acta*. 2005;1756(2):115-125.
69. Cheson BD. Ofatumumab, a novel anti-CD20 monoclonal antibody for the treatment of B-cell malignancies. *J Clin Oncol*. 2010;28(21):3525-3530.
70. Sanford M, McCormack PL. Ofatumumab. *Drugs*. 2010;70(8):1013-1019.
71. Dillman RO. Radiolabeled anti-CD20 monoclonal antibodies for the treatment of B-cell lymphoma. *J Clin Oncol*. 2002;20(16):3545-3557.
72. Hegde S, Schmidt M. Canakinumab. In: Macor JE, ed. *Annual Reports in Medicinal Chemistry*. Vol 45. Academic Press; 2010:484-485.
73. Ng SC, Shi HY, Hamidi N, et al. Worldwide incidence and prevalence of inflammatory bowel disease in the 21st century: a systematic review of population-based studies. *Lancet*. 2018;390(10114):2769-2778.
74. Panes J, Gomollon F, Taxonera C, Hinojosa J, Clofent J, Nos P. Crohn's disease: a review of current treatment with a focus on biologics. *Drugs*. 2007;67(17):2511-2537.
75. Rivkin A. Certolizumab pegol for the management of Crohn's disease in adults. *Clin Ther*. 2009;31(6):1158-1176.
76. Hegde S, Schmidt M. Golimumab. In: Macor JE, ed. *Annual Reports in Medicinal Chemistry*. Vol 45. Academic Press; 2010:503-505.
77. Charneski L, Patel PN. Eculizumab in paroxysmal nocturnal haemoglobinuria. *Drugs*. 2008;68(10):1341-1346.
78. Hegde S, Schmidt M. Eculizumab. In: Macor JE, ed. *Annual Reports in Medicinal Chemistry*. Vol 43. Academic Press; 2008:468-469.
79. Wright NC, Looker AC, Saag KG, et al. The recent prevalence of osteoporosis and low bone mass in the United States based on bone mineral density at the femoral neck or lumbar spine. *J Bone Miner Res*. 2014;29(11):2520-2526.
80. Portell CA, Wenzell CM, Advani AS. Clinical and pharmacologic aspects of blinatumomab in the treatment of B-cell acute lymphoblastic leukemia. *Clin Pharmacol*. 2013;5(Suppl 1):5-11.
81. Sevigny J, Chiao P, Bussière T, et al. The antibody aducanumab reduces Aβ plaques in Alzheimer's disease. *Nature*. 2016;537(7618):50-56.
82. Ghazi A, Trikha A, Calhoun WJ. Benralizumab—a humanized mAb to IL-5Rα with enhanced antibody-dependent cell-mediated cytotoxicity—a novel approach for the treatment of asthma. *Expert Opin Biol Ther*. 2012;12(1):113-118.
83. Tadayoni R, Sararols L, Weissgerber G, Verma R, Clemens A, Holz FG. Brolucizumab: a newly developed anti-VEGF molecule for the treatment of neovascular age-related macular degeneration. *Ophthalmologica*. 2021;244(2):93-101.
84. Ataga KI, Kutlar A, Kanter J, et al. Crizanlizumab for the prevention of pain crises in sickle cell disease. *N Engl J Med*. 2017;376(5):429-439.
85. Piel FB, Patil AP, Howes RE, et al. Global distribution of the sickle cell gene and geographical confirmation of the malaria hypothesis. *Nat Commun*. 2010;1(1):104.
86. Kumar S, Ghosh S, Sharma G, et al. Preclinical characterization of dostarlimab, a therapeutic anti-PD-1 antibody with potent activity to enhance immune function in in vitro cellular assays and in vivo animal models. *MAbs*. 2021;13(1):1954136.
87. Schmitt C, Adamkewicz JI, Xu J, et al. Pharmacokinetics and pharmacodynamics of emicizumab in persons with hemophilia A with factor VIII inhibitors: HAVEN 1 study. *Thromb Haemost*. 2021;121(3):351-360.
88. Scuteri D, Corasaniti MT, Tonin P, Bagetta G. Eptinezumab for the treatment of migraine. *Drugs Today (Barc)*. 2019;55(11):695-703.
89. Yeh WZ, Blizzard L, Taylor BV. What is the actual prevalence of migraine? *Brain Behav*. 2018;8(6):e00950.
90. Raal FJ, Rosenson RS, Reeskamp LF, et al. Evinacumab for homozygous familial hypercholesterolemia. *N Engl J Med*. 2020;383(8):711-720.
91. Jacobson JM, Kuritzkes DR, Godofsky E, et al. Safety, pharmacokinetics, and antiretroviral activity of multiple doses of ibalizumab (formerly TNX-355), an anti-CD4 monoclonal antibody, in human immunodeficiency virus type 1-infected adults. *Antimicrob Agents Chemother*. 2009;53(2):450-457.
92. Blair HA. Spesolimab: first approval. *Drugs*. 2022;82(17):1681-1686.
93. Thakkar S, Chopra A, Nagendra L, Kalra S, Bhattacharya S. Teplizumab in type 1 diabetes mellitus: an updated review. *touchREV Endocrinol*. 2023;19(2):22-30.
94. Markham A. Teprotumumab: first approval. *Drugs*. 2020;80(5):509-512.
95. Lee A. Ublituximab: first approval. *Drugs*. 2023;83(5):455-459.
96. van Dyck CH, Swanson CJ, Aisen P, et al. Lecanemab in early Alzheimer's disease. *N Engl J Med*. 2023;388(1):9-21.
97. Doran SJ, Sawyer RP. Risk factors in developing amyloid related imaging abnormalities (ARIA) and clinical implications. *Front Neurosci*. 2024;18:1326784.
98. Sims JR, Zimmer JA, Evans CD, et al. Donanemab in early symptomatic Alzheimer disease: the TRAILBLAZER-ALZ 2 randomized clinical trial. *JAMA*. 2023;330(6):512-527.
99. Okeley NM, Miyamoto JB, Zhang X, et al. Intracellular activation of SGN-35, a potent anti-CD30 antibody-drug conjugate. *Clin Cancer Res*. 2010;16(3):888-897.

100. Chari RV, Miller ML, Widdison WC. Antibody-drug conjugates: an emerging concept in cancer therapy. *Angew Chem Int Ed Engl.* 2014;53(15):3796-3827.
101. Verma S, Miles D, Gianni L, et al. Trastuzumab emtansine for HER2-positive advanced breast cancer. *N Engl J Med.* 2012; 367(19):1783-1791.
102. Erickson HK, Lewis Phillips GD, Leipold DD, et al. The effect of different linkers on target cell catabolism and pharmacokinetics/pharmacodynamics of trastuzumab maytansinoid conjugates. *Mol Cancer Ther.* 2012;11(5):1133-1142.
103. Dilawari A, Shah M, Ison G, et al. FDA approval summary: mirvetuximab soravtansine-gynx for FRα-positive, platinum-resistant ovarian cancer. *Clin Cancer Res.* 2023;29(19):3835-3840.
104. Ab O, Whiteman KR, Bartle LM, et al. IMGN853, a folate receptor-α (FRα)-targeting antibody-drug conjugate, exhibits potent targeted antitumor activity against FRα-expressing tumors. *Mol Cancer Ther.* 2015;14(7):1605-1613.
105. Markham A. Tisotumab vedotin: first approval. *Drugs.* 2021; 81(18):2141-2147.
106. Chang E, Weinstock C, Zhang L, et al. FDA approval summary: enfortumab vedotin for locally advanced or metastatic urothelial carcinoma. *Clin Cancer Res.* 2021;27(4):922-927.
107. Li C, Zhang C, Li Z, et al. Clinical pharmacology of vc-MMAE antibody-drug conjugates in cancer patients: learning from eight first-in-human Phase 1 studies. *MAbs.* 2020;12(1):1699768.
108. Lee A. Loncastuximab tesirine: first approval. *Drugs.* 2021; 81(10):1229-1233.
109. Starodub AN, Ocean AJ, Shah MA, et al. First-in-human trial of a novel anti-trop-2 antibody-SN-38 conjugate, sacituzumab govitecan, for the treatment of diverse metastatic solid tumors. *Clin Cancer Res.* 2015;21(17):3870-3878.
110. Syed YY. Sacituzumab govitecan: first approval. *Drugs.* 2020; 80(10):1019-1025.
111. Shitara K, Baba E, Fujitani K, Oki E, Fujii S, Yamaguchi K. Discovery and development of trastuzumab deruxtecan and safety management for patients with HER2-positive gastric cancer. *Gastric Cancer.* 2021;24(4):780-789.
112. Quemener AM, Bachelot L, Forestier A, Donnou-Fournet E, Gilot D, Galibert MD. The powerful world of antisense oligonucleotides: from bench to bedside. *Wiley Interdiscip Rev RNA.* 2020;11(5):e1594.
113. Angrish N, Khare G. Antisense oligonucleotide based therapeutics and its applications against bacterial infections. *Med Drug Discov.* 2023;20:100166.
114. Egli M, Manoharan M. Chemistry, structure and function of approved oligonucleotide therapeutics. *Nucleic Acids Res.* 2023;51(6):2529-2573.
115. Kim J, Hu C, Moufawad El Achkar C, et al. Patient-customized oligonucleotide therapy for a rare genetic disease. *N Engl J Med.* 2019;381(17):1644-1652.
116. Xiong H, Veedu RN, Diermeier SD. Recent advances in oligonucleotide therapeutics in oncology. *Int J Mol Sci.* 2021;22(7):3295.
117. Zanetta C, Nizzardo M, Simone C, et al. Molecular therapeutic strategies for spinal muscular atrophies: current and future clinical trials. *Clin Ther.* 2014;36(1):128-140.
118. Chiriboga CA, Swoboda KJ, Darras BT, et al. Results from a phase 1 study of nusinersen (ISIS-SMN(Rx)) in children with spinal muscular atrophy. *Neurology.* 2016;86(10):890-897.
119. Shirley M. Casimersen: first approval. *Drugs.* 2021;81(7):875-879.
120. Heo YA. Golodirsen: first approval. *Drugs.* 2020;80(3):329-333.
121. Keam SJ. Inotersen: first global approval. *Drugs.* 2018;78(13): 1371-1376.
122. Hu B, Zhong L, Weng Y, et al. Therapeutic siRNA: state of the art. *Signal Transduct Target Ther.* 2020;5(1):101.
123. Zogg H, Singh R, Ro S. Current advances in RNA therapeutics for human diseases. *Int J Mol Sci.* 2022;23(5):2736.
124. Scott LJ, Keam SJ. Lumasiran: first approval. *Drugs.* 2021;81(2): 277-282.
125. Scott LJ. Givosiran: first approval. *Drugs.* 2020;80(3):335-339.
126. Hoy SM. Patisiran: first global approval. *Drugs.* 2018;78(15): 1625-1631.
127. Keam SJ. Vutrisiran: first approval. *Drugs.* 2022;82(13):1419-1425.
128. Zhang Y, Chen H, Hong L, et al. Inclisiran: a new generation of lipid-lowering siRNA therapeutic. *Front Pharmacol.* 2023; 14:1260921.
129. Guo F, Li Y, Yu W, Fu Y, Zhang J, Cao H. Recent progress of small interfering RNA delivery on the market and clinical stage. *Mol Pharm.* 2024; 21:2081-2096.

Structure Challenge Answers

1. Brentuximab vedotin contains a protease-sensitive valine-citrulline dipeptide cleavable linker that contains a self-immolative *para*-aminobenzyl carbamate spacer.
2. The valine-citrulline dipeptide undergoes cleavage by lysosomal enzymes such as cathepsin B, which leads to self-immolation of *para*-aminobenzyl carbamate and release of payload, MMAE.
3. MMAE exerts its cytotoxicity by inhibiting the polymerization of tubulin.

APPENDIX

A

Predicted pK_a and cLog P Values of Commonly Prescribed Drugs

Predicted pK_a and cLog P Values of Commonly Prescribed Drugs

Drug	pK_a (Unionized Acid)[a]	pK_a (Ionized Acid)[a]	cLog P[a]
Acetaminophen	9.46		0.91
Acyclovir	11.98	3.02	−1
Albuterol	10.12	9.4	0.34
Alendronate	0.69	9.91	−4.2
Alfuzosin		7.3	1.19
Allopurinol	8.47	1.25	0.03
Alprazolam		5.01	3.02
Amitriptyline		9.76	4.81
Amlodipine		9.45	1.64
Amoxicillin	3.23	7.22	−2.3
Apixaban			1.83
Aspirin	3.41		1.24
Atenolol		9.67	0.43
Atomoxetine		9.8	3.81
Atorvastatin	4.31		5.39
Azithromycin		9.57	2.44
Baclofen	3.89	9.79	−0.78
Benztropine		9.54	4.19
Betamethasone	12.42		1.68
Bisoprolol		9.67	2.2
Buprenorphine	10.42	9.63	3.55
Butalbital	7.48		1.59
Caffeine			−0.55
Canagliflozin			3.52
Carbidopa	2.35	5.66	−1.2

Predicted pK_a and cLog P Values of Commonly Prescribed Drugs (*continued*)

Drug	pK_a (Unionized Acid)[a]	pK_a (Ionized Acid)[a]	cLog P[a]
Carvedilol		8.74	3.42
Cefdinir	2.73	3.61	−0.89
Cefuroxime	2.96		−0.9
Celecoxib	10.6		4.01
Cephalexin	3.26	7.23	−2.1
Chlorhexidine		10.52	4.51
Chlorphen-iramine		9.47	3.58
Cinacalcet		10.01	6.27
Ciprofloxacin	5.56	8.77	−0.86
Citalopram		9.78	3.76
Clarithromycin		9	3.24
Clavulanic acid	3.32		−1.5
Clindamycin		7.55	1.04
Clonazepam	11.65	1.89	3.15
Clopidogrel		4.77	4.03
Clotrimazole		6.26	5.84
Clozapine		7.35	3.4
Colchicine			1.46
Conjugated estrogens	10[b]		3.7[c]
Cyclosporin			3.64
Dabigatran	3.18	12.52	0.08
Dextrometh-orphan		9.85	3.49
Diazepam		2.92	3.08

(*continued*)

Predicted pK_a and cLog *P* Values of Commonly Prescribed Drugs (*continued*)

Drug	pK_a (Unionized Acid)[a]	pK_a (Ionized Acid)[a]	cLog *P*[a]
Diclofenac	4		4.26
Dicyclomine		8.96	4.93
Diphenhydramine		8.87	3.65
Donepezil		9.12	4.21
Doxazosin		7.24	2.14
Doxycycline	3.27	8.33	−3.3
Drospirenone			3.37
Dutasteride			5.79
Efavirenz			4.46
Eletriptan		8.37	3.77
Emtricitabine	5.47		0.08
Enalapril	3.67	5.2	0.59
Entacapone	6.09		1.63
Escitalopram		9.78	3.76
Esomeprazole	9.68	4.77	2.43
Eszopiclone	8.04	6.86	0.52
Ethinyl estradiol	10.33		3.9
Ezetimibe	9.48		4.56
Famotidine	9.29	8.38	−2
Fenofibrate			5.28
Fentanyl		8.77	3.82
Finasteride			3.07
Fingolimod		9.38	4.06
Fluconazole	12.68	2.3	0.56
Fluoxetine		9.8	4.17
Fluticasone	12.19		2.58
Fluticasone propionate	13.61		3.72
Fluvoxamine		8.86	2.8
Furosemide	4.25		1.75
Gabapentin	4.63	9.91	−1.3
Gemfibrozil	4.42		4.39
Glimepiride	4.32		3.12
Glipizide	4.32		1.43
Glyburide	4.32		3.79
Granisetron		9	1.88
Guaifenesin			0.34

Predicted pK_a and cLog *P* Values of Commonly Prescribed Drugs (*continued*)

Drug	pK_a (Unionized Acid)[a]	pK_a (Ionized Acid)[a]	cLog *P*[a]
Haloperidol		8.05	3.66
Hydralazine		8.88	0.75
Hydrochlorothiazide	9.09		−0.58
Hydrocodone		9.17	1.96
Hydrocortisone			1.28
Hydroxychloroquine		9.76	2.89
Ibandronate	0.66	9.93	−2.5
Ibuprofen	4.85		3.84
Imipramine		9.2	4.28
Ipratropium			−1.8
Irbesartan	5.85	4.12	5.39
Isosorbide mononitrate			−1.4
Ketoconazole		6.42	4.19
Lactulose			−4.5
Lamotrigine		5.89	1.93
Lansoprazole	9.35	4.16	3.03
Levetiracetam			−0.59
Levodopa	1.65	9.06	−1.8
Levofloxacin	5.35	6.72	0.09
Levothyroxine	0.27	9.43	3.73
Lidocaine		7.75	2.84
Lisdexamfetamine		10.21	1.14
Lisinopril	3.17	10.21	−3.1
Lorazepam	10.61		3.53
Losartan	5.85	3.85	5
Lovastatin			3.9
Meloxicam	4.47	0.47	1.6
Memantine		10.7	2.07
Metformin		12.33	−0.92
Methadone		9.12	5.01
Methocarbamol			0.45
Methotrexate	2.95	5.48[d]	−2.3
Methylphenidate		9.09	2.25
Metoclopramide		9.04	1.4

Predicted pK_a and cLog *P* Values of Commonly Prescribed Drugs (*continued*)

Drug	pK_a (Unionized Acid)[a]	pK_a (Ionized Acid)[a]	cLog P[a]
Metoprolol		9.67	1.76
Metronidazole		3.03	−0.46
Montelukast	4.4	3.12	8.49
Moxifloxacin	5.49	9.51	−0.51
Mupirocin	4.83		2.45
Nabumetone			3.22
Naloxone	10.07	7.84	1.62
Naproxen	4.19		2.99
Niacin	2.79	4.19	−0.17
Nitrofurantoin	8.23		−0.22
Nitroglycerin			0.26
Nortriptyline		10.47	4.43
Olanzapine		7.24	3.39
Olmesartan	0.89	5.33	2.16
Omeprazole	9.29	4.77	2.43
Ondansetron		7.34	2.35
Oseltamivir		9.31	1.16
Oxycodone		8.77	1.03
Pantoprazole	9.15	3.55	2.18
Paroxetine		9.77	3.15
Pemetrexed	3.39	2.43	1.2
Penicillin G	3.53		1.08
Perindopril	3.79	5.48	0.63
Phenazopyridine		6.86	2.69
Phenytoin	8.49		2.15
Pioglitazone	6.66	5.6	3.33
Pravastatin	4.21		1.65
Prednisolone			1.27
Prednisone			1.66
Pregabalin	4.8	10.23	−1.3
Quetiapine		7.06	2.81
Rabeprazole	9.35	4.24	2.09
Raloxifene	9	8.42	5.46
Raltegravir	7.02		−0.39
Ramipril	3.75	5.2	1.47
Ranitidine		7.8	0.99
Risedronate	0.68	4.91	−3.3
Risperidone		8.76	2.63
Rivaroxaban			1.9

Predicted pK_a and cLog *P* Values of Commonly Prescribed Drugs (*continued*)

Drug	pK_a (Unionized Acid)[a]	pK_a (Ionized Acid)[a]	cLog P[a]
Ropinirole		10.17	3.06
Rosuvastatin	4		1.92
Salmeterol	10.12	9.4	3.61
Sennosides	3.23		1.19
Sertraline		9.56	5.15
Sildenafil	11.14	5.99	1.87
Simvastatin			4.46
Sitagliptin		8.78	1.26
Sofosbuvir	9.7		1.28
Solifenacin		8.88	3.96
Spironolactone			3.64
Sumatriptan	11.24	9.54	0.74
Tadalafil			1.64
Temazepam	10.68		2.79
Tenofovir	1.35	3.74	−3.4
Terazosin		7.24	1.18
Tetracycline	3.26	9.25	−3.5
Tiotropium	10.35		−1.8
Tizanidine		7.49	2.02
Tramadol		9.23	2.45
Trazodone		7.09	3.13
Triamcinolone	11.75		0.24
Triamterene		1.86	1.11
Valganciclovir	11.98	7.48	−0.69
Valproic acid	5.14		2.8
Vardenafil	11.75	6.21	1.43
Venlafaxine		8.91	2.74
Warfarin	5.56		2.74
Zaleplon		0.28	1.53
Zoledronic acid	0.66	6.67	−3.9
Zolmitriptan		9.55	2.04
Zolpidem		5.39	3.02

DrugBank Online. Accessed September 9, 2024. https://go.drugbank.com

[a]Chemaxon unless otherwise noted.

[b]Hurwitz AR, Liu ST. Determination of aqueous solubility and pKa values of estrogens. *J Pharm Sci*. 1977;66:624-627.

[c]Hsieh RW, Rajan SS, Sharma SK, Greene GL. Molecular characterization of a B-ring unsaturated estrogen: implications for conjugated equine estrogen components of Premarin. *Steroids*. 2008;73:59-68.

[d]Alva-Ensastegui JC, Morales-Avila E, de la Luz AP, Bernad-Bernad MJ. Determination of pKa values and deprotonation order of methotrexate using a combined experimental-theoretical study and binding constants of the methotrexate-Laponite complex at different pH values. *J Photochem Photobiol A*. 2024;449:115406.

APPENDIX

B

pH Values of Biologic Fluids

pH Values of Biologic Fluids

Fluid	pH
Aqueous humor	7.2
Blood, arterial	7.4
Blood, venous	7.4
Blood, maternal umbilical	7.3
Cerebrospinal fluid	7.4
Colon[a]	
Fasting	5-8
Fed	5-8
Duodenum[a]	
Fasting	4.4-6.6
Fed	5.2-6.2
Feces[b]	7.1 (4.6-8.8)
Ileum[a]	
Fasting	6.8-8.6
Fed	6.8-8.0
Intestine, microsurface	5.3
Lacrimal fluid (tears)	7.4
Milk, breast	7.0
Muscle, skeletal[c]	6.0
Nasal secretions	6.0
Prostatic fluid	6.5
Saliva	6.4
Semen	7.2
Stomach[a]	
Fasting	1.4-2.1
Fed	3-7
Sweat	5.4
Urine	5.8 (5.5-7.0)
Vaginal secretions, premenopausal	4.5
Vaginal secretions, postmenopausal	7.0

[a]Dressman JB, Amidon GL, Reppas C, et al. Dissolution testing as a prognostic tool for oral drug absorption. *Pharm Res*. 1998;15:11-22.
[b]Value for normal, soft, formed stools. Hard stools tend to be more alkaline, whereas watery, unformed stools are acidic.
[c]Studies conducted intracellularly on the rat.

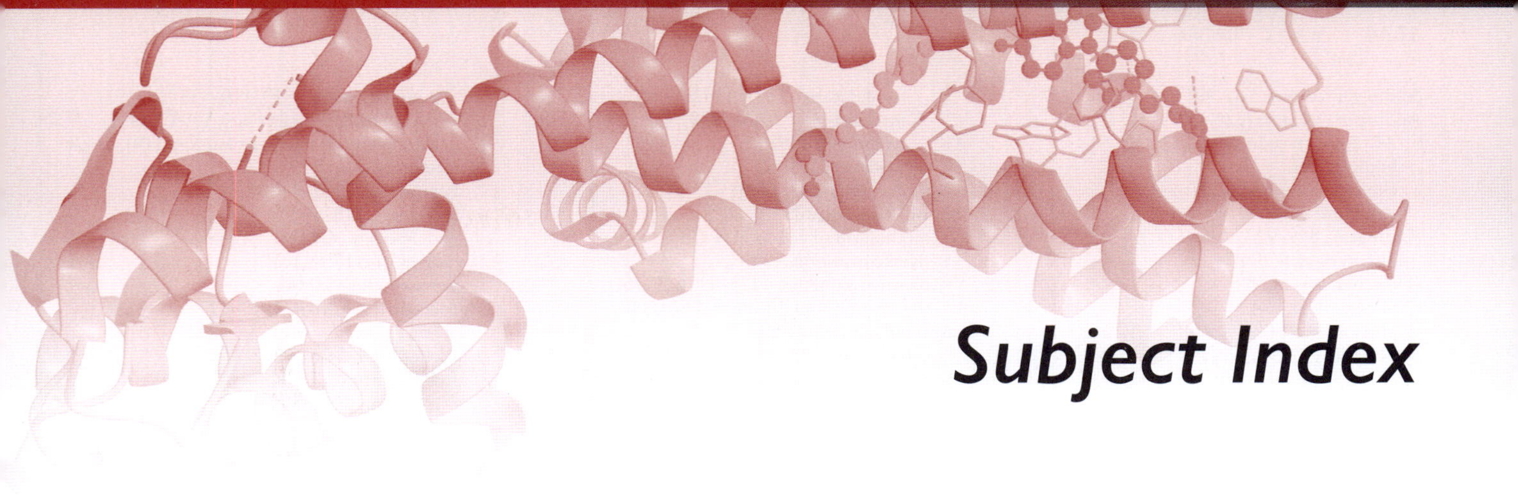

Subject Index

Note: Page numbers followed by "f" indicate figures, "t" indicate tables, and "b" indicate boxes.

A

B

C

E

F

G

H

I

N

Q

R

S

T

U

V

W

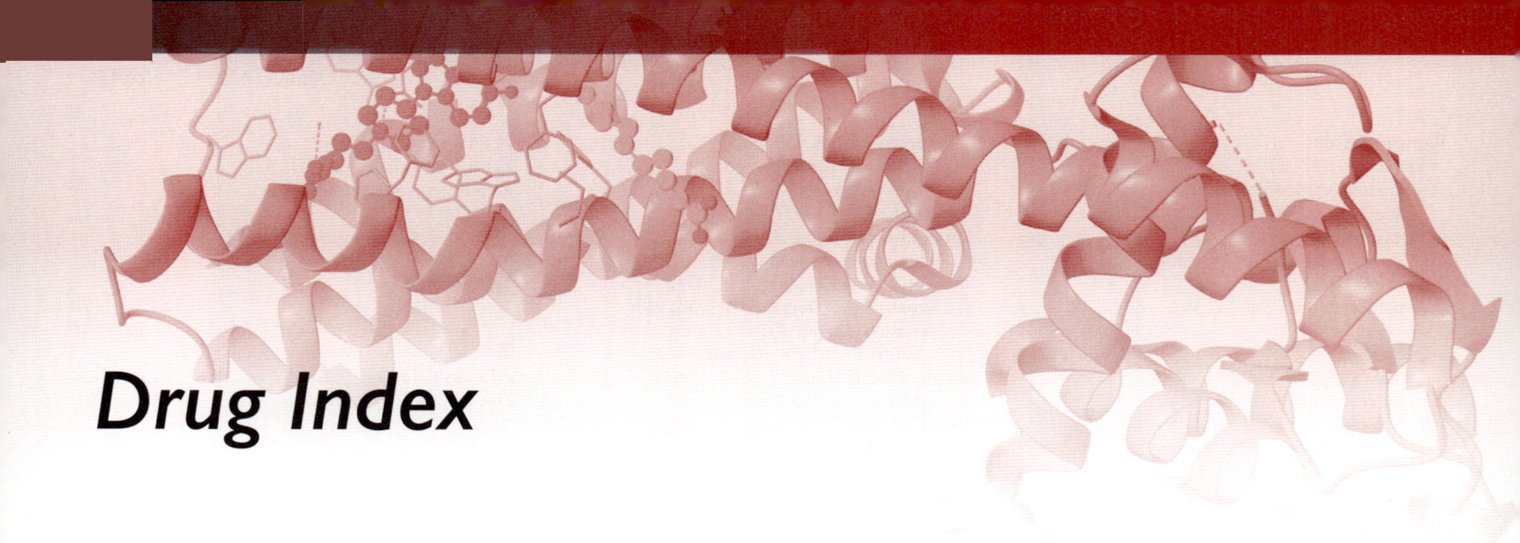

Drug Index

Note: Page numbers followed by "f" denotes figures, "t" denotes tables and "b" denotes boxes

B

C

D

E

F

G

H

I

J

K

N

O

T

QUADM0925